www.shopingenix.com

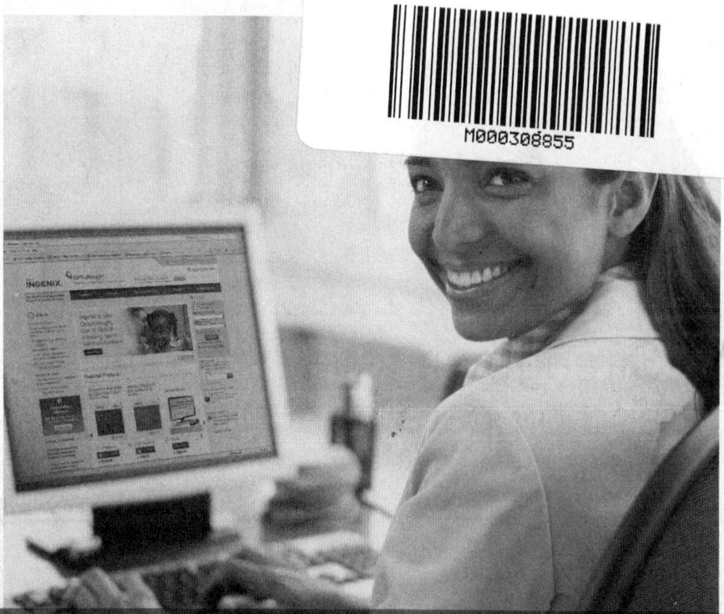

Ordering online at ShopIngenix.com is a snap.

- Find the products you need quickly and easily with our powerful search engine
- View all available formats and edition years on the same page with consolidated product pages
- Browse our eCatalog online
- Chat live with a customer service representative; ask questions about the site or the checkout process
- Visit Coding Central for expert resources including articles, the ICD-10 Coders' Corner, and coding scenarios to test your knowledge

Register on ShopIngenix.com for a customized website experience:

- **View special website promotions/ discounts**
- **Get product recommendations based on your order history**
- **Research your order history**
- **Check on shipment status and tracking**
- **View Invoices and payment history**
- **Pay outstanding invoices online**
- **Manage your address book**
- **Ship orders to multiple locations**
- **Renew your order with a single click**
- **Compile a wish list of the products you want and purchase when you're ready**
- **Receive a $50 coupon for every $500 you spend on ShopIngenix.com (for customers who are not a part of our Medallion or Reseller programs). When logged in, the eRewards meter keeps track of purchases towards your next reward**

Don't have a ShopIngenix.com account yet?

It's easy to create one:

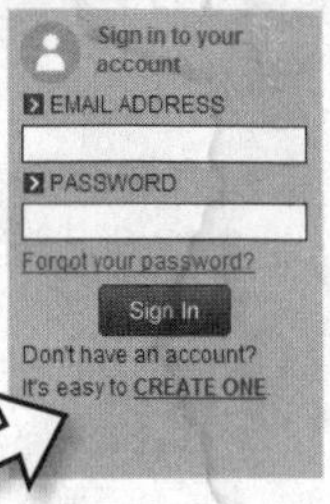

REGISTER TO SAVE 15% ON YOUR NEXT ONLINE ORDER.

INGENIX®

www.shopingenix.com

OPTUMInsight™

Ingenix is now OptumInsight™, part of Optum™—a leading health services business.

Ingenix is now OptumInsight™, part of Optum™—a leading health services business | Call toll-free 1.800.464.3649, option 1.

FOBA12L

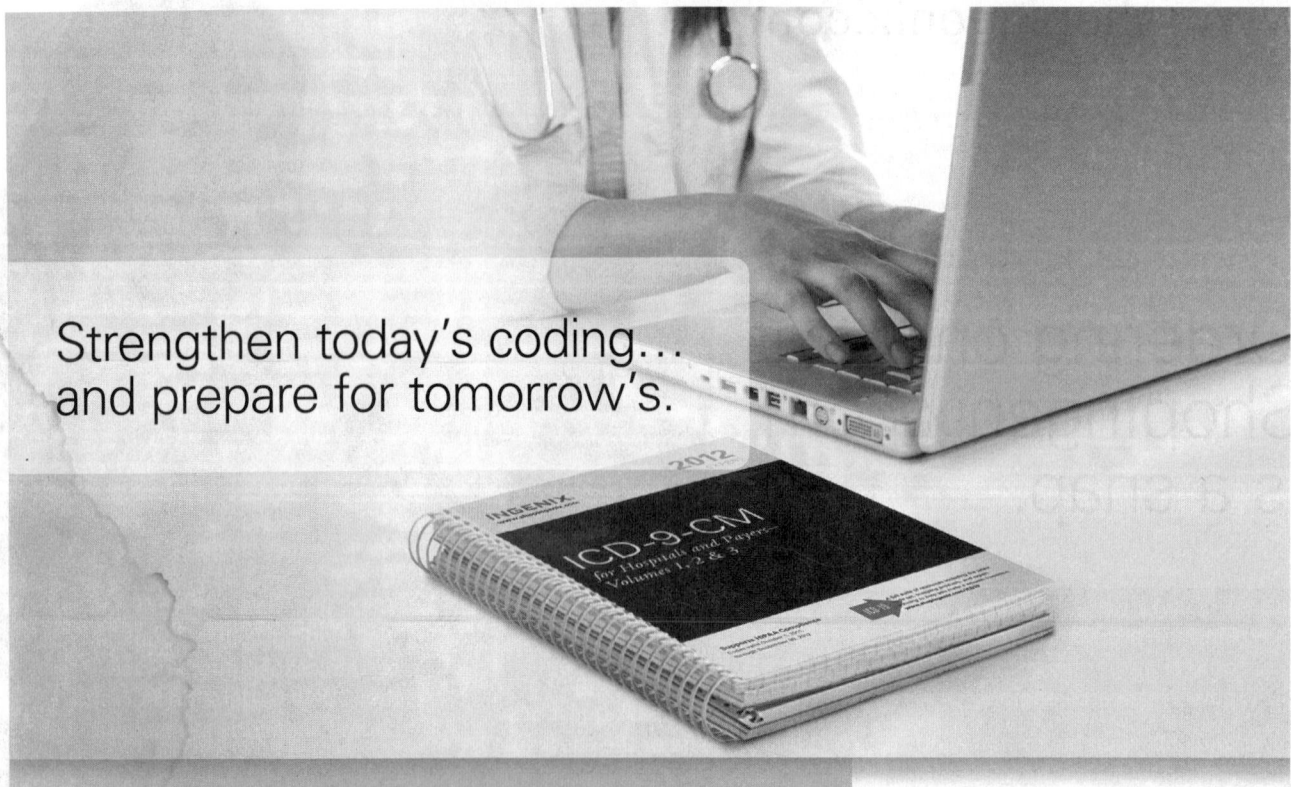

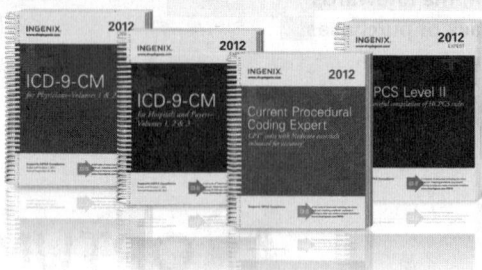

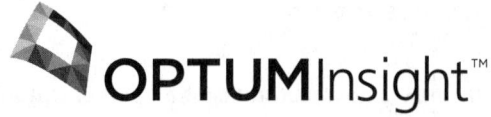

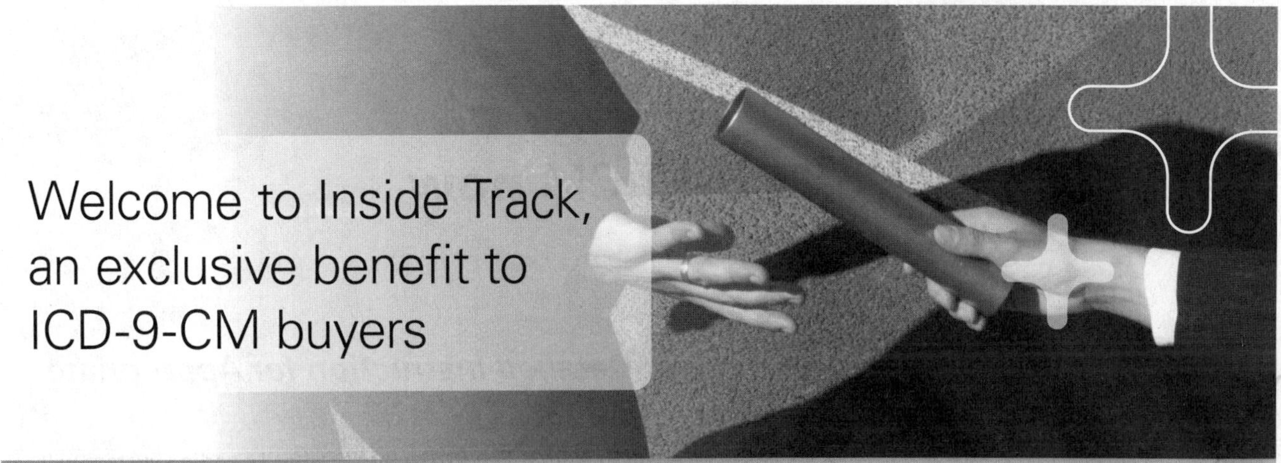

Ingenix Inside Track, your new ICD-9 and ICD-10 hub.

Stay informed with Inside Track. Automatically gain exclusive access to ICD-9-CM news and special reports via email, in addition to ICD-10-CM/PCS training and transition information when you purchase any of the Ingenix ICD-9-CM code books.

← **ICD-9-CM and ICD-10-CM/PCS updates and news**

← **Quarterly e-newsletter**

← **Exclusive offers**

Be sure to opt-in for Inside Track (and pass this great benefit along).

Visit ShopIngenix.com/InsideTrack to sign up today.

Key Features and Benefits

For no additional cost, become a member of Inside Track, and share this benefit with your colleagues! Gain access to the latest tools and updates, conveniently delivered to your inbox to meet your organization's diagnosis coding needs.

- **Stay on top of changing health care, code sets and regulations with Inside Track.**
- **Take advantage of the opportunity to participate in customer surveys and forums to help improve Ingenix diagnosis coding products.**
- **Learn what's going on in the industry with our quarterly e-newsletter, covering ICD-9-CM news and ICD-10-CM/PCS transition updates and tips.**
- **Link right to our ICD-10 Coder's Corner through Inside Track communications.**
- **Learn about new tools available to help with your ICD-10 transition.**

INGENIX®
www.shopingenix.com

OPTUMInsight™
Ingenix is now OptumInsight™, part of Optum™—a leading health services business.

Ingenix is now OptumInsight™, part of Optum™ – a leading health services business| Call toll-free 1.800.464.3649, option 1.

FOBA12J

Learn the basics of ICD-10-CM **now**

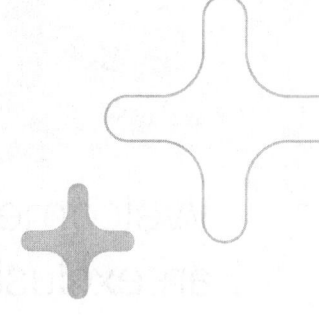

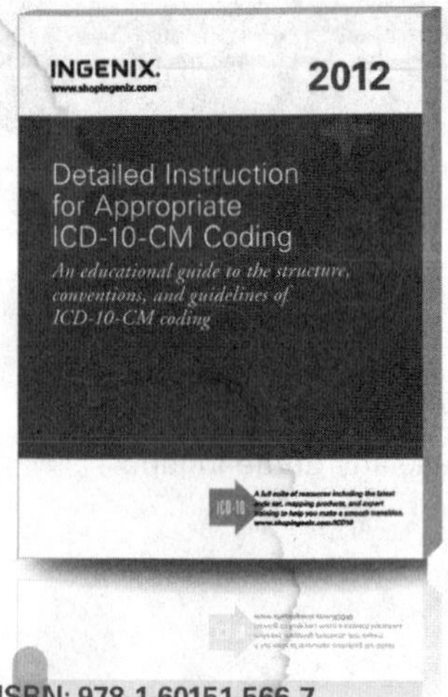

ISBN: 978-1-60151-566-7
Item Number: ITCE12
Available: July, 2011
Price: $99.95

SAVE 25%

SAVE MORE WHEN YOU ORDER ONLINE.

Visit **www.shopingenix.com** and enter promo code FOBA12D to save an additional 5%—that's 30% off.

Or, place your order by calling **1.800.464.3649**, option 1.

Introducing *Detailed Instruction for Appropriate ICD-10-CM Coding*

A successful transition from ICD-9-CM to the ICD-10-CM coding system will require focused training for individuals and organizations. The first step in transitioning to the new coding system is to develop a firm foundation in understanding the coding conventions and guidelines in ICD-10-CM.

This new resource will help create a solid foundation for all levels of ICD-10 CM coding with examples and case studies to explain key coding concepts. The knowledge gleaned from this book will help you evaluate the impact of the new coding system in all aspects of your business.

→ **Learn the coding conventions and guidelines in ICD-10-CM**

→ **Coding examples and case studies**

→ **Knowledge assessments**

Key Features and Benefits

Start your ICD-10-CM training with this easy-to-follow guide.

- This easy-to-follow guide to ICD-10-CM explains the content, structure, and key features of each chapter of the ICD-10-CM coding system
- Detailed review of the official draft ICD-10-CM coding and reporting guidelines provides essential insight into coding concepts and classification changes
- Helpful coding examples illustrate key contrasts and similarities between the ICD-9-CM and ICD-10-CM systems
- Knowledge assessments help quantify understanding of the ICD-10-CM system and feature real-life coding scenarios with the answers explained at length to help sharpen the coding skills of beginner and expert coders
- In-depth review of all 21 chapters of ICD-10-CM, focusing on coding guidelines and conventions

INGENIX®

www.shopingenix.com

OPTUMInsight™

Ingenix is now OptumInsight™, part of Optum™—a leading health services business.

100% money back guarantee. If our merchandise ever fails to meet your expectations, please contact our Customer Service Department toll-free at 1.800.464.3649, option 1, for an immediate response. Software: Credit will be granted for unopened packages only.

Resources are also available from your medical bookstore or distributor.

FOBA12D

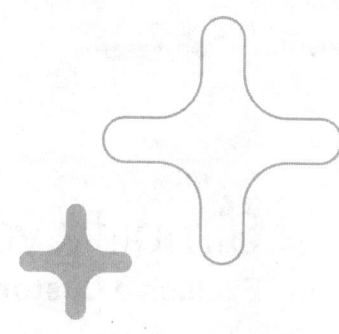

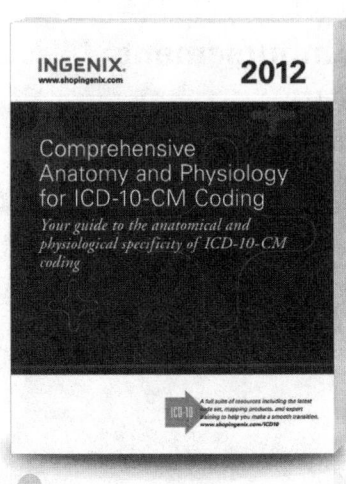

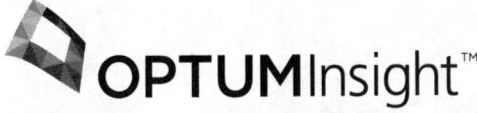

*e*solutions

Simplify your transition to ICD-10 with eSolutions

Exclusive Customer Offer!

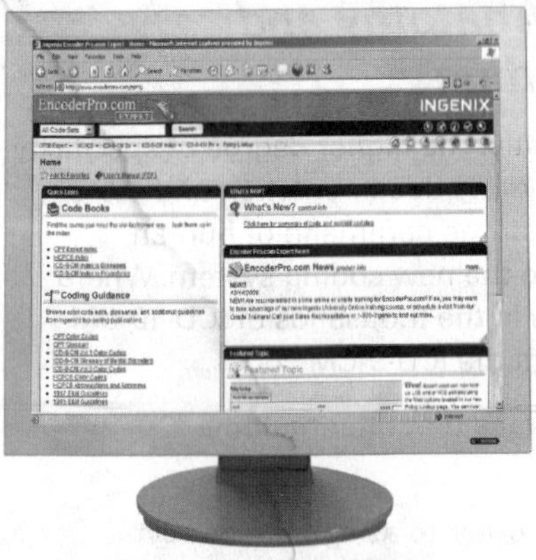

Electronic coding, billing and reimbursement products.

Ingenix provides a robust suite of eSolutions to solve a wide variety of coding, billing and reimbursement issues. As the industry moves to electronic products, to help with the transition to ICD-10, you can rely on Ingenix to help support you through the transition.

→ **Web-based applications for all markets**

→ **Dedicated support and training**

→ **Updated automatically**

→ **ICD-10 code content and mapping**

Exclusive Customer Offer:

Save $150 off a one-year subscription to any eSolution with source code FOBA12L

Visit **www.shopingenix.com** and enter the source code to save $150 off a one-year subscription to any eSolution.

Call toll-free **1.800.464.3649**, option 1 and save $150 off a one-year subscription to any eSolution by mentioning source code FOBA12L.

Key Features and Benefits

Using eSolutions is a step in the right direction when it comes to streamlining your coding, billing and reimbursement practices. Ingenix eSolutions can help you save time and increase your efficiency with accurate and on-time content.

- **Simplify ICD-10 transition.** ICD-10 code content and mapping tools help you understand how your coding will change, and prepare you for coding with ICD-10
- **Save time and money.** Ingenix eSolutions combine the content of over 37 code books and data files
- **Increase accuracy.** Electronic solutions are updated regularly so you know you're always working with the most current content available
- **Get the training and support you need.** Convenient, monthly webinars and customized training programs are available to meet your specific needs
- **Rely on a leader in health care.** Ingenix has been producing quality coding products for over 26 years. All of the expert content that goes into our books goes into our electronic resources
- **Get Started.** Visit **shopingenix.com/ eSolutions** for product listing

INGENIX®

www.shopingenix.com

OPTUMInsight™

Ingenix is now OptumInsight™, part of Optum™— a leading health services business.

Ingenix is now OptumInsight™, part of Optum™ – a leading health services business | Call toll-free 1.800.464.3649, option 1.

Also available from your medical bookstore or distributor.

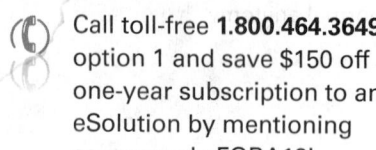

FOBA12L

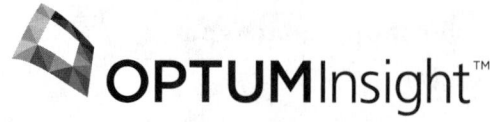

INGENIX.
www.shopingenix.com

OPTUMInsight™
Ingenix is now OptumInsight, part of Optum.

Dear OptumInsight Customer:

Enclosed is the 2012 pre-release draft of the International Classification of Diseases, 10th Revision, Clinical Modification (ICD-10-CM) as written by the World Health Organization (WHO) and National Center for Healthcare Statistics (NCHS). These codes will replace the current ICD-9-CM system for medical documentation and reimbursement. Our new ICD-10-CM code book will help you get a head start with training programs and system conversion.

The Department of Health and Human Services (HHS) published the final rule regarding the adoption of both ICD-10-CM and ICD-10-PCS in the January 16, 2009, *Federal Register* (45 CFR part 162 [CMS—0013—FJ]). The compliance date for implementation of ICD-10-CM and ICD-10-PCS as a replacement for ICD-9-CM is October 1, 2013.

Features and benefits include:

- **Exclusive OptumInsight Edge Color Coding and Icons:**
  - check digit icons to alert coders to required 4th, 5th, 6th, and 7th characters, including a separate icon for placeholder "x" requirements
  - manifestation color coding to ensure appropriate etiology/manifestation code sequencing with no manifestation code sequenced as a first-listed or principal diagnosis
  - color-coded instructional notes that appear in red font
  - color-coded deactivated codes that appear in blue font
- **ICD-10-CM Tabular List of Diseases and Injuries 2012 Addendum:** The complete and official ICD-10-CM Tabular List of Diseases and Injuries 2012 Addendum is available on our website. Log on to www.ShopIngenix.com/productalerts then click on "ICD-9-CM News and Code Book Alerts" to review, download, and print the addendum.
- **Official Preface (2012):** Official preface provided by National Center for Health Statistics (NCHS) as guidance concerning this pre-release draft of ICD-10-CM.
- **Guidelines and Conventions (2012):** The Draft ICD-10-CM Official Guidelines for Coding and Reporting for Acute Short-term and Long-term Hospital Inpatient and Physician Office and Other Outpatient Encounters has been included to assist you with appropriate and consistent code assignment.
- **Index (2012):** Official alphabetic index to the tabular sections.
- **Neoplasm Table (2012):** The Neoplasm Table assists in the indexing and classification of neoplasms within ICD-10-CM.
- **Complete set of ICD-10-CM codes (2012):** All 21 chapters — Infectious and Parasitic Diseases through Injuries, including External Causes and Reasons for Visit.
- **Table of Drugs and Chemicals (2012):** This is a classification of drugs and other chemical substances to assist in the coding of poisoning, overdose states, underdosing, and external causes of adverse effects.

The codes in ICD-10-CM are not currently valid for coding and reporting of medical services for reimbursement purposes. However, the United States began using ICD-10 in 1999 to classify mortality data from death certificates to ensure the international comparability of health statistics.

Thank you for choosing to be an OptumInsight customer. If you have any questions about your *ICD-10-CM Draft 2012* or about any OptumInsight publication, please call our customer service department toll free at (800) 464-3649.

Although this draft of ICD-10-CM is available, the codes in ICD-10-CM are not currently valid for any purpose or use. Updates to this draft are anticipated prior to implementation of ICD-10-CM.

2525 Lake Park Boulevard • Salt Lake City, UT 84120 • 800.464.3649 • Fax 801.982.4033

INGENIX
www.shopingenix.com

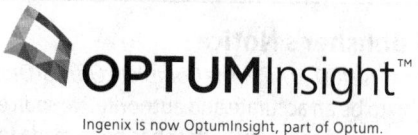

OPTUMInsight™
Ingenix is now OptumInsight, part of Optum.

ICD-10-CM

The Complete Official Draft Code Set

2012

Publisher's Notice

The *ICD-10-CM The Complete Official Draft Code Set* is designed to be an accurate and authoritative source regarding coding and every reasonable effort has been made to ensure accuracy and completeness of the content. However, OptumInsight makes no guarantee, warranty, or representation that this publication is accurate, complete or without errors. It is understood that OptumInsight is not rendering any legal or other professional services or advice in this publication and that OptumInsight bears no liability for any results or consquences that may arise from the use of this book.

Our Commitment to Accuracy

OptumInsight is committed to producing accurate and reliable materials.

To report corrections, please visit www.shopingenix.com/accuracy or email accuracy@ingenix.com. You can also reach customer service by calling 1.800.464.3649, option 1.

Acknowledgments

Anita C. Hart, RHIA, CCS, CCS-P *Product Manager*
Karen Schmidt, BSN, *Technical Director*
Stacy Perry, *Manager, Desktop Publishing*
Lisa Singley, *Project Manager*
Beth Ford, RHIT, CCS, *Clinical/Technical Editor*
Melinda Stegman, MBA, CCS, *Clinical/Technical Editor*
Tracy Betzler, *Desktop Publishing Specialist*
Hope M. Dunn, *Desktop Publishing Specialist*
Katie Russell, *Desktop Publishing Specialist*
Kate Holden, *Editor*

Copyright

Made in the USA
ISBN 1-978-1-60151-605-3

Anita Hart, RHIA,CCS, CCS-P

Product Manager, OptumInsight

Ms. Hart's experience includes 15 years conducting and publishing research in clinical medicine and human genetics for Yale University, Massachusetts General Hospital, and Massachusetts Institute of Technology. Her research conclusions have been published in several peer-reviewed journals. In addition, Ms. Hart has supervised medical records management, health information management, coding and reimbursement, and workers' compensation issues as the office manager for a physical therapy rehabilitation clinic. Ms. Hart is an expert in physician and facility coding, reimbursement systems, and compliance issues. She is also the author of several OptumInsight publications and has served as subject matter advisor on numerous other publications for hospital and physician practices. Ms. Hart is the ICD-9-CM and ICD-10-CM/PCS subject matter expert for OptumInsight, has served as product manager for that product line for 15 years, and has presented at numerous national conferences. Ms. Hart is a member of the American Academy of Professional Coders (AAPC) and is a fully credentialed active member of the American Health Information Management Association (AHIMA). Ms. Hart is a current AHIMA Approved ICD-10-CM/PCS Trainer and leads the training initiatives within OptumInsight Coding Solutions business unit.

Beth Ford, RHIT, CCS

Clinical/Technical Editor

Ms. Ford has more than 25 years experience in physician and facility ICD-9-CM and CPT/HCPCS coding and compliance. She has extensive experience in a variety of health care settings, including acute and post-acute facilities, occupational health, and ambulatory care. Ms. Ford has provided coding education and consulting services to hospitals and physician practices, and has developed curriculum for medical terminology and ICD-9-CM and CPT coding education for a large health care system and multi-specialty physician groups. Formerly, she served as a coding specialist, coding manager, coding trainer/educator, coding consultant, and a health information management director. Her areas of specialization include coding, auditing, and training for DRG, inpatient, outpatient, and physician coding. She is credentialed by the American Health Information Management Association (AHIMA) as a Registered Health Information Technologist (RHIT) and a Certified Coding Specialist (CCS). She is an active member of AHIMA and is an AHIMA-approved ICD-10-CM/PCS trainer.

Melinda Stegman, MBA, CCS

Clinical/Technical Editor

Ms. Stegman has more than 25 years of experience in the HIM profession and has been responsible for the update and maintenance of the ICD-9-CM, ICD-10, DRG resources and some cross coder products for OptumInsight. In the past, she also managed the clinical aspects of the HSS/OptumInsight HIM Consulting practice in the Washington, DC area office. Her areas of specialization include training on inpatient and DRG coding, outpatient coding, and Ambulatory Payment Classifications (APC) for HIM professionals, software developers, and other clients; developing an outpatient billing/coding compliance tool for a major accounting firm; and managing HIM consulting practices. Ms. Stegman is a regular contributing author for Advance for Health Information Management Professionals and for the Journal of Health Care Compliance. She has performed coding assessments and educational sessions throughout the country. Ms. Stegman is credentialed by the American Health Information Management Association (AHIMA) as a Certified Coding Specialist (CCS), is an AHIMA-approved ICD-10-CM/PCS trainer, and holds a Master of Business Administration degree with a concentration in health care management from the University of New Mexico – Albuquerque.

Contents

Preface

ICD-10-CM Official Preface DRAFT

This 2012 pre-release draft of the International Classification of Diseases, 10th Revision, Clinical Modification (ICD-10-CM) is being published by the United States Government in recognition of its responsibility to promulgate this classification throughout the United States for morbidity coding. The International Statistical Classification of Diseases and Related Health Problems, 10th Revision (ICD-10), published by the World Health Organization (WHO), is the foundation of ICD-10-CM. ICD-10 continues to be the classification used in cause-of-death coding in the United States. The ICD-10-CM is comparable with the ICD-10. The WHO Collaborating Center for the Family of International Classifications in North America, housed at the National Center for Health Statistics (NCHS), has responsibility for the implementation of ICD and other WHO-FIC classifications and serves as a liaison with WHO, fulfilling international obligations for comparable classifications and the national health data needs of the United States. The historical background of ICD and ICD-10 can be found in the Introduction to the International Classification of Diseases and Related Health Problems (ICD-10), Second Edition, World Health Organization, Geneva, Switzerland, 2005.

ICD-10-CM is the United States' clinical modification of the World Health Organization's ICD-10. The term clinical is used to emphasize the modification's intent: to serve as a useful tool in the area of classification of morbidity data for indexing of medical records, medical care review, and ambulatory and other medical care programs, as well as for basic health statistics. To describe the clinical picture of the patient, the codes must be more precise than those needed only for statistical groupings and trend analysis.

Characteristics of ICD-10-CM

ICD-10-CM far exceeds its predecessors in the number of concepts and codes provided. The disease classification has been expanded to include health-related conditions and to provide greater specificity at the sixth character level and with a seventh character extension. The sixth and seventh characters are not optional; they are intended for use in recording the information documented in the clinical record.

Introduction

History and Future of ICD-10-CM

The ICD-10-CM classification system was developed by the National Center for Health Statistics (NCHS) as a clinical modification to the ICD-10 system developed by the World Health Organization (WHO), primarily as a unique system for use in the United States for morbidity and mortality reporting. Although ICD-10-CM has not yet been implemented for use in the United States, ICD-10 has been adopted for use in the coding and classification of mortality data from death certificates. ICD-10 replaced ICD-9 for this purpose as of January 1, 1999. Upon legislative approval, ICD-10-CM is planned as the replacement for ICD-9-CM, volumes 1 and 2.

ICD-10 is the copyrighted product of the World Health Organization (WHO), which has authorized the development of a clinical modification (CM) of ICD-10 for use in the United States. However, all modifications to the ICD-10 must conform to WHO conventions for ICD. The development of ICD-10-CM included comprehensive evaluation by a Technical Advisory Panel and extensive consultation with physician groups, clinical coders, and other industry experts.

The ICD-10-CM draft and crosswalk between ICD-9-CM and ICD-10-CM have been made available on the NCHS website for public comment. The initial public comment period extended from December 1997 through February 1998. A field test for ICD-10-CM was conducted in the summer of 2003 jointly by The American Hospital Association (AMA) and the American Health Information Management Association (AHIMA). Public comments and suggestions were reviewed and additional modifications to ICD-10-CM were made. Revisions were made to ICD-10-CM based on the established update process for ICD-9-CM (the ICD-9-CM Coordination and Maintenance Committee) and the World Health Organization's ICD-10 (the Update and Revision Committee).

These revisions to ICD-10-CM have included:

- information relevant to ambulatory and managed care encounters
- expanded injury codes
- creation of combination diagnosis/symptom codes to reduce the number of codes needed to fully describe a condition
- the addition of sixth and seventh character classifications
- incorporation of common 4th and 5th character classifications
- classifications specific to laterality
- classification refinement for increased data granularity

This new structure allows for further expansion than was possible with the ICD-9-CM classification system.

This new 2012 draft update release is available for public viewing. ICD-10-CM codes are not currently valid for any purpose or use other than the reporting of mortality data for death certificates.

The Department of Health and Human Services (HHS) published the final rule regarding the adoption of both ICD-10-CM and ICD-10-PCS in the January 16, 2009 *Federal Register* (45 CFR part 162 [CMS—0013—F]). The compliance date for implementation of ICD-10-CM and ICD-10-PCS as a replacement for ICD-9-CM is October 1, 2013.

How to Use the ICD-10-CM (Draft 2012)

This draft of the International Classification of Diseases, 10th Revision, Clinical Modification (ICD-10-CM) is being published by the United States Government in recognition of its responsibility to promulgate this classification throughout the United States for morbidity coding. This code book represents an adaptation of ICD-10 which was created specifically for use in the United States. Future revisions to ICD-10-CM will be made based on the established update process for ICD-9-CM (the ICD-9-CM Coordination and Maintenance Committee) and the World Health Organization's ICD-10 (the Update and Revision Committee). Upon legislative approval, ICD-10-CM is planned as the replacement for ICD-9-CM, volumes 1 and 2.

Steps to Correct Coding

1. Before beginning to use this code book, review section 1.A., "Conventions," and section 1.B., "General Coding Guidelines of the ICD-10-CM Draft Official Guidelines for Coding and Reporting 2011."
2. Look up the main term in the Alphabetic Index and scan the subterm entries as appropriate. Review continued lines and additional subterms that may appear in the next column or on the next page.
3. Note all parenthetical terms (nonessential modifiers) that help in code selection but do not affect code assignment. Shaded guidelines in the Index are provided to help determine the indentation level for each subterm in relation to the main terms.
4. Pay close attention to the following instructions in the Index:
   - "see," "see also," and "see category" cross-references
   - "with"/"without" notes
   - "omit code" notes
   - "due to" subterms
   - other instructions found in note boxes, such as "code by site"
5. Do not code from the Alphabetic Index without verifying the accuracy of the code in the Tabular List. Locate the code in the alphanumerically arranged Tabular List.
6. To determine the appropriateness of the code selection and proper coding, read all instructional material:
   - "includes" and "excludes" notes
   - "use additional code" and "code first underlying disease" instructions
   - "code also"
   - fourth-, fifth-, and sixth-character requirements and seventh-character extension requirements
7. Consult the official Draft ICD-10-CM guidelines, which govern the use of specific codes. These guidelines provide both general and chapter-specific coding guidance.
8. Confirm and assign the correct code.

Organization

This book is organized in the following manner:

Introduction

The introductory material in this book includes the ICD-10-CM Official Preface, the history and future of ICD-10-CM as well as an overview of the classification system.

Draft Official ICD-10-CM Conventions and Guidelines

This section provides an explanation of the conventions and guidelines regulating the appropriate assignment and reporting of ICD-10-CM codes. This coding guidance is presented by the National Center for Health Statistics (NCHS), a governmental agency of the Centers for Disease Control and Prevention (CDC), within the United States Department of Health and Human Services (DHHS).

Alphabetic Index to Diseases

The Alphabetic Index to Diseases is arranged in alphabetic order by disease — by specific illness, injury, eponym, abbreviation, or other descriptive diagnostic term. The Index also lists diagnostic terms for other reasons for encounters with health care professionals.

Neoplasm Table

The Neoplasm Table provides the proper code based upon histolog the neoplasm and site.

Table of Drugs and Chemicals

The Table of Drugs and Chemicals is also included within the Alpha Index.

The Table of Drugs and Chemicals lists the drug and the specific co that identify the drug and the intent. No additional external cause c injury and poisoning code is assigned in ICD-10-CM.

Index to External Causes

The Alphabetic Index to External Causes of injuries is arranged in alphabetic order by main term indicating the event.

Tabular List of Diseases

ICD-10-CM codes and descriptors are arranged numerically within the Tabular List of Diseases within 21 separate chapters according to body system or nature of injury and disease. Classifications which were previously considered supplemental to ICD-9-CM (e.g., V codes and E codes) are incorporated into the Tabular Listing of ICD-10-CM as individual chapters. Chapters 20 External Causes of Morbidity and 21 Factors Influencing Health Status and Contact with Health Services include chapter-specific guidelines.

ICD-1Ø-CM Draft Conventions

The ICD-1Ø-CM conventions are general rules for the use of the classification system, independent of the guidelines. These conventions are incorporated within the Index and Tabular List as instructional notes and are applicable regardless of the health care setting.

Format

ICD-1Ø-CM is divided into two main parts: the Index, an alphabetical list of terms and their corresponding code, and the Tabular List, a sequential, alphanumeric list of codes divided into chapters based on body system or condition. The Index contains the Index to Diseases and Injuries (main index) and the Index to External Causes of Injury. Also included in the main Index is the Neoplasm Table and a Table of Drugs and Chemicals.

The Tabular List contains categories, subcategories, and valid codes. ICD-1Ø-CM is an alphanumeric classification system. The first character of a three-character category is a letter. The second and third characters may be numbers or alpha characters. A three-character category without further subclassification is equivalent to a valid three-character code. Subcategories are either four or five characters. Subcategory characters include either letters or numbers. Codes may be four, five, or six characters in length, in which each level of subdivision after a category is a subcategory. The final level of subdivision is a valid code. The final character in a code may be either a letter or a number.

The ICD-1Ø-CM used the letter "X" as a place-holder. A placeholder "X" is used as a fifth character place-holder at certain six-character codes to allow for future expansion, without disturbing the sixth-character structure. For instance, an initial encounter for accidental poisoning by penicillin is coded to T36.ØX1A. The "X" in the fifth character position is a place-holder, or filler character.

Similarly, certain categories have applicable seventh-character extensions. In these cases, the seventh-character extension is required for all codes within the category, or as otherwise instructed in the Tabular List notations. Seventh-character extensions must always be the last character in the data field. If a code is not a full six characters in length, a dummy place-holder "X" must be used to fill in the empty characters when a seventh character extension is required.

Punctuation

[ ] In the Tabular List, brackets are used to enclose synonyms, alternative wording, or explanatory phrases. In the Index, brackets are used to identify manifestation codes.

( ) Parentheses are used in both the Index and Tabular List to enclose nonessential modifiers; supplementary words that may be present or absent in the statement of a disease or procedure without affecting the code number to which it is assigned.

: Colons are used in the Tabular List after an incomplete term that needs one or more of the modifiers following the colon to make it assignable to a given category.

Abbreviations

NEC

The abbreviation NEC, "Not elsewhere classifiable" represents "other specified" in the ICD-1Ø-CM. An index entry that states NEC directs the coder to an "other specified" code in the Tabular List. Codes titled "Other" or "Other specified" in the Tabular List (usually a code with a fourth or sixth character 8 or z and fifth character 9) are for use when the information in the medical record provides detail for which a specific code does not exist.

NOS

The abbreviation NOS, "Not otherwise specified," in the Tabular List may be interpreted as "unspecified." Codes in the Tabular List with "Unspecified" in the title (usually a code with a fourth or sixth character 9 and fifth character Ø) are for use when the information in the medical record is insufficient to assign a more specific code.

Typeface

Boldface

Boldface type is used for main term entries in the Alphabetic Index, and all codes and descriptions in the Tabular List.

Italicized

Italicized type is used for all exclusion notes and to identify manifestation codes, those codes that should not be reported as first-listed (principal) diagnoses.

General Notes

The following conventions and notes appear only in the Tabular List of Diseases:

Includes Notes

The word "Includes" appears immediately under certain categories to further define, clarify, or give examples of the content of a code category.

Inclusion Terms

Lists of inclusion terms are included under certain codes. These terms indicate some of the conditions for which that code number may be used. Inclusion terms may be synonyms with the code title, or, in the case of "other specified" codes, the terms may also provide a list of various conditions included within a classification code. The inclusion terms are not exhaustive. The Index may provide additional terms that may also be assigned to a given code.

Excludes Notes

ICD-1Ø-CM has two types of excludes notes. Each note has a different definition for use. However, they are similar in that they both indicate that codes excluded from each other are independent of each other.

Excludes1

An excludes1 note is a "pure" excludes. It means "NOT CODED HERE!" An excludes1 note indicates mutually exclusive codes; two conditions that cannot be reported together. For example, a congenital form of a disease may not be reported with the acquired form of the same condition. The code excluded should never be reported with the applicable codes listed above the excludes notation.

Excludes2

An excludes2 note means "NOT INCLUDED HERE." An excludes2 note indicates that although the excluded condition is not part of the condition it is excluded from, a patient may have both conditions at the same time. Therefore, when an excludes2 note appears under a code, it may be acceptable to use both the code and the excluded code together if supported by the medical documentation.

Instructional Notes in the Alphabetic Index

See/See Also

In the index, the "see" instruction following a main term or subterm refers the coder to an alternate entry to locate the correct code.

Similarly, a "see also" instruction following a main term or subterm indicates that an additional term should be referenced to provide additional information

Default Codes

In the index, the default code is the code listed next to the main term. The default code represents the condition most commonly associated with the main term. This code may be assigned when documentation does not facilitate reporting a more specific code. Alternately, it may provide an unspecified code for the condition.

Syndromes

Follow the Alphabetic Index guidance when coding syndromes. In the absence of index guidance, assign codes for the documented manifestations of the syndrome.

And

When the term "and" is used in a narrative statement it may be interpreted as "and/or."

With/Without

When "with" and "without" are the two options for the final character of a set of codes, the default is always "without." For five-character codes, a "Ø" as the fifth-position character represents "without", and "1" represents "with." For six-character codes, the sixth-position character "1" represents "with" and "9" represents "without."

Instructional Notes Used in the Tabular List

In the tabular section, the following instructional notes appear in red type for emphasis:

Code First/Use additional code:

These instructional notes are in red type and provide sequencing instruction. They may appear independently of each other or to designate certain etiology/manifestation paired codes. These instructions signal the coder that an additional code should be reported to provide a more complete picture of that diagnosis.

In etiology/manifestation coding, ICD-1Ø-CM requires the underlying condition to be sequenced first, followed by the manifestation. In these situations, codes with "In diseases classified elsewhere" in the code description are never permitted as a first-listed or principal diagnosis code and must be sequenced following the underlying condition code.

Code Also:

A code also note alerts the coder that more than one code may be required to fully describe the condition. Code sequencing is discretionary. Factors that may determine sequencing include severity and reason for the encounter. These coding notes appear in red type.

Additional Conventions

Additional Characters Required

√4th This symbol indicates that the code requires a fourth character.

√5th This symbol indicates that the code requires a fifth character.

√6th This symbol indicates that the code requires a sixth character.

√7th This symbol indicates that the code requires a seventh character.

√x7th This symbol indicates that the code requires a seventh character following the placeholder X. Codes less than six characters that require a seventh character must contain placeholder x to fill the missing characters. The seventh character must always be a valid seventh character for that code.

Boldface

Note

The term "Note:" appears enclosed within a red icon and precedes the instructional information. These notes function as an alert, to highlight coding instruction within the text.

Color Coding

Manifestation Code

These codes appear in italic type, with a blue color bar over the title. A manifestation code cannot be reported as a first-listed or principal diagnosis. By definition, a manifestation code represents a demonstration of some aspect of an underlying disease, which is separately classifiable. In the Alphabetic Index, these codes are listed as the secondary code in brackets. The underlying disease code is listed first.

Summary of Code Changes

- ● A41.Ø1 Sepsis due to Methicillin susceptible Staphylococcus aureus
- ● A41.Ø2 Sepsis due to Methicillin resistant Staphylococcus aureus
- ▲ A41.9 Sepsis, unspecified organism
- ● A49.Ø1 Methicillin susceptible Staphylococcus aureus infection, unspecified site
- ● A49.Ø2 Methicillin resistant Staphylococcus aureus infection, unspecified site
- ● B95.61 Methicillin susceptible Staphylococcus aureus infection as the cause of diseases classified elsewhere
- ● B95.62 Methicillin resistant Staphylococcus aureus infection as the cause of diseases classified elsewhere
- ● B96.2Ø Unspecified Escherichia coli [E. coli] as the cause of diseases classified elsewhere
- ● B96.21 Shiga toxin-producing Escherichia coli [E. coli] (STEC) O157 as the cause of diseases classified elsewhere
- ● B96.22 Other specified Shiga toxin-producing Escherichia coli [E. coli] (STEC) as the cause of diseases classified elsewhere
- ● B96.23 Unspecified Shiga toxin-producing Escherichia coli [E. coli] (STEC) as the cause of diseases classified elsewhere
- ● B96.29 Other Escherichia coli [E. coli] as the cause of diseases classified elsewhere
- ▲ C44 Other and unspecified malignant neoplasm of skin
- ▲ C44.Ø Other and unspecified malignant neoplasm of skin of lip
- ● C44.ØØ Unspecified malignant neoplasm of skin of lip
- ● C44.Ø1 Basal cell carcinoma of skin of lip
- ● C44.Ø2 Squamous cell carcinoma of skin of lip
- ● C44.Ø9 Other specified malignant neoplasm of skin of lip
- ▲ C44.1 Other and unspecified malignant neoplasm of skin of eyelid, including canthus
- ▲ C44.1Ø Malignant neoplasm of skin unspecified Unspecified malignant neoplasm of skin of eyelid, including canthus
- ● C44.1Ø1 Unspecified malignant neoplasm of skin of unspecified eyelid, including canthus
- ● C44.1Ø2 Unspecified malignant neoplasm of skin of right eyelid, including canthus
- ● C44.1Ø9 Unspecified malignant neoplasm of skin of left eyelid, including canthus
- ▲ C44.11 Malignant neoplasm of skin of right Basal cell carcinoma of skin of eyelid, including canthus
- ● C44.111 Basal cell carcinoma of skin of unspecified eyelid, including canthus
- ● C44.112 Basal cell carcinoma of skin of right eyelid, including canthus
- ● C44.119 Basal cell carcinoma of skin of left eyelid, including canthus
- ▲ C44.12 Malignant neoplasm of skin of left Squamous cell carcinoma of skin of eyelid, including canthus
- ● C44.121 Squamous cell carcinoma of skin of unspecified eyelid, including canthus
- ● C44.122 Squamous cell carcinoma of skin of right eyelid, including canthus
- ● C44.129 Squamous cell carcinoma of skin of left eyelid, including canthus
- ● C44.19 Other specified malignant neoplasm of skin of eyelid, including canthus
- ● C44.191 Other specified malignant neoplasm of skin of unspecified eyelid, including canthus
- ● C44.192 Other specified malignant neoplasm of skin of right eyelid, including canthus
- ● C44.199 Other specified malignant neoplasm of skin of left eyelid, including canthus
- ▲ C44.2 Other and unspecified malignant neoplasm of skin of ear and external auricular canal
- ▲ C44.2Ø Malignant neoplasm of skin unspecified Unspecified malignant neoplasm of skin of ear and external auricular canal
- ● C44.2Ø1 Unspecified malignant neoplasm of skin of unspecified ear and external auricular canal
- ● C44.2Ø2 Unspecified malignant neoplasm of skin of right ear and external auricular canal
- ● C44.2Ø9 Unspecified malignant neoplasm of skin of left ear and external auricular canal
- ▲ C44.21 Malignant neoplasm of skin right Basal cell carcinoma of skin of ear and external auricular canal
- ● C44.211 Basal cell carcinoma of skin of unspecified ear and external auricular canal
- ● C44.212 Basal cell carcinoma of skin of right ear and external auricular canal
- ● C44.219 Basal cell carcinoma of skin of left ear and external auricular canal
- ▲ C44.22 Malignant neoplasm of skin left Squamous cell carcinoma of skin of ear and external auricular canal
- ● C44.221 Squamous cell carcinoma of skin of unspecified ear and external auricular canal
- ● C44.222 Squamous cell carcinoma of skin of right ear and external auricular canal
- ● C44.229 Squamous cell carcinoma of skin of left ear and external auricular canal
- ● C44.29 Other specified malignant neoplasm of skin of ear and external auricular canal
- ● C44.291 Other specified malignant neoplasm of skin of unspecified ear and external auricular canal
- ● C44.292 Other specified malignant neoplasm of skin of right ear and external auricular canal
- ● C44.299 Other specified malignant neoplasm of skin of left ear and external auricular canal
- ▲ C44.3 Other and unspecified malignant neoplasm of skin of other and unspecified parts of face
- ▲ C44.3Ø Malignant neoplasm of skin of unspecified part Unspecified malignant neoplasm of skin of other and unspecified parts of face
- ● C44.3ØØ Unspecified malignant neoplasm of skin of unspecified part of face
- ● C44.3Ø1 Unspecified malignant neoplasm of skin of nose
- ● C44.3Ø9 Unspecified malignant neoplasm of skin of other parts of face
- ▲ C44.31 Malignant neoplasm of nose Basal cell carcinoma of skin of other and unspecified parts of face
- ● C44.31Ø Basal cell carcinoma of skin of unspecified parts of face
- ● C44.311 Basal cell carcinoma of skin of nose
- ● C44.319 Basal cell carcinoma of skin of other parts of face
- ● C44.32 Squamous cell carcinoma of skin of other and unspecified parts of face
- ● C44.32Ø Squamous cell carcinoma of skin of unspecified parts of face
- ● C44.321 Squamous cell carcinoma of skin of nose
- ● C44.329 Squamous cell carcinoma of skin of other parts of face
- ▲ C44.39 Malignant neoplasm of skin of other Other specified malignant neoplasm of skin of other and unspecified parts of face
- ● C44.39Ø Other specified malignant neoplasm of skin of unspecified parts of face
- ● C44.391 Other specified malignant neoplasm of skin of nose
- ● C44.399 Other specified malignant neoplasm of skin of other parts of face
- ▲ C44.4 Other and unspecified malignant neoplasm of skin of scalp and neck
- ● C44.4Ø Unspecified malignant neoplasm of skin of scalp and neck
- ● C44.41 Basal cell carcinoma of skin of scalp and neck
- ● C44.42 Squamous cell carcinoma of skin of scalp and neck
- ● C44.49 Other specified malignant neoplasm of skin of scalp and neck
- ▲ C44.5 Other and unspecified malignant neoplasm of skin of trunk
- ● C44.5Ø Unspecified malignant neoplasm of skin of trunk
- ● C44.5ØØ Unspecified malignant neoplasm of anal skin
- ● C44.5Ø1 Unspecified malignant neoplasm of skin of breast
- ● C44.5Ø9 Unspecified malignant neoplasm of skin of other part of trunk
- ▲ C44.51 Malignant neoplasm of anal skin Basal cell carcinoma of skin of trunk
- ● C44.51Ø Basal cell carcinoma of anal skin
- ● C44.511 Basal cell carcinoma of skin of breast
- ● C44.519 Basal cell carcinoma of skin of other part of trunk
- ▲ C44.52 Malignant neoplasm of skin of breast Squamous cell carcinoma of skin of trunk
- ● C44.52Ø Squamous cell carcinoma of anal skin
- ● C44.521 Squamous cell carcinoma of skin of breast
- ● C44.529 Squamous cell carcinoma of skin of other part of trunk
- ▲ C44.59 Malignant neoplasm of other part Other specified malignant neoplasm of skin of trunk
- ● C44.59Ø Other specified malignant neoplasm of anal skin
- ● C44.591 Other specified malignant neoplasm of skin of breast
- ● C44.599 Other specified malignant neoplasm of skin of other part of trunk

● New Code ▲ Revised Code

- ▲ C44.6 Other and unspecified malignant neoplasm of skin of upper limb, including shoulder
- ▲ C44.60 Malignant neoplasm of skin of unspecified Unspecified malignant neoplasm of skin of upper limb, including shoulder
- ● C44.601 Unspecified malignant neoplasm of skin of unspecified upper limb, including shoulder
- ● C44.602 Unspecified malignant neoplasm of skin of right upper limb, including shoulder
- ● C44.609 Unspecified malignant neoplasm of skin of left upper limb, including shoulder
- ▲ C44.61 Malignant neoplasm of skin of right Basal cell carcinoma of skin of upper limb, including shoulder
- ● C44.611 Basal cell carcinoma of skin of unspecified upper limb, including shoulder
- ● C44.612 Basal cell carcinoma of skin of right upper limb, including shoulder
- ● C44.619 Basal cell carcinoma of skin of left upper limb, including shoulder
- ▲ C44.62 Malignant neoplasm of skin of left Squamous cell carcinoma of skin of upper limb, including shoulder
- ● C44.621 Squamous cell carcinoma of skin of unspecified upper limb, including shoulder
- ● C44.622 Squamous cell carcinoma of skin of right upper limb, including shoulder
- ● C44.629 Squamous cell carcinoma of skin of left upper limb, including shoulder
- ● C44.69 Other specified malignant neoplasm of skin of upper limb, including shoulder
- ● C44.691 Other specified malignant neoplasm of skin of unspecified upper limb, including shoulder
- ● C44.692 Other specified malignant neoplasm of skin of right upper limb, including shoulder
- ● C44.699 Other specified malignant neoplasm of skin of left upper limb, including shoulder
- ▲ C44.7 Other and unspecified malignant neoplasm of skin of lower limb, including hip
- ▲ C44.70 Malignant neoplasm of skin of unspecified Unspecified malignant neoplasm of skin of lower limb, including hip
- ● C44.701 Unspecified malignant neoplasm of skin of unspecified lower limb, including hip
- ● C44.702 Unspecified malignant neoplasm of skin of right lower limb, including hip
- ● C44.709 Unspecified malignant neoplasm of skin of left lower limb, including hip
- ▲ C44.71 Malignant neoplasm of skin of rightBasal cell carcinoma of skin of lower limb, including hip
- ● C44.711 Basal cell carcinoma of skin of unspecified lower limb, including hip
- ● C44.712 Basal cell carcinoma of skin of right lower limb, including hip
- ● C44.719 Basal cell carcinoma of skin of left lower limb, including hip
- ▲ C44.72 Malignant neoplasm of skin of left Squamous cell carcinoma of skin of lower limb, including hip
- ● C44.721 Squamous cell carcinoma of skin of unspecified lower limb, including hip
- ● C44.722 Squamous cell carcinoma of skin of right lower limb, including hip
- ● C44.729 Squamous cell carcinoma of skin of left lower limb, including hip
- ● C44.79 Other specified malignant neoplasm of skin of lower limb, including hip
- ● C44.791 Other specified malignant neoplasm of skin of unspecified lower limb, including hip
- ● C44.792 Other specified malignant neoplasm of skin of right lower limb, including hip
- ● C44.799 Other specified malignant neoplasm of skin of left lower limb, including hip
- ▲ C44.8 Other and unspecified malignant neoplasm of overlapping sites of skin
- ● C44.80 Unspecified malignant neoplasm of overlapping sites of skin
- ● C44.81 Basal cell carcinoma of overlapping sites of skin
- ● C44.82 Squamous cell carcinoma of overlapping sites of skin
- ● C44.89 Other specified malignant neoplasm of overlapping sites of skin
- ▲ C44.9 Other and unspecified malignant neoplasm of skin, unspecified
- ● C44.90 Unspecified malignant neoplasm of skin, unspecified
- ● C44.91 Basal cell carcinoma of skin, unspecified
- ● C44.92 Squamous cell carcinoma of skin, unspecified
- ● C44.99 Other specified malignant neoplasm of skin, unspecified
- ▲ C83.9 Non-follicular (diffuse) lymphoma, unspecified
- ▲ C83.90 Non-follicular (diffuse) lymphoma, unspecified, unspecified site
- ▲ C83.91 Non-follicular (diffuse) lymphoma, unspecified, lymph nodes of head, face, and neck
- ▲ C83.92 Non-follicular (diffuse) lymphoma, unspecified, intrathoracic lymph nodes
- ▲ C83.93 Non-follicular (diffuse) lymphoma, unspecified, intra-abdominal lymph nodes
- ▲ C83.94 Non-follicular (diffuse) lymphoma, unspecified, lymph nodes of axilla and upper limb
- ▲ C83.95 Non-follicular (diffuse) lymphoma, unspecified, lymph nodes of inguinal region and lower limb
- ▲ C83.96 Non-follicular (diffuse) lymphoma, unspecified, intrapelvic lymph nodes
- ▲ C83.97 Non-follicular (diffuse) lymphoma, unspecified, spleen
- ▲ C83.98 Non-follicular (diffuse) lymphoma, unspecified, lymph nodes of multiple sites
- ▲ C83.99 Non-follicular (diffuse) lymphoma, unspecified, extranodal and solid organ sites
- ▲ C93.Z0 Other monocytic leukemia, not in having achieved remission
- ● C93.Z2 Other monocytic leukemia, in relapse
- ● D17.71 Benign lipomatous neoplasm of kidney
- ● D17.72 Benign lipomatous neoplasm of other genitourinary organ
- ● D17.79 Benign lipomatous neoplasm of other sites
- ▲ D23.70 Other benign neoplasm of skin of unspecified lower limb, including hip
- ● D56.5 Hemoglobin E-beta thalassemia
- ● D61.810 Antineoplastic chemotherapy induced pancytopenia
- ● D61.811 Other drug-induced pancytopenia
- ● D61.818 Other pancytopenia
- ▲ D68.31 Hemorrhagic disorder due to intrinsic circulating anticoagulants, antibodies, or inhibitors
- ● D68.311 Acquired hemophilia
- ● D68.312 Antiphospholipid antibody with hemorrhagic disorder
- ● D68.318 Other hemorrhagic disorder due to intrinsic circulating anticoagulants, antibodies, or inhibitors
- ▲ D68.61 Anticardiolipinphospholipid syndrome
- ▲ D78.0 Intraoperative hemorrhage and hematoma of the spleen complicating a procedure
- ▲ D78.01 Intraoperative hemorrhage and hematoma of the spleen complicating a procedure on the spleen
- ▲ D78.02 Intraoperative hemorrhage and hematoma of the spleen complicating other procedure
- ▲ D78.1 Accidental puncture and laceration of the spleen during a procedure
- ▲ D78.11 Accidental puncture and laceration of the spleen during a procedure on the spleen
- ▲ D78.12 Accidental puncture and laceration of the spleen during other procedure
- ▲ D78.2 Postprocedural hemorrhage and hematoma of the spleen following a procedure
- ▲ D78.21 Postprocedural hemorrhage and hematoma of the spleen following a procedure on the spleen
- ▲ D78.22 Postprocedural hemorrhage and hematoma of the spleen following other procedure
- ▲ D78.8 Other intraoperative and postprocedural complications of the spleen
- ▲ D78.81 Other intraoperative complications of the spleen
- ▲ D78.89 Other postprocedural complications of the spleen
- ▲ F02.80 Dementia in other diseases classified elsewhere, without behavioral disturbance
- ▲ F02.81 Dementia in other diseases classified elsewhere, with behavioral disturbance
- ● F03.9 Unspecified dementia
- ● F03.90 Unspecified dementia without behavioral disturbance
- ● F03.91 Unspecified dementia with behavioral disturbance
- ● F48.2 Pseudobulbar affect
- ▲ F70 Mild mental retardation intellectual disabilities
- ▲ F71 Moderate mental retardation intellectual disabilities
- ▲ F72 Severe mental retardation intellectual disabilities
- ▲ F73 Profound mental retardation intellectual disabilities
- ▲ F78 Other mental retardation intellectual disabilities
- ▲ F79 Unspecified mental retardation intellectual disabilities

▲ G04.00 Postinfectious acute disseminated encephalitis and encephalomyelitis, (postinfectious ADEM) Acute disseminated encephalitis and encephalomyelitis, unspecified
▲ G04.01 Postimmunization acute encephalitis, myelitis and encephalomyelitis Postinfectious acute disseminated encephalitis and encephalomyelitis (postinfectious ADEM)
● G04.02 Postimmunization acute disseminated encephalitis, myelitis and encephalomyelitis
▲ G04.30 Postinfectious acute necrotizing hemorrhagic encephalopathy Acute necrotizing hemorrhagic encephalopathy, unspecified
▲ G04.31 Postimmunization Postinfectious acute necrotizing hemorrhagic encephalopathy
● G04.32 Postimmunization acute necrotizing hemorrhagic encephalopathy
● G04.39 Other acute necrotizing hemorrhagic encephalopathy
● G13.2 Systemic atrophy primarily affecting the central nervous system in myxedema
● G25.83 Benign shuddering attacks
● G31.85 Corticobasal degeneration
● G32.81 Cerebellar ataxia in diseases classified elsewhere
● G32.89 Other specified degenerative disorders of nervous system in diseases classified elsewhere
● G40.A Absence epileptic syndrome
● G40.A0 Absence epileptic syndrome, not intractable
● G40.A01 Absence epileptic syndrome, not intractable, with status epilepticus
● G40.A09 Absence epileptic syndrome, not intractable, without status epilepticus
● G40.A1 Absence epileptic syndrome, intractable
● G40.A11 Absence epileptic syndrome, intractable, with status epilepticus
● G40.A19 Absence epileptic syndrome, intractable, without status epilepticus
● G40.B Juvenile myoclonic epilepsy [impulsive petit mal]
● G40.B0 Juvenile myoclonic epilepsy, not intractable
● G40.B01 Juvenile myoclonic epilepsy, not intractable, with status epilepticus
● G40.B09 Juvenile myoclonic epilepsy, not intractable, without status epilepticus
● G40.B1 Juvenile myoclonic epilepsy, intractable
● G40.B11 Juvenile myoclonic epilepsy, intractable, with status epilepticus
● G40.B19 Juvenile myoclonic epilepsy, intractable, without status epilepticus
▲ G40.5 Special epileptic syndromes Epileptic seizures related to external causes
▲ G40.50 Special epileptic syndromes Epileptic seizures related to external causes, not intractable
▲ G40.501 Special epileptic syndromes Epileptic seizures related to external causes, not intractable, with status epilepticus
▲ G40.509 Special epileptic syndromes Epileptic seizures related to external causes, not intractable, without status epilepticus
▲ G40.8 Other epilepsy and recurrent seizures
▲ G40.80 Other epilepsy, not intractable
● G40.802 Other epilepsy, not intractable, without status epilepticus
● G40.803 Other epilepsy, intractable, with status epilepticus
● G40.804 Other epilepsy, intractable, without status epilepticus
▲ G40.81 Other epilepsy, intractable Lennox-Gastaut syndrome
▲ G40.811 Other epilepsy, Lennox-Gastaut syndrome, not intractable, with status epilepticus
● G40.812 Lennox-Gastaut syndrome, not intractable, without status epilepticus
● G40.813 Lennox-Gastaut syndrome, intractable, with status epilepticus
● G40.814 Lennox-Gastaut syndrome, intractable, without status epilepticus
● G40.82 Epileptic spasms
● G40.821 Epileptic spasms, not intractable, with status epilepticus
● G40.822 Epileptic spasms, not intractable, without status epilepticus
● G40.823 Epileptic spasms, intractable, with status epilepticus
● G40.824 Epileptic spasms, intractable, without status epilepticus
▲ G43.D Menstrual Abdominal migraine
▲ G43.D0 Menstrual Abdominal migraine, not intractable
▲ G43.D1 Menstrual Abdominal migraine, intractable
● G43.82 Menstrual migraine, not intractable
● G43.821 Menstrual migraine, not intractable, with status migrainosus
● G43.829 Menstrual migraine, not intractable, without status migrainosus
● G43.83 Menstrual migraine, intractable
● G43.831 Menstrual migraine, intractable, with status migrainosus
● G43.839 Menstrual migraine, intractable, without status migrainosus
● G70.80 Lambert-Eaton syndrome, unspecified
● G70.81 Lambert-Eaton syndrome in disease classified elsewhere
● G70.89 Other specified myoneural disorders
▲ G73.1 Lambert-Eaton syndrome in neoplastic disease
● G89.29 Other chronic pain
● G93.82 Brain death
▲ H35.30 Unspecified macular degeneration (age-related)
● H40.00 Preglaucoma, unspecified
● H40.001 Preglaucoma, unspecified, right eye
● H40.002 Preglaucoma, unspecified, left eye
● H40.003 Preglaucoma, unspecified, bilateral
● H40.009 Preglaucoma, unspecified, unspecified eye
● H40.01 Open angle with borderline findings, low risk
● H40.011 Open angle with borderline findings, low risk, right eye
● H40.012 Open angle with borderline findings, low risk, left eye
● H40.013 Open angle with borderline findings, low risk, bilateral
● H40.019 Open angle with borderline findings, low risk, unspecified eye
● H40.02 Open angle with borderline findings, high risk
● H40.021 Open angle with borderline findings, high risk, right eye
● H40.022 Open angle with borderline findings, high risk, left eye
● H40.023 Open angle with borderline findings, high risk, bilateral
● H40.029 Open angle with borderline findings, high risk, unspecified eye
● H40.03 Anatomical narrow angle
● H40.031 Anatomical narrow angle, right eye
● H40.032 Anatomical narrow angle, left eye
● H40.033 Anatomical narrow angle, bilateral
● H40.039 Anatomical narrow angle, unspecified eye
● H40.04 Steroid responder
● H40.041 Steroid responder, right eye
● H40.042 Steroid responder, left eye
● H40.043 Steroid responder, bilateral
● H40.049 Steroid responder, unspecified eye
● H40.05 Ocular hypertension
● H40.051 Ocular hypertension, right eye
● H40.052 Ocular hypertension, left eye
● H40.053 Ocular hypertension, bilateral
● H40.059 Ocular hypertension, unspecified eye
● H40.06 Primary angle closure without glaucoma damage
● H40.061 Primary angle closure without glaucoma damage, right eye
● H40.062 Primary angle closure without glaucoma damage, left eye
● H40.063 Primary angle closure without glaucoma damage, bilateral
● H40.069 Primary angle closure without glaucoma damage, unspecified eye
● H40.10X0 Unspecified open-angle glaucoma, stage unspecified
● H40.10X1 Unspecified open-angle glaucoma, mild stage
● H40.10X2 Unspecified open-angle glaucoma, moderate stage
● H40.10X3 Unspecified open-angle glaucoma, severe stage
● H40.10X4 Unspecified open-angle glaucoma, indeterminate stage
● H40.11X0 Primary open-angle glaucoma, stage unspecified
● H40.11X1 Primary open-angle glaucoma, mild stage
● H40.11X2 Primary open-angle glaucoma, moderate stage
● H40.11X3 Primary open-angle glaucoma, severe stage
● H40.11X4 Primary open-angle glaucoma, indeterminate stage
● H40.1210 Low-tension glaucoma, right eye, stage unspecified
● H40.1211 Low-tension glaucoma, right eye, mild stage
● H40.1212 Low-tension glaucoma, right eye, moderate stage
● H40.1213 Low-tension glaucoma, right eye, severe stage
● H40.1214 Low-tension glaucoma, right eye, indeterminate stage
● H40.1220 Low-tension glaucoma, left eye, stage unspecified
● H40.1221 Low-tension glaucoma, left eye, mild stage
● H40.1222 Low-tension glaucoma, left eye, moderate stage
● H40.1223 Low-tension glaucoma, left eye, severe stage
● H40.1224 Low-tension glaucoma, left eye, indeterminate stage

- ● H4Ø.123Ø Low-tension glaucoma, bilateral, stage unspecified
- ● H4Ø.1231 Low-tension glaucoma, bilateral, mild stage
- ● H4Ø.1232 Low-tension glaucoma, bilateral, moderate stage
- ● H4Ø.1233 Low-tension glaucoma, bilateral, severe stage
- ● H4Ø.1234 Low-tension glaucoma, bilateral, indeterminate stage
- ● H4Ø.129Ø Low-tension glaucoma, unspecified eye, stage unspecified
- ● H4Ø.1291 Low-tension glaucoma, unspecified eye, mild stage
- ● H4Ø.1292 Low-tension glaucoma, unspecified eye, moderate stage
- ● H4Ø.1293 Low-tension glaucoma, unspecified eye, severe stage
- ● H4Ø.1294 Low-tension glaucoma, unspecified eye, indeterminate stage
- ● H4Ø.131Ø Pigmentary glaucoma, right eye, stage unspecified
- ● H4Ø.1311 Pigmentary glaucoma, right eye, mild stage
- ● H4Ø.1312 Pigmentary glaucoma, right eye, moderate stage
- ● H4Ø.1313 Pigmentary glaucoma, right eye, severe stage
- ● H4Ø.1314 Pigmentary glaucoma, right eye, indeterminate stage
- ● H4Ø.132Ø Pigmentary glaucoma, left eye, stage unspecified
- ● H4Ø.1321 Pigmentary glaucoma, left eye, mild stage
- ● H4Ø.1322 Pigmentary glaucoma, left eye, moderate stage
- ● H4Ø.1323 Pigmentary glaucoma, left eye, severe stage
- ● H4Ø.1324 Pigmentary glaucoma, left eye, indeterminate stage
- ● H4Ø.133Ø Pigmentary glaucoma, bilateral, stage unspecified
- ● H4Ø.1331 Pigmentary glaucoma, bilateral, mild stage
- ● H4Ø.1332 Pigmentary glaucoma, bilateral, moderate stage
- ● H4Ø.1333 Pigmentary glaucoma, bilateral, severe stage
- ● H4Ø.1334 Pigmentary glaucoma, bilateral, indeterminate stage
- ● H4Ø.139Ø Pigmentary glaucoma, unspecified eye, stage unspecified
- ● H4Ø.1391 Pigmentary glaucoma, unspecified eye, mild stage
- ● H4Ø.1392 Pigmentary glaucoma, unspecified eye, moderate stage
- ● H4Ø.1393 Pigmentary glaucoma, unspecified eye, severe stage
- ● H4Ø.1394 Pigmentary glaucoma, unspecified eye, indeterminate stage
- ● H4Ø.151Ø Residual stage of open-angle glaucoma, right eye, stage unspecified
- ● H4Ø.1511 Residual stage of open-angle glaucoma, right eye, mild stage
- ● H4Ø.1512 Residual stage of open-angle glaucoma, right eye, moderate stage
- ● H4Ø.1513 Residual stage of open-angle glaucoma, right eye, severe stage
- ● H4Ø.1514 Residual stage of open-angle glaucoma, right eye, indeterminate stage
- ● H4Ø.152Ø Residual stage of open-angle glaucoma, left eye, stage unspecified
- ● H4Ø.1521 Residual stage of open-angle glaucoma, left eye, mild stage
- ● H4Ø.1522 Residual stage of open-angle glaucoma, left eye, moderate stage
- ● H4Ø.1523 Residual stage of open-angle glaucoma, left eye, severe stage
- ● H4Ø.1524 Residual stage of open-angle glaucoma, left eye, indeterminate stage
- ● H4Ø.153Ø Residual stage of open-angle glaucoma, bilateral, stage unspecified
- ● H4Ø.1531 Residual stage of open-angle glaucoma, bilateral, mild stage
- ● H4Ø.1532 Residual stage of open-angle glaucoma, bilateral, moderate stage
- ● H4Ø.1533 Residual stage of open-angle glaucoma, bilateral, severe stage
- ● H4Ø.1534 Residual stage of open-angle glaucoma, bilateral, indeterminate stage
- ● H4Ø.159Ø Residual stage of open-angle glaucoma, unspecified eye, stage unspecified
- ● H4Ø.1591 Residual stage of open-angle glaucoma, unspecified eye, mild stage
- ● H4Ø.1592 Residual stage of open-angle glaucoma, unspecified eye, moderate stage
- ● H4Ø.1593 Residual stage of open-angle glaucoma, unspecified eye, severe stage
- ● H4Ø.1594 Residual stage of open-angle glaucoma, unspecified eye, indeterminate stage
- ● H4Ø.2ØXØ Unspecified primary angle-closure glaucoma, stage unspecified
- ● H4Ø.2ØX1 Unspecified primary angle-closure glaucoma, mild stage
- ● H4Ø.2ØX2 Unspecified primary angle-closure glaucoma, moderate stage
- ● H4Ø.2ØX3 Unspecified primary angle-closure glaucoma, severe stage
- ● H4Ø.2ØX4 Unspecified primary angle-closure glaucoma, indeterminate stage
- ● H4Ø.221Ø Chronic angle-closure glaucoma, right eye, stage unspecified
- ● H4Ø.2211 Chronic angle-closure glaucoma, right eye, mild stage
- ● H4Ø.2212 Chronic angle-closure glaucoma, right eye, moderate stage
- ● H4Ø.2213 Chronic angle-closure glaucoma, right eye, severe stage
- ● H4Ø.2214 Chronic angle-closure glaucoma, right eye, indeterminate stage
- ● H4Ø.222Ø Chronic angle-closure glaucoma, left eye, stage unspecified
- ● H4Ø.2221 Chronic angle-closure glaucoma, left eye, mild stage
- ● H4Ø.2222 Chronic angle-closure glaucoma, left eye, moderate stage
- ● H4Ø.2223 Chronic angle-closure glaucoma, left eye, severe stage
- ● H4Ø.2224 Chronic angle-closure glaucoma, left eye, indeterminate stage
- ● H4Ø.223Ø Chronic angle-closure glaucoma, bilateral, stage unspecified
- ● H4Ø.2231 Chronic angle-closure glaucoma, bilateral, mild stage
- ● H4Ø.2232 Chronic angle-closure glaucoma, bilateral, moderate stage
- ● H4Ø.2233 Chronic angle-closure glaucoma, bilateral, severe stage
- ● H4Ø.2234 Chronic angle-closure glaucoma, bilateral, indeterminate stage
- ● H4Ø.229Ø Chronic angle-closure glaucoma, unspecified eye, stage unspecified
- ● H4Ø.2291 Chronic angle-closure glaucoma, unspecified eye, mild stage
- ● H4Ø.2292 Chronic angle-closure glaucoma, unspecified eye, moderate stage
- ● H4Ø.2293 Chronic angle-closure glaucoma, unspecified eye, severe stage
- ● H4Ø.2294 Chronic angle-closure glaucoma, unspecified eye, indeterminate stage
- ● H4Ø.3ØXØ Glaucoma secondary to eye trauma, unspecified eye, stage unspecified
- ● H4Ø.3ØX1 Glaucoma secondary to eye trauma, unspecified eye, mild stage
- ● H4Ø.3ØX2 Glaucoma secondary to eye trauma, unspecified eye, moderate stage
- ● H4Ø.3ØX3 Glaucoma secondary to eye trauma, unspecified eye, severe stage
- ● H4Ø.3ØX4 Glaucoma secondary to eye trauma, unspecified eye, indeterminate stage
- ● H4Ø.31XØ Glaucoma secondary to eye trauma, right eye, stage unspecified
- ● H4Ø.31X1 Glaucoma secondary to eye trauma, right eye, mild stage
- ● H4Ø.31X2 Glaucoma secondary to eye trauma, right eye, moderate stage
- ● H4Ø.31X3 Glaucoma secondary to eye trauma, right eye, severe stage
- ● H4Ø.31X4 Glaucoma secondary to eye trauma, right eye, indeterminate stage
- ● H4Ø.32XØ Glaucoma secondary to eye trauma, left eye, stage unspecified
- ● H4Ø.32X1 Glaucoma secondary to eye trauma, left eye, mild stage
- ● H4Ø.32X2 Glaucoma secondary to eye trauma, left eye, moderate stage
- ● H4Ø.32X3 Glaucoma secondary to eye trauma, left eye, severe stage
- ● H4Ø.32X4 Glaucoma secondary to eye trauma, left eye, indeterminate stage
- ● H4Ø.33XØ Glaucoma secondary to eye trauma, bilateral, stage unspecified
- ● H4Ø.33X1 Glaucoma secondary to eye trauma, bilateral, mild stage
- ● H4Ø.33X2 Glaucoma secondary to eye trauma, bilateral, moderate stage
- ● H4Ø.33X3 Glaucoma secondary to eye trauma, bilateral, severe stage
- ● H4Ø.33X4 Glaucoma secondary to eye trauma, bilateral, indeterminate stage
- ● H4Ø.4ØXØ Glaucoma secondary to eye inflammation, unspecified eye, stage unspecified
- ● H4Ø.4ØX1 Glaucoma secondary to eye inflammation, unspecified eye, mild stage
- ● H4Ø.4ØX2 Glaucoma secondary to eye inflammation, unspecified eye, moderate stage
- ● H4Ø.4ØX3 Glaucoma secondary to eye inflammation, unspecified eye, severe stage
- ● H4Ø.4ØX4 Glaucoma secondary to eye inflammation, unspecified eye, indeterminate stage
- ● H4Ø.41XØ Glaucoma secondary to eye inflammation, right eye, stage unspecified
- ● H4Ø.41X1 Glaucoma secondary to eye inflammation, right eye, mild stage
- ● H4Ø.41X2 Glaucoma secondary to eye inflammation, right eye, moderate stage
- ● H4Ø.41X3 Glaucoma secondary to eye inflammation, right eye, severe stage
- ● H4Ø.41X4 Glaucoma secondary to eye inflammation, right eye, indeterminate stage

- ● H4Ø.42XØ Glaucoma secondary to eye inflammation, left eye, stage unspecified
- ● H4Ø.42X1 Glaucoma secondary to eye inflammation, left eye, mild stage
- ● H4Ø.42X2 Glaucoma secondary to eye inflammation, left eye, moderate stage
- ● H4Ø.42X3 Glaucoma secondary to eye inflammation, left eye, severe stage
- ● H4Ø.42X4 Glaucoma secondary to eye inflammation, left eye, indeterminate stage
- ● H4Ø.43XØ Glaucoma secondary to eye inflammation, bilateral, stage unspecified
- ● H4Ø.43X1 Glaucoma secondary to eye inflammation, bilateral, mild stage
- ● H4Ø.43X2 Glaucoma secondary to eye inflammation, bilateral, moderate stage
- ● H4Ø.43X3 Glaucoma secondary to eye inflammation, bilateral, severe stage
- ● H4Ø.43X4 Glaucoma secondary to eye inflammation, bilateral, indeterminate stage
- ● H4Ø.5ØXØ Glaucoma secondary to other eye disorders, unspecified eye, stage unspecified
- ● H4Ø.5ØX1 Glaucoma secondary to other eye disorders, unspecified eye, mild stage
- ● H4Ø.5ØX2 Glaucoma secondary to other eye disorders, unspecified eye, moderate stage
- ● H4Ø.5ØX3 Glaucoma secondary to other eye disorders, unspecified eye, severe stage
- ● H4Ø.5ØX4 Glaucoma secondary to other eye disorders, unspecified eye, indeterminate stage
- ● H4Ø.51XØ Glaucoma secondary to other eye disorders, right eye, stage unspecified
- ● H4Ø.51X1 Glaucoma secondary to other eye disorders, right eye, mild stage
- ● H4Ø.51X2 Glaucoma secondary to other eye disorders, right eye, moderate stage
- ● H4Ø.51X3 Glaucoma secondary to other eye disorders, right eye, severe stage
- ● H4Ø.51X4 Glaucoma secondary to other eye disorders, right eye, indeterminate stage
- ● H4Ø.52XØ Glaucoma secondary to other eye disorders, left eye, stage unspecified
- ● H4Ø.52X1 Glaucoma secondary to other eye disorders, left eye, mild stage
- ● H4Ø.52X2 Glaucoma secondary to other eye disorders, left eye, moderate stage
- ● H4Ø.52X3 Glaucoma secondary to other eye disorders, left eye, severe stage
- ● H4Ø.52X4 Glaucoma secondary to other eye disorders, left eye, indeterminate stage
- ● H4Ø.53XØ Glaucoma secondary to other eye disorders, bilateral, stage unspecified
- ● H4Ø.53X1 Glaucoma secondary to other eye disorders, bilateral, mild stage
- ● H4Ø.53X2 Glaucoma secondary to other eye disorders, bilateral, moderate stage
- ● H4Ø.53X3 Glaucoma secondary to other eye disorders, bilateral, severe stage
- ● H4Ø.53X4 Glaucoma secondary to other eye disorders, bilateral, indeterminate stage
- ● H4Ø.6ØXØ Glaucoma secondary to drugs, unspecified eye, stage unspecified
- ● H4Ø.6ØX1 Glaucoma secondary to drugs, unspecified eye, mild stage
- ● H4Ø.6ØX2 Glaucoma secondary to drugs, unspecified eye, moderate stage
- ● H4Ø.6ØX3 Glaucoma secondary to drugs, unspecified eye, severe stage
- ● H4Ø.6ØX4 Glaucoma secondary to drugs, unspecified eye, indeterminate stage
- ● H4Ø.61XØ Glaucoma secondary to drugs, right eye, stage unspecified
- ● H4Ø.61X1 Glaucoma secondary to drugs, right eye, mild stage
- ● H4Ø.61X2 Glaucoma secondary to drugs, right eye, moderate stage
- ● H4Ø.61X3 Glaucoma secondary to drugs, right eye, severe stage
- ● H4Ø.61X4 Glaucoma secondary to drugs, right eye, indeterminate stage
- ● H4Ø.62XØ Glaucoma secondary to drugs, left eye, stage unspecified
- ● H4Ø.62X1 Glaucoma secondary to drugs, left eye, mild stage
- ● H4Ø.62X2 Glaucoma secondary to drugs, left eye, moderate stage
- ● H4Ø.62X3 Glaucoma secondary to drugs, left eye, severe stage
- ● H4Ø.62X4 Glaucoma secondary to drugs, left eye, indeterminate stage
- ● H4Ø.63XØ Glaucoma secondary to drugs, bilateral, stage unspecified
- ● H4Ø.63X1 Glaucoma secondary to drugs, bilateral, mild stage
- ● H4Ø.63X2 Glaucoma secondary to drugs, bilateral, moderate stage
- ● H4Ø.63X3 Glaucoma secondary to drugs, bilateral, severe stage
- ● H4Ø.63X4 Glaucoma secondary to drugs, bilateral, indeterminate stage
- ● H43.82 Vitreomacular adhesion
- ● H43.821 Vitreomacular adhesion, right eye
- ● H43.822 Vitreomacular adhesion, left eye
- ● H43.823 Vitreomacular adhesion, bilateral
- ● H43.829 Vitreomacular adhesion, unspecified eye
- ● I25.84 Coronary atherosclerosis due to calcified coronary lesion
- ● I26.Ø2 Saddle embolus of pulmonary artery with acute cor pulmonale
- ● I26.92 Saddle embolus of pulmonary artery without acute cor pulmonale
- ▲ I48.Ø Paroxysmal atrial fibrillation
- ▲ I48.1 Atrial flutterPersistent atrial fibrillation
- ● I48.2 Chronic atrial fibrillation
- ● I48.3 Typical atrial flutter
- ● I48.4 Atypical atrial flutter
- ● I48.9 Unspecified atrial fibrillation and atrial flutter
- ● I48.91 Unspecified atrial fibrillation
- ● I48.92 Unspecified atrial flutter
- ● I67.81 Acute cerebrovascular insufficiency
- ● I67.82 Cerebral ischemia
- ● I67.83 Posterior reversible encephalopathy syndrome
- ● I67.84 Cerebral vasospasm and vasoconstriction
- ● I67.841 Reversible cerebrovascular vasoconstriction syndrome
- ● I67.848 Other cerebrovascular vasospasm and vasoconstriction
- ● I67.89 Other cerebrovascular disease
- ▲ I72.Ø Aneurysm of carotid artery (common) (external) (internal, extracranial portion)
- ● I74.Ø1 Saddle embolus of abdominal aorta
- ● I74.Ø9 Other arterial embolism and thrombosis of abdominal aorta
- ● JØ9.X Influenza due to identified novel influenza A virus
- ● JØ9.X1 Influenza due to identified novel influenza A virus with pneumonia
- ● JØ9.X2 Influenza due to identified novel influenza A virus with other respiratory manifestations
- ● JØ9.X3 Influenza due to identified novel influenza A virus with gastrointestinal manifestations
- ● JØ9.X9 Influenza due to identified novel influenza A virus with other manifestations
- ● J15.211 Pneumonia due to Methicillin susceptible Staphylococcus aureus
- ● J15.212 Pneumonia due to Methicillin resistant Staphylococcus aureus
- ● J7Ø.5 Respiratory conditions due to smoke inhalation
- ● J84.Ø1 Alveolar proteinosis
- ● J84.Ø2 Pulmonary alveolar microlithiasis
- ● J84.Ø3 Idiopathic pulmonary hemosiderosis
- ● J84.Ø9 Other alveolar and parieto-alveolar conditions
- ● J84.1Ø Pulmonary fibrosis, unspecified
- ● J84.11 Idiopathic interstitial pneumonia
- ● J84.111 Idiopathic interstitial pneumonia, not otherwise specified
- ● J84.112 Idiopathic pulmonary fibrosis
- ● J84.113 Idiopathic non-specific interstitial pneumonitis
- ● J84.114 Acute interstitial pneumonitis
- ● J84.115 Respiratory bronchiolitis interstitial lung disease
- ● J84.116 Cryptogenic organizing pneumonia
- ● J84.117 Desquamative interstitial pneumonia
- ● J84.17 Other interstitial pulmonary diseases with fibrosis in diseases classified elsewhere
- ● J84.81 Lymphangioleiomyomatosis
- ● J84.82 Adult pulmonary Langerhans cell histiocytosis
- ● J84.83 Surfactant mutations of the lung
- ● J84.84 Other interstitial lung diseases of childhood
- ● J84.841 Neuroendocrine cell hyperplasia of infancy
- ● J84.842 Pulmonary interstitial glycogenosis
- ● J84.843 Alveolar capillary dysplasia with vein misalignment
- ● J84.848 Other interstitial lung diseases of childhood
- ● J84.89 Other specified interstitial pulmonary diseases
- ▲ J93 Pneumothorax and air leak
- ● J93.11 Primary spontaneous pneumothorax
- ● J93.12 Secondary spontaneous pneumothorax
- ▲ J93.8 Other pneumothorax and air leak
- ● J93.81 Chronic pneumothorax
- ● J93.82 Other air leak
- ● J93.83 Other pneumothorax
- ▲ J95.4 Chemical pneumonitis due to anesthesia [Mendelson's syndrome]
- ▲ J95.81 Postprocedural pneumothorax and air leak
- ● J95.811 Postprocedural pneumothorax
- ● J95.812 Postprocedural air leak
- ● J95.821 Acute postprocedural respiratory failure
- ● J95.822 Acute and chronic postprocedural respiratory failure
- ● K31.84 Gastroparesis

● New Code ▲ Revised Code

- ▲ K43.Ø Ventral Incisional hernia with obstruction, without gangrene
- ▲ K43.1 Ventral Incisional hernia with gangrene
- ● K43.2 Incisional hernia without obstruction or gangrene
- ● K43.3 Parastomal hernia with obstruction, without gangrene
- ● K43.4 Parastomal hernia with gangrene
- ● K43.5 Parastomal hernia without obstruction or gangrene
- ● K43.6 Other and unspecified ventral hernia with obstruction, without gangrene
- ● K43.7 Other and unspecified ventral hernia with gangrene
- ● K64 Hemorrhoids and perianal venous thrombosis
- ● K64.Ø First degree hemorrhoids
- ● K64.1 Second degree hemorrhoids
- ● K64.2 Third degree hemorrhoids
- ● K64.3 Fourth degree hemorrhoids
- ● K64.4 Residual hemorrhoidal skin tags
- ● K64.5 Perianal venous thrombosis
- ● K64.8 Other hemorrhoids
- ● K64.9 Unspecified hemorrhoids
- ● K76.81 Hepatopulmonary syndrome
- ● K76.89 Other specified diseases of liver
- ● K91.86 Retained cholelithiasis following cholecystectomy
- ● K95 Complications of bariatric procedures
- ● K95.Ø Complications of gastric band procedure
- ● K95.Ø1 Infection due to gastric band procedure
- ● K95.Ø9 Other complications of gastric band procedure
- ● K95.8 Complications of other bariatric procedure
- ● K95.81 Infection due to other bariatric procedure
- ● K95.89 Other complications of other bariatric procedure
- ▲ L72.1 Pilar and trichodermal cyst
- ● L72.11 Pilar cyst
- ● L72.12 Trichodermal cyst
- ● L72.3 Sebaceous cyst
- ▲ MØ1.X Direct infection of joint in infectious and parasitic diseases classified elsewhere
- ▲ M13.88 Other specified arthritis, vertebra other site
- ● M21.Ø5 Valgus deformity, not elsewhere classified, hip
- ● M21.Ø51 Valgus deformity, not elsewhere classified, right hip
- ● M21.Ø52 Valgus deformity, not elsewhere classified, left hip
- ● M21.Ø59 Valgus deformity, not elsewhere classified, unspecified hip
- ● M21.15 Varus deformity, not elsewhere classified, hip
- ● M21.151 Varus deformity, not elsewhere classified, right hip
- ● M21.152 Varus deformity, not elsewhere classified, left hip
- ● M21.159 Varus deformity, not elsewhere classified, unspecified
- ▲ M75.1 Rotator cuff syndrome tear or rupture, not specified as traumatic
- ▲ M75.1Ø Rotator cuff syndrome, unspecified shoulder Unspecified rotator cuff tear or rupture, not specified as traumatic
- ● M75.1ØØ Unspecified rotator cuff tear or rupture of unspecified shoulder, not specified as traumatic
- ● M75.1Ø1 Unspecified rotator cuff tear or rupture of right shoulder, not specified as traumatic
- ● M75.1Ø2 Unspecified rotator cuff tear or rupture of left shoulder, not specified as traumatic
- ▲ M75.11 Rotator cuff syndrome, right shoulder Incomplete rotator cuff tear or rupture not specified as traumatic
- ● M75.11Ø Incomplete rotator cuff tear or rupture of unspecified shoulder, not specified as traumatic
- ● M75.111 Incomplete rotator cuff tear or rupture of right shoulder, not specified as traumatic
- ● M75.112 Incomplete rotator cuff tear or rupture of left shoulder, not specified as traumatic
- ▲ M75.12 Rotator cuff syndrome, right shoulder Complete rotator cuff tear or rupture not specified as traumatic
- ● M75.12Ø Complete rotator cuff tear or rupture of unspecified shoulder, not specified as traumatic
- ● M75.121 Complete rotator cuff tear or rupture of right shoulder, not specified as traumatic
- ● M75.122 Complete rotator cuff tear or rupture of left shoulder, not specified as traumatic
- ▲ M85.38 Osteitis condensans, vertebra other site
- ▲ M86.43 Chronic osteomyelitis with draining sinus, forearm radius and ulna
- ▲ M86.431 Chronic osteomyelitis with draining sinus, right forearm radius and ulna
- ▲ M86.432 Chronic osteomyelitis with draining sinus, left forearm radius and ulna
- ▲ M86.439 Chronic osteomyelitis with draining sinus, unspecified forearm radius and ulna
- ▲ M86.46 Chronic osteomyelitis with draining sinus, lower leg tibia and fibula
- ▲ M86.461 Chronic osteomyelitis with draining sinus, right lower leg tibia and fibula
- ▲ M86.462 Chronic osteomyelitis with draining sinus, left lower leg tibia and fibula
- ▲ M86.469 Chronic osteomyelitis with draining sinus, unspecified lower leg tibia and fibula
- ▲ M86.53 Other chronic hematogenous osteomyelitis, forearm radius and ulna
- ▲ M86.531 Other chronic hematogenous osteomyelitis, right forearm radius and ulna
- ▲ M86.532 Other chronic hematogenous osteomyelitis, left forearm radius and ulna
- ▲ M86.539 Other chronic hematogenous osteomyelitis, unspecified forearm radius and ulna
- ▲ M86.56 Other chronic hematogenous osteomyelitis, lower leg tibia and fibula
- ▲ M86.561 Other chronic hematogenous osteomyelitis, right lower leg tibia and fibula
- ▲ M86.562 Other chronic hematogenous osteomyelitis, left lower leg tibia and fibula
- ▲ M86.569 Other chronic hematogenous osteomyelitis, unspecified lower leg tibia and fibula
- ▲ M86.62 Other chronic osteomyelitis, upper arm humerus
- ▲ M86.621 Other chronic osteomyelitis, right upper arm humerus
- ▲ M86.622 Other chronic osteomyelitis, left upper arm humerus
- ▲ M86.629 Other chronic osteomyelitis, unspecified upper arm humerus
- ▲ M86.63 Other chronic osteomyelitis, forearm radius and ulna
- ▲ M86.631 Other chronic osteomyelitis, right forearm radius and ulna
- ▲ M86.632 Other chronic osteomyelitis, left forearm radius and ulna
- ▲ M86.639 Other chronic osteomyelitis, unspecified forearm radius and ulna
- ▲ M86.66 Other chronic osteomyelitis, lower leg tibia and fibula
- ▲ M86.661 Other chronic osteomyelitis, lower leg tibia and fibula
- ▲ M86.662 Other chronic osteomyelitis, left lower leg tibia and fibula
- ▲ M86.669 Other chronic osteomyelitis, unspecified lower leg tibia and fibula
- ● N36.5 Urethral false passage
- ▲ N4Ø Enlarged prostate (EP)
- ▲ N4Ø.Ø Enlarged prostate without lower urinary tract symptoms (LUTS)
- ▲ N4Ø.1 Enlarged prostate with lower urinary tract symptoms (LUTS)
- ● N4Ø.2 Nodular prostate without lower urinary tract symptoms
- ● N4Ø.3 Nodular prostate with lower urinary tract symptoms
- ● N42.83 Cyst of prostate
- ● N48.82 Acquired torsion of penis
- ● N48.83 Acquired buried penis
- ● N5Ø.3 Cyst of epididymis
- ● OØ2.81 Inappropriate change in quantitative human chorionic gonadotropin (hCG) in early pregnancy
- ● OØ2.89 Other abnormal products of conception
- ▲ O14.2 HELLP syndrome (HELLP)
- ▲ O22 Venous complications and hemorrhoids in pregnancy
- ▲ O26.6 Liver and biliary tract disorders in pregnancy, childbirth and the puerperium
- ▲ O26.61 Liver and biliary tract disorders in pregnancy
- ▲ O26.611 Liver and biliary tract disorders in pregnancy, first trimester
- ▲ O26.612 Liver and biliary tract disorders in pregnancy, second trimester
- ▲ O26.613 Liver and biliary tract disorders in pregnancy, third trimester
- ▲ O26.619 Liver and biliary tract disorders in pregnancy, unspecified trimester
- ▲ O26.62 Liver and biliary tract disorders in childbirth
- ▲ O26.63 Liver and biliary tract disorders in the puerperium
- ▲ O3Ø.Ø2 Conjoined twin pregnancy
- ▲ O3Ø.Ø21 Conjoined twin pregnancy, first trimester
- ▲ O3Ø.Ø22 Conjoined twin pregnancy, second trimester
- ▲ O3Ø.Ø23 Conjoined twin pregnancy, third trimester
- ▲ O3Ø.Ø29 Conjoined twin pregnancy, unspecified trimester
- ● O36.8ØXØ Pregnancy with inconclusive fetal viability, not applicable or unspecified
- ● O36.8ØX1 Pregnancy with inconclusive fetal viability, fetus 1

- ● O36.8ØX2 Pregnancy with inconclusive fetal viability, fetus 2
- ● O36.8ØX3 Pregnancy with inconclusive fetal viability, fetus 3
- ● O36.8ØX4 Pregnancy with inconclusive fetal viability, fetus 4
- ● O36.8ØX5 Pregnancy with inconclusive fetal viability, fetus 5
- ● O36.8ØX9 Pregnancy with inconclusive fetal viability, other fetus
- ● O75.82 Onset (spontaneous) of labor after 37 completed weeks of gestation but before 39 completed weeks gestation, with delivery by (planned) cesarean section
- ▲ O87 Venous complications and hemorrhoids in the puerperium
- ▲ O98.7 Human immunodeficiency virus [HIV] disease complicating pregnancy, childbirth and the puerperium
- ▲ O98.71 Human immunodeficiency virus [HIV] disease complicating pregnancy
- ▲ O98.711 Human immunodeficiency virus [HIV] disease complicating pregnancy, first trimester
- ▲ O98.712 Human immunodeficiency virus [HIV] disease complicating pregnancy, second trimester
- ▲ O98.713 Human immunodeficiency virus [HIV] disease complicating pregnancy, third trimester
- ▲ O98.719 Human immunodeficiency virus [HIV] disease complicating pregnancy, unspecified trimester
- ▲ O98.72 Human immunodeficiency virus [HIV] disease complicating childbirth
- ▲ O98.73 Human immunodeficiency virus [HIV] disease complicating the puerperium
- ▲ PØ7.2Ø Extreme immaturity of newborn, unspecified weeks of gestation
- ▲ PØ7.21 Extreme immaturity of newborn, less than 24 gestational age less than 23 completed weeks
- ▲ PØ7.22 Extreme immaturity of newborn, 24 - 26 gestational age 23 completed weeks
- ▲ PØ7.23 Extreme immaturity of newborn, 27gestational age 24 completed weeks
- ● PØ7.24 Extreme immaturity of newborn, gestational age 25 completed weeks
- ● PØ7.25 Extreme immaturity of newborn, gestational age 26 completed weeks
- ● PØ7.26 Extreme immaturity of newborn, gestational age 27 completed weeks
- ▲ PØ7.3 Other preterm newborn Preterm [premature] newborn [other]
- ▲ PØ7.3Ø Other preterm newborn, unspecified weeks Preterm newborn, unspecified weeks of gestation
- ▲ PØ7.31 Other preterm newborn, 28-31 Preterm newborn, gestational age 28 completed weeks
- ▲ PØ7.32 Other preterm newborn, 32-36 Preterm newborn, gestational age 29 completed weeks
- ● PØ7.33 Preterm newborn, gestational age 3Ø completed weeks
- ● PØ7.34 Preterm newborn, gestational age 31 completed weeks
- ● PØ7.35 Preterm newborn, gestational age 32 completed weeks
- ● PØ7.36 Preterm newborn, gestational age 33 completed weeks
- ● PØ7.37 Preterm newborn, gestational age 34 completed weeks
- ● PØ7.38 Preterm newborn, gestational age 35 completed weeks
- ● PØ7.39 Preterm newborn, gestational age 36 completed weeks
- ● Q25.71 Coarctation of pulmonary artery
- ● Q25.72 Congenital pulmonary arteriovenous malformation
- ● Q25.79 Other congenital malformations of pulmonary artery
- ● Q55.63 Congenital torsion of penis
- ● Q55.64 Hidden penis
- ● Q65.81 Congenital coxa valga
- ● Q65.82 Congenital coxa vara
- ● Q65.89 Other specified congenital deformities of hip
- ● Q66.5Ø Congenital pes planus, unspecified foot
- ● Q66.51 Congenital pes planus, right foot
- ● Q66.52 Congenital pes planus, left foot
- ● Q66.8Ø Congenital vertical talus deformity, unspecified foot
- ● Q66.81 Congenital vertical talus deformity, right foot
- ● Q66.82 Congenital vertical talus deformity, left foot
- ● Q66.89 Other specified congenital deformities of feet
- ● R4Ø.24 Glasgow coma scale, total score
- ● R4Ø.241 Glasgow coma scale score 13-15
- ● R4Ø.242 Glasgow coma scale score 9-12
- ● R4Ø.243 Glasgow coma scale score 3-8
- ● R4Ø.244 Other coma, without documented Glasgow coma scale score, or with partial score reported
- ● R48.3 Visual agnosia
- ▲ R76.1 Abnormal reaction to tuberculin test Nonspecific reaction to test for tuberculosis
- ● R76.11 Nonspecific reaction to tuberculin skin test without active tuberculosis
- ● R76.12 Nonspecific reaction to cell mediated immunity measurement of gamma interferon antigen response without active tuberculosis
- ● R91.1 Solitary pulmonary nodule
- ● R91.8 Other nonspecific abnormal finding of lung field
- ● S32.82XA Multiple fractures of pelvis without disruption of pelvic ring, initial encounter for closed fracture
- ● S32.82XB Multiple fractures of pelvis without disruption of pelvic ring, initial encounter for open fracture
- ● S32.82XD Multiple fractures of pelvis without disruption of pelvic ring, subsequent encounter for fracture with routine healing
- ● S32.82XG Multiple fractures of pelvis without disruption of pelvic ring, subsequent encounter for fracture with delayed healing
- ● S32.82XK Multiple fractures of pelvis without disruption of pelvic ring, subsequent encounter for fracture with nonunion
- ● S32.82XS Multiple fractures of pelvis without disruption of pelvic ring, sequela
- ▲ S62.62 Displaced fracture of middle medial phalanx of finger
- ▲ S62.62ØA Displaced fracture of middle medial phalanx of right index finger, initial encounter for closed fracture
- ▲ S62.62ØB Displaced fracture of middle medial phalanx of right index finger, initial encounter for open fracture
- ▲ S62.62ØD Displaced fracture of middle medial l phalanx of right index finger, subsequent encounter for fracture with routine healing
- ▲ S62.62ØG Displaced fracture of middle medial phalanx of right index finger, subsequent encounter for fracture with delayed healing
- ▲ S62.62ØK Displaced fracture of middle medial phalanx of right index finger, subsequent encounter for fracture with nonunion
- ▲ S62.62ØP Displaced fracture of middle medial phalanx of right index finger, subsequent encounter for fracture with malunion
- ▲ S62.62ØS Displaced fracture of middle medial phalanx of right index finger, sequela
- ▲ S62.621A Displaced fracture of middle medial phalanx of left index finger, initial encounter for closed fracture
- ▲ S62.621B Displaced fracture of middle medial phalanx of left index finger, initial encounter for open fracture
- ▲ S62.621D Displaced fracture of middle medial phalanx of left index finger, subsequent encounter for fracture with routine healing
- ▲ S62.621G Displaced fracture of middle medial phalanx of left index finger, subsequent encounter for fracture with delayed healing
- ▲ S62.621K Displaced fracture of middle medial phalanx of left index finger, subsequent encounter for fracture with nonunion
- ▲ S62.621P Displaced fracture of middle medial phalanx of left index finger, subsequent encounter for fracture with malunion
- ▲ S62.621S Displaced fracture of middle medial phalanx of left index finger, sequela
- ▲ S62.622A Displaced fracture of middle medial phalanx of right middle finger, initial encounter for closed fracture
- ▲ S62.622B Displaced fracture of middle medial phalanx of right middle finger, initial encounter for open fracture
- ▲ S62.622D Displaced fracture of middle medial phalanx of right middle finger, subsequent encounter for fracture with routine healing
- ▲ S62.622G Displaced fracture of middle medial phalanx of right middle finger, subsequent encounter for fracture with delayed healing
- ▲ S62.622K Displaced fracture of middle medial phalanx of right middle finger, subsequent encounter for fracture with nonunion
- ▲ S62.622P Displaced fracture of middle medial phalanx of right middle finger, subsequent encounter for fracture with malunion
- ▲ S62.622S Displaced fracture of middle medial phalanx of right middle finger, sequela
- ▲ S62.623A Displaced fracture of middle medial phalanx of left middle finger, initial encounter for closed fracture
- ▲ S62.623B Displaced fracture of middle medial phalanx of left middle finger, initial encounter for open fracture

● New Code ▲ Revised Code

▲ S62.623D Displaced fracture of middle medial phalanx of left middle finger, subsequent encounter for fracture with routine healing
▲ S62.623G Displaced fracture of middle medial phalanx of left middle finger, subsequent encounter for fracture with delayed healing
▲ S62.623K Displaced fracture of middle medial phalanx of left middle finger, subsequent encounter for fracture with nonunion
▲ S62.623P Displaced fracture of middle medial phalanx of left middle finger, subsequent encounter for fracture with malunion
▲ S62.623S Displaced fracture of middle medial phalanx of left middle finger, sequela
▲ S62.624A Displaced fracture of middle medial phalanx of right ring finger, initial encounter for closed fracture
▲ S62.624B Displaced fracture of middle medial phalanx of right ring finger, initial encounter for open fracture
▲ S62.624D Displaced fracture of middle medial phalanx of right ring finger, subsequent encounter for fracture with routine healing
▲ S62.624G Displaced fracture of middle medial phalanx of right ring finger, subsequent encounter for fracture with delayed healing
▲ S62.624K Displaced fracture of middle medial phalanx of right ring finger, subsequent encounter for fracture with nonunion
▲ S62.624P Displaced fracture of middle medial phalanx of right ring finger, subsequent encounter for fracture with malunion
▲ S62.624S Displaced fracture of middle medial phalanx of right ring finger, sequela
▲ S62.625A Displaced fracture of middle medial phalanx of left ring finger, initial encounter for closed fracture
▲ S62.625B Displaced fracture of middle medial phalanx of left ring finger, initial encounter for open fracture
▲ S62.625D Displaced fracture of middle medial phalanx of left ring finger, subsequent encounter for fracture with routine healing
▲ S62.625G Displaced fracture of middle medial phalanx of left ring finger, subsequent encounter for fracture with delayed healing
▲ S62.625K Displaced fracture of middle medial phalanx of left ring finger, subsequent encounter for fracture with nonunion
▲ S62.625P Displaced fracture of middle medial phalanx of left ring finger, subsequent encounter for fracture with malunion
▲ S62.625S Displaced fracture of middle medial phalanx of left ring finger, sequela
▲ S62.626A Displaced fracture of middle medial phalanx of right little finger, initial encounter for closed fracture
▲ S62.626B Displaced fracture of middle medial phalanx of right little finger, initial encounter for open fracture
▲ S62.626D Displaced fracture of middle medial phalanx of right little finger, subsequent encounter for fracture with routine healing
▲ S62.626G Displaced fracture of middle medial phalanx of right little finger, subsequent encounter for fracture with delayed healing
▲ S62.626K Displaced fracture of middle medial phalanx of right little finger, subsequent encounter for fracture with nonunion
▲ S62.626P Displaced fracture of middle medial phalanx of right little finger, subsequent encounter for fracture with malunion
▲ S62.626S Displaced fracture of middle medial phalanx of right little finger, sequela
▲ S62.627A Displaced fracture of middle medial phalanx of left little finger, initial encounter for closed fracture
▲ S62.627B Displaced fracture of middle medial phalanx of left little finger, initial encounter for open fracture
▲ S62.627D Displaced fracture of middle medial phalanx of left little finger, subsequent encounter for fracture with routine healing
▲ S62.627G Displaced fracture of middle medial phalanx of left little finger, subsequent encounter for fracture with delayed healing
▲ S62.627K Displaced fracture of middle medial phalanx of left little finger, subsequent encounter for fracture with nonunion
▲ S62.627P Displaced fracture of middle medial phalanx of left little finger, subsequent encounter for fracture with malunion
▲ S62.627S Displaced fracture of middle medial phalanx of left little finger, sequela
▲ S62.628A Displaced fracture of middle medial phalanx of other finger, initial encounter for closed fracture
▲ S62.628B Displaced fracture of middle medial phalanx of other finger, initial encounter for open fracture
▲ S62.628D Displaced fracture of middle medial phalanx of other finger, subsequent encounter for fracture with routine healing
▲ S62.628G Displaced fracture of middle medial phalanx of other finger, subsequent encounter for fracture with delayed healing
▲ S62.628K Displaced fracture of middle medial phalanx of other finger, subsequent encounter for fracture with nonunion
▲ S62.628P Displaced fracture of middle medial phalanx of other finger, subsequent encounter for fracture with malunion
▲ S62.628S Displaced fracture of middle medial phalanx of other finger, sequela
▲ S62.629A Displaced fracture of middle medial phalanx of unspecified finger, initial encounter for closed fracture
▲ S62.629B Displaced fracture of middle medial phalanx of unspecified finger, initial encounter for open fracture
▲ S62.629D Displaced fracture of middle medial phalanx of unspecified finger, subsequent encounter for fracture with routine healing
▲ S62.629G Displaced fracture of middle medial phalanx of unspecified finger, subsequent encounter for fracture with delayed healing
▲ S62.629K Displaced fracture of middle medial phalanx of unspecified finger, subsequent encounter for fracture with nonunion
▲ S62.629P Displaced fracture of middle medial phalanx of unspecified finger, subsequent encounter for fracture with malunion
▲ S62.629S Displaced fracture of middle medial phalanx of unspecified finger, sequela
▲ S62.65 Nondisplaced fracture of middle medial phalanx of finger
▲ S62.650A Nondisplaced fracture of middle medial phalanx of right index finger, initial encounter for closed fracture
▲ S62.650B Nondisplaced fracture of middle medial phalanx of right index finger, initial encounter for open fracture
▲ S62.650D Nondisplaced fracture of middle medial phalanx of right index finger, subsequent encounter for fracture with routine healing
▲ S62.650G Nondisplaced fracture of middle medial phalanx of right index finger, subsequent encounter for fracture with delayed healing
▲ S62.650K Nondisplaced fracture of middle medial phalanx of right index finger, subsequent encounter for fracture with nonunion
▲ S62.650P Nondisplaced fracture of middle medial phalanx of right index finger, subsequent encounter for fracture with malunion
▲ S62.650S Nondisplaced fracture of middle medial phalanx of right index finger, sequela
▲ S62.651A Nondisplaced fracture of middle medial phalanx of left index finger, initial encounter for closed fracture
▲ S62.651B Nondisplaced fracture of middle medial phalanx of left index finger, initial encounter for open fracture
▲ S62.651D Nondisplaced fracture of middle medial phalanx of left index finger, subsequent encounter for fracture with routine healing
▲ S62.651G Nondisplaced fracture of middle medial phalanx of left index finger, subsequent encounter for fracture with delayed healing
▲ S62.651K Nondisplaced fracture of middle medial phalanx of left index finger, subsequent encounter for fracture with nonunion
▲ S62.651P Nondisplaced fracture of middle medial phalanx of left index finger, subsequent encounter for fracture with malunion
▲ S62.651S Nondisplaced fracture of middle medial phalanx of left index finger, sequela
▲ S62.652A Nondisplaced fracture of middle medial phalanx of right middle finger, initial encounter for closed fracture
▲ S62.652B Nondisplaced fracture of middle medial phalanx of right middle finger, initial encounter for open fracture
▲ S62.652D Nondisplaced fracture of middle medial phalanx of right middle finger, subsequent encounter for fracture with routine healing

- ▲ S62.652G Nondisplaced fracture of middle medial phalanx of right middle finger, subsequent encounter for fracture with delayed healing
- ▲ S62.652K Nondisplaced fracture of middle medial phalanx of right middle finger, subsequent encounter for fracture with nonunion
- ▲ S62.652P Nondisplaced fracture of middle medial phalanx of right middle finger, subsequent encounter for fracture with malunion
- ▲ S62.652S Nondisplaced fracture of middle medial phalanx of right middle finger, sequela
- ▲ S62.653A Nondisplaced fracture of middle medial phalanx of left middle finger, initial encounter for closed fracture
- ▲ S62.653B Nondisplaced fracture of middle medial phalanx of left middle finger, initial encounter for open fracture
- ▲ S62.653D Nondisplaced fracture of middle medial phalanx of left middle finger, subsequent encounter for fracture with routine healing
- ▲ S62.653G Nondisplaced fracture of middle medial phalanx of left middle finger, subsequent encounter for fracture with delayed healing
- ▲ S62.653K Nondisplaced fracture of middle medial phalanx of left middle finger, subsequent encounter for fracture with nonunion
- ▲ S62.653P Nondisplaced fracture of middle medial phalanx of left middle finger, subsequent encounter for fracture with malunion
- ▲ S62.653S Nondisplaced fracture of middle medial phalanx of left middle finger, sequela
- ▲ S62.654A Nondisplaced fracture of middle medial phalanx of right ring finger, initial encounter for closed fracture
- ▲ S62.654B Nondisplaced fracture of middle medial phalanx of right ring finger, initial encounter for open fracture
- ▲ S62.654D Nondisplaced fracture of middle medial phalanx of right ring finger, subsequent encounter for fracture with routine healing
- ▲ S62.654G Nondisplaced fracture of middle medial phalanx of right ring finger, subsequent encounter for fracture with delayed healing
- ▲ S62.654K Nondisplaced fracture of middle medial phalanx of right ring finger, subsequent encounter for fracture with nonunion
- ▲ S62.654P Nondisplaced fracture of middle medial phalanx of right ring finger, subsequent encounter for fracture with malunion
- ▲ S62.654S Nondisplaced fracture of middle medial phalanx of right ring finger, sequela
- ▲ S62.655A Nondisplaced fracture of middle medial phalanx of left ring finger, initial encounter for closed fracture
- ▲ S62.655B Nondisplaced fracture of middle medial phalanx of left ring finger, initial encounter for open fracture
- ▲ S62.655D Nondisplaced fracture of middle medial phalanx of left ring finger, subsequent encounter for fracture with routine healing
- ▲ S62.655G Nondisplaced fracture of middle medial phalanx of left ring finger, subsequent encounter for fracture with delayed healing
- ▲ S62.655K Nondisplaced fracture of middle medial phalanx of left ring finger, subsequent encounter for fracture with nonunion
- ▲ S62.655P Nondisplaced fracture of middle medial phalanx of left ring finger, subsequent encounter for fracture with malunion
- ▲ S62.655S Nondisplaced fracture of middle medial phalanx of left ring finger, sequela
- ▲ S62.656A Nondisplaced fracture of middle medial phalanx of right little finger, initial encounter for closed fracture
- ▲ S62.656B Nondisplaced fracture of middle medial phalanx of right little finger, initial encounter for open fracture
- ▲ S62.656D Nondisplaced fracture of middle medial phalanx of right little finger, subsequent encounter for fracture with routine healing
- ▲ S62.656G Nondisplaced fracture of middle medial phalanx of right little finger, subsequent encounter for fracture with delayed healing
- ▲ S62.656K Nondisplaced fracture of middle medial phalanx of right little finger, subsequent encounter for fracture with nonunion
- ▲ S62.656P Nondisplaced fracture of middle medial phalanx of right little finger, subsequent encounter for fracture with malunion
- ▲ S62.656S Nondisplaced fracture of middle medial phalanx of right little finger, sequela
- ▲ S62.657A Nondisplaced fracture of middle medial phalanx of left little finger, initial encounter for closed fracture
- ▲ S62.657B Nondisplaced fracture of middle medial phalanx of left little finger, initial encounter for open fracture
- ▲ S62.657D Nondisplaced fracture of middle medial phalanx of left little finger, subsequent encounter for fracture with routine healing
- ▲ S62.657G Nondisplaced fracture of middle medial phalanx of left little finger, subsequent encounter for fracture with delayed healing
- ▲ S62.657K Nondisplaced fracture of middle medial phalanx of left little finger, subsequent encounter for fracture with nonunion
- ▲ S62.657P Nondisplaced fracture of middle medial phalanx of left little finger, subsequent encounter for fracture with malunion
- ▲ S62.657S Nondisplaced fracture of middle medial phalanx of left little finger, sequela
- ▲ S62.658A Nondisplaced fracture of middle medial phalanx of other finger, initial encounter for closed fracture
- ▲ S62.658B Nondisplaced fracture of middle medial phalanx of other finger, initial encounter for open fracture
- ▲ S62.658D Nondisplaced fracture of middle medial phalanx of other finger, subsequent encounter for fracture with routine healing
- ▲ S62.658G Nondisplaced fracture of middle medial phalanx of other finger, subsequent encounter for fracture with delayed healing
- ▲ S62.658K Nondisplaced fracture of middle medial phalanx of other finger, subsequent encounter for fracture with nonunion
- ▲ S62.658P Nondisplaced fracture of middle medial phalanx of other finger, subsequent encounter for fracture with malunion
- ▲ S62.658S Nondisplaced fracture of middle medial phalanx of other finger, sequela
- ▲ S62.659A Nondisplaced fracture of middle medial phalanx of unspecified finger, initial encounter for closed fracture
- ▲ S62.659B Nondisplaced fracture of middle medial phalanx of unspecified finger, initial encounter for open fracture
- ▲ S62.659D Nondisplaced fracture of middle medial phalanx of unspecified finger, subsequent encounter for fracture with routine healing
- ▲ S62.659G Nondisplaced fracture of middle medial phalanx of unspecified finger, subsequent encounter for fracture with delayed healing
- ▲ S62.659K Nondisplaced fracture of middle medial phalanx of unspecified finger, subsequent encounter for fracture with nonunion
- ▲ S62.659P Nondisplaced fracture of middle medial phalanx of unspecified finger, subsequent encounter for fracture with malunion
- ▲ S62.659S Nondisplaced fracture of middle medial phalanx of unspecified finger, sequela
- ▲ T4Ø.1 Poisoning by ,adverse effect of and underfosing and adverse effect of heroin
- ▲ T4Ø.8 Poisoning by and adverse effect of lysergide [LSD]
- ▲ T78.Ø Anaphylactic shock due to adverse food reaction reaction due to food
- ▲ T78.ØØXA Anaphylactic shock reaction due to unspecified food, initial encounter
- ▲ T78.ØØXD Anaphylactic shock reaction due to unspecified food, subsequent encounter
- ▲ T78.ØØXS Anaphylactic shock reaction due to unspecified food, sequela
- ▲ T78.Ø1XA Anaphylactic shock reaction due to peanuts, initial encounter
- ▲ T78.Ø1XD Anaphylactic shock reaction due to peanuts, subsequent encounter
- ▲ T78.Ø1XS Anaphylactic shock reaction due to peanuts, sequela
- ▲ T78.Ø2XA Anaphylactic shock reaction due to shellfish (crustaceans), initial encounter
- ▲ T78.Ø2XD Anaphylactic shock reaction due to shellfish (crustaceans), subsequent encounter
- ▲ T78.Ø2XS Anaphylactic shock reaction due to shellfish (crustaceans), sequela
- ▲ T78.Ø3XA Anaphylactic shock reaction due to other fish, initial encounter
- ▲ T78.Ø3XD Anaphylactic shock reaction due to other fish, subsequent encounter
- ▲ T78.Ø3XS Anaphylactic shock reaction due to other fish, sequela

▲ T78.04XA Anaphylactic shock reaction due to fruits and vegetables, initial encounter
▲ T78.04XD Anaphylactic shock reaction due to fruits and vegetables, subsequent encounter
▲ T78.04XS Anaphylactic shock reaction due to fruits and vegetables, sequela
▲ T78.05XA Anaphylactic shock reaction due to tree nuts and seeds, initial encounter
▲ T78.05XD Anaphylactic shock reaction due to tree nuts and seeds, subsequent encounter
▲ T78.05XS Anaphylactic shock reaction due to tree nuts and seeds, sequela
▲ T78.06XA Anaphylactic shock reaction due to food additives, initial encounter
▲ T78.06XD Anaphylactic shock reaction due to food additives, subsequent encounter
▲ T78.06XS Anaphylactic shock reaction due to food additives, sequela
▲ T78.07XA Anaphylactic shock reaction due to milk and dairy products, initial encounter
▲ T78.07XD Anaphylactic shock reaction due to milk and dairy products, subsequent encounter
▲ T78.07XS Anaphylactic shock reaction due to milk and dairy products, sequela
▲ T78.08XA Anaphylactic shock reaction due to eggs, initial encounter
▲ T78.08XD Anaphylactic shock reaction due to eggs, subsequent encounter
▲ T78.08XS Anaphylactic shock reaction due to eggs, sequela
▲ T78.09XA Anaphylactic shock reaction due to other food products, initial encounter
▲ T78.09XD Anaphylactic shock reaction due to other food products, subsequent encounter
▲ T78.09XS Anaphylactic shock reaction due to other food products, sequela
● T80.211A Bloodstream infection due to central venous catheter, initial encounter
● T80.211D Bloodstream infection due to central venous catheter, subsequent encounter
● T80.211S Bloodstream infection due to central venous catheter, sequela
● T80.212A Local infection due to central venous catheter, initial encounter
● T80.212D Local infection due to central venous catheter, subsequent encounter
● T80.212S Local infection due to central venous catheter, sequela
● T80.218A Other infection due to central venous catheter, initial encounter
● T80.218D Other infection due to central venous catheter, subsequent encounter
● T80.218S Other infection due to central venous catheter, sequela
● T80.219A Unspecified infection due to central venous catheter, initial encounter
● T80.219D Unspecified infection due to central venous catheter, subsequent encounter
● T80.219S Unspecified infection due to central venous catheter, sequela
● T80.22XA Acute infection following transfusion, infusion, or injection of blood and blood products, initial encounter
● T80.22XD Acute infection following transfusion, infusion, or injection of blood and blood products, subsequent encounter
● T80.22XS Acute infection following transfusion, infusion, or injection of blood and blood products, sequela
▲ T80.5 Anaphylactic shock reaction due to serum
● T80.51XA Anaphylactic shock reaction due to administration of blood and blood products, initial encounter
● T80.51XD Anaphylactic shock reaction due to administration of blood and blood products, subsequent encounter
● T80.51XS Anaphylactic shock reaction due to administration of blood and blood products, sequela
● T80.52XA Anaphylactic shock reaction due to vaccination, initial encounter
● T80.52XD Anaphylactic shock reaction due to vaccination, subsequent encounter
● T80.52XS Anaphylactic shock reaction due to vaccination, sequela
● T80.59XA Anaphylactic shock reaction due to other serum, initial encounter
● T80.59XD Anaphylactic shock reaction due to other serum, subsequent encounter
● T80.59XS Anaphylactic shock reaction due to other serum, sequela
● T80.61XA Other serum reaction due to administration of blood and blood products, initial encounter
● T80.61XD Other serum reaction due to administration of blood and blood products, subsequent encounter
● T80.61XS Other serum reaction due to administration of blood and blood products, sequela
● T80.62XA Other serum reaction due to vaccination, initial encounter
● T80.62XD Other serum reaction due to vaccination, subsequent encounter
● T80.62XS Other serum reaction due to vaccination, sequela
● T80.69XA Other serum reaction due to other serum, initial encounter
● T80.69XD Other serum reaction due to other serum, subsequent encounter
● T80.69XS Other serum reaction due to other serum, sequela
▲ T81.1 Shock during or resulting from a procedure, not elsewhere classified Postprocedural shock
● T81.10XA Postprocedural shock unspecified, initial encounter
● T81.10XD Postprocedural shock unspecified, subsequent encounter
● T81.10XS Postprocedural shock unspecified, sequela
● T81.11XA Postprocedural cardiogenic shock, initial encounter
● T81.11XD Postprocedural cardiogenic shock, subsequent encounter
● T81.11XS Postprocedural cardiogenic shock, sequela
● T81.12XA Postprocedural septic shock, initial encounter
● T81.12XD Postprocedural septic shock, subsequent encounter
● T81.12XS Postprocedural septic shock, sequela
● T81.19XA Other postprocedural shock, initial encounter
● T81.19XD Other postprocedural shock, subsequent encounter
● T81.19XS Other postprocedural shock, sequela
● T83.7 Complications due to implanted mesh and other prosthetic materials
● T83.71 Erosion of implanted mesh and other prosthetic materials to surrounding organ or tissue
● T83.711A Erosion of implanted vaginal mesh and other prosthetic materials to surrounding organ or tissue, initial encounter
● T83.711D Erosion of implanted vaginal mesh and other prosthetic materials to surrounding organ or tissue, subsequent encounter
● T83.711S Erosion of implanted vaginal mesh and other prosthetic materials to surrounding organ or tissue, sequela
● T83.718A Erosion of other implanted mesh and other prosthetic materials to surrounding organ or tissue, initial encounter
● T83.718D Erosion of other implanted mesh and other prosthetic materials to surrounding organ or tissue, subsequent encounter
● T83.718S Erosion of other implanted mesh and other prosthetic materials to surrounding organ or tissue, sequela
● T83.72 Exposure of implanted mesh and other prosthetic materials into surrounding organ or tissue
● T83.721A Exposure of implanted vaginal mesh and other prosthetic materials into vagina, initial encounter
● T83.721D Exposure of implanted vaginal mesh and other prosthetic materials into vagina, subsequent encounter
● T83.721S Exposure of implanted vaginal mesh and other prosthetic materials into vagina, sequela
● T83.728A Exposure of other implanted mesh and other prosthetic materials to surrounding organ or tissue, initial encounter
● T83.728D Exposure of other implanted mesh and other prosthetic materials to surrounding organ or tissue, subsequent encounter
● T83.728S Exposure of other implanted mesh and other prosthetic materials to surrounding organ or tissue, sequela
▲ T84.022A Dislocation Instability of internal right knee prosthesis, initial encounter
▲ T84.022D Dislocation Instability of internal right knee prosthesis, subsequent encounter
▲ T84.022S Dislocation Instability of internal right knee prosthesis, sequela
▲ T84.023A Dislocation Instability of internal left knee prosthesis, initial encounter
▲ T84.023D Dislocation Instability of internal left knee prosthesis, subsequent encounter
▲ T84.023S Dislocation Instability of internal left knee prosthesis, sequela
● T86.5 Complications of stem cell transplant
● T87.81 Dehiscence of amputation stump
● T87.89 Other complications of amputation stump
▲ T88.6XXA Anaphylactic shock reaction due to adverse effect of correct drug or medicament properly administered, initial encounter
▲ T88.6XXD Anaphylactic shock reaction due to adverse effect of correct drug or medicament properly administered, subsequent encounter

▲ T88.6XXS Anaphylactic shock reaction due to adverse effect of correct drug or medicament properly administered, sequela
● Y92.000 Kitchen of unspecified non-institutional (private) residence as the place of occurrence of the external cause
● Y92.001 Dining room of unspecified non-institutional (private) residence as the place of occurrence of the external cause
● Y92.002 Bathroom of unspecified non-institutional private) residence single-family (private) house as the place of occurrence of the external cause
● Y92.003 Bedroom of unspecified non-institutional (private) residence as the place of occurrence of the external cause
● Y92.007 Garden or yard of unspecified non-institutional (private) residence as the place of occurrence of the external cause
● Y92.008 Other place in unspecified non-institutional (private) residence as the place of occurrence of the external cause
● Y92.009 Unspecified place in unspecified non-institutional (private) residence as the place of occurrence of the external cause
▲ Z16 Infection with drug resistant microorganism Resistance to antimicrobial drugs
● Z16.1 Resistance to beta lactam antibiotics
● Z16.10 Resistance to unspecified beta lactam antibiotics
● Z16.11 Resistance to penicillins
● Z16.12 Extended spectrum beta lactamase (ESBL) resistance
● Z16.19 Resistance to other specified beta lactam antibiotics
● Z16.2 Resistance to other antibiotics
● Z16.20 Resistance to unspecified antibiotic
● Z16.21 Resistance to vancomycin
● Z16.22 Resistance to vancomycin related antibiotics
● Z16.23 Resistance to quinolones and fluoroquinolones
● Z16.24 Resistance to multiple antibiotics
● Z16.29 Resistance to other single specified antibiotic
● Z16.3 Resistance to other antimicrobial drugs
● Z16.30 Resistance to unspecified antimicrobial drugs
● Z16.31 Resistance to antiparasitic drug(s)
● Z16.32 Resistance to antifungal drug(s)
● Z16.33 Resistance to antiviral drug(s)
● Z16.34 Resistance to antimycobacterial drug(s)
● Z16.341 Resistance to single antimycobacterial drug
● Z16.342 Resistance to multiple antimycobacterial drugs
● Z16.35 Resistance to multiple antimicrobial drugs
● Z16.39 Resistance to other specified antimicrobial drug
● Z22.321 Carrier or suspected carrier of Methicillin susceptible Staphylococcus aureus
● Z22.322 Carrier or suspected carrier of Methicillin resistant Staphylococcus aureus
● Z3A Weeks of gestation
● Z3A.0 Weeks of gestation of pregnancy, unspecified or less than 10 weeks
● Z3A.00 Weeks of gestation of pregnancy not specified
● Z3A.01 Less than 8 weeks gestation of pregnancy
● Z3A.08 8 weeks gestation of pregnancy
● Z3A.09 9 weeks gestation of pregnancy
● Z3A.1 Weeks of gestation of pregnancy, weeks 10-19
● Z3A.10 10 weeks gestation of pregnancy
● Z3A.11 11 weeks gestation of pregnancy
● Z3A.12 12 weeks gestation of pregnancy
● Z3A.13 13 weeks gestation of pregnancy
● Z3A.14 14 weeks gestation of pregnancy
● Z3A.15 15 weeks gestation of pregnancy
● Z3A.16 16 weeks gestation of pregnancy
● Z3A.17 17 weeks gestation of pregnancy
● Z3A.18 18 weeks gestation of pregnancy
● Z3A.19 19 weeks gestation of pregnancy
● Z3A.2 Weeks of gestation of pregnancy, weeks 20-29
● Z3A.20 20 weeks gestation of pregnancy
● Z3A.21 21 weeks gestation of pregnancy
● Z3A.22 22 weeks gestation of pregnancy
● Z3A.23 23 weeks gestation of pregnancy
● Z3A.24 24 weeks gestation of pregnancy
● Z3A.25 25 weeks gestation of pregnancy
● Z3A.26 26 weeks gestation of pregnancy
● Z3A.27 27 weeks gestation of pregnancy
● Z3A.28 28 weeks gestation of pregnancy
● Z3A.29 29 weeks gestation of pregnancy
● Z3A.3 Weeks of gestation of pregnancy, weeks 30-39
● Z3A.30 30 weeks gestation of pregnancy
● Z3A.31 31 weeks gestation of pregnancy
● Z3A.32 32 weeks gestation of pregnancy
● Z3A.33 33 weeks gestation of pregnancy
● Z3A.34 34 weeks gestation of pregnancy
● Z3A.35 35 weeks gestation of pregnancy
● Z3A.36 36 weeks gestation of pregnancy
● Z3A.37 37 weeks gestation of pregnancy
● Z3A.38 38 weeks gestation of pregnancy
● Z3A.39 39 weeks gestation of pregnancy
● Z3A.4 Weeks of gestation of pregnancy, weeks 40 or greater
● Z3A.40 40 weeks gestation of pregnancy
● Z3A.41 41 weeks gestation of pregnancy
● Z3A.42 42 weeks gestation of pregnancy
● Z3A.49 Greater than 42 weeks gestation of pregnancy
● Z47.3 Aftercare following explantation of joint prosthesis
● Z47.31 Aftercare following explantation of shoulder joint prosthesis
● Z47.32 Aftercare following explantation of hip joint prosthesis
● Z47.33 Aftercare following explantation of knee joint prosthesis
▲ Z68 Body mass index (BMI) [BMI]
● Z77.012 Contact with and (suspected) exposure to uranium
● Z79.83 Long term (current) use of bisphosphonates
▲ Z81.0 Family history of mental retardation intellectual disabilities
● Z83.51 Family history of eye disorders
● Z83.511 Family history of glaucoma
● Z83.518 Family history of other specified eye disorder
● Z83.52 Family history of ear disorders
● Z85.54 Personal history of malignant neoplasm of ureter
● Z86.14 Personal history of Methicillin resistant Staphylococcus aureus infection
● Z86.32 Personal history of gestational diabetes
● Z86.711 Personal history of pulmonary embolism
● Z86.718 Personal history of other venous thrombosis and embolism
● Z87.892 Personal history of anaphylaxis
▲ Z89.51 Acquired absence of right leg below knee
● Z89.511 Acquired absence of right leg below knee
● Z89.512 Acquired absence of left leg below knee
● Z89.519 Acquired absence of unspecified leg below knee
▲ Z89.52 Acquired absence of left leg below knee
● Z89.521 Acquired absence of right knee
● Z89.522 Acquired absence of left knee
● Z89.529 Acquired absence of unspecified knee
▲ Z89.621 Acquired absence of right hip joint
▲ Z89.622 Acquired absence of left hip joint
▲ Z89.629 Acquired absence of unspecified hip joint
● Z91.83 Wandering in diseases classified elsewhere

● New Code ▲ Revised Code

ICD-10-CM Draft Official Guidelines for Coding and Reporting 2012

Narrative changes appear in bold text

Items <u>underlined</u> have been moved within the guidelines since the 2011 version

***Italics* are used to indicate revisions to heading changes**

The Centers for Medicare and Medicaid Services (CMS) and the National Center for Health Statistics (NCHS), two departments within the U.S. Federal Government's Department of Health and Human Services (DHHS) provide the following guidelines for coding and reporting using the International Classification of Diseases, 10th Revision, Clinical Modification (ICD-10-CM). These guidelines should be used as a companion document to the official version of the ICD-10-CM as published on the NCHS website. The ICD-10-CM is a morbidity classification published by the United States for classifying diagnoses and reason for visits in all health care settings. The ICD-10-CM is based on the ICD-10, the statistical classification of disease published by the World Health Organization (WHO).

These guidelines have been approved by the four organizations that make up the Cooperating Parties for the ICD-10-CM: the American Hospital Association (AHA), the American Health Information Management Association (AHIMA), CMS, and NCHS.

These guidelines are a set of rules that have been developed to accompany and complement the official conventions and instructions provided within the ICD-10-CM itself. The instructions and conventions of the classification take precedence over guidelines. These guidelines are based on the coding and sequencing instructions in the Tabular List and Alphabetic Index of ICD-10-CM, but provide additional instruction. Adherence to these guidelines when assigning ICD-10-CM diagnosis codes is required under the Health Insurance Portability and Accountability Act (HIPAA). The diagnosis codes (Tabular List and Alphabetic Index) have been adopted under HIPAA for all healthcare settings. A joint effort between the healthcare provider and the coder is essential to achieve complete and accurate documentation, code assignment, and reporting of diagnoses and procedures. These guidelines have been developed to assist both the healthcare provider and the coder in identifying those diagnoses and procedures that are to be reported. The importance of consistent, complete documentation in the medical record cannot be overemphasized. Without such documentation accurate coding cannot be achieved. The entire record should be reviewed to determine the specific reason for the encounter and the conditions treated.

The term encounter is used for all settings, including hospital admissions. In the context of these guidelines, the term provider is used throughout the guidelines to mean physician or any qualified health care practitioner who is legally accountable for establishing the patient's diagnosis. Only this set of guidelines, approved by the Cooperating Parties, is official.

The guidelines are organized into sections. Section I includes the structure and conventions of the classification and general guidelines that apply to the entire classification, and chapter-specific guidelines that correspond to the chapters as they are arranged in the classification. Section II includes guidelines for selection of principal diagnosis for non-outpatient settings. Section III includes guidelines for reporting additional diagnoses in non-outpatient settings. Section IV is for outpatient coding and reporting. It is necessary to review all sections of the guidelines to fully understand all of the rules and instructions needed to code properly.

Section I. Conventions, general coding guidelines and chapter specific guidelines

The conventions, general guidelines and chapter-specific guidelines are applicable to all health care settings unless otherwise indicated. The conventions and instructions of the classification take precedence over guidelines.

A. Conventions for the ICD-10-CM

The conventions for the ICD-10-CM are the general rules for use of the classification independent of the guidelines. These conventions are incorporated within the Alphabetic Index and Tabular List of the ICD-10-CM as instructional notes.

1. **The Alphabetic Index and Tabular List**
   The ICD-10-CM is divided into the Alphabetic Index, an alphabetical list of terms and their corresponding code, and the Tabular List, a chronological list of codes divided into chapters based on body system or condition. The Alphabetic Index consists of the following parts: the Index of Diseases and Injury, the Index of External Causes of Injury, the Table of Neoplasms and the Table of Drugs and Chemicals.

   See Section I.C2. General guidelines

   See Section I.C.19. Adverse effects, poisoning, underdosing and toxic effects

2. **Format and Structure:**
   The ICD-10-CM Tabular List contains categories, subcategories and codes. Characters for categories, subcategories and codes may be either a letter or a number. All categories are 3 characters. A three-character category that has no further subdivision is equivalent to a code. Subcategories are either 4 or 5 characters. Codes may be 3, 4, 5, 6 or 7 characters. That is, each level of subdivision after a category is a subcategory. The final level of subdivision is a code. Codes that have applicable 7th characters are still referred to as codes, not subcategories. A code that has an applicable 7th character is considered invalid without the 7th character.

   The ICD-10-CM uses an indented format for ease in reference.

3. **Use of codes for reporting purposes**
   For reporting purposes only codes are permissible, not categories or subcategories, and any applicable 7th character is required.

4. **Placeholder character**
   The ICD-10-CM utilizes a placeholder character "x". The "x" is used as a placeholder at certain codes to allow for future expansion. An example of this is at the poisoning, adverse effect and underdosing codes, categories T36-T50.

   Where a placeholder exists, the x must be used in order for the code to be considered a valid code.

5. **7th Characters**
   Certain ICD-10-CM categories have applicable 7th characters. The applicable 7th character is required for all codes within the category, or as the notes in the Tabular List instruct. The 7th character must always be the 7th character in the data field. If a code that requires a 7th character is not 6 characters, a placeholder X must be used to fill in the empty characters.

6. **Abbreviations**
   a. **Alphabetic Index abbreviations**
      NEC "Not elsewhere classifiable"
      This abbreviation in the Alphabetic Index represents "other specified". When a specific code is not available for a condition, the Alphabetic Index directs the coder to the "other specified" code in the Tabular List.
      NOS "Not otherwise specified"
      This abbreviation is the equivalent of unspecified.

   b. **Tabular List abbreviations**
      NEC "Not elsewhere classifiable"
      This abbreviation in the Tabular List represents "other specified". When a specific code is not available for a condition the Tabular List includes an NEC entry under a code to identify the code as the "other specified" code.
      NOS "Not otherwise specified"
      This abbreviation is the equivalent of unspecified.

7. **Punctuation**
   [ ] Brackets are used in the Tabular List to enclose synonyms, alternative wording or explanatory phrases. Brackets are used in the Alphabetic Index to identify manifestation codes.
   ( ) Parentheses are used in both the Alphabetic Index and Tabular List to enclose supplementary words that may be present or absent in the statement of a disease or procedure without affecting the code number to which it is assigned. The terms within the parentheses are referred to as nonessential modifiers.
   : Colons are used in the Tabular List after an incomplete term which needs one or more of the modifiers following the colon to make it assignable to a given category.

8. **Use of "and"**
   When the term "and" is used in a narrative statement it represents and/or.

9. **Other and Unspecified codes**
   a. **"Other" codes**
      Codes titled "other" or "other specified" are for use when the information in the medical record provides detail for which a specific code does not exist. Alphabetic Index entries with NEC in the line designate "other" codes in the Tabular List. These Alphabetic Index entries represent specific disease entities for which no specific code exists so the term is included within an "other" code.

   b. **"Unspecified" codes**
      Codes titled "unspecified" are for use when the information in the medical record is insufficient to assign a more specific code. For those categories for which an unspecified code is not provided, the "other specified" code may represent both other and unspecified.

10. **Includes Notes**
    This note appears immediately under a three character code title to further define, or give examples of, the content of the category.

11. **Inclusion Terms**
    List of terms is included under some codes. These terms are the conditions for which that code is to be used. The terms may be synonyms of the code title, or, in the case of "other specified" codes, the terms are a list of the various conditions assigned to that code. The inclusion terms are not necessarily exhaustive. Additional terms found only in the Alphabetic Index may also be assigned to a code.

12. **Excludes Notes**
    The ICD-10-CM has two types of excludes notes. Each type of note has a different definition for use but they are all similar in that they indicate that codes excluded from each other are independent of each other.

    a. **Excludes1**
       A type 1 Excludes note is a pure excludes note. It means "NOT CODED HERE!" An Excludes1 note indicates that the code excluded should never be used at the same time as the code above the Excludes1 note. An Excludes1 is used when two conditions cannot occur together, such as a congenital form versus an acquired form of the same condition.

    b. **Excludes2**
       A type 2 excludes note represents "Not included here". An excludes2 note indicates that the condition excluded is not part of the condition represented by the code, but a patient may have both conditions at the same time. When an Excludes2 note appears under a code, it is acceptable to use both the code and the excluded code together, when appropriate.

13. **Etiology/manifestation convention ("code first", "use additional code" and "in diseases classified elsewhere" notes)**
    Certain conditions have both an underlying etiology and multiple body system manifestations due to the underlying etiology. For such conditions, the ICD-10-CM has a coding convention that requires the

underlying condition be sequenced first followed by the manifestation. Wherever such a combination exists, there is a "use additional code" note at the etiology code, and a "code first" note at the manifestation code. These instructional notes indicate the proper sequencing order of the codes, etiology followed by manifestation.

In most cases the manifestation codes will have in the code title, "in diseases classified elsewhere." Codes with this title are a component of the etiology/ manifestation convention. The code title indicates that it is a manifestation code. "In diseases classified elsewhere" codes are never permitted to be used as first-listed or principal diagnosis codes. They must be used in conjunction with an underlying condition code and they must be listed following the underlying condition. See category FØ2, Dementia in other diseases classified elsewhere, for an example of this convention.

There are manifestation codes that do not have "in diseases classified elsewhere" in the title. For such codes a "use additional code" note will still be present and the rules for sequencing apply.

In addition to the notes in the Tabular List, these conditions also have a specific Alphabetic Index entry structure. In the Alphabetic Index both conditions are listed together with the etiology code first followed by the manifestation codes in brackets. The code in brackets is always to be sequenced second.

An example of the etiology/manifestation convention is dementia in Parkinson's disease. In the Alphabetic Index, code G2Ø is listed first, followed by code FØ2.8Ø or FØ2.81 in brackets. Code G2Ø represents the underlying etiology, Parkinson's disease, and must be sequenced first, whereas codes FØ2.8Ø and FØ2.81 represent the manifestation of dementia in diseases classified elsewhere, with or without behavioral disturbance.

"Code first" and "Use additional code" notes are also used as sequencing rules in the classification for certain codes that are not part of an etiology/ manifestation combination.

See Section I.B.7. Multiple coding for a single condition.

14. "And"

The word "and" should be interpreted to mean either "and" or "or" when it appears in a title.

15. "With"

The word "with" should be interpreted to mean "associated with" or "due to" when it appears in a code title, the Alphabetic Index, or an instructional note in the Tabular List.

The word "with" in the Alphabetic Index is sequenced immediately following the main term, not in alphabetical order.

16. "See" and "See Also"

The "see" instruction following a main term in the Alphabetic Index indicates that another term should be referenced. It is necessary to go to the main term referenced with the "see" note to locate the correct code.

A "see also" instruction following a main term in the Alphabetic Index instructs that there is another main term that may also be referenced that may provide additional Alphabetic Index entries that may be useful. It is not necessary to follow the "see also" note when the original main term provides the necessary code.

17. "Code also note"

A "code also" note instructs that two codes may be required to fully describe a condition, but this note does not provide sequencing direction.

18. Default codes

A code listed next to a main term in the ICD-1Ø-CM Alphabetic Index is referred to as a default code. The default code represents that condition that is most commonly associated with the main term, or is the unspecified code for the condition. If a condition is documented in a medical record (for example, appendicitis) without any additional information, such as acute or chronic, the default code should be assigned.

B. General Coding Guidelines

1. Locating a code in the ICD-1Ø-CM

To select a code in the classification that corresponds to a diagnosis or reason for visit documented in a medical record, first locate the term in the Alphabetic Index, and then verify the code in the Tabular List. Read and be guided by instructional notations that appear in both the Alphabetic Index and the Tabular List.

It is essential to use both the Alphabetic Index and Tabular List when locating and assigning a code. The Alphabetic Index does not always provide the full code. Selection of the full code, including laterality and any applicable 7th character can only be done in the Tabular List. A dash (-) at the end of an Alphabetic Index entry indicates that additional characters are required. Even if a dash is not included at the Alphabetic Index entry, it is necessary to refer to the Tabular List to verify that no 7th character is required.

2. Level of Detail in Coding

Diagnosis codes are to be used and reported at their highest number of characters available.

ICD-1Ø-CM diagnosis codes are composed of codes with 3, 4, 5, 6 or 7 characters. Codes with three characters are included in ICD-1Ø-CM as the heading of a category of codes that may be further subdivided by the use of fourth and/or fifth characters and/or sixth characters, which provide greater detail.

A three-character code is to be used only if it is not further subdivided. A code is invalid if it has not been coded to the full number of characters required for that code, including the 7th character, if applicable.

3. Code or codes from AØØ.Ø through T88.9, ZØØ-Z99.8

The appropriate code or codes from AØØ.Ø through T88.9, ZØØ-Z99.8 must be used to identify diagnoses, symptoms, conditions, problems, complaints or other reason(s) for the encounter/visit.

4. Signs and symptoms

Codes that describe symptoms and signs, as opposed to diagnoses, are acceptable for reporting purposes when a related definitive diagnosis has not been established (confirmed) by the provider. Chapter 18 of ICD-1Ø-CM, Symptoms, Signs, and Abnormal Clinical and Laboratory Findings, Not Elsewhere Classified (codes RØØ.Ø - R99) contains many, but not all codes for symptoms.

5. Conditions that are an integral part of a disease process

Signs and symptoms that are associated routinely with a disease process should not be assigned as additional codes, unless otherwise instructed by the classification.

6. Conditions that are not an integral part of a disease process

Additional signs and symptoms that may not be associated routinely with a disease process should be coded when present.

7. Multiple coding for a single condition

In addition to the etiology/manifestation convention that requires two codes to fully describe a single condition that affects multiple body systems, there are other single conditions that also require more than one code. "Use additional code" notes are found in the Tabular List at codes that are not part of an etiology/manifestation pair where a secondary code is useful to fully describe a condition. The sequencing rule is the same as the etiology/manifestation pair, "use additional code" indicates that a secondary code should be added.

For example, for bacterial infections that are not included in chapter 1, a secondary code from category B95, Streptococcus, Staphylococcus, and Enterococcus, as the cause of diseases classified elsewhere, or B96, Other bacterial agents as the cause of diseases classified elsewhere, may be required to identify the bacterial organism causing the infection. A "use additional code" note will normally be found at the infectious disease code, indicating a need for the organism code to be added as a secondary code.

"Code first" notes are also under certain codes that are not specifically manifestation codes but may be due to an underlying cause. When there is a "code first" note and an underlying condition is present, the underlying condition should be sequenced first.

"Code, if applicable, any causal condition first", notes indicate that this code may be assigned as a principal diagnosis when the causal condition is unknown or not applicable. If a causal condition is known, then the code for that condition should be sequenced as the principal or first-listed diagnosis.

Multiple codes may be needed for **sequela**, complication codes and obstetric codes to more fully describe a condition. See the specific guidelines for these conditions for further instruction.

8. Acute and Chronic Conditions

If the same condition is described as both acute (subacute) and chronic, and separate subentries exist in the Alphabetic Index at the same indentation level, code both and sequence the acute (subacute) code first.

9. Combination Code

A combination code is a single code used to classify:

Two diagnoses, or

A diagnosis with an associated secondary process (manifestation)

A diagnosis with an associated complication

Combination codes are identified by referring to subterm entries in the Alphabetic Index and by reading the inclusion and exclusion notes in the Tabular List.

Assign only the combination code when that code fully identifies the diagnostic conditions involved or when the Alphabetic Index so directs. Multiple coding should not be used when the classification provides a combination code that clearly identifies all of the elements documented in the diagnosis. When the combination code lacks necessary specificity in describing the manifestation or complication, an additional code should be used as a secondary code.

1Ø. Sequela (Late Effects)

A **sequela** is the residual effect (condition produced) after the acute phase of an illness or injury has terminated. There is no time limit on when a **sequela** code can be used. The residual may be apparent early, such as in cerebral infarction, or it may occur months or years later, such as that due to a previous injury. Coding of **sequela** generally requires two codes sequenced in the following order: The condition or nature of the **sequela** is sequenced first. The **sequela** code is sequenced second.

An exception to the above guidelines are those instances where the code for **the sequela** is followed by a manifestation code identified in the Tabular List and title, or the **sequela** code has been expanded (at the fourth, fifth or sixth character levels) to include the manifestation(s). The code for the acute phase of an illness or injury that led to the **sequela** is never used with a code for the late effect.

See Section I.C.9. Sequelae of cerebrovascular disease

See Section I.C.15. Sequelae of complication of pregnancy, childbirth and the puerperium

See Section I.C.19. ***Application of 7th characters for Chapter 19***

11. Impending or Threatened Condition

Code any condition described at the time of discharge as "impending" or "threatened" as follows:

If it did occur, code as confirmed diagnosis.

If it did not occur, reference the Alphabetic Index to determine if the condition has a subentry term for "impending" or "threatened" and also reference main term entries for "Impending" and for "Threatened."

If the subterms are listed, assign the given code.

If the subterms are not listed, code the existing underlying condition(s) and not the condition described as impending or threatened.

12. Reporting Same Diagnosis Code More than Once

Each unique ICD-1Ø-CM diagnosis code may be reported only once for an encounter. This applies to bilateral conditions when there are no distinct codes identifying laterality or two different conditions classified to the same ICD-1Ø-CM diagnosis code.

13. Laterality

For bilateral sites, the final character of the codes in the ICD-1Ø-CM indicates laterality. An unspecified side code is also provided should the side not be identified in the medical record. If no bilateral code is provided and the condition is bilateral, assign separate codes for both the left and right side.

14. Documentation for BMI and Pressure Ulcer Stages

For the Body Mass Index (BMI) and pressure ulcer stage codes, code assignment may be based on medical record documentation from clinicians who are not the patient's provider (i.e., physician or other qualified healthcare practitioner legally accountable for establishing the patient's diagnosis), since this information is typically documented by other clinicians involved in the care of the patient (e.g., a dietitian often documents the BMI and nurses often documents the pressure ulcer stages). However, the associated diagnosis (such as overweight, obesity, or pressure ulcer) must be documented by the patient's provider. If there is conflicting medical record documentation, either from the same clinician or different clinicians, the patient's attending provider should be queried for clarification.

The BMI codes should only be reported as secondary diagnoses. As with all other secondary diagnosis codes, the BMI codes should only be assigned when they meet the definition of a reportable additional diagnosis (see Section III, Reporting Additional Diagnoses).

15. Syndromes

Follow the Alphabetic Index guidance when coding syndromes. In the absence of Alphabetic Index guidance, assign codes for the documented manifestations of the syndrome.

16. Documentation of Complications of Care

Code assignment is based on the provider's documentation of the relationship between the condition and the care or procedure. The guideline extends to any complications of care, regardless of the chapter the code is located in. It is important to note that not all conditions that occur during or following medical care or surgery are classified as complications. There must be a cause-and-effect relationship between the care provided and the condition, and an indication in the documentation that it is a complication. Query the provider for clarification, if the complication is not clearly documented.

C. Chapter-Specific Coding Guidelines

In addition to general coding guidelines, there are guidelines for specific diagnoses and/or conditions in the classification. Unless otherwise indicated, these guidelines apply to all health care settings. Please refer to Section II for guidelines on the selection of principal diagnosis.

1. Chapter 1: Certain Infectious and Parasitic Diseases (AØØ-B99)

a. Human immunodeficiency virus (HIV) infections

1) Code only confirmed cases

Code only confirmed cases of HIV infection/illness. This is an exception to the hospital inpatient guideline Section II, H.

In this context, "confirmation" does not require documentation of positive serology or culture for HIV; the provider's diagnostic statement that the patient is HIV positive, or has an HIV-related illness is sufficient.

2) Selection and sequencing of HIV codes

(a) Patient admitted for HIV-related condition

If a patient is admitted for an HIV-related condition, the principal diagnosis should be B2Ø, **Human immunodeficiency virus [HIV] disease** followed by additional diagnosis codes for all reported HIV-related conditions.

(b) Patient with HIV disease admitted for unrelated condition

If a patient with HIV disease is admitted for an unrelated condition (such as a traumatic injury), the code for the unrelated condition (e.g., the nature of injury code) should be the principal diagnosis. Other diagnoses would be B2Ø followed by additional diagnosis codes for all reported HIV-related conditions.

(c) **Whether the patient is newly diagnosed**
Whether the patient is newly diagnosed or has had previous admissions/encounters for HIV conditions is irrelevant to the sequencing decision.

(d) **Asymptomatic human immunodeficiency virus**
Z21, Asymptomatic human immunodeficiency virus [HIV] infection status, is to be applied when the patient without any documentation of symptoms is listed as being "HIV positive," "known HIV," "HIV test positive," or similar terminology. Do not use this code if the term "AIDS" is used or if the patient is treated for any HIV-related illness or is described as having any condition(s) resulting from his/her HIV positive status; use B2Ø in these cases.

(e) **Patients with inconclusive HIV serology**
Patients with inconclusive HIV serology, but no definitive diagnosis or manifestations of the illness, may be assigned code R75, Inconclusive laboratory evidence of human immunodeficiency virus [HIV].

(f) **Previously diagnosed HIV-related illness**
Patients with any known prior diagnosis of an HIV-related illness should be coded to B2Ø. Once a patient has developed an HIV-related illness, the patient should always be assigned code B2Ø on every subsequent admission/encounter. Patients previously diagnosed with any HIV illness (B2Ø) should never be assigned to R75 or Z21, Asymptomatic human immunodeficiency virus [HIV] infection status.

(g) **HIV infection in pregnancy, childbirth and the puerperium**
During pregnancy, childbirth or the puerperium, a patient admitted (or presenting for a health care encounter) because of an HIV-related illness should receive a principal diagnosis code of O98.7-, Human immunodeficiency [HIV] disease complicating pregnancy, childbirth and the puerperium, followed by B2Ø and the code(s) for the HIV-related illness(es). Codes from Chapter 15 always take sequencing priority.

Patients with asymptomatic HIV infection status admitted (or presenting for a health care encounter) during pregnancy, childbirth, or the puerperium should receive codes of O98.7- and Z21.

(h) **Encounters for testing for HIV**
If a patient is being seen to determine his/her HIV status, use code Z11.4, Encounter for screening for human immunodeficiency virus [HIV]. Use additional codes for any associated high risk behavior.

If a patient with signs or symptoms is being seen for HIV testing, code the signs and symptoms. An additional counseling code Z71.7, Human immunodeficiency virus [HIV] counseling, may be used if counseling is provided during the encounter for the test.

When a patient returns to be informed of his/her HIV test results and the test result is negative, use code Z71.7, Human immunodeficiency virus [HIV] counseling.

If the results are positive, see previous guidelines and assign codes as appropriate.

b. Infectious agents as the cause of diseases classified to other chapters
Certain infections are classified in chapters other than Chapter 1 and no organism is identified as part of the infection code. In these instances, it is necessary to use an additional code from Chapter 1 to identify the organism. A code from category B95, Streptococcus, Staphylococcus, and Enterococcus as the cause of diseases classified to other chapters, B96, Other bacterial agents as the cause of diseases classified to other chapters, or B97, Viral agents as the cause of diseases classified to other chapters, is to be used as an additional code to identify the organism. An instructional note will be found at the infection code advising that an additional organism code is required.

c. Infections resistant to antibiotics
Many bacterial infections are resistant to current antibiotics. It is necessary to identify all infections documented as antibiotic resistant. Assign **a** code **from category** Z16, **Resistance to antimicrobial drugs,** following the infection code **only if the infection code does not identify drug resistance.**

d. Sepsis, severe sepsis, and septic shock

1) Coding of sepsis and severe sepsis

(a) **Sepsis**
For a diagnosis of sepsis, assign the appropriate code for the underlying systemic infection. If the type of infection or causal organism is not further specified, assign code A41.9, Sepsis, unspecified **organism**.

A code from subcategory R65.2, Severe sepsis, should not be assigned unless severe sepsis or an associated acute organ dysfunction is documented.

(i) Negative or inconclusive blood cultures and sepsis
Negative or inconclusive blood cultures do not preclude a diagnosis of sepsis in patients with clinical evidence of the condition, however, the provider should be queried.

(ii) Urosepsis
The term urosepsis is a nonspecific term. It is not to be considered synonymous with sepsis. It has no default code in the Alphabetic Index. Should a provider use this term, he/she must be queried for clarification.

(iii) Sepsis with organ dysfunction
If a patient has sepsis and associated acute organ dysfunction or multiple organ dysfunction (MOD), follow the instructions for coding severe sepsis.

(iv) Acute organ dysfunction that is not clearly associated with the sepsis
If a patient has sepsis and an acute organ dysfunction, but the medical record documentation indicates that the acute organ dysfunction is related to a medical condition other than the sepsis, do not assign a code from subcategory R65.2, Severe sepsis. An acute organ dysfunction must be associated with the sepsis in order to assign the severe sepsis code. If the documentation is not clear as to whether an acute organ dysfunction is related to the sepsis or another medical condition, query the provider.

(b) **Severe sepsis**
The coding of severe sepsis requires a minimum of 2 codes: first a code for the underlying systemic infection, followed by a code from subcategory R65.2, Severe sepsis. If the causal organism is not documented, assign code A41.9, Sepsis, unspecified **organism**, for the infection. Additional code(s) for the associated acute organ dysfunction are also required.
Due to the complex nature of severe sepsis, some cases may require querying the provider prior to assignment of the codes.

2) Septic shock

(a) Septic shock **generally refers to** circulatory failure associated with severe sepsis, and therefore, it represents a type of acute organ dysfunction. For all cases of septic shock, the code for the underlying systemic infection should be sequenced first, followed by code R65.21, Severe sepsis with septic shock. Any additional codes for the other acute organ dysfunctions should also be assigned.
For cases of septic shock, the code for the systemic infection should be sequenced first, followed by code R65.21, Severe sepsis with septic shock **or code T81.12, Postprocedural septic shock.** Any additional codes for the other acute organ dysfunctions should also be assigned. **As noted in the sequencing instructions in**

the Tabular List, the code for septic shock cannot be assigned as a principal diagnosis.

3) **Sequencing of severe sepsis**
If severe sepsis is present on admission, and meets the definition of principal diagnosis, the underlying systemic infection should be assigned as principal diagnosis followed by the appropriate code from subcategory R65.2 as required by the sequencing rules in the Tabular List. A code from subcategory R65.2 can never be assigned as a principal diagnosis.

When severe sepsis develops during an encounter (it was not present on admission) the underlying systemic infection and the appropriate code from subcategory R65.2 should be assigned as secondary diagnoses.

Severe sepsis may be present on admission but the diagnosis may not be confirmed until sometime after admission. If the documentation is not clear whether severe sepsis was present on admission, the provider should be queried.

4) **Sepsis and severe sepsis with a localized infection**
If the reason for admission is both sepsis or severe sepsis and a localized infection, such as pneumonia or cellulitis, a code(s) for the underlying systemic infection should be assigned first and the code for the localized infection should be assigned as a secondary diagnosis. If the patient has severe sepsis, a code from subcategory R65.2 should also be assigned as a secondary diagnosis. If the patient is admitted with a localized infection, such as pneumonia, and sepsis/severe sepsis doesn't develop until after admission, the localized infection should be assigned first, followed by the appropriate sepsis/severe sepsis codes.

5) **Sepsis due to a postprocedural infection**

(a) Documentation of causal relationship
As with all postprocedural complications, code assignment is based on the provider's documentation of the relationship between the infection and the procedure.

(b) Sepsis due to a postprocedural infection
For such cases, the postprocedural infection code, such as, T8Ø.2, Infections following infusion, transfusion, and therapeutic injection, T81.4, Infection following a procedure, T88.Ø, Infection following immunization, or O86.Ø, Infection of obstetric surgical wound, should be coded first, followed by the code for the specific infection. If the patient has severe sepsis the appropriate code from subcategory R65.2 should also be assigned with the additional code(s) for any acute organ dysfunction.

(c) Postprocedural infection and postprocedural septic shock
In cases where a postprocedural infection has occurred and has resulted in severe sepsis and postprocedural septic shock, the code for the precipitating complication such as code T81.4, Infection following a procedure, or O86.Ø, Infection of obstetrical surgical wound should be coded first followed by code R65.21, Severe sepsis with septic shock and a code for the systemic infection.

6) **Sepsis and severe sepsis associated with a noninfectious process (condition)**
In some cases a noninfectious process (condition), such as trauma, may lead to an infection which can result in sepsis or severe sepsis. If sepsis or severe sepsis is documented as associated with a noninfectious condition, such as a burn or serious injury, and this condition meets the definition for principal diagnosis, the code for the noninfectious condition should be sequenced first, followed by the code for the resulting infection. If severe sepsis, is present a code from subcategory R65.2 should also be assigned with any associated organ dysfunction(s) codes. It is not necessary to assign a code from subcategory R65.1, Systemic inflammatory response syndrome (SIRS) of non-infectious origin, for these cases.

If the infection meets the definition of principal diagnosis it should be sequenced before the non-infectious condition. When both the associated non-infectious condition and the infection meet the definition of principal diagnosis either may be assigned as principal diagnosis.

Only one code from category R65, Symptoms and signs specifically associated with systemic inflammation and infection, should be assigned. Therefore, when a non-infectious condition leads to an infection resulting in severe sepsis, assign the appropriate code from subcategory R65.2, Severe sepsis. Do not additionally assign a code from subcategory R65.1, Systemic inflammatory response syndrome (SIRS) of non-infectious origin.

See Section I.C.18. SIRS due to non-infectious process

7) **Sepsis and septic shock complicating abortion, pregnancy, childbirth, and the puerperium**
See Section I.C.15. Sepsis and septic shock complicating abortion, pregnancy, childbirth and the puerperium

8) **Newborn sepsis**
See Section I.C.16. ***f. Bacterial sepsis of*** *Newborn*

e. Methicillin resistant *Staphylococcus aureus* (MRSA) conditions

1) **Selection and sequencing of MRSA codes**

(a) Combination codes for MRSA infection
When a patient is diagnosed with an infection that is due to methicillin resistant *Staphylococcus aureus* (MRSA), and that infection has a combination code that includes the causal organism (e.g., sepsis, pneumonia) assign the appropriate combination code for the condition (e.g., code A41.Ø2, Sepsis due to Methicillin resistant *Staphylococcus aureus* or code J15.212, Pneumonia due to Methicillin resistant *Staphylococcus aureus*). Do not assign code B95.62, Methicillin resistant *Staphylococcus aureus* infection as the cause of diseases classified elsewhere, as an additional code because the combination code includes the type of infection and the MRSA organism. Do not assign a code from subcategory Z16.11, Resistance to penicillins, as an additional diagnosis.
See Section C.1. for instructions on coding and sequencing of sepsis and severe sepsis.

(b) Other codes for MRSA infection
When there is documentation of a current infection (e.g., wound infection, stitch abscess, urinary tract infection) due to MRSA, and that infection does not have a combination code that includes the causal organism, assign the appropriate code to identify the condition along with code B95.62, Methicillin resistant *Staphylococcus aureus* infection as the cause of diseases classified elsewhere for the MRSA infection. Do not assign a code from subcategory Z16.11, Resistance to penicillins.

(c) Methicillin susceptible *Staphylococcus aureus* (MSSA) and MRSA colonization
The condition or state of being colonized or carrying MSSA or MRSA is called colonization or carriage, while an individual person is described as being colonized or being a carrier. Colonization means that MSSA or MSRA is present on or in the body without necessarily causing illness. A positive MRSA colonization test might be documented by the provider as "MRSA screen positive" or "MRSA nasal swab positive".

Assign code Z22.322, Carrier or suspected carrier of Methicillin resistant *Staphylococcus aureus*, for patients documented as having MRSA colonization. Assign code Z22.321, Carrier or suspected carrier of Methicillin susceptible *Staphylococcus aureus*, for patient documented as having MSSA colonization. Colonization is not necessarily indicative of a disease process or as the cause of a specific

condition the patient may have unless documented as such by the provider.

(d) MRSA colonization and infection

If a patient is documented as having both MRSA colonization and infection during a hospital admission, code Z22.322, Carrier or suspected carrier of Methicillin resistant *Staphylococcus aureus*, and a code for the MRSA infection may both be assigned.

2. **Chapter 2: Neoplasms (CØØ-D49)**

General guidelines

Chapter 2 of the ICD-1Ø-CM contains the codes for most benign and all malignant neoplasms. Certain benign neoplasms, such as prostatic adenomas, may be found in the specific body system chapters. To properly code a neoplasm it is necessary to determine from the record if the neoplasm is benign, in-situ, malignant, or of uncertain histologic behavior. If malignant, any secondary (metastatic) sites should also be determined.

Primary malignant neoplasms overlapping site boundaries

A primary malignant neoplasm that overlaps two or more contiguous (next to each other) sites should be classified to the subcategory/code .8 ('overlapping lesion'), unless the combination is specifically indexed elsewhere. For multiple neoplasms of the same site that are not contiguous such as tumors in different quadrants of the same breast, codes for each site should be assigned.

Malignant neoplasm of ectopic tissue

Malignant neoplasms of ectopic tissue are to be coded to the site mentioned, e.g., ectopic pancreatic malignant neoplasms are coded to pancreas, unspecified (C25.9).

The neoplasm table in the Alphabetic Index should be referenced first. However, if the histological term is documented, that term should be referenced first, rather than going immediately to the Neoplasm Table, in order to determine which column in the Neoplasm Table is appropriate. For example, if the documentation indicates "adenoma," refer to the term in the Alphabetic Index to review the entries under this term and the instructional note to "see also neoplasm, by site, benign." The table provides the proper code based on the type of neoplasm and the site. It is important to select the proper column in the table that corresponds to the type of neoplasm. The Tabular List should then be referenced to verify that the correct code has been selected from the table and that a more specific site code does not exist.

See Section I.C.21. Factors influencing health status and contact with health services, Status, for information regarding Z15.Ø, codes for genetic susceptibility to cancer.

a. **Treatment directed at the malignancy**

If the treatment is directed at the malignancy, designate the malignancy as the principal diagnosis.

The only exception to this guideline is if a patient admission/encounter is solely for the administration of chemotherapy, immunotherapy or radiation therapy, assign the appropriate Z51.-- code as the first-listed or principal diagnosis, and the diagnosis or problem for which the service is being performed as a secondary diagnosis.

b. **Treatment of secondary site**

When a patient is admitted because of a primary neoplasm with metastasis and treatment is directed toward the secondary site only, the secondary neoplasm is designated as the principal diagnosis even though the primary malignancy is still present.

c. **Coding and sequencing of complications**

Coding and sequencing of complications associated with the malignancies or with the therapy thereof are subject to the following guidelines:

1) **Anemia associated with malignancy**

When admission/encounter is for management of an anemia associated with the malignancy, and the treatment is only for anemia, the appropriate code for the malignancy is sequenced as the principal or first-listed diagnosis followed by **the appropriate code for the anemia (such as** code D63.Ø, Anemia in neoplastic disease).

2) **Anemia associated with chemotherapy, immunotherapy and radiation therapy**

When the admission/encounter is for management of an anemia associated with an adverse effect **of the administration** of chemotherapy or immunotherapy and the only treatment is for the anemia, **the anemia code is sequenced first** followed by the appropriate codes for the neoplasm **and the adverse effect (T45.1X5, Adverse effect of antineoplastic and immunosuppressive drugs).**

When the admission/encounter is for management of an anemia associated with an adverse effect of radiotherapy, the anemia code should be sequenced first, followed by the appropriate neoplasm code and code Y84.2, Radiological procedure and radiotherapy as the cause of abnormal reaction of the patient, or of later complication, without mention of misadventure at the time of the procedure.

3) **Management of dehydration due to the malignancy**

When the admission/encounter is for management of dehydration due to the malignancy and only the dehydration is being treated (intravenous rehydration), the dehydration is sequenced first, followed by the code(s) for the malignancy.

4) **Treatment of a complication resulting from a surgical procedure**

When the admission/encounter is for treatment of a complication resulting from a surgical procedure, designate the complication as the principal or first-listed diagnosis if treatment is directed at resolving the complication.

d. **Primary malignancy previously excised**

When a primary malignancy has been previously excised or eradicated from its site and there is no further treatment directed to that site and there is no evidence of any existing primary malignancy, a code from category Z85, Personal history of malignant neoplasm, should be used to indicate the former site of the malignancy. Any mention of extension, invasion, or metastasis to another site is coded as a secondary malignant neoplasm to that site. The secondary site may be the principal or first-listed with the Z85 code used as a secondary code.

e. **Admissions/Encounters involving chemotherapy, immunotherapy and radiation therapy**

1) **Episode of care involves surgical removal of neoplasm**

When an episode of care involves the surgical removal of a neoplasm, primary or secondary site, followed by adjunct chemotherapy or radiation treatment during the same episode of care, the code for the neoplasm should be assigned as principal or first-listed diagnosis.

2) **Patient admission/encounter solely for administration of chemotherapy, immunotherapy and radiation therapy**

If a patient admission/encounter is solely for the administration of chemotherapy, immunotherapy or radiation therapy assign code Z51.Ø, Encounter for antineoplastic radiation therapy, or Z51.11, Encounter for antineoplastic chemotherapy, or Z51.12, Encounter for antineoplastic immunotherapy as the first-listed or principal diagnosis. If a patient receives more than one of these therapies during the same admission more than one of these codes may be assigned, in any sequence.

The malignancy for which the therapy is being administered should be assigned as a secondary diagnosis.

3) **Patient admitted for radiation therapy, chemotherapy or immunotherapy and develops complications**

When a patient is admitted for the purpose of radiotherapy, immunotherapy or chemotherapy and develops complications such as uncontrolled nausea and vomiting or dehydration, the principal or first-listed diagnosis is Z51.Ø, Encounter for antineoplastic radiation therapy, or Z51.11, Encounter for antineoplastic chemotherapy, or Z51.12,

Encounter for antineoplastic immunotherapy followed by any codes for the complications.

f. Admission/encounter to determine extent of malignancy
When the reason for admission/encounter is to determine the extent of the malignancy, or for a procedure such as paracentesis or thoracentesis, the primary malignancy or appropriate metastatic site is designated as the principal or first-listed diagnosis, even though chemotherapy or radiotherapy is administered.

g. Symptoms, signs, and abnormal findings listed in Chapter 18 associated with neoplasms
Symptoms, signs, and ill-defined conditions listed in Chapter 18 characteristic of, or associated with, an existing primary or secondary site malignancy cannot be used to replace the malignancy as principal or first-listed diagnosis, regardless of the number of admissions or encounters for treatment and care of the neoplasm.

See section I.C.21. Factors influencing health status and contact with health services, Encounter for prophylactic organ removal.

h. Admission/encounter for pain control/management
See Section I.C.6. for information on coding admission/encounter for pain control/management.

i. Malignancy in two or more noncontiguous sites
A patient may have more than one malignant tumor in the same organ. These tumors may represent different primaries or metastatic disease, depending on the site. Should the documentation be unclear, the provider should be queried as to the status of each tumor so that the correct codes can be assigned.

j. Disseminated malignant neoplasm, unspecified
Code C80.Ø, Disseminated malignant neoplasm, unspecified, is for use only in those cases where the patient has advanced metastatic disease and no known primary or secondary sites are specified. It should not be used in place of assigning codes for the primary site and all known secondary sites.

k. Malignant neoplasm without specification of site
Code C8Ø.1, Malignant (primary) neoplasm, unspecified, equates to Cancer, unspecified. This code should only be used when no determination can be made as to the primary site of a malignancy. This code should rarely be used in the inpatient setting.

l. Sequencing of neoplasm codes

1) Encounter for treatment of primary malignancy
If the reason for the encounter is for treatment of a primary malignancy, assign the malignancy as the principal/first-listed diagnosis. The primary site is to be sequenced first, followed by any metastatic sites.

2) Encounter for treatment of secondary malignancy
When an encounter is for a primary malignancy with metastasis and treatment is directed toward the metastatic (secondary) site(s) only, the metastatic site(s) is designated as the principal/first-listed diagnosis. The primary malignancy is coded as an additional code.

3) Malignant neoplasm in a pregnant patient
When a pregnant woman has a malignant neoplasm, a code from subcategory O9A.1-, Malignant neoplasm complicating pregnancy, childbirth, and the puerperium, should be sequenced first, followed by the appropriate code from Chapter 2 to indicate the type of neoplasm.

4) Encounter for complication associated with a neoplasm
When an encounter is for management of a complication associated with a neoplasm, such as dehydration, and the treatment is only for the complication, the complication is coded first, followed by the appropriate code(s) for the neoplasm.

The exception to this guideline is anemia. When the admission/encounter is for management of an anemia associated with the malignancy, and the treatment is only for anemia, the appropriate code for the malignancy is sequenced as the principal or first-listed diagnosis followed by code D63.Ø, Anemia in neoplastic disease.

5) Complication from surgical procedure for treatment of a neoplasm
When an encounter is for treatment of a complication resulting from a surgical procedure performed for the treatment of the neoplasm, designate the complication as the principal/first-listed diagnosis. See guideline regarding the coding of a current malignancy versus personal history to determine if the code for the neoplasm should also be assigned.

6) Pathologic fracture due to a neoplasm
When an encounter is for a pathological fracture due to a neoplasm, **and** the focus of treatment is the fracture, a code from subcategory M84.5, Pathological fracture in neoplastic disease, should be sequenced first, followed by the code for the neoplasm.

If the focus of treatment is the neoplasm with an associated pathological fracture, the neoplasm code should be sequenced first, followed by a code from M84.5 for the pathological fracture.

m. Current malignancy versus personal history of malignancy
When a primary malignancy has been excised but further treatment, such as an additional surgery for the malignancy, radiation therapy or chemotherapy is directed to that site, the primary malignancy code should be used until treatment is completed.

When a primary malignancy has been previously excised or eradicated from its site, there is no further treatment (of the malignancy) directed to that site, and there is no evidence of any existing primary malignancy, a code from category Z85, Personal history of malignant neoplasm, should be used to indicate the former site of the malignancy.

See Section I.C.21. Factors influencing health status and contact with health services, History (of)

n. Leukemia, multiple myeloma, and malignant plasma cell neoplasms in remission versus personal history
The categories for leukemia, and category C9Ø, Multiple myeloma and malignant plasma cell neoplasms, have codes **indicating whether or not the leukemia has achieved** remission. There are also codes Z85.6, Personal history of leukemia, and Z85.79, Personal history of other malignant neoplasms of lymphoid, hematopoietic and related tissues. If the documentation is unclear, as to whether the **leukemia has achieved** remission, the provider should be queried.

See Section I.C.21. Factors influencing health status and contact with health services, History (of)

o. Aftercare following surgery for neoplasm
See Section I.C.21. Factors influencing health status and contact with health services, Aftercare

p. Follow-up care for completed treatment of a malignancy
See Section I.C.21. Factors influencing health status and contact with health services, Follow-up

q. Prophylactic organ removal for prevention of malignancy
See Section I.C. 21, Factors influencing health status and contact with health services, Prophylactic organ removal

r. Malignant neoplasm associated with transplanted organ
A malignant neoplasm of a transplanted organ should be coded as a transplant complication. Assign first the appropriate code from category T86.-, Complications of transplanted organs and tissue, followed by code C8Ø.2, Malignant neoplasm associated with transplanted organ. Use an additional code for the specific malignancy.

3. Chapter 3: Disease of the Blood and Blood-forming Organs and Certain Disorders Involving the Immune Mechanism (D5Ø-D89)
Reserved for future guideline expansion

4. Chapter 4: Endocrine, Nutritional, and Metabolic Diseases (EØØ-E89)

a. Diabetes mellitus

The diabetes mellitus codes are combination codes that include the type of diabetes mellitus, the body system affected, and the complications affecting that body system. As many codes within a particular category as are necessary to describe all of the complications of the disease may be used. They should be sequenced based on the reason for a particular encounter. Assign as many codes from categories EØ8 – E13 as needed to identify all of the associated conditions that the patient has.

1) Type of diabetes

The age of a patient is not the sole determining factor, though most type 1 diabetics develop the condition before reaching puberty. For this reason type 1 diabetes mellitus is also referred to as juvenile diabetes.

2) Type of diabetes mellitus not documented

If the type of diabetes mellitus is not documented in the medical record the default is E11.-, Type 2 diabetes mellitus.

3) Diabetes mellitus and the use of insulin

If the documentation in a medical record does not indicate the type of diabetes but does indicate that the patient uses insulin, code E11, Type 2 diabetes mellitus, should be assigned. Code Z79.4, Long-term (current) use of insulin, should also be assigned to indicate that the patient uses insulin. Code Z79.4 should not be assigned if insulin is given temporarily to bring a type 2 patient's blood sugar under control during an encounter.

4) Diabetes mellitus in pregnancy and gestational diabetes

See Section I.C.15. Diabetes mellitus in pregnancy.

See Section I.C.15. Gestational (pregnancy induced) diabetes

5) Complications due to insulin pump malfunction

(a) Underdose of insulin due to insulin pump failure

An underdose of insulin due to an insulin pump failure should be assigned to a code from subcategory T85.6, Mechanical complication of other specified internal and external prosthetic devices, implants and grafts, that specifies the type of pump malfunction, as the principal or first-listed code, followed by code T38.3x6-, Underdosing of insulin and oral hypoglycemic [antidiabetic] drugs. Additional codes for the type of diabetes mellitus and any associated complications due to the underdosing should also be assigned.

(b) Overdose of insulin due to insulin pump failure

The principal or first-listed code for an encounter due to an insulin pump malfunction resulting in an overdose of insulin, should also be T85.6-, Mechanical complication of other specified internal and external prosthetic devices, implants and grafts, followed by code T38.3X1-, Poisoning by insulin and oral hypoglycemic [antidiabetic] drugs, accidental (unintentional).

6) Secondary diabetes mellitus

Codes under categories EØ8, Diabetes mellitus due to underlying condition, and EØ9, Drug or chemical induced diabetes mellitus, identify complications/manifestations associated with secondary diabetes mellitus. Secondary diabetes is always caused by another condition or event (e.g., cystic fibrosis, malignant neoplasm of pancreas, pancreatectomy, adverse effect of drug, or poisoning).

(a) Secondary diabetes mellitus and the use of insulin

For patients who routinely use insulin, code Z79.4, Long-term (current) use of insulin, should also be assigned. Code Z79.4 should not be assigned if insulin is given temporarily to bring a patient's blood sugar under control during an encounter.

(b) Assigning and sequencing secondary diabetes codes and its causes

The sequencing of the secondary diabetes codes in relationship to codes for the cause of the diabetes is based on the Tabular List instructions for categories EØ8 and EØ9. For example, for category EØ8, Diabetes mellitus due to underlying condition, code first the underlying condition; for category EØ9, Drug or chemical induced diabetes mellitus, code first the drug or chemical (T36-T65).

(i) Secondary diabetes mellitus due to pancreatectomy

For postpancreatectomy diabetes mellitus (lack of insulin due to the surgical removal of all or part of the pancreas), assign code E89.1, Postprocedural hypoinsulinemia. Assign a code from category E13 and a code from subcategory Z9Ø.41-, Acquired absence of pancreas, as additional codes.

(ii) Secondary diabetes due to drugs

Secondary diabetes may be caused by an adverse effect of correctly administered medications, poisoning or **sequela** of poisoning.

See section I.C.19.e for coding of adverse effects and poisoning, and section I.C.2Ø for external cause code reporting.

5. Chapter 5: Mental and behavioral disorders (FØ1 – F99)

a. Pain disorders related to psychological factors

Assign code F45.41, for pain that is exclusively **related to psychological disorders. As indicated by the Excludes 1 note under category G89, a code from category G89 should not be assigned with code F45.41**

Code F45.42, Pain disorders with related psychological factors, should be used with a code from category G89, Pain, not elsewhere classified, if there is documentation of a psychological component for a patient with acute or chronic pain.

See Section I.C.6. Pain

b. Mental and behavioral disorders due to psychoactive substance use

1) In remission

Selection of codes for "in remission" for categories F1Ø-F19, Mental and behavioral disorders due to psychoactive substance use (categories F1Ø-F19 with -.21) requires the provider's clinical judgment. The appropriate codes for "in remission" are assigned only on the basis of provider documentation (as defined in the Official Guidelines for Coding and Reporting).

2) Psychoactive substance use, abuse and dependence

When the provider documentation refers to use, abuse and dependence of the same substance (e.g. alcohol, opioid, cannabis, etc.), only one code should be assigned to identify the pattern of use based on the following hierarchy:

- If both use and abuse are documented, assign only the code for abuse
- If both abuse and dependence are documented, assign only the code for dependence
- If use, abuse and dependence are all documented, assign only the code for dependence
- If both use and dependence are documented, assign only the code for dependence.

3) Psychoactive substance use

As with all other diagnoses, the codes for psychoactive substance use (F1Ø.9-, F11.9-, F12.9-, F13.9-, F14.9-, F15.9-, F16.9-) should only be assigned based on provider documentation and when they meet the definition of a reportable diagnosis (see Section III, Reporting Additional Diagnoses). The codes are to be used only when the psychoactive substance use is associated with a mental or behavioral disorder, and such a relationship is documented by the provider.

6. Chapter 6: Diseases of Nervous System (GØØ-G99)

a. Dominant/nondominant side

Codes from category G81, Hemiplegia and hemiparesis, and subcategories, G83.1, Monoplegia of lower limb, G83.2, Monoplegia of upper limb, and G83.3, Monoplegia, unspecified, identify whether the dominant or nondominant side is affected. Should the affected side be documented, but not specified as dominant or nondominant, and the classification system does not indicate a default, code selection is as follows:

- For ambidextrous patients, the default should be dominant.
- If the left side is affected, the default is non-dominant.
- If the right side is affected, the default is dominant.

b. Pain - Category G89

1) General coding information

Codes in category G89, Pain, not elsewhere classified, may be used in conjunction with codes from other categories and chapters to provide more detail about acute or chronic pain and neoplasm-related pain, unless otherwise indicated below.

If the pain is not specified as acute or chronic, post-thoracotomy, postprocedural, or neoplasm-related, do not assign codes from category G89.

A code from category G89 should not be assigned if the underlying (definitive) diagnosis is known, unless the reason for the encounter is pain control/ management and not management of the underlying condition.

When an admission or encounter is for a procedure aimed at treating the underlying condition (e.g., spinal fusion, kyphoplasty), a code for the underlying condition (e.g., vertebral fracture, spinal stenosis) should be assigned as the principal diagnosis. No code from category G89 should be assigned.

(a) Category G89 codes as principal or first-listed diagnosis

Category G89 codes are acceptable as principal diagnosis or the first-listed code:

- When pain control or pain management is the reason for the admission/encounter (e.g., a patient with displaced intervertebral disc, nerve impingement and severe back pain presents for injection of steroid into the spinal canal). The underlying cause of the pain should be reported as an additional diagnosis, if known.
- When a patient is admitted for the insertion of a neurostimulator for pain control, assign the appropriate pain code as the principal or first-listed diagnosis. When an admission or encounter is for a procedure aimed at treating the underlying condition and a neurostimulator is inserted for pain control during the same admission/encounter, a code for the underlying condition should be assigned as the principal diagnosis and the appropriate pain code should be assigned as a secondary diagnosis.

(b) Use of category G89 codes in conjunction with site specific pain codes

(i) Assigning category G89 and site-specific pain codes

Codes from category G89 may be used in conjunction with codes that identify the site of pain (including codes from chapter 18) if the category G89 code provides additional information. For example, if the code describes the site of the pain, but does not fully describe whether the pain is acute or chronic, then both codes should be assigned.

(ii) Sequencing of category G89 codes with site-specific pain codes

The sequencing of category G89 codes with site-specific pain codes (including chapter 18 codes), is dependent on the circumstances of the encounter/admission as follows:

- If the encounter is for pain control or pain management, assign the code from category G89 followed by the code identifying the specific site of pain (e.g., encounter for pain management for acute neck pain from trauma is assigned code G89.11, Acute pain due to trauma, followed by code M54.2, Cervicalgia, to identify the site of pain).
- If the encounter is for any other reason except pain control or pain management, and a related definitive diagnosis has not been established (confirmed) by the provider, assign the code for the specific site of pain first, followed by the appropriate code from category G89.

2) Pain due to devices, implants and grafts

See Section I.C.19. Pain due to medical devices

3) Postoperative pain

The provider's documentation should be used to guide the coding of postoperative pain, as well as *Section III. Reporting Additional Diagnoses* and *Section IV. Diagnostic Coding and Reporting in the Outpatient Setting.*

The default for post-thoracotomy and other postoperative pain not specified as acute or chronic is the code for the acute form.

Routine or expected postoperative pain immediately after surgery should not be coded.

(a) Postoperative pain not associated with specific postoperative complication

Postoperative pain not associated with a specific postoperative complication is assigned to the appropriate postoperative pain code in category G89.

(b) Postoperative pain associated with specific postoperative complication

Postoperative pain associated with a specific postoperative complication (such as painful wire sutures) is assigned to the appropriate code(s) found in Chapter 19, Injury, poisoning, and certain other consequences of external causes. If appropriate, use additional code(s) from category G89 to identify acute or chronic pain (G89.18 or G89.28).

4) Chronic pain

Chronic pain is classified to subcategory G89.2. There is no time frame defining when pain becomes chronic pain. The provider's documentation should be used to guide use of these codes.

5) Neoplasm related pain

Code G89.3 is assigned to pain documented as being related, associated or due to cancer, primary or secondary malignancy, or tumor. This code is assigned regardless of whether the pain is acute or chronic.

This code may be assigned as the principal or first-listed code when the stated reason for the admission/encounter is documented as pain control/pain management. The underlying neoplasm should be reported as an additional diagnosis.

When the reason for the admission/encounter is management of the neoplasm and the pain associated with the neoplasm is also documented, code G89.3 may be assigned as an additional diagnosis. It is not necessary to assign an additional code for the site of the pain.

See Section I.C.2 for instructions on the sequencing of neoplasms for all other stated reasons for the admission/encounter (except for pain control/pain management).

6) Chronic pain syndrome

Central pain syndrome (G89.Ø) and chronic pain syndrome (G89.4) are different than the term "chronic pain," and therefore codes should only be used when the provider has specifically documented this condition.

See Section I.C.5. Pain disorders related to psychological factors

7. **Chapter 7: Diseases of Eye and Adnexa (H00-H59)**
   a. **Glaucoma**
      1) **Assigning glaucoma codes**
         Assign as many codes from category H40, Glaucoma, as needed to identify the type of glaucoma, the affected eye, and the glaucoma stage.
      2) **Bilateral glaucoma with same type and stage**
         When a patient has bilateral glaucoma and both eyes are documented as being the same type and stage, and there is a code for bilateral glaucoma, report only the code for the type of glaucoma, bilateral, with the seventh character for the stage.

         When a patient has bilateral glaucoma and both eyes are documented as being the same type and stage, and the classification does not provide a code for bilateral glaucoma (i.e. subcategories H40.10, H40.11 and H40.20) report only one code for the type of glaucoma with the appropriate seventh character for the stage.
      3) **Bilateral glaucoma stage with different types or stages**
         When a patient has bilateral glaucoma and each eye is documented as having a different type or stage, and the classification distinguishes laterality, assign the appropriate code for each eye rather than the code for bilateral glaucoma.

         When a patient has bilateral glaucoma and each eye is documented as having a different type, and the classification does not distinguish laterality (i.e. subcategories H40.10, H40.11 and H40.20), assign one code for each type of glaucoma with the appropriate seventh character for the stage.

         When a patient has bilateral glaucoma and each eye is documented as having the same type, but different stage, and the classification does not distinguish laterality (i.e. subcategories H40.10, H40.11 and H40.20), assign a code for the type of glaucoma for each eye with the seventh character for the specific glaucoma stage documented for each eye.
      4) **Patient admitted with glaucoma and stage evolves during the admission**
         If a patient is admitted with glaucoma and the stage progresses during the admission, assign the code for highest stage documented.
      5) **Indeterminate stage glaucoma**
         Assignment of the seventh character "4" for "indeterminate stage" should be based on the clinical documentation. The seventh character "4" is used for glaucomas whose stage cannot be clinically determined. This seventh character should not be confused with the seventh character "0", unspecified, which should be assigned when there is no documentation regarding the stage of the glaucoma.
8. **Chapter 8: Diseases of Ear and Mastoid Process (H60-H95)**
   Reserved for future guideline expansion
9. **Chapter 9: Diseases of Circulatory System (I00-I99)**
   a. **Hypertension**
      1) **Hypertension with heart disease**
         Heart conditions classified to I50.- or I51.4-I51.9, are assigned to, a code from category I11, Hypertensive heart disease, when a causal relationship is stated (due to hypertension) or implied (hypertensive). Use an additional code from category I50, Heart failure, to identify the type of heart failure in those patients with heart failure.

         The same heart conditions (I50.-, I51.4-I51.9) with hypertension, but without a stated causal relationship, are coded separately. Sequence according to the circumstances of the admission/encounter.
      2) **Hypertensive chronic kidney disease**
         Assign codes from category I12, Hypertensive chronic kidney disease, when both hypertension and a condition classifiable to category N18, Chronic kidney disease (CKD), are present. Unlike hypertension with heart disease, ICD-10-CM presumes a cause-and-effect relationship and classifies chronic kidney disease with hypertension as hypertensive chronic kidney disease.

         The appropriate code from category N18 should be used as a secondary code with a code from category I12 to identify the stage of chronic kidney disease.

         See Section I.C.14. Chronic kidney disease.

         If a patient has hypertensive chronic kidney disease and acute renal failure, an additional code for the acute renal failure is required.
      3) **Hypertensive heart and chronic kidney disease**
         Assign codes from combination category I13, Hypertensive heart and chronic kidney disease, when both hypertensive kidney disease and hypertensive heart disease are stated in the diagnosis. Assume a relationship between the hypertension and the chronic kidney disease, whether or not the condition is so designated. If heart failure is present, assign an additional code from category I50 to identify the type of heart failure.

         The appropriate code from category N18, Chronic kidney disease, should be used as a secondary code with a code from category I13 to identify the stage of chronic kidney disease.

         See Section I.C.14. Chronic kidney disease.

         The codes in category I13, Hypertensive heart and chronic kidney disease, are combination codes that include hypertension, heart disease and chronic kidney disease. The Includes note at I13 specifies that the conditions included at I11 and I12 are included together in I13. If a patient has hypertension, heart disease and chronic kidney disease then a code from I13 should be used, not individual codes for hypertension, heart disease and chronic kidney disease, or codes from I11 or I12.

         For patients with both acute renal failure and chronic kidney disease an additional code for acute renal failure is required.
      4) **Hypertensive cerebrovascular disease**
         For hypertensive cerebrovascular disease, first assign the appropriate code from categories I60-I69, followed by the appropriate hypertension code.
      5) **Hypertensive retinopathy**
         Subcategory H35.0, Background retinopathy and retinal vascular changes, should be used with **a** code **from category** I10 – **I15, Hypertensive disease** to include the systemic hypertension. The sequencing is based on the reason for the encounter.
      6) **Hypertension, secondary**
         Secondary hypertension is due to an underlying condition. Two codes are required: one to identify the underlying etiology and one from category I15 to identify the hypertension. Sequencing of codes is determined by the reason for admission/encounter.
      7) **Hypertension, transient**
         Assign code R03.0, Elevated blood pressure reading without diagnosis of hypertension, unless patient has an established diagnosis of hypertension. Assign code O13.-, Gestational [pregnancy-induced] hypertension without significant proteinuria, or O14.-, Pre-eclampsia, for transient hypertension of pregnancy.
      8) **Hypertension, controlled**
         This diagnostic statement usually refers to an existing state of hypertension under control by therapy. Assign the

appropriate code from categories I10-I15, Hypertensive diseases.

9) **Hypertension, uncontrolled**
Uncontrolled hypertension may refer to untreated hypertension or hypertension not responding to current therapeutic regimen. In either case, assign the appropriate code from categories I10-I15, Hypertensive diseases.

b. **Atherosclerotic coronary artery disease and angina**
ICD-10-CM has combination codes for atherosclerotic heart disease with angina pectoris. The subcategories for these codes are I25.11, Atherosclerotic heart disease of native coronary artery with angina pectoris and I25.7, Atherosclerosis of coronary artery bypass graft(s) and coronary artery of transplanted heart with angina pectoris.

When using one of these combination codes it is not necessary to use an additional code for angina pectoris. A causal relationship can be assumed in a patient with both atherosclerosis and angina pectoris, unless the documentation indicates the angina is due to something other than the atherosclerosis.

If a patient with coronary artery disease is admitted due to an acute myocardial infarction (AMI), the AMI should be sequenced before the coronary artery disease.

See Section I.C.9. Acute myocardial infarction (AMI)

c. **Intraoperative and postprocedural cerebrovascular accident**
Medical record documentation should clearly specify the cause-and-effect relationship between the medical intervention and the cerebrovascular accident in order to assign a code for intraoperative or postprocedural cerebrovascular accident.

Proper code assignment depends on whether it was an infarction or hemorrhage and whether it occurred intraoperatively or postoperatively. If it was a cerebral hemorrhage, code assignment depends on the type of procedure performed.

d. **Sequelae of cerebrovascular disease**

1) **Category I69, sequelae of cerebrovascular disease**
Category I69 is used to indicate conditions classifiable to categories I60-I67 as the causes of **sequela** (neurologic deficits), themselves classified elsewhere. These "late effects" include neurologic deficits that persist after initial onset of conditions classifiable to categories I60-I67. The neurologic deficits caused by cerebrovascular disease may be present from the onset or may arise at any time after the onset of the condition classifiable to categories I60-I67.

2) **Codes from category I69 with codes from I60-I67**
Codes from category I69 may be assigned on a health care record with codes from I60-I67, if the patient has a current cerebrovascular disease and deficits from an old cerebrovascular disease.

3) **Code Z86.73**
Assign code Z86.73, Personal history of transient ischemic attack (TIA), and cerebral infarction without residual deficits (and not a code from category I69) as an additional code for history of cerebrovascular disease when no neurologic deficits are present.

e. **Acute myocardial infarction (AMI)**

1) **ST elevation myocardial infarction (STEMI) and non ST elevation myocardial infarction (NSTEMI)**
The ICD-10-CM codes for acute myocardial infarction (AMI) identify the site, such as anterolateral wall or true posterior wall. Subcategories I21.0-I21.2 and code I21.3 are used for ST elevation myocardial infarction (STEMI). Code I21.4, Non-ST elevation (NSTEMI) myocardial infarction, is used for non ST elevation myocardial infarction (NSTEMI) and nontransmural MIs.

If NSTEMI evolves to STEMI, assign the STEMI code. If STEMI converts to NSTEMI due to thrombolytic therapy, it is still coded as STEMI.

For encounters occurring while the myocardial infarction is equal to, or less than, four weeks old, including transfers to another acute setting or a postacute setting, and the patient requires continued care for the myocardial infarction, codes from category I21 may continue to be reported. For encounters after the 4 week time frame and the patient **is still receiving** care related to the myocardial infarction, the appropriate aftercare code should be assigned, rather than a code from category I21. **For old or healed myocardial infarctions not requiring further care,** code I25.2, Old myocardial infarction, may be assigned.

2) **Acute myocardial infarction, unspecified**
Code I21.3, ST elevation (STEMI) myocardial infarction of unspecified site, is the default for the unspecified term acute myocardial infarction. If only STEMI or transmural MI without the site is documented, query the provider as to the site, or assign code I21.3.

3) **AMI documented as nontransmural or subendocardial but site provided**
If an AMI is documented as nontransmural or subendocardial, but the site is provided, it is still coded as a subendocardial AMI.

See Section I.C.21.3 for information on coding status post administration of tPA in a different facility within the last 24 hrs.

4) **Subsequent acute myocardial infarction**
A code from category I22, Subsequent ST elevation (STEMI) and non ST elevation (NSTEMI) myocardial infarction, is to be used when a patient who has suffered an AMI has a new AMI within the 4 week time frame of the initial AMI. A code from category I22 must be used in conjunction with a code from category I21. The sequencing of the I22 and I21 codes depends on the circumstances of the encounter.

10. **Chapter 10: Diseases of *the* Respiratory System (J00-J99)**

a. **Chronic Obstructive Pulmonary Disease [COPD] and Asthma**

1) **Acute exacerbation of chronic obstructive bronchitis and asthma**
The codes in categories J44 and J45 distinguish between uncomplicated cases and those in acute exacerbation. An acute exacerbation is a worsening or a decompensation of a chronic condition. An acute exacerbation is not equivalent to an infection superimposed on a chronic condition, though an exacerbation may be triggered by an infection.

b. **Acute Respiratory Failure**

1) **Acute respiratory failure as principal diagnosis**
A code from subcategory J96.0, Acute respiratory failure, or subcategory J96.2, Acute and chronic respiratory failure, may be assigned as a principal diagnosis when it is the condition established after study to be chiefly responsible for occasioning the admission to the hospital, and the selection is supported by the Alphabetic Index and Tabular List. However, chapter-specific coding guidelines (such as obstetrics, poisoning, HIV, newborn) that provide sequencing direction take precedence.

2) **Acute respiratory failure as secondary diagnosis**
Respiratory failure may be listed as a secondary diagnosis if it occurs after admission, or if it is present on admission, but does not meet the definition of principal diagnosis.

3) **Sequencing of acute respiratory failure and another acute condition**
When a patient is admitted with respiratory failure and another acute condition, (e.g., myocardial infarction, cerebrovascular accident, aspiration pneumonia), the principal diagnosis will not be the same in every situation. This applies whether the other acute condition is a respiratory or nonrespiratory condition. Selection of the principal diagnosis will be dependent on the circumstances of admission. If both the respiratory failure and the other acute condition are equally responsible for occasioning the admission to the hospital, and there are no chapter-specific sequencing rules, the guideline regarding two or more

diagnoses that equally meet the definition for principal diagnosis (Section II, C.) may be applied in these situations.

If the documentation is not clear as to whether acute respiratory failure and another condition are equally responsible for occasioning the admission, query the provider for clarification.

c. **Influenza due to certain identified influenza viruses**

Code only confirmed cases of influenza **due to certain identified influenza viruses (category JØ9).** This is an exception to the hospital inpatient guideline Section II, H. (Uncertain Diagnosis).

In this context, "confirmation" does not require documentation of positive laboratory testing specific for avian or **other** novel influenza **A**. However, coding should be based on the provider's diagnostic statement that the patient has avian influenza**, or other novel influenza A.**

If the provider records "suspected" or "possible" or "probable" avian influenza," the appropriate influenza code from category J11, Influenza due to **unidentified** influenza virus, should be assigned. A code from category JØ9, Influenza due to certain identified influenza viruses, should not be assigned.

d. **Ventilator associated pneumonia**

1) **Documentation of ventilator associated pneumonia**

As with all procedural or postprocedural complications, code assignment is based on the provider's documentation of the relationship between the condition and the procedure.

Code J95.851, Ventilator associated pneumonia, should be assigned only when the provider has documented ventilator associated pneumonia (VAP). An additional code to identify the organism (e.g., Pseudomonas aeruginosa, code B96.5) should also be assigned. Do not assign an additional code from categories J12-J18 to identify the type of pneumonia.

Code J95.851 should not be assigned for cases where the patient has pneumonia and is on a mechanical ventilator **and** the provider has not specifically stated that the pneumonia is ventilator-associated pneumonia. If the documentation is unclear as to whether the patient has a pneumonia that is a complication attributable to the mechanical ventilator, query the provider.

2) **Ventilator associated pneumonia develops after admission**

A patient may be admitted with one type of pneumonia (e.g., code J13, Pneumonia due to Streptococcus pneu- monia) and subsequently develop VAP. In this instance, the principal diagnosis would be the appro- priate code from categories J12-J18 for the pneumonia diagnosed at the time of admission. Code J95.851, Ventilator assoc- iated pneumonia, would be assigned as an additional diagnosis when the provider has also documented the presence of ventilator associated pneumonia.

11. **Chapter 11: Diseases of *the* Digestive System (KØØ-K95)**

Reserved for future guideline expansion

12. **Chapter 12: Diseases of *the* Skin and Subcutaneous Tissue (LØØ-L99)**

a. **Pressure ulcer stage codes**

1) **Pressure ulcer stages**

Codes from category L89, Pressure ulcer, are combination codes that identify the site of the pressure ulcer as well as the stage of the ulcer.

The ICD-1Ø-CM classifies pressure ulcer stages based on severity, which is designated by stages 1-4, unspecified stage and unstageable.

Assign as many codes from category L89 as needed to identify all the pressure ulcers the patient has, if applicable.

2) **Unstageable pressure ulcers**

Assignment of the code for unstageable pressure ulcer (L89.--Ø) should be based on the clinical documentation. These codes are used for pressure ulcers whose stage cannot be clinically determined (e.g., the ulcer is covered by eschar or has been treated with a skin or muscle graft) and pressure ulcers that are documented as deep tissue injury but not documented as due to trauma. This code should not be confused with the codes for unspecified stage (L89.--9). When there is no documentation regarding the stage of the pressure ulcer, assign the appropriate code for unspecified stage (L89.--9).

3) **Documented pressure ulcer stage**

Assignment of the pressure ulcer stage code should be guided by clinical documentation of the stage or documentation of the terms found in the Alphabetic Index. For clinical terms describing the stage that are not found in the Alphabetic Index, and there is no documentation of the stage, the provider should be queried.

4) **Patients admitted with pressure ulcers documented as healed**

No code is assigned if the documentation states that the pressure ulcer is completely healed.

5) **Patients admitted with pressure ulcers documented as healing**

Pressure ulcers described as healing should be assigned the appropriate pressure ulcer stage code based on the documentation in the medical record. If the documentation does not provide information about the stage of the healing pressure ulcer, assign the appropriate code for unspecified stage.

If the documentation is unclear as to whether the patient has a current (new) pressure ulcer or if the patient is being treated for a healing pressure ulcer, query the provider.

6) **Patient admitted with pressure ulcer evolving into another stage during the admission**

If a patient is admitted with a pressure ulcer at one stage and it progresses to a higher stage, assign the code for the highest stage reported for that site.

13. **Chapter 13: Diseases of the Musculoskeletal System and Connective Tissue (MØØ-M99)**

a. **Site and laterality**

Most of the codes within Chapter 13 have site and laterality designations. The site represents the bone, joint or the muscle involved. For some conditions where more than one bone, joint or muscle is usually involved, such as osteoarthritis, there is a "multiple sites" code available. For categories where no multiple site code is provided and more than one bone, joint or muscle is involved, multiple codes should be used to indicate the different sites involved.

1) **Bone versus joint**

For certain conditions, the bone may be affected at the upper or lower end, (e.g., avascular necrosis of bone, M87, Osteoporosis, M8Ø, M81). Though the portion of the bone affected may be at the joint, the site designation will be the bone, not the joint.

b. **Acute traumatic versus chronic or recurrent musculoskeletal conditions**

Many musculoskeletal conditions are a result of previous injury or trauma to a site, or are recurrent conditions. Bone, joint or muscle conditions that are the result of a healed injury are usually found in chapter 13. Recurrent bone, joint or muscle conditions are also usually found in chapter 13. Any current, acute injury should be coded to the appropriate injury code from chapter 19. Chronic or recurrent conditions should generally be coded with a code from chapter 13. If it is difficult to determine from the documentation in the record which code is best to describe a condition, query the provider.

c. **Coding of Pathologic Fractures**

7th character A is for use as long as the patient is receiving active treatment for the fracture. Examples of active treatment are: surgical treatment, emergency department encounter, evaluation and treatment by a new physician. 7th character, D is to be used for encounters after the patient has completed active treatment.

The other 7th characters, listed under each subcategory in the Tabular List, are to be used for subsequent encounters for treatment of problems associated with the healing, such as malunions, nonunions, and sequelae.

Care for complications of surgical treatment for fracture repairs during the healing or recovery phase should be coded with the appropriate complication codes.

See Section I.C.19. Coding of traumatic fractures.

d. Osteoporosis

Osteoporosis is a systemic condition, meaning that all bones of the musculoskeletal system are affected. Therefore, site is not a component of the codes under category M81, Osteoporosis without current pathological fracture. The site codes under category M8Ø, Osteoporosis with current pathological fracture, identify the site of the fracture, not the osteoporosis.

1) Osteoporosis without pathological fracture

Category M81, Osteoporosis without current pathological fracture, is for use for patients with osteoporosis who do not currently have a pathologic fracture due to the osteoporosis, even if they have had a fracture in the past. For patients with a history of osteoporosis fractures, status code Z87.31Ø, Personal history of (healed) osteoporosis fracture, should follow the code from M81.

2) Osteoporosis with current pathological fracture

Category M8Ø, Osteoporosis with current pathological fracture, is for patients who have a current pathologic fracture at the time of an encounter. The codes under M8Ø identify the site of the fracture. A code from category M8Ø, not a traumatic fracture code, should be used for any patient with known osteoporosis who suffers a fracture, even if the patient had a minor fall or trauma, if that fall or trauma would not usually break a normal, healthy bone.

14. Chapter 14: Diseases of Genitourinary System (NØØ-N99)

a. Chronic kidney disease

1) Stages of chronic kidney disease (CKD)

The ICD-1Ø-CM classifies CKD based on severity. The severity of CKD is designated by stages 1-5. Stage 2, code N18.2, equates to mild CKD; stage 3, code N18.3, equates to moderate CKD; and stage 4, code N18.4, equates to severe CKD. Code N18.6, End stage renal disease (ESRD), is assigned when the provider has documented end-stage-renal disease (ESRD).

If both a stage of CKD and ESRD are documented, assign code N18.6 only.

2) Chronic kidney disease and kidney transplant status

Patients who have undergone kidney transplant may still have some form of chronic kidney disease (CKD) because the kidney transplant may not fully restore kidney function. Therefore, the presence of CKD alone does not constitute a transplant complication. Assign the appropriate N18 code for the patient's stage of CKD and code Z94.Ø, Kidney transplant status. If a transplant complication such as failure or rejection or other transplant complication is documented, see section I.C.19.g for information on coding complications of a kidney transplant. If the documentation is unclear as to whether the patient has a complication of the transplant, query the provider.

3) Chronic kidney disease with other conditions

Patients with CKD may also suffer from other serious conditions, most commonly diabetes mellitus and hypertension. The sequencing of the CKD code in relationship to codes for other contributing conditions is based on the conventions in the Tabular List.

See I.C.9. Hypertensive chronic kidney disease.

See I.C.19. Chronic kidney disease and kidney transplant complications.

15. Chapter 15: Pregnancy, Childbirth, and the Puerperium (OØØ-O9A)

a. General Rules for Obstetric Cases

1) Codes from chapter 15 and sequencing priority

Obstetric cases require codes from chapter 15, codes in the range OØØ-O9A, Pregnancy, Childbirth, and the Puerperium. Chapter 15 codes have sequencing priority over codes from other chapters. Additional codes from other chapters may be used in conjunction with chapter 15 codes to further specify conditions. Should the provider document that the pregnancy is incidental to the encounter, then code Z33.1, Pregnant state, incidental, should be used in place of any chapter 15 codes. It is the provider's responsibility to state that the condition being treated is not affecting the pregnancy.

2) Chapter 15 codes used only on the maternal record

Chapter 15 codes are to be used only on the maternal record, never on the record of the newborn.

3) Final character for trimester

The majority of codes in Chapter 15 have a final character indicating the trimester of pregnancy. The timeframes for the trimesters are indicated at the beginning of the chapter. If trimester is not a component of a code it is because the condition always occurs in a specific trimester, or the concept of trimester of pregnancy is not applicable. Certain codes have characters for only certain trimesters because the condition does not occur in all trimesters, but it may occur in more than just one.

Assignment of the final character for trimester should be based on the provider's documentation of the trimester (or number of weeks) for the current admission/encounter. This applies to the assignment of trimester for pre-existing conditions as well as those that develop during or are due to the pregnancy. The provider's documentation of the number of weeks may be used to assign the appropriate code identifying the trimester.

Whenever delivery occurs during the current admission, and there is an "in childbirth" option for the obstetric complication being coded, the "in childbirth" code should be assigned.

4) Selection of trimester for inpatient admissions that encompass more than one trimesters

In instances when a patient is admitted to a hospital for complications of pregnancy during one trimester and remains in the hospital into a subsequent trimester, the trimester character for the antepartum complication code should be assigned on the basis of the trimester when the complication developed, not the trimester of the discharge. If the condition developed prior to the current admission/encounter or represents a pre-existing condition, the trimester character for the trimester at the time of the admission/encounter should be assigned.

5) Unspecified trimester

Each category that includes codes for trimester has a code for "unspecified trimester." The "unspecified trimester" code should rarely be used, such as when the documentation in the record is insufficient to determine the trimester and it is not possible to obtain clarification.

6) 7th character for fetus identification

Where applicable, a 7th character is to be assigned for certain categories (O31, O32, O33.3 - O33.6, O35, O36, O4Ø, O41, O6Ø.1, O6Ø.2, O64, and O69) to identify the fetus for which the complication code applies.

Assign 7th character "Ø":

- For single gestations
- When the documentation in the record is insufficient to determine the fetus affected and it is not possible to obtain clarification.

- When it is not possible to clinically determine which fetus is affected.

b. Selection of OB principal or first-listed diagnosis

1) Routine outpatient prenatal visits

For routine outpatient prenatal visits when no complications are present, a code from category Z34, Encounter for supervision of normal pregnancy, should be used as the first-listed diagnosis. These codes should not be used in conjunction with chapter 15 codes.

2) Prenatal outpatient visits for high-risk patients

For routine prenatal outpatient visits for patients with high-risk pregnancies, a code from category O09, Supervision of high-risk pregnancy, should be used as the first-listed diagnosis. Secondary chapter 15 codes may be used in conjunction with these codes if appropriate.

3) Episodes when no delivery occurs

In episodes when no delivery occurs, the principal diagnosis should correspond to the principal complication of the pregnancy which necessitated the encounter. Should more than one complication exist, all of which are treated or monitored, any of the complications codes may be sequenced first.

4) When a delivery occurs

When a delivery occurs, the principal diagnosis should correspond to the main circumstances or complication of the delivery. In cases of cesarean delivery, the selection of the principal diagnosis should be the condition established after study that was responsible for the patient's admission. If the patient was admitted with a condition that resulted in the performance of a cesarean procedure, that condition should be selected as the principal diagnosis. If the reason for the admission/encounter was unrelated to the condition resulting in the cesarean delivery, the condition related to the reason for the admission/encounter should be selected as the principal diagnosis.

5) Outcome of delivery

A code from category Z37, Outcome of delivery, should be included on every maternal record when a delivery has occurred. These codes are not to be used on subsequent records or on the newborn record.

c. Pre-existing conditions versus conditions due to the pregnancy

Certain categories in Chapter 15 distinguish between conditions of the mother that existed prior to pregnancy (pre-existing) and those that are a direct result of pregnancy. When assigning codes from Chapter 15, it is important to assess if a condition was pre-existing prior to pregnancy or developed during or due to the pregnancy in order to assign the correct code.

Categories that do not distinguish between pre-existing and pregnancy-related conditions may be used for either. It is acceptable to use codes specifically for the puerperium with codes complicating pregnancy and childbirth if a condition arises postpartum during the delivery encounter.

d. Pre-existing hypertension in pregnancy

Category O1Ø, Pre-existing hypertension complicating pregnancy, childbirth and the puerperium, includes codes for hypertensive heart and hypertensive chronic kidney disease. When assigning one of the O1Ø codes that includes hypertensive heart disease or hypertensive chronic kidney disease, it is necessary to add a secondary code from the appropriate hypertension category to specify the type of heart failure or chronic kidney disease.

See Section I.C.9. Hypertension.

e. Fetal conditions affecting the management of the mother

1) Codes from categories O35 and O36

Codes from categories O35, Maternal care for known or suspected fetal abnormality and damage, and O36, Maternal care for other fetal problems, are assigned only when the fetal condition is actually responsible for modifying the management of the mother, i.e., by requiring diagnostic studies, additional observation, special care, or termination of pregnancy. The fact that the fetal condition exists does not justify assigning a code from this series to the mother's record.

2) In utero surgery

In cases when surgery is performed on the fetus, a diagnosis code from category O35, Maternal care for known or suspected fetal abnormality and damage, should be assigned identifying the fetal condition. Assign the appropriate procedure code for the procedure performed.

No code from Chapter 16, the perinatal codes, should be used on the mother's record to identify fetal conditions. Surgery performed in utero on a fetus is still to be coded as an obstetric encounter.

f. HIV Infection in pregnancy, childbirth and the puerperium

During pregnancy, childbirth or the puerperium, a patient admitted because of an HIV-related illness should receive a principal diagnosis from subcategory O98.7-, Human immunodeficiency [HIV] disease complicating pregnancy, childbirth and the puerperium, followed by the code(s) for the HIV-related illness(es).

Patients with asymptomatic HIV infection status admitted during pregnancy, childbirth, or the puerperium should receive codes of O98.7- and Z21, Asymptomatic human immunodeficiency virus [HIV] infection status.

g. Diabetes mellitus in pregnancy

Diabetes mellitus is a significant complicating factor in pregnancy. Pregnant women who are diabetic should be assigned a code from category O24, Diabetes mellitus in pregnancy, childbirth, and the puerperium, first, followed by the appropriate diabetes code(s) (EØ8-E13) from Chapter 4.

h. Long term use of insulin

Code Z79.4, Long-term (current) use of insulin, should also be assigned if the diabetes mellitus is being treated with insulin.

i. Gestational (pregnancy induced) diabetes

Gestational (pregnancy induced) diabetes can occur during the second and third trimester of pregnancy in women who were not diabetic prior to pregnancy. Gestational diabetes can cause complications in the pregnancy similar to those of pre-existing diabetes mellitus. It also puts the woman at greater risk of developing diabetes after the pregnancy. Codes for gestational diabetes are in subcategory O24.4, Gestational diabetes mellitus. No other code from category O24, Diabetes mellitus in pregnancy, childbirth, and the puerperium, should be used with a code from O24.4.

The codes under subcategory O24.4 include diet controlled and insulin controlled. If a patient with gestational diabetes is treated with both diet and insulin, only the code for insulin-controlled is required.

Code Z79.4, Long-term (current) use of insulin, should not be assigned with codes from subcategory O24.4.

An abnormal glucose tolerance in pregnancy is assigned a code from subcategory O99.81, Abnormal glucose complicating pregnancy, childbirth, and the puerperium.

j. Sepsis and septic shock complicating abortion, pregnancy, childbirth and the puerperium

When assigning a chapter 15 code for sepsis complicating abortion, pregnancy, childbirth, and the puerperium, a code for the specific type of infection should be assigned as an additional diagnosis. If severe sepsis is present, a code from subcategory R65.2, Severe sepsis, and code(s) for associated organ dysfunction(s) should also be assigned as additional diagnoses.

k. Puerperal sepsis

Code O85, Puerperal sepsis, should be assigned with a secondary code to identify the causal organism (e.g., for a bacterial infection, assign a code from category B95-B96, Bacterial infections in conditions classified elsewhere). A code from category A4Ø, Streptococcal sepsis, or A41, Other sepsis, should not be used for puerperal sepsis. If applicable, use additional codes to identify severe sepsis (R65.2-) and any associated acute organ dysfunction.

l. Alcohol and tobacco use during pregnancy, childbirth and the puerperium

1) Alcohol use during pregnancy, childbirth and the puerperium

Codes under subcategory O99.31, Alcohol use complicating pregnancy, childbirth, and the puerperium, should be assigned for any pregnancy case when a mother uses alcohol during the pregnancy or postpartum. A secondary code from category F1Ø, Alcohol related disorders, should also be assigned to identify manifestations of the alcohol use.

2) Tobacco use during pregnancy, childbirth and the puerperium

Codes under subcategory O99.33, Smoking (tobacco) complicating pregnancy, childbirth, and the puerperium, should be assigned for any pregnancy case when a mother uses any type of tobacco product during the pregnancy or postpartum. A secondary code from category F17, Nicotine dependence, or code Z72.Ø, Tobacco use, should also be assigned to identify the type of nicotine dependence.

m. Poisoning, toxic effects, adverse effects and underdosing in a pregnant patient

A code from subcategory O9A.2, Injury, poisoning and certain other consequences of external causes complicating pregnancy, childbirth, and the puerperium, should be sequenced first, followed by the appropriate **injury,** poisoning, toxic effect, adverse effect or underdosing code, and then the additional code(s) that specifies the condition caused by the poisoning, toxic effect, adverse effect or underdosing.

See Section I.C.19. Adverse effects, poisoning, underdosing and toxic effects.

n. Normal delivery, code O8Ø

1) Encounter for full term uncomplicated delivery

Code O8Ø should be assigned when a woman is admitted for a full-term normal delivery and delivers a single, healthy infant without any complications antepartum, during the delivery, or postpartum during the delivery episode. Code O8Ø is always a principal diagnosis. It is not to be used if any other code from chapter 15 is needed to describe a current complication of the antenatal, delivery, or perinatal period. Additional codes from other chapters may be used with code O8Ø if they are not related to or are in any way complicating the pregnancy.

2) Uncomplicated delivery with resolved antepartum complication

Code O8Ø may be used if the patient had a complication at some point during the pregnancy, but the complication is not present at the time of the admission for delivery.

3) Outcome of delivery for O8Ø

Z37.Ø, Single live birth, is the only outcome of delivery code appropriate for use with O8Ø.

o. The peripartum and postpartum periods

1) Peripartum and postpartum periods

The postpartum period begins immediately after delivery and continues for six weeks following delivery. The peripartum period is defined as the last month of pregnancy to five months postpartum.

2) Peripartum and postpartum complication

A postpartum complication is any complication occurring within the six-week period.

3) Pregnancy-related complications after 6 week period

Chapter 15 codes may also be used to describe pregnancy-related complications after the peripartum or postpartum period if the provider documents that a condition is pregnancy related.

4) Admission for routine postpartum care following delivery outside hospital

When the mother delivers outside the hospital prior to admission and is admitted for routine postpartum care and no complications are noted, code Z39.Ø, Encounter for care and examination of mother immediately after delivery, should be assigned as the principal diagnosis.

5) Pregnancy associated cardiomyopathy

Pregnancy associated cardiomyopathy, code O9Ø.3, is unique in that it may be diagnosed in the third trimester of pregnancy but may continue to progress months after delivery. For this reason, it is referred to as peripartum cardiomyopathy. Code O9Ø.3 is only for use when the cardiomyopathy develops as a result of pregnancy in a woman who did not have pre-existing heart disease.

p. Code O94, Sequelae of complication of pregnancy, childbirth, and the puerperium

1) Code O94

Code O94, Sequelae of complication of pregnancy, childbirth, and the puerperium, is for use in those cases when an initial complication of a pregnancy develops a sequelae requiring care or treatment at a future date.

2) After the initial postpartum period

This code may be used at any time after the initial postpartum period.

3) Sequencing of code O94

This code, like all late effect codes, is to be sequenced following the code describing the sequelae of the complication.

q. Abortions

1) Abortion with liveborn fetus

When an attempted termination of pregnancy results in a liveborn fetus, assign a code from subcategory O6Ø.1, Preterm labor with preterm delivery, and a code from category Z37, Outcome of Delivery. The procedure code for the attempted termination of pregnancy should also be assigned.

2) Retained products of conception following an abortion

Subsequent encounters for retained products of conception following a spontaneous abortion or elective termination of pregnancy are assigned the appropriate code from category OØ3, Spontaneous abortion, or codes OØ7.4, Failed attempted termination of pregnancy without complication and Z33.2, Encounter for elective termination of pregnancy. This advice is appropriate even when the patient was discharged previously with a discharge diagnosis of complete abortion.

r. Abuse in a pregnant patient

For suspected or confirmed cases of abuse of a pregnant patient, a code(s) from subcategories O9A.3, Physical abuse complicating pregnancy, childbirth, and the puerperium, O9A.4, Sexual abuse complicating pregnancy, childbirth, and the puerperium, and O9A.5, Psychological abuse complicating pregnancy, childbirth, and the puerperium, should be sequenced first, followed by the appropriate codes (if applicable) to identify any associated current injury due to physical abuse, sexual abuse, and the perpetrator of abuse.

See Section I.C.19.f. Adult and child abuse, neglect and other maltreatment.

16. Chapter 16: *Certain Conditions Origination in the Perinatal Period* (PØØ-P96)

For coding and reporting purposes the perinatal period is defined as before birth through the 28th day following birth. The following guidelines are provided for reporting purposes

a. General Perinatal Rules

1) Use of Chapter 16 codes

Codes in this chapter are <u>never</u> for use on the maternal record. Codes from Chapter 15, the obstetric chapter, are never permitted on the newborn record. Chapter 16 codes may be used throughout the life of the patient if the condition is still present.

2) Principal diagnosis for birth record

When coding the birth episode in a newborn record, assign a code from category Z38, Liveborn infants according to place of birth and type of delivery, as the principal diagnosis. A code from category Z38 is assigned only once, to a newborn at the time of birth. If a newborn is transferred to another institution, a code from category Z38 should not be used at the receiving hospital.

A code from category Z38 is used only on the newborn record, not on the mother's record.

3) Use of codes from other chapters with codes from Chapter 16

Codes from other chapters may be used with codes from chapter 16 if the codes from the other chapters provide more specific detail. Codes for signs and symptoms may be assigned when a definitive diagnosis has not been established. If the reason for the encounter is a perinatal condition, the code from chapter 16 should be sequenced first.

4) Use of Chapter 16 codes after the perinatal period

Should a condition originate in the perinatal period, and continue throughout the life of the patient, the perinatal code should continue to be used regardless of the patient's age.

5) Birth process or community acquired conditions

If a newborn has a condition that may be either due to the birth process or community acquired and the documentation does not indicate which it is, the default is due to the birth process and the code from Chapter 16 should be used. If the condition is community-acquired, a code from Chapter 16 should not be assigned.

6) Code all clinically significant conditions

All clinically significant conditions noted on routine newborn examination should be coded. A condition is clinically significant if it requires:

- clinical evaluation; or
- therapeutic treatment; or
- diagnostic procedures; or
- extended length of hospital stay; or
- increased nursing care and/or monitoring; or
- has implications for future health care needs

Note: The perinatal guidelines listed above are the same as the general coding guidelines for "additional diagnoses", except for the final point regarding implications for future health care needs. Codes should be assigned for conditions that have been specified by the provider as having implications for future health care needs.

b. Observation and evaluation of newborns for suspected conditions not found

Assign a code from categories PØØ-PØ4 to identify those instances when a healthy newborn is evaluated for a suspected condition that is determined after study not to be present. Do not use a code from categories PØØ-PØ4 when the patient has identified signs or symptoms of a suspected problem; in such cases, code the sign or symptom.

c. Coding Additional Perinatal Diagnoses

1) Assigning codes for conditions that require treatment

Assign codes for conditions that require treatment or further investigation, prolong the length of stay, or require resource utilization.

2) Codes for conditions specified as having implications for future health care needs

Assign codes for conditions that have been specified by the provider as having implications for future health care needs.

Note: This guideline should not be used for adult patients.

d. Prematurity and fetal growth retardation

Providers utilize different criteria in determining prematurity. A code for prematurity should not be assigned unless it is documented. Assignment of codes in categories PØ5, Disorders of newborn related to slow fetal growth and fetal malnutrition, and PØ7, Disorders of newborn related to short gestation and low birth weight, not elsewhere classified, should be based on the recorded birth weight and estimated gestational age. Codes from category PØ5 should not be assigned with codes from category PØ7.

When both birth weight and gestational age are available, two codes from category PØ7 should be assigned, with the code for birth weight sequenced before the code for gestational age.

A code from PØ5 and codes from PØ7.2 and PØ7.3 may be used to specify weeks of gestation as documented by the provider in the record.

e. Low birth weight and immaturity status

Codes from category PØ7, Disorders of newborn related to short gestation and low birth weight, not elsewhere classified, are for use for a child or adult who was premature or had a low birth weight as a newborn and this is affecting the patient's current health status.

See Section I.C.21. Factors influencing health status and contact with health services, Status.

f. Bacterial sepsis of newborn

Category P36, Bacterial sepsis of newborn, includes congenital sepsis. If a perinate is documented as having sepsis without documentation of congenital or community acquired, the default is congenital and a code from category P36 should be assigned. If the P36 code includes the causal organism, an additional code from category B95, Streptococcus, Staphylococcus, and Enterococcus as the cause of diseases classified elsewhere, or B96, Other bacterial agents as the cause of diseases classified elsewhere, should not be assigned. If the P36 code does not include the causal organism, assign an additional code from category B96. If applicable, use additional codes to identify severe sepsis (R65.2-) and any associated acute organ dysfunction.

g. Stillbirth

Code P95, Stillbirth, is only for use in institutions that maintain separate records for stillbirths. No other code should be used with P95. Code P95 should not be used on the mother's record.

17. Chapter 17: Congenital Malformations, Deformations, and Chromosomal Abnormalities (QØØ-Q99)

Assign an appropriate code(s) from categories QØØ-Q99, Congenital malformations, deformations, and chromosomal abnormalities when a malformation/deformation or chromosomal abnormality is documented. A malformation/deformation/or chromosomal abnormality may be the principal/first-listed diagnosis on a record or a secondary diagnosis.

When a malformation/deformation/or chromosomal abnormality does not have a unique code assignment, assign additional code(s) for any manifestations that may be present.

When the code assignment specifically identifies the malformation/deformation/or chromosomal abnormality, manifestations that are an inherent component of the anomaly should not be coded separately. Additional codes should be assigned for manifestations that are not an inherent component.

Codes from Chapter 17 may be used throughout the life of the patient. If a congenital malformation or deformity has been corrected, a personal history code should be used to identify the history of the malformation or deformity. Although present at birth, malformation/deformation/or chromosomal abnormality may not be identified until later in life. Whenever the condition is diagnosed by the physician, it is appropriate to assign a code from codes QØØ-Q99.

For the birth admission, the appropriate code from category Z38, Liveborn infants, according to place of birth and type of delivery, should be sequenced as the principal diagnosis, followed by any congenital anomaly codes, QØØ- Q99.

18. Chapter 18: Symptoms, Signs, and Abnormal Clinical and Laboratory Findings, Not Elsewhere Classified (RØØ-R99)

Chapter 18 includes symptoms, signs, abnormal results of clinical or other investigative procedures, and ill-defined conditions regarding which no diagnosis classifiable elsewhere is recorded. Signs and symptoms that point to a specific diagnosis have been assigned to a category in other chapters of the classification.

a. **Use of symptom codes**

Codes that describe symptoms and signs are acceptable for reporting purposes when a related definitive diagnosis has not been established (confirmed) by the provider.

b. **Use of a symptom code with a definitive diagnosis code**

Codes for signs and symptoms may be reported in addition to a related definitive diagnosis when the sign or symptom is not routinely associated with that diagnosis, such as the various signs and symptoms associated with complex syndromes. The definitive diagnosis code should be sequenced before the symptom code.

Signs or symptoms that are associated routinely with a disease process should not be assigned as additional codes, unless otherwise instructed by the classification.

c. **Combination codes that include symptoms**

ICD-10-CM contains a number of combination codes that identify both the definitive diagnosis and common symptoms of that diagnosis. When using one of these combination codes, an additional code should not be assigned for the symptom.

d. **Repeated falls**

Code R29.6, Repeated falls, is for use for encounters when a patient has recently fallen and the reason for the fall is being investigated.

Code Z91.81, History of falling, is for use when a patient has fallen in the past and is at risk for future falls. When appropriate, both codes R29.6 and Z91.81 may be assigned together.

e. ***Coma* scale**

The coma scale codes (R40.2-) can be used in conjunction with traumatic brain injury codes, acute cerebrovascular disease or sequelae of cerebrovascular disease codes. These codes are primarily for use by trauma registries, but they may be used in any setting where this information is collected. The coma scale codes should be sequenced after the diagnosis code(s).

These codes, one from each subcategory, are needed to complete the scale. The 7th character indicates when the scale was recorded. The 7th character should match for all three codes.

At a minimum, report the initial score documented on presentation at your facility. This may be a score from the emergency medicine technician (EMT) or in the emergency department. If desired, a facility may choose to capture multiple Glasgow coma scale scores.

Assign code R40.24, Glasgow coma scale, total score, when only the total score is documented in the medical record and not the individual score(s).

f. **Functional quadriplegia**

Functional quadriplegia (code R53.2) is the lack of ability to use one's limbs or to ambulate due to extreme debility. It is not associated with neurologic deficit or injury, and code R53.2 should not be used for cases of neurologic quadriplegia. It should only be assigned if functional quadriplegia is specifically documented in the medical record.

g. **SIRS due to non-infectious process**

The systemic inflammatory response syndrome (SIRS) can develop as a result of certain non-infectious disease processes, such as trauma, malignant neoplasm, or pancreatitis. When SIRS is documented with a noninfectious condition, and no subsequent infection is documented, the code for the underlying condition, such as an injury, should be assigned, followed by code R65.10, Systemic inflammatory response syndrome (SIRS) of non-infectious origin without acute organ dysfunction, or code R65.11, Systemic inflammatory response syndrome (SIRS) of non-infectious origin with acute organ dysfunction. If an associated acute organ dysfunction is documented, the appropriate code(s) for the specific type of organ dysfunction(s) should be assigned in addition to code R65.11. If acute organ dysfunction is documented, but it cannot be determined if the acute organ dysfunction is associated with SIRS or due to another condition (e.g., directly due to the trauma), the provider should be queried.

h. **Death NOS**

Code R99, Ill-defined and unknown cause of mortality, is only for use in the very limited circumstance when a patient who has already died is brought into an emergency department or other healthcare facility and is pronounced dead upon arrival. It does not represent the discharge disposition of death.

19. Chapter 19: Injury, Poisoning, and Certain Other Consequences of External Causes (S00-T88)

a. ***Application of 7th Characters* in Chapter 19**

Most categories in chapter 19 have **a** 7th character requirement for each applicable code. Most categories in this chapter have three **7th character values** (with the exception of fractures): A, initial encounter, D, subsequent encounter and S, sequela. **Categories for traumatic fractures have additional 7th character values.**

7th character "A", initial encounter is used while the patient is receiving active treatment for the **condition**. Examples of active treatment are: surgical treatment, emergency department encounter, and evaluation and treatment by a new physician.

7th character "D" subsequent encounter is used for encounters after the patient has received active treatment of the **condition** and is receiving routine care for the **condition** during the healing or recovery phase. Examples of subsequent care are: cast change or removal, removal of external or internal fixation device, medication adjustment, other aftercare and follow up visits following **treatment of the injury or condition.**

The aftercare Z codes should not be used for aftercare for **conditions such as** injuries **or poisonings, where 7th characters are provided to identify subsequent care. For example, f**or aftercare of an injury, assign the acute injury code with the 7th character "D" (subsequent encounter).

7th character "S", sequela, is for use for complications or conditions that arise as a direct result of a **condition**, such as scar formation after a burn. The scars are sequelae of the burn. When using **7th character** "S", it is necessary to use both the injury code that precipitated the sequela and the code for the sequela itself. The "S" is added only to the injury code, not the sequela code. The **7th character** "S" identifies the injury responsible for the sequela. The specific type of sequela (e.g. scar) is sequenced first, followed by the injury code.

b. **Coding of injuries**

When coding injuries, assign separate codes for each injury unless a combination code is provided, in which case the combination code is assigned. Code T07, Unspecified multiple injuries should not be assigned **in the inpatient setting** unless information for a more specific code is not available. Traumatic injury codes (S00-T14.9) are not to be used for normal, healing surgical wounds or to identify complications of surgical wounds.

The code for the most serious injury, as determined by the provider and the focus of treatment, is sequenced first.

1) **Superficial injuries**

Superficial injuries such as abrasions or contusions are not coded when associated with more severe injuries of the same site.

2) **Primary injury with damage to nerves/blood vessels**

When a primary injury results in minor damage to peripheral nerves or blood vessels, the primary injury is sequenced first with additional code(s) for injuries to nerves and spinal cord (such as category S04), and/or injury to blood vessels (such as category S15). When the primary injury is to the blood vessels or nerves, that injury should be sequenced first.

c. **Coding of traumatic fractures**

The principles of multiple coding of injuries should be followed in coding fractures. Fractures of specified sites are coded individually by site in accordance with both the provisions within categories S02, S12, S22, S32, S42, S49, S52, S59, S62, S72, S79, S82, S89, S92 and the level of detail furnished by medical record content.

A fracture not indicated as open or closed should be coded to closed. A fracture not indicated whether displaced or not displaced should be coded to displaced.

More specific guidelines are as follows:

1) Initial vs. subsequent encounter for fractures

Traumatic fractures are coded using the appropriate 7th character extension for initial encounter (A, B, C) while the patient is receiving active treatment for the fracture. Examples of active treatment are: surgical treatment, emergency department encounter, and evaluation and treatment by a new physician. The appropriate 7th character for initial encounter should also be assigned for a patient who delayed seeking treatment for the fracture or nonunion.

Fractures are coded using the appropriate 7th character extension for subsequent care for encounters after the patient has completed active treatment of the fracture and is receiving routine care for the fracture during the healing or recovery phase. Examples of fracture aftercare are: cast change or removal, removal of external or internal fixation device, medication adjustment, and follow-up visits following fracture treatment.

Care for complications of surgical treatment for fracture repairs during the healing or recovery phase should be coded with the appropriate complication codes.

Care of complications of fractures, such as malunion and nonunion, should be reported with the appropriate 7th character extensions for subsequent care with nonunion (K, M, N,) or subsequent care with malunion (P, Q, R).

A code from category M8Ø, not a traumatic fracture code, should be used for any patient with known osteoporosis who suffers a fracture, even if the patient had a minor fall or trauma, if that fall or trauma would not usually break a normal, healthy bone.

See Section I.C.13. Osteoporosis.

The aftercare Z codes should not be used for aftercare for traumatic fractures. For aftercare of a traumatic fracture, assign the acute fracture code with the appropriate 7th character.

2) Multiple fractures sequencing

Multiple fractures are sequenced in accordance with the severity of the fracture.

d. Coding of burns and corrosions

The ICD-1Ø-CM makes a distinction between burns and corrosions. The burn codes are for thermal burns, except sunburns, that come from a heat source, such as a fire or hot appliance. The burn codes are also for burns resulting from electricity and radiation. Corrosions are burns due to chemicals. The guidelines are the same for burns and corrosions.

Current burns (T2Ø-T25) are classified by depth, extent and by agent (X code). Burns are classified by depth as first degree (erythema), second degree (blistering), and third degree (full-thickness involvement). Burns of the eye and internal organs (T26-T28) are classified by site, but not by degree.

1) Sequencing of burn and related condition codes

Sequence first the code that reflects the highest degree of burn when more than one burn is present.

a. When the reason for the admission or encounter is for treatment of external multiple burns, sequence first the code that reflects the burn of the highest degree.

b. When a patient has both internal and external burns, the circumstances of admission govern the selection of the principal diagnosis or first-listed diagnosis.

c. When a patient is admitted for burn injuries and other related conditions such as smoke inhalation and/or respiratory failure, the circumstances of admission govern the selection of the principal or first-listed diagnosis.

2) Burns of the same local site

Classify burns of the same local site (three-character category level, T2Ø-T28) but of different degrees to the subcategory identifying the highest degree recorded in the diagnosis.

3) Non-healing burns

Non-healing burns are coded as acute burns.

Necrosis of burned skin should be coded as a non-healed burn.

4) Infected burn

For any documented infected burn site, use an additional code for the infection.

5) Assign separate codes for each burn site

When coding burns, assign separate codes for each burn site. Category T3Ø, Burn and corrosion, body region unspecified is extremely vague and should rarely be used.

6) Burns and corrosions classified according to extent of body surface involved

Assign codes from category T31, Burns classified according to extent of body surface involved, or T32, Corrosions classified according to extent of body surface involved, when the site of the burn is not specified or when there is a need for additional data. It is advisable to use category T31 as additional coding when needed to provide data for evaluating burn mortality, such as that needed by burn units. It is also advisable to use category T31 as an additional code for reporting purposes when there is mention of a third-degree burn involving 2Ø percent or more of the body surface.

Categories T31 and T32 are based on the classic "rule of nines" in estimating body surface involved: head and neck are assigned nine percent, each arm nine percent, each leg 18 percent, the anterior trunk 18 percent, posterior trunk 18 percent, and genitalia one percent. Providers may change these percentage assignments where necessary to accommodate infants and children who have proportionately larger heads than adults, and patients who have large buttocks, thighs, or abdomen that involve burns.

7) Encounters for treatment of *sequela* of burns

Encounters for the treatment of the late effects of burns or corrosions (i.e., scars or joint contractures) should be coded with a burn or corrosion code with the 7th character "S" **for** sequela.

8) Sequelae with a late effect code and current burn

When appropriate, both a code for a current burn or corrosion with 7th character "A" or "D" and a burn or corrosion code with **7th character** "S" may be assigned on the same record (when both a current burn and sequelae of an old burn exist). Burns and corrosions do not heal at the same rate and a current healing wound may still exist with sequela of a healed burn or corrosion.

9) Use of an external cause code with burns and corrosions

An external cause code should be used with burns and corrosions to identify the source and intent of the burn, as well as the place where it occurred.

e. Adverse effects, poisoning , underdosing and toxic effects

Codes in categories T36-T65 are combination codes that include the substance **that was taken** as well as the **intent**. No additional external cause code is required for poisonings, toxic effects, adverse effects and underdosing codes.

1) Do not code directly from the Table of Drugs

Do not code directly from the Table of Drugs and Chemicals. Always refer back to the Tabular List.

2) Use as many codes as necessary to describe

Use as many codes as necessary to describe completely all drugs, medicinal or biological substances.

3) If the same code would describe the causative agent

If the same code would describe the causative agent for more than one adverse reaction, poisoning, toxic effect or underdosing, assign the code only once.

4) If two or more drugs, medicinal or biological substances

If two or more drugs, medicinal or biological substances are reported, code each individually unless a combination code is listed in the Table of Drugs and Chemicals.

5) **The occurrence of drug toxicity is classified in ICD-10-CM as follows:**

(a) **Adverse effect**

When coding an adverse effect of a drug that has been correctly prescribed and properly administered, assign the appropriate code for **the nature of the adverse effect followed by the appropriate code for the** adverse effect **of the drug** (T36-T50). **The code for the drug should have a 5th or 6th character "5" (for example T36.0X5-)** Examples of **the nature of an adverse effect** are tachycardia, delirium, gastrointestinal hemorrhaging, vomiting, hypokalemia, hepatitis, renal failure, or respiratory failure.

(b) **Poisoning**

When coding a poisoning or reaction to the improper use of a medication (e.g., overdose, wrong substance given or taken in error, wrong route of administration), **first** assign the appropriate code from categories T36-T50. **The p**oisoning codes have an associated intent **as their 5th or 6th character** (accidental, intentional self-harm, assault and undetermined. Use additional code(s) for all manifestations of poisonings.

If there is also a diagnosis of abuse or dependence **of** the substance, the abuse or dependence is **assigned** as an additional code.

Examples of poisoning include:

(i) Error was made in drug prescription

Errors made in drug prescription or in the administration of the drug by provider, nurse, patient, or other person.

(ii) Overdose of a drug intentionally taken

If an overdose of a drug was intentionally taken or administered and resulted in drug toxicity, it would be coded as a poisoning.

(iii) Nonprescribed drug taken with correctly prescribed and properly administered drug

If a nonprescribed drug or medicinal agent was taken in combination with a correctly prescribed and properly administered drug, any drug toxicity or other reaction resulting from the interaction of the two drugs would be classified as a poisoning.

(iv) Interaction of drug(s) and alcohol

When a reaction results from the interaction of a drug(s) and alcohol, this would be classified as poisoning.

See Section I.C.4. if poisoning is the result of insulin pump malfunctions.

(c) **Underdosing**

Underdosing refers to taking less of a medication than is prescribed by a provider or a manufacturer's instruction. For underdosing, assign the code from categories T36-T50 (fifth or sixth character "6").

Codes for underdosing should never be assigned as principal or first-listed codes. If a patient has a relapse or exacerbation of the medical condition for which the drug is prescribed because of the reduction in dose, then the medical condition itself should be coded.

Noncompliance (Z91.12-, Z91.13-) or complication of care (Y63.61, Y63.8-Y63.9) codes are to be used with an underdosing code to indicate intent, if known.

(d) **Toxic effects**

When a harmful substance is ingested or comes in contact with a person, this is classified as a toxic effect. The toxic effect codes are in categories T51-T65.

Toxic effect codes have an associated intent: accidental, intentional self-harm, assault and undetermined.

f. **Adult and child abuse, neglect and other maltreatment**

Sequence first the appropriate code from categories T74.- (Adult and child abuse, neglect and other maltreatment, confirmed) or T76.- (Adult and child abuse, neglect and other maltreatment, suspected) for abuse, neglect and other maltreatment, followed by any accompanying mental health or injury code(s).

If the documentation in the medical record states abuse or neglect it is coded as confirmed (T74.-). It is coded as suspected if it is documented as suspected (T76.-).

For cases of confirmed abuse or neglect an external cause code from the assault section (X92-Y08) should be added to identify the cause of any physical injuries. A perpetrator code (Y07) should be added when the perpetrator of the abuse is known. For suspected cases of abuse or neglect, do not report external cause or perpetrator code.

If a suspected case of abuse, neglect or mistreatment is ruled out during an encounter code Z04.71, **Encounter for examination and observation following alleged physical adult abuse,** ruled out, or code Z04.72, **Encounter for examination and observation following alleged child physical abuse,** ruled out, should be used, not a code from T76.

If a suspected case of alleged rape or sexual abuse is ruled out during an encounter code Z04.41, Encounter for examination and observation following alleged physical adult abuse, ruled out, or code Z04.42, Encounter for examination and observation following alleged rape or sexual abuse, ruled out, should be used, not a code from T76.

See Section I.C.15. Abuse in a pregnant patient.

g. **Complications of care**

1) ***General guidelines for* complications of care**

(a) **Documentation of complications of care**

See Section I.B.16. for information on documentation of complications of care.

2) **Pain due to medical devices**

Pain associated with devices, implants or grafts left in a surgical site (for example painful hip prosthesis) is assigned to the appropriate code(s) found in Chapter 19, Injury, poisoning, and certain other consequences of external causes. Specific codes for pain due to medical devices are found in the T code section of the ICD-10-CM. Use additional code(s) from category G89 to identify acute or chronic pain due to presence of the device, implant or graft (G89.18 or G89.28).

3) **Transplant complications**

(a) **Transplant complications other than kidney**

Codes under category T86, Complications of transplanted organs and tissues, are for use for both complications and rejection of transplanted organs. A transplant complication code is only assigned if the complication affects the function of the transplanted organ. Two codes are required to fully describe a transplant complication: the appropriate code from category T86 and a secondary code that identifies the complication.

Pre-existing conditions or conditions that develop after the transplant are not coded as complications unless they affect the function of the transplanted organs.

See I.C.21. for transplant organ removal status

See I.C.2. for malignant neoplasm associated with transplanted organ.

(b) ***Kidney transplant complications***

Patients who have undergone kidney transplant may still have some form of chronic kidney disease (CKD) because the kidney transplant may not fully restore kidney function. Code T86.1- should be assigned for documented complications of a kidney transplant, such as transplant failure or rejection or other transplant complication. Code T86.1- should not be assigned for post kidney transplant patients who have chronic kidney (CKD) unless a transplant complication such as transplant failure or rejection is documented. If the documentation is unclear as to whether the patient has a complication of the transplant, query the provider.

Conditions that affect the function of the transplanted kidney, other than CKD, should be assigned a code from subcategory T86.1, Complications of transplanted organ, Kidney, and a secondary code that identifies the complication.

For patients with CKD following a kidney transplant, but who do not have a complication such as failure or rejection, *see section I.C.14. Chronic kidney disease and kidney transplant status.*

4) Complication codes that include the external cause

As with certain other T codes, some of the complications of care codes have the external cause included in the code. The code includes the nature of the complication as well as the type of procedure that caused the complication. No external cause code indicating the type of procedure is necessary for these codes.

5) Complications of care codes within the body system chapters

Intraoperative and postprocedural complication codes are found within the body system chapters with codes specific to the organs and structures of that body system. These codes should be sequenced first, followed by a code(s) for the specific complication, if applicable.

20. Chapter 20: External Causes of Morbidity (V01-Y99)

Introduction: These guidelines are provided for the reporting of external causes of morbidity codes in order that there will be standardization in the process. These codes are secondary codes for use in any health care setting.

External cause codes are intended to provide data for injury research and evaluation of injury prevention strategies. These codes capture how the injury or health condition happened (cause), the intent (unintentional or accidental; or intentional, such as suicide or assault), the place where the event occurred the activity of the patient at the time of the event, and the person's status (e.g., civilian, military).

a. General external cause coding guidelines

1) Used with any code in the range of A00.0-T88.9, Z00-Z99

An external cause code may be used with any code in the range of A00.0-T88.9, Z00-Z99, classification that is a health condition due to an external cause. Though they are most applicable to injuries, they are also valid for use with such things as infections or diseases due to an external source, and other health conditions, such as a heart attack that occurs during strenuous physical activity.

2) External cause code used for length of treatment

Assign the external cause code, with the appropriate 7th character (initial encounter, subsequent encounter or sequela) for each encounter for which the injury or condition is being treated.

3) Use the full range of external cause codes

Use the full range of external cause codes to completely describe the cause, the intent, the place of occurrence, and if applicable, the activity of the patient at the time of the event, and the patient's status, for all injuries, and other health conditions due to an external cause.

4) Assign as many external cause codes as necessary

Assign as many external cause codes as necessary to fully explain each cause. If only one external code can be recorded, assign the code most related to the principal diagnosis.

5) The selection of the appropriate external cause code

The selection of the appropriate external cause code is guided by the Alphabetic Index of External Causes and by Inclusion and Exclusion notes in the Tabular List.

6) External cause code can never be a principal diagnosis

An external cause code can never be a principal (first-listed) diagnosis.

7) Combination external cause codes

Certain of the external cause codes are combination codes that identify sequential events that result in an injury, such as a fall which results in striking against an object. The injury may be due to either event or both. The combination external cause code used should correspond to the sequence of events regardless of which caused the most serious injury.

8) No external cause code needed in certain circumstances

No external cause code from Chapter 20 is needed if the external cause and intent are included in a code from another chapter (e.g. T36.0x1- Poisoning by penicillins, accidental (unintentional)).

b. Place of occurrence guideline

Codes from category Y92, Place of occurrence of the external cause, are secondary codes for use after other external cause codes to identify the location of the patient at the time of injury or other condition.

A place of occurrence code is used only once, at the initial encounter for treatment. No 7th characters are used for Y92. Only one code from Y92 should be recorded on a medical record. A place of occurrence code should be used in conjunction with an activity code, Y93.

Do not use place of occurrence code Y92.9 if the place is not stated or is not applicable.

c. Activity code

Assign a code from category Y93, Activity code, to describe the activity of the patient at the time the injury or other health condition occurred.

An activity code is used only once, at the initial encounter for treatment. Only one code from Y93 should be recorded on a medical record. An activity code should be used in conjunction with a place of occurrence code, Y92.

The activity codes are not applicable to poisonings, adverse effects, misadventures or **sequela**.

Do not assign Y93.9, Unspecified activity, if the activity is not stated.

A code from category Y93 is appropriate for use with external cause and intent codes if identifying the activity provides additional information about the event.

d. Place of occurrence, activity, and status codes used with other external cause code

When applicable, place of occurrence, activity, and external cause status codes are sequenced after the main external cause code(s). Regardless of the number of external cause codes assigned, there should be only one place of occurrence code, one activity code, and one external cause status code assigned to an encounter.

e. If the reporting format limits the number of external cause codes

If the reporting format limits the number of external cause codes that can be used in reporting clinical data, report the code for the cause/intent most related to the principal diagnosis. If the format permits capture of additional external cause codes, the cause/intent, including medical misadventures, of the additional events should be reported rather than the codes for place, activity, or external status.

f. Multiple external cause coding guidelines

More than one external cause code is required to fully describe the external cause of an illness or injury. The assignment of external cause codes should be sequenced in the following priority:

If two or more events cause separate injuries, an external cause code should be assigned for each cause. The first-listed external cause code will be selected in the following order:

External codes for child and adult abuse take priority over all other external cause codes.

See Section I.C.19., Child and Adult abuse guidelines.

External cause codes for terrorism events take priority over all other external cause codes except child and adult abuse.

External cause codes for cataclysmic events take priority over all other external cause codes except child and adult abuse and terrorism.

External cause codes for transport accidents take priority over all other external cause codes except cataclysmic events, child and adult abuse and terrorism.

Activity and external cause status codes are assigned following all causal (intent) external cause codes.

The first-listed external cause code should correspond to the cause of the most serious diagnosis due to an assault, accident, or self-harm, following the order of hierarchy listed above.

g. Child and adult abuse guideline

Adult and child abuse, neglect and maltreatment are classified as assault. Any of the assault codes may be used to indicate the external cause of any injury resulting from the confirmed abuse.

For confirmed cases of abuse, neglect and maltreatment, when the perpetrator is known, a code from YØ7, Perpetrator of maltreatment and neglect, should accompany any other assault codes.

See Section I.C.19. Adult and child abuse, neglect and other maltreatment

h. Unknown or undetermined intent guideline

If the intent (accident, self-harm, assault) of the cause of an injury or other condition is unknown or unspecified, code the intent as accidental intent. All transport accident categories assume accidental intent.

1) Use of undetermined intent

External cause codes for events of undetermined intent are only for use if the documentation in the record specifies that the intent cannot be determined.

i. *Sequelae* (Late Effects) of external cause guidelines

1) *Sequelae* external cause codes

Sequela are reported using the external cause code with the 7th character extension "S" for sequela. These codes should be used with any report of a late effect or sequela resulting from a previous injury.

2) *Sequela* external cause code with a related current injury

A **sequela** external cause code should never be used with a related current nature of injury code.

3) Use of *sequela* external cause codes for subsequent visits

Use a late effect external cause code for subsequent visits when a late effect of the initial injury is being treated. Do not use a late effect external cause code for subsequent visits for follow-up care (e.g., to assess healing, to receive rehabilitative therapy) of the injury when no late effect of the injury has been documented.

j. Terrorism guidelines

1) Cause of injury identified by the Federal Government (FBI) as terrorism

When the cause of an injury is identified by the Federal Government (FBI) as terrorism, the first-listed external cause code should be a code from category Y38, Terrorism. The definition of terrorism employed by the FBI is found at the inclusion note at the beginning of category Y38. Use additional code for place of occurrence (Y92.-). More than one Y38 code may be assigned if the injury is the result of more than one mechanism of terrorism.

2) Cause of an injury is suspected to be the result of terrorism

When the cause of an injury is suspected to be the result of terrorism a code from category Y38 should not be assigned. Suspected cases should be classified as assault.

3) Code Y38.9, terrorism, secondary effects

Assign code Y38.9, Terrorism, secondary effects, for conditions occurring subsequent to the terrorist event. This code should not be assigned for conditions that are due to the initial terrorist act.

It is acceptable to assign code Y38.9 with another code from Y38 if there is an injury due to the initial terrorist event and an injury that is a subsequent result of the terrorist event.

k. External cause status

A code from category Y99, External cause status, should be assigned whenever any other external cause code is assigned for an encounter, including an Activity code, except for the events noted below. Assign a code from category Y99, External cause status, to indicate the work status of the person at the time the event occurred. The status code indicates whether the event occurred during military activity, whether a non-military person was at work, whether an individual including a student or volunteer was involved in a non-work activity at the time of the causal event.

A code from Y99, External cause status, should be assigned, when applicable, with other external cause codes, such as transport accidents and falls. The external cause status codes are not applicable to poisonings, adverse effects, misadventures or late effects.

Do not assign a code from category Y99 if no other external cause codes (cause, activity) are applicable for the encounter.

An external cause status code is used only once, at the initial encounter for treatment. Only one code from Y99 should be recorded on a medical record.

Do not assign code Y99.9, Unspecified external cause status, if the status is not stated.

21. Chapter 21: Factors Influencing Health Status and Contact with Health Services (ZØØ-Z99)

Note: The chapter specific guidelines provide additional information about the use of Z codes for specified encounters.

a. Use of Z codes in any healthcare setting

Z codes are for use in any healthcare setting. Z codes may be used as either a first-listed (principal diagnosis code in the inpatient setting) or secondary code, depending on the circumstances of the encounter. Certain Z codes may only be used as first-listed or principal diagnosis.

b. Z Codes indicate a reason for an encounter

Z codes are not procedure codes. A corresponding procedure code must accompany a Z code to describe any procedure performed.

c. Categories of Z codes

1) Contact/exposure

Category Z2Ø indicates contact with, and suspected exposure to, communicable diseases. These codes are for patients who do not show any sign or symptom of a disease but are suspected to have been exposed to it by close personal contact with an infected individual or are in an area where a disease is epidemic.

Category Z77, indicates contact with and suspected exposures hazardous to health.

Contact/exposure codes may be used as a first-listed code to explain an encounter for testing, or, more commonly, as a secondary code to identify a potential risk.

2) Inoculations and vaccinations

Code Z23 is for encounters for inoculations and vaccinations. It indicates that a patient is being seen to receive a prophylactic inoculation against a disease. Procedure codes are required to identify the actual administration of the injection and the type(s) of immunizations given. Code Z23 may be used as a secondary code if the inoculation is given as a routine part of preventive health care, such as a well-baby visit.

3) Status

Status codes indicate that a patient is either a carrier of a disease or has the sequelae or residual of a past disease or condition. This includes such things as the presence of prosthetic or mechanical devices resulting from past treatment. A status code is informative, because the status may affect the course of treatment and its outcome. A status code is distinct from a history code. The history code indicates that the patient no longer has the condition.

A status code should not be used with a diagnosis code from one of the body system chapters, if the diagnosis code includes the information provided by the status code. For example, code Z94.1, Heart transplant status, should not be used with a code from subcategory T86.2, Complications of heart transplant. The status code does not provide additional information. The complication code indicates that the patient is a heart transplant patient.

For encounters for weaning from a mechanical ventilator, assign a code from subcategory J96.1, Chronic respiratory failure, followed by code Z99.11, Dependence on respirator [ventilator] status.

The status Z codes/categories are:

Z14 Genetic carrier

Genetic carrier status indicates that a person carries a gene, associated with a particular disease, which may be passed to offspring who may develop that disease. The person does not have the disease and is not at risk of developing the disease.

Z15 Genetic susceptibility to disease

Genetic susceptibility indicates that a person has a gene that increases the risk of that person developing the disease.

Codes from category Z15 should not be used as principal or first-listed codes. If the patient has the condition to which he/she is susceptible, and that condition is the reason for the encounter, the code for the current condition should be sequenced first. If the patient is being seen for follow-up after completed treatment for this condition, and the condition no longer exists, a follow-up code should be sequenced first, followed by the appropriate personal history and genetic susceptibility codes. If the purpose of the encounter is genetic counseling associated with procreative management, code Z31.5, Encounter for genetic counseling, should be assigned as the first-listed code, followed by a code from category Z15. Additional codes should be assigned for any applicable family or personal history.

Z16 Resistance to antimicrobial drugs

This code indicates that a patient has **a condition that** is resistant to **antimicrobial** drug treatment. Sequence the infection code first.

Z17 Estrogen receptor status

Z18 Retained foreign body fragments

Z21 Asymptomatic HIV infection status

This code indicates that a patient has tested positive for HIV but has manifested no signs or symptoms of the disease.

Z22 Carrier of infectious disease

Carrier status indicates that a person harbors the specific organisms of a disease without manifest symptoms and is capable of transmitting the infection.

Z28.3 Underimmunization status

Z33.1 Pregnant state, incidental

This code is a secondary code only for use when the pregnancy is in no way complicating the reason for visit. Otherwise, a code from the obstetric chapter is required.

Z66 Do not resuscitate

This code may be used when it is documented by the provider that a patient is on do not resuscitate status at any time during the stay.

Z67 Blood type

Z68 Body mass index (BMI)

Z74.01 Bed confinement status

Z76.82 Awaiting organ transplant status

Z78 Other specified health status

Code Z78.1, Physical restraint status, may be used when it is documented by the provider that a patient has been put in restraints during the current encounter. Please note that this code should not be reported when it is documented by the provider that a patient is temporarily restrained during a procedure.

Z79 Long-term (current) drug therapy

Codes from this category indicate a patient's continuous use of a prescribed drug (including such things as aspirin therapy) for the long-term treatment of a condition or for prophylactic use. It is not for use for patients who have addictions to drugs. This subcategory is not for use of medications for detoxification or maintenance programs to prevent withdrawal symptoms in patients with drug dependence (e.g., methadone maintenance for opiate dependence). Assign the appropriate code for the drug dependence instead.

Assign a code from Z79 if the patient is receiving a medication for an extended period as a prophylactic measure (such as for the prevention of deep vein thrombosis) or as treatment of a chronic condition (such as arthritis) or a disease requiring a lengthy course of treatment (such as cancer). Do not assign a code from category Z79 for medication being administered for a brief period of time to treat an acute illness or injury (such as a course of antibiotics to treat acute bronchitis).

Z88 Allergy status to drugs, medicaments and biological substances

Except: Z88.9, Allergy status to unspecified drugs, medicaments and biological substances status

Z89 Acquired absence of limb

Z90 Acquired absence of organs, not elsewhere classified

Z91.0- Allergy status, other than to drugs and biological substances

Z92.82 Status post administration of tPA (rtPA) in a different facility within the last 24 hours prior to admission to a current facility

Assign code Z92.82, Status post administration of tPA (rtPA) in a different facility within the last 24 hours prior to admission to current facility, as a secondary diagnosis when a patient is received by transfer into a facility and documentation indicates they were administered tissue plasminogen activator (tPA) within the last 24 hours prior to admission to the current facility.

This guideline applies even if the patient is still receiving the tPA at the time they are received into the current facility.

The appropriate code for the condition for which the tPA was administered (such as cerebrovascular disease or myocardial infarction) should be assigned first.

Code Z92.82 is only applicable to the receiving facility record and not to the transferring facility record.

Z93 Artificial opening status

Z94 Transplanted organ and tissue status

Z95 Presence of cardiac and vascular implants and grafts

Z96 Presence of other functional implants

Z97 Presence of other devices

Z98 Other postprocedural states

Assign code Z98.85, Transplanted organ removal status, to indicate that a transplanted organ has been previously removed. This code should not be assigned for the encounter in which the transplanted organ is removed. The complication necessitating removal of the transplant organ should be assigned for that encounter.

See section I.C19.g.3. for information on the coding of organ transplant complications.

Z99 Dependence on enabling machines and devices, not elsewhere classified

Note: Categories Z89-Z9Ø and Z93-Z99 are for use only if there are no complications or malfunctions of the organ or tissue replaced, the amputation site or the equipment on which the patient is dependent.

4) History (of)

There are two types of history Z codes, personal and family. Personal history codes explain a patient's past medical condition that no longer exists and is not receiving any treatment, but that has the potential for recurrence, and therefore may require continued monitoring.

Family history codes are for use when a patient has a family member(s) who has had a particular disease that causes the patient to be at higher risk of also contracting the disease.

Personal history codes may be used in conjunction with follow-up codes and family history codes may be used in conjunction with screening codes to explain the need for a test or procedure. History codes are also acceptable on any medical record regardless of the reason for visit. A history of an illness, even if no longer present, is important information that may alter the type of treatment ordered.

The history Z code categories are:

Z8Ø Family history of primary malignant neoplasm

Z81 Family history of mental and behavioral disorders

Z82 Family history of certain disabilities and chronic diseases (leading to disablement)

Z83 Family history of other specific disorders

Z84 Family history of other conditions

Z85 Personal history of malignant neoplasm

Z86 Personal history of certain other diseases

Z87 Personal history of other diseases and conditions

Z91.4- Personal history of psychological trauma, not elsewhere classified

Z91.5 Personal history of self-harm

Z91.8- Other specified personal risk factors, not elsewhere classified

Exception: Z91.83, Wandering in diseases classified elsewhere

Z92 Personal history of medical treatment

Except: Z92.Ø, Personal history of contraception

Except: Z92.82, Status post administration of tPA (rtPA) in a different facility within the last 24 hours prior to admission to a current facility

5) Screening

Screening is the testing for disease or disease precursors in seemingly well individuals so that early detection and treatment can be provided for those who test positive for the disease (e.g., screening mammogram).

The testing of a person to rule out or confirm a suspected diagnosis because the patient has some sign or symptom is a diagnostic examination, not a screening. In these cases, the sign or symptom is used to explain the reason for the test.

A screening code may be a first-listed code if the reason for the visit is specifically the screening exam. It may also be used as an additional code if the screening is done during an office visit for other health problems. A screening code is not necessary if the screening is inherent to a routine examination, such as a pap smear done during a routine pelvic examination.

Should a condition be discovered during the screening then the code for the condition may be assigned as an additional diagnosis.

The Z code indicates that a screening exam is planned. A procedure code is required to confirm that the screening was performed.

The screening Z codes/categories:

Z11 Encounter for screening for infectious and parasitic diseases

Z12 Encounter for screening for malignant neoplasms

Z13 Encounter for screening for other diseases and disorders

Except: Z13.9, Encounter for screening, unspecified

Z36 Encounter for antenatal screening for mother

6) Observation

There are two observation Z code categories. They are for use in very limited circumstances when a person is being observed for a suspected condition that is ruled out. The observation codes are not for use if an injury or illness or any signs or symptoms related to the suspected condition are present. In such cases the diagnosis/symptom code is used with the corresponding external cause code.

The observation codes are to be used as principal diagnosis only. Additional codes may be used in addition to the observation code but only if they are unrelated to the suspected condition being observed.

Codes from subcategory ZØ3.7, Encounter for suspected maternal and fetal conditions ruled out, may either be used as a first-listed or as an additional code assignment depending on the case. They are for use in very limited circumstances on a maternal record when an encounter is for a suspected maternal or fetal condition that is ruled out during that encounter (for example, a maternal or fetal condition may be suspected due to an abnormal test result). These codes should not be used when the condition is confirmed. In those cases, the confirmed condition should be coded. In addition, these codes are not for use if an illness or any signs or symptoms related to the suspected condition or problem are present. In such cases the diagnosis/symptom code is used.

Additional codes may be used in addition to the code from subcategory ZØ3.7, but only if they are unrelated to the suspected condition being evaluated.

Codes from subcategory ZØ3.7 may not be used for encounters for antenatal screening of mother. *See Section I.C.21.c.5, Screening.*

For encounters for suspected fetal condition that are inconclusive following testing and evaluation, assign the appropriate code from category O35, O36, O4Ø or O41.

The observation Z code categories:

ZØ3 Encounter for medical observation for suspected diseases and conditions ruled out

ZØ4 Encounter for examination and observation for other reasons

Except: ZØ4.9, Encounter for examination and observation for unspecified reason

7) Aftercare

Aftercare visit codes cover situations when the initial treatment of a disease has been performed and the patient requires continued care during the healing or recovery phase, or for the long-term consequences of the disease. The aftercare Z code should not be used if treatment is directed at a current, acute disease. The diagnosis code is to be used in these cases. Exceptions to this rule are codes Z51.Ø, Encounter for antineoplastic radiation therapy, and codes from subcategory Z51.1, Encounter for antineoplastic chemotherapy and immunotherapy. These codes are to be first-listed, followed by the diagnosis code when a patient's encounter is solely to receive radiation therapy, chemotherapy, or immunotherapy for the treatment of a neoplasm. If the reason for the encounter is more than one type of antineoplastic therapy, code Z51.Ø and a code from subcategory Z51.1 may be assigned together, in which case one of these codes would be reported as a secondary diagnosis.

The aftercare Z codes should also not be used for aftercare for injuries. For aftercare of an injury, assign the acute injury code with the appropriate 7th character (for subsequent encounter).

The aftercare codes are generally first-listed to explain the specific reason for the encounter. An aftercare code may be used as an additional code when some type of aftercare is provided in addition to the reason for admission and no diagnosis code is applicable. An example of this would be the closure of a colostomy during an encounter for treatment of another condition.

Aftercare codes should be used in conjunction with other aftercare codes or diagnosis codes to provide better detail on the specifics of an aftercare encounter visit, unless otherwise directed by the classification. Should a patient receive multiple types of antineoplastic therapy during the same encounter, code Z51.Ø, Encounter for antineoplastic radiation therapy, and codes from subcategory Z51.1, Encounter for antineoplastic chemotherapy and immunotherapy, may be used together on a record. The sequencing of multiple aftercare codes depends on the circumstances of the encounter.

Certain aftercare Z code categories need a secondary diagnosis code to describe the resolving condition or sequelae. For others, the condition is included in the code title.

Additional Z code aftercare category terms include fitting and adjustment, and attention to artificial openings.

Status Z codes may be used with aftercare Z codes to indicate the nature of the aftercare. For example code Z95.1, Presence of aortocoronary bypass graft, may be used with code Z48.812, Encounter for surgical aftercare following surgery on the circulatory system, to indicate the surgery for which the aftercare is being performed. A status code should not be used when the aftercare code indicates the type of status, such as using Z43.Ø, Encounter for attention to tracheostomy, with Z93.Ø, Tracheostomy status.

The aftercare Z category/codes:

Z42	Encounter for plastic and reconstructive surgery following medical procedure or healed injury
Z43	Encounter for attention to artificial openings
Z44	Encounter for fitting and adjustment of external prosthetic device
Z45	Encounter for adjustment and management of implanted device
Z46	Encounter for fitting and adjustment of other devices
Z47	Orthopedic aftercare
Z48	Encounter for other postprocedural aftercare
Z49	Encounter for care involving renal dialysis
Z51	Encounter for other aftercare

8) Follow-up

The follow-up codes are used to explain continuing surveillance following completed treatment of a disease, condition, or injury. They imply that the condition has been fully treated and no longer exists. They should not be confused with aftercare codes, or injury codes with a 7th character for subsequent encounter, that explain ongoing care of a healing condition or its sequelae. Follow-up codes may be used in conjunction with history codes to provide the full picture of the healed condition and its treatment. The follow-up code is sequenced first, followed by the history code.

A follow-up code may be used to explain multiple visits. Should a condition be found to have recurred on the follow-up visit, then the diagnosis code for the condition should be assigned in place of the follow-up code.

The follow-up Z code categories:

ZØ8	Encounter for follow-up examination after completed treatment for malignant neoplasm
ZØ9	Encounter for follow-up examination after completed treatment for conditions other than malignant neoplasm
Z39	Encounter for maternal postpartum care and examination

9) Donor

Codes in category Z52, Donors of organs and tissues, are used for living individuals who are donating blood or other body tissue. These codes are only for individuals donating for others, not for self-donations. They are not used to identify cadaveric donations.

1Ø) Counseling

Counseling Z codes are used when a patient or family member receives assistance in the aftermath of an illness or injury, or when support is required in coping with family or social problems. They are not used in conjunction with a diagnosis code when the counseling component of care is considered integral to standard treatment.

The counseling Z codes/categories:

Z3Ø.Ø-	Encounter for general counseling and advice on contraception
Z31.5	Encounter for genetic counseling
Z31.6-	Encounter for general counseling and advice on procreation
Z32.2	Encounter for childbirth instruction
Z32.3	Encounter for childcare instruction
Z69	Encounter for mental health services for victim and perpetrator of abuse
Z7Ø	Counseling related to sexual attitude, behavior and orientation
Z71	Persons encountering health services for other counseling and medical advice, not elsewhere classified
Z76.81	Expectant mother prebirth pediatrician visit

11) Encounters for obstetrical and reproductive services

See Section I.C.15. Pregnancy, Childbirth, and the Puerperium, for further instruction on the use of these codes.

Z codes for pregnancy are for use in those circumstances when none of the problems or complications included in the codes from the Obstetrics chapter exist (a routine prenatal visit or postpartum care). Codes in category Z34, Encounter for supervision of normal pregnancy, are always first-listed and are not to be used with any other code from the OB chapter. **Codes in category Z3A, Weeks of gestation, may be assigned to provide additional information about the pregnancy.**

The outcome of delivery, category Z37, should be included on all maternal delivery records. It is always a secondary code. Codes in category Z37 should not be used on the newborn record.

Z codes for family planning (contraceptive) or procreative management and counseling should be included on an obstetric record either during the pregnancy or the postpartum stage, if applicable.

Z codes/categories for obstetrical and reproductive services:

Z3Ø	Encounter for contraceptive management
Z31	Encounter for procreative management
Z32.2	Encounter for childbirth instruction
Z32.3	Encounter for childcare instruction
Z33	Pregnant state
Z34	Encounter for supervision of normal pregnancy
Z36	Encounter for antenatal screening of mother
Z3A	**Weeks of gestation**
Z37	Outcome of delivery

Z39 Encounter for maternal postpartum care and examination
Z76.81 Expectant mother prebirth pediatrician visit

12) Newborns and Infants

See Section I.C.16. Newborn (Perinatal) Guidelines, for further instruction on the use of these codes.

Newborn Z codes/categories:

Z76.1 Encounter for health supervision and care of foundling
Z00.1- Encounter for routine child health examination
Z38 Liveborn infants according to place of birth and type of delivery

13) Routine and administrative examinations

The Z codes allow for the description of encounters for routine examinations, such as, a general check-up, or, examinations for administrative purposes, such as, a pre-employment physical. The codes are not to be used if the examination is for diagnosis of a suspected condition or for treatment purposes. In such cases the diagnosis code is used. During a routine exam, should a diagnosis or condition be discovered, it should be coded as an additional code. Pre-existing and chronic conditions and history codes may also be included as additional codes as long as the examination is for administrative purposes and not focused on any particular condition.

Some of the codes for routine health examinations distinguish between "with" and "without" abnormal findings. Code assignment depends on the information that is known at the time the encounter is being coded. For example, if no abnormal findings were found during the examination, but the encounter is being coded before test results are back, it is acceptable to assign the code for "without abnormal findings." When assigning a code for "with abnormal findings," additional code(s) should be assigned to identify the specific abnormal finding(s).

Pre-operative examination and pre-procedural laboratory examination Z codes are for use only in those situations when a patient is being cleared for a procedure or surgery and no treatment is given.

The Z codes/categories for routine and administrative examinations:

Z00 Encounter for general examination without complaint, suspected or reported diagnosis
Z01 Encounter for other special examination without complaint, suspected or reported diagnosis
Z02 Encounter for administrative examination
Except: Z02.9, Encounter for administrative examinations, unspecified
Z32.0- Encounter for pregnancy test

14) Miscellaneous Z codes

The miscellaneous Z codes capture a number of other health care encounters that do not fall into one of the other categories. Certain of these codes identify the reason for the encounter; others are for use as additional codes that provide useful information on circumstances that may affect a patient's care and treatment.

Prophylactic Organ Removal

For encounters specifically for prophylactic removal of an organ (such as prophylactic removal of breasts due to a genetic susceptibility to cancer or a family history of cancer), the principal or first-listed code should be a code from category Z40, Encounter for prophylactic surgery, followed by the appropriate codes to identify the associated risk factor (such as genetic susceptibility or family history).

If the patient has a malignancy of one site and is having prophylactic removal at another site to prevent either a new primary malignancy or metastatic disease, a code for the malignancy should also be assigned in addition to a code from subcategory Z40.0, Encounter for prophylactic surgery for risk factors related to malignant neoplasms. A Z40.0 code should not be assigned if the patient is having organ removal for treatment of a malignancy, such as the removal of the testes for the treatment of prostate cancer.

Miscellaneous Z codes/categories:

Z28 Immunization not carried out
Except: Z28.3, Underimmunization status
Z40 Encounter for prophylactic surgery
Z41 Encounter for procedures for purposes other than remedying health state
Except: Z41.9, Encounter for procedure for purposes other than remedying health state, unspecified
Z53 Persons encountering health services for specific procedures and treatment, not carried out
Z55 Problems related to education and literacy
Z56 Problems related to employment and unemployment
Z57 Occupational exposure to risk factors
Z58 Problems related to physical environment
Z59 Problems related to housing and economic circumstances
Z60 Problems related to social environment
Z62 Problems related to upbringing
Z63 Other problems related to primary support group, including family circumstances
Z64 Problems related to certain psychosocial circumstances
Z65 Problems related to other psychosocial circumstances
Z72 Problems related to lifestyle
Z73 Problems related to life management difficulty
Z74 Problems related to care provider dependency
Except: Z74.01, Bed confinement status
Z75 Problems related to medical facilities and other health care
Z76.0 Encounter for issue of repeat prescription
Z76.3 Healthy person accompanying sick person
Z76.4 Other boarder to healthcare facility
Z76.5 Malingerer [conscious simulation]
Z91.1- Patient's noncompliance with medical treatment and regimen
Z91.83 Wandering in diseases classified elsewhere
Z91.89 Other specified personal risk factors, not elsewhere classified

15) Nonspecific Z codes

Certain Z codes are so non-specific, or potentially redundant with other codes in the classification, that there can be little justification for their use in the inpatient setting. Their use in the outpatient setting should be limited to those instances when there is no further documentation to permit more precise coding. Otherwise, any sign or symptom or any other reason for visit that is captured in another code should be used.

Nonspecific Z codes/categories:

Z02.9 Encounter for administrative examinations, unspecified
Z04.9 Encounter for examination and observation for unspecified reason
Z13.9 Encounter for screening, unspecified
Z41.9 Encounter for procedure for purposes other than remedying health state, unspecified
Z52.9 Donor of unspecified organ or tissue
Z86.59 Personal history of other mental and behavioral disorders
Z88.9 Allergy status to unspecified drugs, medicaments and biological substances status
Z92.0 Personal history of contraception

16) Z codes that may only be principal/first-listed diagnosis

The following Z codes/categories may only be reported as the principal/first-listed diagnosis, except when there are multiple encounters on the same day and the medical records for the encounters are combined:

Z00	Encounter for general examination without complaint, suspected or reported diagnosis
Z01	Encounter for other special examination without complaint, suspected or reported diagnosis
Z02	Encounter for administrative examination
Z03	Encounter for medical observation for suspected diseases and conditions ruled out
Z04	Encounter for examination and observation for other reasons
Z31.81	Encounter for male factor infertility in female patient
Z31.82	Encounter for Rh incompatibility status
Z31.83	Encounter for assisted reproductive fertility procedure cycle
Z31.84	Encounter for fertility preservation procedure
Z33.2	Encounter for elective termination of pregnancy
Z34	Encounter for supervision of normal pregnancy
Z38	Liveborn infants according to place of birth and type of delivery
Z39	Encounter for maternal postpartum care and examination
Z42	Encounter for plastic and reconstructive surgery following medical procedure or healed injury
Z51.0	Encounter for antineoplastic radiation therapy
Z51.1-	Encounter for antineoplastic chemotherapy and immunotherapy
Z52	Donors of organs and tissues Except: Z52.9, Donor of unspecified organ or tissue
Z76.1	Encounter for health supervision and care of foundling
Z76.2	Encounter for health supervision and care of other healthy infant and child
Z99.12	Encounter for respirator [ventilator] dependence during power failure

Section II. Selection of Principal Diagnosis

The circumstances of inpatient admission always govern the selection of principal diagnosis. The principal diagnosis is defined in the Uniform Hospital Discharge Data Set (UHDDS) as "that condition established after study to be chiefly responsible for occasioning the admission of the patient to the hospital for care."

The UHDDS definitions are used by hospitals to report inpatient data elements in a standardized manner. These data elements and their definitions can be found in the July 31, 1985, Federal Register (Vol. 50, No, 147), pp. 31038-40.

Since that time the application of the UHDDS definitions has been expanded to include all non-outpatient settings (acute care, short term, long term care and psychiatric hospitals; home health agencies; rehab facilities; nursing homes, etc).

In determining principal diagnosis the coding conventions in the ICD-10-CM, the Tabular List and Alphabetic Index take precedence over these official coding guidelines.

(See Section I.A., Conventions for the ICD-10-CM)

The importance of consistent, complete documentation in the medical record cannot be overemphasized. Without such documentation the application of all coding guidelines is a difficult, if not impossible, task.

A. Codes for symptoms, signs, and ill-defined conditions

Codes for symptoms, signs, and ill-defined conditions from Chapter 18 are not to be used as principal diagnosis when a related definitive diagnosis has been established.

B. Two or more interrelated conditions, each potentially meeting the definition for principal diagnosis

When there are two or more interrelated conditions (such as diseases in the same ICD-10-CM chapter or manifestations characteristically associated with a certain disease) potentially meeting the definition of principal diagnosis, either condition may be sequenced first, unless the circumstances of the admission, the therapy provided, the Tabular List, or the Alphabetic Index indicate otherwise.

C. Two or more diagnoses that equally meet the definition for principal diagnosis

In the unusual instance when two or more diagnoses equally meet the criteria for principal diagnosis as determined by the circumstances of admission, diagnostic workup and/or therapy provided, and the Alphabetic Index, Tabular List, or another coding guidelines does not provide sequencing direction, any one of the diagnoses may be sequenced first.

D. Two or more comparative or contrasting conditions

In those rare instances when two or more contrasting or comparative diagnoses are documented as "either/or" (or similar terminology), they are coded as if the diagnoses were confirmed and the diagnoses are sequenced according to the circumstances of the admission. If no further determination can be made as to which diagnosis should be principal, either diagnosis may be sequenced first.

E. A symptom(s) followed by contrasting/comparative diagnoses

When a symptom(s) is followed by contrasting/comparative diagnoses, the symptom code is sequenced first. All the contrasting/comparative diagnoses should be coded as additional diagnoses.

F. Original treatment plan not carried out

Sequence as the principal diagnosis the condition, which after study occasioned the admission to the hospital, even though treatment may not have been carried out due to unforeseen circumstances.

G. Complications of surgery and other medical care

When the admission is for treatment of a complication resulting from surgery or other medical care, the complication code is sequenced as the principal diagnosis. If the complication is classified to the T80-T88 series and the code lacks the necessary specificity in describing the complication, an additional code for the specific complication should be assigned.

H. Uncertain diagnosis

If the diagnosis documented at the time of discharge is qualified as "probable", "suspected", "likely", "questionable", "possible", or "still to be ruled out", or other similar terms indicating uncertainty, code the condition as if it existed or was established. The bases for these guidelines are the diagnostic workup, arrangements for further workup or observation, and initial therapeutic approach that correspond most closely with the established diagnosis.

Note: This guideline is applicable only to inpatient admissions to short-term, acute, long-term care and psychiatric hospitals.

I. Admission from observation unit

1. **Admission Following Medical Observation**
   When a patient is admitted to an observation unit for a medical condition, which either worsens or does not improve, and is subsequently admitted as an inpatient of the same hospital for this same medical condition, the principal diagnosis would be the medical condition which led to the hospital admission.
2. **Admission Following Post-Operative Observation**
   When a patient is admitted to an observation unit to monitor a condition (or complication) that develops following outpatient surgery, and then is subsequently admitted as an inpatient of the same hospital, hospitals should apply the Uniform Hospital Discharge Data Set (UHDDS) definition of principal diagnosis as "that condition established after study to be chiefly responsible for occasioning the admission of the patient to the hospital for care."

J. Admission from outpatient surgery

When a patient receives surgery in the hospital's outpatient surgery department and is subsequently admitted for continuing inpatient care at the same hospital, the following guidelines should be followed in selecting the principal diagnosis for the inpatient admission:

- If the reason for the inpatient admission is a complication, assign the complication as the principal diagnosis.
- If no complication, or other condition, is documented as the reason for the inpatient admission, assign the reason for the outpatient surgery as the principal diagnosis.
- If the reason for the inpatient admission is another condition unrelated to the surgery, assign the unrelated condition as the principal diagnosis.

Section III. Reporting Additional Diagnoses

GENERAL RULES FOR OTHER (ADDITIONAL) DIAGNOSES

For reporting purposes the definition for "other diagnoses" is interpreted as additional conditions that affect patient care in terms of requiring:

clinical evaluation; or

therapeutic treatment; or

diagnostic procedures; or

extended length of hospital stay; or

increased nursing care and/or monitoring.

The UHDDS item #11-b defines Other Diagnoses as "all conditions that coexist at the time of admission, that develop subsequently, or that affect the treatment received and/or the length of stay. Diagnoses that relate to an earlier episode which have no bearing on the current hospital stay are to be excluded." UHDDS definitions apply to inpatients in acute care, short-term, long term care and psychiatric hospital setting. The UHDDS definitions are used by acute care short-term hospitals to report inpatient data elements in a standardized manner. These data elements and their definitions can be found in the July 31, 1985, Federal Register (Vol. 5Ø, No, 147), pp. 31Ø38-4Ø.

Since that time the application of the UHDDS definitions has been expanded to include all non-outpatient settings (acute care, short term, long term care and psychiatric hospitals; home health agencies; rehab facilities; nursing homes, etc).

The following guidelines are to be applied in designating "other diagnoses" when neither the Alphabetic Index nor the Tabular List in ICD-1Ø-CM provide direction. The listing of the diagnoses in the patient record is the responsibility of the attending provider.

A. Previous conditions

If the provider has included a diagnosis in the final diagnostic statement, such as the discharge summary or the face sheet, it should ordinarily be coded. Some providers include in the diagnostic statement resolved conditions or diagnoses and status-post procedures from previous admission that have no bearing on the current stay. Such conditions are not to be reported and are coded only if required by hospital policy.

However, history codes (categories Z8Ø-Z87) may be used as secondary codes if the historical condition or family history has an impact on current care or influences treatment.

B. Abnormal findings

Abnormal findings (laboratory, x-ray, pathologic, and other diagnostic results) are not coded and reported unless the provider indicates their clinical significance. If the findings are outside the normal range and the attending provider has ordered other tests to evaluate the condition or prescribed treatment, it is appropriate to ask the provider whether the abnormal finding should be added.

Please note: This differs from the coding practices in the outpatient setting for coding encounters for diagnostic tests that have been interpreted by a provider.

C. Uncertain Diagnosis

If the diagnosis documented at the time of discharge is qualified as "probable", "suspected", "likely", "questionable", "possible", or "still to be ruled out" or other similar terms indicating uncertainty, code the condition as if it existed or was established. The bases for these guidelines are the diagnostic workup, arrangements for further workup or observation, and initial therapeutic approach that correspond most closely with the established diagnosis.

Note: This guideline is applicable only to inpatient admissions to short-term, acute, long-term care and psychiatric hospitals.

Section IV. Diagnostic Coding and Reporting Guidelines for Outpatient Services

These coding guidelines for outpatient diagnoses have been approved for use by hospitals/ providers in coding and reporting hospital-based outpatient services and provider-based office visits.

Information about the use of certain abbreviations, punctuation, symbols, and other conventions used in the ICD-1Ø-CM Tabular List (code numbers and titles), can be found in Section IA of these guidelines, under "Conventions Used in the Tabular List." Information about the correct sequence to use in finding a code is also described in Section I.

The terms encounter and visit are often used interchangeably in describing outpatient service contacts and, therefore, appear together in these guidelines without distinguishing one from the other.

Though the conventions and general guidelines apply to all settings, coding guidelines for outpatient and provider reporting of diagnoses will vary in a number of instances from those for inpatient diagnoses, recognizing that:

The Uniform Hospital Discharge Data Set (UHDDS) definition of principal diagnosis applies only to inpatients in acute, short-term, long-term care and psychiatric hospitals.

Coding guidelines for inconclusive diagnoses (probable, suspected, rule out, etc.) were developed for inpatient reporting and do not apply to outpatients.

A. Selection of first-listed condition

In the outpatient setting, the term first-listed diagnosis is used in lieu of principal diagnosis.

In determining the first-listed diagnosis the coding conventions of ICD-1Ø-CM, as well as the general and disease specific guidelines take precedence over the outpatient guidelines.

Diagnoses often are not established at the time of the initial encounter/visit. It may take two or more visits before the diagnosis is confirmed.

The most critical rule involves beginning the search for the correct code assignment through the Alphabetic Index. Never begin searching initially in the Tabular List as this will lead to coding errors.

1. **Outpatient surgery**
   When a patient presents for outpatient surgery (same day surgery), code the reason for the surgery as the first-listed

diagnosis (reason for the encounter), even if the surgery is not performed due to a contraindication.

2. **Observation stay**

When a patient is admitted for observation for a medical condition, assign a code for the medical condition as the first-listed diagnosis.

When a patient presents for outpatient surgery and develops complications requiring admission to observation, code the reason for the surgery as the first reported diagnosis (reason for the encounter), followed by codes for the complications as secondary diagnoses.

B. Codes from AØØ.Ø through T88.9, ZØØ-Z99

The appropriate code(s) from AØØ.Ø through T88.9, ZØØ-Z99 must be used to identify diagnoses, symptoms, conditions, problems, complaints, or other reason(s) for the encounter/visit.

C. Accurate reporting of ICD-1Ø-CM diagnosis codes

For accurate reporting of ICD-1Ø-CM diagnosis codes, the documentation should describe the patient's condition, using terminology which includes specific diagnoses as well as symptoms, problems, or reasons for the encounter. There are ICD-1Ø-CM codes to describe all of these.

D. Codes that describe symptoms and signs

Codes that describe symptoms and signs, as opposed to diagnoses, are acceptable for reporting purposes when a diagnosis has not been established (confirmed) by the provider. Chapter 18 of ICD-1Ø-CM, Symptoms, Signs, and Abnormal Clinical and Laboratory Findings Not Elsewhere Classified (codes RØØ-R99) contain many, but not all codes for symptoms.

E. Encounters for circumstances other than a disease or injury

ICD-1Ø-CM provides codes to deal with encounters for circumstances other than a disease or injury. The Factors Influencing Health Status and Contact with Health Services codes (ZØØ-Z99) are provided to deal with occasions when circumstances other than a disease or injury are recorded as diagnosis or problems.

See Section I.C.21. Factors influencing health status and contact with health services.

F. Level of Detail in Coding

1. **ICD-1Ø-CM codes with *3, 4, 5, 6 or 7 characters***

ICD-1Ø-CM is composed of codes with 3, 4, 5, 6 or 7 characters. Codes with three characters are included in ICD-1Ø-CM as the heading of a category of codes that may be further subdivided by the use of fourth, fifth, sixth or seventh characters to provide greater specificity.

2. **Use of full number of *characters* required for a code**

A three-**character** code is to be used only if it is not further subdivided. A code is invalid if it has not been coded to the full number of characters required for that code, including the 7th character extension, if applicable.

G. ICD-1Ø-CM code for the diagnosis, condition, problem, or other reason for encounter/visit

List first the ICD-1Ø-CM code for the diagnosis, condition, problem, or other reason for encounter/visit shown in the medical record to be chiefly responsible for the services provided. List additional codes that describe any coexisting conditions. In some cases the first-listed diagnosis may be a symptom when a diagnosis has not been established (confirmed) by the physician.

H. Uncertain diagnosis

Do not code diagnoses documented as "probable", "suspected," "questionable," "rule out," or "working diagnosis" or other similar terms indicating uncertainty. Rather, code the condition(s) to the highest degree of certainty for that encounter/visit, such as symptoms, signs, abnormal test results, or other reason for the visit.

Please note: This differs from the coding practices used by short-term, acute care, long-term care and psychiatric hospitals.

I. Chronic diseases

Chronic diseases treated on an ongoing basis may be coded and reported as many times as the patient receives treatment and care for the condition(s)

J. Code all documented conditions that coexist

Code all documented conditions that coexist at the time of the encounter/visit, and require or affect patient care treatment or management. Do not code conditions that were previously treated and no longer exist. However, history codes (categories Z8Ø-Z87) may be used as secondary codes if the historical condition or family history has an impact on current care or influences treatment.

K. Patients receiving diagnostic services only

For patients receiving diagnostic services only during an encounter/visit, sequence first the diagnosis, condition, problem, or other reason for encounter/visit shown in the medical record to be chiefly responsible for the outpatient services provided during the encounter/visit. Codes for other diagnoses (e.g., chronic conditions) may be sequenced as additional diagnoses.

For encounters for routine laboratory/radiology testing in the absence of any signs, symptoms, or associated diagnosis, assign ZØ1.89, Encounter for other specified special examinations. If routine testing is performed during the same encounter as a test to evaluate a sign, symptom, or diagnosis, it is appropriate to assign both the **Z** code and the code describing the reason for the non-routine test.

For outpatient encounters for diagnostic tests that have been interpreted by a physician, and the final report is available at the time of coding, code any confirmed or definitive diagnosis(es) documented in the interpretation. Do not code related signs and symptoms as additional diagnoses.

Please note: This differs from the coding practice in the hospital inpatient setting regarding abnormal findings on test results.

L. Patients receiving therapeutic services only

For patients receiving therapeutic services only during an encounter/visit, sequence first the diagnosis, condition, problem, or other reason for encounter/visit shown in the medical record to be chiefly responsible for the outpatient services provided during the encounter/visit. Codes for other diagnoses (e.g., chronic conditions) may be sequenced as additional diagnoses.

The only exception to this rule is that when the primary reason for the admission/encounter is chemotherapy or radiation therapy, the appropriate Z code for the service is listed first, and the diagnosis or problem for which the service is being performed listed second.

M. Patients receiving preoperative evaluations only

For patients receiving preoperative evaluations only, sequence first a code from subcategory ZØ1.81, Encounter for pre-procedural examinations, to describe the pre-op consultations. Assign a code for the condition to describe the reason for the surgery as an additional diagnosis. Code also any findings related to the pre-op evaluation.

N. Ambulatory surgery

For ambulatory surgery, code the diagnosis for which the surgery was performed. If the postoperative diagnosis is known to be different from the preoperative diagnosis at the time the diagnosis is confirmed, select the postoperative diagnosis for coding, since it is the most definitive.

O. Routine outpatient prenatal visits

See Section I.C.15. Routine outpatient prenatal visits.

P. Encounters for general medical examinations with abnormal findings

The subcategories for encounters for general medical examinations, ZØØ.Ø-, provide codes for with and without abnormal findings. Should a general medical examination result in an abnormal finding, the code for general medical examination with abnormal finding should be assigned as the first-listed diagnosis. A secondary code for the abnormal finding should also be coded.

Q. Encounters for routine health screenings

See Section I.C.21. Factors influencing health status and contact with health services, Screening

Appendix I. Present on Admission Reporting Guidelines

(Effective with 2011 update)

Introduction

These guidelines are to be used as a supplement to the *ICD-10-CM Official Guidelines for Coding and Reporting* to facilitate the assignment of the Present on Admission (POA) indicator for each diagnosis and external cause of injury code reported on claim forms (UB-04 and 837 Institutional).

These guidelines are not intended to replace any guidelines in the main body of the *ICD-10-CM Official Guidelines for Coding and Reporting.* The POA guidelines are not intended to provide guidance on when a condition should be coded, but rather, how to apply the POA indicator to the final set of diagnosis codes that have been assigned in accordance with Sections I, II, and III of the official coding guidelines. Subsequent to the assignment of the ICD-10-CM codes, the POA indicator should then be assigned to those conditions that have been coded.

As stated in the Introduction to the *ICD-10-CM Official Guidelines for Coding and Reporting,* a joint effort between the healthcare provider and the coder is essential to achieve complete and accurate documentation, code assignment, and reporting of diagnoses and procedures. The importance of consistent, complete documentation in the medical record cannot be overemphasized. Medical record documentation from any provider involved in the care and treatment of the patient may be used to support the determination of whether a condition was present on admission or not. In the context of the official coding guidelines, the term "provider" means a physician or any qualified healthcare practitioner who is legally accountable for establishing the patient's diagnosis.

These guidelines are not a substitute for the provider's clinical judgment as to the determination of whether a condition was/was not present on admission. The provider should be queried regarding issues related to the linking of signs/symptoms, timing of test results, and the timing of findings.

General Reporting Requirements

All claims involving inpatient admissions to general acute care hospitals or other facilities that are subject to a law or regulation mandating collection of present on admission information.

Present on admission is defined as present at the time the order for inpatient admission occurs -- conditions that develop during an outpatient encounter, including emergency department, observation, or outpatient surgery, are considered as present on admission.

POA indicator is assigned to principal and secondary diagnoses (as defined in Section II of the Official Guidelines for Coding and Reporting) and the external cause of injury codes.

Issues related to inconsistent, missing, conflicting or unclear documentation must still be resolved by the provider.

If a condition would not be coded and reported based on UHDDS definitions and current official coding guidelines, then the POA indicator would not be reported.

Reporting Options

- Y – Yes
- N – No
- U – Unknown
- W – Clinically undetermined
- Unreported/Not used (or "1" for Medicare usage) – (Exempt from POA reporting)

Reporting Definitions

- Y – present at the time of inpatient admission
- N – not present at the time of inpatient admission
- U – documentation is insufficient to determine if condition is present on admission
- W – provider is unable to clinically determine whether condition was present on admission or not

Timeframe for POA Identification and Documentation

There is no required timeframe as to when a provider (per the definition of "provider" used in these guidelines) must identify or document a condition to be present on admission. In some clinical situations, it may not be possible for a provider to make a definitive diagnosis (or a condition may not be recognized or reported by the patient) for a period of time after admission. In some cases it may be several days before the provider arrives at a definitive diagnosis. This does not mean that the condition was not present on admission. Determination of whether the condition was present on admission or not will be based on the applicable POA guideline as identified in this document, or on the provider's best clinical judgment.

If at the time of code assignment the documentation is unclear as to whether a condition was present on admission or not, it is appropriate to query the provider for clarification.

Assigning the POA Indicator

Condition is on the "Exempt from Reporting" list

Leave the "present on admission" field blank if the condition is on the list of ICD-10-CM codes for which this field is not applicable. This is the only circumstance in which the field may be left blank.

POA Explicitly Documented

Assign "Y" for any condition the provider explicitly documents as being present on admission.

Assign "N" for any condition the provider explicitly documents as not present at the time of admission.

Conditions diagnosed prior to inpatient admission

Assign "Y" for conditions that were diagnosed prior to admission (example: hypertension, diabetes mellitus, asthma).

Conditions diagnosed during the admission but clearly present before admission

Assign "Y" for conditions diagnosed during the admission that were clearly present but not diagnosed until after admission occurred.

Diagnoses subsequently confirmed after admission are considered present on admission if at the time of admission they are documented as suspected, possible, rule out, differential diagnosis, or constitute an underlying cause of a symptom that is present at the time of admission.

Condition develops during outpatient encounter prior to inpatient admission

Assign "Y" for any condition that develops during an outpatient encounter prior to a written order for inpatient admission.

Documentation does not indicate whether condition was present on admission

Assign "U" when the medical record documentation is unclear as to whether the condition was present on admission. "U" should not be routinely assigned and used only in very limited circumstances. Coders are encouraged to query the providers when the documentation is unclear.

Documentation states that it cannot be determined whether the condition was or was not present on admission

Assign "W" when the medical record documentation indicates that it cannot be clinically determined whether or not the condition was present on admission.

Chronic condition with acute exacerbation during the admission

If a single code identifies both the chronic condition and the acute exacerbation, see POA guidelines pertaining to combination codes.

If a single code only identifies the chronic condition and not the acute exacerbation (e.g., acute exacerbation of chronic leukemia), assign "Y."

Conditions documented as possible, probable, suspected, or rule out at the time of discharge

If the final diagnosis contains a possible, probable, suspected, or rule out diagnosis, and this diagnosis was based on signs, symptoms or clinical findings suspected at the time of inpatient admission, assign "Y."

If the final diagnosis contains a possible, probable, suspected, or rule out diagnosis, and this diagnosis was based on signs, symptoms or clinical findings that were not present on admission, assign "N".

Conditions documented as impending or threatened at the time of discharge

If the final diagnosis contains an impending or threatened diagnosis, and this diagnosis is based on symptoms or clinical findings that were present on admission, assign "Y".

If the final diagnosis contains an impending or threatened diagnosis, and this diagnosis is based on symptoms or clinical findings that were not present on admission, assign "N".

Acute and Chronic Conditions

Assign "Y" for acute conditions that are present at time of admission and N for acute conditions that are not present at time of admission.

Assign "Y" for chronic conditions, even though the condition may not be diagnosed until after admission.

If a single code identifies both an acute and chronic condition, see the POA guidelines for combination codes.

Combination Codes

Assign "N" if any part of the combination code was not present on admission (e.g., COPD with acute exacerbation and the exacerbation was not present on admission; gastric ulcer that does not start bleeding until after admission; asthma patient develops status asthmaticus after admission).

Assign "Y" if all parts of the combination code were present on admission (e.g., patient with acute prostatitis admitted with hematuria).

If the final diagnosis includes comparative or contrasting diagnoses, and both were present, or suspected, at the time of admission, assign "Y".

For infection codes that include the causal organism, assign "Y" if the infection (or signs of the infection) was present on admission, even though the culture results may not be known until after admission (e.g., patient is admitted with pneumonia and the provider documents pseudomonas as the causal organism a few days later).

Same Diagnosis Code for Two or More Conditions

When the same ICD-10-CM diagnosis code applies to two or more conditions during the same encounter (e.g. two separate conditions classified to the same ICD-10-CM diagnosis code):

> Assign "Y" if all conditions represented by the single ICD-10-CM code were present on admission (e.g. bilateral unspecified age-related cataracts).
>
> Assign "N" if any of the conditions represented by the single ICD-10-CM code was not present on admission (e.g. traumatic secondary and recurrent hemorrhage and seroma is assigned to a single code T79.2, but only one of the conditions was present on admission).

Obstetrical conditions

Whether or not the patient delivers during the current hospitalization does not affect assignment of the POA indicator. The determining factor for POA assignment is whether the pregnancy complication or obstetrical condition described by the code was present at the time of admission or not.

If the pregnancy complication or obstetrical condition was present on admission (e.g., patient admitted in preterm labor), assign "Y".

If the pregnancy complication or obstetrical condition was not present on admission (e.g., 2nd degree laceration during delivery, postpartum hemorrhage that occurred during current hospitalization, fetal distress develops after admission), assign "N".

If the obstetrical code includes more than one diagnosis and any of the diagnoses identified by the code were not present on admission assign "N". (e.g., Category O11, Pre-existing hypertension with pre-eclampsia).

Perinatal conditions

Newborns are not considered to be admitted until after birth. Therefore, any condition present at birth or that developed in utero is considered present at admission and should be assigned "Y". This includes conditions that occur during delivery (e.g., injury during delivery, meconium aspiration, exposure to streptococcus B in the vaginal canal).

Congenital conditions and anomalies

Assign "Y" for congenital conditions and anomalies except for **categories** Q00-Q99, **Congenital anomalies,** which are **on the** exempt **list.** Congenital conditions are always considered present on admission.

External cause of injury codes

Assign "Y" for any external cause code representing an external cause of morbidity that occurred prior to inpatient admission (e.g., patient fell out of bed at home, patient fell out of bed in emergency room prior to admission).

Assign "N" for any external cause code representing an external cause of morbidity that occurred during inpatient hospitalization (e.g., patient fell out of hospital bed during hospital stay, patient experienced an adverse reaction to a medication administered after inpatient admission).

Categories and Codes Exempt from Diagnosis Present on Admission Requirement

Note: "Diagnosis present on admission" for these code categories are exempt because they represent circumstances regarding the healthcare encounter or factors influencing health status that do not represent a current disease or injury or are always present on admission.

B90–B94	Sequelae of infectious and parasitic diseases
E64	Sequelae of malnutrition and other nutritional deficiences
I25.2	Old myocardial infarction
I69	Sequelae of cerebrovascular disease
O09	Supervision of high risk pregnancy
O66.5	Attempted application of vacuum extractor and forceps
O80	Encounter for full-term uncomplicated delivery
O94	Sequelae of complication of pregnancy, childbirth, and the puerperium
P00	Newborn (suspected to be) affected by maternal conditions that may be unrelated to present pregnancy
Q00 – Q99	Congenital malformations, deformations and chromosomal abnormalities
S00-T88.9	Injury, poisoning and certain other consequences of external causes with 7th character representing subsequent encounter or sequela
V00.121	Fall from non-in-line roller-skates
V00.131	Fall from skateboard
V00.141	Fall from scooter (nonmotorized)
V00.311	Fall from snowboard
V00.321	Fall from snow-skis
V40-V49	Car occupant injured in transport accident
V80-V89	Other land transport accidents
V90-V94	Water transport accidents
V95-V97	Air and space transport accidents
W03	Other fall on same level due to collision with another person
W09	Fall on and from playground equipment
W15	Fall from cliff
W17.0	Fall into well
W17.1	Fall into storm drain or manhole
W18.01	Striking against sports equipment with subsequent fall
W20.8	Other cause of strike by thrown, projected or falling object
W21	Striking against or struck by sports equipment
W30	Contact with agricultural machinery
W31	Contact with other and unspecified machinery
W32-W34	Accidental handgun discharge and malfunction

W35- W4Ø	Exposure to inanimate mechanical forces
W52	Crushed, pushed or stepped on by crowd or human stampede
W89	Exposure to man-made visible and ultraviolet light
XØ2	Exposure to controlled fire in building or structure
XØ3	Exposure to controlled fire, not in building or structure
XØ4	Exposure to ignition of highly flammable material
X52	Prolonged stay in weightless environment
X71-X83	Intentional self-harm
Y21	Drowning and submersion, undetermined intent
Y22	Handgun discharge, undetermined intent
Y23	Rifle, shotgun and larger firearm discharge, undetermined intent
Y24	Other and unspecified firearm discharge, undetermined intent
Y3Ø	Falling, jumping or pushed from a high place, undetermined intent
Y35	Legal intervention
Y36	Operations of war
Y37	Military operations
Y38	Terrorism
Y92	Place of occurrence of the external cause
Y93	Activity code
Y99	External cause status
ZØØ	Encounter for general examination without complaint, suspected or reported diagnosis
ZØ1	Encounter for other special examination without complaint, suspected or reported diagnosis
ZØ2	Encounter for administrative examination
ZØ3	Encounter for medical observation for suspected diseases and conditions ruled out
ZØ8	Encounter for follow-up examination following completed treatment for malignant neoplasm
ZØ9	Encounter for follow-up examination after completed treatment for conditions other than malignant neoplasm
Z11	Encounter for screening for infectious and parasitic diseases
Z11.8	Encounter for screening for other infectious and parasitic diseases
Z12	Encounter for screening for malignant neoplasms
Z13	Encounter for screening for other diseases and disorders
Z13.4	Encounter for screening for certain developmental disorders in childhood
Z13.5	Encounter for screening for eye and ear disorders
Z13.6	Encounter for screening for cardiovascular disorders
Z13.83	Encounter for screening for respiratory disorder NEC
Z13.89	Encounter for screening for other disorder
Z14	Genetic carrier
Z15	Genetic susceptibility to disease
Z17	Estrogen receptor status
Z18	Retained foreign body fragments
Z22	Carrier of infectious disease
Z23	Encounter for immunization
Z28	Immunization not carried out and underimmunization status
Z28.3	Underimmunization status
Z3Ø	Encounter for contraceptive management
Z31	Encounter for procreative management
Z34	Encounter for supervision of normal pregnancy
Z36	Encounter for antenatal screening of mother
Z37	Outcome of delivery
Z38	Liveborn infants according to place of birth and type of delivery
Z39	Encounter for maternal postpartum care and examination
Z41	Encounter for procedures for purposes other than remedying health state
Z42	Encounter for plastic and reconstructive surgery following medical procedure or healed injury
Z43	Encounter for attention to artificial openings
Z44	Encounter for fitting and adjustment of external prosthetic device
Z45	Encounter for adjustment and management of implanted device
Z46	Encounter for fitting and adjustment of other devices
Z47.8	Encounter for other orthopedic aftercare
Z49	Encounter for care involving renal dialysis
Z51	Encounter for other aftercare
Z51.5	Encounter for palliative care
Z51.8	Encounter for other specified aftercare
Z52	Donors of organs and tissues
Z59	Problems related to housing and economic circumstances
Z63	Other problems related to primary support groupincluding family circumstances
Z65	Problems related to other psychosocial circumstances
Z65.8	Other specified problems related to psychosocial circumstances
Z67.1-Z67.9	Blood type
Z68	Body mass index (BMI)
Z72	Problems related to lifestyle
Z74.Ø1	Bed confinement status
Z76	Persons encountering health services in other circumstances
Z77.11Ø-Z77.128	Environmental pollution and hazards in the physical environment
Z78	Other specified health status
Z79	Long term (current) drug therapy
Z8Ø	Family history of primary malignant neoplasm
Z81	Family history of mental and behavioral disorders
Z82	Family history of certain disabilities and chronic diseases (leading to disablement)
Z83	Family history of other specific disorders
Z84	Family history of other conditions
Z85	Personal history of primary malignant neoplasm
Z86	Personal history of certain other diseases
Z87	Personal history of other diseases and conditions
Z87.828	Personal history of other (healed) physical injury and trauma
Z87.891	Personal history of nicotine dependence
Z88	Allergy status to drugs, medicaments and biological substances
Z89	Acquired absence of limb
Z9Ø.71Ø	Acquired absence of both cervix and uterus
Z91.Ø	Allergy status, other than to drugs and biological substances
Z91.4	Personal history of psychological trauma, not elsewhere classified
Z91.5	Personal history of self-harm
Z91.8	Other specified risk factors, not elsewhere classified
Z92	Personal history of medical treatment
Z93	Artificial opening status
Z94	Transplanted organ and tissue status
Z95	Presence of cardiac and vascular implants and grafts
Z97	Presence of other devices
Z98	Other postprocedural states
Z99	Dependence on enabling machines and devices, not elsewhere classified

ICD-1Ø-CM Index to Diseases and Injuries

A

- **Aarskog's syndrome** Q87.1
- **Abandonment** — *see* Maltreatment
- **Abasia** (-astasia) (hysterical) F44.4
- **Abderhalden-Kaufmann-Lignac syndrome** (cystinosis) E72.Ø4
- **Abdomen, abdominal** (*see also* condition)
  - acute R1Ø.Ø
  - angina K55.1
  - muscle deficiency syndrome Q79.4
- **Abdominalgia** — *see* Pain, abdominal
- **Abduction contracture, hip or other joint** — *see* Contraction, joint
- **Aberrant** (congenital) (*see also* Malposition, congenital)
  - adrenal gland Q89.1
  - artery (peripheral) Q27.8
    - basilar NEC Q28.1
    - cerebral Q28.3
    - coronary Q24.5
    - digestive system Q27.8
    - eye Q15.8
    - lower limb Q27.8
    - precerebral Q28.1
    - pulmonary Q25.79
    - renal Q27.2
    - retina Q14.1
    - specified site NEC Q27.8
    - subclavian Q27.8
    - upper limb Q27.8
    - vertebral Q28.1
  - breast Q83.8
  - endocrine gland NEC Q89.2
  - hepatic duct Q44.5
  - pancreas Q45.3
  - parathyroid gland Q89.2
  - pituitary gland Q89.2
  - sebaceous glands, mucous membrane, mouth, congenital Q38.6
  - spleen Q89.Ø9
  - subclavian artery Q27.8
  - thymus (gland) Q89.2
  - thyroid gland Q89.2
  - vein (peripheral) NEC Q27.8
    - cerebral Q28.3
    - digestive system Q27.8
    - lower limb Q27.8
    - precerebral Q28.1
    - specified site NEC Q27.8
    - upper limb Q27.8
- **Aberration**
  - distantial — *see* Disturbance, visual
  - mental F99
- **Abetalipoproteinemia** E78.6
- **Abiotrophy** R68.89
- **Ablatio, ablation**
  - retinae — *see* Detachment, retina
- **Ablepharia, ablepharon** Q1Ø.3
- **Abnormal, abnormality, abnormalities** (*see also* Anomaly)
  - acid-base balance (mixed) E87.4
  - albumin R77.Ø
  - alphafetoprotein R77.2
  - alveolar ridge KØ8.9
  - anatomical relationship Q89.9
  - apertures, congenital, diaphragm Q79.1
  - auditory perception H93.29-
    - diplacusis — *see* Diplacusis
    - hyperacusis — *see* Hyperacusis
    - recruitment — *see* Recruitment, auditory
    - threshold shift — *see* Shift, auditory threshold
  - autosomes Q99.9
    - fragile site Q95.5
  - basal metabolic rate R94.8
  - biosynthesis, testicular androgen E29.1
  - bleeding time R79.1
  - blood-gas level R79.81

Abnormal, abnormality, abnormalities — *continued*

  - blood level (of)
    - cobalt R79.Ø
    - copper R79.Ø
    - iron R79.Ø
    - lithium R78.89
    - magnesium R79.Ø
    - mineral NEC R79.Ø
    - zinc R79.Ø
  - blood pressure
    - elevated RØ3.Ø
    - low reading (nonspecific) RØ3.1
  - blood sugar R73.Ø9
  - bowel sounds R19.15
    - absent R19.11
    - hyperactive R19.12
  - brain scan R94.Ø2
  - breathing RØ6.9
  - caloric test R94.138
  - cerebrospinal fluid R83.9
    - cytology R83.6
    - drug level R83.2
    - enzyme level R83.Ø
    - hormones R83.1
    - immunology R83.4
    - microbiology R83.5
    - nonmedicinal level R83.3
    - specified type NEC R83.8
  - chemistry, blood R79.9
    - C-reactive protein R79.82
    - drugs — *see* Findings, abnormal, in blood
    - gas level R79.81
    - minerals R79.Ø
    - pancytopenia D61.818
    - specified NEC R79.89
    - PTT R79.1
    - toxins — *see* Findings, abnormal, in blood
  - chest sounds (friction) (rales) RØ9.89
  - chromosome, chromosomal Q99.9
    - with more than three X chromosomes, female Q97.1
    - analysis result R89.8
      - bronchial washings R84.8
      - cerebrospinal fluid R83.8
      - cervix uteri NEC R87.89
      - nasal secretions R84.8
      - nipple discharge R89.8
      - peritoneal fluid R85.89
      - pleural fluid R84.8
      - prostatic secretions R86.8
      - saliva R85.89
      - seminal fluid R86.8
      - sputum R84.8
      - synovial fluid R89.8
      - throat scrapings R84.8
      - vagina R87.89
      - vulva R87.89
      - wound secretions R89.8
    - dicentric replacement Q93.2
    - ring replacement Q93.2
    - sex Q99.8
      - female phenotype Q97.9
        - specified NEC Q97.8
      - male phenotype Q98.9
        - specified NEC Q98.8
      - structural male Q98.6
    - specified NEC Q99.8
  - clinical findings NEC R68.89
  - coagulation D68.9
    - newborn, transient P61.6
    - profile R79.1
    - time R79.1
  - communication — *see* Fistula
  - conjunctiva, vascular H11.41-
  - coronary artery Q24.5
  - cortisol-binding globulin E27.8
  - course, eustachian tube Q17.8
  - creatinine clearance R94.4

Abnormal, abnormality, abnormalities — *continued*

  - cytology
    - anus R85.619
      - atypical squamous cells cannot exclude high grade squamous intraepithelial lesion (ASC-H) R85.611
      - atypical squamous cells of undetermined significance (ASC-US) R85.61Ø
      - cytologic evidence of malignancy R85.614
      - high grade squamous intraepithelial lesion (HGSIL) R85.613
      - human papillomavirus (HPV) DNA test
        - high risk positive R85.81
        - low risk postive R85.82
      - inadequate smear R85.615
      - low grade squamous intraepithelial lesion (LGSIL) R85.612
      - satisfactory anal smear but lacking transformation zone R85.616
      - specified NEC R85.618
      - unsatisfactory smear R85.615
    - female genital organs — *see* Abnormal, Papanicolaou (smear)
  - dark adaptation curve H53.61
  - dentofacial NEC — *see* Anomaly, dentofacial
  - development, developmental Q89.9
    - central nervous system QØ7.9
  - diagnostic imaging
    - abdomen, abdominal region NEC R93.5
    - biliary tract R93.2
    - breast R92.8
    - central nervous system NEC R9Ø.89
    - cerebrovascular NEC R9Ø.89
    - coronary circulation R93.1
    - digestive tract NEC R93.3
    - gastrointestinal (tract) R93.3
    - genitourinary organs R93.8
    - head R93.Ø
    - heart R93.1
    - intrathoracic organ NEC R93.8
    - limbs R93.6
    - liver R93.2
    - lung (field) R91.8
    - musculoskeletal system NEC R93.7
    - retroperitoneum R93.5
    - site specified NEC R93.8
    - skin and subcutaneous tissue R93.8
    - skull R93.Ø
    - urinary organs R93.4
  - direction, teeth, fully erupted M26.3Ø
  - ear ossicles, acquired NEC H74.39-
    - ankylosis — *see* Ankylosis, ear ossicles
    - discontinuity — *see* Discontinuity, ossicles, ear
    - partial loss — *see* Loss, ossicles, ear (partial)
  - Ebstein Q22.5
  - echocardiogram R93.1
  - echoencephalogram R9Ø.81
  - echogram — *see* Abnormal, diagnostic imaging
  - electrocardiogram [ECG] [EKG] R94.31
  - electroencephalogram [EEG] R94.Ø1
  - electrolyte — *see* Imbalance, electrolyte
  - electromyogram [EMG] R94.131
  - electro-oculogram [EOG] R94.11Ø
  - electrophysiological intracardiac studies R94.39
  - electroretinogram [ERG] R94.111
  - erythrocytes
    - congenital, with perinatal jaundice D58.9
  - feces (color) (contents) (mucus) R19.5
  - finding — *see* Findings, abnormal, without diagnosis
  - fluid
    - amniotic — *see* Abnormal, specimen, specified
    - cerebrospinal — *see* Abnormal, cerebrospinal fluid
    - peritoneal — *see* Abnormal, specimen, digestive organs
    - pleural — *see* Abnormal, specimen, respiratory organs

Abnormal, abnormality, abnormalities — *continued*
- fluid — *continued*
  - synovial — *see* Abnormal, specimen, specified
  - thorax (bronchial washings) (pleural fluid) — *see* Abnormal, specimen, respiratory organs
  - vaginal — *see* Abnormal, specimen, female genital organs
- form
  - teeth KØØ.2
  - uterus — *see* Anomaly, uterus
- function studies
  - auditory R94.12Ø
  - bladder R94.8
  - brain R94.Ø9
  - cardiovascular R94.3Ø
  - ear R94.128
  - endocrine NEC R94.7
  - eye NEC R94.118
  - kidney R94.4
  - liver R94.5
  - nervous system
    - central NEC R94.Ø9
    - peripheral NEC R94.138
  - pancreas R94.8
  - placenta R94.8
  - pulmonary R94.2
  - special senses NEC R94.128
  - spleen R94.8
  - thyroid R94.6
  - vestibular R94.121
- gait — *see* Gait
  - hysterical F44.4
- gastrin secretion E16.4
- globulin R77.1
  - cortisol-binding E27.8
  - thyroid-binding EØ7.89
- glomerular, minor (*see also* NØØ-NØ7 with fourth character .Ø) NØ5.Ø
- glucagon secretion E16.3
- glucose tolerance (test) (non-fasting) R73.Ø9
- gravitational (G) forces or states (effect of) T75.81
- hair (color) (shaft) L67.9
  - specified NEC L67.8
- hard tissue formation in pulp (dental) KØ4.3
- head movement R25.Ø
- heart
  - rate RØØ.9
    - specified NEC RØØ.8
  - shadow R93.1
  - sounds NEC RØ1.2
- hemoglobin (disease) (*see also* Disease, hemoglobin) D58.2
  - trait — *see* Trait, hemoglobin, abnormal
- histology NEC R89.7
- immunological findings R89.4
  - in serum R76.9
    - specified NEC R76.8
- increase in appetite R63.2
- involuntary movement — *see* Abnormal, movement, involuntary
- jaw closure M26.51
- karyotype R89.8
- kidney function test R94.4
- knee jerk R29.2
- leukocyte (cell) (differential) NEC D72.9
- liver
- loss of
  - height R29.89Ø
  - weight R63.4
- mammogram NEC R92.8
  - calcification (calculus) R92.1
  - microcalcification R92.Ø
- Mantoux test R76.11
- movement (disorder) (*see also* Disorder, movement)
  - head R25.Ø
  - involuntary R25.9
    - fasciculation R25.3
    - of head R25.Ø
    - spasm R25.2
    - specified type NEC R25.8
    - tremor R25.1
- myoglobin (Aberdeen) (Annapolis) R89.7

Abnormal, abnormality, abnormalities — *continued*
- neonatal screening PØ9
- oculomotor study R94.113
- palmar creases Q82.8
- Papanicolaou (smear)
  - anus R85.619
    - atypical squamous cells cannot exclude high grade squamous intraepithelial lesion (ASC-H) R85.611
    - atypical squamous cells of undetermined significance (ASC-US) R85.61Ø
    - cytologic evidence of malignancy R85.614
    - high grade squamous intraepithelial lesion (HGSIL) R85.613
    - human papillomavirus (HPV) DNA test
      - high risk positive R85.81
      - low risk postive R85.82
    - inadequate smear R85.615
    - low grade squamous intraepithelial lesion (LGSIL) R85.612
    - satisfactory anal smear but lacking transformation zone R85.616
    - specified NEC R85.618
    - unsatisfactory smear R85.615
  - bronchial washings R84.6
  - cerebrospinal fluid R83.6
  - cervix R87.619
    - atypical squamous cells cannot exclude high grade squamous intraepithelial lesion (ASC-H) R87.611
    - atypical squamous cells of undetermined significance (ASC-US) R87.61Ø
    - cytologic evidence of malignancy R87.614
    - high grade squamous intraepithelial lesion (HGSIL) R87.613
    - inadequate smear R87.615
    - low grade squamous intraepithelial lesion (LGSIL) R87.612 l
    - non-atypical endometrial cells R87.618
    - satisfactory cervical smear but lacking transformation zone R87.616
    - specified NEC R87.618
    - thin preparaton R87.619
    - unsatisfactory smear R87.615
  - nasal secretions R84.6
  - nipple discharge R89.6
  - peritoneal fluid R85.69
  - pleural fluid R84.6
  - prostatic secretions R86.6
  - saliva R85.69
  - seminal fluid R86.6
  - sites NEC R89.6
  - sputum R84.6
  - synovial fluid R89.6
  - throat scrapings R84.6
  - vagina R87.629
    - atypical squamous cells cannot exclude high grade squamous intraepithelial lesion (ASC-H) R87.621
    - atypical squamous cells of undetermined significance (ASC-US) R87.62Ø
    - cytologic evidence of malignancy R87.624
    - high grade squamous intraepithelial lesion (HGSIL) R87.623
    - inadequate smear R87.625
    - low grade squamous intraepithelial lesion (LGSIL) R87.622
    - specified NEC R87.628
    - thin preparation R87.629
    - unsatisfactory smear R87.625
  - vulva R87.69
  - wound secretions R89.6
- partial thromboplastin time (PTT) R79.1
- plantar reflex R29.2
- pelvis (bony) — *see* Deformity, pelvis
- percussion, chest (tympany) RØ9.89
- periods (grossly) — *see* Menstruation
- phonocardiogram R94.39
- plasma
  - protein R77.9
    - specified NEC R77.8
  - viscosity R7Ø.1
- pleural (folds) Q34.Ø

Abnormal, abnormality, abnormalities — *continued*
- posture R29.3
- product of conception OØ2.9
  - specified type NEC OØ2.89
- prothrombin time (PT) R79.1
- pulmonary
  - artery, congenital Q25.79
  - function, newborn P28.89
  - test results R94.2
- pulsations in neck RØØ.2
- pupillary H21.56-
  - function (reaction) (reflex) — *see* Anomaly, pupil, function
- radiological examination — *see* Abnormal, diagnostic imaging
- red blood cell(s) (morphology) (volume) R71.8
- reflex — *see* Reflex
- renal function test R94.4
- response to nerve stimulation R94.13Ø
- retinal correspondence H53.31
- retinal function study R94.111
- rhythm, heart (*see also* Arrhythmia)
- saliva — *see* Abnormal, specimen, digestive organs
- scan
  - kidney R94.4
  - liver R93.2
  - thyroid R94.6
- secretion
  - gastrin E16.4
  - glucagon E16.3
- semen, seminal fluid — *see* Abnormal, specimen, male genital organs
- serum level (of)
  - acid phosphatase R74.8
  - alkaline phosphatase R74.8
  - amylase R74.8
  - enzymes R74.9
    - specified NEC R74.8
  - lipase R74.8
  - triacylglycerol lipase R74.8
- shape
  - gravid uterus — *see* Anomaly, uterus
- sinus venosus Q21.1
- size, tooth, teeth KØØ.2
- spacing, tooth, teeth, fully erupted M26.3Ø
- specimen
  - digestive organs (peritoneal fluid) (saliva) R85.9
    - cytology R85.69
    - drug level R85.2
    - enzyme level R85.Ø
    - histology R85.7
    - hormones R85.1
    - immunology R85.4
    - microbiology R85.5
    - nonmedicinal level R85.3
    - specified type NEC R85.89
  - female genital organs (secretions) (smears) R87.9
    - cytology R87.69
      - cervix R87.619
        - inadequate (unsatisfactory) smear R87.615
        - human papillomavirus (HPV) DNA test
          - high risk positive R87.81Ø
          - low risk positive R87.82Ø
        - non-atypical endometrial cells R87.618
        - specified NEC R87.89
      - vagina R87.629
        - inadequate (unsatisfactory) smear R87.625
        - human papillomavirus (HPV) DNA test
          - high risk positive R87.811
          - low risk positive R87.821
      - vulva R87.69
    - drug level R87.2
    - enzyme level R87.Ø
    - histological R87.7
    - hormones R87.1
    - immunology R87.4
    - microbiology R87.5
    - nonmedicinal level R87.3
    - specified type NEC R87.89
  - male genital organs (prostatic secretions) (semen) R86.9

Abortion — *continued*
- induced — *continued*
  - complicated by — *continued*
    - urinary tract infection O04.88
    - venous complication NEC O04.85
      - embolism (air) (amniotic fluid) (blood clot) (fat) (pulmonary) (septic) (soap) O04.7
- missed O02.1
- spontaneous — *see* Abortion (complete) (spontaneous)
  - threatened O20.0
- threatened (spontaneous) O20.0
- tubal O00.1
- with retained products of conception — *see* Abortion, incomplete

Abortus fever A23.1

Aboulomania F60.7

Abrami's disease D59.8

Abramov-Fiedler myocarditis (acute isolated myocarditis) I40.1

Abrasion T14.8
- abdomen, abdominal (wall) S30.811
- alveolar process S00.512
- ankle S90.51-
- antecubital space — *see* Abrasion, elbow
- anus S30.817
- arm (upper) S40.81-
- auditory canal — *see* Abrasion, ear
- auricle — *see* Abrasion, ear
- axilla — *see* Abrasion, arm
- back, lower S30.810
- breast S20.11-
- brow S00.81
- buttock S30.810
- calf — *see* Abrasion, leg
- canthus — *see* Abrasion, eyelid
- cheek S00.81
  - internal S00.512
- chest wall — *see* Abrasion, thorax
- chin S00.81
- clitoris S30.814
- cornea S05.0-
- costal region — *see* Abrasion, thorax
- dental K03.1
- digit(s)
  - foot — *see* Abrasion, toe
  - hand — *see* Abrasion, finger
- ear S00.41-
- elbow S50.31-
- epididymis S30.813
- epigastric region S30.811
- epiglottis S10.11
- esophagus (thoracic) S27.818
  - cervical S10.11
- eyebrow — *see* Abrasion, eyelid
- eyelid S00.21-
- face S00.81
- finger(s) S60.41-
  - index S60.41-
  - little S60.41-
  - middle S60.41-
  - ring S60.41-
- flank S30.811
- foot (except toe(s) alone) S90.81-
  - toe — *see* Abrasion, toe
- forearm S50.81-
  - elbow only — *see* Abrasion, elbow
- forehead S00.81
- genital organs, external
  - female S30.816
  - male S30.815
- groin S30.811
- gum S00.512
- hand S60.51-
- head S00.91
  - ear — *see* Abrasion, ear
  - eyelid — *see* Abrasion, eyelid
  - lip S00.511
  - nose S00.31
  - oral cavity S00.512
  - scalp S00.01
  - specified site NEC S00.81

Abrasion — *continued*
- heel — *see* Abrasion, foot
- hip S70.21-
- inguinal region S30.811
- interscapular region S20.419
- jaw S00.81
- knee S80.21-
- labium (majus) (minus) S30.814
- larynx S10.11
- leg (lower) S80.81-
  - knee — *see* Abrasion, knee
  - upper — *see* Abrasion, thigh
- lip S00.511
- lower back S30.810
- lumbar region S30.810
- malar region S00.81
- mammary — *see* Abrasion, breast
- mastoid region S00.81
- mouth S00.512
- nail
  - finger — *see* Abrasion, finger
  - toe — *see* Abrasion, toe
- nape S10.81
- nasal S00.31
- neck S10.91
  - specified site NEC S10.81
  - throat S10.11
- nose S00.31
- occipital region S00.01
- oral cavity S00.512
- orbital region — *see* Abrasion, eyelid
- palate S00.512
- palm — *see* Abrasion, hand
- parietal region S00.01
- pelvis S30.810
- penis S30.812
- perineum
  - female S30.814
  - male S30.810
- periocular area — *see* Abrasion, eyelid
- phalanges
  - finger — *see* Abrasion, finger
  - toe — *see* Abrasion, toe
- pharynx S10.11
- pinna — *see* Abrasion, ear
- popliteal space — *see* Abrasion, knee
- prepuce S30.812
- pubic region S30.810
- pudendum
  - female S30.816
  - male S30.815
- sacral region S30.810
- scalp S00.01
- scapular region — *see* Abrasion, shoulder
- scrotum S30.813
- shin — *see* Abrasion, leg
- shoulder S40.21-
- skin NEC T14.8
- sternal region S20.319
- submaxillary region S00.81
- submental region S00.81
- subungual
  - finger(s) — *see* Abrasion, finger
  - toe(s) — *see* Abrasion, toe
- supraclavicular fossa S10.81
- supraorbital S00.81
- temple S00.81
- temporal region S00.81
- testis S30.813
- thigh S70.31-
- thorax, thoracic (wall) S20.91
  - back S20.41-
  - front S20.31-
- throat S10.11
- thumb S60.31-
- toe(s) (lesser) S90.416
  - great S90.41-
- tongue S00.512
- tooth, teeth (dentifrice) (habitual) (hard tissues) (occupational) (ritual) (traditional) K03.1
- trachea S10.11
- tunica vaginalis S30.813 tympanum, tympanic membrane — *see* Abrasion, ear

Abrasion— *continued*
- uvula S00.512
- vagina S30.814
- vocal cords S10.11
- vulva S30.814
- wrist S60.81-

Abrism — *see* Poisoning, food, noxious, plant

Abruptio placentae O45.9-
- with
  - afibrinogenemia O45.01-
  - coagulation defect O45.00-
    - specified NEC O45.09-
  - disseminated intravascular coagulation O45.02-
  - hypofibrinogenemia O45.01-
- specified NEC O45.8-

Abruption, placenta — *see* Abruptio placentae

Abscess (connective tissue) (embolic) (fistulous) (infective) (metastatic) (multiple) (pernicious) (pyogenic) (septic) L02.91
- with
  - diverticular disease (intestine) K57.80
    - with bleeding K57.81
    - large intestine K57.20
      - with
        - bleeding K57.21
        - small intestine K57.40
          - with bleeding K57.41
    - small intestine K57.00
      - with
        - bleeding K57.01
        - large intestine K57.40
          - with bleeding K57.41
  - lymphangitis—code by site under Abscess
- abdomen, abdominal
  - cavity K65.1
  - wall L02.211
- abdominopelvic K65.1
- accessory sinus — *see* Sinusitis
- adrenal (capsule) (gland) E27.8
- alveolar K04.7
  - with sinus K04.6
- amebic A06.4
  - brain (and liver or lung abscess) A06.6
  - genitourinary tract A06.82
  - liver (without mention of brain or lung abscess) A06.4
  - lung (and liver) (without mention of brain abscess) A06.5
  - specified site NEC A06.89
  - spleen A06.89
- anerobic A48.0
- ankle — *see* Abscess, lower limb
- anorectal K61.2
- antecubital space — *see* Abscess, upper limb
- antrum (chronic) (Highmore) — *see* Sinusitis, maxillary
- anus K61.0
- apical (tooth) K04.7
  - with sinus (alveolar) K04.6
- appendix K35.3
- areola (acute) (chronic) (nonpuerperal) N61
  - puerperal, postpartum or gestational — *see* Infection, nipple
- arm (any part) — *see* Abscess, upper limb
- artery (wall) I77.89
- atheromatous I77.2
- auricle, ear — *see* Abscess, ear, external
- axilla (region) L02.41-
  - lymph gland or node L04.2
- back (any part, except buttock) L02.212
- Bartholin's gland N75.1
  - with
    - abortion — *see* Abortion, by type complicated by, sepsis
    - ectopic or molar pregnancy O08.0
  - following ectopic or molar pregnancy O08.0
- Bezold's — *see* Mastoiditis, acute
- bilharziasis B65.1
- bladder (wall) — *see* Cystitis, specified type NEC
- bone (subperiosteal) (*see also* Osteomyelitis, specified type NEC)
  - accessory sinus (chronic) — *see* Sinusitis
  - chronic or old — *see* Osteomyelitis, chronic

- **Abscess** — *continued*
  - bone — *continued*
    - jaw (lower) (upper) M27.2
    - mastoid — *see* Mastoiditis, acute, subperiosteal
    - petrous — *see* Petrositis
    - spinal (tuberculous) A18.Ø1
      - nontuberculous — *see* Osteomyelitis, vertebra
  - bowel K63.Ø
  - brain (any part) (cystic) (otogenic) GØ6.Ø
    - amebic (with abscess of any other site) AØ6.6
    - gonococcal A54.82
    - pheomycotic (chromomycotic) B43.1
    - tuberculous A17.81
  - breast (acute) (chronic) (nonpuerperal) N61
    - newborn P39.Ø
    - puerperal, postpartum, gestational — *see* Mastitis, obstetric, purulent
  - broad ligament N73.2
    - acute N73.Ø
    - chronic N73.1
  - Brodie's (localized) (chronic) M86.8x-
  - bronchi J98.Ø9
  - buccal cavity K12.2
  - bulbourethral gland N34.Ø
  - bursa M71.ØØ
    - ankle M71.Ø7-
    - elbow M71.Ø2-
    - foot M71.Ø7-
    - hand M71.Ø4-
    - hip M71.Ø5-
    - knee M71.Ø6-
    - multiple sites M71.Ø9
    - pharyngeal J39.1
    - shoulder M71.Ø1-
    - specified site NEC M71.Ø8
    - wrist M71.Ø3-
  - buttock LØ2.31
  - canthus — *see* Blepharoconjunctivitis
  - cartilage — *see* Disorder, cartilage, specified type NEC
  - cecum K35.3
  - cerebellum, cerebellar GØ6.Ø
    - sequelae GØ9
  - cerebral (embolic) GØ6.Ø
    - sequelae GØ9
  - cervical (meaning neck) LØ2.11
    - lymph gland or node LØ4.Ø
  - cervix (stump) (uteri) — *see* Cervicitis
  - cheek (external) LØ2.Ø1
    - inner K12.2
  - chest J86.9
    - with fistula J86.Ø
    - wall LØ2.213
  - chin LØ2.Ø1
  - choroid — *see* Inflammation, chorioretinal
  - circumtonsillar J36
  - cold (lung) (tuberculous) (*see also* Tuberculosis, abscess, lung)
    - articular — *see* Tuberculosis, joint
  - colon (wall) K63.Ø
  - colostomy K94.Ø2
  - conjunctiva — *see* Conjunctivitis, acute
  - cornea H16.31-
  - corpus
    - cavernosum N48.21
    - luteum — *see* Oophoritis
  - Cowper's gland N34.Ø
  - cranium GØ6.Ø
  - cul-de-sac (Douglas') (posterior) — *see* Peritonitis, pelvic, female
  - cutaneous — *see* Abscess, by site
  - dental KØ4.7
    - with sinus (alveolar) KØ4.6
  - dentoalveolar KØ4.7
    - with sinus KØ4.6
  - diaphragm, diaphragmatic K65.1
  - Douglas' cul-de-sac or pouch — *see* Peritonitis, pelvic, female
  - Dubois A5Ø.59
  - ear (middle) (*see also* Otitis, media, suppurative)
    - acute — *see* Otitis, media, suppurative, acute
    - external H6Ø.Ø-
  - entamebic — *see* Abscess, amebic

- **Abscess** — *continued*
  - enterostomy K94.12
  - epididymis N45.4
  - epidural GØ6.2
    - brain GØ6.Ø
    - spinal cord GØ6.1
  - epiglottis J38.7
  - epiploon, epiploic K65.1
  - erysipelatous — *see* Erysipelas
  - esophagus K2Ø.8
  - ethmoid (bone) (chronic) (sinus) J32.2
  - external auditory canal — *see* Abscess, ear, external
  - extradural GØ6.2
    - brain GØ6.Ø
      - sequelae GØ9
    - spinal cord GØ6.1
  - extraperitoneal K68.19
  - eye — *see* Endophthalmitis, purulent
  - eyelid HØØ.Ø3-
  - face (any part, except ear, eye and nose) LØ2.Ø1
  - fallopian tube — *see* Salpingitis
  - fascia M72.8
  - fauces J39.1
  - fecal K63.Ø
  - femoral (region) — *see* Abscess, lower limb
  - filaria, filarial — *see* Infestation, filarial
  - finger (any) (*see also* Abscess, hand)
    - nail — *see* Cellulitis, finger
  - foot LØ2.61-
  - forehead LØ2.Ø1
  - frontal sinus (chronic) J32.1
  - gallbladder K81.Ø
  - genital organ or tract
    - female (external) N76.4
    - male N49.9
      - multiple sites N49.8
      - specified NEC N49.8
  - gestational mammary O91.11-
  - gestational subareolar O91.11-
  - gingival KØ5.21
  - gland, glandular (lymph) (acute) — *see* Lymphadenitis, acute
  - gluteal (region) LØ2.31
  - gonorrheal — *see* Gonococcus
  - groin LØ2.214
  - gum KØ5.21
  - hand LØ2.51-
  - head NEC LØ2.811
    - face (any part, except ear, eye and nose) LØ2.Ø1
  - heart — *see* Carditis
  - heel — *see* Abscess, foot
  - helminthic — *see* Infestation, helminth
  - hepatic (cholangitic) (hematogenic) (lymphogenic) (pylephlebitic) K75.Ø
    - amebic AØ6.4
  - hip (region) — *see* Abscess, lower limb
  - ileocecal K35.3
  - ileostomy (bud) K94.12
  - iliac (region) LØ2.214
    - fossa K35.3
  - infraclavicular (fossa) — *see* Abscess, upper limb
  - inguinal (region) LØ2.214
    - lymph gland or node LØ4.1
  - intestine, intestinal NEC K63.Ø
    - rectal K61.1
  - intra-abdominal (*see also* Abscess, peritoneum) K65.1
    - postoperative T81.4
      - retroperitoneal K68.11
  - intracranial GØ6.Ø
  - intramammary — *see* Abscess, breast
  - intraorbital — *see* Abscess, orbit
  - intraperitoneal K65.1
  - intrasphincteric (anus) K61.4
  - intraspinal GØ6.1
  - intratonsillar J36
  - ischiorectal (fossa) K61.3
  - jaw (bone) (lower) (upper) M27.2
  - joint — *see* Arthritis, pyogenic or pyemic
    - spine (tuberculous) A18.Ø1
      - nontuberculous — *see* Spondylopathy, infective

- **Abscess** — *continued*
  - kidney N15.1
    - with calculus N2Ø.Ø
      - with hydronephrosis N13.6
    - puerperal (postpartum) O86.21
  - knee (*see also* Abscess, lower limb)
    - joint MØØ.9
  - labium (majus) (minus) N76.4
  - lacrimal
    - caruncle — *see* Inflammation, lacrimal, passages, acute
    - gland — *see* Dacryoadenitis
    - passages (duct) (sac) — *see* Inflammation, lacrimal, passages, acute
  - lacunar N34.Ø
  - larynx J38.7
  - lateral (alveolar) KØ4.7
    - with sinus KØ4.6
  - leg (any part) — *see* Abscess, lower limb
  - lens H27.8
  - lingual K14.Ø
    - tonsil J36
  - lip K13.Ø
  - Littre's gland N34.Ø
  - liver (cholangitic) (hematogenic) (lymphogenic) (pylephlebitic) (pyogenic) K75.Ø
    - amebic (due to Entamoeba histolytica) (dysenteric) (tropical) AØ6.4
      - with
        - brain abscess (and liver or lung abscess) AØ6.6
        - lung abscess AØ6.5
  - loin (region) LØ2.211
  - lower limb LØ2.41-
  - lumbar (tuberculous) A18.Ø1
    - nontuberculous LØ2.212
  - lung (miliary) (putrid) J85.2
    - with pneumonia J85.1
      - due to specified organism (see Pneumonia, in (due to))
    - amebic (with liver abscess) AØ6.5
      - with
        - brain abscess AØ6.6
        - pneumonia AØ6.5
  - lymph, lymphatic, gland or node (acute) (*see also* Lymphadenitis, acute)
    - mesentery I88.Ø
  - malar M27.2
  - mammary gland — *see* Abscess, breast
  - marginal, anus K61.Ø
  - mastoid — *see* Mastoiditis, acute
  - maxilla, maxillary M27.2
    - molar (tooth) KØ4.7
      - with sinus KØ4.6
    - premolar KØ4.7
    - sinus (chronic) J32.Ø
  - mediastinum J85.3
  - meibomian gland — *see* Hordeolum
  - meninges GØ6.2
  - mesentery, mesenteric K65.1
  - mesosalpinx — *see* Salpingitis
  - mons pubis LØ2.215
  - mouth (floor) K12.2
  - muscle — *see* Myositis, infective
  - myocardium I4Ø.Ø
  - nabothian (follicle) — *see* Cervicitis
  - nasal J32.9
  - nasopharyngeal J39.1
  - navel LØ2.216
    - newborn P38.9
      - with mild hemorrhage P38.1
      - without hemorrhage P38.9
  - neck (region) LØ2.11
    - lymph gland or node LØ4.Ø
  - nephritic — *see* Abscess, kidney
  - nipple N61
    - associated with
      - lactation — *see* Pregnancy, complicated by,
      - pregnancy — *see* Pregnancy, complicated by
  - nose (external) (fossa) (septum) J34.Ø
    - sinus (chronic) — *see* Sinusitis
  - omentum K65.1
  - operative wound T81.4

- **Abscess** — *continued*
  - vas deferens N49.1
  - vermiform appendix K35.3
  - vertebra (column) (tuberculous) A18.Ø1
    - nontuberculous — *see* Osteomyelitis, vertebra
  - vesical — *see* Cystitis, specified type NEC
  - vesico-uterine pouch — *see* Peritonitis, pelvic, female
  - vitreous (humor) — *see* Endophthalmitis, purulent
  - vocal cord J38.3
  - von Bezold's — *see* Mastoiditis, acute
  - vulva N76.4
  - vulvovaginal gland N75.1
  - web space — *see* Abscess, hand
  - wound T81.4
  - wrist — *see* Abscess, upper limb
- **Absence** (of) (organ or part) (complete or partial)
  - adrenal (gland) (congenital) Q89.1
    - acquired E89.6
  - albumin in blood E88.Ø9
  - alimentary tract (congenital) Q45.8
    - upper Q4Ø.8
  - alveolar process (acquired) — *see* Anomaly, alveolar
  - ankle (acquired) Z89.44-
  - anus (congenital) Q42.3
    - with fistula Q42.2
  - aorta (congenital) Q25.4
  - appendix, congenital Q42.8
  - arm (acquired) Z89.2Ø-
    - above elbow Z89.22-
      - congenital (with hand present) — *see* Agenesis, arm, with hand present
        - and hand — *see* Agenesis, forearm, and hand
    - below elbow Z89.21-
      - congenital (with hand present) — *see* Agenesis, arm, with hand present
        - and hand — *see* Agenesis, forearm, and hand
    - congenital — *see* Defect, reduction, upper limb
    - shoulder (following explantation of shoulder joint prosthesis) (joint) (with or without presence of antibiotic-impregnated cement spacer) Z89.23-
      - congenital (with hand present) — *see* Agenesis, arm, with hand present
  - artery (congenital) (peripheral) Q27.8
    - brain Q28.3
    - coronary Q24.5
    - pulmonary Q25.79
    - specified NEC Q27.8
    - umbilical Q27.Ø
  - atrial septum (congenital) Q21.1
  - auditory canal (congenital) (external) Q16.1
  - auricle (ear), congenital Q16.Ø
  - bile, biliary duct, congenital Q44.5
  - bladder (acquired) Z9Ø.6
    - congenital Q64.5
  - bowel sounds R19.11
  - brain QØØ.Ø
    - part of QØ4.3
  - breast(s) (and nipple(s)) (acquired) Z9Ø.1-
    - congenital Q83.8
  - broad ligament Q5Ø.6
  - bronchus (congenital) Q32.4
  - canaliculus lacrimalis, congenital Q1Ø.4
  - cerebellum (vermis) QØ4.3
  - cervix (acquired) (with uterus) Z9Ø.71Ø
    - with remaining uterus Z9Ø.712
    - congenital Q51.5
  - chin, congenital Q18.8
  - cilia (congenital) Q1Ø.3
    - acquired — *see* Madarosis
  - clitoris (congenital) Q52.6
  - coccyx, congenital Q76.49
  - cold sense R2Ø.8
  - congenital
    - lumen — *see* Atresia
    - organ or site NEC — *see* Agenesis
    - septum — *see* Imperfect, closure
  - corpus callosum QØ4.Ø
  - cricoid cartilage, congenital Q31.8
  - diaphragm (with hernia), congenital Q79.1

- **Absence** — *continued*
  - digestive organ(s) or tract, congenital Q45.8
    - acquired NEC Z9Ø.49
    - upper Q4Ø.8
  - ductus arteriosus Q28.8
  - duodenum (acquired) Z9Ø.49
    - congenital Q41.Ø
  - ear, congenital Q16.9
    - acquired H93.8-
    - auricle Q16.Ø
    - external Q16.Ø
    - inner Q16.5
    - lobe, lobule Q17.8
    - middle, except ossicles Q16.4
      - ossicles Q16.3
    - ossicles Q16.3
  - ejaculatory duct (congenital) Q55.4
  - endocrine gland (congenital) NEC Q89.2
    - acquired E89.89
  - epididymis (congenital) Q55.4
    - acquired Z9Ø.79
  - epiglottis, congenital Q31.8
  - esophagus (congenital) Q39.8
    - acquired (partial) Z9Ø.49
  - eustachian tube (congenital) Q16.2
  - extremity (acquired) Z89.9
    - congenital Q73.Ø
    - knee (following explantation of knee joint prosthesis) (joint) (with or without presence of antibiotic-impregnated cement spacer) Z89.52-
    - lower (above knee) Z89.619
      - below knee Z89.51-
    - upper — *see* Absence, arm
  - eye (acquired) Z9Ø.Ø1
    - congenital Q11.1
    - muscle (congenital) Q1Ø.3
  - eyeball (acquired) Z9Ø.Ø1
  - eyelid (fold) (congenital) Q1Ø.3
    - acquired Z9Ø.Ø1
  - face, specified part NEC Q18.8
  - fallopian tube(s) (acquired) Z9Ø.79
    - congenital Q5Ø.6
  - family member (causing problem in home) NEC Z63.32 (*see also* Disruption, family)
  - femur, congenital — *see* Defect, reduction, lower limb, longitudinal, femur
  - fibrinogen (congenital) D68.2
    - acquired D65
  - finger(s) (acquired) Z89.Ø2-
    - congenital — *see* Agenesis, hand
  - foot (acquired) Z89.43-
    - congenital — *see* Agenesis, foot
  - forearm (acquired) — *see* Absence, arm, below elbow
  - gallbladder (acquired) Z9Ø.49
    - congenital Q44.Ø
  - gamma globulin in blood D8Ø.1
    - hereditary D8Ø.Ø
  - genital organs
    - acquired (female) (male) Z9Ø.79
    - female, congenital Q52.8
      - external Q52.71
      - internal NEC Q52.8
    - male, congenital Q55.8
  - genitourinary organs, congenital NEC
    - female Q52.8
    - male Q55.8
  - globe (acquired) Z9Ø.Ø1
    - congenital Q11.1
  - glottis, congenital Q31.8
  - hand and wrist (acquired) Z89.11-
    - congenital — *see* Agenesis, hand
  - head, part (acquired) NEC Z9Ø.Ø9
  - heat sense R2Ø.8
  - hip (following explantation of hip joint prosthesis) (joint) (with or without presence of antibiotic-impregnated cement spacer) Z89.62-
  - hymen (congenital) Q52.4
  - ileum (acquired) Z9Ø.49
    - congenital Q41.2

- **Absence** — *continued*
  - immunoglobulin, isolated NEC D8Ø.3
    - IgA D8Ø.2
    - IgG D8Ø.3
    - IgM D8Ø.4
  - incus (acquired) — *see* Loss, ossicles, ear
    - congenital Q16.3
  - inner ear, congenital Q16.5
  - intestine (acquired) (small) Z9Ø.49
    - congenital Q41.9
      - specified NEC Q41.8
    - large Z9Ø.49
      - congenital Q42.9
        - specified NEC Q42.8
  - iris, congenital Q13.1
  - jejunum (acquired) Z9Ø.49
    - congenital Q41.1
  - joint
    - acquired
      - hip (following explantation of hip joint prosthesis) (with or without presence of antibiotic-impregnated cement spacer) Z89.62-
      - knee (following explantation of knee joint prosthesis) (with or without presence of antibiotic-impregnated cement spacer) Z89.52-
      - shoulder (following explantation of shoulder joint prosthesis) (with or without presence of antibiotic-impregnated cement spacer) Z89.23-
    - congenital NEC Q74.8
  - knee (following explantation of knee joint prosthesis) (joint) (with or without presence of antibiotic-impregnated cement spacer) Z89.52-
  - kidney(s) (acquired) Z9Ø.5
    - congenital Q6Ø.2
      - bilateral Q6Ø.1
      - unilateral Q6Ø.Ø
  - labyrinth, membranous Q16.5
  - larynx (congenital) Q31.8
    - acquired Z9Ø.Ø2
  - leg (acquired) (above knee) Z89.61-
    - below knee (acquired) Z89.51-
    - congenital — *see* Defect, reduction, lower limb
  - lens (acquired) (*see also* Aphakia)
    - congenital Q12.3
    - post cataract extraction Z98.4-
  - limb (acquired) — *see* Absence, extremity
  - lip Q38.6
  - liver (congenital) Q44.7
  - lung (fissure) (lobe) (bilateral) (unilateral) (congenital) Q33.3
    - acquired (any part) Z9Ø.2
  - menstruation — *see* Amenorrhea
  - muscle (congenital) (pectoral) Q79.8
    - ocular Q1Ø.3
  - neck, part Q18.8
  - neutrophil — *see* Agranulocytosis
  - nipple(s) (with breast(s)) (acquired) Z9Ø.1-
    - congenital Q83.2
  - nose (congenital) Q3Ø.1
    - acquired Z9Ø.Ø9
  - organ
    - of Corti, congenital Q16.5
    - or site, congenital NEC Q89.8
      - acquired NEC Z9Ø.89
  - osseous meatus (ear) Q16.4
  - ovary (acquired)
    - bilateral Z9Ø.722
    - congenital
      - bilateral Q5Ø.Ø2
      - unilateral Q5Ø.Ø1
    - unilateral Z9Ø.721
  - oviduct (acquired)
    - bilateral Z9Ø.722
    - congenital Q5Ø.6
    - unilateral Z9Ø.721
  - pancreas (congenital) Q45.Ø
    - acquired Z9Ø.41Ø
      - complete Z9Ø.41Ø
      - partial Z9Ø.411

- **Absence** — *continued*
  - pancreas— *continued*
    - acquired— *continued*
      - total Z9Ø.41Ø
  - parathyroid gland (acquired) E89.2
    - congenital Q89.2
  - patella, congenital Q74.1
  - penis (congenital) Q55.5
    - acquired Z9Ø.79
  - pericardium (congenital) Q24.8
  - pituitary gland (congenital) Q89.2
    - acquired E89.3
  - prostate (acquired) Z9Ø.79
    - congenital Q55.4
  - pulmonary valve Q22.Ø
  - punctum lacrimale (congenital) Q1Ø.4
  - radius, congenital — *see* Defect, reduction, upper limb, longitudinal, radius
  - rectum (congenital) Q42.1
    - with fistula Q42.Ø
    - acquired Z9Ø.49
  - respiratory organ NOS Q34.9
  - rib (acquired) Z9Ø.89
    - congenital Q76.6
  - sacrum, congenital Q76.49
  - salivary gland(s), congenital Q38.4
  - scrotum, congenital Q55.29
  - seminal vesicles (congenital) Q55.4
    - acquired Z9Ø.79
  - septum
    - atrial (congenital) Q21.1
    - between aorta and pulmonary artery Q21.4
    - ventricular (congenital) Q2Ø.4
  - sex chromosome
    - female phenotype Q97.8
    - male phenotype Q98.8
  - skull bone (congenital) Q75.8
    - with
      - anencephaly QØØ.Ø
      - encephalocele — *see* Encephalocele
      - hydrocephalus QØ3.9
        - with spina bifida — *see* Spina bifida, by site, with hydrocephalus
      - microcephaly QØ2
  - spermatic cord, congenital Q55.4
  - spine, congenital Q76.49
  - spleen (congenital) Q89.Ø1
    - acquired Z9Ø.81
  - sternum, congenital Q76.7
  - stomach (acquired) (partial) Z9Ø.3
    - congenital Q4Ø.2
  - superior vena cava, congenital Q26.8
  - teeth, tooth (congenital) KØØ.Ø
    - acquired (complete) KØ8.1Ø9
      - class I KØ8.1Ø1
      - class II KØ8.1Ø2
      - class III KØ8.1Ø3
      - class IV KØ8.1Ø4
      - due to
        - caries KØ8.139
          - class I KØ8.131
          - class II KØ8.132
          - class III KØ8.133
          - class IV KØ8.134
        - periodontal disease KØ8.129
          - class I KØ8.121
          - class II KØ8.122
          - class III KØ8.123
          - class IV KØ8.124
        - specified NEC KØ8.199
          - class I KØ8.191
          - class II KØ8.192
          - class III KØ8.193
          - class IV KØ8.194
        - trauma KØ8.119
          - class I KØ8.111
          - class II KØ8.112
          - class III KØ8.113
          - class IV KØ8.114
      - partial KØ8.4Ø9
        - class I KØ8.4Ø1
        - class II KØ8.4Ø2
        - class III KØ8.4Ø3

- **Absence** — *continued*
  - teeth — *continued*
    - acquired — *continued*
      - partial — *continued*
        - class IV KØ8.4Ø4
        - due to
          - caries KØ8.439
            - class I KØ8.431
            - class II KØ8.432
            - class III KØ8.433
            - class IV KØ8.434
          - periodontal disease KØ8.429
            - class I KØ8.421
            - class II KØ8.422
            - class III KØ8.423
            - class IV KØ8.424
          - specified NEC KØ8.499
            - class I KØ8.491
            - class II KØ8.492
            - class III KØ8.493
            - class IV KØ8.494
          - trauma KØ8.419
            - class I KØ8.411
            - class II KØ8.412
            - class III KØ8.413
            - class IV KØ8.414
  - tendon (congenital) Q79.8
  - testis (congenital) Q55.Ø
    - acquired Z9Ø.79
  - thumb (acquired) Z89.Ø1-
    - congenital — *see* Agenesis, hand
  - thymus gland Q89.2
  - thyroid (gland) (acquired) E89.Ø
    - cartilage, congenital Q31.8
    - congenital EØ3.1
  - toe(s) (acquired) Z89.42-
    - with foot — *see* Absence, foot and ankle
    - congenital — *see* Agenesis, foot
    - great Z89.41-
  - tongue, congenital Q38.3
  - trachea (cartilage), congenital Q32.1
  - transverse aortic arch, congenital Q25.4
  - tricuspid valve Q22.4
  - umbilical artery, congenital Q27.Ø
  - upper arm and forearm with hand present, congenital — *see* Agenesis, arm, with hand present
  - ureter (congenital) Q62.4
    - acquired Z9Ø.6
  - urethra, congenital Q64.5
  - uterus (acquired) Z9Ø.71Ø
    - with cervix Z9Ø.71Ø
    - with remaining cervical stump Z9Ø.711
    - congenital Q51.Ø
  - uvula, congenital Q38.5
  - vagina, congenital Q52.Ø
  - vas deferens (congenital) Q55.4
    - acquired Z9Ø.79
  - vein (peripheral) congenital NEC Q27.8
    - cerebral Q28.3
    - digestive system Q27.8
    - great Q26.8
    - lower limb Q27.8
    - portal Q26.5
    - precerebral Q28.1
    - specified site NEC Q27.8
    - upper limb Q27.8
  - vena cava (inferior) (superior), congenital Q26.8
  - ventricular septum Q2Ø.4
  - vertebra, congenital Q76.49
  - vulva, congenital Q52.71
  - wrist (acquired) Z89.12-
- **Absorbent system disease** I87.8
- **Absorption**
  - carbohydrate, disturbance K9Ø.4
  - chemical — *see* Table of Drugs and Chemicals
    - through placenta (newborn) PØ4.9
      - environmental substance PØ4.6
      - nutritional substance PØ4.5
      - obstetric anesthetic or analgesic drug PØ4.Ø
  - drug NEC — *see* Table of Drugs and Chemicals

- **Absorption** — *continued*
  - drug NEC — *continued*
    - addictive
      - through placenta (newborn) PØ4.49
        - cocaine PØ4.41
    - medicinal
      - through placenta (newborn) PØ4.1
    - through placenta (newborn) PØ4.1
      - obstetric anesthetic or analgesic drug PØ4.Ø
  - fat, disturbance K9Ø.4
    - pancreatic K9Ø.3
  - noxious substance — *see* Table of Drugs and Chemicals
  - protein, disturbance K9Ø.4
  - starch, disturbance K9Ø.4
  - toxic substance — *see* Table of Drugs and Chemicals
  - uremic — *see* Uremia
- **Abstinence symptoms, syndrome**
  - alcohol F1Ø.239
    - with delirium F1Ø.231
  - cocaine F14.23
  - neonatal P96.1
  - nicotine — *see* Dependence, drug, nicotine, with, withdrawal
  - opioid F11.93
    - with dependence F11.23
  - psychoactive NEC F19.939
    - with
      - delirium F19.931
      - dependence F19.239
        - with
          - delirium F19.231
          - perceptual disturbance F19.232
        - uncomplicated F19.23Ø
      - perceptual disturbance F19.932
    - uncomplicated F19.93Ø
  - sedative F13.939
    - with
      - delirium F13.931
      - dependence F13.239
        - with
          - delirium F13.231
          - perceptual disturbance F13.232
        - uncomplicated F13.23Ø
      - perceptual disturbance F13.932
    - uncomplicated F13.93Ø
  - stimulant NEC F15.93
    - with dependence F15.23
- **Abulia** R68.89
- **Abulomania** F6Ø.7
- **Abuse**
  - adult — *see* Maltreatment, adult
    - as reason for
      - couple seeking advice (including offender) Z63.Ø
  - alcohol (non-dependent) F1Ø.1Ø
    - with
      - anxiety disorder F1Ø.18Ø
      - intoxication F1Ø.129
        - with delirium F1Ø.121
        - uncomplicated F1Ø.12Ø
      - mood disorder F1Ø.14
      - other specified disorder F1Ø.188
      - psychosis F1Ø.159
        - delusions F1Ø.15Ø
        - hallucinations F1Ø.151
      - sexual dysfunction F1Ø.181
      - sleep disorder F1Ø.182
      - unspecified disorder F1Ø.19
    - counseling and surveillance Z71.41
  - amphetamine (or related substance) — *see* Abuse, drug, stimulant NEC
  - analgesics (non-prescribed) (over the counter) F55.8
  - antacids F55.Ø
  - antidepressants — *see* Abuse, drug, psychoactive NEC
  - anxiolytic — *see* Abuse, drug, sedative
  - barbiturates — *see* Abuse, drug, sedative
  - caffeine — *see* Abuse, drug, stimulant NEC
  - cannabis, cannabinoids — *see* Abuse, drug, cannabis
  - child — *see* Maltreatment, child
  - cocaine — *see* Abuse, drug, cocaine

Accessory — *continued*
- eye muscle Q10.3
- eyelid Q10.3
- face bone(s) Q75.8
- fallopian tube (fimbria) (ostium) Q50.6
- finger(s) Q69.0
- foreskin N47.8
- frontonasal process Q75.8
- gallbladder Q44.1
- genital organ(s)
  - female Q52.8
    - external Q52.79
    - internal NEC Q52.8
  - male Q55.8
- genitourinary organs NEC Q89.8
  - female Q52.8
  - male Q55.8
- hallux Q69.2
- heart Q24.8
  - valve NEC Q24.8
    - pulmonary Q22.3
- hepatic ducts Q44.5
- hymen Q52.4
- intestine (large) (small) Q43.4
- kidney Q63.0
- lacrimal canal Q10.6
- leaflet, heart valve NEC Q24.8
- ligament, broad Q50.6
- liver Q44.7
  - duct Q44.5
- lobule (ear) Q17.0
- lung (lobe) Q33.1
- muscle Q79.8
- navicular of carpus Q74.0
- nervous system, part NEC Q07.8
- nipple Q83.3
- nose Q30.8
- organ or site not listed — *see* Anomaly, by site
- ovary Q50.31
- oviduct Q50.6
- pancreas Q45.3
- parathyroid gland Q89.2
- parotid gland (and duct) Q38.4
- pituitary gland Q89.2
- preauricular appendage Q17.0
- prepuce N47.8
- renal arteries (multiple) Q27.2
- rib Q76.6
  - cervical Q76.5
- roots (teeth) K00.2
- salivary gland Q38.4
- sesamoid bones Q74.8
  - foot Q74.2
  - hand Q74.0
- skin tags Q82.8
- spleen Q89.09
- sternum Q76.7
- submaxillary gland Q38.4
- tarsal bones Q74.2
- teeth, tooth K00.1
- tendon Q79.8
- thumb Q69.1
- thymus gland Q89.2
- thyroid gland Q89.2
- toes Q69.2
- tongue Q38.3
- tooth, teeth K00.1
- tragus Q17.0
- ureter Q62.5
- urethra Q64.79
- urinary organ or tract NEC Q64.8
- uterus Q51.2
- vagina Q52.10
- valve, heart NEC Q24.8
  - pulmonary Q22.3
- vertebra Q76.49
- vocal cords Q31.8
- vulva Q52.79

Accident
- birth — *see* Birth, injury
- cardiac — *see* Infarct, myocardium
- cerebral I63.9
- cerebrovascular (embolic) (ischemic) (thrombotic) I63.9
  - aborted I63.9
  - hemorrhagic — *see* Hemorrhage, intracranial, intracerebral
  - old (without sequelae) Z86.73
    - with sequelae (of) — *see* Sequelae, infarction, cerebral
- coronary — *see* Infarct, myocardium
- craniovascular I63.9
- vascular, brain I63.9

Accidental — *see* condition

Accommodation (disorder) (*see also* condition)
- hysterical paralysis of F44.89
- insufficiency of H52.4
- paresis — *see* Paresis, of accommodation
- spasm — *see* Spasm, of accommodation

Accouchement — *see* Delivery

Accreta placenta O43.21-

Accretio cordis (nonrheumatic) I31.0

Accretions, tooth, teeth K03.6

Acculturation difficulty Z60.3

Accumulation secretion, prostate N42.89

Acephalia, acephalism, acephalus, acephaly Q00.0

Acephalobrachia monster Q89.8

Acephalochirus monster Q89.8

Acephalogaster Q89.8

Acephalostomus monster Q89.8

Acephalothorax Q89.8

Acerophobia F40.298

Acetonemia R79.89
- in Type 1 diabetes E10.10
  - with coma E10.11

Acetonuria R82.4

Achalasia (cardia) (esophagus) K22.0
- congenital Q39.5
- pylorus Q40.0
- sphincteral NEC K59.8

Ache(s) — *see* Pain

Acheilia Q38.6

Achillobursitis — *see* Tendinitis, Achilles

Achillodynia — *see* Tendinitis, Achilles

Achlorhydria, achlorhydric (neurogenic) K31.83
- anemia D50.8
- diarrhea K31.83
- psychogenic F45.8
- secondary to vagotomy K91.1

Achluophobia F40.228

Acholia K82.8

Acholuric jaundice (familial) (splenomegalic) (*see also* Spherocytosis)
- acquired D59.8

Achondrogenesis Q77.0

Achondroplasia (osteosclerosis congenita) Q77.4

Achroma, cutis L80

Achromat(ism), achromatopsia (acquired) (congenital) H53.51

Achromia, congenital — *see* Albinism

Achromia parasitica B36.0

Achylia gastrica K31.89
- psychogenic F45.8

Acid
- burn — *see* Corrosion
- deficiency
  - amide nicotinic E52
  - ascorbic E54
  - folic E53.8
  - nicotinic E52
  - pantothenic E53.8
- intoxication E87.2
- peptic disease K30
- phosphatase deficiency E83.39
- stomach K30
  - psychogenic F45.8

Acidemia E87.2
- argininosuccinic E72.22
- isovaleric E71.110
- metabolic (newborn) P19.9
  - first noted before onset of labor P19.0
  - first noted during labor P19.1
  - noted at birth P19.2
- methylmalonic E71.120
- pipecolic E72.3
- propionic E71.121

Acidity, gastric (high) K30
- psychogenic F45.8

Acidocytopenia — *see* Agranulocytosis

Acidocytosis D72.1

Acidopenia — *see* Agranulocytosis

Acidosis (lactic) (respiratory) E87.2
- in Type 1 diabetes E10.10
  - with coma E10.11
- kidney, tubular N25.89
- lactic E87.2
- metabolic NEC E87.2
  - with respiratory acidosis E87.4
  - late, of newborn P74.0
- mixed metabolic and respiratory, newborn P84
- newborn P84
- renal (hyperchloremic) (tubular) N25.89
- respiratory E87.2
  - complicated by
    - metabolic
      - acidosis E87.4
      - alkalosis E87.4

Aciduria
- argininosuccinic E72.22
- glutaric (type I) E72.3
  - type II E71.313
  - type III E71.5-
- orotic (congenital) (hereditary) (pyrimidine deficiency) E79.8
  - anemia D53.0

Acladiosis (skin) B36.0

Aclasis, diaphyseal Q78.6

Acleistocardia Q21.1

Aclusion — *see* Anomaly, dentofacial, malocclusion

Acne L70.9
- artificialis L70.8
- atrophica L70.2
- cachecticorum (Hebra) L70.8
- conglobata L70.1
- cystic L70.0
- decalvans L66.2
- excoriée des jeunes filles L70.5
- frontalis L70.2
- indurata L70.0
- infantile L70.4
- keloid L73.0
- lupoid L70.2
- necrotic, necrotica (miliaris) L70.2
- neonatal L70.4
- nodular L70.0
- occupational L70.8
- picker's L70.5
- pustular L70.0
- rodens L70.2
- rosacea L71.9
- specified NEC L70.8
- tropica L70.3
- varioliformis L70.2
- vulgaris L70.0

Acnitis (primary) A18.4

Acosta's disease T70.29

Acoustic — *see* condition

Acousticophobia F40.298

Acquired (*see also* condition)
- immunodeficiency syndrome (AIDS) B20

Acrania Q00.0

Acroangiodermatitis I78.9

Acroasphyxia, chronic I73.89

Acrobystitis N47.7

Acrocephalopolysyndactyly Q87.0

Acrocephalosyndactyly Q87.0

Acrocephaly Q75.0

Acrochondrohyperplasia — *see* Syndrome, Marfan's

Acrocyanosis I73.8
- newborn P28.2
- meaning transient blue hands and feet—*omit code*

Acrodermatitis L30.8
- atrophicans (chronica) L90.4
- continua (Hallopeau) L40.2
- enteropathica (hereditary) E83.2

- **Acrodermatitis** — *continued*
  - Hallopeau's L4Ø.2
  - infantile papular L44.4
  - perstans L4Ø.2
  - pustulosa continua L4Ø.2
  - recalcitrant pustular L4Ø.2
- **Acrodynia** — *see* Poisoning, mercury
- **Acromegaly, acromegalia** E22.Ø
- **Acromelalgia** I73.81
- **Acromicria, acromikria** Q79.8
- **Acronyx** L6Ø.Ø
- **Acropachy, thyroid** — *see* Thyrotoxicosis
- **Acroparesthesia** (simple) (vasomotor) I73.89
- **Acropathy, thyroid** — *see* Thyrotoxicosis
- **Acrophobia** F4Ø.241
- **Acroposthitis** N47.7
- **Acroscleriasis, acroscleroderma, acrosclerosis** — *see* Sclerosis, systemic
- **Acrosphacelus** I96
- **Acrospiroma, eccrine** — *see* Neoplasm, skin, benign
- **Acrostealgia** — *see* Osteochondropathy
- **Acrotrophodynia** — *see* Immersion
- **ACTH ectopic syndrome** E24.3
- **Actinic** — *see* condition
- **Actinobacillosis, actinobacillus** A28.8
  - mallei A24.Ø
  - muris A25.1
- **Actinomyces israelii** (infection) — *see* Actinomycosis
- **Actinomycetoma** (foot) B47.1
- **Actinomycosis, actinomycotic** A42.9
  - with pneumonia A42.Ø
  - abdominal A42.1
  - cervicofacial A42.2
  - cutaneous A42.89
  - gastrointestinal A42.1
  - pulmonary A42.Ø
  - sepsis A42.7
  - specified site NEC A42.89
- **Actinoneuritis** G62.82
- **Action, heart**
  - disorder I49.9
  - irregular I49.9
    - psychogenic F45.8
- **Active** — *see* condition
- **Activated protein C resistance** D68.51
- **Acute** (*see also* condition)
  - abdomen R1Ø.Ø
  - gallbladder — *see* Cholecystitis, acute
- **Acyanotic heart disease** (congenital) Q24.9
- **Acystia** Q64.5
- **Adair-Dighton syndrome** (brittle bones and blue sclera, deafness) Q78.Ø
- **Adamantinoblastoma** — *see* Ameloblastoma
- **Adamantinoma** (*see also* Cyst, calcifying odontogenic)
  - long bones C4Ø.9Ø
    - lower limb C4Ø.2-
    - upper limb C4Ø.Ø-
  - malignant C41.1
    - jaw (bone) (lower) C41.1
      - upper C41.Ø
  - tibial C4Ø.2-
- **Adamantoblastoma** — *see* Ameloblastoma
- **Adams-Stokes (-Morgagni) disease or syndrome** I45.9
- **Adaption reaction** — *see* Disorder, adjustment
- **Addiction** (*see also* Dependence) F19.2Ø
  - alcohol, alcoholic (ethyl) (methyl) (wood) (without remission) F1Ø.2Ø
    - with remission F1Ø.21
  - drug — *see* Dependence, drug
  - ethyl alcohol (without remission) F1Ø.2Ø
    - with remission F1Ø.21
  - heroin — *see* Dependence, drug, opioid
  - methyl alcohol (without remission) F1Ø.2Ø
    - with remission F1Ø.21
  - methylated spirit (without remission) F1Ø.2Ø
    - with remission F1Ø.21
  - morphine(-like substances) — *see* Dependence, drug, opioid
  - nicotine — *see* Dependence, drug, nicotine
  - opium and opioids — *see* Dependence, drug, opioid
  - tobacco — *see* Dependence, drug, nicotine
- **Addisonian crisis** E27.2
- **Addison's**
  - anemia (pernicious) D51.Ø
  - disease (bronze) or syndrome E27.1
    - tuberculous A18.7
  - keloid L94.Ø
- **Addison-Biermer anemia** (pernicious) D51.Ø
- **Addison-Schilder complex** E71.528
- **Additional** (*see also* Accessory)
  - chromosome(s) Q99.8
    - sex — *see* Abnormal, chromosome, sex
    - 21 — *see* Trisomy, 21
- **Adduction contracture, hip or other joint** — *see* Contraction, joint
- **Adenitis** (*see also* Lymphadenitis)
  - acute, unspecified site LØ4.9
  - axillary I88.9
    - acute LØ4.2
    - chronic or subacute I88.1
  - Bartholin's gland N75.8
  - bulbourethral gland — *see* Urethritis
  - cervical I88.9
    - acute LØ4.Ø
    - chronic or subacute I88.1
  - chancroid (Hemophilus ducreyi) A57
  - chronic, unspecified site I88.1
  - Cowper's gland — *see* Urethritis
  - due to Pasteurella multocida (P. septica) A28.Ø
  - epidemic, acute B27.Ø9
  - gangrenous LØ4.9
  - gonorrheal NEC A54.89
  - groin I88.9
    - acute LØ4.1
    - chronic or subacute I88.1
  - infectious (acute) (epidemic) B27.Ø9
  - inguinal I88.9
    - acute LØ4.1
    - chronic or subacute I88.1
  - lymph gland or node, except mesenteric I88.9
    - acute — *see* Lymphadenitis, acute
    - chronic or subacute I88.1
  - mesenteric (acute) (chronic) (nonspecific) (subacute) I88.Ø
  - parotid gland (suppurative) — *see* Sialoadenitis
  - salivary gland (any) (suppurative) — *see* Sialoadenitis
  - scrofulous (tuberculous) A18.2
  - Skene's duct or gland — *see* Urethritis
  - strumous, tuberculous A18.2
  - subacute, unspecified site I88.1
  - sublingual gland (suppurative) — *see* Sialoadenitis
  - submandibular gland (suppurative) — *see* Sialoadenitis
  - submaxillary gland (suppurative) — *see* Sialoadenitis
  - tuberculous — *see* Tuberculosis, lymph gland
  - urethral gland — *see* Urethritis
  - Wharton's duct (suppurative) — *see* Sialoadenitis
- **Adenoacanthoma** — *see* Neoplasm, malignant, by site
- **Adenoameloblastoma** — *see* Cyst, calcifying odontogenic
- **Adenocarcinoid** (tumor) — *see* Neoplasm, malignant, by site
- **Adenocarcinoma** (*see also* Neoplasm, malignant, by site)
  - acidophil
    - specified site — *see* Neoplasm, malignant, by site
    - unspecified site C75.1
  - adrenal cortical C74.Ø-
  - alveolar — *see* Neoplasm, lung, malignant
  - apocrine
    - breast — *see* Neoplasm, breast, malignant
    - in situ
      - breast DØ5.8-
      - specified site NEC — *see* Neoplasm, skin, in situ
      - unspecified site DØ4.9
    - specified site NEC — *see* Neoplasm, skin, malignant
    - unspecified site C44.99
  - basal cell
    - specified site — *see* Neoplasm, skin, malignant
    - unspecified site CØ8.9
- **Adenocarcinoma** — *continued*
  - basophil
    - specified site — *see* Neoplasm, malignant, by site
    - unspecified site C75.1
  - bile duct type C22.1
    - liver C22.1
    - specified site NEC — *see* Neoplasm, malignant, by site
    - unspecified site C22.1
  - bronchiolar — *see* Neoplasm, lung, malignant
  - bronchioloalveolar — *see* Neoplasm, lung, malignant
  - ceruminous C44.29-
  - cervix, in situ (*see also* Carcinoma, cervix uteri, in situ) DØ6.9
  - chromophobe
    - specified site — *see* Neoplasm, malignant, by site
    - unspecified site C75.1
  - diffuse type
    - specified site — *see* Neoplasm, malignant, by site
    - unspecified site C16.9
  - duct
    - infiltrating
      - with Paget's disease — *see* Neoplasm, breast, malignant, by site
      - specified site — *see* Neoplasm, malignant, by site
      - unspecified site (female) C5Ø.91-
        - male C5Ø.92-
    - specified site — *see* Neoplasm, malignant, by site
    - unspecified site
      - female C56.9
      - male C61
  - eosinophil
    - specified site — *see* Neoplasm, malignant, by site
    - unspecified site C75.1
  - follicular
    - with papillary C73
    - moderately differentiated C73
    - specified site — *see* Neoplasm, malignant, by site
    - trabecular C73
    - unspecified site C73
    - well differentiated C73
  - Hurthle cell C73
  - in
    - adenomatous
      - polyposis coli C18.9
  - infiltrating duct
    - with Paget's disease — *see* Neoplasm, breast, malignant
    - specified site — *see* Neoplasm, malignant, by site
    - unspecified site (female) C5Ø.91-
      - male C5Ø.92-
  - inflammatory
    - specified site — *see* Neoplasm, malignant, by site
    - unspecified site (female) C5Ø.91-
      - male C5Ø.92-
  - intestinal type
    - specified site — *see* Neoplasm, malignant, by site
    - unspecified site C16.9
  - intracystic papillary
  - intraductal
    - breast DØ5.1-
    - noninfiltrating
      - breast DØ5.1-
      - papillary
        - with invasion
          - specified site — *see* Neoplasm, malignant, by site
          - unspecified site (female) C5Ø.91-
            - male C5Ø.92-
        - breast DØ5.1-
        - specified site NEC — *see* Neoplasm, in situ, by site
        - unspecified site DØ5.1-
      - specified site NEC — *see* Neoplasm, in situ, by site
      - unspecified site DØ5.1-
    - papillary
      - with invasion
        - specified site — *see* Neoplasm, malignant, by site

Adenocarcinoma — *continued*
- intraductal — *continued*
  - papillary — *continued*
    - with invasion — *continued*
      - unspecified site (female) C5Ø.91-
        - male C5Ø.92-
    - breast DØ5.1-
    - specified site — *see* Neoplasm, in situ, by site
    - unspecified site DØ5.1-
  - specified site NEC — *see* Neoplasm, in situ, by site
  - unspecified site DØ5.1-
- islet cell
  - with exocrine, mixed
    - specified site — *see* Neoplasm, malignant, by site
    - unspecified site C25.9
  - pancreas C25.4
  - specified site NEC — *see* Neoplasm, malignant, by site
  - unspecified site C25.4
- lobular
  - in situ
    - breast DØ5.Ø-
    - specified site NEC — *see* Neoplasm, in situ, by site
    - unspecified site DØ5.Ø-
  - specified site — *see* Neoplasm, malignant, by site
  - unspecified site (female) C5Ø.91-
    - male C5Ø.92-
- mucoid (*see also* Neoplasm, malignant, by site)
  - cell
    - specified site — *see* Neoplasm, malignant, by site
    - unspecified site C75.1
- nonencapsulated sclerosing C73
- papillary
  - with follicular C73
  - follicular variant C73
  - intraductal (noninfiltrating)
    - with invasion
      - specified site — *see* Neoplasm, malignant, by site
      - unspecified site (female) C5Ø.91-
        - male C5Ø.92-
    - breast DØ5.1-
    - specified site NEC — *see* Neoplasm, in situ, by site
    - unspecified site DØ5.1-
  - serous
    - specified site — *see* Neoplasm, malignant, by site
    - unspecified site C56.9
- papillocystic
  - specified site — *see* Neoplasm, malignant, by site
  - unspecified site C56.9
- pseudomucinous
  - specified site — *see* Neoplasm, malignant, by site
  - unspecified site C56.9
- renal cell C64-
- sebaceous — *see* Neoplasm, skin, malignant
- serous (*see also* Neoplasm, malignant, by site)
  - papillary
    - specified site — *see* Neoplasm, malignant, by site
    - unspecified site C56.9
- sweat gland — *see* Neoplasm, skin, malignant
- water-clear cell C75.Ø

Adenocarcinoma-in-situ (*see also* Neoplasm, in situ, by site)
- breast DØ5.9-

Adenofibroma
- clear cell — *see* Neoplasm, benign, by site
- endometrioid D27.9
  - borderline malignancy D39.1Ø
  - malignant C56-
- mucinous
  - specified site — *see* Neoplasm, benign, by site
  - unspecified site D27.9
- papillary
  - specified site — *see* Neoplasm, benign, by site
  - unspecified site D27.9
- prostate — *see* Enlargement, enlarged, prostate

Adenofibroma — *continued*
- serous
  - specified site — *see* Neoplasm, benign, by site
  - unspecified site D27.9
- specified site — *see* Neoplasm, benign, by site
- unspecified site D27.9

Adenofibrosis
- breast — *see* Fibroadenosis, breast
- endometrioid N8Ø.Ø

Adenoiditis (chronic) J35.Ø2
- with tonsillitis J35.Ø3
- acute JØ3.9Ø
  - recurrent JØ3.91
  - specified organism NEC JØ3.8Ø
    - recurrent JØ3.81
  - staphylococcal JØ3.8Ø
    - recurrent JØ3.81
  - streptococcal JØ3.ØØ
    - recurrent JØ3.Ø1

Adenoids — *see* condition

Adenolipoma — *see* Neoplasm, benign, by site

Adenolipomatosis, Launois-Bensaude E88.89

Adenolymphoma
- specified site — *see* Neoplasm, benign, by site
- unspecified site D11.9

Adenoma (*see also* Neoplasm, benign, by site)
- acidophil
  - specified site — *see* Neoplasm, benign, by site
  - unspecified site D35.2
- acidophil-basophil, mixed
  - specified site — *see* Neoplasm, benign, by site
  - unspecified site D35.2
- adrenal (cortical) D35.ØØ
  - clear cell D35.ØØ
  - compact cell D35.ØØ
  - glomerulosa cell D35.ØØ
  - heavily pigmented variant D35.ØØ
  - mixed cell D35.ØØ
- alpha-cell
  - pancreas D13.7
  - specified site NEC — *see* Neoplasm, benign, by site
  - unspecified site D13.7
- alveolar D14.3Ø
- apocrine
  - breast D24-
  - specified site NEC — *see* Neoplasm, skin, benign, by site
  - unspecified site D23.9
- basal cell D11.9
- basophil
  - specified site — *see* Neoplasm, benign, by site
  - unspecified site D35.2
- basophil-acidophil, mixed
  - specified site — *see* Neoplasm, benign, by site
  - unspecified site D35.2
- beta-cell
  - pancreas D13.7
  - specified site NEC — *see* Neoplasm, benign, by site
  - unspecified site D13.7
- bile duct D13.4
  - common D13.5
  - extrahepatic D13.5
  - intrahepatic D13.4
  - specified site NEC — *see* Neoplasm, benign, by site
  - unspecified site D13.4
- black D35.ØØ
- bronchial D38.1
  - cylindroid type — *see* Neoplasm, lung, malignant
- ceruminous D23.2-
- chief cell D35.1
- chromophobe
  - specified site — *see* Neoplasm, benign, by site
  - unspecified site D35.2
- colloid
  - specified site — *see* Neoplasm, benign, by site
  - unspecified site D34
- duct
- eccrine, papillary — *see* Neoplasm, skin, benign

Adenoma — *continued*
- endocrine, multiple
  - single specified site — *see* Neoplasm, uncertain behavior, by site
  - two or more specified sites D44-
  - unspecified site D44.9
- endometrioid (*see also* Neoplasm, benign)
  - borderline malignancy — *see* Neoplasm, uncertain behavior, by site
- eosinophil
  - specified site — *see* Neoplasm, benign, by site
  - unspecified site D35.2
- fetal
  - specified site — *see* Neoplasm, benign, by site
  - unspecified site D34
- follicular
  - specified site — *see* Neoplasm, benign, by site
  - unspecified site D34
- hepatocellular D13.4
- Hurthle cell D34
- islet cell
  - pancreas D13.7
  - specified site NEC — *see* Neoplasm, benign, by site
  - unspecified site D13.7
- liver cell D13.4
- macrofollicular
  - specified site — *see* Neoplasm, benign, by site
  - unspecified site D34
- malignant, malignum — *see* Neoplasm, malignant, by site
- microcystic
  - pancreas D13.7
  - specified site NEC — *see* Neoplasm, benign, by site
  - unspecified site D13.7
- microfollicular
  - specified site — *see* Neoplasm, benign, by site
  - unspecified site D34
- mucoid cell
  - specified site — *see* Neoplasm, benign, by site
  - unspecified site D35.2
- multiple endocrine
  - single specified site — *see* Neoplasm, uncertain behavior, by site
  - two or more specified sites D44-
  - unspecified site D44.9
- nipple D24-
- papillary (*see also* Neoplasm, benign, by site)
  - eccrine — *see* Neoplasm, skin, benign, by site
- Pick's tubular
  - specified site — *see* Neoplasm, benign, by site
  - unspecified site
    - female D27.9
    - male D29.2Ø
- pleomorphic
  - carcinoma in — *see* Neoplasm, salivary gland, malignant
    - specified site — *see* Neoplasm, malignant, by site
    - unspecified site CØ8.9
- polypoid (*see also* Neoplasm, benign)
  - adenocarcinoma in — *see* Neoplasm, malignant, by site
  - adenocarcinoma in situ — *see* Neoplasm, in situ, by site
- prostate — *see* Neoplasm, benign, prostate
- rete cell D29.2Ø
- sebaceous — *see* Neoplasm, skin, benign
- Sertoli cell
  - specified site — *see* Neoplasm, benign, by site
  - unspecified site
    - female D27.9
    - male D29.2Ø
- skin appendage — *see* Neoplasm, skin, benign
- sudoriferous gland — *see* Neoplasm, skin, benign
- sweat gland — *see* Neoplasm, skin, benign
- testicular
  - specified site — *see* Neoplasm, benign, by site
  - unspecified site
    - female D27.9
    - male D29.2Ø

- **Admission** — *continued*
  - adjustment — *continued*
    - brain neuropacemaker Z46.2
      - implanted Z45.42
    - breast
      - implant Z45.81
      - prosthesis (external) Z44.3
    - colostomy belt Z46.89
    - contact lenses Z46.Ø
    - cystostomy device Z46.6
    - dental prosthesis Z46.3
    - device NEC
      - abdominal Z46.89
      - implanted Z45.89
        - cardiac Z45.Ø9
          - defibrillator (with synchronous cardiac pacemaker) Z45.Ø2
          - pacemaker Z45.Ø18
            - pulse generator Z45.Ø1Ø
        - hearing device Z45.328
          - bone conduction Z45.32Ø
          - cochlear Z45.321
        - infusion pump Z45.1
        - nervous system Z45.49
          - CSF drainage Z45.41
          - hearing device — *see* Admission, adjustment, device, implanted, hearing device
          - neuropacemaker Z45.42
          - visual substitution Z45.31
        - specified NEC Z45.89
        - vascular access Z45.2
        - visual substitution Z45.31
      - nervous system Z46.2
        - implanted — *see* Admission, adjustment, device, implanted, nervous system
      - orthodontic Z46.4
      - prosthetic Z44.9
        - arm — *see* Admission, adjustment, artificial, arm
        - breast Z44.3
        - dental Z46.3
        - eye Z44.2
        - leg — *see* Admission, adjustment, artificial, leg
        - specified type NEC Z44.8
      - substitution
        - auditory Z46.2
          - implanted — *see* Admission, adjustment, device, implanted, hearing device
        - nervous system Z46.2
          - implanted — *see* Admission, adjustment, device, implanted, nervous system
        - visual Z46.2
          - implanted Z45.31
      - urinary Z46.6
    - hearing aid Z46.1
      - implanted — *see* Admission, adjustment, device, implanted, hearing device
    - ileostomy device Z46.89
    - intestinal appliance or device NEC Z46.89
    - neuropacemaker (brain) (peripheral nerve) (spinal cord) Z46.2
      - implanted Z45.42
    - orthodontic device Z46.4
    - orthopedic (brace) (cast) (device) (shoes) Z46.89
    - pacemaker
      - cardiac Z45.Ø18
        - pulse generator Z45.Ø1Ø
      - nervous system Z46.2
        - implanted Z45.42
    - portacath (port-a-cath) Z45.2
    - prosthesis Z44.9
      - arm — *see* Admission, adjustment, artificial, arm
      - breast Z44.3
      - dental Z46.3
      - eye Z44.2
      - leg — *see* Admission, adjustment, artificial, leg
      - specified NEC Z44.8

- **Admission** — *continued*
  - adjustment — *continued*
    - spectacles Z46.Ø
  - aftercare (*see also* Aftercare) Z51.89
    - postpartum
      - immediately after delivery Z39.Ø
      - routine follow-up Z39.2
    - radiation therapy (antineoplastic) Z51.Ø
  - attention to artificial opening (of) Z43.9
    - artificial vagina Z43.7
    - colostomy Z43.3
    - cystostomy Z43.5
    - enterostomy Z43.4
    - gastrostomy Z43.1
    - ileostomy Z43.2
    - jejunostomy Z43.4
    - nephrostomy Z43.6
    - specified site NEC Z43.8
      - intestinal tract Z43.4
      - urinary tract Z43.6
    - tracheostomy Z43.Ø
    - ureterostomy Z43.6
    - urethrostomy Z43.6
  - breast augmentation or reduction Z41.1
  - breast reconstruction following mastectomy Z42.1
  - change of
    - dressing (nonsurgical) Z48.ØØ
    - neuropacemaker device (brain) (peripheral nerve) (spinal cord) Z46.2
      - implanted Z45.42
    - surgical dressing Z48.Ø1
  - circumcision, ritual or routine (in absence of diagnosis) Z41.2
  - clinical research investigation (control) (normal comparison) (participant) ZØØ.6
  - contraceptive management Z3Ø.9
  - cosmetic surgery NEC Z41.1
  - counseling (*see also* Counseling)
    - dietary Z71.3
    - HIV Z71.7
    - human immunodeficiency virus Z71.7
    - nonattending third party Z71.Ø
    - procreative management NEC Z31.69
  - delivery, full-term, uncomplicated O8Ø
    - cesarean, without indication O82
  - dietary surveillance and counseling Z71.3
  - ear piercing Z41.3
  - examination (*see also* Examination) at health care facility (adult) ZØØ.ØØ
    - with abnormal findings ZØØ.Ø1
    - clinical research investigation (control) (normal comparison) (participant) ZØØ.6
    - dental ZØ1.2Ø
      - with abnormal findings ZØ1.21
    - donor (potential) ZØØ.5
    - ear ZØ1.1Ø
      - with abnormal findings NEC ZØ1.118
    - eye ZØ1.ØØ
      - with abnormal findings ZØ1.Ø1
    - general, specified reason NEC ZØØ.8
    - hearing ZØ1.1Ø
      - with abnormal findings NEC ZØ1.118
    - postpartum checkup Z39.2
    - psychiatric (general) ZØØ.8
      - requested by authority ZØ4.6
    - vision ZØ1.ØØ
      - with abnormal findings ZØ1.Ø1
  - fitting (of)
    - artificial
      - arm — *see* Admission, adjustment, artificial, arm
      - eye Z44.2
      - leg — *see* Admission, adjustment, artificial, leg
    - brain neuropacemaker Z46.2
      - implanted Z45.42
    - breast prosthesis (external) Z44.3
    - colostomy belt Z46.89
    - contact lenses Z46.Ø
    - cystostomy device Z46.6
    - dental prosthesis Z46.3
    - dentures Z46.3

- **Admission** — *continued*
  - fitting (of) — *continued*
    - device NEC
      - abdominal Z46.89
      - nervous system Z46.2
        - implanted — *see* Admission, adjustment, device, implanted, nervous system
      - orthodontic Z46.4
      - prosthetic Z44.9
        - breast Z44.3
        - dental Z46.3
        - eye Z44.2
      - substitution
        - auditory Z46.2
          - implanted — *see* Admission, adjustment, device, implanted, hearing device
        - nervous system Z46.2
          - implanted — *see* Admission, adjustment, device, implanted, nervous system
        - visual Z46.2
          - implanted Z45.31
    - hearing aid Z46.1
    - ileostomy device Z46.89
    - intestinal appliance or device NEC Z46.89
    - neuropacemaker (brain) (peripheral nerve) (spinal cord) Z46.2
      - implanted Z45.42
    - orthodontic device Z46.4
    - orthopedic device (brace) (cast) (shoes) Z46.89
    - prosthesis Z44.9
      - arm — *see* Admission, adjustment, artificial, arm
      - breast Z44.3
      - dental Z46.3
      - eye Z44.2
      - leg — *see* Admission, adjustment, artificial, leg
      - specified type NEC Z44.8
    - spectacles Z46.Ø
  - follow-up examination ZØ9
  - intrauterine device management Z3Ø.431
    - initial prescription Z3Ø.Ø14
  - mental health evaluation ZØØ.8
    - requested by authority ZØ4.6
  - observation — *see* Observation
  - Papanicolaou smear, cervix Z12.4
    - for suspected malignant neoplasm Z12.4
  - plastic surgery, cosmetic NEC Z41.1
  - postpartum observation
    - immediately after delivery Z39.Ø
    - routine follow-up Z39.2
  - poststerilization (for restoration) Z31.Ø
    - aftercare Z31.42
  - plastic and reconstructive surgery following medical procedure or healed injury NEC Z42.8
  - procreative management Z31.9
  - prophylactic (measure)
    - organ removal Z4Ø.ØØ
      - breast Z4Ø.Ø1
      - ovary Z4Ø.Ø2
      - specified organ NEC Z4Ø.Ø9
      - testes Z4Ø.Ø9
    - vaccination Z23
  - psychiatric examination (general) ZØØ.8
    - requested by authority ZØ4.6
  - radiation therapy (antineoplastic) Z51.Ø
  - reconstructive surgery following medical procedure or healed injury NEC Z42.8
  - removal of
    - cystostomy catheter Z43.5
    - drains Z48.Ø3
    - dressing (nonsurgical) Z48.ØØ
    - intrauterine contraceptive device Z3Ø.432
    - neuropacemaker (brain) (peripheral nerve) (spinal cord) Z46.2
      - implanted Z45.42
    - staples Z48.Ø2
    - surgical dressing Z48.Ø1
    - sutures Z48.Ø2
    - ureteral stent Z46.6

Admission — *continued*
- respirator [ventilator] use during power failure Z99.12
- restoration of organ continuity (poststerilization) Z31.Ø
  - aftercare Z31.42
- sensitivity test (*see also* Test, skin)
  - allergy NEC ZØ1.82
  - Mantoux Z11.1
- tuboplasty following previous sterilization Z31.Ø
  - aftercare Z31.42
- vasoplasty following previous sterilization Z31.Ø
  - aftercare Z31.42
- vision examination ZØ1.ØØ
  - with abnormal findings ZØ1.Ø1
- waiting period for admission to other facility Z75.1

Adnexitis (suppurative) — *see* Salpingo-oophoritis
Adolescent X-linked adrenoleukodystrophy E71.521
AIPHI RØ4.81
Albers-Schönberg syndrome Q78.2
Adrenal (gland) — *see* condition
Adrenalism, tuberculous A18.7
Adrenalitis, adrenitis E27.8
- autoimmune E27.1
- meningococcal, hemorrhagic A39.1

Adrenarche, premature E27.Ø
Adrenocortical syndrome — *see* Cushing's, syndrome
Adrenogenital syndrome E25.9
- acquired E25.8
- congenital E25.Ø
- salt loss E25.Ø

Adrenogenitalism, congenital E25.Ø
Adrenoleukodystrophy E71.529
- neonatal E71.511
- X-linked E71.529
  - Addison only phenotype E71.528
  - Addison-Schilder E71.528
  - adolescent E71.521
  - adrenomyeloneuropathy E71.522
  - childhood cerebral E71.52Ø
  - other specified E71.528

Adrenomyeloneuropathy E71.522
Adventitious bursa — *see* Bursopathy, specified type NEC
Adverse effect — *see* Table of Drugs and Chemicals, categories T36-T5Ø, with 6th character 5
Advice — *see* Counseling
Adynamia (episodica) (hereditary) (periodic) G72.3
Aeration lung imperfect, newborn — *see* Atelectasis
Aerobullosis T7Ø.3
Aerocele — *see* Embolism, air
Aerodermectasia
- subcutaneous (traumatic) T79.7

Aerodontalgia T7Ø.29
Aeroembolism T7Ø.3
Aerogenes capsulatus infection A48.Ø
Aero-otitis media T7Ø.Ø
Aerophagy, aerophagia (psychogenic) F45.8
Aerophobia F4Ø.228
Aerosinusitis T7Ø.1
Aerotitis T7Ø.Ø
Affection — *see* Disease
Afibrinogenemia (*see also* Defect, coagulation) D68.8
- acquired D65
- congenital D68.2
- following ectopic or molar pregnancy OØ8.1
- in abortion — *see* Abortion, by type, complicated by, afibrinogenemia
- puerperal O72.3

African
- sleeping sickness B56.9
- tick fever A68.1
- trypanosomiasis B56.9
  - gambian B56.Ø
  - rhodesian B56.1

Aftercare (*see also* Care) Z51.89
- following surgery (for) (on)
  - amputation Z47.81
  - attention to
    - drains Z48.Ø3
    - dressings (nonsurgical) Z48.ØØ
      - surgical Z48.Ø1

Aftercare — *continued*
- following surgery — *continued*
  - attention to — *continued*
    - sutures Z48.Ø2
  - circulatory system Z48.812
  - delayed (planned) wound closure Z48.1
  - digestive system Z48.815
  - explantation of joint prosthesis (staged procedure)
    - hip Z47.32
    - knee Z47.33
    - shoulder Z47.31
  - genitourinary system Z48.816
  - joint replacement Z47.1
  - neoplasm Z48.3
  - nervous system Z48.811
  - oral cavity Z48.814
  - organ transplant
    - bone marrow Z48.29Ø
    - heart Z48.21
    - heart-lung Z48.28Ø
    - kidney Z48.22
    - liver Z48.23
    - lung Z48.24
    - multiple organs NEC Z48.288
    - specified NEC Z48.298
  - orthopedic NEC Z47.89
  - planned wound closure Z48.1
  - removal of internal fixation device Z47.2
  - respiratory system Z48.813
  - scoliosis Z47.82
  - sense organs Z48.81Ø
  - skin and subcutaneous tissue Z48.817
  - specified body system
    - circulatory Z48.812
    - digestive Z48.815
    - genitourinary Z48.816
    - nervous Z48.811
    - oral cavity Z48.814
    - respiratory Z48.813
    - sense organs Z48.81Ø
    - skin and subcutaneous tissue Z48.817
    - teeth Z48.814
  - specified NEC Z48.89
  - spinal Z48.89
  - teeth Z48.814
- fracture—code to fracture with seventh character D
- involving
  - removal of
    - drains Z48.Ø3
    - dressings (nonsurgical) Z48.ØØ
    - staples Z48.Ø2
    - surgical dressings Z48.Ø1
    - sutures Z48.Ø2
- neuropacemaker (brain) (peripheral nerve) (spinal cord) Z46.2
  - implanted Z45.42
- orthopedic NEC Z47.89
- postprocedural — *see* Aftercare, following surgery

After-cataract — *see* Cataract, secondary
Agalactia (primary) O92.3
- elective, secondary or therapeutic O92.5

Agammaglobulinemia (acquired (secondary)) (nonfamilial) D8Ø.1
- with
  - immunoglobulin-bearing B-lymphocytes D8Ø.1
  - lymphopenia D81.9
- autosomal recessive (Swiss type) D8Ø.Ø
- Bruton's X-linked D8Ø.Ø
- common variable (CVAgamma) D8Ø.1
- congenital sex-linked D8Ø.Ø
- hereditary D8Ø.Ø
- lymphopenic D81.9
- Swiss type (autosomal recessive) D8Ø.Ø
- X-linked (with growth hormone deficiency)(Bruton) D8Ø.Ø

Aganglionosis (bowel) (colon) Q43.1
Age (old) — *see* Senility
Agenesis
- adrenal (gland) Q89.1
- alimentary tract (complete) (partial) NEC Q45.8
  - upper Q4Ø.8
- anus, anal (canal) Q42.3

Agenesis — *continued*
- anus, anal — *continued*
  - with fistula Q42.2
- aorta Q25.4
- appendix Q42.8
- arm (complete) Q71.Ø-
  - with hand present Q71.1-
- artery (peripheral) Q27.9
  - brain Q28.3
  - coronary Q24.5
  - pulmonary Q25.79
  - specified NEC Q27.8
  - umbilical Q27.Ø
- auditory (canal) (external) Q16.1
- auricle (ear) Q16.Ø
- bile duct or passage Q44.5
- bladder Q64.5
- bone Q79.9
- brain QØØ.Ø
  - part of QØ4.3
- breast (with nipple present) Q83.8
  - with absent nipple Q83.Ø
- bronchus Q32.4
- canaliculus lacrimalis Q1Ø.4
- carpus — *see* Agenesis, hand
- cartilage Q79.9
- cecum Q42.8
- cerebellum QØ4.3
- cervix Q51.5
- chin Q18.8
- cilia Q1Ø.3
- circulatory system, part NOS Q28.9
- clavicle Q74.Ø
- clitoris Q52.6
- coccyx Q76.49
- colon Q42.9
  - specified NEC Q42.8
- corpus callosum QØ4.Ø
- cricoid cartilage Q31.8
- diaphragm (with hernia) Q79.1
- digestive organ(s) or tract (complete) (partial) NEC Q45.8
  - upper Q4Ø.8
- ductus arteriosus Q28.8
- duodenum Q41.Ø
- ear Q16.9
  - auricle Q16.Ø
  - lobe Q17.8
- ejaculatory duct Q55.4
- endocrine (gland) NEC Q89.2
- epiglottis Q31.8
- esophagus Q39.8
- eustachian tube Q16.2
- eye Q11.1
  - adnexa Q15.8
- eyelid (fold) Q1Ø.3
- face
  - bones NEC Q75.8
  - specified part NEC Q18.8
- fallopian tube Q5Ø.6
- femur — *see* Defect, reduction, lower limb, longitudinal, femur
- fibula — *see* Defect, reduction, lower limb, longitudinal, fibula
- finger (complete) (partial) — *see* Agenesis, hand
- foot (and toes) (complete) (partial) Q72.3-
- forearm (with hand present) — *see* Agenesis, arm, with hand present
  - and hand Q71.2-
- gallbladder Q44.Ø
- gastric Q4Ø.2
- genitalia, genital (organ(s))
  - female Q52.8
    - external Q52.71
    - internal NEC Q52.8
  - male Q55.8
- glottis Q31.8
- hair Q84.Ø
- hand (and fingers) (complete) (partial) Q71.3-
- heart Q24.8
  - valve NEC Q24.8
    - pulmonary Q22.Ø
- hepatic Q44.7

- **Albuminuria** — *continued*
  - pre-eclamptic — *see* Pre-eclampsia
  - scarlatinal A38.8
- **Albuminurophobia** F4Ø.298
- **Alcaptonuria** E7Ø.29
- **Alcohol, alcoholic, alcohol-induced**
  - addiction (without remission) F1Ø.2Ø
    - with remission F1Ø.21
  - amnestic disorder, persisting F1Ø.96
    - with dependence F1Ø.26
  - brain syndrome, chronic F1Ø.97
    - with dependence F1Ø.27
  - cardiopathy I42.6
  - counseling and surveillance Z71.41
    - family member Z71.42
  - delirium (acute) (tremens) (withdrawal) F1Ø.231
    - with intoxication F1Ø.921
      - in
        - abuse F1Ø.121
        - dependence F1Ø.221
  - dementia F1Ø.97
    - with dependence F1Ø.27
  - deterioration F1Ø.97
    - with dependence F1Ø.27
  - hallucinosis (acute) F1Ø.951
    - in
      - abuse F1Ø.151
      - dependence F1Ø.251
  - insanity F1Ø.959
  - intoxication (acute) (without dependence) F1Ø.129
    - with
      - delirium F1Ø.121
      - dependence F1Ø.229
        - with delirium F1Ø.221
        - uncomplicated F1Ø.22Ø
    - uncomplicated F1Ø.12Ø
  - jealousy F1Ø.988
  - Korsakoff's, Korsakov's, Korsakow's F1Ø.26
  - liver K7Ø.9
    - acute — *see* Disease, liver, alcoholic, hepatitis
  - mania (acute) (chronic) F1Ø.959
  - paranoia, paranoid (type) psychosis F1Ø.95Ø
  - pellagra E52
  - poisoning, accidental (acute) NEC — *see* Table of Drugs and Chemicals, alcohol, poisoning
  - psychosis — *see* Psychosis, alcoholic
  - withdrawal (without convulsions) F1Ø.239
    - with delirium F1Ø.231
- **Alcoholism** (chronic) (without remission) F1Ø.2Ø
  - with
    - psychosis — *see* Psychosis, alcoholic
    - remission F1Ø.21
  - Korsakov's F1Ø.96
    - with dependence F1Ø.26
- **Alder** (-Reilly) **anomaly or syndrome** (leukocyte granulation) D72.Ø
- **Aldosteronism** E26.9
  - familial (type I) E26.Ø2
  - glucocorticoid-remediable E26.Ø2
  - primary (due to (bilateral) adrenal hyperplasia) E26.Ø9
  - primary NEC E26.Ø9
  - secondary E26.1
  - specified NEC E26.89
- **Aldosteronoma** D44.1Ø
- **Aldrich**(-Wiskott) **syndrome** (eczema-thrombocytopenia) D82.Ø
- **Alektorophobia** F4Ø.218
- **Aleppo boil** B55.1
- **Aleukemic** — *see* condition
- **Aleukia**
  - congenital D7Ø.Ø
  - hemorrhagica D61.9
    - congenital D61.Ø9
  - splenica D73.1
- **Alexia** R48.Ø
  - developmental F81.Ø
  - secondary to organic lesion R48.Ø
- **Algoneurodystrophy** M89.ØØ
  - ankle M89.Ø7-
  - foot M89.Ø7-
  - forearm M89.Ø3-
  - hand M89.Ø4-
- **Algoneurodystrophy** — *continued*
  - lower leg M89.Ø6-
  - multiple sites M89.Ø-
  - shoulder M89.Ø1-
  - specified site NEC M89.Ø8
  - thigh M89.Ø5-
  - upper arm M89.Ø2-
- **Algophobia** F4Ø.298
- **Alienation, mental** — *see* Psychosis
- **Alkalemia** E87.3
- **Alkalosis** E87.3
  - metabolic E87.3
    - with respiratory acidosis E87.4
  - respiratory E87.3
- **Alkaptonuria** E7Ø.29
- **Allen-Masters syndrome** N83.8
- **Allergy, allergic** (reaction) (to) T78.4Ø
  - air-borne substance NEC (rhinitis) J3Ø.89
  - alveolitis (extrinsic) J67.9
    - due to
      - Aspergillus clavatus J67.4
      - Cryptostroma corticale J67.5
      - organisms (fungal, thermophilic actinomycete) growing in ventilation (air conditioning) systems J67.7
    - specified type NEC J67.8
  - anaphylactic reaction or shock T78.2
  - angioneurotic edema T78.3
  - animal (dander) (epidermal) (hair) (rhinitis) J3Ø.81
  - bee sting (anaphylactic shock) — *see* Toxicity, venom, arthropod, bee
  - biological — *see* Allergy, drug
  - colitis K52.2
  - dander (animal) (rhinitis) J3Ø.81
  - dandruff (rhinitis) J3Ø.81
  - dental restorative material (existing) KØ8.55
  - dermatitis — *see* Dermatitis, contact, allergic
  - diathesis — *see* History, allergy
  - drug, medicament & biological (any) (external) (internal) T78.4Ø
    - correct substance properly administered — *see* Table of Drugs and Chemicals, by drug, adverse effect
    - wrong substance given or taken NEC (by accident) — *see* Table of Drugs and Chemicals, by drug, poisoning
  - due to pollen J3Ø.1
  - dust (house) (stock) (rhinitis) J3Ø.89
    - with asthma — *see* Asthma, allergic extrinsic
  - eczema — *see* Dermatitis, contact, allergic
  - epidermal (animal) (rhinitis) J3Ø.81
  - feathers (rhinitis) J3Ø.89
  - food (any) (ingested) NEC T78.1
    - anaphylactic shock — *see* Shock, anaphylactic, due to food
    - dermatitis — *see* Dermatitis, due to, food
    - dietary counseling and surveillance Z71.3
    - in contact with skin L23.6
    - rhinitis J3Ø.5
    - status (without reaction) Z91.Ø18
      - eggs Z91.Ø12
      - milk products Z91.Ø11
      - peanuts Z91.Ø1Ø
      - seafood Z91.Ø13
      - specified NEC Z91.Ø18
  - gastrointestinal K52.2
  - grain J3Ø.1
  - grass (hay fever) (pollen) J3Ø.1
    - asthma — *see* Asthma, allergic extrinsic
  - hair (animal) (rhinitis) J3Ø.81
  - history (of) — *see* History, allergy
  - horse serum — *see* Allergy, serum
  - inhalant (rhinitis) J3Ø.89
    - pollen J3Ø.1
  - kapok (rhinitis) J3Ø.89
  - medicine — *see* Allergy, drug
  - milk protein K52.2
  - nasal, seasonal due to pollen J3Ø.1
  - pneumonia J82
  - pollen (any) (hay fever) J3Ø.1
    - asthma — *see* Asthma, allergic extrinsic
  - primrose J3Ø.1
  - primula J3Ø.1
- **Allergy** — *continued*
  - purpura D69.Ø
  - ragweed (hay fever) (pollen) J3Ø.1
    - asthma — *see* Asthma, allergic extrinsic
  - rose (pollen) J3Ø.1
  - seasonal NEC J3Ø.2
  - Senecio jacobae (pollen) J3Ø.1
  - serum (*see also* Reaction, serum) T8Ø.69
    - anaphylactic shock T8Ø.59
  - shock (anaphylactic) T78.2
    - due to
      - administration of blood and blood products T8Ø.51
      - adverse effect of correct medicinal substance properly administered T88.6
      - immunization T8Ø.52
      - serum NEC T8Ø.59
      - vaccination T8Ø.52
  - specific NEC T78.49
  - tree (any) (hay fever) (pollen) J3Ø.1
    - asthma — *see* Asthma, allergic extrinsic
  - upper respiratory J3Ø.9
  - urticaria L5Ø.Ø
  - vaccine — *see* Allergy, serum
- **Allescheriasis** B48.2
- **Alligator skin disease** Q8Ø.9
- **Allocheiria, allochiria** R2Ø.8
- **Almeida's disease** — *see* Paracoccidioidomycosis
- **Alopecia** (hereditaria) (seborrheica) L65.9
  - androgenic L64.9
    - drug-induced L64.Ø
    - specified NEC L64.8
  - areata L63.9
    - ophiasis L63.2
    - specified NEC L63.8
    - totalis L63.Ø
    - universalis L63.1
  - cicatricial L66.9
    - specified NEC L66.8
  - circumscripta L63.9
  - congenital, congenitalis Q84.Ø
  - due to cytotoxic drugs NEC L65.8
  - mucinosa L65.2
  - postinfective NEC L65.8
  - postpartum L65.Ø
  - premature L64.8
  - specific (syphilitic) A51.32
  - specified NEC L65.8
  - syphilitic (secondary) A51.32
  - totalis (capitis) L63.Ø
  - universalis (entire body) L63.1
  - X-ray L58.1
- **Alpers' disease** G31.81
- **Alpine sickness** T7Ø.29
- **Alport syndrome** Q87.81
- **ALTE** (apparent life threatening event) **in newborn and infant** R68.13
- **Alteration** (of)**, Altered**
  - awareness, transient R4Ø.4
  - mental status R41.82
  - pattern of family relationships affecting child Z62.898
  - sensation
    - following
      - cerebrovascular disease I69.998
        - cerebral infarction I69.398
        - intracerebral hemorrhage I69.198
        - nontraumatic intracranial hemorrhage NEC I69.298
        - specified disease NEC I69.898
        - subarachnoid hemorrhage I69.Ø98
- **Alternating** — *see* condition
- **Altitude, high** (effects) — *see* Effect, adverse, high altitude
- **Aluminosis** (of lung) J63.Ø
- **Alveolitis**
  - allergic (extrinsic) — *see* Pneumonitis, hypersensitivity
  - due to
    - Aspergillus clavatus J67.4
    - Cryptostroma corticale J67.6
  - fibrosing (cryptogenic) (idiopathic) J84.112
  - jaw M27.3

Alveolitis — *continued*
  sicca dolorosa M27.3
Alveolus, alveolar — *see* condition
Alymphocytosis D72.820
  thymic (with immunodeficiency) D82.1
Alymphoplasia, thymic D82.1
Alzheimer's disease or sclerosis — *see* Disease, Alzheimer's
Amastia (with nipple present) Q83.8
  with absent nipple Q83.0
Amathophobia F40.228
Amaurosis (acquired) (congenital) (*see also* Blindness)
  fugax G45.3
  hysterical F44.6
  Leber's congenital H35.50
  uremic — *see* Uremia
Amaurotic idiocy (infantile) (juvenile) (late) E75.4
Amaxophobia F40.248
Ambiguous genitalia Q56.4
Amblyopia (congenital) (ex anopsia) (partial) (suppression) H53.00-
  anisometropic — *see* Amblyopia, refractive
  deprivation H53.01-
  hysterical F44.6
  nocturnal (*see also* Blindness, night)
    vitamin A deficiency E50.5
  refractive H53.02-
  strabismic H53.03-
  tobacco H53.8
  toxic NEC H53.8
  uremic — *see* Uremia
Ameba, amebic (histolytica) (*see also* Amebiasis)
  abscess (liver) A06.4
Amebiasis A06.9
  with abscess — *see* Abscess, amebic
  acute A06.0
  chronic (intestine) A06.1
    with abscess — *see* Abscess, amebic
  cutaneous A06.7
  cutis A06.7
  cystitis A06.81
  genitourinary tract NEC A06.82
  hepatic — *see* Abscess, liver, amebic
  intestine A06.0
  nondysenteric colitis A06.2
  skin A06.7
  specified site NEC A06.89
Ameboma (of intestine) A06.3
Amelia Q73.0
  lower limb — *see* Agenesis, leg
  upper limb — *see* Agenesis, arm
Ameloblastoma (*see also* Cyst, calcifying odontogenic)
  long bones C40.9-
    lower limb C40.2-
    upper limb C40.0-
  malignant C41.1
    jaw (bone) (lower) C41.1
      upper C41.0
  tibial C40.2-
Amelogenesis imperfecta K00.5
  nonhereditaria (segmentalis) K00.4
Amenorrhea N91.2
  hyperhormonal E28.8
  primary N91.0
  secondary N91.1
Amentia — *see* Disability, intellectual
  Meynert's (nonalcoholic) F04
American
  leishmaniasis B55.2
  mountain tick fever A93.2
Ametropia — *see* Disorder, refraction
Amianthosis J61
Amimia R48.8
Amino-acid disorder E72.9
  anemia D53.0
Aminoacidopathy E72.9
Aminoaciduria E72.9
Amnes(t)ic syndrome (post-traumatic) F04
  induced by
    alcohol F10.96
      with dependence F10.26
    psychoactive NEC F19.96

Amnes(t)ic syndrome — *continued*
  induced by — *continued*
    psychoactive NEC — *continued*
      with
        abuse F19.16
        dependence F19.26
    sedative F13.96
      with dependence F13.26
Amnesia R41.3
  anterograde R41.1
  auditory R48.8
  dissociative F44.0
  hysterical F44.0
  postictal in epilepsy — *see* Epilepsy
  psychogenic F44.0
  retrograde R41.2
  transient global G45.4
Amnion, amniotic — *see* condition
Amnionitis — *see* Pregnancy, complicated by
Amok F68.8
Amoral traits F60.89
Ampulla
  lower esophagus K22.8
  phrenic K22.8
Amputation (*see also* Absence, by site, acquired)
  neuroma (postoperative) (traumatic) — *see* Complications, amputation stump, neuroma
  stump (surgical)
    abnormal, painful, or with complication (late) — *see* Complications, amputation stump
    healed or old NOS Z89.9
  traumatic (complete) (partial)
    arm (upper) (complete) S48.91-
      at
        elbow S58.01-
          partial S58.02-
        shoulder joint (complete) S48.01-
          partial S48.02-
      between
        elbow and wrist (complete) S58.11-
          partial S58.12-
        shoulder and elbow (complete) S48.11-
          partial S48.12-
      partial S48.92-
    breast (complete) S28.21-
      partial S28.22-
    clitoris (complete) S38.211
      partial S38.212
    ear (complete) S08.11-
      partial S08.12-
    finger (complete) (metacarpophalangeal) S68.11-
      index S68.11-
      little S68.11-
      middle S68.11-
      partial S68.12-
        index S68.12-
        little S68.12-
        middle S68.12-
        ring S68.12-
      ring S68.11-
      thumb — *see* Amputation, traumatic, thumb
      transphalangeal (complete) S68.61-
        index S68.61-
        little S68.61-
        middle S68.61-
        partial S68.62-
          index S68.62-
          little S68.62-
          middle S68.62-
          ring S68.62-
        ring S68.61-
    foot (complete) S98.91-
      at ankle level S98.01-
        partial S98.02-
      midfoot S98.31-
        partial S98.32-
      partial S98.92-
    forearm (complete) S58.91-
      at elbow level (complete) S58.01-
        partial S58.02-
      between elbow and wrist (complete) S58.11-
        partial S58.12-

Amputation — *continued*
  traumatic — *continued*
    forearm — *continued*
      partial S58.92-
    genital organ(s) (external)
      female (complete) S38.211
        partial S38.212
      male
        penis (complete) S38.221
          partial S38.222
        scrotum (complete) S38.231
          partial S38.232
        testes (complete) S38.231
          partial S38.232
    hand (complete) (wrist level) S68.41-
      finger(s) alone — *see* Amputation, traumatic, finger
      partial S68.42-
      thumb alone — *see* Amputation, traumatic, thumb
      transmetacarpal (complete) S68.71-
        partial S68.72-
    head
      ear — *see* Amputation, traumatic, ear
      nose (partial) S08.812
        complete S08.811
      part S08.89
        scalp S08.0
    hip (and thigh) (complete) S78.91-
      at hip joint (complete) S78.01-
        partial S78.02-
      between hip and knee (complete) S78.11-
        partial S78.12-
      partial S78.92-
    labium (majus) (minus) (complete) S38.21-
      partial S38.21-
    leg (lower) S88.91-
      at knee level S88.01-
        partial S88.02-
      between knee and ankle S88.11-
        partial S88.12-
      partial S88.92-
    nose (partial) S08.812
      complete S08.811
    penis (complete) S38.221
      partial S38.222
    scrotum (complete) S38.231
      partial S38.232
    shoulder — *see* Amputation, traumatic, arm
      at shoulder joint — *see* Amputation, traumatic, arm, at shoulder joint
    testes (complete) S38.231
      partial S38.232
    thigh — *see* Amputation, traumatic, hip
    thorax, part of S28.1
      breast — *see* Amputation, traumatic, breast
    thumb (complete) (metacarpophalangeal) S68.01-
      partial S68.02-
      transphalangeal (complete) S68.51-
        partial S68.52-
    toe (lesser) S98.13-
      great S98.11-
        partial S98.12-
      more than one S98.21-
        partial S98.22-
      partial S98.14-
    vulva (complete) S38.211
      partial S38.212
Amputee (bilateral) (old) Z89.9
Amsterdam dwarfism Q87.1
Amusia R48.8
  developmental F80.89
Amyelencephalus, amyelencephaly Q00.0
Amyelia Q06.0
Amygdalitis — *see* Tonsillitis
Amygdalolith J35.8
Amyloid heart (disease) E85.4 *[I43]*
Amyloidosis (generalized) (primary) E85.9
  with lung involvement E85.4 *[J99]*
  familial E85.2
  genetic E85.2
  heart E85.4 *[I43]*

- **Amyloidosis** — *continued*
  - hemodialysis-associated E85.3
  - liver E85.4 *[K77]*
  - localized E85.4
  - neuropathic heredofamilial E85.1
  - non-neuropathic heredofamilial E85.Ø
  - organ limited E85.4
  - Portuguese E85.1
  - pulmonary E85.4 *[J99]*
  - secondary systemic E85.3
  - skin (lichen) (macular) E85.4 *[L99]*
  - specified NEC E85.8
  - subglottic E85.4 *[J99]*
- **Amylopectinosis** (brancher enzyme deficiency) E74.Ø3
- **Amylophagia** — *see* Pica
- **Amyoplasia congenita** Q79.8
- **Amyotonia** M62.89
  - congenita G7Ø.2
- **Amyotrophia, amyotrophy, amyotrophic** G71.8
  - congenita Q79.8
  - diabetic — *see* Diabetes, amyotrophy
  - lateral sclerosis G12.21
  - neuralgic G54.5
  - spinal progressive G12.21
- **Anacidity, gastric** K31.83
  - psychogenic F45.8
- **Anaerosis of newborn** P28.89
- **Analbuminemia** E88.Ø9
- **Analgesia** — *see* Anesthesia
- **Analphalipoproteinemia** E78.6
- **Anaphylactic**
  - purpura D69.Ø
  - shock or reaction — *see* Shock, anaphylactic
- **Anaphylactoid shock or reaction** — *see* Shock, anaphylactic
- **Anaphylactoid syndrome of pregnancy** O88.Ø1-
- **Anaphylaxis** — *see* **Shock, anaphylactic**
- **Anaplasia cervix** (*see also* Dysplasia, cervix) N87.9
- **Anaplasmosis, human** A77.49
- **Anarthria** R47.1
- **Anasarca** R6Ø.1
  - cardiac — *see* Failure, heart, congestive
  - lung J18.2
  - newborn P83.2
  - nutritional E43
  - pulmonary J18.2
  - renal NØ4.9
- **Anastomosis**
  - aneurysmal — *see* Aneurysm
  - arteriovenous ruptured brain I6Ø.8
  - intestinal K63.89
    - complicated NEC K91.89
      - involving urinary tract N99.89
  - retinal and choroidal vessels (congenital) Q14.8
- **Anatomical narrow angle** H4Ø.Ø3-
- **Ancylostoma, ancylostomiasis** (braziliense) (caninum) (ceylanicum) (duodenale) B76.Ø
  - Necator americanus B76.1
- **Andersen's disease** (glycogen storage) E74.Ø9
- **Anderson-Fabry disease** E75.21
- **Andes disease** T7Ø.29
- **Andrews' disease** (bacterid) LØ8.89
- **Androblastoma**
  - benign
    - specified site — *see* Neoplasm, benign, by site
    - unspecified site
      - female D27.9
      - male D29.2Ø
  - malignant
    - specified site — *see* Neoplasm, malignant, by site
    - unspecified site
      - female C56.9
      - male C62.9Ø
  - specified site — *see* Neoplasm, uncertain behavior, by site
  - tubular
    - with lipid storage
      - specified site — *see* Neoplasm, benign, by site
      - unspecified site
        - female D27.9
        - male D29.2Ø
    - specified site — *see* Neoplasm, benign, by site
- **Androblastoma** — *continued*
  - tubular — *continued*
    - unspecified site
      - female D27.9
      - male D29.2Ø
  - unspecified site
    - female D39.1Ø
    - male D4Ø.1Ø
- **Androgen insensitivity syndrome** (*see also* Syndrome, androgen insensitivity) E34.5Ø
- **Androgen resistance syndrome** (*see also* Syndrome, androgen insensitivity) E34.5Ø
- **Android pelvis** Q74.2
  - with disproportion (fetopelvic) O33.3
    - causing obstructed labor O65.3
- **Androphobia** F4Ø.29Ø
- **Anectasis, pulmonary** (newborn) — *see* Atelectasis
- **Anemia** (essential) (general) (hemoglobin deficiency) (infantile) (primary) (profound) D64.9
  - with (due to) (in)
    - disorder of
      - anaerobic glycolysis D55.2
      - pentose phosphate pathway D55.1
    - koilonychia D5Ø.9
  - achlorhydric D5Ø.8
  - achrestic D53.1
  - Addison(-Biermer) (pernicious) D51.Ø
  - agranulocytic — *see* Agranulocytosis
  - amino-acid-deficiency D53.Ø
  - aplastic D61.9
    - congenital D61.Ø9
    - drug-induced D61.1
    - due to
      - drugs D61.1
      - external agents NEC D61.2
      - infection D61.2
      - radiation D61.2
    - idiopathic D61.3
    - red cell (pure) D6Ø.9
      - chronic D6Ø.Ø
      - congenital D61.Ø1
      - specified type NEC D6Ø.8
      - transient D6Ø.1
    - specified type NEC D61.89
    - toxic D61.2
  - aregenerative
    - congenital D61.Ø9
  - asiderotic D5Ø.9
  - atypical (primary) D64.9
  - Baghdad spring D55.Ø
  - Balantidium coli AØ7.Ø
  - Biermer's (pernicious) D51.Ø
  - blood loss (chronic) D5Ø.Ø
    - acute D62
  - bothriocephalus B7Ø.Ø *[D63.8]*
  - brickmaker's B76.9 *[D63.8]*
  - cerebral I67.89
  - childhood D58.9
  - chlorotic D5Ø.8
  - chronic
    - blood loss D5Ø.Ø
    - hemolytic D58.9
      - idiopathic D59.9
    - simple D53.9
  - chronica congenita aregenerativa D61.Ø9
  - combined system disease NEC D51.Ø *[G32.Ø]*
    - due to dietary vitamin B12 deficiency D51.3 *[G32.Ø]*
  - complicating pregnancy, childbirth or puerperium — *see* Pregnancy, complicated by (management affected by), anemia
  - congenital P61.4
    - aplastic D61.Ø9
    - due to isoimmunization NOS P55.9
    - dyserythropoietic, dyshematopoietic D64.4
    - following fetal blood loss P61.3
    - Heinz body D58.2
    - hereditary hemolytic NOS D58.9
    - pernicious D51.Ø
    - spherocytic D58.Ø
  - Cooley's (erythroblastic) D56.1
  - cytogenic D51.Ø
  - deficiency D53.9
- **Anemia** — *continued*
  - deficiency — *continued*
    - 2, 3 diphosphoglycurate mutase D55.2
    - 2, 3 PG D55.2
    - 6 phosphogluconate dehydrogenase D55.1
    - 6-PGD D55.1
    - amino-acid D53.Ø
    - combined B12 and folate D53.1
    - enzyme D55.9
      - drug-induced (hemolytic) D59.2
      - glucose-6-phosphate dehydrogenase (G6PD) D55.Ø
      - glycolytic D55.2
      - nucleotide metabolism D55.3
      - related to hexose monophosphate (HMP) shunt pathway NEC D55.1
      - specified type NEC D55.8
    - erythrocytic glutathione D55.1
    - folate D52.9
      - dietary D52.Ø
      - drug-induced D52.1
    - folic acid D52.9
      - dietary D52.Ø
      - drug-induced D52.1
    - G SH D55.1
    - GGS-R D55.1
    - glucose-6-phosphate dehydrogenase D55.Ø
    - glutathione reductase D55.1
    - glyceraldehyde phosphate dehydrogenase D55.2
    - G6PD D55.Ø
    - hexokinase D55.2
    - iron D5Ø.9
      - secondary to blood loss (chronic) D5Ø.Ø
    - nutritional D53.9
      - with
        - poor iron absorption D5Ø.8
        - specified deficiency NEC D53.8
    - phosphofructo-aldolase D55.2
    - phosphoglycerate kinase D55.2
    - PK D55.2
    - protein D53.Ø
    - pyruvate kinase D55.2
    - transcobalamin II D51.2
    - triose-phosphate isomerase D55.2
    - vitamin B12 NOS D51.9
      - dietary D51.3
      - due to
        - intrinsic factor deficiency D51.Ø
        - selective vitamin B12 malabsorption with proteinuria D51.1
      - pernicious D51.Ø
      - specified type NEC D51.8
  - Diamond-Blackfan (congenital hypoplastic) D61.Ø1
  - dibothriocephalus B7Ø.Ø *[D63.8]*
  - dimorphic D53.1
  - diphasic D53.1
  - Diphyllobothrium (Dibothriocephalus) B7Ø.Ø *[D63.8]*
  - due to (in) (with)
    - antineoplastic chemotherapy D64.81
    - blood loss (chronic) D5Ø.Ø
      - acute D62
    - chemotherapy, antineoplastic D64.81
    - chronic disease classified elsewhere NEC D63.8
    - chronic kidney disease D63.1
    - deficiency
      - amino-acid D53.Ø
      - copper D53.8
      - folate (folic acid) D52.9
        - dietary D52.Ø
        - drug-induced D52.1
      - molybdenum D53.8
      - protein D53.Ø
      - zinc D53.8
    - dietary vitamin B12 deficiency D51.3
    - disorder of
      - glutathione metabolism D55.1
      - nucleotide metabolism D55.3
    - drug — *see* Anemia, by type (*see also* Table of Drugs and Chemicals)
    - end stage renal disease D63.1
    - enzyme disorder D55.9
    - fetal blood loss P61.3

DRAFT

Anemia — *continued*
- due to — *continued*
  - fish tapeworm (D.latum) infestation B7Ø.Ø *[D63.8]*
  - hemorrhage (chronic) D5Ø.Ø
    - acute D62
  - impaired absorption D5Ø.9
  - loss of blood (chronic) D5Ø.Ø
    - acute D62
  - myxedema EØ3.9 *[D63.8]*
  - Necator americanus B76.1 *[D63.8]*
  - prematurity P61.2
  - selective vitamin B12 malabsorption with proteinuria D51.1
  - transcobalamin II deficiency D51.2
- Dyke-Young type (secondary) (symptomatic) D59.1
- dyserythropoietic (congenital) D64.4
- dyshematopoietic (congenital) D64.4
- Egyptian B76.9 *[D63.8]*
- elliptocytosis — *see* Elliptocytosis
- enzyme-deficiency, drug-induced D59.2
- epidemic (*see also* Ancylostomiasis) B76.9 *[D63.8]*
- erythroblastic
  - familial D56.1
  - newborn (*see also* Disease, hemolytic) P55.9
  - of childhood D56.1
- erythrocytic glutathione deficiency D55.1
- erythropoietin-resistant anemia (EPO resistant anemia) D63.1
- Faber's (achlorhydric anemia) D5Ø.9
- factitious (self-induced blood letting) D5Ø.Ø
- familial erythroblastic D56.1
- Fanconi's (congenital pancytopenia) D61.Ø9
- favism D55.Ø
- fish tapeworm (D. latum) infestation B7Ø.Ø *[D63.8]*
- folate (folic acid) deficiency D52.9
- glucose-6-phosphate dehydrogenase (G6PD) deficiency D55.Ø
- glutathione-reductase deficiency D55.1
- goat's milk D52.Ø
- granulocytic — *see* Agranulocytosis
- Heinz body, congenital D58.2
- hemolytic D58.9
  - acquired D59.9
    - with hemoglobinuria NEC D59.6
    - autoimmune NEC D59.1
    - infectious D59.4
    - specified type NEC D59.8
    - toxic D59.4
  - acute D59.9
    - due to enzyme deficiency specified type NEC D55.8
    - Lederer's D59.1
  - autoimmune D59.1
    - drug-induced D59.Ø
  - chronic D58.9
    - idiopathic D59.9
  - cold type (secondary) (symptomatic) D59.1
  - congenital (spherocytic) — *see* Spherocytosis
  - due to
    - cardiac conditions D59.4
    - drugs (nonautoimmune) D59.2
      - autoimmune D59.Ø
    - enzyme disorder D55.9
      - drug-induced D59.2
    - presence of shunt or other internal prosthetic device D59.4
  - familial D58.9
  - hereditary D58.9
    - due to enzyme disorder D55.9
      - specified type NEC D55.8
    - specified type NEC D58.8
  - idiopathic (chronic) D59.9
  - mechanical D59.4
  - microangiopathic D59.4
  - nonautoimmune D59.4
    - drug-induced D59.2
  - nonspherocytic
    - congenital or hereditary NEC D55.8
      - glucose-6-phosphate dehydrogenase deficiency D55.Ø
      - pyruvate kinase deficiency D55.2

Anemia — *continued*
- hemolytic — *continued*
  - nonspherocytic — *continued*
    - congenital or hereditary NEC — *continued*
      - type
        - I D55.1
        - II D55.2
    - type
      - I D55.1
      - II D55.2
  - secondary D59.4
    - autoimmune D59.1
  - specified (hereditary) type NEC D58.8
  - Stransky-Regala type (*see also* Hemoglobinopathy) D58.8
  - symptomatic D59.4
    - autoimmune D59.1
  - toxic D59.4
  - warm type (secondary) (symptomatic) D59.1
- hemorrhagic (chronic) D5Ø.Ø
  - acute D62
- Herrick's D57.1
- hexokinase deficiency D55.2
- hookworm B76.9 *[D63.8]*
- hypochromic (idiopathic) (microcytic) (normoblastic) D5Ø.9
  - due to blood loss (chronic) D5Ø.Ø
    - acute D62
  - familial sex-linked D64.Ø
  - pyridoxine-responsive D64.3
  - sideroblastic, sex-linked D64.Ø
- hypoplasia, red blood cells D61.9
  - congenital or familial D61.Ø1
- hypoplastic (idiopathic) D61.9
  - congenital or familial (of childhood) D61.Ø1
- hypoproliferative (refractive) D61.9
- idiopathic D64.9
  - aplastic D61.3
  - hemolytic, chronic D59.9
- in (due to) (with)
  - chronic kidney disease D63.1
  - end stage renal disease D63.1
  - failure, kidney (renal) D63.1
  - neoplastic disease (*see also* Neoplasm) D63.Ø
- intertropical (*see also* Ancylostomiasis) D63.8
- iron deficiency D5Ø.9
  - secondary to blood loss (chronic) D5Ø.Ø
    - acute D62
  - specified type NEC D5Ø.8
- Joseph-Diamond-Blackfan (congenital hypoplastic) D61.Ø1
- Lederer's (hemolytic) D59.1
- leukoerythroblastic D61.82
- macrocytic D53.9
  - nutritional D52.Ø
  - tropical D52.8
- malarial (*see also* Malaria) B54 *[D63.8]*
- malignant (progressive) D51.Ø
- malnutrition D53.9
- marsh (*see also* Malaria) B54 *[D63.8]*
- Mediterranean (with other hemoglobinopathy) D56.9
- megaloblastic D53.1
  - combined B12 and folate deficiency D53.1
  - hereditary D51.1
  - nutritional D52.Ø
  - orotic aciduria D53.Ø
  - refractory D53.1
  - specified type NEC D53.1
- megalocytic D53.1
- microcytic (hypochromic) D5Ø.9
  - due to blood loss (chronic) D5Ø.Ø
    - acute D62
  - familial D56.8
- microdrepanocytosis D57.4Ø
- microelliptopoikilocytic (Rietti-GreppiMicheli) D56.9
- miner's B76.9 *[D63.8]*
- myelodysplastic D46.9
- myelofibrosis D75.81
- myelogenous D64.89
- myelopathic D64.89
- myelophthisic D61.82
- myeloproliferative D47.Z9

Anemia — *continued*
- newborn P61.4
  - due to
    - ABO (antibodies, isoimmunization, maternal/fetal incompatibility) P55.1
    - Rh (antibodies, isoimmunization, maternal/fetal incompatibility) P55.Ø
  - following fetal blood loss P61.3
  - posthemorrhagic (fetal) P61.3
- nonspherocytic hemolytic — *see* Anemia, hemolytic, nonspherocytic
- normocytic (infectional) D64.9
  - due to blood loss (chronic) D5Ø.Ø
    - acute D62
  - myelophthisic D61.82
- nutritional (deficiency) D53.9
  - with
    - poor iron absorption D5Ø.8
    - specified deficiency NEC D53.8
  - megaloblastic D52.Ø
- of prematurity P61.2
- orotaciduric (congenital) (hereditary) D53.Ø
- osteosclerotic D64.89
- ovalocytosis (hereditary) — *see* Elliptocytosis
- paludal (*see also* Malaria) B54 *[D63.8]*
- pernicious (congenital) (malignant) (progressive) D51.Ø
- pleochromic D64.89
  - of sprue D52.8
- posthemorrhagic (chronic) D5Ø.Ø
  - acute D62
  - newborn P61.3
- postoperative (postprocedural)
  - due to (acute) blood loss D62
    - chronic blood loss D5Ø.Ø
  - specified NEC D64.9
- postpartum O9Ø.81
- pressure D64.89
- progressive D64.9
  - malignant D51.Ø
  - pernicious D51.Ø
- protein-deficiency D53.Ø
- pseudoleukemica infantum D64.89
- pure red cell D6Ø.9
  - congenital D61.Ø1
- pyridoxine-responsive D64.3
- pyruvate kinase deficiency D55.2
- refractory D46.4
  - with
    - excess of blasts D46.2Ø
      - 1 (RAEB 1) D46.21
      - 2 (RAEB 2) D46.22
      - in transformation (RAEB T) — *see* Leukemia, acute myeloblastic
    - hemochromatosis D46.1
    - sideroblasts (ring) (RARS) D46.1
  - megaloblastic D53.1
  - sideroblastic D46.1
  - sideropenic D5Ø.8
  - without ring sideroblasts, so stated D46.Ø
  - without sideroblasts without excess of blasts D46.Ø
- Rietti-Greppi-Micheli D56.9
- scorbutic D53.2
- secondary to
  - blood loss (chronic) D5Ø.Ø
    - acute D62
  - hemorrhage (chronic) D5Ø.Ø
    - acute D62
- semiplastic D61.89
- sickle-cell — *see* Disease, sickle-cell
- sideroblastic D64.3
  - hereditary D64.Ø
  - hypochromic, sex-linked D64.Ø
  - pyridoxine-responsive NEC D64.3
  - refractory D46.1
  - secondary (due to)
    - disease D64.1
    - drugs and toxins D64.2
  - specified type NEC D64.3
- sideropenic (refractory) D5Ø.9
  - due to blood loss (chronic) D5Ø.Ø
    - acute D62

- **Anemia** — *continued*
  - simple chronic D53.9
  - specified type NEC D64.89
  - spherocytic (hereditary) — *see* Spherocytosis
  - splenic D64.89
  - splenomegalic D64.89
  - stomatocytosis D58.8
  - syphilitic (acquired) (late) A52.79 *[D63.8]*
  - target cell D64.89
  - thalassemia D56.9
  - thrombocytopenic — *see* Thrombocytopenia
  - toxic D61.2
  - tropical B76.9 *[D63.8]*
    - macrocytic D52.8
  - tuberculous A18.89 *[D63.8]*
  - vegan D51.3
  - vitamin
    - B6-responsive D64.3
    - B12 deficiency (dietary) pernicious D51.Ø
  - von Jaksch's D64.89
  - Witts' (achlorhydric anemia) D5Ø.8
- **Anencephalus, anencephaly** QØØ.Ø
- **Anemophobia** F4Ø.228
- **Anergasia** — *see* Psychosis, organic
- **Anesthesia, anesthetic** R2Ø.Ø
  - complication or reaction NEC (*see also* Complications, anesthesia) T88.59
    - due to
      - correct substance properly administered — *see* Table of Drugs and Chemicals, by drug, adverse effect
      - overdose or wrong substance given — *see* Table of Drugs and Chemicals, by drug, poisoning
  - cornea H18.81-
  - dissociative F44.6
  - functional (hysterical) F44.6
  - hyperesthetic, thalamic G89.Ø
  - hysterical F44.6
  - local skin lesion R2Ø.Ø
  - sexual (psychogenic) F52.1
  - shock (due to) T88.2
  - skin R2Ø.Ø
  - testicular N5Ø.9
- **Anetoderma** (maculosum) (of) L9Ø.8
  - Jadassohn-Pellizzari L9Ø.2
  - Schweniger-Buzzi L9Ø.1
- **Aneurin deficiency** E51.9
- **Aneurysm** (anastomotic) (artery) (cirsoid) (diffuse) (false) (fusiform) (multiple) (saccular) I72.9
  - abdominal (aorta) I71.4
    - ruptured I71.3
    - syphilitic A52.Ø1
  - aorta, aortic (nonsyphilitic) I71.9
    - abdominal I71.4
      - ruptured I71.3
    - arch I71.2
      - ruptured I71.1
    - arteriosclerotic I71.9
      - ruptured I71.8
    - ascending I71.2
      - ruptured I71.1
    - congenital Q25.4
    - descending I71.9
      - abdominal I71.4
        - ruptured I71.3
      - ruptured I71.8
      - thoracic I71.2
        - ruptured I71.1
    - ruptured I71.8
    - sinus, congenital Q25.4
    - syphilitic A52.Ø1
    - thoracic I71.2
      - ruptured I71.1
    - thoracoabdominal I71.6
      - ruptured I71.5
    - thorax, thoracic (arch) I71.2
      - ruptured I71.1
    - transverse I71.2
      - ruptured I71.1
    - valve (heart) (*see also* Endocarditis, aortic) I35.8
  - arteriosclerotic I72.9
    - cerebral I67.1

- **Aneurysm** — *continued*
  - arteriosclerotic — *continued*
    - cerebral — *continued*
      - ruptured — *see* Hemorrhage, intracranial, subarachnoid
  - arteriovenous (congenital) (*see also* Malformation, arteriovenous)
    - acquired I77.Ø
      - brain I67.1
      - coronary I25.41
      - pulmonary I28.Ø
    - brain Q28.2
      - ruptured I6Ø.8
    - peripheral — *see* Malformation, arteriovenous, peripheral
    - precerebral vessels Q28.Ø
    - specified site NEC (*see also* Malformation, arteriovenous)
      - acquired I77.Ø
  - basal — *see* Aneurysm, brain
  - berry (congenital) (nonruptured) I67.1
    - ruptured I6Ø.7
  - brain I67.1
    - arteriosclerotic I67.1
      - ruptured — *see* Hemorrhage, intracranial, subarachnoid
    - arteriovenous (congenital) (nonruptured) Q28.2
      - acquired I67.1
        - ruptured I6Ø.8
      - ruptured I6Ø.8
    - berry (congenital) (nonruptured) I67.1
      - ruptured (*see also* Hemorrhage, intracranial, subarachnoid) I6Ø.7
    - congenital Q28.3
      - ruptured I6Ø.7
    - meninges I67.1
      - ruptured I6Ø.8
    - miliary (congenital) (nonruptured) I67.1
      - ruptured (*see also* Hemorrhage, intracranial, subarachnoid) I6Ø.7
    - mycotic I33.Ø
    - ruptured — *see* Hemorrhage, intracranial, subarachnoid
    - syphilitic (hemorrhage) A52.Ø5
  - cardiac (false) (*see also* Aneurysm, heart) I25.3
  - carotid artery (common) (external) I72.Ø
    - internal (intracranial) I67.1
      - extracranial portion I72.Ø
    - ruptured into brain I6Ø.Ø-
    - syphilitic A52.Ø9
      - intracranial A52.Ø5
  - cavernous sinus I67.1
    - arteriovenous (congenital) (nonruptured) Q28.3
      - ruptured I6Ø.8
  - celiac I72.8
  - central nervous system, syphilitic A52.Ø5
  - cerebral — *see* Aneurysm, brain
  - chest — *see* Aneurysm, thorax
  - circle of Willis I67.1
    - congenital Q28.3
      - ruptured I6Ø.6
    - ruptured I6Ø.6
  - common iliac artery I72.3
  - congenital (peripheral) Q27.8
    - brain Q28.3
      - ruptured I6Ø.7
    - coronary Q24.5
    - digestive system Q27.8
    - lower limb Q27.8
    - pulmonary Q25.79
    - retina Q14.1
    - specified site NEC Q27.8
    - upper limb Q27.8
  - conjunctiva — *see* Abnormality, conjunctiva, vascular
  - conus arteriosus — *see* Aneurysm, heart
  - coronary (arteriosclerotic) (artery) I25.41
    - arteriovenous, congenital Q24.5
    - congenital Q24.5
    - ruptured — *see* Infarct, myocardium
    - syphilitic A52.Ø6
    - vein I25.89
  - cylindroid (aorta) I71.9

- **Aneurysm** — *continued*
  - cylindroid (aorta) — *continued*
    - ruptured I71.8
    - syphilitic A52.Ø1
  - ductus arteriosus Q25.Ø
  - endocardial, infective (any valve) I33.Ø
  - femoral (artery) (ruptured) I72.4
  - gastroduodenal I72.8
  - gastroepiploic I72.8
  - heart (wall) (chronic or with a stated duration of over 4 weeks) I25.3
    - valve — *see* Endocarditis
  - hepatic I72.8
  - iliac (common) (artery) (ruptured) I72.3
  - infective I72.9
    - endocardial (any valve) I33.Ø
  - innominate (nonsyphilitic) I72.8
    - syphilitic A52.Ø9
  - interauricular septum — *see* Aneurysm, heart
  - interventricular septum — *see* Aneurysm, heart
  - intrathoracic (nonsyphilitic) I71.2
    - ruptured I71.1
    - syphilitic A52.Ø1
  - lower limb I72.4
  - lung (pulmonary artery) I28.1
  - mediastinal (nonsyphilitic) I72.8
    - syphilitic A52.Ø9
  - miliary (congenital) I67.1
    - ruptured — *see* Hemorrhage, intracerebral, subarachnoid, intracranial
  - mitral (heart) (valve) I34.8
  - mural — *see* Aneurysm, heart
  - mycotic I72.9
    - endocardial (any valve) I33.Ø
    - ruptured, brain — *see* Hemorrhage, intracerebral, subarachnoid
  - myocardium — *see* Aneurysm, heart
  - neck I72.Ø
  - pancreaticoduodenal I72.8
  - patent ductus arteriosus Q25.Ø
  - peripheral NEC I72.8
    - congenital Q27.8
      - digestive system Q27.8
      - lower limb Q27.8
      - specified site NEC Q27.8
      - upper limb Q27.8
  - popliteal (artery) (ruptured) I72.4
  - precerebral, congenital (nonruptured) Q28.1
  - pulmonary I28.1
    - arteriovenous Q25.72
      - acquired I28.Ø
    - syphilitic A52.Ø9
    - valve (heart) — *see* Endocarditis, pulmonary
  - racemose (peripheral) I72.9
    - congenital — *see* Aneurysm, congenital
  - radial I72.1
  - Rasmussen NEC A15.Ø
  - renal (artery) I72.2
  - retina (*see also* Disorder, retina, microaneurysms)
    - congenital Q14.1
    - diabetic — *see* Diabetes, microaneurysms, retinal
  - sinus of Valsalva Q25.4
  - specified NEC I72.8
  - spinal (cord) I72.8
    - syphilitic (hemorrhage) A52.Ø9
  - splenic I72.8
  - subclavian (artery) (ruptured) I72.8
    - syphilitic A52.Ø9
  - superior mesenteric I72.8
  - syphilitic (aorta) A52.Ø1
    - central nervous system A52.Ø5
    - congenital (late) A5Ø.54 *[I79.Ø]*
    - spine, spinal A52.Ø9
  - thoracoabdominal (aorta) I71.6
    - ruptured I71.5
    - syphilitic A52.Ø1
  - thorax, thoracic (aorta) (arch) (nonsyphilitic) I71.2
    - ruptured I71.1
    - syphilitic A52.Ø1
  - traumatic (complication) (early), specified site — *see* Injury, blood vessel
  - tricuspid (heart) (valve) IØ7.8
  - ulnar I72.1

- **Aneurysm** — *continued*
  - upper limb (ruptured) I72.1
  - valve, valvular — *see* Endocarditis
  - venous (*see also* Varix) I86.8
    - congenital Q27.8
      - digestive system Q27.8
      - lower limb Q27.8
      - specified site NEC Q27.8
      - upper limb Q27.8
  - ventricle — *see* Aneurysm, heart
  - visceral NEC I72.8
- **Angelman syndrome** Q93.5
- **Anger** R45.4
- **Angiectasis, angiectopia** I99.8
- **Angiitis** I77.6
  - allergic granulomatous M3Ø.1
  - hypersensitivity M31.Ø
  - necrotizing M31.9
    - specified NEC M31.8
  - nervous system, granulomatous I67.7
- **Angina** (attack) (cardiac) (chest) (heart) (pectoris) (syndrome) (vasomotor) I2Ø.9
  - with
    - atherosclerotic heart disease — *see* Arteriosclerosis, coronary (artery),
    - documented spasm I2Ø.1
  - abdominal K55.1
  - accelerated — *see* Angina, unstable
  - agranulocytic — *see* Agranulocytosis
  - angiospastic — *see* Angina, with documented spasm
  - aphthous BØ8.5
  - crescendo — *see* Angina, unstable
  - croupous JØ5.Ø
  - cruris I73.9
  - de novo effort — *see* Angina, unstable
  - diphtheritic, membranous A36.Ø
  - equivalent I2Ø.8
  - exudative, chronic J37.Ø
  - following acute myocardial infarction I23.7
  - gangrenous diphtheritic A36.Ø
  - intestinal K55.1
  - Ludovici K12.2
  - Ludwig's K12.2
  - malignant diphtheritic A36.Ø
  - membranous JØ5.Ø
    - diphtheritic A36.Ø
    - Vincent's A69.1
  - mesenteric K55.1
  - monocytic — *see* Mononucleosis, infectious
  - of effort — *see* Angina, specified NEC
  - phlegmonous J36
    - diphtheritic A36.Ø
  - post-infarctional I23.7
  - pre-infarctional — *see* Angina, unstable
  - Prinzmetal — *see* Angina, with documented spasm
  - progressive — *see* Angina, unstable
  - pseudomembranous A69.1
  - pultaceous, diphtheritic A36.Ø
  - spasm-induced — *see* Angina, with documented spasm
  - specified NEC I2Ø.8
  - stable I2Ø.9
  - stenocardia — *see* Angina, specified NEC
  - stridulous, diphtheritic A36.2
  - tonsil J36
  - trachealis JØ5.Ø
  - unstable I2Ø.Ø
  - variant — *see* Angina, with documented spasm
  - Vincent's A69.1
  - worsening effort — *see* Angina, unstable
- **Angioblastoma** — *see* Neoplasm, connective tissue, uncertain behavior
- **Angiocholecystitis** — *see* Cholecystitis, acute
- **Angiocholitis** (*see also* Cholecystitis, acute) K83.Ø
- **Angiodysgenesis spinalis** G95.19
- **Angiodysplasia** (cecum) (colon) K55.2Ø
  - with bleeding K55.21
  - duodenum (and stomach) K31.819
    - with bleeding K31.811
  - stomach (and duodenum) K31.819
    - with bleeding K31.811
- **Angioedema** (allergic) (any site) (with urticaria) T78.3
  - hereditary D84.1
- **Angioendothelioma** — *see* Neoplasm, uncertain behavior, by site
  - benign D18.ØØ
    - intra-abdominal D18.Ø3
    - intracranial D18.Ø2
    - skin D18.Ø1
    - specified site NEC D18.Ø9
  - bone — *see* Neoplasm, bone, malignant
  - Ewing's — *see* Neoplasm, bone, malignant
- **Angioendotheliomatosis** C85.8-
- **Angiofibroma** (*see also* Neoplasm, benign, by site)
  - juvenile
    - specified site — *see* Neoplasm, benign, by site
    - unspecified site D1Ø.6
- **Angiohemophilia** (A) (B) D68.Ø
- **Angioid streaks** (choroid) (macula) (retina) H35.33
- **Angiokeratoma** — *see* Neoplasm, skin, benign
  - corporis diffusum E75.21
- **Angioleiomyoma** — *see* Neoplasm, connective tissue, benign
- **Angiolipoma** (*see also* Lipoma)
  - infiltrating — *see* Lipoma
- **Angioma** (*see also* Hemangioma, by site)
  - capillary I78.1
  - hemorrhagicum hereditaria I78.Ø
  - intra-abdominal D18.Ø3
  - intracranial D18.Ø2
  - malignant — *see* Neoplasm, connective tissue, malignant
  - plexiform D18.ØØ
    - intra-abdominal D18.Ø3
    - intracranial D18.Ø2
    - skin D18.Ø1
    - specified site NEC D18.Ø9
  - senile I78.1
  - serpiginosum L81.7
  - skin D18.Ø1
  - specified site NEC D18.Ø9
  - spider I78.1
  - stellate I78.1
  - venous Q28.3
- **Angiomatosis** Q82.8
  - bacillary A79.89
  - encephalotrigeminal Q85.8
  - hemorrhagic familial I78.Ø
  - hereditary familial I78.Ø
  - liver K76.4
- **Angiomyolipoma** — *see* Lipoma
- **Angiomyoliposarcoma** — *see* Neoplasm, connective tissue, malignant
- **Angiomyoma** — *see* Neoplasm, connective tissue, benign
- **Angiomyosarcoma** — *see* Neoplasm, connective tissue, malignant
- **Angiomyxoma**
- — *see* Neoplasm, connective tissue, uncertain behavior
- **Angioneurosis** F45.8
- **Angioneurotic edema** (allergic) (any site) (with urticaria) T78.3
  - hereditary D84.1
- **Angiopathia, angiopathy** I99.9
  - cerebral I67.9
    - amyloid E85.4 *[I68.0]*
  - diabetic (peripheral) — *see* Diabetes, angiopathy
  - peripheral I73.9
    - diabetic — *see* Diabetes, angiopathy
    - specified type NEC I73.89
  - retinae syphilitica A52.Ø5
  - retinalis (juvenilis)
    - diabetic — *see* Diabetes, retinopathy
    - proliferative — *see* Retinopathy, proliferative
- **Angiosarcoma** (*see also* Neoplasm, connective tissue, malignant)
  - liver C22.3
- **Angiosclerosis** — *see* Arteriosclerosis
- **Angiospasm** (peripheral) (traumatic) (vessel) I73.9
  - brachial plexus G54.Ø
  - cerebral G45.9
  - cervical plexus G54.2
  - nerve
    - arm — *see* Mononeuropathy, upper limb
- **Angiospasm** — *continued*
  - nerve — *continued*
    - arm — *continued*
      - axillary G54.Ø
      - median — *see* Lesion, nerve, median
      - ulnar — *see* Lesion, nerve, ulnar
    - axillary G54.Ø
    - leg — *see* Mononeuropathy, lower limb
    - median — *see* Lesion, nerve, median
    - plantar — *see* Lesion, nerve, plantar
    - ulnar — *see* Lesion, nerve, ulnar
- **Angiospastic disease or edema** I73.9
- **Angiostrongyliasis**
  - due to
    - Parastrongylus
      - cantonensis B83.2
      - costaricensis B81.3
  - intestinal B81.3
- **Anguillulosis** — *see* Strongyloidiasis
- **Angulation**
  - cecum — *see* Obstruction, intestine
  - coccyx (acquired) (*see also* subcategory) M43.8
    - congenital NEC Q76.49
  - femur (acquired) (*see also* Deformity, limb, specified type NEC, thigh)
    - congenital Q74.2
  - intestine (large) (small) — *see* Obstruction, intestine
  - sacrum (acquired) (*see also* subcategory) M43.8
    - congenital NEC Q76.49
  - sigmoid (flexure) — *see* Obstruction, intestine
  - spine — *see* Dorsopathy, deforming, specified NEC
  - tibia (acquired) (*see also* Deformity, limb, specified type NEC, lower leg)
    - congenital Q74.2
  - ureter N13.5
    - with infection N13.6
  - wrist (acquired) (*see also* Deformity, limb, specified type NEC, forearm)
    - congenital Q74.Ø
- **Angulus infectiosus** (lips) K13.Ø
- **Anhedonia** R45.84
- **Anhidrosis** L74.4
- **Anhydration, anhydremia** E86.Ø
  - with
    - hypernatremia E87.Ø
    - hyponatremia E87.1
- **Anhydremia** E86.Ø
  - with
    - hypernatremia E87.Ø
    - hyponatremia E87.1
- **Anidrosis** L74.4
- **Aniridia** (congenital) Q13.1
- **Anisakiasis** (infection) (infestation) B81.Ø
- **Anisakis larvae infestation** B81.Ø
- **Aniseikonia** H52.32
- **Anisocoria** (pupil) H57.Ø2
  - congenital Q13.2
- **Anisocytosis** R71.8
- **Anisometropia** (congenital) H52.31
- **Ankle** — *see* condition
- **Ankyloblepharon** (eyelid) (acquired) (*see also* Blepharophimosis)
  - filiforme (adnatum) (congenital) Q1Ø.3
  - total Q1Ø.3
- **Ankyloglossia** Q38.1
- **Ankylosis** (fibrous) (osseous) (joint) M24.6Ø
  - ankle M24.67-
  - arthrodesis status Z98.1
  - cricoarytenoid (cartilage) (joint) (larynx) J38.7
  - dental KØ3.5
  - ear ossicles H74.31-
  - elbow M24.62-
  - foot M24.67-
  - hand M24.64-
  - hip M24.65-
  - incostapedial joint (infectional) — *see* Ankylosis, ear ossicles
  - jaw (temporomandibular) M26.61
  - knee M24.66-
  - lumbosacral (joint) M43.27
  - postoperative (status) Z98.1
  - produced by surgical fusion, status Z98.1
  - sacro-iliac (joint) M43.28

Anthracosis (lung) (occupational) J6Ø
- lingua K14.3

Anthrax A22.9
- with pneumonia A22.1
- cerebral A22.8
- colitis A22.2
- cutaneous A22.Ø
- gastrointestinal A22.2
- inhalation A22.1
- intestinal A22.2
- meningitis A22.8
- pulmonary A22.1
- respiratory A22.1
- sepsis A22.7
- specified manifestation NEC A22.8

Anthropoid pelvis Q74.2
- with disproportion (fetopelvic) O33.Ø

Anthropophobia F4Ø.1Ø
- generalized F4Ø.11

Antibodies, maternal (blood group) — *see* Isoimmunization, affecting management of pregnancy
- anti-D — *see* Isoimmunization, affecting management of pregnancy, Rh
  - newborn P55.Ø

Antibody
- anticardiolipin R76.Ø
  - with
    - hemorrhagic disorder D68.312
    - hypercoagulable state D68.61
- antiphosphatidylglycerol R76.Ø
  - with
    - hemorrhagic disorder D68.312
    - hypercoagulable state D68.61
- antiphosphatidylinositol R76.Ø
  - with
    - hemorrhagic disorder D68.312
    - hypercoagulable state D68.61
- antiphosphatidylserine R76.Ø
  - with
    - hemorrhagic disorder D68.312
    - hypercoagulable state D68.61
- antiphospholipid R76.Ø
  - with
    - hemorrhagic disorder D68.312
    - hypercoagulable state D68.61

Anticardiolipin syndrome D68.61

Anticoagulant, circulating (intrinsic) (*see also* Disorder, hemorrhagic) D68.318
- drug-induced (extrinsic) (*see also* Disorder, hemorrhagic) D68.32

Antidiuretic hormone syndrome E22.2

Antimonial cholera — *see* Poisoning, antimony

Antiphospholipid
- antibody
  - with hemorrhagic disorder D68.312
  - syndrome D68.61

Antisocial personality F6Ø.2

Antithrombinemia — *see* Circulating anticoagulants

Antithromboplastinemia D68.318

Antithromboplastinogenemia D68.318

Antitoxin complication or reaction — *see* Complications, vaccination

Antlophobia F4Ø.228

Antritis J32.Ø
- maxilla J32.Ø
  - acute JØ1.ØØ
    - recurrent JØ1.Ø1
- stomach K29.6Ø
  - with bleeding K29.61

Antrum, antral — *see* condition

Anuria R34
- calculous (impacted) (recurrent) (*see also* Calculus, urinary) N2Ø.9
- following
  - abortion - see Abortion by type complicated by, renal failure
  - ectopic or molar pregnancy OØ8.4
- newborn P96.Ø
- postprocedural N99.Ø
- postrenal N13.8
- traumatic (following crushing) T79.5

Anus, anal — *see* condition

Anusitis K62.89

Anxiety F41.9
- depression F41.8
- episodic paroxysmal F41.Ø
- generalized F41.1
- hysteria F41.8
- neurosis F41.1
- panic type F41.Ø
- reaction F41.1
- separation, abnormal (of childhood) F93.Ø
- specified NEC F41.8
- state F41.1

Aorta, aortic — *see* condition

Aortectasia — *see* Ectasia, aorta
- with aneurysm — *see* Aneurysm, aorta

Aortitis (nonsyphilitic) (calcific) I77.6
- arteriosclerotic I7Ø.Ø
- Doehle-Heller A52.Ø2
- luetic A52.Ø2
- rheumatic — *see* Endocarditis, acute, rheumatic
- specific (syphilitic) A52.Ø2
- syphilitic A52.Ø2
  - congenital A5Ø.54 *[I79.1]*

Apathetic thyroid storm — *see* Thyrotoxicosis

Apathy R45.3

Apeirophobia F4Ø.228

Apepsia K3Ø
- psychogenic F45.8

Aperistalsis, esophagus K22.Ø

Apertognathia M26.29

Apert's syndrome Q87.Ø

Aphagia R13.Ø
- psychogenic F5Ø.9

Aphakia (acquired) (postoperative) H27.Ø-
- congenital Q12.3

Aphasia (amnestic) (global) (nominal) (semantic) (syntactic) R47.Ø1
- acquired, with epilepsy (Landau-Kleffner syndrome) — *see* Epilepsy, specified NEC
- auditory (developmental) F8Ø.2
- developmental (receptive type) F8Ø.2
  - expressive type F8Ø.1
  - Wernicke's F8Ø.2
- following
  - cerebrovascular disease I69.92Ø
    - cerebral infarction I69.32Ø
    - intracerebral hemorrhage I69.12Ø
    - nontraumatic intracranial hemorrhage NEC I69.22Ø
    - specified disease NEC I69.82Ø
    - subarachnoid hemorrhage I69.Ø2Ø
- primary progressive G31.Ø1 *[FØ2.8Ø]*
  - with behavioral disturbance G31.Ø1 *[FØ2.81]*
- progressive isolated G31.Ø1 *[FØ2.8Ø]*
  - with behavioral disturbance G31.Ø1 *[FØ2.81]*
- sensory F8Ø.2
- syphilis, tertiary A52.19
- Wernicke's (developmental) F8Ø.2

Aphonia (organic) R49.1
- hysterical F44.4
- psychogenic F44.4

Aphthae, aphthous (*see also* condition)
- Bednar's K12.Ø
- cachectic K14.Ø
- epizootic BØ8.8
- fever BØ8.8
- oral (recurrent) K12.Ø
- stomatitis (major) (minor) K12.Ø
- thrush B37.Ø
- ulcer (oral) (recurrent) K12.Ø
  - genital organ(s) NEC
    - female N76.6
    - male N5Ø.8
- larynx J38.7

Apical — *see* condition

Apiphobia F4Ø.218

Aplasia (*see also* Agenesis)
- abdominal muscle syndrome Q79.4
- alveolar process (acquired) — *see* Anomaly, alveolar
  - congenital Q38.6
- aorta (congenital) Q25.4
- axialis extracorticalis (congenita) E75.29
- bone marrow (myeloid) D61.9
  - congenital D61.Ø1
- brain QØØ.Ø
  - part of QØ4.3
- bronchus Q32.4
- cementum KØØ.4
- cerebellum QØ4.3
- cervix (congenital) Q51.5
- congenital pure red cell D61.Ø1
- corpus callosum QØ4.Ø
- cutis congenita Q84.8
- erythrocyte congenital D61.Ø1
- extracortical axial E75.29
- eye Q11.1
- fovea centralis (congenital) Q14.1
- gallbladder, congenital Q44.Ø
- iris Q13.1
- labyrinth, membranous Q16.5
- limb (congenital) Q73.8
  - lower — *see* Defect, reduction, lower limb
  - upper — *see* Agenesis, arm
- lung, congenital (bilateral) (unilateral) Q33.3
- pancreas Q45.Ø
- parathyroid-thymic D82.1
- Pelizaeus-Merzbacher E75.29
- penis Q55.5
- prostate Q55.4
- red cell (with thymoma) D6Ø.9
  - acquired D6Ø.9
    - due to drugs D6Ø.9
  - adult D6Ø.9
  - chronic D6Ø.Ø
  - congenital D61.Ø1
  - constitutional D61.Ø1
  - due to drugs D6Ø.9
  - hereditary D61.Ø1
  - of infants D61.Ø1
  - primary D61.Ø1
  - pure D61.Ø1
    - due to drugs D6Ø.9
  - specified type NEC D6Ø.8
  - transient D6Ø.1
- round ligament Q52.8
- skin Q84.8
- spermatic cord Q55.4
- spleen Q89.Ø1
- testicle Q55.Ø
- thymic, with immunodeficiency D82.1
- thyroid (congenital) (with myxedema) EØ3.1
- uterus Q51.Ø
- ventral horn cell QØ6.1

Apnea, apneic (of) (spells) RØ6.81
- newborn NEC P28.4
  - obstructive P28.4
  - sleep (central) (obstructive) (primary) P28.3
- prematurity P28.4
- sleep G47.3Ø
  - central (primary) G47.31
    - in conditions classified elsewhere G47.37
  - obstructive (adult) (pediatric) G47.33
  - primary central G47.31
  - specified NEC G47.39

Apneumatosis, newborn P28.Ø

Apocrine metaplasia (breast) — *see* Dysplasia, mammary, specified type NEC

Apophysitis (bone) (*see also* Osteochondropathy)
- calcaneus M92.8
- juvenile M92.9

Apoplectiform convulsions (cerebral ischemia) I67.82

Apoplexia, apoplexy, apoplectic
- adrenal A39.1
- heart (auricle) (ventricle) — *see* Infarct, myocardium
- heat T67.Ø
- hemorrhagic (stroke) — *see* Hemorrhage, intracranial
- meninges, hemorrhagic — *see* Hemorrhage, intracranial, subarachnoid
- uremic N18.9 *[I68.8]*

Appearance
- bizarre R46.1
- specified NEC R46.89
- very low level of personal hygiene R46.Ø

Appendage
- epididymal (organ of Morgagni) Q55.4
- intestine (epiploic) Q43.8
- preauricular Q17.Ø
- testicular (organ of Morgagni) Q55.29

Appendicitis (pneumococcal) (retrocecal) K37
- with
  - perforation or rupture K35.2
  - peritoneal abscess K35.3
    - with peritonitis K35.2
  - peritonitis K35.2
    - with perforation or rupture K35.2
    - localized K35.3
    - generalized K35.2
- acute (catarrhal) (fulminating) (gangrenous) (obstructive) (retrocecal) (suppurative) K35.8Ø
  - with
    - perforation or rupture K35.2
    - peritoneal abscess K35.3
      - with peritonitis K35.2
    - peritonitis K35.2
      - with perforation or rupture K35.2
      - localized K35.3
      - generalized K35.2
  - specified NEC K35.89
- amebic AØ6.89
- chronic (recurrent) K36
- exacerbation — *see* Appendicitis, acute
- gangrenous — *see* Appendicitis, acute
- healed (obliterative) K36
- interval K36
- neurogenic K36
- obstructive K36
- recurrent K36
- relapsing K36
- subacute (adhesive) K36
- subsiding K36
- suppurative — *see* Appendicitis, acute
- tuberculous A18.32

Appendix, appendicular (*see also* condition)
- epididymis Q55.4
- Morgagni
  - female Q5Ø.5
  - male (epididymal) Q55.4
    - testicular Q55.29
- testis Q55.29

Appendicopathia oxyurica B8Ø

Appetite
- depraved — *see* Pica
- excessive R63.2
- lack or loss (*see also* Anorexia) R63.Ø
  - nonorganic origin F5Ø.8
  - psychogenic F5Ø.8
- perverted (hysterical) — *see* Pica

Apple peel syndrome Q41.1

Apprehension state F41.1

Apprehensiveness, abnormal F41.9

Approximal wear KØ3.Ø

Apraxia (classic) (ideational) (ideokinetic) (ideomotor) (motor) (verbal) R48.2
- following
  - cerebrovascular disease I69.99Ø
    - specified disease NEC I69.89Ø
    - cerebral infarction I69.39Ø
    - intracerebral hemorrhage I69.19Ø
    - nontraumatic intracranial hemorrhage NEC I69.29Ø
    - specified disease NEC I69.89Ø
    - subarachnoid hemorrhage I69.Ø9Ø
- oculomotor, congenital H51.8

Aptyalism K11.7

Apudoma — *see* Neoplasm, uncertain behavior, by site

Aqueous misdirection H4Ø.83-

Arabicum elephantiasis — *see* Infestation, filarial

Arachnitis — *see* Meningitis

Arachnodactyly — *see* Syndrome, Marfan's

Arachnoiditis (acute) (adhesive) (basal) (brain) (cerebrospinal) — *see* Meningitis

Arachnophobia F4Ø.21Ø

Arboencephalitis, Australian A83.4

Arborization block (heart) I45.5

ARC (AIDS-related complex) B2Ø

Arches — *see* condition

Arcuate uterus Q51.81Ø

Arcuatus uterus Q51.81Ø

Arcus (cornea) senilis — *see* Degeneration, cornea, senile

Arc-welder's lung J63.4

Areflexia R29.2

Areola — *see* condition

Argentaffinoma (*see also* Neoplasm, uncertain behavior , by site)
- malignant — *see* Neoplasm, malignant, by site
- syndrome E34.Ø

Argininemia E72.21

Arginosuccinic aciduria E72.22

Argyll Robertson phenomenon, pupil or syndrome (syphilitic) A52.19
- atypical H57.Ø9
- nonsyphilitic H57.Ø9

Argyria, argyriasis
- conjunctival H11.13-
- from drug or medicament — *see* Table of Drugs and Chemicals, by substance

Argyrosis, conjunctival H11.13-

Arhinencephaly QØ4.1

Ariboflavinosis E53.Ø

Arm — *see* condition

Arnold-Chiari disease, obstruction or syndrome (type II) QØ7.ØØ
- with
  - hydrocephalus QØ7.Ø2
    - with spina bifida QØ7.Ø3
  - spina bifida QØ7.Ø1
    - with hydrocephalus QØ7.Ø3
- type III — *see* Encephalocele
- type IV QØ4.8

Aromatic amino-acid metabolism disorder E7Ø.9
- specified NEC E7Ø.8

Arousals, confusional G47.51

Arrest, arrested
- cardiac I46.9
  - complicating
    - abortion — *see* Abortion, by type, complicated by, cardiac arrest
    - anesthesia (general) (local) or other sedation — *see* Table of Drugs and Chemicals, by drug,
      - in labor and delivery O74.2
      - in pregnancy O29.11-
      - postpartum, puerperal O89.1
    - delivery (cesarean) (instrumental) O75.4
  - due to
    - cardiac condition I46.2
    - specified condition NEC I46.8
  - intraoperative I97.71-
  - newborn P29.81
  - postprocedural I97.12-
    - obstetric procedure O75.4
- cardiorespiratory — *see* Arrest, cardiac
- circulatory — *see* Arrest, cardiac
- deep transverse O64.Ø
- development or growth
  - bone — *see* Disorder, bone, development or growth
  - child R62.5Ø
  - tracheal rings Q32.1
- epiphyseal
  - complete
    - femur M89.15-
    - humerus M89.12-
    - tibia M89.16-
    - ulna M89.13-
  - forearm M89.13-
    - specified NEC M89.13-
    - ulna — *see* Arrest, epiphyseal, by type, ulna
  - lower leg M89.16-
    - specified NEC M89.168
    - tibia — *see* Arrest, epiphyseal, by type, tibia
  - partial
    - femur M89.15-
    - humerus M89.12-
    - tibia M89.16-
    - ulna M89.13-
  - specified NEC M89.18

Arrest, arrested — *continued*
- granulopoiesis — *see* Agranulocytosis
- growth plate — *see* Arrest, epiphyseal
- heart — *see* Arrest, cardiac
- legal, anxiety concerning Z65.3
- physeal — *see* Arrest, epiphyseal
- respiratory RØ9.2
  - newborn P28.81
- sinus I45.5
- spermatogenesis (complete) — *see* Azoospermia
  - incomplete — *see* Oligospermia
- transverse (deep) O64.Ø

Arrhenoblastoma
- benign
  - specified site — *see* Neoplasm, benign, by site
  - unspecified site
    - female D27.9
    - male D29.2Ø
- malignant
  - specified site — *see* Neoplasm, malignant, by site
  - unspecified site
    - female C56.9
    - male C62.9Ø
- specified site — *see* Neoplasm, uncertain behavior, by site
- unspecified site
  - female D39.1Ø
  - male D4Ø.1Ø

Arrhythmia (auricle)(cardiac)(juvenile)(nodal) (reflex)(sinus)(supraventricular)(transitory) (ventricle) I49.9
- block I45.9
- extrasystolic I49.49
- newborn
  - bradycardia P29.12
  - tachycardia P29.11
  - occurring before birth PØ3.819
    - before onset of labor PØ3.81Ø
    - during labor PØ3.811
- psychogenic F45.8
- specified NEC I49.8
- vagal R55
- ventricular re-entry I47.Ø

Arrillaga-Ayerza syndrome (pulmonary sclerosis with pulmonary hypertension) I27.Ø

Arsenical pigmentation L81.8
- from drug or medicament — *see* Table of drugs and medicaments

Arsenism — *see* Poisoning, arsenic

Arterial — *see* **condition**

Arteriofibrosis — *see* Arteriosclerosis

Arteriolar sclerosis — *see* Arteriosclerosis

Arteriolith — *see* Arteriosclerosis

Arteriolitis I77.6
- necrotizing, kidney I77.5
- renal — *see* Hypertension, kidney

Arteriolosclerosis — *see* Arteriosclerosis

Arterionephrosclerosis — *see* Hypertension, kidney

Arteriopathy I77.9

Arteriosclerosis, arteriosclerotic (diffuse) (obliterans) (of) (senile) (with calcification) I7Ø.9Ø
- aorta I7Ø.Ø
- arteries of extremities — *see* Arteriosclerosis, extremities
- brain I67.2
- bypass graft
  - coronary — *see* Arteriosclerosis, coronary, bypass graft
  - extremities — *see* Arteriosclerosis, extremities, bypass graft
- cardiac — *see* Disease, heart, ischemic, atherosclerotic
- cardiopathy — *see* Disease, heart, ischemic, atherosclerotic
- cardiorenal — *see* Hypertension, cardiorenal
- cardiovascular — *see* Disease, heart, ischemic, atherosclerotic
- carotid (*see also* Occlusion, artery, carotid) I65.2-
- central nervous system I67.2
- cerebral I67.2
- cerebrovascular I67.2
- coronary (artery) I25.1Ø

- **Arteriosclerosis, arteriosclerotic** — *continued*
  - coronary (artery) — *continued*
    - due to
      - calcified coronary lesion (severely) I25.84
      - lipid rich plaque I25.83
    - native vessel
      - with
        - angina pectoris I25.119
          - specified type NEC I25.118
          - unstable I25.11Ø
          - with documented spasm I25.111
        - ischemic chest pain I25.119
    - bypass graft I25.81Ø
      - with
        - angina pectoris I25.7Ø9
          - specified type NEC I25.7Ø8
          - unstable I25.7ØØ
          - with documented spasm I25.7Ø1
        - ischemic chest pain I25.7Ø9
      - autologous artery I25.81Ø
        - with
          - angina pectoris I25.729
            - specified type I25.728
            - unstable I25.72Ø
            - with documented spasm I25.721
          - ischemic chest pain I25.729
      - autologous vein I25.81Ø
        - with
          - angina pectoris I25.719
            - specified type I25.718
            - unstable I25.71Ø
            - with documented spasm I25.711
          - ischemic chest pain I25.719
      - nonautologous biological I25.81Ø
        - with
          - angina pectoris I25.739
            - specified type I25.738
            - unstable I25.73Ø
            - with documented spasm I25.731
          - ischemic chest pain I25.739
      - specified type NEC I25.81Ø
        - with
          - angina pectoris I25.799
            - specified type I25.798
            - unstable I25.79Ø
            - with documented spasm I25.791
          - ischemic chest pain I25.799
    - transplanted heart I25.811
      - native coronary artery I25.811
        - with
          - angina pectoris I25.759
            - specified type I25.758
            - unstable I25.75Ø
            - with documented spasm I25.751
          - ischemic chest pain I25.759
      - bypass graft I25.812
        - with
          - angina pectoris I25.769
            - specified type I25.768
            - unstable I25.76Ø
            - with documented spasm I25.761
          - ischemic chest pain I25.769
  - extremities (native arteries) I7Ø.2Ø9
    - bypass graft I7Ø.3Ø9
      - autologous vein graft I7Ø.4Ø9
        - leg I7Ø.4Ø9
          - with
            - gangrene (and intermittent claudication, rest pain and ulcer) I7Ø.469
            - intermittent claudication I7Ø.419
            - rest pain (and intermittent claudication) I7Ø.429
          - bilateral I7Ø.4Ø3
            - with
              - gangrene (and intermittent claudication, rest pain and ulcer) I7Ø.463
              - intermittent claudication I7Ø.413
              - rest pain (and intermittent claudication) I7Ø.423
            - specified type NEC I7Ø.493

- **Arteriosclerosis, arteriosclerotic** — *continued*
  - extremities (native arteries) — *continued*
    - bypass graft — *continued*
      - autologous vein graft — *continued*
        - leg — *continued*
          - left I7Ø.4Ø2
            - with
              - gangrene (and intermittent claudication, rest pain and ulcer) I7Ø.462
              - intermittent claudication I7Ø.412
              - rest pain (and intermittent claudication) I7Ø.422
              - ulceration (and intermittent claudication and rest pain) I7Ø.449
                - ankle I7Ø.443
                - calf I7Ø.442
                - foot site NEC I7Ø.445
                - heel I7Ø.444
                - lower leg NEC I7Ø.448
                - midfoot I7Ø.444
                - thigh I7Ø.441
            - specified type NEC I7Ø.492
          - right I7Ø.4Ø1
            - with
              - gangrene (and intermittent claudication, rest pain and ulcer) I7Ø.461
              - intermittent claudication I7Ø.411
              - rest pain (and intermittent claudication) I7Ø.421
              - ulceration (and intermittent claudication and rest pain) I7Ø.439
                - ankle I7Ø.433
                - calf I7Ø.432
                - foot site NEC I7Ø.435
                - heel I7Ø.434
                - lower leg NEC I7Ø.438
                - midfoot I7Ø.434
                - thigh I7Ø.431
            - specified type NEC I7Ø.491
          - specified type NEC I7Ø.499
        - specified NEC I7Ø.4Ø8
          - with
            - gangrene (and intermittent claudication, rest pain and ulcer) I7Ø.468
            - intermittent claudication I7Ø.418
            - rest pain (and intermittent claudication) I7Ø.428
            - ulceration (and intermittent claudication and rest pain) I7Ø.45
          - specified type NEC I7Ø.498
      - leg I7Ø.3Ø9
        - with
          - gangrene (and intermittent claudication, rest pain and ulcer) I7Ø.369
          - intermittent claudication I7Ø.319
          - rest pain (and intermittent claudication) I7Ø.329
        - bilateral I7Ø.3Ø3
          - with
            - gangrene (and intermittent claudication, rest pain and ulcer) I7Ø.363
            - intermittent claudication I7Ø.313
            - rest pain (and intermittent claudication) I7Ø.323
          - specified type NEC I7Ø.393
        - left I7Ø.3Ø2
          - with
            - gangrene (and intermittent claudication, rest pain and ulcer) I7Ø.362
            - intermittent claudication I7Ø.312
            - rest pain (and intermittent claudication) I7Ø.322

- **Arteriosclerosis, arteriosclerotic** — *continued*
  - extremities (native arteries) — *continued*
    - bypass graft — *continued*
      - leg — *continued*
        - left — *continued*
          - with — *continued*
            - ulceration (and intermittent claudication and rest pain) I7Ø.349
              - ankle I7Ø.343
              - calf I7Ø.342
              - foot site NEC I7Ø.345
              - heel I7Ø.344
              - lower leg NEC I7Ø.348
              - midfoot I7Ø.344
              - thigh I7Ø.341
          - specified type NEC I7Ø.392
        - right I7Ø.3Ø1
          - with
            - gangrene (and intermittent claudication, rest pain and ulcer) I7Ø.361
            - intermittent claudication I7Ø.311
            - rest pain (and intermittent claudication) I7Ø.321
            - ulceration (and intermittent claudication and rest pain) I7Ø.339
              - ankle I7Ø.333
              - calf I7Ø.332
              - foot site NEC I7Ø.335
              - heel I7Ø.334
              - lower leg NEC I7Ø.338
              - midfoot I7Ø.334
              - thigh I7Ø.331
          - specified type NEC I7Ø.391
        - specified type NEC I7Ø.399
      - nonautologous biological graft I7Ø.5Ø9
        - leg I7Ø.5Ø9
          - with
            - gangrene (and intermittent claudication, rest pain and ulcer) I7Ø.569
            - intermittent claudication I7Ø.519
            - rest pain (and intermittent claudication) I7Ø.529
          - bilateral I7Ø.5Ø3
            - with
              - gangrene (and intermittent claudication, rest pain and ulcer) I7Ø.563
              - intermittent claudication I7Ø.513
              - rest pain (and intermittent claudication) I7Ø.523
            - specified type NEC I7Ø.593
          - left I7Ø.5Ø2
            - with
              - gangrene (and intermittent claudication, rest pain and ulcer) I7Ø.562
              - intermittent claudication I7Ø.512
              - rest pain (and intermittent claudication) I7Ø.522
              - ulceration (and intermittent claudication and rest pain) I7Ø.549
                - ankle I7Ø.543
                - calf I7Ø.542
                - foot site NEC I7Ø.545
                - heel I7Ø.544
                - lower leg NEC I7Ø.548
                - midfoot I7Ø.544
                - thigh I7Ø.541
            - specified type NEC I7Ø.592
          - right I7Ø.5Ø1
            - with
              - gangrene (and intermittent claudication, rest pain and ulcer) I7Ø.561
              - intermittent claudication I7Ø.511

- **Arteriosclerosis, arteriosclerotic** *— continued*
  - extremities (native arteries) *— continued*
    - leg *— continued*
      - right *— continued*
        - with *— continued*
          - rest pain (and intermittent claudication) I7Ø.221
          - ulceration (and intermittent claudication and rest pain) I7Ø.239
            - ankle I7Ø.233
            - calf I7Ø.232
            - foot site NEC I7Ø.235
            - heel I7Ø.234
            - lower leg NEC I7Ø.238
            - midfoot I7Ø.234
            - thigh I7Ø.231
        - specified type NEC I7Ø.291
      - specified type NEC I7Ø.299
    - specified site NEC I7Ø.2Ø8
      - with
        - gangrene (and intermittent claudication, rest pain and ulcer) I7Ø.268
        - intermittent claudication I7Ø.218
        - rest pain (and intermittent claudication) I7Ø.228
        - ulceration (and intermittent claudication and rest pain) I7Ø.25
      - specified type NEC I7Ø.298
  - generalized I7Ø.91
  - heart (disease) *— see* Arteriosclerosis, coronary (artery),
  - kidney *— see* Hypertension, kidney
  - medial *— see* Arteriosclerosis, extremities
  - mesenteric (artery) K55.1
  - Mönckeberg's *— see* Arteriosclerosis, extremities
  - myocarditis I51.4
  - peripheral (of extremities) *— see* Arteriosclerosis, extremities
  - pulmonary (idiopathic) I27.Ø
  - renal (arterioles) (*see also* Hypertension, kidney artery I7Ø.1)
  - retina (vascular) I7Ø.8 *[H35.Ø-]*
  - specified artery NEC I7Ø.8
  - spinal (cord) G95.19
  - vertebral (artery) I67.2
- **Arteriospasm** I73.9
- **Arteriovenous** *— see* condition
- **Arteritis** I77.6
  - allergic M31.Ø
  - aorta (nonsyphilitic) I77.6
    - syphilitic A52.Ø2
  - aortic arch M31.4
  - brachiocephalic M31.4
  - brain I67.7
    - syphilitic A52.Ø4
  - cerebral I67.7
    - in systemic lupus erythematosus M32.19
    - listerial A32.89
    - syphilitic A52.Ø4
    - tuberculous A18.89
  - coronary (artery) I25.89
    - rheumatic IØ1.8
      - chronic IØ9.89
    - syphilitic A52.Ø6
  - cranial (left) (right), giant cell M31.6
  - deformans *— see* Arteriosclerosis
  - giant cell NEC M31.6
    - with polymyalgia rheumatica M31.5
  - necrosing or necrotizing M31.9
    - specified NEC M31.8
  - nodosa M3Ø.Ø
  - obliterans *— see* Arteriosclerosis
  - pulmonary I28.8
  - rheumatic *— see* Fever, rheumatic
  - senile *— see* Arteriosclerosis
  - suppurative I77.2
  - syphilitic (general) A52.Ø9
    - brain A52.Ø4
    - coronary A52.Ø6
    - spinal A52.Ø9
  - temporal, giant cell M31.6
  - young female aortic arch syndrome M31.4
- **Artery, arterial** (*see also* condition)
  - abscess I77.89
  - single umbilical Q27.Ø
- **Arthralgia** (allergic) (*see also* Pain, joint)
  - in caisson disease T7Ø.3
  - temporomandibular M26.62
- **Arthritis, arthritic** (acute) (chronic) (nonpyogenic) (subacute) M19.9Ø
  - meaning osteoarthritis *— see* Osteoarthritis
  - allergic *— see* Arthritis, specified form NEC
  - ankylosing (crippling) (spine) (*see also* Spondylitis, ankylosing)
    - sites other than spine *— see* Arthritis, specified form NEC
  - atrophic *— see* Osteoarthritis
    - spine *— see* Spondylitis, ankylosing
  - back *— see* Spondylopathy, inflammatory
  - blennorrhagic (gonococcal) A54.42
  - Charcot's *— see* Arthropathy, neuropathic
    - diabetic *— see* Diabetes, arthropathy, neuropathic
    - syringomyelic G95.Ø
  - chylous (filarial) B74.9 (*see also* category MØ1)
  - climacteric (any site) NEC *— see* Arthritis, specified form NEC
  - crystal(-induced) *— see* Arthritis, in, crystals
  - deformans *— see* Osteoarthritis
  - degenerative *— see* Osteoarthritis
  - due to or associated with
    - acromegaly E22.Ø
    - brucellosis *— see* Brucellosis
    - caisson disease T7Ø.3
    - diabetes *— see* Diabetes, arthropathy
    - dracontiasis B72 (*see also* category MØ1)
    - enteritis NEC
      - regional *— see* Enteritis, regional
    - erysipelas (*see also* category MØ1) A46
    - erythema
      - epidemic A25.1
      - nodosum L52
    - filariasis NOS B74.9
    - glanders A24.Ø
    - helminthiasis (*see also* category MØ1) B83.9
    - hemophilia D66 *[M36.2]*
    - Henoch (-Schönlein) purpura D69.Ø *[M36.4]*
    - human parvovirus (*see also* category MØ1) B97.6
    - infectious disease NEC *— see* category MØ1
    - leprosy (*see also* category MØ1) (*see also* Leprosy) A3Ø.9
    - Lyme disease A69.23
    - mycobacteria (*see also* category MØ1) A31.8
    - parasitic disease NEC B89 (*see also* category MØ1)
    - paratyphoid fever (*see also* Fever, paratyphoid) AØ1.4 (*see also* category MØ1)
    - rat bite fever (*see also* category MØ1) A25.1
    - regional enteritis *— see* Enteritis, regional
    - respiratory disorder NOS J98.9
    - serum sickness (*see also* Reaction, serum) T8Ø.69
    - syringomyelia G95.Ø
    - typhoid fever AØ1.Ø4
  - epidemic erythema A25.1
  - febrile *— see* Fever, rheumatic
  - gonococcal A54.42
  - gouty (acute) *— see* Gout, idiopathic
  - in (due to)
    - acromegaly (*see also* subcategory M14.8-) E22.Ø
    - amyloidosis (*see also* subcategory M14.8-) E85.4
    - bacterial disease (*see also* subcategory MØ1) A49.9
    - Behçet's syndrome M35.2
    - caisson disease (*see also* subcategory M14.8-) T7Ø.3
    - coliform bacilli (Escherichia coli) *— see* Arthritis, in, pyogenic organism NEC
    - crystals M11.9
      - dicalcium phosphate *— see* Arthritis, in, crystals, specified type NEC
      - hydroxyapatite M11.Ø-
      - pyrophosphate *— see* Arthritis, in, crystals, specified type NEC
      - specified type NEC M11.8Ø
        - ankle M11.87-

- **Arthritis, arthritic** *— continued*
  - in (due to) *— continued*
    - crystals *— continued*
      - specified type NEC *— continued*
        - elbow M11.82-
        - foot joint M11.87-
        - hand joint M11.84-
        - hip M11.85-
        - knee M11.86-
        - multiple sites M11.8-
        - shoulder M11.81-
        - vertebrae M11.88
        - wrist M11.83-
    - dermatoarthritis, lipoid E78.81
    - dracontiasis (dracunculiasis) B72 (*see also* category MØ1)
    - endocrine disorder NEC (*see also* subcategory M14.8-) E34.9
    - enteritis, infectious NEC AØ9 (*see also* category MØ1)
      - specified organism NEC AØ8.8 (*see also* category MØ1)
    - erythema
      - multiforme (*see also* subcategory M14.8-) L51.9
      - nodosum (*see also* subcategory M14.8-) L52
    - gout *— see* Gout, idiopathic
    - Hemophilus influenzae MØØ.8- *[B96.3]*
    - helminthiasis NEC B83.9 (*see also* category MØ1)
    - hemochromatosis (*see also* subcategory M14.8-) E83.118
    - hemoglobinopathy NEC D58.2 *[M36.3]*
    - hemophilia NEC D66 *[M36.2]*
    - hemophilus influenzae MØØ.8- *[B96.3]*
    - Henoch(-Schönlein) purpura D69.Ø *[M36.4]*
    - hyperparathyroidism NEC (*see also* subcategory M14.8-) E21.3
    - hypersensitivity reaction NEC T78.49 *[M36.4]*
    - hypogammaglobulinemia (*see also* subcategory M14.8-) D8Ø.1
    - hypothyroidism NEC (*see also* subcategory M14.8-) EØ3.9
    - infection *— see* Arthritis, pyogenic or pyemic
      - spine *— see* Spondylopathy, infective
    - infectious disease NEC *— see* category MØ1
    - leprosy A3Ø.9 (*see also* category MØ1)
    - leukemia NEC C95.9- *[M36.1]*
    - lipoid dermatoarthritis E78.81
    - Lyme disease A69.23
    - Mediterranean fever, familial (*see also* subcategory M14.8-) E85.Ø
    - Meningococcus A39.83
    - metabolic disorder NEC (*see also* subcategory M14.8-) E88.9
    - multiple myelomatosis C9Ø.Ø- *[M36.1]*
    - mumps B26.85
    - mycosis NEC B49 (*see also* category MØ1)
    - myelomatosis (multiple) C9Ø.Ø- *[M36.1]*
    - neurological disorder NEC G98.Ø
    - ochronosis (*see also* subcategory M14.8-) E7Ø.29
    - O'nyong-nyong A92.1 (*see also* category MØ1)
    - parasitic disease NEC B89 (*see also* category MØ1)
    - paratyphoid fever AØ1.4 (*see also* category MØ1)
    - Pseudomonas *— see* Arthritis, pyogenic, bacterial NEC
    - psoriasis L4Ø.5Ø
    - pyogenic organism NEC *— see* Arthritis, pyogenic, bacterial NEC
    - Reiter's disease *— see* Reiter's disease
    - respiratory disorder NEC (*see also* subcategory M14.8-) J98.9
    - reticulosis, malignant (*see also* subcategory M14.8-) C86.Ø
    - rubella BØ6.82
    - Salmonella (arizonae) (cholerae-suis) (enteritidis) (typhimurium) AØ2.23
    - sarcoidosis D86.86
    - specified bacteria NEC *— see* Arthritis, pyogenic, bacterial NEC
    - sporotrichosis B42.82
    - syringomyelia G95.Ø
    - thalassemia NEC D56.9 *[M36.3]*
    - tuberculosis *— see* Tuberculosis, arthritis

Arthrodesis status Z98.1
Arthrodynia (*see also* Pain, joint)
Arthrofibrosis, joint — *see* Ankylosis
Arthrodysplasia Q74.9
Arthrogryposis (congenital) Q68.8
   multiplex congenita Q74.3
Arthrokatadysis M24.7
Arthropathy (*see also* Arthritis) M12.9
   Charcot's — *see* Arthropathy, neuropathic
     diabetic — *see* Diabetes, arthropathy,
       neuropathic
     syringomyelic G95.0
   cricoarytenoid J38.7
   crystal(-induced) — *see* Arthritis, in, crystals
   diabetic NEC — *see* Diabetes, arthropathy
   distal interphalangeal, psoriatic L40.51
   enteropathic M07.60
     ankle M07.67-
     elbow M07.62-
     foot joint M07.67-
     hand joint M07.64-
     hip M07.65-
     knee M07.66-
     multiple site M07.69
     shoulder M07.61-
     vertebra M07.68
     wrist M07.63-
   following intestinal bypass M02.00
     ankle M02.07-
     elbow M02.02-
     foot joint M02.07-
     hand joint M02.04-
     hip M02.05-
     knee M02.06-
     multiple site M02.09
     shoulder M02.01-
     vertebra M02.08
     wrist M02.03-
   gouty (*see also* Gout, idiopathic)
     in (due to)
       Lesch-Nyhan syndrome E79.1 *[M14.8-]*
       sickle-cell disorders D57- *[M14.8-]*
   hemophilic NEC D66 *[M36.2]*
     in (due to)
       hyperparathyroidism NEC E21.3 *[M14.8-]*
       metabolic disease NOS E88.9 *[M14.8-]*
   in (due to)
     acromegaly E22.0 *[M14.8-]*
     amyloidosis E85.4 *[M14.8-]*
     blood disorder NOS D75.9 *[M36.3]*
     diabetes — *see* Diabetes, arthropathy
     endocrine disease NOS E34.9 *[M14.8-]*
     erythema
       multiforme L51.9 *[M14.8-]*
       nodosum L52 *[M14.8-]*
     hemochromatosis E83.118 *[M14.8-]*
     hemoglobinopathy NEC D58.2 *[M36.3]*
     hemophilia NEC D66 *[M36.2]*
     Henoch-Schönlein purpura D69.0 *[M36.4]*
     hyperthyroidism E05.90 *[M14.8-]*
     hypothyroidism E03.9 *[M14.8-]*
     infective endocarditis I33.0 *[M12.80]*
     leukemia NEC C95.9- *[M36.1]*
     malignant histiocytosis C96.A *[M36.1]*
     metabolic disease NOS E88.9 *[M14.8-]*
     multiple myeloma C90.0- *[M36.1]*
     neoplastic disease NOS (*see also* Neoplasm)
       D49.9 *[M36.1]*
     nutritional deficiency (*see also* subcategory
       M14.8-) E63.9
     psoriasis NOS L40.50
     sarcoidosis D86.86
     syphilis (late) A52.77
       congenital A50.55 *[M12.80]*
     thyrotoxicosis (*see also* subcategory
       M14.8- E05.90
     ulcerative colitis K51.90 *[M07.60]*
     viral hepatitis (postinfectious) NEC B19.9
       [M12.80]
     Whipple's disease (*see also* subcategory M14.8-)
       K90.81
   Jaccoud — *see* Arthropathy, postrheumatic, chronic
   juvenile — *see* Arthritis, juvenile

Arthropathy — *continued*
   juvenile — *continued*
     psoriatic L40.54
   mutilans (psoriatic) L40.52
   neuropathic (Charcot) M14.60
     ankle M14.67-
     diabetic — *see* Diabetes, arthropathy,
       neuropathic
     elbow M14.62-
     foot joint M14.67-
     hand joint M14.64-
     hip M14.65-
     knee M14.66-
     multiple site M14.69
     nonsyphilitic NEC G98.0
     shoulder M14.61-
     syringomyelic G95.0
     vertebra M14.68
     wrist M14.63-
   osteopulmonary — *see* Osteoarthropathy,
     hypertrophic, specified NEC
   postdysenteric M02.10
     ankle M02.17-
     elbow M02.12-
     foot joint M02.17-
     hand joint M02.14-
     hip M02.15-
     knee M02.16-
     multiple site M02.19
     shoulder M02.11-
     vertebra M02.18
     wrist M02.13-
   postimmunization M02.20
     ankle M02.27-
     elbow M02.22-
     foot joint M02.27-
     hand joint M02.24-
     hip M02.25-
     knee M02.26-
     multiple site M02.29
     shoulder M02.21-
     vertebra M02.28
     wrist M02.23-
   postinfectious NEC B99 *[M12.80]*
     in (due to)
       enteritis due to Yersinia enterocolitica A04.6
        [M12.80]
       syphilis A52.77
       viral hepatitis NEC B19.9 *[M12.80]*
   postrheumatic, chronic (Jaccoud) M12.00
     ankle M12.07-
     elbow M12.02-
     foot joint M12.07-
     hand joint M12.04-
     hip M12.05-
     knee M12.06-
     multiple site M12.09
     shoulder M12.01-
     specified joint NEC M12.08
     wrist M12.03-
   psoriatic NEC L40.59
     interphalangeal, distal L40.51
   reactive M02.9
     in (due to)
       infective endocarditis I33.0 *[M02.9]*
     specified type NEC M02.80
       ankle M02.87-
       elbow M02.82-
       foot joint M02.87-
       hand joint M02.84-
       hip M02.85-
       knee M02.86-
       multiple site M02.89
       shoulder M02.81-
       vertebra M02.88
       wrist M02.83-
   specified form NEC M12.80
     ankle M12.87-
     elbow M12.82-
     foot joint M12.87-
     hand joint M12.84-
     hip M12.85-
     knee M12.86-

Arthropathy — *continued*
   specific form NEC — *continued*
     multiple site M12.89
     shoulder M12.81-
     specified joint NEC M12.88
     wrist M12.83-
   syringomyelic G95.0
   tabes dorsalis A52.16
   tabetic A52.16
   transient — *see* Arthropathy, specified form NEC
   traumatic M12.50
     ankle M12.57-
     elbow M12.52-
     foot joint M12.57-
     hand joint M12.54-
     hip M12.55-
     knee M12.56-
     multiple site M12.59
     shoulder M12.51-
     specified joint NEC M12.58
     wrist M12.53-
Arthropyosis — *see* Arthritis, pyogenic or pyemic
Arthrosis (deformans) (degenerative) (localized)
   M19.90 (*see also* Osteoarthritis)
   spine — *see* Spondylosis
Arthus' phenomenon or reaction T78.41
   due to
     drug — *see* Table of Drugs and Chemicals, by
       drug
Articular — *see* condition
Articulation, reverse (teeth) M26.24
Artificial
   insemination complication — *see* Complications,
     artificial, fertilization
   opening status (functioning) (without complication)
     Z93.9
     anus (colostomy) Z93.3
     colostomy Z93.3
     cystostomy Z93.50
       appendico-vesicostomy Z93.52
       cutaneous Z93.51
       specified NEC Z93.59
     enterostomy Z93.4
     gastrostomy Z93.1
     ileostomy Z93.2
     intestinal tract NEC Z93.4
     jejunostomy Z93.4
     nephrostomy Z93.6
     specified site NEC Z93.8
     tracheostomy Z93.0
     ureterostomy Z93.6
     urethrostomy Z93.6
     urinary tract NEC Z93.6
     vagina Z93.8
   vagina status Z93.8
Arytenoid — *see* condition
Asbestosis (occupational) J61
ASC-H (atypical squamous cells cannot exclude high
   grade squamous intraepithelial lesion on
   cytologic smear)
   anus R85.611
   cervix R87.611
   vagina R87.621
ASC-US (atypical squamous cells of undetermined
   significance on cytologic smear)
   anus R85.610
   cervix R87.610
   vagina R87.620
Ascariasis B77.9
   with
     complications NEC B77.89
     intestinal complications B77.0
     pneumonia, pneumonitis B77.81
Ascaridosis, ascaridiasis — *see* Ascariasis
Ascaris (infection) (infestation) (lumbricoides) — *see*
   Ascariasis
Ascending — *see* condition
Aschoff's bodies — *see* Myocarditis, rheumatic
Ascites (abdominal) R18.8
   cardiac I50.9
   chylous (nonfilarial) I89.8
     filarial — *see* Infestation, filarial

- **Ascites** — *continued*
  - due to
    - cirrhosis, alcoholic K7Ø.31
    - hepatitis
      - alcoholic K7Ø.11
      - chronic active K71.51
    - S. japonicum B65.2
  - heart I5Ø.9
  - malignant R18.Ø
  - pseudochylous R18.8
  - syphilitic A52.74
  - tuberculous A18.31
- **Aseptic** — *see* condition
- **Asherman's syndrome** N85.6
- **Asialia** K11.7
- **Asiatic cholera** — *see* Cholera
- **Asimultagnosia** (simultanagnosia) R48.3
- **Askin's tumor** — *see* Neoplasm, connective tissue, malignant
- **Asocial personality** F6Ø.2
- **Asomatognosia** R41.4
- **Aspartylglucosaminuria** E77.1
- **Asperger's disease or syndrome** F84.5
- **Aspergilloma** — *see* Aspergillosis
- **Aspergillosis** (with pneumonia) B44.9
  - bronchopulmonary, allergic B44.81
  - disseminated B44.7
  - generalized B44.7
  - pulmonary NEC B44.1
    - allergic B44.81
    - invasive B44.Ø
  - specified NEC B44.89
  - tonsillar B44.2
- **Aspergillus** (flavus) (fumigatus) (infection) (terreus) — *see* Aspergillosis
- **Aspermatogenesis** — *see* Azoospermia
- **Aspermia** (testis) — *see* Azoospermia
- **Asphyxia, asphyxiation** (by) RØ9.Ø1
  - antenatal P84
  - birth P84
  - bunny bag — *see* Asphyxia, due to, mechanical threat to breathing, trapped in bed clothes
  - crushing S28.Ø
  - drowning T75.1
  - gas, fumes, or vapor — *see* Table of Drugs and Chemicals
  - inhalation — *see* Inhalation
  - intrauterine P84
  - local I73.ØØ
    - with gangrene I73.Ø1
  - mucus (*see also* Foreign body, respiratory tract, causing asphyxia)
    - newborn P84
  - pathological RØ9.Ø1
  - postnatal P84
    - mechanical — *see* Asphyxia, due to, mechanical threat to breathing
  - prenatal P84
  - reticularis R23.1
  - strangulation — *see* Asphyxia, due to, mechanical threat to breathing
  - submersion T75.1
  - traumatic T71.9
    - due to
      - crushed chest S28.Ø
      - foreign body (in) — *see* Foreign body, respiratory tract, causing asphyxia
      - low oxygen content of ambient air T71.2Ø
        - due to
          - being trapped in
            - low oxygen environment T71.29
              - in car trunk T71.221
                - circumstances undetermined T71.224
                - done with intent to harm by another person T71.223
                - self T71.222
              - in refrigerator T71.231
                - circumstances undetermined T71.234
                - done with intent to harm by another person T71.233

- **Asphyxia, asphyxiation** — *continued*
  - traumatic — *continued*
    - due to — *continued*
      - low oxygen content of ambient air — *continued*
        - due to — *continued*
          - being trapped in — *continued*
            - low oxygen environment — *continued*
              - in refrigerator — *continued*
                - done with intent to harm by another person — *continued*
                  - self T71.232
          - cave-in T71.21
      - mechanical threat to breathing (accidental) T71.191
        - circumstances undetermined T71.194
        - done with intent to harm by another person T71.193
        - self T71.192
        - hanging T71.161
          - circumstances undetermined T71.164
          - done with intent to harm by another person T71.163
          - self T71.162
        - plastic bag T71.121
          - circumstances undetermined T71.124
          - done with intent to harm by another person T71.123
          - self T71.122
        - smothering
          - in furniture T71.151
            - circumstances undetermined T71.154
            - done with intent to harm by another person T71.153
            - self T71.152
          - under
            - another person's body T71.141
              - circumstances undetermined T71.144
              - done with intent to harm T71.143
            - pillow T71.111
              - circumstances undetermined T71.114
              - done with intent to harm by another person T71.113
              - self T71.112
        - trapped in bed clothes T71.131
          - circumstances undetermined T71.134
          - done with intent to harm by another person T71.133
          - self T71.132
  - vomiting, vomitus — *see* Foreign body, respiratory tract, causing asphyxia
- **Aspiration**
  - amniotic (clear) fluid (newborn) P24.1Ø
    - with
      - pneumonia (pneumonitis) P24.11
      - respiratory symptoms P24.11
  - blood
    - newborn (without respiratory symptoms) P24.2Ø
      - with
        - pneumonia (pneumonitis) P24.21
        - respiratory symptoms P24.21
    - specified age NEC — *see* Foreign body, respiratory tract
  - bronchitis J69.Ø
  - food or foreign body (with asphyxiation) — *see* Asphyxia, food
  - liquor (amnii) (newborn) P24.1Ø
    - with
      - pneumonia (pneumonitis) P24.11
      - respiratory symptoms P24.11
  - meconium (newborn) (without respiratory symptoms) P24.ØØ
    - with
      - pneumonitis (pneumonitis) P24.Ø1
      - respiratory symptoms P24.Ø1
  - milk (newborn) (without respiratory symptoms) P24.3Ø

- **Aspiration** — *continued*
  - milk (newborn) (without respiratory symptoms) — *continued*
    - with
      - pneumonia (pneumonitis) P24.31
      - respiratory symptoms P24.31
    - specified age NEC — *see* Foreign body, respiratory tract
  - mucus (*see also* Foreign body, by site, causing asphyxia)
    - newborn P24.1Ø
      - with
        - pneumonia (pneumonitis) P24.11
        - respiratory symptoms P24.11
  - neonatal P24.9
    - specific NEC (without respiratory symptoms) P24.8Ø
      - with
        - pneumonia (pneumonitis) P24.81
        - respiratory symptoms P24.81
  - newborn P24.9
    - specific NEC (without respiratory symptoms) P24.8Ø
      - with
        - pneumonia (pneumonitis) P24.81
        - respiratory symptoms P24.81
  - pneumonia J69.Ø
  - pneumonitis J69.Ø
  - syndrome of newborn — *see* Aspiration, by substance, with pneumonia
  - vernix caseosa (newborn) P24.8Ø
    - with
      - pneumonia (pneumonitis) P24.81
      - respiratory symptoms P24.81
  - vomitus (*see also* Foreign body, respiratory tract)
    - newborn (without respiratory symptoms) P24.3Ø
      - with
        - pneumonia (pneumonitis) P24.31
        - respiratory symptoms P24.31
- **Asplenia** (congenital) Q89.Ø1
  - postsurgical Z9Ø.81
- **Assam fever** B55.Ø
- **Assault, sexual** — *see* Maltreatment
- **Assmann's focus NEC** A15.Ø
- **Astasia** (-abasia) (hysterical) F44.4
- **Asteatosis cutis** L85.3
- **Astereognosia, astereognosis** R48.1
- **Asterixis** R27.8
  - in liver disease K71.3
- **Asteroid hyalitis** — *see* Deposit, crystalline
- **Asthenia, asthenic** R53.1
  - cardiac (*see also* Failure, heart) I5Ø.9
    - psychogenic F45.8
  - cardiovascular (*see also* Failure, heart) I5Ø.9
    - psychogenic F45.8
  - heart (*see also* Failure, heart) I5Ø.9
    - psychogenic F45.8
  - hysterical F44.4
  - myocardial (*see also* Failure, heart) I5Ø.9
    - psychogenic F45.8
  - nervous F48.8
  - neurocirculatory F45.8
  - neurotic F48.8
  - psychogenic F48.8
  - psychoneurotic F48.8
  - psychophysiologic F48.8
  - reaction (psychophysiologic) F48.8
  - senile R54
- **Asthenopia** (*see also* Discomfort, visual)
  - hysterical F44.6
  - psychogenic F44.6
- **Asthenospermia** — *see* Abnormal, specimen, male genital organs
- **Asthma, asthmatic** (bronchial) (catarrh) (spasmodic) J45.9Ø9
  - with
    - chronic obstructive bronchitis J44.9
      - with
        - acute lower respiratory infection J44.Ø
        - exacerbation (acute) J44.1
    - chronic obstructive pulmonary disease J44.9
      - with
        - acute lower respiratory infection J44.Ø

- **Asthma, asthmatic** — *continued*
  - with — *continued*
    - chronic obstructive pulmonary disease — *continued*
      - with — *continued*
        - exacerbation (acute) J44.1
    - exacerbation (acute) J45.9Ø1
    - hay fever — *see* Asthma, allergic extrinsic
    - rhinitis, allergic — *see* Asthma, allergic extrinsic
    - status asthmaticus J45.9Ø2
  - allergic extrinsic J45.9Ø9
    - with
      - exacerbation (acute) J45.9Ø1
      - status asthmaticus J45.9Ø2
  - atopic — *see* Asthma, allergic extrinsic
  - cardiac — *see* Failure, ventricular, left
  - cardiobronchial I5Ø.1
  - childhood J45.9Ø9
    - with
      - exacerbation (acute) J45.9Ø1
      - status asthmaticus J45.9Ø2
  - chronic obstructive J44.9
    - with
      - acute lower respiratory infection J44.Ø
      - exacerbation (acute) J44.1
  - collier's J6Ø
  - cough variant J45.991
  - detergent J69.8
  - due to
    - detergent J69.8
    - inhalation of fumes J68.3
  - eosinophilic J82
  - extrinsic, allergic — *see* Asthma, allergic extrinsic
  - grinder's J62.8
  - hay — *see* Asthma, allergic extrinsic
  - heart I5Ø.1
  - idiosyncratic — *see* Asthma, nonallergic
  - intermittent (mild) J45.2Ø
    - with
      - exacerbation (acute) J45.21
      - status asthmaticus J45.22
  - intrinsic, nonallergic — *see* Asthma, nonallergic
  - Kopp's E32.8
  - late-onset J45.9Ø9
    - with
      - exacerbation (acute) J45.9Ø1
      - status asthmaticus J45.9Ø2
  - mild intermittent J45.2Ø
    - with
      - exacerbation (acute) J45.21
      - status asthmaticus J45.22
  - mild persistent J45.3Ø
    - with
      - exacerbation (acute) J45.31
      - status asthmaticus J45.32
  - Millar's (laryngismus stridulus) J38.5
  - miner's J6Ø
  - mixed J45.9Ø9
    - with
      - exacerbation (acute) J45.9Ø1
      - status asthmaticus J45.9Ø2
  - moderate persistent J45.4Ø
    - with
      - exacerbation (acute) J45.41
      - status asthmaticus J45.42
  - nervous — *see* Asthma, nonallergic
  - nonallergic (intrinsic) J45.9Ø9
    - with
      - exacerbation (acute) J45.9Ø1
      - status asthmaticus J45.9Ø2
  - persistent
    - mild J45.3Ø
      - with
        - exacerbation (acute) J45.31
        - status asthmaticus J45.32
    - moderate J45.4Ø
      - with
        - exacerbation (acute) J45.41
        - status asthmaticus J45.42
    - severe J45.5Ø
      - with
        - exacerbation (acute) J45.51
        - status asthmaticus J45.52
  - platinum J45.998
  - pneumoconiotic NEC J64
  - potter's J62.8
  - predominantly allergic J45.9Ø9
  - psychogenic F54
  - pulmonary eosinophilic J82
  - red cedar J67.8
  - Rostan's I5Ø.1
  - sandblaster's J62.8
  - sequoiosis J67.8
  - severe persistent J45.5Ø
    - with
      - exacerbation (acute) J45.51
      - status asthmaticus J45.52
  - specified NEC J45.998
  - stonemason's J62.8
  - thymic E32.8
  - tuberculous — *see* Tuberculosis, pulmonary
  - Wichmann's (laryngismus stridulus) J38.5
  - wood J67.8
- **Astigmatism** (compound) (congenital) H52.2Ø-
  - irregular H52.21-
  - regular H52.22-
- **Astraphobia** F4Ø.22Ø
- **Astroblastoma**
  - specified site — *see* Neoplasm, malignant, by site
  - unspecified site C71.9
- **Astrocytoma** (cystic)
  - anaplastic
    - specified site — *see* Neoplasm, malignant, by site
    - unspecified site C71.9
  - fibrillary
    - specified site — *see* Neoplasm, malignant, by site
    - unspecified site C71.9
  - fibrous
    - specified site — *see* Neoplasm, malignant, by site
    - unspecified site C71.9
  - gemistocytic
    - specified site — *see* Neoplasm, malignant, by site
    - unspecified site C71.9
  - juvenile
    - specified site — *see* Neoplasm, malignant, by site
    - unspecified site C71.9
  - pilocytic
    - specified site — *see* Neoplasm, malignant, by site
    - unspecified site C71.9
  - piloid
    - specified site — *see* Neoplasm, malignant, by site
    - unspecified site C71.9
  - protoplasmic
    - specified site — *see* Neoplasm, malignant, by site
    - unspecified site C71.9
  - specified site NEC — *see* Neoplasm, malignant, by site
  - subependymal D43.2
    - giant cell
      - specified site — *see* Neoplasm, uncertain behavior, by site
      - unspecified site D43.2
    - specified site — *see* Neoplasm, uncertain behavior, by site
    - unspecified site D43.2
  - unspecified site C71.9
- **Astroglioma**
  - specified site — *see* Neoplasm, malignant, by site
  - unspecified site C71.9
- **Asymbolia** R48.8
- **Asymmetry** (*see also* Distortion)
  - between native and reconstructed breast N65.1
  - face Q67.Ø
  - jaw (lower) — *see* Anomaly, dentofacial, jaw-cranial base relationship, asymmetry
- **Asynergia, asynergy** R27.8
  - ventricular I51.89
- **Asystole** (heart) — *see* Arrest, cardiac
- **At risk**
  - for falling Z91.81
- **Ataxia, ataxy, ataxic** R27.Ø
  - acute R27.8
  - brain (hereditary) G11.9
  - cerebellar (hereditary) G11.9
    - with defective DNA repair G11.3
- **Ataxia, ataxy, ataxic** — *continued*
  - cerebellar (hereditary) — *continued*
    - alcoholic G31.2
    - early-onset G11.1
    - in
      - alcoholism G31.2
      - myxedema EØ3.9 *[G13.2]*
      - neoplastic disease (*see also* Neoplasm) D49.9 *[G13.1]*
      - specified disease NEC G32.81
    - late-onset (Marie's) G11.2
  - cerebral (hereditary) G11.9
  - congenital nonprogressive G11.Ø
  - family, familial — *see* Ataxia, hereditary
  - following
    - cerebrovascular disease I69.993
      - cerebral infarction I69.393
      - intracerebral hemorrhage I69.193
      - nontraumatic intracranial hemorrhage NEC I69.293
      - specified disease NEC I69.893
      - subarachnoid hemorrhage I69.Ø93
  - Friedreich's (heredofamilial) (cerebellar) (spinal) G11.1
  - gait R26.Ø
    - hysterical F44.4
  - general R27.8
  - hereditary G11.9
    - with neuropathy G6Ø.2
    - cerebellar — *see* Ataxia, cerebellar
    - spastic G11.4
    - specified NEC G11.8
    - spinal (Friedreich's) G11.1
  - heredofamilial — *see* Ataxia, hereditary
  - Hunt's G11.1
  - hysterical F44.4
  - locomotor (progressive) (syphilitic) (partial) (spastic) A52.11
    - diabetic — *see* Diabetes, ataxia
  - Marie's (cerebellar) (heredofamilial) (lateonset) G11.2
  - nonorganic origin F44.4
  - nonprogressive, congenital G11.Ø
  - psychogenic F44.4
  - Roussy-Lévy G6Ø.Ø
  - Sanger-Brown's (hereditary) G11.2
  - spastic hereditary G11.4
  - spinal
    - hereditary (Friedreich's) G11.1
    - progressive (syphilitic) A52.11
  - spinocerebellar, X-linked recessive G11.1
  - telangiectasia (Louis-Bar) G11.3
- **Ataxia-telangiectasia** (Louis-Bar) G11.3
- **Atelectasis** (massive) (partial) (pressure) (pulmonary) J98.11
  - newborn P28.1Ø
    - due to resorption P28.11
    - partial P28.19
    - primary P28.Ø
    - secondary P28.19
  - primary (newborn) P28.Ø
  - tuberculous — *see* Tuberculosis, pulmonary
- **Atelocardia** Q24.9
- **Atelomyelia** QØ6.1
- **Atheroembolism**
  - of
    - extremities
      - lower I75.Ø2-
      - upper I75.Ø1-
    - kidney I75.81
    - specified NEC I75.89
- **Atheroma, atheromatous** (*see also* Arteriosclerosis) I7Ø.9Ø
  - aorta, aortic I7Ø.Ø
    - valve (*see also* Endocarditis, aortic) I35.8
  - aorto-iliac I7Ø.Ø
  - artery — *see* Arteriosclerosis
  - basilar (artery) I67.2
  - carotid (artery) (common) (internal) I67.2
  - cerebral (arteries) I67.2
- **Atheroma, atheromatous**
  - coronary (artery) I25.1Ø

B

- **Behavior** — *continued*
  - verbosity and circumstantial detail obscuring reason for contact R46.7
- **Behçet's disease or syndrome** M35.2
- **Behr's disease** — *see* Degeneration, macula
- **Beigel's disease or morbus** (white piedra) B36.2
- **Bejel** A65
- **Bekhterev's syndrome** — *see* Spondylitis, ankylosing
- **Belching** — *see* Eructation
- **Bell's**
  - mania F3Ø.8
  - palsy, paralysis G51.Ø
    - infant or newborn P11.3
  - spasm G51.3
- **Bence Jones albuminuria or proteinuria NEC** R8Ø.3
- **Bends** T7Ø.3
- **Benedikt's paralysis or syndrome** G46.3
- **Benign** (*see also* condition)
  - prostatic hyperplasia — *see* Hyperplasia, prostate
- **Bennett's fracture** (displaced) S62.21-
- **Benson's disease** — *see* Deposit, crystalline
- **Bent**
  - back (hysterical) F44.4
  - nose M95.Ø
    - congenital Q67.4
- **Bereavement** (uncomplicated) Z63.4
- **Bergeron's disease** (hysterical chorea) F44.4
- **Berger's disease** — *see* Nephropathy, IgA
- **Beriberi** (dry) E51.11
  - heart (disease) E51.12
  - polyneuropathy E51.11
  - wet E51.12
    - involving circulatory system E51.11
- **Berlin's disease or edema** (traumatic) SØ5.8X-
- **Berlock** (berloque) **dermatitis** L56.2
- **Bernard-Horner syndrome** G9Ø.2
- **Bernard-Soulier disease or thrombopathia** D69.1
- **Bernhardt** (-Roth) **disease** — *see* Mononeuropathy, lower limb, meralgia paresthetica
- **Bernheim's syndrome** — *see* Failure, heart, congestive
- **Bertielliasis** B71.8
- **Berylliosis** (lung) J63.2
- **Besnier-Boeck** (-Schaumann) **disease** — *see* Sarcoidosis
- **Besnier's**
  - lupus pernio D86.3
  - prurigo L2Ø.Ø
- **Bestiality** F65.89
- **Best's disease** H35.5Ø
- **Beta-mercaptolactate-cysteine disulfiduria** E72.Ø9
- **Betalipoproteinemia, broad or floating** E78.2
- **Betting and gambling** Z72.6
  - pathological (compulsive) F63.Ø
- **Bezoar** T18.9
  - intestine T18.3
  - stomach T18.2
- **Bezold's abscess** — *see* Mastoiditis, acute
- **Bianchi's syndrome** R48.8
- **Bicornate or bicornis uterus** Q51.3
  - in pregnancy or childbirth O34.59-
    - causing obstructed labor O65.5
- **Bicuspid aortic valve** Q23.1
- **Biedl-Bardet syndrome** Q87.89
- **Bielschowsky** (-Jansky) **disease** E75.4
- **Biermer's** (pernicious) **anemia or disease** D51.Ø
- **Biett's disease** L93.Ø
- **Bifid** (congenital)
  - apex, heart Q24.8
  - clitoris Q52.6
  - kidney Q63.8
  - nose Q3Ø.2
  - patella Q74.1
  - scrotum Q55.29
  - toe NEC Q74.2
  - tongue Q38.3
  - ureter Q62.8
  - uterus Q51.3
  - uvula Q35.7
- **Biforis uterus** (suprasimplex) Q51.3
- **Bifurcation** (congenital)
  - gallbladder Q44.1
- **Bifurcation** — *continued*
  - kidney pelvis Q63.8
  - renal pelvis Q63.8
  - rib Q76.6
  - tongue, congenital Q38.3
  - trachea Q32.1
  - ureter Q62.8
  - urethra Q64.74
  - vertebra Q76.49
- **Big spleen syndrome** D73.1
- **Bigeminal pulse** RØØ.8
- **Bilateral** — *see* condition
- **Bile**
  - duct — *see* condition
  - pigments in urine R82.2
- **Bilharziasis** (*see also* Schistosomiasis)
  - chyluria B65.Ø
  - cutaneous B65.3
  - galacturia B65.Ø
  - hematochyluria B65.Ø
  - intestinal B65.1
  - lipemia B65.9
  - lipuria B65.Ø
  - oriental B65.2
  - piarhemia B65.9
  - pulmonary NOS B65.9 *[J99]*
    - pneumonia B65.9 *[J17]*
  - tropical hematuria B65.Ø
  - vesical B65.Ø
- **Biliary** — *see* condition
- **Bilirubin metabolism disorder** E8Ø.7
  - specified NEC E8Ø.6
- **Bilirubinemia, familial nonhemolytic** E8Ø.4
- **Bilirubinuria** R82.2
- **Biliuria** R82.2
- **Bilocular stomach** K31.2
- **Binswanger's disease** I67.3
- **Biparta, bipartite**
  - carpal scaphoid Q74.Ø
  - patella Q74.1
  - vagina Q52.1Ø
- **Bird**
  - face Q75.8
  - fancier's disease or lung J67.2
- **Birt-Hogg-Dube syndrome** Q87.89
- **Birth**
  - complications in mother — *see* Delivery, complicated
  - compression during NOS P15.9
  - defect — *see* Anomaly
  - immature (less than 37 completed weeks) — *see* Preterm, newborn
    - extremely (less than 28 completed weeks) — *see* Immaturity, extreme
  - inattention, at or after — *see* Maltreatment, child, neglect
  - injury NOS P15.9
    - basal ganglia P11.1
    - brachial plexus NEC P14.3
    - brain (compression) (pressure) P11.2
    - central nervous system NOS P11.9
    - cerebellum P11.1
    - cerebral hemorrhage P1Ø.1
    - external genitalia P15.5
    - eye P15.3
    - face P15.4
    - fracture
      - bone P13.9
        - specified NEC P13.8
      - clavicle P13.4
      - femur P13.2
      - humerus P13.3
      - long bone, except femur P13.3
      - radius and ulna P13.3
      - skull P13.Ø
      - spine P11.5
      - tibia and fibula P13.3
    - intracranial P11.2
      - laceration or hemorrhage P1Ø.9
        - specified NEC P1Ø.8
    - intraventricular hemorrhage P1Ø.2
    - laceration
      - brain P1Ø.1
- **Birth** — *continued*
  - injury NOS — *continued*
    - laceration — *continued*
      - by scalpel P15.8
      - peripheral nerve P14.9
    - liver P15.Ø
    - meninges
      - brain P11.1
      - spinal cord P11.5
    - nerve
      - brachial plexus P14.3
      - cranial NEC (except facial) P11.4
      - facial P11.3
      - peripheral P14.9
      - phrenic (paralysis) P14.2
    - paralysis
      - facial nerve P11.3
      - spinal P11.5
    - penis P15.5
    - rupture
      - spinal cord P11.5
    - scalp P12.9
    - scalpel wound P15.8
    - scrotum P15.5
    - skull NEC P13.1
      - fracture P13.Ø
    - specified type NEC P15.8
    - spinal cord P11.5
    - spine P11.5
    - spleen P15.1
    - sternomastoid (hematoma) P15.2
    - subarachnoid hemorrhage P1Ø.3
    - subcutaneous fat necrosis P15.6
    - subdural hemorrhage P1Ø.Ø
    - tentorial tear P1Ø.4
    - testes P15.5
    - vulva P15.5
  - lack of care, at or after — *see* Maltreatment, child, neglect
  - neglect, at or after — *see* Maltreatment, child, neglect
  - palsy or paralysis, newborn, NOS (birth injury) P14.9
  - premature (infant) — *see* Preterm, newborn
  - shock, newborn P96.89
  - trauma — *see* Birth, injury
  - weight
    - low (2499 grams or less) — *see* Low, birthweight
      - extremely (999 grams or less) — *see* Low, birthweight, extreme
    - 4ØØØ grams to 4499 grams PØ8.1
    - 45ØØ grams or more PØ8.Ø
- **Birthmark** Q82.5
- **Bisalbuminemia** E88.Ø9
- **Biskra's button** B55.1
- **Bite(s)** (animal) (human)
  - abdomen, abdominal
    - wall S31.159
      - with penetration into peritoneal cavity S31.659
      - epigastric region S31.152
        - with penetration into peritoneal cavity S31.652
      - left
        - lower quadrant S31.154
          - with penetration into peritoneal cavity S31.654
        - upper quadrant S31.151
          - with penetration into peritoneal cavity S31.651
      - periumbilic region S31.155
        - with penetration into peritoneal cavity S31.655
      - right
        - lower quadrant S31.153
          - with penetration into peritoneal cavity S31.653
        - upper quadrant S31.15Ø
          - with penetration into peritoneal cavity S31.65Ø
      - superficial NEC S3Ø.871
        - insect S3Ø.861
  - alveolar (process) — *see* Bite, oral cavity

- **Bite(s)** — *continued*
  - amphibian (venomous) — *see* Venom, bite, amphibian
  - animal (*see also* Bite, by site)
    - venomous — *see* Venom
  - ankle S91.Ø5-
    - superficial NEC S9Ø.57-
      - insect S9Ø.56-
  - antecubital space — *see* Bite, elbow
  - anus S31.835
    - superficial NEC S3Ø.877
      - insect S3Ø.867
  - arm (upper) S41.15-
    - lower — *see* Bite, forearm
    - superficial NEC S4Ø.87-
      - insect S4Ø.86-
  - arthropod NEC — *see* Venom, bite, arthropod
  - auditory canal (external) (meatus) — *see* Bite, ear
  - auricle, ear — *see* Bite, ear
  - axilla — *see* Bite, arm
  - back (*see also* Bite, thorax, back)
    - lower S31.Ø5Ø
      - with penetration into retroperitoneal space S31.Ø51
      - superficial NEC S3Ø.87Ø
        - insect S3Ø.86Ø
  - bedbug — *see* Bite(s), by site, superficial, insect
  - breast S21.Ø5-
    - superficial NEC S2Ø.17-
      - insect S2Ø.16-
  - brow — *see* Bite, head, specified site NEC
  - buttock S31.8Ø5
    - left S31.825
    - right S31.815
    - superficial NEC S3Ø.87Ø
      - insect S3Ø.86Ø
  - calf — *see* Bite, leg
  - canaliculus lacrimalis — *see* Bite, eyelid
  - canthus, eye — *see* Bite, eyelid
  - centipede — *see* Toxicity, venom, arthropod, centipede
  - cheek (external) SØ1.45-
    - superficial NEC SØØ.87
      - insect SØØ.86
    - internal — *see* Bite, oral cavity
  - chest wall — *see* Bite, thorax
  - chigger B88.Ø
  - chin — *see* Bite, head, specified site NEC
  - clitoris — *see* Bite, vulva
  - costal region — *see* Bite, thorax
  - digit(s)
    - hand — *see* Bite, finger
    - toe — *see* Bite, toe
  - ear (canal) (external) SØ1.35-
    - superficial NEC SØØ.47-
      - insect SØØ.46-
  - elbow S51.Ø5-
    - superficial NEC S5Ø.37-
      - insect S5Ø.36-
  - epididymis — *see* Bite, testis
  - epigastric region — *see* Bite, abdomen
  - epiglottis — *see* Bite, neck, specified site NEC
  - esophagus, cervical S11.25
    - superficial NEC S1Ø.17
      - insect S1Ø.16
  - eyebrow — *see* Bite, eyelid
  - eyelid SØ1.15-
    - superficial NEC SØØ.27-
      - insect SØØ.26-
  - face NEC — *see* Bite, head, specified site NEC
  - finger(s) S61.259
    - with
      - damage to nail S61.359
    - index S61.258
      - with
        - damage to nail S61.358
      - left S61.251
        - with
          - damage to nail S61.351
      - right S61.25Ø
        - with
          - damage to nail S61.35Ø
      - superficial NEC S6Ø.478

- **Bite(s)** — *continued*
  - finger(s) — *continued*
    - index — *continued*
      - superficial NEC — *continued*
        - insect S6Ø.46-
    - little S61.25-
      - with
        - damage to nail S61.35-
      - superficial NEC S6Ø.47-
        - insect S6Ø.46-
    - middle S61.25-
      - with
        - damage to nail S61.35-
      - superficial NEC S6Ø.47-
        - insect S6Ø.46-
    - ring S61.25-
      - with
        - damage to nail S61.35-
      - superficial NEC S6Ø.47-
        - insect S6Ø.46-
    - superficial NEC S6Ø.479
      - insect S6Ø.469
    - thumb — *see* Bite, thumb
  - flank — *see* Bite, abdomen, wall
  - flea — *see* Bite, by site, superficial, insect
  - foot (except toe(s) alone) S91.35-
    - superficial NEC S9Ø.87-
      - insect S9Ø.86-
    - toe — *see* Bite, toe
  - forearm S51.85-
    - elbow only — *see* Bite, elbow
    - superficial NEC S5Ø.87-
      - insect S5Ø.86-
  - forehead — *see* Bite, head, specified site NEC
  - genital organs, external
    - female S31.552
      - superficial NEC S3Ø.876
        - insect S3Ø.866
      - vagina and vulva — *see* Bite, vulva
    - male S31.551
      - penis — *see* Bite, penis
      - scrotum — *see* Bite, scrotum
      - superficial NEC S3Ø.875
        - insect S3Ø.865
      - testes — *see* Bite, testis
  - groin — *see* Bite, abdomen, wall
  - gum — *see* Bite, oral cavity
  - hand S61.45-
    - finger — *see* Bite, finger
    - superficial NEC S6Ø.57-
      - insect S6Ø.56-
    - thumb — *see* Bite, thumb
  - head SØ1.95
    - cheek — *see* Bite, cheek
    - ear — *see* Bite, ear
    - eyelid — *see* Bite, eyelid
    - lip — *see* Bite, lip
    - nose — *see* Bite, nose
    - oral cavity — *see* Bite, oral cavity
    - scalp — *see* Bite, scalp
    - specified site NEC SØ1.85
      - superficial NEC SØØ.87
        - insect SØØ.86
    - superficial NEC SØØ.97
      - insect SØØ.96
    - temporomandibular area — *see* Bite, cheek
  - heel — *see* Bite, foot
  - hip S71.Ø5-
    - superficial NEC S7Ø.27-
      - insect S7Ø.26-
  - hymen S31.45
  - hypochondrium — *see* Bite, abdomen, wall
  - hypogastric region — *see* Bite, abdomen, wall
  - inguinal region — *see* Bite, abdomen, wall
  - insect — *see* Bite, by site, superficial, insect
  - instep — *see* Bite, foot
  - interscapular region — *see* Bite, thorax, back
  - jaw — *see* Bite, head, specified site NEC
  - knee S81.Ø5-
    - superficial NEC S8Ø.27-
      - insect S8Ø.26-
  - labium (majus) (minus) — *see* Bite, vulva
  - lacrimal duct — *see* Bite, eyelid

- **Bite(s)** — *continued*
  - larynx S11.Ø15
    - superficial NEC S1Ø.17
      - insect S1Ø.16
  - leg (lower) S81.85-
    - ankle — *see* Bite, ankle
    - foot — *see* Bite, foot
    - knee — *see* Bite, knee
    - superficial NEC S8Ø.87-
      - insect S8Ø.86-
    - toe — *see* Bite, toe
    - upper — *see* Bite, thigh
  - lip SØ1.551
    - superficial NEC SØØ.571
      - insect SØØ.561
  - lizard (venomous) — *see* Venom, bite, reptile
  - loin — *see* Bite, abdomen, wall
  - lower back — *see* Bite, back, lower
  - lumbar region — *see* Bite, back, lower
  - malar region — *see* Bite, head, specified site NEC
  - mammary — *see* Bite, breast
  - marine animals (venomous) — *see* Toxicity, venom, marine animal
  - mastoid region — *see* Bite, head, specified site NEC
  - mouth — *see* Bite, oral cavity
  - nail
    - finger — *see* Bite, finger
    - toe — *see* Bite, toe
  - nape — *see* Bite, neck, specified site NEC
  - nasal (septum) (sinus) — *see* Bite, nose
  - nasopharynx — *see* Bite, head, specified site NEC
  - neck S11.95
    - involving
      - cervical esophagus — *see* Bite, esophagus, cervical
      - larynx — *see* Bite, larynx
      - pharynx — *see* Bite, pharynx
      - thyroid gland S11.15
      - trachea — *see* Bite, trachea
    - specified site NEC S11.85
      - superficial NEC S1Ø.87
        - insect S1Ø.86
    - superficial NEC S1Ø.97
      - insect S1Ø.96
    - throat S11.85
      - superficial NEC S1Ø.17
        - insect S1Ø.16
  - nose (septum) (sinus) SØ1.25
    - superficial NEC SØØ.37
      - insect SØØ.36
  - occipital region — *see* Bite, scalp
  - oral cavity SØ1.552
    - superficial NEC SØØ.572
      - insect SØØ.562
  - orbital region — *see* Bite, eyelid
  - palate — *see* Bite, oral cavity
  - palm — *see* Bite, hand
  - parietal region — *see* Bite, scalp
  - pelvis S31.Ø5Ø
    - with penetration into retroperitoneal space S31.Ø51
    - superficial NEC S3Ø.87Ø
      - insect S3Ø.86Ø
  - penis S31.25
    - superficial NEC S3Ø.872
      - insect S3Ø.862
  - perineum
    - female — *see* Bite, vulva
    - male — *see* Bite, pelvis
  - periocular area (with or without lacrimal passages) — *see* Bite, eyelid
  - phalanges
    - finger — *see* Bite, finger
    - toe — *see* Bite, toe
  - pharynx S11.25
    - superficial NEC S1Ø.17
      - insect S1Ø.16
  - pinna — *see* Bite, ear
  - poisonous — *see* Venom
  - popliteal space — *see* Bite, knee
  - prepuce — *see* Bite, penis
  - pubic region — *see* Bite, abdomen, wall
  - rectovaginal septum — *see* Bite, vulva

Bite(s) — *continued*
- red bug B88.Ø
- reptile NEC (*see also* Venom, bite, reptile)
  - nonvenomous — *see* Bite, by site
  - snake — *see* Venom, bite, snake
- sacral region — *see* Bite, back, lower
- sacroiliac region — *see* Bite, back, lower
- salivary gland — *see* Bite, oral cavity
- scalp SØ1.Ø5
  - superficial NEC SØØ.Ø7
    - insect SØØ.Ø6
- scapular region — *see* Bite, shoulder
- scrotum S31.35
  - superficial NEC S3Ø.873
    - insect S3Ø.863
- sea-snake (venomous) — *see* Toxicity, venom, snake, sea snake
- shin — *see* Bite, leg
- shoulder S41.Ø5-
  - superficial NEC S4Ø.27-
    - insect S4Ø.26-
- snake (*see also* Venom, bite, snake)
  - nonvenomous — *see* Bite, by site
- spermatic cord — *see* Bite, testis
- spider (venomous) — *see* Toxicity, venom, spider
  - nonvenomous — *see* Bite, by site, superficial, insect
- sternal region — *see* Bite, thorax, front
- submaxillary region — *see* Bite, head, specified site NEC
- submental region — *see* Bite, head, specified site NEC
- subungual
  - finger(s) — *see* Bite, finger
  - toe — *see* Bite, toe
- superficial — *see* Bite, by site, superficial
- supraclavicular fossa S11.85
- supraorbital — *see* Bite, head, specified site NEC
- temple, temporal region — *see* Bite, head, specified site NEC
- temporomandibular area — *see* Bite, cheek
- testis S31.35
  - superficial NEC S3Ø.873
    - insect S3Ø.863
- thigh S71.15-
  - superficial NEC S7Ø.37-
    - insect S7Ø.36-
- thorax, thoracic (wall) S21.95
  - back S21.25-
    - with penetration into thoracic cavity S21.45-
  - breast — *see* Bite, breast
  - front S21.15-
    - with penetration into thoracic cavity S21.35-
  - superficial NEC S2Ø.97
    - back S2Ø.47-
    - front S2Ø.37-
    - insect S2Ø.96
      - back S2Ø.46-
      - front S2Ø.36-
- throat — *see* Bite, neck, throat
- thumb S61.Ø5-
  - with
    - damage to nail S61.15-
  - superficial NEC S6Ø.37-
    - insect S6Ø.36-
- thyroid S11.15
  - superficial NEC S1Ø.87
    - insect S1Ø.86
- toe(s) S91.15-
  - with
    - damage to nail S91.25-
  - great S91.15-
    - with
      - damage to nail S91.25-
  - lesser S91.15-
    - with
      - damage to nail S91.25-
  - superficial NEC S9Ø.47-
    - great S9Ø.47-
    - insect S9Ø.46-
      - great S9Ø.46-
- tongue SØ1.552
- trachea S11.Ø25

Bite(s) — *continued*
- trachea — *continued*
  - superficial NEC S1Ø.17
    - insect S1Ø.16
- tunica vaginalis — *see* Bite, testis
- tympanum, tympanic membrane — *see* Bite, ear
- umbilical region S31.155
- uvula — *see* Bite, oral cavity
- vagina — *see* Bite, vulva
- venomous — *see* Venom
- vocal cords S11.Ø35
  - superficial NEC S1Ø.17
    - insect S1Ø.16
- vulva S31.45
  - superficial NEC S3Ø.874
    - insect S3Ø.864
- wrist S61.55-
  - superficial NEC S6Ø.87-
    - insect S6Ø.86-

Biting, cheek or lip K13.1

Biventricular failure (heart) I5Ø.9

Björck (-Thorson) **syndrome** (malignant carcinoid) E34.Ø

Black
- death A2Ø.9
- eye SØØ.1-
- hairy tongue K14.3
- heel (foot) S9Ø.3-
- lung (disease) J6Ø
- palm (hand) S6Ø.22-

Blackfan-Diamond anemia or syndrome (congenital hypoplastic anemia) D61.Ø1

Blackhead L7Ø.Ø

Blackout R55

Bladder — *see* condition

Blast (air) (hydraulic) (immersion) (underwater)
- blindness SØ5.8x-
- injury
  - abdomen or thorax — *see* Injury, by site
  - ear (acoustic nerve trauma) — *see* Injury, nerve, acoustic, specified type NEC
- syndrome NEC T7Ø.8

Blastoma — *see* Neoplasm, malignant, by site
- pulmonary — *see* Neoplasm, lung, malignant

Blastomycosis, blastomycotic B4Ø.9
- Brazilian — *see* Paracoccidioidomycosis
- cutaneous B4Ø.3
- disseminated B4Ø.7
- European — *see* Cryptococcosis
- generalized B4Ø.7
- keloidal B48.Ø
- North American B4Ø.9
- primary pulmonary B4Ø.Ø
- pulmonary B4Ø.2
  - acute B4Ø.Ø
  - chronic B4Ø.1
- skin B4Ø.3
- South American — *see* Paracoccidioidomycosis
- specified NEC B4Ø.89

Bleb(s) R23.8
- emphysematous (lung) (solitary) J43.9
- endophthalmitis H59.43
- filtering (vitreous), after glaucoma surgery Z98.83
- inflammed (infected), postprocedural H59.4Ø
  - stage 1 H59.41
  - stage 2 H59.42
  - stage 3 H59.43
- lung (ruptured) J43.9
  - congenital — *see* Atelectasis
  - newborn P25.8
- subpleural (emphysematous) J43.9

Blebitis, postprocedural H59.4Ø
- stage 1 H59.41
- stage 2 H59.42
- stage 3 H59.43

Bleeder (familial) (hereditary) — *see* Hemophilia

Bleeding (*see also* Hemorrhage)
- anal K62.5
- anovulatory N97.Ø
- atonic, following delivery O72.1
- capillary I78.8
  - puerperal O72.2
- contact (postcoital) N93.Ø

Bleeding — *continued*
- due to uterine subinvolution N85.3
- ear — *see* Otorrhagia
- excessive, associated with menopausal onset N92.4
- familial — *see* Defect, coagulation
- following intercourse N93.Ø
- gastrointestinal K92.2
- hemorrhoids — *see* Hemorrhoids
- intermenstrual (regular) N92.3
  - irregular N92.1
- intraoperative — *see* Complication, intraoperative, hemorrhage
- irregular N92.6
- menopausal N92.4
- newborn, intraventricular — *see* Newborn, affected by, hemorrhage, intraventricular
- nipple N64.59
- nose RØ4.Ø
- ovulation N92.3
- postclimacteric N95.Ø
- postcoital N93.Ø
- postmenopausal N95.Ø
- postoperative — *see* Complication, postprocedural, hemorrhage
- preclimacteric N92.4
- puberty (excessive, with onset of menstrual periods) N92.2
- rectum, rectal K62.5
  - newborn P54.2
- tendencies — *see* Defect, coagulation
- throat RØ4.1
- tooth socket (post-extraction) K91.84Ø
- umbilical stump P51.9
- uterus, uterine NEC N93.9
  - climacteric N92.4
  - dysfunctional of functional N93.8
  - menopausal N92.4
  - preclimacteric or premenopausal N92.4
  - unrelated to menstrual cycle N93.9
- vagina, vaginal (abnormal) N93.9
  - dysfunctional or functional N93.8
  - newborn P54.6
- vicarious N94.89

Blennorrhagia, blennorrhagic — *see* Gonorrhea

Blennorrhea (acute) (chronic) (*see also* Gonorrhea)
- inclusion (neonatal) (newborn) P39.1
- lower genitourinary tract (gonococcal) A54.ØØ
- neonatorum (gonococcal ophthalmia) A54.31

Blepharelosis — *see* Entropion

Blepharitis (angularis) (ciliaris) (eyelid) (marginal) (nonulcerative) HØ1.ØØ9
- herpes zoster BØ2.39
- left HØ1.ØØ6
  - lower HØ1.ØØ5
  - upper HØ1.ØØ4
- right HØ1.ØØ3
  - lower HØ1.ØØ2
  - upper HØ1.ØØ1
- squamous HØ1.Ø29
  - left HØ1.Ø26
    - lower HØ1.Ø25
    - upper HØ1.Ø24
  - right HØ1.Ø23
    - lower HØ1.Ø22
    - upper HØ1.Ø21
- ulcerative HØ1.Ø19
  - left HØ1.Ø16
    - lower HØ1.Ø15
    - upper HØ1.Ø14
  - right HØ1.Ø13
    - lower HØ1.Ø12
    - upper HØ1.Ø11

Blepharochalasis HØ2.3Ø
- congenital Q1Ø.Ø
- left HØ2.36
  - lower HØ2.35
  - upper HØ2.34
- right HØ2.33
  - lower HØ2.32
  - upper HØ2.31

Blepharoclonus HØ2.59

Blepharoconjunctivitis H1Ø.5Ø-
- angular H1Ø.52-

Blepharoconjunctivitis — *continued*
  contact H10.53-
  ligneous H10.51-
Blepharophimosis (eyelid) H02.529
  congenital Q10.3
  left H02.526
    lower H02.525
    upper H02.524
  right H02.523
    lower H02.522
    upper H02.521
Blepharoptosis H02.40-
  congenital Q10.0
  mechanical H02.41-
  myogenic H02.42-
  neurogenic H02.43-
  paralytic H02.43-
Blepharopyorrhea, gonococcal A54.39
Blepharospasm G24.5
  drug induced G24.01
Blighted ovum O02.0
Blind (*see also* Blindness)
  bronchus (congenital) Q32.4
  loop syndrome K90.2
    congenital Q43.8
  sac, fallopian tube (congenital) Q50.6
  spot, enlarged — *see* Defect, visual field, localized, scotoma, blind spot area
  tract or tube, congenital NEC — *see* Atresia, by site
Blindness (acquired) (congenital) (both eyes) H54.0
  blast S05.8X-
  color — *see* Deficiency, color vision
  concussion S05.8x-
  cortical H47.619
    left brain H47.612
    right brain H47.611
  day H53.11
  due to injury (current episode) S05.9-
    sequelae — code to injury with seventh character S
  eclipse (total) — *see* Retinopathy, solar
  emotional (hysterical) F44.6
  face H53.16
  hysterical F44.6
  legal (both eyes) (USA definition) H54.8
  mind R48.8
  night H53.60
    abnormal dark adaptation curve H53.61
    acquired H53.62
    congenital H53.63
    specified type NEC H53.69
    vitamin A deficiency E50.5
  one eye (other eye normal) H54.40
    left (normal vision on right) H54.42
      low vision on right H54.12
    low vision, other eye H54.10
    right (normal vision on left) H54.41
      low vision on left H54.11
  psychic R48.8
  river B73.01
  snow — *see* Photokeratitis
  sun, solar — *see* Retinopathy, solar
  transient — *see* Disturbance, vision, subjective, loss, transient
  traumatic (current episode) S05.9-
  word (developmental) F81.0
    acquired R48.0
    secondary to organic lesion R48.0
Blister (nonthermal)
  abdominal wall S30.821
  alveolar process S00.522
  ankle S90.52-
  antecubital space — *see* Blister, elbow
  anus S30.827
  arm (upper) S40.82-
  auditory canal — *see* Blister, ear
  auricle — *see* Blister, ear
  axilla — *see* Blister, arm
  back, lower S30.820
  beetle dermatitis L24.89
  breast S20.12-
  brow S00.82
  calf — *see* Blister, leg

Blister — *continued*
  canthus — *see* Blister, eyelid
  cheek S00.82
    internal S00.522
  chest wall — *see* Blister, thorax
  chin S00.82
  costal region — *see* Blister, thorax
  digit(s)
    foot — *see* Blister, toe
    hand — *see* Blister, finger
  due to burn — *see* Burn, by site, second degree
  ear S00.42-
  elbow S50.32-
  epiglottis S10.12
  esophagus, cervical S10.12
  eyebrow — *see* Blister, eyelid
  eyelid S00.22-
  face S00.82
  fever B00.1
  finger(s) S60.429
    index S60.42-
    little S60.42-
    middle S60.42-
    ring S60.42-
  foot (except toe(s) alone) S90.82-
    toe — *see* Blister, toe
  forearm S50.82-
    elbow only — *see* Blister, elbow
  forehead S00.82
  fracture — *omit code*
  genital organ
    female S30.826
    male S30.825
  gum S00.522
  hand S60.52-
  head S00.92
    ear — *see* Blister, ear
    eyelid — *see* Blister, eyelid
    lip S00.521
    nose S00.32
    oral cavity S00.522
    scalp S00.02
    specified site NEC S00.82
  heel — *see* Blister, foot
  hip S70.22-
  interscapular region S20.429
  jaw S00.82
  knee S80.22-
  larynx S10.12
  leg (lower) S80.82-
    knee — *see* Blister, knee
    upper — *see* Blister, thigh
  lip S00.521
  malar region S00.82
  mammary — *see* Blister, breast
  mastoid region S00.82
  mouth S00.522
  multiple, skin, nontraumatic R23.8
  nail
    finger — *see* Blister, finger
    toe — *see* Blister, toe
  nasal S00.32
  neck S10.92
    specified site NEC S10.82
    throat S10.12
  nose S00.32
  occipital region S00.02
  oral cavity S00.522
  orbital region — *see* Blister, eyelid
  palate S00.522
  palm — *see* Blister, hand
  parietal region S00.02
  pelvis S30.820
  penis S30.822
  periocular area — *see* Blister, eyelid
  phalanges
    finger — *see* Blister, finger
    toe — *see* Blister, toe
  pharynx S10.12
  pinna — *see* Blister, ear
  popliteal space — *see* Blister, knee
  scalp S00.02
  scapular region — *see* Blister, shoulder

Blister — *continued*
  scrotum S30.823
  shin — *see* Blister, leg
  shoulder S40.22-
  sternal region S20.329
  submaxillary region S00.82
  submental region S00.82
  subungual
    finger(s) — *see* Blister, finger
    toe(s) — *see* Blister, toe
  supraclavicular fossa S10.82
  supraorbital S00.82
  temple S00.82
  temporal region S00.82
  testis S30.823
  thermal — *see* Burn, second degree, by site
  thigh S70.32-
  thorax, thoracic (wall) S20.92
    back S20.42-
    front S20.32-
  throat S10.12
  thumb S60.32-
  toe(s) S90.42-
    great S90.42-
  tongue S00.522
  trachea S10.12
  tympanum, tympanic membrane — *see* Blister, ear
  upper arm — *see* Blister, arm (upper)
  uvula S00.522
  vagina S30.824
  vocal cords S10.12
  vulva S30.824
  wrist S60.82-
Bloating R14.0
Bloch-Sulzberger disease or syndrome Q82.3
Block, blocked
  alveolocapillary J84.10
  arborization (heart) I45.5
  arrhythmic I45.9
  atrioventricular (incomplete) (partial) I44.30
    with atrioventricular dissociation I44.2
    complete I44.2
      congenital Q24.6
    congenital Q24.6
    first degree I44.0
    second degree (types I and II) I44.1
    specified NEC I44.39
    third degree I44.2
    types I and II I44.1
  auriculoventricular - see Block, atrioventricular
  bifascicular (cardiac) I45.2
  bundle-branch (complete) (false) (incomplete) I45.4
    bilateral I45.2
    left I44.7
      with right bundle branch block I45.2
      hemiblock I44.60
        anterior I44.4
        posterior I44.5
      incomplete I44.7
        with right bundle branch block I45.2
    right I45.10
      with
        left bundle branch block I45.2
        left fascicular block I45.2
      specified NEC I45.19
    Wilson's type I45.19
  cardiac I45.9
  conduction I45.9
    complete I44.2
  fascicular (left) I44.60
    anterior I44.4
    posterior I44.5
    right I45.0
    specified NEC I44.69
  foramen Magendie (acquired) G91.1
    congenital Q03.1
      with spina bifida - see Spina bifida, by site, with hydrocephalus
  heart I45.9
    bundle branch I45.4
      bilateral I45.2
    complete (atrioventricular) I44.2
    congenital Q24.6

Block, blocked — *continued*
- heart — *continued*
  - first degree (atrioventricular) I44.Ø
  - second degree (atrioventricular) I44.1
  - specified type NEC I45.5
  - third degree (atrioventricular) I44.2
- hepatic vein I82.Ø
- intraventricular (nonspecific) I45.4
  - bundle branch
    - bilateral I45.2
- kidney N28.9
  - postcystoscopic or postprocedural N99.Ø
- Mobitz (types I and II) I44.1
- myocardial — *see* Block, heart
- nodal I45.5
- organ or site, congenital NEC — *see* Atresia, by site
- portal (vein) I81
- second degree (types I and II) I44.1
- sinoatrial I45.5
- sinoauricular I45.5
- third degree I44.2
- trifascicular I45.3
- tubal N97.1
- vein NOS I82.9Ø
- Wenckebach (types I and II) I44.1

Blockage — *see* Obstruction

Blocq's disease F44.4

Blood
- constituents, abnormal R78.9
- disease D75.9
- donor — *see* Donor, blood
- dyscrasia D75.9
  - with
    - abortion — *see* Abortion, by type, complicated by, hemorrhage
    - ectopic pregnancy OØ8.1
    - molar pregnancy OØ8.1
  - following ectopic or molar pregnancy OØ8.1
  - newborn P61.9
  - puerperal, postpartum O72.3
- flukes NEC — *see* Schistosomiasis
- in
  - feces K92.1
    - occult R19.5
  - urine — *see* Hematuria
- mole OØ2.Ø
- occult in feces R19.5
- pressure
  - decreased, due to shock following injury T79.4
  - examination only ZØ1.3Ø
  - fluctuating I99.8
  - high — *see* Hypertension
    - borderline RØ3.Ø
    - incidental reading, without diagnosis of hypertension RØ3.Ø
  - low (*see also* Hypotension)
    - incidental reading, without diagnosis of hypotension RØ3.1
- spitting — *see* Hemoptysis
- staining cornea — *see* Pigmentation, cornea, stromal
- transfusion
  - reaction or complication — *see* Complications, transfusion
- type
  - A (Rh positive) Z67.1Ø
    - Rh negative Z67.11
  - AB (Rh positive) Z67.3Ø
    - Rh negative Z67.31
  - B (Rh positive) Z67.2Ø
    - Rh negative Z67.21
  - O (Rh positive) Z67.4Ø
    - Rh negative Z67.41
  - Rh (positive) Z67.9Ø
    - negative Z67.91
- vessel rupture — *see* Hemorrhage
- vomiting — *see* Hematemesis

Blood-forming organs, disease D75.9

Bloodgood's disease — *see* Mastopathy, cystic

Bloom (-Machacek)(-Torre) **syndrome** Q82.8

Blount's disease or osteochondrosis — *see* Osteochondrosis, juvenile, tibia

Blue
- baby Q24.9
- diaper syndrome E72.Ø9
- dome cyst (breast) — *see* Cyst, breast
- dot cataract Q12.Ø
- nevus D22.9
- sclera Q13.5
  - with fragility of bone and deafness Q78.Ø
- toe syndrome I75.Ø2-

Blueness — *see* Cyanosis

Blues, postpartal O9Ø.6
- baby O9Ø.6

Blurring, visual H53.8

Blushing (abnormal) (excessive) R23.2

BMI — *see* Body, mass index

Boarder, hospital NEC Z76.4
- accompanying sick person Z76.3
- healthy infant or child Z76.2
  - foundling Z76.1

Bockhart's impetigo LØ1.Ø2

Bodechtel-Guttman disease (subacute sclerosing panencephalitis) A81.1

Boder-Sedgwick syndrome (ataxia-telangiectasia) G11.3

Body, bodies
- Aschoff's — *see* Myocarditis, rheumatic
- asteroid, vitreous — *see* Deposit, crystalline
- cytoid (retina) — *see* Occlusion, artery, retina
- drusen (degenerative) (macula) (retinal) (*see also* Degeneration, macula, drusen)
  - optic disc — *see* Drusen, optic disc
- foreign — *see* Foreign body
- loose
  - joint, except knee — *see* Loose, body, joint
    - knee M23.4-
  - sheath, tendon — *see* Disorder, tendon, specified type NEC
- mass index (BMI)
  - adult
    - 19 or less Z68.1
    - 2Ø.Ø-2Ø.9 Z68.2Ø
    - 21.Ø-21.9 Z68.21
    - 22.Ø-22.9 Z68.22
    - 23.Ø-23.9 Z68.23
    - 24.Ø-24.9 Z68.24
    - 25.Ø-25.9 Z68.25
    - 26.Ø-26.9 Z68.26
    - 27.Ø-27.9 Z68.27
    - 28.Ø-28.9 Z68.28
    - 29.Ø-29.9 Z68.29
    - 3Ø.Ø-3Ø.9 Z68.3Ø
    - 31.Ø-31.9 Z68.31
    - 32.Ø-32.9 Z68.32
    - 33.Ø-33.9 Z68.33
    - 34.Ø-34.9 Z68.34
    - 35.Ø-35.9 Z68.35
    - 36.Ø-36.9 Z68.36
    - 37.Ø-37.9 Z68.37
    - 38.Ø-38.9 Z68.38
    - 39.Ø-39.9 Z68.39
    - 4Ø.Ø-44.9 Z68.41
    - 45.Ø-49.9 Z68.42
    - 5Ø.Ø-59.9 Z68.43
    - 6Ø.Ø-69.9 Z68.44
    - 7Ø and over Z68.45
  - pediatric
    - 5th percentile to less than 85th percentile for age Z68.52
    - 85th percentile to less than 95th percentile for age Z68.53
    - greater than or equal to ninety-fifth percentile for age Z68.54
    - less than fifth percentile for age Z68.51
- Mooser's A75.2
- rice (*see also* Loose, body, joint)
  - knee M23.4-
- rocking F98.4

Boeck's
- disease or sarcoid — *see* Sarcoidosis
- lupoid (miliary) D86.3

Boerhaave's syndrome (spontaneous esophageal rupture) K22.3

Boggy
- cervix N88.8
- uterus N85.8

Boil (*see also* Furuncle, by site)
- Aleppo B55.1
- Baghdad B55.1
- Delhi B55.1
- lacrimal
  - gland — *see* Dacryoadenitis
  - passages (duct) (sac) — *see* Inflammation, lacrimal, passages, acute
- Natal B55.1
- orbit, orbital — *see* Abscess, orbit
- tropical B55.1

Bold hives — *see* Urticaria

Bombé, iris — *see* Membrane, pupillary

Bone — *see* condition

Bonnevie-Ullrich syndrome Q87.1

Bonnier's syndrome — *see* subcategory H81.8

Bonvale dam fever T73.3

Bony block of joint — *see* Ankylosis

BOOP (bronchiolitis obliterans organized pneumonia) J84.89

Borderline
- diabetes mellitus R73.Ø9
- hypertension RØ3.Ø
- osteopenia M85.8-
- pelvis, with obstruction during labor O65.1
- personality F6Ø.3

Borna disease A83.9

Bornholm disease B33.Ø

Boston exanthem A88.0

Botalli, ductus (patent) (persistent) Q25.Ø

Bothriocephalus latus infestation B7Ø.Ø

Botulism (foodborne intoxication) AØ5.1
- infant A48.51
- non-foodborne A48.52
- wound A48.52

Bouba — *see* Yaws

Bouchard's nodes (with arthropathy) M15.2

Bouffée délirante F23

Bouillaud's disease or syndrome (rheumatic heart disease) IØ1.9

Bourneville's disease Q85.1

Boutonniere deformity (finger) — *see* Deformity, finger, boutonniere

Bouveret (-Hoffmann) **syndrome** (paroxysmal tachycardia) I47.9

Bovine heart — *see* Hypertrophy, cardiac

Bowel — *see* condition

Bowen's
- dermatosis (precancerous) — *see* Neoplasm, skin, in situ
- disease — *see* Neoplasm, skin, in situ
- epithelioma — *see* Neoplasm, skin, in situ
- type
  - epidermoid carcinoma-in-situ — *see* Neoplasm, skin, in situ
  - intraepidermal squamous cell carcinoma — *see* Neoplasm, skin, in situ

Bowing
- femur (*see also* Deformity, limb, specified type NEC, thigh)
  - congenital Q68.3
- fibula (*see also* Deformity, limb, specified type NEC, lower leg)
  - congenital Q68.4
- forearm — *see* Deformity, limb, specified type NEC, forearm
- leg(s), long bones, congenital Q68.5
- radius — *see* Deformity, limb, specified type NEC, forearm
- tibia (*see also* Deformity, limb, specified type NEC, lower leg)
  - congenital Q68.4

Bowleg(s) (acquired) M21.16-
- congenital Q68.5
- rachitic E64.3

Boyd's dysentery AØ3.2

Brachial — *see* condition

Brachycardia RØØ.1

Brachycephaly Q75.Ø

Bradley's disease AØ8.19

Bradyarrhythmia, cardiac I49.8
Bradycardia (sinoatrial) (sinus) (vagal) RØØ.1
neonatal P29.12
reflex G9Ø.Ø9
tachycardia syndrome I49.5
Bradykinesia R25.8
Bradypnea RØ6.89
Bradytachycardia I49.5
Brailsford's disease or osteochondrosis — *see* Osteochondrosis, juvenile, radius
Brain (*see also* condition)
death G93.82
syndrome — *see* Syndrome, brain
Branched-chain amino-acid disorder E71.2
Branchial — *see* condition
cartilage, congenital Q18.2
Branchiogenic remnant (in neck) Q18.Ø
Brandt's syndrome (acrodermatitis enteropathica) E83.2
Brash (water) R12
Bravais-jacksonian epilepsy — *see* Epilepsy, localization-related, symptomatic, with simple partial seizures
Braxton Hicks contractions — *see* False, labor
Brazilian leishmaniasis B55.2
Break, retina (without detachment) H33.3Ø-
with retinal detachment — *see* Detachment, retina
horseshoe tear H33.31-
multiple H33.33-
round hole H33.32-
Breakage, prosthetic join — *see* Complications, joint prosthesis, mechanical, by site
Breakdown
device, graft or implant (*see also* Complications, by site and type, mechanical) T85.618
arterial graft NEC — *see* Complication, cardiovascular device, mechanical, vascular
breast (implant) T85.41
catheter NEC T85.618
cystostomy T83.Ø1Ø
dialysis (renal) T82.41
intraperitoneal T85.611
infusion NEC T82.514
spinal (epidural) (subdural) T85.61Ø
urinary (indwelling) T83.Ø18
electronic (electrode) (pulse generator) (stimulator)
bone T84.31Ø
cardiac T82.119
electrode T82.11Ø
pulse generator T82.111
specified type NEC T82.118
nervous system — *see* Complication, prosthetic device, mechanical, electronic nervous system stimulator
urinary — *see* Complication, genitourinary, device, urinary, mechanical
fixation, internal (orthopedic) NEC — *see* Complication, fixation device, mechanical
gastrointestinal — *see* Complications, prosthetic device, mechanical, gastrointestinal device
genital NEC T83.418
intrauterine contraceptive device T83.31
penile prosthesis T83.41Ø
heart NEC — *see* Complication, cardiovascular device, mechanical
joint prosthesis — *see* Complications, joint prosthesis,internal, mechanical, by site
ocular NEC — *see* Complications, prosthetic device, mechanical, ocular device
orthopedic NEC — *see* Complication, orthopedic, device, mechanical
specified NEC T85.618
sutures, permanent T85.612
used in bone repair — *see* Complications, fixation device, internal (orthopedic), mechanical
urinary NEC (*see also* Complication, genitourinary, device, urinary, mechanical)
graft T83.21
vascular NEC — *see* Complication, cardiovascular device, mechanical
ventricular intracranial shunt T85.Ø1

Breakdown — *continued*
nervous F48.8
perineum O9Ø.1
respirator J95.85Ø
specified NEC J95.859
ventilator J95.85Ø
specified NEC J95.859
Breast (*see also* condition)
buds E3Ø.1
in newborn P96.89
dense R92.2
nodule N63
Breath
foul R19.6
holder, child RØ6.89
holding spell RØ6.89
shortness RØ6.Ø2
Breathing
labored — *see* Hyperventilation
mouth RØ6.5
causing malocclusion M26.5
periodic RØ6.3
high altitude G47.32
Breathlessness RØ6.81
Breda's disease — *see* Yaws
Breech presentation (mother) O32.1
causing obstructed labor O64.1
footling O32.8
causing obstructed labor O64.8
incomplete O32.8
causing obstructed labor O64.8
Breisky's disease N9Ø.4
Brennemann's syndrome I88.Ø
Brenner
tumor (benign) D27.9
borderline malignancy D39.1-
malignant C56
proliferating D39.1-
Bretonneau's disease or angina A36.Ø
Breus' mole OØ2.Ø
Brevicollis Q76.49
Brickmakers' anemia B76.9
Bridge, myocardial Q24.5
BRBPR K62.5
Bright red blood per rectum (BRBPR) K62.5
Bright's disease (*see also* Nephritis)
arteriosclerotic — *see* Hypertension, kidney
Brill(-Zinsser) **disease** (recrudescent typhus) A75.1
flea-borne A75.2
louse-borne A75.1
Brill-Symmers' disease C82.9Ø
Brion-Kayser disease — *see* Fever, parathyroid
Briquet's disorder or syndrome F45.Ø
Brissaud's
infantilism or dwarfism E23.Ø
motor-verbal tic F95.2
Brittle
bones disease Q78.Ø
nails L6Ø.3
congenital Q84.6
Broad (*see also* condition)
beta disease E78.2
ligament laceration syndrome N83.8
Broador floating-betalipoproteinemia E78.2
Brock's syndrome (atelectasis due to enlarged lymph nodes) J98.19
Brocq-Duhring disease (dermatitis herpetiformis) L13.Ø
Brodie's abscess or disease M86.8x-
Broken
arches (*see also* Deformity, limb, flat foot)
arm (meaning upper limb) — *see* Fracture, arm
back — *see* Fracture, vertebra
bone — *see* Fracture
implant or internal device — *see* Complications, by site and type, mechanical
leg (meaning lower limb) — *see* Fracture, leg
nose SØ2.2
tooth, teeth — *see* Fracture, tooth
Bromhidrosis, bromidrosis L75.Ø

Bromidism, bromism G92
due to
correct substance properly administered — *see* Table of Drugs and Chemicals, by drug, adverse effect
overdose or wrong substance given or taken — *see* Table of Drugs and Chemicals, by drug, poisoning
chronic (dependence) F13.2Ø
Bromidrosiphobia F4Ø.298
Bronchi, bronchial — *see* condition
Bronchiectasis (cylindrical) (diffuse) (fusiform) (localized) (saccular) J47.9
with
acute
bronchitis J47.Ø
lower respiratory infection J47.Ø
exacerbation (acute) J47.1
congenital Q33.4
tuberculous NEC — *see* Tuberculosis, pulmonary
Bronchiolectasis — *see* Bronchiectasis
Bronchiolitis (acute) (infective) (subacute) J21.9
with
bronchospasm or obstruction J21.9
influenza, flu or grippe — *see* Influenza, with, respiratory manifestations NEC
chemical (chronic) J68.4
acute J68.Ø
chronic (fibrosing) (obliterative) J44.9
due to
external agent — *see* Bronchitis, acute, due to
human metapneumovirus J21.1
respiratory syncytial virus J21.Ø
specified organism NEC J21.8
fibrosa obliterans J44.9
influenzal — *see* Influenza, with, respiratory manifestations NEC
obliterans J42
with organizing pneumonia (BOOP) J84.89
obliterative (chronic) (subacute) J44.9
due to fumes or vapors J68.4
due to chemicals, gases, fumes or vapors (inhalation) J68.4
respiratory, interstitial lung disease J84.115
Bronchitis (diffuse) (fibrinous) (hypostatic) (infective) (membranous) J4Ø
with
influenza, flu or grippe — *see* Influenza, with, respiratory manifestations NEC
obstruction (airway) (lung) J44.9
tracheitis (l5 years of age and above) J4Ø
acute or subacute J2Ø.9
chronic J42
under l5 years of age J2Ø.9
acute or subacute (with bronchospasm or obstruction) J2Ø.9
with
bronchiectasis J47.Ø
chronic obstructive pulmonary disease J44.Ø
chemical (due to gases, fumes or vapors) J68.Ø
due to
fumes or vapors J68.Ø
Haemophilus influenzae J2Ø.1
Mycoplasma pneumoniae J2Ø.Ø
radiation J7Ø.Ø
specified organism NEC J2Ø.8
Streptococcus J2Ø.2
virus
coxsackie J2Ø.3
echovirus J2Ø.7
parainfluenzae J2Ø.4
respiratory syncytial J2Ø.5
rhinovirus J2Ø.6
viral NEC J2Ø.8
allergic (acute) J45.9Ø9
with
exacerbation (acute) J45.9Ø1
status asthmaticus J45.9Ø2
arachidic T17.528
aspiration (due to fumes or vapors) J68.Ø
asthmatic J45.9
chronic J44.9

- **Bronchitis** — *continued*
  - asthmatic — *continued*
    - chronic — *continued*
      - with
        - acute lower respiratory infection J44.Ø
        - exacerbation (acute) J44.1
  - capillary — *see* Pneumonia, broncho
  - caseous (tuberculous) A15.5
  - Castellani's A69.8
  - catarrhal (l5 years of age and above) J4Ø
    - acute — *see* Bronchitis, acute
    - chronic J41.Ø
    - under l5 years of age J2Ø.9
  - chemical (acute) (subacute) J68.Ø
    - chronic J68.4
    - due to fumes or vapors J68.Ø
      - chronic J68.4
  - chronic J42
    - with
      - airways obstruction J44.9
      - tracheitis (chronic) J42
    - asthmatic (obstructive) J44.9
    - catarrhal J41.Ø
    - chemical (due to fumes or vapors) J68.4
    - due to
      - chemicals, gases, fumes or vapors (inhalation) J68.4
      - radiation J7Ø.1
      - tobacco smoking J41.Ø
    - emphysematous J44.9
    - mucopurulent J41.1
    - non-obstructive J41.Ø
    - obliterans J44.9
    - obstructive J44.9
    - purulent J41.1
    - simple J41.Ø
  - croupous — *see* Bronchitis, acute
  - due to gases, fumes or vapors (chemical) J68.Ø
  - emphysematous (obstructive) J44.9
  - exudative — *see* Bronchitis, acute
  - fetid J41.1
  - grippal — *see* Influenza, with, respiratory manifestations NEC
  - in those under l5 years age — *see* Bronchitis, acute
    - chronic — *see* Bronchitis, chronic
  - influenzal — *see* Influenza, with, respiratory manifestations NEC
  - mixed simple and mucopurulent J41.8
  - moulder's J62.8
  - mucopurulent (chronic) (recurrent) J41.1
    - acute or subacute J2Ø.9
    - simple (mixed) J41.8
  - obliterans (chronic) J44.9
  - obstructive (chronic) (diffuse) J44.9
  - pituitous J41.1
  - pneumococcal, acute or subacute J2Ø.2
  - pseudomembranous, acute or subacute — *see* Bronchitis, acute
  - purulent (chronic) (recurrent) J41.1
    - acute or subacute — *see* Bronchitis, acute
  - putrid J41.1
  - senile (chronic) J42
  - simple and mucopurulent (mixed) J41.8
  - smokers' J41.Ø
  - spirochetal NEC A69.8
  - subacute — *see* Bronchitis, acute
  - suppurative (chronic) J41.1
    - acute or subacute — *see* Bronchitis, acute
  - tuberculous A15.5
  - under l5 years of age — *see* Bronchitis, acute
    - chronic — *see* Bronchitis, chronic
  - viral NEC, acute or subacute (*see also* Bronchitis, acute) J2Ø.8
- **Bronchoalveolitis** J18.Ø
- **Bronchoaspergillosis** B44.1
- **Bronchocele meaning goiter** EØ4.Ø
- **Broncholithiasis** J98.Ø9
  - tuberculous NEC A15.5
- **Bronchomalacia** J98.Ø9
  - congenital Q32.2
- **Bronchomycosis NOS** B49 *[J99]*
  - candidal B37.1
- **Bronchopleuropneumonia** — *see* Pneumonia, broncho
- **Bronchopneumonia** — *see* Pneumonia, broncho
- **Bronchopneumonitis** — *see* Pneumonia, broncho
- **Bronchopulmonary** — *see* condition
- **Bronchopulmonitis** — *see* Pneumonia, broncho
- **Bronchorrhagia** (see Hemoptysis)
- **Bronchorrhea** J98.Ø9
  - acute J2Ø.9
  - chronic (infective) (purulent) J42
- **Bronchospasm** (acute) J98.Ø1
  - with
    - bronchiolitis, acute J21.9
    - bronchitis, acute (conditions in J2Ø) — *see* Bronchitis, acute
  - due to external agent — *see* condition, respiratory, acute, due to
  - exercise induced J45.99Ø
- **Bronchospirochetosis** A69.8
  - Castellani A69.8
- **Bronchostenosis** J98.Ø9
- **Bronchus** — *see* condition
- **Brontophobia** F4Ø.22Ø
- **Bronze baby syndrome** P83.8
- **Brooke's tumor** — *see* Neoplasm, skin, benign
- **Brown enamel of teeth** (hereditary) KØØ.5
- **Brown's sheath syndrome** H5Ø.61-
- **Brown-Séquard disease, paralysis or syndrome** G83.81
- **Bruce sepsis** A23.Ø
- **Brucellosis** (infection) A23.9
  - abortus A23.1
  - canis A23.3
  - dermatitis A23.9
  - melitensis A23.Ø
  - mixed A23.8
  - sepsis A23.9
    - melitensis A23.Ø
    - specified NEC A23.8
  - suis A23.2
- **Bruck-de Lange disease** Q87.1
- **Bruck's disease** — *see* Deformity, limb
- **Brugsch's syndrome** Q82.8
- **Bruise** (skin surface intact) (*see also* Contusion)
  - with
    - open wound — *see* Wound, open
  - internal organ — *see* Injury, by site
  - newborn P54.5
  - scalp, due to birth injury, newborn P12.3
  - umbilical cord O69.5
- **Bruit** (arterial) RØ9.89
  - cardiac RØ1.1
- **Brush burn** — *see* Abrasion, by site
- **Bruton's X-linked agammaglobulinemia** D8Ø.Ø
- **Bruxism**
  - psychogenic F45.8
  - sleep related G47.63
- **Bubbly lung syndrome** P27.Ø
- **Bubo** I88.8
  - blennorrhagic (gonococcal) A54.89
  - chancroidal A57
  - climatic A55
  - due to Haemophilus ducreyi A57
  - gonococcal A54.89
  - indolent (nonspecific) I88.8
  - inguinal (nonspecific) I88.8
    - chancroidal A57
    - climatic A55
    - due to H. ducreyi A57
    - infective I88.8
  - scrofulous (tuberculous) A18.2
  - soft chancre A57
  - suppurating — *see* Lymphadenitis, acute
  - syphilitic (primary) A51.Ø
    - congenital A5Ø.Ø7
  - tropical A55
  - virulent (chancroidal) A57
- **Bubonic plague** A2Ø.Ø
- **Bubonocele** — *see* Hernia, inguinal
- **Buccal** — *see* condition
- **Buchanan's disease or osteochondrosis** M91.Ø
- **Buchem's syndrome** (hyperostosis corticalis) M85.2
- **Bucket-handle fracture or tear** (semilunar cartilage) — *see* Tear, meniscus
- **Budd-Chiari syndrome** (hepatic vein thrombosis) I82.Ø
- **Budgerigar fancier's disease or lung** J67.2
- **Buds**
  - breast E3Ø.1
    - in newborn P96.89
- **Buerger's disease** (thromboangiitis obliterans) I73.1
- **Bulbar** — *see* condition
- **Bulbus cordis** (left ventricle) (persistent) Q21.8
- **Bulimia** (nervosa) F5Ø.2
  - atypical F5Ø.9
  - normal weight F5Ø.9
- **Bulky**
  - stools R19.5
  - uterus N85.2
- **Bulla(e)** R23.8
  - lung (emphysematous) (solitary) J43.9
    - newborn P25.8
- **Bullet wound** (*see also* Wound, open)
  - fracture—code as Fracture, by site
  - internal organ — *see* Injury, by site
- **Bundle**
  - branch block (complete) (false) (incomplete) — *see* Block, bundle-branch
  - of His — *see* condition
- **Bunion** — *see* Deformity, toe, hallux valgus
- **Buphthalmia, buphthalmos** (congenital) Q15.Ø
- **Burdwan fever** B55.Ø
- **Bürger-Grütz disease or syndrome** E78.3
- **Buried**
  - penis (congenital) Q55.64
    - acquired N48.83
  - roots KØ8.3
- **Burke's syndrome** K86.8
- **Burkitt**
  - cell leukemia C91.Ø-
  - lymphoma (malignant) C83.7-
    - small noncleaved, diffuse C83.7-
    - spleen C83.77
    - undifferentiated C83.7-
  - tumor C83.7-
  - type
    - acute lymphoblastic leukemia C91.Ø-
    - undifferentiated C83.7-
- **Burn** (electricity) (flame) (hot gas, liquid or hot object) (radiation) (steam) (thermal) T3Ø.Ø
  - abdomen, abdominal (muscle) (wall) T21.Ø2
    - first degree T21.12
    - second degree T21.22
    - third degree T21.32
  - above elbow T22.Ø39
    - first degree T22.139
    - left T22.Ø32
      - first degree T22.132
      - second degree T22.232
      - third degree T22.332
    - right T22.Ø31
      - first degree T22.131
      - second degree T22.231
      - third degree T22.331
    - second degree T22.239
    - third degree T22.339
  - acid (caustic) (external) (internal) — *see* Corrosion, by site
  - alimentary tract NEC T28.2
    - esophagus T28.1
    - mouth T28.Ø
    - pharynx T28.Ø
  - alkaline (caustic) (external) (internal) — *see* Corrosion, by site
  - ankle T25.Ø19
    - first degree T25.119
    - left T25.Ø12
      - first degree T25.112
      - second degree T25.212
      - third degree T25.312
    - multiple with foot — *see* Burn, lower, limb, multiple, ankle and foot
    - right T25.Ø11
      - first degree T25.111
      - second degree T25.211

- **Burn** — *continued*
  - ankle — *continued*
    - right — *continued*
      - third degree T25.311
    - second degree T25.219
    - third degree T25.319
  - anus — *see* Burn, buttock
  - arm (lower) (upper) — *see* Burn, upper, limb
  - axilla T22.049
    - first degree T22.149
    - left T22.042
      - first degree T22.142
      - second degree T22.242
      - third degree T22.342
    - right T22.041
      - first degree T22.141
      - second degree T22.241
      - third degree T22.341
    - second degree T22.249
    - third degree T22.349
  - back (lower) T21.04
    - first degree T21.14
    - second degree T21.24
    - third degree T21.34
    - upper T21.03
      - first degree T21.13
      - second degree T21.23
      - third degree T21.33
  - blisters—code as Burn, second degree, by site
  - breast(s) — *see* Burn, chest wall
  - buttock(s) T21.05
    - first degree T21.15
    - second degree T21.25
    - third degree T21.35
  - calf T24.039
    - first degree T24.139
    - left T24.032
      - first degree T24.132
      - second degree T24.232
      - third degree T24.332
    - right T24.031
      - first degree T24.131
      - second degree T24.231
      - third degree T24.331
    - second degree T24.239
    - third degree T24.339
  - canthus (eye) — *see* Burn, eyelid
  - caustic acid or alkaline — *see* Corrosion, by site
  - cervix T28.3
  - cheek T20.06
    - first degree T20.16
    - second degree T20.26
    - third degree T20.36
  - chemical (acids) (alkalines) (caustics) (external) (internal) — *see* Corrosion, by site
  - chest wall T21.01
    - first degree T21.11
    - second degree T21.21
    - third degree T21.31
  - chin T20.03
    - first degree T20.13
    - second degree T20.23
    - third degree T20.33
  - colon T28.2
  - conjunctiva (and cornea) — *see* Burn, cornea
  - cornea (and conjunctiva) T26.1-
    - chemical — *see* Corrosion, cornea
  - corrosion (external) (internal) — *see* Corrosion, by site
  - deep necrosis of underlying tissue — code as Burn, third degree, by site
  - dorsum of hand T23.069
    - first degree T23.169
    - left T23.062
      - first degree T23.162
      - second degree T23.262
      - third degree T23.362
    - right T23.061
      - first degree T23.161
      - second degree T23.261
      - third degree T23.361
    - second degree T23.269
    - third degree T23.369

- **Burn** — *continued*
  - due to ingested chemical agent — *see* Corrosion, by site
  - ear (auricle) (external) (canal) T20.01
    - first degree T20.11
    - second degree T20.21
    - third degree T20.31
  - elbow T22.029
    - first degree T22.129
    - left T22.022
      - first degree T22.122
      - second degree T22.222
      - third degree T22.322
    - right T22.021
      - first degree T22.121
      - second degree T22.221
      - third degree T22.321
    - second degree T22.229
    - third degree T22.329
  - epidermal loss—code as Burn, second degree, by site
  - erythema, erythematous—code as Burn, first degree, by site
  - esophagus T28.1
  - extent (percentage of body surface)
    - less than 10 percent T31.0
    - 10-19 percent T31.10
      - with 0-9 percent third degree burns T31.10
      - with 10-19 percent third degree burns T31.11
    - 20-29 percent T31.20
      - with 0-9 percent third degree burns T31.20
      - with 10-19 percent third degree burns T31.21
      - with 20-29 percent third degree burns T31.22
    - 30-39 percent T31.30
      - with 0-9 percent third degree burns T31.30
      - with 10-19 percent third degree burns T31.31
      - with 20-29 percent third degree burns T31.32
      - with 30-39 percent third degree burns T31.33
    - 40-49 percent T31.40
      - with 0-9 percent third degree burns T31.40
      - with 10-19 percent third degree burns T31.41
      - with 20-29 percent third degree burns T31.42
      - with 30-39 percent third degree burns T31.43
      - with 40-49 percent third degree burns T31.44
    - 50-59 percent T31.50
      - with 0-9 percent third degree burns T31.50
      - with 10-19 percent third degree burns T31.51
      - with 20-29 percent third degree burns T31.52
      - with 30-39 percent third degree burns T31.53
      - with 40-49 percent third degree burns T31.54
      - with 50-59 percent third degree burns T31.55
    - 60-69 percent T31.60
      - with 0-9 percent third degree burns T31.60
      - with 10-19 percent third degree burns T31.61
      - with 20-29 percent third degree burns T31.62
      - with 30-39 percent third degree burns T31.63
      - with 40-49 percent third degree burns T31.64
      - with 50-59 percent third degree burns T31.65
      - with 60-69 percent third degree burns T31.66
    - 70-79 percent T31.70
      - with 0-9 percent third degree burns T31.70
      - with 10-19 percent third degree burns T31.71
      - with 20-29 percent third degree burns T31.72
      - with 30-39 percent third degree burns T31.73
      - with 40-49 percent third degree burns T31.74
      - with 50-59 percent third degree burns T31.75
      - with 60-69 percent third degree burns T31.76
      - with 70-79 percent third degree burns T31.77
    - 80-89 percent T31.80
      - with 0-9 percent third degree burns T31.80
      - with 10-19 percent third degree burns T31.81
      - with 20-29 percent third degree burns T31.82
      - with 30-39 percent third degree burns T31.83
      - with 40-49 percent third degree burns T31.84
      - with 50-59 percent third degree burns T31.85
      - with 60-69 percent third degree burns T31.86
      - with 70-79 percent third degree burns T31.87
      - with 80-89 percent third degree burns T31.88
    - 90 percent or more T31.90
      - with 0-9 percent third degree burns T31.90
      - with 10-19 percent third degree burns T31.91
      - with 20-29 percent third degree burns T31.92
      - with 30-39 percent third degree burns T31.93

- **Burn** — *continued*
  - extent (percentage of body surface) — *continued*
    - 90 percent or more — *continued*
      - with 40-49 percent third degree burns T31.94
      - with 50-59 percent third degree burns T31.95
      - with 60-69 percent third degree burns T31.96
      - with 70-79 percent third degree burns T31.97
      - with 80-89 percent third degree burns T31.98
      - with 90 percent or more third degree burns T31.99
  - extremity — *see* Burn, limb
  - eye(s) and adnexa T26.4-
    - with resulting rupture and destruction of eyeball T26.2-
    - conjunctival sac — *see* Burn, cornea
    - cornea — *see* Burn, cornea
    - lid — *see* Burn, eyelid
    - periocular area — *see* Burn eyelid
    - specified site NEC T26.3-
  - eyeball — *see* Burn, eye
  - eyelid(s) T26.0-
    - chemical — *see* Corrosion, eyelid
  - face — *see* Burn, head
  - finger T23.029
    - first degree T23.129
    - left T23.022
      - first degree T23.122
      - second degree T23.222
      - third degree T23.322
    - multiple sites (without thumb) T23.039
      - with thumb T23.049
        - first degree T23.149
        - left T23.042
          - first degree T23.142
          - second degree T23.242
          - third degree T23.342
        - right T23.041
          - first degree T23.141
          - second degree T23.241
          - third degree T23.341
        - second degree T23.249
        - third degree T23.349
      - first degree T23.139
      - left T23.032
        - first degree T23.132
        - second degree T23.232
        - third degree T23.332
      - right T23.031
        - first degree T23.131
        - second degree T23.231
        - third degree T23.331
      - second degree T23.239
      - third degree T23.339
    - right T23.021
      - first degree T23.121
      - second degree T23.221
      - third degree T23.321
    - second degree T23.229
    - third degree T23.329
  - flank — *see* Burn, abdominal wall
  - foot T25.029
    - first degree T25.129
    - left T25.022
      - first degree T25.122
      - second degree T25.222
      - third degree T25.322
    - multiple with ankle — *see* Burn, lower, limb, multiple, ankle and foot
    - right T25.021
      - first degree T25.121
      - second degree T25.221
      - third degree T25.321
    - second degree T25.229
    - third degree T25.329
  - forearm T22.019
    - first degree T22.119
    - left T22.012
      - first degree T22.112
      - second degree T22.212
      - third degree T22.312
    - right T22.011
      - first degree T22.111
      - second degree T22.211

- **Burn** — *continued*
  - forearm — *continued*
    - right — *continued*
      - third degree T22.311
    - second degree T22.219
    - third degree T22.319
  - forehead T2Ø.Ø6
    - first degree T2Ø.16
    - second degree T2Ø.26
    - third degree T2Ø.36
  - fourth degree—code as Burn, third degree, by site
  - friction — *see* Burn, by site
  - from swallowing caustic or corrosive substance NEC — *see* Corrosion, by site
  - full thickness skin loss—code as Burn, third degree, by site
  - gastrointestinal tract NEC T28.2
    - from swallowing caustic or corrosive substance T28.7
  - genital organs
    - external
      - female T21.Ø7
        - first degree T21.17
        - second degree T21.27
        - third degree T21.37
      - male T21.Ø6
        - first degree T21.16
        - second degree T21.26
        - third degree T21.36
    - internal T28.3
      - from caustic or corrosive substance T28.8
  - groin — *see* Burn, abdominal wall
  - hand(s) T23.ØØ9
    - back — *see* Burn, dorsum of hand
    - finger — *see* Burn, finger
    - first degree T23.1Ø9
    - left T23.ØØ2
      - first degree T23.1Ø2
      - second degree T23.2Ø2
      - third degree T23.3Ø2
    - multiple sites with wrist T23.Ø99
      - first degree T23.199
      - left T23.Ø92
        - first degree T23.192
        - second degree T23.292
        - third degree T23.392
      - right T23.Ø91
        - first degree T23.191
        - second degree T23.291
        - third degree T23.391
      - second degree T23.299
      - third degree T23.399
    - palm — *see* Burn, palm
    - right T23.ØØ1
      - first degree T23.1Ø1
      - second degree T23.2Ø1
      - third degree T23.3Ø1
    - second degree T23.2Ø9
    - third degree T23.3Ø9
    - thumb — *see* Burn, thumb
  - head (and face) (and neck) T2Ø.ØØ
    - cheek — *see* Burn, cheek
    - chin — *see* Burn, chin
    - ear — *see* Burn, ear
    - eye(s) only — *see* Burn, eye
    - first degree T2Ø.1Ø
    - forehead — *see* Burn, forehead
    - lip — *see* Burn, lip
    - multiple sites T2Ø.Ø9
      - first degree T2Ø.19
      - second degree T2Ø.29
      - third degree T2Ø.39
    - neck — *see* Burn, neck
    - nose — *see* Burn, nose
    - scalp — *see* Burn, scalp
    - second degree T2Ø.2Ø
    - third degree T2Ø.3Ø
  - hip(s) — *see* Burn, lower, limb
  - inhalation — *see* Burn, respiratory tract
    - caustic or corrosive substance (fumes) — *see* Corrosion, respiratory tract
  - internal organ(s) T28.4Ø
    - alimentary tract T28.2

- **Burn** — *continued*
  - internal organ(s) — *continued*
    - alimentary tract — *continued*
      - esophagus T28.1
    - eardrum T28.41
    - esophagus T28.1
    - from caustic or corrosive substance (swallowing) NEC — *see* Corrosion, by site
    - genitourinary T28.3
    - mouth T28.Ø
    - pharynx T28.Ø
    - respiratory tract — *see* Burn, respiratory tract
    - specified organ NEC T28.49
  - interscapular region — *see* Burn, back, upper
  - intestine (large) (small) T28.2
  - knee T24.Ø29
    - first degree T24.129
    - left T24.Ø22
      - first degree T24.122
      - second degree T24.222
      - third degree T24.322
    - right T24.Ø21
      - first degree T24.121
      - second degree T24.221
      - third degree T24.321
    - second degree T24.229
    - third degree T24.329
  - labium (majus) (minus) — *see* Burn, genital organs, external, female
  - lacrimal apparatus, duct, gland or sac — *see* Burn, eye, specified site NEC
  - larynx T27.Ø
    - with lung T27.1
  - leg(s) (lower) (upper) — *see* Burn, lower, limb
  - lightning — *see* Burn, by site
  - limb(s)
    - lower (except ankle or foot alone) — *see* Burn, lower, limb
    - upper — *see* Burn, upper limb
  - lip(s) T2Ø.Ø2
    - first degree T2Ø.12
    - second degree T2Ø.22
    - third degree T2Ø.32
  - lower
    - back — *see* Burn, back
    - limb T24.ØØ9
      - ankle — *see* Burn, ankle
      - calf — *see* Burn, calf
      - first degree T24.1Ø9
      - foot — *see* Burn, foot
      - knee — *see* Burn, knee
      - left T24.ØØ2
        - first degree T24.1Ø2
        - second degree T24.2Ø2
        - third degree T24.3Ø2
      - multiple sites, except ankle and foot T24.Ø99
        - ankle and foot T25.Ø99
          - first degree T25.199
          - left T25.Ø92
            - first degree T25.192
            - second degree T25.292
            - third degree T25.392
          - right T25.Ø91
            - first degree T25.191
            - second degree T25.291
            - third degree T25.391
          - second degree T25.299
          - third degree T25.399
        - first degree T24.199
        - left T24.Ø92
          - first degree T24.192
          - second degree T24.292
          - third degree T24.392
        - right T24.Ø91
          - first degree T24.191
          - second degree T24.291
          - third degree T24.391
        - second degree T24.299
        - third degree T24.399
      - right T24.ØØ1
        - first degree T24.1Ø1
        - second degree T24.2Ø1
        - third degree T24.3Ø1

- **Burn** — *continued*
  - lower — *continued*
    - limb — *continued*
      - second degree T24.2Ø9
      - hip — *see* Burn, thigh
      - thigh — *see* Burn, thigh
      - third degree T24.3Ø9
      - toe — *see* Burn, toe
  - lung (with larynx and trachea) T27.1
  - mouth T28.Ø
  - neck T2Ø.Ø7
    - first degree T2Ø.17
    - second degree T2Ø.27
    - third degree T2Ø.37
  - nose (septum) T2Ø.Ø4
    - first degree T2Ø.14
    - second degree T2Ø.24
    - third degree T2Ø.34
  - ocular adnexa — *see* Burn, eye
  - orbit region — *see* Burn, eyelid
  - palm T23.Ø59
    - first degree T23.159
    - left T23.Ø52
      - first degree T23.152
      - second degree T23.252
      - third degree T23.352
    - right T23.Ø51
      - first degree T23.151
      - second degree T23.251
      - third degree T23.351
    - second degree T23.259
    - third degree T23.359
  - partial thickness—code as Burn, unspecified degree, by site
  - pelvis — *see* Burn, trunk
  - penis — *see* Burn, genital organs, external, male
  - perineum
    - female — *see* Burn, genital organs, external, female
    - male — *see* Burn, genital organs, external, male
  - periocular area — *see* Burn, eyelid
  - pharynx T28.Ø
  - rectum T28.2
  - respiratory tract T27.3
    - larynx — *see* Burn, larynx
    - specified part NEC T27.2
    - trachea — *see* Burn, trachea
  - sac, lacrimal — *see* Burn, eye, specified site NEC
  - scalp T2Ø.Ø5
    - first degree T2Ø.15
    - second degree T2Ø.25
    - third degree T2Ø.35
  - scapular region T22.Ø69
    - first degree T22.169
    - left T22.Ø62
      - first degree T22.162
      - second degree T22.262
      - third degree T22.362
    - right T22.Ø61
      - first degree T22.161
      - second degree T22.261
      - third degree T22.361
    - second degree T22.269
    - third degree T22.369
  - sclera — *see* Burn, eye, specified site NEC
  - scrotum — *see* Burn, genital organs, external, male
  - shoulder T22.Ø59
    - first degree T22.159
    - left T22.Ø52
      - first degree T22.152
      - second degree T22.252
      - third degree T22.352
    - right T22.Ø51
      - first degree T22.151
      - second degree T22.251
      - third degree T22.351
    - second degree T22.259
    - third degree T22.359
  - stomach T28.2
  - temple — *see* Burn, head
  - testis — *see* Burn, genital organs, external, male
  - thigh T24.Ø19
    - first degree T24.119
    - left T24.Ø12

- **Burn** — *continued*
  - thigh — *continued*
    - left — *continued*
      - first degree T24.112
      - second degree T24.212
      - third degree T24.312
    - right T24.Ø11
      - first degree T24.111
      - second degree T24.211
      - third degree T24.311
    - second degree T24.219
    - third degree T24.319
  - thorax (external) — *see* Burn, trunk
  - throat (meaning pharynx) T28.Ø
  - thumb(s) T23.Ø19
    - first degree T23.119
    - left T23.Ø12
      - first degree T23.112
      - second degree T23.212
      - third degree T23.312
    - multiple sites with fingers T23.Ø49
      - first degree T23.149
      - left T23.Ø42
        - first degree T23.142
        - second degree T23.242
        - third degree T23.342
      - right T23.Ø41
        - first degree T23.141
        - second degree T23.241
        - third degree T23.341
      - second degree T23.249
      - third degree T23.349
    - right T23.Ø11
      - first degree T23.111
      - second degree T23.211
      - third degree T23.311
    - second degree T23.219
    - third degree T23.319
  - toe T25.Ø39
    - first degree T25.139
    - left T25.Ø32
      - first degree T25.132
      - second degree T25.232
      - third degree T25.332
    - right T25.Ø31
      - first degree T25.131
      - second degree T25.231
      - third degree T25.331
    - second degree T25.239
    - third degree T25.339
  - tongue T28.Ø
  - tonsil(s) T28.Ø
  - trachea T27.Ø
    - with lung T27.1
  - trunk T21.ØØ
    - abdominal wall — *see* Burn, abdominal wall
    - anus — *see* Burn, buttock
    - axilla — *see* Burn, upper limb
    - back — *see* Burn, back
    - breast — *see* Burn, chest wall
    - buttock — *see* Burn, buttock
    - chest wall — *see* Burn, chest wall
    - first degree T21.1Ø
    - flank — *see* Burn, abdominal wall
    - genital
      - female — *see* Burn, genital organs, external, female
      - male — *see* Burn, genital organs, external, male
    - groin — *see* Burn, abdominal wall
    - interscapular region — *see* Burn, back, upper
    - labia — *see* Burn, genital organs, external, female
    - lower back — *see* Burn, back
    - penis — *see* Burn, genital organs, external, male
    - perineum
      - female — *see* Burn, genital organs, external, female
      - male — *see* Burn, genital organs, external, male
    - scapula region — *see* Burn, scapular region
    - scrotum — *see* Burn, genital organs, external, male
    - second degree T21.2Ø
    - specified site NEC T21.Ø9
      - first degree T21.19
      - second degree T21.29

- **Burn** — *continued*
  - trunk — *continued*
    - specified site NEC — *continued*
      - third degree T21.39
    - testes — *see* Burn, genital organs, external, male
    - third degree T21.3Ø
    - upper back — *see* Burn, back, upper
    - vulva — *see* Burn, genital organs, external, female
  - unspecified site with extent of body surface involved specified
    - less than 1Ø per cent T31.Ø
    - 1Ø-19 per cent (Ø-9 percent third degree) T31.1Ø
      - with 1Ø-19 percent third degree T31.11
    - 2Ø-29 per cent (Ø-9 percent third degree) T31.2Ø
      - with
        - 1Ø-19 percent third degree T31.21
        - 2Ø-29 percent third degree T31.22
    - 3Ø-39 per cent (Ø-9 percent third degree) T31.3Ø
      - with
        - 1Ø-19 percent third degree T31.31
        - 2Ø-29 percent third degree T31.32
        - 3Ø-39 percent third degree T31.33
    - 4Ø-49 per cent (Ø-9 percent third degree) T31.4Ø
      - with
        - 1Ø-19 percent third degree T31.41
        - 2Ø-29 percent third degree T31.42
        - 3Ø-39 percent third degree T31.43
        - 4Ø-49 percent third degree T31.44
    - 5Ø-59 per cent (Ø-9 percent third degree) T31.5Ø
      - with
        - 1Ø-19 percent third degree T31.51
        - 2Ø-29 percent third degree T31.52
        - 3Ø-39 percent third degree T31.53
        - 4Ø-49 percent third degree T31.54
        - 5Ø-59 percent third degree T31.55
    - 6Ø-69 per cent (Ø-9 percent third degree) T31.6Ø
      - with
        - 1Ø-19 percent third degree T31.61
        - 2Ø-29 percent third degree T31.62
        - 3Ø-39 percent third degree T31.63
        - 4Ø-49 percent third degree T31.64
        - 5Ø-59 percent third degree T31.65
        - 6Ø-69 percent third degree T31.66
    - 7Ø-79 per cent (Ø-9 percent third degree) T31.7Ø
      - with
        - 1Ø-19 percent third degree T31.71
        - 2Ø-29 percent third degree T31.72
        - 3Ø-39 percent third degree T31.73
        - 4Ø-49 percent third degree T31.74
        - 5Ø-59 percent third degree T31.75
        - 6Ø-69 percent third degree T31.76
        - 7Ø-79 percent third degree T31.77
    - 8Ø-89 per cent (Ø-9 percent third degree) T31.8Ø
      - with
        - 1Ø-19 percent third degree T31.81
        - 2Ø-29 percent third degree T31.82
        - 3Ø-39 percent third degree T31.83
        - 4Ø-49 percent third degree T31.84
        - 5Ø-59 percent third degree T31.85
        - 6Ø-69 percent third degree T31.86
        - 7Ø-79 percent third degree T31.87
        - 8Ø-89 percent third degree T31.88
    - 9Ø per cent or more (Ø-9 percent third degree) T31.9Ø
      - with
        - 1Ø-19 percent third degree T31.91
        - 2Ø-29 percent third degree T31.92
        - 3Ø-39 percent third degree T31.93
        - 4Ø-49 percent third degree T31.94
        - 5Ø-59 percent third degree T31.95
        - 6Ø-69 percent third degree T31.96
        - 7Ø-79 percent third degree T31.97
        - 8Ø-89 percent third degree T31.98
        - 9Ø-99 percent third degree T31.99
  - upper limb T22.ØØ
    - above elbow — *see* Burn, above elbow
    - axilla — *see* Burn, axilla
    - elbow — *see* Burn, elbow
    - first degree T22.1Ø
    - forearm — *see* Burn, forearm

- **Burn** — *continued*
  - upper limb — *continued*
    - hand — *see* Burn, hand
    - interscapular region — *see* Burn, back, upper
    - multiple sites T22.Ø99
      - first degree T22.199
      - left T22.Ø92
        - first degree T22.192
        - second degree T22.292
        - third degree T22.392
      - right T22.Ø91
        - first degree T22.191
        - second degree T22.291
        - third degree T22.391
      - second degree T22.299
      - third degree T22.399
    - second degree T22.2Ø
    - scapular region — *see* Burn, scapular region
    - shoulder — *see* Burn, shoulder
    - third degree T22.3Ø
    - wrist — *see* Burn, wrist
  - uterus T28.3
  - vagina T28.3
  - vulva — *see* Burn, genital organs, external, female
  - wrist T23.Ø79
    - first degree T23.179
    - left T23.Ø72
      - first degree T23.172
      - second degree T23.272
      - third degree T23.372
    - multiple sites with hand T23.Ø99
      - first degree T23.199
      - left T23.Ø92
        - first degree T23.192
        - second degree T23.292
        - third degree T23.392
      - right T23.Ø91
        - first degree T23.191
        - second degree T23.291
        - third degree T23.391
      - second degree T23.299
      - third degree T23.399
    - right T23.Ø71
      - first degree T23.171
      - second degree T23.271
      - third degree T23.371
    - second degree T23.279
    - third degree T23.379
- **Burnett's syndrome** E83.52
- **Burning**
  - feet syndrome E53.9
  - sensation R2Ø.8
  - tongue K14.6
- **Burn-out** (state) Z73.Ø
- **Burns' disease or osteochondrosis** — *see* Osteochondrosis, juvenile, ulna
- **Bursa** — *see* condition
- **Bursitis** M71.9
  - Achilles — *see* Tendinitis, Achilles
  - adhesive — *see* Bursitis, specified NEC
  - ankle — *see* Enthesopathy, lower limb, ankle, specified type NEC
  - calcaneal — *see* Enthesopathy, foot, specified type NEC
  - collateral ligament, tibial — *see* Bursitis, tibial collateral
  - due to use, overuse, pressure (*see also* Disorder, soft tissue, due to use, specified type NEC)
    - specified NEC — *see* Disorder, soft tissue, due to use, specified NEC
  - Duplay's M75.Ø
  - elbow NEC M7Ø.3-
    - olecranon M7Ø.2-
  - finger — *see* Disorder, soft tissue, due to use, specified type NEC, hand
  - foot — *see* Enthesopathy, foot, specified type NEC
  - gonococcal A54.49
  - gouty — *see* Gout, idiopathic
  - hand M7Ø.1-
  - hip NEC M7Ø.7-
    - trochanteric M7Ø.6-
  - infective NEC M71.1Ø
    - abscess — *see* Abscess, bursa

C

- **Calcification** — *continued*
  - intracranial — *see* Calcification, cerebral
  - joint — *see* Disorder, joint, specified type NEC
  - kidney N28.89
    - tuberculous B9Ø.1 *[N29]*
  - larynx (senile) J38.7
  - lens — *see* Cataract, specified NEC
  - lung (active) (postinfectional) J98.4
    - tuberculous B9Ø.9
  - lymph gland or node (postinfectional) I89.8
    - tuberculous (*see also* Tuberculosis, lymph gland) B9Ø.8
  - mammographic R92.1
  - massive (paraplegic) — *see* Myositis, ossificans, in, quadriplegia
  - medial — *see* Arteriosclerosis, extremities
  - meninges (cerebral) (spinal) G96.19
  - metastatic E83.59
  - Mönckeberg's — *see* Arteriosclerosis, extremities
  - muscle M61.9
    - due to burns — *see* Myositis, ossificans, in, burns
    - paralytic — *see* Myositis, ossificans, in, quadriplegia
    - specified type NEC M61.4Ø
      - ankle M61.47-
      - foot M61.47-
      - forearm M61.43-
      - hand M61.44-
      - lower leg M61.46-
      - multiple sites M61.49
      - pelvic region M61.45-
      - shoulder region M61.41-
      - specified site NEC M61.48
      - thigh M61.45-
      - upper arm M61.42-
  - myocardium, myocardial — *see* Degeneration, myocardial
  - ovary N83.8
  - pancreas K86.8
  - penis N48.89
  - periarticular — *see* Disorder, joint, specified type NEC
  - pericardium (*see also* Pericarditis) I31.1
  - pineal gland E34.8
  - pleura J94.8
    - postinfectional J94.8
    - tuberculous NEC B9Ø.9
  - pulpal (dental) (nodular) KØ4.2
  - sclera H15.89
  - spleen D73.89
  - subcutaneous L94.2
  - suprarenal (capsule) (gland) E27.49
  - tendon (sheath) (*see also* Tenosynovitis, specified type NEC)
    - with bursitis, synovitis or tenosynovitis—*see* Tendinitis, calcific
  - trachea J39.8
  - ureter N28.89
  - uterus N85.8
  - vitreous — *see* Deposit, crystalline
- **Calcified** — *see* Calcification
- **Calcinosis** (interstitial) (tumoral) (universalis) E83.59
  - with Raynaud's phenomenon, esophageal dysfunction, sclerodactyly, telangiectasia (CREST syndrome) M34.1
  - circumscripta (skin) L94.2
  - cutis L94.2
- **Calciphylaxis** (*see also* Calcification, by site) E83.59
- **Calcium**
  - deposits — *see* Calcification, by site
  - metabolism disorder E83.5Ø
  - salts or soaps in vitreous — *see* Deposit, crystalline
- **Calciuria** R82.99
- **Calculi** — *see* Calculus
- **Calculosis, intrahepatic** — *see* Calculus, bile duct
- **Calculus, calculi, calculous**
  - ampulla of Vater — *see* Calculus, bile duct
  - anuria (impacted) (recurrent) (*see also* Calculus, urinary) N2Ø.9
  - appendix K38.1
  - bile duct (common) (hepatic) K8Ø.5Ø

- **Calculus, calculi, calculous** — *continued*
  - bile duct (common) (hepatic) — *continued*
    - with
      - alculus of gallbladder — *see* Calculus, gallbladder and bile duct
      - cholangitis K8Ø.3Ø
        - with
          - cholecystitis — *see* Calculus, bile duct, with cholecystitis
          - obstruction K8Ø.31
        - acute K8Ø.32
          - with
            - chronic cholangitis K8Ø.36
              - with obstruction K8Ø.37
            - obstruction K8Ø.33
        - chronic K8Ø.34
          - with
            - acute cholangitis K8Ø.36
              - with obstruction K8Ø.37
            - obstruction K8Ø.35
      - cholecystitis (with cholangitis) K8Ø.4Ø
        - with obstruction K8Ø.41
        - acute K8Ø.42
          - with
            - chronic cholecystitis K8Ø.46
              - with obstruction K8Ø.47
            - obstruction K8Ø.43
        - chronic K8Ø.44
          - with
            - acute cholecystitis K8Ø.46
              - with obstruction K8Ø.47
            - obstruction K8Ø.45
      - obstruction K8Ø.51
  - biliary (*see also* Calculus, gallbladder)
    - specified NEC K8Ø.8Ø
      - with obstruction K8Ø.81
  - bilirubin, multiple — *see* Calculus, gallbladder
  - bladder (encysted) (impacted) (urinary) (diverticulum) N21.Ø
  - bronchus J98.Ø9
  - calyx (kidney) (renal) — *see* Calculus, kidney
  - cholesterol (pure) (solitary) — *see* Calculus, gallbladder
  - common duct (bile) — *see* Calculus, bile duct
  - conjunctiva — *see* Concretion, conjunctiva
  - cystic N21.Ø
    - duct — *see* Calculus, gallbladder
  - dental (subgingival) (supragingival) KØ3.6
  - diverticulum
    - bladder N21.Ø
    - kidney N2Ø.Ø
  - epididymis N5Ø.8
  - gallbladder K8Ø.2Ø
    - with
      - bile duct calculus — *see* Calculus, gallbladder and bile duct
      - cholecystitis K8Ø.1Ø
        - with obstruction K8Ø.11
        - acute K8Ø.ØØ
          - with
            - chronic cholecystitis K8Ø.12
              - with obstruction K8Ø.13
            - obstruction K8Ø.Ø1
        - chronic K8Ø.1Ø
          - with
            - acute cholecystitis K8Ø.12
              - with obstruction K8Ø.13
            - obstruction K8Ø.11
        - specified NEC K8Ø.18
          - with obstruction K8Ø.19
      - obstruction K8Ø.21
  - gallbladder and bile duct K8Ø.7Ø
    - with
      - cholecystitis K8Ø.6Ø
        - with obstruction K8Ø.61
        - acute K8Ø.62
          - with
            - chronic cholecystitis K8Ø.66
              - with obstruction K8Ø.67
            - obstruction K8Ø.63
        - chronic K8Ø.64
          - with
            - acute cholecystitis K8Ø.66

- **Calculus, calculi, calculous** — *continued*
  - gallbladder and bile duct — *continued*
    - with — *continued*
      - cholecystitis — *continued*
        - chronic — *continued*
          - with — *continued*
            - acute cholecystitis
              - with obstruction K8Ø.67
            - obstruction K8Ø.65
      - obstruction K8Ø.71
  - hepatic (duct) — *see* Calculus, bile duct
  - ileal conduit N21.8
  - intestinal (impaction) (obstruction) K56.49
  - kidney (impacted) (multiple) (pelvis) (recurrent) (staghorn) N2Ø.Ø
    - with calculus, ureter N2Ø.2
    - congenital Q63.8
  - lacrimal passages — *see* Dacryolith
  - liver (impacted) — *see* Calculus, bile duct
  - lung J98.4
  - mammographic R92.1
  - nephritic (impacted) (recurrent) — *see* Calculus, kidney
  - nose J34.89
  - pancreas (duct) K86.8
  - parotid duct or gland K11.5
  - pelvis, encysted — *see* Calculus, kidney
  - prostate N42.Ø
  - pulmonary J98.4
  - pyelitis (impacted) (recurrent) N2Ø.Ø
    - with hydronephrosis N13.2
  - pyelonephritis (impacted) (recurrent) — *see* category N2Ø
    - with hydronephrosis N13.2
  - renal (impacted) (recurrent) — *see* Calculus, kidney
  - salivary (duct) (gland) K11.5
  - seminal vesicle N5Ø.8
  - staghorn — *see* Calculus, kidney
  - Stensen's duct K11.5
  - stomach K31.89
  - sublingual duct or gland K11.5
    - congenital Q38.4
  - submandibular duct, gland or region K11.5
  - submaxillary duct, gland or region K11.5
  - suburethral N21.8
  - tonsil J35.8
  - tooth, teeth (subgingival) (supragingival) KØ3.6
  - tunica vaginalis N5Ø.8
  - ureter (impacted) (recurrent) N2Ø.1
    - with calculus, kidney N2Ø.2
      - with hydronephrosis N13.2
        - with infection N13.6
  - urethra (impacted) N21.1
  - urinary (duct) (impacted) (passage) (tract) N2Ø.9
    - with hydronephrosis N13.2
      - with infection N13.6
    - in (due to)
    - lower N21.9
      - specified NEC N21.8
  - vagina N89.8
  - vesical (impacted) N21.Ø
  - Wharton's duct K11.5
  - xanthine E79.8 *[N22]*
- **Calicectasis** N28.89
- **Caliectasis** N28.89
- **California**
  - disease B38.9
  - encephalitis A83.5
- **Caligo cornea** — *see* Opacity, cornea, central
- **Callositas, callosity** (infected) L84
- **Callus** (infected) L84
  - bone — *see* Osteophyte
  - excessive, following fracture—code as Sequelae of fracture
- **Calorie deficiency or malnutrition** (*see also* Malnutrition) E46
- **Calvé-Perthes disease** — *see* Legg-Calvé-Perthes disease
- **Calvé's disease** — *see* Osteochondrosis, juvenile, spine
- **Calvities** — *see* Alopecia, androgenic
- **Cameroon fever** — *see* Malaria
- **Camptocormia** (hysterical) F44.4
- **Camurati-Engelmann syndrome** Q78.3

Canal (*see also* condition)
  atrioventricular common Q21.2
Canaliculitis (lacrimal) (acute) (subacute) HØ4.33-
  Actinomyces A42.89
  chronic HØ4.42-
Canavan's disease E75.29
Canceled procedure (surgical) Z53.9
  because of
    contraindication Z53.Ø9
      smoking Z53.Ø1
    left against medical advice (AMA) Z53.21
    patient's decision Z53.2Ø
      for reasons of belief or group pressure Z53.1
      specified reason NEC Z53.29
    specified reason NEC Z53.8
Cancer (*see also* Neoplasm, malignant, by site)
  bile duct type liver C22.1
  blood — *see* Leukemia
  breast (*see also* Neoplam, breast, malignant) C5Ø.91
  hepatocellular C22.Ø
  lung C34.9Ø (*see also* Neoplasm, lung, malignant)
  ovarian C56.9 (*see also* Neoplasm, ovary, malignant)
  unspecified site (primary) C8Ø.1
Cancer(o)phobia F45.29
Cancerous — *see* Neoplasm, malignant, by site
Cancrum oris A69.Ø
Candidiasis, candidal B37.9
  balanitis B37.42
  bronchitis B37.1
  cheilitis B37.83
  congenital P37.5
  cystitis B37.41
  disseminated B37.7
  endocarditis B37.6
  enteritis B37.82
  esophagitis B37.81
  intertrigo B37.2
  lung B37.1
  meningitis B37.5
  mouth B37.Ø
  nails B37.2
  neonatal P37.5
  onychia B37.2
  oral B37.Ø
  osteomyelitis B37.89
  otitis externa B37.84
  paronychia B37.2
  perionyxis B37.2
  pneumonia B37.1
  proctitis B37.82
  pulmonary B37.1
  pyelonephritis B37.49
  sepsis B37.7
  skin B37.2
  specified site NEC B37.89
  stomatitis B37.Ø
  systemic B37.7
  urethritis B37.41
  urogenital site NEC B37.49
  vagina B37.3
  vulva B37.3
  vulvovaginitis B37.3
Candidid L3Ø.2
Candidosis — *see* Candidiasis
Candiru infection or infestation B88.8
Canities (premature) L67.1
  congenital Q84.2
Canker (mouth) (sore) K12.Ø
  rash A38.9
Cannabinosis J66.2
Canton fever A75.9
Cantrell's syndrome Q87.89
Capillariasis (intestinal) B81.1
  hepatic B83.8
Capillary — *see* condition
Caplan's syndrome — *see* Rheumatoid, lung
Capsule — *see* condition
Capsulitis (joint) (*see also* Enthesopathy)
  adhesive (shoulder) M75.Ø-
  hepatic K65.8
  labyrinthine — *see* Otosclerosis, specified NEC
  thyroid EØ6.9
Caput crepitus Q75.8
  medusae I86.8
  succedaneum P12.81
Car sickness T75.3
Carapata (disease) A68.Ø
Carate — *see* Pinta
Carbon lung J6Ø
Carbuncle LØ2.93
  abdominal wall LØ2.231
  anus K61.Ø
  auditory canal, external — *see* Abscess, ear, external
  auricle ear — *see* Abscess, ear, external
  axilla LØ2.43-
  back (any part) LØ2.232
  breast N61
  buttock LØ2.33
  cheek (external) LØ2.Ø3
  chest wall LØ2.233
  chin LØ2.Ø3
  corpus cavernosum N48.21
  ear (any part) (external) (middle) — *see* Abscess, ear, external
  external auditory canal — *see* Abscess, ear, external
  eyelid — *see* Abscess, eyelid
  face NEC LØ2.Ø3
  femoral (region) — *see* Carbuncle, lower limb
  finger — *see* Carbuncle, hand
  flank LØ2.231
  foot LØ2.63-
  forehead LØ2.Ø3
  genital — *see* Abscess, genital
  gluteal (region) LØ2.33
  groin LØ2.234
  hand LØ2.53-
  head NEC LØ2.831
  heel — *see* Carbuncle, foot
  hip — *see* Carbuncle, lower limb
  kidney — *see* Abscess, kidney
  knee — *see* Carbuncle, lower limb
  labium (majus) (minus) N76.4
  lacrimal
    gland — *see* Dacryoadenitis
    passages (duct) (sac) — *see* Inflammation, lacrimal, passages, acute
  leg — *see* Carbuncle, lower limb
  lower limb LØ2.43-
  malignant A22.Ø
  navel LØ2.236
  neck LØ2.13
  nose (external) (septum) J34.Ø
  orbit, orbital — *see* Abscess, orbit
  palmar (space) — *see* Carbuncle, hand
  partes posteriores LØ2.33
  pectoral region LØ2.233
  penis N48.21
  perineum LØ2.235
  pinna — *see* Abscess, ear, external
  popliteal — *see* Carbuncle, lower limb
  scalp LØ2.831
  seminal vesicle N49.Ø
  shoulder — *see* Carbuncle, upper limb
  specified site NEC LØ2.838
  temple (region) LØ2.Ø3
  thumb — *see* Carbuncle, hand
  toe — *see* Carbuncle, foot
  trunk LØ2.239
    abdominal wall LØ2.231
    back LØ2.232
    chest wall LØ2.233
    groin LØ2.234
    perineum LØ2.235
    umbilicus LØ2.236
  umbilicus LØ2.236
  upper limb LØ2.43-
  urethra N34.Ø
  vulva N76.4
Carbunculus — *see* Carbuncle
Carcinoid (tumor) — *see* Tumor, carcinoid
Carcinoidosis E34.Ø
Carcinoma (malignant) (*see also* Neoplasm, malignant, by site)
  acidophil
    specified site — *see* Neoplasm, malignant, by site
Carcinoma — *continued*
  acidophil — *continued*
    unspecified site C75.1
  acidophil-basophil, mixed
    specified site — *see* Neoplasm, malignant, by site
    unspecified site C75.1
  adnexal (skin) — *see* Neoplasm, skin, malignant
  adrenal cortical C74.Ø-
  alveolar — *see* Neoplasm, lung, malignant
    cell — *see* Neoplasm, lung, malignant
  ameloblastic C41.1
    upper jaw (bone) C41.Ø
  apocrine
    breast — *see* Neoplasm, breast, malignant
    specified site NEC — *see* Neoplasm, skin, malignant
    unspecified site C44.99
  basal cell (pigmented) (*see also* Neoplasm, skin, malignant) C44.91
    fibro-epithelial — *see* Neoplasm, skin, malignant
    morphea — *see* Neoplasm, skin, malignant
    multicentric — *see* Neoplasm, skin, malignant
  basaloid
  basal-squamous cell, mixed — *see* Neoplasm, skin, malignant
  basophil
    specified site — *see* Neoplasm, malignant, by site
    unspecified site C75.1
  basophil-acidophil, mixed
    specified site — *see* Neoplasm, malignant, by site
    unspecified site C75.1
  basosquamous — *see* Neoplasm, skin, malignant
  bile duct
    with hepatocellular, mixed C22.Ø
    liver C22.1
    specified site NEC — *see* Neoplasm, malignant, by site
    unspecified site C22.1
  branchial or branchiogenic C1Ø.4
  bronchial or bronchogenic — *see* Neoplasm, lung, malignant
  bronchiolar — *see* Neoplasm, lung, malignant
  bronchioloalveolar — *see* Neoplasm, lung, malignant
  C cell
    specified site — *see* Neoplasm, malignant, by site
    unspecified site C73
  ceruminous C44.29-
  cervix uteri
    in situ DØ6.9
      endocervix DØ6.Ø
      exocervix DØ6.1
      specified site NEC DØ6.7
  chorionic
    specified site — *see* Neoplasm, malignant, by site
    unspecified site
      female C58
      male C62.9Ø
  chromophobe
    specified site — *see* Neoplasm, malignant, by site
    unspecified site C75.1
  cloacogenic
    specified site — *see* Neoplasm, malignant, by site
    unspecified site C21.2
  diffuse type
    specified site — *see* Neoplasm, malignant, by site
    unspecified site C16.9
  duct (cell)
    with Paget's disease — *see* Neoplasm, breast, malignant
    infiltrating
      with lobular carcinoma (in situ)
        specified site — *see* Neoplasm, malignant, by site
        unspecified site (female) C5Ø.91-
          male C5Ø.92-
      specified site — *see* Neoplasm, malignant, by site
      unspecified site (female) C5Ø.91-
        male C5Ø.92-

Carcinoma — *continued*
- ductal
  - with lobular
    - specified site — *see* Neoplasm, malignant, by site
    - unspecified site (female) C5Ø.91-
      - male C5Ø.92-
- ductular, infiltrating
  - specified site — *see* Neoplasm, malignant, by site
  - unspecified site (female) C5Ø.91-
    - male C5Ø.92-
- embryonal
  - liver C22.7
- endometrioid
  - specified site — *see* Neoplasm, malignant, by site
  - unspecified site
    - female C56.9
    - male C61
- eosinophil
  - specified site — *see* Neoplasm, malignant, by site
  - unspecified site C75.1
- epidermoid (*see also* Carcinoma, squamous cell)
  - in situ, Bowen's type — *see* Neoplasm, skin, in situ
- fibroepithelial, basal cell — *see* Neoplasm, skin, malignant
- follicular
  - with papillary (mixed) C73
  - moderately differentiated C73
  - pure follicle C73
  - specified site — *see* Neoplasm, malignant, by site
  - trabecular C73
  - unspecified site C73
  - well differentiated C73
- generalized, with unspecified primary site C8Ø.Ø
- glycogen-rich — *see* Neoplasm, breast, malignant
- granulosa cell C56-
- hepatic cell C22.Ø
- hepatocellular C22.Ø
  - with bile duct, mixed C22.Ø
  - fibrolamellar C22.Ø
- hepatocholangiolitic C22.Ø
- Hurthle cell C73
- in
  - adenomatous
    - polyposis coli C18.9
  - pleomorphic adenoma — *see* Neoplasm, salivary glands, malignant
  - situ — *see* Carcinoma-in-situ
- infiltrating
  - duct
    - with lobular
      - specified site — *see* Neoplasm, malignant, by site
      - unspecified site (female) C5Ø.91-
        - male C5Ø.92-
    - with Paget's disease — *see* Neoplasm, breast, malignant
    - specified site — *see* Neoplasm, malignant
    - unspecified site (female) C5Ø.91-
      - male C5Ø.92-
  - ductural
    - specified site — *see* Neoplasm, malignant
    - unspecified site (female) C5Ø.91-
      - male C5Ø.92-
  - lobular
    - unspecified site (female) C5Ø.91-
      - male C5Ø.92-
- inflammatory
  - specified site — *see* Neoplasm, malignant
  - unspecified site (female) C5Ø.91-
    - male C5Ø.92-
- intestinal type
  - specified site — *see* Neoplasm, malignant, by site
  - unspecified site C16.9
- intracystic
  - noninfiltrating — *see* Neoplasm, in situ, by site
- intraductal (noninfiltrating)
  - with Paget's disease — *see* Neoplasm, breast, malignant
  - breast DØ5.1-

Carcinoma — *continued*
- intraductal (noninfiltrating) — *continued*
  - papillary
    - with invasion
      - specified site — *see* Neoplasm, malignant, by site
      - unspecified site (female) C5Ø.91-
        - male C5Ø.92-
    - breast DØ5.1-
    - specified site NEC — *see* Neoplasm, in situ, by site
    - unspecified site (female) DØ5.1-
  - specified site NEC — *see* Neoplasm, in situ, by site
  - unspecified site (female) DØ5.1-
- intraepidermal — *see* Neoplasm, in situ
  - squamous cell, Bowen's type — *see* Neoplasm, skin, in situ
- intraepithelial — *see* Neoplasm, in situ, by site
  - squamous cell — *see* Neoplasm, in situ, by site
- intraosseous C41.1
  - upper jaw (bone) C41.Ø
- islet cell
  - with exocrine, mixed
    - specified site — *see* Neoplasm, malignant, by site
    - unspecified site C25.9
  - pancreas C25.4
  - specified site NEC — *see* Neoplasm, malignant, by site
  - unspecified site C25.4
- juvenile, breast — *see* Neoplasm, breast, malignant
- large cell
  - small cell
    - specified site — *see* Neoplasm, malignant, by site
    - unspecified site C34.9Ø
- Leydig cell (testis)
  - specified site — *see* Neoplasm, malignant, by site
  - unspecified site
    - female C56.9
    - male C62.9Ø
- lipid-rich (female) C5Ø.91-
  - male C5Ø.92-
- liver cell C22.Ø
- liver NEC C22.7
- lobular (infiltrating)
  - with intraductal
    - specified site — *see* Neoplasm, malignant, by site
    - unspecified site (female) C5Ø.91-
      - male C5Ø.92-
  - noninfiltrating
    - breast DØ5.Ø-
    - specified site NEC — *see* Neoplasm, in situ, by site
    - unspecified site DØ5.Ø-
  - specified site — *see* Neoplasm, malignant, by site
  - unspecified site (female) C5Ø.91-
    - male C5Ø.92-
- medullary
  - with
    - amyloid stroma
      - specified site — *see* Neoplasm, malignant, by site
      - unspecified site C73
    - lymphoid stroma
      - specified site — *see* Neoplasm, malignant, by site
      - unspecified site (female) C5Ø.91-
        - male C5Ø.92-
- Merkel cell C4A.9
  - anal margin C4A.51
  - anal skin C4A.51
  - canthus C4A.1-
  - ear and external auricular canal C4A.2-
  - external auricular canal C4A.2-
  - eyelid, including canthus C4A.1-
  - face C4A.3Ø
  - hip C4A.7-
  - lip C4A.Ø
  - lower limb, including hip C4A.7-
  - neck C4A.4
  - nodal presentation C7B.1

Carcinoma — *continued*
- Merkel cell — *continued*
  - nose C4A.31
    - specified NEC C4A.39
  - overlapping sites C4A.8
  - perianal skin C4A.51
  - scalp C4A.4
  - secondary C7B.1
  - shoulder C4A.6-
  - skin of breast C4A.52
  - trunk NEC C4A.59
  - upper limb, including shoulder C4A.6-
  - visceral metastatic C7B.1
- metastatic — *see* Neoplasm, secondary, by site
- metatypical — *see* Neoplasm, skin, malignant
- morphea, basal cell — *see* Neoplasm, skin, malignant
- mucoid
  - cell
    - specified site — *see* Neoplasm, malignant, by site
    - unspecified site C75.1
- neuroendocrine (*see also* Tumor, neuroendocrine)
  - high grade, any site C7A.1
  - poorly differentiated, any site C7A.1
- nonencapsulated sclerosing C73
- noninfiltrating
  - intracystic — *see* Neoplasm, in situ, by site
  - intraductal
    - breast DØ5.1-
    - papillary
      - breast DØ5.1-
      - specified site NEC — *see* Neoplasm, in situ, by site
      - unspecified site DØ5.1-
    - specified site — *see* Neoplasm, in situ, by site
    - unspecified site DØ5.1-
  - lobular
    - breast DØ5.Ø-
    - specified site NEC — *see* Neoplasm, in situ, by site
    - unspecified site (female) DØ5.Ø-
- oat cell
  - specified site — *see* Neoplasm, malignant, by site
  - unspecified site C34.9Ø
- odontogenic C41.1
  - upper jaw (bone) C41.Ø
- papillary
  - with follicular (mixed) C73
  - follicular variant C73
  - intraductal (noninfiltrating)
    - with invasion
      - specified site — *see* Neoplasm, malignant, by site
      - unspecified site (female) C5Ø.91-
        - male C5Ø.92-
    - breast DØ5.1-
    - specified site NEC — *see* Neoplasm, in situ, by site
    - unspecified site DØ5.1-
  - serous
    - specified site — *see* Neoplasm, malignant, by site
    - surface
      - specified site — *see* Neoplasm, malignant, by site
      - unspecified site C56.9
    - unspecified site C56.9
- papillocystic
  - specified site — *see* Neoplasm, malignant, by site
  - unspecified site C56.9
- parafollicular cell
  - specified site — *see* Neoplasm, malignant, by site
  - unspecified site C73
- pilomatrix — *see* Neoplasm, skin, malignant
- pseudomucinous
  - specified site — *see* Neoplasm, malignant, by site
  - unspecified site C56.9
- renal cell C64-
- Schmincke — *see* Neoplasm, nasopharynx, malignant
- Schneiderian
  - specified site — *see* Neoplasm, malignant, by site

Carcinoma — *continued*
  Schneiderian — *continued*
    unspecified site C3Ø.Ø
  sebaceous — *see* Neoplasm, skin, malignant
  secondary (*see also* Neoplasm, secondary, by site)
    Merkel cell C7B.1
      specified site NEC — see Neoplasm, in situ
  secretory, breast — *see* Neoplasm, breast, malignant
  serous
    papillary
      specified site — *see* Neoplasm, malignant, by site
      unspecified site C56.9
    surface, papillary
      specified site — *see* Neoplasm, malignant, by site
      unspecified site C56.9
  Sertoli cell
    specified site — *see* Neoplasm, malignant, by site
    unspecified site C62.9Ø
      female C56.9
      male C62.9Ø
  skin appendage — *see* Neoplasm, skin, malignant
  small cell
    fusiform cell
      specified site — *see* Neoplasm, malignant, by site
      unspecified site C34.9Ø
    intermediate cell
      specified site — *see* Neoplasm, malignant, by site
      unspecified site C34.9Ø
    large cell
      specified site — *see* Neoplasm, malignant, by site
      unspecified site C34.9Ø
  solid
    with amyloid stroma
      specified site — *see* Neoplasm, malignant, by site
      unspecified site C73
    microinvasive
      specified site — *see* Neoplasm, malignant, by site
      unspecified site C53.9
  sweat gland — *see* Neoplasm, skin, malignant
  theca cell C56.-
  thymic C37
  unspecified site (primary) C8Ø.1
Carcinoma-in-situ (*see also* Neoplasm, in situ, by site)
  breast NOS DØ5.9-
    specified type NEC DØ5.8-
  epidermoid (*see also* Neoplasm, in situ, by site)
    with questionable stromal invasion
      cervix DØ6.9
      specified site NEC — *see* Neoplasm, in situ, by site
      unspecified site DØ6.9
    Bowen's type — *see* Neoplasm, skin, in situ, by site
  intraductal
    breast DØ5.1-
    specified site NEC — *see* Neoplasm, in situ, by site
    unspecified site DØ5.1-
  lobular
    with
      infiltrating duct
        breast (female) C5Ø.91-
          male C5Ø.92-
        specified site NEC — *see* Neoplasm, malignant
        unspecified site (female) C5Ø.91-
          male C5Ø.92-
      intraductal
        breast DØ5.8-
        specified site NEC — *see* Neoplasm, in situ, by site
        unspecified site (female) DØ5.8-
    breast DØ5.Ø-
    specified site NEC — *see* Neoplasm, in situ, by site
    unspecified site DØ5.Ø-
  squamous cell (*see also* Neoplasm, in situ, by site)
    with questionable stromal invasion
      cervix DØ6.9

Carcinoma-in-situ — *continued*
  squamous cell — *continued*
    with questionable stromal invasion — *continued*
      specified site NEC — *see* Neoplasm, in situ, by site
      unspecified site DØ6.9
Carcinomaphobia F45.29
Carcinomatosis C8Ø.Ø
  peritonei C78.6
  unspecified site (primary) (secondary) C8Ø.Ø
Carcinosarcoma — *see* Neoplasm, malignant, by site
  embryonal — *see* Neoplasm, malignant, by site
Cardia, cardial — *see* condition
Cardiac (*see also* condition)
  death, sudden — *see* Arrest, cardiac
  pacemaker
    in situ Z95.Ø
    management or adjustment Z45.Ø18
  tamponade I31.4
Cardialgia — *see* Pain, precordial
Cardiectasis — *see* Hypertrophy, cardiac
Cardiochalasia K21.9
Cardiomalacia I51.5
Cardiomegalia glycogenica diffusa E74.Ø2 *[I43]*
Cardiomegaly (*see also* Hypertrophy, cardiac)
  congenital Q24.8
  glycogen E74.Ø2 *[I43]*
  idiopathic I51.7
Cardiomyoliposis I51.5
Cardiomyopathy (familial) (idiopathic) I42.9
  alcoholic I42.6
  amyloid E85.4 *[I43]*
  arteriosclerotic — *see* Disease, heart, ischemic, atherosclerotic
  beriberi E51.12
  cobalt-beer I42.6
  congenital I42.4
  congestive I42.Ø
  constrictive NOS I42.5
  dilated I42.Ø
  due to
    alcohol I42.6
    beriberi E51.12
    cardiac glycogenosis E74.Ø2 *[I43]*
    drugs I42.7
    Friedreich's ataxia G11.1
    external agents NEC I42.7
    myotonia atrophica G71.11 *[I43]*
    progressive muscular dystrophy G71.Ø
  glycogen storage E74.Ø2 *[I43]*
  hypertensive — *see* Hypertension, heart
  hypertrophic (nonobstructive) I42.2
    obstructive I42.1
      congenital Q24.8
  in
    Chagas' disease (chronic) B57.2
      acute B57.Ø
    sarcoidosis D86.85
  ischemic I25.5
  metabolic E88.9 *[I43]*
    thyrotoxic EØ5.9Ø *[I43]*
      with thyroid storm EØ5.91 *[I43]*
  newborn I42.8
    congenital I42.4
  nutritional E63.9 *[I43]*
    beriberi E51.12
  obscure of Africa I42.8
  peripartum O9Ø.3
  postpartum O9Ø.3
  restrictive NEC I42.5
  rheumatic IØ9.Ø
  secondary I42.9
  stress induced I51.81
  takotsubo I51.81
  thyrotoxic EØ5.9Ø *[I43]*
    with thyroid storm EØ5.91 *[I43]*
  toxic NEC I42.7
  tuberculous A18.84
  viral B33.24
Cardionephritis — *see* Hypertension, cardiorenal
Cardionephropathy — *see* Hypertension, cardiorenal
Cardionephrosis — *see* Hypertension, cardiorenal
Cardiopathia nigra I27.Ø

Cardiopathy (*see also* Disease, heart) I51.9
  idiopathic I42.9
  mucopolysaccharidosis E76.3 *[I52]*
Cardiopericarditis — *see* Pericarditis
Cardiophobia F45.29
Cardiorenal — *see* condition
Cardiorrhexis — *see* Infarct, myocardium
Cardiosclerosis — *see* Disease, heart, ischemic, atherosclerotic
Cardiosis — *see* Disease, heart
Cardiospasm (esophagus) (reflex) (stomach) K22.Ø
  congenital Q39.5
    with megaesophagus Q39.5
Cardiostenosis — *see* Disease, heart
Cardiosymphysis I31.Ø
Cardiovascular — *see* condition
Carditis (acute) (bacterial) (chronic) (subacute) I51.89
  meningococcal A39.5Ø
  rheumatic — *see* Disease, heart, rheumatic
  rheumatoid — *see* Rheumatoid, carditis
  viral B33.2Ø
Care (of) (for) (following)
  child (routine) Z76.2
  family member (handicapped) (sick)
    creating problem for family Z63.6
    provided away from home for holiday relief Z75.5
    unavailable, due to
      absence (person rendering care) (sufferer) Z74.2
      inability (any reason) of person rendering care Z74.2
  foundling Z76.1
  holiday relief Z75.5
  improper — *see* Maltreatment
  lack of (at or after birth) (infant) — *see* Maltreatment, child, neglect
  lactating mother Z39.1
  palliative Z51.5
  postpartum
    immediately after delivery Z39.Ø
    routine follow-up Z39.2
  respite Z75.5
  unavailable, due to
    absence of person rendering care Z74.2
    inability (any reason) of person rendering care Z74.2
  well-baby Z76.2
Caries
  bone NEC A18.Ø3
  dental KØ2.9
    arrested (coronal) (root) KØ2.3
    chewing surface
      limited to enamel KØ2.51
      penetrating into dentin KØ2.52
      penetrating into pulp KØ2.53
    coronal surface
      chewing surface
        limited to enamel KØ2.51
        penetrating into dentin KØ2.52
        penetrating into pulp KØ2.53
      pit and fissure surface
        limited to enamel KØ2.51
        penetrating into dentin KØ2.52
        penetrating into pulp KØ2.53
      smooth surface
        limited to enamel KØ2.61
        penetrating into dentin KØ2.62
        penetrating into pulp KØ2.63
    pit and fissure surface
      limited to enamel KØ2.51
      penetrating into dentin KØ2.52
      penetrating into pulp KØ2.53
    smooth surface
      limited to enamel KØ2.61
      penetrating into dentin KØ2.62
      penetrating into pulp KØ2.63
    root KØ2.7
  external meatus — *see* Disorder, ear, external, specified type NEC
  hip (tuberculous) A18.Ø2
  initial (tooth)
    chewing surface KØ2.51
    pit and fissure surface KØ2.51

Caries — *continued*
initial (tooth) — *continued*
smooth surface K02.61
knee (tuberculous) A18.02
labyrinth — *see* subcategory H83.8
limb NEC (tuberculous) A18.03
mastoid process (chronic) — *see* Mastoiditis, chronic
tuberculous A18.03
middle ear — *see* subcategory H74.8
nose (tuberculous) A18.03
orbit (tuberculous) A18.03
ossicles, ear — *see* Abnormal, ear ossicles
petrous bone — *see* Petrositis
root (dental) (tooth) K02.7
sacrum (tuberculous) A18.01
spine, spinal (column) (tuberculous) A18.01
syphilitic A52.77
congenital (early) A50.02 *[M90.80]*
tooth, teeth — *see* Caries, dental
tuberculous A18.03
vertebra (column) (tuberculous) A18.01
Carious teeth — *see* Caries, dental
Carneous mole O02.0
Carnitine insufficiency E71.40
Carotid body or sinus syndrome G90.01
Carotidynia G90.01
Carotinemia (dietary) E67.1
Carotinosis (cutis) (skin) E67.1
Carpal tunnel syndrome — *see* Syndrome, carpal tunnel
Carpenter's syndrome Q87.0
Carpopedal spasm — *see* Tetany
Carr-Barr-Plunkett syndrome Q97.1
Carrier (suspected) of
amebiasis Z22.1
bacterial disease NEC Z22.39
diphtheria Z22.2
intestinal infectious NEC Z22.1
typhoid Z22.0
meningococcal Z22.31
sexually transmitted Z22.4
specified NEC Z22.39
staphylococcal (Methicillin susceptible) Z22.321
Methicillin resistant Z22.322
streptococcal Z22.338
group B Z22.330
typhoid Z22.0
cholera Z22.1
diphtheria Z22.2
gastrointestinal pathogens NEC Z22.1
genetic Z14.8
cystic fibrosis Z14.1
hemophilia A (asymptomatic) Z14.01
symptomatic Z14.02
gonorrhea Z22.4
HAA (hepatitis Australian-antigen) Z22.59
HB(c)(s)-AG Z22.51
hepatitis (viral) Z22.50
Australia-antigen (HAA) Z22.59
B surface antigen (HBsAg) Z22.51
with acute delta-(super)infection B17.0
C Z22.52
specified NEC Z22.59
human T-cell lymphotropic virus type-1 (HTLV-1)
infection Z22.6
infectious organism Z22.9
specified NEC Z22.8
meningococci Z22.31
Salmonella typhosa Z22.0
serum hepatitis — *see* Carrier, hepatitis
staphylococci (methicillin susceptible) Z22.321
methicillin resistant Z22.322
streptococci Z22.338
group B Z22.330
syphilis Z22.4
typhoid Z22.0
venereal disease NEC Z22.4
Carrion's disease A44.0
Carter's relapsing fever (Asiatic) A68.1
Cartilage — *see* condition
Caruncle (inflamed)
conjunctiva (acute) — *see* Conjunctivitis, acute
labium (majus) (minus) N90.89
lacrimal — *see* Inflammation, lacrimal, passages

Caruncle — *continued*
myrtiform N89.8
urethral (benign) N36.2
Cascade stomach K31.2
Caseation lymphatic gland (tuberculous) A18.2
Cassidy (-Scholte) **syndrome** (malignant carcinoid)
E34.0
Castellani's disease A69.8
Castration, traumatic, male S38.231
Casts in urine R82.99
Cat
cry syndrome Q93.4
ear Q17.3
eye syndrome Q92.8
Catabolism, senile R54
Catalepsy (hysterical) F44.2
schizophrenic F20.2
Cataplexy (idiopathic)—*see* Narcolepsy
Cataract (cortical) (immature) (incipient) H26.9
with
neovascularization — *see* Cataract, complicated
age-related — *see* Cataract, senile
anterior
and posterior axial embryonal Q12.0
pyramidal Q12.0
associated with
galactosemia E74.21 *[H28]*
myotonic disorders G71.19 *[H28]*
blue Q12.0
central Q12.0
cerulean Q12.0
complicated H26.20
with
neovascularization H26.21-
ocular disorder H26.22-
glaucomatous flecks H26.23-
congenital Q12.0
coraliform Q12.0
coronary Q12.0
crystalline Q12.0
diabetic — *see* Diabetes, cataract
drug-induced H26.3-
due to
ocular disorder — *see* Cataract, complicated
radiation H26.8
electric H26.8
extraction status Z98.4-
glass-blower's H26.8
heat ray H26.8
heterochromic — *see* Cataract, complicated
hypermature — *see* Cataract, senile, morgagnian
type
in (due to)
chronic iridocyclitis — *see* Cataract, complicated
diabetes — *see* Diabetes, cataract
endocrine disease E34.9 *[H28]*
eye disease — *see* Cataract, complicated
hypoparathyroidism E20.9 *[H28]*
malnutrition-dehydration E46 *[H28]*
metabolic disease E88.9 *[H28]*
myotonic disorders G71.19 *[H28]*
nutritional disease E63.9 *[H28]*
infantile — *see* Cataract, presenile
irradiational — *see* Cataract, specified NEC
juvenile — *see* Cataract, presenile
malnutrition-dehydration E46 *[H28]*
morgagnian — *see* Cataract, senile, morgagnian
type
myotonic G71.19 *[H28]*
myxedema E03.9 *[H28]*
nuclear
embryonal Q12.0
sclerosis — *see* Cataract, senile, nuclear
presenile H26.00-
combined forms H26.06-
cortical H26.01-
lamellar — *see* Cataract, presenile, cortical
nuclear H26.03-
specified NEC H26.09
subcapsular polar (anterior) H26.04-
posterior H26.05-
zonular — *see* Cataract, presenile, cortical
secondary H26.40

Cataract — *continued*
secondary — *continued*
Soemmering's ring H26.41-
specified NEC H26.49-
to eye disease — *see* Cataract, complicated
senile H25.9
brunescens — *see* Cataract, senile, nuclear
combined forms H25.81-
coronary — *see* Cataract, senile, incipient
cortical H25.01-
hypermature — *see* Cataract, senile, morgagnian
type
incipient (mature) (total) H25.09-
cortical — *see* Cataract, senile, cortical
subcapsular — *see* Cataract, senile,
subcapsular
morgagnian type (hypermature) H25.2-
nuclear (sclerosis) H25.1-
polar subcapsular (anterior) (posterior) — *see*
Cataract, senile, incipient
punctate — *see* Cataract, senile, incipient
specified NEC H25.89
subcapsular polar (anterior) H25.03-
posterior H25.04-
snowflake — *see* Diabetes, cataract
specified NEC H26.8
toxic — *see* Cataract, drug-induced
traumatic H26.10-
localized H26.11-
partially resolved H26.12-
total H26.13-
zonular (perinuclear) Q12.0
Cataracta (*see also* Cataract)
brunescens — *see* Cataract, senile, nuclear
centralis pulverulenta Q12.0
cerulea Q12.0
complicata — *see* Cataract, complicated
congenita Q12.0
coralliformis Q12.0
coronaria Q12.0
diabetic — *see* Diabetes, cataract
membranacea
accreta — *see* Cataract, secondary
congenita Q12.0
nigra — *see* Cataract, senile, nuclear
sunflower — *see* Cataract, complicated
Catarrh, catarrhal (acute) (febrile) (infectious)
(inflammation) (*see also* condition) J00
bronchial — *see* Bronchitis
chest — *see* Bronchitis
chronic J31.0
due to congenital syphilis A50.03
enteric — *see* Enteritis
eustachian H68.009
fauces — *see* Pharyngitis
gastrointestinal — *see* Enteritis
gingivitis K05.00
plaque induced K05.00
nonplaque induced K05.01
hay — *see* Fever, hay
intestinal — *see* Enteritis
larynx, chronic J37.0
liver B15.9
with hepatic coma B15.0
lung — *see* Bronchitis
middle ear, chronic — *see* Otitis, media,
nonsuppurative, chronic, serous
mouth K12.1
nasal (chronic) — *see* Rhinitis
nasobronchial J31.1
nasopharyngeal (chronic) J31.1
acute J00
pulmonary — *see* Bronchitis
spring (eye) (vernal) — *see* Conjunctivitis, acute,
atopic
summer (hay) — *see* Fever, hay
throat J31.2
tubotympanal (*see also* Otitis, media,
nonsuppurative)
chronic — *see* Otitis, media, nonsuppurative,
chronic, serous
Catatonia (schizophrenic) F20.2

Catatonic disorder due to known physiologic condition F06.1
  schizophrenia F20.2
  stupor R40.1
Cat-scratch (*see also* Abrasion)
  disease or fever A28.1
Cauda equina — *see* condition
Cauliflower ear M95.1-
Causalgia (upper limb) G56.4-
  lower limb G57.7-
Cause
  external, general effects T75.89
Caustic burn — *see* Corrosion, by site
Cavare's disease (familial periodic paralysis) G72.3
Cave-in, injury crushing (severe) — *see* Crush
  suffocation — *see* Asphyxia, traumatic, due to low oxygen, due to cave-in
Cavernitis (penis) N48.29
Cavernositis N48.29
Cavernous — *see* condition
Cavitation of lung (*see also* Tuberculosis, pulmonary)
  nontuberculous J98.4
Cavities, dental — *see* Caries, dental
Cavity
  lung — *see* Cavitation of lung
  optic papilla Q14.2
  pulmonary — *see* Cavitation of lung
Cavovarus foot, congenital Q66.1
Cavus foot (congenital) Q66.7
  acquired — *see* Deformity, limb, foot, specified NEC
Cazenave's disease L10.2
Cecitis K52.9
  with perforation, peritonitis, or rupture K65.8
Cecum — *see* condition
Celiac
  artery compression syndrome I77.4
  disease K90.0
  infantilism K90.0
Cell(s), cellular (*see also* condition)
  in urine R82.99
Cellulitis (diffuse) (phlegmonous) (septic) (suppurative) L03.90
  abdominal wall L03.311
  anaerobic A48.0
  ankle — *see* Cellulitis, lower limb
  anus K61.0
  arm — *see* Cellulitis, upper limb
  auricle (ear) — *see* Cellulitis, ear
  axilla L03.11-
  back (any part) L03.312
  broad ligament
    acute N73.0
  buttock L03.317
  cervical (meaning neck) L03.221
  cervix (uteri) — *see* Cervicitis
  cheek (external) L03.211
    internal K12.2
  chest wall L03.313
  chronic L03.90
  clostridial A48.0
  corpus cavernosum N48.22
  digit
    finger — *see* Cellulitis, finger
    toe — *see* Cellulitis, toe
  Douglas' cul-de-sac or pouch
    acute N73.0
  drainage site (following operation) T81.4
  ear (external) H60.1-
  eosinophilic (granulomatous) L98.3
  erysipelatous — *see* Erysipelas
  external auditory canal — *see* Cellulitis, ear
  eyelid — *see* Abscess, eyelid
  face NEC L03.211
  finger (intrathecal) (periosteal) (subcutaneous) (subcuticular) L03.01-
  foot — *see* Cellulitis, lower limb
  gangrenous — *see* Gangrene
  genital organ NEC
    female (external) N76.4
    male N49.9
      multiple sites N49.8
      specified NEC N49.8
  gluteal (region) L03.317

Cellulitis — *continued*
  gonococcal A54.89
  groin L03.314
  hand — *see* Cellulitis, upper limb
  head NEC L03.811
    face (any part, except ear, eye and nose) L03.211
  heel — *see* Cellulitis, lower limb
  hip — *see* Cellulitis, lower limb
  jaw (region) L03.211
  knee — *see* Cellulitis, lower limb
  labium (majus) (minus) — *see* Vulvitis
  lacrimal passages — *see* Inflammation, lacrimal, passages
  larynx J38.7
  leg — *see* Cellulitis, lower limb
  lip K13.0
  lower limb L03.11-
    toe — *see* Cellulitis, toe
  mouth (floor) K12.2
  multiple sites, so stated L03.90
  nasopharynx J39.1
  navel L03.316
    newborn P38.9
      with mild hemorrhage P38.1
      without hemorrhage P38.9
  neck (region) L03.221
  nose (septum) (external) J34.0
  orbit, orbital H05.01-
  palate (soft) K12.2
  pectoral (region) L03.313
  pelvis, pelvic (chronic)
    female (*see also* Disease, pelvis, inflammatory) N73.2
      acute N73.0
    following ectopic or molar pregnancy O08.0
    male K65.0
  penis N48.22
  perineal, perineum L03.315
  perirectal K61.1
  peritonsillar J36
  periurethral N34.0
  periuterine (*see also* Disease, pelvis, inflammatory) N73.2
    acute N73.0
  pharynx J39.1
  rectum K61.1
  retroperitoneal K68.9
  round ligament
    acute N73.0
  scalp (any part) L03.811
  scrotum N49.2
  seminal vesicle N49.0
  shoulder — *see* Cellulitis, upper limb
  specified site NEC L03.818
  submandibular (region) (space) (triangle) K12.2
    gland K11.3
  submaxillary (region) K12.2
    gland K11.3
  thigh — *see* Cellulitis, lower limb
  thumb (intrathecal) (periosteal) (subcutaneous) (subcuticular) — *see* Cellulitis, finger
  toe (intrathecal) (periosteal) (subcutaneous) (subcuticular) L03.03-
  tonsil J36
  trunk L03.319
    abdominal wall L03.311
    back (any part) L03.312
    buttock L03.317
    chest wall L03.313
    groin L03.314
    perineal, perineum L03.315
    umbilicus L03.316
  tuberculous (primary) A18.4
  umbilicus L03.316
  upper limb L03.11-
    axilla — *see* Cellulitis, axilla
    finger — *see* Cellulitis, finger
    thumb — *see* Cellulitis, finger
  vaccinal T88.0
  vocal cord J38.3
  vulva — *see* Vulvitis
  wrist — *see* Cellulitis, upper limb

Cementoblastoma, benign — *see* Cyst, calcifying odontogenic
Cementoma — *see* Cyst, calcifying odontogenic
Cementoperiostitis — *see* Periodontitis
Cementosis K03.4
Central auditory processing disorder H93.25
Central pain syndrome G89.0
Cephalematocele, cephal(o)hematocele
  newborn P52.8
    birth injury P10.8
  traumatic — *see* Hematoma, brain
Cephalematoma, cephalhematoma (calcified)
  newborn (birth injury) P12.0
  traumatic — *see* Hematoma, brain
Cephalgia, cephalalgia (*see also* Headache)
  histamine G44.009
    intractable G44.001
    not intractable G44.009
  trigeminal autonomic (TAC) NEC G44.099
    intractable G44.091
    not intractable G44.099
Cephalic — *see* condition
Cephalitis — *see* Encephalitis
Cephalocele — *see* Encephalocele
Cephalomenia N94.89
Cephalopelvic — *see* condition
Cerclage (with cervical incompetence) **in pregnancy** — *see* Incompetence, cervix, in pregnancy
Cerebellitis — *see* Encephalitis
Cerebellum, cerebellar — *see* condition
Cerebral — *see* condition
Cerebritis — *see* Encephalitis
Cerebro-hepato-renal syndrome Q87.89
Cerebromalacia — *see* Softening, brain
  sequelae of cerebrovascular disease I69.398
Cerebroside lipidosis E75.22
Cerebrospasticity (congenital) G80.1
Cerebrospinal — *see* condition
Cerebrum — *see* condition
Ceroid-lipofuscinosis, neuronal E75.4
Cerumen (accumulation) (impacted) H61.2-
Cervical (*see also* condition)
  auricle Q18.2
  dysplasia in pregnancy — *see* Abnormal, cervix, in pregnancy or childbirth
  erosion in pregnancy — *see* Abnormal, cervix, in pregnancy or childbirth
  fibrosis in pregnancy — *see* Abnormal, cervix, in pregnancy or childbirth
  fusion syndrome Q76.1
  rib Q76.5
  shortening (complicating pregnancy) O26.87-
Cervicalgia M54.2
Cervicitis (acute) (chronic) (nonvenereal) (senile (atrophic)) (subacute) (with ulceration) N72
  with
    abortion — *see* Abortion, by type complicated by genital tract and pelvic infection
    ectopic pregnancy O08.0
    molar pregnancy O08.0
  chlamydial A56.09
  gonococcal A54.03
  herpesviral A60.03
  puerperal (postpartum) O86.11
  syphilitic A52.76
  trichomonal A59.09
  tuberculous A18.16
Cervicocolpitis (emphysematosa) (*see also* Cervicitis) N72
Cervix — *see* condition
Cesarean delivery, previous, affecting management of pregnancy O34.21
Céstani (-Chenais) **paralysis or syndrome** G46.3
Céstan-Raymond syndrome I65.8
Cestode infestation B71.9
  specified type NEC B71.8
Cestodiasis B71.9
Chabert's disease A22.9
Chacaleh E53.8
Chafing L30.4
Chagas' (-Mazza) **disease** (chronic) B57.2
  with
    cardiovascular involvement NEC B57.2
    digestive system involvement B57.30

- **Chagas' (-Mazza) disease** — *continued*
  - with — *continued*
    - digestive system involvement — *continued*
      - megacolon B57.32
      - megaesophagus B57.31
      - other specified B57.39
    - megacolon B57.32
    - megaesophagus B57.31
    - myocarditis B57.2
    - nervous system involvement B57.4Ø
      - meningitis B57.41
      - meningoencephalitis B57.42
      - other specified B57.49
    - specified organ involvement NEC B57.5
  - acute (with) B57.1
    - cardiovascular NEC B57.Ø
    - myocarditis B57.Ø
- **Chagres fever** B5Ø.9
- **Chairridden** Z74.Ø9
- **Chalasia** (cardiac sphincter) K21.9
- **Chalazion** HØØ.19
  - left HØØ.16
    - lower HØØ.15
    - upper HØØ.14
  - right HØØ.13
    - lower HØØ.12
    - upper HØØ.11
- **Chalcosis** (*see also* Disorder, globe, degenerative, chalcosis)
  - cornea — *see* Deposit, cornea
  - crystalline lens — *see* Cataract, complicated
  - retina H35.89
- **Chalicosis** (pulmonum) J62.8
- **Chancre** (any genital site) (hard) (hunterian) (mixed) (primary) (seronegative) (seropositive) (syphilitic) A51.Ø
  - congenital A5Ø.Ø7
  - conjunctiva NEC A51.2
  - Ducrey's A57
  - extragenital A51.2
  - eyelid A51.2
  - lip A51.2
  - nipple A51.2
  - Nisbet's A57
  - of
    - carate A67.Ø
    - pinta A67.Ø
    - yaws A66.Ø
  - palate, soft A51.2
  - phagedenic A57
  - simple A57
  - soft A57
    - bubo A57
    - palate A51.2
  - urethra A51.Ø
  - yaws A66.Ø
- **Chancroid** (anus) (genital) (penis) (perineum) (rectum) (urethra) (vulva) A57
- **Chandler's disease** (osteochondritis dissecans, hip) — *see* Osteochondritis, dissecans, hip
- **Change(s)** (in) (of) (*see also* Removal)
  - arteriosclerotic — *see* Arteriosclerosis
  - bone (*see also* Disorder, bone)
    - diabetic — *see* Diabetes, bone change
  - bowel habit R19.4
  - cardiorenal (vascular) — *see* Hypertension, cardiorenal
  - cardiovascular — *see* Disease, cardiovascular
  - circulatory I99.9
  - cognitive (mild) (organic) R41.89
  - color, tooth, teeth
    - during formation KØØ.8
    - posteruptive KØ3.7
  - contraceptive device Z3Ø.433
  - corneal membrane H18.3Ø
    - Bowman's membrane fold or rupture H18.31-
    - Descemet's membrane
      - fold H18.32-
      - rupture H18.33-
  - coronary — *see* Disease, heart, ischemic
  - degenerative, spine or vertebra — *see* Spondylosis
  - dental pulp, regressive KØ4.2
  - dressing (nonsurgical) Z48.ØØ
- **Change(s)** (in) (of) — *continued*
  - dressing (nonsurgical) — *continued*
    - surgical Z48.Ø1
  - heart — *see* Disease, heart
  - hip joint — *see* Derangement, joint, hip
  - hyperplastic larynx J38.7
  - hypertrophic
    - nasal sinus J34.89
    - turbinate, nasal J34.3
    - upper respiratory tract J39.8
  - indwelling catheter Z46.6
  - inflammatory (*see also* Inflammation)
    - sacroiliac M46.1
  - job, anxiety concerning Z56.1
  - joint — *see* Derangement, joint
  - life — *see* Menopause
  - mental status R41.82
  - minimal (glomerular) (*see also* NØØ-NØ7 with fourth character .Ø) NØ5.Ø
  - myocardium, myocardial — *see* Degeneration, myocardial
  - of life — *see* Menopause
  - pacemaker Z45.Ø18
    - pulse generator Z45.Ø1Ø
  - personality (enduring) F68.8
    - due to (secondary to)
      - general medical condition FØ7.Ø
    - secondary (nonspecific) F6Ø.89
  - regressive, dental pulp KØ4.2
  - renal — *see* Disease, renal
  - retina H35.9
    - myopic H44.2-
  - sacroiliac joint M53.3
  - senile (*see also* condition) R54
  - sensory R2Ø.8
  - skin R23.9
    - acute, due to ultraviolet radiation L56.9
      - specified NEC L56.8
    - chronic, due to nonionizing radiation L57.9
      - specified NEC L57.8
    - cyanosis R23.Ø
    - flushing R23.2
    - pallor R23.1
    - petechiae R23.3
    - specified change NEC R23.8
    - swelling — *see* Mass, localized
    - texture R23.4
  - trophic
    - arm — *see* Mononeuropathy, upper limb
    - leg — *see* Mononeuropathy, lower limb
  - vascular I99.9
  - vasomotor I73.9
  - voice R49.9
    - psychogenic F44.4
    - specified NEC R49.8
- **Changing sleep-work schedule, affecting sleep** G47.26
- **Changuinola fever** A93.1
- **Chapping skin** T69.8
- **Charcot-Marie-Tooth disease, paralysis or syndrome** G6Ø.Ø
- **Charcot's**
  - arthropathy — *see* Arthropathy, neuropathic
  - cirrhosis K74.3
  - disease (tabetic arthropathy) A52.16
  - joint (disease) (tabetic) A52.16
    - diabetic — *see* Diabetes, with, arthropathy
    - syringomyelic G95.Ø
  - syndrome (intermittent claudication) I73.9
- **CHARGE association** Q89.8
- **Charley-horse** (quadriceps) M62.831
  - traumatic (quadriceps) S76.11-
- **Charlouis' disease** — *see* Yaws
- **Cheadle's disease** E54
- **Checking** (of)
  - cardiac pacemaker (battery) (electrode(s)) Z45.Ø18
    - pulse generator Z45.Ø1Ø
  - intrauterine contraceptive device Z3Ø.431
- **Check-up** — *see* Examination
- **Chédiak-Higashi** (-Steinbrinck) **syndrome** (congenital gigantism of peroxidase granules) E7Ø.33Ø
- **Cheek** — *see* condition
- **Cheese itch** B88.Ø
- **Cheese-washer's lung** J67.8
- **Cheese-worker's lung** J67.8
- **Cheilitis** (acute) (angular) (catarrhal) (chronic) (exfoliative) (gangrenous) (glandular) (infectional) (suppurative) (ulcerative) (vesicular) K13.Ø
  - actinic (due to sun) L56.8
    - other than from sun L59.8
  - candidal B37.83
- **Cheilodynia** K13.Ø
- **Cheiloschisis** — *see* Cleft, lip
- **Cheilosis** (angular) K13.Ø
  - with pellagra E52
  - due to
    - vitamin B2 (riboflavin) deficiency E53.Ø
- **Cheiromegaly** M79.89
- **Cheiropompholyx** L3Ø.1
- **Cheloid** — *see* Keloid
- **Chemical burn** — *see* Corrosion, by site
- **Chemodectoma** — *see* Paraganglioma, nonchromaffin
- **Chemosis, conjunctiva** — *see* Edema, conjunctiva
- **Chemotherapy** (session) (for)
  - cancer Z51.11
  - neoplasm Z51.11
- **Cherubism** M27.8
- **Chest** — *see* condition
- **Cheyne-Stokes breathing** (respiration) RØ6.3
- **Chiari's**
  - disease or syndrome (hepatic vein thrombosis) I82.Ø
  - malformation
    - type I G93.5
    - type II — *see* Spina bifida
  - net Q24.8
- **Chicago disease** B4Ø.9
- **Chickenpox** — *see* Varicella
- **Chiclero ulcer or sore** B55.1
- **Chigger** (infestation) B88.Ø
- **Chignon** (disease) B36.8
  - newborn (from vacuum extraction) (birth injury) P12.1
- **Chilaiditi's syndrome** (subphrenic displacement, colon) Q43.3
- **Chilblain(s)** (lupus) T69.1
- **Child**
  - custody dispute Z65.3
- **Childbirth** — *see* Delivery
- **Childhood**
  - cerebral X-linked adrenoleukodystrophy E71.52Ø
  - period of rapid growth ZØØ.2
- **Chill(s) R68.83** with fever R5Ø.9
  - congestive in malarial regions B54
  - without fever R68.83
- **Chilomastigiasis** AØ7.8
- **Chimera 46,XX/46,XY** Q99.Ø
- **Chin** — *see* condition
- **Chinese dysentery** AØ3.9
- **Chionophobia** F4Ø.228
- **Chitral fever** A93.1
- **Chlamydia, chlamydial** A74.9
  - cervicitis A56.Ø9
  - conjunctivitis A74.Ø
  - cystitis A56.Ø1
  - endometritis A56.11
  - epididymitis A56.19
  - female
    - pelvic inflammatory disease A56.11
    - pelviperitonitis A56.11
  - orchitis A56.19
  - peritonitis A74.81
  - pharyngitis A56.4
  - proctitis A56.3
  - psittaci (infection) A7Ø
  - salpingitis A56.11
  - sexually-transmitted infection NEC A56.8
  - specified NEC A74.89
  - urethritis A56.Ø1
  - vulvovaginitis A56.Ø2
- **Chlamydiosis** — *see* Chlamydia
- **Chloasma** (skin) (idiopathic) (symptomatic) L81.1
  - eyelid HØ2.719
    - hyperthyroid EØ5.9Ø *[HØ2.719]*
      - with thyroid storm EØ5.91 *[HØ2.719]*

- **Chloasma** — *continued*
  - eyelid — *continued*
    - left HØ2.716
      - lower HØ2.715
      - upper HØ2.714
    - right HØ2.713
      - lower HØ2.712
      - upper HØ2.711
- **Chloroma** C92.3-
- **Chlorosis** D5Ø.9
  - Egyptian B76.9 *[D63.8]*
  - miner's B76.9 *[D63.8]*
- **Chlorotic anemia** D5Ø.8
- **Chocolate cyst** (ovary) N8Ø.1
- **Choked**
  - disc or disk — *see* Papilledema
  - on food, phlegm, or vomitus NOS — *see* Foreign body, by site
  - while vomiting NOS — *see* Foreign body, by site
- **Chokes** (resulting from bends) T7Ø.3
- **Choking sensation** RØ9.89
- **Cholangiectasis** K83.8
- **Cholangiocarcinoma**
  - with hepatocellular carcinoma, combined C22.Ø
  - liver C22.1
  - specified site NEC — *see* Neoplasm, malignant, by site
  - unspecified site C22.1
- **Cholangiohepatitis** K83.8
  - due to fluke infestation B66.1
- **Cholangiohepatoma** C22.Ø
- **Cholangiolitis** (acute) (chronic) (extrahepatic) (gangrenous) (intrahepatic) K83.Ø
  - paratyphoidal — *see* Fever, paratyphoid
  - typhoidal AØ1.Ø9
- **Cholangioma** D13.4
  - malignant — *see* Cholangiocarcinoma
- **Cholangitis** (ascending) (primary) (recurrent) (sclerosing) (secondary) (stenosing) (suppurative) K83.Ø
  - with calculus, bile duct — *see* Calculus, bile duct, with cholangitis
  - chronic nonsuppurative destructive K74.3
- **Cholecystectasia** K82.8
- **Cholecystitis** K81.9
  - with
    - calculus, stones in
      - bile duct (common) (hepatic) — *see* Calculus, bile duct, with cholecystitis
      - cystic duct — *see* Calculus, gallbladder, with cholecystitis
      - gallbladder — *see* Calculus, gallbladder, with cholecystitis
    - choledocholithiasis — *see* Calculus, bile duct, with cholecystitis
    - cholelithiasis — *see* Calculus, gallbladder, with cholecystitis
  - acute (emphysematous) (gangrenous) (suppurative) K81.Ø
    - with
      - calculus, stones in
        - cystic duct — *see* Calculus, gallbladder, with cholecystitis, acute
        - gallbladder — *see* Calculus, gallbladder, with cholecystitis, acute
      - choledocholithiasis — *see* Calculus, bile duct, with cholecystitis, acute
      - cholelithiasis — *see* Calculus, gallbladder, with cholecystitis, acute
      - chronic cholecystitis K81.2
        - with gallbladder calculus K8Ø.12
          - with obstruction K8Ø.13
  - chronic K81.1
    - with acute cholecystitis K81.2
      - with gallbladder calculus K8Ø.12
        - with obstruction K8Ø.13
  - emphysematous (acute) — *see* Cholecystitis, acute
  - gangrenous — *see* Cholecystitis, acute
  - paratyphoidal, current AØ1.4
  - suppurative — *see* Cholecystitis, acute
  - typhoidal AØ1.Ø9
- **Cholecystolithiasis** — *see* Calculus, gallbladder
- **Choledochitis** (suppurative) K83.Ø
- **Choledocholith** — *see* Calculus, bile duct
- **Choledocholithiasis** (common duct) (hepatic duct) — *see* Calculus, bile duct
  - cystic — *see* Calculus, gallbladder
  - typhoidal AØ1.Ø9
- **Cholelithiasis** (cystic duct) (gallbladder) (impacted) (multiple) — *see* Calculus, gallbladder
  - bile duct (common) (hepatic) — *see* Calculus, bile duct
  - hepatic duct — *see* Calculus, bile duct
  - specified NEC K8Ø.8Ø
    - with obstruction K8Ø.81
- **Cholemia** (*see also* Jaundice)
  - familial (simple) (congenital) E8Ø.4
  - Gilbert's E8Ø.4
- **Choleperitoneum, choleperitonitis** K65.3
- **Cholera** (Asiatic) (epidemic) (malignant) AØØ.9
  - antimonial — *see* Poisoning, antimony
  - classical AØØ.Ø
  - due to Vibrio cholerae Ø1 AØØ.9
    - biovar cholerae AØØ.Ø
    - biovar eltor AØØ.1
    - el tor AØØ.1
  - el tor AØØ.1
- **Cholerine** — *see* Cholera
- **Cholestasis NEC** K83.1
  - with hepatocyte injury K71.Ø
  - due to total parenteral nutrition (TPN) K76.89
  - pure K71.Ø
- **Cholesteatoma** (ear) (middle) (with reaction) H71.9-
  - attic H71.Ø-
  - external ear (canal) H6Ø.4-
  - mastoid H71.2-
  - postmastoidectomy cavity (recurrent) — *see* Complications, postmastoidectomy, recurrent cholesteatoma
  - recurrent (postmastoidectomy) — *see* Complications, postmastoidectomy, recurrent cholesteatoma
  - tympanum H71.1-
- **Cholesteatosis, diffuse** H71.3-
- **Cholesteremia** E78.Ø
- **Cholesterin in vitreous** — *see* Deposit, crystalline
- **Cholesterol**
  - deposit
    - retina H35.89
    - vitreous — *see* Deposit, crystalline
  - elevated (high) E78.Ø
    - with elevated (high) triglycerides E78.2
    - screening for Z13.22Ø
  - imbibition of gallbladder K82.4
- **Cholesterolemia** (essential) (familial) (hereditary) (pure) E78.Ø
- **Cholesterolosis, cholesterosis** (gallbladder) K82.4
  - cerebrotendinous E75.5
- **Cholocolic fistula** K82.3
- **Choluria** R82.2
- **Chondritis** M94.8x9
  - aurical H61.Ø3-
  - costal (Tietze's) M94.Ø
  - external ear H61.Ø3-
  - patella, posttraumatic — *see* Chondromalacia, patella
  - pinna H61.Ø3-
  - purulent M94.8X-
  - tuberculous NEC A18.Ø2
    - intervertebral A18.Ø1
- **Chondroblastoma** (*see also* Neoplasm, bone, benign)
  - malignant — *see* Neoplasm, bone, malignant
- **Chondrocalcinosis** M11.2Ø
  - ankle M11.27-
  - elbow M11.22-
  - familial M11.1Ø
    - ankle M11.17-
    - elbow M11.12-
    - foot joint M11.17-
    - hand joint M11.14-
    - hip M11.15-
    - knee M11.16-
    - multiple site M11.19
    - shoulder M11.11-
    - vertebrae M11.18
    - wrist M11.13-
- **Chondrocalcinosis** — *continued*
  - foot joint M11.27-
  - hand joint M11.24-
  - hip M11.25-
  - knee M11.26-
  - multiple site M11.29
  - shoulder M11.21-
  - specified type NEC M11.2Ø
    - ankle M11.27-
    - elbow M11.22-
    - foot joint M11.27-
    - hand joint M11.24-
    - hip M11.25-
    - knee M11.26-
    - multiple site M11.29
    - shoulder M11.21-
    - vertebrae M11.28
    - wrist M11.23-
  - vertebrae M11.28
  - wrist M11.23-
- **Chondrodermatitis nodularis helicis or anthelicis** — *see* Perichondritis, ear
- **Chondrodysplasia** Q78.9
  - with hemangioma Q78.4
  - calcificans congenita Q77.3
  - fetalis Q77.4
  - metaphyseal (Jansen's) (McKusick's) (Schmid's) Q78.5
  - punctata Q77.3
- **Chondrodystrophy, chondrodystrophia** (familial) (fetalis) (hypoplastic) Q78.9
  - calcificans congenita Q77.3
  - myotonic (congenital) G71.13
  - punctata Q77.3
- **Chondroectodermal dysplasia** Q77.6
- **Chondrogenesis imperfecta** Q77.4
- **Chondrolysis** M94.35-
- **Chondroma** (*see also* Neoplasm, cartilage, benign)
  - juxtacortical — *see* Neoplasm, bone, benign
  - periosteal — *see* Neoplasm, bone, benign
- **Chondromalacia** (systemic) M94.2Ø
  - acromioclavicular joint M94.21-
  - ankle M94.27-
  - elbow M94.22-
  - foot joint M94.27-
  - glenohumeral joint M94.21-
  - hand joint M94.24-
  - hip M94.25-
  - knee M94.26-
    - patella M22.4-
  - multiple sites M94.29
  - patella M22.4-
  - rib M94.28
  - sacroiliac joint M94.259
  - shoulder M94.21-
  - sternoclavicular joint M94.21-
  - vertebral joint M94.28
  - wrist M94.23-
- **Chondromatosis** (*see also* Neoplasm, cartilage, uncertain behavior)
  - internal Q78.4
- **Chondromyxosarcoma** — *see* Neoplasm, cartilage, malignant
- **Chondro-osteodysplasia** (Morquio-Brailsford type) E76.219
- **Chondro-osteodystrophy** E76.29
- **Chondro-osteoma** — *see* Neoplasm, bone, benign
- **Chondropathia tuberosa** M94.Ø
- **Chondrosarcoma** — *see* Neoplasm, cartilage, malignant
  - juxtacortical — *see* Neoplasm, bone, malignant
  - mesenchymal — *see* Neoplasm, connective tissue, malignant
  - myxoid — *see* Neoplasm, cartilage, malignant
- **Chordee** (nonvenereal) N48.89
  - congenital Q54.4
  - gonococcal A54.Ø9
- **Chorditis** (fibrinous) (nodosa) (tuberosa) J38.2
- **Chordoma** — *see* Neoplasm, vertebral (column), malignant
- **Chorea** (chronic) (gravis) (posthemiplegic) (senile) (spasmodic) G25.5

Chorea — *continued*
- with
  - heart involvement I02.Ø
    - active or acute (conditions in IØ1-) IØ2.Ø
    - rheumatic IØ2.9
      - with valvular disorder IØ2.Ø
  - rheumatic heart disease (chronic) (inactive)(quiescent)—code to rheumatic heart condition involved
- drug-induced G25.4
- habit F95.8
- hereditary G1Ø
- Huntington's G1Ø
- hysterical F44.4
- minor IØ2.9
  - with heart involvement IØ2.Ø
- progressive G25.5
  - hereditary G1Ø
- rheumatic (chronic) IØ2.9
  - with heart involvement IØ2.Ø
- Sydenham's IØ2.9
  - with heart involvement — *see* Chorea, with rheumatic heart disease
  - nonrheumatic G25.5

Choreoathetosis (paroxysmal) G25.5
Chorioadenoma (destruens) D39.2
Chorioamnionitis O41.12-
Chorioangioma D26.7
Choriocarcinoma — *see* Neoplasm, malignant, by site
- combined with
  - embryonal carcinoma — *see* Neoplasm, malignant, by site
  - other germ cell elements — *see* Neoplasm, malignant, by site
  - teratoma — *see* Neoplasm, malignant, by site
- specified site — *see* Neoplasm, malignant, by site
- unspecified site
  - female C58
  - male C62.9Ø

Chorioencephalitis (acute) (lymphocytic) (serous) A87.2
Chorioepithelioma — *see* Choriocarcinoma
Choriomeningitis (acute) (lymphocytic) (serous) A87.2
Chorionepithelioma — *see* Choriocarcinoma
Chorioretinitis (*see also* Inflammation, chorioretinal)
- disseminated (*see also* Inflammation, chorioretinal, disseminated)
  - in neurosyphilis A52.19
- focal (*see also* Inflammation, chorioretinal, focal)
- Egyptian B76.9 *[D63.8]*
- histoplasmic B39.9 *[H32]*
- in (due to)
  - histoplasmosis B39.9 *[H32]*
  - syphilis (secondary) A51.43
    - late A52.71
  - toxoplasmosis (acquired) B58.Ø1
    - congenital (active) P37.1 *[H32]*
  - tuberculosis A18.53
- juxtapapillary, juxtapapillaris — *see* Inflammation, chorioretinal, focal, juxtapapillary
- leprous A3Ø.9 *[H32]*
- miner's B76.9 *[D63.8]*
- progressive myopia (degeneration) H44.2-
- syphilitic (secondary) A51.43
  - congenital (early) A5Ø.Ø1 *[H32]*
    - late A5Ø.32
  - late A52.71
- tuberculous A18.53

Chorioretinopathy, central serous H35.71-
Choroid — *see* condition
Choroideremia H31.21
Choroiditis — *see* Chorioretinitis
Choroidopathy — *see* Disorder, choroid
Choroidoretinitis — *see* Chorioretinitis
Choroidoretinopathy, central serous — *see* Chorioretinopathy, central serous
Christian-Weber disease M35.6
Christmas disease D67
Chromaffinoma (*see also* Neoplasm, benign, by site)
- malignant — *see* Neoplasm, malignant, by site

Chromatopsia — *see* Deficiency, color vision
Chromhidrosis, chromidrosis L75.1
Chromoblastomycosis — *see* Chromomycosis
Chromoconversion R82.91
Chromomycosis B43.9
- brain abscess B43.1
- cerebral B43.1
- cutaneous B43.Ø
- skin B43.Ø
- specified NEC B43.8
- subcutaneous abscess or cyst B43.2

Chromophytosis B36.Ø
Chromosome — *see* condition by chromosome involved
- D(1) — *see* condition, chromosome 13
- E(3) — *see* condition, chromosome 18
- G — *see* condition, chromosome 21

Chromotrichomycosis B36.8
Chronic — *see* condition
- fracture — *see* Fracture, pathological

Churg-Strauss syndrome M3Ø.1
Chyle cyst, mesentery I89.8
Chylocele (nonfilarial) I89.8
- filarial (*see also* Infestation, filarial) B74.9 *[N51]*
- tunica vaginalis N5Ø.8
  - filarial (*see also* Infestation, filarial) B74.9 *[N51]*

Chylomicronemia (fasting) (with hyperprebetalipoproteinemia) E78.3
Chylopericardium I31.3
- acute I3Ø.9

Chylothorax (nonfilarial) I89.8
- filarial (*see also* Infestation, filarial) B74.9 *[J91.8]*

Chylous — *see* condition
Chyluria (nonfilarial) R82.Ø
- due to
  - bilharziasis B65.Ø
  - Brugia (malayi) B74.1
    - timori B74.2
  - schistosomiasis (bilharziasis) B65.Ø
  - Wuchereria (bancrofti) B74.Ø
- filarial — *see* Infestation, filarial

Cicatricial (deformity) — *see* Cicatrix
Cicatrix (adherent) (contracted) (painful) (vicious) (*see also* Scar) L9Ø.5
- adenoid (and tonsil) J35.8
- alveolar process M26.79
- anus K62.89
- auricle — *see* Disorder, pinna, specified type NEC
- bile duct (common) (hepatic) K83.8
- bladder N32.89
- bone — *see* Disorder, bone, specified type NEC
- brain G93.89
- cervix (postoperative) (postpartal) N88.1
- common duct K83.8
- cornea H17.9
  - tuberculous A18.59
- duodenum (bulb), obstructive K31.5
- esophagus K22.2
- eyelid — *see* Disorder, eyelid function
- hypopharynx J39.2
- lacrimal passages — *see* Obstruction, lacrimal
- larynx J38.7
- lung J98.4
- middle ear — *see* subcategory H74.8
- mouth K13.79
- muscle M62.89
  - with contracture *see* Contraction, muscle NEC
- nasopharynx J39.2
- palate (soft) K13.79
- penis N48.89
- pharynx J39.2
- prostate N42.89
- rectum K62.89
- retina — *see* Scar, chorioretinal
- semilunar cartilage — *see* Derangement, meniscus
- seminal vesicle N5Ø.8
- skin L9Ø.5
  - infected LØ8.89
  - postinfective L9Ø.5
  - tuberculous B9Ø.8
- specified site NEC L9Ø.5
- throat J39.2
- tongue K14.8
- tonsil (and adenoid) J35.8
- trachea J39.8

Cicatrix — *continued*
- tuberculous NEC B9Ø.9
- urethra N36.8
- uterus N85.8
- vagina N89.8
  - postoperative N99.2
- vocal cord J38.3
- wrist, constricting (annular) L9Ø.5

CIDP (chronic inflammatory demyelinating polyneuropathy) G61.81
CIN — *see* Neoplasia, intraepithelial, cervix
Cinchonism — *see* Deafness, ototoxic
- correct substance properly administered — *see* Table of Drugs and Chemicals, by drug, adverse effect
- overdose or wrong substance given or taken — *see* Table of Drugs and Chemicals, by drug, poisoning

Circle of Willis — *see* condition
Circular — *see* condition
Circulating anticoagulants (*see also* Disorder, hemorrhagic) D68.318
- due to drugs (*see also* Disorder, hemorrhagic) D68.32
- following childbirth O72.3

Circulation
- collateral, any site I99.8
- defective (lower extremity) I99.8
  - congenital Q28.9
- embryonic Q28.9
- failure (peripheral) R57.9
  - newborn P29.89
- fetal, persistent P29.3
- heart, incomplete Q28.9

Circulatory system — *see* condition
Circulus senilis (cornea) — *see* Degeneration, cornea, senile
Circumcision (in absence of medical indication) (ritual) (routine) Z41.2
Circumscribed — *see* condition
Circumvallate placenta O43.11-
Cirrhosis, cirrhotic (hepatic) (liver) K74.6Ø
- alcoholic K7Ø.3Ø
  - with ascites K7Ø.31
- atrophic — *see* Cirrhosis, liver
- Baumgarten-Cruveilhier K74.69
- biliary (cholangiolitic) (cholangitic) (hypertrophic) (obstructive) (pericholangiolitic) K74.5
  - due to
    - Clonorchiasis B66.1
    - flukes B66.3
  - primary K74.3
  - secondary K74.4
- cardiac (of liver) K76.1
- Charcot's K74.3
- cholangiolitic, cholangitic, cholostatic (primary) K74.3
- congestive K76.1
- Cruveilhier-Baumgarten K74.69
- cryptogenic (liver) K74.69
- due to
  - hepatolenticular degeneration E83.Ø1
  - Wilson's disease E83.Ø1
  - xanthomatosis E78.2
- fatty K76.Ø
  - alcoholic K7Ø.Ø
- Hanot's (hypertrophic) K74.3
- hepatic — *see* Cirrhosis, liver
- hypertrophic K74.3
- Indian childhood K74.69
- kidney — *see* Sclerosis, renal
- Laennec's K7Ø.3Ø
  - with ascites K7Ø.31
  - alcoholic K7Ø.3Ø
    - with ascites K7Ø.31
  - nonalcoholic K74.69
- liver K74.6Ø
  - alcoholic K7Ø.3Ø
    - with ascites K7Ø.31
    - fatty K7Ø.Ø
  - congenital P78.81
  - syphilitic A52.74
- lung (chronic) J84.1Ø

Cirrhosis, cirrhotic — *continued*
- macronodular K74.69
  - alcoholic K70.30
    - with ascites K70.31
- micronodular K74.69
  - alcoholic K70.30
    - with ascites K70.31
- mixed type K74.69
- monolobular K74.3
- nephritis — *see* Sclerosis, renal
- nutritional K74.69
  - alcoholic K70.30
    - with ascites K70.31
- obstructive — *see* Cirrhosis, biliary
- ovarian N83.8
- pancreas (duct) K86.8
- pigmentary E83.110
- portal K74.69
  - alcoholic K70.30
    - with ascites K70.31
- postnecrotic K74.69
  - alcoholic K70.30
    - with ascites K70.31
- pulmonary J84.10
- renal — *see* Sclerosis, renal
- spleen D73.2
- stasis K76.1
- Todd's K74.3
- unilobar K74.3
- xanthomatous (biliary) K74.5
  - due to xanthomatosis (familial) (metabolic) (primary) E78.2

Cistern, subarachnoid R93.0
CitrullinemiaE72.23
Citrullinuria E72.23
Civatte's disease or poikiloderma L57.3
Clam digger's itch B65.3
Clammy skin R23.1
Clap — *see* Gonorrhea
Clarke-Hadfield syndrome (pancreatic infantilism) K86.8
Clark's paralysis G80.9
Clastothrix L67.8
Claude Bernard-Horner syndrome G90.2
- traumatic — *see* Injury, nerve, cervical sympathetic

Claude's disease or syndrome G46.3
Claudication, intermittent I73.9
- cerebral (artery) G45.9
- spinal cord (arteriosclerotic) G95.19
  - syphilitic A52.09
- venous (axillary) I87.8

Claudicatio venosa intermittens I87.8
Claustrophobia F40.240
Clavus (infected) L84
Clawfoot (congenital) Q66.89
- acquired — *see* Deformity, limb, clawfoot

Clawhand (acquired) (*see also* Deformity, limb, clawhand)
- congenital Q68.1

Clawtoe (congenital) Q66.89
- acquired — *see* Deformity, toe, specified NEC

Clay eating — *see* Pica
Cleansing of artificial opening — *see* Attention to, artificial, opening
Cleft (congenital) (*see also* Imperfect, closure)
- alveolar process M26.79
- branchial (cyst) (persistent) Q18.2
- cricoid cartilage, posterior Q31.8
- lip (unilateral) Q36.9
  - with cleft palate Q37.9
    - hard Q37.1
      - with soft Q37.5
    - soft Q37.3
      - with hard Q37.5
  - bilateral Q36.0
    - with cleft palate Q37.8
      - hard Q37.0
        - with soft Q37.4
      - soft Q37.2
        - with hard Q37.4
  - median Q36.1
- nose Q30.2
- palate Q35.9

Cleft — *continued*
- palate — *continued*
  - with cleft lip (unilateral) Q37.9
    - bilateral Q37.8
  - hard Q35.1
    - with
      - cleft lip (unilateral) Q37.1
        - bilateral Q37.0
      - soft Q35.5
        - with cleft lip (unilateral) Q37.5
          - bilateral Q37.4
  - medial Q35.5
  - soft Q35.3
    - with
      - cleft lip (unilateral) Q37.3
        - bilateral Q37.2
        - with cleft lip (unilateral) Q37.5
          - bilateral Q37.4
- penis Q55.69
- scrotum Q55.29
- thyroid cartilage Q31.8
- uvula Q35.7

Cleidocranial dysostosis Q74.0
Cleptomania F63.2
Clicking hip (newborn) R29.4
Climacteric (female) (*see also* Menopause)
- arthritis (any site) NEC — *see* Arthritis, specified form NEC
- depression (single episode) F32.8
- male (symptoms) (syndrome) NEC N50.8
- paranoid state F22
- polyarthritis NEC — *see* Arthritis, specified form NEC
- symptoms (female) N95.1

Clinical research investigation (clinical trial) (control subject) (normal comparison) (participant) Z00.6
Clitoris — *see* condition
Cloaca (persistent) Q43.7
Clonorchiasis, clonorchis infection (liver) B66.1
Clonus R25.8
Closed bite M26.29
Clostridium (C.) perfringens, as cause of disease classified elsewhere B96.7
Closure
- congenital, nose Q30.0
- cranial sutures, premature Q75.0
- defective or imperfect NEC — *see* Imperfect, closure
- fistula, delayed — *see* Fistula
- foramen ovale, imperfect Q21.1
- hymen N89.6
- interauricular septum, defective Q21.1
- interventricular septum, defective Q21.0
- lacrimal duct (*see also* Stenosis, lacrimal, duct)
  - congenital Q10.5
- nose (congenital) Q30.0
  - acquired M95.0
- of artificial opening — *see* Attention to, artificial, opening
- vagina N89.5
- valve — *see* Endocarditis
- vulva N90.5

Clot (blood) (*see also* Embolism)
- artery (obstruction) (occlusion) — *see* Embolism
- bladder N32.89
- brain (intradural or extradural) — *see* Occlusion, artery, cerebral
- circulation I74.9
- heart (*see also* Infarct, myocardium)
  - not resulting in infarction I24.0
- vein — *see* Thrombosis

Clouded state R40.1
- epileptic — *see* Epilepsy, specified NEC
- paroxysmal — *see* Epilepsy, specified NEC

Cloudy antrum, antra J32.0
Clouston's (hidrotic) **ectodermal dysplasia** Q82.4
Clubbed nail pachydermoperiostosis M89.40 *[L62]*
Clubbing of finger(s) (nails) R68.3
Clubfinger R68.3
- congenital Q68.1

Clubfoot (congenital) Q66.89
- acquired — *see* Deformity, limb, clubfoot
- equinovarus Q66.0
- paralytic — *see* Deformity, limb, clubfoot

Clubhand
(congenital) (radial) Q71.4-
- acquired — *see* Deformity, limb, clubhand

Clubnail R68.3
- congenital Q84.6

Clump, kidney Q63.1
Clumsiness, clumsy child syndrome F82
Cluttering F80.81
Clutton's joints A50.51 *[M12.80]*
Coagulation, intravascular (diffuse) (disseminated) (*see also* Defibrination syndrome)
- complicating abortion — *see* Abortion, by type, complicated by, intravascular coagulation
- following ectopic or molar pregnancy O08.1

Coagulopathy (*see also* Defect, coagulation)
- consumption D65
- intravascular D65
  - newborn P60

Coalition
- calcaneo-scaphoid Q66.89
- tarsal Q66.89

Coalminer's
- elbow — *see* Bursitis, elbow, olecranon
- lung or pneumoconiosis J60

Coalworker's lung or pneumoconiosis J60
Coarctation
- aorta (preductal) (postductal) Q25.1
- pulmonary artery Q25.71

Coated tongue K14.3
Coats' disease (exudative retinopathy) — *see* Retinopathy, exudative
Cocainism — *see* Dependence, drug, cocaine
Coccidioidomycosis B38.9
- cutaneous B38.3
- disseminated B38.7
- generalized B38.7
- meninges B38.4
- prostate B38.81
- pulmonary B38.2
  - acute B38.0
  - chronic B38.1
- skin B38.3
- specified NEC B38.89

Coccidioidosis — *see* Coccidioidomycosis
Coccidiosis (intestinal) A07.3
Coccydynia, coccygodynia M53.3
Coccyx — *see* condition
Cochin-China diarrhea K90.1
Cockayne's syndrome Q87.1
Cocked up toe — *see* Deformity, toe, specified NEC
Cock's peculiar tumor L72.3
Codman's tumor — *see* Neoplasm, bone, benign
Coenurosis B71.8
Coffee-worker's lung J67.8
Cogan's syndrome H16.32-
- oculomotor apraxia H51.8

Coitus, painful (female) N94.1
- male N53.12
- psychogenic F52.6

Cold J00
- with influenza, flu, or grippe — *see* Influenza, with, respiratory manifestations NEC
- agglutinin disease or hemoglobinuria (chronic) D59.1
- bronchial — *see* Bronchitis
- chest — *see* Bronchitis
- common (head) J00
- effects of T69.9
  - specified effect NEC T69.8
- excessive, effects of T69.9
  - specified effect NEC T69.8
- exhaustion from T69.8
- exposure to T69.9
  - specified effect NEC T69.8
- head J00
- injury syndrome (newborn) P80.0
- on lung — *see* Bronchitis
- rose J30.1
- sensitivity, auto-immune D59.1
- virus J00

Coldsore B00.1

- **Colibacillosis** A49.8
  - as the cause of other disease (*see also* Escherichia coli) B96.2Ø
  - generalized A41.5Ø
- **Colic** (bilious) (infantile) (intestinal) (recurrent) (spasmodic) R1Ø.83
  - abdomen R1Ø.83
    - psychogenic F45.8
  - appendix, appendicular K38.8
  - bile duct — *see* Calculus, bile duct
  - biliary — *see* Calculus, bile duct
  - common duct — *see* Calculus, bile duct
  - cystic duct — *see* Calculus, gallbladder
  - Devonshire NEC — *see* Poisoning, lead
  - gallbladder — *see* Calculus, gallbladder
  - gallstone — *see* Calculus, gallbladder
    - gallbladder or cystic duct — *see* Calculus, gallbladder
  - hepatic (duct) — *see* Calculus, bile duct
  - hysterical F45.8
  - kidney N23
  - lead NEC — *see* Poisoning, lead
  - mucous K58.9
    - with diarrhea K58.Ø
    - psychogenic F54
  - nephritic N23
  - painter's NEC — *see* Poisoning, lead
  - pancreas K86.8
  - psychogenic F45.8
  - renal N23
  - saturnine NEC — *see* Poisoning, lead
  - ureter N23
  - urethral N36.8
    - due to calculus N21.1
  - uterus NEC N94.89
    - menstrual — *see* Dysmenorrhea
  - worm NOS B83.9
- **Colicystitis** — *see* Cystitis
- **Colitis** (acute) (catarrhal) (chronic) (noninfective) (hemorrhagic) (*see also* Enteritis) K52.9
  - allergic K52.2
  - amebic (acute) (*see also* Amebiasis) AØ6.Ø
    - nondysenteric AØ6.2
  - anthrax A22.2
  - bacillary — *see* Infection, Shigella
  - balantidial AØ7.Ø
  - Clostridium difficile AØ4.7
  - coccidial AØ7.3
  - collagenous K52.89
  - cystica superficialis K52.89
  - dietary counseling and surveillance (for) Z71.3
  - dietetic K52.2
  - drug-induced K52.1
  - due to radiation K52.Ø
  - eosinophilic K52.82
  - food hypersensitivity K52.2
  - giardial AØ7.1
  - granulomatous — *see* Enteritis, regional, large intestine
  - infectious — *see* Enteritis, infectious
  - ischemic K55.9
    - acute (fulminant) (subacute) K55.Ø
    - chronic K55.1
    - due to mesenteric artery insufficiency K55.1
    - fulminant (acute) K55.Ø
  - left sided K51.5Ø
    - with
      - complication K51.519
        - specified NEC K51.518
      - abscess K51.514
      - fistula K51.513
      - obstruction K51.512
      - rectal bleeding K51.511
  - lymphocytic K52.89
  - membranous
    - psychogenic F54
  - microscopic (collagenous) (lymphocytic) K52.89
  - mucous — *see* Syndrome, irritable, bowel
    - psychogenic F54
  - noninfective K52.9
    - specified NEC K52.89
  - polyposa — *see* Polyps, colon, inflammatory
  - protozoal AØ7.9

Colitis — *continued*

  - pseudomembranous AØ4.7
  - pseudomucinous — *see* Syndrome, irritable, bowel
  - regional — *see* Enteritis, regional, large intestine
  - segmental — *see* Enteritis, regional, large intestine
  - septic — *see* Enteritis, infectious
  - spastic K58.9
    - with diarrhea K58.Ø
    - psychogenic F54
  - staphylococcal AØ4.8
    - foodborne AØ5.Ø
  - subacute ischemic K55.Ø
  - thromboulcerative K55.Ø
  - toxic NEC K52.1
    - due to Clostridium difficile AØ4.7
  - transmural — *see* Enteritis, regional, large intestine
  - trichomonal AØ7.8
  - tuberculous (ulcerative) A18.32
  - ulcerative (chronic) K51.9Ø
    - with
      - complication K51.919
        - abscess K51.914
        - fistula K51.913
        - obstruction K51.912
        - rectal bleeding K51.911
        - specified complication NEC K51.918
    - enterocolitis — *see* Enterocolitis, ulcerative
    - ileocolitis — *see* Ileocolitis, ulcerative
    - mucosal proctocolitis — *see* Proctocolitis, mucosal
    - proctitis — *see* Proctitis, ulcerative
    - pseudopolyposis — *see* Polyps, colon, inflammatory
    - psychogenic F54
    - rectosigmoiditis — *see* Rectosigmoiditis, ulcerative
    - specified type NEC K51.8Ø
      - with
        - complication K51.819
          - abscess K51.814
          - fistula K51.813
          - obstruction K51.812
          - rectal bleeding K51.811
          - specified complication NEC K51.818
- **Collagenosis, collagen disease** (nonvascular) (vascular) M35.9
  - cardiovascular I42.8
  - reactive perforating L87.1
  - specified NEC M35.8
- **Collapse** R55
  - adrenal E27.2
  - cardiorespiratory R57.Ø
  - cardiovascular R57.Ø
    - newborn P29.89
  - circulatory (peripheral) R57.9
    - during or after labor and delivery O75.1
    - following ectopic or molar pregnancy OØ8.3
    - newborn P29.89
  - during or
    - after labor and delivery O75.1
    - resulting from a procedure, not elsewhere classified T81.1Ø
  - external ear canal — *see* Stenosis, external ear canal
  - general R55
  - heart — *see* Disease, heart
  - heat T67.1
  - hysterical F44.89
  - labyrinth, membranous (congenital) Q16.5
  - lung (massive) (*see also* Atelectasis) J98.19
    - pressure due to anesthesia (general) (local) or other sedation T88.2
      - during labor and delivery O74.1
      - in pregnancy O29.Ø2-
      - postpartum, puerperal O89.Ø9
  - myocardial — *see* Disease, heart
  - nervous F48.8
  - neurocirculatory F45.8
  - nose M95.Ø
  - postoperative (cardiovascular) T81.11
  - pulmonary (*see also* Atelectasis) J98.19
    - newborn — *see* Atelectasis
  - trachea J39.8
  - tracheobronchial J98.Ø9

Collapse — *continued*

  - valvular — *see* Endocarditis
  - vascular (peripheral) R57.9
    - during or after labor and delivery O75.1
    - following ectopic or molar pregnancy OØ8.3
    - newborn P29.89
  - vertebra M48.5Ø-
    - cervical region M48.52-
    - cervicothoracic region M48.53-
    - in (due to)
      - metastasis — *see* Collapse, vertebra, in, specified disease NEC
      - osteoporosis (*see also* Osteoporosis) M8Ø.88
        - cervical region M8Ø.88
        - cervicothoracic region M8Ø.88
        - lumbar region M8Ø.88
        - lumbosacral region M8Ø.88
        - multiple sites M8Ø.88
        - occipito-atlanto-axial region M8Ø.88
        - sacrococcygeal region M8Ø.88
        - thoracic region M8Ø.88
        - thoracolumbar region M8Ø.88
      - specified disease NEC M48.5Ø-
        - cervical region M48.52-
        - cervicothoracic region M48.53-
        - lumbar region M48.56-
        - lumbosacral region M48.57-
        - occipito-atlanto-axial region M48.51-
        - sacrococcygeal region M48.58-
        - thoracic region M48.54-
        - thoracolumbar region M48.55-
    - lumbar region M48.56-
    - lumbosacral region M48.57-
    - occipito-atlanto-axial region M48.51-
    - sacrococcygeal region M48.58-
    - thoracic region M48.54-
    - thoracolumbar region M48.55-
- **Collateral** (*see also* condition)
  - circulation (venous) I87.8
  - dilation, veins I87.8
- **Colles' fracture** S52.53-
- **Collet** (-Sicard) **syndrome** G52.7
- **Collier's asthma or lung** J6Ø
- **Collodion baby** Q8Ø.2
- **Colloid nodule** (of thyroid) (cystic) EØ4.1
- **Coloboma** (iris) Q13.Ø
  - eyelid Q1Ø.3
  - fundus Q14.8
  - lens Q12.2
  - optic disc (congenital) Q14.2
    - acquired H47.31-
- **Coloenteritis** — *see* Enteritis
- **Colon** — *see* condition
- **Colonization**
  - MRSA (methicillin resistant Staphylococcus aureus) Z22.322
  - MSSA (methicillin susceptible Staphylococcus aureus) Z22.321
  - status — *see* Carrier (suspected) of
- **Coloptosis** K63.4
- **Color blindness** — *see* Deficiency, color vision
- **Colostomy**
  - attention to Z43.3
  - fitting or adjustment Z46.89
  - malfunctioning K94.Ø3
  - status Z93.3
- **Colpitis** (acute) — *see* Vaginitis
- **Colpocele** N81.5
- **Colpocystitis** — *see* Vaginitis
- **Colpospasm** N94.2
- **Column, spinal, vertebral** — *see* condition
- **Coma** R4Ø.2Ø
  - with
    - motor response (none) R4Ø.231
      - abnormal R4Ø.233
      - extension R4Ø.232
      - flexion withdrawal R4Ø.234
      - localizes pain R4Ø.235
      - obeys commands R4Ø.236
    - opening of eyes (never) R4Ø.211
      - in response to
        - pain R4Ø.212
        - sound R4Ø.213

- **Coma** — *continued*
  - with — *continued*
    - opening of eyes (never) — *continued*
      - spontaneous R4Ø.214
    - verbal response (none) R4Ø.221
      - confused conversation R4Ø.224
      - inappropriate words R4Ø.223
      - incomprehensible words R4Ø.222
      - oriented R4Ø.225
  - eclamptic — *see* Eclampsia
  - epileptic — *see* Epilepsy
  - Glasgow, scale score — *see* Glasgow coma scale
  - hepatic — *see* Failure, hepatic, by type, with coma
  - hyperglycemic (diabetic) — *see* Diabetes, coma
  - hyperosmolar (diabetic) — *see* Diabetes, coma
  - hypoglycemic (diabetic) — *see* Diabetes, coma, hypoglycemic
    - nondiabetic E15
  - in diabetes — *see* Diabetes, coma
  - insulin-induced — *see* Coma, hypoglycemic
  - myxedematous EØ3.5
  - newborn P91.5
  - persistent vegetative state R4Ø.3
  - specified NEC, without documented Glasgow coma scale score, or with partial Glasgow coma scale score reported R4Ø.244
- **Comatose** — *see* Coma
- **Combat fatigue** F43.Ø
- **Combined** — *see* condition
- **Comedo, comedones** (giant) L7Ø.Ø
- **Comedocarcinoma** (*see also* Neoplasm, breast, malignant)
  - noninfiltrating
    - breast DØ5.8-
    - specified site — *see* Neoplasm, in situ, by site
    - unspecified site DØ5.8-
- **Comedomastitis** — *see* Ectasia, mammary duct
- **Comminuted fracture**—code as Fracture, closed
- **Common**
  - arterial trunk Q2Ø.Ø
  - atrioventricular canal Q21.2
  - atrium Q21.1
  - cold (head) JØØ
  - truncus (arteriosus) Q2Ø.Ø
  - variable immunodeficiency — *see* Immunodeficiency, common variable
  - ventricle Q2Ø.4
- **Commotio, commotion** (current)
  - brain — *see* Injury, intracranial, concussion
  - cerebri — *see* Injury, intracranial, concussion
  - retinae SØ5.8x-
  - spinal cord — *see* Injury, spinal cord, by region
  - spinalis — *see* Injury, spinal cord, by region
- **Communication**
  - between
    - base of aorta and pulmonary artery Q21.4
    - left ventricle and right atrium Q2Ø.5
    - pericardial sac and pleural sac Q34.8
    - pulmonary artery and pulmonary vein, congenital Q25.72
  - congenital between uterus and digestive or urinary tract Q51.7
- **Compartment syndrome** (deep) (posterior) (traumatic) T79.AØ
  - abdomen T79.A3
  - lower extremity (hip, buttock, thigh, leg, foot, toes) T79.A2
  - nontraumatic
    - abdomen M79.A3
    - lower extremity (hip, buttock, thigh, leg, foot, toes) M79.A2-
    - specified site NEC M79.A9
    - upper extremity (shoulder, arm, forearm, wrist, hand, fingers) M79.A1
  - specified site NEC T79.A9
  - upper extremity (shoulder, arm, forearm, wrist, hand, fingers) T79.A1
- **Compensation**
  - failure — *see* Disease, heart
  - neurosis, psychoneurosis — *see* Disorder, factitious
- **Complaint** (*see also* Disease)
  - bowel, functional K59.9
    - psychogenic F45.8
- **Complaint** — *continued*
  - intestine, functional K59.9
    - psychogenic F45.8
  - kidney — *see* Disease, renal
  - miners' J6Ø
- **Complete** — *see* condition
- **Complex**
  - Addison-Schilder E71.528
  - cardiorenal — *see* Hypertension, cardiorenal
  - Costen's M26.69
  - disseminated mycobacterium aviumintracellulare (DMAC) A31.2
  - Eisenmenger's (ventricular septal defect) I27.89
  - hypersexual F52.8
  - jumped process, spine — *see* Dislocation, vertebra
  - primary, tuberculous A15.7
  - Schilder-Addison E71.528
  - subluxation (vertebral) M99.19
    - abdomen M99.19
    - acromioclavicular M99.17
    - cervical region M99.11
    - cervicothoracic M99.11
    - costochondral M99.18
    - costovertebral M99.18
    - head region M99.1Ø
    - hip M99.15
    - lower extremity M99.16
    - lumbar region M99.13
    - lumbosacral M99.13
    - occipitocervical M99.1Ø
    - pelvic region M99.15
    - pubic M99.15
    - rib cage M99.18
    - sacral region M99.14
    - sacrococcygeal M99.14
    - sacroiliac M99.14
    - specified NEC M99.19
    - sternochondral M99.18
    - sternoclavicular M99.17
    - thoracic region M99.12
    - thoracolumbar M99.12
    - upper extremity M99.17
  - Taussig-Bing (transposition, aorta and overriding pulmonary artery) Q2Ø.1
- **Complication**(s) (from) (of)
  - accidental puncture or laceration during a procedure (of) — *see* Complications, intraoperative (intraprocedural), puncture or laceration
  - amputation stump (surgical) (late) NEC T87.9
    - dehiscence T87.81
    - infection or inflammation T87.4Ø
      - lower limb T87.4-
      - upper limb T87.4-
    - necrosis T87.5Ø
      - lower limb T87.5-
      - upper limb T87.5-
    - neuroma T87.3Ø
      - lower limb T87.3-
      - upper limb T87.3-
    - specified type NEC T87.89
  - anastomosis (and bypass) (*see also* Complications, prosthetic device or implant)
    - intestinal (internal) NEC K91.89
      - involving urinary tract N99.89
    - urinary tract (involving intestinal tract) N99.89
    - vascular — *see* Complications, cardiovascular device or implant
  - anesthesia, anesthetic (*see also* Anesthesia, complication) T88.59
    - brain, postpartum, puerperal O89.2
    - cardiac
      - in
        - labor and delivery O74.2
        - pregnancy O29.19-
      - postpartum, puerperal O89.1
    - central nervous system
      - in
        - labor and delivery O74.3
        - pregnancy O29.29-
      - postpartum, puerperal O89.2
    - difficult or failed intubation T88.4
      - in pregnancy O29.6-
- **Complication** — *continued*
  - anesthesia, anesthetic — *continued*
    - failed sedation (conscious) (moderate) during procedure T88.52
    - hyperthermia, malignant T88.3
    - hypothermia T88.51
    - intubation failure T88.4
    - malignant hyperthermia T88.3
    - pulmonary
      - in
        - labor and delivery O74.1
        - pregnancy NEC O29.Ø9-
      - postpartum, puerperal O89.Ø9
    - shock T88.2
    - spinal and epidural
      - in
        - labor and delivery NEC O74.6
          - headache O74.5
        - pregnancy NEC O29.5x-
      - postpartum, puerperal NEC O89.5
        - headache O89.4
  - anti-reflux device — *see* Complications, esophageal anti-reflux device
  - aortic (bifurcation) graft — *see* Complications, graft, vascular
  - aortocoronary (bypass) graft — *see* Complications, coronary artery (bypass) graft
  - aortofemoral (bypass) graft — *see* Complications, extremity artery (bypass) graft
  - arteriovenous
    - fistula, surgically created T82.9
      - embolism T82.818
      - fibrosis T82.828
      - hemorrhage T82.838
      - infection or inflammation T82.7
      - mechanical
        - breakdown T82.51Ø
        - displacement T82.52Ø
        - leakage T82.53Ø
        - malposition T82.52Ø
        - obstruction T82.59Ø
        - perforation T82.59Ø
        - protrusion T82.59Ø
      - pain T82.848
      - specified type NEC T82.898
      - stenosis T82.858
      - thrombosis T82.868
    - shunt, surgically created T82.9
      - embolism T82.818
      - fibrosis T82.828
      - hemorrhage T82.838
      - infection or inflammation T82.7
      - mechanical
        - breakdown T82.511
        - displacement T82.521
        - leakage T82.531
        - malposition T82.521
        - obstruction T82.591
        - perforation T82.591
        - protrusion T82.591
      - pain T82.848
      - specified type NEC T82.898
      - stenosis T82.858
      - thrombosis T82.868
  - arthroplasty — *see* Complications, joint prosthesis
  - artificial
    - fertilization or insemination N98.9
      - attempted introduction (of)
        - embryo in embryo transfer N98.3
        - ovum following in vitro fertilization N98.2
      - hyperstimulation of ovaries N98.1
      - infection N98.Ø
      - specified NEC N98.8
    - heart T82.9
      - embolism T82.817
      - fibrosis T82.827
      - hemorrhage T82.837
      - infection or inflammation T82.7
      - mechanical
        - breakdown T82.512
        - displacement T82.522
        - leakage T82.532
        - malposition T82.522

- **Complication** — *continued*
  - artificial — *continued*
    - heart — *continued*
      - mechanical — *continued*
        - obstruction T82.592
        - perforation T82.592
        - protrusion T82.592
      - pain T82.847
      - specified type NEC T82.897
      - stenosis T82.857
      - thrombosis T82.867
    - opening
      - cecostomy — *see* Complications, colostomy
      - colostomy — *see* Complications, colostomy
      - cystostomy — *see* Complications, cystostomy
      - enterostomy — *see* Complications, enterostomy
      - gastrostomy — *see* Complications, gastrostomy
      - ileostomy — *see* Complications, enterostomy
      - jejunostomy — *see* Complications, enterostomy
      - nephrostomy — *see* Complications, stoma, urinary tract
      - tracheostomy — *see* Complications, tracheostomy
      - ureterostomy — *see* Complications, stoma, urinary tract
      - urethrostomy — *see* Complications, stoma, urinary tract
  - balloon implant or device
    - gastrointestinal T85.9
      - embolism T85.81
      - fibrosis T85.82
      - hemorrhage T85.83
      - infection and inflammation T85.79
      - pain T85.84
      - specified type NEC T85.89
      - stenosis T85.85
      - thrombosis T85.86
    - vascular (counterpulsation) T82.9
      - embolism T82.818
      - fibrosis T82.828
      - hemorrhage T82.838
      - infection or inflammation T82.7
      - mechanical
        - breakdown T82.513
        - displacement T82.523
        - leakage T82.533
        - malposition T82.523
        - obstruction T82.593
        - perforation T82.593
        - protrusion T82.593
      - pain T82.848
      - specified type NEC T82.898
      - stenosis T82.858
      - thrombosis T82.868
  - bariatric procedure
    - gastric band procedure K95.Ø9
      - infection K95.Ø1
    - specified procedure NEC K95.89
      - infection K95.81
  - bile duct implant (prosthetic) T85.9
    - embolism T85.81
    - fibrosis T85.82
    - hemorrhage T85.83
    - infection and inflammation T85.79
    - mechanical
      - breakdown T85.51Ø
      - displacement T85.52Ø
      - malfunction T85.51Ø
      - malposition T85.52Ø
      - obstruction T85.59Ø
      - perforation T85.59Ø
      - protrusion T85.59Ø
      - specified NEC T85.59Ø
    - pain T85.84
    - specified type NEC T85.89
    - stenosis T85.85
    - thrombosis T85.86
  - bladder device (auxiliary) — *see* Complications, genitourinary, device or implant, urinary system

- **Complication** — *continued*
  - bleeding (postoperative) — *see* Complication, postoperative, hemorrhage
    - intraoperative — *see* Complication, intraoperative, hemorrhage
  - blood vessel graft — *see* Complications, graft, vascular
  - bone
    - device NEC T84.9
      - embolism T84.81
      - fibrosis T84.82
      - hemorrhage T84.83
      - infection or inflammation T84.7
      - mechanical
        - breakdown T84.318
        - displacement T84.328
        - malposition T84.328
        - obstruction T84.398
        - perforation T84.398
        - protrusion T84.398
      - pain T84.84
      - specified type NEC T84.89
      - stenosis T84.85
      - thrombosis T84.86
    - graft — *see* Complications, graft, bone
    - growth stimulator (electrode) — *see* Complications, electronic stimulator device, bone
    - marrow transplant — *see* Complications, transplant, bone, marrow
  - brain neurostimulator (electrode) — *see* Complications, electronic stimulator device, brain
  - breast implant (prosthetic) T85.9
    - capsular contracture T85.44
    - embolism T85.81
    - fibrosis T85.82
    - hemorrhage T85.83
    - infection and inflammation T85.79
    - mechanical
      - breakdown T85.41
      - displacement T85.42
      - leakage T85.43
      - malposition T85.42
      - obstruction T85.49
      - perforation T85.49
      - protrusion T85.49
      - specified NEC T85.49
    - pain T85.84
    - specified type NEC T85.89
    - stenosis T85.85
    - thrombosis T85.86
  - bypass (*see also* Complications, prosthetic device or implant)
    - aortocoronary — *see* Complications, coronary artery (bypass) graft
    - arterial (*see also* Complications, graft, vascular)
      - extremity — *see* Complications, extremity artery (bypass) graft
  - cardiac (*see also* Disease, heart)
    - device, implant or graft T82.9
      - embolism T82.817
      - fibrosis T82.827
      - hemorrhage T82.837
      - infection or inflammation T82.7
        - valve prosthesis T82.6
      - mechanical
        - breakdown T82.519
          - specified device NEC T82.518
        - displacement T82.529
          - specified device NEC T82.528
        - leakage T82.539
          - specified device NEC T82.538
        - malposition T82.529
          - specified device NEC T82.528
        - obstruction T82.599
          - specified device NEC T82.598
        - perforation T82.599
          - specified device NEC T82.598
        - protrusion T82.599
          - specified device NEC T82.598
      - pain T82.847
      - specified type NEC T82.897

- **Complication** — *continued*
  - cardiac — *continued*
    - device, implant or graft — *continued*
      - stenosis T82.857
      - thrombosis T82.867
  - cardiovascular device, graft or implant T82.9
    - arteriovenous
      - fistula, artificial — *see* Complication, arteriovenous, fistula, surgically created
      - shunt — *see* Complication, arteriovenous, shunt, surgically created
    - aortic graft — *see* Complications, graft, vascular
    - artificial heart — *see* Complication, artificial, heart
    - balloon (counterpulsation) device — *see* Complication, balloon implant, vascular
    - carotid artery graft — *see* Complications, graft, vascular
    - coronary bypass graft — *see* Complication, coronary artery (bypass) graft
    - dialysis catheter (vascular) — *see* Complication, catheter, dialysis
    - electronic T82.9
      - electrode T82.9
        - embolism T82.817
        - fibrosis T82.827
        - hemorrhage T82.837
        - infection T82.7
        - mechanical
          - breakdown T82.11Ø
          - displacement T82.12Ø
          - leakage T82.19Ø
          - obstruction T82.19Ø
          - perforation T82.19Ø
          - protrusion T82.19Ø
          - specified type NEC T82.19Ø
        - pain T82.847
        - specified NEC T82.897
        - stenosis T82.857
        - thrombosis T82.867
      - embolism T82.817
      - fibrosis T82.827
      - hemorrhage T82.837
      - infection T82.7
      - mechanical
        - breakdown T82.119
        - displacement T82.129
        - leakage T82.199
        - obstruction T82.199
        - perforation T82.199
        - protrusion T82.199
        - specified type NEC T82.199
      - pain T82.847
      - pulse generator T82.9
        - embolism T82.817
        - fibrosis T82.827
        - hemorrhage T82.837
        - infection T82.7
        - mechanical
          - breakdown T82.111
          - displacement T82.121
          - leakage T82.191
          - obstruction T82.191
          - perforation T82.191
          - protrusion T82.191
          - specified type NEC T82.191
        - pain T82.847
        - specified NEC T82.897
        - stenosis T82.857
        - thrombosis T82.867
      - specified condition NEC T82.897
      - specified device NEC T82.9
        - embolism T82.817
        - fibrosis T82.827
        - hemorrhage T82.837
        - infection T82.7
        - mechanical
          - breakdown T82.118
          - displacement T82.128
          - leakage T82.198
          - obstruction T82.198
          - perforation T82.198
          - protrusion T82.198

- **Complication** — *continued*
  - cardiovascular device, graft or implant — *continued*
    - electronic — *continued*
      - specified device NEC — *continued*
        - mechanical — *continued*
          - specified type NEC T82.198
        - pain T82.847
        - specified NEC T82.897
        - stenosis T82.857
        - thrombosis T82.867
      - stenosis T82.857
      - thrombosis T82.867
    - extremity artery graft — *see* Complication, extremity artery (bypass) graft
    - femoral artery graft — *see* Complication, extremity artery (bypass) graft
    - heart-lung transplant — *see* Complication, transplant, heart, with lung
    - heart
      - transplant — *see* Complication, transplant, heart
      - valve — *see* Complication, prosthetic device, heart valve
        - graft — *see* Complication, heart, valve, graft
    - infection or inflammation T82.7
    - umbrella device — *see* Complication, umbrella device, vascular
    - vascular graft (or anastomosis) — *see* Complication, graft, vascular
  - carotid artery (bypass) graft — *see* Complications, graft, vascular
  - catheter (device) NEC (*see also* Complications, prosthetic device or implant)
    - cystostomy T83.9
      - embolism T83.81
      - fibrosis T83.82
      - hemorrhage T83.83
      - infection and inflammation T83.59
      - mechanical
        - breakdown T83.Ø1Ø
        - displacement T83.Ø2Ø
        - leakage T83.Ø3Ø
        - malposition T83.Ø2Ø
        - obstruction T83.Ø9Ø
        - perforation T83.Ø9Ø
        - protrusion T83.Ø9Ø
        - specified NEC T83.Ø9Ø
      - pain T83.84
      - specified type NEC T83.89
      - stenosis T83.85
      - thrombosis T83.86
    - dialysis (vascular) T82.9
      - embolism T82.818
      - fibrosis T82.828
      - hemorrhage T82.838
      - infection and inflammation T82.7
      - intraperitoneal — *see* Complications, catheter, intraperitoneal
      - mechanical
        - breakdown T82.41
        - displacement T82.42
        - leakage T82.43
        - malposition T82.42
        - obstruction T82.49
        - perforation T82.49
        - protrusion T82.49
      - pain T82.848
      - specified type NEC T82.898
      - stenosis T82.858
      - thrombosis T82.868
    - epidural infusion T85.9
      - embolism T85.81
      - fibrosis T85.82
      - hemorrhage T85.83
      - infection and inflammation T85.79
      - mechanical
        - breakdown T85.61Ø
        - displacement T85.62Ø
        - leakage T85.63Ø
        - malfunction T85.61Ø
        - malposition T85.62Ø
        - obstruction T85.69Ø

- **Complication** — *continued*
  - catheter (device) NEC — *continued*
    - epidural infusion — *continued*
      - mechanical — *continued*
        - perforation T85.69Ø
        - protrusion T85.69Ø
        - specified NEC T85.69Ø
      - pain T85.84
      - specified type NEC T85.89
      - stenosis T85.85
      - thrombosis T85.86
    - intraperitoneal dialysis T85.9
      - embolism T85.81
      - fibrosis T85.82
      - hemorrhage T85.83
      - infection and inflammation T85.71
      - mechanical
        - breakdown T85.611
        - displacement T85.621
        - leakage T85.631
        - malfunction T85.611
        - malposition T85.621
        - obstruction T85.691
        - perforation T85.691
        - protrusion T85.691
        - specified NEC T85.691
      - pain T85.84
      - specified type NEC T85.89
      - stenosis T85.85
      - thrombosis T85.86
    - intravenous infusion T82.9
      - embolism T82.818
      - fibrosis T82.828
      - hemorrhage T82.838
      - infection or inflammation T82.7
      - mechanical
        - breakdown T82.514
        - displacement T82.524
        - leakage T82.534
        - malposition T82.524
        - obstruction T82.594
        - perforation T82.594
        - protrusion T82.594
      - pain T82.848
      - specified type NEC T82.898
      - stenosis T82.858
      - thrombosis T82.868
    - subdural infusion T85.9
      - embolism T85.81
      - fibrosis T85.82
      - hemorrhage T85.83
      - infection and inflammation T85.79
      - mechanical
        - breakdown T85.61Ø
        - displacement T85.62Ø
        - leakage T85.63Ø
        - malfunction T85.61Ø
        - malposition T85.62Ø
        - obstruction T85.69Ø
        - perforation T85.69Ø
        - protrusion T85.69Ø
        - specified NEC T85.69Ø
      - pain T85.84
      - specified type NEC T85.89
      - stenosis T85.85
      - thrombosis T85.86
    - urethral, indwelling T83.9
      - displacement T83.Ø28
      - embolism T83.81
      - fibrosis T83.82
      - hemorrhage T83.83
      - infection and inflammation T83.51
      - leakage T83.Ø38
      - malposition T83.Ø28
      - mechanical
        - breakdown T83.Ø18
      - obstruction (mechanical) T83.Ø98
      - pain T83.84
      - perforation T83.Ø98
      - protrusion T83.Ø98
      - specified type NEC T83.Ø98
      - stenosis T83.85
      - thrombosis T83.86

- **Complication** — *continued*
  - catheter (device) NEC — *continued*
    - urinary (indwelling) — *see* Complications, catheter, urethral, indwelling
  - cecostomy (stoma) — *see* Complications, colostomy
  - cesarean delivery wound NEC O9Ø.89
    - disruption O9Ø.Ø
    - hematoma O9Ø.2
    - infection (following delivery) O86.Ø
  - chemotherapy (antineoplastic) NEC T88.7
  - chin implant (prosthetic) — *see* Complication, prosthetic device or implant, specified NEC
  - circulatory system I99.8
    - intraoperative I97.88
    - postprocedural I97.89
      - following cardiac surgery I97.19-
        - postcardiotomy syndrome I97.Ø
      - lymphedema after mastectomy I97.2
      - hypertension I97.3
      - postcardiotomy syndrome I97.Ø
      - specified NEC I97.89
  - colostomy (stoma) K94.ØØ
    - hemorrhage K94.Ø1
    - infection K94.Ø2
    - malfunction K94.Ø3
    - mechanical K94.Ø3
    - specified complication NEC K94.Ø9
  - contraceptive device, intrauterine — *see* Complications, intrauterine, contraceptive device
  - cord (umbilical) — *see* Complications, umbilical cord
  - corneal graft — *see* Complications, graft, cornea
  - coronary artery (bypass) graft T82.9
    - atherosclerosis — *see* Arteriosclerosis, coronary (artery),
    - embolism T82.818
    - fibrosis T82.828
    - hemorrhage T82.838
    - infection and inflammation T82.7
    - mechanical
      - breakdown T82.211
      - displacement T82.212
      - leakage T82.213
      - malposition T82.212
      - obstruction T82.218
      - perforation T82.218
      - protrusion T82.218
      - specified NEC T82.218
    - pain T82.848
    - specified type NEC T82.897
    - stenosis T82.858
    - thrombosis T82.868
  - counterpulsation device (balloon), intraaortic — *see* Complications, balloon implant, vascular
  - cystostomy (stoma) N99.518
    - catheter — *see* Complications, catheter, cystostomy
    - hemorrhage N99.51Ø
    - infection N99.511
    - malfunction N99.512
    - specified type NEC N99.518
  - delivery (*see also* Complications, obstetric) O75.9
    - procedure (instrumental) (manual) (surgical) O75.4
    - specified NEC O75.89
  - dialysis (peritoneal) (renal) (*see also* Complications, infusion)
    - catheter (vascular) — *see* Complication, catheter, dialysis
      - peritoneal, intraperitoneal — *see* Complications, catheter, intraperitoneal
  - dorsal column (spinal) neurostimulator — *see* Complications, electronic stimulator device, spinal cord
  - drug NEC T88.7
  - ear procedure (*see also* Disorder, ear)
    - intraoperative H95.88-
      - hematoma — *see* Complications, intraoperative, hemorrhage (hematoma) (of), ear
      - hemorrhage — *see* Complications, intraoperative, hemorrhage (hematoma) (of), ear

- **Complication** — *continued*
  - ear — *continued*
    - intraoperative — *continued*
      - laceration — *see* Complications, intraoperative, puncture or laceration, ear
      - specified NEC H95.88-
    - postoperative H95.89-
      - external ear canal stenosis H95.81-
      - hematoma — *see* Complications, postprocedural, hemorrhage (hematoma) (of), ear
      - hemorrhage — *see* Complications, postprocedural, hemorrhage (hematoma) (of), ear
      - postmastoidectomy — *see* Complications, postmastoidectomy
      - specified NEC H95.89-
  - ectopic pregnancy OØ8.9
    - damage to pelvic organs OØ8.6
    - embolism OØ8.2
    - genital infection OØ8.Ø
    - hemorrhage (delayed) (excessive) OØ8.1
    - metabolic disorder OØ8.5
    - renal failure OØ8.4
    - shock OØ8.3
    - specified type NEC OØ8.Ø
    - venous complication NEC OØ8.7
  - electronic stimulator device
    - bladder (urinary) — *see* Complications, electronic stimulator device, urinary
    - bone T84.9
      - breakdown T84.31Ø
      - displacement T84.32Ø
      - embolism T84.81
      - fibrosis T84.82
      - hemorrhage T84.83
      - infection or inflammation T84.7
      - malfunction T84.31Ø
      - malposition T84.32Ø
      - mechanical NEC T84.39Ø
      - obstruction T84.39Ø
      - pain T84.84
      - perforation T84.39Ø
      - protrusion T84.39Ø
      - specified type NEC T84.89
      - stenosis T84.85
      - thrombosis T84.86
    - brain T85.9
      - embolism T85.81
      - fibrosis T85.82
      - hemorrhage T85.83
      - infection and inflammation T85.79
      - mechanical
        - breakdown T85.11Ø
        - displacement T85.12Ø
        - leakage T85.19Ø
        - malposition T85.12Ø
        - obstruction T85.19Ø
        - perforation T85.19Ø
        - protrusion T85.19Ø
        - specified NEC T85.19Ø
      - pain T85.84
      - specified type NEC T85.89
      - stenosis T85.85
      - thrombosis T85.86
    - cardiac (defibrillator) (pacemaker) — *see* Complications, cardiovascular device or implant, electronic
    - muscle T84.9
      - breakdown T84.418
      - displacement T84.428
      - embolism T84.81
      - fibrosis T84.82
      - hemorrhage T84.83
      - infection or inflammation T84.7
      - mechanical NEC T84.498
      - pain T84.84
      - specified type NEC T84.89
      - stenosis T84.85
      - thrombosis T84.86
    - nervous system T85.9

- **Complication** — *continued*
  - electronic stimulator device — *continued*
    - nervous system — *continued*
      - brain — *see* Complications, electronic stimulator device, brain
      - embolism T85.81
      - fibrosis T85.82
      - hemorrhage T85.83
      - infection and inflammation T85.79
      - mechanical
        - breakdown T85.118
        - displacement T85.128
        - leakage T85.199
        - malposition T85.128
        - obstruction T85.199
        - perforation T85.199
        - protrusion T85.199
        - specified NEC T85.199
      - pain T85.84
      - peripheral nerve — *see* Complications, electronic stimulator device, peripheral nerve
      - specified type NEC T85.89
      - spinal cord — *see* Complications, electronic stimulator device, spinal cord
      - stenosis T85.85
      - thrombosis T85.86
    - peripheral nerve T85.9
      - embolism T85.81
      - fibrosis T85.82
      - hemorrhage T85.83
      - infection and inflammation T85.79
      - mechanical
        - breakdown T85.111
        - displacement T85.121
        - leakage T85.191
        - malposition T85.121
        - obstruction T85.191
        - perforation T85.191
        - protrusion T85.191
        - specified NEC T85.191
      - pain T85.84
      - specified type NEC T85.89
      - stenosis T85.85
      - thrombosis T85.86
    - spinal cord T85.9
      - embolism T85.81
      - fibrosis T85.82
      - hemorrhage T85.83
      - infection and inflammation T85.79
      - mechanical
        - breakdown T85.112
        - displacement T85.122
        - leakage T85.192
        - malposition T85.122
        - obstruction T85.192
        - perforation T85.192
        - protrusion T85.192
        - specified NEC T85.192
      - pain T85.84
      - specified type NEC T85.89
      - stenosis T85.85
      - thrombosis T85.86
    - urinary T83.9
      - embolism T83.81
      - fibrosis T83.82
      - hemorrhage T83.83
      - infection and inflammation T83.59
      - mechanical
        - breakdown T83.11Ø
        - displacement T83.12Ø
        - malposition T83.12Ø
        - perforation T83.19Ø
        - protrusion T83.19Ø
        - specified NEC T83.19Ø
      - pain T83.84
      - specified type NEC T83.89
      - stenosis T83.85
      - thrombosis T83.86
  - electroshock therapy T88.9
    - specified NEC T88.8
  - endocrine E34.9
    - postprocedural

- **Complication** — *continued*
  - endocrine — *continued*
    - postprocedural — *continued*
      - adrenal hypofunction E89.6
      - hypoinsulinemia E89.1
      - hypoparathyroidism E89.2
      - hypopituitarism E89.3
      - hypothyroidism E89.Ø
      - ovarian failure E89.4Ø
        - asymptomatic E89.4Ø
        - symptomatic E89.41
      - specified NEC E89.89
      - testicular hypofunction E89.5
  - endodontic treatment NEC M27.59
  - enterostomy (stoma) K94.1Ø
    - hemorrhage K94.11
    - infection K94.12
    - malfunction K94.13
    - mechanical K94.13
    - specified complication NEC K94.19
  - episiotomy, disruption O9Ø.1
  - esophageal anti-reflux device T85.9
    - embolism T85.81
    - fibrosis T85.82
    - hemorrhage T85.83
    - infection and inflammation T85.79
    - mechanical
      - breakdown T85.511
      - displacement T85.521
      - malfunction T85.511
      - malposition T85.521
      - obstruction T85.591
      - perforation T85.591
      - protrusion T85.591
      - specified NEC T85.591
    - pain T85.84
    - specified type NEC T85.89
    - stenosis T85.85
    - thrombosis T85.86
  - esophagostomy K94.3Ø
    - hemorrhage K94.31
    - infection K94.32
    - malfunction K94.33
    - mechanical K94.33
    - specified complication NEC K94.39
  - extracorporeal circulation T8Ø.9Ø
  - extremity artery (bypass) graft T82.9
    - arteriosclerosis — *see* Arteriosclerosis, extremities, bypass graft
    - embolism T82.818
    - fibrosis T82.828
    - hemorrhage T82.838
    - infection and inflammation T82.7
    - mechanical
      - breakdown T82.318
        - femoral artery T82.312
      - displacement T82.328
        - femoral artery T82.322
      - leakage T82.338
        - femoral artery T82.332
      - malposition T82.328
        - femoral artery T82.322
      - obstruction T82.398
        - femoral artery T82.392
      - perforation T82.398
        - femoral artery T82.392
      - protrusion T82.398
        - femoral artery T82.392
    - pain T82.848
    - specified type NEC T82.898
    - stenosis T82.858
    - thrombosis T82.868
  - eye H57.9
    - corneal graft — *see* Complications, graft, cornea
    - implant (prosthetic) T85.9
      - embolism T85.81
      - fibrosis T85.82
      - hemorrhage T85.83
      - infection and inflammation T85.79
      - mechanical
        - breakdown T85.318
        - displacement T85.328
        - leakage T85.398

- **Complication** — *continued*
  - insulin pump — *continued*
    - mechanical
      - breakdown T85.614
      - displacement T85.624
      - leakage T85.633
      - malposition T85.624
      - obstruction T85.694
      - perforation T85.694
      - protrusion T85.694
      - specified NEC T85.694
  - intestinal pouch NEC K91.858
  - intraocular lens (prosthetic) T85.9
    - embolism T85.81
    - fibrosis T85.82
    - hemorrhage T85.83
    - infection and inflammation T85.79
    - mechanical
      - breakdown T85.21
      - displacement T85.22
      - malposition T85.22
      - obstruction T85.29
      - perforation T85.29
      - protrusion T85.29
      - specified NEC T85.29
    - pain T85.84
    - specified type NEC T85.89
    - stenosis T85.85
    - thrombosis T85.86
  - intraoperative (intraprocedural)
    - cardiac arrest
      - during cardiac surgery I97.710
      - during other surgery I97.711
    - cardiac functional disturbance NEC
      - during cardiac surgery I97.790
      - during other surgery I97.791
    - hemorrhage (hematoma) (of)
      - circulatory system organ or structure
        - during cardiac bypass I97.411
        - during cardiac catheterization I97.410
        - during other circulatory system procedure I97.418
        - during other procedure I97.42
      - digestive system organ
        - during procedure on digestive system K91.61
        - during procedure on other organ K91.62
      - ear
        - during procedure on ear and mastoid process H95.21
        - during procedure on other organ H95.22
      - endocrine system organ or structure
        - during procedure on endocrine system organ or structure E36.01
        - during procedure on other organ E36.02
      - eye and adnexa
        - during ophthalmic procedure H59.11-
        - during other procedure H59.12-
      - genitourinary organ or structure
        - during procedure on genitourinary organ or structure N99.61
        - during procedure on other organ N99.62
      - mastoid process
        - during procedure on ear and mastoid process H95.21
        - during procedure on other organ H95.22
      - musculoskeletal structure
        - during musculoskeletal surgery M96.810
        - during non-orthopedic surgery M96.811
        - during orthopedic surgery M96.810
      - nervous system
        - during a nervous system procedure G97.31
        - during other procedure G97.32
      - respiratory system
        - during procedure on respiratory system organ or structure J95.61
        - during other procedure J95.62
      - skin and subcutaneous tissue
        - during a dermatologic procedure L76.01
        - during a procedure on other organ L76.02
      - spleen
        - during a procedure on the spleen D78.01

- **Complication** — *continued*
  - intraoperative (intraprocedural) — *continued*
    - hemorrhage (hematoma) — *continued*
      - spleen — *continued*
        - during a procedure on other organ D78.02
    - puncture or laceration (accidental) (unintentional) (of)
      - brain
        - during a nervous system procedure G97.48
        - during other procedure G97.49
      - circulatory system organ or structure
        - during circulatory system procedure I97.51
        - during other procedure I97.52
      - digestive system
        - during procedure on digestive system K91.71
        - during procedure on other organ K91.72
      - ear
        - during procedure on ear and mastoid process H95.31
        - during procedure on other organ H95.32
      - endocrine system organ or structure
        - during procedure on endocrine system organ or structure E36.11
        - during procedure on other organ E36.12
      - eye and adnexa
        - during ophthalmic procedure H59.21-
        - during other procedure H59.22-
      - genitourinary organ or structure
        - during procedure on genitourinary organ or structure N99.71
        - during procedure on other organ N99.72
      - mastoid process
        - during procedure on ear and mastoid process H95.31
        - during procedure on other organ H95.32
      - musculoskeletal structure
        - during musculoskeletal surgery M96.820
        - during non-orthopedic surgery M96.821
        - during orthopedic surgery M96.820
      - nervous system
        - during a nervous system procedure G97.48
        - during other procedure G97.49
      - respiratory system
        - during procedure on respiratory system organ or structure J95.71
        - during other procedure J95.72
      - skin and subcutaneous tissue
        - during a dermatologic procedure L76.11
        - during a procedure on other organ L76.12
      - spleen
        - during a procedure on the spleen D78.11
        - during a procedure on other organ D78.12
    - specified NEC
      - circulatory system I97.88
      - digestive system K91.81
      - ear H95.88
      - endocrine system E36.8
      - eye and adnexa H59.88
      - genitourinary system N99.81
      - mastoid process H95.88
      - nervous system G97.81
      - respiratory system J95.88
      - skin and subcutaneous tissue L76.81
      - spleen D78.81
  - intraperitoneal catheter (dialysis) (infusion) — *see* Complications, catheter, intraperitoneal
  - intrauterine
    - contraceptive device
      - embolism T83.81
      - fibrosis T83.82
      - hemorrhage T83.83
      - infection and inflammation T83.6
      - mechanical
        - breakdown T83.31
        - displacement T83.32
        - malposition T83.32
        - obstruction T83.39
        - perforation T83.39
        - protrusion T83.39

- **Complication** — *continued*
  - intrauterine — *continued*
    - contraceptive device — *continued*
      - mechanical — *continued*
        - specified NEC T83.39
      - pain T83.84
      - specified type NEC T83.89
      - stenosis T83.85
      - thrombosis T83.86
    - procedure (fetal), to newborn P96.5
  - jejunostomy (stoma) — *see* Complications, enterostomy
  - joint prosthesis, internal T84.9
    - breakage (fracture) T84.01-
    - dislocation T84.02-
    - fracture T84.01-
    - instability T84.02-
    - infection or inflammation T84.50
      - hip T84.5-
      - knee T84.5-
      - specified joint NEC T84.59
    - malposition — *see* Complications, joint prosthesis, mechanical, displacement
    - mechanical
      - breakage, broken T84.01-
      - dislocation T84.02-
      - fracture T84.01-
      - instability T84.02-
      - leakage — *see* Complications, joint prosthesis, mechanical, specified NEC
      - loosening T84.039
        - hip T84.03-
        - knee T84.03-
        - specified joint NEC T84.038
      - obstruction — *see* Complications, joint prosthesis, mechanical, specified NEC
      - perforation — *see* Complications, joint prosthesis, mechanical, specified NEC
      - periprosthetic
        - osteolysis T84.059
          - hip T84.05-
          - knee T84.05-
          - other specified joint T84.058
        - fracture T84.049
          - hip T84.04-
          - knee T84.04-
          - other specified joint T84.048
      - protrusion — *see* Complications, joint prosthesis, mechanical, specified NEC
      - specified complication NEC T84.099
        - hip T84.09-
        - knee T84.09-
        - other specified joint T84.098
      - subluxation T84.02-
      - wear of articular bearing surface T84.069
        - hip T84.06-
        - knee T84.069
        - other specified joint T84.068
    - specified joint NEC T84.9
      - embolism T84.81
      - fibrosis T84.82
      - hemorrhage T84.83
      - pain T84.84
      - specified complication NEC T84.89
      - stenosis T84.85
      - thrombosis T84.86
    - subluxation T84.02-
  - kidney transplant — *see* Complications, transplant, kidney
  - labor O75.9
    - specified NEC O75.89
  - liver transplant (immune or nonimmune) — *see* Complications, transplant, liver
  - lumbar puncture G97.1
    - cerebrospinal fluid leak G97.0
    - headache or reaction G97.1
  - lung transplant — *see* Complications, transplant, lung
    - and heart — *see* Complications, transplant, lung, with heart
  - male genital N50.9

- **Complication** — *continued*
  - postprocedural — *continued*
    - hemorrhage (hematoma) (of) — *continued*
      - ear — *continued*
        - following other procedure H95.42
      - endocrine system
        - following endocrine system procedure E89.81Ø
        - following other procedure E89.811
      - eye and adnexa
        - following ophthalmic procedure H59.31-
        - following other procedure H59.32-
      - genitourinary organ or structure
        - following procedure on genitourinary organ or structure N99.82Ø
        - following procedure on other organ N99.821
      - mastoid process
        - following procedure on ear and mastoid process H95.41
        - following other procedure H95.42
      - musculoskeletal structure
        - following musculoskeletal surgery M96.83Ø
        - following non-orthopedic surgery M96.831
        - following orthopedic surgery M96.83Ø
      - nervous system
        - during a nervous system procedure G97.51
        - during other procedure G97.52
      - respiratory system
        - during procedure on respiratory system organ or structure J95.83Ø
        - during other procedure J95.831
      - skin and subcutaneous tissue
        - following a dermatologic procedure L76.21
        - following a procedure on other organ L76.22
      - spleen
        - following procedure on the spleen D78.21
        - following procedure on other organ D78.22
    - specified NEC
      - circulatory system I97.89
      - digestive K91.89
      - ear H95.89
      - endocrine E89.89
      - eye and adnexa H59.89
      - genitourinary N99.89
      - mastoid process H95.89
      - metabolic E89.89
      - musculoskeletal structure M96.89
      - nervous system G97.82
      - respiratory system J95.89
      - skin and subcutaneous tissue L76.82
      - spleen D78.89
  - pregnancy NEC — *see* Pregnancy, complicated by
  - prosthetic device or implant T85.9
    - bile duct — *see* Complications, bile duct implant
    - breast — *see* Complications, breast implant
    - cardiac and vascular NEC — *see* Complications, cardiovascular device or implant
    - corneal transplant — *see* Complications, graft, cornea
    - electronic nervous system stimulator — *see* Complications, electronic stimulator device
    - epidural infusion catheter — *see* Complications, catheter, epidural
    - esophageal anti-reflux device — *see* Complications, esophageal anti-reflux device
    - genital organ or tract — *see* Complications, genitourinary, device or implant, genital tract
    - heart valve — *see* Complications, heart, valve, prosthesis
    - infection or inflammation T85.79
      - intestine transplant T86.892
      - liver transplant T86.43
      - lung transplant T86.812
      - pancreas transplant T86.892

- **Complication** — *continued*
  - prosthetic device or implant — *continued*
    - infection or inflammation — *continued*
      - skin graft T86.822
    - intraocular lens — *see* Complications, intraocular lens
    - intraperitoneal (dialysis) catheter — *see* Complications, catheter, intraperitoneal
    - joint — *see* Complications, joint prosthesis, internal
    - mechanical NEC T85.698
      - dialysis catheter (vascular) (*see also* Complication, catheter, dialysis, mechanical)
        - peritoneal — *see* Complication, catheter, intraperitoneal, mechanical
      - gastrointestinal device T85.598
      - ocular device T85.398
      - subdural (infusion) catheter T85.69Ø
      - suture, permanent T85.692
        - that for bone repair — *see* Complications, fixation device, internal (orthopedic), mechanical
      - ventricular shunt
        - breakdown T85.Ø1
        - displacement T85.Ø2
        - leakage T85.Ø3
        - malposition T85.Ø2
        - obstruction T85.Ø9
        - perforation T85.Ø9
        - protrusion T85.Ø9
        - specified NEC T85.Ø9
    - mesh
      - erosion (to surrounding organ or tissue) T83.718
        - vaginal (into pelvic floor muscles) T83.711
      - exposure (into surrounding organ or tissue) T83.728
        - vaginal (into vagina) (through vaginal wall) T83.721
    - orbital — *see* Complications, orbital prosthesis
    - penile T83.9
      - embolism T83.81
      - fibrosis T83.82
      - hemorrhage T83.83
      - infection and inflammation T83.6
      - mechanical
        - breakdown T83.41Ø
        - displacement T83.42Ø
        - leakage T83.49Ø
        - malposition T83.42Ø
        - obstruction T83.49Ø
        - perforation T83.49Ø
        - protrusion T83.49Ø
        - specified NEC T83.49Ø
      - pain T83.84
      - specified type NEC T83.89
      - stenosis T83.85
      - thrombosis T83.86
    - prosthetic materials NEC
      - erosion (to surrounding organ or tissue) T83.718
        - vaginal (into pelvic floor muscles) T83.711
      - exposure (into surrounding organ or tissue) T83.728
        - vaginal (into vagina) (through vaginal wall) T83.721
    - skin graft T86.829
      - artificial skin or decellularized allodermis
        - embolism T85.81
        - fibrosis T85.82
        - hemorrhage T85.83
        - infection and inflammation T85.79
        - mechanical
          - breakdown T85.613
          - displacement T85.623
          - malfunction T85.613
          - malposition T85.623
          - obstruction T85.693
          - perforation T85.693
          - protrusion T85.693
          - specified NEC T85.693
        - pain T85.84

- **Complication** — *continued*
  - prosthetic device or implant — *continued*
    - skin graft — *continued*
      - artificial skin or decellularized allodermis — *continued*
        - specified type NEC T85.89
        - stenosis T85.85
        - thrombosis T85.86
      - failure T86.821
      - infection T86.822
      - rejection T86.82Ø
      - specified NEC T86.828
    - specified NEC T85.9
      - embolism T85.81
      - fibrosis T85.82
      - hemorrhage T85.83
      - infection and inflammation T85.79
      - mechanical
        - breakdown T85.618
        - displacement T85.628
        - leakage T85.638
        - malfunction T85.618
        - malposition T85.628
        - obstruction T85.698
        - perforation T85.698
        - protrusion T85.698
        - specified NEC T85.698
      - pain T85.84
      - specified type NEC T85.89
      - stenosis T85.85
      - thrombosis T85.86
    - subdural infusion catheter — *see* Complications, catheter, subdural
    - sutures — *see* Complications, sutures
    - urinary organ or tract NEC — *see* Complications, genitourinary, device or implant, urinary system
    - vascular — *see* Complications, cardiovascular device or implant
    - ventricular shunt — *see* Complications, ventricular shunt (device)
  - puerperium — *see* Puerperal
  - puncture, spinal G97.1
    - cerebrospinal fluid leak G97.Ø
    - headache or reaction G97.1
  - pyelogram N99.89
  - radiation
    - kyphosis M96.2
    - scoliosis M96.5
  - reattached
    - extremity (infection) (rejection)
      - lower T87.1x-
      - upper T87.Øx-
    - specified body part NEC T87.2
  - reconstructed breast
    - asymmetry between native and reconstructed breast N65.1
    - deformity N65.Ø
    - disproportion between native and reconstructed breast N65.1
    - excess tissue N65.Ø
    - misshappen N65.Ø
  - reimplant NEC (*see also* Complications, prosthetic device or implant)
    - limb (infection) (rejection) — *see* Complications, reattached, extremity
    - organ (partial) (total) — *see* Complications, transplant
    - prosthetic device NEC — *see* Complications, prosthetic device
  - renal N28.9
    - allograft — *see* Complications, transplant, kidney
    - dialysis — *see* Complications, dialysis
  - respirator
    - mechancial J95.85Ø
      - specified NEC J95.859
  - respiratory system J98.9
    - device, implant or graft — *see* Complication, prosthetic device or implant, specified NEC
    - lung transplant — *see* Complications, prosthetic device or implant, lung transplant
    - postoperative J95.89
      - air leak J95.812

- **Complication** — *continued*
  - respiratory system — *continued*
    - postoperative — *continued*
      - Mendelson's syndrome (chemical pneumonitis) J95.4
      - pneumothorax J95.811
      - pulmonary insufficiency (acute) (after nonthoracic surgery) J95.2
        - chronic J95.3
        - following thoracic surgery J95.1
      - respiratory failure (acute) J95.821
        - acute and chronic J95.822
      - specified NEC J95.89
      - subglottic stenosis J95.5
      - tracheostomy complication — *see* Complications, tracheostomy
    - therapy T81.89
  - sedation during labor and delivery O74.9
    - cardiac O74.2
    - central nervous system O74.3
    - pulmonary NEC O74.1
  - shunt (*see also* Complications, prosthetic device or implant)
    - arteriovenous — *see* Complications, arteriovenous, shunt
    - ventricular (communicating) — *see* Complications, ventricular shunt
  - skin
    - graft T86.829
      - failure T86.821
      - infection T86.822
      - rejection T86.82Ø
      - specified type NEC T86.828
  - spinal
    - anesthesia — *see* Complications, anesthesia, spinal
    - catheter (epidural) (subdural) — *see* Complications, catheter
    - puncture or tap G97.1
      - cerebrospinal fluid leak G97.Ø
      - headache or reaction G97.1
  - stent
    - bile duct — *see* Complications, bile duct prosthesis
    - urinary T83.9
      - embolism T83.81
      - fibrosis T83.82
      - hemorrhage T83.83
      - infection and inflammation T83.59
      - mechanical
        - breakdown T83.112
        - displacement T83.122
        - leakage T83.192
        - malposition T83.122
        - obstruction T83.192
        - perforation T83.192
        - protrusion T83.192
        - specified NEC T83.192
      - pain T83.84
      - specified type NEC T83.89
      - stenosis T83.85
      - thrombosis T83.86
  - stoma
    - digestive tract
      - colostomy — *see* Complications, colostomy
      - enterostomy — *see* Complications, enterostomy
      - esophagostomy — *see* Complications, esophagostomy
      - gastrostomy — *see* Complications, gastrostomy
    - urinary tract N99.538
      - cystostomy — *see* Complications, cystostomy
      - external NOS N99.528
        - hemorrhage N99.52Ø
        - infection N99.521
        - malfunction N99.522
        - specified type NEC N99.528
      - hemorrhage N99.53Ø
      - infection N99.531
      - malfunction N99.532
      - specified type NEC N99.538

- **Complication** — *continued*
  - stomach banding — *see* Complication(s), bariatric procedure
  - stomach stapling — *see* Complication(s), bariatric procedure
  - surgical material, nonabsorbable — *see* Complication, suture, permanent
  - surgical procedure (on) T81.9
    - amputation stump (late) — *see* Complications, amputation stump
    - cardiac — *see* Complications, circulatory system
    - cholesteatoma, recurrent — *see* Complications, postmastoidectomy, recurrent cholesteatoma
    - circulatory (early) — *see* Complications, circulatory system
    - digestive system — *see* Complications, gastrointestinal
    - dumping syndrome (postgastrectomy) K91.1
    - ear — *see* Complications, ear
    - elephantiasis or lymphedema I97.89
      - postmastectomy I97.2
    - emphysema (surgical) T81.82
    - endocrine — *see* Complications, endocrine
    - eye — *see* Complications, eye
    - fistula (persistent postoperative) T81.83
    - foreign body inadvertently left in wound (sponge) (suture) (swab) — *see* Foreign body, accidentally left during a procedure
    - gastrointestinal — *see* Complications, gastrointestinal
    - genitourinary NEC N99.89
    - hematoma
      - intraoperative — *see* Complication, intraoperative, hemorrhage
      - postprocedural— *see* Complication, postprocedural, hemorrhage
    - hemorrhage
      - intraoperative — *see* Complication, intraoperative, hemorrhage
      - postprocedural — *see* Complication, postprocedural, hemorrhage
    - hepatic failure K91.82
    - hyperglycemia (postpancreatectomy) E89.1
    - hypoinsulinemia (postpancreatectomy) E89.1
    - hypoparathyroidism (postparathyroidectomy) E89.2
    - hypopituitarism (posthypophysectomy) E89.3
    - hypothyroidism (post-thyroidectomy) E89.Ø
    - intestinal obstruction K91.3
    - intracranial hypotension following ventricular shunting (ventriculostomy) G97.2
    - lymphedema I97.89
      - postmastectomy I97.2
    - malabsorption (postsurgical) NEC K91.2
      - osteoporosis — *see* Osteoporosis, postsurgical malabsorption
    - mastoidectomy cavity NEC — *see* Complications, postmastoidectomy
    - metabolic E89.89
      - specified NEC E89.89
    - musculoskeletal — *see* Complications, musculoskeletal system
    - nervous system (central) (peripheral) — *see* Complications, nervous system
    - ovarian failure E89.4Ø
      - asymptomatic E89.4Ø
      - symptomatic E89.41
    - peripheral vascular — *see* Complications, surgical procedure, vascular
    - postcardiotomy syndrome I97.Ø
    - postcholecystectomy syndrome K91.5
    - postcommissurotomy syndrome I97.Ø
    - postgastrectomy dumping syndrome K91.1
    - postlaminectomy syndrome NEC M96.1
      - kyphosis M96.3
    - postmastectomy lymphedema syndrome I97.2
    - postmastoidectomy cholesteatoma — *see* Complications, postmastoidectomy, recurrent cholesteatoma
    - postvagotomy syndrome K91.1
    - postvalvulotomy syndrome I97.Ø
    - pulmonary insufficiency (acute) J95.2

- **Complication** — *continued*
  - surgical procedure (on) — *continued*
    - pulmonary insufficiency (acute) — *continued*
      - chronic J95.3
      - following thoracic surgery J95.1
    - reattached body part — *see* Complications, reattached
    - respiratory — *see* Complications, respiratory system
    - shock (hypovolemic) T81.19
    - spleen (postoperative) D78.89
      - intraoperative D78.81
    - stitch abscess T81.4
    - subglottic stenosis (postsurgical) J95.5
    - testicular hypofunction E89.5
    - transplant — *see* Complications, organ or tissue transplant
    - urinary NEC N99.89
    - vaginal vault prolapse (posthysterectomy) N99.3
    - vascular (peripheral)
      - artery T81.719
        - mesenteric T81.71Ø
        - renal T81.711
        - specified NEC T81.718
      - vein T81.72
    - wound infection T81.4
  - suture, permanent (wire) NEC T85.9
    - with repair of bone — *see* Complications, fixation device, internal
    - embolism T85.81
    - fibrosis T85.82
    - hemorrhage T85.83
    - infection and inflammation T85.79
    - mechanical
      - breakdown T85.612
      - displacement T85.622
      - malfunction T85.612
      - malposition T85.622
      - obstruction T85.692
      - perforation T85.692
      - protrusion T85.692
      - specified NEC T85.692
    - pain T85.84
    - specified type NEC T85.89
    - stenosis T85.85
    - thrombosis T85.86
  - tracheostomy J95.ØØ
    - granuloma J95.Ø9
    - hemorrhage J95.Ø1
    - infection J95.Ø2
    - malfunction J95.Ø3
    - mechanical J95.Ø3
    - obstruction J95.Ø3
    - specified type NEC J95.Ø9
    - tracheo-esophageal fistula J95.Ø4
  - transfusion (blood) (lymphocytes) (plasma) T8Ø.92
    - air embolism T8Ø.Ø
    - circulatory overload E87.71
    - febrile nonhemolytic transfusion reaction R5Ø.84
    - hemochromatosis E83.111
    - hemolysis T8Ø.89
    - hemolytic reaction (antigen unspecified) T8Ø.919
    - incompatibility reaction (antigen unspecified) T8Ø.919
      - ABO T8Ø.3Ø
        - delayed serologic (DSTR) T8Ø.39
        - hemolytic transfusion reaction (HTR) (unspecified time after transfusion) T8Ø.319
          - acute (AHTR) (less than 24 hours after transfusion) T8Ø.31Ø
          - delayed (DHTR) (24 hours or more after transfusion) T8Ø.311
        - specified NEC T8Ø.39
      - acute (antigen unspecified) T8Ø.91Ø
      - delayed (antigen unspecified) T8Ø.911
      - delayed serologic (DSTR) T8Ø.89
      - non-ABO (minor antigens (Duffy) (Kell) (Kidd) (Lewis) (M) (N) (P) (S)) T8Ø.AØ
        - delayed serologic (DSTR) T8Ø.A9
        - hemolytic transfusion reaction (HTR) (unspecified time after transfusion) T8Ø.A19

- **Complication** — *continued*
  - wire suture, permanent (implanted) — *see* Complications, suture, permanent
- **Compressed air disease** T7Ø.3
- **Compression**
  - with injury—code by Nature of injury
  - artery I77.1
    - celiac, syndrome I77.4
  - brachial plexus G54.Ø
  - brain (stem) G93.5
    - due to
      - contusion (diffuse) — *see* Injury, intracranial, diffuse
        - focal — *see* Injury, intracranial, focal
      - injury NEC — *see* Injury, intracranial, diffuse
    - traumatic — *see* Injury, intracranial, diffuse
  - bronchus J98.Ø9
  - cauda equina G83.4
  - celiac (artery) (axis) I77.4
  - cerebral — *see* Compression, brain
  - cervical plexus G54.2
  - cord
    - spinal — *see* Compression, spinal
    - umbilical — *see* Compression, umbilical cord
  - cranial nerve G52.9
    - eighth — *see* subcategory H93.3
    - eleventh G52.8
    - fifth G5Ø.8
    - first G52.Ø
    - fourth — *see* Strabismus, paralytic, fourth nerve
    - ninth G52.1
    - second — *see* Disorder, nerve, optic
    - seventh G52.8
    - sixth — *see* Strabismus, paralytic, sixth nerve
    - tenth G52.2
    - third — *see* Strabismus, paralytic, third nerve
    - twelfth G52.3
  - diver's squeeze T7Ø.3
  - during birth (newborn) P15.9
  - esophagus K22.2
  - eustachian tube — *see* Obstruction, eustachian tube, cartilaginous
  - facies Q67.1
  - fracture — *see* Fracture
  - heart — *see* Disease, heart
  - intestine — *see* Obstruction, intestine
  - laryngeal nerve, recurrent G52.2
    - with paralysis of vocal cords and larynx J38.ØØ
      - bilateral J38.Ø2
      - unilateral J38.Ø1
  - lumbosacral plexus G54.1
  - lung J98.4
  - lymphatic vessel I89.Ø
  - medulla — *see* Compression, brain
  - nerve (*see also* Disorder, nerve) G58.9
    - arm NEC — *see* Mononeuropathy, upper limb
    - axillary G54.Ø
    - cranial — *see* Compression, cranial nerve
    - leg NEC — *see* Mononeuropathy, lower limb
    - median (in carpal tunnel) — *see* Syndrome, carpal tunnel
    - optic — *see* Disorder, nerve, optic
    - plantar — *see* Lesion, nerve, plantar
    - posterior tibial (in tarsal tunnel) — *see* Syndrome, tarsal tunnel
    - root or plexus NOS (in) G54.9
      - intervertebral disc disorder NEC — *see* Disorder, disc, with, radiculopathy
        - with myelopathy — *see* Disorder, disc, with, myelopathy
      - neoplastic disease (*see also* Neoplasm) D49.9 *[G55]*
      - spondylosis — *see* Spondylosis, with radiculopathy
    - sciatic (acute) — *see* Lesion, nerve, sciatic
    - sympathetic G9Ø.8
    - traumatic — *see* Injury, nerve
    - ulnar — *see* Lesion, nerve, ulnar
    - upper extremity NEC — *see* Mononeuropathy, upper limb
  - spinal (cord) G95.2Ø
    - by displacement of intervertebral disc NEC (*see also* Disorder, disc, with, myelopathy)

- **Compression** — *continued*
  - spinal (cord) — *continued*
    - nerve root NOS G54.9
      - due to displacement of intervertebral disc NEC — *see* Disorder, disc, with, radiculopathy
        - with myelopathy — *see* Disorder, disc, with, myelopathy
    - specified NEC G95.29
    - spondylogenic (cervical) (lumbar, lumbosacral) (thoracic) — *see* Spondylosis, with myelopathy NEC
      - anterior — *see* Syndrome, anterior, spinal artery, compression
    - traumatic — *see* Injury, spinal cord, by region
  - subcostal nerve (syndrome) — *see* Mononeuropathy, upper limb, specified NEC
  - sympathetic nerve NEC G9Ø.8
  - syndrome T79.5
  - trachea J39.8
  - ulnar nerve (by scar tissue) — *see* Lesion, nerve, ulnar
  - umbilical cord
    - complicating delivery O69.2
      - cord around neck O69.1
      - prolapse O69.Ø
      - specified NEC O69.2
  - ureter N13.5
  - vein I87.1
  - vena cava (inferior) (superior) I87.1
- **Compulsion, compulsive**
  - gambling F63.Ø
  - neurosis F42
  - personality F6Ø.5
  - states F42
  - swearing F42
    - in Gilles de la Tourette's syndrome F95.2
  - tics and spasms F95.9
- **Concato's disease** (pericardial polyserositis) A19.9
  - nontubercular I31.1
  - pleural — *see* Pleurisy, with effusion
- **Concavity chest wall** M95.4
- **Concealed penis** Q55.69
- **Concern** (normal) **about sick person in family** Z63.6
- **Concrescence** (teeth) KØØ.2
- **Concretio cordis I31.1**
  - rheumatic IØ9.2
- **Concretion** (*see also* Calculus)
  - appendicular K38.1
  - canaliculus — *see* Dacryolith
  - clitoris N9Ø.89
  - conjunctiva H11.12-
  - eyelid — *see* Disorder, eyelid, specified type NEC
  - lacrimal passages — *see* Dacryolith
  - prepuce (male) N47.8
  - salivary gland (any) K11.5
  - seminal vesicle N5Ø.8
  - tonsil J35.8
- **Concussion** (brain) (cerebral) (current) SØ6.Øx-
  - blast (air) (hydraulic) (immersion) (underwater)
    - abdomen or thorax — *see* Injury, blast, by site
    - ear with acoustic nerve injury — *see* Injury, nerve, acoustic, specified type NEC
  - cauda equina S34.3
  - conus medullaris S34.139
  - ocular SØ5.8x-
  - spinal (cord)
    - cervical S14.Ø
    - lumbar S34.Ø1
    - sacral S34.Ø2
    - thoracic S24.Ø
  - syndrome FØ7.81
- **Condition** — *see* Disease
- **Conditions arising in the perinatal period** — *see* Newborn, affected by
- **Conduct disorder** — *see* Disorder, conduct
- **Condyloma** A63.Ø
  - acuminatum A63.Ø
  - gonorrheal A54.Ø9
  - latum A51.31
  - syphilitic A51.31
    - congenital A5Ø.Ø7
  - venereal, syphilitic A51.31

- **Conflagration** (*see also* Burn)
  - asphyxia (by inhalation of gases, fumes or vapors) (*see also* Table of Drugs and Chemicals) T59.9-
- **Conflict** (with) (*see also* Discord)
  - family Z73.9
  - marital Z63.Ø
    - involving divorce or estrangement Z63.5
  - parent-child Z62.82Ø
    - parent-adopted child Z62.821
    - parent-biological child Z62.82Ø
    - parent-foster child Z62.822
  - social role NEC Z73.5
- **Confluent** — *see* condition
- **Confusion, confused** R41.Ø
  - epileptic FØ5
  - mental state (psychogenic) F44.89
  - psychogenic F44.89
  - reactive (from emotional stress, psychological trauma) F44.89
- **Confusional arousals** G47.51
- **Congelation** T69.9
- **Congenital** (*see also* condition)
  - aortic septum Q25.4
  - intrinsic factor deficiency D51.Ø
  - malformation — *see* Anomaly
- **Congestion, congestive**
  - bladder N32.89
  - bowel K63.89
  - brain G93.89
  - breast N64.59
  - bronchial J98.Ø9
  - catarrhal J31.Ø
  - chest RØ9.89
  - chill, malarial — *see* Malaria
  - circulatory NEC I99.8
  - duodenum K31.89
  - eye — *see* Hyperemia, conjunctiva
  - facial, due to birth injury P15.4
  - general R68.89
  - glottis J37.Ø
  - heart — *see* Failure, heart, congestive
  - hepatic K76.1
  - hypostatic (lung) — *see* Edema, lung
  - intestine K63.89
  - kidney N28.89
  - labyrinth — *see* subcategory H83.8
  - larynx J37.Ø
  - liver K76.1
  - lung RØ9.89
    - active or acute — *see* Pneumonia
  - malaria, malarial — *see* Malaria
  - nasal RØ9.81
  - nose RØ9.81
  - orbit, orbital (*see also* Exophthalmos)
    - inflammatory (chronic) — *see* Inflammation, orbit
  - ovary N83.8
  - pancreas K86.8
  - pelvic, female N94.89
  - pleural J94.8
  - prostate (active) N42.1
  - pulmonary — *see* Congestion, lung
  - renal N28.89
  - retina H35.81
  - seminal vesicle N5Ø.1
  - spinal cord G95.19
  - spleen (chronic) D73.2
  - stomach K31.89
  - trachea — *see* Tracheitis
  - urethra N36.8
  - uterus N85.8
    - with subinvolution N85.3
  - venous (passive) I87.8
  - viscera R68.89
- **Congestive** — *see* Congestion
- **Conical**
  - cervix (hypertrophic elongation) N88.4
  - cornea — *see* Keratoconus
  - teeth KØØ.2
- **Conjoined twins** Q89.4
- **Conjugal maladjustment** Z63.Ø
  - involving divorce or estrangement Z63.5
- **Conjunctiva** — *see* condition

- **Conjunctivitis** (staphylococcal) (streptococcal) NOS H1Ø.9
  - Acanthamoeba B6Ø.12
  - acute H1Ø.3-
    - chemical H1Ø.21 (*see also* Corrosion, cornea)
    - atopic H1Ø.1-
    - mucopurulent H1Ø.Ø2-
      - follicular H1Ø.Ø1-
    - pseudomembranous H1Ø.22-
    - serous except viral H1Ø.23-
      - viral — *see* Conjunctivitis, viral
    - toxic H1Ø.21-
  - adenoviral (acute) (follicular) B3Ø.1
  - allergic (acute) — *see* Conjunctivitis, acute, atopic
    - chronic H1Ø.45
      - vernal H1Ø.44
  - anaphylactic — *see* Conjunctivitis, acute, atopic
  - Apollo B3Ø.3
  - atopic (acute) — *see* Conjunctivitis, acute, atopic
  - Béal's B3Ø.2
  - blennorrhagic (gonococcal) (neonatorum) A54.31
  - chemical (acute) H1Ø.21 (*see also* Corrosion, cornea)
  - chlamydial A74.Ø
    - due to trachoma A71.1
    - neonatal P39.1
  - chronic (nodosa) (petrificans) (phlyctenular) H1Ø.4Ø-
    - allergic H1Ø.45
      - vernal H1Ø.44
    - follicular H1Ø.43-
    - giant papillary H1Ø.41-
    - simple H1Ø.42-
    - vernal H1Ø.44
  - coxsackievirus 24 B3Ø.3
  - diphtheritic A36.86
  - due to
    - dust — *see* Conjunctivitis, acute, atopic
    - filariasis B74.9
    - mucocutaneous leishmaniasis B55.2
  - enterovirus type 7Ø (hemorrhagic) B3Ø.3
  - epidemic (viral) B3Ø.9
    - hemorrhagic B3Ø.3
  - gonococcal (neonatorum) A54.31
  - granular (trachomatous) A71.1
    - sequelae (late effect) B94.Ø
  - hemorrhagic (acute) (epidemic) B3Ø.3
  - herpes zoster BØ2.31
  - in (due to)
    - Acanthamoeba B6Ø.12
    - adenovirus (acute) (follicular) B3Ø.1
    - Chlamydia A74.Ø
    - coxsackievirus 24 B3Ø.3
    - diphtheria A36.86
    - enterovirus type 7Ø (hemorrhagic) B3Ø.3
    - filariasis B74.9
    - gonococci A54.31
    - herpes (simplex) virus BØØ.53
      - zoster BØ2.31
    - infectious disease NEC B99
    - meningococci A39.89
    - mucocutaneous leishmaniasis B55.2
    - rosacea L71.9
    - syphilis (late) A52.71
    - zoster BØ2.31
  - inclusion A74.Ø
  - infantile P39.1
    - gonococcal A54.31
  - Koch-Weeks' — *see* Conjunctivitis, acute, mucopurulent
  - light — *see* Conjunctivitis, acute, atopic
  - ligneous — *see* Blepharoconjunctivitis, ligneous
  - meningococcal A39.89
  - mucopurulent — *see* Conjunctivitis, acute, mucopurulent
  - neonatal P39.1
    - gonococcal A54.31
  - Newcastle B3Ø.8
  - of Beal B3Ø.2
  - parasitic
    - filariasis B74.9
    - mucocutaneous leishmaniasis B55.2
  - Parinaud's H1Ø.89
  - petrificans H1Ø.89
  - rosacea L71.9
  - specified NEC H1Ø.89
  - swimming-pool B3Ø.1
  - trachomatous A71.1
    - acute A71.Ø
    - sequelae (late effect) B94.Ø
  - traumatic NEC H1Ø.89
  - tuberculous A18.59
  - tularemic A21.1
  - tularensis A21.1
  - viral B3Ø.9
    - due to
      - adenovirus B3Ø.1
      - enterovirus B3Ø.3
    - specified NEC B3Ø.8
- **Conjunctivochalasis** H11.82-
- **Connective tissue** — *see* condition
- **Conn's syndrome** E26.Ø1
- **Conradi**(-Hunermann) **disease** Q77.3
- **Consanguinity** Z84.3
  - counseling Z71.89
- **Conscious simulation** (of illness) Z76.5
- **Consecutive** — *see* condition
- **Consolidation lung** (base) — *see* Pneumonia, lobar
- **Constipation** (atonic) (neurogenic) (simple) (spastic) K59.ØØ
  - drug-induced — *see* Table of Drugs and Chemicals
  - outlet dysfunction K59.Ø2
  - psychogenic F45.8
  - slow transit K59.Ø1
  - specified NEC K59.Ø9
- **Constitutional** (*see also* condition)
  - substandard F6Ø.7
- **Constitutionally substandard** F6Ø.7
- **Constriction** (*see also* Stricture)
  - auditory canal — *see* Stenosis, external ear canal
  - bronchial J98.Ø9
  - duodenum K31.5
  - esophagus K22.2
  - external
    - abdomen, abdominal (wall) S3Ø.841
    - alveolar process SØØ.542
    - ankle S9Ø.54-
    - antecubital space — *see* Constriction, external, forearm
    - arm (upper) S4Ø.84-
    - auricle — *see* Constriction, external, ear
    - axilla — *see* Constriction, external, arm
    - back, lower S3Ø.84Ø
    - breast S2Ø.14-
    - brow SØØ.84
    - buttock S3Ø.84Ø
    - calf — *see* Constriction, external, leg
    - canthus — *see* Constriction, external, eyelid
    - cheek SØØ.84
      - internal SØØ.542
    - chest wall — *see* Constriction, external, thorax
    - chin SØØ.84
    - clitoris S3Ø.844
    - costal region — *see* Constriction, external, thorax
    - digit(s)
      - hand — *see* Constriction, external, finger
      - foot — *see* Constriction, external, toe
    - ear SØØ.44-
    - elbow S5Ø.34-
    - epididymis S3Ø.843
    - epigastric region S3Ø.841
    - esophagus, cervical S1Ø.14
    - eyebrow — *see* Constriction, external, eyelid
    - eyelid SØØ.24-
    - face SØØ.84
    - finger(s) S6Ø.44-
      - index S6Ø.44-
      - little S6Ø.44-
      - middle S6Ø.44-
      - ring S6Ø.44-
    - flank S3Ø.841
    - foot (except toe(s) alone) S9Ø.84-
      - toe — *see* Constriction, external, toe
    - forearm S5Ø.84-
      - elbow only — *see* Constriction, external, elbow
    - forehead SØØ.84

Constriction — *continued*

- external — *continued*
  - genital organs, external
    - female S3Ø.846
    - male S3Ø.845
  - groin S3Ø.841
  - gum SØØ.542
  - hand S6Ø.54-
  - head SØØ.94
    - ear — *see* Constriction, external, ear
    - eyelid — *see* Constriction, external, eyelid
    - lip SØØ.541
    - nose SØØ.34
    - oral cavity SØØ.542
    - scalp SØØ.Ø4
    - specified site NEC SØØ.84
  - heel — *see* Constriction, external, foot
  - hip S7Ø.24-
  - inguinal region S3Ø.841
  - interscapular region S2Ø.449
  - jaw SØØ.84
  - knee S8Ø.24-
  - labium (majus) (minus) S3Ø.844
  - larynx S1Ø.14
  - leg (lower) S8Ø.84-
    - knee — *see* Constriction, external, knee
    - upper — *see* Constriction, external, thigh
  - lip SØØ.541
  - lower back S3Ø.84Ø
  - lumbar region S3Ø.84Ø
  - malar region SØØ.84
  - mammary — *see* Constriction, external, breast
  - mastoid region SØØ.84
  - mouth SØØ.542
  - nail
    - finger — *see* Constriction, external, finger
    - toe — *see* Constriction, external, toe
  - nasal SØØ.34
  - neck S1Ø.94
    - specified site NEC S1Ø.84
    - throat S1Ø.14
  - nose SØØ.34
  - occipital region SØØ.Ø4
  - oral cavity SØØ.542
  - orbital region — *see* Constriction, external, eyelid
  - palate SØØ.542
  - palm — *see* Constriction, external, hand
  - parietal region SØØ.Ø4
  - pelvis S3Ø.84Ø
  - penis S3Ø.842
  - perineum
    - female S3Ø.844
    - male S3Ø.84Ø
  - periocular area — *see* Constriction, external, eyelid
  - phalanges
    - finger — *see* Constriction, external, finger
    - toe — *see* Constriction, external, toe
  - pharynx S1Ø.14
  - pinna — *see* Constriction, external, ear
  - popliteal space — *see* Constriction, external, knee
  - prepuce S3Ø.842
  - pubic region S3Ø.84Ø
  - pudendum
    - female S3Ø.846
    - male S3Ø.845
  - sacral region S3Ø.84Ø
  - scalp SØØ.Ø4
  - scapular region — *see* Constriction, external, shoulder
  - scrotum S3Ø.843
  - shin — *see* Constriction, external, leg
  - shoulder S4Ø.24-
  - sternal region S2Ø.349
  - submaxillary region SØØ.84
  - submental region SØØ.84
  - subungual
    - finger(s) — *see* Constriction, external, finger
    - toe(s) — *see* Constriction, external, toe
  - supraclavicular fossa S1Ø.84
  - supraorbital SØØ.84
  - temple SØØ.84
  - temporal region SØØ.84
  - testis S3Ø.843

Contraction(s), contracture, contracted — *continued*
- ocular muscle — *see* Strabismus
- organ or site, congenital NEC — *see* Atresia, by site
- outlet (pelvis) — *see* Contraction, pelvis
- palmar fascia M72.Ø
- paralytic
  - joint — *see* Contraction, joint
  - muscle (*see also* Contraction, muscle NEC)
    - ocular — *see* Strabismus, paralytic
- pelvis (acquired) (general) M95.5
  - with disproportion (fetopelvic) O33.1
    - causing obstructed labor O65.1
    - inlet O33.2
    - mid-cavity O33.3
    - outlet O33.3
- plantar fascia M72.2
- premature
  - atrium I49.1
  - auriculoventricular I49.49
  - heart I49.49
  - junctional I49.2
  - supraventricular I49.1
  - ventricular I49.3
- prostate N42.89
- pylorus NEC (*see also* Pylorospasm)
  - psychogenic F45.8
- rectum, rectal (sphincter) K59.8
- ring (Bandl's) (complicating delivery) O62.4
- scar — *see* Cicatrix
- spine — *see* Dorsopathy, deforming
- sternocleidomastoid (muscle), congenital Q68.Ø
- stomach K31.89
  - hourglass K31.89
    - congenital Q4Ø.2
    - psychogenic F45.8
  - psychogenic F45.8
- tendon (sheath) M62.4Ø
  - with contracture of joint — *see* Contraction, joint
  - Achilles — *see* Short, tendon, Achilles
  - ankle M62.47-
    - Achilles — *see* Short, tendon, Achilles
  - foot M62.47-
  - forearm M62.43-
  - hand M62.44-
  - lower leg M62.46-
  - multiple sites M62.49
  - neck M62.48
  - pelvic region M62.45-
  - shoulder region M62.41-
  - specified site NEC M62.48
  - thigh M62.45-
  - thorax M62.48
  - trunk M62.48
  - upper arm M62.42-
- toe — *see* Deformity, toe, specified NEC
- ureterovesical orifice (postinfectional) N13.5
  - with infection N13.6
- urethra (*see also* Stricture, urethra)
  - orifice N32.Ø
- uterus N85.8
  - abnormal NEC O62.9
  - clonic (complicating delivery) O62.4
  - dyscoordinate (complicating delivery) O62.4
  - hourglass (complicating delivery) O62.4
  - hypertonic O62.4
  - hypotonic NEC O62.2
  - inadequate
    - primary O62.Ø
    - secondary O62.1
  - incoordinate (complicating delivery) O62.4
  - poor O62.2
  - tetanic (complicating delivery) O62.4
- vagina (outlet) N89.5
- vesical N32.89
  - neck or urethral orifice N32.Ø
- visual field — *see* Defect, visual field, generalized
- Volkmann's (ischemic) T79.6

Contusion (skin surface intact) T14.8
- abdomen, abdominal (muscle) (wall) S3Ø.1
- adnexa, eye NEC SØ5.8X-
- adrenal gland S37.812
- alveolar process SØØ.532
- ankle S9Ø.Ø-
- antecubital space — *see* Contusion, forearm
- anus S3Ø.3
- arm (upper) S4Ø.Ø2-
  - lower (with elbow) — *see* Contusion, forearm
- auditory canal — *see* Contusion, ear
- auricle — *see* Contusion, ear
- axilla — *see* Contusion, arm, upper
- back (*see also* Contusion, thorax, back)
  - lower S3Ø.Ø
- bile duct S36.13
- bladder S37.22
- bone NEC T14.8
- brain (diffuse) — *see* Injury, intracranial, diffuse
  - focal — *see* Injury, intracranial, focal
- brainstem SØ6.38-
- breast S2Ø.Ø-
- broad ligament S37.892
- brow SØØ.83
- buttock S3Ø.Ø
- canthus, eye SØØ.1-
- cauda equina S34.3
- cerebellar, traumatic SØ6.37-
- cerebral SØ6.33-
  - left side SØ6.32-
  - right side SØ6.31-
- cheek SØØ.83
  - internal SØØ.532
- chest (wall) — *see* Contusion, thorax
- chin SØØ.83
- clitoris S3Ø.23
- colon — *see* Injury, intestine, large, contusion
- common bile duct S36.13
- conjunctiva SØ5.1-
  - with foreign body (in conjunctival sac) — *see* Foreign body, conjunctival sac
- conus medullaris (spine) S34.139
- cornea — *see* Contusion, eyeball
  - with foreign body — *see* Foreign body, cornea
- corpus cavernosum S3Ø.21
- cortex (brain) (cerebral) — *see* Injury, intracranial, diffuse
  - focal — *see* Injury, intracranial, focal
- costal region — *see* Contusion, thorax
- cystic duct S36.13
- diaphragm S27.8Ø2
- duodenum S36.42Ø
- ear SØØ.43-
- elbow S5Ø.Ø-
  - with forearm — *see* Contusion, forearm
- epididymis S3Ø.22
- epigastric region S3Ø.1
- epiglottis S1Ø.Ø
- esophagus (thoracic) S27.812
  - cervical S1Ø.Ø
- eyeball SØ5.1-
- eyebrow SØØ.1-
- eyelid (and periocular area) SØØ.1-
- face NEC SØØ.83
- fallopian tube S37.529
  - bilateral S37.522
  - unilateral S37.521
- femoral triangle S3Ø.1
- finger(s) S6Ø.ØØ
  - with damage to nail (matrix) S6Ø.1Ø
  - index S6Ø.Ø2-
    - with damage to nail S6Ø.12-
  - little S6Ø.Ø5-
    - with damage to nail S6Ø.15-
  - middle S6Ø.Ø3-
    - with damage to nail S6Ø.13-
  - ring S6Ø.Ø4-
    - with damage to nail S6Ø.14-
  - thumb — *see* Contusion, thumb
- flank S3Ø.1
- foot (except toe(s) alone) S9Ø.3-
  - toe — *see* Contusion, toe
- forearm S5Ø.1-
  - elbow only — *see* Contusion, elbow
- forehead SØØ.83
- gallbladder S36.122

Contusion — *continued*
- genital organs, external
  - female S3Ø.2Ø2
  - male S3Ø.2Ø1
- globe (eye) — *see* Contusion, eyeball
- groin S3Ø.1
- gum SØØ.532
- hand S6Ø.22-
  - finger(s) — *see* Contusion, finger
  - wrist — *see* Contusion, wrist
- head SØØ.93
  - ear — *see* Contusion, ear
  - eyelid — *see* Contusion, eyelid
  - lip SØØ.531
  - nose SØØ.33
  - oral cavity SØØ.532
  - scalp SØØ.Ø3
  - specified part NEC SØØ.83
- heel — *see* Contusion, foot
- hepatic duct S36.13
- hip S7Ø.Ø-
- ileum S36.428
- iliac region S3Ø.1
- inguinal region S3Ø.1
- interscapular region S2Ø.229
- intra-abdominal organ S36.92
  - colon — *see* Injury, intestine, large, contusion
  - liver S36.112
  - pancreas — *see* Contusion, pancreas
  - rectum S36.62
  - small intestine — *see* Injury, intestine, small, contusion
  - specified organ NEC S36.892
  - spleen — *see* Contusion, spleen
  - stomach S36.32
- iris (eye) — *see* Contusion, eyeball
- jaw SØØ.83
- jejunum S36.428
- kidney S37.Ø1-
  - major (greater than 2 cm) S37.Ø2-
  - minor (less than 2 cm) S37.Ø1-
- knee S8Ø.Ø-
- labium (majus) (minus) S3Ø.23
- lacrimal apparatus, gland or sac SØ5.8x-
- larynx S1Ø.Ø
- leg (lower) S8Ø.1-
  - knee — *see* Contusion, knee
- lens — *see* Contusion, eyeball
- lip SØØ.531
- liver S36.112
- lower back S3Ø.Ø
- lumbar region S3Ø.Ø
- lung S27.329
  - bilateral S27.322
  - unilateral S27.321
- malar region SØØ.83
- mastoid region SØØ.83
- membrane, brain — *see* Injury, intracranial, diffuse
  - focal — *see* Injury, intracranial, focal
- mesentery S36.892
- mesosalpinx S37.529
  - bilateral S37.522
  - unilateral S37.521
- mouth SØØ.532
- muscle — *see* Contusion, by site
- nail
  - finger — *see* Contusion, finger, with damage to nail
  - toe — *see* Contusion, toe, with damage to nail
- nasal SØØ.33
- neck S1Ø.93
  - specified site NEC S1Ø.83
  - throat S1Ø.Ø
- newborn P54.5
- nerve — *see* Injury, nerve
- nose SØØ.33
- occipital
  - lobe (brain) — *see* Injury, intracranial, diffuse
    - focal — *see* Injury, intracranial, focal
  - region (scalp) SØØ.Ø3
- orbit (region) (tissues) SØ5.1-
- ovary S37.429
  - bilateral S37.422

Contusion — *continued*
ovary — *continued*
unilateral S37.421
palate S00.532
pancreas S36.229
body S36.221
head S36.220
tail S36.222
parietal
lobe (brain) — *see* Injury, intracranial, diffuse
focal — *see* Injury, intracranial, focal
region (scalp) S00.03
pelvic organ S37.92
adrenal gland S37.812
bladder S37.22
fallopian tube — *see* Contusion, fallopian tube
kidney — *see* Contusion, kidney
ovary — *see* Contusion, ovary
prostate S37.823
specified organ NEC S37.892
ureter S37.12
urethra S37.32
uterus S37.62
pelvis S30.0
penis S30.21
perineum
female S30.23
male S30.0
periocular area S00.1-
peritoneum S36.81
periurethral tissue — *see* Contusion, urethra
pharynx S10.0
pinna — *see* Contusion, ear
popliteal space — *see* Contusion, knee
prepuce S30.21
prostate S37.822
pubic region S30.1
pudendum
female S30.202
male S30.201
quadriceps femoris — *see* Contusion, thigh
rectum S36.62
retroperitoneum S36.892
round ligament S37.892
sacral region S30.0
scalp S00.03
due to birth injury P12.3
scapular region — *see* Contusion, shoulder
sclera — *see* Contusion, eyeball
scrotum S30.22
seminal vesicle S37.892
shoulder S40.01-
skin NEC T14.8
small intestine — *see* Injury, intestine, small, contusion
spermatic cord S30.22
spinal cord — *see* Injury, spinal cord, by region
cauda equina S34.3
conus medullaris S34.139
spleen S36.029
major S36.021
minor S36.020
sternal region S20.219
stomach S36.32
subconjunctival S05.1-
subcutaneous NEC T14.8
submaxillary region S00.83
submental region S00.83
subperiosteal NEC T14.8
subungual
finger — *see* Contusion, finger, with damage to nail
toe — *see* Contusion, toe, with damage to nail
supraclavicular fossa S10.83
supraorbital S00.83
suprarenal gland S37.812
temple (region) S00.83
temporal
lobe (brain) — *see* Injury, intracranial, diffuse
focal — *see* Injury, intracranial, focal
region S00.83
testis S30.22
thigh S70.1-

Contusion — *continued*
thorax (wall) S20.20
back S20.22-
front S20.21-
throat S10.0
thumb S60.01-
with damage to nail S60.11-
toe(s) (lesser) S90.12-
with damage to nail S90.22-
great S90.11-
with damage to nail S90.21-
specified type NEC S90.221
tongue S00.532
trachea (cervical) S10.0
thoracic S27.52
tunica vaginalis S30.22
tympanum, tympanic membrane — *see* Contusion, ear
ureter S37.12
urethra S37.32
urinary organ NEC S37.892
uterus S37.62
uvula S00.532
vagina S30.23
vas deferens S37.892
vesical S37.22
vocal cord(s) S10.0
vulva S30.23
wrist S60.21-
Conus (congenital) (any type) Q14.8
cornea — *see* Keratoconus
medullaris syndrome G95.81
Conversion hysteria, neurosis or reaction F44.9
Converter, tuberculosis (test reaction) R76.11
Conviction (legal), **anxiety concerning** Z65.0
with imprisonment Z65.1
Convulsions (idiopathic) (*see also* Seizure(s)) R56.9
apoplectiform (cerebral ischemia) I67.82
benign neonatal (familial) — *see* Epilepsy, generalized, idiopathic
dissociative F44.5
epileptic — *see* Epilepsy
epileptiform, epileptoid — *see* Seizure, epileptiform
ether (anesthetic) — *see* Table of Drugs and Chemicals, by drug
febrile R56.00
with status epilepticus G40.901
complex R56.01
with status epilepticus G40.901
simple R56.00
hysterical F44.5
infantile P90
epilepsy — *see* Epilepsy
jacksonian — *see* Epilepsy, localization-related, symptomatic, with simple partial seizures
myoclonic G25.3
neonatal, benign (familial) — *see* Epilepsy, generalized, idiopathic
newborn P90
obstetrical (nephritic) (uremic) — *see* Eclampsia
paretic A52.17
post traumatic R56.1
psychomotor — *see* Epilepsy, localization-related, symptomatic, with complex partial seizures
recurrent R56.9
reflex R25.8
scarlatinal A38.8
tetanus, tetanic — *see* Tetanus
thymic E32.8
Convulsive (*see also* Convulsions)
Cooley's anemia D56.1
Coolie itch B76.9
Cooper's
disease — *see* Mastopathy, cystic
hernia — *see* Hernia, abdomen, specified site NEC
Copra itch B88.0
Coprophagy F50.8
Coprophobia F40.298
Coproporphyria, hereditary E80.29
Cor
biloculare Q20.8
bovis, bovinum — *see* Hypertrophy, cardiac
pulmonale (chronic) I27.81
acute I26.09

Cor — *continued*
triatriatum, triatrium Q24.2
triloculare Q20.8
biatrium Q20.4
biventriculare Q21.1
Corbus' disease (gangrenous balanitis) N48.1
Cord (*see also* condition)
around neck (tightly) (with compression)
complicating delivery O69.1
bladder G95.89
tabetic A52.19
Cordis ectopia Q24.8
Corditis (spermatic) N49.1
Corectopia Q13.2
Cori's disease (glycogen storage) E74.03
Corkhandler's disease or lung J67.3
Corkscrew esophagus K22.4
Corkworker's disease or lung J67.3
Corn (infected) L84
Cornea (*see also* condition)
donor Z52.5
plana Q13.4
Cornelia de Lange syndrome Q87.1
Cornu cutaneum L85.8
Cornual gestation or pregnancy O00.8
Coronary (artery) — *see* condition
Coronavirus, as cause of disease classified elsewhere B97.29
SARS-associated B97.21
Corpora (*see also* condition)
amylacea, prostate N42.89
cavernosa — *see* condition
Corpulence — *see* Obesity
Corpus — *see* condition
Corrected transposition Q20.5
Corrosion (injury) (acid) (caustic) (chemical) (lime) (external) (internal) T30.4
abdomen, abdominal (muscle) (wall) T21.42
first degree T21.52
second degree T21.62
third degree T21.72
above elbow T22.439
first degree T22.539
left T22.432
first degree T22.532
second degree T22.632
third degree T22.732
right T22.431
first degree T22.531
second degree T22.631
third degree T22.731
second degree T22.639
third degree T22.739
alimentary tract NEC T28.7
ankle T25.419
first degree T25.519
left T25.412
first degree T25.512
second degree T25.612
third degree T25.712
multiple with foot — *see* Corrosion, lower, limb, multiple, ankle and foot
right T25.411
first degree T25.511
second degree T25.611
third degree T25.711
second degree T25.619
third degree T25.719
anus — *see* Corrosion, buttock
arm(s) (meaning upper limb(s)) — *see* Corrosion, upper limb
axilla T22.449
first degree T22.549
left T22.442
first degree T22.542
second degree T22.642
third degree T22.742
right T22.441
first degree T22.541
second degree T22.641
third degree T22.741
second degree T22.649
third degree T22.749

- **Corrosion** — *continued*
  - toe — *continued*
    - left T25.432
      - first degree T25.532
      - second degree T25.632
      - third degree T25.732
    - right T25.431
      - first degree T25.531
      - second degree T25.631
      - third degree T25.731
    - second degree T25.639
    - third degree T25.739
  - tongue T28.5
  - tonsil(s) T28.5
  - total body — *see* Corrosion, multiple body regions
  - trachea T27.4
    - with lung T27.5
  - trunk T21.40
    - abdominal wall — *see* Corrosion, abdominal wall
    - anus — *see* Corrosion, buttock
    - axilla — *see* Corrosion, upper limb
    - back — *see* Corrosion, back
    - breast — *see* Corrosion, chest wall
    - buttock — *see* Corrosion, buttock
    - chest wall — *see* Corrosion, chest wall
    - first degree T21.50
    - flank — *see* Corrosion, abdominal wall
    - genital
      - female — *see* Corrosion, genital organs, external, female
      - male — *see* Corrosion, genital organs, external, male
    - groin — *see* Corrosion, abdominal wall
    - interscapular region — *see* Corrosion, back, upper
    - labia — *see* Corrosion, genital organs, external, female
    - lower back — *see* Corrosion, back
    - penis — *see* Corrosion, genital organs, external, male
    - perineum
      - female — *see* Corrosion, genital organs, external, female
      - male — *see* Corrosion, genital organs, external, male
    - scapular region — *see* Corrosion, upper limb
    - scrotum — *see* Corrosion, genital organs, external, male
    - shoulder — *see* Corrosion, upper limb
    - second degree T21.60
    - specified site NEC T21.49
      - first degree T21.59
      - second degree T21.69
      - third degree T21.79
    - testes — *see* Corrosion, genital organs, external, male
    - third degree T21.70
    - upper back — *see* Corrosion, back, upper
    - vagina T28.8
    - vulva — *see* Corrosion, genital organs, external, female
  - unspecified site with extent of body surface involved specified
    - less than 10 per cent T32.0
    - 10-19 per cent (0-9 percent third degree) T32.10
      - with 10-19 percent third degree T32.11
    - 20-29 per cent (0-9 percent third degree) T32.20
      - with
        - 10-19 percent third degree T32.21
        - 20-29 percent third degree T32.22
    - 30-39 per cent (0-9 percent third degree) T32.30
      - with
        - 10-19 percent third degree T32.31
        - 20-29 percent third degree T32.32
        - 30-39 percent third degree T32.33
    - 40-49 per cent (0-9 percent third degree) T32.40
      - with
        - 10-19 percent third degree T32.41
        - 20-29 percent third degree T32.42
        - 30-39 percent third degree T32.43
        - 40-49 percent third degree T32.44

- **Corrosion** — *continued*
  - unspecified site with extent of body surface involved specified — *continued*
    - 50-59 per cent (0-9 percent third degree)
      - with
        - 10-19 percent third degree T32.51
        - 20-29 percent third degree T32.52
        - 30-39 percent third degree T32.53
        - 40-49 percent third degree T32.54
        - 50-59 percent third degree T32.55
    - 60-69 per cent (0-9 percent third degree) T32.60
      - with
        - 10-19 percent third degree T32.61
        - 20-29 percent third degree T32.62
        - 30-39 percent third degree T32.63
        - 40-49 percent third degree T32.64
        - 50-59 percent third degree T32.65
        - 60-69 percent third degree T32.66
    - 70-79 per cent (0-9 percent third degree) T32.70
      - with
        - 10-19 percent third degree T32.71
        - 20-29 percent third degree T32.72
        - 30-39 percent third degree T32.73
        - 40-49 percent third degree T32.74
        - 50-59 percent third degree T32.75
        - 60-69 percent third degree T32.76
        - 70-79 percent third degree T32.77
    - 80-89 per cent (0-9 percent third degree) T32.80
      - with
        - 10-19 percent third degree T32.81
        - 20-29 percent third degree T32.82
        - 30-39 percent third degree T32.83
        - 40-49 percent third degree T32.84
        - 50-59 percent third degree T32.85
        - 60-69 percent third degree T32.86
        - 70-79 percent third degree T32.87
        - 80-89 percent third degree T32.88
    - 90 per cent or more (0-9 percent third degree) T32.90
      - with
        - 10-19 percent third degree T32.91
        - 20-29 percent third degree T32.92
        - 30-39 percent third degree T32.93
        - 40-49 percent third degree T32.94
        - 50-59 percent third degree T32.95
        - 60-69 percent third degree T32.96
        - 70-79 percent third degree T32.97
        - 80-89 percent third degree T32.98
        - 90-99 percent third degree T32.99
  - upper limb (axilla) (scapular region) T22.40
    - above elbow — *see* Corrosion, above elbow
    - axilla — *see* Corrosion, axilla
    - elbow — *see* Corrosion, elbow
    - first degree T22.50
    - forearm — *see* Corrosion, forearm
    - hand — *see* Corrosion, hand
    - interscapular region — *see* Corrosion, back, upper
    - multiple sites T22.499
      - first degree T22.599
      - left T22.492
        - first degree T22.592
        - second degree T22.692
        - third degree T22.792
      - right T22.491
        - first degree T22.591
        - second degree T22.691
        - third degree T22.791
      - second degree T22.699
      - third degree T22.799
    - scapular region — *see* Corrosion, scapular region
    - second degree T22.60
    - shoulder — *see* Corrosion, shoulder
    - third degree T22.70
    - wrist — *see* Corrosion, hand
  - uterus T28.8
  - vagina T28.8
  - vulva — *see* Corrosion, genital organs, external, female
  - wrist T23.479
    - first degree T23.579
    - left T23.472

- **Corrosion** — *continued*
  - wrist — *continued*
    - left — *continued*
      - first degree T23.572
      - second degree T23.672
      - third degree T23.772
    - multiple sites with hand T23.499
      - first degree T23.599
      - left T23.492
        - first degree T23.592
        - second degree T23.692
        - third degree T23.792
      - right T23.491
        - first degree T23.591
        - second degree T23.691
        - third degree T23.791
      - second degree T23.699
      - third degree T23.799
    - right T23.471
      - first degree T23.571
      - second degree T23.671
      - third degree T23.771
    - second degree T23.679
    - third degree T23.779
- **Corrosive burn** — *see* Corrosion
- **Corsican fever** — *see* Malaria
- **Cortical** — *see* condition
- **Cortico-adrenal** — *see* condition
- **Coryza** (acute) J00
  - with grippe or influenza — *see* Influenza, with, respiratory manifestations NEC
  - syphilitic
    - congenital (chronic) A50.05
- **Costen's syndrome or complex** M26.69
- **Costiveness** — *see* Constipation
- **Costochondritis** M94.0
- **Cotard's syndrome** F22
- **Cot death** R99
- **Cotia virus** B08.8
- **Cotton wool spots** (retinal) H35.81
- **Cotungo's disease** — *see* Sciatica
- **Cough** (affected) (chronic) (epidemic) (nervous) R05
  - with hemorrhage — *see* Hemoptysis
  - bronchial R05
    - with grippe or influenza — *see* Influenza, with, respiratory manifestations NEC
  - functional F45.8
  - hysterical F45.8
  - laryngeal, spasmodic R05
  - psychogenic F45.8
  - smokers' J41.0
  - tea taster's B49
- **Counseling** (for) Z71.9
  - abuse NEC
    - perpetrator Z69.82
    - victim Z69.81
  - alcohol abuser Z71.41
    - family Z71.42
  - child abuse
    - nonparental
      - perpetrator Z69.021
      - victim Z69.020
    - parental
      - perpetrator Z69.011
      - victim Z69.010
  - consanguinity Z71.89
  - contraceptive Z30.09
  - dietary Z71.3
  - drug abuser Z71.51
    - family member Z71.52
  - family Z71.89
  - fertility preservation (prior to cancer therapy) (prior to removal of gonads) Z31.62
  - for non-attending third party Z71.0
    - related to sexual behavior or orientation Z70.2
  - genetic NEC Z31.5
  - health (advice) (education) (instruction) — *see* Counseling, medical
  - human immunodeficiency virus (HIV) Z71.7
  - impotence Z70.1
  - insulin pump use Z46.81
  - medical (for) Z71.9
    - boarding school resident Z59.3

Counseling — *continued*
medical (for) — *continued*
consanguinity Z71.89
feared complaint and no disease found Z71.1
human immunodeficiency virus (HIV) Z71.7
institutional resident Z59.3
on behalf of another Z71.Ø
related to sexual behavior or orientation Z7Ø.2
person living alone Z6Ø.2
specified reason NEC Z71.89
natural family planning
procreative Z31.61
to avoid pregnancy Z3Ø.Ø2
perpetrator (of)
abuse NEC Z69.82
child abuse
non-parental Z69.Ø21
parental Z69.Ø11
spousal abuse Z69.12
rape NEC Z69.82
procreative NEC Z31.69
fertility preservation (prior to cancer therapy) (prior to removal of gonads) Z31.62
using natural family planning Z31.61
promiscuity Z7Ø.1
rape victim Z69.81
religious Z71.81
sex, sexual (related to) Z7Ø.9
attitude(s) Z7Ø.Ø
behavior or orientation Z7Ø.1
combined concerns Z7Ø.3
non-responsiveness Z7Ø.1
on behalf of third party Z7Ø.2
specified reason NEC Z7Ø.8
specified reason NEC Z71.89
spiritual Z71.81
spousal abuse (perpetrator) Z69.12
victim Z69.11
substance abuse Z71.89
alcohol Z71.41
drug Z71.51
tobacco Z71.6
tobacco use Z71.6
use (of)
insulin pump Z46.81
victim (of)
abuse Z69.81
child abuse
by parent Z69.Ø1Ø
non-parental Z69.Ø2Ø
rape NEC Z69.81
Coupled rhythm RØØ.8
Couvelaire syndrome or uterus (complicating delivery) O45.8x-
Cowperitis — *see* Urethritis
Cowper's gland — *see* condition
Cowpox BØ8.Ø1Ø
due to vaccination T88.1
Coxa
magna M91.4-
plana M91.2-
valga (acquired) (*see also* Deformity, limb, specified type NEC, thigh)
congenital Q65.81
sequelae (late effect) of rickets E64.3
vara (acquired) (*see also* Deformity, limb, specified type NEC, thigh)
congenital Q65.82
sequelae (late effect) of rickets E64.3
Coxalgia, coxalgic (nontuberculous) (*see also* Pain, joint, hip)
tuberculous A18.Ø2
Coxitis — *see* Monoarthritis, hip
Coxsackie (virus) (infection) B34.1
as cause of disease classified elsewhere B97.11
carditis B33.2Ø
central nervous system NEC A88.8
endocarditis B33.21
enteritis AØ8.39
meningitis (aseptic) A87.Ø
myocarditis B33.22
pericarditis B33.23
pharyngitis BØ8.5

Coxsackie — *continued*
pleurodynia B33.Ø
specific disease NEC B33.8
Crabs, meaning pubic lice B85.3
Crack baby PØ4.41
Cracked nipple N64.Ø
associated with
lactation O92.13
pregnancy O92.11-
Cracked tooth KØ3.81
Cradle cap L21.Ø
Craft neurosis F48.8
Cramp(s) R25.2
abdominal — *see* Pain, abdominal
bathing T75.1
colic R1Ø.83
psychogenic F45.8
due to immersion T75.1
fireman T67.2
heat T67.2
immersion T75.1
intestinal — *see* Pain, abdominal
psychogenic F45.8
leg, sleep related G47.62
limb (lower) (upper) NEC R25.2
sleep related G47.62
linotypist's F48.8
organic G25.89
muscle (limb) (general) R25.2
due to immersion T75.1
psychogenic F45.8
occupational (hand) F48.8
organic G25.89
salt-depletion E87.1
sleep related, leg G47.62
stoker's T67.2
swimmer's T75.1
telegrapher's F48.8
organic G25.89
typist's F48.8
organic G25.89
uterus N94.89
menstrual — *see* Dysmenorrhea
writer's F48.8
organic G25.89
Cranial — *see* condition
Craniocleidodysostosis Q74.Ø
Craniofenestria (skull) Q75.8
Craniolacunia (skull) Q75.8
Craniopagus Q89.4
Craniopathy, metabolic M85.2
Craniopharyngeal — *see* condition
Craniopharyngioma D44.4
Craniorachischisis (totalis) QØØ.1
Cranioschisis Q75.8
Craniostenosis Q75.Ø
Craniosynostosis Q75.Ø
Craniotabes (cause unknown) M83.8
neonatal P96.3
rachitic E64.3
syphilitic A5Ø.56
Cranium — *see* condition
Craw-craw — *see* Onchocerciasis
Creaking joint — *see* Derangement, joint, specified type NEC
Creeping
eruption B76.9
palsy or paralysis G12.22
Crenated tongue K14.8
Creotoxism AØ5.9
Crepitus
caput Q75.8
joint — *see* Derangement, joint, specified type NEC
Crescent or conus choroid, congenital Q14.3
CREST syndrome M34.1
Cretin, cretinism (congenital) (endemic) (nongoitrous) (sporadic) EØØ.9
pelvis
with disproportion (fetopelvic) O33.Ø
causing obstructed labor O65.Ø
type
hypothyroid EØØ.1
mixed EØØ.2

Cretin, cretinism — *continued*
type — *continued*
myxedematous EØØ.1
neurological EØØ.Ø
Creutzfeldt-Jakob disease or syndrome (with dementia) A81.ØØ
familial A81.Ø9
iatrogenic A81.Ø9
specified NEC A81.Ø9
sporadic A81.Ø9
variant (vCJD) A81.Ø1
Crib death R99
Cribriform hymen Q52.3
Cri-du-chat syndrome Q93.4
Crigler-Najjar disease or syndrome E8Ø.5
Crime, victim of Z65.4
Crimean hemorrhagic fever A98.Ø
Criminalism F6Ø.2
Crisis
abdomen R1Ø.Ø
acute reaction F43.Ø
addisonian E27.2
adrenal (cortical) E27.2
celiac K9Ø.Ø
Dietl's N13.8
emotional (*see also* Disorder, adjustment)
acute reaction to stress F43.Ø
specific to childhood and adolescence F93.8
glaucomatocyclitic — *see* Glaucoma, secondary, inflammation
heart — *see* Failure, heart
nitritoid I95.2
correct substance properly administered — *see* Table of Drugs and Chemicals, by drug, adverse effect
overdose or wrong substance given or taken — *see* Table of Drugs and Chemicals, by drug, poisoning
oculogyric H51.8
psychogenic F45.8
Pel's (tabetic) A52.11
psychosexual identity F64.2
renal N28.Ø
sickle-cell D57.ØØ
with
acute chest syndrome D57.Ø1
splenic sequestration D57.Ø2
state (acute reaction) F43.Ø
tabetic A52.11
thyroid — *see* Thyrotoxicosis with thyroid storm
thyrotoxic — *see* Thyrotoxicosis with thyroid storm
Crocq's disease (acrocyanosis) I73.89
Crohn's disease — *see* Enteritis, regional
Crooked septum, nasal J34.2
Cross syndrome E7Ø.328
Crossbite (anterior) (posterior) M26.24
Cross-eye — *see* Strabismus, convergent concomitant
Croup, croupous (catarrhal) (infectious) (inflammatory) (nondiphtheritic) JØ5.Ø
bronchial J2Ø.9
diphtheritic A36.2
false J38.5
spasmodic J38.5
diphtheritic A36.2
stridulous J38.5
diphtheritic A36.2
Crouzon's disease Q75.1
Crowding, tooth, teeth, fully erupted M26.31
CRST syndrome M34.1
Cruchet's disease A85.8
Cruelty in children —*see* Disorder, conduct
Crural ulcer — *see* Ulcer, lower limb
Crush, crushed, crushing T14.8
abdomen S38.1
ankle S97.Ø-
arm (upper) (and shoulder) S47.-
axilla — *see* Crush, arm
back, lower S38.1
buttock S38.1
cheek SØ7.Ø
chest S28.Ø
cranium SØ7.1
ear SØ7.Ø

Crush, crushed, crushing — *continued*
- elbow S57.Ø-
- extremity
  - lower
    - ankle — *see* Crush, ankle
    - below knee — *see* Crush, leg
    - foot — *see* Crush, foot
    - hip — *see* Crush, hip
    - knee — *see* Crush, knee
    - thigh — *see* Crush, thigh
    - toe — *see* Crush, toe
  - upper
    - below elbow S67.9-
    - elbow — *see* Crush, elbow
    - finger — *see* Crush, finger
    - forearm — *see* Crush, forearm
    - hand — *see* Crush, hand
    - thumb — *see* Crush, thumb
    - upper arm — *see* Crush, arm
    - wrist — *see* Crush, wrist
- face SØ7.Ø
- finger(s) S67.1-
  - with hand (and wrist) — *see* Crush, hand, specified site NEC
  - index S67.19-
  - little S67.19-
  - middle S67.19-
  - ring S67.19-
  - thumb — *see* Crush, thumb
- foot S97.8-
  - toe — *see* Crush, toe
- forearm S57.8-
- genitalia, external
  - female S38.ØØ2
    - vagina S38.Ø3
    - vulva S38.Ø3
  - male S38.ØØ1
    - penis S38.Ø1
    - scrotum S38.Ø2
    - testis S38.Ø2
- hand (except fingers alone) S67.2-
  - with wrist S67.4-
- head
  - specified NEC SØ7.8
- heel — *see* Crush, foot
- hip S77.Ø-
  - with thigh S77.2-
- internal organ (abdomen, chest, or pelvis) NEC T14.8
- knee S87.Ø-
- labium (majus) (minus) S38.Ø3
- larynx S17.Ø
- leg (lower) S87.8-
  - knee — *see* Crush, knee
- lip SØ7.Ø
- lower
  - back S38.1
  - leg — *see* Crush, leg
- neck S17.9
- nerve — *see* Injury, nerve
- nose SØ7.Ø
- pelvis S38.1
- penis S38.Ø1
- scalp SØ7.8
- scapular region — *see* Crush, arm
- scrotum S38.Ø2
- severe, unspecified site T14.8
- shoulder (and upper arm) — *see* Crush, arm
- skull SØ7.1
- syndrome (complication of trauma) T79.5
- testis S38.Ø2
- thigh S77.1-
  - with hip S77.2-
- throat S17.8
- thumb S67.Ø-
  - with hand (and wrist) — *see* Crush, hand, specified site NEC
- toe(s) S97.1Ø-
  - great S97.11-
  - lesser S97.12-
- trachea S17.Ø
- vagina S38.Ø3
- vulva S38.Ø3

Crush, crushed, crushing — *continued*
- wrist S67.3-
  - with hand S67.4-

Crusta lactea L21.Ø

Crusts R23.4

Crutch paralysis — *see* Injury, brachial plexus

Cruveilhier-Baumgarten cirrhosis, disease or syndrome K74.69

Cruveilhier's atrophy or disease G12.8

Crying (constant) (continuous) (excessive)
- child, adolescent, or adult R45.83
- infant (baby) (newborn) R68.11

Cryofibrinogenemia D89.2

Cryoglobulinemia(essential) (idiopathic) (mixed) (primary) (purpura) (secondary) (vasculitis) D89.1
- with lung involvement D89.1 *[J99]*

Cryptitis (anal) (rectal) K62.89

Cryptococcosis, cryptococcus (infection) (neoformans) B45.9
- bone B45.3
- cerebral B45.1
- cutaneous B45.2
- disseminated B45.7
- generalized B45.7
- meningitis B45.1
- meningocerebralis B45.1
- osseous B45.3
- pulmonary B45.Ø
- skin B45.2
- specified NEC B45.8

Cryptopapillitis (anus) K62.89

Cryptophthalmos Q11.2
- syndrome Q87.Ø

Cryptorchid, cryptorchism, cryptorchidism Q53.9
- bilateral Q53.2Ø
  - abdominal Q53.21
  - perineal Q53.22
- unilateral Q53.1Ø
  - abdominal Q53.11
  - perineal Q53.12

Cryptosporidiosis AØ7.2
- hepatobiliary B88.8
- respiratory B88.8

Cryptostromosis J67.6

Crystalluria R82.99

Cubitus
- congenital Q68.8
- valgus (acquired) M21.Ø-
  - congenital Q68.8
  - sequelae (late effect) of rickets E64.3
- varus (acquired) M21.1-
  - congenital Q68.8
  - sequelae (late effect) of rickets E64.3

Cultural deprivation or shock Z6Ø.3

Curling esophagus K22.4

Curling's ulcer — *see* Ulcer, peptic, acute

Curschmann (-Batten) (-Steinert) **disease or syndrome** G71.11

Curse, Ondine's — *see* Apnea, sleep

Curvature
- organ or site, congenital NEC — *see* Distortion
- penis (lateral) Q55.61
- Pott's (spinal) A18.Ø1
- radius, idiopathic, progressive (congenital) Q74.Ø
- spine (acquired) (angular) (idiopathic) (incorrect) (postural) — *see* Dorsopathy, deforming
  - congenital Q67.5
  - due to or associated with
    - Charcot-Marie-Tooth disease (*see also* subcategory M49.8) G6Ø.Ø
    - osteitis
      - deformans M88.88
      - fibrosa cystica (*see also* subcategory M49.8) E21.Ø
    - tuberculosis (Pott's curvature) A18.Ø1
  - sequelae (late effect) of rickets E64.3
  - tuberculous A18.Ø1

Cushingoid due to steroid therapy E24.2
- correct substance properly administered — *see* Table of Drugs and Chemicals, by drug, adverse effect

Cushingoid due to steroid therapy — *continued*
- overdose or wrong substance given or taken — *see* Table of Drugs and Chemicals, by drug, poisoning

Cushing's
- syndrome or disease E24.9
  - drug-induced E24.2
  - iatrogenic E24.2
  - pituitary-dependent E24.Ø
  - specified NEC E24.8
- ulcer — *see* Ulcer, peptic, acute

Cusp, Carabelli —*omit code*

Cut (external) (*see also* Laceration)
- muscle — *see* Injury, muscle

Cutaneous (*see also* condition)
- hemorrhage R23.3
- larva migrans B76.9

Cutis (*see also* condition)
- hyperelastica Q82.8
  - acquired L57.4
- laxa (hyperelastica) — *see* Dermatolysis
- marmorata R23.8
- osteosis L94.2
- pendula — *see* Dermatolysis
- rhomboidalis nuchae L57.2
- verticis gyrata Q82.8
  - acquired L91.8

Cyanosis R23.Ø
- due to
  - patent foramen botalli Q21.1
  - persistent foramen ovale Q21.1
- enterogenous D74.8
- paroxysmal digital — *see* Raynaud's disease
  - with gangrene I73.Ø1
- retina, retinal H35.89

Cyanotic heart disease I24.9
- congenital Q24.9

Cycle
- anovulatory N97.Ø
- menstrual, irregular N92.6

Cyclencephaly QØ4.9

Cyclical vomiting (*see also* Vomiting, cyclical) G43.AØ
- psychogenic F5Ø.8

Cyclitis (*see also* Iridocyclitis) H2Ø.9
- chronic — *see* Iridocyclitis, chronic
- Fuchs' heterochromic H2Ø.81-
- granulomatous — *see* Iridocyclitis, chronic
- lens-induced — *see* Iridocyclitis, lens-induced
- posterior H3Ø.2-

Cycloid personality F34.Ø

Cyclophoria H5Ø.54

Cyclopia, cyclops Q87.Ø

Cyclopism Q87.Ø

Cyclosporiasis AØ7.4

Cyclothymia F34.Ø

Cyclothymic personality F34.Ø

Cyclotropia H5Ø.41-

Cylindroma (*see also* Neoplasm, malignant, by site)
- eccrine dermal — *see* Neoplasm, skin, benign
- skin — *see* Neoplasm, skin, benign

Cylindruria R82.99

Cynanche
- diphtheritic A36.2
- tonsillaris J36

Cynophobia F4Ø.218

Cynorexia R63.2

Cyphosis — *see* Kyphosis

Cyprus fever — *see* Brucellosis

Cyst (colloid) (mucous) (simple) (retention)
- adenoid (infected) J35.8
- adrenal gland E27.8
  - congenital Q89.1
- air, lung J98.4
- allantoic Q64.4
- alveolar process (jaw bone) M27.4Ø
- amnion, amniotic O41.8x-
- anterior
  - chamber (eye) — *see* Cyst, iris
  - nasopalatine KØ9.1
- antrum J34.1
- anus K62.89
- apical (tooth) (periodontal) KØ4.8
- appendix K38.8

Cyst — *continued*
- arachnoid, brain (acquired) G93.Ø
  - congenital QØ4.6
- arytenoid J38.7
- Baker's M71.2-
  - ruptured M66.Ø
  - tuberculous A18.Ø2
- Bartholin's gland N75.Ø
- bile duct (common) (hepatic) K83.5
- bladder (multiple) (trigone) N32.89
- blue dome (breast) — *see* Cyst, breast
- bone (local) NEC M85.6Ø
  - aneurysmal M85.5Ø
    - ankle M85.57-
    - foot M85.57-
    - forearm M85.53-
    - hand M85.54-
    - jaw M27.49
    - lower leg M85.56-
    - multiple site M85.59
    - neck M85.58
    - rib M85.58
    - shoulder M85.51-
    - skull M85.58
    - specified site NEC M85.58
    - thigh M85.55-
    - toe M85.57-
    - upper arm M85.52-
    - vertebra M85.58
  - solitary M85.4Ø
    - ankle M85.47-
    - fibula M85.46-
    - foot M85.47-
    - hand M85.44-
    - humerus M85.42-
    - jaw M27.49
    - neck M85.48
    - pelvis M85.45-
    - radius M85.43-
    - rib M85.48
    - shoulder M85.41-
    - skull M85.48
    - specified site NEC M85.48
    - tibia M85.46-
    - toe M85.47-
    - ulna M85.43-
    - vertebra M85.48
  - specified type NEC M85.6Ø
    - ankle M85.67-
    - foot M85.67-
    - forearm M85.63-
    - hand M85.64-
    - jaw M27.4Ø
      - developmental (nonodontogenic) KØ9.1
        - odontogenic KØ9.Ø
      - latent M27.Ø
    - lower leg M85.66-
    - multiple site M85.69
    - neck M85.68
    - rib M85.68
    - shoulder M85.61-
    - skull M85.68
    - specified site NEC M85.68
    - thigh M85.65-
    - toe M85.67-
    - upper arm M85.62-
    - vertebra M85.68
- brain (acquired) G93.Ø
  - congenital QØ4.6
  - hydatid B67.99 *[G94]*
  - third ventricle (colloid), congenital QØ4.6
- branchial (cleft) Q18.Ø
- branchiogenic Q18.Ø
- breast (benign) (blue dome) (pedunculated) (solitary) N6Ø.Ø-
  - involution — *see* Dysplasia, mammary, specified type NEC
  - sebaceous — *see* Dysplasia, mammary, specified type NEC
- broad ligament (benign) N83.8
- bronchogenic (mediastinal) (sequestration) J98.4
  - congenital Q33.Ø
- buccal KØ9.8

Cyst — *continued*
- bulbourethral gland N36.8
- bursa, bursal NEC M71.3Ø
  - with rupture — *see* Rupture, synovium
  - ankle M71.37-
  - elbow M71.32-
  - foot M71.37-
  - hand M71.34-
  - hip M71.35-
  - multiple sites M71.39
  - pharyngeal J39.2
  - popliteal space — *see* Cyst, Baker's
  - shoulder M71.31-
  - specified site NEC M71.38
  - wrist M71.33-
- calcifying odontogenic D16.5
  - upper jaw (bone) (maxilla) D16.4
- canal of Nuck (female) N94.89
  - congenital Q52.4
- canthus — *see* Cyst, conjunctiva
- carcinomatous — *see* Neoplasm, malignant, by site
- cauda equina G95.89
- cavum septi pellucidi — *see* Cyst, brain
- celomic (pericardium) Q24.8
- cerebellopontine (angle) — *see* Cyst, brain
- cerebellum — *see* Cyst, brain
- cerebral — *see* Cyst, brain
- cervical lateral Q18.1
- cervix NEC N88.8
  - embryonic Q51.6
  - nabothian N88.8
- chiasmal optic NEC — *see* Disorder, optic, chiasm
- chocolate (ovary) N8Ø.1
- choledochus, congenital Q44.4
- chorion O41.8x-
- choroid plexus G93.Ø
- ciliary body — *see* Cyst, iris
- clitoris N9Ø.7
- colon K63.89
- common (bile) duct K83.5
- congenital NEC Q89.8
  - adrenal gland Q89.1
  - epiglottis Q31.8
  - esophagus Q39.8
  - fallopian tube Q5Ø.4
  - kidney Q61.ØØ
    - more than one (multiple) Q61.Ø2
      - specified as polycystic Q61.3
        - adult type Q61.2
        - infantile type NEC Q61.19
          - collecting duct dilation Q61.11
    - solitary Q61.Ø1
  - larynx Q31.8
  - liver Q44.6
  - lung Q33.Ø
  - mediastinum Q34.1
  - ovary Q5Ø.1
  - oviduct Q5Ø.4
  - periurethral (tissue) Q64.79
  - prepuce Q55.69
  - salivary gland (any) Q38.4
  - sublingual Q38.6
  - submaxillary gland Q38.6
  - thymus (gland) Q89.2
  - tongue Q38.3
  - ureterovesical orifice Q62.8
  - vulva Q52.79
- conjunctiva H11.44-
- cornea H18.89-
- corpora quadrigemina G93.Ø
- corpus
  - albicans N83.29
  - luteum (hemorrhagic) (ruptured) N83.1
- Cowper's gland (benign) (infected) N36.8
- cranial meninges G93.Ø
- craniobuccal pouch E23.6
- craniopharyngeal pouch E23.6
- cystic duct K82.8
- Cysticercus — *see* Cysticercosis
- Dandy-Walker QØ3.1
  - with spina bifida — *see* Spina bifida
- dental (root) KØ4.8
  - developmental KØ9.Ø

Cyst — *continued*
- dental (root) — *continued*
  - eruption KØ9.Ø
  - primordial KØ9.Ø
- dentigerous (mandible) (maxilla) KØ9.Ø
- dermoid — *see* Neoplasm, benign, by site
  - with malignant transformation C56.-
  - implantation
    - external area or site (skin) NEC L72.Ø
    - iris — *see* Cyst, iris, implantation
    - vagina N89.8
    - vulva N9Ø.7
  - mouth KØ9.8
  - oral soft tissue KØ9.8
  - sacrococcygeal — *see* Cyst, pilonidal
- developmental KØ9.1
  - odontogenic KØ9.Ø
  - oral region (nonodontogenic) KØ9.1
  - ovary, ovarian Q5Ø.1
- dura (cerebral) G93.Ø
  - spinal G96.19
- ear (external) Q18.1
- echinococcal — *see* Echinococcus
- embryonic
  - cervix uteri Q51.6
  - fallopian tube Q5Ø.4
  - vagina Q51.6
- endometrium, endometrial (uterus) N85.8
  - ectopic — *see* Endometriosis
- enterogenous Q43.8
- epidermal, epidermoid (inclusion) (*see also* Cyst, skin) L72.Ø
  - mouth KØ9.8
  - oral soft tissue KØ9.8
- epididymis N5Ø.3
- epiglottis J38.7
- epiphysis cerebri E34.8
- epithelial (inclusion) L72.Ø
- epoophoron Q5Ø.5
- eruption KØ9.Ø
- esophagus K22.8
- ethmoid sinus J34.1
- external female genital organs NEC N9Ø.7
- eye NEC H57.8
  - congenital Q15.8
- eyelid (sebaceous) HØ2.829
  - infected — *see* Hordeolum
  - left HØ2.826
    - lower HØ2.825
    - upper HØ2.824
  - right HØ2.823
    - lower HØ2.822
    - upper HØ2.821
- fallopian tube N83.8
  - congenital Q5Ø.4
- fimbrial (twisted) Q5Ø.4
- fissural (oral region) KØ9.1
- follicle (graafian) (hemorrhagic) N83.Ø
  - nabothian N88.8
- follicular (atretic) (hemorrhagic) (ovarian) N83.Ø
  - dentigerous KØ9.Ø
  - odontogenic KØ9.Ø
  - skin L72.9
    - specified NEC L72.8
- frontal sinus J34.1
- gallbladder K82.8
- ganglion — *see* Ganglion
- Gartner's duct Q52.4
- gingiva KØ9.Ø
- gland of Moll — *see* Cyst, eyelid
- globulomaxillary KØ9.1
- graafian follicle (hemorrhagic) N83.Ø
- granulosal lutein (hemorrhagic) N83.1
- hemangiomatous D18.ØØ
  - intra-abdominal D18.Ø3
  - intracranial D18.Ø2
  - skin D18.Ø1
  - specified site NEC D18.Ø9
- hydatid (*see also* Echinococcus) B67.9Ø
  - brain B67.99 *[G94]*
  - liver (*see also* Cyst, liver, hydatid) B67.8
  - lung NEC B67.99 *[J99]*

- **Cyst** — *continued*
  - hydatid — *continued*
    - Morgagni
      - female Q5Ø.5
      - male (epididymal) Q55.4
        - testicular Q55.29
    - specified site NEC B67.99
  - hymen N89.8
    - embryonic Q52.4
  - hypopharynx J39.2
  - hypophysis, hypophyseal (duct) (recurrent) E23.6
    - cerebri E23.6
  - implantation (dermoid)
    - external area or site (skin) NEC L72.Ø
    - iris — *see* Cyst, iris, implantation
    - vagina N89.8
    - vulva N9Ø.7
  - incisive canal KØ9.1
  - inclusion (epidermal) (epithelial) (epidermoid) (squamous) L72.Ø
    - not of skin—code under Cyst, by site
  - intestine (large) (small) K63.89
  - intracranial — *see* Cyst, brain
  - intraligamentous (*see also* Disorder, ligament)
    - knee — *see* Derangement, knee
  - intrasellar E23.6
  - iris H21.3Ø9
    - exudative H21.31-
    - idiopathic H21.3Ø-
    - implantation H21.32-
    - parasitic H21.33-
    - pars plana (primary) H21.34-
      - exudative H21.35-
  - jaw (bone) (aneurysmal) (hemorrhagic) (traumatic) M27.4Ø
    - developmental (odontogenic) KØ9.Ø
    - fissural KØ9.1
  - joint NEC — *see* Disorder, joint, specified type NEC
  - kidney (acquired) N28.1
    - calyceal — *see* Hydronephrosis
    - congenital Q61.ØØ
    - more than one (multiple) Q61.Ø2
      - specified as polycystic Q61.3
        - adult type (autosomal dominant) Q61.2
        - infantile type (autosomal recessive) NEC Q61.19
          - collecting duct dilation Q61.11
    - pyelogenic — *see* Hydronephrosis
    - simple N28.1
    - solitary (single) Q61.Ø1
      - acquired N28.1
  - labium (majus) (minus) N9Ø.7
    - sebaceous N9Ø.7
  - lacrimal (*see also* Disorder, lacrimal system, specified NEC)
    - gland HØ4.13-
    - passages or sac — *see* Disorder, lacrimal system, specified NEC
  - larynx J38.7
  - lateral periodontal KØ9.Ø
  - lens H27.8
    - congenital Q12.8
  - lip (gland) K13.Ø
  - liver (idiopathic) (simple) K76.89
    - congenital Q44.6
    - hydatid B67.8
      - granulosus B67.Ø
      - multilocularis B67.5
  - lung J98.4
    - congenital Q33.Ø
    - giant bullous J43.9
  - lutein N83.1
  - lymphangiomatous D18.1
  - lymphoepithelial, oral soft tissue KØ9.8
  - macula — *see* Degeneration, macula, hole
  - malignant — *see* Neoplasm, malignant, by site
  - mammary gland — *see* Cyst, breast
  - mandible M27.4Ø
    - dentigerous KØ9.Ø
    - radicular KØ4.8
  - maxilla M27.4Ø
    - dentigerous KØ9.Ø
    - radicular KØ4.8

- **Cyst** — *continued*
  - medial, face and neck Q18.8
  - median
    - anterior maxillary KØ9.1
    - palatal KØ9.1
  - mediastinum, congenital Q34.1
  - meibomian (gland) — *see* Chalazion
    - infected — *see* Hordeolum
  - membrane, brain G93.Ø
  - meninges (cerebral) G93.Ø
    - spinal G96.19
  - meniscus, knee — *see* Derangement, knee, meniscus, cystic
  - mesentery, mesenteric K66.8
    - chyle I89.8
  - mesonephric duct
    - female Q5Ø.5
    - male Q55.4
  - milk N64.89
  - Morgagni (hydatid)
    - female Q5Ø.5
    - male (epididymal) Q55.4
      - testicular Q55.29
  - mouth KØ9.8
  - Müllerian duct Q5Ø.4
    - appendix testis Q55.29
    - cervix Q51.6
    - fallopian tube Q5Ø.4
    - female Q5Ø.4
    - male Q55.29
    - prostatic utricle Q55.4
    - vagina (embryonal) Q52.4
  - multilocular (ovary) D39.1Ø
    - benign — *see* Neoplasm, benign, by site
  - myometrium N85.8
  - nabothian (follicle) (ruptured) N88.8
  - nasoalveolar KØ9.1
  - nasolabial KØ9.1
  - nasopalatine (anterior) (duct) KØ9.1
  - nasopharynx J39.2
  - neoplastic — *see* Neoplasm, uncertain behavior, by site
    - benign — *see* Neoplasm, benign, by site
  - nervous system NEC G96.8
  - neuroenteric (congenital) QØ6.8
  - nipple — *see* Cyst, breast
  - nose (turbinates) J34.1
    - sinus J34.1
  - odontogenic, developmental KØ9.Ø
  - omentum (lesser) K66.8
    - congenital Q45.8
  - ora serrata — *see* Cyst, retina, ora serrata
  - oral
    - region KØ9.9
      - developmental (nonodontogenic) KØ9.1
      - specified NEC KØ9.8
    - soft tissue KØ9.9
      - specified NEC KØ9.8
  - orbit HØ5.81-
  - ovary, ovarian (twisted) N83.2Ø
    - adherent N83.2Ø
    - chocolate N8Ø.1
    - corpus
      - albicans N83.29
      - luteum (hemorrhagic) N83.1
    - dermoid D27.9
    - developmental Q5Ø.1
    - due to failure of involution NEC N83.2Ø
    - endometrial N8Ø.1
    - follicular (graafian) (hemorrhagic) N83.Ø
    - hemorrhagic N83.2Ø
    - in pregnancy or childbirth O34.8-
      - with obstructed labor O65.5
    - multilocular D39.1Ø
    - pseudomucinous D27.9
    - retention N83.29
    - serous N83.2Ø
    - specified NEC N83.29
    - theca lutein (hemorrhagic) N83.1
    - tuberculous A18.18
  - oviduct N83.8
  - palate (median) (fissural) KØ9.1
  - palatine papilla (jaw) KØ9.1

- **Cyst** — *continued*
  - pancreas, pancreatic (hemorrhagic) (true) K86.2
    - congenital Q45.2
    - false K86.3
  - paralabral
    - hip M24.85-
    - shoulder S43.43-
  - paramesonephric duct Q5Ø.4
    - female Q5Ø.4
    - male Q55.29
  - paranephric N28.1
  - paraphysis, cerebri, congenital QØ4.6
  - parasitic B89
  - parathyroid (gland) E21.4
  - paratubal N83.8
  - paraurethral duct N36.8
  - paroophoron Q5Ø.5
  - parotid gland K11.6
  - parovarian Q5Ø.5
  - pelvis, female N94.89
    - in pregnancy or childbirth O34.8-
      - causing obstructed labor O65.5
  - penis (sebaceous) N48.89
  - periapical KØ4.8
  - pericardial (congenital) Q24.8
    - acquired (secondary) I31.8
  - pericoronal KØ9.Ø
  - periodontal KØ4.8
    - lateral KØ9.Ø
  - peripelvic (lymphatic) N28.1
  - peritoneum K66.8
    - chylous I89.8
  - periventricular, acquired, newborn P91.1
  - pharynx (wall) J39.2
  - pilar L72.11
  - pilonidal (infected) (rectum) LØ5.91
    - with abscess LØ5.Ø1
    - malignant C44.59-
  - pituitary (duct) (gland) E23.6
  - placenta O43.19-
  - pleura J94.8
  - popliteal — *see* Cyst, Baker's
  - porencephalic QØ4.6
    - acquired G93.Ø
  - postanal (infected) — *see* Cyst, pilonidal
  - postmastoidectomy cavity (mucosal) — *see* Complications, postmastoidectomy, cyst
  - preauricular Q18.1
  - prepuce N47.4
    - congenital Q55.69
  - primordial (jaw) KØ9.Ø
  - prostate N42.83
  - pseudomucinous (ovary) D27.9
  - pupillary, miotic H21.27-
  - radicular (residual) KØ4.8
  - radiculodental KØ4.8
  - ranular K11.8
  - Rathke's pouch E23.6
  - rectum (epithelium) (mucous) K62.89
  - renal — *see* Cyst, kidney
  - residual (radicular) KØ4.8
  - retention (ovary) N83.29
    - salivary gland K11.6
  - retina H33.19-
    - ora serrata H33.11-
    - parasitic H33.12-
  - retroperitoneal K68.9
  - sacrococcygeal (dermoid) — *see* Cyst, pilonidal
  - salivary gland or duct (mucous extravasation or retention) K11.6
  - Sampson's N8Ø.1
  - sclera H15.89
  - scrotum L72.9
    - sebaceous L72.3
  - sebaceous (duct) (gland) L72.3
    - breast — *see* Dysplasia, mammary, specified type NEC
    - eyelid — *see* Cyst, eyelid
    - genital organ NEC
      - female N94.89
      - male N5Ø.8
    - scrotum L72.3

- **Cyst** — *continued*
  - semilunar cartilage (knee) (multiple) — *see* Derangement, knee, meniscus, cystic
  - seminal vesicle N5Ø.8
  - serous (ovary) N83.2Ø
  - sinus (accessory) (nasal) J34.1
  - Skene's gland N36.8
  - skin L72.9
    - breast — *see* Dysplasia, mammary, specified type NEC
    - epidermal, epidermoid L72.Ø
    - epithelial L72.Ø
    - eyelid — *see* Cyst, eyelid
    - genital organ NEC
      - female N9Ø.7
      - male N5Ø.8
    - inclusion L72.Ø
    - scrotum L72.9
    - sebaceous L72.3
    - sweat gland or duct L74.8
  - solitary
    - bone — *see* Cyst, bone, solitary
    - jaw M27.4Ø
    - kidney N28.1
  - spermatic cord N5Ø.8
  - sphenoid sinus J34.1
  - spinal meninges G96.19
  - spleen NEC D73.4
    - congenital Q89.Ø9
    - hydatid (*see also* Echinococcus) B67.99 *[D77]*
  - Stafne's M27.Ø
  - subarachnoid intrasellar R93.Ø
  - subcutaneous, pheomycotic (chromomycotic) B43.2
  - subdural (cerebral) G93.Ø
    - spinal cord G96.19
  - sublingual gland K11.6
  - submandibular gland K11.6
  - submaxillary gland K11.6
  - suburethral N36.8
  - suprarenal gland E27.8
  - suprasellar — *see* Cyst, brain
  - sweat gland or duct L74.8
  - synovial (*see also* Cyst, bursa)
    - ruptured *see* Rupture, synovium
  - tarsal — *see* Chalazion
  - tendon (sheath) — *see* Disorder, tendon, specified type NEC
  - testis N44.2
    - tunica albuginea N44.1
  - theca lutein (ovary) N83.1
  - Thornwaldt's J39.2
  - thymus (gland) E32.8
  - thyroglossal duct (infected) (persistent) Q89.2
  - thyroid (gland) EØ4.1
  - tongue K14.8
  - tonsil J35.8
  - tooth — *see* Cyst, dental
  - Tornwaldt's J39.2
  - trichilemmal (proliferating) L72.12
  - trichodermal L72.12
  - tubal (fallopian) N83.8
    - inflammatory — *see* Salpingitis, chronic
  - tubo-ovarian N83.8
    - inflammatory N7Ø.13
  - tunica
    - albuginea testis N44.1
    - vaginalis N5Ø.8
  - turbinate (nose) J34.1
  - Tyson's gland N48.89
  - urachus, congenital Q64.4
  - ureter N28.89
  - ureterovesical orifice N28.89
  - urethra, urethral (gland) N36.8
  - uterine ligament N83.8
  - uterus (body) (corpus) (recurrent) N85.8
    - embryonic Q51.818
      - cervix Q51.6
  - vagina, vaginal (implantation) (inclusion) (squamous cell) (wall) N89.8
    - embryonic Q52.4
  - vallecula, vallecular (epiglottis) J38.7
  - vesical (orifice) N32.89
  - vitreous body H43.89

- **Cyst** — *continued*
  - vulva (implantation) (inclusion) N9Ø.7
    - congenital Q52.79
    - sebaceous gland N9Ø.7
  - vulvovaginal gland N9Ø.7
  - wolffian
    - female Q5Ø.5
    - male Q55.4
- **Cystadenocarcinoma** — *see* Neoplasm, malignant, by site
  - bile duct C22.1
  - endometrioid — *see* Neoplasm, malignant, by site
    - specified site — *see* Neoplasm, malignant, by site
    - unspecified site
      - female C56.9
      - male C61
  - mucinous
    - papillary
      - specified site — *see* Neoplasm, malignant, by site
      - unspecified site C56.9
    - specified site — *see* Neoplasm, malignant, by site
    - unspecified site C56.9
  - papillary
    - mucinous
      - specified site — *see* Neoplasm, malignant, by site
      - unspecified site C56.9
    - pseudomucinous
      - specified site — *see* Neoplasm, malignant, by site
      - unspecified site C56.9
    - serous
      - specified site — *see* Neoplasm, malignant, by site
      - unspecified site C56.9
    - specified site — *see* Neoplasm, malignant, by site
    - unspecified site C56.9
  - pseudomucinous
    - papillary
      - specified site — *see* Neoplasm, malignant, by site
      - unspecified site C56.9
    - specified site — *see* Neoplasm, malignant, by site
    - unspecified site C56.9
  - serous
    - papillary
      - specified site — *see* Neoplasm, malignant, by site
      - unspecified site C56.9
    - specified site — *see* Neoplasm, malignant, by site
    - unspecified site C56.9
- **Cystadenofibroma**
  - clear cell — *see* Neoplasm, benign, by site
  - endometrioid D27.9
    - borderline malignancy D39.1-
    - malignant C56.-
  - mucinous
    - specified site — *see* Neoplasm, benign, by site
    - unspecified site D27.9
  - serous
    - specified site — *see* Neoplasm, benign, by site
    - unspecified site D27.9
  - specified site — *see* Neoplasm, benign, by site
  - unspecified site D27.9
- **Cystadenoma** (*see also* Neoplasm, benign, by site)
  - bile duct D13.4
  - endometrioid — *see* Neoplasm, benign, by site
    - borderline malignancy — *see* Neoplasm, uncertain behavior, by site
  - malignant — *see* Neoplasm, malignant, by site
  - mucinous
    - borderline malignancy
      - ovary C56.-
      - specified site NEC — *see* Neoplasm, uncertain behavior, by site
      - unspecified site C56.9
    - papillary
      - borderline malignancy
        - ovary C56.-
        - specified site NEC — *see* Neoplasm, uncertain behavior, by site

- **Cystadenoma** — *continued*
  - mucinous — *continued*
    - papillary — *continued*
      - borderline malignancy — *continued*
        - unspecified site C56.9
      - specified site — *see* Neoplasm, benign, by site
      - unspecified site D27.9
    - specified site — *see* Neoplasm, benign, by site
    - unspecified site D27.9
  - papillary
    - borderline malignancy
      - ovary C56.-
      - specified site NEC — *see* Neoplasm, uncertain behavior, by site
      - unspecified site C56.9
    - lymphomatosum
      - specified site — *see* Neoplasm, benign, by site
      - unspecified site D11.9
    - mucinous
      - borderline malignancy
        - ovary C56.-
        - specified site NEC — *see* Neoplasm, uncertain behavior, by site
        - unspecified site C56.9
      - specified site — *see* Neoplasm, benign, by site
      - unspecified site D27.9
    - pseudomucinous
      - borderline malignancy
        - ovary C56.-
        - specified site NEC — *see* Neoplasm, uncertain behavior, by site
        - unspecified site C56.9
      - specified site — *see* Neoplasm, benign, by site
      - unspecified site D27.9
    - serous
      - borderline malignancy
        - ovary C56.-
        - specified site NEC — *see* Neoplasm, uncertain behavior, by site
        - unspecified site C56.9
      - specified site — *see* Neoplasm, benign, by site
      - unspecified site D27.9
    - specified site — *see* Neoplasm, benign, by site
    - unspecified site D27.9
  - pseudomucinous
    - borderline malignancy
      - ovary C56.-
      - specified site NEC — *see* Neoplasm, uncertain behavior, by site
      - unspecified site C56.9
    - papillary
      - borderline malignancy
        - ovary C56.-
        - specified site NEC — *see* Neoplasm, uncertain behavior, by site
        - unspecified site C56.9
      - specified site — *see* Neoplasm, benign, by site
      - unspecified site D27.9
    - specified site — *see* Neoplasm, benign, by site
    - unspecified site D27.9
  - serous
    - borderline malignancy
      - specified site NEC — *see* Neoplasm, uncertain behavior, by site
      - unspecified site C56.9
    - papillary
      - borderline malignancy
        - ovary C56.-
        - specified site NEC — *see* Neoplasm, uncertain behavior, by site
        - unspecified site C56.9
      - specified site — *see* Neoplasm, benign, by site
      - unspecified site D27.9
    - specified site — *see* Neoplasm, benign, by site
    - unspecified site D27.9
- **Cystathionine synthase deficiency** E72.11
- **Cystathioninemia** E72.19
- **Cystathioninuria** E72.19
- **Cystic** (*see also* condition)
  - breast (chronic) — *see* Mastopathy, cystic
  - corpora lutea (hemorrhagic) N83.1
  - duct — *see* condition
  - eyeball (congenital) Q11.Ø

- **Cystic** — *continued*
  - fibrosis — *see* Fibrosis, cystic
  - kidney (congenital) Q61.9
    - adult type Q61.2
    - infantile type NEC Q61.19
      - collecting duct dilatation Q61.11
    - medullary Q61.5
  - liver, congenital Q44.6
  - lung disease J98.4
    - congenital Q33.Ø
  - mastitis, chronic — *see* Mastopathy, cystic
  - medullary, kidney Q61.5
  - meniscus — *see* Derangement, knee, meniscus, cystic
  - ovary N83.2Ø
- **Cysticercosis, cysticerciasis** B69.9
  - with
    - epileptiform fits B69.Ø
    - myositis B69.81
  - brain B69.Ø
  - central nervous system B69.Ø
  - cerebral B69.Ø
  - ocular B69.1
  - specified NEC B69.89
- **Cysticercus cellulose infestation** — *see* Cysticercosis
- **Cystinosis** (malignant) E72.Ø4
- **Cystinuria** E72.Ø1
- **Cystitis** (exudative) (hemorrhagic) (septic) (suppurative) N3Ø.9Ø
  - with
    - fibrosis — *see* Cystitis, chronic, interstitial
    - hematuria N3Ø.91
    - leukoplakia — *see* Cystitis, chronic, interstitial
    - malakoplakia — *see* Cystitis, chronic, interstitial
    - metaplasia — *see* Cystitis, chronic, interstitial
    - prostatitis N41.3
  - acute N3Ø.ØØ
    - with hematuria N3Ø.Ø1
    - of trigone N3Ø.3Ø
      - with hematuria N3Ø.31
  - allergic — *see* Cystitis, specified type NEC
  - amebic AØ6.81
  - bilharzial B65.9 *[N33]*
  - blennorrhagic (gonococcal) A54.Ø1
  - bullous — *see* Cystitis, specified type NEC
  - calculous N21.Ø
  - chlamydial A56.Ø1
  - chronic N3Ø.2Ø
    - with hematuria N3Ø.21
- **Cystitis** — *continued*
  - chronic — *continued*
    - interstitial N3Ø.1Ø
      - with hematuria N3Ø.11
    - of trigone N3Ø.3Ø
      - with hematuria N3Ø.31
    - specified NEC N3Ø.2Ø
      - with hematuria N3Ø.21
  - cystic(a) — *see* Cystitis, specified type NEC
  - diphtheritic A36.85
  - echinococcal
    - granulosus B67.39
    - multilocularis B67.69
  - emphysematous — *see* Cystitis, specified type NEC
  - encysted — *see* Cystitis, specified type NEC
  - eosinophilic — *see* Cystitis, specified type NEC
  - follicular — *see* Cystitis, of trigone
  - gangrenous — *see* Cystitis, specified type NEC
  - glandularis — *see* Cystitis, specified type NEC
  - gonococcal A54.Ø1
  - incrusted — *see* Cystitis, specified type NEC
  - interstitial (chronic) — *see* Cystitis, chronic, interstitial
  - irradiation N3Ø.4Ø
    - with hematuria N3Ø.41
  - irritation — *see* Cystitis, specified type NEC
  - malignant — *see* Cystitis, specified type NEC
  - of trigone N3Ø.3Ø
    - with hematuria N3Ø.31
  - panmural — *see* Cystitis, chronic, interstitial
  - polyposa — *see* Cystitis, specified type NEC
  - prostatic N41.3
  - puerperal (postpartum) O86.22
  - radiation — *see* Cystitis, irradiation
  - specified type NEC N3Ø.8Ø
    - with hematuria N3Ø.81
  - subacute — *see* Cystitis, chronic
  - submucous — *see* Cystitis, chronic, interstitial
  - syphilitic (late) A52.76
  - trichomonal A59.Ø3
  - tuberculous A18.12
  - ulcerative — *see* Cystitis, chronic, interstitial
- **Cystocele**(-urethrocele)
  - female N81.1Ø
    - with prolapse of uterus — *see* Prolapse, uterus
    - lateral N81.12
    - midline N81.11
    - paravaginal N81.12
- **Cystocele** — *continued*
  - in pregnancy or childbirth O34.8-
    - causing obstructed labor O65.5
  - male N32.89
- **Cystolithiasis** N21.Ø
- **Cystoma**
- (*see also* Neoplasm, benign, by site)
  - endometrial, ovary N8Ø.1
  - mucinous
    - specified site — *see* Neoplasm, benign, by site
    - unspecified site D27.9
  - serous
    - specified site — *see* Neoplasm, benign, by site
    - unspecified site D27.9
  - simple (ovary) N83.29
- **Cystoplegia** N31.2
- **Cystoptosis** N32.89
- **Cystopyelitis** — *see* Pyelonephritis
- **Cystorrhagia** N32.89
- **Cystosarcoma phyllodes** D48.6-
  - benign D24-
  - malignant — *see* Neoplasm, breast, malignant
- **Cystostomy**
  - attention to Z43.5
  - complication — *see* Complications, cystostomy
  - status Z93.5Ø
    - appendico-vesicostomy Z93.52
    - cutaneous Z93.51
    - specified NEC Z93.59
- **Cystourethritis** — *see* Urethritis
- **Cystourethrocele** (*see also* Cystocele)
  - female N81.1Ø
    - with uterine prolapse — *see* Prolapse, uterus
    - lateral N81.12
    - midline N81.11
    - paravaginal N81.12
  - male N32.89
- **Cytomegalic inclusion disease**
  - congenital P35.1
- **Cytomegalovirus infection** B25.9
- **Cytomycosis** (reticuloendothelial) B39.4
- **Cytopenia** D75.9
  - refractory
    - with multilineage dysplasia D46.A
      - and ring sideroblasts (RCMD RS) D46.B
- **Czerny's disease** (periodic hydrarthrosis of the knee) — *see* Effusion, joint, knee

This page was intentionally left blank

D

Daae (-Finsen) **disease** (epidemic pleurodynia) B33.Ø
Da Costa's syndrome F45.8
Dabney's grip B33.Ø
Dacryoadenitis, dacryadenitis HØ4.ØØ-
  acute HØ4.Ø1-
  chronic HØ4.Ø2-
Dacryocystitis HØ4.3Ø-
  acute HØ4.32-
  chronic HØ4.41-
  neonatal P39.1
  phlegmonous HØ4.31-
  syphilitic A52.71
    congenital (early) A5Ø.Ø1
  trachomatous, active A71.1
    sequelae (late effect) B94.Ø
Dacryocystoblenorrhea — *see* Inflammation, lacrimal, passages, chronic
Dacryocystocele — *see* Disorder, lacrimal system, changes
Dacryolith, dacryolithiasis HØ4.51-
Dacryoma — *see* Disorder, lacrimal system, changes
Dacryopericystitis — *see* Dacryocystitis
Dacryops HØ4.11-
Dacryostenosis (*see also* Stenosis, lacrimal)
  congenital Q1Ø.5
Dactylitis
  bone — *see* Osteomyelitis
  sickle-cell D57.ØØ
    Hb C D57.219
    Hb SS D57.ØØ
    specified NEC D57.819
  skin LØ8.9
  syphilitic A52.77
  tuberculous A18.Ø3
Dactylolysis spontanea (ainhum) L94.6
Dactylosymphysis Q7Ø.9
  fingers — *see* Syndactylism, complex, fingers
  toes — *see* Syndactylism, complex, toes
Damage
  arteriosclerotic — *see* Arteriosclerosis
  brain (nontraumatic) G93.9
    anoxic, hypoxic G93.1
      resulting from a procedure G97.82
    child NEC G8Ø.9
    due to birth injury P11.2
  cardiorenal (vascular) — *see* Hypertension, cardiorenal
  cerebral NEC — *see* Damage, brain
  coccyx, complicating delivery O71.6
  coronary — *see* Disease, heart, ischemic
  eye, birth injury P15.3
  liver (nontraumatic) K76.9
    alcoholic K7Ø.9
    due to drugs — *see* Disease, liver, toxic
    toxic — *see* Disease, liver, toxic
  medication T88.7
  pelvic
    joint or ligament, during delivery O71.6
    organ NEC
      during delivery O71.5
      following ectopic or molar pregnancy OØ8.6
  renal — *see* Disease, renal
  subendocardium, subendocardial — *see* Degeneration, myocardial
  vascular I99.9
Dana-Putnam syndrome (subacute combined sclerosis with pernicious anemia) — *see* Degeneration, combined
Danbolt (-Cross) **syndrome** (acrodermatitis enteropathica) E83.2
Dandruff L21.Ø
Dandy-Walker syndrome QØ3.1
  with spina bifida — *see* Spina bifida
Danlos' syndrome Q79.6
Darier(-White) **disease** (congenital) Q82.8
  meaning erythema annulare centrifugum L53.1
Darier-Roussy sarcoid D86.3
Darling's disease or histoplasmosis B39.4
Darwin's tubercle Q17.8
Dawson's (inclusion body) **encephalitis** A81.1
De Beurmann(-Gougerot) **disease** B42.1
De la Tourette's syndrome F95.2
De Lange's syndrome Q87.1
De Morgan's spots (senile angiomas) I78.1
De Quervain's
  disease (tendon sheath) M65.4
  syndrome E34.51
  thyroiditis (subacute granulomatous thyroiditis) EØ6.1
De Toni-Fanconi(-Debré) **syndrome** E72.Ø9
  with cystinosis E72.Ø4
Dead
  fetus, retained (mother) O36.4
    early pregnancy OØ2.1
  labyrinth — *see* subcategory H83.2
  ovum, retained OØ2.Ø
Deaf nonspeaking NEC H91.3
Deafmutism (acquired) (congenital) NEC H91.3
  hysterical F44.6
  syphilitic, congenital (*see also* subcategory H94.8) A5Ø.Ø9
Deafness (acquired) (complete) (hereditary) (partial) H91.9-
  with blue sclera and fragility of bone Q78.Ø
  auditory fatigue — *see* Deafness, specified type NEC
  aviation T7Ø.Ø
    nerve injury — *see* Injury, nerve, acoustic, specified type NEC
  boilermaker's — *see* subcategory H83.3
  central — *see* Deafness, sensorineural
  conductive H9Ø.2
    and sensorineural, mixed H9Ø.8
      bilateral H9Ø.6
    bilateral H9Ø.Ø
    unilateral H9Ø.1-
  congenital H9Ø.5
    with blue sclera and fragility of bone Q78.Ø
  due to toxic agents — *see* Deafness, ototoxic
  emotional (hysterical) F44.6
  functional (hysterical) F44.6
  high frequency H91.9-
  hysterical F44.6
  low frequency H91.9-
  mental R48.8
  mixed conductive and sensorineural H9Ø.8
    bilateral H9Ø.6
    unilateral H9Ø.7-
  nerve — *see* Deafness, sensorineural
  neural — *see* Deafness, sensorineural
  noise-induced (*see also* subcategory) H83.3
    nerve injury — *see* Injury, nerve, acoustic, specified type NEC
  nonspeaking H91.3
  ototoxic — *see* subcategory H91.Ø
  perceptive — *see* Deafness, sensorineural
  psychogenic (hysterical) F44.6
  sensorineural H9Ø.5
    and conductive, mixed H9Ø.8
      bilateral H9Ø.6
    bilateral H9Ø.3
    unilateral H9Ø.4-
  sensory — *see* Deafness, sensorineural
  specified type NEC — *see* subcategory H91.8
  sudden (idiopathic) H91.2-
  syphilitic A52.15
  transient ischemic H93.Ø1-
  traumatic — *see* Injury, nerve, acoustic, specified type NEC
  word (developmental) H93.25
Death (cause unknown) (of) (unexplained) (unspecified cause) R99
  brain G93.82
  cardiac (sudden) (with successful resuscitation)—code to underlying disease
    family history of Z82.41
    personal history of Z86.74
  family member (assumed) Z63.4
Debility (chronic) (general) (nervous) R53.81
  congenital or neonatal NOS P96.9
  old age R54
  nervous R53.81
  senile R54
Débove's disease (splenomegaly) R16.1
Decalcification
  bone — *see* Osteoporosis
  teeth KØ3.89
Decapsulation, kidney N28.89
Decay
  dental — *see* Caries, dental
  senile R54
  tooth, teeth — *see* Caries, dental
Deciduitis (acute)
  following ectopic or molar pregnancy OØ8.Ø
Decline (general) — *see* Debility
  cognitive, age-associated R41.81
Decompensation
  cardiac (acute) (chronic) — *see* Disease, heart
  cardiovascular — *see* Disease, cardiovascular
  heart — *see* Disease, heart
  hepatic — *see* Failure, hepatic
  myocardial (acute) (chronic) — *see* Disease, heart
  respiratory J98.8
Decompression sickness T7Ø.3
Decrease(d)
  absolute neutrophile count — *see* Neutropenia
  blood
    platelets — *see* Thrombocytopenia
    pressure RØ3.1
      due to shock following
        injury T79.4
        operation T81.19
  estrogen E28.39
    postablative E89.4Ø
      asymptomatic E89.4Ø
      symptomatic E89.41
  fragility of erythrocytes D58.8
  function
    lipase (pancreatic) K9Ø.3
    ovary in hypopituitarism E23.Ø
    parenchyma of pancreas K86.8
    pituitary (gland) (anterior) (lobe) E23.Ø
      posterior (lobe) E23.Ø
  functional activity R68.89
  glucose R73.Ø9
  hematocrit R71.Ø
  hemoglobin R71.Ø
  leukocytes D72.819
    specified NEC D72.818
  libido R68.82
  lymphocytes D72.81Ø
  platelets D69.6
  respiration, due to shock following injury T79.4
  sexual desire R68.82
  tear secretion NEC — *see* Syndrome, dry eye
  tolerance
    fat K9Ø.4
    glucose R73.Ø9
    pancreatic K9Ø.3
    salt and water E87.8
  vision NEC H54.7
  white blood cell count D72.819
    specified NEC D72.818
Decubitus (ulcer) — *see* Ulcer, pressure, by site
  cervix N86
Deepening acetabulum — *see* Derangement, joint, specified type NEC, hip
Defect, defective Q89.9
  3-beta-hydroxysteroid dehydrogenase E25.Ø
  11-hydroxylase E25.Ø
  21-hydroxylase E25.Ø
  abdominal wall, congenital Q79.59
  antibody immunodeficiency D8Ø.9
  aorticopulmonary septum Q21.4
  atrial septal (ostium secundum type) Q21.1
    following acute myocardial infarction (current complication) I23.1
    ostium primum type Q21.2
  atrioventricular
    canal Q21.2
    septum Q21.2
  auricular septal Q21.1
  bilirubin excretion NEC E8Ø.6
  biosynthesis, androgen (testicular) E29.1
  bulbar septum Q21.Ø
  catalase E8Ø.3

- **Defect, defective** — *continued*
  - cell membrane receptor complex (CR3) D71
  - circulation I99.9
    - congenital Q28.9
    - newborn Q28.9
  - coagulation (factor) (*see also* Deficiency, factor) D68.9
    - with
      - ectopic pregnancy OØ8.1
      - molar pregnancy OØ8.1
    - acquired D68.4
    - antepartum with hemorrhage — *see* Hemorrhage, antepartum, with coagulation defect
    - due to
      - liver disease D68.4
      - vitamin K deficiency D68.4
    - hereditary NEC D68.2
    - intrapartum O67.Ø
    - newborn, transient P61.6
    - postpartum O72.3
    - specified type NEC D68.8
  - complement system D84.1
  - conduction (heart) I45.9
    - bone — *see* Deafness, conductive
  - congenital, organ or site not listed — *see* Anomaly, by site
  - coronary sinus Q21.1
  - cushion, endocardial Q21.2
  - degradation, glycoprotein E77.1
  - dental bridge, crown, fillings — *see* Defect, dental restoration
  - dental restoration KØ8.5Ø
    - specified NEC KØ8.59
  - dentin (hereditary) KØØ.5
  - Descemet's membrane, congenital Q13.89
  - developmental (*see also* Anomaly)
    - cauda equina QØ6.3
  - diaphragm
    - with elevation, eventration or hernia — *see* Hernia, diaphragm
    - congenital Q79.1
      - with hernia Q79.Ø
      - gross (with hernia) Q79.Ø
  - ectodermal, congenital Q82.9
  - Eisenmenger's Q21.8
  - enzyme
    - catalase E8Ø.3
    - peroxidase E8Ø.3
  - esophagus, congenital Q39.9
  - extensor retinaculum M62.89
  - fibrin polymerization D68.2
  - filling
    - bladder R93.4
    - kidney R93.4
    - stomach R93.3
    - ureter R93.4
  - Gerbode Q21.Ø
  - glycoprotein degradation E77.1
  - Hageman (factor) D68.2
  - hearing — *see* Deafness
  - high grade F7Ø
  - interatrial septal Q21.1
  - interauricular septal Q21.1
  - interventricular septal Q21.Ø
    - with dextroposition of aorta, pulmonary stenosis and hypertrophy of right ventricle Q21.3
    - in tetralogy of Fallot Q21.3
  - learning (specific) — *see* Disorder, learning
  - lymphocyte function antigen-1 (LFA-1) D84.Ø
  - lysosomal enzyme, post-translational modification E77.Ø
  - major osseous M89.7Ø
    - ankle M89.77-
    - carpus M89.74-
    - clavicle M89.71-
    - femur M89.75-
    - fibula M89.76-
    - fingers M89.74-
    - foot M89.77-
    - forearm M89.73-
    - hand M89.74-

- **Defect, defective** — *continued*
  - major osseous — *continued*
    - humerus M89.72-
    - lower leg M89.76-
    - metacarpus M89.74-
    - metatarsus M89.77-
    - multiple sites M89.79
    - pelvic region M89.75-
    - pelvis M89.75-
    - radius M89.73-
    - scapula M89.71-
    - shoulder region M89.71-
    - specified NEC M89.78
    - tarsus M89.77-
    - thigh M89.75-
    - tibia M89.76-
    - toes M89.77-
    - ulna M89.73-
  - mental — *see* Disability, intellectual
  - modification, lysosomal enzymes, post-translational E77.Ø
  - obstructive, congenital
    - renal pelvis Q62.39
    - ureter Q62.39
      - atresia — *see* Atresia, ureter
      - cecoureterocele Q62.32
      - megaureter Q62.2
      - orthotopic ureterocele Q62.31
  - osseous, major M89.7Ø
    - ankle M89.77-
    - carpus M89.74-
    - clavicle M89.71-
    - femur M89.75-
    - fibula M89.76-
    - fingers M89.74-
    - foot M89.77-
    - forearm M89.73-
    - hand M89.74-
    - humerus M89.72-
    - lower leg M89.76-
    - metacarpus M89.74-
    - metatarsus M89.77-
    - multiple sites M89.79
    - pelvic region M89.75-
    - pelvis M89.75-
    - radius M89.73-
    - scapula M89.71-
    - shoulder region M89.71-
    - specified NEC M89.78
    - tarsus M89.77-
    - thigh M89.75-
    - tibia M89.76-
    - toes M89.77-
    - ulna M89.73-
  - osteochondral NEC (*see also* Deformity) M95.8-
  - ostium
    - primum Q21.2
    - secundum Q21.1
  - peroxidase E8Ø.3
  - placental blood supply — *see* Insufficiency, placental
  - platelets, qualitative D69.1
    - constitutional D68.Ø
  - postural NEC, spine — *see* Dorsopathy, deforming
  - reduction
    - limb Q73.8
      - lower Q72.9-
        - absence — *see* Agenesis, leg
          - foot — *see* Agenesis, foot
        - split foot Q72.7-
        - longitudinal
          - femur Q72.4-
          - fibula Q72.6-
          - tibia Q72.5-
        - specified type NEC Q72.89-
      - specified type NEC Q73.8
      - upper Q71.9-
        - absence — *see* Agenesis, arm
          - forearm — *see* Agenesis, forearm
          - hand — *see* Agenesis, hand
        - lobster-claw hand Q71.6-
        - longitudinal
          - radius Q71.4-

- **Defect, defective** — *continued*
  - reduction— *continued*
    - limb— *continued*
      - upper— *continued*
        - longitudinal— *continued*
          - ulna Q71.5-
        - specified type NEC Q71.89-
  - renal pelvis Q63.8
    - obstructive Q62.39
  - respiratory system, congenital Q34.9
  - restoration, dental KØ8.5Ø
    - specified NEC KØ8.59
  - retinal nerve bundle fibers H35.89
  - septal (heart) NOS Q21.9
    - acquired (atrial) (auricular) (ventricular) (old) I51.Ø
    - atrial Q21.1
      - concurrent with acute myocardial infarction — *see* Infarct, myocardium
      - following acute myocardial infarction (current complication) I23.1
    - ventricular (*see also* Defect, ventricular septal) Q21.Ø
  - sinus venosus Q21.1
  - speech R47.9
    - developmental F8Ø.9
    - specified NEC R47.89
  - Taussig-Bing (aortic transposition and overriding pulmonary artery) Q2Ø.1
  - teeth, wedge KØ3.1
  - vascular (local) I99.9
    - congenital Q27.9
  - ventricular septal Q21.Ø
    - concurrent with acute myocardial infarction — *see* Infarct, myocardium
    - following acute myocardial infarction (current complication) I23.2
    - in tetralogy of Fallot Q21.3
  - vision NEC H54.7
  - visual field H53.4Ø
    - bilateral
      - heteronymous H53.47
      - homonymous H53.46-
    - generalized contraction H53.48-
    - localized
      - arcuate H53.43-
      - scotoma (central area) H53.41-
        - blind spot area H53.42-
      - sector H53.43-
      - specified type NEC H53.45-
  - voice R49.9
    - specified NEC R49.8
- **Deferentitis** N49.1
  - gonorrheal (acute) (chronic) A54.23
- **Defibrination** (syndrome) D65
  - antepartum — *see* Hemorrhage, antepartum, with coagulation defect, disseminated intravascular coagulation
  - following ectopic or molar pregnancy OØ8.1
  - intrapartum O67.Ø
  - newborn P6Ø
  - postpartum O72.3
- **Deficiency, deficient**
  - 3-beta hydroxysteroid dehydrogenase E25.Ø
  - 5-alpha reductase (with male pseudohermaphroditism) E29.1
  - 11-hydroxylase E25.Ø
  - 21-hydroxylase E25.Ø
  - abdominal muscle syndrome Q79.4
  - accelerator globulin (Ac G) (blood) D68.2
  - AC globulin (congenital) (hereditary) D68.2
    - acquired D68.4
  - acid phosphatase E83.39
  - activating factor (blood) D68.2
  - adenosine deaminase (ADA) D81.3
  - aldolase (hereditary) E74.19
  - alpha-1-antitrypsin E88.Ø1
  - amino-acids E72.9
  - anemia — *see* Anemia
  - aneurin E51.9
  - antibody with
    - hyperimmunoglobulinemia D8Ø.6
    - near-normal immunoglobins D8Ø.6

Deficiency, deficient — *continued*
- antidiuretic hormone E23.2
- anti-hemophilic
 - factor (A) D66
 - B D67
 - C D68.1
 - globulin (AHG) NEC D66
- antithrombin (antithrombin III) D68.59
- ascorbic acid E54
- attention (disorder) (syndrome) F98.8
 - with hyperactivity — *see* Disorder, attention-deficit hyperactivity
- autoprothrombin
 - I D68.2
 - II D67
 - C D68.2
- beta-glucuronidase E76.29
- biotin E53.8
- biotin-dependent carboxylase D81.819
- biotinidase D81.810
- brancher enzyme (amylopectinosis) E74.03
- calorie, severe E43
 - with marasmus E41
 - and kwashiorkor E42
- cardiac — *see* Insufficiency, myocardial
- carnitine E71.40
 - due to
 - hemodialysis E71.43
 - inborn errors of metabolism E71.42
 - Valproic acid therapy E71.43
 - iatrogenic E71.43
 - muscle palmityltransferase E71.314
 - primary E71.41
 - secondary E71.448
- carotene E50.9
- central nervous system G96.8
- ceruloplasmin (Wilson) E83.01
- choline E53.8
- Christmas factor D67
- chromium E61.4
- specified NEC D68.8
- cognitive F09
- color vision H53.50
 - achromatopsia H53.51
 - acquired H53.52
 - deuteranomaly H53.53
 - protanomaly H53.54
 - specified type NEC H53.59
 - tritanomaly H53.55
- combined glucocorticoid and mineralocorticoid E27.49
- contact factor D68.2
- copper (nutritional) E61.0
- corticoadrenal E27.40
 - primary E27.1
- craniofacial axis Q75.0
- cyanocobalamin E53.8
- C1 esterase inhibitor (C1-INH) D84.1
- debrancher enzyme (limit dextrinosis) E74.03

Deficiency, deficient — *continued*
- dehydrogenase
 - long chain/very long chain acyl CoA E71.310
 - medium chain acyl CoA E71.311
 - short chain acyl CoA E71.312
- diet E63.9
- dihydropyrimidine dehydrogenase (DPD) E88.89
- disaccharidase E73.9
- edema — *see* Malnutrition, severe
- endocrine E34.9
- energy-supply — *see* Malnutrition
- enzymes, circulating NEC E88.09
- ergosterol E55.9
 - with
 - adult osteomalacia M83.8
 - rickets — *see* Rickets
- essential fatty acid (EFA) E63.0
- factor (*see also* Deficiency, coagulation)
 - Hageman D68.2
 - I (congenital) (hereditary) D68.2
 - II (congenital) (hereditary) D68.2
 - IX (congenital) (functional) (hereditary) (with functional defect) D67
 - multiple (congenital) D68.8
- VIII (congenital) (functional) (hereditary) (with functional defect) D66
 - with vascular defect D68.0
 - X (congenital) (hereditary) D68.2
 - XI (congenital) (hereditary) D68.1
 - XII (congenital) (hereditary) D68.2
 - XIII (congenital) (hereditary) D68.2
- femoral, proximal focal (congenital) — *see* Defect, reduction, lower limb, longitudinal, femur
- fibrin-stabilizing factor (congenital) (hereditary) D68.2
 - acquired D68.4
- fibrinase D68.2
- fibrinogen (congenital) (hereditary) D68.2
 - acquired D65
- folate E53.8
- folic acid E53.8
- foreskin N47.3
- fructokinase E74.11
- fructose 1,6-diphosphatase E74.19
- fructose-1-phosphate aldolase E74.19
- galactokinase E74.29
- galactose-1-phosphate uridyl transferase E74.29
- gammaglobulin in blood D80.1
 - hereditary D80.0
- glass factor D68.2
- glucocorticoid E27.49
 - mineralocorticoid E27.49
- glucose-6-phosphatase E74.01
- glucose-6-phosphate dehydrogenase anemia D55.0
- glucuronyl transferase E80.5
- glycogen synthetase E74.09
- gonadotropin (isolated) E23.0
- growth hormone (idiopathic) (isolated) E23.0
- Hageman factor D68.2
- hemoglobin D64.9
- hepatophosphorylase E74.09
- homogentisate 1,2-dioxygenase E70.29
- hormone
 - anterior pituitary (partial) NEC E23.0
 - growth E23.0
 - growth (isolated) E23.0
 - pituitary E23.0
 - testicular E29.1
- hypoxanthine-(guanine)-phosphoribosyltransferase (HGPRT) (total H-PRT) E79.1
- immunity D84.9
 - cell-mediated D84.8
 - with thrombocytopenia and eczema D82.0
 - combined D81.9
 - humoral D80.9
 - IgA (secretory) D80.2
 - IgG D80.3
 - IgM D80.4
- immuno — *see* Immunodeficiency

Deficiency, deficient — *continued*
- immunoglobulin, selective
 - A (IgA) D80.2
 - G (IgG) (subclasses) D80.3
 - M (IgM) D80.4
- inositol (B complex) E53.8
- intrinsic
 - factor (congenital) D51.0
 - sphincter N36.42
 - with urethral hypermobility N36.43
- iodine E61.8
 - congenital syndrome — *see* Syndrome, iodine-deficiency, congenital
- iron E61.1
 - anemia D50.9
- kalium E87.6
- kappa-light chain D80.8
- labile factor (congenital) (hereditary) D68.2
 - acquired D68.4
- lacrimal fluid (acquired) (*see also* Syndrome, dry eye)
 - congenital Q10.6
- lactase
 - congenital E73.0
 - secondary E73.1
- Laki-Lorand factor D68.2
- lecithin cholesterol acyltransferase E78.6
- lipocaic K86.8
- lipoprotein (familial) (high density) E78.6
- liver phosphorylase E74.09
- lysosomal alpha-1, 4 glucosidase E74.02
- magnesium E61.2
- major histocompatibility complex
 - class I D81.6
 - class II D81.7
- manganese E61.3
- menadione (vitamin K) E56.1
 - newborn P53
- mental (familial) (hereditary) — *see* Disability, intellectual
- methylenetetrahydrofolate reductase (MTHFR) E72.12
- mineral NEC E61.8
- mineralocorticoid E27.49
 - with glucocorticoid E27.49
- molybdenum (nutritional) E61.5
- moral F60.2
- multiple nutrient elements E61.7
- muscle
 - carnitine (palmityltransferase) E71.314
 - phosphofructokinase E74.09
- myoadenylate deaminase E79.2
- myocardial — *see* Insufficiency, myocardial
- myophosphorylase E74.04
- NADH diaphorase or reductase (congenital) D74.0
- NADH-methemoglobin reductase (congenital) D74.0
- natrium E87.1
- niacin (amide) (-tryptophan) E52
- nicotinamide E52
- nicotinic acid E52
- number of teeth — *see* Anodontia
- nutrient element E61.9
 - multiple E61.7
 - specified NEC E61.8
- nutrition, nutritional E63.9
 - sequelae — *see* Sequelae, nutritional deficiency
 - specified NEC E63.8
- ornithine transcarbamylase E72.4
- ovarian E28.39
- oxygen — *see* Anoxia
- pantothenic acid E53.8
- parathyroid (gland) E20.9
- perineum (female) N81.89
- phenylalanine hydroxylase E70.1
- phosphoenolpyruvate carboxykinase E74.4
- phosphofructokinase E74.19
- phosphomannomutuse E74.8
- phosphomannose isomerase E74.8
- phosphomannosyl mutase E74.8
- phosphorylase kinase, liver E74.09
- pituitary hormone (isolated) E23.0
- plasma thromboplastin
 - antecedent (PTA) D68.1
 - component (PTC) D67

Deficiency, deficient — *continued*
- platelet NEC D69.1
  - constitutional D68.Ø
- polyglandular E31.8
  - autoimmune E31.Ø
- potassium (K) E87.6
- prepuce N47.3
- proaccelerin (congenital) (hereditary) D68.2
  - acquired D68.4
- proconvertin factor (congenital) (hereditary) D68.2
  - acquired D68.4
- protein (*see also* Malnutrition) E46
  - anemia D53.Ø
  - C D68.59
  - S D68.59
- prothrombin (congenital) (hereditary) D68.2
  - acquired D68.4
- Prower factor D68.2
- pseudocholinesterase E88.Ø9
- PTA (plasma thromboplastin antecedent) D68.1
- PTC (plasma thromboplastin component) D67
- purine nucleoside phosphorylase (PNP) D81.5
- pyracin (alpha) (beta) E53.1
- pyridoxal E53.1
- pyridoxamine E53.1
- pyridoxine (derivatives) E53.1
- pyruvate
  - carboxylase E74.4
  - dehydrogenase E74.4
- riboflavin (vitamin B2) E53.Ø
- salt E87.1
- secretion
  - ovary E28.39
  - salivary gland (any) K11.7
  - urine R34
- selenium (dietary) E59
- serum antitrypsin, familial E88.Ø1
- short stature homeobox gene (SHOX)
  - with
    - dyschondrosteosis Q78.8
    - short stature (idiopathic) E34.3
    - Turner's syndrome Q96.9
- sodium (Na) E87.1
- SPCA (factor VII) D68.2
- sphincter, intrinsic N36.42
  - with urethral hypermobility N36.43
- stable factor (congenital) (hereditary) D68.2
  - acquired D68.4
- Stuart-Prower (factor X) D68.2
- sucrase E74.39
- sulfatase E75.29
- sulfite oxidase E72.19
- thiamin, thiaminic (chloride) E51.9
  - beriberi (dry) E51.11
    - wet E51.12
- thrombokinase D68.2
  - newborn P53
- thyroid (gland) — *see* Hypothyroidism
- tocopherol E56.Ø
- tooth bud KØØ.Ø
- transcobalamine II (anemia) D51.2
- vanadium E61.6
- vascular I99.9
- vasopressin E23.2
- viosterol — *see* Deficiency, calciferol
- vitamin (multiple) NOS E56.9
  - A E5Ø.9
    - with
      - Bitot's spot (corneal) E5Ø.1
      - follicular keratosis E5Ø.8
      - keratomalacia E5Ø.4
      - manifestations NEC E5Ø.8
      - night blindness E5Ø.5
      - scar of cornea, xerophthalmic E5Ø.6
      - xeroderma E5Ø.8
      - xerophthalmia E5Ø.7
      - xerosis
        - conjunctival E5Ø.Ø
          - and Bitot's spot E5Ø.1
        - cornea E5Ø.2
          - and ulceration E5Ø.3
    - sequelae E64.1

Deficiency, deficient — *continued*
- vitamin (multiple) — *continued*
  - B (complex) NOS E53.9
    - with
      - beriberi (dry) E51.11
        - wet E51.12
      - pellagra E52
  - B1 NOS E51.9
    - beriberi (dry) E51.11
      - with circulatory system manifestations E51.11
      - wet E51.12
  - B12 E53.8
  - B2 (riboflavin) E53.Ø
  - B6 E53.1
  - C E54
    - sequelae E64.2
  - D E55.9
    - with
      - adult osteomalacia M83.8
      - rickets — *see* Rickets
    - 25-hydroxylase E83.32
  - E E56.Ø
  - folic acid E53.8
  - G E53.Ø
  - group B E53.9
    - specified NEC E53.8
  - H (biotin) E53.8
  - K E56.1
    - of newborn P53
  - nicotinic E52
  - P E56.8
  - PP (pellagra-preventing) E52
  - specified NEC E56.8
  - thiamin E51.9
    - beriberi — *see* Beriberi
- zinc, dietary E6Ø

Deficit (*see also* Deficiency)
- attention and concentration R41.84Ø
  - disorder — *see* Attention, deficit
- cognitive communication R41.841
- cognitive NEC R41.89
  - following
    - cerebral infarction I69.31
    - cerebrovascular disease I69.91
      - specified disease NEC I69.8
    - intracerebral hemorrhage I69.11
    - nontraumatic intracranial hemorrhage NEC I69.21
    - subarachnoid hemorrhage I69.Ø1
- cognitive communication R41.841
- concentration R41.84Ø
- executive function R41.844
- frontal lobe R41.844
- neurologic NEC R29.818
  - ischemic
    - reversible (RIND) I63.9
      - prolonged (PRIND) I63.9
- oxygen RØ9.Ø2
- prolonged reversible ischemic neurologic (PRIND) I63.9
- psychomotor R41.843
- visuospatial R41.842

Deflection
- radius — *see* Deformity, limb, specified type NEC, forearm
- septum (acquired) (nasal) (nose) J34.2
- spine — *see* Curvature, spine
- turbinate (nose) J34.2

Defluvium
- capillorum — *see* Alopecia
- ciliorum — *see* Madarosis
- unguium L6Ø.8

Deformity Q89.9
- abdomen, congenital Q89.9
- abdominal wall
  - acquired M95.8
  - congenital Q79.59
- acquired (unspecified site) M95.9
- adrenal gland Q89.1
- alimentary tract, congenital Q45.9
  - upper Q4Ø.9

Deformity — *continued*
- ankle (joint) (acquired) (*see also* Deformity, limb, lower leg)
  - abduction — *see* Contraction, joint, ankle
  - congenital Q68.8
  - contraction — *see* Contraction, joint, ankle
  - specified type NEC — *see* Deformity, limb, foot, specified NEC
- anus (acquired) K62.89
  - congenital Q43.9
- aorta (arch) (congenital) Q25.4
  - acquired I77.89
- aortic
  - arch, acquired I77.89
  - cusp or valve (congenital) Q23.8
    - acquired (*see also* Endocarditis, aortic) I35.8
- arm (acquired) (upper) (*see also* Deformity, limb, upper arm)
  - congenital Q68.8
  - forearm — *see* Deformity, limb, forearm
- artery (congenital) (peripheral) NOS Q27.9
  - acquired I77.89
  - coronary (acquired) I25.9
    - congenital Q24.5
  - umbilical Q27.Ø
- atrial septal Q21.1
- auditory canal (external) (congenital) (*see also* Malformation, ear, external)
  - acquired — *see* Disorder, ear, external, specified type NEC
- auricle
  - ear (congenital) (*see also* Malformation, ear, external)
    - acquired — *see* Disorder, pinna, deformity
- back — *see* Dorsopathy, deforming
- bile duct (common) (congenital) (hepatic) Q44.5
  - acquired K83.8
- biliary duct or passage (congenital) Q44.5
  - acquired K83.8
- bladder (neck) (trigone) (sphincter) (acquired) N32.89
  - congenital Q64.79
- bone (acquired) NOS M95.9
  - congenital Q79.9
  - turbinate M95.Ø
- brain (congenital) QØ4.9
  - acquired G93.89
  - reduction QØ4.3
- breast (acquired) N64.89
  - congenital Q83.9
  - reconstructed N65.Ø
- bronchus (congenital) Q32.4
  - acquired NEC J98.Ø9
- bursa, congenital Q79.9
- canaliculi (lacrimalis) (acquired) (*see also* Disorder, lacrimal system, changes)
  - congenital Q1Ø.6
- canthus, acquired — *see* Disorder, eyelid, specified type NEC
- capillary (acquired) I78.8
- cardiovascular system, congenital Q28.9
- caruncle, lacrimal (acquired) (*see also* Disorder, lacrimal system, changes)
  - congenital Q1Ø.6
- cascade, stomach K31.2
- cecum (congenital) Q43.9
  - acquired K63.89
- cerebral, acquired G93.89
  - congenital QØ4.9
- cervix (uterus) (acquired) NEC N88.8
  - congenital Q51.9
- cheek (acquired) M95.2
  - congenital Q18.9
- chest (acquired) (wall) M95.4
  - congenital Q67.8
  - sequelae (late effect) of rickets E64.3
- chin (acquired) M95.2
  - congenital Q18.9
- choroid (congenital) Q14.3
  - acquired H31.8
  - plexus QØ7.8
    - acquired G96.19
- cicatricial — *see* Cicatrix

Deformity — *continued*
- cilia, acquired — *see* Disorder, eyelid, specified type NEC
- clavicle (acquired) M95.8
 - congenital Q68.8
- clitoris (congenital) Q52.6
 - acquired N90.89
- clubfoot — *see* Clubfoot
- coccyx (acquired) — *see* subcategory M43.8
- colon (congenital) Q43.9
 - acquired K63.89
- concha (ear), congenital (*see also* Malformation, ear, external)
 - acquired — *see* Disorder, pinna, deformity
- cornea (acquired) H18.70
 - congenital Q13.4
 - descemetocele — *see* Descemetocele
 - ectasia — *see* Ectasia, cornea
 - specified NEC H18.79-
 - staphyloma — *see* Staphyloma, cornea
- coronary artery (acquired) I25.9
 - congenital Q24.5
- cranium (acquired) — *see* Deformity, skull
- cricoid cartilage (congenital) Q31.8
 - acquired J38.7
- cystic duct (congenital) Q44.5
 - acquired K82.8
- Dandy-Walker Q03.1
 - with spina bifida — *see* Spina bifida
- diaphragm (congenital) Q79.1
 - acquired J98.6
- digestive organ NOS Q45.9
- ductus arteriosus Q25.0
- duodenal bulb K31.89
- duodenum (congenital) Q43.9
 - acquired K31.89
- dura — *see* Deformity, meninges
- ear (acquired) (*see also* Disorder, pinna, deformity)
 - congenital (external) Q17.9
 - internal Q16.5
 - middle Q16.4
 - ossicles Q16.3
 - ossicles Q16.3
- ectodermal (congenital) NEC Q84.9
- ejaculatory duct (congenital) Q55.4
 - acquired N50.8
- elbow (joint) (acquired) (*see also* Deformity, limb, upper arm)
 - congenital Q68.8
 - contraction — *see* Contraction, joint, elbow
- endocrine gland NEC Q89.2
- epididymis (congenital) Q55.4
 - acquired N50.3
- epiglottis (congenital) Q31.8
 - acquired J38.7
- esophagus (congenital) Q39.9
 - acquired K22.8
- eustachian tube (congenital) NEC Q17.8
- eye, congenital Q15.9
- eyebrow (congenital) Q18.8
- eyelid (acquired) (*see also* Disorder, eyelid, specified type NEC)
 - congenital Q10.3
- face (acquired) M95.2
 - congenital Q18.9
- fallopian tube, acquired N83.8
- femur (acquired) — *see* Deformity, limb, specified type NEC, thigh
- fetal
 - with fetopelvic disproportion O33.7
 - causing obstructed labor O66.3
- finger (acquired) M20.00-
 - boutonniere M20.02-
 - congenital Q68.1
 - flexion contracture — *see* Contraction, joint, hand
 - mallet finger M20.01-
 - specified NEC M20.09-
 - swan-neck M20.03-
- flexion (joint) (acquired) (*see also* Deformity, limb, flexion) M21.20
 - congenital NOS Q74.9
 - hip Q65.89

- foot (acquired) (*see also* Deformity, limb, lower leg)
 - cavovarus (congenital) Q66.1
 - congenital NOS Q66.9
 - specified type NEC Q66.89
 - specified type NEC — *see* Deformity, limb, foot, specified NEC
 - valgus (congenital) Q66.6
 - acquired — *see* Deformity, valgus, ankle
 - varus (congenital) NEC Q66.3
 - acquired — *see* Deformity, varus, ankle
- acquired K82.8
- gastrointestinal tract (congenital) NOS Q45.9
 - acquired K63.89
- genitalia, genital organ(s) or system NEC
 - female (congenital) Q52.9
 - acquired N94.89
 - external Q52.70
 - male (congenital) Q55.9
 - acquired N50.8
- globe (eye) (congenital) Q15.8
 - acquired H44.89
- gum, acquired NEC K06.8
- hand (acquired) — *see* Deformity, limb, hand
 - congenital Q68.1
- head (acquired) M95.2
 - congenital Q75.8
- heart (congenital) Q24.9
 - septum Q21.9
 - auricular Q21.1
 - ventricular Q21.0
 - valve (congenital) NEC Q24.8
 - acquired — *see* Endocarditis
- heel (acquired) — *see* Deformity, foot
- hepatic duct (congenital) Q44.5
 - acquired K83.8
- hip (joint) (acquired) (*see also* Deformity, limb, thigh)
 - congenital Q65.9
 - due to (previous) juvenile osteochondrosis — *see* Coxa, plana
 - flexion — *see* Contraction, joint, hip
- hourglass — *see* Contraction, hourglass
- humerus (acquired) M21.82-
 - congenital Q74.0
- hypophyseal (congenital) Q89.2
- ileocecal (coil) (valve) (acquired) K63.89
 - congenital Q43.9
- ileum (congenital) Q43.9
 - acquired K63.89
- ilium (acquired) M95.5
 - congenital Q74.2
- integument (congenital) Q84.9
- intervertebral cartilage or disc (acquired) — *see* Disorder, disc, specified NEC
- intestine (large) (small) (congenital) NOS Q43.9
 - acquired K63.89
- intrinsic minus or plus (hand) — *see* Deformity, limb, specified type NEC, forearm
- iris (acquired) H21.89
 - congenital Q13.2
- ischium (acquired) M95.5
 - congenital Q74.2
- hand M21.94-
 - hip M21.95-
 - knee M21.96-
 - shoulder M21.92-
 - wrist M21.93-
- kidney(s) (calyx) (pelvis) (congenital) Q63.9
 - acquired N28.89

- kidney(s)— *continued*
 - artery (congenital) Q27.2
 - acquired I77.89
- Klippel-Feil (brevicollis) Q76.1
- knee (acquired) NEC (*see also* Deformity, limb, lower leg)
 - congenital Q68.2
- labium (majus) (minus) (congenital) Q52.79
 - acquired N90.89
- lacrimal passages or duct (congenital) NEC Q10.6
 - acquired — *see* Disorder, lacrimal system, changes
- larynx (muscle) (congenital) Q31.8
 - acquired J38.7
 - web (glottic) Q31.0
- leg (upper) (acquired) NEC (*see also* Deformity, limb, thigh)
 - congenital Q68.8
 - lower leg — *see* Deformity, limb, lower leg
- lens (acquired) H27.8
 - congenital Q12.9
- lid (fold) (acquired) (*see also* Disorder, eyelid, specified type NEC)
 - congenital Q10.3
- ligament (acquired) — *see* Disorder, ligament
 - congenital Q79.9
- limb (acquired) M21.90
 - clawfoot M21.53-
 - clawhand M21.51-
 - clubfoot M21.54-
 - clubhand M21.52-
 - congenital, except reduction deformity Q74.9
 - flat foot M21.4-
 - flexion M21.20
 - ankle M21.27-
 - elbow M21.22-
 - finger M21.24-
 - hip M21.25-
 - knee M21.26-
 - shoulder M21.21-
 - toe M21.27-
 - wrist M21.23-
 - foot
 - claw — *see* Deformity, limb, clawfoot
 - club — *see* Deformity, limb, clubfoot
 - drop M21.37-
 - flat — *see* Deformity, limb, flat foot
 - specified NEC M21.6X-
 - forearm M21.93-
 - hand M21.94-
 - lower leg M21.96-
 - specified type NEC M21.80
 - forearm M21.83-
 - lower leg M21.86-
 - thigh M21.85-
 - upper arm M21.82-
 - thigh M21.95-
 - unequal length M21.70
 - short site is
 - femur M21.75-
 - fibula M21.76-
 - humerus M21.72-
 - radius M21.73-
 - tibia M21.76-
 - ulna M21.73-
 - upper arm M21.92-
 - valgus — *see* Deformity, valgus
 - varus — *see* Deformity, varus
 - wrist drop M21.33-
- lip (acquired) NEC K13.0
 - congenital Q38.0
- liver (congenital) Q44.7
 - acquired K76.89
- lumbosacral (congenital) (joint) (region) Q76.49
 - acquired — *see* subcategory M43.8
- acquired J98.4
- lymphatic system, congenital Q89.9
- Madelung's (radius) Q74.0
- mandible (acquired) (congenital) M26.9

Deformity — *continued*
maxilla (acquired) (congenital) M26.9
meninges or membrane (congenital) QØ7.9
cerebral QØ4.8
acquired G96.19
spinal cord (congenital) G96.19
acquired G96.19
metacarpus (acquired) — *see* Deformity, limb, forearm
congenital Q74.Ø
metatarsus (acquired) — *see* Deformity, foot
congenital Q66.9
middle ear (congenital) Q16.4
ossicles Q16.3
mitral (leaflets) (valve) IØ5.8
parachute Q23.2
stenosis, congenital Q23.2
mouth (acquired) K13.79
congenital Q38.6
multiple, congenital NEC Q89.7
muscle (acquired) M62.89
congenital Q79.9
sternocleidomastoid Q68.Ø
musculoskeletal system (acquired) M95.9
congenital Q79.9
specified NEC M95.8
nail (acquired) L6Ø.8
congenital Q84.6
nasal — *see* Deformity, nose
neck (acquired) M95.3
congenital Q18.9
sternocleidomastoid Q68.Ø
nervous system (congenital) QØ7.9
nipple (congenital) Q83.9
acquired N64.89
nose (acquired) (cartilage) M95.Ø
bone (turbinate) M95.Ø
congenital Q3Ø.9
bent or squashed Q67.4
saddle M95.Ø
syphilitic A5Ø.57
septum (acquired) J34.2
congenital Q3Ø.8
sinus (wall) (congenital) Q3Ø.8
acquired M95.Ø
syphilitic (congenital) A5Ø.57
late A52.73
ocular muscle (congenital) Q1Ø.3
acquired — *see* Strabismus, mechanical
opticociliary vessels (congenital) Q13.2
orbit (eye) (acquired) HØ5.3Ø
atrophy — *see* Atrophy, orbit
congenital Q1Ø.7
due to
bone disease NEC HØ5.32-
trauma or surgery HØ5.33-
enlargement — *see* Enlargement, orbit
exostosis — *see* Exostosis, orbit
organ of Corti (congenital) Q16.5
ovary (congenital) Q5Ø.39
acquired N83.8
oviduct, acquired N83.8
palate (congenital) Q38.5
acquired M27.8
cleft (congenital) — *see* Cleft, palate
pancreas (congenital) Q45.3
acquired K86.8
parathyroid (gland) Q89.2
parotid (gland) (congenital) Q38.4
acquired K11.8
patella (acquired) — *see* Disorder, patella, specified NEC
pelvis, pelvic (acquired) (bony) M95.5
with disproportion (fetopelvic) O33.Ø
causing obstructed labor O65.Ø
congenital Q74.2
rachitic sequelae (late effect) E64.3
penis (glans) (congenital) Q55.69
acquired N48.89
pericardium (congenital) Q24.8
acquired — *see* Pericarditis
pharynx (congenital) Q38.8
acquired J39.2

Deformity — *continued*
pinna, acquired (*see also* Disorder, pinna, deformity)
congenital Q17.9
pituitary (congenital) Q89.2
posture — *see* Dorsopathy, deforming
prepuce (congenital) Q55.69
acquired N47.8
prostate (congenital) Q55.4
acquired N42.89
pupil (congenital) Q13.2
acquired — *see* Abnormality, pupillary
pylorus (congenital) Q4Ø.3
acquired K31.89
rachitic (acquired), old or healed E64.3
radius (acquired) (*see also* Deformity, limb, forearm)
congenital Q68.8
rectum (congenital) Q43.9
acquired K62.89
reduction (extremity) (limb), congenital (*see also* condition and site) Q73.8
brain QØ4.3
lower — *see* Defect, reduction, lower limb
upper — *see* Defect, reduction, upper limb
renal — *see* Deformity, kidney
respiratory system (congenital) Q34.9
rib (acquired) M95.4
congenital Q76.6
cervical Q76.5
rotation (joint) (acquired) *see* Deformity, limb, specified site NEC
congenital Q74.9
hip — *see* Deformity, limb, specified type NEC, thigh
congenital Q65.89
sacroiliac joint (congenital) Q74.2
acquired — *see* subcategory M43.8
sacrum (acquired) — *see* subcategory M43.8
saddle
back — *see* Lordosis
nose M95.Ø
syphilitic A5Ø.57
salivary gland or duct (congenital) Q38.4
acquired K11.8
scapula (acquired) M95.8
congenital Q68.8
scrotum (congenital) (*see also* Malformation, testis and scrotum)
acquired N5Ø.8
seminal vesicles (congenital) Q55.4
acquired N5Ø.8
septum, nasal (acquired) J34.2
shoulder (joint) (acquired) — *see* Deformity, limb, upper arm
congenital Q74.Ø
contraction — *see* Contraction, joint, shoulder
sigmoid (flexure) (congenital) Q43.9
acquired K63.89
skin (congenital) Q82.9
skull (acquired) M95.2
congenital Q75.8
with
anencephaly QØØ.Ø
encephalocele — *see* Encephalocele
hydrocephalus QØ3.9
with spina bifida — *see* Spina bifida, by site, with hydrocephalus
microcephaly QØ2
soft parts, organs or tissues (of pelvis)
in pregnancy or childbirth NEC O34.8-
causing obstructed labor O65.5
spermatic cord (congenital) Q55.4
acquired N5Ø.8
torsion — *see* Torsion, spermatic cord
spinal — *see* Dorsopathy, deforming
column (acquired) — *see* Dorsopathy, deforming
congenital Q67.5
cord (congenital) QØ6.9
acquired G95.89
nerve root (congenital) QØ7.9
spine (acquired) (*see also* Dorsopathy, deforming)
congenital Q67.5
rachitic E64.3

Deformity — *continued*
spine— *continued*
specified NEC — *see* Dorsopathy, deforming, specified NEC
spleen
acquired D73.89
congenital Q89.Ø9
Sprengel's (congenital) Q74.Ø
sternocleidomastoid (muscle), congenital Q68.Ø
sternum (acquired) M95.4
congenital NEC Q76.7
stomach (congenital) Q4Ø.3
acquired K31.89
submandibular gland (congenital) Q38.4
submaxillary gland (congenital) Q38.4
acquired K11.8
talipes — *see* Talipes
testis (congenital) (*see also* Malformation, testis and scrotum)
acquired N44.8
torsion — *see* Torsion, testis
thigh (acquired) (*see also* Deformity, limb, thigh)
congenital NEC Q68.8
thorax (acquired) (wall) M95.4
congenital Q67.8
sequelae of rickets E64.3
thumb (acquired) (*see also* Deformity, finger)
congenital NEC Q68.1
thymus (tissue) (congenital) Q89.2
thyroid (gland) (congenital) Q89.2
cartilage Q31.8
acquired J38.7
tibia (acquired) (*see also* Deformity, limb, specified) type NEC, lower leg
congenital NEC Q68.8
saber (syphilitic) A5Ø.56
toe (acquired) M2Ø.6-
congenital Q66.9
hallux rigidus M2Ø.2-
hallux valgus M2Ø.1-
hallux varus M2Ø.3-
hammer toe M2Ø.4-
specified NEC M2Ø.5X-
tongue (congenital) Q38.3
acquired K14.8
tooth, teeth KØØ.2
trachea (rings) (congenital) Q32.1
acquired J39.8
transverse aortic arch (congenital) Q25.4
tricuspid (leaflets) (valve) IØ7.8
atresia or stenosis Q22.4
Ebstein's Q22.5
trunk (acquired) M95.8
congenital Q89.9
ulna (acquired) (*see also* Deformity, limb, forearm)
congenital NEC Q68.8
urachus, congenital Q64.4
ureter (opening) (congenital) Q62.8
acquired N28.89
urethra (congenital) Q64.79
acquired N36.8
urinary tract (congenital) Q64.9
urachus Q64.4
uterus (congenital) Q51.9
acquired N85.8
uvula (congenital) Q38.5
vagina (acquired) N89.8
congenital Q52.4
valgus NEC M21.ØØ
ankle M21.Ø7-
elbow M21.Ø2-
hip M21.Ø5-
knee M21.Ø6-
valve, valvular (congenital) (heart) Q24.8
acquired — *see* Endocarditis
varus NEC M21.1Ø
ankle M21.17-
elbow M21.12-
hip M21.15
knee M21.16-
tibia — *see* Osteochondrosis, juvenile, tibia
vas deferens (congenital) Q55.4
acquired N5Ø.8

Deformity — *continued*
- vein (congenital) Q27.9
  - great Q26.9
- vertebra — *see* Dorsopathy, deforming
- vertical talus (congenital) Q66.80
  - left foot Q66.82
  - right foot Q66.81
- vesicourethral orifice (acquired) N32.89
  - congenital NEC Q64.79
- vessels of optic papilla (congenital) Q14.2
- visual field (contraction) — *see* Defect, visual field
- vitreous body, acquired H43.89
- vulva (congenital) Q52.79
  - acquired N90.89
- wrist (joint) (acquired) (*see also* Deformity, limb, forearm)
  - congenital Q68.8
  - contraction — *see* Contraction, joint, wrist

Degeneration, degenerative
- adrenal (capsule) (fatty) (gland) (hyaline) (infectional) E27.8
- amyloid (*see also* Amyloidosis) E85.9
- anterior cornua, spinal cord G12.29
- anterior labral S43.49-
- aorta, aortic I70.0
  - fatty I77.89
- aortic valve (heart) — *see* Endocarditis, aortic
- arteriovascular — *see* Arteriosclerosis
- artery, arterial (atheromatous) (calcareous) (*see also* Arteriosclerosis)
  - cerebral, amyloid E85.4 *[I68.0]*
  - medial — *see* Arteriosclerosis, extremities
- articular cartilage NEC — *see* Derangement, joint, articular cartilage, by site
- atheromatous — *see* Arteriosclerosis
- basal nuclei or ganglia G23.9
  - specified NEC G23.8
- bone NEC — *see* Disorder, bone, specified type NEC
- brachial plexus G54.0
- brain (cortical) (progressive) G31.9
  - alcoholic G31.2
  - arteriosclerotic I67.2
  - childhood G31.9
    - specified NEC G31.89
  - cystic G31.89
    - congenital Q04.6
  - in
    - alcoholism G31.2
    - beriberi E51.2
    - cerebrovascular disease I67.9
    - congenital hydrocephalus Q03.9
      - with spina bifida (*see also* Spina bifida)
    - Fabry-Anderson disease E75.21
    - Gaucher's disease E75.22
    - Hunter's syndrome E76.1
    - lipidosis
      - cerebral E75.4
      - generalized E75.6
    - mucopolysaccharidosis — *see* Mucopolysaccharidosis
    - myxedema E03.9 *[G32.89]*
    - neoplastic disease (*see also* Neoplasm) D49.6 *[G32.89]*
    - Niemann-Pick disease E75.249 *[G32.89]*
    - sphingolipidosis E75.3 *[G32.89]*
    - vitamin B12 deficiency E53.8 *[G32.89]*
  - senile NEC G31.1
- breast N64.89
- Bruch's membrane — *see* Degeneration, choroid
- capillaries (fatty) I78.8
  - amyloid E85.8 *[I79.8]*
- cardiac (*see also* Degeneration, myocardial)
  - valve, valvular — *see* Endocarditis
- cardiorenal — *see* Hypertension, cardiorenal
- cardiovascular (*see also* Disease, cardiovascular)
  - renal — *see* Hypertension, cardiorenal
- cerebellar NOS G31.9
  - alcoholic G31.2
  - primary (hereditary) (sporadic) G11.9
- cerebral — *see* Degeneration, brain
- cerebrovascular I67.9
  - due to hypertension I67.4
- cervical plexus G54.2

Degeneration, degenerative — *continued*
- cervix N88.8
  - due to radiation (intended effect) N88.8
    - adverse effect or misadventure N99.89
- chamber angle H21.21-
- changes, spine or vertebra — *see* Spondylosis
- chorioretinal (*see also* Degeneration, choroid)
  - hereditary H31.20
- choroid (colloid) (drusen) H31.10-
  - atrophy — *see* Atrophy, choroidal
  - hereditary — *see* Dystrophy, choroidal, hereditary
- ciliary body H21.22-
- cochlear — *see* subcategory H83.8
- combined (spinal cord) (subacute) E53.8 *[G32.0]*
  - with anemia (pernicious) D51.0 *[G32.0]*
    - due to dietary vitamin B12 deficiency D51.3 *[G32.0]*
  - in (due to)
    - vitamin B12 deficiency E53.8 *[G32.0]*
      - anemia D51.9 *[G32.0]*
- conjunctiva H11.10
  - concretions — *see* Concretion, conjunctiva
  - deposits — *see* Deposit, conjunctiva
  - pigmentations — *see* Pigmentation, conjunctiva
  - pinguecula — *see* Pinguecula
  - xerosis — *see* Xerosis, conjunctiva
- cornea H18.40
  - calcerous H18.43
    - band keratopathy H18.42-
  - familial, hereditary — *see* Dystrophy, cornea
  - hyaline (of old scars) H18.49
  - keratomalacia — *see* Keratomalacia
  - nodular H18.45-
  - peripheral H18.46-
  - senile H18.41-
  - specified type NEC H18.49
- cortical (cerebellar) (parenchymatous) G31.89
  - alcoholic G31.2
  - diffuse, due to arteriopathy I67.2
- corticobasal G31.85
- cutis L98.8
  - amyloid E85.4 *[L99]*
- dental pulp K04.2
- disc disease — *see* Degeneration, intervertebral disc NEC
- dorsolateral (spinal cord) — *see* Degeneration, combined
- extrapyramidal G25.9
- eye, macular (*see also* Degeneration, macula)
  - congenital or hereditary — *see* Dystrophy, retina
- facet joints — *see* Spondylosis
- fatty
  - liver NEC K76.0
    - alcoholic K70.0
- grey matter (brain) (Alpers') G31.81
- heart (*see also* Degeneration, myocardial)
  - amyloid E85.4 *[I43]*
  - atheromatous — *see* Disease, heart, ischemic, atherosclerotic
  - ischemic — *see* Disease, heart, ischemic
- hepatolenticular (Wilson's) E83.01
- hepatorenal K76.7
- hyaline (diffuse) (generalized)
  - localized — *see* Degeneration, by site
- infrapatellar fat pad M79.4
- intervertebral disc NOS
  - with
    - myelopathy — *see* Disorder, disc, with, myelopathy
    - radiculitis or radiculopathy — *see* Disorder, disc, with, radiculopathy
  - cervical, cervicothoracic — *see* Disorder, disc, cervical, degeneration
    - with
      - myelopathy — *see* Disorder, disc, cervical, with myelopathy
      - neuritis, radiculitis or radiculopathy — *see* Disorder, disc, cervical, with neuritis
  - lumbar region M51.36
    - with
      - myelopathy M51.06

Degeneration, degenerative — *continued*
- intervertebral disc — *continued*
  - lumbar region — *continued*
    - with — *continued*
      - neuritis, radiculitis, radiculopathy or sciatica M51.16
  - lumbosacral region M51.37
    - with
      - myelopathy M51.07
      - neuritis, radiculitis, radiculopathy or sciatica M51.17
  - sacrococcygeal region M53.3
  - thoracic region M51.34
    - with
      - myelopathy M51.04
      - neuritis, radiculitis, radiculopathy M51.14
  - thoracolumbar region M51.35
    - with
      - myelopathy M51.05
      - neuritis, radiculitis, radiculopathy M51.15
- intestine, amyloid E85.4
- iris (pigmentary) H21.23-
- ischemic — *see* Ischemia
- joint disease — *see* Osteoarthritis
- kidney N28.89
  - amyloid E85.4 *[N29]*
  - cystic, congenital Q61.9
  - fatty N28.89
  - polycystic Q61.3
    - adult type (autosomal dominant) Q61.2
    - infantile type (autosomal recessive) NEC Q61.19
      - collecting duct dilatation Q61.11
- Kuhnt-Junius (*see also* Degeneration, macula) H35.32
- lens — *see* Cataract
- lenticular (familial) (progressive) (Wilson's) (with cirrhosis of liver) E83.01
- liver (diffuse) NEC K76.89
  - amyloid E85.4 *[K77]*
  - cystic K76.89
    - congenital Q44.6
  - fatty NEC K76.0
    - alcoholic K70.0
  - hypertrophic K76.89
  - parenchymatous, acute or subacute K72.00
    - with coma K72.01
  - pigmentary K76.89
  - toxic (acute) K71.9
- lung J98.4
- lymph gland I89.8
  - hyaline I89.8
- macula, macular (acquired) (age-related) (senile) H35.30
  - angioid streaks H35.33
  - atrophic age-related H35.31
  - congenital or hereditary — *see* Dystrophy, retina
  - cystoid H35.35-
  - drusen H35.36-
  - exudative H35.32
  - hole H35.34-
  - nonexudative H35.31
  - puckering H35.37-
  - toxic H35.38-
- membranous labyrinth, congenital (causing impairment of hearing) Q16.5
- meniscus — *see* Derangement, meniscus
- mitral — *see* Insufficiency, mitral
- Mönckeberg's — *see* Arteriosclerosis, extremities
- motor centers, senile G31.1
- multi-system G90.3
- mural — *see* Degeneration, myocardial
- muscle (fatty) (fibrous) (hyaline) (progressive) M62.89
  - heart — *see* Degeneration, myocardial
- myelin, central nervous system G37.9
- myocardial, myocardium (fatty) (hyaline) (senile) I51.5
  - with rheumatic fever (conditions in I00) I09.0
    - active, acute or subacute I01.2
      - with chorea I02.0
    - inactive or quiescent (with chorea) I09.0
  - hypertensive — *see* Hypertension, heart

- **Delirium, delirious** — *continued*
  - due to — *continued*
    - inhalant intoxication — *continued*
      - in
        - abuse F18.121
        - dependence F18.221
    - multiple etiologies FØ5
    - opioid intoxication (acute) F11.921
      - in
        - abuse F11.121
        - dependence F11.221
    - phencyclidine intoxication (acute) F16.921
      - in
        - abuse F16.121
        - dependence F16.221
    - psychoactive substance NEC intoxication (acute) F19.921
      - in
        - abuse F19.121
        - dependence F19.221
    - sedative
      - intoxication F13.921
        - in
          - abuse F13.121
          - dependence F13.221
      - withdrawal F13.231
    - unknown etiology FØ5
  - exhaustion F43.Ø
  - hysterical F44.89
  - postprocedural (postoperative) FØ5
  - puerperal FØ5
  - thyroid — *see* Thyrotoxicosis with thyroid storm
  - traumatic — *see* Injury, intracranial
  - tremens (alcohol-induced) F1Ø.231
    - sedative-induced F13.231
- **Delivery** (childbirth) (labor)
  - arrested active phase O62.1
  - cesarean (for)
    - abnormal
      - pelvis (bony) (deformity) (major) NEC with disproportion (fetopelvic) O33.Ø
        - with obstructed labor O65.Ø
      - presentation or position O32.9
    - abruptio placentae (*see also* Abruptio placentae) O45.9-
    - acromion presentation O32.2
    - atony, uterus O62.2
    - breech presentation O32.1
      - incomplete O32.8
    - brow presentation O32.3
    - cephalopelvic disproportion O33.9
    - cerclage O34.3-
    - chin presentation O32.3
    - cicatrix of cervix O34.4-
    - contracted pelvis (general)
      - inlet O33.2
      - outlet O33.3
    - cord presentation or prolapse O69.Ø
    - cystocele O34.8-
    - deformity (acquired) (congenital)
      - pelvic organs or tissues NEC O34.8-
      - pelvis (bony) NEC O33.Ø
    - disproportion NOS O33.9
    - eclampsia — *see* Eclampsia
    - face presentation O32.3
    - failed
      - forceps O66.5
      - induction of labor O61.9
        - instrumental O61.1
        - mechanical O61.1
        - medical O61.Ø
        - specified NEC O61.8
        - surgical O61.1
      - trial of labor NOS O66.4Ø
        - following previous cesarean delivery O66.41
      - vacuum extraction O66.5
      - ventouse O66.5
    - fetal-maternal hemorrhage O43.Ø1-
    - hemorrhage (intrapartum) O67.9
      - with coagulation defect O67.Ø
      - specified cause NEC O67.8
    - high head at term O32.4
    - hydrocephalic fetus O33.6

- **Delivery** — *continued*
  - cesarean— *continued*
    - incarceration of uterus O34.51-
    - incoordinate uterine action O62.4
    - increased size, fetus O33.5
    - inertia, uterus O62.2
      - primary O62.Ø
      - secondary O62.1
    - lateroversion, uterus O34.59-
    - mal lie O32.9
    - malposition
      - fetus O32.9
      - pelvic organs or tissues NEC O34.8-
      - uterus NEC O34.59-
    - malpresentation NOS O32.9
    - oblique presentation O32.2
    - occurring after 37 completed weeks of gestation but before 39 completed weeks gestation due to (spontaneous) onset of labor O75.82
    - oversize fetus O33.5
    - pelvic tumor NEC O34.8-
    - placenta previa O44.1-
      - without hemorrhage O44.Ø-
    - placental insufficiency O36.51-
    - planned, occurring after 37 completed weeks of gestation but before 39 completed weeks gestation due to (spontaneous) onset of labor O75.82
    - polyp, cervix O34.4-
      - causing obstructed labor O65.5
    - poor dilatation, cervix O62.Ø
    - pre-eclampsia O14.9-
      - mild O14.Ø-
      - moderate O14.Ø-
      - severe
        - with hemolysis, elevated liver enzymes and low platelet count (HELLP) O14.2-
    - previous
      - cesarean delivery O34.21
      - surgery (to)
        - cervix O34.4-
        - gynecological NEC O34.8-
        - rectum O34.7-
        - uterus O34.29
        - vagina O34.6-
    - prolapse
      - arm or hand O32.2
      - uterus O34.52-
    - prolonged labor NOS O63.9
    - rectocele O34.8-
    - retroversion
      - uterus O34.53-
    - rigid
      - cervix O34.4-
      - pelvic floor O34.8-
      - perineum O34.7-
      - vagina O34.6-
      - vulva O34.7-
    - sacculation, pregnant uterus O34.59-
    - scar(s)
      - cervix O34.4-
      - cesarean delivery O34.21
      - uterus O34.29
    - Shirodkar suture in situ O34.3-
    - shoulder presentation O32.2
    - stenosis or stricture, cervix O34.4-
    - streptococcus B carrier state O99.824
    - transverse presentation or lie O32.2
    - tumor, pelvic organs or tissues NEC O34.8-
      - cervix O34.4-
    - umbilical cord presentation or prolapse O69.Ø
    - without indication O82
  - completely normal case O8Ø
  - complicated O75.9
    - by
      - abnormal, abnormality (of)
        - forces of labor O62.9
          - specified type NEC O62.8
        - glucose O99.814
        - uterine contractions NOS O62.9

- **Delivery** — *continued*
  - complicate d— *continued*
    - by — *continued*
      - abruptio placentae (*see also* Abruptio placentae) O45.9-
      - abuse
        - physical O9A.32
      - abuse— *continued*
        - psychological O9A.52
        - sexual O9A.42
      - adherent placenta O72.Ø
        - without hemorrhage O73.Ø
      - alcohol use O99.314
      - anemia (pre-existing) O99.Ø2
      - anesthetic death O74.8
      - annular detachment of cervix O71.3
      - atony, uterus O62.2
      - attempted vacuum extraction and forceps O66.5
      - Bandl's ring O62.4
      - bariatric surgery status O99.844
      - biliary tract disorder O26.62
      - bleeding — *see* Delivery, complicated by, hemorrhage
      - blood disorder NEC O99.12
      - cervical dystocia (hypotonic) O62.2
        - primary O62.Ø
        - secondary O62.1
      - circulatory system disorder O99.42
      - compression of cord (umbilical) NEC O69.2
      - condition NEC O99.89
      - contraction, contracted ring O62.4
      - cord (umbilical)
        - around neck
          - with compression O69.1
          - without compression O69.81
        - bruising O69.5
        - complication O69.9
          - specified NEC O69.89
        - compression NEC O69.2
        - entanglement O69.2
          - without compression O69.82
        - hematoma O69.5
        - presentation O69.Ø
        - prolapse O69.Ø
        - short O69.3
        - thrombosis (vessels) O69.5
        - vascular lesion O69.5
      - Couvelaire uterus O45.8X-
      - delay following rupture of membranes (spontaneous) — *see* Pregnancy, complicated by, premature rupture of membranes
      - damage to (injury to) NEC
        - perineum O71.82
        - periurethral tissue O71.82
        - vulva O71.82
      - depressed fetal heart tones O76
      - diabetes O24.92
        - gestational O24.429
          - diet controlled O24.42Ø
          - insulin controlled O24.424
        - pre-existing O24.32
          - specified NEC O24.82
          - type 1 O24.Ø2
          - type 2 O24.12
      - diastasis recti (abdominis) O71.89
      - dilatation
        - bladder O66.8
        - cervix incomplete, poor or slow O62.Ø
      - disease NEC O99.89
      - disruptio uteri — *see* Delivery, complicated by, rupture, uterus
      - drug use O99.324
      - dysfunction, uterus NOS O62.9
        - hypertonic O62.4
        - hypotonic O62.2
          - primary O62.Ø
          - secondary O62.1
        - incoordinate O62.4
      - eclampsia O15.1
      - embolism (pulmonary) — *see* Embolism, obstetric

- **Delivery** — *continued*
  - complicated — *continued*
    - by — *continued*
      - endocrine, nutritional or metabolic disease NEC O99.284
      - failed
        - attempted vaginal birth after previous cesarean delivery O66.41
        - induction of labor O61.9
          - instrumental O61.1
          - mechanical O61.1
          - medical O61.0
          - specified NEC O61.8
          - surgical O61.1
        - trial of labor O66.40
      - female genital mutilation O65.5
      - fetal
        - abnormal acid-base balance O68
        - acidemia O68
        - acidosis O68
        - alkalosis O68
        - death, early O02.1
        - deformity O66.3
        - heart rate or rhythm (abnormal) (non-reassuring) O76
        - hypoxia O77.8
        - stress O77.9
          - due to drug administration O77.1
          - electrocardiographic evidence of O77.8
          - ultrasound evidence of O77.8
          - specified NEC O77.8
      - fever during labor O75.2
      - gastric banding status O99.844
      - gastric bypass status O99.844
      - gastrointestinal disease NEC O99.62
      - gestational diabetes O24.429
        - diet controlled O24.420
        - insulin (and diet) controlled O24.424
      - gonorrhea O98.22
      - hematoma O71.7
        - ischial spine O71.7
        - pelvic O71.7
        - vagina O71.7
        - vulva or perineum O71.7
      - hemorrhage (uterine) O67.9
        - associated with
          - afibrinogenemia O67.0
          - coagulation defect O67.0
          - hyperfibrinolysis O67.0
          - hypofibrinogenemia O67.0
        - due to
          - low-lying placenta O44.1-
          - placenta previa O44.1-
          - premature separation of placenta (normally implanted) (*see also* Abruptio placentae) O45.9-
          - retained placenta O72.0
          - uterine leiomyoma O67.8
        - placenta NEC O67.8
        - postpartum NEC (atonic) (immediate) O72.1
          - with retained or trapped placenta O72.0
          - delayed O72.2
          - secondary O72.2
          - third stage O72.0
      - hourglass contraction, uterus O62.4
      - hypertension, hypertensive (pre-existing) — *see* Hypertension, complicated by, childbirth (labor)
      - hypotension O26.5-
      - incomplete dilatation (cervix) O62.0
      - incoordinate uterus contractions O62.4
      - inertia, uterus O62.2
        - during latent phase of labor O62.0
        - primary O62.0
        - secondary O62.1
      - infection (maternal) O98.92
        - carrier state NEC O99.834
        - gonorrhea O98.22
        - human immunodeficiency virus (HIV) O98.72

- **Delivery** — *continued*
  - complicated — *continued*
    - by — *continued*
      - infection — *continued*
        - sexually transmitted NEC O98.32
        - specified NEC O98.82
        - syphilis O98.12
        - tuberculosis O98.02
        - viral hepatitis O98.42
        - viral NEC O98.52
      - injury (to mother) (*see also* Delivery, complicated by, damage to) O71.9
        - nonobstetric O9A.22
          - caused by abuse — *see* Delivery, complicated by, abuse
      - intrauterine fetal death, early O02.1
      - inversion, uterus O71.2
      - laceration (perineal) O70.9
        - anus (sphincter) O70.4
          - with third degree laceration O70.2
            - with mucosa O70.3
          - without third degree laceration O70.4
        - bladder (urinary) O71.5
        - bowel O71.5
        - cervix (uteri) O71.3
        - fourchette O70.0
        - hymen O70.0
        - labia O70.0
        - pelvic
          - floor O70.1
          - organ NEC O71.5
        - perineum, perineal O70.9
          - first degree O70.0
          - fourth degree O70.3
          - muscles O70.1
          - second degree O70.1
          - skin O70.0
          - slight O70.0
          - third degree O70.2
        - peritoneum (pelvic) O71.5
        - rectovaginal (septum) (without perineal laceration) O71.4
          - with perineum O70.2
            - with anal or rectal mucosa O70.3
        - specified NEC O71.89
        - sphincter ani — *see* Delivery, complicated, by, laceration, anus (sphincter)
        - urethra O71.5
        - uterus O71.81
          - before labor O71.81
        - vagina, vaginal (deep) (high) (without perineal laceration) O71.4
          - with perineum O70.0
          - muscles, with perineum O70.1
        - vulva O70.0
      - liver disorder O26.62
      - malignancy O9A.12
      - malnutrition O25.2
      - malposition, malpresentation
        - placenta (with hemorrhage) O44.1-
          - without hemorrhage O44.0-
        - uterus or cervix O65.5
        - without obstruction (*see also* Delivery, complicated by, obstruction) O32.9
          - breech O32.1
          - compound O32.6
          - face (brow) (chin) O32.3
          - footling O32.8
          - high head O32.4
          - oblique O32.2
          - specified NEC O32.8
          - transverse O32.2
          - unstable lie O32.0
      - meconium in amniotic fluid O77.0
      - mental disorder NEC O99.344
      - metrorrhexis — *see* Delivery, complicated by, rupture, uterus
      - nervous system disorder O99.354
      - obesity (pre-existing) O99.214
      - obesity surgery status O99.844
      - obstetric trauma O71.9
        - specified NEC O71.89

- **Delivery** — *continued*
  - complicated — *continued*
    - by — *continued*
      - obstructed labor
        - due to
          - breech (complete) (frank) presentation O64.1
            - incomplete O64.8
          - brow presenation O64.3
          - buttock presentation O64.1
          - chin presentation O64.2
          - compound presentation O64.5
          - contracted pelvis O65.1
          - deep transverse arrest O64.0
          - deformed pelvis O65.0
          - dystocia (fetal) O66.9
            - due to
              - conjoined twins O66.3
              - fetal
                - abnormality NEC O66.3
                - ascites O66.3
                - hydrops O66.3
                - meningomyelocele O66.3
                - sacral teratoma O66.3
                - tumor O66.3
              - hydrocephalic fetus O66.3
            - shoulder O66.0
          - face presentation O64.2
          - fetopelvic disproportion O65.4
          - footling presentation O64.8
          - impacted shoulders O66.0
          - incomplete rotation of fetal head O64.0
          - large fetus O66.2
          - locked twins O66.1
          - malposition O64.9
            - specified NEC O64.8
          - malpresentation O64.9
            - specified NEC O64.8
          - multiple fetuses NEC O66.6
          - pelvic
            - abnormality (maternal) O65.9
              - organ O65.5
              - specified NEC O65.8
            - contraction
              - inlet O65.2
              - mid-cavity O65.3
              - outlet O65.3
          - persistent (position)
            - occipitoiliac O64.0
            - occipitoposterior O64.0
            - occipitosacral O64.0
            - occipitotransverse O64.0
          - prolapsed arm O64.4
          - shoulder presentation O64.4
        - specified NEC O66.8
      - pathological retraction ring, uterus O62.4
      - penetration, pregnant uterus by instrument O71.1
      - perforation — *see* Delivery, complicated by, laceration
      - placenta, placental
        - ablatio (*see also* Abruptio placentae) O45.9-
        - abnormality O43.9-
          - specified NEC O43.89-
        - abruptio (*see also* Abruptio placentae) O45.9-
        - accreta O43.21-
        - adherent (with hemorrhage) O72.0
          - without hemorrhage O73.0
        - detachment (premature) (*see also* Abruptio placentae) O45.9-
        - disorder O43.9-
          - specified NEC O43.89-
        - hemorrhage NEC O67.8
        - increta O43.22-
        - low (implantation) O44.1-
          - without hemorrhage O44.0-
        - malformation O43.10-
        - malposition O44.1-
          - without hemorrhage O44.0-
        - percreta O43.23-

- **Delivery** — *continued*
  - complicated — *continued*
    - by — *continued*
      - placenta, placental — *continued*
        - previa (central) (lateral) (low) (marginal) (partial) (total) O44.1-
          - without hemorrhage O44.Ø-
        - retained (with hemorrhage) O72.Ø
          - without hemorrhage O73.Ø
        - separation (premature) O45.9-
          - specified NEC O45.8X-
        - vicious insertion O44.1-
      - precipitate labor O62.3
      - premature rupture, membranes *(see also* Pregnancy, complicated by, premature rupture of membranes) O42.9Ø
      - prolapse
        - arm or hand O32.2
        - cord (umbilical) O69.Ø
        - foot or leg O32.8
        - uterus O34.52-
      - prolonged labor O63.9
        - first stage O63.Ø
        - second stage O63.1
      - protozoal disease (maternal) O98.62
      - respiratory disease NEC O99.52
      - retained membranes or portions of placenta O72.2
        - without hemorrhage O73.1
      - retarded birth O63.9
      - retention of secundines (with hemorrhage) O72.Ø
        - without hemorrhage O73.Ø
        - partial O72.2
          - without hemorrhage O73.1
      - rupture
        - bladder (urinary) O71.5
        - cervix O71.3
        - pelvic organ NEC O71.5
        - urethra O71.5
        - uterus (during or after labor) O71.1
          - before labor O71.Ø-
      - separation, pubic bone (symphysis pubis) O71.6
      - shock O75.1
      - shoulder presentation O64.4
      - skin disorder NEC O99.72
      - spasm, cervix O62.4
      - stenosis or stricture, cervix O65.5
      - streptococcus B carrier state O99.824
      - subluxation of symphysis (pubis) O26.72
      - syphilis (maternal) O98.12
      - tear — *see* Delivery, complicated by, laceration
      - tetanic uterus O62.4
      - trauma (obstetrical) (*see also* Delivery, complicated, by damage to) O71.9
        - non-obstetric O9A.22
        - periurethral O71.82
      - tuberculosis (maternal) O98.Ø2
      - tumor, pelvic organs or tissues NEC O65.5
      - umbilical cord around neck
        - with compression O69.1
        - without compression O69.81
      - uterine inertia O62.2
        - during latent phase of labor O62.Ø
        - primary O62.Ø
        - secondary O62.1
      - vasa previa O69.4
      - velamentous insertion of cord O43.12-
    - specified complication NEC O75.89
  - delayed NOS O63.9
    - following rupture of membranes
      - artificial O75.5
    - second twin, triplet, etc. O63.2
  - forceps, low following failed vacuum extraction O66.5
  - missed (at or near term) O36.4
  - normal O8Ø
  - obstructed — *see* Delivery, complicated by, obstruction
  - precipitate O62.3
  - preterm (*see also* Pregnancy, complicated by, preterm labor) O6Ø.1Ø

- **Delivery** — *continued*
  - spontaneous O8Ø
  - term pregnancy NOS O8Ø
  - uncomplicated O8Ø
  - vaginal, following previous cesarean delivery O34.21
- **Delusions** (paranoid) — *see* Disorder, delusional
- **Dementia** (degenerative (primary)) (old age) (persisting) FØ3.9Ø
  - with
    - aggressive behavior FØ3.91
    - behavioral disturbance FØ3.91
    - combative behavior FØ3.91
    - Lewy bodies G31.83 *[F02.80]*
      - with behavioral disturbance G31.83 *[F02.81]*
    - Parkinson's disease G2Ø *[F02.80]*
      - with behavioral disturbance G2Ø *[F02.81]*
    - Parkinsonism G31.83 *[F02.80]*
      - with behavioral disturbance G31.83 *[F02.81]*
    - violent behavior FØ3.91
  - alcoholic F1Ø.97
    - with dependence F1Ø.27
  - Alzheimer's type — *see* Disease, Alzheimer's
  - arteriosclerotic — *see* Dementia, vascular
  - atypical, Alzheimer's type — *see* Disease, Alzheimer's, specified NEC
  - congenital — *see* Disability, intellectual
  - frontal (lobe) G31.Ø9 *[F02.80]*
    - with behavioral disturbance G31.Ø9 *[F02.81]*
  - frontotemporal G31.Ø9 *[F02.80]*
    - with behavioral disturbance G31.Ø9 *[F02.81]*
    - specified NEC G31.Ø9 *[F02.80]*
      - with behavioral disturbance G31.Ø9 *[F02.81]*
  - in (due to)
    - alcohol F1Ø.97
      - with dependence F1Ø.27
    - Alzheimer's disease — *see* Disease, Alzheimer's
    - arteriosclerotic brain disease — *see* Dementia, vascular
    - cerebral lipidoses E75. *[F02.80]*
      - with behavioral disturbance E75.*[F02.81]*
    - Creutzfeldt-Jakob disease (*see also* Creutzfeldt-Jakob disease or syndrome (with dementia)) A81.ØØ
    - epilepsy G4Ø. *[F02.80]*
      - with behavioral disturbance G4Ø. *[F02.81]*
    - hepatolenticular degeneration E83.Ø1 *[F02.80]*
      - with behavioral disturbance E83.Ø1 *[F02.81]*
    - human immunodeficiency virus (HIV) disease B2Ø *[F02.80]*
      - with behavioral disturbance B2Ø *[F02.81]*
    - Huntington's disease or chorea G1Ø
    - hypercalcemia E83.52 *[F02.80]*
      - with behavioral disturbance E83.52 *[F02.81]*
    - hypothyroidism, acquired EØ3.9 *[F02.80]*
      - with behavioral disturbance EØ3.9 *[F02.81]*
      - due to iodine deficiency EØ1.8 *[F02.80]*
        - with behavioral disturbance EØ1.8 *[F02.81]*
    - inhalants F18.97
      - with dependence F18.27
    - multiple
      - etiologies FØ3
      - sclerosis G35 *[F02.80]*
        - with behavioral disturbance G35 *[F02.81]*
    - neurosyphilis A52.17 *[F02.80]*
      - with behavioral disturbance A52.17 *[F02.81]*
      - juvenile A5Ø.49 *[F02.80]*
        - with behavioral disturbance A5Ø.49 *[F02.81]*
    - niacin deficiency E52 *[F02.80]*
      - with behavioral disturbance E52 *[F02.81]*
    - paralysis agitans G2Ø *[F02.80]*
      - with behavioral disturbance G2Ø *[F02.81]*
    - Parkinson's disease G2Ø *[F02.80]*
    - pellagra E52 *[F02.80]*
      - with behavioral disturbance E52 *[F02.81]*
    - Pick's G31.Ø1 *[F02.80]*
      - with behavioral disturbance G31.Ø1 *[F02.81]*
    - polyarteritis nodosa M3Ø.Ø *[F02.80]*
      - with behavioral disturbance M3Ø.Ø *[F02.81]*
    - psychoactive drug F19.97
      - with dependence F19.27
      - inhalants F18.97
        - with dependence F18.27

- **Dementia** — *continued*
  - in — *continued*
    - psychoactive drug — *continued*
      - sedatives, hypnotics or anxiolytics F13.97
        - with dependence F13.27
    - sedatives, hypnotics or anxiolytics F13.97
      - with dependence F13.27
    - systemic lupus erythematosus M32.*[F02.80]*
      - with behavioral disturbance M32.*[F02.81]*
    - trypanosomiasis
      - African B56.9 *[F02.80]*
        - with behavioral disturbance B56.9 *[F02.81]*
    - unknown etiology FØ3
    - vitamin B12 deficiency E53.8 *[F02.80]*
      - with behavioral disturbance E53.8 *[F02.81]*
    - volatile solvents F18.97
      - with dependence F18.27
    - with behavioral disturbance G31.83 *[F02.81]*
  - infantile, infantilis F84.3
  - Lewy body G31.83 *[F02.80]*
    - with behavioral disturbance G31.83 *[F02.81]*
  - multi-infarct — *see* Dementia, vascular
  - paralytica, paralytic (syphilitic) A52.17 *[F02.80]*
    - with behavioral disturbance A52.17 *[F02.81]*
    - juvenilis A5Ø.45
  - paretic A52.17
  - praecox — *see* Schizophrenia
  - presenile FØ3
    - Alzheimer's type — *see* Disease, Alzheimer's, early onset
  - primary degenerative FØ3
  - progressive, syphilitic A52.17
  - senile FØ3
    - with acute confusional state FØ5
    - Alzheimer's type — *see* Disease, Alzheimer's, late onset
    - depressed or paranoid type FØ3
  - vascular (acute onset) (mixed) (multi-infarct) (subcortical) FØ1.5Ø
    - with behavioral disturbance FØ1.51
- **Demineralization, bone** — *see* Osteoporosis
- **Demodex folliculorum** (infestation) B88.Ø
- **Demophobia** F4Ø.248
- **Demoralization** R45.3
- **Demyelination, demyelinization**
  - central nervous system G37.9
    - specified NEC G37.8
  - corpus callosum (central) G37.1
  - disseminated, acute G36.9
    - specified NEC G36.8
  - global G35
  - in optic neuritis G36.Ø
- **Dengue** (classical) (fever) A9Ø
  - hemorrhagic A91
  - sandfly A93.1
- **Dennie-Marfan syphilitic syndrome** A5Ø.45
- **Dens evaginatus, in dente or invaginatus** KØØ.2
- **Dense breasts** R92.2
- **Density**
  - increased, bone (disseminated) (generalized) (spotted) — *see* Disorder, bone, density and structure, specified type NEC
  - lung (nodular) J98.4
- **Dental** (*see also* condition)
  - examination ZØ1.2Ø
    - with abnormal findings ZØ1.21
  - restoration
    - aesthetically inadequate or displeasing KØ8.56
    - defective KØ8.5Ø
      - specified NEC KØ8.59
    - failure of marginal integrity KØ8.51
    - failure of periodontal anatomical integrity KØ8.54
- **Dentia praecox** K00.6
- **Denticles** (pulp) KØ4.2
- **Dentigerous cyst** KØ9.0
- **Dentin**
  - irregular (in pulp) KØ4.3
  - opalescent KØØ.5
  - secondary (in pulp) KØ4.3
  - sensitive KØ3.89
- **Dentinogenesis imperfecta** K00.5
- **Dentinoma** — *see* Cyst, calcifying odontogenic

- **Dentition** (syndrome) KØØ.7
  - delayed KØØ.6
  - difficult KØØ.7
  - precocious KØØ.6
  - premature KØØ.6
  - retarded KØØ.6
- **Dependence** (on) (syndrome) F19.2Ø
  - with remission F19.21
  - alcohol (ethyl) (methyl) (without remission) F1Ø.2Ø
    - with
      - amnestic disorder, persisting F1Ø.26
      - anxiety disorder F1Ø.28Ø
      - dementia, persisting F1Ø.27
      - intoxication F1Ø.229
        - with delirium F1Ø.221
        - uncomplicated F1Ø.22Ø
      - mood disorder F1Ø.24
      - psychotic disorder F1Ø.259
        - with
          - delusions F1Ø.25Ø
          - hallucinations F1Ø.251
      - remission F1Ø.21
      - sexual dysfunction F1Ø.281
      - sleep disorder F1Ø.282
      - specified disorder NEC F1Ø.288
      - withdrawal F1Ø.239
        - with
          - delirium F1Ø.231
          - perceptual disturbance F1Ø.232
        - uncomplicated F1Ø.23Ø
    - counseling and surveillance Z71.41
  - amobarbital — *see* Dependence, drug, sedative
  - amphetamine(s) (type) — *see* Dependence, drug, stimulant NEC
  - amytal (sodium) — *see* Dependence, drug, sedative
  - analgesic NEC F55.8
  - anesthetic (agent) (gas) (general) (local) NEC — *see* Dependence, drug, psychoactive NEC
  - anxiolytic NEC — *see* Dependence, drug, sedative
  - barbital(s) — *see* Dependence, drug, sedative
  - barbiturate(s) (compounds) (drugs classifiable to T42) — *see* Dependence, drug, sedative
  - benzedrine — *see* Dependence, drug, stimulant NEC
  - bhang — *see* Dependence, drug, cannabis
  - bromide(s) NEC — *see* Dependence, drug, sedative
  - caffeine — *see* Dependence, drug, stimulant NEC
  - cannabis (sativa) (indica) (resin) (derivatives) (type) — *see* Dependence, drug, cannabis
  - chloral (betaine) (hydrate) — *see* Dependence, drug, sedative
  - chlordiazepoxide — *see* Dependence, drug, sedative
  - coca (leaf) (derivatives) — *see* Dependence, drug, cocaine
  - cocaine — *see* Dependence, drug, cocaine
  - codeine — *see* Dependence, drug, opioid
  - combinations of drugs F19.2Ø
  - dagga — *see* Dependence, drug, cannabis
  - demerol — *see* Dependence, drug, opioid
  - dexamphetamine — *see* Dependence, drug, stimulant NEC
  - dexedrine — *see* Dependence, drug, stimulant NEC
  - dextromethorphan — *see* Dependence, drug, opioid
  - dextromoramide — *see* Dependence, drug, opioid
  - dextro-nor-pseudo-ephedrine — seeDependence, drug, stimulant NEC
  - dextrorphan — *see* Dependence, drug, opioid
  - diazepam — *see* Dependence, drug, sedative
  - dilaudid — *see* Dependence, drug, opioid
  - D-lysergic acid diethylamide — *see* Dependence, drug, hallucinogen
  - drug NEC F19.2Ø
    - with sleep disorder F19.282
    - cannabis F12.2Ø
      - with
        - anxiety disorder F12.28Ø
        - intoxication F12.229
          - with
            - delirium F12.221
            - perceptual disturbance F12.222
          - uncomplicated F12.22Ø
        - other specified disorder F12.288
        - psychosis F12.259
          - delusions F12.25Ø

- **Dependence** — *continued*
  - drug — *continued*
    - cannabis — *continued*
      - with — *continued*
        - psychosis — *continued*
          - hallucinations F12.251
        - unspecified disorder F12.29
      - in remission F12.21
    - cocaine F14.2Ø
      - with
        - anxiety disorder F14.28Ø
        - intoxication F14.229
          - with
            - delirium F14.221
            - perceptual disturbance F14.222
          - uncomplicated F14.22Ø
        - mood disorder F14.24
        - other specified disorder F14.288
        - psychosis F14.259
          - delusions F14.25Ø
          - hallucinations F14.251
        - sexual dysfunction F14.281
        - sleep disorder F14.282
        - unspecified disorder F14.29
        - withdrawal F14.23
      - in remission F14.21
      - withdrawal symptoms in newborn P96.1
    - counseling and surveillance Z71.51
    - hallucinogen F16.2Ø
      - with
        - anxiety disorder F16.28Ø
        - flashbacks F16.283
        - intoxication F16.229
          - with delirium F16.221
          - uncomplicated F16.22Ø
        - mood disorder F16.24
        - other specified disorder F16.288
        - perception disorder, persisting F16.283
        - psychosis F16.259
          - delusions F16.25Ø
          - hallucinations F16.251
        - unspecified disorder F16.29
      - in remission F16.21
    - in remission F19.21
    - inhalant F18.2Ø
      - with
        - anxiety disorder F18.28Ø
        - dementia, persisting F18.27
        - intoxication F18.229
          - with delirium F18.221
          - uncomplicated F18.22Ø
        - mood disorder F18.24
        - other specified disorder F18.288
        - psychosis F18.259
          - delusions F18.25Ø
          - hallucinations F18.251
        - unspecified disorder F18.29
      - in remission F18.21
    - nicotine F17.2ØØ
      - with disorder F17.2Ø9
        - remission F17.2Ø1
        - specified disorder NEC F17.2Ø8
        - withdrawal F17.2Ø3
      - chewing tobacco F17.22Ø
        - with disorder F17.229
          - remission F17.221
          - specified disorder NEC F17.228
          - withdrawal F17.223
      - cigarettes F17.21Ø
        - with disorder F17.219
          - remission F17.211
          - specified disorder NEC F17.218
          - withdrawal F17.213
      - specified product NEC F17.29Ø
        - with disorder F17.299
          - remission F17.291
          - specified disorder NEC F17.298
          - withdrawal F17.293
    - opioid F11.2Ø
      - with
        - intoxication F11.229

- **Dependence** — *continued*
  - drug — *continued*
    - opioid — *continued*
      - with — *continued*
        - intoxication — *continued*
          - with
            - delirium F11.221
            - perceptual disturbance F11.222
          - uncomplicated F11.22Ø
        - mood disorder F11.24
        - other specified disorder F11.288
        - psychosis F11.259
          - delusions F11.25Ø
          - hallucinations F11.251
        - sexual dysfunction F11.281
        - sleep disorder F11.282
        - unspecified disorder F11.29
        - withdrawal F11.23
      - in remission F11.21
    - psychoactive NEC F19.2Ø
      - with
        - amnestic disorder F19.26
        - anxiety disorder F19.28Ø
        - dementia F19.27
        - intoxication F19.229
          - with
            - delirium F19.221
            - perceptual disturbance F19.222
          - uncomplicated F19.22Ø
        - mood disorder F19.24
        - other specified disorder F19.288
        - psychosis F19.259
          - delusions F19.25Ø
          - hallucinations F19.251
        - sexual dysfunction F19.281
        - sleep disorder F19.282
        - unspecified disorder F19.29
        - withdrawal F19.239
          - with
            - delirium F19.231
            - perceptual disturbance F19.232
          - uncomplicated F19.23Ø
    - sedative, hypnotic or anxiolytic F13.2Ø
      - with
        - amnestic disorder F13.26
        - anxiety disorder F13.28Ø
        - dementia, persisting F13.27
        - intoxication F13.229
          - with delirium F13.221
          - uncomplicated F13.22Ø
        - mood disorder F13.24
        - other specified disorder F13.288
        - psychosis F13.259
          - delusions F13.25Ø
          - hallucinations F13.251
        - sexual dysfunction F13.281
        - sleep disorder F13.282
        - unspecified disorder F13.29
        - withdrawal F13.239
          - with
            - delirium F13.231
            - perceptual disturbance F13.232
          - uncomplicated F13.23Ø
      - in remission F13.21
    - stimulant NEC F15.2Ø
      - with
        - anxiety disorder F15.28Ø
        - intoxication F15.229
          - with
            - delirium F15.221
            - perceptual disturbance F15.222
          - uncomplicated F15.22Ø
        - mood disorder F15.24
        - other specified disorder F15.288
        - psychosis F15.259
          - delusions F15.25Ø
          - hallucinations F15.251
        - sexual dysfunction F15.281
        - sleep disorder F15.282
        - unspecified disorder F15.29
        - withdrawal F15.23
      - in remission F15.21

Dependence — *continued*
- ethyl
  - alcohol (without remission) F1Ø.2Ø
    - with remission F1Ø.21
  - bromide — *see* Dependence, drug, sedative
  - carbamate F19.2Ø
  - chloride F19.2Ø
  - morphine — *see* Dependence, drug, opioid
- ganja — *see* Dependence, drug, cannabis
- glue (airplane) (sniffing) — *see* Dependence, drug, inhalant
- glutethimide — *see* Dependence, drug, sedative
- hallucinogenics — *see* Dependence, drug, hallucinogen
- hashish — *see* Dependence, drug, cannabis
- hemp — *see* Dependence, drug, cannabis
- heroin (salt) (any) — *see* Dependence, drug, opioid
- hypnotic NEC — *see* Dependence, drug, sedative
- Indian hemp — *see* Dependence, drug, cannabis
- inhalants — *see* Dependence, drug, inhalant
- khat — *see* Dependence, drug, stimulant NEC
- laudanum — *see* Dependence, drug, opioid
- LSD(-25) (derivatives) — *see* Dependence, drug, hallucinogen
- luminal — *see* Dependence, drug, sedative
- lysergic acid — *see* Dependence, drug, hallucinogen
- maconha — *see* Dependence, drug, cannabis
- marihuana — *see* Dependence, drug, cannabis
- meprobamate — *see* Dependence, drug, sedative
- mescaline — *see* Dependence, drug, hallucinogen
- methadone — *see* Dependence, drug, opioid
- methamphetamine(s) — *see* Dependence, drug, stimulant NEC
- methaqualone — *see* Dependence, drug, sedative
- methyl
  - alcohol (without remission) F1Ø.2Ø
    - with remission F1Ø.21
  - bromide — *see* Dependence, drug, sedative
  - morphine — *see* Dependence, drug, opioid
  - phenidate — *see* Dependence, drug, stimulant NEC
  - sulfonal — *see* Dependence, drug, sedative
- morphine (sulfate) (sulfite) (type) — *see* Dependence, drug, opioid
- narcotic (drug) NEC — *see* Dependence, drug, opioid
- nembutal — *see* Dependence, drug, sedative
- neraval — *see* Dependence, drug, sedative
- neravan — *see* Dependence, drug, sedative
- neurobarb — *see* Dependence, drug, sedative
- nicotine — *see* Dependence, drug, nicotine
- nitrous oxide F19.2Ø
- nonbarbiturate sedatives and tranquilizers with similar effect — *see* Dependence, drug, sedative
- on
  - aspirator Z99.Ø
  - care provider (because of) Z74.9
    - impaired mobility Z74.Ø9
    - need for
      - assistance with personal care Z74.1
      - continuous supervision Z74.3
    - no other household member able to render care Z74.2
    - specified reason NEC Z74.8
  - machine Z99.89
    - enabling NEC Z99.89
    - specified type NEC Z99.89
  - renal dialysis (hemodialysis) (peritoneal) Z99.2
  - respirator Z99.11
  - ventilator Z99.11
  - wheelchair Z99.3
- opiate — *see* Dependence, drug, opioid
- opioids — *see* Dependence, drug, opioid
- opium (alkaloids) (derivatives) (tincture) — *see* Dependence, drug, opioid
- oxygen (long-term) (supplemental) Z99.81
- paraldehyde — *see* Dependence, drug, sedative
- paregoric — *see* Dependence, drug, opioid
- PCP (phencyclidine) (*see also* Abuse, drug, hallucinogen) F16.2Ø
- pentobarbital — *see* Dependence, drug, sedative

Dependence — *continued*
- pentobarbitone (sodium) — *see* Dependence, drug, sedative
- pentothal — *see* Dependence, drug, sedative
- peyote — *see* Dependence, drug, hallucinogen
- phencyclidine (PCP) (and related substances) (*see also* Abuse, drug, hallucinogen) F16.2Ø
- phenmetrazine — seeDependence, drug, stimulant NEC
- phenobarbital — *see* Dependence, drug, sedative
- polysubstance F19.2Ø
- psilocibin, psilocin, psilocyn, psilocyline — *see* Dependence, drug, hallucinogen
- psychostimulant NEC — seeDependence, drug, stimulant NEC
- secobarbital — *see* Dependence, drug, sedative
- seconal — *see* Dependence, drug, sedative
- sedative NEC — *see* Dependence, drug, sedative
- specified drug NEC — *see* Dependence, drug
- stimulant NEC — seeDependence, drug, stimulant NEC
- substance NEC — *see* Dependence, drug
- supplemental oxygen Z99.81
- tobacco — *see* Dependence, drug, nicotine
  - counseling and surveillance Z71.6
- tranquilizer NEC — *see* Dependence, drug, sedative
- vitamin B6 E53.1
- volatile solvents — *see* Dependence, drug, inhalant

Dependency
- care-provider Z74.9
- passive F6Ø.7
- reactions (persistent) F6Ø.7

Depersonalization (in neurotic state) (neurotic) (syndrome) F48.1

Depletion
- extracellular fluid E86.9
- plasma E86.1
- potassium E87.6
  - nephropathy N25.89
- salt or sodium E87.1
  - causing heat exhaustion or prostration T67.4
  - nephropathy N28.9
- volume NOS E86.9

Deployment (current) (military) **status** Z56.82
- in theater or in support of military war, peacekeeping and humanitarian operations Z56.82
- personal history of Z91.82
  - military war, peacekeeping and humanitarian deployment (current or past conflict) Z91.82
- returned from Z91.82

Depolarization, premature I49.40
- atrial I49.1
- junctional I49.2
- specified NEC I49.49
- ventricular I49.3

Deposit
- bone in Boeck's sarcoid D86.89
- calcareous, calcium — *see* Calcification
- cholesterol
  - retina H35.89
  - vitreous (body) (humor) — *see* Deposit, crystalline
- conjunctiva H11.11-
- cornea H18.ØØ-
  - argentous H18.Ø2-
  - due to metabolic disorder H18.Ø3-
  - Kayser-Fleischer ring H18.Ø4-
  - pigmentation — *see* Pigmentation, cornea
- crystalline, vitreous (body) (humor) H43.2-
- hemosiderin in old scars of cornea — *see* Pigmentation, cornea, stromal
- metallic in lens — *see* Cataract, specified NEC
- skin R23.8
- tooth, teeth (betel) (black) (green) (materia alba) (orange) (tobacco) KØ3.6
- urate, kidney — *see* Calculus, kidney

Depraved appetite — *see* Pica

Depressed
- HDL cholesterol E78.6

Depression (acute) (mental) F32.9
- agitated (single episode) F32.2
- anaclitic — *see* Disorder, adjustment
- anxiety F41.8
  - persistent F34.1
- arches (*see also* Deformity, limb, flat foot)
- atypical (single episode) F32.8
- basal metabolic rate R94.8
- bone marrow D75.89
- central nervous system RØ9.2
- cerebral R29.818
  - newborn P91.4
- cerebrovascular I67.9
- chest wall M95.4
- climacteric (single episode) F32.8
- endogenous (without psychotic symptoms) F33.2
  - with psychotic symptoms F33.3
- functional activity R68.89
- hysterical F44.89
- involutional (single episode) F32.8
- major F32.9
  - with psychotic symptoms F32.3
  - recurrent — *see* Disorder, depressive, recurrent
- manic-depressive — *see* Disorder, depressive, recurrent
- masked (single episode) F32.8
- medullary G93.89
- menopausal (single episode) F32.8
- metatarsus — *see* Depression, arches
- monopolar F33.9
- nervous F34.1
- neurotic F34.1
- nose M95.Ø
- postnatal F53
- postpartum F53
- post-psychotic of schizophrenia F32.8
- post-schizophrenic F32.8
- psychogenic (reactive) (single episode) F32.9
- psychoneurotic F34.1
- psychotic (single episode) F32.3
  - recurrent F33.3
- reactive (psychogenic) (single episode) F32.9
  - psychotic (single episode) F32.3
- recurrent — *see* Disorder, depressive, recurrent
- respiratory center G93.89
- seasonal — *see* Disorder, depressive, recurrent
- senile FØ3
- severe, single episode F32.2
- situational F43.21
- skull Q67.4
- specified NEC (single episode) F32.8
- sternum M95.4
- visual field — *see* Defect, visual field
- vital (recurrent) (without psychotic symptoms) F33.2
  - with psychotic symptoms F33.3
  - single episode F32.2

Deprivation
- cultural Z6Ø.3
- effects NOS T73.9
  - specified NEC T73.8
- emotional NEC Z65.8
  - affecting infant or child — *see* Maltreatment, child, psychological
- food T73.Ø
- protein — *see* Malnutrition
- sleep Z72.82Ø
- social Z6Ø.4
  - affecting infant or child — *see* Maltreatment, child, psychological
- specified NEC T73.8
- vitamins — *see* Deficiency, vitamin
- water T73.1

Derangement
- ankle (internal) — *see* Derangement, joint, ankle
- cartilage (articular) NEC — *see* Derangement, joint, articular cartilage, by site
  - recurrent — *see* Dislocation, recurrent
- cruciate ligament, anterior, current injury — *see* Sprain, knee, cruciate, anterior
- elbow (internal) — *see* Derangement, joint, elbow
- hip (joint) (internal) (old) — *see* Derangement, joint, hip

- **Derangement** — *continued*
  - joint (internal) M24.9
    - ankylosis — *see* Ankylosis
    - articular cartilage M24.1Ø
      - ankle M24.17-
      - elbow M24.12-
      - foot M24.17-
      - hand M24.14-
      - hip M24.15-
      - knee NEC M23.9-
      - loose body — *see* Loose, body
      - shoulder M24.11-
      - wrist M24.13-
    - contracture — *see* Contraction, joint
    - current injury (*see also* Dislocation)
      - knee, meniscus or cartilage — *see* Tear, meniscus
    - dislocation
      - pathological — *see* Dislocation, pathological
      - recurrent — *see* Dislocation, recurrent
    - knee — *see* Derangement, knee
    - ligament — *see* Disorder, ligament
    - loose body — *see* Loose, body
    - recurrent — *see* Dislocation, recurrent
    - specified type NEC M24.8Ø
      - ankle M24.87-
      - elbow M24.82-
      - foot joint M24.87-
      - hand joint M24.84-
      - hip M24.85-
      - shoulder M24.81-
      - wrist M24.83-
    - temporomandibular M26.69
  - knee (recurrent) M23.9-
    - ligament disruption, spontaneous M23.6Ø-
      - anterior cruciate M23.61-
      - capsular M23.67-
      - instability, chronic M23.5-
      - lateral collateral M23.64-
      - medial collateral M23.63-
      - posterior cruciate M23.62-
    - loose body M23.4-
    - meniscus M23.3Ø-
      - cystic M23.ØØ-
        - lateral M23.Ø2-
          - anterior horn M23.Ø4-
          - posterior horn M23.Ø5-
          - specified NEC M23.Ø6-
        - medial M23.ØØ-
          - anterior horn M23.Ø1-
          - posterior horn M23.Ø2-
          - specified NEC M23.Ø3-
      - degenerate — *see* Derangement, knee, meniscus, specified NEC
      - detached — *see* Derangement, knee, meniscus, specified NEC
      - due to old tear or injury M23.2Ø-
        - lateral M23.2Ø-
          - anterior horn M23.24-
          - posterior horn M23.25-
          - specified NEC M23.26-
        - medial M23.2Ø-
          - anterior horn M23.21-
          - posterior horn M23.22-
          - specified NEC M23.23-
      - retained — *see* Derangement, knee, meniscus, specified NEC
      - specified NEC M23.3Ø-
        - lateral M23.3Ø-
          - anterior horn M23.34-
          - posterior horn M23.35-
          - specified NEC M23.36-
        - medial M23.3Ø-
          - anterior horn M23.31-
          - posterior horn M23.32-
          - specified NEC M23.33-
    - old M23.8X-
    - specified NEC — *see* subcategory M23.8
  - low back NEC — *see* Dorsopathy, specified NEC
  - meniscus — *see* Derangement, knee, meniscus
  - mental — *see* Psychosis
  - patella, specified NEC — *see* Disorder, patella, derangement NEC
  - semilunar cartilage (knee) — *see* Derangement, knee, meniscus, specified NEC
  - shoulder (internal) — *see* Derangement, joint, shoulder
- **Dercum's disease** E88.2
- **Derealization** (neurotic) F48.1
- **Dermal** — *see* condition
- **Dermaphytid** — *see* Dermatophytosis
- **Dermatitis** (eczematous) L3Ø.9
  - ab igne L59.Ø
  - acarine B88.Ø
  - actinic (due to sun) L57.8
    - other than from sun L59.8
  - allergic — *see* Dermatitis, contact, allergic
  - ambustionis, due to burn or scald — *see* Burn
  - amebic AØ6.7
  - ammonia L22
  - arsenical (ingested) L27.8
  - artefacta L98.1
    - psychogenic F54
  - atopic L2Ø.9
    - psychogenic F54
    - specified NEC L2Ø.89
  - autoimmune progesterone L3Ø.8
  - berlock, berloque L56.2
  - blastomycotic B4Ø.3
  - blister beetle L24.89
  - bullous, bullosa L13.9
    - mucosynechial, atrophic L12.1
    - seasonal L3Ø.8
    - specified NEC L13.8
  - calorica L59.Ø
    - due to burn or scald — *see* Burn
  - caterpillar L24.89
  - cercarial B65.3
  - combustionis L59.Ø
    - due to burn or scald — *see* Burn
  - congelationis T69.1
  - contact (occupational) L25.9
    - allergic L23.9
      - due to
        - adhesives L23.1
        - cement L23.5
        - chemical products NEC L23.5
        - chromium L23.Ø
        - cosmetics L23.2
        - dander (cat) (dog) L23.81
        - drugs in contact with skin L23.3
        - dyes L23.4
        - food in contact with skin L23.6
        - hair (cat) (dog) L23.81
        - insecticide L23.5
        - metals L23.Ø
        - nickel L23.Ø
        - plants, non-food L23.7
        - plastic L23.5
        - rubber L23.5
        - specified agent NEC L23.89
    - due to
      - chemical products NEC L25.3
      - cosmetics L25.Ø
      - dander (cat) (dog) L23.81
      - drugs in contact with skin L25.1
      - dyes L25.2
      - food in contact with skin L25.4
      - hair (cat) (dog) L23.81
      - plants, non-food L25.5
      - specified agent NEC L25.8
    - irritant L24.9
      - due to
        - chemical products NEC L24.5
        - cosmetics L24.3
        - detergents L24.Ø
        - drugs in contact with skin L24.4
        - food in contact with skin L24.6
        - oils and greases L24.1
        - plants, non-food L24.7
        - solvents L24.2
        - specified agent NEC L24.89
  - contusiformis L52
  - diabetic — *see* EØ8-E13 with .62Ø
  - diaper L22
  - diphtheritica A36.3
  - dry skin L85.3
  - due to
    - acetone (contact) (irritant) L24.2
    - acids (contact) (irritant) L24.5
    - adhesive(s) (allergic) (contact) (plaster) L23.1
      - irritant L24.5
    - alcohol (irritant) (skin contact) (substances in T51.ØØ-T51.93) L24.2
      - taken internally L27.8
    - alkalis (contact) (irritant) L24.5
    - arsenic (ingested) L27.8
    - carbon disulfide (contact) (irritant) L24.2
    - caustics (contact) (irritant) L24.5
    - cement (contact) L24.5
    - cereal (ingested) L27.2
    - chemical(s) NEC L24.5
      - taken internally L27.8
    - chlorocompounds L24.2
    - chromium (contact) (irritant) L24.81
    - coffee (ingested) L27.2
    - cold weather L3Ø.8
    - cosmetics (contact) L25.Ø
      - allergic L23.2
      - irritant L24.3
    - cyclohexanes L24.2
    - dander (cat) (dog) L23.81
    - Demodex species B88.Ø
    - Dermanyssus gallinae B88.Ø
    - detergents (contact) (irritant) L24.Ø
    - dichromate L24.81
    - drugs and medicaments (generalized) (internal use) L27.Ø
      - external — *see* Dermatitis, due to, drugs, in contact with skin
      - in contact with skin L25.1
        - allergic L23.3
        - irritant L24.4
      - localized skin eruption L27.1
      - specified substance — *see* Table of Drugs and Chemicals
    - dyes (contact) L25.2
      - allergic L23.4
      - irritant L24.89
    - epidermophytosis — *see* Dermatophytosis
    - esters L24.2
    - external irritant NEC L24.9
    - fish (ingested) L27.2
    - flour (ingested) L27.2
    - food (ingested) L27.2
      - in contact with skin L25.4
    - fruit (ingested) L27.2
    - furs (allergic) (contact) L23.81
    - glues — *see* Dermatitis, due to, adhesives
    - glycols L24.2
    - greases NEC (contact) (irritant) L24.1
    - hair (cat) (dog) L23.81
    - hot
      - objects and materials — *see* Burn
      - weather or places L59.Ø
    - hydrocarbons L24.2
    - infrared rays L59.8
    - ingestion, ingested substance L27.9
      - chemical NEC L27.8
      - drugs and medicaments — *see* Dermatitis, due to, drugs
      - food L27.2
      - specified NEC L27.8
    - insecticide in contact with skin L24.5
    - internal agent L27.9
      - drugs and medicaments (generalized) — *see* Dermatitis, due to, drugs
      - food L27.2
    - irradiation — *see* Dermatitis, due to, radioactive substance
    - ketones L24.2
    - lacquer tree (allergic) (contact) L23.7
    - light (sun) NEC L57.8
      - acute L56.8
      - other L59.8
    - Liponyssoides sanguineus B88.Ø
    - low temperature L3Ø.8

Dermatitis — *continued*
- due to — *continued*
  - meat (ingested) L27.2
  - metals, metal salts (contact) (irritant) L24.81
  - milk (ingested) L27.2
  - nickel (contact) (irritant) L24.81
  - nylon (contact) (irritant) L24.5
  - oils NEC (contact) (irritant) L24.1
  - paint solvent (contact) (irritant) L24.2
  - petroleum products (contact) (irritant) (substances in T52.Ø) L24.2
  - plants NEC (contact) L25.5
    - allergic L23.7
    - irritant L24.7
  - plasters (adhesive) (any) (allergic) (contact) L23.1
    - irritant L24.5
  - plastic (contact) L24.5
  - preservatives (contact) — *see* Dermatitis, due to, chemical, in contact with skin
  - primrose (allergic) (contact) L23.7
  - primula (allergic) (contact) L23.7
  - radiation L59.8
    - nonionizing (chronic exposure) L57.8
    - sun NEC L57.8
      - acute L56.8
  - radioactive substance L58.9
    - acute L58.Ø
    - chronic L58.1
  - radium L58.9
    - acute L58.Ø
    - chronic L58.1
  - ragweed (allergic) (contact) L23.7
  - Rhus (allergic) (contact) (diversiloba) (radicans) (toxicodendron) (venenata) (verniciflua) L23.7
  - rubber (contact) L24.5
  - Senecio jacobaea (allergic) (contact) L23.7
  - solvents (contact) (irritant) (substances in T52.ØØ-T53.93) L24.2
  - specified agent NEC (contact) L25.8
    - allergic L23.89
    - irritant L24.89
  - sunshine NEC L57.8
    - acute L56.8
  - tetrachlorethylene (contact) (irritant) L24.2
  - toluene (contact) (irritant) L24.2
  - turpentine (contact) L24.2
  - ultraviolet rays (sun NEC) (chronic exposure) L57.8
    - acute L56.8
  - vaccine or vaccination L27.Ø
    - specified substance — *see* Table of Drugs and Chemicals
  - varicose veins — *see* Varix, leg, with, inflammation
  - X-rays L58.9
    - acute L58.Ø
    - chronic L58.1
- dyshydrotic L3Ø.1
- dysmenorrheica N94.6
- escharotica — *see* Burn
- exfoliative, exfoliativa (generalized) L26
  - neonatorum LØØ
- eyelid (*see also* Dermatosis, eyelid)
  - allergic HØ1.119
    - left HØ1.116
      - lower HØ1.115
      - upper HØ1.114
    - right HØ1.113
      - lower HØ1.112
      - upper HØ1.111
  - contact — *see* Dermatitis, eyelid, allergic
  - due to
    - Demodex species B88.Ø
    - herpes (zoster) BØ2.39
      - simplex BØØ.59
  - eczematous HØ1.139
    - left HØ1.136
      - lower HØ1.135
      - upper HØ1.134
    - right HØ1.133
      - lower HØ1.132
      - upper HØ1.131

Dermatitis — *continued*
- facta, factitia, factitial L98.1
  - psychogenic F54
- flexural NEC L2Ø.82
- friction L3Ø.4
- fungus B36.9
  - specified type NEC B36.8
- gangrenosa, gangrenous infantum LØ8.Ø
- harvest mite B88.Ø
- heat L59.Ø
- herpesviral, vesicular (ear) (lip) BØØ.1
- herpetiformis (bullous) (erythematous) (pustular) (vesicular) L13.Ø
  - juvenile L12.2
  - senile L12.Ø
- hiemalis L3Ø.8
- hypostatic, hypostatica — *see* Varix, leg, with, inflammation
- infectious eczematoid L3Ø.3
- infective L3Ø.3
- irritant — *see* Dermatitis, contact, irritant
- Jacquet's (diaper dermatitis) L22
- Leptus B88.Ø
- lichenified NEC L28.Ø
- medicamentosa (generalized) (internal use) — *see* Dermatitis, due to drugs
- mite B88.Ø
- multiformis L13.Ø
  - juvenile L12.2
- napkin L22
- neurotica L13.Ø
- nummular L3Ø.Ø
- papillaris capillitii L73.Ø
- pellagrous E52
- perioral L71.Ø
- photocontact L56.2
- polymorpha dolorosa L13.Ø
- pruriginosa L13.Ø
- pruritic NEC L3Ø.8
- psychogenic F54
- purulent LØ8.Ø
- pustular
  - contagious BØ8.Ø2
  - subcorneal L13.1
- pyococcal LØ8.Ø
- pyogenica LØ8.Ø
- repens L4Ø.2
- Ritter's (exfoliativa) LØØ
- Schamberg's L81.7
- schistosome B65.3
- seasonal bullous L3Ø.8
- seborrheic L21.9
  - infantile L21.1
  - specified NEC L21.8
- sensitization NOS L23.9
- septic LØ8.Ø
- solare L57.8
- specified NEC L3Ø.8
- stasis I87.2
  - with varicose ulcer — *see* Varix, leg, with ulcer, with inflammation
  - due to postthrombotic syndrome — *see* Syndrome, postthrombotic
- suppurative LØ8.Ø
- traumatic NEC L3Ø.4
- trophoneurotica L13.Ø
- ultraviolet (sun) (chronic exposure) L57.8
  - acute L56.8
- varicose — *see* Varix, leg, with, inflammation
- vegetans L1Ø.1
- verrucosa B43.Ø
- vesicular, herpesviral BØØ.1

Dermatoarthritis, lipoid E78.81

Dermatochalasis, eyelid HØ2.839
- left HØ2.836
  - lower HØ2.835
  - upper HØ2.834
- right HØ2.833
  - lower HØ2.832
  - upper HØ2.831

Dermatofibroma (lenticulare) — *see* Neoplasm, skin, benign
- protuberans — *see* Neoplasm, skin, uncertain behavior

Dermatofibrosarcoma (pigmented) (protuberans) — *see* Neoplasm, skin, malignant

Dermatographia L5Ø.3

Dermatolysis (exfoliativa) (congenital) Q82.8
- acquired L57.4
- eyelids — *see* Blepharochalasis
- palpebrarum — *see* Blepharochalasis
- senile L57.4

Dermatomegaly NEC Q82.8

Dermatomucosomyositis M33.1Ø
- with
  - myopathy M33.12
  - respiratory involvement M33.11
  - specified organ involvement NEC M33.19

Dermatomycosis B36.9
- furfuracea B36.Ø
- specified type NEC B36.8

Dermatomyositis (acute) (chronic) (*see also* Dermatopolymyositis)
- in (due to) neoplastic disease (*see also* Neoplasm) D49.9 *[M36.0]*

Dermatoneuritis of children — *see* Poisoning, mercury

Dermatophilosis A48.8

Dermatophytid L3Ø.2

Dermatophytide — *see* Dermatophytosis

Dermatophytosis (epidermophyton) (infection) (Microsporum) (tinea) (Trichophyton) B35.9
- beard B35.Ø
- body B35.4
- capitis B35.Ø
- corporis B35.4
- deep-seated B35.8
- disseminated B35.8
- foot B35.3
- granulomatous B35.8
- groin B35.6
- hand B35.2
- nail B35.1
- perianal (area) B35.6
- scalp B35.Ø
- specified NEC B35.8

Dermatopolymyositis M33.9Ø
- with
  - myopathy M33.92
  - respiratory involvement M33.91
  - specified organ involvement NEC M33.99
- in neoplastic disease (*see also* Neoplasm) D49.9 *[M36.0]*
- juvenile M33.ØØ
  - with
    - myopathy M33.Ø2
    - respiratory involvement M33.Ø1
    - specified organ involvement NEC M33.Ø9
- specified NEC M33.1Ø
  - myopathy M33.12
  - respiratory involvement M33.11
  - specified organ involvement NEC M33.19

Dermatopolyneuritis — *see* Poisoning, mercury

Dermatorrhexis Q79.6
- acquired L57.4

Dermatosclerosis (*see also* Scleroderma)
- localized L94.Ø

Dermatosis L98.9
- Andrews' LØ8.89
- Bowen's — *see* Neoplasm, skin, in situ
- bullous L13.9
  - specified NEC L13.8
- exfoliativa L26
- eyelid (noninfectious)
  - dermatitis — *see* Dermatitis, eyelid
  - discoid lupus erythematosus — *see* Lupus, erythematosus, eyelid
  - xeroderma — *see* Xeroderma, acquired, eyelid
- factitial L98.1
- febrile neutrophilic L98.2
- gonococcal A54.89
- herpetiformis L13.Ø
  - juvenile L12.2

- **Dermatosis** — *continued*
  - linear IgA L13.8
  - menstrual NEC L98.8
  - neutrophilic, febrile L98.2
  - occupational — *see* Dermatitis, contact
  - papulosa nigra L82.1
  - pigmentary L81.9
    - progressive L81.7
    - Schamberg's L81.7
  - psychogenic F54
  - purpuric, pigmented L81.7
  - pustular, subcorneal L13.1
  - transient acantholytic L11.1
- **Dermographia, dermographism** L50.3
- **Dermoid** (cyst) (*see also* Neoplasm, benign, by site)
  - with malignant transformation C56-
  - due to radiation (nonionizing) L57.8
- **Dermopathy**
  - infiltrative with thyrotoxicosis — *see* Thyrotoxicosis
  - nephrogenic fibrosing L9Ø.8
- **Dermophytosis** — *see* Dermatophytosis
- **Descemetocele** H18.73-
- **Descemet's membrane** — *see* condition
- **Descending** — *see* condition
- **Descensus uteri** — *see* Prolapse, uterus
- **Desert**
  - rheumatism B38.Ø
  - sore — *see* Ulcer, skin
- **Desertion** (newborn) — *see* Maltreatment
- **Desmoid** (extra-abdominal) (tumor) — *see* Neoplasm, connective tissue, uncertain behavior
  - abdominal D48.1
- **Despondency** F32.9
- **Desquamation, skin** R23.4
- **Destruction, destructive** (*see also* Damage)
  - articular facet (*see also* Derangement, joint, specified type NEC)
    - knee M23.8X-
    - vertebra — *see* Spondylosis
  - bone (*see also* Disorder, bone, specified type NEC)
    - syphilitic A52.77
  - joint (*see also* Derangement, joint, specified type NEC)
    - sacroiliac M53.3
  - rectal sphincter K62.89
  - septum (nasal) J34.89
  - tuberculous NEC — *see* Tuberculosis
  - tympanum, tympanic membrane (nontraumatic) — *see* Disorder, tympanic membrane, specified NEC
  - vertebral disc — *see* Degeneration, intervertebral disc
- **Destructiveness** (*see also* Disorder, conduct)
  - adjustment reaction — *see* Disorder, adjustment
- **Desultory labor** O62.2
- **Detachment**
  - cartilage — *see* Sprain
  - cervix, annular N88.8
    - complicating delivery O71.3
  - choroid (old) (postinfectional) (simple) (spontaneous) H31.4Ø-
    - hemorrhagic H31.41-
    - serous H31.42-
  - ligament — *see* Sprain
  - meniscus (knee) (*see also* Derangement, knee, meniscus, specified NEC)
    - current injury — *see* Tear, meniscus
    - due to old tear or injury — *see* Derangement, knee, meniscus, due to old tear
  - retina (without retinal break) (serous) H33.2-
    - with retinal:
      - break H33.ØØ-
        - giant H33.Ø3-
        - multiple H33.Ø2-
        - single H33.Ø1-
      - dialysis H33.Ø4-
    - pigment epithelium — *see* Degeneration, retina, separation of layers, pigment epithelium detachment
    - rhegmatogenous — *see* Detachment, retina, with retinal, break
    - specified NEC H33.8
    - total H33.Ø5-
- **Detachment** — *continued*
  - retina — *continued*
    - traction H33.4-
  - vitreous (body) H43.81
- **Detergent asthma** J69.8
- **Deterioration**
  - epileptic FØ6.8
  - general physical R53.81
  - heart, cardiac — *see* Degeneration, myocardial
  - mental — *see* Psychosis
  - myocardial, myocardium — *see* Degeneration, myocardial
  - senile (simple) R54
- **Deuteranomaly** (anomalous trichromat) H53.53
- **Deuteranopia** (complete) (incomplete) H53.53
- **Development**
  - abnormal, bone Q79.9
  - arrested R62.5Ø
    - bone — *see* Arrest, development or growth, bone
    - child R62.5Ø
    - due to malnutrition E45
  - defective, congenital (*see also* Anomaly, by site)
    - cauda equina QØ6.3
    - left ventricle Q24.8
      - in hypoplastic left heart syndrome Q23.4
    - valve Q24.8
      - pulmonary Q22.3
  - delayed (*see also* Delay, development) R62.5Ø
    - arithmetical skills F81.2
    - language (skills) (expressive) F8Ø.1
    - learning skill F81.9
    - mixed skills F88
    - motor coordination F82
    - reading F81.Ø
    - specified learning skill NEC F81.89
    - speech F8Ø.9
    - spelling F81.81
    - written expression F81.81
  - imperfect, congenital (*see also* Anomaly, by site)
    - heart Q24.9
    - lungs Q33.6
  - incomplete
    - bronchial tree Q32.4
    - organ or site not listed — *see* Hypoplasia, by site
    - respiratory system Q34.9
  - sexual, precocious NEC E3Ø.1
  - tardy, mental (*see also* Disability, intellectual) F79
- **Developmental** — *see* condition
  - testing, child — *see* Examination, child
- **Devergie's disease** (pityriasis rubra pilaris) L44.Ø
- **Deviation** (in)
  - conjugate palsy (eye) (spastic) H51.Ø
  - esophagus (acquired) K22.8
  - eye, skew H51.8
  - midline (jaw) (teeth) (dental arch) M26.29
    - specified site NEC — *see* Malposition
  - nasal septum J34.2
    - congenital Q67.4
  - opening and closing of the mandible M26.53
  - organ or site, congenital NEC — *see* Malposition, congenital
  - septum (nasal) (acquired) J34.2
    - congenital Q67.4
  - sexual F65.9
    - bestiality F65.89
    - erotomania F52.8
    - exhibitionism F65.2
    - fetishism, fetishistic F65.Ø
      - transvestism F65.1
    - frotteurism F65.81
    - masochism F65.51
    - multiple F65.89
    - necrophilia F65.89
    - nymphomania F52.8
    - pederosis F65.4
    - pedophilia F65.4
    - sadism, sadomasochism F65.52
    - satyriasis F52.8
    - specified type NEC F65.89
    - transvestism F64.1
    - voyeurism F65.3
  - teeth, midline M26.29
- **Deviation** — *continued*
  - trachea J39.8
  - ureter, congenital Q62.61
- **Device**
  - cerebral ventricle (communicating) in situ Z98.2
  - contraceptive — *see* Contraceptive, device
  - drainage, cerebrospinal fluid, in situ Z98.2
- **Devic's disease** G36.0
- **Devil's**
  - grip B33.Ø
  - pinches (purpura simplex) D69.2
- **Devitalized tooth** K04.99
- **Devonshire colic** — *see* Poisoning, lead
- **Dextraposition, aorta** Q2Ø.3
  - in tetralogy of Fallot Q21.3
- **Dextrinosis, limit** (debrancher enzyme deficiency) E74.Ø3
- **Dextrocardia** (true) Q24.Ø
  - with
    - complete transposition of viscera Q89.3
    - situs inversus Q89.3
- **Dextrotransposition, aorta** Q20.3
- **d-glycericacidemia** E72.59
- **Dhat syndrome** F48.8
- **Dhobi itch** B35.6
- **Di George's syndrome** D82.1
- **Di Guglielmo's disease** C94.0-
- **Diabetes, diabetic** (mellitus) (sugar) E11.9
  - with
    - amyotrophy E11.44
    - arthropathy NEC E11.618
    - autonomic (poly)neuropathy E11.43
    - cataract E11.36
    - Charcot's joints E11.61Ø
    - chronic kidney disease E11.22
    - circulatory complication NEC E11.59
    - complication E11.8
      - specified NEC E11.69
    - dermatitis E11.62Ø
    - foot ulcer E11.621
    - gangrene E11.52
    - gastroparesis E11.43
    - glomerulonephrosis, intracapillary E11.21
    - glomerulosclerosis, intercapillary E11.21
    - hyperglycemia E11.65
    - hyperosmolarity E11.ØØ
      - with coma E11.Ø1
    - hypoglycemia E11.649
      - with coma E11.641
    - kidney complications NEC E11.29
    - Kimmelsteil-Wilson disease E11.21
    - loss of protective sensation (LOPS) — Diabetes, by type, with neuropathy
    - mononeuropathy E11.41
    - myasthenia E11.44
    - necrobiosis lipoidica E11.62Ø
    - nephropathy E11.21
    - neuralgia E11.42
    - neurologic complication NEC E11.49
    - neuropathic arthropathy E11.61Ø
    - neuropathy E11.4Ø
    - ophthalmic complication NEC E11.39
    - oral complication NEC E11.638
    - periodontal disease E11.63Ø
    - peripheral angiopathy E11.51
      - with gangrene E11.52
    - polyneuropathy E11.42
    - renal complication NEC E11.29
    - renal tubular degeneration E11.29
    - retinopathy E11.319
      - with macular edema E11.311
      - nonproliferative E11.329
        - with macular edema E11.321
        - mild E11.329
          - with macular edema E11.321
        - moderate E11.339
          - with macular edema E11.331
        - severe E11.349
          - with macular edema E11.341
      - proliferative E11.359
        - with macular edema E11.351
    - skin complication NEC E11.628
    - skin ulcer NEC E11.622

Diabetes, diabetic — *continued*
bronzed E83.110
complicating pregnancy — *see* Pregnancy, complicated by, diabetes
dietary counseling and surveillance Z71.3
due to drug or chemical E09.9
 with
 amyotrophy E09.44
 arthropathy NEC E09.618
 autonomic (poly)neuropathy E09.43
 cataract E09.36
 Charcot's joints E09.610
 chronic kidney disease E09.22
 circulatory complication NEC E09.59
 complication E09.8
 specified NEC E09.69
 dermatitis E09.620
 foot ulcer E09.621
 gangrene E09.52
 gastroparesis E09.43
 glomerulonephrosis, intracapillary E09.21
 glomerulosclerosis, intercapillary E09.21
 hyperglycemia E09.65
 hyperosmolarity E09.00
 with coma E09.01
 hypoglycemia E09.649
 with coma E09.641
 ketoacidosis E09.10
 with coma E09.11
 kidney complications NEC E09.29
 Kimmelsteil-Wilson disease E09.21
 mononeuropathy E09.41
 myasthenia E09.44
 necrobiosis lipoidica E09.620
 nephropathy E09.21
 neuralgia E09.42
 neurologic complication NEC E09.49
 neuropathic arthropathy E09.610
 neuropathy E09.40
 ophthalmic complication NEC E09.39
 oral complication NEC E09.638
 periodontal disease E09.630
 peripheral angiopathy E09.51
 with gangrene E09.52
 polyneuropathy E09.42
 renal complication NEC E09.29
 renal tubular degeneration E09.29
 retinopathy E09.319
 with macular edema E09.311
 nonproliferative E09.329
 with macular edema E09.321
 mild E09.329
 with macular edema E09.321
 moderate E09.339
 with macular edema E09.331
 severe E09.349
 with macular edema E09.341
 proliferative E09.359
 with macular edema E09.351
 skin complication NEC E09.628
 skin ulcer NEC E09.622
due to underlying condition E08.9
 with
 amyotrophy E08.44
 arthropathy NEC E08.618
 autonomic (poly)neuropathy E08.43
 cataract E08.36
 Charcot's joints E08.610
 chronic kidney disease E08.22
 circulatory complication NEC E08.59
 complication E08.8
 specified NEC E08.69
 dermatitis E08.620
 foot ulcer E08.621
 gangrene E08.52
hyperglycemia E08.65
 hyperosmolarity E08.00
 with coma E08.01
 hypoglycemia E08.649
 with coma E08.641

Diabetes, diabetic — *continued*
due to underlying condition — *continued*
 with — *continued*
 ketoacidosis E08.10
 with coma E08.11
 kidney complications NEC E08.29
 Kimmelsteil-Wilson disease E08.21
 mononeuropathy E08.41
 myasthenia E08.44
 necrobiosis lipoidica E08.620
 nephropathy E08.21
 neuralgia E08.42
 neurologic complication NEC E08.49
 neuropathic arthropathy E08.610
 neuropathy E08.40
 ophthalmic complication NEC E08.39
 oral complication NEC E08.638
 periodontal disease E08.630
 peripheral angiopathy E08.51
 with gangrene E08.52
 polyneuropathy E08.42
 renal complication NEC E08.29
 renal tubular degeneration E08.29
 retinopathy E08.319
 with macular edema E08.311
 nonproliferative E08.329
 with macular edema E08.321
 mild E08.329
 with macular edema E08.321
 moderate E08.339
 with macular edema E08.331
 severe E08.349
 with macular edema E08.341
 proliferative E08.359
 with macular edema E08.351
 skin complication NEC E08.628
 skin ulcer NEC E08.622
gestational (in pregnancy) O24.419
 affecting newborn P70.0
 diet controlled O24.410
 in childbirth O24.429
 diet controlled O24.420
 insulin (and diet) controlled O24.424
 insulin (and diet) controlled O24.414
 puerperal O24.439
 diet controlled O24.430
 insulin (and diet) controlled O24.434
hepatogenous E13.9
inadequately controlled—code to Diabetes, by type, with hyperglycemia
insipidus E23.2
 nephrogenic N25.1
 pituitary E23.2
 vasopressin resistant N25.1
insulin dependent—code to type of diabetes
juvenile-onset — *see* Diabetes, type 1
ketosis-prone — *see* Diabetes, type 1
latent R73.09
neonatal (transient) P70.2
non-insulin dependent—code to type of diabetes
out of control—code to Diabetes, by type, with hyperglycemia
phosphate E83.39
poorly controlled—code to Diabetes, by type, with hyperglycemia
postpancreatectomy — *see* Diabetes, specified type NEC
postprocedural — *see* Diabetes, specified type NEC
secondary diabetes mellitus NEC — *see* Diabetes, specified type NEC
specified type NEC E13.9
 with
 amyotrophy E13.44
 arthropathy NEC E13.618
 autonomic (poly)neuropathy E13.43
 cataract E13.36
 Charcot's joints E13.610
 chronic kidney disease E13.22
 circulatory complication NEC E13.59
 complication E13.8
 specified NEC E13.69
 dermatitis E13.620
 foot ulcer E13.621

glomerulosclerosis, intercapillary E13.21
 hyperglycemia E13.65
 hyperosmolarity E13.00
 with coma E13.01
 hypoglycemia E13.649
 with coma E13.641
 ketoacidosis E13.10
mononeuropathy E13.41
 myasthenia E13.44
 necrobiosis lipoidica E13.620
 nephropathy E13.21
 neuralgia E13.42
 neurologic complication NEC E13.49
 neuropathic arthropathy E13.610
 neuropathy E13.40
 ophthalmic complication NEC E13.39
 oral complication NEC E13.638
 periodontal disease E13.630
 peripheral angiopathy E13.51
 with gangrene E13.52
 polyneuropathy E13.42
 renal complication NEC E13.29
 renal tubular degeneration E13.29
 retinopathy E13.319
 with macular edema E13.311
 nonproliferative E13.329
 with macular edema E13.321
 mild E13.329
 with macular edema E13.321
 moderate E13.339
 with macular edema E13.331
 severe E13.349
 with macular edema E13.341
 proliferative E13.359
 with macular edema E13.351
 skin complication NEC E13.628
 skin ulcer NEC E13.622
steroid-induced — *see* Diabetes, due to, drug or chemical
type 1 E10.9
 with
 amyotrophy E10.44
 arthropathy NEC E10.618
 autonomic (poly)neuropathy E10.43
 cataract E10.36
 Charcot's joints E10.610
 chronic kidney disease E10.22
 circulatory complication NEC E10.59
 complication E10.8
 specified NEC E10.69
 dermatitis E10.620
 foot ulcer E10.621
 gangrene E10.52
 gastroparesis E10.43
 glomerulonephrosis, intracapillary E10.21
 glomerulosclerosis, intercapillary E10.21
 hyperglycemia E10.65
 hypoglycemia E10.649
 with coma E10.641
 ketoacidosis E10.10
 with coma E10.11
 kidney complications NEC E10.29
 Kimmelsteil-Wilson disease E10.21
 mononeuropathy E10.41
 myasthenia E10.44
 necrobiosis lipoidica E10.620
 nephropathy E10.21
 neuralgia E10.42
 neurologic complication NEC E10.49
 neuropathic arthropathy E10.610
 neuropathy E10.40
 ophthalmic complication NEC E10.39
 oral complication NEC E10.638
 periodontal disease E10.630

- **Diabetes, diabetic** — *continued*
  - type 1 — *continued*
    - with — *continued*
      - peripheral angiopathy E1Ø.51
        - with gangrene E1Ø.52
      - polyneuropathy E1Ø.42
      - renal complication NEC E1Ø.29
      - renal tubular degeneration E1Ø.29
      - retinopathy E1Ø.319
        - with macular edema E1Ø.311
        - nonproliferative E1Ø.329
          - with macular edema E1Ø.321
          - mild E1Ø.329
            - with macular edema E1Ø.321
          - moderate E1Ø.339
            - with macular edema E1Ø.331
          - severe E1Ø.349
            - with macular edema E1Ø.341
        - proliferative E1Ø.359
          - with macular edema E1Ø.351
      - skin complication NEC E1Ø.628
      - skin ulcer NEC E1Ø.622
  - type 2 E11.9
    - with
      - amyotrophy E11.44
      - arthropathy NEC E11.618
      - autonomic (poly)neuropathy E11.43
      - cataract E11.36
      - Charcot's joints E11.61Ø
      - chronic kidney disease E11.22
      - circulatory complication NEC E11.59
      - complication E11.8
        - specified NEC E11.69
      - dermatitis E11.62Ø
      - foot ulcer E11.621
      - gangrene E11.52
      - gastroparesis E11.43
      - glomerulonephrosis, intracapillary E11.21
      - glomerulosclerosis, intercapillary E11.21
      - hyperglycemia E11.65
      - hyperosmolarity E11.ØØ
        - with coma E11.Ø1
      - hypoglycemia E11.649
        - with coma E11.641
      - kidney complications NEC E11.29
      - Kimmelsteil-Wilson disease E11.21
      - mononeuropathy E11.41
      - myasthenia E11.44
      - necrobiosis lipoidica E11.62Ø
      - nephropathy E11.21
      - neuralgia E11.42
      - neurologic complication NEC E11.49
      - neuropathic arthropathy E11.61Ø
      - neuropathy E11.4Ø
      - ophthalmic complication NEC E11.39
      - oral complication NEC E11.638
      - periodontal disease E11.63Ø
      - peripheral angiopathy E11.51
        - with gangrene E11.52
      - polyneuropathy E11.42
      - renal complication NEC E11.29
      - renal tubular degeneration E11.29
      - retinopathy E11.319
        - with macular edema E11.311
        - nonproliferative E11.329
          - with macular edema E11.321
          - mild E11.329
            - with macular edema E11.321
          - moderate E11.339
            - with macular edema E11.331
          - severe E11.349
            - with macular edema E11.341
        - proliferative E11.359
          - with macular edema E11.351
      - skin complication NEC E11.628
      - skin ulcer NEC E11.622
- **Diacyclothrombopathia** D69.1
- **Diagnosis deferred** R69
- **Dialysis** (intermittent) (treatment)
  - noncompliance (with) Z91.15
  - renal (hemodialysis) (peritoneal), status Z99.2
  - retina, retinal — *see* Detachment, retina, with retinal, dialysis
- **Diamond-Blackfan anemia** (congenital hypoplastic) D61.Ø1
- **Diamond-Gardener syndrome** (autoerythrocytesensitization) D69.2
- **Diaper rash** L22
- **Diaphoresis** (excessive) R61
- **Diaphragm** — *see* condition
- **Diaphragmalgia** R07.1
- **Diaphragmatitis, diaphragmitis** J98.6
- **Diaphysial aclasis** Q78.6
- **Diaphysitis** — *see* Osteomyelitis, specified type NEC
- **Diarrhea, diarrheal** (disease) (infantile) (inflammatory) R19.7
  - achlorhydric K31.83
  - allergic K52.2
  - amebic (*see also* Amebiasis) AØ6.Ø
    - with abscess — *see* Abscess, amebic
    - acute AØ6.Ø
    - chronic AØ6.1
    - nondysenteric AØ6.2
  - bacillary — *see* Dysentery, bacillary
  - balantidial AØ7.Ø
  - cachectic NEC K52.89
  - Chilomastix AØ7.8
  - choleriformis AØØ.1
  - chronic (noninfectious) K52.9
  - coccidial AØ7.3
  - Cochin-China K9Ø.1
    - strongyloidiasis B78.Ø
  - Dientamoeba AØ7.8
  - dietetic K52.2
  - drug-induced K52.1
  - due to
    - bacteria AØ4.9
      - specified NEC AØ4.8
    - Campylobacter AØ4.5
    - Capillaria philippinensis B81.1
    - Clostridium difficile AØ4.7
    - Clostridium perfringens (C) (F) AØ4.8
    - Cryptosporidium AØ7.2
    - drugs K52.1
    - Escherichia coli AØ4.4
      - enteroaggregative AØ4.4
      - enterohemorrhagic AØ4.3
      - enteroinvasive AØ4.2
      - enteropathogenic AØ4.Ø
      - enterotoxigenic AØ4.1
      - specified NEC AØ4.4
    - food hypersensitivity K52.2
    - Necator americanus B76.1
    - S. japonicum B65.2
    - specified organism NEC AØ8.8
      - bacterial AØ4.8
      - viral AØ8.39
    - Staphylococcus AØ4.8
    - Trichuris trichiuria B79
    - virus — *see* Enteritis, viral
    - Yersinia enterocolitica AØ4.6
  - dysenteric AØ9
  - endemic AØ9
  - epidemic AØ9
  - flagellate AØ7.9
  - Flexner's (ulcerative) AØ3.1
  - functional K59.1
    - following gastrointestinal surgery K91.89
    - psychogenic F45.8
  - Giardia lamblia AØ7.1
  - giardial AØ7.1
  - hill K9Ø.1
  - infectious AØ9
  - malarial — *see* Malaria
  - mite B88.Ø
  - mycotic NEC B49
  - neonatal (noninfectious) P78.3
  - nervous F45.8
  - neurogenic K59.1
  - noninfectious K52.9
  - postgastrectomy K91.1
  - postvagotomy K91.1
  - protozoal AØ7.9
    - specified NEC AØ7.8
  - psychogenic F45.8
  - specified
    - bacterium NEC AØ4.8
    - virus NEC AØ8.39
  - strongyloidiasis B78.Ø
  - toxic K52.1
  - trichomonal AØ7.8
  - tropical K9Ø.1
  - tuberculous A18.32
  - viral — *see* Enteritis, viral
- **Diastasis**
  - cranial bones M84.88
    - congenital NEC Q75.8
  - joint (traumatic) — *see* Dislocation
  - muscle M62.ØØ
    - ankle M62.Ø7-
    - congenital Q79.8
    - foot M62.Ø7-
    - forearm M62.Ø3-
    - hand M62.Ø4-
    - lower leg M62.Ø6-
    - pelvic region M62.Ø5-
    - shoulder region M62.Ø1-
    - specified site NEC M62.Ø8
    - thigh M62.Ø5-
    - upper arm M62.Ø2-
  - recti (abdomen)
    - complicating delivery O71.89
    - congenital Q79.59
- **Diastema, tooth, teeth, fully erupted** M26.32
- **Diastematomyelia** Q06.2
- **Diataxia, cerebral** G80.4
- **Diathesis**
  - allergic — *see* History, allergy
  - bleeding (familial) D69.9
  - cystine (familial) E72.ØØ
  - gouty — *see* Gout
  - hemorrhagic (familial) D69.9
    - newborn NEC P53
  - spasmophilic R29.Ø
- **Diaz's disease or osteochondrosis** (juvenile) (talus) — *see* Osteochondrosis, juvenile, tarsus
- **Dibothriocephalus, dibothriocephaliasis** (latus) (infection) (infestation) B7Ø.Ø
  - larval B7Ø.1
- **Dicephalus, dicephaly** Q89.4
- **Dichotomy, teeth** K00.2
- **Dichromat, dichromatopsia** (congenital) — *see* Deficiency, color vision
- **Dichuchwa** A65
- **Dicroceliasis** B66.2
- **Didelphia, didelphys** — *see* Double uterus
- **Didymytis** N45.1
  - with orchitis N45.3
- **Dietary**
  - inadequacy or deficiency E63.9
  - surveillance and counseling Z71.3
- **Dietl's crisis** N13.8
- **Dieulafoy lesion** (hemorrhagic)
  - duodenum K31.82
  - esophagus K22.8
  - intestine (colon) K63.81
  - stomach K31.82
- **Difficult, difficulty** (in)
  - acculturation Z6Ø.3
  - feeding R63.3
    - newborn P92.9
      - breast P92.5
      - specified NEC P92.8
    - nonorganic (infant or child) F98.29
  - intubation, in anesthesia T88.4
  - mechanical, gastroduodenal stoma K91.89
    - causing obstruction K91.3
  - reading (developmental) F81.Ø
    - secondary to emotional disorders F93.9
  - spelling (specific) F81.81
    - with reading disorder F81.89
    - due to inadequate teaching Z55.8
  - swallowing — *see* Dysphagia
  - walking R26.2
  - work
    - conditions NEC Z56.5
    - schedule Z56.3

- **Diffuse** — *see* condition
- **DiGeorge's syndrome** (thymic hypoplasia) D82.1
- **Digestive** — *see* condition
- **Dihydropyrimidine dehydrogenase disease (DPD)** E88.89
- **Diktyoma** — *see* Neoplasm, malignant, by site
- **Dilaceration, tooth** K00.4
- **Dilatation**
  - anus K59.8
    - venule — *see* Hemorrhoids
  - aorta (focal) (general) — *see* Ectasia, aorta
    - with aneurysm — *see* Aneurysm, aorta
  - artery — *see* Aneurysm
  - bladder (sphincter) N32.89
    - congenital Q64.79
  - blood vessel I99.8
  - bronchial J47.9
    - with
      - exacerbation (acute) J47.1
      - lower respiratory infection J47.Ø
  - calyx (due to obstruction) — *see* Hydronephrosis
  - capillaries I78.8
  - cardiac (acute) (chronic) (*see also* Hypertrophy, cardiac)
    - congenital Q24.8
      - valve NEC Q24.8
        - pulmonary Q22.23
    - valve — *see* Endocarditis
  - cavum septi pellucidi QØ6.8
  - cervix (uteri) (*see also* Incompetency, cervix)
    - incomplete, poor, slow complicating delivery O62.Ø
  - colon K59.3
    - congenital Q43.1
    - psychogenic F45.8
  - common duct (acquired) K83.8
    - congenital Q44.5
  - cystic duct (acquired) K82.8
    - congenital Q44.5
  - duct, mammary — *see* Ectasia, mammary duct
  - duodenum K59.8
  - esophagus K22.8
    - congenital Q39.5
    - due to achalasia K22.Ø
  - eustachian tube, congenital Q17.8
  - gallbladder K82.8
  - gastric — *see* Dilatation, stomach
  - heart (acute) (chronic) (*see also* Hypertrophy, cardiac)
    - congenital Q24.8
    - valve — *see* Endocarditis
  - ileum K59.8
    - psychogenic F45.8
  - jejunum K59.8
    - psychogenic F45.8
  - kidney (calyx) (collecting structures) (cystic) (parenchyma) (pelvis) (idiopathic) N28.89
  - lacrimal passages or duct — *see* Disorder, lacrimal system, changes
  - lymphatic vessel I89.Ø
  - mammary duct — *see* Ectasia, mammary duct
  - Meckel's diverticulum (congenital) Q43.Ø
    - malignant — *see* Table of Neoplasms, small intestine, malignant
  - myocardium (acute) (chronic) — *see* Hypertrophy, cardiac
  - organ or site, congenital NEC — *see* Distortion
  - pancreatic duct K86.8
  - pericardium — *see* Pericarditis
  - pharynx J39.2
  - prostate N42.89
  - pulmonary
    - artery (idiopathic) I28.8
    - valve, congenital Q22.3
  - pupil H57.Ø4
  - rectum K59.3
  - saccule, congenital Q16.5
  - salivary gland (duct) K11.8
  - sphincter ani K62.89
  - stomach K31.89
    - acute K31.Ø
    - psychogenic F45.8
  - submaxillary duct K11.8
  - trachea, congenital Q32.1
  - ureter (idiopathic) N28.82
    - congenital Q62.2
    - due to obstruction N13.4
  - urethra (acquired) N36.8
  - vasomotor I73.9
  - vein I86.8
  - ventricular, ventricle (acute) (chronic) (*see also* Hypertrophy, cardiac)
    - cerebral, congenital QØ4.8
  - venule NEC I86.8
  - vesical orifice N32.89
- **Dilated, dilation** — *see* Dilatation
- **Diminished, diminution**
  - hearing (acuity) — *see* Deafness
  - sense or sensation (cold) (heat) (tactile) (vibratory) R2Ø.8
  - vision NEC H54.7
  - vital capacity R94.2
- **Diminuta taenia** B71.0
- **Dimitri-Sturge-Weber disease** Q85.8
- **Dimple**
  - parasacral, pilonidal or postanal — *see* Cyst, pilonidal
- **Dioctophyme renalis** (infection) (infestation) B83.8
- **Dipetalonemiasis** B74.4
- **Diphallus** Q55.69
- **Diphtheria, diphtheritic** (gangrenous) (hemorrhagic) A36.9
  - carrier (suspected) Z22.2
  - cutaneous A36.3
  - faucial A36.Ø
  - infection of wound A36.3
  - laryngeal A36.2
  - myocarditis A36.81
  - nasal, anterior A36.89
  - nasopharyngeal A36.1
  - neurological complication A36.89
  - pharyngeal A36.Ø
  - specified site NEC A36.89
  - tonsillar A36.Ø
- **Diphyllobothriasis** (intestine) B7Ø.Ø
  - larval B7Ø.1
- **Diplacusis** H93.22-
- **Diplegia** (upper limbs) G83.Ø
  - congenital (cerebral) G8Ø.8
  - facial G51.Ø
  - lower limbs G82.2Ø
  - spastic G8Ø.1
- **Diplococcus, diplococcal** — *see* condition
- **Diplopia** H53.2
- **Dipsomania** F10.20
  - with
    - psychosis — *see* Psychosis, alcoholic
    - remission F1Ø.21
- **Dipylidiasis** B71.1
- **Direction, teeth, abnormal, fully erupted** M26.30
- **Dirofilariasis** B74.8
- **Dirt-eating child** F98.3
- **Disability, disabilities**
  - heart— *see* Disease, heart
  - intellectual F79
    - with
      - autistic features F84.9
    - mild (I.Q. 5Ø-69) F7Ø
    - moderate (I.Q. 35-49) F71
    - profound (I.Q. under 2Ø) F73
    - severe (I.Q. 2Ø-34) F72
    - specified level NEC F78
  - knowledge acquisition F81.9
  - learning F81.9
  - limiting activities Z73.6
  - spelling, specific F81.81
- **Disappearance of family member** Z63.4
- **Disarticulation** — *see* Amputation
  - meaning traumatic amputation — *see* Amputation, traumatic
- **Discharge** (from)
  - abnormal finding in — *see* Abnormal, specimen
  - breast (female) (male) N64.52
  - diencephalic autonomic idiopathic — *see* Epilepsy, specified NEC
  - ear (*see also* Otorrhea)
    - blood — *see* Otorrhagia
  - excessive urine R35.8
  - nipple N64.52
  - penile R36.9
  - postnasal RØ9.82
  - prison, anxiety concerning Z65.2
  - urethral R36.9
    - without blood R36.Ø
    - hematospermia R36.1
  - vaginal N89.8
- **Discitis, diskitis** M46.40
  - cervical region M46.42
  - cervicothoracic region M46.43
  - lumbar region M46.46
  - lumbosacral region M46.47
  - multiple sites M46.49
  - occipito-atlanto-axial region M46.41
  - pyogenic — *see* Infection, intervertebral disc, pyogenic
  - sacrococcygeal region M46.48
  - thoracic region M46.44
  - thoracolumbar region M46.45
- **Discoid**
  - meniscus (congenital) Q68.6
  - semilunar cartilage (congenital) — *see* Derangement, knee, meniscus, specified NEC
- **Discoloration**
  - nails L6Ø.8
  - teeth (posteruptive) KØ3.7
    - during formation KØØ.8
- **Discomfort**
  - chest RØ7.89
  - visual H53.14-
- **Discontinuity, ossicles, ear** H74.2-
- **Discord** (with)
  - boss Z56.4
  - classmates Z55.4
  - counselor Z64.4
  - employer Z56.4
  - family Z63.8
  - fellow employees Z56.4
  - in-laws Z63.1
  - landlord Z59.2
  - lodgers Z59.2
  - neighbors Z59.2
  - probation officer Z64.4
  - social worker Z64.4
  - teachers Z55.4
  - workmates Z56.4
- **Discordant connection**
  - atrioventricular (congenital) Q2Ø.5
  - ventriculoarterial Q2Ø.3
- **Discrepancy**
  - centric occlusion maximum intercuspation M26.55
  - leg length (acquired) — *see* Deformity, limb, unequal length
    - congenital — *see* Defect, reduction, lower limb
  - uterine size date O26.84-
- **Discrimination**
  - ethnic Z6Ø.5
  - political Z6Ø.5
  - racial Z6Ø.5
  - religious Z6Ø.5
  - sex Z6Ø.5
- **Disease, diseased** (*see also* Syndrome)
  - absorbent system I87.8
  - acid-peptic K3Ø
  - Acosta's T7Ø.29
  - Adams-Stokes (-Morgagni) (syncope with heart block) I45.9
  - Addison's anemia (pernicious) D51.Ø
  - adenoids (and tonsils) J35.9
  - adrenal (capsule) (cortex) (gland) (medullary) E27.9
    - hyperfunction E27.Ø
    - specified NEC E27.8
  - ainhum L94.6
  - airway
    - obstructive, chronic J44.9
      - due to
        - cotton dust J66.Ø
        - specific organic dusts NEC J66.8
    - reactive — *see* Asthma
  - akamushi (scrub typhus) A75.3
  - Albers-Schönberg's (marble bones) Q78.2

Disease, diseased — *continued*
- Albert's — *see* Tendinitis, Achilles
- alimentary canal K63.9
- alligator-skin Q8Ø.9
  - acquired L85.Ø
- alpha heavy chain C88.3
- alpine T7Ø.29
- altitude T7Ø.2Ø
- alveolar ridge
  - edentulous KØ6.9
    - specified NEC KØ6.8
- alveoli, teeth KØ8.9
- Alzheimer's G3Ø.9 *[F02.80]*
  - with behavioral disturbance G3Ø.9 *[F02.81]*
  - early onset G3Ø.Ø *[F02.80]*
    - with behavioral disturbance G3Ø.Ø *[F02.81]*
  - late onset G3Ø.1 *[F02.80]*
    - with behavioral disturbance G3Ø.1 *[F02.81]*
  - specified NEC G3Ø.8 *[F02.80]*
    - with behavioral disturbance G3Ø.8 *[F02.81]*
- amyloid — *see* Amyloidosis
- Andersen's (glycogenosis IV) E74.Ø9
- Andes T7Ø.29
- Andrews' (bacterid) LØ8.89
- angiospastic I73.9
  - cerebral G45.9
  - vein I87.8
- anterior
  - chamber H21.9
  - horn cell G12.29
- antiglomerular basement membrane (antiGBM) antibody M31.Ø
  - tubulo-interstitial nephritis N12
- antral — *see* Sinusitis, maxillary
- anus K62.9
  - specified NEC K62.89
- aorta (nonsyphilitic) I77.9
  - syphilitic NEC A52.Ø2
- aortic (heart) (valve) I35.9
  - rheumatic IØ6.9
- Apollo B3Ø.3
- aponeuroses — *see* Enthesopathy
- appendix K38.9
  - specified NEC K38.8
- aqueous (chamber) H21.9
- Arnold-Chiari — *see* Arnold-Chiari disease
- arterial I77.9
  - occlusive — *see* Occlusion, by site
    - due to stricture or stenosis I77.1
- arteriocardiorenal — *see* Hypertension, cardiorenal
- arteriolar (generalized) (obliterative) I77.9
- arteriorenal — *see* Hypertension, kidney
- arteriosclerotic (*see also* Arteriosclerosis)
  - cardiovascular — *see* Disease, heart, ischemic, atherosclerotic
  - coronary (artery) — *see* Disease, heart, ischemic, atherosclerotic
  - heart — *see* Disease, heart, ischemic, atherosclerotic
- artery I77.9
  - cerebral I67.9
  - coronary I25.1Ø
    - with angina pectoris — *see* Arteriosclerosis, coronary (artery),
- arthropod-borne NOS (viral) A94
  - specified type NEC A93.8
- atticoantral, chronic H66.2Ø
  - left H66.22
    - with right H66.23
  - right H66.21
    - with left H66.23
- auditory canal — *see* Disorder, ear, external
- auricle, ear NEC — *see* Disorder, pinna
- Australian X A83.4
- autoimmune (systemic) NOS M35.9
  - hemolytic (cold type) (warm type) D59.1
    - drug-induced D59.Ø
  - thyroid EØ6.3
- aviator's — *see* Effect, adverse, high altitude
- Ayala's Q78.5
- Ayerza's (pulmonary artery sclerosis with pulmonary hypertension) I27.Ø

Disease, diseased — *continued*
- Babington's (familial hemorrhagic telangiectasia) I78.Ø
- bacterial A49.9
  - specified NEC A48.8
  - zoonotic A28.9
    - specified type NEC A28.8
- Baelz's (cheilitis glandularis apostematosa) K13.Ø
- bagasse J67.1
- balloon — *see* Effect, adverse, high altitude
- Bang's (brucella abortus) A23.1
- Bannister's T78.3
- barometer makers' — *see* Poisoning, mercury
- Barraquer (-Simons') (progressive lipodystrophy) E88.1
- Barrett's — *see* Barrett's, esophagus
- Bartholin's gland N75.9
- basal ganglia G25.9
  - degenerative G23.9
    - specified NEC G23.8
  - specified NEC G25.89
- Basedow's (exophthalmic goiter) — *see* Hyperthyroidism, with, goiter (diffuse)
- Bateman's BØ8.1
- Batten-Steinert G71.11
- Battey A31.Ø
- Beard's (neurasthenia) F48.8
- Becker
  - idiopathic mural endomyocardial I42.3
  - myotonia congenita G71.12
- Begbie's (exophthalmic goiter) — *see* Hyperthyroidism, with, goiter (diffuse)
- Beigel's (white piedra) B36.2
- behavioral, organic FØ7.9
- Benson's — *see* Deposit, crystalline
- Bernard-Soulier (thrombopathy) D69.1
- Bernhardt (-Roth) — *see* Mononeuropathy, lower limb, meralgia paresthetica
- Biermer's (pernicious anemia) D51.Ø
- bile duct (common) (hepatic) K83.9
  - with calculus, stones — *see* Calculus, bile duct
  - specified NEC K83.8
- biliary (tract) K83.9
  - specified NEC K83.8
- Billroth's — *see* Spina bifida
- bird fancier's J67.2
- black lung J6Ø
- bladder N32.9
  - in (due to)
    - schistosomiasis (bilharziasis) B65.Ø *[N33]*
  - specified NEC N32.89
- bleeder's D66
- blood D75.9
  - forming organs D75.9
  - vessel I99.9
- Bloodgood's — *see* Mastopathy, cystic
- Bodechtel-Guttmann (subacute sclerosing panencephalitis) A81.1
- bone (*see also* Disorder, bone)
  - aluminum M83.4
  - fibrocystic NEC
    - jaw M27.49
- bone-marrow D75.9
- Borna A83.9
- Bornholm (epidemic pleurodynia) B33.Ø
- Bouchard's (myopathic dilatation of the stomach) K31.Ø
- Bouillaud's (rheumatic heart disease) IØ1.9
- Bourneville (-Brissaud) (tuberous sclerosis) Q85.1
- Bouveret (-Hoffmann) (paroxysmal tachycardia) I47.9
- bowel K63.9
  - functional K59.9
    - psychogenic F45.8
- brain G93.9
  - arterial, artery I67.9
  - arteriosclerotic I67.2
  - congenital QØ4.9
  - degenerative — *see* Degeneration, brain
  - inflammatory — *see* Encephalitis
  - organic G93.9
    - arteriosclerotic I67.2
  - parasitic NEC B71.9 *[G94]*

Disease, diseased — *continued*
- brain — *continued*
  - senile NEC G31.1
  - specified NEC G93.89
- breast (*see also* Disorder, breast) N64.9
  - cystic (chronic) — *see* Mastopathy, cystic
  - fibrocystic — *see* Mastopathy, cystic
  - Paget's
    - female, unspecified side C5Ø.91-
    - male, unspecified side C5Ø.92-
  - specified NEC N64.89
- Breda's — *see* Yaws
- Bretonneau's (diphtheritic malignant angina) A36.Ø
- Bright's — *see* Nephritis
  - arteriosclerotic — *see* Hypertension, kidney
- Brill's (recrudescent typhus) A75.1
- Brill-Zinsser (recrudescent typhus) A75.1
- Brion-Kayser — *see* Fever, paratyphoid
- broad
  - beta E78.2
  - ligament (noninflammatory) N83.9
    - inflammatory — *see* Disease, pelvis, inflammatory
    - specified NEC N83.8
- Brocq-Duhring (dermatitis herpetiformis) L13.Ø
- Brocq's
  - meaning
    - dermatitis herpetiformis L13.Ø
    - prurigo L28.2
- bronchopulmonary J98.4
- bronchus NEC J98.Ø9
- bronze Addison's E27.1
  - tuberculous A18.7
- budgerigar fancier's J67.2
- bullous L13.9
  - chronic of childhood L12.2
  - specified NEC L13.8
- Buerger's (thromboangiitis obliterans) I73.1
- Bürger-Grütz (essential familial hyperlipemia) E78.3
- bursa — *see* Bursopathy
- caisson T7Ø.3
- California — *see* Coccidioidomycosis
- capillaries I78.9
  - specified NEC I78.8
- Carapata A68.Ø
- cardiac — *see* Disease, heart
- cardiopulmonary, chronic I27.9
- cardiorenal (hepatic) (hypertensive) (vascular) — *see* Hypertension, cardiorenal
- cardiovascular (atherosclerotic) I25.1Ø
  - with angina pectoris — *see* Arteriosclerosis, coronary (artery),
  - congenital Q28.9
  - newborn P29.9
    - specified NEC P29.89
  - hypertensive — *see* Hypertension, heart
  - renal (hypertensive) — *see* Hypertension, cardiorenal
  - syphilitic (asymptomatic) A52.ØØ
- cartilage — *see* Disorder, cartilage
- Castellani's A69.8
- cat-scratch A28.1
- Cavare's (familial periodic paralysis) G72.3
- cecum K63.9
- celiac (adult) (infantile) K9Ø.Ø
- cellular tissue L98.9
- central core G71.2
- cerebellar, cerebellum — *see* Disease, brain
- cerebral (*see also* Disease, brain)
  - degenerative — *see* Degeneration, brain
- cerebrospinal G96.9
- cerebrovascular I67.9
  - acute I67.89
    - embolic I63.4-
    - thrombotic I63.3-
  - arteriosclerotic I67.2
  - specified NEC I67.89
- cervix (uteri) (noninflammatory) N88.9
  - inflammatory — *see* Cervicitis
  - specified NEC N88.8
- Chabert's A22.9
- Chandler's (osteochondritis dissecans, hip) — *see* Osteochondritis, dissecans, hip

Disease, diseased—Disease, diseased

DRAFT

Disease, diseased — *continued*
- hookworm B76.9
  - specified NEC B76.8
- host-versus-graft D89.813
  - acute D89.81Ø
  - acute on chronic D89.812
  - chronic D89.811
- human immunodeficiency virus (HIV) B2Ø
- Huntington's G1Ø
- Hutchinson's (cheiropompholyx) — *see* Hutchinson's disease
- hyaline (diffuse) (generalized)
  - membrane (lung) (newborn) P22.Ø
    - adult J8Ø
- hydatid — *see* Echinococcus
- hydroxyapatite deposition M11.ØØ
  - ankle M11.Ø7-
  - elbow M11.Ø2-
  - foot joint M11.Ø7-
  - hand joint M11.Ø4-
  - hip M11.Ø5-
  - knee M11.Ø6-
  - multiple site M11.Ø9
  - shoulder M11.Ø1-
  - vertebra M11.Ø8
  - wrist M11.Ø3-
- hyperkinetic — *see* Hyperkinesia
- hypertensive — *see* Hypertension
- hypophysis E23.7
- Iceland G93.3
- I-cell E77.Ø
- immune D89.9
- immunoproliferative (malignant) C88.9
  - small intestinal C88.3
  - specified NEC C88.8
- inclusion B25.9
  - salivary gland B25.9
- infectious, infective B99.9
  - congenital P37.9
    - specified NEC P37.8
    - viral
  - specified NEC B99.8
- inflammatory
  - penis N48.29
    - abscess N48.21
    - cellulitis N48.22
  - prepuce N47.7
    - balanoposthitis N47.6
  - tubo-ovarian — *see* Salpingo-oophoritis
- intervertebral disc (*see also* Disorder, disc)
  - with myelopathy — *see* Disorder, disc, with, myelopathy
  - cervical, cervicothoracic — *see* Disorder, disc, cervical
    - with
      - myelopathy — *see* Disorder, disc, cervical, with myelopathy
      - neuritis, radiculitis or radiculopathy — *see* Disorder, disc, cervical, with neuritis
      - specified NEC — *see* Disorder, disc, cervical, specified type NEC
  - lumbar (with)
    - myelopathy M51.Ø6
    - neuritis, radiculitis, radiculopathy or sciatica M51.16
    - specified NEC M51.86
  - lumbosacral (with)
    - myelopathy M51.Ø7
    - neuritis, radiculitis, radiculopathy or sciatica M51.17
    - specified NEC M51.87
  - specified NEC — *see* Disorder, disc, specified NEC
  - thoracic (with)
    - myelopathy M51.Ø4
    - neuritis, radiculitis or radiculopathy M51.14
    - specified NEC M51.84
  - thoracolumbar (with)
    - myelopathy M51.Ø5
    - neuritis, radiculitis or radiculopathy M51.15
    - specified NEC M51.85
- intestine K63.9
  - functional K59.9
    - psychogenic F45.8

Disease, diseased — *continued*
- intestine — *continued*
  - functional — *continued*
    - specified NEC K59.8
  - organic K63.9
  - protozoal AØ7.9
  - specified NEC K63.89
- iris H21.9
  - specified NEC H21.89
- iron metabolism or storage E83.1Ø
- island (scrub typhus) A75.3
- itai-itai — *see* Poisoning, cadmium
- Jakob-Creutzfeldt — *see* Creutzfeldt-Jakob disease or syndrome
- jaw M27.9
  - fibrocystic M27.49
  - specified NEC M27.8
- jigger B88.1
- joint (*see also* Disorder, joint)
  - Charcot's — *see* Arthropathy, neuropathic (Charcot)
  - degenerative — *see* Osteoarthritis
    - multiple M15.9
    - spine — *see* Spondylosis
  - hypertrophic — *see* Osteoarthritis
  - sacroiliac M53.3
  - specified NEC — *see* Disorder, joint, specified type NEC
  - spine NEC — *see* Dorsopathy
  - suppurative — *see* Arthritis, pyogenic or pyemic
- Jourdain's (acute gingivitis) KØ5.ØØ
  - plaque induced KØ5.ØØ
  - nonplaque induced KØ5.Ø1
- Kaschin-Beck (endemic polyarthritis) M12.1Ø
  - ankle M12.17-
  - elbow M12.12-
  - foot joint M12.17-
  - hand joint M12.14-
  - hip M12.15-
  - knee M12.16-
  - multiple site M12.19
  - shoulder M12.11-
  - vertebra M12.18
  - wrist M12.13-
- Katayama B65.2
- Kedani (scrub typhus) A75.3
- Keshan E59
- kidney (functional) (pelvis) N28.9
  - chronic N18.9
    - hypertensive — *see* Hypertension, kidney
    - stage 1 N18.1
    - stage 2 (mild) N18.2
    - stage 3 (moderate) N18.3
    - stage 4 (severe) N18.4
    - stage 5 N18.5
  - complicating pregnancy — *see* Pregnancy, complicated by, renal disease
  - cystic (congenital) Q61.9
  - fibrocystic (congenital) Q61.8
  - hypertensive — *see* Hypertension, kidney
  - in (due to)
    - schistosomiasis (bilharziasis) B65.9 *[N29]*
  - multicystic Q61.4
  - polycystic Q61.3
    - adult type Q61.2
    - childhood type NEC Q61.19
      - collecting duct dilatation Q61.11
- Kimmelstiel (-Wilson) (intercapillary polycystic (congenital) glomerulosclerosis) — *see* EØ8-E13 with .21
- Kinnier Wilson's (hepatolenticular degeneration) E83.Ø1
- kissing — *see* Mononucleosis, infectious
- Klebs' (*see also* Glomerulonephritis) NØ5.-
- Klippel-Feil (brevicollis) Q76.1
- Köhler-Pellegrini-Stieda (calcification, knee joint) — *see* Bursitis, tibial collateral
- Kok Q89.8
- König's (osteochondritis dissecans) — *see* Osteochondritis, dissecans
- Korsakoff's (nonalcoholic) FØ4
  - alcoholic F1Ø.96
    - with dependence F1Ø.26

Disease, diseased — *continued*
- Kostmann's (infantile genetic agranulocytosis) D7Ø.Ø
- kuru A81.81
- Kyasanur Forest A98.2
- labyrinth, ear — *see* Disorder, ear, inner
- lacrimal system — *see* Disorder, lacrimal system
- Lafora's — *see* Epilepsy, generalized, idiopathic
- Lancereaux-Mathieu (leptospiral jaundice) A27.Ø
- Landry's G61.Ø
- Larrey-Weil (leptospiral jaundice) A27.Ø
- larynx J38.7
- legionnaires' A48.1
  - nonpneumonic A48.2
- Lenegre's I44.2
- lens H27.9
  - specified NEC H27.8
- Lev's (acquired complete heart block) I44.2
- Lewy body (dementia) G31.83 *[FØ2.8Ø]*
  - with behavioral disturbance G31.83 *[FØ2.81]*
- Lichtheim's (subacute combined sclerosis with pernicious anemia) D51.Ø
- Lightwood's (renal tubular acidosis) N25.89
- Lignac's (cystinosis) E72.Ø4
- lip K13.Ø
- lipid-storage E75.6
  - specified NEC E75.5
- Lipschütz's N76.6
- liver (chronic) (organic) K76.9
  - alcoholic (chronic) K7Ø.9
    - acute — *see* Disease, liver, alcoholic, hepatitis
    - cirrhosis K7Ø.3Ø
      - with ascites K7Ø.31
    - failure K7Ø.4Ø
      - with coma K7Ø.41
    - fatty liver K7Ø.Ø
    - fibrosis K7Ø.2
    - hepatitis K7Ø.1Ø
      - with ascites K7Ø.11
    - sclerosis K7Ø.2
  - cystic, congenital Q44.6
  - drug-induced (idiosyncratic) (toxic) (predictable) (unpredictable) — *see* Disease, liver, toxic
  - end stage K72.9Ø
    - due to hepatitis — *see* Hepatitis
  - fatty, nonalcoholic (NAFLD) K76.Ø
    - alcoholic K7Ø.Ø
  - fibrocystic (congenital) Q44.6
  - fluke
    - Chinese B66.1
    - oriental B66.1
    - sheep B66.3
  - glycogen storage E74.Ø9 *[K77]*
  - in (due to)
    - schistosomiasis (bilharziasis) B65.9 *[K77]*
  - inflammatory K75.9
    - alcoholic K7Ø.1
    - specified NEC K75.89
  - polycystic (congenital) Q44.6
  - toxic K71.9
    - with
      - cholestasis K71.Ø
      - cirrhosis (liver) K71.7
      - fibrosis (liver) K71.7
      - focal nodular hyperplasia K71.8
      - hepatic granuloma K71.8
      - hepatic necrosis K71.1Ø
        - with coma K71.11
      - hepatitis NEC K71.6
        - acute K71.2
        - chronic
          - active K71.5Ø
            - with ascites K71.51
          - lobular K71.4
          - persistent K71.3
        - lupoid K71.5Ø
          - with ascites K71.51
      - peliosis hepatis K71.8
      - veno-occlusive disease (VOD) of liver K71.8
  - veno-occlusive K76.5
- Lobo's (keloid blastomycosis) B48.Ø
- Lobstein's (brittle bones and blue sclera) Q78.Ø
- Ludwig's (submaxillary cellulitis) K12.2

Disease, diseased — *continued*
- lumbosacral region M53.87
- lung J98.4
  - black J6Ø
  - congenital Q33.9
  - cystic J98.4
    - congenital Q33.Ø
  - fibroid (chronic) — *see* Fibrosis, lung
  - fluke B66.4
    - oriental B66.4
  - in
    - amyloidosis E85.4 *[J99]*
    - sarcoidosis D86.Ø
    - Sjögren's syndrome M35.Ø2
    - systemic
      - lupus erythematosus M32.13
      - sclerosis M34.81
  - interstitial J84.9
    - of childhood, specified NEC J84.848
    - respiratory bronchiolitis J84.115
    - specified NEC J84.89
  - obstructive (chronic) J44.9
    - with
      - acute
        - bronchitis J44.Ø
        - exacerbation NEC J44.1
        - lower respiratory infection J44.Ø
      - alveolitis, allergic J67.9
      - asthma J44.9
      - bronchiectasis J47.9
        - with
          - exacerbation (acute) J47.1
          - lower respiratory infection J47.Ø
      - bronchitis J44.9
        - with
          - exacerbation (acute) J44.1
          - lower respiratory infection J44.Ø
      - emphysema J44.9
      - hypersensitivity pneumonitis J67.9
    - decompensated J44.1
      - with
        - exacerbation (acute) J44.1
  - polycystic J98.4
    - congenital Q33.Ø
  - rheumatoid (diffuse) (interstitial) — *see* Rheumatoid, lung
- Lutembacher's (atrial septal defect with mitral stenosis) Q21.1
- Lyme A69.2Ø
- lymphatic (gland) (system) (channel) (vessel) I89.9
- lymphoproliferative D47.9
  - specified NEC D47.Z9
  - T-gamma D47.Z9
  - X-linked D82.3
- Magitot's M27.2
- malarial — *see* Malaria
- malignant (*see also* Neoplasm, malignant, by site)
- Manson's B65.1
- maple bark J67.6
- maple-syrup-urine E71.Ø
- Marburg (virus) A98.3
- Marion's (bladder neck obstruction) N32.Ø
- Marsh's (exophthalmic goiter) — *see* Hyperthyroidism, with, goiter (diffuse)
- mastoid (process) — *see* Disorder, ear, middle
- Mathieu's (leptospiral jaundice) A27.Ø
- Maxcy's A75.2
- McArdle (-Schmid-Pearson) (glycogenosis V) E74.Ø4
- mediastinum J98.5
- medullary center (idiopathic) (respiratory) G93.89
- Meige's (chronic hereditary edema) Q82.Ø
- meningococcal — *see* Infection, meningococcal
- mental F99
  - organic FØ9
- mesenchymal M35.9
- mesenteric embolic K55.Ø
- metabolic, metabolism E88.9
  - bilirubin E8Ø.7
- metal-polisher's J62.8
- metastatic (*see also* Neoplasm, secondary, by site) C79.9
- microvascular code to condition

Disease, diseased — *continued*
- microvillus
  - atrophy Q43.8
  - inclusion (MVD) Q43.8
- middle ear — *see* Disorder, ear, middle
- Mikulicz' (dryness of mouth, absent or decreased lacrimation) K11.8
- Milroy's (chronic hereditary edema) Q82.Ø
- Minamata — *see* Poisoning, mercury
- minicore G71.2
- Minor's G95.19
- Minot's (hemorrhagic disease, newborn) P53
- Minot-von Willebrand-Jürgens (angiohemophilia) D68.Ø
- Mitchell's (erythromelalgia) I73.81
- mitral (valve) IØ5.9
  - nonrheumatic I34.9
- mixed connective tissue M35.1
- Monge's T7Ø.29
- Morgagni-Adams-Stokes (syncope with heart block) I45.9
- Morgagni's (syndrome) (hyperostosis frontalis interna) M85.2
- Morton's (with metatarsalgia) — *see* Lesion, nerve, plantar
- Morvan's G6Ø.8
- motor neuron (bulbar) (familial) (mixed type) (spinal) G12.2Ø
  - amyotrophic lateral sclerosis G12.21
  - progressive bulbar palsy G12.22
  - specified NEC G12.29
- moldy hay J67.Ø
- moyamoya I67.5
- mu heavy chain disease C88.2
- multicore G71.2
- muscle *see also* Disorder, muscle
  - inflammatory — *see* Myositis
  - ocular (external) — *see* Strabismus
- musculoskeletal system, soft tissue (*see also* Disorder, soft tissue)
  - specified NEC — *see* Disorder, soft tissue, specified type NEC
- mushroom workers' J67.5
- mycotic B49
- myelodysplastic, not classified C94.6
- myeloproliferative, not classified C94.6
  - chronic D47.1
- myocardium, myocardial (*see also* Degeneration, myocardial) I51.5
  - primary (idiopathic) I42.9
- myoneural G7Ø.9
- Naegeli's D69.1
- nails L6Ø.9
  - specified NEC L6Ø.8
- Nairobi (sheep virus) A93.8
- nasal J34.9
- nemaline body G71.2
- nerve — *see* Disorder, nerve
- nervous system G98.8
  - autonomic G9Ø.9
  - central G96.9
    - specified NEC G96.8
  - congenital QØ7.9
  - parasympathetic G9Ø.9
  - specified NEC G98.8
  - sympathetic G9Ø.9
  - vegetative G9Ø.9
- neuromuscular system G7Ø.9
- Newcastle B3Ø.8
- Nicolas (-Durand)-Favre (climatic bubo) A55
- nipple N64.9
  - Paget's C5Ø.Ø1-
    - female C5Ø.Ø1-
    - male C5Ø.Ø2-
- Nishimoto (-Takeuchi) I67.5
- nonarthropod-borne NOS (viral) B34.9
  - enterovirus NEC B34.1
- nonautoimmune hemolytic D59.4
  - drug-induced D59.2
- Nonne-Milroy-Meige (chronic hereditary edema) Q82.Ø
- nose J34.9
- nucleus pulposus — *see* Disorder, disc

Disease, diseased — *continued*
- nutritional E63.9
- oast-house-urine E72.19
  - ocular
    - herpesviral BØØ.5Ø
    - zoster BØ2.3Ø
- obliterative vascular I77.1
- Ohara's — *see* Tularemia
- Opitz's (congestive splenomegaly) D73.2
- Oppenheim-Urbach (necrobiosis lipoidica diabeticorum) — *see* EØ8-E13 with .62Ø
- optic nerve NEC — *see* Disorder, nerve, optic
- orbit — *see* Disorder, orbit
- Oriental liver fluke B66.1
- Oriental lung fluke B66.4
- Ormond's N13.5
- Oropouche virus A93.Ø
- Osler-Rendu (familial hemorrhagic telangiectasia) I78.Ø
- osteofibrocystic E21.Ø
- Otto's M24.7
- outer ear — *see* Disorder, ear, external
- ovary (noninflammatory) N83.9
  - cystic N83.2Ø
  - inflammatory — *see* Salpingo-oophoritis
  - polycystic E28.2
  - specified NEC N83.8
- Owren's (congenital) — *see* Defect, coagulation
- pancreas K86.9
  - cystic K86.2
  - fibrocystic E84.9
  - specified NEC K86.8
- panvalvular IØ8.9
  - specified NEC IØ8.8
- parametrium (noninflammatory) N83.9
- parasitic B89
  - cerebral NEC B71.9 *[G94]*
  - intestinal NOS B82.9
  - mouth B37.Ø
  - skin NOS B88.9
  - specified type — *see* Infestation
  - tongue B37.Ø
- parathyroid (gland) E21.5
  - specified NEC E21.4
- Parkinson's G2Ø
- parodontal KØ5.6
- Parrot's (syphilitic osteochondritis) A5Ø.Ø2
- Parry's (exophthalmic goiter) — *see* Hyperthyroidism, with, goiter (diffuse)
- Parson's (exophthalmic goiter) — *see* Hyperthyroidism, with, goiter (diffuse)
- Paxton's (white piedra) B36.2
- pearl-worker's — *see* Osteomyelitis, specified type NEC
- Pellegrini-Stieda (calcification, knee joint) — *see* Bursitis, tibial collateral
- pelvis, pelvic
  - female NOS N94.9
    - specified NEC N94.89
  - gonococcal (acute) (chronic) A54.24
  - inflammatory (female) N73.9
    - acute N73.Ø
    - chronic N73.1
    - specified NEC N73.8
    - syphilitic (secondary) A51.42
      - late A52.76
    - tuberculous A18.17
  - organ, female N94.9
  - peritoneum, female NEC N94.89
- penis N48.9
  - inflammatory N48.29
    - abscess N48.21
    - cellulitis N48.22
  - specified NEC N48.89
- periapical tissues NOS KØ4.9Ø
- periodontal KØ5.6
  - specified NEC KØ5.5
- periosteum — *see* Disorder, bone, specified type NEC
- peripheral
  - arterial I73.9
  - autonomic nervous system G9Ø.9
  - nerves — *see* Polyneuropathy

Disease, diseased — *continued*
- peripheral — *continued*
  - vascular NOS I73.9
- peritoneum K66.9
  - pelvic, female NEC N94.89
  - specified NEC K66.8
- persistent mucosal (middle ear) H66.2Ø
  - left H66.22
    - with right H66.23
  - right H66.21
    - with left H66.23
- Petit's — *see* Hernia, abdomen, specified site NEC
- pharynx J39.2
  - specified NEC J39.2
- Phocas' — *see* Mastopathy, cystic
- photochromogenic (acid-fast bacilli) (pulmonary) A31.Ø
  - nonpulmonary A31.9
- Pick's G31.Ø1 *[FØ2.8Ø]*
  - with behavioral disturbance G31.Ø1 *[FØ2.81]*
- pigeon fancier's J67.2
- pineal gland E34.8
- pink — *see* Poisoning, mercury
- Pinkus' (lichen nitidus) L44.1
- pinworm B8Ø
- Piry virus A93.8
- pituitary (gland) E23.7
- pituitary-snuff-taker's J67.8
- pleura (cavity) J94.9
  - specified NEC J94.8
- pneumatic drill (hammer) T75.21
- Pollitzer's (hidradenitis suppurativa) L73.2
- polycystic
  - kidney or renal Q61.3
    - adult type Q61.2
    - childhood type NEC Q61.19
      - collecting duct dilatation Q61.11
  - liver or hepatic Q44.6
  - lung or pulmonary J98.4
    - congenital Q33.Ø
  - ovary, ovaries E28.2
  - spleen Q89.Ø9
- polyethylene T84.Ø5-
- Pompe's (glycogenosis II) E74.Ø2
- Posadas-Wernicke B38.9
- Potain's (pulmonary edema) — *see* Edema, lung
- prepuce N47.8
  - inflammatory N47.7
    - balanoposthitis N47.6
- Pringle's (tuberous sclerosis) Q85.1
- prion, central nervous system A81.9
  - specified NEC A81.89
- prostate N42.9
  - specified NEC N42.89
- protozoal B64
  - acanthamebiasis — *see* Acanthamebiasis
  - African trypanosomiasis — *see* African trypanosomiasis
  - babesiosis B6Ø.Ø
  - Chagas disease — *see* Chagas disease
  - intestine, intestinal AØ7.9
  - leishmaniasis — *see* Leishmaniasis
  - malaria — *see* Malaria
  - naegleriasis B6Ø.2
  - pneumocystosis B59
  - specified organism NEC B6Ø.8
  - toxoplasmosis — *see* Toxoplasmosis
- pseudo-Hurler's E77.Ø
- psychiatric F99
- psychotic — *see* Psychosis
- Puente's (simple glandular cheilitis) K13.Ø
- puerperal (*see also* Puerperal) O9Ø.89
- pulmonary (*see also* Disease, lung)
  - artery I28.9
  - chronic obstructive J44.9
    - with
      - acute bronchitis J44.Ø
      - exacerbation (acute) J44.1
      - lower respiratory infection (acute) J44.Ø
    - decompensated J44.1
      - with
        - exacerbation (acute) J44.1

Disease, diseased — *continued*
- pulmonary — *continued*
  - heart I27.9
    - specified NEC I27.89
  - hypertensive (vascular) I27.Ø
  - valve I37.9
    - rheumatic IØ9.89
- pulp (dental) NOS KØ4.9Ø
- pulseless M31.4
- Putnam's (subacute combined sclerosis with pernicious anemia) D51.Ø
- Pyle (-Cohn) (craniometaphyseal dysplasia) Q78.5
- ragpicker's or ragsorter's A22.1
- Raynaud's — *see* Raynaud's disease
- reactive airway — *see* Asthma
- Reclus' (cystic) — *see* Mastopathy, cystic
- rectum K62.9
  - specified NEC K62.89
- Refsum's (heredopathia atactica polyneuritiformis) G6Ø.1
- renal (functional) (pelvis) (*see also* Disease, kidney) N28.9
  - with
    - edema — *see* Nephrosis
    - glomerular lesion — *see* Glomerulonephritis
      - with edema — *see* Nephrosis
    - interstitial nephritis N12
  - acute N28.9
  - chronic (*see also* Disease, kidney, chronic) N18.9
  - cystic, congenital Q61.9
  - diabetic — *see* EØ8-E13 with .22
  - end-stage (failure) N18.6
    - due to hypertension I12.Ø
  - fibrocystic (congenital) Q61.8
  - hypertensive — *see* Hypertension, kidney
  - lupus M32.14
  - phosphate-losing (tubular) N25.Ø
  - polycystic (congenital) Q61.3
    - adult type Q61.2
    - childhood type NEC Q61.19
      - collecting duct dilatation Q61.11
  - rapidly progressive NØ1.9
  - subacute NØ1.9
- Rendu-Osler-Weber (familial hemorrhagic telangiectasia) I78.Ø
- renovascular (arteriosclerotic) — *see* Hypertension, kidney
- respiratory (tract) J98.9
  - acute or subacute NOS JØ6.9
    - due to
      - chemicals, gases, fumes or vapors (inhalation) J68.3
      - external agent J7Ø.9
        - specified NEC J7Ø.8
      - radiation J7Ø.Ø
      - smoke inhalation J7Ø.5
    - noninfectious J39.8
  - chronic NOS J98.9
    - due to
      - chemicals, gases, fumes or vapors J68.4
      - external agent J7Ø.9
        - specified NEC J7Ø.8
      - radiation J7Ø.1
    - newborn P27.9
      - specified NEC P27.8
  - due to
    - chemicals, gases, fumes or vapors J68.9
      - acute or subacute NEC J68.3
      - chronic J68.4
    - external agent J7Ø.9
      - specified NEC J7Ø.8
  - newborn P28.9
    - specified type NEC P28.89
  - upper J39.9
    - acute or subacute JØ6.9
    - noninfectious NEC J39.8
    - specified NEC J39.8
    - streptococcal JØ6.9
- retina, retinal H35.9
  - Batten's or Batten-Mayou E75.4 *[H36]*
  - specified NEC H35.89
- rheumatoid — *see* Arthritis, rheumatoid

Disease, diseased — *continued*
- rickettsial NOS A79.9
  - specified type NEC A79.89
- Riga (-Fede) (cachectic aphthae) K14.Ø
- Riggs' (compound periodontitis) — *see* Periodontitis
- Ritter's LØØ
- Rivalta's (cervicofacial actinomycosis) A42.2
- Robles' (onchocerciasis) B73.Ø1
- Roger's (congenital interventricular septal defect) Q21.Ø
- Rosenthal's (factor XI deficiency) D68.1
- Rossbach's (hyperchlorhydria) K3Ø
- Ross River B33.1
- Rotes Quérol — *see* Hyperostosis, ankylosing
- Roth (-Bernhardt) — *see* Mononeuropathy, lower limb, meralgia paresthetica
- Runeberg's (progressive pernicious anemia) D51.Ø
- sacroiliac NEC M53.3
- salivary gland or duct K11.9
  - inclusion B25.9
  - specified NEC K11.8
  - virus B25.9
- sandworm B76.9
- Schimmelbusch's — *see* Mastopathy, cystic
- Schmorl's — *see* Schmorl's disease or nodes
- Schönlein (-Henoch) (purpura rheumatica) D69.Ø
- Schottmüller's — *see* Fever, paratyphoid
- Schultz's (agranulocytosis) — *see* Agranulocytosis
- Schwalbe-Ziehen-Oppenheim G24.1
- Schwartz-Jampel G71.13
- sclera H15.9
  - specified NEC H15.89
- scrofulous (tuberculous) A18.2
- scrotum N5Ø.9
- sebaceous glands L73.9
- semilunar cartilage, cystic (*see also* Derangement, knee, meniscus, cystic)
- seminal vesicle N5Ø.9
- serum NEC (*see also* Reaction, serum) T8Ø.69
- sexually transmitted A64
  - anogenital
    - herpesviral infection — *see* Herpes, anogenital
    - warts A63.Ø
  - chancroid A57
  - chlamydial infection — *see* Chlamydia
  - gonorrhea — *see* Gonorrhea
  - granuloma inguinale A58
  - specified organism NEC A63.8
  - syphilis — *see* Syphilis
  - trichomoniasis — *see* Trichmoniasis
- Sézary C84.1-
- shimamushi (scrub typhus) A75.3
- shipyard B3Ø.Ø
- sickle-cell D57.1
  - with crisis (vasoocclusive pain) D57.ØØ
    - with
      - acute chest syndrome D57.Ø1
      - splenic sequestration D57.Ø2
  - elliptocytosis D57.8-
  - Hb-C D57.2Ø
    - with crisis (vasoocclusive pain) D57.219
      - with
        - acute chest syndrome D57.211
        - splenic sequestration D57.212
    - without crisis D57.2Ø
  - Hb-SD D57.8Ø
    - with crisis D57.819
      - with
        - acute chest syndrome D57.811
        - splenic sequestration D57.812
  - Hb-SE D57.8Ø
    - with crisis D57.819
      - with
        - acute chest syndrome D57.811
        - splenic sequestration D57.812
  - specified NEC D57.8Ø
    - with crisis D57.819
      - with
        - acute chest syndrome D57.811
        - splenic sequestration D57.812
  - spherocytosis D57.8Ø
    - with crisis D57.819

Disease, diseased — *continued*
- Wilkinson-Sneddon (subcorneal pustular dermatosis) L13.1
- Willis' — *see* Diabetes
- Wilson's (hepatolenticular degeneration) E83.Ø1
- woolsorter's A22.1
- yaba monkey tumor BØ8.72
- yaba pox (virus) BØ8.72
- zoonotic, bacterial A28.9
  - specified type NEC A28.8

Disfigurement (due to scar) L9Ø.5

Disgerminoma — *see* Dysgerminoma

DISH (diffuse idiopathic skeletal hyperostosis) — *see* Hyperostosis, ankylosing

Disinsertion, retina — *see* Detachment, retina

Dislocatable hip, congenital Q65.6

Dislocation (articular)
- with fracture — *see* Fracture
- acromioclavicular (joint) S43.1Ø-
  - with displacement
    - 1ØØ%-2ØØ% S43.12-
    - more than 2ØØ% S43.13-
  - inferior S43.14-
  - posterior S43.15-
- ankle S93.Ø-
- astragalus — *see* Dislocation, ankle
- atlantoaxial S13.121
- atlantooccipital S13.111
- atloidooccipital S13.111
- breast bone S23.29
- capsule, joint—code by site under Dislocation
- carpal (bone) — *see* Dislocation, wrist
- carpometacarpal (joint) NEC S63.Ø5-
  - thumb S63.Ø4-
- cartilage (joint)—code by site under Dislocation
- cervical spine (vertebra) — *see* Dislocation, vertebra, cervical
- chronic — *see* Dislocation, recurrent
- clavicle — *see* Dislocation, acromioclavicular joint
- coccyx S33.2
- congenital NEC Q68.8
- coracoid — *see* Dislocation, shoulder
- costal cartilage S23.29
- costochondral S23.29
- cricoarytenoid articulation S13.29
- cricothyroid articulation S13.29
- dorsal vertebra — *see* Dislocation, vertebra, thoracic
- ear ossicle — *see* Discontinuity, ossicles, ear
- elbow S53.1Ø-
  - congenital Q68.8
  - pathological — *see* Dislocation, pathological NEC, elbow
  - radial head alone — *see* Dislocation, radial head
  - recurrent — *see* Dislocation, recurrent, elbow
  - traumatic S53.1Ø-
    - anterior S53.11-
    - lateral S53.14-
    - medial S53.13-
    - posterior S53.12-
    - specified type NEC S53.19-
- eye, nontraumatic — *see* Luxation, globe
- eyeball, nontraumatic — *see* Luxation, globe
- femur
  - distal end — *see* Dislocation, knee
  - proximal end — *see* Dislocation, hip
- fibula
  - distal end — *see* Dislocation, ankle
  - proximal end — *see* Dislocation, knee
- finger S63.25-
  - index S63.25-
  - interphalangeal S63.27-
    - distal S63.29-
      - index S63.29-
      - little S63.29-
      - middle S63.29-
      - ring S63.29-
    - index S63.27-
    - little S63.27-
    - middle S63.27-
    - proximal S63.28-
      - index S63.28-
      - little S63.28-
      - middle S63.28-

Dislocation — *continued*
- finger— *continued*
  - interphalangeal— *continued*
    - proximal— *continued*
      - ring S63.28-
    - ring S63.27-
  - little S63.25-
  - metacarpophalangeal S63.26-
    - index S63.26-
    - little S63.26-
    - middle S63.26-
    - ring S63.26-
  - middle S63.25-
  - recurrent — *see* Dislocation, recurrent, finger
  - ring S63.25-
  - thumb — *see* Dislocation, thumb
- foot S93.3Ø-
  - recurrent — *see* Dislocation, recurrent, foot
  - specified site NEC S93.33-
  - tarsal joint S93.31-
  - tarsometatarsal joint S93.32-
  - toe — *see* Dislocation, toe
- fracture — *see* Fracture
- glenohumeral (joint) — *see* Dislocation, shoulder
- glenoid — *see* Dislocation, shoulder
- habitual — *see* Dislocation, recurrent
- hip S73.ØØ-
  - anterior S73.Ø3-
    - obturator S73.Ø2-
  - central S73.Ø4-
  - congenital (total) Q65.2
    - bilateral Q65.1
    - partial Q65.5
      - bilateral Q65.4
      - unilateral Q65.3-
    - unilateral Q65.Ø-
  - developmental M24.85-
  - pathological — *see* Dislocation, pathological NEC, hip
  - posterior S73.Ø1-
  - recurrent — *see* Dislocation, recurrent, hip
- humerus, proximal end — *see* Dislocation, shoulder
- incomplete — *see* Subluxation, by site
- incus — *see* Discontinuity, ossicles, ear
- infracoracoid — *see* Dislocation, shoulder
- innominate (pubic junction) (sacral junction) S33.39
  - acetabulum — *see* Dislocation, hip
- interphalangeal (joint(s))
  - finger S63.279
    - distal S63.29-
      - index S63.29-
      - little S63.29-
      - middle S63.29-
      - ring S63.29-
    - index S63.27-
    - little S63.27-
    - middle S63.27-
    - proximal S63.28-
      - index S63.28-
      - little S63.28-
      - middle S63.28-
      - ring S63.28-
    - ring S63.27-
  - foot or toe — *see* Dislocation, toe
  - thumb S63.12-
    - distal joint S63.14-
    - proximal joint S63.13-
- jaw (cartilage) (meniscus) SØ3.Ø
- joint prosthesis — *see* Complications, joint prosthesis, mechanical, displacement, by site
- knee S83.1Ø6
  - cap — *see* Dislocation, patella
  - congenital Q68.2
  - old M23.8X-
  - patella — *see* Dislocation, patella
  - pathological — *see* Dislocation, pathological NEC, knee
  - proximal tibia
    - anteriorly S83.11-
    - laterally S83.14-
    - medially S83.13-
    - posteriorly S83.12-

Dislocation — *continued*
- knee— *continued*
  - recurrent (*see also* Derangement, knee, specified NEC)
    - specified type NEC S83.19-
- lacrimal gland HØ4.16-
- lens (complete) H27.1Ø-
  - anterior H27.12-
  - congenital Q12.1
  - ocular implant — *see* Complications, intraocular lens
  - partial H27.11-
  - posterior H27.13-
  - traumatic SØ5.8X-
- ligament—code by site under Dislocation
- lumbar (vertebra) — *see* Dislocation, vertebra, lumbar
- lumbosacral (vertebra) (*see also* Dislocation, vertebra, lumbar)
  - congenital Q76.49
- mandible SØ3.Ø
- meniscus (knee) — *see* Tear, meniscus
- other sites—code by site under Dislocation
- metacarpal (bone)
  - distal end — *see* Dislocation, finger
  - proximal end S63.Ø6-
- metacarpophalangeal (joint)
  - finger S63.26-
    - index S63.26-
    - little S63.26-
    - middle S63.26-
    - ring S63.26-
  - thumb S63.11-
- metatarsal (bone) — *see* Dislocation, foot
- metatarsophalangeal (joint(s)) — *see* Dislocation, toe
- midcarpal (joint) S63.Ø3-
- midtarsal (joint) — *see* Dislocation, foot
- neck S13.2Ø
  - specified site NEC S13.29
  - vertebra — *see* Dislocation, vertebra, cervical
- nose (septal cartilage) SØ3.1
- occipitoatloid S13.111
- old — *see* Derangement, joint, specified type NEC
- ossicles, ear — *see* Discontinuity, ossicles, ear
- partial — *see* Subluxation, by site
- patella S83.ØØ6
  - congenital Q74.1
  - lateral S83.Ø1-
  - recurrent (nontraumatic) M22.Ø-
    - incomplete M22.1-
  - specified type NEC S83.Ø9-
- pathological NEC M24.3Ø
  - ankle M24.37-
  - elbow M24.32-
  - foot joint M24.37-
  - hand joint M24.34-
  - hip M24.35-
  - knee M24.36-
  - lumbosacral joint — *see* subcategory M53.2
  - pelvic region — *see* Dislocation, pathological, hip
  - sacroiliac — *see* subcategory M53.2
  - shoulder M24.31-
  - wrist M24.33-
- pelvis NEC S33.3Ø
  - specified NEC S33.39
- phalanx
  - finger or hand — *see* Dislocation, finger
  - foot or toe — *see* Dislocation, toe
- prosthesis, internal — *see* Complications, prosthetic device, by site, mechanical
- radial head S53.ØØ6
  - anterior S53.Ø1-
  - posterior S53.Ø2-
  - specified type NEC S53.Ø9-
- radiocarpal (joint) S63.Ø2-
- radiohumeral (joint) — *see* Dislocation, radial head
- radioulnar (joint)
  - distal S63.Ø1-
  - proximal — *see* Dislocation, elbow
- radius
  - distal end — *see* Dislocation, wrist
  - proximal end — *see* Dislocation, radial head

- **Dislocation** —*continued*
  - recurrent M24.4Ø
    - ankle M24.47-
    - elbow M24.42-
    - finger M24.44-
    - foot joint M24.47-
    - hand joint M24.44-
    - hip M24.45-
    - knee M24.46-
      - patella — *see* Dislocation, patella, recurrent
    - patella — *see* Dislocation, patella, recurrent
    - sacroiliac — *see* subcategory M53.2
    - shoulder M24.41-
    - toe M24.47-
    - vertebra (*see also* subcategory) M43.5
      - atlantoaxial M43.4
        - with myelopathy M43.3
    - wrist M24.43-
  - rib (cartilage) S23.29
  - sacrococcygeal S33.2
  - sacroiliac (joint) (ligament) S33.2
    - congenital Q74.2
    - recurrent — *see* subcategory M53.2
  - sacrum S33.2
  - scaphoid (bone) (hand) (wrist) — *see* Dislocation, wrist
    - foot — *see* Dislocation, foot
  - scapula — *see* Dislocation, shoulder, girdle, scapula
  - semilunar cartilage, knee — *see* Tear, meniscus
  - septal cartilage (nose) SØ3.1
  - septum (nasal) (old) J34.2
  - sesamoid bone—code by site under Dislocation
  - shoulder (blade) (ligament) (joint) (traumatic) S43.ØØ6
    - acromioclavicular — *see* Dislocation, acromioclavicular
    - chronic — *see* Dislocation, recurrent, shoulder
    - congenital Q68.8
    - girdle S43.3Ø-
      - scapula S43.31-
      - specified site NEC S43.39-
    - humerus S43.ØØ-
      - anterior S43.Ø1-
      - inferior S43.Ø3-
      - posterior S43.Ø2-
    - pathological — *see* Dislocation, pathological NEC, shoulder
    - recurrent — *see* Dislocation, recurrent, shoulder
    - specified type NEC S43.Ø8-
  - spine
    - cervical — *see* Dislocation, vertebra, cervical
    - congenital Q76.49
    - due to birth trauma P11.5
    - lumbar — *see* Dislocation, vertebra, lumbar
    - thoracic — *see* Dislocation, vertebra, thoracic
  - spontaneous — *see* Dislocation, pathological
  - sternoclavicular (joint) S43.2Ø6
    - anterior S43.21-
    - posterior S43.22-
  - sternum S23.29
  - subglenoid — *see* Dislocation, shoulder
  - symphysis pubis S33.4
  - talus — *see* Dislocation, ankle
  - tarsal (bone(s)) (joint(s)) — *see* Dislocation, foot
  - tarsometatarsal (joint(s)) — *see* Dislocation, foot
  - temporomandibular (joint) SØ3.Ø
  - thigh, proximal end — *see* Dislocation, hip
  - thorax S23.2Ø
    - specified site NEC S23.29
    - vertebra — *see* Dislocation, vertebra
  - thumb S63.1Ø-
    - interphalangeal joint — *see* Dislocation, interphalangeal (joint), thumb
    - metacarpophalangeal joint — *see* Dislocation, metacarpophalangeal (joint), thumb
  - thyroid cartilage S13.29
  - tibia
    - distal end — *see* Dislocation, ankle
    - proximal end — *see* Dislocation, knee
  - tibiofibular (joint)
    - distal — *see* Dislocation, ankle
    - superior — *see* Dislocation, knee

- **Dislocation** —*continued*
  - toe(s) S93.1Ø6
    - great S93.1Ø-
      - interphalangeal joint S93.11-
      - metatarsophalangeal joint S93.12-
    - interphalangeal joint S93.119
    - lesser S93.1Ø6
      - interphalangeal joint S93.11-
      - metatarsophalangeal joint S93.12-
    - metatarsophalangeal joint S93.12-
  - tooth SØ3.2
  - trachea S23.29
  - ulna
    - distal end S63.Ø7-
    - proximal end — *see* Dislocation, elbow
  - ulnohumeral (joint) — *see* Dislocation, elbow
  - vertebra (articular process) (body) (traumatic)
    - cervical S13.1Ø1
      - atlantoaxial joint S13.121
      - atlantooccipital joint S13.111
      - atloidooccipital joint S13.111
      - joint between
        - CØ and C1 S13.111
        - C1 and C2 S13.121
        - C2 and C3 S13.131
        - C3 and C4 S13.141
        - C4 and C5 S13.151
        - C5and C6 S13.161
        - C6and C7 S13.171
        - C7and T1 S13.181
      - occipitoatloid joint S13.111
    - congenital Q76.49
    - lumbar S33.1Ø1
      - joint between
        - L1and L2 S33.111
        - L2and L3 S33.121
        - L3 and L4 S33.131
        - L4and L5 S33.141
    - nontraumatic — *see* Displacement, intervertebral disc
    - partial — *see* Subluxation, by site
    - recurrent NEC — *see* subcategory M43.5
    - thoracic S23.1Ø1
      - joint between
        - T1 and T2 S23.111
        - T2 and T3 S23.121
        - T3 and T4 S23.123
        - T4 and T5 S23.131
        - T5 and T6 S23.133
        - T6 and T7 S23.141
        - T7 and T8 S23.143
        - T8 and T9 S23.151
        - T9 and T1Ø S23.153
        - T1Ø and T11 S23.161
        - T11 and T12 S23.163
        - T12 and L1 S23.171
  - wrist (carpal bone) S63.ØØ6
    - carpometacarpal joint — *see* Dislocation, carpometacarpal (joint)
    - distal radioulnar joint — *see* Dislocation, radioulnar (joint), distal
    - metacarpal bone, proximal — *see* Dislocation, metacarpal (bone), proximal end
    - midcarpal — *see* Dislocation, midcarpal (joint)
    - radiocarpal joint — *see* Dislocation, radiocarpal (joint)
    - recurrent — *see* Dislocation, recurrent, wrist
    - specified site NEC S63.Ø9-
    - ulna — *see* Dislocation, ulna, distal end
  - xiphoid cartilage S23.29
- **Disorder** (of) (*see also* Disease)
  - acantholytic L11.9
    - specified NEC L11.8
  - acute
    - psychotic — *see* Psychosis, acute
    - stress F43.Ø
  - adjustment (grief) F43.2Ø
    - with
      - anxiety F43.22
        - with depressed mood F43.23
      - conduct disturbance F43.24
        - with emotional disturbance F43.25
      - depressed mood F43.21

- **Disorder** —*continued*
  - adjustment—*continued*
    - with—*continued*
      - depressed mood—*continued*
        - with anxiety F43.23
      - other specified symptom F43.29
  - adrenal (capsule) (gland) (medullary) E27.9
    - specified NEC E27.8
  - adrenogenital E25.9
    - drug-induced E25.8
    - iatrogenic E25.8
    - idiopathic E25.8
  - adult personality (and behavior) F69
    - specified NEC F68.8
  - affective (mood) — *see* Disorder, mood
  - aggressive, unsocialized F91.1
  - alcohol-related F1Ø.99
    - with
      - amnestic disorder, persisting F1Ø.96
      - anxiety disorder F1Ø.98Ø
      - dementia, persisting F1Ø.97
      - intoxication F1Ø.929
        - with delirium F1Ø.921
        - uncomplicated F1Ø.92Ø
      - mood disorder F1Ø.94
      - other specified F1Ø.988
      - psychotic disorder F1Ø.959
        - with
          - delusions F1Ø.95Ø
          - hallucinations F1Ø.951
      - sexual dysfunction F1Ø.981
      - sleep disorder F1Ø.982
  - allergic — *see* Allergy
  - alveolar NEC J84.Ø9
  - amino-acid
    - cystathioninuria E72.19
    - cystinosis E72.Ø4
    - cystinuria E72.Ø1
    - glycinuria E72.Ø9
    - homocystinuria E72.11
    - metabolism — *see* Disturbance, metabolism, amino-acid
    - specified NEC E72.8
    - neonatal, transitory P74.8
    - renal transport NEC E72.Ø9
    - transport NEC E72.Ø9
  - amnesic, amnestic
    - alcohol-induced F1Ø.96
      - with dependence F1Ø.26
    - due to (secondary to) general medical condition FØ4
    - psychoactive NEC-induced F19.96
      - with
        - abuse F19.16
        - dependence F19.26
    - sedative, hypnotic or anxiolytic-induced F13.96
      - with dependence F13.26
  - anaerobic glycolysis with anemia D55.2
  - anxiety F41.9
    - due to (secondary to)
      - alcohol F1Ø.98Ø
      - amphetamine F15.98Ø
        - in
          - abuse F15.18Ø
          - dependence F15.28Ø
      - anxiolytic F13.98Ø
        - in
          - abuse F13.18Ø
          - dependence F13.28Ø
      - caffeine F15.98Ø
        - in
          - abuse F15.18Ø
          - dependence F15.28Ø
      - cannabis F12.98Ø
        - in
          - abuse F12.18Ø
          - dependence F12.28Ø
      - cocaine F14.98Ø
        - in
          - abuse F14.18Ø
          - dependence F14.18Ø
      - general medical condition FØ6.4
      - hallucinogen F16.98Ø

- **Disorder** — *continued*
  - anxiety— *continued*
    - due to— *continued*
      - hallucinogen— *continued*
        - in
          - abuse F16.180
          - dependence F16.280
      - hypnotic F13.980
        - in
          - abuse F13.180
          - dependence F13.280
      - inhalant F18.980
        - in
          - abuse F18.180
          - dependence F18.280
      - phencyclidine F16.980
        - in
          - abuse F16.180
          - dependence F16.280
      - psychoactive substance NEC F19.980
        - in
          - abuse F19.180
          - dependence F19.280
      - sedative F13.980
        - in
          - abuse F13.180
          - dependence F13.280
      - volatile solvents F18.980
        - in
          - abuse F18.180
          - dependence F18.280
    - generalized F41.1
    - mixed
      - with depression (mild) F41.8
      - specified NEC F41.3
    - organic F06.4
    - phobic F40.9
      - of childhood F40.8
    - specified NEC F41.8
  - aortic valve — *see* Endocarditis, aortic
  - aromatic amino-acid metabolism E70.9
    - specified NEC E70.8
  - arteriole NEC I77.89
  - artery NEC I77.89
  - articulation — *see* Disorder, joint
  - attachment (childhood)
    - disinhibited F94.2
    - reactive F94.1
  - attention-deficit hyperactivity (adolescent) (adult) (child) F90.9
    - combined type F90.2
    - hyperactive type F90.1
    - inattentive type F90.0
    - specified type NEC F90.8
  - attention-deficit without hyperactivity (adolescent) (adult) (child) F90.0
  - auditory processing (central) H93.25
  - autistic F84.0
  - autonomic nervous system G90.9
    - specified NEC G90.8
  - avoidant, child or adolescent F40.10
  - balance
    - acid-base E87.8
      - mixed E87.4
    - electrolyte E87.8
    - fluid NEC E87.8
  - behavioral (disruptive) — *see* Disorder, conduct
  - beta-amino-acid metabolism E72.8
  - bile acid and cholesterol metabolism E78.70
    - Barth syndrome E78.71
    - other specified E78.79
    - Smith-Lemli-Opitz syndrome E78.72
  - bilirubin excretion E80.6
  - binocular
    - movement H51.9
      - convergence
        - excess H51.12
        - insufficiency H51.11
      - internuclear ophthalmoplegia — *see* Ophthalmoplegia, internuclear
      - palsy of conjugate gaze H51.0
      - specified type NEC H51.8
    - vision NEC — *see* Disorder, vision, binocular

- **Disorder** — *continued*
  - bipolar (I) F31.9
    - current episode
      - depressed F31.9
        - with psychotic features F31.5
        - without psychotic features F31.30
          - mild F31.31
          - moderate F31.32
          - severe (without psychotic features) F31.4
            - with psychotic features F31.5
      - hypomanic F31.0
      - manic F31.9
        - with psychotic features F31.2
        - without psychotic features F31.10
          - mild F31.11
          - moderate F31.12
          - severe (without psychotic features) F31.13
            - with psychotic features F31.2
      - mixed F31.60
        - mild F31.61
        - moderate F31.62
        - severe (without psychotic features) F31.63
          - with psychotic features F31.64
      - severe depression (without psychotic features) F31.4
        - with psychotic features F31.5
    - in remission (currently) F31.70
      - in full remission
        - most recent episode
          - depressed F31.76
          - hypomanic F31.72
          - manic F31.74
          - mixed F31.78
      - in partial remission
        - most recent episode
          - depressed F31.75
          - hypomanic F31.71
          - manic F31.73
          - mixed F31.77
    - organic F06.30
    - single manic episode F30.9
      - mild F30.11
      - moderate F30.12
      - severe (without psychotic symptoms) F30.13
        - with psychotic symptoms F30.2
    - specified NEC F31.89
  - bipolar II F31.81
  - bladder N32.9
    - functional NEC N31.9
    - in schistosomiasis B65.0 *[N33]*
    - specified NEC N32.89
  - bleeding D68.9
  - blood D75.9
    - in congenital early syphilis A50.09 *[D77]*
  - body dysmorphic F45.22
  - bone M89.9
    - continuity M84.9
      - specified type NEC M84.80
        - ankle M84.87-
        - fibula M84.86-
        - foot M84.87-
        - hand M84.84-
        - humerus M84.82-
        - neck M84.88
        - pelvis M84.859
        - radius M84.83-
        - rib M84.88
        - shoulder M84.81-
        - skull M84.88
        - thigh M84.85-
        - tibia M84.86-
        - ulna M84.83-
        - vertebra M84.88
    - density and structure M85.9
      - cyst (*see also* Cyst, bone, specified type NEC)
        - aneurysmal — *see* Cyst, bone, aneurysmal
        - solitary — *see* Cyst, bone, solitary
      - diffuse idiopathic skeletal hyperostosis — *see* Hyperostosis, ankylosing
      - fibrous dysplasia (monostotic) — *see* Dysplasia, fibrous, bone

- **Disorder** — *continued*
  - bone— *continued*
    - density and structure— *continued*
      - fluorosis — *see* Fluorosis, skeletal
      - hyperostosis of skull M85.2
      - osteitis condensans — *see* Osteitis, condensans
      - specified type NEC M85.8-
        - ankle M85.87-
        - foot M85.87-
        - forearm M85.83-
        - hand M85.84-
        - lower leg M85.86-
        - multiple sites M85.89
        - neck M85.88
        - rib M85.88
        - shoulder M85.81-
        - skull M85.88
        - thigh M85.85-
        - upper arm M85.82-
        - vertebra M85.88
    - development and growth NEC M89.20
      - carpus M89.24-
      - clavicle M89.21-
      - femur M89.25-
      - fibula M89.26-
      - finger M89.24-
      - humerus M89.22-
      - ilium M89.259
      - ischium M89.259
      - metacarpus M89.24-
      - metatarsus M89.27-
      - multiple sites M89.29
      - neck M89.28
      - radius M89.23-
      - rib M89.28
      - scapula M89.21-
      - skull M89.28
      - tarsus M89.27-
      - tibia M89.26-
      - toe M89.27-
      - ulna M89.23-
      - vertebra M89.28
    - specified type NEC M89.8X-
  - brachial plexus G54.0
  - branched-chain amino-acid metabolism E71.2
    - specified NEC E71.19
  - breast N64.9
    - agalactia — *see* Agalactia
    - associated with
      - lactation O92.70
        - specified NEC O92.79
      - pregnancy O92.20
        - specified NEC O92.29
      - puerperium O92.20
        - specified NEC O92.29
    - cracked nipple — *see* Cracked nipple
    - galactorrhea *see* Galactorrhea
    - hypogalactia O92.4
    - lactation disorder NEC O92.79
    - mastitis — *see* Mastitis
    - nipple infection — *see* Infection, nipple
    - retracted nipple — *see* Retraction, nipple
    - specified type NEC N64.89
  - Briquet's F45.0
  - bullous, in diseases classified elsewhere L14
  - cannabis use
    - due to drug abuse — *see* Abuse, drug, cannabis
    - due to drug dependence — *see* Dependend, drug, cannabis
  - carbohydrate
    - absorption, intestinal NEC E74.39
    - metabolism (congenital) E74.9
      - specified NEC E74.8
  - cardiac, functional I51.89
  - carnitine metabolism E71.40
  - cartilage M94.9
    - articular NEC — *see* Derangement, joint, articular cartilage
      - chondrocalcinosis — *see* Chondrocalcinosis
    - specified type NEC M94.8X-
      - articular — *see* Derangement, joint, articular cartilage

- **Disorder** — *continued*
  - cartilage— *continued*
    - specified type NEC— *continued-*
      - multiple sites M94.8XØ
  - catatonic
    - due to (secondary to) known physiological condition FØ6.1
    - organic FØ6.1
  - central auditory processing H93.25
  - cervical
    - region NEC M53.82
    - root (nerve) NEC G54.2
  - character NOS F6Ø.9
  - childhood disintegrative NEC F84.3
  - cholesterol and bile acid metabolism E78.7Ø
    - Barth syndrome E78.71
    - other specified E78.79
    - Smith-Lemli-Opitz syndrome E78.72
  - choroid H31.9
    - atrophy — *see* Atrophy, choroid
    - degeneration — *see* Degeneration, choroid
    - detachment — *see* Detachment, choroid
    - dystrophy — *see* Dystrophy, choroid
    - hemorrhage — *see* Hemorrhage, choroid
    - rupture — *see* Rupture, choroid
    - scar — *see* Scar, chorioretinal
    - solar retinopathy — *see* Retinopathy, solar
    - specified type NEC H31.8
  - ciliary body — *see* Disorder, iris
    - degeneration — *see* Degeneration, ciliary body
  - coagulation (factor) (*see also* Defect, coagulation) D68.9
    - newborn, transient P61.6
  - coccyx NEC M53.3
  - cognitive FØ9
    - due to (secondary to) general medical condition FØ9
    - persisting R41.89
      - due to
        - alcohol F1Ø.97
          - with dependence F1Ø.27
        - anxiolytics F13.97
          - with dependence F13.27
        - hypnotics F13.97
          - with dependence F13.27
        - sedatives F13.97
          - with dependence F13.27
        - specified substance NEC F19.97
          - with
            - abuse F19.17
            - dependence F19.27
  - communication F8Ø.9
  - conduct (childhood) F91.9
    - adjustment reaction — *see* Disorder, adjustment
    - adolescent onset type F91.2
    - childhood onset type F91.1
    - compulsive F63.9
    - confined to family context F91.Ø
    - depressive F91.8
    - group type F91.2
    - hyperkinetic — *see* Disorder, attention-deficit hyperactivity
    - oppositional defiance F91.3
    - socialized F91.2
    - solitary aggressive type F91.1
    - specified NEC F91.8
    - unsocialized (aggressive) F91.1
  - conduction, heart I45.9
  - congenital glycosylation (CDG) E74.8
  - conjunctiva H11.9
    - infection — *see* Conjunctivitis
  - connective tissue, localized L94.9
    - specified NEC L94.8
  - conversion — *see* Disorder, dissociative
  - convulsive (secondary) — *see* Convulsions
  - cornea H18.9
    - deformity — *see* Deformity, cornea
    - degeneration — *see* Degeneration, cornea
    - deposits — *see* Deposit, cornea
    - due to contact lens H18.82-
      - specified as edema — *see* Edema, cornea
    - edema — *see* Edema, cornea
    - keratitis — *see* Keratitis

- **Disorder** — *continued*
  - cornea— *continued*
    - keratoconjunctivitis — *see* Keratoconjunctivitis
    - membrane change — *see* Change, corneal membrane
    - neovascularization — *see* Neovascularization, cornea
    - scar — *see* Opacity, cornea
    - specified type NEC H18.89-
    - ulcer — *see* Ulcer, cornea
  - corpus cavernosum N48.9
  - cranial nerve — *see* Disorder, nerve, cranial
  - cyclothymic F34.Ø
  - defiant oppositional F91.3
  - delusional (persistent) (systematized) F22
    - induced F24
  - depersonalization F48.1
  - depressive F32.9
    - major F32.9
      - with psychotic symptoms F32.3
      - in remission (full) F32.5
        - partial F32.4
      - recurrent F33.9
      - single episode F32.9
        - mild F32.Ø
        - moderate F32.1
        - severe (without psychotic symptoms) F32.2
          - with psychotic symptoms F32.3
    - organic FØ6.31
    - recurrent F33.9
      - current episode
        - mild F33.Ø
        - moderate F33.1
        - severe (without psychotic symptoms) F33.2
          - with psychotic symptoms F33.3
      - in remission F33.4Ø
        - full F33.42
        - partial F33.41
      - specified NEC F33.8
    - single episode — *see* Episode, depressive
  - developmental F89
    - arithmetical skills F81.2
    - coordination (motor) F82
    - expressive writing F81.81
    - language F8Ø.9
      - expressive F8Ø.1
      - mixed receptive and expressive F8Ø.2
      - receptive type F8Ø.2
      - specified NEC F8Ø.89
    - learning F81.9
      - arithmetical F81.2
      - reading F81.Ø
    - mixed F88
    - motor coordination or function F82
    - pervasive F84.9
      - specified NEC F84.8
    - phonological F8Ø.Ø
    - reading F81.Ø
    - scholastic skills (*see also* Disorder, learning)
      - mixed F81.89
    - specified NEC F88
    - speech F8Ø.9
      - articulation F8Ø.Ø
      - specified NEC F8Ø.89
    - written expression F81.81
  - diaphragm J98.6
  - digestive (system) K92.9
    - newborn P78.9
      - specified NEC P78.89
    - postprocedural — *see* Complication, gastrointestinal
    - psychogenic F45.8
  - disc (intervertebral) M51.9
    - with
      - myelopathy
        - cervical region M5Ø.ØØ
        - cervicothoracic region M5Ø.Ø3
        - lumbar region M51.Ø6
        - lumbosacral region M51.Ø7
        - mid-cervical region M5Ø.Ø2
        - occipito-atlanto-axial region M5Ø.Ø1

- **Disorder** — *continued*
  - disc— *continued*
    - with— *continued*
      - myelopathy— *continued*
        - sacrococcygeal region M53.3
        - thoracic region M51.Ø4
        - thoracolumbar region M51.Ø5
      - radiculopathy
        - cervical region M5Ø.1Ø
        - cervicothoracic region M5Ø.13
        - lumbar region M51.16
        - lumbosacral region M51.17
        - mid-cervical region M5Ø.12
        - occipito-atlanto-axial region M5Ø.11
        - sacrococcygeal region M53.3
        - thoracic region M51.14
        - thoracolumbar region M51.15
    - cervical M5Ø.9Ø
      - with
        - myelopathy M5Ø.ØØ
          - cervicothoracic region M5Ø.Ø3
          - mid-cervical region M5Ø.Ø2
          - occipito-atlanto-axial region M5Ø.Ø1
        - neuritis, radiculitis or radiculopathy M5Ø.1Ø
          - cervicothoracic region M5Ø.13
          - mid-cervical region M5Ø.12
          - occipito-atlanto-axial region M5Ø.11
      - cervicothoracic region M5Ø.93
      - degeneration M5Ø.3Ø
        - cervicothoracic region M5Ø.33
        - mid-cervical region M5Ø.32
        - occipito-atlanto-axial region M5Ø.31
      - displacement M5Ø.2Ø
        - cervicothoracic region M5Ø.23
        - mid-cervical region M5Ø.22
        - occipito-atlanto-axial region M5Ø.21
      - mid-cervical region M5Ø.92
      - occipito-atlanto-axial region M5Ø.91
      - specified type NEC M5Ø.8Ø
        - cervicothoracic region M5Ø.83
        - mid-cervical region M5Ø.82
        - occipito-atlanto-axial region M5Ø.81
    - specified NEC
      - lumbar region M51.86
      - lumbosacral region M51.87
      - sacrococcygeal region M53.3
      - thoracic region M51.84
      - thoracolumbar region M51.85
  - disinhibited attachment (childhood) F94.2
  - disintegrative, childhood NEC F84.3
  - disruptive behavior F98.9
  - dissocial personality F6Ø.2
  - dissociative F44.9
    - affecting
      - motor function F44.4
        - and sensation F44.7
      - sensation F44.6
        - and motor function F44.7
    - brief reactive F43.Ø
    - due to (secondary to) general medical condition FØ6.8
    - mixed F44.7
    - organic FØ6.8
    - other specified NEC F44.89
  - double heterozygous sickling See Disease, sickle-cell
  - dream anxiety F51.5
  - drug induced hemorrhagic D68.32
  - drug related F19.99
    - abuse — *see* Abuse, drug
    - dependence — *see* Dependence, drug
  - dysmorphic body F45.1
  - dysthymic F34.1
  - ear H93.9-
    - bleeding — *see* Otorrhagia
    - deafness — *see* Deafness
    - degenerative H93.Ø9-
    - discharge — *see* Otorrhea
    - external H61.9-
      - auditory canal stenosis — *see* Stenosis, external ear canal
      - exostosis — *see* Exostosis, external ear canal

- **Disorder** — *continued*
  - ear— *continued*
    - external— *continued*
      - impacted cerumen — *see* Impaction, cerumen
      - otitis — *see* Otitis, externa
      - perichondritis — *see* Perichondritis, ear
      - pinna — *see* Disorder, pinna
      - specified type NEC H61.89-
    - inner H83.9-
      - vestibular dysfunction — *see* Disorder, vestibular function
    - middle H74.9-
      - adhesive H74.1-
      - ossicle — *see* Abnormal, ear ossicles
      - polyp — *see* Polyp, ear (middle)
      - specified NEC, in diseases classified elsewhere H75.8-
    - postprocedural — *see* Complications, ear, procedure
    - specified NEC, in diseases classified elsewhere H94.8
  - eating (adult) (psychogenic) F5Ø.9
    - anorexia — *see* Anorexia
    - bulimia F5Ø.2
    - child F98.29
      - pica F98.3
      - rumination disorder F98.21
    - pica F5Ø.8
      - childhood F98.3
  - electrolyte (balance) NEC E87.8
    - with
      - abortion — *see* Abortion by type complicated by specified condition NEC
      - ectopic pregnancy OØ8.5
      - molar pregnancy OØ8.5
    - acidosis (metabolic) (respiratory) E87.2
    - alkalosis (metabolic) (respiratory) E87.3
  - elimination, transepidermal L87.9
    - specified NEC L87.8
  - emotional (persistent) F34.9
    - of childhood F93.9
      - specified NEC F93.8
  - endocrine E34.9
    - postprocedural E89.89
      - specified NEC E89.89
  - erectile (male) (organic) (*see also* Dysfunction, sexual, male, erectile) N52.9
    - nonorganic F52.21
  - erythematous — *see* Erythema
  - esophagus K22.9
    - functional K22.4
    - psychogenic F45.8
  - eustachian tube H69.9-
    - infection — *see* Salpingitis, eustachian
    - obstruction — *see* Obstruction, eustachian tube
    - patulous — *see* Patulous, eustachian tube
    - specified NEC H69.8-
  - extrapyramidal G25.9
    - specified type NEC G25.89
  - eye H57.9
    - postprocedural *see* Complication, postprocedural, eye
  - eyelid HØ2.9
    - cyst — *see* Cyst, eyelid
    - degenerative HØ2.7Ø
      - chloasma — *see* Chloasma, eyelid
      - madarosis — *see* Madarosis
      - specified type NEC HØ2.79
      - vitiligo — *see* Vitiligo, eyelid
      - xanthelasma — *see* Xanthelasma
    - dermatochalasis — *see* Dermatochalasis
    - edema — *see* Edema, eyelid
    - elephantiasis — *see* Elephantiasis, eyelid
    - foreign body, retained — *see* Foreign body, retained, eyelid
    - function HØ2.59
      - abnormal innervation syndrome — *see* Syndrome, abnormal innervation
      - blepharochalasis — *see* Blepharochalasis
      - blepharoclonus — *see* Blepharoclonus
      - blepharophimosis — *see* Blepharophimosis
      - blepharoptosis — *see* Blepharoptosis
      - lagophthalmos — *see* Lagophthalmos

- **Disorder** — *continued*
  - eyelid— *continued*
    - function— *continued*
      - lid retraction — *see* Retraction, lid
    - hypertrichosis — *see* Hypertrichosis, eyelid
    - specified type NEC HØ2.89
    - vascular HØ2.879
      - left HØ2.876
        - lower HØ2.875
        - upper HØ2.874
      - right HØ2.873
        - lower HØ2.872
        - upper HØ2.871
  - factitious F68.1Ø
    - with predominantly
      - psychological symptoms F68.11
        - with physical symptoms F68.13
      - physical symptoms F68.12
        - with psychological symptoms F68.13
  - factor, coagulation — *see* Defect, coagulation
  - fatty acid
    - metabolism E71.3Ø
      - specified NEC E71.39
    - oxidation
      - LCAD E71.31Ø
      - MCAD E71.311
      - SCAD E71.312
      - specified deficiency NEC E71.318
  - feeding (infant or child) (*see also* Disorder, eating) R63.3-
  - feigned (with obvious motivation) Z76.5
    - without obvious motivation — *see* Disorder, factitious
  - female
    - hypoactive sexual desire F52.Ø
    - orgasmic F52.31
    - sexual arousal F52.22
  - fibroblastic M72.9
    - specified NEC M72.8
  - fluency
    - adult onset F98.5
    - childhood onset F8Ø.81
    - following
      - cerebral infarction I69.323
      - cerebrovascular disease I69.923
        - specified disease NEC I69.823
      - intracerebral hemorrhage I69.123
      - nontraumatic intracranial hemorrhage NEC I69.223
      - subarachnoid hemorrhage I69.Ø23
    - in conditions classified elsewhere R47.82
  - fluid balance E87.8
  - follicular (skin) L73.9
    - specified NEC L73.8
  - fructose metabolism E74.1Ø
    - essential fructosuria E74.11
    - fructokinase deficiency E74.11
    - fructose-1, 6-diphosphatase deficiency E74.19
    - hereditary fructose intolerance E74.12
    - other specified E74.19
  - functional polymorphonuclear neutrophils D71
  - gallbladder, biliary tract and pancreas in diseases classified elsewhere K87
  - gamma-glutamyl cycle E72.8
  - gastric (functional) K31.9
    - motility K3Ø
    - psychogenic F45.8
    - secretion K3Ø
  - gastrointestinal (functional) NOS K92.9
    - newborn P78.9
    - psychogenic F45.8
  - gender-identity or -role F64.9
    - childhood F64.2
    - effect on relationship F66
    - of adolescence or adulthood (nontranssexual) F64.1
    - specified NEC F64.8
    - uncertainty F66
  - genitourinary system
    - female N94.9
    - male N5Ø.9
    - psychogenic F45.8

- **Disorder** — *continued*
  - globe H44.9
    - degenerated condition H44.5Ø
      - absolute glaucoma H44.51-
      - atrophy H44.52-
      - leucocoria H44.53-
    - degenerative H44.3Ø
      - chalcosis H44.31-
      - myopia H44.2-
      - siderosis H44.32-
      - specified type NEC H44.39-
    - endophthalmitis — *see* Endophthalmitis
    - foreign body, retained — *see* Foreign body, intraocular, old, retained
    - hemophthalmos — *see* Hemophthalmos
    - hypotony H44.4Ø
      - due to
        - ocular fistula H44.42-
        - specified disorder NEC H44.43-
      - flat anterior chamber H44.41-
      - primary H44.44-
    - luxation — *see* Luxation, globe
    - specified type NEC H44.89
  - glomerular (in) NØ5.9
    - amyloidosis E85.4 *[NØ8]*
    - cryoglobulinemia D89.1 *[NØ8]*
    - disseminated intravascular coagulation D65 *[NØ8]*
    - Fabry's disease E75.21 *[NØ8]*
    - familial lecithin cholesterol acyltransferase deficiency E78.6 *[NØ8]*
    - Goodpasture's syndrome M31.Ø
    - hemolytic-uremic syndrome D59.3
    - Henoch (-Schönlein) purpura D69.Ø *[NØ8]*
    - malariae malaria B52.Ø
    - microscopic polyangiitis M31.7 *[NØ8]*
    - multiple myeloma C9Ø.Ø- *[NØ8]*
    - mumps B26.83
    - schistosomiasis B65.9 *[NØ8]*
    - sepsis NEC A41.9- *[NØ8]*
      - streptococcal A4Ø.9- *[NØ8]*
    - sickle-cell disorders D57. *[NØ8]*
    - strongyloidiasis B78.9 *[NØ8]*
    - subacute bacterial endocarditis I33.Ø *[NØ8]*
    - syphilis A52.75
    - systemic lupus erythematosus M32.14
    - thrombotic thrombocytopenic purpura M31.1 *[NØ8]*
    - Waldenström macroglobulinemia C88.Ø *[NØ8]*
    - Wegener's granulomatosis M31.31
  - gluconeogenesis E74.4
  - glucosaminoglycan metabolism — *see* Disorder, metabolism, glucosaminoglycan
  - glycine metabolism E72.5Ø
    - d-glycericacidemia E72.59
    - hyperhydroxyprolinemia E72.59
    - hyperoxaluria E72.53
    - hyperprolinemia E72.59
    - non-ketotic hyperglycinemia E72.51
    - oxalosis E72.53
    - oxaluria E72.53
    - sarcosinemia E72.59
    - trimethylaminuria E72.52
  - glycoprotein metabolism E77.9
    - specified NEC E77.8
  - habit (and impulse) F63.9
    - involving sexual behavior NEC F65.9
    - specified NEC F63.89
  - heart action I49.9
  - hematological D75.9
    - newborn (transient) P61.9
      - specified NEC P61.8
  - hematopoietic organs D75.9
  - hemorrhagic NEC D69.9
    - drug-induced D68.32
    - due to
      - extrinsic circulating anticoagulants D68.32
      - increase in
        - anti-IIa D68.32
        - anti-Xa D68.32
      - intrinsic
        - circulating anticoagulants D68.318

- **Disorder** — *continued*
  - metabolism— *continued*
    - amino-acid— *continued*
      - branched chain— *continued*
        - other specified E71.19
        - proprionate NEC E71.128
        - proprionic acidemia E71.121
      - glycine E72.50
        - d-glycericacidemia E72.59
        - hyperhydroxyprolinemia E72.59
        - hyperoxaluria E72.53
        - hyperprolinemia E72.59
        - non-ketotic hyperglycinemia E72.51
        - other specified E72.59
        - sarcosinemia E72.59
        - trimethylaminuria E72.52
      - hydroxylysine E72.3
      - lysine E72.3
      - ornithine E72.4
      - other specified E72.8
        - beta-amino acid E72.8
        - gamma-glutamyl cycle E72.8
      - straight-chain E72.8
      - sulfur-bearing E72.10
        - homocystinuria E72.11
        - methylenetetrahydrofolate reductase deficiency E72.12
        - other specified E72.19
    - bile acid and cholesterol metabolism E78.70
    - bilirubin E80.7
      - specified NEC E80.6
    - calcium E83.50
      - hypercalcemia E83.52
      - hypocalcemia E83.51
      - other specified E83.59
    - carbohydrate E74.9
      - specified NEC E74.8
    - cholesterol and bile acid metabolism E78.70
    - congenital E88.9
    - copper E83.00
      - Wilson's disease E83.01
      - specified type NEC E83.09
    - cystinuria E72.01
    - fructose E74.10
    - galactose E74.20
    - glucosaminoglycan E76.9
      - mucopolysaccharidosis — *see* Mucopolysaccharidosis
      - specified NEC E76.8
    - glutamine E72.8
    - glycine E72.50
    - glycogen storage (hepatorenal) E74.09
    - glycoprotein E77.9
      - specified NEC E77.8
    - glycosaminoglycan E76.9
      - specified NEC E76.8
    - in labor and delivery O75.89
    - iron E83.10
    - isoleucine E71.19
    - leucine E71.19
    - lipoid E78.9
    - lipoprotein E78.9
      - specified NEC E78.89
    - magnesium E83.40
      - hypermagnesemia E83.41
      - hypomagnesemia E83.42
      - other specified E83.49
    - mineral E83.9
      - specified NEC E83.89
    - mitochondrial E88.40
      - MELAS syndrome E88.41
      - MERRF syndrome (myoclonic epilepsy associated with ragged-red fibers) E88.42
      - other specified E88.49
    - ornithine E72.4
    - phosphatases E83.30
    - phosphorus E83.30
      - acid phosphatase deficiency E83.39
      - hypophosphatasia E83.39
      - hypophosphatemia E83.39
        - familial E83.31

- **Disorder** — *continued*
  - metabolism— *continued*
    - phosphorus— *continued*
      - other specified E83.39
      - pseudovitamin D deficiency E83.32
    - plasma protein NEC E88.09
    - porphyrin — *see* Porphyria
    - postprocedural E89.89
      - specified NEC E89.89
    - purine E79.9
      - specified NEC E79.8
    - pyrimidine E79.9
      - specified NEC E79.8
    - pyruvate E74.4
    - serine E72.8
    - sodium E87.8
    - specified NEC E88.89
    - threonine E72.8
    - valine E71.19
    - zinc E83.2
  - methylmalonic acidemia E71.120
  - micturition NEC R39.19
    - feeling of incomplete emptying R39.14
    - hesitancy R39.11
    - poor stream R39.12
    - psychogenic F45.8
    - split stream R39.13
    - straining R39.16
    - urgency R39.15
  - mitochondrial metabolism E88.40
  - mitral (valve) — *see* Endocarditis, mitral
  - mixed
    - anxiety and depressive F41.8
    - of scholastic skills (developmental) F81.89
    - receptive expressive language F80.2
  - mood F39
    - bipolar — *see* Disorder, bipolar
    - depressive — *see* Disorder, depressive
    - due to (secondary to)
      - alcohol F10.94
      - amphetamine F15.94
        - in
          - abuse F15.14
          - dependence F15.24
      - anxiolytic F13.94
        - in
          - abuse F13.14
          - dependence F13.24
      - cocaine F14.94
        - in
          - abuse F14.14
          - dependence F14.24
      - general medical condition F06.30
      - hallucinogen F16.94
        - in
          - abuse F16.14
          - dependence F16.24
      - hypnotic F13.94
        - in
          - abuse F13.14
          - dependence F13.24
      - inhalant F18.94
        - in
          - abuse F18.14
          - dependence F18.24
      - opioid F11.94
        - in
          - abuse F11.14
          - dependence F11.24
      - phencyclidine (PCP) F16.94
        - in
          - abuse F16.14
          - dependence F16.24
      - physiological condition F06.30
        - with
          - depressive features F06.31
          - major depressive-like episode F06.32
          - manic features F06.33
          - mixed features F06.34
      - psychoactive substance NEC F19.94

- **Disorder** — *continued*
  - mood— *continued*
    - due to (secondary to)— *continued*
      - psychoactive substance NEC F19.94 — *continued*
        - in
          - abuse F19.14
          - dependence F19.24
      - sedative F13.94
        - in
          - abuse F13.14
          - dependence F13.24
      - volatile solvents F18.94
        - in
          - abuse F18.14
          - dependence F18.24
    - manic episode F30.9
      - with psychotic symptoms F30.2
      - in remission (full) F30.4
        - partial F30.3
      - specified type NEC F30.8
      - without psychotic symptoms F30.10
        - mild F30.11
        - moderate F30.12
        - severe F30.13
    - organic F06.30
      - right hemisphere F07.89
    - persistent F34.9
      - cyclothymia F34.0
      - dysthymia F34.1
      - specified type NEC F34.8
    - recurrent F39
    - right hemisphere organic F07.89
  - movement G25.9
    - drug-induced G25.70
      - akathisia G25.71
      - specified NEC G25.79
    - hysterical F44.4
    - periodic limb G47.61
      - sleep related G47.61
    - specified NEC G25.89
    - sleep related NEC G47.69
    - stereotyped F98.4
    - treatment-induced G25.9
  - multiple personality F44.81
  - muscle M62.9
    - attachment, spine — *see* Enthesopathy, spinal
    - in trichinellosis — *see* Trichinellosis, with muscle disorder
    - psychogenic F45.8
    - specified type NEC M62.89
    - tone, newborn P94.9
      - specified NEC P94.8
  - muscular
    - attachments (*see also* Enthesopathy)
      - spine — *see* Enthesopathy, spinal
    - urethra N36.44
  - musculoskeletal system, soft tissue — *see* Disorder, soft tissue
    - postprocedural M96.89
    - psychogenic F45.8
  - myoneural G70.9
    - due to lead G70.1
    - specified NEC G70.89
    - toxic G70.1
  - myotonic NEC G71.19
  - nail, in diseases classified elsewhere L62
  - neck region NEC — *see* Dorsopathy, specified NEC
  - nerve G58.9
    - abducent NEC — *see* Strabismus, paralytic, sixth nerve
    - accessory G52.8
    - acoustic — *see* subcategory H93.3
    - auditory — *see* subcategory H93.3
    - auriculotemporal G50.8
    - axillary G54.0
    - cerebral — *see* Disorder, nerve, cranial
    - cranial G52.9
      - eighth — *see* subcategory H93.3
      - eleventh G52.8
      - fifth G50.9
      - first G52.0

- **Disorder** — *continued*
  - nerve— *continued*
    - cranial— *continued*
      - fourth NEC — *see* Strabismus, paralytic, fourth nerve
      - multiple G52.7
      - ninth G52.1
      - second NEC — *see* Disorder, nerve, optic
      - seventh NEC G51.8
      - sixth NEC — *see* Strabismus, paralytic, sixth nerve
      - specified NEC G52.8
      - tenth G52.2
      - third NEC — *see* Strabismus, paralytic, third nerve
      - twelfth G52.3
    - entrapment — *see* Neuropathy, entrapment
    - facial G51.9
      - specified NEC G51.8
    - femoral — *see* Lesion, nerve, femoral
    - glossopharyngeal NEC G52.1
    - hypoglossal G52.3
    - intercostal G58.Ø
    - lateral
      - cutaneous of thigh — *see* Mononeuropathy, lower limb, meralgia paresthetica
      - popliteal — *see* Lesion, nerve, popliteal
    - lower limb — *see* Mononeuropathy, lower limb
    - medial popliteal — *see* Lesion, nerve, popliteal, medial
    - median NEC — *see* Lesion, nerve, median
    - multiple G58.7
    - oculomotor NEC — *see* Strabismus, paralytic, third nerve
    - olfactory G52.Ø
    - optic NEC H47.Ø9-
      - hemorrhage into sheath — *see* Hemorrhage, optic nerve
      - ischemic H47.Ø1-
    - peroneal — *see* Lesion, nerve, popliteal
    - phrenic G58.8
    - plantar — *see* Lesion, nerve, plantar
    - pneumogastric G52.2
    - posterior tibial — *see* Syndrome, tarsal tunnel
    - radial — *see* Lesion, nerve, radial
    - recurrent laryngeal G52.2
    - root
      - cervical G54.2
      - lumbosacral G54.1
      - specified NEC G54.8
      - thoracic G54.3
    - sciatic NEC — *see* Lesion, nerve, sciatic
    - specified NEC G58.8
      - lower limb — *see* Mononeuropathy, lower limb, specified NEC
      - upper limb — *see* Mononeuropathy, upper limb, specified NEC
    - sympathetic G9Ø.9
    - tibial — *see* Lesion, nerve, popliteal, medial
    - trigeminal G5Ø.9
      - specified NEC G5Ø.8
    - trochlear NEC — *see* Strabismus, paralytic, fourth nerve
    - ulnar — *see* Lesion, nerve, ulnar
    - upper limb — *see* Mononeuropathy, upper limb
    - vagus G52.2
  - nervous system G98.8
    - autonomic (peripheral) G9Ø.9
      - specified NEC G9Ø.8
    - central G96.9
      - specified NEC G96.8
    - parasympathetic G9Ø.9
    - specified NEC G98.8
    - sympathetic G9Ø.9
    - vegetative G9Ø.9
  - neurohypophysis NEC E23.3
  - neurological NEC R29.818
  - neuromuscular G7Ø.9
    - hereditary NEC G71.9
    - specified NEC G7Ø.89
    - toxic G7Ø.1
  - neurotic F48.9
    - specified NEC F48.8

- **Disorder** — *continued*
  - neutrophil, polymorphonuclear D71
  - nicotine use — *see* Dependence, drug, nicotine
  - nightmare F51.5
  - nose J34.9
    - specified NEC J34.89
  - obsessive-compulsive F42
  - odontogenesis NOS KØØ.9
  - oesophagus — *see* Disorder, esophagus
  - opioid use
    - due to drug abuse — *see* Abuse, drug, opioid
    - due to drug dependence — *see* Dependence, drug, opioid
  - oppositional defiant F91.3
  - optic
    - chiasm H47.49
      - due to
        - inflammatory disorder H47.41
        - neoplasm H47.42
        - vascular disorder H47.43
    - disc H47.39-
      - coloboma — *see* Coloboma, optic disc
      - drusen — *see* Drusen, optic disc
      - pseudopapilledema — *see* Pseudopapilledema
    - radiations — *see* Disorder, visual, pathway
    - tracts — *see* Disorder, visual, pathway
  - orbit HØ5.9
    - cyst — *see* Cyst, orbit
    - deformity — *see* Deformity, orbit
    - edema — *see* Edema, orbit
    - enophthalmos — *see* Enophthalmos
    - exophthalmos — *see* Exophthalmos
    - hemorrhage — *see* Hemorrhage, orbit
    - inflammation — *see* Inflammation, orbit
    - myopathy — *see* Myopathy, extraocular muscles
    - retained foreign body — *see* Foreign body, orbit, old
    - specified type NEC HØ5.89
  - organic
    - anxiety FØ6.4
    - catatonic FØ6.1
    - delusional FØ6.2
    - dissociative FØ6.8
    - emotionally labile (asthenic) FØ6.8
    - mood (affective) FØ6.3Ø
    - schizophrenia-like FØ6.2
  - orgasmic (female) F52.31
    - male F52.32
  - ornithine metabolism E72.4
  - overanxious F41.1
    - of childhood F93.8
  - pain
    - with related psychological factors F45.42
    - exclusively related to psychological factors F45.41
  - pancreatic internal secretion E16.9
    - specified NEC E16.8
  - panic F41.Ø
    - with agoraphobia F4Ø.Ø1
  - papulosquamous L44.9
    - in diseases classified elsewhere L45
    - specified NEC L44.8
  - paranoid F22
    - induced F24
    - shared F24
  - parathyroid (gland) E21.5
    - specified NEC E21.4
  - parietoalveolar NEC J84.Ø9
  - paroxysmal, mixed R56.9
  - patella M22.9-
    - chondromalacia — *see* Chondromalacia, patella
    - derangement NEC M22.3X-
    - recurrent
      - dislocation — *see* Dislocation, patella, recurrent
      - subluxation — *see* Dislocation, patella, recurrent, incomplete
    - specified NEC M22.8X-
  - patellofemoral M22.2X-
  - pentose phosphate pathway with anemia D55.1
  - perception, due to hallucinogens F16.983
    - in
      - abuse F16.183

- **Disorder** — *continued*
  - perception, due to hallucinogens — *continued*
    - in — *continued*
      - dependence F16.283
  - peripheral nervous system NEC G64
  - peroxisomal E71.5Ø
    - biogenesis
      - neonatal adrenoleukodystrophy E71.511
      - specified disorder NEC E71.518
      - Zellweger syndrome E71.51Ø
    - rhizomelic chondrodysplasia punctata E71.54Ø
    - specified form NEC E71.548
      - group 1 E71.518
      - group 2 E71.53
      - group 3 E71.542
    - X-linked adrenoleukodystrophy E71.529
      - adolescent E71.521
      - adrenomyeloneuropathy E71.522
      - childhood E71.52Ø
      - specified form NEC E71.528
    - Zellweger-like syndrome E71.541
  - persistent
    - affective (mood) F34.9
    - (somatoform) pain F45.41
  - personality (*see also* Personality) F6Ø.9
    - affective F34.Ø
    - aggressive F6Ø.3
    - amoral F6Ø.2
    - anankastic F6Ø.5
    - antisocial F6Ø.2
    - anxious F6Ø.6
    - asocial F6Ø.2
    - asthenic F6Ø.7
    - avoidant F6Ø.6
    - borderline F6Ø.3
    - change (secondary) due to general medical condition FØ7.Ø
    - compulsive F6Ø.5
    - cyclothymic F34.Ø
    - dependent (passive) F6Ø.7
    - depressive F34.1
    - dissocial F6Ø.2
    - emotional instability F6Ø.3
    - expansive paranoid F6Ø.Ø
    - explosive F6Ø.3
    - following organic brain damage FØ7.9
    - histrionic F6Ø.4
    - hyperthymic F34.Ø
    - hypothymic F34.1
    - hysterical F6Ø.4
    - immature F6Ø.89
    - inadequate F6Ø.7
    - labile F6Ø.3
    - mixed (nonspecific) F6Ø.89
    - moral deficiency F6Ø.2
    - narcissistic F6Ø.81
    - negativistic F6Ø.89
    - obsessional F6Ø.5
    - obsessive(-compulsive) F6Ø.5
    - organic FØ7.9
    - overconscientious F6Ø.5
    - paranoid F6Ø.Ø
    - passive(-dependent) F6Ø.7
    - passive-aggressive F6Ø.89
    - pathological NEC F6Ø.9
    - pseudosocial F6Ø.2
    - psychopathic F6Ø.2
    - schizoid F6Ø.1
    - schizotypal F21
    - self-defeating F6Ø.7
    - specified NEC F6Ø.89
    - type A F6Ø.5
    - unstable (emotional) F6Ø.3
  - pervasive, developmental F84.9
  - phobic anxiety, childhood F4Ø.8
  - phosphate-losing tubular N25.Ø
  - pigmentation L81.9
    - choroid, congenital Q14.3
    - diminished melanin formation L81.6
    - iron L81.8
    - specified NEC L81.8
  - pinna (noninfective) H61.1Ø-
    - deformity, acquired H61.11-

- **Disorder** — *continued*
  - sleep — *continued*
    - circadian rhythm — *continued*
      - due to — *continued*
          - dependence F13.282
          - use F13.982
        - stimulant NEC
          - abuse F15.182
          - dependence F15.282
          - use F15.982
      - free running type G47.24
      - in conditions classified elsewhere G47.27
      - irregular sleep wake type G47.23
      - jet lag type G47.25
      - shift work type G47.26
      - specified NEC G47.29
    - due to
      - alcohol
        - abuse F1Ø.182
        - dependence F1Ø.282
        - use F1Ø.982
      - amphetamine
        - abuse F15.182
        - dependence F15.282
        - use F15.982
      - anxiolytic
        - abuse F13.182
        - dependence F13.282
        - use F13.982
      - caffeine
        - abuse F15.182
        - dependence F15.282
        - use F15.982
      - cocaine
        - abuse F14.182
        - dependence F14.282
        - use F14.982
      - drug NEC
        - abuse F19.182
        - dependence F19.282
        - use F19.982
      - hypnotic
        - abuse F13.182
        - dependence F13.282
        - use F13.982
      - opioid
        - abuse F11.182
        - dependence F11.282
        - use F11.982
      - psychoactive substance NEC
        - abuse F19.182
        - dependence F19.282
        - use F19.982
      - sedative
        - abuse F13.182
        - dependence F13.282
        - use F13.982
      - stimulant NEC
        - abuse F15.182
        - dependence F15.282
        - use F15.982
    - emotional F51.9
    - excessive somnolence — *see* Hypersomnia
    - hypersomnia type — *see* Hypersomnia
    - initiating or maintaining — *see* Insomnia
    - nightmares F51.5
    - nonorganic F51.9
      - specified NEC F51.8
    - parasomnia type G47.5Ø
    - specified NEC G47.8
    - terrors F51.4
    - walking F51.3
  - sleep-wake pattern or schedule — *see* Disorder, sleep, circadian rhythm
  - social
    - anxiety of childhood F4Ø.1Ø
    - functioning in childhood F94.9
      - specified NEC F94.8
  - soft tissue M79.9
    - ankle M79.9
    - due to use, overuse and pressure M7Ø.9Ø
      - ankle M7Ø.97-
      - bursitis — *see* Bursitis

- **Disorder** — *continued*
  - soft tissue— *continued*
    - due to use, overuse and pressure— *continued*
      - foot M7Ø.97-
      - forearm M7Ø.93-
      - hand M7Ø.94-
      - lower leg M7Ø.96-
      - multiple sites M7Ø.99
      - pelvic region M7Ø.95-
      - shoulder region M7Ø.91-
      - specified site NEC M7Ø.98
      - specified type NEC M7Ø.8Ø
        - ankle M7Ø.87-
        - foot M7Ø.87-
        - forearm M7Ø.83-
        - hand M7Ø.84-
        - lower leg M7Ø.86-
        - multiple sites M7Ø.89
        - pelvic region M7Ø.85-
        - shoulder region M7Ø.81-
        - specified site NEC M7Ø.88
        - thigh M7Ø.85-
        - upper arm M7Ø.82-
      - thigh M7Ø.95-
      - upper arm M7Ø.92-
    - foot M79.9
    - forearm M79.9
    - hand M79.9
    - lower leg M79.9
    - multiple sites M79.9
    - occupational — *see* Disorder, soft tissue, due to use, overuse and pressure
    - pelvic region M79.9
    - shoulder region M79.9
    - specified type NEC M79.89
    - thigh M79.9
    - upper arm M79.9
  - somatization F45.Ø
  - somatoform F45.9
    - pain (persistent) F45.41
    - somatization (multiple) (long-lasting) F45.Ø
    - specified NEC F45.8
    - undifferentiated F45.1
  - somnolence, excessive — *see* Hypersomnia
  - specific
    - arithmetical F81.2
    - developmental, of motor F82
    - reading F81.Ø
    - speech and language F8Ø.9
    - spelling F81.81
    - written expression F81.81
  - speech R47.9
    - articulation (functional) (specific) F8Ø.Ø
    - developmental F8Ø.9
    - specified NEC R47.89
  - spelling (specific) F81.81
  - spine (*see also* Dorsopathy)
    - ligamentous or muscular attachments, peripheral — *see* Enthesopathy, spinal
    - specified NEC — *see* Dorsopathy, specified NEC
  - stereotyped, habit or movement F98.4
  - stomach (functional) — *see* Disorder, gastric
  - stress F43.9
    - post-traumatic F43.1Ø
      - acute F43.11
      - chronic F43.12
  - sulfur-bearing amino-acid metabolism E72.1Ø
  - sweat gland (eccrine) L74.9
    - apocrine L75.9
      - specified NEC L75.8
    - specified NEC L74.8
  - synovium M67.9Ø
    - acromioclavicular M67.91-
    - ankle M67.97-
    - elbow M67.92-
    - foot M67.97-
    - forearm M67.93-
    - hand M67.94-
    - hip M67.95-
    - knee M67.96-
    - multiple sites M67.99
    - rupture — *see* Rupture, synovium
    - shoulder M67.91-

- **Disorder** — *continued*
  - synovium— *continued*
    - specified type NEC M67.8Ø
      - acromioclavicular M67.81-
      - ankle M67.87-
      - elbow M67.82-
      - foot M67.87-
      - hand M67.84-
      - hip M67.85-
      - knee M67.86-
      - multiple sites M67.89
      - wrist M67.83-
    - synovitis — *see* Synovitis
    - upper arm M67.92-
    - wrist M67.93-
  - temperature regulation, newborn P81.9
    - specified NEC P81.8
  - temporomandibular joint — *see* Anomaly, dentofacial, temporomandibular joint
  - tendon M67.9Ø
    - acromioclavicular M67.91-
    - ankle M67.97-
    - contracture — *see* Contracture, tendon
    - elbow M67.92-
    - foot M67.97-
    - forearm M67.93-
    - hand M67.94-
    - hip M67.95-
    - knee M67.96-
    - multiple sites M67.99
    - rupture — *see* Rupture, tendon
    - shoulder M67.91-
    - specified type NEC M67.8Ø
      - acromioclavicular M67.81-
      - ankle M67.87-
      - elbow M67.82-
      - foot M67.87-
      - hand M67.84-
      - hip M67.85-
      - knee M67.86-
      - multiple sites M67.89
      - trunk M67.88
      - wrist M67.83-
    - synovitis — *see* Synovitis
    - tendinitis — *see* Tendinitis
    - tenosynovitis — *see* Tenosynovitis
    - upper arm M67.92-
    - trunk M67.98
    - wrist M67.93-
  - thoracic root (nerve) NEC G54.3
  - thyrocalcitonin hypersecretion EØ7.Ø
  - thyroid (gland) EØ7.9
    - function NEC, neonatal, transitory P72.2
    - iodine-deficiency related EØ1.8
    - specified NEC EØ7.89
  - tic — *see* Tic
  - tooth KØ8.9
    - development KØØ.9
      - specified NEC KØØ.8
    - eruption KØØ.6
  - Tourette's F95.2
  - trance and possession F44.89
  - tricuspid (valve) — *see* Endocarditis, tricuspid
  - tryptophan metabolism E7Ø.5
  - tubular, phosphate-losing N25.Ø
  - tubulo-interstitial (in)
    - brucellosis A23.9 *[N16]*
    - cystinosis E72.Ø4
    - diphtheria A36.84
    - glycogen storage disease E74.ØØ *[N16]*
    - leukemia NEC C95.9- *[N16]*
    - lymphoma NEC C85.9- *[N16]*
    - mixed cryoglobulinemia D89.1 *[N16]*
    - multiple myeloma C9Ø.Ø- *[N16]*
    - Salmonella infection AØ2.25
    - sarcoidosis D86.84
    - sepsis A41.9 *[N16]*
      - streptococcal A4Ø.9 *[N16]*
    - systemic lupus erythematosus M32.15
    - toxoplasmosis B58.83
    - transplant rejection T86.91 *[N16]*
    - Wilson's disease E83.Ø1 *[N16]*
  - tubulo-renal function, impaired N25.9

- **Disorder** — *continued*
  - tubulo-renal function, impaired — *continued*
    - specified NEC N25.89
  - tympanic membrane H73.9-
    - atrophy — *see* Atrophy, tympanic membrane
    - infection — *see* Myringitis
    - perforation — *see* Perforation, tympanum
    - specified NEC H73.89-
  - unsocialized aggressive F91.1
  - urea cycle metabolism E72.2Ø
    - argininemia E72.21
    - arginosuccinic aciduria E72.22
    - citrullinemia E72.23
    - ornithine transcarbamylase deficiency E72.4
    - other specified E72.29
  - ureter (in) N28.9
    - schistosomiasis B65.Ø *[N29]*
    - tuberculosis A18.11
  - urethra N36.9
    - specified NEC N36.8
  - urinary system N39.9
    - specified NEC N39.8
  - valve, heart
    - aortic — *see* Endocarditis, aortic
    - mitral — *see* Endocarditis, mitral
    - pulmonary — *see* Endocarditis, pulmonary
    - rheumatic
      - aortic — *see* Endocarditis, aortic, rheumatic
      - mitral — *see* Endocarditis, mitral
      - pulmonary — *see* Endocarditis, pulmonary, rheumatic
      - tricuspid — *see* Endocarditis, tricuspid
    - tricuspid — *see* Endocarditis, tricuspid
  - vestibular function H81.9-
    - specified NEC — *see* subcategory H81.8
      - in diseases classified elsewhere H82.-
    - vertigo — *see* Vertigo
  - vision, binocular H53.3Ø
    - abnormal retinal correspondence H53.31
    - diplopia H53.2
    - fusion with defective stereopsis H53.32
    - simultaneous perception H53.33
    - suppression H53.34
  - visual
    - cortex
      - blindness H47.619
        - left brain H47.612
        - right brain H47.611
      - due to
        - inflammatory disorder H47.629
          - left brain H47.622
          - right brain H47.621
        - neoplasm H47.639
          - left brain H47.632
          - right brain H47.631
        - vascular disorder H47.649
          - left brain H47.642
          - right brain H47.641
    - pathway H47.9
      - due to
        - inflammatory disorder H47.51-
        - neoplasm H47.52-
        - vascular disorder H47.53-
      - optic chiasm — *see* Disorder, optic, chiasm
  - vitreous body H43.9
    - crystalline deposits — *see* Deposit, crystalline
    - degeneration — *see* Degeneration, vitreous
    - hemorrhage — *see* Hemorrhage, vitreous
    - opacities — *see* Opacity, vitreous
    - prolapse — *see* Prolapse, vitreous
    - specified type NEC H43.89
  - voice R49.9
    - specified type NEC R49.8
  - volatile solvent use
    - due to drug abuse — *see* Abuse, drug, inhalant
    - due to drug dependence — *see* Dependence, drug, inhalant
  - white blood cells D72.9
    - specified NEC D72.89
  - withdrawing, child or adolescent F4Ø.1Ø
- **Disorientation** R41.0
- **Displacement, displaced**
  - acquired traumatic of bone, cartilage, joint, tendon NEC — *see* Dislocation
  - adrenal gland (congenital) Q89.1
  - appendix, retrocecal (congenital) Q43.8
  - auricle (congenital) Q17.4
  - bladder (acquired) N32.89
    - congenital Q64.19
  - brachial plexus (congenital) QØ7.8
  - brain stem, caudal (congenital) QØ4.8
  - canaliculus (lacrimalis), congenital Q1Ø.6
  - cardia through esophageal hiatus (congenital) Q4Ø.1
  - cerebellum, caudal (congenital) QØ4.8
  - cervix — *see* Malposition, uterus
  - colon (congenital) Q43.3
  - device, implant or graft (*see also* Complications, by site and type, mechanical) T85.628
    - arterial graft NEC — *see* Complication, cardiovascular device, mechanical, vascular
    - breast (implant) T85.42
    - catheter NEC T85.628
      - dialysis (renal) T82.42
        - intraperitoneal T85.621
      - infusion NEC T82.524
        - spinal (epidural) (subdural) T85.62Ø
      - urinary (indwelling) T83.Ø28
        - cystostomy T83.Ø2Ø
    - electronic (electrode) (pulse generator) (stimulator) — *see* Complication, electronic stimulator
    - fixation, internal (orthopedic) NEC — *see* Complication, fixation device, mechanical
    - gastrointestinal — *see* Complications, prosthetic device, mechanical, gastrointestinal device
    - genital NEC T83.428
      - intrauterine contraceptive device T83.32
      - penile prosthesis T83.42Ø
    - heart NEC — *see* Complication, cardiovascular device, mechanical
    - joint prosthesis — *see* Complications, joint prosthesis, mechanical
    - ocular — *see* Complications, prosthetic device, mechanical, ocular device
    - orthopedic NEC — *see* Complication, orthopedic, device or graft, mechanical
    - specified NEC T85.628
    - urinary NEC (*see also* Complication, genitourinary, device, urinary, mechanical)
      - graft T83.22
    - vascular NEC — *see* Complication, cardiovascular device, mechanical
    - ventricular intracranial shunt T85.Ø2
  - electronic stimulator
    - bone T84.32Ø
    - cardiac — *see* Complications, cardiac device, electronic
    - nervous system — *see* Complication, prosthetic device, mechanical, electronic nervous system stimulator
    - urinary — *see* Complications, electronic stimulator, urinary
  - esophageal mucosa into cardia of stomach, congenital Q39.8
  - esophagus (acquired) K22.8
    - congenital Q39.8
  - eyeball (acquired) (lateral) (old) — *see* Displacement, globe
    - congenital Q15.8
    - current — *see* Avulsion, eye
  - fallopian tube (acquired) N83.4
    - congenital Q5Ø.6
    - opening (congenital) Q5Ø.6
  - gallbladder (congenital) Q44.1
  - gastric mucosa (congenital) Q4Ø.2
  - globe (acquired) (old) (lateral) HØ5.21-
    - current — *see* Avulsion, eye
  - heart (congenital) Q24.8
    - acquired I51.89
  - hymen (upward) (congenital) Q52.4
  - intervertebral disc NEC
    - with myelopathy — *see* Disorder, disc, with, myelopathy
- **Displacement, displaced**— *continued*
  - intervertebral disc— *continued*
    - cervical, cervicothoracic (with) M5Ø.2Ø
      - myelopathy — *see* Disorder, disc, cervical, with myelopathy
      - neuritis, radiculitis or radiculopathy — *see* Disorder, disc, cervical, with neuritis
    - due to trauma — *see* Dislocation, vertebra
    - lumbar region M51.26
      - with
        - myelopathy M51.Ø6
        - neuritis, radiculitis, radiculopathy or sciatica M51.16
    - lumbosacral region M51.27
      - with
        - myelopathy M51.Ø7
        - neuritis, radiculitis, radiculopathy or sciatica M51.17
    - sacrococcygeal region M53.3
    - thoracic region M51.24
      - with
        - myelopathy M51.Ø4
        - neuritis, radiculitis, radiculopathy M51.14
    - thoracolumbar region M51.25
      - with
        - myelopathy M51.Ø5
        - neuritis, radiculitis, radiculopathy M51.15
  - intrauterine device T83.32
  - kidney (acquired) N28.83
    - congenital Q63.2
  - lachrymal, lacrimal apparatus or duct (congenital) Q1Ø.6
  - lens, congenital Q12.1
  - macula (congenital) Q14.1
  - Meckel's diverticulum Q43.Ø
    - malignant — *see* Table of Neoplasms, small intestine, malignant
  - nail (congenital) Q84.6
    - acquired L6Ø.8
  - oesophagus (acquired) — *see* Displacement, esophagus
  - opening of Wharton's duct in mouth Q38.4
  - organ or site, congenital NEC — *see* Malposition, congenital
  - ovary (acquired) N83.4
    - congenital Q5Ø.39
    - free in peritoneal cavity (congenital) Q5Ø.39
    - into hernial sac N83.4
  - oviduct (acquired) N83.4
    - congenital Q5Ø.6
  - parathyroid (gland) E21.4
  - parotid gland (congenital) Q38.4
  - punctum lacrimale (congenital) Q1Ø.6
  - sacro-iliac (joint) (congenital) Q74.2
    - current injury S33.2
    - old — *see* subcategory M53.2
  - salivary gland (any) (congenital) Q38.4
  - spleen (congenital) Q89.Ø9
  - stomach, congenital Q4Ø.2
  - sublingual duct Q38.4
  - tongue (downward) (congenital) Q38.3
  - tooth, teeth, fully erupted M26.3Ø
    - horizontal M26.33
    - vertical M26.34
  - trachea (congenital) Q32.1
  - ureter or ureteric opening or orifice (congenital) Q62.62
  - uterine opening of oviducts or fallopian tubes Q5Ø.6
  - uterus, uterine — *see* Malposition, uterus
  - ventricular septum Q21.Ø
    - with rudimentary ventricle Q2Ø.4
- **Disproportion**
  - between native and reconstructed breast N65.1
  - fiber-type G71.2
- **Disruptio uteri** — *see* Rupture, uterus
- **Disruption** (of)
  - ciliary body NEC H21.89
  - closure of
    - cornea T81.31
    - craniotomy T81.32
    - fascia (muscular) (superficial) T81.32
    - internal organ or tissue T81.32
    - laceration (external) (internal) T81.33
    - ligament T81.32

- **Diverticulitis** — *continued*
  - intestine— *continued*
    - with — *continued*
      - bleeding K57.93
    - congenital Q43.8
    - large K57.32
      - with
        - abscess, perforation or peritonitis K57.20
          - with bleeding K57.21
        - bleeding K57.33
        - small intestine K57.52
          - with
            - abscess, perforation or peritonitis K57.40
              - with bleeding K57.41
            - bleeding K57.53
    - small K57.12
      - with
        - abscess, perforation or peritonitis K57.00
          - with bleeding K57.01
        - bleeding K57.13
        - large intestine K57.52
          - with
            - abscess, perforation or peritonitis K57.40
              - with bleeding K57.41
            - bleeding K57.53
- **Diverticulosis** K57.90
  - with bleeding K57.91
  - large intestine K57.30
    - with
      - bleeding K57.31
      - small intestine K57.50
        - with bleeding K57.51
  - small intestine K57.10
    - with
      - bleeding K57.11
      - large intestine K57.50
        - with bleeding K57.51
- **Diverticulum, diverticula** (multiple) K57.90
  - appendix (noninflammatory) K38.2
  - bladder (sphincter) N32.3
    - congenital Q64.6
  - bronchus (congenital) Q32.4
    - acquired J98.09
  - calyx, calyceal (kidney) N28.89
  - cardia (stomach) K31.4
  - cecum — *see* Diverticulosis, intestine, large
    - congenital Q43.8
  - colon — *see* Diverticulosis, intestine, large
    - congenital Q43.8
  - duodenum — *see* Diverticulosis, intestine, small
    - congenital Q43.8
  - epiphrenic (esophagus) K22.5
  - esophagus (congenital) Q39.6
    - acquired (epiphrenic) (pulsion) (traction) K22.5
  - eustachian tube — *see* Disorder, eustachian tube, specified NEC
  - fallopian tube N83.8
  - gastric K31.4
  - heart (congenital) Q24.8
  - ileum — *see* Diverticulosis, intestine, small
  - jejunum — *see* Diverticulosis, intestine, small
  - kidney (pelvis) (calyces) N28.89
    - with calculus — *see* Calculus, kidney
  - Meckel's (displaced) (hypertrophic) Q43.0
    - malignant — *see* Table of Neoplasms, small intestine, malignant
  - midthoracic K22.5
  - organ or site, congenital NEC — *see* Distortion
  - pericardium (congenital) (cyst) Q24.8
    - acquired I31.8
  - pharyngoesophageal (congenital) Q39.6
    - acquired K22.5
  - pharynx (congenital) Q38.7
  - rectosigmoid — *see* Diverticulosis, intestine, large
    - congenital Q43.8
  - rectum — *see* Diverticulosis, intestine, large
  - Rokitansky's K22.5
  - seminal vesicle N50.8
  - sigmoid — *see* Diverticulosis, intestine, large
    - congenital Q43.8
  - stomach (acquired) K31.4
- **Diverticulum, diverticula** — *continued*
  - stomach (acquired) — *continued*
    - congenital Q40.2
  - trachea (acquired) J39.8
  - ureter (acquired) N28.89
    - congenital Q62.8
  - ureterovesical orifice N28.89
  - urethra (acquired) N36.1
    - congenital Q64.79
  - ventricle, left (congenital) Q24.8
  - vesical N32.3
    - congenital Q64.6
  - Zenker's (esophagus) K22.5
- **Division**
  - cervix uteri (acquired) N88.8
  - glans penis Q55.69
  - labia minora (congenital) Q52.79
  - ligament (partial or complete) (current) (*see also* Sprain)
    - with open wound — *see* Wound, open
  - muscle (partial or complete) (current) (*see also* Injury, muscle)
    - with open wound — *see* Wound, open
  - nerve (traumatic) — *see* Injury, nerve
  - spinal cord — *see* Injury, spinal cord, by region
  - vein I87.8
- **Divorce, causing family disruption** Z63.5
- **Dix-Hallpike neurolabyrinthitis** — *see* Neuronitis, vestibular
- **Dizziness** R42
  - hysterical F44.89
  - psychogenic F45.8
- **DMAC** (disseminated mycobacterium aviumintracellulare complex) A31.2
- **DNR** (do not resuscitate) Z66
- **Doan-Wiseman syndrome** (primary splenic neutropenia) — *see* Agranulocytosis
- **Doehle-Heller aortitis** A52.02
- **Dog bite** — *see* Bite
- **Dohle body panmyelopathic syndrome** D72.0
- **Dolichocephaly** Q67.2
- **Dolichocolon** Q43.8
- **Dolichostenomelia** — *see* Syndrome, Marfan's
- **Donohue's syndrome** E34.8
- **Donor** (organ or tissue) Z52.9
  - blood (whole) Z52.000
    - autologous Z52.010
    - specified donor NEC Z52.090
    - specified component (lymphocytes) (platelets) NEC Z52.008
      - autologous Z52.018
      - specified donor NEC Z52.098
    - stem cells Z52.001
      - autologous Z52.011
      - specified donor NEC Z52.091
  - bone Z52.20
    - autologous Z52.21
    - marrow Z52.3
    - specified type NEC Z52.29
  - cornea Z52.5
  - egg (Oocyte) Z52.819
    - age 35 and over Z52.812
      - anonymous recipient Z52.812
      - designated recipient Z52.813
    - under age 35 Z52.810
      - anonymous recipient Z52.810
      - designated recipient Z52.811
  - kidney Z52.4
  - liver Z52.6
  - lung Z52.89
  - lymphocyte *see* Donor, blood, specified components NEC
  - Oocyte — *see* Donor, egg
  - platelets Z52.008
  - potential, examination of Z00.5
  - semen Z52.89
  - skin Z52.10
    - autologous Z52.11
    - specified type NEC Z52.19
  - specified organ or tissue NEC Z52.89
  - sperm Z52.89
- **Donovanosis** A58
- **Dorsalgia** M54.9
  - psychogenic F45.41
  - specified NEC M54.89
- **Dorsopathy** M53.9
  - deforming M43.9
    - specified NEC — *see* subcategory M43.8
  - specified NEC M53.80
    - cervical region M53.82
    - cervicothoracic region M53.83
    - lumbar region M53.86
    - lumbosacral region M53.87
    - occipito-atlanto-axial region M53.81
    - sacrococcygeal region M53.88
    - thoracic region M53.84
    - thoracolumbar region M53.85
- **Double**
  - albumin E88.09
  - aortic arch Q25.4
  - auditory canal Q17.8
  - auricle (heart) Q20.8
  - bladder Q64.79
  - cervix Q51.820
    - with doubling of uterus (and vagina) Q51.10
      - with obstruction Q51.11
  - inlet ventricle Q20.4
  - kidney with double pelvis (renal) Q63.0
  - meatus urinarius Q64.75
  - monster Q89.4
  - outlet
    - left ventricle Q20.2
    - right ventricle Q20.1
  - pelvis (renal) with double ureter Q62.5
  - tongue Q38.3
  - ureter (one or both sides) Q62.5
    - with double pelvis (renal) Q62.5
  - urethra Q64.74
  - urinary meatus Q64.75
  - uterus Q51.2
    - with
      - doubling of cervix (and vagina) Q51.10
        - with obstruction Q51.11
    - in pregnancy or childbirth O34.59-
      - causing obstructed labor O65.5
  - vagina Q52.10
    - with doubling of uterus (and cervix) Q51.10
      - with obstruction Q51.11
  - vision H53.2
  - vulva Q52.79
- **Down syndrome** Q90.9
  - meiotic nondisjunction Q90.0
  - mitotic nondisjunction Q90.1
  - mosaicism Q90.1
  - translocation Q90.2
- **DPD** (dihydropyrimidine dehydrogenase deficiency) E88.89
- **Dracontiasis** B72
- **Dracunculiasis, dracunculosis** B72
- **Dream state, hysterical** F44.89
- **Dreschlera** (hawaiiensis) (infection) B43.8
- **Drepanocytic anemia** — *see* Disease, sickle-cell
- **Dresbach's syndrome** (elliptocytosis) D58.1
- **Dressler's syndrome** I24.1
- **Drift, ulnar** — *see* Deformity, limb, specified type NEC, forearm
- **Drinking** (alcohol)
  - excessive, to excess NEC (without dependence) F10.10
    - habitual (continual) (without remission) F10.20
      - with remission F10.21
- **Drip, postnasal** (chronic) R09.82
  - due to
    - allergic rhinitis — *see* Rhinitis, allergic
    - common cold J00
    - gastroesophageal reflux — *see* Reflux, gastroesophageal
    - nasopharyngitis — *see* Nasopharyngitis
    - other know condition—code to condition
    - sinusitis — *see* Sinusitis
- **Droop**
  - facial R29.810
    - cerebrovascular disease I69.992
      - cerebral infarction I69.392
      - intracerebral hemorrhage I69.192

- **Droop** — *continued*
  - facial — *continued*
    - cerebrovascular disease — *continued*
      - nontraumatic intracranial hemorrhage NEC I69.292
      - subarachnoid hemorrhage I69.Ø92
- **Drop** (in)
  - attack NEC R55
  - finger — *see* Deformity, finger
  - foot — *see* Deformity, limb, foot, drop
  - hematocrit (precipitous) R71.Ø
  - hemoglobin R71.Ø
  - toe — *see* Deformity, toe, specified NEC
  - wrist — *see* Deformity, limb, wrist drop
- **Dropped heart beats** I45.9
- **Dropsy, dropsical** (*see also* Hydrops)
  - abdomen R18.8
  - brain — *see* Hydrocephalus
  - cardiac, heart — *see* Failure, heart, congestive
  - gangrenous — *see* Gangrene
  - heart — *see* Failure, heart, congestive
  - kidney — *see* Nephrosis
  - lung — *see* Edema, lung
  - newborn due to isoimmunization P56.Ø
  - pericardium — *see* Pericarditis
- **Drowned, drowning** (near) T75.1
- **Drowsiness** R40.0
- **Drug**
  - abuse counseling and surveillance Z71.51
  - addiction — *see* Dependence
  - dependence — *see* Dependence
  - habit — *see* Dependence
  - harmful use — *see* Abuse, drug
  - induced fever R5Ø.2
  - overdose — *see* Table of Drugs and Chemicals, by drug, poisoning
  - poisoning — *see* Table of Drugs and Chemicals, by drug, poisoning
  - resistant organism infection (*see also* Resistant, organism, to, drug) Z16.3Ø
  - therapy
    - long term (current) (prophylactic) — *see* Therapy, drug long-term (current) (prophylactic)
    - short term — *omit code*
  - wrong substance given or taken in error — *see* Table of Drugs and Chemicals, by drug, poisoning
- **Drunkenness** (without dependence) F1Ø.129
  - acute in alcoholism F1Ø.229
  - chronic (without remission) F1Ø.2Ø
    - with remission F1Ø.21
  - pathological (without dependence) F1Ø.129
    - with dependence F1Ø.229
  - sleep F51.9
- **Drusen**
  - macula (degenerative) (retina) — *see* Degeneration, macula, drusen
  - optic disc H47.32-
- **Dry, dryness** (*see also* condition)
  - larynx J38.7
  - mouth R68.2
    - due to dehydration E86.Ø
  - nose J34.89
  - socket (teeth) M27.3
  - throat J39.2
- **DSAP** L56.5
- **Duane's syndrome** H50.81-
- **Dubin-Johnson disease or syndrome** E80.6
- **Dubois' disease** (thymus gland) A5Ø.59 *[E35]*
- **Dubowitz' syndrome** Q87.1
- **Duchenne-Aran muscular atrophy** G12.21
- **Duchenne-Griesinger disease** G71.0
- **Duchenne's**
  - disease or syndrome
    - motor neuron disease G12.22
    - muscular dystrophy G71.Ø
  - locomotor ataxia (syphilitic) A52.11
  - paralysis
    - birth injury P14.Ø
    - due to or associated with
      - motor neuron disease G12.22
      - muscular dystrophy G71.Ø
- **Ducrey's chancre** A57
- **Duct, ductus** — *see* condition
- **Duhring's disease** (dermatitis herpetiformis) L13.Ø
- **Dullness, cardiac** (decreased) (increased) RØ1.2
- **Dumb ague** — *see* Malaria
- **Dumbness** — *see* Aphasia
- **Dumdum fever** B55.0
- **Dumping syndrome** (postgastrectomy) K91.1
- **Duodenitis** (nonspecific) (peptic) K29.8Ø
  - with bleeding K29.81
- **Duodenocholangitis** — *see* Cholangitis
- **Duodenum, duodenal** — *see* condition
- **Duplay's bursitis or periarthritis** — *see* Tendinitis, calcific, shoulder
- **Duplication, duplex** (*see also* Accessory)
  - alimentary tract Q45.8
  - anus Q43.4
  - appendix (and cecum) Q43.4
  - biliary duct (any) Q44.5
  - bladder Q64.79
  - cecum (and appendix) Q43.4
  - cervix Q51.82Ø
  - chromosome NEC
    - with complex rearrangements NEC Q92.5
    - seen only at prometaphase Q92.8
  - cystic duct Q44.5
  - digestive organs Q45.8
  - esophagus Q39.8
  - frontonasal process Q75.8
  - intestine (large) (small) Q43.4
  - kidney Q63.Ø
  - liver Q44.7
  - oesophagus Q39.8
  - pancreas Q45.3
  - penis Q55.69
  - respiratory organs NEC Q34.8
  - salivary duct Q38.4
  - spinal cord (incomplete) QØ6.2
  - stomach Q4Ø.2
- **Dupré's disease** (meningism) R29.1
- **Dupuytren's contraction or disease** M72.0
- **Durand-Nicolas-Favre disease** A55
- **Durotomy** (inadvertent) (incidental) G97.41
- **Duroziez's disease** (congenital mitral stenosis) Q23.2
- **Dutton's relapsing fever** (West African) A68.1
- **Dwarfism** E34.3
  - achondroplastic Q77.4
  - congenital E34.3
  - constitutional E34.3
  - hypochondroplastic Q77.4
  - hypophyseal E23.Ø
  - infantile E34.3
  - Laron-type E34.3
  - Lorain(-Levi) type E23.Ø
  - metatropic Q77.8
  - nephrotic-glycosuric (with hypophosphatemic rickets) E72.Ø9
  - nutritional E45
  - pancreatic K86.8
  - pituitary E23.Ø
  - renal N25.Ø
  - thanatophoric Q77.1
- **Dyke-Young anemia** (secondary) (symptomatic) D59.1
- **Dysacusis** — *see* Abnormal, auditory perception
- **Dysadrenocortism E27.9**
  - hyperfunction E27.Ø
- **Dysarthria** R47.1
  - following
    - cerebral infarction I69.322
    - cerebrovascular disease I69.922
      - specified disease NEC I69.822
    - intracerebral hemorrhage I69.122
    - nontraumatic intracranial hemorrhage NEC I69.222
    - subarachnoid hemorrhage I69.Ø22
- **Dysautonomia** (familial) G9Ø.1
- **Dysbarism** T70.3
- **Dysbasia** R26.2
  - angiosclerotica intermittens I73.9
  - hysterical F44.4
  - lordotica (progressiva) G24.1
  - nonorganic origin F44.4
  - psychogenic F44.4
- **Dysbetalipoproteinemia** (familial) E78.2
- **Dyscalculia** R48.8
  - developmental F81.2
- **Dyschezia** K59.00
- **Dyschondroplasia** (with hemangiomata) Q78.4
- **Dyschromia** (skin) L81.9
- **Dyscollagenosis** M35.9
- **Dyscranio-pygo-phalangy** Q87.0
- **Dyscrasia**
  - blood (with) D75.9
    - antepartum hemorrhage — *see* Hemorrhage, antepartum, with coagulation defect
    - newborn P61.9
      - specified type NEC P61.8
    - intrapartum hemorrhage O67.Ø
    - puerperal, postpartum O72.3
  - polyglandular, pluriglandular E31.9
- **Dysendocrinism** E34.9
- **Dysentery, dysenteric** (catarrhal) (diarrhea) (epidemic) (hemorrhagic) (infectious) (sporadic) (tropical) AØ9
  - abscess, liver AØ6.4
  - amebic (*see also* Amebiasis) AØ6.Ø
    - with abscess — *see* Abscess, amebic
    - acute AØ6.Ø
    - chronic AØ6.1
  - arthritis AØ9 (*see also* category MØ1)
    - bacillary AØ3.9(*see also* category MØ1)
  - bacillary AØ3.9
    - arthritis AØ3.9(*see also* category MØ1)
    - Boyd AØ3.2
    - Flexner AØ3.1
    - Schmitz(-Stutzer) AØ3.Ø
    - Shiga(-Kruse) AØ3.Ø
    - Shigella AØ3.9
      - boydii AØ3.2
      - dysenteriae AØ3.Ø
      - flexneri AØ3.1
      - group A AØ3.Ø
      - group B AØ3.1
      - group C AØ3.2
      - group D AØ3.3
      - sonnei AØ3.3
      - specified type NEC AØ3.8
    - Sonne AØ3.3
    - specified type NEC AØ3.8
  - balantidial AØ7.Ø
  - Balantidium coli AØ7.Ø
  - Boyd's AØ3.2
  - candidal B37.82
  - Chilomastix AØ7.8
  - Chinese AØ3.9
  - coccidial AØ7.3
  - Dientamoeba (fragilis) AØ7.8
  - Embadomonas AØ7.8
  - Entamoeba, entamebic — *see* Dysentery, amebic
  - Flexner-Boyd AØ3.2
  - Flexner's AØ3.1
  - Giardia lamblia AØ7.1
  - Hiss-Russell AØ3.1
  - Lamblia AØ7.1
  - leishmanial B55.Ø
  - malarial — *see* Malaria
  - metazoal B82.Ø
  - monilial B37.82
  - protozoal AØ7.9
  - Salmonella AØ2.Ø
  - schistosomal B65.1
  - Schmitz(-Stutzer) AØ3.Ø
  - Shiga(-Kruse) AØ3.Ø
  - Shigella NOS — *see* Dysentery, bacillary
  - Sonne AØ3.3
  - strongyloidiasis B78.Ø
  - trichomonal AØ7.8
  - viral (*see also* Enteritis, viral) AØ8.4
- **Dysequilibrium** R42
- **Dysesthesia** R20.8
  - hysterical F44.6
- **Dysfibrinogenemia** (congenital) D68.2
- **Dysfunction**
  - adrenal E27.9
    - hyperfunction E27.Ø
  - autonomic
    - due to alcohol G31.2

Dyskinesia— *continued*
- drug induced
  - orofacial G24.Ø1
- esophagus K22.4
- hysterical F44.4
- intestinal K59.8
- nonorganic origin F44.4
- orofacial (idiopathic) G24.4
  - drug induced G24.Ø1
- psychogenic F44.4
- subacute, drug induced G24.Ø1
- tardive G24.Ø1
  - neuroleptic induced G24.Ø1
- trachea J39.8
- tracheobronchial J98.Ø9

Dyslalia (developmental) F8Ø.Ø

Dyslexia R48.0
- developmental F81.Ø

Dyslipidemia E78.5
- depressed HDL cholesterol E78.6
- elevated fasting triglycerides E78.1

Dysmaturity (*see also* Light for dates)
- pulmonary (newborn) (Wilson-Mikity) P27.Ø

Dysmenorrhea (essential) (exfoliative) N94.6
- congestive (syndrome) N94.6
- primary N94.4
- psychogenic F45.8
- secondary N94.5

Dysmetabolic syndrome X E88.81

Dysmetria R27.8

Dysmorphism (due to)
- alcohol Q86.Ø
- exogenous cause NEC Q86.8
- hydantoin Q86.1
- warfarin Q86.2

Dysmorphophobia (nondelusional) F45.22
- delusional F22

Dysnomia R47.01

Dysorexia R63.0
- psychogenic F5Ø.8

Dysostosis
- cleidocranial, cleidocranialis Q74.Ø
- craniofacial Q75.1
- Fairbank's (idiopathic familial generalized osteophytosis) Q78.9
- mandibulofacial (incomplete) Q75.4
- multiplex E76.Ø1
- oculomandibular Q75.5

Dyspareunia (female) N94.1
- male N53.12
- nonorganic F52.6
- psychogenic F52.6
- secondary N94.1

Dyspepsia R1Ø.13
- atonic K3Ø
- functional (allergic) (congenital) (gastrointestinal) (occupational) (reflex) K3Ø
- intestinal K59.8
- nervous F45.8
- neurotic F45.8
- psychogenic F45.8

Dysphagia R13.10
- cervical R13.19
- following
  - cerebral infarction I69.391
  - cerebrovascular disease I69.991
    - specified NEC I69.891
  - intracerebral hemorrhage I69.191
  - nontraumatic intracranial hemorrhage NEC I69.291
  - specified disease NEC I69.891
  - subarachnoid hemorrhage I69.Ø91
- functional (hysterical) F45.8
- hysterical F45.8
- nervous (hysterical) F45.8
- neurogenic R13.19
- oral phase R13.11
- oropharyngeal phase R13.12
- pharyneal phase R13.13
- pharyngoesophageal phase R13.14
- psychogenic F45.8
- sideropenic D5Ø.1
- spastica K22.4

Dysphagia — *continued*
- specified NEC R13.19

Dysphagocytosis, congenital D71

Dysphasia R47.02
- developmental
  - expressive type F8Ø.1

Dysphasia— *continued*
- developmental— *continued*
  - receptive type F8Ø.2
- following
  - cerebrovascular disease I69.921
    - cerebral infarction I69.321
    - intracerebral hemorrhage I69.121
    - nontraumatic intracranial hemorrhage NEC I69.221
    - specified disease NEC I69.821
    - subarachnoid hemorrhage I69.Ø21

Dysphonia R49.0
- functional F44.4
- hysterical F44.4
- psychogenic F44.4
- spastica J38.3

Dysphoria, postpartal O90.6

Dyspituitarism E23.3

Dysplasia (*see also* Anomaly)
- acetabular, congenital Q65.89
- alveolar capillary, with vein misalignment J84.843
- anus (histologically confirmed) (mild) (moderate) K62.82
  - severe DØ1.3
- arrhythmogenic right ventricular I42.8
- arterial, fibromuscular I77.3
- asphyxiating thoracic (congenital) Q77.2
- brain QØ7.9
- bronchopulmonary, perinatal P27.1
- cervix (uteri) N87.9
  - mild N87.Ø
  - moderate N87.1
  - severe DØ6.9
- chondroectodermal Q77.6
- colon D12.6
- craniometaphyseal Q78.5
- dentinal KØØ.5
- diaphyseal, progressive Q78.3
- dystrophic Q77.5
- ectodermal (anhidrotic) (congenital) (hereditary) Q82.4
  - hydrotic Q82.8
- epithelial, uterine cervix — *see* Dysplasia, cervix
- eye (congenital) Q11.2
- fibrous
  - bone NEC (monostotic) M85.ØØ
    - ankle M85.Ø7-
    - foot M85.Ø7-
    - forearm M85.Ø3-
    - hand M85.Ø4-
    - lower leg M85.Ø6-
    - multiple site M85.Ø9
    - neck M85.Ø8
    - rib M85.Ø8
    - shoulder M85.Ø1-
    - skull M85.Ø8
    - specified site NEC M85.Ø8
    - thigh M85.Ø5-
    - toe M85.Ø7-
    - upper arm M85.Ø2-
    - vertebra M85.Ø8
  - diaphyseal, progressive Q78.3
  - jaw M27.8
  - polyostotic Q78.1
- florid osseous (*see also* Cyst, calcifying odontogenic)
- high grade, focal D12.6
- hip, congenital Q65.89
- joint, congenital Q74.8
- kidney Q61.4
  - multicystic Q61.4
- leg Q74.2
- lung, congenital (not associated with short gestation) Q33.6
- mammary (gland) (benign) N6Ø.9-
  - cyst (solitary) — *see* Cyst, breast
  - cystic — *see* Mastopathy, cystic
  - duct ectasia — *see* Ectasia, mammary duct

Dysplasia — *continued*
- mammary (gland) (benign) — *continued*
  - fibroadenosis — *see* Fibroadenosis, breast
  - fibrosclerosis — *see* Fibrosclerosis, breast
  - specified type NEC N6Ø.8-
- metaphyseal (Jansen's) (McKusick's) (Schmid's) Q78.5
- muscle Q79.8

Dysplasia — *continued*
- oculodentodigital Q87.Ø
- periapical (cemental) (cemento-osseous) — *see* Cyst, calcifying odontogenic
- periosteum — *see* Disorder, bone, specified type NEC
- polyostotic fibrous Q78.1
- prostate (*see also* Neoplasia, intraepithelial, prostate) N42.3
  - severe DØ7.5
- renal Q61.4
  - multicystic Q61.4
- retinal, congenital Q14.1
- right ventricular, arrhythmogenic I42.8
- septo-optic QØ4.4
- skin L98.8
- spinal cord QØ6.1
- spondyloepiphyseal Q77.7
- thymic, with immunodeficiency D82.1
- vagina N89.3
  - mild N89.Ø
  - moderate N89.1
  - severe NEC DØ7.2
- vulva N9Ø.3
  - mild N9Ø.Ø
  - moderate N9Ø.1
  - severe NEC DØ7.1

Dyspnea (nocturnal) (paroxysmal) RØ6.ØØ
- asthmatic (bronchial) J45.9Ø9
  - with
    - exacerbation (acute) J45.9Ø1
    - bronchitis J45.9Ø9
      - with
        - exacerbation (acute) J45.9Ø1
        - status asthmaticus J45.9Ø2
      - chronic J44.9
    - status asthmaticus J45.9Ø2
  - cardiac — *see* Failure, ventricular, left
- cardiac — *see* Failure, ventricular, left
- functional F45.8
- hyperventilation RØ6.4
- hysterical F45.8
- newborn P28.89
- orthopnea RØ6.Ø1
- psychogenic F45.8
- shortness of breath RØ6.Ø2
- specified type NEC RØ6.Ø9

Dyspraxia R27.8
- developmental (syndrome) F82

Dysproteinemia E88.09

Dysreflexia, autonomic G90.4

Dysrhythmia
- cardiac I49.9
  - newborn
    - bradycardia P29.12
    - tachycardia P29.11
    - occurring before birth PØ3.819
      - before onset of labor PØ3.81Ø
      - during labor PØ3.811
  - postoperative I97.89
- cerebral or cortical — *see* Epilepsy

Dyssomnia — *see* Disorder, sleep

Dyssynergia
- biliary K83.8
- bladder sphincter N36.44
- cerebellaris myoclonica (Hunt's ataxia) G11.1

Dysthymia F34.1

Dysthyroidism E07.9

Dystocia O66.9
- affecting newborn PØ3.1
- cervical (hypotonic) O62.2
  - affecting newborn PØ3.6
  - primary O62.Ø
  - secondary O62.1
- contraction ring O62.4

E

- **Elephantiasis**— *continued*
  - lymphatic vessel I89.Ø
    - due to mastectomy I97.2
  - scrotum (nonfilarial) I89.Ø
  - streptococcal I89.Ø
  - surgical I97.89
    - postmastectomy I97.2
  - telangiectodes I89.Ø
  - vulva (nonfilarial) N9Ø.89
- **Elevated, elevation**
  - antibody titer R76.Ø
  - basal metabolic rate R94.8
  - blood pressure (*see also* Hypertension)
    - reading (incidental) (isolated) (nonspecific), no diagnosis of hypertension RØ3.Ø
  - blood sugar R73.9
  - body temperature (of unknown origin) R5Ø.9
  - C-reactive protein (CRP) R79.82
  - cancer antigen 125 [CA 125] R97.1
  - carcinoembryonic antigen [CEA] R97.Ø
  - cholesterol E78.Ø
    - with high triglycerides E78.2
  - conjugate, eye H51.Ø
  - diaphragm, congenital Q79.1
  - erythrocyte sedimentation rate R7Ø.Ø
  - fasting glucose R73.Ø1
  - fasting triglycerides E78.1
  - finding on laboratory examination — *see* Findings, abnormal, inconclusive, without diagnosis, by type of exam
  - GFR (glomerular filtration rate) — *see* Findings, abnormal, inconclusive, without diagnosis, by type of exam
  - glucose tolerance (oral) R73.Ø2
  - immunoglobulin level R76.8
  - indoleacetic acid R82.5
  - lactic acid dehydrogenase (LDH) level R74.Ø
  - leukocytes D72.829
  - lipoprotein a level E78.8
  - liver function
    - study R94.5
    - test R79.89
      - alkaline phosphatase R74.8
      - aminotransferase R74.Ø
      - bilirubin R17
      - hepatic enzyme R74.8
      - lactate dehydrogenase R74.Ø
  - lymphocytes D72.82Ø
  - prostate specific antigen [PSA] R97.2
  - Rh titer T8Ø.4 — *see* Complication(s), transfusion, incompatiblity reaction, Rh (factor)
  - scapula, congenital Q74.Ø
  - sedimentation rate R7Ø.Ø
  - SGOT R74.Ø
  - SGPT R74.Ø
  - transaminase level R74.Ø
  - triglycerides E78.1
    - with high cholesterol E78.2
  - tumor associated antigens [TAA] NEC R97.8
  - tumor specific antigens [TSA] NEC R97.8
  - urine level of
    - catecholamine R82.5
    - indoleacetic acid R82.5
    - 17-ketosteroids R82.5
    - steroids R82.5
    - vanillylmandelic acid (VMA) R82.5
  - venous pressure I87.8
  - white blood cell count D72.829
    - specified NEC D72.828
- **Elliptocytosis** (congenital) (hereditary) D58.1 Hb C (disease) D58.1
  - hemoglobin disease D58.1
  - sickle-cell (disease) D57.8-
    - trait D57.3
- **Ellison-Zollinger syndrome** E16.4
- **Ellis-van Creveld syndrome** (chondroectodermal dysplasia) Q77.6
- **Elongated, elongation** (congenital) (*see also* Distortion)
  - bone Q79.9
  - cervix (uteri) Q51.828
    - acquired N88.4
    - hypertrophic N88.4
- **Elongated, elongation**— *continued*
  - colon Q43.8
  - common bile duct Q44.5
  - cystic duct Q44.5
  - frenulum, penis Q55.69
  - labia minora (acquired) N9Ø.6
  - ligamentum patellae Q74.1
  - petiolus (epiglottidis) Q31.8
  - tooth, teeth KØØ.2
  - uvula Q38.6
- **Eltor cholera** A00.1
- **Emaciation** (due to malnutrition) E41
- **Embadomoniasis** A07.8
- **Embedded tooth, teeth** K01.0
  - root only KØ8.3
- **Embolic** — *see* condition
- **Embolism** (multiple) (paradoxical) I74.9
  - air (any site) (traumatic) T79.Ø
    - following
      - abortion — *see* Abortion by type complicated by embolism
      - ectopic pregnancy OØ8.2
      - infusion, therapeutic injection or transfusion T8Ø.Ø
      - molar pregnancy OØ8.2
      - procedure NEC
        - artery T81.719
          - mesenteric T81.71Ø
          - renal T81.711
          - specified NEC T81.718
        - vein T81.72
    - in pregnancy, childbirth or puerperium — *see* Embolism, obstetric
  - amniotic fluid (pulmonary) (*see also* Embolism, obstetric)
    - following
      - abortion — *see* Abortion by type complicated by embolism
      - ectopic pregnancy OØ8.2
      - molar pregnancy OØ8.2
  - aorta, aortic I74.1Ø
    - abdominal I74.Ø9
      - saddle I74.Ø1
    - bifurcation I74.Ø9
    - saddle I74.Ø1
    - thoracic I74.11
  - artery I74.9
    - auditory, internal I65.8
    - basilar — *see* Occlusion, artery, basilar
    - carotid (common) (internal) — *see* Occlusion, artery, carotid
    - cerebellar (anterior inferior) (posterior inferior) (superior) I66.3
    - cerebral — *see* Occlusion, artery, cerebral
    - choroidal (anterior) I66.8
    - communicating posterior I66.8
    - coronary (*see also* Infarct, myocardium)
      - not resulting in infarction I24.Ø
    - extremity I74.4
      - lower I74.3
      - upper I74.2
    - hypophyseal I66.8
    - iliac I74.5
    - limb I74.4
      - lower I74.3
      - upper I74.2
    - mesenteric (with gangrene) K55.Ø
    - ophthalmic — *see* Occlusion, artery, retina
    - peripheral I74.4
    - pontine I66.8
    - precerebral — *see* Occlusion, artery, precerebral
    - pulmonary — *see* Embolism, pulmonary
    - renal N28.Ø
    - retinal — *see* Occlusion, artery, retina
    - septic I76
    - specified NEC I74.8
    - vertebral — *see* Occlusion, artery, vertebral
  - basilar (artery) I65.1
  - blood clot
    - following
      - abortion — *see* Abortion by type complicated by embolism
      - ectopic or molar pregnancy OØ8.2
- **Embolism** — *continued*
  - blood clot— *continued*
    - in pregnancy, childbirth or puerperium — *see* Embolism, obstetric
  - brain (*see also* Occlusion, artery, cerebral)
    - following
      - abortion — *see* Abortion by type complicated by embolism
      - ectopic or molar pregnancy OØ8.2
    - puerperal, postpartum, childbirth — *see* Embolism, obstetric
  - capillary I78.8
  - cardiac (*see also* Infarct, myocardium)
    - not resulting in infarction I24.Ø
  - carotid (artery) (common) (internal) — *see* Occlusion, artery, carotid
  - cavernous sinus (venous) — *see* Embolism, intracranial venous sinus
  - cerebral — *see* Occlusion, artery, cerebral
  - cholesterol — *see* Atheroembolism
  - coronary (artery or vein) (systemic) — *see* Occlusion, coronary
  - due to device, implant or graft (*see also* Complications, by site and type, specified NEC)
    - arterial graft NEC T82.818
    - breast (implant) T85.81
    - catheter NEC T85.81
      - dialysis (renal) T82.818
        - intraperitoneal T85.81
      - infusion NEC T82.818
        - spinal (epidural) (subdural) T85.81
      - urinary (indwelling) T83.81
    - electronic (electrode) (pulse generator) (stimulator)
      - bone T84.81
      - cardiac T82.817
      - nervous system (brain) (peripheral nerve) (spinal) T85.81
      - urinary T83.81
    - fixation, internal (orthopedic) NEC T84.81
    - gastrointestinal (bile duct) (esophagus) T85.81
    - genital NEC T83.81
    - heart (graft) (valve) T82.817
    - joint prosthesis T84.81
    - ocular (corneal graft) (orbital implant) T85.81
    - orthopedic (bone graft) NEC T86.838
    - specified NEC T85.81
    - urinary (graft) NEC T83.81
    - vascular NEC T82.818
    - ventricular intracranial shunt T85.81
  - extremities
    - lower — *see* Embolism, vein, lower extremity
      - arterial I74.3
    - upper I74.2
  - eye H34.9
  - fat (cerebral) (pulmonary) (systemic) T79.1
    - following
      - abortion — *see* Abortion by type complicated by embolism
      - ectopic or molar pregnancy OØ8.2
    - complicating delivery — *see* Embolism, obstetric
  - following
    - abortion — *see* Abortion by type complicated by embolism
    - ectopic or molar pregnancy OØ8.2
    - infusion, therapeutic injection or transfusion
      - air T8Ø.Ø
      - thrombus T8Ø.1
  - heart (fatty) (*see also* Infarct, myocardium)
    - not resulting in infarction I24.Ø
  - hepatic (vein) I82.Ø
  - in pregnancy, childbirth or puerperium — *see* Embolism, obstetric
  - intestine (artery) (vein) (with gangrene) K55.Ø
  - intracranial (*see also* Occlusion, artery, cerebral)
    - venous sinus (any) GØ8
      - nonpyogenic I67.6
  - intraspinal venous sinuses or veins GØ8
    - nonpyogenic G95.19
  - kidney (artery) N28.Ø
  - lateral sinus (venous) — *see* Embolism, intracranial, venous sinus

Embolism — *continued*
- leg — *see* Embolism, vein, lower extremity
  - arterial I74.3
- longitudinal sinus (venous) — *see* Embolism, intracranial, venous sinus
- lung (massive) — *see* Embolism, pulmonary
- meninges I66.8
- mesenteric (artery) (vein) (with gangrene) K55.Ø
- obstetric (in) (pulmonary)
  - childbirth O88.82
    - air O88.Ø2
    - amniotic fluid O88.12
    - blood clot O88.22
    - fat O88.82
    - pyemic O88.32
    - septic O88.32
    - specified type NEC O88.82
  - pregnancy O88.81-
    - air O88.Ø1-
    - amniotic fluid O88.11-
    - blood clot O88.21-
    - fat O88.81-
    - pyemic O88.31-
    - septic O88.31-
    - specified type NEC O88.81-
  - puerperal O88.83
    - air O88.Ø3
    - amniotic fluid O88.13
    - blood clot O88.23
    - fat O88.83
    - pyemic O88.33
    - septic O88.33
    - specified type NEC O88.83
- ophthalmic — *see* Occlusion, artery, retina
- penis N48.81
- peripheral artery NOS I74.4
- pituitary E23.6
- popliteal (artery) I74.3
- portal (vein) I81
- postoperative, postrpocedural
  - artery T81.719
    - mesenteric T81.71Ø
    - renal T81.711
    - specified NEC T81.718
  - vein T81.72
- precerebral artery — *see* Occlusion, artery, precerebral
- puerperal — *see* Embolism, obstetric
- pulmonary (acute) (artery) (vein) I26.99
  - with acute cor pulmonale I26.Ø9
  - chronic I27.82
  - following
    - abortion — *see* Abortion by type complicated by embolism
    - ectopic or molar pregnancy OØ8.2
  - healed or old Z86.711
  - in pregnancy, childbirth or puerperium — *see* Embolism, obstetric
  - personal history of Z86.711
  - saddle I26.92
    - with acute cor pulmonale I26.Ø2
  - septic I26.9Ø
    - with acute cor pulmonale I26.Ø1
- pyemic (multiple) I76
  - following
    - abortion — *see* Abortion by type complicated by embolism
    - ectopic or molar pregnancy OØ8.2
  - Hemophilus influenzae A41.3
  - pneumococcal A4Ø.3
    - with pneumonia J13
  - puerperal, postpartum, childbirth (any organism) — *see* Embolism, obstetric
  - specified organism NEC A41.89
  - staphylococcal A41.2
  - streptococcal A4Ø.9
- renal (artery) N28.Ø
  - vein I82.3
- retina, retinal — *see* Occlusion, artery, retina
- saddle
  - abdominal aorta I74.Ø1
  - pulmonary artery I26.92
    - with acute cor pulmonale I26.Ø2

Embolism — *continued*
- septic (arterial) I76
  - complicating abortion — *see* Abortion, by type, complicated by, embolism
- sinus — *see* Embolism, intracranial, venous sinus
- soap complicating abortion — *see* Abortion, by type, complicated by, embolism
- spinal cord G95.19
  - pyogenic origin GØ6.1
- spleen, splenic (artery) I74.8
- upper extremity I74.2
- vein (acute) I82.9Ø
  - antecubital I82.61-
    - chronic I82.71
  - axillary I82.A1-
    - chronic I82.A2-
  - basilic I82.61-
    - chronic I82.71
  - brachial I82.62-
    - chronic I82.72
  - brachiocephalic (innominate) I82.29Ø
    - chronic I82.291
  - cephalic I82.61-
    - chronic I82.71
  - chronic I82.91
    - upper extremity I82.7Ø
  - deep (DVT) I82.4Ø-
    - calf I82.4Z-
      - chronic I82.5Z-
    - lower leg I82.4Z-
      - chronic I82.5Z-
    - thigh I82.4Y-
      - chronic I82.5Y-
    - upper leg I82.4Y-
      - chronic I82.5Y-
  - femoral I82.41-
    - chronic I82.51
  - iliac (iliofemoral) I82.42-
    - chronic I82.51-
  - innominate I82.29Ø
    - chronic I82.291
  - internal jugular I82.C1-
    - chronic I82.C2-
  - lower extremity
    - deep I82.4Ø-
      - chronic I82.5Ø-
      - specifed NEC I82.49-
        - chronic NEC I82.59-
    - distal
      - deep I82.4Z-
    - proximal
      - deep I82.4Y-
        - chronic I82.5Y-
    - superficial I82.81
  - mesenteric (with gangrene) K55.Ø
  - popliteal I82.43-
    - chronic I82.53-
  - radial I82.62-
    - chronic I82.72-
  - renal I82.3
  - saphenous (greater) (lesser) I82.81-
  - specified NEC I82.89Ø
    - chronic I82.891
  - subclavian I82.B1-
    - chronic I82.B2-
  - thoracic NEC I82.29Ø
    - chronic I82.291
  - tibial I82.44-
    - chronic I82.54-
  - ulnar I82.62-
    - chronic I82.72-
  - upper extremity I82.6Ø-
    - chronic I82.7Ø-
    - deep I82.62-
      - chronic I82.72-
    - superficial I82.61-
      - chronic I82.71
- vena cava
  - inferior (acute) I82.22Ø
    - chronic I82.221
  - superior (acute) I82.21Ø
    - chronic I82.211
- venous sinus GØ8

Embolism — *continued*
- vessels of brain — *see* Occlusion, artery, cerebral

Embolus — *see* Embolism

Embryoma (*see also* Neoplasm, uncertain behavior, by site)
- benign — *see* Neoplasm, benign, by site
- kidney C64.-
- liver C22.Ø
- malignant (*see also* Neoplasm, malignant, by site)
  - kidney C64.-
  - liver C22.Ø
  - testis C62.9-
    - descended (scrotal) C62.1-
    - undescended C62.Ø-
- testis C62.9-
  - descended (scrotal) C62.1-
  - undescended C62.Ø-

Embryonic
- circulation Q28.9
- heart Q28.9
- vas deferens Q55.4

Embryopathia NOS Q89.9

Embryotoxon Q13.4

Emesis — *see* Vomiting

Emotional lability R45.86

Emotionality, pathological F60.3

Emotogenic disease — *see* Disorder, psychogenic

Emphysema (atrophic) (bullous) (chronic) (interlobular) (lung) (obstructive) (pulmonary) (senile) (vesicular) J43.9
- cellular tissue (traumatic) T79.7
  - surgical T81.82
- centrilobular J43.2
- compensatory J98.3
- congenital (interstitial) P25.Ø
- conjunctiva H11.89
- connective tissue (traumatic) T79.7
  - surgical T81.82
- due to chemicals, gases, fumes or vapors J68.4
- eyelid(s) — see Disorder, eyelid, specified type NEC
  - surgical T81.82
  - traumatic T79.7
- interstitial J98.2
  - congenital P25.Ø
  - perinatal period P25.Ø
- laminated tissue T79.7
  - surgical T81.82
- mediastinal J98.2
  - newborn P25.2
- orbit, orbital — see Disorder, orbit, specified type NEC
- panacinar J43.1
- panlobular J43.1
- specified NEC J43.8
- subcutaneous (traumatic) T79.7
  - nontraumatic J98.2
  - postprocedural T81.82
  - surgical T81.82
- surgical T81.82
- thymus (gland) (congenital) E32.8
- traumatic (subcutaneous) T79.7
- unilateral J43.Ø

Empty nest syndrome Z60.0

Empyema (acute) (chest) (double) (pleura) (supradiaphragmatic) (thorax) J86.9
- with fistula J86.Ø
- accessory sinus (chronic) — *see* Sinusitis
- antrum (chronic) — *see* Sinusitis, maxillary
- brain (any part) — *see* Abscess, brain
- ethmoidal (chronic) (sinus) — *see* Sinusitis, ethmoidal
- extradural — *see* Abscess, extradural
- frontal (chronic) (sinus) — *see* Sinusitis, frontal
- gallbladder K81.Ø
- mastoid (process) (acute) — *see* Mastoiditis, acute
- maxilla, maxillary M27.2
  - sinus (chronic) — *see* Sinusitis, maxillary
- nasal sinus (chronic) — *see* Sinusitis
- sinus (accessory) (chronic) (nasal) — *see* Sinusitis
- sphenoidal (sinus) (chronic) — *see* Sinusitis, sphenoidal
- subarachnoid — *see* Abscess, extradural
- subdural — *see* Abscess, subdural
- tuberculous A15.6
- ureter — *see* Ureteritis

- **Empyema**— *continued*
  - ventricular — *see* Abscess, brain
- **En coup de sabre lesion** L94.1
- **Enamel pearls** K00.2
- **Enameloma** K00.2
- **Enanthema, viral** B09
- **Encephalitis** (chronic) (hemorrhagic) (idiopathic) (nonepidemic) (spurious) (subacute) G04.90
  - acute (*see also* Encephalitis, viral) A86
    - disseminated G04.00
      - infectious G04.01
      - noninfectious G04.81
      - postimmunization (postvaccination) G04.02
      - postinfectious G04.01
    - inclusion body A85.8
    - necrotizing hemorrhagic G04.30
      - postimmunization G04.32
      - postinfectious G04.31
      - specified NEC G04.39
  - arboviral, arbovirus NEC A85.2
  - arthropod-borne NEC (viral) A85.2
  - Australian A83.4
  - California (virus) A83.5
  - Central European (tick-borne) A84.1
  - Czechoslovakian A84.1
  - Dawson's (inclusion body) A81.1
  - diffuse sclerosing A81.1
  - disseminated, acute G04.00
  - due to
    - cat scratch disease A28.1
    - human immunodeficiency virus [HIV] disease B20 *[G05]*
    - malaria — *see* Malaria
    - rickettsiosis — *see* Rickettsiosis
    - smallpox inoculation G04.02
    - typhus — *see* Typhus
  - Eastern equine A83.2
  - endemic (viral) A86
  - epidemic NEC (viral) A86
  - equine (acute) (infectious) (viral) A83.9
    - Eastern A83.2
    - Venezuelan A92.2
    - Western A83.1
  - Far Eastern (tick-borne) A84.0
  - following vaccination or other immunization procedure G04.02
  - herpes zoster B02.0
  - herpesviral B00.4
    - due to herpesvirus 6 B10.01
    - due to herpesvirus 7 B10.09
    - specified NEC B10.09
  - Ilheus (virus) A83.8
  - inclusion body A81.1
  - in (due to)
    - actinomycosis A42.82
    - adenovirus A85.1
    - African trypanosomiasis B56.9 *[G05.3]*
    - Chagas' disease (chronic) B57.42
    - cytomegalovirus B25.8
    - enterovirus A85.0
    - herpes (simplex) virus B00.4
      - due to herpesvirus 6 B10.01
      - due to herpesvirus 7 B10.09
    - herpes (simplex) virus— *continued*
      - specified NEC B10.09
    - infectious disease NEC B99 *[G05.3]*
    - influenza — *see* Influenza, with, encephalopathy
    - listeriosis A32.12
    - measles B05.0
    - mumps B26.2
    - naegleriasis B60.2
    - parasitic disease NEC B89 *[G05.3]*
    - poliovirus A80.9 *[G05.3]*
    - rubella B06.01
    - syphilis
      - congenital A50.42
      - late A52.14
    - systemic lupus erythematosus M32.19
    - toxoplasmosis (acquired) B58.2
      - congenital P37.1
    - tuberculosis A17.82
    - zoster B02.0
  - infectious (acute) (virus) NEC A86

- **Encephalitis** — *continued*
  - Japanese (B type) A83.0
  - La Crosse A83.5
  - lead — *see* Poisoning, lead
  - lethargica (acute) (infectious) A85.8
  - louping ill A84.8
  - lupus erythematosus, systemic M32.19
  - lymphatica A87.2
  - Mengo A85.8
  - meningococcal A39.81
  - Murray Valley A83.4
  - otitic NEC H66.40 *[G05.3]*
  - parasitic NOS B71.9
  - periaxial G37.0
  - periaxialis (concentrica) (diffuse) G37.5
  - postchickenpox B01.11
  - postexanthematous NEC B09
  - postimmunization G04.02
  - postinfectious NEC G04.01
  - postmeasles B05.0
  - postvaccinal G04.02
  - postvaricella B01.11
  - postviral NEC A86
  - Powassan A84.8
  - Rasmussen G04.81
  - Rio Bravo A85.8
  - Russian
    - autumnal A83.0
    - spring-summer (taiga) A84.0
  - saturnine — *see* Poisoning, lead
  - specified NEC G04.81
  - St. Louis A83.3
  - subacute sclerosing A81.1
  - summer A83.0
  - suppurative G04.81
  - tick-borne A84.9
  - Torula, torular (cryptococcal) B45.1
  - toxic NEC G92
  - trichinosis B75 *[G05.3]*
  - type
    - B A83.0
    - C A83.3
  - van Bogaert's A81.1
  - Venezuelan equine A92.2
  - Vienna A85.8
  - viral, virus A86
    - arthropod-borne NEC A85.2
      - mosquito-borne A83.9
        - Australian X disease A83.4
        - California virus A83.5
        - Eastern equine A83.2
        - Japanese (B type) A83.0
        - Murray Valley A83.4
        - specified NEC A83.8
        - St. Louis A83.3
        - type B A83.0
        - type C A83.3
        - Western equine A83.1
      - tick-borne A84.9
        - biundulant A84.1
        - central European A84.1
        - Czechoslovakian A84.1
        - diphasic meningoencephalitis A84.1
        - Far Eastern A84.0
        - Russian spring-summer (taiga) A84.0
        - specified NEC A84.8
    - specified type NEC A85.8
  - Western equine A83.1
- **Encephalocele** Q01.9
  - frontal Q01.0
  - nasofrontal Q01.1
  - occipital Q01.2
  - specified NEC Q01.8
- **Encephalocystocele** — *see* Encephalocele
- **Encephaloduroarteriomyosynangiosis** (EDAMS) I67.5
- **Encephalomalacia** (brain) (cerebellar) (cerebral) — *see* Softening, brain
- **Encephalomeningitis** — *see* Meningoencephalitis
- **Encephalomeningocele** — *see* Encephalocele
- **Encephalomeningomyelitis** — *see* Meningoencephalitis

- **Encephalomyelitis** (*see also* Encephalitis) G04.90
  - acute disseminated G04.00
    - infectious G04.01
    - noninfectious G04.81
    - postinfectious G04.01
    - postimmunization G04.02
  - acute necrotizing hemorrhagic (postinfectious) G04.30
    - postimmunization G04.32
    - postinfectious G04.31
    - specified NEC G04.39
  - benign myalgic G93.3
  - equine A83.9
    - Eastern A83.2
    - Venezuelan A92.2
    - Western A83.1
  - in diseases classified elsewhere G05.3
  - myalgic, benign G93.3
  - postchickenpox B01.11
  - postinfectious NEC G04.01
  - postmeasles B05.0
  - postvaccinal G04.02
  - postvaricella B01.11
  - rubella B06.01
  - specified NEC G04.81
  - Venezuelan equine A92.2
- **Encephalomyelocele** — *see* Encephalocele
- **Encephalomyelomeningitis** — *see* Meningoencephalitis
- **Encephalomyelopathy** G96.9
- **Encephalomyeloradiculitis** (acute) G61.0
- **Encephalomyeloradiculoneuritis** (acute) (Guillain-Barré) G61.0
- **Encephalomyeloradiculopathy** G96.9
- **Encephalopathia hyperbilirubinemica, newborn** P57.9
  - due to isoimmunization (conditions in P55) P57.0
- **Encephalopathy** (acute) G93.40
  - acute necrotizing hemorrhagic G04.30
    - postimmunization G04.32
    - postinfectious G04.31
    - specified NEC G04.39
  - alcoholic G31.2
  - anoxic — *see* Damage, brain, anoxic
  - arteriosclerotic I67.2
  - centrolobar progressive (Schilder) G37.0
  - congenital Q07.9
  - degenerative, in specified disease NEC G32.89
  - demyelinating callosal G37.1
  - due to
    - drugs (*see also* Table of Drugs and Chemicals) G92
  - hepatic — *see* Failure, hepatic
  - hyperbilirubinemic, newborn P57.9
    - due to isoimmunization (conditions in P55) P57.0
  - hypertensive I67.4
  - hypoglycemic E16.2
  - hypoxic — *see* Damage, brain, anoxic
  - hypoxic ischemic P91.60
    - mild P91.61
    - moderate P91.62
    - severe P91.63
  - in (due to) (with)
    - birth injury P11.1
    - hyperinsulinism E16.1 *[G94]*
    - influenza — *see* Influenza, with, encephalopathy
    - lack of vitamin (*see also* Deficiency, vitamin) E56.9 *[G32.89]*
    - neoplastic disease (*see also* Neoplasm) D49.9 *[G13.1]*
    - serum (*see also* Reaction, serum) T80.69
    - syphilis A52.17
    - trauma (postconcussional) F07.81
      - current injury — *see* Injury, intracranial
    - vaccination G04.02
  - lead — *see* Poisoning, lead
  - metabolic G93.41
    - drug induced G92
    - toxic G92
  - myoclonic, early, symptomatic — *see* Epilepsy, generalized, specified NEC
  - necrotizing, subacute (Leigh) G31.82
  - pellagrous E52 *[G32.89]*
  - portosystemic — *see* Failure, hepatic

Encephalopathy — *continued*
- postcontusional F07.81
  - current injury — *see* Injury, intracranial, diffuse
- posthypoglycemic (coma) E16.1 *[G94]*
- postradiation G93.89
- saturnine — *see* Poisoning, lead
- septic G93.41
- specified NEC G93.49
- spongiform, subacute (viral) A81.09
- toxic G92
  - metabolic G92
- traumatic (postconcussional) F07.81
  - current injury — *see* Injury, intracranial
- vitamin B deficiency NEC E53.9 *[G32.89]*
  - vitamin B1 E51.2
- Wernicke's E51.2

Encephalorrhagia — *see* Hemorrhage, intracranial, intracerebral

Encephalosis, posttraumatic F07.81

Enchondroma (*see also* Neoplasm, bone, benign)

Enchondromatosis (cartilaginous) (multiple) Q78.4

Encopresis R15.9
- functional F98.1
- nonorganic origin F98.1
- psychogenic F98.1

Encounter (with health service) (for) Z76.89
- adjustment and management (of)
  - breast implant Z45.81
  - implanted device NEC Z45.89
  - myringotomy device (stent) (tube) Z45.82
- administrative purpose only Z02.9
  - examination for
    - adoption Z02.82
    - armed forces Z02.3
    - disability determination Z02.71
    - driving license Z02.4
    - employment Z02.1
    - insurance Z02.6
    - medical certificate NEC Z02.79
    - paternity testing Z02.81
    - residential institution admission Z02.2
    - school admission Z02.0
    - sports Z02.5
  - specified reason NEC Z02.89
- aftercare — *see* Aftercare
- antenatal screening Z36
- assisted reproductive fertility procedure cycle Z31.83
- blood typing Z01.83
  - Rh typing Z01.83
- breast augmentation or reduction Z41.1
- breast implant exchange (different material) (different size) Z45.81
- breast reconstruction following mastectomy Z42.1
- check-up — *see* Examination
- chemotherapy for neoplasm Z51.11
- colonoscopy, screening Z12.11
- counseling — *see* Counseling
- delivery, full-term, uncomplicated O80
  - cesarean, without indication O82
- ear piercing Z41.3
- examination — *see* Examination
- expectant parent(s) (adoptive) pre-birth
  - pediatrician visit Z76.81
- fertility preservation procedure (prior to cancer therapy) (prior to removal of gonads) Z31.84
- fitting (of) — *see* Fitting (and adjustment) (of)
- genetic
  - counseling Z31.5
  - testing — *see* Test, genetic
- hearing conservation and treatment Z01.12
- immunotherapy for neoplasm Z51.12
- in vitro fertilization cycle Z31.83
- instruction (in)
  - childbirth Z32.2
  - child care (postpartal) (prenatal) Z32.3
  - natural family planning
    - procreative Z31.61
    - to avoid pregnancy Z30.02
- insulin pump titration Z46.81
- joint prosthesis insertion following prior explantation of joint prosthesis (staged procedure)
  - hip Z47.32

Encounter — *continued*
- joint prosthesis insertion following prior explantation of joint prosthesis— *continued*
  - knee Z47.33
  - shoulder Z47.31
- laboratory (as part of a general medical examination) Z00.00
  - with abnormal findings Z00.01
- mental health services (for)
  - abuse NEC
    - perpetrator Z69.82
    - victim Z69.81
  - child abuse
    - nonparental
      - perpetrator Z69.021
      - victim Z69.020
    - parental
      - perpetrator Z69.011
      - victim Z69.010
  - spousal or partner abuse
    - perpetrator Z69.12
    - victim Z69.11
- observation (for) (ruled out)
  - exposure to (suspected)
    - anthrax Z03.810
    - biological agent NEC Z03.818
- pediatrician visit, by expectant parent(s) (adoptive) Z76.81
- plastic and reconstructive surgery following medical procedure or healed injury NEC Z42.8
- pregnancy
  - supervision of — *see* Pregnancy, supervision of
  - test Z32.00
    - result negative Z32.02
    - result positive Z32.01
- radiation therapy (antineoplastic) Z51.0
- radiological (as part of a general medical examination) Z00.00
  - with abnormal findings Z00.01
- reconstructive surgery following medical procedure or healed injury NEC Z42.8
- removal (of) (*see also* Removal)
  - artificial
    - arm Z44.00-
      - complete Z44.01-
      - partial Z44.02-
    - eye Z44.2-
    - leg Z44.10-
      - complete Z44.11-
      - partial Z44.12-
  - breast implant Z45.81
    - tissue expander (without synchronous insertion of permanent implant) Z45.81
  - device Z46.9
    - specified NEC Z46.89
    - external
      - fixation device — code to fracture with seventh character D
      - prosthesis, prosthetic device Z44.9
        - breast Z44.3-
        - specified NEC Z44.8
    - implanted device NEC Z45.89
    - internal fixation device Z47.2
    - insulin pump Z46.81
    - myringotomy device (stent) (tube) Z45.82
    - nervous system device NEC Z46.2
      - brain neuropacemaker Z46.2
      - visual substitution device Z46.2
        - implanted Z45.31
    - non-vascular catheter Z46.82
    - orthodontic device Z46.4
    - stent
      - ureteral Z46.6
    - urinary device Z46.6
- repeat cervical smear to confirm findings of recent normal smear following initial abnormal smear Z01.42
- respirator [ventilator] use during power failure Z99.12
- Rh typing Z01.83
- screening — *see* Screening
- specified NEC Z76.89
- sterilization Z30.2

Encounter — *continued*
- suspected condition, ruled out
  - amniotic cavity and membrane Z03.71
  - cervical shortening Z03.75
  - fetal anomaly Z03.73
  - fetal growth Z03.74
  - maternal and fetal conditions NEC Z03.79
  - oligohydramnios Z03.71
  - placental problem Z03.72
  - polyhydramnios Z03.71
- suspected exposure (to), ruled out
  - anthrax Z03.810
  - biological agents NEC Z03.818
- termination of pregnancy, elective Z33.2
- testing — *see* Test
- therapeutic drug level monitoring Z51.81
- titration, insulin pump Z46.81
- to determine fetal viability of pregnancy O36.80
- training
  - insulin pump Z46.81
- X-ray of chest (as part of a general medical examination) Z00.00
  - with abnormal findings Z00.01

Encystment — *see* Cyst

Endarteritis (bacterial, subacute) (infective) I77.6
- brain I67.7
- cerebral or cerebrospinal I67.7
- deformans — *see* Arteriosclerosis
- embolic — *see* Embolism
- obliterans (*see also* Arteriosclerosis)
  - pulmonary I28.8
- pulmonary I28.8
- retina — *see* Vasculitis, retina
- senile — *see* Arteriosclerosis
- syphilitic A52.09
  - brain or cerebral A52.04
  - congenital A50.54 *[I79.8]*
- tuberculous A18.89

Endemic — *see* condition

Endocarditis (chronic) (marantic) (nonbacterial) (thrombotic) (valvular) I38
- with rheumatic fever (conditions in I00)
  - active — *see* Endocarditis, acute, rheumatic
  - inactive or quiescent (with chorea) I09.1
- acute or subacute I33.9
  - infective I33.0
  - rheumatic (aortic) (mitral) (pulmonary) (tricuspid) I01.1
    - with chorea (acute) (rheumatic) (Sydenham's) I02.0
- aortic (heart) (nonrheumatic) (valve) I35.8
  - with
    - mitral disease I08.0
      - with tricuspid (valve) disease I08.3
        - active or acute I01.1
          - with chorea (acute) (rheumatic) (Sydenham's) I02.0
      - rheumatic fever (conditions in I00)
        - active — *see* Endocarditis, acute, rheumatic
        - inactive or quiescent (with chorea) I06.9
    - tricuspid (valve) disease I08.2
      - with mitral (valve) disease I08.3
  - acute or subacute I33.9
  - arteriosclerotic I35.8
  - rheumatic I06.9
    - with mitral disease I08.0
      - with tricuspid (valve) disease I08.3
        - active or acute I01.1
          - with chorea (acute) (rheumatic) (Sydenham's) I02.0
    - active or acute I01.1
      - with chorea (acute) (rheumatic) (Sydenham's) I02.0
    - specified NEC I06.8
  - specified cause NEC I35.8
  - syphilitic A52.03
- arteriosclerotic I38
- atypical verrucous (Libman-Sacks) M32.11
- bacterial (acute) (any valve) (subacute) I33.0
- candidal B37.6
- congenital Q24.8

- **Endocarditis** — *continued*
  - constrictive I33.Ø
  - Coxiella burnetii A78 *[I39]*
  - Coxsackie B33.21
  - due to
    - prosthetic cardiac valve T82.6
    - Q fever A78 *[I39]*
    - Serratia marcescens I33.Ø
    - typhoid (fever) AØ1.Ø2
  - gonococcal A54.83
  - infectious or infective (acute) (any valve) (subacute) I33.Ø
  - lenta (acute) (any valve) (subacute) I33.Ø
  - Libman-Sacks M32.11
  - listerial A32.82
  - Löffler's I42.3
  - malignant (acute) (any valve) (subacute) I33.Ø
  - meningococcal A39.51
  - mitral (chronic) (double) (fibroid) (heart) (inactive) (valve) (with chorea) IØ5.9
    - with
      - aortic (valve) disease IØ8.Ø
        - with tricuspid (valve) disease IØ8.3
        - active or acute IØ1.1
          - with chorea (acute) (rheumatic) (Sydenham's) IØ2.Ø
      - rheumatic fever (conditions in IØØ)
        - active — *see* Endocarditis, acute, rheumatic
        - inactive or quiescent (with chorea) IØ5.9
      - tricuspid (valve) disease IØ8.1
        - with aortic (valve) disease IØ8.3
    - active or acute IØ1.1
      - with chorea (acute) (rheumatic) (Sydenham's) IØ2.Ø
    - bacterial I33.Ø
    - arteriosclerotic I34.8
    - nonrheumatic I34.8
      - acute or subacute I33.9
    - specified NEC IØ5.8
  - monilial B37.6
  - multiple valves IØ8.9
    - specified disorders IØ8.8
  - mycotic (acute) (any valve) (subacute) I33.Ø
  - pneumococcal (acute) (any valve) (subacute) I33.Ø
  - pulmonary (chronic) (heart) (valve) I37.8
    - with rheumatic fever (conditions in IØØ)
      - active — *see* Endocarditis, acute, rheumatic
      - inactive or quiescent (with chorea) IØ9.89
        - with aortic, mitral or tricuspid disease IØ8.8
    - acute or subacute I33.9
      - rheumatic IØ1.1
        - with chorea (acute) (rheumatic) (Sydenham's) IØ2.Ø
    - arteriosclerotic I37.8
    - congenital Q22.2
    - rheumatic (chronic) (inactive) (with chorea) I09.89
      - active or acute IØ1.1
        - with chorea (acute) (rheumatic) (Sydenham's) IØ2.Ø
    - syphilitic A52.Ø3
  - purulent (acute) (any valve) (subacute) I33.Ø
  - Q fever A78 *[I39]*
  - rheumatic (chronic) (inactive) (with chorea) IØ9.1
    - active or acute (aortic) (mitral) (pulmonary) (tricuspid) IØ1.1
      - with chorea (acute) (rheumatic) (Sydenham's) IØ2.Ø
  - rheumatoid — *see* Rheumatoid, carditis
  - septic (acute) (any valve) (subacute) I33.Ø
  - streptococcal (acute) (any valve) (subacute) I33.0
  - subacute — *see* Endocarditis, acute
  - suppurative (acute) (any valve) (subacute) I33.Ø
  - syphilitic A52.Ø3
  - toxic I33.9
  - tricuspid (chronic) (heart) (inactive) (rheumatic) (valve) (with chorea) IØ7.9
    - with
      - aortic (valve) disease IØ8.2
        - mitral (valve) disease IØ8.3
      - mitral (valve) disease IØ8.1
        - aortic (valve) disease IØ8.3
- **Endocarditis** — *continued*
  - tricuspid— *continued*
    - with— *continued*
      - rheumatic fever (conditions in IØØ)
        - active — *see* Endocarditis, acute, rheumatic
        - inactive or quiescent (with chorea) IØ7.8
    - active or acute IØ1.1
      - with chorea (acute) (rheumatic) (Sydenham's) IØ2.Ø
    - arteriosclerotic I36.8
    - nonrheumatic I36.8
      - acute or subacute I33.9
    - specified cause, except rheumatic I36.8
  - tuberculous — *see* Tuberculosis, endocarditis
  - typhoid AØ1.Ø2
  - ulcerative (acute) (any valve) (subacute) I33.Ø
  - vegetative (acute) (any valve) (subacute) I33.Ø
  - verrucous (atypical) (nonbacterial) (nonrheumatic) M32.11
- **Endocardium, endocardial** (*see also* condition)
  - cushion defect Q21.2
- **Endocervicitis** (*see also* Cervicitis)
  - due to intrauterine (contraceptive) device T83.6
  - hyperplastic N72
- **Endocrine** — *see* condition
- **Endocrinopathy, pluriglandular** E31.9
- **Endodontic**
  - overfill M27.52
  - underfill M27.53
- **Endodontitis** K04.0
- **Endomastoiditis** — *see* Mastoiditis
- **Endometrioma** N80.9
- **Endometriosis** N80.9
  - appendix N8Ø.5
  - bladder N8Ø.8
  - bowel N8Ø.5
  - broad ligament N8Ø.3
  - cervix N8Ø.Ø
  - colon N8Ø.5
  - cul-de-sac (Douglas') N8Ø.3
  - exocervix N8Ø.Ø
  - fallopian tube N8Ø.2
  - female genital organ NEC N8Ø.8
  - gallbladder N8Ø.8
  - in scar of skin N8Ø.6
  - internal N8Ø.Ø
  - intestine N8Ø.5
  - lung N8Ø.8
  - myometrium N8Ø.Ø
  - ovary N8Ø.1
  - parametrium N8Ø.3
  - pelvic peritoneum N8Ø.3
  - peritoneal (pelvic) N8Ø.3
  - rectovaginal septum N8Ø.4
  - rectum N8Ø.5
  - round ligament N8Ø.3
  - skin (scar) N8Ø.6
  - specified site NEC N8Ø.8
  - stromal D39.Ø
  - umbilicus N8Ø.8
  - uterus (internal) N8Ø.Ø
  - vagina N8Ø.4
  - vulva N8Ø.8
- **Endometritis** (decidual) (nonspecific) (purulent) (senile) (atrophic) (suppurative) N71.9
  - with ectopic pregnancy OØ8.Ø
  - acute N71.Ø
  - blenorrhagic (gonococcal) (acute) (chronic) A54.24
  - cervix, cervical (with erosion or ectropion) (*see also* Cervicitis)
    - hyperplastic N72
  - chlamydial A56.11
  - chronic N71.1
  - following
    - abortion — *see* Abortion by type complicated by genital infection
    - ectopic or molar pregnancy OØ8.Ø
  - gonococcal, gonorrheal (acute) (chronic) A54.24
  - hyperplastic (*see also* Hyperplasia, endometrial) N85.ØØ
    - cervix N72
  - puerperal, postpartum, childbirth O86.12
- **Endometritis** — *continued*
  - subacute N71.Ø
  - tuberculous A18.17
- **Endometrium** — *see* condition
- **Endomyocarditis** — *see* Endocarditis
- **Endomyocardiopathy, South African** I42.3
- **Endomyofibrosis** I42.3
- **Endomyometritis** — *see* Endometritis
- **Endopericarditis** — *see* Endocarditis
- **Endoperineuritis** — *see* Disorder, nerve
- **Endophlebitis** — *see* Phlebitis
- **Endophthalmia** — *see* Endophthalmitis, purulent
- **Endophthalmitis** (acute) (infective) (metastatic) (subacute) H44.ØØ9
  - bleb associated (*see also* Bleb, inflammed (infected), postprocedural) H59.4
  - gonorrheal A54.39
  - in (due to)
    - cysticercosis B69.1
    - onchocerciasis B73.Ø1
    - toxocariasis B83.Ø
  - panuveitis — *see* Panuveitis
  - parasitic H44.12-
  - purulent H44.ØØ-
    - panophthalmitis — *see* Panophthalmitis
    - vitreous abscess H44.Ø2-
  - specified NEC H44.19
  - sympathetic — *see* Uveitis, sympathetic
- **Endosalpingioma** D28.2
- **Endosalpingiosis** N94.89
- **Endosteitis** — *see* Osteomyelitis
- **Endothelioma, bone** — *see* Neoplasm, bone, malignant
- **Endotheliosis** (hemorrhagic infectional) D69.8
- **Endotoxemia** —code to condition
- **Endotrachelitis** — *see* Cervicitis
- **Engelmann**(-Camurati) syndrome Q78.3
- **English disease** — *see* Rickets
- **Engman's disease** L30.3
- **Engorgement**
  - breast N64.59
    - newborn P83.4
    - puerperal, postpartum O92.79
  - lung (passive) — *see* Edema, lung
  - pulmonary (passive) — *see* Edema, lung
  - stomach K31.89
  - venous, retina — *see* Occlusion, retina, vein, engorgement
- **Enlargement, enlarged** (*see also* Hypertrophy)
  - adenoids J35.2
    - with tonsils J35.3
  - alveolar ridge KØ8.8
    - congenital — *see* Anomaly, alveolar
  - apertures of diaphragm (congenital) Q79.1
  - gingival KØ6.1
  - heart, cardiac — *see* Hypertrophy, cardiac
  - lacrimal gland, chronic HØ4.Ø3-
  - liver — *see* Hypertrophy, liver
  - lymph gland or node R59.9
    - generalized R59.1
    - localized R59.Ø
  - orbit HØ5.34-
  - organ or site, congenital NEC — *see* Anomaly, by site
  - parathyroid (gland) E21.Ø
  - pituitary fossa R93.Ø
  - prostate N4Ø.Ø
    - with lower urinary tract symptoms (LUTS) N4Ø.1
    - without lower urinary tract symtpoms (LUTS) N4Ø.Ø
  - sella turcica R93.Ø
  - spleen — *see* Splenomegaly
  - thymus (gland) (congenital) E32.Ø
  - thyroid (gland) — *see* Goiter
  - tongue K14.8
  - tonsils J35.1
    - with adenoids J35.3
  - uterus N85.2
- **Enophthalmos** HØ5.4Ø-
  - due to
    - orbital tissue atrophy HØ5.41-
    - trauma or surgery HØ5.42-
- **Enostosis** M27.8
- **Entamebic, entamebiasis** — *see* Amebiasis

- **Entanglement**
  - umbilical cord(s) O69.2
    - with compression O69.2
      - without compression O69.82
    - around neck (with compression) O69.1
      - without compression O69.81
    - of twins in monoamniotic sac O69.2
- **Enteralgia** — *see* Pain, abdominal
- **Enteric** — *see* condition
- **Enteritis** (acute) (diarrheal) (hemorrhagic) (noninfective) (septic) K52.9
  - aertrycke infection AØ2.Ø
  - adenovirus AØ8.2
  - allergic K52.2
  - amebic (acute) AØ6.Ø
    - with abscess — *see* Abscess, amebic
    - chronic AØ6.1
      - with abscess — *see* Abscess, amebic
      - nondysenteric AØ6.2
    - nondysenteric AØ6.2
  - astrovirus AØ8.32
  - bacillary NOS AØ3.9
  - bacterial AØ4.9
    - specified NEC AØ4.8
  - calicivirus AØ8.31
  - candidal B37.82
  - Chilomastix AØ7.8
  - choleriformis AØØ.1
  - chronic (noninfectious) K52.9
    - ulcerative — *see* Colitis, ulcerative
  - cicatrizing (chronic) — *see* Enteritis, regional, small intestine
  - Clostridium
    - botulinum (food poisoning) AØ5.1
    - difficile AØ4.7
  - coccidial AØ7.3
  - coxsackie virus AØ8.39
  - dietetic K52.2
  - drug-induced K52.1
  - due to
    - astrovirus AØ8.32
    - calicivirus AØ8.31
    - coxsackie virus AØ8.39
    - drugs K52.1
    - echovirus AØ8.39
    - enterovirus NEC AØ8.39
    - food hypersensitivity K52.2
    - infectious organism (bacterial) (viral) — *see* Enteritis, infectious
    - torovirus AØ8.39
    - Yersinia enterocolitica AØ4.6
  - echovirus AØ8.39
  - eltor AØØ.1
  - enterovirus NEC AØ8.39
  - eosinophilic K52.81
  - epidemic (infectious) AØ9
  - fulminant K55.Ø
  - gangrenous — *see* Enteritis, infectious
  - giardial AØ7.1
  - infectious NOS AØ9
    - due to
      - adenovirus AØ8.2
      - Aerobacter aerogenes AØ4.8
      - Arizona (bacillus) AØ2.Ø
      - bacteria NOS AØ4.9
        - specified NEC AØ4.8
      - Campylobacter AØ4.5
      - Clostridium difficile AØ4.7
      - Clostridium perfringens AØ4.8
      - Enterobacter aerogenes AØ4.8
      - enterovirus AØ8.39
      - Escherichia coli AØ4.4
        - enteroaggregative AØ4.4
        - enterohemorrhagic AØ4.3
        - enteroinvasive AØ4.2
        - enteropathogenic AØ4.Ø
        - enterotoxigenic AØ4.1
        - specified NEC AØ4.4
      - specified
        - bacteria NEC AØ4.8
        - virus NEC AØ8.39
      - Staphylococcus AØ4.8

- **Enteritis**— *continued*
  - infectious— *continued*
    - due to— *continued*
      - virus NEC AØ8.4
        - specified type NEC AØ8.39
      - Yersinia enterocolitica AØ4.6
    - specified organism NEC AØ8.8
  - influenzal — *see* Influenza, with, digestive manifestations
  - ischemic K55.9
    - acute K55.Ø
    - chronic K55.1
  - microsporidial AØ7.8
  - mucomembranous, myxomembranous — *see* Syndrome, irritable bowel
  - mucous — *see* Syndrome, irritable bowel
  - necroticans AØ5.2
  - necrotizing of newborn — *see* Enterocolitis, necrotizing, in newborn
  - neurogenic — *see* Syndrome, irritable bowel
  - newborn necrotizing — *see* Enterocolitis, necrotizing, in newborn
  - noninfectious K52.9
  - norovirus AØ8.11
  - parasitic NEC B82.9
  - paratyphoid (fever) — *see* Fever, paratyphoid
  - protozoal AØ7.9
    - specified NEC AØ7.8
  - radiation K52.Ø
  - regional (of) K5Ø.9Ø
    - with
      - complication K5Ø.919
        - abscess K5Ø.914
        - fistula K5Ø.913
        - intestinal obstruction K5Ø.912
        - rectal bleeding K5Ø.911
        - specified complication NEC K5Ø.918
    - colon — *see* Enteritis, regional, large intestine
    - duodenum — *see* Enteritis, regional, small intestine
    - ileum — *see* Enteritis, regional, small intestine
    - jejunum — *see* Enteritis, regional, small intestine
    - large bowel — *see* Enteritis, regional, large intestine
    - large intestine (colon) (rectum) K5Ø.1Ø
      - with
        - complication K5Ø.119
          - abscess K5Ø.114
          - fistula K5Ø.113
          - intestinal obstruction K5Ø.112
          - rectal bleeding K5Ø.111
          - small intestine (duodenum) (ileum) (jejunum) involvement K5Ø.8Ø
            - with
              - complication K5Ø.819
                - abscess K5Ø.814
                - fistula K5Ø.813
                - intestinal obstruction K5Ø.812
                - rectal bleeding K5Ø.811
                - specified complication NEC K5Ø.818
          - specified complication NEC K5Ø.118
    - rectum — *see* Enteritis, regional, large intestine
    - small intestine (duodenum) (ileum) (jejunum) K5Ø.ØØ
      - with
        - complication K5Ø.Ø19
          - abscess K5Ø.Ø14
          - fistula K5Ø.Ø13
          - intestinal obstruction K5Ø.Ø12
          - large intestine (colon) (rectum) involvement K5Ø.8Ø
            - with
              - complication K5Ø.819
                - abscess K5Ø.814
                - fistula K5Ø.813
                - intestinal obstruction K5Ø.812
                - rectal bleeding K5Ø.811
                - specified complication NEC K5Ø.818

- **Enteritis**— *continued*
  - regional— *continued*
    - small intestine— *continued*
      - with— *continued*
        - complication— *continued*
          - rectal bleeding K5Ø.Ø11
          - specified complication NEC K5Ø.Ø18
  - rotaviral AØ8.Ø
  - Salmonella, salmonellosis (arizonae) (cholerae-suis) (enteritidis) (typhimurium) AØ2.Ø
  - segmental — *see* Enteritis, regional
  - septic AØ9
  - Shigella — *see* Infection, Shigella
  - small round structured NEC AØ8.19
  - spasmodic, spastic — *see* Syndrome, irritable bowel
  - staphylococcal AØ4.8
    - due to food AØ5.Ø
  - torovirus AØ8.39
  - toxic NEC K52.1
    - due to Clostridium difficile AØ4.7
  - trichomonal AØ7.8
  - tuberculous A18.32
  - typhosa AØ1.ØØ
  - ulcerative (chronic) — *see* Colitis, ulcerative
  - viral AØ8.4
    - adenovirus AØ8.2
    - enterovirus AØ8.39
    - Rotavirus AØ8.Ø
    - small round structured NEC AØ8.19
    - specified NEC AØ8.39
    - virus specified NEC AØ8.39
- **Enterobiasis** B8Ø
- **Enterobius vermicularis** (infection) (infestation) B8Ø
- **Enterocele** (*see also* Hernia, abdomen)
  - pelvic, pelvis (acquired) (congenital) N81.5
  - vagina, vaginal (acquired) (congenital) NEC N81.5
- **Enterocolitis** (*see also* Enteritis) K52.9
  - due to Clostridium difficile AØ4.7
  - fulminant ischemic K55.Ø
  - granulomatous — *see* Enteritis, regional
  - hemorrhagic (acute) K55.Ø
    - chronic K55.1
  - infectious NEC AØ9
  - ischemic K55.9
  - necrotizing
    - due to Clostridium difficile AØ4.7
    - in newborn P77.9
      - stage 1 (without pneumatosis, without perforation) P77.1
      - stage 2 (with pneumatosis, without perforation) P77.2
      - stage 3 (with pneumatosis, with perforation) P77.3
  - noninfectious K52.9
    - newborn — *see* Enterocolitis, necrotizing, in newborn
  - pseudomembranous (newborn) AØ4.7
  - radiation K52.Ø
    - newborn — *see* Enterocolitis, necrotizing, in newborn
  - ulcerative (chronic) *see* Pancolitis, ulcerative (chronic)
- **Enterogastritis** — *see* Enteritis
- **Enteropathy** K63.9
  - gluten-sensitive K9Ø.Ø
  - hemorrhagic, terminal K55.Ø
  - protein-losing K9Ø.4
- **Enteroperitonitis** — *see* Peritonitis
- **Enteroptosis** K63.4
- **Enterorrhagia** K92.2
- **Enterospasm** (*see also* Syndrome, irritable, bowel)
  - psychogenic F45.8
- **Enterostenosis** (*see also* Obstruction, intestine) K56.69
- **Enterostomy**
  - complication — *see* Complication, enterostomy
  - status Z93.4
- **Enterovirus, as cause of disease classified elsewhere** B97.1Ø
  - coxsackievirus B97.11
  - echovirus B97.12
  - other specified B97.19

- **Enthesopathy** (peripheral) M77.9
  - Achilles tendinitis — *see* Tendinitis, Achilles
  - ankle and tarsus M77.9
    - specified type NEC — *see* Enthesopathy, foot, specified type NEC
  - anterior tibial syndrome M76.81-
  - calcaneal spur — *see* Spur, bone, calcaneal
  - elbow region M77.8
    - lateral epicondylitis — *see* Epicondylitis, lateral
    - medial epicondylitis — *see* Epicondylitis, medial
  - foot NEC M77.9
    - metatarsalgia — *see* Metatarsalgia
    - specified type NEC M77.5-
  - forearm M77.9
  - gluteal tendinitis — *see* Tendinitis, gluteal
  - hand M77.9
  - hip — *see* Enthesopathy, lower limb, specified type NEC
  - iliac crest spur — *see* Spur, bone, iliac crest
  - iliotibial band syndrome — *see* Syndrome, iliotibial band
  - knee — *see* Enthesopathy, lower limb, lower leg, specified type NEC
  - lateral epicondylitis — *see* Epicondylitis, lateral
  - lower limb (excluding foot) M76.9
    - Achilles tendinitis — *see* Tendinitis, Achilles
    - anterior tibial syndrome M76.81-
    - gluteal tendinitis — *see* Tendinitis, gluteal
    - iliac crest spur — *see* Spur, bone, iliac crest
    - iliotibial band syndrome — *see* Syndrome, iliotibial band
    - patellar tendinitis — *see* Tendinitis, patellar
    - pelvic region — *see* Enthesopathy, lower limb, specified type NEC
    - peroneal tendinitis — *see* Tendinitis, peroneal
    - posterior tibial syndrome M76.82
    - psoas tendinitis — *see* Tendinitis, psoas
    - shoulder M77.9
    - specified type NEC M76.89-
    - tibial collateral bursitis — *see* Bursitis, tibial collateral
  - medial epicondylitis — *see* Epicondylitis, medialmetatarsalgia — *see* Metatarsalgia
  - multiple sites M77.9
  - patellar tendinitis — *see* Tendinitis, patellar
  - pelvis M77.9
  - periarthritis of wrist — *see* Periarthritis, wrist
  - peroneal tendinitis — *see* Tendinitis, peroneal
  - posterior tibial syndrome M76.82-
  - psoas tendinitis — *see* Tendinitis, psoas
  - shoulder region — *see* Lesion, shoulder
  - specified site NEC M77.9
  - specified type NEC M77.8
  - spinal M46.ØØ
    - cervical region M46.Ø2
    - cervicothoracic region M46.Ø3
    - lumbar region M46.Ø6
    - lumbosacral region M46.Ø7
    - multiple sites M46.Ø9
    - occipito-atlanto-axial region M46.Ø1
    - sacrococcygeal region M46.Ø8
    - thoracic region M46.Ø4
    - thoracolumbar region M46.Ø5
  - tibial collateral bursitis — *see* Bursitis, tibial collateral
  - upper arm M77.9
  - wrist and carpus NEC M77.8
    - calcaneal spur — *see* Spur, bone, calcaneal
    - periarthritis of wrist — *see* Periarthritis, wrist
- **Entomophobia** F40.218
- **Entomophthoromycosis** B46.8
- **Entrance, air into vein** — *see* Embolism, air
- **Entrapment, nerve** — *see* Neuropathy, entrapment
- **Entropion** (eyelid) (paralytic) HØ2.ØØ9
  - cicatricial HØ2.Ø19
    - left HØ2.Ø16
      - lower HØ2.Ø15
      - upper HØ2.Ø14
    - right HØ2.Ø13
      - lower HØ2.Ø12
      - upper HØ2.Ø11
  - congenital Q1Ø.2

Entropion — *continued*

  - left HØ2.ØØ6
    - lower HØ2.ØØ5
    - upper HØ2.ØØ4
  - mechanical HØ2.Ø29
    - left HØ2.Ø26
      - lower HØ2.Ø25
      - upper HØ2.Ø24
    - right HØ2.Ø23
      - lower HØ2.Ø22
      - upper HØ2.Ø21
  - right HØ2.ØØ3
    - lower HØ2.ØØ2
    - upper HØ2.ØØ1
  - senile HØ2.Ø39
    - left HØ2.Ø36
      - lower HØ2.Ø35
      - upper HØ2.Ø34
    - right HØ2.Ø33
      - lower HØ2.Ø32
      - upper HØ2.Ø31
  - spastic HØ2.Ø49
    - left HØ2.Ø46
      - lower HØ2.Ø45
      - upper HØ2.Ø44
    - right HØ2.Ø43
      - lower HØ2.Ø42
      - upper HØ2.Ø41
- **Enucleated eye** (traumatic, current) SØ5.7-
- **Enuresis** R32
  - functional F98.Ø
  - habit disturbance F98.Ø
  - nocturnal N39.44
    - psychogenic F98.Ø
  - nonorganic origin F98.Ø
  - psychogenic F98.Ø
- **Eosinopenia** — *see* Agranulocytosis
- **Eosinophilia** (allergic) (hereditary) (idiopathic) (secondary) D72.1
  - with
    - angiolymphoid hyperplasia (ALHE) D18.Ø1
  - infiltrative J82
  - Löffler's J82
  - peritonal — *see* Peritonitis, eosinophilic
  - pulmonary NEC J82
  - tropical (pulmonary) J82
- **Eosinophilia-myalgia syndrome** M35.8
- **Ependymitis** (acute) (cerebral) (chronic) (granular) — *see* Encephalomyelitis
- **Ependymoblastoma**
  - specified site — *see* Neoplasm, malignant, by site
  - unspecified site C71.9
- **Ependymoma** (epithelial) (malignant)
  - anaplastic
    - specified site — *see* Neoplasm, malignant, by site
    - unspecified site C71.9
  - benign
    - specified site — *see* Neoplasm, benign, by site
    - unspecified site D33.2
  - myxopapillary D43.2
    - specified site — *see* Neoplasm, uncertain behavior, by site
    - unspecified site D43.2
  - papillary D43.2
    - specified site — *see* Neoplasm, uncertain behavior, by site
    - unspecified site D43.2
  - specified site — *see* Neoplasm, malignant, by site
  - unspecified site C71.9
- **Ependymopathy** G93.89
- **Ephelis, ephelides** L81.2
- **Epiblepharon** (congenital) Q1Ø.3
- **Epicanthus, epicanthic fold** (eyelid) (congenital) Q1Ø.3
- **Epicondylitis** (elbow)
  - lateral M77.1-
  - medial M77.Ø-
- **Epicystitis** — *see* Cystitis
- **Epidemic** — *see* condition
- **Epidermidalization, cervix** — *see* Dysplasia, cervix
- **Epidermis, epidermal** — *see* condition
- **Epidermodysplasia verruciformis** BØ7.8
- **Epidermolysis**
  - bullosa (congenital) Q81.9
    - acquired L12.3Ø
      - drug-induced L12.31
      - specified cause NEC L12.35
    - dystrophica Q81.2
    - letalis Q81.1
    - simplex Q81.Ø
    - specified NEC Q81.8
  - necroticans combustiformis L51.2
    - due to drug — *see* Table of Drugs and Chemicals, by drug
- **Epidermophytid** — *see* Dermatophytosis
- **Epidermophytosis** (infected) — *see* Dermatophytosis
- **Epididymis** — *see* condition
- **Epididymitis** (acute) (nonvenereal) (recurrent) (residual) N45.1
  - with orchitis N45.3
  - blennorrhagic (gonococcal) A54.23
  - caseous (tuberculous) A18.15
  - chlamydial A56.19
  - filarial B74.9
  - gonococcal A54.23
  - syphilitic A52.76
  - tuberculous A18.15
- **Epididymo-orchitis** (*see also* Epididymitis) N45.3
- **Epidural** — *see* condition
- **Epigastrium, epigastric** — *see* condition
- **Epigastrocele** — *see* Hernia, ventral
- **Epiglottis** — *see* condition
- **Epiglottitis, epiglottiditis** (acute) JØ5.1Ø
  - with obstruction JØ5.11
  - chronic J37.Ø
- **Epignathus** Q89.4
- **Epilepsia partialis continua** (*see also* Kozhevnikof's epilepsy) G4Ø.1-
- **Epilepsy, epileptic, epilepsia** (attack) (cerebral) (convulsion) (fit) (seizure) G4Ø.9Ø9

Note: the following terms are to be considered equivalent to intractable: pharmacoresistant (pharmacologically resistant), treatment resistant, refractory (medically) and poorly controlled

---

  - with
    - complex partial seizures — *see* Epilepsy, localization-related, symptomatic, with complex partial seizures
    - grand mal seizures on awakening — *see* Epilepsy, generalized, specified NEC
    - myoclonic absences — *see* Epilepsy, generalized, specified NEC
    - myoclonic-astatic seizures — *see* Epilepsy, generalized, specified NEC
    - simple partial seizures — *see* Epilepsy, localization-related, symptomatic, with simple partial seizures
  - akinetic — *see* Epilepsy, generalized, specified NEC
  - benign childhood with centrotemporal EEG spikes — *see* Epilepsy, localization-related, idiopathic
  - benign myoclonic in infancy G4Ø.8Ø-
  - Bravais-jacksonian — *see* Epilepsy, localization-related, symptomatic, with simple partial seizures
  - childhood absence G4Ø.AØ9
    - intractable G4Ø.A19
      - with status epilepticus G4Ø.A11
      - without status epilepticus G4Ø.A19
    - not intractable G4Ø.AØ9
      - with status epilepticus G4Ø.AØ1
      - without status epilepticus G4Ø.AØ9
  - childhood with occipital EEG paroxysms — *see* Epilepsy, localization-related, idiopathic
  - climacteric — *see* Epilepsy, specified NEC
  - cysticercosis B69.Ø
  - deterioration (mental) FØ6.8
  - due to syphilis A52.19
  - focal — *see* Epilepsy, localization-related, symptomatic, with simple partial seizures
  - generalized
    - idiopathic G4Ø.3Ø9

- **Epilepsy, epileptic, epilepsia** — *continued*
  - generalized— *continued*
    - idiopathic— *continued*
      - intractable G40.319
        - with status epilepticus G40.311
        - without status epilepticus G40.319
      - not intractable G40.309
        - with status epilepticus G40.301
        - without status epilepticus G40.309
    - specified NEC G40.409
      - intractable G40.419
        - with status epilepticus G40.411
        - without status epilepticus G40.419
      - not intractable G40.409
        - with status epilepticus G40.401
        - without status epilepticus G40.409
  - impulsive petit mal — *see* Epilepsy, juvenile myoclonic
  - intractable G40.919
    - with status epilepticus G40.911
    - without status epilepticus G40.919
  - juvenile absence G40.A09
    - intractable G40.A19
      - with status epilepticus G40.A11
      - without status epilepticus G40.A19
    - not intractable G40.A09
      - with status epilepticus G40.A01
      - without status epilepticus G40.A09
  - juvenile myoclonic G40.B09
    - intractable G40.B19
      - with status epilepticus G40.B11
      - without status epilepticus G40.B19
    - not intractable G40.B09
      - with status epilepticus G40.B01
      - without status epilepticus G40.B09
  - localization-related (focal) (partial)
    - idiopathic G40.009
      - with seizures of localized onset G40.009
        - intractable G40.019
          - with status epilepticus G40.011
          - without status epilepticus G40.019
        - not intractable G40.009
          - with status epilepticus G40.001
          - without status epilepticus G40.009
    - symptomatic
      - with complex partial seizures G40.209
        - intractable G40.219
          - with status epilepticus G40.211
          - without status epilepticus G40.219
        - not intractable G40.209
          - with status epilepticus G40.201
          - without status epilepticus G40.209
      - with simple partial seizures G40.109
        - intractable G40.119
          - with status epilepticus G40.111
          - without status epilepticus G40.119
        - not intractable G40.109
          - with status epilepticus G40.101
          - without status epilepticus G40.109
  - myoclonus, myoclonic (progressive) — *see* Epilepsy, generalized, specified NEC
  - not intractable G40.909
    - with status epilepticus G40.901
    - without status epilepticus G40.909
  - on awakening — *see* Epilepsy, generalized, specified NEC
  - parasitic NOS B71.9 *[G94]*
  - partialis continua (*see also* Kozhevnikof's epilepsy) G40.1-
  - peripheral — *see* Epilepsy, specified NEC
  - procursiva — *see* Epilepsy, localization-related, symptomatic, with simple partial seizures
  - progressive (familial) myoclonic — *see* Epilepsy, generalized, idiopathic
  - reflex — *see* Epilepsy, specified NEC
  - related to
    - alcohol G40.509
      - not intractable G40.509
        - with status epilepticus G40.501
        - without status epliepticus G40.509
    - drugs G40.509
      - not intractable G40.509
        - with status epilepticus G40.501
- **Epilepsy, epileptic, epilepsia** — *continued*
  - related to — *continued*
    - drugs— *continued*
      - not intractable— *continued*
        - without status epliepticus G40.509
    - external causes G40.509
      - not intractable G40.509
        - with status epilepticus G40.501
        - without status epliepticus G40.509
    - hormonal changes G40.509
      - not intractable G40.509
        - with status epilepticus G40.501
        - without status epliepticus G40.509
    - sleep deprivation G40.509
      - not intractable G40.509
        - with status epilepticus G40.501
        - without status epliepticus G40.509
    - stress G40.509
      - not intractable G40.509
        - with status epilepticus G40.501
        - without status epliepticus G40.509
  - somatomotor — *see* Epilepsy, localization-related, symptomatic, with simple partial seizures
  - somatosensory — *see* Epilepsy, localization-related, symptomatic, with simple partial seizures
  - spasms G40.822
    - intractable G40.824
      - with status epilepticus G40.823
      - without status epilepticus G40.824
    - not intractable G40.822
      - with status epilepticus G40.821
      - without status epilepticus G40.822
  - specified NEC G40.802
    - intractable G40.804
      - with status epilepticus G40.803
      - without status epilepticus G40.804
    - not intractable G40.802
      - with status epilepticus G40.801
      - without status epilepticus G40.802
  - syndromes
    - generalized
      - idiopathic G40.309
        - intractable G40.319
          - with status epilepticus G40.311
          - without status epilepticus G40.319
        - not intractable G40.309
          - with status epilepticus G40.301
          - without status epilepticus G40.309
      - specified NEC G40.409
        - intractable G40.419
          - with status epilepticus G40.411
          - without status epilepticus G40.419
        - not intractable G40.409
          - with status epilepticus G40.401
          - without status epilepticus G40.409
    - localization-related (focal) (partial)
      - idiopathic G40.009
        - with seizures of localized onset G40.009
          - intractable G40.019
            - with status epilepticus G40.011
            - without status epilepticus G40.019
          - not intractable G40.009
            - with status epilepticus G40.001
            - without status epilepticus G40.009
      - symptomatic
        - with complex partial seizures G40.209
          - intractable G40.219
            - with status epilepticus G40.211
            - without status epilepticus G40.219
          - not intractable G40.209
            - with status epilepticus G40.201
            - without status epilepticus G40.209
        - with simple partial seizures G40.109
          - intractable G40.119
            - with status epilepticus G40.111
            - without status epilepticus G40.119
          - not intractable G40.109
            - with status epilepticus G40.101
            - without status epilepticus G40.109
    - specified NEC G40.802
      - intractable G40.804
        - with status epilepticus G40.803
        - without status epilepticus G40.804
- **Epilepsy, epileptic, epilepsia** — *continued*
  - syndromes— *continued*
    - specified— *continued*
      - not intractable G40.802
        - with status epilepticus G40.801
        - without status epilepticus G40.802
  - tonic (-clonic) — *see* Epilepsy, generalized, specified NEC
  - twilight F05
  - uncinate (gyrus) — *see* Epilepsy, localization-related, symptomatic, with complex partial seizures
  - Unverricht (-Lundborg) (familial myoclonic) — *see* Epilepsy, generalized, idiopathic
  - visceral — *see* Epilepsy, specified NEC
  - visual — *see* Epilepsy, specified NEC
- **Epiloia** Q85.1
- **Epimenorrhea** N92.0
- **Epipharyngitis** — *see* Nasopharyngitis
- **Epiphora** H04.20-
  - due to
    - excess lacrimation H04.21-
    - insufficient drainage H04.22-
- **Epiphyseal arrest** — *see* Arrest, epiphyseal
- **Epiphyseolysis, epiphysiolysis** — *see* Osteochondropathy
- **Epiphysitis** (*see also* Osteochondropathy)
  - juvenile M92.9
  - syphilitic (congenital) A50.02
- **Epiplocele** — *see* Hernia, abdomen
- **Epiploitis** — *see* Peritonitis
- **Epiplosarcomphalocele** — *see* Hernia, umbilicus
- **Episcleritis** (suppurative) H15.10-
  - in (due to)
    - syphilis A52.71
    - tuberculosis A18.51
  - nodular H15.12-
  - periodica fugax H15.11-
    - angioneurotic — *see* Edema, angioneurotic
  - syphilitic (late) A52.71
  - tuberculous A18.51
- **Episode**
  - affective, mixed F39
  - depersonalization (in neurotic state) F48.1
  - depressive F32.9
    - major F32.9
      - mild F32.0
      - moderate F32.1
      - severe (without psychotic symptoms) F32.2
        - with psychotic symptoms F32.3
    - recurrent F33.9
      - brief F33.8
    - specified NEC F32.8
  - hypomanic F30.8
  - manic F30.9
    - with
      - psychotic symptoms F30.2
      - remission (full) F30.4
        - partial F30.3
    - other specified F30.8
    - recurrent F31.89
    - without psychotic symptoms F30.10
      - mild F30.11
      - moderate F30.12
      - severe (without psychotic symptoms) F30.13
        - with psychotic symptoms F30.2
  - psychotic F23
    - organic F06.8
  - schizophrenic (acute) NEC, brief F23
- **Epispadias** (female) (male) Q64.0
- **Episplenitis** D73.89
- **Epistaxis** (multiple) R04.0
  - hereditary I78.0
  - vicarious menstruation N94.89
- **Epithelioma** (malignant) (*see also* Neoplasm, malignant, by site)
  - adenoides cysticum — *see* Neoplasm, skin, benign
  - basal cell — *see* Neoplasm, skin, malignant
  - benign — *see* Neoplasm, benign, by site
  - Bowen's — *see* Neoplasm, skin, in situ
  - calcifying, of Malherbe — *see* Neoplasm, skin, benign
  - external site — *see* Neoplasm, skin, malignant

Epithelioma— *continued*
- intraepidermal, Jadassohn — *see* Neoplasm, skin, benign
- squamous cell — *see* Neoplasm, malignant, by site

Epitheliomatosis pigmented Q82.1
Epitheliopathy, multifocal placoid pigment H30.14-
Epithelium, epithelial — *see* condition
Epituberculosis (with atelectasis) (allergic) A15.7
Eponychia Q84.6
Epstein's
- nephrosis or syndrome — *see* Nephrosis
- pearl KØ9.8

Epulis (gingiva) (fibrous) (giant cell) KØ6.8
Equinia A24.0
Equinovarus (congenital) (talipes) Q66.Ø
- acquired — *see* Deformity, limb, clubfoot

Equivalent
- convulsive (abdominal) — *see* Epilepsy, specified NEC
- epileptic (psychic) — *see* Epilepsy, localization-related, symptomatic, with complex partial seizures

Erb(-Duchenne) **paralysis** (birth injury) (newborn) P14.Ø
Erb-Goldflam disease or syndrome G70.00
- with exacerbation (acute) G7Ø.Ø1
- in crisis G7Ø.Ø1

Erb's
- disease G71.Ø
- palsy, paralysis (brachial) (birth) (newborn) P14.Ø
  - spinal (spastic) syphilitic A52.17
- pseudohypertrophic muscular dystrophy G71.Ø

Erdheim's syndrome (acromegalic macrospondylitis) E22.Ø
Erection, painful (persistent) — *see* Priapism
Ergosterol deficiency (vitamin D) E55.9
- with
  - adult osteomalacia M83.8
  - rickets — *see* Rickets

Ergotism (*see also* Poisoning, food, noxious, plant)
- from ergot used as drug (migraine therapy) — *see* Table of Drugs and Chemicals

Erosio interdigitalis blastomycetica B37.2
Erosion
- artery I77.2
  - without rupture I77.89
- bone — *see* Disorder, bone, density and structure, specified NEC
- bronchus J98.Ø9
- cartilage (joint) — *see* Disorder, cartilage, specified type NEC
- cervix (uteri) (acquired) (chronic) (congenital) N86
  - with cervicitis N72
- cornea (nontraumatic) — *see* Ulcer, cornea
  - recurrent H18.83-
  - traumatic — *see* Abrasion, cornea
- dental (idiopathic) (occupational) (due to diet, drugs or vomiting) KØ3.2
- duodenum, postpyloric — *see* Ulcer, duodenum
- esophagus K22.1Ø
  - with bleeding K22.11
- gastric — *see* Ulcer, stomach
- gastrojejunal — *see* Ulcer, gastrojejunal
- implanted mesh — *see* Complications, mesh
- intestine K63.3
- lymphatic vessel I89.8
- pylorus, pyloric (ulcer) — *see* Ulcer, stomach
- spine, aneurysmal A52.Ø9
- stomach — *see* Ulcer, stomach
- teeth (idiopathic) (occupational) (due to diet, drugs or vomiting) KØ3.2
- urethra N36.8
- uterus N85.8

Erotomania F52.8
Error
- metabolism, inborn — *see* Disorder, metabolism
- refractive — *see* Disorder, refraction

Eructation R14.2
- nervous or psychogenic F45.8

Eruption
- creeping B76.9
- drug (generalized) (taken internally) L27.Ø
  - fixed L27.1

Eruption— *continued*
- drug— *continued*
  - in contact with skin — *see* Dermatitis, due to drugs
  - localized L27.1
- Hutchinson, summer L56.4
- Kaposi's varicelliform BØØ.Ø
- napkin L22
- polymorphous light (sun) L56.4
- recalcitrant pustular L13.8
- ringed R23.8
- skin (nonspecific) R21
  - creeping (meaning hookworm) B76.9
  - due to inoculation/vaccination (generalized) (*see also* Dermatitis, due to, vaccine) L27.Ø
    - localized L27.1
  - erysipeloid A26.Ø
  - feigned L98.1
  - Kaposi's varicelliform BØØ.Ø
  - lichenoid L28.Ø
  - meaning dermatitis — *see* Dermatitis
  - toxic NEC L53.Ø
- tooth, teeth, abnormal (incomplete) (late) (premature) (sequence) KØØ.6
- vesicular R23.8

Erysipelas (gangrenous) (infantile) (newborn) (phlegmonous) (suppurative) A46
- external ear A46 *[H62.40]*
- puerperal, postpartum O86.89

Erysipeloid A26.9
- cutaneous (Rosenbach's) A26.Ø
- disseminated A26.8
- sepsis A26.7
- specified NEC A26.8

Erythema, erythematous (infectional) (inflammation) L53.9
- ab igne L59.Ø
- annulare (centrifugum) (rheumaticum) L53.1
- arthriticum epidemicum A25.1
- brucellum — *see* Brucellosis
- chronic figurate NEC L53.3
- chronicum migrans (Borrelia burgdorferi) A69.2Ø
- diaper L22
- due to
  - chemical NEC L53.Ø
    - in contact with skin L24.5
  - drug (internal use) — *see* Dermatitis, due to, drugs
- elevatum diutinum L95.1
- endemic E52
- epidemic, arthritic A25.1
- figuratum perstans L53.3
- gluteal L22
- heat—code by site under Burn, first degree
- ichthyosiforme congenitum bullous Q8Ø.3
- in diseases classified elsewhere L54
- induratum (nontuberculous) L52
  - tuberculous A18.4
- infectiosum BØ8.3
- intertrigo L3Ø.4
- iris L51.9
- marginatum L53.2
  - in (due to) acute rheumatic fever IØØ
- medicamentosum — *see* Dermatitis, due to, drugs
- migrans A26.Ø
  - chronicum A69.2Ø
  - tongue K14.1
- multiforme (major) (minor) L51.9
  - bullous, bullosum L51.1
  - conjunctiva L51.1
  - nonbullous L51.Ø
  - pemphigoides L12.Ø
  - specified NEC L51.8
- napkin L22
- neonatorum P83.8
  - toxic P83.1
- nodosum L52
  - tuberculous A18.4
- palmar L53.8
- pernio T69.1
- rash, newborn P83.8
- scarlatiniform (recurrent) (exfoliative) L53.8
- solare L55.Ø

Erythema, erythematous— *continued*
- specified NEC L53.8
- toxic, toxicum NEC L53.Ø
  - newborn P83.1
- tuberculous (primary) A18.4

Erythematous, erythematosus — *see* condition
Erythermalgia (primary) I73.81
Erythralgia I73.81
Erythrasma LØ8.1
Erythredema (polyneuropathy) — *see* Poisoning, mercury
Erythremia (acute) C94.Ø-
- chronic D45
- secondary D75.1

Erythroblastopenia (*see also* Aplasia, red cell) D6Ø.9
- congenital D61.Ø1

Erythroblastophthisis D61.09
Erythroblastosis (fetalis) (newborn) P55.9
- due to
  - ABO (antibodies) (incompatibility) (isoimmunization) P55.1
  - Rh (antibodies) (incompatibility) (isoimmunization) P55.Ø

Erythrocyanosis (crurum) I73.89
Erythrocythemia — *see* Erythremia
Erythrocytosis (megalosplenic) (secondary) D75.1
- familial D75.Ø
- oval, hereditary — *see* Elliptocytosis
- secondary D75.1
- stress D75.1

Erythroderma (secondary) (*see also* Erythema) L53.9
- bullous ichthyosiform, congenital Q8Ø.3
- desquamativum L21.1
- ichthyosiform, congenital (bullous) Q8Ø.3
- neonatorum P83.8
- psoriaticum L4Ø.8

Erythrodysesthesia, palmar plantar (PPE) L27.1
Erythrogenesis imperfecta D61.09
Erythroleukemia C94.0-
Erythromelalgia I73.81
Erythrophagocytosis D75.89
Erythrophobia F40.298
Erythroplakia, oral epithelium, and tongue K13.29
Erythroplasia (Queyrat) DØ7.4
- specified site — *see* Neoplasm, skin, in situ
- unspecified site DØ7.4

Escherichia coli (E. coli), as cause of disease classified elsewhere B96.2Ø
- non-O157 Shiga toxin-producing (with known O group) B96.22
- non-Shiga toxin-producing B96.29
- O157 with confirmation of Shiga toxin when H antigen is unknown, or is not H7 B96.21
- O157:H- (nonmotile) with confirmation of Shiga toxin B96.21
- O157:H7 with or without confirmation of Shiga toxin-production B96.21
- Shiga toxin-producing (with unspecified O group) (STEC) B96.23
  - O157 B96.21
  - O157:H7 with or without confirmation of Shiga toxin-production B96.21
  - specified NEC B96.22
- specified NEC B96.29

Esophagismus K22.4
Esophagitis (acute) (alkaline) (chemical) (chronic) (infectional) (necrotic) (peptic) (postoperative) K2Ø.9
- candidal B37.81
- due to gastrointestinal reflux disease K21.Ø
- eosinophilic K2Ø.Ø
- reflux K21.Ø
- specified NEC K2Ø.8
- tuberculous A18.83
- ulcerative K22.1Ø
  - with bleeding K22.11

Esophagocele K22.5
Esophagomalacia K22.8
Esophagospasm K22.4
Esophagostenosis K22.2
Esophagostomiasis B81.8
Esophagotracheal — *see* condition
Esophagus — *see* condition

- **Esophoria** H5Ø.51
  - convergence, excess H51.12
  - divergence, insufficiency H51.8
- **Esotropia** — *see* Strabismus, convergent concomitant
- **Espundia** B55.2
- **Essential** — *see* condition
- **Esthesioneuroblastoma** C3Ø.Ø
- **Esthesioneurocytoma** C3Ø.Ø
- **Esthesioneuroepithelioma** C3Ø.Ø
- **Esthiomene** A55
- **Estivo-autumnal malaria** (fever) B5Ø.9
- **Estrangement** (marital) Z63.5
  - parent-child NEC Z62.89Ø
- **Estriasis** — *see* Myiasis
- **Ethanolism** — *see* Alcoholism
- **Etherism** — *see* Dependence, drug, inhalant
- **Ethmoid, ethmoidal** — *see* condition
- **Ethmoiditis** (chronic) (nonpurulent) (purulent) (*see also* Sinusitis, ethmoidal)
  - influenzal — *see* Influenza, with, respiratory manifestations NEC
  - Woakes' J33.1
- **Ethylism** — *see* Alcoholism
- **Eulenburg's disease** (congenital paramyotonia) G71.19
- **Eumycetoma** B47.Ø
- **Eunuchoidism** E29.1
  - hypogonadotropic E23.Ø
- **European blastomycosis** — *see* Cryptococcosis
- **Eustachian** — *see* condition
- **Evaluation** (for) (of)
  - development state
    - adolescent ZØØ.3
    - period of
      - delayed growth in childhood ZØØ.7Ø
        - with abnormal findings ZØØ.71
      - rapid growth in childhood ZØØ.2
    - puberty ZØØ.3
  - growth and developmental state (period of rapid growth) ZØØ.2
    - delayed growth ZØØ.7Ø
      - with abnormal findings ZØØ.71
  - mental health (status) ZØØ.8
    - requested by authority ZØ4.6
  - period of
    - delayed growth in childhood ZØØ.7Ø
      - with abnormal findings ZØØ.71
    - rapid growth in childhood ZØØ.2
  - suspected condition — *see* Observation
- **Evans syndrome** D69.41
- **Event apparent life threatening in newborn and infant** (ALTE) R68.13
- **Eventration** (*see also* Hernia, ventral)
  - colon into chest — *see* Hernia, diaphragm
  - diaphragm (congenital) Q79.1
- **Eversion**
  - bladder N32.89
  - cervix (uteri) N86
    - with cervicitis N72
  - foot NEC (*see also* Deformity, valgus, ankle)
    - congenital Q66.6
  - punctum lacrimale (postinfectional) (senile) HØ4.52-
  - ureter (meatus) N28.89
  - urethra (meatus) N36.8
  - uterus N81.4
- **Evidence**
  - cytologic
    - of malignancy on anal smear R85.614
    - of malignancy on cervical smear R87.614
    - of malignancy on vaginal smear R87.624
- **Evisceration**
  - birth injury P15.8
  - traumatic NEC
    - eye — *see* Enucleated eye
- **Evulsion** — *see* Avulsion
- **Ewing's sarcoma or tumor** — *see* Neoplasm, bone, malignant
- **Examination** (for) (following) (general) (of) (routine) ZØØ.ØØ-
  - with abnormal findings ZØØ.Ø1
  - abuse, physical (alleged), ruled out
    - adult ZØ4.71
    - child ZØ4.72
  - adolescent (development state) ZØØ.3
  - alleged rape or sexual assault (victim), ruled out
    - adult ZØ4.41
    - child ZØ4.42
  - allergy ZØ1.82
  - annual (adult) (periodic) (physical) ZØØ.ØØ
    - with abnormal findings ZØØ.Ø1
    - gynecological ZØ1.419
      - with abnormal findings ZØ1.411
  - antibody response ZØ1.84
  - blood — *see* Examination, laboratory
  - blood pressure ZØ1.3Ø
    - with abnormal findings ZØ1.31
  - cancer staging — *see* Neoplasm, malignant, by site
  - cervical Papanicolaou smear Z12.4
    - as part of routine gynecological examination ZØ1.419
      - with abnormal findings ZØ1.411
  - child (over 28 days old) ZØØ.129
    - with abnormal findings ZØØ.121
    - under 28 days old — *see* Newborn, examination
  - clinical research control or normal comparison (control) (participant) ZØØ.6
  - contraceptive (drug) maintenance (routine) Z3Ø.8
    - device (intrauterine) Z3Ø.431
  - developmental — *see* Examination, child
  - dental ZØ1.2Ø
    - with abnormal findings ZØ1.21
  - donor (potential) ZØØ.5
  - ear ZØ1.1Ø
    - with abnormal findings NEC ZØ1.118
  - eye ZØ1.ØØ
    - with abnormal findings ZØ1.Ø1
  - following
    - accident NEC ZØ4.3
      - transport ZØ4.1
      - work ZØ4.2
    - assault, alleged, ruled out
      - adult ZØ4.71
      - child ZØ4.72
    - motor vehicle accident ZØ4.1
    - treatment (for) ZØ9
      - combined NEC ZØ9
        - fracture ZØ9
        - malignant neoplasm ZØ8
      - malignant neoplasm ZØ8
      - mental disorder ZØ9
      - specified condition NEC ZØ9
  - follow-up (routine) (following) ZØ9
    - chemotherapy NEC ZØ9
      - malignant neoplasm ZØ8
    - fracture ZØ9
    - malignant neoplasm ZØ8
    - postpartum Z39.2
    - psychotherapy ZØ9
    - radiotherapy NEC ZØ9
      - malignant neoplasm ZØ8
    - surgery NEC ZØ9
      - malignant neoplasm ZØ8
  - gynecological ZØ1.419
    - with abnormal findings ZØ1.411
    - for contraceptive maintenance Z3Ø.8
  - health — *see* Examination, medical
  - hearing ZØ1.1Ø
    - with abnormal findings NEC ZØ1.118
    - following failed hearing screening ZØ1.11Ø
  - immunity status testing ZØ1.84
  - laboratory (as part of a general medical examination) ZØØ.ØØ
    - with abnormal findings ZØØ.Ø1
    - preprocedural ZØ1.812
  - lactating mother Z39.1
  - medical (adult) (for) (of) ZØØ.ØØ
    - with abnormal findings ZØØ.Ø1
    - administrative purpose only ZØ2.9
      - specified NEC ZØ2.89
    - admission to
      - armed forces ZØ2.3
      - old age home ZØ2.2
      - prison ZØ2.89
      - residential institution ZØ2.2
      - school ZØ2.Ø
        - following illness or medical treatment ZØ2.Ø
      - summer camp ZØ2.89
    - adoption ZØ2.82
    - blood alcohol or drug level ZØ2.83
    - camp (summer) ZØ2.89
    - clinical research, normal subject (control) (partcipant) ZØØ.6
    - control subject in clinical research (normal comparision) (participant) ZØØ.6
    - donor (potential) ZØØ.5
    - driving license ZØ2.4
    - general (adult) ZØØ.ØØ
      - with abnormal findings ZØØ.Ø1
    - immigration ZØ2.89
    - insurance purposes ZØ2.6
    - marriage ZØ2.89
    - medicolegal reasons NEC ZØ4.8
    - naturalization ZØ2.89
    - participation in sport ZØ2.5
    - paternity testing ZØ2.81
    - population survey ZØØ.8
    - pre-employment ZØ2.1
    - pre-operative — *see* Examination, pre-procedural
    - pre-procedural
      - cardiovascular ZØ1.81Ø
      - respiratory ZØ1.811
      - specified NEC ZØ1.818
    - preschool children
      - for admission to school ZØ2.Ø
    - prisoners
      - for entrance into prison ZØ2.89
    - recruitment for armed forces ZØ2.3
    - specified NEC ZØØ.8
    - sport competition ZØ2.5
  - medicolegal reason NEC ZØ4.8
  - newborn — *see* Newborn, examination
  - pelvic (annual) (periodic) ZØ1.419
    - with abnormal findings ZØ1.411
  - period of rapid growth in childhood ZØØ.2
  - periodic (adult) (annual) (routine) ZØØ.ØØ
    - with abnormal findings ZØØ.Ø1
  - physical (adult) (*see also* Examination, medical) ZØØ.ØØ
    - sports ZØ2.5
  - postpartum
    - immediately after delivery Z39.Ø
    - routine follow-up Z39.2
  - prenatal (normal pregnancy) (*see also* Pregnancy, normal) Z34.9-
  - pre-chemotherapy (antineoplastic) ZØ1.818
  - pre-procedural (pre-operative)
    - cardiovascular ZØ1.81Ø
    - laboratory ZØ1.812
    - respiratory ZØ1.811
    - specified NEC ZØ1.818
  - prior to chemotherapy (antineoplastic) ZØ1.818
  - psychiatric NEC ZØØ.8
    - follow-up not needing further care ZØ9
    - requested by authority ZØ4.6
  - radiological (as part of a general medical examination) ZØØ.ØØ
    - with abnormal findings ZØØ.Ø1
  - repeat cervical smear to confirm findings of recent normal smear following initial abnormal smear ZØ1.42
  - skin (hypersensitivity) ZØ1.82
  - special (*see also* Examination, by type) ZØ1.89
    - specified type NEC ZØ1.89
  - specified type or reason NEC ZØ4.8
  - teeth ZØ1.2Ø
    - with abnormal findings ZØ1.21
  - urine — *see* Examination, laboratory
  - vision ZØ1.ØØ
    - with abnormal findings ZØ1.Ø1
- **Exanthem, exanthema** (*see also* Rash)
  - with enteroviral vesicular stomatitis BØ8.4
  - Boston A88.Ø

Exanthem, exanthema— *continued*
- epidemic with meningitis A88.Ø *[G02]*
- subitum BØ8.2Ø
  - due to human herpesvirus 6 BØ8.21
  - due to human herpesvirus 7 BØ8.22
- viral, virus BØ9
  - specified type NEC BØ8.8

Excess, excessive, excessively
- alcohol level in blood R78.Ø
- androgen (ovarian) E28.1
- attrition, tooth, teeth KØ3.Ø
- carotene, carotin (dietary) E67.1
- cold, effects of T69.9
  - specified effect NEC T69.8
- convergence H51.12
- crying
  - in child, adolescent, or adult R45.83
  - in infant R68.11
- development, breast N62
- divergence H51.8
- drinking (alcohol) NEC (without dependence) F1Ø.1Ø
  - habitual (continual) (without remission) F1Ø.2Ø
- eating R63.2
- estrogen E28.Ø
- fat (*see also* Obesity)
  - in heart — *see* Degeneration, myocardial
  - localized E65
- foreskin N47.8
- gas R14.Ø
- glucagon E16.3
- heat — *see* Heat
- intermaxillary vertical dimension of fully erupted teeth M26.37
- interocclusal distance of fully erupted teeth M26.37
- kalium E87.5
- large
  - colon K59.3
    - congenital Q43.8
  - infant PØ8.Ø
  - organ or site, congenital NEC — *see* Anomaly, by site
- long
  - organ or site, congenital NEC — *see* Anomaly, by site
- menstruation (with regular cycle) N92.Ø
  - with irregular cycle N92.1
- napping Z72.821
- natrium E87.Ø
- number of teeth KØØ.1
- nutrient (dietary) NEC R63.2
- potassium (K) E87.5
- salivation K11.7
- secretion (*see also* Hypersecretion)
  - milk O92.6
  - sputum RØ9.3
  - sweat R61
- sexual drive F52.8
- short
  - organ or site, congenital NEC — *see* Anomaly, by site
  - umbilical cord in labor or delivery O69.3
- skin, eyelid (acquired) — *see* Blepharochalasis
  - congenital Q1Ø.3
- sodium (Na) E87.Ø
- spacing of fully erupted teeth M26.32
- sputum RØ9.3
- sweating R61
- thirst R63.1
  - due to deprivation of water T73.1
- tuberosity of jaw M26.Ø7
- vitamin
  - A (dietary) E67.Ø
    - administered as drug (prolonged intake) — *see* Table of Drugs and Chemicals, vitamins, adverse effect
    - overdose or wrong substance given or taken — *see* Table of Drugs and Chemicals, vitamins, poisoning
  - D (dietary) E67.3
    - administered as drug (prolonged intake) — *see* Table of Drugs and Chemicals, vitamins, adverse effect

Excess, excessive, excessively— *continued*
- vitamin— *continued*
  - D— *continued*
    - overdose or wrong substance given or taken — *see* Table of Drugs and Chemicals, vitamins, poisoning
- weight
  - gain R63.5
  - loss R63.4

Excitability, abnormal, under minor stress (personality disorder) F6Ø.3

Excitation
- anomalous atrioventricular I45.6
- psychogenic F3Ø.8
- reactive (from emotional stress, psychological trauma) F3Ø.8

Excitement
- hypomanic F3Ø.8
- manic F3Ø.9
- mental, reactive (from emotional stress, psychological trauma) F3Ø.8
- state, reactive (from emotional stress, psychological trauma) F3Ø.8

Excoriation (traumatic) (*see also* Abrasion)
- neurotic L98.1

Exfoliation
- due to erythematous conditions according to extent of body surface involved L49.Ø
  - 1Ø-19 percent of body surface L49.1
  - 2Ø-29 percent of body surface L49.2
  - 3Ø-39 percent of body surface L49.3
  - 4Ø-49 percent of body surface L49.4
  - 5Ø-59 percent of body surface L49.5
- due to erythematous conditions according to extent of body surface involved— *continued*
  - 6Ø-69 percent of body surface L49.6
  - 7Ø-79 percent of body surface L49.7
  - 8Ø-89 percent of body surface L49.8
  - 9Ø-99 percent of body surface L49.9
  - less than 1Ø percent of body surface L49.Ø
- teeth, due to systemic causes KØ8.Ø

Exfoliative — *see* condition

Exhaustion, exhaustive (physical NEC) R53.83
- battle F43.Ø
- cardiac — *see* Failure, heart
- delirium F43.Ø
- due to
  - cold T69.8
  - excessive exertion T73.3
  - exposure T73.2
  - neurasthenia F48.8
- heart — *see* Failure, heart
- heat (*see also* Heat, exhaustion) T67.5
  - due to
    - salt depletion T67.4
    - water depletion T67.3
- maternal, complicating delivery O75.81
- mental F48.8
- myocardium, myocardial — *see* Failure, heart
- nervous F48.8
- old age R54
- psychogenic F48.8
- psychosis F43.Ø
- senile R54
- vital NEC Z73.Ø

Exhibitionism F65.2

Exocervicitis — *see* Cervicitis

Exomphalos Q79.2
- meaning hernia — *see* Hernia, umbilicus

Exophoria H5Ø.52
- convergence, insufficiency H51.11
- divergence, excess H51.8

Exophthalmos HØ5.2-
- congenital Q15.8
- constant NEC HØ5.24-
- displacement, globe — *see* Displacement, globe
- due to thyrotoxicosis (hyperthyroidism) — *see* Hyperthyroidism, with, goiter (diffuse)
- dysthyroid — *see* Hyperthyroidism, with, goiter (diffuse)
- goiter — *see* Hyperthyroidism, with, goiter (diffuse)
- intermittent NEC HØ5.25-

Exophthalmos— *continued*
- malignant — *see* Hyperthyroidism, with, goiter (diffuse)
- orbital
  - edema — *see* Edema, orbit
  - hemorrhage — *see* Hemorrhage, orbit
- pulsating NEC HØ5.26-
- thyrotoxic, thyrotropic — *see* Hyperthyroidism, with, goiter (diffuse)

Exostosis (*see also* Disorder, bone)
- cartilaginous — *see* Neoplasm, bone, benign
- congenital (multiple) Q78.6
- external ear canal H61.81-
- gonococcal A54.49
- jaw (bone) M27.8
- multiple, congenital Q78.6
- orbit HØ5.35-
- osteocartilaginous — *see* Neoplasm, bone, benign
- syphilitic A52.77

Exotropia — *see* Strabismus, divergent concomitant

Explanation of
- investigation finding Z71.2
- medication Z71.89

Exposure (to) (*see also* Contact, with) T75.89
- acariasis Z2Ø.7
- AIDS virus Z2Ø.6
- air pollution Z77.11Ø
- algae and algae toxins Z77.121
- algae bloom Z77.121
- anthrax Z2Ø.81Ø
- aromatic amines Z77.Ø2Ø
- aromatic (hazardous) compounds NEC Z77.Ø28
- aromatic dyes NOS Z77.Ø28
- arsenic Z77.Ø1Ø
- asbestos Z77.Ø9Ø
- bacterial disease NEC Z2Ø.818
- benzene Z77.Ø21
- blue-green algae bloom Z77.121
- body fluids (potentially hazardous) Z77.21
- brown tide Z77.121
- chemicals (chiefly nonmedicinal) (hazardous) NEC Z77.Ø98
- cholera Z2Ø.Ø9
- chromium compounds Z77.Ø18
- cold, effects of T69.9
  - specified effect NEC T69.8
- communicable disease Z2Ø.9
  - bacterial NEC Z2Ø.818
  - specified NEC Z2Ø.89
  - viral NEC Z2Ø.828
- cyanobacteria bloom Z77.121
- disaster Z65.5
- discrimination Z6Ø.5
- dyes Z77.Ø98
- Escherichia coli (E. coli) Z2Ø.Ø1
- effects of T73.9
- environmental tobacco smoke (acute) (chronic) Z77.22
- exhaustion due to T73.2
- fiberglass — *see* Table of Drugs and Chemicals, fiberglass
- German measles Z2Ø.4
- gonorrhea Z2Ø.2
- hazardous metals NEC Z77.Ø18
- hazardous substances NEC Z77.29
- hazards in the physical environment NEC Z77.128
- hazards to health NEC Z77.9
- human immunodeficiency virus (HIV) Z2Ø.6
- human T-lymphotropic virus type-1 (HTLV-1) Z2Ø.89
- implanted
  - mesh — *see* Complications, mesh
  - prosthetic materials NEC — *see* Complications, prosthetic materials NEC
- infestation (parasitic) NEC Z2Ø.7
- intestinal infectious disease NEC Z2Ø.Ø9
  - Escherichia coli (E. coli) Z2Ø.Ø1
- lead Z77.Ø11
- meningococcus Z2Ø.811
- mold (toxic) Z77.12Ø
- nickel dust Z77.Ø18
- noise Z77.122
- occupational
  - air contaminants NEC Z57.39

F

Fever— *continued*
- hemorrhagic (arthropod-borne) NOS A94
  - with renal syndrome A98.5
  - arenaviral A96.9
    - specified NEC A96.8
  - Argentinian A96.Ø
  - Bangkok A91
  - Bolivian A96.1
  - Central Asian A98.Ø
  - Chikungunya A92.Ø
  - Crimean-Congo A98.Ø
  - dengue (virus) A91
  - epidemic A98.5
  - Junin (virus) A96.Ø
  - Korean A98.5
  - Kyasanur forest A98.2
  - Machupo (virus) A96.1
  - mite-borne A93.8
  - mosquito-borne A92.8
  - Omsk A98.1
  - Philippine A91
  - Russian A98.5
  - Singapore A91
  - Southeast Asia A91
  - Thailand A91
  - tick-borne NEC A93.8
  - viral A99
    - specified NEC A98.8
- hepatic — *see* Cholecystitis
- herpetic — *see* Herpes
- icterohemorrhagic A27.Ø
- Indiana A93.8
- infective B99.9
  - specified NEC B99.8
- intermittent (bilious) (*see also* Malaria)
  - of unknown origin R5Ø.9
  - pernicious B5Ø.9
- iodide R5Ø.2
- Japanese river A75.3
- jungle (*see also* Malaria)
  - yellow A95.Ø
- Junin (virus) hemorrhagic A96.Ø
- Katayama B65.2
- kedani A75.3
- Kenya (tick) A77.1
- Kew Garden A79.1
- Korean hemorrhagic A98.5
- Lassa A96.2
- Lone Star A77.Ø
- Machupo (virus) hemorrhagic A96.1
- malaria, malarial — *see* Malaria
- Malta A23.9
- Marseilles A77.1
- marsh — *see* Malaria
- Mayaro (viral) A92.8
- Mediterranean (*see also* Brucellosis) A23.9
  - familial E85.Ø
  - tick A77.1
- meningeal — *see* Meningitis
- Meuse A79.Ø
- Mexican A75.2
- mianeh A68.1
- miasmatic — *see* Malaria
- mosquito-borne (viral) A92.9
  - hemorrhagic A92.8
- mountain (*see also* Brucellosis)
  - meaning Rocky Mountain spotted fever A77.Ø
  - tick (American) (Colorado) (viral) A93.2
- Mucambo (viral) A92.8
- mud A27.9
- Neapolitan — *see* Brucellosis
- neutropenic D7Ø.9
- newborn P81.9
  - environmental P81.Ø
- Nine-Mile A78
- non-exanthematous tick A93.2
- North Asian tick-borne A77.2
- Omsk hemorrhagic A98.1
- O'nyong-nyong (viral) A92.1
- Oropouche (viral) A93.Ø
- Oroya A44.Ø
- paludal — *see* Malaria
- Panama (malarial) B5Ø.9

Fever— *continued*
- Pappataci A93.1
- paratyphoid AØ1.4
  - A AØ1.1
  - B AØ1.2
  - C AØ1.3
- parrot A7Ø
- periodic (Mediterranean) E85.Ø
- persistent (of unknown origin) R5Ø.9
- petechial A39.Ø
- pharyngoconjunctival B3Ø.2
- Philippine hemorrhagic A91
- phlebotomus A93.1
- Piry (virus) A93.8
- Pixuna (viral) A92.8
- Plasmodium ovale B53.Ø
- polioviral (nonparalytic) A8Ø.4
- Pontiac A48.2
- postimmunization R5Ø.83
- postoperative R5Ø.82
  - due to infection T81.4
- posttoperative R5Ø.82
- posttransfusion R5Ø.84
- postvaccination R5Ø.83
- presenting with conditions classified elsewhere R5Ø.81
- pretibial A27.89
- puerperal O86.4
- Q A78
- quadrilateral A78
- quartan (malaria) B52.9
- Queensland (coastal) (tick) A77.3
- quintan A79.Ø
- rabbit — *see* Tularemia
- rat-bite A25.9
  - due to
    - Spirillum A25.Ø
    - Streptobacillus moniliformis A25.1
- recurrent — *see* Fever, relapsing
- relapsing (Borrelia) A68.9
  - Carter's (Asiatic) A68.1
  - Dutton's (West African) A68.1
  - Koch's A68.9
  - louse-borne A68.Ø
  - Novy's
    - louse-borne A68.Ø
    - tick-borne A68.1
  - Obermeyer's (European) A68.Ø
  - tick-borne A68.1
- remittent (bilious) (congestive) (gastric) — *see* Malaria
- rheumatic (active) (acute) (chronic) (subacute) IØØ
  - with central nervous system involvement IØ2.9
  - active with heart involvement — *see* category IØ1
  - inactive or quiescent with
    - cardiac hypertrophy IØ9.89
    - carditis IØ9.9
    - endocarditis IØ9.1
      - aortic (valve) IØ6.9
        - with mitral (valve) disease IØ8.Ø
      - mitral (valve) IØ5.9
        - with aortic (valve) disease IØ8.Ø
      - pulmonary (valve) IØ9.89
      - tricuspid (valve) IØ7.8
    - heart disease NEC IØ9.89
    - heart failure (congestive) (conditions in I5Ø.9) IØ9.81
    - left ventricular failure (conditions in I5Ø.1) IØ9.81
    - myocarditis, myocardial degeneration (conditions in I51.4) IØ9.Ø
    - pancarditis IØ9.9
    - pericarditis IØ9.2
- Rift Valley (viral) A92.4
- Rocky Mountain spotted A77.Ø
- rose J3Ø.1
- Ross River B33.1
- Russian hemorrhagic A98.5
- San Joaquin (Valley) B38.Ø
- sandfly A93.1
- Sao Paulo A77.Ø
- scarlet A38.9
- seven day (leptospirosis) (autumnal) (Japanese) A27.89
  - dengue A9Ø

Fever— *continued*
- shin-bone A79.Ø
- Singapore hemorrhagic A91
- solar A9Ø
- Songo A98.5
- sore BØØ.1
- South African tick-bite A68.1
- Southeast Asia hemorrhagic A91
- spinal — *see* Meningitis
- spirillary A25.Ø
- splenic — *see* Anthrax
- spotted A77.9
  - American A77.Ø
  - Brazilian A77.Ø
  - cerebrospinal meningitis A39.Ø
  - Colombian A77.Ø
  - due to Rickettsia
    - australis A77.3
    - conorii A77.1
    - rickettsii A77.Ø
    - sibirica A77.2
    - specified type NEC A77.8
  - Ehrlichiosis A77.4Ø
    - due to
      - E. chafeensis A77.41
      - specified organism NEC A77.49
  - Rocky Mountain A77.Ø
- steroid R5Ø.2
- streptobacillary A25.1
- subtertian B5Ø.9
- Sumatran mite A75.3
- sun A9Ø
- swamp A27.9
- swine AØ2.8
- sylvatic, yellow A95.Ø
- Tahyna B33.8
- tertian — *see* Malaria, tertian
- Thailand hemorrhagic A91
- thermic T67.Ø
- three-day A93.1
- tick
  - American mountain A93.2
  - Colorado A93.2
  - Kemerovo A93.8
  - Mediterranean A77.1
  - mountain A93.2
  - nonexanthematous A93.2
  - Quaranfil A93.8
- tick-bite NEC A93.8
- tick-borne (hemorrhagic) NEC A93.8
- trench A79.Ø
- tsutsugamushi A75.3
- typhogastric AØ1.ØØ
- typhoid (abortive) (hemorrhagic) (intermittent) (malignant) AØ1.ØØ
  - complicated by
    - arthritis AØ1.Ø4
    - heart involvement AØ1.Ø2
    - meningitis AØ1.Ø1
    - osteomyelitis AØ1.Ø5
    - pneumonia AØ1.Ø3
    - specified NEC AØ1.Ø9
- typhomalarial — *see* Malaria
- typhus — *see* Typhus (fever)
- undulant — *see* Brucellosis
- unknown origin R5Ø.9
- uveoparotid D86.89
- valley B38.Ø
- Venezuelan equine A92.2
- vesicular stomatitis A93.8
- viral hemorrhagic — *see* Fever, hemorrhagic, by type of virus
- Volhynian A79.Ø
- Wesselsbron (viral) A92.8
- West
  - African B5Ø.8
  - Nile (viral) A92.3Ø
    - with
      - complications NEC A92.39
      - cranial nerve disorders A92.32
      - encephalitis A92.31
      - encephalomyelitis A92.31
      - neurologic manifestation NEC A92.32

- **Fever**— *continued*
  - West— *continued*
    - Nile— *continued*
      - with— *continued*
        - optic neuritis A92.32
        - polyradiculitis A92.32
  - Whitmore's — *see* Melioidosis
  - Wolhynian A79.Ø
  - worm B83.9
  - yellow A95.9
    - jungle A95.Ø
    - sylvatic A95.Ø
    - urban A95.1
  - Zika (viral) A92.8
- **Fibrillation**
  - atrial or auricular (established) I48.91
    - chronic I48.2
    - paroxysmal I48.Ø
    - permanent I48.2
    - persistent I48.1
  - cardiac I49.8
  - heart I49.8
  - muscular M62.89
  - ventricular I49.Ø1
- **Fibrin**
  - ball or bodies, pleural (sac) J94.1
  - chamber, anterior (eye) (gelatinous exudate) — *see* Iridocyclitis, acute
- **Fibrinogenolysis** — *see* Fibrinolysis
- **Fibrinogenopenia** D68.8
  - acquired D65
  - congenital D68.2
- **Fibrinolysis** (hemorrhagic) (acquired) D65
  - antepartum hemorrhage — *see* Hemorrhage, antepartum, with coagulation defect
  - following
    - abortion — *see* Abortion by type complicated by hemorrhage
    - ectopic or molar pregnancy OØ8.1
  - intrapartum O67.Ø
  - newborn, transient P6Ø
  - postpartum O72.3
- **Fibrinopenia** (hereditary) D68.2
  - acquired D68.4
- **Fibrinopurulent** — *see* condition
- **Fibrinous** — *see* condition
- **Fibroadenoma**
  - cellular intracanalicular D24-
  - giant D24-
  - intracanalicular
    - cellular D24-
    - giant D24-
    - specified site — *see* Neoplasm, benign, by site
    - unspecified site D24-
  - juvenile D24.-
  - pericanalicular
    - specified site — *see* Neoplasm, benign, by site
    - unspecified site D24-
  - phyllodes D24-
  - prostate D29.1
  - specified site NEC — *see* Neoplasm, benign, by site
  - unspecified site D24-
- **Fibroadenosis, breast** (chronic) (cystic) (diffuse) (periodic) (segmental) N6Ø.2-
- **Fibroangioma** (*see also* Neoplasm, benign, by site)
  - juvenile
    - specified site — *see* Neoplasm, benign, by site
    - unspecified site D1Ø.6
- **Fibrochondrosarcoma** — *see* Neoplasm, cartilage, malignant
- **Fibrocystic**
  - disease (*see also* Fibrosis, cystic)
    - breast — *see* Mastopathy, cystic
    - jaw M27.49
    - kidney (congenital) Q61.8
    - liver Q44.6
    - pancreas E84.9
  - kidney (congenital) Q61.8
- **Fibrodysplasia ossificans progressiva** — *see* Myositis, ossificans, progressiva
- **Fibroelastosis** (cordis) (endocardial) (endomyocardial) I42.4
- **Fibroid** (tumor) (*see also* Neoplasm, connective tissue, benign)
  - disease, lung (chronic) — *see* Fibrosis, lung
  - heart (disease) — *see* Myocarditis
  - in pregnancy or childbirth O34.1-
    - causing obstructed labor O65.5
  - induration, lung (chronic) — *see* Fibrosis, lung
  - lung — *see* Fibrosis, lung
  - pneumonia (chronic) — *see* Fibrosis, lung
  - uterus D25.9
- **Fibrolipoma** — *see* Lipoma
- **Fibroliposarcoma** — *see* Neoplasm, connective tissue, malignant
- **Fibroma** (*see also* Neoplasm, connective tissue, benign)
  - ameloblastic — *see* Cyst, calcifying odontogenic
  - bone (nonossifying) — *see* Disorder, bone, specified type NEC
    - ossifying — *see* Neoplasm, bone, benign
  - cementifying — *see* Neoplasm, bone, benign
  - chondromyxoid — *see* Neoplasm, bone, benign
  - desmoplastic — *see* Neoplasm, connective tissue, uncertain behavior
  - durum — *see* Neoplasm, connective tissue, benign
  - fascial — *see* Neoplasm, connective tissue, benign
  - invasive — *see* Neoplasm, connective tissue, uncertain behavior
  - molle — *see* Lipoma
  - myxoid — *see* Neoplasm, connective tissue, benign
  - nasopharynx, nasopharyngeal (juvenile) D1Ø.6
  - nonosteogenic (nonossifying) — *see* Dysplasia, fibrous
  - odontogenic (central) — *see* Cyst, calcifying odontogenic
  - ossifying — *see* Neoplasm, bone, benign
  - periosteal — *see* Neoplasm, bone, benign
  - soft — *see* Lipoma
- **Fibromatosis** M72.9
  - abdominal — *see* Neoplasm, connective tissue, uncertain behavior
  - aggressive — *see* Neoplasm, connective tissue, uncertain behavior
  - congenital generalized — *see* Neoplasm, connective tissue, uncertain behavior
  - Dupuytren's M72.Ø
  - gingival KØ6.1
  - palmar (fascial) M72.Ø
  - plantar (fascial) M72.2
  - pseudosarcomatous (proliferative) (subcutaneous) M72.4
  - retroperitoneal D48.3
  - specified NEC M72.8
- **Fibromyalgia** M79.7
- **Fibromyoma** (*see also* Neoplasm, connective tissue, benign)
  - uterus (corpus) (*see also* Leiomyoma, uterus)
    - in pregnancy or childbirth — *see* Fibroid, in pregnancy or childbirth
      - causing obstructed labor O65.5
- **Fibromyositis** M79.7
- **Fibromyxolipoma** D17.9
- **Fibromyxoma** — *see* Neoplasm, connective tissue, benign
- **Fibromyxosarcoma** — *see* Neoplasm, connective tissue, malignant
- **Fibro-odontoma, ameloblastic** — *see* Cyst, calcifying odontogenic
- **Fibro-osteoma** — *see* Neoplasm, bone, benign
- **Fibroplasia, retrolental** H35.17-
- **Fibropurulent** — *see* condition
- **Fibrosarcoma** (*see also* Neoplasm, connective tissue, malignant)
  - ameloblastic C41.1
    - upper jaw (bone) C41.Ø
  - congenital — *see* Neoplasm, connective tissue, malignant
  - fascial — *see* Neoplasm, connective tissue, malignant
  - infantile — *see* Neoplasm, connective tissue, malignant
  - odontogenic C41.1
    - upper jaw (bone) C41.Ø
  - periosteal — *see* Neoplasm, bone, malignant
- **Fibrosclerosis**
  - breast N6Ø.3-
  - multifocal M35.5
  - penis (corpora cavernosa) N48.6
- **Fibrosis, fibrotic**
  - adrenal (gland) E27.8
  - amnion O41.8X-
  - anal papillae K62.89
  - arteriocapillary — *see* Arteriosclerosis
  - bladder N32.89
    - interstitial — *see* Cystitis, chronic, interstitial
    - localized submucosal — *see* Cystitis, chronic, interstitial
    - panmural — *see* Cystitis, chronic, interstitial
  - breast — *see* Fibrosclerosis, breast
  - capillary (*see also* Arteriosclerosis) I7Ø.9Ø
    - lung (chronic) — *see* Fibrosis, lung
  - cardiac — *see* Myocarditis
  - cervix N88.8
  - chorion O41.8X-
  - corpus cavernosum (sclerosing) N48.6
  - cystic (of pancreas) E84.9
    - with
      - distal intestinal obstruction syndrome E84.19
      - fecal impaction E84.19
      - intestinal manifestations NEC E84.19
      - pulmonary manifestations E84.Ø
      - specified manifestations NEC E84.8
  - due to device, implant or graft (*see also* Complications, by site and type, specified NEC) T85.82
    - arterial graft NEC T82.828
    - breast (implant) T85.82
    - catheter NEC T85.82
      - dialysis (renal) T82.828
        - intraperitoneal T85.82
      - infusion NEC T82.828
        - spinal (epidural) (subdural) T85.82
      - urinary (indwelling) T83.82
    - electronic (electrode) (pulse generator) (stimulator)
      - bone T84.82
      - cardiac T82.827
      - nervous system (brain) (peripheral nerve) (spinal) T85.82
      - urinary T83.82
    - fixation, internal (orthopedic) NEC T84.82
    - gastrointestinal (bile duct) (esophagus) T85.82
    - genital NEC T83.82
    - heart NEC T82.827
    - joint prosthesis T84.82
    - ocular (corneal graft) (orbital implant) NEC T85.82
    - orthopedic NEC T84.82
    - specified NEC T85.82
    - urinary NEC T83.82
    - vascular NEC T82.828
    - ventricular intracranial shunt T85.82
  - ejaculatory duct N5Ø.8
  - endocardium — *see* Endocarditis
  - endomyocardial (tropical) I42.3
  - epididymis N5Ø.8
  - eye muscle — *see* Strabismus, mechanical
  - heart — *see* Myocarditis
  - hepatic — *see* Fibrosis, liver
  - hepatolienal (portal hypertension) K76.6
  - hepatosplenic (portal hypertension) K76.6
  - infrapatellar fat pad M79.4
  - intrascrotal N5Ø.8
  - kidney N26.9
  - liver K74.Ø
    - with sclerosis K74.2
    - alcoholic K7Ø.2
  - lung (atrophic) (chronic) (confluent) (massive) (perialveolar) (peribronchial) J84.1Ø
    - with
      - anthracosilicosis J6Ø
      - anthracosis J6Ø
      - asbestosis J61
      - bagassosis J67.1
      - bauxite J63.1
      - berylliosis J63.2
      - byssinosis J66.Ø

- **Fibrosis, fibrotic**— *continued*
  - lung— *continued*
    - with— *continued*
      - calcicosis J62.8
      - chalicosis J62.8
      - dust reticulation J64
      - farmer's lung J67.Ø
      - ganister disease J62.8
      - graphite J63.3
      - pneumoconiosis NOS J64
      - siderosis J63.4
      - silicosis J62.8
    - capillary J84.1Ø
    - congenital P27.8
    - diffuse (idiopathic) J84.1Ø
      - chemicals, gases, fumes or vapors (inhalation) J68.4
      - interstitial J84.1Ø
        - acute J84.114
      - talc J62.Ø
    - following radiation J7Ø.1
    - idiopathic J84.112
    - postinflammatory J84.1Ø
    - silicotic J62.8
    - tuberculous — *see* Tuberculosis, pulmonary
  - lymphatic gland I89.8
  - median bar — *see* Hyperplasia, prostate
  - mediastinum (idiopathic) J98.5
  - meninges G96.19
  - myocardium, myocardial — *see* Myocarditis
  - ovary N83.8
  - oviduct N83.8
  - pancreas K86.8
  - penis NEC N48.6
  - pericardium I31.Ø
  - perineum, in pregnancy or childbirth O34.7-
    - causing obstructed labor O65.5
  - pleura J94.1
  - popliteal fat pad M79.4
  - prostate (chronic) — *see* Hyperplasia, prostate
  - pulmonary (*see also* Fibrosis, lung) J84.1Ø
    - congenital P27.8
    - idiopathic J84.112
  - rectal sphincter K62.89
  - retroperitoneal, idiopathic (with ureteral obstruction) N13.5
    - with infection N13.6
  - sclerosing mesenteric (idiopathic) K65.4
  - scrotum N5Ø.8
  - seminal vesicle N5Ø.8
  - senile R54
  - skin L9Ø.5
  - spermatic cord N5Ø.8
  - spleen D73.89
    - in schistosomiasis (bilharziasis) B65.9 *[D77]*
  - subepidermal nodular — *see* Neoplasm, skin, benign
  - submucous (oral) (tongue) K13.5
  - testis N44.8
    - chronic, due to syphilis A52.76
  - thymus (gland) E32.8
  - tongue, submucous K13.5
  - tunica vaginalis N5Ø.8
  - uterus (non-neoplastic) N85.8
  - vagina N89.8
  - valve, heart — *see* Endocarditis
  - vas deferens N5Ø.8
  - vein I87.8
- **Fibrositis** (periarticular) M79.7
  - nodular, chronic (Jaccoud's) (rheumatoid) — *see* Arthropathy, postrheumatic, chronic
- **Fibrothorax** J94.1
- **Fibrotic** — *see* Fibrosis
- **Fibrous** — *see* condition
- **Fibroxanthoma** (*see also* Neoplasm, connective tissue, benign)
  - atypical — *see* Neoplasm, connective tissue, uncertain behavior
  - malignant — *see* Neoplasm, connective tissue, malignant
- **Fibroxanthosarcoma** — *see* Neoplasm, connective tissue, malignant
- **Fiedler's**
  - disease (icterohemorrhagic leptospirosis) A27.Ø
  - myocarditis (acute) I4Ø.1
- **Fifth disease** B08.3
  - venereal A55
- **Filaria, filarial, filariasis** — *see* Infestation, filarial
- **Filatov's disease** — *see* Mononucleosis, infectious
- **File-cutter's disease** — *see* Poisoning, lead
- **Filling defect**
  - biliary tract R93.2
  - bladder R93.4
  - duodenum R93.3
  - gallbladder R93.2
  - gastrointestinal tract R93.3
  - intestine R93.3
  - kidney R93.4
  - stomach R93.3
  - ureter R93.4
- **Fimbrial cyst** Q50.4
- **Financial problem affecting care NOS** Z59.9
  - bankruptcy Z59.8
  - foreclosure on loan Z59.8
- **Findings, abnormal, inconclusive, without diagnosis** (*see also* Abnormal)
  - 17-ketosteroids, elevated R82.5
  - acetonuria R82.4
  - alcohol in blood R78.Ø
  - anisocytosis R71.8
  - antenatal screening of mother O28.9
    - biochemical O28.1
    - cytological O28.2
    - chromosomal O28.5
    - genetic O28.5
    - hematological O28.Ø
    - radiological O28.4
    - specified NEC O28.8
    - ultrasonic O28.3
  - antibody titer, elevated R76.Ø
  - anticardiolipin antibody R76.Ø
  - antiphosphatidylglycerol antibody R76.Ø
  - antiphosphatidylinositol antibody R76.Ø
  - antiphosphatidylserine antibody R76.Ø
  - antiphospholipid antibody R76.Ø
  - bacteriuria N39.Ø
  - bicarbonate E87.8
  - bile in urine R82.2
  - blood sugar R73.Ø9
    - high R73.9
    - low (transient) E16.2
  - body fluid or substance, specified NEC R88.8
  - casts, urine R82.99
  - catecholamines R82.5
  - cells, urine R82.99
  - chloride E87.8
  - cholesterol E78.9
    - high E78.Ø
      - with high triglycerides E78.2
  - chyluria R82.Ø
  - cloudy
    - dialysis effluent R88.Ø
    - urine R82.9Ø
  - creatinine clearance R94.4
  - crystals, urine R82.99
  - culture
    - blood R78.81
    - positive — *see* Positive, culture
  - echocardiogram R93.1
  - electrolyte level, urinary R82.99
  - function study NEC R94.8
    - bladder R94.8
    - endocrine NEC R94.7
      - thyroid R94.6
    - kidney R94.4
    - liver R94.5
    - pancreas R94.8
    - placenta R94.8
    - pulmonary R94.2
    - spleen R94.8
  - gallbladder, nonvisualization R93.2
  - glucose (tolerance test) (non-fasting) R73.Ø9
  - glycosuria R81
  - heart
    - shadow R93.1

- **Findings, abnormal, inconclusive, without diagnosis** — *continued*
  - heart— *continued*
    - sounds RØ1.2
  - hematinuria R82.3
  - hematocrit drop (precipitous) R71.Ø
  - hemoglobinuria R82.3
  - human papillomavirus (HPV) DNA test positive
    - cervix
      - high risk R87.81Ø
      - low risk R87.82Ø
    - vagina
      - high risk R87.811
      - low risk R87.821
  - in blood (of substance not normally found in blood) R78.9
    - addictive drug NEC R78.4
    - alcohol (excessive level) R78.Ø
    - cocaine R78.2
    - hallucinogen R78.3
    - heavy metals (abnormal level) R78.79
    - lead R78.71
    - lithium (abnormal level) R78.89
    - opiate drug R78.1
    - psychotropic drug R78.5
    - specified substance NEC R78.89
    - steroid agent R78.6
  - indolacetic acid, elevated R82.5
  - ketonuria R82.4
  - lactic acid dehydrogenase (LDH) R74.Ø
  - liver function test R79.89
  - mammogram NEC R92.8
    - calcification (calculus) R92.1
    - inconclusive result (due to dense breasts) R92.2
    - microcalcification R92.Ø
  - mediastinal shift R93.8
  - melanin, urine R82.99
  - myoglobinuria R82.1
  - neonatal screening PØ9
  - nonvisualization of gallbladder R93.2
  - odor of urine NOS R82.9Ø
  - Papanicolaou cervix R87.619
    - non-atypical endometrial cells R87.618
  - pneumoencephalogram R93.Ø
  - poikilocytosis R71.8
  - potassium (deficiency) E87.6
    - excess E87.5
  - PPD R76.11
  - radiologic (X-ray) R93.8
    - abdomen R93.5
    - biliary tract R93.2
    - breast R92.8
    - gastrointestinal tract R93.3
    - genitourinary organs R93.8
    - head R93.Ø
    - inconclusive due to excess body fat of patient R93.9
    - intrathoracic organs NEC R93.1
    - placenta R93.8
    - retroperitoneum R93.5
    - skin R93.8
    - skull R93.Ø
    - subcutaneous tissue R93.8
  - red blood cell (count) (morphology) (sickling) (volume) R71.8
  - scan NEC R94.8
    - bladder R94.8
    - bone R94.8
    - kidney R94.4
    - liver R93.2
    - lung R94.2
    - pancreas R94.8
    - placental R94.8
    - spleen R94.8
    - thyroid R94.6
  - sedimentation rate, elevated R7Ø.Ø
  - SGOT R74.Ø
  - SGPT R74.Ø
  - sodium (deficiency) E87.1
    - excess E87.Ø
  - specified body fluid NEC R88.8
  - stress test R94.39

- **Findings, abnormal, inconclusive, without diagnosis** — *continued*
  - thyroid (function) (metabolic rate) (scan) (uptake) R94.6
  - transaminase (level) R74.Ø
  - triglycerides E78.9
    - high E78.1
      - with high cholesterol E78.2
  - tuberculin skin test (without active tuberculosis) R76.11
  - urine R82.9Ø
    - acetone R82.4
    - bacteria N39.Ø
    - bile R82.2
    - casts or cells R82.99
    - chyle R82.Ø
    - culture positive R82.7
    - glucose R81
    - hemoglobin R82.3
    - ketone R82.4
    - sugar R81
  - vanillylmandelic acid (VMA), elevated R82.5
  - vectorcardiogram (VCG) R94.39
  - ventriculogram R93.Ø
  - white blood cell (count) (differential) (morphology) D72.9
  - xerography R92.8
- **Finger** — *see* condition
- **Fire, Saint Anthony's** — *see* Erysipelas
- **Fire-setting**
  - pathological (compulsive) F63.1
- **Fish hook stomach** K31.89
- **Fishmeal-worker's lung** J67.8
- **Fissure, fissured**
  - anus, anal K6Ø.2
    - acute K6Ø.Ø
    - chronic K6Ø.1
    - congenital Q43.8
  - ear, lobule, congenital Q17.8
  - epiglottis (congenital) Q31.8
  - larynx J38.7
    - congenital Q31.8
  - lip K13.Ø
    - congenital — *see* Cleft, lip
  - nipple N64.Ø
    - associated with
      - lactation O92.13
      - pregnancy O92.11-
      - puerperium O92.12
  - nose Q3Ø.2
  - palate (congenital) — *see* Cleft, palate
  - skin R23.4
  - spine (congenital) (*see also* Spina bifida)
    - with hydrocephalus — *see* Spina bifida, by site, with hydrocephalus
  - tongue (acquired) K14.5
    - congenital Q38.3
- **Fistula** (cutaneous) L98.8
  - abdomen (wall) K63.2
    - bladder N32.2
    - intestine NEC K63.2
    - ureter N28.89
    - uterus N82.5
  - abdominorectal K63.2
  - abdominosigmoidal K63.2
  - abdominothoracic J86.Ø
  - abdominouterine N82.5
    - congenital Q51.7
  - abdominovesical N32.2
  - accessory sinuses — *see* Sinusitis
  - actinomycotic — *see* Actinomycosis
  - alveolar antrum — *see* Sinusitis, maxillary
  - alveolar process KØ4.6
  - anorectal K6Ø.5
  - antrobuccal — *see* Sinusitis, maxillary
  - antrum — *see* Sinusitis, maxillary
  - anus, anal (recurrent) (infectional) K6Ø.3
    - congenital Q43.6
      - with absence, atresia and stenosis Q42.2
    - tuberculous A18.32
  - aorta-duodenal I77.2
  - appendix, appendicular K38.3

- **Fistula** — *continued*
  - arteriovenous (acquired) (nonruptured) I77.Ø
    - brain I67.1
      - congenital Q28.2
        - ruptured I6Ø.8
      - ruptured I6Ø.8
    - cerebral — *see* Fistula, arteriovenous, brain
    - congenital (peripheral) (*see also* Malformation, arteriovenous)
      - brain Q28.2
        - ruptured I6Ø.8
      - coronary Q24.5
      - pulmonary Q25.72
    - coronary I25.41
      - congenital Q24.5
    - pulmonary I28.Ø
      - congenital Q25.72
    - surgically created (for dialysis) Z99.2
      - complication — *see* Complication, arteriovenous, fistula, surgically created
    - traumatic — *see* Injury, blood vessel
  - artery I77.2
  - aural (mastoid) — *see* Mastoiditis, chronic
  - auricle (*see also* Disorder, pinna, specified type NEC)
    - congenital Q18.1
  - Bartholin's gland N82.8
  - bile duct (common) (hepatic) K83.3
    - with calculus, stones — *see* Calculus, bile duct
  - biliary (tract) — *see* Fistula, bile duct
  - bladder (sphincter) NEC (*see also* Fistula, vesico-) N32.2
    - into seminal vesicle N32.82
  - bone (*see also* Disorder, bone, specified type NEC)
    - with osteomyelitis, chronic — *see* Osteomyelitis, chronic, with draining sinus
  - brain G93.89
    - arteriovenous (acquired) I67.1
      - congenital Q28.2
  - branchial (cleft) Q18.Ø
  - branchiogenous Q18.Ø
  - breast N61
    - puerperal, postpartum or gestational, due to mastitis (purulent) — *see* Mastitis, obstetric, purulent
  - bronchial J86.Ø
  - bronchocutaneous, bronchomediastinal, bronchopleural, bronchopleuromediastinal (infective) J86.Ø
    - tuberculous NEC A15.5
  - bronchoesophageal J86.Ø
    - congenital Q39.2
      - with atresia of esophagus Q39.1
  - bronchovisceral J86.Ø
  - buccal cavity (infective) K12.2
  - cecosigmoidal K63.2
  - cecum K63.2
  - cerebrospinal (fluid) G96.Ø
  - cervical, lateral Q18.1
  - cervicoaural Q18.1
  - cervicosigmoidal N82.4
  - cervicovesical N82.1
  - cervix N82.8
  - chest (wall) J86.Ø
  - cholecystenteric — *see* Fistula, gallbladder
  - cholecystocolic — *see* Fistula, gallbladder
  - cholecystocolonic — *see* Fistula, gallbladder
  - cholecystoduodenal — *see* Fistula, gallbladder
  - cholecystogastric — *see* Fistula, gallbladder
  - cholecystointestinal — *see* Fistula, gallbladder
  - choledochoduodenal — *see* Fistula, bile duct
  - cholocolic K82.3
  - coccyx — *see* Sinus, pilonidal
  - colon K63.2
  - colostomy K94.Ø9
  - common duct — *see* Fistula, bile duct
  - congenital, site not listed — *see* Anomaly, by site
  - coronary, arteriovenous I25.41
    - congenital Q24.5
  - costal region J86.Ø
  - cul-de-sac, Douglas' N82.8
  - cystic duct (*see also* Fistula, gallbladder)
    - congenital Q44.5
  - dental KØ4.6

- **Fistula** — *continued*
  - diaphragm J86.Ø
  - duodenum K31.6
  - ear (external) (canal) — *see* Disorder, ear, external, specified type NEC
  - enterocolic K63.2
  - enterocutaneous K63.2
  - enterouterine N82.4
    - congenital Q51.7
  - enterovaginal N82.4
    - congenital Q52.2
    - large intestine N82.3
    - small intestine N82.2
  - enterovesical N32.1
  - epididymis N5Ø.8
    - tuberculous A18.15
  - esophagobronchial J86.Ø
    - congenital Q39.2
      - with atresia of esophagus Q39.1
  - esophagocutaneous K22.8
  - esophagopleural-cutaneous J86.Ø
  - esophagotracheal J86.Ø
    - congenital Q39.2
      - with atresia of esophagus Q39.1
  - esophagus K22.8
    - congenital Q39.2
      - with atresia of esophagus Q39.1
  - ethmoid — *see* Sinusitis, ethmoidal
  - eyeball (cornea) (sclera) — *see* Disorder, globe, hypotony
  - eyelid HØ1.8
  - fallopian tube, external N82.5
  - fecal K63.2
    - congenital Q43.6
  - from periapical abscess KØ4.6
  - frontal sinus — *see* Sinusitis, frontal
  - gallbladder K82.3
    - with calculus, cholelithiasis, stones — *see* Calculus, gallbladder
  - gastric K31.6
  - gastrocolic K31.6
    - congenital Q4Ø.2
    - tuberculous A18.32
  - gastroenterocolic K31.6
  - gastroesophageal K31.6
  - gastrojejunal K31.6
  - gastrojejunocolic K31.6
  - genital tract (female) N82.9
    - specified NEC N82.8
    - to intestine NEC N82.4
    - to skin N82.5
  - hepatic artery-portal vein, congenital Q26.6
  - hepatopleural J86.Ø
  - hepatopulmonary J86.Ø
  - ileorectal or ileosigmoidal K63.2
  - ileovaginal N82.2
  - ileovesical N32.1
  - ileum K63.2
  - in ano K6Ø.3
    - tuberculous A18.32
  - inner ear (labyrinth) — *see* subcategory H83.1
  - intestine NEC K63.2
  - intestinocolonic (abdominal) K63.2
  - intestinoureteral N28.89
  - intestinouterine N82.4
  - intestinovaginal N82.4
    - large intestine N82.3
    - small intestine N82.2
  - intestinovesical N32.1
  - ischiorectal (fossa) K61.3
  - jejunum K63.2
  - joint M25.1Ø
    - ankle M25.17-
    - elbow M25.12-
    - foot joint M25.17-
    - hand joint M25.14-
    - hip M25.15-
    - knee M25.16-
    - shoulder M25.11-
    - specified joint NEC M25.18
    - tuberculous — *see* Tuberculosis, joint
    - wrist M25.13-
  - kidney N28.89

- **Fistula** — *continued*
  - labium (majus) (minus) N82.8
  - labyrinth — *see* subcategory H83.1
  - lacrimal (gland) (sac) HØ4.61-
  - lacrimonasal duct — *see* Fistula, lacrimal
  - laryngotracheal, congenital Q34.8
  - larynx J38.7
  - lip K13.Ø
    - congenital Q38.Ø
  - lumbar, tuberculous A18.Ø1
  - lung J86.Ø
  - lymphatic I89.8
  - mammary (gland) N61
  - mastoid (process) (region) — *see* Mastoiditis, chronic
  - maxillary J32.Ø
  - medial, face and neck Q18.8
  - mediastinal J86.Ø
  - mediastinobronchial J86.Ø
  - mediastinocutaneous J86.Ø
  - middle ear — *see* subcategory H74.8
  - mouth K12.2
  - nasal J34.89
    - sinus — *see* Sinusitis
  - nasopharynx J39.2
  - nipple N64.Ø
  - nose J34.89
  - oral (cutaneous) K12.2
    - maxillary J32.Ø
    - nasal (with cleft palate) — *see* Cleft, palate
  - orbit, orbital — *see* Disorder, orbit, specified type NEC
  - oroantral J32.Ø
  - oviduct, external N82.5
  - palate (hard) M27.8
  - pancreatic K86.8
  - pancreaticoduodenal K86.8
  - parotid (gland) K11.4
    - region K12.2
  - penis N48.89
  - perianal K6Ø.3
  - pericardium (pleura) (sac) — *see* Pericarditis
  - pericecal K63.2
  - perineorectal K6Ø.4
  - perineosigmoidal K63.2
  - perineum, perineal (with urethral involvement) NEC N36.Ø
    - tuberculous A18.13
    - ureter N28.89
  - perirectal K6Ø.4
    - tuberculous A18.32
  - peritoneum K65.9
  - pharyngoesophageal J39.2
  - pharynx J39.2
    - branchial cleft (congenital) Q18.Ø
  - pilonidal (infected) (rectum) — *see* Sinus, pilonidal
  - pleura, pleural, pleurocutaneous, pleuroperitoneal J86.Ø
    - tuberculous NEC A15.6
  - pleuropericardial I31.8
  - portal vein-hepatic artery, congenital Q26.6
  - postauricular H7Ø.81-
  - postoperative, persistent T81.83
    - specified site — *see* Fistula, by site
  - preauricular (congenital) Q18.1
  - prostate N42.89
  - pulmonary J86.Ø
    - arteriovenous I28.Ø
      - congenital Q25.72
    - tuberculous — *see* Tuberculosis, pulmonary
  - pulmonoperitoneal J86.Ø
  - rectolabial N82.4
  - rectosigmoid (intercommunicating) K63.2
  - rectoureteral N28.89
  - rectourethral N36.Ø
    - congenital Q64.73
  - rectouterine N82.4
    - congenital Q51.7
  - rectovaginal N82.3
    - congenital Q52.2
    - tuberculous A18.18
  - rectovesical N32.1
    - congenital Q64.79

- **Fistula** — *continued*
  - rectovesicovaginal N82.3
  - rectovulval N82.4
    - congenital Q52.79
  - rectum (to skin) K6Ø.4
    - congenital Q43.6
      - with absence, atresia and stenosis Q42.Ø
    - tuberculous A18.32
  - renal N28.89
  - retroauricular — *see* Fistula, postauricular
  - salivary duct or gland (any) K11.4
    - congenital Q38.4
  - scrotum (urinary) N5Ø.8
    - tuberculous A18.15
  - semicircular canals — *see* subcategory H83.1
  - sigmoid K63.2
    - to bladder N32.1
  - sinus — *see* Sinusitis
  - skin L98.8
    - to genital tract (female) N82.5
  - splenocolic D73.89
  - stercoral K63.2
  - stomach K31.6
  - sublingual gland K11.4
  - submandibular gland K11.4
  - submaxillary (gland) K11.4
    - region K12.2
  - thoracic J86.Ø
    - duct I89.8
  - thoracoabdominal J86.Ø
  - thoracogastric J86.Ø
  - thoracointestinal J86.Ø
  - thorax J86.Ø
  - thyroglossal duct Q89.2
  - thyroid EØ7.89
  - trachea, congenital (external) (internal) Q32.1
  - tracheoesophageal J86.Ø
    - congenital Q39.2
      - with atresia of esophagus Q39.1
    - following tracheostomy J95.Ø4
  - traumatic arteriovenous — *see* Injury, blood vessel, by site
  - tuberculous—code by site under Tuberculosis
  - typhoid AØ1.Ø9
  - umbilicourinary Q64.8
  - urachus, congenital Q64.4
  - ureter (persistent) N28.89
  - ureteroabdominal N28.89
  - ureterorectal N28.89
  - ureterosigmoido-abdominal N28.89
  - ureterovaginal N82.1
  - ureterovesical N32.2
  - urethra N36.Ø
    - congenital Q64.79
    - tuberculous A18.13
  - urethroperineal N36.Ø
  - urethroperineovesical N32.2
  - urethrorectal N36.Ø
    - congenital Q64.73
  - urethroscrotal N5Ø.8
  - urethrovaginal N82.1
  - urethrovesical N32.2
  - urinary (tract) (persistent) (recurrent) N36.Ø
  - uteroabdominal N82.5
    - congenital Q51.7
  - uteroenteric, uterointestinal N82.4
    - congenital Q51.7
  - uterorectal N82.4
    - congenital Q51.7
  - uteroureteric N82.1
  - uterourethral Q51.7
  - uterovaginal N82.8
  - uterovesical N82.1
    - congenital Q51.7
  - uterus N82.8
  - vagina (postpartal) (wall) N82.8
  - vaginocutaneous (postpartal) N82.5
  - vaginointestinal NEC N82.4
    - large intestine N82.3
    - small intestine N82.2
  - vaginoperineal N82.5
  - vasocutaneous, congenital Q55.7
  - vesical NEC N32.2

- **Fistula** — *continued*
  - vesicoabdominal N32.2
  - vesicocervicovaginal N82.1
  - vesicocolic N32.1
  - vesicocutaneous N32.2
  - vesicoenteric N32.1
  - vesicointestinal N32.1
  - vesicometrorectal N82.4
  - vesicoperineal N32.2
  - vesicorectal N32.1
    - congenital Q64.79
  - vesicosigmoidal N32.1
  - vesicosigmoidovaginal N82.3
  - vesicoureteral N32.2
  - vesicoureterovaginal N82.1
  - vesicourethral N32.2
  - vesicourethrorectal N32.1
  - vesicouterine N82.1
    - congenital Q51.7
  - vesicovaginal N82.Ø
  - vulvorectal N82.4
    - congenital Q52.79
- **Fit** R56.9
  - epileptic — *see* Epilepsy
  - fainting R55
  - hysterical F44.5
  - newborn P9Ø
- **Fitting** (and adjustment) (of)
  - artificial
    - arm — *see* Admission, adjustment, artificial, arm
    - breast Z44.3
    - eye Z44.2
    - leg — *see* Admission, adjustment, artificial, leg
  - automatic implantable cardiac defibrillator (with synchronous cardiac pacemaker) Z45.Ø2
  - brain neuropacemaker Z46.2
    - implanted Z45.42
  - cardiac defibrillator — *see* Fitting (and adjustment) (of), automatic implantable cardiac defibrillator
  - catheter, non-vascular Z46.82
  - colostomy belt Z46.89
  - contact lenses Z46.Ø
  - cystostomy device Z46.6
  - defibrillator, cardiac — *see* Fitting (and adjustment) (of), automatic implantable cardiac defibrillator
  - dentures Z46.3
  - device NOS Z46.9
    - abdominal Z46.89
    - gastrointestinal NEC Z46.59
    - implanted NEC Z45.89
    - nervous system Z46.2
      - implanted — *see* Admission, adjustment, device, implanted, nervous system
    - orthodontic Z46.4
    - orthoptic Z46.Ø
    - orthotic Z46.89
    - prosthetic (external) Z44.9
      - breast Z44.3
      - dental Z46.3
      - eye Z44.2
      - specified NEC Z44.8
    - specified NEC Z46.89
    - substitution
      - auditory Z46.2
        - implanted — *see* Admission, adjustment, device, implanted, hearing device
      - nervous system Z46.2
        - implanted — *see* Admission, adjustment, device, implanted, nervous system
      - visual Z46.2
        - implanted Z45.31
    - urinary Z46.6
  - gastric lap band Z46.51
  - gastrointestinal appliance NEC Z46.59
  - glasses (reading) Z46.Ø
  - hearing aid Z46.1
  - ileostomy device Z46.89
  - insulin pump Z46.81
  - intestinal appliance NEC Z46.89
  - myringotomy device (stent) (tube) Z45.82

- **Foreign body**— *continued*
  - accidentally left following a procedure T81.5Ø9
    - aspiration T81.5Ø6
      - resulting in
        - adhesions T81.516
        - obstruction T81.526
        - perforation T81.536
        - specified complication NEC T81.596
    - cardiac catheterization T81.5Ø5
      - resulting in
        - acute reaction T81.6Ø
          - aseptic peritonitis T81.61
          - specified NEC T81.69
        - adhesions T81.515
        - obstruction T81.525
        - perforation T81.535
        - specified complication NEC T81.595
    - endoscopy T81.5Ø4
      - resulting in
        - adhesions T81.514
        - obstruction T81.524
        - perforation T81.534
        - specified complication NEC T81.594
    - immunization T81.5Ø3
      - resulting in
        - adhesions T81.513
        - obstruction T81.523
        - perforation T81.533
        - specified complication NEC T81.593
    - infusion T81.5Ø1
      - resulting in
        - adhesions T81.511
        - obstruction T81.521
        - perforation T81.531
        - specified complication NEC T81.591
    - injection T81.5Ø3
      - resulting in
        - adhesions T81.513
        - obstruction T81.523
        - perforation T81.533
        - specified complication NEC T81.593
    - kidney dialysis T81.5Ø2
      - resulting in
        - adhesions T81.512
        - obstruction T81.522
        - perforation T81.532
        - specified complication NEC T81.592
    - packing removal T81.5Ø7
      - resulting in
        - acute reaction T81.6Ø
          - aseptic peritonitis T81.61
          - specified NEC T81.69
        - adhesions T81.517
        - obstruction T81.527
        - perforation T81.537
        - specified complication NEC T81.597
    - puncture T81.5Ø6
      - resulting in
        - adhesions T81.516
        - obstruction T81.526
        - perforation T81.536
        - specified complication NEC T81.596
    - specified procedure NEC T81.5Ø8
      - resulting in
        - acute reaction T81.6Ø
          - aseptic peritonitis T81.61
          - specified NEC T81.69
        - adhesions T81.518
        - obstruction T81.528
        - perforation T81.538
        - specified complication NEC T81.598
    - surgical operation T81.5ØØ
      - resulting in
        - acute reaction T81.6Ø
          - aseptic peritonitis T81.61
          - specified NEC T81.69
        - adhesions T81.51Ø
        - obstruction T81.52Ø
        - perforation T81.53Ø
        - specified complication NEC T81.59Ø
    - transfusion T81.5Ø1
      - resulting in
        - adhesions T81.511

- **Foreign body**— *continued*
  - accidentally left following a procedure— *continued*
    - transfusion— *continued*
      - resulting in— *continued*
        - obstruction T81.521
        - perforation T81.531
        - specified complication NEC T81.591
    - causing
      - acute reaction T81.6Ø
        - aseptic peritonitis T81.61
        - specified complication NEC T81.69
      - adhesions T81.519
      - aseptic peritonitis T81.61
      - obstruction T81.529
      - perforation T81.539
      - specified complication NEC T81.599
  - alimentary tract T18.9
    - anus T18.5
    - colon T18.4
    - esophagus — *see* Foreign body, esophagus
    - mouth T18.Ø
    - multiple sites T18.8
    - rectosigmoid (junction) T18.5
    - rectum T18.5
    - small intestine T18.3
    - specified site NEC T18.8
    - stomach T18.2
  - anterior chamber (eye) SØ5.5-
  - auditory canal — *see* Foreign body, entering through orifice, ear
  - bronchus T17.5Ø8
    - causing
      - asphyxiation T17.5ØØ
        - food (bone) (seed) T17.52Ø
        - gastric contents (vomitus) T17.51Ø
        - specified type NEC T17.59Ø
      - injury NEC T17.5Ø8
        - food (bone) (seed) T17.528
        - gastric contents (vomitus) T17.518
        - specified type NEC T17.598
  - canthus — *see* Foreign body, conjunctival sac
  - ciliary body (eye) SØ5.5-
  - conjunctival sac T15.1-
  - cornea T15.Ø-
  - entering through orifice
    - accessory sinus T17.Ø
    - alimentary canal T18.9
      - multiple parts T18.8
      - specified part NEC T18.8
    - alveolar process T18.Ø
    - antrum (Highmore's) T17.Ø
    - anus T18.5
    - appendix T18.4
    - auditory canal — *see* Foreign body, entering through orifice, ear
    - auricle — *see* Foreign body, entering through orifice, ear
    - bladder T19.1
    - bronchioles — *see* Foreign body, respiratory tract, specified site NEC
    - bronchus (main) — *see* Foreign body, bronchus
    - buccal cavity T18.Ø
    - canthus (inner) — *see* Foreign body, conjunctival sac
    - cecum T18.4
    - cervix (canal) (uteri) T19.3
    - colon T18.4
    - conjunctival sac — *see* Foreign body, conjunctival sac
    - cornea — *see* Foreign body, cornea
    - digestive organ or tract NOS T18.9
      - multiple parts T18.8
      - specified part NEC T18.8
    - duodenum T18.3
    - ear (external) T16.-
    - esophagus — *see* Foreign body, esophagus
    - eye (external) NOS T15.9-
      - conjunctival sac — *see* Foreign body, conjunctival sac
      - cornea — *see* Foreign body, cornea
      - specified part NEC T15.8-

- **Foreign body**— *continued*
  - entering through orifice— *continued*
    - eyeball (*see also* Foreign body, entering through orifice, eye, specified part NEC)
      - with penetrating wound — *see* Puncture, eyeball
    - eyelid (*see also* Foreign body, conjunctival sac)
      - with
        - laceration — *see* Laceration, eyelid, with foreign body
        - puncture — *see* Puncture, eyelid, with foreign body
        - superficial injury — *see* Foreign body, superficial, eyelid
    - fragment — *see* Retained, foreign body fragments (type of)
    - gastrointestinal tract T18.9
      - multiple parts T18.8
      - specified part NEC T18.8
    - genitourinary tract T19.9
      - multiple parts T19.8
      - specified part NEC T19.8
    - globe — *see* Foreign body, entering through orifice, eyeball
    - gum T18.Ø
    - Highmore's antrum T17.Ø
    - hypopharynx — *see* Foreign body, pharynx
    - ileum T18.3
    - intestine (small) T18.3
      - large T18.4
    - lacrimal apparatus (punctum) — *see* Foreign body, entering through orifice, eye, specified part NEC
    - large intestine T18.4
    - larynx — *see* Foreign body, larynx
    - lung — *see* Foreign body, respiratory tract, specified site NEC
    - maxillary sinus T17.Ø
    - mouth T18.Ø
    - nasal sinus T17.Ø
    - nasopharynx — *see* Foreign body, pharynx
    - nose (passage) T17.1
    - nostril T17.1
    - oral cavity T18.Ø
    - palate T18.Ø
    - penis T19.4
    - pharynx — *see* Foreign body, pharynx
    - piriform sinus — *see* Foreign body, pharynx
    - rectosigmoid (junction) T18.5
    - rectum T18.5
    - respiratory tract — *see* Foreign body, respiratory tract
    - sinus (accessory) (frontal) (maxillary) (nasal) T17.Ø
      - piriform — *see* Foreign body, pharynx
    - small intestine T18.3
    - stomach T18.2
    - suffocation by — *see* Foreign body, by site
    - tear ducts or glands — *see* Foreign body, entering through orifice, eye, specified part NEC
    - throat — *see* Foreign body, pharynx
    - tongue T18.Ø
    - tonsil, tonsillar (fossa) — *see* Foreign body, pharynx
    - trachea — *see* Foreign body, trachea
    - ureter T19.8
    - urethra T19.Ø
    - uterus (any part) T19.3
    - vagina T19.2
    - vulva T19.2
  - esophagus T18.1Ø8
    - causing
      - injury NEC T18.1Ø8
        - food (bone) (seed) T18.128
        - gastric contents (vomitus) T18.118
        - specified type NEC T18.198
      - tracheal compression T18.1ØØ
        - food (bone) (seed) T18.12Ø
        - gastric contents (vomitus) T18.11Ø
        - specified type NEC T18.19Ø
- felling of, in throat RØ9.89

Foreign body— *continued*
- genitourinary tract T19.9
  - bladder T19.1
  - multiple parts T19.8
  - penis T19.4
  - specified site NEC T19.8
  - urethra T19.Ø
  - uterus T19.3
    - IUD Z97.5
  - vagina T19.2
    - contraceptive device Z97.5
  - vulva T19.2
- granuloma (old) (soft tissue) (*see also* Granuloma, foreign body)
  - skin L92.3
- in
  - laceration — *see* Laceration, by site, with foreign body
  - puncture wound — *see* Puncture, by site, with foreign body
  - soft tissue (residual) M79.5
- inadvertently left in operation wound — *see* Foreign body, accidentally left during a procedure
- ingestion, ingested NOS T18.9
- inhalation or inspiration — *see* Foreign body, by site
- internal organ, not entering through a natural orifice—code as specific injury with foreign body
- intraocular SØ5.5-
  - old, retained (nonmagnetic) H44.7Ø-
    - anterior chamber H44.71-
    - ciliary body H44.72-
    - iris H44.72-
    - lens H44.73-
    - magnetic H44.6Ø-
      - anterior chamber H44.61-
      - ciliary body H44.62-
      - iris H44.62-
      - lens H44.63-
      - posterior wall H44.64-
      - specified site NEC H44.69-
      - vitreous body H44.65-
    - posterior wall H44.74-
    - specified site NEC H44.79-
    - vitreous body H44.75-
- iris — *see* Foreign body, intraocular
- lacrimal punctum — *see* Foreign body, entering through orifice, eye, specified part NEC
- larynx T17.3Ø8
  - causing
    - asphyxiation T17.3ØØ
      - food (bone) (seed) T17.32Ø
      - gastric contents (vomitus) T17.31Ø
      - specified type NEC T17.39Ø
    - injury NEC T17.3Ø8
      - food (bone) (seed) T17.328
      - gastric contents (vomitus) T17.318
      - specified type NEC T17.398
- lens — *see* Foreign body, intraocular
- ocular muscle SØ5.4-
  - old, retained — *see* Foreign body, orbit, old
- old or residual
  - soft tissue (residual) M79.5
- operation wound, left accidentally — *see* Foreign body, accidentally left during a procedure
- orbit SØ5.4-
  - old, retained HØ5.5-
- pharynx T17.2Ø8
  - causing
    - asphyxiation T17.2ØØ
      - food (bone) (seed) T17.22Ø
      - gastric contents (vomitus) T17.21Ø
      - specified type NEC T17.29Ø
    - injury NEC T17.2Ø8
      - food (bone) (seed) T17.228
      - gastric contents (vomitus) T17.218
      - specified type NEC T17.298
- respiratory tract T17.9Ø8
  - bronchioles — *see* Foreign body, respiratory tract, specified site NEC
  - bronchus — *see* Foreign body, bronchus
  - causing

Foreign body— *continued*
- respiratory tract— *continued*
  - causing— *continued*
    - asphyxiation T17.9ØØ
      - food (bone) (seed) T17.92Ø
      - gastric contents (vomitus) T17.91Ø
      - specified type NEC T17.99Ø
    - injury NEC T17.9Ø8
      - food (bone) (seed) T17.928
      - gastric contents (vomitus) T17.918
      - specified type NEC T17.998
  - larynx — *see* Foreign body, larynx
  - lung — *see* Foreign body, respiratory tract, specified site NEC
  - multiple parts — *see* Foreign body, respiratory tract, specified site NEC
  - nasal sinus T17.Ø
  - nasopharynx — *see* Foreign body, pharynx
  - nose T17.1
  - nostril T17.1
  - pharynx — *see* Foreign body, pharynx
  - specified site NEC T17.8Ø8
    - causing
      - asphyxiation T17.8ØØ
        - food (bone) (seed) T17.82Ø
        - gastric contents (vomitus) T17.81Ø
        - specified type NEC T17.89Ø
      - injury NEC T17.8Ø8
        - food (bone) (seed) T17.828
        - gastric contents (vomitus) T17.818
        - specified type NEC T17.898
  - throat — *see* Foreign body, pharynx
  - trachea — *see* Foreign body, trachea
- retained (old) (nonmagnetic) (in)
  - anterior chamber (eye) — *see* Foreign body, intraocular, old, retained, anterior chamber
    - magnetic — *see* Foreign body, intraocular, old, retained, magnetic, anterior chamber
  - ciliary body — *see* Foreign body, intraocular, old, retained, ciliary body
    - magnetic — *see* Foreign body, intraocular, old, retained, magnetic, ciliary body
  - eyelid HØ2.819
    - left HØ2.816
      - lower HØ2.815
      - upper HØ2.814
    - right HØ2.813
      - lower HØ2.812
      - upper HØ2.811
  - fragments — see Retained, foreign body fragments (type of)
  - globe — *see* Foreign body, intraocular, old, retained
    - magnetic — *see* Foreign body, intraocular, old, retained, magnetic
  - intraocular — *see* Foreign body, intraocular, old, retained
    - magnetic — *see* Foreign body, intraocular, old, retained, magnetic
  - iris — *see* Foreign body, intraocular, old, retained, iris
    - magnetic — *see* Foreign body, intraocular, old, retained, magnetic, iris
  - lens — *see* Foreign body, intraocular, old, retained, lens
    - magnetic — *see* Foreign body, intraocular, old, retained, magnetic, lens
  - muscle — *see* Foreign body, retained, soft tissue
  - orbit — *see* Foreign body, orbit, old
  - posterior wall of globe — *see* Foreign body, intraocular, old, retained, posterior wall
    - magnetic — *see* Foreign body, intraocular, old, retained, magnetic, posterior wall
  - retrobulbar — *see* Foreign body, orbit, old, retrobulbar
  - soft tissue M79.5
  - vitreous — *see* Foreign body, intraocular, old, retained, vitreous body
    - magnetic — *see* Foreign body, intraocular, old, retained, magnetic, vitreous body
- retina SØ5.5-

Foreign body— *continued*
- superficial, without open wound
  - abdomen, abdominal (wall) S3Ø.851
  - alveolar process SØØ.552
  - ankle S9Ø.55-
  - antecubital space — *see* Foreign body, superficial, forearm
  - anus S3Ø.857
  - arm (upper) S4Ø.85-
  - auditory canal — *see* Foreign body, superficial, ear
  - auricle — *see* Foreign body, superficial, ear
  - axilla — *see* Foreign body, superficial, arm
  - back, lower S3Ø.85Ø
  - breast S2Ø.15-
  - brow SØØ.85
  - buttock S3Ø.85Ø
  - calf — *see* Foreign body, superficial, leg
  - canthus — *see* Foreign body, superficial, eyelid
  - cheek SØØ.85
    - internal SØØ.552
  - chest wall — *see* Foreign body, superficial, thorax
  - chin SØØ.85
  - clitoris S3Ø.854
  - costal region — *see* Foreign body, superficial, thorax
  - digit(s)
    - hand — *see* Foreign body, superficial, finger
    - foot — *see* Foreign body, superficial, toe
  - ear SØØ.45-
  - elbow S5Ø.35-
  - epididymis S3Ø.853
  - epigastric region S3Ø.851
  - epiglottis S1Ø.15
  - esophagus, cervical S1Ø.15
  - eyebrow — *see* Foreign body, superficial, eyelid
  - eyelid SØØ.25-
  - face SØØ.85
  - finger(s) S6Ø.459
    - index S6Ø.45-
    - little S6Ø.45-
    - middle S6Ø.45-
    - ring S6Ø.45-
  - flank S3Ø.851
  - foot (except toe(s) alone) S9Ø.85-
    - toe — *see* Foreign body, superficial, toe
  - forearm S5Ø.85-
    - elbow only — *see* Foreign body, superficial, elbow
  - forehead SØØ.85
  - genital organs, external
    - female S3Ø.856
    - male S3Ø.855
  - groin S3Ø.851
  - gum SØØ.552
  - hand S6Ø.55-
  - head SØØ.95
    - ear — *see* Foreign body, superficial, ear
    - eyelid — *see* Foreign body, superficial, eyelid
    - lip SØØ.551
    - nose SØØ.35
    - oral cavity SØØ.552
    - scalp SØØ.Ø5
    - specified site NEC SØØ.85
  - heel — *see* Foreign body, superficial, foot
  - hip S7Ø.25-
  - inguinal region S3Ø.851
  - interscapular region S2Ø.459
  - jaw SØØ.85
  - knee S8Ø.25-
  - labium (majus) (minus) S3Ø.854
  - larynx S1Ø.15
  - leg (lower) S8Ø.85-
    - knee — *see* Foreign body, superficial, knee
    - upper — *see* Foreign body, superficial, thigh
  - lip SØØ.551
  - lower back S3Ø.85Ø
  - lumbar region S3Ø.85Ø
  - malar region SØØ.85
  - mammary — *see* Foreign body, superficial, breast
  - mastoid region SØØ.85
  - mouth SØØ.552

Fracture, traumatic — *continued*
  acetabulum — *continued*
    wall
      anterior (displaced) S32.41-
        nondisplaced S32.41-
      medial (displaced) S32.47-
        nondisplaced S32.47-
      posterior (displaced) S32.42-
        with associated transverse fracture (displaced) S32.46-
          nondisplaced S32.46-
        nondisplaced S32.42-
  acromion — *see* Fracture, scapula, acromial process
  ankle S82.899
    bimalleolar (displaced) S82.84-
      nondisplaced S82.84-
    lateral malleolus only (displaced) S82.6-
      nondisplaced S82.6-
    medial malleolus (displaced) S82.5-
      associated with Maisonneuve's fracture — *see* Fracture, Maisonneuve's
      nondisplaced S82.5-
    talus — *see* Fracture, tarsal, talus
    trimalleolar (displaced) S82.85-
      nondisplaced S82.85-
  arm (upper) (*see also* Fracture, humerus, shaft)
    humerus — *see* Fracture, humerus
    radius — *see* Fracture, radius
    ulna — *see* Fracture, ulna
  astragalus — *see* Fracture, tarsal, talus
  atlas — *see* Fracture, neck, cervical vertebra, first
  axis — *see* Fracture, neck, cervical vertebra, second
  back — *see* Fracture, vertebra
  Barton's — *see* Barton's fracture
  base of skull — *see* Fracture, skull, base
  basicervical (basal) (femoral) S72.Ø
  Bennett's — *see* Bennett's fracture
  bimalleolar — *see* Fracture, ankle, bimalleolar
  blow-out SØ2.3
  bone NEC T14.8
    birth injury P13.9
    following insertion of orthopedic implant, joint prosthesis or bone plate — *see* Fracture, following insertion of orthopedic implant, joint prosthesis or bone plate
    in (due to) neoplastic disease NEC — *see* Fracture, pathological, due to, neoplastic disease
    pathological (cause unknown) — *see* Fracture, pathological
  breast bone — *see* Fracture, sternum
  bucket handle (semilunar cartilage) — *see* Tear, meniscus
  burst — *see* Fracture, traumatic, tarsal, by site
  calcaneus — *see* Fracture, tarsal, calcaneus
  carpal bone(s) S62.1Ø-
    capitate (displaced) S62.13-
      nondisplaced S62.13-
    cuneiform — *see* Fracture, carpal bone, triquetrum
    hamate (body) (displaced) S62.143
      hook process (displaced) S62.15-
        nondisplaced S62.15-
      nondisplaced S62.14-
    larger multangular — *see* Fracture, carpal bones, trapezium
    lunate (displaced) S62.12-
      nondisplaced S62.12-
    navicular S62.ØØ-
      distal pole (displaced) S62.Ø1-
        nondisplaced S62.Ø1-
      middle third (displaced) S62.Ø2-
        nondisplaced S62.Ø2-
      proximal third (displaced) S62.Ø3-
        nondisplaced S62.Ø3-
      volar tuberosity — *see* Fracture, carpal bones, navicular, distal pole
    os magnum — *see* Fracture, carpal bones, capitate
    pisiform (displaced) S62.16-
      nondisplaced S62.16-
    semilunar — *see* Fracture, carpal bones, lunate

Fracture, traumatic — *continued*
  carpal bone(s)— *continued*
    smaller multangular — *see* Fracture, carpal bones, trapezoid
    trapezium (displaced) S62.17-
      nondisplaced S62.17-
    trapezoid (displaced) S62.18-
      nondisplaced S62.18-
    triquetrum (displaced) S62.11-
      nondisplaced S62.11-
    unciform — *see* Fracture, carpal bones, hamate
  cervical — *see* Fracture, vertebra, cervical
  clavicle S42.ØØ-
    acromial end (displaced) S42.Ø3-
      nondisplaced S42.Ø3-
    birth injury P13.4
    lateral end — *see* Fracture, clavicle, acromial end
    shaft (displaced) S42.Ø2-
      nondisplaced S42.Ø2-
    sternal end (anterior) (displaced) S42.Ø1-
      nondisplaced S42.Ø1-
      posterior S42.Ø1-
  coccyx S32.2
  collapsed — *see* Collapse, vertebra
  collar bone — *see* Fracture, clavicle
  Colles' — *see* Colles' fracture
  compression, not due to trauma — *see* Collapse, vertebra
  coronoid process — *see* Fracture, ulna, upper end, coronoid process
  corpus cavernosum penis S39.84Ø
  costochondral cartilage S23.41
  costochondral, costosternal junction — *see* Fracture, rib
  cranium — *see* Fracture, skull
  cricoid cartilage S12.8
  cuboid (ankle) — *see* Fracture, tarsal, cuboid
  cuneiform
    foot — *see* Fracture, tarsal, cuneiform
    wrist — *see* Fracture, carpal, triquetrum
  delayed union — *see* Delay, union, fracture
  dental restorative material KØ8.539
    with loss of material KØ8.531
    without loss of material KØ8.53Ø
  due to
    birth injury — *see* Birth, injury, fracture
    osteoporosis — *see* Osteoporosis, with fracture
  Dupuytren's — *see* Fracture, ankle, lateral malleolus
  elbow S42.4Ø-
  ethmoid (bone) (sinus) — *see* Fracture, skull, base
  face bone SØ2.92
  fatigue (*see also* Fracture, stress)
    vertebra M48.4Ø
      cervical region M48.42
      cervicothoracic region M48.43
      lumbar region M48.46
      lumbosacral region M48.47
      occipito-atlanto-axial region M48.41
      sacrococcygeal region M48.48
      thoracic region M48.44
      thoracolumbar region M48.45
  femur, femoral S72.9-
    basicervical (basal) S72.Ø
    birth injury P13.2
    capital epiphyseal S79.Ø1-
    condyles, epicondyles — *see* Fracture, femur, lower end
    distal end — *see* Fracture, femur, lower end
    epiphysis
      head — *see* Fracture, femur, upper end, epiphysis
      lower — *see* Fracture, femur, lower end, epiphysis
      upper — *see* Fracture, femur, upper end, epiphysis
    following insertion of implant, prosthesis or plate M96.66-
    head — *see* Fracture, femur, upper end, head
    intertrochanteric — *see* Fracture, femur, trochanteric
    intratrochanteric — *see* Fracture, femur, trochanteric

Fracture, traumatic — *continued*
  femur, femoral— *continued*
    lower end S72.4Ø-
      condyle (displaced) S72.41-
        lateral (displaced) S72.42-
          nondisplaced S72.42-
        medial (displaced) S72.43-
          nondisplaced S72.43-
        nondisplaced S72.41-
      epiphysis (displaced) S72.44-
        nondisplaced S72.44-
      physeal S79.1Ø-
        Salter-Harris
          Type I S79.11-
          Type II S79.12-
          Type III S79.13-
          Type IV S79.14-
        specified NEC S79.19-
      specified NEC S72.49-
      supracondylar (displaced) S72.45-
        with intracondylar extension (displaced) S72.46-
          nondisplaced S72.46-
        nondisplaced S72.45-
      torus S72.47-
    neck — *see* Fracture, femur, upper end, neck
    pertrochanteric — *see* Fracture, femur, trochanteric
    shaft (lower third) (middle third) (upper third) S72.3Ø-
      comminuted (displaced) S72.35-
        nondisplaced S72.35-
      oblique (displaced) S72.33-
        nondisplaced S72.33-
      segmental (displaced) S72.36-
        nondisplaced S72.36-
      specified NEC S72.39-
      spiral (displaced) S72.34-
        nondisplaced S72.34-
      transverse (displaced) S72.32-
        nondisplaced S72.32-
    specified site NEC — *see* subcategory S72.8
    subcapital (displaced) S72.Ø1-
    subtrochanteric (region) (section) (displaced) S72.2-
      nondisplaced S72.2-
    transcervical — *see* Fracture, femur, upper end, neck
    transtrochanteric — *see* Fracture, femur, trochanteric
    trochanteric S72.1Ø-
      apophyseal (displaced) S72.14-
        nondisplaced S72.14-
      greater trochanter (displaced) S72.11-
        nondisplaced S72.11-
      intertrochanteric (displaced) S72.13-
        nondisplaced S72.13-
      lesser trochanter (displaced) S72.12-
        nondisplaced S72.12-
    upper end S72.ØØ-
      apophyseal (displaced) S72.13-
        nondisplaced S72.13-
      cervicotrochanteric — *see* Fracture, femur, upper end, neck, base
      epiphysis (displaced) S72.Ø2-
        nondisplaced S72.Ø2-
      head S72.Ø5-
        articular (displaced) S72.Ø6-
          nondisplaced S72.Ø6-
        specified NEC S72.Ø9-
      intertrochanteric (displaced) S72.14-
        nondisplaced S72.14-
      intracapsular S72.Ø1-
      midcervical (displaced) S72.Ø3-
        nondisplaced S72.Ø3-
      neck S72.ØØ-
        base (displaced) S72.Ø4-
          nondisplaced S72.Ø4-
        specified NEC S72.Ø9-
      pertrochanteric — *see* Fracture, femur, upper end, trochanteric
      physeal S79.ØØ-
        Salter-Harris type I S79.Ø1-

Fracture, traumatic — *continued*
- femur, femoral— *continued*
  - upper end— *continued*
    - physeal— *continued-*
      - specified NEC S79.Ø9-
    - subcapital (displaced) S72.Ø1-
    - subtrochanteric (displaced) S72.2-
      - nondisplaced S72.2-
    - transcervical — *see* Fracture, femur, upper end, midcervical
    - trochanteric S72.1Ø-
      - greater (displaced) S72.11-
        - nondisplaced S72.11-
      - lesser (displaced) S72.12-
        - nondisplaced S72.12-
- fibula (shaft) (styloid) S82.4Ø-
  - comminuted (displaced) S82.45-
    - nondisplaced S82.45-
  - following insertion of implant, prosthesis or plate M96.67-
  - involving ankle or malleolus — *see* Fracture, fibula, lateral malleolus
  - lateral malleolus (displaced) S82.6-
    - nondisplaced S82.6-
  - lower end
    - physeal S89.3Ø-
      - Salter-Harris
        - Type I S89.31-
        - Type II S89.32-
      - specified NEC S89.39-
    - specified NEC S82.83-
    - torus S82.82-
  - oblique (displaced) S82.43-
    - nondisplaced S82.43-
  - segmental (displaced) S82.46-
    - nondisplaced S82.46-
  - specified NEC S82.49-
  - spiral (displaced) S82.44-
    - nondisplaced S82.44-
  - transverse (displaced) S82.42-
    - nondisplaced S82.42-
  - upper end
    - physeal S89.2Ø-
      - Salter-Harris
        - Type I S89.21-
        - Type II S89.22-
      - specified NEC S89.29-
    - specified NEC S82.83-
    - torus S82.81-
- finger (except thumb) S62.6Ø-
  - distal phalanx (displaced) S62.63-
    - nondisplaced S62.66-
  - index S62.6Ø-
    - distal phalanx (displaced) S62.63-
      - nondisplaced S62.66-
    - medial phalanx (displaced) S62.62-
      - nondisplaced S62.65-
    - proximal phalanx (displaced) S62.61-
      - nondisplaced S62.64-
  - little S62.6Ø-
    - distal phalanx (displaced) S62.63-
      - nondisplaced S62.66-
    - medial phalanx (displaced) S62.62-
      - nondisplaced S62.65-
    - proximal phalanx (displaced) S62.61-
      - nondisplaced S62.64-
  - medial phalanx (displaced) S62.62-
    - nondisplaced S62.65-
  - middle S62.6Ø-
    - distal phalanx (displaced) S62.63-
      - nondisplaced S62.66-
    - medial phalanx (displaced) S62.62-
      - nondisplaced S62.65-
    - proximal phalanx (displaced) S62.61-
      - nondisplaced S62.64-
  - proximal phalanx (displaced) S62.61-
    - nondisplaced S62.64-
  - ring S62.6Ø-
    - distal phalanx (displaced) S62.63-
      - nondisplaced S62.66-
    - medial phalanx (displaced) S62.62-
      - nondisplaced S62.65-

Fracture, traumatic — *continued*
- finger— *continued*
  - ring— *continued*
    - proximal phalanx (displaced) S62.61-
      - nondisplaced S62.64-
  - thumb — *see* Fracture, thumb
- following insertion (intraoperative) (postoperative) of orthopedic implant, joint prosthesis or bone plate M96.69
  - femur M96.66-
  - fibula M96.67-
  - humerus M96.62-
  - pelvis M96.65
  - radius M96.63-
  - specified bone NEC M96.69
  - tibia M96.67-
  - ulna M96.63-
- foot S92.9Ø-
  - astragalus — *see* Fracture, tarsal, talus
  - calcaneus — *see* Fracture, tarsal, calcaneus
  - cuboid — *see* Fracture, tarsal, cuboid
  - cuneiform — *see* Fracture, tarsal, cuneiform
  - metatarsal — *see* Fracture, metatarsal
  - navicular — *see* Fracture, tarsal, navicular
  - talus — *see* Fracture, tarsal, talus
  - tarsal — *see* Fracture, tarsal
  - toe — *see* Fracture, toe
- forearm S52.9-
  - radius — *see* Fracture, radius
  - ulna — *see* Fracture, ulna
- fossa (anterior) (middle) (posterior) SØ2.19
- frontal (bone) (skull) SØ2.Ø
  - sinus SØ2.19
- glenoid (cavity) (scapula) — *see* Fracture, scapula, glenoid cavity
- greenstick — *see* Fracture, by site
- hallux — *see* Fracture, toe, great
- hand S62.9-
  - carpal — *see* Fracture, carpal bone
  - finger (except thumb) — *see* Fracture, finger
  - metacarpal — *see* Fracture, metacarpal
  - navicular (scaphoid) (hand) — *see* Fracture, carpal bone, navicular
  - thumb — *see* Fracture, thumb
- healed or old
  - with complications — code by Nature of the complication
- heel bone — *see* Fracture, tarsal, calcaneus
- Hill-Sachs S42.29-
- hip — *see* Fracture, femur, neck
- humerus S42.3Ø-
  - anatomical neck — seeFracture, humerus, upper end
  - articular process — *see* Fracture, humerus, lower end
  - capitellum — *see* Fracture, humerus, lower end, condyle, lateral
  - distal end — *see* Fracture, humerus, lower end
  - epiphysis
    - lower — *see* Fracture, humerus, lower end, physeal
    - upper — *see* Fracture, humerus, upper end, physeal
  - external condyle — *see* Fracture, humerus, lower end, condyle, lateral
  - following insertion of implant, prosthesis or plate M96.62-
  - great tuberosity — *see* Fracture, humerus, upper end, greater tuberosity
  - intercondylar — *see* Fracture, humerus, lower end
  - internal epicondyle — *see* Fracture, humerus, lower end, epicondyle, medial
  - lesser tuberosity — *see* Fracture, humerus, upper end, lesser tuberosity
  - lower end S42.4Ø-
    - condyle
      - lateral (displaced) S42.45-
        - nondisplaced S42.45-
      - medial (displaced) S42.46-
        - nondisplaced S42.46-
    - epicondyle
      - lateral (displaced) S42.43-

Fracture, traumatic — *continued*
- humerus— *continued*
  - lower end— *continued*
    - epicondyle— *continued*
      - lateral— *continued*
        - nondisplaced S42.43-
      - medial (displaced) S42.44-
        - incarcerated S42.44-
        - nondisplaced S42.44-
    - physeal S49.1Ø-
      - Salter-Harris
        - Type I S49.11-
        - Type II S49.12-
        - Type III S49.13-
        - Type IV S49.14-
      - specified NEC S49.19-
    - specified NEC (displaced) S42.49-
      - nondisplaced S42.49-
    - supracondylar (simple) (displaced) S42.41-
      - comminuted (displaced) S42.42-
        - nondisplaced S42.42-
      - nondisplaced S42.41-
    - torus S42.48-
    - transcondylar (displaced) S42.47-
      - nondisplaced S42.47-
  - proximal end — *see* Fracture, humerus, upper end
  - shaft S42.3Ø-
    - comminuted (displaced) S42.35-
      - nondisplaced S42.35-
    - greenstick S42.31-
    - oblique (displaced) S42.33-
      - nondisplaced S42.33-
    - segmental (displaced) S42.36-
      - nondisplaced S42.36-
    - specified NEC S42.39-
    - spiral (displaced) S42.34-
      - nondisplaced S42.34-
    - transverse (displaced) S42.32-
      - nondisplaced S42.32-
  - supracondylar — *see* Fracture, humerus, lower end
  - surgical neck — *see* Fracture, humerus, upper end, surgical neck
  - trochlea — *see* Fracture, humerus, lower end, condyle, medial
  - tuberosity — *see* Fracture, humerus, upper end
  - upper end S42.2Ø-
    - anatomical neck — *see* Fracture, humerus, upper end, specified NEC
    - articular head — *see* Fracture, humerus, upper end, specified NEC
    - epiphysis — *see* Fracture, humerus, upper end, physeal
    - greater tuberosity (displaced) S42.25-
      - nondisplaced S42.25-
    - lesser tuberosity (displaced) S42.26-
      - nondisplaced S42.26-
    - physeal S49.ØØ-
      - Salter-Harris
        - Type I S49.Ø1-
        - Type II S49.Ø2-
        - Type III S49.Ø3-
        - Type IV S49.Ø4-
      - specified NEC S49.Ø9-
    - specified NEC (displaced) S42.29-
      - nondisplaced S42.29-
    - surgical neck (displaced) S42.21-
      - four-part S42.24-
      - nondisplaced S42.21-
      - three-part S42.23-
      - two-part (displaced) S42.22-
        - nondisplaced S42.22-
    - torus S42.27-
    - transepiphyseal — *see* Fracture, humerus, upper end, physeal
- hyoid bone S12.8
- ilium S32.3Ø-
  - with disruption of pelvic ring — *see* Disruption, pelvic ring
  - avulsion (displaced) S32.31-
    - nondisplaced S32.31-
  - specified NEC S32.39-

- **Fracture, traumatic** — *continued*
  - impaction, impacted—code as Fracture, by site
  - innominate bone — *see* Fracture, ilium
  - instep — *see* Fracture, foot
  - ischium S32.60-
    - with disruption of pelvic ring — *see* Disruption, pelvic ring
    - avulsion (displaced) S32.61-
      - nondisplaced S32.61-
    - specified NEC S32.69-
  - jaw (bone) (lower) — *see* Fracture, mandible
    - upper — *see* Fracture, maxilla
  - joint prosthesis — *see* Complications, joint prosthesis, mechanical, breakdown, by site
    - periprosthetic — *see* Complications, joint prosthesis, mechanical, periprosthesis, fracture, by site
  - knee cap — *see* Fracture, patella
  - larynx S12.8
  - late effects — *see* Sequelae, fracture
  - leg (lower) S82.9-
    - ankle — *see* Fracture, ankle
    - femur — *see* Fracture, femur
    - fibula — *see* Fracture, fibula
    - malleolus — *see* Fracture, ankle
    - patella — *see* Fracture, patella
    - specified site NEC S82.89-
    - tibia — *see* Fracture, tibia
  - lumbar spine — *see* Fracture, vertebra, lumbar
  - lumbosacral spine S32.9
  - Maisonneuve's (displaced) S82.86-
    - nondisplaced S82.86-
  - malar bone (*see also* Fracture, maxilla) S02.400
  - malleolus — *see* Fracture, ankle
  - malunion — *see* Fracture, by site
  - mandible (lower jaw (bone) S02.609
    - alveolous S02.67
    - angle (of jaw) S02.65
    - body, unspecified S02.600
    - condylar process S02.61
    - coronoid process S02.63
    - ramus, unspecified S02.64
    - specified site NEC S02.69
    - subcondylar process S02.62
    - symphysis S02.66
  - manubrium (sterni) S22.21
    - dissociation from sternum S22.23
  - march — *see* Fracture, traumatic, stress, by site
  - maxilla, maxillary (bone) (sinus) (superior) (upper jaw) S02.401
    - alveolus S02.42
    - inferior — *see* Fracture, mandible
    - LeFort I S02.411
    - LeFort II S02.412
    - LeFort III S02.413
  - metacarpal S62.309
    - base (displaced) S62.319
      - nondisplaced S62.349
    - fifth S62.30-
      - base (displaced) S62.31-
        - nondisplaced S62.34-
      - neck (displaced) S62.33-
        - nondisplaced S62.36-
      - shaft (displaced) S62.32-
        - nondisplaced S62.35-
      - specified NEC S62.398
    - first S62.20-
      - base NEC (displaced) S62.23-
        - nondisplaced S62.23-
      - Bennett's — *see* Bennett's fracture
      - neck (displaced) S62.25-
        - nondisplaced S62.25-
      - shaft (displaced) S62.24-
        - nondisplaced S62.24-
      - specified NEC S62.29-
    - fourth S62.30-
      - base (displaced) S62.31-
        - nondisplaced S62.34-
      - neck (displaced) S62.33-
        - nondisplaced S62.36-
      - shaft (displaced) S62.32-
        - nondisplaced S62.35-
      - specified NEC S62.39-

- **Fracture, traumatic** — *continued*
  - metacarpal— *continued*
    - neck (displaced) S62.33-
      - nondisplaced S62.36-
    - Rolando's — *see* Rolando's fracture
    - second S62.30-
      - base (displaced) S62.31-
        - nondisplaced S62.34-
      - neck (displaced) S62.33-
        - nondisplaced S62.36-
      - shaft (displaced) S62.32-
        - nondisplaced S62.35-
      - specified NEC S62.39-
    - shaft (displaced) S62.32-
      - nondisplaced S62.35-
    - third S62.30-
      - base (displaced) S62.31-
        - nondisplaced S62.34-
      - neck (displaced) S62.33-
        - nondisplaced S62.36-
      - shaft (displaced) S62.32-
        - nondisplaced S62.35-
      - specified NEC S62.39-
    - specified NEC S62.399
  - metastatic (*see also* Neoplasm) — *see* Fracture, pathological, due to, neoplastic disease
  - metatarsal bone S92.30-
    - fifth (displaced) S92.35-
      - nondisplaced S92.35-
    - first (displaced) S92.31-
      - nondisplaced S92.31-
    - fourth (displaced) S92.34-
      - nondisplaced S92.34-
    - second (displaced) S92.32-
      - nondisplaced S92.32-
    - third (displaced) S92.33-
      - nondisplaced S92.33-
  - Monteggia's — *see* Monteggia's fracture
  - multiple
    - hand (and wrist) NEC — *see* Fracture, by site
    - ribs — *see* Fracture, rib, multiple
  - nasal (bone(s)) S02.2
  - navicular (scaphoid) (foot) (*see also* Fracture, tarsal, navicular)
    - hand — *see* Fracture, carpal, navicular
  - neck S12.9
    - cervical vertebra S12.9
      - fifth (displaced) S12.400
        - nondisplaced S12.401
        - specified type NEC (displaced) S12.490
          - nondisplaced S12.491
      - first (displaced) S12.000
        - burst (stable) S12.01
          - unstable S12.02
        - lateral mass (displaced) S12.040
          - nondisplaced S12.041
        - nondisplaced S12.001
        - posterior arch (displaced) S12.030
          - nondisplaced S12.031
        - specified type NEC (displaced) S12.090
          - nondisplaced S12.091
      - fourth (displaced) S12.300
        - nondisplaced S12.301
        - specified type NEC (displaced) S12.390
          - nondisplaced S12.391
      - second (displaced) S12.100
        - nondisplaced S12.101
        - dens (anterior) (displaced) (type II) S12.110
          - nondisplaced S12.112
          - posterior S12.111
          - specified type NEC (displaced) S12.120
            - nondisplaced S12.121
        - specified type NEC (displaced) S12.190
          - nondisplaced S12.191
      - seventh (displaced) S12.600
        - nondisplaced S12.601
        - specified type NEC (displaced) S12.690
          - displaced S12.691
      - sixth (displaced) S12.500
        - nondisplaced S12.501
        - specified type NEC (displaced) S12.590
          - displaced S12.591

- **Fracture, traumatic** — *continued*
  - neck— *continued*
    - cervical vertebra— *continued*
      - third (displaced) S12.200
        - nondisplaced S12.201
        - specified type NEC (displaced) S12.290
          - displaced S12.291
    - hyoid bone S12.8
    - larynx S12.8
    - specified site NEC S12.8
    - thyroid cartilage S12.8
    - trachea S12.8
  - neoplastic NEC — *see* Fracture, pathological, due to, neoplastic disease
  - neural arch — *see* Fracture, vertebra
  - newborn — *see* Birth, injury, fracture
  - nontraumatic — *see* Fracture, pathological
  - nonunion — *see* Nonunion, fracture
  - nose, nasal (bone) (septum) S02.2
  - occiput — *see* Fracture, skull, base, occiput
  - odontoid process — *see* Fracture, neck, cervical vertebra, second
  - olecranon (process) (ulna) — *see* Fracture, ulna, upper end, olecranon process
  - orbit, orbital (bone) (region) S02.8
    - floor (blow-out) S02.3
    - roof S02.19
  - os
    - calcis — *see* Fracture, tarsal, calcaneus
    - magnum — *see* Fracture, carpal, capitate
    - pubis — *see* Fracture, pubis
  - palate S02.8
  - parietal bone (skull) S02.0
  - patella S82.00-
    - comminuted (displaced) S82.04-
      - nondisplaced S82.04-
    - longitudinal (displaced) S82.02-
      - nondisplaced S82.02-
    - osteochondral (displaced) S82.01-
      - nondisplaced S82.01-
    - specified NEC S82.09-
    - transverse (displaced) S82.03-
      - nondisplaced S82.03-
  - pedicle (of vertebral arch) — *see* Fracture, vertebra
  - pelvis, pelvic (bone) S32.9
    - acetabulum — *see* Fracture, acetabulum
    - circle — *see* Disruption, pelvic ring
    - following insertion of implant, prosthesis or plate M96.65
    - ilium — *see* Fracture, ilium
    - ischium — *see* Fracture, ischium
    - multiple
      - with disruption of pelvic ring (circle) — *see* Disruption, pelvic ring
      - without disruption of pelvic ring (circle) S32.82
    - pubis — *see* Fracture, pubis
    - specified site NEC S32.89
    - sacrum — *see* Fracture, sacrum
  - phalanx
    - foot — *see* Fracture, toe
    - hand — *see* Fracture, finger
  - pisiform — *see* Fracture, carpal, pisiform
  - pond — *see* Fracture, skull
  - prosthetic device, internal — *see* Complications, prosthetic device, by site, mechanical
  - pubis S32.50-
    - with disruption of pelvic ring — *see* Disruption, pelvic ring
    - specified site NEC S32.59-
    - superior rim S32.51-
  - radius S52.9-
    - distal end — *see* Fracture, radius, lower end
    - following insertion of implant, prosthesis or plate M96.63-
    - head — *see* Fracture, radius, upper end, head
    - lower end S52.50-
      - Barton's — *see* Barton's fracture
      - Colles' — *see* Colles' fracture
      - extraarticular NEC S52.55-
      - intraarticular NEC S52.57-
      - physeal S59.20-

- **Fracture, traumatic** — *continued*
  - thorax— *continued*
    - vertebra— *continued*
      - second S22.029
        - burst (stable) S22.021
          - unstable S22.022
        - specified type NEC S22.028
        - wedge compression S22.020
      - seventh S22.069
        - burst (stable) S22.061
          - unstable S22.062
        - specified type NEC S22.068
        - wedge compression S22.060
      - sixth S22.059
        - burst (stable) S22.051
          - unstable S22.052
        - specified type NEC S22.058
        - wedge compression S22.050
      - specified type NEC S22.008
      - tenth S22.079
        - burst (stable) S22.071
          - unstable S22.072
        - specified type NEC S22.078
        - wedge compression S22.070
      - third S22.039
        - burst (stable) S22.031
          - unstable S22.032
        - specified type NEC S22.038
        - wedge compression S22.030
      - twelfth S22.089
        - burst (stable) S22.081
          - unstable S22.082
        - specified type NEC S22.088
        - wedge compression S22.080
      - wedge compression S22.000
  - thumb S62.50-
    - distal phalanx (displaced) S62.52-
      - nondisplaced S62.52-
    - proximal phalanx (displaced) S62.51-
      - nondisplaced S62.51-
  - thyroid cartilage S12.8
  - tibia (shaft) S82.20-
    - comminuted (displaced) S82.25-
      - nondisplaced S82.25-
    - condyles — *see* Fracture, tibia, upper end
    - distal end — *see* Fracture, tibia, lower end
    - epiphysis
      - lower — *see* Fracture, tibia, lower end
      - upper — *see* Fracture, tibia, upper end
    - following insertion of implant, prosthesis or plate M96.67-
    - head (involving knee joint) — *see* Fracture, tibia, upper end
    - intercondyloid eminence — seeFracture, tibia, upper end
    - involving ankle or malleolus — *see* Fracture, ankle, medial malleolus
    - lower end S82.30-
      - physeal S89.10-
        - Salter-Harris
          - Type I S89.11-
          - Type II S89.12-
          - Type III S89.13-
          - Type IV S89.14-
        - specified NEC S89.19-
      - pilon (displaced) S82.87-
        - nondisplaced S82.87-
      - specified NEC S82.39-
      - torus S82.31-
    - malleolus — *see* Fracture, ankle, medial malleolus
    - oblique (displaced) S82.23-
      - nondisplaced S82.23-
    - pilon — *see* Fracture, tibia, lower end, pilon
    - proximal end — *see* Fracture, tibia, upper end
    - segmental (displaced) S82.26-
      - nondisplaced S82.26-
    - specified NEC S82.29-
    - spine — *see* Fracture, upper end, spine
    - spiral (displaced) S82.24-
      - nondisplaced S82.24-
    - transverse (displaced) S82.22-
      - nondisplaced S82.22-

- **Fracture, traumatic** — *continued*
  - tibia (shaft)— *continued*
    - tuberosity — *see* Fracture, tibia, upper end, tuberosity
    - upper end S82.10-
      - bicondylar (displaced) S82.14-
        - nondisplaced S82.14-
      - lateral condyle (displaced) S82.12-
        - nondisplaced S82.12-
      - medial condyle (displaced) S82.13-
        - nondisplaced S82.13-
      - physeal S89.00-
        - Salter-Harris
          - Type I S89.01-
          - Type II S89.02-
          - Type III S89.03-
          - Type IV S89.04-
        - specified NEC S89.09-
      - plateau — *see* Fracture, tibia, upper end, bicondylar
      - spine (displaced) S82.11-
        - nondisplaced S82.11-
      - torus S82.16-
      - specified NEC S82.19-
      - tuberosity (displaced) S82.15-
        - nondisplaced S82.15-
  - toe S92.91-
    - great (displaced) S92.40-
      - distal phalanx (displaced) S92.42-
        - nondisplaced S92.42-
      - nondisplaced S92.40-
      - proximal phalanx (displaced) S92.41-
        - nondisplaced S92.41-
      - specified NEC S92.49-
    - lesser (displaced) S92.50-
      - distal phalanx (displaced) S92.53-
        - nondisplaced S92.53-
      - medial phalanx (displaced) S92.52-
        - nondisplaced S92.52-
      - nondisplaced S92.50-
      - proximal phalanx (displaced) S92.51-
        - nondisplaced S92.51-
      - specified NEC S92.59-
  - tooth (root) S02.5
  - trachea (cartilage) S12.8
  - transverse process — *see* Fracture, vertebra
  - trapezium or trapezoid bone — *see* Fracture, carpal
  - trimalleolar — *see* Fracture, ankle, trimalleolar
  - triquetrum (cuneiform of carpus) — *see* Fracture, carpal, triquetrum
  - trochanter — *see* Fracture, femur, trochanteric
  - tuberosity (external)—code by site under Fracture
  - ulna (shaft) S52.20-
    - bent bone S52.28-
    - coronoid process — *see* Fracture, ulna, upper end, coronoid process
    - distal end — *see* Fracture, ulna, lower end
    - following insertion of implant, prosthesis or plate M96.63-
    - head S52.00-
    - lower end S52.60-
      - physeal S59.00-
        - Salter-Harris
          - Type I S59.01-
          - Type II S59.02-
          - Type III S59.03-
          - Type IV S59.04-
        - specified NEC S59.09-
      - specified NEC S52.69-
      - styloid process (displaced) S52.61-
        - nondisplaced S52.61-
      - torus S52.62-
    - proximal end — *see* Fracture, ulna, upper end
    - shaft S52.20-
      - comminuted (displaced) S52.25-
        - nondisplaced S52.25-
      - greenstick S52.21-
      - Monteggia's — *see* Monteggia's fracture
      - oblique (displaced) S52.23-
        - nondisplaced S52.23-
      - segmental (displaced) S52.26-
        - nondisplaced S52.26-
      - specified NEC S52.29-

- **Fracture, traumatic** — *continued*
  - ulna (shaft)— *continued*
    - shaft— *continued*
      - spiral (displaced) S52.24-
        - nondisplaced S52.24-
      - transverse (displaced) S52.22-
        - nondisplaced S52.22-
    - upper end S52.00-
      - coronoid process (displaced) S52.04-
        - nondisplaced S52.04-
      - olecranon process (displaced) S52.02-
        - with intraarticular extension S52.03-
        - nondisplaced S52.02-
          - with intraarticular extension S52.03-
      - specified NEC S52.09-
      - torus S52.01-
  - unciform — *see* Fracture, carpal, hamate
  - vault of skull S02.0
  - vertebra, vertebral (arch) (body) (column) (neural arch) (pedicle) (spinous process) (transverse process)
    - atlas — *see* Fracture, neck, cervical vertebra, first
    - axis — *see* Fracture, neck, cervical vertebra, second
    - cervical (teardrop) S12.9
      - axis — *see* Fracture, neck, cervical vertebra, second
      - first (atlas) — *see* Fracture, neck, cervical vertebra, first
      - second (axis) — *see* Fracture, neck, cervical vertebra, second
    - chronic M84.48
    - coccyx S32.2
    - dorsal — *see* Fracture, thorax, vertebra
    - lumbar S32.009
      - burst (stable) S32.001
        - unstable S32.002
      - fifth S32.059
        - burst (stable) S32.051
          - unstable S32.052
        - specified type NEC S32.058
        - wedge compression S32.050
      - first S32.019
        - burst (stable) S32.011
          - unstable S32.012
        - specified type NEC S32.018
        - wedge compression S32.010
      - fourth S32.049
        - burst (stable) S32.041
          - unstable S32.042
        - specified type NEC S32.048
        - wedge compression S32.040
      - second S32.029
        - burst (stable) S32.021
          - unstable S32.022
      - specified type NEC S32.028
        - wedge compression S32.020
      - specified type NEC S32.008
      - third S32.039
        - burst (stable) S32.031
          - unstable S32.032
        - specified type NEC S32.038
        - wedge compression S32.030
      - wedge compression S32.000
    - metastatic (*see also* Neoplasm) — *see* Collapse, vertebra, in, specified disease NEC
    - newborn (birth injury) P11.5
    - sacrum S32.10
      - specified NEC S32.19
      - Type
        - 1 S32.14
        - 2 S32.15
        - 3 S32.16
        - 4 S32.17
      - Zone
        - I S32.119
          - displaced (minimally) S32.111
            - severely S32.112
          - nondisplaced S32.110

G

- **Ganglioneuromatosis** D36.10
- **Ganglionitis**
  - fifth nerve — *see* Neuralgia, trigeminal
  - gasserian (postherpetic) (postzoster) BØ2.21
  - geniculate G51.1
    - newborn (birth injury) P11.3
    - postherpetic, postzoster BØ2.21
  - herpes zoster BØ2.21
  - postherpetic geniculate BØ2.21
- **Gangliosidosis** E75.10
  - GM1 E75.19
  - GM2 E75.ØØ
    - other specified E75.Ø9
    - Sandhoff disease E75.Ø1
    - Tay-Sachs disease E75.Ø2
  - GM3 E75.19
  - mucolipidosis IV E75.11
- **Gangosa** A66.5
- **Gangrene, gangrenous** (connective tissue) (dropsical) (dry) (moist) (skin) (ulcer) (*see also* Necrosis) I96
  - with diabetes (mellitus) — *see* Diabetes, gangrene
  - abdomen (wall) I96
  - alveolar M27.3
  - appendix K35.3
    - with
      - perforation or rupture K35.2
      - peritoneal abscess K35.3
      - peritonitis, localized K35.3
        - with perforation or rupture K35.2
        - generalized K35.2
  - arteriosclerotic (general) (senile) — *see* Arteriosclerosis, extremities, with, gangrene
  - auricle I96
  - Bacillus welchii A48.Ø
  - bladder (infectious) — *see* Cystitis, specified type NEC
  - bowel, cecum, or colon — *see* Gangrene, intestine
  - Clostridium perfringens or welchii A48.Ø
  - cornea H18.89-
  - corpora cavernosa N48.29
    - noninfective N48.89
  - cutaneous, spreading I96
  - decubital — *see* Ulcer, pressure, by site
  - diabetic (any site) — *see* Diabetes, gangrene
  - epidemic — *see* Poisoning, food, noxious, plant
  - epididymis (infectional) N45.1
  - erysipelas — *see* Erysipelas
  - emphysematous — *see* Gangrene, gas
  - extremity (lower) (upper) I96
  - Fournier N49.3
    - female N76.89
  - fusospirochetal A69.Ø
  - gallbladder — *see* Cholecystitis, acute
  - gas (bacillus) A48.Ø
    - following
      - abortion — *see* Abortion by type complicated by infection
      - ectopic or molar pregnancy OØ8.Ø
  - glossitis K14.Ø
  - hernia — *see* Hernia, by site, with gangrene
  - intestine, intestinal (hemorrhagic) (massive) K55.Ø
    - with
      - mesenteric embolism K55.Ø
      - obstruction — *see* Obstruction, intestine
  - laryngitis JØ4.Ø
  - limb (lower) (upper) I96
  - lung J85.Ø
    - spirochetal A69.8
  - lymphangitis I89.1
  - Meleney's (synergistic) — *see* Ulcer, skin
  - mesentery K55.Ø
    - with
      - embolism K55.Ø
      - intestinal obstruction — *see* Obstruction, intestine
  - mouth A69.Ø
  - ovary — *see* Oophoritis
  - pancreas K85.9
  - penis N48.29
    - noninfective N48.89
  - perineum I96
  - pharynx (*see also* Pharyngitis)
    - Vincent's A69.1

- **Gangrene, gangrenous** — *continued*
  - presenile I73.1
  - progressive synergistic — *see* Ulcer, skin
  - pulmonary J85.Ø
  - pulpal (dental) KØ4.1
  - quinsy J36
  - Raynaud's (symmetric gangrene) I73.Ø1
  - retropharyngeal J39.2
  - scrotum N49.3
    - noninfective N5Ø.8
  - senile (atherosclerotic) — *see* Arteriosclerosis, extremities, with, gangrene
  - spermatic cord N49.1
    - noninfective N5Ø.8
  - spine I96
  - spirochetal NEC A69.8
  - spreading cutaneous I96
  - stomatitis A69.Ø
  - symmetrical I73.Ø1
  - testis (infectional) N45.2
    - noninfective N44.8
  - throat (*see also* Pharyngitis)
    - diphtheritic A36.Ø
    - Vincent's A69.1
  - thyroid (gland) EØ7.89
  - tooth (pulp) KØ4.1
  - tuberculous NEC — *see* Tuberculosis
  - tunica vaginalis N49.1
    - noninfective N5Ø.8
  - umbilicus I96
  - uterus — *see* Endometritis
  - uvulitis K12.2
  - vas deferens N49.1
    - noninfective N5Ø.8
  - vulva N76.89
- **Ganister disease** J62.8
- **Ganser's syndrome** (hysterical) F44.89
- **Gardner-Diamond syndrome** (autoerythrocyte sensitization) D69.2
- **Gargoylism** E76.01
- **Garré's disease, osteitis** (sclerosing)**, osteomyelitis** — *see* Osteomyelitis, specified type NEC
- **Garrod's pad, knuckle** M72.1
- **Gartner's duct**
  - cyst Q52.4
  - persistent Q5Ø.6
- **Gas** R14.3
  - asphyxiation, inhalation, poisoning, suffocation NEC — *see* Table of Drugs and Chemicals
  - excessive R14.Ø
  - gangrene A48.Ø
    - following
      - abortion — *see* Abortion by type complicated by infection
      - ectopic or molar pregnancy OØ8.Ø
  - on stomach R14.Ø
  - pains R14.1
- **Gastralgia** (*see also* Pain, abdominal)
- **Gastrectasis** K31.0
  - psychogenic F45.8
- **Gastric** — *see* condition
- **Gastrinoma**
  - malignant
    - pancreas C25.4
    - specified site NEC — *see* Neoplasm, malignant, by site
    - unspecified site C25.4
  - specified site — *see* Neoplasm, uncertain behavior
  - unspecified site D37.9
- **Gastritis** (simple) K29.7Ø
  - with bleeding K29.71
  - acute (erosive) K29.ØØ
    - with bleeding K29.Ø1
  - alcoholic K29.2Ø
    - with bleeding K29.21
  - allergic K29.6Ø
    - with bleeding K29.61
  - atrophic (chronic) K29.4Ø
    - with bleeding K29.41
  - chronic (antral) (fundal) K29.5Ø
    - with bleeding K29.51
    - atrophic K29.4Ø
      - with bleeding K29.41

- **Gastritis**— *continued*
  - chronic— *continued*
    - superficial K29.3Ø
      - with bleeding K29.31
  - dietary counseling and surveillance Z71.3
  - due to diet deficiency E63.9
  - eosinophilic K52.81
  - giant hypertrophic K29.6Ø
    - with bleeding K29.61
  - granulomatous K29.6Ø
    - with bleeding K29.61
  - hypertrophic (mucosa) K29.6Ø
    - with bleeding K29.61
  - nervous F54
  - spastic K29.6Ø
    - with bleeding K29.61
  - specified NEC K29.6Ø
    - with bleeding K29.61
  - superficial chronic K29.3Ø
    - with bleeding K29.31
  - tuberculous A18.83
  - viral NEC AØ8.4
- **Gastrocarcinoma** — *see* Neoplasm, malignant, stomach
- **Gastrocolic** — *see* condition
- **Gastrodisciasis, gastrodiscoidiasis** B66.8
- **Gastroduodenitis** K29.90
  - with bleeding K29.91
  - virus, viral AØ8.4
    - specified type NEC AØ8.39
- **Gastrodynia** — *see* Pain, abdominal
- **Gastroenteritis** (acute) (chronic) (noninfectious) (*see also* Enteritis) K52.9
  - allergic K52.2
  - dietetic K52.2
  - drug-induced K52.1
  - due to
    - Cryptosporidium AØ7.2
    - drugs K52.1
    - food poisoning — *see* Intoxication, foodborne
    - radiation K52.Ø
  - eosinophilic K52.81
  - epidemic (infectious) AØ9
  - food hypersensitivity K52.2
  - infectious — *see* Enteritis, infectious
  - influenzal — *see* Influenza, with gastroenteritis
  - noninfectious K52.9
    - specified NEC K52.89
  - rotaviral AØ8.Ø
  - Salmonella AØ2.Ø
  - toxic K52.1
  - viral NEC AØ8.4
    - acute infectious AØ8.39
      - type Norwalk AØ8.11
    - infantile (acute) AØ8.39
    - Norwalk agent AØ8.11
    - rotaviral AØ8.Ø
    - severe of infants AØ8.39
    - specified type NEC AØ8.39
- **Gastroenteropathy** (*see also* Gastroenteritis) K52.9
  - acute, due to Norwalk agent AØ8.11
  - acute, due to Norovirus AØ8.11
  - infectious AØ9
- **Gastroenteroptosis** K63.4
- **Gastroesophageal laceration hemorrhage syndrome** K22.6
- **Gastrointestinal** — *see* condition
- **Gastrojejunal** — *see* condition
- **Gastrojejunitis** (*see also* Enteritis) K52.9
- **Gastrojejunocolic** — *see* condition
- **Gastroliths** K31.89
- **Gastromalacia** K31.89
- **Gastroparalysis** K31.84
  - diabetic — *see* Diabetes, gastroparalysis
- **Gastroparesis** K31.84
  - diabetic — *see* Diabetes, by type, with gastroparesis
- **Gastropathy** K31.9
  - congestive portal K31.89
  - erythematous K29.7Ø
  - exudative K9Ø.89
  - portal hypertensive K31.89
- **Gastroptosis** K31.89

DRAFT

- **Gastrorrhagia** K92.2
  - psychogenic F45.8
- **Gastroschisis** (congenital) Q79.3
- **Gastrospasm** (neurogenic) (reflex) K31.89
  - neurotic F45.8
  - psychogenic F45.8
- **Gastrostaxis** — *see* Gastritis, with bleeding
- **Gastrostenosis** K31.89
- **Gastrostomy**
  - attention to Z43.1
  - status Z93.1
- **Gastrosuccorrhea** (continuous) (intermittent) K31.89
  - neurotic F45.8
  - psychogenic F45.8
- **Gatophobia** F40.218
- **Gaucher's disease or splenomegaly** (adult) infantile) E75.22
- **Gee** (-Herter)(-Thaysen) **disease** (nontropical sprue) K90.0
- **Gélineau's syndrome** G47.419
  - with cataplexy G47.411
- **Gemination, tooth, teeth** K00.2
- **Gemistocytoma**
  - specified site — *see* Neoplasm, malignant, by site
  - unspecified site C71.9
- **General, generalized** — *see* condition
- **Genetic**
  - carrier (status)
    - cystic fibrosis Z14.1
    - hemophilia A (asymptomatic) Z14.Ø1
      - symptomatic Z14.Ø2
    - specified NEC Z14.8
  - susceptibility to disease NEC Z15.89
    - malignant neoplasm Z15.Ø9
      - breast Z15.Ø1
      - endometrium Z15.Ø4
      - ovary Z15.Ø2
      - prostate Z15.Ø3
      - specified NEC Z15.Ø9
    - multiple endocrine neoplasia Z15.81
- **Genital** — *see* condition
- **Genito-anorectal syndrome** A55
- **Genitourinary system** — *see* condition
- **Genu**
  - congenital Q74.1
  - extrorsum (acquired) (*see also* Deformity, varus, knee)
    - congenital Q74.1
    - sequelae (late effect) of rickets E64.3
  - introrsum (acquired) (*see also* Deformity, valgus, knee)
    - congenital Q74.1
    - sequelae (late effect) of rickets E64.3
  - rachitic (old) E64.3
  - recurvatum (acquired) (*see also* Deformity, limb, specified type NEC, lower leg)
    - congenital Q68.2
    - sequelae (late effect) of rickets E64.3
  - valgum (acquired) (knock-knee) M21.Ø6-
    - congenital Q74.1
    - sequelae (late effect) of rickets E64.3
  - varum (acquired) (bowleg) M21.16-
    - congenital Q74.1
    - sequelae (late effect) of rickets E64.3
- **Geographic tongue** K14.1
- **Geophagia** — *see* Pica
- **Geotrichosis** B48.3
  - stomatitis B48.3
- **Gephyrophobia** F40.242
- **Gerbode defect** Q21.0
- **GERD** (gastroesophageal reflux disease) K21.9
- **Gerhardt's**
  - disease (erythromelalgia) I73.81
  - syndrome (vocal cord paralysis) J38.ØØ
    - bilateral J38.Ø2
    - unilateral J38.Ø1
- **German measles** (*see also* Rubella)
  - exposure to Z2Ø.4
- **Germinoblastoma** (diffuse) C85.9-
  - follicular C82.9-
- **Germinoma** — *see* Neoplasm, malignant, by site
- **Gerontoxon** — *see* Degeneration, cornea, senile
- **Gerstmann-Sträussler-Scheinker syndrome** (GSS) A81.82
- **Gerstmann's syndrome** R48.8
  - developmental F81.2
- **Gestation** (period) (*see also* Pregnancy)
  - ectopic — *see* Pregnancy
  - multiple O3Ø.9-
    - greater than quadruplets — *see* Pregnancy, multiple (gestation), specified NEC
  - specified NEC — *see* Pregnancy, multiple (gestation), specified NEC
- **Gestational**
  - mammary abscess O91.11-
  - purulent mastitis O91.11-
  - subareolar abscess O91.11-
- **Ghon tubercle, primary infection** A15.7
- **Ghost**
  - teeth KØØ.4
  - vessels (cornea) H16.41-
- **Ghoul hand** A66.3
- **Gianotti-Crosti disease** L44.4
- **Giant**
  - cell
    - epulis KØ6.8
    - peripheral granuloma KØ6.8
  - esophagus, congenital Q39.5
  - kidney, congenital Q63.3
  - oesophagus, congenital Q39.5
  - urticaria T78.3
    - hereditary D84.1
- **Giardiasis** A07.1
- **Gibert's disease or pityriasis** L42
- **Giddiness** R42
  - hysterical F44.89
  - psychogenic F45.8
- **Gierke's disease** (glycogenosis I) E74.Ø1
- **Gigantism** (cerebral) (hypophyseal) (pituitary) E22.Ø
  - constitutional E34.4
- **Gilbert's disease or syndrome** E80.4
- **Gilchrist's disease** B40.9
- **Gilford-Hutchinson disease** E34.8
- **Gilles de la Tourette's disease or syndrome** (motor-verbal tic) F95.2
- **Gingivitis** K05.10
  - acute (catarrhal) KØ5.ØØ
    - necrotizing A69.1
    - plaque induced KØ5.ØØ
    - nonplaque induced KØ5.Ø1
  - chronic (desquamative) (hyperplastic) (simple marginal) (ulcerative) KØ5.1Ø
    - plaque induced KØ5.1Ø
    - nonplaque induced KØ5.11
  - expulsiva — *see* Periodontitis
  - necrotizing ulcerative (acute) A69.1
  - pellagrous E52
    - acute necrotizing A69.1
  - Vincent's A69.1
- **Gingivoglossitis** K14.0
- **Gingivopericementitis** — *see* Periodontitis
- **Gingivosis** — *see* Gingivitis, chronic
- **Gingivostomatitis** K05.10
  - herpesviral BØØ.2
  - necrotizing ulcerative (acute) A69.1
- **Gland, glandular** — *see* condition
- **Glanders** A24.0
- **Glanzmann** (-Naegeli) **disease or thrombasthenia** D69.1
- **Glasgow coma scale**
  - total score
    - 3-8 R4Ø.243
    - 9-12 R4Ø.242
    - 13-15 R4Ø.241
- **Glass-blower's disease** (cataract) — *see* Cataract, specified NEC
- **Glaucoma** H40.9
  - with
    - increased episcleral venous pressure H4Ø.81-
    - pseudoexfoliation of lens — *see* Glaucoma, open angle, primary, capsular
  - absolute H44.51-
  - angle-closure (primary) H4Ø.2Ø-
    - acute (attack) (crisis) H4Ø.21-
    - chronic H4Ø.22-
- **Glaucoma** — *continued*
  - angle-closure— *continued*
    - intermittent H4Ø.23-
    - residual stage H4Ø.24-
  - borderline H4Ø.ØØ-
  - capsular (with pseudoexfoliation of lens) — *see* Glaucoma, open angle, primary, capsular
  - childhood Q15.Ø
  - closed angle — *see* Glaucoma, angle-closure
  - congenital Q15.Ø
  - corticosteroid-induced — *see* Glaucoma, secondary, drugs
  - hypersecretion H4Ø.82-
  - in (due to)
    - amyloidosis E85.4 *[H42]*
    - aniridia Q13.1 *[H42]*
    - concussion of globe — *see* Glaucoma, secondary, trauma
    - dislocation of lens — *see* Glaucoma, secondary
    - disorder of lens NEC — *see* Glaucoma, secondary
    - drugs — *see* Glaucoma, secondary, drugs
    - endocrine disease NOS E34.9 *[H42]*
    - eye
      - inflammation — *see* Glaucoma, secondary, inflammation
      - trauma — *see* Glaucoma, secondary, trauma
    - hypermature cataract — *see* Glaucoma, secondary
    - iridocyclitis — *see* Glaucoma, secondary, inflammation
    - lens disorder — *see* Glaucoma, secondary,
    - Lowe's syndrome E72.Ø3 *[H42]*
    - metabolic disease NOS E88.9 *[H42]*
    - ocular disorders NEC — *see* Glaucoma, secondary
    - onchocerciasis B73.Ø2
    - pupillary block — *see* Glaucoma, secondary
    - retinal vein occlusion — *see* Glaucoma, secondary
    - Rieger's anomaly Q13.81 *[H42]*
    - rubeosis of iris — *see* Glaucoma, secondary
    - tumor of globe — *see* Glaucoma, secondary
  - infantile Q15.Ø
  - low tension — *see* Glaucoma, open angle, primary, low-tension
  - malignant H4Ø.83-
  - narrow angle — *see* Glaucoma, angle-closure
  - newborn Q15.Ø
  - noncongestive (chronic) — *see* Glaucoma, open angle
  - nonobstructive — *see* Glaucoma, open angle
  - obstructive (*see also* Glaucoma, angle-closure)
    - due to lens changes — *see* Glaucoma, secondary
  - open angle H4Ø.1Ø-
    - primary H4Ø.11-
      - capsular (with pseudoexfoliation of lens) H4Ø.14-
      - low-tension H4Ø.12-
      - pigmentary H4Ø.13-
      - residual stage H4Ø.15-
  - phacolytic — *see* Glaucoma, secondary
  - pigmentary — *see* Glaucoma, open angle, primary, pigmentary
  - postinfectious — *see* Glaucoma, secondary, inflammation
  - secondary (to) H4Ø.5-
    - drugs H4Ø.6-
    - inflammation H4Ø.4-
    - trauma H4Ø.3-
  - simple (chronic) H4Ø.11
  - simplex H4Ø.11
  - specified type NEC H4Ø.89
  - suspect H4Ø.ØØ-
  - syphilitic A52.71
  - traumatic (*see also* Glaucoma, secondary, trauma)
    - newborn (birth injury) P15.3
  - tuberculous A18.59
- **Glaucomatous flecks** (subcapsular) — *see* Cataract, complicated
- **Glazed tongue** K14.4
- **Gleet** (gonococcal) A54.Ø1
- **Glénard's disease** K63.4

- **Glioblastoma** (multiforme)
  - with sarcomatous component
    - specified site — *see* Neoplasm, malignant, by site
    - unspecified site C71.9
  - giant cell
    - specified site — *see* Neoplasm, malignant, by site
    - unspecified site C71.9
  - specified site — *see* Neoplasm, malignant, by site
  - unspecified site C71.9
- **Glioma** (malignant)
  - astrocytic
    - specified site — *see* Neoplasm, malignant, by site
    - unspecified site C71.9
  - mixed
    - specified site — *see* Neoplasm, malignant, by site
    - unspecified site C71.9
  - nose Q30.8
  - specified site NEC — *see* Neoplasm, malignant, by site
  - subependymal D43.2
    - specified site — *see* Neoplasm, uncertain behavior, by site
    - unspecified site D43.2
  - unspecified site C71.9
- **Gliomatosis cerebri** C71.0
- **Glioneuroma** — *see* Neoplasm, uncertain behavior, by site
- **Gliosarcoma**
  - specified site — *see* Neoplasm, malignant, by site
  - unspecified site C71.9
- **Gliosis** (cerebral) G93.89
  - spinal G95.89
- **Glisson's disease** — *see* Rickets
- **Globinuria** R82.3
- **Globus** (hystericus) F45.8
- **Glomangioma** D18.00
  - intra-abdominal D18.03
  - intracranial D18.02
  - skin D18.01
  - specified site NEC D18.09
- **Glomangiomyoma** D18.00
  - intra-abdominal D18.03
  - intracranial D18.02
  - skin D18.01
  - specified site NEC D18.09
- **Glomangiosarcoma** — *see* Neoplasm, connective tissue, malignant
- **Glomerular**
  - disease in syphilis A52.75
  - nephritis — *see* Glomerulonephritis
- **Glomerulitis** — *see* Glomerulonephritis
- **Glomerulonephritis** (*see also* Nephritis) N05.9
  - with
    - edema — *see* Nephrosis
    - minimal change N05.0
    - minor glomerular abnormality N05.0
  - acute N00.9
  - chronic N03.9
  - crescentic (diffuse) NEC (*see also* N00-N07 with fourth character .7) N05.7
  - dense deposit (*see also* N00-N07 with fourth character .6) N05.6
  - diffuse
    - crescentic (*see also* N00-N07 with fourth character .7) N05.7
    - endocapillary proliferative (*see also* N00-N07 with fourth character .4) N05.4
    - mesangial proliferative (*see also* N00-N07 with fourth character .3) N05.3
  - endocapillary proliferative (*see also* N00-N07 with fourth character .4) N05.4
    - membranous (*see also* N00-N07 with fourth character .2) N05.2
    - mesangial proliferative (*see also* N00-N07 with fourth character .3) N05.3
    - mesangiocapillary (*see also* N00-N07 with fourth character .5) N05.5
    - sclerosing N05.8
      - endocapillary proliferative (diffuse) NEC (*see also* N00-N07 with fourth character .4) N05.4
  - extracapillary NEC (*see also* N00-N07 with fourth character .7) N05.7

- **Glomerulonephritis** — *continued*
  - focal (and segmental) (*see also* N00-N07 with fourth character .1) N05.1
  - hypocomplementemic — *see* Glomerulonephritis, membranoproliferative
  - IgA — *see* Nephropathy, IgA
  - immune complex (circulating) NEC N05.8
  - in (due to)
    - amyloidosis E85.4 *[N08]*
    - bilharziasis B65.9 *[N08]*
    - cryoglobulinemia D89.1 *[N08]*
    - defibrination syndrome D65 *[N08]*
    - diabetes mellitus — *see* Diabetes, glomerulosclerosis
    - disseminated intravascular coagulation D65 *[N08]*
    - Fabry(-Anderson) disease E75.21 *[N08]*
    - Goodpasture's syndrome M31.0
    - hemolytic-uremic syndrome D59.3
    - Henoch(-Schönlein) purpura D69.0 *[N08]*
    - lecithin cholesterol acyltransferase deficiency E78.6 *[N08]*
    - microscopic polyangiitis M31.7 *[N08]*
    - multiple myeloma C90.0- *[N08]*
    - Plasmodium malariae B52.0
    - schistosomiasis B65.9 *[N08]*
    - sepsis A41.9 *[N08]*
      - streptococcal A40- *[N08]*
    - sickle-cell disorders D57.- *[N08]*
    - strongyloidiasis B78.9 *[N08]*
    - subacute bacterial endocarditis I33.0 *[N08]*
    - syphilis (late) congenital A50.59 *[N08]*
    - systemic lupus erythematosus M32.14
    - thrombotic thrombocytopenic purpura M31.1 *[N08]*
    - typhoid fever A01.09
    - Waldenström macroglobulinemia C88.0 *[N08]*
    - Wegener's granulomatosis M31.31
  - latent or quiescent N03.9
  - lobular, lobulonodular — *see* Glomerulonephritis, membranoproliferative
  - membranoproliferative (diffuse)(type 1 or 3)(*see also* N00-N07 with fourth character .5) N05.5
    - dense deposit (type 2) NEC (*see also* N00-N07 with fourth character .6) N05.6
  - membranous (diffuse) NEC (*see also* N00-N07 with fourth character .2) N05.2
  - mesangial
    - IgA/IgG — *see* Nephropathy, IgA
    - proliferative (diffuse) NEC (*see also* N00-N07 with fourth character .3) N05.3
  - mesangiocapillary (diffuse) NEC (*see also* N00-N07 with fourth character .5) N05.5
  - necrotic, necrotizing NEC (*see also* N00N07 with fourth character .8) N05.8
  - nodular — *see* Glomerulonephritis, membranoproliferative
  - poststreptococcal NEC N05.9
    - acute N00.9
    - chronic N03.9
    - rapidly progressive N01.9
  - proliferative NEC (*see also* N00-N07 with fourth character .8) N05.8
    - diffuse (lupus) M32.14
  - rapidly progressive N01.9
  - sclerosing, diffuse N05.8
  - specified pathology NEC (*see also* N00N07 with fourth character .8) N05.8
  - subacute N01.9
- **Glomerulopathy** — *see* Glomerulonephritis
- **Glomerulosclerosis** (*see also* Sclerosis, renal)
  - intercapillary (nodular) (with diabetes) — *see* Diabetes, glomerulosclerosis
  - intracapillary — *see* Diabetes, glomerulosclerosis
- **Glossagra** K14.6
- **Glossalgia** K14.6
- **Glossitis** (chronic superficial) (gangrenous) (Moeller's) K14.0
  - areata exfoliativa K14.1
  - atrophic K14.4
  - benign migratory K14.1
  - cortical superficial, sclerotic K14.0
  - Hunter's D51.0

- **Glossitis**— *continued*
  - interstitial, sclerous K14.0
  - median rhomboid K14.2
  - pellagrous E52
  - superficial, chronic K14.0
- **Glossocele** K14.8
- **Glossodynia** K14.6
  - exfoliativa K14.4
- **Glossoncus** K14.8
- **Glossopathy** K14.9
- **Glossophytia** K14.3
- **Glossoplegia** K14.8
- **Glossoptosis** K14.8
- **Glossopyrosis** K14.6
- **Glossotrichia** K14.3
- **Glossy skin** L90.8
- **Glottis** — *see* condition
- **Glottitis** (*see also* Laryngitis) J04.0
- **Glucagonoma**
  - pancreas
    - benign D13.7
    - malignant C25.4
    - uncertain behavior D37.8
  - specified site NEC
    - benign — *see* Neoplasm, benign, by site
    - malignant — *see* Neoplasm, malignant, by site
    - uncertain behavior — *see* Neoplasm, uncertain behavior, by site
  - unspecified site
    - benign D13.7
    - malignant C25.4
    - uncertain behavior D37.8
- **Glucoglycinuria** E72.51
- **Glucose-galactose malabsorption** E74.39
- **Glue**
  - ear — *see* Otitis, media, nonsuppurative, chronic, mucoid
  - sniffing (airplane) — *see* Abuse, drug, inhalant
    - dependence — *see* Dependence, drug, inhalant
- **Glutaric aciduria** E72.3
- **Glycinemia** E72.51
- **Glycinuria** (renal) (with ketosis) E72.09
- **Glycogen**
  - infiltration — *see* Disease, glycogen storage
  - storage disease — *see* Disease, glycogen storage
- **Glycogenosis** (diffuse) (generalized) (*see also* Disease, glycogen storage)
  - cardiac E74.02 *[I43]*
  - diabetic, secondary — *see* Diabetes, glycogenosis, secondary
  - pulmonary interstitial J84.842
- **Glycopenia** E16.2
- **Glycosuria** R81
  - renal E74.8
- **Gnathostoma spinigerum** (infection) (infestation), **gnathostomiasis** (wandering swelling) B83.1
- **Goiter** (plunging) (substernal) E04.9
  - with
    - hyperthyroidism (recurrent) — *see* Hyperthyroidism, with, goiter
    - thyrotoxicosis — *see* Hyperthyroidism, with, goiter
  - adenomatous — *see* Goiter, nodular
  - cancerous C73
  - congenital (nontoxic) E03.0
    - diffuse E03.0
    - parenchymatous E03.0
    - transitory, with normal functioning P72.0
  - cystic E04.2
    - due to iodine-deficiency E01.1
  - due to
    - enzyme defect in synthesis of thyroid hormone E07.1
    - iodine-deficiency (endemic) E01.2
  - dyshormonogenetic (familial) E07.1
  - endemic (iodine-deficiency) E01.2
    - diffuse E01.0
    - multinodular E01.1
  - exophthalmic — *see* Hyperthyroidism, with, goiter
  - iodine-deficiency (endemic) E01.2
    - diffuse E01.0
    - multinodular E01.1
    - nodular E01.1

- **Goiter**— *continued*
  - lingual Q89.2
  - lymphadenoid EØ6.3
  - malignant C73
  - multinodular (cystic) (nontoxic) EØ4.2
    - toxic or with hyperthyroidism EØ5.2Ø
      - with thyroid storm EØ5.21
  - neonatal NEC P72.Ø
  - nodular (nontoxic) (due to) EØ4.9
    - with
      - hyperthyroidism EØ5.2Ø
        - with thyroid storm EØ5.21
      - thyrotoxicosis EØ5.2Ø
        - with thyroid storm EØ5.21
    - endemic EØ1.1
    - iodine-deficiency EØ1.1
    - sporadic EØ4.9
    - toxic EØ5.2Ø
      - with thyroid storm EØ5.21
  - nontoxic EØ4.9
    - diffuse (colloid) EØ4.Ø
    - multinodular EØ4.2
    - simple EØ4.Ø
    - specified NEC EØ4.8
    - uninodular EØ4.1
  - simple EØ4.Ø
  - toxic — *see* Hyperthyroidism, with, goiter
  - uninodular (nontoxic) EØ4.1
    - toxic or with hyperthyroidism EØ5.1Ø
      - with thyroid storm EØ5.11
- **Goiter-deafness syndrome** EØ7.1
- **Goldberg syndrome** Q89.8
- **Goldberg-Maxwell syndrome** E34.51
- **Goldblatt's hypertension or kidney** I7Ø.1
- **Goldenhar** (-Gorlin) **syndrome** Q87.Ø
- **Goldflam-Erb disease or syndrome** G7Ø.ØØ
  - with exacerbation (acute) G7Ø.Ø1
  - in crisis G7Ø.Ø1
- **Goldscheider's disease** Q81.8
- **Goldstein's disease** (familial hemorrhagic telangiectasia) I78.Ø
- **Golfer's elbow** — *see* Epicondylitis, medial
- **Gonadoblastoma**
  - specified site — *see* Neoplasm, uncertain behavior, by site
  - unspecified site
    - female D39.1Ø
    - male D4Ø.1Ø
- **Gonecystitis** — *see* Vesiculitis
- **Gongylonemiasis** B83.8
- **Goniosynechiae** — *see* Adhesions, iris, goniosynechiae
- **Gonococcemia** A54.86
- **Gonococcus, gonococcal** (disease) (infection) (*see also* condition) A54.9
  - anus A54.6
  - bursa, bursitis A54.49
  - conjunctiva, conjunctivitis (neonatorum) A54.31
  - endocardium A54.83
  - eye A54.3Ø
    - conjunctivitis A54.31
    - iridocyclitis A54.32
    - keratitis A54.33
    - newborn A54.31
    - other specified A54.39
  - fallopian tubes (acute) (chronic) A54.24
  - genitourinary (organ) (system) (tract) (acute)
    - lower A54.ØØ
      - with abscess (accessory gland) (periurethral) A54.1
    - upper (*see also* condition) A54.29
  - heart A54.83
  - iridocyclitis A54.32
  - joint A54.42
  - lymphatic (gland) (node) A54.89
  - meninges, meningitis A54.81
  - musculoskeletal A54.4Ø
    - arthritis A54.42
    - osteomyelitis A54.43
    - other specified A54.49
    - spondylopathy A54.41
  - pelviperitonitis A54.24
  - pelvis (acute) (chronic) A54.24
- **Gonococcus, gonococcal**— *continued*
  - pharynx A54.5
  - proctitis A54.6
  - pyosalpinx (acute) (chronic) A54.24
  - rectum A54.6
  - skin A54.89
  - specified site NEC A54.89
  - tendon sheath A54.49
  - throat A54.5
  - urethra (acute) (chronic) A54.Ø1
    - with abscess (accessory gland) (periurethral) A54.1
  - vulva (acute) (chronic) A54.Ø2
- **Gonocytoma**
  - specified site — *see* Neoplasm, uncertain behavior, by site
  - unspecified site
    - female D39.1Ø
    - male D4Ø.1Ø
- **Gonorrhea** (acute) (chronic) A54.9
  - Bartholin's gland (acute) (chronic) (purulent) A54.Ø2
    - with abscess (accessory gland) (periurethral) A54.1
  - bladder A54.Ø1
  - cervix A54.Ø3
  - conjunctiva, conjunctivitis (neonatorum) A54.31
  - contact Z2Ø.2
  - Cowper's gland (with abscess) A54.1
  - exposure to Z2Ø.2
  - fallopian tube (acute) (chronic) A54.24
  - kidney (acute) (chronic) A54.21
  - lower genitourinary tract A54.ØØ
    - with abscess (accessory gland) (periurethral) A54.1
  - ovary (acute) (chronic) A54.24
  - pelvis (acute) (chronic) A54.24
    - female pelvic inflammatory disease A54.24
  - penis A54.Ø9
  - prostate (acute) (chronic) A54.22
  - seminal vesicle (acute) (chronic) A54.23
  - specified site not listed (*see also* Gonococcus) A54.89
  - spermatic cord (acute) (chronic) A54.23
  - urethra A54.Ø1
    - with abscess (accessory gland) (periurethral) A54.1
  - vagina A54.Ø2
  - vas deferens (acute) (chronic) A54.23
  - vulva A54.Ø2
- **Goodall's disease** AØ8.19
- **Goodpasture's syndrome** M31.0
- **Gopalan's syndrome** (burning feet) E53.Ø
- **Gorlin-Chaudry-Moss syndrome** Q87.0
- **Gottron's papules** L94.4
- **Gougerot's syndrome** (trisymptomatic) L81.7
- **Gougerot-Blum syndrome** (pigmented purpuric lichenoid dermatitis) L81.7
- **Gougerot-Carteaud disease or syndrome** (confluent reticulate papillomatosis**)** L83
- **Gouley's syndrome** (constrictive pericarditis) I31.1
- **Goundou** A66.6
- **Gout, gouty** (acute) (attack) (flare) (*see also* Gout, chronic) M1Ø.9-
  - drug-induced M1Ø.2Ø
    - ankle M1Ø.27-
    - elbow M1Ø.22-
    - foot joint M1Ø.27-
    - hand joint M1Ø.24-
    - hip M1Ø.25-
    - knee M1Ø.26-
    - multiple site M1Ø.29
    - shoulder M1Ø.21-
    - vertebrae M1Ø.28
    - wrist M1Ø.23-
  - idiopathic M1Ø.ØØ
    - ankle M1Ø.Ø7-
    - elbow M1Ø.Ø2-
    - foot joint M1Ø.Ø7-
    - hand joint M1Ø.Ø4-
    - hip M1Ø.Ø5-
    - knee M1Ø.Ø6-
    - multiple site M1Ø.Ø9
- **Gout, gouty**— *continued*
  - idiopathic— *continued*
    - shoulder M1Ø.Ø1-
    - vertebrae M1Ø.Ø8
    - wrist M1Ø.Ø3-
  - in (due to) renal impairment M1Ø.3Ø
    - ankle M1Ø.37-
    - elbow M1Ø.32-
    - foot joint M1Ø.37-
    - hand joint M1Ø.34-
    - hip M1Ø.35-
    - knee M1Ø.36-
    - multiple site M1Ø.39
    - shoulder M1Ø.31-
    - vertebrae M1Ø.38
    - wrist M1Ø.33-
  - lead-induced M1Ø.1Ø
    - ankle M1Ø.17-
    - elbow M1Ø.12-
    - foot joint M1Ø.17-
    - hand joint M1Ø.14-
    - hip M1Ø.15-
    - knee M1Ø.16-
    - multiple site M1Ø.19
    - shoulder M1Ø.11-
    - vertebrae M1Ø.18
    - wrist M1Ø.13-
  - primary — *see* Gout, idiopathic
  - saturnine — *see* Gout, lead-induced
  - secondary NEC M1Ø.4Ø
    - ankle M1Ø.47-
    - elbow M1Ø.42-
    - foot joint M1Ø.47-
    - hand joint M1Ø.44-
    - hip M1Ø.45-
    - knee M1Ø.46-
    - multiple site M1Ø.49
    - shoulder M1Ø.41-
    - vertebrae M1Ø.48
    - wrist M1Ø.43-
  - syphilitic (*see also* subcategory M14.8-) A52.77
  - tophi — *see* Gout by type
- **Gout, chronic** (*see also* Gout, gouty) M1A.9
  - drug-induced M1A.2Ø
    - ankle M1A.27-
    - elbow M1A.22-
    - foot joint M1A.27-
    - hand joint M1A.24-
    - hip M1A.25-
    - knee M1A.26-
    - multiple site M1A.29-
    - shoulder M1A.21-
    - vertebrae M1A.28
    - wrist M1A.23-
  - idiopathic M1A.ØØ
    - ankle M1A.Ø7-
    - elbow M1A.Ø2-
    - foot joint M1A.Ø7-
    - hand joint M1A.Ø4-
    - hip M1A.Ø5-
    - knee M1A.Ø6-
    - multiple site M1A.Ø9
    - shoulder M1A.Ø1-
    - vertebrae M1A.Ø8
    - wrist M1A.Ø3-
  - in (due to) renal impairment M1A.3Ø
    - ankle M1A.37-
    - elbow M1A.32-
    - foot joint M1A.37-
    - hand joint M1A.34-
    - hip M1A.35-
    - knee M1A.36-
    - multiple site M1A.39
    - shoulder M1A.31-
    - vertebrae M1A.38
    - wrist M1A.33
  - lead-induced M1A.1Ø
    - ankle M1A.17-
    - elbow M1A.12-
    - foot joint M1A.17-
    - hand joint M1A.14-
    - hip M1A.15-
    - knee M1A.16

Gout, chronic — *continued*
lead-induced— *continued*
multiple site M1A.19
shoulder M1A.11-
vertebrae M1A.18
wrist M1A.13
primary — *see* Gout, chronic, idiopathic
saturnine — *see* Gout, chronic, lead-induced
secondary NEC M1A.4Ø
ankle M1A.47-
elbow M1A.42-
foot joint M1A.47-
hand joint M1A.44-
hip M1A.45-
knee M1A.46-
multiple site M1A.49
shoulder M1A.41-
vertebrae M1A.48
wrist M1A.43-
syphilitic (*see also* subcategory M14.8-) A52.77
tophi — *see* Gout by type
Gower's
muscular dystrophy G71.Ø
syndrome (vasovagal attack) R55
Gradenigo's syndrome — *see* Otitis, media, suppurative, acute
Graefe's disease — *see* Strabismus, paralytic, ophthalmoplegia, progressive
Graft-versus-host disease D89.813
acute D89.81Ø
acute on chronic D89.812
chronic D89.811
Grainhandler's disease or lung J67.8
Grain mite (itch) B88.Ø
Grand mal — *see* Epilepsy, generalized, specified NEC
Grand multipara status only (not pregnant) Z64.1
pregnant — *see* Pregnancy, complicated by, grand multiparity
Granite worker's lung J62.8
Granular *(see also* condition)
inflammation, pharynx J31.2
kidney (contracting) — *see* Sclerosis, renal
liver K74.69
Granulation tissue (abnormal) (excessive) L92.9
postmastoidectomy cavity — *see* Complications, postmastoidectomy, granulation
Granulocytopenia (primary) (malignant) — *see* Aganulocytosis
Granuloma L92.9
abdomen K66.8
from residual foreign body L92.3
pyogenicum L98.Ø
actinic L57.5
annulare (perforating) L92.Ø
apical KØ4.5
aural — *see* Otitis, externa, specified NEC
beryllium (skin) L92.3
bone
eosinophilic C96.6
from residual foreign body — *see* Osteomyelitis, specified type NEC
lung C96.6
brain (any site) GØ6.Ø
schistosomiasis B65.9 *[G07]*
canaliculus lacrimalis — *see* Granuloma, lacrimal
candidal (cutaneous) B37.2
cerebral (any site) GØ6.Ø
coccidioidal (primary) (progressive) B38.7
lung B38.1
meninges B38.4
colon K63.89
conjunctiva H11.22-
dental KØ4.5
ear, middle — *see* Cholesteatoma
eosinophilic C96.6
bone C96.6
lung C96.6
oral mucosa K13.4
skin L92.2
eyelid HØ1.8
facial(e) L92.2
foreign body (in soft tissue) NEC M6Ø.2Ø
ankle M6Ø.27-

Granuloma — *continued*
foreign body— *continued*
forearm M6Ø.23-
hand M6Ø.24-
in operation wound — *see* Foreign body, accidentally left during a procedure
lower leg M6Ø.26-
pelvic region M6Ø.25-
shoulder region M6Ø.21-
skin L92.3
specified site NEC M6Ø.28
subcutaneous tissue L92.3
thigh M6Ø.25-
upper arm M6Ø.22-
gangraenescens M31.2
genito-inguinale A58
giant cell (central) (reparative) (jaw) M27.1
gingiva (peripheral) KØ6.8
gland (lymph) I88.8
hepatic NEC K75.3
in (due to)
berylliosis J63.2 *[K77]*
sarcoidosis D86.89
Hodgkin C81.9
ileum K63.89
infectious B99.9
specified NEC B99.8
inguinale (Donovan) (venereal) A58
intestine NEC K63.89
intracranial (any site) GØ6.Ø
intraspinal (any part) GØ6.1
iridocyclitis — *see* Iridocyclitis, chronic
jaw (bone) (central) M27.1
reparative giant cell M27.1
kidney (*see also* Infection, kidney) N15.8
lacrimal HØ4.81-
larynx J38.7
lethal midline (faciale(e)) M31.2
liver NEC — *see* Granuloma, hepatic
lung (infectious) (*see also* Fibrosis, lung)
coccidioidal B38.1
eosinophilic C96.6
Majocchi's B35.8
malignant (facial(e)) M31.2
mandible (central) M27.1
midline (lethal) M31.2
monilial (cutaneous) B37.2
nasal sinus — *see* Sinusitis
operation wound T81.89
foreign body — *see* Foreign body, accidentally left during a procedure
stitch T81.89
talc — *see* Foreign body, accidentally left during a procedure
oral mucosa K13.4
orbit, orbital HØ5.11-
paracoccidioidal B41.8
penis, venereal A58
periapical KØ4.5
peritoneum K66.8
due to ova of helminths NOS (*see also* Helminthiasis) B83.9 *[K67]*
postmastoidectomy cavity — *see* Complications, postmastoidectomy, recurrent cholesteatoma
prostate N42.89
pudendi (ulcerating) A58
pulp, internal (tooth) KØ3.3
pyogenic, pyogenicum (of) (skin) L98.Ø
gingiva KØ6.8
maxillary alveolar ridge KØ4.5
oral mucosa K13.4
rectum K62.89
reticulohistiocytic D76.3
rubrum nasi L74.8
Schistosoma — *see* Schistosomiasis
septic (skin) L98.Ø
silica (skin) L92.3
sinus (accessory) (infective) (nasal) — *see* Sinusitis
skin L92.9
from residual foreign body L92.3
pyogenicum L98.Ø
spine
syphilitic (epidural) A52.19

Granuloma — *continued*
spine— *continued*
tuberculous A18.Ø1
stitch (postoperative) T81.89
suppurative (skin) L98.Ø
swimming pool A31.1
talc (*see also* Granuloma, foreign body)
in operation wound — *see* Foreign body, accidentally left during a procedure
telangiectaticum (skin) L98.Ø
tracheostomy J95.Ø9
trichophyticum B35.8
tropicum A66.4
umbilicus L92.9
urethra N36.8
uveitis — *see* Iridocyclitis, chronic
vagina A58
venereum A58
vocal cord J38.3
Granulomatosis L92.9
lymphoid C83.8-
miliary (listerial) A32.89
necrotizing, respiratory M31.3Ø
progressive septic D71
specified NEC L92.8
Wegener's M31.3Ø
with renal involvement M31.31
Granulomatous tissue (abnormal) (excessive) L92.9
Granulosis rubra nasi L74.8
Graphite fibrosis (of lung) J63.3
Graphospasm F48.8
organic G25.89
Grating scapula M89.8x1
Gravel (urinary) — *see* Calculus, urinary
Graves' disease — *see* Hyperthyroidism, with, goiter
Gravis — *see* condition
Grawitz tumor C64.-
Gray syndrome (newborn) P93.Ø
Grayness, hair (premature) L67.1
congenital Q84.2
Green sickness D50.8
Greenfield's disease
meaning
concentric sclerosis (encephalitis periaxialis concentrica) G37.5
metachromatic leukodystrophy E75.25
Greenstick fracture—code as Fracture, by site
Grey syndrome (newborn) P93.Ø
Grief F43.21
prolonged F43.29
reaction (*see also* Disorder, adjustment) F43.2Ø
Griesinger's disease B76.9
Grinder's lung or pneumoconiosis J62.8
Grinding, teeth
psychogenic F45.8
sleep related G47.63
Grip
Dabney's B33.Ø
devil's B33.Ø
Grippe, grippal (*see also* Influenza)
Balkan A78
summer, of Italy A93.1
Grisel's disease M43.6
Groin — *see* condition
Grooved tongue K14.5
Ground itch B76.9
Grover's disease or syndrome L11.1
Growing pains, children R29.898
Growth (fungoid) (neoplastic) (new) (*see also* Neoplasm)
adenoid (vegetative) J35.8
benign — *see* Neoplasm, benign, by site
malignant — *see* Neoplasm, malignant, by site
rapid, childhood ZØØ.2
secondary — *see* Neoplasm, secondary, by site
Gruby's disease B35.0
Gubler-Millard paralysis or syndrome G46.3
Guerin-Stern syndrome Q74.3
Guidance, insufficient anterior (occlusal) M26.54
Guillain-Barré disease or syndrome G61.0
sequelae G65.Ø
Guinea worms (infection) (infestation) B72
Guinon's disease (motor-verbal tic) F95.2

H

H (Hartnup's) **disease** E72.Ø2
Haas' disease or osteochondrosis (juvenile) (head of humerus) — *see* Osteochondrosis, juvenile, humerus
Habit, habituation
  bad sleep Z72.821
  chorea F95.8
  disturbance, child F98.9
  drug — *see* Dependence, drug
  irregular sleep Z72.821
  laxative F55.2
  spasm — *see* Tic
  tic — *see* Tic
Haemophilus (H.) **influenzae, as cause of disease classified elsewhere** B96.3
Haff disease — *see* Poisoning, mercury
Hageman's factor defect, deficiency or disease D68.2
Haglund's disease or osteochondrosis (juvenile) (os tibiale externum) — *see* Osteochondrosis, juvenile, tarsus
Hailey-Hailey disease Q82.8
Hair (*see also* condition)
  plucking F63.3
    in stereotyped movement disorder F98.4
  tourniquet syndrome (*see also* Constriction, external, by site)
    finger S6Ø.44-
    penis S3Ø.842
    thumb S6Ø.34-
    toe S9Ø.44-
Hairball in stomach T18.2
Hair-pulling, pathological (compulsive) F63.3
Hairy black tongue K14.3
Half vertebra Q76.49
Halitosis R19.6
Hallerman-Streiff syndrome Q87.Ø
Hallervorden-Spatz disease G23.Ø
Hallopeau's acrodermatitis or disease L4Ø.2
Hallucination R44.3
  auditory R44.Ø
  gustatory R44.2
  olfactory R44.2
  specified NEC R44.2
  tactile R44.2
  visual R44.1
Hallucinosis (chronic) F28
  alcoholic (acute) F1Ø.951
    in
      abuse F1Ø.151
      dependence F1Ø.251
  drug-induced F19.951
    cannabis F12.951
    cocaine F14.951
    hallucinogen F16.151
    in
      abuse F19.151
        cannabis F12.151
        cocaine F14.151
        hallucinogen F16.151
        inhalant F18.151
        opioid F11.151
        sedative, anxiolytic or hypnotic F13.151
        stimulant NEC F15.151
      dependence F19.251
        cannabis F12.251
        cocaine F14.251
        hallucinogen F16.251
        inhalant F18.251
        opioid F11.251
        sedative, anxiolytic or hypnotic F13.251
        stimulant NEC F15.251
    inhalant F18.951
    opioid F11.951
    sedative, anxiolytic or hypnotic F13.951
Hallucinosis (chronic) F28
    stimulant NEC F15.951
  organic FØ6.Ø
Hallux
  deformity (acquired) NEC M2Ø.5X-
  limitus M2Ø.5X-
  malleus (acquired) NEC M2Ø.3-
  rigidus (acquired) M2Ø.2-
    congenital Q74.2
    sequelae (late effect) of rickets E64.3
  valgus (acquired) M2Ø.1-
    congenital Q66.6
  varus (acquired) M2Ø.3-
    congenital Q66.3
Halo, visual H53.19
Hamartoma, hamartoblastoma Q85.9
  epithelial (gingival), odontogenic, central or peripheral — *see* Cyst, calcifying odontogenic
Hamartosis Q85.9
Hamman-Rich syndrome J84.114
Hammer toe (acquired) NEC (*see also* Deformity, toe, hammer toe)
  congenital Q66.89
  sequelae (late effect) of rickets E64.3
Hand — *see* condition
Hand-foot syndrome L27.1
Handicap, handicapped
  educational Z55.9
    specified NEC Z55.8
Hand-Schüller-Christian disease or syndrome C96.5
Hanging (asphyxia) (strangulation) (suffocation) — *see* Asphyxia, traumatic, due to mechanical threat
Hangnail (*see also* Cellulitis, digit)
  with lymphangitis — *see* Lymphangitis, acute, digit
Hangover (alcohol) F1Ø.129
Hanhart's syndrome Q87.Ø
Hanot-Chauffard(-Troisier) **syndrome** E83.19
Hanot's cirrhosis or disease K74.3
Hansen's disease — *see* Leprosy
Hantaan virus disease (Korean hemorrhagic fever) A98.5
Hantavirus disease (with renal manifestations) (Dobrava) (Puumala) (Seoul) A98.5
  with pulmonary manifestations (Andes) (Bayou) (Bermejo) (Black Creek Canal) (Choclo) (Juquitiba) (Laguna negra) (Lechiguanas) (New York) (Oran) (Sin nombre) B33.4
Happy puppet syndrome Q93.5
Harada's disease or syndrome H3Ø.81-
Hardening
  artery — *see* Arteriosclerosis
  brain G93.89
Harelip (complete) (incomplete) — *see* Cleft, lip
Harlequin (newborn) Q8Ø.4
Harley's disease D59.6
Harmful use (of)
  alcohol F1Ø.1Ø
  anxiolytics — *see* Abuse, drug, sedative
  cannabinoids — *see* Abuse, drug, cannabis
  cocaine — *see* Abuse, drug, cocaine
  drug — *see* Abuse, drug
  hallucinogens — *see* Abuse, drug, hallucinogen
  hypnotics — *see* Abuse, drug, sedative
  opioids — *see* Abuse, drug, opioid
  PCP (phencyclidine) — *see* Abuse, drug, hallucinogen
  sedatives — *see* Abuse, drug, sedative
  stimulants NEC — *see* Abuse, drug, stimulant
Harris' lines — *see* Arrest, epiphyseal
Hartnup's disease E72.Ø2
Harvester's lung J67.Ø
Harvesting ovum for in vitro fertilization Z31.83
Hashimoto's disease or thyroiditis EØ6.3
Hashitoxicosis (transient) EØ6.3
Hassal-Henle bodies or warts (cornea) H18.49
Haut mal — *see* Epilepsy, generalized, specified NEC
Haverhill fever A25.1
Hay fever (*see also* Fever, hay) J3Ø.1
Hayem-Widal syndrome D59.8
Haygarth's nodes M15.8
Haymaker's lung J67.Ø
Hb (abnormal)
  Bart's disease D56.Ø
  disease — *see* Disease, hemoglobin
  trait — *see* Trait
Head — *see* condition
Headache R51
  allergic NEC G44.89
  associated with sexual activity G44.82
  chronic daily R51
  cluster G44.ØØ9
    chronic G44.Ø29
      intractable G44.Ø21
      not intractable G44.Ø29
    episodic G44.Ø19
      intractable G44.Ø11
      not intractable G44.Ø19
    intractable G44.ØØ1
    not intractable G44.ØØ9
  cough (primary) G44.83
  daily chronic R51
  drug-induced NEC G44.4Ø
    intractable G44.41
    not intractable G44.4Ø
  exertional (primary) G44.84
  histamine G44.ØØ9
    intractable G44.ØØ1
    not intractable G44.ØØ9
  hypnic G44.81
  lumbar puncture G97.1
  medication overuse G44.4Ø
    intractable G44.41
    not intractable G44.4Ø
  menstrual — *see* Migraine, menstrual
  migraine (type) (*see also* Migraine) G43.9Ø9
  nasal septum R51
  neuralgiform, short lasting unilateral, with conjunctival injection and tearing (SUNCT) G44.Ø59
    intractable G44.Ø51
    not intractable G44.Ø59
  new daily persistent (NDPH) G44.52
  orgasmic G44.82
  periodic syndromes in adults and children G43.CØ9
    with refractory migraine G43.C1
    intractable G43.C19
    not intractable G43.CØ9
    without refractory migraine G43.CØ
  postspinal puncture G97.1
  post-traumatic G44.3Ø9
    acute G44.319
      intractable G44.311
      not intractable G44.319
    chronic G44.329
      intractable G44.321
      not intractable G44.329
    intractable G44.3Ø1
    not intractable G44.3Ø9
  pre-menstrual — *see* Migraine, menstrual
  preorgasmic G44.82
  primary
    cough G44.83
    exertional G44.84
    stabbing G44.85
    thunderclap G44.53
  rebound G44.4Ø
    intractable G44.41
    not intractable G44.4Ø
  short lasting unilateral neuralgiform, with conjunctival injection and tearing (SUNCT) G44.Ø59
    intractable G44.Ø51
    not intractable G44.Ø59
  specified syndrome NEC G44.89
  spinal and epidural anesthesia induced T88.59
    in labor and delivery O74.5
    in pregnancy O29.4-
    postpartum, puerperal O89.4
  spinal fluid loss (from puncture) G97.1
  stabbing (primary) G44.85
  tension(-type) G44.2Ø9
    chronic G44.229
      intractable G44.221
      not intractable G44.229

Headache — *continued*
tension(-type)— *continued*
episodic G44.219
intractable G44.211
not intractable G44.219
intractable G44.2Ø1
not intractable G44.2Ø9
thunderclap (primary) G44.53
vascular NEC G44.1Ø
intractable G44.11
not intractable G44.1Ø
Healthy
infant
accompanying sick mother Z76.3
receiving care Z76.2
person accompanying sick person Z76.3
Hearing examination ZØ1.1Ø
with abnormal findings NEC ZØ1.118
following failed hearing screening ZØ1.11Ø
for hearing conservation and treatment ZØ1.12
Heart — *see* condition
Heart beat
abnormality RØØ.9
specified NEC RØØ.8
awareness RØØ.2
rapid RØØ.Ø
slow RØØ.1
Heartburn R12
psychogenic F45.8
Heat (effects) T67.9
apoplexy T67.Ø
burn (*see also* Burn) L55.9
collapse T67.1
cramps T67.2
dermatitis or eczema L59.Ø
edema T67.7
erythema—code by site under Burn, first degree
excessive T67.9
specified effect NEC T67.8
exhaustion T67.5
anhydrotic T67.3
due to
salt (and water) depletion T67.4
water depletion T67.3
with salt depletion T67.4
fatigue (transient) T67.6
fever T67.Ø
hyperpyrexia T67.Ø
prickly L74.Ø
prostration — *see* Heat, exhaustion
pyrexia T67.Ø
rash L74.Ø
specified effect NEC T67.8
stroke T67.Ø
sunburn — *see* Sunburn
syncope T67.1
Heavy-for-dates NEC (infant) (4ØØØg to 4499g) PØ8.1
exceptionally (45ØØg or more) PØ8.Ø
Hebephrenia, hebephrenic (schizophrenia) F2Ø.1
Heberden's disease or nodes (with arthropathy) M15.1
Hebra's
pityriasis L26
prurigo L28.2
Heel — *see* condition
Heerfordt's disease D86.89
Hegglin's anomaly or syndrome D72.Ø
Heilmeyer-Schoner disease D45
Heine-Medin disease A8Ø.9
Heinz body anemia, congenital D58.2
Heliophobia F4Ø.228
Heller's disease or syndrome F84.3
HELLP syndrome (hemolysis, elevated liver enzymes and low platelet count) O14.2-
Helminthiasis (*see also* Infestation, helminth)
Ancylostoma B76.Ø
intestinal B82.Ø
mixed types (types classifiable to more than one of the titles B65.Ø-B81.3 and B81.8) B81.4
specified type NEC B81.8
mixed types (intestinal) (types classifiable to more than one of the titles B65.Ø-B81.3 and B81.8) B81.4

Helminthiasis — *continued*
Necator (americanus) B76.1
specified type NEC B83.8
Heloma L84
Hemangioblastoma — *see* Neoplasm, connective tissue, uncertain behavior
malignant — *see* Neoplasm, connective tissue, malignant
Hemangioendothelioma (*see also* Neoplasm, uncertain behavior, by site)
benign D18.ØØ
intra-abdominal D18.Ø3
intracranial D18.Ø2
skin D18.Ø1
specified site NEC D18.Ø9
bone (diffuse) — *see* Neoplasm, bone, malignant
epithelioid (*see also* Neoplasm, uncertain behavior, by site)
malignant — *see* Neoplasm, malignant, by site
malignant — *see* Neoplasm, connective tissue, malignant
Hemangiofibroma — *see* Neoplasm, benign, by site
Hemangiolipoma — *see* Lipoma
Hemangioma D18.ØØ
arteriovenous D18.ØØ
intra-abdominal D18.Ø3
intracranial D18.Ø2
skin D18.Ø1
specified site NEC D18.Ø9
capillary D18.ØØ
intra-abdominal D18.Ø3
intracranial D18.Ø2
skin D18.Ø1
specified site NEC D18.Ø9
cavernous D18.ØØ
intra-abdominal D18.Ø3
intracranial D18.Ø2
skin D18.Ø1
specified site NEC D18.Ø9
epithelioid D18.ØØ
intra-abdominal D18.Ø3
intracranial D18.Ø2
skin D18.Ø1
specified site NEC D18.Ø9
histiocytoid D18.ØØ
intra-abdominal D18.Ø3
intracranial D18.Ø2
skin D18.Ø1
specified site NEC D18.Ø9
infantile D18.ØØ
intra-abdominal D18.Ø3
intracranial D18.Ø2
skin D18.Ø1
specified site NEC D18.Ø9
intra-abdominal D18.Ø3
intracranial D18.Ø2
intramuscular D18.ØØ
intra-abdominal D18.Ø3
intracranial D18.Ø2
skin D18.Ø1
specified site NEC D18.Ø9
juvenile D18.ØØ
malignant — *see* Neoplasm, connective tissue, malignant
plexiform D18.ØØ
intra-abdominal D18.Ø3
intracranial D18.Ø2
skin D18.Ø1
specified site NEC D18.Ø9
racemose D18.ØØ
intra-abdominal D18.Ø3
intracranial D18.Ø2
skin D18.Ø1
specified site NEC D18.Ø9
sclerosing — *see* Neoplasm,skin, benign
simplex D18.ØØ
intra-abdominal D18.Ø3
intracranial D18.Ø2
skin D18.Ø1
specified site NEC D18.Ø9
skin D18.Ø1
specified site NEC D18.Ø9
venous D18.ØØ

Hemangioma — *continued*
venous— *continued*
intra-abdominal D18.Ø3
intracranial D18.Ø2
skin D18.Ø1
specified site NEC D18.Ø9
verrucous keratotic D18.ØØ
intra-abdominal D18.Ø3
intracranial D18.Ø2
skin D18.Ø1
specified site NEC D18.Ø9
Hemangiomatosis (systemic) I78.8
involving single site — *see* Hemangioma
Hemangiopericytoma (*see also* Neoplasm, connective tissue, uncertain behavior)
benign — *see* Neoplasm, connective tissue, benign
malignant — *see* Neoplasm, connective tissue, malignant
Hemangiosarcoma — *see* Neoplasm, connective tissue, malignant
Hemarthrosis (nontraumatic) M25.ØØ
ankle M25.Ø7-
elbow M25.Ø2-
foot joint M25.Ø7-
hand joint M25.Ø4-
hip M25.Ø5-
in hemophilic arthropathy — *see* Arthropathy, hemophilic
knee M25.Ø6-
shoulder M25.Ø1-
specified joint NEC M25.Ø8
traumatic — *see* Sprain, by site
wrist M25.Ø3-
Hematemesis K92.Ø
with ulcer—code by site under Ulcer, with hemorrhage K27.4
newborn, neonatal P54.Ø
due to swallowed maternal blood P78.2
Hematidrosis L74.8
Hematinuria (*see also* Hemoglobinuria)
malarial B5Ø.8
Hematobilia K83.8
Hematocele
female NEC N94.89
with ectopic pregnancy OØØ.9
ovary N83.8
male N5Ø.1
Hematochezia (*see also* Melena) K92.1
Hematochyluria (*see also* Infestation, filarial)
schistosomiasis (bilharziasis) B65.Ø
Hematocolpos (with hematometra or hematosalpinx) N89.7
Hematocornea — *see* Pigmentation, cornea, stromal
Hematogenous — *see* condition
Hematoma (traumatic) (skin surface intact) (*see also* Contusion)
with
injury of internal organs — *see* Injury, by site
open wound — *see* Wound, open
amputation stump (surgical) (late) T87.8
aorta, dissecting I71.ØØ
abdominal I71.Ø2
thoracic I71.Ø1
thoracoabdominal I71.Ø3
aortic intramural — *see* Dissection, aorta
arterial (complicating trauma) — *see* Injury, blood vessel, by site
auricle — *see* Contusion, ear
nontraumatic — *see* Disorder, pinna, hematoma
birth injury NEC P15.8
brain (traumatic)
with
cerebral laceration or contusion (diffuse) — *see* Injury, intracranial, diffuse
focal — *see* Injury, intracranial, focal
cerebellar, traumatic SØ6.37-
newborn NEC P52.4
birth injury P1Ø.1
intracerebral, traumatic — *see* Injury, intracranial, intracerebral hemorrhage
nontraumatic — *see* Hemorrhage, intracranial
subarachnoid, arachnoid, traumatic — *see* Injury, intracranial, subarachnoid hemorrhage

- **Hematoma** — *continued*
  - brain (traumatic) — *continued*
    - subdural, traumatic — *see* Injury, intracranial, subdural hemorrhage
  - breast (nontraumatic) N64.89
  - broad ligament (nontraumatic) N83.7
    - traumatic S37.892
  - cerebellar, traumatic SØ6.37-
  - cerebral — *see* Hematoma, brain
  - cerebrum SØ6.36-
    - left SØ6.35-
    - right SØ6.34-
  - cesarean delivery wound O9Ø.2
  - complicating delivery (perineal) (pelvic) (vagina) (vulva) O71.7
  - corpus cavernosum (nontraumatic) N48.89
  - epididymis (nontraumatic) N5Ø.1
  - epidural (traumatic) — *see* Injury, intracranial, epidural hemorrhage
    - spinal — *see* Injury, spinal cord, by region
  - episiotomy O9Ø.2
  - face, birth injury P15.4
  - genital organ NEC (nontraumatic)
    - female (nonobstetric) N94.89
      - traumatic S3Ø.2Ø2
    - male N5Ø.1
      - traumatic S3Ø.2Ø1
  - internal organs — *see* Injury, by site
  - intracerebral, traumatic — *see* Injury, intracranial, intracerebral hemorrhage
  - intraoperative — *see* Complications, intraoperative, hemorrhage
  - labia (nontraumatic) (nonobstetric) N9Ø.89
  - liver (subcapsular) (nontraumatic) K76.89
    - birth injury P15.Ø
  - perianal (nontraumatic) K64.5
  - mediastinum — *see* Injury, intrathoracic
  - mesosalpinx (nontraumatic) N83.7
    - traumatic S37.529
      - bilateral S37.522
      - unilateral S37.521
  - muscle—code by site under Contusion
  - nontraumatic
    - muscle M79.81
    - soft tissue M79.81
  - obstetrical surgical wound O9Ø.2
  - orbit, orbital (nontraumatic) (*see also* Hemorrhage, orbit)
    - traumatic — *see* Contusion, orbit
  - pelvis (female) (nontraumatic) (nonobstetric) N94.89
    - obstetric O71.7
    - traumatic — *see* Injury, by site
  - penis (nontraumatic) N48.89
    - birth injury P15.5
  - perineal S3Ø.23
    - complicating delivery O71.7
  - perirenal — *see* Injury, kidney
  - pinna — *see* Contusion, ear
    - nontraumatic — *see* Disorder, pinna, hematoma
  - placenta O43.89-
  - postoperative (postprocedural) — *see* Complication, postprocedural, hemorrhage
  - retroperitoneal (nontraumatic) K66.1
    - traumatic S36.892
  - scrotum, superficial S3Ø.22
    - birth injury P15.5
  - seminal vesicle (nontraumatic) N5Ø.1
    - traumatic S37.892
  - spermatic cord (traumatic) S37.892
    - nontraumatic N5Ø.1
  - spinal (cord) (meninges) (*see also* Injury, spinal cord, by region)
    - newborn (birth injury) P11.5
  - spleen D73.5
    - intraoperative *see* Complications, intraoperative, hemorrhage, spleen
    - postprocedural (postoperative) *see* Complications, postprocedural, hemorrhage, spleen
  - sternocleidomastoid, birth injury P15.2
  - sternomastoid, birth injury P15.2

- **Hematoma** — *continued*
  - subarachnoid (traumatic) — *see* Injury, intracranial, subarachnoid hemorrhage
    - newborn (nontraumatic) P52.5
      - due to birth injury P1Ø.3
    - nontraumatic — *see* Hemorrhage, intracranial, subarachnoid
  - subdural (traumatic) — *see* Injury, intracranial, subdural hemorrhage
    - newborn (localized) P52.8
      - birth injury P1Ø.Ø
    - nontraumatic — *see* Hemorrhage, intracranial, subdural
  - superficial, newborn P54.5
  - testis (nontraumatic) N5Ø.1
    - birth injury P15.5
  - tunica vaginalis (nontraumatic) N5Ø.1
  - umbilical cord, complicating delivery O69.5
  - uterine ligament (broad) (nontraumatic) N83.7
    - traumatic S37.62
  - vagina (ruptured) (nontraumatic) N89.8
    - complicating delivery O71.7
  - vas deferens (nontraumatic) N5Ø.1
    - traumatic S37.892
  - vitreous — *see* Hemorrhage, vitreous
  - vulva (nontraumatic) (nonobstetric) N9Ø.89
    - complicating delivery O71.7
    - newborn (birth injury) P15.5
- **Hematometra** N85.7
  - with hematocolpos N89.7
- **Hematomyelia** (central) G95.19
  - newborn (birth injury) P11.5
  - traumatic T14.8
- **Hematomyelitis** GØ4.9Ø
- **Hematoperitoneum** — *see* Hemoperitoneum
- **Hematophobia** F4Ø.23Ø
- **Hematopneumothorax** (see Hemothorax)
- **Hematopoiesis, cyclic** D7Ø.4
- **Hematoporphyria** — *see* Porphyria
- **Hematorachis, hematorrhachis** G95.19
  - newborn (birth injury) P11.5
- **Hematosalpinx** N83.6
  - with
    - hematocolpos N89.7
    - hematometra N85.7
      - with hematocolpos N89.7
  - infectional — *see* Salpingitis
- **Hematospermia** R36.1
- **Hematothorax** (see Hemothorax)
- **Hematuria** R31.9
  - due to sulphonamide, sulfonamide — *see* Table of Drugs and Chemicals, by drug
  - benign (familial) (of childhood) (*see also* Hematuria, idiopathic)
    - essential microscopic R31.1
  - endemic (*see also* Schistosomiasis) B65.Ø
  - gross R31.Ø
  - idiopathic NØ2.9
    - with glomerular lesion
      - crescentic (diffuse) glomerulonephritis NØ2.7
      - dense deposit disease NØ2.6
      - endocapillary proliferative glomerulonephritis NØ2.4
      - focal and segmental hyalinosis or sclerosis NØ2.1
      - membranoproliferative (diffuse) NØ2.5
      - membranous (diffuse) NØ2.2
      - mesangial proliferative (diffuse) NØ2.3
      - mesangiocapillary (diffuse) NØ2.5
      - minor abnormality NØ2.Ø
      - proliferative NEC NØ2.8
      - specified pathology NEC NØ2.8
  - intermittent — *see* Hematuria, idiopathic
  - malarial B5Ø.8
  - microscopic NEC R31.2
    - benign essential R31.1
  - paroxysmal (*see also* Hematuria, idiopathic)
    - nocturnal D59.5
  - persistent — *see* Hematuria, idiopathic
  - recurrent — *see* Hematuria, idiopathic
  - tropical (*see also* Schistosomiasis) B65.Ø
  - tuberculous A18.13

- **Hemeralopia** (day blindness) H53.11
  - vitamin A deficiency E5Ø.5
- **Hemi-akinesia** R41.4
- **Hemianalgesia** R2Ø.Ø
- **Hemianencephaly** Q00.0
- **Hemianesthesia** R2Ø.Ø
- **Hemianopia, hemianopsia** (heteronymous) H53.47
  - homonymous H53.46-
  - syphilitic A52.71
- **Hemiathetosis** R25.8
- **Hemiatrophy** R68.89
  - cerebellar G31.9
  - face, facial, progressive (Romberg) G51.8
  - tongue K14.8
- **Hemiballism**(us) G25.5
- **Hemicardia** Q24.8
- **Hemicephalus, hemicephaly** QØØ.Ø
- **Hemichorea** G25.5
- **Hemicolitis, left** — *see* Colitis, left sided
- **Hemicrania**
  - congenital malformation QØØ.Ø
  - continua G44.51
  - meaning migraine (*see also* Migraine) G43.9Ø9
  - paroxysmal G44.Ø39
    - chronic G44.Ø49
      - intractable G44.Ø41
      - not intractable G44.Ø49
    - episodic G44.Ø39
      - intractable G44.Ø31
      - not intractable G44.Ø39
    - intractable G44.Ø31
    - not intractable G44.Ø39
- **Hemidystrophy** — *see* Hemiatrophy
- **Hemiectromelia** Q73.8
- **Hemihypalgesia** R2Ø.8
- **Hemihypesthesia** R2Ø.1
- **Hemi-inattention** R41.4
- **Hemimelia** Q73.8
  - lower limb — *see* Defect, reduction, lower limb, specified type NEC
  - upper limb — *see* Defect, reduction, upper limb, specified type NEC
- **Hemiparalysis** — *see* Hemiplegia
- **Hemiparesis** — *see* Hemiplegia
- **Hemiparesthesia** R2Ø.2
- **Hemiparkinsonism** G2Ø
- **Hemiplegia** G81.9-
  - alternans facialis G83.89
  - ascending NEC G81.9Ø
    - spinal G95.89
  - congenital (cerebral) G8Ø.8
    - spastic G8Ø.2
  - embolic (current episode) I63.4-
  - flaccid G81.Ø-
  - following
    - cerebrovascular disease I69.959
      - cerebral infarction I69.35-
      - intracerebral hemorrhage I69.15-
      - nontraumatic intracranial hemorrhage NEC I69.25-
      - specified disease NEC I69.85-
      - stroke NOS I69.35-
      - subarachnoid hemorrhage I69.Ø5-
  - hysterical F44.4
  - newborn NEC P91.8
    - birth injury P11.9
  - spastic G81.1-
    - congenital G8Ø.2
  - thrombotic (current episode) I63.3
- **Hemisection, spinal cord** — *see* Injury, spinal cord, by region
- **Hemispasm** (facial) R25.2
- **Hemisporosis** B48.8
- **Hemitremor** R25.1
- **Hemivertebra** Q76.49
  - failure of segmentation with scoliosis Q76.3
  - fusion with scoliosis Q76.3
- **Hemochromatosis** E83.119
  - with refractory anemia D46.1
  - due to repeated red blood cell transfusion E83.111
  - hereditary (primary) E83.11Ø
  - primary E83.11Ø

- **Hemochromatosis** — *continued*
  - specified NEC E83.118
- **Hemoglobin** (*see also* condition)
  - abnormal (disease) — *see* Disease, hemoglobin
  - AS genotype D57.3
  - Constant Spring D58.2
  - E-beta thalassemia D56.5
  - fetal, hereditary persistence (HPFH) D56.4
  - H Constant Spring D56.Ø
  - low NOS D64.9
  - S (Hb S), heterozygous D57.3
- **Hemoglobinemia** D59.9
  - due to blood transfusion T8Ø.89
  - paroxysmal D59.6
    - nocturnal D59.5
- **Hemoglobinopathy** (mixed) D58.2
  - with thalassemia D56.8
  - sickle-cell D57.1
    - with thalassemia D57.4Ø
      - with crisis (vasoocclusive pain) D57.419
        - with
          - acute chest syndrome D57.411
          - splenic sequestration D57.412
      - without crisis D57.4Ø
- **Hemoglobinuria** R82.3
  - with anemia, hemolytic, acquired (chronic) NEC D59.6
  - cold (agglutinin) (paroxysmal) (with Raynaud's syndrome) D59.6
  - due to exertion or hemolysis NEC D59.6
  - intermittent D59.6
  - malarial B5Ø.8
  - march D59.6
  - nocturnal (paroxysmal) D59.5
  - paroxysmal (cold) D59.6
    - nocturnal D59.5
- **Hemolymphangioma** D18.1
- **Hemolysis**
  - intravascular
    - with
      - abortion — *see* Abortion, by type, complicated by, hemorrhage
      - ectopic or molar pregnancy OØ8.1
      - hemorrhage
        - antepartum — *see* Hemorrhage, antepartum, with coagulation defect
        - intrapartum (*see also* Hemorrhage, complicating, delivery) O67.Ø
    - postpartum O72.3
  - neonatal (excessive) P58.9
    - specified NEC P58.8
- **Hemolytic** — *see* condition
- **Hemopericardium** I31.2
  - following acute myocardial infarction (current complication) I23.Ø
  - newborn P54.8
  - traumatic — *see* Injury, heart, with hemopericardium
- **Hemoperitoneum** K66.1
  - infectional K65.9
  - traumatic S36.899
    - with open wound — *see* Wound, open, with penetration into peritoneal cavity
- **Hemophilia** (classical) (familial) (hereditary) D66
  - A D66
  - acquired D68.311
  - autoimmune D68.311
  - B D67
  - C D68.1
  - calcipriva (*see also* Defect, coagulation) D68.4
  - nonfamilial (*see also* Defect, coagulation) D68.4
  - secondary D68.311
  - vascular D68.Ø
- **Hemophthalmos** H44.81-
- **Hemopneumothorax** (*see also* Hemothorax)
  - traumatic S27.2
- **Hemoptysis** RØ4.2
  - newborn P26.9
  - tuberculous — *see* Tuberculosis, pulmonary
- **Hemorrhage, hemorrhagic** (concealed) R58
  - abdomen R58
  - accidental antepartum — *see* Hemorrhage, antepartum
  - acute idiopathic pulmonary, in infants RØ4.81
  - adenoid J35.8
  - adrenal (capsule) (gland) E27.49
    - medulla E27.8
    - newborn P54.4
  - after delivery — *see* Hemorrhage, postpartum
  - alveolar
    - lung, newborn P26.8
    - process KØ8.8
  - alveolus KØ8.8
  - amputation stump (surgical) T87.89
  - anemia (chronic) D5Ø.Ø
    - acute D62
  - antepartum (with) O46.9Ø
    - with coagulation defect O46.ØØ-
      - afibrinogenemia O46.Ø1-
      - disseminated intravascular coagulation O46.Ø2-
      - hypofibrinogenemia O46.Ø1-
      - specified defect NEC O46.Ø9-
    - before 2Ø weeks gestation O2Ø.9
      - specified type NEC O2Ø.8
      - threatened abortion O2Ø.Ø
    - due to
      - abruptio placenta (*see also* Abruptio placentae) O45.9-
      - leiomyoma, uterus — *see* Hemorrhage, antepartum, specified cause NEC
      - placenta previa O44.1-
    - specified cause NEC — *see* subcategory O46.8X-
  - anus (sphincter) K62.5
  - apoplexy (stroke) — *see* Hemorrhage, intracranial, intracerebral
  - arachnoid — *see* Hemorrhage, intracranial, subarachnoid
  - artery R58
    - brain — *see* Hemorrhage, intracranial, intracerebral
  - basilar (ganglion) I61.Ø
  - bladder N32.89
  - bowel K92.2
    - newborn P54.3
  - brain (miliary) (nontraumatic) — *see* Hemorrhage, intracranial, intracerebral
    - due to
      - birth injury P1Ø.1
      - syphilis A52.Ø5
    - epidural or extradural (traumatic) — *see* Injury, intracranial, epidural hemorrhage
    - newborn P52.4
      - birth injury P1Ø.1
    - subarachnoid — *see* Hemorrhage, intracranial, subarachnoid
    - subdural — *see* Hemorrhage, intracranial, subdural
  - brainstem (nontraumatic) I61.3
    - traumatic SØ6.38-
  - breast N64.59
  - bronchial tube — *see* Hemorrhage, lung
  - bronchopulmonary — *see* Hemorrhage, lung
  - bronchus — *see* Hemorrhage, lung
  - bulbar I61.5
  - capillary I78.8
    - primary D69.8
  - cecum K92.2
  - cerebellar, cerebellum (nontraumatic) I61.4
    - newborn P52.6
    - traumatic SØ6.37-
  - cerebral, cerebrum (*see also* Hemorrhage, intracranial, intracerebral)
    - newborn (anoxic) P52.4
      - birth injury P1Ø.1
    - lobe I61.1
  - cerebromeningeal I61.8
  - cerebrospinal — *see* Hemorrhage, intracranial, intracerebral
  - cervix (uteri) (stump) NEC N88.8
  - chamber, anterior (eye) — *see* Hyphema
  - childbirth — *see* Hemorrhage, complicating, delivery
  - choroid H31.3Ø-
    - expulsive H31.31-
  - ciliary body — *see* Hyphema
  - cochlea — *see* subcategory H83.8
  - colon K92.2
  - complicating
    - abortion — *see* Abortion, by type, complicated by, hemorrhage
    - delivery O67.9
      - associated with coagulation defect (afibrinogenemia) (DIC) (hyperfibrinolysis) O67.Ø
      - specified cause NEC O67.8
    - surgical procedure — *see* Hemorrhage, intraoperative
  - conjunctiva H11.3-
    - newborn P54.8
  - cord, newborn (stump) P51.9
  - corpus luteum (ruptured) cyst N83.1
  - cortical (brain) I61.1
  - cranial — *see* Hemorrhage, intracranial
  - cutaneous R23.3
    - due to autosensitivity, erythrocyte D69.2
    - newborn P54.5
  - delayed
    - following ectopic or molar pregnancy OØ8.1
    - postpartum O72.2
  - diathesis (familial) D69.9
  - disease D69.9
    - newborn P53
    - specified type NEC D69.8
  - due to or associated with
    - afibrinogenemia or other coagulation defect (conditions in categories D65D69)
      - antepartum — *see* Hemorrhage, antepartum, with coagulation defect
      - intrapartum O67.Ø
    - dental implant M27.61
    - device, implant or graft (*see also* Complications, by site and type, specified NEC) T85.83
      - arterial graft NEC T82.838
      - breast T85.83
      - catheter NEC T85.83
        - dialysis (renal) T82.838
          - intraperitoneal T85.83
        - infusion NEC T82.838
          - spinal (epidural) (subdural) T85.83
        - urinary (indwelling) T83.83
      - electronic (electrode) (pulse generator) (stimulator)
        - bone T84.83
        - cardiac T82.837
        - nervous system (brain) (peripheral nerve) (spinal) T85.83
        - urinary T83.83
      - fixation, internal (orthopedic) NEC T84.83
      - gastrointestinal (bile duct) (esophagus) T85.83
      - genital NEC T83.83
      - heart NEC T82.837
      - joint prosthesis T84.83
      - ocular (corneal graft) (orbital implant) NEC T85.83
      - orthopedic NEC T84.83
        - bone graft T86.838
      - specified NEC T85.83
      - urinary NEC T83.83
      - vascular NEC T82.838
      - ventricular intracranial shunt T85.83
  - duodenum, duodenal K92.2
    - ulcer — *see* Ulcer, duodenum, with hemorrhage
  - dura mater — *see* Hemorrhage, intracranial, subdural
  - endotracheal — *see* Hemorrhage, lung
  - epicranial subaponeurotic (massive), birth injury P12.2
  - epidural (traumatic) (*see also* Injury, intracranial, epidural hemorrhage)
    - nontraumatic I62.1

- **Hemorrhage, hemorrhagic** — *continued*
  - esophagus K22.8
    - varix I85.Ø1
      - secondary I85.11
  - excessive, following ectopic gestation (subsequent episode) OØ8.1
  - extradural (traumatic) — *see* Injury, intracranial, epidural hemorrhage
    - birth injury P1Ø.8
    - newborn (anoxic) (nontraumatic) P52.8
    - nontraumatic I62.1
  - eye NEC H57.8
    - fundus — *see* Hemorrhage, retina
    - lid — *see* Disorder, eyelid, specified type NEC
  - fallopian tube N83.6
  - fibrinogenolysis — *see* Fibrinolysis
  - fibrinolytic (acquired) — *see* Fibrinolysis
  - from
    - ear (nontraumatic) — *see* Otorrhagia
    - tracheostomy stoma J95.Ø1
  - fundus, eye — *see* Hemorrhage, retina
  - funis — *see* Hemorrhage, umbilicus, cord
  - gastric — *see* Hemorrhage, stomach
  - gastroenteric K92.2
    - newborn P54.3
  - gastrointestinal (tract) K92.2
    - newborn P54.3
  - genital organ, male N5Ø.1
  - genitourinary (tract) NOS R31.9
  - gingiva KØ6.8
  - globe (eye) — *see* Hemophthalmos
  - graafian follicle cyst (ruptured) N83.Ø
  - gum KØ6.8
  - heart I51.89
  - hypopharyngeal (throat) RØ4.1
  - intermenstrual (regular) N92.3
    - irregular N92.1
  - internal (organs) NEC R58
    - capsule I61.Ø
    - ear — *see* subcategory H83.8
    - newborn P54.8
  - intestine K92.2
    - newborn P54.3
  - intra-abdominal R58
  - intra-alveolar (lung), newborn P26.8
  - intracerebral (nontraumatic) — *see* Hemorrhage, intracranial, intracerebral
  - intracranial (nontraumatic) I62.9
    - birth injury P1Ø.9
    - epidural, nontraumatic I62.1
    - extradural, nontraumatic I62.1
    - newborn P52.9
      - specified NEC P52.8
    - intracerebral (nontraumatic) (in) I61.9
      - brain stem I61.3
      - cerebellum I61.4
      - newborn P52.4
        - birth injury P1Ø.1
      - hemisphere I61.2
        - cortical (superficial) I61.1
        - subcortical (deep) I61.Ø
      - intraoperative
        - during a nervous system procedure G97.31
        - during other procedure G97.32
      - intraventricular I61.5
      - multiple localized I61.6
      - postprocedural
        - during a nervous system procedure G97.51
        - during other procedure G97.52
      - specified NEC I61.8
      - superficial I61.1
      - traumatic (diffuse) — *see* Injury, intracranial, diffuse
        - focal — *see* Injury, intracranial, focal
    - subarachnoid (nontraumatic) (from) I6Ø.9
      - newborn P52.5
        - birth injury P1Ø.3
      - intracranial (cerebral) artery I6Ø.7
        - anterior communicating I6Ø.2-
        - basilar I6Ø.4
        - carotid siphon and bifurcation I6Ø.Ø-

- **Hemorrhage, hemorrhagic** — *continued*
  - intracranial (nontraumatic)— *continued*
    - subarachnoid (nontraumatic) (from)— *continued*
      - intracranial (cerebral) artery — *continued*
        - communicating I6Ø.7
          - anterior I6Ø.2-
          - posterior I6Ø.3-
        - middle cerebral I6Ø.1-
        - posterior communicating I6Ø.3-
        - specified artery NEC I6Ø.6
        - vertebral I6Ø.5-
      - specified NEC I6Ø.8
      - traumatic SØ6.6X-
    - subdural (nontraumatic) I62.ØØ
      - acute I62.Ø1
      - birth injury P1Ø.Ø
      - chronic I62.Ø3
      - newborn (anoxic) (hypoxic) P52.8
        - birth injury P1Ø.Ø
      - spinal G95.19
      - subacute I62.Ø2
      - traumatic — *see* Injury, intracranial, subdural hemorrhage
    - traumatic — *see* Injury, intracranial, focal brain injury
  - intramedullary NEC G95.19
  - intraocular — *see* Hemophthalmos
  - intraoperative, intraprocedural — *see* Complication, hemorrhage (hematoma), intraoperative (intraprocedural), by site
  - intrapartum — *see* Hemorrhage, complicating, delivery
  - intrapelvic
    - female N94.89
    - male K66.1
  - intraperitoneal K66.1
  - intrapontine I61.3
  - intraprocedural — *see* Complication, hemorrhage (hematoma), intraoperative (intraprocedural), by site
  - intrauterine N85.7
    - complicating delivery (*see also* Hemorrhage, complicating, delivery) O67.9
    - postpartum — *see* Hemorrhage, postpartum
  - intraventricular I61.5
    - newborn (nontraumatic) (*see also* Newborn, affected by, hemorrhage) P52.3
      - due to birth injury P1Ø.2
      - grade
        - 1 P52.Ø
        - 2 P52.1
        - 3 P52.21
        - 4 P52.22
  - intravesical N32.89
  - iris (postinfectional) (postinflammatory) (toxic) — *see* Hyphema
  - joint (nontraumatic) — *see* Hemarthrosis
  - kidney N28.89
  - knee (joint) (nontraumatic) — *see* Hemarthrosis, knee
  - labyrinth — *see* subcategory H83.8
  - lenticular striate artery I61.Ø
  - ligature, vessel — *see* Hemorrhage, postoperative
  - liver K76.89
  - lung RØ4.89
    - newborn P26.9
      - massive P26.1
      - specified NEC P26.8
    - tuberculous — *see* Tuberculosis, pulmonary
  - massive umbilical, newborn P51.Ø
  - mediastinum — *see* Hemorrhage, lung
  - medulla I61.3
  - membrane (brain) I6Ø.8
    - spinal cord — *see* Hemorrhage, spinal cord
  - meninges, meningeal (brain) (middle) I6Ø.8
    - spinal cord — *see* Hemorrhage, spinal cord
  - mesentery K66.1
  - metritis — *see* Endometritis
  - mouth K13.79
  - mucous membrane NEC R58
    - newborn P54.8
  - muscle M62.89
  - nail (subungual) L6Ø.8

- **Hemorrhage, hemorrhagic** — *continued*
  - nasal turbinate RØ4.Ø
    - newborn P54.8
  - navel, newborn P51.9
  - newborn P54.9
    - specified NEC P54.8
  - nipple N64.59
  - nose RØ4.Ø
    - newborn P54.8
  - omentum K66.1
  - optic nerve (sheath) H47.Ø2-
  - orbit, orbital HØ5.23-
  - ovary NEC N83.8
  - oviduct N83.6
  - pancreas K86.8
  - parathyroid (gland) (spontaneous) E21.4
  - parturition — *see* Hemorrhage, complicating, delivery
  - penis N48.89
  - pericardium, pericarditis I31.2
  - peritoneum, peritoneal K66.1
  - peritonsillar tissue J35.8
    - due to infection J36
  - petechial R23.3
    - due to autosensitivity, erythrocyte D69.2
  - pituitary (gland) E23.6
  - pleura — *see* Hemorrhage, lung
  - polioencephalitis, superior E51.2
  - polymyositis — *see* Polymyositis
  - pons, pontine I61.3
  - posterior fossa (nontraumatic) I61.8
    - newborn P52.6
  - postmenopausal N95.Ø
  - postnasal RØ4.Ø
  - postoperative — *see* Complications, postprocedural, hemorrhage, by site
  - postpartum NEC (following delivery of placenta) O72.1
    - delayed or secondary O72.2
    - retained placenta O72.Ø
    - third stage O72.Ø
  - pregnancy — *see* Hemorrhage, antepartum
  - preretinal — *see* Hemorrhage, retina
  - prostate N42.1
  - puerperal — *see* Hemorrhage, postpartum
    - delayed or secondary O72.2
  - pulmonary RØ4.89
    - newborn P26.9
      - massive P26.1
      - specified NEC P26.8
    - tuberculous — *see* Tuberculosis, pulmonary
  - purpura (primary) D69.3
  - rectum (sphincter) K62.5
    - newborn P54.2
  - recurring, following initial hemorrhage at time of injury T79.2
  - renal N28.89
  - respiratory passage or tract RØ4.9
    - specified NEC RØ4.89
  - retina, retinal (vessels) H35.6-
    - diabetic — *see* Diabetes, retinal, hemorrhage
  - retroperitoneal R58
  - scalp R58
  - scrotum N5Ø.1
  - secondary (nontraumatic) R58
    - following initial hemorrhage at time of injury T79.2
  - seminal vesicle N5Ø.1
  - skin R23.3
    - newborn P54.5
  - slipped umbilical ligature P51.8
  - spermatic cord N5Ø.1
  - spinal (cord) G95.19
    - newborn (birth injury) P11.5
  - spleen D73.5
    - intraoperative — *see* Complications, intraoperative, hemorrhage, spleen
    - postprocedural — *see* Complications, postprocedural, hemorrhage, spleen
  - stomach K92.2
    - newborn P54.3
    - ulcer — *see* Ulcer, stomach, with hemorrhage

Hemorrhage, hemorrhagic — *continued*
- subarachnoid (nontraumatic) — *see* Hemorrhage, intracranial, subarachnoid
- subconjunctival (*see also* Hemorrhage, conjunctiva)
  - birth injury P15.3
- subcortical (brain) I61.Ø
- subcutaneous R23.3
- subdiaphragmatic R58
- subdural (acute) (nontraumatic) — *see* Hemorrhage, intracranial, subdural
- subependymal
  - newborn P52.Ø
    - with intraventricular extension P52.1
      - and intracerebral extension P52.22
- subhyaloid — *see* Hemorrhage, retina
- subperiosteal — *see* Disorder, bone, specified type NEC
- subretinal — *see* Hemorrhage, retina
- subtentorial — *see* Hemorrhage, intracranial, subdural
- subungual L6Ø.8
- suprarenal (capsule) (gland) E27.49
  - newborn P54.4
- tentorium (traumatic) NEC — *see* Hemorrhage, brain
  - newborn (birth injury) P1Ø.4
- testis N5Ø.1
- third stage (postpartum) O72.Ø
- thorax — *see* Hemorrhage, lung
- throat RØ4.1
- thymus (gland) E32.8
- thyroid (cyst) (gland) EØ7.89
- tongue K14.8
- tonsil J35.8
- trachea — *see* Hemorrhage, lung
- tracheobronchial RØ4.89
  - newborn P26.Ø
- traumatic—code to specific injury
  - cerebellar — *see* Hemorrhage, brain
  - intracranial — *see* Hemorrhage, brain
  - recurring or secondary (following initial hemorrhage at time of injury) T79.2
- tuberculous NEC (*see also* Tuberculosis, pulmonary) A15.Ø
- tunica vaginalis N5Ø.1
- ulcer—code by site under Ulcer, with hemorrhage K27.4
- umbilicus, umbilical
  - cord
    - after birth, newborn P51.9
    - complicating delivery O69.5
  - newborn P51.9
    - massive P51.Ø
    - slipped ligature P51.8
  - stump P51.9
- urethra (idiopathic) N36.8
- uterus, uterine (abnormal) N93.9
  - climacteric N92.4
  - complicating delivery — *see* Hemorrhage, complicating, delivery
  - dysfunctional or functional N93.8
  - intermenstrual (regular) N92.3
    - irregular N92.1
  - postmenopausal N95.Ø
  - postpartum — *see* Hemorrhage, postpartum
  - preclimacteric or premenopausal N92.4
  - prepubertal N93.8
  - pubertal N92.2
- vagina (abnormal) N93.9
  - newborn P54.6
- vas deferens N5Ø.1
- vasa previa O69.4
- ventricular I61.5
- vesical N32.89
- viscera NEC R58
  - newborn P54.8
- vitreous (humor) (intraocular) H43.1-
- vulva N9Ø.89

Hemorrhoids (bleeding) (without mention of degree) K64.9
- 1st degree (grade/stage I) (without prolapse outside of anal canal) K64.Ø
- 2nd degree (grade/stage II) (that prolapse with straining but retract spontaneously) K64.1

Hemorrhoids — *continued*
- 3rd degree (grade/stage III) (that prolapse with straining and require manual replacement back inside anal canal) K64.2
- 4th degree (grade/stage IV) (with prolapsed tissue that cannot be manually replaced) K64.3
- complicating
  - pregnancy O22.4
  - puerperium O87.2
- external K64.4
  - with
    - thrombosis K64.5
- internal (without mention of degree) K64.8
- prolapsed K64.8
- skin tags
  - anus K64.4
  - residual K64.4
- specified NEC K64.8
- strangulated (*see also* Hemorrhoids, by degree) K64.8
- thrombosed (*see also* Hemorrhoids, by degree) K64.5
- ulcerated (*see also* Hemorrhoids, by degree) K64.8

Hemosalpinx N83.6
- with
  - hematocolpos N89.7
  - hematometra N85.7
    - with hematocolpos N89.7

Hemosiderosis (dietary) E83.19
- pulmonary, idiopathic E83.1 *[J84.03]*
- transfusion T8Ø.89

Hemothorax (bacterial) (nontuberculous) J94.2
- newborn P54.8
- traumatic S27.1
  - with pneumothorax S27.2
- tuberculous NEC A15.6

Henoch(-Schönlein) disease or syndrome (purpura) D69.Ø

Henpue, henpuye A66.6

Hepar lobatum (syphilitic) A52.74

Hepatalgia K76.89

Hepatitis K75.9
- acute B17.9
  - with coma K72.Ø1
  - with hepatic failure — *see* Failure, hepatic
  - alcoholic — *see* Hepatitis, alcoholic
  - infectious B15.9
    - with hepatic coma B15.Ø
  - viral B17.9
- alcoholic (acute) (chronic) K7Ø.1Ø
  - with ascites K7Ø.11
- amebic — *see* Abscess, liver, amebic
- anicteric (viral) — *see* Hepatitis, viral
- antigen-associated (HAA) — *see* Hepatitis, B
- Australia-antigen (positive) — *see* Hepatitis, B
- autoimmune K75.4
- B B19.1Ø
  - with hepatic coma B19.11
  - acute B16.9
    - with
      - delta-agent (coinfection) (without hepatic coma) B16.1
        - with hepatic coma B16.Ø
      - hepatic coma (without delta-agent coinfection) B16.2
  - chronic B18.1
    - with delta-agent B18.Ø
- bacterial NEC K75.89
- C (viral) B19.2Ø
  - with hepatic coma B19.21
  - acute B17.1Ø
    - with hepatic coma B17.11
  - chronic B18.2
- catarrhal (acute) B15.9
  - with hepatic coma B15.Ø
- cholangiolitic K75.89
- cholestatic K75.89
- chronic K73.9
  - active NEC K73.2
  - lobular NEC K73.1
  - persistent NEC K73.Ø

Hepatitis — *continued*
- chronic — *continued*
  - specified NEC K73.8
- cytomegaloviral B25.1
- due to ethanol (acute) (chronic) — *see* Hepatitis, alcoholic
- epidemic B15.9
  - with hepatic coma B15.Ø
- fulminant NEC (viral) — *see* Hepatitis, viral
- granulomatous NEC K75.3
- herpesviral BØØ.81
- history of
  - B Z86.19
  - C Z86.19
- homologous serum — *see* Hepatitis, viral, type B
- in (due to)
  - mumps B26.81
  - toxoplasmosis (acquired) B58.1
    - congenital (active) P37.1 *[K77]*
- infectious, infective (acute) (chronic) (subacute) B15.9
  - with hepatic coma B15.Ø
- inoculation — *see* Hepatitis, viral, type B
- interstitial (chronic) K74.69
- lupoid NEC K75.4
- malignant NEC (with hepatic failure) K72.9Ø
  - with coma K72.91
- neonatal giant cell P59.29
- neonatal (idiopathic) (toxic) P59.29
- newborn P59.29
- postimmunization — *see* Hepatitis, viral, type B
- post-transfusion — *see* Hepatitis, viral, type B
- reactive, nonspecific K75.2
- serum — *see* Hepatitis, viral, type B
- specified type NEC
  - with hepatic failure — *see* Failure, hepatic
- syphilitic (late) A52.74
  - congenital (early) A5Ø.Ø8 *[K77]*
    - late A5Ø.59 *[K77]*
  - secondary A51.45
- toxic (*see also* Disease, liver, toxic) K71.6
- tuberculous A18.83
- viral, virus B19.9
  - with hepatic coma B19.Ø
  - acute B17.9
  - chronic B18.9
    - specified NEC B18.8
    - type
      - B B18.1
        - with delta-agent B18.Ø
      - C B18.2
  - congenital P35.3
  - coxsackie B33.8 *[K77]*
  - cytomegalic inclusion B25.1
  - in remission, any type—code to Hepatitis, chronic, by type
  - non-A, non-B B17.8
  - specified type NEC (with or without coma) B17.8
  - type
    - A B15.9
      - with hepatic coma B15.Ø
    - B B19.1Ø
      - with hepatic coma B19.11
      - acute B16.9
        - with
          - delta-agent (coinfection) (without hepatic coma) B16.1
            - with hepatic coma B16.Ø
          - hepatic coma (without delta-agent coinfection) B16.2
      - chronic B18.1
        - with delta-agent B18.Ø
    - C B19.2Ø
      - with hepatic coma B19.21
      - acute B17.1Ø
        - with hepatic coma B17.11
      - chronic B18.2
    - E B17.2
    - non-A, non-B B17.8

Hepatization lung (acute) — *see* Pneumonia, lobar

Hepatoblastoma C22.2

Hepatocarcinoma C22.Ø

Hepatocholangiocarcinoma C22.Ø

- **Hepatocholangioma, benign** D13.4
- **Hepatocholangitis** K75.89
- **Hepatolenticular degeneration** E83.Ø1
- **Hepatoma** (malignant) C22.Ø
  - benign D13.4
  - embryonal C22.Ø
- **Hepatomegaly** (*see also* Hypertrophy, liver)
  - with splenomegaly R16.2
  - congenital Q44.7
  - in mononucleosis
    - gammaherpesviral B27.Ø9
    - infectious specified NEC B27.89
- **Hepatoptosis** K76.89
- **Hepatorenal syndrome following labor and delivery** O9Ø.4
- **Hepatosis** K76.89
- **Hepatosplenomegaly** R16.2
  - hyperlipemic (Bürger-Grütz type) E78.3 *[K77]*
- **Hereditary** — *see* condition
- **Heredodegeneration, macular** — *see* Dystrophy, retina
- **Heredopathia atactica polyneuritiformis** G6Ø.1
- **Heredosyphilis** — *see* Syphilis, congenital
- **Herlitz' syndrome** Q81.1
- **Hermansky-Pudlak syndrome** E7Ø.331
- **Hermaphrodite, hermaphroditism** (true) Q56.Ø
  - 46,XX with streak gonads Q99.1
  - 46,XX/46,XY Q99.Ø
  - 46,XY with streak gonads Q99.1
  - chimera 46,XX/46,XY Q99.Ø
- **Hernia, hernial** (acquired) (recurrent) K46.9
  - with
    - gangrene — *see* Hernia, by site, with, gangrene
    - incarceration — *see* Hernia, by site, with, obstruction
    - irreducible — *see* Hernia, by site, with, obstruction
    - obstruction — *see* Hernia, by site, with, obstruction
    - strangulation — *see* Hernia, by site, with, obstruction
  - abdomen, abdominal K46.9
    - with
      - gangrene (and obstruction) K46.1
      - obstruction K46.Ø
    - femoral — *see* Hernia, femoral
    - incisional — *see* Hernia, incisional
    - inguinal — *see* Hernia, inguinal
    - specified site NEC K45.8
      - with
        - gangrene (and obstruction) K45.1
        - obstruction K45.Ø
    - umbilical — *see* Hernia, umbilical
    - wall — *see* Hernia, ventral
  - appendix — *see* Hernia, abdomen
  - bladder (mucosa) (sphincter)
    - congenital (female) (male) Q79.51
    - female — *see* Cystocele
    - male N32.89
  - brain, congenital — *see* Encephalocele
  - cartilage, vertebra — *see* Displacement, intervertebral disc
  - cerebral, congenital (*see also* Encephalocele)
    - endaural QØ1.8
  - ciliary body (traumatic) SØ5.2-
  - colon — *see* Hernia, abdomen
  - Cooper's — *see* Hernia, abdomen, specified site NEC
  - crural — *see* Hernia, femoral
  - diaphragm, diaphragmatic K44.9
    - with
      - gangrene (and obstruction) K44.1
      - obstruction K44.Ø
    - congenital Q79.Ø
  - direct (inguinal) — *see* Hernia, inguinal
  - diverticulum, intestine — *see* Hernia, abdomen
  - double (inguinal) — *see* Hernia, inguinal, bilateral
  - due to adhesions (with obstruction) K56.5
  - epigastric (*see also* Hernia, ventral) K43.9
  - esophageal hiatus — *see* Hernia, hiatal
  - external (inguinal) — *see* Hernia, inguinal
  - fallopian tube N83.4
  - fascia M62.89

- **Hernia, hernial**— *continued*
  - femoral K41.9Ø
    - with
      - gangrene (and obstruction) K41.4Ø
        - not specified as recurrent K41.4Ø
        - recurrent K41.41
      - obstruction K41.3Ø
        - not specified as recurrent K41.3Ø
        - recurrent K41.31
    - bilateral K41.2Ø
      - with
        - gangrene (and obstruction) K41.1Ø
          - not specified as recurrent K41.1Ø
          - recurrent K41.11
        - obstruction K41.ØØ
          - not specified as recurrent K41.ØØ
          - recurrent K41.Ø1
      - not specified as recurrent K41.2Ø
      - recurrent K41.21
    - unilateral K41.9Ø
      - with
        - gangrene (and obstruction) K41.4Ø
          - not specified as recurrent K41.4Ø
          - recurrent K41.41
        - obstruction K41.3Ø
          - not specified as recurrent K41.3Ø
          - recurrent K41.31
      - not specified as recurrent K41.9Ø
      - recurrent K41.91
    - not specified as recurrent K41.9Ø
    - recurrent K41.91
  - foramen magnum G93.5
    - congenital QØ1.8
  - funicular (umbilical) (*see also* Hernia, umbilicus)
    - spermatic (cord) — *see* Hernia, inguinal
  - gastrointestinal tract — *see* Hernia, abdomen
  - Hesselbach's — *see* Hernia, femoral, specified site NEC
  - hiatal (esophageal) (sliding) K44.9
    - with
      - gangrene (and obstruction) K44.1
      - obstruction K44.Ø
    - congenital Q4Ø.1
  - hypogastric — *see* Hernia, ventral
  - incarcerated (*see also* Hernia, by site, with obstruction)
    - with gangrene — *see* Hernia, by site, with gangrene
  - incisional K43.2
    - with
      - gangrene (and obstruction) K43.1
      - obstruction K43.Ø
  - indirect (inguinal) — *see* Hernia, inguinal
  - inguinal (direct) (external) (funicular) (indirect) (internal) (oblique) (scrotal) (sliding) K4Ø.9Ø
    - with
      - gangrene (and obstruction) K4Ø.4Ø
        - not specified as recurrent K4Ø.4Ø
        - recurrent K4Ø.41
      - obstruction K4Ø.3Ø
        - not specified as recurrent K4Ø.3Ø
        - recurrent K4Ø.31
    - not specified as recurrent K4Ø.9Ø
    - recurrent K4Ø.91
    - bilateral K4Ø.2Ø
      - with
        - gangrene (and obstruction) K4Ø.1Ø
          - not specified as recurrent K4Ø.1Ø
          - recurrent K4Ø.11
        - obstruction K4Ø.ØØ
          - not specified as recurrent K4Ø.ØØ
          - recurrent K4Ø.Ø1
      - not specified as recurrent K4Ø.2Ø
      - recurrent K4Ø.21
    - unilateral K4Ø.9Ø
      - with
        - gangrene (and obstruction) K4Ø.4Ø
          - not specified as recurrent K4Ø.4Ø
          - recurrent K4Ø.41
        - obstruction K4Ø.3Ø
          - not specified as recurrent K4Ø.3Ø
          - recurrent K4Ø.31

- **Hernia, hernial**— *continued*
  - inguinal (direct) (external) (funicular) (indirect) (internal) (oblique) (scrotal) (sliding) — *continued*
    - unilateral — *continued*
      - not specified as recurrent K4Ø.9Ø
      - recurrent K4Ø.91
  - internal (*see also* Hernia, abdomen)
    - inguinal — *see* Hernia, inguinal
  - interstitial — *see* Hernia, abdomen
  - intervertebral cartilage or disc — *see* Displacement, intervertebral disc
  - intestine, intestinal — *see* Hernia, by site
  - intra-abdominal — *see* Hernia, abdomen
  - iris (traumatic) SØ5.2-
  - irreducible (*see also* Hernia, by site, with obstruction)
    - with gangrene — *see* Hernia, by site, with gangrene
  - ischiatic — *see* Hernia, abdomen, specified site NEC
  - ischiorectal — *see* Hernia, abdomen, specified site NEC
  - lens (traumatic) SØ5.2-
  - linea (alba) (semilunaris) — *see* Hernia, ventral
  - Littre's — *see* Hernia, abdomen
  - lumbar — *see* Hernia, abdomen, specified site NEC
  - lung (subcutaneous) J98.4
  - mediastinum J98.5
  - mesenteric (internal) — *see* Hernia, abdomen
  - midline — *see* Hernia, ventral
  - muscle (sheath) M62.89
  - nucleus pulposus — *see* Displacement, intervertebral disc
  - oblique (inguinal) — *see* Hernia, inguinal
  - obstructive (*see also* Hernia, by site, with obstruction)
    - with gangrene — *see* Hernia, by site, with gangrene
  - obturator — *see* Hernia, abdomen, specified site NEC
  - omental — *see* Hernia, abdomen
  - ovary N83.4
  - oviduct N83.4
  - paraesophageal (*see also* Hernia, diaphragm
    - congenital) Q4Ø.1
  - parastomal K43.5
    - with
      - gangrene (and obstruction) K43.4
      - obstruction K43.3
  - paraumbilical — *see* Hernia, umbilicus
  - perineal — *see* Hernia, abdomen, specified site NEC
  - Petit's — *see* Hernia, abdomen, specified site NEC
  - postoperative — *see* Hernia, incisional
  - pregnant uterus — *see* Abnormal, uterus in pregnancy or childbirth
  - prevesical N32.89
  - properitoneal — *see* Hernia, abdomen, specified site NEC
  - pudendal — *see* Hernia, abdomen, specified site NEC
  - rectovaginal N81.6
  - retroperitoneal — *see* Hernia, abdomen, specified site NEC
  - Richter's — *see* Hernia, abdomen, with obstruction
  - Rieux's, Riex's — *see* Hernia, abdomen, specified site NEC
  - sac condition (adhesion) (dropsy) (inflammation) (laceration) (suppuration)—code by site under Hernia
  - sciatic — *see* Hernia, abdomen, specified site NEC
  - scrotum, scrotal — *see* Hernia, inguinal
  - sliding (inguinal) (*see also* Hernia, inguinal)
    - hiatus — *see* Hernia, hiatal
  - spigelian — *see* Hernia, ventral
  - spinal — *see* Spina bifida
  - strangulated (*see also* Hernia, by site, with obstruction)
    - with gangrene — *see* Hernia, by site, with gangrene
  - subxiphoid — *see* Hernia, ventral
  - supra-umbilicus — *see* Hernia, ventral
  - tendon — *see* Disorder, tendon, specified type NEC

NEC
 tunica vaginalis Q55.29
 umbilicus, umbilical K42.9
 with
 gangrene (and obstruction) K42.1
 obstruction K42.0
 ureter N28.89
 urethra, congenital Q64.79
 urinary meatus, congenital Q64.79
 uterus N81.4
 pregnant — *see* Abnormal, uterus in pregnancy
 or childbirth
 vaginal (anterior) (wall) — *see* Cystocele
 Velpeau's — *see* Hernia, femoral
 ventral K43.9
 with
 gangrene (and obstruction) K43.7
 obstruction K43.6
 recurrent — *see* Hernia, incisional
 incisional K43.2
 with
 gangrene (and obstruction) K43.1
 obstruction K43.0
 specified NEC K43.9
 with
 gangrene (and obstruction) K43.7
 obstruction K43.6
 vesical
 congenital (female) (male) Q79.51
 female — *see* Cystocele
 male N32.89
 vitreous (into wound) S05.2-
 into anterior chamber — *see* Prolapse, vitreous
Herniation (*see also* Hernia)
 brain (stem) G93.5
 cerebral G93.5
 mediastinum J98.5
 nucleus pulposus — *see* Displacement,
 intervertebral disc
Herpangina B08.5
Herpes, herpesvirus, herpetic B00.9
 anogenital A60.9
 perianal skin A60.1
 rectum A60.1
 urogenital tract A60.00
 cervix A60.03
 male genital organ NEC A60.02
 penis A60.01
 specified site NEC A60.09
 vagina A60.04
 vulva A60.04
 blepharitis (zoster) B02.39
 simplex B00.59
 circinatus B35.4
 bullosus L12.0
 conjunctivitis (simplex) B00.53
 zoster B02.31
 cornea B02.33
 encephalitis B00.4
 due to herpesvirus 6 B10.01
 due to herpesvirus 7 B10.09
 specified NEC B10.09
 eye (zoster) B02.30
 simplex B00.50
 eyelid (zoster) B02.39
 simplex B00.59
 facialis B00.1
 febrilis B00.1
 geniculate ganglionitis B02.21
 genital, genitalis A60.00
 female A60.09
 male A60.02
 gestational, gestationis O26.4-
 gingivostomatitis B00.2
 human B00.9
 1 — *see* Herpes, simplex
 2 — *see* Herpes, simplex
 3 — *see* Varicella
 4 — *see* Mononucleosis, Epstein-Barr (virus)
 5 — *see* Disease, cytomegalic inclusion
 (generalized)

Herpes, herpesvirus, herpetic — *continued*
 human — *continued*
 6
 encephalitis B10.01
 specified NEC B10.81
 7
 encephalitis B10.09
 specified NEC B10.82
 8 B10.89
 infection NEC B10.89
 Kaposi's sarcoma associated B10.89
 iridocyclitis (simplex) B00.51
 zoster B02.32
 iris (vesicular erythema multiforme) L51.9
 iritis (simplex) B00.51
 Kaposi's sarcoma associated B10.89
 keratitis (simplex) (dendritic) (disciform) (interstitial)
 B00.52
 zoster (interstitial) B02.33
 keratoconjunctivitis (simplex) B00.52
 zoster B02.33
 labialis B00.1
 lip B00.1
 meningitis (simplex) B00.3
 zoster B02.1
 ophthalmicus (zoster) NEC B02.30
 simplex B00.50
 penis A60.01
 perianal skin A60.1
 pharyngitis, pharyngotonsillitis B00.2
 rectum A60.1
 scrotum A60.02
 sepsis B00.7
 simplex B00.9
 complicated NEC B00.89
 congenital P35.2
 conjunctivitis B00.53
 external ear B00.1
 eyelid B00.59
 hepatitis B00.81
 keratitis (interstitial) B00.52
 myelitis B00.82
 specified complication NEC B00.89
 visceral B00.89
 stomatitis B00.2
 tonsurans B35.0
 visceral B00.89
 vulva A60.04
 whitlow B00.89
 zoster (*see also* condition) B02.9
 auricularis B02.21
 complicated NEC B02.8
 conjunctivitis B02.31
 disseminated B02.7
 encephalitis B02.0
 eye(lid) B02.39
 geniculate ganglionitis B02.21
 keratitis (interstitial) B02.33
 meningitis B02.1
 myelitis B02.24
 neuritis, neuralgia B02.29
 ophthalmicus NEC B02.30
 oticus B02.21
 polyneuropathy B02.23
 specified complication NEC B02.8
 trigeminal neuralgia B02.22
Herpesvirus (human) — *see* Herpes
Herpetophobia F40.218
Herrick's anemia — *see* Disease, sickle-cell
Hers' disease E74.09
Herter-Gee syndrome K90.0
Herxheimer's reaction R68.89
Hesitancy
 of micturition R39.11
 urinary R39.11
Hesselbach's hernia — *see* Hernia, femoral, specified
 site NEC
Heterochromia (congenital) Q13.2
 cataract — *see* Cataract, complicated
 cyclitis (Fuchs) — *see* Cyclitis, Fuchs' heterochromic
 hair L67.1
 iritis — *see* Cyclitis, Fuchs' heterochromic

Heterochromia (congenital) — *continued*
 retained metallic foreign body (nonmagnetic) — *see*
 Foreign body, intraocular, old, retained
 magnetic — *see* Foreign body, intraocular, old,
 retained, magnetic
 uveitis — *see* Cyclitis, Fuchs' heterochromic
Heterophoria — *see* Strabismus, heterophoria
Heterophyes, heterophyiasis (small intestine) B66.8
Heterotopia, heterotopic (*see also* Malposition,
 congenital)
 cerebralis Q04.8
Heterotropia — *see* Strabismus
Heubner-Herter disease K90.0
Hexadactylism Q69.9
HGSIL
 (cytology finding) (high grade squamous
 intraepithelial lesion on cytologic smear) (Pap
 smear finding)
 anus R85.613
 cervix R87.613
 biopsy (histology) finding—code to CIN II or CIN
 III
 vagina R87.623
 biopsy (histology) finding—code to VAIN II or
 VAIN III
Hibernoma — *see* Lipoma
Hiccup, hiccough R06.6
 epidemic B33.0
 psychogenic F45.8
Hidden penis (congenital) Q55.64
 acquired N48.83
Hidradenitis (axillaris) (suppurative) L73.2
Hidradenoma (nodular) (*see also* Neoplasm, skin,
 benign)
 clear cell — *see* Neoplasm, skin, benign
 papillary — *see* Neoplasm, skin, benign
Hidrocystoma — *see* Neoplasm, skin, benign
High
 altitude effects T70.20
 anoxia T70.29
 on
 ears T70.0
 sinuses T70.1
 polycythemia D75.1
 arch
 foot Q66.7
 palate, congenital Q38.5
 arterial tension — *see* Hypertension
 basal metabolic rate R94.8
 blood pressure (*see also* Hypertension)
 borderline R03.0
 reading (incidental) (isolated) (nonspecific),
 without diagnosis of hypertension R03.0
 cholesterol E78.0
 with high triglycerides E78.2
 diaphragm (congenital) Q79.1
 expressed emotional level within family Z63.8
 head at term O32.4
 palate, congenital Q38.5
 risk
 infant NEC Z76.2
 sexual behavior (heterosexual) Z72.51
 bisexual Z72.53
 homosexual Z72.52
 temperature (of unknown origin) R50.9
 thoracic rib Q76.6
 triglycerides E78.1
 with high cholesterol E78.2
Hildenbrand's disease A75.0
Hilum — *see* condition
Hip— *see* condition
Hippel's disease Q85.8
Hippophobia F40.218
Hippus H57.09
Hirschsprung's disease or megacolon Q43.1
Hirsutism, hirsuties L68.0
Hirudiniasis
 external B88.3
 internal B83.4
Hiss-Russell dysentery A03.1
Histidinemia, histidinuria E70.41

Index Histiocytoma—History

DRAFT

- **History**— *continued*
  - personal (of)— *continued*
    - disease or disorder (of) — *continued*
      - digestive system— *continued*
        - specified condition NEC Z87.19
      - ear Z86.69
      - endocrine Z86.39
        - diabetic foot ulcer Z86.31
        - gestational diabetes Z86.32
        - specified type NEC Z86.39
      - eye Z86.69
      - genital system (track) system NEC
        - female Z87.42
        - male Z87.438
      - hematological Z86.2
      - Hodgkin Z85.71
      - immune mechanism Z86.2
      - infectious Z86.19
        - malaria Z86.13
        - methicillin resistant Staphylococcus aureus (MRSA) Z86.14
        - poliomyelitis Z86.12
        - specified NEC Z86.19
        - tuberculosis Z86.11
      - mental NEC Z86.59
      - metabolic Z86.39
        - diabetic foot ulcer Z86.31
        - gestational diabetes Z86.32
        - specified type NEC Z86.39
      - musculoskeletal NEC Z87.39
      - nervous system Z86.69
      - nutritional Z86.39
      - parasitic Z86.19
      - respiratory system NEC Z87.Ø9
      - sense organs Z86.69
      - skin Z87.2
      - specified site or type NEC Z87.898
      - subcutaneous tissue Z87.2
      - trophoblastic Z87.59
      - urinary system NEC Z87.448
    - drug dependence — *see* Dependence, drug, by type, in remission
    - drug therapy
      - antineoplastic chemotherapy Z92.21
      - estrogen Z92.23
      - immunosupression Z92.25
      - inhaled steroids Z92.24Ø
      - monoclonal drug Z92.22
      - specified NEC Z92.29
      - steroid Z92.241
      - systemic steroids Z92.241
    - dysplasia
      - cervical Z87.41Ø
      - prostatic Z87.43Ø
      - vaginal Z87.411
      - vulvar Z87.412
    - embolism (venous) Z86.718
      - pulmonary Z86.711
    - encephalitis Z86.61
    - estrogen therapy Z92.23
    - extracorporeal membrane oxygenation (ECMO) Z92.81
    - failed moderate sedation Z92.83
    - failed conscious sedation Z92.83
    - fall, falling Z91.81
    - fracture (healed)
      - fatigue Z87.312
      - fragility Z87.31Ø
      - osteoporosis Z87.31Ø
      - pathological NEC Z87.311
      - stress Z87.312
      - traumatic Z87.81
    - gestational diabetes Z86.32
    - hepatitis
      - B Z86.19
      - C Z86.19
    - Hodgkin disease Z85.71
    - hyperthermia, malignant Z88.4
    - hypospadias (corrected) Z87.71Ø
    - hysterectomy Z9Ø.71Ø
    - immunosupression therapy Z92.25
    - in situ neoplasm
      - breast Z86.ØØØ

- **History**— *continued*
  - personal (of)— *continued*
    - in situ neoplasm — *continued*
      - cervix uteri Z86.ØØ1
      - specified NEC Z86.ØØ8
    - infection NEC Z86.19
      - central nervous system Z86.61
      - methicillin resistant Staphylococcus aureus (MRSA) Z86.14
      - urinary (recurrent) (tract) Z87.44Ø
    - injury NEC Z87.828
    - in utero procedure during pregnancy Z98.87Ø
    - in utero procedure while a fetus Z98.871
    - irradiation Z92.3
    - kidney stones Z87.442
    - leukemia Z85.6
    - lymphoma (non-Hodgkin) Z85.72
    - malignant melanoma (skin) Z85.82Ø
    - malignant neoplasm (of) Z85.9
      - accessory sinuses Z85.22
      - anus NEC Z85.Ø48
        - carcinoid Z85.Ø4Ø
      - bladder Z85.51
      - bone Z85.83Ø
      - brain Z85.841
      - breast Z85.3
      - bronchus NEC Z85.118
        - carcinoid Z85.11Ø
      - carcinoid — *see* History, personal (of), malignant neoplasm, by site, carcinioid
      - cervix Z85.41
      - colon NEC Z85.Ø38
        - carcinoid Z85.Ø3Ø
      - digestive organ Z85.ØØ
        - specified NEC Z85.Ø9
      - endocrine gland NEC Z85.858
      - epididymis Z85.48
      - esophagus Z85.Ø1
      - eye Z85.84Ø
      - gastrointestinal tract — *see* History, malignant neoplasm, digestive organ
      - genital organ
        - female Z85.4Ø
          - specified NEC Z85.44
        - male Z85.45
          - specified NEC Z85.49
      - hematopoietic NEC Z85.79
      - intrathoracic organ Z85.2Ø
      - kidney NEC Z85.528
        - carcinoid Z85.52Ø
      - large intestine NEC Z85.Ø38
        - carcinoid Z85.Ø3Ø
      - larynx Z85.21
      - liver Z85.Ø5
      - lung NEC Z85.118
        - carcinoid Z85.11Ø
      - mediastinum Z85.29
      - Merkel cell Z85.821
      - Methicillin resistant Staphylococcus aureus (MRSA) Z86.14
      - middle ear Z85.22
      - nasal cavities Z85.22
      - nervous system NEC Z85.848
      - oral cavity Z85.819
        - specified site NEC Z85.818
      - ovary Z85.43
      - pancreas Z85.Ø7
      - pharynx Z85.819
        - specified site NEC Z85.818
      - pelvis Z85.53
      - pleura Z85.29
      - prostate Z85.46
      - rectosigmoid junction NEC Z85.Ø48
        - carcinoid Z85.Ø4Ø
      - rectum NEC Z85.Ø48
        - carcinoid Z85.Ø4Ø
      - respiratory organ Z85.2Ø
      - sinuses, accessory Z85.22
      - skin NEC Z85.828
        - melanoma Z85.82Ø
        - Merkel cell Z85.821
      - small intestine NEC Z85.Ø68
        - carcinoid Z85.Ø6Ø

- **History**— *continued*
  - personal (of)— *continued*
    - malignant neoplasm (of)— *continued*
      - soft tissue Z85.831
      - specified site NEC Z85.89
      - stomach NEC Z85.Ø28
        - carcinoid Z85.Ø2Ø
      - testis Z85.47
      - thymus NEC Z85.238
        - carcinoid Z85.23Ø
      - thyroid Z85.85Ø
      - tongue Z85.81Ø
      - trachea Z85.12
      - urinary organ or tract Z85.5Ø
        - specified NEC Z85.59
      - uterus Z85.42
    - maltreatment Z91.89
    - medical treatment NEC Z92.89
    - melanoma (malignant) (skin) Z85.82Ø
    - meningitis Z86.61
    - mental disorder Z86.59
    - Merkel cell carcinoma (skin) Z85.821
    - methicillin resistant Staphylococcus aureus (MRSA) Z86.14
    - military deployment Z91.82
    - military war, peacekeeping and humanitarian deployment (current or past conflict) Z91.82
    - myocardial infarction (old) I25.2
    - neglect (in)
      - adult Z91.412
      - childhood Z62.812
    - neoplasm
      - benign Z86.Ø18
        - brain Z86.Ø11
        - colon polyp Z86.Ø1Ø
      - in situ
        - breast Z86.ØØØ
        - cervix uteri Z86.ØØ1
        - specified NEC Z86.ØØ8
      - malignant — *see* History of, malignant neoplasm
      - uncertain behavior Z86.Ø3
    - nephrotic syndrome Z87.441
    - nicotine dependence Z87.891
    - noncompliance with medical treatment or regimen — *see* Noncompliance
    - nutritional deficiency Z86.39
    - obstetric complications Z87.59
      - childbirth Z87.59
      - pregnancy Z87.59
      - pre-term labor Z87.51
      - puerperium Z87.59
    - osteoporosis fractures Z87.31
    - parasuicide (attempt) Z91.5
    - physical trauma NEC Z87.828
      - self-harm or suicide attempt Z91.5
    - poisoning NEC Z91.89
      - self-harm or suicide attempt Z91.5
    - poor personal hygiene Z91.89
    - pneumonia (recurrent) Z87.Ø1
    - preterm labor Z87.51
    - prolonged reversible ischemic neurologic deficit (PRIND) Z86.73
    - procedure during pregnancy Z98.87Ø
    - procedure while a fetus Z98.871
    - prostatic dysplasia Z87.43Ø
    - psychological
      - abuse
        - adult Z91.411
        - child Z62.811
      - trauma, specified NEC Z91.49
    - radiation therapy Z92.3
    - removal
      - implant
        - breast Z98.86
    - renal calculi Z87.442
    - respiratory condition NEC Z87.Ø9
    - retained foreign body fully removed Z87.821
    - risk factors NEC Z91.89
    - self-harm Z91.5
    - self-poisoning attempt Z91.5
    - sex reassignment Z87.89Ø

- **Hypercorticosteronism** E24.2
  - correct substance properly administered — *see* Table of Drugs and Chemicals, by drug, adverse effect
  - overdose or wrong substance given or taken — *see* Table of Drugs and Chemicals, by drug, poisoning
- **Hypercortisonism** E24.2
  - correct substance properly administered — *see* Table of Drugs and Chemicals, by drug, adverse effect
  - overdose or wrong substance given or taken — *see* Table of Drugs and Chemicals, by drug, poisoning
- **Hyperekplexia** Q89.8
- **Hyperelectrolytemia** E87.8
- **Hyperemesis** R11.1Ø
  - with nausea R11.2
  - gravidarum (mild) O21.Ø
    - with
      - carbohydrate depletion O21.1
      - dehydration O21.1
      - electrolyte imbalance O21.1
      - metabolic disturbance O21.1
    - severe (with metabolic disturbance) O21.1
  - projectile R11.12
  - psychogenic F45.8
- **Hyperemia** (acute) (passive) R68.89
  - anal mucosa K62.89
  - bladder N32.89
  - cerebral I67.89
  - conjunctiva H11.43-
  - ear internal, acute — *see* subcategory H83.Ø
  - enteric K59.8
  - eye — *see* Hyperemia, conjunctiva
  - eyelid (active) (passive) — *see* Disorder, eyelid, specified type NEC
  - intestine K59.8
  - iris — *see* Disorder, iris, vascular
  - kidney N28.89
  - labyrinth — *see* subcategory H83.Ø
  - liver (active) K76.89
  - lung (passive) — *see* Edema, lung
  - pulmonary (passive) — *see* Edema, lung
  - renal N28.89
  - retina H35.89
  - stomach K31.89
- **Hyperesthesia** (body surface) R2Ø.3
  - larynx (reflex) J38.7
    - hysterical F44.89
  - pharynx (reflex) J39.2
    - hysterical F44.89
- **Hyperestrogenism** (drug-induced) (iatrogenic) E28.Ø
- **Hyperexplexia** Q89.8
- **Hyperfibrinolysis** — *see* Fibrinolysis
- **Hyperfructosemia** E74.19
- **Hyperfunction** adrenal cortex, not associated with Cushing's syndrome E27.Ø
    - medulla E27.5
      - adrenomedullary E27.5
    - virilism E25.9
      - congenital E25.Ø
  - ovarian E28.8
  - pancreas K86.8
  - parathyroid (gland) E21.3
  - pituitary (gland) (anterior) E22.9
    - specified NEC E22.8
  - polyglandular E31.1
  - testicular E29.Ø
- **Hypergammaglobulinemia** D89.2
  - polyclonal D89.Ø
  - Waldenström D89.Ø
- **Hypergastrinemia** E16.4
- **Hyperglobulinemia** R77.1
- **Hyperglycemia, hyperglycemic** (transient) R73.9
  - coma — *see* Diabetes, by type, with coma
  - postpancreatectomy E89.1
- **Hyperglyceridemia** (endogenous) (essential) (familial) (hereditary) (pure) E78.1
  - mixed E78.3
- **Hyperglycinemia** (non-ketotic) E72.51
- **Hypergonadism**
  - ovarian E28.8
  - testicular (primary) (infantile) E29.Ø
- **Hyperheparinemia** D68.32
- **Hyperhidrosis, hyperidrosis** R61
  - focal
    - primary L74.519
      - axilla L74.51Ø
      - face L74.511
      - palms L74.512
      - soles L74.513
    - secondary L74.52
  - generalized R61
  - localized
    - primary L74.519
      - axilla L74.51Ø
      - face L74.511
      - palms L74.512
      - soles L74.513
    - secondary L74.52
  - psychogenic F45.8
  - secondary R61
    - focal L74.52
- **Hyperhistidinemia** E7Ø.41
- **Hyperhomocysteinemia** E72.11
- **Hyperhydroxyprolinemia** E72.59
- **Hyperinsulinism** (functional) E16.1
  - with
    - coma (hypoglycemic) E15
    - encephalopathy E16.1 *[G94]*
  - ectopic E16.1
  - therapeutic misadventure (from administration of insulin) — *see* subcategory T38.3
- **Hyperkalemia** E87.5
- **Hyperkeratosis** (*see also* Keratosis) L85.9
  - cervix N88.Ø
  - due to yaws (early) (late) (palmar or plantar) A66.3
  - follicularis Q82.8
    - penetrans (in cutem) L87.Ø
  - palmoplantaris climacterica L85.1
  - pinta A67.1
  - senile (with pruritus) L57.Ø
  - universalis congenita Q8Ø.8
  - vocal cord J38.3
  - vulva N9Ø.4
- **Hyperkinesia, hyperkinetic** (disease) (reaction) (syndrome) (childhood) (adolescence) (*see also* Disorder, attention-deficit hyperactivity)
  - heart I51.89
- **Hyperleucine-isoleucinemia** E71.19
- **Hyperlipemia, hyperlipidemia** E78.5
  - combined E78.2
    - familial E78.4
  - group
    - A E78.Ø
    - B E78.1
    - C E78.2
    - D E78.3
  - mixed E78.2
  - specified NEC E78.4
- **Hyperlipidosis** E75.6
  - hereditary NEC E75.5
- **Hyperlipoproteinemia** E78.5
  - Fredrickson's type
    - I E78.3
    - IIa E78.Ø
    - IIb E78.2
    - III E78.2
    - IV E78.1
    - V E78.3
  - low-density-lipoprotein-type (LDL) E78.Ø
  - very-low-density-lipoprotein-type (VLDL) E78.1
- **Hyperlucent lung, unilateral** J43.Ø
- **Hyperlysinemia** E72.3
- **Hypermagnesemia** E83.41
  - neonatal P71.8
- **Hypermenorrhea** N92.Ø
- **Hypermethioninemia** E72.19
- **Hypermetropia** (congenital) H52.Ø-
- **Hypermobility, hypermotility**
  - cecum — *see* Syndrome, irritable bowel
  - coccyx — *see* subcategory M53.2
  - colon — *see* Syndrome, irritable bowel
- **Hypermobility, hypermotility** — *continued*
  - colon — *continued*
    - psychogenic F45.8
  - ileum K58.9
  - intestine (*see also* Syndrome, irritable bowel) K58.9
    - psychogenic F45.8
  - meniscus (knee) — *see* Derangement, knee, meniscus
  - scapula — *see* Instability, joint, shoulder
  - stomach K31.89
    - psychogenic F45.8
  - syndrome M35.7
  - urethra N36.41
    - with intrinsic sphincter deficiency N36.43
- **Hypernasality** R49.21
- **Hypernatremia** E87.Ø
- **Hypernephroma** C64.-
- **Hyperopia** — *see* Hypermetropia
- **Hyperorexia nervosa** F5Ø.2
- **Hyperornithinemia** E72.4
- **Hyperosmia** R43.1
- **Hyperosmolality** E87.Ø
- **Hyperostosis** (monomelic) (*see also* Disorder, bone, density and structure, specified NEC)
  - ankylosing (spine) M48.1Ø
    - cervical region M48.12
    - cervicothoracic region M48.13
    - lumbar region M48.16
    - lumbosacral region M48.17
    - multiple sites M48.19
    - occipito-atlanto-axial region M48.11
    - sacrococcygeal region M48.18
    - thoracic region M48.14
    - thoracolumbar region M48.15
  - cortical (skull) M85.2
    - infantile M89.8X-
  - frontal, internal of skull M85.2
  - interna frontalis M85.2
  - skeletal, diffuse idiopathic — *see* Hyperostosis, ankylosing
  - skull M85.2
    - congenital Q75.8
  - vertebral, ankylosing — *see* Hyperostosis, ankylosing
- **Hyperovarism** E28.8
- **Hyperoxaluria** (primary) E72.53
- **Hyperparathyroidism** E21.3
  - primary E21.Ø
  - secondary (renal) N25.81
    - non-renal E21.1
  - specified NEC E21.2
  - tertiary E21.2
- **Hyperpathia** R2Ø.8
- **Hyperperistalsis** R19.2
  - psychogenic F45.8
- **Hyperpermeability, capillary** I78.8
- **Hyperphagia** R63.2
- **Hyperphenylalaninemia NEC** E7Ø.1
- **Hyperphoria** (alternating) H5Ø.53
- **Hyperphosphatemia** E83.39
- **Hyperpiesis, hyperpiesia** — *see* Hypertension
- **Hyperpigmentation** (*see also* Pigmentation)
  - melanin NEC L81.4
  - postinflammatory L81.Ø
- **Hyperpinealism** E34.8
- **Hyperpituitarism** E22.9
- **Hyperplasia, hyperplastic**
  - adenoids J35.2
  - adrenal (capsule) (cortex) (gland) E27.8
    - with
      - sexual precocity (male) E25.9
        - congenital E25.Ø
      - virilism, adrenal E25.9
        - congenital E25.Ø
      - virilization (female) E25.9
        - congenital E25.Ø
    - congenital E25.Ø
      - salt-losing E25.Ø
  - adrenomedullary E27.5
  - angiolymphoid, eosinophilia (ALHE) D18.Ø1
  - appendix (lymphoid) K38.Ø
  - artery, fibromuscular I77.3

Hyperplasia, hyperplastic— *continued*
- bone (*see also* Hypertrophy, bone)
  - marrow D75.89
- breast (*see also* Hypertrophy, breast)
  - ductal (atypical) N6Ø.9-
- C-cell, thyroid EØ7.Ø
- cementation (tooth) (teeth) KØ3.4
- cervical gland R59.Ø
- cervix (uteri) (basal cell) (endometrium) (polypoid) (*see also* Dysplasia, cervix)
  - congenital Q51.828
- clitoris, congenital Q52.6
- denture KØ6.2
- endocervicitis N72
- endometrium, endometrial (adenomatous) (benign) (cystic) (glandular) (glandular-cystic) (polypoid) N85.ØØ
  - with atypia N85.Ø2
  - cervix — *see* Dysplasia, cervix
  - complex (without atypia) N85.Ø1
  - simple (without atypia) N85.Ø1
- epithelial L85.9
  - focal, oral, including tongue K13.29
  - nipple N62
  - skin L85.9
  - tongue K13.29
  - vaginal wall N89.3
- erythroid D75.89
- fibromuscular of artery (carotid) (renal) I77.3
- genital
  - female NEC N94.89
  - male N5Ø.8
- gingiva KØ6.1
- glandularis cystica uteri (interstitialis) *(see also* Hyperplasia, endometrial) N85.ØØ
- gum KØ6.1
- hymen, congenital Q52.4
- irritative, edentulous (alveolar) KØ6.2
- jaw M26.Ø9
  - alveolar M26.79
  - lower M26.Ø3
    - alveolar M26.72
  - upper M26.Ø1
    - alveolar M26.71
- kidney (congenital) Q63.3
- labia N9Ø.6
  - epithelial N9Ø.3
- liver (congenital) Q44.7
  - nodular, focal K76.89
- lymph gland or node R59.9
- mandible, mandibular M26.Ø3
  - alveolar M26.72
  - unilateral condylar M27.8
- maxilla, maxillary M26.Ø1
  - alveolar M26.71
- myometrium, myometrial N85.2
- neuroendocrine cell, of infancy J84.841
- nose
  - lymphoid J34.89
  - polypoid J33.9
- oral mucosa (irritative) K13.6
- organ or site, congenital NEC — *see* Anomaly, by site
- ovary N83.8
- palate, papillary (irritative) K13.6
- pancreatic islet cells E16.9
  - alpha E16.8
    - with excess
      - gastrin E16.4
      - glucagon E16.3
  - beta E16.1
- parathyroid (gland) E21.Ø
- pharynx (lymphoid) J39.2
- prostate (adenofibromatous) (nodular) N4Ø.Ø
  - with lower urinary tract symptoms (LUTS) N4Ø.1
  - without lower urinary tract symtpoms (LUTS) N4Ø.Ø
- renal artery I77.89
- reticulo-endothelial (cell) D75.89
- salivary gland (any) K11.1
- Schimmelbusch's — *see* Mastopathy, cystic
- suprarenal capsule (gland) E27.8
- thymus (gland) (persistent) E32.Ø
- thyroid (gland) — *see* Goiter

Hyperplasia, hyperplastic— *continued*
- tonsils (faucial) (infective) (lingual) (lymphoid) J35.1
  - with adenoids J35.3
- unilateral condylar M27.8
- uterus, uterine N85.2
  - endometrium (glandular)(*see also* Hyperplasia, endometrial) N85.ØØ
- vulva N9Ø.6
  - epithelial N9Ø.3

Hyperpnea — *see* Hyperventilation

Hyperpotassemia E87.5

Hyperprebetalipoproteinemia (familial) E78.1

Hyperprolactinemia E22.1

Hyperprolinemia (type I) (type II) E72.59

Hyperproteinemia E88.Ø9

Hyperprothrombinemia, causing coagulation factor deficiency D68.4

Hyperpyrexia R5Ø.9
- heat (effects) T67.Ø
- malignant, due to anesthetic T88.3
- rheumatic — *see* Fever, rheumatic
- unknown origin R5Ø.9

Hyper-reflexia R29.2

Hypersalivation K11.7

Hypersecretion
- ACTH (not associated with Cushing's syndrome) E27.Ø
  - pituitary E24.Ø
- adrenaline E27.5
- adrenomedullary E27.5
- androgen (testicular) E29.Ø
  - ovarian (drug-induced) (iatrogenic) E28.1
- calcitonin EØ7.Ø
- catecholamine E27.5
- corticoadrenal E24.9
- cortisol E24.9
- epinephrine E27.5
- estrogen E28.Ø
- gastric K31.89
  - psychogenic F45.8
- gastrin E16.4
- glucagon E16.3
- hormone(s)
  - ACTH (not associated with Cushing's syndrome) E27.Ø
    - pituitary E24.Ø
  - antidiuretic E22.2
  - growth E22.Ø
  - intestinal NEC E34.1
  - ovarian androgen E28.1
  - pituitary E22.9
  - testicular E29.Ø
  - thyroid stimulating EØ5.8Ø
    - with thyroid storm EØ5.81
- insulin — *see* Hyperinsulinism
- lacrimal glands — *see* Epiphora
- medulloadrenal E27.5
- milk O92.6
- ovarian androgens E28.1
- salivary gland (any) K11.7
- thyrocalcitonin EØ7.Ø
- upper respiratory J39.8

Hypersegmentation, leukocytic, hereditary D72.Ø

Hypersensitive, hypersensitiveness, hypersensitivity (*see also* Allergy)
- carotid sinus G9Ø.Ø1
- colon — *see* Irritable, colon
- drug T88.7
- gastrointestinal K52.2
  - psychogenic F45.8
- labyrinth — *see* subcategory H83.2
- pain R2Ø.8
- pneumonitis — *see* Pneumonitis, allergic
- reaction T78.4Ø
  - upper respiratory tract NEC J39.3

Hypersomnia (organic) G47.1Ø
- due to
  - alcohol
    - abuse F1Ø.182
    - dependence F1Ø.282
    - use F1Ø.982
  - amphetamines
    - abuse F15.182

Hypersomnia — *continued*
- due to — *continued*
  - amphetamines — *continued*
    - dependence F15.282
    - use F15.982
  - caffeine
    - abuse F15.182
    - dependence F15.282
    - use F15.982
  - cocaine
    - abuse F14.182
    - dependence F14.282
    - use F14.982
  - drug NEC
    - abuse F19.182
    - dependence F19.282
    - use F19.982
  - medical condition G47.14
  - mental disorder F51.13
  - opioid
    - abuse F11.182
    - dependence F11.282
    - use F11.982
  - psychoactive substance NEC
    - abuse F19.182
    - dependence F19.282
    - use F19.982
  - sedative, hypnotic, or anxiolytic
    - abuse F13.182
    - dependence F13.282
    - use F13.982
  - stimulant NEC
    - abuse F15.182
    - dependence F15.282
    - use F15.982
- idiopathic G47.11
  - with long sleep time G47.11
  - without long sleep time G47.12
- menstrual related G47.13
- nonorganic origin F51.11
  - specified NEC F51.19
- not due to a substance or known physiological condition F51.11
  - specified NEC F51.19
- primary F51.11
- recurrent G47.13
- specified NEC G47.19

Hypersplenia, hypersplenism D73.1

Hyperstimulation, ovaries (associated with induced ovulation) N98.1

Hypersusceptibility — *see* Allergy

Hypertelorism (ocular) (orbital) Q75.2

Hypertension, hypertensive (accelerated) (benign) (essential) (idiopathic) (malignant) (systemic) I1Ø
- with
  - heart involvement (conditions in I51.4 - I51.9 due to hypertension) — *see* Hypertension, heart
  - kidney involvement — *see* Hypertension, kidney
- benign, intracranial G93.2
- borderline RØ3.Ø
- cardiorenal (disease) I13.1Ø
  - with heart failure I13.Ø
    - with stage 1 through stage 4 chronic kidney disease I13.Ø
    - with stage 5 or end stage renal disease I13.2
  - without heart failure I13.1Ø
    - with stage 1 through stage 4 chronic kidney disease I13.1Ø
    - with stage 5 or end stage renal disease I13.11
  - disease (arteriosclerotic) (sclerotic) — *see* Hypertension, heart
- cardiovascular
  - renal (disease) — *see* Hypertension, cardiorenal
- chronic venous — *see* Hypertension, venous (chronic)
- complicating
  - childbirth (labor) O1Ø.92
    - with
      - heart disease O1Ø.12
        - with renal disease O1Ø.32
      - renal disease O1Ø.22
        - with heart disease O1Ø.32
    - essential O1Ø.Ø2

- **Hypertension, hypertensive** — *continued*
  - complicating — *continued*
    - childbirth (labor) — *continued*
      - secondary O1Ø.42
    - pregnancy O16.-
      - with edema (*see also* Pre-eclampsia) O14.9-
      - gestational (pregnancy induced) (transient) (without proteinuria) O13.-
        - with proteinuria O14.9-
          - mild pre-eclampsia O14.Ø-
          - moderate pre-eclampsia O14.Ø-
          - severe pre-eclampsia O14.1-
            - with hemolysis, elevated liver enzymes and low platelet count (HELLP) O14.2-
      - pre-existing O1Ø.91-
        - with
          - heart disease O1Ø.11-
            - with renal disease O1Ø.31-
          - pre-eclampsia O11.-
          - renal disease O1Ø.21-
            - with heart disease O1Ø.31-
        - essential O1Ø.Ø1-
        - secondary O1Ø.41-
    - puerperium O1Ø.93
      - with
        - heart disease O1Ø.13
          - with renal disease O1Ø.33
        - renal disease O1Ø.23
          - with heart disease O1Ø.33
      - essential O1Ø.Ø3
      - secondary O1Ø.43
  - due to
    - endocrine disorders I15.2
    - pheochromocytoma I15.2
    - renal disorders NEC I15.1
      - arterial I15.Ø
    - renovascular disorders I15.Ø
    - specified disease NEC I15.8
  - encephalopathy I67.4
  - gestational (without significant proteinuria) (pregnancy-induced) (transient) O13.-
    - with significant proteinuria — *see* Pre-eclampsia
  - Goldblatt's I7Ø.1
  - heart (disease) (conditions in I51.4-I51.9 due to hypertension) I11.9
    - with
      - heart failure (congestive) I11.Ø
      - kidney disease (chronic) — *see* Hypertension, cardiorenal
  - intracranial (benign) G93.2
  - kidney I12.9
    - with
      - heart disease — *see* Hypertension, cardiorenal
      - stage 5 chronic kidney disease (CKD) or end stage renal disease (ESRD) I12.Ø
      - stage 1 through stage 4 chronic kidney disease I12.9
  - lesser circulation I27.Ø
  - newborn P29.2
    - pulmonary (persistent) P29.3
  - ocular H4Ø.Ø5-
  - pancreatic duct—code to underlying condition
    - with chronic pancreatitis K86.1
  - portal (due to chronic liver disease) (idiopathic) K76.6
    - gastropathy K31.89
    - in (due to) schistosomiasis (bilharziasis) B65.9 *[K77]*
  - postoperative I97.3
  - psychogenic F45.8
  - pulmonary (artery) (secondary) NEC I27.2
    - with
      - cor pulmonale (chronic) I27.2
        - acute I26.Ø9
      - right heart ventricular strain/failure I27.2
        - acute I26.Ø9
    - of newborn (persistent) P29.3
    - primary (idiopathic) I27.Ø
  - renal — *see* Hypertension, kidney
  - renovascular I15.Ø
  - secondary NEC I15.9

- **Hypertension, hypertensive** — *continued*
  - secondary NEC — *continued*
    - due to
      - endocrine disorders I15.2
      - pheochromocytoma I15.2
      - renal disorders NEC I15.1
        - arterial I15.Ø
      - renovascular disorders I15.Ø
    - specified NEC I15.8
  - venous (chronic)
    - due to
      - deep vein thrombosis — *see* Syndrome, postthrombotic
    - idiopathic I87.3Ø9
      - with
        - inflammation I87.32-
          - with ulcer I87.33-
        - specified complication NEC I87.39-
        - ulcer I87.31-
          - with inflammation I87.33-
      - asymptomatic I87.3Ø-
- **Hypertensive urgency** — see Hypertension
- **Hyperthecosis ovary** E28.8
- **Hyperthermia** (of unknown origin) (*see also* Hyperpyrexia)
  - malignant, due to anesthesia T88.3
  - newborn P81.9
    - environmental P81.Ø
- **Hyperthyroid** (recurrent) — *see* Hyperthyroidism
- **Hyperthyroidism** (latent) (pre-adult) (recurrent) EØ5.9Ø
  - with
    - goiter (diffuse) EØ5.ØØ
      - with thyroid storm EØ5.Ø1
      - nodular (multinodular) EØ5.2Ø
        - with thyroid storm EØ5.21
        - uninodular EØ5.1Ø
          - with thyroid storm EØ5.11
    - storm EØ5.91
  - due to ectopic thyroid tissue EØ5.3Ø
    - with thyroid storm EØ5.31
  - neonatal, transitory P72.1
  - specified NEC EØ5.8Ø
    - with thyroid storm EØ5.81
- **Hypertony, hypertonia, hypertonicity**
  - bladder N31.8
  - congenital P94.1
  - stomach K31.89
    - psychogenic F45.8
  - uterus, uterine (contractions) (complicating delivery) O62.4
- **Hypertrichosis** L68.9
  - congenital Q84.2
  - eyelid HØ2.869
    - left HØ2.866
      - lower HØ2.865
      - upper HØ2.864
    - right HØ2.863
      - lower HØ2.862
      - upper HØ2.861
  - lanuginosa Q84.2
    - acquired L68.1
  - localized L68.2
  - specified NEC L68.8
- **Hypertriglyceridemia, essential** E78.1
- **Hypertrophy, hypertrophic**
  - adenofibromatous, prostate — *see* Enlargement, enlarged, prostate
  - adenoids (infective) J35.2
    - with tonsils J35.3
  - adrenal cortex E27.8
  - alveolar process or ridge — *see* Anomaly, alveolar
  - anal papillae K62.89
  - artery I77.89
    - congenital NEC Q27.8
      - digestive system Q27.8
      - lower limb Q27.8
      - specified site NEC Q27.8
      - upper limb Q27.8
  - auricular — *see* Hypertrophy, cardiac
  - Bartholin's gland N75.8
  - bile duct (common) (hepatic) K83.8
  - bladder (sphincter) (trigone) N32.89

- **Hypertrophy, hypertrophic** — *continued*
  - bone M89.3Ø
    - carpus M89.34-
    - clavicle M89.31-
    - femur M89.35-
    - fibula M89.36-
    - finger M89.34-
    - humerus M89.32-
    - ilium M89.359
    - ischium M89.359
    - metacarpus M89.34-
    - metatarsus M89.37-
    - multiple sites M89.39
    - neck M89.38
    - radius M89.33-
    - rib M89.38
    - scapula M89.31-
    - skull M89.38
    - tarsus M89.37-
    - tibia M89.36-
    - toe M89.37-
    - ulna M89.33-
    - vertebra M89.38
  - brain G93.89
  - breast N62
    - cystic — *see* Mastopathy, cystic
    - newborn P83.4
    - pubertal, massive N62
    - puerperal, postpartum — *see* Disorder, breast, specified type NEC
    - senile (parenchymatous) N62
  - cardiac (chronic) (idiopathic) I51.7
    - with rheumatic fever (conditions in IØØ)
      - active IØ1.8
      - inactive or quiescent (with chorea) IØ9.89
    - congenital NEC Q24.8
    - fatty — *see* Degeneration, myocardial
    - hypertensive — *see* Hypertension, heart
    - rheumatic (with chorea) IØ9.89
      - active or acute IØ1.8
        - with chorea IØ2.Ø
    - valve — *see* Endocarditis
  - cartilage — *see* Disorder, cartilage, specified type NEC
  - cecum — *see* Megacolon
  - cervix (uteri) N88.8
    - congenital Q51.828
    - elongation N88.4
  - clitoris (cirrhotic) N9Ø.89
    - congenital Q52.6
  - colon (*see also* Megacolon)
    - congenital Q43.2
  - conjunctiva, lymphoid H11.89
  - corpora cavernosa N48.89
  - cystic duct K82.8
  - duodenum K31.89
  - endometrium (glandular) (*see also* Hyperplasia, endometrial) N85.ØØ
    - cervix N88.8
  - epididymis N5Ø.8
  - esophageal hiatus (congenital) Q79.1
    - with hernia — *see* Hernia, hiatal
  - eyelid — *see* Disorder, eyelid, specified type NEC
  - fat pad E65
    - knee (infrapatellar) (popliteal) (prepatellar) (retropatellar) M79.4
  - foot (congenital) Q74.2
  - frenulum, frenum (tongue) K14.8
    - lip K13.Ø
  - gallbladder K82.8
  - gastric mucosa K29.6Ø
    - with bleeding K29.61
  - gland, glandular R59.9
    - generalized R59.1
    - localized R59.Ø
  - gum (mucous membrane) KØ6.1
  - heart (idiopathic) (*see also* Hypertrophy, cardiac)
    - valve (*see also* Endocarditis) I38
  - hemifacial Q67.4
  - hepatic — *see* Hypertrophy, liver
  - hiatus (esophageal) Q79.1
  - hilus gland R59.Ø
  - hymen, congenital Q52.4

Hypogonadism
 female E28.39
 hypogonadotropic E23.0
 male E29.1
 ovarian (primary) E28.39
 pituitary E23.0
 testicular (primary) E29.1
Hypohidrosis, hypoidrosis L74.4
Hypoinsulinemia, postprocedural E89.1
Hypokalemia E87.6
Hypoleukocytosis — *see* Agranulocytosis
Hypolipoproteinemia (alpha) (beta) E78.6
Hypomagnesemia E83.42
 neonatal P71.2
Hypomania, hypomanic reaction F30.8
Hypomenorrhea — *see* Oligomenorrhea
Hypometabolism R63.8
Hypomotility
 gastrointestinal (tract) K31.89
 psychogenic F45.8
 intestine K59.8
 psychogenic F45.8
 stomach K31.89
 psychogenic F45.8
Hyponasality R49.22
Hyponatremia E87.1
Hypo-osmolality E87.1
Hypo-ovarianism, hypo-ovarism E28.39
Hypoparathyroidism E20.9
 familial E20.8
 idiopathic E20.0
 neonatal, transitory P71.4
 postprocedural E89.2
 specified NEC E20.8
Hypoperfusion (in)
 newborn P96.89
Hypopharyngitis — *see* Laryngopharyngitis
Hypophoria H50.53
Hypophosphatemia, hypophosphatasia (acquired)
 (congenital) (renal) E83.39
 familial E83.31
Hypophyseal, hypophysis (*see also* condition)
 dwarfism E23.0
 gigantism E22.0
Hypopiesis — *see* Hypotension
Hypopinealism E34.8
Hypopituitarism (juvenile) E23.0
 drug-induced E23.1
 due to
 hypophysectomy E89.3
 radiotherapy E89.3
 iatrogenic NEC E23.1
 postirradiation E89.3
 postpartum E23.0
 postprocedural E89.3
Hypoplasia, hypoplastic
 adrenal (gland), congenital Q89.1
 alimentary tract, congenital Q45.8
 upper Q40.8
 anus, anal (canal) Q42.3
 with fistula Q42.2
 aorta, aortic Q25.4
 ascending, in hypoplastic left heart syndrome
 Q23.4
 valve Q23.1
 in hypoplastic left heart syndrome Q23.4
 areola, congenital Q83.8
 arm (congenital) — *see* Defect, reduction, upper
 limb
 artery (peripheral) Q27.8
 brain (congenital) Q28.3
 coronary Q24.5
 digestive system Q27.8
 lower limb Q27.8
 pulmonary Q25.79
 functional, unilateral J43.0
 retinal (congenital) Q14.1
 specified site NEC Q27.8
 umbilical Q27.0
 upper limb Q27.8
 auditory canal Q17.8
 causing impairment of hearing Q16.9
 biliary duct or passage Q44.5

Hypoplasia, hypoplastic — *continued*
 bone NOS
 face Q75.8
 marrow D61.9
 megakaryocytic D69.49
 skull — *see* Hypoplasia, skull
 brain Q02
 gyri Q04.3
 part of Q04.3
 breast (areola) N64.82
 bronchus Q32.4
 cardiac Q24.8
 carpus — *see* Defect, reduction, upper limb,
 specified type NEC
 cartilage hair Q78.5
 cecum Q42.8
 cementum K00.4
 cephalic Q02
 cerebellum Q04.3
 cervix (uteri), congenital Q51.821
 clavicle (congenital) Q74.0
 coccyx Q76.49
 colon Q42.9
 specified NEC Q42.8
 corpus callosum Q04.0
 cricoid cartilage Q31.2
 digestive organ(s) or tract NEC Q45.8
 upper (congenital) Q40.8
 ear (auricle) (lobe) Q17.2
 middle Q16.4
 enamel of teeth (neonatal) (postnatal) (prenatal)
 K00.4
 endocrine (gland) NEC Q89.2
 endometrium N85.8
 epididymis (congenital) Q55.4
 epiglottis Q31.2
 erythroid, congenital D61.01
 esophagus (congenital) Q39.8
 eustachian tube Q17.8
 eye Q11.2
 eyelid (congenital) Q10.3
 face Q18.8
 bone(s) Q75.8
 femur (congenital) — *see* Defect, reduction, lower
 limb, specified type NEC
 fibula (congenital) — *see* Defect, reduction, lower
 limb, specified type NEC
 finger (congenital) — *see* Defect, reduction, upper
 limb, specified type NEC
 focal dermal Q82.8
 foot — *see* Defect, reduction, lower limb, specified
 type NEC
 gallbladder Q44.0
 genitalia, genital organ(s)
 female, congenital Q52.8
 external Q52.79
 internal NEC Q52.8
 in adiposogenital dystrophy E23.6
 glottis Q31.2
 hair Q84.2
 hand (congenital) — *see* Defect, reduction, upper
 limb, specified type NEC
 heart Q24.8
 humerus (congenital) — *see* Defect, reduction,
 upper limb, specified type NEC
 intestine (small) Q41.9
 large Q42.9
 specified NEC Q42.8
 jaw M26.09
 alveolar M26.79
 lower M26.04
 alveolar M26.74
 upper M26.02
 alveolar M26.73
 kidney(s) Q60.5
 bilateral Q60.4
 unilateral Q60.3
 labium (majus) (minus), congenital Q52.79
 larynx Q31.2
 left heart syndrome Q23.4
upper limb
 liver Q44.7
 lung (lobe) (not associated with short gestation)
 Q33.6
 associated with immaturity, low birth weight,
 prematurity, or short gestation P28.0
 mammary (areola), congenital Q83.8
 mandible, mandibular M26.04
 alveolar M26.74
 unilateral condylar M27.8
 maxillary M26.02
 alveolar M26.73
 medullary D61.9
 megakaryocytic D69.49
 metacarpus — *see* Defect, reduction, upper limb,
 specified type NEC
 metatarsus — *see* Defect, reduction, lower limb,
 specified type NEC
 muscle Q79.8
 nail(s) Q84.6
 nose, nasal Q30.1
 optic nerve H47.03-
 osseous meatus (ear) Q17.8
 ovary, congenital Q50.39
 pancreas Q45.0
 parathyroid (gland) Q89.2
 parotid gland Q38.4
 patella Q74.1
 pelvis, pelvic girdle Q74.2
 penis (congenital) Q55.62
 peripheral vascular system Q27.8
 digestive system Q27.8
 lower limb Q27.8
 specified site NEC Q27.8
 upper limb Q27.8
 pituitary (gland) (congenital) Q89.2
 pulmonary (not associated with short gestation)
 Q33.6
 artery, functional J43.0
 associated with short gestation P28.0
 radioulnar — *see* Defect, reduction, upper limb,
 specified type NEC
 radius — *see* Defect, reduction, upper limb
 rectum Q42.1
 with fistula Q42.0
 respiratory system NEC Q34.8
 rib Q76.6
 right heart syndrome Q22.6
 sacrum Q76.49
 scapula Q74.0
 scrotum Q55.1
 shoulder girdle Q74.0
 skin Q82.8
 skull (bone) Q75.8
 with
 anencephaly Q00.0
 encephalocele — *see* Encephalocele
 hydrocephalus Q03.9
 with spina bifida — *see* Spina bifida, by
 site, with hydrocephalus
 microcephaly Q02
 spinal (cord) (ventral horn cell) Q06.1
 spine Q76.49
 sternum Q76.7
 tarsus — *see* Defect, reduction, lower limb, specified
 type NEC
 testis Q55.1
 thymic, with immunodeficiency D82.1
 thymus (gland) Q89.2
 with immunodeficiency D82.1
 thyroid (gland) E03.1
 cartilage Q31.2
 tibiofibular (congenital) — *see* Defect, reduction,
 lower limb, specified type NEC
 toe — *see* Defect, reduction, lower limb, specified
 type NEC
 tongue Q38.3
 Turner's K00.4

Hypoplasia, hypoplastic — *continued*
- ulna (congenital) — *see* Defect, reduction, upper limb
- umbilical artery Q27.Ø
- unilateral condylar M27.8
- ureter Q62.8
- uterus, congenital Q51.811
- vagina Q52.4
- vascular NEC peripheral Q27.8
  - brain Q28.3
  - digestive system Q27.8
  - lower limb Q27.8
  - specified site NEC Q27.8
  - upper limb Q27.8
- vein(s) (peripheral) Q27.8
  - brain Q28.3
  - digestive system Q27.8
  - great Q26.8
  - lower limb Q27.8
  - specified site NEC Q27.8
  - upper limb Q27.8
- vena cava (inferior) (superior) Q26.8
- vertebra Q76.49
- vulva, congenital Q52.79
- zonule (ciliary) Q12.8

Hypopotassemia E87.6

Hypoproconvertinemia, congenital (hereditary) D68.2

Hypoproteinemia E77.8

Hypoprothrombinemia (congenital) (hereditary) (idiopathic) D68.2
- acquired D68.4
- newborn, transient P61.6

Hypoptyalism K11.7

Hypopyon (eye) (anterior chamber) — *see* Iridocyclitis, acute, hypopyon

Hypopyrexia R68.Ø

Hyporeflexia R29.2

Hyposecretion
- ACTH E23.Ø
- antidiuretic hormone E23.2
- ovary E28.39
- salivary gland (any) K11.7
- vasopressin E23.2

Hyposegmentation, leukocytic, hereditary D72.Ø

Hyposiderinemia D5Ø.9

Hypospadias Q54.9
- balanic Q54.Ø
- coronal Q54.Ø
- glandular Q54.Ø
- penile Q54.1
- penoscrotal Q54.2
- perineal Q54.3
- specified NEC Q54.8

Hypospermatogenesis — *see* Oligospermia

Hyposplenism D73.Ø

Hypostasis pulmonary, passive — *see* Edema, lung

Hypostatic — *see* condition

Hyposthenuria N28.89

Hypotension (arterial) (constitutional) I95.9
- chronic I95.89
- due to (of) hemodialysis I95.3
- drug-induced I95.2
- iatrogenic I95.89
- idiopathic (permanent) I95.Ø
- intracranial, following ventricular shunting (ventriculostomy) G97.2
- intra-dialytic I95.3
- maternal, syndrome (following labor and delivery) O26.5-
- neurogenic, orthostatic G9Ø.3
- orthostatic (chronic) I95.1
  - due to drugs I95.2
  - neurogenic G9Ø.3
- postoperative I95.81
- postural I95.1
- specified NEC I95.89

Hypothermia (accidental) T68
- due to anesthesia, anesthetic T88.51
- low environmental temperature T68
- neonatal P8Ø.9
  - environmental (mild) NEC P8Ø.8
  - mild P8Ø.8

Hypothermia (accidental) — *continued*
- neonatal — *continued*
  - severe (chronic) (cold injury syndrome) P8Ø.Ø
  - specified NEC P8Ø.8
- not associated with low environmental temperature R68.Ø

Hypothyroidism (acquired) EØ3.9
- congenital (without goiter) EØ3.1
  - with goiter (diffuse) EØ3.Ø
- due to
  - exogenous substance NEC EØ3.2
  - iodine-deficiency, acquired EØ1.8
    - subclinical EØ2
  - irradiation therapy E89.Ø
  - medicament NEC EØ3.2
  - P-aminosalicylic acid (PAS) EØ3.2
  - phenylbutazone EØ3.2
  - resorcinol EØ3.2
  - sulfonamide EØ3.2
  - surgery E89.Ø
  - thiourea group drugs EØ3.2
- iatrogenic NEC EØ3.2
- iodine-deficiency (acquired) EØ1.8
- congenital — *see* Syndrome, iodine deficiency, congenital
- subclinical EØ2
- neonatal, transitory P72.2
- postinfectious EØ3.3
- postirradiation E89.Ø
- postprocedural E89.Ø
- postsurgical E89.Ø
- specified NEC EØ3.8
- subclinical, iodine-deficiency related EØ2

Hypotonia, hypotonicity, hypotony
- bladder N31.2
- congenital (benign) P94.2
- eye — *see* Disorder, globe, hypotony

Hypotrichosis — *see* Alopecia

Hypotropia H5Ø.2-

Hypoventilation RØ6.89
- congenital central alveolar G47.35
- sleep related
  - idiopathic nonobstructive alveolar G47.34
  - in conditions classified elsewhere G47.36

Hypovitaminosis — *see* Deficiency, vitamin

Hypovolemia E86.1
- surgical shock T81.19
- traumatic (shock) T79.4

Hypoxemia RØ9.Ø2
- newborn P84
- sleep related, in conditions classified elsewhere G47.36

Hypoxia (*see also* Anoxia) RØ9.Ø2
- cerebral, during a procedure NEC G97.81
  - postprocedural NEC G97.82
- intrauterine P84
- myocardial — *see* Insufficiency, coronary
- newborn P84
- sleep-related G47.34

Hypsarhythmia — *see* Epilepsy, generalized, specified NEC

Hysteralgia, pregnant uterus O26.89-

Hysteria, hysterical (conversion) (dissociative state) F44.9
- anxiety F41.8
- convulsions F44.5
- psychosis, acute F44.9

Hysteroepilepsy F44.5

I

Ichthyoparasitism due to Vandellia cirrhosa B88.8

Ichthyosis (congenital) Q8Ø.9
- acquired L85.Ø
- fetalis Q8Ø.4
- hystrix Q8Ø.8
- lamellar Q8Ø.2
- lingual K13.29
- palmaris and plantaris Q82.8
- simplex Q8Ø.Ø
- vera Q8Ø.8
- vulgaris Q8Ø.Ø
- X-linked Q8Ø.1

Ichthyotoxism — *see* Poisoning, fish
- bacterial — *see* Intoxication, foodborne

Icteroanemia, hemolytic (acquired) D59.9
- congenital — *see* Spherocytosis

Icterus (*see also* Jaundice)
- conjunctiva R17
- newborn P59.9
- gravis, newborn P55.Ø
- hematogenous (acquired) D59.9
- hemolytic (acquired) D59.9
  - congenital — *see* Spherocytosis
- hemorrhagic (acute) (leptospiral) (spirochetal) A27.Ø
  - newborn P53
- infectious B15.9
  - with hepatic coma B15.Ø
  - leptospiral A27.Ø
  - spirochetal A27.Ø
- neonatorum — *see* Jaundice, newborn
- spirochetal A27.Ø

Ictus solaris, solis T67.Ø

Ideation
- homicidal R45.85Ø
- suicidal R45.851

Identity disorder (child) F64.9
- gender role F64.2
- psychosexual F64.2

Id reaction (due to bacteria) L3Ø.2

Idioglossia F8Ø.Ø

Idiopathic — *see* condition

Idiot, idiocy (congenital) F73
- amaurotic (Bielschowsky(-Jansky)) (family) (infantile) (late)) (juvenile (late)) (Vogt-Spielmeyer) E75.4
- microcephalic QØ2

IgE asthma J45.9Ø9

IIAC (idiopathic infantile arterial calcification) Q28.8

Ileitis (chronic) (noninfectious) (*see also* Enteritis) K52.9
- backwash — *see* Pancolitis, ulcerative (chronic)
- infectious AØ9
- regional (ulcerative) — *see* Enteritis, regional, small intestine
- segmental — *see* Enteritis, regional
- terminal (ulcerative) — *see* Enteritis, regional, small intestine

Ileocolitis (*see also* Enteritis) K52.9
- regional — *see* Enteritis, regional
- infectious AØ9

Ileostomy
- attention to Z43.2
- malfunctioning K94.13
- status Z93.2
  - with complication — *see* Complications, enterostomy

Ileotyphus — *see* Typhoid

Ileum — *see* condition

Ileus (bowel) (colon) (inhibitory) (intestine) K56.7
- adynamic K56.Ø
- due to gallstone (in intestine) K56.3
- duodenal (chronic) K31.5
- gallstone K56.3
- mechanical NEC K56.69
- meconium P76.Ø
  - in cystic fibrosis E84.11
  - meaning meconium plug (without cystic fibrosis) P76.Ø
- myxedema K59.8

Ileus— *continued*
- neurogenic K56.Ø
  - Hirschsprung's disease or megacolon Q43.1
- newborn
  - due to meconium P76.Ø
    - in cystic fibrosis E84.11
    - meaning meconium plug (without cystic fibrosis) P76.Ø
  - transitory P76.1
- obstructive K56.69
- paralytic K56.Ø

Iliac — *see* condition

Iliotibial band syndrome M76.3-

Illiteracy Z55.Ø

Illness (*see also* Disease) R69
- manic-depressive — *see* Disorder, bipolar

Imbalance R26.89
- autonomic G9Ø.8
- constituents of food intake E63.1
- electrolyte E87.8
  - with
    - abortion — *see* Abortion by type, complicated by, electrolyte imbalance
    - molar pregnancy OØ8.5
  - due to hyperemesis gravidarum O21.1
  - following ectopic or molar pregnancy OØ8.5
  - neonatal, transitory NEC P74.4
    - potassium P74.3
    - sodium P74.2
- endocrine E34.9
- eye muscle NOS H5Ø.9
- hormone E34.9
- hysterical F44.4
- labyrinth — *see* subcategory H83.2
- posture R29.3
- protein-energy — *see* Malnutrition
- sympathetic G9Ø.8

Imbecile, imbecility (I.Q. 35-49) F71

Imbedding, intrauterine device T83.39

Imbibition, cholesterol (gallbladder) K82.4

Imbrication, teeth,, fully erupted M26.3Ø

Imerslund (-Gräsbeck) **syndrome** D51.1

Immature (*see also* Immaturity)
- birth (less than 37 completed weeks) — *see* Preterm, newborn
  - extremely (less than 28 completed weeks) — *see* Immaturity, extreme
- personality F6Ø.89

Immaturity (less than 37 completed weeks) (*see also* Preterm, newborn)
- extreme of newborn (less than 28 completed weeks of gestation) (less than 196 completed days of gestation) (unspecified weeks of gestation) PØ7.2Ø
  - gestational age
    - 23 completed weeks (23 weeks, Ø days through 23 weeks, 6 days) PØ7.22
    - 24 completed weeks (24 weeks, Ø days through 24 weeks, 6 days) PØ7.23
    - 25 completed weeks (25 weeks, Ø days through 25 weeks, 6 days) PØ7.24
    - 26 completed weeks (26 weeks, Ø days through 26 weeks, 6 days) PØ7.25
    - 27 completed weeks (27 weeks, Ø days through 27 weeks, 6 days) PØ7.26
    - less than 23 completed weeks PØ7.21
- fetus or infant light-for-dates — *see* Light-for-dates
- lung, newborn P28.Ø
- organ or site NEC — *see* Hypoplasia
- pulmonary, newborn P28.Ø
- reaction F6Ø.89
- sexual (female) (male), after puberty E3Ø.Ø

Immersion T75.1
- hand T69.Ø1-
- foot T69.Ø2-

Immobile, immobility
- complete, due to severe physical disability or frailty R53.2
- intestine K59.8
- syndrome (paraplegic) M62.3

Immune reconstitution (inflammatory) syndrome [IRIS] D89.3

Immunization (*see also* Vaccination)
- ABO — *see* Incompatibility, ABO
  - in newborn P55.1
- complication — *see* Complications, vaccination
- encounter for Z23
- not done (not carried out) Z28.9
  - because (of)
    - acute illness of patient Z28.Ø1
    - allergy to vaccine (or component) Z28.Ø4
    - caregiver refusal Z28.82
    - chronic illness of patient Z28.Ø2
    - contraindication NEC Z28.Ø9
    - group pressure Z28.1
    - guardian refusal Z28.82
    - immune compromised state of patient Z28.Ø3
    - parent refusal Z28.82
    - patient's belief Z28.1
    - patient had disease being vaccinated against Z28.81
    - patient refusal Z28.21
    - religious beliefs of patient Z28.1
    - specified reason NEC Z28.89
      - of patient Z28.29
    - unspecified patient reason Z28.2Ø
- Rh factor
  - affecting management of pregnancy NEC O36.Ø9-
    - anti-D antibody O36.Ø1-
  - from transfusion — *see* Complication(s) transfusion, incompatibility reaction, Rh (factor)

Immunocytoma C83.Ø-

Immunodeficiency D84.9
- with
  - adenosine-deaminase deficiency D81.3
  - antibody defects D8Ø.9
    - specified type NEC D8Ø.8
  - hyperimmunoglobulinemia D8Ø.6
  - increased immunoglobulin M (IgM) D8Ø.5
  - major defect D82.9
    - specified type NEC D82.8
  - partial albinism D82.8
  - short-limbed stature D82.2
  - thrombocytopenia and eczema D82.Ø
- antibody with
  - hyperimmunoglobulinemia D8Ø.6
  - near-normal immunoglobulins D8Ø.6
- autosomal recessive, Swiss type D8Ø.Ø
- combined D81.9
  - biotin-dependent carboxylase D81.819
    - biotinidase D81.81Ø
    - holocarboxylase synthetase D81.818
    - specified type NEC D81.818
  - severe (SCID) D81.9
    - with
      - low or normal B-cell numbers D81.2
      - low T- and B-cell numbers D81.1
      - reticular dysgenesis D81.Ø
  - specified type NEC D81.89
- common variable D83.9
  - with
    - abnormalities of B-cell numbers and function D83.Ø
    - autoantibodies to B- or T-cells D83.2
    - immunoregulatory T-cell disorders D83.1
  - specified type NEC D83.8
- following hereditary defective response to Epstein-Barr virus (EBV) D82.3
- selective, immunoglobulin
  - A (IgA) D8Ø.2
  - G (IgG) (subclasses) D8Ø.3
  - M (IgM) D8Ø.4
- severe combined (SCID) D81.9
- specified type NEC D84.8
- X-linked, with increased IgM D8Ø.5

Immunotherapy (encounter for)
- antineoplastic Z51.12

Impaction, impacted
- bowel, colon, rectum (*see also* Impaction, fecal) K56.49
  - by gallstone K56.3
- calculus — *see* Calculus
- cerumen (ear) (external) H61.2-

Impaction, impacted— *continued*
- cuspid — *see* Impaction, tooth
- dental (same or adjacent tooth) KØ1.1
- fecal, feces K56.41
- fracture — *see* Fracture, by site
- gallbladder — *see* Calculus, gallbladder
- gallstone(s) — *see* Calculus, gallbladder
  - bile duct (common) (hepatic) — *see* Calculus, bile duct
  - cystic duct — *see* Calculus, gallbladder
  - in intestine, with obstruction (any part) K56.3
- intestine (calculous) NEC (*see also* impaction, fecal) K56.49
  - gallstone, with ileus K56.3
- intrauterine device (IUD) T83.39
- molar — *see* Impaction, tooth
- shoulder, causing obstructed labor O66.Ø
- tooth, teeth KØ1.1
- turbinate J34.89

Impaired, impairment (function)
- auditory discrimination — *see* Abnormal, auditory perception
- cognitive, mild, so stated G31.84
- dual sensory Z73.82
- fasting glucose R73.Ø1
- glucose tolerance (oral) R73.Ø2
- hearing — *see* Deafness
- heart — *see* Disease, heart
- kidney N28.9
  - disorder resulting from N25.9
    - specified NEC N25.89
- liver K72.9Ø
  - with coma K72.91
- mastication KØ8.8
- mild cognitive, so stated G31.84
- mobility
  - ear ossicles — *see* Ankylosis, ear ossicles
  - requiring care provider Z74.Ø9
- myocardium, myocardial — *see* Insufficiency, myocardial
- rectal sphincter R19.8
- renal (acute) (chronic) N28.9
  - disorder resulting from N25.9
    - specified NEC N25.89
- vision NEC H54.7
  - both eyes H54.3

Impediment, speech R47.9
- psychogenic (childhood) F98.8
- slurring R47.81
- specified NEC R47.89

Impending
- coronary syndrome I2Ø.Ø
- delirium tremens F1Ø.239
- myocardial infarction I2Ø.Ø

Imperception auditory (acquired) (*see also* Deafness)
- congenital H93.25

Imperfect
- aeration, lung (newborn) NEC — *see* Atelectasis
- closure (congenital)
  - alimentary tract NEC Q45.8
    - lower Q43.8
    - upper Q4Ø.8
  - atrioventricular ostium Q21.2
  - atrium (secundum) Q21.1
  - branchial cleft or sinus Q18.Ø
  - choroid Q14.3
  - cricoid cartilage Q31.8
  - cusps, heart valve NEC Q24.8
    - pulmonary Q22.3
  - ductus
    - arteriosus Q25.Ø
    - Botalli Q25.Ø
  - ear drum (causing impairment of hearing) Q16.4
  - esophagus with communication to bronchus or trachea Q39.1
  - eyelid Q1Ø.3
  - foramen
    - botalli Q21.1
    - ovale Q21.1
  - genitalia, genital organ(s) or system
    - female Q52.8
      - external Q52.79

- **Infarct, infarction**— *continued*
  - cerebral — *continued*
    - cortical I63.9
    - due to
      - cerebral venous thrombosis, nonpyogenic I63.6
      - embolism
        - cerebral arteries I63.4-
        - precerebral arteries I63.1-
      - occlusion NEC
        - cerebral arteries I63.5-
        - precerebral arteries I63.2-
      - stenosis NEC
        - cerebral arteries I63.5-
        - precerebral arteries I63.2-
      - thrombosis
        - cerebral artery I63.3-
        - precerebral artery I63.Ø-
    - intraoperative
      - during cardiac surgery I97.81Ø
      - during other surgery I97.811
    - postprocedural
      - following cardiac surgery I97.82Ø
      - following other surgery I97.821
    - specified NEC I63.8
  - colon (acute) (agnogenic) (embolic) (hemorrhagic) (nonocclusive) (nonthrombotic) (occlusive) (segmental) (thrombotic) (with gangrene) K55.Ø
  - coronary artery — *see* Infarct, myocardium
  - embolic — *see* Embolism
  - fallopian tube N83.8
  - gallbladder K82.8
  - heart — *see* Infarct, myocardium
  - hepatic K76.3
  - hypophysis (anterior lobe) E23.6
  - impending (myocardium) I2Ø.Ø
  - intestine (acute) (agnogenic) (embolic) (hemorrhagic) (nonocclusive) (nonthrombotic) (occlusive) (thrombotic) (with gangrene) K55.Ø
  - kidney N28.Ø
  - liver K76.3
  - lung (embolic) (thrombotic) — *see* Embolism, pulmonary
  - lymph node I89.8
  - mesentery, mesenteric (embolic) (thrombotic) (with gangrene) K55.Ø
  - muscle (ischemic) M62.2Ø
    - ankle M62.27-
    - foot M62.27-
    - forearm M62.23-
    - hand M62.24-
    - lower leg M62.26-
    - pelvic region M62.25-
    - shoulder region M62.21-
    - specified site NEC M62.28
    - thigh M62.25-
    - upper arm M62.22-
  - myocardium, myocardial (acute) (with stated duration of 4 weeks or less) I21.3
    - diagnosed on ECG, but presenting no symptoms I25.2
    - healed or old I25.2
    - intraoperative
      - during cardiac surgery I97.79Ø
      - during other surgery I97.791
    - non-Q wave I21.4
    - non-ST elevation (NSTEMI) I21.4
      - subsequent I22.2
    - nontransmural I21.4
    - past (diagnosed on ECG or other investigation, but currently presenting no symptoms) I25.2
    - postprocedural
      - following cardiac surgery I97.19Ø
      - following other surgery I97.191
    - Q wave (*see also*, Infarct, myocardium, by site) I21.3
    - ST elevation (STEMI) I21.3
      - anterior (anteroapical) (anterolateral) (anteroseptal) (Q wave) (wall) I21.Ø9
        - subsequent I22.Ø

- **Infarct, infarction**— *continued*
  - myocardium, myocardial— *continued*
    - ST elevation — *continued*
      - inferior (diaphragmatic) (inferolateral) (inferoposterior) (wall) NEC I21.19
        - subsequent I22.1
      - inferoposterior transmural (Q wave) I21.11
      - involving
        - coronary artery of anterior wall NEC I21.Ø9
        - coronary artery of inferior wall NEC I21.19
        - diagonal coronary artery I21.Ø2
        - left anterior descending coronary artery I21.Ø2
        - left circumflex coronary artery I21.21
        - left main coronary artery I21.Ø1
        - oblique marginal coronary artery I21.21
        - right coronary artery I21.11
      - lateral (apical-lateral) (basal-lateral) (high) I21.29
        - subsequent I22.8
      - posterior (posterobasal) (posterolateral) (posteroseptal) (true) I21.29
        - subsequent I22.8
      - septal I21.29
        - subsequent I22.8
      - specified NEC I21.29
        - subsequent I22.8
      - subsequent I22.9
    - subsequent (recurrent) (reinfarction) I22.9
      - anterior (anteroapical) (anterolateral) (anteroseptal) (wall) I22.Ø
      - diaphragmatic (wall) I22.1
      - inferior (diaphragmatic) (inferolateral) (inferoposterior) (wall) I22.1
      - lateral (apical-lateral) (basal-lateral) (high) I22.8
      - non-ST elevation (NSTEMI) I22.2
      - posterior (posterobasal) (posterolateral) (posteroseptal) (true) I22.8
      - septal I22.8
      - specified NEC I22.8
      - ST elevation I22.9
        - anterior (anteroapical) (anterolateral) (anteroseptal) (wall) I22.Ø
        - inferior (diaphragmatic) (inferolateral) (inferoposterior) (wall) I22.1
        - specified NEC I22.8
      - subendocardial I22.2
      - transmural I22.9
        - anterior (anteroapical) (anterolateral) (anteroseptal) (wall) I22.Ø
        - diaphragmatic (wall) I22.1
        - inferior (diaphragmatic) (inferolateral) (inferoposterior) (wall) I22.1
        - lateral (apical-lateral) (basal-lateral) (high) I22.8
        - posterior (posterobasal) (posterolateral) (posteroseptal) (true) I22.8
        - specified NEC I22.8
    - syphilitic A52.Ø6
    - transmural I21.3
      - anterior (anteroapical) (anterolateral) (anteroseptal) (Q wave) (wall) NEC I21.Ø9
      - inferior (diaphragmatic) (inferolateral) (inferoposterior) (Q wave) (wall) NEC I21.19
      - inferoposterior (Q wave) I21.11
      - lateral (apical-lateral) (basal-lateral) (high) NEC I21.29
      - posterior (posterobasal) (posterolateral) (posteroseptal) (true) NEC I21.29
      - septal NEC I21.29
      - specified NEC I21.29
  - nontransmural I21.4
  - omentum K55.Ø
  - ovary N83.8
  - pancreas
  - papillary muscle — *see* Infarct, myocardium
  - parathyroid gland E21.4
  - pituitary (gland) E23.6
  - placenta O43.81-
  - prostate N42.89

- **Infarct, infarction**— *continued*
  - pulmonary (artery) (vein) (hemorrhagic) — *see* Embolism, pulmonary
  - renal (embolic) (thrombotic) N28.Ø
  - retina, retinal (artery) — *see* Occlusion, artery, retina
  - spinal (cord) (acute) (embolic) (nonembolic) G95.11
  - spleen D73.5
    - embolic or thrombotic I74.8
  - subendocardial (acute) (nontransmural) I21.4
  - suprarenal (capsule) (gland) E27.49
  - testis N5Ø.1
  - thrombotic (*see also* Thrombosis)
    - artery, arterial — *see* Embolism
  - thyroid (gland) EØ7.89
  - ventricle (heart) — *see* Infarct, myocardium
- **Infecting** — *see* condition
- **Infection, infected, infective** (opportunistic) B99.9
  - with
    - drug resistant organism (*see also* specific organism) — *see* Resistance (to) drug
    - lymphangitis — *see* Lymphangitis
    - organ dysfunction (acute) R65.2Ø
      - with septic shock R65.21
  - abscess (skin) code by site under Abscess
  - Absidia — *see* Mucormycosis
  - Acanthamoeba — *see* Acanthamebiasis
  - Acanthocheilonema (perstans) (streptocerca) B74.4
  - accessory sinus (chronic) — *see* Sinusitis
  - achorion — *see* Dermatophytosis
  - Acremonium falciforme B47.Ø
  - acromioclavicular MØØ.9
  - Actinobacillus (actinomycetem-comitans) A28.8
    - mallei A24.Ø
    - muris A25.1
  - Actinomadura B47.1
  - Actinomyces (israelii) (*see also* Actinomycosis) A42.9
  - Actinomycetales — *see* Actinomycosis
  - actinomycotic NOS — *see* Actinomycosis
  - adenoid (and tonsil) JØ3.9Ø
    - chronic J35.Ø2
  - adenovirus NEC
    - as cause of disease classified elsewhere B97.Ø
    - unspecified nature or site B34.Ø
  - aerogenes capsulatus A48.Ø
  - aertrycke — *see* Infection, salmonella
  - alimentary canal NOS — *see* Enteritis, infectious
  - Allescheria boydii B48.2
  - Alternaria B48.8
  - alveolus, alveolar (process) KØ4.7
  - Ameba, amebic (histolytica) — *see* Amebiasis
  - amniotic fluid, sac or cavity O41.1Ø-
    - chorioamnionitis O41.12-
    - placentitis O41.14-
  - amputation stump (surgical) — *see* Complication, amputation stump, infection
  - Ancylostoma (duodenalis) B76.Ø
  - Anisakiasis, Anisakis larvae B81.Ø
  - anthrax — *see* Anthrax
  - antrum (chronic) — *see* Sinusitis, maxillary
  - anus, anal (papillae) (sphincter) K62.89
  - arbovirus (arbor virus) A94
    - specified type NEC A93.8
  - artificial insemination N98.Ø
  - Ascaris lumbricoides — *see* Ascariasis
  - Ascomycetes B47.Ø
  - Aspergillus (flavus) (fumigatus) (terreus) — *see* Aspergillosis
  - atypical
    - acid-fast (bacilli) — *see* Mycobacterium, atypical
    - mycobacteria — *see* Mycobacterium, atypical
    - virus A81.9
      - specified type NEC A81.89
  - auditory meatus (external) — *see* Otitis, externa, infective
  - auricle (ear) — *see* Otitis, externa, infective
  - axillary gland (lymph) LØ4.2
  - Bacillus A49.9
    - abortus A23.1
    - anthracis — *see* Anthrax
    - Ducrey's (any location) A57
    - Flexner's AØ3.1
    - Friedländer's NEC A49.8
    - gas (gangrene) A48.Ø

- **Infection, infected, infective** — *continued*
  - Bacillus — *continued*
    - mallei A24.Ø
    - melitensis A23.Ø
    - paratyphoid, paratyphosus AØ1.4
      - A AØ1.1
      - B AØ1.2
      - C AØ1.3
    - Shiga(-Kruse) AØ3.Ø
    - suipestifer — *see* Infection, salmonella
    - swimming pool A31.1
    - typhosa AØ1.ØØ
    - welchii — *see* Gangrene, gas
  - bacterial NOS A49.9
    - as cause of disease classified elsewhere B96.89
      - Clostridium perfringens [C. perfringens] B96.7
      - Bacteroides fragilis [B. fragilis] B96.6
      - Enterobacter sakazakii B96.89
      - Enterococcus B95.2
      - Escherichia coli [E. coli] (*see also* Escherichia coli) B96.2Ø
      - Helicobacter pylori [H.pylori] B96.81
      - Hemophilus influenzae [H. influenzae] B96.3
      - Klebsiella pneumoniae [K. pneumoniae] B96.1
      - Mycoplasma pneumoniae [M. pneumoniae] B96.Ø
      - Proteus (mirabilis) (morganii) B96.4
      - Pseudomonas (aeruginosa) (mallei) (pseudomallei) B96.5
      - Staphylococcus B95.8
        - aureus (methicillin susceptible) (MSSA) B95.61
          - methicillin resistant (MRSA) B95.62
        - specified NEC B95.7
      - Streptococcus B95.5
        - group A B95.Ø
        - group B B95.1
        - pneumoniae B95.3
        - specified NEC B95.4
      - Vibrio vulnificus B96.82
    - specified NEC A48.8
  - Bacterium
    - paratyphosum AØ1.4
      - A AØ1.1
      - B AØ1.2
      - C AØ1.3
    - typhosum AØ1.ØØ
  - Bacteroides NEC A49.8
    - fragilis, as cause of disease classified elsewhere B96.6
  - Balantidium coli AØ7.Ø
  - Bartholin's gland N75.8
  - Basidiobolus B46.8
  - bile duct (common) (hepatic) — *see* Cholangitis
  - bladder — *see* Cystitis
  - Blastomyces, blastomycotic (*see also* Blastomycosis)
    - brasiliensis — *see* Paracoccidioidomycosis
    - dermatitidis — *see* Blastomycosis
    - European — *see* Cryptococcosis
    - Loboi B48.Ø
    - North American B4Ø.9
    - South American — *see* Paracoccidioidomycosis
  - bleb, postprocedure — *see* Blebitis
  - bone — *see* Osteomyelitis
  - Bordetella — *see* Whooping cough
  - Borrelia bergdorfi A69.2Ø
  - brain (*see also* Encephalitis) GØ4.9Ø
    - membranes — *see* Meningitis
    - septic GØ6.Ø
      - meninges — *see* Meningitis, bacterial
  - branchial cyst Q18.Ø
  - breast — *see* Mastitis
  - bronchus — *see* Bronchitis
  - Brucella A23.9
    - abortus A23.1
    - canis A23.3
    - melitensis A23.Ø
    - mixed A23.8
    - specified NEC A23.8
    - suis A23.2
  - Brugia (malayi) B74.1
    - timori B74.2
  - bursa — *see* Bursitis, infective

- **Infection, infected, infective** — *continued*
  - buttocks (skin) LØ8.9
  - Campylobacter, intestinal AØ4.5
    - as cause of disease classified elsewhere B96.81
  - Candida (albicans) (tropicalis) — *see* Candidiasis
  - candiru B88.8
  - Capillaria (intestinal) B81.1
    - hepatica B83.8
    - philippinensis B81.1
  - cartilage — *see* Disorder, cartilage, specified type NEC
  - catheter-related bloodstream (CRBSI) T8Ø.211
  - cat liver fluke B66.Ø
  - cellulitis code by site under Cellulitis
  - central line-associated T8Ø.219
    - bloodstream (CLABSI) T8Ø.211
    - specified NEC T8Ø.218
  - Cephalosporium falciforme B47.Ø
  - cerebrospinal — *see* Meningitis
  - cervical gland (lymph) LØ4.Ø
  - cervix — *see* Cervicitis
  - cesarean delivery wound (puerperal) O86.Ø
  - cestodes — *see* Infestation, cestodes
  - chest J22
  - Chilomastix (intestinal) AØ7.8
  - Chlamydia, chlamydial A74.9
    - anus A56.3
    - genitourinary tract A56.2
      - lower A56.ØØ
      - specified NEC A56.19
    - lymphogranuloma A55
    - pharynx A56.4
    - psittaci A7Ø
    - rectum A56.3
    - sexually transmitted NEC A56.8
  - cholera — *see* Cholera
  - Cladosporium
    - bantianum (brain abscess) B43.1
    - carrionii B43.Ø
    - castellanii B36.1
    - trichoides (brain abscess) B43.1
    - werneckii B36.1
  - Clonorchis (sinensis) (liver) B66.1
  - Clostridium NEC
    - bifermentans A48.Ø
    - botulinum (food poisoning) AØ5.1
      - infant A48.51
      - wound A48.52
    - difficile
      - as cause of disease classified elsewhere B96.89
      - foodborne (disease) AØ4.7
      - gas gangrene A48.Ø
      - necrotizing enterocolitis AØ4.7
      - sepsis A41.4
    - gas-forming NEC A48.Ø
    - histolyticum A48.Ø
    - novyi, causing gas gangrene A48.Ø
    - oedematiens A48.Ø
    - perfringens
      - as cause of disease classified elsewhere B96.7
      - due to food AØ5.2
      - foodborne (disease) AØ5.2
      - gas gangrene A48.Ø
      - sepsis A41.4
    - septicum, causing gas gangrene A48.Ø
    - sordellii, causing gas gangrene A48.Ø
    - welchii
      - as cause of disease classified elsewhere B96.7
      - foodborne (disease) AØ5.2
      - gas gangrene A48.Ø
      - necrotizing enteritis AØ5.2
      - sepsis A41.4
  - Coccidioides (immitis) — *see* Coccidioidomycosis
  - colon — *see* Enteritis, infectious
  - colostomy K94.Ø2
  - common duct — *see* Cholangitis
  - congenital P39.9
    - Candida (albicans) P37.5
    - cytomegalovirus P35.1
    - hepatitis, viral P35.3
    - herpes simplex P35.2
    - infectious or parasitic disease P37.9
      - specified NEC P37.8

- **Infection, infected, infective** — *continued*
  - congenital — *continued*
    - listeriosis (disseminated) P37.2
    - malaria NEC P37.4
      - falciparum P37.3
    - Plasmodium falciparum P37.3
    - poliomyelitis P35.8
    - rubella P35.Ø
    - skin P39.4
    - toxoplasmosis (acute) (subacute) (chronic) P37.1
    - tuberculosis P37.Ø
    - urinary (tract) P39.3
    - vaccinia P35.8
    - virus P35.9
      - specified type NEC P35.8
  - Conidiobolus B46.8
  - coronavirus NEC B34.2
    - as cause of disease classified elsewhere B97.29
    - severe acute respiratory syndrome (SARS associated) B97.21
  - corpus luteum — *see* Salpingo-oophoritis
  - Corynebacterium diphtheriae — *see* Diphtheria
  - cotia virus BØ8.8
  - Coxiella burnetii A78
  - coxsackie — *see* Coxsackie
  - Cryptococcus neoformans — *see* Cryptococcosis
  - Cryptosporidium AØ7.2
  - Cunninghamella — *see* Mucormycosis
  - cyst — *see* Cyst
  - cystic duct (*see also* Cholecystitis) K81.9
  - Cysticercus cellulosae — *see* Cysticercosis
  - cytomegalovirus, cytomegaloviral B25.9
    - congenital P35.1
    - maternal, maternal care for (suspected) damage to fetus O35.3
    - mononucleosis B27.1Ø
      - with
        - complication NEC B27.19
        - meningitis B27.12
        - polyneuropathy B27.11
  - delta-agent (acute), in hepatitis B carrier B17.Ø
  - dental (pulpal origin) KØ4.7
  - Deuteromycetes B47.Ø
  - Dicrocoelium dendriticum B66.2
  - Dipetalonema (perstans) (streptocerca) B74.4
  - diphtherial — *see* Diphtheria
  - Diphyllobothrium (adult) (latum) (pacificum) B7Ø.Ø
    - larval B7Ø.1
  - Diplogonoporus (grandis) B71.8
  - Dipylidium caninum B67.4
  - Dirofilaria B74.8
  - Dracunculus medinensis B72
  - Drechslera (hawaiiensis) B43.8
  - Ducrey Haemophilus (any location) A57
  - due to or resulting from
    - artificial insemination N98.Ø
    - central venous catheter T8Ø.219
      - bloodstream T8Ø.211
      - exit or insertion site T8Ø.212
      - localized T8Ø.212
      - port or reservoir T8Ø.212
      - specified NEC T8Ø.218
      - tunnel T8Ø.212
    - device, implant or graft (*see also* Complications, by site and type, infection or inflammation) T85.79
      - arterial graft NEC T82.7
      - breast (implant) T85.79
      - catheter NEC T85.79
        - dialysis (renal) T82.7
          - intraperitoneal T85.71
        - infusion NEC T82.7
          - spinal (epidural) (subdural) T85.79
        - urinary (indwelling) T83.51
      - electronic (electrode) (pulse generator) (stimulator)
        - bone T84.7
        - cardiac T82.7
        - nervous system (brain) (peripheral nerve) (spinal) T85.79
        - urinary T83.59
      - fixation, internal (orthopedic) NEC — *see* Complication, fixation device, infection

- **Infection, infected, infective** — *continued*
  - due to or resulting from— *continued*
    - device, implant or graft— *continued*
      - gastrointestinal (bile duct) (esophagus) T85.79
      - genital NEC T83.6
      - heart NEC T82.7
        - valve (prosthesis) T82.6
          - graft T82.7
      - joint prosthesis — *see* Complication, joint prosthesis, infection
      - ocular (corneal graft) (orbital implant) NEC T85.79
      - orthopedic NEC T84.7
      - specified NEC T85.79
      - urinary NEC T83.59
      - vascular NEC T82.7
      - ventricular intracranial shunt T85.79
    - Hickman catheter T8Ø.219
      - bloodstream T8Ø.211
      - localized T8Ø.212
      - specified NEC T8Ø.218
    - immunization or vaccination T88.Ø
    - infusion, injection or transfusion NEC T8Ø.29
    - injury NEC code by site under Wound, open
    - portacath (port-a-cath) T8Ø.21
    - peripherally inserted central catheter (PICC) T8Ø.219
      - bloodstream T8Ø.211
      - localized T8Ø.212
      - specified NEC T8Ø.218
    - portacath (port-a-cath) T8Ø.219
      - bloodstream T8Ø.211
      - localized T8Ø.212
      - specified NEC T8Ø.218
    - surgery T81.4
    - triple lumen catheter T8Ø.219
      - bloodstream T8Ø.211
      - localized T8Ø.212
      - specified NEC T8Ø.218
    - umbilical venous catheter T8Ø.219
      - bloodstream T8Ø.211
      - localized T8Ø.212
      - specified NEC T8Ø.218
  - during labor NEC O75.3
  - ear (middle) (*see also* Otitis media)
    - external — *see* Otitis, externa, infective
    - inner — *see* subcategory H83.Ø
  - Eberthella typhosa AØ1.ØØ
  - Echinococcus — *see* Echinococcus
  - echovirus
    - as cause of disease classified elsewhere B97.12
    - unspecified nature or site B34.1
  - endocardium I33.Ø
  - endocervix — *see* Cervicitis
  - Entamoeba — *see* Amebiasis
  - enteric — *see* Enteritis, infectious
  - Enterobacter sakazakii B96.89
  - Enterobius vermicularis B8Ø
  - enterostomy K94.12
  - enterovirus B34.1
    - as cause of disease classified elsewhere B97.1Ø
      - coxsackievirus B97.11
      - echovirus B97.12
      - specified NEC B97.19
  - Entomophthora B46.8
  - Epidermophyton — *see* Dermatophytosis
  - epididymis — *see* Epididymitis
  - episiotomy (puerperal) O86.Ø
  - Erysipelothrix (insidiosa) (rhusiopathiae) — *see* Erysipeloid
  - erythema infectiosum BØ8.3
  - Escherichia (E.) coli NEC A49.8
    - as cause of disease classified elsewhere (*see also* Escherichia coli) B96.2Ø
    - congenital P39.8
      - sepsis P36.4
    - generalized A41.51
    - intestinal — *see* Enteritis, infectious, due to, Escherichia coli
  - ethmoidal (chronic) (sinus) — *see* Sinusitis, ethmoidal
  - eustachian tube (ear) — *see* Salpingitis, eustachian
- **Infection, infected, infective** — *continued*
  - external auditory canal (meatus) NEC — *see* Otitis, externa, infective
  - eye (purulent) — *see* Endophthalmitis, purulent
  - eyelid — *see* Inflammation, eyelid
  - fallopian tube — *see* Salpingo-oophoritis
  - Fasciola (gigantica) (hepatica) (indica) B66.3
  - Fasciolopsis (buski) B66.5
  - filarial — *see* Infestation, filarial
  - finger (skin) LØ8.9
    - nail LØ3.Ø1-
      - fungus B35.1
  - fish tapeworm B7Ø.Ø
    - larval B7Ø.1
  - flagellate, intestinal AØ7.9
  - fluke — *see* Infestation, fluke
  - focal
    - teeth (pulpal origin) KØ4.7
    - tonsils J35.Ø1
  - Fonsecaea (compactum) (pedrosoi) B43.Ø
  - food — *see* Intoxication, foodborne
  - foot (skin) LØ8.9
    - dermatophytic fungus B35.3
  - Francisella tularensis — *see* Tularemia
  - frontal (sinus) (chronic) — *see* Sinusitis, frontal
  - fungus NOS B49
    - beard B35.Ø
    - dermatophytic — *see* Dermatophytosis
    - foot B35.3
    - groin B35.6
    - hand B35.2
    - nail B35.1
    - pathogenic to compromised host only B48.8
    - perianal (area) B35.6
    - scalp B35.Ø
    - skin B36.9
      - foot B35.3
      - hand B35.2
      - toenails B35.1
  - Fusarium B48.8
  - gallbladder — *see* Cholecystitis
  - gas bacillus — *see* Gangrene, gas
  - gastrointestinal — *see* Enteritis, infectious
  - generalized NEC — *see* Sepsis
  - genital organ or tract
    - female — *see* Disease, pelvis, inflammatory
    - male N49.9
      - multiple sites N49.8
      - specified NEC N49.8
  - Ghon tubercle, primary A15.7
  - Giardia lamblia AØ7.1
  - gingiva (chronic) KØ5.1Ø
    - acute KØ5.ØØ
      - plaque induced KØ5.ØØ
      - nonplaque induced KØ5.Ø1
    - plaque induced KØ5.1Ø
    - nonplaque induced KØ5.11
  - glanders A24.Ø
  - glenosporopsis B48.Ø
  - Gnathostoma (spinigerum) B83.1
  - Gongylonema B83.8
  - gonococcal — *see* Gonococcus
  - gram-negative bacilli NOS A49.9
  - guinea worm B72
  - gum (chronic) KØ5.1Ø
    - acute KØ5.ØØ
      - plaque induced KØ5.ØØ
      - nonplaque induced KØ5.Ø1
    - plaque induced KØ5.1Ø
    - nonplaque induced KØ5.11
  - Haemophilus — *see* Infection, Hemophilus
  - heart — *see* Carditis
  - Helicobacter pylori AØ4.5
    - as cause of disease classified elsewhere B96.81
  - helminths B83.9
    - intestinal B82.Ø
      - mixed (types classifiable to more than one of the titles B65.Ø-B81.3 and B81.8) B81.4
      - specified type NEC B81.8
    - specified type NEC B83.8
  - Hemophilus
    - aegyptius, systemic A48.4
    - ducrey (any location) A57
- **Infection, infected, infective** — *continued*
  - Hemophilus — *continued*
    - influenzae NEC A49.2
      - as cause of disease classified elsewhere B96.3
    - generalized A41.3
  - herpes (simplex) (*see also* Herpes)
    - congenital P35.2
    - disseminated BØØ.7
    - zoster BØ2.9
  - herpesvirus, herpesviral — *see* Herpes
  - Heterophyes (heterophyes) B66.8
  - hip (joint) NEC MØØ.9
    - due to internal joint prosthesis
      - left T84.52
      - right T84.51
    - skin NEC LØ8.9
  - Histoplasma — *see* Histoplasmosis
    - American B39.4
    - capsulatum B39.4
  - hookworm B76.9
  - human
    - papilloma virus A63.Ø
    - T-cell lymphotropic virus type-1 (HTLV-1) B33.3
  - hydrocele N43.Ø
  - Hymenolepis B71.Ø
  - hypopharynx — *see* Pharyngitis
  - inguinal (lymph) glands LØ4.1
    - due to soft chancre A57
  - intervertebral disc, pyogenic M46.3Ø
    - cervical region M46.32
    - cervicothoracic region M46.33
    - lumbar region M46.36
    - lumbosacral region M46.37
    - multiple sites M46.39
    - occipito-atlanto-axial region M46.31
    - sacrococcygeal region M46.38
    - thoracic region M46.34
    - thoracolumbar region M46.35
  - intestine, intestinal — *see* Enteritis, infectious
    - specified NEC AØ8.8
  - intra-amniotic affecting newborn NEC P39.2
  - Isospora belli or hominis AØ7.3
  - Japanese B encephalitis A83.Ø
  - jaw (bone) (lower) (upper) M27.2
  - joint NEC MØØ.9
    - due to internal joint prosthesis T84.5Ø
  - kidney (cortex) (hematogenous) N15.9
    - with calculus N2Ø.Ø
      - with hydronephrosis N13.6
    - following ectopic gestation OØ8.89
    - pelvis and ureter (cystic) N28.85
    - puerperal (postpartum) O86.21
    - specified NEC N15.8
  - Klebsiella (K.) pneumoniae NEC A49.8
    - as cause of disease classified elsewhere B96.1
  - knee (joint) NEC MØØ.9
    - due to internal joint prosthesis
      - left T84.54
      - right T84.53
    - skin LØ8.9
  - Koch's — *see* Tuberculosis
  - labia (majora) (minora) (acute) — *see* Vulvitis
  - lacrimal
    - gland — *see* Dacryoadenitis
    - passages (duct) (sac) — *see* Inflammation, lacrimal, passages
  - lancet fluke B66.2
  - larynx NEC J38.7
  - leg (skin) NOS LØ8.9
  - Legionella pneumophila A48.1
    - nonpneumonic A48.2
  - Leishmania (*see also* Leishmaniasis)
    - aethiopica B55.1
    - braziliensis B55.2
    - chagasi B55.Ø
    - donovani B55.Ø
    - infantum B55.Ø
    - major B55.1
    - mexicana B55.1
    - tropica B55.1
  - lentivirus, as cause of disease classified elsewhere B97.31
  - Leptosphaeria senegalensis B47.Ø

- **Infection, infected, infective** — *continued*
  - respiratory (tract) NEC — *continued*
    - upper (acute) NOS — *continued*
      - chronic J39.8
      - streptococcal JØ6.9
      - viral NOS JØ6.9
  - resulting from
    - presence of internal prosthesis, implant, graft — *see* Complications, by site and type, infection
  - retortamoniasis AØ7.8
  - retroperitoneal NEC K68.9
  - retrovirus B33.3
    - as cause of disease classified elsewhere B97.3Ø
      - human
        - immunodeficiency, type 2 (HIV 2) B97.35
        - T-cell lymphotropic
          - type I (HTLV-I) B97.33
          - type II (HTLV-II) B97.34
      - lentivirus B97.31
      - oncovirus B97.32
      - specified NEC B97.39
  - Rhinosporidium (seeberi) B48.1
  - rhinovirus
    - as cause of disease classified elsewhere B97.89
    - unspecified nature or site B34.8
  - Rhizopus — *see* Mucormycosis
  - rickettsial NOS A79.9
  - roundworm (large) NEC B82.Ø
    - Ascariasis (*see also* Ascariasis) B77.9
  - rubella — *see* Rubella
  - Saccharomyces — *see* Candidiasis
  - salivary duct or gland (any) — *see* Sialoadenitis
  - Salmonella (aertrycke) (arizonae) (callinarum) (cholerae-suis) (enteritidis) (suipestifer) (typhimurium) AØ2.9
    - with
      - (gastro) enteritis AØ2.Ø
      - sepsis AØ2.1
      - specified manifestation NEC AØ2.8
    - due to food (poisoning) AØ2.9
    - hirschfeldii AØ1.3
    - localized AØ2.2Ø
      - arthritis AØ2.23
      - meningitis AØ2.21
      - osteomyelitis AØ2.24
      - pneumonia AØ2.22
      - pyelonephritis AØ2.25
      - specified NEC AØ2.29
    - paratyphi AØ1.4
      - A AØ1.1
      - B AØ1.2
      - C AØ1.3
    - schottmuelleri AØ1.2
    - typhi, typhosa — *see* Typhoid
  - Sarcocystis AØ7.8
  - scabies B86
  - Schistosoma — *see* Infestation, Schistosoma
  - scrotum (acute) NEC N49.2
  - seminal vesicle — *see* Vesiculitis
  - septic
    - localized, skin — *see* Abscess
  - sheep liver fluke B66.3
  - Shigella AØ3.9
    - boydii AØ3.2
    - dysenteriae AØ3.Ø
    - flexneri AØ3.1
    - group
      - A AØ3.Ø
      - B AØ3.1
      - C AØ3.2
      - D AØ3.3
    - Schmitz (-Stutzer) AØ3.Ø
    - schmitzii AØ3.Ø
    - shigae AØ3.Ø
    - sonnei AØ3.3
    - specified NEC AØ3.8
  - shoulder (joint) NEC MØØ.9
    - due to internal joint prosthesis T84.59
    - skin NEC LØ8.9
  - sinus (accessory) (chronic) (nasal) (*see also* Sinusitis)
    - pilonidal — *see* Sinus, pilonidal
    - skin NEC LØ8.89

- **Infection, infected, infective** — *continued*
  - Skene's duct or gland — *see* Urethritis
  - skin (local) (staphylococcal) (streptococcal) LØ8.9
    - abscess code by site under Abscess
    - cellulitis code by site under Cellulitis
    - due to fungus B36.9
      - specified type NEC B36.8
    - mycotic B36.9
      - specified type NEC B36.8
    - newborn P39.4
    - ulcer — *see* Ulcer, skin
  - slow virus A81.9
    - specified NEC A81.89
  - Sparganum (mansoni) (proliferum) (baxteri) B7Ø.1
  - specific (*see also* Syphilis)
    - to perinatal period — *see* Infection, congenital
  - specified NEC B99.8
  - spermatic cord NEC N49.1
  - sphenoidal (sinus) — *see* Sinusitis, sphenoidal
  - spinal cord NOS (*see also* Myelitis) GØ4.91
    - abscess GØ6.1
    - meninges — *see* Meningitis
    - streptococcal GØ4.89
  - Spirillum A25.Ø
  - spirochetal NOS A69.9
    - lung A69.8
    - specified NEC A69.8
  - Spirometra larvae B7Ø.1
  - spleen D73.89
  - Sporotrichum, Sporothrix (schenckii) — *see* Sporotrichosis
  - staphylococcal, unspecified site
    - aureus (methicillin susceptible) (MSSA) A49.Ø1
      - methicillin resistant (MRSA) A49.Ø2
    - as cause of disease classified elsewhere B95.8
      - aureus (methicillin susceptible) (MSSA) B95.61
        - methicillin resistant (MRSA) B95.62
      - specified NEC B95.7
    - food poisoning AØ5.Ø
    - generalized (purulent) A41.2
    - pneumonia — *see* Pneumonia, staphylococcal
  - Stellantchasmus falcatus B66.8
  - streptobacillus moniliformis A25.1
  - streptococcal NEC A49.1
    - as cause of disease classified elsewhere B95.5
    - B genitourinary complicating
      - childbirth O98.82
      - pregnancy O98.81-
      - puerperium O98.83
    - congenital
      - sepsis P36.1Ø
        - group B P36.Ø
        - specified NEC P36.19
    - generalized (purulent) A4Ø.9
  - Streptomyces B47.1
  - Strongyloides (stercoralis) — *see* Strongyloidiasis
  - stump (amputation) (surgical) — *see* Complication, amputation stump, infection
  - subcutaneous tissue, local LØ8.9
  - suipestifer — *see* Infection, salmonella
  - swimming pool bacillus A31.1
  - Taenia — *see* Infestation, Taenia
  - Taeniarhynchus saginatus B68.1
  - tapeworm — *see* Infestation, tapeworm
  - tendon (sheath) — *see* Tenosynovitis, infective NEC
  - Ternidens diminutus B81.8
  - testis — *see* Orchitis
  - threadworm B8Ø
  - throat — *see* Pharyngitis
  - thyroglossal duct K14.8
  - toe (skin) LØ8.9
    - cellulitis LØ3.Ø3-
      - fungus B35.1
    - nail LØ3.Ø3-
      - fungus B35.1
  - tongue NEC K14.Ø
    - parasitic B37.Ø
  - tonsil (and adenoid) (faucial) (lingual) (pharyngeal) — *see* Tonsillitis
  - tooth, teeth KØ4.7
    - periapical KØ4.7
    - peridental, periodontal KØ5.2Ø
      - generalized KØ5.22

- **Infection, infected, infective** — *continued*
  - tooth, teeth — *continued*
    - peridental, periodontal — *continued*
      - localized KØ5.21
    - pulp KØ4.Ø
    - socket M27.3
  - TORCH — *see* Infection, congenital
    - without active infection PØØ.2
  - Torula histolytica — *see* Cryptococcosis
  - Toxocara (canis) (cati) (felis) B83.Ø
  - Toxoplasma gondii — *see* Toxoplasma
  - trachea, chronic J42
  - trematode NEC — *see* Infestation, fluke
  - trench fever A79.Ø
  - Treponema pallidum — *see* Syphilis
  - Trichinella (spiralis) B75
  - Trichomonas A59.9
    - cervix A59.Ø9
    - intestine AØ7.8
    - prostate A59.Ø2
    - specified site NEC A59.8
    - urethra A59.Ø3
    - urogenitalis A59.ØØ
    - vagina A59.Ø1
    - vulva A59.Ø1
  - Trichophyton, trichophytic — *see* Dermatophytosis
  - Trichosporon (beigelii) cutaneum B36.2
  - Trichostrongylus B81.2
  - Trichuris (trichiura) B79
  - Trombicula (irritans) B88.Ø
  - Trypanosoma
    - brucei
      - gambiense B56.Ø
      - rhodesiense B56.1
    - cruzi — *see* Chagas' disease
  - tubal — *see* Salpingo-oophoritis
  - tuberculous NEC — *see* Tuberculosis
  - tubo-ovarian — *see* Salpingo-oophoritis
  - tunica vaginalis N49.1
  - tunnel T8Ø.212
  - tympanic membrane NEC — *see* Myringitis
  - typhoid (abortive) (ambulant) (bacillus) — *see* Typhoid
  - typhus A75.9
    - flea-borne A75.2
    - mite-borne A75.3
    - recrudescent A75.1
    - tick-borne A77.9
      - African A77.1
      - North Asian A77.2
  - umbilicus LØ8.82
  - ureter N28.86
  - urethra — *see* Urethritis
  - urinary (tract) N39.Ø
    - bladder — *see* Cystitis
    - complicating
      - pregnancy O23.4-
        - specified type NEC O23.3-
    - kidney — *see* Infection, kidney
    - newborn P39.3
    - puerperal (postpartum) O86.2Ø
    - tuberculous A18.13
    - urethra — *see* Urethritis
  - uterus, uterine — *see* Endometritis
  - vaccination T88.Ø
  - vaccinia not from vaccination BØ8.Ø11
  - vagina (acute) — *see* Vaginitis
  - varicella BØ1.9
  - varicose veins — *see* Varix
  - vas deferens NEC N49.1
  - vesical — *see* Cystitis
  - Vibrio
    - cholerae AØØ.Ø
      - El Tor AØØ.1
    - parahaemolyticus (food poisoning) AØ5.3
    - vulnificus
      - as cause of disease classified elsewhere B96.82
      - foodborne intoxication AØ5.5
  - Vincent's (gum) (mouth) (tonsil) A69.1

- **Infection, infected, infective** — *continued*
  - virus, viral NOS B34.9
    - adenovirus
      - as cause of disease classified elsewhere B97.Ø
      - unspecified nature or site B34.Ø
    - arborvirus, arbovirus arthropod-borne A94
    - as cause of disease classified elsewhere B97.89
      - adenovirus B97.Ø
      - coronavirus B97.29
        - SARS-associated B97.21
      - coxsackievirus B97.11
      - echovirus B97.12
      - enterovirus B97.1Ø
        - coxsackievirus B97.11
        - echovirus B97.12
        - specified NEC B97.19
      - human
        - immunodeficiency, type 2 (HIV 2) B97.35
        - metapneumovirus B97.81
        - T-cell lymphotropic,
          - type I (HTLV-I) B97.33
          - type II (HTLV-II) B97.34
      - papillomavirus B97.7
      - parvovirus B97.6
      - reovirus B97.5
      - respiratory syncytial B97.4
      - retrovirus B97.3Ø
        - human
          - immunodeficiency, type 2 (HIV 2) B97.35
          - T-cell lymphotropic,
            - type I (HTLV-I)B97.33
            - type II (HTLV-II)B97.34
        - lentivirus B97.31
        - oncovirus B97.32
        - specified NEC B97.39
      - specified NEC B97.89
    - central nervous system A89
      - atypical A81.9
        - specified NEC A81.89
      - enterovirus NEC A88.8
        - meningitis A87.Ø
      - slow virus A81.9
        - specified NEC A81.89
      - specified NEC A88.8
    - chest J98.8
    - cotia BØ8.8
    - coxsackie (*see also* Infection, coxsackie) B34.1
      - as cause of disease classified elsewhere B97.11
    - ECHO
      - as cause of disease classified elsewhere B97.12
      - unspecified nature or site B34.1
    - encephalitis, tick-borne A84.9
    - enterovirus, as cause of disease classified elsewhere B97.1Ø
      - coxsackievirus B97.11
      - echovirus B97.12
      - specified NEC B97.19
    - exanthem NOS BØ9
    - human metapneumovirus as cause of disease classified elsewhere B97.81
    - human papilloma as cause of disease classified elsewhere B97.7
    - intestine — *see* Enteritis, viral
    - respiratory syncytial
      - as cause of disease classified elsewhere B97.4
      - bronchopneumonia J12.1
      - common cold syndrome JØØ
      - nasopharyngitis (acute) JØØ
    - rhinovirus
      - as cause of disease classified elsewhere B97.89
      - unspecified nature or site B34.8
    - slow A81.9
      - specified NEC A81.89
    - specified type NEC B33.8
      - as cause of disease classified elsewhere B97.89
      - unspecified nature or site B34.8
    - unspecified nature or site B34.9

- **Infection, infected, infective** — *continued*
  - virus, viral NOS — *continued*
    - West Nile — *see* Virus, West Nile
  - vulva (acute) — *see* Vulvitis
  - whipworm B79
  - worms B83.9
    - specified type NEC B83.8
  - Wuchereria (bancrofti) B74.Ø
    - malayi B74.1
  - yatapoxvirus BØ8.7Ø
    - specified NEC BØ8.79
  - yeast (*see also* Candidiasis) B37.9
  - yellow fever — *see* Fever, yellow
  - Yersinia
    - enterocolitica (intestinal) AØ4.6
    - pestis — *see* Plague
    - pseudotuberculosis A28.2
  - Zeis' gland — *see* Hordeolum
  - zoonotic bacterial NOS A28.9
  - Zopfia senegalensis B47.Ø
- **Infective, infectious** — *see* condition
- **Infertility**
  - female N97.9
    - age-related N97.8
    - associated with
      - anovulation N97.Ø
      - cervical (mucus) disease or anomaly N88.3
      - congenital anomaly
        - cervix N88.3
        - fallopian tube N97.1
        - uterus N97.2
        - vagina N97.8
      - dysmucorrhea N88.3
      - fallopian tube disease or anomaly N97.1
      - pituitary-hypothalamic origin E23.Ø
      - specified origin NEC N97.8
      - Stein-Leventhal syndrome E28.2
      - uterine disease or anomaly N97.2
      - vaginal disease or anomaly N97.8
    - due to
      - cervical anomaly N88.3
      - fallopian tube anomaly N97.1
      - ovarian failure E28.39
      - Stein-Leventhal syndrome E28.2
      - uterine anomaly N97.2
      - vaginal anomaly N97.8
    - nonimplantation N97.2
    - origin
      - cervical N88.3
      - tubal (block) (occlusion) (stenosis) N97.1
      - uterine N97.2
      - vaginal N97.8
  - male N46.9
    - azoospermia N46.Ø1
      - extratesticular cause N46.Ø29
        - drug therapy N46.Ø21
        - efferent duct obstruction N46.Ø23
        - infection N46.Ø22
        - radiation N46.Ø24
        - specified cause NEC N46.Ø29
        - systemic disease N46.Ø25
    - oligospermia N46.11
      - extratesticular cause N46.129
        - drug therapy N46.121
        - efferent duct obstruction N46.123
        - infection N46.122
        - radiation N46.124
        - specified cause NEC N46.129
        - systemic disease N46.125
    - specified type NEC N46.8
- **Infestation** B88.9
  - Acanthocheilonema (perstans) (streptocerca) B74.4
  - Acariasis B88.Ø
    - demodex folliculorum B88.Ø
    - sarcoptes scabiei B86
    - trombiculae B88.Ø
  - Agamofilaria streptocerca B74.4
  - Ancylostoma, ankylostoma (braziliense) (caninum) (ceylanicum) (duodenale) B76.Ø
    - americanum B76.1
    - new world B76.1
  - Anisakis larvae, anisakiasis B81.Ø
  - arthropod NEC B88.2

- **Infestation** — *continued*
  - Ascaris lumbricoides — *see* Ascariasis
  - Balantidium coli AØ7.Ø
  - beef tapeworm B68.1
  - Bothriocephalus (latus) B7Ø.Ø
    - larval B7Ø.1
  - broad tapeworm B7Ø.Ø
    - larval B7Ø.1
  - Brugia (malayi) B74.1
    - timori B74.2
  - candiru B88.8
  - Capillaria
    - hepatica B83.8
    - philippinensis B81.1
  - cat liver fluke B66.Ø
  - cestodes B71.9
    - diphyllobothrium — *see* Infestation, diphyllobothrium
    - dipylidiasis B71.1
    - hymenolepiasis B71.Ø
    - specified type NEC B71.8
  - chigger B88.Ø
  - chigo, chigoe B88.1
  - Clonorchis (sinensis) (liver) B66.1
  - coccidial AØ7.3
  - crab-lice B85.3
  - Cysticercus cellulosae — *see* Cysticercosis
  - Demodex (folliculorum) B88.Ø
  - Dermanyssus gallinae B88.Ø
  - Dermatobia (hominis) — *see* Myiasis
  - Dibothriocephalus (latus) B7Ø.Ø
    - larval B7Ø.1
  - Dicrocoelium dendriticum B66.2
  - Diphyllobothrium (adult) (latum) (intestinal) (pacificum) B7Ø.Ø
    - larval B7Ø.1
  - Diplogonoporus (grandis) B71.8
  - Dipylidium caninum B67.4
  - Distoma hepaticum B66.3
  - dog tapeworm B67.4
  - Dracunculus medinensis B72
  - dragon worm B72
  - dwarf tapeworm B71.Ø
  - Echinococcus — *see* Echinococcus
  - Echinostomum ilocanum B66.8
  - Entamoeba (histolytica) — *see* Infection, Ameba
  - Enterobius vermicularis B8Ø
  - eyelid
    - in (due to)
      - leishmaniasis B55.1
      - loiasis B74.3
      - onchocerciasis B73.Ø9
      - phthiriasis B85.3
    - parasitic NOS B89
  - eyeworm B74.3
  - Fasciola (gigantica) (hepatica) (indica) B66.3
  - Fasciolopsis (buski) (intestine) B66.5
  - filarial B74.9
    - bancroftian B74.Ø
    - conjunctiva B74.9
    - due to
      - Acanthocheilonema (perstans) (streptocerca) B74.4
      - Brugia (malayi) B74.1
        - timori B74.2
      - Dracunculus medinensis B72
      - guinea worm B72
      - loa loa B74.3
      - Mansonella (ozzardi) (perstans) (streptocerca) B74.4
      - Onchocerca volvulus B73.ØØ
        - eye B73.ØØ
        - eyelid B73.Ø9
      - Wuchereria (bancrofti) B74.Ø
    - Malayan B74.1
    - ozzardi B74.4
    - specified type NEC B74.8
  - fish tapeworm B7Ø.Ø
    - larval B7Ø.1
  - fluke B66.9
    - blood NOS — *see* Schistosomiasis
    - cat liver B66.Ø
    - intestinal B66.5

- **Infestation** — *continued*
  - fluke— *continued*
    - liver (sheep) B66.3
      - cat B66.Ø
      - Chinese B66.1
      - due to clonorchiasis B66.1
      - oriental B66.1
    - lancet B66.2
    - lung (oriental) B66.4
    - sheep liver B66.3
    - specified type NEC B66.8
  - fly larvae — *see* Myiasis
  - Gasterophilus (intestinalis) — *see* Myiasis
  - Gastrodiscoides hominis B66.8
  - Giardia lamblia AØ7.1
  - Gnathostoma (spinigerum) B83.1
  - Gongylonema B83.8
  - guinea worm B72
  - helminth B83.9
    - angiostrongyliasis B83.2
      - intestinal B81.3
    - gnathostomiasis B83.1
    - hirudiniasis, internal B83.4
    - intestinal B82.Ø
      - angiostrongyliasis B81.3
      - anisakiasis B81.Ø
      - ascariasis — *see* Ascariasis
      - capillariasis B81.1
      - cysticercosis — *see* Cysticercosis
      - diphyllobothriasis — *see* Infestation, diphyllobothriasis
      - dracunculiasis B72
      - echinococcus — *see* Echinococcosis
      - enterobiasis B8Ø
      - filariasis — *see* Infestation, filarial
      - fluke — *see* Infestation, fluke
      - hookworm — *see* Infestation, hookworm
      - mixed (types classifiable to more than one of the titles B65.Ø-B81.3 and B81.8) B81.4
      - onchocerciasis — *see* Onchocerciasis
      - schistosomiasis — *see* Infestation, schistosoma
      - specified
        - cestode NEC — *see* Infestation, cestode
        - type NEC B81.8
      - strongyloidiasis — *see* Strongyloidiasis
      - taenia — *see* Infestation, taenia
      - trichinellosis B75
      - trichostrongyliasis B81.2
      - trichuriasis B79
    - specified type NEC B83.8
    - syngamiasis B83.3
    - visceral larva migrans B83.Ø
  - Heterophyes (heterophyes) B66.8
  - hookworm B76.9
    - ancylostomiasis B76.Ø
    - necatoriasis B76.1
    - specified type NEC B76.8
  - Hymenolepis (diminuta) (nana) B71.Ø
  - intestinal NEC B82.9
  - leeches (aquatic) (land) — *see* Hirudiniasis
  - Leishmania — *see* Leishmaniasis
  - lice, louse — *see* Infestation, Pediculus
  - Linguatula B88.8
  - Liponyssoides sanguineus B88.Ø
  - Loa loa B74.3
    - conjunctival B74.3
    - eyelid B74.3
  - louse — *see* Infestation, Pediculus
  - maggots — *see* Myiasis
  - Mansonella (ozzardi) (perstans) (streptocerca) B74.4
  - Medina (worm) B72
  - Metagonimus (yokogawai) B66.8
  - microfilaria streptocerca (*see also* Onchocerciasis)
    - eye B73.ØØ
    - eyelid B73.Ø9
  - mites B88.9
    - scabic B86
  - Monilia (albicans) — *see* Candidiasis
  - mouth B37.Ø
  - Necator americanus B76.1
  - nematode NEC (intestinal) B82.Ø
    - Ancylostoma B76.Ø

- **Infestation** — *continued*
  - nematode NEC— *continued*
    - conjunctiva NEC B83.9
    - Enterobius vermicularis B8Ø
    - Gnathostoma spinigerum B83.1
    - physaloptera B8Ø
    - specified NEC B81.8
    - trichostrongylus B81.2
    - trichuris (trichuria) B79
  - Oesophagostomum (apiostomum) B81.8
  - Oestrus ovis (*see also* Myiasis) B87.9
  - Onchocerca (volvulus) — *see* Onchocerciasis
  - Opisthorchis (felineus) (viverrini) B66.Ø
  - orbit, parasitic NOS B89
  - Oxyuris vermicularis B8Ø
  - Paragonimus (westermani) B66.4
  - parasite, parasitic B89
    - eyelid B89
    - intestinal NOS B82.9
    - mouth B37.Ø
    - skin B88.9
    - tongue B37.Ø
  - Parastrongylus
    - cantonensis B83.2
    - costaricensis B81.3
  - Pediculus B85.2
    - body B85.1
    - capitis (humanus) (any site) B85.Ø
    - corporis (humanus) (any site) B85.1
    - head B85.Ø
    - mixed (classifiable to more than one of the titles B85.Ø - B85.3) B85.4
    - pubis (any site) B85.3
  - Pentastoma B88.8
  - Phthirus (pubis) (any site) B85.3
    - with any infestation classifiable to B85.Ø - B85.2 B85.4
  - pinworm B8Ø
  - pork tapeworm (adult) B68.Ø
  - protozoal NEC B64
    - intestinal AØ7.9
      - specified NEC AØ7.8
    - specified NEC B6Ø.8
  - pubic, louse B85.3
  - rat tapeworm B71.Ø
  - red bug B88.Ø
  - roundworm (large) NEC B82.Ø
    - Ascariasis (*see also* Ascariasis) B77.9
  - sandflea B88.1
  - Sarcoptes scabiei B86
  - scabies B86
  - Schistosoma B65.9
    - bovis B65.8
    - cercariae B65.3
    - haematobium B65.Ø
    - intercalatum B65.8
    - japonicum B65.2
    - mansoni B65.1
    - mattheei B65.8
    - mekongi B65.8
    - specified type NEC B65.8
    - spindale B65.8
  - screw worms — *see* Myiasis
  - skin NOS B88.9
  - Sparganum (mansoni) (proliferum) (baxteri) B7Ø.1
    - larval B7Ø.1
  - specified type NEC B88.8
  - Spirometra larvae B7Ø.1
  - Stellantchasmus falcatus B66.8
  - Strongyloides stercoralis — *see* Strongyloidiasis
  - Taenia B68.9
    - diminuta B71.Ø
    - echinococcus — *see* Echinococcus
    - mediocanellata B68.1
    - nana B71.Ø
    - saginata B68.1
    - solium (intestinal form) B68.Ø
      - larval form — *see* Cysticercosis
  - Taeniarhynchus saginatus B68.1
  - tapeworm B71.9
    - beef B68.1
    - broad B7Ø.Ø
      - larval B7Ø.1

- **Infestation** — *continued*
  - tapeworm— *continued*
    - dog B67.4
    - dwarf B71.Ø
    - fish B7Ø.Ø
      - larval B7Ø.1
    - pork B68.Ø
    - rat B71.Ø
  - Ternidens diminutus B81.8
  - Tetranychus molestissimus B88.Ø
  - threadworm B8Ø
  - tongue B37.Ø
  - Toxocara (canis) (cati) (felis) B83.Ø
  - trematode(s) NEC — *see* Infestation, fluke
  - Trichinella (spiralis) B75
  - Trichocephalus B79
  - Trichomonas — *see* Trichomoniasis
  - Trichostrongylus B81.2
  - Trichuris (trichiura) B79
  - Trombicula (irritans) B88.Ø
  - Tunga penetrans B88.1
  - Uncinaria americana B76.1
  - Vandellia cirrhosa B88.8
  - whipworm B79
  - worms B83.9
    - intestinal B82.Ø
  - Wuchereria (bancrofti) B74.Ø
- **Infiltrate, infiltration**
  - amyloid (generalized) (localized) — *see* Amyloidosis
  - calcareous NEC R89.7
    - localized — *see* Degeneration, by site
  - calcium salt R89.7
  - cardiac
    - fatty — *see* Degeneration, myocardial
    - glycogenic E74.Ø2 *[I43]*
  - corneal — *see* Edema, cornea
  - eyelid — *see* Inflammation, eyelid
  - glycogen, glycogenic — *see* Disease, glycogen storage
  - heart, cardiac
    - fatty — *see* Degeneration, myocardial
    - glycogenic E74.Ø2 *[I43]*
  - inflammatory in vitreous H43.89
  - kidney N28.89
  - leukemic — *see* Leukemia
  - liver K76.89
    - fatty — *see* Fatty, liver NEC
    - glycogen (*see also* Disease, glycogen storage) E74.Ø3 *[K77]*
  - lung R91.8
    - eosinophilic J82
  - lymphatic (*see also* Leukemia, lymphatic) C91.9-
    - gland I88.9
  - muscle, fatty M62.89
  - myocardium, myocardial
    - fatty — *see* Degeneration, myocardial
    - glycogenic E74.Ø2 *[I43]*
  - on chest x-ray R91.8
  - pulmonary R91.8
    - with eosinophilia J82
  - skin (lymphocytic) L98.6
  - thymus (gland) (fatty) E32.8
  - urine R39.Ø
  - vesicant agent
    - antineoplastic chemotherapy T8Ø.81Ø
    - other agent NEC T8Ø.818
  - vitreous body H43.89
- **Infirmity** R68.89
  - senile R54
- **Inflammation, inflamed, inflammatory** (with exudation)
  - abducent (nerve) — *see* Strabismus, paralytic, sixth nerve
  - accessory sinus (chronic) — *see* Sinusitis
  - adrenal (gland) E27.8
  - alveoli, teeth M27.3
    - scorbutic E54
  - anal canal, anus K62.89
  - antrum (chronic) — *see* Sinusitis, maxillary
  - appendix — *see* Appendicitis
  - arachnoid — *see* Meningitis
  - areola N61

- **Inflammation, inflamed, inflammatory** — *continued*
  - trochlear (nerve) — *see* Strabismus, paralytic, fourth nerve
  - tubal — *see* Salpingo-oophoritis
  - tuberculous NEC — *see* Tuberculosis
  - tubo-ovarian — *see* Salpingo-oophoritis
  - tunica vaginalis N49.1
  - tympanic membrane — *see* Tympanitis
  - umbilicus, umbilical LØ8.82
  - uterine ligament — *see* Disease, pelvis, inflammatory
  - uterus (catarrhal) — *see* Endometritis
  - uveal tract (anterior) NOS (*see also* Iridocyclitis)
    - posterior — *see* Chorioretinitis
  - vagina — *see* Vaginitis
  - vas deferens N49.1
  - vein (*see also* Phlebitis)
    - intracranial or intraspinal (septic) GØ8
    - thrombotic I8Ø.9
      - leg — *see* Phlebitis, leg
      - lower extremity — *see* Phlebitis, leg
  - vocal cord J38.3
  - vulva — *see* Vulvitis
  - Wharton's duct (suppurative) — *see* Sialoadenitis
- **Inflation, lung, imperfect** (newborn) — *see* Atelectasis
- **Influenza** (bronchial) (epidemic) (respiratory (upper) (unidentified influenza virus) J11.1
  - with
    - digestive manifestations J11.2
    - encephalopathy J11.81
    - enteritis J11.2
    - gastroenteritis J11.2
    - gastrointestinal manifestations J11.2
    - laryngitis J11.1
    - myocarditis J11.82
    - otitis media J11.83
    - pharyngitis J11.1
    - pneumonia J11.ØØ
      - specified type J11.Ø8
    - respiratory manifestations NEC J11.1
    - specified manifestation NEC J11.89
  - A/H5N1 (*see also* Influenza, due to, identified novel influenza A virus) JØ9.X2
  - avian (*see also* Influenza, due to, identified novel influenza A virus) JØ9.X2
  - bird (*see also* Influenza, due to, identified novel influenza A virus) JØ9.X2
  - due to
    - avian (*see also* Influenza, due to, identified novel influenza A virus) JØ9.X2
    - identified influenza virus NEC J1Ø.1
      - with
        - digestive manifestations J1Ø.2
        - encephalopathy J1Ø.81
        - enteritis J1Ø.2
        - gastroenteritis J1Ø.2
        - gastrointestinal manifestations J1Ø.2
        - laryngitis J1Ø.1
        - myocarditis J1Ø.82
        - otitis media J1Ø.83
        - pharyngitis J1Ø.1
        - pneumonia (unspecified type) J1Ø.ØØ
          - with same identified influenza virus J1Ø.Ø1
          - specified type NEC J1Ø.Ø8
        - respiratory manifestations NEC J1Ø.1
        - specified manifestation NEC J1Ø.89
    - identified novel influenza A virus JØ9.X2
      - with
        - digestive manifestations JØ9.X3
        - encephalopathy JØ9.X9
        - enteritis JØ9.X3
        - gastroenteritis JØ9.X3
        - gastrointestinal manifestations JØ9.X3
        - laryngitis JØ9.X2
        - myocarditis JØ9.X9
        - otitis media JØ9.X9
        - pharyngitis JØ9.X2
        - pneumonia JØ9.X1
        - respiratory manifestations NEC JØ9.X2
        - specified manifestation NEC JØ9.X9
        - upper respiratory symptoms JØ9.X2
- **Influenza** — *continued*
  - novel (2ØØ9) H1N1 influenza (*see also* Influenza, due to, identified influenza virus NEC) J1Ø.
  - novel influenza A/H1N1(*see also* Influenza, due to, identified influenza virus NEC) J1Ø.1
  - of other animal origin, not bird or swine (*see also* Influenza, due to, identified novel influenza A virus) JØ9.X2
  - swine (viruses that normally cause infections in pigs) (*see also* Influenza, due to, identified novel influenza A virus) JØ9.X2
- **Influenza-like disease** — *see* Influenza
- **Influenzal**— *see* Influenza
- **Infraction, Freiberg's** (metatarsal head) — *see* Osteochondrosis, juvenile, metatarsus
- **Infraeruption of tooth** (teeth) M26.34
- **Infusion complication, misadventure, or reaction** — *see* Complications, infusion
- **Ingestion**
  - chemical — *see* Table of Drugs and Chemicals, by substance, poisoning
  - drug or medicament
    - correct substance properly administered — seeTable of Drugs and Chemicals, by drug, adverse effect
    - overdose or wrong substance given or taken — *see* Table of Drugs and Chemicals, by drug, poisoning
  - foreign body — *see* Foreign body, alimentary tract
  - tularemia A21.3
- **Ingrowing**
  - hair (beard) L73.1
  - nail (finger) (toe) L6Ø.Ø
- **Inguinal** (*see also* condition)
  - testicle Q53.9
    - bilateral Q53.21
    - unilateral Q53.11
- **Inhalation**
  - anthrax A22.1
  - flame T27.3
  - food or foreign body — *see* Foreign body, by site
  - gases, fumes, or vapors NEC T59.9-
    - specified agent — *see* Table of Drugs and Chemicals, by substance
  - liquid or vomitus — *see* Asphyxia
  - meconium (newborn) P24.ØØ
    - with
      - pneumonia (pneumonitis) P24.Ø1
      - with respiratory symptoms P24.Ø1
  - mucus — *see* Asphyxia, mucus
  - oil or gasoline (causing suffocation) — *see* Foreign body, by site
  - smoke J7Ø.5
    - due to chemicals, gases, fumes and vapors J68.9
  - steam — *see* Toxicity, vapors
  - stomach contents or secretions — *see* Foreign body, by site
    - due to anesthesia (general) (local) or other sedation T88.59
    - in labor and delivery O74.Ø
    - in pregnancy O29.Ø1-
    - postpartum, puerperal O89.Ø1
- **Inhibition, orgasm**
  - female F52.31
  - male F52.32
- **Inhibitor, systemic lupus erythematosus** (presence of) D68.62
- **Iniencephalus, iniencephaly** QØØ.2
- **Injection, traumatic jet** (air) (industrial) (water) (paint or dye) T7Ø.4
- **Injury** (*see also* specified injury type) T14.9Ø
  - abdomen, abdominal S39.91
    - blood vessel — *see* Injury, blood vessel, abdomen
    - cavity — *see* Injury, intra-abdominal
    - contusion S3Ø.1
    - internal — *see* Injury, intra-abdominal
    - intra-abdominal organ — *see* Injury, intra-abdominal
    - nerve — *see* Injury, nerve, abdomen
    - open — *see* Wound, open, abdomen
    - specified NEC S39.81
    - superficial — *see* Injury, superficial, abdomen
- **Injury** — *continued*
  - Achilles tendon S86.ØØ-
    - laceration S86.Ø2-
    - specified type NEC S86.Ø9-
    - strain S86.Ø1-
  - acoustic, resulting in deafness — *see* Injury, nerve, acoustic
  - adrenal (gland) S37.819
    - contusion S37.812
    - laceration S37.813
    - specified type NEC S37.818
  - alveolar (process) SØ9.93
  - ankle S99.91-
    - contusion — *see* Contusion, ankle
    - dislocation — *see* Dislocation, ankle
    - fracture — *see* Fracture, ankle
    - nerve — *see* Injury, nerve, ankle
    - open — *see* Wound, open, ankle
    - specified type NEC S99.81-
    - sprain — *see* Sprain, ankle
    - superficial — *see* Injury, superficial, ankle
  - anterior chamber, eye — *see* Injury, eye, specified site NEC
  - anus — *see* Injury, abdomen
  - aorta (thoracic) S25.ØØ
    - abdominal S35.ØØ
      - laceration (minor) (superficial) S35.Ø1
        - major S35.Ø2
      - specified type NEC S35.Ø9
    - laceration (minor) (superficial) S25.Ø1
      - major S25.Ø2
    - specified type NEC S25.Ø9
  - arm (upper) S49.9-
    - blood vessel — *see* Injury, blood vessel, arm
    - contusion — *see* Contusion, arm, upper
    - fracture — *see* Fracture, humerus
    - lower — *see* Injury, forearm
    - muscle — *see* Injury, muscle, shoulder
    - nerve — *see* Injury, nerve, arm
    - open — *see* Wound, open, arm
    - specified type NEC S49.8-
    - superficial — *see* Injury, superficial, arm
  - artery (complicating trauma) (*see also* Injury, blood vessel, by site)
    - cerebral or meningeal — *see* Injury, intracranial
  - auditory canal (external) (meatus) SØ9.91
  - auricle, auris, ear SØ9.91
  - axilla — *see* Injury, shoulder
  - back — *see* Injury, back, lower
  - bile duct — *see* Injury, gallbladder
  - birth (*see also* Birth, injury) P15.9
  - bladder (sphincter) S37.2Ø
    - at delivery O71.5
    - contusion S37.22
    - laceration S37.23
    - obstetrical trauma O71.5
    - specified type NEC S37.29
  - blast (air) (hydraulic) (immersion) (underwater) NEC T14.8
    - acoustic nerve trauma — *see* Injury, nerve, acoustic
    - bladder — *see* Injury, bladder, blast injury
    - brain — *see* Concussion
    - colon — *see* Injury, intestine, large, blast injury
    - ear (primary) SØ9.31-
      - secondary SØ9.39-
    - generalized T7Ø.8
    - lung — *see* Injury, intrathoracic, lung, blast injury
    - multiple body organs T7Ø.8
    - peritoneum S36.81
    - rectum S36.61
    - retroperitoneum S36.898
    - small intestine S36.419
      - duodenum S36.41Ø
      - specified site NEC S36.418
    - specified
      - intra-abdominal organ NEC S36.898
      - pelvic organ NEC S37.899
  - blood vessel NEC T14.8
    - abdomen S35.9Ø
      - aorta — *see* Injury, aorta, abdominal
      - celiac artery — *see* Injury, blood vessel, celiac artery

- **Injury** — *continued*
  - blood vessel — *continued*
    - abdomen — *continued*
      - iliac vessel — *see* Injury, blood vessel, iliac
      - laceration S35.91
      - mesenteric vessel — *see* Injury, mesenteric
      - portal vein — *see* Injury, blood vessel, portal vein
      - renal vessel — *see* Injury, blood vessel, renal
      - specified T14.8
        - site NEC — *see* subcategory S35.8
        - type NEC S35.99
      - splenic vessel — *see* Injury, blood vessel, splenic
      - vena cava — *see* Injury, vena cava, inferior
    - ankle — *see* Injury, blood vessel, foot
    - aorta (abdominal) (thoracic) — *see* Injury, aorta
    - arm (upper) NEC S45.90-
      - forearm — *see* Injury, blood vessel, forearm
      - laceration S45.91-
      - specified
        - site NEC S45.80-
          - laceration S45.81-
          - specified type NEC S45.89-
        - type NEC S45.99-
      - superficial vein S45.30-
        - laceration S45.31-
        - specified type NEC S45.39-
    - axillary
      - artery S45.00-
        - laceration S45.01-
        - specified type NEC S45.09-
      - vein S45.20-
        - laceration S45.21-
        - specified type NEC S45.29-
    - azygos vein — *see* Injury, blood vessel, thoracic, specified site NEC
    - brachial
      - artery S45.10-
        - laceration S45.11-
        - specified type NEC S45.19-
      - vein S45.20-
        - laceration S45.219
        - specified type NEC S45.29-
    - carotid artery (common) (external) (internal, extracranial) S15.00-
      - internal, intracranial S06.8-
      - laceration (minor) (superficial) S15.01-
        - major S15.02-
      - specified type NEC S15.09-
    - celiac artery S35.219
      - branch S35.299
        - laceration (minor) (superficial) S35.291
          - major S35.292
        - specified NEC S35.298
      - laceration (minor) (superficial) S35.211
        - major S35.212
      - specified type NEC S35.218
    - cerebral — *see* Injury, intracranial
    - deep plantar — *see* Injury, nerve, medial plantar
    - digital (hand) — *see* Injury, blood vessel, finger
    - dorsal
      - artery (foot) S95.00-
        - laceration S95.01-
        - specified type NEC S95.09-
      - vein (foot) S95.20-
        - laceration S95.21-
        - specified type NEC S95.29-
    - due to accidental laceration during procedure — *see* Laceration, accidental complicating surgery
    - extremity — *see* Injury, blood vessel, limb
    - femoral
      - artery (common) (superficial) S75.00-
        - laceration (minor) (superficial) S75.01-
          - major S75.02-
        - specified type NEC S75.09-
      - vein (hip level) (thigh level) S75.10-
        - laceration (minor) (superficial) S75.11-
          - major S75.12-
        - specified type NEC S75.19-
    - finger S65.50-

- **Injury** — *continued*
  - blood vessel— *continued*
    - finger— *continued*
      - index S65.50-
        - laceration S65.51-
        - specified type NEC S65.59-
      - laceration S65.51-
      - little S65.50-
        - laceration S65.51-
        - specified type NEC S65.59-
      - middle S65.50-
        - laceration S65.51-
        - specified type NEC S65.59-
      - specified type NEC S65.59-
      - thumb — *see* Injury, blood vessel, thumb
    - foot S95.90-
      - dorsal
        - artery — *see* Injury, blood vessel, dorsal, artery
        - vein — *see* Injury, blood vessel, dorsal, vein
      - laceration S95.91-
      - plantar artery — *see* Injury, blood vessel, plantar artery
      - specified
        - site NEC S95.80-
          - laceration S95.81-
          - specified type NEC S95.89-
        - specified type NEC S95.99-
    - forearm S55.90-
      - laceration S55.91-
      - radial artery — *see* Injury, blood vessel, radial artery
      - specified
        - site NEC S55.80-
          - laceration S55.81-
          - specified type NEC S55.89-
        - type NEC S55.99-
      - ulnar artery — *see* Injury, blood vessel, ulnar artery
      - vein S55.20-
        - laceration S55.21-
        - specified type NEC S55.29-
    - gastric
      - artery — *see* Injury, mesenteric, artery, branch
      - vein — *see* Injury, blood vessel, abdomen
    - gastroduodenal artery — *see* Injury, mesenteric, artery, branch
    - greater saphenous vein (lower leg level) S85.30-
      - hip (and thigh) level S75.20-
        - laceration (minor) (superficial) S75.21-
          - major S75.22-
        - specified type NEC S75.29-
      - laceration S85.31-
      - specified type NEC S85.39-
    - hand (level) S65.90-
      - finger — *see* Injury, blood vessel, finger
      - laceration S65.91-
      - palmar arch — *see* Injury, blood vessel, palmar arch
      - radial artery — *see* Injury, blood vessel, radial artery, hand
      - specified
        - site NEC S65.80-
          - laceration S65.81-
          - specified type NEC S65.89-
        - type NEC S65.99-
      - thumb — *see* Injury, blood vessel, thumb
      - ulnar artery — *see* Injury, blood vessel, ulnar artery, hand
    - head S09.0
      - intracranial — *see* Injury, intracranial
      - multiple S09.0
    - hepatic
      - artery — *see* Injury, mesenteric, artery
      - vein — *see* Injury, vena cava, inferior
    - hip S75.90-
      - femoral artery — *see* Injury, blood vessel, femoral, artery
      - femoral vein — *see* Injury, blood vessel, femoral, vein
      - greater saphenous vein — *see* Injury, blood vessel, greater saphenous, hip level

- **Injury** — *continued*
  - blood vessel — *continued*
    - hip — *continued*
      - laceration S75.91-
      - specified
        - site NEC S75.80-
          - laceration S75.81-
          - specified type NEC S75.89-
        - type NEC S75.99-
    - hypogastric (artery) (vein) — *see* Injury, blood vessel, iliac
    - iliac S35.5-
      - artery S35.51-
      - specified vessel NEC S35.5-
      - uterine vessel — *see* Injury, blood vessel, uterine
      - vein S35.51-
    - innominate — *see* Injury, blood vessel, thoracic, innominate
    - intercostal (artery) (vein) — *see* Injury, blood vessel, thoracic, intercostal
    - jugular vein (external) S15.20-
      - internal S15.30-
        - laceration (minor) (superficial) S15.31-
          - major S15.32-
        - specified type NEC S15.39-
      - laceration (minor) (superficial) S15.21-
        - major S15.22-
      - specified type NEC S15.29-
    - leg (level) (lower) S85.90-
      - greater saphenous — *see* Injury, blood vessel, greater saphenous
      - laceration S85.91-
      - lesser saphenous — *see* Injury, blood vessel, lesser saphenous
      - peroneal artery — *see* Injury, blood vessel, peroneal artery
      - popliteal
        - artery — *see* Injury, blood vessel, popliteal, artery
        - vein — *see* Injury, blood vessel, popliteal, vein
      - specified
        - site NEC S85.80-
          - laceration S85.81-
          - specified type NEC S85.89-
        - type NEC S85.99-
      - thigh — *see* Injury, blood vessel, hip
      - tibial artery — *see* Injury, blood vessel, tibial artery
    - lesser saphenous vein (lower leg level) S85.40-
      - laceration S85.41-
      - specified type NEC S85.49-
    - limb
      - lower — *see* Injury, blood vessel, leg
      - upper — *see* Injury, blood vessel, arm
    - lower back — *see* Injury, blood vessel, abdomen
      - specified NEC — *see* Injury, blood vessel, abdomen, specified, site NEC
    - mammary (artery) (vein) — *see* Injury, blood vessel, thoracic, specified site NEC
    - mesenteric (inferior) (superior)
      - artery — *see* Injury, mesenteric, artery
      - vein — *see* Injury, blood vessel, portal vein
    - neck S15.9
      - specified site NEC S15.8
    - ovarian (artery) (vein) — *see* subcategory S35.8
    - palmar arch (superficial) S65.20-
      - deep S65.30-
        - laceration S65.31-
        - specified type NEC S65.39-
      - laceration S65.21-
      - specified type NEC S65.29-
    - pelvis — *see* Injury, blood vessel, abdomen
      - specified NEC — *see* Injury, blood vessel, abdomen, specified, site NEC
    - peroneal artery S85.20-
      - laceration S85.21-
      - specified type NEC S85.29-
    - plantar artery (deep) (foot) S95.10-
      - laceration S95.11-
      - specified type NEC S95.19-

- **Injury** — *continued*
  - blood vessel— *continued*
    - popliteal
      - artery S85.ØØ-
        - laceration S85.Ø1-
        - specified type NEC S85.Ø9-
      - vein S85.5Ø-
        - laceration S85.51-
        - specified type NEC S85.59-
    - portal vein S35.319
      - laceration S35.311
      - specified type NEC S35.318
    - precerebral — *see* Injury, blood vessel, neck
    - pulmonary (artery) (vein) — *see* Injury, blood vessel, thoracic, pulmonary
    - radial artery (forearm level) S55.1Ø-
      - hand and wrist (level) S65.1Ø-
        - laceration S65.11-
        - specified type NEC S65.19-
      - laceration S55.11-
      - specified type NEC S55.19-
    - renal
      - artery S35.4Ø-
        - laceration S35.41-
        - specified NEC S35.49-
      - vein S35.4Ø-
        - laceration S35.41-
        - specified NEC S35.49-
    - saphenous vein (greater) (lower leg level) — *see* Injury, blood vessel, greater saphenous
      - hip and thigh level — *see* Injury, blood vessel, greater saphenous, hip level
      - lesser — *see* Injury, blood vessel, lesser saphenous
    - shoulder
      - specified NEC — *see* Injury, blood vessel, arm, specified site NEC
      - superficial vein — *see* Injury, blood vessel, arm, superficial vein
    - specified NEC
    - splenic
      - artery — *see* Injury, blood vessel, celiac artery, branch
      - vein S35.329
        - laceration S35.321
        - specified NEC S35.328
    - subclavian — *see* Injury, blood vessel, thoracic, innominate
    - thigh — *see* Injury, blood vessel, hip
    - thoracic S25.9Ø
      - aorta S25.ØØ
        - laceration (minor) (superficial) S25.Ø1
          - major S25.Ø2
        - specified type NEC S25.Ø9
      - azygos vein — *see* Injury, blood vessel, thoracic, specified, site NEC
      - innominate
        - artery S25.1Ø-
          - laceration (minor) (superficial) S25.11-
            - major S25.12-
          - specified type NEC S25.19-
        - vein S25.3Ø-
          - laceration (minor) (superficial) S25.31-
            - major S25.32-
          - specified type NEC S25.39-
      - intercostal S25.5Ø-
        - laceration S25.51-
        - specified type NEC S25.59-
      - laceration S25.91
      - mammary vessel — *see* Injury, blood vessel, thoracic, specified, site NEC
      - pulmonary S25.4Ø-
        - laceration (minor) (superficial) S25.41-
          - major S25.42-
        - specified type NEC S25.49-
      - specified
        - site NEC S25.8Ø-
          - laceration S25.81-
          - specified type NEC S25.89-
        - type NEC S25.99
      - subclavian — *see* Injury, blood vessel, thoracic, innominate

- **Injury** — *continued*
  - blood vessel— *continued*
    - thoracic— *continued*
      - vena cava (superior) S25.2Ø
        - laceration (minor) (superficial) S25.21
          - major S25.22
        - specified type NEC S25.29
    - thumb S65.4Ø-
      - laceration S65.41-
      - specified type NEC S65.49-
    - tibial artery S85.1Ø-
      - anterior S85.13-
        - laceration S85.14-
        - specified injury NEC S85.15-
      - laceration S85.11-
      - posterior S85.16-
        - laceration S85.17-
        - specified injury NEC S85.18-
      - specified injury NEC S85.12-
    - ulnar artery (forearm level) S55.ØØ-
      - hand and wrist (level) S65.ØØ-
        - laceration S65.Ø1-
        - specified type NEC S65.Ø9-
      - laceration S55.Ø1-
      - specified type NEC S55.Ø9-
    - upper arm (level) — *see* Injury, blood vessel, arm
      - superficial vein — *see* Injury, blood vessel, arm, superficial vein
    - uterine S35.5-
      - artery S35.53-
      - vein S35.53-
    - vena cava — *see* Injury, vena cava
    - vertebral artery S15.1Ø-
      - laceration (minor) (superficial) S15.11-
        - major S15.12-
      - specified type NEC S15.19-
    - wrist (level) — *see* Injury, blood vessel, hand
  - brachial plexus S14.3
    - newborn P14.3
  - brain (traumatic) SØ6.9-
    - diffuse (axonal) SØ6.2X-
    - focal SØ6.3Ø-
    - traumatic — *see* category SØ6
  - brainstem SØ6.38-
  - breast NOS S29.9
  - broad ligament — *see* Injury, pelvic organ, specified site NEC
  - bronchus, bronchi — *see* Injury, intrathoracic, bronchus
  - brow SØ9.9Ø
  - buttock S39.92
  - canthus, eye SØ5.9Ø
  - cardiac plexus — *see* Injury, nerve, thorax, sympathetic
  - cauda equina S34.3
  - cavernous sinus — *see* Injury, intracranial
  - cecum — *see* Injury, colon
  - celiac ganglion or plexus — *see* Injury, nerve, lumbosacral, sympathetic
  - cerebellum — *see* Injury, intracranial
  - cerebral — *see* Injury, intracranial
  - cervix (uteri) — *see* Injury, uterus
  - cheek (wall) SØ9.93
  - chest — *see* Injury, thorax
  - childbirth (newborn) (*see also* Birth, injury)
    - maternal NEC O71.9
  - chin SØ9.93
  - choroid (eye) — *see* Injury, eye, specified site NEC
  - clitoris S39.94
  - coccyx (*see also* Injury, back, lower)
    - complicating delivery O71.6
  - colon — *see* Injury, intestine, large
  - common bile duct — *see* Injury, liver
  - conjunctiva (superficial) — *see* Injury, eye, conjunctiva
  - conus medullaris — *see* Injury, spinal, sacral
  - cord
    - spermatic (pelvic region) S37.898
      - scrotal region S39.848
    - spinal — *see* Injury, spinal cord, by region
  - cornea — *see* Injury, eye, specified site NEC
    - abrasion — *see* Injury, eye, cornea, abrasion
  - cortex (cerebral) (*see also* Injury, intracranial)
    - visual — *see* Injury, nerve, optic

- **Injury** — *continued*
  - costal region NEC S29.9
  - costochondral NEC S29.9
  - cranial
    - cavity — *see* Injury, intracranial
    - nerve — *see* Injury, nerve, cranial
  - crushing — *see* Crush
  - cutaneous sensory nerve
  - cystic duct — *see* Injury, liver
  - deep tissue — *see* Contusion, by site
    - meaning pressure ulcer — *see* Ulcer, pressure, unstageable, by site
  - delivery (newborn) P15.9
    - maternal NEC O71.9
  - Descemet's membrane — *see* Injury, eyeball, penetrating
  - diaphragm — *see* Injury, intrathoracic, diaphragm
  - duodenum — *see* Injury, intestine, small, duodenum
  - ear (auricle) (external) (canal) SØ9.91
    - abrasion — *see* Abrasion, ear
    - bite — *see* Bite, ear
    - blister — *see* Blister, ear
    - bruise — *see* Contusion, ear
    - contusion — *see* Contusion, ear
    - external constriction — *see* Constriction, external, ear
    - hematoma — *see* Hematoma, ear
    - inner — *see* Injury, ear, middle
    - laceration — *see* Laceration, ear
    - middle SØ9.3Ø-
      - blast — *see* Injury, blast, ear
      - specified NEC SØ9.39-
    - puncture — *see* Puncture, ear
    - superficial — *see* Injury, superficial, ear
  - eighth cranial nerve (acoustic or auditory) — *see* Injury, nerve, acoustic
  - elbow S59.9Ø-
    - contusion — *see* Contusion, elbow
    - dislocation — *see* Dislocation, elbow
    - fracture — *see* Fracture, ulna, upper end
    - open — *see* Wound, open, elbow
    - specified NEC S59.8Ø-
    - sprain — *see* Sprain, elbow
    - superficial — *see* Injury, superficial, elbow
  - eleventh cranial nerve (accessory) — *see* Injury, nerve, accessory
  - epididymis S39.94
  - epigastric region S39.91
  - epiglottis NEC S19.89
  - esophageal plexus — *see* Injury, nerve, thorax, sympathetic
  - esophagus (thoracic part) (*see also* Injury, intrathoracic, esophagus)
    - cervical NEC S19.85
  - eustachian tube SØ9.91
  - eye SØ5.9-
    - avulsion SØ5.7-
    - ball — *see* Injury, eyeball
    - conjunctiva SØ5.Ø-
    - cornea
      - abrasion SØ5.Ø-
    - laceration SØ5.3-
      - with prolapse SØ5.2-
    - lacrimal apparatus SØ5.8X-
    - orbit penetration SØ5.4-
    - specified site NEC SØ5.8X-
  - eyeball SØ5.8X-
    - contusion SØ5.1-
    - penetrating SØ5.6-
      - with
        - foreign body SØ5.5-
        - prolapse or loss of intraocular tissue SØ5.2-
      - without prolapse or loss of intraocular tissue SØ5.3-
    - specified type NEC SØ5.8-
  - eyebrow SØ9.93
  - eyelid SØ9.93
    - abrasion — *see* Abrasion, eyelid
    - contusion — *see* Contusion, eyelid
    - open — *see* Wound, open, eyelid
  - face SØ9.93
  - fallopian tube S37.5Ø9
    - bilateral S37.5Ø2

Injury — *continued*
- fallopian tube — *continued*
  - bilateral — *continued*
    - blast injury S37.512
    - contusion S37.522
    - laceration S37.532
    - specified type NEC S37.592
  - blast injury (primary) S37.519
    - bilateral S37.512
    - secondary — *see* Injury, fallopian tube, specified type NEC
    - unilateral S37.511
  - contusion S37.529
    - bilateral S37.522
    - unilateral S37.521
  - laceration S37.539
    - bilateral S37.532
    - unilateral S37.531
  - specified type NEC S37.599
    - bilateral S37.592
    - unilateral S37.591
  - unilateral S37.5Ø1
    - blast injury S37.511
    - contusion S37.521
    - laceration S37.531
    - specified type NEC S37.591
- fascia — *see* Injury, muscle
- fifth cranial nerve (trigeminal) — *see* Injury, nerve, trigeminal
- finger (nail) S69.9-
  - blood vessel — *see* Injury, blood vessel, finger
  - contusion — *see* Contusion, finger
  - dislocation — *see* Dislocation, finger
  - fracture — *see* Fracture, finger
  - muscle — *see* Injury, muscle, finger
  - nerve — *see* Injury, nerve, digital, finger
  - open — *see* Wound, open, finger
  - specified NEC S69.8-
  - sprain — *see* Sprain, finger
  - superficial — *see* Injury, superficial, finger
- first cranial nerve (olfactory) — *see* Injury, nerve, olfactory
- flank — *see* Injury, abdomen
- foot S99.92-
  - blood vessel — *see* Injury, blood vessel, foot
  - contusion — *see* Contusion, foot
  - dislocation — *see* Dislocation, foot
  - fracture — *see* Fracture, foot
  - muscle — *see* Injury, muscle, foot
  - open — *see* Wound, open, foot
  - specified type NEC S99.82-
  - sprain — *see* Sprain, foot
  - superficial — *see* Injury, superficial, foot
- forceps NOS P15.9
- forearm S59.91-
  - blood vessel — *see* Injury, blood vessel, forearm
  - contusion — *see* Contusion, forearm
  - fracture — *see* Fracture, forearm
  - muscle — *see* Injury, muscle, forearm
  - nerve — *see* Injury, nerve, forearm
  - open — *see* Wound, open, forearm
  - specified NEC S59.81-
  - superficial — *see* Injury, superficial, forearm
- forehead SØ9.9Ø
- fourth cranial nerve (trochlear) — *see* Injury, nerve, trochlear
- gallbladder S36.129
  - contusion S36.122
  - laceration S36.123
  - specified NEC S36.128
- ganglion
  - celiac, coeliac — *see* Injury, nerve, lumbosacral, sympathetic
  - gasserian — *see* Injury, nerve, trigeminal
  - stellate — *see* Injury, nerve, thorax, sympathetic
  - thoracic sympathetic — *see* Injury, nerve, thorax, sympathetic
- gasserian ganglion — *see* Injury, nerve, trigeminal
- gastric artery — *see* Injury, blood vessel, celiac artery, branch
- gastroduodenal artery — *see* Injury, blood vessel, celiac artery, branch

Injury — *continued*
- gastrointestinal tract — *see* Injury, intra-abdominal
  - with open wound into abdominal cavity — *see* Wound, open, with penetration into peritoneal cavity
  - colon — *see* Injury, intestine, large
  - rectum — *see* Injury, intestine, large, rectum
    - with open wound into abdominal cavity S36.61
  - specified site NEC — *see* Injury, intra-abdominal, specified, site NEC
  - stomach — *see* Injury, stomach
  - small intestine — *see* Injury, intestine, small
- genital organ(s)
  - external S39.94
    - specified NEC S39.848
  - internal S37.9Ø
    - fallopian tube — *see* Injury, fallopian tube
    - ovary — *see* Injury, ovary
    - prostate — *see* Injury, prostate
    - seminal vesicle — *see* Injury, pelvis, organ, specified site NEC
    - uterus — *see* Injury, uterus
    - vas deferens — *see* Injury, pelvis, organ, specified site NEC
  - obstetrical trauma O71.9
- gland
  - lacrimal laceration — *see* Injury, eye, specified site NEC
  - salivary SØ9.9Ø
  - thyroid NEC S19.84
- globe (eye) SØ5.9Ø
  - specified NEC SØ5.8X-
- groin — *see* Injury, abdomen
- gum SØ9.9Ø
- hand S69.9-
  - blood vessel — *see* Injury, blood vessel, hand
  - contusion — *see* Contusion, hand
  - fracture — *see* Fracture, hand
  - muscle — *see* Injury, muscle, hand
  - nerve — *see* Injury, nerve, hand
  - open — *see* Wound, open, hand
  - specified NEC S69.8-
  - sprain — *see* Sprain, hand
  - superficial — *see* Injury, superficial, hand
- head SØ9.9Ø
  - with loss of consciousness SØ6.9-
  - specified NEC SØ9.8
- heart S26.9Ø
  - with hemopericardium S26.ØØ
    - contusion S26.Ø1
    - laceration (mild) S26.Ø2Ø
      - moderate S26.Ø21
      - major S26.Ø22
    - specified type NEC S26.Ø9
  - contusion S26.91
  - laceration S26.92
  - specified type NEC S26.99
  - without hemopericardium S26.1Ø
    - contusion S26.11
    - laceration S26.12
    - specified type NEC S26.19
- heel — *see* Injury, foot
- hepatic
  - artery — *see* Injury, blood vessel, celiac artery, branch
  - duct — *see* Injury, liver
  - vein — *see* Injury, vena cava, inferior
- hip S79.91-
  - blood vessel — *see* Injury, blood vessel, hip
  - contusion — *see* Contusion, hip
  - dislocation — *see* Dislocation, hip
  - fracture — *see* Fracture, femur, neck
  - muscle — *see* Injury, muscle, hip
  - nerve — *see* Injury, nerve, hip
  - open — *see* Wound, open, hip
  - sprain — *see* Sprain, hip
  - superficial — *see* Injury, superficial, hip
  - specified NEC S79.81-
- hymen S39.94
- hypogastric
  - blood vessel — *see* Injury, blood vessel, iliac

Injury — *continued*
- hypogastric — *continued*
  - plexus — *see* Injury, nerve, lumbosacral, sympathetic
- ileum — *see* Injury, intestine, small
- iliac region S39.91
- instrumental (during surgery) — *see* Laceration, accidental complicating surgery
  - birth injury — *see* Birth, injury
  - nonsurgical — *see* Injury, by site
  - obstetrical O71.9
    - bladder O71.5
    - cervix O71.3
    - high vaginal O71.4
    - perineal NOS O7Ø.9
    - urethra O71.5
    - uterus O71.5
      - with rupture or perforation O71.1
- internal T14.8
  - aorta — *see* Injury, aorta
  - bladder (sphincter) — *see* Injury, bladder
    - with
      - ectopic or molar pregnancy OØ8.6
    - following ectopic or molar pregnancy OØ8.6
    - obstetrical trauma O71.5
  - bronchus, bronchi — *see* Injury, intrathoracic, bronchus
  - cecum — *see* Injury, intestine, large
  - cervix (uteri) (*see also* Injury, uterus)
    - with ectopic or molar pregnancy OØ8.6
    - following ectopic or molar pregnancy OØ8.6
    - obstetrical trauma O71.3
  - chest — *see* Injury, intrathoracic
  - gastrointestinal tract — *see* Injury, intra-abdominal
  - heart — *see* Injury, heart
  - intestine NEC — *see* Injury, intestine
  - intrauterine — *see* Injury, uterus
  - mesentery — *see* Injury, intra-abdominal, specified, site NEC
  - pelvis, pelvic (organ) S37.9Ø
    - following ectopic or molar pregnancy (subsequent episode) OØ8.6
    - obstetrical trauma NEC O71.5
      - rupture or perforation O71.1
    - specified NEC S39.83
  - rectum — *see* Injury, intestine, large, rectum
  - stomach — *see* Injury, stomach
  - ureter — *see* Injury, ureter
  - urethra (sphincter) following ectopic or molar pregnancy OØ8.6
  - uterus — *see* Injury, uterus
- interscapular area — *see* Injury, thorax
- intestine
  - large S36.5Ø9
    - ascending (right) S36.5ØØ
      - blast injury (primary) S36.51Ø
        - secondary S36.59Ø
      - contusion S36.52Ø
      - laceration S36.53Ø
      - specified type NEC S36.59Ø
    - blast injury (primary) S36.519
      - ascending (right) S36.51Ø
      - descending (left) S36.512
      - rectum S36.61
      - sigmoid S36.513
      - specified site NEC S36.518
      - transverse S36.511
    - contusion S36.529
      - ascending (right) S36.52Ø
      - descending (left) S36.522
      - rectum S36.62
      - sigmoid S36.523
      - specified site NEC S36.528
      - transverse S36.521
    - descending (left) S36.5Ø2
      - blast injury (primary) S36.512
        - secondary S36.592
      - contusion S36.522
      - laceration S36.532
      - specified type NEC S36.592
    - laceration S36.539
      - ascending (right) S36.53Ø

- **Injury** — *continued*
  - intestine — *continued*
    - large— *continued*
      - laceration— *continued*
        - descending (left) S36.532
        - rectum S36.63
        - sigmoid S36.533
        - specified site NEC S36.538
        - transverse S36.531
      - rectum S36.6Ø
        - blast injury (primary) S36.61
          - secondary S36.69
        - contusion S36.62
        - laceration S36.63
        - specified type NEC S36.69
      - sigmoid S36.5Ø3
        - blast injury (primary) S36.513
          - secondary S36.593
        - contusion S36.523
        - laceration S36.533
        - specified type NEC S36.593
      - specified
        - site NEC S36.5Ø8
          - blast injury (primary) S36.518
            - secondary S36.598
          - contusion S36.528
          - laceration S36.538
          - specified type NEC S36.598
        - type NEC S36.599
          - ascending (right) S36.59Ø
          - descending (left) S36.592
          - rectum S36.69
          - sigmoid S36.593
          - specified site NEC S36.598
          - transverse S36.591
      - transverse S36.5Ø1
        - blast injury (primary) S36.511
          - secondary S36.591
        - contusion S36.521
        - laceration S36.531
        - specified type NEC S36.591
    - small S36.4Ø9
      - blast injury (primary) S36.419
        - duodenum S36.41Ø
        - secondary S36.499
          - duodenum S36.49Ø
          - specified site NEC S36.498
        - specified site NEC S36.418
      - contusion S36.429
        - duodenum S36.42Ø
        - specified site NEC S36.428
      - duodenum S36.4ØØ
        - blast injury (primary) S36.41Ø
          - secondary S36.49Ø
        - contusion S36.42Ø
        - laceration S36.43Ø
        - specified NEC S36.49Ø
      - laceration S36.439
        - duodenum S36.43Ø
        - specified site NEC S36.438
      - specified
        - type NEC S36.499
          - duodenum S36.49Ø
          - specified site NEC S36.498
        - site NEC S36.4Ø8
  - intra-abdominal S36.9Ø
    - adrenal gland — *see* Injury, adrenal gland
    - bladder — *see* Injury, bladder
    - colon — *see* Injury, intestine, large
    - contusion S36.92
    - fallopian tube — *see* Injury, fallopian tube
    - gallbladder — *see* Injury, gallbladder
    - intestine — *see* Injury, intestine
    - laceration S36.93
    - liver — *see* Injury, liver
    - kidney — *see* Injury, kidney
    - ovary — *see* Injury, ovary
    - pancreas — *see* Injury, pancreas
    - pelvic NOS S37.9Ø
    - peritoneum — *see* Injury, intra-abdominal, specified, site NEC
    - prostate — *see* Injury, prostate
    - rectum — *see* Injury, intestine, large, rectum

- **Injury** — *continued*
  - intra-abdominal— *continued*
    - retroperitoneum — *see* Injury, intra-abdominal, specified, site NEC
    - seminal vesicle — *see* Injury, pelvis, organ, specified site NEC
    - small intestine — *see* Injury, intestine, small
    - specified
      - site NEC S36.899
        - contusion S36.892
        - laceration S36.893
        - specified type NEC S36.898
      - type NEC S36.99
      - pelvic S37.9Ø
        - specified
          - site NEC S37.899
            - specified type NEC S37.898
          - type NEC S37.99
    - spleen — *see* Injury, spleen
    - stomach — *see* Injury, stomach
    - ureter — *see* Injury, ureter
    - urethra — *see* Injury, urethra
    - uterus — *see* Injury, uterus
    - vas deferens — *see* Injury, pelvis, organ, specified site NEC
  - intracranial (traumatic) SØ6.9-
    - cerebellar hemorrhage, traumatic — *see* Injury, intracranial, focal
    - cerebral edema, traumatic SØ6.1X-
      - diffuse SØ6.1X-
      - focal SØ6.1X-
    - diffuse (axonal) SØ6.2X-
    - epidural hemorrhage (traumatic) SØ6.4X-
    - focal brain injury SØ6.3Ø-
      - contusion — *see* Contusion, cerebral
      - laceration — *see* Laceration, cerebral
    - intracerebral hemorrhage, traumatic SØ6.36-
      - left side SØ6.35-
      - right side SØ6.34-
    - subarachnoid hemorrhage, traumatic SØ6.6X-
    - subdural hemorrhage, traumatic SØ6.5X-
  - intraocular — *see* Injury, eyeball, penetrating
  - intrathoracic S27.9
    - bronchus S27.4Ø9
      - bilateral S27.4Ø2
      - blast injury (primary) S27.419
        - bilateral S27.412
        - secondary — *see* Injury, intrathoracic, bronchus, specified type NEC
        - unilateral S27.411
      - contusion S27.429
        - bilateral S27.422
        - unilateral S27.421
      - laceration S27.439
        - bilateral S27.432
        - unilateral S27.431
      - specified type NEC S27.499
        - bilateral S27.492
        - unilateral S27.491
      - unilateral S27.4Ø1
    - diaphragm S27.8Ø9
      - contusion S27.8Ø2
      - laceration S27.8Ø3
      - specified type NEC S27.8Ø8
    - esophagus (thoracic) S27.819
      - contusion S27.812
      - laceration S27.813
      - specified type NEC S27.818
    - heart — *see* Injury, heart
    - hemopneumothorax S27.2
    - hemothorax S27.1
    - lung S27.3Ø9
      - aspiration J69.Ø
      - bilateral S27.3Ø2
      - blast injury (primary) S27.319
        - bilateral S27.312
        - secondary — *see* Injury, intrathoracic, lung, specified type NEC
        - unilateral S27.311
      - contusion S27.329
        - bilateral S27.322
        - unilateral S27.321

- **Injury** — *continued*
  - intrathoracic— *continued*
    - lung — *continued*
      - laceration S27.339
        - bilateral S27.332
        - unilateral S27.331
      - specified type NEC S27.399
        - bilateral S27.392
        - unilateral S27.391
      - unilateral S27.3Ø1
    - pleura S27.6Ø
      - laceration S27.63
      - specified type NEC S27.69
    - pneumothorax S27.Ø
    - specified organ NEC S27.899
      - contusion S27.892
      - laceration S27.893
      - specified type NEC S27.898
    - thoracic duct — *see* Injury, intrathoracic, specified organ NEC
    - thymus gland — *see* Injury, intrathoracic, specified organ NEC
    - trachea, thoracic S27.5Ø
      - blast (primary) S27.51
      - contusion S27.52
      - laceration S27.53
      - specified type NEC S27.59
  - iris — *see* Injury, eye, specified site NEC
    - penetrating — *see* Injury, eyeball, penetrating
  - jaw SØ9.93
  - jejunum — *see* Injury, intestine, small
  - joint NOS T14.8
    - old or residual — *see* Disorder, joint, specified type NEC
  - kidney S37.ØØ-
    - contusion — *see* Contusion, kidney
    - laceration — *see* Laceration, kidney
    - specified NEC S37.Ø9-
  - knee S89.9-
    - contusion — *see* Contusion, knee
    - dislocation — *see* Dislocation, knee
    - meniscus (lateral) (medial) — *see* Sprain, knee, specified site NEC
      - old injury or tear — *see* Derangement, knee, meniscus, due to old injury
    - open — *see* Wound, open, knee
    - specified NEC S89.8-
    - sprain — *see* Sprain, knee
    - superficial — *see* Injury, superficial, knee
  - labium (majus) (minus) S39.94
  - labyrinth, ear SØ9.91
  - lacrimal apparatus, duct, gland, or sac — *see* Injury, eye, specified site NEC
  - larynx NEC S19.81
  - leg (lower) S89.9-
    - blood vessel — *see* Injury, blood vessel, leg
    - contusion — *see* Contusion, leg
    - fracture — *see* Fracture, leg
    - muscle — *see* Injury, muscle, leg
    - nerve — *see* Injury, nerve, leg
    - open — *see* Wound, open, leg
    - specified NEC S89.8-
    - superficial — *see* Injury, superficial, leg
  - lens, eye — *see* Injury, eye, specified site NEC
    - penetrating — *see* Injury, eyeball, penetrating
  - limb NEC T14.8
  - lip SØ9.93
  - liver S36.119
    - contusion S36.112
    - laceration S36.113
      - major (stellate) S36.116
      - minor S36.114
      - moderate S36.115
    - specified NEC S36.118
  - lower back S39.92
    - specified NEC S39.82
  - lumbar, lumbosacral (region) S39.92
    - plexus — *see* Injury, lumbosacral plexus
  - lumbosacral plexus S34.4
  - lung (*see also* Injury, intrathoracic, lung)
    - aspiration J69.Ø
    - transfusion-related (TRALI) J95.84

- **Injury** — *continued*
  - lymphatic thoracic duct — *see* Injury, intrathoracic, specified organ NEC
  - malar region SØ9.93
  - mastoid region SØ9.9Ø
  - maxilla SØ9.93
  - mediastinum — *see* Injury, intrathoracic, specified organ NEC
  - membrane, brain — *see* Injury, intracranial
  - meningeal artery — *see* Injury, intracranial, subdural hemorrhage
  - meninges (cerebral) — *see* Injury, intracranial
  - mesenteric
    - artery
      - branch S35.299
        - laceration (minor) (superficial) S35.291
          - major S35.292
        - specified NEC S35.298
      - inferior S35.239
        - laceration (minor) (superficial) S35.231
          - major S35.232
        - specified NEC S35.238
      - superior S35.229
        - laceration (minor) (superficial) S35.221
          - major S35.222
        - specified NEC S35.228
    - plexus (inferior) (superior) — *see* Injury, nerve, lumbosacral, sympathetic
    - vein
      - inferior S35.349
        - laceration S35.341
        - specified NEC S35.348
      - superior S35.339
        - laceration S35.331
        - specified NEC S35.338
  - mesentery — *see* Injury, intra-abdominal, specified site NEC
  - mesosalpinx — *see* Injury, pelvic organ, specified site NEC
  - middle ear SØ9.91
  - midthoracic region NOS S29.9
  - mouth SØ9.93
  - multiple NOS TØ7
  - muscle (and fascia) (and tendon)
    - abdomen S39.ØØ1
      - laceration S39.Ø21
      - specified type NEC S39.Ø91
      - strain S39.Ø11
    - abductor
      - thumb, forearm level — *see* Injury, muscle, thumb, abductor
    - adductor
      - thigh S76.2Ø-
        - laceration S76.22-
        - specified type NEC S76.29-
        - strain S76.21-
    - ankle — *see* Injury, muscle, foot
    - anterior muscle group, at leg level (lower) S86.2Ø-
      - laceration S86.22-
      - specified type NEC S86.29-
      - strain S86.21-
    - arm (upper) — *see* Injury, muscle, shoulder
    - biceps (parts NEC) S46.2Ø-
      - laceration S46.22-
      - long head S46.1Ø-
        - laceration S46.12-
        - strain S46.11-
        - specified type NEC S46.19-
      - specified type NEC S46.29-
      - strain S46.21-
    - extensor
      - finger(s) (other than thumb) — *see* Injury, muscle, finger by site, extensor
      - forearm level, specified NEC — *see* Injury, muscle, forearm, extensor
      - thumb — *see* Injury, muscle, thumb, extensor
      - toe (large) (ankle level) (foot level) — *see* Injury, muscle, toe, extensor
    - finger
      - extensor (forearm level) S56.4Ø-
        - hand level S66.3Ø9
          - laceration S66.329

- **Injury** — *continued*
  - muscle — *continued*
    - finger — *continued*
      - extensor— *continued*
        - hand level — *continued*
          - specified type NEC S66.399
          - strain S66.319
        - laceration S56.429
        - specified type NEC S56.499
        - strain S56.419
      - flexor (forearm level) S56.1Ø-
        - hand level S66.1Ø9
          - laceration S66.129
          - specified type NEC S66.199
          - strain S66.119
        - laceration S56.129
        - specified type NEC S56.199
        - strain S56.119
      - intrinsic S66.5Ø9
        - laceration S66.529
        - specified type NEC S66.599
        - strain S66.519
      - index
        - extensor (forearm level)
          - hand level S66.3Ø8
            - laceration S66.32-
            - specified type NEC S66.39-
            - strain S66.31-
          - specified type NEC S56.492-
        - flexor (forearm level)
          - hand level S66.1Ø8
            - laceration S66.12-
            - specified type NEC S66.19-
            - strain S66.11-
          - specified type NEC S56.19-
          - strain S56.11-
        - intrinsic S66.5Ø-
          - laceration S66.52-
          - specified type NEC S66.59-
          - strain S66.51-
      - little
        - extensor (forearm level)
          - hand level S66.3Ø-
            - laceration S66.32-
            - specified type NEC S66.39-
            - strain S66.31-
          - laceration S56.42-
          - specified type NEC S56.49-
          - strain S56.41-
        - flexor (forearm level)
          - hand level S66.1Ø-
            - laceration S66.12-
            - specified type NEC S66.19-
            - strain S66.11-
          - laceration S56.12-
          - specified type NEC S56.19-
          - strain S56.11-
        - intrinsic S66.5Ø-
          - laceration S66.52-
          - specified type NEC S66.59-
          - strain S66.51-
      - middle
        - extensor (forearm level)
          - hand level S66.3Ø-
            - laceration S66.32-
            - specified type NEC S66.39-
            - strain S66.31-
          - laceration S56.42-
          - specified type NEC S56.49-
          - strain S56.41-
        - flexor (forearm level)
          - hand level S66.1Ø-
            - laceration S66.12-
            - specified type NEC S66.19-
            - strain S66.11-
          - laceration S56.12-
          - specified type NEC S56.19-
          - strain S56.11-
        - intrinsic S66.5Ø-
          - laceration S66.52-
          - specified type NEC S66.59-
          - strain S66.51-

- **Injury** — *continued*
  - muscle — *continued*
    - finger— *continued*
      - ring
        - extensor (forearm level)
          - hand level S66.3Ø-
            - laceration S66.32-
            - specified type NEC S66.39-
            - strain S66.31-
          - laceration S56.42-
          - specified type NEC S56.49-
      - strain S56.41-
        - flexor (forearm level)
          - hand level S66.1Ø-
            - laceration S66.12-
            - specified type NEC S66.19-
            - strain S66.11-
          - laceration S56.12-
          - specified type NEC S56.19-
          - strain S56.11-
        - intrinsic S66.5Ø-
          - laceration S66.52-
          - specified type NEC S66.59-
          - strain S66.51-
    - flexor
      - finger(s) (other than thumb) — *see* Injury, muscle, finger
      - forearm level, specified NEC — *see* Injury, muscle, forearm, flexor
      - thumb — *see* Injury, muscle, thumb, flexor
      - toe (long) (ankle level) (foot level) — *see* Injury, muscle, toe, flexor
    - foot S96.9Ø-
      - intrinsic S96.2Ø-
        - laceration S96.22-
        - specified type NEC S96.29-
        - strain S96.21-
      - laceration S96.92-
      - long extensor, toe — *see* Injury, muscle, toe, extensor
      - long flexor, toe — *see* Injury, muscle, toe, flexor
      - specified
        - site NEC S96.8Ø-
          - laceration S96.82-
          - specified type NEC S96.89-
          - strain S96.81-
        - type NEC S96.99-
      - strain S96.91-
    - forearm (level) S56.9Ø-
      - extensor S56.5Ø-
        - laceration S56.52-
        - specified type NEC S56.59-
        - strain S56.51-
      - flexor S56.2Ø-
        - laceration S56.22-
        - specified type NEC S56.29-
        - strain S56.21-
      - laceration S56.92-
      - specified S56.99-
        - site NEC S56.8Ø-
          - laceration S56.82-
          - strain S56.81-
        - type NEC S56.89-
      - strain S56.91-
    - hand (level) S66.9Ø-
      - laceration S66.92-
      - specified
        - site NEC S66.8Ø-
          - laceration S66.82-
          - specified type NEC S66.89-
          - strain S66.81-
        - type NEC S66.99-
      - strain S66.91-
    - head SØ9.1Ø
      - laceration SØ9.12
      - specified type NEC SØ9.19
      - strain SØ9.11
    - hip NEC S76.ØØ-
      - laceration S76.Ø2-
      - specified type NEC S76.Ø9-
      - strain S76.Ø1-

- **Injury** — *continued*
  - muscle — *continued*
    - intrinsic
      - ankle and foot level — *see* Injury, muscle, foot, intrinsic
      - finger (other than thumb) — *see* Injury, muscle, finger by site, intrinsic
      - foot (level) — *see* Injury, muscle, foot, intrinsic
      - thumb — *see* Injury, muscle, thumb, intrinsic
    - leg (level) (lower) S86.9Ø-
      - Achilles tendon — *see* Injury, Achilles tendon
      - anterior muscle group — *see* Injury, muscle, anterior muscle group
      - laceration S86.92-
      - peroneal muscle group — *see* Injury, muscle, peroneal muscle group
      - posterior muscle group — *see* Injury, muscle, posterior muscle group, leg level
      - specified
        - site NEC S86.8Ø-
          - laceration S86.82-
          - specified type NEC S86.89-
          - strain S86.81-
        - type NEC S86.99-
      - strain S86.91-
    - long
      - extensor toe, at ankle and foot level — *see* Injury, muscle, toe, extensor
      - flexor, toe, at ankle and foot level — *see* Injury, muscle, toe, flexor
      - head, biceps — *see* Injury, muscle, biceps, long head
    - lower back S39.ØØ2
      - laceration S39.Ø22
      - specified type NEC S39.Ø92
      - strain S39.Ø12
    - neck (level) S16.9
      - laceration S16.2
      - specified type NEC S16.8
      - strain S16.1
    - pelvis S39.ØØ3
      - laceration S39.Ø23
      - specified type NEC S39.Ø93
      - strain S39.Ø13
    - peroneal muscle group, at leg level (lower) S86.3Ø-
      - laceration S86.32-
      - specified type NEC S86.39-
      - strain S86.31-
    - posterior muscle (group)
      - leg level (lower) S86.1Ø-
        - laceration S86.12-
        - specified type NEC S86.19-
        - strain S86.11-
      - thigh level S76.3Ø-
        - laceration S76.32-
        - specified type NEC S76.39-
        - strain S76.31-
    - quadriceps (thigh) S76.1Ø-
      - laceration S76.12-
      - specified type NEC S76.19-
      - strain S76.11-
    - shoulder S46.9Ø-
      - laceration S46.92-
      - rotator cuff — *see* Injury, rotator cuff
      - specified site NEC S46.8Ø-
        - laceration S46.82-
        - strain S46.81-
        - specified type NEC S46.89-
      - strain S46.91-
      - specified type NEC S46.99-
    - thigh NEC (level) S76.9Ø-
      - adductor — *see* Injury, muscle, adductor, thigh
      - laceration S76.92-
      - posterior muscle (group) — *see* Injury, muscle, posterior muscle, thigh level
      - quadriceps — *see* Injury, muscle, quadriceps
      - specified
        - site NEC S76.8Ø-
          - laceration S76.82-
          - specified type NEC S76.89-
          - strain S76.81-

- **Injury** — *continued*
  - muscle — *continued*
    - thigh NEC— *continued*
      - specified — *continued*
        - type NEC S76.99-
      - strain S76.91-
    - thorax (level) S29.ØØ9
      - back wall S29.ØØ2
      - front wall S29.ØØ1
      - laceration S29.Ø29
        - back wall S29.Ø22
        - front wall S29.Ø21
      - specified type NEC S29.Ø99
        - back wall S29.Ø92
        - front wall S29.Ø91
      - strain S29.Ø19
        - back wall S29.Ø12
        - front wall S29.Ø11
    - thumb
      - abductor (forearm level) S56.3Ø-
        - laceration S56.32-
        - specified type NEC S56.39-
        - strain S56.31-
      - extensor (forearm level) S56.3Ø-
        - hand level S66.2Ø-
          - laceration S66.22-
          - specified type NEC S66.29-
          - strain S66.21-
        - laceration S56.32-
        - specified type NEC S56.39-
        - strain S56.31-
      - flexor (forearm level) S56.ØØ-
        - hand level S66.ØØ-
          - laceration S66.Ø2-
          - specified type NEC S66.Ø9-
          - strain S66.Ø1-
        - laceration S56.Ø2-
        - specified type NEC S56.Ø9-
        - strain S56.Ø1-
        - wrist level — *see* Injury, muscle, thumb, flexor, hand level
      - intrinsic S66.4Ø-
        - laceration S66.42-
        - specified type NEC S66.49-
        - strain S66.41-
    - toe (*see also* Injury, muscle, foot)
      - extensor, long S96.1Ø-
        - laceration S96.12-
        - specified type NEC S96.19-
        - strain S96.11-
      - flexor, long S96.ØØ-
        - laceration S96.Ø2-
        - specified type NEC S96.Ø9-
        - strain S96.Ø1-
    - triceps S46.3Ø-
      - laceration S46.32-
      - specified type NEC S46.39-
      - strain S46.31-
    - wrist (and hand) level — *see* Injury, muscle, hand
  - musculocutaneous nerve — *see* Injury, nerve, musculocutaneous
  - myocardium — *see* Injury, heart
  - nape — *see* Injury, neck
  - nasal (septum) (sinus) SØ9.92
  - nasopharynx SØ9.92
  - neck S19.9
    - specified NEC S19.8Ø
      - specified site NEC S19.89
  - nerve NEC T14.8
    - abdomen S34.9
      - peripheral S34.6
      - specified site NEC S34.8
    - abducens SØ4.4-
      - contusion SØ4.4-
      - laceration SØ4.4-
      - specified type NEC SØ4.4-
    - abducent — *see* Injury, nerve, abducens
    - accessory SØ4.7-
      - contusion SØ4.7-
      - laceration SØ4.7-
      - specified type NEC SØ4.7-

- **Injury** — *continued*
  - nerve — *continued*
    - acoustic SØ4.6-
      - contusion SØ4.6-
      - laceration SØ4.6-
      - specified type NEC SØ4.6-
    - ankle S94.9-
      - cutaneous sensory S94.3-
      - specified site NEC — *see* subcategory S94.8
    - anterior crural, femoral — *see* Injury, nerve, femoral
    - arm (upper) S44.9-
      - axillary — *see* Injury, nerve, axillary
      - cutaneous — *see* Injury, nerve, cutaneous, arm
      - median — *see* Injury, nerve, median, upper arm
      - musculocutaneous — *see* Injury, nerve, musculocutaneous
      - radial — *see* Injury, nerve, radial, upper arm
      - specified site NEC — *see* subcategory S44.8
      - ulnar — *see* Injury, nerve, ulnar, arm
    - auditory — *see* Injury, nerve, acoustic
    - axillary S44.3-
    - brachial plexus — *see* Injury, brachial plexus
    - cervical sympathetic S14.5
    - cranial SØ4.9
      - contusion SØ4.9
      - eighth (acoustic or auditory) — *see* Injury, nerve, acoustic
      - eleventh (accessory) — *see* Injury, nerve, accessory
      - fifth (trigeminal) — *see* Injury, nerve, trigeminal
      - first (olfactory) — *see* Injury, nerve, olfactory
      - fourth (trochlear) — *see* Injury, nerve, trochlear
      - laceration SØ4.9
      - ninth (glossopharyngeal) — *see* Injury, nerve, glossopharyngeal
      - second (optic) — *see* Injury, nerve, optic
      - seventh (facial) — *see* Injury, nerve, facial
      - sixth (abducent) — *see* Injury, nerve, abducens
      - specified
        - nerve NEC SØ4.89-
          - contusion SØ4.89-
          - laceration SØ4.89-
          - specified type NEC SØ4.89-
        - type NEC SØ4.9
      - tenth (pneumogastric or vagus) — *see* Injury, nerve, vagus
      - third (oculomotor) — *see* Injury, nerve, oculomotor
      - twelfth (hypoglossal) — *see* Injury, nerve, hypoglossal
    - cutaneous sensory
      - ankle (level) S94.3-
      - arm (upper) (level) S44.5-
      - foot (level) — *see* Injury, nerve, cutaneous sensory, ankle
      - forearm (level) S54.3-
      - hip (level) S74.2-
      - leg (lower level) S84.2-
      - shoulder (level) — *see* Injury, nerve, cutaneous sensory, arm
      - thigh (level) — *see* Injury, nerve, cutaneous sensory, hip
    - deep peroneal — *see* Injury, nerve, peroneal, foot
    - digital
      - finger S64.4-
        - index S64.49-
        - little S64.49-
        - middle S64.49-
        - ring S64.49-
      - thumb S64.3-
      - toe — *see* Injury, nerve, ankle, specified site NEC
    - eighth cranial (acoustic or auditory) — *see* Injury, nerve, acoustic
    - eleventh cranial (accessory) — *see* Injury, nerve, accessory

- **Injury** — *continued*
  - nerve — *continued*
    - facial SØ4.5-
      - contusion SØ4.5-
      - laceration SØ4.5-
      - newborn P11.3
      - specified type NEC SØ4.5-
    - femoral (hip level) (thigh level) S74.1-
    - fifth cranial (trigeminal) — *see* Injury, nerve, trigeminal
    - finger (digital) — *see* Injury, nerve, digital, finger
    - first cranial (olfactory) — *see* Injury, nerve, olfactory
    - foot S94.9-
      - cutaneous sensory S94.3-
      - deep peroneal S94.2-
      - lateral plantar S94.Ø-
      - medial plantar S94.1-
      - specified site NEC — *see* subcategory S94.8
    - forearm (level) S54.9-
      - cutaneous sensory — *see* Injury, nerve, cutaneous sensory, forearm
      - median — *see* Injury, nerve, median
      - radial — *see* Injury, nerve, radial
      - specified site NEC — *see* subcategory S54.8
      - ulnar — *see* Injury, nerve, ulnar
    - fourth cranial (trochlear) — *see* Injury, nerve, trochlear
    - glossopharyngeal SØ4.89-
      - specified type NEC SØ4.89-
    - hand S64.9-
      - median — *see* Injury, nerve, median, hand
      - radial — *see* Injury, nerve, radial, hand
      - specified NEC — *see* subcategory S64.8
      - ulnar — *see* Injury, nerve, ulnar, hand
    - hip (level) S74.9-
      - cutaneous sensory — *see* Injury, nerve, cutaneous sensory, hip
      - femoral — *see* Injury, nerve, femoral
      - sciatic — *see* Injury, nerve, sciatic
      - specified site NEC — *see* subcategory S74.8
    - hypoglossal SØ4.89-
      - specified type NEC SØ4.89-
    - lateral plantar S94.Ø-
    - leg (lower) S84.9-
      - cutaneous sensory — *see* Injury, nerve, cutaneous sensory, leg
      - peroneal — *see* Injury, nerve, peroneal
      - specified site NEC — *see* subcategory S84.8
      - tibial — *see* Injury, nerve, tibial
      - upper — *see* Injury, nerve, thigh
    - lower
      - back — *see* Injury, nerve, abdomen, specified site NEC
        - peripheral — *see* Injury, nerve, abdomen, peripheral
      - limb — *see* Injury, nerve, leg
    - lumbar plexus — *see* Injury, nerve, lumbosacral, sympathetic
    - lumbar spinal — *see* Injury, nerve spinal, lumbar
    - lumbosacral
      - plexus — *see* Injury, nerve, lumbosacral, sympathetic
      - sympathetic S34.5
    - medial plantar S94.1-
    - median (forearm level) S54.1-
      - hand (level) S64.1-
      - upper arm (level) S44.1-
      - wrist (level) — *see* Injury, nerve, median, hand
    - musculocutaneous S44.4-
    - musculospiral (upper arm level) — *see* Injury, nerve, radial, upper arm
    - neck S14.9
      - peripheral S14.4
      - specified site NEC S14.8
      - sympathetic S14.5
    - ninth cranial (glossopharyngeal) — *see* Injury, nerve, glossopharyngeal
    - oculomotor SØ4.1-
      - contusion SØ4.1-
      - laceration SØ4.1-
      - specified type NEC SØ4.1-

- **Injury** — *continued*
  - nerve — *continued*
    - olfactory SØ4.81-
      - specified type NEC SØ4.81-
    - optic SØ4.Ø1-
      - contusion SØ4.Ø1-
      - laceration SØ4.Ø1-
      - specified type NEC SØ4.Ø1-
    - pelvic girdle — *see* Injury, nerve, hip
    - pelvis — *see* Injury, nerve, abdomen, specified site NEC
      - peripheral — *see* Injury, nerve, abdomen, peripheral
    - peripheral NEC T14.8
      - abdomen — *see* Injury, nerve, abdomen, peripheral
      - lower back — *see* Injury, nerve, abdomen, peripheral
      - neck — *see* Injury, nerve, neck, peripheral
      - pelvis — *see* Injury, nerve, abdomen, peripheral
      - specified NEC T14.8
    - peroneal (lower leg level) S84.1-
      - foot S94.2-
    - plexus
      - brachial — *see* Injury, brachial plexus
      - celiac, coeliac — *see* Injury, nerve, lumbosacral, sympathetic
      - mesenteric, inferior — *see* Injury, nerve, lumbosacral, sympathetic
      - sacral — *see* Injury, lumbosacral plexus
      - spinal
        - brachial — *see* Injury, brachial plexus
        - lumbosacral — *see* Injury, lumbosacral plexus
    - pneumogastric — *see* Injury, nerve, vagus
    - radial (forearm level) S54.2-
      - hand (level) S64.2-
      - upper arm (level) S44.2-
      - wrist (level) — *see* Injury, nerve, radial, hand
    - root — *see* Injury, nerve, spinal, root
    - sacral plexus — *see* Injury, lumbosacral plexus
    - sacral spinal — *see* Injury, nerve, spinal. sacral
    - sciatic (hip level) (thigh level) S74.Ø-
    - second cranial (optic) — *see* Injury, nerve, optic
    - seventh cranial (facial) — *see* Injury, nerve, facial
    - shoulder — *see* Injury, nerve, arm
    - sixth cranial (abducent) — *see* Injury, nerve, abducens
    - spinal
      - plexus — *see* Injury, nerve, plexus, spinal
      - root
        - cervical S14.2
        - dorsal S24.2
        - lumbar S34.21
        - sacral S34.22
        - thoracic — *see* Injury, nerve, spinal, root, dorsal
    - splanchnic — *see* Injury, nerve, lumbosacral, sympathetic
    - sympathetic NEC — *see* Injury, nerve, lumbosacral, sympathetic
      - cervical — *see* Injury, nerve, cervical sympathetic
    - tenth cranial (pneumogastric or vagus) — *see* Injury, nerve, vagus
    - thigh (level) — *see* Injury, nerve, hip
      - cutaneous sensory — *see* Injury, nerve, cutaneous sensory, hip
      - femoral — *see* Injury, nerve, femoral
      - sciatic — *see* Injury, nerve, sciatic
      - specified NEC — *see* Injury, nerve, hip
    - third cranial (oculomotor) — *see* Injury, nerve, oculomotor
    - thorax S24.9
      - peripheral S24.3
      - specified site NEC S24.8
      - sympathetic S24.4
    - thumb, digital — *see* Injury, nerve, digital, thumb
    - tibial (lower leg level) (posterior) S84.Ø-
    - toe — *see* Injury, nerve, ankle

- **Injury** — *continued*
  - nerve — *continued*
    - trigeminal SØ4.3-
      - contusion SØ4.3-
      - laceration SØ4.3-
      - specified type NEC SØ4.3-
    - trochlear SØ4.2-
      - contusion SØ4.2-
      - laceration SØ4.2-
      - specified type NEC SØ4.2-
    - twelfth cranial (hypoglossal) — *see* Injury, nerve, hypoglossal
    - ulnar (forearm level) S54.Ø-
      - arm (upper) (level) S44.Ø-
      - hand (level) S64.Ø-
      - wrist (level) — *see* Injury, nerve, ulnar, hand
    - vagus SØ4.89-
      - specified type NEC SØ4.89-
    - wrist (level) — *see* Injury, nerve, hand
  - ninth cranial nerve (glossopharyngeal) — *see* Injury, nerve, glossopharyngeal
  - nose (septum) SØ9.92
  - obstetrical O71.9
    - specified NEC O71.89
  - occipital (region) (scalp) SØ9.9Ø
    - lobe — *see* Injury, intracranial
  - optic chiasm SØ4.Ø2
  - optic radiation SØ4.Ø3-
  - optic tract and pathways SØ4.Ø3-
  - orbit, orbital (region) — *see* Injury, eye
    - penetrating (with foreign body) — *see* Injury, eye, orbit, penetrating
    - specified NEC — *see* Injury, eye, specified site NEC
  - ovary, ovarian S37.4Ø9
    - bilateral S37.4Ø2
      - contusion S37.422
      - laceration S37.432
      - specified type NEC S37.492
    - blood vessel — *see* Injury, blood vessel, ovarian
    - contusion S37.429
      - bilateral S37.422
      - unilateral S37.421
    - laceration S37.439
      - bilateral S37.432
      - unilateral S37.431
    - specified type NEC S37.499
      - bilateral S37.492
      - unilateral S37.491
    - unilateral S37.4Ø1
      - contusion S37.421
      - laceration S37.431
      - specified type NEC S37.491
  - palate (hard) (soft) SØ9.93
  - pancreas S36.2Ø9
    - body S36.2Ø1
      - contusion S36.221
      - laceration S36.239
        - major S36.269
        - minor S36.249
        - moderate S36.259
      - specified type NEC S36.291
    - contusion S36.229
    - head S36.2ØØ
      - contusion S36.22Ø
      - laceration S36.23Ø
        - major S36.26Ø
        - minor S36.24Ø
        - moderate S36.25Ø
      - specified type NEC S36.29Ø
    - laceration S36.239
      - major S36.269
      - minor S36.249
      - moderate S36.259
    - specified type NEC S36.299
    - tail S36.2Ø2
      - contusion S36.222
      - laceration S36.232
        - major S36.262
        - minor S36.242
        - moderate S36.252
      - specified type NEC S36.292

Insufficiency, insufficient— *continued*
- cardiovascular — *see* Disease, cardiovascular
- cerebrovascular (acute) I67.81
  - with transient focal neurological signs and symptoms G45.8
- circulatory NEC I99.8
  - newborn P29.89
- convergence H51.11
- coronary (acute or subacute) I24.8
  - chronic or with a stated duration of over 4 weeks I25.89
- corticoadrenal E27.4Ø
  - primary E27.1
- dietary E63.9
- divergence H51.8
- food T73.Ø
- gastroesophageal K22.8
- gonadal
  - ovary E28.39
  - testis E29.1
- heart (*see also* Insufficiency, myocardial)
  - newborn P29.Ø
  - valve — *see* Endocarditis
- hepatic — *see* Failure, hepatic
- idiopathic autonomic G9Ø.Ø9
- interocclusal distance of fully erupted teeth (ridge) M26.36
- kidney N28.9
  - acute N28.9
  - chronic N18.9
- lacrimal (secretion) HØ4.12-
  - passages — *see* Stenosis, lacrimal
- liver — *see* Failure, hepatic
- lung — *see* Insufficiency, pulmonary
- mental (congenital) — *see* Disability, intellectual
- mesenteric K55.1
- mitral (valve) I34.Ø
  - with
    - aortic valve disease IØ8.Ø
      - with tricuspid (valve) disease IØ8.3
    - obstruction or stenosis IØ5.2
      - with aortic valve disease IØ8.Ø
  - congenital Q23.3
  - rheumatic IØ5.1
    - with
      - aortic valve disease IØ8.Ø
        - with tricuspid (valve) disease IØ8.3
      - obstruction or stenosis IØ5.2
        - with aortic valve disease IØ8.Ø
          - with tricuspid (valve) disease IØ8.3
      - tricuspid (valve) disease IØ8.1
      - tricuspid (valve) disease IØ8.1
        - with aortic (valve) disease IØ8.3
    - active or acute IØ1.1
      - with chorea, rheumatic (Sydenham's) IØ2.Ø
  - specified cause, except rheumatic I34.Ø
- muscle (*see also* Disease, muscle)
  - heart — *see* Insufficiency, myocardial
  - ocular NEC H5Ø.9
- myocardial, myocardium (with arteriosclerosis) I5Ø.9
  - with
    - rheumatic fever (conditions in IØØ) IØ9.Ø
      - active, acute or subacute IØ1.2
        - with chorea IØ2.Ø
      - inactive or quiescent (with chorea) IØ9.Ø
  - congenital Q24.8
  - hypertensive — *see* Hypertension, heart
  - newborn P29.Ø
  - rheumatic IØ9.Ø
    - active, acute, or subacute IØ1.2
  - syphilitic A52.Ø6
- nourishment T73.Ø
- pancreatic K86.8
- parathyroid (gland) E2Ø.9
- peripheral vascular (arterial) I73.9
- pituitary E23.Ø
- placental (mother) O36.51-
- platelets D69.6
- prenatal care affecting management of pregnancy OØ9.3-
- progressive pluriglandular E31.Ø

Insufficiency, insufficient— *continued*
- pulmonary J98.4
  - acute, following surgery (nonthoracic) J95.2
    - thoracic J95.1
  - chronic, following surgery J95.3
  - following
    - shock J8Ø
    - trauma J8Ø
  - newborn P28.5
  - valve I37.1
    - with stenosis I37.2
    - congenital Q22.2
    - rheumatic IØ9.89
      - with aortic, mitral or tricuspid (valve) disease IØ8.8
- pyloric K31.89
- renal (acute) N28.9
  - chronic N18.9
- respiratory RØ6.89
  - newborn P28.5
- rotation — *see* Malrotation
- sleep syndrome F51.12
- social insurance Z59.7
- suprarenal E27.4Ø
  - primary E27.1
- tarso-orbital fascia, congenital Q1Ø.3
- testis E29.1
- thyroid (gland) (acquired) EØ3.9
  - congenital EØ3.1
- tricuspid (valve) (rheumatic) IØ7.1
  - with
    - aortic (valve) disease IØ8.2
      - with mitral (valve) disease IØ8.3
    - mitral (valve) disease IØ8.1
      - with aortic (valve) disease IØ8.3
    - obstruction or stenosis IØ7.2
      - with aortic (valve) disease IØ8.2
        - with mitral (valve) disease IØ8.3
  - congenital Q22.8
  - nonrheumatic I36.1
    - with stenosis I36.2
- urethral sphincter R32
- valve, valvular (heart) — *see* Endocarditis
  - congenital Q24.8
- vascular I99.8
  - intestine K55.9
    - acute K55.Ø
  - mesenteric K55.1
  - peripheral I73.9
  - renal — *see* Hypertension, kidney
- velopharyngeal
  - acquired K13.79
  - congenital Q38.8
- venous (chronic) (peripheral) I87.2
- ventricular — *see* Insufficiency, myocardial
- welfare support Z59.7

Insufflation, fallopian Z31.41

Insular — *see* condition

Insulinoma
- pancreas
  - benign D13.7
  - malignant C25.4
  - uncertain behavior D37.8
- specified site
  - benign — *see* Neoplasm, by site, benign
  - malignant — *see* Neoplasm, by site, malignant
  - uncertain behavior — *see* Neoplasm, by site, uncertain behavior
- unspecified site
  - benign D13.7
  - malignant C25.4
  - uncertain behavior D37.8

Insuloma — *see* Insulinoma

Interference
- balancing side M26.56
- non-working side M26.56

Intermenstrual — *see* condition

Intermittent — *see* condition

Internal — *see* condition

Interrogation
- cardiac defibrillator (automatic) (implantable) Z45.Ø2
- cardiac pacemaker Z45.Ø18

Interrogation— *continued*
- cardiac (event) (loop) recorder Z45.Ø9
- infusion pump (implanted) (intrathecal) Z45.1
- neurostimulator Z46.2

Interruption
- bundle of His I44.3Ø
- phase-shift, sleep cycle — *see* Disorder, sleep, circadian rhythm
- sleep phase-shift, or 24 hour sleep-wake cycle — *see* Disorder, sleep, circadian rhythm

Interstitial — *see* condition

Intertrigo L30.4
- labialis K13.Ø

Intervertebral disc — *see* condition

Intestine, intestinal — *see* condition

Intolerance
- carbohydrate K9Ø.4
- disaccharide, hereditary E73.Ø
- fat NEC K9Ø.4
  - pancreatic K9Ø.3
- food K9Ø.4
  - dietary counseling and surveillance Z71.3
- fructose E74.1Ø
  - hereditary E74.12
- glucose(-galactose) E74.39
- gluten K9Ø.Ø
- lactose E73.9
  - specified NEC E73.8
- lysine E72.3
- milk NEC K9Ø.4
  - lactose E73.9
- protein K9Ø.4
- starch NEC K9Ø.4
- sucrose(-isomaltose) E74.31

Intoxicated NEC (without dependence) — *see* Alcohol, intoxication

Intoxication
- acid E87.2
- alcoholic (acute) (without dependence) — *see* Alcohol, intoxication
- alimentary canal K52.1
- amphetamine (without dependence) — *see* Abuse, drug, stimulant, with intoxication
  - with dependence — *see* Dependence, drug, stimulant, with intoxication
- anxiolytic (acute) (without dependence) — *see* Abuse, drug, sedative, with intoxication
  - with dependence — *see* Dependence, drug, sedative, with intoxication
- caffeine (acute) (without dependence) — *see* Abuse, drug, stimulant, with intoxication
  - with dependence — *see* Dependence, drug, stimulant, with intoxication
- cannabinoids (acute) (without dependence) — *see* Abuse, drug, cannabis, with intoxication
  - with dependence — *see* Dependence, drug, cannabis, with intoxication
- chemical — *see* Table of Drugs and Chemicals
  - via placenta or breast milk — *see* Absorption, chemical, through placenta
- cocaine (acute) (without dependence) — *see* Abuse, drug, cocaine, with intoxication
  - with dependence — *see* Dependence, drug, cocaine, with intoxication
- drug
  - acute (without dependence) — *see* Abuse, drug, by type with intoxication
    - with dependence — *see* Dependence, drug, by type with intoxication
  - addictive
    - via placenta or breast milk — *see* Absorption, drug, addictive, through placenta
  - newborn P93.8
    - gray baby syndrome P93.Ø
  - overdose or wrong substance given or taken — *see* Table of Drugs and Chemicals, by drug, poisoning
- enteric K52.1
- foodborne AØ5.9
  - bacterial AØ5.9
  - classical (Clostridium botulinum) AØ5.1

- **Intoxication**— *continued*
  - foodborne — *continued*
    - due to
      - Bacillus cereus AØ5.4
      - bacterium AØ5.9
        - specified NEC AØ5.8
      - Clostridium
        - botulinum AØ5.1
        - perfringens AØ5.2
        - welchii AØ5.2
      - Salmonella AØ2.9
        - with
          - (gastro) enteritis AØ2.Ø
          - localized infection(s) AØ2.2Ø
            - arthritis AØ2.23
            - meningitis AØ2.21
            - osteomyelitis AØ2.24
            - pneumonia AØ2.22
            - pyelonephritis AØ2.25
            - specified NEC AØ2.29
          - sepsis AØ2.1
          - specified manifestation NEC AØ2.8
      - Staphylococcus AØ5.Ø
      - Vibrio
        - parahaemolyticus AØ5.3
        - vulnificus AØ5.5
    - enterotoxin, staphylococcal AØ5.Ø
    - noxious — *see* Poisoning, food, noxious
  - gastrointestinal K52.1
  - hallucinogenic (without dependence) — *see* Abuse, drug, hallucinogen, with intoxication
    - with dependence — *see* Dependence, drug, hallucinogen, with intoxication
  - hypnotic (acute) (without dependence) — *see* Abuse, drug, sedative, with intoxication
    - with dependence — *see* Dependence, drug, sedative, with intoxication
  - inhalant (acute) (without dependence) — *see* Abuse, drug, inhalant, with intoxication
    - with dependence — *see* Dependence, drug, inhalant, with intoxication
  - meaning
    - inebriation — *see* category F1Ø
    - poisoning — *see* Table of Drugs and Chemicals
  - methyl alcohol (acute) (without dependence) — *see* Alcohol, intoxication
  - opioid (acute) (without dependence) — *see* Abuse, drug, opioid, with intoxication
    - with dependence — *see* Dependence, drug, opioid, with intoxication
  - pathologic NEC (without dependence) — *see* Alcohol, intoxication
  - phencyclidine (without dependence) — *see* Abuse, drug, psychoactive NEC, with intoxication
    - with dependence — *see* Dependence, drug, psychoactive NEC, with intoxication
  - potassium (K) E87.5
  - psychoactive substance NEC (without dependence) — *see* Abuse, drug, psychoactive NEC, with intoxication
    - with dependence — *see* Dependence, drug, psychoactive NEC, with intoxication
  - sedative (acute) (without dependence) — *see* Abuse, drug, sedative, with intoxication
    - with dependence — *see* Dependence, drug, sedative, with intoxication
  - serum (*see also* Reaction, serum) T8Ø.69
  - uremic — *see* Uremia
  - volatile solvents (acute) (without dependence) — *see* Abuse, drug, inhalant, with intoxication
    - with dependence — *see* Dependence, drug, inhalant, with intoxication
  - water E87.79
- **Intracranial** — *see* condition
- **Intrahepatic gallbladder** Q44.1
- **Intraligamentous** — *see* condition
- **Intrathoracic** (*see also* condition)
  - kidney Q63.2
- **Intrauterine contraceptive device**
  - checking, Z3Ø.431
  - insertion Z3Ø.43Ø
    - immediately following removal Z3Ø.433
- **Intrauterine contraceptive device**— *continued*
  - in situ Z97.5
  - management Z3Ø.431
  - reinsertion Z3Ø.433
  - removal Z3Ø.432
  - replacement Z3Ø.433
  - retention in pregnancy O26.3-
- **Intraventricular** — *see* condition
- **Intrinsic deformity** — *see* Deformity
- **Intubation, difficult or failed** T88.4
- **Intumescence, lens** (eye) (cataract) — *see* Cataract
- **Intussusception** (bowel) (colon) (enteric) (ileocecal) (ileocolic) (intestine) (rectum) K56.1
  - appendix K38.8
  - congenital Q43.8
  - ureter (with obstruction) N13.5
- **Invagination** (bowel, colon, intestine or rectum) K56.1
- **Inversion**
  - albumin-globulin (A-G) ratio E88.Ø9
  - bladder N32.89
  - cecum — *see* Intussusception
  - cervix N88.8
  - chromosome in normal individual Q95.1
  - circadian rhythm — *see* Disorder, sleep, circadian rhythm
  - nipple N64.59
    - congenital Q83.8
    - gestational — *see* Retraction, nipple
    - puerperal, postpartum — *see* Retraction, nipple
  - nyctohemeral rhythm — *see* Disorder, sleep, circadian rhythm
  - optic papilla Q14.2
  - organ or site, congenital NEC — *see* Anomaly, by site
  - sleep rhythm — *see* Disorder, sleep, circadian rhythm
  - testis (congenital) Q55.29
  - uterus (chronic) (postinfectional) (postpartal, old) N85.5
    - postpartum O71.2
  - vagina (posthysterectomy) N99.3
  - ventricular Q2Ø.5
- **Investigation** (*see also* Examination) ZØ4.9
  - clinical research subject (control) (normal comparison) (participant) ZØØ.6
- **Involuntary movement, abnormal** R25.9
- **Involution, involutional** (*see also* condition)
  - breast, cystic — *see* Dysplasia, mammary, specified type NEC
  - depression (single episode) F32.8
    - recurrent episode F33.9
  - melancholia (recurrent episode) (single episode) F32.8
  - ovary, senile — *see* Atrophy, ovary
  - thymus failure E32.8
- **I.Q.**
  - under 2Ø F73
  - 2Ø-34 F72
  - 35-49 F71
  - 5Ø-69 F7Ø
- **IRDS** (type I) P22.Ø
  - type II P22.1
- **Irideremia** Q13.1
- **Iridis rubeosis** — *see* Disorder, iris, vascular
- **Iridochoroiditis** (panuveitis) — *see* Panuveitis
- **Iridocyclitis** H2Ø.9-
  - acute H2Ø.Ø-
    - hypopyon H2Ø.Ø5-
    - primary H2Ø.Ø1-
    - recurrent H2Ø.Ø2-
    - secondary (noninfectious) H2Ø.Ø4-
      - infectious H2Ø.Ø3-
  - chronic H2Ø.1-
  - due to allergy — *see* Iridocyclitis, acute, secondary
  - endogenous — *see* Iridocyclitis, acute, primary
  - Fuchs' — *see* Cyclitis, Fuchs' heterochromic
  - gonococcal A54.32
  - granulomatous — *see* Iridocyclitis, chronic
  - herpes, herpetic (simplex) BØØ.51
    - zoster BØ2.32
  - hypopyon — *see* Iridocyclitis, acute, hypopyon
- **Iridocyclitis** — *continued*
  - in (due to)
    - ankylosing spondylitis M45.9
    - gonococcal infection A54.32
    - herpes (simplex) virus BØØ.51
      - zoster BØ2.32
    - infectious disease NOS B99
    - parasitic disease NOS B89 *[H22]*
    - sarcoidosis D86.83
    - syphilis A51.43
    - tuberculosis A18.54
    - zoster BØ2.32
  - lens-induced H2Ø.2-
  - nongranulomatous — *see* Iridocyclitis, acute
  - recurrent — *see* Iridocyclitis, acute, recurrent
  - rheumatic — *see* Iridocyclitis, chronic
  - subacute — *see* Iridocyclitis, acute
  - sympathetic — *see* Uveitis, sympathetic
  - syphilitic (secondary) A51.43
  - tuberculous (chronic) A18.54
  - Vogt-Koyanagi H2Ø.82-
- **Iridocyclochoroiditis** (panuveitis) — *see* Panuveitis
- **Iridodialysis** H21.53-
- **Iridodonesis** H21.89
- **Iridoplegia** (complete) (partial) (reflex) H57.Ø9
- **Iridoschisis** H21.25-
- **Iris** (*see also* condition)
  - bombé — *see* Membrane, pupillary
- **Iritis** (*see also* Iridocyclitis)
  - chronic — *see* Iridocyclitis, chronic
  - diabetic — *see* EØ8-E13 with .39
  - due to
    - herpes simplex BØØ.51
    - leprosy A3Ø.9 *[H22]*
  - gonococcal A54.32
  - gouty M1Ø.9
  - granulomatous — *see* Iridocyclitis, chronic
  - lens induced — *see* Iridocyclitis, lens-induced
  - papulosa (syphilitic) A52.71
  - rheumatic — *see* Iridocyclitis, chronic
  - syphilitic (secondary) A51.43
    - congenital (early) A5Ø.Ø1
    - late A52.71
  - tuberculous A18.54
- **Iron** — *see* condition
- **Iron-miner's lung** J63.4
- **Irradiated enamel** (tooth, teeth) KØ3.89
- **Irradiation effects, adverse** T66
- **Irreducible, irreducibility** — *see* condition
- **Irregular, irregularity**
  - action, heart I49.9
  - alveolar process KØ8.8
  - bleeding N92.6
  - breathing RØ6.89
  - contour of cornea (acquired) — *see* Deformity, cornea
    - congenital Q13.4
  - contour, reconstructed breast N65.Ø
  - dentin (in pulp) KØ4.3
  - eye movements H55.89
    - nystagmus — *see* Nystagmus
    - saccadic H55.81
  - labor O62.2
  - menstruation (cause unknown) N92.6
  - periods N92.6
  - prostate N42.9
  - pupil — *see* Abnormality, pupillary
  - reconstructed breast N65.Ø
  - respiratory RØ6.89
  - septum (nasal) J34.2
  - shape, organ or site, congenital NEC — *see* Distortion
  - sleep-wake pattern (rhythm) G47.23
- **Irritable, irritability** R45.4
  - bladder N32.89
  - bowel (syndrome) K58.9
    - with diarrhea K58.Ø
    - psychogenic F45.8
  - bronchial — *see* Bronchitis
  - cerebral, in newborn P91.3
  - colon K58.9
    - with diarrhea K58.Ø
    - psychogenic F45.8

- **Irritable, irritability**— *continued*
  - duodenum K59.8
  - heart (psychogenic) F45.8
  - hip — *see* Derangement, joint, specified type NEC, hip
  - ileum K59.8
  - infant R68.12
  - jejunum K59.8
  - rectum K59.8
  - stomach K31.89
    - psychogenic F45.8
  - sympathetic G9Ø.8
  - urethra N36.8
- **Irritation**
  - anus K62.89
  - axillary nerve G54.Ø
  - bladder N32.89
  - brachial plexus G54.Ø
  - bronchial — *see* Bronchitis
  - cervical plexus G54.2
  - cervix — *see* Cervicitis
  - choroid, sympathetic — *see* Endophthalmitis
  - cranial nerve — *see* Disorder, nerve, cranial
  - gastric K31.89
    - psychogenic F45.8
  - globe, sympathetic — *see* Uveitis, sympathetic
  - labyrinth — *see* subcategory H83.2
  - lumbosacral plexus G54.1
  - meninges (traumatic) — *see* Injury, intracranial
    - nontraumatic — *see* Meningismus
  - nerve — *see* Disorder, nerve
  - nervous R45.Ø
  - penis N48.89
  - perineum NEC L29.3
  - peripheral autonomic nervous system G9Ø.8
  - peritoneum — *see* Peritonitis
  - pharynx J39.2
  - plantar nerve — *see* Lesion, nerve, plantar
  - spinal (cord) (traumatic) (*see also* Injury, spinal cord, by region)
    - nerve G58.9
      - root NEC — *see* Radiculopathy
    - nontraumatic — *see* Myelopathy
  - stomach K31.89
    - psychogenic F45.8
  - sympathetic nerve NEC G9Ø.8
  - ulnar nerve — *see* Lesion, nerve, ulnar
  - vagina N89.8
- **Ischemia, ischemic** I99.8
  - brain — *see* Ischemia, cerebral
  - bowel (transient)
    - acute K55.Ø
    - chronic K55.1
    - due to mesenteric artery insufficiency K55.1
  - cardiac (see Disease, heart, ischemic)
  - cardiomyopathy I25.5
  - cerebral (chronic) (generalized) I67.82
    - arteriosclerotic I67.2
    - intermittent G45.9
    - newborn P91.Ø
    - recurrent focal G45.8
    - transient G45.9
- **Ischemia, ischemic** — *continued*
  - colon chronic (due to mesenteric artery insufficiency) K55.1
  - coronary — *see* Disease, heart, ischemic
  - demand (coronary) (*see also* Angina) I24.8
  - heart (chronic or with a stated duration of over 4 weeks) I25.9
    - acute or with a stated duration of 4 weeks or less I24.9
    - subacute I24.9
  - infarction, muscle — *see* Infarct, muscle
  - intestine (large) (small) (transient) K55.9
    - acute K55.Ø
    - chronic K55.1
    - due to mesenteric artery insufficiency K55.1
  - kidney N28.Ø
  - mesenteric, acute K55.Ø
  - muscle, traumatic T79.6
  - myocardium, myocardial (chronic or with a stated duration of over 4 weeks) I25.9
    - acute, without myocardial infarction I24.Ø
    - silent (asymptomatic) I25.6
    - transient of newborn P29.4
  - renal N28.Ø
  - retina, retinal — *see* Occlusion, artery, retina
  - small bowel
    - acute K55.Ø
    - chronic K55.1
    - due to mesenteric artery insufficiency K55.1
  - spinal cord G95.11
  - subendocardial — *see* Insufficiency, coronary
  - supply (coronary) (*see also* Angina) I25.9
    - due to vasospasm I2Ø.1
- **Ischial spine** — *see* condition
- **Ischialgia** — *see* Sciatica
- **Ischiopagus** Q89.4
- **Ischium, ischial** — *see* condition
- **Ischuria** R34
- **Iselin's disease or osteochondrosis** — *see* Osteochondrosis, juvenile, metatarsus
- **Islands of**
  - parotid tissue in
    - lymph nodes Q38.6
    - neck structures Q38.6
  - submaxillary glands in
    - fascia Q38.6
    - lymph nodes Q38.6
    - neck muscles Q38.6
- **Islet cell tumor, pancreas** D13.7
- **Isoimmunization NEC** (*see also* Incompatibility)
  - affecting management of pregnancy (ABO) (with hydrops fetalis) O36.11-
    - anti-A sensitization O36.11-
    - anti-B sensitization O36.19-
    - anti-c sensitization O36.Ø9-
    - anti-C sensitization O36.Ø9-
    - anti-e sensitization O36.Ø9-
    - anti-E sensitization O36.Ø9-
    - Rh NEC O36.Ø9-
      - anti-D antibody O36.Ø1-
    - specified NEC O36.19-
- **Isoimmunization NEC** — *continued*
  - newborn P55.9
    - with
      - hydrops fetalis P56.Ø
      - kernicterus P57.Ø
    - ABO (blood groups) P55.1
    - Rhesus (Rh) factor P55.Ø
    - specified type NEC P55.8
- **Isolation, isolated**
  - dwelling Z59.8
  - family Z63.79
  - social Z6Ø.4
- **Isoleucinosis** E71.19
- **Isomerism atrial appendages** (with asplenia or polysplenia) Q2Ø.6
- **Isosporiasis, isosporosis** AØ7.3
- **Isovaleric acidemia** E71.11Ø
- **Issue of**
  - medical certificate ZØ2.79
    - for disability determination ZØ2.71
  - repeat prescription (appliance) (glasses) (medicinal substance, medicament, medicine) Z76.Ø
    - contraception — *see* Contraception
- **Itch, itching** (*see also* Pruritus)
  - baker's L23.6
  - barber's B35.Ø
  - bricklayer's L24.5
  - cheese B88.Ø
  - clam digger's B65.3
  - coolie B76.9
  - copra B88.Ø
  - dew B76.9
  - dhobi B35.6
  - filarial — *see* Infestation, filarial
  - grain B88.Ø
  - grocer's B88.Ø
  - ground B76.9
  - harvest B88.Ø
  - jock B35.6
  - Malabar B35.5
    - beard B35.Ø
    - foot B35.3
    - scalp B35.Ø
  - meaning scabies B86
  - Norwegian B86
  - perianal L29.Ø
  - poultrymen's B88.Ø
  - sarcoptic B86
  - scabies B86
  - scrub B88.Ø
  - straw B88.Ø
  - swimmer's B65.3
  - water B76.9
  - winter L29.8
- **Ivemark's syndrome** (asplenia with congenital heart disease) Q89.Ø1
- **Ivory bones** Q78.2
- **Ixodiasis NEC** B88.8

J

K

L

Laceration— *continued*
- lip SØ1.511
  - with foreign body SØ1.521
- liver S36.113
  - major (stellate) S36.116
  - minor S36.114
  - moderate S36.115
- loin — *see* Laceration, abdomen, wall
- lower back — *see* Laceration, back, lower
- lumbar region — *see* Laceration, back, lower
- lung S27.339
  - bilateral S27.332
  - unilateral S27.331
- malar region — *see* Laceration, head, specified site NEC
- mammary — *see* Laceration, breast
- mastoid region — *see* Laceration, head, specified site NEC
- meninges — *see* Injury, intracranial, diffuse
- meniscus — *see* Tear, meniscus
- mesentery S36.893
- mesosalpinx S37.539
  - bilateral S37.532
  - unilateral S37.531
- mouth — *see* Laceration, oral cavity
- muscle — *see* Injury, muscle, by site, laceration
- nail
  - finger — *see* Laceration, finger, with damage to nail
  - toe — *see* Laceration, toe, with damage to nail
- nasal (septum) (sinus) — *see* Laceration, nose
- nasopharynx — *see* Laceration, head, specified site NEC
- neck S11.91
  - with foreign body S11.92
  - involving
    - cervical esophagus S11.21
      - with foreign body S11.22
    - larynx — *see* Laceration, larynx
    - pharynx — *see* Laceration, pharynx
    - thyroid gland — *see* Laceration, thyroid gland
    - trachea — *see* Laceration, trachea
  - specified site NEC S11.81
    - with foreign body S11.82
- nerve — *see* Injury, nerve
- nose (septum) (sinus) SØ1.21
  - with foreign body SØ1.22
- ocular NOS SØ5.3-
  - adnexa NOS SØ1.11-
- oral cavity SØ1.512
  - with foreign body SØ1.522
- orbit (eye) — *see* Wound, open, ocular, orbit
- ovary S37.439
  - bilateral S37.432
  - unilateral S37.431
- palate — *see* Laceration, oral cavity
- palm — *see* Laceration, hand
- pancreas S36.239
  - body S36.231
    - major S36.261
    - minor S36.241
    - moderate S36.251
  - head S36.23Ø
    - major S36.26Ø
    - minor S36.24Ø
    - moderate S36.25Ø
  - major S36.269
  - minor S36.249
  - moderate S36.259
  - tail S36.232
    - major S36.262
    - minor S36.242
    - moderate S36.252
- pelvic S31.Ø1Ø
  - with
    - foreign body S31.Ø2Ø
      - penetration into retroperitoneal cavity S31.Ø21
    - penetration into retroperitoneal cavity S31.Ø11
  - floor (*see also* Laceration, back, lower)
    - with ectopic or molar pregnancy OØ8.6
    - complicating delivery O7Ø.1

Laceration— *continued*
- pelvic — *continued*
  - floor — *continued*
    - following ectopic or molar pregnancy OØ8.6
    - old (postpartal) N81.89
  - organ S37.93
    - with ectopic or molar pregnancy OØ8.6
    - adrenal gland S37.813
    - bladder S37.23
    - fallopian tube — *see* Laceration, fallopian tube
    - following ectopic or molar pregnancy OØ8.6
    - kidney — *see* Laceration, kidney
    - obstetrical trauma O71.5
    - ovary — *see* Laceration, ovary
    - prostate S37.823
    - specified site NEC S37.893
    - ureter S37.13
    - urethra S37.33
    - uterus S37.63
- penis S31.21
  - with foreign body S31.22
- perineum
  - female S31.41
    - with
      - ectopic or molar pregnancy OØ8.6
      - foreign body S31.42
    - during delivery O7Ø.9
      - first degree O7Ø.Ø
      - fourth degree O7Ø.3
      - second degree O7Ø.1
      - third degree O7Ø.2
    - old (postpartal) N81.89
    - postpartal N81.89
    - secondary (postpartal) O9Ø.1
  - male S31.119
    - with foreign body S31.129
- periocular area (with or without lacrimal passages) — *see* Laceration, eyelid
- peritoneum S36.893
- periumbilic region — *see* Laceration, abdomen, wall, periumbilic
- periurethral tissue — *see* Laceration, urethra
- phalanges
  - finger — *see* Laceration, finger
  - toe — *see* Laceration, toe
- pharynx S11.21
  - with foreign body S11.22
- pinna — *see* Laceration, ear
- popliteal space — *see* Laceration, knee
- prepuce — *see* Laceration, penis
- prostate S37.823
- pubic region S31.119
  - with foreign body S31.129
- pudendum — *see* Laceration, genital organs, external
- rectovaginal septum — *see* Laceration, vagina
- rectum S36.63
- retroperitoneum S36.893
- round ligament S37.893
- sacral region — *see* Laceration, back, lower
- sacroiliac region — *see* Laceration, back, lower
- salivary gland — *see* Laceration, oral cavity
- scalp SØ1.Ø1
  - with foreign body SØ1.Ø2
- scapular region — *see* Laceration, shoulder
- scrotum S31.31
  - with foreign body S31.32
- seminal vesicle S37.893
- shin — *see* Laceration, leg
- shoulder S41.Ø19
  - with foreign body S41.Ø29
  - left S41.Ø12
    - with foreign body S41.Ø22
  - right S41.Ø11
    - with foreign body S41.Ø21
- small intestine — *see* Laceration, intestine, small
- spermatic cord — *see* Laceration, testis
- spinal cord (meninges) (*see also* Injury, spinal cord, by region)
  - due to injury at birth P11.5
  - newborn (birth injury) P11.5

Laceration— *continued*
- spleen S36.Ø39
  - major (massive) (stellate) S36.Ø32
  - moderate S36.Ø31
  - superficial (minor) S36.Ø3Ø
- sternal region — *see* Laceration, thorax, front
- stomach S36.33
- submaxillary region — *see* Laceration, head, specified site NEC
- submental region — *see* Laceration, head, specified site NEC
- subungual
  - finger(s) — *see* Laceration, finger, with damage to nail
  - toe(s) — *see* Laceration, toe, with damage to nail
- suprarenal gland — *see* Laceration, adrenal gland
- temple, temporal region — *see* Laceration, head, specified site NEC
- temporomandibular area — *see* Laceration, cheek
- tendon — *see* Injury, muscle, by site, laceration
  - Achilles S86.Ø2-
- tentorium cerebelli — *see* Injury, intracranial, diffuse
- testis S31.31
  - with foreign body S31.32
- thigh S71.11-
  - with foreign body S71.12-
- thorax, thoracic (wall) S21.91
  - with foreign body S21.92
    - back S21.22-
      - with penetration into thoracic cavity S21.42-
    - front S21.12-
      - with penetration into thoracic cavity S21.32-
  - back S21.21-
    - with
      - foreign body S21.22-
        - with penetration into thoracic cavity S21.42-
      - penetration into thoracic cavity S21.41-
  - breast — *see* Laceration, breast
  - front S21.11-
    - foreign body S21.12-
      - with penetration into thoracic cavity S21.32-
    - penetration into thoracic cavity S21.31-
- thumb S61.Ø19
  - with
    - damage to nail S61.119
      - with
        - foreign body S61.129
    - foreign body S61.Ø29
  - left S61.Ø12
    - with
      - damage to nail S61.112
        - with
          - foreign body S61.122
      - foreign body S61.Ø22
  - right S61.Ø11
    - with
      - damage to nail S61.111
        - with
          - foreign body S61.121
      - foreign body S61.Ø21
- thyroid gland S11.11
  - with foreign body S11.12
- toe(s) S91.119
  - with
    - damage to nail S91.219
      - with
        - foreign body S91.229
    - foreign body S91.129
  - great S91.113
    - with
      - damage to nail S91.213
        - with
          - foreign body S91.223
      - foreign body S91.123

Laryngitis— *continued*
  Hemophilus influenzae J04.Ø
  H. influenzae J04.Ø
  hypertrophic J37.Ø
  influenzal — *see* Influenza, with, respiratory manifestations NEC
  obstructive J05.Ø
  sicca J37.Ø
  spasmodic J05.Ø
    acute J04.Ø
  streptococcal J04.Ø
  stridulous J05.Ø
  syphilitic (late) A52.73
    congenital A50.59 *[J99]*
      early A50.03 *[J99]*
  tuberculous A15.5
  Vincent's A69.1
Laryngocele (congenital) (ventricular) Q31.3
Laryngofissure J38.7
  congenital Q31.8
Laryngomalacia (congenital) Q31.5
Laryngopharyngitis (acute) J06.Ø
  chronic J37.Ø
  due to external agent — *see* Inflammation, respiratory, upper, due to
Laryngoplegia J38.ØØ
  bilateral J38.Ø2
  unilateral J38.Ø1
Laryngoptosis J38.7
Laryngospasm J38.5
Laryngostenosis J38.6
Laryngotracheitis (acute) (Infectional) (infective) (viral) J04.2
  atrophic J37.1
  catarrhal J37.1
  chronic J37.1
  diphtheritic A36.2
  due to external agent — *see* Inflammation, respiratory, upper, due to
  Hemophilus influenzae J04.2
  hypertrophic J37.1
  influenzal — *see* Influenza, with, respiratory manifestations NEC
  pachydermic J38.7
  sicca J37.1
  spasmodic J38.5
    acute J05.Ø
  streptococcal J04.2
  stridulous J38.5
  syphilitic (late) A52.73
    congenital A50.59 *[J99]*
      early A50.03 *[J99]*
  tuberculous A15.5
  Vincent's A69.1
Laryngotracheobronchitis — *see* Bronchitis
Larynx, laryngeal — *see* condition
Lassa fever A96.2
Lassitude — *see* Weakness
Late
  talker R62.Ø
  walker R62.Ø
Late effect(s) — *see* Sequelae
Latent — *see* condition
Laterocession — *see* Lateroversion
Lateroflexion — *see* Lateroversion
Lateroversion
  cervix — *see* Lateroversion, uterus
  uterus, uterine (cervix) (postinfectional) (postpartal, old) N85.4
    congenital Q51.818
    in pregnancy or childbirth O34.59-
Lathyrism — *see* Poisoning, food, noxious, plant
Launois' syndrome (pituitary gigantism) E22.Ø
Launois-Bensaude adenolipomatosis E88.89
Laurence-Moon(-Bardet)-Biedl syndrome Q87.89
Lax, laxity (*see also* Relaxation)
  ligament(ous) (*see also* Disorder, ligament)
    familial M35.7
    knee — *see* Derangement, knee
  skin (acquired) L57.4
    congenital Q82.8
Laxative habit F55.2
Lazy leukocyte syndrome D70.8
Lead miner's lung J63.6
Leak, leakage
  air NEC J93.82
    postprocedural J95.812
  amniotic fluid — *see* Rupture, membranes, premature
  blood (microscopic), fetal, into maternal circulation affecting management of pregnancy — *see* Pregnancy, complicated by
  cerebrospinal fluid G96.Ø
    from spinal (lumbar) puncture G97.Ø
  device, implant or graft (*see also* Complications, by site and type, mechanical)
    arterial graft NEC — *see* Complication, cardiovascular device, mechanical, vascular
    breast (implant) T85.43
    catheter NEC T85.638
      dialysis (renal) T82.43
        intraperitoneal T85.631
      infusion NEC T82.534
        spinal (epidural) (subdural) T85.63Ø
      urinary, indwelling T83.Ø38
        cystostomy T83.Ø3Ø
    gastrointestinal — *see* Complications, prosthetic device, mechanical, gastrointestinal device
    genital NEC T83.498
      penile prosthesis T83.49Ø
    heart NEC — *see* Complication, cardiovascular device, mechanical
    ocular NEC — *see* Complications, prosthetic device, mechanical, ocular device
    orthopedic NEC — *see* Complication, orthopedic, device, mechanical
    persistent air J93.82
    specified NEC T85.638
    urinary NEC (*see also* Complication, genitourinary, device, urinary, mechanical)
     graft T83.23
    vascular NEC — *see* Complication, cardiovascular device, mechanical
    ventricular intracranial shunt T85.Ø3
    joint prosthesis — *see* Complications, joint prosthesis, mechanical, specified NEC, by site
  urine — *see* Incontinence
Leaky heart — *see* Endocarditis
Learning defect (specific) F81.9
Leather bottle stomach C16.9
Leber's
  congenital amaurosis H35.5Ø
  optic atrophy (hereditary) H47.22
Lederer's anemia D59.1
Leeches (external) — *see* Hirudiniasis
Leg — *see* condition
Legg(-Calvé)**-Perthes disease, syndrome or osteochondrosis** M91.1-
Legionellosis A48.1
  nonpneumonic A48.2
Legionnaires'
  disease A48.1
    nonpneumonic A48.2
  pneumonia A48.1
Leigh's disease G31.82
Leiner's disease L21.1
Leiofibromyoma — *see* Leiomyoma
Leiomyoblastoma — *see* Neoplasm, connective tissue, benign
Leiomyofibroma (*see also* Neoplasm, connective tissue, benign)
  uterus (cervix) (corpus) D25.9
Leiomyoma (*see also* Neoplasm, connective tissue, benign)
  bizarre — *see* Neoplasm, connective tissue, benign
  cellular — *see* Neoplasm, connective tissue, benign
  epithelioid — *see* Neoplasm, connective tissue, benign
  uterus (cervix) (corpus) D25.9
    intramural D25.1
    submucous D25.Ø
    subserosal D25.2
  vascular — *see* Neoplasm, connective tissue, benign
Leiomyoma, leiomyomatosis (intravascular) — *see* Neoplasm, connective tissue, uncertain behavior
Leiomyosarcoma (*see also* Neoplasm, connective tissue, malignant)
  epithelioid — *see* Neoplasm, connective tissue, malignant
  myxoid — *see* Neoplasm, connective tissue, malignant
Leishmaniasis B55.9
  American (mucocutaneous) B55.2
    cutaneous B55.1
  Asian Desert B55.1
  Brazilian B55.2
  cutaneous (any type) B55.1
  dermal (*see also* Leishmaniasis, cutaneous)
    post-kala-azar B55.Ø
  eyelid B55.1
  infantile B55.Ø
  Mediterranean B55.Ø
  mucocutaneous (American) (New World) B55.2
  naso-oral B55.2
  nasopharyngeal B55.2
  old world B55.1
  tegumentaria diffusa B55.1
  visceral B55.Ø
Leishmanoid, dermal (*see also* Leishmaniasis, cutaneous)
  post-kala-azar B55.Ø
Lenegre's disease I44.2
Lengthening, leg — *see* Deformity, limb, unequal length
Lennert's lymphoma — *see* Lymphoma, Lennert's
Lennox-Gastaut syndrome G40.812
  intractable G40.814
    with status epilepticus G40.813
    without status epilepticus G40.814
  not intractable G40.812
    with status epilepticus G40.811
    without status epilepticus G40.812
Lens — *see* condition
Lenticonus (anterior) (posterior) (congenital) Q12.8
Lenticular degeneration, progressive E83.Ø1
Lentiglobus (posterior) (congenital) Q12.8
Lentigo (congenital) L81.4
  maligna (*see also* Melanoma, in situ)
    melanoma — *see* Melanoma
Lentivirus, as cause of disease classified elsewhere B97.31
Leontiasis
  ossium M85.2
  syphilitic (late) A52.78
    congenital A50.59
Lepothrix A48.8
Lepra — *see* Leprosy
Leprechaunism E34.8
Leprosy A30.-
  with muscle disorder A30.9 *[M63.80]*
    ankle A30.9 *[M63.87-]*
    foot A30.9 *[M63.87-]*
    forearm A30.9 *[M63.83-]*
    hand A30.9 *[M63.84-]*
    lower leg A30.9 *[M63.86-]*
    multiple sites A30.9 *[M63.89]*
    pelvic region A30.9 *[M63.85-]*
    shoulder region A30.9 *[M63.81-]*
    specified site NEC A30.9 *[M63.88]*
    thigh A30.9 *[M63.85-]*
    upper arm A30.9 *[M63.82-]*
  anesthetic A30.9
  BB A30.3
  BL A30.4
  borderline (infiltrated) (neuritic) A30.3
    lepromatous A30.4
    tuberculoid A30.2
  BT A30.2
  dimorphous (infiltrated) (neuritic) A30.3
  I A30.Ø
  indeterminate (macular) (neuritic) A30.Ø
  lepromatous (diffuse) (infiltrated) (macular) (neuritic) (nodular) A30.5
  LL A30.5
  macular (early) (neuritic) (simple) A30.9
  maculoanesthetic A30.9

Leprosy — *continued*
- mixed A3Ø.3
- neural A3Ø.9
- nodular A3Ø.5
- primary neuritic A3Ø.3
- specified type NEC A3Ø.8
- TT A3Ø.1
- tuberculoid (major) (minor) A3Ø.1

Leptocytosis, hereditary D56.9
Leptomeningitis (chronic) (circumscribed) (hemorrhagic) (nonsuppurative) — *see* Meningitis
Leptomeningopathy G96.19
Leptospiral — *see* condition
Leptospirochetal — *see* condition
Leptospirosis A27.9
- canicola A27.89
- due to Leptospira interrogans serovar icterohaemorrhagiae A27.Ø
- icterohemorrhagica A27.Ø
- pomona A27.89
- Weil's disease A27.Ø

Leptus dermatitis B88.Ø
Leriche's syndrome (aortic bifurcation occlusion) I74.Ø9
Leri's pleonosteosis Q78.8
Leri-Weill syndrome Q77.8
Lermoyez' syndrome — *see* Vertigo, peripheral NEC
Lesch-Nyhan syndrome E79.1
Leser-Trélat disease L82.1
- inflamed L82.Ø

Lesion(s) (nontraumatic)
- abducens nerve — *see* Strabismus, paralytic, sixth nerve
- alveolar process KØ8.9
- angiocentric immunoproliferative D47.Z9
- anorectal K62.9
- aortic (valve) I35.9
- auditory nerve — *see* subcategory H93.3
- basal ganglion G25.9
- bile duct — *see* Disease, bile duct
- biomechanical M99.9
  - specified type NEC M99.89
    - abdomen M99.89
    - acromioclavicular M99.87
    - cervical region M99.81
    - cervicothoracic M99.81
    - costochondral M99.88
    - costovertebral M99.88
    - head region M99.8Ø
    - hip M99.85
    - lower extremity M99.86
    - lumbar region M99.83
    - lumbosacral M99.83
    - occipitocervical M99.8Ø
    - pelvic region M99.85
    - pubic M99.85
    - rib cage M99.88
    - sacral region M99.84
    - sacrococcygeal M99.84
    - sacroiliac M99.84
    - specified NEC M99.89
    - sternochondral M99.88
    - sternoclavicular M99.87
    - thoracic region M99.82
    - thoracolumbar M99.82
    - upper extremity M99.87
- bladder N32.9
- bone — *see* Disorder, bone
- brachial plexus G54.Ø
- brain G93.9
  - congenital QØ4.9
  - vascular I67.9
    - degenerative I67.9
    - hypertensive I67.4
- buccal cavity K13.79
- calcified — *see* Calcification
- canthus — *see* Disorder, eyelid
- carate — *see* Pinta, lesions
- cardia K22.9
- cardiac (*see also* Disease, heart) I51.9
  - congenital Q24.9
  - valvular — *see* Endocarditis

Lesion(s)— *continued*
- cauda equina G83.4
- cecum K63.9
- cerebral — *see* Lesion, brain
- cerebrovascular I67.9
  - degenerative I67.9
  - hypertensive I67.4
- cervical (nerve) root NEC G54.2
- chiasmal — *see* Disorder, optic, chiasm
- chorda tympani G51.8
- coin, lung R91.1
- colon K63.9
- congenital — *see* Anomaly, by site
- conjunctiva H11.9
- conus medullaris — *see* Injury, conus medullaris
- coronary artery — *see* Ischemia, heart
- cranial nerve G52.9
  - eighth — *see* Disorder, ear
  - eleventh G52.9
  - fifth G5Ø.9
  - first G52.Ø
  - fourth — *see* Strabismus, paralytic, fourth nerve
  - seventh G51.9
  - sixth — *see* Strabismus, paralytic, sixth nerve
  - tenth G52.2
  - twelfth G52.3
- cystic — *see* Cyst
- degenerative — *see* Degeneration
- duodenum K31.9
- edentulous (alveolar) ridge, associated with trauma, due to traumatic occlusion KØ6.2
- en coup de sabre L94.1
- eyelid — *see* Disorder, eyelid
- gasserian ganglion G5Ø.8
- gastric K31.9
- gastroduodenal K31.9
- gastrointestinal K63.9
- gingiva, associated with trauma KØ6.2
- glomerular
  - focal and segmental (*see also* NØØ-NØ7 with fourth character .1) NØ5.1
  - minimal change (*see also* NØØ-NØ7 with fourth character .Ø) NØ5.Ø
- heart (organic) — *see* Disease, heart
- hyperchromic, due to pinta (carate) A67.1
- hyperkeratotic — *see* Hyperkeratosis
- hypothalamic E23.7
- ileocecal K63.9
- ileum K63.9
- iliohypogastric nerve G57.8-
- inflammatory — *see* Inflammation
- intestine K63.9
- intracerebral — *see* Lesion, brain
- intrachiasmal (optic) — *see* Disorder, optic, chiasm
- intracranial, space-occupying R9Ø.Ø
- joint — *see* Disorder, joint
  - sacroiliac (old) M53.3
- keratotic — *see* Keratosis
- kidney — *see* Disease, renal
- laryngeal nerve (recurrent) G52.2
- lip K13.Ø
- liver K76.9
- lumbosacral
  - plexus G54.1
  - root (nerve) NEC G54.4
- lung (coin) R91.2
- maxillary sinus J32.Ø
- mitral IØ5.9
- Morel-Lavallée — *see* Hematoma, by site
- motor cortex NEC G93.89
- mouth K13.79
- nerve G58.9
  - femoral G57.2-
  - median G56.1-
    - carpal tunnel syndrome — *see* Syndrome, carpal tunnel
  - plantar G57.6-
  - popliteal (lateral) G57.3-
    - medial G57.4-
  - radial G56.3-
  - sciatic G57.Ø-
  - spinal — *see* Injury, nerve, spinal
  - ulnar G56.2-

Lesion(s)— *continued*
- nervous system, congenital QØ7.9
- nonallopathic — *see* Lesion, biomechanical
- nose (internal) J34.89
- obstructive — *see* Obstruction
- obturator nerve G57.8-
- oral mucosa K13.7Ø
- organ or site NEC — *see* Disease, by site
- osteolytic — *see* Osteolysis
- peptic K27.9
- periodontal, due to traumatic occlusion KØ5.5
- pharynx J39.2
- pigment, pigmented (skin) L81.9
- pinta — *see* Pinta, lesions
- polypoid — *see* Polyp
- prechiasmal (optic) — *see* Disorder, optic, chiasm
- primary (*see also* Syphilis, primary) A51.Ø
  - carate A67.Ø
  - pinta A67.Ø
  - yaws A66.Ø
- pulmonary J98.4
  - valve I37.9
- pylorus K31.9
- rectosigmoid K63.9
- retina, retinal H35.9
- sacroiliac (joint) (old) M53.3
- salivary gland K11.9
  - benign lymphoepithelial K11.8
- saphenous nerve G57.8-
- sciatic nerve G57.Ø-
- secondary — *see* Syphilis, secondary
- shoulder (region) M75.9-
  - specified NEC M75.8-
- sigmoid K63.9
- sinus (accessory) (nasal) J34.89
- skin L98.9
  - suppurative LØ8.Ø
- SLAP S43.43-
- spinal cord G95.9
  - congenital QØ6.9
- spleen D73.89
- stomach K31.9
- superior glenoid labrum S43.43-
- syphilitic — *see* Syphilis
- tertiary — *see* Syphilis, tertiary
- thoracic root (nerve) NEC G54.3
- tonsillar fossa J35.9
- tooth, teeth KØ8.9
  - white spot
    - chewing surface KØ2.51
    - pit and fissure surface KØ2.51
    - smooth surface KØ2.61
- traumatic — *see* specific type of injury by site
- tricuspid (valve) IØ7.9
  - nonrheumatic I36.9
- trigeminal nerve G5Ø.9
- ulcerated or ulcerative — *see* Ulcer, skin
- uterus N85.9
- vagus nerve G52.2
- valvular — *see* Endocarditis
- vascular I99.9
  - affecting central nervous system I67.9
  - following trauma NEC T14.8
  - umbilical cord, complicating delivery O69.5
- warty — *see* Verruca
- white spot (tooth)
  - chewing surface KØ2.51
  - pit and fissure surface KØ2.51
  - smooth surface KØ2.61

Lethargic — *see* condition
Lethargy R53.83
Letterer-Siwe's disease C96.Ø
Leuc(o) — *see* Leuk(o)
Leukemia, leukemic C95.9-
- acute basophilic C94.8-
- acute bilineal C95.Ø-
- acute erythroid C94.Ø-
- acute lymphoblastic C91.Ø-
- acute megakaryoblastic C94.2-
- acute megakaryocytic C94.2-
- acute mixed lineage C95.Ø-
- acute monoblastic (monoblastic/monocytic) C93.Ø-
- acute monocytic (monoblastic/monocytic) C93.Ø-

Leukemia, leukemic— *continued*
- acute myeloblastic (minimal differentiation) (with maturation) C92.Ø-
- acute myeloid
  - with
    - 11q23-abnormality C92.6-
    - dysplasia of remaining hematopoesis and/or myelodysplastic disease in its history C92.A-
    - multilineage dysplasia C92.A-
    - variation of MLL-gene C92.6-
  - M6(a)(b) C94.Ø-
  - M7 C94.2-
- acute myelomonocytic C92.5-
- acute promyelocytic C92.4-
- adult T-cell (HTLV-1-associated) (acute variant) (chronic variant) (lymphomatoid variant) (smouldering variant) C91.5-
- aggressive NK-cell C94.8-
- AML (1/ETO) (MØ) (M1) (M2) (without a FAB classification) C92.Ø-
- AML M3 C92.4-
- AML M4 (Eo with inv(16) or t(16;16)) C92.5-
- AML M5 C93.Ø-
- AML M5a C93.Ø-
- AML M5b C93.Ø-
- AML Me with t(15;17) and variants C92.4-
- atypical chronic myeloid, BCR/ABL-negative C92.2-
- biphenotypic acute C95.Ø-
- blast cell C95.Ø-
- Burkitt-type, mature B-cell C91.A-
- chronic lymphocytic, of B-cell type C91.1-
- chronic monocytic C93.1-
- chronic myelogenous (Philadelphia chromosome (Ph1) positive) (t(9;22) (q34;q11) (with crisis of blast cells) C92.1-
- chronic myeloid, BCR/ABL-positive C92.1-
  - atypical, BCR/ABL-negative C92.2-
- chronic myelomonocytic C93.1-
- chronic neutrophilic D47.1
- CMML (-1) (-2) (with eosinophilia) C93.1-
- granulocytic (*see also* Category C92) C92.9-
- hairy cell C91.4-
- juvenile myelomonocytic C93.3-
- lymphoid C91.9-
  - specified NEC C91.Z-
- mast cell C94.3-
- mature B-cell, Burkitt-type C91.A-
- monocytic (subacute) C93.9-
  - specified NEC C93.Z-
- myelogenous (*see also* Category C92) C92.9-
- myeloid C92.9-
  - specified NEC C92.Z-
- plasma cell C9Ø.1-
- plasmacytic C9Ø.1-
- prolymphocytic
  - of B-cell type C91.3-
  - of T-cell type C91.6-
- specified NEC C94.8-
- stem cell, of unclear lineage C95.Ø-
- subacute lymphocytic C91.9-
- T-cell large granular lymphocytic C91.Z-
- unspecified cell type C95.9-
  - acute C95.Ø-
  - chronic C95.1-

Leukemoid reaction (*see also* Reaction, leukemoid) D72.823

Leukoaraiosis (hypertensive) I67.81

Leukoariosis — *see* Leukoaraiosis

Leukocoria — *see* Disorder, globe, degenerated condition, leucocoria

Leukocytopenia D72.819

Leukocytosis D72.829
- eosinophilic D72.1

Leukoderma, leukodermia NEC L81.5
- syphilitic A51.39
  - late A52.79

Leukodystrophy E75.29

Leukoedema, oral epithelium K13.29

Leukoencephalitis GØ4.81
- acute (subacute) hemorrhagic G36.1
  - postimmunization or postvaccinal GØ4.Ø2
- postinfectious GØ4.Ø1

Leukoencephalitis — *continued*
- subacute sclerosing A81.1
- van Bogaert's (sclerosing) A81.1

Leukoencephalopathy (*see also* Encephalopathy) G93.49
- Binswanger's I67.3
- heroin vapor G92
- metachromatic E75.25
- multifocal (progressive) A81.2
- postimmunization and postvaccinal GØ4.Ø2
- progressive multifocal A81.2
- reversible, posterior G93.6
- van Bogaert's (sclerosing) A81.1
- vascular, progressive I67.3

Leukoerythroblastosis D75.9

Leukokeratosis (*see also* Leukoplakia)
- mouth K13.21
- nicotina palati K13.24
- oral mucosa K13.21
- tongue K13.21
- vocal cord J38.3

Leukokraurosis vulva(e) N9Ø.4

Leukoma (cornea) (*see also* Opacity, cornea)
- adherent H17.Ø-
- interfering with central vision — *see* Opacity, cornea, central

Leukomalacia, cerebral, newborn P91.2
- periventricular P91.2

Leukomelanopathy, hereditary D72.Ø

Leukonychia (punctata) (striata) L6Ø.8
- congenital Q84.4

Leukopathia unguium L6Ø.8
- congenital Q84.4

Leukopenia D72.819
- basophilic D72.818
- chemotherapy (cancer) induced D7Ø.1
- congenital D7Ø.Ø
- cyclic D7Ø.Ø
- drug induced NEC D7Ø.2
  - due to cytoreductive cancer chemotherapy D7Ø.1
- eosinophilic D72.818
- familial D7Ø.Ø
- infantile genetic D7Ø.Ø
- malignant D7Ø.9
- periodic D7Ø.Ø
- transitory neonatal P61.5

Leukopenic — *see* condition

Leukoplakia
- anus K62.89
- bladder (postinfectional) N32.89
- buccal K13.21
- cervix (uteri) N88.Ø
- esophagus K22.8
- gingiva K13.21
- hairy (oral mucosa) (tongue) K13.3
- kidney (pelvis) N28.89
- larynx J38.7
- lip K13.21
- mouth K13.21
- oral epithelium, including tongue (mucosa) K13.21
- palate K13.21
- pelvis (kidney) N28.89
- penis (infectional) N48.Ø
- rectum K62.89
- syphilitic (late) A52.79
- tongue K13.21
- ureter (postinfectional) N28.89
- urethra (postinfectional) N36.8
- uterus N85.8
- vagina N89.4
- vocal cord J38.3
- vulva N9Ø.4

Leukorrhea N89.8
- due to Trichomonas (vaginalis) A59.ØØ
- trichomonal A59.ØØ

Leukosarcoma C85.9-

Levocardia (isolated) Q24.1
- with situs inversus Q89.3

Levotransposition Q2Ø.5

Lev's disease or syndrome (acquired complete heart block) I44.2

Levulosuria — *see* Fructosuria

Levurid L3Ø.2

Lewy body(ies) (dementia) (disease) G31.83

Leyden-Moebius dystrophy G71.Ø

Leydig cell
- carcinoma
  - specified site — *see* Neoplasm, malignant, by site
  - unspecified site
    - female C56.9-
    - male C62.9-
- tumor
  - benign
    - specified site — *see* Neoplasm, benign, by site
    - unspecified site
      - female D27.-
      - male D29.2-
  - malignant
    - specified site — *see* Neoplasm, malignant, by site
    - unspecified site
      - female C56.-
      - male C62.9-
  - specified site — *see* Neoplasm, uncertain behavior, by site
  - unspecified site
    - female D39.1-
    - male D4Ø.1-

Leydig-Sertoli cell tumor
- specified site — *see* Neoplasm, benign, by site
- unspecified site
  - female D27.-
  - male D29.2-

LGSIL (Low grade squamous intraepithelial lesion on cytologic smear of)
- anus R85.612
- cervix R87.612
- vagina R87.622

Liar, pathologic F6Ø.2

Libido
- decreased R68.82

Libman-Sacks disease M32.11

Lice (infestation) B85.2
- body (Pediculus corporis) B85.1
- crab B85.3
- head (Pediculus capitis) B85.Ø
- mixed (classifiable to more than one of the titles B85.Ø-B85.3) B85.4
- pubic (Phthirus pubis) B85.3

Lichen L28.Ø
- albus L9Ø.Ø
  - penis N48.Ø
  - vulva N9Ø.4
- amyloidosis E85.4 *[L99]*
- atrophicus L9Ø.Ø
  - penis N48.Ø
  - vulva N9Ø.4
- congenital Q82.8
- myxedematosus L98.5
- nitidus L44.1
- pilaris Q82.8
  - acquired L85.8
- planopilaris L66.1
- planus (chronicus) L43.9
  - annularis L43.8
  - bullous L43.1
  - follicular L66.1
  - hypertrophic L43.Ø
  - moniliformis L44.3
  - of Wilson L43.9
  - specified NEC L43.8
  - subacute (active) L43.3
  - tropicus L43.3
- ruber
  - acuminatus L44.Ø
  - moniliformis L44.3
  - planus L43.9
- sclerosus (et atrophicus) L9Ø.Ø
  - penis N48.Ø
  - vulva N9Ø.4
- scrofulosus (primary) (tuberculous) A18.4
- simplex (chronicus) (circumscriptus) L28.Ø
- striatus L44.2
- urticatus L28.2

Lichenification L28.Ø

Lichenoides tuberculosis (primary) A18.4
Lichtheim's disease or syndrome — *see* Degeneration, combined
Lien migrans D73.89
Ligament — *see* condition
Light
for gestational age — *see* Light for dates
headedness R42
Light-for-dates (infant) P05.00
with weight of
499 grams or less P05.01
500-749 grams P05.02
750-999 grams P05.03
1000-1249 grams P05.04
1250-1499 grams P05.05
1500-1749 grams P05.06
1750-1999 grams P05.07
2000-2499 grams P05.08
and small-for-dates — *see* Small for dates
affecting management of pregnancy O36.59-
Lightning (effects) (stroke) (struck by) T75.00
burn — *see* Burn
foot E53.8
shock T75.01
specified effect NEC T75.09
Lightwood-Albright syndrome N25.89
Lightwood's disease or syndrome (renal tubular acidosis) N25.89
Lignac (-de Toni) (-Fanconi) (-Debré) **disease or syndrome** E72.09
with cystinosis E72.04
Ligneous thyroiditis E06.5
Likoff's syndrome I20.8
Limb — *see* condition
Limbic epilepsy personality syndrome F07.0
Limitation, limited
activities due to disability Z73.6
cardiac reserve — *see* Disease, heart
eye muscle duction, traumatic — *see* Strabismus, mechanical
mandibular range of motion M26.52
Lindau (-von Hippel) **disease** Q85.8
Line(s)
Beau's L60.4
Harris' — *see* Arrest, epiphyseal
Hudson's (cornea) — *see* Pigmentation, cornea, anterior
Stähli's (cornea) — *see* Pigmentation, cornea, anterior
Linea corneae senilis — *see* Change, cornea, senile
Lingua
geographica K14.1
nigra (villosa) K14.3
plicata K14.5
tylosis K13.29
Lingual — *see* condition
Linguatulosis B88.8
Linitis (gastric) **plastica** C16.9
Lip — *see* condition
Lipedema — *see* Edema
Lipemia (*see also* Hyperlipidemia)
retina, retinalis E78.3
Lipidosis E75.6
cerebral (infantile) (juvenile) (late) E75.4
cerebroretinal E75.4
cerebroside E75.22
cholesterol (cerebral) E75.5
glycolipid E75.21
hepatosplenomegalic E78.3
sphingomyelin — *see* Niemann-Pick disease or syndrome
sulfatide E75.29
Lipoadenoma — *see* Neoplasm, benign, by site
Lipoblastoma — *see* Lipoma
Lipoblastomatosis — *see* Lipoma
Lipochondrodystrophy E76.01
Lipodermatosclerosis — *see* Varix, leg, with, inflammation
ulcerated — *see* Varix, leg, with, ulcer, with inflammation by site
Lipochrome histiocytosis (familial) D71
Lipodystrophia progressiva E88.1
Lipodystrophy (progressive) E88.1
insulin E88.1
intestinal K90.81
mesenteric K65.4
Lipofibroma — *see* Lipoma
Lipofuscinosis, neuronal (with ceroidosis) E75.4
Lipogranuloma, sclerosing L92.8
Lipogranulomatosis E78.89
Lipoid (*see also* condition)
histiocytosis D76.3
essential E75.29
nephrosis N04.9
proteinosis of Urbach E78.89
Lipoidemia — *see* Hyperlipidemia
Lipoidosis — *see* Lipidosis
Lipoma D17.9
fetal D17.9
fat cell D17.9
infiltrating D17.9
intramuscular D17.9
pleomorphic D17.9
site classification
arms (skin) (subcutaneous) D17.2-
connective tissue D17.30
intra-abdominal D17.5
intrathoracic D17.4
peritoneum D17.79
retroperitoneum D17.79
specified site NEC D17.39
spermatic cord D17.6
face (skin) (subcutaneous) D17.0
genitourinary organ NEC D17.72
head (skin) (subcutaneous) D17.0
intra-abdominal D17.5
intrathoracic D17.4
kidney D17.71
legs (skin) (subcutaneous) D17.2-
neck (skin) (subcutaneous) D17.0
peritoneum D17.79
retroperitoneum D17.79
skin D17.30
specified site NEC D17.39
specified site NEC D17.79
spermatic cord D17.6
subcutaneous D17.30
specified site NEC D17.39
trunk (skin) (subcutaneous) D17.1
unspecified D17.9
spindle cell D17.9
Lipomatosis E88.2
dolorosa (Dercum) E88.2
fetal — *see* Lipoma
Launois-Bensaude E88.89
Lipomyoma — *see* Lipoma
Lipomyxoma — *see* Lipoma
Lipomyxosarcoma — *see* Neoplasm, connective tissue, malignant
Lipoprotein metabolism disorder E78.9
Lipoproteinemia E78.5
broad-beta E78.2
floating-beta E78.2
hyper-pre-beta E78.1
Liposarcoma (*see also* Neoplasm, connective tissue, malignant)
dedifferentiated — *see* Neoplasm, connective tissue, malignant
differentiated type — *see* Neoplasm, connective tissue, malignant
embryonal — *see* Neoplasm, connective tissue, malignant
mixed type — *see* Neoplasm, connective tissue, malignant
myxoid — *see* Neoplasm, connective tissue, malignant
pleomorphic — *see* Neoplasm, connective tissue, malignant
round cell — *see* Neoplasm, connective tissue, malignant
well differentiated type — *see* Neoplasm, connective tissue, malignant
Liposynovitis prepatellaris E88.89
Lipping, cervix N86
Lipschütz disease or ulcer N76.6
Lipuria R82.0
schistosomiasis (bilharziasis) B65.0
Lisping F80.0
Lissauer's paralysis A52.17
Lissencephalia, lissencephaly Q04.3
Listeriosis, listerellosis A32.9
congenital (disseminated) P37.2
cutaneous A32.0
neonatal, newborn (disseminated) P37.2
oculoglandular A32.81
specified NEC A32.89
Lithemia E79.0
Lithiasis — *see* Calculus
Lithosis J62.8
Lithuria R82.99
Litigation, anxiety concerning Z65.3
Little leaguer's elbow — *see* Epicondylitis, medial
Little's disease G80.9
Littre's
gland — *see* condition
hernia — *see* Hernia, abdomen
Littritis — *see* Urethritis
Livedo (annularis) (racemosa) (reticularis) R23.1
Liver — *see* condition
Living alone (problems with) Z60.2
with handicapped person Z74.2
Lloyd's syndrome — *see* Adenomatosis, endocrine
Loa loa, loaiasis, loasis B74.3
Lobar — *see* condition
Lobomycosis B48.0
Lobo's disease B48.0
Lobotomy syndrome F07.0
Lobstein (-Ekman) **disease or syndrome** Q78.0
Lobster-claw hand Q71.6-
Lobulation (congenital) (*see also* Anomaly, by site)
kidney, Q63.1
liver, abnormal Q44.7
spleen Q89.09
Lobule, lobular — *see* condition
Local, localized — *see* condition
Locked-in state G83.5
Locked twins causing obstructed labor O66.1
Locking
joint — *see* Derangement, joint, specified type NEC
knee — *see* Derangement, knee
Lockjaw — *see* Tetanus
Löffler's
endocarditis I42.3
eosinophilia J82
pneumonia J82
syndrome (eosinophilic pneumonitis) J82
Loiasis (with conjunctival infestation) (eyelid) B74.3
Lone Star fever A77.0
Long
labor O63.9
first stage O63.0
second stage O63.1
QT syndrome I45.81
Long-term (current) (prophylactic) **drug therapy** (use of)
agents affecting estrogen receptors and estrogen levels NEC Z79.818
anastrozole (Arimidex) Z79.811
antibiotics Z79.2
short-term use — *omit code*
anticoagulants Z79.01
anti-inflammatory, non-steroidal (NSAID) Z79.1
antiplatelet Z79.02
antithrombotics Z79.02
aromatase inhibitors Z79.811
aspirin Z79.82
birth control pill or patch Z79.3
bisphosphonates Z79.83
contraceptive, oral Z79.3
drug, specified NEC Z79.899
estrogen receptor downregulators Z79.818
Evista Z79.810
exemestane (Aromasin) Z79.811
Fareston Z79.810
fulvestrant (Faslodex) Z79.818
gonadotropin-releasing hormone (GnRH) agonist Z79.818

- **Long-term drug therapy** — *continued*
  - goserelin acetate (Zoladex) Z79.818
  - hormone replacement (postmenopausal) Z79.89Ø
  - insulin Z79.4
  - letrozole (Femara) Z79.811
  - leuprolide acetate (leuprorelin) (Lupron) Z79.818
  - megestrol acetate (Megace) Z79.818
  - methadone for pain management Z79.891
  - Nolvadex Z79.81Ø
  - non-steroidal anti-inflammatories (NSAID) Z79.1
  - opiate analgesic Z79.891
  - oral contraceptive Z79.3
  - raloxifene (Evista) Z79.81Ø
  - selective estrogen receptor modulators (SERMs) Z79.81Ø
  - steroids
    - inhaled Z79.51
    - systemic Z79.52
  - tamoxifen (Nolvadex) Z79.81Ø
  - toremifene (Fareston) Z79.81Ø
- **Longitudinal stripes or grooves, nails** L6Ø.8
  - congenital Q84.6
- **Loop**
  - intestine — *see* Volvulus
  - vascular on papilla (optic) Q14.2
- **Loose** (*see also* condition)
  - body
    - joint M24.ØØ
      - ankle M24.Ø7-
      - elbow M24.Ø2-
      - hand M24.Ø4-
      - hip M24.Ø5-
      - knee M23.4-
      - shoulder (region) M24.Ø1-
      - specified site NEC M24.Ø8
      - vertebra M24.Ø8
      - toe M24.Ø7-
      - wrist M24.Ø3-
    - knee M23.4-
    - sheath, tendon — *see* Disorder, tendon, specified type NEC
  - cartilage — *see* Loose, body, joint
  - tooth, teeth KØ8.8
- **Loosening**
  - aseptic
    - joint prosthesis — *see* Complications, joint prosthesis, mechanical, loosening, by site
  - epiphysis — *see* Osteochondropathy
  - mechanical
    - joint prosthesis — *see* Complications, joint prosthesis, mechanical, loosening, by site
- **Looser-Milkman** (-Debray) **syndrome** M83.8
- **Lop ear** (deformity) Q17.3
- **Lorain** (-Levi) **short stature syndrome** E23.Ø
- **Lordosis** M4Ø.5Ø
  - acquired — *see* Lordosis, specified type NEC
  - congenital Q76.429
    - lumbar region Q76.426
    - lumbosacral region Q76.427
    - sacral region Q76.428
    - sacrococcygeal region Q76.428
    - thoracolumbar region Q76.425
  - lumbar region M4Ø.56
  - lumbosacral region M4Ø.57
  - postsurgical M96.4
  - postural — *see* Lordosis, specified type NEC
  - rachitic (late effect) (sequelae) E64.3
  - sequelae of rickets E64.3
  - specified type NEC M4Ø.4Ø
    - lumbar region M4Ø.46
    - lumbosacral region M4Ø.47
    - thoracolumbar region M4Ø.45
  - thoracolumbar region M4Ø.55
  - tuberculous A18.Ø1
- **Loss** (of)
  - appetite (*see also* Anorexia) R63.Ø
    - hysterical F5Ø.8
    - nonorganic origin F5Ø.8
    - psychogenic F5Ø.8
  - blood — *see* Hemorrhage
  - control, sphincter, rectum R15.9
    - nonorganic origin F98.1
- **Loss** — *continued*
  - consciousness, transient R55
    - traumatic — *see* Injury, intracranial
  - elasticity, skin R23.4
  - family (member) in childhood Z62.898
  - fluid (acute) E86.9
    - with
      - hypernatremia E87.Ø
      - hyponatremia E87.1
  - function of labyrinth — *see* subcategory H83.2
  - hair, nonscarring — *see* Alopecia
  - hearing (*see also* Deafness)
    - central NOS H9Ø.5
    - neural NOS H9Ø.5
    - perceptive NOS H9Ø.5
    - sensorineural NOS H9Ø.5
    - sensory NOS H9Ø.5
  - height R29.89Ø
  - limb or member, traumatic, current — *see* Amputation, traumatic
  - love relationship in childhood Z62.898
  - memory (*see also* Amnesia)
    - mild, following organic brain damage FØ6.8
  - mind — *see* Psychosis
  - occlusal vertical dimension of fully erupted teeth M26.37
  - organ or part — *see* Absence, by site, acquired
  - ossicles, ear (partial) H74.32-
  - parent in childhood Z63.4
  - pregnancy, recurrent N46
    - care in current pregnancy O26.2-
    - without current pregnancy N96
  - recurrent pregnancy — *see* Loss, pregnancy, recurrent
  - self-esteem, in childhood Z62.898
  - sense of
    - smell — *see* Disturbance, sensation, smell
    - taste — *see* Disturbance, sensation, taste
    - touch R2Ø.8
  - sensory R44.9
    - dissociative F44.6
  - sexual desire F52.Ø
  - sight (acquired) (complete) (congenital) — *see* Blindness
  - substance of
    - bone — *see* Disorder, bone, density and structure, specified NEC
    - cartilage — *see* Disorder, cartilage, specified type NEC
      - auricle (ear) — *see* Disorder, pinna, specified type NEC
    - vitreous (humor) H15.89
  - tooth, teeth *see* Absence, teeth, acquired
  - vision, visual H54.7
    - both eyes H54.3
    - one eye H54.6Ø
      - left (normal vision on right) H54.62
      - right (normal vision on left) H54.61
    - specified as blindness — *see* Blindness
    - subjective
      - sudden H53.13-
      - transient H53.12-
  - vitreous — *see* Prolapse, vitreous
  - voice — *see* Aphonia
  - weight (abnormal) (cause unknown) R63.4
- **Louis-Bar syndrome** (ataxia-telangiectasia) G11.3
- **Louping ill** (encephalitis) A84.8
- **Louse, lousiness** — *see* Lice
- **Low**
  - achiever, school Z55.3
  - back syndrome M54.5
  - basal metabolic rate R94.8
  - birthweight (2499 grams or less) PØ7.1Ø
    - with weight of
      - 1ØØØ-1249 grams PØ7.14
      - 125Ø-1499 grams PØ7.15
      - 15ØØ-1749 grams PØ7.16
      - 175Ø-1999 grams PØ7.17
      - 2ØØØ-2499 grams PØ7.18
    - extreme (999 grams or less) PØ7.ØØ
      - with weight of
        - 499 grams or less PØ7.Ø1
        - 5ØØ-749 grams PØ7.Ø2
- **Low** — *continued*
  - birthweight — *continued*
    - extreme — *continued*
      - with weight of — *continued*
        - 75Ø-999 grams PØ7.Ø3
    - for gestational age — *see* Light for dates
  - blood pressure (*see also* Hypotension)
    - reading (incidental) (isolated) (nonspecific) RØ3.1
  - cardiac reserve — *see* Disease, heart
  - function (*see also* Hypofunction)
    - kidney N28.9
  - hematocrit D64.9
  - hemoglobin D64.9
  - income Z59.6
  - level of literacy Z55.Ø
  - lying
    - kidney N28.89
    - organ or site, congenital — *see* Malposition, congenital
  - output syndrome (cardiac) — *see* Failure, heart
  - platelets (blood) — *see* Thrombocytopenia
  - reserve, kidney N28.89
  - salt syndrome E87.1
  - self esteem R45.81
  - set ears Q17.4
  - vision H54.2
    - one eye (other eye normal) H54.5Ø
      - left (normal vision on right) H54.52
      - other eye blind — *see* Blindness
      - right (normal vision on left) H54.51
- **Low-density-lipoprotein-type** (LDL) **hyperlipoproteinemia** E78.Ø
- **Lowe's syndrome** E72.Ø3
- **Lown-Ganong-Levine syndrome** I45.6
- **LSD reaction** (acute) (without dependence) F16.9Ø
  - with dependence F16.2Ø
- **L-shaped kidney** Q63.8
- **Ludwig's angina or disease** K12.2
- **Lues** (venerea), **luetic** — *see* Syphilis
- **Luetscher's syndrome** (dehydration) E86.Ø
- **Lumbago, lumbalgia M54.5**
  - with sciatica M54.4-
    - due to intervertebral disc disorder M51.17
  - due to displacement, intervertebral disc M51.27
    - with sciatica M51.17
- **Lumbar** — *see* condition
- **Lumbarization, vertebra, congenital** Q76.49
- **Lumbermen's itch** B88.Ø
- **Lump** — *see* Mass
- **Lunacy** — *see* Psychosis
- **Lung** — *see* condition
- **Lupoid** (miliary) **of Boeck** D86.3
- **Lupus**
  - anticoagulant D68.62
    - with
      - hemorrhagic disorder D68.312
      - hypercoagulable state D68.62
    - finding without diagnosis R76.Ø
  - discoid (local) L93.Ø
  - erythematosus (discoid) (local) L93.Ø
    - disseminated — *see* Lupus, erythematosus, systemic
    - eyelid HØ1.129
      - left HØ1.126
        - lower HØ1.125
        - upper HØ1.124
      - right HØ1.123
        - lower HØ1.122
        - upper HØ1.121
    - profundus L93.2
    - specified NEC L93.2
    - subacute cutaneous L93.1
    - systemic M32.9
      - with organ or system involvement M32.1Ø
        - endocarditis M32.11
        - lung M32.13
        - pericarditis M32.12
        - renal (glomerular) M32.14
          - tubulo-interstitial M32.15
        - specified organ or system NEC M32.19
      - drug-induced M32.Ø

- **Malabsorption** — *continued*
  - galactose E74.2Ø
  - glucose(-galactose) E74.39
  - intestinal K9Ø.9
    - specified NEC K9Ø.89
  - isomaltose E74.31
  - lactose E73.9
  - methionine E72.19
  - monosaccharide E74.39
  - postgastrectomy K91.2
  - postsurgical K91.2
  - protein K9Ø.4
  - starch K9Ø.4
  - sucrose E74.39
  - syndrome K9Ø.9
    - postsurgical K91.2
- **Malacia, bone** (adult) M83.9
  - juvenile — *see* Rickets
- **Malacoplakia**
  - bladder N32.89
  - pelvis (kidney) N28.89
  - ureter N28.89
  - urethra N36.8
- **Malacosteon, juvenile** — *see* Rickets
- **Maladaptation** — *see* Maladjustment
- **Maladie de Roger** Q21.Ø
- **Maladjustment**
  - conjugal Z63.Ø
    - involving divorce or estrangement Z63.5
  - educational Z55.4
  - family Z63.9
  - marital Z63.Ø
    - involving divorce or estrangement Z63.5
  - occupational NEC Z56.89
  - simple, adult — *see* Disorder, adjustment
  - situational — *see* Disorder, adjustment
  - social Z6Ø.9
    - due to
      - acculturation difficulty Z6Ø.3
      - discrimination and persecution (perceived) Z6Ø.5
      - exclusion and isolation Z6Ø.4
      - life-cycle (phase of life) transition Z6Ø.Ø
      - rejection Z6Ø.4
      - specified reason NEC Z6Ø.8
- **Malaise** R53.81
- **Malakoplakia** — *see* Malacoplakia
- **Malaria, malarial** (fever) B54
  - with
    - blackwater fever B5Ø.8
      - hemoglobinuric (bilious) B5Ø.8
    - hemoglobinuria B5Ø.8
  - accidentally induced (therapeutically)—code by type under Malaria
  - algid B5Ø.9
  - cerebral B5Ø.Ø *[G94]*
  - clinically diagnosed (without parasitological confirmation) B54
  - congenital NEC P37.4
    - falciparum P37.3
  - congestion, congestive B54
  - continued (fever) B5Ø.9
  - estivo-autumnal B5Ø.9
  - falciparum B5Ø.9
    - with complications NEC B5Ø.8
      - cerebral B5Ø.Ø *[G94]*
      - severe B5Ø.8
  - hemorrhagic B54
  - malariae B52.9
    - with
      - complications NEC B52.8
      - glomerular disorder B52.Ø
  - malignant (tertian) — *see* Malaria, falciparum
  - mixed infections—code to first listed type in B5Ø-B53
  - ovale B53.Ø
  - parasitologically confirmed NEC B53.8
  - pernicious, acute — *see* Malaria, falciparum
  - Plasmodium (P.)
    - falciparum NEC — *see* Malaria, falciparum
    - malariae NEC B52.9

- **Malaria, malarial**— *continued*
  - Plasmodium— *continued*
    - malariae NEC — *continued*
      - with Plasmodium
        - falciparum (and or vivax) — *see* Malaria, falciparum
        - vivax (*see also* Malaria, vivax)
          - and falciparum — *see* Malaria, falciparum
    - ovale B53.Ø
      - with Plasmodium malariae (*see also* Malaria, malariae)
        - and vivax (*see also* Malaria, vivax)
          - and falciparum — *see* Malaria, falciparum
    - simian B53.1
      - with Plasmodium malariae (*see also* Malaria, malariae)
        - and vivax (*see also* Malaria, vivax)
          - and falciparum — *see* Malaria, falciparum
    - vivax NEC B51.9
      - with Plasmodium falciparum — *see* Malaria, falciparum
  - quartan — *see* Malaria, malariae
  - quotidian — *see* Malaria, falciparum
  - recurrent B54
  - remittent B54
  - specified type NEC (parasitologically confirmed) B53.8
  - spleen B54
  - subtertian (fever) — *see* Malaria, falciparum
  - tertian (benign) (*see also* Malaria, vivax)
    - malignant B5Ø.9
  - tropical B5Ø.9
  - typhoid B54
  - vivax B51.9
    - with
      - complications NEC B51.8
      - ruptured spleen B51.Ø
- **Malassimilation** K9Ø.9
- **Malassez's disease** (cystic) N5Ø.8
- **Mal de los pintos** — *see* Pinta
- **Mal de mer** T75.3
- **Maldescent, testis** Q53.9
  - bilateral Q53.2Ø
    - abdominal Q53.21
    - perineal Q53.22
  - unilateral Q53.1Ø
    - abdominal Q53.11
    - perineal Q53.12
- **Maldevelopment** (*see also* Anomaly)
  - brain Q07.9
  - colon Q43.9
  - hip Q74.2
    - congenital dislocation Q65.2
      - bilateral Q65.1
      - unilateral Q65.Ø-
  - mastoid process Q75.8
  - middle ear Q16.4
    - except ossicles Q16.4
    - ossicles Q16.3
  - ossicles Q16.3
  - spine Q76.49
  - toe Q74.2
- **Male type pelvis** Q74.2
  - with disproportion (fetopelvic) O33.3
    - causing obstructed labor O65.3
- **Malformation** (congenital) (*see also* Anomaly)
  - adrenal gland Q89.1
  - affecting multiple systems with skeletal changes NEC Q87.5
  - alimentary tract Q45.9
    - specified type NEC Q45.8
    - upper Q4Ø.9
      - specified type NEC Q4Ø.8
  - aorta Q25.9
    - atresia Q25.2
    - coarctation (preductal) (postductal) Q25.1
    - patent ductus arteriosus Q25.Ø
    - specified type NEC Q25.4
    - stenosis (supravalvular) Q25.3

- **Malformation** — *continued*
  - aortic valve Q23.9
    - specified NEC Q23.8
  - arteriovenous, aneurysmatic (congenital) Q27.3Ø
    - brain Q28.2
    - cerebral Q28.2
    - peripheral Q27.3Ø
      - digestive system Q27.33
      - lower limb Q27.32
      - other specified site Q27.39
      - renal vessel Q27.34
      - upper limb Q27.31
    - precerebral vessels (nonruptured) Q28.Ø
  - auricle
    - ear (congenital) Q17.3
      - acquired H61.119
        - left H61.112
          - with right H61.113
        - right H61.111
          - with left H61.113
  - bile duct Q44.5
  - bladder Q64.79
    - aplasia Q64.5
    - diverticulum Q64.6
    - exstrophy — *see* Exstrophy, bladder
    - neck obstruction Q64.31
  - bone Q79.9
    - face Q75.9
      - specified type NEC Q75.8
    - skull Q75.9
      - specified type NEC Q75.8
  - brain (multiple) QØ4.9
    - arteriovenous Q28.2
    - specified type NEC QØ4.8
  - branchial cleft Q18.2
  - breast Q83.9
    - specified type NEC Q83.8
  - broad ligament Q5Ø.6
  - bronchus Q32.4
  - bursa Q79.9
  - cardiac
    - chambers Q2Ø.9
      - specified type NEC Q2Ø.8
    - septum Q21.9
      - specified type NEC Q21.8
  - cerebral QØ4.9
    - vessels Q28.3
  - cervix uteri Q51.9
    - specified type NEC Q51.828
  - Chiari
    - Type I G93.5
    - Type II QØ7.Ø1
  - choroid (congenital) Q14.3
    - plexus QØ7.8
  - circulatory system Q28.9
  - cochlea Q16.5
  - cornea Q13.4
  - coronary vessels Q24.5
  - corpus callosum (congenital) QØ4.Ø
  - diaphragm Q79.1
  - digestive system NEC, specified type NEC Q45.8
  - dura QØ7.9
    - brain QØ4.9
    - spinal QØ6.9
  - ear Q17.9
    - causing impairment of hearing Q16.9
    - external Q17.9
      - accessory auricle Q17.Ø
      - causing impairment of hearing Q16.9
        - absence of
          - auditory canal Q16.1
          - auricle Q16.Ø
      - macrotia Q17.1
      - microtia Q17.2
      - misplacement Q17.4
      - misshapen NEC Q17.3
      - prominence Q17.5
      - specified type NEC Q17.8
    - inner Q16.5
    - middle Q16.4
      - absence of eustachian tube Q16.2
      - ossicles (fusion) Q16.3

- **Malta fever** — *see* Brucellosis
- **Maltworker's lung** J67.4
- **Malunion, fracture** — *see* Fracture, by site
- **Mammillitis** N61
  - puerperal, postpartum O91.Ø2
- **Mammitis** — *see* Mastitis
- **Mammogram** (examination) Z12.39
  - routine Z12.31
- **Mammoplasia** N62
- **Management** (of)
  - bone conduction hearing device (implanted) Z45.32Ø
  - cardiac pacemaker NEC Z45.Ø18
  - cerebrospinal fluid drainage device Z45.41
  - cochlear device (implanted) Z45.321
  - contraceptive Z3Ø.9
    - specified NEC Z3Ø.8
  - implanted device Z45.9
    - specified NEC Z45.89
  - infusion pump Z45.1
  - procreative Z31.9
    - male factor infertility in female Z31.81
    - specified NEC Z31.89
  - prosthesis (external) (*see also* Fitting) Z44.9
    - implanted Z45.9
      - specified NEC Z45.89
  - renal dialysis catheter Z49.Ø1
  - vascular access device Z45.2
- **Mangled** — *see* specified injury by site
- **Mania** (monopolar) (*see also* Disorder, mood, manic episode
  - with psychotic symptoms F3Ø.2
  - without psychotic symptoms F3Ø.1Ø
    - mild F3Ø.11
    - moderate F3Ø.12
    - severe F3Ø.13
  - Bell's F3Ø.8
  - chronic (recurrent) F31.89
  - hysterical F44.89
  - puerperal F3Ø.8
  - recurrent F31.89
- **Manic-depressive insanity, psychosis, or syndrome** — *see* Disorder, bipolar
- **Mannosidosis** E77.1
- **Mansonelliasis, mansonellosis** B74.4
- **Manson's**
  - disease B65.1
  - schistosomiasis B65.1
- **Manual** — *see* condition
- **Maple-bark-stripper's lung** (disease) J67.6
- **Maple-syrup-urine disease** E71.Ø
- **Marable's syndrome** (celiac artery compression) I77.4
- **Marasmus** E41
  - due to malnutrition E41
  - intestinal E41
  - nutritional E41
  - senile R54
  - tuberculous NEC — *see* Tuberculosis
- **Marble**
  - bones Q78.2
  - skin R23.8
- **Marburg virus disease** A98.3
- **March**
  - fracture — *see* Fracture, traumatic, stress, by site
  - hemoglobinuria D59.6
- **Marchesani**(-Weill) **syndrome** Q87.Ø
- **Marchiafava**(-Bignami) **syndrome or disease** G37.1
- **Marchiafava-Micheli syndrome** D59.5
- **Marcus Gunn's syndrome** QØ7.8
- **Marfan's syndrome**
- — *see* Syndrome, Marfan's
- **Marie-Bamberger disease** — *see* Osteoarthropathy, hypertrophic, specified NEC
- **Marie-Charcot-Tooth neuropathic muscular atrophy** G6Ø.Ø
- **Marie's**
  - cerebellar ataxia (late-onset) G11.2
  - disease or syndrome (acromegaly) E22.Ø
- **Marie-Strümpell arthritis, disease or spondylitis** — *see* Spondylitis, ankylosing
- **Marion's disease** (bladder neck obstruction) N32.Ø
- **Marital conflict** Z63.Ø
- **Mark**
  - port wine Q82.5
  - raspberry Q82.5
  - strawberry Q82.5
  - stretch L9Ø.6
  - tattoo L81.8
- **Marker heterochromatin** — *see* Extra, marker chromosomes
- **Maroteaux-Lamy syndrome** (mild) (severe) E76.29
- **Marrow** (bone)
  - arrest D61.9
  - poor function D75.89
- **Marseilles fever** A77.1
- **Marsh fever** — *see* Malaria
- **Marshall's** (hidrotic) **ectodermal dysplasia** Q82.4
- **Marsh's disease** (exophthalmic goiter) EØ5.ØØ
  - with storm EØ5.Ø1
- **Masculinization** (female) **with adrenal hyperplasia** E25.9
  - congenital E25.Ø
- **Masculinovoblastoma** D27.-
- **Masochism** (sexual) F65.51
- **Mason's lung** J62.8
- **Mass**
  - abdominal R19.ØØ
    - epigastric R19.Ø6
    - generalized R19.Ø7
    - left lower quadrant R19.Ø4
    - left upper quadrant R19.Ø2
    - periumbilic R19.Ø5
    - right lower quadrant R19.Ø3
    - right upper quadrant R19.Ø1
    - specified site NEC R19.Ø9
  - breast N63
  - chest R22.2
  - cystic — *see* Cyst
  - ear H93.8-
  - head R22.Ø
  - intra-abdominal (diffuse) (generalized) — *see* Mass, abdominal
  - kidney N28.89
  - liver R16.Ø
  - localized (skin) R22.9
    - chest R22.2
    - head R22.Ø
    - limb
      - lower R22.4-
      - upper R22.3-
    - neck R22.1
    - trunk R22.2
  - lung R91.8
  - malignant — *see* Neoplasm, malignant, by site
  - neck R22.1
  - pelvic (diffuse) (generalized) — *see* Mass, abdominal
  - specified organ NEC — *see* Disease, by site
  - splenic R16.1
  - substernal thyroid — *see* Goiter
  - superficial (localized) R22.9
  - umbilical (diffuse) (generalized) R19.Ø9
- **Massive** — *see* condition
- **Mast cell**
  - disease, systemic tissue D47.Ø
  - leukemia C94.3-
  - sarcoma C96.2
  - tumor D47.Ø
    - malignant C96.2-
- **Mastalgia** N64.4
- **Masters-Allen syndrome** N83.8
- **Mastitis** (acute) (diffuse) (nonpuerperal) (subacute) N61
  - chronic (cystic) — *see* Mastopathy, cystic
  - cystic (Schimmelbusch's type) — *see* Mastopathy, cystic
  - fibrocystic — *see* Mastopathy, cystic
  - infective N61
    - newborn P39.Ø
  - interstitial, gestational or puerperal — *see* Mastitis, obstetric
  - neonatal (noninfective) P83.4
    - infective P39.Ø
  - obstetric (interstitial) (nonpurulent)
    - associated with
      - lactation O91.23
- **Mastitis** — *continued*
  - obstetric — *continued*
    - associated with — *continued*
      - pregnancy O91.21-
      - puerperium O91.22
    - purulent
      - associated with
        - lactation O91.13
        - pregnancy O91.11-
        - puerperium O91.12
  - periductal — *see* Ectasia, mammary duct
  - phlegmonous — *see* Mastopathy, cystic
  - plasma cell — *see* Ectasia, mammary duct
- **Mastocytoma** D47.Ø
  - malignant C96.2
- **Mastocytosis** Q82.2
  - aggressive systemic C96.2
  - indolent systemic D47.Ø
  - malignant C96.2
  - systemic, associated with clonal hematopoetic non-mast-cell disease (SM-AHNMD) D47.Ø
- **Mastodynia** N64.4
- **Mastoid** — *see* condition
- **Mastoidalgia** — *see* subcategory H92.Ø
- **Mastoiditis** (coalescent) (hemorrhagic) (suppurative) H7Ø.9-
  - acute, subacute H7Ø.ØØ-
    - complicated NEC H7Ø.Ø9-
    - subperiosteal H7Ø.Ø1-
  - chronic (necrotic) (recurrent) H7Ø.1-
  - in (due to)
    - infectious disease NEC B99 *[H75.0-]*
    - parasitic disease NEC B89 *[H75.0-]*
    - tuberculosis A18.Ø3
  - petrositis — *see* Petrositis
  - postauricular fistula — *see* Fistula, postauricular
  - specified NEC H7Ø.89-
  - tuberculous A18.Ø3
- **Mastopathy, mastopathia** N64.9
  - chronica cystica — *see* Mastopathy, cystic
  - cystic (chronic) (diffuse) N6Ø.1-
    - with epithelial proliferation N6Ø.3-
  - diffuse cystic — *see* Mastopathy, cystic
  - estrogenic, oestrogenica N64.89
  - ovarian origin N64.89
- **Mastoplasia, mastoplastia** N62
- **Masturbation** (excessive) F98.8
- **Maternal care** (for) — *see* Pregnancy (complicated by) (management affected by)
- **Matheiu's disease** (leptospiral jaundice) A27.Ø
- **Mauclaire's disease or osteochondrosis** — *see* Osteochondrosis, juvenile, hand, metacarpal
- **Maxcy's disease** A75.2
- **Maxilla, maxillary** — *see* condition
- **May**(-Hegglin) **anomaly or syndrome** D72.Ø
- **McArdle**(-Schmid)(-Pearson) **disease** (glycogen storage) E74.Ø4
- **McCune-Albright syndrome** Q78.1
- **McQuarrie's syndrome** (idiopathic familial hypoglycemia) E16.2
- **Meadow's syndrome** Q86.1
- **Measles** (black) (hemorrhagic) (suppressed) BØ5.9
  - with
    - complications NEC BØ5.89
    - encephalitis BØ5.Ø
    - intestinal complications BØ5.4
    - keratitis (keratoconjunctivitis) BØ5.81
    - meningitis BØ5.1
    - otitis media BØ5.3
    - pneumonia BØ5.2
  - French — *see* Rubella
  - German — *see* Rubella
  - Liberty — *see* Rubella
- **Meatitis, urethral** — *see* Urethritis
- **Meatus, meatal** — *see* condition
- **Meat-wrappers' asthma** J68.9
- **Meckel-Gruber syndrome** Q61.9
- **Meckel's diverticulitis, diverticulum** (displaced) (hypertrophic) Q43.Ø
  - malignant — *see* Table of Neoplasms, small intestine, malignant

- **Meningitis**— *continued*
  - in (due to)
    - adenovirus A87.1
    - African trypanosomiasis B56.9 *[G02]*
    - anthrax A22.8
    - bacterial disease NEC A48.8 *[G01]*
    - Chagas' disease (chronic) B57.41
    - chickenpox B01.0
    - coccidioidomycosis B38.4
    - Diplococcus pneumoniae G00.1
    - enterovirus A87.0
    - herpes (simplex) virus B00.3
      - zoster B02.1
    - infectious mononucleosis B27.92
    - leptospirosis A27.81
    - Listeria monocytogenes A32.11
    - Lyme disease A69.21
    - measles B05.1
    - mumps (virus) B26.1
    - neurosyphilis (late) A52.13
    - parasitic disease NEC B89 *[G02]*
    - poliovirus A80.9 *[G02]*
    - preventive immunization, inoculation or vaccination G03.8
    - rubella B06.02
    - Salmonella infection A02.21
    - specified cause NEC G03.8
    - typhoid fever A01.01
    - varicella B01.0
    - viral disease NEC A87.8
    - whooping cough A37.90
    - zoster B02.1
  - infectious G00.9
  - influenzal (H. influenzae) G00.0
  - Klebsiella G00.8
  - leptospiral (aseptic) A27.81
  - lymphocytic (acute) (benign) (serous) A87.2
  - meningococcal A39.0
  - Mima polymorpha G00.8
  - Mollaret (benign recurrent) G03.2
  - monilial B37.5
  - mycotic NEC B49 *[G02]*
  - Neisseria A39.0
  - nonbacterial G03.0
  - nonpyogenic NEC G03.0
  - ossificans G96.19
  - pneumococcal G00.1
  - poliovirus A80.9 *[G02]*
  - postmeasles B05.1
  - purulent G00.9
    - specified organism NEC G00.8
  - pyogenic G00.9
    - specified organism NEC G00.8
  - Salmonella (arizonae) (Cholerae-Suis) (enteritidis) (typhimurium) A02.21
  - septic G00.9
    - specified organism NEC G00.8
  - serosa circumscripta NEC G03.0
  - serous NEC G93.2
  - specified organism NEC G00.8
  - sporotrichosis B42.81
  - staphylococcal G00.3
  - sterile G03.0
  - streptococcal (acute) G00.2
  - suppurative G00.9
    - specified organism NEC G00.8
  - syphilitic (late) (tertiary) A52.13
    - acute A51.41
    - congenital A50.41
    - secondary A51.41
  - Torula histolytica (cryptococcal) B45.1
  - traumatic (complication of injury) T79.8
  - tuberculous A17.0
  - typhoid A01.01
  - viral NEC A87.9
  - Yersinia pestis A20.3
- **Meningocele** (spinal) (*see also* Spina bifida)
  - with hydrocephalus — *see* Spina bifida, by site, with hydrocephalus
  - acquired (traumatic) G96.19
  - cerebral — *see* Encephalocele
- **Meningocerebritis** — *see* Meningoencephalitis
- **Meningococcemia** A39.4
  - acute A39.2
  - chronic A39.3
- **Meningococcus, meningococcal** (*see also* condition) A39.9
  - adrenalitis, hemorrhagic A39.1
  - carrier (suspected) of Z22.31
  - meningitis (cerebrospinal) A39.0
- **Meningoencephalitis** (*see also* Encephalitis) G04.90
  - acute NEC (*see also* Encephalitis, viral) A86
  - bacterial NEC G04.2
  - California A83.5
  - diphasic A84.1
  - eosinophilic B83.2
  - epidemic A39.81
  - herpesviral, herpetic B00.4
    - due to herpesvirus 6 B10.01
    - due to herpesvirus 7 B10.09
    - specified NEC B10.09
  - in (due to)
    - blastomycosis NEC B40.81
    - diseases classified elsewhere G05.3
    - free-living amebae B60.2
    - Hemophilus influenzae (H. influenzae) G04.2
    - herpes B00.4
      - due to herpesvirus 6 B10.01
      - due to herpesvirus 7 B10.09
      - specified NEC B10.09
    - H. influenzae G00.0
    - Lyme disease A69.22
    - mercury — *see* subcategory T56.1
    - mumps B26.2
    - Naegleria (amebae) (organisms) (fowleri) B60.2
    - Parastrongylus cantonensis B83.2
    - toxoplasmosis (acquired) B58.2
      - congenital P37.1
  - infectious (acute) (viral) A86
  - influenzal (H. influenzae) G04.2
  - Listeria monocytogenes A32.12
  - lymphocytic (serous) A87.2
  - mumps B26.2
  - parasitic NEC B89 *[G05.3]*
  - pneumococcal G00.1
  - primary amebic B60.2
  - specific (syphilitic) A52.14
  - specified organism NEC G04.81
  - staphylococcal G04.2
  - streptococcal G04.2
  - syphilitic A52.14
  - toxic NEC G92
    - due to mercury — *see* subcategory T56.1
  - tuberculous A17.82
  - virus NEC A86
- **Meningoencephalocele** (*see also* Encephalocele)
  - syphilitic A52.19
    - congenital A50.49
- **Meningoencephalomyelitis** (*see also* Meningoencephalitis)
  - acute NEC (viral) A86
    - disseminated G04.00
      - postimmunization or postvaccination G04.02
      - postinfectious G04.01
  - due to
    - actinomycosis A42.82
    - Toxoplasma or toxoplasmosis (acquired) B58.2
      - congenital P37.1
  - postimmunization or postvaccination G04.02
- **Meningoencephalomyelopathy** G96.9
- **Meningoencephalopathy** G96.9
- **Meningomyelitis** (*see also* Meningoencephalitis)
  - bacterial NEC G04.2
  - blastomycotic NEC B40.81
  - cryptococcal B45.1
  - in diseases classified elsewhere G05.4
  - meningococcal A39.81
  - syphilitic A52.14
  - tuberculous A17.82
- **Meningomyelocele** (*see also* Spina bifida)
  - syphilitic A52.19
- **Meningomyeloneuritis** — *see* Meningoencephalitis
- **Meningoradiculitis** — *see* Meningitis
- **Meningovascular** — *see* condition
- **Menkes' disease or syndrome** E83.09
  - meaning maple-syrup-urine disease E71.0
- **Menometrorrhagia** N92.1
- **Menopause, menopausal** (asymptomatic) (state) Z78.0
  - arthritis (any site) NEC — *see* Arthritis, specified form NEC
  - bleeding N92.4
  - depression (single episode) F32.8
    - agitated (single episode) F32.2
      - recurrent episode F33.9
    - psychotic (single episode) F32.8
      - recurrent episode F33.9
    - recurrent episode F33.9
  - melancholia (single episode) F32.8
    - recurrent episode F33.9
  - paranoid state F22
  - premature E28.319
    - asymptomatic E28.319
      - postirradiation E89.40
      - postsurgical E89.40
    - symptomatic E28.310
      - postirradiation E89.41
      - postsurgical E89.41
  - psychosis NEC F28
  - symptomatic N95.1
  - toxic polyarthritis NEC — *see* Arthritis, specified form NEC
- **Menorrhagia** (primary) N92.0
  - climacteric N92.4
    - menopausal N92.4
  - menopausal N92.4
  - postclimacteric N95.0
  - postmenopausal N95.0
  - preclimacteric or premenopausal N92.4
  - pubertal (menses retained) N92.2
- **Menostaxis** N92.0
- **Menses, retention** N94.89
- **Menstrual** — *see* Menstruation
- **Menstruation**
  - absent — *see* Amenorrhea
  - anovulatory N97.0
  - cycle, irregular N92.6
  - delayed N91.0
  - disorder N93.9
    - psychogenic F45.8
  - during pregnancy O20.8
  - excessive (with regular cycle) N92.0
    - with irregular cycle N92.1
    - at puberty N92.2
  - frequent N92.0
  - infrequent — *see* Oligomenorrhea
  - irregular N92.6
    - specified NEC N92.5
  - latent N92.5
  - membranous N92.5
  - painful (*see also* Dysmenorrhea) N94.6
    - primary N94.4
    - psychogenic F45.8
    - secondary N94.5
  - passage of clots N92.0
  - precocious E30.1
  - protracted N92.5
  - rare — *see* Oligomenorrhea
  - retained N94.89
  - retrograde N92.5
  - scanty — *see* Oligomenorrhea
  - suppression N94.89
  - vicarious (nasal) N94.89
- **Mental** (*see also* condition)
  - deficiency — *see* Disability, intellectual
  - deterioration — *see* Psychosis
  - disorder — *see* Disorder, mental
  - exhaustion F48.8
  - insufficiency (congenital) — *see* Disability, intellectual
  - observation without need for further medical care Z03.89
  - retardation — *see* Disability, intellectual
  - subnormality — *see* Disability, intellectual
  - upset — *see* Disorder, mental

Migraine (idiopathic) G43.9Ø9
- with aura (acute-onset) (prolonged) (typical) (without headache) G43.1Ø9
  - with refractory migraine G43.119
    - with status migrainosus G43.111
    - without status migrainosus G43.119
  - intractable G43.119
    - with status migrainosus G43.111
    - without status migrainosus G43.119
  - not intractable G43.1Ø9
    - with status migrainosus G43.1Ø1
    - without status migrainosus G43.1Ø9
  - persistent G43.5Ø9
    - with cerebral infarction G43.6Ø9
      - with refractory migraine G43.619
        - with status migrainosus G43.611
        - without status migrainosus G43.619
      - without refractory migraine G43.6Ø9
        - with status migrainosus G43.6Ø1
        - without status migrainosus G43.6Ø9
      - intractable G43.619
        - with status migrainosus G43.611
        - without status migrainosus G43.619
      - not intractable G43.6Ø9
        - with status migrainosus G43.6Ø1
        - without status migrainosus G43.6Ø9
    - without cerebral infarction G43.5Ø9
      - with refractory migraine G43.519
        - with status migrainosus G43.511
        - without status migrainosus G43.519
      - without refractory migraine G43.5Ø9
        - with status migrainosus G43.5Ø1
        - without status migrainosus G43.5Ø9
      - intractable G43.519
        - with status migrainosus G43.511
        - without status migrainosus G43.519
      - not intractable G43.5Ø9
        - with status migrainosus G43.5Ø1
        - without status migrainosus G43.5Ø9
  - without mention of refractory migraine G43.1Ø9
    - with status migrainosus G43.1Ø1
    - without status migrainosus G43.1Ø9
- with refractory migraine G43.919
  - with status migrainosus G43.911
  - without status migrainosus G43.919
- without aura G43.ØØ9
  - with refractory migraine G43.Ø19
    - with status migrainosus G43.Ø11
    - without status migrainosus G43.Ø19
  - without mention of refractory migraine G43.ØØ9
    - with status migrainosus G43.ØØ1
    - without status migrainosus G43.ØØ9
  - without status migrainosus G43.ØØ9
    - with refractory migraine G43.719
      - with status migrainosus G43.711
      - without status migrainosus G43.719
    - without refractory migraine G43.7Ø9
      - with status migrainosus G43.7Ø1
      - without status migrainosus G43.7Ø9
  - chronic G43.7Ø9
    - with refractory migraine G43.719
      - with status migrainosus G43.711
      - without status migrainosus G43.719
    - without refractory migraine G43.7Ø9
      - with status migrainosus G43.7Ø1
      - without status migrainosus G43.7Ø9
    - intractable
      - with status migrainosus G43.711
      - without status migrainosus G43.719
    - not intractable
      - with status migrainosus G43.7Ø1
      - without status migrainosus G43.7Ø9
  - intractable
    - with status migrainosus G43.Ø11
    - without status migrainosus G43.Ø19
  - not intractable
    - with status migrainosus G43.ØØ1
- without refractory migraine G43.9Ø9
  - with status migrainosus G43.9Ø1
  - without status migrainosus G43.919
- abdominal G43.DØ
  - with refractory migraine G43.D1
  - without refractory migraine G43.DØ

Migraine — *continued*
- abdominal — *continued*
  - intractable G43.D1
  - not intractable G43.DØ
- basilar — *see* Migraine, with aura
- classical — *see* Migraine, with aura
- common — *see* Migraine, without aura
- complicated G43.1Ø9
- equivalents — *see* Migraine, with aura
- familiar — *see* Migraine, hemiplegic
- hemiplegic G43.4Ø9
  - with refractory migraine G43.419
    - with status migrainosus G43.411
    - without status migrainosus G43.419
  - without refractory migraine G43.4Ø9
    - with status migrainosus G43.4Ø1
    - without status migrainosus G43.4Ø9
  - intractable G43.419
    - with status migrainosus G43.411
    - without status migrainosus G43.419
  - not intractable G43.4Ø9
    - with status migrainosus G43.4Ø1
    - without status migrainosus G43.4Ø9
- intractable G43.919
  - with status migrainosus G43.911
  - without status migrainosus G43.919
- menstrual G43.829
  - with refractory migraine G43.839
    - with status migrainosus G43.831
    - without status migrainosus G43.839
  - without refractory migraine G43.829
    - with status migrainosus G43.821
    - without status migrainosus G43.829
  - intractable G43.839
    - with status migrainosus G43.831
    - without status migrainosus G43.839
  - not intractable G43.829
    - with status migrainosus G43.821
    - without status migrainosus G43.829
- menstrually related — *see* Migraine, menstrual
- not intractable G43.9Ø9
  - with status migrainosus G43.9Ø1
  - without status migrainosus G43.919
- ophthalmoplegic G43.BØ9
  - with refractory migraine G43.B1
  - without refractory migraine G43.BØ
  - intractable G43.B1
  - not intractable G43.BØ9
- persistent aura (with, without) cerebral infarction — *see* Migraine, with aura, persistent
- preceded or accompanied by transient focal neurological phenomena — *see* Migraine, with aura
- pre-menstrual — *see* Migraine, menstrual
- pure menstrual — *see* Migraine, menstrual
- retinal — *see* Migraine, with aura
- specified NEC G43.8Ø9
  - intractable G43.819
    - with status migrainosus G43.811
    - without status migrainosus G43.819
  - not intractable G43.8Ø9
    - with status migrainosus G43.8Ø1
    - without status migrainosus G43.8Ø9
- sporadic — *see* Migraine, hemiplegic
- transformed — *see* Migraine, without aura, chronic
- triggered seizures — *see* Migraine, with aura

Migrant, social Z59.Ø
Migration, anxiety concerning Z6Ø.3
Migratory, migrating (*see also* condition)
- person Z59.Ø
- testis Q55.29

Mikity-Wilson disease or syndrome P27.Ø
Mikulicz' disease or syndrome K11.8
Miliaria L74.3
- alba L74.1
- apocrine L75.2
- crystallina L74.1
- profunda L74.2
- rubra L74.Ø
- tropicalis L74.2

Miliary — *see* condition
Milium L72.Ø
- colloid L57.8

Milk
- crust L21.Ø
- excessive secretion O92.6
- poisoning — *see* Poisoning, food, noxious
- retention O92.79
- sickness — *see* Poisoning, food, noxious
- spots I31.Ø

Milk-alkali disease or syndrome E83.52
Milk-leg (deep vessels) (nonpuerperal) — *see* Embolism, vein, lower extremity
- complicating pregnancy O22.3-
- puerperal, postpartum, childbirth O87.1

Milkman's disease or syndrome M83.8
Milky urine — *see* Chyluria
Millard-Gubler(-Foville) **paralysis or syndrome** G46.3
Millar's asthma J38.5
Miller Fisher syndrome G61.Ø
Mills' disease — *see* Hemiplegia
Millstone maker's pneumoconiosis J62.8
Milroy's disease (chronic hereditary edema) Q82.Ø
Minamata disease T26.1-
Minkowski-Chauffard syndrome — *see* Spherocytosis
Miners' asthma or lung J6Ø
Minkowski-Chauffard syndrome — *see* Spherocytosis
Minor — *see* condition
Minor's disease (hematomyelia) G95.19
Minot's disease (hemorrhagic disease), newborn P53
Minot-von Willebrand-Jurgens disease or syndrome (angiohemophilia) D68.Ø
Minus (and plus) **hand** (intrinsic) — *see* Deformity, limb, specified type NEC, forearm
Miosis (pupil) H57.Ø3
Mirizzi's syndrome (hepatic duct stenosis) K83.1
Mirror writing F81.Ø
Misadventure (of) (prophylactic) (therapeutic)(*see also* Complications) T88.9
- administration of insulin (by accident) — *see* subcategory T38.3
- infusion — *see* Complications, infusion
- local applications (of fomentations, plasters, etc.) T88.9
  - burn or scald — *see* Burn
  - specified NEC T88.8
- medical care (early) (late) T88.9
  - adverse effect of drugs or chemicals — *see* Table of Drugs and Chemicals
- medical care (early) (late)
  - burn or scald — *see* Burn
  - specified NEC T88.8
- specified NEC T88.8
- surgical procedure (early) (late) — *see* Complications, surgical procedure
- transfusion — *see* Complications, transfusion
- vaccination or other immunological procedure — *see* Complications, vaccination

Miscarriage OØ3.9
Misdirection, aqueous H4Ø.83-
Misperception, sleep state F51.Ø2
Misplaced, misplacement
- ear Q17.4
- kidney (acquired) N28.89
  - congenital Q63.2
- organ or site, congenital NEC — *see* Malposition, congenital

Missed
- abortion OØ2.1
- delivery O36.4

Missing — *see* Absence
Misuse of drugs F19.99
Mitchell's disease (erythromelalgia) I73.81
Mite(s) (infestation) B88.9
- diarrhea B88.Ø
- grain (itch) B88.Ø
- hair follicle (itch) B88.Ø
- in sputum B88.Ø

Mitral — *see* condition
Mittelschmerz N94.Ø
Mixed — *see* condition
MNGIE (Mitochondrial Neurogastrointestinal Encephalopathy) syndrome E88.49

- **Morton's metatarsalgia** (neuralgia)(neuroma) (syndrome) G57.6-
- **Morvan's disease or syndrome** G6Ø.8
- **Mosaicism, mosaic** (autosomal) (chromosomal)
  - 45,X/other cell lines NEC with abnormal sex chromosome Q96.4
  - 45,X/46,XX Q96.3
  - sex chromosome
    - female Q97.8
    - lines with various numbers of X chromosomes Q97.2
    - male Q98.7
  - XY Q96.3
- **Moschowitz' disease** M31.1
- **Mother yaw** A66.Ø
- **Motion sickness** (from travel, any vehicle) (from roundabouts or swings) T75.3
- **Mottled, mottling, teeth** (enamel) (endemic) (nonendemic) KØØ.3
- **Mounier-Kuhn syndrome** Q32.4
  - with bronchiectasis J47.9
    - exacerbation (acute) J47.1
    - lower respiratory infection J47.Ø
  - acquired J98.Ø9
    - with bronchiectasis J47.9
      - with
        - exacerbation (acute) J47.1
        - lower respiratory infection J47.Ø
- **Mountain**
  - sickness T7Ø.29
    - with polycythemia , acquired (acute) D75.1
  - tick fever A93.2
- **Mouse, joint** — *see* Loose, body, joint
  - knee M23.4-
- **Mouth** — *see* condition
- **Movable**
  - coccyx — *see* subcategory M53.2
  - kidney N28.89
    - congenital Q63.8
  - spleen D73.89
- **Movements, dystonic** R25.8
- **Moyamoya disease** I67.5
- **MRSA** (methicillin resistant Staphylococcus aureus)
  - infection A49.Ø2
    - as the cause of diseases classified elsewhere B95.62
  - sepsis A41.Ø2
- **MSSA** (methicillin susceptible Staphylococcus aureus)
  - infection A49.Ø1
    - as the cause of diseases classified elsewhere B95.61
  - sepsis A41.Ø1
- **Mucha-Habermann disease** L41.Ø
- **Mucinosis** (cutaneous) (focal) (papular) (skin) L98.5
  - oral K13.79
- **Mucocele**
  - appendix K38.8
  - buccal cavity K13.79
  - gallbladder K82.1
  - lacrimal sac, chronic HØ4.43-
  - nasal sinus J34.1
  - nose J34.1
  - salivary gland (any) K11.6
  - sinus (accessory) (nasal) J34.1
  - turbinate (bone) (middle) (nasal) J34.1
  - uterus N85.8
- **Mucolipidosis**
  - I E77.1
  - II, III E77.Ø
  - IV E75.11
- **Mucopolysaccharidosis** E76.3
  - beta-gluduronidase deficiency E76.29
  - cardiopathy E76.3 *[I52]*
  - Hunter's syndrome E76.1
  - Hurler's syndrome E76.Ø1
  - Hurler-Scheie syndrome E76.Ø2
  - Maroteaux-Lamy syndrome E76.29
  - Morquio syndrome E76.219
    - A E76.21Ø
    - B E76.211
    - classic E76.21Ø
  - Sanfilippo syndrome E76.22
  - Scheie's syndrome E76.Ø3
- **Mucopolysaccharidosis** — *continued*
  - specified NEC E76.29
  - type
    - I
      - Hurler's syndrome E76.Ø1
      - Hurler-Scheie syndrome E76.Ø2
      - Scheie's syndrome E76.Ø3
    - II E76.1
    - III E76.22
    - IV E76.219
    - IVA E76.21Ø
    - IVB E76.211
    - VI E76.29
    - VII E76.29
- **Mucormycosis** B46.5
  - cutaneous B46.3
  - disseminated B46.4
  - gastrointestinal B46.2
  - generalized B46.4
  - pulmonary B46.Ø
  - rhinocerebral B46.1
  - skin B46.3
  - subcutaneous B46.3
- **Mucositis** (ulcerative) K12.3Ø
  - due to drugs NEC K12.32
  - gastrointestinal K92.81
  - mouth (oral) (oropharyngeal) K12.3Ø
    - due to antineoplastic therapy K12.31
    - due to drugs NEC K12.32
    - due to radiation K12.33
    - specified NEC K12.39
    - viral K12.39
  - nasal J34.81
  - oral cavity — *see* Mucositis, mouth
  - oral soft tissues — *see* Mucositis, mouth
  - vagina and vulva N76.81
- **Mucositis necroticans agranulocytica** — *see* Agranulocytosis
- **Mucous** (*see also* condition)
  - patches (syphilitic) A51.39
    - congenital A5Ø.Ø7
- **Mucoviscidosis** E84.9
  - with meconium obstruction E84.11
- **Mucus**
  - asphyxia or suffocation — *see* Asphyxia, mucus
  - in stool R19.5
  - plug — *see* Asphyxia, mucus
- **Muguet** B37.Ø
- **Mulberry molars** (congenital syphilis) A5Ø.52
- **Müllerian mixed tumor**
  - specified site — *see* Neoplasm, malignant, by site
  - unspecified site C54.9
- **Multicystic kidney** (development) Q61.4
- **Multiparity** (grand) Z64.1
  - affecting management of pregnancy, labor and delivery (supervision only) OØ9.4-
  - requiring contraceptive management — *see* Contraception
- **Multipartita placenta** O43.19-
- **Multiple, multiplex** (*see also* condition)
  - digits (congenital) Q69.9
  - endocrine neoplasia — *see* Neoplasia, endocrine, multiple (MEN)
  - personality F44.81
- **Mumps** B26.9
  - arthritis B26.85
  - complication NEC B26.89
  - encephalitis B26.2
  - hepatitis B26.81
  - meningitis (aseptic) B26.1
  - meningoencephalitis B26.2
  - myocarditis B26.82
  - oophoritis B26.89
  - orchitis B26.Ø
  - pancreatitis B26.3
  - polyneuropathy B26.84
- **Mumu** (*see also* Infestation, filarial) B74.9 *[N51]*
- **Münchhausen's syndrome** — *see* Disorder, factitious
- **Münchmeyer's syndrome** — *see* Myositis, ossificans, progressiva
- **Mural** — *see* condition
- **Murmur** (cardiac) (heart) (organic) RØ1.1
  - abdominal R19.15
  - aortic (valve) — *see* Endocarditis, aortic
  - benign RØ1.Ø
  - diastolic — *see* Endocarditis
  - Flint I35.1
  - functional RØ1.Ø
  - Graham Steell I37.1
  - innocent RØ1.Ø
  - mitral (valve) — *see* Insufficiency, mitral
  - nonorganic RØ1.Ø
  - presystolic, mitral — *see* Insufficiency, mitral
  - pulmonic (valve) I37.8
  - systolic (valvular) — *see* Endocarditis
  - tricuspid (valve) IØ7.9
  - valvular — *see* Endocarditis
- **Murri's disease** (intermittent hemoglobinuria) D59.6
- **Muscle, muscular** (*see also* condition)
  - carnitine (palmityltransferase) deficiency E71.314
- **Musculoneuralgia** — *see* Neuralgia
- **Mushroom-workers'** (pickers') **disease or lung** J67.5
- **Mushrooming hip** — *see* Derangement, joint, specified NEC, hip
- **Mutation(s)**
  - factor V Leiden D68.51
  - prothrombin gene D68.52
  - surfactant, of lung J84.83
- **Mutism** (*see also* Aphasia)
  - deaf (acquired) (congenital) NEC H91.3
  - elective (adjustment reaction) (childhood) F94.Ø
  - hysterical F44.4
  - selective (childhood) F94.Ø
- **MVD** (microvillus inclusion disease) Q43.8
- **MVID** (microvillus inclusion disease) Q43.8
- **Myalgia** M79.1
  - epidemic (cervical) B33.Ø
  - traumatic NEC T14.8
- **Myasthenia** G7Ø.9
  - congenital G7Ø.2
  - cordis — *see* Failure, heart
  - developmental G7Ø.2
  - gravis G7Ø.ØØ
    - with exacerbation (acute)G7Ø.Ø1
    - in crisis G7Ø.Ø1
    - neonatal, transient P94.Ø
    - pseudoparalytica G7Ø.ØØ
      - with exacerbation (acute) G7Ø.Ø1
      - in crisis G7Ø.Ø1
  - stomach, psychogenic F45.8
  - syndrome
    - in
      - diabetes mellitus — *see* EØ8-E13 with .44
      - neoplastic disease (*see also* Neoplasm) D49.9 *[G73.3]*
      - pernicious anemia D51.Ø *[G73.3]*
      - thyrotoxicosis EØ5.9Ø *[G73.3]*
        - with thyroid storm EØ5.91 *[G73.3]*
- **Myasthenic** M62.81
- **Mycelium infection** B49
- **Mycetismus** — *see* Poisoning, food, noxious, mushroom
- **Mycetoma** B47.9
  - actinomycotic B47.1
  - bone (mycotic) B47.9 *[M9Ø.8Ø]*
  - eumycotic B47.Ø
  - foot B47.9
    - actinomycotic B47.1
    - mycotic B47.Ø
  - madurae NEC B47.9
    - mycotic B47.Ø
  - maduromycotic B47.Ø
  - mycotic B47.Ø
  - nocardial B47.1
- **Mycobacteriosis** — *see* Mycobacterium
- **Mycobacterium, mycobacterial** (infection) A31.9
  - anonymous A31.9
  - atypical A31.9
    - cutaneous A31.1
    - pulmonary A31.Ø
      - tuberculous — *see* Tuberculosis, pulmonary
    - specified site NEC A31.8
  - avium (intracellulare complex) A31.Ø

This page was intentionally left blank

N

- **Naegeli's**
  - disease Q82.8
  - leukemia, monocytic C93.1-
- **Naegleriasis** (with meningoencephalitis) B6Ø.2
- **Naffziger's syndrome** G54.Ø
- **Naga sore** — *see* Ulcer, skin
- **Nägele's pelvis** M95.5
  - with disproportion (fetopelvic) O33.Ø
    - causing obstructed labor O65.Ø
- **Nail** (*see also* condition)
  - biting F98.8
  - patella syndrome Q87.2
- **Nanism, nanosomia** — *see* Dwarfism
- **Nanophyetiasis** B66.8
- **Nanukayami** A27.89
- **Napkin rash** L22
- **Narcolepsy** G47.419
  - with cataplexy G47.411
  - in conditions classified elsewhere G47.429
    - with cataplexy G47.421
- **Narcosis** RØ6.89
- **Narcotism** — *see* Dependence
- **NARP** (Neuropathy, Ataxia and Retinitis pigmentosa) syndrome E88.49
- **Narrow**
  - anterior chamber angle H4Ø.Ø3-
  - pelvis — *see* Contraction, pelvis
- **Narrowing** (*see also* Stenosis)
  - artery I77.1
    - auditory, internal I65.8
    - basilar — *see* Occlusion, artery, basilar
    - carotid — *see* Occlusion, artery, carotid
    - cerebellar — *see* Occlusion, artery, cerebellar
    - cerebral — *see* Occlusion artery, cerebral
    - choroidal — *see* Occlusion, artery, cerebral, specified NEC
    - communicating posterior — *see* Occlusion, artery, cerebral, specified NEC
    - coronary (*see also* Disease, heart, ischemic, atherosclerotic)
      - congenital Q24.5
        - syphilitic A5Ø.54 *[I52]*
      - due to syphilis NEC A52.Ø6
    - hypophyseal — *see* Occlusion, artery, cerebral, specified NEC
    - pontine — *see* Occlusion, artery, cerebral, specified NEC
    - precerebral — *see* Occlusion, artery, precerebral
    - vertebral — *see* Occlusion, artery, vertebral
  - auditory canal (external) — *see* Stenosis, external ear canal
  - eustachian tube — *see* Obstruction, eustachian tube
  - eyelid — *see* Disorder, eyelid function
  - larynx J38.6
  - mesenteric artery K55.Ø
  - palate M26.89
  - palpebral fissure — *see* Disorder, eyelid function
  - ureter N13.5
    - with infection N13.6
  - urethra — *see* Stricture, urethra
- **Narrowness, abnormal, eyelid** Q1Ø.3
- **Nasal** — *see* condition
- **Nasolachrymal, nasolacrimal** — *see* condition
- **Nasopharyngeal** (*see also* condition)
  - pituitary gland Q89.2
  - torticollis M43.6
- **Nasopharyngitis** (acute) (infective) (streptococcal) (subacute) JØØ
  - chronic (suppurative) (ulcerative) J31.1
- **Nasopharynx, nasopharyngeal** — *see* condition
- **Natal tooth, teeth** KØØ.6
- **Nausea** (without vomiting) R11.Ø
  - with vomiting R11.2
  - gravidarum — *see* Hyperemesis, gravidarum
  - marina T75.3
  - navalis T75.3
- **Navel** — *see* condition
- **Neapolitan fever** — *see* Brucellosis
- **Near drowning** T75.1
- **Nearsightedness** — *see* Myopia
- **Near-syncope** R55
- **Nebula, cornea** — *see* Opacity, cornea
- **Necator americanus infestation** B76.1
- **Necatoriasis** B76.1
- **Neck** — *see* condition
- **Necrobiosis** R68.89
  - lipoidica NEC L92.1
    - with diabetes — *see* EØ8-E13 with .62Ø
- **Necrolysis, toxic epidermal** L51.2
  - due to drug
    - correct substance properly administered — *see* Table of Drugs and Chemicals, by drug, adverse effect
    - overdose or wrong substance given or taken — *see* Table of Drugs and Chemicals, by drug, poisoning
- **Necrophilia** F65.89
- **Necrosis, necrotic** (ischemic) (*see also* Gangrene)
  - adrenal (capsule) (gland) E27.49
  - amputation stump (surgical) (late) T87.5Ø
    - arm T87.5-
    - leg T87.5-
  - antrum J32.Ø
  - aorta (hyaline) (*see also* Aneurysm, aorta)
    - cystic medial — *see* Dissection, aorta
  - artery I77.5
  - bladder (aseptic) (sphincter) N32.89
  - bone (*see also* Osteonecrosis) M87.9
    - aseptic or avascular — *see* Osteonecrosis
      - idiopathic M87.ØØ
    - ethmoid J32.2
    - jaw M27.2
    - tuberculous — *see* Tuberculosis, bone
  - brain I67.89
  - breast (aseptic) (fat) (segmental) N64.1
  - bronchus J98.Ø9
  - central nervous system NEC I67.89
  - cerebellar I67.89
  - cerebral I67.89
  - colon K55.Ø
  - cornea H18.4Ø
  - cortical (acute) (renal) N17.1
  - cystic medial (aorta) — *see* Dissection, aorta
  - dental pulp KØ4.1
  - esophagus K22.8
  - ethmoid (bone) J32.2
  - eyelid — *see* Disorder, eyelid, degenerative
  - fat, fatty (generalized) (*see also* Disorder, soft tissue, specified type NEC)
    - abdominal wall K65.4
    - breast (aseptic) (segmental) N64.1
    - localized — *see* Degeneration, by site, fatty
    - mesentery K65.4
    - omentum K65.4
    - pancreas K86.8
    - peritoneum K65.4
    - skin (subcutaneous), newborn P83.Ø
    - subcutaneous, due to birth injury P15.6
  - gallbladder — *see* Cholecystitis, acute
  - heart — *see* Infarct, myocardium
  - hip, aseptic or avascular — *see* Osteonecrosis, by type, femur
  - intestine (acute) (hemorrhagic) (massive) K55.Ø
  - jaw M27.2
  - kidney (bilateral) N28.Ø
    - acute N17.9
    - cortical (acute) (bilateral) N17.1
      - with ectopic or molar pregnancy OØ8.4
    - medullary (bilateral) (in acute renal failure) (papillary) N17.2
    - papillary (bilateral) (in acute renal failure) N17.2
    - tubular N17.Ø
      - with ectopic or molar pregnancy OØ8.4
      - complicating
        - abortion — *see* Abortion, by type, complicated by, tubular necrosis
        - ectopic or molar pregnancy OØ8.4
        - pregnancy — *see* Pregnancy, complicated by, diseases of, specified type or system NEC
      - following ectopic or molar pregnancy OØ8.4
      - traumatic T79.5

Necrosis, necrotic— *continued*

  - larynx J38.7
  - liver (with hepatic failure) (cell)—*see* Failure, hepatic
    - hemorrhagic, central K76.2
  - lung J85.Ø
  - lymphatic gland — *see* Lymphadenitis, acute
  - mammary gland (fat) (segmental) N64.1
  - mastoid (chronic) — *see* Mastoiditis, chronic
  - medullary (acute) (renal) N17.2
  - mesentery K55.Ø
    - fat K65.4
  - mitral valve — *see* Insufficiency, mitral
  - myocardium, myocardial — *see* Infarct, myocardium
  - nose J34.Ø
  - omentum (with mesenteric infarction) K55.Ø
    - fat K65.4
  - orbit, orbital — *see* Osteomyelitis, orbit
  - ossicles, ear — *see* Abnormal, ear ossicles
  - ovary N7Ø.92
  - pancreas (aseptic) (duct) (fat) K86.8
    - acute (infective) — *see* Pancreatitis, acute
    - infective — *see* Pancreatitis, acute
  - papillary (acute) (renal) N17.2
  - perineum N9Ø.89
  - peritoneum (with mesenteric infarction) K55.Ø
    - fat K65.4
  - pharynx JØ2.9
    - in granulocytopenia — *see* Neutropenia
    - Vincent's A69.1
  - phosphorus — *see* subcategory T54.2
  - pituitary (gland) (postpartum) (Sheehan) E23.Ø
  - pressure — *see* Ulcer, pressure, by site
  - pulmonary J85.Ø
  - pulp (dental) KØ4.1
  - radiation — *see* Necrosis, by site
  - radium — *see* Necrosis, by site
  - renal — *see* Necrosis, kidney
  - sclera H15.89
  - scrotum N5Ø.8
  - skin or subcutaneous tissue NEC I96
  - spine, spinal (column) (*see also* Osteonecrosis, by type, vertebra)
    - cord G95.19
  - spleen D73.5
  - stomach K31.89
  - stomatitis (ulcerative) A69.Ø
  - subcutaneous fat, newborn P83.8
  - subendocardial (acute) I21.4
    - chronic I25.89
  - suprarenal (capsule) (gland) E27.49
  - testis N5Ø.8
  - thymus (gland) E32.8
  - tonsil J35.8
  - trachea J39.8
  - tuberculous NEC — *see* Tuberculosis
  - tubular (acute) (anoxic) (renal) (toxic) N17.Ø
    - postprocedural N99.Ø
  - vagina N89.8
  - vertebra (*see also* Osteonecrosis, by type, vertebra)
    - tuberculous A18.Ø1
  - vulva N9Ø.89
  - X-ray — *see* Necrosis, by site
- **Necrospermia** — *see* Infertility, male
- **Need** (for)
  - care provider because (of)
    - assistance with personal care Z74.1
    - continuous supervision required Z74.3
    - impaired mobility Z74.Ø9
    - no other household member able to render care Z74.2
    - specified reason NEC Z74.8
  - immunization — *see* Vaccination
  - vaccination — *see* Vaccination
- **Neglect**
  - adult
    - confirmed T74.Ø1
    - history of Z91.412
    - suspected T76.Ø1
  - child (childhood)
    - confirmed T74.Ø2
    - history of Z62.812
    - suspected T76.Ø2

- **Neglect**— *continued*
  - emotional, in childhood Z62.898
  - hemispatial R41.4
  - left-sided R41.4
  - sensory R41.4
  - visuospatial R41.4
- **Neisserian infection NEC** — *see* Gonococcus
- **Nelaton's syndrome** G6Ø.8
- **Nelson's syndrome** E24.1
- **Nematodiasis** (intestinal) B82.Ø
  - Ancylostoma B76.Ø
- **Neonatal** (*see also* Newborn)
  - acne L7Ø.4
  - bradycardia P29.12
  - tachycardia P29.11
  - screening, abnormal findings on PØ9
  - tooth, teeth KØØ.6
- **Neonatorum** — *see* condition
- **Neoplasia**
  - endocrine, multiple (MEN) E31.2Ø
    - type I E31.21
    - type IIA E31.22
    - type IIB E31.23
  - intraepithelial (histologically confirmed)
    - anal (AIN)
      - grade I K62.82
      - grade II K62.82
      - severe DØ1.3
    - cervical glandular (histologically confirmed) DØ6.9
    - cervix (uteri) (CIN) (histologically confirmed) N87.9
      - glandular DØ6.9
      - grade I N87.Ø
      - grade II N87.1
      - grade III (severe dysplasia) (*see also* Carcinoma, cervix uteri, in situ) DØ6.9
    - vagina (histologically confirmed) (VAIN) N89.3
      - grade I N89.Ø
      - grade II N89.1
      - grade III (severe dysplasia) DØ7.2
    - prostate (histologically confirmed) (PIN I) (PIN II) N42.3
      - grade I N42.3
      - grade II N42.3
      - severe DØ7.5
    - vulva (histologically confirmed) (VIN) N9Ø.3
      - grade I N9Ø.Ø
      - grade II N9Ø.1
      - grade III (severe dysplasia) DØ7.1
- **Neoplasm, neoplastic** (*see also* Table of Neoplasms)
  - lipomatous, benign — *see* Lipoma
- **Neovascularization**
  - ciliary body — *see* Disorder, iris, vascular
  - cornea H16.4Ø-
    - deep H16.44-
    - ghost vessels — *see* Ghost, vessels
    - localized H16.43-
    - pannus — *see* Pannus
  - iris — *see* Disorder, iris, vascular
  - retina H35.Ø5-
- **Nephralgia** N23
- **Nephritis, nephritic** (albuminuric) (azotemic) (congenital) (disseminated) (epithelial) (familial) (focal) (granulomatous) (hemorrhagic) (infantile) (nonsuppurative, excretory) (uremic) NØ5.9
  - with
    - dense deposit disease NØ5.6
    - diffuse
      - crescentic glomerulonephritis NØ5.7
      - endocapillary proliferative glomerulonephritis NØ5.4
      - membranous glomerulonephritis NØ5.2
      - mesangial proliferative glomerulonephritis NØ5.3
      - mesangiocapillary glomerulonephritis NØ5.5
    - edema — *see* Nephrosis
    - focal and segmental glomerular lesions NØ5.1
    - foot process disease NØ4.9
    - glomerular lesion
      - diffuse sclerosing NØ5.8
      - hypocomplementemic — *see* Nephritis, membranoproliferative

- **Nephritis, nephritic**— *continued*
  - with — *continued*
    - glomerular lesion — *continued*
      - IgA — *see* Nephropathy, IgA
    - glomerular lesion— *continued*
      - lobular, lobulonodular — *see* Nephritis, membranoproliferative
      - nodular — *see* Nephritis, membranoproliferative
    - lesion of
      - glomerulonephritis, proliferative NØ5.8
      - renal necrosis NØ5.9
    - minor glomerular abnormality NØ5.Ø
    - specified morphological changes NEC NØ5.8
  - acute NØØ.9
    - with
      - dense deposit disease NØØ.6
      - diffuse
        - crescentic glomerulonephritis NØØ.7
        - endocapillary proliferative glomerulonephritis NØØ.4
        - membranous glomerulonephritis NØØ.2
        - mesangial proliferative glomerulonephritis NØØ.3
        - mesangiocapillary glomerulonephritis NØØ.5
      - focal and segmental glomerular lesions NØØ.1
      - minor glomerular abnormality NØØ.Ø
      - specified morphological changes NEC NØØ.8
  - amyloid E85.4 *[N08]*
  - antiglomerular basement membrane (anti-GBM) antibody NEC
    - in Goodpasture's syndrome M31.Ø
  - antitubular basement membrane (tubulo-interstitial) NEC N12
    - toxic — *see* Nephropathy, toxic
  - arteriolar — *see* Hypertension, kidney
  - arteriosclerotic — *see* Hypertension, kidney
  - ascending — *see* Nephritis, tubulo-interstitial
  - atrophic NØ3.9
  - Balkan (endemic) N15.Ø
  - calculous, calculus — *see* Calculus, kidney
  - cardiac — *see* Hypertension, kidney
  - cardiovascular — *see* Hypertension, kidney
  - chronic NØ3.9
    - with
      - dense deposit disease NØ3.6
      - diffuse
        - crescentic glomerulonephritis NØ3.7
        - endocapillary proliferative glomerulonephritis NØ3.4
        - membranous glomerulonephritis NØ3.2
        - mesangial proliferative glomerulonephritis NØ3.3
        - mesangiocapillary glomerulonephritis NØ3.5
      - focal and segmental glomerular lesions NØ3.1
      - minor glomerular abnormality NØ3.Ø
      - specified morphological changes NEC NØ3.8
    - arteriosclerotic — *see* Hypertension, kidney
  - cirrhotic N26.9
  - complicating pregnancy O26.83-
  - croupous NØØ.9
  - degenerative — *see* Nephrosis
  - diffuse sclerosing NØ5.8
  - due to
    - diabetes mellitus — *see* EØ8-E13 with .21
    - subacute bacterial endocarditis I33.Ø
    - systemic lupus erythematosus (chronic) M32.14
    - typhoid fever AØ1.Ø9
  - gonococcal (acute) (chronic) A54.21
  - hypocomplementemic — *see* Nephritis, membranoproliferative
  - IgA — *see* Nephropathy, IgA
  - immune complex (circulating) NEC NØ5.8
  - infective — *see* Nephritis, tubulo-interstitial
  - interstitial — *see* Nephritis, tubulo-interstitial
  - lead N14.3
  - membranoproliferative (diffuse) (type 1 or 3) (*see also* NØØ-NØ7 with fourth character .5) NØ5.5
    - type 2 (*see also* NØØ-NØ7 with fourth character .6) NØ5.6
  - minimal change NØ5.Ø

- **Nephritis, nephritic**— *continued*
  - necrotic, necrotizing NEC (*see also* NØØ-NØ7 with fourth character .8) NØ5.8
  - nephrotic — *see* Nephrosis
  - nodular — *see* Nephritis, membranoproliferative
  - polycystic Q61.3
    - adult type Q61.2
    - autosomal
      - dominant Q61.2
      - recessive NEC Q61.19
    - childhood type NEC Q61.19
    - infantile type NEC Q61.19
  - poststreptococcal NØ5.9
    - acute NØØ.9
    - chronic NØ3.9
    - rapidly progressive NØ1.9
  - proliferative NEC (*see also* NØØ-NØ7 with fourth character .8) NØ5.8
  - purulent — *see* Nephritis, tubulo-interstitial
  - rapidly progressive NØ1.9
    - with
      - dense deposit disease NØ1.6
      - diffuse
        - crescentic glomerulonephritis NØ1.7
        - endocapillary proliferative glomerulonephritis NØ1.4
        - membranous glomerulonephritis NØ1.2
        - mesangial proliferative glomerulonephritis NØ1.3
        - mesangiocapillary glomerulonephritis NØ1.5
      - focal and segmental glomerular lesions NØ1.1
      - minor glomerular abnormality NØ1.Ø
      - specified morphological changes NEC NØ1.8
  - salt losing or wasting NEC N28.89
  - saturnine N14.3
  - sclerosing, diffuse NØ5.8
  - septic — *see* Nephritis, tubulo-interstitial
  - specified pathology NEC (*see also* NØØ-NØ7 with fourth character .8) NØ5.8
  - subacute NØ1.9
  - suppurative — *see* Nephritis, tubulo-interstitial
  - syphilitic (late) A52.75
    - congenital A5Ø.59 *[N08]*
    - early (secondary) A51.44
  - toxic — *see* Nephropathy, toxic
  - tubal, tubular — *see* Nephritis, tubulo-interstitial
  - tuberculous A18.11
  - tubulo-interstitial (in) N12
    - acute (infectious) N1Ø
    - chronic (infectious) N11.9
      - nonobstructive N11.8
        - reflux-associated N11.Ø
      - obstructive N11.1
      - specified NEC N11.8
    - due to
      - brucellosis A23.9 *[N16]*
      - cryoglobulinemia D89.1 *[N16]*
      - glycogen storage disease E74.ØØ *[N16]*
    - Sjögren's syndrome M35.Ø4
  - vascular — *see* Hypertension, kidney
  - war NØØ.9
- **Nephroblastoma** (epithelial) (mesenchymal) C64-
- **Nephrocalcinosis** E83.59 *[N29]*
- **Nephrocystitis, pustular** — *see* Nephritis, tubulo-interstitial
- **Nephrolithiasis** (congenital) (pelvis) (recurrent) (*see also* Calculus, kidney)
- **Nephroma** C64-
  - mesoblastic D41.Ø-
- **Nephronephritis** — *see* Nephrosis
- **Nephronophthisis** Q61.5
- **Nephropathia epidemica** A98.5
- **Nephropathy** (*see also* Nephritis) N28.9
  - with
    - edema — *see* Nephrosis
    - glomerular lesion — *see* Glomerulonephritis
  - amyloid, hereditary E85.Ø
  - analgesic N14.Ø
    - with medullary necrosis, acute N17.2
  - Balkan (endemic) N15.Ø
  - chemical — *see* Nephropathy, toxic
  - diabetic — *see* EØ8-E13 with .21

Nephropathy — *continued*
- drug-induced N14.2
  - specified NEC N14.1
- focal and segmental hyalinosis or sclerosis NØ2.1
- heavy metal-induced N14.3
- hereditary NEC NØ7.9
  - with
    - dense deposit disease NØ7.6
    - diffuse
      - crescentic glomerulonephritis NØ7.7
      - endocapillary proliferative glomerulonephritis NØ7.4
      - membranous glomerulonephritis NØ7.2
      - mesangial proliferative glomerulonephritis NØ7.3
      - mesangiocapillary glomerulonephritis NØ7.5
    - focal and segmental glomerular lesions NØ7.1
    - minor glomerular abnormality NØ7.Ø
    - specified morphological changes NEC NØ7.8
- hypercalcemic N25.89
- hypertensive — *see* Hypertension, kidney
- hypokalemic (vacuolar) N25.89
- IgA NØ2.8
  - with glomerular lesion NØ2.9
    - focal and segmental hyalinosis or sclerosis N02.1
    - membranoproliferative (diffuse) NØ2.5
    - membranous (diffuse) NØ2.2
    - mesangial proliferative (diffuse) NØ2.3
    - mesangiocapillary (diffuse) NØ2.5
    - proliferative NEC NØ2.8
    - specified pathology NEC NØ2.8
- lead N14.3
- membranoproliferative (diffuse) NØ2.5
- membranous (diffuse) NØ2.2
- mesangial (IgA/IgG) — *see* Nephropathy, IgA
  - proliferative (diffuse) NØ2.3
- mesangiocapillary (diffuse) NØ2.5
- obstructive N13.8
- phenacetin N17.2
- phosphate-losing N25.Ø
- potassium depletion N25.89
- pregnancy-related O26.83-
- proliferative NEC (*see also* NØØ-NØ7 with fourth character .8) NØ5.8
- protein-losing N25.89
- saturnine N14.3
- sickle-cell D57.*[N08]*
- toxic NEC N14.4
  - due to
    - drugs N14.2
      - analgesic N14.Ø
      - specified NEC N14.1
    - heavy metals N14.3
- vasomotor N17.Ø
- water-losing N25.89

Nephroptosis N28.83

Nephropyosis — *see* Abscess, kidney

Nephrorrhagia N28.89

Nephrosclerosis (arteriolar)(arteriosclerotic) (chronic) (hyaline) (*see also* Hypertension, kidney)
- hyperplastic — *see* Hypertension, kidney
- senile N26.9

Nephrosis, nephrotic (Epstein's) (syndrome) (congenital) NØ4.9
- with
  - foot process disease NØ4.9
  - glomerular lesion NØ4.1
  - hypocomplementemic NØ4.5
- acute NØ4.9
- anoxic — *see* Nephrosis, tubular
- chemical — *see* Nephrosis, tubular
- cholemic K76.7
- diabetic — *see* EØ8-E13 with .21
- Finnish type (congenital) Q89.8
- hemoglobin N1Ø
- hemoglobinuric — *see* Nephrosis, tubular
- in
  - amyloidosis E85.4 *[N08]*
  - diabetes mellitus — *see* EØ8-E13 with .21
  - epidemic hemorrhagic fever A98.5
  - malaria (malariae) B52.Ø
- ischemic — *see* Nephrosis, tubular

Nephrosis, nephrotic— *continued*
- lipoid NØ4.9
- lower nephron — *see* Nephrosis, tubular
- malarial (malariae) B52.Ø
- minimal change NØ4.Ø
- myoglobin N1Ø
- necrotizing — *see* Nephrosis, tubular
- osmotic (sucrose) N25.89
- radiation NØ4.9
- syphilitic (late) A52.75
- toxic — *see* Nephrosis, tubular
- tubular (acute) N17.Ø
  - postprocedural N99.Ø
  - radiation NØ4.9

Nephrosonephritis, hemorrhagic (endemic) A98.5

Nephrostomy
- attention to Z43.6
- status Z93.6

Nerve (*see also* condition)
- injury — *see* Injury, nerve, by body site

Nerves R45.Ø

Nervous (*see also* condition) R45.Ø
- heart F45.8
- stomach F45.8
- tension R45.Ø

Nervousness R45.Ø

Nesidioblastoma
- pancreas D13.7
- specified site NEC — *see* Neoplam, benign, by site
- unspecified site D13.7

Nettleship's syndrome Q82.2

Neumann's disease or syndrome L1Ø.1

Neuralgia, neuralgic (acute) M79.2
- accessory (nerve) G52.8
- acoustic (nerve) — *see* subcategory H93.3
- auditory (nerve) — *see* subcategory H93.3
- ciliary G44.ØØ9
  - intractable G44.ØØ1
  - not intractable G44.ØØ9
- cranial
  - nerve (*see also* Disorder, nerve, cranial)
    - fifth or trigeminal — *see* Neuralgia, trigeminal
  - postherpetic, postzoster BØ2.29
- ear — *see* subcategory H92.Ø
- facialis vera G51.1
- Fothergill's — *see* Neuralgia, trigeminal
- glossopharyngeal (nerve) G52.1
- Horton's G44.Ø99
  - intractable G44.Ø91
  - not intractable G44.Ø99
- Hunt's BØ2.21
- hypoglossal (nerve) G52.3
- infraorbital — *see* Neuralgia, trigeminal
- malarial — *see* Malaria
- migrainous G44.ØØ9
  - intractable G44.ØØ1
  - not intractable G44.ØØ9
- Morton's G57.6-
- nerve, cranial — *see* Disorder, nerve, cranial
- nose G52.Ø
- occipital M54.81
- olfactory G52.Ø
- penis N48.9
- perineum R1Ø.2
- postherpetic NEC BØ2.29
  - trigeminal BØ2.22
- pubic region R1Ø.2
- scrotum R1Ø.2
- Sluder's G44.89
- specified nerve NEC G58.8
- spermatic cord R1Ø.2
- sphenopalatine (ganglion) G9Ø.Ø9
- trifacial — *see* Neuralgia, trigeminal
- trigeminal G5Ø.Ø
  - postherpetic, postzoster BØ2.22
- vagus (nerve) G52.2
- writer's F48.8
  - organic G25.89

Neurapraxia — *see* Injury, nerve

Neurasthenia F48.8
- cardiac F45.8
- gastric F45.8
- heart F45.8

Neurilemmoma (*see also* Neoplasm, nerve, benign)
- acoustic (nerve) D33.3
- malignant (*see also* Neoplasm, nerve, malignant)
  - acoustic (nerve) C72.4-

Neurilemmosarcoma — *see* Neoplasm, nerve, malignant

Neurinoma — *see* Neoplasm, nerve, benign

Neurinomatosis — *see* Neoplasm, nerve, uncertain behavior

Neuritis (rheumatoid) M79.2
- abducens (nerve) — *see* Strabismus, paralytic, sixth nerve
- accessory (nerve) G52.8
- acoustic (nerve) (*see also* subcategory) H93.3
  - in (due to)
    - infectious disease NEC B99 *[H94.0-]*
    - parasitic disease NEC B89 *[H94.0-]*
  - syphilitic A52.15
- alcoholic G62.1
  - with psychosis — *see* Psychosis, alcoholic
- amyloid, any site E85.4 *[G63]*
- auditory (nerve) — *see* subcategory H93.3
- brachial — *see* Radiculopathy
  - due to displacement, intervertebral disc — *see* Disorder, disc, cervical, with neuritis
- cranial nerve
  - due to Lyme disease A69.22
  - eighth or acoustic or auditory — *see* subcategory H93.3
  - eleventh or accessory G52.8
  - fifth or trigeminal G51.Ø
  - first or olfactory G52.Ø
  - fourth or trochlear — *see* Strabismus, paralytic, fourth nerve
  - second or optic — *see* Neuritis, optic
  - seventh or facial G51.8
    - newborn (birth injury) P11.3
  - sixth or abducent — *see* Strabismus, paralytic, sixth nerve
  - tenth or vagus G52.2
  - third or oculomotor — *see* Strabismus, paralytic, third nerve
  - twelfth or hypoglossal G52.3
- Déjérine-Sottas G6Ø.Ø
- diabetic (mononeuropathy) — *see* EØ8-E13 with .41
  - polyneuropathy — *see* EØ8-E13 with .42
- due to
  - beriberi E51.11
  - displacement, prolapse or rupture, intervertebral disc — *see* Disorder, disc, with, radiculopathy
  - herniation, nucleus pulposus M51.9 *[G55]*
- endemic E51.11
- facial G51.8
  - newborn (birth injury) P11.3
- general — *see* Polyneuropathy
- geniculate ganglion G51.1
  - due to herpes (zoster) BØ2.21
- gouty M1Ø.ØØ *[G63]*
- hypoglossal (nerve) G52.3
- ilioinguinal (nerve) G57.9-
- infectious (multiple) NEC G61.Ø
- interstitial hypertrophic progressive G6Ø.Ø
- lumbar M54.16
- lumbosacral M54.17
- multiple (*see also* Polyneuropathy)
  - endemic E51.11
  - infective, acute G61.Ø
- multiplex endemica E51.11
- nerve root — *see* Radiculopathy
- oculomotor (nerve) — *see* Strabismus, paralytic, third nerve
- olfactory nerve G52.Ø
- optic (nerve) (hereditary) (sympathetic) H46.9
  - with demyelination G36.Ø
  - in myelitis G36.Ø
  - nutritional H46.2
  - papillitis — *see* Papillitis, optic
  - retrobulbar H46.1-
  - specified type NEC H46.8
  - toxic H46.3

Neuritis — *continued*
- peripheral (nerve) G62.9
  - multiple — *see* Polyneuropathy
  - single — *see* Mononeuritis
- pneumogastric (nerve) G52.2
- postherpetic, postzoster BØ2.29
- progressive hypertrophic interstitial G6Ø.Ø
- retrobulbar (*see also* Neuritis, optic, retrobulbar)
  - in (due to)
    - late syphilis A52.15
    - meningococcal infection A39.82
  - meningococcal A39.82
  - syphilitic A52.15
- sciatic (nerve) (*see also* Sciatica)
  - due to displacement of intervertebral disc — *see* Disorder, disc, with, radiculopathy
- serum (*see also* Reaction, serum) T8Ø.69
- shoulder-girdle G54.5
- specified nerve NEC G58.8
- spinal (nerve) root — *see* Radiculopathy
- syphilitic A52.15
- thenar (median) G56.1-
- thoracic M54.14
- toxic NEC G62.2
- trochlear (nerve) — *see* Strabismus, paralytic, fourth nerve
- vagus (nerve) G52.2

Neuroastrocytoma — *see* Neoplasm, uncertain behavior, by site

Neuroavitaminosis E56.9 *[G99.8]*

Neuroblastoma
- olfactory C3Ø.Ø
- specified site — *see* Neoplasm, malignant, by site
- unspecified site C74.9Ø

Neurochorioretinitis — *see* Chorioretinitis

Neurocirculatory asthenia F45.8

Neurocysticercosis B69.Ø

Neurocytoma — *see* Neoplasm, benign, by site

Neurodermatitis (circumscribed) (circumscripta) (local) L28.Ø
- atopic L2Ø.81
- diffuse (Brocq) L2Ø.81
- disseminated L2Ø.81

Neuroencephalomyelopathy, optic G36.Ø

Neuroepithelioma (*see also* Neoplasm, malignant, by site)
- olfactory C3Ø.Ø

Neurofibroma (*see also* Neoplasm, nerve, benign)
- melanotic — *see* Neoplasm, nerve, benign
- multiple — *see* Neurofibromatosis
- plexiform — *see* Neoplasm, nerve, benign

Neurofibromatosis (multiple) (nonmalignant) Q85.ØØ
- acoustic Q85.Ø2
- malignant — *see* Neoplasm, nerve, malignant
- specified NEC Q85.Ø9
- type 1 (von Recklinghausen) Q85.Ø1
- type 2 Q85.Ø2

Neurofibrosarcoma — *see* Neoplasm, nerve, malignant

Neurogenic (*see also* condition)
- bladder (*see also* Dysfunction, bladder, neuromuscular) N31.9
  - cauda equina syndrome G83.4
- bowel NEC K59.2
- heart F45.8

Neuroglioma — *see* Neoplasm, uncertain behavior, by site

Neurolabyrinthitis (of Dix and Hallpike) — *see* Neuronitis, vestibular

Neurolathyrism — *see* Poisoning, food, noxious, plant

Neuroleprosy A3Ø.9

Neuroma (*see also* Neoplasm, nerve, benign)
- acoustic (nerve) D33.3
- amputation (stump) (traumatic) (surgical complication) (late) T87.3-
  - arm T87.3-
  - leg T87.3-
- digital (toe) G57.6-
- interdigital (toe) G58.8
  - lower limb G57.8-
  - upper limb G56.8-
- intermetatarsal G57.8-
- Morton's G57.6-

Neuroma — *continued*
- nonneoplastic
  - arm G56.9-
  - leg G57.9-
  - lower extremity G57.9-
  - upper extremity G56.9-
- optic (nerve) D33.3
- plantar G57.6-
- plexiform — *see* Neoplasm, nerve, benign
- surgical (nonneoplastic)
  - arm G56.9-
  - leg G57.9-
  - lower extremity G57.9-
  - upper extremity G56.9-

Neuromyalgia — *see* Neuralgia

Neuromyasthenia (epidemic) (postinfectious) G93.3

Neuromyelitis G36.9
- ascending G61.Ø
- optica G36.Ø

Neuromyopathy G7Ø.9
- paraneoplastic D49.9 *[G13.Ø]*

Neuromyotonia (Isaacs) G71.19

Neuronevus — *see* Nevus

Neuronitis G58.9
- ascending (acute) G57.2-
- vestibular H81.2-

Neuroparalytic — *see* condition

Neuropathy, neuropathic G62.9
- acute motor G62.81
- alcoholic G62.1
  - with psychosis — *see* Psychosis, alcoholic
- arm G56.9-
- autonomic, peripheral — *see* Neuropathy, peripheral, autonomic
- axillary G56.9-
- bladder N31.9
  - atonic (motor) (sensory) N31.2
  - autonomous N31.2
  - flaccid N31.2
  - nonreflex N31.2
  - reflex N31.1
  - uninhibited N31.Ø
- brachial plexus G54.Ø
- cervical plexus G54.2
- chronic
  - progressive segmentally demyelinating G62.89
  - relapsing demyelinating G62.89
- Déjérine-Sottas G6Ø.Ø
- diabetic — *see* EØ8-E13 with .4Ø
  - mononeuropathy — *see* EØ8-E13 with .41
  - polyneuropathy — *see* EØ8-E13 with .42
- entrapment G58.9
  - iliohypogastric nerve G57.8-
  - ilioinguinal nerve G57.8-
  - lateral cutaneous nerve of thigh G57.1-
  - median nerve G56.Ø-
  - obturator nerve G57.8-
  - peroneal nerve G57.3-
  - posterior tibial nerve G57.5-
  - saphenous nerve G57.8-
  - ulnar nerve G56.2-
- facial nerve G51.9
- hereditary G6Ø.9
  - motor and sensory (types I-IV) G6Ø.Ø
  - sensory G6Ø.8
  - specified NEC G6Ø.8
- hypertrophic G6Ø.Ø
  - Charcot-Marie-Tooth G6Ø.Ø
  - Déjérine-Sottas G6Ø.Ø
  - interstitial progressive G6Ø.Ø
  - of infancy G6Ø.Ø
  - Refsum G6Ø.1
- idiopathic G6Ø.9
  - progressive G6Ø.3
  - specified NEC G6Ø.8
- in association with hereditary ataxia G6Ø.2
- intercostal G58.Ø
- ischemic — *see* Disorder, nerve
- Jamaica (ginger) G62.2
- leg NEC G57.9-
- lower extremity G57.9-
- lumbar plexus G54.1
- median nerve G56.1-

Neuropathy, neuropathic — *continued*
- motor and sensory (*see also* Polyneuropathy hereditary (types I-IV) G6Ø.Ø
- multiple (acute) (chronic) — *see* Polyneuropathy
- optic (nerve) (*see also* Neuritis, optic)
  - ischemic H47.Ø1-
- paraneoplastic (sensorial) (Denny Brown) D49.9 *[G13.Ø]*
- peripheral (nerve) (*see also* Polyneuropathy) G62.9
  - autonomic G9Ø.9
    - idiopathic G9Ø.Ø9
    - in (due to)
      - amyloidosis E85.4 *[G99.Ø]*
      - diabetes mellitus — *see* EØ8-E13 with .43
      - endocrine disease NEC E34.9 *[G99.Ø]*
      - gout M1Ø.ØØ *[G99.Ø]*
      - hyperthyroidism EØ5.9Ø *[G99.Ø]*
        - with thyroid storm EØ5.91 *[G99.Ø]*
      - metabolic disease NEC E88.9 *[G99.Ø]*
  - idiopathic G6Ø.9
    - progressive G6Ø.3
  - in (due to)
    - antitetanus serum G62.Ø
    - arsenic G62.2
    - drugs NEC G62.Ø
    - lead G62.2
    - organophosphate compounds G62.2
    - toxic agent NEC G62.2
- plantar nerves G57.6-
- progressive
  - hypertrophic interstitial G6Ø.Ø
  - inflammatory G62.81
- radicular NEC — *see* Radiculopathy
- sacral plexus G54.1
- sciatic G57.Ø-
- serum G61.1
- toxic NEC G62.2
- trigeminal sensory G5Ø.8
- ulnar nerve G56.2-
- uremic N18.9 *[G63]*
- vitamin B12 E53.8 *[G63]*
  - with anemia (pernicious) D51.Ø *[G63]*
    - due to dietary deficiency D51.3 *[G63]*

Neurophthisis (*see also* Disorder, nerve)
- peripheral, diabetic — *see* EØ8-E13 with .42

Neuroretinitis — *see* Chorioretinitis

Neuroretinopathy, hereditary optic H47.22

Neurosarcoma — *see* Neoplasm, nerve, malignant

Neurosclerosis — *see* Disorder, nerve

Neurosis, neurotic F48.9
- anankastic F42
- anxiety (state) F41.1
  - panic type F41.Ø
- asthenic F48.8
- bladder F45.8
- cardiac (reflex) F45.8
- cardiovascular F45.8
- character F6Ø.9
- colon F45.8
- compensation F68.1
- compulsive, compulsion F42
- conversion F44.9
- craft F48.8
- cutaneous F45.8
- depersonalization F48.1
- depressive (reaction) (type) F34.1
- environmental F48.8
- excoriation L98.1
- fatigue F48.8
- functional — *see* Disorder, somatoform
- gastric F45.8
- gastrointestinal F45.8
- heart F45.8
- hypochondriacal F45.21
- hysterical F44.9
- incoordination F45.8
  - larynx F45.8
  - vocal cord F45.8
- intestine F45.8
- larynx (sensory) F45.8
  - hysterical F44.4
- mixed NEC F48.8
- musculoskeletal F45.8

Neurosis, neurotic — *continued*
- obsessional F42
- obsessive-compulsive F42
- occupational F48.8
- ocular NEC F45.8
- organ — *see* Disorder, somatoform
- pharynx F45.8
- phobic F4Ø.9
- posttraumatic (situational) F43.1Ø
  - acute F43.11
  - chronic F43.12
- psychasthenic (type) F48.8
- railroad F48.8
- rectum F45.8
- respiratory F45.8
- rumination F45.8
- sexual F65.9
- situational F48.8
- social F4Ø.1Ø
  - generalized F4Ø.11
- specified type NEC F48.8
- state F48.9
  - with depersonalization episode F48.1
- stomach F45.8
- traumatic F43.1Ø
  - acute F43.11
  - chronic F43.12
- vasomotor F45.8
- visceral F45.8
- war F48.8

Neurospongioblastosis diffusa Q85.1

Neurosyphilis (arrested) (early) (gumma) (late) (latent) (recurrent) (relapse) A52.3
- with ataxia (cerebellar) (locomotor) (spastic) (spinal) A52.19
- aneurysm (cerebral) A52.Ø5
- arachnoid (adhesive) A52.13
- arteritis (any artery) (cerebral) A52.Ø4
- asymptomatic A52.2
- congenital A5Ø.4Ø
- dura (mater) A52.13
- general paresis A52.17
- hemorrhagic A52.Ø5
- juvenile (asymptomatic) (meningeal) A5Ø.4Ø
- leptomeninges (aseptic) A52.13
- meningeal, meninges (adhesive) A52.13
- meningitis A52.13
- meningovascular (diffuse) A52.13
- optic atrophy A52.15
- parenchymatous (degenerative) A52.19
- paresis, paretic A52.17
  - juvenile A5Ø.45
- remission in (sustained) A52.3
- serological (without symptoms) A52.2
- specified nature or site NEC A52.19
- tabes, tabetic (dorsalis) A52.11
  - juvenile A5Ø.45
- taboparesis A52.17
  - juvenile A5Ø.45
- thrombosis (cerebral) A52.Ø5
- vascular (cerebral) NEC A52.Ø5

Neurothekeoma — *see* Neoplasm, nerve, benign

Neurotic — *see* Neurosis

Neurotoxemia — *see* Toxemia

Neutroclusion M26.211

Neutropenia, neutropenic (chronic) (genetic) (idiopathic) (immune) (infantile) (malignant) (pernicious) (splenic) D7Ø.9
- congenital (primary) D7Ø.Ø
- cyclic D7Ø.4
- cytoreductive cancer chemotherapy sequela D7Ø.1
- drug-induced D7Ø.2
  - due to cytoreductive cancer chemotherapy D7Ø.1
- due to infection D7Ø.3
- fever D7Ø.9
- neonatal, transitory (isoimmune) (maternal transfer) P61.5
- periodic D7Ø.4
- secondary (cyclic) (periodic) (splenic) D7Ø.4
  - drug-induced D7Ø.2
    - due to cytoreductive cancer chemotherapy D7Ø.1

Neutropenia, neutropenic — *continued*
- toxic D7Ø.8

Neutrophilia, hereditary giant D72.Ø

Nevocarcinoma — *see* Melanoma

Nevus D22.9
- achromic — *see* Neoplasm, skin, benign
- amelanotic — *see* Neoplasm, skin, benign
- angiomatous D18.ØØ
  - intra-abdominal D18.Ø3
  - intracranial D18.Ø2
  - skin D18.Ø1
  - specified site NEC D18.Ø9
- araneus I78.1
- balloon cell — *see* Neoplasm, skin, benign
- bathing trunk D48.5
- blue — *see* Neoplasm, skin, benign
  - cellular — *see* Neoplasm, skin, benign
  - giant — *see* Neoplasm, skin, benign
  - Jadassohn's — *see* Neoplasm, skin, benign
  - malignant — *see* Melanoma
- capillary D18.ØØ
  - intra-abdominal D18.Ø3
  - intracranial D18.Ø2
  - skin D18.Ø1
  - specified site NEC D18.Ø9
- cavernous D18.ØØ
  - intra-abdominal D18.Ø3
  - intracranial D18.Ø2
  - skin D18.Ø1
  - specified site NEC D18.Ø9
- cellular — *see* Neoplasm, skin, benign
  - blue — *see* Neoplasm, skin, benign
- choroid D31.3-
- comedonicus Q82.5
- conjunctiva D31.Ø-
- dermal — *see* Neoplasm, skin, benign
  - with epidermal nevus — *see* Neoplasm, skin, benign
- dysplastic — *see* Neoplasm, skin, benign
- eye D31.9-
- flammeus Q82.5
- hemangiomatous D18.ØØ
  - intra-abdominal D18.Ø3
  - intracranial D18.Ø2
  - skin D18.Ø1
  - specified site NEC D18.Ø9
- iris D31.4-
- lacrimal gland D31.5-
- lymphatic D18.1
- magnocellular
  - specified site — *see* Neoplasm, benign, by site
  - unspecified site D31.4Ø
- malignant — *see* Melanoma
- meaning hemangioma D18.ØØ
  - intra-abdominal D18.Ø3
  - intracranial D18.Ø2
  - skin D18.Ø1
  - specified site NEC D18.Ø9
- mouth (mucosa) D1Ø.3Ø
  - specified site NEC D1Ø.39
  - white sponge Q38.6
- multiplex Q85.1
- non-neoplastic I78.1
- oral mucosa D1Ø.3Ø
  - specified site NEC D1Ø.39
  - white sponge Q38.6
- orbit D31.6-
- pigmented
  - giant (*see also* Neoplasm, skin, uncertain behavior) D48.5
    - malignant melanoma in — *see* Melanoma
- portwine Q82.5
- retina D31.2-
- retrobulbar D31.6-
- sanguineous Q82.5
- senile I78.1
- skin D22.9
  - abdominal wall D22.5
  - ala nasi D22.39
  - ankle D22.7-
  - anus, anal D22.5
  - arm D22.6-
  - auditory canal (external) D22.2-

Nevus — *continued*
- skin— *continued*
  - auricle (ear) D22.2-
  - auricular canal (external) D22.2-
  - axilla, axillary fold D22.5
  - back D22.5
  - breast D22.5
  - brow D22.39
  - buttock D22.5
  - canthus (eye) D22.1-
  - cheek (external) D22.39
  - chest wall D22.5
  - chin D22.39
  - ear (external) D22.2-
  - external meatus (ear) D22.2-
  - eyebrow D22.39
  - eyelid (lower) (upper) D22.1-
  - face D22.3Ø
    - specified NEC D22.39
  - female genital organ (external) NEC D28.Ø
  - finger D22.6-
  - flank D22.5
  - foot D22.7-
  - forearm D22.6-
  - forehead D22.39
  - foreskin D29.Ø
  - genital organ (external) NEC
    - female D28.Ø
    - male D29.9
  - gluteal region D22.5
  - groin D22.5
  - hand D22.6-
  - heel D22.7-
  - helix D22.2-
  - hip D22.7-
  - interscapular region D22.5
  - jaw D22.39
  - knee D22.7-
  - labium (majus) (minus) D28.Ø
  - leg D22.7-
  - lip (lower) (upper) D22.Ø
  - lower limb D22.7-
  - male genital organ (external) D29.9
  - nail D22.9
    - finger D22.6-
    - toe D22.7-
  - nasolabial groove D22.39
  - nates D22.5
  - neck D22.4
  - nose (external) D22.39
  - palpebra D22.1-
  - penis D29.Ø
  - perianal skin D22.5
  - perineum D22.5
  - pinna D22.2-
  - popliteal fossa or space D22.7-
  - prepuce D29.Ø
  - pudendum D28.Ø
  - scalp D22.4
  - scrotum D29.4
  - shoulder D22.6-
  - submammary fold D22.5
  - temple D22.39
  - thigh D22.7-
  - toe D22.7-
  - trunk NEC D22.5
  - umbilicus D22.5
  - upper limb D22.6-
  - vulva D28.Ø
- specified site NEC — *see* Neoplasm, benign, by site
- spider I78.1
- stellar I78.1
- strawberry Q82.5
- Sutton's — *see* Neoplasm, skin, benign,
- unius lateris Q82.5
- Unna's Q82.5
- vascular Q82.5
- verrucous Q82.5

Newborn (infant) (liveborn) (singleton) Z38.2
- acne L7Ø.4
- abstinence syndrome P96.1

- **Nicotine** — *see* Tobacco
- **Nicotinic acid deficiency** E52
- **Niemann-Pick disease or syndrome** E75.249
  - specified NEC E75.248
  - type
    - A E75.24Ø
    - B E75.241
    - C E75.242
    - D E75.243
- **Night**
  - blindness — *see* Blindness, night
  - sweats R61
  - terrors (child) F51.4
- **Nightmares** (REM sleep type) F51.5
- **Nipple** — *see* condition
- **Nisbet's chancre** A57
- **Nishimoto** (-Takeuchi) **disease** I67.5
- **Nitritoid crisis or reaction** — *see* Crisis, nitritoid
- **Nitrosohemoglobinemia** D74.8
- **Njovera** A65
- **Nocardiosis, nocardiasis** A43.9
  - cutaneous A43.1
  - lung A43.Ø
  - pneumonia A43.Ø
  - pulmonary A43.Ø
  - specified site NEC A43.8
- **Nocturia** R35.1
  - psychogenic F45.8
- **Nocturnal** — *see* condition
- **Nodal rhythm** I49.8
- **Node(s)** (*see also* Nodule)
  - Bouchard's (with arthropathy) M15.2
  - Haygarth's M15.8
  - Heberden's (with arthropathy) M15.1
  - larynx J38.7
  - lymph — *see* condition
  - milker's BØ8.Ø3
  - Osler's I33.Ø
  - Schmorl's — *see* Schmorl's disease
  - singer's J38.2
  - teacher's J38.2
  - tuberculous — *see* Tuberculosis, lymph gland
  - vocal cord J38.2
- **Nodule(s), nodular**
  - actinomycotic — *see* Actinomycosis
  - breast NEC N63
  - colloid (cystic), thyroid EØ4.1
  - cutaneous — *see* Swelling, localized
  - endometrial (stromal) D26.1
  - Haygarth's M15.8
  - inflammatory — *see* Inflammation
  - juxta-articular
    - syphilitic A52.77
    - yaws A66.7
  - larynx J38.7
  - lung, solitary (subsegmental branch of the bronchial tree) R91.1
    - multiple R91.8
  - milker's BØ8.Ø3
  - prostate N4Ø.2
    - with lower urinary tract symptoms (LUTS) N4Ø.3
    - without lower urinary tract symtpoms (LUTS) N4Ø.2
  - pulmonary, solitary (subsegmental branch of the bronchial tree) R91.1
  - retrocardiac RØ9.89
  - rheumatoid MØ6.3Ø
    - ankle MØ6.37-
    - elbow MØ6.32-
    - foot joint MØ6.37-
    - hand joint MØ6.34-
    - hip MØ6.35-
    - knee MØ6.36-
    - multiple site MØ6.39
    - shoulder MØ6.31-
    - vertebra MØ6.38
    - wrist MØ6.33-
  - scrotum (inflammatory) N49.2
  - singer's J38.2
  - solitary, lung (subsegmental branch of the bronchial tree) R91.1
    - multiple R91.8
- **Nodule(s), nodular**— *continued*
  - subcutaneous — *see* Swelling, localized
  - teacher's J38.2
  - thyroid (cold) (gland) (nontoxic) EØ4.1
    - with thyrotoxicosis EØ5.2Ø
      - with thyroid storm EØ5.21
    - toxic or with hyperthyroidism EØ5.2Ø
      - with thyroid storm EØ5.21
  - vocal cord J38.2
- **Noma** (gangrenous) (hospital) (infective) A69.Ø
  - auricle I96
  - mouth A69.Ø
  - pudendi N76.89
  - vulvae N76.89
- **Nomad, nomadism** Z59.Ø
- **Nonautoimmune hemolytic anemia** D59.4
  - drug-induced D59.2
- **Nonclosure** (*see also* Imperfect, closure)
  - ductus arteriosus (Botallo's) Q25.Ø
  - foramen
    - botalli Q21.1
    - ovale Q21.1
- **Noncompliance** Z91.19
  - with
    - dietary regimen Z91.11
    - dialysis Z91.15
    - medical treatment Z91.19
    - medication regimen NEC Z91.14
      - underdosing (*see also* Table of Drugs and Chemicals, categories T36-T5Ø, with final character 6) Z91.14
        - intentional NEC Z91.128
          - due to financial hardship of patient Z91.12Ø
        - unintentional NEC Z91.138
          - due to patient's age related debility Z91.13Ø
    - renal dialysis Z91.15
- **Nondescent** (congenital) (*see also* Malposition, congenital)
  - cecum Q43.3
  - colon Q43.3
  - testicle Q53.9
    - bilateral Q53.2Ø
      - abdominal Q53.21
      - perineal Q53.22
    - unilateral Q53.1Ø
      - abdominal Q53.11
      - perineal Q53.12
- **Nondevelopment**
  - brain QØ2
    - part of QØ4.3
  - heart Q24.8
  - organ or site, congenital NEC — *see* Hypoplasia
- **Nonengagement**
  - head NEC O32.4
    - in labor, causing obstructed labor O64.8
- **Nonexanthematous tick fever** A93.2
- **Nonexpansion, lung** (newborn) P28.Ø
- **Nonfunctioning**
  - cystic duct (*see also* Disease, gallbladder) K82.8
  - gallbladder (*see also* Disease, gallbladder) K82.8
  - kidney N28.9
  - labyrinth — *see* subcategory H83.2
- **Non-Hodgkin lymphoma NEC** — *see* Lymphoma, non-Hodgkin
- **Non-working side interference** M26.56
- **Nonimplantation, ovum** N97.2
- **Noninsufflation, fallopian tube** N97.1
- **Non-ketotic hyperglycinemia** E72.51
- **Nonne-Milroy syndrome** Q82.Ø
- **Nonovulation** N97.Ø
- **Nonpatent fallopian tube** N97.1
- **Nonpneumatization, lung NEC** P28.Ø
- **Nonrotation** — *see* Malrotation
- **Nonsecretion, urine** — *see* Anuria
- **Nonunion**
  - fracture — *see* Fracture, by site
  - organ or site, congenital NEC — *see* Imperfect, closure
  - symphysis pubis, congenital Q74.2
- **Nonvisualization, gallbladder** R93.2
- **Nonvital, nonvitalized tooth** KØ4.99
- **Noonan's syndrome** Q87.1
- **Normocytic anemia** (infectional) due to blood loss (chronic) D5Ø.Ø
  - acute D62
- **Norrie's disease** (congenital) Q15.8
- **North American blastomycosis** B4Ø.9
- **Norwegian itch** B86
- **Nose, nasal** — *see* condition
- **Nosebleed** RØ4.Ø
- **Nose-picking** F98.8
- **Nosomania** F45.21
- **Nosophobia** F45.22
- **Nostalgia** F43.2Ø
- **Notch of iris** Q13.2
- **Notching nose, congenital** (tip) Q3Ø.2
- **Nothnagel's** syndrome — *see* Strabismus, paralytic, third nerve
  - vasomotor acroparesthesia I73.89
- **Novy's relapsing fever** A68.9
  - louse-borne A68.Ø
  - tick-borne A68.1
- **Noxious**
  - foodstuffs, poisoning by — *see* Poisoning, food, noxious, plant
  - substances transmitted through placenta or breast milk PØ4.9
- **Nucleus pulposus** — *see* condition
- **Numbness** R2Ø.Ø
- **Nuns' knee** — *see* Bursitis, prepatellar
- **Nursemaid's elbow** S53.Ø3-
- **Nutcracker esophagus** K22.4
- **Nutmeg liver** K76.1
- **Nutrient element deficiency** E61.9
  - specified NEC E61.8
- **Nutrition deficient or insufficient** (*see also* Malnutrition) E46
  - due to
    - insufficient food T73.Ø
    - lack of
      - care (child) T76.Ø2
        - adult T76.Ø1
      - food T73.Ø
- **Nutritional stunting** E45
- **Nyctalopia** (night blindness) — *see* Blindness, night
- **Nycturia** R35.1
  - psychogenic F45.8
- **Nymphomania** F52.8
- **Nystagmus** H55.ØØ
  - benign paroxysmal — *see* Vertigo, benign paroxysmal
  - central positional H81.4-
  - congenital H55.Ø1
  - dissociated H55.Ø4
  - latent H55.Ø2
  - miners' H55.Ø9
  - positional
    - benign paroxysmal H81.4-
    - central H81.4-
  - specified form NEC H55.Ø9
  - visual deprivation H55.Ø3

O

- **Obermeyer's relapsing fever** (European) A68.Ø
- **Obesity** E66.9
  - with alveolar hyperventilation E66.2
  - adrenal E27.8
  - complicating
    - childbirth O99.214
    - pregnancy O99.21-
    - puerperium O99.215
  - constitutional E66.8
  - dietary counseling and surveillance Z71.3
  - drug-induced E66.1
  - due to
    - drug E66.1
    - excess calories E66.Ø9
      - morbid E66.Ø1
      - severe E66.Ø1
  - endocrine E66.8
  - endogenous E66.8
  - familial E66.8
  - glandular E66.8
  - hypothyroid — *see* Hypothyroidism
  - morbid E66.Ø1
    - with alveolar hypoventilation E66.2
    - due to excess calories E66.Ø1
  - nutritional E66.Ø9
  - pituitary E23.6
  - severe E66.Ø1
  - specified type NEC E66.8
- **Oblique** — *see* condition
- **Obliteration**
  - appendix (lumen) K38.8
  - artery I77.1
  - bile duct (noncalculous) K83.1
  - common duct (noncalculous) K83.1
  - cystic duct — *see* Obstruction, gallbladder
  - disease, arteriolar I77.1
  - endometrium N85.8
  - eye, anterior chamber — *see* Disorder, globe, hypotony
  - fallopian tube N97.1
  - lymphatic vessel I89.Ø
    - due to mastectomy I97.2
  - organ or site, congenital NEC — *see* Atresia, by site
  - ureter N13.5
    - with infection N13.6
  - urethra — *see* Stricture, urethra
  - vein I87.8
  - vestibule (oral) KØ8.8
- **Observation** (following) (for) (without need for further medical care) ZØ4.9
  - accident NEC ZØ4.3
    - at work ZØ4.2
    - transport ZØ4.1
  - adverse effect of drug ZØ3.6
  - alleged rape or sexual assault (victim), ruled out
    - adult ZØ4.41
    - child ZØ4.42
  - criminal assault ZØ4.8
  - development state
    - adolescent ZØØ.3
    - period of rapid growth in childhood ZØØ.2
    - puberty ZØØ.3
  - disease, specified NEC ZØ3.89
  - following work accident ZØ4.2
  - growth and development state — *see* Observation, development state
  - injuries (accidental) NEC (*see also* Observation, accident)
  - newborn (for suspected condition, ruled out)—*see* Newborn, affected by (suspected to be), maternal (complication of) (use of)
  - postpartum
    - immediately after delivery Z39.Ø
    - routine follow-up Z39.2
  - pregnancy (normal) (without complication) Z34.9-
    - high risk OØ9.9-
  - suicide attempt, alleged NEC ZØ3.89
    - self-poisoning ZØ3.6
- **Observation** — *continued*
  - suspected, ruled out (*see also* Suspected condition, ruled out)
    - abuse, physical
      - adult ZØ4.71
      - child ZØ4.72
    - accident at work ZØ4.2
    - adult battering victim ZØ4.71
    - child battering victim ZØ4.72
    - condition NEC ZØ3.89
  - newborn *see* Newborn, affected by (suspected to be), maternal (complication of) (use of)
    - drug poisoning or adverse effect ZØ3.6
    - exposure (to)
      - anthrax ZØ3.81Ø
      - biological agent NEC ZØ3.818
    - inflicted injury NEC ZØ4.8
    - suicide attempt, alleged ZØ3.89
      - self-poisoning ZØ3.6
    - toxic effects from ingested substance (drug) (poison) ZØ3.6
  - toxic effects from ingested substance (drug) (poison) ZØ3.6
- **Obsession, obsessional state** F42
- **Obsessive-compulsive neurosis or reaction** F42
- **Obstetric embolism, septic** — *see* Embolism, obstetric, septic
- **Obstetrical trauma** (complicating delivery) O71.9
  - with or following ectopic or molar pregnancy OØ8.6
  - specified type NEC O71.89
- **Obstipation** — *see* Constipation
- **Obstruction, obstructed, obstructive**
  - airway J98.8
    - with
      - allergic alveolitis J67.9
      - asthma J45.9Ø9
        - with
          - exacerbation (acute) J45.9Ø1
          - status asthmaticus J45.9Ø2
      - bronchiectasis J47.9
        - with
          - exacerbation (acute) J47.1
          - lower respiratory infection J47.Ø
      - bronchitis (chronic) J44.9
      - emphysema J43.9
    - chronic J44.9
      - with
        - allergic alveolitis — *see* Pneumonitis, hypersensitivity
        - bronchiectasis J47.9
          - with
            - exacerbation (acute) J47.1
            - lower respiratory infection J47.Ø
      - foreign body — *see* Foreign body, by site, causing asphyxia
      - inhalation of fumes or vapors J68.9
      - laryngospasm J38.5
  - ampulla of Vater K83.1
  - aortic (heart) (valve) — *see* Stenosis, aortic
  - aortoiliac I74.Ø9
  - aqueduct of Sylvius G91.1
    - congenital QØ3.Ø
      - with spina bifida — *see* Spina bifida, by site, with hydrocephalus
  - Arnold-Chiari — *see* Arnold-Chiari disease
  - artery (*see also* Embolism, artery) I74.9
    - basilar (complete) (partial) — *see* Occlusion, artery, basilar
    - carotid (complete) (partial) — *see* Occlusion, artery, carotid
    - cerebellar — *see* Occlusion, artery, cerebellar
    - cerebral (anterior) (middle) (posterior) — *see* Occlusion, artery, cerebral
    - precerebral — *see* Occlusion, artery, precerebral
    - renal N28.Ø
    - retinal NEC — *see* Occlusion, artery, retina
    - vertebral (complete) (partial) — *see* Occlusion, artery, vertebral
  - band (intestinal) K56.69
  - bile duct or passage (common) (hepatic) (noncalculous) K83.1
    - with calculus K8Ø.51
    - congenital (causing jaundice) Q44.3
- **Obstruction, obstructed, obstructive** — *continued*
  - biliary (duct) (tract) K83.1
    - gallbladder K82.Ø
  - bladder-neck (acquired) N32.Ø
    - congenital Q64.31
    - due to hyperplasia (hypertrophy) of prostate — *see* Hyperplasia, prostate
  - bowel — *see* Obstruction, intestine
  - bronchus J98.Ø9
  - canal, ear — *see* Stenosis, external ear canal
  - cardia K22.2
  - caval veins (inferior) (superior) I87.1
  - cecum — *see* Obstruction, intestine
  - circulatory I99.8
  - colon — *see* Obstruction, intestine
  - common duct (noncalculous) K83.1
  - coronary (artery) — *see* Occlusion, coronary
  - cystic duct (*see also* Obstruction, gallbladder)
    - with calculus K8Ø.21
  - device, implant or graft (*see also* Complications, by site and type, mechanical) T85.698
    - arterial graft NEC — *see* Complication, cardiovascular device, mechanical, vascular
    - catheter NEC T85.628
      - cystostomy T83.Ø9Ø
      - dialysis (renal) T82.49
        - intraperitoneal T85.691
      - infusion NEC T82.594
        - spinal (epidural) (subdural) T85.69Ø
      - urinary, indwelling T83.Ø98
    - due to infection T85.79
    - gastrointestinal — *see* Complications, prosthetic device, mechanical, gastrointestinal device
    - genital NEC T83.498
      - intrauterine contraceptive device T83.39
      - penile prosthesis T83.49Ø
    - heart NEC — *see* Complication, cardiovascular device, mechanical
    - joint prosthesis — *see* Complications, joint prosthesis, mechanical, specified NEC, by site
    - orthopedic NEC — *see* Complication, orthopedic, device, mechanical
    - specified NEC T85.628
    - urinary NEC (*see also* Complication, genitourinary, device, urinary, mechanical)
      - graft T83.29
    - vascular NEC — *see* Complication, cardiovascular device, mechanical
    - ventricular intracranial shunt T85.Ø9
  - due to foreign body accidentally left in operative wound T81.529
  - duodenum K31.5
  - ejaculatory duct N5Ø.8
  - esophagus K22.2
  - eustachian tube (complete) (partial) H68.1Ø-
    - cartilagenous (extrinsic) H68.13-
      - intrinsic H68.12-
    - osseous H68.11-
  - fallopian tube (bilateral) N97.1
  - fecal K56.41
    - with hernia — *see* Hernia, by site, with obstruction
  - foramen of Monro (congenital) QØ3.8
    - with spina bifida — *see* Spina bifida, by site, with hydrocephalus
  - foreign body — *see* Foreign body
  - gallbladder K82.Ø
    - with calculus, stones K8Ø.21
    - congenital Q44.1
  - gastric outlet K31.1
  - gastrointestinal — *see* Obstruction, intestine
  - hepatic K76.89
    - duct (noncalculous) K83.1
  - ileum — *see* Obstruction, intestine
  - iliofemoral (artery) I74.5
  - intestine K56.6Ø
    - with
      - adhesions (intestinal) (peritoneal) K56.5
    - adynamic K56.Ø
    - by gallstone K56.3
    - congenital (small) Q41.9

Occlusion, occluded— *continued*
- bowel — *see* Obstruction, intestine
- carotid (artery) (common) (internal) — *see* Occlusion, artery, carotid
- centric (of teeth) M26.59
  - maximum intercuspation discrepancy M26.55
- cerebellar (artery) — *see* Occlusion, artery, cerebellar
- cerebral (artery) — *see* Occlusion, artery, cerebral
- cerebrovascular (*see also* Occlusion, artery, cerebral)
  - with infarction I63.5
- cervical canal — *see* Stricture, cervix
- cervix (uteri) — *see* Stricture, cervix
- choanal Q30.Ø
- choroidal (artery) — *see* Occlusion, artery, precerebral, specified NEC
- colon — *see* Obstruction, intestine
- communicating posterior artery — *see* Occlusion, artery, precerebral, specified NEC
- coronary (artery) (vein) (thrombotic) (*see also* Infarct, myocardium)
  - chronic total I25.82
  - healed or old I25.2
  - not resulting in infarction I24.Ø
  - total (chronic) I25.82
- cystic duct — *see* Obstruction, gallbladder
- embolic — *see* Embolism
- fallopian tube N97.1
  - congenital Q5Ø.6
- gallbladder (*see also* Obstruction, gallbladder)
  - congenital (causing jaundice) Q44.1
- gingiva, traumatic KØ6.2
- hymen N89.6
  - congenital Q52.3
- hypophyseal (artery) — *see* Occlusion, artery, precerebral, specified NEC
- iliac artery I74.5
- intestine — *see* Obstruction, intestine
- lacrimal passages — *see* Obstruction, lacrimal
- lung J98.4
- lymph or lymphatic channel I89.Ø
- mammary duct N64.89
- mesenteric artery (embolic) (thrombotic) K55.Ø
- nose J34.89
  - congenital Q3Ø.Ø
- organ or site, congenital NEC — *see* Atresia, by site
- oviduct N97.1
  - congenital Q5Ø.6
- peripheral arteries
  - due to stricture or stenosis I77.1
  - upper extremity I74.2
- pontine (artery) — *see* Occlusion, artery, precerebral, specified NEC
- posterior lingual, of mandibular teeth M26.29
- precerebral artery — *see* Occlusion, artery, precerebral
- punctum lacrimale — *see* Obstruction, lacrimal
- pupil — *see* Membrane, pupillary
- pylorus, adult (*see also* Stricture, pylorus) K31.1
- renal artery N28.Ø
- retina, retinal
  - artery — *see* Occlusion, artery, retinal
  - vein (central) H34.81-
    - engorgement H34.82-
    - tributary H34.83-
  - vessels H34.9
- spinal artery — *see* Occlusion, artery, precerebral, vertebral
- teeth (mandibular) (posterior lingual) M26.29
- thoracic duct I89.Ø
- thrombotic — *see* Thrombosis, artery
- traumatic
  - edentulous (alveolar) ridge KØ6.2
  - gingiva KØ6.2
  - periodontal KØ5.5
- tubal N97.1
- ureter (complete) (partial) N13.5
  - congenital Q62.1Ø
- ureteropelvic junction N13.5
  - congenital Q62.11
- ureterovesical orifice N13.5
  - congenital Q62.12
- urethra — *see* Stricture, urethra
- uterus N85.8
- vagina N89.5
- vascular NEC I99.8
- vein — *see* Thrombosis
  - retinal — *see* Occlusion, retinal, vein
- vena cava (inferior) (superior) — *see* Embolism, vena cava
- ventricle (brain) NEC G91.1
- vertebral (artery) — *see* Occlusion, artery, vertebral
- vessel (blood) I99.8
- vulva N9Ø.5

Occult
- blood in feces (stools) R19.5

Occupational
- problems NEC Z56.89

Ochlophobia — *see* Agoraphobia

Ochronosis (endogenous) E7Ø.29

Ocular muscle — *see* condition

Oculogyric crisis or disturbance H51.8
- psychogenic F45.8

Oculomotor syndrome H51.9

Oculopathy
- syphilitic NEC A52.71
  - congenital
    - early A5Ø.Ø1
    - late A5Ø.3Ø
  - early (secondary) A51.43
  - late A52.71

Oddi's sphincter spasm K83.4

Odontalgia KØ8.8

Odontoameloblastoma — *see* Cyst, calcifying odontogenic

Odontoclasia KØ3.89

Odontodysplasia, regional KØØ.4

Odontogenesis imperfecta KØØ.5

Odontoma (ameloblastic) (complex) (compound) (fibroameloblastic) — *see* Cyst, calcifying odontogenic

Odontomyelitis (closed) (open) KØ4.Ø

Odontorrhagia KØ8.8

Odontosarcoma, ameloblastic C41.1
- upper jaw (bone) C41.Ø

Oedema, oedematous — *see* Edema

Oesophag(o) — *see* Esophag(o)-

Oestriasis — *see* Myiasis

Oguchi's disease H53.63

Ohara's disease — *see* Tularemia

Oidiomycosis — *see* Candidiasis

Oidium albicans infection — *see* Candidiasis

Old age (without mention of debility) R54
- dementia FØ3

Old (previous) myocardial infarction I25.2

Olfactory — *see* condition

Oligemia — *see* Anemia

Oligoastrocytoma
- specified site — *see* Neoplasm, malignant, by site
- unspecified site C71.9

Oligocythemia D64.9

Oligodendroblastoma
- specified site — *see* Neoplasm, malignant, by site
- unspecified site C71.9

Oligodendroglioma
- anaplastic type
  - specified site — *see* Neoplasm, malignant, by site
  - unspecified site C71.9
- specified site — *see* Neoplasm, malignant, by site
- unspecified site C71.9

Oligodontia — *see* Anodontia

Oligoencephalon QØ2

Oligohidrosis L74.4

Oligohydramnios O41.Ø-

Oligohydrosis L74.4

Oligomenorrhea N91.5
- primary N91.3
- secondary N91.4

Oligophrenia (*see also* Disability, intellectual)
- phenylpyruvic E7Ø.Ø

Oligospermia N46.11
- due to
  - drug therapy N46.121
  - efferent duct obstruction N46.123
  - infection N46.122
  - radiation N46.124
  - specified cause NEC N46.129
  - systemic disease N46.125

Oligotrichia — *see* Alopecia

Oliguria R34
- with, complicating or following ectopic or molar pregnancy OØ8.4
- postprocedural N99.Ø

Ollier's disease Q78.4

Omentitis — *see* Peritonitis

Omenotocele — *see* Hernia, abdomen, specified site NEC

Omentum, omental — *see* condition

Omphalitis (congenital) (newborn) P38.9
- with mild hemorrhage P38.1
- without hemorrhage P38.9
- not of newborn LØ8.82
- tetanus A33

Omphalocele Q79.2

Omphalomesenteric duct, persistent Q43.Ø

Omphalorrhagia, newborn P51.9

Omsk hemorrhagic fever A98.1

Onanism (excessive) F98.8

Onchocerciasis, onchocercosis B73.1
- with
  - eye disease B73.ØØ
    - endophthalmitis B73.Ø1
    - eyelid B73.Ø9
    - glaucoma B73.Ø2
    - specified NEC B73.Ø9
- eye NEC B73.ØØ
- eyelid B73.Ø9

Oncocytoma — *see* Neoplasm, benign, by site

Oncovirus, as cause of disease classified elsewhere B97.32

Ondine's curse — *see* Apnea, sleep

Oneirophrenia F23

Onychauxis L6Ø.2
- congenital Q84.5

Onychia (*see also* Cellulitis, digit)
- with lymphangitis — *see* Lymphangitis, acute, digit
- candidal B37.2
- dermatophytic B35.1

Onychitis (*see also* Cellulitis, digit)
- with lymphangitis — *see* Lymphangitis, acute, digit

Onychocryptosis L6Ø.Ø

Onychodystrophy L6Ø.3
- congenital Q84.6

Onychogryphosis, onychogryposis L6Ø.2

Onycholysis L6Ø.1

Onychomadesis L6Ø.8

Onychomalacia L6Ø.3

Onychomycosis (finger) (toe) B35.1

Onycho-osteodysplasia Q79.8

Onychophagia F98.8

Onychophosis L6Ø.8

Onychoptosis L6Ø.8

Onychorrhexis L6Ø.3
- congenital Q84.6

Onychoschizia L6Ø.3

Onyxis (finger) (toe) L6Ø.Ø

Onyxitis (*see also* Cellulitis, digit)
- with lymphangitis — *see* Lymphangitis, acute, digit

Oophoritis (cystic) (infectional) (interstitial) N7Ø.92
- with salpingitis N7Ø.93
- acute N7Ø.Ø2
  - with salpingitis N7Ø.Ø3
- chronic N7Ø.12
  - with salpingitis N7Ø.13
- complicating abortion — *see* Abortion, by type, complicated by, oophoritis

Oophorocele N83.4

Opacity, opacities
- cornea H17.-
  - central H17.1-
  - congenital Q13.3
  - degenerative — *see* Degeneration, cornea
  - hereditary — *see* Dystrophy, cornea
  - inflammatory — *see* Keratitis
  - minor H17.81-
  - peripheral H17.82-

Osteochondrosis — *continued*
- juvenile, juvenilis— *continued*
  - after congenital dislocation of hip reduction — *see* Osteochondrosis, juvenile, hip, specified NEC
  - arm — *see* Osteochondrosis, juvenile, upper limb NEC
  - capitular epiphysis (femur) — *see* Legg-Calvé-Perthes disease
  - clavicle, sternal epiphysis — *see* Osteochondrosis, juvenile, upper limb NEC
  - coxae — *see* Legg-Calvé-Perthes disease
  - deformans M92.9
  - fibula M92.5-
  - foot NEC M92.8
  - hand M92.2Ø-
    - carpal lunate M92.21-
    - metacarpal head M92.22-
    - specified site NEC M92.29-
  - head of femur — *see* Legg-Calvé-Perthes disease
  - hip and pelvis M91.9-
    - coxa plana — *see* Coxa, plana
    - femoral head — *see* Legg-Calvé-Perthes disease
    - pelvis M91.Ø
    - pseudocoxalgia — *see* Pseudocoxalgia
    - specified NEC M91.8-
  - humerus M92.Ø-
  - limb
    - lower NEC M92.8
    - upper NEC — *see* Osteochondrosis, juvenile, upper limb NEC
  - medial cuneiform bone — *see* Osteochondrosis, juvenile, tarsus
  - metatarsus M92.7-
  - patella M92.4-
  - radius M92.1-
  - specified site NEC M92.8
  - spine M42.ØØ
    - cervical region M42.Ø2
    - cervicothoracic region M42.Ø3
    - lumbar region M42.Ø6
    - lumbosacral region M42.Ø7
    - multiple sites M42.Ø9
    - occipito-atlanto-axial region M42.Ø1
    - sacrococcygeal region M42.Ø8
    - thoracic region M42.Ø4
    - thoracolumbar region M42.Ø5
  - tarsus M92.6-
  - tibia M92.5-
  - ulna M92.1-
  - upper limb NEC M92.3-
  - vertebra (body) (epiphyseal plates) (Calvé's) (Scheuermann's) — *see* Osteochondrosis, juvenile, spine
- Kienböck's — *see* Osteochondrosis, juvenile, hand, carpal lunate
  - adult M93.1
- Köhler's
  - patellar — *see* Osteochondrosis, juvenile, patella
  - tarsal navicular — *see* Osteochondrosis, juvenile, tarsus
- Legg-Perthes(-Calvé)(-Waldenström) — *see* Legg-Calvé-Perthes disease
- limb
  - lower NEC (juvenile) M92.8
  - upper NEC (juvenile) — *see* Osteochondrosis, juvenile, upper limb NEC
- lunate bone (carpal) (juvenile) (*see also* Osteochondrosis, juvenile, hand, carpal lunate)
  - adult M93.1
- Mauclaire's — *see* Osteochondrosis, juvenile, hand, metacarpal
- metacarpal (head) (juvenile) — *see* Osteochondrosis, juvenile, hand, metacarpal
- metatarsus (fifth) (head) (juvenile) (second) — *see* Osteochondrosis, juvenile, metatarsus
- navicular (juvenile) — *see* Osteochondrosis, juvenile, tarsus
- os
  - calcis (juvenile) — *see* Osteochondrosis, juvenile, tarsus

Osteochondrosis — *continued*
- os — *continued*
  - tibiale externum (juvenile) — *see* Osteochondrosis, juvenile, tarsus
- Osgood-Schlatter — *see* Osteochondrosis, juvenile, tibia
- Panner's — *see* Osteochondrosis, juvenile, humerus
- patellar center (juvenile) (primary) (secondary) — *see* Osteochondrosis, juvenile, patella
- pelvis (juvenile) M91.Ø
- Pierson's M91.Ø
- radius (head) (juvenile) — *see* Osteochondrosis, juvenile, radius
- Scheuermann's — *see* Osteochondrosis, juvenile, spine
- Sever's — *see* Osteochondrosis, juvenile, tarsus
- Sinding-Larsen — *see* Osteochondrosis, juvenile, patella
- spine M42.9
  - adult M42.1Ø
    - cervical region M42.12
    - cervicothoracic region M42.13
    - lumbar region M42.16
    - lumbosacral region M42.17
    - multiple sites M42.19
    - occipito-atlanto-axial region M42.11
    - sacrococcygeal region M42.18
    - thoracic region M42.14
    - thoracolumbar region M42.15
  - juvenile — *see* Osteochondrosis, juvenile, spine
- symphysis pubis (juvenile) M91.Ø
- syphilitic (congenital) A5Ø.Ø2
- talus (juvenile) — *see* Osteochondrosis, juvenile, tarsus
- tarsus (navicular) (juvenile) — *see* Osteochondrosis, juvenile, tarsus
- tibia (proximal) (tubercle) (juvenile) — *see* Osteochondrosis, juvenile, tibia
- tuberculous — *see* Tuberculosis, bone
- ulna (lower) (juvenile) — *see* Osteochondrosis, juvenile, ulna
- van Neck's M91.Ø
- vertebral — *see* Osteochondrosis, spine

Osteoclastoma D48.Ø
- malignant — *see* Neoplasm, bone, malignant

Osteodynia — *see* Disorder, bone, specified type NEC

Osteodystrophy Q78.9
- azotemic N25.Ø
- congenital Q78.9
- parathyroid, secondary E21.1
- renal N25.Ø

Osteofibroma — *see* Neoplasm, bone, benign

Osteofibrosarcoma — *see* Neoplasm, bone, malignant

Osteogenesis imperfecta Q78.Ø

Osteogenic — *see* condition

Osteolysis M89.5Ø
- carpus M89.54-
- clavicle M89.51-
- femur M89.55-
- fibula M89.56-
- finger M89.54-
- humerus M89.52-
- ilium M89.559
- ischium M89.559
- joint prosthesis (periprosthetic) — *see* Complications, joint prosthesis, mechanical, periprosthetic, osteolysis, by site
- metacarpus M89.54-
- metatarsus M89.57-
- multiple sites M89.59
- neck M89.58
- periprosthetic — *see* Complications, joint prosthesis, mechanical, periprosthetic, osteolysis, by site
- radius M89.53-
- rib M89.58
- scapula M89.51-
- skull M89.58
- tarsus M89.57-
- tibia M89.56-
- toe M89.57-
- ulna M89.53-
- vertebra M89.58

Osteoma (*see also* Neoplasm, bone, benign)
- osteoid (*see also* Neoplasm, bone, benign)
  - giant — *see* Neoplasm, bone, benign

Osteomalacia M83.9
- adult M83.9
  - drug-induced NEC M83.5
  - due to
    - malabsorption (postsurgical) M83.2
    - malnutrition M83.3
  - specified NEC M83.8
- aluminium-induced M83.4
- infantile — *see* Rickets
- juvenile — *see* Rickets
- oncogenic E83.89
- pelvis M83.8
- puerperal M83.Ø
- senile M83.1
- vitamin-D-resistant in adults E83.31 *[M90.8-]*
  - carpus E83.31 *[M90.84-]*
  - clavicle E83.31 *[M90.81-]*
  - femur E83.31 *[M90.85-]*
  - fibula E83.31 *[M90.86-]*
  - finger E83.31 *[M90.84-]*
  - humerus E83.31 *[M90.82-]*
  - ilium E83.31 *[M90.859]*
  - ischium E83.31 *[M90.859]*
  - metacarpus E83.31 *[M90.84-]*
  - metatarsus E83.31 *[M90.87-]*
  - multiple sites E83.31 *[M90.89]*
  - neck E83.31 *[M90.88]*
  - radius E83.31 *[M90.83-]*
  - rib E83.31 *[M90.88]*
  - scapula E83.31 *[M90.819]*
  - skull E83.31 *[M90.88]*
  - tarsus E83.31 *[M90.879]*
  - tibia E83.31 *[M90.869]*
  - toe E83.31 *[M90.879]*
  - ulna E83.31 *[M90.839]*
  - vertebra E83.31 *[M90.88]*

Osteomyelitis (general) (infective) (localized) (neonatal) (purulent) (septic) (staphylococcal) (streptococcal) (suppurative) (with periostitis) M86.9
- acute M86.1Ø
  - carpus M86.14-
  - clavicle M86.11-
  - femur M86.15-
  - fibula M86.16-
  - finger M86.14-
  - hematogenous M86.ØØ
    - carpus M86.Ø4-
    - clavicle M86.Ø1-
    - femur M86.Ø5-
    - fibula M86.Ø6-
    - finger M86.Ø4-
    - humerus M86.Ø2-
    - ilium M86.Ø59
    - ischium M86.Ø59
    - mandible M27.2
    - metacarpus M86.Ø4-
    - metatarsus M86.Ø7-
    - multiple sites M86.Ø9
    - neck M86.Ø8
    - orbit HØ5.Ø2-
    - petrous bone — *see* Petrositis
    - radius M86.Ø3-
    - rib M86.Ø8
    - scapula M86.Ø1-
    - skull M86.Ø8
    - tarsus M86.Ø7-
    - tibia M86.Ø6-
    - toe M86.Ø7-
    - ulna M86.Ø3-
    - vertebra — *see* Osteomyelitis, vertebra
  - humerus M86.12-
  - ilium M86.159
  - ischium M86.159
  - mandible M27.2
  - metacarpus M86.14-
  - metatarsus M86.17-
  - multiple sites M86.19
  - neck M86.18
  - orbit HØ5.Ø2-

- **Osteomyelitis** — *continued*
  - acute — *continued*
    - petrous bone — *see* Petrositis
    - radius M86.13-
    - rib M86.18
    - scapula M86.11-
    - skull M86.18
    - tarsus M86.17-
    - tibia M86.16-
    - toe M86.17-
    - ulna M86.13-
    - vertebra — *see* Osteomyelitis, vertebra
  - chronic (or old) M86.6Ø
    - with draining sinus M86.4Ø
      - carpus M86.44-
      - clavicle M86.41-
      - femur M86.45-
      - fibula M86.46-
      - finger M86.44-
      - humerus M86.42-
      - ilium M86.459
      - ischium M86.459
      - mandible M27.2
      - metacarpus M86.44-
      - metatarsus M86.47-
      - multiple sites M86.49
      - neck M86.48
      - orbit HØ5.Ø2-
      - petrous bone — *see* Petrositis
      - radius M86.43-
      - rib M86.48
      - scapula M86.41-
      - skull M86.48
      - tarsus M86.47-
      - tibia M86.46-
      - toe M86.47-
      - ulna M86.43-
      - vertebra — *see* Osteomyelitis, vertebra
    - carpus M86.64-
    - clavicle M86.61-
    - femur M86.65-
    - fibula M86.66-
    - finger M86.64-
    - hematogenous NEC M86.5Ø
      - carpus M86.54-
      - clavicle M86.51-
      - femur M86.55-
      - fibula M86.56-
      - finger M86.54-
      - humerus M86.52-
      - ilium M86.559
      - ischium M86.559
      - mandible M27.2
      - metacarpus M86.54-
      - metatarsus M86.57-
      - multifocal M86.3Ø
        - carpus M86.34-
        - clavicle M86.31-
        - femur M86.35-
        - fibula M86.36-
        - finger M86.34-
        - humerus M86.32-
        - ilium M86.359
        - ischium M86.359
        - metacarpus M86.34-
        - metatarsus M86.37-
        - multiple sites M86.39
        - neck M86.38
        - radius M86.33-
        - rib M86.38
        - scapula M86.31-
        - skull M86.38
        - tarsus M86.37-
        - tibia M86.36-
        - toe M86.37-
        - ulna M86.33-
        - vertebra — *see* Osteomyelitis, vertebra
      - multiple sites M86.59
      - neck M86.58
      - orbit HØ5.Ø2-
      - petrous bone — *see* Petrositis
      - radius M86.53-
      - rib M86.58

- **Osteomyelitis** — *continued*
  - chronic (or old)— *continued*
    - hematogenous — *continued*
      - scapula M86.51-
      - skull M86.58
      - tarsus M86.57-
      - tibia M86.56-
      - toe M86.57-
      - ulna M86.53-
      - vertebra — *see* Osteomyelitis, vertebra
    - humerus M86.62-
    - ilium M86.659
    - ischium M86.659
    - mandible M27.2
    - metacarpus M86.64-
    - metatarsus M86.67-
    - multifocal — *see* Osteomyelitis, chronic, hematogenous, multifocal
    - multiple sites M86.69
    - neck M86.68
    - orbit HØ5.Ø2-
    - petrous bone — *see* Petrositis
    - radius M86.63-
    - rib M86.68
    - scapula M86.61-
    - skull M86.68
    - tarsus M86.67-
    - tibia M86.66-
    - toe M86.67-
    - ulna M86.63-
    - vertebra — *see* Osteomyelitis, vertebra
  - echinococcal B67.2
  - Garr's — *see* Osteomyelitis, specified type NEC
  - jaw (acute) (chronic) (lower) (neonatal) (suppurative) (upper) M27.2
  - nonsuppurating — *see* Osteomyelitis, specified type NEC
  - orbit HØ5.Ø2-
  - petrous bone — *see* Petrositis
  - Salmonella (arizonae) (cholerae-suis) (enteritidis) (typhimurium) AØ2.24
  - sclerosing, nonsuppurative — *see* Osteomyelitis, specified type NEC
  - specified type NEC (*see also* subcategory) M86.8x-
    - mandible M27.2
    - orbit HØ5.Ø2-
    - petrous bone — *see* Petrositis
    - vertebra — *see* Osteomyelitis, vertebra
  - subacute M86.2Ø
    - carpus M86.24-
    - clavicle M86.21-
    - femur M86.25-
    - fibula M86.26-
    - finger M86.24-
    - humerus M86.22-
    - mandible M27.2
    - metacarpus M86.24-
    - metatarsus M86.27-
    - multiple sites M86.29
    - neck M86.28
    - orbit HØ5.Ø2-
    - petrous bone — *see* Petrositis
    - radius M86.23-
    - rib M86.28
    - scapula M86.21-
    - skull M86.28
    - tarsus M86.27-
    - tibia M86.26-
    - toe M86.27-
    - ulna M86.23-
    - vertebra — *see* Osteomyelitis, vertebra
  - syphilitic A52.77
    - congenital (early) A5Ø.Ø2 *[M90.80]*
  - tuberculous — *see* Tuberculosis, bone
  - typhoid AØ1.Ø5
  - vertebra M46.2Ø
    - cervical region M46.22
    - cervicothoracic region M46.23
    - lumbar region M46.26
    - lumbosacral region M46.27
    - occipito-atlanto-axial region M46.21
    - sacrococcygeal region M46.28
    - thoracic region M46.24

- **Osteomyelitis** — *continued*
  - vertebra— *continued*
    - thoracolumbar region M46.25
- **Osteomyelofibrosis** D75.89
- **Osteomyelosclerosis** D75.89
- **Osteonecrosis** M87.9
  - due to
    - drugs — *see* Osteonecrosis, secondary, due to, drugs
    - trauma — *see* Osteonecrosis, secondary, due to, trauma
  - idiopathic aseptic M87.ØØ
    - ankle M87.Ø7-
    - carpus M87.Ø3-
    - clavicle M87.Ø1-
    - femur M87.Ø5-
    - fibula M87.Ø6-
    - finger M87.Ø4-
    - humerus M87.Ø2-
    - ilium M87.Ø5Ø
    - ischium M87.Ø5Ø
    - metacarpus M87.Ø4-
    - metatarsus M87.Ø7-
    - multiple site M87.Ø9
    - neck M87.Ø8
    - pelvis M87.Ø5Ø
    - radius M87.Ø3-
    - rib M87.Ø8
    - scapula M87.Ø1-
    - skull M87.Ø8
    - tarsus M87.Ø7-
    - tibia M87.Ø6-
    - toe M87.Ø7-
    - ulna M87.Ø3-
    - vertebra M87.Ø8
  - secondary NEC M87.3Ø
    - carpus M87.33-
    - clavicle M87.31-
    - due to
      - drugs M87.1Ø
        - carpus M87.13-
        - clavicle M87.11-
        - femur M87.15-
        - fibula M87.16-
        - finger M87.14-
        - humerus M87.12-
        - ilium M87.159
        - ischium M87.159
        - jaw M87.18Ø
        - metacarpus M87.14-
        - metatarsus M87.17-
        - multiple sites M87.19
        - neck M87.18
        - radius M87.13-
        - rib M87.18
        - scapula M87.11-
        - skull M87.18
        - tarsus M87.17-
        - tibia M87.16-
        - toe M87.17-
        - ulna M87.13-
        - vertebra M87.18
      - hemoglobinopathy NEC D58.2 *[M90.50]*
        - carpus D58.2 *[M90.54-]*
        - clavicle D58.2 *[M90.51-]*
        - femur D58.2 *[M90.55-]*
        - fibula D58.2 *[M90.56-]*
        - finger D58.2 *[M90.54-]*
        - humerus D58.2 *[M90.52-]*
        - ilium D58.2 *[M90.55-]*
        - ischium D58.2 *[M90.55-]*
        - metacarpus D58.2 *[M90.54-]*
        - metatarsus D58.2 *[M90.57-]*
        - multiple sites D58.2 *[M90.58]*
        - neck D58.2 *[M90.58]*
        - radius D58.2 *[M90.53-]*
        - rib D58.2 *[M90.58]*
        - scapula D58.2 *[M90.51-]*
        - skull D58.2 *[M90.58]*
        - tarsus D58.2 *[M90.57-]*
        - tibia D58.2 *[M90.56-]*
        - toe D58.2 *[M90.57-]*
        - ulna D58.2 *[M90.53-]*

- **Osteonecrosis**— *continued*
  - secondary— *continued*
    - due to— *continued*
      - hemoglobinopathy NEC — *continued*
        - vertebra D58.2 *[M90.58]*
      - trauma (previous) M87.2Ø
        - carpus M87.23-
        - clavicle M87.21-
        - femur M87.25-
        - fibula M87.26-
        - finger M87.24-
        - humerus M87.22-
        - ilium M87.25-
        - ischium M87.25-
        - metacarpus M87.24-
        - metatarsus M87.27-
        - multiple sites M87.29
        - neck M87.28
        - radius M87.23-
        - rib M87.28
        - scapula M87.21-
        - skull M87.28
        - tarsus M87.27-
        - tibia M87.26-
        - toe M87.27-
        - ulna M87.23-
        - vertebra M87.28
    - femur M87.35-
    - fibula M87.36-
    - finger M87.34-
    - humerus M87.32-
    - ilium M87.35Ø
    - in
      - caisson disease T7Ø.3 *[M90.50]*
        - carpus T7Ø.3 *[M90.54-]*
        - clavicle T7Ø.3 *[M90.51-]*
        - femur T7Ø.3 *[M90.55-]*
        - fibula T7Ø.3 *[M90.56-]*
        - finger T7Ø.3 *[M90.54-]*
        - humerus T7Ø.3 *[M90.52-]*
        - ilium T7Ø.3 *[M90.55-]*
        - ischium T7Ø.3 *[M90.55-]*
        - metacarpus T7Ø.3 *[M90.54-]*
        - metatarsus T7Ø.3 *[M90.57-]*
        - multiple sites T7Ø.3 *[M90.59]*
        - neck T7Ø.3 *[M90.58]*
        - radius T7Ø.3 *[M90.53-]*
        - rib T7Ø.3 *[M90.58]*
        - scapula T7Ø.3 *[M90.51-]*
        - skull T7Ø.3 *[M90.58]*
        - tarsus T7Ø.3 *[M90.57-]*
        - tibia T7Ø.3 *[M90.56-]*
        - toe T7Ø.3 *[M90.57-]*
        - ulna T7Ø.3 *[M90.53-]*
        - vertebra T7Ø.3 *[M90.58]*
    - ischium M87.35Ø
    - metacarpus M87.34-
    - metatarsus M87.37-
    - multiple site M87.39
    - neck M87.38
    - radius M87.33-
    - rib M87.38
    - scapula M87.319
    - skull M87.38
    - tarsus M87.379
    - tibia M87.366
    - toe M87.379
    - ulna M87.33-
    - vertebra M87.38
  - specified type NEC M87.8Ø
    - carpus M87.83-
    - clavicle M87.81-
    - femur M87.85-
    - fibula M87.86-
    - finger M87.84-
    - humerus M87.82-
    - ilium M87.85-
    - ischium M87.85-
    - metacarpus M87.84-
    - metatarsus M87.87-
    - multiple sites M87.89
    - neck M87.88
    - radius M87.83-

- **Osteonecrosis**— *continued*
  - specified type NEC— *continued*
    - rib M87.88-
    - scapula M87.81-
    - skull M87.88
    - tarsus M87.87-
    - tibia M87.86-
    - toe M87.87-
    - ulna M87.83-
    - vertebra M87.88
- **Osteo-onycho-arthro-dysplasia** Q79.8
- **Osteo-onychodysplasia, hereditary** Q79.8
- **Osteopathia condensans disseminata** Q78.8
- **Osteopathy** (*see also* Osteomyelitis, Osteonecrosis, Osteoporosis)
  - after poliomyelitis M89.6Ø
    - carpus M89.64-
    - clavicle M89.61-
    - femur M89.65-
    - fibula M89.66-
    - finger M89.64-
    - humerus M89.62-
    - ilium M89.659
    - ischium M89.659
    - metacarpus M89.64-
    - metatarsus M89.67-
    - multiple sites M89.69
    - neck M89.68
    - radius M89.63-
    - rib M89.68
    - scapula M89.61-
    - skull M89.68
    - tarsus M89.67-
    - tibia M89.66-
    - toe M89.67-
    - ulna M89.63-
    - vertebra M89.68
  - in (due to)
    - renal osteodystrophy N25.Ø
    - specified diseases classified elsewhere — *see* subcategory M90.8
- **Osteopenia** M85.8-
  - borderline M85.8-
- **Osteoperiostitis** — *see* Osteomyelitis, specified type NEC
- **Osteopetrosis** (familial) Q78.2
- **Osteophyte** M25.7Ø
  - ankle M25.77-
  - elbow M25.72-
  - foot joint M25.77-
  - hand joint M25.74-
  - hip M25.75-
  - knee M25.76-
  - shoulder M25.71-
  - spine M25.78
  - vertebrae M25.78
  - wrist M25.73-
- **Osteopoikilosis** Q78.8
- **Osteoporosis** (female) (male) M81.Ø
  - with current pathological fracture M8Ø.ØØ
  - age-related M81.Ø
    - with current pathologic fracture M8Ø.ØØ
      - carpus M8Ø.Ø4-
      - clavicle M8Ø.Ø1-
      - fibula M8Ø.Ø6-
      - finger M8Ø.Ø4-
      - humerus M8Ø.Ø2-
      - ilium M8Ø.Ø5-
      - ischium M8Ø.Ø5-
      - metacarpus M8Ø.Ø4-
      - metatarsus M8Ø.Ø7-
      - pelvis M8Ø.Ø5-
      - radius M8Ø.Ø3-
      - scapula M8Ø.Ø1-
      - tarsus M8Ø.Ø7-
      - tibia M8Ø.Ø6-
      - toe M8Ø.Ø7-
      - ulna M8Ø.Ø3-
      - vertebra M8Ø.Ø8
  - disuse M81.8
    - with current pathological fracture M8Ø.8Ø
      - carpus M8Ø.84-
      - clavicle M8Ø.81-

- **Osteoporosis**— *continued*
  - disuse — *continued*
    - with current pathological fracture — *continued*
      - fibula M8Ø.86-
      - finger M8Ø.84-
      - humerus M8Ø.82-
      - ilium M8Ø.85-
      - ischium M8Ø.85-
      - metacarpus M8Ø.84-
      - metatarsus M8Ø.87-
      - pelvis M8Ø.85-
      - radius M8Ø.83-
      - scapula M8Ø.81-
      - tarsus M8Ø.87-
      - tibia M8Ø.86-
      - toe M8Ø.87-
      - ulna M8Ø.83-
      - vertebra M8Ø.88
  - drug-induced — *see* Osteoporosis, specified type NEC
  - idiopathic — *see* Osteoporosis, specified type NEC
  - involutional — *see* Osteoporosis, age-related
  - Lequesne M81.6
  - localized M81.6
  - postmenopausal M81.Ø
    - with pathological fracture M8Ø.ØØ
      - carpus M8Ø.Ø4-
      - clavicle M8Ø.Ø1-
      - fibula M8Ø.Ø6-
      - finger M8Ø.Ø4-
      - humerus M8Ø.Ø2-
      - ilium M8Ø.Ø5-
      - ischium M8Ø.Ø5-
      - metacarpus M8Ø.Ø4-
      - metatarsus M8Ø.Ø7-
      - pelvis M8Ø.Ø5-
      - radius M8Ø.Ø3-
      - scapula M8Ø.Ø1-
      - tarsus M8Ø.Ø7-
      - tibia M8Ø.Ø6-
      - toe M8Ø.Ø7-
      - ulna M8Ø.Ø3-
      - vertebra M8Ø.Ø8
  - postoophorectomy — *see* Osteoporosis, specified type NEC
  - postsurgical malabsorption — *see* Osteoporosis, specified type NEC
  - post-traumatic — *see* Osteoporosis, specified type NEC
  - senile — *see* Osteoporosis, age-related
  - specified type NEC M81.8
    - with pathological fracture M8Ø.8Ø
      - carpus M8Ø.84-
      - clavicle M8Ø.81-
      - fibula M8Ø.86-
      - finger M8Ø.84-
      - humerus M8Ø.82-
      - ilium M8Ø.85-
      - ischium M8Ø.85-
      - metacarpus M8Ø.84-
      - metatarsus M8Ø.87-
      - pelvis M8Ø.85-
      - radius M8Ø.83-
      - scapula M8Ø.81-
      - tarsus M8Ø.87-
      - tibia M8Ø.86-
      - toe M8Ø.87-
      - ulna M8Ø.83-
      - vertebra M8Ø.88
- **Osteopsathyrosis** (idiopathica) Q78.Ø
- **Osteoradionecrosis, jaw** (acute) (chronic) (lower) (suppurative) (upper) M27.2
- **Osteosarcoma** (any form) — *see* Neoplasm, bone, malignant
- **Osteosclerosis** Q78.2
  - acquired M85.8-
  - congenita Q77.4
  - fragilitas (generalisata) Q78.2
  - myelofibrosis D75.81
- **Osteosclerotic anemia** D64.89
- **Osteosis**
  - cutis L94.2
  - renal fibrocystic N25.Ø

- **Österreicher-Turner syndrome** Q87.2
- **Ostium**
  - atrioventriculare commune Q21.2
  - primum (arteriosum) (defect) (persistent) Q21.2
  - secundum (arteriosum) (defect) (patent) (persistent) Q21.1
- **Ostrum-Furst syndrome** Q75.8
- **Otalgia** — *see* subcategory H92.Ø
- **Otitis** (acute) H66.9Ø
  - with effusion (*see also* Otitis, media, nonsuppurative)
    - purulent — *see* Otitis, media, suppurative
  - adhesive — *see* subcategory H74.1
  - chronic (*see also* Otitis, media, chronic)
    - with effusion (*see also* Otitis, media, nonsuppurative, chronic)
  - externa H6Ø.9Ø-
    - abscess — *see* Abscess, ear, external
    - acute (noninfective) H6Ø.5Ø-
      - actinic H6Ø.51-
      - chemical H6Ø.52-
      - contact H6Ø.53-
      - eczematoid H6Ø.54-
      - infective — *see* Otitis, externa, infective
      - reactive H6Ø.55-
      - specified NEC H6Ø.59-
    - cellulitis — *see* Cellulitis, ear
    - chronic H6Ø.6-
    - diffuse — *see* Otitis, externa, infective, diffuse
    - hemorrhagic — *see* Otitis, externa, infective, hemorrhagic
    - in (due to)
      - aspergillosis B44.89
      - candidiasis B37.84
      - erysipelas A46 *[H62.40]*
      - herpes (simplex) virus infection BØØ.1
        - zoster BØ2.8
      - impetigo LØ1.ØØ *[H62.40]*
      - infectious disease NEC B99 *[H62.4-]*
      - mycosis NEC B36.9 *[H62.40]*
      - parasitic disease NEC B89 *[H62.40]*
      - viral disease NEC B34.9 *[H62.40]*
      - zoster BØ2.8
    - infective NEC H6Ø.39-
      - abscess — *see* Abscess, ear, external
      - cellulitis — *see* Cellulitis, ear
      - diffuse H6Ø.31-
      - hemorrhagic H6Ø.32-
      - swimmer's ear — *see* Swimmer's, ear
    - malignant H6Ø.2-
    - mycotic B36.9 *[H62.40]*
    - necrotizing — *see* Otitis, externa, malignant
    - Pseudomonas aeruginosa — *see* Otitis, externa, malignant
    - reactive — *see* Otitis, externa, acute, reactive
    - specified NEC — *see* subcategory H6Ø.8
    - tropical B36.8
  - insidiosa — *see* Otosclerosis
  - interna — *see* subcategory H83.Ø
  - media (hemorrhagic) (staphylococcal) (streptococcal) H66.9-
    - with effusion (nonpurulent) — *see* Otitis, media, nonsuppurative
    - acute, subacute H66.9Ø
      - allergic — *see* Otitis, media, nonsuppurative, acute, allergic
      - exudative — *see* Otitis, media, nonsuppurative, acute
      - mucoid — *see* Otitis, media, nonsuppurative, acute
      - necrotizing (*see also* Otitis, media, suppurative, acute)
        - in
          - measles BØ5.3
          - scarlet fever A38.Ø
      - nonsuppurative NEC — *see* Otitis, media, nonsuppurative, acute
      - purulent — *see* Otitis, media, suppurative, acute
      - sanguinous — *see* Otitis, media, nonsuppurative, acute
      - secretory — *see* Otitis, media, nonsuppurative, acute, serous

Otitis — *continued*
- media— *continued*
  - acute, subacute — *continued*
    - seromucinous — *see* Otitis, media, nonsuppurative, acute
    - serous — *see* Otitis, media, nonsuppurative, acute, serous
    - suppurative — *see* Otitis, media, suppurative, acute
  - allergic — *see* Otitis, media, nonsuppurative
  - catarrhal — *see* Otitis, media, nonsuppurative
  - chronic H66.9Ø
    - with effusion (nonpurulent) — *see* Otitis, media, nonsuppurative, chronic
    - allergic — *see* Otitis, media, nonsuppurative, chronic, allergic
    - benign suppurative — *see* Otitis, media, suppurative, chronic, tubotympanic
    - catarrhal — *see* Otitis, media, nonsuppurative, chronic, serous
    - exudative — *see* Otitis, media, nonsuppurative, chronic
    - mucinous — *see* Otitis, media, nonsuppurative, chronic, mucoid
    - mucoid — *see* Otitis, media, nonsuppurative, chronic, mucoid
    - nonsuppurative NEC — *see* Otitis, media, nonsuppurative, chronic
    - purulent — *see* Otitis, media, suppurative, chronic
    - secretory — *see* Otitis, media, nonsuppurative, chronic, mucoid
    - seromucinous — *see* Otitis, media, nonsuppurative, chronic
    - serous — *see* Otitis, media, nonsuppurative, chronic, serous
    - suppurative — *see* Otitis, media, suppurative, chronic
    - transudative — *see* Otitis, media, nonsuppurative, chronic, mucoid
  - exudative — *see* Otitis, media, nonsuppurative
  - in (due to) (with)
    - influenza — *see* Influenza, with, otitis media
    - measles BØ5.3
    - scarlet fever A38.Ø
    - tuberculosis A18.6
    - viral disease NEC B34.- *[H67.-]*
  - mucoid — *see* Otitis, media, nonsuppurative
  - nonsuppurative H65.9-
    - acute or subacute NEC H65.19-
      - allergic H65.11-
        - recurrent H65.11-
      - recurrent H65.19-
      - secretory — *see* Otitis, media, nonsuppurative, serous
      - serous H65.Ø-
        - recurrent H65.Ø-
    - chronic H65.49-
      - allergic H65.41-
      - mucoid H65.3-
      - serous H65.2-
  - postmeasles BØ5.3
  - purulent — *see* Otitis, media, suppurative
  - secretory — *see* Otitis, media, nonsuppurative
  - seromucinous — *see* Otitis, media, nonsuppurative
  - serous — *see* Otitis, media, nonsuppurative
  - suppurative H66.4-
    - acute H66.ØØ-
      - with rupture of ear drum H66.Ø1-
      - recurrent H66.ØØ-
        - with rupture of ear drum H66.Ø1-
    - chronic (*see also* subcategory) H66.3
      - atticoantral H66.2-
      - benign — *see* Otitis, media, suppurative, chronic, tubotympanic
      - tubotympanic H66.1-
  - transudative — *see* Otitis, media, nonsuppurative
- **Otocephaly** Q18.2
- **Otolith syndrome** — *see* subcategory H81.8
- **Otomycosis** (diffuse) **NEC** B36.9 *[H62.40]*
  - in
    - aspergillosis B44.89
    - candidiasis B37.84
    - moniliasis B37.84
- **Otoporosis** — *see* Otosclerosis
- **Otorrhagia** (nontraumatic) H92.2-
  - traumatic — code by Type of injury
- **Otorrhea** H92.1-
  - cerebrospinal G96.Ø
- **Otosclerosis** (general) H8Ø.9-
  - cochlear (endosteal) H8Ø.2-
  - involving
    - otic capsule — *see* Otosclerosis, cochlear
    - oval window
      - nonobliterative H8Ø.Ø-
      - obliterative H8Ø.1-
    - round window — *see* Otosclerosis, cochlear
  - nonobliterative — *see* Otosclerosis, involving, oval window, nonobliterative
  - obliterative — *see* Otosclerosis, involving, oval window, obliterative
  - specified NEC H8Ø.8-
- **Otospongiosis** — *see* Otosclerosis
- **Otto's disease or pelvis** M24.7
- **Outcome of delivery** Z37.9
  - multiple births Z37.9
    - all liveborn Z37.5Ø
      - quadruplets Z37.52
      - quintuplets Z37.53
      - sextuplets Z37.54
      - specified number NEC Z37.59
      - triplets Z37.51
    - all stillborn Z37.7
    - some liveborn Z37.6Ø
      - quadruplets Z37.62
      - quintuplets Z37.63
      - sextuplets Z37.64
      - specified number NEC Z37.69
      - triplets Z37.61
  - single NEC Z37.9
    - liveborn Z37.Ø
    - stillborn Z37.1
  - twins NEC Z37.9
    - both liveborn Z37.2
    - both stillborn Z37.4
    - one liveborn, one stillborn Z37.3
- **Outlet** — *see* condition
- **Ovalocytosis** (congenital) (hereditary) — *see* Elliptocytosis
- **Ovarian** — *see* Condition
- **Ovariocele** N83.4
- **Ovaritis** (cystic) — *see* Oophoritis
- **Ovary, ovarian** (*see also* condition)
  - resistant syndrome E28.39
  - vein syndrome N13.8
- **Overactive** (*see also* Hyperfunction)
  - adrenal cortex NEC E27.Ø
  - bladder N32.81
  - hypothalamus E23.3
  - thyroid — *see* Hyperthyroidism
- **Overactivity** R46.3
  - child — *see* Disorder, attention-deficit hyperactivity
- **Overbite** (deep) (excessive) (horizontal) (vertical) M26.29
- **Overbreathing** — *see* Hyperventilation
- **Overconscientious personality** F6Ø.5
- **Overdevelopment** — *see* Hypertrophy
- **Overdistension** — *see* Distension
- **Overdose, overdosage** (drug) — *see* Table of Drugs and Chemicals, by drug, poisoning
- **Overeating** R63.2
  - nonorganic origin F5Ø.8
  - psychogenic F5Ø.8
- **Overexertion** (effects) (exhaustion) T73.3
- **Overexposure** (effects) T73.9
  - exhaustion T73.2
- **Overfeeding** — *see* Overeating
  - newborn P92.4
- **Overfill, endodontic** M27.52
- **Overgrowth, bone** — *see* Hypertrophy, bone

Overhanging of dental restorative material (unrepairable) KØ8.52
Overheated (places) (effects) — *see* Heat
Overjet (excessive horizontal) M26.23
Overlaid, overlying (suffocation) — *see* Asphyxia, traumatic, due to mechanical threat
Overlap, excessive horizontal (teeth) M26.23
Overlapping toe (acquired) (*see also* Deformity, toe, specified NEC)
- congenital (fifth toe) Q66.89

Overload
- circulatory, due to transfusion (blood) (blood components) (TACO) E87.71
- fluid E87.7Ø
  - due to transfusion (blood) (blood components) E87.71
  - specified NEC E87.79
- iron, due to repeated red blood cell transfusions E83.111
- potassium (K) E87.5
- sodium (Na) E87.Ø

Overnutrition — *see* Hyperalimentation
Overproduction (*see also* Hypersecretion)
- ACTH E27.Ø
- catecholamine E27.5
- growth hormone E22.Ø

Overprotection, child by parent Z62.1
Overriding
- aorta Q25.4
- finger (acquired) — *see* Deformity, finger
  - congenital Q68.1
- toe (acquired) (*see also* Deformity, toe, specified NEC)
  - congenital Q66.89

Overstrained R53.83
- heart — *see* Hypertrophy, cardiac

Overuse, muscle NEC M7Ø.8-
Overweight E66.3
Overworked R53.83
Oviduct — *see* condition
Ovotestis Q56.Ø
Ovulation (cycle)
- failure or lack of N97.Ø
- pain N94.Ø

Ovum — *see* condition
Owren's disease or syndrome (parahemophilia) D68.2
Ox heart — *see* Hypertrophy, cardiac
Oxalosis E72.53
Oxaluria E72.53
Oxycephaly, oxycephalic Q75.Ø
- syphilitic, congenital A5Ø.Ø2

Oxyuriasis B8Ø
Oxyuris vermicularis (infestation) B8Ø
Ozena J31.Ø

P

Pachyderma, pachydermia L85.9
- larynx (verrucosa) J38.7

Pachydermatocele (congenital) Q82.8
Pachydermoperiostosis (*see also* Osteoarthropathy, hypertrophic, specified type NEC)
- clubbed nail M89.4Ø *[L62]*

Pachygyria QØ4.3
Pachymeningitis (adhesive) (basal) (brain) (cervical) (chronic)(circumscribed) (external) (fibrous) (hemorrhagic) (hypertrophic) (internal) (purulent) (spinal) (suppurative) — *see* Meningitis
Pachyonychia (congenital) Q84.5
Pacinian tumor — *see* Neoplasm, skin, benign
Pad, knuckle or Garrod's M72.1
Paget-Schroetter syndrome I82.89Ø
Paget's disease
- with infiltrating duct carcinoma — *see* Neoplasm, breast, malignant
- bone M88.9
  - carpus M88.84-
  - clavicle M88.81-
  - femur M88.85-
  - fibula M88.86-
  - finger M88.84-
  - humerus M88.82-
  - ilium M88.85-
  - in neoplastic disease — *see* Osteitis, deformans, in neoplastic disease
  - ischium M88.85-
  - metacarpus M88.84-
  - metatarsus M88.87-
  - multiple sites M88.89
  - neck M88.88
  - radius M88.83-
  - rib M88.88
  - scapula M88.81-
  - skull M88.Ø
  - tarsus M88.87-
  - tibia M88.86-
  - toe M88.87-
  - ulna M88.83-
  - vertebra M88.88
- breast (female) C5Ø.Ø1-
  - male C5Ø.Ø2-
- extramammary (*see also* Neoplasm, skin, malignant)
  - anus C21.Ø
    - margin C44.59Ø
    - skin C44.59Ø
- intraductal carcinoma — *see* Neoplasm, breast, malignant
- malignant — *see* Neoplasm, skin, malignant
  - breast (female) C5Ø.Ø1-
    - male C5Ø.Ø2-
  - unspecified site (female) C5Ø.Ø1-
    - male C5Ø.Ø2-
- mammary — *see* Paget's disease, breast
- nipple — *see* Paget's disease, breast
- osteitis deformans — *see* Paget's disease, bone

Pain(s) (*see also* Painful) R52
- abdominal R1Ø.9
  - colic R1Ø.83
  - generalized R1Ø.84
    - with acute abdomen R1Ø.Ø
  - lower R1Ø.3Ø
    - left quadrant R1Ø.32
    - pelvic or perineal R1Ø.2
    - periumbilical R1Ø.33
    - right quadrant R1Ø.31
  - rebound — *see* Tenderness, abdominal, rebound
  - severe with abdominal rigidity R1Ø.Ø
  - tenderness — *see* Tenderness, abdominal
  - upper R1Ø.1Ø
    - epigastric R1Ø.13
    - left quadrant R1Ø.12
    - right quadrant R1Ø.11
- acute R52
  - due to trauma G89.11
  - neoplasm related G89.3
  - postprocedural NEC G89.18

Pain(s) — *continued*
- acute— *continued*
  - post-thoracotomy G89.12
  - specified by site code to Pain, by site
- adnexa (uteri) R1Ø.2
- anginoid — *see* Pain, precordial
- anus K62.89
- arm — *see* Pain, limb, upper
- axillary (axilla) M79.62-
- back (postural) M54.9
- bladder R39.89
  - associated with micturition — *see* Micturition, painful
- bone — *see* Disorder, bone, specified type NEC
- breast N64.4
- broad ligament R1Ø.2
- cancer associated (acute) (chronic) G89.3
- cecum — *see* Pain, abdominal
- cervicobrachial M53.1
- chest (central) RØ7.9
  - anterior wall RØ7.89
  - atypical RØ7.89
  - ischemic I2Ø.9
  - musculoskeletal RØ7.89
  - non-cardiac RØ7.89
  - on breathing RØ7.1
  - pleurodynia RØ7.81
  - precordial RØ7.2
  - wall (anterior) RØ7.89
- chronic G89.29
  - associated with significant psychosocial dysfunction G89.4
  - due to trauma G89.21
  - neoplasm related G89.3
  - postoperative NEC G89.28
  - postprocedural NEC G89.28
  - post-thoracotomy G89.22
  - specified NEC G89.29
- coccyx M53.3
- colon — *see* Pain, abdominal
- coronary — *see* Angina
- costochondral RØ7.1
- diaphragm RØ7.1
- due to cancer G89.3
- due to device, implant or graft (*see also* Complications, by site and type, specified NEC) T85.84
  - arterial graft NEC T82.848
  - breast (implant) T85.84
  - catheter NEC T85.84
    - dialysis (renal) T82.848
      - intraperitoneal T85.84
    - infusion NEC T82.848
      - spinal (epidural) (subdural) T85.84
    - urinary (indwelling) T83.84
  - electronic (electrode) (pulse generator) (stimulator)
    - bone T84.84
    - cardiac T82.847
    - nervous system (brain) (peripheral nerve) (spinal) T85.84
    - urinary T83.84
  - fixation, internal (orthopedic) NEC T84.84
  - gastrointestinal (bile duct) (esophagus) T85.84
  - genital NEC T83.84
  - heart NEC T82.847
  - infusion NEC T85.84
  - joint prosthesis T84.84
  - ocular (corneal graft) (orbital implant) NEC T85.84
  - orthopedic NEC T84.84
  - specified NEC T85.84
  - urinary NEC T83.84
  - vascular NEC T82.848
  - ventricular intracranial shunt T85.84
- due to malignancy (primary) (secondary) G89.3
- ear — *see* subcategory H92.Ø
- epigastric, epigastrium R1Ø.13
- eye — *see* Pain, ocular
- face, facial R51
  - atypical G5Ø.1
- female genital organs NEC N94.89
- finger — *see* Pain, limb, upper

- **Pancolitis, ulcerative** — *continued*
  - with — *continued*
    - obstruction K51.Ø12
    - rectal bleeding K51.Ø11
    - specified complication NEC K51.Ø18
- **Pancreas, pancreatic** — *see* condition
- **Pancreatitis** (annular) (apoplectic) (calcareous) (edematous) (hemorrhagic) (malignant) (recurrent) (subacute) (suppurative) K85.9
  - acute K85.9
    - alcohol induced K85.2
    - biliary K85.1
    - drug induced K85.3
    - gallstone K85.1
    - idiopathic K85.Ø
    - specified NEC K85.8
  - chronic (infectious) K86.1
    - alcohol-induced K86.Ø
    - recurrent K86.1
    - relapsing K86.1
  - cystic (chronic) K86.1
  - cytomegaloviral B25.2
  - fibrous (chronic) K86.1
  - gangrenous K85.8
  - gallstone K85.1
  - interstitial (chronic) K86.1
    - acute K85.8
  - mumps B26.3
  - recurrent (chronic) K86.1
  - relapsing, chronic K86.1
  - syphilitic A52.74
- **Pancreatoblastoma** — *see* Neoplasm, pancreas, malignant
- **Pancreolithiasis** K86.8
- **Pancytolysis** D75.89
- **Pancytopenia** (acquired) D61.818
  - with
    - malformations D61.Ø9
    - myelodysplastic syndrome — *see* Syndrome, myelodysplastic
  - antineoplastic chemotherapy induced D61.81Ø
  - congenital D61.Ø9
  - drug-induced NEC D61.811
- **Panencephalitis, subacute, sclerosing** A81.1
- **Panhematopenia** D61.9
  - congenital D61.Ø9
  - constitutional D61.Ø9
  - splenic, primary D73.1
- **Panhemocytopenia** D61.9
  - congenital D61.Ø9
  - constitutional D61.Ø9
- **Panhypogonadism** E29.1
- **Panhypopituitarism** E23.Ø
  - prepubertal E23.Ø
- **Panic** (attack) (state) F41.Ø
  - reaction to exceptional stress (transient) F43.Ø
- **Panmyelopathy, familial, constitutional** D61.Ø9
- **Panmyelophthisis** D61.82
  - congenital D61.Ø9
- **Panmyelosis** (acute) (with myelofibrosis) C94.4-
- **Panner's disease** — *see* Osteochondrosis, juvenile, humerus
- **Panneuritis endemica** E51.11
- **Panniculitis** (nodular) (nonsuppurative) M79.3
  - back M54.ØØ
    - cervical region M54.Ø2
    - cervicothoracic region M54.Ø3
    - lumbar region M54.Ø6
    - lumbosacral region M54.Ø7
    - multiple sites M54.Ø9
    - occipito-atlanto-axial region M54.Ø1
    - sacrococcygeal region M54.Ø8
    - thoracic region M54.Ø4
    - thoracolumbar region M54.Ø5
  - lupus L93.2
  - mesenteric K65.4
  - neck M54.Ø2
    - cervicothoracic region M54.Ø3
    - occipito-atlanto-axial region M54.Ø1
  - relapsing M35.6
- **Panniculus adiposus** (abdominal) E65
- **Pannus** (allergic) (cornea) (degenerativus) (keratic) H16.42-
  - abdominal (symptomatic) E65
  - trachomatosus, trachomatous (active) A71.1
- **Panophthalmitis** H44.Ø1-
- **Pansinusitis** (chronic) (hyperplastic) (nonpurulent) (purulent) J32.4
  - acute JØ1.4Ø
    - recurrent JØ1.41
  - tuberculous A15.8
- **Panuveitis** (sympathetic) H44.11-
- **Panvalvular disease** IØ8.9
  - specified NEC IØ8.8
- **Papanicolaou smear, cervix** Z12.4
  - as part of routine gynecological examination ZØ1.419
    - with abnormal findings ZØ1.411
  - for suspected neoplasm Z12.4
  - nonspecific abnormal finding R87.619
  - routine ZØ1.419
    - with abnormal findings ZØ1.411
- **Papilledema** (choked disc) H47.1Ø
  - associated with
    - decreased ocular pressure H47.12
    - increased intracranial pressure H47.11
    - retinal disorder H47.13
  - Foster-Kennedy syndrome H47.14-
- **Papillitis** H46.ØØ
  - anus K62.89
  - chronic lingual K14.4
  - necrotizing, kidney N17.2
  - optic H46.Ø-
  - rectum K62.89
  - renal, necrotizing N17.2
  - tongue K14.Ø
- **Papilloma** (*see also* Neoplasm, benign, by site)
  - acuminatum (female) (male) (anogenital) A63.Ø
  - benign pinta (primary) A67.Ø
  - bladder (urinary) (transitional cell) D41.4
  - choroid plexus (lateral ventricle) (third ventricle) D33.Ø
    - anaplastic C71.5
    - fourth ventricle D33.1
    - malignant C71.5
  - renal pelvis (transitional cell) D41.1-
    - benign D3Ø.1-
  - Schneiderian
    - specified site — *see* Neoplasm, benign, by site
    - unspecified stie D14.Ø
  - serous surface
    - borderline malignancy
      - specified site — *see* Neoplasm, uncertain behavior, by site
      - unspecified
    - specified site — see Neoplasm, benign, by site
    - unspecified site D27.9
  - transitional (cell)
    - bladder (urinary) D41.4
    - inverted type — *see* Neoplasm, uncertain behavior, by site
    - renal pelvis D41.1-
    - ureter D41.2-
  - ureter (transitional cell) D41.2-
    - benign D3Ø.2-
  - urothelial — *see* Neoplasm, uncertain behavior, by site
  - villous — *see* Neoplasm, uncertain behavior, by site
    - adenocarcinoma in — *see* Neoplasm, malignant by site
    - in situ — *see* Neoplasm, in situ
  - yaws, plantar or palmar A66.1
- **Papillomata, multiple, of yaws** A66.1
- **Papillomatosis** (*see also* Neoplasm, benign, by site)
  - confluent and reticulated L83
  - cystic, breast — *see* Mastopathy, cystic
  - ductal, breast — *see* Mastopathy, cystic
  - intraductal (diffuse) — *see* Neoplasm, benign, by site
  - subareolar duct D24-
- **Papillomavirus, as cause of disease classified elsewhere** B97.7
- **Papillon-Léage and Psaume syndrome** Q87.Ø
- **Papule(s)** R23.8
  - carate (primary) A67.Ø
  - fibrous, of nose D22.39
  - Gottron's L94.4
  - pinta (primary) A67.Ø
- **Papulosis**
  - lymphomatoid C86.6
  - malignant I77.89
- **Papyraceous fetus** O31.Ø-
- **Para-albuminemia** E88.Ø9
- **Paracephalus** Q89.7
- **Parachute mitral valve** Q23.2
- **Paracoccidioidomycosis** B41.9
  - disseminated B41.7
  - generalized B41.7
  - mucocutaneous-lymphangitic B41.8
  - pulmonary B41.Ø
  - specified NEC B41.8
  - visceral B41.8
- **Paradentosis** KØ5.4
- **Paraffinoma** T88.8
- **Paraganglioma** D44.7
  - adrenal D35.Ø-
    - malignant C74.1-
  - aortic body D44.7
    - malignant C75.5
  - carotid body D44.6
    - malignant C75.4
  - chromaffin (*see also* Neoplasm, benign, by site)
    - malignant — *see* Neoplasm, malignant, by site
  - extra-adrenal D44.7
    - malignant C75.5
      - specified site — *see* Neoplasm
    - specified site — *see* Neoplasm, uncertain behavior, by site
  - gangliocytic D13.2
    - specified site — *see* Neoplasm, benign, by site
  - glomus jugulate D44.7
  - jugular D44.7
  - malignant C75.5
    - specified site — *see* Neoplasm, malignant, by site
  - nonchromaffin D44.7
    - malignant C75.5
      - specifed site — *see* Neoplasm, malignant, by site
    - specifed site — *see* Neoplasm, uncertain behavior, by site
  - parasympathetic D44.7
    - specified site — *see* Neoplasm, uncertain behavior, by site
  - specified site — *see* Neoplasm, uncertain behavior, by site
  - sympathetic D44.7
    - specified site — *see* Neoplasm, uncertain behavior, by site
    - unspecified site D44.7
  - unspecified site D44.7
- **Parageusia** R43.2
  - psychogenic F45.8
- **Paragonimiasis** B66.4
- **Paragranuloma, Hodgkin** — *see* Lymphoma, Hodgkin, classical, specified NEC
- **Parahemophilia** (*see also* Defect, coagulation) D68.2
- **Parakeratosis** R23.4
  - variegata L41.Ø
- **Paralysis, paralytic** (complete) (incomplete) G83.9
  - with
    - syphilis A52.17
  - abducens, abducent (nerve) — *see* Strabismus, paralytic, sixth nerve
  - abductor, lower extremity G57.9-
  - accessory nerve G52.8
  - accommodation (*see also* Paresis, of accommodation)
    - hysterical F44.89
  - acoustic nerve (except Deafness) — *see* subcategory H93.3
  - agitans (*see also* Parkinsonism) G2Ø
    - arteriosclerotic G21.4
  - alternating (oculomotor) G83.89
  - amyotrophic G12.21
  - ankle G57.9-

Paresthesia *(see also* Disturbance, sensation)
  Bernhardt G57.1-
Paretic — *see* condition
Parinaud's
  conjunctivitis H1Ø.89
  oculoglandular syndrome H1Ø.89
  ophthalmoplegia H49.88-
Parkinsonism (idiopathic) (primary) G2Ø
  with neurogenic orthostatic hypotension (symptomatic) G9Ø.3
  arteriosclerotic G21.4
  dementia G31.83 *[F02.80]*
    with behavioral disturbance G31.83 *[F02.81]*
  due to
    drugs NEC G21.19
      neuroleptic G21.11
  neuroleptic induced G21.11
  postencephalitic G21.3
  secondary G21.9
    due to
      arteriosclerosis G21.4
      drugs NEC G21.19
        neuroleptic G21.11
      encephalitis G21.3
      external agents NEC G21.2
      syphilis A52.19
    specified NEC G21.8
  syphilitic A52.19
  treatment-induced NEC G21.19
  vascular G21.4
Parkinson's disease, syndrome or tremor — *see* Parkinsonism
Parodontitis — *see* Periodontitis
Parodontosis KØ5.4
Paronychia *(see also* Cellulitis, digit)
  with lymphangitis — *see* Lymphangitis, acute, digit
  candidal (chronic) B37.2
  tuberculous (primary) A18.4
Parorexia (psychogenic) F5Ø.8
Parosmia R43.1
  psychogenic F45.8
Parotid gland — *see* condition
Parotitis, parotiditis (allergic)(nonspecific toxic) (purulent) (septic) (suppurative) *(see also* Sialoadenitis)
  epidemic — *see* Mumps
  infectious — *see* Mumps
  postoperative K91.89
  surgical K91.89
Parrot fever A7Ø
Parrot's disease (early congenital syphilitic pseudoparalysis) A5Ø.Ø2
Parry-Romberg syndrome G51.8
Parry's disease or syndrome EØ5.ØØ
  with thyroid storm EØ5.Ø1
Pars planitis — *see* Cyclitis
Parsonage(-Aldren)-**Turner syndrome** G54.5
Parson's disease (exophthalmic goiter) EØ5.ØØ
  with thyroid storm EØ5.Ø1
Particolored infant Q82.8
Parturition — *see* Delivery
Parulis KØ4.7
  with sinus KØ4.6
Parvovirus, as cause of disease classified elsewhere B97.6
Pasini and Pierini's atrophoderma L9Ø.3
Passage
  false, urethra N36.5
  meconium (newborn) during delivery PØ3.82
  of sounds or bougies — *see* Attention to, artificial, opening
Passive — *see* condition
  smoking Z77.22
Pasteurella septica A28.Ø
Pasteurellosis — *see* Infection, Pasteurella
PAT (paroxysmal atrial tachycardia) I47.1
Patau's syndrome — *see* Trisomy, 13
Patches
  mucous (syphilitic) A51.39
    congenital A5Ø.Ø7
  smokers' (mouth) K13.24
Patellar — *see* condition
Patent *(see also* Imperfect, closure)
  canal of Nuck Q52.4
  cervix N88.3
  ductus arteriosus or Botallo's Q25.Ø
  foramen
    botalli Q21.1
    ovale Q21.1
  interauricular septum Q21.1
  interventricular septum Q21.Ø
  omphalomesenteric duct Q43.Ø
  os (uteri) — *see* Patent, cervix
  ostium secundum Q21.1
  urachus Q64.4
  vitelline duct Q43.Ø
Paterson(-Brown)(-Kelly) **syndrome or web** D5Ø.1
Pathologic, pathological *(see also* condition)
  asphyxia RØ9.Ø1
  fire-setting F63.1
  gambling F63.Ø
  ovum OØ2.Ø
  resorption, tooth KØ3.3
  stealing F63.2
Pathology (of) — *see* Disease
  periradicular, associated with previous endodontic treatment NEC M27.59
Pattern, sleep-wake, irregular G47.23
Patulous *(see also* Imperfect, closure (congenital))
  alimentary tract Q45.8
    lower Q43.8
    upper Q4Ø.8
  eustachian tube H69.Ø-
Pause, sinoatrial I49.5
Paxton's disease B36.2
Pearl(s)
  enamel KØØ.2
  Epstein's KØ9.8
Pearl-worker's disease — *see* Osteomyelitis, specified type NEC
Pectenosis K62.4
Pectoral — *see* condition
Pectus
  carinatum (congenital) Q67.7
    acquired M95.4
    rachitic sequelae (late effect) E64.3
  excavatum (congenital) Q67.6
    acquired M95.4
    rachitic sequelae (late effect) E64.3
  recurvatum (congenital) Q67.6
Pedatrophia E41
Pederosis F65.4
Pediculosis (infestation) B85.2
  capitis (head-louse) (any site) B85.Ø
  corporis (body-louse) (any site) B85.1
  eyelid B85.Ø
  mixed (classifiable to more than one of the titles B85.Ø-B85.3) B85.4
  pubis (pubic louse) (any site) B85.3
  vestimenti B85.1
  vulvae B85.3
Pediculus (infestation) — *see* Pediculosis
Pedophilia F65.4
Peg-shaped teeth KØØ.2
Pelade — *see* Alopecia, areata
Pelger-Huët anomaly or syndrome D72.Ø
Peliosis (rheumatica) D69.Ø
  hepatis K76.4
    with toxic liver disease K71.8
Pelizaeus-Merzbacher disease E75.29
Pellagra (alcoholic) (with polyneuropathy) E52
Pellagra-cerebellar-ataxia-renal aminoaciduria syndrome E72.Ø2
Pellegrini (-Stieda) **disease or syndrome** — *see* Bursitis, tibial collateral
Pellizzi's syndrome E34.8
Pel's crisis A52.11
Pelvic *(see also* condition)
  examination (periodic) (routine) ZØ1.419
    with abnormal findings ZØ1.411
  kidney, congenital Q63.2
Pelviolithiasis — *see* Calculus, kidney
Pelviperitonitis *(see also* Peritonitis, pelvic)
  gonococcal A54.24
  puerperal O85
Pelvis — *see* condition or type
Pemphigoid L12.9
  benign, mucous membrane L12.1
  bullous L12.Ø
  cicatricial L12.1
  juvenile L12.2
  ocular L12.1
  specified NEC L12.8
Pemphigus L1Ø.9
  benign familial (chronic) Q82.8
  Brazilian L1Ø.3
  circinatus L13.Ø
  conjunctiva L12.1
  drug-induced L1Ø.5
  erythematosus L1Ø.4
  foliaceous L1Ø.2
  gangrenous — *see* Gangrene
  neonatorum LØ1.Ø3
  ocular L12.1
  paraneoplastic L1Ø.81
  specified NEC L1Ø.89
  syphilitic (congenital) A5Ø.Ø6
  vegetans L1Ø.1
  vulgaris L1Ø.Ø
  wildfire L1Ø.3
Pendred's syndrome EØ7.1
Pendulous
  abdomen, in pregnancy — *see* Pregnancy, complicated by, abnormal, pelvic organs or tissues NEC
  breast N64.89
Penetrating wound *(see also* Puncture)
  with internal injury — *see* Injury, by site
  eyeball — *see* Puncture, eyeball
  orbit (with or without foreign body) — *see* Puncture, orbit
  uterus by instrument with or following ectopic or molar pregnancy OØ8.6
Penicillosis B48.4
Penis — *see* condition
Penitis N48.29
Pentalogy of Fallot Q21.8
Pentasomy X syndrome Q97.1
Pentosuria (essential) E74.8
Percreta placenta O43.23
Peregrinating patient — *see* Disorder, factitious
Perforation, perforated (nontraumatic) (of)
  accidental during procedure (blood vessel) (nerve) (organ) — *see* Complication, accidental puncture or laceration
  antrum — *see* Sinusitis, maxillary
  appendix K35.2
  atrial septum, multiple Q21.1
  attic, ear — *see* Perforation, tympanum, attic
  bile duct (common) (hepatic) K83.2
    cystic K82.2
  bladder (urinary)
    with or following ectopic or molar pregnancy OØ8.6
    obstetrical trauma O71.5
    traumatic S37.29
      at delivery O71.5
  bowel K63.1
    with or following ectopic or molar pregnancy OØ8.6
    newborn P78.Ø
    obstetrical trauma O71.5
    traumatic — *see* Laceration, intestine
  broad ligament N83.8
    with or following ectopic or molar pregnancy OØ8.6
    obstetrical trauma O71.6
  by
    device, implant or graft *(see also* Complications, by site and type, mechanical) T85.628
      arterial graft NEC — *see* Complication, cardiovascular device, mechanical, vascular
      breast (implant) T85.49
      catheter NEC T85.698
        cystostomy T83.Ø9Ø

Pericarditis— *continued*
- fibrinopurulent I3Ø.1
- fibrinous I3Ø.8
- fibrous I31.Ø
- gonococcal A54.83
- idiopathic I3Ø.Ø
- in systemic lupus erythematosus M32.12
- infective I3Ø.1
- meningococcal A39.53
- neoplastic (chronic) I31.8
  - acute I3Ø.9
- obliterans, obliterating I31.Ø
- plastic I31.Ø
- pneumococcal I3Ø.1
- postinfarction I24.1
- purulent I3Ø.1
- rheumatic (active) (acute) (with effusion) (with pneumonia) IØ1.Ø
  - with chorea (acute) (rheumatic) (Sydenham's) IØ2.Ø
  - chronic or inactive (with chorea) IØ9.2
- rheumatoid — *see* Rheumatoid, carditis
- septic I3Ø.1
- serofibrinous I3Ø.8
- staphylococcal I3Ø.1
- streptococcal I3Ø.1
- suppurative I3Ø.1
- syphilitic A52.Ø6
- tuberculous A18.84
- uremic N18.9 *[I32]*
- viral I3Ø.1

Pericardium, pericardial — *see* condition
Pericellulitis — *see* Cellulitis
Pericementitis (chronic) (suppurative) *(see also* Periodontitis)
- acute KØ5.2Ø
  - generalized KØ5.22
  - localized KØ5.21

Perichondritis
- auricle — *see* Perichondritis, ear
- bronchus J98.Ø9
- ear (external) H61.ØØ-
  - acute H61.Ø1-
  - chronic H61.Ø2-
- external auditory canal — *see* Perichondritis, ear
- larynx J38.7
  - syphilitic A52.73
  - typhoid AØ1.Ø9
- nose J34.89
- pinna — *see* Perichondritis, ear
- trachea J39.8

Periclasia KØ5.4
Pericoronitis — *see* Periodontitis
Pericystitis N3Ø.9Ø
- with hematuria N3Ø.91

Peridiverticulitis (intestine) K57.92
- cecum — *see* Diverticulitis, intestine, large
- colon — *see* Diverticulitis, intestine, large
- duodenum — *see* Diverticulitis, intestine, small
- intestine — *see* Diverticulitis, intestine
- jejunum — *see* Diverticulitis, intestine, small
- rectosigmoid — *see* Diverticulitis, intestine, large
- rectum — *see* Diverticulitis, intestine, large
- sigmoid — *see* Diverticulitis, intestine, large

Periendocarditis — *see* Endocarditis
Periepididymitis N45.1
Perifolliculitis LØ1.Ø2
- abscedens, caput, scalp L66.3
- capitis, abscedens (et suffodiens) L66.3
- superficial pustular LØ1.Ø2

Perihepatitis K65.8
Perilabyrinthitis (acute) — *see* subcategory H83.Ø
Perimeningitis — *see* Meningitis
Perimetritis — *see* Endometritis
Perimetrosalpingitis — *see* Salpingo-oophoritis
Perineocele N81.81
Perinephric, perinephritic — *see* condition
Perinephritis *(see also* Infection, kidney)
- purulent — *see* Abscess, kidney

Perineum, perineal — *see* condition
Perineuritis NEC — *see* Neuralgia
Periodic — *see* condition
Periodontitis (chronic) (complex) (compound) (local) (simplex) KØ5.3Ø
- acute KØ5.2Ø
  - generalized KØ5.22
  - localized KØ5.21
- apical KØ4.5
  - acute (pulpal origin) KØ4.4
- generalized KØ5.32
- localized KØ5.31

Periodontoclasia KØ5.4
Periodontosis (juvenile) KØ5.4
Periods *(see also* Menstruation)
- heavy N92.Ø
- irregular N92.6
- shortened intervals (irregular) N92.1

Perionychia *(see also* Cellulitis, digit)
- with lymphangitis — *see* Lymphangitis, acute, digit

Perioophoritis — *see* Salpingo-oophoritis
Periorchitis N45.2
Periosteum, periosteal — *see* condition
Periostitis (albuminosa) (circumscribed) (diffuse) (infective) (monomelic) *(see also* Osteomyelitis)
- alveolar M27.3
- alveolodental M27.3
- dental M27.3
- gonorrheal A54.43
- jaw (lower) (upper) M27.2
- orbit HØ5.Ø3-
- syphilitic A52.77
  - congenital (early) A5Ø.Ø2 *[M9Ø.8Ø]*
  - secondary A51.46
- tuberculous — *see* Tuberculosis, bone
- yaws (hypertrophic) (early) (late) A66.6 *[M9Ø.8Ø]*

Periostosis (hyperplastic) *(see also* Disorder, bone, specified type NEC)
- with osteomyelitis — *see* Osteomyelitis, specified type NEC

Peripartum
- cardiomyopathy O9Ø.3

Periphlebitis — *see* Phlebitis
Periproctitis K62.89
Periprostatitis — *see* Prostatitis
Perirectal — *see* condition
Perirenal — *see* condition
Perisalpingitis — *see* Salpingo-oophoritis
Perisplenitis (infectional) D73.89
Peristalsis, visible or reversed R19.2
Peritendinitis — *see* Enthesopathy
Peritoneum, peritoneal — *see* condition
Peritonitis (adhesive) (bacterial) (fibrinous) (hemorrhagic) (idiopathic) (localized) (perforative) (primary) (with adhesions) (with effusion) K65.9
- with or following
  - abscess K65.1
  - appendicitis K35.2
    - with perforation or rupture K35.2
    - localized K35.3
    - generalized K35.2
  - diverticular disease (intestine) K57.8Ø
    - with bleeding K57.81
    - large intestine K57.2Ø
      - with
        - bleeding K57.21
        - small intestine K57.4Ø
          - with bleeding K57.41
    - small intestine K57.ØØ
      - with
        - bleeding K57.Ø1
        - large intestine K57.4Ø
          - with bleeding K57.41
  - ectopic or molar pregnancy OØ8.Ø
- acute (generalized) K65.Ø
- aseptic T81.61
- bile, biliary K65.3
- chemical T81.61
- chlamydial A74.81
- complicating abortion — *see* Abortion, by type, complicated by, pelvic peritonitis
- congenital P78.1
- chronic proliferative K65.8
- diaphragmatic K65.Ø
- diffuse K65.Ø

Peritonitis— *continued*
- diphtheritic A36.89
- disseminated K65.Ø
- due to
  - bile K65.3
  - foreign
    - body or object accidentally left during a procedure (instrument) (sponge) (swab) T81.599
    - substance accidentally left during a procedure (chemical) (powder) (talc) T81.61
  - talc T81.61
  - urine K65.8
- eosinophilic K65.8
  - acute K65.Ø
- fibrocaseous (tuberculous) A18.31
- fibropurulent K65.Ø
- following ectopic or molar pregnancy OØ8.Ø
- general(ized) K65.Ø
- gonococcal A54.85
- meconium (newborn) P78.Ø
- neonatal P78.1
  - meconium P78.Ø
- pancreatic K65.Ø
- paroxysmal, familial E85.Ø
  - benign E85.Ø
- pelvic
  - female N73.5
    - acute N73.3
    - chronic N73.4
      - with adhesions N73.6
  - male K65.Ø
- periodic, familial E85.Ø
- proliferative, chronic K65.8
- puerperal, postpartum, childbirth O85
- purulent K65.Ø
- septic K65.Ø
- specified NEC K65.8
- spontaneous bacterial K65.2
- subdiaphragmatic K65.Ø
- subphrenic K65.Ø
- suppurative K65.Ø
- syphilitic A52.74
  - congenital (early) A5Ø.Ø8 *[K67]*
- talc T81.61
- tuberculous A18.31
- urine K65.8

Peritonsillar — *see* condition
Peritonsillitis J36
Perityphlitis K37
Periureteritis N28.89
Periurethral — *see* condition
Periurethritis (gangrenous) — *see* Urethritis
Periuterine — *see* condition
Perivaginitis — *see* Vaginitis
Perivasculitis, retinal H35.Ø6-
Perivasitis (chronic) N49.1
Perivesiculitis (seminal) — *see* Vesiculitis
Perlèche NEC K13.Ø
- due to
  - candidiasis B37.83
  - moniliasis B37.83
  - riboflavin deficiency E53.Ø
  - vitamin B2 (riboflavin) deficiency E53.Ø

Pernicious — *see* condition
Pernio, perniosis T69.1
Perpetrator (of abuse) — *see* Index to External Cause of Injury, Perpetrator
Persecution
- delusion F22
- social Z6Ø.5

Perseveration (tonic) R48.8
Persistence, persistent (congenital)
- anal membrane Q42.3
  - with fistula Q42.2
- arteria stapedia Q16.3
- atrioventricular canal Q21.2
- branchial cleft Q18.Ø
- bulbus cordis in left ventricle Q21.8
- canal of Cloquet Q14.Ø
- capsule (opaque) Q12.8
- cilioretinal artery or vein Q14.8
- cloaca Q43.7

Persistence, persistent— *continued*
- communication — *see* Fistula, congenital
- convolutions
  - aortic arch Q25.4
  - fallopian tube Q5Ø.6
  - oviduct Q5Ø.6
  - uterine tube Q5Ø.6
- double aortic arch Q25.4
- ductus arteriosus (Botalli) Q25.Ø
- fetal
  - circulation P29.3
  - form of cervix (uteri) Q51.828
  - hemoglobin, hereditary (HPFH) D56.4
- foramen
  - Botalli Q21.1
  - ovale Q21.1
- Gartner's duct Q52.4
- hemoglobin, fetal (hereditary) (HPFH) D56.4
- hyaloid
  - artery (generally incomplete) Q14.Ø
  - system Q14.8
- hymen, in pregnancy or childbirth — *see* Pregnancy, complicated by, abnormal, vulva
- lanugo Q84.2
- left
  - posterior cardinal vein Q26.8
  - root with right arch of aorta Q25.4
  - superior vena cava Q26.1
- Meckel's diverticulum Q43.Ø
  - malignant — *see* Table of Neoplams, small intestine, malignant
- mucosal disease (middle ear) — *see* Otitis, media, suppurative, chronic, tubotympanic
- nail(s), anomalous Q84.6
- omphalomesenteric duct Q43.Ø
- organ or site not listed — *see* Anomaly, by site
- ostium
  - atrioventriculare commune Q21.2
  - primum Q21.2
  - secundum Q21.1
- ovarian rests in fallopian tube Q5Ø.6
- pancreatic tissue in intestinal tract Q43.8
- primary (deciduous)
  - teeth KØØ.6
  - vitreous hyperplasia Q14.Ø
- pupillary membrane Q13.89
- right aortic arch Q25.4
- rhesus (Rh) titer — *see* Complication(s), transfusion, incompatibility reaction, Rh (factor)
- sinus
  - urogenitalis
    - female Q52.8
    - male Q55.8
  - venosus with imperfect incorporation in right auricle Q26.8
- thymus (gland) (hyperplasia) E32.Ø
- thyroglossal duct Q89.2
- thyrolingual duct Q89.2
- truncus arteriosus or communis Q2Ø.Ø
- tunica vasculosa lentis Q12.2
- umbilical sinus Q64.4
- urachus Q64.4
- vitelline duct Q43.Ø

Person (with)
- admitted for clinical research, as a control subject (normal comparison) (participant) ZØØ.6
- awaiting admission to adequate facility elsewhere Z75.1
- concern (normal) about sick person in family Z63.6
- consulting on behalf of another Z71.Ø
- feigning illness Z76.5
- living (in)
  - alone Z6Ø.2
  - boarding school Z59.3
  - residential institution Z59.3
  - without
    - adequate housing (heating) (space) Z59.1
    - housing (permanent) (temporary) Z59.Ø
    - person able to render necessary care Z74.2
    - shelter Z59.Ø
- on waiting list Z75.1
- sick or handicapped in family Z63.6

Personality (disorder) F6Ø.9
- accentuation of traits (type A pattern) Z73.1
- affective F34.Ø
- aggressive F6Ø.3
- amoral F6Ø.2
- anacastic, anankastic F6Ø.5
- antisocial F6Ø.2
- anxious F6Ø.6
- asocial F6Ø.2
- asthenic F6Ø.7
- avoidant F6Ø.6
- borderline F6Ø.3
- change due to organic condition (enduring) FØ7.Ø
- compulsive F6Ø.5
- cycloid F34.Ø
- cyclothymic F34.Ø
- dependent F6Ø.7
- depressive F34.1
- dissocial F6Ø.2
- dual F44.81
- eccentric F6Ø.89
- emotionally unstable F6Ø.3
- expansive paranoid F6Ø.Ø
- explosive F6Ø.3
- fanatic F6Ø.Ø
- haltlose type F6Ø.89
- histrionic F6Ø.4
- hyperthymic F34.Ø
- hypothymic F34.1
- hysterical F6Ø.4
- immature F6Ø.89
- inadequate F6Ø.7
- labile (emotional) F6Ø.3
- mixed (nonspecific) F6Ø.81
- morally defective F6Ø.2
- multiple F44.81
- narcissistic F6Ø.81
- obsessional F6Ø.5
- obsessive(-compulsive) F6Ø.5
- organic FØ7.Ø
- overconscientious F6Ø.5
- paranoid F6Ø.Ø
- passive(-dependent) F6Ø.7
- passive-aggressive F6Ø.89
- pathologic F6Ø.9
- pattern defect or disturbance F6Ø.9
- pseudopsychopathic (organic) FØ7.Ø
- pseudoretarded (organic) FØ7.Ø
- psychoinfantile F6Ø.4
- psychoneurotic NEC F6Ø.89
- psychopathic F6Ø.2
- querulant F6Ø.Ø
- sadistic F6Ø.89
- schizoid F6Ø.1
- self-defeating F6Ø.7
- sensitive paranoid F6Ø.Ø
- sociopathic (amoral) (antisocial) (asocial) (dissocial) F6Ø.2
- specified NEC F6Ø.89
- type A Z73.1
- unstable (emotional) F6Ø.3

Perthes' disease — *see* Legg-Calvé-Perthes disease

Pertussis *(see also* Whooping cough) A37.9Ø

Perversion, perverted
- appetite F5Ø.8
  - psychogenic F5Ø.8
- function
  - pituitary gland E23.2
    - posterior lobe E22.2
- sense of smell and taste R43.8
  - psychogenic F45.8
- sexual — *see* Deviation, sexual

Pervious, congenital *(see also* Imperfect, closure)
- ductus arteriosus Q25.Ø

Pes (congenital) *(see also* Talipes)
- acquired *(see also* Deformity, limb, foot, specified NEC)
  - planus — *see* Deformity, limb, flat foot
- adductus Q66.89
- cavus Q66.7
- deformity NEC, acquired — *see* Deformity, limb, foot, specified NEC

Pes — *continued*
- planus (acquired) (any degree) *(see also* Deformity, limb, flat foot)
  - rachitic sequelae (late effect) E64.3
- valgus Q66.6

Pest, pestis — *see* Plague

Petechia, petechiae R23.3
- newborn P54.5

Petechial typhus A75.9

Peter's anomaly Q13.4

Petit mal seizure — *see* Epilepsy, generalized, specified NEC

Petit's hernia — *see* Hernia, abdomen, specified site NEC

Petrellidosis B48.2

Petrositis H7Ø.2Ø-
- acute H7Ø.21-
- chronic H7Ø.22-

Peutz-Jeghers disease or syndrome Q85.8

Peyronie's disease N48.6

Pfeiffer's disease — *see* Mononucleosis, infectious

Phagedena (dry) (moist) (sloughing) *(see also* Gangrene)
- geometric L88
- penis N48.29
- tropical — *see* Ulcer, skin
- vulva N76.6

Phagedenic — *see* condition

Phakoma H35.89

Phakomatosis *(see also* specific eponymous syndromes) Q85.9
- Bourneville's Q85.1
- specified NEC Q85.8

Phantom limb syndrome (without pain) G54.7
- with pain G54.6

Pharyngeal pouch syndrome D82.1

Pharyngitis (acute) (catarrhal)(gangrenous) (infective) (malignant) (membranous) (phlegmonous) (pseudomembranous) (simple) (subacute) (suppurative) (ulcerative) (viral) JØ2.9
- with influenza, flu, or grippe — *see* Influenza, with, pharyngitis
- aphthous BØ8.5
- atrophic J31.2
- chlamydial A56.4
- chronic (atrophic) (granular) (hypertrophic) J31.2
- coxsackievirus BØ8.5
- diphtheritic A36.Ø
- enteroviral vesicular BØ8.5
- follicular (chronic) J31.2
- fusospirochetal A69.1
- gonococcal A54.5
- granular (chronic) J31.2
- herpesviral BØØ.2
- hypertrophic J31.2
- infectional, chronic J31.2
- influenzal — *see* Influenza, with, respiratory manifestations NEC
- lymphonodular, acute (enteroviral) BØ8.8
- pneumococcal JØ2.8
- purulent JØ2.9
- putrid JØ2.9
- septic JØ2.Ø
- sicca J31.2
- specified organism NEC JØ2.8
- staphylococcal JØ2.8
- streptococcal JØ2.Ø
- syphilitic, congenital (early) A5Ø.Ø3
- tuberculous A15.8
- vesicular, enteroviral BØ8.5
- viral NEC JØ2.8

Pharyngoconjunctivitis, viral B3Ø.2

Pharyngolaryngitis (acute) JØ6.Ø
- chronic J37.Ø

Pharyngoplegia J39.2

Pharyngotonsillitis, herpesviral BØØ.2

Pharyngotracheitis, chronic J42

Pharynx, pharyngeal — *see* condition

Phenomenon
- Arthus' — *see* Arthus' phenomenon
- jaw-winking QØ7.8
- lupus erythematosus (LE) cell M32.9

- **Phenomenon**— *continued*
  - Raynaud's (secondary) I73.ØØ
    - with gangrene I73.Ø1
  - vasomotor R55
  - vasospastic I73.9
  - vasovagal R55
  - Wenckebach's I44.1
- **Phenylketonuria** E7Ø.1
  - classical E7Ø.Ø
  - maternal E7Ø.1
- **Pheochromoblastoma**
  - specified site — *see* Neoplasm, malignant, by site
  - unspecfied site C74.1Ø
- **Pheochromocytoma**
  - malignant
    - specified site — *see* Neoplasm, malignant, by site
    - unspecified site C74.1Ø
  - specified site — *see* Neoplasm, benign, by site
  - unspecified site D35.ØØ
- **Pheohyphomycosis** — *see* Chromomycosis
- **Pheomycosis** — *see* Chromomycosis
- **Phimosis** (congenital) (due to infection) N47.1
  - chancroidal A57
- **Phlebectasia** *(see also* Varix)
  - congenital Q27.4
- **Phlebitis** (infective) (pyemic) (septic) (suppurative) I8Ø.9
  - antepartum — *see* Thrombophlebitis, antepartum
  - blue — *see* Phlebitis, leg, deep
  - breast, superficial I8Ø.8
  - cavernous (venous) sinus — *see* Phlebitis, intracranial (venous) sinus
  - cerebral (venous) sinus — *see* Phlebitis, intracranial (venous) sinus
  - chest wall, superficial I8Ø.8
  - cranial (venous) sinus — *see* Phlebitis, intracranial (venous) sinus
  - deep (vessels) — *see* Phlebitis, leg, deep
  - due to implanted device — *see* Complications, by site and type, specified NEC
  - during or resulting from a procedure T81.72
  - femoral vein (superficial) I8Ø.1-
  - femoropopliteal vein I8Ø.Ø-
  - gestational — *see* Phlebopathy, gestational
  - hepatic veins I8Ø.8
  - iliofemoral — *see* Phlebitis, femoral vein
  - intracranial (venous) sinus (any) GØ8
    - nonpyogenic I67.6
  - intraspinal venous sinuses and veins GØ8
    - nonpyogenic G95.19
  - lateral (venous) sinus — *see* Phlebitis, intracranial (venous) sinus
  - leg I8Ø.3
    - antepartum — *see* Thrombophlebitis, antepartum
    - deep (vessels) NEC I8Ø.2Ø-
      - iliac I8Ø.21-
      - popliteal vein I8Ø.22-
      - specified vessel NEC I8Ø.29-
      - tibial vein I8Ø.23-
    - femoral vein (superficial) I8Ø.1-
    - superficial (vessels) I8Ø.Ø-
  - longitudinal sinus — *see* Phlebitis, intracranial (venous) sinus
  - lower limb — *see* Phlebitis, leg
  - migrans, migrating (superficial) I82.1
  - pelvic
    - with ectopic or molar pregnancy OØ8.Ø
    - following ectopic or molar pregnancy OØ8.Ø
    - puerperal, postpartum O87.1
  - popliteal vein — *see* Phlebitis, leg, deep, popliteal
  - portal (vein) K75.1
  - postoperative T81.72
  - pregnancy — *see* Thrombophlebitis, antepartum
  - puerperal, postpartum, childbirth O87.Ø
    - deep O87.1
    - pelvic O87.1
    - superficial O87.Ø
  - retina — *see* Vasculitis, retina
  - saphenous (accessory) (great) (long) (small) — *see* Phlebitis, leg, superficial
  - sinus (meninges) — *see* Phlebitis, intracranial (venous) sinus
- **Phlebitis** — *continued*
  - specified site NEC I8Ø.8
  - syphilitic A52.Ø9
  - tibial vein — *see* Phlebitis, leg, deep, tibial
  - ulcerative I8Ø.9
    - leg — *see* Phlebitis, leg
  - umbilicus I8Ø.8
  - uterus (septic) — *see* Endometritis
  - varicose (leg) (lower limb) — *see* Varix, leg, with, inflammation
- **Phlebofibrosis** I87.8
- **Phleboliths** I87.8
- **Phlebopathy,**
  - gestational O22.9-
  - puerperal O87.9
- **Phlebosclerosis** I87.8
- **Phlebothrombosis** *(see also* Thrombosis)
  - antepartum — *see* Thrombophlebitis, antepartum
  - pregnancy — *see* Thrombophlebitis, antepartum
  - puerperal — *see* Thrombophlebitis, puerperal
- **Phlebotomus fever** A93.1
- **Phlegmasia**
  - alba dolens O87.1
    - nonpuerperal — *see* Phlebitis, femoral vein
  - cerulea dolens — *see* Phlebitis, leg, deep
- **Phlegmon** — *see* Abscess
- **Phlegmonous** — *see* condition
- **Phlyctenulosis** (allergic) (keratoconjunctivitis) (nontuberculous) *(see also* Keratoconjunctivitis)
  - cornea — *see* Keratoconjunctivitis
  - tuberculous A18.52
- **Phobia, phobic** F4Ø.9
  - animal F4Ø.218
    - spiders F4Ø.21Ø
  - examination F4Ø.298
  - reaction F4Ø.9
  - simple F4Ø.298
  - social F4Ø.1Ø
    - generalized F4Ø.11
  - specific (isolated) F4Ø.298
    - animal F4Ø.218
      - spiders F4Ø.21Ø
    - blood F4Ø.23Ø
    - injection F4Ø.231
    - injury F4Ø.233
    - men F4Ø.29Ø
    - natural environment F4Ø.228
      - thunderstorms F4Ø.22Ø
    - situational F4Ø.248
      - bridges F4Ø.242
      - closed in spaces F4Ø.24Ø
      - flying F4Ø.243
      - heights F4Ø.241
    - specified focus NEC F4Ø.298
    - transfusion F4Ø.231
    - women F4Ø.291
  - specified NEC F4Ø.8
    - medical care NEC F4Ø.232
  - state F4Ø.9
- **Phocas' disease** — *see* Mastopathy, cystic
- **Phocomelia** Q73.1
  - lower limb — *see* Agenesis, leg, with foot present
  - upper limb — *see* Agenesis, arm, with hand present
- **Phoria** H5Ø.5Ø
- **Phosphate-losing tubular disorder** N25.Ø
- **Phosphatemia** E83.39
- **Phosphaturia** E83.39
- **Photodermatitis** (sun) L56.8
  - chronic L57.8
  - due to drug L56.8
  - light other than sun L59.8
- **Photokeratitis** H16.13-
- **Photophobia** H53.14-
- **Photophthalmia** — *see* Photokeratitis
- **Photopsia** H53.19
- **Photoretinitis** — *see* Retinopathy, solar
- **Photosensitivity, photosensitization** (sun) skin L56.8
  - light other than sun L59.8
- **Phrenitis** — *see* Encephalitis
- **Phrynoderma** (vitamin A deficiency) E5Ø.8
- **Phthiriasis** (pubis) B85.3
  - with any infestation classifiable to B85.Ø-B85.2 B85.4
- **Phthirus infestation** — *see* Phthiriasis
- **Phthisis** *(see also* Tuberculosis)
  - bulbi (infectional) — *see* Disorder, globe, degenerated condition, atrophy
  - eyeball (due to infection) — *see* Disorder, globe, degenerated condition, atrophy
- **Phycomycosis** — *see* Zygomycosis
- **Physalopteriasis** B81.8
- **Physical restraint status** Z78.1
- **Phytobezoar** T18.9
  - intestine T18.3
  - stomach T18.2
- **Pian** — *see* Yaws
- **Pianoma** A66.1
- **Pica** F5Ø.8
  - in adults F5Ø.8
  - infant or child F98.3
- **Picking, nose** F98.8
- **Pick-Niemann disease** — *see* Niemann-Pick disease or syndrome
- **Pick's**
  - cerebral atrophy G31.Ø1 *[F02.80]*
    - with behavioral disturbance G31.Ø1 *[F02.81]*
  - disease or syndrome (brain) G31.Ø1 *[F02.80]*
    - with behavioral disturbance G31.Ø1 *[F02.81]*
- **Pickwickian syndrome** E66.2
- **Piebaldism** E7Ø.39
- **Piedra** (beard) (scalp) B36.8
  - black B36.3
  - white B36.2
- **Pierre Robin deformity or syndrome** Q87.Ø
- **Pierson's disease or osteochondrosis** M91.Ø
- **Pig-bel** AØ5.2
- **Pigeon**
  - breast or chest (acquired) M95.4
    - congenital Q67.7
    - rachitic sequelae (late effect) E64.3
  - breeder's disease or lung J67.2
  - fancier's disease or lung J67.2
  - toe — *see* Deformity, toe, specified NEC
- **Pigmentation** (abnormal) (anomaly) L81.9
  - conjunctiva H11.13-
  - cornea (anterior) H18.Ø1-
    - posterior H18.Ø5-
    - stromal H18.Ø6-
  - diminished melanin formation NEC L81.6
  - iron L81.8
  - lids, congenital Q82.8
  - limbus corneae — *see* Pigmentation, cornea
  - metals L81.8
  - optic papilla, congenital Q14.2
  - retina, congenital (grouped) (nevoid) Q14.1
  - scrotum, congenital Q82.8
  - tattoo L81.8
- **Piles** *(see also* Hemorrhoids) K64.9
- **Pili**
  - annulati or torti (congenital) Q84.1
  - incarnati L73.1
- **Pill roller hand** (intrinsic) — *see* Parkinsonism
- **Pilomatrixoma** — *see* Neoplasm, skin, benign
  - malignant — *see* Neoplasm, skin, malignant
- **Pilonidal** — *see* condition
- **Pimple** R23.8
- **Pinched nerve** — *see* Neuropathy, entrapment
- **Pindborg tumor** — *see* Cyst, calcifying odontogenic
- **Pineal body or gland** — *see* condition
- **Pinealoblastoma** C75.3
- **Pinealoma** D44.5
  - malignant C75.3
- **Pineoblastoma** C75.3
- **Pineocytoma** D44.5
- **Pinguecula** H11.15-
- **Pingueculitis** H1Ø.81-
- **Pinhole meatus** *(see also* Stricture, urethra) N35.9
- **Pink**
  - disease — *see* subcategory T56.1
  - eye — *see* Conjunctivitis, acute, mucopurulent
- **Pinkus' disease** (lichen nitidus) L44.1
- **Pinpoint**
  - meatus — *see* Stricture, urethra
  - os (uteri) — *see* Stricture, cervix

Pins and needles R2Ø.2
Pinta A67.9
- cardiovascular lesions A67.2
- chancre (primary) A67.Ø
- erythematous plaques A67.1
- hyperchromic lesions A67.1
- hyperkeratosis A67.1
- lesions A67.9
  - cardiovascular A67.2
  - hyperchromic A67.1
  - intermediate A67.1
  - late A67.2
  - mixed A67.3
  - primary A67.Ø
  - skin (achromic) (cicatricial) (dyschromic) A67.2
    - hyperchromic A67.1
    - mixed (achromic and hyperchromic) A67.3
- papule (primary) A67.Ø
- skin lesions (achromic) (cicatricial) (dyschromic) A67.2
  - hyperchromic A67.1
  - mixed (achromic and hyperchromic) A67.3
- vitiligo A67.2

Pintids A67.1
Pinworm (disease) (infection) (infestation) B8Ø
Piroplasmosis B6Ø.Ø
Pistol wound — *see* Gunshot wound
Pitchers' elbow — *see* Derangement, joint, specified type NEC, elbow
Pithecoid pelvis Q74.2
- with disproportion (fetopelvic) O33.Ø
  - causing obstructed labor O65.Ø

Pithiatism F48.8
Pitted — *see* Pitting
Pitting (*see also* Edema) R6Ø.9
- lip R6Ø.Ø
- nail L6Ø.8
- teeth KØØ.4

Pituitary gland — *see* condition
Pituitary-snuff-taker's disease J67.8
Pityriasis (capitis) L21.Ø
- alba L3Ø.5
- circinata (et maculata) L42
- furfuracea L21.Ø
- Hebra's L26
- lichenoides L41.Ø
  - chronica L41.1
  - et varioliformis (acuta) L41.Ø
- maculata (et circinata) L3Ø.5
- nigra B36.1
- pilaris, Hebra's L44.Ø
- rosea L42
- rotunda L44.8
- rubra (Hebra) pilaris L44.Ø
- simplex L3Ø.5
- specified type NEC L3Ø.5
- streptogenes L3Ø.5
- versicolor (scrotal) B36.Ø

Placenta, placental — *see* Pregnancy, complicated by (care of) (management affected by), specified condition
Placentitis O41.14-
Plagiocephaly Q67.3
Plague A2Ø.9
- abortive A2Ø.8
- ambulatory A2Ø.8
- asymptomatic A2Ø.8
- bubonic A2Ø.Ø
- cellulocutaneous A2Ø.1
- cutaneobubonic A2Ø.1
- lymphatic gland A2Ø.Ø
- meningitis A2Ø.3
- pharyngeal A2Ø.8
- pneumonic (primary) (secondary) A2Ø.2
- pulmonary, pulmonic A2Ø.2
- septicemic A2Ø.7
- tonsillar A2Ø.8
  - septicemic A2Ø.7

Planning, family
- contraception Z3Ø.9
- procreation Z31.69

Plaque(s) artery, arterial — *see* Arteriosclerosis
- calcareous — *see* Calcification
- coronary, lipid rich I25.83
- epicardial I31.8
- erythematous, of pinta A67.1
- Hollenhorst's — *see* Occlusion, artery, retina
- lipid rich, coronary I25.83
- pleural (without asbestos) J92.9
  - with asbestos J92.Ø
- tongue K13.29

Plasmacytoma C9Ø.3-
- extramedullary C9Ø.2-
- medullary C9Ø.Ø-
- solitary C9Ø.3-

Plasmacytopenia D72.818
Plasmacytosis D72.822
Plaster ulcer — *see* Ulcer, pressure, by site
Plateau iris syndrome (post-iridectomy) (postprocedural) (without glaucoma) H21.82
- with glaucoma H4Ø.22-

Platybasia Q75.8
Platyonychia (congenital) Q84.6
- acquired L6Ø.8

Platypelloid pelvis M95.5
- with disproportion (fetopelvic) O33.Ø
  - causing obstructed labor O65.Ø
- congenital Q74.2

Platyspondylisis Q76.49
Plaut(-Vincent) **disease** (*see also* Vincent's) A69.1
Plethora R23.2
- newborn P61.1

Pleura, pleural — *see* condition
Pleuralgia RØ7.89
Pleurisy (acute) (adhesive) (chronic) (costal) (diaphragmatic) (double) (dry) (fibrinous) (fibrous) (interlobar) (latent) (plastic) (primary) (residual) (sicca) (sterile) (subacute) (unresolved) RØ9.1
- with
  - adherent pleura J86.Ø
  - effusion J9Ø
    - chylous, chyliform J94.Ø
    - tuberculous (non primary) A15.6
      - primary (progressive) A15.7
  - tuberculosis — *see* Pleurisy, tuberculous (non primary)
- encysted — *see* Pleurisy, with effusion
- exudative — *see* Pleurisy, with effusion
- fibrinopurulent, fibropurulent — *see* Pyothorax
- hemorrhagic — *see* Hemothorax
- pneumococcal J9Ø
- purulent — *see* Pyothorax
- septic — *see* Pyothorax
- serofibrinous — *see* Pleurisy, with effusion
- seropurulent — *see* Pyothorax
- serous — *see* Pleurisy, with effusion
- staphylococcal J86.9
- streptococcal J9Ø
- suppurative — *see* Pyothorax
- traumatic (post) (current) — *see* Injury, intrathoracic, pleura
- tuberculous (with effusion) (non primary) A15.6
  - primary (progressive) A15.7

Pleuritis sicca — *see* Pleurisy
Pleurobronchopneumonia — *see* Pneumonia, broncho-
Pleurodynia RØ7.81
- epidemic B33.Ø
- viral B33.Ø

Pleuropericarditis (*see also* Pericarditis)
- acute I3Ø.9

Pleuropneumonia (acute) (bilateral) (double) (septic) (*see also* Pneumonia) J18.8
- chronic — *see* Fibrosis, lung

Pleuro-pneumonia-like-organism (PPLO), **as cause of disease classified elsewhere** B96.Ø
Pleurorrhea — *see* Pleurisy, with effusion
Plexitis, brachial G54.Ø
Plica
- polonica B85.Ø
- syndrome, knee M67.5-
- tonsil J35.8

Plicated tongue K14.5
Plug
- bronchus NEC J98.Ø9
- meconium (newborn) NEC syndrome P76.Ø
- mucus — *see* Asphyxia, mucus

Plumbism — *see* subcategory T56.Ø
Plummer's disease EØ5.2Ø
- with thyroid storm EØ5.21

Plummer-Vinson syndrome D5Ø.1
Pluricarential syndrome of infancy E4Ø
Plus (and minus) **hand** (intrinsic) — *see* Deformity, limb, specified type NEC, forearm
Pneumathemia — *see* Air, embolism
Pneumatic hammer (drill) syndrome T75.21
Pneumatocele (lung) J98.4
- intracranial G93.89
- tension J44.9

Pneumatosis
- cystoides intestinalis K63.89
- intestinalis K63.89
- peritonei K66.8

Pneumaturia R39.89
Pneumoblastoma — *see* Neoplasm, lung, malignant
Pneumocephalus G93.89
Pneumococcemia A4Ø.3
Pneumococcus, pneumococcal — *see* condition
Pneumoconiosis (due to) (inhalation of) J64
- with tuberculosis (any type in A15) J65
- aluminum J63.Ø
- asbestos J61
- bagasse, bagassosis J67.1
- bauxite J63.1
- beryllium J63.2
- coal miners' (simple) J6Ø
- coalworkers' (simple) J6Ø
- collier's J6Ø
- cotton dust J66.Ø
- diatomite (diatomaceous earth) J62.8
- dust
  - inorganic NEC J63.6
  - lime J62.8
  - marble J62.8
  - organic NEC J66.8
- fumes or vapors (from silo) J68.9
- graphite J63.3
- grinder's J62.8
- kaolin J62.8
- mica J62.8
- millstone maker's J62.8
- mineral fibers NEC J61
- miner's J6Ø
- moldy hay J67.Ø
- potter's J62.8
- rheumatoid — *see* Rheumatoid, lung
- sandblaster's J62.8
- silica, silicate NEC J62.8
  - with carbon J6Ø
- stonemason's J62.8
- talc (dust) J62.Ø

Pneumocystis carinii pneumonia B59
Pneumocystis jiroveci (pneumonia) B59
Pneumocystosis (with pneumonia) B59
Pneumohemopericardium I31.2
Pneumohemothorax J94.2
- traumatic S27.2

Pneumohydropericardium — *see* Pericarditis
Pneumohydrothorax — *see* Hydrothorax
Pneumomediastinum J98.2
- congenital or perinatal P25.2

Pneumomycosis B49 *[J99]*
Pneumonia (acute) (double) (migratory) (purulent) (septic) (unresolved) J18.9
- with
  - influenza — *see* Influenza, with, pneumonia
  - lung abscess J85.1
    - due to specified organism — *see* Pneumonia, in (due to)
- adenoviral J12.Ø
- adynamic J18.2
- alba A5Ø.Ø4
- allergic (eosinophilic) J82
- alveolar — *see* Pneumonia, lobar
- anaerobes J15.8
- anthrax A22.1

- **Pneumonia** — *continued*
  - apex, apical — *see* Pneumonia, lobar
  - Ascaris B77.81
  - aspiration J69.Ø
    - due to
      - aspiration of microorganisms
        - bacterial J15.9
        - viral J12.9
      - food (regurgitated) J69.Ø
      - gastric secretions J69.Ø
      - milk (regurgitated) J69.Ø
      - oils, essences J69.1
      - solids, liquids NEC J69.8
      - vomitus J69.Ø
    - newborn P24.81
      - amniotic fluid (clear) P24.11
      - blood P24.21
      - liquor (amnii) P24.11
      - meconium P24.Ø1
      - milk P24.31
      - mucus P24.11
      - food (regurgitated) P24.31
      - specified NEC P24.81
      - stomach contents P24.31
    - postprocedural J95.4
  - atypical NEC J18.9
  - bacillus J15.9
    - specified NEC J15.8
  - bacterial J15.9
    - specified NEC J15.8
  - Bacteroides (fragilis) (oralis) (melaninogenicus) J15.8
  - basal, basic, basilar — *see* Pneumonia, by type
  - bronchiolitis obliterans organized (BOOP) J84.89
  - broncho-, bronchial (confluent) (croupous) (diffuse) (disseminated) (hemorrhagic) (involving lobes) (lobar) (terminal) J18.Ø
    - allergic (eosinophilic) J82
    - aspiration — *see* Pneumonia, aspiration
    - bacterial J15.9
      - specified NEC J15.8
    - chronic — *see* Fibrosis, lung
    - diplococcal J13
    - Eaton's agent J15.7
    - Escherichia coli (E. coli) J15.5
    - Friedländer's bacillus J15.Ø
    - Hemophilus influenzae J14
    - hypostatic J18.2
    - inhalation (*see also* Pneumonia, aspiration
      - due to fumes or vapors (chemical) J68.Ø
      - of oils or essences J69.1
    - Klebsiella (pneumoniae) J15.Ø
    - lipid, lipoid J69.1
      - endogenous J84.89
    - Mycoplasma (pneumoniae) J15.7
    - pleuro-pneumonia-like-organisms (PPLO) J15.7
    - pneumococcal J13
    - Proteus J15.6
    - Pseudomonas J15.1
    - Serratia marcescens J15.6
    - specified organism NEC J16.8
    - staphylococcal — *see* Pneumonia, staphylococcal
    - streptococcal NEC J15.4
      - group B J15.3
      - pneumoniae J13
    - viral, virus — *see* Pneumonia, viral
  - Butyrivibrio (fibriosolvens) J15.8
  - Candida B37.1
  - caseous — *see* Tuberculosis, pulmonary
  - catarrhal — *see* Pneumonia, broncho
  - chlamydial J16.Ø
    - congenital P23.1
  - cholesterol J84.89
  - cirrhotic (chronic) — *see* Fibrosis, lung
  - Clostridium (haemolyticum) (novyi) J15.8
  - confluent — *see* Pneumonia, broncho
  - congenital (infective) P23.9
    - due to
      - bacterium NEC P23.6
      - Chlamydia P23.1
      - Escherichia coli P23.4
      - Haemophilus influenzae P23.6
      - infective organism NEC P23.8

- **Pneumonia**— *continued*
  - congenital — *continued*
    - due to — *continued*
      - Klebsiella pneumoniae P23.6
      - Mycoplasma P23.6
      - Pseudomonas P23.5
      - Staphylococcus P23.2
      - Streptococcus (except group B) P23.6
        - group B P23.3
      - viral agent P23.Ø
    - specified NEC P23.8
  - croupous — *see* Pneumonia, lobar
  - cryptogenic organizing J84.116
  - cytomegalic inclusion B25.Ø
  - cytomegaloviral B25.Ø
  - deglutition — *see* Pneumonia, aspiration
  - desquamative interstitial J84.117
  - diffuse — *see* Pneumonia, broncho
  - diplococcal, diplococcus (broncho) (lobar) J13
  - disseminated (focal) — *see* Pneumonia, broncho
  - Eaton's agent J15.7
  - embolic, embolism — *see* Embolism, pulmonary
  - Enterobacter J15.6
  - eosinophilic J82
  - Escherichia coli (E. coli) J15.5
  - Eubacterium J15.8
  - fibrinous — *see* Pneumonia, lobar
  - fibroid, fibrous (chronic) — *see* Fibrosis, lung
  - Friedländer's bacillus J15.Ø
  - Fusobacterium (nucleatum) J15.8
  - gangrenous J85.Ø
  - giant cell (measles) BØ5.2
  - gonococcal A54.84
  - gram-negative bacteria NEC J15.6
    - anaerobic J15.8
  - Hemophilus influenzae (broncho) (lobar) J14
  - human metapneumovirus J12.3
  - hypostatic (broncho) (lobar) J18.2
  - in (due to)
    - actinomycosis A42.Ø
    - adenovirus J12.Ø
    - anthrax A22.1
    - ascariasis B77.81
    - aspergillosis B44.9
    - Bacillus anthracis A22.1
    - Bacterium anitratum J15.6
    - candidiasis B37.1
    - chickenpox BØ1.2
    - Chlamydia J16.Ø
      - neonatal P23.1
    - coccidioidomycosis B38.2
      - acute B38.Ø
      - chronic B38.1
    - cytomegalovirus disease B25.Ø
    - Diplococcus (pneumoniae) J13
    - Eaton's agent J15.7
    - Enterobacter J15.6
    - Escherichia coli (E. coli) J15.5
    - Friedländer's bacillus J15.Ø
    - fumes and vapors (chemical) (inhalation) J68.Ø
    - gonorrhea A54.84
    - Hemophilus influenzae (H. influenzae) J14
    - Herellea J15.6
    - histoplasmosis B39.2
      - acute B39.Ø
      - chronic B39.1
    - human metapneumovirus J12.3
    - Klebsiella (pneumoniae) J15.Ø
    - measles BØ5.2
    - Mycoplasma (pneumoniae) J15.7
    - nocardiosis, nocardiasis A43.Ø
    - ornithosis A7Ø
    - parainfluenza virus J12.2
    - pleuro-pneumonia-like-organism (PPLO) J15.7
    - pneumococcus J13
    - pneumocystosis (Pneumocystis carinii) (Pneumocystis jiroveci) B59
    - Proteus J15.6
    - Pseudomonas NEC J15.1
      - pseudomallei A24.1
    - psittacosis A7Ø
    - Q fever A78
    - respiratory syncytial virus J12.1

- **Pneumonia**— *continued*
  - in (due to)— *continued*
    - rheumatic fever IØØ *[J17]*
    - rubella BØ6.81
    - Salmonella (infection) AØ2.22
      - typhi AØ1.Ø3
    - schistosomiasis B65.9 *[J17]*
    - Serratia marcescens J15.6
    - specified
      - bacterium NEC J15.8
      - organism NEC J16.8
    - spirochetal NEC A69.8
    - Staphylococcus J15.2Ø
      - aureus (methicillin susceptible) (MSSA) J15.211
        - methicillin resistant (MRSA) J15.212
      - specified NEC J15.29
    - Streptococcus J15.4
      - group B J15.3
      - pneumoniae J13
      - specified NEC J15.4
    - toxoplasmosis B58.3
    - tularemia A21.2
    - typhoid (fever) AØ1.Ø3
    - varicella BØ1.2
    - virus — *see* Pneumonia, viral
    - whooping cough A37.91
      - due to
        - Bordetella parapertussis A37.11
        - Bordetella pertussis A37.Ø1
        - specified NEC A37.81
    - Yersinia pestis A2Ø.2
  - inhalation of food or vomit — *see* Pneumonia, aspiration
  - interstitial J84.9
    - chronic J84.111
    - desquamative J84.117
    - due to
      - collagen vascular disease J84.17
      - known underlying cause J84.17
    - idiopathic NOS J84.111
    - in disease classified elsewhere J84.17
    - lymphocytic (due to collagen vascular disease) (in diseases classified elsewhere) J84.17
    - lymphoid J84.2
    - non-specific J84.89
      - due to
        - collagen vascular disease J84.17
        - known underlying cause J84.17
      - idiopathic J84.113
      - in diseases classified elsewhere J84.17
    - plasma cell B59
    - pseudomonas J15.1
    - usual J84.112
      - due to collagen vascular disease J84.17
      - idiopathic J84.112
      - in diseases classified elsewhere J84.17
  - Klebsiella (pneumoniae) J15.Ø
  - lipid, lipoid (exogenous) J69.1
    - endogenous J84.89
  - lobar (disseminated) (double) (interstitial) J18.1
    - bacterial J15.9
      - specified NEC J15.8
    - chronic — *see* Fibrosis, lung
    - Escherichia coli (E. coli) J15.5
    - Friedländer's bacillus J15.Ø
    - Hemophilus influenzae J14
    - hypostatic J18.2
    - Klebsiella (pneumoniae) J15.Ø
    - lymphocytic (due to collagen vascular disease) (in diseases classified elsewhere) J84.17
    - non-specific J84.89
    - pneumococcal J13
    - Proteus J15.6
    - Pseudomonas J15.1
    - specified organism NEC J16.8
    - staphylococcal — *see* Pneumonia, staphylococcal
    - streptococcal NEC J15.4
    - Streptococcus pneumoniae J13
    - viral, virus — *see* Pneumonia, viral
  - lobular — *see* Pneumonia, broncho
  - Löffler's J82

Poisoning— *continued*
- food— *continued*
  - due to— *continued*
    - Clostridium (perfringens) (Welchii) AØ5.2
    - salmonella (aertrycke) (callinarum) (choleraesuis) (enteritidis) (paratyphi) (suipestifer) AØ2.9
      - with
        - gastroenteritis AØ2.Ø
        - sepsis AØ2.1
    - staphylococcus AØ5.Ø
    - Vibrio
      - parahaemolyticus AØ5.3
      - vulnificus AØ5.5
  - noxious or naturally toxic T62.9-
    - berries — *see* subcategory T62.1-
    - fish — *see* Poisoning, seafood
    - mushrooms — *see* subcategory T62.ØX-
    - plants NEC — *see* subcategory T62.2X-
    - seafood — *see* Poisoning, seafood
    - specified NEC — *see* subcategory T62.8X-
- ichthyotoxism — *see* Poisoning, seafood
- kreotoxism, food AØ5.9
- latex T65.81-
- lead T56.Ø-
- mushroom — *see* Poisoning, food, noxious, mushroom
- mussels (*see also* Poisoning, shellfish)
  - bacterial — *see* Intoxication, foodborne, by agent
- nicotine (tobacco) T65.2-
- noxious foodstuffs — *see* Poisoning, food, noxious
- plants, noxious — *see* Poisoning, food, noxious, plants NEC
- ptomaine — *see* Poisoning, food
- radiation J7Ø.Ø
- Salmonella (arizonae) (cholerae-suis) (enteritidis) (typhimurium) AØ2.9
- scombroid fish T61.1-
- seafood (noxious) T61.9-
  - bacterial — *see* Intoxication, foodborne, by agent
  - fish — *see* Poisoning, fish
  - shellfish — *see* Poisoning, shellfish
  - specified NEC — *see* subcategory T61.8X-
- shellfish (amnesic) (azaspiracid) (diarrheic) (neurotoxic) (noxious) (paralytic) T61.78-
  - bacterial — *see* Intoxication, foodborne, by agent
  - ciguatera mollusk — *see* Poisoning, ciguatera fish
- specified substance NEC T65.891
- Staphylococcus, food AØ5.Ø
- tobacco (nicotine) T65.2-
- water E87.79

Poker spine — *see* Spondylitis, ankylosing

Poland syndrome Q79.8

Polioencephalitis (acute) (bulbar) A8Ø.9
- inferior G12.22
- influenzal — *see* Influenza, with, encephalopathy
- superior hemorrhagic (acute) (Wernicke's) E51.2
- Wernicke's E51.2

Polioencephalomyelitis (acute) (anterior) A8Ø.9
- with beriberi E51.2

Polioencephalopathy, superior hemorrhagic E51.2
- with
  - beriberi E51.11
  - pellagra E52

Poliomeningoencephalitis — *see* Meningoencephalitis

Poliomyelitis (acute) (anterior) (epidemic) A8Ø.9
- with paralysis (bulbar) — *see* Poliomyelitis, paralytic
- abortive A8Ø.4
- ascending (progressive) — *see* Poliomyelitis, paralytic
- bulbar (paralytic) — *see* Poliomyelitis, paralytic
- congenital P35.8
- nonepidemic A8Ø.9
- nonparalytic A8Ø.4
- paralytic A8Ø.3Ø
  - specified NEC A8Ø.39
  - vaccine-associated A8Ø.Ø
  - wild virus
    - imported A8Ø.1
    - indigenous A8Ø.2
- spinal, acute A8Ø.9

Poliosis (eyebrow) (eyelashes) L67.1 circumscripta, acquired L67.1

Pollakiuria R35.Ø
- psychogenic F45.8

Pollinosis J3Ø.1

Pollitzer's disease L73.2

Polyadenitis (*see also* Lymphadenitis)
- malignant A2Ø.Ø

Polyalgia M79.89

Polyangiitis M3Ø.Ø
- microscopic M31.7
- overlap syndrome M3Ø.8

Polyarteritis
- microscopic M31.7
- nodosa M3Ø.Ø
  - with lung involvement M3Ø.1
  - juvenile M3Ø.2
  - related condition NEC M3Ø.8

Polyarthralgia — *see* Pain, joint

Polyarthritis, polyarthropathy (*see also* Arthritis) M13.Ø
- due to or associated with other specified conditions — *see* Arthritis
- epidemic (Australian) (with exanthema) B33.1
- infective — *see* Arthritis, pyogenic or pyemic
- inflammatory MØ6.4
- juvenile (chronic) (seronegative) MØ8.3
- migratory — *see* Fever, rheumatic
- rheumatic, acute — *see* Fever, rheumatic

Polyarthrosis M15.9
- post-traumatic M15.3
- primary M15.Ø
- specified NEC M15.8

Polycarential syndrome of infancy E4Ø

Polychondritis (atrophic) (chronic) (*see also* Disorder, cartilage, specified type NEC)
- relapsing M94.1

Polycoria Q13.2

Polycystic (disease)
- degeneration, kidney Q61.3
  - autosomal dominant (adult type) Q61.2
  - autosomal recessive (infantile type) NEC Q61.19
- kidney Q61.3
  - autosomal
    - dominant Q61.2
    - recessive NEC Q61.19
  - autosomal dominant (adult type) Q61.2
  - autosomal recessive (childhood type) NEC Q61.19
  - infantile type NEC Q61.19
- liver Q44.6
- lung J98.4
  - congenital Q33.Ø
- ovary, ovaries E28.2
- spleen Q89.Ø9

Polycythemia (secondary) D75.1
- acquired D75.1
- benign (familial) D75.Ø
- due to
  - donor twin P61.1
  - erythropoietin D75.1
  - fall in plasma volume D75.1
  - high altitude D75.1
  - maternal-fetal transfusion P61.1
  - stress D75.1
- emotional D75.1
- erythropoietin D75.1
- familial (benign) D75.Ø
- Gaisböck's (hypertonica) D75.1
- high altitude D75.1
- hypertonica D75.1
- hypoxemic D75.1
- neonatorum P61.1
- nephrogenous D75.1
- relative D75.1
- secondary D75.1
- spurious D75.1
- stress D75.1
- vera D45

Polycytosis cryptogenica D75.1

Polydactylism, polydactyly Q69.9
- toes Q69.2

Polydipsia R63.1

Polydystrophy, pseudo-Hurler E77.Ø

Polyembryoma — *see* Neoplasm, malignant, by site

Polyglandular
- deficiency E31.Ø
- dyscrasia E31.9
- dysfunction E31.9
- syndrome E31.8

Polyhydramnios O4Ø.-

Polymastia Q83.1

Polymenorrhea N92.Ø

Polymyalgia M35.3
- arteritica, giant cell M31.5
- rheumatica M35.3
  - with giant cell arteritis M31.5

Polymyositis (acute) (chronic) (hemorrhagic) M33.2Ø
- with
  - myopathy M33.22
  - respiratory involvement M33.21
  - skin involvement — *see* Dermatopolymyositis
  - specified organ involvement NEC M33.29
- ossificans (generalisata) (progressiva) — *see* Myositis, ossificans, progressiva

Polyneuritis, polyneuritic (*see also* Polyneuropathy)
- acute (post-) infective G61.Ø
- alcoholic G62.1
- cranialis G52.7
- demyelinating, chronic inflammatory (CIDP) G61.81
- diabetic — *see* Diabetes, polyneuropathy
- diphtheritic A36.83
- due to lack of vitamin NEC E56.9 *[G63]*
- endemic E51.11
- erythredema — *see* subcategory T56.1
- febrile, acute G61.Ø
- hereditary ataxic G6Ø.1
- idiopathic, acute G61.Ø
- infective (acute) G61.Ø
- inflammatory, chronic demyelinating (CIDP) G61.81
- nutritional E63.9 *[G63]*
- postinfective (acute) G61.Ø
- specified NEC G62.89

Polyneuropathy (peripheral) G62.9
- alcoholic G62.1
- amyloid (Portuguese) E85.1 *[G63]*
- arsenical G62.2
- critical illness G62.81
- demyelinating, chronic inflammatory (CIDP) G61.81
- diabetic — *see* Diabetes, polyneuropathy
- drug-induced G62.Ø
- hereditary G6Ø.9
  - specified NEC G6Ø.8
- idiopathic G6Ø.9
  - progressive G6Ø.3
- in (due to)
  - alcohol G62.1
    - sequelae G65.2
  - amyloidosis, familial (Portuguese) E85.1 *[G63]*
  - antitetanus serum G61.1
  - arsenic G62.2
    - sequelae G65.2
  - avitaminosis NEC E56.9 *[G63]*
  - beriberi E51.11
  - collagen vascular disease NEC M35.9 *[G63]*
  - deficiency (of)
    - B(-complex) vitamins E53.9 *[G63]*
    - vitamin B6 E53.1 *[G63]*
  - diabetes — *see* Diabetes, polyneuropathy
  - diphtheria A36.83
  - drug or medicament G62.Ø
    - correct substance properly administered — *see* Table of Drugs and Chemicals, by drug, adverse effect
    - overdose or wrong substance given or taken — *see* Table of Drugs and Chemicals, by drug, poisoning
  - endocrine disease NEC E34.9 *[G63]*
  - herpes zoster BØ2.23
  - hypoglycemia E16.2 *[G63]*
  - infectious
    - disease NEC B99 *[G63]*
    - mononucleosis B27.91
  - lack of vitamin NEC E56.9 *[G63]*

Positive
culture (nonspecific)
blood R78.81
bronchial washings R84.5
cerebrospinal fluid R83.5
cervix uteri R87.5
nasal secretions R84.5
nipple discharge R89.5
nose R84.5
staphylococcus (methicillin susceptible) Z22.321
methicillin resistant Z22.322
peritoneal fluid R85.5
pleural fluid R84.5
prostatic secretions R86.5
saliva R85.5
seminal fluid R86.5
sputum R84.5
synovial fluid R89.5
throat scrapings R84.5
urine R82.7
vagina R87.5
vulva R87.5
wound secretions R89.5
PPD (skin test) R76.11
serology for syphilis A53.Ø
false R76.8
with signs or symptoms code as Syphilis, by site and stage
skin test, tuberculin (without active tuberculosis) R76.11
test, human immunodeficiency virus (HIV) R75
VDRL A53.Ø
with signs or symptoms code by site and stage under Syphilis A53.9
Wassermann reaction A53.Ø
Postcardiotomy syndrome I97.Ø
Postcaval ureter Q62.62
Postcholecystectomy syndrome K91.5
Postclimacteric bleeding N95.Ø
Postcommissurotomy syndrome I97.Ø
Postconcussional syndrome FØ7.81
Postcontusional syndrome FØ7.81
Postcricoid region — *see* condition
Post-dates (4Ø-42 weeks) (pregnancy) (mother) O48.Ø
more than 42 weeks gestation O48.1
Postencephalitic syndrome FØ7.89
Posterior — *see* condition
Posterolateral sclerosis (spinal cord) — *see* Degeneration, combined
Postexanthematous — *see* condition
Postfebrile — *see* condition
Postgastrectomy dumping syndrome K91.1
Posthemiplegic chorea — *see* Monoplegia
Posthemorrhagic anemia (chronic) D5Ø.Ø
acute D62
newborn P61.3
Postherpetic neuralgia (zoster) BØ2.29
trigeminal BØ2.22
Posthitis N47.7
Postimmunization complication or reaction — *see* Complications, vaccination
Postinfectious — *see* condition
Postlaminectomy syndrome NEC M96.1
Postleukotomy syndrome FØ7.Ø
Postmastectomy lymphedema (syndrome) I97.2
Postmaturity, postmature (over 42 weeks)
maternal (over 42 weeks gestation) O48.1
newborn PØ8.22
Postmeasles complication NEC (*see also* condition) BØ5.89
Postmenopausal
endometrium (atrophic) N95.8
suppurative (*see also* Endometritis) N71.9
osteoporosis — *see* Osteoporosis, postmenopausal
Postnasal drip RØ9.82
due to
allergic rhinitis — *see* Rhinitis, allergic
common cold JØØ
gastroesophageal reflux — *see* Reflux, gastroesophageal
nasopharyngitis — *see* Nasopharyngitis
other known condition code to condition

Postnasal drip — *continued*
sinusitis — *see* Sinusitis
Postnatal — *see* condition
Postoperative (postprocedural) — *see* Complication, postoperative
pneumothorax, therapeutic Z98.3
state NEC Z98.89
Postpancreatectomy hyperglycemia E89.1
Postpartum — *see* Puerperal
Postphlebitic syndrome — *see* Syndrome, postthrombotic
Postpoliomyelitic (*see also* condition)
osteopathy — *see* Osteopathy, after poliomyelitis
Postpolio (myelitic) **syndrome** G14
Postprocedural (*see also* Postoperative)
hypoinsulinemia E89.1
Postschizophrenic depression F32.8
Postsurgery status (*see also* Status (post))
pneumothorax, therapeutic Z98.3
Post-term (4Ø-42 weeks) (pregnancy) (mother) O48.Ø
infant PØ8.21
more than 42 weeks gestation (mother) O48.1
Post-traumatic brain syndrome, nonpsychotic FØ7.81
Post-typhoid abscess AØ1.Ø9
Postures, hysterical F44.2
Postvaccinal reaction or complication — *see* Complications, vaccination
Postvalvulotomy syndrome I97.Ø
Potain's
disease (pulmonary edema) — *see* Edema, lung
syndrome (gastrectasis with dyspepsia) K31.Ø
Potter's
asthma J62.8
facies Q6Ø.6
lung J62.8
syndrome (with renal agenesis) Q6Ø.6
Pott's
curvature (spinal) A18.Ø1
disease or paraplegia A18.Ø1
spinal curvature A18.Ø1
tumor, puffy — *see* Osteomyelitis, specified type NEC
Pouch
bronchus Q32.4
Douglas' — *see* condition
esophagus, esophageal, congenital Q39.6
acquired K22.5
gastric K31.4
Hartmann's K82.8
pharynx, pharyngeal (congenital) Q38.7
Pouchitis K91.85Ø
Poultrymen's itch B88.Ø
Poverty NEC Z59.6
extreme Z59.5
Poxvirus NEC BØ8.8
Prader-Willi syndrome Q87.1
Preauricular appendage or tag Q17.Ø
Prebetalipoproteinemia (acquired) (essential) (familial) (hereditary) (primary) (secondary) E78.1
with chylomicronemia E78.3
Precipitate labor or delivery O62.3
Preclimacteric bleeding (menorrhagia) N92.4
Precocious
adrenarche E3Ø.1
menarche E3Ø.1
menstruation E3Ø.1
pubarche E3Ø.1
puberty E3Ø.1
central E22.8
sexual development NEC E3Ø.1
thelarche E3Ø.8
Precocity, sexual (constitutional) (cryptogenic) (female) (idiopathic) (male) E3Ø.1
with adrenal hyperplasia E25.9
congenital E25.Ø
Precordial pain RØ7.2
Predeciduous teeth KØØ.2
Prediabetes, prediabetic R73.Ø9
complicating
pregnancy — *see* Pregnancy, complicated by, diseases of, specified type or system NEC

Prediabetes, prediabetic — *continued*
complicating — *continued*
puerperium O99.89
Predislocation status of hip at birth Q65.6
Pre-eclampsia O14.9-
with pre-existing hypertension — *see* Hypertension, complicating pregnancy, pre-existing, with, pre-eclampsia
moderate O14.Ø-
severe O14.1-
with hemolysis, elevated liver enzymes and low platelet count (HELLP) O14.2-
Pre-eruptive color change, teeth, tooth KØØ.8
Pre-excitation atrioventricular conduction I45.6
Preglaucoma H4Ø.ØØ-
Pregnancy (childbirth) (labor) (puerperium) (*see also* Delivery and Puerperal)

Note: The Tabular must be reviewed for assignment of the appropriate character indicating the trimester of the pregnancy

Note:The Tabular must be reviewed for assignment of appropriate seventh character for multiple gestation codes in Chapter 15

abdominal (ectopic) OØØ.Ø
with viable fetus O36.7-
ampullar OØØ.1
biochemical OØ2.81
broad ligament OØØ.8
cervical OØØ.8
chemical OØ2.81
complicated by (care of) (management affected by)
abnormal, abnormality
cervix O34.4-
causing obstructed labor O65.5
cord (umbilical) O69.9
findings on antenatal screening of mother O28.9
biochemical O28.1
cytological O28.2
chromosomal O28.5
genetic O28.5
hematological O28.Ø
radiological O28.4
specified NEC O28.8
ultrasonic O28.3
glucose (tolerance) NEC O99.81Ø
pelvic organs O34.9-
specified NEC O34.8-
causing obstructed labor O65.5
pelvis (bony) (major) NEC O33.Ø
perineum O34.7-
position
placenta O44.1-
without hemorrhage O44.Ø-
uterus O34.59-
uterus O34.59-
causing obstructed labor O65.5
congenital O34.Ø-
vagina O34.6-
causing obstructed labor O65.5
vulva O34.7-
causing obstructed labor O65.5
abruptio placentae — *see* Abruptio placentae
abscess or cellulitis
bladder O23.1-
breast O91.11-
genital organ or tract O23.9-
abuse
physical O9A.31
psychological O9A.51
sexual O9A.41
adverse effect anesthesia O29.9-
aspiration pneumonitis O29.Ø1-
cardiac arrest O29.11-
cardiac complication NEC O29.19-
cardiac failure O29.12-
central nervous system complication NEC O29.29-
cerebral anoxia O29.21-
failed or difficult intubation O29.6-

- **Pregnancy** — *continued*
  - complicated by— *continued*
    - hydrorrhea O42.9Ø
    - hyperemesis (gravidarum) (mild) (*see also* Hyperemesis, gravidarum) O21.Ø
    - hypertension — *see* Hypertension, complicating pregnancy
    - hypertensive
      - heart and renal disease, pre-existing — *see* Hypertension, complicating, pregnancy, pre-existing, with, heart disease, with renal disease
      - heart disease, pre-existing — *see* Hypertension, complicating, pregnancy, pre-existing, with, heart disease
      - renal disease, pre-existing — *see* Hypertension, complicating, pregnancy, pre-existing, with, renal disease
    - hypotension O26.5-
    - immune disorders NEC (conditions in D8Ø-D89) O99.11-
    - incarceration, uterus O34.51-
    - incompetent cervix O34.3-
    - inconclusive fetal viability O36.8Ø
    - infection(s) O98.91-
      - amniotic fluid or sac O41.1Ø-
      - bladder O23.1-
      - carrier state NEC O99.83Ø
        - streptococcus B O99.82Ø
      - genital organ or tract O23.9-
        - specified NEC O23.59-
      - genitourinary tract O23.9-
      - gonorrhea O98.21-
      - hepatitis (viral) O98.41-
      - HIV O98.71-
      - human immunodeficiency virus (HIV) O98.71-
      - kidney O23.Ø-
      - nipple O91.Ø1-
      - parasitic disease O98.91-
        - specified NEC O98.81-
      - protozoal disease O98.61-
      - sexually transmitted NEC O98.31-
      - specified type NEC O98.81-
      - syphilis O98.11-
      - tuberculosis O98.Ø1-
      - urethra O23.2-
      - urinary (tract) O23.4-
        - specified NEC O23.3-
      - viral disease O98.51-
    - injury or poisoning (conditions in SØØ-T88) O9A.21-
      - due to abuse
        - physical O9A.31-
        - psychological O9A.51-
        - sexual O9A.41-
    - insufficient
      - prenatal care OØ9.3-
      - weight gain O26.1-
    - insulin resistance O26.89
    - isoimmunization O36.11-
      - anti-A sensitization O36.11-
      - anti-B sensitization O36.19-
      - Rh O36.Ø9-
        - anti-D antibody O36.Ø1-
      - specified NEC O36.19-
    - intrauterine fetal death (near term) O36.4
      - early pregnancy OØ2.1
      - multiple gestation (one fetus or more) O31.2-
    - laceration of uterus NEC O71.81
    - malformation
      - placenta, placental (vessel) O43.1Ø-
        - specified NEC O43.19-
      - uterus (congenital) O34.Ø-
    - malnutrition (conditions in E4Ø-E46) O25.1-
    - maternal hypotension syndrome O26.5-
    - mental disorders (conditions in FØ1-FØ9, F2Ø-F99) O99.34-
      - alcohol use O99.31-
      - drug use O99.32-
      - smoking O99.33-
    - mentum presentation O32.3
    - metabolic disorders O99.28-
    - missed
      - abortion OØ2.1
      - delivery O36.4
    - multiple gestations O3Ø.9-
      - conjoined twins O3Ø.Ø2-
      - specified number of multiples NEC — *see* Pregnancy, multiple (gestation), specified NEC
      - quadruplet — *see* Pregnancy, quadruplet
      - specified complication NEC O31.8X-
      - triplet— *see* Pregnancy, triplet
      - twin— *see* Pregnancy, twin
    - musculoskeletal condition (conditions is MØØ-M99) O99.89
    - necrosis, liver (conditions in K72) O26.61-
    - neoplasm
      - benign
        - cervix O34.4-
        - corpus uteri O34.1-
        - uterus O34.1-
      - malignant O9A.11-
    - nephropathy NEC O26.83-
    - nervous system condition (conditions in GØØ-G99) O99.35-
    - nutritional diseases NEC O99.28-
    - obesity (pre-existing) O99.21-
    - obesity surgery status O99.84-
    - oblique lie or presentation O32.2
    - older mother— *see* Pregnancy, complicated by, elderly
    - oligohydramnios O41.Ø-
      - with premature rupture of membranes (*see also* Pregnancy, complicated by, premature rupture of membranes) O42.
    - onset (spontaneous) of labor after 37 completed weeks of gestation but before 39 completed weeks gestation, with delivery by (planned) cesarean section O75.82
    - oophoritis O23.52-
    - overdose, drug (*see also* Table of Drugs and Chemicals, by drug, poisoning) O9A.21
    - oversize fetus O33.5
    - papyraceous fetus O31.Ø-
    - pelvic inflammatory disease O99.89
    - periodontal disease O99.61-
    - peripheral neuritis O26.82-
    - peritoneal (pelvic) adhesions O99.89
    - phlebitis O22.9-
    - phlebopathy O22.9-
    - phlebothrombosis (superficial) O22.2-
      - deep O22.3-
    - placenta accreta O43.21-
    - placenta increta O43.22-
    - placenta percreta O43.23-
    - placenta previa O44.1-
      - without hemorrhage O44.Ø-
    - placental disorder O43.9-
      - specified NEC O43.89-
    - placental dysfunction O43.89-
    - placental infarction O43.81-
    - placental insufficiency O36.51-
    - placental transfusion syndromes
      - fetomaternal O43.Ø1-
      - fetus to fetus O43.Ø2-
      - maternofetal O43.Ø1-
    - placentitis O41.14-
    - pneumonia O99.51-
    - poisoning (*see also* Table of Drugs and Chemicals) O9A.21-
    - polyhydramnios O4Ø-
    - polymorphic eruption of pregnency O26.86
    - poor obstetric history NEC OØ9.29-
    - postmaturity (post-term) (4Ø to 42 weeks) O48.Ø
      - more than 42 completed weeks gestation (prolonged) O48.1
    - pre-eclampsia O14.9-
      - mild O14.Ø-
      - moderate O14.Ø-
      - severe O14.1-
        - with hemolysis, elevated liver enzymes and low platelet count (HELLP) O14.2-
    - premature labor — *see* Pregnancy, complicated by, preterm labor
    - premature rupture of membranes O42.9Ø
      - full-term O42.92
      - with onset of labor
        - within 24 hours O42.ØØ
          - after 37 weeks gestation O42.Ø2
          - pre-term (before 37 completed weeks of gestation) O42.Ø1-
        - after 24 hours O42.1Ø
          - after 37 weeks gestation O42.12
          - pre-term (before 37 completed weeks of gestation) O42.11-
      - after 37 weeks gestation O42.92
      - pre-term (before 37 completed weeks of gestation) O42.91-
    - premature separation of placenta (*see also* Abruptio placentae) O45.9-
    - presentation, fetal — *see* Delivery (childbirth) (labor) (complicated by)
    - preterm delivery O6Ø.1Ø
    - preterm labor
      - with delivery O6Ø.1Ø
        - preterm O6Ø.1Ø
        - term O6Ø.2Ø
      - second trimester
        - with term delivery O6Ø.22
        - without delivery O6Ø.Ø2
        - with preterm delivery
          - second trimester O6Ø.12
          - third trimester O6Ø.13
      - third trimester
        - with term delivery O6Ø.23
        - without delivery O6Ø.Ø3
        - with third trimester preterm delivery O6Ø.14
      - without delivery O6Ø.ØØ
        - second trimester O6Ø.Ø2
        - third trimester O6Ø.Ø3
    - previous history of — *see* Pregnancy, supervision of, high-risk
    - prolapse, uterus O34.52-
    - proteinuria (gestational) O12.1-
      - with edema O12.2-
    - pruritic urticarial papules and plaques of pregnancy (PUPPP) O26.86
    - pruritus (neurogenic) O26.89-
    - psychosis or psychoneurosis (puerperal) F53
    - ptyalism O26.89-
    - PUPPP (pruritic urticarial papules and plaques of pregnancy) O26.86
    - pyelitis O23.Ø-
    - recurrent pregnancy loss O26.2-
    - renal disease or failure NEC O26.83-
      - with secondary hypertension, pre-existing — *see* Hypertension, complicating, pregnancy, pre-existing, secondary
      - hypertensive, pre-existing — *see* Hypertension, complicating, pregnancy, pre-existing, with, renal disease
    - respiratory condition (conditions in JØØ-J99) O99.51-
    - retained, retention
      - dead ovum OØ2.Ø
      - intrauterine contraceptive device O26.3-
    - retroversion, uterus O34.53-
    - Rh immunization, incompatibility or sensitization NEC O36.Ø9-
      - anti-D antibody O36.Ø1-
    - rupture
      - amnion (premature) (*see also* Pregnancy, complicated by, premature rupture of membranes) O42-
      - membranes (premature) (*see also* Pregnancy, complicated by, premature rupture of membranes) O42-

- **Pregnancy** — *continued*
  - supervision of — *continued*
    - elderly mother — *continued*
      - due to (history of) — *continued*
        - very young mother
          - multigravida OØ9.62-
          - primigravida OØ9.61-
      - resulting from in vitro fertilization OØ9.81-
    - hidden pregnancy OØ9.3-
    - high-risk OØ9.9-
      - due to (history of)
        - elderly — *see* Pregnancy, supervision, elderly mother
        - older mother — *see* Pregnancy, supervision of, elderly mother
        - very young mother — *see* Pregnancy, supervision, young mother
    - normal Z34.9-
      - first Z34.Ø-
      - specified NEC Z34.8-
    - young mother
      - multigravida OØ9.62-
      - primigravida OØ9.61-
  - triplet O3Ø.1Ø-
    - with
      - two or more monoamniotic fetuses O3Ø.12-
      - two or more monochrorionic fetuses O3Ø.11-
    - two or more monoamniotic fetuses O3Ø.12-
    - two or more monochrorionic fetuses O3Ø.11-
    - unable to determine number of placenta and number of amniotic sacs O3Ø.19-
    - unspecified number of placenta and unspecified number of amniotic sacs O3Ø.1Ø-
  - tubal (with abortion) (with rupture) OØØ.1
  - twin O3Ø.ØØ-
    - conjoined O3Ø.Ø2-
    - dichorionic/diamniotic (two placenta, two amniotic sacs) O3Ø.Ø4-
    - monochorionic/diamniotic (one placenta, two amniotic sacs) O3Ø.Ø3-
    - monochorionic/monoamniotic (one placenta, one amniotic sac) O3Ø.Ø1-
    - unable to determine number of placenta and number of amniotic sacs O3Ø.Ø9-
    - unspecified number of placenta and unspecified number of amniotic sacs O3Ø.ØØ-
  - weeks of gestation
    - 8 weeks Z3A.Ø8
    - 9 weeks Z3A.Ø9
    - 1Ø weeks Z3A.1Ø
    - 11 weeks Z3A.11
    - 12 weeks Z3A.12
    - 13 weeks Z3A.13
    - 14 weeks Z3A.14
    - 15 weeks Z3A.15
    - 16 weeks Z3A.16
    - 17 weeks Z3A.17
    - 18 weeks Z3A.18
    - 19 weeks Z3A.19
    - 2Ø weeks Z3A.2Ø
    - 21 weeks Z3A.21
    - 22 weeks Z3A.22
    - 23 weeks Z3A.23
    - 24 weeks Z3A.24
    - 25 weeks Z3A.25
    - 26 weeks Z3A.26
    - 27 weeks Z3A.27
    - 28 weeks Z3A.28
    - 29 weeks Z3A.29
    - 3Ø weeks Z3A.3Ø
    - 31 weeks Z3A.31
    - 32 weeks Z3A.32
    - 33 weeks Z3A.33
    - 34 weeks Z3A.34
    - 35 weeks Z3A.35
    - 36 weeks Z3A.36
    - 37 weeks Z3A.37
    - 38 weeks Z3A.38
    - 39 weeks Z3A.39
    - 4Ø weeks Z3A.4Ø
    - 41 weeks Z3A.41
    - 42 weeks Z3A.42
    - greater than 42 weeks Z3A.49

- **Pregnancy** — *continued*
  - weeks of gestation — *continued*
    - less than 8 weeks Z3A.Ø1
    - not specified Z3A.ØØ
- **Preiser's disease** — *see* Osteonecrosis, secondary, due to, trauma, metacarpus
- **Pre-kwashiorkor** — *see* Malnutrition, severe
- **Preleukemia** (syndrome) D46.9
- **Preluxation, hip, congenital** Q65.6
- **Premature** (*see also* condition)
  - adrenarche E27.Ø
  - aging E34.8
  - beats I49.4Ø
    - atrial I49.1
    - auricular I49.1
    - supraventricular I49.1
  - birth NEC — *see* Preterm, newborn
  - closure, foramen ovale Q21.8
  - contraction
    - atrial I49.1
    - atrioventricular I49.49
    - auricular I49.1
    - auriculoventricular I49.49
    - heart (extrasystole) I49.49
    - junctional I49.2
    - ventricular I49.3
  - delivery (*see also* Pregnancy, complicated by, preterm labor) O6Ø.1Ø
  - ejaculation F52.4
  - infant NEC — *see* Preterm, newborn
    - light-for-dates — *see* Light for dates
  - labor — *see* Pregnancy, complicated by, preterm labor
  - lungs P28.Ø
  - menopause E28.319
    - asymptomatic E28.319
    - symptomatic E28.31Ø
  - newborn
    - extreme (less than 28 completed weeks) — *see* Immaturity, extreme
    - less than 37 completed weeks — *see* Preterm, newborn
  - puberty E3Ø.1
  - rupture membranes or amnion — *see* Pregnancy, complicated by, premature rupture of membranes
  - senility E34.8
  - thelarche E3Ø.8
  - ventricular systole I49.3
- **Prematurity NEC** (less than 37 completed weeks) — *see* Preterm, newborn
  - extreme (less than 28 completed weeks) — *see* Immaturity, extreme
- **Premenstrual**
  - dysphoric disorder (PMDD) N94.3
  - tension (syndrome) N94.3
- **Premolarization, cuspids** KØØ.2
- **Prenatal**
  - care, normal pregnancy — *see* Pregnancy, normal
  - screening of mother Z36
  - teeth KØØ.6
- **Preparatory care for subsequent treatment NEC**
  - for dialysis Z49.Ø1
    - peritoneal Z49.Ø2
- **Prepartum** — *see* condition
- **Preponderance, left or right ventricular** I51.7
- **Prepuce** — *see* condition
- **PRES** (posterior reversible encephalopathy syndrome) I67.83
- **Presbycardia** R54
- **Presbycusis, presbyacusia** H91.1-
- **Presbyesophagus** K22.8
- **Presbyophrenia** FØ3
- **Presbyopia** H52.4
- **Prescription of contraceptives** (initial) Z3Ø.Ø19
  - emergency (postcoital) Z3Ø.Ø12
  - implantable subdermal Z3Ø.Ø19
  - injectable Z3Ø.Ø13
  - intrauterine contraceptive device Z3Ø.Ø14
  - pills Z3Ø.Ø11
  - postcoital (emergency) Z3Ø.Ø12
  - repeat Z3Ø.4Ø
    - implantable subdermal Z3Ø.49

- **Prescription of contraceptives** — *continued*
  - repeat — *continued*
    - injectable Z3Ø.42
    - pills Z3Ø.41
    - specified type NEC Z3Ø.49
  - specified type NEC Z3Ø.Ø18
- **Presence** (of)
  - ankle-joint implant (functional) (prosthesis) Z96.66-
  - aortocoronary (bypass) graft Z95.1
  - arterial-venous shunt (dialysis) Z99.2
  - artificial
    - eye (globe) Z97.Ø
    - heart (fully implantable) (mechanical) Z95.812
      - valve Z95.2
    - larynx Z96.3
    - lens (intraocular) Z96.1
    - limb (complete) (partial) Z97.1-
      - arm Z97.1-
        - bilateral Z97.15
      - leg Z97.1-
        - bilateral Z97.16
  - audiological implant (functional) Z96.29
  - bladder implant (functional) Z96.Ø
  - bone
    - conduction hearing device Z96.29
    - implant (functional) NEC Z96.7
    - joint (prosthesis) — *see* Presence, joint implant
  - cardiac
    - defibrillator (functional) (with synchronous cardiac pacemaker) Z95.81Ø
    - implant or graft Z95.9
      - specified type NEC Z95.818
    - pacemaker Z95.Ø
  - cerebrospinal fluid drainage device Z98.2
  - cochlear implant (functional) Z96.21
  - contact lens(es) Z97.3
  - coronary artery graft or prosthesis Z95.5
  - CSF shunt Z98.2
  - dental prosthesis device Z97.2
  - dentures Z97.2
  - device (external) NEC Z97.8
    - cardiac NEC Z95.818
    - heart assist Z95.811
    - implanted (functional) Z96.9
      - specified NEC Z96.89
    - prosthetic Z97.8
  - ear implant Z96.2Ø
    - cochlear implant Z96.21
    - myringotomy tube Z96.22
    - specified type NEC Z96.29
  - elbow-joint implant (functional) (prosthesis) Z96.62-
  - endocrine implant (functional) NEC Z96.49
  - eustachian tube stent or device (functional) Z96.29
  - external hearing-aid or device Z97.4
  - finger-joint implant (functional) (prosthetic) Z96.69-
  - functional implant Z96.9
    - specified NEC Z96.89
  - graft
    - cardiac NEC Z95.818
    - vascular NEC Z95.828
  - hearing-aid or device (external) Z97.4
    - implant (bone) (cochlear) (functional) Z96.21
  - heart assist device Z95.811
  - heart valve implant (functional) Z95.2
    - prosthetic Z95.2
    - specified type NEC Z95.4
    - xenogenic Z95.3
  - hip-joint implant (functional) (prosthesis) Z96.64-
  - implanted device (artificial) (functional) (prosthetic) Z96.9
    - automatic cardiac defibrillator (with synchronous cardiac pacemaker) Z95.81Ø
    - cardiac pacemaker Z95.Ø
    - cochlear Z96.21
    - dental Z96.5
    - heart Z95.812
    - heart valve Z95.2
      - prosthetic Z95.2
      - specified NEC Z95.4
      - xenogenic Z95.3
    - insulin pump Z96.41
    - intraocular lens Z96.1

Presence — *continued*
implanted device— *continued*
joint Z96.6Ø
ankle Z96.66-
elbow Z96.62-
finger Z96.69-
hip Z96.64-
knee Z96.65-
shoulder Z96.61-
specified NEC Z96.698
wrist Z96.63-
larynx Z96.3
myringotomy tube Z96.22
otological Z96.2Ø
cochlear Z96.21
eustachian stent Z96.29
myringotomy Z96.22
specified NEC Z96.29
stapes Z96.29
skin Z96.81
skull plate Z96.7
specified NEC Z96.89
urogenital Z96.Ø
insulin pump (functional) Z96.41
intestinal bypass or anastomosis Z98.Ø
intraocular lens (functional) Z96.1
intrauterine contraceptive device (IUD) Z97.5
intravascular implant (functional) (prosthetic) NEC Z95.9
coronary artery Z95.5
defibrillator (with synchronous cardiac pacemaker) Z95.81Ø
peripheral vessel (with angioplasty) Z95.82Ø
joint implant (prosthetic) (any) Z96.6Ø
ankle — *see* Presence, ankle joint implant
elbow — *see* Presence, elbow joint implant
finger — *see* Presence, finger joint implant
hip — *see* Presence, hip joint implant
knee — *see* Presence, knee joint implant
shoulder — *see* Presence, shoulder joint implant
specified joint NEC Z96.698
wrist — *see* Presence, wrist joint implant
knee-joint implant (functional) (prosthesis) Z96.65-
laryngeal implant (functional) Z96.3
mandibular implant (dental) Z96.5
myringotomy tube(s) Z96.22
orthopedic-joint implant (prosthetic) (any) — *see* Presence, joint implant
otological implant (functional) Z96.29
shoulder-joint implant (functional) (prosthesis) Z96.61-
skull-plate implant Z96.7
spectacles Z97.3
stapes implant (functional) Z96.29
systemic lupus erythematosus [SLE] inhibitor D68.62
tendon implant (functional) (graft) Z96.7
tooth root(s) implant Z96.5
ureteral stent Z96.Ø
urethral stent Z96.Ø
urogenital implant (functional) Z96.Ø
vascular implant or device Z95.9
access port device Z95.828
specified type NEC Z95.828
wrist-joint implant (functional) (prosthesis) Z96.63-
Presenile (*see also* condition)
dementia FØ3
premature aging E34.8
Presentation, fetal — *see* Delivery (childbirth) (labor) (complicated by), malposition, malpresentation
Prespondylolisthesis (congenital) Q76.2
Pressure
area, skin — *see* Ulcer, pressure, by site
brachial plexus G54.Ø
brain G93.5
injury at birth NEC P11.1
cerebral — *see* Pressure, brain
chest RØ7.89
cone, tentorial G93.5
hyposystolic (*see also* Hypotension)
incidental reading, without diagnosis of hypotension RØ3.1

Pressure— *continued*
increased
intracranial (benign) G93.2
injury at birth P11.Ø
intraocular H4Ø.Ø5-
lumbosacral plexus G54.1
mediastinum J98.5
necrosis (chronic) — *see* Ulcer, pressure, by site
parental, inappropriate (excessive) Z62.6
sore (chronic) — *see* Ulcer, pressure, by site
spinal cord G95.2Ø
ulcer (chronic) — *see* Ulcer, pressure, by site
venous, increased I87.8
Pre-syncope R55
Preterm
delivery (*see also* Pregnancy, complicated by, preterm labor) O6Ø.1Ø
labor — *see* Pregnancy, complicated by, preterm labor
newborn (infant) PØ7.3Ø
gestational age
28 completed weeks (28 weeks, Ø days through 28 weeks, 6 days) PØ7.31
29 completed weeks (29 weeks, Ø days through 29 weeks, 6 days) PØ7.32
3Ø completed weeks (3Ø weeks, Ø days through 3Ø weeks, 6 days) PØ7.33
31 completed weeks (31 weeks, Ø days through 31 weeks, 6 days) PØ7.34
32 completed weeks (32 weeks, Ø days through 32 weeks, 6 days) PØ7.35
33 completed weeks (33 weeks, Ø days through 33 weeks, 6 days) PØ7.36
34 completed weeks (34 weeks, Ø days through 34 weeks, 6 days) PØ7.37
35 completed weeks (35 weeks, Ø days through 35 weeks, 6 days) PØ7.38
36 completed weeks (36 weeks, Ø days through 36 weeks, 6 days) PØ7.39
Previa
placenta (low) (marginal) (partial) (total) (with hemorrhage) O44.1-
without hemorrhage O44.Ø-
vasa O69.4
Priapism N48.3Ø
due to
disease classified elsewhere N48.32
drug N48.33
specified cause NEC N48.39
trauma N48.31
Prickling sensation (skin) R2Ø.2
Prickly heat L74.Ø
Primary — *see* condition
Primigravida
elderly, affecting management of pregnancy, labor and delivery (supervision only) — *see* Pregnancy, complicated by, elderly, primigravida
older, affecting management of pregnancy, labor and delivery (supervision only) — *see* Pregnancy, complicated by, elderly, primigravida
very young, affecting management of pregnancy, labor and delivery (supervision only) — *see* Pregnancy, complicated by, young mother, primigravida
Primipara
elderly, affecting management of pregnancy, labor and delivery (supervision only) — *see* Pregnancy, complicated by, elderly, primigravida
older, affecting management of pregnancy, labor and delivery (supervision only) — *see* Pregnancy, complicated by, elderly, primigravida
very young, affecting management of pregnancy, labor and delivery (supervision only) — *see* Pregnancy, complicated by, young mother, primigravida
Primus varus (bilateral) Q66.2
PRIND (Prolonged reversible ischemic neurologic deficit) I63.9
Pringle's disease (tuberous sclerosis) Q85.1

Prinzmetal angina I2Ø.1
Prizefighter ear — *see* Cauliflower ear
Problem (with) (related to)
academic Z55.8
acculturation Z6Ø.3
adjustment (to)
change of job Z56.1
life-cycle transition Z6Ø.Ø
pension Z6Ø.Ø
retirement Z6Ø.Ø
adopted child Z62.821
alcoholism in family Z63.72
atypical parenting situation Z62.9
bankruptcy Z59.8
behavioral (adult) F69
drug seeking Z72.89
birth of sibling affecting child Z62.898
care (of)
provider dependency Z74.9
specified NEC Z74.8
sick or handicapped person in family or household Z63.6
child
abuse (affecting the child) — *see* Maltreatment, child
custody or support proceedings Z65.3
in welfare custody Z62.21
in care of non-parental family member Z62.21
in foster care Z62.21
living in orphanage or group home Z62.22
child-rearing Z62.9
specified NEC Z62.898
communication (developmental) F8Ø.9
conflict or discord (with)
boss Z56.4
classmates Z55.4
counselor Z64.4
employer Z56.4
family Z63.9
specified NEC Z63.8
probation officer Z64.4
social worker Z64.4
teachers Z55.4
workmates Z56.4
conviction in legal proceedings Z65.Ø
with imprisonment Z65.1
counselor Z64.4
creditors Z59.8
digestive K92.9
drug addict in family Z63.72
ear — *see* Disorder, ear
economic Z59.9
affecting care Z59.9
specified NEC Z59.8
education Z55.9
specified NEC Z55.8
employment Z56.9
change of job Z56.1
discord Z56.4
environment Z56.5
sexual harassment Z56.81
specified NEC Z56.89
stress NEC Z56.6
stressful schedule Z56.3
threat of job loss Z56.2
unemployment Z56.Ø
enuresis, child F98.Ø
eye H57.9
failed examinations (school) Z55.2
falling Z91.81
family (*see also* Disruption, family) Z63.9
specified NEC Z63.8
feeding (elderly) (infant) R63.3
newborn P92.9
breast P92.5
overfeeding P92.4
slow P92.2
specified NEC P92.8
underfeeding P92.3
nonorganic F5Ø.8
finance Z59.9
specified NEC Z59.8
foreclosure on loan Z59.8

- **Problem**— *continued*
  - foster child Z62.822
  - frightening experience(s) in childhood Z62.898
  - genital NEC
    - female N94.9
    - male N5Ø.9
  - health care Z75.9
    - specified NEC Z75.8
  - hearing — *see* Deafness
  - homelessness Z59.Ø
  - housing Z59.9
    - inadequate Z59.1
    - isolated Z59.8
    - specified NEC Z59.8
  - identity (of childhood) F93.8
  - illegitimate pregnancy (unwanted) Z64.Ø
  - illiteracy Z55.Ø
  - impaired mobility Z74.Ø9
  - imprisonment or incarceration Z65.1
  - inadequate teaching affecting education Z55.8
  - inappropriate (excessive) parental pressure Z62.6
  - influencing health status NEC Z78.9
  - in-law Z63.1
  - institutionalization, affecting child Z62.22
  - intrafamilial communication Z63.8
  - jealousy, child F93.8
  - landlord Z59.2
  - language (developmental) F8Ø.9
  - learning (developmental) F81.9
  - legal Z65.3
    - conviction without imprisonment Z65.Ø
    - imprisonment Z65.1
    - release from prison Z65.2
  - life-management Z73.9
    - specified NEC Z73.89
  - life-style Z72.9
    - gambling Z72.6
    - high-risk sexual behavior (heterosexual) Z72.51
      - bisexual Z72.53
      - homosexual Z72.52
    - inappropriate eating habits Z72.4
    - self-damaging behavior NEC Z72.89
    - specified NEC Z72.89
    - tobacco use Z72.Ø
  - literacy Z55.9
    - low level Z55.Ø
    - specified NEC Z55.8
  - living alone Z6Ø.2
  - lodgers Z59.2
  - loss of love relationship in childhood Z62.898
  - marital Z63.Ø
    - involving
      - divorce Z63.5
      - estrangement Z63.5
      - gender identity F66
  - mastication KØ8.8
  - medical
    - care, within family Z63.6
    - facilities Z75.9
      - specified NEC Z75.8
  - mental F48.9
  - multiparity Z64.1
  - negative life events in childhood Z62.9
    - altered pattern of family relationships Z62.898
    - frightening experience Z62.898
    - loss of
      - love relationship Z62.898
      - self-esteem Z62.898
    - physical abuse (alleged) — *see* Maltreatment, child
    - removal from home Z62.29
    - specified event NEC Z62.898
  - neighbor Z59.2
  - neurological NEC R29.818
  - new step-parent affecting child Z62.898
  - none (feared complaint unfounded) Z71.1
  - occupational NEC Z56.89
  - parent-child — *see* Conflict, parent-child
  - personal hygiene Z91.89
  - personality F69
  - phase-of-life transition, adjustment Z6Ø.Ø
  - presence of sick or disabled person in family or household Z63.79

- **Problem**— *continued*
  - presence of sick or disabled person in family or household — *continued*
    - needing care Z63.6
  - primary support group (family) Z63.9
    - specified NEC Z63.8
  - probation officer Z64.4
  - psychiatric F99
  - psychosexual (development) F66
  - psychosocial Z65.9
    - specified NEC Z65.8
  - relationship Z63.9
    - childhood F93.8
  - release from prison Z65.2
  - removal from home affecting child Z62.29
  - seeking and accepting known hazardous and harmful
    - behavioral or psychological interventions Z65.8
    - chemical, nutritional or physical interventions Z65.8
  - sexual function (nonorganic) F52.9
  - sight H54.7
  - sleep disorder, child F51.9
  - smell — *see* Disturbance, sensation, smell
  - social
    - environment Z6Ø.9
      - specified NEC Z6Ø.8
    - exclusion and rejection Z6Ø.4
    - worker Z64.4
  - speech R47.9
    - developmental F8Ø.9
    - specified NEC R47.89
  - swallowing — *see* Dysphagia
  - taste — *see* Disturbance, sensation, taste
  - tic, child F95.Ø
  - underachievement in school Z55.3
  - unemployment Z56.Ø
    - threatened Z56.2
  - unwanted pregnancy Z64.Ø
  - upbringing Z62.9
    - specified NEC Z62.898
  - urinary N39.9
  - voice production R47.89
  - work schedule (stressful) Z56.3
- **Procedure** (surgical)
  - elective — *see* Surgery, elective
  - for purpose other than remedying health state Z41.9
    - specified NEC Z41.8
  - not done Z53.9
    - because of
      - administrative reasons Z53.8
      - contraindication Z53.Ø9
        - smoking Z53.Ø1
      - patient's decision Z53.2Ø
        - for reasons of belief or group pressure Z53.1
        - left against medical advice (AMA) Z53.21
        - specified reason NEC Z53.29
      - specified reason NEC Z53.8
- **Procidentia** (uteri) N81.3
- **Proctalgia** K62.89
  - fugax K59.4
  - spasmodic K59.4
- **Proctitis** K62.89
  - amebic (acute) AØ6.Ø
  - chlamydial A56.3
  - gonococcal A54.6
  - granulomatous — *see* Enteritis, regional, large intestine
  - herpetic A6Ø.1
  - radiation K62.7
  - tuberculous A18.32
  - ulcerative (chronic) K51.2Ø
    - with
      - complication K51.219
        - abscess K51.214
        - fistula K51.213
        - obstruction K51.212
        - rectal bleeding K51.211
        - specified NEC K51.218
- **Proctocele**
  - female (without uterine prolapse) N81.6

- **Proctocele** — *continued*
  - female (without uterine prolapse) — *continued*
    - with uterine prolapse N81.2
      - complete N81.3
  - male K62.3
- **Proctocolitis, mucosal** — *see* Rectosigmoiditis, ulcerative
- **Proctoptosis** K62.3
- **Proctorrhagia** K62.5
- **Proctosigmoiditis** K63.89
  - ulcerative (chronic) — *see* Rectosigmoiditis, ulcerative
- **Proctospasm** K59.4
  - psychogenic F45.8
- **Profichet's disease** — *see* Disorder, soft tissue, specified type NEC
- **Progeria** E34.8
- **Prognathism** (mandibular) (maxillary) M26.19
- **Progonoma** (melanotic) — *see* Neoplasm, benign, by site
- **Progressive** — *see* condition
- **Prolactinoma**
  - specified site — *see* Neoplasm, benign, by site
  - unspecified site D35.2
- **Prolapse, prolapsed**
  - anus, anal (canal) (sphincter) K62.2
  - arm or hand O32.2
    - causing obstructed labor O64.4
  - bladder (mucosa) (sphincter) (acquired)
    - congenital Q79.4
    - female — *see* Cystocele
    - male N32.89
  - breast implant (prosthetic) T85.49
  - cecostomy K94.Ø9
  - cecum K63.4
  - cervix, cervical (hypertrophied) N81.2
    - anterior lip, obstructing labor O65.5
    - congenital Q51.828
    - postpartal, old N81.2
    - stump N81.85
  - ciliary body (traumatic) — *see* Laceration, eye(ball), with prolapse or loss of interocular tissue
  - colon (pedunculated) K63.4
  - colostomy K94.Ø9
  - disc (intervertebral) — *see* Displacement, intervertebral disc
  - eye implant (orbital) T85.398
    - lens (ocular) — *see* Complications, intraocular lens
  - fallopian tube N83.4
  - gastric (mucosa) K31.89
  - genital, female N81.9
    - specified NEC N81.89
  - globe, nontraumatic — *see* Luxation, globe
  - ileostomy bud K94.19
  - intervertebral disc — *see* Displacement, intervertebral disc
  - intestine (small) K63.4
  - iris (traumatic) — *see* Laceration, eye(ball), with prolapse or loss of interocular tissue
    - nontraumatic H21.89
  - kidney N28.83
    - congenital Q63.2
  - laryngeal muscles or ventricle J38.7
  - liver K76.89
  - meatus urinarius N36.8
  - mitral (valve) I34.1
  - ocular lens implant — *see* Complications, intraocular lens
  - organ or site, congenital NEC — *see* Malposition, congenital
  - ovary N83.4
  - pelvic floor, female N81.89
  - perineum, female N81.89
  - rectum (mucosa) (sphincter) K62.3
    - due to trichuris trichuria B79
  - spleen D73.89
  - stomach K31.89
  - umbilical cord
    - complicating delivery O69.Ø
  - urachus, congenital Q64.4
  - ureter N28.89
    - with obstruction N13.5

Prolapse, prolapsed — *continued*
- ureter — *continued*
  - with obstruction — *continued*
    - with infection N13.6
- ureterovesical orifice N28.89
- urethra (acquired) (infected) (mucosa) N36.8
  - congenital Q64.71
- urinary meatus N36.8
  - congenital Q64.72
- uterovaginal N81.4
  - complete N81.3
  - incomplete N81.2
- uterus (with prolapse of vagina) N81.4
  - complete N81.3
  - congenital Q51.818
  - first degree N81.2
  - in pregnancy or childbirth — *see* Pregnancy, complicated by, abnormal, uterus
  - incomplete N81.2
  - postpartal (old) N81.4
  - second degree N81.2
  - third degree N81.3
- uveal (traumatic) — *see* Laceration, eye(ball), with prolapse or loss of interocular tissue
- vagina (anterior) (wall) — *see* Cystocele
  - with prolapse of uterus N81.4
    - complete N81.3
    - incomplete N81.2
  - posterior wall N81.6
  - posthysterectomy N99.3
- vitreous (humor) H43.Ø-
  - in wound — *see* Laceration, eye(ball), with prolapse or loss of interocular tissue
- womb — *see* Prolapse, uterus

Prolapsus, female N81.9
- specified NEC N81.89

Proliferation(s)
- primary cutaneous CD3Ø-positive large T-cell C86.6

Proliferative — *see* condition

Prolonged, prolongation (of)
- bleeding (time) (idiopathic) R79.1
- coagulation (time) R79.1
- gestation (over 42 completed weeks)
  - mother O48.1
  - newborn PØ8.22
- interval I44.Ø
- labor O63.9
  - first stage O63.Ø
  - second stage O63.1
- partial thromboplastin time (PTT) R79.1
- pregnancy (more than 42 weeks gestation) O48.1
- prothrombin time R79.1
- QT interval I45.81
- uterine contractions in labor O62.4

Prominence, prominent
- auricle (congenital) (ear) Q17.5
- ischial spine or sacral promontory
  - with disproportion (fetopelvic) O33.Ø
    - causing obstructed labor O65.Ø
- nose (congenital) acquired M95.Ø

Promiscuity — *see* High, risk, sexual behavior

Pronation
- ankle — *see* Deformity, limb, foot, specified NEC
- foot (*see also* Deformity, limb, foot, specified NEC)
  - congenital Q74.2

Prophylactic
- administration of
  - antibiotics, long-term Z79.2
    - short-term use — *omit code*
  - drug (*see also* Long-term (current) drug therapy (use of)) Z79.899
- medication Z79.899
- organ removal (for neoplasia management) Z4Ø.ØØ
  - breast Z4Ø.Ø1
  - ovary Z4Ø.Ø2
  - specified site NEC Z4Ø.Ø9
- surgery Z4Ø.9
  - for risk factors related to malignant neoplasm — *see* Prophylactic, organ removal
  - specified NEC Z4Ø.8
- vaccination Z23

Propionic acidemia E71.121

Proptosis (ocular) (*see also* Exophthalmos)
- thyroid — *see* Hyperthyroidism, with goiter

Prosecution, anxiety concerning Z65.3

Prosopagnosia R48.3

Prostadynia N42.81

Prostate, prostatic — *see* condition

Prostatism — *see* Hyperplasia, prostate

Prostatitis (congestive) (suppurative) (with cystitis) N41.9
- acute N41.ØØ
- cavitary N41.8
- chronic N41.1Ø
- diverticular N41.8
- due to Trichomonas (vaginalis) A59.Ø2
- fibrous N41.1Ø
  - with hematuria N41.11
- gonococcal (acute) (chronic) A54.22
- granulomatous N41.4
- hypertrophic N41.1Ø
  - with hematuria N41.11
- subacute N41.1Ø
  - with hematuria N41.11
- trichomonal A59.Ø2
- tuberculous A18.14

Prostatocystitis N41.3

Prostatorrhea N42.89

Prostatosis N42.82

Prostration R53.83
- heat (*see also* Heat, exhaustion)
  - anhydrotic T67.3
  - due to
    - salt (and water) depletion T67.4
    - water depletion T67.3
- nervous F48.8
- senile R54

Protanomaly (anomalous trichromat) H53.54

Protanopia (complete) (incomplete) H53.54

Protection (against) (from) — *see* Prophylactic

Protein
- deficiency NEC — *see* Malnutrition
- malnutrition — *see* Malnutrition
- sickness (*see also* Reaction, serum) TØ8.69

Proteinemia R77.9

Proteinosis
- alveolar (pulmonary) J84.Ø1
- lipid or lipoid (of Urbach) E78.89

Proteinuria R8Ø.9
- Bence Jones R8Ø.3
- complicating pregnancy — *see* Proteinuria, gestational
- gestational O12.1-
  - with edema O12.2-
- idiopathic R8Ø.Ø
- isolated R8Ø.Ø
  - with glomerular lesion NØ6.9
    - dense deposit disease NØ6.6
    - diffuse
      - crescentic glomerulonephritis NØ6.7
      - endocapillary proliferative glomerulonephritis NØ6.4
      - mesangiocapillary glomerulonephritis NØ6.5
    - focal and segmental hyalinosis or sclerosis NØ6.1
    - membranous (diffuse) NØ6.2
    - mesangial proliferative (diffuse) NØ6.3
    - minimal change NØ6.Ø
    - specified pathology NEC NØ6.8
- orthostatic R8Ø.2
  - with glomerular lesion — *see* Proteinuria, isolated, with glomerular lesion
- persistent R8Ø.1
  - with glomerular lesion — *see* Proteinuria, isolated, with glomerular lesion
- postural R8Ø.2
  - with glomerular lesion — *see* Proteinuria, isolated, with glomerular lesion
- pre-eclamptic — *see* Pre-eclampsia
- specified type NEC R8Ø.8

Proteolysis, pathologic D65

Proteus (mirabilis) (morganii), **as cause of disease classified elsewhere** B96.4

Prothrombin gene mutation D68.52

Protoporphyria, erythropoietic E8Ø.Ø

Protozoal (*see also* condition)
- disease B64
  - specified NEC B6Ø.8

Protrusion, protrusio
- acetabuli M24.7
- acetabulum (into pelvis) M24.7
- device, implant or graft (*see also* Complications, by site and type, mechanical) T85.698
  - arterial graft NEC — *see* Complication, cardiovascular device, mechanical, vascular
  - breast (implant) T85.49
  - catheter NEC T85.698
    - cystostomy T83.Ø9Ø
    - dialysis (renal) T82.49
      - intraperitoneal T85.691
    - infusion NEC T82.594
      - spinal (epidural) (subdural) T85.69Ø
    - urinary, indwelling T83.Ø98
  - electronic (electrode) (pulse generator) (stimulator)
    - bone T84.39Ø
    - nervous system — *see* Complication, prosthetic device, mechanical, electronic nervous system stimulator
  - fixation, internal (orthopedic) NEC — *see* Complication, fixation device, mechanical
  - gastrointestinal — *see* Complications, prosthetic device, mechanical, gastrointestinal device
  - genital NEC T83.498
    - intrauterine contraceptive device T83.39
    - penile prosthesis T83.49Ø
  - heart NEC — *see* Complication, cardiovascular device, mechanical
  - joint prosthesis — *see* Complications, joint prosthesis, mechanical, specified NEC, by site
  - ocular NEC — *see* Complications, prosthetic device, mechanical, ocular device
  - orthopedic NEC — *see* Complication, orthopedic, device, mechanical
  - specified NEC T85.628
  - urinary NEC (*see also* Complication, genitourinary, device, urinary, mechanical)
    - graft T83.29
  - vascular NEC — *see* Complication, cardiovascular device, mechanical
  - ventricular intracranial shunt T85.Ø9
- intervertebral disc — *see* Displacement, intervertebral disc
- joint prosthesis — *see* Complications, joint prosthesis, mechanical, specified NEC, by site
- nucleus pulposus — *see* Displacement, intervertebral disc

Prune belly (syndrome) Q79.4

Prurigo (ferox) (gravis) (Hebrae) (Hebra's) (mitis) (simplex) L28.2
- Besnier's L2Ø.Ø
- estivalis L56.4
- nodularis L28.1
- psychogenic F45.8

Pruritus, pruritic (essential) L29.9
- ani, anus L29.Ø
  - psychogenic F45.8
- anogenital L29.3
  - psychogenic F45.8
- due to onchocerca volvulus B73.1
- gravidarum — *see* Pregnancy, complicated by, specified pregnancy-related condition NEC
- hiemalis L29.8
- neurogenic (any site) F45.8
- perianal L29.Ø
- psychogenic (any site) F45.8
- scroti, scrotum L29.1
  - psychogenic F45.8
- senile, senilis L29.8
- specified NEC L29.8
  - psychogenic F45.8
- Trichomonas A59.9

Psychosis, psychotic — *continued*
- Korsakoff's — *continued*
  - induced by other psychoactive substance — *see* categories F11-F19 with .x5x
- mania, manic (single episode) F3Ø.2
  - recurrent type F31.89
- manic-depressive — *see* Disorder, mood
- menopausal — *see* Psychosis, involutional
- mixed schizophrenic and affective F25.8
- multi-infarct (cerebrovascular) FØ1.5Ø
  - with behavioral disturbance FØ1.51
- nonorganic F29
  - specified NEC F28
- organic FØ9
  - due to or associated with
    - arteriosclerosis (cerebral) — *see* Psychosis, arteriosclerotic
    - cerebrovascular disease, arteriosclerotic — *see* Psychosis, arteriosclerotic
    - childbirth — *see* Psychosis, puerperal
    - Creutzfeldt-Jakob disease or syndrome — *see* Creutzfeldt-Jakob disease or syndrome
    - dependence, alcohol F1Ø.259
    - disease
      - alcoholic liver F1Ø.259
      - brain, arteriosclerotic — *see* Psychosis, arteriosclerotic
      - cerebrovascular FØ1.5Ø
        - with behavioral disturbance FØ1.51
      - Creutzfeldt-Jakob — *see* Creutzfeldt-Jakob disease or syndrome
      - endocrine or metabolic FØ6.8
        - acute or subacute FØ5
      - liver, alcoholic F1Ø.259
    - epilepsy transient (acute) FØ5
    - infection
      - brain (intracranial) FØ6.8
        - acute or subacute FØ5
    - intoxication
      - alcoholic (acute) F1Ø.259
      - drug F11-F19 with .x59
    - ischemia, cerebrovascular (generalized) — *see* Psychosis, arteriosclerotic
    - puerperium — *see* Psychosis, puerperal
    - trauma, brain (birth) (from electric current) (surgical) FØ6.8
      - acute or subacute FØ5
  - infective FØ6.8
    - acute or subacute FØ5
  - post-traumatic FØ6.8
    - acute or subacute FØ5
- paranoiac F22
- paranoid (climacteric) (involutional) (menopausal) F22
  - psychogenic (acute) F23
  - schizophrenic F2Ø.Ø
  - senile FØ3
- postpartum F53
- presbyophrenic (type) FØ3
- presenile FØ3
- psychogenic (paranoid) F23
  - depressive F32.3
- puerperal F53
  - specified type — *see* Psychosis, by type
- reactive (brief) (transient) (emotional stress) (psychological trauma) F23
  - depressive F32.3
    - recurrent F33.3
  - excitative type F3Ø.8
- schizoaffective F25.9
  - depressive type F25.1
  - manic type F25.Ø
- schizophrenia, schizophrenic — *see* Schizophrenia
- schizophrenia-like, in epilepsy FØ6.2
- schizophreniform F2Ø.81
  - affective type F25.9
  - brief F23
  - confusional type F23
  - depressive type F25.1
  - manic type F25.Ø
  - mixed type F25.Ø
- senile NEC FØ3
  - depressed or paranoid type FØ3

Psychosis, psychotic — *continued*
- senile NEC — *continued*
  - simple deterioration FØ3
- specified type code to condition
- shared F24
- situational (reactive) F23
- symbiotic (childhood) F84.3
- symptomatic FØ9

Psychosomatic — *see* Disorder, psychosomatic

Psychosyndrome, organic FØ7.9

Psychotic episode due to or associated with physical condition FØ6.8

Pterygium (eye) H11.ØØ-
- amyloid H11.Ø1-
- central H11.Ø2-
- colli Q18.3
- double H11.Ø3-
- peripheral
  - progressive H11.Ø5-
  - stationary H11.Ø4-
- recurrent H11.Ø6-

Ptilosis (eyelid) — *see* Madarosis

Ptomaine (poisoning) — *see* Poisoning, food

Ptosis (*see also* Blepharoptosis)
- adiposa (false) — *see* Blepharoptosis
- breast N64.81
- cecum K63.4
- colon K63.4
- congenital (eyelid) Q1Ø.Ø
  - specified site NEC — *see* Anomaly, by site
- eyelid — *see* Blepharoptosis
  - congenital Q1Ø.Ø
- gastric K31.89
- intestine K63.4
- kidney N28.83
- liver K76.89
- renal N28.83
- splanchnic K63.4
- spleen D73.89
- stomach K31.89
- viscera K63.4

PTP D69.51

Ptyalism (periodic) K11.7
- hysterical F45.8
- pregnancy — *see* Pregnancy, complicated by, specified pregnancy-related condition NEC
- psychogenic F45.8

Ptyalolithiasis K11.5

Pubarche, precocious E3Ø.1

Pubertas praecox E3Ø.1

Puberty (development state) ZØØ.3
- bleeding (excessive) N92.2
- delayed E3Ø.Ø
- precocious (constitutional) (cryptogenic) (idiopathic) E3Ø.1
  - central E22.8
  - due to
    - ovarian hyperfunction E28.1
      - estrogen E28.Ø
    - testicular hyperfunction E29.Ø
- premature E3Ø.1
  - due to
    - adrenal cortical hyperfunction E25.8
    - pineal tumor E34.8
    - pituitary (anterior) hyperfunction E22.8

Puckering, macula — *see* Degeneration, macula, puckering

Pudenda, pudendum — *see* condition

Puente's disease (simple glandular cheilitis) K13.Ø

Puerperal, puerperium (complicated by, complications)
- abnormal glucose (tolerance test) O99.815
- abscess
  - areola O91.Ø2
    - associated with lactation O91.Ø3
  - Bartholin's gland O86.19
  - breast O91.12
    - associated with lactation O91.13
  - cervix (uteri) O86.11
  - genital organ NEC O86.19
  - kidney O86.21
  - mammary O91.12
    - associated with lactation O91.13

Puerperal, puerperium — *continued*
- abscess — *continued*
  - nipple O91.Ø2
    - associated with lactation O91.Ø3
  - peritoneum O85
  - subareolar O91.12
    - associated with lactation O91.13
  - urinary tract — *see* Puerperal, infection, urinary
  - uterus O86.12
  - vagina (wall) O86.13
  - vaginorectal O86.13
  - vulvovaginal gland O86.13
- adnexitis O86.19
- afibrinogenemia, or other coagulation defect O72.3
- albuminuria (acute) (subacute) — *see* Proteinuria, gestational
- alcohol use O99.315
- anemia O9Ø.81
  - pre-existing (pre-pregnancy) O99.Ø3
- anesthetic death O89.8
- apoplexy O99.43
- bariatric surgery status O99.845
- blood disorder NEC O99.13
- blood dyscrasia O72.3
- cardiomyopathy O9Ø.3
- cerebrovascular disorder (conditions in I6Ø-I69) O99.43
- cervicitis O86.11
- circulatory system disorder O99.43
- coagulopathy (any) O72.3
- complications O9Ø.9
  - specified NEC O9Ø.89
- convulsions — *see* Eclampsia
- cystitis O86.22
- cystopyelitis O86.29
- delirium NEC FØ5
- diabetes O24.93
  - gestational — *see* Puerperal, gestational diabetes
  - pre-existing O24.33
    - specified NEC O24.83
    - type 1 O24.Ø3
    - type 2 O24.13
- digestive system disorder O99.63
- disease O9Ø.9
  - breast NEC O92.29
  - cerebrovascular (acute) O99.43
  - nonobstetric NEC O99.89
  - tubo-ovarian O86.19
  - Valsuani's O99.Ø3
- disorder O9Ø.9
  - biliary tract O26.63
  - lactation O92.79
  - liver O26.63
  - nonobstetric NEC O99.89
- disruption
  - cesarean wound O9Ø.Ø
  - episiotomy wound O9Ø.1
  - perineal laceration wound O9Ø.1
- drug use O99.325
- eclampsia (with pre-existing hypertension) O15.2
- embolism (pulmonary) (blood clot) — *see* Embolism, obstetric, puerperal
- endocrine, nutritional or metabolic disease NEC O99.285
- endophlebitis — *see* Puerperal, phlebitis
- endotrachelitis O86.19
- failure
  - lactation (complete) O92.3
    - partial O92.4
  - renal, acute O9Ø.4
- fever (of unknown origin) O86.4
  - septic O85
- fissure, nipple O92.12
  - associated with lactation O92.13
- fistula
  - breast (due to mastitis) O91.12
    - associated with lactation O91.13
  - nipple O91.Ø2
    - associated with lactation O91.Ø3
- galactophoritis O91.22
  - associated with lactation O91.23
- galactorrhea O92.6
- gastric banding status O99.845

- **Puerperal, puerperium** — *continued*
  - gastric bypass status O99.845
  - gastrointestinal disease NEC O99.63
  - gestational diabetes O24.439
    - diet controlled O24.43Ø
    - insulin (and diet) controlled O24.434
  - gonorrhea O98.23
  - hematoma, subdural O99.43
  - hemiplegia, cerebral O99.355-
    - due to cerbrovascular disorder O99.43
  - hemorrhage O72.1
    - brain O99.43
    - bulbar O99.43
    - cerebellar O99.43
    - cerebral O99.43
    - cortical O99.43
    - delayed or secondary O72.2
    - extradural O99.43
    - internal capsule O99.43
    - intracranial O99.43
    - intrapontine O99.43
    - meningeal O99.43
    - pontine O99.43
    - retained placenta O72.Ø
    - subarachnoid O99.43
    - subcortical O99.43
    - subdural O99.43
    - third stage O72.Ø
    - uterine, delayed O72.2
    - ventricular O99.43
  - hemorrhoids O87.2
  - hepatorenal syndrome O9Ø.4
  - hypertension — *see* Hypertension, complicating, puerperium
  - hypertrophy, breast O92.29
  - induration breast (fibrous) O92.29
  - infection O86.4
    - cervix O86.11
    - generalized O85
    - genital tract NEC O86.19
      - obstetric surgical wound O86.Ø
    - kidney (bacillus coli) O86.21
    - maternal O98.93
      - carrier state NEC O99.835
      - gonorrhea O98.23
      - human immunodeficiency virus (HIV) O98.73
      - protozoal O98.63
      - sexually transmitted NEC O98.33
      - specified NEC O98.83
      - streptococcus B carrier state O99.825
      - syphilis O98.13
      - tuberculosis O98.Ø3
      - viral hepatitis O98.43
      - viral NEC O98.53
    - nipple O91.Ø2
      - associated with lactation O91.Ø3
    - peritoneum O85
    - renal O86.21
    - specified NEC O86.89
    - urinary (asymptomatic) (tract) NEC O86.2Ø
      - bladder O86.22
      - kidney O86.21
      - specified site NEC O86.29
      - urethra O86.22
    - vagina O86.13
    - vein — *see* Puerperal, phlebitis
  - ischemia, cerebral O99.43
  - lymphangitis O86.89
    - breast O91.22
      - associated with lactation O91.23
  - malignancy O9A.13
  - malnutrition O25.3
  - mammillitis O91.Ø2
    - associated with lactation O91.Ø3
  - mammitis O91.22
    - associated with lactation O91.23
  - mania F3Ø.8
  - mastitis O91.22
    - associated with lactation O91.23
    - purulent O91.12
      - associated with lactation O91.13
  - melancholia — *see* Disorder, depressive
  - mental disorder NEC O99.345

- **Puerperal, puerperium** — *continued*
  - metroperitonitis O85
  - metrorrhagia — *see* Hemorrhage, postpartum
  - metrosalpingitis O86.19
  - metrovaginitis O86.13
  - milk leg O87.1
  - monoplegia, cerebral O99.43
  - mood disturbance O9Ø.6
  - necrosis, liver (acute) (subacute) (conditions in subcategory K72.Ø) O26.63
    - with renal failure O9Ø.4
  - nervous system disorder O99.355
  - obesity (pre-existing prior to pregnancy) O99.215
  - obesity surgery status O99.845
  - occlusion, precerebral artery O99.43
  - paralysis
    - bladder (sphincter) O9Ø.89
    - cerebral O99.43
  - paralytic stroke O99.43
  - parametritis O85
  - paravaginitis O86.13
  - pelviperitonitis O85
  - perimetritis O86.19
  - perimetrosalpingitis O86.19
  - perinephritis O86.21
  - periphlebitis — *see* Puerperal phlebitis
  - peritoneal infection O85
  - peritonitis (pelvic) O85
  - perivaginitis O86.13
  - phlebitis O87.Ø
    - deep O87.1
    - pelvic O87.1
    - superficial O87.Ø
  - phlebothrombosis, deep O87.1
  - phlegmasia alba dolens O87.1
  - placental polyp O9Ø.89
  - pneumonia, embolic — *see* Embolism, obstetric, puerperal
  - pre-eclampsia — *see* Pre-eclampsia
  - psychosis F53
  - pyelitis O86.21
  - pyelocystitis O86.29
  - pyelonephritis O86.21
  - pyelonephrosis O86.21
  - pyemia O85
  - pyocystitis O86.29
  - pyohemia O85
  - pyometra O86.19
  - pyonephritis O86.21
  - pyosalpingitis O86.19
  - pyrexia (of unknown origin) O86.4
  - renal
    - disease NEC O9Ø.89
    - failure O9Ø.4
  - respiratory disease NEC O99.53
  - retention
    - decidua — *see* Retention, decidua
    - placenta O72.Ø
    - secundines — *see* Retention, secundines
  - retrated nipple O92.Ø2
  - salpingo-ovaritis O86.19
  - salpingoperitonitis O85
  - secondary perineal tear O9Ø.1
  - sepsis (pelvic) O85
  - sepsis O85
  - septic thrombophlebitis O86.81
  - skin disorder NEC O99.73
  - specified condition NEC O99.89
  - stroke O99.43
  - subinvolution (uterus) O9Ø.89
  - subluxation of symphysis (pubis) O26.73
  - suppuration — *see* Puerperal, abscess
  - tetanus A34
  - thelitis O91.Ø2
    - associated with lactation O91.Ø3
  - thrombocytopenia O72.3
  - thrombophlebitis (superficial) O87.Ø
    - deep O87.1
    - pelvic O87.1
    - septic O86.81
  - thrombosis (venous) — *see* Thrombosis, puerperal
  - thyroiditis O9Ø.5

- **Puerperal, puerperium** — *continued*
  - toxemia (eclamptic) (pre-eclamptic) (with convulsions) O15.2
  - trauma, non-obstetric O9A.23
    - caused by abuse (physical) (suspected) O9A.33
      - confirmed O9A.33
      - psychological (suspected) O9A.53
        - confirmed O9A.53
      - sexual (suspected) O9A.43
        - confirmed O9A.43
  - uremia (due to renal failure) O9Ø.4
  - urethritis O86.22
  - vaginitis O86.13
  - varicose veins (legs) O87.4
    - vulva or perineum O87.8
  - venous O87.9
  - vulvitis O86.19
  - vulvovaginitis O86.13
  - white leg O87.1
- **Puerperium** — *see* Puerperal
- **Pulmolithiasis** J98.4
- **Pulmonary** — *see* condition
- **Pulpitis** (acute) (anachoretic) (chronic) (hyperplastic) (irreversible) (putrescent) (reversible) (suppurative) (ulcerative) KØ4.Ø
- **Pulpless tooth** KØ4.99
- **Pulse** alternating RØØ.8
  - bigeminal RØØ.8
  - fast RØØ.Ø
  - feeble, rapid due to shock following injury T79.4
  - rapid RØØ.Ø
  - weak RØ9.89
- **Pulsus alternans or trigeminus** RØØ.8
- **Punch drunk** FØ7.81
- **Punctum lacrimale occlusion** — *see* Obstruction, lacrimal
- **Puncture**
  - abdomen, abdominal wall S31.139
    - with
      - foreign body S31.149
      - penetration into peritoneal cavity S31.639
        - with foreign body S31.649
    - epigastric region S31.132
      - with
        - foreign body S31.142
        - penetration into peritoneal cavity S31.632
          - with foreign body S31.642
    - left
      - lower quadrant S31.134
        - with
          - foreign body S31.144
          - penetration into peritoneal cavity S31.634
            - with foreign body S31.644
      - upper quadrant S31.131
        - with
          - foreign body S31.141
          - penetration into peritoneal cavity S31.631
            - with foreign body S31.641
    - periumbilic region S31.135
      - with
        - foreign body S31.145
        - penetration into peritoneal cavity S31.635
          - with foreign body S31.645
    - right
      - lower quadrant S31.133
        - with
          - foreign body S31.143
          - penetration into peritoneal cavity S31.633
            - with foreign body S31.643
      - upper quadrant S31.13Ø
        - with
          - foreign body S31.14Ø
          - penetration into peritoneal cavity S31.63Ø
            - with foreign body S31.64Ø

Puncture— *continued*
- accidental, complicating surgery — *see* Complication, accidental puncture or laceration
- alveolar (process) — *see* Puncture, oral cavity
- ankle S91.Ø39
  - with
    - foreign body S91.Ø49
  - left S91.Ø32
    - with
      - foreign body S91.Ø42
  - right S91.Ø31
    - with
      - foreign body S91.Ø41
- anus S31.833
  - with foreign body S31.834
- arm (upper) S41.139
  - with foreign body S41.149
  - left S41.132
    - with foreign body S41.142
  - lower — *see* Puncture, forearm
  - right S41.131
    - with foreign body S41.141
- auditory canal (external) (meatus) — *see* Puncture, ear
- auricle, ear — *see* Puncture, ear
- axilla — *see* Puncture, arm
- back (*see also* Puncture, thorax, back)
  - lower S31.Ø3Ø
    - with
      - foreign body S31.Ø4Ø
        - with penetration into retroperitoneal space S31.Ø41
      - penetration into retroperitoneal space S31.Ø31
- bladder (traumatic) S37.29
  - nontraumatic N32.89
- breast S21.Ø39
  - with foreign body S21.Ø49
  - left S21.Ø32
    - with foreign body S21.Ø42
  - right S21.Ø31
    - with foreign body S21.Ø41
- buttock S31.8Ø3
  - with foreign body S31.8Ø4
  - left S31.823
    - with foreign body S31.824
  - right S31.813
    - with foreign body S31.814
- by
  - device, implant or graft — *see* Complications, by site and type, mechanical
  - foreign body left accidentally in operative wound T81.539
  - instrument (any) during a procedure, accidental — *see* Puncture, accidental complicating surgery
- calf — *see* Puncture, leg
- canaliculus lacrimalis — *see* Puncture, eyelid
- canthus, eye — *see* Puncture, eyelid
- cervical esophagus S11.23
  - with foreign body S11.24
- cheek (external) SØ1.439
  - with foreign body SØ1.449
  - left SØ1.432
    - with foreign body SØ1.442
  - right SØ1.431
    - with foreign body SØ1.441
  - internal — *see* Puncture, oral cavity
- chest wall — *see* Puncture, thorax
- chin — *see* Puncture, head, specified site NEC
- clitoris — *see* Puncture, vulva
- costal region — *see* Puncture, thorax
- digit(s)
  - hand — *see* Puncture, finger
  - foot — *see* Puncture, toe
- ear (canal) (external) SØ1.339
  - with foreign body SØ1.349
  - left SØ1.332
    - with foreign body SØ1.342
  - right SØ1.331
    - with foreign body SØ1.341
  - drum SØ9.2-

Puncture— *continued*
- elbow S51.Ø39
  - with
    - foreign body S51.Ø49
  - left S51.Ø32
    - with
      - foreign body S51.Ø42
  - right S51.Ø31
    - with
      - foreign body S51.Ø41
- epididymis — *see* Puncture, testis
- epigastric region — *see* Puncture, abdomen, wall, epigastric
- epiglottis S11.83
  - with foreign body S11.84
- esophagus
  - cervical S11.23
    - with foreign body S11.24
  - thoracic S27.818
- eyeball SØ5.6-
  - with foreign body SØ5.5-
- eyebrow — *see* Puncture, eyelid
- eyelid SØ1.13-
  - with foreign body SØ1.14-
  - left SØ1.132
    - with foreign body SØ1.142
  - right SØ1.131
    - with foreign body SØ1.141
- face NEC — *see* Puncture, head, specified site NEC
- finger(s) S61.239
  - with
    - damage to nail S61.339
      - with
        - foreign body S61.349
    - foreign body S61.249
  - index S61.238
    - with
      - damage to nail S61.338
        - with
          - foreign body S61.348
      - foreign body S61.248
    - left S61.231
      - with
        - damage to nail S61.331
          - with
            - foreign body S61.341
        - foreign body S61.241
    - right S61.23Ø
      - with
        - damage to nail S61.33Ø
          - with
            - foreign body S61.34Ø
        - foreign body S61.24Ø
  - little S61.238
    - with
      - damage to nail S61.338
        - with
          - foreign body S61.348
      - foreign body S61.248
    - left S61.237
      - with
        - damage to nail S61.337
          - with
            - foreign body S61.347
        - foreign body S61.247
    - right S61.236
      - with
        - damage to nail S61.336
          - with
            - foreign body S61.346
        - foreign body S61.246
  - middle S61.238
    - with
      - damage to nail S61.338
        - with
          - foreign body S61.348
      - foreign body S61.248
    - left S61.233
      - with
        - damage to nail S61.333
          - with
            - foreign body S61.343
        - foreign body S61.243

Puncture— *continued*
- finger(s) — *continued*
  - middle — *continued*
    - right S61.232
      - with
        - damage to nail S61.332
          - with
            - foreign body S61.342
        - foreign body S61.242
  - ring S61.238
    - with
      - damage to nail S61.338
        - with
          - foreign body S61.348
      - foreign body S61.248
    - left S61.235
      - with
        - damage to nail S61.335
          - with
            - foreign body S61.345
        - foreign body S61.245
    - right S61.234
      - with
        - damage to nail S61.334
          - with
            - foreign body S61.344
        - foreign body S61.244
- flank S31.139
  - with foreign body S31.149
- foot (except toe(s) alone) S91.339
  - with foreign body S91.349
  - left S91.332
    - with foreign body S91.342
  - right S91.331
    - with foreign body S91.341
  - toe — *see* Puncture, toe
- forearm S51.839
  - with
    - foreign body S51.849
  - elbow only — *see* Puncture, elbow
  - left S51.832
    - with
      - foreign body S51.842
  - right S51.831
    - with
      - foreign body S51.841
- forehead — *see* Puncture, head, specified site NEC
- genital organs, external
  - female S31.532
    - with foreign body S31.542
    - vagina — *see* Puncture, vagina
    - vulva — *see* Puncture, vulva
  - male S31.531
    - with foreign body S31.541
    - penis — *see* Puncture, penis
    - scrotum — *see* Puncture, scrotum
    - testis — *see* Puncture, testis
- groin — *see* Puncture, abdomen, wall
- gum — *see* Puncture, oral cavity
- hand S61.439
  - with
    - foreign body S61.449
  - finger — *see* Puncture, finger
  - left S61.432
    - with
      - foreign body S61.442
  - right S61.431
    - with
      - foreign body S61.441
  - thumb — *see* Puncture, thumb
- head SØ1.93
  - with foreign body SØ1.94
  - cheek — *see* Puncture, cheek
  - ear — *see* Puncture, ear
  - eyelid — *see* Puncture, eyelid
  - lip — *see* Puncture, oral cavity
  - nose — *see* Puncture, nose
  - oral cavity — *see* Puncture, oral cavity
  - scalp SØ1.Ø3
    - with foreign body SØ1.Ø4
  - specified site NEC SØ1.83
    - with foreign body SØ1.84
  - temporomandibular area — *see* Puncture, cheek

Puncture— *continued*
- uvula — *see* Puncture, oral cavity
- vagina S31.43
  - with foreign body S31.44
- vocal cords S11.Ø33
  - with foreign body S11.Ø34
- vulva S31.43
  - with foreign body S31.44
- wrist S61.539
  - with
    - foreign body S61.549
  - left S61.532
    - with
      - foreign body S61.542
  - right S61.531
    - with
      - foreign body S61.541

PUO (pyrexia of unknown origin) R5Ø.9
Pupillary membrane (persistent) Q13.89
Pupillotonia — *see* Anomaly, pupil, function, tonic pupil
Purpura D69.2
- abdominal D69.Ø
- allergic D69.Ø
- anaphylactoid D69.Ø
- annularis telangiectodes L81.7
- arthritic D69.Ø
- autoerythrocyte sensitization D69.2
- autoimmune D69.Ø
- bacterial D69.Ø
- Bateman's (senile) D69.2
- capillary fragility (hereditary) (idiopathic)D69.8
- cryoglobulinemic D89.1
- Devil's pinches D69.2
- fibrinolytic — *see* Fibrinolysis
- fulminans, fulminous D65
- gangrenous D65
- hemorrhagic, hemorrhagica D69.3
  - not due to thrombocytopenia D69.Ø
- Henoch(-Schönlein) (allergic) D69.Ø
- hypergammaglobulinemic (benign) (Waldenström) D89.Ø
- idiopathic (thrombocytopenic) D69.3
  - nonthrombocytopenic D69.Ø
- immune thrombocytopenic D69.3
- infectious D69.Ø
- malignant D69.Ø
- neonatorum P54.5
- nervosa D69.Ø
- newborn P54.5
- nonthrombocytopenic D69.2
  - hemorrhagic D69.Ø
  - idiopathic D69.Ø
- nonthrombopenic D69.2
- peliosis rheumatica D69.Ø
- posttransfusion (post-transfusion) (from (fresh) whole blood or blood products) D69.51
- primary D69.49
- red cell membrane sensitivity D69.2
- rheumatica D69.Ø
- Schönlein(-Henoch) (allergic) D69.Ø
- scorbutic E54 *[D77]*
- senile D69.2
- simplex D69.2
- symptomatica D69.Ø
- telangiectasia annularis L81.7
- thrombocytopenic D69.49
  - congenital D69.42
  - hemorrhagic D69.3
  - hereditary D69.42
  - idiopathic D69.3
  - immune D69.3
  - neonatal, transitory P61.Ø
  - thrombotic M31.1
- thrombohemolytic — *see* Fibrinolysis
- thrombolytic — *see* Fibrinolysis
- thrombopenic D69.49
- thrombotic, thrombocytopenic M31.1
- toxic D69.Ø
- vascular D69.Ø
- visceral symptoms D69.Ø

Purpuric spots R23.3
Purulent — *see* condition
Pus
- in
  - stool R19.5
  - urine N39.Ø
- tube (rupture) — *see* Salpingo-oophoritis

Pustular rash LØ8.Ø
Pustule (nonmalignant) LØ8.9
- malignant A22.Ø

Pustulosis palmaris et plantaris L4Ø.3
Putnam(-Dana) **disease or syndrome** — *see* Degeneration, combined
Putrescent pulp (dental) KØ4.1
Pyarthritis, pyarthrosis — *see* Arthritis, pyogenic or pyemic
- tuberculous — *see* Tuberculosis, joint

Pyelectasis — *see* Hydronephrosis
Pyelitis (congenital) (uremic) *(see also* Pyelonephritis)
- with
  - calculus — *see* category N2Ø
    - with hydronephrosis N13.2
  - contracted kidney N11.9
- acute N1Ø
- chronic N11.9
  - with calculus — *see* category N2Ø
    - with hydronephrosis N13.2
- cystica N28.84
- puerperal (postpartum) O86.21
- tuberculous A18.11

Pyelocystitis — *see* Pyelonephritis
Pyelonephritis *(see also* Nephritis, tubulo-interstitial)
- with
  - calculus — *see* category N2Ø
    - with hydronephrosis N13.2
  - contracted kidney N11.9
- acute N1Ø
- calculous — *see* category N2Ø
  - with hydronephrosis N13.2
- chronic N11.9
  - with calculus — *see* category N2Ø
    - with hydronephrosis N13.2
  - associated with ureteral obstruction or stricture N11.1
  - nonobstructive N11.8
    - with reflux (vesicoureteral) N11.Ø
  - obstructive N11.1
  - specified NEC N11.8
- in (due to)
  - brucellosis A23.9 *[N16]*
  - cryoglobulinemia (mixed) D89.1 *[N16]*
  - cystinosis E72.Ø4
  - diphtheria A36.84
  - glycogen storage disease E74.Ø9 *[N16]*
  - leukemia NEC C95.9- *[N16]*
  - lymphoma NEC C85.9Ø *[N16]*
  - multiple myeloma C9Ø.Ø- *[N16]*
  - obstruction N11.1
  - Salmonella infection AØ2.25
  - sarcoidosis D86.84
  - sepsis A41.9 *[N16]*
  - Sjögren's disease M35.Ø4
  - toxoplasmosis B58.83
  - transplant rejection T86.91 *[N16]*
  - Wilson's disease E83.Ø1 *[N16]*
- nonobstructive N12
  - with reflux (vesicoureteral) N11.Ø
  - chronic N11.8
- syphilitic A52.75

Pyelonephrosis (obstructive) N11.1
- chronic N11.9

Pyelophlebitis I8Ø.8
Pyeloureteritis cystica N28.85
Pyemia, pyemic (fever) (infection) (purulent) *(see also* Sepsis)
- joint — *see* Arthritis, pyogenic or pyemic
- liver K75.1
- pneumococcal A4Ø.3
- portal K75.1
- postvaccinal T88.Ø
- puerperal, postpartum, childbirth O85
- specified organism NEC A41.89
- tuberculous — *see* Tuberculosis, miliary

Pygopagus Q89.4
Pyknoepilepsy (idiopathic) — *see* Pyknolepsy
Pyknolepsy G4Ø.AØ9
- intractable G4Ø.A19
  - with status epilepticus G4Ø.A11
  - without status epilepticus G4Ø.A19
- not intractable G4Ø.AØ9
  - with status epilepticus G4Ø.AØ1
  - without status epilepticus G4Ø.AØ9

Pylephlebitis K75.1
Pyle's syndrome Q78.5
Pylethrombophlebitis K75.1
Pylethrombosis K75.1
Pyloritis K29.9Ø
- with bleeding K29.91

Pylorospasm (reflex) NEC K31.3
- congenital or infantile Q4Ø.Ø
- newborn Q4Ø.Ø

Q

R

- **Reaction** — *continued*
  - drug NEC — *continued*
    - addictive — *see* Dependence, drug — *continued*
      - transmitted via placenta or breast milk — *see* Absorption, drug, addictive, through placenta
    - allergic — *see* Allergy, drug
    - lichenoid L43.2
    - newborn P93.8
      - gray baby syndrome P93.Ø
    - overdose or poisoning (by accident) — *see* Table of Drugs and Chemicals, by drug, poisoning
    - photoallergic L56.1
    - phototoxic L56.Ø
    - withdrawal— *see* Dependence, by drug, with, withdrawal
      - infant of dependent mother P96.1
      - newborn P96.1
    - wrong substance given or taken (by accident) — *see* Table of Drugs and Chemicals, by drug, poisoning
  - fear F4Ø.9
    - child (abnormal) F93.8
  - febrile nonhemolytic transfusion (FNHTR) R5Ø.84
  - fluid loss, cerebrospinal G97.1
  - foreign
    - body NEC — *see* Granuloma, foreign body
      - in operative wound (inadvertently left) — *see* Foreign body, accidentally left during a procedure
    - substance accidentally left during a procedure (chemical) (powder) (talc) T81.6Ø
      - aseptic peritonitis T81.61
      - body or object (instrument) (sponge) (swab) — *see* Foreign body, accidentally left during a procedure
      - specified reaction NEC T81.69
  - grief — *see* Disorder, adjustment
  - Herxheimer's R68.89
  - hyperkinetic — *see* Hyperkinesia
  - hypochondriacal F45.2Ø
  - hypoglycemic, due to insulin E16.Ø
    - with coma (diabetic) — *see* Diabetes, coma
      - nondiabetic E15
    - therapeutic misadventure — *see* subcategory T38.3
  - hypomanic F3Ø.8
  - hysterical F44.9
  - immunization — *see* Complications, vaccination
  - incompatibility
    - ABO blood group (infusion) (transfusion) — *see* Complication(s), transfusion, incompatiblity reaction, ABO
      - delayed serologic T8Ø.39
    - minor blood group (Duffy) (E) (K(ell)) (Kidd) (Lewis) (M) (N) (P) (S) T8Ø.89
    - Rh (factor) (infusion) (transfusion) T8Ø.4 — see Complication(s), transfusion, incompatibility reaction, Rh (factor)
  - inflammatory — *see* Infection
  - infusion — *see* Complications, infusion
  - inoculation (immune serum) — *see* Complications, vaccination
  - insulin T38.3-
  - involutional psychotic — *see* Disorder, depressive
  - leukemoid D72.823
    - basophilic D72.823
    - lymphocytic D72.823
    - monocytic D72.823
    - myelocytic D72.823
    - neutrophilic D72.823
  - LSD (acute)
    - due to drug abuse — *see* Abuse, drug, hallucinogen
    - due to drug dependence — *see* Dependence, drug, hallucinogen
  - lumbar puncture G97.1
  - manic-depressive — *see* Disorder, bipolar
  - neurasthenic F48.8
  - neurogenic — *see* Neurosis
  - neurotic F48.9
  - neurotic-depressive F34.1

- **Reaction** — *continued*
  - nitritoid — *see* Crisis, nitritoid
  - nonspecific
    - to
      - cell mediated immunity measurement of gamma interferon antigen response without active tuberculosis R76.12
      - QuantiFERON-TB test (QFT) without active tuberculosis R76.12
      - tuberculin test (*see also* Reaction, tuberculin skin test) R76.11
  - obsessive-compulsive F42
  - organic, acute or subacute — *see* Delirium
  - paranoid (acute) F23
    - chronic F22
    - senile FØ3
  - passive dependency F6Ø.7
  - phobic F4Ø.9
  - post-traumatic stress, uncomplicated Z73.3
  - psychogenic F99
  - psychoneurotic (*see also* Neurosis)
    - compulsive F42
    - depersonalization F48.1
    - depressive F34.1
    - hypochondriacal F45.2Ø
    - neurasthenic F48.8
    - obsessive F42
  - psychophysiologic — *see* Disorder, somatoform
  - psychosomatic — *see* Disorder, somatoform
  - psychotic — *see* Psychosis
  - scarlet fever toxin — *see* Complications, vaccination
  - schizophrenic F23
    - acute (brief) (undifferentiated) F23
    - latent F21
    - undifferentiated (acute) (brief) F23
  - serological for syphilis — *see* Serology for syphilis
  - serum T8Ø.69
    - anaphylactic (immediate) (*see also* Shock, anaphylactic) T8Ø.59
    - specified reaction NEC
      - due to
        - administration of blood and blood products T8Ø.61
        - immunization T8Ø.62
        - serum specified NEC T8Ø.69
        - vaccination T8Ø.62
  - situational — *see* Disorder, adjustment
  - somatization — *see* Disorder, somatoform
  - spinal puncture G97.1
  - stress (severe) F43.9
    - acute (agitation) ("daze") (disorientation) (disturbance of consciousness) (flight reaction) (fugue) F43.Ø
    - specified NEC F43.8
  - surgical procedure — *see* Complications, surgical procedure
  - tetanus antitoxin — *see* Complications, vaccination
  - toxic, to local anesthesia T81.89
    - in labor and delivery O74.4
    - in pregnancy O29.3x-
    - postpartum, puerperal O89.3
  - toxin-antitoxin — *see* Complications, vaccination
  - transfusion (blood) (bone marrow) (lymphocytes) (allergic) — *see* Complications, transfusion
  - tuberculin skin test, abnormal R76.11
  - vaccination (any) — *see* Complications, vaccination
  - withdrawing, child or adolescent F93.8
- **Reactive airway disease** — *see* Asthma
- **Reactive depression** — *see* Reaction, depressive
- **Rearrangement**
  - chromosomal
    - balanced (in) Q95.9
      - abnormal individual (autosomal) Q95.2
        - non-sex (autosomal) chromosomes Q95.2
        - sex/non-sex chromosomes Q95.3
      - specified NEC Q95.8
- **Recalcitrant patient** — *see* Noncompliance
- **Recanalization, thrombus** — *see* Thrombosis
- **Recession, receding**
  - chamber angle (eye) H21.55-
  - chin M26.Ø9
  - gingival (generalized) (localized) (postinfective) (postoperative) KØ6.Ø

- **Recklinghausen disease** Q85.Ø1
  - bones E21.Ø
- **Reclus' disease** (cystic) — *see* Mastopathy, cystic
- **Recrudescent typhus** (fever) A75.1
- **Recruitment, auditory** H93.21-
- **Rectalgia** K62.89
- **Rectitis** K62.89
- **Rectocele**
  - female (without uterine prolapse) N81.6
    - with uterine prolapse N81.4
      - incomplete N81.2
  - in pregnancy — *see* Pregnancy, complicated by, abnormal, pelvic organs or tissues NEC
  - male K62.3
- **Rectosigmoid junction** — *see* condition
- **Rectosigmoiditis** K63.89
  - ulcerative (chronic) K51.3Ø
    - with
      - complication K51.319
        - abscess K51.314
        - fistula K51.313
        - obstruction K51.312
        - rectal bleeding K51.311
        - specified NEC K51.318
- **Rectourethral**— *see* condition
- **Rectovaginal** — *see* condition
- **Rectovesical** — *see* condition
- **Rectum, rectal** — *see* condition
- **Recurrent** — *see* condition
  - pregnancy loss — *see* Loss (of), pregnancy, recurrent
- **Red bugs** B88.Ø
- **Red-cedar lung or pneumonitis** J67.8
- **Red tide** (*see also* Table of Drugs and Chemicals) T65.82
- **Reduced**
  - mobility Z74.Ø9
  - ventilatory or vital capacity R94.2
- **Redundant, redundancy**
  - anus (congenital) Q43.8
  - clitoris N9Ø.89
  - colon (congenital) Q43.8
  - foreskin (congenital) N47.8
  - intestine (congenital) Q43.8
  - labia N9Ø.6
  - organ or site, congenital NEC — *see* Accessory
  - panniculus (abdominal) E65
  - prepuce (congenital) N47.8
  - pylorus K31.89
  - rectum (congenital) Q43.8
  - scrotum N5Ø.8
  - sigmoid (congenital) Q43.8
  - skin (of face) L57.4
    - eyelids — *see* Blepharochalasis
  - stomach K31.89
- **Reduplication** — *see* Duplication
- **Reflex** R29.2
  - hyperactive gag J39.2
  - pupillary, abnormal — *see* Anomaly, pupil, function
  - vasoconstriction I73.9
  - vasovagal R55
- **Reflux** K21.9
  - acid K21.9
  - esophageal K21.9
    - with esophagitis K21.Ø
    - newborn P78.83
  - gastroesophageal K21.9
    - with esophagitis K21.Ø
  - mitral — *see* Insufficiency, mitral
  - ureteral — *see* Reflux, vesicoureteral
  - vesicoureteral (with scarring) N13.7Ø
    - with
      - nephropathy N13.729
        - with hydroureter N13.739
          - bilateral N13.732
          - unilateral N13.731
        - bilateral N13.722
        - unilateral N13.721
        - without hydroureter N13.729
          - bilateral N13.722
          - unilateral N13.721
      - pyelonephritis (chronic) N11.Ø
    - congenital Q62.7
    - without nephropathy N13.71

- **Reforming, artificial openings** — *see* Attention to, artificial, opening
- **Refractive error** — *see* Disorder, refraction
- **Refsum's disease or syndrome** G6Ø.1
- **Refusal of**
  - food, psychogenic F5Ø.8
  - treatment (because of) Z53.2Ø
    - left against medical advice (AMA) Z53.21
    - patient's decision NEC Z53.29
    - reasons of belief or group pressure Z53.1
- **Regional** — *see* condition
- **Regurgitation** R11.1Ø
  - aortic (valve) — *see* Insufficiency, aortic
  - food (*see also* Vomiting)
    - with reswallowing — *see* Rumination
    - newborn P92.1
  - gastric contents — *see* Vomiting
  - heart — *see* Endocarditis
  - mitral (valve) — *see* Insufficiency, mitral
    - congenital Q23.3
  - myocardial — *see* Endocarditis
  - pulmonary (valve) (heart) I37.1
    - congenital Q22.2
    - syphilitic A52.Ø3
  - tricuspid — *see* Insufficiency, tricuspid
  - valve, valvular — *see* Endocarditis
    - congenital Q24.8
  - vesicoureteral — *see* Reflux, vesicoureteral
- **Reifenstein syndrome** E34.52
- **Reinsertion, contraceptive device** Z3Ø.433
- **Reiter's disease, syndrome, or urethritis** MØ2.3Ø
  - ankle MØ2.37-
  - elbow MØ2.32-
  - foot joint MØ2.37-
  - hand joint MØ2.34-
  - hip MØ2.35-
  - knee MØ2.36-
  - multiple site MØ2.39
  - shoulder MØ2.31-
  - vertebra MØ2.38
  - wrist MØ2.33-
- **Reichmann's disease or syndrome** K31.89
- **Rejection**
  - food, psychogenic F5Ø.8
  - transplant T86.91
    - bone T86.83Ø
      - marrow T86.Ø1
    - cornea T86.84Ø
    - heart T86.21
      - with lung(s) T86.31
    - intestine T86.85Ø
    - kidney T86.11
    - liver T86.41
    - lung(s) T86.81Ø
      - with heart T86.31
    - organ (immune or nonimmune cause) T86.91
    - pancreas T86.89Ø
    - skin (allograft) (autograft) T86.82Ø
    - specified NEC T86.89Ø
    - stem cell (peripheral blood) (umbilical cord) T86.5
- **Relapsing fever** A68.9
  - Carter's (Asiatic) A68.1
  - Dutton's (West African) A68.1
  - Koch's A68.9
  - louse-borne (epidemic) A68.Ø
  - Novy's (American) A68.1
  - Obermeyers's (European) A68.Ø
  - Spirillum A68.9
  - tick-borne (endemic) A68.1
- **Relationship**
  - occlusal
    - open anterior M26.22Ø
    - open posterior M26.221
- **Relaxation**
  - anus (sphincter) K62.89
    - psychogenic F45.8
  - arch (foot) (*see also* Deformity, limb, flat foot)
  - back ligaments — *see* Instability, joint, spine
  - bladder (sphincter) N31.2
  - cardioesophageal K21.9
  - cervix — *see* Incompetency, cervix
  - diaphragm J98.6
- **Relaxation** — *continued*
  - joint (capsule) (ligament) (paralytic) — *see* Flail, joint
    - congenital NEC Q74.8
  - lumbosacral (joint) — *see* subcategory M53.2
  - pelvic floor N81.89
  - perineum N81.89
  - posture R29.3
  - rectum (sphincter) K62.89
  - sacroiliac (joint) — *see* subcategory M53.2
  - scrotum N5Ø.8
  - urethra (sphincter) N36.44
  - vesical N31.2
- **Release from prison, anxiety concerning** Z65.2
- **Remains**
  - canal of Cloquet Q14.Ø
  - capsule (opaque) Q14.8
- **Remittent fever** (malarial) B54
- **Remnant** canal of Cloquet Q14.Ø
  - capsule (opaque) Q14.8
  - cervix, cervical stump (acquired) (postoperative) N88.8
  - cystic duct, postcholecystectomy K91.5
  - fingernail L6Ø.8
    - congenital Q84.6
  - meniscus, knee — *see* Derangement, knee, meniscus, specified NEC
  - thyroglossal duct Q89.2
  - tonsil J35.8
    - infected (chronic) J35.Ø1
  - urachus Q64.4
- **Removal** (from) (of)
  - artificial
    - arm Z44.ØØ-
      - complete Z44.Ø1-
      - partial Z44.Ø2-
    - eye Z44.2-
    - leg Z44.1Ø-
      - complete Z44.11-
      - partial Z44.12-
  - breast implant Z45.81
  - cardiac pulse generator (battery) (end-of-life) Z45.Ø1Ø
  - catheter (urinary) (indwelling) Z46.6
    - from artificial opening — *see* Attention to, artificial, opening
    - non-vascular Z46.82
    - vascular NEC Z45.2
  - drains Z48.Ø3
  - device Z46.9
    - contraceptive Z3Ø.432
    - implanted NEC Z45.89
    - specified NEC Z46.89
  - dressing (nonsurgical) Z48.ØØ
    - surgical Z48.Ø1
  - external
    - fixation device — code to fracture with seventh character D
    - prosthesis, prosthetic device Z44.9
      - breast Z44.3-
      - specified NEC Z44.8
  - home in childhood (to foster home or institution) Z62.29
  - ileostomy Z43.2
  - insulin pump Z46.81
  - myringotomy device (stent) (tube) Z45.82
  - nervous system device NEC Z46.2
    - brain neuropacemaker Z46.2
    - visual substitution device Z46.2
      - implanted Z45.31
  - non-vascular catheter Z46.82
  - orthodontic device Z46.4
  - organ, prophylactic (for neoplasia management) — *see* Prophylactic, organ removal
  - staples Z48.Ø2
  - stent
    - ureteral Z46.6
  - suture Z48.Ø2
  - urinary device Z46.6
  - vascular access device or catheter Z45.2
- **Ren**
  - arcuatus Q63.1
  - mobile, mobilis N28.89
    - congenital Q63.8
- **Ren** — *continued*
  - unguliformis Q63.1
- **Renal** — *see* condition
- **Rendu-Osler-Weber disease or syndrome** I78.Ø
- **Reninoma** D41.Ø-
- **Renon-Delille syndrome** E23.3
- **Reovirus, as cause of disease classified elsewhere** B97.5
- **Repeated falls NEC** R29.6
- **Replaced chromosome by dicentric ring** Q93.2
- **Replacement by artificial or mechanical device or prosthesis of**
  - bladder Z96.Ø
  - blood vessel NEC Z95.828
  - bone NEC Z96.7
  - cochlea Z96.21
  - coronary artery Z95.5
  - eustachian tube Z96.29
  - eye globe Z97.Ø
  - heart Z95.812
    - valve Z95.2
      - prosthetic Z95.2
      - specified NEC Z95.4
      - xenogenic Z95.3
  - intestine Z96.89
  - joint Z96.6Ø
    - hip — *see* Presence, hip joint implant
    - knee — *see* Presence, knee joint implant
    - specified site NEC Z96.698
  - larynx Z96.3
  - lens Z96.1
  - limb(s) — *see* Presence, artificial, limb
  - mandible NEC (for tooth root implant(s)) Z96.5
  - organ NEC Z96.89
  - peripheral vessel NEC Z95.828
  - stapes Z96.29
  - teeth Z97.2
  - tendon Z96.7
  - tissue NEC Z96.89
  - tooth root(s) Z96.5
  - vessel NEC Z95.828
    - coronary (artery) Z95.5
- **Request for expert evidence** ZØ4.8
- **Reserve, decreased or low**
  - cardiac — *see* Disease, heart
  - kidney N28.89
- **Residual** (*see also* condition)
  - ovary syndrome N99.83
  - state, schizophrenic F2Ø.5
  - urine R39.19
- **Resistance, resistant**
  - activated protein C (to) D68.51
  - complicating pregnancy O26.89
  - insulin E88.81
  - organism(s)
    - to
      - drug
        - aminoglycosides Z16.29
        - amoxicillin Z16.11
        - ampicillin Z16.11
        - antibiotic(s) Z16.2Ø
          - multiple Z16.24
          - specified NEC Z16.29
        - antifungal Z16.32
        - antimicrobial (single) Z16.3Ø
          - multiple Z16.35
          - specified NEC Z16.39
        - antimycobacterial (single) Z16.341
          - multiple Z16.342
        - antiparasitic Z16.31
        - antiviral Z16.33
        - beta lactam antibiotics Z16.1Ø
          - specified NEC Z16.19
        - cephalosporins Z16.19
        - extended beta lactamase (ESBL) Z16.12
        - fluoroquinolones Z16.23
        - macrolides Z16.29
        - methicillin — *see* MRSA
        - multiple drugs (MDRO)
          - antibiotics Z16.24
        - penicillins Z16.11
        - quinine (and related compounds) Z16.31
        - quinolones Z16.23

        - sulfonamides Z16.29
- **Resistance, resistant** — *continued*
  - organism(s) — *continued*
    - to — *continued*
      - drug — *continued*
        - tetracyclines Z16.29
        - tuberculostatics (single) Z16.341
          - multiple Z16.342
        - vancomycin Z16.21
          - related antibiotics Z16.22
  - thyroid hormone EØ7.89
- **Resorption**
  - dental (roots) KØ3.3
    - alveoli M26.79
  - teeth (external) (internal) (pathological) (roots) KØ3.3
- **Respiration**
  - Cheyne-Stokes RØ6.3
  - decreased due to shock, following injury T79.4
  - disorder of, psychogenic F45.8
  - insufficient, or poor RØ6.89
    - newborn P28.5
  - painful RØ7.1
  - sighing, psychogenic F45.8
- **Respiratory** (*see also* condition)
  - distress syndrome (newborn) (type I) P22.Ø
    - type II P22.1
  - syncytial virus, as cause of disease classified elsewhere B97.4
- **Respite care** Z75.5
- **Response** (drug)
  - photoallergic L56.1
  - phototoxic L56.Ø
- **Restless legs** (syndrome) G25.81
- **Restlessness** R45.1
- **Restriction of housing space** Z59.1
- **Restoration** (of)
  - dental
    - aesthetically inadequate or displeasing KØ8.56
    - defective KØ8.5Ø
      - specified NEC KØ8.59
    - failure of marginal integrity KØ8.51
    - failure of periodontal anatomical intergrity KØ8.54
  - organ continuity from previous sterilization (tuboplasty) (vasoplasty) Z31.Ø
    - aftercare Z31.42
  - tooth (existing)
    - contours biologically incompatible with oral health KØ8.54
    - open margins KØ8.51
    - overhanging KØ8.52
    - poor aesthetic KØ8.56
    - poor gingival margins KØ8.51
  - unsatisfactory, of tooth KØ8.5Ø
    - specified NEC KØ8.59
- **Restorative material** (dental)
  - allergy to KØ8.55
  - fractured KØ8.539
    - with loss of material KØ8.531
    - without loss of material KØ8.53Ø
  - unrepairable overhanging of KØ8.52
- **Rests, ovarian, in fallopian tube** Q5Ø.6
- **Restzustand** (schizophrenic) F2Ø.5
- **Retained** (*see also* Retention)
  - cholelithiasis following cholecystectomy K91.86
  - foreign body fragments (type of) Z18.9
    - acrylics Z18.2
    - animal quill(s) or spines Z18.31
    - cement Z18.83
    - concrete Z18.83
    - crystalline Z18.83
    - depleted isotope Z18.Ø9
    - depleted uranium Z18.Ø1
    - diethylhexylphthalates Z18.2
    - glass Z18.81
    - isocyanate Z18.2
    - magnetic metal Z18.11
    - metal Z18.1Ø
    - nonmagnetic metal Z18.12
    - nontherapeutic radioactive Z18.Ø9
    - organic NEC Z18.39
    - plastic Z18.2
- **Retained**— *continued*
  - foreign body fragments (type of) — *continued*
    - quill(s) (animal) Z18.31
    - radioactive (nontherapeutic) NEC Z18.Ø9
    - specified NEC Z18.89
    - spine(s) (animal) Z18.31
    - stone Z18.83
    - tooth (teeth) Z18.32
    - wood Z18.33
  - fragments (type of) Z18.9
    - acrylics Z18.2
    - animal quill(s) or spines Z18.31
    - cement Z18.83
    - concrete Z18.83
    - crystalline Z18.83
    - depleted isotope Z18.Ø9
    - depleted uranium Z18.Ø1
    - diethylhexylphthalates Z18.2
    - glass Z18.81
    - isocyanate Z18.2
    - magnetic metal Z18.11
    - metal Z18.1Ø
    - nonmagnetic metal Z18.12
    - nontherapeutic radioactive Z18.Ø9
    - organic NEC Z18.39
    - plastic Z18.2
    - quill(s) (animal) Z18.31
    - radioactive (nontherapeutic) NEC Z18.Ø9
    - specified NEC Z18.89
    - spine(s) (animal) Z18.31
    - stone Z18.83
    - tooth (teeth) Z18.32
    - wood Z18.33
  - gallstones, following cholecystectomy K91.86
- **Retardation**
  - development, developmental, specific — *see* Disorder, developmental
  - endochondral bone growth — *see* Disorder, bone, development or growth
  - growth R62.5Ø
    - due to malnutrition E45
  - mental — *see* Disability, intellectual
  - motor function, specific F82
  - physical (child) R62.52
    - due to malnutrition E45
  - reading (specific) F81.Ø
  - spelling (specific) (without reading disorder) F81.81
- **Retching** — *see* Vomiting
- **Retention** (*see also* Retained)
  - bladder — *see* Retention, urine
  - carbon dioxide E87.2
  - cholelithiasis following cholecystectomy K91.86
  - cyst — *see* Cyst
  - dead
    - fetus (at or near term) (mother) O36.4
      - early fetal death OØ2.1
    - ovum OØ2.Ø
  - decidua (fragments) (following delivery) (with hemorrhage) O72.2
    - without hemorrhage O73.1
  - deciduous tooth KØØ.6
  - dental root KØ8.3
  - fecal — *see* Constipation
  - fetus
    - dead O36.4
      - early OØ2.1
  - fluid R6Ø.9
  - foreign body (*see also* Foreign body, retained)
    - current trauma — code as Foreign body, by site or type
  - gallstones, following cholecystectomy K91.86
  - gastric K31.89
  - intrauterine contraceptive device, in pregnancy — *see* Pregnancy, complicated by, retention, intrauterine device
  - membranes (complicating delivery) (with hemorrhage) O72.2
    - with abortion — *see* Abortion, by type
    - without hemorrhage O73.1
  - meniscus — *see* Derangement, meniscus
  - menses N94.89
  - milk (puerperal, postpartum) O92.79
  - nitrogen, extrarenal R39.2
- **Retention** — *continued*
  - ovary syndrome N99.83
  - placenta (total) (with hemorrhage) O72.Ø
    - without hemorrhage O73.Ø
    - portions or fragments (with hemorrhage) O72.2
      - without hemorrhage O73.1
  - products of conception
    - early pregnancy (dead fetus) OØ2.1
    - following
      - delivery (with hemorrhage) O72.2
        - without hemorrhage O73.1
  - secundines (following delivery) (with hemorrhage) O72.Ø
    - without hemorrhage O73.Ø
    - complicating puerperium (delayed hemorrhage) O72.2
    - partial O72.2
      - without hemorrhage O73.1
  - smegma, clitoris N9Ø.89
  - urine R33.9
    - due to hyperplasia (hypertrophy) of prostate — *see* Hyperplasia, prostate
    - drug-induced R33.Ø
    - organic R33.8
      - drug-induced R33.Ø
    - psychogenic F45.8
    - specified NEC R33.8
  - water (in tissues) — *see* Edema
- **Reticulation, dust** — *see* Pneumoconiosis
- **Reticulocytosis** R7Ø.1
- **Reticuloendotheliosis**
  - acute infantile C96.Ø
  - leukemic C91.4-
  - malignant C96.9
  - nonlipid C96.Ø
- **Reticulohistiocytoma** (giant-cell) D76.3
- **Reticuloid, actinic** L57.1
- **Reticulosis** (skin)
  - acute of infancy C96.Ø
  - hemophagocytic, familial D76.1
  - histiocytic medullary C96.9
  - lipomelanotic I89.8
  - malignant (midline) C86.Ø
  - nonlipid C96.Ø
  - polymorphic C83.8-
  - Sézary — *see* Sézary disease
- **Retina, retinal** (*see also* condition)
  - dark area D49.81
- **Retinitis** (*see also* Inflammation, chorioretinal)
  - albuminurica N18.9 *[H32]*
  - diabetic — *see* Diabetes, retinitis
  - disciformis — *see* Degeneration, macula
  - focal — *see* Inflammation, chorioretinal, focal
  - gravidarum — *see* Pregnancy, complicated by, specified pregnancy-related condition NEC
  - juxtapapillaris — *see* Inflammation, chorioretinal, focal, juxtapapillary
  - luetic — *see* Retinitis, syphilitic
  - pigmentosa H35.52
  - proliferans — *see* Disorder, globe, degenerative, specified type NEC
  - proliferating — *see* Disorder, globe, degenerative, specified type NEC
  - renal N18.9 *[H32]*
  - syphilitic (early) (secondary) A51.43
    - central, recurrent A52.71
    - congenital (early) A5Ø.Ø1 *[H32]*
    - late A52.71
  - tuberculous A18.53
- **Retinoblastoma** C69.2-
  - differentiated C69.2-
  - undifferentiated C69.2-
- **Retinochoroiditis** (*see also* Inflammation, chorioretinal)
  - disseminated — *see* Inflammation, chorioretinal, disseminated
    - syphilitic A52.71
  - focal — *see* Inflammation, chorioretinal
  - juxtapapillaris — *see* Inflammation, chorioretinal, focal, juxtapapillary
- **Retinopathy** (background) H35.ØØ
  - arteriosclerotic I7Ø.8 *[H35.0-]*
  - atherosclerotic I7Ø.8 *[H35.0-]*

- **Rhinitis** — *continued*
  - allergic J3Ø.9
    - with asthma J45.9Ø9
      - with
        - exacerbation (acute) J45.9Ø1
        - status asthmaticus J45.9Ø2
    - due to
      - food J3Ø.5
      - pollen J3Ø.1
    - nonseasonal J3Ø.89
    - perennial J3Ø.89
    - seasonal NEC J3Ø.2
    - specified NEC J3Ø.89
  - infective JØØ
  - pneumococcal JØØ
  - syphilitic A52.73
    - congenital A5Ø.Ø5 *[J99]*
  - tuberculous A15.8
  - vasomotor J3Ø.Ø
- **Rhinoantritis** (chronic) — *see* Sinusitis, maxillary
- **Rhinodacryolith** — *see* Dacryolith
- **Rhinolith** (nasal sinus) J34.89
- **Rhinomegaly** J34.89
- **Rhinopharyngitis** (acute) (subacute) (*see also* Nasopharyngitis)
  - chronic J31.1
  - destructive ulcerating A66.5
  - mutilans A66.5
- **Rhinophyma** L71.1
- **Rhinorrhea** J34.89
  - cerebrospinal (fluid) G96.Ø
  - paroxysmal — *see* Rhinitis, allergic
  - spasmodic — *see* Rhinitis, allergic
- **Rhinosalpingitis** — *see* Salpingitis, eustachian
- **Rhinoscleroma** A48.8
- **Rhinosporidiosis** B48.1
- **Rhinovirus infection NEC** B34.8
- **Rhizomelic chondrodysplasia punctata** E71.54Ø
- **Rhythm**
  - atrioventricular nodal I49.8
  - disorder I49.9
    - coronary sinus I49.8
    - ectopic I49.8
    - nodal I49.8
  - escape I49.9
  - heart, abnormal I49.9
  - idioventricular I44.2
  - nodal I49.8
  - sleep, inversion G47.2-
    - nonorganic origin — *see* Disorder, sleep, circadian rhythm, psychogenic
- **Rhytidosis facialis** L98.8
- **Rib** (*see also* condition)
  - cervical Q76.5
- **Riboflavin deficiency** E53.Ø
- **Rice bodies** (*see also* Loose, body, joint)
  - knee M23.4-
- **Richter syndrome** — *see* Leukemia, chronic lymphocytic, B-cell type
- **Richter's hernia** — *see* Hernia, abdomen, with obstruction
- **Ricinism** — *see* Poisoning, food, noxious, plant
- **Rickets** (active) (acute) (adolescent) (chest wall) (congenital) (current) (infantile) (intestinal) E55.Ø
  - adult — *see* Osteomalacia
  - celiac K9Ø.Ø
  - hypophosphatemic with nephrotic-glycosuric dwarfism E72.Ø9
  - inactive E64.3
  - kidney N25.Ø
  - renal N25.Ø
  - sequelae, any E64.3
  - vitamin-D-resistant E83.31 *[M9Ø.8Ø]*
- **Rickettsial disease** A79.9
  - specified type NEC A79.89
- **Rickettsialpox** (Rickettsia akari) A79.1
- **Rickettsiosis** A79.9
  - due to
    - Ehrlichia sennetsu A79.81
    - Rickettsia akari (rickettsialpox) A79.1
  - specified type NEC A79.89
  - tick-borne A77.9
  - vesicular A79.1
- **Rider's bone** — *see* Ossification, muscle, specified NEC
- **Ridge, alveolus** (*see also* condition)
  - flabby KØ6.8
- **Ridged ear, congenital** Q17.3
- **Riedel's**
  - lobe, liver Q44.7
  - struma, thyroiditis or disease EØ6.5
- **Rieger's anomaly or syndrome** Q13.81
- **Riehl's melanosis** L81.4
- **Rietti-Greppi-Micheli anemia** D56.9
- **Rieux's hernia** — *see* Hernia, abdomen, specified site NEC
- **Riga** (-Fede) **disease** K14.Ø
- **Riggs' disease** — *see* Periodontitis
- **Right middle lobe syndrome** J98.11
- **Rigid, rigidity** (*see also* condition)
  - abdominal R19.3Ø
    - with severe abdominal pain R1Ø.Ø
    - epigastric R19.36
    - generalized R19.37
    - left lower quadrant R19.34
    - left upper quadrant R19.32
    - periumbilic R19.35
    - right lower quadrant R19.33
    - right upper quadrant R19.31
  - articular, multiple, congenital Q68.8
  - cervix (uteri) in pregnancy — *see* Pregnancy, complicated by, abnormal, cervix
  - hymen (acquired) (congenital) N89.6
  - nuchal R29.1
  - pelvic floor in pregnancy — *see* Pregnancy, complicated by, abnormal, pelvic organs or tissues NEC
  - perineum or vulva in pregnancy — *see* Pregnancy, complicated by, abnormal, vulva
  - spine — *see* Dorsopathy, specified NEC
  - vagina in pregnancy — *see* Pregnancy, complicated by, abnormal, vagina
- **Rigors** R68.89
  - with fever R5Ø.9
- **Riley-Day syndrome** G9Ø.1
- **RIND** (reversible ischemic neurologic deficit) I63.9
- **Ring(s)**
  - aorta (vascular) Q25.4
  - Bandl's O62.4
  - contraction, complicating delivery O62.4
  - esophageal, lower (muscular) K22.2
  - Fleischer's (cornea) H18.Ø4-
  - hymenal, tight (acquired) (congenital) N89.6
  - Kayser-Fleischer (cornea) H18.Ø4-
  - retraction, uterus, pathological O62.4
  - Schatzki's (esophagus) (lower) K22.2
    - congenital Q39.3
  - Soemmerring's — *see* Cataract, secondary
  - vascular (congenital) Q25.8
    - aorta Q25.4
- **Ringed hair** (congenital) Q84.1
- **Ringworm** B35.9
  - beard B35.Ø
  - black dot B35.Ø
  - body B35.4
  - Burmese B35.5
  - corporeal B35.4
  - foot B35.3
  - groin B35.6
  - hand B35.2
  - honeycomb B35.Ø
  - nails B35.1
  - perianal (area) B35.6
  - scalp B35.Ø
  - specified NEC B35.8
  - Tokelau B35.5
- **Rise, venous pressure** I87.8
- **Risk, suicidal**
  - meaning personal history of attempted suicide Z91.5
  - meaning suicidal ideation — *see* Ideation, suicidal
- **Ritter's disease** LØØ
- **Rivalry, sibling** Z62.891
- **Rivalta's disease** A42.2
- **River blindness** B73.Ø1
- **Robert's pelvis** Q74.2
  - with disproportion (fetopelvic) O33.Ø
- **Robert's pelvis** — *continued*
  - with disproportion (fetopelvic) — *continued*
    - causing obstructed labor O65.Ø
- **Robin**(-Pierre) **syndrome** Q87.Ø
- **Robinow-Silvermann-Smith syndrome** Q87.1
- **Robinson's** (hidrotic) **ectodermal dysplasia or syndrome** Q82.4
- **Robles' disease** B73.Ø1
- **Rocky Mountain** (spotted) fever A77.Ø
- **Roetheln** — *see* Rubella
- **Roger's disease** Q21.Ø
- **Rokitansky-Aschoff sinuses** (gallbladder) K82.8
- **Rolando's fracture** (displaced) S62.22-
  - nondisplaced S62.22-
- **Romano-Ward** (prolonged QT interval) syndrome I45.81
- **Romberg's disease or syndrome** G51.8
- **Roof, mouth** — *see* condition
- **Rosacea** L71.9
  - acne L71.9
  - keratitis L71.8
  - specified NEC L71.8
- **Rosary, rachitic** E55.Ø
- **Rose**
  - cold J3Ø.1
  - fever J3Ø.1
  - rash R21
    - epidemic BØ6.9
- **Rosenbach's erysipeloid** A26.Ø
- **Rosenthal's disease or syndrome** D68.1
- **Roseola** BØ9
  - infantum BØ8.2Ø
    - due to human herpesvirus 6 BØ8.21
    - due to human herpesvirus 7 BØ8.22
- **Rossbach's disease** K31.89
  - psychogenic F45.8
- **Ross River disease or fever** B33.1
- **Rostan's asthma** (cardiac) — *see* Failure, ventricular, left
- **Rotation**
  - anomalous, incomplete or insufficient, intestine Q43.3
  - cecum (congenital) Q43.3
  - colon (congenital) Q43.3
  - spine, incomplete or insufficient — *see* Dorsopathy, deforming, specified NEC
  - tooth, teeth, fully erupted M26.35
  - vertebra, incomplete or insufficient — *see* Dorsopathy, deforming, specified NEC
- **Rotes Quérol disease or syndrome** — *see* Hyperostosis, ankylosing
- **Roth**(-Bernhardt) **disease or syndrome** — *see* Meralgia paraesthetica
- **Rothmund**(-Thomson) **syndrome** Q82.8
- **Rotor's disease or syndrome** E8Ø.6
- **Round**
  - back (with wedging of vertebrae) — *see* Kyphosis
    - sequelae (late effect) of rickets E64.3
  - worms (large) (infestation) NEC B82.Ø
    - Ascariasis (*see also* Ascariasis) B77.9
- **Roussy-Lévy syndrome** G6Ø.Ø
- **Rubella** (German measles) BØ6.9
  - complication NEC BØ6.Ø9
    - neurological BØ6.ØØ
  - congenital P35.Ø
  - contact Z2Ø.4
  - exposure to Z2Ø.4
  - maternal
    - manifest rubella in infant P35.Ø
    - care for (suspected) damage to fetus O35.3
    - suspected damage to fetus affecting management of pregnancy O35.3
  - specified complications NEC BØ6.89
- **Rubeola** (meaning measles) — *see* Measles
  - meaning rubella — *see* Rubella
- **Rubeosis, iris** — *see* Disorder, iris, vascular
- **Rubinstein-Taybi syndrome** Q87.2
- **Rudimentary** (congenital) (*see also* Agenesis)
  - arm — *see* Defect, reduction, upper limb
  - bone Q79.9
  - cervix uteri Q51.828
  - eye Q11.2
  - lobule of ear Q17.3

S

Saber, sabre shin or tibia (syphilitic) A50.56 *[M90.8-]*
Sac lacrimal — *see* condition
Saccharomyces infection B37.9
Saccharopinuria E72.3
Saccular — *see* condition
Sacculation aorta (nonsyphilitic) — *see* Aneurysm, aorta
- bladder N32.3
- intralaryngeal (congenital) (ventricular) Q31.3
- larynx (congenital) (ventricular) Q31.3
- organ or site, congenital — *see* Distortion
- pregnant uterus — *see* Pregnancy, complicated by, abnormal, uterus
- ureter N28.89
- urethra N36.1
- vesical N32.3

Sachs' amaurotic familial idiocy or disease E75.02
Sachs-Tay disease E75.02
Sacks-Libman disease M32.11
Sacralgia M53.3
Sacralization Q76.49
Sacrodynia M53.3
Sacroiliac joint — *see* condition
Sacroiliitis NEC M46.1
Sacrum — *see* condition
Saddle
- back — *see* Lordosis
- embolus
  - abdominal aorta I74.01
  - pulmonary artery I26.92
    - with acute cor pulmonale I26.02
- injury — code to condition
- nose M95.0
  - due to syphilis A50.57

Sadism (sexual) F65.52
Sadness, postpartal O90.6
Sadomasochism F65.50
Saemisch's ulcer (cornea) — *see* Ulcer, cornea, central
Sahib disease B55.0
Sailors' skin L57.8
Saint
- Anthony's fire — *see* Erysipelas
- triad — *see* Hernia, diaphragm
- Vitus' dance — *see* Chorea, Sydenham's

Salaam
- attack(s) — *see* Epilepsy, spasms
- tic R25.8

Salicylism
- abuse F55.8
- overdose or wrong substance given — *see* Table of Drugs and Chemicals, by drug, poisoning

Salivary duct or gland — *see* condition
Salivation, excessive K11.7
Salmonella — *see* Infection, Salmonella
Salmonellosis A02.0
Salpingitis (catarrhal) (fallopian tube) (nodular) (pseudofollicular) (purulent) (septic) N70.91
- with oophoritis N70.93
- acute N70.01
  - with oophoritis N70.03
- chlamydial A56.11
- chronic N70.11
  - with oophoritis N70.13
- complicating abortion — *see* Abortion, by type, complicated by, salpingitis
- ear — *see* Salpingitis, eustachian
- eustachian (tube) H68.00-
  - acute H68.01-
  - chronic H68.02-
- follicularis N70.11
  - with oophoritis N70.13
- gonococcal (acute) (chronic) A54.24
- interstitial, chronic N70.11
  - with oophoritis N70.13
- isthmica nodosa N70.11
  - with oophoritis N70.13
- specific (gonococcal) (acute) (chronic) A54.24
- tuberculous (acute) (chronic) A18.17
- venereal (gonococcal) (acute) (chronic) A54.24

Salpingocele N83.4
Salpingo-oophoritis (catarrhal) (purulent) (ruptured) (septic) (suppurative) N70.93
- acute N70.03
  - with ectopic or molar pregnancy O08.0
  - following ectopic or molar pregnancy O08.0
  - gonococcal A54.24
- chronic N70.13
- following ectopic or molar pregnancy O08.0
- gonococcal (acute) (chronic) A54.24
- puerperal O86.19
- specific (gonococcal) (acute) (chronic) A54.24
- subacute N70.03
- tuberculous (acute) (chronic) A18.17
- venereal (gonococcal) (acute) (chronic) A54.24

Salpingo-ovaritis — *see* Salpingo-oophoritis
Salpingoperitonitis — *see* Salpingo-oophoritis
Salzmann's nodular dystrophy — *see* Degeneration, cornea, nodular
Sampson's cyst or tumor N80.1
San Joaquin (Valley) **fever** B38.0
Sandblaster's asthma, lung or pneumoconiosis J62.8
Sander's disease (paranoia) F22
Sandfly fever A93.1
Sandhoff's disease E75.01
Sanfilippo (Type B) (Type C) (Type D) **syndrome** E76.22
Sanger-Brown ataxia G11.2
Sao Paulo fever or typhus A77.0
Saponification, mesenteric K65.8
Sarcocele (benign)
- syphilitic A52.76
  - congenital A50.59

Sarcocystosis A07.8
Sarcoepiplocele — *see* Hernia
Sarcoepiplomphalocele Q79.2
Sarcoid (*see also* Sarcoidosis)
- arthropathy D86.86
- Boeck's D86.9
- Darier-Roussy D86.3
- iridocyclitis D86.83
- meningitis D86.81
- myocarditis D86.85
- myositis D86.87
- pyelonephritis D86.84
- Spiegler-Fendt L08.89

Sarcoidosis D86.9
- with
  - cranial nerve palsies D86.82
  - hepatic granuloma D86.89
  - polyarthritis D86.86
  - tubulo-interstitial nephropathy D86.84
- combined sites NEC D86.89
- lung D86.0
  - and lymph nodes D86.2
- lymph nodes D86.1
  - and lung D86.2
- meninges D86.81
- skin D86.3
- specified type NEC D86.89

Sarcoma (of) (*see also* Neoplasm, connective tissue, malignant)
- alveolar soft part — *see* Neoplasm, connective tissue, malignant
- ameloblastic C41.1
  - upper jaw (bone) C41.0
- botryoid — *see* Neoplasm, connective tissue, malignant
- botryoides — *see* Neoplasm, connective tissue, malignant
- cerebellar C71.6
  - circumscribed (arachnoidal) C71.6
- circumscribed (arachnoidal) cerebellar C71.6
- clear cell (*see also* Neoplasm, connective tissue, malignant)
  - kidney C64.-
- dendritic cells (accessory cells) C96.4
- embryonal — *see* Neoplasm, connective tissue, malignant
- endometrial (stromal) C54.1
  - isthmus C54.0
- epithelioid (cell) — *see* Neoplasm, connective tissue, malignant

Sarcoma (of) — *continued*
- Ewing's — *see* Neoplasm, bone, malignant
- follicular dendritic cell C96.4
- germinoblastic (diffuse) — *see* Lymphoma, diffuse large cell
  - follicular — *see* Lymphoma, follicular, specified NEC
- giant cell (except of bone) (*see also* Neoplasm, connective tissue, malignant)
  - bone — *see* Neoplasm, bone, malignant
- glomoid — *see* Neoplasm, connective tissue, malignant
- granulocytic C92.3-
- hemangioendothelial — *see* Neoplasm, connective tissue, malignant
- hemorrhagic, multiple — *see* Sarcoma, Kaposi's
- histiocytic C96.A
- Hodgkin — *see* Lymphoma, Hodgkin
- immunoblastic (diffuse) — *see* Lymphoma, diffuse large cell
- interdigitating dendritic cell C96.4
- Kaposi's
  - colon C46.4
  - connective tissue C46.1
  - gastrointestinal organ C46.4
  - lung C46.5-
  - lymph node(s) C46.3
  - palate (hard) (soft) C46.2
  - rectum C46.4
  - skin C46.0
  - specified site NEC C46.7
  - stomach C46.4
  - unspecified site C46.9
- Kupffer cell C22.3
- Langerhans cell C96.4
- leptomeningeal — *see* Neoplasm, meninges, malignant
- liver NEC C22.4
- lymphangioendothelial — *see* Neoplasm, connective tissue, malignant
- lymphoblastic — *see* Lymphoma, lymphoblastic (diffuse)
- lymphocytic — *see* Lymphoma, small cell B-cell
- mast cell C96.2
- melanotic — *see* Melanoma
- meningeal — *see* Neoplasm, meninges, malignant
- meningothelial — *see* Neoplasm, meninges, malignant
- mesenchymal (*see also* Neoplasm, connective tissue, malignant)
  - mixed — *see* Neoplasm, connective tissue, malignant
- mesothelial — *see* Mesothelioma
- monstrocellular
  - specified site — *see* Neoplasm, malignant, by site
  - unspecified site C71.9
- myeloid C92.3-
- neurogenic — *see* Neoplasm, nerve, malignant
- odontogenic C41.1
  - upper jaw (bone) C41.0
- osteoblastic — *see* Neoplasm, bone, malignant
- osteogenic (*see also* Neoplasm, bone, malignant)
  - juxtacortical — *see* Neoplasm, bone, malignant
  - periosteal — *see* Neoplasm, bone, malignant
- periosteal (*see also* Neoplasm, bone, malignant)
  - osteogenic — *see* Neoplasm, bone, malignant
- pleomorphic cell — *see* Neoplasm, connective tissue, malignant
- reticulum cell (diffuse) — *see* Lymphoma, diffuse large cell
  - nodular — *see* Lymphoma, follicular
  - pleomorphic cell type — *see* Lymphoma, diffuse large cell
- rhabdoid — *see* Neoplasm, malignant, by site
- round cell — *see* Neoplasm, connective tissue, malignant
- small cell — *see* Neoplasm, connective tissue, malignant
- soft tissue — *see* Neoplasm, connective tissue, malignant
- spindle cell — *see* Neoplasm, connective tissue, malignant
- stromal (endometrial) C54.1

Secondary dentin (in pulp) KØ4.3
- neoplasm, secondaries — *see* Table of Neoplasms, secondary

Secretion
- antidiuretic hormone, inappropriate E22.2
- catecholamine, by pheochromocytoma E27.5
- hormone
  - antidiuretic, inappropriate (syndrome) E22.2
  - by
    - carcinoid tumor E34.Ø
    - pheochromocytoma E27.5
  - ectopic NEC E34.2
- urinary
  - excessive R35.8
  - suppression R34

Section
- nerve, traumatic — *see* Injury, nerve

Segmentation, incomplete (congenital) (*see also* Fusion)
- bone NEC Q78.8
- lumbosacral (joint) (vertebra) Q76.49

Seitelberger's syndrome (infantile neuraxonal dystrophy) G31.89

Seizure(s) (*see also* Convulsions) R56.9
- akinetic — *see* Epilepsy, generalized, specified NEC
- atonic — *see* Epilepsy, generalized, specified NEC
- autonomic (hysterical) F44.5
- convulsive — *see* Convulsions
- cortical (focal) (motor) — *see* Epilepsy, localization-related, symptomatic, with simple partial seizures
- disorder (*see also* Epilepsy) G4Ø.9Ø9
- due to stroke — *see* Sequelae (of), disease, cerebrovascular, by type, specified NEC
- epileptic — *see* Epilepsy
- febrile (simple) R56.ØØ
  - with status epilepticus G4Ø.9Ø1
  - complex (atypical) (complicated) R56.Ø1
    - with status epilepticus G4Ø.9Ø1
- grand mal G4Ø.4Ø9
  - intractable G4Ø.419
    - with status epilepticus G4Ø.411
    - without status epilepticus G4Ø.419
  - not intractable G4Ø.4Ø9
    - with status epilepticus G4Ø.4Ø1
    - without status epilepticus G4Ø.4Ø9
- heart — *see* Disease, heart
- hysterical F44.5
- intractable G4Ø.919
  - with status epilepticus G4Ø.911
- Jacksonian (focal) (motor type) (sensory type) — *see* Epilepsy, localization-related, symptomatic, with simple partial seizures
- newborn P9Ø
- nonspecific epileptic
  - atonic — *see* Epilepsy, generalized, specified NEC
  - clonic — *see* Epilepsy, generalized, specified NEC
  - myoclonic — *see* Epilepsy, generalized, specified NEC
  - tonic — *see* Epilepsy, generalized, specified NEC
  - tonic-clonic — *see* Epilepsy, generalized, specified NEC
- partial, developing into secondarily generalized seizures
  - complex — *see* Epilepsy, localization-related, symptomatic, with complex partial seizures
  - simple — *see* Epilepsy, localization-related, symptomatic, with simple partial seizures
- petit mal G4Ø.4Ø9
  - intractable G4Ø.419
    - with status epilepticus G4Ø.411
    - without status epilepticus G4Ø.419
  - not intractable G4Ø.4Ø9
    - with status epilepticus G4Ø.4Ø1
    - without status epilepticus G4Ø.4Ø9
- post traumatic R56.1
- recurrent G4Ø.9Ø9
- specified NEC G4Ø.89
- uncinate — *see* Epilepsy, localization-related, symptomatic, with complex partial seizures

Selenium deficiency, dietary E59

Self-damaging behavior (life-style) Z72.89

Self-harm (attempted)
- history (personal) Z91.5
  - in family Z81.8

Self-mutilation (attempted)
- history (personal) Z91.5
  - in family Z81.8

Self-poisoning
- history (personal) Z91.5
  - in family Z81.8
- observation following (alleged) attempt ZØ3.6

Semicoma R4Ø.1

Seminal vesiculitis N49.Ø

Seminoma C62.9-
- specified site — *see* Neoplasm, malignant, by site

Senear-Usher disease or syndrome L1Ø.4

Senectus R54

Senescence (without mention of psychosis) R54

Senile, senility (*see also* condition) R41.81
- with
  - acute confusional state FØ5
  - mental changes NOS FØ3
  - psychosis NEC — *see* Psychosis, senile
- asthenia R54
- cervix (atrophic) N88.8
- debility R54
- endometrium (atrophic) N85.8
- fallopian tube (atrophic) — *see* Atrophy, fallopian tube
- heart (failure) R54
- ovary (atrophic) — *see* Atrophy, ovary
- premature E34.8
- vagina, vaginitis (atrophic) N95.2
- wart L82.1

Sensation
- burning (skin) R2Ø.8
  - tongue K14.6
- loss of R2Ø.8
- prickling (skin) R2Ø.2
- tingling (skin) R2Ø.2

Sense loss
- smell — *see* Disturbance, sensation, smell
- taste — *see* Disturbance, sensation, taste
- touch R2Ø.8

Sensibility disturbance (cortical) (deep) (vibratory) R2Ø.9

Sensitive, sensitivity (*see also* Allergy)
- carotid sinus G9Ø.Ø1
- child (excessive) F93.8
- cold, autoimmune D59.1
- dentin KØ3.89
- latex Z91.Ø4Ø
- methemoglobin D74.8
- tuberculin, without clinical or radiological symptoms R76.11
- visual
  - glare H53.71
  - impaired contrast H53.72

Sensitiver Beziehungswahn F22

Sensitization, auto-erythrocytic D69.2

Separation
- anxiety, abnormal (of childhood) F93.Ø
- apophysis, traumatic code as Fracture, by site
- choroid — *see* Detachment, choroid
- epiphysis, epiphyseal
  - nontraumatic (*see also* Osteochondropathy, specified type NEC)
    - upper femoral — *see* Slipped, epiphysis, upper femoral
  - traumatic code as Fracture, by site
- fracture — *see* Fracture
- infundibulum cardiac from right ventricle by a partition Q24.3
- joint (traumatic) (current) code by site under Dislocation
- pubic bone, obstetrical trauma O71.6
- retina, retinal — *see* Detachment, retina
- symphysis pubis, obstetrical trauma O71.6
- tracheal ring, incomplete, congenital Q32.1

Sepsis (generalized) (unspecified organism) A41.9
- with
  - organ dysfunction (acute) (multiple) R65.2Ø
    - with septic shock R65.21
- actinomycotic A42.7

Sepsis (generalized) — *continued*
- adrenal hemorrhage syndrome (meningococcal) A39.1
- anaerobic A41.4
- Bacillus anthracis A22.7
- Brucella (*see also* Brucellosis) A23.9
- candidal B37.7
- cryptogenic A41.9
- due to device, implant or graft T85.79
  - arterial graft NEC T82.7
  - breast (implant) T85.79
  - catheter NEC T85.79
    - dialysis (renal) T82.7
      - intraperitoneal T85.71
    - infusion NEC T82.7
      - spinal (epidural) (subdural) T85.79
    - urinary (indwelling) T83.51
  - ectopic or molar pregnancy OØ8.82
  - electronic (electrode) (pulse generator) (stimulator)
    - bone T84.7
    - cardiac T82.7
    - nervous system (brain) (peripheral nerve) (spinal) T85.79
    - urinary T83.59
  - fixation, internal (orthopedic) — *see* Complication, fixation device, infection
  - gastrointestinal (bile duct) (esophagus) T85.79
  - genital T83.6
  - heart NEC T82.7
    - valve (prosthesis) T82.6
      - graft T82.7
  - joint prosthesis — *see* Complication, joint prosthesis, infection
  - ocular (corneal graft) (orbital implant) T85.79
  - orthopedic NEC T84.7
    - fixation device, internal — *see* Complication, fixation device, infection
  - specified NEC T85.79
  - vascular T82.7
  - ventricular intracranial shunt T85.79
- during labor O75.3
- Enterococcus A41.81
- Erysipelothrix (rhusiopathiae) (erysipeloid) A26.7
- Escherichia coli (E. coli) A41.5
- extraintestinal yersiniosis A28.2
- following
  - abortion (subsequent episode) OØ8.Ø
    - current episode — *see* Abortion
  - ectopic or molar pregnancy OØ8.82
  - immunization T88.Ø
  - infusion, therapeutic injection or transfusion NEC T8Ø.29
- gangrenous A41.9
- gonococcal A54.86
- gram-negative (organism) A41.5
  - anaerobic A41.4
- Haemophilus influenzae A41.3
- herpesviral BØØ.7
- intra-abdominal K65.1
- intraocular — *see* Endophthalmitis, purulent
- Listeria monocytogenes A32.7
- localized — code to specific localized infection
  - in operation wound T81.4
  - skin — *see* Abscess
- malleus A24.Ø
- melioidosis A24.1
- meningeal — *see* Meningitis
- meningococcal A39.4
  - acute A39.2
  - chronic A39.3
  - specified NEC P36.8
- MSSA (methicillin susceptible Staphylococcus aureus) A41.Ø1
- newborn P36.9
  - due to
    - anaerobes NEC P36.5
    - Escherichia coli P36.4
    - Staphylococcus P36.3Ø
      - aureus P36.2
      - specified NEC P36.39
    - Streptococcus P36.1Ø
      - group B P36.Ø

- **Sepsis** (generalized) — *continued*
  - newborn — *continued*
    - due to — *continued*
      - Streptococcus — *continued*
        - specified NEC P36.19
    - specified NEC P36.8
  - Pasteurella multocida A28.Ø
  - pelvic, puerperal, postpartum, childbirth O85
  - postprocedural T81.4
  - pneumococcal A4Ø.3
  - puerperal, postpartum, childbirth (pelvic) O85
  - Salmonella (arizonae) (cholerae-suis) (enteritidis) (typhimurium) AØ2.1
  - severe R65.2Ø
    - with septic shock R65.21
  - skin, localized — *see* Abscess
  - Shigella (*see also* Dysentery, bacillary) AØ3.9
  - specified organism NEC A41.89
  - Staphylococcus, staphylococcal A41.2
    - aureus (methicillin susceptible) (MSSA) A41.Ø1
      - methicillin resistant (MRSA) A41.Ø2
    - coagulase-negative A41.1
    - specified NEC A41.1
  - Streptococcus, streptococcal A4Ø.9
    - agalactiae A4Ø.1
    - group
      - A A4Ø.Ø
      - B A4Ø.1
      - D A41.81
    - neonatal P36.1Ø
      - group B P36.Ø
      - specified NEC P36.19
    - pneumoniae A4Ø.3
    - pyogenes A4Ø.Ø
    - specified NEC A4Ø.8
  - tracheostomy stoma J95.Ø2
  - tularemic A21.7
  - umbilical, umbilical cord (newborn) — *see* Sepsis, newborn
  - Yersinia pestis A2Ø.7
- **Septate** — *see* Septum
- **Septic** — *see* condition
  - arm — *see* Cellulitis, upper limb
    - with lymphangitis — *see* Lymphangitis, acute, upper limb
  - embolus — *see* Embolism
  - finger — *see* Cellulitis, digit
    - with lymphangitis — *see* Lymphangitis, acute, digit
  - foot — *see* Cellulitis, lower limb
    - with lymphangitis — *see* Lymphangitis, acute, lower limb
  - gallbladder (acute) K81.Ø
  - hand — *see* Cellulitis, upper limb
    - with lymphangitis — *see* Lymphangitis, acute, upper limb
  - joint — *see* Arthritis, pyogenic or pyemic
  - leg — *see* Cellulitis, lower limb
    - with lymphangitis — *see* Lymphangitis, acute, lower limb
  - nail (*see also* Cellulitis, digit)
    - with lymphangitis — *see* Lymphangitis, acute, digit
  - sore (*see also* Abscess)
    - throat JØ2.Ø
      - streptococcal JØ2.Ø
  - spleen (acute) D73.89
  - teeth, tooth (pulpal origin) KØ4.4
  - throat — *see* Pharyngitis
  - thrombus — *see* Thrombosis
  - toe — *see* Cellulitis, digit
    - with lymphangitis — *see* Lymphangitis, acute, digit
  - tonsils, chronic J35.Ø1
    - with adenoiditis J35.Ø3
  - uterus — *see* Endometritis
- **Septicemia** A41.9
  - meaning sepsis — *see* Sepsis
- **Septum, septate** (congenital) (*see also* Anomaly, by site)
  - anal Q42.3
    - with fistula Q42.2
- **Septum, septate** — *continued*
  - aqueduct of Sylvius QØ3.Ø
    - with spina bifida — *see* Spina bifida, by site, with hydrocephalus
  - uterus (complete) (partial) Q51.2
  - vagina Q52.1Ø
    - in pregnancy (*see also* Pregnancy, complicated by, abnormal vagina)
      - causing obstructed labor O65.5
    - longitudinal (with or without obstruction) Q52.12
    - transverse Q52.11
- **Sequelae** (of) (*see also* condition)
  - abscess, intracranial or intraspinal (conditions in GØ6) GØ9
  - amputation — code to injury with seventh character S
  - burn and corrosion — code to injury with seventh character S
  - calcium deficiency E64.8
  - cerebrovascular disease — *see* Sequelae, disease, cerebrovascular
  - childbirth O94
  - contusion — code to injury with seventh character S
  - corrosion — *see* Sequelae, burn and corrosion
  - crushing injury — code to injury with seventh character S
  - disease
    - cerebrovascular I69.9Ø
      - alteration of sensation I69.998
      - aphasia I69.92Ø
      - apraxia I69.99Ø
      - ataxia I69.993
      - cognitive deficits I69.91
      - disturbance of vision I69.998
      - dysarthria I69.922
      - dysphagia I69.991
      - dysphasia I69.921
      - facial droop I69.992
      - facial weakness I69.992
      - fluency disorder I69.923
      - hemiplegia I69.95-
      - hemorrhage
        - intracerebral — *see* Sequelae, hemorrhage, intracerebral
        - intracranial, nontraumatic NEC — *see* Sequelae, hemorrhage, intracranial, nontraumatic
        - subarachnoid — *see* Sequelae, hemorrhage, subarachnoid
      - language deficit I69.928
      - monoplegia
        - lower limb I69.84-
        - upper limb I69.93-
      - paralytic syndrome I69.96-
      - specified effect NEC I69.998
      - specified type NEC I69.8Ø
        - alteration of sensation I69.898
        - aphasia I69.82Ø
        - apraxia I69.89Ø
        - ataxia I69.893
        - cognitive deficits I69.81
        - disturbance of vision I69.898
        - dysarthria I69.822
        - dysphagia I69.891
        - dysphasia I69.821
        - facial droop I69.892
        - facial weakness I69.892
        - fluency disorder I69.823
        - hemiplegia I69.85-
        - language deficit I69.828
        - monoplegia
          - lower limb I69.84-
          - upper limb I69.83-
        - paralytic syndrome I69.86-
        - specified effect NEC I69.898
      - speech deficit I69.928
        - speech deficit I69.828
      - stroke NOS — *see* Sequelae, stroke NOS
  - dislocation — code to injury with seventh character S
  - encephalitis or encephalomyelitis (conditions in GØ4) GØ9
- **Sequelae** (of) — *continued*
  - encephalitis or encephalomyelitis — *continued*
    - in infectious disease NEC B94.8
    - viral B94.1
  - external cause — code to injury with seventh character S
  - foreign body entering natural orifice — code to injury with seventh character S
  - fracture — code to injury with seventh character S
  - frostbite — code to injury with seventh character S
  - Hansen's disease B92
  - hemorrhage
    - intracerebral I69.1Ø
      - alteration of sensation I69.198
      - aphasia I69.12Ø
      - apraxia I69.19Ø
      - ataxia I69.193
      - cognitive deficits I69.11
      - disturbance of vision I69.198
      - dysarthria I69.122
      - dysphagia I69.191
      - dysphasia I69.121
      - facial droop I69.192
      - facial weakness I69.192
      - fluency disorder I69.123
      - hemiplegia I69.15-
      - language deficit NEC I69.128
      - monoplegia
        - lower limb I69.14-
        - upper limb I69.13-
      - paralytic syndrome I69.16-
      - specified effect NEC I69.198
      - speech deficit NEC I69.128
    - intracranial, nontraumatic NEC I69.2Ø
      - alteration of sensation I69.298
      - aphasia I69.22Ø
      - apraxia I69.29Ø
      - ataxia I69.293
      - cognitive deficits I69.21
      - disturbance of vision I69.298
      - dysarthria I69.222
      - dysphagia I69.291
      - dysphasia I69.221
      - facial droop I69.292
      - facial weakness I69.292
      - fluency disorder I69.223
      - hemiplegia I69.25-
      - language deficit NEC I69.228
      - monoplegia
        - lower limb I69.24-
        - upper limb I69.23-
      - paralytic syndrome I69.26-
      - specified effect NEC I69.298
      - speech deficit NEC I69.228
    - subarachnoid I69.ØØ
      - alteration of sensation I69.Ø98
      - aphasia I69.Ø2Ø
      - apraxia I69.Ø9Ø
      - ataxia I69.Ø93
      - cognitive deficits I69.Ø1
      - disturbance of vision I69.Ø98
      - dysarthria I69.Ø22
      - dysphagia I69.Ø91
      - dysphasia I69.Ø21
      - facial droop I69.Ø92
      - facial weakness I69.Ø92
      - fluency disorder I69.Ø23
      - hemiplegia I69.Ø5-
      - language deficit NEC I69.Ø28
      - monoplegia
        - lower limb I69.Ø4-
        - upper limb I69.Ø3-
      - paralytic syndrome I69.Ø6-
      - specified effect NEC I69.Ø98
      - speech deficit NEC I69.Ø28
  - hepatitis, viral B94.2
  - hyperalimentation E68
  - infarction
    - cerebral I69.3Ø
      - alteration of sensation I69.398
      - aphasia I69.32Ø
      - apraxia I69.39Ø
      - ataxia I69.393

- **Sequelae** (of) — *continued*
  - infarction — *continued*
    - cerebral — *continued*
      - cognitive deficits I69.31
      - disturbance of vision I69.398
      - dysarthria I69.322
      - dysphagia I69.391
      - dysphasia I69.321
      - facial droop I69.392
      - facial weakness I69.392
      - fluency disorder I69.323
      - hemiplegia I69.35-
      - language deficit NEC I69.328
      - monoplegia
        - lower limb I69.34-
        - upper limb I69.33-
      - paralytic syndrome I69.36-
      - specified effect NEC I69.398
      - speech deficit NEC I69.328
  - infection, pyogenic, intracranial or intraspinal GØ9
  - infectious disease B94.9
    - specified NEC B94.8
  - injury — code to injury with seventh character S
  - leprosy B92
  - meningitis
    - bacterial (conditions in GØØ) GØ9
    - other or unspecified cause (conditions in GØ3) GØ9
  - muscle (and tendon) injury — code to injury with seventh character S
  - myelitis — *see* Sequelae, encephalitis
  - niacin deficiency E64.8
  - nutritional deficiency E64.9
    - specified NEC E64.8
  - obstetrical condition O94
  - parasitic disease B94.9
  - phlebitis or thrombophlebitis of intracranial or intraspinal venous sinuses and veins (conditions in GØ8) GØ9
  - poisoning — code to poisoning with seventh character S
    - nonmedicinal substance — *see* Sequelae, toxic effect, nonmedicinal substance
  - poliomyelitis (acute) B91
  - pregnancy O94
  - protein-energy malnutrition E64.Ø
  - puerperium O94
  - rickets E64.3
  - selenium deficiency E64.8
  - sprain and strain — code to injury with seventh character S
  - stroke NOS I69.3Ø
    - alteration in sensation I69.398
    - aphasia I69.32Ø
    - apraxia I69.39Ø
    - ataxia I69.393
    - cognitive deficits I69.31
    - disturbance of vision I69.398
    - dysarthria I69.322
    - dysphagia I69.391
    - dysphasia I69.321
    - facial droop I69.392
    - facial weakness I69.392
    - hemiplegia I69.35-
    - language deficit NEC I69.328
    - monoplegia
      - lower limb I69.34-
      - upper limb I69.33-
    - paralytic syndrome I69.36-
    - specified effect NEC I69.398
    - speech deficit NEC I69.328
  - tendon and muscle injury — code to injury with seventh character S
  - thiamine deficiency E64.8
  - trachoma B94.Ø
  - tuberculosis B9Ø.9
    - bones and joints B9Ø.2
    - central nervous system B9Ø.Ø
    - genitourinary B9Ø.1
    - pulmonary (respiratory) B9Ø.9
    - specified organs NEC B9Ø.8
  - viral
    - encephalitis B94.1
- **Sequelae** (of) — *continued*
  - viral — *continued*
    - hepatitis B94.2
  - vitamin deficiency NEC E64.8
    - A E64.1
    - B E64.8
    - C E64.2
  - wound, open — code to injury with seventh character S
- **Sequestration** (*see also* Sequestrum)
  - lung, congenital Q33.2
- **Sequestrum**
  - bone — *see* Osteomyelitis, chronic
  - dental M27.2
  - jaw bone M27.2
  - orbit — *see* Osteomyelitis, orbit
  - sinus (accessory) (nasal) — *see* Sinusitis
- **Sequoiosis lung or pneumonitis** J67.8
- **Serology for syphilis** doubtful
    - with signs or symptoms code by site and stage under Syphilis
    - follow-up of latent syphilis — *see* Syphilis, latent
  - negative, with signs or symptoms code by site and stage under Syphilis
  - positive A53.Ø
    - with signs or symptoms code by site and stage under Syphilis
  - reactivated A53.Ø
- **Seroma** (*see also* Hematoma)
  - traumatic, secondary and recurrent T79.2
- **Seropurulent** — *see* condition
- **Serositis, multiple** K65.8
  - pericardial I31.1
  - peritoneal K65.8
- **Serous** — *see* condition
- **Sertoli cell**
  - adenoma
    - specified site — *see* Neoplasm, benign, by site
    - unspecified site
      - female D27.9
      - male D29.2Ø
  - carcinoma
    - specified site — *see* Neoplasm, malignant, by site
    - unspecified site (male) C62.9-
      - female C56.9
  - tumor
    - with lipid storage
      - specified site — *see* Neoplasm, benign, by site
      - unspecified site
        - female D27.9
        - male D29.2Ø
    - specified site — *see* Neoplasm, benign, by site
    - unspecified site
      - female D27.9
      - male D29.2Ø
- **Sertoli-Leydig cell tumor** — *see* Neoplasm, benign, by site
  - specified site — *see* Neoplasm, benign, by site
  - unspecified site
    - female D27.9
    - male D29.2Ø
- **Serum**
  - allergy, allergic reaction (*see also* Reaction, serum) T8Ø.69
    - shock (*see also* Shock, anaphylactic) T8Ø.59
  - arthritis (*see also* Reaction, serum) T8Ø.69
  - complication or reaction NEC (*see also* Reaction, serum) T8Ø.69
  - disease NEC (*see also* Reaction, serum) T8Ø.69
  - hepatitis (*see also* Hepatitis, viral, type B)
    - carrier (suspected) of Z22.51
  - intoxication (*see also* Reaction, serum) T8Ø.69
  - neuritis (*see also* Reaction, serum) T8Ø.69
  - neuropathy G61.1
  - poisoning NEC (*see also* Reaction, serum) T8Ø.69
  - rash NEC (*see also* Reaction, serum) T8Ø.69
  - reaction NEC (*see also* Reaction, serum) T8Ø.69
  - sickness NEC (*see also* Reaction, serum) T8Ø.69
  - urticaria (*see also* Reaction, serum) T8Ø.69
- **Sesamoiditis** — *see* Osteomyelitis, specified type NEC
- **Sever's disease or osteochondrosis** — *see* Osteochondrosis, juvenile, tarsus
- **Severe sepsis** R65.2Ø
  - with septic shock R65.21
- **Sex**
  - chromosome mosaics Q97.8
    - lines with various numbers of X chromosomes Q97.2
  - education Z7Ø.8
  - reassignment surgery status Z87.89Ø
- **Sextuplet pregnancy** — *see* Pregnancy, sextuplet
- **Sexual**
  - function, disorder of (psychogenic) F52.9
  - immaturity (female) (male) E3Ø.Ø
  - impotence (psychogenic) organic origin NEC — *see* Dysfunction, sexual, male
  - precocity (constitutional) (cryptogenic)(female) (idiopathic) (male) E3Ø.1
- **Sexuality, pathologic** — *see* Deviation, sexual
- **Sézary disease** C84.1-
- **Shadow, lung** R91.8
- **Shaking palsy or paralysis** — *see* Parkinsonism
- **Shallowness, acetabulum** — *see* Derangement, joint, specified type NEC, hip
- **Shaver's disease** J63.1
- **Sheath** (tendon) — *see* condition
- **Sheathing, retinal vessels** H35.Ø1-
- **Shedding** nail L6Ø.8
  - premature, primary (deciduous) teeth KØØ.6
- **Sheehan's disease or syndrome** E23.Ø
- **Shelf, rectal** K62.89
- **Shell teeth** KØØ.5
- **Shellshock** (current) F43.Ø
  - lasting state — *see* Disorder, post-traumatic stress
- **Shield kidney** Q63.1
- **Shift**
  - auditory threshold (temporary) H93.24-
  - mediastinal R93.8
- **Shifting sleep-work schedule** (affecting sleep) G47.26
- **Shiga**(-Kruse) **dysentery** AØ3.Ø
- **Shiga's bacillus** AØ3.Ø
- **Shigella** (dysentery) — *see* Dysentery, bacillary
- **Shigellosis** AØ3.9
  - Group A AØ3.Ø
  - Group B AØ3.1
  - Group C AØ3.2
  - Group D AØ3.3
- **Shin splints** T79.6
- **Shingles** — *see* Herpes, zoster
- **Shipyard disease or eye** B3Ø.Ø
- **Shirodkar suture, in pregnancy** — *see* Pregnancy, complicated by, incompetent cervix
- **Shock** R57.9
  - with ectopic or molar pregnancy OØ8.3
  - adrenal (cortical) (Addisonian) E27.2
  - adverse food reaction (anaphylactic) — *see* Shock, anaphylactic, due to food
  - allergic — *see* Shock, anaphylactic
  - anaphylactic T78.2
    - chemical — *see* Table of Drugs and Chemicals
    - due to drug or medicinal substance
      - correct substance properly administered T88.6
      - overdose or wrong substance given or taken (by accident) — *see* Table of Drugs and Chemicals, by drug, poisoning
    - due to food (nonpoisonous) T78.ØØ
      - additives T78.Ø6
      - dairy products T78.Ø7
      - eggs T78.Ø8
      - fish T78.Ø3
        - shellfish T78.Ø2
      - fruit T78.Ø4
      - milk T78.Ø7
      - nuts T78.Ø5
        - peanuts T78.Ø1
      - peanuts T78.Ø1
      - seeds T78.Ø5
      - specified type NEC T78.Ø9
      - vegetable T78.Ø4
    - following sting(s) — *see* Venom
    - immunization T8Ø.52
    - serum T8Ø.59
      - blood and blood products T8Ø.51

- **Silo-fillers' disease** J68.8
  - bronchitis J68.Ø
  - pneumonitis J68.Ø
  - pulmonay edema J68.1
- **Silver's syndrome** Q87.1
- **Simian malaria** B53.1
- **Simmonds' cachexia or disease** E23.0
- **Simons' disease or syndrome** (progressive lipodystrophy) E88.1
- **Simple, simplex** — *see* condition
- **Simulation, conscious** (of illness) Z76.5
- **Simultanagnosia** (asimultagnosia) R48.3
- **Sin Nombre virus disease** (Hantavirus (cardio)-pulmonary syndrome) B33.4
- **Sinding-Larsen disease or osteochondrosis** — *see* Osteochondrosis, juvenile, patella
- **Singapore hemorrhagic fever** A91
- **Singer's node or nodule** J38.2
- **Single**
  - atrium Q21.2
  - coronary artery Q24.5
  - umbilical artery Q27.Ø
  - ventricle Q2Ø.4
- **Singultus** R06.6
  - epidemicus B33.Ø
- **Sinus** (*see also* Fistula)
  - abdominal K63.89
  - arrest I45.5
  - arrhythmia I49.8
  - bradycardia RØØ.1
  - branchial cleft (internal) (external) Q18.Ø
  - coccygeal — *see* Sinus, pilonidal
  - dental KØ4.6
  - dermal (congenital) QØ6.8
    - with abscess QØ6.8
    - coccygeal, pilonidal — *see* Sinus, coccygeal
  - infected, skin NEC LØ8.89
  - marginal, ruptured or bleeding — *see* Hemorrhage, antepartum, specified cause NEC
  - medial, face and neck Q18.8
  - pause I45.5
  - pericranii QØ1.9
  - pilonidal (infected) (rectum) LØ5.92
    - with abscess LØ5.Ø2
  - preauricular Q18.1
  - rectovaginal N82.3
  - Rokitansky-Aschoff (gallbladder) K82.8
  - sacrococcygeal (dermoid) (infected) — *see* Sinus, pilonidal
  - tachycardia RØØ.Ø
    - paroxysmal I47.1
  - tarsi syndrome — *see* Syndrome, tarsal tunnel
  - testis N5Ø.8
  - tract (postinfective) — *see* Fistula
  - urachus Q64.4
- **Sinusitis** (accessory) (chronic) (hyperplastic) (nasal) (nonpurulent) (purulent) J32.9
  - acute JØ1.9Ø
    - ethmoidal JØ1.2Ø
      - recurrent JØ1.21
    - frontal JØ1.1Ø
      - recurrent JØ1.11
    - involving more than one sinus, other than pansinusitis JØ1.8Ø
      - recurrent JØ1.81
    - maxillary JØ1.ØØ
      - recurrent JØ1.Ø1
    - pansinusitis JØ1.4Ø
      - recurrent JØ1.41
    - recurrent JØ1.91
    - specified NEC JØ1.8Ø
      - recurrent JØ1.81
    - sphenoidal JØ1.3Ø
      - recurrent JØ1.31
  - allergic — *see* Rhinitis, allergic
  - due to high altitude T7Ø.1
  - ethmoidal J32.2
    - acute JØ1.2Ø
      - recurrent JØ1.21
  - frontal J32.1
    - acute JØ1.1Ø
      - recurrent JØ1.11

- **Sinusitis** — *continued*
  - influenzal — *see* Influenza, with, respiratory manifestations NEC
  - involving more than one sinus but not pansinusitis J32.8
    - acute JØ1.8Ø
      - recurrent JØ1.81
  - maxillary J32.Ø
    - acute JØ1.ØØ
      - recurrent JØ1.Ø1
  - sphenoidal J32.3
    - acute JØ1.3Ø
      - recurrent JØ1.31
  - tuberculous, any sinus A15.8
- **Sinusitis-bronchiectasis-situs inversus** (syndrome) (triad) Q89.3
- **Sipple's syndrome** E31.22
- **Sirenomelia** (syndrome) Q87.2
- **Siriasis** T67.0
- **Sirkari's disease** B55.0
- **Siti** A65
- **Situation, psychiatric** F99
- **Situational**
  - disturbance (transient) — *see* Disorder, adjustment
    - acute F43.Ø
  - maladjustment — *see* Disorder, adjustment
  - reaction — *see* Disorder, adjustment
    - acute F43.Ø
- **Situs inversus or transversus** (abdominalis) (thoracis) Q89.3
- **Sixth disease** B08.20
  - due to human herpesvirus 6 BØ8.21
  - due to human herpesvirus 7 BØ8.22
- **Sjögren-Larsson syndrome** Q87.1
- **Sjögren's syndrome or disease** — *see* Sicca syndrome
- **Skeletal** — *see* condition
- **Skene's gland** — *see* condition
- **Skenitis** — *see* Urethritis
- **Skerljevo** A65
- **Skevas-Zerfus disease** — *see* Toxicity, venom, marine animal, sea anemone
- **Skin** (*see also* condition)
  - clammy R23.1
  - donor — *see* Donor, skin
  - hidebound M35.9
- **Slate-dressers' or slate-miners' lung** J62.8
- **Sleep**
  - apnea — *see* Apnea, sleep
  - deprivation Z72.82Ø
  - disorder or disturbance G47.9
    - child F51.9
    - nonorganic origin F51.9
    - specified NEC G47.8
  - disturbance G47.9
    - nonorganic origin F51.9
  - drunkenness F51.9
  - rhythm inversion G47.2-
  - terrors F51.4
  - walking F51.3
    - hysterical F44.89
- **Sleep hygiene**
  - abuse Z72.821
  - inadequate Z72.821
  - poor Z72.821
- **Sleeping sickness** — *see* Sickness, sleeping
- **Sleeplessness** — *see* Insomnia
  - menopausal N95.1
- **Sleep-wake schedule disorder** G47.2Ø
- **Slim disease** (in HIV infection) B2Ø
- **Slipped, slipping**
  - epiphysis (traumatic) (*see also* Osteochondropathy, specified type NEC)
    - capital femoral (traumatic)
      - acute (on chronic) S79.Ø1-
    - current traumatic code as Fracture, by site
    - upper femoral (nontraumatic) M93.ØØ-
      - acute M93.Ø1-
        - on chronic M93.Ø3-
      - chronic M93.Ø2-
  - intervertebral disc — *see* Displacement, intervertebral disc
  - ligature, umbilical P51.8
  - patella — *see* Disorder, patella, derangement NEC

- **Slipped, slipping** — *continued*
  - rib M89.8x8
  - sacroiliac joint — *see* subcategory M53.2
  - tendon — *see* Disorder, tendon
  - ulnar nerve, nontraumatic — *see* Lesion, nerve, ulnar
  - vertebra NEC — *see* Spondylolisthesis
- **Slocumb's syndrome** E27.0
- **Sloughing** (multiple) (phagedena) (skin) (*see also* Gangrene)
  - abscess — *see* Abscess
  - appendix K38.8
  - fascia — *see* Disorder, soft tissue, specified type NEC
  - scrotum N5Ø.8
  - tendon — *see* Disorder, tendon
  - transplanted organ — *see* Rejection, transplant
  - ulcer — *see* Ulcer, skin
- **Slow**
  - feeding, newborn P92.2
  - flow syndrome, coronary I2Ø.8
  - heart(beat) RØØ.1
- **Slowing, urinary stream** R39.19
- **Sluder's neuralgia** (syndrome) G44.89
- **Slurred, slurring speech** R47.81
- **Small**(ness)
  - for gestational age — *see* Small for dates
  - introitus, vagina N89.6
  - kidney (unknown cause) N27.9
    - bilateral N27.1
    - unilateral N27.Ø
  - ovary (congenital) Q5Ø.39
  - pelvis
    - with disproportion (fetopelvic) O33.1
      - causing obstructed labor O65.1
  - uterus N85.8
  - white kidney NØ3.9
- **Small-and-light-for-dates** — *see* Small for dates
- **Small-for-dates** (infant) PØ5.1Ø
  - with weight of
    - 499 grams or less PØ5.11
    - 5ØØ-749 grams PØ5.12
    - 75Ø-999 grams PØ5.13
    - 1ØØØ-1249 grams PØ5.14
    - 125Ø-1499 grams PØ5.15
    - 15ØØ-1749 grams PØ5.16
    - 175Ø-1999 grams PØ5.17
    - 2ØØØ-2499 grams PØ5.18
- **Smallpox** B03
- **Smearing, fecal** R15.1
- **Smith-Lemli-Opitz syndrome** E78.72
- **Smith's fracture** S52.54-
- **Smoker** — *see* Dependence, drug, nicotine
- **Smoker's**
  - bronchitis J41.Ø
  - cough J41.Ø
  - palate K13.24
  - throat J31.2
  - tongue K13.24
- **Smoking**
  - passive Z77.22
- **Smothering spells** R06.81
- **Snaggle teeth, tooth** M26.39
- **Snapping**
  - finger — *see* Trigger finger
  - hip — *see* Derangement, joint, specified type NEC, hip
    - involving the iliotiblial band M76.3-
  - knee — *see* Derangement, knee
    - involving the iliotiblial band M76.3-
- **Sneddon-Wilkinson disease or syndrome** (sub-corneal pustular dermatosis) L13.1
- **Sneezing** (intractable) RØ6.7
- **Sniffing**
  - cocaine
    - abuse — *see* Abuse, drug, cocaine
    - dependence — *see* Dependence, drug, cocaine
  - gasoline
    - abuse — *see* Abuse, drug, inhalant
    - dependence — *see* Dependence, drug, inhalant
  - glue (airplane)
    - abuse — *see* Abuse, drug, inhalant
    - drug dependence — *see* Dependence, drug, inhalant

Sniffles
- newborn P28.89

Snoring R06.83
Snow blindness — *see* Photokeratitis
Snuffles (non-syphilitic) RØ6.5
- newborn P28.89
- syphilitic (infant) A5Ø.Ø5 *[J99]*

Social exclusion Z6Ø.4
- due to discrimination or persecution (perceived) Z6Ø.5
- migrant Z59.Ø
  - acculturation difficulty Z6Ø.3
- rejection Z6Ø.4
  - due to discrimination or persecution Z6Ø.5
- role conflict NEC Z73.5
- skills inadequacy NEC Z73.4
- transplantation Z6Ø.3

Sodoku A25.0
Soemmerring's ring — *see* Cataract, secondary
Soft (*see also* condition)
- nails L6Ø.3

Softening
- bone — *see* Osteomalacia
- brain (necrotic) (progressive) G93.89
  - congenital QØ4.8
  - embolic I63.4
  - hemorrhagic — *see* Hemorrhage, intracranial, intracerebral
  - occlusive I63.5
  - thrombotic I63.3
- cartilage M94.2-
  - patella M22.4-
- cerebellar — *see* Softening, brain
- cerebral — *see* Softening, brain
- cerebrospinal — *see* Softening, brain
- myocardial, heart — *see* Degeneration, myocardial
- spinal cord G95.89
- stomach K31.89

Soldier's
- heart F45.8
- patches I31.Ø

Solitary
- cyst, kidney N28.1
- kidney, congenital Q6Ø.Ø

Solvent abuse — *see* Abuse, drug, inhalant
- dependence — *see* Dependence, drug, inhalant

Somatization reaction, somatic reaction — *see* Disorder, somatoform
Somnambulism F51.3
- hysterical F44.89

Somnolence R40.0
- nonorganic origin F51.11

Sonne dysentery A03.3
Soor B37.0
Sore
- bed — *see* Ulcer, pressure, by site
- chiclero B55.1
- Delhi B55.1
- desert — *see* Ulcer, skin
- eye H57.1-
- Lahore B55.1
- mouth K13.79
  - canker K12.Ø
- muscle M79.1
- Naga — *see* Ulcer, skin
- of skin — *see* Ulcer, skin
- oriental B55.1
- pressure — *see* Ulcer, pressure, by site
- skin L98.9
- soft A57
- throat (acute) (*see also* Pharyngitis)
  - with influenza, flu, or grippe — *see* Influenza, with, respiratory manifestations NEC
  - chronic J31.2
  - coxsackie (virus) BØ8.5
  - diphtheritic A36.Ø
  - herpesviral BØØ.2
  - influenzal — *see* Influenza, with, respiratory manifestations NEC
  - septic JØ2.Ø
  - streptococcal (ulcerative) JØ2.Ø
  - viral NEC JØ2.8
    - coxsackie BØ8.5

Sore — *continued*
- tropical — *see* Ulcer, skin
- veldt — *see* Ulcer, skin

Soto's syndrome (cerebral gigantism) Q87.3
South African cardiomyopathy syndrome I42.8
Southeast Asian hemorrhagic fever A91
Spacing abnormal, tooth, teeth, fully erupted M26.3Ø
- excessive, tooth, fully erupted M26.32

Spade-like hand (congenital) Q68.1
Spading nail L60.8
- congenital Q84.6

Spanish collar N47.1
Sparganosis B70.1
Spasm(s), **spastic, spasticity** (*see also* condition) R25.2
- accommodation — *see* Spasm, of accommodation
- ampulla of Vater K83.4
- anus, ani (sphincter) (reflex) K59.4
  - psychogenic F45.8
- artery I73.9
  - cerebral G45.9
- Bell's G51.3
- bladder (sphincter, external or internal) N32.89
  - psychogenic F45.8
- bronchus, bronchiole J98.Ø1
- cardia K22.Ø
- cardiac I2Ø.1
- carpopedal — *see* Tetany
- cerebral (arteries) (vascular) G45.9
- cervix, complicating delivery O62.4
- ciliary body (of accommodation) — *see* Spasm, of accommodation
- colon K58.9
  - with diarrhea K58.Ø
  - psychogenic F45.8
- common duct K83.8
- compulsive — *see* Tic
- conjugate H51.8
- coronary (artery) I2Ø.1
- diaphragm (reflex) RØ6.6
  - epidemic B33.Ø
  - psychogenic F45.8
- duodenum K59.8
- epidemic diaphragmatic (transient) B33.Ø
- esophagus (diffuse) K22.4
  - psychogenic F45.8
- facial G51.3
- fallopian tube N83.8
- gastrointestinal (tract) K31.89
  - psychogenic F45.8
- glottis J38.5
  - hysterical F44.4
  - psychogenic F45.8
    - conversion reaction F44.4
  - reflex through recurrent laryngeal nerve J38.5
- habit — *see* Tic
- heart I2Ø.1
- hemifacial (clonic) G51.3
- hourglass — *see* Contraction, hourglass
- hysterical F44.4
- infantile — *see* Epilepsy, spasms
- inferior oblique, eye H51.8
- intestinal (*see also* Syndrome, irritable bowel) K58.9
  - psychogenic F45.8
- larynx, laryngeal J38.5
  - hysterical F44.4
  - psychogenic F45.8
    - conversion reaction F44.4
- levator palpebrae superioris — *see* Disorder, eyelid function
- muscle NEC M62.838
  - back M62.83Ø
- nerve, trigeminal G51.Ø
- nervous F45.8
- nodding F98.4
- occupational F48.8
- oculogyric H51.8
  - psychogenic F45.8
- of accommodation H52.53-
- ophthalmic artery — *see* Occlusion, artery, retina
- perineal, female N94.89
- peroneo-extensor (*see also* Deformity, limb, flat foot)
- pharynx (reflex) J39.2

Spasm(s), **spastic, spasticity** — *continued*
- pharynx (reflex) — *continued*
  - hysterical F45.8
  - psychogenic F45.8
- psychogenic F45.8
- pylorus NEC K31.3
  - adult hypertrophic K31.89
  - congenital or infantile Q4Ø.Ø
  - psychogenic F45.8
- rectum (sphincter) K59.4
  - psychogenic F45.8
- retinal (artery) — *see* Occlusion, artery, retina
- sigmoid (*see also* Syndrome, irritable bowel)K58.9
  - psychogenic F45.8
- sphincter of Oddi K83.4
- stomach K31.89
  - neurotic F45.8
- throat J39.2
  - hysterical F45.8
  - psychogenic F45.8
- tic F95.9
  - chronic F95.1
  - transient of childhood F95.Ø
- tongue K14.8
- torsion (progressive) G24.1
- trigeminal nerve — *see* Neuralgia, trigeminal
- ureter N13.5
- urethra (sphincter) N35.9
- uterus N85.8
  - complicating labor O62.4
- vagina N94.2
  - psychogenic F52.5
- vascular I73.9
- vasomotor I73.9
- vein NEC I87.8
- viscera — *see* Pain, abdominal

Spasmodic — *see* condition
Spasmophilia — *see* Tetany
Spasmus nutans F98.4
Spastic, spasticity (*see also* Spasm)
- child (cerebral) (congenital) (paralysis) G8Ø.1

Speaker's throat R49.8
Specific, specified — *see* condition
Speech
- defect, disorder, disturbance, impediment R47.9
  - psychogenic, in childhood and adolescence F98.8
  - slurring R47.81
  - specified NEC R47.89

Spencer's disease A08.19
Spens' syndrome (syncope with heart block) I45.9
Sperm counts (fertility testing) Z31.41
- postvasectomy Z3Ø.8
  - reversal Z31.42

Spermatic cord — *see* condition
Spermatocele N43.40
- congenital Q55.4
- multiple N43.42
- single N43.41

Spermatocystitis N49.0
Spermatocytoma C62.9-
- specified site — *see* Neoplasm, malignant, by site

Spermatorrhea N50.8
Sphacelus — *see* Gangrene
Sphenoidal — *see* condition
Sphenoiditis (chronic) — *see* Sinusitis, sphenoidal
Sphenopalatine ganglion neuralgia G90.09
Sphericity, increased, lens (congenital) Q12.4
Spherocytosis (congenital) (familial) (hereditary) D58.Ø
- hemoglobin disease D58.Ø
- sickle-cell (disease) D57.8-

Spherophakia Q12.4
Sphincter — *see* condition
Sphincteritis, sphincter of Oddi — *see* Cholangitis
Sphingolipidosis E75.3
- specified NEC E75.29

Sphingomyelinosis E75.3
Spicule tooth K00.2
Spider
- bite — *see* Toxicity, venom, spider
- fingers — *see* Syndrome, Marfan's
- nevus I78.1

- **Spider** — *continued*
  - toes — *see* Syndrome, Marfan's
  - vascular I78.1
- **Spiegler-Fendt**
  - benign lymphocytoma L98.8
  - sarcoid LØ8.89
- **Spielmeyer-Vogt disease** E75.4
- **Spina bifida** (aperta) QØ5.9
  - with hydrocephalus NEC QØ5.4
  - cervical QØ5.5
    - with hydrocephalus QØ5.Ø
  - dorsal QØ5.6
    - with hydrocephalus QØ5.1
  - lumbar QØ5.7
    - with hydrocephalus QØ5.2
  - lumbosacral QØ5.7
    - with hydrocephalus QØ5.2
  - occulta Q76.Ø
  - sacral QØ5.8
    - with hydrocephalus QØ5.3
  - thoracic QØ5.6
    - with hydrocephalus QØ5.1
  - thoracolumbar QØ5.6
    - with hydrocephalus QØ5.1
- **Spindle, Krukenberg's** — *see* Pigmentation, cornea, posterior
- **Spine, spinal** — *see* condition
- **Spiradenoma** (eccrine) — *see* Neoplasm, skin, benign
- **Spirillosis** A25.0
- **Spirillum**
  - minus A25.Ø
  - obermeieri infection A68.Ø
- **Spirochetal** — *see* condition
- **Spirochetosis** A69.9
  - arthritic, arthritica A69.9
  - bronchopulmonary A69.8
  - icterohemorrhagic A27.Ø
  - lung A69.8
- **Spirometrosis** B70.1
- **Spitting blood** — *see* Hemoptysis
- **Splanchnoptosis** K63.4
- **Spleen, splenic** — *see* condition
- **Splenectasis** — *see* Splenomegaly
- **Splenitis** (interstitial) (malignant) (nonspecific) D73.89
  - malarial B54
  - tuberculous A18.85
- **Splenocele** D73.89
- **Splenomegaly, splenomegalia** (Bengal) (cryptogenic) (idiopathic) (tropical) R16.1
  - with hepatomegaly R16.2
  - cirrhotic D73.2
  - congenital Q89.Ø9
  - congestive, chronic D73.2
  - Egyptian B65.1
  - Gaucher's E75.22
  - malarial (*see also* Malaria) B54 *[D77]*
  - neutropenic D73.81
  - Niemann-Pick — *see* Niemann-Pick disease or syndrome
  - siderotic D73.2
  - syphilitic A52.79
    - congenital (early) A5Ø.Ø8 *[D77]*
- **Splenopathy** D73.9
- **Splenoptosis** D73.89
- **Splenosis** D73.89
- **Splinter** — *see* Foreign body, superficial, by site
- **Split, splitting**
  - foot Q72.7-
  - heart sounds RØ1.2
  - lip, congenital — *see* Cleft, lip
  - nails L6Ø.3
  - urinary stream R39.13
- **Spondylarthrosis** — *see* Spondylosis
- **Spondylitis** (chronic) (*see also* Spondylopathy, inflammatory)
  - ankylopoietica — *see* Spondylitis, ankylosing
  - ankylosing (chronic) M45.9
    - with lung involvement M45.9 *[J99]*
    - cervical region M45.2
    - cervicothoracic region M45.3
    - juvenile MØ8.1
    - lumbar region M45.6
    - lumbosacral region M45.7
- **Spondylitis** (chronic) — *continued*
  - ankylosing (chronic) — *continued*
    - multiple sites M45.Ø
    - occipito-atlanto-axial region M45.1
    - sacrococcygeal region M45.8
    - thoracic region M45.4
    - thoracolumbar region M45.5
  - atrophic (ligamentous) — *see* Spondylitis, ankylosing
  - deformans (chronic) — *see* Spondylosis
  - gonococcal A54.41
  - gouty M1Ø.Ø8
  - in (due to)
    - brucellosis A23.9 *[M49.80]*
      - cervical region A23.9 *[M49.82]*
      - cervicothoracic region A23.9 *[M49.83]*
      - lumbar region A23.9 *[M49.86]*
      - lumbosacral region A23.9 *[M49.87]*
      - multiple sites A23.9 *[M49.89]*
      - occipito-atlanto-axial region A23.9 *[M49.81]*
      - sacrococcygeal region A23.9 *[M49.88]*
      - thoracic region A23.9 *[M49.84]*
      - thoracolumbar region A23.9 *[M49.85]*
    - enterobacteria (*see also* subcategory M49.8) AØ4.9
    - tuberculosis A18.Ø1
  - infectious NEC — *see* Spondylopathy, infective
  - juvenile ankylosing (chronic) MØ8.1
  - Kümmell's — *see* Spondylopathy, traumatic
  - Marie-Strümpell — *see* Spondylitis, ankylosing
  - muscularis — *see* Spondylopathy, specified NEC
  - psoriatic L4Ø.53
  - rheumatoid — *see* Spondylitis, ankylosing
  - rhizomelica — *see* Spondylitis, ankylosing
  - sacroiliac NEC M46.1
  - senescent, senile — *see* Spondylosis
  - traumatic (chronic) or post-traumatic — *see* Spondylopathy, traumatic
  - tuberculous A18.Ø1
  - typhosa AØ1.Ø5
- **Spondylarthrosis** — *see* Spondylosis
- **Spondylolisthesis** (acquired) (degenerative) M43.1Ø
  - with disproportion (fetopelvic) O33.Ø
    - causing obstructed labor O65.Ø
  - cervical region M43.12
  - cervicothoracic region M43.13
  - congenital Q76.2
  - lumbar region M43.16
  - lumbosacral region M43.17
  - multiple sites M43.19
  - occipito-atlanto-axial region M43.11
  - sacrococcygeal region M43.18
  - thoracic region M43.14
  - thoracolumbar region M43.15
  - traumatic (old) M43.1Ø
    - acute
      - fifth cervical (displaced) S12.43Ø
        - nondisplaced S12.431
        - specified type NEC (displaced) S12.45Ø
          - nondisplaced S12.451
        - type III S12.44
      - fourth cervical (displaced) S12.33Ø
        - nondisplaced S12.331
        - specified type NEC (displaced) S12.35Ø
          - nondisplaced S12.351
        - type III S12.34
      - second cervical (displaced) S12.13Ø
        - nondisplaced S12.131
        - specified type NEC (displaced) S12.15Ø
          - nondisplaced S12.151
        - type III S12.14
      - seventh cervical (displaced) S12.63Ø
        - nondisplaced S12.631
        - specified type NEC (displaced) S12.65Ø
          - nondisplaced S12.651
        - type III S12.64
      - sixth cervical (displaced) S12.53Ø
        - nondisplaced S12.531
        - specified type NEC (displaced) S12.55Ø
          - nondisplaced S12.551
        - type III S12.54
      - third cervical (displaced) S12.23Ø
        - nondisplaced S12.231
- **Spondylolisthesis** — *continued*
  - traumatic (old) — *continued*
    - acute — *continued*
      - third cervical (displaced) — *continued*
        - specified type NEC (displaced) S12.25Ø
          - nondisplaced S12.251
        - type III S12.24
- **Spondylolysis** (acquired) M43.ØØ
  - cervical region M43.Ø2
  - cervicothoracic region M43.Ø3
  - congenital Q76.2
  - lumbar region M43.Ø6
  - lumbosacral region M43.Ø7
    - with disproportion (fetopelvic) O33.Ø
      - causing obstructed labor O65.8
  - multiple sites M43.Ø9
  - occipito-atlanto-axial region M43.Ø1
  - sacrococcygeal region M43.Ø8
  - thoracic region M43.Ø4
  - thoracolumbar region M43.Ø5
- **Spondylopathy** M48.9
  - infective NEC M46.5Ø
    - cervical region M46.52
    - cervicothoracic region M46.53
    - lumbar region M46.56
    - lumbosacral region M46.57
    - multiple sites M46.59
    - occipito-atlanto-axial region M46.51
    - sacrococcygeal region M46.58
    - thoracic region M46.54
    - thoracolumbar region M46.55
  - inflammatory M46.9Ø
    - cervical region M46.92
    - cervicothoracic region M46.93
    - lumbar region M46.96
    - lumbosacral region M46.97
    - multiple sites M46.99
    - occipito-atlanto-axial region M46.91
    - sacrococcygeal region M46.98
    - specified type NEC M46.8Ø
      - cervical region M46.82
      - cervicothoracic region M46.83
      - lumbar region M46.86
      - lumbosacral region M46.87
      - multiple sites M46.89
      - occipito-atlanto-axial region M46.81
      - sacrococcygeal region M46.88
      - thoracic region M46.84
      - thoracolumbar region M46.85
    - thoracic region M46.94
    - thoracolumbar region M46.95
  - neuropathic, in
    - syringomyelia and syringobulbia G95.Ø
    - tabes dorsalis A52.11
  - specified NEC — *see* subcategory M48.8
  - traumatic M48.3Ø
    - cervical region M48.32
    - cervicothoracic region M48.33
    - lumbar region M48.36
    - lumbosacral region M48.37
    - occipito-atlanto-axial region M48.31
    - sacrococcygeal region M48.38
    - thoracic region M48.34
    - thoracolumbar region M48.35
- **Spondylosis** M47.9
  - with
    - disproportion (fetopelvic) O33.Ø
      - causing obstructed labor O65.Ø
    - myelopathy NEC M47.1Ø
      - cervical region M47.12
      - cervicothoracic region M47.13
      - lumbar region M47.16
      - lumbosacral region M47.17
      - occipito-atlanto-axial region M47.11
      - sacrococcygeal region M47.18
      - thoracic region M47.14
      - thoracolumbar region M47.15
    - radiculopathy M47.2Ø
      - cervical region M47.22
      - cervicothoracic region M47.23
      - lumbar region M47.26
      - lumbosacral region M47.27
      - occipito-atlanto-axial region M47.21

- **Spondylosis** — *continued*
  - with — *continued*
    - radiculopathy — *continued*
      - sacrococcygeal region M47.28
      - thoracic region M47.24
      - thoracolumbar region M47.25
  - specified NEC M47.899
    - cervical region M47.892
    - cervicothoracic region M47.893
    - lumbar region M47.896
    - lumbosacral region M47.897
    - occipito-atlanto-axial region M47.891
    - sacrococcygeal region M47.898
    - thoracic region M47.894
    - thracolumbar region M47.895
  - traumatic — *see* Spondylopathy, traumatic
  - without myelopathy or radiculopathy M47.819
    - cervical region M47.812
    - cervicothoracic region M47.813
    - lumbar region M47.816
    - lumbosacral region M47.817
    - occipito-atlanto-axial region M47.811
    - sacrococcygeal region M47.818
    - thoracic region M47.814
    - thoracolumbar region M47.815
- **Sponge**
  - inadvertently left in operation wound — *see* Foreign body, accidentally left during a procedure
  - kidney (medullary) Q61.5
- **Sponge-diver's disease** — *see* Toxicity, venom, marine animal, sea anemone
- **Spongioblastoma** (any type) — *see* Neoplasm, malignant, by site
  - specified site — *see* Neoplasm, malignant, by site
  - unspecified site C71.9
- **Spongioneuroblastoma** — *see* Neoplasm, malignant by site
- **Spontaneous** (*see also* condition)
  - fracture (cause unknown) — *see* Fracture, pathological
- **Spoon nail** L60.3
  - congenital Q84.6
- **Sporadic** — *see* condition
- **Sporothrix schenckii infection** — *see* Sporotrichosis
- **Sporotrichosis** B42.9
  - arthritis B42.82
  - disseminated B42.7
  - generalized B42.7
  - lymphocutaneous (fixed) (progressive) B42.1
  - pulmonary B42.Ø
  - specified NEC B42.89
- **Spots, spotting** (in) (of)
  - Bitot's (*see also* Pigmentation, conjunctiva)
    - in the young child E5Ø.1
    - vitamin A deficiency E5Ø.1
  - café, au lait L81.3
  - Cayenne pepper I78.1
  - cotton wool, retina — *see* Occlusion, artery, retina
  - de Morgan's (senile angiomas) I78.1
  - Fuchs' black (myopic) H44.2-
  - intermenstrual (regular) N92.Ø
    - irregular N92.1
  - Koplik's BØ5.9
  - liver L81.4
  - pregnancy O26.85-
  - purpuric R23.3
  - ruby I78.1
- **Spotted fever** — *see* Fever, spotted N92.3
- **Sprain** (joint) (ligament)
  - acromioclavicular joint or ligament S43.5-
  - ankle S93.4Ø-
    - calcaneofibular ligament S93.41-
    - deltoid ligament S93.42-
    - internal collateral ligament — *see* Sprain, ankle, specified ligament NEC
    - specified ligament NEC S93.49-
    - talofibular ligament — *see* Sprain, ankle, specified ligament NEC
    - tibiofibular ligament S93.43-
  - anterior longitudinal, cervical S13.4
  - atlas, atlanto-axial, atlanto-occipital S13.4
  - breast bone — *see* Sprain, sternum
  - calcaneofibular — *see* Sprain, ankle

- **Sprain** (joint) (ligament) — *continued*
  - carpal — *see* Sprain, wrist
  - carpometacarpal — *see* Sprain, hand, specified site NEC
  - cartilage
    - costal S23.41
    - semilunar (knee) — *see* Sprain, knee, specified site NEC
      - with current tear — *see* Tear, meniscus
    - thyroid region S13.5
    - xiphoid — *see* Sprain, sternum
  - cervical, cervicodorsal, cervicothoracic S13.4
  - chondrosternal S23.421
  - coracoclavicular S43.8-
  - coracohumeral S43.41-
  - coronary, knee — *see* Sprain, knee, specified site NEC
  - costal cartilage S23.41
  - cricoarytenoid articulation or ligament S13.5
  - cricothyroid articulation S13.5
  - cruciate, knee — *see* Sprain, knee, cruciate
  - deltoid, ankle — *see* Sprain, ankle
  - dorsal (spine) S23.3
  - elbow S53.4Ø-
    - radial collateral ligament S53.43-
    - radiohumeral S53.41-
    - rupture
      - radial collateral ligament — *see* Rupture, traumatic, ligament, radial collateral
      - ulnar collateral ligament — *see* Rupture, traumatic, ligament, ulnar collateral
    - specified type NEC S53.49-
    - ulnar collateral ligament S53.44-
    - ulnohumeral S53.42-
  - femur, head — *see* Sprain, hip
  - fibular collateral, knee — *see* Sprain, knee, collateral
  - fibulocalcaneal — *see* Sprain, ankle
  - finger(s) S63.61-
    - index S63.61-
    - interphalangeal (joint) S63.63-
      - index S63.63-
      - little S63.63-
      - middle S63.63-
      - ring S63.63-
    - little S63.61-
    - metacarpophalangeal (joint) S63.65-
    - middle S63.61-
    - ring S63.61-
    - specified site NEC S63.69-
      - index S63.69-
      - little S63.69-
      - middle S63.69-
      - ring S63.69-
  - foot S93.6Ø-
    - specified ligament NEC S93.69-
    - tarsal ligament S93.61-
    - tarsometatarsal ligament S93.62-
    - toe — *see* Sprain, toe
  - hand S63.9-
    - finger — *see* Sprain, finger
    - specified site NEC — *see* subcategory S63.8
    - thumb — *see* Sprain, thumb
  - head SØ3.9
  - hip S73.1Ø-
    - iliofemoral ligament S73.11-
    - ischiocapsular (ligament) S73.12-
    - specified NEC S73.19-
  - iliofemoral — *see* Sprain, hip
  - innominate
    - acetabulum — *see* Sprain, hip
    - sacral junction S33.6
  - internal
    - collateral, ankle — *see* Sprain, ankle
    - semilunar cartilage — *see* Sprain, knee, specified site NEC
  - interphalangeal
    - finger — *see* Sprain, finger, interphalangeal (joint)
    - toe — *see* Sprain, toe, interphalangeal joint
  - ischiocapsular — *see* Sprain, hip
  - ischiofemoral — *see* Sprain, hip
  - jaw (articular disc) (cartilage) (meniscus) SØ3.4
    - old M26.69

- **Sprain** (joint) (ligament) — *continued*
  - knee S83.9-
    - collateral ligament S83.4Ø-
      - lateral (fibular) S83.42-
      - medial (tibial) S83.41-
    - cruciate ligament S83.5Ø-
      - anterior S83.51-
      - posterior S83.52-
    - lateral (fibular) collateral ligament S83.42-
    - medial (tibial) collateral ligament S83.41-
    - patellar ligament S76.11-
    - specified site NEC S83.8x-
    - superior tibiofibular joint (ligament) S83.6-
  - lateral collateral, knee — *see* Sprain, knee, collateral
  - lumbar (spine) S33.5
  - lumbosacral S33.9
  - mandible (articular disc) SØ3.4
    - old M26.69
  - medial collateral, knee — *see* Sprain, knee, collateral
  - meniscus
    - jaw SØ3.4
      - old M26.69
    - knee (*see also* Sprain, knee, specified site NEC)
      - with current tear — *see* Tear, meniscus
        - old — *see* Derangement, knee, meniscus, due to old tear
    - mandible SØ3.4
      - old M26.69
  - metacarpal (distal) (proximal) — *see* Sprain, hand, specified site NEC
  - metacarpophalangeal — *see* Sprain, finger, metacarpophalangeal (joint)
  - metatarsophalangeal — *see* Sprain, toe, metatarsophalangeal joint
  - midcarpal — *see* Sprain, hand, specified site NEC
  - midtarsal — *see* Sprain, foot, specified site NEC
  - neck S13.9
    - anterior longitudinal cervical ligament S13.4
    - atlanto-axial joint S13.4
    - atlanto-occipital joint S13.4
    - cervical spine S13.4
    - cricoarytenoid ligament S13.5
    - cricothyroid ligament S13.5
    - specified site NEC S13.8
    - thyroid region (cartilage) S13.5
  - nose SØ3.8
  - orbicular, hip — *see* Sprain, hip
  - patella — *see* Sprain, knee, specified site NEC
  - patellar ligament S76.11-
  - pelvis NEC S33.8
  - phalanx
    - finger — *see* Sprain, finger
    - toe — *see* Sprain, toe
  - pubofemoral — *see* Sprain, hip
  - radiocarpal — *see* Sprain, wrist
  - radiohumeral — *see* Sprain, elbow
  - radius, collateral — *see* Rupture, traumatic, ligament, radial collateral
  - rib (cage) S23.41
  - rotator cuff (capsule) S43.42-
  - sacroiliac (region)
    - chronic or old — *see* subcategory M53.2
    - joint S33.6
  - scaphoid (hand) — *see* Sprain, hand, specified site NEC
  - scapula(r) — *see* Sprain, shoulder girdle, specified site NEC
  - semilunar cartilage (knee) (*see also* Sprain, knee, specified site NEC)
    - with current tear — *see* Tear, meniscus
      - old — *see* Derangement, knee, meniscus, due to old tear
  - shoulder joint S43.4Ø-
    - acromioclavicular joint (ligament) — *see* Sprain, acromioclavicular joint
    - blade — *see* Sprain, shoulder, girdle, specified site NEC
    - coracoclavicular joint (ligament) — *see* Sprain, coracoclavicular joint
    - coracohumeral ligament — *see* Sprain, coracohumeral joint
    - girdle S43.9-
      - specified site NEC S43.8-

- **Sprain** (joint) (ligament) — *continued*
  - shoulder joint — *continued*
    - rotator cuff — *see* Sprain, rotator cuff
    - specified site NEC S43.49-
    - sternoclavicular joint (ligament) — *see* Sprain, sternoclavicular joint
  - spine
    - cervical S13.4
    - lumbar S33.5
    - thoracic S23.3
  - sternoclavicular joint S43.6-
  - sternum S23.429
    - chondrosternal joint S23.421
    - specified site NEC S23.428
    - sternoclavicular (joint) (ligament) S23.42Ø
  - symphysis
    - jaw SØ3.4
      - old M26.69
    - mandibular SØ3.4
      - old M26.69
  - talofibular — *see* Sprain, ankle
  - tarsal — *see* Sprain, foot, specified site NEC
  - tarsometatarsal — *see* Sprain, foot, specified site NEC
  - temporomandibular SØ3.4
    - old M26.69
  - thorax S23.9
    - ribs S23.41
    - specified site NEC S23.8
    - spine S23.3
    - sternum — *see* sprain, sternum
  - thumb S63.6Ø-
    - interphalangeal (joint) S63.62-
    - metacarpophalangeal (joint) S63.64-
    - specified site NEC S63.68-
  - thyroid cartilage or region S13.5
  - tibia (proximal end) — *see* Sprain, knee, specified site NEC
  - tibial collateral, knee — *see* Sprain, knee, collateral
  - tibiofibular
    - distal — *see* Sprain, ankle
    - superior — *see* Sprain, knee, specified site NEC
  - toe(s) S93.5Ø-
    - great S93.5Ø-
    - interphalangeal joint S93.51-
      - great S93.51-
      - lesser S93.51-
    - lesser S93.5Ø-
    - metatarsophalangeal joint S93.52-
      - great S93.52-
      - lesser S93.52-
  - ulna, collateral — *see* Rupture, traumatic, ligament, ulnar collateral
  - ulnohumeral — *see* Sprain, elbow
  - wrist S63.5Ø-
    - carpal S63.51-
    - radiocarpal S63.52-
    - specified site NEC S63.59-
  - xiphoid cartilage — *see* Sprain, sternum
- **Sprengel's deformity** (congenital) Q74.Ø
- **Sprue** (tropical) K9Ø.1
  - celiac K9Ø.Ø
  - idiopathic K9Ø.Ø
  - meaning thrush B37.Ø
  - nontropical K9Ø.Ø
- **Spur, bone** (*see also* Enthesopathy)
  - calcaneal M77.3-
  - iliac crest M76.2-
  - nose (septum) J34.89
- **Spurway's syndrome** Q78.0
- **Sputum**
  - abnormal (amount) (color) (odor) (purulent) RØ9.3
  - blood-stained RØ4.2
  - excessive (cause unknown) RØ9.3
- **Squamous** (*see also* condition)
  - epithelium in
    - cervical canal (congenital) Q51.828
    - uterine mucosa (congenital) Q51.818
- **Squashed nose** M95.0
  - congenital Q67.4
- **Squeeze, diver's** T70.3
- **Squint** (*see also* Strabismus)
  - accommodative — *see* Strabismus, convergent concomitant
- **St. Hubert's disease** A82.9
- **Stab** (*see also* Laceration)
  - internal organs — *see* Injury, by site
- **Stafne's cyst or cavity** M27.0
- **Staggering gait** R26.0
  - hysterical F44.4
- **Staghorn calculus** — *see* Calculus, kidney
- **Stähli's line** (cornea) (pigment) — *see* Pigmentation, cornea, anterior
- **Stain, staining**
  - meconium (newborn) P96.83
  - port wine Q82.5
  - tooth, teeth (hard tissues) (extrinsic) KØ3.6
    - due to
      - accretions KØ3.6
      - deposits (betel) (black) (green) (materia alba) (orange) (soft) (tobacco) KØ3.6
      - metals (copper) (silver) KØ3.7
      - nicotine KØ3.6
      - pulpal bleeding KØ3.7
      - tobacco KØ3.6
    - intrinsic KØØ.8
- **Stammering** (*see also* Disorder, fluency) F80.81
- **Standstill**
  - auricular I45.5
  - cardiac — *see* Arrest, cardiac
  - sinoatrial I45.5
  - ventricular — *see* Arrest, cardiac
- **Stannosis** J63.5
- **Stanton's disease** — *see* Melioidosis
- **Staphylitis** (acute) (catarrhal) (chronic) (gangrenous) (membranous) (suppurative) (ulcerative) K12.2
- **Staphylococcal scalded skin syndrome** L00
- **Staphylococcemia** A41.2
- **Staphylococcus, staphylococcal** (*see also* condition)
  - as cause of disease classified elsewhere B95.8
    - aureus (methicillin susceptible) (MSSA) B95.61
      - methicillin resistant (MRSA) B95.62
  - specified NEC, as cause of disease classified elsewhere B95.7
- **Staphyloma** (sclera)
  - cornea H18.72-
  - equatorial H15.81-
  - localized (anterior) H15.82-
  - posticum H15.83-
  - ring H15.85-
- **Stargardt's disease** — *see* Dystrophy, retina
- **Starvation** (inanition) (due to lack of food) T73.Ø
  - edema — *see* Malnutrition, severe
- **Stasis**
  - bile (noncalculous) K83.1
  - bronchus J98.Ø9
    - with infection — *see* Bronchitis
  - cardiac — *see* Failure, heart, congestive
  - cecum K59.8
  - colon K59.8
  - dermatitis — *see* Varix, leg, with, inflammation
  - duodenal K31.5
  - eczema — *see* Varix, leg, with, inflammation
  - edema — *see* Hypertension, venous (chronic), idiopathic
  - foot T69.Ø-
  - ileocecal coil K59.8
  - ileum K59.8
  - intestinal K59.8
  - jejunum K59.8
  - kidney N19
  - liver (cirrhotic) K76.1
  - lymphatic I89.8
  - pneumonia J18.2
  - pulmonary — *see* Edema, lung
  - rectal K59.8
  - renal N19
    - tubular N17.Ø
  - ulcer — *see* Varix, leg, with, ulcer
    - without varicose veins I87.2
  - urine — *see* Retention, urine
  - venous I87.8
- **State** (of)
  - affective and paranoid, mixed, organic psychotic FØ6.8
  - agitated R45.1
    - acute reaction to stress F43.Ø
- **State** (of) — *continued*
  - anxiety (neurotic) F41.1
  - apprehension F41.1
  - burn-out Z73.Ø
  - climacteric, female Z78.Ø
    - symptomatic N95.1
  - compulsive F42
    - mixed with obsessional thoughts F42
  - confusional (psychogenic) F44.89
    - acute (*see also* Delirium)
      - with
        - arteriosclerotic dementia FØ1.5Ø
          - with behavioral disturbance FØ1.51
        - senility or dementia FØ5
      - alcoholic F1Ø.231
    - epileptic FØ5
    - reactive (from emotional stress, psychological trauma) F44.89
    - subacute — *see* Delirium
  - convulsive — *see* Convulsions
  - crisis F43.Ø
  - depressive F32.9
    - neurotic F34.1
  - dissociative F44.9
  - emotional shock (stress) R45.7
  - hypercoagulation — *see* Hypercoagulable
  - locked-in G83.5
  - menopausal Z78.Ø
    - symptomatic N95.1
  - neurotic F48.9
    - with depersonalization F48.1
  - obsessional F42
  - oneiroid (schizophrenia-like) F23
  - organic
    - hallucinatory (nonalcoholic) FØ6.Ø
    - paranoid(-hallucinatory) FØ6.2
  - panic F41.Ø
  - paranoid F22
    - climacteric F22
    - involutional F22
    - menopausal F22
    - organic FØ6.2
    - senile FØ3
    - simple F22
  - persistent vegetative R4Ø.3
  - phobic F4Ø.9
  - postleukotomy FØ7.Ø
  - pregnant, incidental Z33.1
  - psychogenic, twilight F44.89
  - psychopathic (constitutional) F6Ø.2
  - psychotic, organic (*see also* Psychosis, organic)
    - mixed paranoid and affective FØ6.8
    - senile or presenile FØ3
    - transient NEC FØ6.8
      - with
        - hallucinations FØ6.Ø
        - depression FØ6.31
  - residual schizophrenic F2Ø.5
  - restlessness R45.1
  - stress (emotional) R45.7
  - tension (mental) F48.9
    - specified NEC F48.8
  - transient organic psychotic NEC FØ6.8
    - depressive type FØ6.31
    - hallucinatory type FØ6.3Ø
  - twilight
    - epileptic FØ5
    - psychogenic F44.89
  - vegetative, persistent R4Ø.3
  - vital exhaustion Z73.Ø
  - withdrawal, *see* Withdrawal, state
- **Status** (post) (*see also* Presence (of))
  - absence, epileptic — *see* Epilepsy, by type, with status epilepticus
  - administration of tPA (rtPA) in a different facility within the last 24 hours prior to admission to current facility Z92.82
  - adrenalectomy (unilateral) (bilateral) E89.6
  - anastomosis Z98.Ø
  - angioplasty (peripheral) Z98.62
    - with implant Z95.82Ø
    - coronary artery Z98.61
      - with implant Z95.5

Status (post) — *continued*
- anginosus I2Ø.9
- aortocoronary bypass Z95.1
- arthrodesis Z98.1
- artificial opening (of) Z93.9
  - gastrointestinal tract Z93.4
  - specified NEC Z93.8
  - urinary tract Z93.6
  - vagina Z93.8
- asthmaticus — *see* Asthma, by type, with status asthmaticus
- awaiting organ transplant Z76.82
- bariatric surgery Z98.84
- bed confinement Z74.Ø1
- bleb, filtering (vitreous), after glaucoma surgery Z98.83
- breast implant Z98.82
  - removal Z98.86
- cataract extraction Z98.4-
- cholecystectomy Z9Ø.49
- clitorectomy N9Ø.811
  - with excision of labia minora N9Ø.812
- colectomy (complete) (partial) Z9Ø.49
- colonization — *see* Carrier (suspected) of
- colostomy Z93.3
- convulsivus idiopathicus — *see* Epilepsy, by type, with status epilepticus
- coronary artery angioplasty — *see* Status, angioplasty, coronary artery
- cystectomy (urinary bladder) Z9Ø.6
- cystostomy Z93.5Ø
  - appendico-vesicostomy Z93.52
  - cutaneous Z93.51
  - specified NEC Z93.59
- delinquent immunization Z28.3
- dental Z98.818
  - crown Z98.811
  - fillings Z98.811
  - restoration Z98.811
  - sealant Z98.81Ø
  - specified NEC Z98.818
- deployment (current) (military) Z56.82
- dialysis (hemodialysis) (peritoneal) Z99.2
- do not resuscitate (DNR) Z66
- donor — *see* Donor
- embedded fragments — *see* Retained, foreign body fragments (type of)
- embedded splinter — *see* Retained, foreign body fragments (type of)
- enterostomy Z93.4
- epileptic, epilepticus (*see also* Epilepsy, by type, with status epilepticus) G4Ø.9Ø1
- estrogen receptor
  - negative Z17.Ø
  - positive Z17.1
- female genital cutting — *see* Female genital mutilation status
- female genital mutilation — *see* Female genital mutilation status
- filtering (vitreous) bleb after glaucoma surgery Z98.83
- gastrectomy (complete) (partial) Z9Ø.3
- gastric banding Z98.84
- gastric bypass for obesity Z98.84
- gastrostomy Z93.1
- human immunodeficiency virus (HIV) infection, asymptomatic Z21
- hysterectomy (complete) (total) Z9Ø.71Ø
  - partial (with remaining cervial stump) Z9Ø.711
- ileostomy Z93.2
- implant
  - breast Z98.82
- infibulation N9Ø.813
- intestinal bypass Z98.Ø
- jejunostomy Z93.4
- laryngectomy Z9Ø.Ø2
- lapsed immunization schedule Z28.3
- lymphaticus E32.8
- marmoratus G8Ø.3
- mastectomy (unilateral) (bilateral) Z9Ø.1-

Status (post) — *continued*
- military deployment status (current) Z56.82
  - in theater or in support of military war, peacekeeping and humanitarian operations Z56.82
- nephrectomy (unilateral) (bilateral) Z9Ø.5
- nephrostomy Z93.6
- obesity surgery Z98.84
- oophorectomy
  - bilateral Z9Ø.722
  - unilateral Z9Ø.721
- organ replacement
  - by artificial or mechanical device or prosthesis of
    - artery Z95.828
    - bladder Z96.Ø
    - blood vessel Z95.828
    - breast Z97.8
    - eye globe Z97.Ø
    - heart Z95.812
      - valve Z95.2
    - intestine Z97.8
    - joint Z96.6Ø
      - hip — *see* Presence, hip joint implant
      - knee — *see* Presence, knee joint implant
      - specified site NEC Z96.698
    - kidney Z97.8
    - larynx Z96.3
    - lens Z96.1
    - limbs — *see* Presence, artificial, limb
    - liver Z97.8
    - lung Z97.8
    - pancreas Z97.8
  - by organ transplant (heterologous)(homologous) — *see* Transplant
- pacemaker
  - brain Z96.89
  - cardiac Z95.Ø
  - specified NEC Z96.89
- pancreatectomy Z9Ø.41Ø
  - complete Z9Ø.41Ø
  - partial Z9Ø.411
  - total Z9Ø.41Ø
- physical restraint Z78.1
- pneumonectomy (complete) (partial) Z9Ø.2
- pneumothorax, therapeutic Z98.3
- postcommotio cerebri FØ7.81
- postoperative (postprocedural) NEC Z98.89
  - breast implant Z98.82
  - dental Z98.818
    - crown Z98.811
    - fillings Z98.811
    - restoration Z98.811
    - sealant Z98.81Ø
    - specified NEC Z98.818
  - pneumothorax, therapeutic Z98.3
- postpartum (routine follow-up) Z39.2
  - care immediately after delivery Z39.Ø
- postsurgical (postprocedural) NEC Z98.89
  - pneumothorax, therapeutic Z98.3
- pregnancy, incidental Z33.1
- prosthesis coronary angioplasty Z95.5
- pseudophakia Z96.1
- renal dialysis (hemodialysis) (peritoneal) Z99.2
- retained foreign body — *see* Retained, foreign body fragments (type of)
- reversed jejunal transposition (for bypass) Z98.Ø
- salpingo-oophorectomy
  - bilateral Z9Ø.722
  - unilateral Z9Ø.721
- sex reassignment surgery status Z87.89Ø
- shunt
  - arteriovenous (for dialysis) Z99.2
  - cerebrospinal fluid Z98.2
  - ventricular (communicating) (for drainage) Z98.2
- splenectomy Z9Ø.81
- thymicolymphaticus E32.8
- thymicus E32.8
- thymolymphaticus E32.8
- thyroidectomy (hypothyroidism) E89.Ø
- tooth (teeth) extraction (*see also* Absence, teeth, acquired) KØ8.4Ø9

Status (post) — *continued*
- tPA (rtPA) administration in a different facility within the last 24 hours prior to admission to current facility Z92.82
- tracheostomy Z93.Ø
- transplant — *see* Transplant
  - organ removed Z98.85
- tubal ligation Z98.51
- underimmunization Z28.3
- ureterostomy Z93.6
- urethrostomy Z93.6
- vagina, artificial Z93.8
- vasectomy Z98.52
- wheelchair confinement Z99.3

Stealing
- child problem F91.8
  - in company with others Z72.81Ø
- pathological (compulsive) F63.2

Steam burn — *see* Burn

Steatocystoma multiplex L72.2

Steatohepatitis (nonalcoholic) (NASH) K75.81

Steatoma L72.3
- eyelid (cystic) — *see* Dermatosis, eyelid
  - infected — *see* Hordeolum

Steatorrhea (chronic) K9Ø.4
- with lacteal obstruction K9Ø.2
- idiopathic (adult) (infantile) K9Ø.Ø
- pancreatic K9Ø.3
- primary K9Ø.Ø
- tropical K9Ø.1

Steatosis E88.89
- heart — *see* Degeneration, myocardial
- kidney N28.89
- liver NEC K76.Ø

Steele-Richardson-Olszewski disease or syndrome G23.1

Steinbrocker's syndrome G9Ø.8

Steinert's disease G71.11

Stein-Leventhal syndrome E28.2

Stein's syndrome E28.2
- STEMI I21.3 (*see also* Infarct, myocardium, ST elevation)

Stenocardia I2Ø.8

Stenocephaly Q75.8

Stenosis, stenotic (cicatricial) (*see also* Stricture)
- ampulla of Vater K83.1
- anus, anal (canal) (sphincter) K62.4
  - and rectum K62.4
  - congenital Q42.3
    - with fistula Q42.2
- aorta (ascending) (supraventricular) (congenital) Q25.3
  - arteriosclerotic I7Ø.Ø
  - calcified I7Ø.Ø
- aortic (valve) I35.Ø
  - with insufficiency I35.2
  - congenital Q23.Ø
  - rheumatic IØ6.Ø
    - with
      - incompetency, insufficiency or regurgitation IØ6.2
        - with mitral (valve) disease IØ8.Ø
          - with tricuspid (valve) disease IØ8.3
      - mitral (valve) disease IØ8.Ø
        - with tricuspid (valve) disease IØ8.3
      - tricuspid (valve) disease IØ8.2
        - with mitral (valve) disease IØ8.3
  - specified cause NEC I35.Ø
  - syphilitic A52.Ø3
- aqueduct of Sylvius (congenital) QØ3.Ø
  - with spina bifida — *see* Spina bifida, by site, with hydrocephalus
  - acquired G91.1
- artery NEC (*see also* Arteriosclerosis) I77.1
  - celiac I77.4
  - cerebral — *see* Occlusion, artery, cerebral
  - extremities — *see* Arteriosclerosis, extremities
  - precerebral — *see* Occlusion, artery, precerebral
  - pulmonary (congenital) Q25.6
    - acquired I28.8
  - renal I7Ø.1
- bile duct (common) (hepatic) K83.1
  - congenital Q44.3

- **Stenosis, stenotic**— *continued*
  - bladder-neck (acquired) N32.0
    - congenital Q64.31
  - brain G93.89
  - bronchus J98.09
    - congenital Q32.3
    - syphilitic A52.72
  - cardia (stomach) K22.2
    - congenital Q39.3
  - cardiovascular — *see* Disease, cardiovascular
  - caudal M48.08
  - cervix, cervical (canal) N88.2
    - congenital Q51.828
    - in pregnancy or childbirth — *see* Pregnancy, complicated by, abnormal cervix
  - colon (*see also* Obstruction, intestine)
    - congenital Q42.9
      - specified NEC Q42.8
  - colostomy K94.03
  - common (bile) duct K83.1
    - congenital Q44.3
  - coronary (artery) — *see* Disease, heart, ischemic, atherosclerotic
  - cystic duct — *see* Obstruction, gallbladder
  - due to presence of device, implant or graft (*see also* Complications, by site and type, specified NEC) T85.85
    - arterial graft NEC T82.858
    - breast (implant) T85.85
    - catheter T85.85
      - dialysis (renal) T82.858
        - intraperitoneal T85.85
      - infusion NEC T82.858
        - spinal (epidural) (subdural) T85.85
      - urinary (indwelling) T83.85
    - fixation, internal (orthopedic) NEC T84.85
    - gastrointestinal (bile duct) (esophagus) T85.85
    - genital NEC T83.85
    - heart NEC T82.857
    - joint prosthesis T84.85
    - ocular (corneal graft) (orbital implant) NEC T85.85
    - orthopedic NEC T84.85
    - specified NEC T85.85
    - urinary NEC T83.85
    - vascular NEC T82.858
    - ventricular intracranial shunt T85.85
  - duodenum K31.5
    - congenital Q41.0
  - ejaculatory duct NEC N50.8
  - endocervical os — *see* Stenosis, cervix
  - enterostomy K94.13
  - esophagus K22.2
    - congenital Q39.3
    - syphilitic A52.79
      - congenital A50.59 *[K23]*
  - eustachian tube — *see* Obstruction, eustachian tube
  - external ear canal (acquired) H61.30-
    - congenital Q16.1
    - due to
      - inflammation H61.32-
      - trauma H61.31-
    - postprocedural H95.81-
    - specified cause NEC H61.39-
  - gallbladder — *see* Obstruction, gallbladder
  - glottis J38.6
  - heart valve (congenital) Q24.8
    - aortic Q23.0
    - mitral Q23.2
    - pulmonary Q22.1
    - tricuspid Q22.4
  - hepatic duct K83.1
  - hymen N89.6
  - hypertrophic subaortic (idiopathic) I42.1
  - ileum K56.69
    - congenital Q41.2
  - infundibulum cardia Q24.3
  - intervertebral foramina (*see also* Lesion, biomechanical, specified NEC)
    - connective tissue M99.79
      - abdomen M99.79
      - cervical region M99.71
      - cervicothoracic M99.71

- **Stenosis, stenotic**— *continued*
  - intervertebral foramina — *continued*
    - connective tissue — *continued*
      - head region M99.70
      - lumbar region M99.73
      - lumbosacral M99.73
      - occipitocervical M99.70
      - sacral region M99.74
      - sacrococcygeal M99.74
      - sacroiliac M99.74
      - specified NEC M99.79
      - thoracic region M99.72
      - thoracolumbar M99.72
    - disc M99.79
      - abdomen M99.79
      - cervical region M99.71
      - cervicothoracic M99.71
      - head region M99.70
      - lower extremity M99.76
      - lumbar region M99.73
      - lumbosacral M99.73
      - occipitocervical M99.70
      - pelvic M99.75
      - rib cage M99.78
      - sacral region M99.74
      - sacrococcygeal M99.74
      - sacroiliac M99.74
      - specified NEC M99.79
      - thoracic region M99.72
      - thoracolumbar M99.72
      - upper extremity M99.77
    - osseous M99.69
      - abdomen M99.69
      - cervical region M99.61
      - cervicothoracic M99.61
      - head region M99.60
      - lower extremity M99.66
      - lumbar region M99.63
      - lumbosacral M99.63
      - occipitocervical M99.60
      - pelvic M99.65
      - rib cage M99.68
      - sacral region M99.64
      - sacrococcygeal M99.64
      - sacroiliac M99.64
      - specified NEC M99.69
      - thoracic region M99.62
      - thoracolumbar M99.62
      - upper extremity M99.67
    - subluxation — *see* Stenosis, intervertebral foramina, osseous
  - intestine (*see also* Obstruction, intestine)
    - congenital (small) Q41.9
      - large Q42.9
        - specified NEC Q42.8
      - specified NEC Q41.8
  - jejunum K56.69
    - congenital Q41.1
  - lacrimal (passage)
    - canaliculi H04.54-
    - congenital Q10.5
    - duct H04.55-
    - punctum H04.56-
    - sac H04.57-
  - lacrimonasal duct — *see* Stenosis, lacrimal, duct
    - congenital Q10.5
  - larynx J38.6
    - congenital NEC Q31.8
      - subglottic Q31.1
    - syphilitic A52.73
      - congenital A50.59 *[J99]*
  - mitral (chronic) (inactive) (valve) I05.0
    - with
      - aortic valve disease I08.0
      - incompetency, insufficiency or regurgitation I05.2
    - active or acute I01.1
      - with rheumatic or Sydenham's chorea I02.0
    - congenital Q23.2
    - specified cause, except rheumatic I34.2
    - syphilitic A52.03

- **Stenosis, stenotic**— *continued*
  - myocardium, myocardial (*see also* Degeneration, myocardial)
    - hypertrophic subaortic (idiopathic) I42.1
  - nares (anterior) (posterior) J34.89
    - congenital Q30.0
  - nasal duct (*see also* Stenosis, lacrimal, duct)
    - congenital Q10.5
  - nasolacrimal duct (*see also* Stenosis, lacrimal, duct)
    - congenital Q10.5
  - neural canal (*see also* Lesion, biomechanical, specified NEC)
    - connective tissue M99.49
      - abdomen M99.49
      - cervical region M99.41
      - cervicothoracic M99.41
      - head region M99.40
      - lower extremity M99.46
      - lumbar region M99.43
      - lumbosacral M99.43
      - occipitocervical M99.40
      - pelvic M99.45
      - rib cage M99.48
      - sacral region M99.44
      - sacrococcygeal M99.44
      - sacroiliac M99.44
      - specified NEC M99.49
      - thoracic region M99.42
      - thoracolumbar M99.42
      - upper extremity M99.47
    - intervertebral disc M99.59
      - abdomen M99.59
      - cervical region M99.51
      - cervicothoracic M99.51
      - head region M99.50
      - lower extremity M99.56
      - lumbar region M99.53
      - lumbosacral M99.53
      - occipitocervical M99.50
      - pelvic M99.55
      - rib cage M99.58
      - sacral region M99.54
      - sacrococcygeal M99.54
      - sacroiliac M99.54
      - specified NEC M99.59
      - thoracic region M99.52
      - thoracolumbar M99.52
      - upper extremity M99.57
    - osseous M99.39
      - abdomen M99.39
      - cervical region M99.31
      - cervicothoracic M99.31
      - head region M99.30
      - lower extremity M99.36
      - lumbar region M99.33
      - lumbosacral M99.33
      - pelvic M99.35
      - rib cage M99.38
      - occipitocervical M99.30
      - sacral region M99.34
      - sacrococcygeal M99.34
      - sacroiliac M99.34
      - specified NEC M99.39
      - thoracic region M99.32
      - thoracolumbar M99.32
      - upper extremity M99.37
    - subluxation M99.29
      - cervical region M99.21
      - cervicothoracic M99.21
      - head region M99.20
      - lower extremity M99.26
      - lumbar region M99.23
      - lumbosacral M99.23
      - occipitocervical M99.20
      - pelvic M99.25
      - rib cage M99.28
      - sacral region M99.24
      - sacrococcygeal M99.24
      - sacroiliac M99.24
      - specified NEC M99.29
      - thoracic region M99.22
      - thoracolumbar M99.22
      - upper extremity M99.27

- **Stenosis, stenotic**— *continued*
  - oesophagus — *see* Stenosis, esophagus
  - organ or site, congenital NEC — *see* Atresia, by site
  - papilla of Vater K83.1
  - pulmonary (artery) (congenital) Q25.6
    - with ventricular septal defect, transposition of aorta, and hypertrophy of right ventricle Q21.3
    - acquired I28.8
    - in tetralogy of Fallot Q21.3
    - infundibular Q24.3
    - valve I37.Ø
      - with insufficiency I37.2
      - congenital Q22.1
      - rheumatic IØ9.89
        - with aortic, mitral or tricuspid (valve) disease IØ8.8
    - subvalvular Q24.3
    - supravalvular Q25.6
    - vein, acquired I28.8
    - vessel NEC I28.8
  - pulmonic (congenital) Q22.1
    - infundibular Q24.3
    - subvalvular Q24.3
  - pylorus (hypertrophic) (acquired) K31.1
    - adult K31.1
    - congenital Q4Ø.Ø
    - infantile Q4Ø.Ø
  - rectum (sphincter) — *see* Stricture, rectum
  - renal artery I7Ø.1
    - congenital Q27.1
  - salivary duct (any) K11.8
  - sphincter of Oddi K83.1
  - spinal M48.ØØ
    - cervical region M48.Ø2
    - cervicothoracic region M48.Ø3
    - lumbar region M48.Ø6
    - lumbosacral region M48.Ø7
    - occipito-atlanto-axial region M48.Ø1
    - sacrococcygeal region M48.Ø8
    - thoracic region M48.Ø4
    - thoracolumbar region M48.Ø5
  - stomach, hourglass K31.2
  - subaortic (congenital) Q24.4
    - hypertrophic (idiopathic) I42.1
  - subglottic J38.6
    - congenital Q31.1
    - postprocedural J95.5
  - trachea J39.8
    - congenital Q32.1
    - syphilitic A52.73
    - tuberculous NEC A15.5
  - tracheostomy J95.Ø3
  - tricuspid (valve) IØ7.Ø
    - with
      - aortic (valve) disease IØ8.2
      - incompetency, insufficiency or regurgitation IØ7.2
        - with aortic (valve) disease IØ8.2
          - with mitral (valve) disease IØ8.3
      - mitral (valve) disease IØ8.1
        - with aortic (valve) disease IØ8.3
    - congenital Q22.4
    - nonrheumatic I36.Ø
      - with insufficiency I36.2
  - tubal N97.1
  - ureter — *see* Atresia, ureter
  - ureteropelvic junction, congenital Q62.11
  - ureterovesical orifice, congenital Q62.12
  - urethra (valve) (*see also* Stricture, urethra)
    - congenital Q64.32
  - urinary meatus, congenital Q64.33
  - vagina N89.5
    - congenital Q52.4
    - in pregnancy — *see* Pregnancy, complicated by, abnormal vagina
      - causing obstructed labor O65.5
  - valve (cardiac) (heart) (*see also* Endocarditis) I38
    - congenital Q24.8
      - aortic Q23.Ø
      - mitral Q23.2
      - pulmonary Q22.1
      - tricuspid Q22.4
- **Stenosis, stenotic**— *continued*
  - vena cava (inferior) (superior) I87.1
    - congenital Q26.Ø
  - vesicourethral orifice Q64.31
  - vulva N9Ø.5
- **Stent jail** T82.897
- **Stercolith** (impaction) K56.41
  - appendix K38.1
- **Stercoraceous, stercoral ulcer** K63.3
  - anus or rectum K62.6
- **Stereotypies NEC** F98.4
- **Sterility** — *see* Infertility
- **Sterilization** — *see* Encounter (for), sterilization
- **Sternalgia** — *see* Angina
- **Sternopagus** Q89.4
- **Sternum bifidum** Q76.7
- **Steroid**
  - effects (adverse) (adrenocortical) (iatrogenic)
    - cushingoid E24.2
      - correct substance properly administered — *see* Table of Drugs and Chemicals, by drug, adverse effect
      - overdose or wrong substance given or taken — *see* Table of Drugs and Chemicals, by drug, poisoning
    - diabetes — *see* category EØ9
      - correct substance properly administered Table of Drugs and Chemicals, by drug, adverse effect
        - overdose or wrong substance given or taken — *see* Table of Drugs and Chemicals, by drug, poisoning
    - fever R5Ø.2
    - insufficiency E27.3
      - correct substance properly administered — *see* Table of Drugs and Chemicals, by drug, adverse effect
      - overdose or wrong substance given or taken — *see* Table of Drugs and Chemicals, by drug, poisoning
  - responder H4Ø.Ø4-
- **Stevens-Johnson disease or syndrome** L51.1
  - toxic epidermal necrolysis overlap L51.3
- **Stewart-Morel syndrome** M85.2
- **Sticker's disease** BØ8.3
- **Sticky eye** — *see* Conjunctivitis, acute, mucopurulent
- **Stieda's disease** — *see* Bursitis, tibial collateral
- **Stiff neck** — *see* Torticollis
- **Stiff-man syndrome** G25.82
- **Stiffness, joint NEC** M25.60
  - ankle M25.67-
  - ankylosis — *see* Ankylosis, joint
  - contracture — *see* Contraction, joint
  - elbow M25.6-
  - foot M25.6-
  - hand M25.6-
  - hip M25.6-
  - knee M25.6-
  - shoulder M25.1-
  - wrist M25.3-
- **Stigmata congenital syphilis** A50.59
- **Stillbirth** P95
- **Still-Felty syndrome** — *see* Felty's syndrome
- **Still's disease or syndrome** (juvenile) MØ8.2Ø
  - adult-onset MØ6.1
  - ankle MØ8.27-
  - elbow MØ8.22-
  - foot joint MØ8.27-
  - hand joint MØ8.24-
  - hip MØ8.25-
  - knee MØ8.26-
  - multiple site MØ8.29
  - shoulder MØ8.21-
  - vertebra MØ8.28
  - wrist MØ8.23-
- **Stimulation, ovary** E28.1
- **Sting** (venomous) (with allergic or anaphylactic shock) — *see* Table of Drugs and Chemicals, by animal or substance, poisoning
- **Stippled epiphyses** Q78.8
- **Stitch**
  - abscess T81.4
- **Stitch**— *continued*
  - burst (in operation wound) — *see* Disruption, wound, operation
- **Stokes-Adams disease or syndrome** I45.9
- **Stokes' disease** EØ5.ØØ with thyroid storm EØ5.Ø1
- **Stokvis** (-Talma) **disease** D74.8B
- **Stoma malfunction**
  - colostomy K94.Ø3
  - enterostomy K94.13
  - gastrostomy K94.23
  - ileostomy K94.13
  - tracheostomy J95.Ø3
- **Stomach** — *see* condition
- **Stomatitis** (denture) (ulcerative) K12.1
  - angular K13.Ø
    - due to dietary or vitamin deficiency E53.Ø
  - aphthous K12.Ø
  - bovine BØ8.61
  - candidal B37.Ø
  - catarrhal K12.1
  - diphtheritic A36.89
  - due to
    - dietary deficiency E53.Ø
    - thrush B37.Ø
    - vitamin deficiency
      - B group NEC E53.9
      - B2 (riboflavin) E53.Ø
  - epidemic BØ8.8
  - epizootic BØ8.8
  - follicular K12.1
  - gangrenous A69.Ø
  - Geotrichum B48.3
  - herpesviral, herpetic BØØ.2
  - herpetiformis K12.Ø
  - malignant K12.1
  - membranous acute K12.1
  - monilial B37.Ø
  - mycotic B37.Ø
  - necrotizing ulcerative A69.Ø
  - parasitic B37.Ø
  - septic K12.1
  - spirochetal A69.1
  - suppurative (acute) K12.2
  - ulceromembranous A69.1
  - vesicular K12.1
    - with exanthem (enteroviral) BØ8.4
    - virus disease A93.8
  - Vincent's A69.1
- **Stomatocytosis** D58.8
- **Stomatomycosis** B37.0
- **Stomatorrhagia** K13.79
- **Stone**(s) (*see also* Calculus)
  - bladder (diverticulum) N21.Ø
  - cystine E72.Ø9
  - heart syndrome I5Ø.1
  - kidney N2Ø.Ø
  - prostate N42.Ø
  - pulpal (dental) KØ4.2
  - renal N2Ø.Ø
  - salivary gland or duct (any) K11.5
  - urethra (impacted) N21.1
  - urinary (duct) (impacted) (passage) N2Ø.9
    - bladder (diverticulum) N21.Ø
    - lower tract N21.9
    - specified NEC N21.8
  - xanthine E79.8 *[N22]*
- **Stonecutter's lung** J62.8
- **Stonemason's asthma, disease, lung or pneumoconiosis** J62.8
- **Stoppage**
  - heart — *see* Arrest, cardiac
  - urine — *see* Retention, urine
- **Storm, thyroid** — *see* Thyrotoxicosis
- **Strabismus** (congenital) (nonparalytic) H5Ø.9
  - concomitant H5Ø.4Ø
    - convergent — *see* Strabismus, convergent concomitant
    - divergent — *see* Strabismus, divergent concomitant
  - convergent concomitant H5Ø.ØØ
    - accommodative component H5Ø.43
    - alternating H5Ø.Ø5

- **Subphrenic** — *see* condition
- **Subscapular nerve** — *see* condition
- **Subseptus uterus** Q51.2
- **Subsiding appendicitis** K36
- **Substernal thyroid** E04.9
  - congenital Q89.2
- **Substitution disorder** F44.9
- **Subtentorial** — *see* condition
- **Subthyroidism** (acquired) (*see also* Hypothyroidism)
  - congenital EØ3.1
- **Succenturiate placenta** O43.19-
- **Sucking thumb, child** (excessive) F98.8
- **Sudamen, sudamina** L74.1
- **Sudanese kala-azar** B55.0
- **Sudden**
  - heart failure — *see* Failure, heart
  - hearing loss — *see* Deafness, sudden
- **Sudeck's atrophy, disease, or syndrome** — *see* Algoneurodystrophy
- **Suffocation** — *see* Asphyxia, traumatic
- **Sugar**
  - blood
    - high (transient) R73.9
    - low (transient) E16.2
  - in urine R81
- **Suicide, suicidal** (attempted) T14.91
  - by poisoning — *see* Table of Drugs and Chemicals
  - history of (personal) Z91.5
    - in family Z81.8
  - ideation — *see* Ideation, suicidal
  - risk
    - meaning personal history of attempted suicide Z91.5
    - meaning suicidal ideation — *see* Ideation, suicidal
  - tendencies
    - meaning personal history of attempted suicide Z91.5
    - meaning suicidal ideation — *see* Ideation, suicidal
  - trauma — *see* nature of injury by site
- **Suipestifer infection** — *see* Infection, salmonella
- **Sulfhemoglobinemia, sulphemoglobinemia** (acquired) (with methemoglobinemia) D74.8
- **Sumatran mite fever** A75.3
- **Summer** — *see* condition
- **Sunburn** L55.9
  - first degree L55.Ø
  - second degree L55.1
  - third degree L55.2
- **SUNCT** (short lasting unilateral neuralgiform headache with conjunctival injection and tearing) G44.Ø59
  - intractable G44.Ø51
  - not intractable G44.Ø59
- **Sunken acetabulum** — *see* Derangement, joint, specified type NEC, hip
- **Sunstroke** T67.0
- **Superfecundation** — *see* Pregnancy, multiple
- **Superfetation** — *see* Pregnancy, multiple
- **Superinvolution** (uterus) N85.8
- **Supernumerary** (congenital)
  - aortic cusps Q23.8
  - auditory ossicles Q16.3
  - bone Q79.8
  - breast Q83.1
  - carpal bones Q74.Ø
  - cusps, heart valve NEC Q24.8
    - aortic Q23.8
    - mitral Q23.2
    - pulmonary Q22.3
  - digit(s) Q69.9
  - ear (lobule) Q17.Ø
  - fallopian tube Q5Ø.6
  - finger Q69.Ø
  - hymen Q52.4
  - kidney Q63.Ø
  - lacrimonasal duct Q1Ø.6
  - lobule (ear) Q17.Ø
  - mitral cusps Q23.2
  - muscle Q79.8
  - nipple(s) Q83.3
  - organ or site not listed — *see* Accessory
  - ossicles, auditory Q16.3
- **Supernumerary** (congenital) — *continued*
  - ovary Q5Ø.31
  - oviduct Q5Ø.6
  - pulmonary, pulmonic cusps Q22.3
  - rib Q76.6
    - cervical or first (syndrome) Q76.5
  - roots (of teeth) KØØ.2
  - spleen Q89.Ø9
  - tarsal bones Q74.2
  - teeth KØØ.1
  - testis Q55.29
  - thumb Q69.1
  - toe Q69.2
  - uterus Q51.2
  - vagina Q52.1
  - vertebra Q76.49
- **Supervision** (of)
  - contraceptive — *see* Prescription, contraceptives
  - dietary (for) Z71.3
    - allergy (food) Z71.3
    - colitis Z71.3
    - diabetes mellitus Z71.3
    - food allergy or intolerance Z71.3
    - gastritis Z71.3
    - hypercholesterolemia Z71.3
    - hypoglycemia Z71.3
    - intolerance (food) Z71.3
    - obesity Z71.3
    - specified NEC Z71.3
  - healthy infant or child Z76.2
    - foundling Z76.1
  - high-risk pregnancy — *see* Pregnancy, complicated by, high, risk
  - lactation Z39.1
  - pregnancy — *see* Pregnancy, supervision of
- **Supplemental teeth** K00.1
- **Suppression**
  - binocular vision H53.34
  - lactation O92.5
  - menstruation N94.89
  - ovarian secretion E28.39
  - renal N28.9
  - urine, urinary secretion R34
- **Suppuration, suppurative** (*see also* condition)
  - accessory sinus (chronic) — *see* Sinusitis
  - adrenal gland
  - antrum (chronic) — *see* Sinusitis, maxillary
  - bladder — *see* Cystitis
  - brain GØ6.Ø
    - sequelae GØ9
  - breast N61
    - puerperal, postpartum or gestational — *see* Mastitis, obstetric, purulent
  - dental periosteum M27.3
  - ear (middle) (*see also* Otitis, media)
    - external NEC — *see* Otitis, externa, infective
    - internal — *see* subcategory H83.Ø
  - ethmoidal (chronic) (sinus) — *see* Sinusitis, ethmoidal
  - fallopian tube — *see* Salpingo-oophoritis
  - frontal (chronic) (sinus) — *see* Sinusitis, frontal
  - gallbladder (acute) K81.Ø
  - gum KØ5.2Ø
    - generalized KØ5.22
    - localized KØ5.21
  - intracranial GØ6.Ø
  - joint — *see* Arthritis, pyogenic or pyemic
  - labyrinthine — *see* subcategory H83.Ø
  - lung — *see* Abscess, lung
  - mammary gland N61
    - puerperal, postpartum O91.12
      - associated with lactation O91.13
  - maxilla, maxillary M27.2
    - sinus (chronic) — *see* Sinusitis, maxillary
  - muscle — *see* Myositis, infective
  - nasal sinus (chronic) — *see* Sinusitis
  - pancreas, acute K85.8
  - parotid gland — *see* Sialoadenitis
  - pelvis, pelvic
    - female — *see* Disease, pelvis, inflammatory
    - male K65.Ø
  - pericranial — *see* Osteomyelitis
  - salivary duct or gland (any) — *see* Sialoadenitis
- **Suppuration, suppurative** — *continued*
  - sinus (accessory) (chronic) (nasal) — *see* Sinusitis
  - sphenoidal sinus (chronic) — *see* Sinusitis, sphenoidal
  - thymus (gland) E32.1
  - thyroid (gland) EØ6.Ø
  - tonsil — *see* Tonsillitis
  - uterus — *see* Endometritis
- **Supraeruption of tooth** (teeth) M26.34
- **Supraglottitis** J04.30
  - with obstruction JØ4.31
- **Suprarenal** (gland) — *see* condition
- **Suprascapular nerve** — *see* condition
- **Suprasellar** — *see* condition
- **Surfer's knots or nodules** S89.8-
- **Surgical**
  - emphysema T81.82
  - procedures, complication or misadventure — *see* Complications, surgical procedures
  - shock T81.1Ø
- **Surveillance** (of) (for) (*see also* Observation)
  - alcohol abuse Z71.41
  - contraceptive — *see* Prescription, contraceptives
  - dietary Z71.3
  - drug abuse Z71.51
- **Susceptibility to disease, genetic** Z15.89
  - malignant neoplasm Z15.Ø9
    - breast Z15.Ø1
    - endometrium Z15.Ø4
    - ovary Z15.Ø2
    - prostate Z15.Ø3
    - specified NEC Z15.Ø9
  - multiple endocrine neoplasia Z15.81
- **Suspected condition, ruled out** (*see also* Observation, suspected)
  - amniotic cavity and membrane ZØ3.71
  - cervical shortening ZØ3.75
  - fetal anomaly ZØ3.73
  - fetal growth ZØ3.74
  - maternal and fetal conditions NEC ZØ3.79
  - oligohydramnios ZØ3.71
  - placental problem ZØ3.72
  - polyhydramnios ZØ3.71
- **Suspended uterus**
  - in pregnancy or childbirth — *see* Pregnancy, complicated by, abnormal uterus
- **Sutton's nevus** D22.9
- **Suture**
  - burst (in operation wound) T81.31
    - external operation wound T81.31
    - internal operation wound T81.32
  - inadvertently left in operation wound — *see* Foreign body, accidentally left during a procedure
  - removal Z48.Ø2
- **Swab inadvertently left in operation wound** — *see* Foreign body, accidentally left during a procedure
- **Swallowed, swallowing**
  - difficulty — *see* Dysphagia
  - foreign body — *see* Foreign body, alimentary tract
- **Swan-neck deformity** (finger) — *see* Deformity, finger, swan-neck
- **Swearing, compulsive** F42
  - in Gilles de la Tourette's syndrome F95.2
- **Sweat, sweats**
  - fetid L75.Ø
  - night R61
- **Sweating, excessive** R61
- **Sweeley-Klionsky disease** E75.21
- **Sweet's disease or dermatosis** L98.2
- **Swelling** (of) R6Ø.9
  - abdomen, abdominal (not referable to any particular organ) — *see* Mass, abdominal
  - ankle — *see* Effusion, joint, ankle
  - arm M79.89
    - forearm M79.89
  - breast N63
  - Calabar B74.3
  - cervical gland R59.Ø
  - chest, localized R22.2
  - ear H93.8-
  - extremity (lower) (upper) — *see* Disorder, soft tissue, specified type NEC

Swelling (of) — *continued*
- finger M79.89
- foot M79.89
- glands R59.9
  - generalized R59.1
  - localized R59.Ø
- hand M79.89
- head (localized) R22.Ø
- inflammatory — *see* Inflammation
- intra-abdominal — *see* Mass, abdominal
- joint — *see* Effusion, joint
- leg M79.89
  - lower M79.89
- limb — *see* Disorder, soft tissue, specified type NEC
- localized (skin) R22.9
  - chest R22.2
  - head R22.Ø
  - limb
    - lower — *see* Mass, localized, limb, lower
    - upper — *see* Mass, localized, limb, upper
  - neck R22.1
  - trunk R22.2
- neck (localized) R22.1
- pelvic — *see* Mass, abdominal
- scrotum N5Ø.8
- splenic — *see* Splenomegaly
- testis N5Ø.8
- toe M79.89
- umbilical R19.Ø9
- wandering, due to Gnathostoma (spinigerum) B83.1
- white — *see* Tuberculosis, arthritis

Swift(-Feer) **disease**
- overdose or wrong substance given or taken — *see* Table of Drugs and Chemicals, by drug, poisoning

Swimmer's
- cramp T75.1
- ear H6Ø.33-
- itch B65.3

Swimming in the head R42
Swollen — *see* Swelling
Swyer syndrome Q99.1
Sycosis L73.8
- barbae (not parasitic) L73.8
- contagiosa (mycotic) B35.Ø
- lupoides L73.8
- mycotic B35.Ø
- parasitic B35.Ø
- vulgaris L73.8

Sydenham's chorea — *see* Chorea, Sydenham's
Sylvatic yellow fever A95.0
Sylvest's disease B33.0
Symblepharon H11.23-
- congenital Q1Ø.3

Symond's syndrome G93.2
Sympathetic — *see* condition
Sympatheticotonia G90.8
Sympathicoblastoma
- specified site — *see* Neoplasm, malignant, by site
- unspecified site C74.9Ø

Sympathogonioma — *see* Sympathicoblastoma
Symphalangy (fingers) (toes) Q7Ø.9
Symptoms NEC R68.89
- breast NEC N64.59
- development NEC R63.8
- factitious, self-induced — *see* Disorder, factitious
- genital organs, female R1Ø.2
- involving
  - abdomen NEC R19.8
  - appearance NEC R46.89
  - awareness R41.9
    - altered mental status R41.82
    - amnesia — *see* Amnesia
    - borderline intellectual functioning R41.83
    - coma — *see* Coma
    - disorientation R41.Ø
    - neurologic neglect syndrome R41.4
    - senile cognitive decline R41.81
    - specified symptom NEC R41.89
  - behavior NEC R46.89
  - cardiovascular system NEC RØ9.89
  - chest NEC RØ9.89
  - circulatory system NEC RØ9.89

Symptoms NEC — *continued*
- involving — *continued*
  - cognitive functions R41.9
    - altered mental status R41.82
    - amnesia — *see* Amnesia
    - borderline intellectual functioning R41.83
    - coma — *see* Coma
    - disorientation R41.Ø
    - neurologic neglect syndrome R41.4
    - senile cognitive decline R41.81
    - specified symptom NEC R41.89
  - development NEC R62.5Ø
  - digestive system NEC R19.8
  - emotional state NEC R45.89
    - emotional lability R45.86
  - food and fluid intake R63.8
  - general perceptions and sensations R44.9
    - specified NEC R44.8
  - musculoskeletal system R29.91
    - specified NEC R29.898
  - nervous system R29.9Ø
    - specified NEC R29.818
  - pelvis NEC R19.8
  - respiratory system NEC RØ9.89
  - skin and integument R23.9
  - urinary system R39.9
- menopausal N95.1
- metabolism NEC R63.8
- neurotic F48.8
- of infancy R68.19
- pelvis NEC, female R1Ø.2
- skin and integument NEC R23.8
- subcutaneous tissue NEC R23.8

Sympus Q74.2
Syncephalus Q89.4
Synchondrosis
- abnormal (congenital) Q78.8
- ischiopubic M91.Ø

Synchysis (scintillans) (senile) (vitreous body) H43.89
Syncope (near) (pre-) R55
- anginosa I2Ø.8
- bradycardia RØØ.1
- cardiac R55
- carotid sinus G9Ø.Ø1
- due to spinal (lumbar) puncture G97.1
- heart R55
- heat T67.1
- laryngeal RØ5
- psychogenic F48.8
- tussive RØ5
- vasoconstriction R55
- vasodepressor R55
- vasomotor R55
- vasovagal R55

Syndactylism, syndactyly Q70.9
- complex (with synostosis)
  - fingers Q7Ø.Ø-
  - toes Q7Ø.2-
- simple (without synostosis)
  - fingers Q7Ø.1-
  - toes Q7Ø.3-

Syndrome (*see also* Disease)
- 5q minus NOS D46.C
- 48,XXXX Q97.1
- 49,XXXXX Q97.1
- abdominal
  - acute R1Ø.Ø
  - muscle deficiency Q79.4
- abnormal innervation HØ2.519
  - left HØ2.516
    - lower HØ2.515
    - upper HØ2.514
  - right HØ2.513
    - lower HØ2.512
    - upper HØ2.511
- abstinence, neonatal P96.1
- acid pulmonary aspiration, obstetric O74.Ø
- acquired immunodeficiency — *see* Human, immunodeficiency virus (HIV) disease
- acute abdominal R1Ø.Ø
- acute respiratory distress (adult) (child) J8Ø
- Adair-Dighton Q78.Ø
- Adams-Stokes(-Morgagni) I45.9

Syndrome — *continued*
- adiposogenital E23.6
- adrenal
  - hemorrhage (meningococcal) A39.1
  - meningococcic A39.1
- adrenocortical — *see* Cushing's, syndrome
- adrenogenital E25.9
  - congenital, associated with enzyme deficiency E25.Ø
- afferent loop NEC K91.89
- Alagille's Q44.7
- alcohol withdrawal (without convulsions) — *see* Dependence, alcohol, with, withdrawal
- Alder's D72.Ø
- Aldrich(-Wiskott) D82.Ø
- alien hand R41.4
- Alport Q87.81
- alveolar hypoventilation E66.2
- alveolocapillary block J84.1Ø
- amnesic, amnestic (confabulatory) (due to) — *see* Disorder, amnesic
- amyostatic (Wilson's disease) E83.Ø1
- androgen insensitivity E34.5Ø
  - complete E34.51
  - partial E34.52
- androgen resistance (*see also* Syndrome, androgen insensitivity) E34.5Ø
- Angelman Q93.5
- anginal — *see* Angina
- ankyloglossia superior Q38.1
- anterior
  - chest wall RØ7.89
  - cord G83.82
  - spinal artery G95.19
    - compression M47.Ø19
      - cervical region M47.Ø12
      - cervicothoracic region M47.Ø13
      - lumbar region M47.Ø16
      - occipito-atlanto-axial region M47.Ø11
      - thoracic region M47.Ø14
      - thoracolumbar region M47.Ø15
  - tibial M76.81-
- antibody deficiency D8Ø.9
  - agammaglobulinemic D8Ø.1
    - hereditary D8Ø.Ø
  - congenital D8Ø.Ø
  - hypogammaglobulinemic D8Ø.1
    - hereditary D8Ø.Ø
- anticardiolipin (-antibody) D68.61
- antiphospholipid (-antibody) D68.61
- aortic
  - arch M31.4
  - bifurcation I74.Ø9
- aortomesenteric duodenum occlusion K31.5
- apical ballooning (transient left ventricular) I51.81
- arcuate ligament I77.4
- argentaffin, argintaffinoma E34.Ø
- Arnold-Chiari — *see* Arnold-Chiari disease
- Arrillaga-Ayerza I27.Ø
- Asherman's N85.6
- aspiration, of newborn — *see* Aspiration, by substance, with pneumonia
  - meconium P24.Ø1
- ataxia-telangiectasia G11.3
- auriculotemporal G5Ø.8
- autoerythrocyte sensitization (Gardner-Diamond) D69.2
- autoimmune lymphoproliferative [ALPS] D89.82
- autoimmune polyglandular E31.Ø
- autosomal — *see* Abnormal, autosomes
- Avellis' G46.8
- Ayerza(-Arrillaga) I27.Ø
- Babinski-Nageotte G83.89
- Bakwin-Krida Q79.8
- bare lymphocyte D81.6
- Barré-Guillain G61.Ø
- Barré-Liéou M53.Ø
- Barrett's — *see* Barrett's, esophagus
- Barsony-Polgar K22.4
- Barsony-Teschendorf K22.4
- Barth E78.71
- Bartter's E26.81
- basal cell nevus Q87.89

Syndrome — *continued*
- interspinous ligament — *see* Spondylopathy, specified NEC
- intestinal
  - carcinoid E34.Ø
  - knot K56.2
- intravascular coagulation-fibrinolysis (ICF) D65
- iodine-deficiency, congenital EØØ.9
  - type
    - mixed EØØ.2
    - myxedematous EØØ.1
    - neurological EØØ.Ø
- IRDS (idiopathic respiratory distress, newborn) P22.Ø
- irritable
  - bowel K58.9
    - with diarrhea K58.Ø
    - psychogenic F45.8
  - heart (psychogenic) F45.8
  - weakness F48.8
- ischemic bowel (transient) K55.9
  - chronic K55.1
  - due to mesenteric artery insufficiency K55.1
- IVC (intravascular coagulopathy) D65
- Ivemark's Q89.Ø1
- Jaccoud's — *see* Arthropathy, postrheumatic, chronic
- Jackson's G83.89
- Jakob-Creutzfeldt — *see* Creutzfeldt-Jakob disease or syndrome
- jaw-winking QØ7.8
- Jervell-Lange-Nielsen I45.81
- jet lag G47.25
- Job's D71
- Joseph-Diamond-Blackfan D61.Ø1
- jugular foramen G52.7
- Kabuki Q89.8
- Kanner's (autism) F84.Ø
- Kartagener's Q89.3
- Kelly's D5Ø.1
- Kimmelsteil-Wilson — *see* Diabetes, specified type, with Kimmelsteil-Wilson disease
- Klein(e)-Levine G47.13
- Klippel-Feil (brevicollis) Q76.1
- Köhler-Pellegrini-Steida — *see* Bursitis, tibial collateral
- König's K59.8
- Korsakoff (-Wernicke) (nonalcoholic) FØ4
  - alcoholic F1Ø.26
- Kostmann's D7Ø.Ø
- Krabbe's congenital muscle hypoplasia Q79.8
- labyrinthine — *see* subcategory H83.2
- lacunar NEC G46.7
- Lambert-Eaton G7Ø.8Ø
  - in
    - neoplastic disease G73.1
    - specified disease NEC G7Ø.81
- Landau-Kleffner — *see* Epilepsy, specified NEC
- Larsen's Q74.8
- lateral
  - cutaneous nerve of thigh G57.1-
  - medullary G46.4
- Launois' E22.Ø
- lazy
  - leukocyte D7Ø.8
  - posture M62.3
- Lemiere I8Ø.8
- Lennox-Gastaut G4Ø.812
  - intractable G4Ø.814
    - with status epilepticus G4Ø.813
    - without status epilepticus G4Ø.814
  - not intractable G4Ø.812
    - with status epilepticus G4Ø.811
    - without status epilepticus G4Ø.812
- lenticular, progressive E83.Ø1
- Leopold-Levi's EØ5.9Ø
- Lev's I44.2
- Li-Fraumeni Z15.Ø1
- Lichtheim's D51.Ø
- Lightwood's N25.89
- Lignac (de Toni) (-Fanconi) (-Debré) E72.Ø9
  - with cystinosis E72.Ø4
- Likoff's I2Ø.8
- limbic epilepsy personality FØ7.Ø

Syndrome — *continued*
- liver-kidney K76.7
- lobotomy FØ7.Ø
- Loffler's J82
- long arm 18 or 21 deletion Q93.89
- long QT I45.81
- Louis-Barré G11.3
- low
  - atmospheric pressure T7Ø.29
  - back M54.5
  - output (cardiac) I5Ø.9
- lower radicular, newborn (birth injury) P14.8
- Luetscher's (dehydration) E86.Ø
- Lupus anticoagulant D68.62
- Lutembacher's Q21.1
- macrophage activation D76.1
  - due to infection D76.2
- Mal de Debarquement R42
- magnesium-deficiency R29.Ø
- malabsorption K9Ø.9
  - postsurgical K91.2
- malformation, congenital, due to
  - alcohol Q86.Ø
  - exogenous cause NEC Q86.8
  - hydantoin Q86.1
  - warfarin Q86.2
- malignant
  - carcinoid E34.Ø
  - neuroleptic G21.Ø
- Mallory-Weiss K22.6
- mandibulofacial dysostosis Q75.4
- manic-depressive — *see* Disorder, bipolar, affective
- maple-syrup-urine E71.Ø
- Marable's I77.4
- Marfan's Q87.4Ø
  - with
    - cardiovascular manifestations Q87.418
      - aortic dilation Q87.41Ø
    - ocular manifestations Q87.42
    - skeletal manifestations Q87.43
- Marie's (acromegaly) E22.Ø
- maternal hypotension — *see* Syndrome, hypotension, maternal
- May (-Hegglin) D72.Ø
- McArdle (-Schmidt) (-Pearson) E74.Ø4
- McQuarrie's E16.2
- meconium plug (newborn) P76.Ø
- median arcuate ligament I77.4
- Meekeren-Ehlers-Danlos Q79.6
- megavitamin-B6 E67.2
- Meige G24.4
- MELAS E88.41
- Mendelson's O74.Ø
- MERRF (myoclonic epilepsy associated with ragged-red fibers) E88.42
- mesenteric
  - artery (superior) K55.1
  - vascular insufficiency K55.1
- metabolic E88.81
- metastatic carcinoid E34.Ø
- micrognathia-glossoptosis Q87.Ø
- midbrain NEC G93.89
- middle lobe (lung) J98.19
- middle radicular G54.Ø
- migraine (*see also* Migraine) G43.9Ø9
- Mikulicz' K11.8
- milk-alkali E83.52
- Millard-Gubler G46.3
- Miller-Dieker Q93.88
- Miller-Fisher G61.Ø
- Minkowski-Chauffard D58.Ø
- Mirizzi's K83.1
- MNGIE (Mitochondrial Neurogastrointestinal Encephalopathy) E88.49
- Möbius, ophthalmoplegic migraine — *see* Migraine, ophthalmoplegic
- monofixation H5Ø.42
- Morel-Moore M85.2
- Morel-Morgagni M85.2
- Morgagni (-Morel) (-Stewart) M85.2
- Morgagni-Adams-Stokes I45.9
- mucocutaneous lymph node (acute febrile) (MCLS) M3Ø.3

Syndrome — *continued*
- multiple endocrine neoplasia (MEN) — *see* Neoplasia, endocrine, multiple (MEN)
- multiple operations — *see* Disorder, factitious
- Mounier-Kuhn Q32.4
  - with bronchiectasis J47.9
    - with
      - exacerbation (acute) J47.1
      - lower respiratory infection J47.Ø
  - acquired J98.Ø9
    - with bronchiectasis J47.9
      - with
        - exacerbation (acute) J47.1
        - lower respiratory infection J47.Ø
- myasthenic G7Ø.9
  - in
    - diabetes mellitus — *see* Diabetes, amyotrophy
    - endocrine disease NEC E34.9 *[G73.3]*
    - neoplastic disease (*see also* Neoplasm) D49.9 *[G73.3]*
    - thyrotoxicosis (hyperthyroidism) EØ5.9Ø *[G73.3]*
      - with thyroid storm EØ5.91 *[G73.3]*
- myelodysplastic D46.9
  - with
    - 5q deletion D46.C
    - isolated del (5q) chromosomal abnormality D46.C
  - lesions, low grade D46.2Ø
  - specified NEC D46.Z
- myelopathic pain G89.Ø
- myeloproliferative (chronic) D47.1
- myofascial pain M79.1
- Naffziger's G54.Ø
- nail patella Q87.2
- NARP (Neuropathy, Ataxia and Retinitis pigmentosa) E88.49
- neonatal abstinence P96.1
- nephritic (*see also* Nephritis)
  - with edema — *see* Nephrosis
  - acute NØØ.9
  - chronic NØ3.9
  - rapidly progressive NØ1.9
- nephrotic (congenital) (*see also* Nephrosis) NØ4.9
  - with
    - dense deposit disease NØ4.6
    - diffuse
      - crescentic glomerulonephritis NØ4.7
      - endocapillary proliferative glomerulonephritis NØ4.4
      - membranous glomerulonephritis NØ4.2
      - mesangial proliferative glomerulonephritis NØ4.3
      - mesangiocapillary glomerulonephritis NØ4.5
    - focal and segmental glomerular lesions NØ4.1
    - minor glomerular abnormality NØ4.Ø
    - specified morphological changes NEC NØ4.8
  - diabetic — *see* Diabetes, nephrosis
- neurologic neglect R41.4
- Nezelof's D81.4
- Nonne-Milroy-Meige Q82.Ø
- Nothnagel's vasomotor acroparesthesia I73.89
- oculomotor H51.9
- ophthalmoplegia-cerebellar ataxia — *see* Strabismus, paralytic, third nerve
- oral-facial-digital Q87.Ø
- organic
  - affective FØ6.3Ø
  - amnesic (not alcoholor drug-induced) FØ4
  - brain FØ9
  - depressive FØ6.31
  - hallucinosis FØ6.Ø
  - personality FØ7.Ø
- Ormond's N13.5
- oro-facial-digital Q87.Ø
- os trigonum Q68.8
- Osler-Weber-Rendu I78.Ø
- osteoporosis-osteomalacia M83.8
- Osterreicher-Turner Q79.8
- otolith — *see* subcategory H81.8
- oto-palatal-digital Q87.Ø

Syndrome — *continued*
- outlet (thoracic) G54.Ø
- ovary
  - polycystic E28.2
  - resistant E28.39
  - sclerocystic E28.2
- Owren's D68.2
- Paget-Schroetter I82.89Ø
- pain (*see also* Pain)
  - complex regional I G9Ø.5Ø
    - lower limb G9Ø.52-
    - specified site NEC G9Ø.59
    - upper limb G9Ø.51-
  - complex regional II — *see* Causalgia
- painful
  - bruising D69.2
  - feet E53.8
  - prostate N42.81
- paralysis agitans — *see* Parkinsonism
- paralytic G83.9
  - specified NEC G83.89
- Parinaud's H51.Ø
- parkinsonian — *see* Parkinsonism
- Parkinson's — *see* Parkinsonism
- paroxysmal facial pain G5Ø.Ø
- Parry's EØ5.ØØ
  - with thyroid storm EØ5.Ø1
- Parsonage (-Aldren)-Turner G54.5
- patella clunk M25.86-
- Paterson(-Brown) (-Kelly) D5Ø.1
- pectoral girdle I77.89
- pectoralis minor I77.89
- Pelger-Huet D72.Ø
- pellagra-cerebellar ataxia-renal aminoaciduria E72.Ø2
- pellagroid E52
- Pellegrini-Stieda — *see* Bursitis, tibial collateral
- pelvic congestion-fibrosis, female N94.89
- penta X Q97.1
- peptic ulcer — *see* Ulcer, peptic
- perabduction I77.89
- periodic headache, in adults and children — *see* Headache, periodic syndromes in adults and children
- periurethral fibrosis N13.5
- phantom limb (without pain) G54.7
  - with pain G54.6
- pharyngeal pouch D82.1
- Pick's (heart) (liver) I31.1
- Pickwickian E66.2
- PIE (pulmonary infiltration with eosinophilia) J82
- pigmentary pallidal degeneration (progressive) G23.Ø
- pineal E34.8
- pituitary E22.Ø
- plantar fascia M72.2
- placental transfusion — *see* Pregnancy, complicated by, placental transfusion syndromes
- plateau iris (post-iridectomy) (postprocedural) H21.82
- Plummer-Vinson D5Ø.1
- pluricarential of infancy E4Ø
- plurideficiency E4Ø
- pluriglandular (compensatory) E31.8
  - autoimmune E31.Ø
- pneumatic hammer T75.21
- polyangiitis overlap M3Ø.8
- polycarential of infancy E4Ø
- polyglandular E31.8
  - autoimmune E31.Ø
- polysplenia Q89.Ø9
- pontine NEC G93.89
- popliteal
  - artery entrapment I77.89
  - web Q87.89
- post chemoembolization — code to associated conditions
- postcardiac injury
  - postcardiotomy I97.Ø
  - postmyocardial infarction I24.1
- postcardiotomy I97.Ø
- postcholecystectomy K91.5
- postcommissurotomy I97.Ø

Syndrome — *continued*
- postconcussional FØ7.81
- postcontusional FØ7.81
- postencephalitic FØ7.89
- posterior
  - cervical sympathetic M53.Ø
  - cord G83.83
  - fossa compression G93.5
  - reversible encephalopathy (PRES) I67.83
- postgastrectomy (dumping) K91.1
- postgastric surgery K91.1
- postinfarction I24.1
- postlaminectomy NEC M96.1
- postleukotomy FØ7.Ø
- postmastectomy lymphedema I97.2
- postmyocardial infarction I24.1
- postoperative NEC T81.9
  - blind loop K9Ø.2
- postpartum panhypopituitary (Sheehan) E23.Ø
- postpolio (myelitic) G14
- postthrombotic I87.ØØ9
  - with
    - inflammation I87.Ø2-
      - with ulcer I87.Ø3-
    - specified complication NEC I87.Ø9-
    - ulcer I87.Ø1-
      - with inflammation I87.Ø3-
  - asymptomatic I87.ØØ-
- postvagotomy K91.1
- postvalvulotomy I97.Ø
- postviral NEC G93.3
  - fatigue G93.3
- Potain's K31.Ø
- potassium intoxication E87.5
- precerebral artery (multiple) (bilateral) G45.2
- preinfarction I2Ø.Ø
- preleukemic D46.9
- premature senility E34.8
- premenstrual dysphoric N94.3
- premenstrual tension N94.3
- Prinzmetal-Massumi RØ7.1
- prune belly Q79.4
- pseudocarpal tunnel (sublimis) — *see* Syndrome, carpal tunnel
- pseudoparalytica G7Ø.ØØ
  - with exacerbation (acute) G7Ø.Ø1
  - in crisis G7Ø.Ø1
- pseudo -Turner's Q87.1
- psycho-organic (nonpsychotic severity) FØ7.9
  - acute or subacute FØ5
  - depressive type FØ6.31
  - hallucinatory type FØ6.Ø
  - nonpsychotic severity FØ7.Ø
  - specified NEC FØ7.89
- pulmonary
  - arteriosclerosis I27.Ø
  - dysmaturity (Wilson-Mikity) P27.Ø
  - hypoperfusion (idiopathic) P22.Ø
  - renal (hemorrhagic) (Goodpasture's) M31.Ø
- pure
  - motor lacunar G46.5
  - sensory lacunar G46.6
- Putnam-Dana D51.Ø
- pyramidopallidonigral G2Ø
- pyriformis — *see* Lesion, nerve, sciatic
- QT interval prolongation I45.81
- radicular NEC — *see* Radiculopathy
  - upper limbs, newborn (birth injury) P14.3
- rapid time-zone change G47.25
- Rasmussen GØ4.81
- Raymond (-Céstan) I65.8
- Raynaud's I73.ØØ
  - with gangrene I73.Ø1
- RDS (respiratory distress syndrome, newborn) P22.Ø
- reactive airways dysfunction J68.3
- Refsum's G6Ø.1
- Reifenstein E34.52
- renal glomerulohyalinosis-diabetic — *see* Diabetes, nephrosis
- Rendu-Osler-Weber I78.Ø
- residual ovary N99.83
- resistant ovary E28.39

Syndrome — *continued*
- respiratory
  - distress
    - acute J8Ø
      - adult J8Ø
      - child J8Ø
    - newborn (idiopathic) (type I) P22.Ø
      - type II P22.1
- restless legs G25.81
- retinoblastoma (familial) C69.2
- retroperitoneal fibrosis N13.5
- retroviral seroconversion (acute) Z21
- Reye's G93.7
- Richter — *see* Leukemia, chronic lymphocytic, B-cell type
- Ridley's I5Ø.1
- right
  - heart, hypoplastic Q22.6
  - ventricular obstruction — *see* Failure, heart, congestive
- Romano-Ward (prolonged QT interval) I45.81
- rotator cuff, shoulder (*see also* Tear, rotator cuff) M75.1Ø-
- Rotes Quérol — *see* Hyperostosis, ankylosing
- Roth — *see* Meralgia paresthetica
- rubella (congenital) P35.Ø
- Ruvalcaba-Myhre-Smith E71.44Ø
- Rytand-Lipsitch I44.2
- salt
  - depletion E87.1
    - due to heat NEC T67.8
      - causing heat exhaustion or prostration T67.4
  - low E87.1
- salt-losing N28.89
- Scaglietti-Dagnini E22.Ø
- scalenus anticus (anterior) G54.Ø
- scapulocostal — *see* Mononeuropathy, upper limb, specified site NEC
- scapuloperoneal G71.Ø
- schizophrenic, of childhood NEC F84.5
- Schnitzler D47.2
- Scholte's E34.Ø
- Schroeder's E27.Ø
- Schüller-Christian C96.5
- Schwachman's — *see* Syndrome, Shwachman's
- Schwartz (-Jampel) G71.13
- Schwartz-Bartter E22.2
- scimitar Q26.8
- sclerocystic ovary E28.2
- Seitelberger's G31.89
- septicemic adrenal hemorrhage A39.1
- seroconversion, retroviral (acute) Z21
- serous meningitis G93.2
- severe acute respiratory (SARS) J12.81
- shaken infant T74.4
- shock (traumatic) T79.4
  - kidney N17.Ø
    - following crush injury T79.5
  - toxic A48.3
- shock-lung J8Ø
- Shone's code to specific anomalies
- short
  - bowel K91.2
  - rib Q77.2
- shoulder-hand — *see* Algoneurodystrophy
- Shwachman's D7Ø.4
- sicca — *see* Sicca syndrome
- sick
  - cell E87.1
  - sinus I49.5
- sick-euthyroid EØ7.81
- sideropenic D5Ø.1
- Siemens' ectodermal dysplasia Q82.4
- Silfverskóld's Q78.9
- Simons' E88.1
- sinus tarsi — *see* Syndrome, tarsal tunnel
- sinusitis-bronchiectasis-situs inversus Q89.3
- Sipple's E31.22
- sirenomelia Q87.2
- Slocumb's E27.Ø
- slow flow, coronary I2Ø.8
- Sluder's G44.89

T

Tabacism, tabacosis, tabagism (*see also* Poisoning, tobacco)
- meaning dependence (without remission) F17.2ØØ
  - with
    - disorder F17.299
      - remission F17.211
      - specified disorder NEC F17.298
      - withdrawal F17.2Ø3

Tabardillo A75.9
- flea-borne A75.2
- louse-borne A75.Ø

Tabes, tabetic A52.10
- with
  - central nervous system syphilis A52.1Ø
  - Charcot's joint A52.16
  - cord bladder A52.19
  - crisis, viscera (any) A52.19
  - paralysis, general A52.17
  - paresis (general) A52.17
  - perforating ulcer (foot) A52.19
- arthropathy (Charcot) A52.16
- bladder A52.19
- bone A52.11
- cerebrospinal A52.12
- congenital A5Ø.45
- conjugal A52.1Ø
- dorsalis A52.11
  - juvenile A5Ø.49
- juvenile A5Ø.49
- latent A52.19
- mesenterica A18.39
- paralysis, insane, general A52.17
- spasmodic A52.17
- syphilis (cerebrospinal) A52.12

Taboparalysis A52.17

Taboparesis (remission) A52.17
- juvenile A5Ø.45

TAC (trigeminal autonomic cephalgia) **NEC** G44.Ø99
- intractable G44.Ø91
- not intractable G44.Ø99

Tache noir S60.22-

Tachyalimentation K91.2

Tachyarrhythmia, tachyrhythmia — *see* Tachycardia

Tachycardia R00.0
- atrial (paroxysmal) I47.1
- auricular I47.1
- AV nodal re-entry (re-entrant) I47.1
- junctional (paroxysmal) I47.1
- newborn P29.11
- nodal (paroxysmal) I47.1
- non-paroxysmal AV nodal I45.89
- paroxysmal (sustained) (nonsustained) I47.9
  - with sinus bradycardia I49.5
  - atrial (PAT) I47.1
  - atrioventricular (AV) (re-entrant) I47.1
    - psychogenic F54
  - junctional I47.1
    - ectopic I47.1
  - nodal I47.1
  - psychogenic (atrial) (supraventricular) (ventricular) F54
  - supraventricular (sustained) I47.1
    - psychogenic F54
  - ventricular I47.2
    - psychogenic F54
- psychogenic F45.8
- sick sinus I49.5
- sinoauricular NOS RØØ.Ø
  - paroxysmal I47.1
- sinus [sinusal] NOS RØØ.Ø
  - paroxysmal I47.1
- supraventricular I47.1
- ventricular (paroxysmal) (sustained) I47.2
  - psychogenic F54

Tachygastria K31.89

Tachypnea R06.82
- hysterical F45.8
- newborn (idiopathic) (transitory) P22.1
- psychogenic F45.8
- transitory, of newborn P22.1

TACO (transfusion associated circulatory overload) E87.71

Taenia (infection) (infestation) B68.9
- diminuta B71.Ø
- echinococcal infestation B67.9Ø
- mediocanellata B68.1
- nana B71.Ø
- saginata B68.1
- solium (intestinal form) B68.Ø
  - larval form — *see* Cysticercosis

Taeniasis (intestine) — *see* Taenia

Tag (hypertrophied skin) (infected) L91.8
- adenoid J35.8
- anus K64.4
- hemorrhoidal K64.4
- hymen N89.8
- perineal N9Ø.89
- preauricular Q17.Ø
- sentinel K64.4
- skin L91.8
  - accessory (congenital) Q82.8
  - anus K64.4
  - congenital Q82.8
  - preauricular Q17.Ø
- tonsil J35.8
- urethra, urethral N36.8
- vulva N9Ø.89

Tahyna fever B33.8

Takahara's disease E80.3

Takayasu's disease or syndrome M31.4

Talcosis (pulmonary) J62.Ø

Talipes (congenital) Q66.89
- acquired, planus — *see* Deformity, limb, flat foot
- asymmetric Q66.89
- calcaneovalgus Q66.4
- calcaneovarus Q66.1
- calcaneus Q66.89
- cavus Q66.7
- equinovalgus Q66.6
- equinovarus Q66.Ø
- equinus Q66.89
- percavus Q66.7
- planovalgus Q66.6
- planus (acquired) (any degree) (*see also* Deformity, limb, flat foot)
  - congenital Q66.5-
  - due to rickets (sequelae) E64.3
- valgus Q66.6
- varus Q66.3

Tall stature, constitutional E34.4

Talma's disease M62.89

Talon noir S90.3-
- hand S6Ø.22-
- heel S9Ø.3-
- toe S9Ø.1-

Tamponade, heart I31.4

Tanapox (virus disease) BØ8.71

Tangier disease E78.6

Tantrum, child problem F91.8

Tapeworm (infection) (infestation) — *see* Infestation, tapeworm

Tapia's syndrome G52.7

TAR (thrombocytopenia with absent radius) **syndrome** Q87.2

Tarral-Besnier disease L44.0

Tarsal tunnel syndrome — *see* Syndrome, tarsal tunnel

Tarsalgia — *see* Pain, limb, lower

Tarsitis (eyelid) HØ1.8
- syphilitic A52.71
- tuberculous A18.4

Tartar (teeth) (dental calculus) KØ3.6

Tattoo (mark) L81.8

Tauri's disease E74.09

Taurodontism K00.2

Taussig-Bing syndrome Q20.1

Taybi's syndrome Q87.2

Tay-Sachs amaurotic familial idiocy or disease E75.02

TBI (traumatic brain injury) — *see* category SØ6

Teacher's node or nodule J38.2

Tear, torn (traumatic) (*see also* Laceration)
- with abortion — *see* Abortion
- annular fibrosis M51.35
- anus, anal (sphincter) S31.831
  - complicating delivery
    - with third degree perineal laceration O7Ø.2
      - with mucosa O7Ø.3
    - without third degree perineal laceration O7Ø.4
  - nontraumatic (healed) (old) K62.81
- articular cartilage, old — *see* Derangement, joint, articular cartilage, by site
- bladder
  - with ectopic or molar pregnancy OØ8.6
  - following ectopic or molar pregnancy OØ8.6
  - obstetrical O71.5
  - traumatic — *see* Injury, bladder
- bowel
  - with ectopic or molar pregnancy OØ8.6
  - following ectopic or molar pregnancy OØ8.6
  - obstetrical trauma O71.5
- broad ligament
  - with ectopic or molar pregnancy OØ8.6
  - following ectopic or molar pregnancy OØ8.6
  - obstetrical trauma O71.6
- bucket handle (knee) (meniscus) — *see* Tear, meniscus
- capsule, joint — *see* Sprain
- cartilage (*see also* Sprain)
  - articular, old — *see* Derangement, joint, articular cartilage, by site
- cervix
  - with ectopic or molar pregnancy OØ8.6
  - following ectopic or molar pregnancy OØ8.6
  - obstetrical trauma (current) O71.3
  - old N88.1
  - traumatic *see* Injury, uterus
- dural G97.41
  - nontraumatic G96.11
- internal organ — *see* Injury, by site
- knee cartilage
  - articular (current) S83.3-
  - old — *see* Derangement, knee, meniscus, due to old tear
- ligament — *see* Sprain
- meniscus (knee) (current injury) S83.2Ø9
  - bucket-handle S83.2Ø-
  - lateral
    - bucket-handle S83.25-
    - complex S83.27-
    - peripheral S83.26-
    - specified type NEC S83.28-
  - medial
    - bucket-handle S83.21-
    - complex S83.23-
    - peripheral S83.22-
    - specified type NEC S83.24-
  - old — *see* Derangement, knee, meniscus, due to old tear
  - site other than knee code as Sprain
  - specified type NEC S83.2Ø-
- muscle — *see* Strain
- pelvic
  - floor, complicating delivery O7Ø.1
  - organ NEC, obstetrical trauma O71.5
    - with ectopic or molar pregnancy OØ8.6
    - following ectopic or molar pregnancy OØ8.6
- perineal, secondary O9Ø.1
- periurethral tissue, obstetrical trauma O71.82
  - with ectopic or molar pregnancy OØ8.6
  - following ectopic or molar pregnancy OØ8.6
- rectovaginal septum — *see* Laceration, vagina
- retina, retinal (without detachment) (horseshoe) (*see also* Break, retina, horseshoe)
  - with detachment — *see* Detachment, retina, with retinal, break
- rotator cuff (nontraumatic) M75.1Ø-
  - complete M75.12-
  - incomplete M75.11-
  - traumatic S46.Ø1-
    - capsule S43.42-
- semilunar cartilage, knee — *see* Tear, meniscus

Test, tests, testing — *continued*
- immunity status Z01.84
- intelligence NEC Z01.89
- laboratory (as part of a general medical examination) Z00.00
  - with abnormal finding Z00.01
  - for medicolegal reason NEC Z04.8
- male partner of patient with recurrent pregnancy loss Z31.411
- Mantoux (for tuberculosis) Z11.1
  - abnormal result R76.11
- pregnancy, positive first pregnancy — *see* Pregnancy, normal, first
- procreative Z31.49
  - fertility Z31.41
- skin, diagnostic
  - allergy Z01.82
    - special screening examination — *see* Screening, by name of disease
  - Mantoux Z11.1
  - tuberculin Z11.1
- specified NEC Z01.89
- tuberculin Z11.1
  - abnormal result R76.11
- vision Z01.00
  - with abnormal findings Z01.01
- Wassermann Z11.3
  - positive — *see* Serology for syphilis, positive

Testicle, testicular, testis (*see also* condition)
- feminization syndrome (*see also* Syndrome, androgen insensitivity) E34.51
- migrans Q55.29

Tetanus, tetanic (cephalic) (convulsions) A35
- with
  - abortion A34
  - ectopic or molar pregnancy O08.0
- following ectopic or molar pregnancy O08.0
- inoculation reaction (due to serum) — *see* Complications, vaccination
- neonatorum A33
- obstetrical A34
- puerperal, postpartum, childbirth A34

Tetany (due to) R29.0
- alkalosis E87.3
- associated with rickets E55.0
- convulsions R29.0
  - hysterical F44.5
- functional (hysterical) F44.5
- hyperkinetic R29.0
  - hysterical F44.5
- hyperpnea R06.4
  - hysterical F44.5
  - psychogenic F45.8
- hyperventilation (*see also* Hyperventilation) R06.4
  - hysterical F44.5
- neonatal (without calcium or magnesium deficiency) P71.3
- parathyroid (gland) E20.9
- parathyroprival E89.2
- post- (para)thyroidectomy E89.2
- postoperative E89.2
- pseudotetany R29.0
- psychogenic (conversion reaction) F44.5

Tetralogy of Fallot Q21.3

Tetraplegia (chronic) (*see also* Quadriplegia) G82.50

Thailand hemorrhagic fever A91

Thalassanemia — *see* Thalassemia

Thalassemia (anemia) (disease) D56.9
- with other hemoglobinopathy D56.8
- alpha (major) (severe) (triple gene defect) D56.0
  - minor D56.3
  - silent carrier D56.3
  - trait D56.3
- beta (severe) D56.1
  - homozygous D56.1
  - major D56.1
  - minor D56.3
  - trait D56.3
- delta-beta (homozygous) D56.2
  - minor D56.3
  - trait D56.3
- dominant D56.8

Thalassemia — *continued*
- hemoglobin
  - C D56.8
  - E-beta D56.5
- intermedia D56.1
- major D56.1
- minor D56.3
- mixed D56.8
- sickle-cell — *see* Disease, sickle-cell, thalassemia
- specified type NEC D56.8
- trait D56.3
- variants D56.8

Thanatophoric dwarfism or short stature Q77.1

Thaysen-Gee disease (nontropical sprue) K90.0

Thaysen's disease K90.0

Thecoma D27-
- luteinized D27-
- malignant C56-

Thelarche, premature E30.8

Thelaziasis B83.8

Thelitis N61
- puerperal, postpartum or gestational — *see* Infection, nipple

Therapeutic — *see* condition

Therapy
- drug, long-term (current) (prophylactic)
  - agents affecting estrogen receptors and estrogen levels NEC Z79.818
  - anastrozole (Arimidex) Z79.811
  - antibiotics Z79.2
    - short-term use — *omit code*
  - anticoagulants Z79.01
  - anti-inflammatory Z79.1
  - antiplatelet Z79.02
  - antithrombotics Z79.02
  - aromatase inhibitors Z79.811
  - aspirin Z79.82
  - birth control pill or patch Z79.3
  - bisphosphonates Z79.83
  - contraceptive, oral Z79.3
  - drug, specified NEC Z79.899
  - estrogen receptor downregulators Z79.818
  - Evista Z79.810
  - exemestane (Aromasin) Z79.811
  - Fareston Z79.810
  - fulvestrant (Faslodex) Z79.818
  - gonadotropin-releasing hormone (GnRH) agonist Z79.818
  - goserelin acetate (Zoladex) Z79.818
  - hormone replacement (postmenopausal) Z79.890
  - insulin Z79.4
  - letrozole (Femara) Z79.811
  - leuprolide acetate (leuprorelin) (Lupron) Z79.818
  - megestrol acetate (Megace) Z79.818
  - methadone
    - for pain management Z79.891
    - maintenance therapy F11.20
  - Nolvadex Z79.810
  - opiate analgesic Z79.891
  - oral contraceptive Z79.3
  - raloxifene (Evista) Z79.810
  - short term — *omit code*
  - selective estrogen receptor modulators (SERMs) Z79.810
  - steroids
    - inhaled Z79.51
    - systemic Z79.52
  - tamoxifen (Nolvadex) Z79.810
  - toremifene (Fareston) Z79.810

Thermic — *see* condition

Thermography (abnormal) (*see also* Abnormal, diagnostic imaging) R93.8
- breast R92.8

Thermoplegia T67.0

Thesaurismosis, glycogen — *see* Disease, glycogen storage

Thiamin deficiency E51.9
- specified NEC E51.8

Thiaminic deficiency with beriberi E51.11

Thibierge-Weissenbach syndrome — *see* Sclerosis, systemic

Thickening
- bone — *see* Hypertrophy, bone
- breast N64.59
- endometrium R93.8
- epidermal L85.9
  - specified NEC L85.8
- hymen N89.6
- larynx J38.7
- nail L60.2
  - congenital Q84.5
- periosteal — *see* Hypertrophy, bone
- pleura J92.9
  - with asbestos J92.0
- skin R23.4
- subepiglottic J38.7
- tongue K14.8
- valve, heart — *see* Endocarditis

Thigh — *see* condition

Thinning vertebra — *see* Spondylopathy, specified NEC

Thirst, excessive R63.1
- due to deprivation of water T73.1

Thomsen disease G71.12

Thoracic (*see also* condition)
- kidney Q63.2
- outlet syndrome G54.0

Thoracogastroschisis (congenital) Q79.8

Thoracopagus Q89.4

Thorax — *see* condition

Thorn's syndrome N28.89

Thorson-Björck syndrome E34.0

Threadworm (infection) (infestation) B80

Threatened
- abortion O20.0
  - with subsequent abortion O03.9
- job loss, anxiety concerning Z56.2
- labor (without delivery) O47.9
  - after 37 completed weeks of gestation O47.1
  - before 37 completed weeks of gestation O47.0-
- loss of job, anxiety concerning Z56.2
- miscarriage O20.0
- unemployment, anxiety concerning Z56.2

Three-day fever A93.1

ThresHers' lung J67.0

Thrix annulata (congenital) Q84.1

Throat — *see* condition

Thrombasthenia (Glanzmann) (hemorrhagic) (hereditary) D69.1

Thromboangiitis I73.1
- obliterans (general) I73.1
  - cerebral I67.89
  - vessels
    - brain I67.89
    - spinal cord I67.89

Thromboarteritis — *see* Arteritis

Thromboasthenia (Glanzmann) (hemorrhagic) (hereditary) D69.1

Thrombocytasthenia (Glanzmann) D69.1

Thrombocythemia (essential) (hemorrhagic) (idiopathic) (primary) D47.3

Thrombocytopathy (dystrophic) (granulopenic) D69.1

Thrombocytopenia, thrombocytopenic D69.6
- with absent radius (TAR) Q87.2
- congenital D69.42
- dilutional D69.59
- due to
  - drugs D69.59
  - extracorporeal circulation of blood D69.59
  - (massive) blood transfusion D69.59
  - platelet alloimmunization D69.59
- essential D69.3
- heparin induced (HIT) D75.82
- hereditary D69.42
- idiopathic D69.3
- neonatal, transitory P61.0
  - due to
    - exchange transfusion P61.0
    - idiopathic maternal thrombocytopenia P61.0
    - isoimmunization P61.0
- primary NEC D69.49
  - idiopathic D69.3
- puerperal, postpartum O72.3
- secondary D69.59

Thrombocytopenia — *continued*
- transient neonatal P61.Ø

Thrombocytosis, essential D47.3
- primary D47.3

Thromboembolism — *see* Embolism

Thrombopathy (Bernard-Soulier) D69.1
- constitutional D68.Ø
- Willebrand-Jurgens D68.Ø

Thrombopenia — *see* Thrombocytopenia

Thrombophilia D68.59
- primary NEC D68.59
- secondary NEC D68.69
- specified NEC D68.69

Thrombophlebitis I80.9
- antepartum O22.2-
  - deep O22.3-
  - superficial O22.2-
- cavernous (venous) sinus GØ8
  - complicating pregnancy O22.5-
  - nonpyogenic I67.6
- cerebral (sinus) (vein) GØ8
- cerebral (sinus) (vein) GØ8
  - nonpyogenic I67.6
  - sequelae GØ9
- due to implanted device — *see* Complications, by site and type, specified NEC
- during or resulting from a procedure NEC T81.72
- femoral vein (superficial) I8Ø.1-
- femoropopliteal vein I8Ø.Ø-
- hepatic (vein) I8Ø.8
- idiopathic, recurrent I82.1
- iliofemoral I8Ø.1-
- intracranial venous sinus (any) GØ8
  - nonpyogenic I67.6
  - sequelae GØ9
- intraspinal venous sinuses and veins GØ8
  - nonpyogenic G95.19
- lateral (venous) sinus GØ8
  - nonpyogenic I67.6
- leg I8Ø.299
  - superficial I8Ø.Ø-
- longitudinal (venous) sinus GØ8
  - nonpyogenic I67.6
- lower extremity I8Ø.299
- migrans, migrating I82.1
- pelvic
  - with ectopic or molar pregnancy OØ8.Ø
  - following ectopic or molar pregnancy OØ8.Ø
  - puerperal O87.1
- popliteal vein — *see* Phlebitis, leg, deep, popliteal
- portal (vein) K75.1
- postoperative T81.72
- pregnancy — *see* Thrombophlebitis, antepartum
- puerperal, postpartum, childbirth O87.Ø
  - deep O87.1
  - pelvic O87.1
  - septic O86.81
  - superficial O87.Ø
- saphenous (greater) (lesser) I8Ø.Ø-
- sinus (intracranial) GØ8
  - nonpyogenic I67.6
- specified site NEC I8Ø.8
- tibial vein I8Ø.23-

Thrombosis, thrombotic (bland) (multiple) (progressive) (silent) (vessel) I82.9Ø
- anal K64.5
- antepartum — *see* Thrombophlebitis, antepartum
- aorta, aortic I74.1Ø
  - abdominal I74.Ø9
    - saddle I74.Ø1
  - bifurcation I74.Ø9
  - saddle I74.Ø1
  - specified site NEC I74.19
  - terminal I74.Ø9
  - thoracic I74.11
  - valve — *see* Endocarditis, aortic
- apoplexy I63.3
- artery, arteries (postinfectional) I74.9
  - auditory, internal — *see* Occlusion, artery, precerebral, specified NEC
  - basilar — *see* Occlusion, artery, basilar
  - carotid (common) (internal) — *see* Occlusion, artery, carotid

Thrombosis, thrombotic — *continued*
- artery, arteries — *continued*
  - cerebellar (anterior inferior) (posterior inferior) (superior) — *see* Occlusion, artery, cerebellar
  - cerebral — *see* Occlusion, artery, cerebral
  - choroidal (anterior) — *see* Occlusion, artery, cerebral, specified NEC
  - communicating, posterior — *see* Occlusion, artery, cerebral, specified NEC
  - coronary (*see also* Infarct, myocardium)
    - not resulting in infarction I24.Ø
  - hepatic I74.8
  - hypophyseal — *see* Occlusion, artery, cerebral, specified NEC
  - iliac I74.5
  - limb I74.4
    - lower I74.3
    - upper I74.2
  - meningeal, anterior or posterior — *see* Occlusion, artery, cerebral, specified NEC
  - mesenteric (with gangrene) K55.Ø
  - ophthalmic — *see* Occlusion, artery, retina
  - pontine — *see* Occlusion, artery, cerebral, specified NEC
  - precerebral — *see* Occlusion, artery, precerebral
  - pulmonary (iatrogenic) — *see* Embolism, pulmonary
  - renal N28.Ø
  - retinal — *see* Occlusion, artery, retina
  - spinal, anterior or posterior G95.11
  - traumatic NEC T14.8
  - vertebral — *see* Occlusion, artery, vertebral
- atrium, auricular (*see also* Infarct, myocardium)
  - following acute myocardial infarction (current complication) I23.6
  - not resulting in infarction I24.Ø
- basilar (artery) — *see* Occlusion, artery, basilar
- brain (artery) (stem) (*see also* Occlusion, artery, cerebral)
  - due to syphilis A52.Ø5
  - puerperal O99.43
  - sinus — *see* Thrombosis, intracranial venous sinus
- capillary I78.8
- cardiac (*see also* Infarct, myocardium)
  - not resulting in infarction I24.Ø
  - valve — *see* Endocarditis
- carotid (artery) (common) (internal) — *see* Occlusion, artery, carotid
- cavernous (venous) sinus — *see* Thrombosis, intracranial venous sinus
- cerebellar artery (anterior inferior) (posterior inferior) (superior) I66.3
- cerebral (artery) — *see* Occlusion, artery, cerebral
- cerebrovenous sinus (*see also* Thrombosis, intracranial venous sinus)
  - puerperium O87.3
- chronic I82.91
- coronary (artery) (vein) (*see also* Infarct, myocardium)
  - not resulting in infarction I24.Ø
- corpus cavernosum N48.89
- cortical I66.9
- deep — *see* Embolism, vein, lower extremity
- due to device, implant or graft (*see also* Complications, by site and type, specified NEC) T85.86
  - arterial graft NEC T82.868
  - breast (implant) T85.86
  - catheter NEC T85.86
    - dialysis (renal) T82.868
      - intraperitoneal T85.86
    - infusion NEC T82.868
      - spinal (epidural) (subdural) T85.86
    - urinary (indwelling) T83.86
  - electronic (electrode) (pulse generator) (stimulator)
    - bone T84.86
    - cardiac T82.867
    - nervous system (brain) (peripheral nerve) (spinal) T85.86
    - urinary T83.86

Thrombosis, thrombotic — *continued*
- due to device, implant or graft — *continued*
  - fixation, internal (orthopedic) NEC T84.86
  - gastrointestinal (bile duct) (esophagus) T85.86
  - genital NEC T83.86
  - heart T82.867
  - joint prosthesis T84.86
  - ocular (corneal graft) (orbital implant) NEC T85.86
  - orthopedic NEC T84.86
  - specified NEC T85.86
  - urinary NEC T83.86
  - vascular NEC T82.868
  - ventricular intracranial shunt T85.86
- during the puerperium — *see* Thrombosis, puerperal
- endocardial (*see also* Infarct, myocardium)
  - not resulting in infarction I24.Ø
- eye — *see* Occlusion, retina
- genital organ
  - female NEC N94.89
    - pregnancy — *see* Thrombophlebitis, antepartum
  - male N5Ø.1
- gestational — *see* Phlebopathy, gestational
- heart (chamber) (*see also* Infarct, myocardium)
  - not resulting in infarction I24.Ø
- hepatic (vein) I82.Ø
  - artery I74.8
- history (of) Z86.718
- intestine (with gangrene) K55.Ø
- intracardiac NEC (apical) (atrial) (auricular) (ventricular) (old) I51.3
- intracranial (arterial) I66.9
  - venous sinus (any) GØ8
    - nonpyogenic origin I67.6
    - puerperium O87.3
- intramural (*see also* Infarct, myocardium)
  - not resulting in infarction I24.Ø
- intraspinal venous sinuses and veins GØ8
  - nonpyogenic G95.19
- kidney (artery) N28.Ø
- lateral (venous) sinus — *see* Thrombosis, intracranial venous sinus
- leg — *see* Thrombosis, vein, lower extremity
  - arterial I74.3
- liver (venous) I82.Ø
  - artery I74.8
  - portal vein I81
- longitudinal (venous) sinus — *see* Thrombosis, intracranial venous sinus
- lower limb — *see* Thrombosis, vein, lower extremity
- lung (iatrogenic) (postoperative) — *see* Embolism, pulmonary
- meninges (brain) (arterial) I66.8
- mesenteric (artery) (with gangrene) K55.Ø
  - vein (inferior) (superior) I81
- mitral I34.8
- mural (*see also* Infarct, myocardium)
  - due to syphilis A52.Ø6
  - not resulting in infarction I24.Ø
- omentum (with gangrene) K55.Ø
- ophthalmic — *see* Occlusion, retina
- pampiniform plexus (male) N5Ø.1
- parietal (*see also* Infarct, myocardium)
  - not resulting in infarction I24.Ø
- penis, superficial vein N48.81
- perianal venous K64.5
- peripheral arteries I74.4
  - upper I74.2
- personal history (of) Z86.718
- portal I81
  - due to syphilis A52.Ø9
- precerebral artery — *see* Occlusion, artery, precerebral
- puerperal, postpartum O87.Ø
  - brain (artery) O99.43
    - venous (sinus) O87.3
  - cardiac O99.43
  - cerebral (artery) O99.43
    - venous (sinus) O87.3
  - superficial O87.Ø

Tight, tightness — *continued*
- foreskin (congenital) N47.1
- hymen, hymenal ring N89.6
- introitus (acquired) (congenital) N89.6
- rectal sphincter K62.89
- tendon — *see* Short, tendon
- urethral sphincter N35.9

Tilting vertebra — *see* Dorsopathy, deforming, specified NEC
Timidity, child F93.8
Tin-miner's lung J63.5
Tinea (intersecta) (tarsi) B35.9
- amiantacea L44.8
- asbestina B35.Ø
- barbae B35.Ø
- beard B35.Ø
- black dot B35.Ø
- blanca B36.2
- capitis B35.Ø
- corporis B35.4
- cruris B35.6
- flava B36.Ø
- foot B35.3
- furfuracea B36.Ø
- imbricata (Tokelau) B35.5
- kerion B35.Ø
- manuum B35.2
- microsporic — *see* Dermatophytosis
- nigra B36.1
- nodosa — *see* Piedra
- pedis B35.3
- scalp B35.Ø
- specified site NEC B35.8
- sycosis B35.Ø
- tonsurans B35.Ø
- trichophytic — *see* Dermatophytosis
- unguium B35.1
- versicolor B36.Ø

Tingling sensation (skin) R2Ø.2
Tinnitus (audible) (aurium) (subjective) — *see* subcategory H93.1
Tipped tooth (teeth) M26.33
Tipping
- pelvis M95.5
  - with disproportion (fetopelvic) O33.Ø
    - causing obstructed labor O65.Ø
- tooth (teeth), fully erupted M26.33

Tiredness R53.83
Tissue — *see* condition
Tobacco (nicotine)
- dependence — *see* Dependence, drug, nicotine
- harmful use Z72.Ø
- heart — *see* Tobacco, toxic effect
- maternal use, affecting newborn PØ4.2
- toxic effect — *see* Table of Drugs and Chemicals, by substance, poisoning
  - chewing tobacco — *see* Table of Drugs and Chemicals, by substance, poisoning
  - cigarettes — *see* Table of Drugs and Chemicals, by substance, poisoning
- use Z72.Ø
  - complicating
    - childbirth O99.334
    - pregnancy O99.33-
    - puerperium O99.335
  - counseling and surveillance Z71.6
- withdrawal state — *see* Dependence, drug, nicotine

Tocopherol deficiency E56.0
Todd's
- cirrhosis K74.3
- paralysis (postepileptic) (transitory) G83.84

Toe — *see* condition
Toilet, artificial opening — *see* Attention to, artificial, opening
Tokelau (ringworm) B35.5
Tollwut — *see* Rabies
Tommaselli's disease R31.9
- correct substance properly administered — *see* Table of Drugs and Chemicals, by drug, adverse effect
- overdose or wrong substance given or taken — *see* Table of Drugs and Chemicals, by drug, poisoning

Tongue (*see also* condition)
- tie Q38.1

Tonic pupil — *see* Anomaly, pupil, function, tonic pupil
Toni-Fanconi syndrome (cystinosis) E72.Ø9
- with cystinosis E72.Ø4

Tonsil — *see* condition
Tonsillitis (acute) (catarrhal) (croupous) (follicular) (gangrenous) (infective) (lacunar) (lingual) (malignant) (membranous) (parenchymatous) (phlegmonous) (pseudomembranous) (purulent) (septic) (subacute) (suppurative) (toxic) (ulcerative) (vesicular) (viral) JØ3.9Ø
- chronic J35.Ø1
  - with adenoiditis J35.Ø3
- diphtheritic A36.Ø
- hypertrophic J35.Ø1
  - with adenoiditis J35.Ø3
- recurrent JØ3.91
- specified organism NEC JØ3.8Ø
  - recurrent JØ3.81
- staphylococcal JØ3.8Ø
  - recurrent JØ3.81
- streptococcal JØ3.ØØ
  - recurrent JØ3.Ø1
- tuberculous A15.8
- Vincent's A69.1

Tooth, teeth — *see* condition
Toothache KØ8.8
Topagnosis R2Ø.8
Tophi — *see* Gout
TORCH infection — *see* Infection, congenital
- without active infection PØØ.2

Torn — *see* Tear
Tornwaldt's cyst or disease J39.2
Torsion
- accessory tube — *see* Torsion, fallopian tube
- adnexa (female) — *see* Torsion, fallopian tube
- aorta, acquired I77.1
- appendix epididymis N44.Ø4
- appendix testis N44.Ø3
- bile duct (common) (hepatic) K83.8
  - congenital Q44.5
- bowel, colon or intestine K56.2
- cervix — *see* Malposition, uterus
- cystic duct K82.8
- dystonia — *see* Dystonia, torsion
- epididymis (appendix) N44.Ø4
- fallopian tube N83.52
  - with ovary N83.53
- gallbladder K82.8
  - congenital Q44.1
- hydatid of Morgagni
  - female N83.52
  - male N44.Ø3
- kidney (pedicle) (leading to infarction) N28.Ø
- Meckel's diverticulum (congenital) Q43.Ø
  - malignant — *see* Table of Neoplasms, small intestine, malignant
- mesentery K56.2
- omentum K56.2
- organ or site, congenital NEC — *see* Anomaly, by site
- ovary (pedicle) N83.51
  - with fallopian tube N83.53
  - congenital Q5Ø.2
- oviduct — *see* Torsion, fallopian tube
- penis (acquired) N48.82
  - congenital Q55.63
- spasm — *see* Dystonia, torsion
- spermatic cord N44.Ø2
  - extravaginal N44.Ø1
  - intravaginal N44.Ø2
- spleen D73.5
- testis, testicle N44.ØØ
  - appendix N44.Ø3
- tibia — *see* Deformity, limb, specified type NEC, lower leg
- uterus — *see* Malposition, uterus

Torticollis (intermittent) (spastic) M43.6
- congenital (sternomastoid) Q68.Ø
- due to birth injury P15.8
- hysterical F44.4
- ocular R29.891
- psychogenic F45.8

Torticollis — *continued*
- psychogenic — *continued*
  - conversion reaction F44.4
- rheumatic M43.6
- rheumatoid MØ6.88
- spasmodic G24.3
- traumatic, current S13.4

Tortipelvis G24.1
Tortuous
- artery I77.1
- organ or site, congenital NEC — *see* Distortion
- retinal vessel, congenital Q14.1
- ureter N13.8
- urethra N36.8
- vein — *see* Varix

Torture, victim of Z65.4
Torula, torular (histolytica) (infection) — *see* Cryptococcosis
Torulosis — *see* Cryptococcosis
Torus (mandibularis) (palatinus) M27.Ø
- fracture — *see* Fracture, by site, torus

Touraine's syndrome Q79.8
Tourette's syndrome F95.2
Tourniquet syndrome — *see* Constriction, external, by site
Tower skull Q75.0
- with exophthalmos Q87.Ø

Toxemia R68.89
- bacterial — *see* Sepsis
- burn — *see* Burn
- eclamptic (with pre-existing hypertension) — *see* Eclampsia
- erysipelatous — *see* Erysipelas
- fatigue R68.89
- food — *see* Poisoning, food
- gastrointestinal K52.1
- intestinal K52.1
- kidney — *see* Uremia
- malarial — *see* Malaria
- myocardial — *see* Myocarditis, toxic
- of pregnancy — *see* Pre-eclampsia
- pre-eclamptic — *see* Pre-eclampsia
- small intestine K52.1
- staphylococcal, due to food AØ5.Ø
- stasis R68.89
- uremic — *see* Uremia
- urinary — *see* Uremia

Toxemica cerebropathia psychica (nonalcoholic) FØ4
- alcoholic — *see* Alcohol, amnestic disorder

Toxic (poisoning) (*see also* condition) T65.91
- effect — *see* Table of Drugs and Chemicals, by substance, poisoning
- shock syndrome A48.3
- thyroid (gland) — *see* Thyrotoxicosis

Toxicemia — *see* Toxemia
Toxicity — *see* Table of Drugs and Chemicals, by substance, poisoning
- fava bean D55.Ø
- food, noxious — *see* Poisoning, food
- from drug or nonmedicinal substance — *see* Table of Drugs and Chemicals, by drug

Toxicosis (*see also* Toxemia)
- capillary, hemorrhagic D69.Ø

Toxinfection, gastrointestinal K52.1
Toxocariasis B83.0
Toxoplasma, toxoplasmosis (acquired) B58.9
- with
  - hepatitis B58.1
  - meningoencephalitis B58.2
  - ocular involvement B58.ØØ
  - other organ involvement B58.89
  - pneumonia, pneumonitis B58.3
- congenital (acute) (subacute) (chronic) P37.1
- maternal, manifest toxoplasmosis in infant (acute) (subacute) (chronic) P37.1

tPA (rtPA) **administration in a different facility within the last 24 hours prior to admission to current facility** Z92.82
Trabeculation, bladder N32.89
Trachea — *see* condition
Tracheitis (catarrhal) (infantile) (membranous) (plastic) (septal) (suppurative) (viral) JØ4.1Ø

- **Tracheitis** — *continued*
  - with
    - bronchitis (15 years of age and above) J4Ø
      - acute or subacute — *see* Bronchitis, acute
      - chronic J42
      - tuberculous NEC A15.5
      - under 15 years of age J2Ø.9
    - laryngitis (acute) JØ4.2
      - chronic J37.1
      - tuberculous NEC A15.5
  - acute JØ4.1Ø
    - with obstruction JØ4.11
  - chronic J42
    - with
      - bronchitis (chronic) J42
      - laryngitis (chronic) J37.1
  - diphtheritic (membranous) A36.89
  - due to external agent — *see* Inflammation, respiratory, upper, due to
  - syphilitic A52.73
  - tuberculous A15.5
- **Trachelitis** (nonvenereal) — *see* Cervicitis
- **Tracheobronchial** — *see* condition
- **Tracheobronchitis** (15 years of age and above) (*see also*) Bronchitis
  - due to
    - Bordetella bronchiseptica A37.8Ø
      - with pneumonia A37.81
    - Francisella tularensis A21.8
- **Tracheobronchomegaly** Q32.4
  - with bronchiectasis J47.9
    - with
      - exacerbation (acute) J47.1
      - lower respiratory infection J47.Ø
  - acquired J98.Ø9
    - with bronchiectasis J47.9
      - with
        - exacerbation (acute) J47.1
        - lower respiratory infection J47.Ø
- **Tracheobronchopneumonitis** — *see* Pneumonia, broncho-
- **Tracheocele** (external) (internal) J39.8
  - congenital Q32.1
- **Tracheomalacia** J39.8
  - congenital Q32.Ø
- **Tracheopharyngitis** (acute) JØ6.9
  - due to external agent — *see* Inflammation, respiratory, upper, due to
- **Tracheostenosis** J39.8
- **Tracheostomy**
  - complication — *see* Complication, tracheostomy
  - status Z93.Ø
    - attention to Z43.Ø
    - malfunctioning J95.Ø3
- **Trachoma, trachomatous** A71.9
  - active (stage) A71.1
  - contraction of conjunctiva A71.1
  - dubium A71.Ø
  - initial (stage) A71.Ø
  - healed or sequelae B94.Ø
  - pannus A71.1
  - Türck's J37.Ø
- **Traction, vitreomacular** H43.82-
- **Train sickness** T75.3
- **Trait(s)**
  - Hb-S D57.3
  - hemoglobin
    - abnormal NEC D58.2
      - with thalassemia D56.3
    - C — *see* Disease, hemoglobin C
    - S (Hb-S) D57.3
  - Lepore D56.3
  - personality, accentuated Z73.1
  - sickle-cell D57.3
    - with elliptocytosis or spherocytosis D57.3
  - type A personality Z73.1
- **Tramp** Z59.0
- **Trance** R41.89
  - hysterical F44.89
- **Transection**
  - abdomen (partial) S38.3
  - aorta (incomplete) (*see also* Injury, aorta)
    - complete — *see* Injury, aorta, laceration, major
- **Transection** — *continued*
  - carotid artery (incomplete) (*see also* Injury, blood vessel, carotid, laceration)
    - complete — *see* Injury, blood vessel, carotid, laceration, major
  - celiac artery (incomplete) S35.211
    - branch (incomplete) S35.291
      - complete S35.292
    - complete S35.212
  - innominate
    - artery (incomplete) (*see also* Injury, blood vessel, thoracic, innominate, artery, laceration)
      - complete — *see* Injury, blood vessel, thoracic, innominate, artery, laceration, major
    - vein (incomplete) (*see also* Injury, blood vessel, thoracic, innominate, vein, laceration)
      - complete — *see* Injury, blood vessel, thoracic, innominate, vein, laceration, major
  - jugular vein (external) (incomplete) (*see also* Injury, blood vessel, jugular vein, laceration)
    - complete — *see* Injury, blood vessel, jugular vein, laceration, major
    - internal (incomplete) (*see also* Injury, blood vessel, jugular vein, internal, laceration)
      - complete — *see* Injury, blood vessel, jugular vein, internal, laceration, major
  - mesenteric artery (incomplete) (*see also* Injury, mesenteric, artery, laceration)
    - complete — *see* Injury, mesenteric artery, laceration, major
  - pulmonary vessel (incomplete) (*see also* Injury, blood vessel, thoracic, pulmonary, laceration)
    - complete — *see* Injury, blood vessel, thoracic, pulmonary, laceration, major
  - subclavian — *see* Transection, innominate
  - vena cava (incomplete) (*see also* Injury, vena cava)
    - complete — *see* Injury, vena cava, laceration, major
  - vertebral artery (incomplete) (*see also* Injury, blood vessel, vertebral, laceration)
    - complete — *see* Injury, blood vessel, vertebral, laceration, major
- **Transaminasemia** R74.0
- **Transfusion**
  - associated (red blood bell) hemochromatosis E83.111
  - blood
    - ABO incompatible — *see* Complication(s), transfusion, incompatibility reaction, ABO
    - minor blood group (Duffy) (E) (K(ell)) (Kidd) (Lewis) (M) (N) (P) (S) T8Ø.89
    - reaction or complication — *see* Complications, transfusion
  - fetomaternal (mother) — *see* Pregnancy, complicated by, placenta, transfusion syndrome
  - maternofetal (mother) — *see* Pregnancy, complicated by, placenta, transfusion syndrome
  - placental (syndrome) (mother) — *see* Pregnancy, complicated by, placenta, transfusion syndrome
  - reaction (adverse) — *see* Complications, transfusion
  - related acute lung injury (TRALI) J95.84
  - twin-to-twin — *see* Pregnancy, complicated by, placenta, transfusion syndrome, fetus to fetus
- **Transient** (meaning homeless) (*see also* condition) Z59.Ø
- **Translocation**
  - balanced autosomal Q95.9
    - in normal individual Q95.Ø
  - chromosomes NEC Q99.8
    - balanced and insertion in normal individual Q95.Ø
  - Down syndrome Q9Ø.2
  - trisomy
    - 13 Q91.6
    - 18 Q91.2
    - 21 Q9Ø.2
- **Translucency, iris** — *see* Degeneration, iris
- **Transmission of chemical substances through the placenta** — *see* Absorption, chemical, through placenta
- **Transparency, lung, unilateral** J43.0
- **Transplant**(ed) (status) Z94.9
  - awaiting organ Z76.82
  - bone Z94.6
    - marrow Z94.81
  - candidate Z76.82
  - complication — *see* Complication, transplant
  - cornea Z94.7
  - heart Z94.1
    - and lung(s) Z94.3
    - valve Z95.2
      - prosthetic Z95.2
      - specified NEC Z95.4
      - xenogenic Z95.3
  - intestine Z94.82
  - kidney Z94.Ø
  - liver Z94.4
  - lung(s) Z94.2
    - and heart Z94.3
  - organ (failure) (infection) (rejection) Z94.9
    - removal status Z98.85
  - pancreas Z94.83
  - skin Z94.5
  - social Z6Ø.3
  - specified organ or tissue NEC Z94.89
  - stem cells Z94.84
  - tissue Z94.9
- **Transplants, ovarian, endometrial** N80.1
- **Transposed** — *see* Transposition
- **Transposition** (congenital) (*see also* Malposition, congenital)
  - abdominal viscera Q89.3
  - aorta (dextra) Q2Ø.3
  - appendix Q43.8
  - colon Q43.8
  - corrected Q2Ø.5
  - great vessels (complete) (partial) Q2Ø.3
  - heart Q24.Ø
    - with complete transposition of viscera Q89.3
  - intestine (large) (small) Q43.8
  - reversed jejunal (for bypass) (status) Z98.Ø
  - scrotum Q55.23
  - stomach Q4Ø.2
    - with general transposition of viscera Q89.3
  - tooth, teeth, fully erupted M26.3Ø
  - vessels, great (complete) (partial) Q2Ø.3
  - viscera (abdominal) (thoracic) Q89.3
- **Transsexualism** F64.1
- **Transverse** (*see also* condition)
  - arrest (deep), in labor O64.Ø
  - lie (mother) O32.2
    - causing obstructed labor O64.8
- **Transvestism, transvestitism** (dual-role) F64.1
  - fetishistic F65.1
- **Trapped placenta** (with hemorrhage) O72.Ø
  - without hemorrhage O73.Ø
- **Trauma, traumatism** (*see also* Injury)
  - acoustic — *see* subcategory H83.3
  - birth — *see* Birth, injury
  - complicating ectopic or molar pregnancy OØ8.6
  - during delivery O71.9
  - following ectopic or molar pregnancy OØ8.6
  - obstetric O71.9
    - specified NEC O71.89
- **Traumatic** (*see also* condition)
  - brain injury — *see* category SØ6
- **Treacher Collins syndrome** Q75.4
- **Treitz's hernia** — *see* Hernia, abdomen, specified site NEC
- **Trematode infestation** — *see* Infestation, fluke
- **Trematodiasis** — *see* Infestation, fluke
- **Trembling paralysis** — *see* Parkinsonism
- **Tremor**(s) R25.1
  - drug induced G25.1
  - essential (benign) G25.Ø
  - familial G25.Ø
  - hereditary G25.Ø
  - hysterical F44.4
  - intention G25.2
  - medication induced postural G25.1
  - mercurial — *see* subcategory T56.1
  - Parkinson's — *see* Parkinsonism
  - psychogenic (conversion reaction) F44.4
  - senilis R54

Tumor — *continued*
- aortic body D44.7
  - malignant C75.5
- Askin's — *see* Neoplasm, connective tissue, malignant
- basal cell (*see also* Neoplasm, skin, uncertain behavior) D48.5
- Bednar — *see* Neoplasm, skin, malignant
- benign (unclassified) — *see* Neoplasm, benign, by site
- beta-cell
  - malignant
    - pancreas C25.4
    - specified site NEC — *see* Neoplasm, malignant, by site
    - unspecified site C25.4
  - pancreas D13.7
  - specified site NEC — *see* Neoplasm, benign, by site
  - unspecified site D13.7
- Brenner D27.9
  - borderline malignancy D39.1-
  - malignant C56-
  - proliferating D39.1-
- bronchial alveolar, intravascular D38.1
- Brooke's — *see* Neoplasm, skin, benign
- brown fat — *see* Lipoma
- Burkitt — *see* Lymphoma, Burkitt
- calcifying epithelial odontogenic — *see* Cyst, calcifying odontogenic
- carcinoid
  - benign D3A.ØØ
    - appendix D3A.Ø2Ø
    - ascending colon D3A.Ø22
    - bronchus (lung) D3A.Ø9Ø
    - cecum D3A.Ø21
    - colon D3A.Ø29
    - descending colon D3A.Ø24
    - duodenum D3A.Ø1Ø
    - foregut NOS D3A.Ø94
    - hindgut NOS D3A.Ø96
    - ileum D3A.Ø12
    - jejunum D3A.Ø11
    - kidney D3A.Ø93
    - large intestine D3A.Ø29
    - lung (bronchus) D3A.Ø9Ø
    - midgut NOS D3A.Ø95
    - rectum D3A.Ø26
    - sigmoid colon D3A.Ø25
    - small intestine D3A.Ø19
    - specified NEC D3A.Ø98
    - stomach D3A.Ø92
    - thymus D3A.Ø91
    - transverse colon D3A.Ø23
  - malignant C7A.ØØ
    - appendix C7A.Ø2Ø
    - ascending colon C7A.Ø22
    - bronchus (lung) C7A.Ø9Ø
    - cecum C7A.Ø21
    - colon C7A.Ø29
    - descending colon C7A.Ø24
    - duodenum C7A.Ø1Ø
    - foregut NOS C7A.Ø94
    - hindgut NOS C7A.Ø96
    - ileum C7A.Ø12
    - jejunum C7A.Ø11
    - kidney C7A.Ø93
    - large intestine C7A.Ø29
    - lung (bronchus) C7A.Ø9Ø
    - midgut NOS C7A.Ø95
    - rectum C7A.Ø26
    - sigmoid colon C7A.Ø25
    - small intestine C7A.Ø19
    - specified NEC C7A.Ø98
    - stomach C7A.Ø92
    - thymus C7A.Ø91
    - transverse colon C7A.Ø23
  - mesentery metastasis C7B.Ø4
  - secondary C7B.ØØ
    - bone C7B.Ø3
    - distant lymph nodes C7B.Ø1
    - liver C7B.Ø2
    - peritoneum C7B.Ø4

Tumor — *continued*
- carcinoid— *continued*
  - secondary— *continued*
    - specified NEC C7B.Ø9
- carotid body D44.6
  - malignant C75.4
- cells (*see also* Neoplasm, unspecified behavior, by site)
  - benign — *see* Neoplasm, benign, by site
  - malignant — *see* Neoplasm, malignant, by site
  - uncertain whether benign or malignant — *see* Neoplasm, uncertain behavior, by site
- cervix, in pregnancy or childbirth — *see* Pregnancy, complicated by, tumor, cervix
- chondromatous giant cell — *see* Neoplasm, bone, benign
- chromaffin (*see also* Neoplasm, benign, by site)
  - malignant — *see* Neoplasm, malignant
- Cock's peculiar L72.3
- Codman's — *see* Neoplasm, bone, benign
- dentigerous, mixed — *see* Cyst, calcifying odontogenic
- dermoid (*see also* Neoplasm, benign, by site)
  - with malignant transformation C56-
- desmoid (extra-abdominal) (*see also* Neoplasm, connective tissue, uncertain behavior)
  - abdominal — *see* Neoplasm, connective tissue, uncertain behavior
- embolus — *see* Neoplasm, secondary, by site
- embryonal (mixed) (*see also* Neoplasm, uncertain behavior, by site)
  - liver C22.7
  - unspecified site
    - female C56.-
    - male C62.9Ø
- endodermal sinus
  - specified site — *see* Neoplasm, malignant, by site
- epithelial
  - benign — *see* Neoplasm, benign by site
  - malignant — *see* Neoplasm, malignant by site
- Ewing's — *see* Neoplasm, bone, malignant by site
- fatty — *see* Lipoma
- fibroid — *see* Leiomyoma
  - specified site — *see* Neoplasm, uncertain behavior, by site
  - unspecified site D37.9
- G cell
  - malignant
    - pancreas C25.4
    - specified site NEC — *see* Neoplasm, malignant, by site
    - unspecified site C25.4
  - unspecified site D37.8
- germ cell (*see also* Neoplasm, malignant, by site)
  - mixed — *see* Neoplasm, malignant, by site
- ghost cell, odontogenic — *see* Cyst, calcifying odontogenic
- giant cell (*see also* Neoplasm, uncertain behavior, by site)
  - bone D48.Ø
    - malignant — *see* Neoplasm, bone, malignant, by site
  - chondromatous — *see* Neoplasm, bone, benign
  - malignant — *see* Neoplasm, malignant, by site
  - soft parts (*see also* Neoplasm, connective tissue, uncertain behavior)
    - malignant — *see* Neoplasm, connective tissue, malignant
- glomus D18.ØØ
  - intra-abdominal D18.Ø3
  - intracranial D18.Ø2
  - jugulare D44.7
    - malignant C75.5
  - skin D18.Ø1
  - specified site NEC D18.Ø9
- gonadal stromal — *see* Neoplasm, uncertain behavior, by site
- granular cell (*see also* Neoplasm, connective tissue, benign)
  - malignant — *see* Neoplasm, connective tissue, malignant
- granulosa cell D39.1-
  - juvenile D39.1-

Tumor — *continued*
- granulosa cell— *continued*
  - malignant C56-
- granulosa cell-theca cell D39.1-
  - malignant C56.-
- Grawitz's C64-
- hemorrhoidal — *see* Hemorrhoids
- hilar cell D27-
- hilus cell D27-
- Hurthle cell (benign) D34
  - malignant C73
- hydatid — *see* Echinococcus
- hypernephroid — *see* Neoplasm, uncertain behavior, by site
- interstitial cell (*see also* Neoplasm, uncertain behavior, by site)
  - benign — *see* Neoplasm, benign, by site
  - malignant — *see* Neoplasm, malignant, by site
- intravascular bronchial alveolar D38.1
- islet cell (*see also* Neoplasm, benign, by site)
  - malignant (*see also* Neoplasm, malignant, by site)
    - pancreas C25.4
    - specified site NEC — *see* Neoplasm, malignant, by site
    - unspecified site C25.4
  - pancreas D13.7
  - specified site NEC — *see* Neoplasm, benign, by site
  - unspecified site D13.7
- juxtaglomerular D41.Ø-
- Klatskin's C22.1
- Krukenberg's C79.6-
- Leydig cell (*see also* Neoplasm, uncertain behavior, by site)
  - benign (*see also* Neoplasm, benign, by site)
    - specified site — *see* Neoplasm, benign, by site
    - unspecified site
      - female D27.9
      - male D29.2Ø
  - malignant (*see also* Neoplasm, malignant, by site)
    - specified site — *see* Neoplasm, malignant, by site
    - unspecified site
      - female C56.9
      - male C62.9Ø
  - specified site — *see* Neoplasm, uncertain behavior , by site
  - unspecified site
    - female D39.1Ø
    - male D4Ø.1Ø
- lipid cell, ovary D27-
- lipoid cell, ovary D27-
- malignant (*see also* Neoplasm, malignant, by site) C8Ø.1
  - fusiform cell (type) C8Ø.1
  - giant cell (type) C8Ø.1
  - localized, plasma cell — *see* Plasmacytoma, solitary
  - mixed NEC C8Ø.1
  - small cell (type) C8Ø.1
  - spindle cell (type) C8Ø.1
  - unclassified C8Ø.1
- mast cell D47.Ø
  - malignant C96.2
- melanotic, neuroectodermal — *see* Neoplasm, benign, by site
- Merkel cell — *see* Carcinoma, Merkel cell
- mesenchymal
  - malignant — *see* Neoplasm, connective tissue, malignant
  - mixed — *see* Neoplasm, connective tissue, uncertain behavior
- mesodermal, mixed (*see also* Neoplasm, malignant, by site)
  - liver C22.4
- mesonephric (*see also* Neoplasm, uncertain behavior, by site)
  - malignant — *see* Neoplasm, malignant, by site
- metastatic
  - from specified site — *see* Neoplasm, malignant, by site
  - of specified site — *see* Neoplasm, malignant, by site

- **Tumor** — *continued*
  - metastatic— *continued*
    - to specified site — *see* Neoplasm, secondary, by site
  - mixed NEC (*see also* Neoplasm, benign, by site)
    - malignant — *see* Neoplasm, malignant, by site
    - unspecified site C56.9
  - mucinous of low malignant potential
    - specified site — *see* Neoplasm, malignant, by site
    - unspecified site C18.1
  - mucocarcinoid
    - specified site — *see* Neoplasm, malignant, by site
  - mucoepidermoid — *see* Neoplasm, uncertain behavior, by site
  - Müllerian, mixed
    - specified site — *see* Neoplasm, malignant, by site
    - unspecified site C54.9
  - myoepithelial — *see* Neoplasm, benign, by site
  - neuroectodermal (peripheral) (*see also* Neoplasm, malignant, by site)
    - primitive
      - specified site — *see* Neoplasm, malignant, by site
      - unspecified site C71.9
  - neuroendocrine D3A.8
    - malignant poorly differentiated C7A.1
    - secondary NEC C7B.8
    - specified NEC C7A.8
  - neurogenic olfactory C3Ø.Ø
  - nonencapsulated sclerosing C73
  - odontogenic (adenomatoid) (benign) (calcifying epithelial) (keratocystic) (squamous) *(see also* Cyst, calcifying odontogenic)
    - malignant C41.1
      - upper jaw (bone) C41.Ø
  - ovarian stromal D39.1-
  - ovary, in pregnancy — *see* Pregnancy, complicated by
  - pacinian — *see* Neoplasm, skin, benign
  - Pancoast's — *see* Pancoast's syndrome
  - papillary (*see also* Papilloma)
    - cystic D37.9
    - mucinous of low malignant potential C56-
      - specified site — *see* Neoplasm, malignant, by site
      - unspecified site C56.9
    - serous of low malignant potential
      - specified site — *see* Neoplasm, malignant, by site
      - unspecified site C56.9
  - pelvic, in pregnancy or childbirth — *see* Pregnancy, complicated by
  - phantom F45.8
  - phyllodes D48.6-
    - benign D24-
    - malignant — *see* Neoplasm, breast, malignant
  - Pindborg — *see* Cyst, calcifying odontogenic
  - placental site trophoblastic D39.2
  - plasma cell (malignant) (localized) — *see* Plasmacytoma, solitary
  - polyvesicular vitelline
    - specifed site — *see* Neoplasm, malignant, by site
    - unspecified site
      - female C56.9
      - male C62.9Ø
  - Pott's puffy — *see* Osteomyelitis, specified NEC
  - Rathke's pouch D44.3
  - retinal anlage — *see* Neoplasm, benign, by site
  - salivary gland type, mixed (*see also* Neoplasm, salivary gland, benign)
    - malignant — *see* Neoplasm, salivary gland, malignant
  - Sampson's N8Ø.1
  - Schmincke's — *see* Neoplasm, nasopharynx, malignant
  - sclerosing stromal D27-
  - sebaceous — *see* Cyst, sebaceous
  - secondary (*see also* Neoplasm, secondary, by site)
    - carcinoid C7B.ØØ
      - bone C7B.Ø3
      - distant lymph nodes C7B.Ø1
      - liver C7B.Ø2

- **Tumor** — *continued*
  - secondary— *continued*
    - carcinoid— *continued*
      - peritoneum C7B.Ø4
      - specified NEC C7B.Ø9
    - neuroendocrine NEC C7B.8
  - serous of low malignant potential
    - specified site — *see* Neoplasm, malignant, by site
    - unspecified site C56.9
  - Sertoli cell (*see also* Neoplasm, benign, by site)
    - with lipid storage
      - specified stie — *see* Neoplasm, benign, by site
    - specified site — *see* Neoplasm, benign, by site
    - unspecified site
      - female D27.9
      - male D29.2Ø
  - Sertoli-Leydig cell *(see also* Neoplasm, benign, by site)
    - specified site — *see* Neoplasm, benign, by site
    - unspecified site
      - female D27.9
      - male D29.2Ø
  - sex cord(-stromal) *(see also* Neoplasm, uncertain behavior, by site)
    - with annular tubules D39.1-
  - skin appendage — *see* Neoplasm, skin, benign
  - smooth muscle — *see* Neoplasm, connective tissue, uncertain behavior
  - soft tissue
    - benign — *see* Neoplasm, connective tissue, benign
    - malignant — *see* Neoplasm, connective tissue, malignant
  - sternomastoid (congenital) Q68.Ø
  - stromal
    - endometrial D39.Ø
    - gastric D48.1
      - benign D21.4
      - malignant C16.9
      - uncertain behavior D48.1
    - gastrointestinal
      - benign D21.4
      - malignant C49.4
      - uncertain behavior D48.1
    - intestine
      - benign D21.4
      - malignant C49.4
      - uncertain behavior D48.1
    - ovarian D39.1-
    - stomach
      - benign D21.4
      - malignant C16.9
      - uncertain behavior D48.1
  - testicular D4Ø.1Ø
  - sweat gland (*see also* Neoplasm, skin, uncertain behavior)
    - benign — *see* Neoplasm, skin, benign
    - malignant — *see* Neoplasm, skin, malignant
  - syphilitic, brain A52.17
  - testicular stromal D4Ø.1-
  - theca cell D27.-
  - theca cell-granulosa cell D39.1-
  - Triton, malignant — *see* Neoplasm, nerve, malignant
  - trophoblastic, placental site D39.2
  - turban D23.4
  - uterus (body), in pregnancy or childbirth — *see* Pregnancy, complicated by, tumor, uterus
  - vagina, in pregnancy or childbirth — *see* Pregnancy, complicated by
  - varicose — *see* Varix
  - von Recklinghausen's — *see* Neurofibromatosis
  - vulva or perineum, in pregnancy or childbirth — *see* Pregnancy, complicated by
    - causing obstructed labor O65.5
  - Warthin's — *see* Neoplasm, salivary gland, benign
  - Wilms' C64-
  - yolk sac (*see also* Neoplasm, malignant, by site)
    - specified site — *see* Neoplasm, malignant, by site
    - unspecified site
      - female C56.9
      - male C62.9Ø

- **Tumor lysis syndrome** (following antineoplastic chemotherapy) (spontaneous) NEC E88.3
- **Tumorlet** — *see* Neoplasm, uncertain behavior, by site
- **Tungiasis** B88.1
- **Tunica vasculosa lentis** Q12.2
- **Turban tumor** D23.4
- **Türck's trachoma** J37.0
- **Turner-Kieser syndrome** Q79.8
- **Turner-like syndrome** Q87.1
- **Turner's**
  - hypoplasia (tooth) KØØ.4
  - syndrome Q96.9
    - specified NEC Q96.8
  - tooth KØØ.4
- **Turner-Ullrich syndrome** Q96.9
- **Tussis convulsiva** — *see* Whooping cough
- **Twiddler's syndrome** (due to)
  - automatic implantable defibrillatorT82.198
  - cardiac pacemaker T82.198
- **Twilight state**
  - epileptic FØ5
  - psychogenic F44.89
- **Twin** (newborn) (*see also* Newborn, twin
  - conjoined) Q89.4
    - pregnancy — *see* Pregnancy, twin, conjoined
- **Twinning, teeth** K00.2
- **Twist, twisted**
  - bowel, colon or intestine K56.2
  - hair (congenital) Q84.1
  - mesentery K56.2
  - omentum K56.2
  - organ or site, congenital NEC — *see* Anomaly, by site
  - ovarian pedicle — *see* Torsion, ovary
- **Twitching** R25.3
- **Tylosis** (acquired) L84
  - buccalis K13.29
  - linguae K13.29
  - palmaris et plantaris (congenital) (inherited) Q82.8
    - acquired L85.1
- **Tympanism** R14.0
- **Tympanites** (abdominal) (intestinal) R14.Ø
- **Tympanitis** — *see* Myringitis
- **Tympanosclerosis** — *see* subcategory H74.Ø
- **Tympanum** — *see* condition
- **Tympany**
  - abdomen R14.Ø
  - chest RØ9.89
- **Type A behavior pattern** Z73.1
- **Typhlitis** — *see* Appendicitis
- **Typhoenteritis** — *see* Typhoid
- **Typhoid** (abortive) (ambulant) (any site) (clinical) (fever) (hemorrhagic) (infection) (intermittent) (malignant) (rheumatic) (Widalnegative) AØ1.ØØ
  - with pneumonia AØ1.Ø3
  - abdominal AØ1.Ø9
  - arthritis AØ1.Ø4
  - carrier (suspected) of Z22.Ø
  - cholecystitis (current) AØ1.Ø9
  - endocarditis AØ1.Ø2
  - heart involvement AØ1.Ø2
  - inoculation reaction — *see* Complications, vaccination
  - meningitis AØ1.Ø1
  - mesenteric lymph nodes AØ1.Ø9
  - myocarditis AØ1.Ø2
  - osteomyelitis AØ1.Ø5
  - perichondritis, larynx AØ1.Ø9
  - pneumonia AØ1.Ø3
  - spine AØ1.Ø5
  - specified NEC AØ1.Ø9
  - ulcer (perforating) AØ1.Ø9
- **Typhomalaria** (fever) — *see* Malaria
- **Typhomania** A01.00
- **Typhoperitonitis** A01.09
- **Typhus** (fever) A75.9
  - abdominal, abdominalis — *see* Typhoid
  - African tick A77.1
  - amarillic A95.9
  - brain A75.9 *[G94]*
  - cerebral A75.9 *[G94]*
  - classical A75.Ø

- **Typhus** (fever) — *continued*
  - due to Rickettsia
    - prowazekii A75.Ø
      - recrudescent A75.1
    - tsutsugamushi A75.3
    - typhi A75.2
  - endemic (flea-borne) A75.2
  - epidemic (louse-borne) A75.Ø
  - exanthematic NEC A75.Ø
  - exanthematicus SAI A75.Ø
    - brillii SAI A75.1
    - mexicanus SAI A75.2
    - typhus murinus A75.2
  - flea-borne A75.2
  - India tick A77.1
  - Kenya (tick) A77.1
  - louse-borne A75.Ø
  - Mexican A75.2
  - mite-borne A75.3
  - murine A75.2
  - North Asian tick-borne A77.2
  - petechial A75.9
  - Queensland tick A77.3
  - rat A75.2
  - recrudescent A75.1
  - recurrens — *see* Fever, relapsing
  - Sao Paulo A77.Ø
  - scrub (China) (India) (Malaysia) (New Guinea) A75.3
  - shop (of Malaysia) A75.2
  - Siberian tick A77.2
- **Typhus** (fever) A75.9
  - tick-borne A77.9
  - tropical (mite-borne) A75.3
- **Tyrosinemia** E70.21
  - newborn, transitory P74.5
- **Tyrosinosis** E70.21
- **Tyrosinuria** E70.29

U

- **Uhl's anomaly or disease** Q24.8
- **Ulcer, ulcerated, ulcerating, ulceration, ulcerative**
  - alveolar process M27.3
  - amebic (intestine) AØ6.1
    - skin AØ6.7
  - anastomotic — *see* Ulcer, gastrojejunal
  - anorectal K62.6
  - antral — *see* Ulcer, stomach
  - anus (sphincter) (solitary) K62.6
  - aorta — *see* Aneurysm
  - aphthous (oral) (recurrent) K12.Ø
    - genital organ(s)
      - female N76.6
      - male N5Ø.8
  - artery I77.2
  - atrophic — *see* Ulcer, skin
    - decubitus — *see* Ulcer, pressure, by site
  - back L98.429
    - with
      - bone necrosis L98.424
      - exposed fat layer L98.422
      - muscle necrosis L98.423
      - skin breakdown only L98.421
  - Barrett's (esophagus) K22.1Ø
    - with bleeding K22.11
  - bile duct (common) (hepatic) K83.8
  - bladder (solitary) (sphincter) NEC N32.89
    - bilharzial B65.9 *[N33]*
    - in schistosomiasis (bilharzial) B65.9 *[N33]*
    - submucosal — *see* Cystitis, interstitial
    - tuberculous A18.12
  - bleeding K27.4
  - bone — *see* Osteomyelitis, specified type NEC
  - bowel — *see* Ulcer, intestine
  - breast N61
  - bronchus J98.Ø9
  - buccal (cavity) (traumatic) K12.1
  - Buruli A31.1
  - buttock L98.419
    - bone necrosis L98.414
    - exposed fat layer L98.412
    - muscle necrosis L98.413
    - skin breakdown L98.411
  - cancerous — *see* Neoplasm, malignant, by site
  - cardia K22.1Ø
    - with bleeding K22.11
  - cardioesophageal (peptic) K22.1Ø
    - with bleeding K22.11
  - cecum — *see* Ulcer, intestine
  - cervix (uteri) (decubitus) (trophic) N86
    - with cervicitis N72
  - chancroidal A57
  - chiclero B55.1
  - chronic (cause unknown) — *see* Ulcer, skin
  - Cochin-China B55.1
  - colon — *see* Ulcer, intestine
  - conjunctiva H1Ø.89
  - cornea H16.ØØ-
    - with hypopyon H16.Ø3-
    - central H16.Ø1-
    - dendritic (herpes simplex) BØØ.52
    - marginal H16.Ø4-
    - Mooren's H16.Ø5-
    - mycotic H16.Ø6-
    - perforated H16.Ø7-
    - ring H16.Ø2-
    - tuberculous (phlyctenular) A18.52
  - corpus cavernosum (chronic) N48.5
  - crural — *see* Ulcer, lower limb
  - Curling's — *see* Ulcer, peptic, acute
  - Cushing's — *see* Ulcer, peptic, acute
  - cystic duct K82.8
  - cystitis (interstitial) — *see* Cystitis, interstitial
  - decubitus — *see* Ulcer, pressure, by site
  - dendritic, cornea (herpes simplex) BØØ.52
  - diabetes, diabetic — *see* Diabetes, ulcer
  - Dieulafoy's K25.Ø
  - due to
    - infection NEC — *see* Ulcer, skin
    - radiation NEC L59.8

- **Ulcer** — *continued*
  - due to — *continued*
    - trophic disturbance (any region) — *see* Ulcer, skin
    - X-ray L58.1
  - duodenum, duodenal (eroded) (peptic) K26.9
    - with
      - hemorrhage K26.4
        - and perforation K26.6
      - perforation K26.5
    - acute K26.3
      - with
        - hemorrhage K26.Ø
          - and perforation K26.2
        - perforation K26.1
    - chronic K26.7
      - with
        - hemorrhage K26.4
          - and perforation K26.6
        - perforation K26.5
  - dysenteric AØ9
  - elusive — *see* Cystitis, interstitial
  - endocarditis (acute) (chronic) (subacute) I28.8
  - epiglottis J38.7
  - esophagus (peptic) K22.1Ø
    - with bleeding K22.11
    - due to
      - aspirin K22.1Ø
        - with bleeding K22.11
      - gastrointestinal reflux disease K21.Ø
      - ingestion of chemical or medicament K22.1Ø
        - with bleeding K22.11
    - fungal K22.1Ø
      - with bleeding K22.11
    - infective K22.1Ø
      - with bleeding K22.11
    - varicose — *see* Varix, esophagus
  - eyelid (region) HØ1.8
  - fauces J39.2
  - Fenwick (-Hunner) (solitary) — *see* Cystitis, interstitial
  - fistulous — *see* Ulcer, skin
  - foot (indolent) (trophic) — *see* Ulcer, lower limb
  - frambesial, initial A66.Ø
  - frenum (tongue) K14.Ø
  - gallbladder or duct K82.8
  - gangrenous — *see* Gangrene
  - gastric — *see* Ulcer, stomach
  - gastrocolic — *see* Ulcer, gastrojejunal
  - gastroduodenal — *see* Ulcer, peptic
  - gastroesophageal — *see* Ulcer, stomach
  - gastrointestinal — *see* Ulcer, gastrojejunal
  - gastrojejunal (peptic) K28.9
    - with
      - hemorrhage K28.4
        - and perforation K28.6
      - perforation K28.5
    - acute K28.3
      - with
        - hemorrhage K28.Ø
          - and perforation K28.2
        - perforation K28.1
    - chronic K28.7
      - with
        - hemorrhage K28.4
          - and perforation K28.6
        - perforation K28.5
  - gastrojejunocolic — *see* Ulcer, gastrojejunal
  - gingiva KØ6.8
  - gingivitis KØ5.1Ø
    - plaque induced KØ5.1Ø
    - nonplaque induced KØ5.11
  - glottis J38.7
  - granuloma of pudenda A58
  - gum KØ6.8
  - gumma, due to yaws A66.4
  - heel — *see* Ulcer, lower limb
  - hemorrhoid (*see also* Hemorrhoids, by degree) K64.8
  - Hunner's — *see* Cystitis, interstitial
  - hypopharynx J39.2
  - hypopyon (chronic) (subacute) — *see* Ulcer, cornea, with hypopyon
  - hypostaticum — *see* Ulcer, varicose

- **Ulcer** — *continued*
  - ileum — *see* Ulcer, intestine
  - intestine, intestinal K63.3
    - with perforation K63.1
    - amebic AØ6.1
    - duodenal — *see* Ulcer, duodenum
    - granulocytopenic (with hemorrhage) — *see* Neutropenia
    - marginal — *see* Ulcer, gastrojejunal
    - perforating K63.1
      - newborn P78.Ø
    - primary, small intestine K63.3
    - rectum K62.6
    - stercoraceous, stercoral K63.3
    - tuberculous A18.32
    - typhoid (fever) — *see* Typhoid
    - varicose I86.8
  - jejunum, jejunal — *see* Ulcer, gastrojejunal
  - keratitis — *see* Ulcer, cornea
  - knee — *see* Ulcer, lower limb
  - labium (majus) (minus) N76.6
  - laryngitis — *see* Laryngitis
  - larynx (aphthous) (contact) J38.7
    - diphtheritic A36.2
  - leg — *see* Ulcer, lower limb
  - lip K13.Ø
  - Lipschütz's N76.6
  - lower limb (atrophic) (chronic) (neurogenic) (perforating) (pyogenic) (trophic) (tropical) L97.9Ø9
    - with
      - bone necrosis L97.9Ø4
      - exposed fat layer L97.9Ø2
      - muscle necrosis L97.9Ø3
      - skin breakdown only L97.9Ø1
    - ankle L97.3Ø9
      - with
        - bone necrosis L97.3Ø4
        - exposed fat layer L97.3Ø2
        - muscle necrosis L97.3Ø3
        - skin breakdown only L97.3Ø1
      - left L97.329
        - with
          - bone necrosis L97.324
          - exposed fat layer L97.322
          - muscle necrosis L97.323
          - skin breakdown only L97.321
      - right L97.319
        - with
          - bone necrosis L97.314
          - exposed fat layer L97.312
          - muscle necrosis L97.313
          - skin breakdown only L97.311
    - calf L97.2Ø9
      - with
        - bone necrosis L97.2Ø4
        - exposed fat layer L97.2Ø2
        - muscle necrosis L97.2Ø3
        - skin breakdown only L97.2Ø1
      - left L97.229
        - with
          - bone necrosis L97.224
          - exposed fat layer L97.222
          - muscle necrosis L97.223
          - skin breakdown only L97.221
      - right L97.219
        - with
          - bone necrosis L97.214
          - exposed fat layer L97.212
          - muscle necrosis L97.213
          - skin breakdown only L97.211
    - decubitus — *see* Ulcer, pressure, by site
    - foot specified NEC L97.5Ø9
      - with
        - bone necrosis L97.5Ø4
        - exposed fat layer L97.5Ø2
        - muscle necrosis L97.5Ø3
        - skin breakdown only L97.5Ø1
      - left L97.529
        - with
          - bone necrosis L97.524
          - exposed fat layer L97.522
          - muscle necrosis L97.523

- **Ulcer** — *continued*
  - lower limb — *continued*
    - foot specified NEC — *continued*
      - left — *continued*
        - with — *continued*
          - skin breakdown only L97.521
      - right L97.519
        - with
          - bone necrosis L97.514
          - exposed fat layer L97.512
          - muscle necrosis L97.513
          - skin breakdown only L97.511
    - heel L97.4Ø9
      - with
        - bone necrosis L97.4Ø4
        - exposed fat layer L97.4Ø2
        - muscle necrosis L97.4Ø3
        - skin breakdown only L97.4Ø1
      - left L97.429
        - with
          - bone necrosis L97.424
          - exposed fat layer L97.422
          - muscle necrosis L97.423
          - skin breakdown only L97.421
      - right L97.419
        - with
          - bone necrosis L97.414
          - exposed fat layer L97.412
          - muscle necrosis L97.413
          - skin breakdown only L97.411
    - left L97.929
      - with
        - bone necrosis L97.924
        - exposed fat layer L97.922
        - muscle necrosis L97.923
        - skin breakdown only L97.921
    - lower leg NOS L97.9Ø9
      - with
        - bone necrosis L97.9Ø4
        - exposed fat layer L97.9Ø2
        - muscle necrosis L97.9Ø3
        - skin breakdown only L97.9Ø1
      - left L97.929
        - with
          - bone necrosis L97.924
          - exposed fat layer L97.922
          - muscle necrosis L97.923
          - skin breakdown only L97.921
      - right L97.919
        - with
          - bone necrosis L97.914
          - exposed fat layer L97.912
          - muscle necrosis L97.913
          - skin breakdown only L97.911
      - specified site NEC L97.8Ø9
        - with
          - bone necrosis L97.8Ø4
          - exposed fat layer L97.8Ø2
          - muscle necrosis L97.8Ø3
          - skin breakdown only L97.8Ø1
        - left L97.829
          - with
            - bone necrosis L97.824
            - exposed fat layer L97.822
            - muscle necrosis L97.823
            - skin breakdown only L97.821
        - right L97.819
          - with
            - bone necrosis L97.814
            - exposed fat layer L97.812
            - muscle necrosis L97.813
            - skin breakdown only L97.811
    - midfoot L97.4Ø9
      - with
        - bone necrosis L97.4Ø4
        - exposed fat layer L97.4Ø2
        - muscle necrosis L97.4Ø3
        - skin breakdown only L97.4Ø1
      - left L97.429
        - with
          - bone necrosis L97.424
          - exposed fat layer L97.422
          - muscle necrosis L97.423

- **Ulcer** — *continued*
  - lower limb — *continued*
    - midfoot — *continued*
      - left — *continued*
        - with — *continued*
          - skin breakdown only L97.421
      - right L97.419
        - with
          - bone necrosis L97.414
          - exposed fat layer L97.412
          - muscle necrosis L97.413
          - skin breakdown only L97.411
    - right L97.919
      - with
        - bone necrosis L97.914
        - exposed fat layer L97.912
        - muscle necrosis L97.913
        - skin breakdown only L97.911
    - thigh L97.1Ø9
      - with
        - bone necrosis L97.1Ø4
        - exposed fat layer L97.1Ø2
        - muscle necrosis L97.1Ø3
        - skin breakdown only L97.1Ø1
      - left L97.129
        - with
          - bone necrosis L97.124
          - exposed fat layer L97.122
          - muscle necrosis L97.123
          - skin breakdown only L97.121
      - right L97.119
        - with
          - bone necrosis L97.114
          - exposed fat layer L97.112
          - muscle necrosis L97.113
          - skin breakdown only L97.111
    - toe L97.5Ø9
      - with
        - bone necrosis L97.5Ø4
        - exposed fat layer L97.5Ø2
        - muscle necrosis L97.5Ø3
        - skin breakdown only L97.5Ø1
      - left L97.529
        - with
          - bone necrosis L97.524
          - exposed fat layer L97.522
          - muscle necrosis L97.523
          - skin breakdown only L97.521
      - right L97.519
        - with
          - bone necrosis L97.514
          - exposed fat layer L97.512
          - muscle necrosis L97.513
          - skin breakdown only L97.511
    - leprous A3Ø.1
    - syphilitic A52.19
    - varicose — *see* Varix, leg, with, ulcer
  - luetic — *see* Ulcer, syphilitic
  - lung J98.4
    - tuberculous — *see* Tuberculosis, pulmonary
  - malignant — *see* Neoplasm, malignant, by site
  - marginal NEC — *see* Ulcer, gastrojejunal
  - meatus (urinarius) N34.2
  - Meckel's diverticulum Q43.Ø
    - malignant — *see* Table of Neoplasms, small intestine, malignant
  - Meleney's (chronic undermining) — *see* Ulcer, skin
  - Mooren's (cornea) — *see* Ulcer, cornea, Mooren's
  - mycobacterial (skin) A31.1
  - nasopharynx J39.2
  - neck, uterus N86
  - neurogenic NEC — *see* Ulcer, skin
  - nose, nasal (passage) (infective) (septum) J34.Ø
    - skin — *see* Ulcer, skin
    - spirochetal A69.8
    - varicose (bleeding) I86.8
  - oral mucosa (traumatic) K12.1
  - palate (soft) K12.1
  - penis (chronic) N48.5
  - peptic (site unspecified) K27.9
    - with
      - hemorrhage K27.4
        - and perforation K27.6

- **Ulcer** — *continued*
  - peptic (site unspecified) — *continued*
    - with — *continued*
      - perforation K27.5
    - acute K27.3
      - with
        - hemorrhage K27.Ø
          - and perforation K27.2
        - perforation K27.1
    - chronic K27.7
      - with
        - hemorrhage K27.4
          - and perforation K27.6
        - perforation K27.5
    - esophagus K22.1Ø
      - with bleeding K22.11
    - newborn P78.82
  - perforating K27.5
    - skin — *see* Ulcer, skin
  - peritonsillar J35.8
  - phagedenic (tropical) — *see* Ulcer, skin
  - pharynx J39.2
  - phlebitis — *see* Phlebitis
  - plaster — *see* Ulcer, pressure, by site
  - popliteal space — *see* Ulcer, lower limb
  - postpyloric — *see* Ulcer, duodenum
  - prepuce N47.7
  - prepyloric — *see* Ulcer, stomach
  - pressure (pressure area) L89.9-
    - ankle L89.5-
    - back L89.1-
    - buttock L89.3-
    - coccyx L89.15-
    - contiguous site of back, buttock, hip L89.4-
    - elbow L89.Ø-
    - face L89.81-
    - head L89.81-
    - heel L89.6-
    - hip L89.2-
    - sacral region (tailbone) L89.15-
    - specified site NEC L89.89-
    - stage 1 (healing) (pre-ulcer skin changes limited to persistent focal edema)
      - ankle L89.5-
      - back L89.1-
      - buttock L89.3-
      - coccyx L89.15-
      - contiguous site of back, buttock, hip L89.4-
      - elbow L89.Ø-
      - face L89.81-
      - head L89.81-
      - heel L89.6-
      - hip L89.2-
      - sacral region (tailbone) L89.15-
      - specified site NEC L89.89-
    - stage 2 (healing) (abrasion, blister, partial thickness skin loss involving epidermis and/or dermis)
      - ankle L89.5-
      - back L89.1-
      - buttock L89.3-
      - coccyx L89.15-
      - contiguous site of back, buttock, hip L89.4-
      - elbow L89.Ø-
      - face L89.81-
      - head L89.81-
      - heel L89.6-
      - hip L89.2-
      - sacral region (tailbone) L89.15-
      - specified site NEC L89.89-
    - stage 3 (healing) (full thickness skin loss involving damage or necrosis of subcutaneous tissue)
      - ankle L89.5-
      - back L89.1-
      - buttock L89.3-
      - coccyx L89.15-
      - contiguous site of back, buttock, hip L89.4-
      - elbow L89.Ø-
      - face L89.81-
      - head L89.81-
      - heel L89.6-
      - hip L89.2-

- **Ulcer** — *continued*
  - pressure — *continued*
    - stage 3 — *continued*
      - sacral region (tailbone) L89.15-
      - specified site NEC L89.89-
    - stage 4 (healing) (necrosis of soft tissues through to underlying muscle, tendon, or bone)
      - ankle L89.5-
      - back L89.1-
      - buttock L89.3-
      - coccyx L89.15-
      - contiguous site of back, buttock, hip L89.4-
      - elbow L89.Ø-
      - face L89.81-
      - head L89.81-
      - heel L89.6-
      - hip L89.2-
      - sacral region (tailbone) L89.15-
      - specified site NEC L89.89-
    - unspecified stage
      - ankle L89.5-
      - back L89.1-
      - buttock L89.3-
      - coccyx L89.15-
      - contiguous site of back, buttock, hip L89.4-
      - elbow L89.Ø-
      - face L89.81-
      - head L89.81-
      - heel L89.6-
      - hip L89.2-
      - sacral region (tailbone) L89.15-
      - specified site NEC L89.89-
    - unstageable
      - ankle L89.5-
      - back L89.1-
      - buttock L89.3-
      - coccyx L89.15-
      - contiguous site of back, buttock, hip L89.4-
      - elbow L89.Ø-
      - face L89.81-
      - head L89.81-
      - heel L89.6-
      - hip L89.2-
      - sacral region (tailbone) L89.15-
      - specified site NEC L89.89-
  - primary of intestine K63.3
    - with perforation K63.1
  - prostate N41.9
  - pyloric — *see* Ulcer, stomach
  - rectosigmoid K63.3
    - with perforation K63.1
  - rectum (sphincter) (solitary) K62.6
    - stercoraceous, stercoral K62.6
  - retina — *see* Inflammation, chorioretinal
  - rodent (*see also* Neoplasm, skin, malignant)
  - sclera — *see* Scleritis
  - scrofulous (tuberculous) A18.2
  - scrotum N5Ø.8
    - tuberculous A18.15
    - varicose I86.1
  - seminal vesicle N5Ø.8
  - sigmoid — *see* Ulcer, intestine
  - skin (atrophic) (chronic) (neurogenic) (non-healing) (perforating) (pyogenic) (trophic) (tropical) L98.499
    - with gangrene — *see* Gangrene
    - amebic AØ6.7
    - back — *see* Ulcer, back
    - buttock — *see* Ulcer, buttock
    - decubitus — *see* Ulcer, pressure
    - lower limb — *see* Ulcer, lower limb
    - mycobacterial A31.1
    - specified site NEC L98.499
      - with
        - bone necrosis L98.494
        - exposed fat layer L98.492
        - muscle necrosis L98.493
        - skin breakdown only L98.491
    - tuberculous (primary) A18.4
    - varicose — *see* Ulcer, varicose
  - sloughing — *see* Ulcer, skin
  - solitary, anus or rectum (sphincter) K62.6
  - sore throat JØ2.9

- **Ulcer** — *continued*
  - sore throat — *continued*
    - streptococcal JØ2.Ø
  - spermatic cord N5Ø.8
  - spine (tuberculous) A18.Ø1
  - stasis (venous) — *see* Varix, leg, with, ulcer
    - without varicose veins I87.2
  - stercoraceous, stercoral K63.3
    - with perforation K63.1
    - anus or rectum K62.6
  - stoma, stomal — *see* Ulcer, gastrojejunal
  - stomach (eroded) (peptic) (round) K25.9
    - with
      - hemorrhage K25.4
        - and perforation K25.6
      - perforation K25.5
    - acute K25.3
      - with
        - hemorrhage K25.Ø
          - and perforation K25.2
        - perforation K25.1
    - chronic K25.7
      - with
        - hemorrhage K25.4
          - and perforation K25.6
        - perforation K25.5
  - stomal — *see* Ulcer, gastrojejunal
  - stomatitis K12.1
  - stress — *see* Ulcer, peptic
  - strumous (tuberculous) A18.2
  - submucosal, bladder — *see* Cystitis, interstitial
  - syphilitic (any site) (early) (secondary) A51.39
    - late A52.79
    - perforating A52.79
      - foot A52.11
  - testis N5Ø.8
  - thigh — *see* Ulcer, lower limb
  - throat J39.2
    - diphtheritic A36.Ø
  - toe — *see* Ulcer, lower limb
  - tongue (traumatic) K14.Ø
  - tonsil J35.8
    - diphtheritic A36.Ø
  - trachea J39.8
  - trophic — *see* Ulcer, skin
  - tropical — *see* Ulcer, skin
  - tuberculous — *see* Tuberculosis, ulcer
  - tunica vaginalis N5Ø.8
  - turbinate J34.89
  - typhoid (perforating) — *see* Typhoid
  - unspecified site — *see* Ulcer, skin
  - urethra (meatus) — *see* Urethritis
  - uterus N85.8
    - cervix N86
      - with cervicitis N72
    - neck N86
      - with cervicitis N72
  - vagina N76.5
    - in Behçet's disease M35.2 *[N77.0]*
    - pessary N89.8
  - valve, heart I33.Ø
  - varicose (lower limb, any part) (*see also* Varix, leg, with, ulcer)
    - broad ligament I86.2
    - esophagus — *see* Varix, esophagus
    - inflamed or infected — *see* Varix, leg, with ulcer, with inflammation
    - nasal septum I86.8
    - perineum I86.3
    - scrotum I86.1
    - specified site NEC I86.8
    - sublingual I86.Ø
    - vulva I86.3
  - vas deferens N5Ø.8
  - vulva (acute) (infectional) N76.6
    - in (due to)
      - Behçet's disease M35.2 *[N77.0]*
      - herpesviral (herpes simplex) infection A6Ø.Ø4
      - tuberculosis A18.18
  - vulvobuccal, recurring N76.6
  - X-ray L58.1
  - yaws A66.4
- **Ulcerosa scarlatina** A38.8

- **Urinemia** — *see* Uremia
- **Urinoma, urethra** N36.8
- **Uroarthritis, infectious** (Reiter's) — *see* Reiter's disease
- **Urodialysis** R34
- **Urolithiasis** — *see* Calculus, urinary
- **Uronephrosis** — *see* Hydronephrosis
- **Uropathy** N39.9
  - obstructive N13.9
    - specified NEC N13.8
  - reflux N13.9
    - specified NEC N13.8
  - vesicoureteral reflux-associated — *see* Reflux, vesicoureteral
- **Urosepsis** — code to condition
- **Urticaria** L50.9
  - with angioneurotic edema T78.3
    - hereditary D84.1
  - allergic L50.0
  - cholinergic L50.5
  - chronic L50.8
  - cold, familial L50.2
  - contact L50.6
  - dermatographic L50.3
  - due to
    - cold or heat L50.2
    - drugs L50.0
    - food L50.0
    - inhalants L50.0
    - plants L50.6
    - serum (*see also* Reaction, serum) T80.69
  - factitial L50.3
  - giant T78.3
    - hereditary D84.1
  - gigantea T78.3
  - idiopathic L50.1
  - larynx T78.3
    - hereditary D84.1
  - neonatorum P83.8
  - nonallergic L50.1
  - papulosa (Hebra) L28.2
  - pigmentosa Q82.2
  - recurrent periodic L50.8
  - serum (*see also* Reaction, serum) T80.69
  - solar L56.3
  - specified type NEC L50.8
  - thermal (cold) (heat) L50.2
  - vibratory L50.4
  - xanthelasmoidea Q82.2
- **Use** (of)
  - alcohol F10.99
    - with sleep disorder F10.982
    - harmful — *see* Abuse, alcohol
  - amphetamines — *see* Use, stimulant NEC
  - caffeine — *see* Use, stimulant NEC
  - cannabis F12.90
    - with
      - anxiety disorder F12.980
      - intoxication F12.929
        - with
          - delirium F12.921
          - perceptual disturbance F12.922
        - uncomplicated F12.920
      - other specified disorder F12.988
      - psychosis F12.959
        - delusions F12.950
        - hallucinations F12.951
      - unspecified disorder F12.99
  - cocaine F14.90
    - with
      - anxiety disorder F14.980
      - intoxication F14.929
        - with
          - delirium F14.921
          - perceptual disturbance F14.922
        - uncomplicated F14.920
      - other specified disorder F14.988
      - psychosis F14.959
        - delusions F14.950
        - hallucinations F14.951
      - sexual dysfunction F14.981
      - sleep disorder F14.982
      - unspecifed disorder F14.99

- **Use** (of) — *continued*
  - cocaine — *continued*
    - harmful — *see* Abuse, drug, cocaine
  - drug(s) NEC F19.90
    - with sleep disorder F19.982
    - harmful — *see* Abuse, drug, by type
  - hallucinogen NEC F16.90
    - with
      - anxiety disorder F16.980
      - intoxication F16.929
        - with
          - delirium F16.921
        - uncomplicated F16.920
      - mood disorder F16.94
      - other specified disorder F16.988
      - perception disorder (flashbacks) F16.983
      - psychosis F16.959
        - delusion(s) F16.950
        - hallucinations F16.951
      - unspecified disorder F16.99
    - harmful — *see* Abuse, drug, hallucinogen NEC
  - inhalants F18.90
    - with
      - anxiety disorder F18.980
      - intoxication F18.929
        - with delirium F18.921
        - uncomplicated F18.920
      - mood disorder F18.94
      - other specified disorder F18.988
      - persisting dementia F18.97
      - psychosis F18.959
        - delusions F18.950
        - hallucinations F18.951
      - unspecified disorder F18.99
    - harmful — *see* Abuse, drug, inhalant
  - methadone F11.20
  - nonprescribed drugs F19.90
    - harmful — *see* Abuse, non-psychoactive substance
  - opioid F11.90
    - with
      - disorder F11.99
        - mood F11.94
        - sleep F11.982
        - specified type NEC F11.988
      - intoxication F11.929
        - with
          - delirium F11.921
          - perceptual disturbance F11.922
        - uncomplicated F11.920
      - withdrawal F11.93
    - harmful — *see* Abuse, drug, opioid
  - patent medicines F19.90
    - harmful — *see* Abuse, non-psychoactive substance
  - psychoactive drug NEC F19.90
    - with
      - anxiety disorder F19.980
      - intoxication F19.929
        - with
          - delirium F19.921
          - perceptual disturbance F19.922
        - uncomplicated F19.920
      - mood disorder F19.94
      - other specifed disorder F19.988
      - persisting
        - amnestic disorder F19.96
        - dementia F19.97
      - psychosis F19.959
        - delusions F19.950
        - hallucinations F19.951
      - sexual dysfunction F19.981
      - sleep disorder F19.982
      - unspecified disorder F19.99
      - withdrawal F19.939
        - with
          - delirium F19.931
          - perceptual disturbance F19.932
        - uncomplicated F19.930
    - with sleep disorder F19.982
    - harmful — *see* Abuse, drug NEC, psychoactive NEC

- **Use** (of) — *continued*
  - sedative, hypnotic, or anxiolytic F13.90
    - with
      - anxiety disorder F13.980
      - intoxication F13.929
        - with
          - delirium F13.921
        - uncomplicated F13.920
      - other specified disorder F13.988
      - persisting
        - amnestic disorder F13.96
          - dementia F13.97
        - psychosis F13.959
          - delusions F13.950
          - hallucinations F13.951
        - sexual dysfunction F13.981
        - sleep disorder F13.982
        - unspecified disorder F13.99
    - harmful — *see* Abuse, drug, sedative, hypnotic, or anxiolytic
  - stimulant NEC F15.90
    - with
      - anxiety disorder F15.980
      - intoxication F15.929
        - with
          - delirium F15.921
          - perceptual disturbance F15.922
        - uncomplicated F15.920
      - mood disorder F19.94
      - other specified disorder F15.988
      - psychosis F15.959
        - delusions F15.950
        - hallucinations F15.951
      - sexual dysfunction F15.982
      - sleep disorder F15.982
      - unspecified disorder F15.99
      - withdrawal F15.93
    - harmful — *see* Abuse, drug, stimulant NEC
  - tobacco Z72.0
  - volatile solvents (*see also* Use, inhalant F18.90
    - harmful — *see* Abuse, drug, inhalant
  - tobacco Z72.0
- **Usher-Senear disease or syndrome** L10.4
- **Uta** B55.1
- **Uteromegaly** N85.2
- **Uterovaginal** — *see* condition
- **Uterovesical** — *see* condition
- **Uveal** — *see* condition
- **Uveitis** (anterior) (*see also* Iridocyclitis
  - acute) — *see* Iridocyclitis, acute
  - chronic — *see* Iridocyclitis, chronic
  - due to toxoplasmosis (acquired) B58.09
    - congenital P37.1
  - granulomatous — *see* Iridocyclitis, chronic
  - heterochromic — *see* Cyclitis, Fuchs' heterochromic
  - lens-induced — *see* Iridocyclitis, lens-induced
  - posterior — *see* Chorioretinitis
  - sympathetic H44.13-
  - syphilitic (secondary) A51.43
    - congenital (early) A50.01
    - late A52.71
  - tuberculous A18.54
- **Uveoencephalitis** — *see* Inflammation, chorioretinal
- **Uveokeratitis** — *see* Iridocyclitis
- **Uveoparotitis** D86.89
- **Uvula** — *see* condition
- **Uvulitis** (acute) (catarrhal) (chronic) (membranous) (suppurative) (ulcerative) K12.2

V

W

Weak, weakening, weakness — *continued*
- facial — *continued*
  - following — *continued*
    - cerebrovascular disease — *continued*
      - subarachnoid hemorrhage I69.Ø92
- foot (double) — *see* Weak, arches
- heart, cardiac — *see* Failure, heart
- mind F7Ø
- muscle M62.81
- myocardium — *see* Failure, heart
- newborn P96.89
- pelvic fundus N81.89
- pubocervical tissue N81.82
- senile R54
- rectovaginal tissue N81.83
- urinary stream R39.12
- valvular — *see* Endocarditis

Wear, worn (with normal or routine use)
- articular bearing surface of internal joint prosthesis — *see* Complications, joint prosthesis, mechanical, wear of articular bearing surfaces, by site
- device, implant or graft — *see* Complications, by site, mechanical complication
- tooth, teeth (approximal) (hard tissues) (interproximal) (occlusal) KØ3.Ø

Weather, weathered
- effects of
  - cold T69.9
    - specified effect NEC T69.8
  - hot — *see* Heat
- skin L57.8

Weaver's syndrome Q87.3
Web, webbed (congenital)
- duodenal Q43.8
- esophagus Q39.4
- fingers Q7Ø.1
- larynx (glottic) (subglottic) Q31.Ø
- neck (pterygium colli) Q18.3
- Paterson-Kelly D5Ø.1
- popliteal syndrome Q87.89
- toes Q7Ø.3-

Weber-Christian disease M35.6
Weber-Cockayne syndrome (epidermolysis bullosa) Q81.8
Weber-Gubler syndrome G46.3
Weber-Leyden syndrome G46.3
Weber-Osler syndrome I78.0
Weber's paralysis or syndrome G46.3
Wedge-shaped or wedging vertebra — *see* Collapse, vertebra NEC
Wegener's granulomatosis or syndrome M31.30
- with
  - kidney involvement M31.31
  - lung involvement M31.3Ø
    - with kidney involvement M31.31

Wegner's disease A50.02
Weight
- 1ØØØ-2499 grams at birth (low) — *see* Low, birthweight
- 999 grams or less at birth (extremely low) — *see* Low, birthweight, extreme
- gain (abnormal) (excessive) R63.5
  - in pregnancy — *see* Pregnancy, complicated by, excessive weight gain
    - low — *see* Pregnancy, complicated by, insufficient, weight gain
- loss (abnormal) (cause unknown) R63.4

Weightlessness (effect of) T75.82
Weil(l)**-Marchesani syndrome** Q87.1
Weil's disease A27.0
Weingarten's syndrome J82
Weir Mitchell's disease I73.81
Weiss-Baker syndrome G90.09
Wells' disease L98.3
Wen — *see* Cyst, sebaceous
Wenckebach's block or phenomenon I44.1
Werdnig-Hoffmann syndrome (muscular atrophy) G12.Ø
Werlhof's disease D69.3
Wermer's disease or syndrome E31.21
Werner-His disease A79.0
Werner's disease or syndrome E34.8
Wernicke-Korsakoff's syndrome or psychosis (alcoholic) F10.96
- with dependence F1Ø.26 drug-induced
  - due to drug abuse — *see* Abuse, drug, by type, with amnestic disorder
  - due to drug dependence — *see* Dependence, drug, by type, with amnestic disorder
- nonalcoholic FØ4

Wernicke-Posadas disease B38.9
Wernicke's
- developmental aphasia F8Ø.2
- disease or syndrome E51.2
- encephalopathy E51.2
- polioencephalitis, superior E51.2

West African fever B50.8
Westphal-Strümpell syndrome E83.01
West's syndrome — *see* Epilepsy, spasms
Wet
- feet, tropical (maceration) (syndrome) — *see* Immersion, foot
- lung (syndrome), newborn P22.1

Wharton's duct — *see* condition
Wheal — *see* Urticaria
Wheezing R06.2
Whiplash injury S13.4
Whipple's disease (*see also* subcategory) M14.8- K9Ø.81
Whipworm (disease) (infection) (infestation) B79
Whistling face Q87.0
White (*see also* condition)
- kidney, small NØ3.9
- leg, puerperal, postpartum, childbirth O87.1
- mouth B37.Ø
- patches of mouth K13.29
- spot lesions, teeth
  - chewing surface KØ2.51
  - pit and fissure surface KØ2.51
  - smooth surface KØ2.61

Whitehead L70.0
Whitlow (*see also* Cellulitis, digit)
- with lymphangitis — *see* Lymphangitis, acute, digit
- herpesviral BØØ.89

Whitmore's disease or fever — *see* Melioidosis
Whooping cough A37.90
- with pneumonia A37.91
  - due to Bordetella
    - bronchiseptica A37.81
    - parapertussis A37.11
    - pertussis A37.Ø1
  - specified organism NEC A37.81
- due to
  - Bordetella
    - bronchiseptica A37.8Ø
      - with pneumonia A37.81
    - parapertussis A37.1Ø
      - with pneumonia A37.11
    - pertussis A37.ØØ
      - with pneumonia A37.Ø1
    - specified NEC A37.8Ø
      - with pneumonia A37.81

Wichman's asthma J38.5
Wide cranial sutures, newborn P96.3
Widening aorta — *see* Ectasia, aorta
- with aneurysm — *see* Aneurysm, aorta

Wilkie's disease or syndrome K55.1
Wilkinson-Sneddon disease or syndrome L13.1
Willebrand (-Jürgens) **thrombopathy** D68.Ø
Willige-Hunt disease or syndrome G23.1
Wilms' tumor C64-
Wilson-Mikity syndrome P27.0
Wilson's
- disease or syndrome E83.Ø1
- hepatolenticular degeneration E83.Ø1
- lichen ruber L43.9

Window (*see also* Imperfect, closure)
- aorticopulmonary Q21.4

Winter — *see* condition
Wiskott-Aldrich syndrome D82.0
Withdrawal state (*see also* Dependence, drug by type, with withdrawal)
- newborn
  - correct therapeutic substance properly administered P96.2
  - infant of dependent mother P96.1
- therapeutic substance, neonatal P96.2

Witts' anemia D50.8
Witzelsucht F07.0
Woakes' ethmoiditis or syndrome J33.1
Wolff-Hirschorn syndrome Q93.3
Wolff-Parkinson-White syndrome I45.6
Wolhynian fever A79.0
Wolman's disease E75.5
Wood lung or pneumonitis J67.8
Woolly, wooly hair (congenital) (nevus) Q84.1
Woolsorter's disease A22.1
Word
- blindness (congenital) (developmental) F81.Ø
- deafness (congenital) (developmental) H93.25

Worm(s) (infection) (infestation) (*see also* Infestation, helminth)
- guinea B72
- in intestine NEC B82.Ø

Worm-eaten soles A66.3
Worn out (*see also* Exhaustion)
- cardiac
  - defibrillator (with synchronous cardiace pacemaker) Z45.Ø2
  - pacemaker
    - battery Z45.Ø1Ø
    - lead Z45.Ø18
- device, implant or graft — *see* Complications, by site, mechanical

Worried well Z71.1
Worries R45.82
Wound, open
- abdomen, abdominal
  - wall S31.1Ø9
    - with penetration into peritoneal cavity S31.6Ø9
    - bite — *see* Bite, abdomen, wall
    - epigastric region S31.1Ø2
      - with penetration into peritoneal cavity S31.6Ø2
      - bite — *see* Bite, abdomen, wall, epigastric region
      - laceration — *see* Laceration, abdomen, wall, epigastric region
      - puncture — *see* Puncture, abdomen, wall, epigastric region
    - laceration — *see* Laceration, abdomen, wall
    - left
      - lower quadrant S31.1Ø4
        - with penetration into peritoneal cavity S31.6Ø4
        - bite — *see* Bite, abdomen, wall, left, lower quadrant
        - laceration — *see* Laceration, abdomen, wall, left, lower quadrant
        - puncture — *see* Puncture, abdomen, wall, left, lower quadrant
      - upper quadrant S31.1Ø1
        - with penetration into peritoneal cavity S31.6Ø1
        - bite — *see* Bite, abdomen, wall, left, upper quadrant
        - laceration — *see* Laceration, abdomen, wall, left, upper quadrant
        - puncture — *see* Puncture, abdomen, wall, left, upper quadrant
    - periumbilic region S31.1Ø5
      - with penetration into peritoneal cavity S31.6Ø5
      - bite — *see* Bite, abdomen, wall, periumbilic region
      - laceration — *see* Laceration, abdomen, wall, periumbilic region
      - puncture — *see* Puncture, abdomen, wall, periumbilic region
    - puncture — *see* Puncture, abdomen, wall
    - right
      - lower quadrant S31.1Ø3

X

Y

Z

ICD-1Ø-CM Neoplasm Table

Notes—

The list below gives the code numbers for neoplasms by anatomical site. For each site there are six possible code numbers according to whether the neoplasm in question is malignant, benign, in situ, of uncertain behavior, or of unspecified nature. The description of the neoplasm will often indicate which of the six columns is appropriate; e.g., malignant melanoma of skin, benign fibroadenoma of breast, carcinoma in situ of cervix uteri.

Where such descriptors are not present, the remainder of the Index should be consulted where guidance is given to the appropriate column for each morphological (histological) variety listed; e.g., Mesonephroma — *see* Neoplasm, malignant; Embryoma (*see also* Neoplasm, uncertain behavior); Disease, Bowen's — *see* Neoplasm, skin, in situ. However, the guidance in the Index can be overridden if one of the descriptors mentioned above is present; e.g., malignant adenoma of colon is coded to C18.9 and not to D12.6 as the adjective "malignant" overrides the Index entry "Adenoma (*see also* Neoplasm, benign)."

Codes listed with a dash -, following the code have a required 5th character for laterality. The tablular list must be reviewed for the complete code.

	Malignant Primary	Malignant Secondary	Ca in situ	Benign	Uncertain Behavior	Unspecified Behavior
Neoplasm, neoplastic	C8Ø.1	C79.9	DØ9.9	D36.9	D48.9	D49.9
abdomen, abdominal	C76.2	C79.8-	DØ9.8	D36.7	D48.7	D49.89
cavity	C76.2	C79.8-	DØ9.8	D36.7	D48.7	D49.89
organ	C76.2	C79.8-	DØ9.8	D36.7	D48.7	D49.89
viscera	C76.2	C79.8-	DØ9.8	D36.7	D48.7	D49.89
wall (*see also* Neoplasm, abdomen, wall, skin)	C44.5Ø9	C79.2	DØ4.5	D23.5	D48.5	D49.2
connective tissue	C49.4	C79.8-	—	D21.4	D48.1	D49.2
skin	C44.5Ø9					
basal cell carcinoma	C44.519	—	—	—	—	—
specified type NEC	C44.599	—	—	—	—	—
squamous cell carcinoma	C44.529	—	—	—	—	—
abdominopelvic	C76.8	C79.8-	—	D36.7	D48.7	D49.89
accessory sinus — *see* Neoplasm, sinus						
acoustic nerve	C72.4-	C79.49	—	D33.3	D43.3	D49.7
adenoid (pharynx) (tissue)	C11.1	C79.89	DØØ.Ø8	D1Ø.6	D37.Ø5	D49.Ø
adipose tissue (*see also* Neoplasm, connective tissue)	C49.4	C79.89	—	D21.9	D48.1	D49.2
adnexa (uterine)	C57.4	C79.89	DØ7.39	D28.7	D39.8	D49.5
adrenal	C74.9-	C79.7-	DØ9.3	D35.Ø-	D44.1-	D49.7
capsule	C74.9-	C79.7-	DØ9.3	D35.Ø-	D44.1-	D49.7
cortex	C74.Ø-	C79.7-	DØ9.3	D35.Ø-	D44.1-	D49.7
gland	C74.9-	C79.7-	DØ9.3	D35.Ø-	D44.1-	D49.7
medulla	C74.1-	C79.7-	DØ9.3	D35.Ø-	D44.1-	D49.7
ala nasi (external) (*see also* Neoplasm, skin, nose)	C44.3Ø1	C79.2	DØ4.39	D23.39	D48.5	D49.2
alimentary canal or tract NEC	C26.9	C78.8Ø	DØ1.9	D13.9	D37.9	D49.Ø
alveolar	CØ3.9	C79.89	DØØ.Ø3	D1Ø.39	D37.Ø9	D49.Ø
mucosa	CØ3.9	C79.89	DØØ.Ø3	D1Ø.39	D37.Ø9	D49.Ø
lower	CØ3.1	C79.89	DØØ.Ø3	D1Ø.39	D37.Ø9	D49.Ø
upper	CØ3.Ø	C79.89	DØØ.Ø3	D1Ø.39	D37.Ø9	D49.Ø
ridge or process	C41.1	C79.51	—	D16.5-	D48.Ø	D49.2
carcinoma	CØ3.9	C79.8-	—	—	—	—
lower	CØ3.1	C79.8-	—	—	—	—
upper	CØ3.Ø	C79.8-	—	—	—	—
lower	C41.1	C79.51	—	D16.5-	D48.Ø	D49.2
mucosa	CØ3.9	C79.89	DØØ.Ø3	D1Ø.39	D37.Ø9	D49.Ø
lower	CØ3.1	C79.89	DØØ.Ø3	D1Ø.39	D37.Ø9	D49.Ø
upper	CØ3.Ø	C79.89	DØØ.Ø3	D1Ø.39	D37.Ø9	D49.Ø
upper	C41.Ø	C79.51	—	D16.4-	D48.Ø	D49.2
sulcus	CØ6.1	C79.89	DØØ.Ø2	D1Ø.39	D37.Ø9	D49.Ø
alveolus	CØ3.9	C79.89	DØØ.Ø3	D1Ø.39	D37.Ø9	D49.Ø
lower	CØ3.1	C79.89	DØØ.Ø3	D1Ø.39	D37.Ø9	D49.Ø
upper	CØ3.Ø	C79.89	DØØ.Ø3	D1Ø.39	D37.Ø9	D49.Ø
ampulla of Vater	C24.1	C78.89	DØ1.5	D13.5	D37.6	D49.Ø
ankle NEC	C76.5-	C79.89	DØ4.7-	D36.7	D48.7	D49.89
anorectum, anorectal (junction)	C21.8	C78.5	DØ1.3	D12.9	D37.8	D49.Ø
antecubital fossa or space	C76.4-	C79.89	DØ4.6-	D36.7	D48.7	D49.89
antrum (Highmore) (maxillary)	C31.Ø	C78.39	DØ2.3	D14.Ø	D38.5	D49.1
pyloric	C16.3	C78.89	DØØ.2	D13.1	D37.1	D49.Ø
tympanicum	C3Ø.1	C78.39	DØ2.3	D14.Ø	D38.5	D49.1
anus, anal	C21.Ø	C78.5	DØ1.3	D12.9	D37.8	D49.Ø
canal	C21.1	C78.5	DØ1.3	D12.9	D37.8	D49.Ø
cloacogenic zone	C21.2	C78.5	DØ1.3	D12.9	D37.8	D49.Ø

	Malignant Primary	Malignant Secondary	Ca in situ	Benign	Uncertain Behavior	Unspecified Behavior
Neoplasm, neoplastic — *continued*						
anus, anal — *continued*						
margin (*see also* Neoplasm, anus, skin)	C44.5ØØ	C79.2	DØ4.5	D23.5	D48.5	D49.2
overlapping lesion with rectosigmoid junction or rectum	C21.8	—	—	—	—	—
skin	C44.5ØØ	C79.2	DØ4.5	D23.5	D48.5	D49.2
basal cell carcinoma	C44.51Ø	—	—	—	—	—
specified type NEC	C44.59Ø	—	—	—	—	—
squamous cell carcinoma	C44.52Ø	—	—	—	—	—
sphincter	C21.1	C78.5	DØ1.3	D12.9	D37.8	D49.Ø
aorta (thoracic)	C49.3	C79.89	—	D21.3	D48.1	D49.2
abdominal	C49.4	C79.89	—	D21.4	D48.1	D49.2
aortic body	C75.5	C79.89	—	D35.6	D44.7	D49.7
aponeurosis	C49.9	C79.89	—	D21.9	D48.1	D49.2
palmar	C49.1-	C79.89	—	D21.1-	D48.1	D49.2
plantar	C49.2-	C79.89	—	D21.2-	D48.1	D49.2
appendix	C18.1	C78.5	DØ1.Ø	D12.1	D37.3	D49.Ø
arachnoid	C7Ø.9	C79.49	—	D32.9	D42.9	D49.7
cerebral	C7Ø.Ø	C79.32	—	D32.Ø	D42.Ø	D49.7
spinal	C7Ø.1	C79.49	—	D32.1	D42.1	D49.7
areola	C5Ø.Ø-	C79.81	DØ5.-	D24.-	D48.6-	D49.3
arm NEC	C76.4-	C79.89	DØ4.6-	D36.7	D48.7	D49.89
artery — *see* Neoplasm, connective tissue						
aryepiglottic fold	C13.1	C79.89	DØØ.Ø8	D1Ø.7	D37.Ø5	D49.Ø
hypopharyngeal aspect	C13.1	C79.89	DØØ.Ø8	D1Ø.7	D37.Ø5	D49.Ø
laryngeal aspect	C32.1	C78.39	DØ2.Ø	D14.1	D38.Ø	D49.1
marginal zone	C13.1	C79.89	DØØ.Ø8	D1Ø.7	D37.Ø5	D49.Ø
arytenoid (cartilage)	C32.3	C78.39	DØ2.Ø	D14.1	D38.Ø	D49.1
fold — *see* Neoplasm, aryepiglottic						
associated with transplanted organ	C8Ø.2	—	—	—	—	—
atlas	C41.2	C79.51	—	D16.6-	D48.Ø	D49.2
atrium, cardiac	C38.Ø	C79.89	—	D15.1	D48.7	D49.89
auditory						
canal (external) (skin) A81	C44.2Ø-	C79.2	DØ4.2-	D23.2-	D48.5	D49.2
internal	C3Ø.1	C78.39	DØ2.3	D14.Ø	D38.5	D49.1
nerve	C72.4-	C79.49	—	D33.3	D43.3	D49.7
tube	C3Ø.1	C78.39	DØ2.3	D14.Ø	D38.5	D49.1
opening	C11.2	C79.89	DØØ.Ø8	D1Ø.6	D37.Ø5	D49.Ø
auricle, ear (*see also* Neoplasm, skin, ear)	C44.2Ø-	C79.2	DØ4.2-	D23.2-	D48.5	D49.2
auricular canal (external) (*see also* Neoplasm, skin, ear)	C44.2Ø-	C79.2	DØ4.2-	D23.2-	D48.5	D49.2
internal	C3Ø.1	C78.39	DØ2.3	D14.Ø	D38.5	D49.2
autonomic nerve or nervous system NEC — *see* Neoplasm, nerve, peripheral						
axilla, axillary	C76.1	C79.89	DØ9.8	D36.7	D48.7	D49.89
fold (*see also* Neoplasm, skin, trunk)	C44.5Ø9	C79.2	DØ4.5	D23.5	D48.5	D49.2
back NEC	C76.8	C79.89	DØ4.5	D36.7	D48.7	D49.89
Bartholin's gland	C51.Ø	C79.82	DØ7.1	D28.Ø	D39.8	D49.5
basal ganglia	C71.Ø	C79.31	—	D33.Ø	D43.Ø	D49.6
basis pedunculi	C71.7	C79.31	—	D33.1	D43.1	D49.6
bile or biliary (tract)	C24.9	C78.89	DØ1.5	D13.5	D37.6	D49.Ø
canaliculi (biliferi) (intrahepatic)	C22.1	C78.7	DØ1.5	D13.4	D37.6	D49.Ø
canals, interlobular	C22.1	C78.89	DØ1.5	D13.4	D37.6	D49.Ø
duct or passage (common) (cystic) (extrahepatic)	C24.Ø	C78.89	DØ1.5	D13.5	D37.6	D49.Ø
interlobular	C22.1	C78.89	DØ1.5	D13.4	D37.6	D49.Ø
intrahepatic	C22.1	C78.7	DØ1.5	D13.4	D37.6	D49.Ø
and extrahepatic	C24.8	C78.89	DØ1.5	D13.5	D37.6	D49.Ø
bladder (urinary)	C67.9	C79.11	DØ9.Ø	D3Ø.3	D41.4	D49.4
dome	C67.1	C79.11	DØ9.Ø	D3Ø.3	D41.4	D49.4
neck	C67.5	C79.11	DØ9.Ø	D3Ø.3	D41.4	D49.4
orifice	C67.9	C79.11	DØ9.Ø	D3Ø.3	D41.4	D49.4

	Malignant Primary	Malignant Secondary	Ca in situ	Benign	Uncertain Behavior	Unspecified Behavior
Neoplasm, neoplastic — *continued*						
bladder — *continued*						
orifice — *continued*						
ureteric	C67.6	C79.11	D09.0	D30.3	D41.4	D49.4
urethral	C67.5	C79.11	D09.0	D30.3	D41.4	D49.4
overlapping lesion	C67.8	—	—	—	—	—
sphincter	C67.8	C79.11	D09.0	D30.3	D41.4	D49.4
trigone	C67.0	C79.11	D09.0	D30.3	D41.4	D49.4
urachus	C67.7	C79.11	D09.0	D30.3	D41.4	D49.4
wall	C67.9	C79.11	D09.0	D30.3	D41.4	D49.4
anterior	C67.3	C79.11	D09.0	D30.3	D41.4	D49.4
lateral	C67.2	C79.11	D09.0	D30.3	D41.4	D49.4
posterior	C67.4	C79.11	D09.0	D30.3	D41.4	D49.4
blood vessel — *see* Neoplasm, connective tissue						
bone (periosteum)	C41.9	C79.51	—	D16.9-	D48.0	D49.2
acetabulum	C41.4	C79.51	—	D16.8-	D48.0	D49.2
ankle	C40.3-	C79.51	—	D16.3-	—	—
arm NEC	C40.0-	C79.51	—	D16.0-	—	—
astragalus	C40.3-	C79.51	—	D16.3-	—	—
atlas	C41.2	C79.51	—	D16.6-	D48.0	D49.2
axis	C41.2	C79.51	—	D16.6-	D48.0	D49.2
back NEC	C41.2	C79.51	—	D16.6-	D48.0	D49.2
calcaneus	C40.3-	C79.51	—	D16.3-	—	—
calvarium	C41.0	C79.51	—	D16.4-	D48.0	D49.2
carpus (any)	C40.1-	C79.51	—	D16.1-	—	—
cartilage NEC	C41.9	C79.51	—	D16.9-	D48.0	D49.2
clavicle	C41.3	C79.51	—	D16.7-	D48.0	D49.2
clivus	C41.0	C79.51	—	D16.4-	D48.0	D49.2
coccygeal vertebra	C41.4	C79.51	—	D16.8-	D48.0	D49.2
coccyx	C41.4	C79.51	—	D16.8-	D48.0	D49.2
costal cartilage	C41.3	C79.51	—	D16.7-	D48.0	D49.2
costovertebral joint	C41.3	C79.51	—	D16.7-	D48.0	D49.2
cranial	C41.0	C79.51	—	D16.4-	D48.0	D49.2
cuboid	C40.3	C79.51	—	D16.3-	—	—
cuneiform	C41.9	C79.51	—	D16.9-	D48.0	D49.2
elbow	C40.0-	C79.51	—	D16.0-	—	—
ethmoid (labyrinth)	C41.0	C79.51	—	D16.4-	D48.0	D49.2
face	C41.0	C79.51	—	D16.4-	D48.0	D49.2
femur (any part)	C40.2-	C79.51	—	D16.2-	—	—
fibula (any part)	C40.2-	C79.51	—	D16.2-	—	—
finger (any)	C40.1-	C79.51	—	D16.1-	—	—
foot	C40.3-	C79.51	—	D16.3-	—	—
forearm	C40.0-	C79.51	—	D16.0-	—	—
frontal	C41.0	C79.51	—	D16.4-	D48.0	D49.2
hand	C40.1	C79.51	—	D16.1-	—	—
heel	C40.3-	C79.51	—	D16.3-	—	—
hip	C41.4	C79.51	—	D16.8-	D48.0	D49.2
humerus (any part)	C40.0-	C79.51	—	D16.0-	—	—
hyoid	C41.0	C79.51	—	D16.4-	D48.0	D49.2
ilium	C41.4	C79.51	—	D16.8-	D48.0	D49.2
innominate	C41.4	C79.51	—	D16.8-	D48.0	D49.2
intervertebral cartilage or disc	C41.2	C79.51	—	D16.6-	D48.0	D49.2
ischium	C41.4	C79.51	—	D16.8-	D48.0	D49.2
jaw (lower)	C41.1	C79.51	—	D16.5-	D48.0	D49.2
knee	C40.2-	C79.51	—	D16.2-	—	—
leg NEC	C40.2-	C79.51	—	D16.2-	—	—
limb NEC	C40.9-	C79.51	—	D16.9-	—	—
lower (long bones)	C40.2-	C79.51	—	D16.2-	—	—
short bones	C40.3-	C79.51	—	D16.3-	—	—
upper (long bones)	C40.0-	C79.51	—	D16.0-	—	—
short bones	C40.1-	C79.51	—	D16.1-	—	—
malar	C41.0	C79.51	—	D16.4-	D48.0	D49.2
mandible	C41.1	C79.51	—	D16.5-	D48.0	D49.2
marrow NEC (any bone)	C96.9	C79.52	—	—	D47.9	D49.89
mastoid	C41.0	C79.51	—	D16.4-	D48.0	D49.2
maxilla, maxillary (superior)	C41.0	C79.51	—	D16.4-	D48.0	D49.2
inferior	C41.1	C79.51	—	D16.5-	D48.0	D49.2
metacarpus (any)	C40.1-	C79.51	—	D16.1-	—	—
metatarsus (any)	C40.3-	C79.51	—	D16.3-	—	—
overlapping sites	C40.8-	—	—	—	—	—
navicular			—	—	—	—
Neoplasm, neoplastic — *continued*						
bone — *continued*						
navicular — *continued*						
ankle	C40.3-	C79.51	—	—	—	—
hand	C40.1-	C79.51	—	—	—	—
nose, nasal	C41.0	C79.51	—	D16.4-	D48.0	D49.2
occipital	C41.0	C79.51	—	D16.4-	D48.0	D49.2
orbit	C41.0	C79.51	—	D16.4-	D48.0	D49.2
parietal	C41.0	C79.51	—	D16.4-	D48.0	D49.2
patella	C40.2-	C79.51	—	—	—	—
pelvic	C41.4	C79.51	—	D16.8-	D48.0	D49.2
phalanges			—			
foot	C40.3-	C79.51	—	—	—	—
hand	C40.1-	C79.51	—	—	—	—
pubic	C41.4	C79.51	—	D16.8-	D48.0	D49.2
radius (any part)	C40.0-	C79.51	—	D16.0-	—	—
rib	C41.3	C79.51	—	D16.7-	D48.0	D49.2
sacral vertebra	C41.4	C79.51	—	D16.8-	D48.0	D49.2
sacrum	C41.4	C79.51	—	D16.8-	D48.0	D49.2
scaphoid					—	—
of ankle	C40.3-	C79.51	—	—	—	—
of hand	C40.1-	C79.51	—	—	—	—
scapula (any part)	C40.0-	C79.51	—	D16.0-	—	—
sella turcica	C41.0	C79.51	—	D16.4-	D48.0	D49.2
shoulder	C40.0-	C79.51	—	D16.0-	—	—
skull	C41.0	C79.51	—	D16.4-	D48.0	D49.2
sphenoid	C41.0	C79.51	—	D16.4-	D48.0	D49.2
spine, spinal (column)	C41.2	C79.51	—	D16.6-	D48.0	D49.2
coccyx	C41.4	C79.51	—	D16.8-	D48.0	D49.2
sacrum	C41.4	C79.51	—	D16.8-	D48.0	D49.2
sternum	C41.3	C79.51	—	D16.7-	D48.0	D49.2
tarsus (any)	C40.3-	C79.51	—	—	—	—
temporal	C41.0	C79.51	—	D16.4-	D48.0	D49.2
thumb	C40.1-	C79.51	—	—	—	—
tibia (any part)	C40.2-	C79.51	—	—	—	—
toe (any)	C40.3-	C79.51	—	—	—	—
trapezium	C40.1-	C79.51	—	—	—	—
trapezoid	C40.1-	C79.51	—	—	—	—
turbinate	C41.0	C79.51	—	D16.4-	D48.0	D49.2
ulna (any part)	C40.0-	C79.51	—	D16.0-	—	—
unciform	C40.1-	C79.51	—	—	—	—
vertebra (column)	C41.2	C79.51	—	D16.6-	D48.0	D49.2
coccyx	C41.4	C79.51	—	D16.8-	D48.0	D49.2
sacrum	C41.4	C79.51	—	D16.8-	D48.0	D49.2
vomer	C41.0	C79.51	—	D16.4-	D48.0	D49.2
wrist	C40.1-	C79.51	—	—	—	—
xiphoid process	C41.3	C79.51	—	D16.7-	D48.0	D49.2
zygomatic	C41.0	C79.51	—	D16.4-	D48.0	D49.2
book-leaf (mouth) (ventral surface of tongue and floor of mouth)	C06.89	C79.89	D00.00	D10.39	D37.09	D49.0
bowel — *see* Neoplasm, intestine						
brachial plexus	C47.1-	C79.89	—	D36.12	D48.2	D49.2
brain NEC	C71.9	C79.31	—	D33.2	D43.2	D49.6
basal ganglia	C71.0	C79.31	—	D33.0	D43.0	D49.6
cerebellopontine angle	C71.6	C79.31	—	D33.1	D43.1	D49.6
cerebellum NOS	C71.6	C79.31	—	D33.1	D43.1	D49.6
cerebrum	C71.0	C79.31	—	D33.0	D43.0	D49.6
choroid plexus	C71.7	C79.31	—	D33.1	D43.1	D49.6
corpus callosum	C71.8	C79.31	—	D33.2	D43.2	D49.6
corpus striatum	C71.0	C79.31	—	D33.0	D43.0	D49.6
cortex (cerebral)	C71.0	C79.31	—	D33.0	D43.0	D49.6
frontal lobe	C71.1	C79.31	—	D33.0	D43.0	D49.6
globus pallidus	C71.0	C79.31	—	D33.0	D43.0	D49.6
hippocampus	C71.2	C79.31	—	D33.0	D43.0	D49.6
hypothalamus	C71.0	C79.31	—	D33.0	D43.0	D49.6
internal capsule	C71.0	C79.31	—	D33.0	D43.0	D49.6
medulla oblongata	C71.7	C79.31	—	D33.1	D43.1	D49.6
meninges	C70.0	C79.32	—	D32.0	D42.0	D49.7
midbrain	C71.7	C79.31	—	D33.1	D43.1	D49.6
occipital lobe	C71.4	C79.31	—	D33.0	D43.0	D49.6
overlapping lesion	C71.8	C79.31	—	—	—	—

	Malignant Primary	Malignant Secondary	Ca in situ	Benign	Uncertain Behavior	Unspecified Behavior
Neoplasm, neoplastic — *continued*						
brain NEC — *continued*						
parietal lobe	C71.3	C79.31	—	D33.Ø	D43.Ø	D49.6
peduncle	C71.7	C79.31	—	D33.1	D43.1	D49.6
pons	C71.7	C79.31	—	D33.1	D43.1	D49.6
stem	C71.7	C79.31	—	D33.1	D43.1	D49.6
tapetum	C71.8	C79.31	—	D33.2	D43.2	D49.6
temporal lobe	C71.2	C79.31	—	D33.Ø	D43.Ø	D49.6
thalamus	C71.Ø	C79.31	—	D33.Ø	D43.Ø	D49.6
uncus	C71.2	C79.31	—	D33.Ø	D43.Ø	D49.6
ventricle (floor)	C71.5	C79.31	—	D33.Ø	D43.Ø	D49.6
fourth	C71.7	C79.31	—	D33.1	D43.1	D49.6
branchial (cleft) (cyst) (vestiges)	C1Ø.4	C79.89	DØØ.Ø8	D1Ø.5	D37.Ø5	D49.Ø
breast (connective tissue) (glandular tissue) (soft parts)	C5Ø.9-	C79.81	DØ5.-	D24.-	D48.6-	D49.3
areola	C5Ø.Ø-	C79.81	DØ5.-	D24.-	D48.6-	D49.3
axillary tail	C5Ø.6-	C79.81	DØ5.-	D24.-	D48.6-	D49.3
central portion	C5Ø.1-	C79.81	DØ5.-	D24.-	D48.6-	D49.3
inner	C5Ø.8-	C79.81	DØ5.-	D24.-	D48.6-	D49.3
lower	C5Ø.8-	C79.81	DØ5.-	D24.-	D48.6-	D49.3
lower-inner quadrant	C5Ø.3	C79.81	DØ5.-	D24.-	D48.6-	D49.3
lower-outer quadrant	C5Ø.5-	C79.81	DØ5.-	D24.-	D48.6-	D49.3
mastectomy site (skin) (*see also* Neoplasm, breast, skin)	C44.5Ø1	C79.2	—	—	—	—
specified as breast tissue	C5Ø.8-	C79.81	—	—	—	—
midline	C5Ø.8-	C79.81	DØ5.-	D24.-	D48.6-	D49.3
nipple	C5Ø.Ø-	C79.81	DØ5.-	D24.-	D48.6-	D49.3
outer	C5Ø.8-	C79.81	DØ5.-	D24.-	D48.6-	D49.3
overlapping lesion	C5Ø.8-	—	—	—	—	—
skin	C44.5Ø1	C79.2	DØ4.5	D23.5	D48.5	D49.2
basal cell carcinoma	C44.511	—	—	—	—	—
specified type NEC	C44.591	—	—	—	—	—
squamous cell carcinoma	C44.521	—	—	—	—	—
tail (axillary)	C5Ø.6-	C79.81	DØ5.-	D24.-	D48.6-	D49.3
upper	C5Ø.8-	C79.81	DØ5.-	D24.-	D48.6-	D49.3
upper-inner quadrant	C5Ø.2-	C79.81	DØ5.-	D24.-	D48.6-	D49.3
upper-outer quadrant	C5Ø.4-	C79.81	DØ5.-	D24.-	D48.6-	D49.3
broad ligament	C57.1	C79.82	DØ7.39	D28.2	D39.8	D49.5
bronchiogenic, bronchogenic (lung)	C34.9-	C78.Ø-	DØ2.2-	D14.3-	D38.1	D49.1
bronchiole	C34.9-	C78.Ø-	DØ2.2-	D14.3-	D38.1	D49.1
bronchus	C34.9-	C78.Ø-	DØ2.2-	D14.3-	D38.1	D49.1
carina	C34.Ø-	C78.Ø-	DØ2.2-	D14.3-	D38.1	D49.1
lower lobe of lung	C34.3-	C78.Ø-	DØ2.2-	D14.3-	D38.1	D49.1
main	C34.Ø-	C78.Ø-	DØ2.2-	D14.3-	D38.1	D49.1
middle lobe of lung	C34.2	C78.Ø-	DØ2.21	D14.31	D38.1	D49.1
overlapping lesion	C34.8-	—	—	—	—	—
upper lobe of lung	C34.1-	C78.Ø-	DØ2.2-	D14.3-	D38.1	D49.1
brow	C44.3Ø9	C79.2	DØ4.39	D23.39	D48.5	D49.2
basal cell carcinoma	C44.319	—	—	—	—	—
specified type NEC	C44.399	—	—	—	—	—
squamous cell carcinoma	C44.329	—	—	—	—	—
buccal (cavity)	CØ6.9	C79.89	DØØ.ØØ	D1Ø.39	D37.Ø9	D49.Ø
commissure	CØ6.Ø	C79.89	DØØ.Ø2	D1Ø.39	D37.Ø9	D49.Ø
groove (lower) (upper)	CØ6.1	C79.89	DØØ.Ø2	D1Ø.39	D37.Ø9	D49.Ø
mucosa	CØ6.Ø	C79.89	DØØ.Ø2	D1Ø.39	D37.Ø9	D49.Ø
sulcus (lower) (upper)	CØ6.1	C79.89	DØØ.Ø2	D1Ø.39	D37.Ø9	D49.Ø
bulbourethral gland	C68.Ø	C79.19	DØ9.19	D3Ø.4	D41.3	D49.5
bursa — *see* Neoplasm, connective tissue						
buttock NEC	C76.3	C79.89	DØ4.5	D36.7	D48.7	D49.89
calf	C76.5-	C79.89	DØ4.7-	D36.7	D48.7	D49.89
calvarium	C41.Ø	C79.51	—	D16.4-	D48.Ø	D49.2
calyx, renal	C65.-	C79.Ø-	DØ9.19	D3Ø.1-	D41.1-	D49.5
canal						
anal	C21.1	C78.5	DØ1.3	D12.9	D37.8	D49.Ø
auditory (external) (*see also* Neoplasm, skin, ear)	C44.2Ø-	C79.2	DØ4.2-	D23.2-	D48.5	D49.2
auricular (external) (*see also* Neoplasm, skin, ear)	C44.2Ø-	C79.2	DØ4.2-	D23.2-	D48.5	D49.2
canaliculi, biliary (biliferi) (intrahepatic)	C22.1	C78.7	DØ1.5	D13.4	D37.6	D49.Ø

	Malignant Primary	Malignant Secondary	Ca in situ	Benign	Uncertain Behavior	Unspecified Behavior
Neoplasm, neoplastic — *continued*						
canthus (eye) (inner) (outer)	C44.1Ø-	C79.2	DØ4.1-	D23.1-	D48.5	D49.2
basal cell carcinoma	C44.11-	—	—	—	—	—
specified type NEC	C44.19-	—	—	—	—	—
squamous cell carcinoma	C44.12-	—	—	—	—	—
capillary — *see* Neoplasm, connective tissue						
caput coli	C18.Ø	C78.5	DØ1.Ø	D12.Ø	D37.4	D49.Ø
carcinoid *see* Tumor, carcinoid						
cardia (gastric)	C16.Ø	C78.89	DØØ.2	D13.1	D37.1	D49.Ø
cardiac orifice (stomach)	C16.Ø	C78.89	DØØ.2	D13.1	D37.1	D49.Ø
cardio-esophageal junction	C16.Ø	C78.89	DØØ.2	D13.1	D37.1	D49.Ø
cardio-esophagus	C16.Ø	C78.89	DØØ.2	D13.1	D37.1	D49.Ø
carina (bronchus)	C34.Ø-	C78.Ø-	DØ2.2-	D14.3-	D38.1	D49.1
carotid (artery)	C49.Ø	C79.89	—	D21.Ø	D48.1	D49.2
body	C75.4	C79.89	—	D35.5	D44.6-	D49.7
carpus (any bone)	C4Ø.1-	C79.51	—	D16.1-	—	—
cartilage (articular) (joint) NEC (*see also* Neoplasm, bone)	C41.9	C79.51	—	D16.9-	D48.Ø	D49.2
arytenoid	C32.3	C78.39	DØ2.Ø	D14.1	D38.Ø	D49.1
auricular	C49.Ø	C79.89	—	D21.Ø	D48.1	D49.2
bronchi	C34.Ø-	C78.39	—	D14.3-	D38.1	D49.1
costal	C41.3	C79.51	—	D16.7-	D48.Ø	D49.2
cricoid	C32.3	C78.39	DØ2.Ø	D14.1	D38.Ø	D49.1
cuneiform	C32.3	C78.39	DØ2.Ø	D14.1	D38.Ø	D49.1
ear (external)	C49.Ø	C79.89	—	D21.Ø	D48.1	D49.2
ensiform	C41.3	C79.51	—	D16.7-	D48.Ø	D49.2
epiglottis	C32.1	C78.39	DØ2.Ø	D14.1	D38.Ø	D49.1
anterior surface	C1Ø.1	C79.89	DØØ.Ø8	D1Ø.5	D37.Ø5	D49.Ø
eyelid	C49.Ø	C79.89	—	D21.Ø	D48.1	D49.2
intervertebral	C41.2	C79.51	—	D16.6-	D48.Ø	D49.2
larynx, laryngeal	C32.3	C78.39	DØ2.Ø	D14.1	D38.Ø	D49.1
nose, nasal	C3Ø.Ø	C78.39	DØ2.3	D14.Ø	D38.5	D49.1
pinna	C49.Ø	C79.89	—	D21.Ø	D48.1	D49.2
rib	C41.3	C79.51	—	D16.7-	D48.Ø	D49.2
semilunar (knee)	C4Ø.2-	C79.51	—	D16.2-	D48.Ø	D49.2
thyroid	C32.3	C78.39	DØ2.Ø	D14.1	D38.Ø	D49.1
trachea	C33	C78.39	DØ2.1	D14.2	D38.1	D49.1
cauda equina	C72.1	C79.49	—	D33.4	D43.4	D49.7
cavity						
buccal	CØ6.9	C79.89	DØØ.ØØ	D1Ø.3Ø	D37.Ø9	D49.Ø
nasal	C3Ø.Ø	C78.39	DØ2.3	D14.Ø	D38.5	D49.1
oral	CØ6.9	C79.89	DØØ.ØØ	D1Ø.3Ø	D37.Ø9	D49.Ø
peritoneal	C48.2	C78.6	—	D2Ø.1	D48.4	D49.Ø
tympanic	C3Ø.1	C78.39	DØ2.3	D14.Ø	D38.5	D49.1
cecum	C18.Ø	C78.5	DØ1.Ø	D12.Ø	D37.4	D49.Ø
central nervous system	C72.9	C79.4Ø	—	—	—	—
cerebellopontine (angle)	C71.6	C79.31	—	D33.1	D43.1	D49.6
cerebellum, cerebellar	C71.6	C79.31	—	D33.1	D43.1	D49.6
cerebrum, cerebral (cortex) (hemisphere) (white matter)	C71.Ø	C79.31	—	D33.Ø	D43.Ø	D49.6
meninges	C7Ø.Ø	C79.32	—	D32.Ø	D42.Ø	D49.7
peduncle	C71.7	C79.31	—	D33.1	D43.1	D49.6
ventricle	C71.5	C79.31	—	D33.Ø	D43.Ø	D49.6
fourth	C71.7	C79.31	—	D33.1	D43.1	D49.6
cervical region	C76.Ø	C79.89	DØ9.8	D36.7	D48.7	D49.89
cervix (cervical) (uteri) (uterus)	C53.9	C79.82	DØ6.9	D26.Ø	D39.Ø	D49.5
canal	C53.Ø	C79.82	DØ6.Ø	D26.Ø	D39.Ø	D49.5
endocervix (canal) (gland)	C53.Ø	C79.82	DØ6.Ø	D26.Ø	D39.Ø	D49.5
exocervix	C53.1	C79.82	DØ6.1	D26.Ø	D39.Ø	D49.5
external os	C53.1	C79.82	DØ6.1	D26.Ø	D39.Ø	D49.5
internal os	C53.Ø	C79.82	DØ6.Ø	D26.Ø	D39.Ø	D49.5
nabothian gland	C53.Ø	C79.82	DØ6.Ø	D26.Ø	D39.Ø	D49.5
overlapping lesion	C53.8	—	—	—	—	—
squamocolumnar junction	C53.8	C79.82	DØ6.7	D26.Ø	D39.Ø	D49.5
stump	C53.8	C79.82	DØ6.7	D26.Ø	D39.Ø	D49.5
cheek	C76.Ø	C79.89	DØ9.8	D36.7	D48.7	D49.89
external	C44.3Ø9	C79.2	DØ4.39	D23.39	D48.5	D49.2
basal cell carcinoma	C44.319	—	—	—	—	—
specified type NEC	C44.399	—	—	—	—	—
squamous cell carcinoma	C44.329	—	—	—	—	—

	Malignant Primary	Malignant Secondary	Ca in situ	Benign	Uncertain Behavior	Unspecified Behavior
Neoplasm, neoplastic — *continued*						
cheek — *continued*						
inner aspect	C06.Ø	C79.89	DØØ.02	D1Ø.39	D37.Ø9	D49.Ø
internal	C06.Ø	C79.89	DØØ.02	D1Ø.39	D37.Ø9	D49.Ø
mucosa	C06.Ø	C79.89	DØØ.02	D1Ø.39	D37.Ø9	D49.Ø
chest (wall) NEC	C76.1	C79.89	DØ9.8	D36.7	D48.7	D49.89
chiasma opticum	C72.3-	C79.49	—	D33.3	D43.3	D49.7
chin	C44.309	C79.2	DØ4.39	D23.39	D48.5	D49.2
basal cell carcinoma	C44.319	—	—	—	—	—
specified type NEC	C44.399	—	—	—	—	—
squamous cell carcinoma	C44.329	—	—	—	—	—
choana	C11.3	C79.89	DØØ.Ø8	D1Ø.6	D37.Ø5	D49.Ø
cholangiole	C22.1	C78.89	DØ1.5	D13.4	D37.6	D49.Ø
choledochal duct	C24.Ø	C78.89	DØ1.5	D13.5	D37.6	D49.Ø
choroid	C69.3-	C79.49	DØ9.2-	D31.3-	D48.7	D49.81
plexus	C71.5	C79.31	—	D33.Ø	D43.Ø	D49.6
ciliary body	C69.4-	C79.49	DØ9.2-	D31.4-	D48.7	D49.89
clavicle	C41.3	C79.51	—	D16.7-	D48.Ø	D49.2
clitoris	C51.2	C79.82	DØ7.1	D28.Ø	D39.8	D49.5
clivus	C41.Ø	C79.51	—	D16.4-	D48.Ø	D49.2
cloacogenic zone	C21.2	C78.5	DØ1.3	D12.9	D37.8	D49.Ø
coccygeal						
body or glomus	C75.5	C79.89	—	D35.6	D44.7	D49.7
vertebra	C41.4	C79.51	—	D16.8-	D48.Ø	D49.2
coccyx	C41.4	C79.51	—	D16.8-	D48.Ø	D49.2
colon	C18.9	C78.5	—	—	—	—
with rectum	C19	C78.5	DØ1.1	D12.7	D37.5	D49.Ø
column, spinal — *see* Neoplasm, spine						
columnella (*see also* Neoplasm, skin, face)	C44.39Ø	C79.2	DØ4.39	D23.39	D48.5	D49.2
commissure						
labial, lip	CØØ.6	C79.89	DØØ.Ø1	D1Ø.39	D37.Ø1	D49.Ø
laryngeal	C32.Ø	C78.39	DØ2.Ø	D14.1	D38.Ø	D49.1
common (bile) duct	C24.Ø	C78.89	DØ1.5	D13.5	D37.6	D49.Ø
concha (*see also* Neoplasm, skin, ear)	C44.2Ø-	C79.2	DØ4.2-	D23.2-	D48.5	D49.2
nose	C3Ø.Ø	C78.39	DØ2.3	D14.Ø	D38.5	D49.1
conjunctiva	C69.Ø-	C79.49	DØ9.2-	D31.Ø	D48.7	D49.89

Note: For neoplasms of connective tissue (blood vessel, bursa, fascia, ligament, muscle, peripheral nerves, sympathetic and parasympathetic nerves and ganglia, synovia, tendon, etc.) or of morphological types that indicate connective tissue, code according to the list under "Neoplasm, connective tissue". For sites that do not appear in this list, code to neoplasm of that site; e.g., fibrosarcoma, pancreas (C25.9)

Note: Morphological types that indicate connective tissue appear in their proper place in the alphabetic index with the instruction "*see* Neoplasm, connective tissue ...."

	Malignant Primary	Malignant Secondary	Ca in situ	Benign	Uncertain Behavior	Unspecified Behavior
connective tissue NEC	C49.9	C79.89	—	D21.9	D48.1	D49.2
abdomen	C49.4	C79.89	—	D21.4	D48.1	D49.2
abdominal wall	C49.4	C79.89	—	D21.4	D48.1	D49.2
ankle	C49.2-	C79.89	—	D21.2-	D48.1	D49.2
antecubital fossa or space	C49.1-	C79.89	—	D21.1-	D48.1	D49.2
arm	C49.1-	C79.89	—	D21.1-	D48.1	D49.2
auricle (ear)	C49.Ø	C79.89	—	D21.Ø	D48.1	D49.2
axilla	C49.3	C79.89	—	D21.3	D48.1	D49.2
back	C49.6	C79.89	—	D21.6	D48.1	D49.2
breast — *see* Neoplasm, breast						
buttock	C49.5	C79.89	—	D21.5	D48.1	D49.2
calf	C49.2-	C79.89	—	D21.2-	D48.1	D49.2
cervical region	C49.Ø	C79.89	—	D21.Ø	D48.1	D49.2
cheek	C49.Ø	C79.89	—	D21.Ø	D48.1	D49.2
chest (wall)	C49.3	C79.89	—	D21.3	D48.1	D49.2
chin	C49.Ø	C79.89	—	D21.Ø	D48.1	D49.2
diaphragm	C49.3	C79.89	—	D21.3	D48.1	D49.2
ear (external)	C49.Ø	C79.89	—	D21.Ø	D48.1	D49.2
elbow	C49.1-	C79.89	—	D21.1-	D48.1	D49.2
extrarectal	C49.5	C79.89	—	D21.5	D48.1	D49.2
extremity	C49.9	C79.89	—	D21.9	D48.1	D49.2
lower	C49.2-	C79.89	—	D21.2-	D48.1	D49.2
upper	C49.1-	C79.89	—	D21.1-	D48.1	D49.2
eyelid	C49.Ø	C79.89	—	D21.Ø	D48.1	D49.2
face.	C49.Ø	C79.89	—	D21.Ø	D48.1	D49.2
finger	C49.1-	C79.89	—	D21.1-	D48.1	D49.2

	Malignant Primary	Malignant Secondary	Ca in situ	Benign	Uncertain Behavior	Unspecified Behavior
Neoplasm, neoplastic — *continued*						
connective tissue NEC — *continued*						
flank	C49.6	C79.89	—	D21.6	D48.1	D49.2
foot	C49.2-	C79.89	—	D21.2-	D48.1	D49.2
forearm	C49.1-	C79.89	—	D21.1-	D48.1	D49.2
forehead	C49.Ø	C79.89	—	D21.Ø	D48.1	D49.2
gastric	C49.4	C79.89	—	D21.4	D48.1	D49.2
gastrointestinal	C49.4	C79.89	—	D21.4	D48.1	D49.2
gluteal region	C49.5	C79.89	—	D21.5	D48.1	D49.2
great vessels NEC	C49.3	C79.89	—	D21.3	D48.1	D49.2
groin	C49.5	C79.89	—	D21.5	D48.1	D49.2
hand	C49.1-	C79.89	—	D21.1-	D48.1	D49.2
head	C49.Ø	C79.89	—	D21.Ø	D48.1	D49.2
heel	C49.2-	C79.89	—	D21.2-	D48.1	D49.2
hip	C49.2-	C79.89	—	D21.2-	D48.1	D49.2
hypochondrium	C49.4	C79.89	—	D21.4	D48.1	D49.2
iliopsoas muscle	C49.5	C79.89	—	D21.5	D48.1	D49.2
infraclavicular region	C49.3	C79.89	—	D21.3	D48.1	D49.2
inguinal (canal) (region)	C49.5	C79.89	—	D21.5	D48.1	D49.2
intestinal	C49.4	C79.89	—	D21.4	D48.1	D49.2
intrathoracic	C49.3	C79.89	—	D21.3	D48.1	D49.2
ischiorectal fossa	C49.5	C79.89	—	D21.5	D48.1	D49.2
jaw	CØ3.9	C79.89	DØØ.Ø3	D1Ø.39	D48.1	D49.Ø
knee	C49.2-	C79.89	—	D21.2-	D48.1	D49.2
leg	C49.2-	C79.89	—	D21.2-	D48.1	D49.2
limb NEC	C49.9	C79.89	—	D21.9	D48.1	D49.2
lower	C49.2-	C79.89	—	D21.2-	D48.1	D49.2
upper	C49.1-	C79.89	—	D21.1-	D48.1	D49.2
nates	C49.5	C79.89	—	D21.5	D48.1	D49.2
neck	C49.Ø	C79.89	—	D21.Ø	D48.1	D49.2
orbit	C69.6-	C79.49	DØ9.2-	D31.6-	D48.1	D49.89
overlapping lesion	C49.8	—	—	—	—	—
pararectal	C49.5	C79.89	—	D21.5	D48.1	D49.2
para-urethral	C49.5	C79.89	—	D21.5	D48.1	D49.2
paravaginal	C49.5	C79.89	—	D21.5	D48.1	D49.2
pelvis (floor)	C49.5	C79.89	—	D21.5	D48.1	D49.2
pelvo-abdominal	C49.8	C79.89	—	D21.6	D48.1	D49.2
perineum	C49.5	C79.89	—	D21.5	D48.1	D49.2
perirectal (tissue)	C49.5	C79.89	—	D21.5	D48.1	D49.2
periurethral (tissue)	C49.5	C79.89	—	D21.5	D48.1	D49.2
popliteal fossa or space	C49.2-	C79.89	—	D21.2-	D48.1	D49.2
presacral	C49.5	C79.89	—	D21.5	D48.1	D49.2
psoas muscle	C49.4	C79.89	—	D21.4	D48.1	D49.2
pterygoid fossa	C49.Ø	C79.89	—	D21.Ø	D48.1	D49.2
rectovaginal septum or wall	C49.5	C79.89	—	D21.5	D48.1	D49.2
rectovesical	C49.5	C79.89	—	D21.5	D48.1	D49.2
retroperitoneum	C48.Ø	C78.6	—	D2Ø.Ø	D48.3	D49.Ø
sacrococcygeal region	C49.5	C79.89	—	D21.5	D48.1	D49.2
scalp	C49.Ø	C79.89	—	D21.Ø	D48.1	D49.2
scapular region	C49.3	C79.89	—	D21.3	D48.1	D49.2
shoulder	C49.1-	C79.89	—	D21.1-	D48.1	D49.2
skin (dermis) NEC (*see also* Neoplasm, skin, by site)	C44.9Ø	C79.2	DØ4.9	D23.9	D48.5	D49.2
stomach	C49.4	C79.89	—	D21.4	D48.1	D49.2
submental	C49.Ø	C79.89	—	D21.Ø	D48.1	D49.2
supraclavicular region	C49.Ø	C79.89	—	D21.Ø	D48.1	D49.2
temple	C49.Ø	C79.89	—	D21.Ø	D48.1	D49.2
temporal region	C49.Ø	C79.89	—	D21.Ø	D48.1	D49.2
thigh	C49.2-	C79.89	—	D21.2-	D48.1	D49.2
thoracic (duct) (wall)	C49.3	C79.89	—	D21.3	D48.1	D49.2
thorax	C49.3	C79.89	—	D21.3	D48.1	D49.2
thumb	C49.1-	C79.89	—	D21.1-	D48.1	D49.2
toe	C49.2-	C79.89	—	D21.2-	D48.1	D49.2
trunk	C49.6	C79.89	—	D21.6	D48.1	D49.2
umbilicus	C49.4	C79.89	—	D21.4	D48.1	D49.2
vesicorectal	C49.5	C79.89	—	D21.5	D48.1	D49.2
wrist	C49.1-	C79.89	—	D21.1-	D48.1	D49.2
conus medullaris	C72.Ø	C79.49	—	D33.4	D43.4	D49.7
cord (true) (vocal)	C32.Ø	C78.39	DØ2.Ø	D14.1	D38.Ø	D49.1
false	C32.1	C78.39	DØ2.Ø	D14.1	D38.Ø	D49.1

	Malignant Primary	Malignant Secondary	Ca in situ	Benign	Uncertain Behavior	Unspecified Behavior
Neoplasm, neoplastic — *continued*						
cord — *continued*						
spermatic	C63.1-	C79.82	DØ7.69	D29.8	D4Ø.8	D49.5
spinal (cervical) (lumbar) (thoracic)	C72.Ø	C79.49	—	D33.4	D43.4	D49.7
cornea (limbus)	C69.1-	C79.49	DØ9.2-	D31.1-	D48.7	D49.89
corpus						
albicans	C56.-	C79.6-	DØ7.39	D27.-	D39.1-	D49.5
callosum, brain	C71.Ø	C79.31	—	D33.2	D43.2	D49.6
cavernosum	C6Ø.2	C79.82	DØ7.4	D29.Ø	D4Ø.8	D49.5
gastric	C16.2	C78.89	DØØ.2	D13.1	D37.1	D49.Ø
overlapping sites	C54.8	—	—	—	—	—
penis	C6Ø.2	C79.82	DØ7.4	D29.Ø	D4Ø.8	D49.5
striatum, cerebrum	C71.Ø	C79.31	—	D33.Ø	D43.Ø	D49.6
uteri	C54.9	C79.82	DØ7.Ø	D26.1	D39.Ø	D49.5
isthmus	C54.Ø	C79.82	DØ7.Ø	D26.1	D39.Ø	D49.5
cortex						
adrenal	C74.Ø-	C79.7-	DØ9.3	D35.Ø-	D44.1-	D49.7
cerebral	C71.Ø	C79.31	—	D33.Ø	D43.Ø	D49.6
costal cartilage	C41.3	C79.51	—	D16.7-	D48.Ø	D49.2
costovertebral joint	C41.3	C79.51	—	D16.7-	D48.Ø	D49.2
Cowper's gland	C68.Ø	C79.19	DØ9.19	D3Ø.4	D41.3	D49.5
cranial (fossa, any)	C71.9	C79.31	—	D33.2	D43.2	D49.6
meninges	C7Ø.Ø	C79.32	—	D32.Ø	D42.Ø	D49.7
nerve	C72.5Ø	C79.49	—	D33.3	D43.3	D49.7
specified NEC	C72.59	C79.49	—	D33.3	D43.3	D49.7
craniobuccal pouch	C75.2	C79.89	DØ9.3	D35.2	D44.3	D49.7
craniopharyngeal (duct) (pouch)	C75.2	C79.89	DØ9.3	D35.3	D44.4	D49.7
cricoid	C13.Ø	C79.89	DØØ.Ø8	D1Ø.7	D37.Ø5	D49.Ø
cartilage	C32.3	C79.89	DØ2.Ø	D14.1	D38.Ø	D49.1
cricopharynx	C13.Ø	C79.89	DØØ.Ø8	D1Ø.7	D37.Ø5	D49.Ø
crypt of Morgagni	C21.8	C78.5	DØ1.3	D12.9	D37.8	D49.Ø
crystalline lens	C69.4-	C79.49	DØ9.2-	D31.4-	D48.7	D49.89
cul-de-sac (Douglas')	C48.1	C78.6	—	D2Ø.1	D48.4	D49.Ø
cuneiform cartilage	C32.3	C78.39	DØ2.Ø	D14.1	D38.Ø	D49.1
cutaneous — *see* Neoplasm, skin						
cutis — *see* Neoplasm, skin						
cystic (bile) duct (common)	C24.Ø	C78.89	DØ1.5	D13.5	D37.6	D49.Ø
dermis — *see* Neoplasm, skin						
diaphragm	C49.3	C79.89	—	D21.3	D48.1	D49.2
digestive organs, system, tube, or tract NEC	C26.9	C78.89	DØ1.9	D13.9	D37.9	D49.Ø
disc, intervertebral	C41.2	C79.51	—	D16.6-	D48.Ø	D49.2
disease, generalized	C8Ø.Ø	—	—	—	—	—
disseminated	C8Ø.Ø	—	—	—	—	—
Douglas' cul-de-sac or pouch	C48.1	C78.6	—	D2Ø.1	D48.4	D49.Ø
duodenojejunal junction	C17.8	C78.4	DØ1.49	D13.39	D37.2	D49.Ø
duodenum	C17.Ø	C78.4	DØ1.49	D13.2	D37.2	D49.Ø
dura (cranial) (mater)	C7Ø.9	C79.49	—	D32.9	D42.9	D49.7
cerebral	C7Ø.Ø	C79.32	—	D32.Ø	D42.Ø	D49.7
spinal	C7Ø.1	C79.49	—	D32.1	D42.1	D49.7
ear (external) (*see also* Neoplasm, skin, ear)	C44.2Ø-	C79.2	DØ4.2	D23.2-	D48.5	D49.2
auricle or auris (*see also* Neoplasm, skin, ear)	C44.2Ø-	C79.2	DØ4.2-	D23.2-	D48.5	D49.2
canal, external (*see also* Neoplasm, skin, ear)	C44.2Ø-	C79.2	DØ4.2-	D23.2-	D48.5	D49.2
cartilage	C49.Ø	C79.89	-	D21.Ø	D48.1	D49.2
external meatus (*see also* Neoplasm, skin, ear)	C44.2Ø-	C79.2	DØ4.2-	D23.2-	D48.5	D49.2
inner	C3Ø.1	C78.39	DØ2.3	D14.Ø	D38.5	D49.1
lobule (*see also* Neoplasm, skin, ear)	C44.2Ø-	C79.2	DØ4.2-	D23.2-	D48.5	D49.2
middle	C3Ø.1	C78.39	DØ2.3	D14.Ø	D38.5	D49.1
overlapping lesion with accessory sinuses	C31.8	—	—	—	—	—
skin	C44.2Ø-	C79.2	DØ4.2-	D23.2-	D48.5	D49.2
basal cell carcinoma	C44.21-	—	—	—	—	—
specified type NEC	C44.29-	—	—	—	—	—
squamous cell carcinoma	C44.22-	—	—	—	—	—

	Malignant Primary	Malignant Secondary	Ca in situ	Benign	Uncertain Behavior	Unspecified Behavior
Neoplasm, neoplastic — *continued*						
earlobe	C44.2Ø-	C79.2	DØ4.2-	D23.2-	D48.5	D49.2
basal cell carcinoma	C44.21-	—	—	—	—	—
specified type NEC	C44.29-	—	—	—	—	—
squamous cell carcinoma	C44.22-	—	—	—	—	—
ejaculatory duct	C63.7	C79.82	DØ7.69	D29.8	D4Ø.8	D49.5
elbow NEC	C76.4-	C79.89	DØ4.6-	D36.7	D48.7	D49.89
endocardium	C38.Ø	C79.89	—	D15.1	D48.7	D49.89
endocervix (canal) (gland)	C53.Ø	C79.82	DØ6.Ø	D26.Ø	D39.Ø	D49.5
endocrine gland NEC	C75.9	C79.89	DØ9.3	D35.9	D44.9	D49.7
pluriglandular	C75.8	C79.89	DØ9.3	D35.7	D44.9	D49.7
endometrium (gland) (stroma)	C54.1	C79.82	DØ7.Ø	D26.1	D39.Ø	D49.5
ensiform cartilage	C41.3	C79.51	—	D16.7-	D48.Ø	D49.2
enteric — *see* Neoplasm, intestine						
ependyma (brain)	C71.5	C79.31	—	D33.Ø	D43.Ø	D49.6
fourth ventricle	C71.7	C79.31	—	D33.1	D43.1	D49.6
epicardium	C38.Ø	C79.89	—	D15.1	D48.7	D49.89
epididymis	C63.Ø-	C79.82	DØ7.69	D29.3-	D4Ø.8	D49.5
epidural	C72.9	C79.49	—	D33.9	D43.9	D49.7
epiglottis	C32.1	C78.39	DØ2.Ø	D14.1	D38.Ø	D49.1
anterior aspect or surface	C1Ø.1	C79.89	DØØ.Ø8	D1Ø.5	D37.Ø5	D49.Ø
cartilage	C32.3	C78.39	DØ2.Ø	D14.1	D38.Ø	D49.1
free border (margin)	C1Ø.1	C79.89	DØØ.Ø8	D1Ø.5	D37.Ø5	D49.Ø
junctional region	C1Ø.8	C79.89	DØØ.Ø8	D1Ø.5	D37.Ø5	D49.Ø
posterior (laryngeal) surface	C32.1	C78.39	DØ2.Ø	D14.1	D38.Ø	D49.1
suprahyoid portion	C32.1	C78.39	DØ2.Ø	D14.1	D38.Ø	D49.1
esophagogastric junction	C16.Ø	C78.89	DØØ.2	D13.1	D37.1	D49.Ø
esophagus	C15.9	C78.89	DØØ.1	D13.Ø	D37.8	D49.Ø
abdominal	C15.5	C78.89	DØØ.1	D13.Ø	D37.8	D49.Ø
cervical	C15.3	C78.89	DØØ.1	D13.Ø	D37.8	D49.Ø
distal (third)	C15.5	C78.89	DØØ.1	D13.Ø	D37.8	D49.Ø
lower (third)	C15.5	C78.89	DØØ.1	D13.Ø	D37.8	D49.Ø
middle (third)	C15.4	C78.89	DØØ.1	D13.Ø	D37.8	D49.Ø
overlapping lesion	C15.8	—	—	—	—	—
proximal (third)	C15.3	C78.89	DØØ.1	D13.Ø	D37.8	D49.Ø
thoracic	C15.4	C78.89	DØØ.1	D13.Ø	D37.8	D49.Ø
upper (third)	C15.3	C78.89	DØØ.1	D13.Ø	D37.8	D49.Ø
ethmoid (sinus)	C31.1	C78.39	DØ2.3	D14.Ø	D38.5	D49.1
bone or labyrinth	C41.Ø	C79.51	—	D16.4-	D48.Ø	D49.2
eustachian tube	C3Ø.1	C78.39	DØ2.3	D14.Ø	D38.5	D49.1
exocervix	C53.1	C79.82	DØ6.1	D26.Ø	D39.Ø	D49.5
external						
meatus (ear) (*see also* Neoplasm, skin, ear)	C44.2Ø-	C79.2	DØ4.2-	D23.2-	D48.5	D49.2
os, cervix uteri	C53.1	C79.82	DØ6.1	D26.Ø	D39.Ø	D49.5
extradural	C72.9	C79.49	—	D33.9	D43.9	D49.7
extrahepatic (bile) duct	C24.Ø	C78.89	DØ1.5	D13.5	D37.6	D49.Ø
overlapping lesion with gallbladder	C24.8	—	—	—	—	—
extraocular muscle	C69.6-	C79.49	DØ9.2-	D31.6-	D48.7	D49.89
extrarectal	C76.3	C79.89	DØ9.8	D36.7	D48.7	D49.89
extremity	C76.8	C79.89	DØ4.8	D36.7	D48.7	D49.89
lower	C76.5-	C79.89	DØ4.7-	D36.7	D48.7	D49.89
upper	C76.4-	C79.89	DØ4.6-	D36.7	D48.7	D49.89
eye NEC	C69.9	C79.49	DØ9.2-	D31.9	D48.7	D49.89
eyeball	C69.4-	C79.49	DØ9.2-	D31.4-	D48.7	D49.89
overlapping sites	C69.8	—	—	—	—	—
eyebrow	C44.3Ø9	C79.2	DØ4.39	D23.39	D48.5	D49.2
basal cell carcinoma	C44.319	—	—	—	—	—
specified type NEC	C44.399	—	—	—	—	—
squamous cell carcinoma	C44.329	—	—	—	—	—
eyelid (lower) (skin) (upper)	C44.1Ø-	—	—	—	—	—
basal cell carcinoma	C44.11-	—	—	—	—	—
specified type NEC	C44.19-	—	—	—	—	—
squamous cell carcinoma	C44.12-	—	—	—	—	—
cartilage	C49.Ø	C79.89	—	D21.Ø	D48.1	D49.2
face NEC	C76.Ø	C79.89	DØ4.39	D36.7	D48.7	D49.89
fallopian tube (accessory)	C57.Ø-	C79.82	DØ7.39	D28.2	D39.8	D49.5
falx (cerebella) (cerebri)	C7Ø.Ø	C79.32	—	D32.Ø	D42.Ø	D49.7

	Malignant Primary	Malignant Secondary	Ca in situ	Benign	Uncertain Behavior	Unspecified Behavior
Neoplasm, neoplastic — *continued*						
fascia (*see also* Neoplasm, connective tissue)						
palmar	C49.1-	C79.89	—	D21.1-	D48.1	D49.2
plantar	C49.2-	C79.89	—	D21.2-	D48.1	D49.2
fatty tissue — *see* Neoplasm, connective tissue						
fauces, faucial NEC	C1Ø.9	C79.89	DØØ.Ø8	D1Ø.5	D37.Ø5	D49.Ø
pillars	CØ9.1	C79.89	DØØ.Ø8	D1Ø.5	D37.Ø5	D49.Ø
tonsil	CØ9.9	C79.89	DØØ.Ø8	D1Ø.4	D37.Ø5	D49.Ø
femur (any part)	C4Ø.2-	—	—	D16.2-	—	—
fetal membrane	C58	C79.82	DØ7.Ø	D26.7	D39.2	D49.5
fibrous tissue — *see* Neoplasm, connective tissue						
fibula (any part)	C4Ø.2-	C79.51	—	D16.2-	—	—
filum terminale	C72.Ø	C79.49	—	D33.4	D43.4	D49.7
finger NEC	C76.4-	C79.89	DØ4.6-	D36.7	D48.7	D49.89
flank NEC	C76.8	C79.89	DØ4.5	D36.7	D48.7	D49.89
follicle, nabothian	C53.Ø	C79.82	DØ6.Ø	D26.Ø	D39.Ø	D49.5
foot NEC	C76.5-	C79.89	DØ4.7-	D36.7	D48.7	D49.89
forearm NEC	C76.4-	C79.89	DØ4.6-	D36.7	D48.7	D49.89
forehead (skin)	C44.3Ø9	C79.2	DØ4.39	D23.39	D48.5	D49.2
basal cell carcinoma	C44.319	—	—	—	—	—
specified type NEC	C44.399	—	—	—	—	—
squamous cell carcinoma	C44.329	—	—	—	—	—
foreskin	C6Ø.Ø	C79.82	DØ7.4	D29.Ø	D4Ø.8	D49.5
fornix						
pharyngeal	C11.3	C79.89	DØØ.Ø8	D1Ø.6	D37.Ø5	D49.Ø
vagina	C52	C79.82	DØ7.2	D28.1	D39.8	D49.5
fossa (of)						
anterior (cranial)	C71.9	C79.31	—	D33.2	D43.2	D49.6
cranial	C71.9	C79.31	—	D33.2	D43.2	D49.6
ischiorectal	C76.3	C79.89	DØ9.8	D36.7	D48.7	D49.89
middle (cranial)	C71.9	C79.31	—	D33.2	D43.2	D49.6
piriform	C12	C79.89	DØØ.Ø8	D1Ø.7	D37.Ø5	D49.Ø
pituitary	C75.1	C79.89	DØ9.3	D35.2	D44.3	D49.7
posterior (cranial)	C71.9	C79.31	—	D33.2	D43.2	D49.6
pterygoid	C49.Ø	C79.89	—	D21.Ø	D48.1	D49.2
pyriform	C12	C79.89	DØØ.Ø8	D1Ø.7	D37.Ø5	D49.Ø
Rosenmüller	C11.2	C79.89	DØØ.Ø8	D1Ø.6	D37.Ø5	D49.Ø
tonsillar	CØ9.Ø	C79.89	DØØ.Ø8	D1Ø.5	D37.Ø5	D49.Ø
fourchette	C51.9	C79.82	DØ7.1	D28.Ø	D39.8	D49.5
frenulum						
labii — *see* Neoplasm, lip, internal						
linguae	CØ2.2	C79.89	DØØ.Ø7	D1Ø.1	D37.Ø2	D49.Ø
frontal						
bone	C41.Ø	C79.51	—	D16.4-	D48.Ø	D49.2
lobe, brain	C71.1	C79.31	—	D33.Ø	D43.Ø	D49.6
pole	C71.1	C79.31	—	D33.Ø	D43.Ø	D49.6
sinus	C31.2	C78.39	DØ2.3	D14.Ø	D38.5	D49.1
fundus						
stomach	C16.1	C78.89	DØØ.2	D13.1	D37.1	D49.Ø
uterus	C54.3	C79.82	DØ7.Ø	D26.1	D39.Ø	D49.5
gall duct (extrahepatic)	C24.Ø	C78.89	DØ1.5	D13.5	D37.6	D49.Ø
intrahepatic	C22.1	C78.7	DØ1.5	D13.4	D37.6	D49.Ø
gallbladder	C23	C78.89	DØ1.5	D13.5	D37.6	D49.Ø
overlapping lesion with extrahepatic bile ducts	C24.8	—	—	—	—	—
ganglia (*see also* Neoplasm, nerve, peripheral)	C47.9	C79.89	—	D36.1Ø	D48.2	D49.2
basal	C71.Ø	C79.31	—	D33.Ø	D43.Ø	D49.6
cranial nerve	C72.5Ø	C79.49	—	D33.3	D43.3	D49.7
Gartner's duct	C52	C79.82	DØ7.2	D28.1	D39.8	D49.5
gastric — *see* Neoplasm, stomach						
gastrocolic	C26.9	C78.89	DØ1.9	D13.9	D37.9	D49.Ø
gastroesophageal junction	C16.Ø	C78.89	DØØ.2	D13.1	D37.1	D49.Ø
gastrointestinal (tract) NEC	C26.9	C78.89	DØ1.9	D13.9	D37.9	D49.Ø
generalized	C8Ø.Ø	—	—	—	—	—
genital organ or tract						
female NEC	C57.9	C79.82	DØ7.3Ø	D28.9	D39.9	D49.5
overlapping lesion	C57.8	—	—	—	—	—
Neoplasm, neoplastic — *continued*						
genital organ or tract — *continued*						
female NEC — *continued*						
specified site NEC	C57.7	C79.82	DØ7.39	D28.7	D39.8	D49.5
male NEC	C63.9	C79.82	DØ7.6Ø	D29.9	D4Ø.9	D49.5
overlapping lesion	C63.8	—	—	—	—	—
specified site NEC	C63.7	C79.82	DØ7.69	D29.8	D4Ø.8	D49.5
genitourinary tract						
female	C57.9	C79.82	DØ7.3Ø	D28.9	D39.9	D49.5
male	C63.9	C79.82	DØ7.6Ø	D29.9	D4Ø.9	D49.5
gingiva (alveolar) (marginal)	CØ3.9	C79.89	DØØ.Ø3	D1Ø.39	D37.Ø9	D49.Ø
lower	CØ3.1	C79.89	DØØ.Ø3	D1Ø.39	D37.Ø9	D49.Ø
mandibular	CØ3.1	C79.89	DØØ.Ø3	D1Ø.39	D37.Ø9	D49.Ø
maxillary	CØ3.Ø	C79.89	DØØ.Ø3	D1Ø.39	D37.Ø9	D49.Ø
gingiva (alveolar) (marginal)						
upper	CØ3.Ø	C79.89	DØØ.Ø3	D1Ø.39	D37.Ø9	D49.Ø
gland, glandular (lymphatic) (system) (*see also* Neoplasm, lymph gland)						
endocrine NEC	C75.9	C79.89	DØ9.3	D35.9	D44.9	D49.7
salivary — *see* Neoplasm, salivary gland						
glans penis	C6Ø.1	C79.82	DØ7.4	D29.Ø	D4Ø.8	D49.5
globus pallidus	C71.Ø	C79.31	—	D33.Ø	D43.Ø	D49.6
glomus						
coccygeal	C75.5	C79.89	—	D35.6	D44.7	D49.7
jugularis	C75.5	C79.89	—	D35.6	D44.7	D49.7
glosso-epiglottic fold (s)	C1Ø.1	C79.89	DØØ.Ø8	D1Ø.5	D37.Ø5	D49.Ø
glossopalatine fold	CØ9.1	C79.89	DØØ.Ø8	D1Ø.5	D37.Ø5	D49.Ø
glossopharyngeal sulcus	CØ9.Ø	C79.89	DØØ.Ø8	D1Ø.5	D37.Ø5	D49.Ø
glottis	C32.Ø	C78.39	DØ2.Ø	D14.1	D38.Ø	D49.1
gluteal region	C76.3	C79.89	DØ4.5	D36.7	D48.7	D49.89
great vessels NEC	C49.3	C79.89	—	D21.3	D48.1	D49.2
groin NEC	C76.3	C79.89	DØ4.5	D36.7	D48.7	D49.89
gum	CØ3.9	C79.89	DØØ.Ø3	D1Ø.39	D37.Ø9	D49.Ø
lower	CØ3.1	C79.89	DØØ.Ø3	D1Ø.39	D37.Ø9	D49.Ø
upper	CØ3.Ø	C79.89	DØØ.Ø3	D1Ø.39	D37.Ø9	D49.Ø
hand NEC	C76.4-	C79.89	DØ4.6-	D36.7	D48.7	D49.89
head NEC	C76.Ø	C79.89	DØ4.4	D36.7	D48.7	D49.89
heart	C38.Ø	C79.89	—	D15.1	D48.7	D49.89
heel NEC	C76.5-	C79.89	DØ4.7-	D36.7	D48.7	D49.89
helix (*see also* Neoplasm, skin, ear)	C44.2Ø-	C79.2	DØ4.2-	D23.2-	D48.5	D49.2
hematopoietic, hemopoietic tissue NEC	C96.9	—	—	—	—	—
specified NEC	C96.Z	—	—	—	—	—
hemisphere, cerebral	C71.Ø	C79.31	—	D33.Ø	D43.Ø	D49.6
hemorrhoidal zone	C21.1	C78.5	DØ1.3	D12.9	D37.8	D49.Ø
hepatic— *see also* Index to disease, by histology	C22.9	C78.7	DØ1.5	D13.4	D37.6	D49.Ø
duct (bile)	C24.Ø	C78.89	DØ1.5	D13.5	D37.6	D49.Ø
flexure (colon)	C18.3	C78.5	DØ1.Ø	D12.3	D37.4	D49.Ø
primary	C22.8	C78.7	DØ1.5	D13.4	D37.6	D49.Ø
hepatoblastoma	C22.2	C78.7	DØ1.5	D13.4	D37.6	D49.Ø
hepatoma	C22.Ø	C78.7	DØ1.5	D13.4	D37.6	D49.Ø
hilus of lung	C34.Ø-	C78.Ø-	DØ2.2-	D14.3-	D38.1	D49.1
hip NEC	C76.5-	C79.89	DØ4.7-	D36.7	D48.7	D49.89
hippocampus, brain	C71.2	C79.31	—	D33.Ø	D43.Ø	D49.6
humerus (any part)	C4Ø.Ø-	C79.51	—	D16.Ø-	—	—
hymen	C52	C79.82	DØ7.2	D28.1	D39.8	D49.5
hypopharynx, hypopharyngeal NEC	C13.9	C79.89	DØØ.Ø8	D1Ø.7	D37.Ø5	D49.Ø
overlapping lesion	C13.8	—	—	—	—	—
postcricoid region	C13.Ø	C79.89	DØØ.Ø8	D1Ø.7	D37.Ø5	D49.Ø
posterior wall	C13.2	C79.89	DØØ.Ø8	D1Ø.7	D37.Ø5	D49.Ø
pyriform fossa (sinus)	C12	C79.89	DØØ.Ø8	D1Ø.7	D37.Ø5	D49.Ø
hypophysis	C75.1	C79.89	DØ9.3	D35.2	D44.3	D49.7
hypothalamus	C71.Ø	C79.31	—	D33.Ø	D43.Ø	D49.6
ileocecum, ileocecal (coil) (junction) (valve)	C18.Ø	C78.5	DØ1.Ø	D12.Ø	D37.4	D49.Ø
ileum	C17.2	C78.4	DØ1.49	D13.39	D37.2	D49.Ø
ilium	C41.4	C79.51	—	D16.8-	D48.Ø	D49.2

	Malignant Primary	Malignant Secondary	Ca in situ	Benign	Uncertain Behavior	Unspecified Behavior
Neoplasm, neoplastic — *continued*						
immunoproliferative NEC	C88.9	—	—	—	—	—
infraclavicular (region)	C76.1	C79.89	DØ4.5	D36.7	D48.7	D49.89
inguinal (region)	C76.3	C79.89	DØ4.5	D36.7	D48.7	D49.89
insula	C71.Ø	C79.31	—	D33.Ø	D43.Ø	D49.6
insular tissue (pancreas)	C25.4	C78.89	DØ1.7	D13.7	D37.8	D49.Ø
brain	C71.Ø	C79.31	—	D33.Ø	D43.Ø	D49.6
interarytenoid fold	C13.1	C79.89	DØØ.Ø8	D1Ø.7	D37.Ø5	D49.Ø
hypopharyngeal aspect	C13.1	C79.89	DØØ.Ø8	D1Ø.7	D37.Ø5	D49.Ø
laryngeal aspect	C32.1	C79.89	DØ2.Ø	D14.1	D38.Ø	D49.1
marginal zone	C13.1	C79.89	DØØ.Ø8	D1Ø.7	D37.Ø5	D49.Ø
interdental papillae	CØ3.9	C79.89	DØØ.Ø3	D1Ø.39	D37.Ø9	D49.Ø
lower	CØ3.1	C79.89	DØØ.Ø3	D1Ø.39	D37.Ø9	D49.Ø
upper	CØ3.Ø	C79.89	DØØ.Ø3	D1Ø.39	D37.Ø9	D49.Ø
internal						
capsule	C71.Ø	C79.31	—	D33.Ø	D43.Ø	D49.6
os (cervix)	C53.Ø	C79.82	DØ6.Ø	D26.Ø	D39.Ø	D49.5
intervertebral cartilage or disc	C41.2	C79.51	—	D16.6-	D48.Ø	D49.2
intestine, intestinal	C26.Ø	C78.8Ø	DØ1.4Ø	D13.9	D37.8	D49.Ø
large	C18.9	C78.5	DØ1.Ø	D12.6	D37.4	D49.Ø
appendix	C18.1	C78.5	DØ1.Ø	D12.1	D37.3	D49.Ø
caput coli	C18.Ø	C78.5	DØ1.Ø	D12.Ø	D37.4	D49.Ø
cecum	C18.Ø	C78.5	DØ1.Ø	D12.Ø	D37.4	D49.Ø
colon	C18.9	C78.5	DØ1.Ø	D12.6	D37.4	D49.Ø
and rectum	C19	C78.5	DØ1.1	D12.7	D37.5	D49.Ø
ascending	C18.2	C78.5	DØ1.Ø	D12.2	D37.4	D49.Ø
caput	C18.Ø	C78.5	DØ1.Ø	D12.Ø	D37.4	D49.Ø
descending	C18.6	C78.5	DØ1.Ø	D12.4	D37.4	D49.Ø
distal	C18.6	C78.5	DØ1.Ø	D12.4	D37.4	D49.Ø
left	C18.6	C78.5	DØ1.Ø	D12.4	D37.4	D49.Ø
overlapping lesion	C18.8	—	—	—	—	—
pelvic	C18.7	C78.5	DØ1.Ø	D12.5	D37.4	D49.Ø
right	C18.2	C78.5	DØ1.Ø	D12.2	D37.4	D49.Ø
sigmoid (flexure)	C18.7	C78.5	DØ1.Ø	D12.5	D37.4	D49.Ø
transverse	C18.4	C78.5	DØ1.Ø	D12.3	D37.4	D49.Ø
hepatic flexure	C18.3	C78.5	DØ1.Ø	D12.3	D37.4	D49.Ø
ileocecum, ileocecal (coil) (valve)	C18.Ø	C78.5	DØ1.Ø	D12.Ø	D37.4	D49.Ø
overlapping lesion	C18.8	—	—	—	—	—
sigmoid flexure (lower) (upper)	C18.7	C78.5	DØ1.Ø	D12.5	D37.4	D49.Ø
splenic flexure	C18.5	C78.5	DØ1.Ø	D12.3	D37.4	D49.Ø
small	C17.9	C78.4	DØ1.4Ø	D13.3Ø	D37.2	D49.Ø
duodenum	C17.Ø	C78.4	DØ1.49	D13.2	D37.2	D49.Ø
ileum	C17.2	C78.4	DØ1.49	D13.39	D37.2	D49.Ø
jejunum	C17.1	C78.4	DØ1.49	D13.39	D37.2	D49.Ø
overlapping lesion	C17.8	—	—	—	—	—
tract NEC	C26.Ø	C78.89	DØ1.4Ø	D13.9	D37.8	D49.Ø
intra-abdominal	C76.2	C79.89	DØ9.8	D36.7	D48.7	D49.89
intracranial NEC	C71.9	C79.31	—	D33.2	D43.2	D49.6
intrahepatic (bile) duct	C22.1	C78.7	DØ1.5	D13.4	D37.6	D49.Ø
intraocular	C69.4-	C79.49	DØ9.2-	D31.4-	D48.7	D49.89
intraorbital	C69.6-	C79.49	DØ9.2-	D31.6-	D48.7	D49.89
intrasellar	C75.1	C79.89	DØ9.3	D35.2	D44.3	D49.7
intrathoracic (cavity) (organs)	C76.1	C79.89	DØ9.8	D15.9	D48.7	D49.89
specified NEC	C76.1	C79.89	DØ9.8	D15.7	—	—
iris	C69.4-	C79.49	DØ9.2-	D31.4-	D48.7	D49.89
ischiorectal (fossa)	C76.3	C79.89	DØ9.8	D36.7	D48.7	D49.89
ischium	C41.4	C79.51	—	D16.8-	D48.Ø	D49.2
island of Reil	C71.Ø	C79.31	—	D33.Ø	D43.Ø	D49.6
islands or islets of Langerhans	C25.4	C78.89	DØ1.7	D13.7	D37.8	D49.Ø
isthmus uteri	C54.Ø	C79.82	DØ7.Ø	D26.1	D39.Ø	D49.5
jaw	C76.Ø	C79.89	DØ9.8	D36.7	D48.7	D49.89
bone	C41.1	C79.51	—	D16.5-	D48.Ø	D49.2
lower	C41.1	C79.51	—	D16.5-	—	—
upper	C41.Ø	C79.51	—	D16.4-	—	—
carcinoma (any type) (lower) (upper)	C76.Ø	C79.89	—	—	—	—
skin (*see also* Neoplasm, skin, face)	C44.3Ø9	C79.2	DØ4.39	D23.39	D48.5	D49.2
soft tissues	CØ3.9	C79.89	DØØ.Ø3	D1Ø.39	D37.Ø9	D49.Ø
lower	CØ3.1	C79.89	DØØ.Ø3	D1Ø.39	D37.Ø9	D49.Ø

	Malignant Primary	Malignant Secondary	Ca in situ	Benign	Uncertain Behavior	Unspecified Behavior
Neoplasm, neoplastic — *continued*						
soft tissues — *continued*						
upper	CØ3.Ø	C79.89	DØØ.Ø3	D1Ø.39	D37.Ø9	D49.Ø
jejunum	C17.1	C78.4	DØ1.49	D13.39	D37.2	D49.Ø
joint NEC (*see also* Neoplasm, bone)	C41.9	C79.51	—	D16.9-	D48.Ø	D49.2
acromioclavicular	C4Ø.Ø-	C79.51	—	D16.Ø-	—	—
bursa or synovial membrane — *see* Neoplasm, connective tissue						
costovertebral	C41.3	C79.51	—	D16.7-	D48.Ø	D49.2
sternocostal	C41.3	C79.51	—	D16.7-	D48.Ø	D49.2
temporomandibular	C41.1	C79.51	—	D16.5-	D48.Ø	D49.2
junction						
anorectal	C21.8	C78.5	DØ1.3	D12.9	D37.8	D49.Ø
cardioesophageal	C16.Ø	C78.89	DØØ.2	D13.1	D37.1	D49.Ø
esophagogastric	C16.Ø	C78.89	DØØ.2	D13.1	D37.1	D49.Ø
gastroesophageal	C16.Ø	C78.89	DØØ.2	D13.1	D37.1	D49.Ø
hard and soft palate	CØ5.9	C79.89	DØØ.ØØ	D1Ø.39	D37.Ø9	D49.Ø
ileocecal	C18.Ø	C78.5	DØ1.Ø	D12.Ø	D37.4	D49.Ø
pelvirectal	C19	C78.5	DØ1.1	D12.7	D37.5	D49.Ø
pelviureteric	C65.-	C79.Ø-	DØ9.19	D3Ø.1-	D41.1-	D49.5
rectosigmoid	C19	C78.5	DØ1.1	D12.7	D37.5	D49.Ø
squamocolumnar, of cervix	C53.8	C79.82	DØ6.7	D26.Ø	D39.Ø	D49.5
Kaposi's sarcoma — *see* Kaposi's, sarcoma						
kidney (parenchymal)	C64.-	C79.Ø-	DØ9.19	D3Ø.Ø-	D41.Ø-	D49.5
calyx	C65.-	C79.Ø-	DØ9.19	D3Ø.1-	D41.1-	D49.5
hilus	C65.-	C79.Ø-	DØ9.19	D3Ø.1-	D41.1-	D49.5
pelvis	C65.-	C79.Ø-	DØ9.19	D3Ø.1-	D41.1-	D49.5
knee NEC	C76.5-	C79.89	DØ4.7-	D36.7	D48.7	D49.89
labia (skin)	C51.9	C79.82	DØ7.1	D28.Ø	D39.8	D49.5
majora	C51.Ø	C79.82	DØ7.1	D28.Ø	D39.8	D49.5
minora	C51.1	C79.82	DØ7.1	D28.Ø	D39.8	D49.5
labial (*see also* Neoplasm, lip)	CØØ.9	C79.89	DØØ.Ø1	D1Ø.Ø	D37.Ø1	D49.Ø
sulcus (lower) (upper)	CØ6.1	C79.89	DØØ.Ø2	D1Ø.39	D37.Ø9	D49.Ø
labium (skin)	C51.9	C79.82	DØ7.1	D28.Ø	D39.8	D49.5
majus	C51.Ø	C79.82	DØ7.1	D28.Ø	D39.8	D49.5
minus	C51.1	C79.82	DØ7.1	D28.Ø	D39.8	D49.5
lacrimal						
canaliculi	C69.5-	C79.49	DØ9.2-	D31.5-	D48.7	D49.89
duct (nasal)	C69.5-	C79.49	DØ9.2-	D31.5-	D48.7	D49.89
gland	C69.5-	C79.49	DØ9.2-	D31.5-	D48.7	D49.89
punctum	C69.5-	C79.49	DØ9.2-	D31.5-	D48.7	D49.89
sac	C69.5-	C79.49	DØ9.2-	D31.5-	D48.7	D49.89
Langerhans, islands or islets	C25.4	C78.89	DØ1.7	D13.7	D37.8	D49.Ø
laryngopharynx	C13.9	C79.89	DØØ.Ø8	D1Ø.7	D37.Ø5	D49.Ø
larynx, laryngeal NEC	C32.9	C78.39	DØ2.Ø	D14.1	D38.Ø	D49.1
aryepiglottic fold	C32.1	C78.39	DØ2.Ø	D14.1	D38.Ø	D49.1
cartilage (arytenoid) (cricoid) (cuneiform) (thyroid)	C32.3	C78.39	DØ2.Ø	D14.1	D38.Ø	D49.1
commissure (anterior) (posterior)	C32.Ø	C78.39	DØ2.Ø	D14.1	D38.Ø	D49.1
extrinsic NEC	C32.1	C78.39	DØ2.Ø	D14.1	D38.Ø	D49.1
meaning hypopharynx	C13.9	C79.89	DØØ.Ø8	D1Ø.7	D37.Ø5	D49.Ø
interarytenoid fold	C32.1	C78.39	DØ2.Ø	D14.1	D38.Ø	D49.1
intrinsic	C32.Ø	C78.39	DØ2.Ø	D14.1	D38.Ø	D49.1
overlapping lesion	C32.8	—	—	—	—	—
ventricular band	C32.1	C78.39	DØ2.Ø	D14.1	D38.Ø	D49.1
leg NEC	C76.5-	C79.89	DØ4.7-	D36.7	D48.7	D49.89
lens, crystalline	C69.4-	C79.49	DØ9.2-	D31.4-	D48.7	D49.89
lid (lower) (upper)	C44.1Ø-	C79.2	DØ4.1-	D23.1-	D48.5	D49.2
basal cell carcinoma	C44.11-	—	—	—	—	—
specified type NEC	C44.19-	—	—	—	—	—
squamous cell carcinoma	C44.12-	—	—	—	—	—
ligament (*see also* Neoplasm, connective tissue)						
broad	C57.1	C79.82	DØ7.39	D28.2	D39.8	D49.5
Mackenrodt's	C57.7	C79.82	DØ7.39	D28.7	D39.8	D49.5
non-uterine — *see* Neoplasm, connective tissue						
round	C57.2	C79.82	—	D28.2	D39.8	D49.5
sacro-uterine	C57.3	C79.82	—	D28.2	D39.8	D49.5

	Malignant Primary	Malignant Secondary	Ca in situ	Benign	Uncertain Behavior	Unspecified Behavior
Neoplasm, neoplastic — *continued*						
ligament — *continued*						
uterine	C57.3	C79.82	—	D28.2	D39.8	D49.5
utero-ovarian	C57.7	C79.82	DØ7.39	D28.2	D39.8	D49.5
uterosacral	C57.3	C79.82	—	D28.2	D39.8	D49.5
limb	C76.8	C79.89	DØ4.8	D36.7	D48.7	D49.89
lower	C76.5-	C79.89	DØ4.7-	D36.7	D48.7	D49.89
upper	C76.4-	C79.89	DØ4.6-	D36.7	D48.7	D49.89
limbus of cornea	C69.1-	C79.49	DØ9.2-	D31.1-	D48.7	D49.89
lingual NEC (*see also* Neoplasm, tongue)	CØ2.9	C79.89	DØØ.Ø7	D1Ø.1	D37.Ø2	D49.Ø
lingula, lung	C34.1-	C78.Ø-	DØ2.2-	D14.3-	D38.1	D49.1
lip	CØØ.9	C79.89	DØØ.Ø1	D1Ø.Ø	D37.Ø1	D49.Ø
buccal aspect — *see* Neoplasm, lip, internal						
commissure	CØØ.6	C79.89	DØØ.Ø1	D1Ø.Ø	D37.Ø1	D49.Ø
external	CØØ.2	C79.89	DØØ.Ø1	D1Ø.Ø	D37.Ø1	D49.Ø
lower	CØØ.1	C79.89	DØØ.Ø1	D1Ø.Ø	D37.Ø1	D49.Ø
upper	CØØ.Ø	C79.89	DØØ.Ø1	D1Ø.Ø	D37.Ø1	D49.Ø
frenulum — *see* Neoplasm, lip, internal						
inner aspect — *see* Neoplasm, lip, internal						
internal	CØØ.5	C79.89	DØØ.Ø1	D1Ø.Ø	D37.Ø1	D49.Ø
lower	CØØ.4	C79.89	DØØ.Ø1	D1Ø.Ø	D37.Ø1	D49.Ø
upper	CØØ.3	C79.89	DØØ.Ø1	D1Ø.Ø	D37.Ø1	D49.Ø
lipstick area	CØØ.2	C79.89	DØØ.Ø1	D1Ø.Ø	D37.Ø1	D49.Ø
lower	CØØ.1	C79.89	DØØ.Ø1	D1Ø.Ø	D37.Ø1	D49.Ø
upper	CØØ.Ø	C79.89	DØØ.Ø1	D1Ø.Ø	D37.Ø1	D49.Ø
lower	CØØ.1	C79.89	DØØ.Ø1	D1Ø.Ø	D37.Ø1	D49.Ø
internal	CØØ.4	C79.89	DØØ.Ø1	D1Ø.Ø	D37.Ø1	D49.Ø
mucosa — *see* Neoplasm, lip, internal						
oral aspect — *see* Neoplasm, lip, internal						
overlapping lesion	CØØ.8	—	—	—	—	—
with oral cavity or pharynx	C14.8	—	—	—	—	—
skin (commissure) (lower) (upper)	C44.ØØ	C79.2	DØ4.Ø	D23.Ø	D48.5	D49.2
basal cell carcinoma	C44.Ø1	—	—	—	—	—
specified type NEC	C44.Ø9	—	—	—	—	—
squamous cell carcinoma	C44.Ø2	—	—	—	—	—
upper	CØØ.Ø	C79.89	DØØ.Ø1	D1Ø.Ø	D37.Ø1	D49.Ø
internal	CØØ.3	C79.89	DØØ.Ø1	D1Ø.Ø	D37.Ø1	D49.Ø
vermilion border	CØØ.2	C79.89	DØØ.Ø1	D1Ø.Ø	D37.Ø1	D49.Ø
lower	CØØ.1	C79.89	DØØ.Ø1	D1Ø.Ø	D37.Ø1	D49.Ø
upper	CØØ.Ø	C79.89	DØØ.Ø1	D1Ø.Ø	D37.Ø1	D49.Ø
lipomatous — *see* Lipoma, by site						
liver (*see also* Index to disease, by histology)	C22.9	C78.7	DØ1.5	D13.4	D37.6	D49.Ø
primary	C22.8	C78.7	DØ1.5	D13.4	D37.6	D49.Ø
lumbosacral plexus	C47.5	C79.89	—	D36.16	D48.2	D49.2
lung	C34.9-	C78.Ø-	DØ2.2-	D14.3-	D38.1	D49.1
azygos lobe	C34.1-	C78.Ø-	DØ2.2-	D14.3-	D38.1	D49.1
carina	C34.Ø-	C78.Ø-	DØ2.2-	D14.3-	D38.1	D49.1
hilus	C34.Ø-	C78.Ø-	DØ2.2-	D14.3-	D38.1	D49.1
linqula	C34.1-	C78.Ø-	DØ2.2-	D14.3-	D38.1	D49.1
lobe NEC	C34.9-	C78.Ø-	DØ2.2-	D14.3-	D38.1	D49.1
lower lobe	C34.3-	C78.Ø-	DØ2.2-	D14.3-	D38.1	D49.1
main bronchus	C34.Ø-	C78.Ø-	DØ2.2-	D14.3-	D38.1	D49.1
mesothelioma — *see* Mesothelioma						
middle lobe	C34.2	C78.Ø-	DØ2.21	D14.31	D38.1	D49.1
overlapping lesion	C34.8-	—	—	—	—	—
upper lobe	C34.1-	C78.Ø-	DØ2.2-	D14.3-	D38.1	D49.1
lymph, lymphatic channel NEC	C49.9	C79.89	—	D21.9	D48.1	D49.2
gland (secondary)	—	C77.9	—	D36.Ø	D48.7	D49.89
abdominal	—	C77.2	—	D36.Ø	D48.7	D49.89
aortic	—	C77.2	—	D36.Ø	D48.7	D49.89
arm	—	C77.3	—	D36.Ø	D48.7	D49.89
auricular (anterior) (posterior)	—	C77.Ø	—	D36.Ø	D48.7	D49.89

	Malignant Primary	Malignant Secondary	Ca in situ	Benign	Uncertain Behavior	Unspecified Behavior
Neoplasm, neoplastic — *continued*						
lymph, lymphatic channel NEC — *continued*						
gland (secondary) — *continued*						
axilla, axillary	—	C77.3	—	D36.Ø	D48.7	D49.89
brachial	—	C77.3	—	D36.Ø	D48.7	D49.89
bronchial	—	C77.1	—	D36.Ø	D48.7	D49.89
bronchopulmonary	—	C77.1	—	D36.Ø	D48.7	D49.89
celiac	—	C77.2	—	D36.Ø	D48.7	D49.89
cervical	—	C77.Ø	—	D36.Ø	D48.7	D49.89
cervicofacial	—	C77.Ø	—	D36.Ø	D48.7	D49.89
Cloquet	—	C77.4	—	D36.Ø	D48.7	D49.89
colic	—	C77.2	—	D36.Ø	D48.7	D49.89
common duct	—	C77.2	—	D36.Ø	D48.7	D49.89
cubital	—	C77.3	—	D36.Ø	D48.7	D49.89
diaphragmatic	—	C77.1	—	D36.Ø	D48.7	D49.89
epigastric, inferior	—	C77.1	—	D36.Ø	D48.7	D49.89
epitrochlear	—	C77.3	—	D36.Ø	D48.7	D49.89
esophageal	—	C77.1	—	D36.Ø	D48.7	D49.89
face	—	C77.Ø	—	D36.Ø	D48.7	D49.89
femoral	—	C77.4	—	D36.Ø	D48.7	D49.89
gastric	—	C77.2	—	D36.Ø	D48.7	D49.89
groin	—	C77.4	—	D36.Ø	D48.7	D49.89
head	—	C77.Ø	—	D36.Ø	D48.7	D49.89
hepatic	—	C77.2	—	D36.Ø	D48.7	D49.89
hilar (pulmonary)	—	C77.1	—	D36.Ø	D48.7	D49.89
splenic	—	C77.2	—	D36.Ø	D48.7	D49.89
hypogastric	—	C77.5	—	D36.Ø	D48.7	D49.89
ileocolic	—	C77.2	—	D36.Ø	D48.7	D49.89
iliac	—	C77.5	—	D36.Ø	D48.7	D49.89
infraclavicular	—	C77.3	—	D36.Ø	D48.7	D49.89
inguina, inguinal	—	C77.4	—	D36.Ø	D48.7	D49.89
innominate	—	C77.1	—	D36.Ø	D48.7	D49.89
intercostal	—	C77.1	—	D36.Ø	D48.7	D49.89
intestinal	—	C77.2	—	D36.Ø	D48.7	D49.89
intrabdominal	—	C77.2	—	D36.Ø	D48.7	D49.89
intrapelvic	—	C77.5	—	D36.Ø	D48.7	D49.89
intrathoracic	—	C77.1	—	D36.Ø	D48.7	D49.89
jugular	—	C77.Ø	—	D36.Ø	D48.7	D49.89
leg	—	C77.4	—	D36.Ø	D48.7	D49.89
limb						
lower	—	C77.4	—	D36.Ø	D48.7	D49.89
upper	—	C77.3	—	D36.Ø	D48.7	D49.89
lower limb	—	C77.4	—	D36.Ø	D48.7	D49.89
lumbar	—	C77.2	—	D36.Ø	D48.7	D49.89
mandibular	—	C77.Ø	—	D36.Ø	D48.7	D49.89
mediastinal	—	C77.1	—	D36.Ø	D48.7	D49.89
mesenteric (inferior) (superior)	—	C77.2	—	D36.Ø	D48.7	D49.89
midcolic	—	C77.2	—	D36.Ø	D48.7	D49.89
multiple sites in categories C77.0–C77.5	—	C77.8	—	D36.Ø	D48.7	D49.89
neck	—	C77.Ø	—	D36.Ø	D48.7	D49.89
obturator	—	C77.5	—	D36.Ø	D48.7	D49.89
occipital	—	C77.Ø	—	D36.Ø	D48.7	D49.89
pancreatic	—	C77.2	—	D36.Ø	D48.7	D49.89
para-aortic	—	C77.2	—	D36.Ø	D48.7	D49.89
paracervical	—	C77.5	—	D36.Ø	D48.7	D49.89
parametrial	—	C77.5	—	D36.Ø	D48.7	D49.89
parasternal	—	C77.1	—	D36.Ø	D48.7	D49.89
parotid	—	C77.Ø	—	D36.Ø	D48.7	D49.89
pectoral	—	C77.3	—	D36.Ø	D48.7	D49.89
pelvic	—	C77.5	—	D36.Ø	D48.7	D49.89
peri-aortic	—	C77.2	—	D36.Ø	D48.7	D49.89
peripancreatic	—	C77.2	—	D36.Ø	D48.7	D49.89
popliteal	—	C77.4	—	D36.Ø	D48.7	D49.89
porta hepatis	—	C77.2	—	D36.Ø	D48.7	D49.89
portal	—	C77.2	—	D36.Ø	D48.7	D49.89
preauricular	—	C77.Ø	—	D36.Ø	D48.7	D49.89
prelaryngeal	—	C77.Ø	—	D36.Ø	D48.7	D49.89
presymphysial	—	C77.5	—	D36.Ø	D48.7	D49.89
pretracheal	—	C77.Ø	—	D36.Ø	D48.7	D49.89

	Malignant Primary	Malignant Secondary	Ca in situ	Benign	Uncertain Behavior	Unspecified Behavior
Neoplasm, neoplastic — *continued*						
lymph, lymphatic channel NEC — *continued*						
gland (secondary) — *continued*						
primary (any site) NEC	C96.9	—	—	—	—	—
pulmonary (hiler)	—	C77.1	—	D36.Ø	D48.7	D49.89
pyloric	—	C77.2	—	D36.Ø	D48.7	D49.89
retroperitoneal	—	C77.2	—	D36.Ø	D48.7	D49.89
retropharyngeal	—	C77.Ø	—	D36.Ø	D48.7	D49.89
Rosenmüller's	—	C77.4	—	D36.Ø	D48.7	D49.89
sacral	—	C77.5	—	D36.Ø	D48.7	D49.89
scalene	—	C77.Ø	—	D36.Ø	D48.7	D49.89
site NEC	—	C77.9	—	D36.Ø	D48.7	D49.89
splenic (hilar)	—	C77.2	—	D36.Ø	D48.7	D49.89
subclavicular	—	C77.3	—	D36.Ø	D48.7	D49.89
subinguinal	—	C77.4	—	D36.Ø	D48.7	D49.89
sublingual	—	C77.Ø	—	D36.Ø	D48.7	D49.89
submandibular	—	C77.Ø	—	D36.Ø	D48.7	D49.89
submaxillary	—	C77.Ø	—	D36.Ø	D48.7	D49.89
submental	—	C77.Ø	—	D36.Ø	D48.7	D49.89
subscapular	—	C77.3	—	D36.Ø	D48.7	D49.89
supraclavicular	—	C77.Ø	—	D36.Ø	D48.7	D49.89
thoracic	—	C77.1	—	D36.Ø	D48.7	D49.89
tibial	—	C77.4	—	D36.Ø	D48.7	D49.89
tracheal	—	C77.1	—	D36.Ø	D48.7	D49.89
tracheobronchial	—	C77.1	—	D36.Ø	D48.7	D49.89
upper limb	—	C77.3	—	D36.Ø	D48.7	D49.89
Virchow's	—	C77.Ø	—	D36.Ø	D48.7	D49.89
node (*see also* Neoplasm, lymph gland)						
primary NEC	C96.9	—	—	—	—	—
vessel (*see also* Neoplasm, connective tissue)	C49.9	C79.89	—	D21.9	D48.1	D49.2
Mackenrodt's ligament	C57.7	C79.82	DØ7.39	D28.7	D39.8	D49.5
malar	C41.Ø	C79.51	—	D16.4-	D48.Ø	D49.2
region — *see* Neoplasm, cheek						
mammary gland — *see* Neoplasm, breast						
mandible	C41.1	C79.51	—	D16.5-	D48.Ø	D49.2
alveolar						
mucosa (carcinoma)	CØ3.1	C79.89	DØØ.Ø3	D1Ø.39	D37.Ø9	D49.Ø
ridge or process	C41.1	C79.51	—	D16.5-	D48.Ø	D49.2
marrow (bone) NEC	C96.9	C79.52	—	—	D47.9	D49.89
mastectomy site (skin) (*see also* Neoplasm, breast, skin)	C44.Ø1	C79.2	—	—	—	—
specified as breast tissue	C5Ø.8-	C79.81	—	—	—	—
mastoid (air cells) (antrum) (cavity)	C3Ø.1	C78.39	DØ2.3	D14.Ø	D38.5	D49.1
bone or process	C41.Ø	C79.51	—	D16.4-	D48.Ø	D49.2
maxilla, maxillary (superior)	C41.Ø	C79.51	—	D16.4-	D48.Ø	D49.2
alveolar						
mucosa	CØ3.Ø	C79.89	DØØ.Ø3	D1Ø.39	D37.Ø9	D49.Ø
ridge or process (carcinoma)	C41.Ø	C79.51	—	D16.4-	D48.Ø	D49.2
antrum	C31.Ø	C78.39	DØ2.3	D14.Ø	D38.5	D49.1
carcinoma	CØ3.Ø	C79.51	—	—	—	—
inferior — *see* Neoplasm, mandible						
sinus	C31.Ø	C78.39	DØ2.3	D14.Ø	D38.5	D49.1
meatus external (ear) (*see also* Neoplasm, skin, ear)	C44.2Ø-	C79.2	DØ4.2-	D23.2-	D48.5	D49.2
Meckel diverticulum, malignant	C17.3	C78.4	DØ1.49	D13.39	D37.2	D49.Ø
mediastinum, mediastinal	C38.3	C78.1	—	D15.2	D38.3	D49.89
anterior	C38.1	C78.1	—	D15.2	D38.3	D49.89
posterior	C38.2	C78.1	—	D15.2	D38.3	D49.89
medulla						
adrenal	C74.1-	C79.7-	DØ9.3	D35.Ø-	D44.1-	D49.7
oblongata	C71.7	C79.31	—	D33.1	D43.1	D49.6
meibomian gland	C44.1Ø-	C79.2	DØ4.1-	D23.1-	D48.5	D49.2
basal cell carcinoma	C44.11-	—	—	—	—	—
specified type NEC	C44.19-	—	—	—	—	—
squamous cell carcinoma	C44.12-	—	—	—	—	—
melanoma — *see* Melanoma						

	Malignant Primary	Malignant Secondary	Ca in situ	Benign	Uncertain Behavior	Unspecified Behavior
Neoplasm, neoplastic — *continued*						
meninges	C7Ø.9	C79.49	—	D32.9	D42.9	D49.7
brain	C7Ø.Ø	C79.32	—	D32.Ø	D42.Ø	D49.7
cerebral	C7Ø.Ø	C79.32	—	D32.Ø	D42.Ø	D49.7
crainial	C7Ø.Ø	C79.32	—	D32.Ø	D42.Ø	D49.7
intracranial	C7Ø.Ø	C79.32	—	D32.Ø	D42.Ø	D49.7
spinal (cord)	C7Ø.1	C79.49	—	D32.1	D42.1	D49.7
meniscus, knee joint (lateral) (medial)	C4Ø.2-	C79.51	—	D16.2-	D48.Ø	D49.2
Merkel cell — *see* Carcinoma, Merkel cell						
mesentery, mesenteric	C48.1	C78.6	—	D2Ø.1	D48.4	D49.Ø
mesoappendix	C48.1	C78.6	—	D2Ø.1	D48.4	D49.Ø
mesocolon	C48.1	C78.6	—	D2Ø.1	D48.4	D49.Ø
mesopharynx — *see* Neoplasm, oropharynx						
mesosalpinx	C57.1	C79.82	DØ7.39	D28.2	D39.8	D49.5
mesothelial tissue — *see* Mesothelioma						
mesothelioma — *see* Mesothelioma						
mesovarium	C57.1	C79.82	DØ7.39	D28.2	D39.8	D49.5
metacarpus (any bone)	C4Ø.1-	C79.51	—	D16.1-	—	—
metastatic NEC (*see also* Neoplasm, by site, secondary)	—	C79.9	—	—	—	—
metatarsus (any bone)	C4Ø.3-	C79.51	—	D16.3-	—	—
midbrain	C71.7	C79.31	—	D33.1	D43.1	D49.6
milk duct — *see* Neoplasm, breast						
mons						
pubis	C51.9	C79.82	DØ7.1	D28.Ø	D39.8	D49.5
veneris	C51.9	C79.82	DØ7.1	D28.Ø	D39.8	D49.5
motor tract	C72.9	C79.49	—	D33.9	D43.9	D49.7
brain	C71.9	C79.31	—	D33.2	D43.2	D49.6
cauda equina	C72.1	C79.49	—	D33.4	D43.4	D49.7
spinal	C72.Ø	C79.49	—	D33.4	D43.4	D49.7
mouth	CØ6.9	C79.89	DØØ.ØØ	D1Ø.3Ø	D37.Ø9	D49.Ø
book-leaf	CØ6.89	C79.89	—	—	—	—
floor	CØ4.9	C79.89	DØØ.Ø6	D1Ø.2	D37.Ø9	D49.Ø
anterior portion	CØ4.Ø	C79.89	DØØ.Ø6	D1Ø.2	D37.Ø9	D49.Ø
lateral portion	CØ4.1	C79.89	DØØ.Ø6	D1Ø.2	D37.Ø9	D49.Ø
overlapping lesion	CØ4.8	—	—	—	—	—
overlapping NEC	CØ6.8Ø	—	—	—	—	—
roof	CØ5.9	C79.89	DØØ.ØØ	D1Ø.39	D37.Ø9	D49.Ø
specified part NEC	CØ6.89	C79.89	DØØ.ØØ	D1Ø.39	D37.Ø9	D49.Ø
vestibule	CØ6.1	C79.89	DØØ.ØØ	D1Ø.39	D37.Ø9	D49.Ø
mucosa						
alveolar (ridge or process)	CØ3.9	C79.89	DØØ.Ø3	D1Ø.39	D37.Ø9	D49.Ø
lower	CØ3.1	C79.89	DØØ.Ø3	D1Ø.39	D37.Ø9	D49.Ø
upper	CØ3.Ø	C79.89	DØØ.Ø3	D1Ø.39	D37.Ø9	D49.Ø
buccal	CØ6.Ø	C79.89	DØØ.Ø2	D1Ø.39	D37.Ø9	D49.Ø
cheek	CØ6.Ø	C79.89	DØØ.Ø2	D1Ø.39	D37.Ø9	D49.Ø
lip — *see* Neoplasm, lip, internal						
nasal	C3Ø.Ø	C78.39	DØ2.3	D14.Ø	D38.5	D49.1
oral	CØ6.Ø	C79.89	DØØ.Ø2	D1Ø.39	D37.Ø9	D49.Ø
Müllerian duct						
female	C57.7	C79.82	DØ7.39	D28.7	D39.8	D49.5
male	C63.7	C79.82	DØ7.69	D29.8	D4Ø.8	D49.5
muscle (*see also* Neoplasm, connective tissue)						
extraocular	C69.6-	C79.49	DØ9.2-	D31.6-	D48.7	D49.89
myocardium	C38.Ø	C79.89	—	D15.1	D48.7	D49.89
myometrium	C54.2	C79.82	DØ7.Ø	D26.1	D39.Ø	D49.5
myopericardium	C38.Ø	C79.89	—	D15.1	D48.7	D49.89
nabothian gland (follicle)	C53.Ø	C79.82	DØ6.Ø	D26.Ø	D39.Ø	D49.5
nail (*see also* Neoplasm, skin, limb)	C44.9Ø	C79.2	DØ4.9	D23.9	D48.5	D49.2
finger (*see also* Neoplasm, skin, limb, upper)	C44.6Ø-	C79.2	DØ4.6-	D23.6-	D48.5	D49.2
toe (*see also* Neoplasm, skin, limb, lower)	C44.7Ø-	C79.2	DØ4.7-	D23.7-	D48.5	D49.2
nares, naris (anterior) (posterior)	C3Ø.Ø	C78.39	DØ2.3	D14.Ø	D38.5	D49.1
nasal — *see* Neoplasm, nose						
nasolabial groove (*see also* Neoplasm, skin, face)	C44.3Ø9	C79.2	DØ4.39	D23.39	D48.5	D49.2

	Malignant Primary	Malignant Secondary	Ca in situ	Benign	Uncertain Behavior	Unspecified Behavior
Neoplasm, neoplastic — *continued*						
nasolacrimal duct	C69.5-	C79.49	DØ9.2-	D31.5-	D48.7	D49.89
nasopharynx, nasopharyngeal	C11.9	C79.89	DØØ.Ø8	D1Ø.6	D37.Ø5	D49.Ø
floor	C11.3	C79.89	DØØ.Ø8	D1Ø.6	D37.Ø5	D49.Ø
overlapping lesion	C11.8	—	—	—	—	—
roof	C11.Ø	C79.89	DØØ.Ø8	D1Ø.6	D37.Ø5	D49.Ø
wall	C11.9	C79.89	DØØ.Ø8	D1Ø.6	D37.Ø5	D49.Ø
anterior	C11.3	C79.89	DØØ.Ø8	D1Ø.6	D37.Ø5	D49.Ø
lateral	C11.2	C79.89	DØØ.Ø8	D1Ø.6	D37.Ø5	D49.Ø
posterior	C11.1	C79.89	DØØ.Ø8	D1Ø.6	D37.Ø5	D49.Ø
superior	C11.Ø	C79.89	DØØ.Ø8	D1Ø.6	D37.Ø5	D49.Ø
nates (*see also* Neoplasm, skin, trunk)	C44.509	C79.2	DØ4.5	D23.5	D48.5	D49.2
neck NEC	C76.Ø	C79.89	DØ9.8	D36.7	D48.7	D49.89
skin	C44.4Ø	—	—	—	—	—
basal cell carcinoma	C44.41	—	—	—	—	—
specified type NEC	C44.49	—	—	—	—	—
squamous cell carcinoma	C44.42	—	—	—	—	—
nerve (ganglion)	C47.9	C79.89	—	D36.1Ø	D48.2	D49.2
abducens	C72.59	C79.49	—	D33.3	D43.3	D49.7
accessory (spinal)	C72.59	C79.49	—	D33.3	D43.3	D49.7
acoustic	C72.4-	C79.49	—	D33.3	D43.3	D49.7
auditory	C72.4-	C79.49	—	D33.3	D43.3	D49.7
autonomic NEC (*see also* Neoplasm, nerve, peripheral)	C47.9	C79.89	—	D36.1Ø	D48.2	D49.2
brachial	C47.1-	C79.89	—	D36.12	D48.2	D49.2
cranial	C72.5Ø	C79.49	—	D33.3	D43.3	D49.7
specified NEC	C72.59	C79.49	—	D33.3	D43.3	D49.7
facial	C72.59	C79.49	—	D33.3	D43.3	D49.7
femoral	C47.2-	C79.89	—	D36.13	D48.2	D49.2
ganglion NEC (*see also* Neoplasm, nerve, peripheral)	C47.9	C79.89	—	D36.1Ø	D48.2	D49.2
glossopharyngeal	C72.59	C79.49	—	D33.3	D43.3	D49.7
hypoglossal	C72.59	C79.49	—	D33.3	D43.3	D49.7
intercostal	C47.3	C79.89	—	D36.14	D48.2	D49.2
lumbar	C47.6	C79.89	—	D36.17	D48.2	D49.2
median	C47.1-	C79.89	—	D36.12	D48.2	D49.2
obturator	C47.2-	C79.89	—	D36.13	D48.2	D49.2
oculomotor	C72.59	C79.49	—	D33.3	D43.3	D49.7
olfactory	C72.2-	C79.49	—	D33.3	D43.3	D49.7
optic	C72.3-	C79.49	—	D33.3	D43.3	D49.7
parasympathetic NEC	C47.9	C79.89	—	D36.1Ø	D48.2	D49.2
peripheral NEC	C47.9	C79.89	—	D36.1Ø	D48.2	D49.2
abdomen	C47.4	C79.89	—	D36.15	D48.2	D49.2
abdominal wall	C47.4	C79.89	—	D36.15	D48.2	D49.2
ankle	C47.2-	C79.89	—	D36.13	D48.2	D49.2
antecubital fossa or space	C47.1-	C79.89	—	D36.12	D48.2	D49.2
arm	C47.1-	C79.89	—	D36.12	D48.2	D49.2
auricle (ear)	C47.Ø	C79.89	—	D36.11	D48.2	D49.2
axilla	C47.3	C79.89	—	D36.12	D48.2	D49.2
back	C47.6	C79.89	—	D36.17	D48.2	D49.2
buttock	C47.5	C79.89	—	D36.16	D48.2	D49.2
calf	C47.2-	C79.89	—	D36.13	D48.2	D49.2
cervical region	C47.Ø	C79.89	—	D36.11	D48.2	D49.2
cheek	C47.Ø	C79.89	—	D36.11	D48.2	D49.2
chest (wall)	C47.3	C79.89	—	D36.14	D48.2	D49.2
chin	C47.Ø	C79.89	—	D36.11	D48.2	D49.2
ear (external)	C47.Ø	C79.89	—	D36.11	D48.2	D49.2
elbow	C47.1-	C79.89	—	D36.12	D48.2	D49.2
extrarectal	C47.5	C79.89	—	D36.16	D48.2	D49.2
extremity	C47.9	C79.89	—	D36.1Ø	D48.2	D49.2
lower	C47.2-	C79.89	—	D36.13	D48.2	D49.2
upper	C47.1-	C79.89	—	D36.12	D48.2	D49.2
eyelid	C47.Ø	C79.89	—	D36.11	D48.2	D49.2
face	C47.Ø	C79.89	—	D36.11	D48.2	D49.2
finger	C47.1-	C79.89	—	D36.12	D48.2	D49.2
flank	C47.6	C79.89	—	D36.17	D48.2	D49.2
foot	C47.2-	C79.89	—	D36.13	D48.2	D49.2
forearm	C47.1-	C79.89	—	D36.12	D48.2	D49.2
forehead	C47.Ø	C79.89	—	D36.11	D48.2	D49.2

	Malignant Primary	Malignant Secondary	Ca in situ	Benign	Uncertain Behavior	Unspecified Behavior
Neoplasm, neoplastic — *continued*						
nerve (ganglion) — *continued*						
peripheral NEC — *continued*						
gluteal region	C47.5	C79.89	—	D36.16	D48.2	D49.2
groin	C47.5	C79.89	—	D36.16	D48.2	D49.2
hand	C47.1-	C79.89	—	D36.12	D48.2	D49.2
head	C47.Ø	C79.89	—	D36.11	D48.2	D49.2
heel	C47.2-	C79.89	—	D36.13	D48.2	D49.2
hip	C47.2-	C79.89	—	D36.13	D48.2	D49.2
infraclavicular region	C47.3	C79.89	—	D36.14	D48.2	D49.2
inguinal (canal) (region)	C47.5	C79.89	—	D36.16	D48.2	D49.2
intrathoracic	C47.3	C79.89	—	D36.14	D48.2	D49.2
ischiorectal fossa	C47.5	C79.89	—	D36.16	D48.2	D49.2
knee	C47.2-	C79.89	—	D36.13	D48.2	D49.2
leg	C47.2-	C79.89	—	D36.13	D48.2	D49.2
limb NEC	C47.9	C79.89	—	D36.1Ø	D48.2	D49.2
lower	C47.2-	C79.89	—	D36.13	D48.2	D49.2
upper	C47.1-	C79.89	—	D36.12	D48.2	D49.2
nates	C47.5	C79.89	—	D36.16	D48.2	D49.2
neck	C47.Ø	C79.89	—	D36.11	D48.2	D49.2
orbit	C69.6-	C79.49	—	D31.6-	D48.7	D49.2
pararectal	C47.5	C79.89	—	D36.16	D48.2	D49.2
paraurethral	C47.5	C79.89	—	D36.16	D48.2	D49.2
paravaginal	C47.5	C79.89	—	D36.16	D48.2	D49.2
pelvis (floor)	C47.5	C79.89	—	D36.16	D48.2	D49.2
pelvoabdominal	C47.8	C79.89	—	D36.17	D48.2	D49.2
perineum	C47.5	C79.89	—	D36.16	D48.2	D49.2
perirectal (tissue)	C47.5	C79.89	—	D36.16	D48.2	D49.2
periurethral (tissue)	C47.5	C79.89	—	D36.16	D48.2	D49.2
popliteal fossa or space	C47.2-	C79.89	—	D36.13	D48.2	D49.2
presacral	C47.5	C79.89	—	D36.16	D48.2	D49.2
pterygoid fossa	C47.Ø	C79.89	—	D36.11	D48.2	D49.2
rectovaginal septum or wall	C47.5	C79.89	—	D36.16	D48.2	D49.2
rectovesical	C47.5	C79.89	—	D36.16	D48.2	D49.2
sacrococcygeal region	C47.5	C79.89	—	D36.16	D48.2	D49.2
scalp	C47.Ø	C79.89	—	D36.11	D48.2	D49.2
scapular region	C47.3	C79.89	—	D36.14	D48.2	D49.2
shoulder	C47.1-	C79.89	—	D36.12	D48.2	D49.2
submental	C47.Ø	C79.89	—	D36.11	D48.2	D49.2
supraclavicular region	C47.Ø	C79.89	—	D36.11	D48.2	D49.2
temple	C47.Ø	C79.89	—	D36.11	D48.2	D49.2
temporal region	C47.Ø	C79.89	—	D36.11	D48.2	D49.2
thigh	C47.2-	C79.89	—	D36.13	D48.2	D49.2
thoracic (duct) (wall)	C47.3	C79.89	—	D36.14	D48.2	D49.2
thorax	C47.3	C79.89	—	D36.14	D48.2	D49.2
thumb	C47.1-	C79.89	—	D36.12	D48.2	D49.2
toe	C47.2-	C79.89	—	D36.13	D48.2	D49.2
trunk	C47.6	C79.89	—	D36.17	D48.2	D49.2
umbilicus	C47.4	C79.89	—	D36.15	D48.2	D49.2
vesicorectal	C47.5	C79.89	—	D36.16	D48.2	D49.2
wrist	C47.1-	C79.89	—	D36.12	D48.2	D49.2
radial	C47.1-	C79.89	—	D36.12	D48.2	D49.2
sacral	C47.5	C79.89	—	D36.16	D48.2	D49.2
sciatic	C47.2-	C79.89	—	D36.13	D48.2	D49.2
spinal NEC	C47.9	C79.89	—	D36.1Ø	D48.2	D49.2
accessory	C72.59	C79.49	—	D33.3	D43.3	D49.7
sympathetic NEC (*see also* Neoplasm, nerve, peripheral)	C47.9	C79.89	—	D36.1Ø	D48.2	D49.2
trigeminal	C72.59	C79.49	—	D33.3	D43.3	D49.7
trochlear	C72.59	C79.49	—	D33.3	D43.3	D49.7
ulnar	C47.1-	C79.89	—	D36.12	D48.2	D49.2
vagus	C72.59	C79.49	—	D33.3	D43.3	D49.7
nervous system (central)	C72.9	C79.4Ø	—	D33.9	D43.9	D49.7
autonomic — *see* Neoplasm, nerve, peripheral						
nevus — *see* Nevus						
parasympathetic — *see* Neoplasm, nerve, peripheral						
specified site NEC	—	C79.49	—	D33.7	D43.8	—

	Malignant Primary	Malignant Secondary	Ca in situ	Benign	Uncertain Behavior	Unspecified Behavior
Neoplasm, neoplastic — *continued*						
nervous system (central) — *continued*						
sympathetic — *see* Neoplasm, nerve, peripheral						
nipple	C5Ø.Ø-	C79.81	DØ5.-	D24.-	—	—
nose, nasal	C76.Ø	C79.89	DØ9.8	D36.7	D48.7	D49.89
ala (external) (nasi) (*see also* Neoplasm, nose, skin)	C44.3Ø1	C79.2	DØ4.39	D23.39	D48.5	D49.2
bone	C41.Ø	C79.51	—	D16.4-	D48.Ø	D49.2
cartilage	C3Ø.Ø	C78.39	DØ2.3	D14.Ø	D38.5	D49.1
cavity	C3Ø.Ø	C78.39	DØ2.3	D14.Ø	D38.5	D49.1
choana	C11.3	C79.89	DØØ.Ø8	D1Ø.6	D37.Ø5	D49.Ø
external (skin) (*see also* Neoplasm, nose, skin)	C44.3Ø1	C79.2	DØ4.39	D23.39	D48.5	D49.2
fossa	C3Ø.Ø	C78.39	DØ2.3	D14.Ø	D38.5	D49.1
internal	C3Ø.Ø	C78.39	DØ2.3	D14.Ø	D38.5	D49.1
mucosa	C3Ø.Ø	C78.39	DØ2.3	D14.Ø	D38.5	D49.1
septum	C3Ø.Ø	C78.39	DØ2.3	D14.Ø	D38.5	D49.1
posterior margin	C11.3	C79.89	DØØ.Ø8	D1Ø.6	D37.Ø5	D49.Ø
sinus — *see* Neoplasm, sinus						
skin	C44.3Ø1	C79.2	DØ4.39	D23.39	D48.5	D49.2
basal cell carcinoma	C44.311	—	—	—	—	—
specified type NEC	C44.391	—	—	—	—	—
squamous cell carcinoma	C44.321	—	—	—	—	—
turbinate (mucosa)	C3Ø.Ø	C78.39	DØ2.3	D14.Ø	D38.5	D49.1
bone	C41.Ø	C79.51	—	D16.4-	D48.Ø	D49.2
vestibule	C3Ø.Ø	C78.39	DØ2.3	D14.Ø	D38.5	D49.1
nostril	C3Ø.Ø	C78.39	DØ2.3	D14.Ø	D38.5	D49.1
nucleus pulposus	C41.2	C79.51	—	D16.6-	D48.Ø	D49.2
occipital			—			
bone	C41.Ø	C79.51	—	D16.4-	D48.Ø	D49.2
lobe or pole, brain	C71.4	C79.31	—	D33.Ø	D43.Ø	D49.6
odontogenic — *see* Neoplasm, jaw bone			—			
olfactory nerve or bulb	C72.2-	C79.49	—	D33.3	D43.3	D49.7
olive (brain)	C71.7	C79.31	—	D33.1	D43.1	D49.6
omentum	C48.1	C78.6	—	D2Ø.1	D48.4	D49.Ø
operculum (brain)	C71.Ø	C79.31	—	D33.Ø	D43.Ø	D49.6
optic nerve, chiasm, or tract	C72.3-	C79.49	—	D33.3	D43.3	D49.7
oral (cavity)	CØ6.9	C79.89	DØØ.ØØ	D1Ø.3Ø	D37.Ø9	D49.Ø
ill-defined	C14.8	C79.89	DØØ.ØØ	D1Ø.3Ø	D37.Ø9	D49.Ø
mucosa	CØ6.Ø	C79.89	DØØ.Ø2	D1Ø.39	D37.Ø9	D49.Ø
orbit	C69.6-	C79.49	DØ9.2-	D31.6-	D48.7	D49.89
autonomic nerve	C69.6-	C79.49	—	D31.6-	D48.7	D49.2
bone	C41.Ø	C79.51	—	D16.4-	D48.Ø	D49.2
eye	C69.6-	C79.49	DØ9.2-	D31.6-	D48.7	D49.89
peripheral nerves	C69.6-	C79.49	—	D31.6-	D48.7	D49.2
soft parts	C69.6-	C79.49	DØ9.2-	D31.6-	D48.7	D49.89
organ of Zuckerkandl	C75.5	C79.89	—	D35.6	D44.7	D49.7
oropharynx	C1Ø.9	C79.89	DØØ.Ø8	D1Ø.5	D37.Ø5	D49.Ø
branchial cleft (vestige)	C1Ø.4	C79.89	DØØ.Ø8	D1Ø.5	D37.Ø5	D49.Ø
junctional region	C1Ø.8	C79.89	DØØ.Ø8	D1Ø.5	D37.Ø5	D49.Ø
lateral wall	C1Ø.2	C79.89	DØØ.Ø8	D1Ø.5	D37.Ø5	D49.Ø
overlapping lesion	C1Ø.8	—	—	—	—	—
pillars or fauces	CØ9.1	C79.89	DØØ.Ø8	D1Ø.5	D37.Ø5	D49.Ø
posterior wall	C1Ø.3	C79.89	DØØ.Ø8	D1Ø.5	D37.Ø5	D49.Ø
vallecula	C1Ø.Ø	C79.89	DØØ.Ø8	D1Ø.5	D37.Ø5	D49.Ø
os						
external	C53.1	C79.82	DØ6.1	D26.Ø	D39.Ø	D49.5
internal	C53.Ø	C79.82	DØ6.Ø	D26.Ø	D39.Ø	D49.5
ovary	C56.-	C79.6-	DØ7.39	D27.-	D39.1-	D49.5
oviduct	C57.Ø-	C79.82	DØ7.39	D28.2	D39.8	D49.5
palate	CØ5.9	C79.89	DØØ.ØØ	D1Ø.39	D37.Ø9	D49.Ø
hard	CØ5.Ø	C79.89	DØØ.Ø5	D1Ø.39	D37.Ø9	D49.Ø
junction of hard and soft palate	CØ5.9	C79.89	DØØ.ØØ	D1Ø.39	D37.Ø9	D49.Ø
overlapping lesions	CØ5.8	—	—	—	—	—
soft	CØ5.1	C79.89	DØØ.Ø4	D1Ø.39	D37.Ø9	D49.Ø
nasopharyngeal surface	C11.3	C79.89	DØØ.Ø8	D1Ø.6	D37.Ø5	D49.Ø
posterior surface	C11.3	C79.89	DØØ.Ø8	D1Ø.6	D37.Ø5	D49.Ø
superior surface	C11.3	C79.89	DØØ.Ø8	D1Ø.6	D37.Ø5	D49.Ø
palatoglossal arch	CØ9.1	C79.89	DØØ.ØØ	D1Ø.5	D37.Ø9	D49.Ø

	Malignant Primary	Malignant Secondary	Ca in situ	Benign	Uncertain Behavior	Unspecified Behavior
Neoplasm, neoplastic — *continued*						
palatopharyngeal arch	CØ9.1	C79.89	DØØ.ØØ	D1Ø.5	D37.Ø9	D49.Ø
pallium	C71.Ø	C79.31	—	D33.Ø	D43.Ø	D49.6
palpebra	C44.1Ø-	C79.2	DØ4.1-	D23.1-	D48.5	D49.2
basal cell carcinoma	C44.11-	—	—	—	—	—
specified type NEC	C44.19-	—	—	—	—	—
squamous cell carcinoma	C44.12-	—	—	—	—	—
pancreas	C25.9	C78.89	DØ1.7	D13.6	D37.8	D49.Ø
body	C25.1	C78.89	DØ1.7	D13.6	D37.8	D49.Ø
duct (of Santorini) (of Wirsung)	C25.3	C78.89	DØ1.7	D13.6	D37.8	D49.Ø
ectopic tissue	C25.7	C78.89	-	D13.6	D37.8	D49.Ø
head	C25.Ø	C78.89	DØ1.7	D13.6	D37.8	D49.Ø
islet cells	C25.4	C78.89	DØ1.7	D13.7	D37.8	D49.Ø
neck	C25.7	C78.89	DØ1.7	D13.6	D37.8	D49.Ø
overlapping lesion	C25.8	—	—	—	—	—
tail	C25.2	C78.89	DØ1.7	D13.6	D37.8	D49.Ø
para-aortic body	C75.5	C79.89	—	D35.6	D44.7	D49.7
paraganglion NEC	C75.5	C79.89	—	D35.6	D44.7	D49.7
parametrium	C57.3	C79.82	—	D28.2	D39.8	D49.5
paranephric	C48.Ø	C78.6	—	D2Ø.Ø	D48.3	D49.Ø
pararectal	C76.3	C79.89	—	D36.7	D48.7	D49.89
parasagittal (region)	C76.Ø	C79.89	DØ9.8	D36.7	D48.7	D49.89
parasellar	C72.9	C79.49	—	D33.9	D43.8	D49.7
parathyroid (gland)	C75.Ø	C79.89	DØ9.3	D35.1	D44.2-	D49.7
paraurethral	C76.3	C79.89	—	D36.7	D48.7	D49.89
gland	C68.1	C79.19	DØ9.19	D3Ø.8	D41.8	D49.5
paravaginal	C76.3	C79.89	—	D36.7	D48.7	D49.89
parenchyma, kidney	C64.-	C79.Ø-	DØ9.19	D3Ø.Ø-	D41.Ø-	D49.5
parietal						
bone	C41.Ø	C79.51	—	D16.4-	D48.Ø	D49.2
lobe, brain	C71.3	C79.31	—	D33.Ø	D43.Ø	D49.6
paroophoron	C57.1	C79.82	DØ7.39	D28.2	D39.8	D49.5
parotid (duct) (gland)	CØ7	C79.89	DØØ.ØØ	D11.Ø	D37.Ø3Ø	D49.Ø
parovarium	C57.1	C79.82	DØ7.39	D28.2	D39.8	D49.5
patella	C4Ø.2Ø	C79.51	—	—	—	—
peduncle, cerebral	C71.7	C79.31	—	D33.1	D43.1	D49.6
pelvirectal junction	C19	C78.5	DØ1.1	D12.7	D37.5	D49.Ø
pelvis, pelvic	C76.3	C79.89	DØ9.8	D36.7	D48.7	D49.89
bone	C41.4	C79.51	—	D16.8-	D48.Ø	D49.2
floor	C76.3	C79.89	DØ9.8	D36.7	D48.7	D49.89
renal	C65.-	C79.Ø-	DØ9.19	D3Ø.1-	D41.1-	D49.5
viscera	C76.3	C79.89	DØ9.8	D36.7	D48.7	D49.89
wall	C76.3	C79.89	DØ9.8	D36.7	D48.7	D49.89
pelvo-abdominal	C76.8	C79.89	DØ9.8	D36.7	D48.7	D49.89
penis	C6Ø.9	C79.82	DØ7.4	D29.Ø	D4Ø.8	D49.5
body	C6Ø.2	C79.82	DØ7.4	D29.Ø	D4Ø.8	D49.5
corpus (cavernosum)	C6Ø.2	C79.82	DØ7.4	D29.Ø	D4Ø.8	D49.5
glans	C6Ø.1	C79.82	DØ7.4	D29.Ø	D4Ø.8	D49.5
overlapping sites	C6Ø.8	—	—	—	—	—
skin NEC	C6Ø.9	C79.82	DØ7.4	D29.Ø	D4Ø.8	D49.5
periadrenal (tissue)	C48.Ø	C78.6	—	D2Ø.Ø	D48.3	D49.Ø
perianal (skin) (*see also* Neoplasm, anus, skin)	C44.5ØØ	C79.2	DØ4.5	D23.5	D48.5	D49.2
pericardium	C38.Ø	C79.89	—	D15.1	D48.7	D49.89
perinephric	C48.Ø	C78.6	—	D2Ø.Ø	D48.3	D49.Ø
perineum	C76.3	C79.89	DØ9.8	D36.7	D48.7	D49.89
periodontal tissue NEC	CØ3.9	C79.89	DØØ.Ø3	D1Ø.39	D37.Ø9	D49.Ø
periosteum — *see* Neoplasm, bone						
peripancreatic	C48.Ø	C78.6	—	D2Ø.Ø	D48.3	D49.Ø
peripheral nerve NEC	C47.9	C79.89	—	D36.1Ø	D48.2	D49.2
perirectal (tissue)	C76.3	C79.89	—	D36.7	D48.7	D49.89
perirenal (tissue)	C48.Ø	C78.6	—	D2Ø.Ø	D48.3	D49.Ø
peritoneum, peritoneal (cavity)	C48.2	C78.6	—	D2Ø.1	D48.4	D49.Ø
benign mesothelial tissue — *see* Mesothelioma, benign						
overlapping lesion	C48.8	—	—	—	—	—
with digestive organs	C26.9	—	—	—	—	—
parietal	C48.1	C78.6	—	D2Ø.1	D48.4	D49.Ø
pelvic	C48.1	C78.6	—	D2Ø.1	D48.4	D49.Ø
specified part NEC	C48.1	C78.6	—	D2Ø.1	D48.4	D49.Ø
peritonsillar (tissue)	C76.Ø	C79.89	DØ9.8	D36.7	D48.7	D49.89

	Malignant Primary	Malignant Secondary	Ca in situ	Benign	Uncertain Behavior	Unspecified Behavior
Neoplasm, neoplastic — *continued*						
periurethral tissue	C76.3	C79.89	—	D36.7	D48.7	D49.89
phalanges						
foot	C4Ø.3-	C79.51	—	D16.3-	—	—
hand	C4Ø.1-	C79.51	—	D16.1-	—	—
pharynx, pharyngeal	C14.Ø	C79.89	DØØ.Ø8	D1Ø.9	D37.Ø5	D49.Ø
bursa	C11.1	C79.89	DØØ.Ø8	D1Ø.6	D37.Ø5	D49.Ø
fornix	C11.3	C79.89	DØØ.Ø8	D1Ø.6	D37.Ø5	D49.Ø
recess	C11.2	C79.89	DØØ.Ø8	D1Ø.6	D37.Ø5	D49.Ø
region	C14.Ø	C79.89	DØØ.Ø8	D1Ø.9	D37.Ø5	D49.Ø
tonsil	C11.1	C79.89	DØØ.Ø8	D1Ø.6	D37.Ø5	D49.Ø
wall (lateral) (posterior)	C14.Ø	C79.89	DØØ.Ø8	D1Ø.9	D37.Ø5	D49.Ø
pia mater	C7Ø.9	C79.4Ø	—	D32.9	D42.9	D49.7
cerebral	C7Ø.Ø	C79.32	—	D32.Ø	D42.Ø	D49.7
cranial	C7Ø.Ø	C79.32	—	D32.Ø	D42.Ø	D49.7
spinal	C7Ø.1	C79.49	—	D32.1	D42.1	D49.7
pillars of fauces	CØ9.1	C79.89	DØØ.Ø8	D1Ø.5	D37.Ø5	D49.Ø
pineal (body) (gland)	C75.3	C79.89	DØ9.3	D35.4	D44.5	D49.7
pinna (ear) NEC (*see also* Neoplasm, skin, ear)	C44.2Ø-	C79.2	DØ4.2-	D23.2-	D48.5	D49.2
piriform fossa or sinus	C12	C79.89	DØØ.Ø8	D1Ø.7	D37.Ø5	D49.Ø
pituitary (body) (fossa) (gland) (lobe)	C75.1	C79.89	DØ9.3	D35.2	D44.3	D49.7
placenta	C58	C79.82	DØ7.Ø	D26.7	D39.2	D49.5
pleura, pleural (cavity)	C38.4	C78.2	—	D19.Ø	D38.2	D49.1
overlapping lesion with heart or mediastinum	C38.8	—	—	—	—	—
parietal	C38.4	C78.2	—	D19.Ø	D38.2	D49.1
visceral	C38.4	C78.2	—	D19.Ø	D38.2	D49.1
plexus			—			
brachial	C47.1-	C79.89	—	D36.12	D48.2	D49.2
cervical	C47.Ø	C79.89	—	D36.11	D48.2	D49.2
choroid	C71.5	C79.31	—	D33.Ø	D43.Ø	D49.6
lumbosacral	C47.5	C79.89	—	D36.16	D48.2	D49.2
sacral	C47.5	C79.89	—	D36.16	D48.2	D49.2
pluriendocrine	C75.8	C79.89	DØ9.3	D35.7	D44.9	D49.7
pole						
frontal	C71.1	C79.31	—	D33.Ø	D43.Ø	D49.6
occipital	C71.4	C79.31	—	D33.Ø	D43.Ø	D49.6
pons (varolii)	C71.7	C79.31	—	D33.1	D43.1	D49.6
popliteal fossa or space	C76.5-	C79.89	DØ4.7-	D36.7	D48.7	D49.89
postcricoid (region)	C13.Ø	C79.89	DØØ.Ø8	D1Ø.7	D37.Ø5	D49.Ø
posterior fossa (cranial)	C71.9	C79.31	—	D33.2	D43.2	D49.6
postnasal space	C11.9	C79.89	DØØ.Ø8	D1Ø.6	D37.Ø5	D49.Ø
prepuce	C6Ø.Ø	C79.82	DØ7.4	D29.Ø	D4Ø.8	D49.5
prepylorus	C16.4	C78.89	DØØ.2	D13.1	D37.1	D49.Ø
presacral (region)	C76.3	C79.89	—	D36.7	D48.7	D49.89
prostate (gland)	C61	C79.82	DØ7.5	D29.1	D4Ø.Ø-	D49.5
utricle	C68.Ø	C79.19	DØ9.19	D3Ø.4	D41.3	D49.5
pterygoid fossa	C49.Ø	C79.89	—	D21.Ø	D48.1	D49.2
pubic bone	C41.4	C79.51	—	D16.8-	D48.Ø	D49.2
pudenda, pudendum (femaie)	C51.9	C79.82	DØ7.1	D28.Ø	D39.8	D49.5
pulmonary (*see also* Neoplasm, lung)	C34.9-	C78.Ø-	DØ2.2-	D14.3-	D38.1	D49.1
putamen	C71.Ø	C79.31	—	D33.Ø	D43.Ø	D49.6
pyloric						
antrum	C16.3	C78.89	DØØ.2	D13.1	D37.1	D49.Ø
canal	C16.4	C78.89	DØØ.2	D13.1	D37.1	D49.Ø
pylorus	C16.4	C78.89	DØØ.2	D13.1	D37.1	D49.Ø
pyramid (brain)	C71.7	C79.31	—	D33.1	D43.1	D49.6
pyriform fossa or sinus	C12	C79.89	DØØ.Ø8	D1Ø.7	D37.Ø5	D49.Ø
radius (any part)	C4Ø.Ø-	C79.51	—	D16.Ø-	—	—
Rathke's pouch	C75.1	C79.89	DØ9.3	D35.2	D44.3	D49.7
rectosigmoid (junction)	C19	C78.5	DØ1.1	D12.7	D37.5	D49.Ø
overlapping lesion with anus or rectum	C21.8	—	—	—	—	—
rectouterine pouch	C48.1	C78.6	—	D2Ø.1	D48.4	D49.Ø
rectovaginal septum or wall	C76.3	C79.89	DØ9.8	D36.7	D48.7	D49.89
rectovesical septum	C76.3	C79.89	DØ9.8	D36.7	D48.7	D49.89
rectum (ampulla)	C2Ø	C78.5	DØ1.2	D12.8	D37.5	D49.Ø
and colon	C19	C78.5	DØ1.1	D12.7	D37.5	D49.Ø

	Malignant Primary	Malignant Secondary	Ca in situ	Benign	Uncertain Behavior	Unspecified Behavior
Neoplasm, neoplastic — *continued*						
rectum (ampulla) — *continued*						
overlapping lesion with anus or rectosigmoid junction	C21.8	—	—	—	—	—
renal	C64.-	C79.Ø-	DØ9.19	D3Ø.Ø-	D41.Ø-	D49.5
calyx	C65.-	C79.Ø-	DØ9.19	D3Ø.1-	D41.1-	D49.5
hilus	C65.-	C79.Ø-	DØ9.19	D3Ø.1-	D41.1-	D49.5
parenchyma	C64.-	C79.Ø-	DØ9.19	D3Ø.Ø--	D41.Ø-	D49.5
pelvis	C65.-	C79.Ø-	DØ9.19	D3Ø.1-	D41.1-	D49.5
respiratory						
organs or system NEC	C39.9	C78.3Ø	DØ2.4	D14.4	D38.6	D49.1
tract NEC	C39.9	C78.3Ø	DØ2.4	D14.4	D38.5	D49.1
upper	C39.Ø	C78.3Ø	DØ2.4	D14.4	D38.5	D49.1
retina	C69.2-	C79.49	DØ9.2-	D31.2	D48.7	D49.81
retrobulbar	C69.6-	C79.49	—	D31.6-	D48.7	D49.89
retrocecal	C48.Ø	C78.6	—	D2Ø.Ø	D48.3	D49.Ø
retromolar (area) (triangle) (trigone)	CØ6.2	C79.89	DØØ.ØØ	D1Ø.39	D37.Ø9	D49.Ø
retro-orbital	C76.Ø	C79.89	DØ9.8	D36.7	D48.7	D49.89
retroperitoneal (space) (tissue)	C48.Ø	C78.6	—	D2Ø.Ø	D48.3	D49.Ø
retroperitoneum	C48.Ø	C78.6	—	D2Ø.Ø	D48.3	D49.Ø
retropharyngeal	C14.Ø	C79.89	DØØ.Ø8	D1Ø.9	D37.Ø5	D49.Ø
retrovesical (septum)	C76.3	C79.89	DØ9.8	D36.7	D48.7	D49.89
rhinencephalon	C71.Ø	C79.31	—	D33.Ø	D43.Ø	D49.6
rib	C41.3	C79.51	—	D16.7-	D48.Ø	D49.2
Rosenmüller's fossa	C11.2	C79.89	DØØ.Ø8	D1Ø.6	D37.Ø5	D49.Ø
round ligament	C57.2	C79.82	—	D28.2	D39.8	D49.5
sacrococcyx, sacrococcygeal	C41.4	C79.51	—	D16.8-	D48.Ø	D49.2
region	C76.3	C79.89	DØ9.8	D36.7	D48.7	D49.89
sacrouterine ligament	C57.3	C79.82	—	D28.2	D39.8	D49.5
sacrum, sacral (vertebra)	C41.4	C79.51	—	D16.8-	D48.Ø	D49.2
salivary gland or duct (major)	CØ8.9	C79.89	DØØ.ØØ	D11.9	D37.Ø39	D49.Ø
minor NEC	CØ6.9	C79.89	DØØ.ØØ	D1Ø.39	D37.Ø4	D49.Ø
overlapping lesion	CØ8.9	—	—	—	—	—
parotid	CØ7	C79.89	DØØ.ØØ	D11.Ø	D37.Ø3Ø	D49.Ø
pluriglandular	CØ8.9	C79.89	DØØ.ØØ	D11.9	D37.Ø39	D49.Ø
sublingual	CØ8.1	C79.89	DØØ.ØØ	D11.7	D37.Ø31	D49.Ø
submandibular	CØ8.Ø	C79.89	DØØ.ØØ	D11.7	D37.Ø32	D49.Ø
submaxillary	CØ8.Ø	C79.89	DØØ.ØØ	D11.7	D37.Ø32	D49.Ø
salpinx (uterine)	C57.Ø-	C79.82	DØ7.39	D28.2	D39.8	D49.5
Santorini's duct	C25.3	C78.89	DØ1.7	D13.6	D37.8	D49.Ø
scalp	C44.4Ø	C79.2	DØ4.4	D23.4	D48.5	D49.2
basal cell carcinoma	C44.41	—	—	—	—	—
specified type NEC	C44.49	—	—	—	—	—
squamous cell carcinoma	C44.42	—	—	—	—	—
scapula (any part)	C4Ø.Ø-	C79.51	—	D16.Ø-	—	—
scapular region	C76.1	C79.89	DØ9.8	D36.7	D48.7	D49.89
scar NEC (*see also* Neoplasm, skin, by site)	C44.9Ø	C79.2	DØ4.9	D23.9	D48.5	D49.2
sciatic nerve	C47.2-	C79.89	—	D36.13	D48.2	D49.2
sclera	C69.4-	C79.49	DØ9.2-	D31.4-	D48.7	D49.89
scrotum (skin)	C63.2	C79.82	DØ7.61	D29.4	D4Ø.8	D49.5
sebaceous gland — *see* Neoplasm, skin						
sella turcica	C75.1	C79.89	DØ9.3	D35.2	D44.3	D49.7
bone	C41.Ø	C79.51	—	D16.4-	D48.Ø	D49.2
seminal vesicle	C63.7	C79.82	DØ7.69	D29.8	D4Ø.8	D49.5
semilunar cartilage (knee)	C4Ø.2-	C79.51	—	D16.2-	D48.Ø	D49.2
septum						
nasal	C3Ø.Ø	C78.39	DØ2.3	D14.Ø	D38.5	D49.1
posterior margin	C11.3	C79.89	DØØ.Ø8	D1Ø.6	D37.Ø5	D49.Ø
rectovaginal	C76.3	C79.89	DØ9.8	D36.7	D48.7	D49.89
rectovesical	C76.3	C79.89	DØ9.8	D36.7	D48.7	D49.89
urethrovaginal	C57.9	C79.82	DØ7.3Ø	D28.9	D39.9	D49.5
vesicovaginal	C57.9	C79.82	DØ7.3Ø	D28.9	D39.9	D49.5
shoulder NEC	C76.4-	C79.89	DØ4.6-	D36.7	D48.7	D49.89
sigmoid flexure (lower) (upper)	C18.7	C78.5	DØ1.Ø	D12.5	D37.4	D49.Ø
sinus (accessory)	C31.9	C78.39	DØ2.3	D14.Ø	D38.5	D49.1
bone (any)	C41.Ø	C79.51	—	D16.4-	D48.Ø	D49.2
ethmoidal	C31.1	C78.39	DØ2.3	D14.Ø	D38.5	D49.1
frontal	C31.2	C78.39	DØ2.3	D14.Ø	D38.5	D49.1
maxillary	C31.Ø	C78.39	DØ2.3	D14.Ø	D38.5	D49.1

	Malignant Primary	Malignant Secondary	Ca in situ	Benign	Uncertain Behavior	Unspecified Behavior
Neoplasm, neoplastic — *continued*						
sinus (accessory) — *continued*						
nasal, paranasal NEC	C31.9	C78.39	DØ2.3	D14.Ø	D38.5	D49.1
overlapping lesion	C31.8	—	—	—	—	—
pyriform	C12	C79.89	DØØ.Ø8	D1Ø.7	D37.Ø5	D49.Ø
sphenoid	C31.3	C78.39	DØ2.3	D14.Ø	D38.5	D49.1
skeleton, skeletal NEC	C41.9	C79.51	—	D16.9-	D48.Ø	D49.2
Skene's gland	C68.1	C79.19	DØ9.19	D3Ø.8	D41.8	D49.5
skin NOS	C44.9Ø	C79.2	DØ4.9	D23.9	D48.5	D49.2
abdominal wall	C44.5Ø9	C79.2	DØ4.5	D23.5	D48.5	D49.2
basal cell carcinoma	C44.519	—	—	—	—	—
specified type NEC	C44.599	—	—	—	—	—
squamous cell carcinoma	C44.529	—	—	—	—	—
ala nasi (*see also* Neoplasm, nose, skin)	C44.3Ø1	C79.2	DØ4.39	D23.39	D48.5	D49.2
ankle (*see also* Neoplasm, skin, limb, lower)	C44.7Ø-	C79.2	DØ4.7-	D23.7-	D48.5	D49.2
antecubital space (*see also* Neoplasm, skin,limb, upper)	C44.6Ø-	C79.2	DØ4.6-	D23.6-	D48.5	D49.2
anus	C44.5ØØ	C79.2	DØ4.5	D23.5	D48.5	D49.2
basal cell carcinoma	C44.51Ø	—	—	—	—	—
specified type NEC	C44.59Ø	—	—	—	—	—
squamous cell carcinoma	C44.52Ø	—	—	—	—	—
arm (*see also* Neoplasm, skin, limb, upper)	C44.6Ø-	C79.2	DØ4.6-	D23.6-	D48.5	D49.2
auditory canal (external) (*see also* Neoplasm,skin, ear)	C44.2Ø-	C79.2	DØ4.2-	D23.2-	D48.5	D49.2
auricle (ear) (*see also* Neoplasm, skin, ear)	C44.2Ø-	C79.2	DØ4.2-	D23.2-	D48.5	D49.2
auricular canal (external) (*see also* Neoplasm, skin, ear)	C44.2Ø-	C79.2	DØ4.2-	D23.2-	D48.5	D49.2
axilla, axillary fold (*see also* Neoplasm, skin, trunk)	C44.5Ø9	C79.2	DØ4.5	D23.5	D48.5	D49.2
back (*see also* Neoplasm, skin, trunk)	C44.5Ø9	C79.2	DØ4.5	D23.5	D48.5	D49.2
basal cell carcinoma	C44.91					
breast	C44.5Ø1	C79.2	DØ4.5	D23.5	D48.5	D49.2
basal cell carcinoma	C44.511	—	—	—	—	—
specified type NEC	C44.591	—	—	—	—	—
squamous cell carcinoma	C44.521	—	—	—	—	—
brow (*see also* Neoplasm, skin, face)	C44.3Ø9	C79.2	DØ4.39	D23.39	D48.5	D49.2
buttock (*see also* Neoplasm, skin, trunk)	C44.5Ø9	C79.2	DØ4.5	D23.5	D48.5	D49.2
calf (*see also* Neoplasm, skin, limb, lower)	C44.7Ø-	C79.2	DØ4.7-	D23.7-	D48.5	D49.2
canthus (eye) (inner) (outer)	C44.1Ø-	C79.2	DØ4.1-	D23.1-	D48.5	D49.2
basal cell carcinoma	C44.11-	—	—	—	—	—
specified type NEC	C44.19-	—	—	—	—	—
squamous cell carcinoma	C44.12-	—	—	—	—	—
cervical region (*see also* Neoplasm, skin, neck)	C44.4Ø	C79.2	DØ4.4	D23.4	D48.5	D49.2
cheek (external) (*see also* Neoplasm, skin, face)	C44.3Ø9	C79.2	DØ4.39	D23.39	D48.5	D49.2
chest (wall) (*see also* Neoplasm, skin, trunk)	C44.5Ø9	C79.2	DØ4.5	D23.5	D48.5	D49.2
chin (*see also* Neoplasm, skin, face)	C44.3Ø9	C79.2	DØ4.39	D23.39	D48.5	D49.2
clavicular area (*see also* Neoplasm, skin, trunk)	C44.5Ø9	C79.2	DØ4.5	D23.5	D48.5	D49.2
clitoris	C51.2	C79.82	DØ7.1	D28.Ø	D39.8	D49.5
columnella (*see also* Neoplasm, skin, face)	C44.3Ø9	C79.2	DØ4.39	D23.39	D48.5	D49.2
concha (*see also* Neoplasm, skin, ear)	C44.2Ø-	C79.2	DØ4.2-	D23.2-	D48.5	D49.2
ear (external)	C44.2Ø-	C79.2	DØ4.2-	D23.2-	D48.5	D49.2
basal cell carcinoma	C44.21-	—	—	—	—	—
specified type NEC	C44.29-	—	—	—	—	—
squamous cell carcinoma	C44.22-	—	—	—	—	—
elbow (*see also* Neoplasm, skin, limb, upper)	C44.6Ø-	C79.2	DØ4.6-	D23.6-	D48.5	D49.2
eyebrow (*see also* Neoplasm, skin, face)	C44.3Ø9	C79.2	DØ4.39	D23.39	D48.5	D49.2

	Malignant Primary	Malignant Secondary	Ca in situ	Benign	Uncertain Behavior	Unspecified Behavior
Neoplasm, neoplastic — *continued*						
skin NOS — *continued*						
eyelid	C44.1Ø-	C79.2	DØ4.1-	D23.1-	D48.5	D49.2
basal cell carcinoma	C44.11-	—	—	—	—	—
specified type NEC	C44.19-	—	—	—	—	—
squamous cell carcinoma	C44.12-	—	—	—	—	—
face NOS	C44.3ØØ	C79.2	DØ4.3Ø	D23.3Ø	D48.5	D49.2
basal cell carcinoma	C44.31Ø	—	—	—	—	—
specified type NEC	C44.39Ø	—	—	—	—	—
squamous cell carcinoma	C44.32Ø	—	—	—	—	—
female genital organs (external)	C51.9	C79.82	DØ7.1	D28.Ø	D39.8	D49.5
clitoris	C51.2	C79.82	DØ7.1	D28.Ø	D39.8	D49.5
labium NEC	C51.9	C79.82	DØ7.1	D28.Ø	D39.8	D49.5
majus	C51.Ø	C79.82	DØ7.1	D28.Ø	D39.8	D49.5
minus	C51.1	C79.82	DØ7.1	D28.Ø	D39.8	D49.5
pudendum	C51.9	C79.82	DØ7.1	D28.Ø	D39.8	D49.5
vulva	C51.9	C79.82	DØ7.1	D28.Ø	D39.8	D49.5
finger (*see also* Neoplasm, skin, limb, upper)	C44.6Ø-	C79.2	DØ4.6-	D23.6-	D48.5	D49.2
flank (*see also* Neoplasm, skin, trunk)	C44.5Ø9	C79.2	DØ4.5	D23.5	D48.5	D49.2
foot (*see also* Neoplasm, skin, limb, lower)	C44.7Ø-	C79.2	DØ4.7-	D23.7-	D48.5	D49.2
forearm (*see also* Neoplasm, skin, limb, upper)	C44.6Ø-	C79.2	DØ4.6-	D23.6-	D48.5	D49.2
forehead (*see also* Neoplasm, skin, face)	C44.3Ø9	C79.2	DØ4.39	D23.39	D48.5	D49.2
glabella (*see also* Neoplasm, skin, face)	C44.3Ø9	C79.2	DØ4.39	D23.39	D48.5	D49.2
gluteal region (*see also* Neoplasm, skin, trunk)	C44.5Ø9	C79.2	DØ4.5	D23.5	D48.5	D49.2
groin (*see also* Neoplasm, skin, trunk)	C44.5Ø9	C79.2	DØ4.5	D23.5	D48.5	D49.2
hand (*see also* Neoplasm, skin, limb, upper)	C44.6Ø-	C79.2	DØ4.6-	D23.6-	D48.5	D49.2
head NEC (*see also* Neoplasm, skin, scalp)	C44.4Ø	C79.2	DØ4.4	D23.4	D48.5	D49.2
heel (*see also* Neoplasm, skin, limb, lower)	C44.7Ø-	C79.2	DØ4.7-	D23.7-	D48.5	D49.2
helix (*see also* Neoplasm, skin, ear)	C44.2Ø-	C79.2	DØ4.2-	D23.2-	D48.5	D49.2
hip (*see also* Neoplasm, skin, limb, lower)	C44.7Ø-	C79.2	DØ4.7-	D23.7-	D48.5	D49.2
infraclavicular region (*see also* Neoplasm, skin, trunk)	C44.5Ø9	C79.2	DØ4.5	D23.5	D48.5	D49.2
inguinal region (*see also* Neoplasm, skin,trunk)	C44.5Ø9	C79.2	DØ4.5	D23.5	D48.5	D49.2
jaw (*see also* Neoplasm, skin, face)	C44.3Ø9	C79.2	DØ4.39	D23.39	D48.5	D49.2
Kaposi's sarcoma — *see* Kaposi's, sarcoma, skin						
knee (*see also* Neoplasm, skin, limb, lower)	C44.7Ø-	C79.2	DØ4.7-	D23.7-	D48.5	D49.2
labia						
majora	C51.Ø	C79.82	DØ7.1	D28.Ø	D39.8	D49.5
minora	C51.1	C79.82	DØ7.1	D28.Ø	D39.8	D49.5
leg (*see also* Neoplasm, skin, limb, lower)	C44.7Ø-	C79.2	DØ4.7-	D23.7-	D48.5	D49.2
lid (lower) (upper)	C44.1Ø-	C79.2	DØ4.1-	D23.1-	D48.5	D49.2
basal cell carcinoma	C44.11-	—	—	—	—	—
specified type NEC	C44.19-	—	—	—	—	—
squamous cell carcinoma	C44.12-	—	—	—	—	—
limb NEC	C44.9Ø	C79.2	DØ4.9	D23.9	D48.5	D49.2
basal cell carcinoma	C44.91					
lower	C44.7Ø-	C79.2	DØ4.7-	D23.7-	D48.5	D49.2
basal cell carcinoma	C44.71-	—	—	—	—	—
specified type NEC	C44.79-	—	—	—	—	—
squamous cell carcinoma	C44.72-	—	—	—	—	—
upper	C44.6Ø-	C79.2	DØ4.6-	D23.6-	D48.5	D49.2
basal cell carcinoma	C44.61-	—	—	—	—	—
specified type NEC	C44.69-	—	—	—	—	—
squamous cell carcinoma	C44.62-	—	—	—	—	—

	Malignant Primary	Malignant Secondary	Ca in situ	Benign	Uncertain Behavior	Unspecified Behavior
Neoplasm, neoplastic — *continued*						
skin NOS — *continued*						
lip (lower) (upper)	C44.ØØ	C79.2	DØ4.Ø	D23.Ø	D48.5	D49.2
basal cell carcinoma	C44.Ø1	—	—	—	—	—
specified type NEC	C44.Ø9	—	—	—	—	—
squamous cell carcinoma	C44.Ø2	—	—	—	—	—
male genital organs	C63.9	C79.82	DØ7.6Ø	D29.9	D4Ø.8	D49.5
penis	C6Ø.9	C79.82	DØ7.4	D29.Ø	D4Ø.8	D49.5
prepuce	C6Ø.Ø	C79.82	DØ7.4	D29.Ø	D4Ø.8	D49.5
scrotum	C63.2	C79.82	DØ7.61	D29.4	D4Ø.8	D49.5
mastectomy site (skin) (*see also* Neoplasm, skin, breast)	C44.5Ø1	C79.2	—	—	—	—
specified as breast tissue	C5Ø.8-	C79.81	—	—	—	—
meatus, acoustic (external) (*see also* Neoplasm, skin, ear)	C44.2Ø-	C79.2	DØ4.2-	D23.2-	D48.5	D49.2
melanotic — *see* Melanoma						
Merkel cell — *see* Carcinoma, Merkel cell						
nates (*see also* Neoplasm, skin, trunk)	C44.5Ø9	C79.2	DØ4.5	D23.5	D48.5	D49.2
neck	C44.4Ø	C79.2	DØ4.4	D23.4	D48.5	D49.2
basal cell carcinoma	C44.41	—	—	—	—	—
specified type NEC	C44.49	—	—	—	—	—
squamous cell carcinoma	C44.42	—	—	—	—	—
nevus — *see* Nevus, skin						
nose (external) (*see also* Neoplasm, nose, skin)	C44.3Ø1	C79.2	DØ4.39	D23.39	D48.5	D49.2
overlapping lesion	C44.8Ø	—	—	—	—	—
basal cell carcinoma	C44.81	—	—	—	—	—
specified type NEC	C44.89	—	—	—	—	—
squamous cell carcinoma	C44.82	—	—	—	—	—
palm (*see also* Neoplasm, skin, limb, upper)	C44.6Ø-	C79.2	DØ4.6-	D23.6-	D48.5	D49.2
palpebra	C44.1Ø-	C79.2	DØ4.1-	D23.1-	D48.5	D49.2
basal cell carcinoma	C44.11-	—	—	—	—	—
specified type NEC	C44.19-	—	—	—	—	—
squamous cell carcinoma	C44.12-	—	—	—	—	—
penis NEC	C6Ø.9	C79.82	DØ7.4	D29.Ø	D4Ø.8	D49.5
perianal (*see also* Neoplasm, skin, anus)	C44.5ØØ	C79.2	DØ4.5	D23.5	D48.5	D49.2
perineum (*see also* Neoplasm, skin, anus)	C44.5ØØ	C79.2	DØ4.5	D23.5	D48.5	D49.2
pinna (*see also* Neoplasm, skin, ear)	C44.2Ø-	C79.2	DØ4.2-	D23.2-	D48.5	D49.2
plantar (*see also* Neoplasm, skin, limb, lower)	C44.7Ø-	C79.2	DØ4.7-	D23.7-	D48.5	D49.2
popliteal fossa or space (*see also* Neoplasm, skin, limb, lower)	C44.7Ø-	C79.2	DØ4.7-	D23.7-	D48.5	D49.2
prepuce	C6Ø.Ø	C79.82	DØ7.4	D29.Ø	D4Ø.8	D49.5
pubes (*see also* Neoplasm, skin, trunk)	C44.5Ø9	C79.2	DØ4.5	D23.5	D48.5	D49.2
sacrococcygeal region (*see also* Neoplasm, skin, trunk)	C44.5Ø9	C79.2	DØ4.5	D23.5	D48.5	D49.2
scalp	C44.4Ø	C79.2	DØ4.4	D23.4	D48.5	D49.2
basal cell carcinoma	C44.41	—	—	—	—	—
specified type NEC	C44.49	—	—	—	—	—
squamous cell carcinoma	C44.42	—	—	—	—	—
scapular region (*see also* Neoplasm, skin, trunk)	C44.5Ø9	C79.2	DØ4.5	D23.5	D48.5	D49.2
scrotum	C63.2	C79.82	DØ7.61	D29.4	D4Ø.8	D49.5
shoulder (*see also* Neoplasm, skin, limb, upper)	C44.6Ø-	C79.2	DØ4.6-	D23.6-	D48.5	D49.2
sole (foot) (*see also* Neoplasm, skin, limb, lower)	C44.7Ø-	C79.2	DØ4.7-	D23.7-	D48.5	D49.2
specified sites NEC	C44.8Ø	C79.2	DØ4.8	D23.9	D48.5	D49.2
basal cell carcinoma	C44.81	—	—	—	—	—
specified type NEC	C44.89	—	—	—	—	—
squamous cell carcinoma	C44.82	—	—	—	—	—
specified type NEC	C44.99	—	—	—	—	—
squamous cell carcinoma	C44.92	—	—	—	—	—
submammary fold (*see also* Neoplasm, skin, trunk)	C44.5Ø9	C79.2	DØ4.5	D23.5	D48.5	D49.2

	Malignant Primary	Malignant Secondary	Ca in situ	Benign	Uncertain Behavior	Unspecified Behavior
Neoplasm, neoplastic — *continued*						
skin NOS — *continued*						
supraclavicular region (*see also* Neoplasm, skin, neck)	C44.4Ø	C79.2	DØ4.4	D23.4	D48.5	D49.2
temple (*see also* Neoplasm, skin, face)	C44.3Ø9	C79.2	DØ4.39	D23.39	D48.5	D49.2
thigh (*see also* Neoplasm, skin, limb, lower)	C44.7Ø-	C79.2	DØ4.7-	D23.7-	D48.5	D49.2
thoracic wall (*see also* Neoplasm, skin, trunk)	C44.5Ø9	C79.2	DØ4.5	D23.5	D48.5	D49.2
thumb (*see also* Neoplasm, skin, limb, upper)	C44.6Ø-	C79.2	DØ4.6-	D23.6-	D48.5	D49.2
toe (*see also* Neoplasm, skin, limb, lower)	C44.7Ø-	C79.2	DØ4.7-	D23.7-	D48.5	D49.2
tragus (*see also* Neoplasm, skin, ear)	C44.2Ø-	C79.2	DØ4.2-	D23.2-	D48.5	D49.2
trunk	C44.5Ø9	C79.2	DØ4.5	D23.5	D48.5	D49.2
basal cell carcinoma	C44.519	—	—	—	—	—
specified type NEC	C44.599	—	—	—	—	—
squamous cell carcinoma	C44.529	—	—	—	—	—
umbilicus (*see also* Neoplasm, skin, trunk)	C44.5Ø9	C79.2	DØ4.5	D23.5	D48.5	D49.2
vulva	C51.9	C79.82	DØ7.1	D28.Ø	D39.8	D49.5
overlapping lesion	C51.8	—	—	—	—	—
wrist (*see also* Neoplasm, skin, limb, upper)	C44.6Ø-	C79.2	DØ4.6-	D23.6-	D48.5	D49.2
skull	C41.Ø	C79.51	—	D16.4-	D48.Ø	D49.2
soft parts or tissues — *see* Neoplasm, connective tissue						
specified site NEC	C76.8	C79.89	DØ9.8	D36.7	D48.7	D49.89
spermatic cord	C63.1-	C79.82	DØ7.69	D29.8	D4Ø.8	D49.5
sphenoid	C31.3	C78.39	DØ2.3	D14.Ø	D38.5	D49.1
bone	C41.Ø	C79.51	—	D16.4-	D48.Ø	D49.2
sinus	C31.3	C78.39	DØ2.3	D14.Ø	D38.5	D49.1
sphincter						
anal	C21.1	C78.5	DØ1.3	D12.9	D37.8	D49.Ø
of Oddi	C24.Ø	C78.89	DØ1.5	D13.5	D37.6	D49.Ø
spine, spinal (column)	C41.2	C79.51	—	D16.6	D48.Ø	D49.2
bulb	C71.7	C79.31	—	D33.1	D43.1	D49.6
coccyx	C41.4	C79.51	—	D16.8-	D48.Ø	D49.2
cord (cervical) (lumbar) (sacral) (thoracic)	C72.Ø	C79.49	—	D33.4	D43.4	D49.7
dura mater	C7Ø.1	C79.49	—	D32.1	D42.1	D49.7
lumbosacral	C41.2	C79.51	—	D16.6	D48.Ø	D49.2
marrow NEC	C96.9	C79.52	—	—	D47.9	D49.89
membrane	C7Ø.1	C79.49	—	D32.1	D42.1	D49.7
meninges	C7Ø.1	C79.49	—	D32.1	D42.1	D49.7
nerve (root)	C47.9	C79.89	—	D36.1Ø	D48.2	D49.2
pia mater	C7Ø.1	C79.49	—	D32.1	D42.1	D49.7
root	C47.9	C79.89	—	D36.1Ø	D48.2	D49.2
sacrum	C41.4	C79.51	—	D16.8-	D48.Ø	D49.2
spleen, splenic NEC	C26.1	C78.89	DØ1.7	D13.9	D37.8	D49.Ø
flexure (colon)	C18.5	C78.5	DØ1.Ø	D12.3	D37.4	D49.Ø
stem, brain	C71.7	C79.31	—	D33.1	D43.1	D49.6
Stensen's duct	CØ7	C79.89	DØØ.ØØ	D11.Ø	D37.Ø3Ø	D49.Ø
sternum	C41.3	C79.51	—	D16.7-	D48.Ø	D49.2
stomach	C16.9	C78.89	DØØ.2	D13.1	D37.1	D49.Ø
antrum (pyloric)	C16.3	C78.89	DØØ.2	D13.1	D37.1	D49.Ø
body	C16.2	C78.89	DØØ.2	D13.1	D37.1	D49.Ø
cardia	C16.Ø	C78.89	DØØ.2	D13.1	D37.1	D49.Ø
cardiac orifice	C16.Ø	C78.89	DØØ.2	D13.1	D37.1	D49.Ø
corpus	C16.2	C78.89	DØØ.2	D13.1	D37.1	D49.Ø
fundus	C16.1	C78.89	DØØ.2	D13.1	D37.1	D49.Ø
greater curvature NEC	C16.6	C78.89	DØØ.2	D13.1	D37.1	D49.Ø
lesser curvature NEC	C16.5	C78.89	DØØ.2	D13.1	D37.1	D49.Ø
overlapping lesion	C16.8	—	—	—	—	—
prepylorus	C16.4	C78.89	DØØ.2	D13.1	D37.1	D49.Ø
pylorus	C16.4	C78.89	DØØ.2	D13.1	D37.1	D49.Ø
wall NEC	C16.9	C78.89	DØØ.2	D13.1	D37.1	D49.Ø
anterior NEC	C16.8	C78.89	DØØ.2	D13.1	D37.1	D49.Ø
posterior NEC	C16.8	C78.89	DØØ.2	D13.1	D37.1	D49.Ø
stroma, endometrial	C54.1	C79.82	DØ7.Ø	D26.1	D39.Ø	D49.5

	Malignant Primary	Malignant Secondary	Ca in situ	Benign	Uncertain Behavior	Unspecified Behavior
Neoplasm, neoplastic — *continued*						
stump, cervical	C53.8	C79.82	D06.7	D26.0	D39.0	D49.5
subcutaneous (nodule) (tissue) NEC — *see* Neoplasm, connective tissue						
subdural	C70.9	C79.32	—	D32.9	D42.9	D49.7
subglottis, subglottic	C32.2	C78.39	D02.0	D14.1	D38.0	D49.1
sublingual	C04.9	C79.89	D00.06	D10.2	D37.09	D49.0
gland or duct	C08.1	C79.89	D00.00	D11.7	D37.031	D49.0
submandibular gland	C08.0	C79.89	D00.00	D11.7	D37.032	D49.0
submaxillary gland or duct	C08.0	C79.89	D00.00	D11.7	D37.032	D49.0
submental	C76.0	C79.89	D09.8	D36.7	D48.7	D49.89
subpleural	C34.9-	C78.0-	D02.2-	D14.3-	D38.1	D49.1
substernal	C38.1	C78.1	—	D15.2	D38.3	D49.89
sudoriferous, sudoriparous gland, site unspecified	C44.90	C79.2	D04.9	D23.9	D48.5	D49.2
specified site — *see* Neoplasm, skin						
supraclavicular region	C76.0	C79.89	D09.8	D36.7	D48.7	D49.89
supraglottis	C32.1	C78.39	D02.0	D14.1	D38.0	D49.1
suprarenal	C74.9-	C79.7-	D09.3	D35.0-	D44.1-	D49.7
capsule	C74.9-	C79.7-	D09.3	D35.0-	D44.1-	D49.7
cortex	C74.0-	C79.7-	D09.3	D35.0-	D44.1-	D49.7
gland	C74.9-	C79.7-	D09.3	D35.0-	D44.1-	D49.7
medulla	C74.1-	C79.7-	D09.3	D35.0-	D44.1-	D49.7
suprasellar (region)	C71.9	C79.31	—	D33.2	D43.2	D49.6
supratentorial (brain) NEC	C71.0	C79.31	—	D33.0	D43.0	D49.6
sweat gland (apocrine) (eccrine), site unspecified	C44.90	C79.2	D04.9	D23.9	D48.5	D49.2
specified site — *see* Neoplasm, skin						
sympathetic nerve or nervous system NEC	C47.9	C79.89	—	D36.10	D48.2	D49.2
symphysis pubis	C41.4	C79.51	—	D16.8-	D48.0	D49.2
synovial membrane — *see* Neoplasm, connective tissue						
tapetum, brain	C71.8	C79.31	—	D33.2	D43.2	D49.6
tarsus (any bone)	C40.3-	C79.51	—	D16.3-	—	—
temple (skin) (*see also* Neoplasm, skin, face)	C44.309	C79.2	D04.39	D23.39	D48.5	D49.2
temporal						
bone	C41.0	C79.51	—	D16.4-	D48.0	D49.2
lobe or pole	C71.2	C79.31	—	D33.0	D43.0	D49.6
region	C76.0	C79.89	D09.8	D36.7	D48.7	D49.89
skin (*see also* Neoplasm, skin, face)	C44.309	C79.2	D04.39	D23.39	D48.5	D49.2
tendon (sheath) — *see* Neoplasm, connective tissue						
tentorium (cerebelli)	C70.0	C79.32	—	D32.0	D42.0	D49.7
testis, testes	C62.9	C79.82	D07.69	D29.2	D40.1-	D49.5
descended	C62.1-	C79.82	D07.69	D29.2	D40.1-	D49.5
ectopic	C62.0	C79.82	D07.69	D29.2	D40.1-	D49.5
retained	C62.0	C79.82	D07.69	D29.2	D40.1-	D49.5
scrotal	C62.1-	C79.82	D07.69	D29.2	D40.1-	D49.5
undescended	C62.0	C79.82	D07.69	D29.2	D40.1-	D49.5
unspecified whether descended or undescended	C62.9	C79.82	D07.69	D29.2	D40.1-	D49.5
thalamus	C71.0	C79.31	—	D33.0	D43.0	D49.6
thigh NEC	C76.5-	C79.89	D04.7-	D36.7	D48.7	D49.89
thorax, thoracic (cavity) (organs NEC)	C76.1	C79.89	D09.8	D36.7	D48.7	D49.89
duct	C49.3	C79.89	—	D21.3	D48.1	D49.2
wall NEC	C76.1	C79.89	D09.8	D36.7	D48.7	D49.89
throat	C14.0	C79.89	D00.08	D10.9	D37.05	D49.0
thumb NEC	C76.4-	C79.89	D04.6-	D36.7	D48.7	D49.89
thymus (gland)	C37	C79.89	D09.3	D15.0	D38.4	D49.89
thyroglossal duct	C73	C79.89	D09.3	D34	D44.0	D49.7
thyroid (gland)	C73	C79.89	D09.3	D34	D44.0	D49.7
cartilage	C32.3	C78.39	D02.0	D14.1	D38.0	D49.1
tibia (any part)	C40.2-	C79.51	—	D16.2-	—	—
toe NEC	C76.5-	C79.89	D04.7-	D36.7	D48.7	D49.89

	Malignant Primary	Malignant Secondary	Ca in situ	Benign	Uncertain Behavior	Unspecified Behavior
Neoplasm, neoplastic — *continued*						
tongue	C02.9	C79.89	D00.07	D10.1	D37.02	D49.0
anterior (two-thirds) NEC	C02.3	C79.89	D00.07	D10.1	D37.02	D49.0
dorsal surface	C02.0	C79.89	D00.07	D10.1	D37.02	D49.0
ventral surface	C02.2	C79.89	D00.07	D10.1	D37.02	D49.0
base (dorsal surface)	C01	C79.89	D00.07	D10.1	D37.02	D49.0
border (lateral)	C02.1	C79.89	D00.07	D10.1	D37.02	D49.0
dorsal surface NEC	C02.0	C79.89	D00.07	D10.1	D37.02	D49.0
fixed part NEC	C01	C79.89	D00.07	D10.1	D37.02	D49.0
foreamen cecum	C02.0	C79.89	D00.07	D10.1	D37.02	D49.0
frenulum linguae	C02.2	C79.89	D00.07	D10.1	D37.02	D49.0
junctional zone	C02.8	C79.89	D00.07	D10.1	D37.02	D49.0
margin (lateral)	C02.1	C79.89	D00.07	D10.1	D37.02	D49.0
midline NEC	C02.0	C79.89	D00.07	D10.1	D37.02	D49.0
mobile part NEC	C02.3	C79.89	D00.07	D10.1	D37.02	D49.0
overlapping lesion	C02.8	—	—	—	—	—
posterior (third)	C01	C79.89	D00.07	D10.1	D37.02	D49.0
root	C01	C79.89	D00.07	D10.1	D37.02	D49.0
surface (dorsal)	C02.0	C79.89	D00.07	D10.1	D37.02	D49.0
base	C01	C79.89	D00.07	D10.1	D37.02	D49.0
ventral	C02.2	C79.89	D00.07	D10.1	D37.02	D49.0
tip	C02.1	C79.89	D00.07	D10.1	D37.02	D49.0
tonsil	C02.4	C79.89	D00.07	D10.1	D37.02	D49.0
tonsil	C09.9	C79.89	D00.08	D10.4	D37.05	D49.0
fauces, faucial	C09.9	C79.89	D00.08	D10.4	D37.05	D49.0
lingual	C02.4	C79.89	D00.07	D10.1	D37.02	D49.0
overlapping sites	C09.8	—	—	—	—	—
palatine	C09.9	C79.89	D00.08	D10.4	D37.05	D49.0
pharyngeal	C11.1	C79.89	D00.08	D10.6	D37.05	D49.0
pillar (anterior) (posterior)	C09.1	C79.89	D00.08	D10.5	D37.05	D49.0
tonsillar fossa	C09.0	C79.89	D00.08	D10.5	D37.05	D49.0
tooth socket NEC	C03.9	C79.89	D00.03	D10.39	D37.09	D49.0
trachea (cartilage) (mucosa)	C33	C78.39	D02.1	D14.2	D38.1	D49.1
overlapping lesion with bronchus or lung	C34.8-	—	—	—	—	—
tracheobronchial	C34.8-	C78.39	D02.1	D14.2	D38.1	D49.1
overlapping lesion with lung	C34.8-	—	—	—	—	—
tragus (*see also* Neoplasm, skin, ear)	C44.20-	C79.2	D04.2-	D23.2-	D48.5	D49.2
trunk NEC	C76.8	C79.89	D04.5	D36.7	D48.7	D49.89
tubo-ovarian	C57.8	C79.82	D07.39	D28.7	D39.8	D49.5
tunica vaginalis	C63.7	C79.82	D07.69	D29.8	D40.8	D49.5
turbinate (bone)	C41.0	C79.51	—	D16.4-	D48.0	D49.2
nasal	C30.0	C78.39	D02.3	D14.0	D38.5	D49.1
tympanic cavity	C30.1	C78.39	D02.3	D14.0	D38.5	D49.1
ulna (any part)	C40.0-	C79.51	—	D16.0-	—	—
umbilicus, umbilical (*see also* Neoplasm, skin, trunk)	C44.509	C79.2	D04.5	D23.5	D48.5	D49.2
uncus, brain	C71.2	C79.31	—	D33.0	D43.0	D49.6
unknown site or unspecified	C80.1	C79.9	D09.9	D36.9	D48.9	D49.9
urachus	C67.7	C79.11	D09.0	D30.3	D41.4	D49.4
ureter, ureteral	C66.-	C79.19	D09.19	D30.2-	D41.2-	D49.5
orifice (bladder)	C67.6	C79.11	D09.0	D30.3	D41.4	D49.4
ureter-bladder (junction)	C67.6	C79.11	D09.0	D30.3	D41.4	D49.4
urethra, urethral (gland)	C68.0	C79.19	D09.19	D30.4	D41.3	D49.5
orifice, internal	C67.5	C79.11	D09.0	D30.3	D41.4	D49.4
urethrovaginal (septum)	C57.9	C79.82	D07.30	D28.9	D39.8	D49.5
urinary organ or system	C68.9	C79.10	D09.10	D30.9	D41.9	D49.5
bladder — *see* Neoplasm, bladder						
overlapping lesion	C68.8	—	—	—	—	—
specified sites NEC	C68.8	C79.19	D09.19	D30.8	D41.8	D49.5
utero-ovarian	C57.8	C79.82	D07.39	D28.7	D39.8	D49.5
ligament	C57.1	C79.82	D07.39	D28.2	D39.8	D49.5
uterosacral ligament	C57.3	C79.82	—	D28.2	D39.8	D49.5
uterus, uteri, uterine	C55	C79.82	D07.0	D26.9	D39.0	D49.5
adnexa NEC	C57.4	C79.82	D07.39	D28.7	D39.8	D49.5
body	C54.9	C79.82	D07.0	D26.1	D39.0	D49.5
cervix	C53.9	C79.82	D06.9	D26.0	D39.0	D49.5
cornu	C54.9	C79.82	D07.0	D26.1	D39.0	D49.5

	Malignant Primary	Malignant Secondary	Ca in situ	Benign	Uncertain Behavior	Unspecified Behavior
Neoplasm, neoplastic — *continued*						
uterus, uteri, uterine — *continued*						
corpus	C54.9	C79.82	DØ7.Ø	D26.1	D39.Ø	D49.5
endocervix (canal) (gland)	C53.Ø	C79.82	DØ6.Ø	D26.Ø	D39.Ø	D49.5
endometrium	C54.1	C79.82	DØ7.Ø	D26.1	D39.Ø	D49.5
exocervix	C53.1	C79.82	DØ6.1	D26.Ø	D39.Ø	D49.5
external os	C53.1	C79.82	DØ6.1	D26.Ø	D39.Ø	D49.5
fundus	C54.3	C79.82	DØ7.Ø	D26.1	D39.Ø	D49.5
internal os	C53.Ø	C79.82	DØ6.Ø	D26.Ø	D39.Ø	D49.5
isthmus	C54.Ø	C79.82	DØ7.Ø	D26.1	D39.Ø	D49.5
ligament	C57.3	C79.82	—	D28.2	D39.8	D49.5
broad	C57.1	C79.82	DØ7.39	D28.2	D39.8	D49.5
round	C57.2	C79.82	—	D28.2	D39.8	D49.5
lower segment	C54.Ø	C79.82	DØ7.Ø	D26.1	D39.Ø	D49.5
myometrium	C54.2	C79.82	DØ7.Ø	D26.1	D39.Ø	D49.5
overlapping sites	C54.8	—	—	—	—	—
squamocolumnar junction	C53.8	C79.82	DØ6.7	D26.Ø	D39.Ø	D49.5
tube	C57.Ø-	C79.82	DØ7.39	D28.2	D39.8	D49.5
utricle, prostatic	C68.Ø	C79.19	DØ9.19	D3Ø.4	D41.3	D49.5
uveal tract	C69.4-	C79.49	DØ9.2-	D31.4-	D48.7	D49.89
uvula	CØ5.2	C79.89	DØØ.Ø4	D1Ø.39	D37.Ø9	D49.Ø
vagina, vaginal (fornix) (vault) (wall)	C52	C79.82	DØ7.2	D28.1	D39.8	D49.5
vaginovesical	C57.9	C79.82	DØ7.3Ø	D28.9	D39.9	D49.5
septum	C57.9	C79.82	DØ7.3Ø	D28.9	D39.9	D49.5
vallecula (epigiottis)	C1Ø.Ø	C79.89	DØØ.Ø8	D1Ø.5	D37.Ø5	D49.Ø
vas deferens	C63.1-	C79.82	DØ7.69	D29.8	D4Ø.8	D49.5
vascular — *see* Neoplasm, connective tissue						
Vater's ampulla	C24.1	C78.89	DØ1.5	D13.5	D37.6	D49.Ø
vein, venous — *see* Neoplasm, connective tissue						
vena cava (abdominal) (inferior)	C49.4	C79.89	—	D21.4	D48.1	D49.2
superior	C49.3	C79.89	—	D21.3	D48.1	D49.2
ventricle (cerebral) (floor) (lateral) (third)	C71.5	C79.31	—	D33.Ø	D43.Ø	D49.6
cardiac (left) (right)	C38.Ø	C79.89	—	D15.1	D48.7	D49.89
fourth	C71.7	C79.31	—	D33.1	D43.1	D49.6
ventricular band of larynx	C32.1	C78.39	DØ2.Ø	D14.1	D38.Ø	D49.1
ventriculus — *see* Neoplasm, stomach						

	Malignant Primary	Malignant Secondary	Ca in situ	Benign	Uncertain Behavior	Unspecified Behavior
Neoplasm, neoplastic — *continued*						
vermillion border — *see* Neoplasm, lip						
vermis, cerebellum	C71.6	C79.31	—	D33.1	D43.1	D49.6
vertebra (column)	C41.2	C79.51	—	D16.6	D47.9	D49.89
coccyx	C41.4	C79.51	—	D16.8-	D48.Ø	D49.2
marrow NEC	C96.9	C79.52	—	—	D47.9	D49.89
sacrum	C41.4	C79.51	—	D16.8-	D48.Ø	D49.2
vesical — *see* Neoplasm, bladder						
vesicle, seminal	C63.7	C79.82	DØ7.69	D29.8	D4Ø.8	D49.5
vesicocervical tissue	C57.9	C79.82	DØ7.3Ø	D28.9	D39.9	D49.5
vesicorectal	C76.3	C79.82	DØ9.8	D36.7	D48.7	D49.89
vesicovaginal	C57.9	C79.82	DØ7.3Ø	D28.9	D39.9	D49.5
septum	C57.9	C79.82	DØ7.3Ø	D28.9	D39.8	D49.5
vessel (blood) — *see* Neoplasm, connective tissue						
vestibular gland, greater	C51.Ø	C79.82	DØ7.1	D28.Ø	D39.8	D49.5
vestibule						
mouth	CØ6.1	C79.89	DØØ.ØØ	D1Ø.39	D37.Ø9	D49.Ø
nose	C3Ø.Ø	C78.39	DØ2.3	D14.Ø	D38.5	D49.1
Virchow's gland	C77.Ø	C77.Ø	—	D36.Ø	D48.7	D49.89
viscera NEC	C76.8	C79.89	DØ9.8	D36.7	D48.7	D49.89
vocal cords (true)	C32.Ø	C78.39	DØ2.Ø	D14.1	D38.Ø	D49.1
false	C32.1	C78.39	DØ2.Ø	D14.1	D38.Ø	D49.1
vomer	C41.Ø	C79.51	—	D16.4-	D48.Ø	D49.2
vulva	C51.9	C79.82	DØ7.1	D28.Ø	D39.8	D49.5
vulvovaginal gland	C51.Ø	C79.82	DØ7.1	D28.Ø	D39.8	D49.5
Waldeyer's ring	C14.2	C79.89	DØØ.Ø8	D1Ø.9	D37.Ø5	D49.Ø
Wharton's duct	CØ8.Ø	C79.89	DØØ.ØØ	D11.7	D37.Ø32	D49.Ø
white matter (central) (cerebral)	C71.Ø	C79.31	—	D33.Ø	D43.Ø	D49.6
windpipe	C33	C78.39	DØ2.1	D14.2	D38.1	D49.1
Wirsung's duct	C25.3	C78.89	DØ1.7	D13.6	D37.8	D49.Ø
wolffian (body) (duct)						
female	C57.7	C79.82	DØ7.39	D28.7	D39.8	D49.5
male	C63.7	C79.82	DØ7.69	D29.8	D4Ø.8	D49.5
womb — *see* Neoplasm, uterus						
wrist NEC	C76.4-	C79.89	DØ4.6-	D36.7	D48.7	D49.89
xiphoid process	C41.3	C79.51	—	D16.7-	D48.Ø	D49.2
Zuckerkandl organ	C75.5	C79.89	—	D35.6	D44.7	D49.7

ICD-1Ø-CM Table of Drugs and Chemicals

Substance	Poisoning, Accidental (unintentional)	Poisoning, Intentional Self-harm	Poisoning, Assault	Poisoning, Undetermined	Adverse Effect	Under-dosing
1-Propanol	T51.3X1	T51.3X2	T51.3X3	T51.3X4	—	—
2-Propanol	T51.2X1	T51.2X2	T51.2X3	T51.2X4	—	—
2,4-D (dichlorophen oxyacetic acid)	T6Ø.3X1	T6Ø.3X2	T6Ø.3X3	T6Ø.3X4	—	—
2,4-toluene diisocyanate	T65.ØX1	T65.ØX2	T65.ØX3	T65.ØX4	—	—
2,4,5-T (trichlorophenoxyacetic acid)	T6Ø.1X1	T6Ø.1X2	T6Ø.1X3	T6Ø.1X4	—	—
14-hydroxydihydro-morphinone	T4Ø.2X1	T4Ø.2X2	T4Ø.2X3	T4Ø.2X4	T4Ø.2X5	T4Ø.2X6
A						
ABOB	T37.5X1	T37.5X2	T37.5X3	T37.5X4	T37.5X5	T37.5X6
Abrine	T62.2X1	T62.2X2	T62.2X3	T62.2X4	—	—
Abrus (seed)	T62.2X1	T62.2X2	T62.2X3	T62.2X4	—	—
Absinthe	T51.ØX1	T51.ØX2	T51.ØX3	T51.ØX4	—	—
beverage	T51.ØX1	T51.ØX2	T51.ØX3	T51.ØX4	—	—
Acaricide	T6Ø.8X1	T6Ø.8X2	T6Ø.8X3	T6Ø.8X4	—	—
Acebutolol	T44.7X1	T44.7X2	T44.7X3	T44.7X4	T44.7X5	T44.7X6
Acecarbromal	T42.6X1	T42.6X2	T42.6X3	T42.6X4	T42.6X5	T42.6X6
Aceclidine	T44.1X1	T44.1X2	T44.1X3	T44.1X4	T44.1X5	T44.1X6
Acedapsone	T37.ØX1	T37.ØX2	T37.ØX3	T37.ØX4	T37.ØX5	T37.ØX6
Acefylline piperazine	T48.6X1	T48.6X2	T48.6X3	T48.6X4	T48.6X5	T48.6X6
Acemorphan	T4Ø.2X1	T4Ø.2X2	T4Ø.2X3	T4Ø.2X4	T4Ø.2X5	T4Ø.2X6
Acenocoumarin	T45.511	T45.512	T45.513	T45.514	T45.515	T45.516
Acenocoumarol	T45.511	T45.512	T45.513	T45.514	T45.515	T45.516
Acepifylline	T48.6X1	T48.6X2	T48.6X3	T48.6X4	T48.6X5	T48.6X6
Acepromazine	T43.3X1	T43.3X2	T43.3X3	T43.3X4	T43.3X5	T43.3X6
Acesulfamethoxypyridazine	T37.ØX1	T37.ØX2	T37.ØX3	T37.ØX4	T37.ØX5	T37.ØX6
Acetal	T52.8X1	T52.8X2	T52.8X3	T52.8X4	—	—
Acetaldehyde (vapor)	T52.8X1	T52.8X2	T52.8X3	T52.8X4	—	—
liquid	T65.891	T65.892	T65.893	T65.894	—	—
P-Acetamidophenol	T39.1X1	T39.1X2	T39.1X3	T39.1X4	T39.1X5	T39.1X6
Acetaminophen	T39.1X1	T39.1X2	T39.1X3	T39.1X4	T39.1X5	T39.1X6
Acetaminosalol	T39.1X1	T39.1X2	T39.1X3	T39.1X4	T39.1X5	T39.1X6
Acetanilide	T39.1X1	T39.1X2	T39.1X3	T39.1X4	T39.1X5	T39.1X6
Acetarsol	T37.3X1	T37.3X2	T37.3X3	T37.3X4	T37.3X5	T37.3X6
Acetazolamide	T5Ø.2X1	T5Ø.2X2	T5Ø.2X3	T5Ø.2X4	T5Ø.2X5	T5Ø.2X6
Acetiamine	T45.2X1	T45.2X2	T45.2X3	T45.2X4	T45.2X5	T45.2X6
Acetic						
acid	T54.2X1	T54.2X2	T54.2X3	T54.2X4	—	—
with sodium acetate (ointment)	T49.3X1	T49.3X2	T49.3X3	T49.3X4	T49.3X5	T49.3X6
ester (solvent)(vapor)	T52.8X1	T52.8X2	T52.8X3	T52.8X4	—	—
irrigating solution	T5Ø.3X1	T5Ø.3X2	T5Ø.3X3	T5Ø.3X4	T5Ø.3X5	T5Ø.3X6
medicinal (lotion)	T49.2X1	T49.2X2	T49.2X3	T49.2X4	T49.2X5	T49.2X6
anhydride	T65.891	T65.892	T65.893	T65.894	—	—
ether (vapor)	T52.8X1	T52.8X2	T52.8X3	T52.8X4	—	—
Acetohexamide	T38.3X1	T38.3X2	T38.3X3	T38.3X4	T38.3X5	T38.3X6
Acetohydroxamic acid	T5Ø.991	T5Ø.992	T5Ø.993	T5Ø.994	T5Ø.995	T5Ø.996
Acetomenaphthone	T45.7X1	T45.7X2	T45.7X3	T45.7X4	T45.7X5	T45.7X6
Acetomorphine	T4Ø.1X1	T4Ø.1X2	T4Ø.1X3	T4Ø.1X4	T4Ø.1X5	—
Acetone (oils)	T52.4X1	T52.4X2	T52.4X3	T52.4X4	—	—
chlorinated	T52.4X1	T52.4X2	T52.4X3	T52.4X4	—	—
vapor	T52.4X1	T52.4X2	T52.4X3	T52.4X4	—	—
Acetonitrile	T52.8X1	T52.8X2	T52.8X3	T52.8X4	—	—
Acetophenazine	T43.3X1	T43.3X2	T43.3X3	T43.3X4	T43.3X5	T43.3X6
Acetophenetedin	T39.1X1	T39.1X2	T39.1X3	T39.1X4	T39.1X5	T39.1X6
Acetophenone	T52.4X1	T52.4X2	T52.4X3	T52.4X4	—	—
Acetorphine	T4Ø.2X1	T4Ø.2X2	T4Ø.2X3	T4Ø.2X4	—	—
Acetosulfone (sodium)	T37.1X1	T37.1X2	T37.1X3	T37.1X4	T37.1X5	T37.1X6
Acetrizoate (sodium)	T5Ø.8X1	T5Ø.8X2	T5Ø.8X3	T5Ø.8X4	T5Ø.8X5	T5Ø.8X6
Acetrizoic acid	T5Ø.8X1	T5Ø.8X2	T5Ø.8X3	T5Ø.8X4	T5Ø.8X5	T5Ø.8X6
Acetylcarbromal	T42.6X1	T42.6X2	T42.6X3	T42.6X4	T42.6X5	T42.6X6
Acetyl						
bromide	T53.6X1	T53.6X2	T53.6X3	T53.6X4	—	—
chloride	T53.6X1	T53.6X2	T53.6X3	T53.6X4	—	—
Acetylcholine						
chloride	T44.1X1	T44.1X2	T44.1X3	T44.1X4	T44.1X5	T44.1X6
derivative	T44.1X1	T44.1X2	T44.1X3	T44.1X4	T44.1X5	T44.1X6
Acetylcysteine	T48.4X1	T48.4X2	T48.4X3	T48.4X4	T48.4X5	T48.4X6
Acetyldigitoxin	T46.ØX1	T46.ØX2	T46.ØX3	T46.ØX4	T46.ØX5	T46.ØX6
Acetyldigoxin	T46.ØX1	T46.ØX2	T46.ØX3	T46.ØX4	T46.ØX5	T46.ØX6
Acetyldihydrocodeine	T4Ø.2X1	T4Ø.2X2	T4Ø.2X3	T4Ø.2X4	—	—
Acetyldihydrocodeinone	T4Ø.2X1	T4Ø.2X2	T4Ø.2X3	T4Ø.2X4	—	—
Acetylene (gas)	T59.891	T59.892	T59.893	T59.894	—	—
dichloride	T53.6X1	T53.6X2	T53.6X3	T53.6X4	—	—
incomplete combustion of	T58.11	T58.12	T58.13	T58.14	—	—
industrial	T59.891	T59.892	T59.893	T59.894	—	—
tetrachloride	T53.6X1	T53.6X2	T53.6X3	T53.6X4	—	—
vapor	T53.6X1	T53.6X2	T53.6X3	T53.6X4	—	—
Acetylphenylhydrazine	T39.8X1	T39.8X2	T39.8X3	T39.8X4	T39.8X5	T39.8X6
Acetylpheneturide	T42.6X1	T42.6X2	T42.6X3	T42.6X4	T42.6X5	T42.6X6
Acetylsalicylic acid (salts)	T39.Ø11	T39.Ø12	T39.Ø13	T39.Ø14	T39.Ø15	T39.Ø16
enteric coated	T39.Ø11	T39.Ø12	T39.Ø13	T39.Ø14	T39.Ø15	T39.Ø16
Acetylsulfamethoxypyridazine	T37.ØX1	T37.ØX2	T37.ØX3	T37.ØX4	T37.ØX5	T37.ØX6
Achromycin	T36.4X1	T36.4X2	T36.4X3	T36.4X4	T36.4X5	T36.4X6
ophthalmic preparation	T49.5X1	T49.5X2	T49.5X3	T49.5X4	T49.5X5	T49.5X6
topical NEC	T49.ØX1	T49.ØX2	T49.ØX3	T49.ØX4	T49.ØX5	T49.ØX6
Aciclovir	T37.5X1	T37.5X2	T37.5X3	T37.5X4	T37.5X5	T37.5X6
Acid (corrosive) **NEC**	T54.2X1	T54.2X2	T54.2X3	T54.2X4	—	—
Acidifying agent NEC	T5Ø.9Ø1	T5Ø.9Ø2	T5Ø.9Ø3	T5Ø.9Ø4	T5Ø.9Ø5	T5Ø.9Ø6
Acipimox	T46.6X1	T46.6X2	T46.6X3	T46.6X4	T46.6X5	T46.6X6
Acitretin	T5Ø.991	T5Ø.992	T5Ø.993	T5Ø.994	T5Ø.995	T5Ø.996
Aclarubicin	T45.1X1	T45.1X2	T45.1X3	T45.1X4	T45.1X5	T45.1X6
Aclatonium napadisilate	T48.1X1	T48.1X2	T48.1X3	T48.1X4	T48.1X5	T48.1X6
Aconite (wild)	T46.991	T46.992	T46.993	T46.994	T46.995	T46.996
Aconitine	T46.991	T46.992	T46.993	T46.994	T46.995	T46.996
Aconitum ferox	T46.991	T46.992	T46.993	T46.994	T46.995	T46.996
Acridine	T65.6X1	T65.6X2	T65.6X3	T65.6X4	—	—
vapor	T59.891	T59.892	T59.893	T59.894	—	—
Acriflavine	T37.91	T37.92	T37.93	T37.94	T37.95	T37.96
Acriflavinium chloride	T49.ØX1	T49.ØX2	T49.ØX3	T49.ØX4	T49.ØX5	T49.ØX6
Acrinol	T49.ØX1	T49.ØX2	T49.ØX3	T49.ØX4	T49.ØX5	T49.ØX6
Acrisorcin	T49.ØX1	T49.ØX2	T49.ØX3	T49.ØX4	T49.ØX5	T49.ØX6
Acrivastine	T45.ØX1	T45.ØX2	T45.ØX3	T45.ØX4	T45.ØX5	T45.ØX6
Acrolein (gas)	T59.891	T59.892	T59.893	T59.894	—	—
liquid	T54.1X1	T54.1X2	T54.1X3	T54.1X4	—	—
Acrylamide	T65.891	T65.892	T65.893	T65.894	—	—
Acrylic resin	T49.3X1	T49.3X2	T49.3X3	T49.3X4	T49.3X5	T49.3X6
Acrylonitrile	T65.891	T65.892	T65.893	T65.894	—	—
Actaea spicata	T62.2X1	T62.2X2	T62.2X3	T62.2X4	—	—
berry	T62.1X1	T62.1X2	T62.1X3	T62.1X4	—	—
Acterol	T37.3X1	T37.3X2	T37.3X3	T37.3X4	T37.3X5	T37.3X6
ACTH	T38.811	T38.812	T38.813	T38.814	T38.815	T38.816
Actinomycin C	T45.1X1	T45.1X2	T45.1X3	T45.1X4	T45.1X5	T45.1X6
Actinomycin D	T45.1X1	T45.1X2	T45.1X3	T45.1X4	T45.1X5	T45.1X6
Activated charcoal (*see also* Charcoal, medicinal)	T47.6X1	T47.6X2	T47.6X3	T47.6X4	T47.6X5	T47.6X6
Acyclovir	T37.5X1	T37.5X2	T37.5X3	T37.5X4	T37.5X5	T37.5X6
Adenine	T45.2X1	T45.2X2	T45.2X3	T45.2X4	T45.2X5	T45.2X6
arabinoside	T37.5X1	T37.5X2	T37.5X3	T37.5X4	T37.5X5	T37.5X6
Adenosine (phosphate)	T46.2X1	T46.2X2	T46.2X3	T46.2X4	T46.2X5	T46.2X6
ADH	T38.891	T38.892	T38.893	T38.894	T38.895	T38.896
Adhesive NEC	T65.891	T65.892	T65.893	T65.894	—	—
Adicillin	T36.ØX1	T36.ØX2	T36.ØX3	T36.ØX4	T36.ØX5	T36.ØX6
Adiphenine	T44.3X1	T44.3X2	T44.3X3	T44.3X4	T44.3X5	T44.3X6
Adipiodone	T5Ø.8X1	T5Ø.8X2	T5Ø.8X3	T5Ø.8X4	T5Ø.8X5	T5Ø.8X6
Adjunct, pharmaceutical	T5Ø.9Ø1	T5Ø.9Ø2	T5Ø.9Ø3	T5Ø.9Ø4	T5Ø.9Ø5	T5Ø.9Ø6
Adrenal (extract, cortex or medulla) (glucocorticoids) (hormones) (mineralocorticoids)	T38.ØX1	T38.ØX2	T38.ØX3	T38.ØX4	T38.ØX5	T38.ØX6
ENT agent	T49.6X1	T49.6X2	T49.6X3	T49.6X4	T49.6X5	T49.6X6
ophthalmic preparation	T49.5X1	T49.5X2	T49.5X3	T49.5X4	T49.5X5	T49.5X6
topical NEC	T49.ØX1	T49.ØX2	T49.ØX3	T49.ØX4	T49.ØX5	T49.ØX6
Adrenaline	T44.5X1	T44.5X2	T44.5X3	T44.5X4	T44.5X5	T44.5X6
Adrenalin—*see* Adrenaline						

Substance	Poisoning, Accidental (unintentional)	Poisoning, Intentional Self-harm	Poisoning, Assault	Poisoning, Undetermined	Adverse Effect	Under-dosing
Adrenergic NEC	T44.9Ø1	T44.9Ø2	T44.9Ø3	T44.9Ø4	T44.9Ø5	T44.9Ø6
blocking agent NEC	T44.8X1	T44.8X2	T44.8X3	T44.8X4	T44.8X5	T44.8X6
beta, heart	T44.7X1	T44.7X2	T44.7X3	T44.7X4	T44.7X5	T44.7X6
specified NEC	T44.991	T44.992	T44.993	T44.994	T44.995	T44.996
Adrenochrome						
(mono) semicarbazone	T46.991	T46.992	T46.993	T46.994	T46.995	T46.996
derivative	T46.991	T46.992	T46.993	T46.994	T46.995	T46.996
Adrenocorticotrophic hormone	T38.811	T38.812	T38.813	T38.814	T38.815	T38.816
Adrenocorticotrophin	T38.811	T38.812	T38.813	T38.814	T38.815	T38.816
Adriamycin	T45.1X1	T45.1X2	T45.1X3	T45.1X4	T45.1X5	T45.1X6
Aerosol spray NEC	T65.91	T65.92	T65.93	T65.94	—	—
Aerosporin	T36.8X1	T36.8X2	T36.8X3	T36.8X4	T36.8X5	T36.8X6
ENT agent	T49.6X1	T49.6X2	T49.6X3	T49.6X4	T49.6X5	T49.6X6
ophthalmic preparation	T49.5X1	T49.5X2	T49.5X3	T49.5X4	T49.5X5	T49.5X6
topical NEC	T49.ØX1	T49.ØX2	T49.ØX3	T49.ØX4	T49.ØX5	T49.ØX6
Aethusa cynapium	T62.2X1	T62.2X2	T62.2X3	T62.2X4	—	—
Afghanistan black	T4Ø.7X1	T4Ø.7X2	T4Ø.7X3	T4Ø.7X4	T4Ø.7X5	T4Ø.7X6
Aflatoxin	T64.Ø1	T64.Ø2	T64.Ø3	T64.Ø4	—	—
Afloqualone	T42.8X1	T42.8X2	T42.8X3	T42.8X4	T42.8X5	T42.8X6
African boxwood	T62.2X1	T62.2X2	T62.2X3	T62.2X4	—	—
Agar	T47.4X1	T47.4X2	T47.4X3	T47.4X4	T47.4X5	T47.4X6
Agonist						
predominantly						
alpha-adrenoreceptor	T44.4X1	T44.4X2	T44.4X3	T44.4X4	T44.4X5	T44.4X6
beta-adrenoreceptor	T44.5X1	T44.5X2	T44.5X3	T44.5X4	T44.5X5	T44.5X6
Agricultural agent NEC	T65.91	T65.92	T65.93	T65.94	—	—
Agrypnal	T42.3X1	T42.3X2	T42.3X3	T42.3X4	T42.3X5	T42.3X6
AHLG	T5Ø.Z11	T5Ø.Z12	T5Ø.Z13	T5Ø.Z14	T5Ø.Z15	T5Ø.Z16
Air contaminant(s), source/type NOS	T65.91	T65.92	T65.93	T65.94	—	—
Ajmaline	T46.2X1	T46.2X2	T46.2X3	T46.2X4	T46.2X5	T46.2X6
Akritoin	T37.8X1	T37.8X2	T37.8X3	T37.8X4	T37.8X5	T37.8X6
Akee	T62.1X1	T62.1X2	T62.1X3	T62.1X4	—	—
Akrinol	T49.ØX1	T49.ØX2	T49.ØX3	T49.ØX4	T49.ØX5	T49.ØX6
Alacepril	T46.4X1	T46.4X2	T46.4X3	T46.4X4	T46.4X5	T46.4X6
Alantolactone	T37.4X1	T37.4X2	T37.4X3	T37.4X4	T37.4X5	T37.4X6
Albamycin	T36.8X1	T36.8X2	T36.8X3	T36.8X4	T36.8X5	T36.8X6
Albendazole	T37.4X1	T37.4X2	T37.4X3	T37.4X4	T37.4X5	T37.4X6
Albumin						
bovine	T45.8X1	T45.8X2	T45.8X3	T45.8X4	T45.8X5	T45.8X6
human serum	T45.8X1	T45.8X2	T45.8X3	T45.8X4	T45.8X5	T45.8X6
salt-poor	T45.8X1	T45.8X2	T45.8X3	T45.8X4	T45.8X5	T45.8X6
normal human serum	T45.8X1	T45.8X2	T45.8X3	T45.8X4	T45.8X5	T45.8X6
Albuterol	T48.6X1	T48.6X2	T48.6X3	T48.6X4	T48.6X5	T48.6X6
Albutoin	T42.ØX1	T42.ØX2	T42.ØX3	T42.ØX4	T42.ØX5	T42.ØX6
Alclometasone	T49.ØX1	T49.ØX2	T49.ØX3	T49.ØX4	T49.ØX5	T49.ØX6
Alcohol	T51.91	T51.92	T51.93	T51.94	—	—
absolute	T51.ØX1	T51.ØX2	T51.ØX3	T51.ØX4	—	—
beverage	T51.ØX1	T51.ØX2	T51.ØX3	T51.ØX4	—	—
allyl	T51.8X1	T51.8X2	T51.8X3	T51.8X4	—	—
antifreeze	T51.1X1	T51.1X2	T51.1X3	T51.1X4	—	—
amyl	T51.3X1	T51.3X2	T51.3X3	T51.3X4	—	—
beverage	T51.ØX1	T51.ØX2	T51.ØX3	T51.ØX4	—	—
butyl	T51.3X1	T51.3X2	T51.3X3	T51.3X4	—	—
dehydrated	T51.ØX1	T51.ØX2	T51.ØX3	T51.ØX4	—	—
beverage	T51.ØX1	T51.ØX2	T51.ØX3	T51.ØX4	—	—
denatured	T51.ØX1	T51.ØX2	T51.ØX3	T51.ØX4	—	—
deterrent NEC	T5Ø.6X1	T5Ø.6X2	T5Ø.6X3	T5Ø.6X4	T5Ø.6X5	T5Ø.6X6
diagnostic (gastric function)	T5Ø.8X1	T5Ø.8X2	T5Ø.8X3	T5Ø.8X4	T5Ø.8X5	T5Ø.8X6
ethyl	T51.ØX1	T51.ØX2	T51.ØX3	T51.ØX4	—	—
beverage	T51.ØX1	T51.ØX2	T51.ØX3	T51.ØX4	—	—
grain	T51.ØX1	T51.ØX2	T51.ØX3	T51.ØX4	—	—
beverage	T51.ØX1	T51.ØX2	T51.ØX3	T51.ØX4	—	—
industrial	T51.ØX1	T51.ØX2	T51.ØX3	T51.ØX4	—	—
isopropyl	T51.2X1	T51.2X2	T51.2X3	T51.2X4	—	—
methyl	T51.1X1	T51.1X2	T51.1X3	T51.1X4	—	—
preparation for consumption	T51.ØX1	T51.ØX2	T51.ØX3	T51.ØX4	—	—
propyl	T51.3X1	T51.3X2	T51.3X3	T51.3X4	—	—
secondary	T51.2X1	T51.2X2	T51.2X3	T51.2X4	—	—
radiator	T51.1X1	T51.1X2	T51.1X3	T51.1X4	—	—

Substance	Poisoning, Accidental (unintentional)	Poisoning, Intentional Self-harm	Poisoning, Assault	Poisoning, Undetermined	Adverse Effect	Under-dosing
Alcohol—*continued*						
rubbing	T51.2X1	T51.2X2	T51.2X3	T51.2X4	—	—
specified type NEC	T51.8X1	T51.8X2	T51.8X3	T51.8X4	—	—
surgical	T51.ØX1	T51.ØX2	T51.ØX3	T51.ØX4	—	—
vapor (from any type of Alcohol)	T59.891	T59.892	T59.893	T59.894	—	—
wood	T51.1X1	T51.1X2	T51.1X3	T51.1X4	—	—
Alcuronium (chloride)	T48.1X1	T48.1X2	T48.1X3	T48.1X4	T48.1X5	T48.1X6
Aldactone	T5Ø.ØX1	T5Ø.ØX2	T5Ø.ØX3	T5Ø.ØX4	T5Ø.ØX5	T5Ø.ØX6
Aldesulfone sodium	T37.1X1	T37.1X2	T37.1X3	T37.1X4	T37.1X5	T37.1X6
Aldicarb	T6Ø.ØX1	T6Ø.ØX2	T6Ø.ØX3	T6Ø.ØX4	—	—
Aldomet	T46.5X1	T46.5X2	T46.5X3	T46.5X4	T46.5X5	T46.5X6
Aldosterone	T5Ø.ØX1	T5Ø.ØX2	T5Ø.ØX3	T5Ø.ØX4	T5Ø.ØX5	T5Ø.ØX6
Aldrin (dust)	T6Ø.1X1	T6Ø.1X2	T6Ø.1X3	T6Ø.1X4	—	—
Aleve—*see* Naproxen						
Alexitol sodium	T47.1X1	T47.1X2	T47.1X3	T47.1X4	T47.1X5	T47.1X6
Alfacalcidol	T45.2X1	T45.2X2	T45.2X3	T45.2X4	T45.2X5	T45.2X6
Alfadolone	T41.1X1	T41.1X2	T41.1X3	T41.1X4	T41.1X5	T41.1X6
Alfaxalone	T41.1X1	T41.1X2	T41.1X3	T41.1X4	T41.1X5	T41.1X6
Alfentanil	T4Ø.4X1	T4Ø.4X2	T4Ø.4X3	T4Ø.4X4	T4Ø.4X5	T4Ø.4X6
Alfuzosin (hydrochloride)	T44.8X1	T44.8X2	T44.8X3	T44.8X4	T44.8X5	T44.8X6
Algae (harmful) (toxin)	T65.821	T65.822	T65.823	T65.824	—	—
Algeldrate	T47.1X1	T47.1X2	T47.1X3	T47.1X4	T47.1X5	T47.1X6
Algin	T47.8X1	T47.8X2	T47.8X3	T47.8X4	T47.8X5	T47.8X6
Alglucerase	T45.3X1	T45.3X2	T45.3X3	T45.3X4	T45.3X5	T45.3X6
Alidase	T45.3X1	T45.3X2	T45.3X3	T45.3X4	T45.3X5	T45.3X6
Alimemazine	T43.3X1	T43.3X2	T43.3X3	T43.3X4	T43.3X5	T43.3X6
Aliphatic thiocyanates	T65.ØX1	T65.ØX2	T65.ØX3	T65.ØX4	—	—
Alizapride	T45.ØX1	T45.ØX2	T45.ØX3	T45.ØX4	T45.ØX5	T45.ØX6
Alkali (caustic)	T54.3X1	T54.3X2	T54.3X3	T54.3X4	—	—
Alkalizing agent NEC	T5Ø.9Ø1	T5Ø.9Ø2	T5Ø.9Ø3	T5Ø.9Ø4	T5Ø.9Ø5	T5Ø.9Ø6
Alkaline antiseptic solution (aromatic)	T49.6X1	T49.6X2	T49.6X3	T49.6X4	T49.6X5	T49.6X6
Alkalinizing agents (medicinal)	T5Ø.9Ø1	T5Ø.9Ø2	T5Ø.9Ø3	T5Ø.9Ø4	T5Ø.9Ø5	T5Ø.9Ø6
Alka-seltzer	T39.Ø11	T39.Ø12	T39.Ø13	T39.Ø14	T39.Ø15	T39.Ø16
Alkavervir	T46.5X1	T46.5X2	T46.5X3	T46.5X4	T46.5X5	T46.5X6
Alkonium (bromide)	T49.ØX1	T49.ØX2	T49.ØX3	T49.ØX4	T49.ØX5	T49.ØX6
Alkylating drug NEC	T45.1X1	T45.1X2	T45.1X3	T45.1X4	T45.1X5	T45.1X6
antimyeloproliferative	T45.1X1	T45.1X2	T45.1X3	T45.1X4	T45.1X5	T45.1X6
lymphatic	T45.1X1	T45.1X2	T45.1X3	T45.1X4	T45.1X5	T45.1X6
Alkylisocyanate	T65.ØX1	T65.ØX2	T65.ØX3	T65.ØX4	—	—
Allantoin	T49.4X1	T49.4X2	T49.4X3	T49.4X4	T49.4X5	T49.4X6
Allegron	T43.Ø11	T43.Ø12	T43.Ø13	T43.Ø14	T43.Ø15	T43.Ø16
Allethrin	T49.ØX1	T49.ØX2	T49.ØX3	T49.ØX4	T49.ØX5	T49.ØX6
Allobarbital	T42.3X1	T42.3X2	T42.3X3	T42.3X4	T42.3X5	T42.3X6
Allopurinol	T5Ø.4X1	T5Ø.4X2	T5Ø.4X3	T5Ø.4X4	T5Ø.4X5	T5Ø.4X6
Allyl						
Alcohol	T51.8X1	T51.8X2	T51.8X3	T51.8X4	—	—
disulfide	T46.6X1	T46.6X2	T46.6X3	T46.6X4	T46.6X5	T46.6X6
Allylestrenol	T38.5X1	T38.5X2	T38.5X3	T38.5X4	T38.5X5	T38.5X6
Allylisopropylacetylurea	T42.6X1	T42.6X2	T42.6X3	T42.6X4	T42.6X5	T42.6X6
Allylisopropylmalonylurea	T42.3X1	T42.3X2	T42.3X3	T42.3X4	T42.3X5	T42.3X6
Allylthiourea	T49.3X1	T49.3X2	T49.3X3	T49.3X4	T49.3X5	T49.3X6
Allyltribromide	T42.6X1	T42.6X2	T42.6X3	T42.6X4	T42.6X5	T42.6X6
Allypropymal	T42.3X1	T42.3X2	T42.3X3	T42.3X4	T42.3X5	T42.3X6
Almagate	T47.1X1	T47.1X2	T47.1X3	T47.1X4	T47.1X5	T47.1X6
Almasilate	T47.1X1	T47.1X2	T47.1X3	T47.1X4	T47.1X5	T47.1X6
Almitrine	T5Ø.7X1	T5Ø.7X2	T5Ø.7X3	T5Ø.7X4	T5Ø.7X5	T5Ø.7X6
Aloes	T47.2X1	T47.2X2	T47.2X3	T47.2X4	T47.2X5	T47.2X6
Aloglutamol	T47.1X1	T47.1X2	T47.1X3	T47.1X4	T47.1X5	T47.1X6
Aloin	T47.2X1	T47.2X2	T47.2X3	T47.2X4	T47.2X5	T47.2X6
Aloxidone	T42.2X1	T42.2X2	T42.2X3	T42.2X4	T42.2X5	T42.2X6
Alpha						
acetyldigoxin	T46.ØX1	T46.ØX2	T46.ØX3	T46.ØX4	T46.ØX5	T46.ØX6
adrenergic blocking drug	T44.6X1	T44.6X2	T44.6X3	T44.6X4	T44.6X5	T44.6X6
amylase	T45.3X1	T45.3X2	T45.3X3	T45.3X4	T45.3X5	T45.3X6
tocoferol(acetate)	T45.2X1	T45.2X2	T45.2X3	T45.2X4	T45.2X5	T45.2X6
tocopherol	T45.2X1	T45.2X2	T45.2X3	T45.2X4	T45.2X5	T45.2X6
Alphadolone	T41.1X1	T41.1X2	T41.1X3	T41.1X4	T41.1X5	T41.1X6
Alphaprodine	T4Ø.4X1	T4Ø.4X2	T4Ø.4X3	T4Ø.4X4	T4Ø.4X5	T4Ø.4X6
Alphaxalone	T41.1X1	T41.1X2	T41.1X3	T41.1X4	T41.1X5	T41.1X6
Alprazolam	T42.4X1	T42.4X2	T42.4X3	T42.4X4	T42.4X5	T42.4X6

Substance	Poisoning, Accidental (unintentional)	Poisoning, Intentional Self-harm	Poisoning, Assault	Poisoning, Undetermined	Adverse Effect	Under-dosing
Alprenolol	T44.7X1	T44.7X2	T44.7X3	T44.7X4	T44.7X5	T44.7X6
Alprostadil	T46.7X1	T46.7X2	T46.7X3	T46.7X4	T46.7X5	T46.7X6
Alsactide	T38.811	T38.812	T38.813	T38.814	T38.815	T38.816
Alseroxylon	T46.5X1	T46.5X2	T46.5X3	T46.5X4	T46.5X5	T46.5X6
Alteplase	T45.611	T45.612	T45.613	T45.614	T45.615	T45.616
Altizide	T5Ø.2X1	T5Ø.2X2	T5Ø.2X3	T5Ø.2X4	T5Ø.2X5	T5Ø.2X6
Altretamine	T45.1X1	T45.1X2	T45.1X3	T45.1X4	T45.1X5	T45.1X6
Alum (medicinal)	T49.4X1	T49.4X2	T49.4X3	T49.4X4	T49.4X5	T49.4X6
nonmedicinal (ammonium) (potassium)	T56.891	T56.892	T56.893	T56.894	—	—
Aluminium, aluminum						
acetate	T49.2X1	T49.2X2	T49.2X3	T49.2X4	T49.2X5	T49.2X6
solution	T49.ØX1	T49.ØX2	T49.ØX3	T49.ØX4	T49.ØX5	T49.ØX6
aspirin	T39.Ø11	T39.Ø12	T39.Ø13	T39.Ø14	T39.Ø15	T39.Ø16
bis (acetylsalicylate)	T39.Ø11	T39.Ø12	T39.Ø13	T39.Ø14	T39.Ø15	T39.Ø16
carbonate (gel, basic)	T47.1X1	T47.1X2	T47.1X3	T47.1X4	T47.1X5	T47.1X6
chlorhydroxide-complex	T47.1X1	T47.1X2	T47.1X3	T47.1X4	T47.1X5	T47.1X6
chloride	T49.2X1	T49.2X2	T49.2X3	T49.2X4	T49.2X5	T49.2X6
clofibrate	T46.6X1	T46.6X2	T46.6X3	T46.6X4	T46.6X5	T46.6X6
diacetate	T49.2X1	T49.2X2	T49.2X3	T49.2X4	T49.2X5	T49.2X6
glycinate	T47.1X1	T47.1X2	T47.1X3	T47.1X4	T47.1X5	T47.1X6
hydroxide (gel)	T47.1X1	T47.1X2	T47.1X3	T47.1X4	T47.1X5	T47.1X6
hydroxide-magnesium carb. gel	T47.1X1	T47.1X2	T47.1X3	T47.1X4	T47.1X5	T47.1X6
magnesium silicate	T47.1X1	T47.1X2	T47.1X3	T47.1X4	T47.1X5	T47.1X6
nicotinate	T46.7X1	T46.7X2	T46.7X3	T46.7X4	T46.7X5	T46.7X6
ointment (surgical) (topical)	T49.3X1	T49.3X2	T49.3X3	T49.3X4	T49.3X5	T49.3X6
phosphate	T47.1X1	T47.1X2	T47.1X3	T47.1X4	T47.1X5	T47.1X6
salicylate	T39.Ø91	T39.Ø92	T39.Ø93	T39.Ø94	T39.Ø95	T39.Ø96
silicate	T47.1X1	T47.1X2	T47.1X3	T47.1X4	T47.1X5	T47.1X6
sodium silicate	T47.1X1	T47.1X2	T47.1X3	T47.1X4	T47.1X5	T47.1X6
subacetate	T49.2X1	T49.2X2	T49.2X3	T49.2X4	T49.2X5	T49.2X6
sulfate	T49.ØX1	T49.ØX2	T49.ØX3	T49.ØX4	T49.ØX5	T49.ØX6
tannate	T47.6X1	T47.6X2	T47.6X3	T47.6X4	T47.6X5	T47.6X6
topical NEC	T49.3X1	T49.3X2	T49.3X3	T49.3X4	T49.3X5	T49.3X6
Alurate	T42.3X1	T42.3X2	T42.3X3	T42.3X4	T42.3X5	T42.3X6
Alverine	T44.3X1	T44.3X2	T44.3X3	T44.3X4	T44.3X5	T44.3X6
Alvodine	T4Ø.2X1	T4Ø.2X2	T4Ø.2X3	T4Ø.2X4	T4Ø.2X5	T4Ø.2X6
Amanita phalloides	T62.ØX1	T62.ØX2	T62.ØX3	T62.ØX4	—	—
Amanitine	T62.ØX1	T62.ØX2	T62.ØX3	T62.ØX4	—	—
Amantadine	T42.8X1	T42.8X2	T42.8X3	T42.8X4	T42.8X5	T42.8X6
Ambazone	T49.6X1	T49.6X2	T49.6X3	T49.6X4	T49.6X5	T49.6X6
Ambenonium (chloride)	T44.ØX1	T44.ØX2	T44.ØX3	T44.ØX4	T44.ØX5	T44.ØX6
Ambroxol	T48.4X1	T48.4X2	T48.4X3	T48.4X4	T48.4X5	T48.4X6
Ambuphylline	T48.6X1	T48.6X2	T48.6X3	T48.6X4	T48.6X5	T48.6X6
Ambutonium bromide	T44.3X1	T44.3X2	T44.3X3	T44.3X4	T44.3X5	T44.3X6
Amcinonide	T49.ØX1	T49.ØX2	T49.ØX3	T49.ØX4	T49.ØX5	T49.ØX6
Amdinocilline	T36.ØX1	T36.ØX2	T36.ØX3	T36.ØX4	T36.ØX5	T36.ØX6
Ametazole	T5Ø.8X1	T5Ø.8X2	T5Ø.8X3	T5Ø.8X4	T5Ø.8X5	T5Ø.8X6
Amethocaine	T41.3X1	T41.3X2	T41.3X3	T41.3X4	T41.3X5	T41.3X6
regional	T41.3X1	T41.3X2	T41.3X3	T41.3X4	T41.3X5	T41.3X6
spinal	T41.3X1	T41.3X2	T41.3X3	T41.3X4	T41.3X5	T41.3X6
Amethopterin	T45.1X1	T45.1X2	T45.1X3	T45.1X4	T45.1X5	T45.1X6
Amezinium metilsulfate	T44.991	T44.992	T44.993	T44.994	T44.995	T44.996
Amfebutamone	T43.291	T43.292	T43.293	T43.294	T43.295	T43.296
Amfepramone	T5Ø.5X1	T5Ø.5X2	T5Ø.5X3	T5Ø.5X4	T5Ø.5X5	T5Ø.5X6
Amfetamine	T43.621	T43.622	T43.623	T43.624	T43.625	T43.626
Amfetaminil	T43.621	T43.622	T43.623	T43.624	T43.625	T43.626
Amfomycin	T36.8X1	T36.8X2	T36.8X3	T36.8X4	T36.8X5	T36.8X6
Amidefrine mesilate	T48.5X1	T48.5X2	T48.5X3	T48.5X4	T48.5X5	T48.5X6
Amidone	T4Ø.3X1	T4Ø.3X2	T4Ø.3X3	T4Ø.3X4	T4Ø.3X5	T4Ø.3X6
Amidopyrine	T39.2X1	T39.2X2	T39.2X3	T39.2X4	T39.2X5	T39.2X6
Amidotrizoate	T5Ø.8X1	T5Ø.8X2	T5Ø.8X3	T5Ø.8X4	T5Ø.8X5	T5Ø.8X6
Amiflamine	T43.1X1	T43.1X2	T43.1X3	T43.1X4	T43.1X5	T43.1X6
Amikacin	T36.5X1	T36.5X2	T36.5X3	T36.5X4	T36.5X5	T36.5X6
Amikhelline	T46.3X1	T46.3X2	T46.3X3	T46.3X4	T46.3X5	T46.3X6
Amiloride	T5Ø.2X1	T5Ø.2X2	T5Ø.2X3	T5Ø.2X4	T5Ø.2X5	T5Ø.2X6
Aminacrine	T49.ØX1	T49.ØX2	T49.ØX3	T49.ØX4	T49.ØX5	T49.ØX6
Amineptine	T43.Ø11	T43.Ø12	T43.Ø13	T43.Ø14	T43.Ø15	T43.Ø16
Aminitrozole	T37.3X1	T37.3X2	T37.3X3	T37.3X4	T37.3X5	T37.3X6
Aminoacetic acid (derivatives)	T5Ø.3X1	T5Ø.3X2	T5Ø.3X3	T5Ø.3X4	T5Ø.3X5	T5Ø.3X6
Amino acids	T5Ø.3X1	T5Ø.3X2	T5Ø.3X3	T5Ø.3X4	T5Ø.3X5	T5Ø.3X6

Substance	Poisoning, Accidental (unintentional)	Poisoning, Intentional Self-harm	Poisoning, Assault	Poisoning, Undetermined	Adverse Effect	Under-dosing
Aminoacridine	T49.ØX1	T49.ØX2	T49.ØX3	T49.ØX4	T49.ØX5	T49.ØX6
Aminobenzoic acid (-p)	T49.3X1	T49.3X2	T49.3X3	T49.3X4	T49.3X5	T49.3X6
4-Aminobutyric acid	T43.8X1	T43.8X2	T43.8X3	T43.8X4	T43.8X5	T43.8X6
Aminocaproic acid	T45.621	T45.622	T45.623	T45.624	T45.625	T45.626
Aminofenazone	T39.2X1	T39.2X2	T39.2X3	T39.2X4	T39.2X5	T39.2X6
Aminoethylisothiourium	T45.8X1	T45.8X2	T45.8X3	T45.8X4	T45.8X5	T45.8X6
Aminoglutethimide	T45.1X1	T45.1X2	T45.1X3	T45.1X4	T45.1X5	T45.1X6
Aminohippuric acid	T5Ø.8X1	T5Ø.8X2	T5Ø.8X3	T5Ø.8X4	T5Ø.8X5	T5Ø.8X6
Aminomethylbenzoic acid	T45.691	T45.692	T45.693	T45.694	T45.695	T45.696
Aminometradine	T5Ø.2X1	T5Ø.2X2	T5Ø.2X3	T5Ø.2X4	T5Ø.2X5	T5Ø.2X6
Aminopentamide	T44.3X1	T44.3X2	T44.3X3	T44.3X4	T44.3X5	T44.3X6
Aminophenazone	T39.2X1	T39.2X2	T39.2X3	T39.2X4	T39.2X5	T39.2X6
Aminophenol	T54.ØX1	T54.ØX2	T54.ØX3	T54.ØX4	—	—
4-Aminophenol derivatives	T39.1X1	T39.1X2	T39.1X3	T39.1X4	T39.1X5	T39.1X6
Aminophenylpyridone	T43.591	T43.592	T43.593	T43.594	T43.595	T43.596
Aminophylline	T48.6X1	T48.6X2	T48.6X3	T48.6X4	T48.6X5	T48.6X6
Aminopterin sodium	T45.1X1	T45.1X2	T45.1X3	T45.1X4	T45.1X5	T45.1X6
Aminopyrine	T39.2X1	T39.2X2	T39.2X3	T39.2X4	T39.2X5	T39.2X6
8-Aminoquinoline drugs	T37.2X1	T37.2X2	T37.2X3	T37.2X4	T37.2X5	T37.2X6
Aminorex	T5Ø.5X1	T5Ø.5X2	T5Ø.5X3	T5Ø.5X4	T5Ø.5X5	T5Ø.5X6
Aminosalicylic acid	T37.1X1	T37.1X2	T37.1X3	T37.1X4	T37.1X5	T37.1X6
Aminosalylum	T37.1X1	T37.1X2	T37.1X3	T37.1X4	T37.1X5	T37.1X6
Amiodarone	T46.2X1	T46.2X2	T46.2X3	T46.2X4	T46.2X5	T46.2X6
Amiphenazole	T5Ø.7X1	T5Ø.7X2	T5Ø.7X3	T5Ø.7X4	T5Ø.7X5	T5Ø.7X6
Amiquinsin	T46.5X1	T46.5X2	T46.5X3	T46.5X4	T46.5X5	T46.5X6
Amisometradine	T5Ø.2X1	T5Ø.2X2	T5Ø.2X3	T5Ø.2X4	T5Ø.2X5	T5Ø.2X6
Amisulpride	T43.591	T43.592	T43.593	T43.594	T43.595	T43.596
Amitriptyline	T43.Ø11	T43.Ø12	T43.Ø13	T43.Ø14	T43.Ø15	T43.Ø16
Amitriptylinoxide	T43.Ø11	T43.Ø12	T43.Ø13	T43.Ø14	T43.Ø15	T43.Ø16
Amlexanox	T48.6X1	T48.6X2	T48.6X3	T48.6X4	T48.6X5	T48.6X6
Ammonia (fumes) (gas) (vapor)	T59.891	T59.892	T59.893	T59.894	—	—
aromatic spirit	T48.991	T48.992	T48.993	T48.994	T48.995	T48.996
liquid (household)	T54.3X1	T54.3X2	T54.3X3	T54.3X4	—	—
Ammoniated mercury	T49.ØX1	T49.ØX2	T49.ØX3	T49.ØX4	T49.ØX5	T49.ØX6
Ammonium						
acid tartrate	T49.5X1	T49.5X2	T49.5X3	T49.5X4	T49.5X5	T49.5X6
bromide	T42.6X1	T42.6X2	T42.6X3	T42.6X4	T42.6X5	T42.6X6
carbonate	T54.3X1	T54.3X2	T54.3X3	T54.3X4	—	—
chloride	T5Ø.991	T5Ø.992	T5Ø.993	T5Ø.994	T5Ø.995	T5Ø.996
expectorant	T48.4X1	T48.4X2	T48.4X3	T48.4X4	T48.4X5	T48.4X6
compounds (household) NEC	T54.3X1	T54.3X2	T54.3X3	T54.3X4	—	—
fumes (any usage)	T59.891	T59.892	T59.893	T59.894	—	—
industrial	T54.3X1	T54.3X2	T54.3X3	T54.3X4	—	—
ichthyosulronate	T49.4X1	T49.4X2	T49.4X3	T49.4X4	T49.4X5	T49.4X6
mandelate	T37.91	T37.92	T37.93	T37.94	T37.95	T37.96
sulfamate	T6Ø.3X1	T6Ø.3X2	T6Ø.3X3	T6Ø.3X4	—	—
sulfonate resin	T47.8X1	T47.8X2	T47.8X3	T47.8X4	T47.8X5	T47.8X6
Amobarbital (sodium)	T42.3X1	T42.3X2	T42.3X3	T42.3X4	T42.3X5	T42.3X6
Amodiaquine	T37.2X1	T37.2X2	T37.2X3	T37.2X4	T37.2X5	T37.2X6
Amopyroquin(e)	T37.2X1	T37.2X2	T37.2X3	T37.2X4	T37.2X5	T37.2X6
Amoxapine	T43.Ø11	T43.Ø12	T43.Ø13	T43.Ø14	T43.Ø15	T43.Ø16
Amoxicillin	T36.ØX1	T36.ØX2	T36.ØX3	T36.ØX4	T36.ØX5	T36.ØX6
Amperozide	T43.591	T43.592	T43.593	T43.594	T43.595	T43.596
Amphenidone	T43.591	T43.592	T43.593	T43.594	T43.595	T43.596
Amphetamine NEC	T43.621	T43.622	T43.623	T43.624	T43.625	T43.626
Amphomycin	T36.8X1	T36.8X2	T36.8X3	T36.8X4	T36.8X5	T36.8X6
Amphotalide	T37.4X1	T37.4X2	T37.4X3	T37.4X4	T37.4X5	T37.4X6
Amphotericin B	T36.7X1	T36.7X2	T36.7X3	T36.7X4	T36.7X5	T36.7X6
topical	T49.ØX1	T49.ØX2	T49.ØX3	T49.ØX4	T49.ØX5	T49.ØX6
Ampicillin	T36.ØX1	T36.ØX2	T36.ØX3	T36.ØX4	T36.ØX5	T36.ØX6
Amprotropine	T44.3X1	T44.3X2	T44.3X3	T44.3X4	T44.3X5	T44.3X6
Amsacrine	T45.1X1	T45.1X2	T45.1X3	T45.1X4	T45.1X5	T45.1X6
Amygdaline	T62.2X1	T62.2X2	T62.2X3	T62.2X4	—	—
Amyl						
acetate	T52.8X1	T52.8X2	T52.8X3	T52.8X4	—	—
vapor	T59.891	T59.892	T59.893	T59.894	—	—
alcohol	T51.3X1	T51.3X2	T51.3X3	T51.3X4	—	—
chloride	T53.6X1	T53.6X2	T53.6X3	T53.6X4	—	—
formate	T52.8X1	T52.8X2	T52.8X3	T52.8X4	—	—
nitrite	T46.3X1	T46.3X2	T46.3X3	T46.3X4	T46.3X5	T46.3X6
propionate	T65.891	T65.892	T65.893	T65.894	—	—

Substance	Poisoning, Accidental (unintentional)	Poisoning, Intentional Self-harm	Poisoning, Assault	Poisoning, Undetermined	Adverse Effect	Under-dosing
Amylase	T47.5X1	T47.5X2	T47.5X3	T47.5X4	T47.5X5	T47.5X6
Amyleine, regional	T41.3X1	T41.3X2	T41.3X3	T41.3X4	T41.3X5	T41.3X6
Amylene						
dichloride	T53.6X1	T53.6X2	T53.6X3	T53.6X4	—	—
hydrate	T51.3X1	T51.3X2	T51.3X3	T51.3X4	—	—
Amylmetacresol	T49.6X1	T49.6X2	T49.6X3	T49.6X4	T49.6X5	T49.6X6
Amylobarbitone	T42.3X1	T42.3X2	T42.3X3	T42.3X4	T42.3X5	T42.3X6
Amylocaine, regional	T41.3X1	T41.3X2	T41.3X3	T41.3X4	T41.3X5	T41.3X6
infiltration (subcutaneous)	T41.3X1	T41.3X2	T41.3X3	T41.3X4	T41.3X5	T41.3X6
nerve block (peripheral) (plexus)	T41.3X1	T41.3X2	T41.3X3	T41.3X4	T41.3X5	T41.3X6
spinal	T41.3X1	T41.3X2	T41.3X3	T41.3X4	T41.3X5	T41.3X6
topical (surface)	T41.3X1	T41.3X2	T41.3X3	T41.3X4	T41.3X5	T41.3X6
Amylopectin	T47.6X1	T47.6X2	T47.6X3	T47.6X4	T47.6X5	T47.6X6
Amytal (sodium)	T42.3X1	T42.3X2	T42.3X3	T42.3X4	T42.3X5	T42.3X6
Anabolic steroid	T38.7X1	T38.7X2	T38.7X3	T38.7X4	T38.7X5	T38.7X6
Analeptic NEC	T5Ø.7X1	T5Ø.7X2	T5Ø.7X3	T5Ø.7X4	T5Ø.7X5	T5Ø.7X6
Analgesic	T39.91	T39.92	T39.93	T39.94	T39.95	T39.96
anti-inflammatory NEC	T39.91	T39.92	T39.93	T39.94	T39.95	T39.96
propionic acid derivative	T39.311	T39.312	T39.313	T39.314	T39.315	T39.316
antirheumatic NEC	T39.4X1	T39.4X2	T39.4X3	T39.4X4	T39.4X5	T39.4X6
aromatic NEC	T39.1X1	T39.1X2	T39.1X3	T39.1X4	T39.1X5	T39.1X6
narcotic NEC	T4Ø.6Ø1	T4Ø.6Ø2	T4Ø.6Ø3	T4Ø.6Ø4	T4Ø.6Ø5	T4Ø.6Ø6
combination	T4Ø.6Ø1	T4Ø.6Ø2	T4Ø.6Ø3	T4Ø.6Ø4	T4Ø.6Ø5	T4Ø.6Ø6
obstetric	T4Ø.6Ø1	T4Ø.6Ø2	T4Ø.6Ø3	T4Ø.6Ø4	T4Ø.6Ø5	T4Ø.6Ø6
non-narcotic NEC	T39.91	T39.92	T39.93	T39.94	T39.95	T39.96
combination	T39.91	T39.92	T39.93	T39.94	T39.95	T39.96
pyrazole	T39.2X1	T39.2X2	T39.2X3	T39.2X4	T39.2X5	T39.2X6
specified NEC	T39.8X1	T39.8X2	T39.8X3	T39.8X4	T39.8X5	T39.8X6
Analgin	T39.2X1	T39.2X2	T39.2X3	T39.2X4	T39.2X5	T39.2X6
Anamirta cocculus	T62.1X1	T62.1X2	T62.1X3	T62.1X4	—	—
Ancillin	T36.ØX1	T36.ØX2	T36.ØX3	T36.ØX4	T36.ØX5	T36.ØX6
Ancrod	T45.691	T45.692	T45.693	T45.694	T45.695	T45.696
Androgen	T38.7X1	T38.7X2	T38.7X3	T38.7X4	T38.7X5	T38.7X6
Androgen-estrogen mixture	T38.7X1	T38.7X2	T38.7X3	T38.7X4	T38.7X5	T38.7X6
Androstalone	T38.7X1	T38.7X2	T38.7X3	T38.7X4	T38.7X5	T38.7X6
Androstanolone	T38.7X1	T38.7X2	T38.7X3	T38.7X4	T38.7X5	T38.7X6
Androsterone	T38.7X1	T38.7X2	T38.7X3	T38.7X4	T38.7X5	T38.7X6
Anemone pulsatilla	T62.2X1	T62.2X2	T62.2X3	T62.2X4	—	—
Anesthesia						
caudal	T41.3X1	T41.3X2	T41.3X3	T41.3X4	T41.3X5	T41.3X6
endotracheal	T41.ØX1	T41.ØX2	T41.ØX3	T41.ØX4	T41.ØX5	T41.ØX6
epidural	T41.3X1	T41.3X2	T41.3X3	T41.3X4	T41.3X5	T41.3X6
inhalation	T41.ØX1	T41.ØX2	T41.ØX3	T41.ØX4	T41.ØX5	T41.ØX6
local	T41.3X1	T41.3X2	T41.3X3	T41.3X4	T41.3X5	T41.3X6
mucosal	T41.3X1	T41.3X2	T41.3X3	T41.3X4	T41.3X5	T41.3X6
muscle relaxation	T48.1X1	T48.1X2	T48.1X3	T48.1X4	T48.1X5	T48.1X6
nerve blocking	T41.3X1	T41.3X2	T41.3X3	T41.3X4	T41.3X5	T41.3X6
plexus blocking	T41.3X1	T41.3X2	T41.3X3	T41.3X4	T41.3X5	T41.3X6
potentiated	T41.2Ø1	T41.2Ø2	T41.2Ø3	T41.2Ø4	T41.2Ø5	T41.2Ø6
rectal	T41.2Ø1	T41.2Ø2	T41.2Ø3	T41.2Ø4	T41.2Ø5	T41.2Ø6
general	T41.2Ø1	T41.2Ø2	T41.2Ø3	T41.2Ø4	T41.2Ø5	T41.2Ø6
local	T41.3X1	T41.3X2	T41.3X3	T41.3X4	T41.3X5	T41.3X6
regional	T41.3X1	T41.3X2	T41.3X3	T41.3X4	T41.3X5	T41.3X6
surface	T41.3X1	T41.3X2	T41.3X3	T41.3X4	T41.3X5	T41.3X6
Anesthetic NEC (*see also* Anesthesia)	T41.41	T41.42	T41.43	T41.44	T41.45	T41.46
with muscle relaxant	T41.2Ø1	T41.2Ø2	T41.2Ø3	T41.2Ø4	T41.2Ø5	T41.2Ø6
general	T41.2Ø1	T41.2Ø2	T41.2Ø3	T41.2Ø4	T41.2Ø5	T41.2Ø6
local	T41.3X1	T41.3X2	T41.3X3	T41.3X4	T41.3X5	T41.3X6
gaseous NEC	T41.ØX1	T41.ØX2	T41.ØX3	T41.ØX4	T41.ØX5	T41.ØX6
general NEC	T41.2Ø1	T41.2Ø2	T41.2Ø3	T41.2Ø4	T41.2Ø5	T41.2Ø6
halogenated hydrocarbon derivatives NEC	T41.ØX1	T41.ØX2	T41.ØX3	T41.ØX4	T41.ØX5	T41.ØX6
infiltration NEC	T41.3X1	T41.3X2	T41.3X3	T41.3X4	T41.3X5	T41.3X6
intravenous NEC	T41.1X1	T41.1X2	T41.1X3	T41.1X4	T41.1X5	T41.1X6
local NEC	T41.3X1	T41.3X2	T41.3X3	T41.3X4	T41.3X5	T41.3X6
rectal	T41.2Ø1	T41.2Ø2	T41.2Ø3	T41.2Ø4	T41.2Ø5	T41.2Ø6
general	T41.2Ø1	T41.2Ø2	T41.2Ø3	T41.2Ø4	T41.2Ø5	T41.2Ø6
local	T41.3X1	T41.3X2	T41.3X3	T41.3X4	T41.3X5	T41.3X6
regional NEC	T41.3X1	T41.3X2	T41.3X3	T41.3X4	T41.3X5	T41.3X6
spinal NEC	T41.3X1	T41.3X2	T41.3X3	T41.3X4	T41.3X5	T41.3X6

Substance	Poisoning, Accidental (unintentional)	Poisoning, Intentional Self-harm	Poisoning, Assault	Poisoning, Undetermined	Adverse Effect	Under-dosing
Anesthetic NEC— *continued*						
thiobarbiturate	T41.1X1	T41.1X2	T41.1X3	T41.1X4	T41.1X5	T41.1X6
topical	T41.3X1	T41.3X2	T41.3X3	T41.3X4	T41.3X5	T41.3X6
Aneurine	T45.2X1	T45.2X2	T45.2X3	T45.2X4	T45.2X5	T45.2X6
Angio-Conray	T5Ø.8X1	T5Ø.8X2	T5Ø.8X3	T5Ø.8X4	T5Ø.8X5	T5Ø.8X6
Angiotensin	T44.5X1	T44.5X2	T44.5X3	T44.5X4	T44.5X5	T44.5X6
Angiotensinamide	T44.991	T44.992	T44.993	T44.994	T44.995	T44.996
Anhydrohydroxy progesterone	T38.5X1	T38.5X2	T38.5X3	T38.5X4	T38.5X5	T38.5X6
Anhydron	T5Ø.2X1	T5Ø.2X2	T5Ø.2X3	T5Ø.2X4	T5Ø.2X5	T5Ø.2X6
Anileridine	T4Ø.4X1	T4Ø.4X2	T4Ø.4X3	T4Ø.4X4	T4Ø.4X5	T4Ø.4X6
Aniline (dye) (liquid)	T65.3X1	T65.3X2	T65.3X3	T65.3X4	—	—
analgesic	T39.1X1	T39.1X2	T39.1X3	T39.1X4	T39.1X5	T39.1X6
derivatives, therapeutic NEC	T39.1X1	T39.1X2	T39.1X3	T39.1X4	T39.1X5	T39.1X6
vapor	T65.3X1	T65.3X2	T65.3X3	T65.3X4	—	—
Anise oil	T47.5X1	T47.5X2	T47.5X3	T47.5X4	T47.5X5	T47.5X6
Aniscoropine	T44.3X1	T44.3X2	T44.3X3	T44.3X4	T44.3X5	T44.3X6
Anisidine	T65.3X1	T65.3X2	T65.3X3	T65.3X4	—	—
Anisindione	T45.511	T45.512	T45.513	T45.514	T45.515	T45.516
Anisotropine methyl-bromide	T44.3X1	T44.3X2	T44.3X3	T44.3X4	T44.3X5	T44.3X6
Anistreplase	T45.611	T45.612	T45.613	T45.614	T45.615	T45.616
Anorexiant (central)	T5Ø.5X1	T5Ø.5X2	T5Ø.5X3	T5Ø.5X4	T5Ø.5X5	T5Ø.5X6
Anorexic agents	T5Ø.5X1	T5Ø.5X2	T5Ø.5X3	T5Ø.5X4	T5Ø.5X5	T5Ø.5X6
Ansamycin	T36.6X1	T36.6X2	T36.6X3	T36.6X4	T36.6X5	T36.6X6
Ant (bite) (sting)	T63.421	T63.422	T63.423	T63.424	—	—
Antabuse	T5Ø.6X1	T5Ø.6X2	T5Ø.6X3	T5Ø.6X4	T5Ø.6X5	T5Ø.6X6
Antacid NEC	T47.1X1	T47.1X2	T47.1X3	T47.1X4	T47.1X5	T47.1X6
Antagonist						
Aldosterone	T5Ø.ØX1	T5Ø.ØX2	T5Ø.ØX3	T5Ø.ØX4	T5Ø.ØX5	T5Ø.ØX6
alpha-adrenoreceptor	T44.6X1	T44.6X2	T44.6X3	T44.6X4	T44.6X5	T44.6X6
anticoagulant	T45.7X1	T45.7X2	T45.7X3	T45.7X4	T45.7X5	T45.7X6
beta-adrenoreceptor	T44.7X1	T44.7X2	T44.7X3	T44.7X4	T44.7X5	T44.7X6
extrapyramidal NEC	T44.3X1	T44.3X2	T44.3X3	T44.3X4	T44.3X5	T44.3X6
folic acid	T45.1X1	T45.1X2	T45.1X3	T45.1X4	T45.1X5	T45.1X6
heavy metal	T45.8X1	T45.8X2	T45.8X3	T45.8X4	T45.8X5	T45.8X6
H2 receptor	T47.ØX1	T47.ØX2	T47.ØX3	T47.ØX4	T47.ØX5	T47.ØX6
narcotic analgesic	T5Ø.7X1	T5Ø.7X2	T5Ø.7X3	T5Ø.7X4	T5Ø.7X5	T5Ø.7X6
opiate	T5Ø.7X1	T5Ø.7X2	T5Ø.7X3	T5Ø.7X4	T5Ø.7X5	T5Ø.7X6
pyrimidine	T45.1X1	T45.1X2	T45.1X3	T45.1X4	T45.1X5	T45.1X6
serotonin	T46.5X1	T46.5X2	T46.5X3	T46.5X4	T46.5X5	T46.5X6
Antazolin(e)	T45.ØX1	T45.ØX2	T45.ØX3	T45.ØX4	T45.ØX5	T45.ØX6
Anterior pituitary hormone NEC	T38.811	T38.812	T38.813	T38.814	T38.815	T38.816
Anthelmintic NEC	T37.4X1	T37.4X2	T37.4X3	T37.4X4	T37.4X5	T37.4X6
Anthiolimine	T37.4X1	T37.4X2	T37.4X3	T37.4X4	T37.4X5	T37.4X6
Anthralin	T49.4X1	T49.4X2	T49.4X3	T49.4X4	T49.4X5	T49.4X6
Anthramycin	T45.1X1	T45.1X2	T45.1X3	T45.1X4	T45.1X5	T45.1X6
Antiadrenergic NEC	T44.8X1	T44.8X2	T44.8X3	T44.8X4	T44.8X5	T44.8X6
Antiallergic NEC	T45.ØX1	T45.ØX2	T45.ØX3	T45.ØX4	T45.ØX5	T45.ØX6
Antiandrogen NEC	T38.6X1	T38.6X2	T38.6X3	T38.6X4	T38.6X5	T38.6X6
Anti-anemic (drug) (preparation)	T45.8X1	T45.8X2	T45.8X3	T45.8X4	T45.8X5	T45.8X6
Antianxiety drug NEC	T43.5Ø1	T43.5Ø2	T43.5Ø3	T43.5Ø4	T43.5Ø5	T43.5Ø6
Antiaris toxicaria	T65.891	T65.892	T65.893	T65.894	—	—
Antiarteriosclerotic drug	T46.6X1	T46.6X2	T46.6X3	T46.6X4	T46.6X5	T46.6X6
Antiasthmatic drug NEC	T48.6X1	T48.6X2	T48.6X3	T48.6X4	T48.6X5	T48.6X6
Antibiotic NEC	T36.91	T36.92	T36.93	T36.94	T36.95	T36.96
aminoglycoside	T36.5X1	T36.5X2	T36.5X3	T36.5X4	T36.5X5	T36.5X6
anticancer	T45.1X1	T45.1X2	T45.1X3	T45.1X4	T45.1X5	T45.1X6
antifungal	T36.7X1	T36.7X2	T36.7X3	T36.7X4	T36.7X5	T36.7X6
antimycobacterial	T36.5X1	T36.5X2	T36.5X3	T36.5X4	T36.5X5	T36.5X6
antineoplastic	T45.1X1	T45.1X2	T45.1X3	T45.1X4	T45.1X5	T45.1X6
cephalosporin (group)	T36.1X1	T36.1X2	T36.1X3	T36.1X4	T36.1X5	T36.1X6
chloramphenicol (group)	T36.2X1	T36.2X2	T36.2X3	T36.2X4	T36.2X5	T36.2X6
ENT	T49.6X1	T49.6X2	T49.6X3	T49.6X4	T49.6X5	T49.6X6
eye	T49.5X1	T49.5X2	T49.5X3	T49.5X4	T49.5X5	T49.5X6
fungicidal (local)	T49.ØX1	T49.ØX2	T49.ØX3	T49.ØX4	T49.ØX5	T49.ØX6
intestinal	T36.8X1	T36.8X2	T36.8X3	T36.8X4	T36.8X5	T36.8X6
b-lactam NEC	T36.1X1	T36.1X2	T36.1X3	T36.1X4	T36.1X5	T36.1X6
local	T49.ØX1	T49.ØX2	T49.ØX3	T49.ØX4	T49.ØX5	T49.ØX6
macrolides	T36.3X1	T36.3X2	T36.3X3	T36.3X4	T36.3X5	T36.3X6
polypeptide	T36.8X1	T36.8X2	T36.8X3	T36.8X4	T36.8X5	T36.8X6
specified NEC	T36.8X1	T36.8X2	T36.8X3	T36.8X4	T36.8X5	T36.8X6
tetracycline (group)	T36.4X1	T36.4X2	T36.4X3	T36.4X4	T36.4X5	T36.4X6

Substance	Poisoning, Accidental (unintentional)	Poisoning, Intentional Self-harm	Poisoning, Assault	Poisoning, Undetermined	Adverse Effect	Under-dosing
Antibiotic NEC — *continued*						
throat	T49.6X1	T49.6X2	T49.6X3	T49.6X4	T49.6X5	T49.6X6
Anticancer agents NEC	T45.1X1	T45.1X2	T45.1X3	T45.1X4	T45.1X5	T45.1X6
Anticholesterolemic drug NEC	T46.6X1	T46.6X2	T46.6X3	T46.6X4	T46.6X5	T46.6X6
Anticholinergic NEC	T44.3X1	T44.3X2	T44.3X3	T44.3X4	T44.3X5	T44.3X6
Anticholinesterase	T44.ØX1	T44.ØX2	T44.ØX3	T44.ØX4	T44.ØX5	T44.ØX6
organophosphorus	T44.ØX1	T44.ØX2	T44.ØX3	T44.ØX4	T44.ØX5	T44.ØX6
insecticide	T6Ø.ØX1	T6Ø.ØX2	T6Ø.ØX3	T6Ø.ØX4	—	—
nerve gas	T59.891	T59.892	T59.893	T59.894	—	—
reversible	T44.ØX1	T44.ØX2	T44.ØX3	T44.ØX4	T44.ØX5	T44.ØX6
ophthalmological	T49.5X1	T49.5X2	T49.5X3	T49.5X4	T49.5X5	T49.5X6
Anticoagulant NEC	T45.511	T45.512	T45.513	T45.514	T45.515	T45.516
antagonist	T45.7X1	T45.7X2	T45.7X3	T45.7X4	T45.7X5	T45.7X6
Anti-common-cold drug NEC	T48.5X1	T48.5X2	T48.5X3	T48.5X4	T48.5X5	T48.5X6
Anticonvulsant	T42.71	T42.72	T42.73	T42.74	T42.75	T42.76
barbiturate	T42.3X1	T42.3X2	T42.3X3	T42.3X4	T42.3X5	T42.3X6
combination (with barbiturate)	T42.3X1	T42.3X2	T42.3X3	T42.3X4	T42.3X5	T42.3X6
hydantoin	T42.ØX1	T42.ØX2	T42.ØX3	T42.ØX4	T42.ØX5	T42.ØX6
hypnotic NEC	T42.6X1	T42.6X2	T42.6X3	T42.6X4	T42.6X5	T42.6X6
oxazolidinedione	T42.2X1	T42.2X2	T42.2X3	T42.2X4	T42.2X5	T42.2X6
pyrimidinedione	T42.6X1	T42.6X2	T42.6X3	T42.6X4	T42.6X5	T42.6X6
specified NEC	T42.6X1	T42.6X2	T42.6X3	T42.6X4	T42.6X5	T42.6X6
succinimide	T42.2X1	T42.2X2	T42.2X3	T42.2X4	T42.2X5	T42.2X6
Anti-D immunoglobulin (human)	T5Ø.Z11	T5Ø.Z12	T5Ø.Z13	T5Ø.Z14	T5Ø.Z15	T5Ø.Z16
Antidepressant	T43.2Ø1	T43.2Ø2	T43.2Ø3	T43.2Ø4	T43.2Ø5	T43.2Ø6
monoamine oxidase inhibitor	T43.1X1	T43.1X2	T43.1X3	T43.1X4	T43.1X5	T43.1X6
selective serotonin norepinephrine reuptake inhibitor	T43.211	T43.212	T43.213	T43.214	T43.215	T43.216
selective serotonin reuptake inhibitor	T43.221	T43.222	T43.223	T43.224	T43.225	T43.226
specified NEC	T43.291	T43.292	T43.293	T43.294	T43.295	T43.296
triazolopyridine	T43.211	T43.212	T43.213	T43.214	T43.215	T43.216
tetracyclic	T43.Ø21	T43.Ø22	T43.Ø23	T43.Ø24	T43.Ø25	T43.Ø26
tricyclic	T43.Ø11	T43.Ø12	T43.Ø13	T43.Ø14	T43.Ø15	T43.Ø16
Antidiabetic NEC	T38.3X1	T38.3X2	T38.3X3	T38.3X4	T38.3X5	T38.3X6
biguanide	T38.3X1	T38.3X2	T38.3X3	T38.3X4	T38.3X5	T38.3X6
and sulfonyl combined	T38.3X1	T38.3X2	T38.3X3	T38.3X4	T38.3X5	T38.3X6
combined	T38.3X1	T38.3X2	T38.3X3	T38.3X4	T38.3X5	T38.3X6
sulfonylurea	T38.3X1	T38.3X2	T38.3X3	T38.3X4	T38.3X5	T38.3X6
Antidiarrheal drug NEC	T47.6X1	T47.6X2	T47.6X3	T47.6X4	T47.6X5	T47.6X6
absorbent	T47.6X1	T47.6X2	T47.6X3	T47.6X4	T47.6X5	T47.6X6
Antidiphtheria serum	T5Ø.Z11	T5Ø.Z12	T5Ø.Z13	T5Ø.Z14	T5Ø.Z15	T5Ø.Z16
Antidiuretic hormone	T38.891	T38.892	T38.893	T38.894	T38.895	T38.896
Antidote NEC	T5Ø.6X1	T5Ø.6X2	T5Ø.6X3	T5Ø.6X4	T5Ø.6X5	T5Ø.6X6
heavy metal	T45.8X1	T45.8X2	T45.8X3	T45.8X4	T45.8X5	T45.8X6
Antidysrhythmic NEC	T46.2X1	T46.2X2	T46.2X3	T46.2X4	T46.2X5	T46.2X6
Antiemetic drug	T45.ØX1	T45.ØX2	T45.ØX3	T45.ØX4	T45.ØX5	T45.ØX6
Antiepilepsy agent	T42.71	T42.72	T42.73	T42.74	T42.75	T42.76
combination	T42.5X1	T42.5X2	T42.5X3	T42.5X4	T42.5X5	T42.5X6
mixed	T42.5X1	T42.5X2	T42.5X3	T42.5X4	T42.5X5	T42.5X6
specified, NEC	T42.6X1	T42.6X2	T42.6X3	T42.6X4	T42.6X5	T42.6X6
Antiestrogen NEC	T38.6X1	T38.6X2	T38.6X3	T38.6X4	T38.6X5	T38.6X6
Antifertility pill	T38.4X1	T38.4X2	T38.4X3	T38.4X4	T38.4X5	T38.4X6
Antifibrinolytic drug	T45.621	T45.622	T45.623	T45.624	T45.625	T45.626
Antifilarial drug	T37.4X1	T37.4X2	T37.4X3	T37.4X4	T37.4X5	T37.4X6
Antiflatulent	T47.5X1	T47.5X2	T47.5X3	T47.5X4	T47.5X5	T47.5X6
Antifreeze	T65.91	T65.92	T65.93	T65.94	—	—
alcohol	T51.1X1	T51.1X2	T51.1X3	T51.1X4	—	—
ethylene glycol	T51.8X1	T51.8X2	T51.8X3	T51.8X4	—	—
Antifungal						
antibiotic (systemic)	T36.7X1	T36.7X2	T36.7X3	T36.7X4	T36.7X5	T36.7X6
anti-infective NEC	T37.91	T37.92	T37.93	T37.94	T37.95	T37.96
disinfectant, local	T49.ØX1	T49.ØX2	T49.ØX3	T49.ØX4	T49.ØX5	T49.ØX6
nonmedicinal (spray)	T6Ø.3X1	T6Ø.3X2	T6Ø.3X3	T6Ø.3X4	—	—
topical	T49.ØX1	T49.ØX2	T49.ØX3	T49.ØX4	T49.ØX5	T49.ØX6
Anti-gastric-secretion drug NEC	T47.1X1	T47.1X2	T47.1X3	T47.1X4	T47.1X5	T47.1X6
Antigonadotrophin NEC	T38.6X1	T38.6X2	T38.6X3	T38.6X4	T38.6X5	T38.6X6
Antihallucinogen	T43.5Ø1	T43.5Ø2	T43.5Ø3	T43.5Ø4	T43.5Ø5	T43.5Ø6
Antihelmintics	T37.4X1	T37.4X2	T37.4X3	T37.4X4	T37.4X5	T37.4X6
Antihemophilic						
factor	T45.8X1	T45.8X2	T45.8X3	T45.8X4	T45.8X5	T45.8X6
fraction	T45.8X1	T45.8X2	T45.8X3	T45.8X4	T45.8X5	T45.8X6
globulin concentrate	T45.7X1	T45.7X2	T45.7X3	T45.7X4	T45.7X5	T45.7X6
human plasma	T45.8X1	T45.8X2	T45.8X3	T45.8X4	T45.8X5	T45.8X6
plasma, dried	T45.7X1	T45.7X2	T45.7X3	T45.7X4	T45.7X5	T45.7X6
Antihemorrhoidal preparation	T49.2X1	T49.2X2	T49.2X3	T49.2X4	T49.2X5	T49.2X6
Antiheparin drug	T45.7X1	T45.7X2	T45.7X3	T45.7X4	T45.7X5	T45.7X6
Antihistamine	T45.ØX1	T45.ØX2	T45.ØX3	T45.ØX4	T45.ØX5	T45.ØX6
Antihookworm drug	T37.4X1	T37.4X2	T37.4X3	T37.4X4	T37.4X5	T37.4X6
Anti-human lymphocytic globulin	T5Ø.Z11	T5Ø.Z12	T5Ø.Z13	T5Ø.Z14	T5Ø.Z15	T5Ø.Z16
Antihyperlipidemic drug	T46.6X1	T46.6X2	T46.6X3	T46.6X4	T46.6X5	T46.6X6
Antihypertensive drug NEC	T46.5X1	T46.5X2	T46.5X3	T46.5X4	T46.5X5	T46.5X6
Anti-infective NEC	T37.91	T37.92	T37.93	T37.94	T37.95	T37.96
antibiotics	T36.91	T36.92	T36.93	T36.94	T36.95	T36.96
specified NEC	T36.8X1	T36.8X2	T36.8X3	T36.8X4	T36.8X5	T36.8X6
anthelmintic	T37.4X1	T37.4X2	T37.4X3	T37.4X4	T37.4X5	T37.4X6
antimalarial	T37.2X1	T37.2X2	T37.2X3	T37.2X4	T37.2X5	T37.2X6
antimycobacterial NEC	T37.1X1	T37.1X2	T37.1X3	T37.1X4	T37.1X5	T37.1X6
antibiotics	T36.5X1	T36.5X2	T36.5X3	T36.5X4	T36.5X5	T36.5X6
antiprotozoal NEC	T37.3X1	T37.3X2	T37.3X3	T37.3X4	T37.3X5	T37.3X6
blood	T37.2X1	T37.2X2	T37.2X3	T37.2X4	T37.2X5	T37.2X6
antiviral	T37.5X1	T37.5X2	T37.5X3	T37.5X4	T37.5X5	T37.5X6
arsenical	T37.8X1	T37.8X2	T37.8X3	T37.8X4	T37.8X5	T37.8X6
bismuth, local	T49.ØX1	T49.ØX2	T49.ØX3	T49.ØX4	T49.ØX5	T49.ØX6
ENT	T49.6X1	T49.6X2	T49.6X3	T49.6X4	T49.6X5	T49.6X6
eye NEC	T49.5X1	T49.5X2	T49.5X3	T49.5X4	T49.5X5	T49.5X6
heavy metals NEC	T37.8X1	T37.8X2	T37.8X3	T37.8X4	T37.8X5	T37.8X6
local NEC	T49.ØX1	T49.ØX2	T49.ØX3	T49.ØX4	T49.ØX5	T49.ØX6
specified NEC	T49.ØX1	T49.ØX2	T49.ØX3	T49.ØX4	T49.ØX5	T49.ØX6
mixed	T37.91	T37.92	T37.93	T37.94	T37.95	T37.96
ophthalmic preparation	T49.5X1	T49.5X2	T49.5X3	T49.5X4	T49.5X5	T49.5X6
topical NEC	T49.ØX1	T49.ØX2	T49.ØX3	T49.ØX4	T49.ØX5	T49.ØX6
Anti-inflammatory drug NEC	T39.391	T39.392	T39.393	T39.394	T39.395	T39.396
local	T49.ØX1	T49.ØX2	T49.ØX3	T49.ØX4	T49.ØX5	T49.ØX6
nonsteroidal NEC	T39.391	T39.392	T39.393	T39.394	T39.395	T39.396
propionic acid derivative	T39.311	T39.312	T39.313	T39.314	T39.315	T39.316
specified NEC	T39.391	T39.392	T39.393	T39.394	T39.395	T39.396
Antikaluretic	T5Ø.3X1	T5Ø.3X2	T5Ø.3X3	T5Ø.3X4	T5Ø.3X5	T5Ø.3X6
Antiknock (tetraethyl lead)	T56.ØX1	T56.ØX2	T56.ØX3	T56.ØX4	—	—
Antilipemic drug NEC	T46.6X1	T46.6X2	T46.6X3	T46.6X4	T46.6X5	T46.6X6
Antimalarial	T37.2X1	T37.2X2	T37.2X3	T37.2X4	T37.2X5	T37.2X6
prophylactic NEC	T37.2X1	T37.2X2	T37.2X3	T37.2X4	T37.2X5	T37.2X6
pyrimidine derivative	T37.2X1	T37.2X2	T37.2X3	T37.2X4	T37.2X5	T37.2X6
Antimetabolite	T45.1X1	T45.1X2	T45.1X3	T45.1X4	T45.1X5	T45.1X6
Antimitotic agent	T45.1X1	T45.1X2	T45.1X3	T45.1X4	T45.1X5	T45.1X6
Antimony (compounds) (vapor) NEC	T56.891	T56.892	T56.893	T56.894	—	—
anti-infectives	T37.8X1	T37.8X2	T37.8X3	T37.8X4	T37.8X5	T37.8X6
dimercaptosuccinate	T37.3X1	T37.3X2	T37.3X3	T37.3X4	T37.3X5	T37.3X6
hydride	T56.891	T56.892	T56.893	T56.894	—	—
pesticide (vapor)	T6Ø.8X1	T6Ø.8X2	T6Ø.8X3	T6Ø.8X4	—	—
potassium (sodium) tartrate	T37.8X1	T37.8X2	T37.8X3	T37.8X4	T37.8X5	T37.8X6
tartrated	T37.8X1	T37.8X2	T37.8X3	T37.8X4	T37.8X5	T37.8X6
sodium dimercaptosuccinate	T37.3X1	T37.3X2	T37.3X3	T37.3X4	T37.3X5	T37.3X6
Antimuscarinic NEC	T44.3X1	T44.3X2	T44.3X3	T44.3X4	T44.3X5	T44.3X6
Antimycobacterial drug NEC	T37.1X1	T37.1X2	T37.1X3	T37.1X4	T37.1X5	T37.1X6
antibiotics	T36.5X1	T36.5X2	T36.5X3	T36.5X4	T36.5X5	T36.5X6
combination	T37.1X1	T37.1X2	T37.1X3	T37.1X4	T37.1X5	T37.1X6
Antinausea drug	T45.ØX1	T45.ØX2	T45.ØX3	T45.ØX4	T45.ØX5	T45.ØX6
Antinematode drug	T37.4X1	T37.4X2	T37.4X3	T37.4X4	T37.4X5	T37.4X6
Antineoplastic NEC	T45.1X1	T45.1X2	T45.1X3	T45.1X4	T45.1X5	T45.1X6
antibiotics	T45.1X1	T45.1X2	T45.1X3	T45.1X4	T45.1X5	T45.1X6
alkaloidal	T45.1X1	T45.1X2	T45.1X3	T45.1X4	T45.1X5	T45.1X6
combination	T45.1X1	T45.1X2	T45.1X3	T45.1X4	T45.1X5	T45.1X6
estrogen	T38.5X1	T38.5X2	T38.5X3	T38.5X4	T38.5X5	T38.5X6
steroid	T38.7X1	T38.7X2	T38.7X3	T38.7X4	T38.7X5	T38.7X6
Antiparasitic drug (systemic)	T37.91	T37.92	T37.93	T37.94	T37.95	T37.96
local	T49.ØX1	T49.ØX2	T49.ØX3	T49.ØX4	T49.ØX5	T49.ØX6
specified NEC	T37.8X1	T37.8X2	T37.8X3	T37.8X4	T37.8X5	T37.8X6

Substance	Poisoning, Accidental (unintentional)	Poisoning, Intentional Self-harm	Poisoning, Assault	Poisoning, Undetermined	Adverse Effect	Under-dosing
Antiparkinsonism drug NEC	T42.8X1	T42.8X2	T42.8X3	T42.8X4	T42.8X5	T42.8X6
Antiperspirant NEC	T49.2X1	T49.2X2	T49.2X3	T49.2X4	T49.2X5	T49.2X6
Antiphlogistic NEC	T39.4X1	T39.4X2	T39.4X3	T39.4X4	T39.4X5	T39.4X6
Antiplatyhelmintic drug	T37.4X1	T37.4X2	T37.4X3	T37.4X4	T37.4X5	T37.4X6
Antiprotozoal drug NEC	T37.3X1	T37.3X2	T37.3X3	T37.3X4	T37.3X5	T37.3X6
blood	T37.2X1	T37.2X2	T37.2X3	T37.2X4	T37.2X5	T37.2X6
local	T49.ØX1	T49.ØX2	T49.ØX3	T49.ØX4	T49.ØX5	T49.ØX6
Antipruritic drug NEC	T49.1X1	T49.1X2	T49.1X3	T49.1X4	T49.1X5	T49.1X6
Antipsychotic drug	T43.5Ø1	T43.5Ø2	T43.5Ø3	T43.5Ø4	T43.5Ø5	T43.5Ø6
specified NEC	T43.591	T43.592	T43.593	T43.594	T43.595	T43.596
Antipyretic	T39.91	T39.92	T39.93	T39.94	T39.95	T39.96
specified NEC	T39.8X1	T39.8X2	T39.8X3	T39.8X4	T39.8X5	T39.8X6
Antipyrine	T39.2X1	T39.2X2	T39.2X3	T39.2X4	T39.2X5	T39.2X6
Antirabies hyperimmune serum	T5Ø.Z11	T5Ø.Z12	T5Ø.Z13	T5Ø.Z14	T5Ø.Z15	T5Ø.Z16
Antirheumatic NEC	T39.4X1	T39.4X2	T39.4X3	T39.4X4	T39.4X5	T39.4X6
Antirigidity drug NEC	T42.8X1	T42.8X2	T42.8X3	T42.8X4	T42.8X5	T42.8X6
Antischistosomal drug	T37.4X1	T37.4X2	T37.4X3	T37.4X4	T37.4X5	T37.4X6
Antiscorpion sera	T5Ø.Z11	T5Ø.Z12	T5Ø.Z13	T5Ø.Z14	T5Ø.Z15	T5Ø.Z16
Antiseborrheics	T49.4X1	T49.4X2	T49.4X3	T49.4X4	T49.4X5	T49.4X6
Antiseptics (external) (medicinal)	T49.ØX1	T49.ØX2	T49.ØX3	T49.ØX4	T49.ØX5	T49.ØX6
Antistine	T45.ØX1	T45.ØX2	T45.ØX3	T45.ØX4	T45.ØX5	T45.ØX6
Antitapeworm drug	T37.4X1	T37.4X2	T37.4X3	T37.4X4	T37.4X5	T37.4X6
Antitetanus immunoglobulin	T5Ø.Z11	T5Ø.Z12	T5Ø.Z13	T5Ø.Z14	T5Ø.Z15	T5Ø.Z16
Antithyroid drug NEC	T38.2X1	T38.2X2	T38.2X3	T38.2X4	T38.2X5	T38.2X6
Antitoxin	T5Ø.Z11	T5Ø.Z12	T5Ø.Z13	T5Ø.Z14	T5Ø.Z15	T5Ø.Z16
diphtheria	T5Ø.Z11	T5Ø.Z12	T5Ø.Z13	T5Ø.Z14	T5Ø.Z15	T5Ø.Z16
gas gangrene	T5Ø.Z11	T5Ø.Z12	T5Ø.Z13	T5Ø.Z14	T5Ø.Z15	T5Ø.Z16
tetanus	T5Ø.Z11	T5Ø.Z12	T5Ø.Z13	T5Ø.Z14	T5Ø.Z15	T5Ø.Z16
Antitrichomonal drug	T37.3X1	T37.3X2	T37.3X3	T37.3X4	T37.3X5	T37.3X6
Antituberculars	T37.1X1	T37.1X2	T37.1X3	T37.1X4	T37.1X5	T37.1X6
antibiotics	T36.5X1	T36.5X2	T36.5X3	T36.5X4	T36.5X5	T36.5X6
Antitussive NEC	T48.3X1	T48.3X2	T48.3X3	T48.3X4	T48.3X5	T48.3X6
codeine mixture	T4Ø.2X1	T4Ø.2X2	T4Ø.2X3	T4Ø.2X4	T4Ø.2X5	T4Ø.2X6
opiate	T4Ø.2X1	T4Ø.2X2	T4Ø.2X3	T4Ø.2X4	T4Ø.2X5	T4Ø.2X6
Antivaricose drug	T46.8X1	T46.8X2	T46.8X3	T46.8X4	T46.8X5	T46.8X6
Antivenin, antivenom (sera)	T5Ø.Z11	T5Ø.Z12	T5Ø.Z13	T5Ø.Z14	T5Ø.Z15	T5Ø.Z16
crotaline	T5Ø.Z11	T5Ø.Z12	T5Ø.Z13	T5Ø.Z14	T5Ø.Z15	T5Ø.Z16
spider bite	T5Ø.Z11	T5Ø.Z12	T5Ø.Z13	T5Ø.Z14	T5Ø.Z15	T5Ø.Z16
Antivertigo drug	T45.ØX1	T45.ØX2	T45.ØX3	T45.ØX4	T45.ØX5	T45.ØX6
Antiviral drug NEC	T37.5X1	T37.5X2	T37.5X3	T37.5X4	T37.5X5	T37.5X6
eye	T49.5X1	T49.5X2	T49.5X3	T49.5X4	T49.5X5	T49.5X6
Antiwhipworm drug	T37.4X1	T37.4X2	T37.4X3	T37.4X4	T37.4X5	T37.4X6
Ant poisons—*see* Pesticides						
Antrol (*see also* by specific chemical substance)	T6Ø.91	T6Ø.92	T6Ø.93	T6Ø.94	—	—
fungicide	T6Ø.91	T6Ø.92	T6Ø.93	T6Ø.94	—	—
ANTU (alpha naphthylthiourea)	T6Ø.4X1	T6Ø.4X2	T6Ø.4X3	T6Ø.4X4	—	—
Apalcillin	T36.ØX1	T36.ØX2	T36.ØX3	T36.ØX4	T36.ØX5	T36.ØX6
APC	T48.5X1	T48.5X2	T48.5X3	T48.5X4	T48.5X5	T48.5X6
Aplonidine	T44.4X1	T44.4X2	T44.4X3	T44.4X4	T44.4X5	T44.4X6
Apomorphine	T47.7X1	T47.7X2	T47.7X3	T47.7X4	T47.7X5	T47.7X6
Appetite depressants, central	T5Ø.5X1	T5Ø.5X2	T5Ø.5X3	T5Ø.5X4	T5Ø.5X5	T5Ø.5X6
Apraclonidine (hydrochloride)	T44.4X1	T44.4X2	T44.4X3	T44.4X4	T44.4X5	T44.4X6
Apresoline	T46.5X1	T46.5X2	T46.5X3	T46.5X4	T46.5X5	T46.5X6
Aprindine	T46.2X1	T46.2X2	T46.2X3	T46.2X4	T46.2X5	T46.2X6
Aprobarbital	T42.3X1	T42.3X2	T42.3X3	T42.3X4	T42.3X5	T42.3X6
Apronalide	T42.6X1	T42.6X2	T42.6X3	T42.6X4	T42.6X5	T42.6X6
Aprotinin	T45.621	T45.622	T45.623	T45.624	T45.625	T45.626
Aptocaine	T41.3X1	T41.3X2	T41.3X3	T41.3X4	T41.3X5	T41.3X6
Aqua fortis	T54.2X1	T54.2X2	T54.2X3	T54.2X4	—	—
Ara-A	T37.5X1	T37.5X2	T37.5X3	T37.5X4	T37.5X5	T37.5X6
Ara-C	T45.1X1	T45.1X2	T45.1X3	T45.1X4	T45.1X5	T45.1X6
Arachis oil	T49.3X1	T49.3X2	T49.3X3	T49.3X4	T49.3X5	T49.3X6
cathartic	T47.4X1	T47.4X2	T47.4X3	T47.4X4	T47.4X5	T47.4X6
Aralen	T37.2X1	T37.2X2	T37.2X3	T37.2X4	T37.2X5	T37.2X6
Arecoline	T44.1X1	T44.1X2	T44.1X3	T44.1X4	T44.1X5	T44.1X6
Arginine	T5Ø.991	T5Ø.992	T5Ø.993	T5Ø.994	T5Ø.995	T5Ø.996
glutamate	T5Ø.991	T5Ø.992	T5Ø.993	T5Ø.994	T5Ø.995	T5Ø.996
Argyrol	T49.ØX1	T49.ØX2	T49.ØX3	T49.ØX4	T49.ØX5	T49.ØX6
ENT agent	T49.6X1	T49.6X2	T49.6X3	T49.6X4	T49.6X5	T49.6X6
ophthalmic preparation	T49.5X1	T49.5X2	T49.5X3	T49.5X4	T49.5X5	T49.5X6

Substance	Poisoning, Accidental (unintentional)	Poisoning, Intentional Self-harm	Poisoning, Assault	Poisoning, Undetermined	Adverse Effect	Under-dosing
Aristocort	T38.ØX1	T38.ØX2	T38.ØX3	T38.ØX4	T38.ØX5	T38.ØX6
ENT agent	T49.6X1	T49.6X2	T49.6X3	T49.6X4	T49.6X5	T49.6X6
ophthalmic preparation	T49.5X1	T49.5X2	T49.5X3	T49.5X4	T49.5X5	T49.5X6
topical NEC	T49.ØX1	T49.ØX2	T49.ØX3	T49.ØX4	T49.ØX5	T49.ØX6
Aromatics, corrosive	T54.1X1	T54.1X2	T54.1X3	T54.1X4	—	—
disinfectants	T54.1X1	T54.1X2	T54.1X3	T54.1X4	—	—
Arsenate of lead	T57.ØX1	T57.ØX2	T57.ØX3	T57.ØX4	—	—
herbicide	T57.ØX1	T57.ØX2	T57.ØX3	T57.ØX4	—	—
Arsenic, arsenicals (compounds) (dust) (vapor) **NEC**	T57.ØX1	T57.ØX2	T57.ØX3	T57.ØX4	—	—
anti-infectives	T37.8X1	T37.8X2	T37.8X3	T37.8X4	T37.8X5	T37.8X6
pesticide (dust) (fumes)	T57.ØX1	T57.ØX2	T57.ØX3	T57.ØX4	—	—
Arsine (gas)	T57.ØX1	T57.ØX2	T57.ØX3	T57.ØX4	—	—
Arsphenamine (silver)	T37.8X1	T37.8X2	T37.8X3	T37.8X4	T37.8X5	T37.8X6
Arsthinol	T37.3X1	T37.3X2	T37.3X3	T37.3X4	T37.3X5	T37.3X6
Artane	T44.3X1	T44.3X2	T44.3X3	T44.3X4	T44.3X5	T44.3X6
Arthropod (venomous) **NEC**	T63.481	T63.482	T63.483	T63.484	—	—
Articaine	T41.3X1	T41.3X2	T41.3X3	T41.3X4	T41.3X5	T41.3X6
Asbestos	T57.8X1	T57.8X2	T57.8X3	T57.8X4	—	—
Ascaridole	T37.4X1	T37.4X2	T37.4X3	T37.4X4	T37.4X5	T37.4X6
Ascorbic acid	T45.2X1	T45.2X2	T45.2X3	T45.2X4	T45.2X5	T45.2X6
Asiaticoside	T49.ØX1	T49.ØX2	T49.ØX3	T49.ØX4	T49.ØX5	T49.ØX6
Asparaginase	T45.1X1	T45.1X2	T45.1X3	T45.1X4	T45.1X5	T45.1X6
Aspidium (oleoresin)	T37.4X1	T37.4X2	T37.4X3	T37.4X4	T37.4X5	T37.4X6
Aspirin (aluminum) (soluble)	T39.Ø11	T39.Ø12	T39.Ø13	T39.Ø14	T39.Ø15	T39.Ø16
Aspoxicillin	T36.ØX1	T36.ØX2	T36.ØX3	T36.ØX4	T36.ØX5	T36.ØX6
Astemizole	T45.ØX1	T45.ØX2	T45.ØX3	T45.ØX4	T45.ØX5	T45.ØX6
Astringent (local)	T49.2X1	T49.2X2	T49.2X3	T49.2X4	T49.2X5	T49.2X6
specified NEC	T49.2X1	T49.2X2	T49.2X3	T49.2X4	T49.2X5	T49.2X6
Astromicin	T36.5X1	T36.5X2	T36.5X3	T36.5X4	T36.5X5	T36.5X6
Ataractic drug NEC	T43.5Ø1	T43.5Ø2	T43.5Ø3	T43.5Ø4	T43.5Ø5	T43.5Ø6
Atenolol	T44.7X1	T44.7X2	T44.7X3	T44.7X4	T44.7X5	T44.7X6
Atonia drug, intestinal	T47.4X1	T47.4X2	T47.4X3	T47.4X4	T47.4X5	T47.4X6
Atophan	T5Ø.4X1	T5Ø.4X2	T5Ø.4X3	T5Ø.4X4	T5Ø.4X5	T5Ø.4X6
Atracurium besilate	T48.1X1	T48.1X2	T48.1X3	T48.1X4	T48.1X5	T48.1X6
Atropine	T44.3X1	T44.3X2	T44.3X3	T44.3X4	T44.3X5	T44.3X6
derivative	T44.3X1	T44.3X2	T44.3X3	T44.3X4	T44.3X5	T44.3X6
methonitrate	T44.3X1	T44.3X2	T44.3X3	T44.3X4	T44.3X5	T44.3X6
Attapulgite	T47.6X1	T47.6X2	T47.6X3	T47.6X4	T47.6X5	T47.6X6
Auramine	T65.891	T65.892	T65.893	T65.894	—	—
dye	T65.6X1	T65.6X2	T65.6X3	T65.6X4	—	—
fungicide	T6Ø.3X1	T6Ø.3X2	T6Ø.3X3	T6Ø.3X4	—	—
Auranofin	T39.4X1	T39.4X2	T39.4X3	T39.4X4	T39.4X5	T39.4X6
Aurantiin	T46.991	T46.992	T46.993	T46.994	T46.995	T46.996
Aureomycin	T36.4X1	T36.4X2	T36.4X3	T36.4X4	T36.4X5	T36.4X6
ophthalmic preparation	T49.5X1	T49.5X2	T49.5X3	T49.5X4	T49.5X5	T49.5X6
topical NEC	T49.ØX1	T49.ØX2	T49.ØX3	T49.ØX4	T49.ØX5	T49.ØX6
Aurothioglucose	T39.4X1	T39.4X2	T39.4X3	T39.4X4	T39.4X5	T39.4X6
Aurothioglycanide	T39.4X1	T39.4X2	T39.4X3	T39.4X4	T39.4X5	T39.4X6
Aurothiomalate sodium	T39.4X1	T39.4X2	T39.4X3	T39.4X4	T39.4X5	T39.4X6
Aurotioprol	T39.4X1	T39.4X2	T39.4X3	T39.4X4	T39.4X5	T39.4X6
Automobile fuel	T52.ØX1	T52.ØX2	T52.ØX3	T52.ØX4	—	—
Autonomic nervous system agent NEC	T44.9Ø1	T44.9Ø2	T44.9Ø3	T44.9Ø4	T44.9Ø5	T44.9Ø6
Avlosulfon	T37.1X1	T37.1X2	T37.1X3	T37.1X4	T37.1X5	T37.1X6
Avomine	T42.6X1	T42.6X2	T42.6X3	T42.6X4	T42.6X5	T42.6X6
Axerophthol	T45.2X1	T45.2X2	T45.2X3	T45.2X4	T45.2X5	T45.2X6
Azacitidine	T45.1X1	T45.1X2	T45.1X3	T45.1X4	T45.1X5	T45.1X6
Azacyclonol	T43.591	T43.592	T43.593	T43.594	T43.595	T43.596
Azadirachta	T6Ø.2X1	T6Ø.2X2	T6Ø.2X3	T6Ø.2X4	—	—
Azanidazole	T37.3X1	T37.3X2	T37.3X3	T37.3X4	T37.3X5	T37.3X6
Azapetine	T46.7X1	T46.7X2	T46.7X3	T46.7X4	T46.7X5	T46.7X6
Azapropazone	T39.2X1	T39.2X2	T39.2X3	T39.2X4	T39.2X5	T39.2X6
Azaribine	T45.1X1	T45.1X2	T45.1X3	T45.1X4	T45.1X5	T45.1X6
Azaserine	T45.1X1	T45.1X2	T45.1X3	T45.1X4	T45.1X5	T45.1X6
Azatadine	T45.ØX1	T45.ØX2	T45.ØX3	T45.ØX4	T45.ØX5	T45.ØX6
Azatepa	T45.1X1	T45.1X2	T45.1X3	T45.1X4	T45.1X5	T45.1X6
Azathioprine	T45.1X1	T45.1X2	T45.1X3	T45.1X4	T45.1X5	T45.1X6
Azelaic acid	T49.ØX1	T49.ØX2	T49.ØX3	T49.ØX4	T49.ØX5	T49.ØX6
Azelastine	T45.ØX1	T45.ØX2	T45.ØX3	T45.ØX4	T45.ØX5	T45.ØX6
Azidocillin	T36.ØX1	T36.ØX2	T36.ØX3	T36.ØX4	T36.ØX5	T36.ØX6

Substance	Poisoning, Accidental (unintentional)	Poisoning, Intentional Self-harm	Poisoning, Assault	Poisoning, Undetermined	Adverse Effect	Under-dosing
Azidothymidine	T37.5X1	T37.5X2	T37.5X3	T37.5X4	T37.5X5	T37.5X6
Azinphos (ethyl) (methyl)	T6Ø.ØX1	T6Ø.ØX2	T6Ø.ØX3	T6Ø.ØX4	—	—
Aziridine (chelating)	T54.1X1	T54.1X2	T54.1X3	T54.1X4	—	—
Azithromycin	T36.3X1	T36.3X2	T36.3X3	T36.3X4	T36.3X5	T36.3X6
Azlocillin	T36.ØX1	T36.ØX2	T36.ØX3	T36.ØX4	T36.ØX5	T36.ØX6
Azobenzene smoke	T65.3X1	T65.3X2	T65.3X3	T65.3X4	—	—
acaricide	T6Ø.8X1	T6Ø.8X2	T6Ø.8X3	T6Ø.8X4	—	—
Azosulfamide	T37.ØX1	T37.ØX2	T37.ØX3	T37.ØX4	T37.ØX5	T37.ØX6
AZT	T37.5X1	T37.5X2	T37.5X3	T37.5X4	T37.5X5	T37.5X6
Aztreonam	T36.1X1	T36.1X2	T36.1X3	T36.1X4	T36.1X5	T36.1X6
Azulfidine	T37.ØX1	T37.ØX2	T37.ØX3	T37.ØX4	T37.ØX5	T37.ØX6
Azuresin	T5Ø.8X1	T5Ø.8X2	T5Ø.8X3	T5Ø.8X4	T5Ø.8X5	T5Ø.8X6
B						
Bacampicillin	T36.ØX1	T36.ØX2	T36.ØX3	T36.ØX4	T36.ØX5	T36.ØX6
Bacillus						
lactobacillus	T47.8X1	T47.8X2	T47.8X3	T47.8X4	T47.8X5	T47.8X6
subtilis	T47.6X1	T47.6X2	T47.6X3	T47.6X4	T47.6X5	T47.6X6
Bacimycin	T49.ØX1	T49.ØX2	T49.ØX3	T49.ØX4	T49.ØX5	T49.ØX6
ophthalmic preparation	T49.5X1	T49.5X2	T49.5X3	T49.5X4	T49.5X5	T49.5X6
Bacitracin zinc	T49.ØX1	T49.ØX2	T49.ØX3	T49.ØX4	T49.ØX5	T49.ØX6
with neomycin	T49.ØX1	T49.ØX2	T49.ØX3	T49.ØX4	T49.ØX5	T49.ØX6
ENT agent	T49.6X1	T49.6X2	T49.6X3	T49.6X4	T49.6X5	T49.6X6
ophthalmic preparation	T49.5X1	T49.5X2	T49.5X3	T49.5X4	T49.5X5	T49.5X6
topical NEC	T49.ØX1	T49.ØX2	T49.ØX3	T49.ØX4	T49.ØX5	T49.ØX6
Baclofen	T42.8X1	T42.8X2	T42.8X3	T42.8X4	T42.8X5	T42.8X6
Baking soda	T5Ø.991	T5Ø.992	T5Ø.993	T5Ø.994	T5Ø.995	T5Ø.996
BAL	T45.8X1	T45.8X2	T45.8X3	T45.8X4	T45.8X5	T45.8X6
Bambuterol	T48.6X1	T48.6X2	T48.6X3	T48.6X4	T48.6X5	T48.6X6
Bamethan (sulfate)	T46.7X1	T46.7X2	T46.7X3	T46.7X4	T46.7X5	T46.7X6
Bamifylline	T48.6X1	T48.6X2	T48.6X3	T48.6X4	T48.6X5	T48.6X6
Bamipine	T45.ØX1	T45.ØX2	T45.ØX3	T45.ØX4	T45.ØX5	T45.ØX6
Baneberry—*see* Actaea spicata						
Banewort—*see* Belladonna						
Barbenyl	T42.3X1	T42.3X2	T42.3X3	T42.3X4	T42.3X5	T42.3X6
Barbexaclone	T42.6X1	T42.6X2	T42.6X3	T42.6X4	T42.6X5	T42.6X6
Barbital	T42.3X1	T42.3X2	T42.3X3	T42.3X4	T42.3X5	T42.3X6
sodium	T42.3X1	T42.3X2	T42.3X3	T42.3X4	T42.3X5	T42.3X6
Barbitone	T42.3X1	T42.3X2	T42.3X3	T42.3X4	T42.3X5	T42.3X6
Barbiturate NEC	T42.3X1	T42.3X2	T42.3X3	T42.3X4	T42.3X5	T42.3X6
with tranquilizer	T42.3X1	T42.3X2	T42.3X3	T42.3X4	T42.3X5	T42.3X6
anesthetic (intravenous)	T41.1X1	T41.1X2	T41.1X3	T41.1X4	T41.1X5	T41.1X6
Barium (carbonate) (chloride) (sulfite)	T57.8X1	T57.8X2	T57.8X3	T57.8X4	—	—
diagnostic agent	T5Ø.8X1	T5Ø.8X2	T5Ø.8X3	T5Ø.8X4	T5Ø.8X5	T5Ø.8X6
pesticide	T6Ø.4X1	T6Ø.4X2	T6Ø.4X3	T6Ø.4X4	—	—
rodenticide	T6Ø.4X1	T6Ø.4X2	T6Ø.4X3	T6Ø.4X4	—	—
sulfate (medicinal)	T5Ø.8X1	T5Ø.8X2	T5Ø.8X3	T5Ø.8X4	T5Ø.8X5	T5Ø.8X6
Barrier cream	T49.3X1	T49.3X2	T49.3X3	T49.3X4	T49.3X5	T49.3X6
Basic fuchsin	T49.ØX1	T49.ØX2	T49.ØX3	T49.ØX4	T49.ØX5	T49.ØX6
Battery acid or fluid	T54.2X1	T54.2X2	T54.2X3	T54.2X4	—	—
Bay rum	T51.8X1	T51.8X2	T51.8X3	T51.8X4	—	—
BCG (vaccine)	T5Ø.A91	T5Ø.A92	T5Ø.A93	T5Ø.A94	T5Ø.A95	T5Ø.A96
BCNU	T45.1X1	T45.1X2	T45.1X3	T45.1X4	T45.1X5	T45.1X6
Bearsfoot	T62.2X1	T62.2X2	T62.2X3	T62.2X4	—	—
Beclamide	T42.6X1	T42.6X2	T42.6X3	T42.6X4	T42.6X5	T42.6X6
Beclomethasone	T44.5X1	T44.5X2	T44.5X3	T44.5X4	T44.5X5	T44.5X6
Bee (sting) (venom)	T63.441	T63.442	T63.443	T63.444	—	—
Befunolol	T49.5X1	T49.5X2	T49.5X3	T49.5X4	T49.5X5	T49.5X6
Bekanamycin	T36.5X1	T36.5X2	T36.5X3	T36.5X4	T36.5X5	T36.5X6
Belladonna (*see also* Nightshade)						
alkaloids	T44.3X1	T44.3X2	T44.3X3	T44.3X4	T44.3X5	T44.3X6
extract	T44.3X1	T44.3X2	T44.3X3	T44.3X4	T44.3X5	T44.3X6
herb	T44.3X1	T44.3X2	T44.3X3	T44.3X4	T44.3X5	T44.3X6
Bemegride	T5Ø.7X1	T5Ø.7X2	T5Ø.7X3	T5Ø.7X4	T5Ø.7X5	T5Ø.7X6
Benactyzine	T44.3X1	T44.3X2	T44.3X3	T44.3X4	T44.3X5	T44.3X6
Benadryl	T45.ØX1	T45.ØX2	T45.ØX3	T45.ØX4	T45.ØX5	T45.ØX6
Benaprizine	T44.3X1	T44.3X2	T44.3X3	T44.3X4	T44.3X5	T44.3X6
Benazepril	T46.4X1	T46.4X2	T46.4X3	T46.4X4	T46.4X5	T46.4X6
Bencyclane	T46.7X1	T46.7X2	T46.7X3	T46.7X4	T46.7X5	T46.7X6
Bendazol	T46.3X1	T46.3X2	T46.3X3	T46.3X4	T46.3X5	T46.3X6
Bendrofluazide	T5Ø.2X1	T5Ø.2X2	T5Ø.2X3	T5Ø.2X4	T5Ø.2X5	T5Ø.2X6
Bendroflumethiazide	T5Ø.2X1	T5Ø.2X2	T5Ø.2X3	T5Ø.2X4	T5Ø.2X5	T5Ø.2X6
Benemid	T5Ø.4X1	T5Ø.4X2	T5Ø.4X3	T5Ø.4X4	T5Ø.4X5	T5Ø.4X6
Benethamine penicillin	T36.ØX1	T36.ØX2	T36.ØX3	T36.ØX4	T36.ØX5	T36.ØX6
Benisone	T49.ØX1	T49.ØX2	T49.ØX3	T49.ØX4	T49.ØX5	T49.ØX6
Benexate	T47.1X1	T47.1X2	T47.1X3	T47.1X4	T47.1X5	T47.1X6
Benfluorex	T46.6X1	T46.6X2	T46.6X3	T46.6X4	T46.6X5	T46.6X6
Benfotiamine	T45.2X1	T45.2X2	T45.2X3	T45.2X4	T45.2X5	T45.2X6
Benomyl	T6Ø.ØX1	T6Ø.ØX2	T6Ø.ØX3	T6Ø.ØX4	—	—
Benoquin	T49.8X1	T49.8X2	T49.8X3	T49.8X4	T49.8X5	T49.8X6
Benoxinate	T41.3X1	T41.3X2	T41.3X3	T41.3X4	T41.3X5	T41.3X6
Benperidol	T43.4X1	T43.4X2	T43.4X3	T43.4X4	T43.4X5	T43.4X6
Benproperine	T48.3X1	T48.3X2	T48.3X3	T48.3X4	T48.3X5	T48.3X6
Benserazide	T42.8X1	T42.8X2	T42.8X3	T42.8X4	T42.8X5	T42.8X6
Bentazepam	T42.4X1	T42.4X2	T42.4X3	T42.4X4	T42.4X5	T42.4X6
Bentiromide	T5Ø.8X1	T5Ø.8X2	T5Ø.8X3	T5Ø.8X4	T5Ø.8X5	T5Ø.8X6
Bentonite	T49.3X1	T49.3X2	T49.3X3	T49.3X4	T49.3X5	T49.3X6
Benzalbutyramide	T46.6X1	T46.6X2	T46.6X3	T46.6X4	T46.6X5	T46.6X6
Benzalkonium (chloride)	T49.ØX1	T49.ØX2	T49.ØX3	T49.ØX4	T49.ØX5	T49.ØX6
ophthalmic preparation	T49.5X1	T49.5X2	T49.5X3	T49.5X4	T49.5X5	T49.5X6
Benzamine	T41.3X1	T41.3X2	T41.3X3	T41.3X4	T41.3X5	T41.3X6
lactate	T49.1X1	T49.1X2	T49.1X3	T49.1X4	T49.1X5	T49.1X6
Benzamidosalicylate (calcium)	T37.1X1	T37.1X2	T37.1X3	T37.1X4	T37.1X5	T37.1X6
Benzamphetamine	T5Ø.5X1	T5Ø.5X2	T5Ø.5X3	T5Ø.5X4	T5Ø.5X5	T5Ø.5X6
Benzapril hydrochloride	T46.5X1	T46.5X2	T46.5X3	T46.5X4	T46.5X5	T46.5X6
Benzathine benzylpenicillin	T36.ØX1	T36.ØX2	T36.ØX3	T36.ØX4	T36.ØX5	T36.ØX6
Benzathine penicillin	T36.ØX1	T36.ØX2	T36.ØX3	T36.ØX4	T36.ØX5	T36.ØX6
Benzatropine	T42.8X1	T42.8X2	T42.8X3	T42.8X4	T42.8X5	T42.8X6
Benzbromarone	T5Ø.4X1	T5Ø.4X2	T5Ø.4X3	T5Ø.4X4	T5Ø.4X5	T5Ø.4X6
Benzcarbimine	T45.1X1	T45.1X2	T45.1X3	T45.1X4	T45.1X5	T45.1X6
Benzedrex	T44.991	T44.992	T44.993	T44.994	T44.995	T44.996
Benzedrine (amphetamine)	T43.621	T43.622	T43.623	T43.624	T43.625	T43.626
Benzenamine	T65.3X1	T65.3X2	T65.3X3	T65.3X4	—	—
Benzene	T52.1X1	T52.1X2	T52.1X3	T52.1X4	—	—
homologues (acetyl) (dimethyl)(methyl)(solvent)	T52.2X1	T52.2X2	T52.2X3	T52.2X4	—	—
Benzethonium (chloride)	T49.ØX1	T49.ØX2	T49.ØX3	T49.ØX4	T49.ØX5	T49.ØX6
Benzfetamine	T5Ø.5X1	T5Ø.5X2	T5Ø.5X3	T5Ø.5X4	T5Ø.5X5	T5Ø.5X6
Benzhexol	T44.3X1	T44.3X2	T44.3X3	T44.3X4	T44.3X5	T44.3X6
Benzhydramine (chloride)	T45.ØX1	T45.ØX2	T45.ØX3	T45.ØX4	T45.ØX5	T45.ØX6
Benzidine	T65.891	T65.892	T65.893	T65.894	—	—
Benzilonium bromide	T44.3X1	T44.3X2	T44.3X3	T44.3X4	T44.3X5	T44.3X6
Benzimidazole	T6Ø.3X1	T6Ø.3X2	T6Ø.3X3	T6Ø.3X4	—	—
Benzin(e)—*see* Ligroin						
Benziodarone	T46.3X1	T46.3X2	T46.3X3	T46.3X4	T46.3X5	T46.3X6
Benznidazole	T37.3X1	T37.3X2	T37.3X3	T37.3X4	T37.3X5	T37.3X6
Benzocaine	T41.3X1	T41.3X2	T41.3X3	T41.3X4	T41.3X5	T41.3X6
Benzodiapin	T42.4X1	T42.4X2	T42.4X3	T42.4X4	T42.4X5	T42.4X6
Benzodiazepine NEC	T42.4X1	T42.4X2	T42.4X3	T42.4X4	T42.4X5	T42.4X6
Benzoic acid	T49.ØX1	T49.ØX2	T49.ØX3	T49.ØX4	T49.ØX5	T49.ØX6
with salicylic acid	T49.ØX1	T49.ØX2	T49.ØX3	T49.ØX4	T49.ØX5	T49.ØX6
Benzoin (tincture)	T48.5X1	T48.5X2	T48.5X3	T48.5X4	T48.5X5	T48.5X6
Benzol (benzene)	T52.1X1	T52.1X2	T52.1X3	T52.1X4	—	—
vapor	T52.ØX1	T52.ØX2	T52.ØX3	T52.ØX4	—	—
Benzomorphan	T4Ø.2X1	T4Ø.2X2	T4Ø.2X3	T4Ø.2X4	T4Ø.2X5	T4Ø.2X6
Benzonatate	T48.3X1	T48.3X2	T48.3X3	T48.3X4	T48.3X5	T48.3X6
Benzophenones	T49.3X1	T49.3X2	T49.3X3	T49.3X4	T49.3X5	T49.3X6
Benzopyrone	T46.991	T46.992	T46.993	T46.994	T46.995	T46.996
Benzothiadiazides	T5Ø.2X1	T5Ø.2X2	T5Ø.2X3	T5Ø.2X4	T5Ø.2X5	T5Ø.2X6
Benzoxonium chloride	T49.ØX1	T49.ØX2	T49.ØX3	T49.ØX4	T49.ØX5	T49.ØX6
Benzoyl peroxide	T49.ØX1	T49.ØX2	T49.ØX3	T49.ØX4	T49.ØX5	T49.ØX6
Benzoylpas calcium	T37.1X1	T37.1X2	T37.1X3	T37.1X4	T37.1X5	T37.1X6
Benzperidin	T43.591	T43.592	T43.593	T43.594	T43.595	T43.596
Benzperidol	T43.591	T43.592	T43.593	T43.594	T43.595	T43.596
Benzphetamine	T5Ø.5X1	T5Ø.5X2	T5Ø.5X3	T5Ø.5X4	T5Ø.5X5	T5Ø.5X6
Benzpyrinium bromide	T44.1X1	T44.1X2	T44.1X3	T44.1X4	T44.1X5	T44.1X6
Benzquinamide	T45.ØX1	T45.ØX2	T45.ØX3	T45.ØX4	T45.ØX5	T45.ØX6
Benzthiazide	T5Ø.2X1	T5Ø.2X2	T5Ø.2X3	T5Ø.2X4	T5Ø.2X5	T5Ø.2X6
Benztropine						
anticholinergic	T44.3X1	T44.3X2	T44.3X3	T44.3X4	T44.3X5	T44.3X6
antiparkinson	T42.8X1	T42.8X2	T42.8X3	T42.8X4	T42.8X5	T42.8X6
Benzydamine	T49.ØX1	T49.ØX2	T49.ØX3	T49.ØX4	T49.ØX5	T49.ØX6

Substance	Poisoning, Accidental (unintentional)	Poisoning, Intentional Self-harm	Poisoning, Assault	Poisoning, Undetermined	Adverse Effect	Under-dosing
Benzyl						
acetate	T52.8X1	T52.8X2	T52.8X3	T52.8X4	—	—
alcohol	T49.ØX1	T49.ØX2	T49.ØX3	T49.ØX4	T49.ØX5	T49.ØX6
benzoate	T49.ØX1	T49.ØX2	T49.ØX3	T49.ØX4	T49.ØX5	T49.ØX6
Benzoic acid	T49.ØX1	T49.ØX2	T49.ØX3	T49.ØX4	T49.ØX5	T49.ØX6
morphine	T4Ø.2X1	T4Ø.2X2	T4Ø.2X3	T4Ø.2X4	—	—
nicotinate	T46.6X1	T46.6X2	T46.6X3	T46.6X4	T46.6X5	T46.6X6
penicillin	T36.ØX1	T36.ØX2	T36.ØX3	T36.ØX4	T36.ØX5	T36.ØX6
Benzylhydrochlorthiazide	T5Ø.2X1	T5Ø.2X2	T5Ø.2X3	T5Ø.2X4	T5Ø.2X5	T5Ø.2X6
Benzylpenicillin	T36.ØX1	T36.ØX2	T36.ØX3	T36.ØX4	T36.ØX5	T36.ØX6
Benzylthiouracil	T38.2X1	T38.2X2	T38.2X3	T38.2X4	T38.2X5	T38.2X6
Bephenium hydroxy-naphthoate	T37.4X1	T37.4X2	T37.4X3	T37.4X4	T37.4X5	T37.4X6
Bepridil	T46.1X1	T46.1X2	T46.1X3	T46.1X4	T46.1X5	T46.1X6
Bergamot oil	T65.891	T65.892	T65.893	T65.894	—	—
Bergapten	T5Ø.991	T5Ø.992	T5Ø.993	T5Ø.994	T5Ø.995	T5Ø.996
Berries, poisonous	T62.1X1	T62.1X2	T62.1X3	T62.1X4	—	—
Beryllium (compounds)	T56.7X1	T56.7X2	T56.7X3	T56.7X4	—	—
b-acetyldigoxin	T46.ØX1	T46.ØX2	T46.ØX3	T46.ØX4	T46.ØX5	T46.ØX6
beta adrenergic blocking agent, heart	T44.7X1	T44.7X2	T44.7X3	T44.7X4	T44.7X5	T44.7X6
b-benzalbutyramide	T46.6X1	T46.6X2	T46.6X3	T46.6X4	T46.6X5	T46.6X6
Betacarotene	T45.2X1	T45.2X2	T45.2X3	T45.2X4	T45.2X5	T45.2X6
Beta-Chlor	T42.6X1	T42.6X2	T42.6X3	T42.6X4	T42.6X5	T42.6X6
b-eucaine	T49.1X1	T49.1X2	T49.1X3	T49.1X4	T49.1X5	T49.1X6
b-galactosidase	T47.5X1	T47.5X2	T47.5X3	T47.5X4	T47.5X5	T47.5X6
Betahistine	T46.7X1	T46.7X2	T46.7X3	T46.7X4	T46.7X5	T46.7X6
Betaine	T47.5X1	T47.5X2	T47.5X3	T47.5X4	T47.5X5	T47.5X6
Betamethasone	T49.ØX1	T49.ØX2	T49.ØX3	T49.ØX4	T49.ØX5	T49.ØX6
topical	T49.ØX1	T49.ØX2	T49.ØX3	T49.ØX4	T49.ØX5	T49.ØX6
Betamicin	T36.8X1	T36.8X2	T36.8X3	T36.8X4	T36.8X5	T36.8X6
Betanidine	T46.5X1	T46.5X2	T46.5X3	T46.5X4	T46.5X5	T46.5X6
b-sitosterol(s)	T46.6X1	T46.6X2	T46.6X3	T46.6X4	T46.6X5	T46.6X6
Betaxolol	T44.7X1	T44.7X2	T44.7X3	T44.7X4	T44.7X5	T44.7X6
Betazole	T5Ø.8X1	T5Ø.8X2	T5Ø.8X3	T5Ø.8X4	T5Ø.8X5	T5Ø.8X6
Bethanechol	T44.1X1	T44.1X2	T44.1X3	T44.1X4	T44.1X5	T44.1X6
chloride	T44.1X1	T44.1X2	T44.1X3	T44.1X4	T44.1X5	T44.1X6
Bethanidine	T46.5X1	T46.5X2	T46.5X3	T46.5X4	T46.5X5	T46.5X6
Betoxycaine	T41.3X1	T41.3X2	T41.3X3	T41.3X4	T41.3X5	T41.3X6
Betula oil	T49.3X1	T49.3X2	T49.3X3	T49.3X4	T49.3X5	T49.3X6
Bevantolol	T44.7X1	T44.7X2	T44.7X3	T44.7X4	T44.7X5	T44.7X6
Bevonium metilsulfate	T44.3X1	T44.3X2	T44.3X3	T44.3X4	T44.3X5	T44.3X6
Bezafibrate	T46.6X1	T46.6X2	T46.6X3	T46.6X4	T46.6X5	T46.6X6
Bezitramide	T4Ø.4X1	T4Ø.4X2	T4Ø.4X3	T4Ø.4X4	T4Ø.4X5	T4Ø.4X6
BHA	T5Ø.991	T5Ø.992	T5Ø.993	T5Ø.994	T5Ø.995	T5Ø.996
Bhang	T4Ø.7X1	T4Ø.7X2	T4Ø.7X3	T4Ø.7X4	T4Ø.7X5	T4Ø.7X6
BHC (medicinal)	T49.ØX1	T49.ØX2	T49.ØX3	T49.ØX4	T49.ØX5	T49.ØX6
nonmedicinal (vapor)	T53.6X1	T53.6X2	T53.6X3	T53.6X4	—	—
Bialamicol	T37.3X1	T37.3X2	T37.3X3	T37.3X4	T37.3X5	T37.3X6
Bibenzonium bromide	T48.3X1	T48.3X2	T48.3X3	T48.3X4	T48.3X5	T48.3X6
Bibrocathol	T49.5X1	T49.5X2	T49.5X3	T49.5X4	T49.5X5	T49.5X6
Bichloride of mercury—*see* Mercury, chloride						
Bichromates (calcium) (potassium) (sodium) (crystals)	T57.8X1	T57.8X2	T57.8X3	T57.8X4	—	—
fumes	T56.2X1	T56.2X2	T56.2X3	T56.2X4	—	—
Biclotymol	T49.6X1	T49.6X2	T49.6X3	T49.6X4	T49.6X5	T49.6X6
Bicucculine	T5Ø.7X1	T5Ø.7X2	T5Ø.7X3	T5Ø.7X4	T5Ø.7X5	T5Ø.7X6
Bifemelane	T43.291	T43.292	T43.293	T43.294	T43.295	T43.296
Biguanide derivatives, oral	T38.3X1	T38.3X2	T38.3X3	T38.3X4	T38.3X5	T38.3X6
Biligrafin	T5Ø.8X1	T5Ø.8X2	T5Ø.8X3	T5Ø.8X4	T5Ø.8X5	T5Ø.8X6
Bile salts	T47.5X1	T47.5X2	T47.5X3	T47.5X4	T47.5X5	T47.5X6
Bilopaque	T5Ø.8X1	T5Ø.8X2	T5Ø.8X3	T5Ø.8X4	T5Ø.8X5	T5Ø.8X6
Binifibrate	T46.6X1	T46.6X2	T46.6X3	T46.6X4	T46.6X5	T46.6X6
Binitrobenzol	T65.3X1	T65.3X2	T65.3X3	T65.3X4		
Bioflavonoid(s)	T46.991	T46.992	T46.993	T46.994	T46.995	T46.996
Biological substance NEC	T5Ø.9Ø1	T5Ø.9Ø2	T5Ø.9Ø3	T5Ø.9Ø4	T5Ø.9Ø5	T5Ø.9Ø6
Biotin	T45.2X1	T45.2X2	T45.2X3	T45.2X4	T45.2X5	T45.2X6
Biperiden	T44.3X1	T44.3X2	T44.3X3	T44.3X4	T44.3X5	T44.3X6
Bisacodyl	T47.2X1	T47.2X2	T47.2X3	T47.2X4	T47.2X5	T47.2X6
Bisbentiamine	T45.2X1	T45.2X2	T45.2X3	T45.2X4	T45.2X5	T45.2X6
Bisbutiamine	T45.2X1	T45.2X2	T45.2X3	T45.2X4	T45.2X5	T45.2X6
Bisdequalinium (salts) (diacetate)	T49.6X1	T49.6X2	T49.6X3	T49.6X4	T49.6X5	T49.6X6
Bishydroxycoumarin	T45.511	T45.512	T45.513	T45.514	T45.515	T45.516
Bismarsen	T37.8X1	T37.8X2	T37.8X3	T37.8X4	T37.8X5	T37.8X6
Bismuth salts	T47.6X1	T47.6X2	T47.6X3	T47.6X4	T47.6X5	T47.6X6
aluminate	T47.1X1	T47.1X2	T47.1X3	T47.1X4	T47.1X5	T47.1X6
anti-infectives	T37.8X1	T37.8X2	T37.8X3	T37.8X4	T37.8X5	T37.8X6
formic iodide	T49.ØX1	T49.ØX2	T49.ØX3	T49.ØX4	T49.ØX5	T49.ØX6
glycolylarsenate	T49.ØX1	T49.ØX2	T49.ØX3	T49.ØX4	T49.ØX5	T49.ØX6
nonmedicinal (compounds) NEC	T65.91	T65.92	T65.93	T65.94	—	—
subcarbonate	T47.6X1	T47.6X2	T47.6X3	T47.6X4	T47.6X5	T47.6X6
subsalicylate	T37.8X1	T37.8X2	T37.8X3	T37.8X4	T37.8X5	T37.8X6
sulfarsphenamine	T37.8X1	T37.8X2	T37.8X3	T37.8X4	T37.8X5	T37.8X6
Bisoprolol	T44.7X1	T44.7X2	T44.7X3	T44.7X4	T44.7X5	T44.7X6
Bisoxatin	T47.2X1	T47.2X2	T47.2X3	T47.2X4	T47.2X5	T47.2X6
Bisulepin (hydrochloride)	T45.ØX1	T45.ØX2	T45.ØX3	T45.ØX4	T45.ØX5	T45.ØX6
Bithionol	T37.8X1	T37.8X2	T37.8X3	T37.8X4	T37.8X5	T37.8X6
anthelminthic	T37.4X1	T37.4X2	T37.4X3	T37.4X4	T37.4X5	T37.4X6
Bitolterol	T48.6X1	T48.6X2	T48.6X3	T48.6X4	T48.6X5	T48.6X6
Bitoscanate	T37.4X1	T37.4X2	T37.4X3	T37.4X4	T37.4X5	T37.4X6
Bitter almond oil	T62.8X1	T62.8X2	T62.8X3	T62.8X4	—	—
Bittersweet	T62.2X1	T62.2X2	T62.2X3	T62.2X4	—	—
Black						
flag	T6Ø.91	T6Ø.92	T6Ø.93	T6Ø.94	—	—
henbane	T62.2X1	T62.2X2	T62.2X3	T62.2X4	—	—
leaf (40)	T6Ø.91	T6Ø.92	T6Ø.93	T6Ø.94	—	—
widow spider (bite)	T63.311	T63.312	T63.313	T63.314	—	—
antivenin	T5Ø.Z11	T5Ø.Z12	T5Ø.Z13	T5Ø.Z14	T5Ø.Z15	T5Ø.Z16
Blast furnace gas (carbon monoxide from)	T58.8X1	T58.8X2	T58.8X3	T58.8X4	—	—
Bleach	T54.91	T54.92	T54.93	T54.94	—	—
Bleaching agent (medicinal)	T49.4X1	T49.4X2	T49.4X3	T49.4X4	T49.4X5	T49.4X6
Bleomycin	T45.1X1	T45.1X2	T45.1X3	T45.1X4	T45.1X5	T45.1X6
Blockain	T41.3X1	T41.3X2	T41.3X3	T41.3X4	T41.3X5	T41.3X6
infiltration (subcutaneous)	T41.3X1	T41.3X2	T41.3X3	T41.3X4	T41.3X5	T41.3X6
nerve block (peripheral) (plexus)	T41.3X1	T41.3X2	T41.3X3	T41.3X4	T41.3X5	T41.3X6
topical (surface)	T41.3X1	T41.3X2	T41.3X3	T41.3X4	T41.3X5	T41.3X6
Blockers, calcium channel	T46.1X1	T46.1X2	T46.1X3	T46.1X4	T46.1X5	T46.1X6
Blood (derivatives) (natural) (plasma) (whole)	T45.8X1	T45.8X2	T45.8X3	T45.8X4	T45.8X5	T45.8X6
dried	T45.8X1	T45.8X2	T45.8X3	T45.8X4	T45.8X5	T45.8X6
drug affecting NEC	T45.91	T45.92	T45.93	T45.94	T45.95	T45.96
expander NEC	T45.8X1	T45.8X2	T45.8X3	T45.8X4	T45.8X5	T45.8X6
fraction NEC	T45.8X1	T45.8X2	T45.8X3	T45.8X4	T45.8X5	T45.8X6
substitute (macromolecular)	T45.8X1	T45.8X2	T45.8X3	T45.8X4	T45.8X5	T45.8X6
Blue velvet	T4Ø.2X1	T4Ø.2X2	T4Ø.2X3	T4Ø.2X4	—	—
Bone meal	T62.8X1	T62.8X2	T62.8X3	T62.8X4	—	—
Bonine	T45.ØX1	T45.ØX2	T45.ØX3	T45.ØX4	T45.ØX5	T45.ØX6
Bopindolol	T44.7X1	T44.7X2	T44.7X3	T44.7X4	T44.7X5	T44.7X6
Boracic acid	T49.ØX1	T49.ØX2	T49.ØX3	T49.ØX4	T49.ØX5	T49.ØX6
ENT agent	T49.6X1	T49.6X2	T49.6X3	T49.6X4	T49.6X5	T49.6X6
ophthalmic preparation	T49.5X1	T49.5X2	T49.5X3	T49.5X4	T49.5X5	T49.5X6
Borane complex	T57.8X1	T57.8X2	T57.8X3	T57.8X4	—	—
Borate(s)	T57.8X1	T57.8X2	T57.8X3	T57.8X4	—	—
buffer	T5Ø.991	T5Ø.992	T5Ø.993	T5Ø.994	T5Ø.995	T5Ø.996
cleanser	T54.91	T54.92	T54.93	T54.94	—	—
sodium	T57.8X1	T57.8X2	T57.8X3	T57.8X4	—	—
Borax (cleanser)	T54.91	T54.92	T54.93	T54.94	—	—
Bordeaux mixture	T6Ø.3X1	T6Ø.3X2	T6Ø.3X3	T6Ø.3X4	—	—
Boric acid	T49.ØX1	T49.ØX2	T49.ØX3	T49.ØX4	T49.ØX5	T49.ØX6
ENT agent	T49.6X1	T49.6X2	T49.6X3	T49.6X4	T49.6X5	T49.6X6
ophthalmic preparation	T49.5X1	T49.5X2	T49.5X3	T49.5X4	T49.5X5	T49.5X6
Bornaprine	T44.3X1	T44.3X2	T44.3X3	T44.3X4	T44.3X5	T44.3X6
Boron	T57.8X1	T57.8X2	T57.8X3	T57.8X4	—	—
hydride NEC	T57.8X1	T57.8X2	T57.8X3	T57.8X4	—	—
fumes or gas	T57.8X1	T57.8X2	T57.8X3	T57.8X4	—	—
trifluoride	T59.891	T59.892	T59.893	T59.894	—	—
Botox	T48.291	T48.292	T48.293	T48.294	T48.295	T48.296
Botulinus anti-toxin (type A, B)	T5Ø.Z11	T5Ø.Z12	T5Ø.Z13	T5Ø.Z14	T5Ø.Z15	T5Ø.Z16
Brake fluid vapor	T59.891	T59.892	T59.893	T59.894	—	—
Brallobarbital	T42.3X1	T42.3X2	T42.3X3	T42.3X4	T42.3X5	T42.3X6

Substance	Poisoning, Accidental (unintentional)	Poisoning, Intentional Self-harm	Poisoning, Assault	Poisoning, Undetermined	Adverse Effect	Under-dosing
Bran (wheat)	T47.4X1	T47.4X2	T47.4X3	T47.4X4	T47.4X5	T47.4X6
Brass (fumes)	T56.891	T56.892	T56.893	T56.894	—	—
Brasso	T52.ØX1	T52.ØX2	T52.ØX3	T52.ØX4	—	—
Bretylium tosilate	T46.2X1	T46.2X2	T46.2X3	T46.2X4	T46.2X5	T46.2X6
Brevital (sodium)	T41.1X1	T41.1X2	T41.1X3	T41.1X4	T41.1X5	T41.1X6
Brinase	T45.3X1	T45.3X2	T45.3X3	T45.3X4	T45.3X5	T45.3X6
British antilewisite	T45.8X1	T45.8X2	T45.8X3	T45.8X4	T45.8X5	T45.8X6
Brodifacoum	T6Ø.4X1	T6Ø.4X2	T6Ø.4X3	T6Ø.4X4	—	—
Bromal (hydrate)	T42.6X1	T42.6X2	T42.6X3	T42.6X4	T42.6X5	T42.6X6
Bromazepam	T42.4X1	T42.4X2	T42.4X3	T42.4X4	T42.4X5	T42.4X6
Bromazine	T45.ØX1	T45.ØX2	T45.ØX3	T45.ØX4	T45.ØX5	T45.ØX6
Brombenzylcyanide	T59.3X1	T59.3X2	T59.3X3	T59.3X4	—	—
Bromelains	T45.3X1	T45.3X2	T45.3X3	T45.3X4	T45.3X5	T45.3X6
Bromethalin	T6Ø.4X1	T6Ø.4X2	T6Ø.4X3	T6Ø.4X4	—	—
Bromhexine	T48.4X1	T48.4X2	T48.4X3	T48.4X4	T48.4X5	T48.4X6
Bromide salts	T42.6X1	T42.6X2	T42.6X3	T42.6X4	T42.6X5	T42.6X6
Bromindione	T45.511	T45.512	T45.513	T45.514	T45.515	T45.516
Bromine						
compounds (medicinal)	T42.6X1	T42.6X2	T42.6X3	T42.6X4	T42.6X5	T42.6X6
sedative	T42.6X1	T42.6X2	T42.6X3	T42.6X4	T42.6X5	T42.6X6
vapor	T59.891	T59.892	T59.893	T59.894	—	—
Bromisovalum	T42.6X1	T42.6X2	T42.6X3	T42.6X4	T42.6X5	T42.6X6
Bromisoval	T42.6X1	T42.6X2	T42.6X3	T42.6X4	T42.6X5	T42.6X6
Bromobenzylcyanide	T59.3X1	T59.3X2	T59.3X3	T59.3X4	—	—
Bromochlorosalicylanilide	T49.ØX1	T49.ØX2	T49.ØX3	T49.ØX4	T49.ØX5	T49.ØX6
Bromocriptine	T42.8X1	T42.8X2	T42.8X3	T42.8X4	T42.8X5	T42.8X6
Bromodiphenhydramine	T45.ØX1	T45.ØX2	T45.ØX3	T45.ØX4	T45.ØX5	T45.ØX6
Bromoform	T42.6X1	T42.6X2	T42.6X3	T42.6X4	T42.6X5	T42.6X6
Bromophenol blue reagent	T5Ø.991	T5Ø.992	T5Ø.993	T5Ø.994	T5Ø.995	T5Ø.996
Bromopride	T47.8X1	T47.8X2	T47.8X3	T47.8X4	T47.8X5	T47.8X6
Bromosalicylchloranitide	T49.ØX1	T49.ØX2	T49.ØX3	T49.ØX4	T49.ØX5	T49.ØX6
Bromosalicylhydroxamic acid	T37.1X1	T37.1X2	T37.1X3	T37.1X4	T37.1X5	T37.1X6
Bromo-Seltzer	T39.1X1	T39.1X2	T39.1X3	T39.1X4	T39.1X5	T39.1X6
Bromoxynil	T6Ø.3X1	T6Ø.3X2	T6Ø.3X3	T6Ø.3X4	—	—
Bromperidol	T43.4X1	T43.4X2	T43.4X3	T43.4X4	T43.4X5	T43.4X6
Brompheniramine	T45.ØX1	T45.ØX2	T45.ØX3	T45.ØX4	T45.ØX5	T45.ØX6
Bromsulfophthalein	T5Ø.8X1	T5Ø.8X2	T5Ø.8X3	T5Ø.8X4	T5Ø.8X5	T5Ø.8X6
Bromural	T42.6X1	T42.6X2	T42.6X3	T42.6X4	T42.6X5	T42.6X6
Bromvaletone	T42.6X1	T42.6X2	T42.6X3	T42.6X4	T42.6X5	T42.6X6
Bronchodilator NEC	T48.6X1	T48.6X2	T48.6X3	T48.6X4	T48.6X5	T48.6X6
Brotizolam	T42.4X1	T42.4X2	T42.4X3	T42.4X4	T42.4X5	T42.4X6
Brovincamine	T46.7X1	T46.7X2	T46.7X3	T46.7X4	T46.7X5	T46.7X6
Brown spider (bite) (venom)	T63.391	T63.392	T63.393	T63.394	—	—
Brown recluse spider (bite) (venom)	T63.331	T63.332	T63.333	T63.334	—	—
Broxaterol	T48.6X1	T48.6X2	T48.6X3	T48.6X4	T48.6X5	T48.6X6
Broxuridine	T45.1X1	T45.1X2	T45.1X3	T45.1X4	T45.1X5	T45.1X6
Broxyquinoline	T37.8X1	T37.8X2	T37.8X3	T37.8X4	T37.8X5	T37.8X6
Bruceine	T48.291	T48.292	T48.293	T48.294	T48.295	T48.296
Brucia	T62.2X1	T62.2X2	T62.2X3	T62.2X4	—	—
Brucine	T65.1X1	T65.1X2	T65.1X3	T65.1X4	—	—
Brunswick green—*see* Copper						
Bruten—*see* Ibuprofen						
Bryonia	T47.2X1	T47.2X2	T47.2X3	T47.2X4	T47.2X5	T47.2X6
Buclizine	T45.ØX1	T45.ØX2	T45.ØX3	T45.ØX4	T45.ØX5	T45.ØX6
Buclosamide	T49.ØX1	T49.ØX2	T49.ØX3	T49.ØX4	T49.ØX5	T49.ØX6
Budesonide	T44.5X1	T44.5X2	T44.5X3	T44.5X4	T44.5X5	T44.5X6
Budralazine	T46.5X1	T46.5X2	T46.5X3	T46.5X4	T46.5X5	T46.5X6
Bufferin	T39.Ø11	T39.Ø12	T39.Ø13	T39.Ø14	T39.Ø15	T39.Ø16
Buflomedil	T46.7X1	T46.7X2	T46.7X3	T46.7X4	T46.7X5	T46.7X6
Buformin	T38.3X1	T38.3X2	T38.3X3	T38.3X4	T38.3X5	T38.3X6
Bufotenine	T4Ø.991	T4Ø.992	T4Ø.993	T4Ø.994	—	—
Bufrolin	T48.6X1	T48.6X2	T48.6X3	T48.6X4	T48.6X5	T48.6X6
Bufylline	T48.6X1	T48.6X2	T48.6X3	T48.6X4	T48.6X5	T48.6X6
Bulk filler	T5Ø.5X1	T5Ø.5X2	T5Ø.5X3	T5Ø.5X4	T5Ø.5X5	T5Ø.5X6
cathartic	T47.4X1	T47.4X2	T47.4X3	T47.4X4	T47.4X5	T47.4X6
Bumetanide	T5Ø.1X1	T5Ø.1X2	T5Ø.1X3	T5Ø.1X4	T5Ø.1X5	T5Ø.1X6
Bunaftine	T46.2X1	T46.2X2	T46.2X3	T46.2X4	T46.2X5	T46.2X6
Bunamiodyl	T5Ø.8X1	T5Ø.8X2	T5Ø.8X3	T5Ø.8X4	T5Ø.8X5	T5Ø.8X6
Bunazosin	T44.6X1	T44.6X2	T44.6X3	T44.6X4	T44.6X5	T44.6X6
Bunitrolol	T44.7X1	T44.7X2	T44.7X3	T44.7X4	T44.7X5	T44.7X6

Substance	Poisoning, Accidental (unintentional)	Poisoning, Intentional Self-harm	Poisoning, Assault	Poisoning, Undetermined	Adverse Effect	Under-dosing
Buphenine	T46.7X1	T46.7X2	T46.7X3	T46.7X4	T46.7X5	T46.7X6
Bupivacaine	T41.3X1	T41.3X2	T41.3X3	T41.3X4	T41.3X5	T41.3X6
infiltration (subcutaneous)	T41.3X1	T41.3X2	T41.3X3	T41.3X4	T41.3X5	T41.3X6
nerve block (peripheral) (plexus)	T41.3X1	T41.3X2	T41.3X3	T41.3X4	T41.3X5	T41.3X6
spinal	T41.3X1	T41.3X2	T41.3X3	T41.3X4	T41.3X5	T41.3X6
Bupranolol	T44.7X1	T44.7X2	T44.7X3	T44.7X4	T44.7X5	T44.7X6
Buprenorphine	T4Ø.4X1	T4Ø.4X2	T4Ø.4X3	T4Ø.4X4	T4Ø.4X5	T4Ø.4X6
Bupropion	T43.291	T43.292	T43.293	T43.294	T43.295	T43.296
Burimamide	T47.1X1	T47.1X2	T47.1X3	T47.1X4	T47.1X5	T47.1X6
Buserelin	T38.891	T38.892	T38.893	T38.894	T38.895	T38.896
Buspirone	T43.591	T43.592	T43.593	T43.594	T43.595	T43.596
Busulfan, busulphan	T45.1X1	T45.1X2	T45.1X3	T45.1X4	T45.1X5	T45.1X6
Butabarbital (sodium)	T42.3X1	T42.3X2	T42.3X3	T42.3X4	T42.3X5	T42.3X6
Butabarbitone	T42.3X1	T42.3X2	T42.3X3	T42.3X4	T42.3X5	T42.3X6
Butabarpal	T42.3X1	T42.3X2	T42.3X3	T42.3X4	T42.3X5	T42.3X6
Butacaine	T41.3X1	T41.3X2	T41.3X3	T41.3X4	T41.3X5	T41.3X6
Butalamine	T46.7X1	T46.7X2	T46.7X3	T46.7X4	T46.7X5	T46.7X6
Butalbital	T42.3X1	T42.3X2	T42.3X3	T42.3X4	T42.3X5	T42.3X6
Butallylonal	T42.3X1	T42.3X2	T42.3X3	T42.3X4	T42.3X5	T42.3X6
Butamben	T41.3X1	T41.3X2	T41.3X3	T41.3X4	T41.3X5	T41.3X6
Butamirate	T48.3X1	T48.3X2	T48.3X3	T48.3X4	T48.3X5	T48.3X6
Butane (distributed in mobile container)	T59.891	T59.892	T59.893	T59.894	—	—
distributed through pipes	T59.891	T59.892	T59.893	T59.894	—	—
incomplete combustion	T58.11	T58.12	T58.13	T58.14	—	—
Butanilicaine	T41.3X1	T41.3X2	T41.3X3	T41.3X4	T41.3X5	T41.3X6
Butanol	T51.3X1	T51.3X2	T51.3X3	T51.3X4	—	—
Butanone, 2-butanone	T52.4X1	T52.4X2	T52.4X3	T52.4X4	—	—
Butantrone	T49.4X1	T49.4X2	T49.4X3	T49.4X4	T49.4X5	T49.4X6
Butaperazine	T43.3X1	T43.3X2	T43.3X3	T43.3X4	T43.3X5	T43.3X6
Butazolidin	T39.2X1	T39.2X2	T39.2X3	T39.2X4	T39.2X5	T39.2X6
Butetamate	T48.6X1	T48.6X2	T48.6X3	T48.6X4	T48.6X5	T48.6X6
Butethal	T42.3X1	T42.3X2	T42.3X3	T42.3X4	T42.3X5	T42.3X6
Butethamate	T44.3X1	T44.3X2	T44.3X3	T44.3X4	T44.3X5	T44.3X6
Buthalitone (sodium)	T41.1X1	T41.1X2	T41.1X3	T41.1X4	T41.1X5	T41.1X6
Butisol (sodium)	T42.3X1	T42.3X2	T42.3X3	T42.3X4	T42.3X5	T42.3X6
Butizide	T5Ø.2X1	T5Ø.2X2	T5Ø.2X3	T5Ø.2X4	T5Ø.2X5	T5Ø.2X6
Butobarbital	T42.3X1	T42.3X2	T42.3X3	T42.3X4	T42.3X5	T42.3X6
sodium	T42.3X1	T42.3X2	T42.3X3	T42.3X4	T42.3X5	T42.3X6
Butobarbitone	T42.3X1	T42.3X2	T42.3X3	T42.3X4	T42.3X5	T42.3X6
Butoconazole (nitrate)	T49.ØX1	T49.ØX2	T49.ØX3	T49.ØX4	T49.ØX5	T49.ØX6
Butorphanol	T4Ø.4X1	T4Ø.4X2	T4Ø.4X3	T4Ø.4X4	T4Ø.4X5	T4Ø.4X6
Butriptyline	T43.Ø11	T43.Ø12	T43.Ø13	T43.Ø14	T43.Ø15	T43.Ø16
Butropium bromide	T44.3X1	T44.3X2	T44.3X3	T44.3X4	T44.3X5	T44.3X6
Buttercups	T62.2X1	T62.2X2	T62.2X3	T62.2X4	—	—
Butter of antimony—*see* Antimony						
Butyl						
acetate (secondary)	T52.8X1	T52.8X2	T52.8X3	T52.8X4	—	—
alcohol	T51.3X1	T51.3X2	T51.3X3	T51.3X4	—	—
aminobenzoate	T41.3X1	T41.3X2	T41.3X3	T41.3X4	T41.3X5	T41.3X6
butyrate	T52.8X1	T52.8X2	T52.8X3	T52.8X4	—	—
carbinol	T51.3X1	T51.3X2	T51.3X3	T51.3X4	—	—
carbitol	T52.3X1	T52.3X2	T52.3X3	T52.3X4	—	—
cellosolve	T52.3X1	T52.3X2	T52.3X3	T52.3X4	—	—
chloral (hydrate)	T42.6X1	T42.6X2	T42.6X3	T42.6X4	T42.6X5	T42.6X6
formate	T52.8X1	T52.8X2	T52.8X3	T52.8X4	—	—
lactate	T52.8X1	T52.8X2	T52.8X3	T52.8X4	—	—
propionate	T52.8X1	T52.8X2	T52.8X3	T52.8X4	—	—
scopolamine bromide	T44.3X1	T44.3X2	T44.3X3	T44.3X4	T44.3X5	T44.3X6
thiobarbital sodium	T41.1X1	T41.1X2	T41.1X3	T41.1X4	T41.1X5	T41.1X6
Butylated hydroxy-anisole	T5Ø.991	T5Ø.992	T5Ø.993	T5Ø.994	T5Ø.995	T5Ø.996
Butylchloral hydrate	T42.6X1	T42.6X2	T42.6X3	T42.6X4	T42.6X5	T42.6X6
Butyltoluene	T52.2X1	T52.2X2	T52.2X3	T52.2X4	—	—
Butyn	T41.3X1	T41.3X2	T41.3X3	T41.3X4	T41.3X5	T41.3X6
Butyrophenone (-based tranquilizers)	T43.4X1	T43.4X2	T43.4X3	T43.4X4	T43.4X5	T43.4X6
C						
Cabergoline	T42.8X1	T42.8X2	T42.8X3	T42.8X4	T42.8X5	T42.8X6
Cacodyl, cacodylic acid	T57.ØX1	T57.ØX2	T57.ØX3	T57.ØX4	—	—
Cactinomycin	T45.1X1	T45.1X2	T45.1X3	T45.1X4	T45.1X5	T45.1X6

Substance	Poisoning, Accidental (unintentional)	Poisoning, Intentional Self-harm	Poisoning, Assault	Poisoning, Undetermined	Adverse Effect	Under-dosing
Cade oil	T49.4X1	T49.4X2	T49.4X3	T49.4X4	T49.4X5	T49.4X6
Cadexomer iodine	T49.ØX1	T49.ØX2	T49.ØX3	T49.ØX4	T49.ØX5	T49.ØX6
Cadmium (chloride) (fumes) (oxide)	T56.3X1	T56.3X2	T56.3X3	T56.3X4	—	—
sulfide (medicinal) NEC	T49.4X1	T49.4X2	T49.4X3	T49.4X4	T49.4X5	T49.4X6
Cadralazine	T46.5X1	T46.5X2	T46.5X3	T46.5X4	T46.5X5	T46.5X6
Caffeine	T43.611	T43.612	T43.613	T43.614	T43.615	T43.616
Calabar bean	T62.2X1	T62.2X2	T62.2X3	T62.2X4	—	—
Caladium seguinum	T62.2X1	T62.2X2	T62.2X3	T62.2X4	—	—
Calamine (lotion)	T49.3X1	T49.3X2	T49.3X3	T49.3X4	T49.3X5	T49.3X6
Calcifediol	T45.2X1	T45.2X2	T45.2X3	T45.2X4	T45.2X5	T45.2X6
Calciferol	T45.2X1	T45.2X2	T45.2X3	T45.2X4	T45.2X5	T45.2X6
Calcitonin	T5Ø.991	T5Ø.992	T5Ø.993	T5Ø.994	T5Ø.995	T5Ø.996
Calcitriol	T45.2X1	T45.2X2	T45.2X3	T45.2X4	T45.2X5	T45.2X6
Calcium	T5Ø.3X1	T5Ø.3X2	T5Ø.3X3	T5Ø.3X4	T5Ø.3X5	T5Ø.3X6
actylsalicylate	T39.Ø11	T39.Ø12	T39.Ø13	T39.Ø14	T39.Ø15	T39.Ø16
benzamidosalicylate	T37.1X1	T37.1X2	T37.1X3	T37.1X4	T37.1X5	T37.1X6
bromide	T42.6X1	T42.6X2	T42.6X3	T42.6X4	T42.6X5	T42.6X6
bromolactobionate	T42.6X1	T42.6X2	T42.6X3	T42.6X4	T42.6X5	T42.6X6
carbaspirin	T39.Ø11	T39.Ø12	T39.Ø13	T39.Ø14	T39.Ø15	T39.Ø16
carbimide	T5Ø.6X1	T5Ø.6X2	T5Ø.6X3	T5Ø.6X4	T5Ø.6X5	T5Ø.6X6
carbonate	T47.1X1	T47.1X2	T47.1X3	T47.1X4	T47.1X5	T47.1X6
chloride	T5Ø.991	T5Ø.992	T5Ø.993	T5Ø.994	T5Ø.995	T5Ø.996
anhydrous	T5Ø.991	T5Ø.992	T5Ø.993	T5Ø.994	T5Ø.995	T5Ø.996
cyanide	T57.8X1	T57.8X2	T57.8X3	T57.8X4	—	—
dioctyl sulfosuccinate	T47.4X1	T47.4X2	T47.4X3	T47.4X4	T47.4X5	T47.4X6
disodium edathamil	T45.8X1	T45.8X2	T45.8X3	T45.8X4	T45.8X5	T45.8X6
disodium edetate	T45.8X1	T45.8X2	T45.8X3	T45.8X4	T45.8X5	T45.8X6
dobesilate	T46.991	T46.992	T46.993	T46.994	T46.995	T46.996
EDTA	T45.8X1	T45.8X2	T45.8X3	T45.8X4	T45.8X5	T45.8X6
ferrous citrate	T45.4X1	T45.4X2	T45.4X3	T45.4X4	T45.4X5	T45.4X6
folinate	T45.8X1	T45.8X2	T45.8X3	T45.8X4	T45.8X5	T45.8X6
glubionate	T5Ø.3X1	T5Ø.3X2	T5Ø.3X3	T5Ø.3X4	T5Ø.3X5	T5Ø.3X6
gluconate	T5Ø.3X1	T5Ø.3X2	T5Ø.3X3	T5Ø.3X4	T5Ø.3X5	T5Ø.3X6
gluconogalactogluconate	T5Ø.3X1	T5Ø.3X2	T5Ø.3X3	T5Ø.3X4	T5Ø.3X5	T5Ø.3X6
hydrate, hydroxide	T54.3X1	T54.3X2	T54.3X3	T54.3X4	—	—
hypochlorite	T54.3X1	T54.3X2	T54.3X3	T54.3X4	—	—
iodide	T48.4X1	T48.4X2	T48.4X3	T48.4X4	T48.4X5	T48.4X6
ipodate	T5Ø.8X1	T5Ø.8X2	T5Ø.8X3	T5Ø.8X4	T5Ø.8X5	T5Ø.8X6
lactate	T5Ø.3X1	T5Ø.3X2	T5Ø.3X3	T5Ø.3X4	T5Ø.3X5	T5Ø.3X6
leucovorin	T45.8X1	T45.8X2	T45.8X3	T45.8X4	T45.8X5	T45.8X6
mandelate	T37.91	T37.92	T37.93	T37.94	T37.95	T37.96
oxide	T54.3X1	T54.3X2	T54.3X3	T54.3X4	—	—
pantothenate	T45.2X1	T45.2X2	T45.2X3	T45.2X4	T45.2X5	T45.2X6
phosphate	T5Ø.3X1	T5Ø.3X2	T5Ø.3X3	T5Ø.3X4	T5Ø.3X5	T5Ø.3X6
salicylate	T39.Ø91	T39.Ø92	T39.Ø93	T39.Ø94	T39.Ø95	T39.Ø96
salts	T5Ø.3X1	T5Ø.3X2	T5Ø.3X3	T5Ø.3X4	T5Ø.3X5	T5Ø.3X6
Calculus-dissolving drug	T5Ø.991	T5Ø.992	T5Ø.993	T5Ø.994	T5Ø.995	T5Ø.996
Calomel	T49.ØX1	T49.ØX2	T49.ØX3	T49.ØX4	T49.ØX5	T49.ØX6
Caloric agent	T5Ø.3X1	T5Ø.3X2	T5Ø.3X3	T5Ø.3X4	T5Ø.3X5	T5Ø.3X6
Calusterone	T38.7X1	T38.7X2	T38.7X3	T38.7X4	T38.7X5	T38.7X6
Camazepam	T42.4X1	T42.4X2	T42.4X3	T42.4X4	T42.4X5	T42.4X6
Camomile	T49.ØX1	T49.ØX2	T49.ØX3	T49.ØX4	T49.ØX5	T49.ØX6
Camoquin	T37.2X1	T37.2X2	T37.2X3	T37.2X4	T37.2X5	T37.2X6
Camphor						
insecticide	T6Ø.2X1	T6Ø.2X2	T6Ø.2X3	T6Ø.2X4	—	—
medicinal	T49.8X1	T49.8X2	T49.8X3	T49.8X4	T49.8X5	T49.8X6
Camylofin	T44.3X1	T44.3X2	T44.3X3	T44.3X4	T44.3X5	T44.3X6
Cancer chemotherapy drug regimen	T45.1X1	T45.1X2	T45.1X3	T45.1X4	T45.1X5	T45.1X6
Candeptin	T49.ØX1	T49.ØX2	T49.ØX3	T49.ØX4	T49.ØX5	T49.ØX6
Candicidin	T49.ØX1	T49.ØX2	T49.ØX3	T49.ØX4	T49.ØX5	T49.ØX6
Cannabinol	T4Ø.7X1	T4Ø.7X2	T4Ø.7X3	T4Ø.7X4	T4Ø.7X5	T4Ø.7X6
Cannabis (derivatives)	T4Ø.7X1	T4Ø.7X2	T4Ø.7X3	T4Ø.7X4	T4Ø.7X5	T4Ø.7X6
Canned heat	T51.1X1	T51.1X2	T51.1X3	T51.1X4	—	—
Canrenoic acid	T5Ø.ØX1	T5Ø.ØX2	T5Ø.ØX3	T5Ø.ØX4	T5Ø.ØX5	T5Ø.ØX6
Canrenone	T5Ø.ØX1	T5Ø.ØX2	T5Ø.ØX3	T5Ø.ØX4	T5Ø.ØX5	T5Ø.ØX6
Cantharides, cantharidin, cantharis	T49.8X1	T49.8X2	T49.8X3	T49.8X4	T49.8X5	T49.8X6
Canthaxanthin	T5Ø.991	T5Ø.992	T5Ø.993	T5Ø.994	T5Ø.995	T5Ø.996
Capillary-active drug NEC	T46.9Ø1	T46.9Ø2	T46.9Ø3	T46.9Ø4	T46.9Ø5	T46.9Ø6
Capreomycin	T36.8X1	T36.8X2	T36.8X3	T36.8X4	T36.8X5	T36.8X6

Substance	Poisoning, Accidental (unintentional)	Poisoning, Intentional Self-harm	Poisoning, Assault	Poisoning, Undetermined	Adverse Effect	Under-dosing
Capsicum	T49.4X1	T49.4X2	T49.4X3	T49.4X4	T49.4X5	T49.4X6
Captafol	T6Ø.3X1	T6Ø.3X2	T6Ø.3X3	T6Ø.3X4	—	—
Captan	T6Ø.3X1	T6Ø.3X2	T6Ø.3X3	T6Ø.3X4	—	—
Captodiame, captodiamine	T43.591	T43.592	T43.593	T43.594	T43.595	T43.596
Captopril	T46.4X1	T46.4X2	T46.4X3	T46.4X4	T46.4X5	T46.4X6
Caramiphen	T44.3X1	T44.3X2	T44.3X3	T44.3X4	T44.3X5	T44.3X6
Carazolol	T44.7X1	T44.7X2	T44.7X3	T44.7X4	T44.7X5	T44.7X6
Carbachol	T44.1X1	T44.1X2	T44.1X3	T44.1X4	T44.1X5	T44.1X6
Carbacrylamine (resin)	T5Ø.3X1	T5Ø.3X2	T5Ø.3X3	T5Ø.3X4	T5Ø.3X5	T5Ø.3X6
Carbamate (insecticide)	T6Ø.ØX1	T6Ø.ØX2	T6Ø.ØX3	T6Ø.ØX4	—	—
Carbamate (sedative)	T42.6X1	T42.6X2	T42.6X3	T42.6X4	T42.6X5	T42.6X6
herbicide	T6Ø.ØX1	T6Ø.ØX2	T6Ø.ØX3	T6Ø.ØX4	—	—
insecticide	T6Ø.ØX1	T6Ø.ØX2	T6Ø.ØX3	T6Ø.ØX4	—	—
Carbamazepine	T42.1X1	T42.1X2	T42.1X3	T42.1X4	T42.1X5	T42.1X6
Carbamide	T47.3X1	T47.3X2	T47.3X3	T47.3X4	T47.3X5	T47.3X6
peroxide	T49.ØX1	T49.ØX2	T49.ØX3	T49.ØX4	T49.ØX5	T49.ØX6
topical	T49.8X1	T49.8X2	T49.8X3	T49.8X4	T49.8X5	T49.8X6
Carbamylcholine chloride	T44.1X1	T44.1X2	T44.1X3	T44.1X4	T44.1X5	T44.1X6
Carbaril	T6Ø.ØX1	T6Ø.ØX2	T6Ø.ØX3	T6Ø.ØX4	T6Ø.ØX5	T6Ø.ØX6
Carbarsone	T37.3X1	T37.3X2	T37.3X3	T37.3X4	T37.3X5	T37.3X6
Carbaryl	T6Ø.ØX1	T6Ø.ØX2	T6Ø.ØX3	T6Ø.ØX4	—	—
Carbaspirin	T39.Ø11	T39.Ø12	T39.Ø13	T39.Ø14	T39.Ø15	T39.Ø16
Carbazochrome (salicylate) (sodium sulfonate)	T49.4X1	T49.4X2	T49.4X3	T49.4X4	T49.4X5	T49.4X6
Carbenicillin	T36.ØX1	T36.ØX2	T36.ØX3	T36.ØX4	T36.ØX5	T36.ØX6
Carbenoxolone	T47.1X1	T47.1X2	T47.1X3	T47.1X4	T47.1X5	T47.1X6
Carbetapentane	T48.3X1	T48.3X2	T48.3X3	T48.3X4	T48.3X5	T48.3X6
Carbethyl salicylate	T39.Ø91	T39.Ø92	T39.Ø93	T39.Ø94	T39.Ø95	T39.Ø96
Carbidopa (with levodopa)	T42.8X1	T42.8X2	T42.8X3	T42.8X4	T42.8X5	T42.8X6
Carbimazole	T38.2X1	T38.2X2	T38.2X3	T38.2X4	T38.2X5	T38.2X6
Carbinol	T51.1X1	T51.1X2	T51.1X3	T51.1X4	—	—
Carbinoxamine	T45.ØX1	T45.ØX2	T45.ØX3	T45.ØX4	T45.ØX5	T45.ØX6
Carbiphene	T39.8X1	T39.8X2	T39.8X3	T39.8X4	T39.8X5	T39.8X6
Carbitol	T52.3X1	T52.3X2	T52.3X3	T52.3X4	—	—
Carbocaine	T41.3X1	T41.3X2	T41.3X3	T41.3X4	T41.3X5	T41.3X6
infiltration (subcutaneous)	T41.3X1	T41.3X2	T41.3X3	T41.3X4	T41.3X5	T41.3X6
nerve block (peripheral) (plexus)	T41.3X1	T41.3X2	T41.3X3	T41.3X4	T41.3X5	T41.3X6
topical (surface)	T41.3X1	T41.3X2	T41.3X3	T41.3X4	T41.3X5	T41.3X6
Carbo medicinalis	T47.6X1	T47.6X2	T47.6X3	T47.6X4	T47.6X5	T47.6X6
Carbomycin	T36.8X1	T36.8X2	T36.8X3	T36.8X4	T36.8X5	T36.8X6
Carbocisteine	T48.4X1	T48.4X2	T48.4X3	T48.4X4	T48.4X5	T48.4X6
Carbocromen	T46.3X1	T46.3X2	T46.3X3	T46.3X4	T46.3X5	T46.3X6
Carbol fuchsin	T49.ØX1	T49.ØX2	T49.ØX3	T49.ØX4	T49.ØX5	T49.ØX6
Carbolic acid (*see also* Phenol)	T54.ØX1	T54.ØX2	T54.ØX3	T54.ØX4	—	—
Carbolonium (bromide)	T48.1X1	T48.1X2	T48.1X3	T48.1X4	T48.1X5	T48.1X6
Carbon						
bisulfide (liquid)	T65.4X1	T65.4X2	T65.4X3	T65.4X4	—	—
vapor	T65.4X1	T65.4X2	T65.4X3	T65.4X4	—	—
dioxide (gas)	T59.7X1	T59.7X2	T59.7X3	T59.7X4	—	—
medicinal	T41.5X1	T41.5X2	T41.5X3	T41.5X4	T41.5X5	T41.5X6
nonmedicinal	T59.7X1	T59.7X2	T59.7X3	T59.7X4	—	—
snow	T49.4X1	T49.4X2	T49.4X3	T49.4X4	T49.4X5	T49.4X6
disulfide (liquid)	T65.4X1	T65.4X2	T65.4X3	T65.4X4	—	—
vapor	T65.4X1	T65.4X2	T65.4X3	T65.4X4	—	—
monoxide (from incomplete combustion)	T58.91	T58.92	T58.93	T58.94	—	—
blast furnace gas	T58.8X1	T58.8X2	T58.8X3	T58.8X4	—	—
butane (distributed in mobile container)	T58.11	T58.12	T58.13	T58.14	—	—
distributed through pipes	T58.11	T58.12	T58.13	T58.14	—	—
charcoal fumes	T58.2X1	T58.2X2	T58.2X3	T58.2X4	—	—
coal	T58.2X1	T58.2X2	T58.2X3	T58.2X4	—	—
coke (in domestic stoves, fireplaces)	T58.2X1	T58.2X2	T58.2X3	T58.2X4	—	—
exhaust gas (motor) not in transit	T58.Ø1	T58.Ø2	T58.Ø3	T58.Ø4	—	—
combustion engine, any not in watercraft	T58.Ø1	T58.Ø2	T58.Ø3	T58.Ø4	—	—
farm tractor, not in transit	T58.Ø1	T58.Ø2	T58.Ø3	T58.Ø4	—	—
gas engine	T58.Ø1	T58.Ø2	T58.Ø3	T58.Ø4	—	—
motor pump	T58.Ø1	T58.Ø2	T58.Ø3	T58.Ø4	—	—
motor vehicle, not in transit	T58.Ø1	T58.Ø2	T58.Ø3	T58.Ø4	—	—

Substance	Poisoning, Accidental (unintentional)	Poisoning, Intentional Self-harm	Poisoning, Assault	Poisoning, Undetermined	Adverse Effect	Under-dosing
Carbon—*continued*						
monoxide—*continued*						
fuel (in domestic use)	T58.2X1	T58.2X2	T58.2X3	T58.2X4	—	—
gas (piped)	T58.11	T58.12	T58.13	T58.14	—	—
in mobile container	T58.11	T58.12	T58.13	T58.14	—	—
utility	T58.11	T58.12	T58.13	T58.14	—	—
in mobile container	T58.11	T58.12	T58.13	T58.14	—	—
piped (natural)	T58.11	T58.12	T58.13	T58.14	—	—
gas (piped)	T58.11	T58.12	T58.13	T58.14	—	—
illuminating gas	T58.11	T58.12	T58.13	T58.14	—	—
industrial fuels or gases, any	T58.8X1	T58.8X2	T58.8X3	T58.8X4	—	—
kerosene (in domestic stoves, fireplaces)	T58.2X1	T58.2X2	T58.2X3	T58.2X4	—	—
kiln gas or vapor	T58.8X1	T58.8X2	T58.8X3	T58.8X4	—	—
motor exhaust gas, not in transit	T58.Ø1	T58.Ø2	T58.Ø3	T58.Ø4	—	—
piped gas (manufactured) (natural)	T58.11	T58.12	T58.13	T58.14	—	—
producer gas	T58.8X1	T58.8X2	T58.8X3	T58.8X4	—	—
propane (distributed in mobile container)	T58.11	T58.12	T58.13	T58.14	—	—
distributed through pipes	T58.11	T58.12	T58.13	T58.14	—	—
solid (in domestic stoves, fireplaces)	T58.2X1	T58.2X2	T58.2X3	T58.2X4	—	—
specified source NEC	T58.8X1	T58.8X2	T58.8X3	T58.8X4	—	—
stove gas	T58.11	T58.12	T58.13	T58.14	—	—
piped	T58.11	T58.12	T58.13	T58.14	—	—
utility gas	T58.11	T58.12	T58.13	T58.14	—	—
piped	T58.11	T58.12	T58.13	T58.14	—	—
water gas	T58.1X1	T58.1X2	T58.1X3	T58.1X4	—	—
wood (in domestic stoves, fireplaces)	T58.2X1	T58.2X2	T58.2X3	T58.2X4	—	—
tetrachloride (vapor) NEC	T53.ØX1	T53.ØX2	T53.ØX3	T53.ØX4	—	—
liquid (cleansing agent) NEC	T53.ØX1	T53.ØX2	T53.ØX3	T53.ØX4	—	—
solvent	T53.ØX1	T53.ØX2	T53.ØX3	T53.ØX4	—	—
Carbonic acid gas	T59.7X1	T59.7X2	T59.7X3	T59.7X4	—	—
anhydrase inhibitor NEC	T5Ø.2X1	T5Ø.2X2	T5Ø.2X3	T5Ø.2X4	T5Ø.2X5	T5Ø.2X6
Carbophenothion	T6Ø.ØX1	T6Ø.ØX2	T6Ø.ØX3	T6Ø.ØX4	—	—
Carboplatin	T45.1X1	T45.1X2	T45.1X3	T45.1X4	T45.1X5	T45.1X6
Carboprost	T48.ØX1	T48.ØX2	T48.ØX3	T48.ØX4	T48.ØX5	T48.ØX6
Carboquone	T45.1X1	T45.1X2	T45.1X3	T45.1X4	T45.1X5	T45.1X6
Carbowax	T49.3X1	T49.3X2	T49.3X3	T49.3X4	T49.3X5	T49.3X6
Carboxymethyl-cellulose	T47.4X1	T47.4X2	T47.4X3	T47.4X4	T47.4X5	T47.4X6
S-Carboxymethyl-cysteine	T47.4X1	T47.4X2	T47.4X3	T47.4X4	T47.4X5	T47.4X6
Carbrital	T42.3X1	T42.3X2	T42.3X3	T42.3X4	T42.3X5	T42.3X6
Carbromal	T42.6X1	T42.6X2	T42.6X3	T42.6X4	T42.6X5	T42.6X6
Carbutamide	T38.3X1	T38.3X2	T38.3X3	T38.3X4	T38.3X5	T38.3X6
Carbuterol	T48.6X1	T48.6X2	T48.6X3	T48.6X4	T48.6X5	T48.6X6
Cardiac						
depressants	T46.2X1	T46.2X2	T46.2X3	T46.2X4	T46.2X5	T46.2X6
rhythm regulator	T46.2X1	T46.2X2	T46.2X3	T46.2X4	T46.2X5	T46.2X6
specified NEC	T46.2X1	T46.2X2	T46.2X3	T46.2X4	T46.2X5	T46.2X6
Cardiografin	T5Ø.8X1	T5Ø.8X2	T5Ø.8X3	T5Ø.8X4	T5Ø.8X5	T5Ø.8X6
Cardio-green	T5Ø.8X1	T5Ø.8X2	T5Ø.8X3	T5Ø.8X4	T5Ø.8X5	T5Ø.8X6
Cardiotonic (glycoside) **NEC**	T46.ØX1	T46.ØX2	T46.ØX3	T46.ØX4	T46.ØX5	T46.ØX6
Cardiovascular drug NEC	T46.9Ø1	T46.9Ø2	T46.9Ø3	T46.9Ø4	T46.9Ø5	T46.9Ø6
Cardrase	T5Ø.2X1	T5Ø.2X2	T5Ø.2X3	T5Ø.2X4	T5Ø.2X5	T5Ø.2X6
Carfusin	T49.ØX1	T49.ØX2	T49.ØX3	T49.ØX4	T49.ØX5	T49.ØX6
Carfecillin	T36.ØX1	T36.ØX2	T36.ØX3	T36.ØX4	T36.ØX5	T36.ØX6
Carfenazine	T43.3X1	T43.3X2	T43.3X3	T43.3X4	T43.3X5	T43.3X6
Carindacillin	T36.ØX1	T36.ØX2	T36.ØX3	T36.ØX4	T36.ØX5	T36.ØX6
Carisoprodol	T42.8X1	T42.8X2	T42.8X3	T42.8X4	T42.8X5	T42.8X6
Carmellose	T47.4X1	T47.4X2	T47.4X3	T47.4X4	T47.4X5	T47.4X6
Carminative	T47.5X1	T47.5X2	T47.5X3	T47.5X4	T47.5X5	T47.5X6
Carmofur	T45.1X1	T45.1X2	T45.1X3	T45.1X4	T45.1X5	T45.1X6
Carmustine	T45.1X1	T45.1X2	T45.1X3	T45.1X4	T45.1X5	T45.1X6
Carotene	T45.2X1	T45.2X2	T45.2X3	T45.2X4	T45.2X5	T45.2X6
Carphenazine	T43.3X1	T43.3X2	T43.3X3	T43.3X4	T43.3X5	T43.3X6
Carpipramine	T42.4X1	T42.4X2	T42.4X3	T42.4X4	T42.4X5	T42.4X6
Carprofen	T39.311	T39.312	T39.313	T39.314	T39.315	T39.316
Carpronium chloride	T44.3X1	T44.3X2	T44.3X3	T44.3X4	T44.3X5	T44.3X6
Carrageenan	T47.8X1	T47.8X2	T47.8X3	T47.8X4	T47.8X5	T47.8X6

Substance	Poisoning, Accidental (unintentional)	Poisoning, Intentional Self-harm	Poisoning, Assault	Poisoning, Undetermined	Adverse Effect	Under-dosing
Carteolol	T44.7X1	T44.7X2	T44.7X3	T44.7X4	T44.7X5	T44.7X6
Carter's Little Pills	T47.2X1	T47.2X2	T47.2X3	T47.2X4	T47.2X5	T47.2X6
Cascara (sagrada)	T47.2X1	T47.2X2	T47.2X3	T47.2X4	T47.2X5	T47.2X6
Cassava	T62.2X1	T62.2X2	T62.2X3	T62.2X4	—	—
Castellani's paint	T49.ØX1	T49.ØX2	T49.ØX3	T49.ØX4	T49.ØX5	T49.ØX6
Castor						
bean	T62.2X1	T62.2X2	T62.2X3	T62.2X4	—	—
oil	T47.2X1	T47.2X2	T47.2X3	T47.2X4	T47.2X5	T47.2X6
Catalase	T45.3X1	T45.3X2	T45.3X3	T45.3X4	T45.3X5	T45.3X6
Caterpillar (sting)	T63.431	T63.432	T63.433	T63.434	—	—
Catha (edulis) (tea)	T43.691	T43.692	T43.693	T43.694	—	—
Cathartic NEC	T47.4X1	T47.4X2	T47.4X3	T47.4X4	T47.4X5	T47.4X6
anthacene derivative	T47.2X1	T47.2X2	T47.2X3	T47.2X4	T47.2X5	T47.2X6
bulk	T47.4X1	T47.4X2	T47.4X3	T47.4X4	T47.4X5	T47.4X6
contact	T47.2X1	T47.2X2	T47.2X3	T47.2X4	T47.2X5	T47.2X6
emollient NEC	T47.4X1	T47.4X2	T47.4X3	T47.4X4	T47.4X5	T47.4X6
irritant NEC	T47.2X1	T47.2X2	T47.2X3	T47.2X4	T47.2X5	T47.2X6
mucilage	T47.4X1	T47.4X2	T47.4X3	T47.4X4	T47.4X5	T47.4X6
saline	T47.3X1	T47.3X2	T47.3X3	T47.3X4	T47.3X5	T47.3X6
vegetable	T47.2X1	T47.2X2	T47.2X3	T47.2X4	T47.2X5	T47.2X6
Cathine	T5Ø.5X1	T5Ø.5X2	T5Ø.5X3	T5Ø.5X4	T5Ø.5X5	T5Ø.5X6
Cathomycin	T36.8X1	T36.8X2	T36.8X3	T36.8X4	T36.8X5	T36.8X6
Cation exchange resin	T5Ø.3X1	T5Ø.3X2	T5Ø.3X3	T5Ø.3X4	T5Ø.3X5	T5Ø.3X6
Caustic(s) NEC	T54.91	T54.92	T54.93	T54.94	—	—
alkali	T54.3X1	T54.3X2	T54.3X3	T54.3X4	—	—
hydroxide	T54.3X1	T54.3X2	T54.3X3	T54.3X4	—	—
potash	T54.3X1	T54.3X2	T54.3X3	T54.3X4	—	—
specified NEC	T54.91	T54.92	T54.93	T54.94	—	—
soda	T54.3X1	T54.3X2	T54.3X3	T54.3X4	—	—
Ceepryn	T49.ØX1	T49.ØX2	T49.ØX3	T49.ØX4	T49.ØX5	T49.ØX6
ENT agent	T49.6X1	T49.6X2	T49.6X3	T49.6X4	T49.6X5	T49.6X6
lozenges	T49.6X1	T49.6X2	T49.6X3	T49.6X4	T49.6X5	T49.6X6
Cefacetrile	T36.1X1	T36.1X2	T36.1X3	T36.1X4	T36.1X5	T36.1X6
Cefaclor	T36.1X1	T36.1X2	T36.1X3	T36.1X4	T36.1X5	T36.1X6
Cefadroxil	T36.1X1	T36.1X2	T36.1X3	T36.1X4	T36.1X5	T36.1X6
Cefalexin	T36.1X1	T36.1X2	T36.1X3	T36.1X4	T36.1X5	T36.1X6
Cefaloglycin	T36.1X1	T36.1X2	T36.1X3	T36.1X4	T36.1X5	T36.1X6
Cefaloridine	T36.1X1	T36.1X2	T36.1X3	T36.1X4	T36.1X5	T36.1X6
Cefalosporins	T36.1X1	T36.1X2	T36.1X3	T36.1X4	T36.1X5	T36.1X6
Cefalotin	T36.1X1	T36.1X2	T36.1X3	T36.1X4	T36.1X5	T36.1X6
Cefamandole	T36.1X1	T36.1X2	T36.1X3	T36.1X4	T36.1X5	T36.1X6
Cefamycin antibiotic	T36.1X1	T36.1X2	T36.1X3	T36.1X4	T36.1X5	T36.1X6
Cefapirin	T36.1X1	T36.1X2	T36.1X3	T36.1X4	T36.1X5	T36.1X6
Cefatrizine	T36.1X1	T36.1X2	T36.1X3	T36.1X4	T36.1X5	T36.1X6
Cefazedone	T36.1X1	T36.1X2	T36.1X3	T36.1X4	T36.1X5	T36.1X6
Cefazolin	T36.1X1	T36.1X2	T36.1X3	T36.1X4	T36.1X5	T36.1X6
Cefbuperazone	T36.1X1	T36.1X2	T36.1X3	T36.1X4	T36.1X5	T36.1X6
Cefetamet	T36.1X1	T36.1X2	T36.1X3	T36.1X4	T36.1X5	T36.1X6
Cefixime	T36.1X1	T36.1X2	T36.1X3	T36.1X4	T36.1X5	T36.1X6
Cefmenoxime	T36.1X1	T36.1X2	T36.1X3	T36.1X4	T36.1X5	T36.1X6
Cefmetazole	T36.1X1	T36.1X2	T36.1X3	T36.1X4	T36.1X5	T36.1X6
Cefminox	T36.1X1	T36.1X2	T36.1X3	T36.1X4	T36.1X5	T36.1X6
Cefonicid	T36.1X1	T36.1X2	T36.1X3	T36.1X4	T36.1X5	T36.1X6
Cefoperazone	T36.1X1	T36.1X2	T36.1X3	T36.1X4	T36.1X5	T36.1X6
Ceforanide	T36.1X1	T36.1X2	T36.1X3	T36.1X4	T36.1X5	T36.1X6
Cefotaxime	T36.1X1	T36.1X2	T36.1X3	T36.1X4	T36.1X5	T36.1X6
Cefotetan	T36.1X1	T36.1X2	T36.1X3	T36.1X4	T36.1X5	T36.1X6
Cefotiam	T36.1X1	T36.1X2	T36.1X3	T36.1X4	T36.1X5	T36.1X6
Cefoxitin	T36.1X1	T36.1X2	T36.1X3	T36.1X4	T36.1X5	T36.1X6
Cefpimizole	T36.1X1	T36.1X2	T36.1X3	T36.1X4	T36.1X5	T36.1X6
Cefpiramide	T36.1X1	T36.1X2	T36.1X3	T36.1X4	T36.1X5	T36.1X6
Cefradine	T36.1X1	T36.1X2	T36.1X3	T36.1X4	T36.1X5	T36.1X6
Cefroxadine	T36.1X1	T36.1X2	T36.1X3	T36.1X4	T36.1X5	T36.1X6
Cefsulodin	T36.1X1	T36.1X2	T36.1X3	T36.1X4	T36.1X5	T36.1X6
Ceftazidime	T36.1X1	T36.1X2	T36.1X3	T36.1X4	T36.1X5	T36.1X6
Cefteram	T36.1X1	T36.1X2	T36.1X3	T36.1X4	T36.1X5	T36.1X6
Ceftezole	T36.1X1	T36.1X2	T36.1X3	T36.1X4	T36.1X5	T36.1X6
Ceftizoxime	T36.1X1	T36.1X2	T36.1X3	T36.1X4	T36.1X5	T36.1X6
Ceftriaxone	T36.1X1	T36.1X2	T36.1X3	T36.1X4	T36.1X5	T36.1X6
Cefuroxime	T36.1X1	T36.1X2	T36.1X3	T36.1X4	T36.1X5	T36.1X6
Cefuzonam	T36.1X1	T36.1X2	T36.1X3	T36.1X4	T36.1X5	T36.1X6

Substance	Poisoning, Accidental (unintentional)	Poisoning, Intentional Self-harm	Poisoning, Assault	Poisoning, Undetermined	Adverse Effect	Under-dosing
Celestone	T38.0X1	T38.0X2	T38.0X3	T38.0X4	T38.0X5	T38.0X6
topical	T49.0X1	T49.0X2	T49.0X3	T49.0X4	T49.0X5	T49.0X6
Celiprolol	T44.7X1	T44.7X2	T44.7X3	T44.7X4	T44.7X5	T44.7X6
Cellosolve	T52.91	T52.92	T52.93	T52.94	—	—
Cell stimulants and proliferants	T49.8X1	T49.8X2	T49.8X3	T49.8X4	T49.8X5	T49.8X6
Cellulose						
cathartic	T47.4X1	T47.4X2	T47.4X3	T47.4X4	T47.4X5	T47.4X6
hydroxyethyl	T47.4X1	T47.4X2	T47.4X3	T47.4X4	T47.4X5	T47.4X6
nitrates (topical)	T49.3X1	T49.3X2	T49.3X3	T49.3X4	T49.3X5	T49.3X6
oxidized	T49.4X1	T49.4X2	T49.4X3	T49.4X4	T49.4X5	T49.4X6
Centipede (bite)	T63.411	T63.412	T63.413	T63.414	—	—
Central nervous system						
depressants	T42.71	T42.72	T42.73	T42.74	T42.75	T42.76
anesthetic (general) NEC	T41.201	T41.202	T41.203	T41.204	T41.205	T41.206
gases NEC	T41.0X1	T41.0X2	T41.0X3	T41.0X4	T41.0X5	T41.0X6
intravenous	T41.1X1	T41.1X2	T41.1X3	T41.1X4	T41.1X5	T41.1X6
barbiturates	T42.3X1	T42.3X2	T42.3X3	T42.3X4	T42.3X5	T42.3X6
benzodiazepines	T42.4X1	T42.4X2	T42.4X3	T42.4X4	T42.4X5	T42.4X6
bromides	T42.6X1	T42.6X2	T42.6X3	T42.6X4	T42.6X5	T42.6X6
cannabis sativa	T40.7X1	T40.7X2	T40.7X3	T40.7X4	T40.7X5	T40.7X6
chloral hydrate	T42.6X1	T42.6X2	T42.6X3	T42.6X4	T42.6X5	T42.6X6
ethanol	T51.0X1	T51.0X2	T51.0X3	T51.0X4	—	—
hallucinogenics	T40.901	T40.902	T40.903	T40.904	T40.905	T40.906
hypnotics	T42.71	T42.72	T42.73	T42.74	T42.75	T42.76
specified NEC	T42.6X1	T42.6X2	T42.6X3	T42.6X4	T42.6X5	T42.6X6
muscle relaxants	T42.8X1	T42.8X2	T42.8X3	T42.8X4	T42.8X5	T42.8X6
paraldehyde	T42.6X1	T42.6X2	T42.6X3	T42.6X4	T42.6X5	T42.6X6
sedatives; sedative-hypnotics	T42.71	T42.72	T42.73	T42.74	T42.75	T42.76
mixed NEC	T42.6X1	T42.6X2	T42.6X3	T42.6X4	T42.6X5	T42.6X6
specified NEC	T42.6X1	T42.6X2	T42.6X3	T42.6X4	T42.6X5	T42.6X6
muscle-tone depressants	T42.8X1	T42.8X2	T42.8X3	T42.8X4	T42.8X5	T42.8X6
stimulants	T43.601	T43.602	T43.603	T43.604	T43.605	T43.606
amphetamines	T43.621	T43.622	T43.623	T43.624	T43.625	T43.626
analeptics	T50.7X1	T50.7X2	T50.7X3	T50.7X4	T50.7X5	T50.7X6
antidepressants	T43.201	T43.202	T43.203	T43.204	T43.205	T43.206
opiate antagonists	T50.7X1	T50.7X2	T50.7X3	T50.7X4	T50.7X5	T50.7X6
specified NEC	T43.691	T43.692	T43.693	T43.694	T43.695	T43.696
Cephalexin	T36.1X1	T36.1X2	T36.1X3	T36.1X4	T36.1X5	T36.1X6
Cephaloglycin	T36.1X1	T36.1X2	T36.1X3	T36.1X4	T36.1X5	T36.1X6
Cephaloridine	T36.1X1	T36.1X2	T36.1X3	T36.1X4	T36.1X5	T36.1X6
Cephalosporins	T36.1X1	T36.1X2	T36.1X3	T36.1X4	T36.1X5	T36.1X6
N (adicillin)	T36.0X1	T36.0X2	T36.0X3	T36.0X4	T36.0X5	T36.0X6
Cephalothin	T36.1X1	T36.1X2	T36.1X3	T36.1X4	T36.1X5	T36.1X6
Cephalotin	T36.1X1	T36.1X2	T36.1X3	T36.1X4	T36.1X5	T36.1X6
Cephradine	T36.1X1	T36.1X2	T36.1X3	T36.1X4	T36.1X5	T36.1X6
Cerbera (odallam)	T62.2X1	T62.2X2	T62.2X3	T62.2X4	—	—
Cerberin	T46.0X1	T46.0X2	T46.0X3	T46.0X4	T46.0X5	T46.0X6
Cerebral stimulants	T43.601	T43.602	T43.603	T43.604	T43.605	T43.606
psychotherapeutic	T43.601	T43.602	T43.603	T43.604	T43.605	T43.606
specified NEC	T43.691	T43.692	T43.693	T43.694	T43.695	T43.696
Cerium oxalate	T45.0X1	T45.0X2	T45.0X3	T45.0X4	T45.0X5	T45.0X6
Cerous oxalate	T45.0X1	T45.0X2	T45.0X3	T45.0X4	T45.0X5	T45.0X6
Ceruletide	T50.8X1	T50.8X2	T50.8X3	T50.8X4	T50.8X5	T50.8X6
Cetalkonium (chloride)	T49.0X1	T49.0X2	T49.0X3	T49.0X4	T49.0X5	T49.0X6
Cethexonium chloride	T49.0X1	T49.0X2	T49.0X3	T49.0X4	T49.0X5	T49.0X6
Cetiedil	T46.7X1	T46.7X2	T46.7X3	T46.7X4	T46.7X5	T46.7X6
Cetirizine	T45.0X1	T45.0X2	T45.0X3	T45.0X4	T45.0X5	T45.0X6
Cetomacrogol	T50.991	T50.992	T50.993	T50.994	T50.995	T50.996
Cetotiamine	T45.2X1	T45.2X2	T45.2X3	T45.2X4	T45.2X5	T45.2X6
Cetoxime	T45.0X1	T45.0X2	T45.0X3	T45.0X4	T45.0X5	T45.0X6
Cetraxate	T47.1X1	T47.1X2	T47.1X3	T47.1X4	T47.1X5	T47.1X6
Cetrimide	T49.0X1	T49.0X2	T49.0X3	T49.0X4	T49.0X5	T49.0X6
Cetrimonium (bromide)	T49.0X1	T49.0X2	T49.0X3	T49.0X4	T49.0X5	T49.0X6
Cetylpyridinium chloride	T49.0X1	T49.0X2	T49.0X3	T49.0X4	T49.0X5	T49.0X6
ENT agent	T49.6X1	T49.6X2	T49.6X3	T49.6X4	T49.6X5	T49.6X6
lozenges	T49.6X1	T49.6X2	T49.6X3	T49.6X4	T49.6X5	T49.6X6
Cevadilla—*see* Sabadilla						
Cevitamic acid	T45.2X1	T45.2X2	T45.2X3	T45.2X4	T45.2X5	T45.2X6
Chalk, precipitated	T47.1X1	T47.1X2	T47.1X3	T47.1X4	T47.1X5	T47.1X6
Chamomile	T49.0X1	T49.0X2	T49.0X3	T49.0X4	T49.0X5	T49.0X6
Ch'an su	T46.0X1	T46.0X2	T46.0X3	T46.0X4	T46.0X5	T46.0X6
Charcoal	T47.6X1	T47.6X2	T47.6X3	T47.6X4	T47.6X5	T47.6X6
activated (*see also* Charcoal, medicinal)	T47.6X1	T47.6X2	T47.6X3	T47.6X4	T47.6X5	T47.6X6
fumes (Carbon monoxide)	T58.2X1	T58.2X2	T58.2X3	T58.2X4	—	—
industrial	T58.8X1	T58.8X2	T58.8X3	T58.8X4	—	—
medicinal (activated)	T47.6X1	T47.6X2	T47.6X3	T47.6X4	T47.6X5	T47.6X6
antidiarrheal	T47.6X1	T47.6X2	T47.6X3	T47.6X4	T47.6X5	T47.6X6
poison control	T47.8X1	T47.8X2	T47.8X3	T47.8X4	T47.8X5	T47.8X6
specified use other than for diarrhea	T47.8X1	T47.8X2	T47.8X3	T47.8X4	T47.8X5	T47.8X6
topical	T49.8X1	T49.8X2	T49.8X3	T49.8X4	T49.8X5	T49.8X6
Chaulmosulfone	T37.1X1	T37.1X2	T37.1X3	T37.1X4	T37.1X5	T37.1X6
Chelating agent NEC	T50.6X1	T50.6X2	T50.6X3	T50.6X4	T50.6X5	T50.6X6
Chelidonium majus	T62.2X1	T62.2X2	T62.2X3	T62.2X4	—	—
Chemical substance NEC	T65.91	T65.92	T65.93	T65.94	—	—
Chenodeoxycholic acid	T47.5X1	T47.5X2	T47.5X3	T47.5X4	T47.5X5	T47.5X6
Chenodiol	T47.5X1	T47.5X2	T47.5X3	T47.5X4	T47.5X5	T47.5X6
Chenopodium	T37.4X1	T37.4X2	T37.4X3	T37.4X4	T37.4X5	T37.4X6
Cherry laurel	T62.2X1	T62.2X2	T62.2X3	T62.2X4	—	—
Chinidin(e)	T46.2X1	T46.2X2	T46.2X3	T46.2X4	T46.2X5	T46.2X6
Chiniofon	T37.8X1	T37.8X2	T37.8X3	T37.8X4	T37.8X5	T37.8X6
Chlophedianol	T48.3X1	T48.3X2	T48.3X3	T48.3X4	T48.3X5	T48.3X6
Chloral	T42.6X1	T42.6X2	T42.6X3	T42.6X4	T42.6X5	T42.6X6
derivative	T42.6X1	T42.6X2	T42.6X3	T42.6X4	T42.6X5	T42.6X6
hydrate	T42.6X1	T42.6X2	T42.6X3	T42.6X4	T42.6X5	T42.6X6
Chloralamide	T42.6X1	T42.6X2	T42.6X3	T42.6X4	T42.6X5	T42.6X6
Chloralodol	T42.6X1	T42.6X2	T42.6X3	T42.6X4	T42.6X5	T42.6X6
Chloralose	T60.4X1	T60.4X2	T60.4X3	T60.4X4	—	—
Chlorambucil	T45.1X1	T45.1X2	T45.1X3	T45.1X4	T45.1X5	T45.1X6
Chloramine	T57.8X1	T57.8X2	T57.8X3	T57.8X4	—	—
T	T49.0X1	T49.0X2	T49.0X3	T49.0X4	T49.0X5	T49.0X6
topical	T49.0X1	T49.0X2	T49.0X3	T49.0X4	T49.0X5	T49.0X6
Chloramphenicol	T36.2X1	T36.2X2	T36.2X3	T36.2X4	T36.2X5	T36.2X6
ENT agent	T49.6X1	T49.6X2	T49.6X3	T49.6X4	T49.6X5	T49.6X6
ophthalmic preparation	T49.5X1	T49.5X2	T49.5X3	T49.5X4	T49.5X5	T49.5X6
topical NEC	T49.0X1	T49.0X2	T49.0X3	T49.0X4	T49.0X5	T49.0X6
Chlorate (potassium) (sodium) NEC	T60.3X1	T60.3X2	T60.3X3	T60.3X4	—	—
herbicide	T60.3X1	T60.3X2	T60.3X3	T60.3X4	—	—
Chlorazanil	T50.2X1	T50.2X2	T50.2X3	T50.2X4	T50.2X5	T50.2X6
Chlorbenzene, chlorbenzol	T53.7X1	T53.7X2	T53.7X3	T53.7X4	—	—
Chlorbenzoxamine	T44.3X1	T44.3X2	T44.3X3	T44.3X4	T44.3X5	T44.3X6
Chlorbutol	T42.6X1	T42.6X2	T42.6X3	T42.6X4	T42.6X5	T42.6X6
Chlorcyclizine	T45.0X1	T45.0X2	T45.0X3	T45.0X4	T45.0X5	T45.0X6
Chlordan(e) (dust)	T60.1X1	T60.1X2	T60.1X3	T60.1X4	—	—
Chlordantoin	T49.0X1	T49.0X2	T49.0X3	T49.0X4	T49.0X5	T49.0X6
Chlordiazepoxide	T42.4X1	T42.4X2	T42.4X3	T42.4X4	T42.4X5	T42.4X6
Chlordiethyl benzamide	T49.3X1	T49.3X2	T49.3X3	T49.3X4	T49.3X5	T49.3X6
Chloresium	T49.8X1	T49.8X2	T49.8X3	T49.8X4	T49.8X5	T49.8X6
Chlorethiazol	T42.6X1	T42.6X2	T42.6X3	T42.6X4	T42.6X5	T42.6X6
Chlorethyl—*see* Ethyl chloride						
Chloretone	T42.6X1	T42.6X2	T42.6X3	T42.6X4	T42.6X5	T42.6X6
Chlorex	T53.6X1	T53.6X2	T53.6X3	T53.6X4	—	—
insecticide	T60.1X1	T60.1X2	T60.1X3	T60.1X4	—	—
Chlorfenvinphos	T60.0X1	T60.0X2	T60.0X3	T60.0X4	—	—
Chlorhexadol	T42.6X1	T42.6X2	T42.6X3	T42.6X4	T42.6X5	T42.6X6
Chlorhexamide	T45.1X1	T45.1X2	T45.1X3	T45.1X4	T45.1X5	T45.1X6
Chlorhexidine	T49.0X1	T49.0X2	T49.0X3	T49.0X4	T49.0X5	T49.0X6
Chlorhydroxyquinolin	T49.0X1	T49.0X2	T49.0X3	T49.0X4	T49.0X5	T49.0X6
Chloride of lime (bleach)	T54.3X1	T54.3X2	T54.3X3	T54.3X4	—	—
Chlorimipramine	T43.011	T43.012	T43.013	T43.014	T43.015	T43.016
Chlorinated						
camphene	T53.6X1	T53.6X2	T53.6X3	T53.6X4	—	—
diphenyl	T53.7X1	T53.7X2	T53.7X3	T53.7X4	—	—
hydrocarbons NEC	T53.91	T53.92	T53.93	T53.94	—	—
solvents	T53.91	T53.92	T53.93	T53.94	—	—
lime (bleach)	T54.3X1	T54.3X2	T54.3X3	T54.3X4	—	—
and boric acid solution	T49.0X1	T49.0X2	T49.0X3	T49.0X4	T49.0X5	T49.0X6
naphthalene (insecticide)	T60.1X1	T60.1X2	T60.1X3	T60.1X4	—	—
industrial (non-pesticide)	T53.7X1	T53.7X2	T53.7X3	T53.7X4	—	—
pesticide NEC	T60.8X1	T60.8X2	T60.8X3	T60.8X4	—	—

Substance	Poisoning, Accidental (unintentional)	Poisoning, Intentional Self-harm	Poisoning, Assault	Poisoning, Undetermined	Adverse Effect	Under-dosing
Chlorinated — *continued*						
soda (*see also* sodium hypochlorite)						
solution	T49.ØX1	T49.ØX2	T49.ØX3	T49.ØX4	T49.ØX5	T49.ØX6
Chlorine (fumes) (gas)	T59.4X1	T59.4X2	T59.4X3	T59.4X4	—	—
bleach	T54.3X1	T54.3X2	T54.3X3	T54.3X4	—	—
compound gas NEC	T59.4X1	T59.4X2	T59.4X3	T59.4X4	—	—
disinfectant	T59.4X1	T59.4X2	T59.4X3	T59.4X4	—	—
releasing agents NEC	T59.4X1	T59.4X2	T59.4X3	T59.4X4	—	—
Chlorisondamine chloride	T46.991	T46.992	T46.993	T46.994	T46.995	T46.996
Chlormadinone	T38.5X1	T38.5X2	T38.5X3	T38.5X4	T38.5X5	T38.5X6
Chlormephos	T6Ø.ØX1	T6Ø.ØX2	T6Ø.ØX3	T6Ø.ØX4	—	—
Chlormerodrin	T5Ø.2X1	T5Ø.2X2	T5Ø.2X3	T5Ø.2X4	T5Ø.2X5	T5Ø.2X6
Chlormethiazole	T42.6X1	T42.6X2	T42.6X3	T42.6X4	T42.6X5	T42.6X6
Chlormethine	T45.1X1	T45.1X2	T45.1X3	T45.1X4	T45.1X5	T45.1X6
Chlormethylenecycline	T36.4X1	T36.4X2	T36.4X3	T36.4X4	T36.4X5	T36.4X6
Chlormezanone	T42.6X1	T42.6X2	T42.6X3	T42.6X4	T42.6X5	T42.6X6
Chloroacetic acid	T6Ø.3X1	T6Ø.3X2	T6Ø.3X3	T6Ø.3X4	—	—
Chloroacetone	T59.3X1	T59.3X2	T59.3X3	T59.3X4	—	—
Chloroacetophenone	T59.3X1	T59.3X2	T59.3X3	T59.3X4	—	—
Chloroaniline	T53.7X1	T53.7X2	T53.7X3	T53.7X4	—	—
Chlorobenzene, chlorobenzol	T53.7X1	T53.7X2	T53.7X3	T53.7X4	—	—
Chlorobromomethane (fire extinguisher)	T53.6X1	T53.6X2	T53.6X3	T53.6X4	—	—
Chlorobutanol	T49.ØX1	T49.ØX2	T49.ØX3	T49.ØX4	T49.ØX5	T49.ØX6
Chlorocresol	T49.ØX1	T49.ØX2	T49.ØX3	T49.ØX4	T49.ØX5	T49.ØX6
Chlorodehydro-methyltestosterone	T38.7X1	T38.7X2	T38.7X3	T38.7X4	T38.7X5	T38.7X6
Chlorodinitrobenzene	T53.7X1	T53.7X2	T53.7X3	T53.7X4	—	—
dust or vapor	T53.7X1	T53.7X2	T53.7X3	T53.7X4	—	—
Chlorodiphenyl	T53.7X1	T53.7X2	T53.7X3	T53.7X4	—	—
Chloroethane—*see* Ethyl chloride						
Chloroethylene	T53.6X1	T53.6X2	T53.6X3	T53.6X4	—	—
Chlorofluorocarbons	T53.5X1	T53.5X2	T53.5X3	T53.5X4	—	—
Chloroform (fumes) (vapor)	T53.1X1	T53.1X2	T53.1X3	T53.1X4	—	—
anesthetic	T41.ØX1	T41.ØX2	T41.ØX3	T41.ØX4	T41.ØX5	T41.ØX6
solvent	T53.1X1	T53.1X2	T53.1X3	T53.1X4	—	—
water, concentrated	T41.ØX1	T41.ØX2	T41.ØX3	T41.ØX4	T41.ØX5	T41.ØX6
Chloroguanide	T37.2X1	T37.2X2	T37.2X3	T37.2X4	T37.2X5	T37.2X6
Chloromycetin	T36.2X1	T36.2X2	T36.2X3	T36.2X4	T36.2X5	T36.2X6
ENT agent	T49.6X1	T49.6X2	T49.6X3	T49.6X4	T49.6X5	T49.6X6
ophthalmic preparation	T49.5X1	T49.5X2	T49.5X3	T49.5X4	T49.5X5	T49.5X6
otic solution	T49.6X1	T49.6X2	T49.6X3	T49.6X4	T49.6X5	T49.6X6
topical NEC	T49.ØX1	T49.ØX2	T49.ØX3	T49.ØX4	T49.ØX5	T49.ØX6
Chloronitrobenzene	T53.7X1	T53.7X2	T53.7X3	T53.7X4	—	—
dust or vapor	T53.7X1	T53.7X2	T53.7X3	T53.7X4	—	—
Chlorophacinone	T6Ø.4X1	T6Ø.4X2	T6Ø.4X3	T6Ø.4X4	—	—
Chlorophenol	T53.7X1	T53.7X2	T53.7X3	T53.7X4	—	—
Chlorophenothane	T6Ø.1X1	T6Ø.1X2	T6Ø.1X3	T6Ø.1X4	—	—
Chlorophyll	T5Ø.991	T5Ø.992	T5Ø.993	T5Ø.994	T5Ø.995	T5Ø.996
Chloropicrin (fumes)	T53.6X1	T53.6X2	T53.6X3	T53.6X4	—	—
fumigant	T6Ø.8X1	T6Ø.8X2	T6Ø.8X3	T6Ø.8X4	—	—
fungicide	T6Ø.3X1	T6Ø.3X2	T6Ø.3X3	T6Ø.3X4	—	—
pesticide	T6Ø.8X1	T6Ø.8X2	T6Ø.8X3	T6Ø.8X4	—	—
Chloroprocaine	T41.3X1	T41.3X2	T41.3X3	T41.3X4	T41.3X5	T41.3X6
infiltration (subcutaneous)	T41.3X1	T41.3X2	T41.3X3	T41.3X4	T41.3X5	T41.3X6
nerve block (peripheral) (plexus)	T41.3X1	T41.3X2	T41.3X3	T41.3X4	T41.3X5	T41.3X6
spinal	T41.3X1	T41.3X2	T41.3X3	T41.3X4	T41.3X5	T41.3X6
Chloroptic	T49.5X1	T49.5X2	T49.5X3	T49.5X4	T49.5X5	T49.5X6
Chloropurine	T45.1X1	T45.1X2	T45.1X3	T45.1X4	T45.1X5	T45.1X6
Chloropyramine	T45.ØX1	T45.ØX2	T45.ØX3	T45.ØX4	T45.ØX5	T45.ØX6
Chloropyrifos	T6Ø.ØX1	T6Ø.ØX2	T6Ø.ØX3	T6Ø.ØX4	—	—
Chloropyrilene	T45.ØX1	T45.ØX2	T45.ØX3	T45.ØX4	T45.ØX5	T45.ØX6
Chloroquine	T37.2X1	T37.2X2	T37.2X3	T37.2X4	T37.2X5	T37.2X6
Chlorothalonil	T6Ø.3X1	T6Ø.3X2	T6Ø.3X3	T6Ø.3X4	—	—
Chlorothen	T45.ØX1	T45.ØX2	T45.ØX3	T45.ØX4	T45.ØX5	T45.ØX6
Chlorothiazide	T5Ø.2X1	T5Ø.2X2	T5Ø.2X3	T5Ø.2X4	T5Ø.2X5	T5Ø.2X6
Chlorothymol	T49.4X1	T49.4X2	T49.4X3	T49.4X4	T49.4X5	T49.4X6
Chlorotrianisene	T38.5X1	T38.5X2	T38.5X3	T38.5X4	T38.5X5	T38.5X6
Chlorovinyldichloroarsine, not in war	T57.ØX1	T57.ØX2	T57.ØX3	T57.ØX4	—	—
Chloroxine	T49.4X1	T49.4X2	T49.4X3	T49.4X4	T49.4X5	T49.4X6
Chloroxylenol	T49.ØX1	T49.ØX2	T49.ØX3	T49.ØX4	T49.ØX5	T49.ØX6
Chlorphenamine	T45.ØX1	T45.ØX2	T45.ØX3	T45.ØX4	T45.ØX5	T45.ØX6
Chlorphenesin	T42.8X1	T42.8X2	T42.8X3	T42.8X4	T42.8X5	T42.8X6
topical (antifungal)	T49.ØX1	T49.ØX2	T49.ØX3	T49.ØX4	T49.ØX5	T49.ØX6
Chlorpheniramine	T45.ØX1	T45.ØX2	T45.ØX3	T45.ØX4	T45.ØX5	T45.ØX6
Chlorphenoxamine	T45.ØX1	T45.ØX2	T45.ØX3	T45.ØX4	T45.ØX5	T45.ØX6
Chlorphentermine	T5Ø.5X1	T5Ø.5X2	T5Ø.5X3	T5Ø.5X4	T5Ø.5X5	T5Ø.5X6
Chlorprocaine—*see* Chloroprocaine						
Chlorproguanil	T37.2X1	T37.2X2	T37.2X3	T37.2X4	T37.2X5	T37.2X6
Chlorpromazine	T43.3X1	T43.3X2	T43.3X3	T43.3X4	T43.3X5	T43.3X6
Chlorpropamide	T38.3X1	T38.3X2	T38.3X3	T38.3X4	T38.3X5	T38.3X6
Chlorprothixene	T43.4X1	T43.4X2	T43.4X3	T43.4X4	T43.4X5	T43.4X6
Chlorquinaldol	T49.ØX1	T49.ØX2	T49.ØX3	T49.ØX4	T49.ØX5	T49.ØX6
Chlorquinol	T49.ØX1	T49.ØX2	T49.ØX3	T49.ØX4	T49.ØX5	T49.ØX6
Chlortalidone	T5Ø.2X1	T5Ø.2X2	T5Ø.2X3	T5Ø.2X4	T5Ø.2X5	T5Ø.2X6
Chlortetracycline	T36.4X1	T36.4X2	T36.4X3	T36.4X4	T36.4X5	T36.4X6
Chlorthalidone	T5Ø.2X1	T5Ø.2X2	T5Ø.2X3	T5Ø.2X4	T5Ø.2X5	T5Ø.2X6
Chlorthiophos	T6Ø.ØX1	T6Ø.ØX2	T6Ø.ØX3	T6Ø.ØX4	—	—
Chlorotrianisene	T38.5X1	T38.5X2	T38.5X3	T38.5X4	T38.5X5	T38.5X6
Chlor-Trimeton	T45.ØX1	T45.ØX2	T45.ØX3	T45.ØX4	T45.ØX5	T45.ØX6
Chlorthion	T6Ø.ØX1	T6Ø.ØX2	T6Ø.ØX3	T6Ø.ØX4	—	—
Chlorzoxazone	T42.8X1	T42.8X2	T42.8X3	T42.8X4	T42.8X5	T42.8X6
Choke damp	T59.7X1	T59.7X2	T59.7X3	T59.7X4	—	—
Cholagogues	T47.5X1	T47.5X2	T47.5X3	T47.5X4	T47.5X5	T47.5X6
Cholebrine	T5Ø.8X1	T5Ø.8X2	T5Ø.8X3	T5Ø.8X4	T5Ø.8X5	T5Ø.8X6
Cholecalciferol	T45.2X1	T45.2X2	T45.2X3	T45.2X4	T45.2X5	T45.2X6
Cholecystokinin	T5Ø.8X1	T5Ø.8X2	T5Ø.8X3	T5Ø.8X4	T5Ø.8X5	T5Ø.8X6
Cholera vaccine	T5Ø.A91	T5Ø.A92	T5Ø.A93	T5Ø.A94	T5Ø.A95	T5Ø.A96
Choleretic	T47.5X1	T47.5X2	T47.5X3	T47.5X4	T47.5X5	T47.5X6
Cholesterol-lowering agents	T46.6X1	T46.6X2	T46.6X3	T46.6X4	T46.6X5	T46.6X6
Cholestyramine (resin)	T46.6X1	T46.6X2	T46.6X3	T46.6X4	T46.6X5	T46.6X6
Cholic acid	T47.5X1	T47.5X2	T47.5X3	T47.5X4	T47.5X5	T47.5X6
Choline	T48.6X1	T48.6X2	T48.6X3	T48.6X4	T48.6X5	T48.6X6
chloride	T5Ø.991	T5Ø.992	T5Ø.993	T5Ø.994	T5Ø.995	T5Ø.996
dihydrogen citrate	T5Ø.991	T5Ø.992	T5Ø.993	T5Ø.994	T5Ø.995	T5Ø.996
salicylate	T39.Ø91	T39.Ø92	T39.Ø93	T39.Ø94	T39.Ø95	T39.Ø96
theophyllinate	T48.6X1	T48.6X2	T48.6X3	T48.6X4	T48.6X5	T48.6X6
Cholinergic (drug) **NEC**	T44.1X1	T44.1X2	T44.1X3	T44.1X4	T44.1X5	T44.1X6
muscle tone enhancer	T44.1X1	T44.1X2	T44.1X3	T44.1X4	T44.1X5	T44.1X6
organophosphorus	T44.ØX1	T44.ØX2	T44.ØX3	T44.ØX4	T44.ØX5	T44.ØX6
insecticide	T6Ø.ØX1	T6Ø.ØX2	T6Ø.ØX3	T6Ø.ØX4	—	—
nerve gas	T59.891	T59.892	T59.893	T59.894	—	—
trimethyl ammonium propanediol	T44.1X1	T44.1X2	T44.1X3	T44.1X4	T44.1X5	T44.1X6
Cholinesterase reactivator	T5Ø.6X1	T5Ø.6X2	T5Ø.6X3	T5Ø.6X4	T5Ø.6X5	T5Ø.6X6
Cholografin	T5Ø.8X1	T5Ø.8X2	T5Ø.8X3	T5Ø.8X4	T5Ø.8X5	T5Ø.8X6
Chorionic gonadotropin	T38.891	T38.892	T38.893	T38.894	T38.895	T38.896
Chromate	T56.2X1	T56.2X2	T56.2X3	T56.2X4	—	—
dust or mist	T56.2X1	T56.2X2	T56.2X3	T56.2X4	—	—
lead (*see also* lead)	T56.ØX1	T56.ØX2	T56.ØX3	T56.ØX4	—	—
paint	T56.ØX1	T56.ØX2	T56.ØX3	T56.ØX4	—	—
Chromic						
acid	T56.2X1	T56.2X2	T56.2X3	T56.2X4	—	—
dust or mist	T56.2X1	T56.2X2	T56.2X3	T56.2X4	—	—
phosphate 32P	T45.1X1	T45.1X2	T45.1X3	T45.1X4	T45.1X5	T45.1X6
Chromium	T56.2X1	T56.2X2	T56.2X3	T56.2X4	—	—
compounds—*see* Chromate						
sesquioxide	T5Ø.8X1	T5Ø.8X2	T5Ø.8X3	T5Ø.8X4	T5Ø.8X5	T5Ø.8X6
Chromomycin A3	T45.1X1	T45.1X2	T45.1X3	T45.1X4	T45.1X5	T45.1X6
Chromonar	T46.3X1	T46.3X2	T46.3X3	T46.3X4	T46.3X5	T46.3X6
Chromyl chloride	T56.2X1	T56.2X2	T56.2X3	T56.2X4	—	—
Chrysarobin	T49.4X1	T49.4X2	T49.4X3	T49.4X4	T49.4X5	T49.4X6
Chrysazin	T47.2X1	T47.2X2	T47.2X3	T47.2X4	T47.2X5	T47.2X6
Chymar	T45.3X1	T45.3X2	T45.3X3	T45.3X4	T45.3X5	T45.3X6
ophthalmic preparation	T49.5X1	T49.5X2	T49.5X3	T49.5X4	T49.5X5	T49.5X6
Chymopapain	T45.3X1	T45.3X2	T45.3X3	T45.3X4	T45.3X5	T45.3X6
Chymotrypsin	T45.3X1	T45.3X2	T45.3X3	T45.3X4	T45.3X5	T45.3X6
ophthalmic preparation	T49.5X1	T49.5X2	T49.5X3	T49.5X4	T49.5X5	T49.5X6
Cianidanol	T5Ø.991	T5Ø.992	T5Ø.993	T5Ø.994	T5Ø.995	T5Ø.996

Substance	Poisoning, Accidental (unintentional)	Poisoning, Intentional Self-harm	Poisoning, Assault	Poisoning, Undetermined	Adverse Effect	Under-dosing
Cianopramine	T43.Ø11	T43.Ø12	T43.Ø13	T43.Ø14	T43.Ø15	T43.Ø16
Cibenzoline	T46.2X1	T46.2X2	T46.2X3	T46.2X4	T46.2X5	T46.2X6
Ciclacillin	T36.ØX1	T36.ØX2	T36.ØX3	T36.ØX4	T36.ØX5	T36.ØX6
Ciclobarbital—*see* Hexobarbital						
Ciclonicate	T46.7X1	T46.7X2	T46.7X3	T46.7X4	T46.7X5	T46.7X6
Ciclopirox (olamine)	T49.ØX1	T49.ØX2	T49.ØX3	T49.ØX4	T49.ØX5	T49.ØX6
Ciclosporin	T45.1X1	T45.1X2	T45.1X3	T45.1X4	T45.1X5	T45.1X6
Cicuta maculata or virosa	T62.2X1	T62.2X2	T62.2X3	T62.2X4	—	—
Cicutoxin	T62.2X1	T62.2X2	T62.2X3	T62.2X4	—	—
Cigarette lighter fluid	T52.ØX1	T52.ØX2	T52.ØX3	T52.ØX4	—	—
Cigarettes (tobacco)	T65.221	T65.222	T65.223	T65.224	—	—
Ciguatoxin	T61.Ø1	T61.Ø2	T61.Ø3	T61.Ø4	—	—
Cilazapril	T46.4X1	T46.4X2	T46.4X3	T46.4X4	T46.4X5	T46.4X6
Cimetidine	T47.ØX1	T47.ØX2	T47.ØX3	T47.ØX4	T47.ØX5	T47.ØX6
Cimetropium bromide	T44.3X1	T44.3X2	T44.3X3	T44.3X4	T44.3X5	T44.3X6
Cinchocaine	T41.3X1	T41.3X2	T41.3X3	T41.3X4	T41.3X5	T41.3X6
topical (surface)	T41.3X1	T41.3X2	T41.3X3	T41.3X4	T41.3X5	T41.3X6
Cinchona	T37.2X1	T37.2X2	T37.2X3	T37.2X4	T37.2X5	T37.2X6
Cinchonine alkaloids	T37.2X1	T37.2X2	T37.2X3	T37.2X4	T37.2X5	T37.2X6
Cinchophen	T5Ø.4X1	T5Ø.4X2	T5Ø.4X3	T5Ø.4X4	T5Ø.4X5	T5Ø.4X6
Cinepazide	T46.7X1	T46.7X2	T46.7X3	T46.7X4	T46.7X5	T46.7X6
Cinnamedrine	T48.5X1	T48.5X2	T48.5X3	T48.5X4	T48.5X5	T48.5X6
Cinnarizine	T45.ØX1	T45.ØX2	T45.ØX3	T45.ØX4	T45.ØX5	T45.ØX6
Cinoxacin	T37.8X1	T37.8X2	T37.8X3	T37.8X4	T37.8X5	T37.8X6
Ciprofibrate	T46.6X1	T46.6X2	T46.6X3	T46.6X4	T46.6X5	T46.6X6
Ciprofloxacin	T36.8X1	T36.8X2	T36.8X3	T36.8X4	T36.8X5	T36.8X6
Cisapride	T47.8X1	T47.8X2	T47.8X3	T47.8X4	T47.8X5	T47.8X6
Cisplatin	T45.1X1	T45.1X2	T45.1X3	T45.1X4	T45.1X5	T45.1X6
Citalopram	T43.221	T43.222	T43.223	T43.224	T43.225	T43.226
Citanest	T41.3X1	T41.3X2	T41.3X3	T41.3X4	T41.3X5	T41.3X6
infiltration (subcutaneous)	T41.3X1	T41.3X2	T41.3X3	T41.3X4	T41.3X5	T41.3X6
nerve block (peripheral) (plexus)	T41.3X1	T41.3X2	T41.3X3	T41.3X4	T41.3X5	T41.3X6
Citric acid	T47.5X1	T47.5X2	T47.5X3	T47.5X4	T47.5X5	T47.5X6
Citrovorum (factor)	T45.8X1	T45.8X2	T45.8X3	T45.8X4	T45.8X5	T45.8X6
Claviceps purpurea	T62.2X1	T62.2X2	T62.2X3	T62.2X4	—	—
Clavulanic acid	T36.1X1	T36.1X2	T36.1X3	T36.1X4	T36.1X5	T36.1X6
Cleaner, cleansing agent, type not specified	T65.891	T65.892	T65.8933	T65.894	—	—
of paint or varnish	T52.91	T52.92	T52.93	T52.94	—	—
specified type NEC	T65.891	T65.892	T65.893	T65.894	—	—
Clebopride	T47.8X1	T47.8X2	T47.8X3	T47.8X4	T47.8X5	T47.8X6
Clefamide	T37.3X1	T37.3X2	T37.3X3	T37.3X4	T37.3X5	T37.3X6
Clemastine	T45.ØX1	T45.ØX2	T45.ØX3	T45.ØX4	T45.ØX5	T45.ØX6
Clematis vitalba	T62.2X1	T62.2X2	T62.2X3	T62.2X4	—	—
Clemizole	T45.ØX1	T45.ØX2	T45.ØX3	T45.ØX4	T45.ØX5	T45.ØX6
penicillin	T36.ØX1	T36.ØX2	T36.ØX3	T36.ØX4	T36.ØX5	T36.ØX6
Clenbuterol	T48.6X1	T48.6X2	T48.6X3	T48.6X4	T48.6X5	T48.6X6
Clidinium bromide	T44.3X1	T44.3X2	T44.3X3	T44.3X4	T44.3X5	T44.3X6
Clindamycin	T36.8X1	T36.8X2	T36.8X3	T36.8X4	T36.8X5	T36.8X6
Clinofibrate	T46.6X1	T46.6X2	T46.6X3	T46.6X4	T46.6X5	T46.6X6
Clioquinol	T37.8X1	T37.8X2	T37.8X3	T37.8X4	T37.8X5	T37.8X6
Cliradon	T4Ø.2X1	T4Ø.2X2	T4Ø.2X3	T4Ø.2X4	—	—
Clobazam	T42.4X1	T42.4X2	T42.4X3	T42.4X4	T42.4X5	T42.4X6
Clobenzorex	T5Ø.5X1	T5Ø.5X2	T5Ø.5X3	T5Ø.5X4	T5Ø.5X5	T5Ø.5X6
Clobetasol	T49.ØX1	T49.ØX2	T49.ØX3	T49.ØX4	T49.ØX5	T49.ØX6
Clobetasone	T49.ØX1	T49.ØX2	T49.ØX3	T49.ØX4	T49.ØX5	T49.ØX6
Clobutinol	T48.3X1	T48.3X2	T48.3X3	T48.3X4	T48.3X5	T48.3X6
Clocortolone	T38.ØX1	T38.ØX2	T38.ØX3	T38.ØX4	T38.ØX5	T38.ØX6
Clodantoin	T49.ØX1	T49.ØX2	T49.ØX3	T49.ØX4	T49.ØX5	T49.ØX6
Clodronic acid	T5Ø.991	T5Ø.992	T5Ø.993	T5Ø.994	T5Ø.995	T5Ø.996
Clofazimine	T37.1X1	T37.1X2	T37.1X3	T37.1X4	T37.1X5	T37.1X6
Clofedanol	T48.3X1	T48.3X2	T48.3X3	T48.3X4	T48.3X5	T48.3X6
Clofenamide	T5Ø.2X1	T5Ø.2X2	T5Ø.2X3	T5Ø.2X4	T5Ø.2X5	T5Ø.2X6
Clofenotane	T49.ØX1	T49.ØX2	T49.ØX3	T49.ØX4	T49.ØX5	T49.ØX6
Clofezone	T39.2X1	T39.2X2	T39.2X3	T39.2X4	T39.2X5	T39.2X6
Clofibrate	T46.6X1	T46.6X2	T46.6X3	T46.6X4	T46.6X5	T46.6X6
Clofibride	T46.6X1	T46.6X2	T46.6X3	T46.6X4	T46.6X5	T46.6X6
Cloforex	T5Ø.5X1	T5Ø.5X2	T5Ø.5X3	T5Ø.5X4	T5Ø.5X5	T5Ø.5X6
Clomethiazole	T42.6X1	T42.6X2	T42.6X3	T42.6X4	T42.6X5	T42.6X6
Clometocillin	T36.ØX1	T36.ØX2	T36.ØX3	T36.ØX4	T36.ØX5	T36.ØX6
Clomifene	T38.5X1	T38.5X2	T38.5X3	T38.5X4	T38.5X5	T38.5X6
Clomiphene	T38.5X1	T38.5X2	T38.5X3	T38.5X4	T38.5X5	T38.5X6
Clomipramine	T43.Ø11	T43.Ø12	T43.Ø13	T43.Ø14	T43.Ø15	T43.Ø16
Clomocycline	T36.4X1	T36.4X2	T36.4X3	T36.4X4	T36.4X5	T36.4X6
Clonazepam	T42.4X1	T42.4X2	T42.4X3	T42.4X4	T42.4X5	T42.4X6
Clonidine	T46.5X1	T46.5X2	T46.5X3	T46.5X4	T46.5X5	T46.5X6
Clonixin	T39.8X1	T39.8X2	T39.8X3	T39.8X4	T39.8X5	T39.8X6
Clopamide	T5Ø.2X1	T5Ø.2X2	T5Ø.2X3	T5Ø.2X4	T5Ø.2X5	T5Ø.2X6
Clopenthixol	T43.4X1	T43.4X2	T43.4X3	T43.4X4	T43.4X5	T43.4X6
Cloperastine	T48.3X1	T48.3X2	T48.3X3	T48.3X4	T48.3X5	T48.3X6
Clophedianol	T48.3X1	T48.3X2	T48.3X3	T48.3X4	T48.3X5	T48.3X6
Cloponone	T36.2X1	T36.2X2	T36.2X3	T36.2X4	T36.2X5	T36.2X6
Cloprednol	T38.ØX1	T38.ØX2	T38.ØX3	T38.ØX4	T38.ØX5	T38.ØX6
Cloral betaine	T42.6X1	T42.6X2	T42.6X3	T42.6X4	T42.6X5	T42.6X6
Cloramfenicol	T36.2X1	T36.2X2	T36.2X3	T36.2X4	T36.2X5	T36.2X6
Clorazepate (dipotassium)	T42.4X1	T42.4X2	T42.4X3	T42.4X4	T42.4X5	T42.4X6
Clorexolone	T5Ø.2X1	T5Ø.2X2	T5Ø.2X3	T5Ø.2X4	T5Ø.2X5	T5Ø.2X6
Clorox (bleach)	T54.91	T54.92	T54.93	T54.94	—	—
Clorfenamine	T45.ØX1	T45.ØX2	T45.ØX3	T45.ØX4	T45.ØX5	T45.ØX6
Clorgiline	T43.1X1	T43.1X2	T43.1X3	T43.1X4	T43.1X5	T43.1X6
Clorotepine	T44.3X1	T44.3X2	T44.3X3	T44.3X4	T44.3X5	T44.3X6
Clorprenaline	T48.6X1	T48.6X2	T48.6X3	T48.6X4	T48.6X5	T48.6X6
Clortermine	T5Ø.5X1	T5Ø.5X2	T5Ø.5X3	T5Ø.5X4	T5Ø.5X5	T5Ø.5X6
Clotiapine	T43.591	T43.592	T43.593	T43.594	T43.595	T43.596
Clotiazepam	T42.4X1	T42.4X2	T42.4X3	T42.4X4	T42.4X5	T42.4X6
Clotibric acid	T46.6X1	T46.6X2	T46.6X3	T46.6X4	T46.6X5	T46.6X6
Clotrimazole	T49.ØX1	T49.ØX2	T49.ØX3	T49.ØX4	T49.ØX5	T49.ØX6
Cloxacillin	T36.ØX1	T36.ØX2	T36.ØX3	T36.ØX4	T36.ØX5	T36.ØX6
Cloxazolam	T42.4X1	T42.4X2	T42.4X3	T42.4X4	T42.4X5	T42.4X6
Cloxiquine	T49.ØX1	T49.ØX2	T49.ØX3	T49.ØX4	T49.ØX5	T49.ØX6
Clozapine	T42.4X1	T42.4X2	T42.4X3	T42.4X4	T42.4X5	T42.4X6
Coagulant NEC	T45.7X1	T45.7X2	T45.7X3	T45.7X4	T45.7X5	T45.7X6
Coal (carbon monoxide from) (*see also* Carbon, monoxide, coal)	T58.2X1	T58.2X2	T58.2X3	T58.2X4	—	—
oil—*see* Kerosene						
tar	T49.1X1	T49.1X2	T49.1X3	T49.1X4	T49.1X5	T49.1X6
fumes	T59.891	T59.892	T59.893	T59.894	—	—
medicinal (ointment)	T49.4X1	T49.4X2	T49.4X3	T49.4X4	T49.4X5	T49.4X6
analgesics NEC	T39.2X1	T39.2X2	T39.2X3	T39.2X4	T39.2X5	T39.2X6
naphtha (solvent)	T52.ØX1	T52.ØX2	T52.ØX3	T52.ØX4	—	—
Cobalamine	T45.2X1	T45.2X2	T45.2X3	T45.2X4	T45.2X5	T45.2X6
Cobalt (nonmedicinal) (fumes) (industrial)	T56.891	T56.892	T56.893	T56.894	—	—
medicinal (trace) (chloride)	T45.8X1	T45.8X2	T45.8X3	T45.8X4	T45.8X5	T45.8X6
Cobra (venom)	T63.Ø41	T63.Ø42	T63.Ø43	T63.Ø44		
Coca (leaf)	T4Ø.5X1	T4Ø.5X2	T4Ø.5X3	T4Ø.5X4	T4Ø.5X5	T4Ø.5X6
Cocaine	T4Ø.5X1	T4Ø.5X2	T4Ø.5X3	T4Ø.5X4	T4Ø.5X5	T4Ø.5X6
topical anesthetic	T41.3X1	T41.3X2	T41.3X3	T41.3X4	T41.3X5	T41.3X6
Cocarboxylase	T45.3X1	T45.3X2	T45.3X3	T45.3X4	T45.3X5	T45.3X6
Coccidioidin	T5Ø.8X1	T5Ø.8X2	T5Ø.8X3	T5Ø.8X4	T5Ø.8X5	T5Ø.8X6
Cocculus indicus	T62.1X1	T62.1X2	T62.1X3	T62.1X4	—	—
Cochineal	T65.6X1	T65.6X2	T65.6X3	T65.6X4	—	—
medicinal products	T5Ø.991	T5Ø.992	T5Ø.993	T5Ø.994	T5Ø.995	T5Ø.996
Codeine	T4Ø.2X1	T4Ø.2X2	T4Ø.2X3	T4Ø.2X4	T4Ø.2X5	T4Ø.2X6
Cod-liver oil	T45.2X1	T45.2X2	T45.2X3	T45.2X4	T45.2X5	T45.2X6
Coenzyme A	T5Ø.991	T5Ø.992	T5Ø.993	T5Ø.994	T5Ø.995	T5Ø.996
Coffee	T62.8X1	T62.8X2	T62.8X3	T62.8X4	—	—
Cogalactoisomerase	T5Ø.991	T5Ø.992	T5Ø.993	T5Ø.994	T5Ø.995	T5Ø.996
Cogentin	T44.3X1	T44.3X2	T44.3X3	T44.3X4	T44.3X5	T44.3X6
Coke fumes or gas (carbon monoxide)	T58.2X1	T58.2X2	T58.2X3	T58.2X4	—	—
industrial use	T58.8X1	T58.8X2	T58.8X3	T58.8X4	—	—
Colace	T47.4X1	T47.4X2	T47.4X3	T47.4X4	T47.4X5	T47.4X6
Colaspase	T45.1X1	T45.1X2	T45.1X3	T45.1X4	T45.1X5	T45.1X6
Colchicine	T5Ø.4X1	T5Ø.4X2	T5Ø.4X3	T5Ø.4X4	T5Ø.4X5	T5Ø.4X6
Colchicum	T62.2X1	T62.2X2	T62.2X3	T62.2X4	—	—
Cold cream	T49.3X1	T49.3X2	T49.3X3	T49.3X4	T49.3X5	T49.3X6
Colecalciferol	T45.2X1	T45.2X2	T45.2X3	T45.2X4	T45.2X5	T45.2X6
Colestipol	T46.6X1	T46.6X2	T46.6X3	T46.6X4	T46.6X5	T46.6X6
Colestyramine	T46.6X1	T46.6X2	T46.6X3	T46.6X4	T46.6X5	T46.6X6
Colimycin	T36.8X1	T36.8X2	T36.8X3	T36.8X4	T36.8X5	T36.8X6
Colistimethate	T36.8X1	T36.8X2	T36.8X3	T36.8X4	T36.8X5	T36.8X6

Substance	Poisoning, Accidental (unintentional)	Poisoning, Intentional Self-harm	Poisoning, Assault	Poisoning, Undetermined	Adverse Effect	Under-dosing
Colistin	T36.8X1	T36.8X2	T36.8X3	T36.8X4	T36.8X5	T36.8X6
sulfate (eye preparation)	T49.5X1	T49.5X2	T49.5X3	T49.5X4	T49.5X5	T49.5X6
Collagen	T5Ø.991	T5Ø.992	T5Ø.993	T5Ø.994	T5Ø.995	T5Ø.996
Collagenase	T49.4X1	T49.4X2	T49.4X3	T49.4X4	T49.4X5	T49.4X6
Collodion	T49.3X1	T49.3X2	T49.3X3	T49.3X4	T49.3X5	T49.3X6
Colocynth	T47.2X1	T47.2X2	T47.2X3	T47.2X4	T47.2X5	T47.2X6
Colophony adhesive	T49.3X1	T49.3X2	T49.3X3	T49.3X4	T49.3X5	T49.3X6
Colorant (*see also* Dye)	T5Ø.991	T5Ø.992	T5Ø.993	T5Ø.994	T5Ø.995	T5Ø.996
Coloring matter—*see* Dye(s)						
Combustion gas (after combustion)—*see* Carbon, monoxide						
prior to combustion	T59.891	T59.892	T59.893	T59.894	—	—
Compazine	T43.3X1	T43.3X2	T43.3X3	T43.3X4	T43.3X5	T43.3X6
Compound						
42 (warfarin)	T6Ø.4X1	T6Ø.4X2	T6Ø.4X3	T6Ø.4X4	—	—
269 (endrin)	T6Ø.1X1	T6Ø.1X2	T6Ø.1X3	T6Ø.1X4	—	—
497 (dieldrin)	T6Ø.1X1	T6Ø.1X2	T6Ø.1X3	T6Ø.1X4	—	—
1080 (sodium fluoroacetate)	T6Ø.4X1	T6Ø.4X2	T6Ø.4X3	T6Ø.4X4	—	—
3422 (parathion)	T6Ø.ØX1	T6Ø.ØX2	T6Ø.ØX3	T6Ø.ØX4	—	—
3911 (phorate)	T6Ø.ØX1	T6Ø.ØX2	T6Ø.ØX3	T6Ø.ØX4	—	—
3956 (toxaphene)	T6Ø.1X1	T6Ø.1X2	T6Ø.1X3	T6Ø.1X4	—	—
4049 (malathion)	T6Ø.ØX1	T6Ø.ØX2	T6Ø.ØX3	T6Ø.ØX4	—	—
4069 (malathion)	T6Ø.ØX1	T6Ø.ØX2	T6Ø.ØX3	T6Ø.ØX4	—	—
4124 (dicapthon)	T6Ø.ØX1	T6Ø.ØX2	T6Ø.ØX3	T6Ø.ØX4	—	—
E (cortisone)	T38.ØX1	T38.ØX2	T38.ØX3	T38.ØX4	T38.ØX5	T38.ØX6
F (hydrocortisone)	T38.ØX1	T38.ØX2	T38.ØX3	T38.ØX4	T38.ØX5	T38.ØX6
Congener, anabolic	T38.7X1	T38.7X2	T38.7X3	T38.7X4	T38.7X5	T38.7X6
Congo red	T5Ø.8X1	T5Ø.8X2	T5Ø.8X3	T5Ø.8X4	T5Ø.8X5	T5Ø.8X6
Coniine, conine	T62.2X1	T62.2X2	T62.2X3	T62.2X4	—	—
Conium (maculatum)	T62.2X1	T62.2X2	T62.2X3	T62.2X4	—	—
Conjugated estrogenic substances	T38.5X1	T38.5X2	T38.5X3	T38.5X4	T38.5X5	T38.5X6
Contac	T48.5X1	T48.5X2	T48.5X3	T48.5X4	T48.5X5	T48.5X6
Contact lens solution	T49.5X1	T49.5X2	T49.5X3	T49.5X4	T49.5X5	T49.5X6
Contraceptive (oral)	T38.4X1	T38.4X2	T38.4X3	T38.4X4	T38.4X5	T38.4X6
vaginal	T49.8X1	T49.8X2	T49.8X3	T49.8X4	T49.8X5	T49.8X6
Contrast medium, radiography	T5Ø.8X1	T5Ø.8X2	T5Ø.8X3	T5Ø.8X4	T5Ø.8X5	T5Ø.8X6
Convallaria glycosides	T46.ØX1	T46.ØX2	T46.ØX3	T46.ØX4	T46.ØX5	T46.ØX6
Convallaria majalis	T62.2X1	T62.2X2	T62.2X3	T62.2X4	—	—
berry	T62.1X1	T62.1X2	T62.1X3	T62.1X4	—	—
Copper (dust) (fumes) (nonmedicinal) **NEC**	T56.4X1	T56.4X2	T56.4X3	T56.4X4	—	—
arsenate, arsenite	T57.ØX1	T57.ØX2	T57.ØX3	T57.ØX4	—	—
insecticide	T6Ø.2X1	T6Ø.2X2	T6Ø.2X3	T6Ø.2X4	—	—
emetic	T47.7X1	T47.7X2	T47.7X3	T47.7X4	T47.7X5	T47.7X6
fungicide	T6Ø.3X1	T6Ø.3X2	T6Ø.3X3	T6Ø.3X4	—	—
gluconate	T49.ØX1	T49.ØX2	T49.ØX3	T49.ØX4	T49.ØX5	T49.ØX6
insecticide	T6Ø.2X1	T6Ø.2X2	T6Ø.2X3	T6Ø.2X4	—	—
medicinal (trace)	T45.8X1	T45.8X2	T45.8X3	T45.8X4	T45.8X5	T45.8X6
oleate	T49.ØX1	T49.ØX2	T49.ØX3	T49.ØX4	T49.ØX5	T49.ØX6
sulfate	T56.4X1	T56.4X2	T56.4X3	T56.4X4	—	—
cupric	T56.4X1	T56.4X2	T56.4X3	T56.4X4	—	—
fungicide	T6Ø.3X1	T6Ø.3X2	T6Ø.3X3	T6Ø.3X4	—	—
medicinal						
ear	T49.6X1	T49.6X2	T49.6X3	T49.6X4	T49.6X5	T49.6X6
emetic	T47.7X1	T47.7X2	T47.7X3	T47.7X4	T47.7X5	T47.7X6
eye	T49.5X1	T49.5X2	T49.5X3	T49.5X4	T49.5X5	T49.5X6
cuprous	T56.4X1	T56.4X2	T56.4X3	T56.4X4	—	—
fungicide	T6Ø.3X1	T6Ø.3X2	T6Ø.3X3	T6Ø.3X4	—	—
medicinal						
ear	T49.6X1	T49.6X2	T49.6X3	T49.6X4	T49.6X5	T49.6X6
emetic	T47.7X1	T47.7X2	T47.7X3	T47.7X4	T47.7X5	T47.7X6
eye	T49.5X1	T49.5X2	T49.5X3	T49.5X4	T49.5X5	T49.5X6
Copperhead snake (bite) (venom)	T63.Ø61	T63.Ø62	T63.Ø63	T63.Ø64	—	—
Coral (sting)	T63.691	T63.692	T63.693	T63.694	—	—
snake (bite) (venom)	T63.Ø21	T63.Ø22	T63.Ø23	T63.Ø24	—	—
Corbadrine	T49.6X1	T49.6X2	T49.6X3	T49.6X4	T49.6X5	T49.6X6
Cordran	T49.ØX1	T49.ØX2	T49.ØX3	T49.ØX4	T49.ØX5	T49.ØX6
Cordite	T65.891	T65.892	T65.893	T65.894	—	—
vapor	T59.891	T59.892	T59.893	T59.894	—	—

Substance	Poisoning, Accidental (unintentional)	Poisoning, Intentional Self-harm	Poisoning, Assault	Poisoning, Undetermined	Adverse Effect	Under-dosing
Corn cures	T49.4X1	T49.4X2	T49.4X3	T49.4X4	T49.4X5	T49.4X6
Cornhusker's lotion	T49.3X1	T49.3X2	T49.3X3	T49.3X4	T49.3X5	T49.3X6
Corn starch	T49.3X1	T49.3X2	T49.3X3	T49.3X4	T49.3X5	T49.3X6
Coronary vasodilator NEC	T46.3X1	T46.3X2	T46.3X3	T46.3X4	T46.3X5	T46.3X6
Corrosive NEC	T54.91	T54.92	T54.93	T54.94	—	—
acid NEC	T54.2X1	T54.2X2	T54.2X3	T54.2X4	—	—
aromatics	T54.1X1	T54.1X2	T54.1X3	T54.1X4	—	—
disinfectant	T54.1X1	T54.1X2	T54.1X3	T54.1X4	—	—
fumes NEC	T54.91	T54.92	T54.93	T54.94	—	—
specified NEC	T54.91	T54.92	T54.93	T54.94	—	—
sublimate	T56.1X1	T56.1X2	T56.1X3	T56.1X4	—	—
Cortate	T38.ØX1	T38.ØX2	T38.ØX3	T38.ØX4	T38.ØX5	T38.ØX6
Cort-Dome	T38.ØX1	T38.ØX2	T38.ØX3	T38.ØX4	T38.ØX5	T38.ØX6
ENT agent	T49.6X1	T49.6X2	T49.6X3	T49.6X4	T49.6X5	T49.6X6
ophthalmic preparation	T49.5X1	T49.5X2	T49.5X3	T49.5X4	T49.5X5	T49.5X6
topical NEC	T49.ØX1	T49.ØX2	T49.ØX3	T49.ØX4	T49.ØX5	T49.ØX6
Cortef	T38.ØX1	T38.ØX2	T38.ØX3	T38.ØX4	T38.ØX5	T38.ØX6
ENT agent	T49.6X1	T49.6X2	T49.6X3	T49.6X4	T49.6X5	T49.6X6
ophthalmic preparation	T49.5X1	T49.5X2	T49.5X3	T49.5X4	T49.5X5	T49.5X6
topical NEC	T49.ØX1	T49.ØX2	T49.ØX3	T49.ØX4	T49.ØX5	T49.ØX6
Corticosteroid	T38.ØX1	T38.ØX2	T38.ØX3	T38.ØX4	T38.ØX5	T38.ØX6
ENT agent	T49.6X1	T49.6X2	T49.6X3	T49.6X4	T49.6X5	T49.6X6
mineral	T5Ø.ØX1	T5Ø.ØX2	T5Ø.ØX3	T5Ø.ØX4	T5Ø.ØX5	T5Ø.ØX6
ophthalmic	T49.5X1	T49.5X2	T49.5X3	T49.5X4	T49.5X5	T49.5X6
topical NEC	T49.ØX1	T49.ØX2	T49.ØX3	T49.ØX4	T49.ØX5	T49.ØX6
Corticotropin	T38.811	T38.812	T38.813	T38.814	T38.815	T38.816
Cortisol	T49.ØX1	T49.ØX2	T49.ØX3	T49.ØX4	T49.ØX5	T49.ØX6
ENT agent	T49.6X1	T49.6X2	T49.6X3	T49.6X4	T49.6X5	T49.6X6
ophthalmic preparation	T49.5X1	T49.5X2	T49.5X3	T49.5X4	T49.5X5	T49.5X6
topical NEC	T49.ØX1	T49.ØX2	T49.ØX3	T49.ØX4	T49.ØX5	T49.ØX6
Cortisone (acetate)	T38.ØX1	T38.ØX2	T38.ØX3	T38.ØX4	T38.ØX5	T38.ØX6
ENT agent	T49.6X1	T49.6X2	T49.6X3	T49.6X4	T49.6X5	T49.6X6
ophthalmic preparation	T49.5X1	T49.5X2	T49.5X3	T49.5X4	T49.5X5	T49.5X6
topical NEC	T49.ØX1	T49.ØX2	T49.ØX3	T49.ØX4	T49.ØX5	T49.ØX6
Cortivazol	T38.ØX1	T38.ØX2	T38.ØX3	T38.ØX4	T38.ØX5	T38.ØX6
Cortogen	T38.ØX1	T38.ØX2	T38.ØX3	T38.ØX4	T38.ØX5	T38.ØX6
ENT agent	T49.6X1	T49.6X2	T49.6X3	T49.6X4	T49.6X5	T49.6X6
ophthalmic preparation	T49.5X1	T49.5X2	T49.5X3	T49.5X4	T49.5X5	T49.5X6
Cortone	T38.ØX1	T38.ØX2	T38.ØX3	T38.ØX4	T38.ØX5	T38.ØX6
ENT agent	T49.6X1	T49.6X2	T49.6X3	T49.6X4	T49.6X5	T49.6X6
ophthalmic preparation	T49.5X1	T49.5X2	T49.5X3	T49.5X4	T49.5X5	T49.5X6
Cortril	T38.ØX1	T38.ØX2	T38.ØX3	T38.ØX4	T38.ØX5	T38.ØX6
ENT agent	T49.6X1	T49.6X2	T49.6X3	T49.6X4	T49.6X5	T49.6X6
ophthalmic preparation	T49.5X1	T49.5X2	T49.5X3	T49.5X4	T49.5X5	T49.5X6
topical NEC	T49.ØX1	T49.ØX2	T49.ØX3	T49.ØX4	T49.ØX5	T49.ØX6
Corynebacterium parvum	T45.1X1	T45.1X2	T45.1X3	T45.1X4	T45.1X5	T45.1X6
Cosmetic preparation	T49.8X1	T49.8X2	T49.8X3	T49.8X4	T49.8X5	T49.8X6
Cosmetics	T49.8X1	T49.8X2	T49.8X3	T49.8X4	T49.8X5	T49.8X6
Cosyntropin	T38.811	T38.812	T38.813	T38.814	T38.815	T38.816
Cotarnine	T45.7X1	T45.7X2	T45.7X3	T45.7X4	T45.7X5	T45.7X6
Co-trimoxazole	T36.8X1	T36.8X2	T36.8X3	T36.8X4	T36.8X5	T36.8X6
Cottonseed oil	T49.3X1	T49.3X2	T49.3X3	T49.3X4	T49.3X5	T49.3X6
Cough mixture (syrup)	T48.4X1	T48.4X2	T48.4X3	T48.4X4	T48.4X5	T48.4X6
containing opiates	T4Ø.2X1	T4Ø.2X2	T4Ø.2X3	T4Ø.2X4	T4Ø.2X5	T4Ø.2X6
expectorants	T48.4X1	T48.4X2	T48.4X3	T48.4X4	T48.4X5	T48.4X6
Coumadin	T45.511	T45.512	T45.513	T45.514	T45.515	T45.516
rodenticide	T6Ø.4X1	T6Ø.4X2	T6Ø.4X3	T6Ø.4X4	—	—
Coumaphos	T6Ø.ØX1	T6Ø.ØX2	T6Ø.ØX3	T6Ø.ØX4	—	—
Coumarin	T45.511	T45.512	T45.513	T45.514	T45.515	T45.516
Coumetarol	T45.511	T45.512	T45.513	T45.514	T45.515	T45.516
Cowbane	T62.2X1	T62.2X2	T62.2X3	T62.2X4	—	—
Cozyme	T45.2X1	T45.2X2	T45.2X3	T45.2X4	T45.2X5	T45.2X6
Crack	T4Ø.5X1	T4Ø.5X2	T4Ø.5X3	T4Ø.5X4	—	—
Crataegus extract	T46.ØX1	T46.ØX2	T46.ØX3	T46.ØX4	T46.ØX5	T46.ØX6
Creolin	T54.1X1	T54.1X2	T54.1X3	T54.1X4	—	—
disinfectant	T54.1X1	T54.1X2	T54.1X3	T54.1X4	—	—
Creosol (compound)	T49.ØX1	T49.ØX2	T49.ØX3	T49.ØX4	T49.ØX5	T49.ØX6
Creosote (coal tar) (beechwood)	T49.ØX1	T49.ØX2	T49.ØX3	T49.ØX4	T49.ØX5	T49.ØX6
medicinal (expectorant)	T48.4X1	T48.4X2	T48.4X3	T48.4X4	T48.4X5	T48.4X6
syrup	T48.4X1	T48.4X2	T48.4X3	T48.4X4	T48.4X5	T48.4X6

Substance	Poisoning, Accidental (unintentional)	Poisoning, Intentional Self-harm	Poisoning, Assault	Poisoning, Undetermined	Adverse Effect	Under-dosing
Cresol(s)	T49.ØX1	T49.ØX2	T49.ØX3	T49.ØX4	T49.ØX5	T49.ØX6
and soap solution	T49.ØX1	T49.ØX2	T49.ØX3	T49.ØX4	T49.ØX5	T49.ØX6
Cresyl acetate	T49.ØX1	T49.ØX2	T49.ØX3	T49.ØX4	T49.ØX5	T49.ØX6
Cresylic acid	T49.ØX1	T49.ØX2	T49.ØX3	T49.ØX4	T49.ØX5	T49.ØX6
Crimidine	T6Ø.4X1	T6Ø.4X2	T6Ø.4X3	T6Ø.4X4	—	—
Croconazole	T37.8X1	T37.8X2	T37.8X3	T37.8X4	T37.8X5	T37.8X6
Cromoglicic acid	T48.6X1	T48.6X2	T48.6X3	T48.6X4	T48.6X5	T48.6X6
Cromolyn	T48.6X1	T48.6X2	T48.6X3	T48.6X4	T48.6X5	T48.6X6
Cromonar	T46.3X1	T46.3X2	T46.3X3	T46.3X4	T46.3X5	T46.3X6
Cropropamide	T39.8X1	T39.8X2	T39.8X3	T39.8X4	T39.8X5	T39.8X6
with crotethamide	T5Ø.7X1	T5Ø.7X2	T5Ø.7X3	T5Ø.7X4	T5Ø.7X5	T5Ø.7X6
Crotamiton	T49.ØX1	T49.ØX2	T49.ØX3	T49.ØX4	T49.ØX5	T49.ØX6
Crotethamide	T39.8X1	T39.8X2	T39.8X3	T39.8X4	T39.8X5	T39.8X6
with cropropamide	T5Ø.7X1	T5Ø.7X2	T5Ø.7X3	T5Ø.7X4	T5Ø.7X5	T5Ø.7X6
Croton (oil)	T47.2X1	T47.2X2	T47.2X3	T47.2X4	T47.2X5	T47.2X6
chloral	T42.6X1	T42.6X2	T42.6X3	T42.6X4	T42.6X5	T42.6X6
Crude oil	T52.ØX1	T52.ØX2	T52.ØX3	T52.ØX4	—	—
Cryogenine	T39.8X1	T39.8X2	T39.8X3	T39.8X4	T39.8X5	T39.8X6
Cryolite (vapor)	T6Ø.1X1	T6Ø.1X2	T6Ø.1X3	T6Ø.1X4	—	—
insecticide	T6Ø.1X1	T6Ø.1X2	T6Ø.1X3	T6Ø.1X4	—	—
Cryptenamine (tannates)	T46.5X1	T46.5X2	T46.5X3	T46.5X4	T46.5X5	T46.5X6
Crystal violet	T49.ØX1	T49.ØX2	T49.ØX3	T49.ØX4	T49.ØX5	T49.ØX6
Cuckoopint	T62.2X1	T62.2X2	T62.2X3	T62.2X4	—	—
Cumetharol	T45.511	T45.512	T45.513	T45.514	T45.515	T45.516
Cupric						
acetate	T6Ø.3X1	T6Ø.3X2	T6Ø.3X3	T6Ø.3X4	—	—
acetoarsenite	T57.ØX1	T57.ØX2	T57.ØX3	T57.ØX4	—	—
arsenate	T57.ØX1	T57.ØX2	T57.ØX3	T57.ØX4	—	—
gluconate	T49.ØX1	T49.ØX2	T49.ØX3	T49.ØX4	T49.ØX5	T49.ØX6
oleate	T49.ØX1	T49.ØX2	T49.ØX3	T49.ØX4	T49.ØX5	T49.ØX6
sulfate	T56.4X1	T56.4X2	T56.4X3	T56.4X4	—	—
Cuprous sulfate (*see also* Copper sulfate)	T56.4X1	T56.4X2	T56.4X3	T56.4X4	—	—
Curare, curarine	T48.1X1	T48.1X2	T48.1X3	T48.1X4	T48.1X5	T48.1X6
Cyamemazine	T43.3X1	T43.3X2	T43.3X3	T43.3X4	T43.3X5	T43.3X6
Cyamopsis tetragono-loba	T46.6X1	T46.6X2	T46.6X3	T46.6X4	T46.6X5	T46.6X6
Cyanacetyl hydrazide	T37.1X1	T37.1X2	T37.1X3	T37.1X4	T37.1X5	T37.1X6
Cyanic acid (gas)	T59.891	T59.892	T59.893	T59.894	—	—
Cyanide(s) (compounds) (potassium) (sodium) **NEC**	T65.ØX1	T65.ØX2	T65.ØX3	T65.ØX4	—	—
dust or gas (inhalation) NEC	T57.3X1	T57.3X2	T57.3X3	T57.3X4	—	—
fumigant	T65.ØX1	T65.ØX2	T65.ØX3	T65.ØX4	—	—
hydrogen	T57.3X1	T57.3X2	T57.3X3	T57.3X4	—	—
mercuric—*see* Mercury						
pesticide (dust) (fumes)	T65.ØX1	T65.ØX2	T65.ØX3	T65.ØX4	—	—
Cyanoacrylate adhesive	T49.3X1	T49.3X2	T49.3X3	T49.3X4	T49.3X5	T49.3X6
Cyanocobalamin	T45.8X1	T45.8X2	T45.8X3	T45.8X4	T45.8X5	T45.8X6
Cyanogen (chloride) (gas) **NEC**	T59.891	T59.892	T59.893	T59.894	—	—
Cyclacillin	T36.ØX1	T36.ØX2	T36.ØX3	T36.ØX4	T36.ØX5	T36.ØX6
Cyclaine	T41.3X1	T41.3X2	T41.3X3	T41.3X4	T41.3X5	T41.3X6
Cyclamate	T5Ø.991	T5Ø.992	T5Ø.993	T5Ø.994	T5Ø.995	T5Ø.996
Cyclamen europaeum	T62.2X1	T62.2X2	T62.2X3	T62.2X4	—	—
Cyclandelate	T46.7X1	T46.7X2	T46.7X3	T46.7X4	T46.7X5	T46.7X6
Cyclazocine	T5Ø.7X1	T5Ø.7X2	T5Ø.7X3	T5Ø.7X4	T5Ø.7X5	T5Ø.7X6
Cyclizine	T45.ØX1	T45.ØX2	T45.ØX3	T45.ØX4	T45.ØX5	T45.ØX6
Cyclobarbital	T42.3X1	T42.3X2	T42.3X3	T42.3X4	T42.3X5	T42.3X6
Cyclobarbitone	T42.3X1	T42.3X2	T42.3X3	T42.3X4	T42.3X5	T42.3X6
Cyclobenzaprine	T48.1X1	T48.1X2	T48.1X3	T48.1X4	T48.1X5	T48.1X6
Cyclodrine	T44.3X1	T44.3X2	T44.3X3	T44.3X4	T44.3X5	T44.3X6
Cycloguanil embonate	T37.2X1	T37.2X2	T37.2X3	T37.2X4	T37.2X5	T37.2X6
Cyclohexane	T52.8X1	T52.8X2	T52.8X3	T52.8X4	—	—
Cyclohexanol	T51.8X1	T51.8X2	T51.8X3	T51.8X4	—	—
Cyclohexanone	T52.4X1	T52.4X2	T52.4X3	T52.4X4	—	—
Cycloheximide	T6Ø.3X1	T6Ø.3X2	T6Ø.3X3	T6Ø.3X4	—	—
Cyclohexyl acetate	T52.8X1	T52.8X2	T52.8X3	T52.8X4	—	—
Cycloleucin	T45.1X1	T45.1X2	T45.1X3	T45.1X4	T45.1X5	T45.1X6
Cyclomethycaine	T41.3X1	T41.3X2	T41.3X3	T41.3X4	T41.3X5	T41.3X6
Cyclopentamine	T44.4X1	T44.4X2	T44.4X3	T44.4X4	T44.4X5	T44.4X6
Cyclopenthiazide	T5Ø.2X1	T5Ø.2X2	T5Ø.2X3	T5Ø.2X4	T5Ø.2X5	T5Ø.2X6
Cyclopentolate	T44.3X1	T44.3X2	T44.3X3	T44.3X4	T44.3X5	T44.3X6
Cyclophosphamide	T45.1X1	T45.1X2	T45.1X3	T45.1X4	T45.1X5	T45.1X6

Substance	Poisoning, Accidental (unintentional)	Poisoning, Intentional Self-harm	Poisoning, Assault	Poisoning, Undetermined	Adverse Effect	Under-dosing
Cycloplegic drug	T49.5X1	T49.5X2	T49.5X3	T49.5X4	T49.5X5	T49.5X6
Cyclopropane	T41.291	T41.292	T41.293	T41.294	T41.295	T41.296
Cyclopyrabital	T39.8X1	T39.8X2	T39.8X3	T39.8X4	T39.8X5	T39.8X6
Cycloserine	T37.1X1	T37.1X2	T37.1X3	T37.1X4	T37.1X5	T37.1X6
Cyclosporin	T45.1X1	T45.1X2	T45.1X3	T45.1X4	T45.1X5	T45.1X6
Cyclothiazide	T5Ø.2X1	T5Ø.2X2	T5Ø.2X3	T5Ø.2X4	T5Ø.2X5	T5Ø.2X6
Cycrimine	T44.3X1	T44.3X2	T44.3X3	T44.3X4	T44.3X5	T44.3X6
Cyhalothrin	T6Ø.1X1	T6Ø.1X2	T6Ø.1X3	T6Ø.1X4	—	—
Cymarin	T46.ØX1	T46.ØX2	T46.ØX3	T46.ØX4	T46.ØX5	T46.ØX6
Cypermethrin	T6Ø.1X1	T6Ø.1X2	T6Ø.1X3	T6Ø.1X4	—	—
Cyphenothrin	T6Ø.2X1	T6Ø.2X2	T6Ø.2X3	T6Ø.2X4	—	—
Cyproheptadine	T45.ØX1	T45.ØX2	T45.ØX3	T45.ØX4	T45.ØX5	T45.ØX6
Cyproterone	T38.6X1	T38.6X2	T38.6X3	T38.6X4	T38.6X5	T38.6X6
Cysteamine	T5Ø.6X1	T5Ø.6X2	T5Ø.6X3	T5Ø.6X4	T5Ø.6X5	T5Ø.6X6
Cytarabine	T45.1X1	T45.1X2	T45.1X3	T45.1X4	T45.1X5	T45.1X6
Cytisus						
laburnum	T62.2X1	T62.2X2	T62.2X3	T62.2X4	—	—
scoparius	T62.2X1	T62.2X2	T62.2X3	T62.2X4	—	—
Cytochrome C	T47.5X1	T47.5X2	T47.5X3	T47.5X4	T47.5X5	T47.5X6
Cytomel	T38.1X1	T38.1X2	T38.1X3	T38.1X4	T38.1X5	T38.1X6
Cytosine arabinoside	T45.1X1	T45.1X2	T45.1X3	T45.1X4	T45.1X5	T45.1X6
Cytoxan	T45.1X1	T45.1X2	T45.1X3	T45.1X4	T45.1X5	T45.1X6
Cytozyme	T45.7X1	T45.7X2	T45.7X3	T45.7X4	T45.7X5	T45.7X6
D						
2,4-D	T6Ø.3X1	T6Ø.3X2	T6Ø.3X3	T6Ø.3X4	—	—
Dacarbazine	T45.1X1	T45.1X2	T45.1X3	T45.1X4	T45.1X5	T45.1X6
Dactinomycin	T45.1X1	T45.1X2	T45.1X3	T45.1X4	T45.1X5	T45.1X6
DADPS	T37.1X1	T37.1X2	T37.1X3	T37.1X4	T37.1X5	T37.1X6
Dakin's solution	T49.ØX1	T49.ØX2	T49.ØX3	T49.ØX4	T49.ØX5	T49.ØX6
Dalapon (sodium)	T6Ø.3X1	T6Ø.3X2	T6Ø.3X3	T6Ø.3X4	—	—
Dalmane	T42.4X1	T42.4X2	T42.4X3	T42.4X4	T42.4X5	T42.4X6
Danazol	T38.6X1	T38.6X2	T38.6X3	T38.6X4	T38.6X5	T38.6X6
Danilone	T45.511	T45.512	T45.513	T45.514	T45.515	T45.516
Danthron	T47.2X1	T47.2X2	T47.2X3	T47.2X4	T47.2X5	T47.2X6
Dantrolene	T42.8X1	T42.8X2	T42.8X3	T42.8X4	T42.8X5	T42.8X6
Dantron	T47.2X1	T47.2X2	T47.2X3	T47.2X4	T47.2X5	T47.2X6
Daphne (gnidium) (mezereum)	T62.2X1	T62.2X2	T62.2X3	T62.2X4	—	—
berry	T62.1X1	T62.1X2	T62.1X3	T62.1X4	—	—
Dapsone	T37.1X1	T37.1X2	T37.1X3	T37.1X4	T37.1X5	T37.1X6
Daraprim	T37.2X1	T37.2X2	T37.2X3	T37.2X4	T37.2X5	T37.2X6
Darnel	T62.2X1	T62.2X2	T62.2X3	T62.2X4	—	—
Darvon	T39.8X1	T39.8X2	T39.8X3	T39.8X4	T39.8X5	T39.8X6
Daunomycin	T45.1X1	T45.1X2	T45.1X3	T45.1X4	T45.1X5	T45.1X6
Daunorubicin	T45.1X1	T45.1X2	T45.1X3	T45.1X4	T45.1X5	T45.1X6
DBI	T38.3X1	T38.3X2	T38.3X3	T38.3X4	T38.3X5	T38.3X6
D-Con	T6Ø.91	T6Ø.92	T6Ø.93	T6Ø.94	—	—
insecticide	T6Ø.2X1	T6Ø.2X2	T6Ø.2X3	T6Ø.2X4	—	—
rodenticide	T6Ø.4X1	T6Ø.4X2	T6Ø.4X3	T6Ø.4X4	—	—
DDAVP	T38.891	T38.892	T38.893	T38.894	T38.895	T38.896
DDE (bis(chlorophenyl)-dichloroethylene)	T6Ø.2X1	T6Ø.2X2	T6Ø.2X3	T6Ø.2X4	—	—
DDS	T37.1X1	T37.1X2	T37.1X3	T37.1X4	T37.1X5	T37.1X6
DDT (dust)	T6Ø.1X1	T6Ø.1X2	T6Ø.1X3	T6Ø.1X4	—	—
Deadly nightshade (*see also* Belladonna)	T62.2X1	T62.2X2	T62.2X3	T62.2X4	—	—
berry	T62.1X1	T62.1X2	T62.1X3	T62.1X4	—	—
Deamino-D-arginine vasopressin	T38.891	T38.892	T38.893	T38.894	T38.895	T38.896
Deanol (aceglumate)	T5Ø.991	T5Ø.992	T5Ø.993	T5Ø.994	T5Ø.995	T5Ø.996
Debrisoquine	T46.5X1	T46.5X2	T46.5X3	T46.5X4	T46.5X5	T46.5X6
Decaborane	T57.8X1	T57.8X2	T57.8X3	T57.8X4	—	—
fumes	T59.891	T59.892	T59.893	T59.894	—	—
Decadron	T38.ØX1	T38.ØX2	T38.ØX3	T38.ØX4	T38.ØX5	T38.ØX6
ENT agent	T49.6X1	T49.6X2	T49.6X3	T49.6X4	T49.6X5	T49.6X6
ophthalmic preparation	T49.5X1	T49.5X2	T49.5X3	T49.5X4	T49.5X5	T49.5X6
topical NEC	T49.ØX1	T49.ØX2	T49.ØX3	T49.ØX4	T49.ØX5	T49.ØX6
Decahydronaphthalene	T52.8X1	T52.8X2	T52.8X3	T52.8X4	—	—
Decalin	T52.8X1	T52.8X2	T52.8X3	T52.8X4	—	—
Decamethonium (bromide)	T48.1X1	T48.1X2	T48.1X3	T48.1X4	T48.1X5	T48.1X6
Decholin	T47.5X1	T47.5X2	T47.5X3	T47.5X4	T47.5X5	T47.5X6
Declomycin	T36.4X1	T36.4X2	T36.4X3	T36.4X4	T36.4X5	T36.4X6

Substance	Poisoning, Accidental (unintentional)	Poisoning, Intentional Self-harm	Poisoning, Assault	Poisoning, Undetermined	Adverse Effect	Under-dosing
Decongestant, nasal (mucosa)	T48.5X1	T48.5X2	T48.5X3	T48.5X4	T48.5X5	T48.5X6
combination	T48.5X1	T48.5X2	T48.5X3	T48.5X4	T48.5X5	T48.5X6
Deet	T6Ø.8X1	T6Ø.8X2	T6Ø.8X3	T6Ø.8X4	—	—
Deferoxamine	T45.8X1	T45.8X2	T45.8X3	T45.8X4	T45.8X5	T45.8X6
Deflazacort	T38.ØX1	T38.ØX2	T38.ØX3	T38.ØX4	T38.ØX5	T38.ØX6
Deglycyrrhizinized extract of licorice	T48.4X1	T48.4X2	T48.4X3	T48.4X4	T48.4X5	T48.4X6
Dehydrocholic acid	T47.5X1	T47.5X2	T47.5X3	T47.5X4	T47.5X5	T47.5X6
Dehydroemetine	T37.3X1	T37.3X2	T37.3X3	T37.3X4	T37.3X5	T37.3X6
Dekalin	T52.8X1	T52.8X2	T52.8X3	T52.8X4	—	—
Delalutin	T38.5X1	T38.5X2	T38.5X3	T38.5X4	T38.5X5	T38.5X6
Delphinium	T62.2X1	T62.2X2	T62.2X3	T62.2X4	—	—
Deltasone	T38.ØX1	T38.ØX2	T38.ØX3	T38.ØX4	T38.ØX5	T38.ØX6
Deltra	T38.ØX1	T38.ØX2	T38.ØX3	T38.ØX4	T38.ØX5	T38.ØX6
Delvinal	T42.3X1	T42.3X2	T42.3X3	T42.3X4	T42.3X5	T42.3X6
Delorazepam	T42.4X1	T42.4X2	T42.4X3	T42.4X4	T42.4X5	T42.4X6
Deltamethrin	T6Ø.1X1	T6Ø.1X2	T6Ø.1X3	T6Ø.1X4	—	—
Demecarium (bromide)	T49.5X1	T49.5X2	T49.5X3	T49.5X4	T49.5X5	T49.5X6
Demeclocycline	T36.4X1	T36.4X2	T36.4X3	T36.4X4	T36.4X5	T36.4X6
Demecolcine	T45.1X1	T45.1X2	T45.1X3	T45.1X4	T45.1X5	T45.1X6
Demegestone	T38.5X1	T38.5X2	T38.5X3	T38.5X4	T38.5X5	T38.5X6
Demelanizing agents	T49.8X1	T49.8X2	T49.8X3	T49.8X4	T49.8X5	T49.8X6
Demephion -O and -S	T6Ø.ØX1	T6Ø.ØX2	T6Ø.ØX3	T6Ø.ØX4	—	—
Demerol	T4Ø.2X1	T4Ø.2X2	T4Ø.2X3	T4Ø.2X4	T4Ø.2X5	T4Ø.2X6
Demethylchlortetracycline	T36.4X1	T36.4X2	T36.4X3	T36.4X4	T36.4X5	T36.4X6
Demethyltetracycline	T36.4X1	T36.4X2	T36.4X3	T36.4X4	T36.4X5	T36.4X6
Demeton -O and -S	T6Ø.ØX1	T6Ø.ØX2	T6Ø.ØX3	T6Ø.ØX4	—	—
Demulcent (external)	T49.3X1	T49.3X2	T49.3X3	T49.3X4	T49.3X5	T49.3X6
specified NEC	T49.3X1	T49.3X2	T49.3X3	T49.3X4	T49.3X5	T49.3X6
Demulen	T38.4X1	T38.4X2	T38.4X3	T38.4X4	T38.4X5	T38.4X6
Denatured alcohol	T51.ØX1	T51.ØX2	T51.ØX3	T51.ØX4	—	—
Dendrid	T49.5X1	T49.5X2	T49.5X3	T49.5X4	T49.5X5	T49.5X6
Dental drug, topical application NEC	T49.7X1	T49.7X2	T49.7X3	T49.7X4	T49.7X5	T49.7X6
Dentifrice	T49.7X1	T49.7X2	T49.7X3	T49.7X4	T49.7X5	T49.7X6
Deodorant spray (feminine hygiene)	T49.8X1	T49.8X2	T49.8X3	T49.8X4	T49.8X5	T49.8X6
Deoxycortone	T5Ø.ØX1	T5Ø.ØX2	T5Ø.ØX3	T5Ø.ØX4	T5Ø.ØX5	T5Ø.ØX6
2-Deoxy-5-fluorouridine	T45.1X1	T45.1X2	T45.1X3	T45.1X4	T45.1X5	T45.1X6
5-Deoxy-5-fluorouridine	T45.1X1	T45.1X2	T45.1X3	T45.1X4	T45.1X5	T45.1X6
Deoxyribonuclease (pancreatic)	T45.3X1	T45.3X2	T45.3X3	T45.3X4	T45.3X5	T45.3X6
Depilatory	T49.4X1	T49.4X2	T49.4X3	T49.4X4	T49.4X5	T49.4X6
Deprenalin	T42.8X1	T42.8X2	T42.8X3	T42.8X4	T42.8X5	T42.8X6
Deprenyl	T42.8X1	T42.8X2	T42.8X3	T42.8X4	T42.8X5	T42.8X6
Depressant, appetite	T5Ø.5X1	T5Ø.5X2	T5Ø.5X3	T5Ø.5X4	T5Ø.5X5	T5Ø.5X6
Depressant						
appetite, central	T5Ø.5X1	T5Ø.5X2	T5Ø.5X3	T5Ø.5X4	T5Ø.5X5	T5Ø.5X6
cardiac	T46.2X1	T46.2X2	T46.2X3	T46.2X4	T46.2X5	T46.2X6
central nervous system (anesthetic) (*see also* Central nervous system, depressants)	T42.71	T42.72	T42.73	T42.74	T42.75	T42.76
general anesthetic	T41.2Ø1	T41.2Ø2	T41.2Ø3	T41.2Ø4	T41.2Ø5	T41.2Ø6
muscle tone	T42.8X1	T42.8X2	T42.8X3	T42.8X4	T42.8X5	T42.8X6
muscle tone, central	T42.8X1	T42.8X2	T42.8X3	T42.8X4	T42.8X5	T42.8X6
psychotherapeutic	T43.5Ø1	T43.5Ø2	T43.5Ø3	T43.5Ø4	T43.5Ø5	T43.5Ø6
Deptropine	T45.ØX1	T45.ØX2	T45.ØX3	T45.ØX4	T45.ØX5	T45.ØX6
Dequalinium (chloride)	T49.ØX1	T49.ØX2	T49.ØX3	T49.ØX4	T49.ØX5	T49.ØX6
Derris root	T6Ø.2X1	T6Ø.2X2	T6Ø.2X3	T6Ø.2X4	—	—
Deserpidine	T46.5X1	T46.5X2	T46.5X3	T46.5X4	T46.5X5	T46.5X6
Desferrioxamine	T45.8X1	T45.8X2	T45.8X3	T45.8X4	T45.8X5	T45.8X6
Desipramine	T43.Ø11	T43.Ø12	T43.Ø13	T43.Ø14	T43.Ø15	T43.Ø16
Deslanoside	T46.ØX1	T46.ØX2	T46.ØX3	T46.ØX4	T46.ØX5	T46.ØX6
Desloughing agent	T49.4X1	T49.4X2	T49.4X3	T49.4X4	T49.4X5	T49.4X6
Desmethylimipramine	T43.Ø11	T43.Ø12	T43.Ø13	T43.Ø14	T43.Ø15	T43.Ø16
Desmopressin	T38.891	T38.892	T38.893	T38.894	T38.895	T38.896
Desocodeine	T4Ø.2X1	T4Ø.2X2	T4Ø.2X3	T4Ø.2X4	T4Ø.2X5	T4Ø.2X6
Desogestrel	T38.5X1	T38.5X2	T38.5X3	T38.5X4	T38.5X5	T38.5X6
Desomorphine	T4Ø.2X1	T4Ø.2X2	T4Ø.2X3	T4Ø.2X4	—	—
Desonide	T49.ØX1	T49.ØX2	T49.ØX3	T49.ØX4	T49.ØX5	T49.ØX6
Desoximetasone	T49.ØX1	T49.ØX2	T49.ØX3	T49.ØX4	T49.ØX5	T49.ØX6
Desoxycorticosteroid	T5Ø.ØX1	T5Ø.ØX2	T5Ø.ØX3	T5Ø.ØX4	T5Ø.ØX5	T5Ø.ØX6
Desoxycortone	T5Ø.ØX1	T5Ø.ØX2	T5Ø.ØX3	T5Ø.ØX4	T5Ø.ØX5	T5Ø.ØX6
Desoxyephedrine	T43.621	T43.622	T43.623	T43.624	T43.625	T43.626
Detaxtran	T46.6X1	T46.6X2	T46.6X3	T46.6X4	T46.6X5	T46.6X6
Detergent	T49.2X1	T49.2X2	T49.2X3	T49.2X4	T49.2X5	T49.2X6
external medication	T49.2X1	T49.2X2	T49.2X3	T49.2X4	T49.2X5	T49.2X6
local	T49.2X1	T49.2X2	T49.2X3	T49.2X4	T49.2X4	T49.2X6
medicinal	T49.2X1	T49.2X2	T49.2X3	T49.2X4	T49.2X4	T49.2X6
nonmedicinal	T55.1X1	T55.1X2	T55.1X3	T55.1X4	—	—
specified NEC	T55.1X1	T55.1X2	T55.1X3	T55.1X4	—	—
Deterrent, alcohol	T5Ø.6X1	T5Ø.6X2	T5Ø.6X3	T5Ø.6X4	T5Ø.6X5	T5Ø.6X6
Detoxifying agent	T5Ø.6X1	T5Ø.6X2	T5Ø.6X3	T5Ø.6X4	T5Ø.6X5	T5Ø.6X6
Detrothyronine	T38.1X1	T38.1X2	T38.1X3	T38.1X4	T38.1X5	T38.1X6
Dettol (external medication)	T49.ØX1	T49.ØX2	T49.ØX3	T49.ØX4	T49.ØX5	T49.ØX6
Dexamethasone	T38.ØX1	T38.ØX2	T38.ØX3	T38.ØX4	T38.ØX5	T38.ØX6
ENT agent	T49.6X1	T49.6X2	T49.6X3	T49.6X4	T49.6X5	T49.6X6
ophthalmic preparation	T49.5X1	T49.5X2	T49.5X3	T49.5X4	T49.5X5	T49.5X6
topical NEC	T49.ØX1	T49.ØX2	T49.ØX3	T49.ØX4	T49.ØX5	T49.ØX6
Dexamfetamine	T43.621	T43.622	T43.623	T43.624	T43.625	T43.626
Dexamphetamine	T43.621	T43.622	T43.623	T43.624	T43.625	T43.626
Dexbrompheniramine	T45.ØX1	T45.ØX2	T45.ØX3	T45.ØX4	T45.ØX5	T45.ØX6
Dexchlorpheniramine	T45.ØX1	T45.ØX2	T45.ØX3	T45.ØX4	T45.ØX5	T45.ØX6
Dexedrine	T43.621	T43.622	T43.623	T43.624	T43.625	T43.626
Dexetimide	T44.3X1	T44.3X2	T44.3X3	T44.3X4	T44.3X5	T44.3X6
Dexfenfluramine	T5Ø.5X1	T5Ø.5X2	T5Ø.5X3	T5Ø.5X4	T5Ø.5X5	T5Ø.5X6
Dexpanthenol	T45.2X1	T45.2X2	T45.2X3	T45.2X4	T45.2X5	T45.2X6
Dextran (40) (70) (150)	T45.8X1	T45.8X2	T45.8X3	T45.8X4	T45.8X5	T45.8X6
Dextriferron	T45.4X1	T45.4X2	T45.4X3	T45.4X4	T45.4X5	T45.4X6
Dextroamphetamine	T43.621	T43.622	T43.623	T43.624	T43.625	T43.626
Dextro calcium pantothenate	T45.2X1	T45.2X2	T45.2X3	T45.2X4	T45.2X5	T45.2X6
Dextromethorphan	T48.3X1	T48.3X2	T48.3X3	T48.3X4	T48.3X5	T48.3X6
Dextromoramide	T4Ø.4X1	T4Ø.4X2	T4Ø.4X3	T4Ø.4X4	—	—
topical	T49.8X1	T49.8X2	T49.8X3	T49.8X4	T49.8X5	T49.8X6
Dextro pantothenyl alcohol	T45.2X1	T45.2X2	T45.2X3	T45.2X4	T45.2X5	T45.2X6
Dextropropoxyphene	T4Ø.4X1	T4Ø.4X2	T4Ø.4X3	T4Ø.4X4	T4Ø.4X5	T4Ø.4X6
Dextrorphan	T4Ø.2X1	T4Ø.2X2	T4Ø.2X3	T4Ø.2X4	T4Ø.2X5	T4Ø.2X6
Dextrose	T5Ø.3X1	T5Ø.3X2	T5Ø.3X3	T5Ø.3X4	T5Ø.3X5	T5Ø.3X6
concentrated solution, intravenous	T46.8X1	T46.8X2	T46.8X3	T46.8X4	T46.8X5	T46.8X6
Dextrothyroxin	T38.1X1	T38.1X2	T38.1X3	T38.1X4	T38.1X5	T38.1X6
Dextrothyroxine sodium	T38.1X1	T38.1X2	T38.1X3	T38.1X4	T38.1X5	T38.1X6
DFP	T44.ØX1	T44.ØX2	T44.ØX3	T44.ØX4	T44.ØX5	T44.ØX6
DHE	T37.3X1	T37.3X2	T37.3X3	T37.3X4	T37.3X5	T37.3X6
45	T46.5X1	T46.5X2	T46.5X3	T46.5X4	T46.5X5	T46.5X6
Diabinese	T38.3X1	T38.3X2	T38.3X3	T38.3X4	T38.3X5	T38.3X6
Diacetone alcohol	T52.4X1	T52.4X2	T52.4X3	T52.4X4	—	—
Diacetyl monoxime	T5Ø.991	T5Ø.992	T5Ø.993	T5Ø.994	—	—
Diacetylmorphine	T4Ø.1X1	T4Ø.1X2	T4Ø.1X3	T4Ø.1X4	T4Ø.1X5	—
Diachylon plaster	T49.4X1	T49.4X2	T49.4X3	T49.4X4	T49.4X5	T49.4X6
Diaethylstilboestrolum	T38.5X1	T38.5X2	T38.5X3	T38.5X4	T38.5X5	T38.5X6
Diagnostic agent NEC	T5Ø.8X1	T5Ø.8X2	T5Ø.8X3	T5Ø.8X4	T5Ø.8X5	T5Ø.8X6
Dial (soap)	T49.2X1	T49.2X2	T49.2X3	T49.2X4	T49.2X5	T49.2X6
sedative	T42.3X1	T42.3X2	T42.3X3	T42.3X4	T42.3X5	T42.3X6
Dialkyl carbonate	T52.91	T52.92	T52.93	T52.94	—	—
Diallylbarbituric acid	T42.3X1	T42.3X2	T42.3X3	T42.3X4	T42.3X5	T42.3X6
Diallymal	T42.3X1	T42.3X2	T42.3X3	T42.3X4	T42.3X5	T42.3X6
Dialysis solution (intraperitoneal)	T5Ø.3X1	T5Ø.3X2	T5Ø.3X3	T5Ø.3X4	T5Ø.3X5	T5Ø.3X6
Diaminodiphenylsulfone	T37.1X1	T37.1X2	T37.1X3	T37.1X4	T37.1X5	T37.1X6
Diamorphine	T4Ø.1X1	T4Ø.1X2	T4Ø.1X3	T4Ø.1X4	T4Ø.1X5	—
Diamox	T5Ø.2X1	T5Ø.2X2	T5Ø.2X3	T5Ø.2X4	T5Ø.2X5	T5Ø.2X6
Diamthazole	T49.ØX1	T49.ØX2	T49.ØX3	T49.ØX4	T49.ØX5	T49.ØX6
Dianthone	T47.2X1	T47.2X2	T47.2X3	T47.2X4	T47.2X5	T47.2X6
Diaphenylsulfone	T37.ØX1	T37.ØX2	T37.ØX3	T37.ØX4	T37.ØX5	T37.ØX6
Diasone (sodium)	T37.1X1	T37.1X2	T37.1X3	T37.1X4	T37.1X5	T37.1X6
Diastase	T47.5X1	T47.5X2	T47.5X3	T47.5X4	T47.5X5	T47.5X6
Diatrizoate	T5Ø.8X1	T5Ø.8X2	T5Ø.8X3	T5Ø.8X4	T5Ø.8X5	T5Ø.8X6
Diazepam	T42.4X1	T42.4X2	T42.4X3	T42.4X4	T42.4X5	T42.4X6
Diazinon	T6Ø.ØX1	T6Ø.ØX2	T6Ø.ØX3	T6Ø.ØX4	—	—
Diazomethane (gas)	T59.891	T59.892	T59.893	T59.894	—	—
Diazoxide	T46.5X1	T46.5X2	T46.5X3	T46.5X4	T46.5X5	T46.5X6
Dibekacin	T36.5X1	T36.5X2	T36.5X3	T36.5X4	T36.5X5	T36.5X6
Dibenamine	T44.6X1	T44.6X2	T44.6X3	T44.6X4	T44.6X5	T44.6X6

Substance	Poisoning, Accidental (unintentional)	Poisoning, Intentional Self-harm	Poisoning, Assault	Poisoning, Undetermined	Adverse Effect	Under-dosing
Dibenzepin	T43.Ø11	T43.Ø12	T43.Ø13	T43.Ø14	T43.Ø15	T43.Ø16
Dibenzheptropine	T45.ØX1	T45.ØX2	T45.ØX3	T45.ØX4	T45.ØX5	T45.ØX6
Dibenzyline	T44.6X1	T44.6X2	T44.6X3	T44.6X4	T44.6X5	T44.6X6
Diborane (gas)	T59.891	T59.892	T59.893	T59.894	—	—
Dibromochloropropane	T6Ø.8X1	T6Ø.8X2	T6Ø.8X3	T6Ø.8X4	—	—
Dibromodulcitol	T45.1X1	T45.1X2	T45.1X3	T45.1X4	T45.1X5	T45.1X6
Dibromoethane	T53.6X1	T53.6X2	T53.6X3	T53.6X4	—	—
Dibromomannitol	T45.1X1	T45.1X2	T45.1X3	T45.1X4	T45.1X5	T45.1X6
Dibromopropamidine isethionate	T49.ØX1	T49.ØX2	T49.ØX3	T49.ØX4	T49.ØX5	T49.ØX6
Dibrompropamidine	T49.ØX1	T49.ØX2	T49.ØX3	T49.ØX4	T49.ØX5	T49.ØX6
Dibucaine	T41.3X1	T41.3X2	T41.3X3	T41.3X4	T41.3X5	T41.3X6
topical (surface)	T41.3X1	T41.3X2	T41.3X3	T41.3X4	T41.3X5	T41.3X6
Dibunate sodium	T48.3X1	T48.3X2	T48.3X3	T48.3X4	T48.3X5	T48.3X6
Dibutoline sulfate	T44.3X1	T44.3X2	T44.3X3	T44.3X4	T44.3X5	T44.3X6
Dicamba	T6Ø.3X1	T6Ø.3X2	T6Ø.3X3	T6Ø.3X4	—	—
Dicapthon	T6Ø.ØX1	T6Ø.ØX2	T6Ø.ØX3	T6Ø.ØX4	—	—
Dichlobenil	T6Ø.3X1	T6Ø.3X2	T6Ø.3X3	T6Ø.3X4	—	—
Dichlone	T6Ø.3X1	T6Ø.3X2	T6Ø.3X3	T6Ø.3X4	—	—
Dichloralphenozone	T42.6X1	T42.6X2	T42.6X3	T42.6X4	T42.6X5	T42.6X6
Dichlorbenzidine	T65.3X1	T65.3X2	T65.3X3	T65.3X4	—	—
Dichlorhydrin	T52.8X1	T52.8X2	T52.8X3	T52.8X4	—	—
Dichlorhydroxyquinoline	T37.8X1	T37.8X2	T37.8X3	T37.8X4	T37.8X5	T37.8X6
Dichlorobenzene	T53.7X1	T53.7X2	T53.7X3	T53.7X4	—	—
Dichlorobenzyl alcohol	T49.6X1	T49.6X2	T49.6X3	T49.6X4	T49.6X5	T49.6X6
Dichlorodifluoromethane	T53.5X1	T53.5X2	T53.5X3	T53.5X4	—	—
Dichloroethane	T52.8X1	T52.8X2	T52.8X3	T52.8X4	—	—
Sym-Dichloroethyl ether	T53.6X1	T53.6X2	T53.6X3	T536X4	—	—
Dichloroethyl sulfide, not in war	T59.891	T59.892	T59.893	T59.894	—	—
Dichloroethylene	T53.6X1	T53.6X2	T53.6X3	T53.6X4	—	—
Dichloroformoxine, not in war	T59.891	T59.892	T59.893	T59.894	—	—
Dichlorohydrin, alpha-dichlorohydrin	T52.8X1	T52.8X2	T52.8X3	T52.8X4	—	—
Dichloromethane (solvent)	T53.4X1	T53.4X2	T53.4X3	T53.4X4	—	—
vapor	T53.4X1	T53.4X2	T53.4X3	T53.4X4	—	—
Dichloronaphthoquinone	T6Ø.3X1	T6Ø.3X2	T6Ø.3X3	T6Ø.3X4	—	—
Dichlorophen	T37.4X1	T37.4X2	T37.4X3	T37.4X4	T37.4X5	T37.4X6
2,4-Dichlorophenoxyacetic acid	T6Ø.3X1	T6Ø.3X2	T6Ø.3X3	T6Ø.3X4	—	—
Dichloropropene	T6Ø.3X1	T6Ø.3X2	T6Ø.3X3	T6Ø.3X4	—	—
Dichloropropionic acid	T6Ø.3X1	T6Ø.3X2	T6Ø.3X3	T6Ø.3X4	—	—
Dichlorphenamide	T5Ø.2X1	T5Ø.2X2	T5Ø.2X3	T5Ø.2X4	T5Ø.2X5	T5Ø.2X6
Dichlorvos	T6Ø.ØX1	T6Ø.ØX2	T6Ø.ØX3	T6Ø.ØX4	—	—
Diclofenac	T39.391	T39.392	T39.393	T39.394	T39.395	T39.396
Diclofenamide	T5Ø.2X1	T5Ø.2X2	T5Ø.2X3	T5Ø.2X4	T5Ø.2X5	T5Ø.2X6
Diclofensine	T43.291	T43.292	T43.293	T43.294	T43.295	T43.296
Diclonixine	T39.8X1	T39.8X2	T39.8X3	T39.8X4	T39.8X5	T39.8X6
Dicloxacillin	T36.ØX1	T36.ØX2	T36.ØX3	T36.ØX4	T36.ØX5	T36.ØX6
Dicophane	T49.ØX1	T49.ØX2	T49.ØX3	T49.ØX4	T49.ØX5	T49.ØX6
Dicoumarol, dicoumarin, dicumarol	T45.511	T45.512	T45.513	T45.514	T45.515	T45.516
Dicrotophos	T6Ø.ØX1	T6Ø.ØX2	T6Ø.ØX3	T6Ø.ØX4	—	—
Dicyanogen (gas)	T65.ØX1	T65.ØX2	T65.ØX3	T65.ØX4	—	—
Dicyclomine	T44.3X1	T44.3X2	T44.3X3	T44.3X4	T44.3X5	T44.3X6
Dicycloverine	T44.3X1	T44.3X2	T44.3X3	T44.3X4	T44.3X5	T44.3X6
Dideoxycytidine	T37.5X1	T37.5X2	T37.5X3	T37.5X4	T37.5X5	T37.5X6
Dideoxyinosine	T37.5X1	T37.5X2	T37.5X3	T37.5X4	T37.5X5	T37.5X6
Dieldrin (vapor)	T6Ø.1X1	T6Ø.1X2	T6Ø.1X3	T6Ø.1X4	—	—
Diemal	T42.3X1	T42.3X2	T42.3X3	T42.3X4	T42.3X5	T42.3X6
Dienestrol	T38.5X1	T38.5X2	T38.5X3	T38.5X4	T38.5X5	T38.5X6
Dienoestrol	T38.5X1	T38.5X2	T38.5X3	T38.5X4	T38.5X5	T38.5X6
Dietetic drug NEC	T5Ø.9Ø1	T5Ø.9Ø2	T5Ø.9Ø3	T5Ø.9Ø4	T5Ø.9Ø5	T5Ø.9Ø6
Diethazine	T42.8X1	T42.8X2	T42.8X3	T42.8X4	T42.8X5	T42.8X6
Diethyl						
barbituric acid	T42.3X1	T42.3X2	T42.3X3	T42.3X4	T42.3X5	T42.3X6
carbamazine	T37.4X1	T37.4X2	T37.4X3	T37.4X4	T37.4X5	T37.4X6
carbinol	T51.3X1	T51.3X2	T51.3X3	T51.3X4	—	—
carbonate	T52.8X1	T52.8X2	T52.8X3	T52.8X4	—	—
ether (vapor) (*see also* ether)	T41.ØX1	T41.ØX2	T41.ØX3	T41.ØX4	T41.ØX5	T41.ØX6
Diethyl— *continued*						
oxide	T52.8X1	T52.8X2	T52.8X3	T52.8X4	—	—
propion	T5Ø.5X1	T5Ø.5X2	T5Ø.5X3	T5Ø.5X4	T5Ø.5X5	T5Ø.5X6
stilbestrol	T38.5X1	T38.5X2	T38.5X3	T38.5X4	T38.5X5	T38.5X6
toluamide (nonmedicinal)	T6Ø.8X1	T6Ø.8X2	T6Ø.8X3	T6Ø.8X4	—	—
medicinal	T49.3X1	T49.3X2	T49.3X3	T49.3X4	T49.3X5	T49.3X6
Diethylcarbamazine	T37.4X1	T37.4X2	T37.4X3	T37.4X4	T37.4X5	T37.4X6
Diethylene						
dioxide	T52.8X1	T52.8X2	T52.8X3	T52.8X4	—	—
glycol (monoacetate) (monobutyl ether) (monoethyl ether)	T52.3X1	T52.3X2	T52.3X3	T52.3X4	—	—
Diethylhexylphthalate	T65.891	T65.892	T65.893	T65.894	—	—
Diethylpropion	T5Ø.5X1	T5Ø.5X2	T5Ø.5X3	T5Ø.5X4	T5Ø.5X5	T5Ø.5X6
Diethylstilbestrol	T38.5X1	T38.5X2	T38.5X3	T38.5X4	T38.5X5	T38.5X6
Diethylstilboestrol	T38.5X1	T38.5X2	T38.5X3	T38.5X4	T38.5X5	T38.5X6
Diethylsulfone-diethylmethane	T42.6X1	T42.6X2	T42.6X3	T42.6X4	T42.6X5	T42.6X6
Diethyltoluamide	T49.ØX1	T49.ØX2	T49.ØX3	T49.ØX4	T49.ØX5	T49.ØX6
Diethyltryptamine (DET)	T4Ø.991	T4Ø.992	T4Ø.993	T4Ø.994	—	—
Difebarbamate	T42.3X1	T42.3X2	T42.3X3	T42.3X4	T42.3X5	T42.3X6
Difencloxazine	T4Ø.2X1	T4Ø.2X2	T4Ø.2X3	T4Ø.2X4	T4Ø.2X5	T4Ø.2X6
Difenidol	T45.ØX1	T45.ØX2	T45.ØX3	T45.ØX4	T45.ØX5	T45.ØX6
Difenoxin	T47.6X1	T47.6X2	T47.6X3	T47.6X4	T47.6X5	T47.6X6
Difetarsone	T37.3X1	T37.3X2	T37.3X3	T37.3X4	T37.3X5	T37.3X6
Diffusin	T45.3X1	T45.3X2	T45.3X3	T45.3X4	T45.3X5	T45.3X6
Diflorasone	T49.ØX1	T49.ØX2	T49.ØX3	T49.ØX4	T49.ØX5	T49.ØX6
Diflubenzuron	T6Ø.1X1	T6Ø.1X2	T6Ø.1X3	T6Ø.1X4	—	—
Diflos	T44.ØX1	T44.ØX2	T44.ØX3	T44.ØX4	T44.ØX5	T44.ØX6
Diflucortolone	T49.ØX1	T49.ØX2	T49.ØX3	T49.ØX4	T49.ØX5	T49.ØX6
Diflunisal	T39.Ø91	T39.Ø92	T39.Ø93	T39.Ø94	T39.Ø95	T39.Ø96
Difluoromethyldopa	T42.8X1	T42.8X2	T42.8X3	T42.8X4	T42.8X5	T42.8X6
Difluorophate	T44.ØX1	T44.ØX2	T44.ØX3	T44.ØX4	T44.ØX5	T44.ØX6
Digestant NEC	T47.5X1	T47.5X2	T47.5X3	T47.5X4	T47.5X5	T47.5X6
Digitalin(e)	T46.ØX1	T46.ØX2	T46.ØX3	T46.ØX4	T46.ØX5	T46.ØX6
Digitalis (leaf)(glycoside)	T46.ØX1	T46.ØX2	T46.ØX3	T46.ØX4	T46.ØX5	T46.ØX6
lanata	T46.ØX1	T46.ØX2	T46.ØX3	T46.ØX4	T46.ØX5	T46.ØX6
purpurea	T46.ØX1	T46.ØX2	T46.ØX3	T46.ØX4	T46.ØX5	T46.ØX6
Digitoxin	T46.ØX1	T46.ØX2	T46.ØX3	T46.ØX4	T46.ØX5	T46.ØX6
Digitoxose	T46.ØX1	T46.ØX2	T46.ØX3	T46.ØX4	T46.ØX5	T46.ØX6
Digoxin	T46.ØX1	T46.ØX2	T46.ØX3	T46.ØX4	T46.ØX5	T46.ØX6
Digoxine	T46.ØX1	T46.ØX2	T46.ØX3	T46.ØX4	T46.ØX5	T46.ØX6
Dihydralazine	T46.5X1	T46.5X2	T46.5X3	T46.5X4	T46.5X5	T46.5X6
Dihydrazine	T46.5X1	T46.5X2	T46.5X3	T46.5X4	T46.5X5	T46.5X6
Dihydrocodeine	T4Ø.2X1	T4Ø.2X2	T4Ø.2X3	T4Ø.2X4	T4Ø.2X5	T4Ø.2X6
Dihydrocodeinone	T4Ø.2X1	T4Ø.2X2	T4Ø.2X3	T4Ø.2X4	T4Ø.2X5	T4Ø.2X6
Dihydroergocornine	T46.7X1	T46.7X2	T46.7X3	T46.7X4	T46.7X5	T46.7X6
Dihydroergocristine (mesilate)	T46.7X1	T46.7X2	T46.7X3	T46.7X4	T46.7X5	T46.7X6
Dihydroergokryptine	T46.7X1	T46.7X2	T46.7X3	T46.7X4	T46.7X5	T46.7X6
Dihydroergotamine	T46.5X1	T46.5X2	T46.5X3	T46.5X4	T46.5X5	T46.5X6
Dihydroergotoxine	T46.7X1	T46.7X2	T46.7X3	T46.7X4	T46.7X5	T46.7X6
mesilate	T46.7X1	T46.7X2	T46.7X3	T46.7X4	T46.7X5	T46.7X6
Dihydrohydroxycodeinone	T4Ø.2X1	T4Ø.2X2	T4Ø.2X3	T4Ø.2X4	T4Ø.2X5	T4Ø.2X6
Dihydrohydroxymorphinone	T4Ø.2X1	T4Ø.2X2	T4Ø.2X3	T4Ø.2X4	T4Ø.2X5	T4Ø.2X6
Dihydroisocodeine	T4Ø.2X1	T4Ø.2X2	T4Ø.2X3	T4Ø.2X4	T4Ø.2X5	T4Ø.2X6
Dihydromorphine	T4Ø.2X1	T4Ø.2X2	T4Ø.2X3	T4Ø.2X4	—	—
Dihydromorphinone	T4Ø.2X1	T4Ø.2X2	T4Ø.2X3	T4Ø.2X4	T4Ø.2X5	T4Ø.2X6
Dihydrostreptomycin	T36.5X1	T36.5X2	T36.5X3	T36.5X4	T36.5X5	T36.5X6
Dihydrotachysterol	T45.2X1	T45.2X2	T45.2X3	T45.2X4	T45.2X5	T45.2X6
Dihydroxyaluminum aminoacetate	T47.1X1	T47.1X2	T47.1X3	T47.1X4	T47.1X5	T47.1X6
Dihydroxyaluminum sodium carbonate	T47.1X1	T47.1X2	T47.1X3	T47.1X4	T47.1X5	T47.1X6
Dihydroxyanthraquinone	T47.2X1	T47.2X2	T47.2X3	T47.2X4	T47.2X5	T47.2X6
Dihydroxycodeinone	T4Ø.2X1	T4Ø.2X2	T4Ø.2X3	T4Ø.2X4	T4Ø.2X5	T4Ø.2X6
Dihydroxypropyl theophylline	T5Ø.2X1	T5Ø.2X2	T5Ø.2X3	T5Ø.2X4	T5Ø.2X5	T5Ø.2X6
Diiodohydroxyquin	T37.8X1	T37.8X2	T37.8X3	T37.8X4	T37.8X5	T37.8X6
topical	T49.ØX1	T49.ØX2	T49.ØX3	T49.ØX4	T49.ØX5	T49.ØX6
Diiodohydroxyquinoline	T37.8X1	T37.8X2	T37.8X3	T37.8X4	T37.8X5	T37.8X6
Diiodotyrosine	T38.2X1	T38.2X2	T38.2X3	T38.2X4	T38.2X5	T38.2X6
Diisopromine	T44.3X1	T44.3X2	T44.3X3	T44.3X4	T44.3X5	T44.3X6
Diisopropylamine	T46.3X1	T46.3X2	T46.3X3	T46.3X4	T46.3X5	T46.3X6

Substance	Poisoning, Accidental (unintentional)	Poisoning, Intentional Self-harm	Poisoning, Assault	Poisoning, Undetermined	Adverse Effect	Under-dosing
Diisopropylfluorophosphonate	T44.ØX1	T44.ØX2	T44.ØX3	T44.ØX4	T44.ØX5	T44.ØX6
Dilantin	T42.ØX1	T42.ØX2	T42.ØX3	T42.ØX4	T42.ØX5	T42.ØX6
Dilaudid	T4Ø.2X1	T4Ø.2X2	T4Ø.2X3	T4Ø.2X4	T4Ø.2X5	T4Ø.2X6
Dilazep	T46.3X1	T46.3X2	T46.3X3	T46.3X4	T46.3X5	T46.3X6
Dill	T47.5X1	T47.5X2	T47.5X3	T47.5X4	T47.5X5	T47.5X6
Diloxanide	T37.3X1	T37.3X2	T37.3X3	T37.3X4	T37.3X5	T37.3X6
Diltiazem	T46.1X1	T46.1X2	T46.1X3	T46.1X4	T46.1X5	T46.1X6
Dimazole	T49.ØX1	T49.ØX2	T49.ØX3	T49.ØX4	T49.ØX5	T49.ØX6
Dimefline	T5Ø.7X1	T5Ø.7X2	T5Ø.7X3	T5Ø.7X4	T5Ø.7X5	T5Ø.7X6
Dimefox	T6Ø.ØX1	T6Ø.ØX2	T6Ø.ØX3	T6Ø.ØX4	—	—
Dimemorfan	T48.3X1	T48.3X2	T48.3X3	T48.3X4	T48.3X5	T48.3X6
Dimenhydrinate	T45.ØX1	T45.ØX2	T45.ØX3	T45.ØX4	T45.ØX5	T45.ØX6
Dimercaprol (British anti-lewisite)	T45.8X1	T45.8X2	T45.8X3	T45.8X4	T45.8X5	T45.8X6
Dimercaptopropanol	T45.8X1	T45.8X2	T45.8X3	T45.8X4	T45.8X5	T45.8X6
Dimestrol	T38.5X1	T38.5X2	T38.5X3	T38.5X4	T38.5X5	T38.5X6
Dimetane	T45.ØX1	T45.ØX2	T45.ØX3	T45.ØX4	T45.ØX5	T45.ØX6
Dimethicone	T47.1X1	T47.1X2	T47.1X3	T47.1X4	T47.1X5	T47.1X6
Dimethindene	T45.ØX1	T45.ØX2	T45.ØX3	T45.ØX4	T45.ØX5	T45.ØX6
Dimethisoquin	T49.1X1	T49.1X2	T49.1X3	T49.1X4	T49.1X5	T49.1X6
Dimethisterone	T38.5X1	T38.5X2	T38.5X3	T38.5X4	T38.5X5	T38.5X6
Dimethoate	T6Ø.ØX1	T6Ø.ØX2	T6Ø.ØX3	T6Ø.ØX4	—	—
Dimethocaine	T41.3X1	T41.3X2	T41.3X3	T41.3X4	T41.3X5	T41.3X6
Dimethoxanate	T48.3X1	T48.3X2	T48.3X3	T48.3X4	T48.3X5	T48.3X6
Dimethyl						
arsine, arsinic acid	T57.ØX1	T57.ØX2	T57.ØX3	T57.ØX4	—	—
carbinol	T51.2X1	T51.2X2	T51.2X3	T51.2X4	—	—
carbonate	T52.8X1	T52.8X2	T52.8X3	T52.8X4	—	—
diguanide	T38.3X1	T38.3X2	T38.3X3	T38.3X4	T38.3X5	T38.3X6
ketone	T52.4X1	T52.4X2	T52.4X3	T52.4X4	—	—
vapor	T52.4X1	T52.4X2	T52.4X3	T52.4X4	—	—
meperidine	T4Ø.2X1	T4Ø.2X2	T4Ø.2X3	T4Ø.2X4	T4Ø.2X5	T4Ø.2X6
parathion	T6Ø.ØX1	T6Ø.ØX2	T6Ø.ØX3	T6Ø.ØX4	—	—
phthlate	T49.3X1	T49.3X2	T49.3X3	T49.3X4	T49.3X5	T49.3X6
polysiloxane	T47.8X1	T47.8X2	T47.8X3	T47.8X4	T47.8X5	T47.8X6
sulfate (fumes)	T59.891	T59.892	T59.893	T59.894	—	—
liquid	T65.891	T65.892	T65.893	T65.894	—	—
sulfoxide (nonmedicinal)	T52.8X1	T52.8X2	T52.8X3	T52.8X4	—	—
medicinal	T49.4X1	T49.4X2	T49.4X3	T49.4X4	T49.4X5	T49.4X6
tryptamine	T4Ø.991	T4Ø.992	T4Ø.993	T4Ø.994	—	—
tubocurarine	T48.1X1	T48.1X2	T48.1X3	T48.1X4	T48.1X5	T48.1X6
Dimethylamine sulfate	T49.4X1	T49.4X2	T49.4X3	T49.4X4	T49.4X5	T49.4X6
Dimethylformamide	T52.8X1	T52.8X2	T52.8X3	T52.8X4	—	—
Dimethyltubocurarinium chloride	T48.1X1	T48.1X2	T48.1X3	T48.1X4	T48.1X5	T48.1X6
Dimeticone	T47.1X1	T47.1X2	T47.1X3	T47.1X4	T47.1X5	T47.1X6
Dimetilan	T6Ø.ØX1	T6Ø.ØX2	T6Ø.ØX3	T6Ø.ØX4	—	—
Dimetindene	T45.ØX1	T45.ØX2	T45.ØX3	T45.ØX4	T45.ØX5	T45.ØX6
Dimetotiazine	T43.3X1	T43.3X2	T43.3X3	T43.3X4	T43.3X5	T43.3X6
Dimorpholamine	T5Ø.7X1	T5Ø.7X2	T5Ø.7X3	T5Ø.7X4	T5Ø.7X5	T5Ø.7X6
Dimoxyline	T46.3X1	T46.3X2	T46.3X3	T46.3X4	T46.3X5	T46.3X6
Dinitrobenzene	T65.3X1	T65.3X2	T65.3X3	T65.3X4	—	—
vapor	T59.891	T59.892	T59.893	T59.894	—	—
Dinitrobenzol	T65.3X1	T65.3X2	T65.3X3	T65.3X4	—	—
vapor	T59.891	T59.892	T59.893	T59.894	—	—
Dinitrobutylphenol	T65.3X1	T65.3X2	T65.3X3	T65.3X4	—	—
Dinitro(-ortho-)cresol (pesticide) (spray)	T65.3X1	T65.3X2	T65.3X3	T65.3X4	—	—
Dinitrocyclohexylphenol	T65.3X1	T65.3X2	T65.3X3	T65.3X4	—	—
Dinitrophenol	T65.3X1	T65.3X2	T65.3X3	T65.3X4	—	—
Dinoprost	T48.ØX1	T48.ØX2	T48.ØX3	T48.ØX4	T48.ØX5	T48.ØX6
Dinoprostone	T48.ØX1	T48.ØX2	T48.ØX3	T48.ØX4	T48.ØX5	T48.ØX6
Dinoseb	T6Ø.3X1	T6Ø.3X2	T6Ø.3X3	T6Ø.3X4	—	—
Dioctyl sulfosuccinate (calcium) (sodium)	T47.4X1	T47.4X2	T47.4X3	T47.4X4	T47.4X5	T47.4X6
Diodone	T5Ø.8X1	T5Ø.8X2	T5Ø.8X3	T5Ø.8X4	T5Ø.8X5	T5Ø.8X6
Diodoquin	T37.8X1	T37.8X2	T37.8X3	T37.8X4	T37.8X5	T37.8X6
Dionin	T4Ø.2X1	T4Ø.2X2	T4Ø.2X3	T4Ø.2X4	T4Ø.2X5	T4Ø.2X6
Diosmin	T46.991	T46.992	T46.993	T46.994	T46.995	T46.996
Dioxane	T52.8X1	T52.8X2	T52.8X3	T52.8X4	—	—
Dioxathion	T6Ø.ØX1	T6Ø.ØX2	T6Ø.ØX3	T6Ø.ØX4	—	—
Dioxin	T53.7X1	T53.7X2	T53.7X3	T53.7X4	—	—
Dioxopromethazine	T43.3X1	T43.3X2	T43.3X3	T43.3X4	T43.3X5	T43.3X6
Dioxyline	T46.3X1	T46.3X2	T46.3X3	T46.3X4	T46.3X5	T46.3X6
Dipentene	T52.8X1	T52.8X2	T52.8X3	T52.8X4	—	—
Diperodon	T41.3X1	T41.3X2	T41.3X3	T41.3X4	T41.3X5	T41.3X6
Diphacinone	T6Ø.4X1	T6Ø.4X2	T6Ø.4X3	T6Ø.4X4	—	—
Diphemanil	T44.3X1	T44.3X2	T44.3X3	T44.3X4	T44.3X5	T44.3X6
metilsulfate	T44.3X1	T44.3X2	T44.3X3	T44.3X4	T44.3X5	T44.3X6
Diphenadione	T45.511	T45.512	T45.513	T45.514	T45.515	T45.516
rodenticide	T6Ø.4X1	T6Ø.4X2	T6Ø.4X3	T6Ø.4X4	—	—
Diphenhydramine	T45.ØX1	T45.ØX2	T45.ØX3	T45.ØX4	T45.ØX5	T45.ØX6
Diphenidol	T45.ØX1	T45.ØX2	T45.ØX3	T45.ØX4	T45.ØX5	T45.ØX6
Diphenoxylate	T47.6X1	T47.6X2	T47.6X3	T47.6X4	T47.6X5	T47.6X6
Diphenylamine	T65.3X1	T65.3X2	T65.3X3	T65.3X4	—	—
Diphenylbutazone	T39.2X1	T39.2X2	T39.2X3	T39.2X4	T39.2X5	T39.2X6
Diphenylchloroarsine, not in war	T57.ØX1	T57.ØX2	T57.ØX3	T57.ØX4	—	—
Diphenylhydantoin	T42.ØX1	T42.ØX2	T42.ØX3	T42.ØX4	T42.ØX5	T42.ØX6
Diphenylmethane dye	T52.1X1	T52.1X2	T52.1X3	T52.1X4	—	—
Diphenylpyraline	T45.ØX1	T45.ØX2	T45.ØX3	T45.ØX4	T45.ØX5	T45.ØX6
Diphtheria						
antitoxin	T5Ø.Z11	T5Ø.Z12	T5Ø.Z13	T5Ø.Z14	T5Ø.Z15	T5Ø.Z16
toxoid	T5Ø.A91	T5Ø.A92	T5Ø.A93	T5Ø.A94	T5Ø.A95	T5Ø.A96
with tetanus toxoid	T5Ø.A21	T5Ø.A22	T5Ø.A23	T5Ø.A24	T5Ø.A25	T5Ø.A26
with pertussis component	T5Ø.A11	T5Ø.A12	T5Ø.A13	T5Ø.A14	T5Ø.A15	T5Ø.A16
vaccine	T5Ø.A91	T5Ø.A92	T5Ø.A93	T5Ø.A94	T5Ø.A95	T5Ø.A96
combination						
including pertussis	T5Ø.A11	T5Ø.A12	T5Ø.A13	T5Ø.A14	T5Ø.A15	T5Ø.A16
without pertussis	T5Ø.A21	T5Ø.A22	T5Ø.A23	T5Ø.A24	T5Ø.A25	T5Ø.A26
Diphylline	T5Ø.2X1	T5Ø.2X2	T5Ø.2X3	T5Ø.2X4	T5Ø.2X5	T5Ø.2X6
Dipipanone	T4Ø.4X1	T4Ø.4X2	T4Ø.4X3	T4Ø.4X4	—	—
Dipivefrine	T49.5X1	T49.5X2	T49.5X3	T49.5X4	T49.5X5	T49.5X6
Diplovax	T5Ø.B91	T5Ø.B92	T5Ø.B93	T5Ø.B94	T5Ø.B95	T5Ø.B96
Diprophylline	T5Ø.2X1	T5Ø.2X2	T5Ø.2X3	T5Ø.2X4	T5Ø.2X5	T5Ø.2X6
Dipropyline	T48.291	T48.292	T48.293	T48.294	T48.295	T48.296
Dipyridamole	T46.3X1	T46.3X2	T46.3X3	T46.3X4	T46.3X5	T46.3X6
Dipyrone	T39.2X1	T39.2X2	T39.2X3	T39.2X4	T39.2X5	T39.2X6
Diquat (dibromide)	T6Ø.3X1	T6Ø.3X2	T6Ø.3X3	T6Ø.3X4	—	—
Disinfectant	T65.891	T65.892	T65.893	T65.894	—	—
alkaline	T54.3X1	T54.3X2	T54.3X3	T54.3X4	—	—
aromatic	T54.1X1	T54.1X2	T54.1X3	T54.1X4	—	—
intestinal	T37.8X1	T37.8X2	T37.8X3	T37.8X4	T37.8X5	T37.8X6
Disipal	T42.8X1	T42.8X2	T42.8X3	T42.8X4	T42.8X5	T42.8X6
Disodium edetate	T5Ø.6X1	T5Ø.6X2	T5Ø.6X3	T5Ø.6X4	T5Ø.6X5	T5Ø.6X6
Disoprofol	T41.291	T41.292	T41.293	T41.294	T41.295	T41.296
Disopyramide	T46.2X1	T46.2X2	T46.2X3	T46.2X4	T46.2X5	T46.2X6
Distigmine (bromide)	T44.ØX1	T44.ØX2	T44.ØX3	T44.ØX4	T44.ØX5	T44.ØX6
Disulfamide	T5Ø.2X1	T5Ø.2X2	T5Ø.2X3	T5Ø.2X4	T5Ø.2X5	T5Ø.2X6
Disulfanilamide	T37.ØX1	T37.ØX2	T37.ØX3	T37.ØX4	T37.ØX5	T37.ØX6
Disulfiram	T5Ø.6X1	T5Ø.6X2	T5Ø.6X3	T5Ø.6X4	T5Ø.6X5	T5Ø.6X6
Disulfoton	T6Ø.ØX1	T6Ø.ØX2	T6Ø.ØX3	T6Ø.ØX4	—	—
Dithiazanine iodide	T37.4X1	T37.4X2	T37.4X3	T37.4X4	T37.4X5	T37.4X6
Dithiocarbamate	T6Ø.ØX1	T6Ø.ØX2	T6Ø.ØX3	T6Ø.ØX4	—	—
Dithranol	T49.4X1	T49.4X2	T49.4X3	T49.4X4	T49.4X5	T49.4X6
Diucardin	T5Ø.2X1	T5Ø.2X2	T5Ø.2X3	T5Ø.2X4	T5Ø.2X5	T5Ø.2X6
Diupres	T5Ø.2X1	T5Ø.2X2	T5Ø.2X3	T5Ø.2X4	T5Ø.2X5	T5Ø.2X6
Diuretic NEC	T5Ø.2X1	T5Ø.2X2	T5Ø.2X3	T5Ø.2X4	T5Ø.2X5	T5Ø.2X6
carbonic acid anhydrase inhibitors	T5Ø.2X1	T5Ø.2X2	T5Ø.2X3	T5Ø.2X4	T5Ø.2X5	T5Ø.2X6
benzothiadiazine	T5Ø.2X1	T5Ø.2X2	T5Ø.2X3	T5Ø.2X4	T5Ø.2X5	T5Ø.2X6
furfuryl NEC	T5Ø.2X1	T5Ø.2X2	T5Ø.2X3	T5Ø.2X4	T5Ø.2X5	T5Ø.2X6
loop (high-ceiling)	T5Ø.1X1	T5Ø.1X2	T5Ø.1X3	T5Ø.1X4	T5Ø.1X5	T5Ø.1X6
mercurial NEC	T5Ø.2X1	T5Ø.2X2	T5Ø.2X3	T5Ø.2X4	T5Ø.2X5	T5Ø.2X6
osmotic	T5Ø.2X1	T5Ø.2X2	T5Ø.2X3	T5Ø.2X4	T5Ø.2X5	T5Ø.2X6
purine NEC	T5Ø.2X1	T5Ø.2X2	T5Ø.2X3	T5Ø.2X4	T5Ø.2X5	T5Ø.2X6
saluretic NEC	T5Ø.2X1	T5Ø.2X2	T5Ø.2X3	T5Ø.2X4	T5Ø.2X5	T5Ø.2X6
sulfonamide	T5Ø.2X1	T5Ø.2X2	T5Ø.2X3	T5Ø.2X4	T5Ø.2X5	T5Ø.2X6
thiazide NEC	T5Ø.2X1	T5Ø.2X2	T5Ø.2X3	T5Ø.2X4	T5Ø.2X5	T5Ø.2X6
xanthine	T5Ø.2X1	T5Ø.2X2	T5Ø.2X3	T5Ø.2X4	T5Ø.2X5	T5Ø.2X6
Diurgin	T5Ø.2X1	T5Ø.2X2	T5Ø.2X3	T5Ø.2X4	T5Ø.2X5	T5Ø.2X6
Diuril	T5Ø.2X1	T5Ø.2X2	T5Ø.2X3	T5Ø.2X4	T5Ø.2X5	T5Ø.2X6

Substance	Poisoning, Accidental (unintentional)	Poisoning, Intentional Self-harm	Poisoning, Assault	Poisoning, Undetermined	Adverse Effect	Under-dosing
Diuron	T60.3X1	T60.3X2	T60.3X3	T60.3X4	—	—
Divalproex	T42.6X1	T42.6X2	T42.6X3	T42.6X4	T42.6X5	T42.6X6
Divinyl ether	T41.0X1	T41.0X2	T41.0X3	T41.0X4	T41.0X5	T41.0X6
Dixanthogen	T49.0X1	T49.0X2	T49.0X3	T49.0X4	T49.0X5	T49.0X6
Dixyrazine	T43.3X1	T43.3X2	T43.3X3	T43.3X4	T43.3X5	T43.3X6
D-lysergic acid diethylamide	T40.8X1	T40.8X2	T40.8X3	T40.8X4	T40.8X5	—
DMCT	T36.4X1	T36.4X2	T36.4X3	T36.4X4	T36.4X5	—
DMSO—*see* Dimethyl sulfoxide						
DNBP	T60.3X1	T60.3X2	T60.3X3	T60.3X4	—	—
DNOC	T65.3X1	T65.3X2	T65.3X3	T65.3X4	—	—
DOCA	T38.0X1	T38.0X2	T38.0X3	T38.0X4	T38.0X5	T38.0X6
Dobutamine	T44.5X1	T44.5X2	T44.5X3	T44.5X4	T44.5X5	T44.5X6
Docusate sodium	T47.4X1	T47.4X2	T47.4X3	T47.4X4	T47.4X5	T47.4X6
Dodicin	T49.0X1	T49.0X2	T49.0X3	T49.0X4	T49.0X5	T49.0X6
Dofamium chloride	T49.0X1	T49.0X2	T49.0X3	T49.0X4	T49.0X5	T49.0X6
Dolophine	T40.3X1	T40.3X2	T40.3X3	T40.3X4	T40.3X5	T40.3X6
Doloxene	T39.8X1	T39.8X2	T39.8X3	T39.8X4	T39.8X5	T39.8X6
Domestic gas (after combustion)—*see* Gas, utility						
prior to combustion	T59.891	T59.892	T59.893	T59.894	—	—
Domiodol	T48.4X1	T48.4X2	T48.4X3	T48.4X4	T48.4X5	T48.4X6
Domiphen (bromide)	T49.0X1	T49.0X2	T49.0X3	T49.0X4	T49.0X5	T49.0X6
Domperidone	T45.0X1	T45.0X2	T45.0X3	T45.0X4	T45.0X5	T45.0X6
Dopa	T42.8X1	T42.8X2	T42.8X3	T42.8X4	T42.8X5	T42.8X6
Dopamine	T44.991	T44.992	T44.993	T44.994	T44.995	T44.996
Doriden	T42.6X1	T42.6X2	T42.6X3	T42.6X4	T42.6X5	T42.6X6
Dormiral	T42.3X1	T42.3X2	T42.3X3	T42.3X4	T42.3X5	T42.3X6
Dormison	T42.6X1	T42.6X2	T42.6X3	T42.6X4	T42.6X5	T42.6X6
Dornase	T48.4X1	T48.4X2	T48.4X3	T48.4X4	T48.4X5	T48.4X6
Dorsacaine	T41.3X1	T41.3X2	T41.3X3	T41.3X4	T41.3X5	T41.3X6
Dosulepin	T43.011	T43.012	T43.013	T43.014	T43.015	T43.016
Dothiepin	T43.011	T43.012	T43.013	T43.014	T43.015	T43.016
Doxantrazole	T48.6X1	T48.6X2	T48.6X3	T48.6X4	T48.6X5	T48.6X6
Doxapram	T50.7X1	T50.7X2	T50.7X3	T50.7X4	T50.7X5	T50.7X6
Doxazosin	T44.6X1	T44.6X2	T44.6X3	T44.6X4	T44.6X5	T44.6X6
Doxepin	T43.011	T43.012	T43.013	T43.014	T43.015	T43.016
Doxifluridine	T45.1X1	T45.1X2	T45.1X3	T45.1X4	T45.1X5	T45.1X6
Doxorubicin	T45.1X1	T45.1X2	T45.1X3	T45.1X4	T45.1X5	T45.1X6
Doxycycline	T36.4X1	T36.4X2	T36.4X3	T36.4X4	T36.4X5	T36.4X6
Doxylamine	T45.0X1	T45.0X2	T45.0X3	T45.0X4	T45.0X5	T45.0X6
Dramamine	T45.0X1	T45.0X2	T45.0X3	T45.0X4	T45.0X5	T45.0X6
Drano (drain cleaner)	T54.3X1	T54.3X2	T54.3X3	T54.3X4	—	—
Dressing, live pulp	T49.7X1	T49.7X2	T49.7X3	T49.7X4	T49.7X5	T49.7X6
Drocode	T40.2X1	T40.2X2	T40.2X3	T40.2X4	T40.2X5	T40.2X6
Dromoran	T40.2X1	T40.2X2	T40.2X3	T40.2X4	T40.2X5	T40.2X6
Dromostanolone	T38.7X1	T38.7X2	T38.7X3	T38.7X4	T38.7X5	T38.7X6
Dronabinol	T40.7X1	T40.7X2	T40.7X3	T40.7X4	T40.7X5	T40.7X6
Droperidol	T43.591	T43.592	T43.593	T43.594	T43.595	T43.596
Dropropizine	T48.3X1	T48.3X2	T48.3X3	T48.3X4	T48.3X5	T48.3X6
Drostanolone	T38.7X1	T38.7X2	T38.7X3	T38.7X4	T38.7X5	T38.7X6
Drotaverine	T44.3X1	T44.3X2	T44.3X3	T44.3X4	T44.3X5	T44.3X6
Drotrecogin alfa	T45.511	T45.512	T45.513	T45.514	T45.515	T45.516
Drug NEC	T50.901	T50.902	T50.903	T50.904	T50.905	T50.906
specified NEC	T50.991	T50.992	T50.993	T50.994	T50.995	T50.996
DTIC	T45.1X1	T45.1X2	T45.1X3	T45.1X4	T45.1X5	T45.1X6
Duboisine	T44.3X1	T44.3X2	T44.3X3	T44.3X4	T44.3X5	T44.3X6
Dulcolax	T47.2X1	T47.2X2	T47.2X3	T47.2X4	T47.2X5	T47.2X6
Duponol (C) (EP)	T49.2X1	T49.2X2	T49.2X3	T49.2X4	T49.2X5	T49.2X6
Durabolin	T38.7X1	T38.7X2	T38.7X3	T38.7X4	T38.7X5	T38.7X6
Dyclone	T41.3X1	T41.3X2	T41.3X3	T41.3X4	T41.3X5	T41.3X6
Dyclonine	T41.3X1	T41.3X2	T41.3X3	T41.3X4	T41.3X5	T41.3X6
Dydrogesterone	T38.5X1	T38.5X2	T38.5X3	T38.5X4	T38.5X5	T38.5X6
Dye NEC	T65.6X1	T65.6X2	T65.6X3	T65.6X4	—	—
antiseptic	T49.0X1	T49.0X2	T49.0X3	T49.0X4	T49.0X5	T49.0X6
diagnostic agents	T50.8X1	T50.8X2	T50.8X3	T50.8X4	T50.8X5	T50.8X6
pharmaceutical NEC	T50.901	T50.902	T50.903	T50.904	T50.905	T50.906
Dyflos	T44.0X1	T44.0X2	T44.0X3	T44.0X4	T44.0X5	T44.0X6
Dymelor	T38.3X1	T38.3X2	T38.3X3	T38.3X4	T38.3X5	T38.3X6
Dynamite	T65.3X1	T65.3X2	T65.3X3	T65.3X4	—	—
fumes	T59.891	T59.892	T59.893	T59.894	—	—

Substance	Poisoning, Accidental (unintentional)	Poisoning, Intentional Self-harm	Poisoning, Assault	Poisoning, Undetermined	Adverse Effect	Under-dosing
Dyphylline	T44.3X1	T44.3X2	T44.3X3	T44.3X4	T44.3X5	T44.3X6
E						
Ear drug NEC	T49.6X1	T49.6X2	T49.6X3	T49.6X4	T49.6X5	T49.6X6
Ear preparations	T49.6X1	T49.6X2	T49.6X3	T49.6X4	T49.6X5	T49.6X6
Econazole	T49.0X1	T49.0X2	T49.0X3	T49.0X4	T49.0X5	T49.0X6
Ecothiopate iodide	T49.5X1	T49.5X2	T49.5X3	T49.5X4	T49.5X5	T49.5X6
Echothiophate, echothiopate, ecothiopate	T49.5X1	T49.5X2	T49.5X3	T49.5X4	T49.5X5	T49.5X6
Ecstasy	T43.621	T43.622	T43.623	T43.624	T43.625	T43.626
Ectylurea	T42.6X1	T42.6X2	T42.6X3	T42.6X4	T42.6X5	T42.6X6
Edathamil disodium	T45.8X1	T45.8X2	T45.8X3	T45.8X4	T45.8X5	T45.8X6
Edecrin	T50.1X1	T50.1X2	T50.1X3	T50.1X4	T50.1X5	T50.1X6
Edetate, disodium (calcium)	T45.8X1	T45.8X2	T45.8X3	T45.8X4	T45.8X5	T45.8X6
Edoxudine	T49.5X1	T49.5X2	T49.5X3	T49.5X4	T49.5X5	T49.5X6
Edrophonium	T44.0X1	T44.0X2	T44.0X3	T44.0X4	T44.0X5	T44.0X6
chloride	T44.0X1	T44.0X2	T44.0X3	T44.0X4	T44.0X5	T44.0X6
EDTA	T50.6X1	T50.6X2	T50.6X3	T50.6X4	T50.6X5	T50.6X6
Eflornithine	T37.2X1	T37.2X2	T37.2X3	T37.2X4	T37.2X5	T37.2X6
Efloxate	T46.3X1	T46.3X2	T46.3X3	T46.3X4	T46.3X5	T46.3X6
Elase	T49.8X1	T49.8X2	T49.8X3	T49.8X4	T49.8X5	T49.8X6
Elastase	T47.5X1	T47.5X2	T47.5X3	T47.5X4	T47.5X5	T47.5X6
Elaterium	T47.2X1	T47.2X2	T47.2X3	T47.2X4	T47.2X5	T47.2X6
Elcatonin	T50.991	T50.992	T50.993	T50.994	T50.995	T50.996
Elder	T62.2X1	T62.2X2	T62.2X3	T62.2X4	—	—
berry, (unripe)	T62.1X1	T62.1X2	T62.1X3	T62.1X4	—	—
Electrolyte balance drug	T50.3X1	T50.3X2	T50.3X3	T50.3X4	T50.3X5	T50.3X6
Electrolytes NEC	T50.3X1	T50.3X2	T50.3X3	T50.3X4	T50.3X5	T50.3X6
Electrolytic agent NEC	T50.3X1	T50.3X2	T50.3X3	T50.3X4	T50.3X5	T50.3X6
Elemental diet	T50.901	T50.902	T50.903	T50.904	T50.905	T50.906
Elliptinium acetate	T45.1X1	T45.1X2	T45.1X3	T45.1X4	T45.1X5	T45.1X6
Embramine	T45.0X1	T45.0X2	T45.0X3	T45.0X4	T45.0X5	T45.0X6
Emepronium (salts)	T44.3X1	T44.3X2	T44.3X3	T44.3X4	T44.3X5	T44.3X6
bromide	T44.3X1	T44.3X2	T44.3X3	T44.3X4	T44.3X5	T44.3X6
Emetic NEC	T47.7X1	T47.7X2	T47.7X3	T47.7X4	T47.7X5	T47.7X6
Emetine	T37.3X1	T37.3X2	T37.3X3	T37.3X4	T37.3X5	T37.3X6
Emollient NEC	T49.3X1	T49.3X2	T49.3X3	T49.3X4	T49.3X5	T49.3X6
Emorfazone	T39.8X1	T39.8X2	T39.8X3	T39.8X4	T39.8X5	T39.8X6
Emylcamate	T43.591	T43.592	T43.593	T43.594	T43.595	T43.596
Enalapril	T46.4X1	T46.4X2	T46.4X3	T46.4X4	T46.4X5	T46.4X6
Enalaprilat	T46.4X1	T46.4X2	T46.4X3	T46.4X4	T46.4X5	T46.4X6
Encainide	T46.2X1	T46.2X2	T46.2X3	T46.2X4	T46.2X5	T46.2X6
Endocaine	T41.3X1	T41.3X2	T41.3X3	T41.3X4	T41.3X5	T41.3X6
Endosulfan	T60.2X1	T60.2X2	T60.2X3	T60.2X4	—	—
Endothall	T60.3X1	T60.3X2	T60.3X3	T60.3X4	—	—
Endralazine	T46.5X1	T46.5X2	T46.5X3	T46.5X4	T46.5X5	T46.5X6
Endrin	T60.1X1	T60.1X2	T60.1X3	T60.1X4	—	—
Enflurane	T41.0X1	T41.0X2	T41.0X3	T41.0X4	T41.0X5	T41.0X6
Enhexymal	T42.3X1	T42.3X2	T42.3X3	T42.3X4	T42.3X5	T42.3X6
Enocitabine	T45.1X1	T45.1X2	T45.1X3	T45.1X4	T45.1X5	T45.1X6
Enovid	T38.4X1	T38.4X2	T38.4X3	T38.4X4	T38.4X5	T38.4X6
Enoxacin	T36.8X1	T36.8X2	T36.8X3	T36.8X4	T36.8X5	T36.8X6
Enoxaparin (sodium)	T45.511	T45.512	T45.513	T45.514	T45.515	T45.516
Enpiprazole	T43.591	T43.592	T43.593	T43.594	T43.595	T43.596
Enprofylline	T48.6X1	T48.6X2	T48.6X3	T48.6X4	T48.6X5	T48.6X6
Enprostil	T47.1X1	T47.1X2	T47.1X3	T47.1X4	T47.1X5	T47.1X6
Enterogastrone	T38.891	T38.892	T38.893	T38.894	T38.895	T38.896
ENT preparations (anti-infectives)	T49.6X1	T49.6X2	T49.6X3	T49.6X4	T49.6X5	T49.6X6
Enviomycin	T36.8X1	T36.8X2	T36.8X3	T36.8X4	T36.8X5	T36.8X6
Enzodase	T45.3X1	T45.3X2	T45.3X3	T45.3X4	T45.3X5	T45.3X6
Enzyme NEC	T45.3X1	T45.3X2	T45.3X3	T45.3X4	T45.3X5	T45.3X6
depolymerizing	T49.8X1	T49.8X2	T49.8X3	T49.8X4	T49.8X5	T49.8X6
fibrolytic	T45.3X1	T45.3X2	T45.3X3	T45.3X4	T45.3X5	T45.3X6
gastric	T47.5X1	T47.5X2	T47.5X3	T47.5X4	T47.5X5	T47.5X6
intestinal	T47.5X1	T47.5X2	T47.5X3	T47.5X4	T47.5X5	T47.5X6
local action	T49.4X1	T49.4X2	T49.4X3	T49.4X4	T49.4X5	T49.4X6
proteolytic	T49.4X1	T49.4X2	T49.4X3	T49.4X4	T49.4X5	T49.4X6
thrombolytic	T45.3X1	T45.3X2	T45.3X3	T45.3X4	T45.3X5	T45.3X6
EPAB	T41.3X1	T41.3X2	T41.3X3	T41.3X4	T41.3X5	T41.3X6
Epanutin	T42.0X1	T42.0X2	T42.0X3	T42.0X4	T42.0X5	T42.0X6
Ephedra	T44.991	T44.992	T44.993	T44.994	T44.995	T44.996
Ephedrine	T44.991	T44.992	T44.993	T44.994	T44.995	T44.996

Substance	Poisoning, Accidental (unintentional)	Poisoning, Intentional Self-harm	Poisoning, Assault	Poisoning, Undetermined	Adverse Effect	Under-dosing
Epichlorhydrin, epichlorohydrin	T52.8X1	T52.8X2	T52.8X3	T52.8X4	—	—
Epicillin	T36.ØX1	T36.ØX2	T36.ØX3	T36.ØX4	T36.ØX5	T36.ØX6
Epiestriol	T38.5X1	T38.5X2	T38.5X3	T38.5X4	T38.5X5	T38.5X6
Epilim—*see* Sodium valproate						
Epimestrol	T38.5X1	T38.5X2	T38.5X3	T38.5X4	T38.5X5	T38.5X6
Epinephrine	T44.5X1	T44.5X2	T44.5X3	T44.5X4	T44.5X5	T44.5X6
Epirubicin	T45.1X1	T45.1X2	T45.1X3	T45.1X4	T45.1X5	T45.1X6
Epitiostanol	T38.7X1	T38.7X2	T38.7X3	T38.7X4	T38.7X5	T38.7X6
Epitizide	T5Ø.2X1	T5Ø.2X2	T5Ø.2X3	T5Ø.2X4	T5Ø.2X5	T5Ø.2X6
EPN	T6Ø.ØX1	T6Ø.ØX2	T6Ø.ØX3	T6Ø.ØX4	—	—
EPO	T45.8X1	T45.8X2	T45.8X3	T45.8X4	T45.8X5	T45.8X6
Epoetin alpha	T45.8X1	T45.8X2	T45.8X3	T45.8X4	T45.8X5	T45.8X6
Epomediol	T5Ø.991	T5Ø.992	T5Ø.993	T5Ø.994	T5Ø.995	T5Ø.996
Epoprostenol	T45.521	T45.522	T45.523	T45.524	T45.525	T45.526
Epoxy resin	T65.891	T65.892	T65.893	T65.894	—	—
Eprazinone	T48.4X1	T48.4X2	T48.4X3	T48.4X4	T48.4X5	T48.4X6
Epsilon amino-caproic acid	T45.621	T45.622	T45.623	T45.624	T45.625	T45.626
Epsom salt	T47.3X1	T47.3X2	T47.3X3	T47.3X4	T47.3X5	T47.3X6
Eptazocine	T4Ø.4X1	T4Ø.4X2	T4Ø.4X3	T4Ø.4X4	T4Ø.4X5	T4Ø.4X6
Equanil	T43.591	T43.592	T43.593	T43.594	T43.595	T43.596
Equisetum	T62.2X1	T62.2X2	T62.2X3	T62.2X4	—	—
diuretic	T5Ø.2X1	T5Ø.2X2	T5Ø.2X3	T5Ø.2X4	T5Ø.2X5	T5Ø.2X6
Ergobasine	T48.ØX1	T48.ØX2	T48.ØX3	T48.ØX4	T48.ØX5	T48.ØX6
Ergocalciferol	T45.2X1	T45.2X2	T45.2X3	T45.2X4	T45.2X5	T45.2X6
Ergoloid mesylates	T46.7X1	T46.7X2	T46.7X3	T46.7X4	T46.7X5	T46.7X6
Ergometrine	T48.ØX1	T48.ØX2	T48.ØX3	T48.ØX4	T48.ØX5	T48.ØX6
Ergonovine	T48.ØX1	T48.ØX2	T48.ØX3	T48.ØX4	T48.ØX5	T48.ØX6
Ergot NEC	T64.81	T64.82	T64.83	T64.84	—	—
derivative	T48.ØX1	T48.ØX2	T48.ØX3	T48.ØX4	T48.ØX5	T48.ØX6
medicinal (alkaloids)	T48.ØX1	T48.ØX2	T48.ØX3	T48.ØX4	T48.ØX5	T48.ØX6
prepared	T48.ØX1	T48.ØX2	T48.ØX3	T48.ØX4	T48.ØX5	T48.ØX6
Ergotamine	T46.5X1	T46.5X2	T46.5X3	T46.5X4	T46.5X5	T46.5X6
Ergotocine	T48.ØX1	T48.ØX2	T48.ØX3	T48.ØX4	T48.ØX5	T48.ØX6
Ergotrate	T48.ØX1	T48.ØX2	T48.ØX3	T48.ØX4	T48.ØX5	T48.ØX6
Eritrityl tetranitrate	T46.3X1	T46.3X2	T46.3X3	T46.3X4	T46.3X5	T46.3X6
Erythrityl tetranitrate	T46.3X1	T46.3X2	T46.3X3	T46.3X4	T46.3X5	T46.3X6
Erythrol tetranitrate	T46.3X1	T46.3X2	T46.3X3	T46.3X4	T46.3X5	T46.3X6
Erythromycin (salts)	T36.3X1	T36.3X2	T36.3X3	T36.3X4	T36.3X5	T36.3X6
ophthalmic preparation	T49.5X1	T49.5X2	T49.5X3	T49.5X4	T49.5X5	T49.5X6
topical NEC	T49.ØX1	T49.ØX2	T49.ØX3	T49.ØX4	T49.ØX5	T49.ØX6
Erythropoietin	T45.8X1	T45.8X2	T45.8X3	T45.8X4	T45.8X5	T45.8X6
human	T45.8X1	T45.8X2	T45.8X3	T45.8X4	T45.8X5	T45.8X6
Escin	T46.991	T46.992	T46.993	T46.994	T46.995	T46.996
Esculin	T45.2X1	T45.2X2	T45.2X3	T45.2X4	T45.2X5	T45.2X6
Esculoside	T45.2X1	T45.2X2	T45.2X3	T45.2X4	T45.2X5	T45.2X6
ESDT (ether-soluble tar distillate)	T49.1X1	T49.1X2	T49.1X3	T49.1X4	T49.1X5	T49.1X6
Eserine	T49.5X1	T49.5X2	T49.5X3	T49.5X4	T49.5X5	T49.5X6
Esflurbiprofen	T39.311	T39.312	T39.313	T39.314	T39.315	T39.316
Eskabarb	T42.3X1	T42.3X2	T42.3X3	T42.3X4	T42.3X5	T42.3X6
Eskalith	T43.8X1	T43.8X2	T43.8X3	T43.8X4	T43.8X5	T43.8X6
Esmolol	T44.7X1	T44.7X2	T44.7X3	T44.7X4	T44.7X5	T44.7X6
Estanozolol	T38.7X1	T38.7X2	T38.7X3	T38.7X4	T38.7X5	T38.7X6
Estazolam	T42.4X1	T42.4X2	T42.4X3	T42.4X4	T42.4X5	T42.4X6
Estradiol	T38.5X1	T38.5X2	T38.5X3	T38.5X4	T38.5X5	T38.5X6
with testosterone	T38.7X1	T38.7X2	T38.7X3	T38.7X4	T38.7X5	T38.7X6
benzoate	T38.5X1	T38.5X2	T38.5X3	T38.5X4	T38.5X5	T38.5X6
Estramustine	T45.1X1	T45.1X2	T45.1X3	T45.1X4	T45.1X5	T45.1X6
Estriol	T38.5X1	T38.5X2	T38.5X3	T38.5X4	T38.5X5	T38.5X6
Estrogen	T38.5X1	T38.5X2	T38.5X3	T38.5X4	T38.5X5	T38.5X6
with progesterone	T38.5X1	T38.5X2	T38.5X3	T38.5X4	T38.5X5	T38.5X6
conjugated	T38.5X1	T38.5X2	T38.5X3	T38.5X4	T38.5X5	T38.5X6
Estrone	T38.5X1	T38.5X2	T38.5X3	T38.5X4	T38.5X5	T38.5X6
Estropipate	T38.5X1	T38.5X2	T38.5X3	T38.5X4	T38.5X5	T38.5X6
Etacrynate sodium	T5Ø.1X1	T5Ø.1X2	T5Ø.1X3	T5Ø.1X4	T5Ø.1X5	T5Ø.1X6
Etacrynic acid	T5Ø.1X1	T5Ø.1X2	T5Ø.1X3	T5Ø.1X4	T5Ø.1X5	T5Ø.1X6
Etafedrine	T48.6X1	T48.6X2	T48.6X3	T48.6X4	T48.6X5	T48.6X6
Etafenone	T46.3X1	T46.3X2	T46.3X3	T46.3X4	T46.3X5	T46.3X6
Etambutol	T37.1X1	T37.1X2	T37.1X3	T37.1X4	T37.1X5	T37.1X6
Etamiphyllin	T48.6X1	T48.6X2	T48.6X3	T48.6X4	T48.6X5	T48.6X6
Etamivan	T5Ø.7X1	T5Ø.7X2	T5Ø.7X3	T5Ø.7X4	T5Ø.7X5	T5Ø.7X6
Etamsylate	T45.7X1	T45.7X2	T45.7X3	T45.7X4	T45.7X5	T45.7X6

Substance	Poisoning, Accidental (unintentional)	Poisoning, Intentional Self-harm	Poisoning, Assault	Poisoning, Undetermined	Adverse Effect	Under-dosing
Etebenecid	T5Ø.4X1	T5Ø.4X2	T5Ø.4X3	T5Ø.4X4	T5Ø.4X5	T5Ø.4X6
Ethacridine	T49.ØX1	T49.ØX2	T49.ØX3	T49.ØX4	T49.ØX5	T49.ØX6
Ethacrynic acid	T5Ø.1X1	T5Ø.1X2	T5Ø.1X3	T5Ø.1X4	T5Ø.1X5	T5Ø.1X6
Ethadione	T42.2X1	T42.2X2	T42.2X3	T42.2X4	T42.2X5	T42.2X6
Ethambutol	T37.1X1	T37.1X2	T37.1X3	T37.1X4	T37.1X5	T37.1X6
Ethamide	T5Ø.2X1	T5Ø.2X2	T5Ø.2X3	T5Ø.2X4	T5Ø.2X5	T5Ø.2X6
Ethamivan	T5Ø.7X1	T5Ø.7X2	T5Ø.7X3	T5Ø.7X4	T5Ø.7X5	T5Ø.7X6
Ethamsylate	T45.7X1	T45.7X2	T45.7X3	T45.7X4	T45.7X5	T45.7X6
Ethanol	T51.ØX1	T51.ØX2	T51.ØX3	T51.ØX4	—	—
beverage	T51.ØX1	T51.ØX2	T51.ØX3	T51.ØX4	—	—
Ethanolamine oleate	T46.8X1	T46.8X2	T46.8X3	T46.8X4	T46.8X5	T46.8X6
Ethaverine	T44.3X1	T44.3X2	T44.3X3	T44.3X4	T44.3X5	T44.3X6
Ethchlorvynol	T42.6X1	T42.6X2	T42.6X3	T42.6X4	T42.6X5	T42.6X6
Ethebenecid	T5Ø.4X1	T5Ø.4X2	T5Ø.4X3	T5Ø.4X4	T5Ø.4X5	T5Ø.4X6
Ether (vapor)	T41.ØX1	T41.ØX2	T41.ØX3	T41.ØX4	T41.ØX5	T41.ØX6
anesthetic	T41.ØX1	T41.ØX2	T41.ØX3	T41.ØX4	T41.ØX5	T41.ØX6
divinyl	T41.ØX1	T41.ØX2	T41.ØX3	T41.ØX4	T41.ØX5	T41.ØX6
ethyl (medicinal)	T41.ØX1	T41.ØX2	T41.ØX3	T41.ØX4	T41.ØX5	T41.ØX6
nonmedicinal	T52.8X1	T52.8X2	T52.8X3	T52.8X4	—	—
petroleum—*see* Ligroin						
solvent	T52.8X1	T52.8X2	T52.8X3	T52.8X4	—	—
Ethiazide	T5Ø.2X1	T5Ø.2X2	T5Ø.2X3	T5Ø.2X4	T5Ø.2X5	T5Ø.2X6
Ethidium chloride (vapor)	T59.891	T59.892	T59.893	T59.894	—	—
Ethinamate	T42.6X1	T42.6X2	T42.6X3	T42.6X4	T42.6X5	T42.6X6
Ethinylestradiol, ethinyloestradiol	T38.5X1	T38.5X2	T38.5X3	T38.5X4	T38.5X5	T38.5X6
with						
levonorgestrel	T38.4X1	T38.4X2	T38.4X3	T38.4X4	T38.4X5	T38.4X6
norethisterone	T38.4X1	T38.4X2	T38.4X3	T38.4X4	T38.4X5	T38.4X6
Ethiodized oil (131 I)	T5Ø.8X1	T5Ø.8X2	T5Ø.8X3	T5Ø.8X4	T5Ø.8X5	T5Ø.8X6
Ethion	T6Ø.ØX1	T6Ø.ØX2	T6Ø.ØX3	T6Ø.ØX4	—	—
Ethionamide	T37.1X1	T37.1X2	T37.1X3	T37.1X4	T37.1X5	T37.1X6
Ethioniamide	T37.1X1	T37.1X2	T37.1X3	T37.1X4	T37.1X5	T37.1X6
Ethisterone	T38.5X1	T38.5X2	T38.5X3	T38.5X4	T38.5X5	T38.5X6
Ethobral	T42.3X1	T42.3X2	T42.3X3	T42.3X4	T42.3X5	T42.3X6
Ethocaine (infiltration) (topical)	T41.3X1	T41.3X2	T41.3X3	T41.3X4	T41.3X5	T41.3X6
nerve block (peripheral) (plexus)	T41.3X1	T41.3X2	T41.3X3	T41.3X4	T41.3X5	T41.3X6
spinal	T41.3X1	T41.3X2	T41.3X3	T41.3X4	T41.3X5	T41.3X6
Ethoheptazine	T4Ø.4X1	T4Ø.4X2	T4Ø.4X3	T4Ø.4X4	T4Ø.4X5	T4Ø.4X6
Ethopropazine	T44.3X1	T44.3X2	T44.3X3	T44.3X4	T44.3X5	T44.3X6
Ethosuximide	T42.2X1	T42.2X2	T42.2X3	T42.2X4	T42.2X5	T42.2X6
Ethotoin	T42.ØX1	T42.ØX2	T42.ØX3	T42.ØX4	T42.ØX5	T42.ØX6
Ethoxazene	T37.91	T37.92	T37.93	T37.94	T37.95	T37.96
Ethoxazorutoside	T46.991	T46.992	T46.993	T46.994	T46.995	T46.996
2-Ethoxyethanol	T52.3X1	T52.3X2	T52.3X3	T52.3X4	—	—
Ethoxzolamide	T5Ø.2X1	T5Ø.2X2	T5Ø.2X3	T5Ø.2X4	T5Ø.2X5	T5Ø.2X6
Ethyl						
acetate	T52.8X1	T52.8X2	T52.8X3	T52.8X4	—	—
alcohol	T51.ØX1	T51.ØX2	T51.ØX3	T51.ØX4	—	—
beverage	T51.ØX1	T51.ØX2	T51.ØX3	T51.ØX4	—	—
aldehyde (vapor)	T59.891	T59.892	T59.893	T59.894	—	—
liquid	T52.8X1	T52.8X2	T52.8X3	T52.8X4	—	—
aminobenzoate	T41.3X1	T41.3X2	T41.3X3	T41.3X4	T41.3X5	T41.3X6
aminophenothiazine	T43.3X1	T43.3X2	T43.3X3	T43.3X4	T43.3X5	T43.3X6
benzoate	T52.8X1	T52.8X2	T52.8X3	T52.8X4	—	—
biscoumacetate	T45.511	T45.512	T45.513	T45.514	T45.515	T45.516
bromide (anesthetic)	T41.ØX1	T41.ØX2	T41.ØX3	T41.ØX4	T41.ØX5	T41.ØX6
carbamate	T45.1X1	T45.1X2	T45.1X3	T45.1X4	T45.1X5	T45.1X6
carbinol	T51.3X1	T51.3X2	T51.3X3	T51.3X4	—	—
carbonate	T52.8X1	T52.8X2	T52.8X3	T52.8X4	—	—
chaulmoograte	T37.1X1	T37.1X2	T37.1X3	T37.1X4	T37.1X5	T37.1X6
chloride (anesthetic)	T41.ØX1	T41.ØX2	T41.ØX3	T41.ØX4	T41.ØX5	T41.ØX6
anesthetic (local)	T41.3X1	T41.3X2	T41.3X3	T41.3X4	T41.3X5	T41.3X6
inhaled	T41.ØX1	T41.ØX2	T41.ØX3	T41.ØX4	T41.ØX5	T41.ØX6
local	T49.4X1	T49.4X2	T49.4X3	T49.4X4	T49.4X5	T49.4X6
solvent	T53.6X1	T53.6X2	T53.6X3	T53.6X4	—	—
dibunate	T48.3X1	T48.3X2	T48.3X3	T48.3X4	T48.3X5	T48.3X6
dichloroarsine (vapor)	T57.ØX1	T57.ØX2	T57.ØX3	T57.ØX4	—	—
estranol	T38.7X1	T38.7X2	T38.7X3	T38.7X4	T38.7X5	T38.7X6
ether (*see also* ether)	T52.8X1	T52.8X2	T52.8X3	T52.8X4	—	—
formate NEC (solvent)	T52.ØX1	T52.ØX2	T52.ØX3	T52.ØX4	—	—

Substance	Poisoning, Accidental (unintentional)	Poisoning, Intentional Self-harm	Poisoning, Assault	Poisoning, Undetermined	Adverse Effect	Under-dosing
Ethyl—*continued*						
fumarate	T49.4X1	T49.4X2	T49.4X3	T49.4X4	T49.4X5	T49.4X6
hydroxyisobutyrate NEC (solvent)	T52.8X1	T52.8X2	T52.8X3	T52.8X4	—	—
iodoacetate	T59.3X1	T59.3X2	T59.3X3	T59.3X4	—	—
lactate NEC (solvent)	T52.8X1	T52.8X2	T52.8X3	T52.8X4	—	—
loflazepate	T42.4X1	T42.4X2	T42.4X3	T42.4X4	T42.4X5	T42.4X6
mercuric chloride	T56.1X1	T56.1X2	T56.1X3	T56.1X4	—	—
methylcarbinol	T51.8X1	T51.8X2	T51.8X3	T51.8X4	—	—
morphine	T4Ø.2X1	T4Ø.2X2	T4Ø.2X3	T4Ø.2X4	T4Ø.2X5	T4Ø.2X6
noradrenaline	T48.6X1	T48.6X2	T48.6X3	T48.6X4	T48.6X5	T48.6X6
oxybutyrate NEC (solvent)	T52.8X1	T52.8X2	T52.8X3	T52.8X4	—	—
Ethylene (gas)	T59.891	T59.892	T59.893	T59.894	—	—
anesthetic (general)	T41.ØX1	T41.ØX2	T41.ØX3	T41.ØX4	T41.ØX5	T41.ØX6
chlorohydrin	T52.8X1	T52.8X2	T52.8X3	T52.8X4	—	—
vapor	T53.6X1	T53.6X2	T53.6X3	T53.6X4	—	—
dichloride	T52.8X1	T52.8X2	T52.8X3	T52.8X4	—	—
vapor	T53.6X1	T53.6X2	T53.6X3	T53.6X4	—	—
dinitrate	T52.3X1	T52.3X2	T52.3X3	T52.3X4	—	—
glycol(s)	T52.8X1	T52.8X2	T52.8X3	T52.8X4	—	—
dinitrate	T52.3X1	T52.3X2	T52.3X3	T52.3X4	—	—
monobutyl ether	T52.3X1	T52.3X2	T52.3X3	T52.3X4	—	—
imine	T54.1X1	T54.1X2	T54.1X3	T54.1X4	—	—
oxide (fumigant) (nonmedicinal)	T59.891	T59.892	T59.893	T59.894	—	—
medicinal	T49.ØX1	T49.ØX2	T49.ØX3	T49.ØX4	T49.ØX5	T49.ØX6
Ethylenediamine theophylline	T48.6X1	T48.6X2	T48.6X3	T48.6X4	T48.6X5	T48.6X6
Ethylenediaminetetraacetic acid	T5Ø.6X1	T5Ø.6X2	T5Ø.6X3	T5Ø.6X4	T5Ø.6X5	T5Ø.6X6
Ethylenedinitrilotetra-acetate	T5Ø.6X1	T5Ø.6X2	T5Ø.6X3	T5Ø.6X4	T5Ø.6X5	T5Ø.6X6
Ethylestrenol	T38.7X1	T38.7X2	T38.7X3	T38.7X4	T38.7X5	T38.7X6
Ethylhydroxycellulose	T47.4X1	T47.4X2	T47.4X3	T47.4X4	T47.4X5	T47.4X6
Ethylidene						
chloride NEC	T53.6X1	T53.6X2	T53.6X3	T53.6X4	—	—
diacetate	T6Ø.3X1	T6Ø.3X2	T6Ø.3X3	T6Ø.3X4	—	—
dicoumarin	T45.511	T45.512	T45.513	T45.514	T45.515	T45.516
dicoumarol	T45.511	T45.512	T45.513	T45.514	T45.515	T45.516
diethyl ether	T52.ØX1	T52.ØX2	T52.ØX3	T52.ØX4	—	—
Ethylmorphine	T4Ø.2X1	T4Ø.2X2	T4Ø.2X3	T4Ø.2X4	T4Ø.2X5	T4Ø.2X6
Ethylnorepinephrine	T48.6X1	T48.6X2	T48.6X3	T48.6X4	T48.6X5	T48.6X6
Ethylparachlorophen-oxyisobutyrate	T46.6X1	T46.6X2	T46.6X3	T46.6X4	T46.6X5	T46.6X6
Ethynodiol	T38.4X1	T38.4X2	T38.4X3	T38.4X4	T38.4X5	T38.4X6
with mestranol diacetate	T38.4X1	T38.4X2	T38.4X3	T38.4X4	T38.4X5	T38.4X6
Etidocaine	T41.3X1	T41.3X2	T41.3X3	T41.3X4	T41.3X5	T41.3X6
infiltration (subcutaneous)	T41.3X1	T41.3X2	T41.3X3	T41.3X4	T41.3X5	T41.3X6
nerve (peripheral) (plexus)	T41.3X1	T41.3X2	T41.3X3	T41.3X4	T41.3X5	T41.3X6
Etidronate	T5Ø.991	T5Ø.992	T5Ø.993	T5Ø.994	T5Ø.995	T5Ø.996
Etidronic acid (disodium salt)	T5Ø.991	T5Ø.992	T5Ø.993	T5Ø.994	T5Ø.995	T5Ø.996
Etifoxine	T42.6X1	T42.6X2	T42.6X3	T42.6X4	T42.6X5	T42.6X6
Etilefrine	T44.4X1	T44.4X2	T44.4X3	T44.4X4	T44.4X5	T44.4X6
Etilfen	T42.3X1	T42.3X2	T42.3X3	T42.3X4	T42.3X5	T42.3X6
Etinodiol	T38.4X1	T38.4X2	T38.4X3	T38.4X4	T38.4X5	T38.4X6
Etiroxate	T46.6X1	T46.6X2	T46.6X3	T46.6X4	T46.6X5	T46.6X6
Etizolam	T42.4X1	T42.4X2	T42.4X3	T42.4X4	T42.4X5	T42.4X6
Etodolac	T39.391	T39.392	T39.393	T39.394	T39.395	T39.396
Etofamide	T37.3X1	T37.3X2	T37.3X3	T37.3X4	T37.3X5	T37.3X6
Etofibrate	T46.6X1	T46.6X2	T46.6X3	T46.6X4	T46.6X5	T46.6X6
Etofylline	T46.7X1	T46.7X2	T46.7X3	T46.7X4	T46.7X5	T46.7X6
clofibrate	T46.6X1	T46.6X2	T46.6X3	T46.6X4	T46.6X5	T46.6X6
Etoglucid	T45.1X1	T45.1X2	T45.1X3	T45.1X4	T45.1X5	T45.1X6
Etomidate	T41.1X1	T41.1X2	T41.1X3	T41.1X4	T41.1X5	T41.1X6
Etomide	T39.8X1	T39.8X2	T39.8X3	T39.8X4	T39.8X5	T39.8X6
Etomidoline	T44.3X1	T44.3X2	T44.3X3	T44.3X4	T44.3X5	T44.3X6
Etoposide	T45.1X1	T45.1X2	T45.1X3	T45.1X4	T45.1X5	T45.1X6
Etorphine	T4Ø.2X1	T4Ø.2X2	T4Ø.2X3	T4Ø.2X4	T4Ø.2X5	T4Ø.2X6
Etozolin	T5Ø.1X1	T5Ø.1X2	T5Ø.1X3	T5Ø.1X4	T5Ø.1X5	T5Ø.1X6
Etretinate	T5Ø.991	T5Ø.992	T5Ø.993	T5Ø.994	T5Ø.995	T5Ø.996
Etryptamine	T43.691	T43.692	T43.693	T43.694	T43.695	T43.696
Etybenzatropine	T44.3X1	T44.3X2	T44.3X3	T44.3X4	T44.3X5	T44.3X6
Etynodiol	T38.4X1	T38.4X2	T38.4X3	T38.4X4	T38.4X5	T38.4X6
Eucaine	T41.3X1	T41.3X2	T41.3X3	T41.3X4	T41.3X5	T41.3X6
Eucalyptus oil	T49.7X1	T49.7X2	T49.7X3	T49.7X4	T49.7X5	T49.7X6
Eucatropine	T49.5X1	T49.5X2	T49.5X3	T49.5X4	T49.5X5	T49.5X6
Eucodal	T4Ø.2X1	T4Ø.2X2	T4Ø.2X3	T4Ø.2X4	T4Ø.2X5	T4Ø.2X6
Euneryl	T42.3X1	T42.3X2	T42.3X3	T42.3X4	T42.3X5	T42.3X6
Euphthalmine	T44.3X1	T44.3X2	T44.3X3	T44.3X4	T44.3X5	T44.3X6
Eurax	T49.ØX1	T49.ØX2	T49.ØX3	T49.ØX4	T49.ØX5	T49.ØX6
Euresol	T49.4X1	T49.4X2	T49.4X3	T49.4X4	T49.4X5	T49.4X6
Euthroid	T38.1X1	T38.1X2	T38.1X3	T38.1X4	T38.1X5	T38.1X6
Evans blue	T5Ø.8X1	T5Ø.8X2	T5Ø.8X3	T5Ø.8X4	T5Ø.8X5	T5Ø.8X6
Evipal	T42.3X1	T42.3X2	T42.3X3	T42.3X4	T42.3X5	T42.3X6
sodium	T41.1X1	T41.1X2	T41.1X3	T41.1X4	T41.1X5	T41.1X6
Evipan	T42.3X1	T42.3X2	T42.3X3	T42.3X4	T42.3X5	T42.3X6
sodium	T41.1X1	T41.1X2	T41.1X3	T41.1X4	T41.1X5	T41.1X6
Exalamide	T49.ØX1	T49.ØX2	T49.ØX3	T49.ØX4	T49.ØX5	T49.ØX6
Exalgin	T39.1X1	T39.1X2	T39.1X3	T39.1X4	T39.1X5	T39.1X6
Excipients, pharmaceutical	T5Ø.9Ø1	T5Ø.9Ø2	T5Ø.9Ø3	T5Ø.9Ø4	T5Ø.9Ø5	T5Ø.9Ø6
Exhaust gas (engine) (motor vehicle)	T58.Ø1	T58.Ø2	T58.Ø3	T58.Ø4	—	—
Ex-Lax (phenolphthalein)	T47.2X1	T47.2X2	T47.2X3	T47.2X4	T47.2X5	T47.2X6
Expectorant NEC	T48.4X1	T48.4X2	T48.4X3	T48.4X4	T48.4X5	T48.4X6
Extended insulin zinc suspension	T38.3X1	T38.3X2	T38.3X3	T38.3X4	T38.3X5	T38.3X6
External medications (skin) (mucous membrane)	T49.91	T49.92	T49.93	T49.94	T49.95	T49.96
dental agent	T49.7X1	T49.7X2	T49.7X3	T49.7X4	T49.7X5	T49.7X6
ENT agent	T49.6X1	T49.6X2	T49.6X3	T49.6X4	T49.6X5	T49.6X6
ophthalmic preparation	T49.5X1	T49.5X2	T49.5X3	T49.5X4	T49.5X5	T49.5X6
specified NEC	T49.8X1	T49.8X2	T49.8X3	T49.8X4	T49.8X5	T49.8X6
Extrapyramidal antagonist NEC	T44.3X1	T44.3X2	T44.3X3	T44.3X4	T44.3X5	T44.3X6
Eye agents (anti-infective)	T49.5X1	T49.5X2	T49.5X3	T49.5X4	T49.5X5	T49.5X6
Eye drug NEC	T49.5X1	T49.5X2	T49.5X3	T49.5X4	T49.5X5	T49.5X6
F						
FAC (fluorouracil + doxorubicin + cyclophosphamide)	T45.1X1	T45.1X2	T45.1X3	T45.1X4	T45.1X5	T45.1X6
Factor						
I (fibrinogen)	T45.8X1	T45.8X2	T45.8X3	T45.8X4	T45.8X5	T45.8X6
III (thromboplastin)	T45.8X1	T45.8X2	T45.8X3	T45.8X4	T45.8X5	T45.8X6
VIII (antihemophilic factor) (concentrate)	T45.8X1	T45.8X2	T45.8X3	T45.8X4	T45.8X5	T45.8X6
IX complex	T45.7X1	T45.7X2	T45.7X3	T45.7X4	T45.7X5	T45.7X6
human	T45.8X1	T45.8X2	T45.8X3	T45.8X4	T45.8X5	T45.8X6
Famotidine	T47.ØX1	T47.ØX2	T47.ØX3	T47.ØX4	T47.ØX5	T47.ØX6
Fat suspension, intravenous	T5Ø.991	T5Ø.992	T5Ø.993	T5Ø.994	T5Ø.995	T5Ø.996
Fazadinium bromide	T48.1X1	T48.1X2	T48.1X3	T48.1X4	T48.1X5	T48.1X6
Febarbamate	T42.3X1	T42.3X2	T42.3X3	T42.3X4	T42.3X5	T42.3X6
Fecal softener	T47.4X1	T47.4X2	T47.4X3	T47.4X4	T47.4X5	T47.4X6
Fedrilate	T48.3X1	T48.3X2	T48.3X3	T48.3X4	T48.3X5	T48.3X6
Felodipine	T46.1X1	T46.1X2	T46.1X3	T46.1X4	T46.1X5	T46.1X6
Felypressin	T38.891	T38.892	T38.893	T38.894	T38.895	T38.896
Femoxetine	T43.221	T43.222	T43.223	T43.224	T43.225	T43.226
Fenalcomine	T46.3X1	T46.3X2	T46.3X3	T46.3X4	T46.3X5	T46.3X6
Fenamisal	T37.1X1	T37.1X2	T37.1X3	T37.1X4	T37.1X5	T37.1X6
Fenazone	T39.2X1	T39.2X2	T39.2X3	T39.2X4	T39.2X5	T39.2X6
Fenbendazole	T37.4X1	T37.4X2	T37.4X3	T37.4X4	T37.4X5	T37.4X6
Fenbutrazate	T5Ø.5X1	T5Ø.5X2	T5Ø.5X3	T5Ø.5X4	T5Ø.5X5	T5Ø.5X6
Fencamfamine	T43.691	T43.692	T43.693	T43.694	T43.695	T43.696
Fendiline	T46.1X1	T46.1X2	T46.1X3	T46.1X4	T46.1X5	T46.1X6
Fenetylline	T43.691	T43.692	T43.693	T43.694	T43.695	T43.696
Fenflumizole	T39.391	T39.392	T39.393	T39.394	T39.395	T39.396
Fenfluramine	T5Ø.5X1	T5Ø.5X2	T5Ø.5X3	T5Ø.5X4	T5Ø.5X5	T5Ø.5X6
Fenobarbital	T42.3X1	T42.3X2	T42.3X3	T42.3X4	T42.3X5	T42.3X6
Fenofibrate	T46.6X1	T46.6X2	T46.6X3	T46.6X4	T46.6X5	T46.6X6
Fenoprofen	T39.311	T39.312	T39.313	T39.314	T39.315	T39.316
Fenoterol	T48.6X1	T48.6X2	T48.6X3	T48.6X4	T48.6X5	T48.6X6
Fenoverine	T44.3X1	T44.3X2	T44.3X3	T44.3X4	T44.3X5	T44.3X6
Fenoxazoline	T48.5X1	T48.5X2	T48.5X3	T48.5X4	T48.5X5	T48.5X6
Fenproporex	T5Ø.5X1	T5Ø.5X2	T5Ø.5X3	T5Ø.5X4	T5Ø.5X5	T5Ø.5X6
Fenquizone	T5Ø.2X1	T5Ø.2X2	T5Ø.2X3	T5Ø.2X4	T5Ø.2X5	T5Ø.2X6
Fentanyl	T4Ø.4X1	T4Ø.4X2	T4Ø.4X3	T4Ø.4X4	T4Ø.4X5	T4Ø.4X6
Fentazin	T43.3X1	T43.3X2	T43.3X3	T43.3X4	T43.3X5	T43.3X6
Fenthion	T6Ø.ØX1	T6Ø.ØX2	T6Ø.ØX3	T6Ø.ØX4	—	—
Fenticlor	T49.ØX1	T49.ØX2	T49.ØX3	T49.ØX4	T49.ØX5	T49.ØX6

Substance	Poisoning, Accidental (unintentional)	Poisoning, Intentional Self-harm	Poisoning, Assault	Poisoning, Undetermined	Adverse Effect	Under-dosing
Fenylbutazone	T39.2X1	T39.2X2	T39.2X3	T39.2X4	T39.2X5	T39.2X6
Feprazone	T39.2X1	T39.2X2	T39.2X3	T39.2X4	T39.2X5	T39.2X6
Fer de lance (bite) (venom)	T63.Ø61	T63.Ø62	T63.Ø63	T63.Ø64	—	—
Ferric (*see also* Iron)						
chloride	T45.4X1	T45.4X2	T45.4X3	T45.4X4	T45.4X5	T45.4X6
citrate	T45.4X1	T45.4X2	T45.4X3	T45.4X4	T45.4X5	T45.4X6
hydroxide						
colloidal	T45.4X1	T45.4X2	T45.4X3	T45.4X4	T45.4X5	T45.4X6
polymaltose	T45.4X1	T45.4X2	T45.4X3	T45.4X4	T45.4X5	T45.4X6
pyrophosphate	T45.4X1	T45.4X2	T45.4X3	T45.4X4	T45.4X5	T45.4X6
Ferritin	T45.4X1	T45.4X2	T45.4X3	T45.4X4	T45.4X5	T45.4X6
Ferrocholinate	T45.4X1	T45.4X2	T45.4X3	T45.4X4	T45.4X5	T45.4X6
Ferrodextrane	T45.4X1	T45.4X2	T45.4X3	T45.4X4	T45.4X5	T45.4X6
Ferropolimaler	T45.4X1	T45.4X2	T45.4X3	T45.4X4	T45.4X5	T45.4X6
Ferrous (*see also* Iron)						
phosphate	T45.4X1	T45.4X2	T45.4X3	T45.4X4	T45.4X5	T45.4X6
salt	T45.4X1	T45.4X2	T45.4X3	T45.4X4	T45.4X5	T45.4X6
with folic acid	T45.4X1	T45.4X2	T45.4X3	T45.4X4	T45.4X5	T45.4X6
Ferrous fumerate, gluconate, lactate, salt NEC, sulfate (medicinal)	T45.4X1	T45.4X2	T45.4X3	T45.4X4	T45.4X5	T45.4X6
Ferrovanadium (fumes)	T59.891	T59.892	T59.893	T59.894	—	—
Ferrum—*see* Iron						
Fertilizers NEC	T65.891	T65.892	T65.893	T65.894	—	—
with herbicide mixture	T6Ø.3X1	T6Ø.3X2	T6Ø.3X3	T6Ø.3X4	—	—
Fetoxilate	T47.6X1	T47.6X2	T47.6X3	T47.6X4	T47.6X5	T47.6X6
Fiber, dietary	T47.4X1	T47.4X2	T47.4X3	T47.4X4	T47.4X5	T47.4X6
Fiberglass	T65.831	T65.832	T65.833	T65.834	—	—
Fibrinogen (human)	T45.8X1	T45.8X2	T45.8X3	T45.8X4	T45.8X5	T45.8X6
Fibrinolysin (human)	T45.691	T45.692	T45.693	T45.694	T45.695	T45.696
Fibrinolysis						
affecting drug	T45.6Ø1	T45.6Ø2	T45.6Ø3	T45.6Ø4	T45.6Ø5	T45.6Ø6
inhibitor NEC	T45.621	T45.622	T45.623	T45.624	T45.625	T45.626
Fibrinolytic drug	T45.611	T45.612	T45.613	T45.614	T45.615	T45.616
Filix mas	T37.4X1	T37.4X2	T37.4X3	T37.4X4	T37.4X5	T37.4X6
Filtering cream	T49.3X1	T49.3X2	T49.3X3	T49.3X4	T49.3X5	T49.3X6
Fiorinal	T39.Ø11	T39.Ø12	T39.Ø13	T39.Ø14	T39.Ø15	T39.Ø16
Firedamp	T59.891	T59.892	T59.893	T59.894	—	—
Fish, noxious, nonbacterial	T61.91	T61.92	T61.93	T61.94	—	—
ciguatera	T61.Ø1	T61.Ø2	T61.Ø3	T61.Ø4	—	—
scombroid	T61.11	T61.12	T61.13	T61.14	—	—
shell	T61.781	T61.782	T61.783	T61.784	—	—
specified NEC	T61.771	T61.772	T61.773	T61.774	—	—
Flagyl	T37.3X1	T37.3X2	T37.3X3	T37.3X4	T37.3X5	T37.3X6
Flavine adenine dinucleotide	T45.2X1	T45.2X2	T45.2X3	T45.2X4	T45.2X5	T45.2X6
Flavodic acid	T46.991	T46.992	T46.993	T46.994	T46.995	T46.996
Flavoxate	T44.3X1	T44.3X2	T44.3X3	T44.3X4	T44.3X5	T44.3X6
Flaxedil	T48.1X1	T48.1X2	T48.1X3	T48.1X4	T48.1X5	T48.1X6
Flaxseed (medicinal)	T49.3X1	T49.3X2	T49.3X3	T49.3X4	T49.3X5	T49.3X6
Flecainide	T46.2X1	T46.2X2	T46.2X3	T46.2X4	T46.2X5	T46.2X6
Fleroxacin	T36.8X1	T36.8X2	T36.8X3	T36.8X4	T36.8X5	T36.8X6
Floctafenine	T39.8X1	T39.8X2	T39.8X3	T39.8X4	T39.8X5	T39.8X6
Flomax	T44.6X1	T44.6X2	T44.6X3	T44.6X4	T44.6X5	T44.6X6
Flomoxef	T36.1X1	T36.1X2	T36.1X3	T36.1X4	T36.1X5	T36.1X6
Flopropione	T44.3X1	T44.3X2	T44.3X3	T44.3X4	T44.3X5	T44.3X6
Florantyrone	T47.5X1	T47.5X2	T47.5X3	T47.5X4	T47.5X5	T47.5X6
Floraquin	T37.8X1	T37.8X2	T37.8X3	T37.8X4	T37.8X5	T37.8X6
Florinef	T38.ØX1	T38.ØX2	T38.ØX3	T38.ØX4	T38.ØX5	T38.ØX6
ENT agent	T49.6X1	T49.6X2	T49.6X3	T49.6X4	T49.6X5	T49.6X6
ophthalmic preparation	T49.5X1	T49.5X2	T49.5X3	T49.5X4	T49.5X5	T49.5X6
topical NEC	T49.ØX1	T49.ØX2	T49.ØX3	T49.ØX4	T49.ØX5	T49.ØX6
Flowers of sulfur	T49.4X1	T49.4X2	T49.4X3	T49.4X4	T49.4X5	T49.4X6
Floxuridine	T45.1X1	T45.1X2	T45.1X3	T45.1X4	T45.1X5	T45.1X6
Fluanisone	T43.4X1	T43.4X2	T43.4X3	T43.4X4	T43.4X5	T43.4X6
Flubendazole	T37.4X1	T37.4X2	T37.4X3	T37.4X4	T37.4X5	T37.4X6
Fluclorolone acetonide	T49.ØX1	T49.ØX2	T49.ØX3	T49.ØX4	T49.ØX5	T49.ØX6
Flucloxacillin	T36.ØX1	T36.ØX2	T36.ØX3	T36.ØX4	T36.ØX5	T36.ØX6
Fluconazole	T37.8X1	T37.8X2	T37.8X3	T37.8X4	T37.8X5	T37.8X6
Flucytosine	T37.8X1	T37.8X2	T37.8X3	T37.8X4	T37.8X5	T37.8X6
Fludeoxyglucose (18F)	T5Ø.8X1	T5Ø.8X2	T5Ø.8X3	T5Ø.8X4	T5Ø.8X5	T5Ø.8X6
Fludiazepam	T42.4X1	T42.4X2	T42.4X3	T42.4X4	T42.4X5	T42.4X6

Substance	Poisoning, Accidental (unintentional)	Poisoning, Intentional Self-harm	Poisoning, Assault	Poisoning, Undetermined	Adverse Effect	Under-dosing
Fludrocortisone	T5Ø.ØX1	T5Ø.ØX2	T5Ø.ØX3	T5Ø.ØX4	T5Ø.ØX5	T5Ø.ØX6
ENT agent	T49.6X1	T49.6X2	T49.6X3	T49.6X4	T49.6X5	T49.6X6
ophthalmic preparation	T49.5X1	T49.5X2	T49.5X3	T49.5X4	T49.5X5	T49.5X6
topical NEC	T49.ØX1	T49.ØX2	T49.ØX3	T49.ØX4	T49.ØX5	T49.ØX6
Fludroxycortide	T49.ØX1	T49.ØX2	T49.ØX3	T49.ØX4	T49.ØX5	T49.ØX6
Flufenamic acid	T39.391	T39.392	T39.393	T39.394	T39.395	T39.396
Fluindione	T45.511	T45.512	T45.513	T45.514	T45.515	T45.516
Flumequine	T37.8X1	T37.8X2	T37.8X3	T37.8X4	T37.8X5	T37.8X6
Flumethasone	T49.ØX1	T49.ØX2	T49.ØX3	T49.ØX4	T49.ØX5	T49.ØX6
Flumethiazide	T5Ø.2X1	T5Ø.2X2	T5Ø.2X3	T5Ø.2X4	T5Ø.2X5	T5Ø.2X6
Flumidin	T37.5X1	T37.5X2	T37.5X3	T37.5X4	T37.5X5	T37.5X6
Flunarizine	T46.7X1	T46.7X2	T46.7X3	T46.7X4	T46.7X5	T46.7X6
Flunidazole	T37.8X1	T37.8X2	T37.8X3	T37.8X4	T37.8X5	T37.8X6
Flunisolide	T48.6X1	T48.6X2	T48.6X3	T48.6X4	T48.6X5	T48.6X6
Flunitrazepam	T42.4X1	T42.4X2	T42.4X3	T42.4X4	T42.4X5	T42.4X6
Fluocinolone (acetonide)	T49.ØX1	T49.ØX2	T49.ØX3	T49.ØX4	T49.ØX5	T49.ØX6
Fluocinonide	T49.ØX1	T49.ØX2	T49.ØX3	T49.ØX4	T49.ØX5	T49.ØX6
Fluocortin (butyl)	T49.ØX1	T49.ØX2	T49.ØX3	T49.ØX4	T49.ØX5	T49.ØX6
Fluocortolone	T49.ØX1	T49.ØX2	T49.ØX3	T49.ØX4	T49.ØX5	T49.ØX6
Fluohydrocortisone	T38.ØX1	T38.ØX2	T38.ØX3	T38.ØX4	T38.ØX5	T38.ØX6
ENT agent	T49.6X1	T49.6X2	T49.6X3	T49.6X4	T49.6X5	T49.6X6
ophthalmic preparation	T49.5X1	T49.5X2	T49.5X3	T49.5X4	T49.5X5	T49.5X6
topical NEC	T49.ØX1	T49.ØX2	T49.ØX3	T49.ØX4	T49.ØX5	T49.ØX6
Fluonid	T49.ØX1	T49.ØX2	T49.ØX3	T49.ØX4	T49.ØX5	T49.ØX6
Fluopromazine	T43.3X1	T43.3X2	T43.3X3	T43.3X4	T43.3X5	T43.3X6
Fluoracetate	T6Ø.8X1	T6Ø.8X2	T6Ø.8X3	T6Ø.8X4	—	—
Fluorescein	T5Ø.8X1	T5Ø.8X2	T5Ø.8X3	T5Ø.8X4	T5Ø.8X5	T5Ø.8X6
Fluorhydrocortisone	T5Ø.ØX1	T5Ø.ØX2	T5Ø.ØX3	T5Ø.ØX4	T5Ø.ØX5	T5Ø.ØX6
Fluoride (nonmedicinal) (pesticide) (sodium) **NEC**	T6Ø.8X1	T6Ø.8X2	T6Ø.8X3	T6Ø.8X4	—	—
hydrogen—*see* Hydrofluoric acid						
medicinal NEC	T5Ø.991	T5Ø.992	T5Ø.993	T5Ø.994	T5Ø.995	T5Ø.996
dental use	T49.7X1	T49.7X2	T49.7X3	T49.7X4	T49.7X5	T49.7X6
not pesticide NEC	T54.91	T54.92	T54.93	T54.94	—	—
stannous	T49.7X1	T49.7X2	T49.7X3	T49.7X4	T49.7X5	T49.7X6
Fluorinated corticosteroids	T38.ØX1	T38.ØX2	T38.ØX3	T38.ØX4	T38.ØX5	T38.ØX6
Fluorine (gas)	T59.5X1	T59.5X2	T59.5X3	T59.5X4	—	—
salt—*see* Fluoride(s)						
Fluoristan	T49.7X1	T49.7X2	T49.7X3	T49.7X4	T49.7X5	T49.7X6
Fluormetholone	T49.ØX1	T49.ØX2	T49.ØX3	T49.ØX4	T49.ØX5	T49.ØX6
Fluoroacetate	T6Ø.8X1	T6Ø.8X2	T6Ø.8X3	T6Ø.8X4	—	—
Fluorocarbon monomer	T53.6X1	T53.6X2	T53.6X3	T53.6X4	—	—
Fluorocytosine	T37.8X1	T37.8X2	T37.8X3	T37.8X4	T37.8X5	T37.8X6
Fluorodeoxyuridine	T45.1X1	T45.1X2	T45.1X3	T45.1X4	T45.1X5	T45.1X6
Fluorometholone	T49.ØX1	T49.ØX2	T49.ØX3	T49.ØX4	T49.ØX5	T49.ØX6
ophthalmic preparation	T49.5X1	T49.5X2	T49.5X3	T49.5X4	T49.5X5	T49.5X6
Fluorophosphate insecticide	T6Ø.ØX1	T6Ø.ØX2	T6Ø.ØX3	T6Ø.ØX4	—	—
Fluorosol	T46.3X1	T46.3X2	T46.3X3	T46.3X4	T46.3X5	T46.3X6
Fluorouracil	T45.1X1	T45.1X2	T45.1X3	T45.1X4	T45.1X5	T45.1X6
Fluorphenylalanine	T49.5X1	T49.5X2	T49.5X3	T49.5X4	T49.5X5	T49.5X6
Fluothane	T41.ØX1	T41.ØX2	T41.ØX3	T41.ØX4	T41.ØX5	T41.ØX6
Fluoxetine	T43.221	T43.222	T43.223	T43.224	T43.225	T43.226
Fluoxymesterone	T38.7X1	T38.7X2	T38.7X3	T38.7X4	T38.7X5	T38.7X6
Flupenthixol	T43.4X1	T43.4X2	T43.4X3	T43.4X4	T43.4X5	T43.4X6
Flupentixol	T43.4X1	T43.4X2	T43.4X3	T43.4X4	T43.4X5	T43.4X6
Fluphenazine	T43.3X1	T43.3X2	T43.3X3	T43.3X4	T43.3X5	T43.3X6
Fluprednidene	T49.ØX1	T49.ØX2	T49.ØX3	T49.ØX4	T49.ØX5	T49.ØX6
Fluprednisolone	T38.ØX1	T38.ØX2	T38.ØX3	T38.ØX4	T38.ØX5	T38.ØX6
Fluradoline	T39.8X1	T39.8X2	T39.8X3	T39.8X4	T39.8X5	T39.8X6
Flurandrenolide	T49.ØX1	T49.ØX2	T49.ØX3	T49.ØX4	T49.ØX5	T49.ØX6
Flurandrenolone	T49.ØX1	T49.ØX2	T49.ØX3	T49.ØX4	T49.ØX5	T49.ØX6
Flurazepam	T42.4X1	T42.4X2	T42.4X3	T42.4X4	T42.4X5	T42.4X6
Flurbiprofen	T39.311	T39.312	T39.313	T39.314	T39.315	T39.316
Flurobate	T49.ØX1	T49.ØX2	T49.ØX3	T49.ØX4	T49.ØX5	T49.ØX6
Fluroxene	T41.ØX1	T41.ØX2	T41.ØX3	T41.ØX4	T41.ØX5	T41.ØX6
Fluspirilene	T43.591	T43.592	T43.593	T43.594	T43.595	T43.596
Flutamide	T38.6X1	T38.6X2	T38.6X3	T38.6X4	T38.6X5	T38.6X6
Flutazolam	T42.4X1	T42.4X2	T42.4X3	T42.4X4	T42.4X5	T42.4X6
Fluticasone propionate	T49.1X1	T49.1X2	T49.1X3	T49.1X4	T49.1X5	T49.1X6
Flutoprazepam	T42.4X1	T42.4X2	T42.4X3	T42.4X4	T42.4X5	T42.4X6
Flutropium bromide	T48.6X1	T48.6X2	T48.6X3	T48.6X4	T48.6X5	T48.6X6

Substance	Poisoning, Accidental (unintentional)	Poisoning, Intentional Self-harm	Poisoning, Assault	Poisoning, Undetermined	Adverse Effect	Under-dosing
Fluvoxamine	T43.221	T43.222	T43.223	T43.224	T43.225	T43.226
Folacin	T45.8X1	T45.8X2	T45.8X3	T45.8X4	T45.8X5	T45.8X6
Folic acid	T45.8X1	T45.8X2	T45.8X3	T45.8X4	T45.8X5	T45.8X6
with ferrous salt	T45.2X1	T45.2X2	T45.2X3	T45.2X4	T45.2X5	T45.2X6
antagonist	T45.1X1	T45.1X2	T45.1X3	T45.1X4	T45.1X5	T45.1X6
Folinic acid	T45.8X1	T45.8X2	T45.8X3	T45.8X4	T45.8X5	T45.8X6
Folium stramoniae	T48.6X1	T48.6X2	T48.6X3	T48.6X4	T48.6X5	T48.6X6
Follicle-stimulating hormone, human	T38.811	T38.812	T38.813	T38.814	T38.815	T38.816
Folpet	T6Ø.3X1	T6Ø.3X2	T6Ø.3X3	T6Ø.3X4	—	—
Fominoben	T48.3X1	T48.3X2	T48.3X3	T48.3X4	T48.3X5	T48.3X6
Food, foodstuffs, noxious, nonbacterial, NEC	T62.91	T62.92	T62.93	T62.94	—	—
berries	T62.1X1	T62.1X2	T62.1X3	T62.1X4	—	—
fish (*see also* Fish)	T61.91	T61.92	T61.93	T61.94	—	—
mushrooms	T62.ØX1	T62.ØX2	T62.ØX3	T62.ØX4	—	—
plants	T62.2X1	T62.2X2	T62.2X3	T62.2X4	—	—
seafood	T61.91	T61.92	T61.93	T61.94	—	—
specified NEC	T61.8X1	T61.8X2	T61.8X3	T61.8X4	—	—
seeds	T62.2X1	T62.2X2	T62.2X3	T62.2X4	—	—
shellfish	T61.781	T61.782	T61.783	T61.784	—	—
specified NEC	T62.8X1	T62.8X2	T62.8X3	T62.8X4	—	—
Fool's parsley	T62.2X1	T62.2X2	T62.2X3	T62.2X4	—	—
Formaldehyde (solution), **gas or vapor**	T59.2X1	T59.2X2	T59.2X3	T59.2X4	—	—
fungicide	T6Ø.3X1	T6Ø.3X2	T6Ø.3X3	T6Ø.3X4	—	—
Formalin	T59.2X1	T59.2X2	T59.2X3	T59.2X4	—	—
fungicide	T6Ø.3X1	T6Ø.3X2	T6Ø.3X3	T6Ø.3X4	—	—
vapor	T59.2X1	T59.2X2	T59.2X3	T59.2X4	—	—
Formic acid	T54.2X1	T54.2X2	T54.2X3	T54.2X4	—	—
vapor	T59.891	T59.892	T59.893	T59.894	—	—
Foscarnet sodium	T37.5X1	T37.5X2	T37.5X3	T37.5X4	T37.5X5	T37.5X6
Fosfestrol	T38.5X1	T38.5X2	T38.5X3	T38.5X4	T38.5X5	T38.5X6
Fosfomycin	T36.8X1	T36.8X2	T36.8X3	T36.8X4	T36.8X5	T36.8X6
Fosfonet sodium	T37.5X1	T37.5X2	T37.5X3	T37.5X4	T37.5X5	T37.5X6
Fosinopril	T46.4X1	T46.4X2	T46.4X3	T46.4X4	T46.4X5	T46.4X6
sodium	T46.4X1	T46.4X2	T46.4X3	T46.4X4	T46.4X5	T46.4X6
Fowler's solution	T57.ØX1	T57.ØX2	T57.ØX3	T57.ØX4	—	—
Foxglove	T62.2X1	T62.2X2	T62.2X3	T62.2X4	—	—
Framycetin	T36.5X1	T36.5X2	T36.5X3	T36.5X4	T36.5X5	T36.5X6
Frangula	T47.2X1	T47.2X2	T47.2X3	T47.2X4	T47.2X5	T47.2X6
extract	T47.2X1	T47.2X2	T47.2X3	T47.2X4	T47.2X5	T47.2X6
Frei antigen	T5Ø.8X1	T5Ø.8X2	T5Ø.8X3	T5Ø.8X4	T5Ø.8X5	T5Ø.8X6
Freon	T53.5X1	T53.5X2	T53.5X3	T53.5X4	—	—
Fructose	T5Ø.3X1	T5Ø.3X2	T5Ø.3X3	T5Ø.3X4	T5Ø.3X5	T5Ø.3X6
Frusemide	T5Ø.1X1	T5Ø.1X2	T5Ø.1X3	T5Ø.1X4	T5Ø.1X5	T5Ø.1X6
FSH	T38.811	T38.812	T38.813	T38.814	T38.815	T38.816
Ftorafur	T45.1X1	T45.1X2	T45.1X3	T45.1X4	T45.1X5	T45.1X6
Fuel						
automobile	T52.ØX1	T52.ØX2	T52.ØX3	T52.ØX4	—	—
exhaust gas, not in transit	T58.Ø1	T58.Ø2	T58.Ø3	T58.Ø4	—	—
vapor NEC	T52.ØX1	T52.ØX2	T52.ØX3	T52.ØX4	—	—
gas (domestic use) (*see also* Carbon, monoxide, fuel, utility)	T59.891	T59.892	T59.893	T59.894	—	—
utility	T59.891	T59.892	T59.893	T59.894	—	—
incomplete combustion of—*see* Carbon, monoxide, fuel, utility						
in mobile container	T59.891	T59.892	T59.893	T59.894	—	—
piped (natural)	T59.891	T59.892	T59.893	T59.894	—	—
industrial, incomplete combustion	T58.8X1	T58.8X2	T58.8X3	T58.8X4	—	—
Fugillin	T36.8X1	T36.8X2	T36.8X3	T36.8X4	T36.8X5	T36.8X6
Fulminate of mercury	T56.1X1	T56.1X2	T56.1X3	T56.1X4	—	—
Fulvicin	T36.7X1	T36.7X2	T36.7X3	T36.7X4	T36.7X5	T36.7X6
Fumadil	T36.8X1	T36.8X2	T36.8X3	T36.8X4	T36.8X5	T36.8X6
Fumagillin	T36.8X1	T36.8X2	T36.8X3	T36.8X4	T36.8X5	T36.8X6
Fumaric acid	T49.4X1	T49.4X2	T49.4X3	T49.4X4	T49.4X5	T49.4X6
Fumes (from)	T59.91	T59.92	T59.93	T59.94	—	—
carbon monoxide—*see* Carbon, monoxide						

Substance	Poisoning, Accidental (unintentional)	Poisoning, Intentional Self-harm	Poisoning, Assault	Poisoning, Undetermined	Adverse Effect	Under-dosing
Fumes—*continued*						
charcoal (domestic use)—*see* Charcoal, fumes						
chloroform—*see* Chloroform						
coke (in domestic stoves, fireplaces)—*see* Coke fumes						
corrosive NEC	T54.91	T54.92	T54.93	T54.94	—	—
ether—*see* Ether						
freons	T53.5X1	T53.5X2	T53.5X3	T53.5X4	—	—
hydrocarbons	T59.891	T59.892	T59.893	T59.894	—	—
petroleum (liquefied)	T59.891	T59.892	T59.893	T59.894	—	—
distributed through pipes (pure or mixed with air)	T59.891	T59.892	T59.893	T59.894	—	—
lead—*see* Lead						
metal—*see* Metals, or the specified metal						
nitrogen dioxide	T59.ØX1	T59.ØX2	T59.ØX3	T59.ØX4	—	—
pesticides—*see* Pesticides						
petroleum (liquefied)	T59.891	T59.892	T59.893	T59.894	—	—
distributed through pipes (pure or mixed with air)	T59.891	T59.892	T59.893	T59.894	—	—
polyester	T59.891	T59.892	T59.893	T59.894	—	—
specified source NEC (*see also* substance specified)	T59.891	T59.892	T59.893	T59.894	—	—
sulfur dioxide	T59.1X1	T59.1X2	T59.1X3	T59.1X4	—	—
Fumigant NEC	T6Ø.91	T6Ø.92	T6Ø.93	T6Ø.94	—	—
Fungi, noxious, used as food	T62.ØX1	T62.ØX2	T62.ØX3	T62.ØX4	—	—
Fungicide NEC (nonmedicinal)	T6Ø.3X1	T6Ø.3X2	T6Ø.3X3	T6Ø.3X4	—	—
Fungizone	T36.7X1	T36.7X2	T36.7X3	T36.7X4	T36.7X5	T36.7X6
topical	T49.ØX1	T49.ØX2	T49.ØX3	T49.ØX4	T49.ØX5	T49.ØX6
Furacin	T49.ØX1	T49.ØX2	T49.ØX3	T49.ØX4	T49.ØX5	T49.ØX6
Furadantin	T37.91	T37.92	T37.93	T37.94	T37.95	T37.96
Furazolidone	T37.8X1	T37.8X2	T37.8X3	T37.8X4	T37.8X5	T37.8X6
Furazolium chloride	T49.ØX1	T49.ØX2	T49.ØX3	T49.ØX4	T49.ØX5	T49.ØX6
Furfural	T52.8X1	T52.8X2	T52.8X3	T52.8X4	—	—
Furnace (coal burning) (domestic), **gas from**	T58.2X1	T58.2X2	T58.2X3	T58.2X4	—	—
industrial	T58.8X1	T58.8X2	T58.8X3	T58.8X4	—	—
Furniture polish	T65.891	T65.892	T65.893	T65.894	—	—
Furosemide	T5Ø.1X1	T5Ø.1X2	T5Ø.1X3	T5Ø.1X4	T5Ø.1X5	T5Ø.1X6
Furoxone	T37.91	T37.92	T37.93	T37.94	T37.95	T37.96
Fursultiamine	T45.2X1	T45.2X2	T45.2X3	T45.2X4	T45.2X5	T45.2X6
Fusafungine	T36.8X1	T36.8X2	T36.8X3	T36.8X4	T36.8X5	T36.8X6
Fusel oil (any) (amyl) (butyl) (propyl), **vapor**	T51.3X1	T51.3X2	T51.3X3	T51.3X4	—	—
Fusidate (ethanolamine) (sodium)	T36.8X1	T36.8X2	T36.8X3	T36.8X4	T36.8X5	T36.8X6
Fusidic acid	T36.8X1	T36.8X2	T36.8X3	T36.8X4	T36.8X5	T36.8X6
Fytic acid, nonasodium	T5Ø.6X1	T5Ø.6X2	T5Ø.6X3	T5Ø.6X4	T5Ø.6X5	T5Ø.6X6
G						
GABA	T43.8X1	T43.8X2	T43.8X3	T43.8X4	T43.8X5	T43.8X6
Gadopentetic acid	T5Ø.8X1	T5Ø.8X2	T5Ø.8X3	T5Ø.8X4	T5Ø.8X5	T5Ø.8X6
Galactose	T5Ø.3X1	T5Ø.3X2	T5Ø.3X3	T5Ø.3X4	T5Ø.3X5	T5Ø.3X6
b-Galactosidase	T47.5X1	T47.5X2	T47.5X3	T47.5X4	T47.5X5	T47.5X6
Galantamine	T44.ØX1	T44.ØX2	T44.ØX3	T44.ØX4	T44.ØX5	T44.ØX6
Gallamine (triethiodide)	T48.1X1	T48.1X2	T48.1X3	T48.1X4	T48.1X5	T48.1X6
Gallium citrate	T5Ø.991	T5Ø.992	T5Ø.993	T5Ø.994	T5Ø.995	T5Ø.996
Gallopamil	T46.1X1	T46.1X2	T46.1X3	T46.1X4	T46.1X5	T46.1X6
Gamboge	T47.2X1	T47.2X2	T47.2X3	T47.2X4	T47.2X5	T47.2X6
Gamimune	T5Ø.Z11	T5Ø.Z12	T5Ø.Z13	T5Ø.Z14	T5Ø.Z15	T5Ø.Z16
Gamma-aminobutyric acid	T43.8X1	T43.8X2	T43.8X3	T43.8X4	T43.8X5	T43.8X6
Gamma-benzene hexachloride (medicinal)	T49.ØX1	T49.ØX2	T49.ØX3	T49.ØX4	T49.ØX5	T49.ØX6
nonmedicinal, vapor	T53.6X1	T53.6X2	T53.6X3	T53.6X4	—	—
Gamma-BHC (medicinal) (*see also* Gamma-benzene hexachloride)	T49.ØX1	T49.ØX2	T49.ØX3	T49.ØX4	T49.ØX5	T49.ØX6
Gamma globulin	T5Ø.Z11	T5Ø.Z12	T5Ø.Z13	T5Ø.Z14	T5Ø.Z15	T5Ø.Z16
Gamulin	T5Ø.Z11	T5Ø.Z12	T5Ø.Z13	T5Ø.Z14	T5Ø.Z15	T5Ø.Z16
Ganciclovir (sodium)	T37.5X1	T37.5X2	T37.5X3	T37.5X4	T37.5X5	T37.5X6
Ganglionic blocking drug NEC	T44.2X1	T44.2X2	T44.2X3	T44.2X4	T44.2X5	T44.2X6
specified NEC	T44.2X1	T44.2X2	T44.2X3	T44.2X4	T44.2X5	T44.2X6

Substance	Poisoning, Accidental (unintentional)	Poisoning, Intentional Self-harm	Poisoning, Assault	Poisoning, Undetermined	Adverse Effect	Under-dosing
Ganja	T4Ø.7X1	T4Ø.7X2	T4Ø.7X3	T4Ø.7X4	T4Ø.7X5	T4Ø.7X6
Garamycin	T36.5X1	T36.5X2	T36.5X3	T36.5X4	T36.5X5	T36.5X6
ophthalmic preparation	T49.5X1	T49.5X2	T49.5X3	T49.5X4	T49.5X5	T49.5X6
topical NEC	T49.ØX1	T49.ØX2	T49.ØX3	T49.ØX4	T49.ØX5	T49.ØX6
Gardenal	T42.3X1	T42.3X2	T42.3X3	T42.3X4	T42.3X5	T42.3X6
Gardepanyl	T42.3X1	T42.3X2	T42.3X3	T42.3X4	T42.3X5	T42.3X6
Gas	T59.91	T59.92	T59.93	T59.94	—	—
acetylene	T59.891	T59.892	T59.893	T59.894	—	—
incomplete combustion of	T58.11	T58.12	T58.13	T58.14	—	—
air contaminants, source or type not specified	T59.91	T59.92	T59.93	T59.94	—	—
anesthetic	T41.ØX1	T41.ØX2	T41.ØX3	T41.ØX4	T41.ØX5	T41.ØX6
blast furnace	T58.8X1	T58.8X2	T58.8X3	T58.8X4	—	—
butane—*see* butane						
carbon monoxide—*see* Carbon, monoxide						
chlorine	T59.4X1	T59.4X2	T59.4X3	T59.4X4	—	—
coal	T58.2X1	T58.2X2	T58.2X3	T58.2X4	—	—
cyanide	T57.3X1	T57.3X2	T57.3X3	T57.3X4	—	—
dicyanogen	T65.ØX1	T65.ØX2	T65.ØX3	T65.ØX4	—	—
domestic—*see* Domestic gas						
exhaust	T58.Ø1	T58.Ø2	T58.Ø3	T58.Ø4	—	—
from utility (for cooking, heating, or lighting) (after combustion)—*see* Carbon, monoxide, fuel, utility						
prior to combustion	T59.891	T59.892	T59.893	T59.894	—	—
from wood or coal-burning stove or fireplace	T58.2X1	T58.2X2	T58.2X3	T58.2X4	—	—
fuel (domestic use) (after combustion) (*see also* Carbon, monoxide, fuel)						
industrial use	T58.8X1	T58.8X2	T58.8X3	T58.8X4	—	—
prior to combustion	T59.891	T59.892	T59.893	T59.894	—	—
utility	T59.891	T59.892	T59.893	T59.894	—	—
incomplete combustion of—*see* Carbon, monoxide, fuel, utility						
in mobile container	T59.891	T59.892	T59.893	T59.894	—	—
piped (natural)	T59.891	T59.892	T59.893	T59.894	—	—
garage	T58.Ø1	T58.Ø2	T58.Ø3	T58.Ø4	—	—
hydrocarbon NEC	T59.891	T59.892	T59.893	T59.894	—	—
incomplete combustion of—*see* Carbon, monoxide, fuel, utility						
liquefied—*see* butane						
piped	T59.891	T59.892	T59.893	T59.894	—	—
hydrocyanic acid	T65.ØX1	T65.ØX2	T65.ØX3	T65.ØX4	—	—
illuminating (after combustion)	T58.11	T58.12	T58.13	T58.14	—	—
prior to combustion	T59.891	T59.892	T59.893	T59.894	—	—
incomplete combustion, any—*see* Carbon, monoxide						
kiln	T58.8X1	T58.8X2	T58.8X3	T58.8X4	—	—
lacrimogenic	T59.3X1	T59.3X2	T59.3X3	T59.3X4	—	—
liquefied petroleum—*see* Butane						
marsh	T59.891	T59.892	T59.893	T59.894	—	—
motor exhaust, not in transit	T58.Ø1	T58.Ø2	T58.Ø3	T58.Ø4	—	—
mustard, not in war	T59.891	T59.892	T59.893	T59.894	—	—
natural	T59.891	T59.892	T59.893	T59.894	—	—
nerve, not in war	T59.91	T59.92	T59.93	T59.94	—	—
oil	T52.ØX1	T52.ØX2	T52.ØX3	T52.ØX4	—	—
petroleum (liquefied) (distributed in mobile containers)	T59.891	T59.892	T59.893	T59.894	—	—
piped (pure or mixed with air)	T59.891	T59.892	T59.893	T59.894	—	—
piped (manufactured) (natural) NEC	T59.891	T59.892	T59.893	T59.894	—	—
producer	T58.8X1	T58.8X2	T58.8X3	T58.8X4	—	—
propane—*see* propane						
refrigerant (chlorofluorocarbon)	T53.5X1	T53.5X2	T53.5X3	T53.5X4	—	—
not chlorofluorocarbon	T59.891	T59.892	T59.893	T59.894	—	—
sewer	T59.91	T59.92	T59.93	T59.94	—	—
specified source NEC	T59.91	T59.92	T59.93	T59.94	—	—

Substance	Poisoning, Accidental (unintentional)	Poisoning, Intentional Self-harm	Poisoning, Assault	Poisoning, Undetermined	Adverse Effect	Under-dosing
Gas—*continued*						
stove (after combustion)	T58.11	T58.12	T58.13	T58.14	—	—
prior to combustion	T59.891	T59.892	T59.893	T59.894	—	—
tear	T59.3X1	T59.3X2	T59.3X3	T59.3X4	—	—
therapeutic	T41.5X1	T41.5X2	T41.5X3	T41.5X4	T41.5X5	T41.5X6
utility (for cooking, heating, or lighting) (piped) NEC	T59.891	T59.892	T59.893	T59.894	—	—
incomplete combustion of—*see* Carbon, monoxide, fuel, utilty						
in mobile container	T59.891	T59.892	T59.893	T59.894	—	—
piped (natural)	T59.891	T59.892	T59.893	T59.894	—	—
water	T58.1X1	T58.1X2	T58.1X3	T58.1X4	—	—
incomplete combustion of—*see* Carbon, monoxide, fuel, utility						
Gaseous substance—*see* Gas						
Gasoline, gasoline	T52.ØX1	T52.ØX2	T52.ØX3	T52.ØX4	—	—
vapor	T52.ØX1	T52.ØX2	T52.ØX3	T52.ØX4	—	—
Gastric enzymes	T47.5X1	T47.5X2	T47.5X3	T47.5X4	T47.5X5	T47.5X6
Gastrografin	T5Ø.8X1	T5Ø.8X2	T5Ø.8X3	T5Ø.8X4	T5Ø.8X5	T5Ø.8X6
Gastrointestinal drug	T47.91	T47.92	T47.93	T47.94	T47.95	T47.96
biological	T47.8X1	T47.8X2	T47.8X3	T47.8X4	T47.8X5	T47.8X6
specified NEC	T47.8X1	T47.8X2	T47.8X3	T47.8X4	T47.8X5	T47.8X6
Gaultheria procumbens	T62.2X1	T62.2X2	T62.2X3	T62.2X4	—	—
Gelatin (intravenous)	T45.8X1	T45.8X2	T45.8X3	T45.8X4	T45.8X5	T45.8X6
absorbable (sponge)	T45.7X1	T45.7X2	T45.7X3	T45.7X4	T45.7X5	T45.7X6
Gefarnate	T44.3X1	T44.3X2	T44.3X3	T44.3X4	T44.3X5	T44.3X6
Gelfilm	T49.8X1	T49.8X2	T49.8X3	T49.8X4	T49.8X5	T49.8X6
Gelfoam	T45.7X1	T45.7X2	T45.7X3	T45.7X4	T45.7X5	T45.7X6
Gelsemine	T5Ø.991	T5Ø.992	T5Ø.993	T5Ø.994	T5Ø.995	T5Ø.996
Gelsemium (sempervirens)	T62.2X1	T62.2X2	T62.2X3	T62.2X4	—	—
Gemeprost	T48.ØX1	T48.ØX2	T48.ØX3	T48.ØX4	T48.ØX5	T48.ØX6
Gemfibrozil	T46.6X1	T46.6X2	T46.6X3	T46.6X4	T46.6X5	T46.6X6
Gemonil	T42.3X1	T42.3X2	T42.3X3	T42.3X4	T42.3X5	T42.3X6
Gentamicin	T36.5X1	T36.5X2	T36.5X3	T36.5X4	T36.5X5	T36.5X6
ophthalmic preparation	T49.5X1	T49.5X2	T49.5X3	T49.5X4	T49.5X5	T49.5X6
topical NEC	T49.ØX1	T49.ØX2	T49.ØX3	T49.ØX4	T49.ØX5	T49.ØX6
Gentian	T47.5X1	T47.5X2	T47.5X3	T47.5X4	T47.5X5	T47.5X6
violet	T49.ØX1	T49.ØX2	T49.ØX3	T49.ØX4	T49.ØX5	T49.ØX6
Gepefrine	T44.4X1	T44.4X2	T44.4X3	T44.4X4	T44.4X5	T44.4X6
Gestonorone caproate	T38.5X1	T38.5X2	T38.5X3	T38.5X4	T38.5X5	T38.5X6
Gexane	T49.ØX1	T49.ØX2	T49.ØX3	T49.ØX4	T49.ØX5	T49.ØX6
Gila monster (venom)	T63.111	T63.112	T63.113	T63.114	—	—
Ginger	T47.5X1	T47.5X2	T47.5X3	T47.5X4	T47.5X5	T47.5X6
Jamaica — *see* Jamaica , ginger						
Gitalin	T46.ØX1	T46.ØX2	T46.ØX3	T46.ØX4	T46.ØX5	T46.ØX6
amorphous	T46.ØX1	T46.ØX2	T46.ØX3	T46.ØX4	T46.ØX5	T46.ØX6
Gitaloxin	T46.ØX1	T46.ØX2	T46.ØX3	T46.ØX4	T46.ØX5	T46.ØX6
Gitoxin	T46.ØX1	T46.ØX2	T46.ØX3	T46.ØX4	T46.ØX5	T46.ØX6
Glafenine	T39.8X1	T39.8X2	T39.8X3	T39.8X4	T39.8X5	T39.8X6
Glandular extract (medicinal) **NEC**	T5Ø.Z91	T5Ø.Z92	T5Ø.Z93	T5Ø.Z94	T5Ø.Z95	T5Ø.Z96
Glaucarubin	T37.3X1	T37.3X2	T37.3X3	T37.3X4	T37.3X5	T37.3X6
Glibenclamide	T38.3X1	T38.3X2	T38.3X3	T38.3X4	T38.3X5	T38.3X6
Glibornuride	T38.3X1	T38.3X2	T38.3X3	T38.3X4	T38.3X5	T38.3X6
Gliclazide	T38.3X1	T38.3X2	T38.3X3	T38.3X4	T38.3X5	T38.3X6
Glimidine	T38.3X1	T38.3X2	T38.3X3	T38.3X4	T38.3X5	T38.3X6
Glipizide	T38.3X1	T38.3X2	T38.3X3	T38.3X4	T38.3X5	T38.3X6
Gliquidone	T38.3X1	T38.3X2	T38.3X3	T38.3X4	T38.3X5	T38.3X6
Glisolamide	T38.3X1	T38.3X2	T38.3X3	T38.3X4	T38.3X5	T38.3X6
Glisoxepide	T38.3X1	T38.3X2	T38.3X3	T38.3X4	T38.3X5	T38.3X6
Globin zinc insulin	T38.3X1	T38.3X2	T38.3X3	T38.3X4	T38.3X5	T38.3X6
Globulin						
antilymphocytic	T5Ø.Z11	T5Ø.Z12	T5Ø.Z13	T5Ø.Z14	T5Ø.Z15	T5Ø.Z16
antirhesus	T5Ø.Z11	T5Ø.Z12	T5Ø.Z13	T5Ø.Z14	T5Ø.Z15	T5Ø.Z16
antivenin	T5Ø.Z11	T5Ø.Z12	T5Ø.Z13	T5Ø.Z14	T5Ø.Z15	T5Ø.Z16
antiviral	T5Ø.Z11	T5Ø.Z12	T5Ø.Z13	T5Ø.Z14	T5Ø.Z15	T5Ø.Z16
Glucagon	T38.3X1	T38.3X2	T38.3X3	T38.3X4	T38.3X5	T38.3X6
Glucocorticoids	T38.ØX1	T38.ØX2	T38.ØX3	T38.ØX4	T38.ØX5	T38.ØX6
Glucocorticosteroid	T38.ØX1	T38.ØX2	T38.ØX3	T38.ØX4	T38.ØX5	T38.ØX6
Gluconic acid	T5Ø.991	T5Ø.992	T5Ø.993	T5Ø.994	T5Ø.995	T5Ø.996

Substance	Poisoning, Accidental (unintentional)	Poisoning, Intentional Self-harm	Poisoning, Assault	Poisoning, Undetermined	Adverse Effect	Under-dosing
Glucosamine sulfate	T39.4X1	T39.4X2	T39.4X3	T39.4X4	T39.4X5	T39.4X6
Glucose	T5Ø.3X1	T5Ø.3X2	T5Ø.3X3	T5Ø.3X4	T5Ø.3X5	T5Ø.3X6
with sodium chloride	T5Ø.3X1	T5Ø.3X2	T5Ø.3X3	T5Ø.3X4	T5Ø.3X5	T5Ø.3X6
Glucosulfone sodium	T37.1X1	T37.1X2	T37.1X3	T37.1X4	T37.1X5	T37.1X6
Glucurolactone	T47.8X1	T47.8X2	T47.8X3	T47.8X4	T47.8X5	T47.8X6
Glue NEC	T52.8X1	T52.8X2	T52.8X3	T52.8X4	—	—
Glutamic acid	T47.5X1	T47.5X2	T47.5X3	T47.5X4	T47.5X5	T47.5X6
Glutaral (medicinal)	T49.ØX1	T49.ØX2	T49.ØX3	T49.ØX4	T49.ØX5	T49.ØX6
nonmedicinal	T65.891	T65.892	T65.893	T65.894	—	—
Glutaraldehyde (nonmedicinal)	T65.891	T65.892	T65.893	T65.894	—	—
medicinal	T49.ØX1	T49.ØX2	T49.ØX3	T49.ØX4	T49.ØX5	T49.ØX6
Glutathione	T5Ø.6X1	T5Ø.6X2	T5Ø.6X3	T5Ø.6X4	T5Ø.6X5	T5Ø.6X6
Glutethimide	T42.6X1	T42.6X2	T42.6X3	T42.6X4	T42.6X5	T42.6X6
Glyburide	T38.3X1	T38.3X2	T38.3X3	T38.3X4	T38.3X5	T38.3X6
Glycerin	T47.4X1	T47.4X2	T47.4X3	T47.4X4	T47.4X5	T47.4X6
Glycerol	T47.4X1	T47.4X2	T47.4X3	T47.4X4	T47.4X5	T47.4X6
borax	T49.6X1	T49.6X2	T49.6X3	T49.6X4	T49.6X5	T49.6X6
intravenous	T5Ø.3X1	T5Ø.3X2	T5Ø.3X3	T5Ø.3X4	T5Ø.3X5	T5Ø.3X6
iodinated	T48.4X1	T48.4X2	T48.4X3	T48.4X4	T48.4X5	T48.4X6
Glycerophosphate	T5Ø.991	T5Ø.992	T5Ø.993	T5Ø.994	T5Ø.995	T5Ø.996
Glyceryl						
gualacolate	T48.4X1	T48.4X2	T48.4X3	T48.4X4	T48.4X5	T48.4X6
nitrate	T46.3X1	T46.3X2	T46.3X3	T46.3X4	T46.3X5	T46.3X6
triacetate (topical)	T49.ØX1	T49.ØX2	T49.ØX3	T49.ØX4	T49.ØX5	T49.ØX6
trinitrate	T46.3X1	T46.3X2	T46.3X3	T46.3X4	T46.3X5	T46.3X6
Glycine	T5Ø.3X1	T5Ø.3X2	T5Ø.3X3	T5Ø.3X4	T5Ø.3X5	T5Ø.3X6
Glyclopyramide	T38.3X1	T38.3X2	T38.3X3	T38.3X4	T38.3X5	T38.3X6
Glycobiarsol	T37.3X1	T37.3X2	T37.3X3	T37.3X4	T37.3X5	T37.3X6
Glycols (ether)	T52.3X1	T52.3X2	T52.3X3	T52.3X4	—	—
Glyconiazide	T37.1X1	T37.1X2	T37.1X3	T37.1X4	T37.1X5	T37.1X6
Glycopyrrolate	T44.3X1	T44.3X2	T44.3X3	T44.3X4	T44.3X5	T44.3X6
Glycopyrronium	T44.3X1	T44.3X2	T44.3X3	T44.3X4	T44.3X5	T44.3X6
bromide	T44.3X1	T44.3X2	T44.3X3	T44.3X4	T44.3X5	T44.3X6
Glycoside, cardiac (stimulant)	T46.ØX1	T46.ØX2	T46.ØX3	T46.ØX4	T46.ØX5	T46.ØX6
Glycyclamide	T38.3X1	T38.3X2	T38.3X3	T38.3X4	T38.3X5	T38.3X6
Glycyrrhiza extract	T48.4X1	T48.4X2	T48.4X3	T48.4X4	T48.4X5	T48.4X6
Glycyrrhizic acid	T48.4X1	T48.4X2	T48.4X3	T48.4X4	T48.4X5	T48.4X6
Glycyrrhizinate potassium	T48.4X1	T48.4X2	T48.4X3	T48.4X4	T48.4X5	T48.4X6
Glymidine sodium	T38.3X1	T38.3X2	T38.3X3	T38.3X4	T38.3X5	T38.3X6
Glyphosate	T6Ø.3X1	T6Ø.3X2	T6Ø.3X3	T6Ø.3X4	—	—
Glyphylline	T48.6X1	T48.6X2	T48.6X3	T48.6X4	T48.6X5	T48.6X6
Gold						
colloidal (I98Au)	T45.1X1	T45.1X2	T45.1X3	T45.1X4	T45.1X5	T45.1X6
salts	T39.4X1	T39.4X2	T39.4X3	T39.4X4	T39.4X5	T39.4X6
Golden sulfide of antimony	T56.891	T56.892	T56.893	T56.894	—	—
Goldylocks	T62.2X1	T62.2X2	T62.2X3	T62.2X4	—	—
Gonadal tissue extract	T38.9Ø1	T38.9Ø2	T38.9Ø3	T38.9Ø4	T38.9Ø5	T38.9Ø6
female	T38.5X1	T38.5X2	T38.5X3	T38.5X4	T38.5X5	T38.5X6
male	T38.7X1	T38.7X2	T38.7X3	T38.7X4	T38.7X5	T38.7X6
Gonadorelin	T38.891	T38.892	T38.893	T38.894	T38.895	T38.896
Gonadotropin	T38.891	T38.892	T38.893	T38.894	T38.895	T38.896
chorionic	T38.891	T38.892	T38.893	T38.894	T38.895	T38.896
pituitary	T38.811	T38.812	T38.813	T38.814	T38.815	T38.816
Goserelin	T45.1X1	T45.1X2	T45.1X3	T45.1X4	T45.1X5	T45.1X6
Grain alcohol	T51.ØX1	T51.ØX2	T51.ØX3	T51.ØX4	—	—
Gramicidin	T49.ØX1	T49.ØX2	T49.ØX3	T49.ØX4	T49.ØX5	T49.ØX6
Granisetron	T45.ØX1	T45.ØX2	T45.ØX3	T45.ØX4	T45.ØX5	T45.ØX6
Gratiola officinalis	T62.2X1	T62.2X2	T62.2X3	T62.2X4	—	—
Grease	T65.891	T65.892	T65.893	T65.894	—	—
Green hellebore	T62.2X1	T62.2X2	T62.2X3	T62.2X4	—	—
Green soap	T49.2X1	T49.2X2	T49.2X3	T49.2X4	T49.2X5	T49.2X6
Grifulvin	T36.7X1	T36.7X2	T36.7X3	T36.7X4	T36.7X5	T36.7X6
Griseofulvin	T36.7X1	T36.7X2	T36.7X3	T36.7X4	T36.7X5	T36.7X6
Growth hormone	T38.811	T38.812	T38.813	T38.814	T38.815	T38.816
Guaiacol derivatives	T48.4X1	T48.4X2	T48.4X3	T48.4X4	T48.4X5	T48.4X6
Guaiac reagent	T5Ø.991	T5Ø.992	T5Ø.993	T5Ø.994	T5Ø.995	T5Ø.996
Guaifenesin	T48.4X1	T48.4X2	T48.4X3	T48.4X4	T48.4X5	T48.4X6
Guaimesal	T48.4X1	T48.4X2	T48.4X3	T48.4X4	T48.4X5	T48.4X6
Guaiphenesin	T48.4X1	T48.4X2	T48.4X3	T48.4X4	T48.4X5	T48.4X6
Guamecycline	T36.4X1	T36.4X2	T36.4X3	T36.4X4	T36.4X5	T36.4X6
Guanabenz	T46.5X1	T46.5X2	T46.5X3	T46.5X4	T46.5X5	T46.5X6

Substance	Poisoning, Accidental (unintentional)	Poisoning, Intentional Self-harm	Poisoning, Assault	Poisoning, Undetermined	Adverse Effect	Under-dosing
Guanacline	T46.5X1	T46.5X2	T46.5X3	T46.5X4	T46.5X5	T46.5X6
Guanadrel	T46.5X1	T46.5X2	T46.5X3	T46.5X4	T46.5X5	T46.5X6
Guanatol	T37.2X1	T37.2X2	T37.2X3	T37.2X4	T37.2X5	T37.2X6
Guanethidine	T46.5X1	T46.5X2	T46.5X3	T46.5X4	T46.5X5	T46.5X6
Guanfacine	T46.5X1	T46.5X2	T46.5X3	T46.5X4	T46.5X5	T46.5X6
Guano	T65.891	T65.892	T65.893	T65.894	—	—
Guanochlor	T46.5X1	T46.5X2	T46.5X3	T46.5X4	T46.5X5	T46.5X6
Guanoclor	T46.5X1	T46.5X2	T46.5X3	T46.5X4	T46.5X5	T46.5X6
Guanoctine	T46.5X1	T46.5X2	T46.5X3	T46.5X4	T46.5X5	T46.5X6
Guanoxabenz	T46.5X1	T46.5X2	T46.5X3	T46.5X4	T46.5X5	T46.5X6
Guanoxan	T46.5X1	T46.5X2	T46.5X3	T46.5X4	T46.5X5	T46.5X6
Guar gum (medicinal)	T46.6X1	T46.6X2	T46.6X3	T46.6X4	T46.6X5	T46.6X6
H						
Hachimycin	T36.7X1	T36.7X2	T36.7X3	T36.7X4	T36.7X5	T36.7X6
Hair						
dye	T49.4X1	T49.4X2	T49.4X3	T49.4X4	T49.4X5	T49.4X6
preparation NEC	T49.4X1	T49.4X2	T49.4X3	T49.4X4	T49.4X5	T49.4X6
Halazepam	T42.4X1	T42.4X2	T42.4X3	T42.4X4	T42.4X5	T42.4X6
Halcinolone	T49.ØX1	T49.ØX2	T49.ØX3	T49.ØX4	T49.ØX5	T49.ØX6
Halcinonide	T49.ØX1	T49.ØX2	T49.ØX3	T49.ØX4	T49.ØX5	T49.ØX6
Halethazole	T49.ØX1	T49.ØX2	T49.ØX3	T49.ØX4	T49.ØX5	T49.ØX6
Hallucinogen NEC	T4Ø.9Ø1	T4Ø.9Ø2	T4Ø.9Ø3	T4Ø.9Ø4	T4Ø.9Ø5	T4Ø.9Ø6
Halofantrine	T37.2X1	T37.2X2	T37.2X3	T37.2X4	T37.2X5	T37.2X6
Halofenate	T46.6X1	T46.6X2	T46.6X3	T46.6X4	T46.6X5	T46.6X6
Halometasone	T49.ØX1	T49.ØX2	T49.ØX3	T49.ØX4	T49.ØX5	T49.ØX6
Haloperidol	T43.4X1	T43.4X2	T43.4X3	T43.4X4	T43.4X5	T43.4X6
Haloprogin	T49.ØX1	T49.ØX2	T49.ØX3	T49.ØX4	T49.ØX5	T49.ØX6
Halotex	T49.ØX1	T49.ØX2	T49.ØX3	T49.ØX4	T49.ØX5	T49.ØX6
Halothane	T41.ØX1	T41.ØX2	T41.ØX3	T41.ØX4	T41.ØX5	T41.ØX6
Haloxazolam	T42.4X1	T42.4X2	T42.4X3	T42.4X4	T42.4X5	T42.4X6
Halquinols	T49.ØX1	T49.ØX2	T49.ØX3	T49.ØX4	T49.ØX5	T49.ØX6
Hamamelis	T49.2X1	T49.2X2	T49.2X3	T49.2X4	T49.2X5	T49.2X6
Haptendextran	T45.8X1	T45.8X2	T45.8X3	T45.8X4	T45.8X5	T45.8X6
Harmonyl	T46.5X1	T46.5X2	T46.5X3	T46.5X4	T46.5X5	T46.5X6
Hartmann's solution	T5Ø.3X1	T5Ø.3X2	T5Ø.3X3	T5Ø.3X4	T5Ø.3X5	T5Ø.3X6
Hashish	T4Ø.7X1	T4Ø.7X2	T4Ø.7X3	T4Ø.7X4	T4Ø.7X5	T4Ø.7X6
Hawaiian Woodrose seeds	T4Ø.991	T4Ø.992	T4Ø.993	T4Ø.994	—	—
HCB	T6Ø.3X1	T6Ø.3X2	T6Ø.3X3	T6Ø.3X4	—	—
HCH	T53.6X1	T53.6X2	T53.6X3	T53.6X4	—	—
medicinal	T49.ØX1	T49.ØX2	T49.ØX3	T49.ØX4	T49.ØX5	T49.ØX6
HCN	T57.3X1	T57.3X2	T57.3X3	T57.3X4	—	—
Headache cures, drugs, powders NEC	T5Ø.9Ø1	T5Ø.9Ø2	T5Ø.9Ø3	T5Ø.9Ø4	T5Ø.9Ø5	T5Ø.9Ø6
Heavenly Blue (morning glory)	T4Ø.991	T4Ø.992	T4Ø.993	T4Ø.994	—	—
Heavy metal antidote	T45.8X1	T45.8X2	T45.8X3	T45.8X4	T45.8X5	T45.8X6
Hedaquinium	T49.ØX1	T49.ØX2	T49.ØX3	T49.ØX4	T49.ØX5	T49.ØX6
Hedge hyssop	T62.2X1	T62.2X2	T62.2X3	T62.2X4	—	—
Heet	T49.8X1	T49.8X2	T49.8X3	T49.8X4	T49.8X5	T49.8X6
Helium (nonmedicinal) **NEC**	T59.891	T59.892	T59.893	T59.894	—	—
medicinal	T48.991	T48.992	T48.993	T48.994	T48.995	T48.996
Helenin	T37.4X1	T37.4X2	T37.4X3	T37.4X4	T37.4X5	T37.4X6
Hellebore (black) (green) (white)	T62.2X1	T62.2X2	T62.2X3	T62.2X4	—	—
Hematin	T45.8X1	T45.8X2	T45.8X3	T45.8X4	T45.8X5	T45.8X6
Hematinic preparation	T45.8X1	T45.8X2	T45.8X3	T45.8X4	T45.8X5	T45.8X6
Hematological agent	T45.91	T45.92	T45.93	T45.94	T45.95	T45.96
specified NEC	T45.8X1	T45.8X2	T45.8X3	T45.8X4	T45.8X5	T45.8X6
Hemlock	T62.2X1	T62.2X2	T62.2X3	T62.2X4	—	—
Hemostatic	T45.621	T45.622	T45.623	T45.624	T45.625	T45.626
drug, systemic	T45.621	T45.622	T45.623	T45.624	T45.625	T45.626
Hemostyptic	T49.4X1	T49.4X2	T49.4X3	T49.4X4	T49.4X5	T49.4X6
Henbane	T62.2X1	T62.2X2	T62.2X3	T62.2X4	—	—
Heparin (sodium)	T45.511	T45.512	T45.513	T45.514	T45.515	T45.516
action reverser	T45.7X1	T45.7X2	T45.7X3	T45.7X4	T45.7X5	T45.7X6
Heparin-fraction	T45.511	T45.512	T45.513	T45.514	T45.515	T45.516
Heparinoid (systemic)	T45.511	T45.512	T45.513	T45.514	T45.515	T45.516
Hepatic secretion stimulant	T47.8X1	T47.8X2	T47.8X3	T47.8X4	T47.8X5	T47.8X6
Hepatitis B						
immune globulin	T5Ø.Z11	T5Ø.Z12	T5Ø.Z13	T5Ø.Z14	T5Ø.Z15	T5Ø.Z16
vaccine	T5Ø.B91	T5Ø.B92	T5Ø.B93	T5Ø.B94	T5Ø.B95	T5Ø.B96
Hepronicate	T46.7X1	T46.7X2	T46.7X3	T46.7X4	T46.7X5	T46.7X6
Heptabarb	T42.3X1	T42.3X2	T42.3X3	T42.3X4	T42.3X5	T42.3X6

Substance	Poisoning, Accidental (unintentional)	Poisoning, Intentional Self-harm	Poisoning, Assault	Poisoning, Undetermined	Adverse Effect	Under-dosing
Heptabarbital	T42.3X1	T42.3X2	T42.3X3	T42.3X4	T42.3X5	T42.3X6
Heptabarbitone	T42.3X1	T42.3X2	T42.3X3	T42.3X4	T42.3X5	T42.3X6
Heptachlor	T6Ø.1X1	T6Ø.1X2	T6Ø.1X3	T6Ø.1X4	—	—
Heptalgin	T4Ø.2X1	T4Ø.2X2	T4Ø.2X3	T4Ø.2X4	T4Ø.2X5	T4Ø.2X6
Heptaminol	T46.3X1	T46.3X2	T46.3X3	T46.3X4	T46.3X5	T46.3X6
Herbicide NEC	T6Ø.3X1	T6Ø.3X2	T6Ø.3X3	T6Ø.3X4	—	—
Heroin	T4Ø.1X1	T4Ø.1X2	T4Ø.1X3	T4Ø.1X4	T4Ø.1X5	—
Herplex	T49.5X1	T49.5X2	T49.5X3	T49.5X4	T49.5X5	T49.5X6
HES	T45.8X1	T45.8X2	T45.8X3	T45.8X4	T45.8X5	T45.8X6
Hesperidin	T46.991	T46.992	T46.993	T46.994	T46.995	T46.996
Hetacillin	T36.ØX1	T36.ØX2	T36.ØX3	T36.ØX4	T36.ØX5	T36.ØX6
Hetastarch	T45.8X1	T45.8X2	T45.8X3	T45.8X4	T45.8X5	T45.8X6
HETP	T6Ø.ØX1	T6Ø.ØX2	T6Ø.ØX3	T6Ø.ØX4	—	—
Hexachlorobenzene (vapor)	T6Ø.3X1	T6Ø.3X2	T6Ø.3X3	T6Ø.3X4	—	—
Hexachlorocyclohexane	T53.6X1	T53.6X2	T53.6X3	T53.6X4	—	—
Hexachlorophene	T49.ØX1	T49.ØX2	T49.ØX3	T49.ØX4	T49.ØX5	T49.ØX6
Hexadiline	T46.3X1	T46.3X2	T46.3X3	T46.3X4	T46.3X5	T46.3X6
Hexadimethrine (bromide)	T45.7X1	T45.7X2	T45.7X3	T45.7X4	T45.7X5	T45.7X6
Hexadylamine	T46.3X1	T46.3X2	T46.3X3	T46.3X4	T46.3X5	T46.3X6
Hexaethyl tetraphosphate	T6Ø.ØX1	T6Ø.ØX2	T6Ø.ØX3	T6Ø.ØX4	—	—
Hexafluorenium bromide	T48.1X1	T48.1X2	T48.1X3	T48.1X4	T48.1X5	T48.1X6
Hexafluronium (bromide)	T48.1X1	T48.1X2	T48.1X3	T48.1X4	T48.1X5	T48.1X6
Hexahydrobenzol	T52.8X1	T52.8X2	T52.8X3	T52.8X4	—	—
Hexahydrocresol (s)	T51.8X1	T51.8X2	T51.8X3	T51.8X4	—	—
arsenide	T57.ØX1	T57.ØX2	T57.ØX3	T57.ØX4	—	—
arseniurated	T57.ØX1	T57.ØX2	T57.ØX3	T57.ØX4	—	—
cyanide	T57.3X1	T57.3X2	T57.3X3	T57.3X4	—	—
gas	T59.891	T59.892	T59.893	T59.894	—	—
Fluoride (liquid)	T57.8X1	T57.8X2	T57.8X3	T57.8X4	—	—
vapor	T59.891	T59.892	T59.893	T59.894	—	—
phophorated	T6Ø.ØX1	T6Ø.ØX2	T6Ø.ØX3	T6Ø.ØX4	—	—
sulfate	T57.8X1	T57.8X2	T57.8X3	T57.8X4	—	—
sulfide (gas)	T59.6X1	T59.6X2	T59.6X3	T59.6X4	—	—
arseniurated	T57.ØX1	T57.ØX2	T57.ØX3	T57.ØX4	—	—
sulfurated	T57.8X1	T57.8X2	T57.8X3	T57.8X4	—	—
Hexahydrophenol	T51.8X1	T51.8X2	T51.8X3	T51.8X4	—	—
Hexa-germ	T49.2X1	T49.2X2	T49.2X3	T49.2X4	T49.2X5	T49.2X6
Hexalen	T51.8X1	T51.8X2	T51.8X3	T51.8X4	—	—
Hexamethonium bromide	T44.2X1	T44.2X2	T44.2X3	T44.2X4	T44.2X5	T44.2X6
Hexamethylene	T52.8X1	T52.8X2	T52.8X3	T52.8X4	—	—
Hexamethylmelamine	T45.1X1	T45.1X2	T45.1X3	T45.1X4	T45.1X5	T45.1X6
Hexamidine	T49.ØX1	T49.ØX2	T49.ØX3	T49.ØX4	T49.ØX5	T49.ØX6
Hexamine (mandelate)	T37.8X1	T37.8X2	T37.8X3	T37.8X4	T37.8X5	T37.8X6
Hexanone, 2-hexanone	T52.4X1	T52.4X2	T52.4X3	T52.4X4	—	—
Hexanuorenium	T48.1X1	T48.1X2	T48.1X3	T48.1X4	T48.1X5	T48.1X6
Hexapropymate	T42.6X1	T42.6X2	T42.6X3	T42.6X4	T42.6X5	T42.6X6
Hexasonium iodide	T44.3X1	T44.3X2	T44.3X3	T44.3X4	T44.3X5	T44.3X6
Hexcarbacholine bromide	T48.1X1	T48.1X2	T48.1X3	T48.1X4	T48.1X5	T48.1X6
Hexemal	T42.3X1	T42.3X2	T42.3X3	T42.3X4	T42.3X5	T42.3X6
Hexestrol	T38.5X1	T38.5X2	T38.5X3	T38.5X4	T38.5X5	T38.5X6
Hexethal (sodium)	T42.3X1	T42.3X2	T42.3X3	T42.3X4	T42.3X5	T42.3X6
Hexetidine	T37.8X1	T37.8X2	T37.8X3	T37.8X4	T37.8X5	T37.8X6
Hexobarbital	T42.3X1	T42.3X2	T42.3X3	T42.3X4	T42.3X5	T42.3X6
rectal	T41.291	T41.292	T41.293	T41.294	T41.295	T41.296
sodium	T41.1X1	T41.1X2	T41.1X3	T41.1X4	T41.1X5	T41.1X6
Hexobendine	T46.3X1	T46.3X2	T46.3X3	T46.3X4	T46.3X5	T46.3X6
Hexocyclium	T44.3X1	T44.3X2	T44.3X3	T44.3X4	T44.3X5	T44.3X6
metilsulfate	T44.3X1	T44.3X2	T44.3X3	T44.3X4	T44.3X5	T44.3X6
Hexoestrol	T38.5X1	T38.5X2	T38.5X3	T38.5X4	T38.5X5	T38.5X6
Hexone	T52.4X1	T52.4X2	T52.4X3	T52.4X4	—	—
Hexoprenaline	T48.6X1	T48.6X2	T48.6X3	T48.6X4	T48.6X5	T48.6X6
Hexylcaine	T41.3X1	T41.3X2	T41.3X3	T41.3X4	T41.3X5	T41.3X6
Hexylresorcinol	T52.2X1	T52.2X2	T52.2X3	T52.2X4	—	—
HGH (human growth hormone)	T38.811	T38.812	T38.813	T38.814	T38.815	T38.816
Hinkle's pills	T47.2X1	T47.2X2	T47.2X3	T47.2X4	T47.2X5	T47.2X6
Histalog	T5Ø.8X1	T5Ø.8X2	T5Ø.8X3	T5Ø.8X4	T5Ø.8X5	T5Ø.8X6
Histamine (phosphate)	T5Ø.8X1	T5Ø.8X2	T5Ø.8X3	T5Ø.8X4	T5Ø.8X5	T5Ø.8X6
Histoplasmin	T5Ø.8X1	T5Ø.8X2	T5Ø.8X3	T5Ø.8X4	T5Ø.8X5	T5Ø.8X6
Holly berries	T62.2X1	T62.2X2	T62.2X3	T62.2X4	—	—
Homatropine	T44.3X1	T44.3X2	T44.3X3	T44.3X4	T44.3X5	T44.3X6
methylbromide	T44.3X1	T44.3X2	T44.3X3	T44.3X4	T44.3X5	T44.3X6

Substance	Poisoning, Accidental (unintentional)	Poisoning, Intentional Self-harm	Poisoning, Assault	Poisoning, Undetermined	Adverse Effect	Under-dosing
Homochlorcyclizine	T45.ØX1	T45.ØX2	T45.ØX3	T45.ØX4	T45.ØX5	T45.ØX6
Homosalate	T49.3X1	T49.3X2	T49.3X3	T49.3X4	T49.3X5	T49.3X6
Homo-tet	T5Ø.Z11	T5Ø.Z12	T5Ø.Z13	T5Ø.Z14	T5Ø.Z15	T5Ø.Z16
Hormone	T38.8Ø1	T38.8Ø2	T38.8Ø3	T38.8Ø4	T38.8Ø5	T38.8Ø6
adrenal cortical steroids	T38.ØX1	T38.ØX2	T38.ØX3	T38.ØX4	T38.ØX5	T38.ØX6
androgenic	T38.7X1	T38.7X2	T38.7X3	T38.7X4	T38.7X5	T38.7X6
anterior pituitary NEC	T38.811	T38.812	T38.813	T38.814	T38.815	T38.816
antidiabetic agents	T38.3X1	T38.3X2	T38.3X3	T38.3X4	T38.3X5	T38.3X6
antidiuretic	T38.891	T38.892	T38.893	T38.894	T38.895	T38.896
cancer therapy	T45.1X1	T45.1X2	T45.1X3	T45.1X4	T45.1X5	T45.1X6
follicle stimulating	T38.811	T38.812	T38.813	T38.814	T38.815	T38.816
gonadotropic	T38.891	T38.892	T38.893	T38.894	T38.895	T38.896
pituitary	T38.811	T38.812	T38.813	T38.814	T38.815	T38.816
growth	T38.811	T38.812	T38.813	T38.814	T38.815	T38.816
luteinizing	T38.811	T38.812	T38.813	T38.814	T38.815	T38.816
ovarian	T38.5X1	T38.5X2	T38.5X3	T38.5X4	T38.5X5	T38.5X6
oxytocic	T48.ØX1	T48.ØX2	T48.ØX3	T48.ØX4	T48.ØX5	T48.ØX6
parathyroid (derivatives)	T5Ø.991	T5Ø.992	T5Ø.993	T5Ø.994	T5Ø.995	T5Ø.996
pituitary (posterior) NEC	T38.891	T38.892	T38.893	T38.894	T38.895	T38.896
anterior	T38.811	T38.812	T38.813	T38.814	T38.815	T38.816
specified, NEC	T38.891	T38.892	T38.893	T38.894	T38.895	T38.896
thyroid	T38.1X1	T38.1X2	T38.1X3	T38.1X4	T38.1X5	T38.1X6
Hornet (sting)	T63.451	T63.452	T63.453	T63.454	—	—
Horse anti-human lymphocytic serum	T5Ø.Z11	T5Ø.Z12	T5Ø.Z13	T5Ø.Z14	T5Ø.Z15	T5Ø.Z16
Horticulture agent NEC	T65.91	T65.92	T65.93	T65.94	—	—
with pesticide	T6Ø.91	T6Ø.92	T6Ø.93	T6Ø.94	—	—
Human						
albumin	T45.8X1	T45.8X2	T45.8X3	T45.8X4	T45.8X5	T45.8X6
growth hormone (HGH)	T38.811	T38.812	T38.813	T38.814	T38.815	T38.816
immune serum	T5Ø.Z11	T5Ø.Z12	T5Ø.Z13	T5Ø.Z14	T5Ø.Z15	T5Ø.Z16
Hyaluronidase	T45.3X1	T45.3X2	T45.3X3	T45.3X4	T45.3X5	T45.3X6
Hyazyme	T45.3X1	T45.3X2	T45.3X3	T45.3X4	T45.3X5	T45.3X6
Hycodan	T4Ø.2X1	T4Ø.2X2	T4Ø.2X3	T4Ø.2X4	T4Ø.2X5	T4Ø.2X6
Hydantoin derivative NEC	T42.ØX1	T42.ØX2	T42.ØX3	T42.ØX4	T42.ØX5	T42.ØX6
Hydeltra	T38.ØX1	T38.ØX2	T38.ØX3	T38.ØX4	T38.ØX5	T38.ØX6
Hydergine	T44.6X1	T44.6X2	T44.6X3	T44.6X4	T44.6X5	T44.6X6
Hydrabamine penicillin	T36.ØX1	T36.ØX2	T36.ØX3	T36.ØX4	T36.ØX5	T36.ØX6
Hydralazine	T46.5X1	T46.5X2	T46.5X3	T46.5X4	T46.5X5	T46.5X6
Hydrargaphen	T49.ØX1	T49.ØX2	T49.ØX3	T49.ØX4	T49.ØX5	T49.ØX6
Hydrargyri aminochloridum	T49.ØX1	T49.ØX2	T49.ØX3	T49.ØX4	T49.ØX5	T49.ØX6
Hydrastine	T48.291	T48.292	T48.293	T48.294	T48.295	T48.296
Hydrazine	T54.1X1	T54.1X2	T54.1X3	T54.1X4	—	—
monoamine oxidase inhibitors	T43.1X1	T43.1X2	T43.1X3	T43.1X4	T43.1X5	T43.1X6
Hydrazoic acid, azides	T54.2X1	T54.2X2	T54.2X3	T54.2X4	—	—
Hydriodic acid	T48.4X1	T48.4X2	T48.4X3	T48.4X4	T48.4X5	T48.4X6
Hydrocarbon gas	T59.891	T59.892	T59.893	T59.894	—	—
incomplete combustion of— *see* Carbon, monoxide, fuel, utility						
liquefied (mobile container)	T59.891	T59.892	T59.893	T59.894	—	—
piped (natural)	T59.891	T59.892	T59.893	T59.894	—	—
Hydrochloric acid (liquid)	T54.2X1	T54.2X2	T54.2X3	T54.2X4	—	—
medicinal (digestant)	T47.5X1	T47.5X2	T47.5X3	T47.5X4	T47.5X5	T47.5X6
vapor	T59.891	T59.892	T59.893	T59.894	—	—
Hydrochlorothiazide	T5Ø.2X1	T5Ø.2X2	T5Ø.2X3	T5Ø.2X4	T5Ø.2X5	T5Ø.2X6
Hydrocodone	T4Ø.2X1	T4Ø.2X2	T4Ø.2X3	T4Ø.2X4	T4Ø.2X5	T4Ø.2X6
Hydrocortisone (derivatives)	T49.ØX1	T49.ØX2	T49.ØX3	T49.ØX4	T49.ØX5	T49.ØX6
aceponate	T49.ØX1	T49.ØX2	T49.ØX3	T49.ØX4	T49.ØX5	T49.ØX6
ENT agent	T49.6X1	T49.6X2	T49.6X3	T49.6X4	T49.6X5	T49.6X6
ophthalmic preparation	T49.5X1	T49.5X2	T49.5X3	T49.5X4	T49.5X5	T49.5X6
topical NEC	T49.ØX1	T49.ØX2	T49.ØX3	T49.ØX4	T49.ØX5	T49.ØX6
Hydrocortone	T38.ØX1	T38.ØX2	T38.ØX3	T38.ØX4	T38.ØX5	T38.ØX6
ENT agent	T49.6X1	T49.6X2	T49.6X3	T49.6X4	T49.6X5	T49.6X6
ophthalmic preparation	T49.5X1	T49.5X2	T49.5X3	T49.5X4	T49.5X5	T49.5X6
topical NEC	T49.ØX1	T49.ØX2	T49.ØX3	T49.ØX4	T49.ØX5	T49.ØX6
Hydrocyanic acid (liquid)	T57.3X1	T57.3X2	T57.3X3	T57.3X4	—	—
gas	T65.ØX1	T65.ØX2	T65.ØX3	T65.ØX4	—	—
Hydroflumethiazide	T5Ø.2X1	T5Ø.2X2	T5Ø.2X3	T5Ø.2X4	T5Ø.2X5	T5Ø.2X6
Hydrofluoric acid (liquid)	T54.2X1	T54.2X2	T54.2X3	T54.2X4	—	—
vapor	T59.891	T59.892	T59.893	T59.894	—	—

Substance	Poisoning, Accidental (unintentional)	Poisoning, Intentional Self-harm	Poisoning, Assault	Poisoning, Undetermined	Adverse Effect	Under-dosing
Hydrogen	T59.891	T59.892	T59.893	T59.894	—	—
arsenide	T57.ØX1	T57.ØX2	T57.ØX3	T57.ØX4	—	—
arseniureted	T57.ØX1	T57.ØX2	T57.ØX3	T57.ØX4	—	—
cyanide (salts)	T57.3X1	T57.3X2	T57.3X3	T57.3X4	—	—
gas	T57.3X1	T57.3X2	T57.3X3	T57.3X4	—	—
chloride	T57.8X1	T57.8X2	T57.8X3	T57.8X4	—	—
Fluoride	T59.5X1	T59.5X2	T59.5X3	T59.5X4	—	—
vapor	T59.5X1	T59.5X2	T59.5X3	T59.5X4	—	—
peroxide	T49.ØX1	T49.ØX2	T49.ØX3	T49.ØX4	T49.ØX5	T49.ØX6
phosphureted	T57.1X1	T57.1X2	T57.1X3	T57.1X4	—	—
sulfide	T59.6X1	T59.6X2	T59.6X3	T59.6X4	—	—
arseniureted	T57.ØX1	T57.ØX2	T57.ØX3	T57.ØX4	—	—
sulfureted	T59.6X1	T59.6X2	T59.6X3	T59.6X4	—	—
Hydromethylpyridine	T46.7X1	T46.7X2	T46.7X3	T46.7X4	T46.7X5	T46.7X6
Hydromorphinol	T4Ø.2X1	T4Ø.2X2	T4Ø.2X3	T4Ø.2X4	—	—
Hydromorphinone	T4Ø.2X1	T4Ø.2X2	T4Ø.2X3	T4Ø.2X4	T4Ø.2X5	T4Ø.2X6
Hydromorphone	T4Ø.2X1	T4Ø.2X2	T4Ø.2X3	T4Ø.2X4	T4Ø.2X5	T4Ø.2X6
Hydromox	T5Ø.2X1	T5Ø.2X2	T5Ø.2X3	T5Ø.2X4	T5Ø.2X5	T5Ø.2X6
Hydrophilic lotion	T49.3X1	T49.3X2	T49.3X3	T49.3X4	T49.3X5	T49.3X6
Hydroquinidine	T46.2X1	T46.2X2	T46.2X3	T46.2X4	T46.2X5	T46.2X6
Hydroquinone	T52.2X1	T52.2X2	T52.2X3	T52.2X4	—	—
vapor	T59.891	T59.892	T59.893	T59.894	—	—
Hydrosulfuric acid (gas)	T59.6X1	T59.6X2	T59.6X3	T59.6X4	—	—
Hydrotalcite	T47.1X1	T47.1X2	T47.1X3	T47.1X4	T47.1X5	T47.1X6
Hydrous wool fat	T49.3X1	T49.3X2	T49.3X3	T49.3X4	T49.3X5	T49.3X6
Hydroxide, caustic	T54.3X1	T54.3X2	T54.3X3	T54.3X4	—	—
Hydroxocobalamin	T45.8X1	T45.8X2	T45.8X3	T45.8X4	T45.8X5	T45.8X6
Hydroxyamphetamine	T49.5X1	T49.5X2	T49.5X3	T49.5X4	T49.5X5	T49.5X6
Hydroxycarbamide	T45.1X1	T45.1X2	T45.1X3	T45.1X4	T45.1X5	T45.1X6
Hydroxychloroquine	T37.8X1	T37.8X2	T37.8X3	T37.8X4	T37.8X5	T37.8X6
Hydroxydihydrocodeinone	T4Ø.2X1	T4Ø.2X2	T4Ø.2X3	T4Ø.2X4	T4Ø.2X5	T4Ø.2X6
Hydroxyestrone	T38.5X1	T38.5X2	T38.5X3	T38.5X4	T38.5X5	T38.5X6
Hydroxyethyl starch	T45.8X1	T45.8X2	T45.8X3	T45.8X4	T45.8X5	T45.8X6
Hydroxymethylpentanone	T52.4X1	T52.4X2	T52.4X3	T52.4X4	—	—
Hydroxyphenamate	T43.591	T43.592	T43.593	T43.594	T43.595	T43.596
Hydroxyphenylbutazone	T39.2X1	T39.2X2	T39.2X3	T39.2X4	T39.2X5	T39.2X6
Hydroxyprogesterone	T38.5X1	T38.5X2	T38.5X3	T38.5X4	T38.5X5	T38.5X6
caproate	T38.5X1	T38.5X2	T38.5X3	T38.5X4	T38.5X5	T38.5X6
Hydroxyquinoline (derivatives) **NEC**	T37.8X1	T37.8X2	T37.8X3	T37.8X4	T37.8X5	T37.8X6
Hydroxystilbamidine	T37.3X1	T37.3X2	T37.3X3	T37.3X4	T37.3X5	T37.3X6
Hydroxytoluene (nonmedicinal)	T54.ØX1	T54.ØX2	T54.ØX3	T54.ØX4	—	—
medicinal	T49.ØX1	T49.ØX2	T49.ØX3	T49.ØX4	T49.ØX5	T49.ØX6
Hydroxyurea	T45.1X1	T45.1X2	T45.1X3	T45.1X4	T45.1X5	T45.1X6
Hydroxyzine	T43.591	T43.592	T43.593	T43.594	T43.595	T43.596
Hyoscine	T44.3X1	T44.3X2	T44.3X3	T44.3X4	T44.3X5	T44.3X6
Hyoscyamine	T44.3X1	T44.3X2	T44.3X3	T44.3X4	T44.3X5	T44.3X6
Hyoscyamus	T44.3X1	T44.3X2	T44.3X3	T44.3X4	T44.3X5	T44.3X6
dry extract	T44.3X1	T44.3X2	T44.3X3	T44.3X4	T44.3X5	T44.3X6
Hypaque	T5Ø.8X1	T5Ø.8X2	T5Ø.8X3	T5Ø.8X4	T5Ø.8X5	T5Ø.8X6
Hypertussis	T5Ø.Z11	T5Ø.Z12	T5Ø.Z13	T5Ø.Z14	T5Ø.Z15	T5Ø.Z16
Hypnotic	T42.71	T42.72	T42.73	T42.74	T42.75	T42.76
anticonvulsant	T42.71	T42.72	T42.73	T42.74	T42.75	T42.76
specified NEC	T42.6X1	T42.6X2	T42.6X3	T42.6X4	T42.6X5	T42.6X6
Hypochlorite	T49.ØX1	T49.ØX2	T49.ØX3	T49.ØX4	T49.ØX5	T49.ØX6
Hypophysis, posterior	T38.891	T38.892	T38.893	T38.894	T38.895	T38.896
Hypotensive NEC	T46.5X1	T46.5X2	T46.5X3	T46.5X4	T46.5X5	T46.5X6
Hypromellose	T49.5X1	T49.5X2	T49.5X3	T49.5X4	T49.5X5	T49.5X6
I						
Ibacitabine	T37.5X1	T37.5X2	T37.5X3	T37.5X4	T37.5X5	T37.5X6
Ibopamine	T44.991	T44.992	T44.993	T44.994	T44.995	T44.996
Ibufenac	T39.311	T39.312	T39.313	T39.314	T39.315	T39.316
Ibuprofen	T39.311	T39.312	T39.313	T39.314	T39.315	T39.316
Ibuproxam	T39.311	T39.312	T39.313	T39.314	T39.315	T39.316
Ibuterol	T48.6X1	T48.6X2	T48.6X3	T48.6X4	T48.6X5	T48.6X6
Ichthammol	T49.ØX1	T49.ØX2	T49.ØX3	T49.ØX4	T49.ØX5	T49.ØX6
Ichthyol	T49.4X1	T49.4X2	T49.4X3	T49.4X4	T49.4X5	T49.4X6
Idarubicin	T45.1X1	T45.1X2	T45.1X3	T45.1X4	T45.1X5	T45.1X6
Idrocilamide	T42.8X1	T42.8X2	T42.8X3	T42.8X4	T42.8X5	T42.8X6
Ifenprodil	T46.7X1	T46.7X2	T46.7X3	T46.7X4	T46.7X5	T46.7X6

Substance	Poisoning, Accidental (unintentional)	Poisoning, Intentional Self-harm	Poisoning, Assault	Poisoning, Undetermined	Adverse Effect	Under-dosing
Ifosfamide	T45.1X1	T45.1X2	T45.1X3	T45.1X4	T45.1X5	T45.1X6
Iletin	T38.3X1	T38.3X2	T38.3X3	T38.3X4	T38.3X5	T38.3X6
Ilex	T62.2X1	T62.2X2	T62.2X3	T62.2X4	—	—
Illuminating gas (after combustion)	T58.11	T58.12	T58.13	T58.14	—	—
prior to combustion	T59.891	T59.892	T59.893	T59.894	—	—
Ilopan	T45.2X1	T45.2X2	T45.2X3	T45.2X4	T45.2X5	T45.2X6
Iloprost	T46.7X1	T46.7X2	T46.7X3	T46.7X4	T46.7X5	T46.7X6
Ilotycin	T36.3X1	T36.3X2	T36.3X3	T36.3X4	T36.3X5	T36.3X6
ophthalmic preparation	T49.5X1	T49.5X2	T49.5X3	T49.5X4	T49.5X5	T49.5X6
topical NEC	T49.ØX1	T49.ØX2	T49.ØX3	T49.ØX4	T49.ØX5	T49.ØX6
Imidazole-4-carboxamide	T45.1X1	T45.1X2	T45.1X3	T45.1X4	T45.1X5	T45.1X6
Iminostilbene	T42.1X1	T42.1X2	T42.1X3	T42.1X4	T42.1X5	T42.1X6
Imipenem	T36.ØX1	T36.ØX2	T36.ØX3	T36.ØX4	T36.ØX5	T36.ØX6
Imipramine	T43.Ø11	T43.Ø12	T43.Ø13	T43.Ø14	T43.Ø15	T43.Ø16
Immu-G	T5Ø.Z11	T5Ø.Z12	T5Ø.Z13	T5Ø.Z14	T5Ø.Z15	T5Ø.Z16
Immuglobin	T5Ø.Z11	T5Ø.Z12	T5Ø.Z13	T5Ø.Z14	T5Ø.Z15	T5Ø.Z16
Immune						
globulin	T5Ø.Z11	T5Ø.Z12	T5Ø.Z13	T5Ø.Z14	T5Ø.Z15	T5Ø.Z16
serum globulin	T5Ø.Z11	T5Ø.Z12	T5Ø.Z13	T5Ø.Z14	T5Ø.Z15	T5Ø.Z16
Immunoglobin human (intravenous) (normal)	T5Ø.Z11	T5Ø.Z12	T5Ø.Z13	T5Ø.Z14	T5Ø.Z15	T5Ø.Z16
unmodified	T5Ø.Z11	T5Ø.Z12	T5Ø.Z13	T5Ø.Z14	T5Ø.Z15	T5Ø.Z16
Immunosuppressive drug	T45.1X1	T45.1X2	T45.1X3	T45.1X4	T45.1X5	T45.1X6
Immu-tetanus	T5Ø.Z11	T5Ø.Z12	T5Ø.Z13	T5Ø.Z14	T5Ø.Z15	T5Ø.Z16
Indalpine	T43.221	T43.222	T43.223	T43.224	T43.225	T43.226
Indanazoline	T48.5X1	T48.5X2	T48.5X3	T48.5X4	T48.5X5	T48.5X6
Indandione (derivatives)	T45.511	T45.512	T45.513	T45.514	T45.515	T45.516
Indapamide	T46.5X1	T46.5X2	T46.5X3	T46.5X4	T46.5X5	T46.5X6
Indendione (derivatives)	T45.511	T45.512	T45.513	T45.514	T45.515	T45.516
Indenolol	T44.7X1	T44.7X2	T44.7X3	T44.7X4	T44.7X5	T44.7X6
Inderal	T44.7X1	T44.7X2	T44.7X3	T44.7X4	T44.7X5	T44.7X6
Indian						
hemp	T4Ø.7X1	T4Ø.7X2	T4Ø.7X3	T4Ø.7X4	T4Ø.7X5	T4Ø.7X6
tobacco	T62.291	T62.292	T62.293	T62.294	—	—
Indigo carmine	T5Ø.8X1	T5Ø.8X2	T5Ø.8X3	T5Ø.8X4	T5Ø.8X5	T5Ø.8X6
Indobufen	T45.521	T45.522	T45.523	T45.524	T45.525	T45.526
Indocin	T39.2X1	T39.2X2	T39.2X3	T39.2X4	T39.2X5	T39.2X6
Indocyanine green	T5Ø.8X1	T5Ø.8X2	T5Ø.8X3	T5Ø.8X4	T5Ø.8X5	T5Ø.8X6
Indometacin	T39.391	T39.392	T39.393	T39.394	T39.395	T39.396
Indomethacin	T39.391	T39.392	T39.393	T39.394	T39.395	T39.396
farnesil	T39.4X1	T39.4X2	T39.4X3	T39.4X4	T39.4X5	T39.4X6
Indoramin	T44.6X1	T44.6X2	T44.6X3	T44.6X4	T44.6X5	T44.6X6
Industrial						
alcohol	T51.ØX1	T51.ØX2	T51.ØX3	T51.ØX4	—	—
fumes	T59.891	T59.892	T59.893	T59.894	—	—
solvents (fumes) (vapors)	T52.91	T52.92	T52.93	T52.94	—	—
Influenza vaccine	T5Ø.B91	T5Ø.B92	T5Ø.B93	T5Ø.B94	T5Ø.B95	T5Ø.B96
Ingested substance NEC	T65.91	T65.92	T65.93	T65.94	—	—
INH	T37.1X1	T37.1X2	T37.1X3	T37.1X4	T37.1X5	T37.1X6
Inhalation, gas (noxious)—*see* Gas						
Inhibitor						
angiotensin-converting enzyme	T46.4X1	T46.4X2	T46.4X3	T46.4X4	T46.4X5	T46.4X6
carbonic anhydrase	T5Ø.2X1	T5Ø.2X2	T5Ø.2X3	T5Ø.2X4	T5Ø.2X5	T5Ø.2X6
fibrinolysis	T45.621	T45.622	T45.623	T45.624	T45.625	T45.626
monoamine oxidase NEC	T43.1X1	T43.1X2	T43.1X3	T43.1X4	T43.1X5	T43.1X6
hydrazine	T43.1X1	T43.1X2	T43.1X3	T43.1X4	T43.1X5	T43.1X6
postsynaptic	T43.8X1	T43.8X2	T43.8X3	T43.8X4	T43.8X5	T43.8X6
prothrombin synthesis	T45.511	T45.512	T45.513	T45.514	T45.515	T45.516
Ink	T65.891	T65.892	T65.893	T65.894	—	—
Inosine pranobex	T37.5X1	T37.5X2	T37.5X3	T37.5X4	T37.5X5	T37.5X6
Inositol	T5Ø.991	T5Ø.992	T5Ø.993	T5Ø.994	T5Ø.995	T5Ø.996
nicotinate	T46.7X1	T46.7X2	T46.7X3	T46.7X4	T46.7X5	T46.7X6
Inproquone	T45.1X1	T45.1X2	T45.1X3	T45.1X4	T45.1X5	T45.1X6
Insect (sting), **venomous**	T63.481	T63.482	T63.483	T63.484	—	—
ant	T63.421	T63.422	T63.423	T63.424	—	—
bee	T63.441	T63.442	T63.443	T63.444	—	—
caterpillar	T63.431	T63.432	T63.433	T63.434	—	—
hornet	T63.451	T63.452	T63.453	T63.454	—	—
wasp	T63.461	T63.462	T63.463	T63.464	—	—

Substance	Poisoning, Accidental (unintentional)	Poisoning, Intentional Self-harm	Poisoning, Assault	Poisoning, Undetermined	Adverse Effect	Under-dosing
Insecticide NEC	T60.91	T60.92	T60.93	T60.94	—	—
carbamate	T60.0X1	T60.0X2	T60.0X3	T60.0X4	—	—
chlorinated	T60.1X1	T60.1X2	T60.1X3	T60.1X4	—	—
mixed	T60.91	T60.92	T60.93	T60.94	—	—
organochlorine	T60.1X1	T60.1X2	T60.1X3	T60.1X4	—	—
organophosphorus	T60.0X1	T60.0X2	T60.0X3	T60.0X4	—	—
Insular tissue extract	T38.3X1	T38.3X2	T38.3X3	T38.3X4	T38.3X5	T38.3X6
Insulin (amorphous) (globin) (isophane) (Lente) (NPH) (Semilente) (Ultralente)	T38.3X1	T38.3X2	T38.3X3	T38.3X4	T38.3X5	T38.3X6
defalan	T38.3X1	T38.3X2	T38.3X3	T38.3X4	T38.3X5	T38.3X6
human	T38.3X1	T38.3X2	T38.3X3	T38.3X4	T38.3X5	T38.3X6
injection, soluble	T38.3X1	T38.3X2	T38.3X3	T38.3X4	T38.3X5	T38.3X6
biphasic	T38.3X1	T38.3X2	T38.3X3	T38.3X4	T38.3X5	T38.3X6
intermediate acting	T38.3X1	T38.3X2	T38.3X3	T38.3X4	T38.3X5	T38.3X6
protamine zinc	T38.3X1	T38.3X2	T38.3X3	T38.3X4	T38.3X5	T38.3X6
slow acting	T38.3X1	T38.3X2	T38.3X3	T38.3X4	T38.3X5	T38.3X6
zinc						
protamine injection	T38.3X1	T38.3X2	T38.3X3	T38.3X4	T38.3X5	T38.3X6
suspension (amorphous) (crystalline)	T38.3X1	T38.3X2	T38.3X3	T38.3X4	T38.3X5	T38.3X6
Interferon (alpha) (beta) (gamma)	T37.5X1	T37.5X2	T37.5X3	T37.5X4	T37.5X5	T37.5X6
Intestinal motility control drug	T47.6X1	T47.6X2	T47.6X3	T47.6X4	T47.6X5	T47.6X6
biological	T47.8X1	T47.8X2	T47.8X3	T47.8X4	T47.8X5	T47.8X6
Intranarcon	T41.1X1	T41.1X2	T41.1X3	T41.1X4	T41.1X5	T41.1X6
Intravenous						
amino acids	T50.991	T50.992	T50.993	T50.994	T50.995	T50.996
fat suspension	T50.991	T50.992	T50.993	T50.994	T50.995	T50.996
Inulin	T50.8X1	T50.8X2	T50.8X3	T50.8X4	T50.8X5	T50.8X6
Invert sugar	T50.3X1	T50.3X2	T50.3X3	T50.3X4	T50.3X5	T50.3X6
Inza—*see* Naproxen						
Iobenzamic acid	T50.8X1	T50.8X2	T50.8X3	T50.8X4	T50.8X5	T50.8X6
Iocarmic acid	T50.8X1	T50.8X2	T50.8X3	T50.8X4	T50.8X5	T50.8X6
Iocetamic acid	T50.8X1	T50.8X2	T50.8X3	T50.8X4	T50.8X5	T50.8X6
Iodamide	T50.8X1	T50.8X2	T50.8X3	T50.8X4	T50.8X5	T50.8X6
Iodide NEC (*see also* Iodine)	T49.0X1	T49.0X2	T49.0X3	T49.0X4	T49.0X5	T49.0X6
mercury (ointment)	T49.0X1	T49.0X2	T49.0X3	T49.0X4	T49.0X5	T49.0X6
methylate	T49.0X1	T49.0X2	T49.0X3	T49.0X4	T49.0X5	T49.0X6
potassium (expectorant) NEC	T48.4X1	T48.4X2	T48.4X3	T48.4X4	T48.4X5	T48.4X6
Iodinated						
contrast medium	T50.8X1	T50.8X2	T50.8X3	T50.8X4	T50.8X5	T50.8X6
glycerol	T48.4X1	T48.4X2	T48.4X3	T48.4X4	T48.4X5	T48.4X6
human serum albumin (131I)	T50.8X1	T50.8X2	T50.8X3	T50.8X4	T50.8X5	T50.8X6
Iodine (antiseptic, external) (tincture) **NEC**	T49.0X1	T49.0X2	T49.0X3	T49.0X4	T49.0X5	T49.0X6
solution	T49.0X1	T49.0X2	T49.0X3	T49.0X4	T49.0X5	T49.0X6
125 (*see also* Radiation sickness, and Exposure to radioactivce isotopes)	T50.8X1	T50.8X2	T50.8X3	T50.8X4	T50.8X5	T50.8X6
therapeutic	T50.991	T50.992	T50.993	T50.994	T50.995	T50.996
131 (*see also* Radiation sickness, and Exposure to radioactivce isotopes)	T50.8X1	T50.8X2	T50.8X3	T50.8X4	T50.8X5	T50.8X6
therapeutic	T38.2X1	T38.2X2	T38.2X3	T38.2X4	T38.2X5	T38.2X6
diagnostic	T50.8X1	T50.8X2	T50.8X3	T50.8X4	T50.8X5	T50.8X6
for thyroid conditions (antithyroid)	T38.2X1	T38.2X2	T38.2X3	T38.2X4	T38.2X5	T38.2X6
vapor	T59.891	T59.892	T59.893	T59.894	—	—
Iodipamide	T50.8X1	T50.8X2	T50.8X3	T50.8X4	T50.8X5	T50.8X6
Iodized (poppy seed) **oil**	T50.8X1	T50.8X2	T50.8X3	T50.8X4	T50.8X5	T50.8X6
Iodobismitol	T37.8X1	T37.8X2	T37.8X3	T37.8X4	T37.8X5	T37.8X6
Iodochlorhydroxyquin	T37.8X1	T37.8X2	T37.8X3	T37.8X4	T37.8X5	T37.8X6
topical	T49.0X1	T49.0X2	T49.0X3	T49.0X4	T49.0X5	T49.0X6
Iodochlorhydroxyquinoline	T37.8X1	T37.8X2	T37.8X3	T37.8X4	T37.8X5	T37.8X6
Iodocholesterol (131I)	T50.8X1	T50.8X2	T50.8X3	T50.8X4	T50.8X5	T50.8X6
Iodoform	T49.0X1	T49.0X2	T49.0X3	T49.0X4	T49.0X5	T49.0X6
Iodohippuric acid	T50.8X1	T50.8X2	T50.8X3	T50.8X4	T50.8X5	T50.8X6
Iodopanoic acid	T50.8X1	T50.8X2	T50.8X3	T50.8X4	T50.8X5	T50.8X6
Iodophthalein (sodium)	T50.8X1	T50.8X2	T50.8X3	T50.8X4	T50.8X5	T50.8X6
Iodopyracet	T50.8X1	T50.8X2	T50.8X3	T50.8X4	T50.8X5	T50.8X6
Iodoquinol	T37.8X1	T37.8X2	T37.8X3	T37.8X4	T37.8X5	T37.8X6
Iodoxamic acid	T50.8X1	T50.8X2	T50.8X3	T50.8X4	T50.8X5	T50.8X6

Substance	Poisoning, Accidental (unintentional)	Poisoning, Intentional Self-harm	Poisoning, Assault	Poisoning, Undetermined	Adverse Effect	Under-dosing
Iofendylate	T50.8X1	T50.8X2	T50.8X3	T50.8X4	T50.8X5	T50.8X6
Ioglycamic acid	T50.8X1	T50.8X2	T50.8X3	T50.8X4	T50.8X5	T50.8X6
Iohexol	T50.8X1	T50.8X2	T50.8X3	T50.8X4	T50.8X5	T50.8X6
Ion exchange resin						
anion	T47.8X1	T47.8X2	T47.8X3	T47.8X4	T47.8X5	T47.8X6
cation	T50.3X1	T50.3X2	T50.3X3	T50.3X4	T50.3X5	T50.3X6
cholestyramine	T46.6X1	T46.6X2	T46.6X3	T46.6X4	T46.6X5	T46.6X6
intestinal	T47.8X1	T47.8X2	T47.8X3	T47.8X4	T47.8X5	T47.8X6
Iopamidol	T50.8X1	T50.8X2	T50.8X3	T50.8X4	T50.8X5	T50.8X6
Iopanoic acid	T50.8X1	T50.8X2	T50.8X3	T50.8X4	T50.8X5	T50.8X6
Iophenoic acid	T50.8X1	T50.8X2	T50.8X3	T50.8X4	T50.8X5	T50.8X6
Iopodate, sodium	T50.8X1	T50.8X2	T50.8X3	T50.8X4	T50.8X5	T50.8X6
Iopodic acid	T50.8X1	T50.8X2	T50.8X3	T50.8X4	T50.8X5	T50.8X6
Iopromide	T50.8X1	T50.8X2	T50.8X3	T50.8X4	T50.8X5	T50.8X6
Iopydol	T50.8X1	T50.8X2	T50.8X3	T50.8X4	T50.8X5	T50.8X6
Iotalamic acid	T50.8X1	T50.8X2	T50.8X3	T50.8X4	T50.8X5	T50.8X6
Iothalamate	T50.8X1	T50.8X2	T50.8X3	T50.8X4	T50.8X5	T50.8X6
Iothiouracil	T38.2X1	T38.2X2	T38.2X3	T38.2X4	T38.2X5	T38.2X6
Iotrol	T50.8X1	T50.8X2	T50.8X3	T50.8X4	T50.8X5	T50.8X6
Iotrolan	T50.8X1	T50.8X2	T50.8X3	T50.8X4	T50.8X5	T50.8X6
Iotroxate	T50.8X1	T50.8X2	T50.8X3	T50.8X4	T50.8X5	T50.8X6
Iotroxic acid	T50.8X1	T50.8X2	T50.8X3	T50.8X4	T50.8X5	T50.8X6
Ioversol	T50.8X1	T50.8X2	T50.8X3	T50.8X4	T50.8X5	T50.8X6
Ioxaglate	T50.8X1	T50.8X2	T50.8X3	T50.8X4	T50.8X5	T50.8X6
Ioxaglic acid	T50.8X1	T50.8X2	T50.8X3	T50.8X4	T50.8X5	T50.8X6
Ioxitalamic acid	T50.8X1	T50.8X2	T50.8X3	T50.8X4	T50.8X5	T50.8X6
Ipecac	T47.7X1	T47.7X2	T47.7X3	T47.7X4	T47.7X5	T47.7X6
Ipecacuanha	T48.4X1	T48.4X2	T48.4X3	T48.4X4	T48.4X5	T48.4X6
Ipodate, calcium	T50.8X1	T50.8X2	T50.8X3	T50.8X4	T50.8X5	T50.8X6
Ipral	T42.3X1	T42.3X2	T42.3X3	T42.3X4	T42.3X5	T42.3X6
Ipratropium (bromide)	T48.6X1	T48.6X2	T48.6X3	T48.6X4	T48.6X5	T48.6X6
Ipriflavone	T46.3X1	T46.3X2	T46.3X3	T46.3X4	T46.3X5	T46.3X6
Iprindole	T43.011	T43.012	T43.013	T43.014	T43.015	T43.016
Iproclozide	T43.1X1	T43.1X2	T43.1X3	T43.1X4	T43.1X5	T43.1X6
Iprofenin	T50.8X1	T50.8X2	T50.8X3	T50.8X4	T50.8X5	T50.8X6
Iproheptine	T49.2X1	T49.2X2	T49.2X3	T49.2X4	T49.2X5	T49.2X6
Iproniazid	T43.1X1	T43.1X2	T43.1X3	T43.1X4	T43.1X5	T43.1X6
Iproplatin	T45.1X1	T45.1X2	T45.1X3	T45.1X4	T45.1X5	T45.1X6
Iproveratril	T46.1X1	T46.1X2	T46.1X3	T46.1X4	T46.1X5	T46.1X6
Iron (compounds) (medicinal) **NEC**	T45.4X1	T45.4X2	T45.4X3	T45.4X4	T45.4X5	T45.4X6
ammonium	T45.4X1	T45.4X2	T45.4X3	T45.4X4	T45.4X5	T45.4X6
dextran injection	T45.4X1	T45.4X2	T45.4X3	T45.4X4	T45.4X5	T45.4X6
nonmedicinal	T56.891	T56.892	T56.893	T56.894	—	—
salts	T45.4X1	T45.4X2	T45.4X3	T45.4X4	T45.4X5	T45.4X6
sorbitex	T45.4X1	T45.4X2	T45.4X3	T45.4X4	T45.4X5	T45.4X6
sorbitol citric acid complex	T45.4X1	T45.4X2	T45.4X3	T45.4X4	T45.4X5	T45.4X6
Irrigating fluid (vaginal)	T49.8X1	T49.8X2	T49.8X3	T49.8X4	T49.8X5	T49.8X6
eye	T49.5X1	T49.5X2	T49.5X3	T49.5X4	T49.5X5	T49.5X6
Isepamicin	T36.5X1	T36.5X2	T36.5X3	T36.5X4	T36.5X5	T36.5X6
Isoaminile (citrate)	T48.3X1	T48.3X2	T48.3X3	T48.3X4	T48.3X5	T48.3X6
Isoamyl nitrite	T46.3X1	T46.3X2	T46.3X3	T46.3X4	T46.3X5	T46.3X6
Isobenzan	T60.1X1	T60.1X2	T60.1X3	T60.1X4	—	—
Isobutyl acetate	T52.8X1	T52.8X2	T52.8X3	T52.8X4	—	—
Isocarboxazid	T43.1X1	T43.1X2	T43.1X3	T43.1X4	T43.1X5	T43.1X6
Isoconazole	T49.0X1	T49.0X2	T49.0X3	T49.0X4	T49.0X5	T49.0X6
Isocyanate	T65.0X1	T65.0X2	T65.0X3	T65.0X4	—	—
Isoephedrine	T44.991	T44.992	T44.993	T44.994	T44.995	T44.996
Isoetarine	T48.6X1	T48.6X2	T48.6X3	T48.6X4	T48.6X5	T48.6X6
Isoethadione	T42.2X1	T42.2X2	T42.2X3	T42.2X4	T42.2X5	T42.2X6
Isoetharine	T44.5X1	T44.5X2	T44.5X3	T44.5X4	T44.5X5	T44.5X6
Isoflurane	T41.0X1	T41.0X2	T41.0X3	T41.0X4	T41.0X5	T41.0X6
Isoflurophate	T44.0X1	T44.0X2	T44.0X3	T44.0X4	T44.0X5	T44.0X6
Isomaltose, ferric complex	T45.4X1	T45.4X2	T45.4X3	T45.4X4	T45.4X5	T45.4X6
Isometheptene	T44.3X1	T44.3X2	T44.3X3	T44.3X4	T44.3X5	T44.3X6
Isoniazid	T37.1X1	T37.1X2	T37.1X3	T37.1X4	T37.1X5	T37.1X6
with						
rifampicin	T36.6X1	T36.6X2	T36.6X3	T36.6X4	T36.6X5	T36.6X6
thioacetazone	T37.1X1	T37.1X2	T37.1X3	T37.1X4	T37.1X5	T37.1X6
Isonicotinic acid hydrazide	T37.1X1	T37.1X2	T37.1X3	T37.1X4	T37.1X5	T37.1X6
Isonipecaine	T40.4X1	T40.4X2	T40.4X3	T40.4X4	T40.4X5	T40.4X6
Isopentaquine	T37.2X1	T37.2X2	T37.2X3	T37.2X4	T37.2X5	T37.2X6

Substance	Poisoning, Accidental (unintentional)	Poisoning, Intentional Self-harm	Poisoning, Assault	Poisoning, Undetermined	Adverse Effect	Under-dosing
Isophane insulin	T38.3X1	T38.3X2	T38.3X3	T38.3X4	T38.3X5	T38.3X6
Isophorone	T65.891	T65.892	T65.893	T65.894	—	—
Isophosphamide	T45.1X1	T45.1X2	T45.1X3	T45.1X4	T45.1X5	T45.1X6
Isopregnenone	T38.5X1	T38.5X2	T38.5X3	T38.5X4	T38.5X5	T38.5X6
Isoprenaline	T48.6X1	T48.6X2	T48.6X3	T48.6X4	T48.6X5	T48.6X6
Isopromethazine	T43.3X1	T43.3X2	T43.3X3	T43.3X4	T43.3X5	T43.3X6
Isopropamide	T44.3X1	T44.3X2	T44.3X3	T44.3X4	T44.3X5	T44.3X6
iodide	T44.3X1	T44.3X2	T44.3X3	T44.3X4	T44.3X5	T44.3X6
Isopropanol	T51.2X1	T51.2X2	T51.2X3	T51.2X4	—	—
Isopropyl						
acetate	T52.8X1	T52.8X2	T52.8X3	T52.8X4	—	—
alcohol	T51.2X1	T51.2X2	T51.2X3	T51.2X4	—	—
medicinal	T49.4X1	T49.4X2	T49.4X3	T49.4X4	T49.4X5	T49.4X6
ether	T52.8X1	T52.8X2	T52.8X3	T52.8X4	—	—
Isopropylaminophenazone	T39.2X1	T39.2X2	T39.2X3	T39.2X4	T39.2X5	T39.2X6
Isoproterenol	T48.6X1	T48.6X2	T48.6X3	T48.6X4	T48.6X5	T48.6X6
Isosorbide dinitrate	T46.3X1	T46.3X2	T46.3X3	T46.3X4	T46.3X5	T46.3X6
Isothipendyl	T45.ØX1	T45.ØX2	T45.ØX3	T45.ØX4	T45.ØX5	T45.ØX6
Isotretinoin	T5Ø.991	T5Ø.992	T5Ø.993	T5Ø.994	T5Ø.995	T5Ø.996
Isoxazolyl penicillin	T36.ØX1	T36.ØX2	T36.ØX3	T36.ØX4	T36.ØX5	T36.ØX6
Isoxicam	T39.391	T39.392	T39.393	T39.394	T39.395	T39.396
Isoxsuprine	T46.7X1	T46.7X2	T46.7X3	T46.7X4	T46.7X5	T46.7X6
Ispagula	T47.4X1	T47.4X2	T47.4X3	T47.4X4	T47.4X5	T47.4X6
husk	T47.4X1	T47.4X2	T47.4X3	T47.4X4	T47.4X5	T47.4X6
Isradipine	T46.1X1	T46.1X2	T46.1X3	T46.1X4	T46.1X5	T46.1X6
I-thyroxine sodium	T38.1X1	T38.1X2	T38.1X3	T38.1X4	T38.1X5	T38.1X6
Itraconazole	T37.8X1	T37.8X2	T37.8X3	T37.8X4	T37.8X5	T37.8X6
Itramin tosilate	T46.3X1	T46.3X2	T46.3X3	T46.3X4	T46.3X5	T46.3X6
Ivermectin	T37.4X1	T37.4X2	T37.4X3	T37.4X4	T37.4X5	T37.4X6
Izoniazid	T37.1X1	T37.1X2	T37.1X3	T37.1X4	T37.1X5	T37.1X6
with thioacetazone	T37.1X1	T37.1X2	T37.1X3	T37.1X4	T37.1X5	T37.1X6
J						
Jalap	T47.2X1	T47.2X2	T47.2X3	T47.2X4	T47.2X5	T47.2X6
Jamaica						
dogwood (bark)	T39.8X1	T39.8X2	T39.8X3	T39.8X4	T39.8X5	T39.8X6
ginger	T65.891	T65.892	T65.893	T65.894	—	—
root	T62.2X1	T62.2X2	T62.2X3	T62.2X4	—	—
Jatropha	T62.2X1	T62.2X2	T62.2X3	T62.2X4	—	—
curcas	T62.2X1	T62.2X2	T62.2X3	T62.2X4	—	—
Jectofer	T45.4X1	T45.4X2	T45.4X3	T45.4X4	T45.4X5	T45.4X6
Jellyfish (sting)	T63.621	T63.622	T63.623	T63.624	—	—
Jequirity (bean)	T62.2X1	T62.2X2	T62.2X3	T62.2X4	—	—
Jimson weed (stramonium)	T62.2X1	T62.2X2	T62.2X3	T62.2X4	—	—
seeds	T62.2X1	T62.2X2	T62.2X3	T62.2X4	—	—
Josamycin	T36.3X1	T36.3X2	T36.3X3	T36.3X4	T36.3X5	T36.3X6
Juniper tar	T49.1X1	T49.1X2	T49.1X3	T49.1X4	T49.1X5	T49.1X6
K						
Kallidinogenase	T46.7X1	T46.7X2	T46.7X3	T46.7X4	T46.7X5	T46.7X6
Kallikrein	T46.7X1	T46.7X2	T46.7X3	T46.7X4	T46.7X5	T46.7X6
Kanamycin	T36.5X1	T36.5X2	T36.5X3	T36.5X4	T36.5X5	T36.5X6
Kantrex	T36.5X1	T36.5X2	T36.5X3	T36.5X4	T36.5X5	T36.5X6
Kaolin	T47.6X1	T47.6X2	T47.6X3	T47.6X4	T47.6X5	T47.6X6
light	T47.6X1	T47.6X2	T47.6X3	T47.6X4	T47.6X5	T47.6X6
Karaya (gum)	T47.4X1	T47.4X2	T47.4X3	T47.4X4	T47.4X5	T47.4X6
Kebuzone	T39.2X1	T39.2X2	T39.2X3	T39.2X4	T39.2X5	T39.2X6
Kelevan	T6Ø.1X1	T6Ø.1X2	T6Ø.1X3	T6Ø.1X4	—	—
Kemithal	T41.1X1	T41.1X2	T41.1X3	T41.1X4	T41.1X5	T41.1X6
Kenacort	T38.ØX1	T38.ØX2	T38.ØX3	T38.ØX4	T38.ØX5	T38.ØX6
Keratolytic drug NEC	T49.4X1	T49.4X2	T49.4X3	T49.4X4	T49.4X5	T49.4X6
anthracene	T49.4X1	T49.4X2	T49.4X3	T49.4X4	T49.4X5	T49.4X6
Keratoplastic NEC	T49.4X1	T49.4X2	T49.4X3	T49.4X4	T49.4X5	T49.4X6
Kerosene, kerosine (fuel) (solvent) **NEC**	T52.ØX1	T52.ØX2	T52.ØX3	T52.ØX4	—	—
insecticide	T52.ØX1	T52.ØX2	T52.ØX3	T52.ØX4	—	—
vapor	T52.ØX1	T52.ØX2	T52.ØX3	T52.ØX4	—	—
Ketamine	T41.291	T41.292	T41.293	T41.294	T41.295	T41.296
Ketazolam	T42.4X1	T42.4X2	T42.4X3	T42.4X4	T42.4X5	T42.4X6
Ketazon	T39.2X1	T39.2X2	T39.2X3	T39.2X4	T39.2X5	T39.2X6
Ketobemidone	T4Ø.4X1	T4Ø.4X2	T4Ø.4X3	T4Ø.4X4	—	—
Ketoconazole	T49.ØX1	T49.ØX2	T49.ØX3	T49.ØX4	T49.ØX5	T49.ØX6

Substance	Poisoning, Accidental (unintentional)	Poisoning, Intentional Self-harm	Poisoning, Assault	Poisoning, Undetermined	Adverse Effect	Under-dosing
Ketols	T52.4X1	T52.4X2	T52.4X3	T52.4X4	—	—
Ketone oils	T52.4X1	T52.4X2	T52.4X3	T52.4X4	—	—
Ketoprofen	T39.311	T39.312	T39.313	T39.314	T39.315	T39.316
Ketorolac	T39.8X1	T39.8X2	T39.8X3	T39.8X4	T39.8X5	T39.8X6
Ketotifen	T45.ØX1	T45.ØX2	T45.ØX3	T45.ØX4	T45.ØX5	T45.ØX6
Khat	T43.691	T43.692	T43.693	T43.694	—	—
Khellin	T46.3X1	T46.3X2	T46.3X3	T46.3X4	T46.3X5	T46.3X6
Khelloside	T46.3X1	T46.3X2	T46.3X3	T46.3X4	T46.3X5	T46.3X6
Kiln gas or vapor (carbon monoxide)	T58.8X1	T58.8X2	T58.8X3	T58.8X4	—	—
Kitasamycin	T36.3X1	T36.3X2	T36.3X3	T36.3X4	T36.3X5	T36.3X6
Konsyl	T47.4X1	T47.4X2	T47.4X3	T47.4X4	T47.4X5	T47.4X6
Kosam seed	T62.2X1	T62.2X2	T62.2X3	T62.2X4	—	—
Krait (venom)	T63.Ø91	T63.Ø92	T63.Ø93	T63.Ø94	—	—
Kwell (insecticide)	T6Ø.1X1	T6Ø.1X2	T6Ø.1X3	T6Ø.1X4	—	—
anti-infective (topical)	T49.ØX1	T49.ØX2	T49.ØX3	T49.ØX4	T49.ØX5	T49.ØX6
L						
Labetalol	T44.8X1	T44.8X2	T44.8X3	T44.8X4	T44.8X5	T44.8X6
Laburnum (seeds)	T62.2X1	T62.2X2	T62.2X3	T62.2X4	—	—
leaves	T62.2X1	T62.2X2	T62.2X3	T62.2X4	—	—
Lachesine	T49.5X1	T49.5X2	T49.5X3	T49.5X4	T49.5X5	T49.5X6
Lacidipine	T46.5X1	T46.5X2	T46.5X3	T46.5X4	T46.5X5	T46.5X6
Lacquer	T65.6X1	T65.6X2	T65.6X3	T65.6X4	—	—
Lacrimogenic gas	T59.3X1	T59.3X2	T59.3X3	T59.3X4	—	—
Lactated potassic saline	T5Ø.3X1	T5Ø.3X2	T5Ø.3X3	T5Ø.3X4	T5Ø.3X5	T5Ø.3X6
Lactic acid	T49.8X1	T49.8X2	T49.8X3	T49.8X4	T49.8X5	T49.8X6
Lactobacillus						
acidophilus	T47.6X1	T47.6X2	T47.6X3	T47.6X4	T47.6X5	T47.6X6
compound	T47.6X1	T47.6X2	T47.6X3	T47.6X4	T47.6X5	T47.6X6
bifidus, lyophilized	T47.6X1	T47.6X2	T47.6X3	T47.6X4	T47.6X5	T47.6X6
bulgaricus	T47.6X1	T47.6X2	T47.6X3	T47.6X4	T47.6X5	T47.6X6
sporogenes	T47.6X1	T47.6X2	T47.6X3	T47.6X4	T47.6X5	T47.6X6
Lactoflavin	T45.2X1	T45.2X2	T45.2X3	T45.2X4	T45.2X5	T45.2X6
Lactose (as excipient)	T5Ø.9Ø1	T5Ø.9Ø2	T5Ø.9Ø3	T5Ø.9Ø4	T5Ø.9Ø5	T5Ø.9Ø6
Lactuca (virosa) (extract)	T42.6X1	T42.6X2	T42.6X3	T42.6X4	T42.6X5	T42.6X6
Lactucarium	T42.6X1	T42.6X2	T42.6X3	T42.6X4	T42.6X5	T42.6X6
Lactulose	T47.3X1	T47.3X2	T47.3X3	T47.3X4	T47.3X5	T47.3X6
Laevo—*see* Levo						
Lanatosides	T46.ØX1	T46.ØX2	T46.ØX3	T46.ØX4	T46.ØX5	T46.ØX6
Lanolin	T49.3X1	T49.3X2	T49.3X3	T49.3X4	T49.3X5	T49.3X6
Largactil	T43.3X1	T43.3X2	T43.3X3	T43.3X4	T43.3X5	T43.3X6
Larkspur	T62.2X1	T62.2X2	T62.2X3	T62.2X4	—	—
Laroxyl	T43.Ø11	T43.Ø12	T43.Ø13	T43.Ø14	T43.Ø15	T43.Ø16
Lassar's paste	T49.4X1	T49.4X2	T49.4X3	T49.4X4	T49.4X5	T49.4X6
Lasix	T5Ø.1X1	T5Ø.1X2	T5Ø.1X3	T5Ø.1X4	T5Ø.1X5	T5Ø.1X6
Latamoxef	T36.1X1	T36.1X2	T36.1X3	T36.1X4	T36.1X5	T36.1X6
Latex	T65.811	T65.812	T65.813	T65.814	—	—
Lathyrus (seed)	T62.2X1	T62.2X2	T62.2X3	T62.2X4	—	—
Laudanum	T4Ø.ØX1	T4Ø.ØX2	T4Ø.ØX3	T4Ø.ØX4	T4Ø.ØX5	T4Ø.ØX6
Laudexium	T48.1X1	T48.1X2	T48.1X3	T48.1X4	T48.1X5	T48.1X6
Laughing gas	T41.ØX1	T41.ØX2	T41.ØX3	T41.ØX4	T41.ØX5	T41.ØX6
Laurel, black or cherry	T62.2X1	T62.2X2	T62.2X3	T62.2X4	—	—
Laurolinium	T49.ØX1	T49.ØX2	T49.ØX3	T49.ØX4	T49.ØX5	T49.ØX6
Lauryl sulfoacetate	T49.2X1	T49.2X2	T49.2X3	T49.2X4	T49.2X5	T49.2X6
Laxative NEC	T47.4X1	T47.4X2	T47.4X3	T47.4X4	T47.4X5	T47.4X6
osmotic	T47.3X1	T47.3X2	T47.3X3	T47.3X4	T47.3X5	T47.3X6
saline	T47.3X1	T47.3X2	T47.3X3	T47.3X4	T47.3X5	T47.3X6
stimulant	T47.2X1	T47.2X2	T47.2X3	T47.2X4	T47.2X5	T47.2X6
L-dopa	T42.8X1	T42.8X2	T42.8X3	T42.8X4	T42.8X5	T42.8X6
Lead (dust) (fumes) (vapor) **NEC**	T56.ØX1	T56.ØX2	T56.ØX3	T56.ØX4	—	—
acetate	T49.2X1	T49.2X2	T49.2X3	T49.2X4	T49.2X5	T49.2X6
alkyl (fuel additive)	T56.ØX1	T56.ØX2	T56.ØX3	T56.ØX4	—	—
anti-infectives	T37.8X1	T37.8X2	T37.8X3	T37.8X4	T37.8X5	T37.8X6
antiknock compound (tetraethyl)	T56.ØX1	T56.ØX2	T56.ØX3	T56.ØX4	—	—
arsenate, arsenite (dust)(herbicide) (insecticide) (vapor)	T57.ØX1	T57.ØX2	T57.ØX3	T57.ØX4	—	—
carbonate	T56.ØX1	T56.ØX2	T56.ØX3	T56.ØX4	—	—
paint	T56.ØX1	T56.ØX2	T56.ØX3	T56.ØX4	—	—

Substance	Poisoning, Accidental (unintentional)	Poisoning, Intentional Self-harm	Poisoning, Assault	Poisoning, Undetermined	Adverse Effect	Under-dosing
Lead— *continued*						
chromate	T56.ØX1	T56.ØX2	T56.ØX3	T56.ØX4	—	—
paint	T56.ØX1	T56.ØX2	T56.ØX3	T56.ØX4	—	—
dioxide	T56.ØX1	T56.ØX2	T56.ØX3	T56.ØX4	—	—
inorganic	T56.ØX1	T56.ØX2	T56.ØX3	T56.ØX4	—	—
iodide	T56.ØX1	T56.ØX2	T56.ØX3	T56.ØX4	—	—
pigment (paint)	T56.ØX1	T56.ØX2	T56.ØX3	T56.ØX4	—	—
monoxide (dust)	T56.ØX1	T56.ØX2	T56.ØX3	T56.ØX4	—	—
paint	T56.ØX1	T56.ØX2	T56.ØX3	T56.ØX4	—	—
organic	T56.ØX1	T56.ØX2	T56.ØX3	T56.ØX4	—	—
oxide	T56.ØX1	T56.ØX2	T56.ØX3	T56.ØX4	—	—
paint	T56.ØX1	T56.ØX2	T56.ØX3	T56.ØX4	—	—
paint	T56.ØX1	T56.ØX2	T56.ØX3	T56.ØX4	—	—
salts	T56.ØX1	T56.ØX2	T56.ØX3	T56.ØX4	—	—
specified compound NEC	T56.ØX1	T56.ØX2	T56.ØX3	T56.ØX4	—	—
tetra-ethyl	T56.ØX1	T56.ØX2	T56.ØX3	T56.ØX4	—	—
Lebanese red	T4Ø.7X1	T4Ø.7X2	T4Ø.7X3	T4Ø.7X4	T4Ø.7X5	T4Ø.7X6
Lefetamine	T39.8X1	T39.8X2	T39.8X3	T39.8X4	T39.8X5	T39.8X6
Lenperone	T43.4X1	T43.4X2	T43.4X3	T43.4X4	T43.4X5	T43.4X6
Lente lietin (insulin)	T38.3X1	T38.3X2	T38.3X3	T38.3X4	T38.3X5	T38.3X6
Leptazol	T5Ø.7X1	T5Ø.7X2	T5Ø.7X3	T5Ø.7X4	T5Ø.7X5	T5Ø.7X6
Leptophos	T6Ø.ØX1	T6Ø.ØX2	T6Ø.ØX3	T6Ø.ØX4	—	—
Leritine	T4Ø.2X1	T4Ø.2X2	T4Ø.2X3	T4Ø.2X4	T4Ø.2X5	T4Ø.2X6
Letosteine	T48.4X1	T48.4X2	T48.4X3	T48.4X4	T48.4X5	T48.4X6
Letter	T38.1X1	T38.1X2	T38.1X3	T38.1X4	T38.1X5	T38.1X6
Lettuce opium	T42.6X1	T42.6X2	T42.6X3	T42.6X4	T42.6X5	T42.6X6
Leucinocaine	T41.3X1	T41.3X2	T41.3X3	T41.3X4	T41.3X5	T41.3X6
Leucocianidol	T46.991	T46.992	T46.993	T46.994	T46.995	T46.996
Leucovorin (factor)	T45.8X1	T45.8X2	T45.8X3	T45.8X4	T45.8X5	T45.8X6
Leukeran	T45.1X1	T45.1X2	T45.1X3	T45.1X4	T45.1X5	T45.1X6
Leuprolide	T38.891	T38.892	T38.893	T38.894	T38.895	T38.896
Levalbuterol	T48.6X1	T48.6X2	T48.6X3	T48.6X4	T48.6X5	T48.6X6
Levallorphan	T5Ø.7X1	T5Ø.7X2	T5Ø.7X3	T5Ø.7X4	T5Ø.7X5	T5Ø.7X6
Levamisole	T37.4X1	T37.4X2	T37.4X3	T37.4X4	T37.4X5	T37.4X6
Levanil	T42.6X1	T42.6X2	T42.6X3	T42.6X4	T42.6X5	T42.6X6
Levarterenol	T44.4X1	T44.4X2	T44.4X3	T44.4X4	T44.4X5	T44.4X6
Levdropropizine	T48.3X1	T48.3X2	T48.3X3	T48.3X4	T48.3X5	T48.3X6
Levobunolol	T49.5X1	T49.5X2	T49.5X3	T49.5X4	T49.5X5	T49.5X6
Levocabastine (hydrochloride)	T45.ØX1	T45.ØX2	T45.ØX3	T45.ØX4	T45.ØX5	T45.ØX6
Levocarnitine	T5Ø.991	T5Ø.992	T5Ø.993	T5Ø.994	T5Ø.995	T5Ø.996
Levodopa	T42.8X1	T42.8X2	T42.8X3	T42.8X4	T42.8X5	T42.8X6
with carbidopa	T42.8X1	T42.8X2	T42.8X3	T42.8X4	T42.8X5	T42.8X6
Levo-dromoran	T4Ø.2X1	T4Ø.2X2	T4Ø.2X3	T4Ø.2X4	T4Ø.2X5	T4Ø.2X6
Levoglutamide	T5Ø.991	T5Ø.992	T5Ø.993	T5Ø.994	T5Ø.995	T5Ø.996
Levoid	T38.1X1	T38.1X2	T38.1X3	T38.1X4	T38.1X5	T38.1X6
Levo-iso-methadone	T4Ø.3X1	T4Ø.3X2	T4Ø.3X3	T4Ø.3X4	T4Ø.3X5	T4Ø.3X6
Levomepromazine	T43.3X1	T43.3X2	T43.3X3	T43.3X4	T43.3X5	T43.3X6
Levonordefrin	T49.6X1	T49.6X2	T49.6X3	T49.6X4	T49.6X5	T49.6X6
Levonorgestrel	T38.4X1	T38.4X2	T38.4X3	T38.4X4	T38.4X5	T38.4X6
with ethinylestradiol	T38.5X1	T38.5X2	T38.5X3	T38.5X4	T38.5X5	T38.5X6
Levopromazine	T43.3X1	T43.3X2	T43.3X3	T43.3X4	T43.3X5	T43.3X6
Levoprome	T42.6X1	T42.6X2	T42.6X3	T42.6X4	T42.6X5	T42.6X6
Levopropoxyphene	T4Ø.4X1	T4Ø.4X2	T4Ø.4X3	T4Ø.4X4	T4Ø.4X5	T4Ø.4X6
Levopropylhexedrine	T5Ø.5X1	T5Ø.5X2	T5Ø.5X3	T5Ø.5X4	T5Ø.5X5	T5Ø.5X6
Levoproxyphylline	T48.6X1	T48.6X2	T48.6X3	T48.6X4	T48.6X5	T48.6X6
Levorphanol	T4Ø.4X1	T4Ø.4X2	T4Ø.4X3	T4Ø.4X4	T4Ø.4X5	T4Ø.4X6
Levothyroxine	T38.1X1	T38.1X2	T38.1X3	T38.1X4	T38.1X5	T38.1X6
sodium	T38.1X1	T38.1X2	T38.1X3	T38.1X4	T38.1X5	T38.1X6
Levsin	T44.3X1	T44.3X2	T44.3X3	T44.3X4	T44.3X5	T44.3X6
Levulose	T5Ø.3X1	T5Ø.3X2	T5Ø.3X3	T5Ø.3X4	T5Ø.3X5	T5Ø.3X6
Lewisite (gas), **not in war**	T57.ØX1	T57.ØX2	T57.ØX3	T57.ØX4	—	—
Librium	T42.4X1	T42.4X2	T42.4X3	T42.4X4	T42.4X5	T42.4X6
Lidex	T49.ØX1	T49.ØX2	T49.ØX3	T49.ØX4	T49.ØX5	T49.ØX6
Lidocaine	T41.3X1	T41.3X2	T41.3X3	T41.3X4	T41.3X5	T41.3X6
regional	T41.3X1	T41.3X2	T41.3X3	T41.3X4	T41.3X5	T41.3X6
spinal	T41.3X1	T41.3X2	T41.3X3	T41.3X4	T41.3X5	T41.3X6
Lidofenin	T5Ø.8X1	T5Ø.8X2	T5Ø.8X3	T5Ø.8X4	T5Ø.8X5	T5Ø.8X6
Lidoflazine	T46.1X1	T46.1X2	T46.1X3	T46.1X4	T46.1X5	T46.1X6
Lighter fluid	T52.ØX1	T52.ØX2	T52.ØX3	T52.ØX4	—	—
Lignin hemicellulose	T47.6X1	T47.6X2	T47.6X3	T47.6X4	T47.6X5	T47.6X6
Lignocaine	T41.3X1	T41.3X2	T41.3X3	T41.3X4	T41.3X5	T41.3X6
regional	T41.3X1	T41.3X2	T41.3X3	T41.3X4	T41.3X5	T41.3X6
spinal	T41.3X1	T41.3X2	T41.3X3	T41.3X4	T41.3X5	T41.3X6
Ligroin(e) (solvent)	T52.ØX1	T52.ØX2	T52.ØX3	T52.ØX4	—	—
vapor	T59.891	T59.892	T59.893	T59.894	—	—
Ligustrum vulgare	T62.2X1	T62.2X2	T62.2X3	T62.2X4	—	—
Lily of the valley	T62.2X1	T62.2X2	T62.2X3	T62.2X4	—	—
Lime (chloride)	T54.3X1	T54.3X2	T54.3X3	T54.3X4	—	—
Limonene	T52.8X1	T52.8X2	T52.8X3	T52.8X4	—	—
Lincomycin	T36.8X1	T36.8X2	T36.8X3	T36.8X4	T36.8X5	T36.8X6
Lindane (insecticide) (nonmedicinal) (vapor)	T53.6X1	T53.6X2	T53.6X3	T53.6X4	—	—
medicinal	T49.ØX1	T49.ØX2	T49.ØX3	T49.ØX4	T49.ØX5	T49.ØX6
Liniments NEC	T49.91	T49.92	T49.93	T49.94	T49.95	T49.96
Linoleic acid	T46.6X1	T46.6X2	T46.6X3	T46.6X4	T46.6X5	T46.6X6
Linolenic acid	T46.6X1	T46.6X2	T46.6X3	T46.6X4	T46.6X5	T46.6X6
Linseed	T47.4X1	T47.4X2	T47.4X3	T47.4X4	T47.4X5	T47.4X6
Liothyronine	T38.1X1	T38.1X2	T38.1X3	T38.1X4	T38.1X5	T38.1X6
Liotrix	T38.1X1	T38.1X2	T38.1X3	T38.1X4	T38.1X5	T38.1X6
Lipancreatin	T47.5X1	T47.5X2	T47.5X3	T47.5X4	T47.5X5	T47.5X6
Lipo-alprostadil	T46.7X1	T46.7X2	T46.7X3	T46.7X4	T46.7X5	T46.7X6
Lipo-Lutin	T38.5X1	T38.5X2	T38.5X3	T38.5X4	T38.5X5	T38.5X6
Lipotropic drug NEC	T5Ø.9Ø1	T5Ø.9Ø2	T5Ø.9Ø3	T5Ø.9Ø4	T5Ø.9Ø5	T5Ø.9Ø6
Liquefied petroleum gases	T59.891	T59.892	T59.893	T59.894	—	—
piped (pure or mixed with air)	T59.891	T59.892	T59.893	T59.894	—	—
Liquid						
paraffin	T47.4X1	T47.4X2	T47.4X3	T47.4X4	T47.4X5	T47.4X6
petrolatum	T47.4X1	T47.4X2	T47.4X3	T47.4X4	T47.4X5	T47.4X6
topical	T49.3X1	T49.3X2	T49.3X3	T49.3X4	T49.3X5	T49.3X6
specified NEC	T65.891	T65.892	T65.893	T65.894	—	—
substance	T65.91	T65.92	T65.93	T65.94	—	—
Liquor creosolis compositus	T65.891	T65.892	T65.893	T65.894	—	—
Liquorice	T48.4X1	T48.4X2	T48.4X3	T48.4X4	T48.4X5	T48.4X6
extract	T47.8X1	T47.8X2	T47.8X3	T47.8X4	T47.8X5	T47.8X6
Lisinopril	T46.4X1	T46.4X2	T46.4X3	T46.4X4	T46.4X5	T46.4X6
Lisuride	T42.8X1	T42.8X2	T42.8X3	T42.8X4	T42.8X5	T42.8X6
Lithane	T43.8X1	T43.8X2	T43.8X3	T43.8X4	T43.8X5	T43.8X6
Lithium	T56.891	T56.892	T56.893	T56.894	—	—
gluconate	T43.591	T43.592	T43.593	T43.594	T43.595	T43.596
salts (carbonate)	T43.591	T43.592	T43.593	T43.594	T43.595	T43.596
Lithonate	T43.8X1	T43.8X2	T43.8X3	T43.8X4	T43.8X5	T43.8X6
Liver						
extract	T45.8X1	T45.8X2	T45.8X3	T45.8X4	T45.8X5	T45.8X6
for parenteral use	T45.8X1	T45.8X2	T45.8X3	T45.8X4	T45.8X5	T45.8X6
fraction 1	T45.8X1	T45.8X2	T45.8X3	T45.8X4	T45.8X5	T45.8X6
hydrolysate	T45.8X1	T45.8X2	T45.8X3	T45.8X4	T45.8X5	T45.8X6
Lizard (bite) (venom)	T63.121	T63.122	T63.123	T63.124	—	—
LMD	T45.8X1	T45.8X2	T45.8X3	T45.8X4	T45.8X5	T45.8X6
Lobelia	T62.2X1	T62.2X2	T62.2X3	T62.2X4	—	—
Lobeline	T5Ø.7X1	T5Ø.7X2	T5Ø.7X3	T5Ø.7X4	T5Ø.7X5	T5Ø.7X6
Local action drug NEC	T49.8X1	T49.8X2	T49.8X3	T49.8X4	T49.8X5	T49.8X6
Locorten	T49.ØX1	T49.ØX2	T49.ØX3	T49.ØX4	T49.ØX5	T49.ØX6
Lofepramine	T43.Ø11	T43.Ø12	T43.Ø13	T43.Ø14	T43.Ø15	T43.Ø16
Lolium temulentum	T62.2X1	T62.2X2	T62.2X3	T62.2X4	—	—
Lomotil	T47.6X1	T47.6X2	T47.6X3	T47.6X4	T47.6X5	T47.6X6
Lomustine	T45.1X1	T45.1X2	T45.1X3	T45.1X4	T45.1X5	T45.1X6
Lonidamine	T45.1X1	T45.1X2	T45.1X3	T45.1X4	T45.1X5	T45.1X6
Loperamide	T47.6X1	T47.6X2	T47.6X3	T47.6X4	T47.6X5	T47.6X6
Loprazolam	T42.4X1	T42.4X2	T42.4X3	T42.4X4	T42.4X5	T42.4X6
Lorajmine	T46.2X1	T46.2X2	T46.2X3	T46.2X4	T46.2X5	T46.2X6
Loratidine	T45.ØX1	T45.ØX2	T45.ØX3	T45.ØX4	T45.ØX5	T45.ØX6
Lorazepam	T42.4X1	T42.4X2	T42.4X3	T42.4X4	T42.4X5	T42.4X6
Lorcainide	T46.2X1	T46.2X2	T46.2X3	T46.2X4	T46.2X5	T46.2X6
Lormetazepam	T42.4X1	T42.4X2	T42.4X3	T42.4X4	T42.4X5	T42.4X6
Lotions NEC	T49.91	T49.92	T49.93	T49.94	T49.95	T49.96
Lotusate	T42.3X1	T42.3X2	T42.3X3	T42.3X4	T42.3X5	T42.3X6
Lovastatin	T46.6X1	T46.6X2	T46.6X3	T46.6X4	T46.6X5	T46.6X6
Loxapine	T43.591	T43.592	T43.593	T43.594	T43.595	T43.596
Lowila	T49.2X1	T49.2X2	T49.2X3	T49.2X4	T49.2X5	T49.2X6
Lozenges (throat)	T49.6X1	T49.6X2	T49.6X3	T49.6X4	T49.6X5	T49.6X6
LSD	T4Ø.8X1	T4Ø.8X2	T4Ø.8X3	T4Ø.8X4	T4Ø.8X5	—

Substance	Poisoning, Accidental (unintentional)	Poisoning, Intentional Self-harm	Poisoning, Assault	Poisoning, Undetermined	Adverse Effect	Under-dosing
L-tryptophan—*see* amino acid						
Lubricant, eye	T49.5X1	T49.5X2	T49.5X3	T49.5X4	T49.5X5	T49.5X6
Lubricating oil NEC	T52.0X1	T52.0X2	T52.0X3	T52.0X4	—	—
Lucanthone	T37.4X1	T37.4X2	T37.4X3	T37.4X4	T37.4X5	T37.4X6
Luminal	T42.3X1	T42.3X2	T42.3X3	T42.3X4	T42.3X5	T42.3X6
Lung irritant (gas) **NEC**	T59.91	T59.92	T59.93	T59.94	—	—
Luteinizing hormone	T38.811	T38.812	T38.813	T38.814	T38.815	T38.816
Lutocylol	T38.5X1	T38.5X2	T38.5X3	T38.5X4	T38.5X5	T38.5X6
Lutromone	T38.5X1	T38.5X2	T38.5X3	T38.5X4	T38.5X5	T38.5X6
Lututrin	T48.291	T48.292	T48.293	T48.294	T48.295	T48.296
Lye (concentrated)	T54.3X1	T54.3X2	T54.3X3	T54.3X4	—	—
Lygranum (skin test)	T50.8X1	T50.8X2	T50.8X3	T50.8X4	T50.8X5	T50.8X6
Lymecycline	T36.4X1	T36.4X2	T36.4X3	T36.4X4	T36.4X5	T36.4X6
Lymphogranuloma venereum antigen	T50.8X1	T50.8X2	T50.8X3	T50.8X4	T50.8X5	T50.8X6
Lynestrenol	T38.4X1	T38.4X2	T38.4X3	T38.4X4	T38.4X5	T38.4X6
Lypressin	T38.891	T38.892	T38.893	T38.894	T38.895	T38.896
Lyovac sodium edecrin	T50.1X1	T50.1X2	T50.1X3	T50.1X4	T50.1X5	T50.1X6
Lysergic acid diethylamide	T40.8X1	T40.8X2	T40.8X3	T40.8X4	T40.8X5	—
Lysergide	T40.8X1	T40.8X2	T40.8X3	T40.8X4	T40.8X5	—
Lysine vasopressin	T38.891	T38.892	T38.893	T38.894	T38.895	T38.896
Lysol	T54.1X1	T54.1X2	T54.1X3	T54.1X4	—	—
Lysozyme	T49.0X1	T49.0X2	T49.0X3	T49.0X4	T49.0X5	T49.0X6
Lytta (vitatta)	T49.8X1	T49.8X2	T49.8X3	T49.8X4	T49.8X5	T49.8X6
M						
Mace	T59.3X1	T59.3X2	T59.3X3	T59.3X4	—	—
Macrogol	T50.991	T50.992	T50.993	T50.994	T50.995	T50.996
Macrolide						
anabolic drug	T38.7X1	T38.7X2	T38.7X3	T38.7X4	T38.7X5	T38.7X6
antibiotic	T36.3X1	T36.3X2	T36.3X3	T36.3X4	T36.3X5	T36.3X6
Mafenide	T49.0X1	T49.0X2	T49.0X3	T49.0X4	T49.0X5	T49.0X6
Magaldrate	T47.1X1	T47.1X2	T47.1X3	T47.1X4	T47.1X5	T47.1X6
Magic mushroom	T40.991	T40.992	T40.993	T40.994	—	—
Magnamycin	T36.8X1	T36.8X2	T36.8X3	T36.8X4	T36.8X5	T36.8X6
Magnesia magma	T47.1X1	T47.1X2	T47.1X3	T47.1X4	T47.1X5	T47.1X6
Magnesium NEC	T56.891	T56.892	T56.893	T56.894	—	—
carbonate	T47.1X1	T47.1X2	T47.1X3	T47.1X4	T47.1X5	T47.1X6
citrate	T47.4X1	T47.4X2	T47.4X3	T47.4X4	T47.4X5	T47.4X6
hydroxide	T47.1X1	T47.1X2	T47.1X3	T47.1X4	T47.1X5	T47.1X6
oxide	T47.1X1	T47.1X2	T47.1X3	T47.1X4	T47.1X5	T47.1X6
peroxide	T49.0X1	T49.0X2	T49.0X3	T49.0X4	T49.0X5	T49.0X6
salicylate	T39.091	T39.092	T39.093	T39.094	T39.095	T39.096
silicofluoride	T50.3X1	T50.3X2	T50.3X3	T50.3X4	T50.3X5	T50.3X6
sulfate	T47.4X1	T47.4X2	T47.4X3	T47.4X4	T47.4X5	T47.4X6
thiosulfate	T45.0X1	T45.0X2	T45.0X3	T45.0X4	T45.0X5	T45.0X6
trisilicate	T47.1X1	T47.1X2	T47.1X3	T47.1X4	T47.1X5	T47.1X6
Malathion (medicinal)	T49.0X1	T49.0X2	T49.0X3	T49.0X4	T49.0X5	T49.0X6
insecticide	T60.0X1	T60.0X2	T60.0X3	T60.0X4	—	—
Male fern extract	T37.4X1	T37.4X2	T37.4X3	T37.4X4	T37.4X5	T37.4X6
M-AMSA	T45.1X1	T45.1X2	T45.1X3	T45.1X4	T45.1X5	T45.1X6
Mandelic acid	T37.8X1	T37.8X2	T37.8X3	T37.8X4	T37.8X5	T37.8X6
Manganese (dioxide) (salts)	T57.2X1	T57.2X2	T57.2X3	T57.2X4	—	—
medicinal	T50.991	T50.992	T50.993	T50.994	T50.995	T50.996
Mannitol	T47.3X1	T47.3X2	T47.3X3	T47.3X4	T47.3X5	T47.3X6
hexanitrate	T46.3X1	T46.3X2	T46.3X3	T46.3X4	T46.3X5	T46.3X6
Mannomustine	T45.1X1	T45.1X2	T45.1X3	T45.1X4	T45.1X5	T45.1X6
MAO inhibitors	T43.1X1	T43.1X2	T43.1X3	T43.1X4	T43.1X5	T43.1X6
Mapharsen	T37.8X1	T37.8X2	T37.8X3	T37.8X4	T37.8X5	T37.8X6
Maphenide	T49.0X1	T49.0X2	T49.0X3	T49.0X4	T49.0X5	T49.0X6
Maprotiline	T43.021	T43.022	T43.023	T43.024	T43.025	T43.026
Marcaine	T41.3X1	T41.3X2	T41.3X3	T41.3X4	T41.3X5	T41.3X6
infiltration (subcutaneous)	T41.3X1	T41.3X2	T41.3X3	T41.3X4	T41.3X5	T41.3X6
nerve block (peripheral) (plexus)	T41.3X1	T41.3X2	T41.3X3	T41.3X4	T41.3X5	T41.3X6
Marezine	T45.0X1	T45.0X2	T45.0X3	T45.0X4	T45.0X5	T45.0X6
Marihuana	T40.7X1	T40.7X2	T40.7X3	T40.7X4	T40.7X5	T40.7X6
Marijuana	T40.7X1	T40.7X2	T40.7X3	T40.7X4	T40.7X5	T40.7X6
Marine (sting)	T63.691	T63.692	T63.693	T63.694	—	—
animals (sting)	T63.691	T63.692	T63.693	T63.694	—	—
plants (sting)	T63.711	T63.712	T63.713	T63.714	—	—
Marplan	T43.1X1	T43.1X2	T43.1X3	T43.1X4	T43.1X5	T43.1X6
Marsh gas	T59.891	T59.892	T59.893	T59.894	—	—
Marsilid	T43.1X1	T43.1X2	T43.1X3	T43.1X4	T43.1X5	T43.1X6
Matulane	T45.1X1	T45.1X2	T45.1X3	T45.1X4	T45.1X5	T45.1X6
Mazindol	T50.5X1	T50.5X2	T50.5X3	T50.5X4	T50.5X5	T50.5X6
MCPA	T60.3X1	T60.3X2	T60.3X3	T60.3X4	—	—
MDMA	T43.621	T43.622	T43.623	T43.624	T43.625	T43.626
Meadow saffron	T62.2X1	T62.2X2	T62.2X3	T62.2X4	—	—
Measles virus vaccine (attenuated)	T50.B91	T50.B92	T50.B93	T50.B94	T50.B95	T50.B96
Meat, noxious	T62.8X1	T62.8X2	T62.8X3	T62.8X4	—	—
Meballymal	T42.3X1	T42.3X2	T42.3X3	T42.3X4	T42.3X5	T42.3X6
Mebanazine	T43.1X1	T43.1X2	T43.1X3	T43.1X4	T43.1X5	T43.1X6
Mebaral	T42.3X1	T42.3X2	T42.3X3	T42.3X4	T42.3X5	T42.3X6
Mebendazole	T37.4X1	T37.4X2	T37.4X3	T37.4X4	T37.4X5	T37.4X6
Mebeverine	T44.3X1	T44.3X2	T44.3X3	T44.3X4	T44.3X5	T44.3X6
Mebhydrolin	T45.0X1	T45.0X2	T45.0X3	T45.0X4	T45.0X5	T45.0X6
Mebumal	T42.3X1	T42.3X2	T42.3X3	T42.3X4	T42.3X5	T42.3X6
Mebutamate	T43.591	T43.592	T43.593	T43.594	T43.595	T43.596
Mecamylamine	T44.2X1	T44.2X2	T44.2X3	T44.2X4	T44.2X5	T44.2X6
Mechlorethamine	T45.1X1	T45.1X2	T45.1X3	T45.1X4	T45.1X5	T45.1X6
Mecillinam	T36.0X1	T36.0X2	T36.0X3	T36.0X4	T36.0X5	T36.0X6
Meclizine (hydrochloride)	T45.0X1	T45.0X2	T45.0X3	T45.0X4	T45.0X5	T45.0X6
Meclocycline	T36.4X1	T36.4X2	T36.4X3	T36.4X4	T36.4X5	T36.4X6
Meclofenamate	T39.391	T39.392	T39.393	T39.394	T39.395	T39.396
Meclofenamic acid	T39.391	T39.392	T39.393	T39.394	T39.395	T39.396
Meclofenoxate	T43.691	T43.692	T43.693	T43.694	T43.695	T43.696
Meclozine	T45.0X1	T45.0X2	T45.0X3	T45.0X4	T45.0X5	T45.0X6
Mecobalamin	T45.8X1	T45.8X2	T45.8X3	T45.8X4	T45.8X5	T45.8X6
Mecoprop	T60.3X1	T60.3X2	T60.3X3	T60.3X4	—	—
Mecrilate	T49.3X1	T49.3X2	T49.3X3	T49.3X4	T49.3X5	T49.3X6
Mecysteine	T48.4X1	T48.4X2	T48.4X3	T48.4X4	T48.4X5	T48.4X6
Medazepam	T42.4X1	T42.4X2	T42.4X3	T42.4X4	T42.4X5	T42.4X6
Medicament NEC	T50.901	T50.902	T50.903	T50.904	T50.905	T50.906
Medinal	T42.3X1	T42.3X2	T42.3X3	T42.3X4	T42.3X5	T42.3X6
Medomin	T42.3X1	T42.3X2	T42.3X3	T42.3X4	T42.3X5	T42.3X6
Medrogestone	T38.5X1	T38.5X2	T38.5X3	T38.5X4	T38.5X5	T38.5X6
Medroxalol	T44.8X1	T44.8X2	T44.8X3	T44.8X4	T44.8X5	T44.8X6
Medroxyprogesterone acetate (depot)	T38.5X1	T38.5X2	T38.5X3	T38.5X4	T38.5X5	T38.5X6
Medrysone	T49.0X1	T49.0X2	T49.0X3	T49.0X4	T49.0X5	T49.0X6
Mefenamic acid	T39.391	T39.392	T39.393	T39.394	T39.395	T39.396
Mefenorex	T50.5X1	T50.5X2	T50.5X3	T50.5X4	T50.5X5	T50.5X6
Mefloquine	T37.2X1	T37.2X2	T37.2X3	T37.2X4	T37.2X5	T37.2X6
Mefruside	T50.2X1	T50.2X2	T50.2X3	T50.2X4	T50.2X5	T50.2X6
Megahallucinogen	T40.901	T40.902	T40.903	T40.904	T40.905	T40.906
Megestrol	T38.5X1	T38.5X2	T38.5X3	T38.5X4	T38.5X5	T38.5X6
Meglumine						
antimoniate	T37.8X1	T37.8X2	T37.8X3	T37.8X4	T37.8X5	T37.8X6
diatrizoate	T50.8X1	T50.8X2	T50.8X3	T50.8X4	T50.8X5	T50.8X6
iodipamide	T50.8X1	T50.8X2	T50.8X3	T50.8X4	T50.8X5	T50.8X6
iotroxate	T50.8X1	T50.8X2	T50.8X3	T50.8X4	T50.8X5	T50.8X6
MEK (methyl ethyl ketone)	T52.4X1	T52.4X2	T52.4X3	T52.4X4	—	—
Meladrazine	T44.3X1	T44.3X2	T44.3X3	T44.3X4	T44.3X5	T44.3X6
Meladinin	T49.3X1	T49.3X2	T49.3X3	T49.3X4	T49.3X5	T49.3X6
Melaleuca alternifolia oil	T49.0X1	T49.0X2	T49.0X3	T49.0X4	T49.0X5	T49.0X6
Melanizing agents	T49.3X1	T49.3X2	T49.3X3	T49.3X4	T49.3X5	T49.3X6
Melanocyte-stimulating hormone	T38.891	T38.892	T38.893	T38.894	T38.895	T38.896
Melarsonyl potassium	T37.3X1	T37.3X2	T37.3X3	T37.3X4	T37.3X5	T37.3X6
Melarsoprol	T37.3X1	T37.3X2	T37.3X3	T37.3X4	T37.3X5	T37.3X6
Melia azedarach	T62.2X1	T62.2X2	T62.2X3	T62.2X4	—	—
Melitracen	T43.011	T43.012	T43.013	T43.014	T43.015	T43.016
Mellaril	T43.3X1	T43.3X2	T43.3X3	T43.3X4	T43.3X5	T43.3X6
Meloxine	T49.3X1	T49.3X2	T49.3X3	T49.3X4	T49.3X5	T49.3X6
Melperone	T43.4X1	T43.4X2	T43.4X3	T43.4X4	T43.4X5	T43.4X6
Melphalan	T45.1X1	T45.1X2	T45.1X3	T45.1X4	T45.1X5	T45.1X6
Memantine	T43.8X1	T43.8X2	T43.8X3	T43.8X4	T43.8X5	T43.8X6
Menadiol	T45.7X1	T45.7X2	T45.7X3	T45.7X4	T45.7X5	T45.7X6
sodium sulfate	T45.7X1	T45.7X2	T45.7X3	T45.7X4	T45.7X5	T45.7X6
Menadione	T45.7X1	T45.7X2	T45.7X3	T45.7X4	T45.7X5	T45.7X6
sodium bisulfite	T45.7X1	T45.7X2	T45.7X3	T45.7X4	T45.7X5	T45.7X6
Menaphthone	T45.7X1	T45.7X2	T45.7X3	T45.7X4	T45.7X5	T45.7X6

Substance	Poisoning, Accidental (unintentional)	Poisoning, Intentional Self-harm	Poisoning, Assault	Poisoning, Undetermined	Adverse Effect	Under-dosing
Menaquinone	T45.7X1	T45.7X2	T45.7X3	T45.7X4	T45.7X5	T45.7X6
Menatetrenone	T45.7X1	T45.7X2	T45.7X3	T45.7X4	T45.7X5	T45.7X6
Meningococcal vaccine	T5Ø.A91	T5Ø.A92	T5Ø.A93	T5Ø.A94	T5Ø.A95	T5Ø.A96
Menningovax (-AC) (-C)	T5Ø.A91	T5Ø.A92	T5Ø.A93	T5Ø.A94	T5Ø.A95	T5Ø.A96
Menotropins	T38.811	T38.812	T38.813	T38.814	T38.815	T38.816
Menthol	T48.5X1	T48.5X2	T48.5X3	T48.5X4	T48.5X5	T48.5X6
Mepacrine	T37.2X1	T37.2X2	T37.2X3	T37.2X4	T37.2X5	T37.2X6
Meparfynol	T42.6X1	T42.6X2	T42.6X3	T42.6X4	T42.6X5	T42.6X6
Mepartricin	T36.7X1	T36.7X2	T36.7X3	T36.7X4	T36.7X5	T36.7X6
Mepazine	T43.3X1	T43.3X2	T43.3X3	T43.3X4	T43.3X5	T43.3X6
Mepenzolate	T44.3X1	T44.3X2	T44.3X3	T44.3X4	T44.3X5	T44.3X6
bromide	T44.3X1	T44.3X2	T44.3X3	T44.3X4	T44.3X5	T44.3X6
Meperidine	T4Ø.4X1	T4Ø.4X2	T4Ø.4X3	T4Ø.4X4	T4Ø.4X5	T4Ø.4X6
Mephebarbital	T42.3X1	T42.3X2	T42.3X3	T42.3X4	T42.3X5	T42.3X6
Mephenamin(e)	T42.8X1	T42.8X2	T42.8X3	T42.8X4	T42.8X5	T42.8X6
Mephenesin	T42.8X1	T42.8X2	T42.8X3	T42.8X4	T42.8X5	T42.8X6
Mephenhydramine	T45.ØX1	T45.ØX2	T45.ØX3	T45.ØX4	T45.ØX5	T45.ØX6
Mephenoxalone	T42.8X1	T42.8X2	T42.8X3	T42.8X4	T42.8X5	T42.8X6
Mephentermine	T44.991	T44.992	T44.993	T44.994	T44.995	T44.996
Mephenytoin	T42.ØX1	T42.ØX2	T42.ØX3	T42.ØX4	T42.ØX5	T42.ØX6
with phenobarbital	T42.3X1	T42.3X2	T42.3X3	T42.3X4	T42.3X5	T42.3X6
Mephobarbital	T42.3X1	T42.3X2	T42.3X3	T42.3X4	T42.3X5	T42.3X6
Mephosfolan	T6Ø.ØX1	T6Ø.ØX2	T6Ø.ØX3	T6Ø.ØX4	—	—
Mepindolol	T44.7X1	T44.7X2	T44.7X3	T44.7X4	T44.7X5	T44.7X6
Mepiperphenidol	T44.3X1	T44.3X2	T44.3X3	T44.3X4	T44.3X5	T44.3X6
Mepitiostane	T38.7X1	T38.7X2	T38.7X3	T38.7X4	T38.7X5	T38.7X6
Mepivacaine	T41.3X1	T41.3X2	T41.3X3	T41.3X4	T41.3X5	T41.3X6
epidural	T41.3X1	T41.3X2	T41.3X3	T41.3X4	T41.3X5	T41.3X6
Meprednisone	T38.ØX1	T38.ØX2	T38.ØX3	T38.ØX4	T38.ØX5	T38.ØX6
Meprobam	T43.591	T43.592	T43.593	T43.594	T43.595	T43.596
Meprobamate	T43.591	T43.592	T43.593	T43.594	T43.595	T43.596
Meproscillarin	T46.ØX1	T46.ØX2	T46.ØX3	T46.ØX4	T46.ØX5	T46.ØX6
Meprylcaine	T41.3X1	T41.3X2	T41.3X3	T41.3X4	T41.3X5	T41.3X6
Meptazinol	T39.8X1	T39.8X2	T39.8X3	T39.8X4	T39.8X5	T39.8X6
Mepyramine	T45.ØX1	T45.ØX2	T45.ØX3	T45.ØX4	T45.ØX5	T45.ØX6
Mequitazine	T43.3X1	T43.3X2	T43.3X3	T43.3X4	T43.3X5	T43.3X6
Meralluride	T5Ø.2X1	T5Ø.2X2	T5Ø.2X3	T5Ø.2X4	T5Ø.2X5	T5Ø.2X6
Merbaphen	T5Ø.2X1	T5Ø.2X2	T5Ø.2X3	T5Ø.2X4	T5Ø.2X5	T5Ø.2X6
Merbromin	T49.ØX1	T49.ØX2	T49.ØX3	T49.ØX4	T49.ØX5	T49.ØX6
Mercaptobenzothiazole salts	T49.ØX1	T49.ØX2	T49.ØX3	T49.ØX4	T49.ØX5	T49.ØX6
Mercaptomerin	T5Ø.2X1	T5Ø.2X2	T5Ø.2X3	T5Ø.2X4	T5Ø.2X5	T5Ø.2X6
Mercaptopurine	T45.1X1	T45.1X2	T45.1X3	T45.1X4	T45.1X5	T45.1X6
Mercumatilin	T5Ø.2X1	T5Ø.2X2	T5Ø.2X3	T5Ø.2X4	T5Ø.2X5	T5Ø.2X6
Mercuramide	T5Ø.2X1	T5Ø.2X2	T5Ø.2X3	T5Ø.2X4	T5Ø.2X5	T5Ø.2X6
Mercurochrome	T49.ØX1	T49.ØX2	T49.ØX3	T49.ØX4	T49.ØX5	T49.ØX6
Mercurophylline	T5Ø.2X1	T5Ø.2X2	T5Ø.2X3	T5Ø.2X4	T5Ø.2X5	T5Ø.2X6
Mercury, mercurial, mercuric, mercurous (compounds) (cyanide) (fumes) (nonmedicinal) (vapor) NEC	T56.1X1	T56.1X2	T56.1X3	T56.1X4	—	—
ammoniated	T49.ØX1	T49.ØX2	T49.ØX3	T49.ØX4	T49.ØX5	T49.ØX6
anti-infective						
local	T49.ØX1	T49.ØX2	T49.ØX3	T49.ØX4	T49.ØX5	T49.ØX6
systemic	T37.8X1	T37.8X2	T37.8X3	T37.8X4	T37.8X5	T37.8X6
topical	T49.ØX1	T49.ØX2	T49.ØX3	T49.ØX4	T49.ØX5	T49.ØX6
chloride (ammoniated)	T49.ØX1	T49.ØX2	T49.ØX3	T49.ØX4	T49.ØX5	T49.ØX6
fungicide	T56.1X1	T56.1X2	T56.1X3	T56.1X4	—	—
diuretic NEC	T5Ø.2X1	T5Ø.2X2	T5Ø.2X3	T5Ø.2X4	T5Ø.2X5	T5Ø.2X6
fungicide	T56.1X1	T56.1X2	T56.1X3	T56.1X4	—	—
organic (fungicide)	T56.1X1	T56.1X2	T56.1X3	T56.1X4	—	—
oxide, yellow	T49.ØX1	T49.ØX2	T49.ØX3	T49.ØX4	T49.ØX5	T49.ØX6
Mersalyl	T5Ø.2X1	T5Ø.2X2	T5Ø.2X3	T5Ø.2X4	T5Ø.2X5	T5Ø.2X6
Merthiolate	T49.ØX1	T49.ØX2	T49.ØX3	T49.ØX4	T49.ØX5	T49.ØX6
ophthalmic preparation	T49.5X1	T49.5X2	T49.5X3	T49.5X4	T49.5X5	T49.5X6
Meruvax	T5Ø.B91	T5Ø.B92	T5Ø.B93	T5Ø.B94	T5Ø.B95	T5Ø.B96
Mesalazine	T47.8X1	T47.8X2	T47.8X3	T47.8X4	T47.8X5	T47.8X6
Mescal buttons	T4Ø.991	T4Ø.992	T4Ø.993	T4Ø.994	—	—
Mescaline	T4Ø.991	T4Ø.992	T4Ø.993	T4Ø.994	—	—
Mesna	T48.4X1	T48.4X2	T48.4X3	T48.4X4	T48.4X5	T48.4X6
Mesoglycan	T46.6X1	T46.6X2	T46.6X3	T46.6X4	T46.6X5	T46.6X6
Mesoridazine	T43.3X1	T43.3X2	T43.3X3	T43.3X4	T43.3X5	T43.3X6

Substance	Poisoning, Accidental (unintentional)	Poisoning, Intentional Self-harm	Poisoning, Assault	Poisoning, Undetermined	Adverse Effect	Under-dosing
Mestanolone	T38.7X1	T38.7X2	T38.7X3	T38.7X4	T38.7X5	T38.7X6
Mesterolone	T38.7X1	T38.7X2	T38.7X3	T38.7X4	T38.7X5	T38.7X6
Mestranol	T38.5X1	T38.5X2	T38.5X3	T38.5X4	T38.5X5	T38.5X6
Mesulergine	T42.8X1	T42.8X2	T42.8X3	T42.8X4	T42.8X5	T42.8X6
Mesulfen	T49.ØX1	T49.ØX2	T49.ØX3	T49.ØX4	T49.ØX5	T49.ØX6
Mesuximide	T42.2X1	T42.2X2	T42.2X3	T42.2X4	T42.2X5	T42.2X6
Metabutethamine	T41.3X1	T41.3X2	T41.3X3	T41.3X4	T41.3X5	T41.3X6
Metactesylacetate	T49.ØX1	T49.ØX2	T49.ØX3	T49.ØX4	T49.ØX5	T49.ØX6
Metacycline	T36.4X1	T36.4X2	T36.4X3	T36.4X4	T36.4X5	T36.4X6
Metaldehyde (snail killer) **NEC**	T6Ø.8X1	T6Ø.8X2	T6Ø.8X3	T6Ø.8X4	—	—
Metals (heavy) (nonmedicinal)	T56.91	T56.92	T56.93	T56.94	—	—
dust, fumes, or vapor NEC	T56.91	T56.92	T56.93	T56.94	—	—
light NEC	T56.91	T56.92	T56.93	T56.94	—	—
dust, fumes, or vapor NEC	T56.91	T56.92	T56.93	T56.94	—	—
specified NEC	T56.891	T56.892	T56.893	T56.894	—	—
thallium	T56.811	T56.812	T56.813	T56.814	—	—
Metamfetamine	T43.621	T43.622	T43.623	T43.624	T43.625	T43.626
Metamizole sodium	T39.2X1	T39.2X2	T39.2X3	T39.2X4	T39.2X5	T39.2X6
Metampicillin	T36.ØX1	T36.ØX2	T36.ØX3	T36.ØX4	T36.ØX5	T36.ØX6
Metamucil	T47.4X1	T47.4X2	T47.4X3	T47.4X4	T47.4X5	T47.4X6
Metaphen	T49.ØX1	T49.ØX2	T49.ØX3	T49.ØX4	T49.ØX5	T49.ØX6
Metandienone	T38.7X1	T38.7X2	T38.7X3	T38.7X4	T38.7X5	T38.7X6
Metandrostenolone	T38.7X1	T38.7X2	T38.7X3	T38.7X4	T38.7X5	T38.7X6
Metaphos	T6Ø.ØX1	T6Ø.ØX2	T6Ø.ØX3	T6Ø.ØX4	—	—
Metapramine	T43.Ø11	T43.Ø12	T43.Ø13	T43.Ø14	T43.Ø15	T43.Ø16
Metaproterenol	T48.291	T48.292	T48.293	T48.294	T48.295	T48.296
Metaraminol	T44.4X1	T44.4X2	T44.4X3	T44.4X4	T44.4X5	T44.4X6
Metaxalone	T42.8X1	T42.8X2	T42.8X3	T42.8X4	T42.8X5	T42.8X6
Metenolone	T38.7X1	T38.7X2	T38.7X3	T38.7X4	T38.7X5	T38.7X6
Metergoline	T42.8X1	T42.8X2	T42.8X3	T42.8X4	T42.8X5	T42.8X6
Metescufylline	T46.991	T46.992	T46.993	T46.994	T46.995	T46.996
Metetoin	T42.ØX1	T42.ØX2	T42.ØX3	T42.ØX4	T42.ØX5	T42.ØX6
Metformin	T38.3X1	T38.3X2	T38.3X3	T38.3X4	T38.3X5	T38.3X6
Methacholine	T44.1X1	T44.1X2	T44.1X3	T44.1X4	T44.1X5	T44.1X6
Methacycline	T36.4X1	T36.4X2	T36.4X3	T36.4X4	T36.4X5	T36.4X6
Methadone	T4Ø.3X1	T4Ø.3X2	T4Ø.3X3	T4Ø.3X4	T4Ø.3X5	T4Ø.3X6
Methallenestril	T38.5X1	T38.5X2	T38.5X3	T38.5X4	T38.5X5	T38.5X6
Methallenoestril	T38.5X1	T38.5X2	T38.5X3	T38.5X4	T38.5X5	T38.5X6
Methamphetamine	T43.621	T43.622	T43.623	T43.624	T43.625	T43.626
Methampyrone	T39.2X1	T39.2X2	T39.2X3	T39.2X4	T39.2X5	T39.2X6
Methandienone	T38.7X1	T38.7X2	T38.7X3	T38.7X4	T38.7X5	T38.7X6
Methandriol	T38.7X1	T38.7X2	T38.7X3	T38.7X4	T38.7X5	T38.7X6
Methandrostenolone	T38.7X1	T38.7X2	T38.7X3	T38.7X4	T38.7X5	T38.7X6
Methane	T59.891	T59.892	T59.893	T59.894	—	—
Methanethiol	T59.891	T59.892	T59.893	T59.894	—	—
Methaniazide	T37.1X1	T37.1X2	T37.1X3	T37.1X4	T37.1X5	T37.1X6
Methanol (vapor)	T51.1X1	T51.1X2	T51.1X3	T51.1X4	—	—
Methantheline	T44.3X1	T44.3X2	T44.3X3	T44.3X4	T44.3X5	T44.3X6
Methanthelinium bromide	T44.3X1	T44.3X2	T44.3X3	T44.3X4	T44.3X5	T44.3X6
Methaphenilene	T45.ØX1	T45.ØX2	T45.ØX3	T45.ØX4	T45.ØX5	T45.ØX6
Methapyrilene	T45.ØX1	T45.ØX2	T45.ØX3	T45.ØX4	T45.ØX5	T45.ØX6
Methaqualone (compound)	T42.6X1	T42.6X2	T42.6X3	T42.6X4	T42.6X5	T42.6X6
Metharbital	T42.3X1	T42.3X2	T42.3X3	T42.3X4	T42.3X5	T42.3X6
Methazolamide	T5Ø.2X1	T5Ø.2X2	T5Ø.2X3	T5Ø.2X4	T5Ø.2X5	T5Ø.2X6
Methdilazine	T43.3X1	T43.3X2	T43.3X3	T43.3X4	T43.3X5	T43.3X6
Methedrine	T43.621	T43.622	T43.623	T43.624	T43.625	T43.626
Methenamine (mandelate)	T37.8X1	T37.8X2	T37.8X3	T37.8X4	T37.8X5	T37.8X6
Methenolone	T38.7X1	T38.7X2	T38.7X3	T38.7X4	T38.7X5	T38.7X6
Methergine	T48.ØX1	T48.ØX2	T48.ØX3	T48.ØX4	T48.ØX5	T48.ØX6
Methetoin	T42.ØX1	T42.ØX2	T42.ØX3	T42.ØX4	T42.ØX5	T42.ØX6
Methiacil	T38.2X1	T38.2X2	T38.2X3	T38.2X4	T38.2X5	T38.2X6
Methicillin	T36.ØX1	T36.ØX2	T36.ØX3	T36.ØX4	T36.ØX5	T36.ØX6
Methimazole	T38.2X1	T38.2X2	T38.2X3	T38.2X4	T38.2X5	T38.2X6
Methiodal sodium	T5Ø.8X1	T5Ø.8X2	T5Ø.8X3	T5Ø.8X4	T5Ø.8X5	T5Ø.8X6
Methionine	T5Ø.991	T5Ø.992	T5Ø.993	T5Ø.994	T5Ø.995	T5Ø.996
Methisazone	T37.5X1	T37.5X2	T37.5X3	T37.5X4	T37.5X5	T37.5X6
Methisoprinol	T37.5X1	T37.5X2	T37.5X3	T37.5X4	T37.5X5	T37.5X6
Methitural	T42.3X1	T42.3X2	T42.3X3	T42.3X4	T42.3X5	T42.3X6
Methixene	T44.3X1	T44.3X2	T44.3X3	T44.3X4	T44.3X5	T44.3X6
Methobarbital, methobarbitone	T42.3X1	T42.3X2	T42.3X3	T42.3X4	T42.3X5	T42.3X6

Substance	Poisoning, Accidental (unintentional)	Poisoning, Intentional Self-harm	Poisoning, Assault	Poisoning, Undetermined	Adverse Effect	Under-dosing
Methocarbamol	T42.8X1	T42.8X2	T42.8X3	T42.8X4	T42.8X5	T42.8X6
skeletal muscle relaxant	T48.1X1	T48.1X2	T48.1X3	T48.1X4	T48.1X5	T48.1X6
Methohexital	T41.1X1	T41.1X2	T41.1X3	T41.1X4	T41.1X5	T41.1X6
Methohexitone	T41.1X1	T41.1X2	T41.1X3	T41.1X4	T41.1X5	T41.1X6
Methoin	T42.ØX1	T42.ØX2	T42.ØX3	T42.ØX4	T42.ØX5	T42.ØX6
Methopholine	T39.8X1	T39.8X2	T39.8X3	T39.8X4	T39.8X5	T39.8X6
Methopromazine	T43.3X1	T43.3X2	T43.3X3	T43.3X4	T43.3X5	T43.3X6
Methorate	T48.3X1	T48.3X2	T48.3X3	T48.3X4	T48.3X5	T48.3X6
Methoserpidine	T46.5X1	T46.5X2	T46.5X3	T46.5X4	T46.5X5	T46.5X6
Methotrexate	T45.1X1	T45.1X2	T45.1X3	T45.1X4	T45.1X5	T45.1X6
Methotrimeprazine	T43.3X1	T43.3X2	T43.3X3	T43.3X4	T43.3X5	T43.3X6
Methoxa-Dome	T49.3X1	T49.3X2	T49.3X3	T49.3X4	T49.3X5	T49.3X6
Methoxamine	T44.4X1	T44.4X2	T44.4X3	T44.4X4	T44.4X5	T44.4X6
Methoxsalen	T5Ø.991	T5Ø.992	T5Ø.993	T5Ø.994	T5Ø.995	T5Ø.996
Methoxyaniline	T65.3X1	T65.3X2	T65.3X3	T65.3X4	—	—
Methoxybenzyl penicillin	T36.ØX1	T36.ØX2	T36.ØX3	T36.ØX4	T36.ØX5	T36.ØX6
Methoxychlor	T53.7X1	T53.7X2	T53.7X3	T53.7X4	—	—
Methoxy-DDT	T53.7X1	T53.7X2	T53.7X3	T53.7X4	—	—
2-Methoxyethanol	T52.3X1	T52.3X2	T52.3X3	T52.3X4	—	—
Methoxyflurane	T41.ØX1	T41.ØX2	T41.ØX3	T41.ØX4	T41.ØX5	T41.ØX6
Methoxyphenamine	T48.6X1	T48.6X2	T48.6X3	T48.6X4	T48.6X5	T48.6X6
Methoxypromazine	T43.3X1	T43.3X2	T43.3X3	T43.3X4	T43.3X5	T43.3X6
5-Methoxypsoralen (5-MOP)	T5Ø.991	T5Ø.992	T5Ø.993	T5Ø.994	T5Ø.995	T5Ø.996
8-Methoxypsoralen (8-MOP)	T5Ø.991	T5Ø.992	T5Ø.993	T5Ø.994	T5Ø.995	T5Ø.996
Methscopolamine bromide	T44.3X1	T44.3X2	T44.3X3	T44.3X4	T44.3X5	T44.3X6
Methsuximide	T42.2X1	T42.2X2	T42.2X3	T42.2X4	T42.2X5	T42.2X6
Methyclothiazide	T5Ø.2X1	T5Ø.2X2	T5Ø.2X3	T5Ø.2X4	T5Ø.2X5	T5Ø.2X6
Methyl						
acetate	T52.4X1	T52.4X2	T52.4X3	T52.4X4	—	—
acetone	T52.4X1	T52.4X2	T52.4X3	T52.4X4	—	—
acrylate	T65.891	T65.892	T65.893	T65.894	—	—
alcohol	T51.1X1	T51.1X2	T51.1X3	T51.1X4	—	—
aminophenol	T65.3X1	T65.3X2	T65.3X3	T65.3X4	—	—
amphetamine	T43.621	T43.622	T43.623	T43.624	T43.625	T43.626
androstanolone	T38.7X1	T38.7X2	T38.7X3	T38.7X4	T38.7X5	T38.7X6
atropine	T44.3X1	T44.3X2	T44.3X3	T44.3X4	T44.3X5	T44.3X6
benzene	T52.2X1	T52.2X2	T52.2X3	T52.2X4	—	—
benzoate	T52.8X1	T52.8X2	T52.8X3	T52.8X4	—	—
benzol	T52.2X1	T52.2X2	T52.2X3	T52.2X4	—	—
bromide (gas)	T59.891	T59.892	T59.893	T59.894	—	—
fumigant	T6Ø.8X1	T6Ø.8X2	T6Ø.8X3	T6Ø.8X4	—	—
butanol	T51.3X1	T51.3X2	T51.3X3	T51.3X4	—	—
carbonate	T52.8X1	T52.8X2	T52.8X3	T52.8X4	—	—
carbinol	T51.1X1	T51.1X2	T51.1X3	T51.1X4	—	—
CCNU	T45.1X1	T45.1X2	T45.1X3	T45.1X4	T45.1X5	T45.1X6
cellosolve	T52.91	T52.92	T52.93	T52.94	—	—
cellulose	T47.4X1	T47.4X2	T47.4X3	T47.4X4	T47.4X5	T47.4X6
chloride (gas)	T59.891	T59.892	T59.893	T59.894	—	—
chloroformate	T59.3X1	T59.3X2	T59.3X3	T59.3X4	—	—
cyclohexane	T52.8X1	T52.8X2	T52.8X3	T52.8X4	—	—
cyclohexanol	T51.8X1	T51.8X2	T51.8X3	T51.8X4	—	—
cyclohexanone	T52.8X1	T52.8X2	T52.8X3	T52.8X4	—	—
cyclohexyl acetate	T52.8X1	T52.8X2	T52.8X3	T52.8X4	—	—
demeton	T6Ø.ØX1	T6Ø.ØX2	T6Ø.ØX3	T6Ø.ØX4	—	—
dihydromorphinone	T4Ø.2X1	T4Ø.2X2	T4Ø.2X3	T4Ø.2X4	T4Ø.2X5	T4Ø.2X6
ergometrine	T48.ØX1	T48.ØX2	T48.ØX3	T48.ØX4	T48.ØX5	T48.ØX6
ergonovine	T48.ØX1	T48.ØX2	T48.ØX3	T48.ØX4	T48.ØX5	T48.ØX6
ethyl ketone	T52.4X1	T52.4X2	T52.4X3	T52.4X4	—	—
glucamine antimonate	T37.8X1	T37.8X2	T37.8X3	T37.8X4	T37.8X5	T37.8X6
hydrazine	T65.891	T65.892	T65.893	T65.894	—	—
iodide	T65.891	T65.892	T65.893	T65.894	—	—
isobutyl ketone	T52.4X1	T52.4X2	T52.4X3	T52.4X4	—	—
isothiocyanate	T6Ø.3X1	T6Ø.3X2	T6Ø.3X3	T6Ø.3X4	—	—
mercaptan	T59.891	T59.892	T59.893	T59.894	—	—
morphine NEC	T4Ø.2X1	T4Ø.2X2	T4Ø.2X3	T4Ø.2X4	T4Ø.2X5	T4Ø.2X6
nicotinate	T49.4X1	T49.4X2	T49.4X3	T49.4X4	T49.4X5	T49.4X6
paraben	T49.ØX1	T49.ØX2	T49.ØX3	T49.ØX4	T49.ØX5	T49.ØX6
parafynol	T42.6X1	T42.6X2	T42.6X3	T42.6X4	T42.6X5	T42.6X6
parathion	T6Ø.ØX1	T6Ø.ØX2	T6Ø.ØX3	T6Ø.ØX4	—	—
peridol	T43.4X1	T43.4X2	T43.4X3	T43.4X4	T43.4X5	T43.4X6
phenidate	T43.631	T43.632	T43.633	T43.634	T43.635	T43.636

Substance	Poisoning, Accidental (unintentional)	Poisoning, Intentional Self-harm	Poisoning, Assault	Poisoning, Undetermined	Adverse Effect	Under-dosing
Methyl — *continued*						
prednisolone	T38.ØX1	T38.ØX2	T38.ØX3	T38.ØX4	T38.ØX5	T38.ØX6
ENT agent	T49.6X1	T49.6X2	T49.6X3	T49.6X4	T49.6X5	T49.6X6
ophthalmic preparation	T49.5X1	T49.5X2	T49.5X3	T49.5X4	T49.5X5	T49.5X6
topical NEC	T49.ØX1	T49.ØX2	T49.ØX3	T49.ØX4	T49.ØX5	T49.ØX6
rosaniline NEC	T49.ØX1	T49.ØX2	T49.ØX3	T49.ØX4	T49.ØX5	T49.ØX6
salicylate	T49.2X1	T49.2X2	T49.2X3	T49.2X4	T49.2X5	T49.2X6
sulfate (fumes)	T59.891	T59.892	T59.893	T59.894	—	—
liquid	T52.8X1	T52.8X2	T52.8X3	T52.8X4	—	—
sulfonal	T42.6X1	T42.6X2	T42.6X3	T42.6X4	T42.6X5	T42.6X6
testosterone	T38.7X1	T38.7X2	T38.7X3	T38.7X4	T38.7X5	T38.7X6
thiouracil	T38.2X1	T38.2X2	T38.2X3	T38.2X4	T38.2X5	T38.2X6
Methylamphetamine	T43.621	T43.622	T43.623	T43.624	T43.625	T43.626
Methylated spirit	T51.1X1	T51.1X2	T51.1X3	T51.1X4	—	—
Methylatropine nitrate	T44.3X1	T44.3X2	T44.3X3	T44.3X4	T44.3X5	T44.3X6
Methylbenactyzium bromide	T44.3X1	T44.3X2	T44.3X3	T44.3X4	T44.3X5	T44.3X6
Methylbenzethonium chloride	T49.ØX1	T49.ØX2	T49.ØX3	T49.ØX4	T49.ØX5	T49.ØX6
Methylcellulose	T47.4X1	T47.4X2	T47.4X3	T47.4X4	T47.4X5	T47.4X6
laxative	T47.4X1	T47.4X2	T47.4X3	T47.4X4	T47.4X5	T47.4X6
Methylchlorophenoxyacetic acid	T6Ø.3X1	T6Ø.3X2	T6Ø.3X3	T6Ø.3X4	—	—
Methyldopa	T46.5X1	T46.5X2	T46.5X3	T46.5X4	T46.5X5	T46.5X6
Methyldopate	T46.5X1	T46.5X2	T46.5X3	T46.5X4	T46.5X5	T46.5X6
Methylene						
blue	T5Ø.6X1	T5Ø.6X2	T5Ø.6X3	T5Ø.6X4	T5Ø.6X5	T5Ø.6X6
chloride or dichloride (solvent) NEC	T53.4X1	T53.4X2	T53.4X3	T53.4X4	—	—
Methylenedioxyamphetamine	T43.621	T43.622	T43.623	T43.624	T43.625	T43.626
Methylenedioxymethamphetamine	T43.621	T43.622	T43.623	T43.624	T43.625	T43.626
Methylergometrine	T48.ØX1	T48.ØX2	T48.ØX3	T48.ØX4	T48.ØX5	T48.ØX6
Methylergonovine	T48.ØX1	T48.ØX2	T48.ØX3	T48.ØX4	T48.ØX5	T48.ØX6
Methylestrenolone	T38.5X1	T38.5X2	T38.5X3	T38.5X4	T38.5X5	T38.5X6
Methylethyl cellulose	T5Ø.991	T5Ø.992	T5Ø.993	T5Ø.994	T5Ø.995	T5Ø.996
Methylhexabital	T42.3X1	T42.3X2	T42.3X3	T42.3X4	T42.3X5	T42.3X6
Methylmorphine	T4Ø.2X1	T4Ø.2X2	T4Ø.2X3	T4Ø.2X4	T4Ø.2X5	T4Ø.2X6
Methylparaben (ophthalmic)	T49.5X1	T49.5X2	T49.5X3	T49.5X4	T49.5X5	T49.5X6
Methylparafynol	T42.6X1	T42.6X2	T42.6X3	T42.6X4	T42.6X5	T42.6X6
Methylpentynol, methylpenthynol	T42.6X1	T42.6X2	T42.6X3	T42.6X4	T42.6X5	T42.6X6
Methylphenidate	T43.631	T43.632	T43.633	T43.634	T43.635	T43.636
Methylphenobarbital	T42.3X1	T42.3X2	T42.3X3	T42.3X4	T42.3X5	T42.3X6
Methylpolysiloxane	T47.1X1	T47.1X2	T47.1X3	T47.1X4	T47.1X5	T47.1X6
Methylprednisolone — *see* Methyl, prednisolone						
Methylrosaniline	T49.ØX1	T49.ØX2	T49.ØX3	T49.ØX4	T49.ØX5	T49.ØX6
Methylrosanilinium chloride	T49.ØX1	T49.ØX2	T49.ØX3	T49.ØX4	T49.ØX5	T49.ØX6
Methyltestosterone	T38.7X1	T38.7X2	T38.7X3	T38.7X4	T38.7X5	T38.7X6
Methylthionine chloride	T5Ø.6X1	T5Ø.6X2	T5Ø.6X3	T5Ø.6X4	T5Ø.6X5	T5Ø.6X6
Methylthioninium chloride	T5Ø.6X1	T5Ø.6X2	T5Ø.6X3	T5Ø.6X4	T5Ø.6X5	T5Ø.6X6
Methylthiouracil	T38.2X1	T38.2X2	T38.2X3	T38.2X4	T38.2X5	T38.2X6
Methyprylon	T42.6X1	T42.6X2	T42.6X3	T42.6X4	T42.6X5	T42.6X6
Methysergide	T46.5X1	T46.5X2	T46.5X3	T46.5X4	T46.5X5	T46.5X6
Metiamide	T47.1X1	T47.1X2	T47.1X3	T47.1X4	T47.1X5	T47.1X6
Meticillin	T36.ØX1	T36.ØX2	T36.ØX3	T36.ØX4	T36.ØX5	T36.ØX6
Meticrane	T5Ø.2X1	T5Ø.2X2	T5Ø.2X3	T5Ø.2X4	T5Ø.2X5	T5Ø.2X6
Metildigoxin	T46.ØX1	T46.ØX2	T46.ØX3	T46.ØX4	T46.ØX5	T46.ØX6
Metipranolol	T49.5X1	T49.5X2	T49.5X3	T49.5X4	T49.5X5	T49.5X6
Metirosine	T46.5X1	T46.5X2	T46.5X3	T46.5X4	T46.5X5	T46.5X6
Metisazone	T37.5X1	T37.5X2	T37.5X3	T37.5X4	T37.5X5	T37.5X6
Metixene	T44.3X1	T44.3X2	T44.3X3	T44.3X4	T44.3X5	T44.3X6
Metizoline	T48.5X1	T48.5X2	T48.5X3	T48.5X4	T48.5X5	T48.5X6
Metoclopramide	T45.ØX1	T45.ØX2	T45.ØX3	T45.ØX4	T45.ØX5	T45.ØX6
Metofenazate	T43.3X1	T43.3X2	T43.3X3	T43.3X4	T43.3X5	T43.3X6
Metofoline	T39.8X1	T39.8X2	T39.8X3	T39.8X4	T39.8X5	T39.8X6
Metolazone	T5Ø.2X1	T5Ø.2X2	T5Ø.2X3	T5Ø.2X4	T5Ø.2X5	T5Ø.2X6
Metopon	T4Ø.2X1	T4Ø.2X2	T4Ø.2X3	T4Ø.2X4	T4Ø.2X5	T4Ø.2X6
Metoprine	T45.1X1	T45.1X2	T45.1X3	T45.1X4	T45.1X5	T45.1X6
Metoprolol	T44.7X1	T44.7X2	T44.7X3	T44.7X4	T44.7X5	T44.7X6
Metrifonate	T6Ø.ØX1	T6Ø.ØX2	T6Ø.ØX3	T6Ø.ØX4	—	—
Metrizamide	T5Ø.8X1	T5Ø.8X2	T5Ø.8X3	T5Ø.8X4	T5Ø.8X5	T5Ø.8X6

Substance	Poisoning, Accidental (unintentional)	Poisoning, Intentional Self-harm	Poisoning, Assault	Poisoning, Undetermined	Adverse Effect	Under-dosing
Metrizoic acid	T5Ø.8X1	T5Ø.8X2	T5Ø.8X3	T5Ø.8X4	T5Ø.8X5	T5Ø.8X6
Metronidazole	T37.8X1	T37.8X2	T37.8X3	T37.8X4	T37.8X5	T37.8X6
Metycaine	T41.3X1	T41.3X2	T41.3X3	T41.3X4	T41.3X5	T41.3X6
infiltration (subcutaneous)	T41.3X1	T41.3X2	T41.3X3	T41.3X4	T41.3X5	T41.3X6
nerve block (peripheral) (plexus)	T41.3X1	T41.3X2	T41.3X3	T41.3X4	T41.3X5	T41.3X6
topical (surface)	T41.3X1	T41.3X2	T41.3X3	T41.3X4	T41.3X5	T41.3X6
Metyrapone	T5Ø.8X1	T5Ø.8X2	T5Ø.8X3	T5Ø.8X4	T5Ø.8X5	T5Ø.8X6
Mevinphos	T6Ø.ØX1	T6Ø.ØX2	T6Ø.ØX3	T6Ø.ØX4	—	—
Mexazolam	T42.4X1	T42.4X2	T42.4X3	T42.4X4	T42.4X5	T42.4X6
Mexenone	T49.3X1	T49.3X2	T49.3X3	T49.3X4	T49.3X5	T49.3X6
Mexiletine	T46.2X1	T46.2X2	T46.2X3	T46.2X4	T46.2X5	T46.2X6
Mezereon	T62.2X1	T62.2X2	T62.2X3	T62.2X4	—	—
berries	T62.1X1	T62.1X2	T62.1X3	T62.1X4	—	—
Mezlocillin	T36.ØX1	T36.ØX2	T36.ØX3	T36.ØX4	T36.ØX5	T36.ØX6
Mianserin	T43.Ø21	T43.Ø22	T43.Ø23	T43.Ø24	T43.Ø25	T43.Ø26
Micatin	T49.ØX1	T49.ØX2	T49.ØX3	T49.ØX4	T49.ØX5	T49.ØX6
Miconazole	T49.ØX1	T49.ØX2	T49.ØX3	T49.ØX4	T49.ØX5	T49.ØX6
Micronomicin	T36.5X1	T36.5X2	T36.5X3	T36.5X4	T36.5X5	T36.5X6
Midazolam	T42.4X1	T42.4X2	T42.4X3	T42.4X4	T42.4X5	T42.4X6
Midecamycin	T36.3X1	T36.3X2	T36.3X3	T36.3X4	T36.3X5	T36.3X6
Mifepristone	T38.6X1	T38.6X2	T38.6X3	T38.6X4	T38.6X5	T38.6X6
Milk of magnesia	T47.1X1	T47.1X2	T47.1X3	T47.1X4	T47.1X5	T47.1X6
Millipede (tropical) (venomous)	T63.411	T63.412	T63.413	T63.414	—	—
Miltown	T43.591	T43.592	T43.593	T43.594	T43.595	T43.596
Milverine	T44.3X1	T44.3X2	T44.3X3	T44.3X4	T44.3X5	T44.3X6
Minaprine	T43.291	T43.292	T43.293	T43.294	T43.295	T43.296
Minaxolone	T41.291	T41.292	T41.293	T41.294	T41.295	T41.296
Mineral						
acids	T54.2X1	T54.2X2	T54.2X3	T54.2X4	—	—
oil (laxative)(medicinal)	T47.4X1	T47.4X2	T47.4X3	T47.4X4	T47.4X5	T47.4X6
emulsion	T47.2X1	T47.2X2	T47.2X3	T47.2X4	T47.2X5	T47.2X6
nonmedicinal	T52.ØX1	T52.ØX2	T52.ØX3	T52.ØX4	—	—
topical	T49.3X1	T49.3X2	T49.3X3	T49.3X4	T49.3X5	T49.3X6
salt NEC	T5Ø.3X1	T5Ø.3X2	T5Ø.3X3	T5Ø.3X4	T5Ø.3X5	T5Ø.3X6
spirits	T52.ØX1	T52.ØX2	T52.ØX3	T52.ØX4	—	—
Mineralocorticosteroid	T5Ø.ØX1	T5Ø.ØX2	T5Ø.ØX3	T5Ø.ØX4	T5Ø.ØX5	T5Ø.ØX6
Minocycline	T36.4X1	T36.4X2	T36.4X3	T36.4X4	T36.4X5	T36.4X6
Minoxidil	T46.7X1	T46.7X2	T46.7X3	T46.7X4	T46.7X5	T46.7X6
Miokamycin	T36.3X1	T36.3X2	T36.3X3	T36.3X4	T36.3X5	T36.3X6
Miotic drug	T49.5X1	T49.5X2	T49.5X3	T49.5X4	T49.5X5	T49.5X6
Mipafox	T6Ø.ØX1	T6Ø.ØX2	T6Ø.ØX3	T6Ø.ØX4	—	—
Mirex	T6Ø.1X1	T6Ø.1X2	T6Ø.1X3	T6Ø.1X4	—	—
Mirtazapine	T43.Ø21	T43.Ø22	T43.Ø23	T43.Ø24	T43.Ø25	T43.Ø26
Misonidazole	T37.3X1	T37.3X2	T37.3X3	T37.3X4	T37.3X5	T37.3X6
Misoprostol	T47.1X1	T47.1X2	T47.1X3	T47.1X4	T47.1X5	T47.1X6
Mithramycin	T45.1X1	T45.1X2	T45.1X3	T45.1X4	T45.1X5	T45.1X6
Mitobronitol	T45.1X1	T45.1X2	T45.1X3	T45.1X4	T45.1X5	T45.1X6
Mitoguazone	T45.1X1	T45.1X2	T45.1X3	T45.1X4	T45.1X5	T45.1X6
Mitolactol	T45.1X1	T45.1X2	T45.1X3	T45.1X4	T45.1X5	T45.1X6
Mitomycin	T45.1X1	T45.1X2	T45.1X3	T45.1X4	T45.1X5	T45.1X6
Mitopodozide	T45.1X1	T45.1X2	T45.1X3	T45.1X4	T45.1X5	T45.1X6
Mitotane	T45.1X1	T45.1X2	T45.1X3	T45.1X4	T45.1X5	T45.1X6
Mitoxantrone	T45.1X1	T45.1X2	T45.1X3	T45.1X4	T45.1X5	T45.1X6
Mivacurium chloride	T48.1X1	T48.1X2	T48.1X3	T48.1X4	T48.1X5	T48.1X6
Miyari bacteria	T47.6X1	T47.6X2	T47.6X3	T47.6X4	T47.6X5	T47.6X6
Moclobemide	T43.1X1	T43.1X2	T43.1X3	T43.1X4	T43.1X5	T43.1X6
Moderil	T46.5X1	T46.5X2	T46.5X3	T46.5X4	T46.5X5	T46.5X6
Mofebutazone	T39.2X1	T39.2X2	T39.2X3	T39.2X4	T39.2X5	T39.2X6
Mogadon—*see* Nitrazepam						
Molindone	T43.591	T43.592	T43.593	T43.594	T43.595	T43.596
Molsidomine	T46.3X1	T46.3X2	T46.3X3	T46.3X4	T46.3X5	T46.3X6
Mometasone	T49.ØX1	T49.ØX2	T49.ØX3	T49.ØX4	T49.ØX5	T49.ØX6
Monistat	T49.ØX1	T49.ØX2	T49.ØX3	T49.ØX4	T49.ØX5	T49.ØX6
Monkshood	T62.2X1	T62.2X2	T62.2X3	T62.2X4	—	—
Monoamine oxidase inhibitor NEC	T43.1X1	T43.1X2	T43.1X3	T43.1X4	T43.1X5	T43.1X6
hydrazine	T43.1X1	T43.1X2	T43.1X3	T43.1X4	T43.1X5	T43.1X6
Monobenzone	T49.4X1	T49.4X2	T49.4X3	T49.4X4	T49.4X5	T49.4X6
Monochloroacetic acid	T6Ø.3X1	T6Ø.3X2	T6Ø.3X3	T6Ø.3X4	—	—
Monochlorobenzene	T53.7X1	T53.7X2	T53.7X3	T53.7X4	—	—

Substance	Poisoning, Accidental (unintentional)	Poisoning, Intentional Self-harm	Poisoning, Assault	Poisoning, Undetermined	Adverse Effect	Under-dosing
Monoethanolamine	T46.8X1	T46.8X2	T46.8X3	T46.8X4	T46.8X5	T46.8X6
oleate	T46.8X1	T46.8X2	T46.8X3	T46.8X4	T46.8X5	T46.8X6
Monooctanoin	T5Ø.991	T5Ø.992	T5Ø.993	T5Ø.994	T5Ø.995	T5Ø.996
Monophenylbutazone	T39.2X1	T39.2X2	T39.2X3	T39.2X4	T39.2X5	T39.2X6
Monosodium glutamate	T65.891	T65.892	T65.893	T65.894	—	—
Monosulfiram	T49.ØX1	T49.ØX2	T49.ØX3	T49.ØX4	T49.ØX5	T49.ØX6
Monoxide, carbon—*see* Carbon, monoxide						
Monoxidine hydrochloride	T46.1X1	T46.1X2	T46.1X3	T46.1X4	T46.1X5	T46.1X6
Monuron	T6Ø.3X1	T6Ø.3X2	T6Ø.3X3	T6Ø.3X4	—	—
Moperone	T43.4X1	T43.4X2	T43.4X3	T43.4X4	T43.4X5	T43.4X6
Mopidamol	T45.1X1	T45.1X2	T45.1X3	T45.1X4	T45.1X5	T45.1X6
MOPP (mechloreth-amine + vincristine + prednisone + procarbazine)	T45.1X1	T45.1X2	T45.1X3	T45.1X4	T45.1X5	T45.1X6
Morfin	T4Ø.2X1	T4Ø.2X2	T4Ø.2X3	T4Ø.2X4	T4Ø.2X5	T4Ø.2X6
Morinamide	T37.1X1	T37.1X2	T37.1X3	T37.1X4	T37.1X5	T37.1X6
Morning glory seeds	T4Ø.991	T4Ø.992	T4Ø.993	T4Ø.994	—	—
Moroxydine	T37.5X1	T37.5X2	T37.5X3	T37.5X4	T37.5X5	T37.5X6
Morphazinamide	T37.1X1	T37.1X2	T37.1X3	T37.1X4	T37.1X5	T37.1X6
Morphine	T4Ø.2X1	T4Ø.2X2	T4Ø.2X3	T4Ø.2X4	T4Ø.2X5	T4Ø.2X6
antagonist	T5Ø.7X1	T5Ø.7X2	T5Ø.7X3	T5Ø.7X4	T5Ø.7X5	T5Ø.7X6
Morpholinylethylmorphine	T4Ø.2X1	T4Ø.2X2	T4Ø.2X3	T4Ø.2X4	—	—
Morsuximide	T42.2X1	T42.2X2	T42.2X3	T42.2X4	T42.2X5	T42.2X6
Mosapramine	T43.591	T43.592	T43.593	T43.594	T43.595	T43.596
Moth balls (*see also* Pesticides)	T6Ø.2X1	T6Ø.2X2	T6Ø.2X3	T6Ø.2X4	—	—
naphthalene	T6Ø.2X1	T6Ø.2X2	T6Ø.2X3	T6Ø.2X4	—	—
paradichlorobenzene	T6Ø.1X1	T6Ø.1X2	T6Ø.1X3	T6Ø.1X4	—	—
Motor exhaust gas	T58.Ø1	T58.Ø2	T58.Ø3	T58.Ø4	—	—
Mouthwash (antiseptic) (zinc chloride)	T49.6X1	T49.6X2	T49.6X3	T49.6X4	T49.6X5	T49.6X6
Moxastine	T45.ØX1	T45.ØX2	T45.ØX3	T45.ØX4	T45.ØX5	T45.ØX6
Moxaverine	T44.3X1	T44.3X2	T44.3X3	T44.3X4	T44.3X5	T44.3X6
Moxisylyte	T46.7X1	T46.7X2	T46.7X3	T46.7X4	T46.7X5	T46.7X6
Mucilage, plant	T47.4X1	T47.4X2	T47.4X3	T47.4X4	T47.4X5	T47.4X6
Mucolytic drug	T48.4X1	T48.4X2	T48.4X3	T48.4X4	T48.4X5	T48.4X6
Mucomyst	T48.4X1	T48.4X2	T48.4X3	T48.4X4	T48.4X5	T48.4X6
Mucous membrane agents (external)	T49.91	T49.92	T49.93	T49.94	T49.95	T49.96
specified NEC	T49.8X1	T49.8X2	T49.8X3	T49.8X4	T49.8X5	T49.8X6
Mumps						
immune globulin (human)	T5Ø.Z11	T5Ø.Z12	T5Ø.Z13	T5Ø.Z14	T5Ø.Z15	T5Ø.Z16
skin test antigen	T5Ø.8X1	T5Ø.8X2	T5Ø.8X3	T5Ø.8X4	T5Ø.8X5	T5Ø.8X6
vaccine	T5Ø.B91	T5Ø.B92	T5Ø.B93	T5Ø.B94	T5Ø.B95	T5Ø.B96
Mumpsvax	T5Ø.B91	T5Ø.B92	T5Ø.B93	T5Ø.B94	T5Ø.B95	T5Ø.B96
Mupirocin	T49.ØX1	T49.ØX2	T49.ØX3	T49.ØX4	T49.ØX5	T49.ØX6
Muriatic acid—*see* Hydrochloric acid						
Muromonab-CD3	T45.1X1	T45.1X2	T45.1X3	T45.1X4	T45.1X5	T45.1X6
Muscle relaxant—*see* Relaxant, muscle						
Muscle-action drug NEC	T48.2Ø1	T48.2Ø2	T48.2Ø3	T48.2Ø4	T48.2Ø5	T48.2Ø6
Muscle affecting agents NEC	T48.2Ø1	T48.2Ø2	T48.2Ø3	T48.2Ø4	T48.2Ø5	T48.2Ø6
oxytocic	T48.ØX1	T48.ØX2	T48.ØX3	T48.ØX4	T48.ØX5	T48.ØX6
relaxants	T48.2Ø1	T48.2Ø2	T48.2Ø3	T48.2Ø4	T48.2Ø5	T48.2Ø6
central nervous system	T42.8X1	T42.8X2	T42.8X3	T42.8X4	T42.8X5	T42.8X6
skeletal	T48.1X1	T48.1X2	T48.1X3	T48.1X4	T48.1X5	T48.1X6
smooth	T44.3X1	T44.3X2	T44.3X3	T44.3X4	T44.3X5	T44.3X6
Muscle-tone depressant, central NEC	T42.8X1	T42.8X2	T42.8X3	T42.8X4	T42.8X5	T42.8X6
specified NEC	T42.8X1	T42.8X2	T42.8X3	T42.8X4	T42.8X5	T42.8X6
Mushroom, noxious	T62.ØX1	T62.ØX2	T62.ØX3	T62.ØX4	—	—
Mussel, noxious	T61.781	T61.782	T61.783	T61.784	—	—
Mustard (emetic)	T47.7X1	T47.7X2	T47.7X3	T47.7X4	T47.7X5	T47.7X6
black	T47.7X1	T47.7X2	T47.7X3	T47.7X4	T47.7X5	T47.7X6
gas, not in war	T59.91	T59.92	T59.93	T59.94	—	—
nitrogen	T45.1X1	T45.1X2	T45.1X3	T45.1X4	T45.1X5	T45.1X6
Mustine	T45.1X1	T45.1X2	T45.1X3	T45.1X4	T45.1X5	T45.1X6
M-vac	T45.1X1	T45.1X2	T45.1X3	T45.1X4	T45.1X5	T45.1X6
Mycifradin	T36.5X1	T36.5X2	T36.5X3	T36.5X4	T36.5X5	T36.5X6
topical	T49.ØX1	T49.ØX2	T49.ØX3	T49.ØX4	T49.ØX5	T49.ØX6

Substance	Poisoning, Accidental (unintentional)	Poisoning, Intentional Self-harm	Poisoning, Assault	Poisoning, Undetermined	Adverse Effect	Under-dosing
Mycitracin	T36.8X1	T36.8X2	T36.8X3	T36.8X4	T36.8X5	T36.8X6
ophthalmic preparation	T49.5X1	T49.5X2	T49.5X3	T49.5X4	T49.5X5	T49.5X6
Mycostatin	T36.7X1	T36.7X2	T36.7X3	T36.7X4	T36.7X5	T36.7X6
topical	T49.ØX1	T49.ØX2	T49.ØX3	T49.ØX4	T49.ØX5	T49.ØX6
Mycotoxins	T64.81	T64.82	T64.83	T64.84	—	—
aflatoxin	T64.Ø1	T64.Ø2	T64.Ø3	T64.Ø4	—	—
specified NEC	T64.81	T64.82	T64.83	T64.84	—	—
Mydriacyl	T44.3X1	T44.3X2	T44.3X3	T44.3X4	T44.3X5	T44.3X6
Mydriatic drug	T49.5X1	T49.5X2	T49.5X3	T49.5X4	T49.5X5	T49.5X6
Myelobromal	T45.1X1	T45.1X2	T45.1X3	T45.1X4	T45.1X5	T45.1X6
Myleran	T45.1X1	T45.1X2	T45.1X3	T45.1X4	T45.1X5	T45.1X6
Myochrysin(e)	T39.2X1	T39.2X2	T39.2X3	T39.2X4	T39.2X5	T39.2X6
Myoneural blocking agents	T48.1X1	T48.1X2	T48.1X3	T48.1X4	T48.1X5	T48.1X6
Myralact	T49.ØX1	T49.ØX2	T49.ØX3	T49.ØX4	T49.ØX5	T49.ØX6
Myristica fragrans	T62.2X1	T62.2X2	T62.2X3	T62.2X4	—	—
Myristicin	T65.891	T65.892	T65.893	T65.894	—	—
Mysoline	T42.3X1	T42.3X2	T42.3X3	T42.3X4	T42.3X5	T42.3X6
N						
Nabilone	T4Ø.7X1	T4Ø.7X2	T4Ø.7X3	T4Ø.7X4	T4Ø.7X5	T4Ø.7X6
Nabumetone	T39.391	T39.392	T39.393	T39.394	T39.395	T39.396
Nadolol	T44.7X1	T44.7X2	T44.7X3	T44.7X4	T44.7X5	T44.7X6
Nafcillin	T36.ØX1	T36.ØX2	T36.ØX3	T36.ØX4	T36.ØX5	T36.ØX6
Nafoxidine	T38.6X1	T38.6X2	T38.6X3	T38.6X4	T38.6X5	T38.6X6
Naftazone	T46.991	T46.992	T46.993	T46.994	T46.995	T46.996
Naftidrofuryl (oxalate)	T46.7X1	T46.7X2	T46.7X3	T46.7X4	T46.7X5	T46.7X6
Naftifine	T49.ØX1	T49.ØX2	T49.ØX3	T49.ØX4	T49.ØX5	T49.ØX6
Nail polish remover	T52.91	T52.92	T52.93	T52.94	—	—
Nalbuphine	T4Ø.4X1	T4Ø.4X2	T4Ø.4X3	T4Ø.4X4	T4Ø.4X5	T4Ø.4X6
Naled	T6Ø.ØX1	T6Ø.ØX2	T6Ø.ØX3	T6Ø.ØX4	—	—
Nalidixic acid	T37.8X1	T37.8X2	T37.8X3	T37.8X4	T37.8X5	T37.8X6
Nalorphine	T5Ø.7X1	T5Ø.7X2	T5Ø.7X3	T5Ø.7X4	T5Ø.7X5	T5Ø.7X6
Naloxone	T5Ø.7X1	T5Ø.7X2	T5Ø.7X3	T5Ø.7X4	T5Ø.7X5	T5Ø.7X6
Naltrexone	T5Ø.7X1	T5Ø.7X2	T5Ø.7X3	T5Ø.7X4	T5Ø.7X5	T5Ø.7X6
Namenda	T43.8X1	T43.8X2	T43.8X3	T43.8X4	T43.8X5	T43.8X6
Nandrolone	T38.7X1	T38.7X2	T38.7X3	T38.7X4	T38.7X5	T38.7X6
Naphazoline	T48.5X1	T48.5X2	T48.5X3	T48.5X4	T48.5X5	T48.5X6
Naphtha (painters') (petroleum)	T52.ØX1	T52.ØX2	T52.ØX3	T52.ØX4	—	—
solvent	T52.ØX1	T52.ØX2	T52.ØX3	T52.ØX4	—	—
vapor	T52.ØX1	T52.ØX2	T52.ØX3	T52.ØX4	—	—
Naphthalene (non-chlorinated)	T6Ø.2X1	T6Ø.2X2	T6Ø.2X3	T6Ø.2X4	—	—
chlorinated	T6Ø.1X1	T6Ø.1X2	T6Ø.1X3	T6Ø.1X4	—	—
vapor	T6Ø.1X1	T6Ø.1X2	T6Ø.1X3	T6Ø.1X4	—	—
insecticide or moth repellent	T6Ø.2X1	T6Ø.2X2	T6Ø.2X3	T6Ø.2X4	—	—
chlorinated	T6Ø.1X1	T6Ø.1X2	T6Ø.1X3	T6Ø.1X4	—	—
vapor	T6Ø.2X1	T6Ø.2X2	T6Ø.2X3	T6Ø.2X4	—	—
chlorinated	T6Ø.1X1	T6Ø.1X2	T6Ø.1X3	T6Ø.1X4	—	—
Naphthol	T65.891	T65.892	T65.893	T65.894	—	—
Naphthylamine	T65.891	T65.892	T65.893	T65.894	—	—
Naphthylthiourea (ANTU)	T6Ø.4X1	T6Ø.4X2	T6Ø.4X3	T6Ø.4X4	—	—
Naprosyn—*see* Naproxen						
Naproxen	T39.311	T39.312	T39.313	T39.314	T39.315	T39.316
Narcotic (drug)	T4Ø.6Ø1	T4Ø.6Ø2	T4Ø.6Ø3	T4Ø.6Ø4	T4Ø.6Ø5	T4Ø.6Ø6
analgesic NEC	T4Ø.6Ø1	T4Ø.6Ø2	T4Ø.6Ø3	T4Ø.6Ø4	T4Ø.6Ø5	T4Ø.6Ø6
antagonist	T5Ø.7X1	T5Ø.7X2	T5Ø.7X3	T5Ø.7X4	T5Ø.7X5	T5Ø.7X6
specified NEC	T4Ø.691	T4Ø.692	T4Ø.693	T4Ø.694	T4Ø.695	T4Ø.696
synthetic	T4Ø.4X1	T4Ø.4X2	T4Ø.4X3	T4Ø.4X4	T4Ø.4X5	T4Ø.4X6
Narcotine	T48.3X1	T48.3X2	T48.3X3	T48.3X4	T48.3X5	T48.3X6
Nardil	T43.1X1	T43.1X2	T43.1X3	T43.1X4	T43.1X5	T43.1X6
Nasal drug NEC	T49.6X1	T49.6X2	T49.6X3	T49.6X4	T49.6X5	T49.6X6
Natamycin	T49.ØX1	T49.ØX2	T49.ØX3	T49.ØX4	T49.ØX5	T49.ØX6
Natrium cyanide—*see* Cyanide(s)						
Natural						
blood (product)	T45.8X1	T45.8X2	T45.8X3	T45.8X4	T45.8X5	T45.8X6
gas (piped)	T59.891	T59.892	T59.893	T59.894	—	—
incomplete combustion	T58.11	T58.12	T58.13	T58.14	—	—
Nealbarbital	T42.3X1	T42.3X2	T42.3X3	T42.3X4	T42.3X5	T42.3X6
Nectadon	T48.3X1	T48.3X2	T48.3X3	T48.3X4	T48.3X5	T48.3X6
Nedocromil	T48.6X1	T48.6X2	T48.6X3	T48.6X4	T48.6X5	T48.6X6
Nefopam	T39.8X1	T39.8X2	T39.8X3	T39.8X4	T39.8X5	T39.8X6
Nematocyst (sting)	T63.691	T63.692	T63.693	T63.694	—	—
Nembutal	T42.3X1	T42.3X2	T42.3X3	T42.3X4	T42.3X5	T42.3X6
Nemonapride	T43.591	T43.592	T43.593	T43.594	T43.595	T43.596
Neoarsphenamine	T37.8X1	T37.8X2	T37.8X3	T37.8X4	T37.8X5	T37.8X6
Neocinchophen	T5Ø.4X1	T5Ø.4X2	T5Ø.4X3	T5Ø.4X4	T5Ø.4X5	T5Ø.4X6
Neomycin (derivatives)	T36.5X1	T36.5X2	T36.5X3	T36.5X4	T36.5X5	T36.5X6
with						
bacitracin	T49.ØX1	T49.ØX2	T49.ØX3	T49.ØX4	T49.ØX5	T49.ØX6
neostigmine	T44.ØX1	T44.ØX2	T44.ØX3	T44.ØX4	T44.ØX5	T44.ØX6
ENT agent	T49.6X1	T49.6X2	T49.6X3	T49.6X4	T49.6X5	T49.6X6
ophthalmic preparation	T49.5X1	T49.5X2	T49.5X3	T49.5X4	T49.5X5	T49.5X6
topical NEC	T49.ØX1	T49.ØX2	T49.ØX3	T49.ØX4	T49.ØX5	T49.ØX6
Neonal	T42.3X1	T42.3X2	T42.3X3	T42.3X4	T42.3X5	T42.3X6
Neoprontosil	T37.ØX1	T37.ØX2	T37.ØX3	T37.ØX4	T37.ØX5	T37.ØX6
Neosalvarsan	T37.8X1	T37.8X2	T37.8X3	T37.8X4	T37.8X5	T37.8X6
Neosilversalvarsan	T37.8X1	T37.8X2	T37.8X3	T37.8X4	T37.8X5	T37.8X6
Neosporin	T36.8X1	T36.8X2	T36.8X3	T36.8X4	T36.8X5	T36.8X6
ENT agent	T49.6X1	T49.6X2	T49.6X3	T49.6X4	T49.6X5	T49.6X6
ophthalmic preparation	T49.5X1	T49.5X2	T49.5X3	T49.5X4	T49.5X5	T49.5X6
topical NEC	T49.ØX1	T49.ØX2	T49.ØX3	T49.ØX4	T49.ØX5	T49.ØX6
Neostigmine bromide	T44.ØX1	T44.ØX2	T44.ØX3	T44.ØX4	T44.ØX5	T44.ØX6
Neraval	T42.3X1	T42.3X2	T42.3X3	T42.3X4	T42.3X5	T42.3X6
Neravan	T42.3X1	T42.3X2	T42.3X3	T42.3X4	T42.3X5	T42.3X6
Nerium oleander	T62.2X1	T62.2X2	T62.2X3	T62.2X4	—	—
Nerve gas, not in war	T59.91	T59.92	T59.93	T59.94	—	—
Nesacaine	T41.3X1	T41.3X2	T41.3X3	T41.3X4	T41.3X5	T41.3X6
infiltration (subcutaneous)	T41.3X1	T41.3X2	T41.3X3	T41.3X4	T41.3X5	T41.3X6
nerve block (peripheral) (plexus)	T41.3X1	T41.3X2	T41.3X3	T41.3X4	T41.3X5	T41.3X6
Netilmicin	T36.5X1	T36.5X2	T36.5X3	T36.5X4	T36.5X5	T36.5X6
Neurobarb	T42.3X1	T42.3X2	T42.3X3	T42.3X4	T42.3X5	T42.3X6
Neuroleptic drug NEC	T43.5Ø1	T43.5Ø2	T43.5Ø3	T43.5Ø4	T43.5Ø5	T43.5Ø6
Neuromuscular blocking drug	T48.1X1	T48.1X2	T48.1X3	T48.1X4	T48.1X5	T48.1X6
Neutral insulin injection	T38.3X1	T38.3X2	T38.3X3	T38.3X4	T38.3X5	T38.3X6
Neutral spirits	T51.ØX1	T51.ØX2	T51.ØX3	T51.ØX4	—	—
beverage	T51.ØX1	T51.ØX2	T51.ØX3	T51.ØX4	—	—
Niacin	T46.7X1	T46.7X2	T46.7X3	T46.7X4	T46.7X5	T46.7X6
Niacinamide	T45.2X1	T45.2X2	T45.2X3	T45.2X4	T45.2X5	T45.2X6
Nialamide	T43.1X1	T43.1X2	T43.1X3	T43.1X4	T43.1X5	T43.1X6
Niaprazine	T42.6X1	T42.6X2	T42.6X3	T42.6X4	T42.6X5	T42.6X6
Nicametate	T46.7X1	T46.7X2	T46.7X3	T46.7X4	T46.7X5	T46.7X6
Nicardipine	T46.1X1	T46.1X2	T46.1X3	T46.1X4	T46.1X5	T46.1X6
Nicergoline	T46.7X1	T46.7X2	T46.7X3	T46.7X4	T46.7X5	T46.7X6
Nickel (carbonyl) (tetra-carbonyl)(fumes) (vapor)	T56.891	T56.892	T56.893	T56.894	—	—
Nickelocene	T56.891	T56.892	T56.893	T56.894	—	—
Niclosamide	T37.4X1	T37.4X2	T37.4X3	T37.4X4	T37.4X5	T37.4X6
Nicofuranose	T46.7X1	T46.7X2	T46.7X3	T46.7X4	T46.7X5	T46.7X6
Nicomorphine	T4Ø.2X1	T4Ø.2X2	T4Ø.2X3	T4Ø.2X4	—	—
Nicorandil	T46.3X1	T46.3X2	T46.3X3	T46.3X4	T46.3X5	T46.3X6
Nicotiana (plant)	T62.2X1	T62.2X2	T62.2X3	T62.2X4	—	—
Nicotinamide	T45.2X1	T45.2X2	T45.2X3	T45.2X4	T45.2X5	T45.2X6
Nicotine (insecticide) (spray) (sulfate) **NEC**	T6Ø.2X1	T6Ø.2X2	T6Ø.2X3	T6Ø.2X4	—	—
from tobacco	T65.291	T65.292	T65.293	T65.294	—	—
cigarettes	T65.221	T65.222	T65.223	T65.224	—	—
not insecticide	T65.291	T65.292	T65.293	T65.294	—	—
Nicotinic acid	T46.7X1	T46.7X2	T46.7X3	T46.7X4	T46.7X5	T46.7X6
Nicotinyl alcohol	T46.7X1	T46.7X2	T46.7X3	T46.7X4	T46.7X5	T46.7X6
Nicoumalone	T45.511	T45.512	T45.513	T45.514	T45.515	T45.516
Nifedipine	T46.1X1	T46.1X2	T46.1X3	T46.1X4	T46.1X5	T46.1X6
Nifenazone	T39.2X1	T39.2X2	T39.2X3	T39.2X4	T39.2X5	T39.2X6
Nifuraldezone	T37.91	T37.92	T37.93	T37.94	T37.95	T37.96
Nifuratel	T37.8X1	T37.8X2	T37.8X3	T37.8X4	T37.8X5	T37.8X6
Nifurtimox	T37.3X1	T37.3X2	T37.3X3	T37.3X4	T37.3X5	T37.3X6
Nifurtoinol	T37.8X1	T37.8X2	T37.8X3	T37.8X4	T37.8X5	T37.8X6
Nightshade, deadly (solanum) (*see also* Belladonna)	T62.2X1	T62.2X2	T62.2X3	T62.2X4	—	—
berry	T62.1X1	T62.1X2	T62.1X3	T62.1X4	—	—
Nikethamide	T5Ø.7X1	T5Ø.7X2	T5Ø.7X3	T5Ø.7X4	T5Ø.7X5	T5Ø.7X6
Nilstat	T36.7X1	T36.7X2	T36.7X3	T36.7X4	T36.7X5	T36.7X6
topical	T49.ØX1	T49.ØX2	T49.ØX3	T49.ØX4	T49.ØX5	T49.ØX6
Nilutamide	T38.6X1	T38.6X2	T38.6X3	T38.6X4	T38.6X5	T38.6X6

Substance	Poisoning, Accidental (unintentional)	Poisoning, Intentional Self-harm	Poisoning, Assault	Poisoning, Undetermined	Adverse Effect	Under-dosing
Nimesulide	T39.391	T39.392	T39.393	T39.394	T39.395	T39.396
Nimetazepam	T42.4X1	T42.4X2	T42.4X3	T42.4X4	T42.4X5	T42.4X6
Nimodipine	T46.1X1	T46.1X2	T46.1X3	T46.1X4	T46.1X5	T46.1X6
Nimorazole	T37.3X1	T37.3X2	T37.3X3	T37.3X4	T37.3X5	T37.3X6
Nimustine	T45.1X1	T45.1X2	T45.1X3	T45.1X4	T45.1X5	T45.1X6
Niridazole	T37.4X1	T37.4X2	T37.4X3	T37.4X4	T37.4X5	T37.4X6
Nisentil	T4Ø.2X1	T4Ø.2X2	T4Ø.2X3	T4Ø.2X4	T4Ø.2X5	T4Ø.2X6
Nisoldipine	T46.1X1	T46.1X2	T46.1X3	T46.1X4	T46.1X5	T46.1X6
Nitramine	T65.3X1	T65.3X2	T65.3X3	T65.3X4	—	—
Nitrate, organic	T46.3X1	T46.3X2	T46.3X3	T46.3X4	T46.3X5	T46.3X6
Nitrazepam	T42.4X1	T42.4X2	T42.4X3	T42.4X4	T42.4X5	T42.4X6
Nitrefazole	T5Ø.6X1	T5Ø.6X2	T5Ø.6X3	T5Ø.6X4	T5Ø.6X5	T5Ø.6X6
Nitrendipine	T46.1X1	T46.1X2	T46.1X3	T46.1X4	T46.1X5	T46.1X6
Nitric						
acid (liquid)	T54.2X1	T54.2X2	T54.2X3	T54.2X4	—	—
vapor	T59.891	T59.892	T59.893	T59.894	—	—
oxide (gas)	T59.ØX1	T59.ØX2	T59.ØX3	T59.ØX4	—	—
Nitrimidazine	T37.3X1	T37.3X2	T37.3X3	T37.3X4	T37.3X5	T37.3X6
Nitrite, amyl (medicinal) (vapor)	T46.3X1	T46.3X2	T46.3X3	T46.3X4	T46.3X5	T46.3X6
Nitroaniline	T65.3X1	T65.3X2	T65.3X3	T65.3X4	—	—
vapor	T59.891	T59.892	T59.893	T59.894	—	—
Nitrobenzene, nitrobenzol	T65.3X1	T65.3X2	T65.3X3	T65.3X4	—	—
vapor	T65.3X1	T65.3X2	T65.3X3	T65.3X4	—	—
Nitrocellulose	T65.891	T65.892	T65.893	T65.894	—	—
lacquer	T65.891	T65.892	T65.893	T65.894	—	—
Nitrodiphenyl	T65.3X1	T65.3X2	T65.3X3	T65.3X4	—	—
Nitrofural	T49.ØX1	T49.ØX2	T49.ØX3	T49.ØX4	T49.ØX5	T49.ØX6
Nitrofurantoin	T37.8X1	T37.8X2	T37.8X3	T37.8X4	T37.8X5	T37.8X6
Nitrofurazone	T49.ØX1	T49.ØX2	T49.ØX3	T49.ØX4	T49.ØX5	T49.ØX6
Nitrogen	T59.ØX1	T59.ØX2	T59.ØX3	T59.ØX4	—	—
mustard	T45.1X1	T45.1X2	T45.1X3	T45.1X4	T45.1X5	T45.1X6
Nitroglycerin, nitro-glycerol (medicinal)	T46.3X1	T46.3X2	T46.3X3	T46.3X4	T46.3X5	T46.3X6
nonmedicinal	T65.5X1	T65.5X2	T65.5X3	T65.5X4	—	—
fumes	T65.5X1	T65.5X2	T65.5X3	T65.5X4	—	—
Nitroglycol	T52.3X1	T52.3X2	T52.3X3	T52.3X4	—	—
Nitrohydrochloric acid	T54.2X1	T54.2X2	T54.2X3	T54.2X4	—	—
Nitromersol	T49.ØX1	T49.ØX2	T49.ØX3	T49.ØX4	T49.ØX5	T49.ØX6
Nitronaphthalene	T65.891	T65.892	T65.893	T65.894	—	—
Nitrophenol	T54.ØX1	T54.ØX2	T54.ØX3	T54.ØX4	—	—
Nitropropane	T52.8X1	T52.8X2	T52.8X3	T52.8X4	—	—
Nitroprusside	T46.5X1	T46.5X2	T46.5X3	T46.5X4	T46.5X5	T46.5X6
Nitrosodimethylamine	T65.3X1	T65.3X2	T65.3X3	T65.3X4	—	—
Nitrothiazol	T37.4X1	T37.4X2	T37.4X3	T37.4X4	T37.4X5	T37.4X6
Nitrotoluene, nitrotoluol	T65.3X1	T65.3X2	T65.3X3	T65.3X4	—	—
vapor	T65.3X1	T65.3X2	T65.3X3	T65.3X4	—	—
Nitrous						
acid (liquid)	T54.2X1	T54.2X2	T54.2X3	T54.2X4	—	—
fumes	T59.891	T59.892	T59.893	T59.894	—	—
ether spirit	T46.3X1	T46.3X2	T46.3X3	T46.3X4	T46.3X5	T46.3X6
oxide	T41.ØX1	T41.ØX2	T41.ØX3	T41.ØX4	T41.ØX5	T41.ØX6
Nitroxoline	T37.8X1	T37.8X2	T37.8X3	T37.8X4	T37.8X5	T37.8X6
Nitrozone	T49.ØX1	T49.ØX2	T49.ØX3	T49.ØX4	T49.ØX5	T49.ØX6
Nizatidine	T47.ØX1	T47.ØX2	T47.ØX3	T47.ØX4	T47.ØX5	T47.ØX6
Nizofenone	T43.8X1	T43.8X2	T43.8X3	T43.8X4	T43.8X5	T43.8X6
Noctec	T42.6X1	T42.6X2	T42.6X3	T42.6X4	T42.6X5	T42.6X6
Noludar	T42.6X1	T42.6X2	T42.6X3	T42.6X4	T42.6X5	T42.6X6
Noptil	T42.3X1	T42.3X2	T42.3X3	T42.3X4	T42.3X5	T42.3X6
Nomegestrol	T38.5X1	T38.5X2	T38.5X3	T38.5X4	T38.5X5	T38.5X6
Nomifensine	T43.291	T43.292	T43.293	T43.294	T43.295	T43.296
Nonoxinol	T49.8X1	T49.8X2	T49.8X3	T49.8X4	T49.8X5	T49.8X6
Nonylphenoxy (polyethoxy-ethanol)	T49.8X1	T49.8X2	T49.8X3	T49.8X4	T49.8X5	T49.8X6
Noptil	T42.3X1	T42.3X2	T42.3X3	T42.3X4	T42.3X5	T42.3X6
Noradrenaline	T44.4X1	T44.4X2	T44.4X3	T44.4X4	T44.4X5	T44.4X6
Noramidopyrine	T39.2X1	T39.2X2	T39.2X3	T39.2X4	T39.2X5	T39.2X6
methanesulfonate sodium	T39.2X1	T39.2X2	T39.2X3	T39.2X4	T39.2X5	T39.2X6
Norbormide	T6Ø.4X1	T6Ø.4X2	T6Ø.4X3	T6Ø.4X4	—	—
Nordazepam	T42.4X1	T42.4X2	T42.4X3	T42.4X4	T42.4X5	T42.4X6
Norepinephrine	T44.4X1	T44.4X2	T44.4X3	T44.4X4	T44.4X5	T44.4X6
Norethandrolone	T38.7X1	T38.7X2	T38.7X3	T38.7X4	T38.7X5	T38.7X6
Norethindrone	T38.4X1	T38.4X2	T38.4X3	T38.4X4	T38.4X5	T38.4X6
Norethisterone (acetate) (enantate)	T38.4X1	T38.4X2	T38.4X3	T38.4X4	T38.4X5	T38.4X6
with ethinylestradiol	T38.5X1	T38.5X2	T38.5X3	T38.5X4	T38.5X5	T38.5X6
Noretynodrel	T38.5X1	T38.5X2	T38.5X3	T38.5X4	T38.5X5	T38.5X6
Norfenefrine	T44.4X1	T44.4X2	T44.4X3	T44.4X4	T44.4X5	T44.4X6
Norfloxacin	T36.8X1	T36.8X2	T36.8X3	T36.8X4	T36.8X5	T36.8X6
Norgestrel	T38.4X1	T38.4X2	T38.4X3	T38.4X4	T38.4X5	T38.4X6
Norgestrienone	T38.4X1	T38.4X2	T38.4X3	T38.4X4	T38.4X5	T38.4X6
Norlestrin	T38.4X1	T38.4X2	T38.4X3	T38.4X4	T38.4X5	T38.4X6
Norlutin	T38.4X1	T38.4X2	T38.4X3	T38.4X4	T38.4X5	T38.4X6
Normal serum albumin (human), salt-poor	T45.8X1	T45.8X2	T45.8X3	T45.8X4	T45.8X5	T45.8X6
Normethandrone	T38.5X1	T38.5X2	T38.5X3	T38.5X4	T38.5X5	T38.5X6
Normison—*see* Benzodiazepines						
Normorphine	T4Ø.2X1	T4Ø.2X2	T4Ø.2X3	T4Ø.2X4	—	—
Norpseudoephedrine	T5Ø.5X1	T5Ø.5X2	T5Ø.5X3	T5Ø.5X4	T5Ø.5X5	T5Ø.5X6
Nortestosterone (furanpropionate)	T38.7X1	T38.7X2	T38.7X3	T38.7X4	T38.7X5	T38.7X6
Nortriptyline	T43.Ø11	T43.Ø12	T43.Ø13	T43.Ø14	T43.Ø15	T43.Ø16
Noscapine	T48.3X1	T48.3X2	T48.3X3	T48.3X4	T48.3X5	T48.3X6
Nose preparations	T49.6X1	T49.6X2	T49.6X3	T49.6X4	T49.6X5	T49.6X6
Novobiocin	T36.5X1	T36.5X2	T36.5X3	T36.5X4	T36.5X5	T36.5X6
Novocain (infiltration) (topical)	T41.3X1	T41.3X2	T41.3X3	T41.3X4	T41.3X5	T41.3X6
nerve block (peripheral) (plexus)	T41.3X1	T41.3X2	T41.3X3	T41.3X4	T41.3X5	T41.3X6
spinal	T41.3X1	T41.3X2	T41.3X3	T41.3X4	T41.3X5	T41.3X6
Noxious foodstuff	T62.91	T62.92	T62.93	T62.94	—	—
specified NEC	T62.8X1	T62.8X2	T62.8X3	T62.8X4	—	—
Noxiptiline	T43.Ø11	T43.Ø12	T43.Ø13	T43.Ø14	T43.Ø15	T43.Ø16
Noxytiolin	T49.ØX1	T49.ØX2	T49.ØX3	T49.ØX4	T49.ØX5	T49.ØX6
NPH Iletin (insulin)	T38.3X1	T38.3X2	T38.3X3	T38.3X4	T38.3X5	T38.3X6
Numorphan	T4Ø.2X1	T4Ø.2X2	T4Ø.2X3	T4Ø.2X4	T4Ø.2X5	T4Ø.2X6
Nunol	T42.3X1	T42.3X2	T42.3X3	T42.3X4	T42.3X5	T42.3X6
Nupercaine (spinal anesthetic)	T41.3X1	T41.3X2	T41.3X3	T41.3X4	T41.3X5	T41.3X6
topical (surface)	T41.3X1	T41.3X2	T41.3X3	T41.3X4	T41.3X5	T41.3X6
Nutmeg oil (liniment)	T49.3X1	T49.3X2	T49.3X3	T49.3X4	T49.3X5	T49.3X6
Nutritional supplement	T5Ø.9Ø1	T5Ø.9Ø2	T5Ø.9Ø3	T5Ø.9Ø4	T5Ø.9Ø5	T5Ø.9Ø6
Nux vomica	T65.1X1	T65.1X2	T65.1X3	T65.1X4	—	—
Nydrazid	T37.1X1	T37.1X2	T37.1X3	T37.1X4	T37.1X5	T37.1X6
Nylidrin	T46.7X1	T46.7X2	T46.7X3	T46.7X4	T46.7X5	T46.7X6
Nystatin	T36.7X1	T36.7X2	T36.7X3	T36.7X4	T36.7X5	T36.7X6
topical	T49.ØX1	T49.ØX2	T49.ØX3	T49.ØX4	T49.ØX5	T49.ØX6
Nytol	T45.ØX1	T45.ØX2	T45.ØX3	T45.ØX4	T45.ØX5	T45.ØX6
O						
Obidoxime chloride	T5Ø.6X1	T5Ø.6X2	T5Ø.6X3	T5Ø.6X4	T5Ø.6X5	T5Ø.6X6
Octafonium (chloride)	T49.3X1	T49.3X2	T49.3X3	T49.3X4	T49.3X5	T49.3X6
Octamethyl pyrophos-phoramide	T6Ø.ØX1	T6Ø.ØX2	T6Ø.ØX3	T6Ø.ØX4	—	—
Octanoin	T5Ø.991	T5Ø.992	T5Ø.993	T5Ø.994	T5Ø.995	T5Ø.996
Octatropine methylbromide	T44.3X1	T44.3X2	T44.3X3	T44.3X4	T44.3X5	T44.3X6
Octotiamine	T45.2X1	T45.2X2	T45.2X3	T45.2X4	T45.2X5	T45.2X6
Octoxinol (9)	T49.8X1	T49.8X2	T49.8X3	T49.8X4	T49.8X5	T49.8X6
Octreotide	T38.991	T38.992	T38.993	T38.994	T38.995	T38.996
Octyl nitrite	T46.3X1	T46.3X2	T46.3X3	T46.3X4	T46.3X5	T46.3X6
Oestradiol	T38.5X1	T38.5X2	T38.5X3	T38.5X4	T38.5X5	T38.5X6
Oestriol	T38.5X1	T38.5X2	T38.5X3	T38.5X4	T38.5X5	T38.5X6
Oestrogen	T38.5X1	T38.5X2	T38.5X3	T38.5X4	T38.5X5	T38.5X6
Oestrone	T38.5X1	T38.5X2	T38.5X3	T38.5X4	T38.5X5	T38.5X6
Ofloxacin	T36.8X1	T36.8X2	T36.8X3	T36.8X4	T36.8X5	T36.8X6
Oil (of)	T65.891	T65.892	T65.893	T65.894	—	—
bitter almond	T62.8X1	T62.8X2	T62.8X3	T62.8X4	—	—
cloves	T49.7X1	T49.7X2	T49.7X3	T49.7X4	T49.7X5	T49.7X6
colors	T65.6X1	T65.6X2	T65.6X3	T65.6X4	—	—
fumes	T59.891	T59.892	T59.893	T59.894	—	—
lubricating	T52.ØX1	T52.ØX2	T52.ØX3	T52.ØX4	—	—
Niobe	T52.8X1	T52.8X2	T52.8X3	T52.8X4	—	—
vitriol (liquid)	T54.2X1	T54.2X2	T54.2X3	T54.2X4	—	—
fumes	T54.2X1	T54.2X2	T54.2X3	T54.2X4	—	—
wintergreen (bitter) NEC	T49.3X1	T49.3X2	T49.3X3	T49.3X4	T49.3X5	T49.3X6
Oily preparation (for skin)	T49.3X1	T49.3X2	T49.3X3	T49.3X4	T49.3X5	T49.3X6
Ointment NEC	T49.3X1	T49.3X2	T49.3X3	T49.3X4	T49.3X5	T49.3X6

Substance	Poisoning, Accidental (unintentional)	Poisoning, Intentional Self-harm	Poisoning, Assault	Poisoning, Undetermined	Adverse Effect	Under-dosing
Olanzapine	T43.591	T43.592	T43.593	T43.594	T43.595	T43.596
Oleander	T62.2X1	T62.2X2	T62.2X3	T62.2X4	—	—
Oleandomycin	T36.3X1	T36.3X2	T36.3X3	T36.3X4	T36.3X5	T36.3X6
Oleandrin	T46.ØX1	T46.ØX2	T46.ØX3	T46.ØX4	T46.ØX5	T46.ØX6
Oleic acid	T46.6X1	T46.6X2	T46.6X3	T46.6X4	T46.6X5	T46.6X6
Oleovitamin A	T45.2X1	T45.2X2	T45.2X3	T45.2X4	T45.2X5	T45.2X6
Oleum ricini	T47.2X1	T47.2X2	T47.2X3	T47.2X4	T47.2X5	T47.2X6
Olive oil (medicinal) **NEC**	T47.4X1	T47.4X2	T47.4X3	T47.4X4	T47.4X5	T47.4X6
Olivomycin	T45.1X1	T45.1X2	T45.1X3	T45.1X4	T45.1X5	T45.1X6
Olsalazine	T47.8X1	T47.8X2	T47.8X3	T47.8X4	T47.8X5	T47.8X6
Omeprazole	T47.1X1	T47.1X2	T47.1X3	T47.1X4	T47.1X5	T47.1X6
OMPA	T6Ø.ØX1	T6Ø.ØX2	T6Ø.ØX3	T6Ø.ØX4	—	—
Ondansetron	T45.ØX1	T45.ØX2	T45.ØX3	T45.ØX4	T45.ØX5	T45.ØX6
Oncovin	T45.1X1	T45.1X2	T45.1X3	T45.1X4	T45.1X5	T45.1X6
Ophthaine	T41.3X1	T41.3X2	T41.3X3	T41.3X4	T41.3X5	T41.3X6
Ophthetic	T41.3X1	T41.3X2	T41.3X3	T41.3X4	T41.3X5	T41.3X6
Opiate NEC	T4Ø.6Ø1	T4Ø.6Ø2	T4Ø.6Ø3	T4Ø.6Ø4	T4Ø.6Ø5	T4Ø.6Ø6
antagonists	T5Ø.7X1	T5Ø.7X2	T5Ø.7X3	T5Ø.7X4	T5Ø.7X5	T5Ø.7X6
Opioid NEC	T4Ø.2X1	T4Ø.2X2	T4Ø.2X3	T4Ø.2X4	T4Ø.2X5	T4Ø.2X6
Opipramol	T43.Ø11	T43.Ø12	T43.Ø13	T43.Ø14	T43.Ø15	T43.Ø16
Opium alkaloids (total)	T4Ø.ØX1	T4Ø.ØX2	T4Ø.ØX3	T4Ø.ØX4	T4Ø.ØX5	T4Ø.ØX6
standardized powdered	T4Ø.ØX1	T4Ø.ØX2	T4Ø.ØX3	T4Ø.ØX4	T4Ø.ØX5	T4Ø.ØX6
tincture (camphorated)	T4Ø.ØX1	T4Ø.ØX2	T4Ø.ØX3	T4Ø.ØX4	T4Ø.ØX5	T4Ø.ØX6
Oracon	T38.4X1	T38.4X2	T38.4X3	T38.4X4	T38.4X5	T38.4X6
Oragrafin	T5Ø.8X1	T5Ø.8X2	T5Ø.8X3	T5Ø.8X4	T5Ø.8X5	T5Ø.8X6
Oral contraceptives	T38.4X1	T38.4X2	T38.4X3	T38.4X4	T38.4X5	T38.4X6
Oral rehydration salts	T5Ø.3X1	T5Ø.3X2	T5Ø.3X3	T5Ø.3X4	T5Ø.3X5	T5Ø.3X6
Orazamide	T5Ø.991	T5Ø.992	T5Ø.993	T5Ø.994	T5Ø.995	T5Ø.996
Orciprenaline	T48.291	T48.292	T48.293	T48.294	T48.295	T48.296
Organidin	T48.4X1	T48.4X2	T48.4X3	T48.4X4	T48.4X5	T48.4X6
Organonitrate NEC	T46.3X1	T46.3X2	T46.3X3	T46.3X4	T46.3X5	T46.3X6
Organophosphates	T6Ø.ØX1	T6Ø.ØX2	T6Ø.ØX3	T6Ø.ØX4	—	—
Orimune	T5Ø.B91	T5Ø.B92	T5Ø.B93	T5Ø.B94	T5Ø.B95	T5Ø.B96
Orinase	T38.3X1	T38.3X2	T38.3X3	T38.3X4	T38.3X5	T38.3X6
Ormeloxifene	T38.6X1	T38.6X2	T38.6X3	T38.6X4	T38.6X5	T38.6X6
Ornidazole	T37.3X1	T37.3X2	T37.3X3	T37.3X4	T37.3X5	T37.3X6
Ornithine aspartate	T5Ø.991	T5Ø.992	T5Ø.993	T5Ø.994	T5Ø.995	T5Ø.996
Ornoprostil	T47.1X1	T47.1X2	T47.1X3	T47.1X4	T47.1X5	T47.1X6
Orphenadrine (hydrochloride)	T42.8X1	T42.8X2	T42.8X3	T42.8X4	T42.8X5	T42.8X6
Ortal (sodium)	T42.3X1	T42.3X2	T42.3X3	T42.3X4	T42.3X5	T42.3X6
Orthoboric acid	T49.ØX1	T49.ØX2	T49.ØX3	T49.ØX4	T49.ØX5	T49.ØX6
ENT agent	T49.6X1	T49.6X2	T49.6X3	T49.6X4	T49.6X5	T49.6X6
ophthalmic preparation	T49.5X1	T49.5X2	T49.5X3	T49.5X4	T49.5X5	T49.5X6
Orthocaine	T41.3X1	T41.3X2	T41.3X3	T41.3X4	T41.3X5	T41.3X6
Orthodichlorobenzene	T53.7X1	T53.7X2	T53.7X3	T53.7X4	—	—
Ortho-Novum	T38.4X1	T38.4X2	T38.4X3	T38.4X4	T38.4X5	T38.4X6
Orthotolidine (reagent)	T54.2X1	T54.2X2	T54.2X3	T54.2X4	—	—
Osmic acid (liquid)	T54.2X1	T54.2X2	T54.2X3	T54.2X4	—	—
fumes	T54.2X1	T54.2X2	T54.2X3	T54.2X4	—	—
Osmotic diuretics	T5Ø.2X1	T5Ø.2X2	T5Ø.2X3	T5Ø.2X4	T5Ø.2X5	T5Ø.2X6
Otilonium bromide	T44.3X1	T44.3X2	T44.3X3	T44.3X4	T44.3X5	T44.3X6
Otorhinolaryngological drug NEC	T49.6X1	T49.6X2	T49.6X3	T49.6X4	T49.6X5	T49.6X6
Ouabain(e)	T46.ØX1	T46.ØX2	T46.ØX3	T46.ØX4	T46.ØX5	T46.ØX6
Ovarian						
hormone	T38.5X1	T38.5X2	T38.5X3	T38.5X4	T38.5X5	T38.5X6
stimulant	T38.5X1	T38.5X2	T38.5X3	T38.5X4	T38.5X5	T38.5X6
Ovral	T38.4X1	T38.4X2	T38.4X3	T38.4X4	T38.4X5	T38.4X6
Ovulen	T38.4X1	T38.4X2	T38.4X3	T38.4X4	T38.4X5	T38.4X6
Oxacillin	T36.ØX1	T36.ØX2	T36.ØX3	T36.ØX4	T36.ØX5	T36.ØX6
Oxalic acid	T54.2X1	T54.2X2	T54.2X3	T54.2X4	—	—
ammonium salt	T5Ø.991	T5Ø.992	T5Ø.993	T5Ø.994	T5Ø.995	T5Ø.996
Oxamniquine	T37.4X1	T37.4X2	T37.4X3	T37.4X4	T37.4X5	T37.4X6
Oxanamide	T43.591	T43.592	T43.593	T43.594	T43.595	T43.596
Oxandrolone	T38.7X1	T38.7X2	T38.7X3	T38.7X4	T38.7X5	T38.7X6
Oxantel	T37.4X1	T37.4X2	T37.4X3	T37.4X4	T37.4X5	T37.4X6
Oxapium iodide	T44.3X1	T44.3X2	T44.3X3	T44.3X4	T44.3X5	T44.3X6
Oxaprotiline	T43.Ø21	T43.Ø22	T43.Ø23	T43.Ø24	T43.Ø25	T43.Ø26
Oxaprozin	T39.311	T39.312	T39.313	T39.314	T39.315	T39.316
Oxatomide	T45.ØX1	T45.ØX2	T45.ØX3	T45.ØX4	T45.ØX5	T45.ØX6
Oxazepam	T42.4X1	T42.4X2	T42.4X3	T42.4X4	T42.4X5	T42.4X6

Substance	Poisoning, Accidental (unintentional)	Poisoning, Intentional Self-harm	Poisoning, Assault	Poisoning, Undetermined	Adverse Effect	Under-dosing
Oxazimedrine	T5Ø.5X1	T5Ø.5X2	T5Ø.5X3	T5Ø.5X4	T5Ø.5X5	T5Ø.5X6
Oxazolam	T42.4X1	T42.4X2	T42.4X3	T42.4X4	T42.4X5	T42.4X6
Oxazolidine (derivative)	T42.2X1	T42.2X2	T42.2X3	T42.2X4	T42.2X5	T42.2X6
Oxazolidinedione (derivative)	T42.2X1	T42.2X2	T42.2X3	T42.2X4	T42.2X5	T42.2X6
Ox bile extract	T47.5X1	T47.5X2	T47.5X3	T47.5X4	T47.5X5	T47.5X6
Oxcarbazepine	T42.1X1	T42.1X2	T42.1X3	T42.1X4	T42.1X5	T42.1X6
Oxedrine	T44.4X1	T44.4X2	T44.4X3	T44.4X4	T44.4X5	T44.4X6
Oxeladin (citrate)	T48.3X1	T48.3X2	T48.3X3	T48.3X4	T48.3X5	T48.3X6
Oxendolone	T38.5X1	T38.5X2	T38.5X3	T38.5X4	T38.5X5	T38.5X6
Oxetacaine	T41.3X1	T41.3X2	T41.3X3	T41.3X4	T41.3X5	T41.3X6
Oxethazine	T41.3X1	T41.3X2	T41.3X3	T41.3X4	T41.3X5	T41.3X6
Oxetorone	T39.8X1	T39.8X2	T39.8X3	T39.8X4	T39.8X5	T39.8X6
Oxiconazole	T49.ØX1	T49.ØX2	T49.ØX3	T49.ØX4	T49.ØX5	T49.ØX6
Oxidizing agent NEC	T54.91	T54.92	T54.93	T54.94	—	—
Oxipurinol	T5Ø.4X1	T5Ø.4X2	T5Ø.4X3	T5Ø.4X4	T5Ø.4X5	T5Ø.4X6
Oxitriptan	T43.291	T43.292	T43.293	T43.294	T43.295	T43.296
Oxitropium bromide	T48.6X1	T48.6X2	T48.6X3	T48.6X4	T48.6X5	T48.6X6
Oxodipine	T46.1X1	T46.1X2	T46.1X3	T46.1X4	T46.1X5	T46.1X6
Oxolamine	T48.3X1	T48.3X2	T48.3X3	T48.3X4	T48.3X5	T48.3X6
Oxolinic acid	T37.8X1	T37.8X2	T37.8X3	T37.8X4	T37.8X5	T37.8X6
Oxomemazine	T43.3X1	T43.3X2	T43.3X3	T43.3X4	T43.3X5	T43.3X6
Oxophenarsine	T37.3X1	T37.3X2	T37.3X3	T37.3X4	T37.3X5	T37.3X6
Oxprenolol	T44.7X1	T44.7X2	T44.7X3	T44.7X4	T44.7X5	T44.7X6
Oxsoralen	T49.3X1	T49.3X2	T49.3X3	T49.3X4	T49.3X5	T49.3X6
Oxtriphylline	T48.6X1	T48.6X2	T48.6X3	T48.6X4	T48.6X5	T48.6X6
Oxybate sodium	T41.291	T41.292	T41.293	T41.294	T41.295	T41.296
Oxybuprocaine	T41.3X1	T41.3X2	T41.3X3	T41.3X4	T41.3X5	T41.3X6
Oxybutynin	T44.3X1	T44.3X2	T44.3X3	T44.3X4	T44.3X5	T44.3X6
Oxychlorosene	T49.ØX1	T49.ØX2	T49.ØX3	T49.ØX4	T49.ØX5	T49.ØX6
Oxycodone	T4Ø.2X1	T4Ø.2X2	T4Ø.2X3	T4Ø.2X4	T4Ø.2X5	T4Ø.2X6
Oxyfedrine	T46.3X1	T46.3X2	T46.3X3	T46.3X4	T46.3X5	T46.3X6
Oxygen	T41.5X1	T41.5X2	T41.5X3	T41.5X4	T41.5X5	T41.5X6
Oxylone	T49.ØX1	T49.ØX2	T49.ØX3	T49.ØX4	T49.ØX5	T49.ØX6
ophthalmic preparation	T49.5X1	T49.5X2	T49.5X3	T49.5X4	T49.5X5	T49.5X6
Oxymesterone	T38.7X1	T38.7X2	T38.7X3	T38.7X4	T38.7X5	T38.7X6
Oxymetazoline	T48.5X1	T48.5X2	T48.5X3	T48.5X4	T48.5X5	T48.5X6
Oxymetholone	T38.7X1	T38.7X2	T38.7X3	T38.7X4	T38.7X5	T38.7X6
Oxymorphone	T4Ø.2X1	T4Ø.2X2	T4Ø.2X3	T4Ø.2X4	T4Ø.2X5	T4Ø.2X6
Oxypertine	T43.591	T43.592	T43.593	T43.594	T43.595	T43.596
Oxyphenbutazone	T39.2X1	T39.2X2	T39.2X3	T39.2X4	T39.2X5	T39.2X6
Oxyphencyclimine	T44.3X1	T44.3X2	T44.3X3	T44.3X4	T44.3X5	T44.3X6
Oxyphenisatine	T47.2X1	T47.2X2	T47.2X3	T47.2X4	T47.2X5	T47.2X6
Oxyphenonium bromide	T44.3X1	T44.3X2	T44.3X3	T44.3X4	T44.3X5	T44.3X6
Oxypolygelatin	T45.8X1	T45.8X2	T45.8X3	T45.8X4	T45.8X5	T45.8X6
Oxyquinoline (derivatives)	T37.8X1	T37.8X2	T37.8X3	T37.8X4	T37.8X5	T37.8X6
Oxytetracycline	T36.4X1	T36.4X2	T36.4X3	T36.4X4	T36.4X5	T36.4X6
Oxytocic drug NEC	T48.ØX1	T48.ØX2	T48.ØX3	T48.ØX4	T48.ØX5	T48.ØX6
Oxytocin (synthetic)	T48.ØX1	T48.ØX2	T48.ØX3	T48.ØX4	T48.ØX5	T48.ØX6
Ozone	T59.891	T59.892	T59.893	T59.894	—	—
P						
PABA	T49.3X1	T49.3X2	T49.3X3	T49.3X4	T49.3X5	T49.3X6
Packed red cells	T45.8X1	T45.8X2	T45.8X3	T45.8X4	T45.8X5	T45.8X6
Padimate	T49.3X1	T49.3X2	T49.3X3	T49.3X4	T49.3X5	T49.3X6
Paint NEC	T65.6X1	T65.6X2	T65.6X3	T65.6X4	—	—
cleaner	T52.91	T52.92	T52.93	T52.94	—	—
fumes NEC	T59.891	T59.892	T59.893	T59.894	—	—
lead (fumes)	T56.ØX1	T56.ØX2	T56.ØX3	T56.ØX4	—	—
solvent NEC	T52.8X1	T52.8X2	T52.8X3	T52.8X4	—	—
stripper	T52.8X1	T52.8X2	T52.8X3	T52.8X4	—	—
Palfium	T4Ø.2X1	T4Ø.2X2	T4Ø.2X3	T4Ø.2X4	—	—
Palm kernel oil	T5Ø.991	T5Ø.992	T5Ø.993	T5Ø.994	T5Ø.995	T5Ø.996
Paludrine	T37.2X1	T37.2X2	T37.2X3	T37.2X4	T37.2X5	T37.2X6
PAM (pralidoxime)	T5Ø.6X1	T5Ø.6X2	T5Ø.6X3	T5Ø.6X4	T5Ø.6X5	T5Ø.6X6
Pamaquine (naphthoute)	T37.2X1	T37.2X2	T37.2X3	T37.2X4	T37.2X5	T37.2X6
Panadol	T39.1X1	T39.1X2	T39.1X3	T39.1X4	T39.1X5	T39.1X6
Pancreatic						
digestive secretion stimulant	T47.8X1	T47.8X2	T47.8X3	T47.8X4	T47.8X5	T47.8X6
dornase	T45.3X1	T45.3X2	T45.3X3	T45.3X4	T45.3X5	T45.3X6
Pancreatin	T47.5X1	T47.5X2	T47.5X3	T47.5X4	T47.5X5	T47.5X6
Pancrelipase	T47.5X1	T47.5X2	T47.5X3	T47.5X4	T47.5X5	T47.5X6

Substance	Poisoning, Accidental (unintentional)	Poisoning, Intentional Self-harm	Poisoning, Assault	Poisoning, Undetermined	Adverse Effect	Under-dosing
Pancuronium (bromide)	T48.1X1	T48.1X2	T48.1X3	T48.1X4	T48.1X5	T48.1X6
Pangamic acid	T45.2X1	T45.2X2	T45.2X3	T45.2X4	T45.2X5	T45.2X6
Panthenol	T45.2X1	T45.2X2	T45.2X3	T45.2X4	T45.2X5	T45.2X6
topical	T49.8X1	T49.8X2	T49.8X3	T49.8X4	T49.8X5	T49.8X6
Pantopon	T40.ØX1	T40.ØX2	T40.ØX3	T40.ØX4	T40.ØX5	T40.ØX6
Pantothenic acid	T45.2X1	T45.2X2	T45.2X3	T45.2X4	T45.2X5	T45.2X6
Panwarfin	T45.511	T45.512	T45.513	T45.514	T45.515	T45.516
Papain	T47.5X1	T47.5X2	T47.5X3	T47.5X4	T47.5X5	T47.5X6
digestant	T47.5X1	T47.5X2	T47.5X3	T47.5X4	T47.5X5	T47.5X6
Papaveretum	T40.ØX1	T40.ØX2	T40.ØX3	T40.ØX4	T40.ØX5	T40.ØX6
Papaverine	T44.3X1	T44.3X2	T44.3X3	T44.3X4	T44.3X5	T44.3X6
Para-acetamidophenol	T39.1X1	T39.1X2	T39.1X3	T39.1X4	T39.1X5	T39.1X6
Para-aminobenzoic acid	T49.3X1	T49.3X2	T49.3X3	T49.3X4	T49.3X5	T49.3X6
Para-aminophenol derivatives	T39.1X1	T39.1X2	T39.1X3	T39.1X4	T39.1X5	T39.1X6
Para-aminosalicylic acid	T37.1X1	T37.1X2	T37.1X3	T37.1X4	T37.1X5	T37.1X6
Paracetaldehyde	T42.6X1	T42.6X2	T42.6X3	T42.6X4	T42.6X5	T42.6X6
Paracetamol	T39.1X1	T39.1X2	T39.1X3	T39.1X4	T39.1X5	T39.1X6
Parachlorophenol (camphorated)	T49.ØX1	T49.ØX2	T49.ØX3	T49.ØX4	T49.ØX5	T49.ØX6
Paracodin	T40.2X1	T40.2X2	T40.2X3	T40.2X4	T40.2X5	T40.2X6
Paradione	T42.2X1	T42.2X2	T42.2X3	T42.2X4	T42.2X5	T42.2X6
Paraffin(s) (wax)	T52.ØX1	T52.ØX2	T52.ØX3	T52.ØX4	—	—
liquid (medicinal)	T47.4X1	T47.4X2	T47.4X3	T47.4X4	T47.4X5	T47.4X6
nonmedicinal	T52.ØX1	T52.ØX2	T52.ØX3	T52.ØX4	—	—
Paraformaldehyde	T6Ø.3X1	T6Ø.3X2	T6Ø.3X3	T6Ø.3X4	—	—
Paraldehyde	T42.6X1	T42.6X2	T42.6X3	T42.6X4	T42.6X5	T42.6X6
Paramethadione	T42.2X1	T42.2X2	T42.2X3	T42.2X4	T42.2X5	T42.2X6
Paramethasone	T38.ØX1	T38.ØX2	T38.ØX3	T38.ØX4	T38.ØX5	T38.ØX6
acetate	T49.ØX1	T49.ØX2	T49.ØX3	T49.ØX4	T49.ØX5	T49.ØX6
Paraoxon	T6Ø.ØX1	T6Ø.ØX2	T6Ø.ØX3	T6Ø.ØX4	—	—
Paraquat	T6Ø.3X1	T6Ø.3X2	T6Ø.3X3	T6Ø.3X4	—	—
Parasympatholytic NEC	T44.3X1	T44.3X2	T44.3X3	T44.3X4	T44.3X5	T44.3X6
Parasympathomimetic drug NEC	T44.1X1	T44.1X2	T44.1X3	T44.1X4	T44.1X5	T44.1X6
Parathion	T6Ø.ØX1	T6Ø.ØX2	T6Ø.ØX3	T6Ø.ØX4	—	—
Parathormone	T5Ø.991	T5Ø.992	T5Ø.993	T5Ø.994	T5Ø.995	T5Ø.996
Parathyroid extract	T5Ø.991	T5Ø.992	T5Ø.993	T5Ø.994	T5Ø.995	T5Ø.996
Paratyphoid vaccine	T5Ø.A91	T5Ø.A92	T5Ø.A93	T5Ø.A94	T5Ø.A95	T5Ø.A96
Paredrine	T44.4X1	T44.4X2	T44.4X3	T44.4X4	T44.4X5	T44.4X6
Paregoric	T40.ØX1	T40.ØX2	T40.ØX3	T40.ØX4	T40.ØX5	T40.ØX6
Pargyline	T46.5X1	T46.5X2	T46.5X3	T46.5X4	T46.5X5	T46.5X6
Paris green	T57.ØX1	T57.ØX2	T57.ØX3	T57.ØX4	—	—
insecticide	T57.ØX1	T57.ØX2	T57.ØX3	T57.ØX4	—	—
Parnate	T43.1X1	T43.1X2	T43.1X3	T43.1X4	T43.1X5	T43.1X6
Paromomycin	T36.5X1	T36.5X2	T36.5X3	T36.5X4	T36.5X5	T36.5X6
Paroxypropione	T45.1X1	T45.1X2	T45.1X3	T45.1X4	T45.1X5	T45.1X6
Parzone	T40.2X1	T40.2X2	T40.2X3	T40.2X4	T40.2X5	T40.2X6
PAS	T37.1X1	T37.1X2	T37.1X3	T37.1X4	T37.1X5	T37.1X6
Pasiniazid	T37.1X1	T37.1X2	T37.1X3	T37.1X4	T37.1X5	T37.1X6
PBB (polybrominated biphenyls)	T65.891	T65.892	T65.893	T65.894	—	—
PCB	T65.891	T65.892	T65.893	T65.894	—	—
PCP						
meaning pentachlorophenol	T6Ø.1X1	T6Ø.1X2	T6Ø.1X3	T6Ø.1X4	—	—
fungicide	T6Ø.3X1	T6Ø.3X2	T6Ø.3X3	T6Ø.3X4	—	—
herbicide	T6Ø.3X1	T6Ø.3X2	T6Ø.3X3	T6Ø.3X4	—	—
insecticide	T6Ø.1X1	T6Ø.1X2	T6Ø.1X3	T6Ø.1X4	—	—
meaning phencyclidine	T40.991	T40.992	T40.993	T40.994	—	—
Peach kernel oil (emulsion)	T47.4X1	T47.4X2	T47.4X3	T47.4X4	T47.4X5	T47.4X6
Peanut oil (emulsion) **NEC**	T47.4X1	T47.4X2	T47.4X3	T47.4X4	T47.4X5	T47.4X6
topical	T49.3X1	T49.3X2	T49.3X3	T49.3X4	T49.3X5	T49.3X6
Pearly Gates (morning glory seeds)	T40.991	T40.992	T40.993	T40.994	—	—
Pecazine	T43.3X1	T43.3X2	T43.3X3	T43.3X4	T43.3X5	T43.3X6
Pectin	T47.6X1	T47.6X2	T47.6X3	T47.6X4	T47.6X5	T47.6X6
Pefloxacin	T37.8X1	T37.8X2	T37.8X3	T37.8X4	T37.8X5	T37.8X6
Pegademase, bovine	T5Ø.Z91	T5Ø.Z92	T5Ø.Z93	T5Ø.Z94	T5Ø.Z95	T5Ø.Z96
Pelletierine tannate	T37.4X1	T37.4X2	T37.4X3	T37.4X4	T37.4X5	T37.4X6
Pemirolast (potassium)	T48.6X1	T48.6X2	T48.6X3	T48.6X4	T48.6X5	T48.6X6
Pemoline	T5Ø.7X1	T5Ø.7X2	T5Ø.7X3	T5Ø.7X4	T5Ø.7X5	T5Ø.7X6
Pempidine	T44.2X1	T44.2X2	T44.2X3	T44.2X4	T44.2X5	T44.2X6
Penamecillin	T36.ØX1	T36.ØX2	T36.ØX3	T36.ØX4	T36.ØX5	T36.ØX6
Penbutolol	T44.7X1	T44.7X2	T44.7X3	T44.7X4	T44.7X5	T44.7X6

Substance	Poisoning, Accidental (unintentional)	Poisoning, Intentional Self-harm	Poisoning, Assault	Poisoning, Undetermined	Adverse Effect	Under-dosing
Penethamate	T36.ØX1	T36.ØX2	T36.ØX3	T36.ØX4	T36.ØX5	T36.ØX6
Penfluridol	T43.591	T43.592	T43.593	T43.594	T43.595	T43.596
Penflutizide	T5Ø.2X1	T5Ø.2X2	T5Ø.2X3	T5Ø.2X4	T5Ø.2X5	T5Ø.2X6
Pengitoxin	T46.ØX1	T46.ØX2	T46.ØX3	T46.ØX4	T46.ØX5	T46.ØX6
Penicillamine	T5Ø.6X1	T5Ø.6X2	T5Ø.6X3	T5Ø.6X4	T5Ø.6X5	T5Ø.6X6
Penicillin (any)	T36.ØX1	T36.ØX2	T36.ØX3	T36.ØX4	T36.ØX5	T36.ØX6
Penicillinase	T45.3X1	T45.3X2	T45.3X3	T45.3X4	T45.3X5	T45.3X6
Penicilloyl polylysine	T5Ø.8X1	T5Ø.8X2	T5Ø.8X3	T5Ø.8X4	T5Ø.8X5	T5Ø.8X6
Penimepicycline	T36.4X1	T36.4X2	T36.4X3	T36.4X4	T36.4X5	T36.4X6
Pentachloroethane	T53.6X1	T53.6X2	T53.6X3	T53.6X4	—	—
Pentachloronaphthalene	T53.7X1	T53.7X2	T53.7X3	T53.7X4	—	—
Pentachlorophenol (pesticide)	T6Ø.1X1	T6Ø.1X2	T6Ø.1X3	T6Ø.1X4	—	—
herbicide	T6Ø.3X1	T6Ø.3X2	T6Ø.3X3	T6Ø.3X4	—	—
fungicide	T6Ø.3X1	T6Ø.3X2	T6Ø.3X3	T6Ø.3X4	—	—
insecticide	T6Ø.1X1	T6Ø.1X2	T6Ø.1X3	T6Ø.1X4	—	—
Pentaerythritol	T46.3X1	T46.3X2	T46.3X3	T46.3X4	T46.3X5	T46.3X6
chloral	T42.6X1	T42.6X2	T42.6X3	T42.6X4	T42.6X5	T42.6X6
tetranitrate NEC	T46.3X1	T46.3X2	T46.3X3	T46.3X4	T46.3X5	T46.3X6
Pentaerythritol tetranitrate	T46.3X1	T46.3X2	T46.3X3	T46.3X4	T46.3X5	T46.3X6
Pentagastrin	T5Ø.8X1	T5Ø.8X2	T5Ø.8X3	T5Ø.8X4	T5Ø.8X5	T5Ø.8X6
Pentalin	T53.6X1	T53.6X2	T53.6X3	T53.6X4	—	—
Pentamethonium bromide	T44.2X1	T44.2X2	T44.2X3	T44.2X4	T44.2X5	T44.2X6
Pentamidine	T37.3X1	T37.3X2	T37.3X3	T37.3X4	T37.3X5	T37.3X6
Pentanol	T51.3X1	T51.3X2	T51.3X3	T51.3X4	—	—
Pentapyrrolinium (bitartrate)	T44.2X1	T44.2X2	T44.2X3	T44.2X4	T44.2X5	T44.2X6
Pentaquine	T37.2X1	T37.2X2	T37.2X3	T37.2X4	T37.2X5	T37.2X6
Pentazocine	T40.4X1	T40.4X2	T40.4X3	T40.4X4	T40.4X5	T40.4X6
Pentetrazole	T5Ø.7X1	T5Ø.7X2	T5Ø.7X3	T5Ø.7X4	T5Ø.7X5	T5Ø.7X6
Penthienate bromide	T44.3X1	T44.3X2	T44.3X3	T44.3X4	T44.3X5	T44.3X6
Pentifylline	T46.7X1	T46.7X2	T46.7X3	T46.7X4	T46.7X5	T46.7X6
Pentobarbital	T42.3X1	T42.3X2	T42.3X3	T42.3X4	T42.3X5	T42.3X6
sodium	T42.3X1	T42.3X2	T42.3X3	T42.3X4	T42.3X5	T42.3X6
Pentobarbitone	T42.3X1	T42.3X2	T42.3X3	T42.3X4	T42.3X5	T42.3X6
Pentolonium tartrate	T44.2X1	T44.2X2	T44.2X3	T44.2X4	T44.2X5	T44.2X6
Pentosan polysulfate (sodium)	T39.8X1	T39.8X2	T39.8X3	T39.8X4	T39.8X5	T39.8X6
Pentostatin	T45.1X1	T45.1X2	T45.1X3	T45.1X4	T45.1X5	T45.1X6
Pentothal	T41.1X1	T41.1X2	T41.1X3	T41.1X4	T41.1X5	T41.1X6
Pentoxifylline	T46.7X1	T46.7X2	T46.7X3	T46.7X4	T46.7X5	T46.7X6
Pentoxyverine	T48.3X1	T48.3X2	T48.3X3	T48.3X4	T48.3X5	T48.3X6
Pentrinat	T46.3X1	T46.3X2	T46.3X3	T46.3X4	T46.3X5	T46.3X6
Pentylenetetrazole	T5Ø.7X1	T5Ø.7X2	T5Ø.7X3	T5Ø.7X4	T5Ø.7X5	T5Ø.7X6
Pentylsalicylamide	T37.1X1	T37.1X2	T37.1X3	T37.1X4	T37.1X5	T37.1X6
Pentymal	T42.3X1	T42.3X2	T42.3X3	T42.3X4	T42.3X5	T42.3X6
Peplomycin	T45.1X1	T45.1X2	T45.1X3	T45.1X4	T45.1X5	T45.1X6
Peppermint (oil)	T47.5X1	T47.5X2	T47.5X3	T47.5X4	T47.5X5	T47.5X6
Pepsin	T47.5X1	T47.5X2	T47.5X3	T47.5X4	T47.5X5	T47.5X6
digestant	T47.5X1	T47.5X2	T47.5X3	T47.5X4	T47.5X5	T47.5X6
Pepstatin	T47.1X1	T47.1X2	T47.1X3	T47.1X4	T47.1X5	T47.1X6
Peptavlon	T5Ø.8X1	T5Ø.8X2	T5Ø.8X3	T5Ø.8X4	T5Ø.8X5	T5Ø.8X6
Perazine	T43.3X1	T43.3X2	T43.3X3	T43.3X4	T43.3X5	T43.3X6
Percaine (spinal)	T41.3X1	T41.3X2	T41.3X3	T41.3X4	T41.3X5	T41.3X6
topical (surface)	T41.3X1	T41.3X2	T41.3X3	T41.3X4	T41.3X5	T41.3X6
Perchloroethylene	T53.3X1	T53.3X2	T53.3X3	T53.3X4	—	—
vapor	T53.3X1	T53.3X2	T53.3X3	T53.3X4	—	—
medicinal	T37.4X1	T37.4X2	T37.4X3	T37.4X4	T37.4X5	T37.4X6
Percodan	T40.2X1	T40.2X2	T40.2X3	T40.2X4	T40.2X5	T40.2X6
Percogesic (*see also* Acetaminophen)	T45.ØX1	T45.ØX2	T45.ØX3	T45.ØX4	T45.ØX5	T45.ØX6
Percorten	T38.ØX1	T38.ØX2	T38.ØX3	T38.ØX4	T38.ØX5	T38.ØX6
Pergolide	T42.8X1	T42.8X2	T42.8X3	T42.8X4	T42.8X5	T42.8X6
Pergonal	T38.811	T38.812	T38.813	T38.814	T38.815	T38.816
Perhexilene	T46.3X1	T46.3X2	T46.3X3	T46.3X4	T46.3X5	T46.3X6
Perhexiline (maleate)	T46.3X1	T46.3X2	T46.3X3	T46.3X4	T46.3X5	T46.3X6
Periactin	T45.ØX1	T45.ØX2	T45.ØX3	T45.ØX4	T45.ØX5	T45.ØX6
Periciazine	T43.3X1	T43.3X2	T43.3X3	T43.3X4	T43.3X5	T43.3X6
Periclor	T42.6X1	T42.6X2	T42.6X3	T42.6X4	T42.6X5	T42.6X6
Perindopril	T46.4X1	T46.4X2	T46.4X3	T46.4X4	T46.4X5	T46.4X6
Perisoxal	T39.8X1	T39.8X2	T39.8X3	T39.8X4	T39.8X5	T39.8X6
Peritrate	T46.3X1	T46.3X2	T46.3X3	T46.3X4	T46.3X5	T46.3X6
Peritoneal dialysis solution	T5Ø.3X1	T5Ø.3X2	T5Ø.3X3	T5Ø.3X4	T5Ø.3X5	T5Ø.3X6
Perlapine	T42.4X1	T42.4X2	T42.4X3	T42.4X4	T42.4X5	T42.4X6

Substance	Poisoning, Accidental (unintentional)	Poisoning, Intentional Self-harm	Poisoning, Assault	Poisoning, Undetermined	Adverse Effect	Under-dosing
Permanganate	T65.891	T65.892	T65.893	T65.894	—	—
Permethrin	T6Ø.1X1	T6Ø.1X2	T6Ø.1X3	T6Ø.1X4	—	—
Pernocton	T42.3X1	T42.3X2	T42.3X3	T42.3X4	T42.3X5	T42.3X6
Pernoston	T42.3X1	T42.3X2	T42.3X3	T42.3X4	T42.3X5	T42.3X6
Peronine	T4Ø.2X1	T4Ø.2X2	T4Ø.2X3	T4Ø.2X4	—	—
Perphenazine	T43.3X1	T43.3X2	T43.3X3	T43.3X4	T43.3X5	T43.3X6
Pertofrane	T43.Ø11	T43.Ø12	T43.Ø13	T43.Ø14	T43.Ø15	T43.Ø16
Pertussis						
immune serum (human)	T5Ø.Z11	T5Ø.Z12	T5Ø.Z13	T5Ø.Z14	T5Ø.Z15	T5Ø.Z16
vaccine (with diphtheria toxoid) (with tetanus toxoid)	T5Ø.A11	T5Ø.A12	T5Ø.A13	T5Ø.A14	T5Ø.A15	T5Ø.A16
Peruvian balsam	T49.ØX1	T49.ØX2	T49.ØX3	T49.ØX4	T49.ØX5	T49.ØX6
Peruvoside	T46.ØX1	T46.ØX2	T46.ØX3	T46.ØX4	T46.ØX5	T46.ØX6
Pesticide (dust) (fumes) (vapor) **NEC**	T6Ø.91	T6Ø.92	T6Ø.93	T6Ø.94	—	—
arsenic	T57.ØX1	T57.ØX2	T57.ØX3	T57.ØX4	—	—
chlorinated	T6Ø.1X1	T6Ø.1X2	T6Ø.1X3	T6Ø.1X4	—	—
cyanide	T65.ØX1	T65.ØX2	T65.ØX3	T65.ØX4	—	—
kerosene	T52.ØX1	T52.ØX2	T52.ØX3	T52.ØX4	—	—
mixture (of compounds)	T6Ø.91	T6Ø.92	T6Ø.93	T6Ø.94	—	—
naphthalene	T6Ø.2X1	T6Ø.2X2	T6Ø.2X3	T6Ø.2X4	—	—
organochlorine (compounds)	T6Ø.1X1	T6Ø.1X2	T6Ø.1X3	T6Ø.1X4	—	—
petroleum (distillate) (products) NEC	T6Ø.8X1	T6Ø.8X2	T6Ø.8X3	T6Ø.8X4	—	—
specified ingredient NEC	T6Ø.8X1	T6Ø.8X2	T6Ø.8X3	T6Ø.8X4	—	—
strychnine	T65.1X1	T65.1X2	T65.1X3	T65.1X4	—	—
thallium	T6Ø.4X1	T6Ø.4X2	T6Ø.4X3	T6Ø.4X4	—	—
Pethidine*	T4Ø.4X1	T4Ø.4X2	T4Ø.4X3	T4Ø.4X4	T4Ø.4X5	T4Ø.4X6
Petrichloral	T42.6X1	T42.6X2	T42.6X3	T42.6X4	T42.6X5	T42.6X6
Petrol	T52.ØX1	T52.ØX2	T52.ØX3	T52.ØX4	—	—
vapor	T52.ØX1	T52.ØX2	T52.ØX3	T52.ØX4	—	—
Petrolatum	T49.3X1	T49.3X2	T49.3X3	T49.3X4	T49.3X5	T49.3X6
hydrophilic	T49.3X1	T49.3X2	T49.3X3	T49.3X4	T49.3X5	T49.3X6
liquid	T47.4X1	T47.4X2	T47.4X3	T47.4X4	T47.4X5	T47.4X6
topical	T49.3X1	T49.3X2	T49.3X3	T49.3X4	T49.3X5	T49.3X6
nonmedicinal	T52.ØX1	T52.ØX2	T52.ØX3	T52.ØX4	—	—
red veterinary	T49.3X1	T49.3X2	T49.3X3	T49.3X4	T49.3X5	T49.3X6
white	T49.3X1	T49.3X2	T49.3X3	T49.3X4	T49.3X5	T49.3X6
Petroleum (products) **NEC**	T52.ØX1	T52.ØX2	T52.ØX3	T52.ØX4	—	—
benzine(s)—*see* Ligroin						
ether—*see* Ligroin						
jelly—*see* Petrolatum						
naphtha—*see* Ligroin						
pesticide	T6Ø.8X1	T6Ø.8X2	T6Ø.8X3	T6Ø.8X4	—	—
solids	T52.ØX1	T52.ØX2	T52.ØX3	T52.ØX4	—	—
solvents	T52.ØX1	T52.ØX2	T52.ØX3	T52.ØX4	—	—
vapor	T52.ØX1	T52.ØX2	T52.ØX3	T52.ØX4	—	—
Peyote	T4Ø.991	T4Ø.992	T4Ø.993	T4Ø.994	—	—
Phanodorm, phanodorn	T42.3X1	T42.3X2	T42.3X3	T42.3X4	T42.3X5	T42.3X6
Phanquinone	T37.3X1	T37.3X2	T37.3X3	T37.3X4	T37.3X5	T37.3X6
Phanquone	T37.3X1	T37.3X2	T37.3X3	T37.3X4	T37.3X5	T37.3X6
Pharmaceutical						
adjunct NEC	T5Ø.9Ø1	T5Ø.9Ø2	T5Ø.9Ø3	T5Ø.9Ø4	T5Ø.9Ø5	T5Ø.9Ø6
excipient NEC	T5Ø.9Ø1	T5Ø.9Ø2	T5Ø.9Ø3	T5Ø.9Ø4	T5Ø.9Ø5	T5Ø.9Ø6
sweetener	T5Ø.9Ø1	T5Ø.9Ø2	T5Ø.9Ø3	T5Ø.9Ø4	T5Ø.9Ø5	T5Ø.9Ø6
viscous agent	T5Ø.9Ø1	T5Ø.9Ø2	T5Ø.9Ø3	T5Ø.9Ø4	T5Ø.9Ø5	T5Ø.9Ø6
Phemitone	T42.3X1	T42.3X2	T42.3X3	T42.3X4	T42.3X5	T42.3X6
Phenacaine	T41.3X1	T41.3X2	T41.3X3	T41.3X4	T41.3X5	T41.3X6
Phenacemide	T42.6X1	T42.6X2	T42.6X3	T42.6X4	T42.6X5	T42.6X6
Phenacetin	T39.1X1	T39.1X2	T39.1X3	T39.1X4	T39.1X5	T39.1X6
Phenadoxone	T4Ø.2X1	T4Ø.2X2	T4Ø.2X3	T4Ø.2X4	—	—
Phenaglycodol	T43.591	T43.592	T43.593	T43.594	T43.595	T43.596
Phenantoin	T42.ØX1	T42.ØX2	T42.ØX3	T42.ØX4	T42.ØX5	T42.ØX6
Phenaphthazine reagent	T5Ø.991	T5Ø.992	T5Ø.993	T5Ø.994	T5Ø.995	T5Ø.996
Phenazocine	T4Ø.4X1	T4Ø.4X2	T4Ø.4X3	T4Ø.4X4	T4Ø.4X5	T4Ø.4X6
Phenazone	T39.2X1	T39.2X2	T39.2X3	T39.2X4	T39.2X5	T39.2X6
Phenazopyridine	T39.8X1	T39.8X2	T39.8X3	T39.8X4	T39.8X5	T39.8X6
Phenbenicillin	T36.ØX1	T36.ØX2	T36.ØX3	T36.ØX4	T36.ØX5	T36.ØX6
Phenbutrazate	T5Ø.5X1	T5Ø.5X2	T5Ø.5X3	T5Ø.5X4	T5Ø.5X5	T5Ø.5X6
Phencyclidine	T4Ø.991	T4Ø.992	T4Ø.993	T4Ø.994	T4Ø.995	T4Ø.996
Phendimetrazine	T5Ø.5X1	T5Ø.5X2	T5Ø.5X3	T5Ø.5X4	T5Ø.5X5	T5Ø.5X6
Phenelzine	T43.1X1	T43.1X2	T43.1X3	T43.1X4	T43.1X5	T43.1X6
Phenemal	T42.3X1	T42.3X2	T42.3X3	T42.3X4	T42.3X5	T42.3X6
Phenergan	T42.6X1	T42.6X2	T42.6X3	T42.6X4	T42.6X5	T42.6X6
Pheneticillin	T36.ØX1	T36.ØX2	T36.ØX3	T36.ØX4	T36.ØX5	T36.ØX6
Pheneturide	T42.6X1	T42.6X2	T42.6X3	T42.6X4	T42.6X5	T42.6X6
Phenformin	T38.3X1	T38.3X2	T38.3X3	T38.3X4	T38.3X5	T38.3X6
Phenglutarimide	T44.3X1	T44.3X2	T44.3X3	T44.3X4	T44.3X5	T44.3X6
Phenicarbazide	T39.8X1	T39.8X2	T39.8X3	T39.8X4	T39.8X5	T39.8X6
Phenindamine	T45.ØX1	T45.ØX2	T45.ØX3	T45.ØX4	T45.ØX5	T45.ØX6
Phenindione	T45.511	T45.512	T45.513	T45.514	T45.515	T45.516
Pheniprazine	T43.1X1	T43.1X2	T43.1X3	T43.1X4	T43.1X5	T43.1X6
Pheniramine	T45.ØX1	T45.ØX2	T45.ØX3	T45.ØX4	T45.ØX5	T45.ØX6
Phenisatin	T47.2X1	T47.2X2	T47.2X3	T47.2X4	T47.2X5	T47.2X6
Phenmetrazine	T5Ø.5X1	T5Ø.5X2	T5Ø.5X3	T5Ø.5X4	T5Ø.5X5	T5Ø.5X6
Phenobal	T42.3X1	T42.3X2	T42.3X3	T42.3X4	T42.3X5	T42.3X6
Phenobarbital	T42.3X1	T42.3X2	T42.3X3	T42.3X4	T42.3X5	T42.3X6
with						
mephenytoin	T42.3X1	T42.3X2	T42.3X3	T42.3X4	T42.3X5	T42.3X6
phenytoin	T42.3X1	T42.3X2	T42.3X3	T42.3X4	T42.3X5	T42.3X6
sodium	T42.3X1	T42.3X2	T42.3X3	T42.3X4	T42.3X5	T42.3X6
Phenobarbitone	T42.3X1	T42.3X2	T42.3X3	T42.3X4	T42.3X5	T42.3X6
Phenobutiodil	T5Ø.8X1	T5Ø.8X2	T5Ø.8X3	T5Ø.8X4	T5Ø.8X5	T5Ø.8X6
Phenoctide	T49.ØX1	T49.ØX2	T49.ØX3	T49.ØX4	T49.ØX5	T49.ØX6
Phenol	T49.ØX1	T49.ØX2	T49.ØX3	T49.ØX4	T49.ØX5	T49.ØX6
disinfectant	T54.ØX1	T54.ØX2	T54.ØX3	T54.ØX4	—	—
in oil injection	T46.8X1	T46.8X2	T46.8X3	T46.8X4	T46.8X5	T46.8X6
medicinal	T49.1X1	T49.1X2	T49.1X3	T49.1X4	T49.1X5	T49.1X6
nonmedicinal NEC	T54.ØX1	T54.ØX2	T54.ØX3	T54.ØX4	—	—
pesticide	T6Ø.8X1	T6Ø.8X2	T6Ø.8X3	T6Ø.8X4	—	—
red	T5Ø.8X1	T5Ø.8X2	T5Ø.8X3	T5Ø.8X4	T5Ø.8X5	T5Ø.8X6
Phenolic preparation	T49.1X1	T49.1X2	T49.1X3	T49.1X4	T49.1X5	T49.1X6
Phenolphthalein	T47.2X1	T47.2X2	T47.2X3	T47.2X4	T47.2X5	T47.2X6
Phenolsulfonphthalein	T5Ø.8X1	T5Ø.8X2	T5Ø.8X3	T5Ø.8X4	T5Ø.8X5	T5Ø.8X6
Phenomorphan	T4Ø.2X1	T4Ø.2X2	T4Ø.2X3	T4Ø.2X4	—	—
Phenonyl	T42.3X1	T42.3X2	T42.3X3	T42.3X4	T42.3X5	T42.3X6
Phenoperidine	T4Ø.4X1	T4Ø.4X2	T4Ø.4X3	T4Ø.4X4	—	—
Phenopyrazone	T46.991	T46.992	T46.993	T46.994	T46.995	T46.996
Phenoquin	T5Ø.4X1	T5Ø.4X2	T5Ø.4X3	T5Ø.4X4	T5Ø.4X5	T5Ø.4X6
Phenothiazine (psychotropic) **NEC**	T43.3X1	T43.3X2	T43.3X3	T43.3X4	T43.3X5	T43.3X6
insecticide	T6Ø.2X1	T6Ø.2X2	T6Ø.2X3	T6Ø.2X4	—	—
Phenothrin	T49.ØX1	T49.ØX2	T49.ØX3	T49.ØX4	T49.ØX5	T49.ØX6
Phenoxybenzamine	T46.7X1	T46.7X2	T46.7X3	T46.7X4	T46.7X5	T46.7X6
Phenoxyethanol	T49.ØX1	T49.ØX2	T49.ØX3	T49.ØX4	T49.ØX5	T49.ØX6
Phenoxymethyl penicillin	T36.ØX1	T36.ØX2	T36.ØX3	T36.ØX4	T36.ØX5	T36.ØX6
Phenprobamate	T42.8X1	T42.8X2	T42.8X3	T42.8X4	T42.8X5	T42.8X6
Phenprocoumon	T45.511	T45.512	T45.513	T45.514	T45.515	T45.516
Phensuximide	T42.2X1	T42.2X2	T42.2X3	T42.2X4	T42.2X5	T42.2X6
Phentermine	T5Ø.5X1	T5Ø.5X2	T5Ø.5X3	T5Ø.5X4	T5Ø.5X5	T5Ø.5X6
Phenthicillin	T36.ØX1	T36.ØX2	T36.ØX3	T36.ØX4	T36.ØX5	T36.ØX6
Phentolamine	T46.7X1	T46.7X2	T46.7X3	T46.7X4	T46.7X5	T46.7X6
Phenyl						
butazone	T39.2X1	T39.2X2	T39.2X3	T39.2X4	T39.2X5	T39.2X6
enediamine	T65.3X1	T65.3X2	T65.3X3	T65.3X4	—	—
hydrazine	T65.3X1	T65.3X2	T65.3X3	T65.3X4	—	—
antineoplastic	T45.1X1	T45.1X2	T45.1X3	T45.1X4	T45.1X5	T45.1X6
mercuric compounds—*see* Mercury						
salicylate	T49.3X1	T49.3X2	T49.3X3	T49.3X4	T49.3X5	T49.3X6
Phenylalanine mustard	T45.1X1	T45.1X2	T45.1X3	T45.1X4	T45.1X5	T45.1X6
Phenylbutazone	T39.2X1	T39.2X2	T39.2X3	T39.2X4	T39.2X5	T39.2X6
Phenylenediamine	T65.3X1	T65.3X2	T65.3X3	T65.3X4	—	—
Phenylephrine	T44.4X1	T44.4X2	T44.4X3	T44.4X4	T44.4X5	T44.4X6
Phenylethylbiguanide	T38.3X1	T38.3X2	T38.3X3	T38.3X4	T38.3X5	T38.3X6
Phenylmercuric						
acetate	T49.ØX1	T49.ØX2	T49.ØX3	T49.ØX4	T49.ØX5	T49.ØX6
borate	T49.ØX1	T49.ØX2	T49.ØX3	T49.ØX4	T49.ØX5	T49.ØX6
nitrate	T49.ØX1	T49.ØX2	T49.ØX3	T49.ØX4	T49.ØX5	T49.ØX6
Phenylmethylbarbitone	T42.3X1	T42.3X2	T42.3X3	T42.3X4	T42.3X5	T42.3X6
Phenylpropanol	T47.5X1	T47.5X2	T47.5X3	T47.5X4	T47.5X5	T47.5X6
Phenylpropanolamine	T44.991	T44.992	T44.993	T44.994	T44.995	T44.996

Substance	Poisoning, Accidental (unintentional)	Poisoning, Intentional Self-harm	Poisoning, Assault	Poisoning, Undetermined	Adverse Effect	Under-dosing
Phenylsulfthion	T60.0X1	T60.0X2	T60.0X3	T60.0X4	—	—
Phenyltoloxamine	T45.0X1	T45.0X2	T45.0X3	T45.0X4	T45.0X5	T45.0X6
Phenyramidol, phenyramidon	T39.8X1	T39.8X2	T39.8X3	T39.8X4	T39.8X5	T39.8X6
Phenytoin	T42.0X1	T42.0X2	T42.0X3	T42.0X4	T42.0X5	T42.0X6
with Phenobarbital	T42.3X1	T42.3X2	T42.3X3	T42.3X4	T42.3X5	T42.3X6
pHisoHex	T49.2X1	T49.2X2	T49.2X3	T49.2X4	T49.2X5	T49.2X6
Pholcodine	T48.3X1	T48.3X2	T48.3X3	T48.3X4	T48.3X5	T48.3X6
Pholedrine	T46.991	T46.992	T46.993	T46.994	T46.995	T46.996
Phorate	T60.0X1	T60.0X2	T60.0X3	T60.0X4	—	—
Phosdrin	T60.0X1	T60.0X2	T60.0X3	T60.0X4	—	—
Phosfolan	T60.0X1	T60.0X2	T60.0X3	T60.0X4	—	—
Phosgene (gas)	T59.891	T59.892	T59.893	T59.894	—	—
Phosphamidon	T60.0X1	T60.0X2	T60.0X3	T60.0X4	—	—
Phosphate	T65.891	T65.892	T65.893	T65.894	—	—
laxative	T47.4X1	T47.4X2	T47.4X3	T47.4X4	T47.4X5	T47.4X6
Phosphate						
organic	T60.0X1	T60.0X2	T60.0X3	T60.0X4	—	—
solvent	T52.91	T52.92	T52.93	T52.94	—	—
tricresyl	T65.891	T65.892	T65.893	T65.894	—	—
Phosphine	T57.1X1	T57.1X2	T57.1X3	T57.1X4	—	—
fumigant	T57.1X1	T57.1X2	T57.1X3	T57.1X4	—	—
Phospholine	T49.5X1	T49.5X2	T49.5X3	T49.5X4	T49.5X5	T49.5X6
Phosphoric acid	T54.2X1	T54.2X2	T54.2X3	T54.2X4	—	—
Phosphorus (compound) **NEC**	T57.1X1	T57.1X2	T57.1X3	T57.1X4	—	—
pesticide	T60.0X1	T60.0X2	T60.0X3	T60.0X4	—	—
Phthalates	T65.891	T65.892	T65.893	T65.894	—	—
Phthalic anhydride	T65.891	T65.892	T65.893	T65.894	—	—
Phthalimidoglutarimide	T42.6X1	T42.6X2	T42.6X3	T42.6X4	T42.6X5	T42.6X6
Phthalylsulfathiazole	T37.0X1	T37.0X2	T37.0X3	T37.0X4	T37.0X5	T37.0X6
Phylloquinone	T45.7X1	T45.7X2	T45.7X3	T45.7X4	T45.7X5	T45.7X6
Physeptone	T40.3X1	T40.3X2	T40.3X3	T40.3X4	T40.3X5	T40.3X6
Physostigma venenosum	T62.2X1	T62.2X2	T62.2X3	T62.2X4	—	—
Physostigmine	T49.5X1	T49.5X2	T49.5X3	T49.5X4	T49.5X5	T49.5X6
Phytolacca decandra	T62.2X1	T62.2X2	T62.2X3	T62.2X4	—	—
berries	T62.1X1	T62.1X2	T62.1X3	T62.1X4	—	—
Phytomenadione	T45.7X1	T45.7X2	T45.7X3	T45.7X4	T45.7X5	T45.7X6
Phytonadione	T45.7X1	T45.7X2	T45.7X3	T45.7X4	T45.7X5	T45.7X6
Picoperine	T48.3X1	T48.3X2	T48.3X3	T48.3X4	T48.3X5	T48.3X6
Picosulfate (sodium)	T47.2X1	T47.2X2	T47.2X3	T47.2X4	T47.2X5	T47.2X6
Picric (acid)	T54.2X1	T54.2X2	T54.2X3	T54.2X4	—	—
Picrotoxin	T50.7X1	T50.7X2	T50.7X3	T50.7X4	T50.7X5	T50.7X6
Piketoprofen	T49.0X1	T49.0X2	T49.0X3	T49.0X4	T49.0X5	T49.0X6
Pilocarpine	T44.1X1	T44.1X2	T44.1X3	T44.1X4	T44.1X5	T44.1X6
Pilocarpus (jaborandi) **extract**	T44.1X1	T44.1X2	T44.1X3	T44.1X4	T44.1X5	T44.1X6
Pilsicainide (hydrochloride)	T46.2X1	T46.2X2	T46.2X3	T46.2X4	T46.2X5	T46.2X6
Pimaricin	T36.7X1	T36.7X2	T36.7X3	T36.7X4	T36.7X5	T36.7X6
Pimeclone	T50.7X1	T50.7X2	T50.7X3	T50.7X4	T50.7X5	T50.7X6
Pimelic ketone	T52.8X1	T52.8X2	T52.8X3	T52.8X4	—	—
Pimethixene	T45.0X1	T45.0X2	T45.0X3	T45.0X4	T45.0X5	T45.0X6
Piminodine	T40.2X1	T40.2X2	T40.2X3	T40.2X4	T40.2X5	T40.2X6
Pimozide	T43.591	T43.592	T43.593	T43.594	T43.595	T43.596
Pinacidil	T46.5X1	T46.5X2	T46.5X3	T46.5X4	T46.5X5	T46.5X6
Pinaverium bromide	T44.3X1	T44.3X2	T44.3X3	T44.3X4	T44.3X5	T44.3X6
Pinazepam	T42.4X1	T42.4X2	T42.4X3	T42.4X4	T42.4X5	T42.4X6
Pindolol	T44.7X1	T44.7X2	T44.7X3	T44.7X4	T44.7X5	T44.7X6
Pindone	T60.4X1	T60.4X2	T60.4X3	T60.4X4	—	—
Pine oil (disinfectant)	T65.891	T65.892	T65.893	T65.894	—	—
Pinkroot	T37.4X1	T37.4X2	T37.4X3	T37.4X4	T37.4X5	T37.4X6
Pipadone	T40.2X1	T40.2X2	T40.2X3	T40.2X4	—	—
Pipamazine	T45.0X1	T45.0X2	T45.0X3	T45.0X4	T45.0X5	T45.0X6
Pipamperone	T43.4X1	T43.4X2	T43.4X3	T43.4X4	T43.4X5	T43.4X6
Pipazetate	T48.3X1	T48.3X2	T48.3X3	T48.3X4	T48.3X5	T48.3X6
Pipemidic acid	T37.8X1	T37.8X2	T37.8X3	T37.8X4	T37.8X5	T37.8X6
Pipenzolate bromide	T44.3X1	T44.3X2	T44.3X3	T44.3X4	T44.3X5	T44.3X6
Piperacetazine	T43.3X1	T43.3X2	T43.3X3	T43.3X4	T43.3X5	T43.3X6
Piperacillin	T36.0X1	T36.0X2	T36.0X3	T36.0X4	T36.0X5	T36.0X6
Piperazine	T37.4X1	T37.4X2	T37.4X3	T37.4X4	T37.4X5	T37.4X6
estrone sulfate	T38.5X1	T38.5X2	T38.5X3	T38.5X4	T38.5X5	T38.5X6
Piper cubeba	T62.2X1	T62.2X2	T62.2X3	T62.2X4	—	—
Piperidione	T48.3X1	T48.3X2	T48.3X3	T48.3X4	T48.3X5	T48.3X6
Piperidolate	T44.3X1	T44.3X2	T44.3X3	T44.3X4	T44.3X5	T44.3X6
Piperocaine	T41.3X1	T41.3X2	T41.3X3	T41.3X4	T41.3X5	T41.3X6
infiltration (subcutaneous)	T41.3X1	T41.3X2	T41.3X3	T41.3X4	T41.3X5	T41.3X6
nerve block (peripheral) (plexus)	T41.3X1	T41.3X2	T41.3X3	T41.3X4	T41.3X5	T41.3X6
topical (surface)	T41.3X1	T41.3X2	T41.3X3	T41.3X4	T41.3X5	T41.3X6
Piperonyl butoxide	T60.8X1	T60.8X2	T60.8X3	T60.8X4	—	—
Pipethanate	T44.3X1	T44.3X2	T44.3X3	T44.3X4	T44.3X5	T44.3X6
Pipobroman	T45.1X1	T45.1X2	T45.1X3	T45.1X4	T45.1X5	T45.1X6
Pipotiazine	T43.3X1	T43.3X2	T43.3X3	T43.3X4	T43.3X5	T43.3X6
Pipoxizine	T45.0X1	T45.0X2	T45.0X3	T45.0X4	T45.0X5	T45.0X6
Pipradrol	T43.691	T43.692	T43.693	T43.694	T43.695	T43.696
Piprinhydrinate	T45.0X1	T45.0X2	T45.0X3	T45.0X4	T45.0X5	T45.0X6
Pirarubicin	T45.1X1	T45.1X2	T45.1X3	T45.1X4	T45.1X5	T45.1X6
Pirazinamide	T37.1X1	T37.1X2	T37.1X3	T37.1X4	T37.1X5	T37.1X6
Pirbuterol	T48.6X1	T48.6X2	T48.6X3	T48.6X4	T48.6X5	T48.6X6
Pirenzepine	T47.1X1	T47.1X2	T47.1X3	T47.1X4	T47.1X5	T47.1X6
Piretanide	T50.1X1	T50.1X2	T50.1X3	T50.1X4	T50.1X5	T50.1X6
Piribedil	T42.8X1	T42.8X2	T42.8X3	T42.8X4	T42.8X5	T42.8X6
Piridoxilate	T46.3X1	T46.3X2	T46.3X3	T46.3X4	T46.3X5	T46.3X6
Piritramide	T40.4X1	T40.4X2	T40.4X3	T40.4X4	—	—
Piromidic acid	T37.8X1	T37.8X2	T37.8X3	T37.8X4	T37.8X5	T37.8X6
Piroxicam	T39.391	T39.392	T39.393	T39.394	T39.395	T39.396
beta-cyclodextrin complex	T39.8X1	T39.8X2	T39.8X3	T39.8X4	T39.8X5	T39.8X6
Pirozadil	T46.6X1	T46.6X2	T46.6X3	T46.6X4	T46.6X5	T46.6X6
Piscidia (bark) (erythrina)	T39.8X1	T39.8X2	T39.8X3	T39.8X4	T39.8X5	T39.8X6
Pitch	T65.891	T65.892	T65.893	T65.894	—	—
Pitkin's solution	T41.3X1	T41.3X2	T41.3X3	T41.3X4	T41.3X5	T41.3X6
Pitocin	T48.0X1	T48.0X2	T48.0X3	T48.0X4	T48.0X5	T48.0X6
Pitressin (tannate)	T38.891	T38.892	T38.893	T38.894	T38.895	T38.896
Pituitary extracts (posterior)	T38.891	T38.892	T38.893	T38.894	T38.895	T38.896
anterior	T38.811	T38.812	T38.813	T38.814	T38.815	T38.816
Pituitrin	T38.891	T38.892	T38.893	T38.894	T38.895	T38.896
Pivampicillin	T36.0X1	T36.0X2	T36.0X3	T36.0X4	T36.0X5	T36.0X6
Pivmecillinam	T36.0X1	T36.0X2	T36.0X3	T36.0X4	T36.0X5	T36.0X6
Placental hormone	T38.891	T38.892	T38.893	T38.894	T38.895	T38.896
Placidyl	T42.6X1	T42.6X2	T42.6X3	T42.6X4	T42.6X5	T42.6X6
Plague vaccine	T50.A91	T50.A92	T50.A93	T50.A94	T50.A95	T50.A96
Plant						
food or fertilizer NEC	T65.891	T65.892	T65.893	T65.894	—	—
containing herbicide	T60.3X1	T60.3X2	T60.3X3	T60.3X4	—	—
noxious, used as food	T62.2X1	T62.2X2	T62.2X3	T62.2X4	—	—
berries	T62.1X1	T62.1X2	T62.1X3	T62.1X4	—	—
seeds	T62.2X1	T62.2X2	T62.2X3	T62.2X4	—	—
specified type NEC	T62.2X1	T62.2X2	T62.2X3	T62.2X4	—	—
Plasma	T45.8X1	T45.8X2	T45.8X3	T45.8X4	T45.8X5	T45.8X6
expander NEC	T45.8X1	T45.8X2	T45.8X3	T45.8X4	T45.8X5	T45.8X6
protein fraction (human)	T45.8X1	T45.8X2	T45.8X3	T45.8X4	T45.8X5	T45.8X6
Plasmanate	T45.8X1	T45.8X2	T45.8X3	T45.8X4	T45.8X5	T45.8X6
Plasminogen (tissue) **activator**	T45.611	T45.612	T45.613	T45.614	T45.615	T45.616
Plaster dressing	T49.3X1	T49.3X2	T49.3X3	T49.3X4	T49.3X5	T49.3X6
Plastic dressing	T49.3X1	T49.3X2	T49.3X3	T49.3X4	T49.3X5	T49.3X6
Plegicil	T43.3X1	T43.3X2	T43.3X3	T43.3X4	T43.3X5	T43.3X6
Plicamycin	T45.1X1	T45.1X2	T45.1X3	T45.1X4	T45.1X5	T45.1X6
Podophyllotoxin	T49.8X1	T49.8X2	T49.8X3	T49.8X4	T49.8X5	T49.8X6
Podophyllum (resin)	T49.4X1	T49.4X2	T49.4X3	T49.4X4	T49.4X5	T49.4X6
Poison NEC	T65.91	T65.92	T65.93	T65.94	—	—
Poisonous berries	T62.1X1	T62.1X2	T62.1X3	T62.1X4	—	—
Pokeweed (any part)	T62.2X1	T62.2X2	T62.2X3	T62.2X4	—	—
Poldine metilsulfate	T44.3X1	T44.3X2	T44.3X3	T44.3X4	T44.3X5	T44.3X6
Polidexide (sulfate)	T46.6X1	T46.6X2	T46.6X3	T46.6X4	T46.6X5	T46.6X6
Polidocanol	T46.8X1	T46.8X2	T46.8X3	T46.8X4	T46.8X5	T46.8X6
Poliomyelitis vaccine	T50.B91	T50.B92	T50.B93	T50.B94	T50.B95	T50.B96
Polish (car) (floor) (furni-ture) (metal) (porcelain) (silver)	T65.891	T65.892	T65.893	T65.894	—	—
abrasive	T65.891	T65.892	T65.893	T65.894	—	—
porcelain	T65.891	T65.892	T65.893	T65.894	—	—
Poloxalkol	T47.4X1	T47.4X2	T47.4X3	T47.4X4	T47.4X5	T47.4X6
Poloxamer	T47.4X1	T47.4X2	T47.4X3	T47.4X4	T47.4X5	T47.4X6
Polyaminostyrene resins	T50.3X1	T50.3X2	T50.3X3	T50.3X4	T50.3X5	T50.3X6
Polycarbophil	T47.4X1	T47.4X2	T47.4X3	T47.4X4	T47.4X5	T47.4X6
Polychlorinated biphenyl	T65.891	T65.892	T65.893	T65.894	—	—
Polycycline	T36.4X1	T36.4X2	T36.4X3	T36.4X4	T36.4X5	T36.4X6

Substance	Poisoning, Accidental (unintentional)	Poisoning, Intentional Self-harm	Poisoning, Assault	Poisoning, Undetermined	Adverse Effect	Under-dosing
Polyester fumes	T59.891	T59.892	T59.893	T59.894	—	—
Polyester resin hardener	T52.91	T52.92	T52.93	T52.94	—	—
fumes	T59.891	T59.892	T59.893	T59.894	—	—
Polyestradiol phosphate	T38.5X1	T38.5X2	T38.5X3	T38.5X4	T38.5X5	T38.5X6
Polyethanolamine alkyl sulfate	T49.2X1	T49.2X2	T49.2X3	T49.2X4	T49.2X5	T49.2X6
Polyethylene adhesive	T49.3X1	T49.3X2	T49.3X3	T49.3X4	T49.3X5	T49.3X6
Polyferose	T45.4X1	T45.4X2	T45.4X3	T45.4X4	T45.4X5	T45.4X6
Polygeline	T45.8X1	T45.8X2	T45.8X3	T45.8X4	T45.8X5	T45.8X6
Polymyxin	T36.8X1	T36.8X2	T36.8X3	T36.8X4	T36.8X5	T36.8X6
B	T36.8X1	T36.8X2	T36.8X3	T36.8X4	T36.8X5	T36.8X6
ENT agent	T49.6X1	T49.6X2	T49.6X3	T49.6X4	T49.6X5	T49.6X6
ophthalmic preparation	T49.5X1	T49.5X2	T49.5X3	T49.5X4	T49.5X5	T49.5X6
topical NEC	T49.ØX1	T49.ØX2	T49.ØX3	T49.ØX4	T49.ØX5	T49.ØX6
E sulfate (eye preparation)	T49.5X1	T49.5X2	T49.5X3	T49.5X4	T49.5X5	T49.5X6
Polynoxylin	T49.ØX1	T49.ØX2	T49.ØX3	T49.ØX4	T49.ØX5	T49.ØX6
Polyoestradiol phosphate	T38.5X1	T38.5X2	T38.5X3	T38.5X4	T38.5X5	T38.5X6
Polyoxymethyleneurea	T49.ØX1	T49.ØX2	T49.ØX3	T49.ØX4	T49.ØX5	T49.ØX6
Polysilane	T47.8X1	T47.8X2	T47.8X3	T47.8X4	T47.8X5	T47.8X6
Polytetrafluoroethylene (inhaled)	T59.891	T59.892	T59.893	T59.894	—	—
Polythiazide	T5Ø.2X1	T5Ø.2X2	T5Ø.2X3	T5Ø.2X4	T5Ø.2X5	T5Ø.2X6
Polyvidone	T45.8X1	T45.8X2	T45.8X3	T45.8X4	T45.8X5	T45.8X6
Polyvinylpyrrolidone	T45.8X1	T45.8X2	T45.8X3	T45.8X4	T45.8X5	T45.8X6
Pontocaine (hydrochloride) (infiltration) (topical)	T41.3X1	T41.3X2	T41.3X3	T41.3X4	T41.3X5	T41.3X6
nerve block (peripheral) (plexus)	T41.3X1	T41.3X2	T41.3X3	T41.3X4	T41.3X5	T41.3X6
spinal	T41.3X1	T41.3X2	T41.3X3	T41.3X4	T41.3X5	T41.3X6
Porfiromycin	T45.1X1	T45.1X2	T45.1X3	T45.1X4	T45.1X5	T45.1X6
Posterior pituitary hormone NEC	T38.891	T38.892	T38.893	T38.894	T38.895	T38.896
Pot	T4Ø.7X1	T4Ø.7X2	T4Ø.7X3	T4Ø.7X4	T4Ø.7X5	T4Ø.7X6
Potash (caustic)	T54.3X1	T54.3X2	T54.3X3	T54.3X4	—	—
Potassic saline injection (lactated)	T5Ø.3X1	T5Ø.3X2	T5Ø.3X3	T5Ø.3X4	T5Ø.3X5	T5Ø.3X6
Potassium (salts) **NEC**	T5Ø.3X1	T5Ø.3X2	T5Ø.3X3	T5Ø.3X4	T5Ø.3X5	T5Ø.3X6
aminobenzoate	T45.8X1	T45.8X2	T45.8X3	T45.8X4	T45.8X5	T45.8X6
aminosalicylate	T37.1X1	T37.1X2	T37.1X3	T37.1X4	T37.1X5	T37.1X6
antimony 'tartrate'	T37.8X1	T37.8X2	T37.8X3	T37.8X4	T37.8X5	T37.8X6
arsenite (solution)	T57.ØX1	T57.ØX2	T57.ØX3	T57.ØX4	—	—
bichromate	T56.2X1	T56.2X2	T56.2X3	T56.2X4	—	—
bisulfate	T47.3X1	T47.3X2	T47.3X3	T47.3X4	T47.3X5	T47.3X6
bromide	T42.6X1	T42.6X2	T42.6X3	T42.6X4	T42.6X5	T42.6X6
canrenoate	T5Ø.ØX1	T5Ø.ØX2	T5Ø.ØX3	T5Ø.ØX4	T5Ø.ØX5	T5Ø.ØX6
carbonate	T54.3X1	T54.3X2	T54.3X3	T54.3X4	—	—
chlorate NEC	T65.891	T65.892	T65.893	T65.894	—	—
chloride	T5Ø.3X1	T5Ø.3X2	T5Ø.3X3	T5Ø.3X4	T5Ø.3X5	T5Ø.3X6
citrate	T5Ø.991	T5Ø.992	T5Ø.993	T5Ø.994	T5Ø.995	T5Ø.996
cyanide	T65.ØX1	T65.ØX2	T65.ØX3	T65.ØX4	—	—
ferric hexacyanoferrate (medicinal)	T5Ø.6X1	T5Ø.6X2	T5Ø.6X3	T5Ø.6X4	T5Ø.6X5	T5Ø.6X6
nonmedicinal	T65.891	T65.892	T65.893	T65.894	—	—
Fluoride	T57.8X1	T57.8X2	T57.8X3	T57.8X4	—	—
glucaldrate	T47.1X1	T47.1X2	T47.1X3	T47.1X4	T47.1X5	T47.1X6
hydroxide	T54.3X1	T54.3X2	T54.3X3	T54.3X4	—	—
iodate	T49.ØX1	T49.ØX2	T49.ØX3	T49.ØX4	T49.ØX5	T49.ØX6
iodide	T48.4X1	T48.4X2	T48.4X3	T48.4X4	T48.4X5	T48.4X6
nitrate	T57.8X1	T57.8X2	T57.8X3	T57.8X4	—	—
oxalate	T65.891	T65.892	T65.893	T65.894	—	—
perchlorate (nonmedicinal) NEC	T65.891	T65.892	T65.893	T65.894	—	—
antithyroid	T38.2X1	T38.2X2	T38.2X3	T38.2X4	T38.2X5	T38.2X6
medicinal	T38.2X1	T38.2X2	T38.2X3	T38.2X4	T38.2X5	T38.2X6
Permanganate (nonmedicinal)	T65.891	T65.892	T65.893	T65.894	—	—
medicinal	T49.ØX1	T49.ØX2	T49.ØX3	T49.ØX4	T49.ØX5	T49.ØX6
sulfate	T47.2X1	T47.2X2	T47.2X3	T47.2X4	T47.2X5	T47.2X6
Potassium-removing resin	T5Ø.3X1	T5Ø.3X2	T5Ø.3X3	T5Ø.3X4	T5Ø.3X5	T5Ø.3X6
Potassium-retaining drug	T5Ø.3X1	T5Ø.3X2	T5Ø.3X3	T5Ø.3X4	T5Ø.3X5	T5Ø.3X6
Povidone	T45.8X1	T45.8X2	T45.8X3	T45.8X4	T45.8X5	T45.8X6
iodine	T49.ØX1	T49.ØX2	T49.ØX3	T49.ØX4	T49.ØX5	T49.ØX6
Practolol	T44.7X1	T44.7X2	T44.7X3	T44.7X4	T44.7X5	T44.7X6
Prajmalium bitartrate	T46.2X1	T46.2X2	T46.2X3	T46.2X4	T46.2X5	T46.2X6
Pralidoxime (iodide)	T5Ø.6X1	T5Ø.6X2	T5Ø.6X3	T5Ø.6X4	T5Ø.6X5	T5Ø.6X6
chloride	T5Ø.6X1	T5Ø.6X2	T5Ø.6X3	T5Ø.6X4	T5Ø.6X5	T5Ø.6X6
Pramiverine	T44.3X1	T44.3X2	T44.3X3	T44.3X4	T44.3X5	T44.3X6
Pramocaine	T49.1X1	T49.1X2	T49.1X3	T49.1X4	T49.1X5	T49.1X6
Pramoxine	T49.1X1	T49.1X2	T49.1X3	T49.1X4	T49.1X5	T49.1X6
Prasterone	T38.7X1	T38.7X2	T38.7X3	T38.7X4	T38.7X5	T38.7X6
Pravastatin	T46.6X1	T46.6X2	T46.6X3	T46.6X4	T46.6X5	T46.6X6
Prazepam	T42.4X1	T42.4X2	T42.4X3	T42.4X4	T42.4X5	T42.4X6
Praziquantel	T37.4X1	T37.4X2	T37.4X3	T37.4X4	T37.4X5	T37.4X6
Prazitone	T43.291	T43.292	T43.293	T43.294	T43.295	T43.296
Prazosin	T44.6X1	T44.6X2	T44.6X3	T44.6X4	T44.6X5	T44.6X6
Prednicarbate	T49.ØX1	T49.ØX2	T49.ØX3	T49.ØX4	T49.ØX5	T49.ØX6
Prednimustine	T45.1X1	T45.1X2	T45.1X3	T45.1X4	T45.1X5	T45.1X6
Prednisolone	T38.ØX1	T38.ØX2	T38.ØX3	T38.ØX4	T38.ØX5	T38.ØX6
ENT agent	T49.6X1	T49.6X2	T49.6X3	T49.6X4	T49.6X5	T49.6X6
ophthalmic preparation	T49.5X1	T49.5X2	T49.5X3	T49.5X4	T49.5X5	T49.5X6
steaglate	T49.ØX1	T49.ØX2	T49.ØX3	T49.ØX4	T49.ØX5	T49.ØX6
topical NEC	T49.ØX1	T49.ØX2	T49.ØX3	T49.ØX4	T49.ØX5	T49.ØX6
Prednisone	T38.ØX1	T38.ØX2	T38.ØX3	T38.ØX4	T38.ØX5	T38.ØX6
Prednylidene	T38.ØX1	T38.ØX2	T38.ØX3	T38.ØX4	T38.ØX5	T38.ØX6
Pregnandiol	T38.5X1	T38.5X2	T38.5X3	T38.5X4	T38.5X5	T38.5X6
Pregneninolone	T38.5X1	T38.5X2	T38.5X3	T38.5X4	T38.5X5	T38.5X6
Preludin	T43.691	T43.692	T43.693	T43.694	T43.695	T43.696
Premarin	T38.5X1	T38.5X2	T38.5X3	T38.5X4	T38.5X5	T38.5X6
Premedication anesthetic	T41.2Ø1	T41.2Ø2	T41.2Ø3	T41.2Ø4	T41.2Ø5	T41.2Ø6
Prenalterol	T44.5X1	T44.5X2	T44.5X3	T44.5X4	T44.5X5	T44.5X6
Prenoxdiazine	T48.3X1	T48.3X2	T48.3X3	T48.3X4	T48.3X5	T48.3X6
Prenylamine	T46.3X1	T46.3X2	T46.3X3	T46.3X4	T46.3X5	T46.3X6
Preparation, local	T49.4X1	T49.4X2	T49.4X3	T49.4X4	T49.4X5	T49.4X6
Preparation H	T49.8X1	T49.8X2	T49.8X3	T49.8X4	T49.8X5	T49.8X6
Preservative (nonmedicinal)	T65.891	T65.892	T65.893	T65.894	—	—
medicinal	T5Ø.9Ø1	T5Ø.9Ø2	T5Ø.9Ø3	T5Ø.9Ø4	T5Ø.9Ø5	T5Ø.9Ø6
wood	T6Ø.91	T6Ø.92	T6Ø.93	T6Ø.94	—	—
Prethcamide	T5Ø.7X1	T5Ø.7X2	T5Ø.7X3	T5Ø.7X4	T5Ø.7X5	T5Ø.7X6
Pride of China	T62.2X1	T62.2X2	T62.2X3	T62.2X4	—	—
Pridinol	T44.3X1	T44.3X2	T44.3X3	T44.3X4	T44.3X5	T44.3X6
Prifinium bromide	T44.3X1	T44.3X2	T44.3X3	T44.3X4	T44.3X5	T44.3X6
Prilocaine	T41.3X1	T41.3X2	T41.3X3	T41.3X4	T41.3X5	T41.3X6
infiltration (subcutaneous)	T41.3X1	T41.3X2	T41.3X3	T41.3X4	T41.3X5	T41.3X6
nerve block (peripheral) (plexus)	T41.3X1	T41.3X2	T41.3X3	T41.3X4	T41.3X5	T41.3X6
regional	T41.3X1	T41.3X2	T41.3X3	T41.3X4	T41.3X5	T41.3X6
Primaquine	T37.2X1	T37.2X2	T37.2X3	T37.2X4	T37.2X5	T37.2X6
Primidone	T42.6X1	T42.6X2	T42.6X3	T42.6X4	T42.6X5	T42.6X6
Primula (veris)	T62.2X1	T62.2X2	T62.2X3	T62.2X4	—	—
Prinadol	T4Ø.2X1	T4Ø.2X2	T4Ø.2X3	T4Ø.2X4	T4Ø.2X5	T4Ø.2X6
Priscol, Priscoline	T44.6X1	T44.6X2	T44.6X3	T44.6X4	T44.6X5	T44.6X6
Pristinamycin	T36.3X1	T36.3X2	T36.3X3	T36.3X4	T36.3X5	T36.3X6
Privet	T62.2X1	T62.2X2	T62.2X3	T62.2X4	—	—
berries	T62.1X1	T62.1X2	T62.1X3	T62.1X4	—	—
Privine	T44.4X1	T44.4X2	T44.4X3	T44.4X4	T44.4X5	T44.4X6
Pro-Banthine	T44.3X1	T44.3X2	T44.3X3	T44.3X4	T44.3X5	T44.3X6
Probarbital	T42.3X1	T42.3X2	T42.3X3	T42.3X4	T42.3X5	T42.3X6
Probenecid	T5Ø.4X1	T5Ø.4X2	T5Ø.4X3	T5Ø.4X4	T5Ø.4X5	T5Ø.4X6
Probucol	T46.6X1	T46.6X2	T46.6X3	T46.6X4	T46.6X5	T46.6X6
Procainamide	T46.2X1	T46.2X2	T46.2X3	T46.2X4	T46.2X5	T46.2X6
Procaine	T41.3X1	T41.3X2	T41.3X3	T41.3X4	T41.3X5	T41.3X6
benzylpenicillin	T36.ØX1	T36.ØX2	T36.ØX3	T36.ØX4	T36.ØX5	T36.ØX6
nerve block (peripheral) (plexus)	T41.3X1	T41.3X2	T41.3X3	T41.3X4	T41.3X5	T41.3X6
penicillin G	T36.ØX1	T36.ØX2	T36.ØX3	T36.ØX4	T36.ØX5	T36.ØX6
regional	T41.3X1	T41.3X2	T41.3X3	T41.3X4	T41.3X5	T41.3X6
spinal	T41.3X1	T41.3X2	T41.3X3	T41.3X4	T41.3X5	T41.3X6
Procalmidol	T43.591	T43.592	T43.593	T43.594	T43.595	T43.596
Procarbazine	T45.1X1	T45.1X2	T45.1X3	T45.1X4	T45.1X5	T45.1X6
Procaterol	T44.5X1	T44.5X2	T44.5X3	T44.5X4	T44.5X5	T44.5X6
Prochlorperazine	T43.3X1	T43.3X2	T43.3X3	T43.3X4	T43.3X5	T43.3X6
Procyclidine	T44.3X1	T44.3X2	T44.3X3	T44.3X4	T44.3X5	T44.3X6
Producer gas	T58.8X1	T58.8X2	T58.8X3	T58.8X4	—	—
Profadol	T4Ø.4X1	T4Ø.4X2	T4Ø.4X3	T4Ø.4X4	T4Ø.4X5	T4Ø.4X6
Profenamine	T44.3X1	T44.3X2	T44.3X3	T44.3X4	T44.3X5	T44.3X6
Profenil	T44.3X1	T44.3X2	T44.3X3	T44.3X4	T44.3X5	T44.3X6
Proflavine	T49.ØX1	T49.ØX2	T49.ØX3	T49.ØX4	T49.ØX5	T49.ØX6
Progabide	T42.6X1	T42.6X2	T42.6X3	T42.6X4	T42.6X5	T42.6X6

Substance	Poisoning, Accidental (unintentional)	Poisoning, Intentional Self-harm	Poisoning, Assault	Poisoning, Undetermined	Adverse Effect	Under-dosing
Progestin	T38.5X1	T38.5X2	T38.5X3	T38.5X4	T38.5X5	T38.5X6
oral contraceptive	T38.4X1	T38.4X2	T38.4X3	T38.4X4	T38.4X5	T38.4X6
Progesterone	T38.5X1	T38.5X2	T38.5X3	T38.5X4	T38.5X5	T38.5X6
Progestogen NEC	T38.5X1	T38.5X2	T38.5X3	T38.5X4	T38.5X5	T38.5X6
Progestone	T38.5X1	T38.5X2	T38.5X3	T38.5X4	T38.5X5	T38.5X6
Proglumide	T47.1X1	T47.1X2	T47.1X3	T47.1X4	T47.1X5	T47.1X6
Proguanil	T37.2X1	T37.2X2	T37.2X3	T37.2X4	T37.2X5	T37.2X6
Prolactin	T38.811	T38.812	T38.813	T38.814	T38.815	T38.816
Prolintane	T43.691	T43.692	T43.693	T43.694	T43.695	T43.696
Proloid	T38.1X1	T38.1X2	T38.1X3	T38.1X4	T38.1X5	T38.1X6
Proluton	T38.5X1	T38.5X2	T38.5X3	T38.5X4	T38.5X5	T38.5X6
Promacetin	T37.1X1	T37.1X2	T37.1X3	T37.1X4	T37.1X5	T37.1X6
Promazine	T43.3X1	T43.3X2	T43.3X3	T43.3X4	T43.3X5	T43.3X6
Promedol	T40.2X1	T40.2X2	T40.2X3	T40.2X4	—	—
Promegestone	T38.5X1	T38.5X2	T38.5X3	T38.5X4	T38.5X5	T38.5X6
Promethazine (teoclate)	T43.3X1	T43.3X2	T43.3X3	T43.3X4	T43.3X5	T43.3X6
Promin	T37.1X1	T37.1X2	T37.1X3	T37.1X4	T37.1X5	T37.1X6
Pronase	T45.3X1	T45.3X2	T45.3X3	T45.3X4	T45.3X5	T45.3X6
Pronestyl (hydrochloride)	T46.2X1	T46.2X2	T46.2X3	T46.2X4	T46.2X5	T46.2X6
Pronetalol	T44.7X1	T44.7X2	T44.7X3	T44.7X4	T44.7X5	T44.7X6
Prontosil	T37.0X1	T37.0X2	T37.0X3	T37.0X4	T37.0X5	T37.0X6
Propachlor	T60.3X1	T60.3X2	T60.3X3	T60.3X4	—	—
Propafenone	T46.2X1	T46.2X2	T46.2X3	T46.2X4	T46.2X5	T46.2X6
Propallylonal	T42.3X1	T42.3X2	T42.3X3	T42.3X4	T42.3X5	T42.3X6
Propamidine	T49.0X1	T49.0X2	T49.0X3	T49.0X4	T49.0X5	T49.0X6
Propane (distributed in mobile container)	T59.891	T59.892	T59.893	T59.894	—	—
distributed through pipes	T59.891	T59.892	T59.893	T59.894	—	—
incomplete combustion	T58.11	T58.12	T58.13	T58.14	—	—
Propanidid	T41.291	T41.292	T41.293	T41.294	T41.295	T41.296
Propanil	T60.3X1	T60.3X2	T60.3X3	T60.3X4	—	—
1-Propanol	T51.3X1	T51.3X2	T51.3X3	T51.3X4	—	—
2-Propanol	T51.2X1	T51.2X2	T51.2X3	T51.2X4	—	—
Propantheline	T44.3X1	T44.3X2	T44.3X3	T44.3X4	T44.3X5	T44.3X6
bromide	T44.3X1	T44.3X2	T44.3X3	T44.3X4	T44.3X5	T44.3X6
Proparacaine	T41.3X1	T41.3X2	T41.3X3	T41.3X4	T41.3X5	T41.3X6
Propatylnitrate	T46.3X1	T46.3X2	T46.3X3	T46.3X4	T46.3X5	T46.3X6
Propicillin	T36.0X1	T36.0X2	T36.0X3	T36.0X4	T36.0X5	T36.0X6
Propiolactone	T49.0X1	T49.0X2	T49.0X3	T49.0X4	T49.0X5	T49.0X6
Propiomazine	T45.0X1	T45.0X2	T45.0X3	T45.0X4	T45.0X5	T45.0X6
Propionaldehyde (medicinal)	T42.6X1	T42.6X2	T42.6X3	T42.6X4	T42.6X5	T42.6X6
Propionate (calcium) (sodium)	T49.0X1	T49.0X2	T49.0X3	T49.0X4	T49.0X5	T49.0X6
Propion gel	T49.0X1	T49.0X2	T49.0X3	T49.0X4	T49.0X5	T49.0X6
Propitocaine	T41.3X1	T41.3X2	T41.3X3	T41.3X4	T41.3X5	T41.3X6
infiltration (subcutaneous)	T41.3X1	T41.3X2	T41.3X3	T41.3X4	T41.3X5	T41.3X6
nerve block (peripheral) (plexus)	T41.3X1	T41.3X2	T41.3X3	T41.3X4	T41.3X5	T41.3X6
Propofol	T41.291	T41.292	T41.293	T41.294	T41.295	T41.296
Propoxur	T60.0X1	T60.0X2	T60.0X3	T60.0X4	—	—
Propoxycaine	T41.3X1	T41.3X2	T41.3X3	T41.3X4	T41.3X5	T41.3X6
infiltration (subcutaneous)	T41.3X1	T41.3X2	T41.3X3	T41.3X4	T41.3X5	T41.3X6
nerve block (peripheral) (plexus)	T41.3X1	T41.3X2	T41.3X3	T41.3X4	T41.3X5	T41.3X6
topical (surface)	T41.3X1	T41.3X2	T41.3X3	T41.3X4	T41.3X5	T41.3X6
Propoxyphene	T40.4X1	T40.4X2	T40.4X3	T40.4X4	T40.4X5	T40.4X6
Propranolol	T44.7X1	T44.7X2	T44.7X3	T44.7X4	T44.7X5	T44.7X6
Propyl						
alcohol	T51.3X1	T51.3X2	T51.3X3	T51.3X4	—	—
carbinol	T51.3X1	T51.3X2	T51.3X3	T51.3X4	—	—
hexadrine	T44.4X1	T44.4X2	T44.4X3	T44.4X4	T44.4X5	T44.4X6
iodone	T50.8X1	T50.8X2	T50.8X3	T50.8X4	T50.8X5	T50.8X6
thiouracil	T38.2X1	T38.2X2	T38.2X3	T38.2X4	T38.2X5	T38.2X6
Propylaminopheno-thiazine	T43.3X1	T43.3X2	T43.3X3	T43.3X4	T43.3X5	T43.3X6
Propylene	T59.891	T59.892	T59.893	T59.894	—	—
Propylhexedrine	T48.5X1	T48.5X2	T48.5X3	T48.5X4	T48.5X5	T48.5X6
Propyliodone	T50.8X1	T50.8X2	T50.8X3	T50.8X4	T50.8X5	T50.8X6
Propylthiouracil	T38.2X1	T38.2X2	T38.2X3	T38.2X4	T38.2X5	T38.2X6
Propylparaben (ophthalmic)	T49.5X1	T49.5X2	T49.5X3	T49.5X4	T49.5X5	T49.5X6
Propyphenazone	T39.2X1	T39.2X2	T39.2X3	T39.2X4	T39.2X5	T39.2X6
Proquazone	T39.391	T39.392	T39.393	T39.394	T39.395	T39.396
Proscillaridin	T46.0X1	T46.0X2	T46.0X3	T46.0X4	T46.0X5	T46.0X6
Prostacyclin	T45.521	T45.522	T45.523	T45.524	T45.525	T45.526

Substance	Poisoning, Accidental (unintentional)	Poisoning, Intentional Self-harm	Poisoning, Assault	Poisoning, Undetermined	Adverse Effect	Under-dosing
Prostaglandin (I2)	T45.521	T45.522	T45.523	T45.524	T45.525	T45.526
E1	T46.7X1	T46.7X2	T46.7X3	T46.7X4	T46.7X5	T46.7X6
E2	T48.0X1	T48.0X2	T48.0X3	T48.0X4	T48.0X5	T48.0X6
F2 alpha	T48.0X1	T48.0X2	T48.0X3	T48.0X4	T48.0X5	T48.0X6
Prostigmin	T44.0X1	T44.0X2	T44.0X3	T44.0X4	T44.0X5	T44.0X6
Prosultiamine	T45.2X1	T45.2X2	T45.2X3	T45.2X4	T45.2X5	T45.2X6
Protamine sulfate	T45.7X1	T45.7X2	T45.7X3	T45.7X4	T45.7X5	T45.7X6
zinc insulin	T38.3X1	T38.3X2	T38.3X3	T38.3X4	T38.3X5	T38.3X6
Protease	T47.5X1	T47.5X2	T47.5X3	T47.5X4	T47.5X5	T47.5X6
Protectant, skin NEC	T49.3X1	T49.3X2	T49.3X3	T49.3X4	T49.3X5	T49.3X6
Protein hydrolysate	T50.991	T50.992	T50.993	T50.994	T50.995	T50.996
Prothiaden—*see* Dothiepin hydrochloride						
Prothionamide	T37.1X1	T37.1X2	T37.1X3	T37.1X4	T37.1X5	T37.1X6
Prothipendyl	T43.591	T43.592	T43.593	T43.594	T43.595	T43.596
Prothoate	T60.0X1	T60.0X2	T60.0X3	T60.0X4	—	—
Prothrombin						
activator	T45.7X1	T45.7X2	T45.7X3	T45.7X4	T45.7X5	T45.7X6
synthesis inhibitor	T45.511	T45.512	T45.513	T45.514	T45.515	T45.516
Protionamide	T37.1X1	T37.1X2	T37.1X3	T37.1X4	T37.1X5	T37.1X6
Protirelin	T38.891	T38.892	T38.893	T38.894	T38.895	T38.896
Protokylol	T48.6X1	T48.6X2	T48.6X3	T48.6X4	T48.6X5	T48.6X6
Protopam	T50.6X1	T50.6X2	T50.6X3	T50.6X4	T50.6X5	T50.6X6
Protoveratrine(s) (A) (B)	T46.5X1	T46.5X2	T46.5X3	T46.5X4	T46.5X5	T46.5X6
Protriptyline	T43.011	T43.012	T43.013	T43.014	T43.015	T43.016
Provera	T38.5X1	T38.5X2	T38.5X3	T38.5X4	T38.5X5	T38.5X6
Provitamin A	T45.2X1	T45.2X2	T45.2X3	T45.2X4	T45.2X5	T45.2X6
Proxibarbal	T42.3X1	T42.3X2	T42.3X3	T42.3X4	T42.3X5	T42.3X6
Proxymetacaine	T41.3X1	T41.3X2	T41.3X3	T41.3X4	T41.3X5	T41.3X6
Proxyphylline	T48.6X1	T48.6X2	T48.6X3	T48.6X4	T48.6X5	T48.6X6
Prozac—*see* Fluoxetine hydrochloride						
Prunus						
laurocerasus	T62.2X1	T62.2X2	T62.2X3	T62.2X4	—	—
virginiana	T62.2X1	T62.2X2	T62.2X3	T62.2X4	—	—
Prussian blue						
commercial	T65.891	T65.892	T65.893	T65.894	—	—
therapeutic	T50.6X1	T50.6X2	T50.6X3	T50.6X4	T50.6X5	T50.6X6
Prussic acid	T65.0X1	T65.0X2	T65.0X3	T65.0X4	—	—
vapor	T57.3X1	T57.3X2	T57.3X3	T57.3X4	—	—
Pseudoephedrine	T44.991	T44.992	T44.993	T44.994	T44.995	T44.996
Psilocin	T40.991	T40.992	T40.993	T40.994	—	—
Psilocybin	T40.991	T40.992	T40.993	T40.994	—	—
Psilocybine	T40.991	T40.992	T40.993	T40.994	—	—
Psoralene (nonmedicinal)	T65.891	T65.892	T65.893	T65.894	—	—
Psoralens (medicinal)	T50.991	T50.992	T50.993	T50.994	T50.995	T50.996
PSP (phenolsulfonphthalein)	T50.8X1	T50.8X2	T50.8X3	T50.8X4	T50.8X5	T50.8X6
Psychodysleptic drug NEC	T40.901	T40.902	T40.903	T40.904	T40.905	T40.906
Psychostimulant	T43.601	T43.602	T43.603	T43.604	T43.605	T43.606
amphetamine	T43.621	T43.622	T43.623	T43.624	T43.625	T43.626
caffeine	T43.611	T43.612	T43.613	T43.614	T43.615	T43.616
methylphenidate	T43.631	T43.632	T43.633	T43.634	T43.635	T43.636
specified NEC	T43.691	T43.692	T43.693	T43.694	T43.695	T43.696
Psychotherapeutic drug NEC	T43.91	T43.92	T43.93	T43.94	T43.95	T43.96
antidepressants (*see also* Antidepressant)	T43.201	T43.202	T43.203	T43.204	T43.205	T43.206
specified NEC	T43.8X1	T43.8X2	T43.8X3	T43.8X4	T43.8X5	T43.8X6
tranquilizers NEC	T43.501	T43.502	T43.503	T43.504	T43.505	T43.506
Psychotomimetic agents	T40.901	T40.902	T40.903	T40.904	T40.905	T40.906
Psychotropic drug NEC	T43.91	T43.92	T43.93	T43.94	T43.95	T43.96
specified NEC	T43.8X1	T43.8X2	T43.8X3	T43.8X4	T43.8X5	T43.8X6
Psyllium hydrophilic mucilloid	T47.4X1	T47.4X2	T47.4X3	T47.4X4	T47.4X5	T47.4X6
Pteroylglutamic acid	T45.8X1	T45.8X2	T45.8X3	T45.8X4	T45.8X5	T45.8X6
Pteroyltriglutamate	T45.1X1	T45.1X2	T45.1X3	T45.1X4	T45.1X5	T45.1X6
PTFE—*see* Polytetrafluoroethylene						
Pulp						
devitalizing paste	T49.7X1	T49.7X2	T49.7X3	T49.7X4	T49.7X5	T49.7X6
dressing	T49.7X1	T49.7X2	T49.7X3	T49.7X4	T49.7X5	T49.7X6
Pulsatilla	T62.2X1	T62.2X2	T62.2X3	T62.2X4	—	—
Pumpkin seed extract	T37.4X1	T37.4X2	T37.4X3	T37.4X4	T37.4X5	T37.4X6

Substance	Poisoning, Accidental (unintentional)	Poisoning, Intentional Self-harm	Poisoning, Assault	Poisoning, Undetermined	Adverse Effect	Under-dosing
Purex (bleach)	T54.91	T54.92	T54.93	T54.94	—	—
Purgative NEC (*see also* Cathartic)	T47.4X1	T47.4X2	T47.4X3	T47.4X4	T47.4X5	T47.4X6
Purine analogue (antineoplastic)	T45.1X1	T45.1X2	T45.1X3	T45.1X4	T45.1X5	T45.1X6
Purine diuretics	T5Ø.2X1	T5Ø.2X2	T5Ø.2X3	T5Ø.2X4	T5Ø.2X5	T5Ø.2X6
Purinethol	T45.1X1	T45.1X2	T45.1X3	T45.1X4	T45.1X5	T45.1X6
PVP	T45.8X1	T45.8X2	T45.8X3	T45.8X4	T45.8X5	T45.8X6
Pyrabital	T39.8X1	T39.8X2	T39.8X3	T39.8X4	T39.8X5	T39.8X6
Pyramidon	T39.2X1	T39.2X2	T39.2X3	T39.2X4	T39.2X5	T39.2X6
Pyrantel	T37.4X1	T37.4X2	T37.4X3	T37.4X4	T37.4X5	T37.4X6
Pyrathiazine	T45.ØX1	T45.ØX2	T45.ØX3	T45.ØX4	T45.ØX5	T45.ØX6
Pyrazinamide	T37.1X1	T37.1X2	T37.1X3	T37.1X4	T37.1X5	T37.1X6
Pyrazinoic acid (amide)	T37.1X1	T37.1X2	T37.1X3	T37.1X4	T37.1X5	T37.1X6
Pyrazole (derivatives)	T39.2X1	T39.2X2	T39.2X3	T39.2X4	T39.2X5	T39.2X6
Pyrazolone analgesic NEC	T39.2X1	T39.2X2	T39.2X3	T39.2X4	T39.2X5	T39.2X6
Pyrethrin, pyrethrum (nonmedicinal)	T6Ø.2X1	T6Ø.2X2	T6Ø.2X3	T6Ø.2X4	—	—
Pyrethrum extract	T49.ØX1	T49.ØX2	T49.ØX3	T49.ØX4	T49.ØX5	T49.ØX6
Pyribenzamine	T45.ØX1	T45.ØX2	T45.ØX3	T45.ØX4	T45.ØX5	T45.ØX6
Pyridine	T52.8X1	T52.8X2	T52.8X3	T52.8X4	—	—
aldoxime methiodide	T5Ø.6X1	T5Ø.6X2	T5Ø.6X3	T5Ø.6X4	T5Ø.6X5	T5Ø.6X6
aldoxime methyl chloride	T5Ø.6X1	T5Ø.6X2	T5Ø.6X3	T5Ø.6X4	T5Ø.6X5	T5Ø.6X6
vapor	T59.891	T59.892	T59.893	T59.894	—	—
Pyridium	T39.8X1	T39.8X2	T39.8X3	T39.8X4	T39.8X5	T39.8X6
Pyridostigmine bromide	T44.ØX1	T44.ØX2	T44.ØX3	T44.ØX4	T44.ØX5	T44.ØX6
Pyridoxal phosphate	T45.2X1	T45.2X2	T45.2X3	T45.2X4	T45.2X5	T45.2X6
Pyridoxine	T45.2X1	T45.2X2	T45.2X3	T45.2X4	T45.2X5	T45.2X6
Pyrilamine	T45.ØX1	T45.ØX2	T45.ØX3	T45.ØX4	T45.ØX5	T45.ØX6
Pyrimethamine	T37.2X1	T37.2X2	T37.2X3	T37.2X4	T37.2X5	T37.2X6
with sulfadoxine	T37.2X1	T37.2X2	T37.2X3	T37.2X4	T37.2X5	T37.2X6
Pyrimidine antagonist	T45.1X1	T45.1X2	T45.1X3	T45.1X4	T45.1X5	T45.1X6
Pyriminil	T6Ø.4X1	T6Ø.4X2	T6Ø.4X3	T6Ø.4X4	—	—
Pyrithione zinc	T49.4X1	T49.4X2	T49.4X3	T49.4X4	T49.4X5	T49.4X6
Pyrithyldione	T42.6X1	T42.6X2	T42.6X3	T42.6X4	T42.6X5	T42.6X6
Pyrogallic acid	T49.ØX1	T49.ØX2	T49.ØX3	T49.ØX4	T49.ØX5	T49.ØX6
Pyrogallol	T49.ØX1	T49.ØX2	T49.ØX3	T49.ØX4	T49.ØX5	T49.ØX6
Pyroxylin	T49.3X1	T49.3X2	T49.3X3	T49.3X4	T49.3X5	T49.3X6
Pyrrobutamine	T45.ØX1	T45.ØX2	T45.ØX3	T45.ØX4	T45.ØX5	T45.ØX6
Pyrrolizidine alkaloids	T62.8X1	T62.8X2	T62.8X3	T62.8X4	—	—
Pyrvinium chloride	T37.4X1	T37.4X2	T37.4X3	T37.4X4	T37.4X5	T37.4X6
PZI	T38.3X1	T38.3X2	T38.3X3	T38.3X4	T38.3X5	T38.3X6
Q						
Quaalude	T42.6X1	T42.6X2	T42.6X3	T42.6X4	T42.6X5	T42.6X6
Quarternary ammonium						
anti-infective	T49.ØX1	T49.ØX2	T49.ØX3	T49.ØX4	T49.ØX5	T49.ØX6
ganglion blocking	T44.2X1	T44.2X2	T44.2X3	T44.2X4	T44.2X5	T44.2X6
parasympatholytic	T44.3X1	T44.3X2	T44.3X3	T44.3X4	T44.3X5	T44.3X6
Quazepam	T42.4X1	T42.4X2	T42.4X3	T42.4X4	T42.4X5	T42.4X6
Quicklime	T54.3X1	T54.3X2	T54.3X3	T54.3X4	—	—
Quillaja extract	T48.4X1	T48.4X2	T48.4X3	T48.4X4	T48.4X5	T48.4X6
Quinacrine	T37.2X1	T37.2X2	T37.2X3	T37.2X4	T37.2X5	T37.2X6
Quinaglute	T46.2X1	T46.2X2	T46.2X3	T46.2X4	T46.2X5	T46.2X6
Quinalbarbital	T42.3X1	T42.3X2	T42.3X3	T42.3X4	T42.3X5	T42.3X6
Quinalbarbitone sodium	T42.3X1	T42.3X2	T42.3X3	T42.3X4	T42.3X5	T42.3X6
Quinalphos	T6Ø.ØX1	T6Ø.ØX2	T6Ø.ØX3	T6Ø.ØX4	—	—
Quinapril	T46.4X1	T46.4X2	T46.4X3	T46.4X4	T46.4X5	T46.4X6
Quinestradiol	T38.5X1	T38.5X2	T38.5X3	T38.5X4	T38.5X5	T38.5X6
Quinestradol	T38.5X1	T38.5X2	T38.5X3	T38.5X4	T38.5X5	T38.5X6
Quinestrol	T38.5X1	T38.5X2	T38.5X3	T38.5X4	T38.5X5	T38.5X6
Quinethazone	T5Ø.2X1	T5Ø.2X2	T5Ø.2X3	T5Ø.2X4	T5Ø.2X5	T5Ø.2X6
Quingestanol	T38.4X1	T38.4X2	T38.4X3	T38.4X4	T38.4X5	T38.4X6
Quinidine	T46.2X1	T46.2X2	T46.2X3	T46.2X4	T46.2X5	T46.2X6
Quinine	T37.2X1	T37.2X2	T37.2X3	T37.2X4	T37.2X5	T37.2X6
Quiniobine	T37.8X1	T37.8X2	T37.8X3	T37.8X4	T37.8X5	T37.8X6
Quinisocaine	T49.1X1	T49.1X2	T49.1X3	T49.1X4	T49.1X5	T49.1X6
Quinocide	T37.2X1	T37.2X2	T37.2X3	T37.2X4	T37.2X5	T37.2X6
Quinoline (derivatives) **NEC**	T37.8X1	T37.8X2	T37.8X3	T37.8X4	T37.8X5	T37.8X6
Quinupramine	T43.Ø11	T43.Ø12	T43.Ø13	T43.Ø14	T43.Ø15	T43.Ø16
Quotane	T41.3X1	T41.3X2	T41.3X3	T41.3X4	T41.3X5	T41.3X6

Substance	Poisoning, Accidental (unintentional)	Poisoning, Intentional Self-harm	Poisoning, Assault	Poisoning, Undetermined	Adverse Effect	Under-dosing
R						
Rabies						
immune globulin (human)	T5Ø.Z11	T5Ø.Z12	T5Ø.Z13	T5Ø.Z14	T5Ø.Z15	T5Ø.Z16
vaccine	T5Ø.B91	T5Ø.B92	T5Ø.B93	T5Ø.B94	T5Ø.B95	T5Ø.B96
Racemoramide	T4Ø.2X1	T4Ø.2X2	T4Ø.2X3	T4Ø.2X4	—	—
Racemorphan	T4Ø.2X1	T4Ø.2X2	T4Ø.2X3	T4Ø.2X4	T4Ø.2X5	T4Ø.2X6
Racepinefrin	T44.5X1	T44.5X2	T44.5X3	T44.5X4	T44.5X5	T44.5X6
Raclopride	T43.591	T43.592	T43.593	T43.594	T43.595	T43.596
Radiator alcohol	T51.1X1	T51.1X2	T51.1X3	T51.1X4	—	—
Radioactive drug NEC	T5Ø.8X1	T5Ø.8X2	T5Ø.8X3	T5Ø.8X4	T5Ø.8X5	T5Ø.8X6
Radio-opaque (drugs) (materials)	T5Ø.8X1	T5Ø.8X2	T5Ø.8X3	T5Ø.8X4	T5Ø.8X5	T5Ø.8X6
Ramifenazone	T39.2X1	T39.2X2	T39.2X3	T39.2X4	T39.2X5	T39.2X6
Ramipril	T46.4X1	T46.4X2	T46.4X3	T46.4X4	T46.4X5	T46.4X6
Ranitidine	T47.ØX1	T47.ØX2	T47.ØX3	T47.ØX4	T47.ØX5	T47.ØX6
Ranunculus	T62.2X1	T62.2X2	T62.2X3	T62.2X4	—	—
Rat poison NEC	T6Ø.4X1	T6Ø.4X2	T6Ø.4X3	T6Ø.4X4	—	—
Rattlesnake (venom)	T63.Ø11	T63.Ø12	T63.Ø13	T63.Ø14	—	—
Raubasine	T46.7X1	T46.7X2	T46.7X3	T46.7X4	T46.7X5	T46.7X6
Raudixin	T46.5X1	T46.5X2	T46.5X3	T46.5X4	T46.5X5	T46.5X6
Rautensin	T46.5X1	T46.5X2	T46.5X3	T46.5X4	T46.5X5	T46.5X6
Rautina	T46.5X1	T46.5X2	T46.5X3	T46.5X4	T46.5X5	T46.5X6
Rautotal	T46.5X1	T46.5X2	T46.5X3	T46.5X4	T46.5X5	T46.5X6
Rauwiloid	T46.5X1	T46.5X2	T46.5X3	T46.5X4	T46.5X5	T46.5X6
Rauwoldin	T46.5X1	T46.5X2	T46.5X3	T46.5X4	T46.5X5	T46.5X6
Rauwolfia (alkaloids)	T46.5X1	T46.5X2	T46.5X3	T46.5X4	T46.5X5	T46.5X6
Razoxane	T45.1X1	T45.1X2	T45.1X3	T45.1X4	T45.1X5	T45.1X6
Realgar	T57.ØX1	T57.ØX2	T57.ØX3	T57.ØX4	—	—
Recombinant (R)—*see* specific protein						
Red blood cells, packed	T45.8X1	T45.8X2	T45.8X3	T45.8X4	T45.8X5	T45.8X6
Red squill (scilliroside)	T6Ø.4X1	T6Ø.4X2	T6Ø.4X3	T6Ø.4X4	—	—
Reducing agent, industrial NEC	T65.891	T65.892	T65.893	T65.894	—	—
Refrigerant gas (chlorofluoro-carbon)	T53.5X1	T53.5X2	T53.5X3	T53.5X4	—	—
not chlorofluorocarbon	T59.891	T59.892	T59.893	T59.894	—	—
Regroton	T5Ø.2X1	T5Ø.2X2	T5Ø.2X3	T5Ø.2X4	T5Ø.2X5	T5Ø.2X6
Rehydration salts (oral)	T5Ø.3X1	T5Ø.3X2	T5Ø.3X3	T5Ø.3X4	T5Ø.3X5	T5Ø.3X6
Rela	T42.8X1	T42.8X2	T42.8X3	T42.8X4	T42.8X5	T42.8X6
Relaxant, muscle						
anesthetic	T48.1X1	T48.1X2	T48.1X3	T48.1X4	T48.1X5	T48.1X6
central nervous system	T42.8X1	T42.8X2	T42.8X3	T42.8X4	T42.8X5	T42.8X6
skeletal NEC	T48.1X1	T48.1X2	T48.1X3	T48.1X4	T48.1X5	T48.1X6
smooth NEC	T44.3X1	T44.3X2	T44.3X3	T44.3X4	T44.3X5	T44.3X6
Remoxipride	T43.591	T43.592	T43.593	T43.594	T43.595	T43.596
Renese	T5Ø.2X1	T5Ø.2X2	T5Ø.2X3	T5Ø.2X4	T5Ø.2X5	T5Ø.2X6
Renografin	T5Ø.8X1	T5Ø.8X2	T5Ø.8X3	T5Ø.8X4	T5Ø.8X5	T5Ø.8X6
Replacement solution	T5Ø.3X1	T5Ø.3X2	T5Ø.3X3	T5Ø.3X4	T5Ø.3X5	T5Ø.3X6
Reproterol	T48.6X1	T48.6X2	T48.6X3	T48.6X4	T48.6X5	T48.6X6
Rescinnamine	T46.5X1	T46.5X2	T46.5X3	T46.5X4	T46.5X5	T46.5X6
Reserpin(e)	T46.5X1	T46.5X2	T46.5X3	T46.5X4	T46.5X5	T46.5X6
Resorcin, resorcinol (nonmedicinal)	T65.891	T65.892	T65.893	T65.894	—	—
medicinal	T49.4X1	T49.4X2	T49.4X3	T49.4X4	T49.4X5	T49.4X6
Respaire	T48.4X1	T48.4X2	T48.4X3	T48.4X4	T48.4X5	T48.4X6
Respiratory drug NEC	T48.9Ø1	T48.9Ø2	T48.9Ø3	T48.9Ø4	T48.9Ø5	T48.9Ø6
antiasthmatic NEC	T48.6X1	T48.6X2	T48.6X3	T48.6X4	T48.6X5	T48.6X6
anti-common-cold NEC	T48.5X1	T48.5X2	T48.5X3	T48.5X4	T48.5X5	T48.5X6
expectorant NEC	T48.4X1	T48.4X2	T48.4X3	T48.4X4	T48.4X5	T48.4X6
stimulant	T48.9Ø1	T48.9Ø2	T48.9Ø3	T48.9Ø4	T48.9Ø5	T48.9Ø6
Retinoic acid	T49.ØX1	T49.ØX2	T49.ØX3	T49.ØX4	T49.ØX5	T49.ØX6
Retinol	T45.2X1	T45.2X2	T45.2X3	T45.2X4	T45.2X5	T45.2X6
Rh (D) immune globulin (human)	T5Ø.Z11	T5Ø.Z12	T5Ø.Z13	T5Ø.Z14	T5Ø.Z15	T5Ø.Z16
Rhodine	T39.Ø11	T39.Ø12	T39.Ø13	T39.Ø14	T39.Ø15	T39.Ø16
RhoGAM	T5Ø.Z11	T5Ø.Z12	T5Ø.Z13	T5Ø.Z14	T5Ø.Z15	T5Ø.Z16
Rhubarb						
dry extract	T47.2X1	T47.2X2	T47.2X3	T47.2X4	T47.2X5	T47.2X6
tincture, compound	T47.2X1	T47.2X2	T47.2X3	T47.2X4	T47.2X5	T47.2X6
Ribavirin	T37.5X1	T37.5X2	T37.5X3	T37.5X4	T37.5X5	T37.5X6
Riboflavin	T45.2X1	T45.2X2	T45.2X3	T45.2X4	T45.2X5	T45.2X6
Ribostamycin	T36.5X1	T36.5X2	T36.5X3	T36.5X4	T36.5X5	T36.5X6
Ricin	T62.2X1	T62.2X2	T62.2X3	T62.2X4	—	—

Substance	Poisoning, Accidental (unintentional)	Poisoning, Intentional Self-harm	Poisoning, Assault	Poisoning, Undetermined	Adverse Effect	Under-dosing
Ricinus communis	T62.2X1	T62.2X2	T62.2X3	T62.2X4	—	—
Rickettsial vaccine NEC	T5Ø.A91	T5Ø.A92	T5Ø.A93	T5Ø.A94	T5Ø.A95	T5Ø.A96
Rifabutin	T36.6X1	T36.6X2	T36.6X3	T36.6X4	T36.6X5	T36.6X6
Rifamide	T36.6X1	T36.6X2	T36.6X3	T36.6X4	T36.6X5	T36.6X6
Rifampicin	T36.6X1	T36.6X2	T36.6X3	T36.6X4	T36.6X5	T36.6X6
with isoniazid	T37.1X1	T37.1X2	T37.1X3	T37.1X4	T37.1X5	T37.1X6
Rifampin	T36.6X1	T36.6X2	T36.6X3	T36.6X4	T36.6X5	T36.6X6
Rifamycin	T36.6X1	T36.6X2	T36.6X3	T36.6X4	T36.6X5	T36.6X6
Rifaximin	T36.6X1	T36.6X2	T36.6X3	T36.6X4	T36.6X5	T36.6X6
Rimantadine	T37.5X1	T37.5X2	T37.5X3	T37.5X4	T37.5X5	T37.5X6
Rimazolium metilsulfate	T39.8X1	T39.8X2	T39.8X3	T39.8X4	T39.8X5	T39.8X6
Rimifon	T37.1X1	T37.1X2	T37.1X3	T37.1X4	T37.1X5	T37.1X6
Rimiterol	T48.6X1	T48.6X2	T48.6X3	T48.6X4	T48.6X5	T48.6X6
Ringer (lactate) **solution**	T5Ø.3X1	T5Ø.3X2	T5Ø.3X3	T5Ø.3X4	T5Ø.3X5	T5Ø.3X6
Ristocetin	T36.8X1	T36.8X2	T36.8X3	T36.8X4	T36.8X5	T36.8X6
Ritalin	T43.631	T43.632	T43.633	T43.634	T43.635	T43.636
Ritodrine	T44.5X1	T44.5X2	T44.5X3	T44.5X4	T44.5X5	T44.5X6
Roach killer—*see* Insecticide						
Rociverine	T44.3X1	T44.3X2	T44.3X3	T44.3X4	T44.3X5	T44.3X6
Rocky Mountain spotted fever vaccine	T5Ø.A91	T5Ø.A92	T5Ø.A93	T5Ø.A94	T5Ø.A95	T5Ø.A96
Rodenticide NEC	T6Ø.4X1	T6Ø.4X2	T6Ø.4X3	T6Ø.4X4	—	—
Rohypnol	T42.4X1	T42.4X2	T42.4X3	T42.4X4	T42.4X5	T42.4X6
Rokitamycin	T36.3X1	T36.3X2	T36.3X3	T36.3X4	T36.3X5	T36.3X6
Rolaids	T47.1X1	T47.1X2	T47.1X3	T47.1X4	T47.1X5	T47.1X6
Rolitetracycline	T36.4X1	T36.4X2	T36.4X3	T36.4X4	T36.4X5	T36.4X6
Romilar	T48.3X1	T48.3X2	T48.3X3	T48.3X4	T48.3X5	T48.3X6
Ronifibrate	T46.6X1	T46.6X2	T46.6X3	T46.6X4	T46.6X5	T46.6X6
Rosaprostol	T47.1X1	T47.1X2	T47.1X3	T47.1X4	T47.1X5	T47.1X6
Rose bengal sodium (131I)	T5Ø.8X1	T5Ø.8X2	T5Ø.8X3	T5Ø.8X4	T5Ø.8X5	T5Ø.8X6
Rose water ointment	T49.3X1	T49.3X2	T49.3X3	T49.3X4	T49.3X5	T49.3X6
Rosoxacin	T37.8X1	T37.8X2	T37.8X3	T37.8X4	T37.8X5	T37.8X6
Rotenone	T6Ø.2X1	T6Ø.2X2	T6Ø.2X3	T6Ø.2X4	—	—
Rotoxamine	T45.ØX1	T45.ØX2	T45.ØX3	T45.ØX4	T45.ØX5	T45.ØX6
Rough-on-rats	T6Ø.4X1	T6Ø.4X2	T6Ø.4X3	T6Ø.4X4	—	—
Roxatidine	T47.ØX1	T47.ØX2	T47.ØX3	T47.ØX4	T47.ØX5	T47.ØX6
Roxithromycin	T36.3X1	T36.3X2	T36.3X3	T36.3X4	T36.3X5	T36.3X6
Rt-PA	T45.611	T45.612	T45.613	T45.614	T45.615	T45.616
Rubbing alcohol	T51.2X1	T51.2X2	T51.2X3	T51.2X4	—	—
Rubefacient	T49.4X1	T49.4X2	T49.4X3	T49.4X4	T49.4X5	T49.4X6
Rubella vaccine	T5Ø.B91	T5Ø.B92	T5Ø.B93	T5Ø.B94	T5Ø.B95	T5Ø.B96
Rubeola vaccine	T5Ø.B91	T5Ø.B92	T5Ø.B93	T5Ø.B94	T5Ø.B95	T5Ø.B96
Rubidium chloride Rb82	T5Ø.8X1	T5Ø.8X2	T5Ø.8X3	T5Ø.8X4	T5Ø.8X5	T5Ø.8X6
Rubidomycin	T45.1X1	T45.1X2	T45.1X3	T45.1X4	T45.1X5	T45.1X6
Rue	T62.2X1	T62.2X2	T62.2X3	T62.2X4	—	—
Rufocromomycin	T45.1X1	T45.1X2	T45.1X3	T45.1X4	T45.1X5	T45.1X6
Russel's viper venin	T45.7X1	T45.7X2	T45.7X3	T45.7X4	T45.7X5	T45.7X6
Ruta (graveolens)	T62.2X1	T62.2X2	T62.2X3	T62.2X4	—	—
Rutinum	T46.991	T46.992	T46.993	T46.994	T46.995	T46.996
Rutoside	T46.991	T46.992	T46.993	T46.994	T46.995	T46.996
S						
Sabadilla (plant)	T62.2X1	T62.2X2	T62.2X3	T62.2X4	—	—
pesticide	T6Ø.2X1	T6Ø.2X2	T6Ø.2X3	T6Ø.2X4	—	—
Saccharated iron oxide	T45.8X1	T45.8X2	T45.8X3	T45.8X4	T45.8X5	T45.8X6
Saccharin	T5Ø.9Ø1	T5Ø.9Ø2	T5Ø.9Ø3	T5Ø.9Ø4	T5Ø.9Ø5	T5Ø.9Ø6
Saccharomyces boulardii	T47.6X1	T47.6X2	T47.6X3	T47.6X4	T47.6X5	T47.6X6
Safflower oil	T46.6X1	T46.6X2	T46.6X3	T46.6X4	T46.6X5	T46.6X6
Safrazine	T43.1X1	T43.1X2	T43.1X3	T43.1X4	T43.1X5	T43.1X6
Salazosulfapyridine	T37.ØX1	T37.ØX2	T37.ØX3	T37.ØX4	T37.ØX5	T37.ØX6
Salbutamol	T48.6X1	T48.6X2	T48.6X3	T48.6X4	T48.6X5	T48.6X6
Salicylamide	T39.Ø91	T39.Ø92	T39.Ø93	T39.Ø94	T39.Ø95	T39.Ø96
Salicylate NEC	T39.Ø91	T39.Ø92	T39.Ø93	T39.Ø94	T39.Ø95	T39.Ø96
methyl	T49.3X1	T49.3X2	T49.3X3	T49.3X4	T49.3X5	T49.3X6
theobromine calcium	T5Ø.2X1	T5Ø.2X2	T5Ø.2X3	T5Ø.2X4	T5Ø.2X5	T5Ø.2X6
Salicylazosulfapyridine	T37.ØX1	T37.ØX2	T37.ØX3	T37.ØX4	T37.ØX5	T37.ØX6
Salicylhydroxamic acid	T49.ØX1	T49.ØX2	T49.ØX3	T49.ØX4	T49.ØX5	T49.ØX6
Salicylic acid	T49.4X1	T49.4X2	T49.4X3	T49.4X4	T49.4X5	T49.4X6
with benzoic acid	T49.4X1	T49.4X2	T49.4X3	T49.4X4	T49.4X5	T49.4X6
congeners	T39.Ø91	T39.Ø92	T39.Ø93	T39.Ø94	T39.Ø95	T39.Ø96
derivative	T39.Ø91	T39.Ø92	T39.Ø93	T39.Ø94	T39.Ø95	T39.Ø96
salts	T39.Ø91	T39.Ø92	T39.Ø93	T39.Ø94	T39.Ø95	T39.Ø96
Salinazid	T37.1X1	T37.1X2	T37.1X3	T37.1X4	T37.1X5	T37.1X6
Salmeterol	T48.6X1	T48.6X2	T48.6X3	T48.6X4	T48.6X5	T48.6X6
Salol	T49.3X1	T49.3X2	T49.3X3	T49.3X4	T49.3X5	T49.3X6
Salsalate	T39.Ø91	T39.Ø92	T39.Ø93	T39.Ø94	T39.Ø95	T39.Ø96
Salt substitute	T5Ø.9Ø1	T5Ø.9Ø2	T5Ø.9Ø3	T5Ø.9Ø4	T5Ø.9Ø5	T5Ø.9Ø6
Salt-replacing drug	T5Ø.9Ø1	T5Ø.9Ø2	T5Ø.9Ø3	T5Ø.9Ø4	T5Ø.9Ø5	T5Ø.9Ø6
Salt-retaining mineralocorticoid	T5Ø.ØX1	T5Ø.ØX2	T5Ø.ØX3	T5Ø.ØX4	T5Ø.ØX5	T5Ø.ØX6
Saluretic NEC	T5Ø.2X1	T5Ø.2X2	T5Ø.2X3	T5Ø.2X4	T5Ø.2X5	T5Ø.2X6
Saluron	T5Ø.2X1	T5Ø.2X2	T5Ø.2X3	T5Ø.2X4	T5Ø.2X5	T5Ø.2X6
Salvarsan 606 (neosilver) (silver)	T37.8X1	T37.8X2	T37.8X3	T37.8X4	T37.8X5	T37.8X6
Sambucus canadensis	T62.2X1	T62.2X2	T62.2X3	T62.2X4	—	—
berry	T62.1X1	T62.1X2	T62.1X3	T62.1X4	—	—
Sandril	T46.5X1	T46.5X2	T46.5X3	T46.5X4	T46.5X5	T46.5X6
Sanguinaria canadensis	T62.2X1	T62.2X2	T62.2X3	T62.2X4	—	—
Saniflush (cleaner)	T54.2X1	T54.2X2	T54.2X3	T54.2X4	—	—
Santonin	T37.4X1	T37.4X2	T37.4X3	T37.4X4	T37.4X5	T37.4X6
Santyl	T49.8X1	T49.8X2	T49.8X3	T49.8X4	T49.8X5	T49.8X6
Saralasin	T46.5X1	T46.5X2	T46.5X3	T46.5X4	T46.5X5	T46.5X6
Sarcolysin	T45.1X1	T45.1X2	T45.1X3	T45.1X4	T45.1X5	T45.1X6
Sarkomycin	T45.1X1	T45.1X2	T45.1X3	T45.1X4	T45.1X5	T45.1X6
Saroten	T43.Ø11	T43.Ø12	T43.Ø13	T43.Ø14	T43.Ø15	T43.Ø16
Saturnine—*see* Lead						
Savin (oil)	T49.4X1	T49.4X2	T49.4X3	T49.4X4	T49.4X5	T49.4X6
Scammony	T47.2X1	T47.2X2	T47.2X3	T47.2X4	T47.2X5	T47.2X6
Scarlet red	T49.8X1	T49.8X2	T49.8X3	T49.8X4	T49.8X5	T49.8X6
Scheele's green	T57.ØX1	T57.ØX2	T57.ØX3	T57.ØX4	—	—
insecticide	T57.ØX1	T57.ØX2	T57.ØX3	T57.ØX4	—	—
Schizontozide (blood) (tissue)	T37.2X1	T37.2X2	T37.2X3	T37.2X4	T37.2X5	T37.2X6
Schradan	T6Ø.ØX1	T6Ø.ØX2	T6Ø.ØX3	T6Ø.ØX4	—	—
Schweinfurth green	T57.ØX1	T57.ØX2	T57.ØX3	T57.ØX4	—	—
insecticide	T57.ØX1	T57.ØX2	T57.ØX3	T57.ØX4	—	—
Scilla, rat poison	T6Ø.4X1	T6Ø.4X2	T6Ø.4X3	T6Ø.4X4	—	—
Scillaren	T6Ø.4X1	T6Ø.4X2	T6Ø.4X3	T6Ø.4X4	—	—
Sclerosing agent	T46.8X1	T46.8X2	T46.8X3	T46.8X4	T46.8X5	T46.8X6
Scombrotoxin	T61.11	T61.12	T61.13	T61.14	—	—
Scopolamine	T44.3X1	T44.3X2	T44.3X3	T44.3X4	T44.3X5	T44.3X6
Scopolia extract	T44.3X1	T44.3X2	T44.3X3	T44.3X4	T44.3X5	T44.3X6
Scouring powder	T65.891	T65.892	T65.893	T65.894		
Sea						
anemone (sting)	T63.631	T63.632	T63.633	T63.634	—	—
cucumber (sting)	T63.691	T63.692	T63.693	T63.694	—	—
snake (bite) (venom)	T63.Ø91	T63.Ø92	T63.Ø93	T63.Ø94	—	—
urchin spine (puncture)	T63.691	T63.692	T63.693	T63.694	—	—
Seafood	T61.91	T61.92	T61.93	T61.94	—	—
specified NEC	T61.8X1	T61.8X2	T61.8X3	T61.8X4	—	—
Secbutabarbital	T42.3X1	T42.3X2	T42.3X3	T42.3X4	T42.3X5	T42.3X6
Secbutabarbitone	T42.3X1	T42.3X2	T42.3X3	T42.3X4	T42.3X5	T42.3X6
Secnidazole	T37.3X1	T37.3X2	T37.3X3	T37.3X4	T37.3X5	T37.3X6
Secobarbital	T42.3X1	T42.3X2	T42.3X3	T42.3X4	T42.3X5	T42.3X6
Seconal	T42.3X1	T42.3X2	T42.3X3	T42.3X4	T42.3X5	T42.3X6
Secretin	T5Ø.8X1	T5Ø.8X2	T5Ø.8X3	T5Ø.8X4	T5Ø.8X5	T5Ø.8X6
Sedative NEC	T42.71	T42.72	T42.73	T42.74	T42.75	T42.76
mixed NEC	T42.6X1	T42.6X2	T42.6X3	T42.6X4	T42.6X5	T42.6X6
Sedormid	T42.6X1	T42.6X2	T42.6X3	T42.6X4	T42.6X5	T42.6X6
Seed disinfectant or dressing	T6Ø.8X1	T6Ø.8X2	T6Ø.8X3	T6Ø.8X4	—	—
Seeds (poisonous)	T62.2X1	T62.2X2	T62.2X3	T62.2X4	—	—
Selegiline	T42.8X1	T42.8X2	T42.8X3	T42.8X4	T42.8X5	T42.8X6
Selenium NEC	T56.891	T56.892	T56.893	T56.894	—	—
disulfide or sulfide	T49.4X1	T49.4X2	T49.4X3	T49.4X4	T49.4X5	T49.4X6
fumes	T59.891	T59.892	T59.893	T59.894	—	—
sulfide	T49.4X1	T49.4X2	T49.4X3	T49.4X4	T49.4X5	T49.4X6
Selenomethionine (75Se)	T5Ø.8X1	T5Ø.8X2	T5Ø.8X3	T5Ø.8X4	T5Ø.8X5	T5Ø.8X6
Selsun	T49.4X1	T49.4X2	T49.4X3	T49.4X4	T49.4X5	T49.4X6
Semustine	T45.1X1	T45.1X2	T45.1X3	T45.1X4	T45.1X5	T45.1X6
Senega syrup	T48.4X1	T48.4X2	T48.4X3	T48.4X4	T48.4X5	T48.4X6
Senna	T47.2X1	T47.2X2	T47.2X3	T47.2X4	T47.2X5	T47.2X6
Sennoside A+B	T47.2X1	T47.2X2	T47.2X3	T47.2X4	T47.2X5	T47.2X6
Septisol	T49.2X1	T49.2X2	T49.2X3	T49.2X4	T49.2X5	T49.2X6
Seractide	T38.811	T38.812	T38.813	T38.814	T38.815	T38.816
Serax	T42.4X1	T42.4X2	T42.4X3	T42.4X4	T42.4X5	T42.4X6

Substance	Poisoning, Accidental (unintentional)	Poisoning, Intentional Self-harm	Poisoning, Assault	Poisoning, Undetermined	Adverse Effect	Under-dosing
Serenesil	T42.6X1	T42.6X2	T42.6X3	T42.6X4	T42.6X5	T42.6X6
Serenium (hydrochloride)	T37.91	T37.92	T37.93	T37.94	T37.95	T37.96
Serepax—*see* Oxazepam						
Sermorelin	T38.891	T38.892	T38.893	T38.894	T38.895	T38.896
Sernyl	T41.1X1	T41.1X2	T41.1X3	T41.1X4	T41.1X5	T41.1X6
Serotonin	T5Ø.991	T5Ø.992	T5Ø.993	T5Ø.994	T5Ø.995	T5Ø.996
Serpasil	T46.5X1	T46.5X2	T46.5X3	T46.5X4	T46.5X5	T46.5X6
Serrapeptase	T45.3X1	T45.3X2	T45.3X3	T45.3X4	T45.3X5	T45.3X6
Serum						
antibotulinus	T5Ø.Z11	T5Ø.Z12	T5Ø.Z13	T5Ø.Z14	T5Ø.Z15	T5Ø.Z16
anticytotoxic	T5Ø.Z11	T5Ø.Z12	T5Ø.Z13	T5Ø.Z14	T5Ø.Z15	T5Ø.Z16
antidiphtheria	T5Ø.Z11	T5Ø.Z12	T5Ø.Z13	T5Ø.Z14	T5Ø.Z15	T5Ø.Z16
antimeningococcus	T5Ø.Z11	T5Ø.Z12	T5Ø.Z13	T5Ø.Z14	T5Ø.Z15	T5Ø.Z16
anti-Rh	T5Ø.Z11	T5Ø.Z12	T5Ø.Z13	T5Ø.Z14	T5Ø.Z15	T5Ø.Z16
anti-snake-bite	T5Ø.Z11	T5Ø.Z12	T5Ø.Z13	T5Ø.Z14	T5Ø.Z15	T5Ø.Z16
antitetanic	T5Ø.Z11	T5Ø.Z12	T5Ø.Z13	T5Ø.Z14	T5Ø.Z15	T5Ø.Z16
antitoxic	T5Ø.Z11	T5Ø.Z12	T5Ø.Z13	T5Ø.Z14	T5Ø.Z15	T5Ø.Z16
complement (inhibitor)	T45.8X1	T45.8X2	T45.8X3	T45.8X4	T45.8X5	T45.8X6
convalescent	T5Ø.Z11	T5Ø.Z12	T5Ø.Z13	T5Ø.Z14	T5Ø.Z15	T5Ø.Z16
hemolytic complement	T45.8X1	T45.8X2	T45.8X3	T45.8X4	T45.8X5	T45.8X6
immune (human)	T5Ø.Z11	T5Ø.Z12	T5Ø.Z13	T5Ø.Z14	T5Ø.Z15	T5Ø.Z16
protective NEC	T5Ø.Z11	T5Ø.Z12	T5Ø.Z13	T5Ø.Z14	T5Ø.Z15	T5Ø.Z16
Setastine	T45.ØX1	T45.ØX2	T45.ØX3	T45.ØX4	T45.ØX5	T45.ØX6
Setoperone	T43.591	T43.592	T43.593	T43.594	T43.595	T43.596
Sewer gas	T59.91	T59.92	T59.93	T59.94	—	—
Shampoo	T55.ØX1	T55.ØX2	T55.ØX3	T55.ØX4	—	—
Shellfish, noxious, nonbacterial	T61.781	T61.782	T61.783	T61.784	—	—
Sildenafil	T46.7X1	T46.7X2	T46.7X3	T46.7X4	T46.7X5	T46.7X6
Silibinin	T5Ø.991	T5Ø.992	T5Ø.993	T5Ø.994	T5Ø.995	T5Ø.996
Silicone NEC	T65.891	T65.892	T65.893	T65.894	—	—
medicinal	T49.3X1	T49.3X2	T49.3X3	T49.3X4	T49.3X5	T49.3X6
Silvadene	T49.ØX1	T49.ØX2	T49.ØX3	T49.ØX4	T49.ØX5	T49.ØX6
Silver	T49.ØX1	T49.ØX2	T49.ØX3	T49.ØX4	T49.ØX5	T49.ØX6
anti-infectives	T49.ØX1	T49.ØX2	T49.ØX3	T49.ØX4	T49.ØX5	T49.ØX6
arsphenamine	T37.8X1	T37.8X2	T37.8X3	T37.8X4	T37.8X5	T37.8X6
colloidal	T49.ØX1	T49.ØX2	T49.ØX3	T49.ØX4	T49.ØX5	T49.ØX6
nitrate	T49.ØX1	T49.ØX2	T49.ØX3	T49.ØX4	T49.ØX5	T49.ØX6
ophthalmic preparation	T49.5X1	T49.5X2	T49.5X3	T49.5X4	T49.5X5	T49.5X6
toughened (keratolytic)	T49.4X1	T49.4X2	T49.4X3	T49.4X4	T49.4X5	T49.4X6
nonmedicinal (dust)	T56.891	T56.892	T56.893	T56.894	—	—
protein	T49.5X1	T49.5X2	T49.5X3	T49.5X4	T49.5X5	T49.5X6
salvarsan	T37.8X1	T37.8X2	T37.8X3	T37.8X4	T37.8X5	T37.8X6
sulfadiazine	T49.4X1	T49.4X2	T49.4X3	T49.4X4	T49.4X5	T49.4X6
Silymarin	T5Ø.991	T5Ø.992	T5Ø.993	T5Ø.994	T5Ø.995	T5Ø.996
Simaldrate	T47.1X1	T47.1X2	T47.1X3	T47.1X4	T47.1X5	T47.1X6
Simazine	T6Ø.3X1	T6Ø.3X2	T6Ø.3X3	T6Ø.3X4	—	—
Simethicone	T47.1X1	T47.1X2	T47.1X3	T47.1X4	T47.1X5	T47.1X6
Simfibrate	T46.6X1	T46.6X2	T46.6X3	T46.6X4	T46.6X5	T46.6X6
Simvastatin	T46.6X1	T46.6X2	T46.6X3	T46.6X4	T46.6X5	T46.6X6
Sincalide	T5Ø.8X1	T5Ø.8X2	T5Ø.8X3	T5Ø.8X4	T5Ø.8X5	T5Ø.8X6
Sinequan	T43.Ø11	T43.Ø12	T43.Ø13	T43.Ø14	T43.Ø15	T43.Ø16
Singoserp	T46.5X1	T46.5X2	T46.5X3	T46.5X4	T46.5X5	T46.5X6
Sintrom	T45.511	T45.512	T45.513	T45.514	T45.515	T45.516
Sisomicin	T36.5X1	T36.5X2	T36.5X3	T36.5X4	T36.5X5	T36.5X6
Sitosterols	T46.6X1	T46.6X2	T46.6X3	T46.6X4	T46.6X5	T46.6X6
Skeletal muscle relaxants	T48.1X1	T48.1X2	T48.1X3	T48.1X4	T48.1X5	T48.1X6
Skin						
agents (external)	T49.91	T49.92	T49.93	T49.94	T49.95	T49.96
specified NEC	T49.8X1	T49.8X2	T49.8X3	T49.8X4	T49.8X5	T49.8X6
test antigen	T5Ø.8X1	T5Ø.8X2	T5Ø.8X3	T5Ø.8X4	T5Ø.8X5	T5Ø.8X6
Sleep-eze	T45.ØX1	T45.ØX2	T45.ØX3	T45.ØX4	T45.ØX5	T45.ØX6
Sleeping draught, pill	T42.71	T42.72	T42.73	T42.74	T42.75	T42.76
Smallpox vaccine	T5Ø.B11	T5Ø.B12	T5Ø.B13	T5Ø.B14	T5Ø.B15	T5Ø.B16
Smelter fumes NEC	T56.91	T56.92	T56.93	T56.94	—	—
Smog	T59.1X1	T59.1X2	T59.1X3	T59.1X4	—	—
Smoke NEC	T59.811	T59.812	T59.813	T59.814	—	—
Smooth muscle relaxant	T44.3X1	T44.3X2	T44.3X3	T44.3X4	T44.3X5	T44.3X6
Snail killer NEC	T6Ø.8X1	T6Ø.8X2	T6Ø.8X3	T6Ø.8X4	—	—
Snake venom or bite	T63.ØØ1	T63.ØØ2	T63.ØØ3	T63.ØØ4	—	—
hemocoagulase	T45.7X1	T45.7X2	T45.7X3	T45.7X4	T45.7X5	T45.7X6
Snuff	T65.211	T65.212	T65.213	T65.214	—	—

Substance	Poisoning, Accidental (unintentional)	Poisoning, Intentional Self-harm	Poisoning, Assault	Poisoning, Undetermined	Adverse Effect	Under-dosing
Soap (powder) (product)	T55.ØX1	T55.ØX2	T55.ØX3	T55.ØX4	—	—
enema	T47.4X1	T47.4X2	T47.4X3	T47.4X4	T47.4X5	T47.4X6
medicinal, soft	T49.2X1	T49.2X2	T49.2X3	T49.2X4	T49.2X5	T49.2X6
superfatted	T49.2X1	T49.2X2	T49.2X3	T49.2X4	T49.2X5	T49.2X6
Sobrerol	T48.4X1	T48.4X2	T48.4X3	T48.4X4	T48.4X5	T48.4X6
Soda (caustic)	T54.3X1	T54.3X2	T54.3X3	T54.3X4	—	—
bicarb	T47.1X1	T47.1X2	T47.1X3	T47.1X4	T47.1X5	T47.1X6
chlorinated—*see* Sodium, hypochlorite						
Sodium						
acetosulfone	T37.1X1	T37.1X2	T37.1X3	T37.1X4	T37.1X5	T37.1X6
acetrizoate	T5Ø.8X1	T5Ø.8X2	T5Ø.8X3	T5Ø.8X4	T5Ø.8X5	T5Ø.8X6
acid phosphate	T5Ø.3X1	T5Ø.3X2	T5Ø.3X3	T5Ø.3X4	T5Ø.3X5	T5Ø.3X6
alginate	T47.8X1	T47.8X2	T47.8X3	T47.8X4	T47.8X5	T47.8X6
amidotrizoate	T5Ø.8X1	T5Ø.8X2	T5Ø.8X3	T5Ø.8X4	T5Ø.8X5	T5Ø.8X6
aminopterin	T45.1X1	T45.1X2	T45.1X3	T45.1X4	T45.1X5	T45.1X6
amylosulfate	T47.8X1	T47.8X2	T47.8X3	T47.8X4	T47.8X5	T47.8X6
amytal	T42.3X1	T42.3X2	T42.3X3	T42.3X4	T42.3X5	T42.3X6
antimony gluconate	T37.3X1	T37.3X2	T37.3X3	T37.3X4	T37.3X5	T37.3X6
arsenate	T57.ØX1	T57.ØX2	T57.ØX3	T57.ØX4	—	—
aurothiomalate	T39.4X1	T39.4X2	T39.4X3	T39.4X4	T39.4X5	T39.4X6
aurothiosulfate	T39.4X1	T39.4X2	T39.4X3	T39.4X4	T39.4X5	T39.4X6
barbiturate	T42.3X1	T42.3X2	T42.3X3	T42.3X4	T42.3X5	T42.3X6
basic phosphate	T47.4X1	T47.4X2	T47.4X3	T47.4X4	T47.4X5	T47.4X6
bicarbonate	T47.1X1	T47.1X2	T47.1X3	T47.1X4	T47.1X5	T47.1X6
bichromate	T57.8X1	T57.8X2	T57.8X3	T57.8X4	—	—
biphosphate	T5Ø.3X1	T5Ø.3X2	T5Ø.3X3	T5Ø.3X4	T5Ø.3X5	T5Ø.3X6
bisulfate	T65.891	T65.892	T65.893	T65.894	—	—
borate						
cleanser	T57.8X1	T57.8X2	T57.8X3	T57.8X4	—	—
eye	T49.5X1	T49.5X2	T49.5X3	T49.5X4	T49.5X5	T49.5X6
therapeutic	T49.8X1	T49.8X2	T49.8X3	T49.8X4	T49.8X5	T49.8X6
bromide	T42.6X1	T42.6X2	T42.6X3	T42.6X4	T42.6X5	T42.6X6
cacodylate (nonmedicinal) NEC	T5Ø.8X1	T5Ø.8X2	T5Ø.8X3	T5Ø.8X4	T5Ø.8X5	T5Ø.8X6
anti-infective	T37.8X1	T37.8X2	T37.8X3	T37.8X4	T37.8X5	T37.8X6
herbicide	T6Ø.3X1	T6Ø.3X2	T6Ø.3X3	T6Ø.3X4	—	—
calcium edetate	T45.8X1	T45.8X2	T45.8X3	T45.8X4	T45.8X5	T45.8X6
carbonate NEC	T54.3X1	T54.3X2	T54.3X3	T54.3X4	—	—
chlorate NEC	T65.891	T65.892	T65.893	T65.894	—	—
herbicide	T54.91	T54.92	T54.93	T54.94	—	—
chloride	T5Ø.3X1	T5Ø.3X2	T5Ø.3X3	T5Ø.3X4	T5Ø.3X5	T5Ø.3X6
with glucose	T5Ø.3X1	T5Ø.3X2	T5Ø.3X3	T5Ø.3X4	T5Ø.3X5	T5Ø.3X6
chromate	T65.891	T65.892	T65.893	T65.894	—	—
citrate	T5Ø.991	T5Ø.992	T5Ø.993	T5Ø.994	T5Ø.995	T5Ø.996
cromoglicate	T48.6X1	T48.6X2	T48.6X3	T48.6X4	T48.6X5	T48.6X6
cyanide	T65.ØX1	T65.ØX2	T65.ØX3	T65.ØX4	—	—
cyclamate	T5Ø.3X1	T5Ø.3X2	T5Ø.3X3	T5Ø.3X4	T5Ø.3X5	T5Ø.3X6
dehydrocholate	T45.8X1	T45.8X2	T45.8X3	T45.8X4	T45.8X5	T45.8X6
diatrizoate	T5Ø.8X1	T5Ø.8X2	T5Ø.8X3	T5Ø.8X4	T5Ø.8X5	T5Ø.8X6
dibunate	T48.4X1	T48.4X2	T48.4X3	T48.4X4	T48.4X5	T48.4X6
dioctyl sulfosuccinate	T47.4X1	T47.4X2	T47.4X3	T47.4X4	T47.4X5	T47.4X6
dipantoyl ferrate	T45.8X1	T45.8X2	T45.8X3	T45.8X4	T45.8X5	T45.8X6
edetate	T45.8X1	T45.8X2	T45.8X3	T45.8X4	T45.8X5	T45.8X6
ethacrynate	T5Ø.1X1	T5Ø.1X2	T5Ø.1X3	T5Ø.1X4	T5Ø.1X5	T5Ø.1X6
feredetate	T45.8X1	T45.8X2	T45.8X3	T45.8X4	T45.8X5	T45.8X6
fluoride—*see* Fluoride						
fluoroacetate (dust) (pesticide)	T6Ø.4X1	T6Ø.4X2	T6Ø.4X3	T6Ø.4X4	—	—
free salt	T5Ø.3X1	T5Ø.3X2	T5Ø.3X3	T5Ø.3X4	T5Ø.3X5	T5Ø.3X6
fusidate	T36.8X1	T36.8X2	T36.8X3	T36.8X4	T36.8X5	T36.8X6
glucaldrate	T47.1X1	T47.1X2	T47.1X3	T47.1X4	T47.1X5	T47.1X6
glucosulfone	T37.1X1	T37.1X2	T37.1X3	T37.1X4	T37.1X5	T37.1X6
glutamate	T45.8X1	T45.8X2	T45.8X3	T45.8X4	T45.8X5	T45.8X6
hydrogen carbonate	T5Ø.3X1	T5Ø.3X2	T5Ø.3X3	T5Ø.3X4	T5Ø.3X5	T5Ø.3X6
hydroxide	T54.3X1	T54.3X2	T54.3X3	T54.3X4	—	—
hypochlorite (bleach) NEC	T54.3X1	T54.3X2	T54.3X3	T54.3X4	—	—
disinfectant	T54.3X1	T54.3X2	T54.3X3	T54.3X4	—	—
medicinal (anti-infective) (external)	T49.ØX1	T49.ØX2	T49.ØX3	T49.ØX4	T49.ØX5	T49.ØX6
vapor	T54.3X1	T54.3X2	T54.3X3	T54.3X4	—	—
hyposulfite	T49.ØX1	T49.ØX2	T49.ØX3	T49.ØX4	T49.ØX5	T49.ØX6
indigotin disulfonate	T5Ø.8X1	T5Ø.8X2	T5Ø.8X3	T5Ø.8X4	T5Ø.8X5	T5Ø.8X6

Substance	Poisoning, Accidental (unintentional)	Poisoning, Intentional Self-harm	Poisoning, Assault	Poisoning, Undetermined	Adverse Effect	Under-dosing
Sodium— *continued*						
iodide	T5Ø.991	T5Ø.992	T5Ø.993	T5Ø.994	T5Ø.995	T5Ø.996
I-131	T5Ø.8X1	T5Ø.8X2	T5Ø.8X3	T5Ø.8X4	T5Ø.8X5	T5Ø.8X6
therapeutic	T38.2X1	T38.2X2	T38.2X3	T38.2X4	T38.2X5	T38.2X6
iodohippurate (131I)	T5Ø.8X1	T5Ø.8X2	T5Ø.8X3	T5Ø.8X4	T5Ø.8X5	T5Ø.8X6
iopodate	T5Ø.8X1	T5Ø.8X2	T5Ø.8X3	T5Ø.8X4	T5Ø.8X5	T5Ø.8X6
iothalamate	T5Ø.8X1	T5Ø.8X2	T5Ø.8X3	T5Ø.8X4	T5Ø.8X5	T5Ø.8X6
iron edetate	T45.4X1	T45.4X2	T45.4X3	T45.4X4	T45.4X5	T45.4X6
lactate (compound solution)	T45.8X1	T45.8X2	T45.8X3	T45.8X4	T45.8X5	T45.8X6
lauryl (sulfate)	T49.2X1	T49.2X2	T49.2X3	T49.2X4	T49.2X5	T49.2X6
(L) -triiodothyronine	T38.1X1	T38.1X2	T38.1X3	T38.1X4	T38.1X5	T38.1X6
magnesium citrate	T5Ø.991	T5Ø.992	T5Ø.993	T5Ø.994	T5Ø.995	T5Ø.996
mersalate	T5Ø.2X1	T5Ø.2X2	T5Ø.2X3	T5Ø.2X4	T5Ø.2X5	T5Ø.2X6
metasilicate	T65.891	T65.892	T65.893	T65.894	—	—
metrizoate	T5Ø.8X1	T5Ø.8X2	T5Ø.8X3	T5Ø.8X4	T5Ø.8X5	T5Ø.8X6
monofluoroacetate (pesticide)	T6Ø.1X1	T6Ø.1X2	T6Ø.1X3	T6Ø.1X4	—	—
morrhuate	T46.8X1	T46.8X2	T46.8X3	T46.8X4	T46.8X5	T46.8X6
nafcillin	T36.ØX1	T36.ØX2	T36.ØX3	T36.ØX4	T36.ØX5	T36.ØX6
nitrate(oxidizing agent)	T65.891	T65.892	T65.893	T65.894	—	—
nitrite	T5Ø.6X1	T5Ø.6X2	T5Ø.6X3	T5Ø.6X4	T5Ø.6X5	T5Ø.6X6
nitroferricyanide	T46.5X1	T46.5X2	T46.5X3	T46.5X4	T46.5X5	T46.5X6
nitroprusside	T46.5X1	T46.5X2	T46.5X3	T46.5X4	T46.5X5	T46.5X6
oxalate	T65.891	T65.892	T65.893	T65.894	—	—
oxide/peroxide	T65.891	T65.892	T65.893	T65.894	—	—
oxybate	T41.291	T41.292	T41.293	T41.294	T41.295	T41.296
para-aminohippurate	T5Ø.8X1	T5Ø.8X2	T5Ø.8X3	T5Ø.8X4	T5Ø.8X5	T5Ø.8X6
perborate (nonmedicinal) NEC	T65.891	T65.892	T65.893	T65.894	—	—
medicinal	T49.ØX1	T49.ØX2	T49.ØX3	T49.ØX4	T49.ØX5	T49.ØX6
soap	T55.ØX1	T55.ØX2	T55.ØX3	T55.ØX4	—	—
percarbonate—*see* Sodium, perborate						
pertechnetate Tc99m	T5Ø.8X1	T5Ø.8X2	T5Ø.8X3	T5Ø.8X4	T5Ø.8X5	T5Ø.8X6
phosphate						
cellulose	T45.8X1	T45.8X2	T45.8X3	T45.8X4	T45.8X5	T45.8X6
dibasic	T47.2X1	T47.2X2	T47.2X3	T47.2X4	T47.2X5	T47.2X6
monobasic	T47.2X1	T47.2X2	T47.2X3	T47.2X4	T47.2X5	T47.2X6
phytate	T5Ø.6X1	T5Ø.6X2	T5Ø.6X3	T5Ø.6X4	T5Ø.6X5	T5Ø.6X6
picosulfate	T47.2X1	T47.2X2	T47.2X3	T47.2X4	T47.2X5	T47.2X6
polyhydroxyaluminium monocarbonate	T47.1X1	T47.1X2	T47.1X3	T47.1X4	T47.1X5	T47.1X6
polystyrene sulfonate	T5Ø.3X1	T5Ø.3X2	T5Ø.3X3	T5Ø.3X4	T5Ø.3X5	T5Ø.3X6
propionate	T49.ØX1	T49.ØX2	T49.ØX3	T49.ØX4	T49.ØX5	T49.ØX6
propyl hydroxybenzoate	T5Ø.991	T5Ø.992	T5Ø.993	T5Ø.994	T5Ø.995	T5Ø.996
psylliate	T46.8X1	T46.8X2	T46.8X3	T46.8X4	T46.8X5	T46.8X6
removing resins	T5Ø.3X1	T5Ø.3X2	T5Ø.3X3	T5Ø.3X4	T5Ø.3X5	T5Ø.3X6
salicylate	T39.Ø91	T39.Ø92	T39.Ø93	T39.Ø94	T39.Ø95	T39.Ø96
salt NEC	T5Ø.3X1	T5Ø.3X2	T5Ø.3X3	T5Ø.3X4	T5Ø.3X5	T5Ø.3X6
selenate	T6Ø.2X1	T6Ø.2X2	T6Ø.2X3	T6Ø.2X4	—	—
stibogluconate	T37.3X1	T37.3X2	T37.3X3	T37.3X4	T37.3X5	T37.3X6
sulfate	T47.4X1	T47.4X2	T47.4X3	T47.4X4	T47.4X5	T47.4X6
sulfoxone	T37.1X1	T37.1X2	T37.1X3	T37.1X4	T37.1X5	T37.1X6
tetradecyl sulfate	T46.8X1	T46.8X2	T46.8X3	T46.8X4	T46.8X5	T46.8X6
thiopental	T41.1X1	T41.1X2	T41.1X3	T41.1X4	T41.1X5	T41.1X6
thiosalicylate	T39.Ø91	T39.Ø92	T39.Ø93	T39.Ø94	T39.Ø95	T39.Ø96
thiosulfate	T5Ø.6X1	T5Ø.6X2	T5Ø.6X3	T5Ø.6X4	T5Ø.6X5	T5Ø.6X6
tolbutamide	T38.3X1	T38.3X2	T38.3X3	T38.3X4	T38.3X5	T38.3X6
tyropanoate	T5Ø.8X1	T5Ø.8X2	T5Ø.8X3	T5Ø.8X4	T5Ø.8X5	T5Ø.8X6
valproate	T42.6X1	T42.6X2	T42.6X3	T42.6X4	T42.6X5	T42.6X6
versenate	T5Ø.6X1	T5Ø.6X2	T5Ø.6X3	T5Ø.6X4	T5Ø.6X5	T5Ø.6X6
Sodium-free salt	T5Ø.9Ø1	T5Ø.9Ø2	T5Ø.9Ø3	T5Ø.9Ø4	T5Ø.9Ø5	T5Ø.9Ø6
Sodium-removing resin	T5Ø.3X1	T5Ø.3X2	T5Ø.3X3	T5Ø.3X4	T5Ø.3X5	T5Ø.3X6
Soft soap	T55.ØX1	T55.ØX2	T55.ØX3	T55.ØX4	—	—
Solanine	T62.2X1	T62.2X2	T62.2X3	T62.2X4	—	—
berries	T62.1X1	T62.1X2	T62.1X3	T62.1X4	—	—
Solanum dulcamara	T62.2X1	T62.2X2	T62.2X3	T62.2X4	—	—
berries	T62.1X1	T62.1X2	T62.1X3	T62.1X4	—	—
Solapsone	T37.1X1	T37.1X2	T37.1X3	T37.1X4	T37.1X5	T37.1X6
Solar lotion	T49.3X1	T49.3X2	T49.3X3	T49.3X4	T49.3X5	T49.3X6
Solasulfone	T37.1X1	T37.1X2	T37.1X3	T37.1X4	T37.1X5	T37.1X6
Soldering fluid	T65.891	T65.892	T65.893	T65.894	—	—
Solid substance	T65.91	T65.92	T65.93	T65.94	—	—
specified NEC	T65.891	T65.892	T65.893	T65.894	—	—
Solvent, industrial NEC	T52.91	T52.92	T52.93	T52.94	—	—
naphtha	T52.ØX1	T52.ØX2	T52.ØX3	T52.ØX4	—	—
petroleum	T52.ØX1	T52.ØX2	T52.ØX3	T52.ØX4	—	—
specified NEC	T52.8X1	T52.8X2	T52.8X3	T52.8X4	—	—
Soma	T42.8X1	T42.8X2	T42.8X3	T42.8X4	T42.8X5	T42.8X6
Somatorelin	T38.891	T38.892	T38.893	T38.894	T38.895	T38.896
Somatostatin	T38.991	T38.992	T38.993	T38.994	T38.995	T38.996
Somatotropin	T38.811	T38.812	T38.813	T38.814	T38.815	T38.816
Somatrem	T38.811	T38.812	T38.813	T38.814	T38.815	T38.816
Somatropin	T38.811	T38.812	T38.813	T38.814	T38.815	T38.816
Sominex	T45.ØX1	T45.ØX2	T45.ØX3	T45.ØX4	T45.ØX5	T45.ØX6
Somnos	T42.6X1	T42.6X2	T42.6X3	T42.6X4	T42.6X5	T42.6X6
Somonal	T42.3X1	T42.3X2	T42.3X3	T42.3X4	T42.3X5	T42.3X6
Soneryl	T42.3X1	T42.3X2	T42.3X3	T42.3X4	T42.3X5	T42.3X6
Soothing syrup	T5Ø.9Ø1	T5Ø.9Ø2	T5Ø.9Ø3	T5Ø.9Ø4	T5Ø.9Ø5	T5Ø.9Ø6
Sopor	T42.6X1	T42.6X2	T42.6X3	T42.6X4	T42.6X5	T42.6X6
Soporific	T42.71	T42.72	T42.73	T42.74	T42.75	T42.76
Soporific drug	T42.71	T42.72	T42.73	T42.74	T42.75	T42.76
specified type NEC	T42.6X1	T42.6X2	T42.6X3	T42.6X4	T42.6X5	T42.6X6
Sorbide nitrate	T46.3X1	T46.3X2	T46.3X3	T46.3X4	T46.3X5	T46.3X6
Sorbitol	T47.4X1	T47.4X2	T47.4X3	T47.4X4	T47.4X5	T47.4X6
Sotalol	T44.7X1	T44.7X2	T44.7X3	T44.7X4	T44.7X5	T44.7X6
Sotradecol	T46.8X1	T46.8X2	T46.8X3	T46.8X4	T46.8X5	T46.8X6
Soysterol	T46.6X1	T46.6X2	T46.6X3	T46.6X4	T46.6X5	T46.6X6
Spacoline	T44.3X1	T44.3X2	T44.3X3	T44.3X4	T44.3X5	T44.3X6
Spanish fly	T49.8X1	T49.8X2	T49.8X3	T49.8X4	T49.8X5	T49.8X6
Sparine	T43.3X1	T43.3X2	T43.3X3	T43.3X4	T43.3X5	T43.3X6
Sparteine	T48.ØX1	T48.ØX2	T48.ØX3	T48.ØX4	T48.ØX5	T48.ØX6
Spasmolytic						
anticholinergics	T44.3X1	T44.3X2	T44.3X3	T44.3X4	T44.3X5	T44.3X6
autonomic	T44.3X1	T44.3X2	T44.3X3	T44.3X4	T44.3X5	T44.3X6
bronchial NEC	T48.6X1	T48.6X2	T48.6X3	T48.6X4	T48.6X5	T48.6X6
quaternary ammonium	T44.3X1	T44.3X2	T44.3X3	T44.3X4	T44.3X5	T44.3X6
skeletal muscle NEC	T48.1X1	T48.1X2	T48.1X3	T48.1X4	T48.1X5	T48.1X6
Spectinomycin	T36.5X1	T36.5X2	T36.5X3	T36.5X4	T36.5X5	T36.5X6
Speed	T43.621	T43.622	T43.623	T43.624	T43.625	T43.626
Spermicide	T49.8X1	T49.8X2	T49.8X3	T49.8X4	T49.8X5	T49.8X6
Spider (bite) (venom)	T63.391	T63.392	T63.393	T63.394	—	—
antivenin	T5Ø.Z11	T5Ø.Z12	T5Ø.Z13	T5Ø.Z14	T5Ø.Z15	T5Ø.Z16
Spigelia (root)	T37.4X1	T37.4X2	T37.4X3	T37.4X4	T37.4X5	T37.4X6
Spindle inactivator	T5Ø.4X1	T5Ø.4X2	T5Ø.4X3	T5Ø.4X4	T5Ø.4X5	T5Ø.4X6
Spiperone	T43.4X1	T43.4X2	T43.4X3	T43.4X4	T43.4X5	T43.4X6
Spiramycin	T36.3X1	T36.3X2	T36.3X3	T36.3X4	T36.3X5	T36.3X6
Spirapril	T46.4X1	T46.4X2	T46.4X3	T46.4X4	T46.4X5	T46.4X6
Spirilene	T43.591	T43.592	T43.593	T43.594	T43.595	T43.596
Spirit(s) (neutral) **NEC**	T51.ØX1	T51.ØX2	T51.ØX3	T51.ØX4	—	—
beverage	T51.ØX1	T51.ØX2	T51.ØX3	T51.ØX4	—	—
industrial	T51.ØX1	T51.ØX2	T51.ØX3	T51.ØX4	—	—
mineral	T52.ØX1	T52.ØX2	T52.ØX3	T52.ØX4	—	—
of salt—*see* Hydrochloric acid						
surgical	T51.ØX1	T51.ØX2	T51.ØX3	T51.ØX4	—	—
Spironolactone	T5Ø.ØX1	T5Ø.ØX2	T5Ø.ØX3	T5Ø.ØX4	T5Ø.ØX5	T5Ø.ØX6
Spiroperidol	T43.4X1	T43.4X2	T43.4X3	T43.4X4	T43.4X5	T43.4X6
Sponge, absorbable (gelatin)	T45.7X1	T45.7X2	T45.7X3	T45.7X4	T45.7X5	T45.7X6
Sporostacin	T49.ØX1	T49.ØX2	T49.ØX3	T49.ØX4	T49.ØX5	T49.ØX6
Spray (aerosol)	T65.91	T65.92	T65.93	T65.94	—	—
cosmetic	T65.891	T65.892	T65.893	T65.894	—	—
medicinal NEC	T5Ø.9Ø1	T5Ø.9Ø2	T5Ø.9Ø3	T5Ø.9Ø4	T5Ø.9Ø5	T5Ø.9Ø6
pesticides—*see* Pesticides						
specified content—*see* specific substance						
Spurge flax	T62.2X1	T62.2X2	T62.2X3	T62.2X4	—	—
Spurges	T62.2X1	T62.2X2	T62.2X3	T62.2X4	—	—
Sputum viscosity-lowering drug	T48.4X1	T48.4X2	T48.4X3	T48.4X4	T48.4X5	T48.4X6
Squill	T46.ØX1	T46.ØX2	T46.ØX3	T46.ØX4	T46.ØX5	T46.ØX6
rat poison	T6Ø.4X1	T6Ø.4X2	T6Ø.4X3	T6Ø.4X4	—	—
Squirting cucumber (cathartic)	T47.2X1	T47.2X2	T47.2X3	T47.2X4	T47.2X5	T47.2X6
Stains	T65.6X1	T65.6X2	T65.6X3	T65.6X4	—	—
Stannous fluoride	T49.7X1	T49.7X2	T49.7X3	T49.7X4	T49.7X5	T49.7X6

Substance	Poisoning, Accidental (unintentional)	Poisoning, Intentional Self-harm	Poisoning, Assault	Poisoning, Undetermined	Adverse Effect	Under-dosing
Stanolone	T38.7X1	T38.7X2	T38.7X3	T38.7X4	T38.7X5	T38.7X6
Stanozolol	T38.7X1	T38.7X2	T38.7X3	T38.7X4	T38.7X5	T38.7X6
Staphisagria or stavesacre (pediculicide)	T49.ØX1	T49.ØX2	T49.ØX3	T49.ØX4	T49.ØX5	T49.ØX6
Starch	T5Ø.9Ø1	T5Ø.9Ø2	T5Ø.9Ø3	T5Ø.9Ø4	T5Ø.9Ø5	T5Ø.9Ø6
Stelazine	T43.3X1	T43.3X2	T43.3X3	T43.3X4	T43.3X5	T43.3X6
Stemetil	T43.3X1	T43.3X2	T43.3X3	T43.3X4	T43.3X5	T43.3X6
Stepronin	T48.4X1	T48.4X2	T48.4X3	T48.4X4	T48.4X5	T48.4X6
Sterculia	T47.4X1	T47.4X2	T47.4X3	T47.4X4	T47.4X5	T47.4X6
Sternutator gas	T59.891	T59.892	T59.893	T59.894	—	—
Steroid	T38.ØX1	T38.ØX2	T38.ØX3	T38.ØX4	T38.ØX5	T38.ØX6
anabolic	T38.7X1	T38.7X2	T38.7X3	T38.7X4	T38.7X5	T38.7X6
androgenic	T38.7X1	T38.7X2	T38.7X3	T38.7X4	T38.7X5	T38.7X6
antineoplastic, hormone	T38.7X1	T38.7X2	T38.7X3	T38.7X4	T38.7X5	T38.7X6
estrogen	T38.5X1	T38.5X2	T38.5X3	T38.5X4	T38.5X5	T38.5X6
ENT agent	T49.6X1	T49.6X2	T49.6X3	T49.6X4	T49.6X5	T49.6X6
ophthalmic preparation	T49.5X1	T49.5X2	T49.5X3	T49.5X4	T49.5X5	T49.5X6
topical NEC	T49.ØX1	T49.ØX2	T49.ØX3	T49.ØX4	T49.ØX5	T49.ØX6
Stibine	T56.891	T56.892	T56.893	T56.894	—	—
Stibogluconate	T37.3X1	T37.3X2	T37.3X3	T37.3X4	T37.3X5	T37.3X6
Stibophen	T37.4X1	T37.4X2	T37.4X3	T37.4X4	T37.4X5	T37.4X6
Stilbamidine (isetionate)	T37.3X1	T37.3X2	T37.3X3	T37.3X4	T37.3X5	T37.3X6
Stilbestrol	T38.5X1	T38.5X2	T38.5X3	T38.5X4	T38.5X5	T38.5X6
Stilboestrol	T38.5X1	T38.5X2	T38.5X3	T38.5X4	T38.5X5	T38.5X6
Stimulant						
central nervous system (*see also* Psychostimulant)	T43.6Ø1	T43.6Ø2	T43.6Ø3	T43.6Ø4	T43.6Ø5	T43.6Ø6
analeptics	T5Ø.7X1	T5Ø.7X2	T5Ø.7X3	T5Ø.7X4	T5Ø.7X5	T5Ø.7X6
opiate antagonist	T5Ø.7X1	T5Ø.7X2	T5Ø.7X3	T5Ø.7X4	T5Ø.7X5	T5Ø.7X6
psychotherapeutic NEC (*see also* Psychotherapeutic drug)	T43.6Ø1	T43.6Ø2	T43.6Ø3	T43.6Ø4	T43.6Ø5	T43.6Ø6
specified NEC	T43.691	T43.692	T43.693	T43.694	T43.695	T43.696
respiratory	T48.9Ø1	T48.9Ø2	T48.9Ø3	T48.9Ø4	T48.9Ø5	T48.9Ø6
Stone-dissolving drug	T5Ø.9Ø1	T5Ø.9Ø2	T5Ø.9Ø3	T5Ø.9Ø4	T5Ø.9Ø5	T5Ø.9Ø6
Storage battery (cells) (acid)	T54.2X1	T54.2X2	T54.2X3	T54.2X4	—	—
Stovaine	T41.3X1	T41.3X2	T41.3X3	T41.3X4	T41.3X5	T41.3X6
infiltration (subcutaneous)	T41.3X1	T41.3X2	T41.3X3	T41.3X4	T41.3X5	T41.3X6
nerve block (peripheral) (plexus)	T41.3X1	T41.3X2	T41.3X3	T41.3X4	T41.3X5	T41.3X6
spinal	T41.3X1	T41.3X2	T41.3X3	T41.3X4	T41.3X5	T41.3X6
topical (surfuce)	T41.3X1	T41.3X2	T41.3X3	T41.3X4	T41.3X5	T41.3X6
Stovarsal	T37.8X1	T37.8X2	T37.8X3	T37.8X4	T37.8X5	T37.8X6
Stove gas—*see* Gas, stove						
Stoxil	T49.5X1	T49.5X2	T49.5X3	T49.5X4	T49.5X5	T49.5X6
Stramonium	T48.6X1	T48.6X2	T48.6X3	T48.6X4	T48.6X5	T48.6X6
natural state	T62.2X1	T62.2X2	T62.2X3	T62.2X4	—	—
Streptodornase	T45.3X1	T45.3X2	T45.3X3	T45.3X4	T45.3X5	T45.3X6
Streptoduocin	T36.5X1	T36.5X2	T36.5X3	T36.5X4	T36.5X5	T36.5X6
Streptokinase	T45.611	T45.612	T45.613	T45.614	T45.615	T45.616
Streptomycin (derivative)	T36.5X1	T36.5X2	T36.5X3	T36.5X4	T36.5X5	T36.5X6
Streptonivicin	T36.5X1	T36.5X2	T36.5X3	T36.5X4	T36.5X5	T36.5X6
Streptovarycin	T36.5X1	T36.5X2	T36.5X3	T36.5X4	T36.5X5	T36.5X6
Streptozocin	T45.1X1	T45.1X2	T45.1X3	T45.1X4	T45.1X5	T45.1X6
Streptozotocin	T45.1X1	T45.1X2	T45.1X3	T45.1X4	T45.1X5	T45.1X6
Stripper (paint) (solvent)	T52.8X1	T52.8X2	T52.8X3	T52.8X4	—	—
Strobane	T6Ø.1X1	T6Ø.1X2	T6Ø.1X3	T6Ø.1X4	—	—
Strofantina	T46.ØX1	T46.ØX2	T46.ØX3	T46.ØX4	T46.ØX5	T46.ØX6
Strophanthin (g) (k)	T46.ØX1	T46.ØX2	T46.ØX3	T46.ØX4	T46.ØX5	T46.ØX6
Strophanthus	T46.ØX1	T46.ØX2	T46.ØX3	T46.ØX4	T46.ØX5	T46.ØX6
Strophantin	T46.ØX1	T46.ØX2	T46.ØX3	T46.ØX4	T46.ØX5	T46.ØX6
Strophantin-g	T46.ØX1	T46.ØX2	T46.ØX3	T46.ØX4	T46.ØX5	T46.ØX6
Strychnine (nonmedicinal) (pesticide) (salts)	T65.1X1	T65.1X2	T65.1X3	T65.1X4	—	—
medicinal	T48.291	T48.292	T48.293	T48.294	T48.295	T48.296
Strychnos (ignatii)—*see* Strychnine						
Styramate	T42.8X1	T42.8X2	T42.8X3	T42.8X4	T42.8X5	T42.8X6
Styrene	T65.891	T65.892	T65.893	T65.894	—	—
Succinimide, antiepileptic or anticonvulsant	T42.2X1	T42.2X2	T42.2X3	T42.2X4	T42.2X5	T42.2X6
mercuric—*see* Mercury						
Succinylcholine	T48.1X1	T48.1X2	T48.1X3	T48.1X4	T48.1X5	T48.1X6
Succinylsulfathiazole	T37.ØX1	T37.ØX2	T37.ØX3	T37.ØX4	T37.ØX5	T37.ØX6
Sucralfate	T47.1X1	T47.1X2	T47.1X3	T47.1X4	T47.1X5	T47.1X6
Sucrose	T5Ø.3X1	T5Ø.3X2	T5Ø.3X3	T5Ø.3X4	T5Ø.3X5	T5Ø.3X6
Sufentanil	T4Ø.4X1	T4Ø.4X2	T4Ø.4X3	T4Ø.4X4	T4Ø.4X5	T4Ø.4X6
Sulbactam	T36.ØX1	T36.ØX2	T36.ØX3	T36.ØX4	T36.ØX5	T36.ØX6
Sulbenicillin	T36.ØX1	T36.ØX2	T36.ØX3	T36.ØX4	T36.ØX5	T36.ØX6
Sulbentine	T49.ØX1	T49.ØX2	T49.ØX3	T49.ØX4	T49.ØX5	T49.ØX6
Sulfacetamide	T49.ØX1	T49.5ØX2	T49.ØX3	T49.ØX4	T49.ØX5	T49.ØX6
ophthalmic preparation	T49.5X1	T49.5X2	T49.5X3	T49.5X4	T49.5X5	T49.5X6
Sulfachlorpyridazine	T37.ØX1	T37.ØX2	T37.ØX3	T37.ØX4	T37.ØX5	T37.ØX6
Sulfacitine	T37.ØX1	T37.ØX2	T37.ØX3	T37.ØX4	T37.ØX5	T37.ØX6
Sulfadiasulfone sodium	T37.ØX1	T37.ØX2	T37.ØX3	T37.ØX4	T37.ØX5	T37.ØX6
Sulfadiazine	T37.ØX1	T37.ØX2	T37.ØX3	T37.ØX4	T37.ØX5	T37.ØX6
silver (topical)	T49.ØX1	T49.ØX2	T49.ØX3	T49.ØX4	T49.ØX5	T49.ØX6
Sulfadimethoxine	T37.ØX1	T37.ØX2	T37.ØX3	T37.ØX4	T37.ØX5	T37.ØX6
Sulfadimidine	T37.ØX1	T37.ØX2	T37.ØX3	T37.ØX4	T37.ØX5	T37.ØX6
Sulfadoxine	T37.ØX1	T37.ØX2	T37.ØX3	T37.ØX4	T37.ØX5	T37.ØX6
with pyrimethamine	T37.2X1	T37.2X2	T37.2X3	T37.2X4	T37.2X5	T37.2X6
Sulfaethidole	T37.ØX1	T37.ØX2	T37.ØX3	T37.ØX4	T37.ØX5	T37.ØX6
Sulfafurazole	T37.ØX1	T37.ØX2	T37.ØX3	T37.ØX4	T37.ØX5	T37.ØX6
Sulfaguanidine	T37.ØX1	T37.ØX2	T37.ØX3	T37.ØX4	T37.ØX5	T37.ØX6
Sulfalene	T37.ØX1	T37.ØX2	T37.ØX3	T37.ØX4	T37.ØX5	T37.ØX6
Sulfaloxate	T37.ØX1	T37.ØX2	T37.ØX3	T37.ØX4	T37.ØX5	T37.ØX6
Sulfaloxic acid	T37.ØX1	T37.ØX2	T37.ØX3	T37.ØX4	T37.ØX5	T37.ØX6
Sulfamazone	T39.2X1	T39.2X2	T39.2X3	T39.2X4	T39.2X5	T39.2X6
Sulfamerazine	T37.ØX1	T37.ØX2	T37.ØX3	T37.ØX4	T37.ØX5	T37.ØX6
Sulfameter	T37.ØX1	T37.ØX2	T37.ØX3	T37.ØX4	T37.ØX5	T37.ØX6
Sulfamethazine	T37.ØX1	T37.ØX2	T37.ØX3	T37.ØX4	T37.ØX5	T37.ØX6
Sulfamethizole	T37.ØX1	T37.ØX2	T37.ØX3	T37.ØX4	T37.ØX5	T37.ØX6
Sulfamethoxazole	T37.ØX1	T37.ØX2	T37.ØX3	T37.ØX4	T37.ØX5	T37.ØX6
with trimethoprim	T36.8X1	T36.8X2	T36.8X3	T36.8X4	T36.8X5	T36.8X6
Sulfamethoxydiazine	T37.ØX1	T37.ØX2	T37.ØX3	T37.ØX4	T37.ØX5	T37.ØX6
Sulfamethoxypyridazine	T37.ØX1	T37.ØX2	T37.ØX3	T37.ØX4	T37.ØX5	T37.ØX6
Sulfamethylthiazole	T37.ØX1	T37.ØX2	T37.ØX3	T37.ØX4	T37.ØX5	T37.ØX6
Sulfametoxydiazine	T37.ØX1	T37.ØX2	T37.ØX3	T37.ØX4	T37.ØX5	T37.ØX6
Sulfamidopyrine	T39.2X1	T39.2X2	T39.2X3	T39.2X4	T39.2X5	T39.2X6
Sulfamonomethoxine	T37.ØX1	T37.ØX2	T37.ØX3	T37.ØX4	T37.ØX5	T37.ØX6
Sulfamoxole	T37.ØX1	T37.ØX2	T37.ØX3	T37.ØX4	T37.ØX5	T37.ØX6
Sulfamylon	T49.ØX1	T49.ØX2	T49.ØX3	T49.ØX4	T49.ØX5	T49.ØX6
Sulfan blue (diagnostic dye)	T5Ø.8X1	T5Ø.8X2	T5Ø.8X3	T5Ø.8X4	T5Ø.8X5	T5Ø.8X6
Sulfanilamide	T37.ØX1	T37.ØX2	T37.ØX3	T37.ØX4	T37.ØX5	T37.ØX6
Sulfanilylguanidine	T37.ØX1	T37.ØX2	T37.ØX3	T37.ØX4	T37.ØX5	T37.ØX6
Sulfaperin	T37.ØX1	T37.ØX2	T37.ØX3	T37.ØX4	T37.ØX5	T37.ØX6
Sulfaphenazole	T37.ØX1	T37.ØX2	T37.ØX3	T37.ØX4	T37.ØX5	T37.ØX6
Sulfaphenylthiazole	T37.ØX1	T37.ØX2	T37.ØX3	T37.ØX4	T37.ØX5	T37.ØX6
Sulfaproxyline	T37.ØX1	T37.ØX2	T37.ØX3	T37.ØX4	T37.ØX5	T37.ØX6
Sulfapyridine	T37.ØX1	T37.ØX2	T37.ØX3	T37.ØX4	T37.ØX5	T37.ØX6
Sulfapyrimidine	T37.ØX1	T37.ØX2	T37.ØX3	T37.ØX4	T37.ØX5	T37.ØX6
Sulfarsphenamine	T37.8X1	T37.8X2	T37.8X3	T37.8X4	T37.8X5	T37.8X6
Sulfasalazine	T37.ØX1	T37.ØX2	T37.ØX3	T37.ØX4	T37.ØX5	T37.ØX6
Sulfasuxidine	T37.ØX1	T37.ØX2	T37.ØX3	T37.ØX4	T37.ØX5	T37.ØX6
Sulfasymazine	T37.ØX1	T37.ØX2	T37.ØX3	T37.ØX4	T37.ØX5	T37.ØX6
Sulfated amylopectin	T47.8X1	T47.8X2	T47.8X3	T47.8X4	T47.8X5	T47.8X6
Sulfathiazole	T37.ØX1	T37.ØX2	T37.ØX3	T37.ØX4	T37.ØX5	T37.ØX6
Sulfatostearate	T49.2X1	T49.2X2	T49.2X3	T49.2X4	T49.2X5	T49.2X6
Sulfinpyrazone	T5Ø.4X1	T5Ø.4X2	T5Ø.4X3	T5Ø.4X4	T5Ø.4X5	T5Ø.4X6
Sulfiram	T49.ØX1	T49.ØX2	T49.ØX3	T49.ØX4	T49.ØX5	T49.ØX6
Sulfisomidine	T37.ØX1	T37.ØX2	T37.ØX3	T37.ØX4	T37.ØX5	T37.ØX6
Sulfisoxazole	T37.ØX1	T37.ØX2	T37.ØX3	T37.ØX4	T37.ØX5	T37.ØX6
ophthalmic preparation	T49.5X1	T49.5X2	T49.5X3	T49.5X4	T49.5X5	T49.5X6
Sulfobromophthalein (sodium)	T5Ø.8X1	T5Ø.8X2	T5Ø.8X3	T5Ø.8X4	T5Ø.8X5	T5Ø.8X6
Sulfobromphthalein	T5Ø.8X1	T5Ø.8X2	T5Ø.8X3	T5Ø.8X4	T5Ø.8X5	T5Ø.8X6
Sulfogaiacol	T48.4X1	T48.4X2	T48.4X3	T48.4X4	T48.4X5	T48.4X6
Sulfomyxin	T36.8X1	T36.8X2	T36.8X3	T36.8X4	T36.8X5	T36.8X6
Sulfonal	T42.6X1	T42.6X2	T42.6X3	T42.6X4	T42.6X5	T42.6X6
Sulfonamide NEC	T37.ØX1	T37.ØX2	T37.ØX3	T37.ØX4	T37.ØX5	T37.ØX6
eye	T49.5X1	T49.5X2	T49.5X3	T49.5X4	T49.5X5	T49.5X6
Sulfonazide	T37.1X1	T37.1X2	T37.1X3	T37.1X4	T37.1X5	T37.1X6
Sulfones	T37.1X1	T37.1X2	T37.1X3	T37.1X4	T37.1X5	T37.1X6
Sulfonethylmethane	T42.6X1	T42.6X2	T42.6X3	T42.6X4	T42.6X5	T42.6X6
Sulfonmethane	T42.6X1	T42.6X2	T42.6X3	T42.6X4	T42.6X5	T42.6X6

Substance	Poisoning, Accidental (unintentional)	Poisoning, Intentional Self-harm	Poisoning, Assault	Poisoning, Undetermined	Adverse Effect	Under-dosing
Sulfonphthal, sulfonphthol	T5Ø.8X1	T5Ø.8X2	T5Ø.8X3	T5Ø.8X4	T5Ø.8X5	T5Ø.8X6
Sulfonylurea derivatives, oral	T38.3X1	T38.3X2	T38.3X3	T38.3X4	T38.3X5	T38.3X6
Sulforidazine	T43.3X1	T43.3X2	T43.3X3	T43.3X4	T43.3X5	T43.3X6
Sulfoxone	T37.1X1	T37.1X2	T37.1X3	T37.1X4	T37.1X5	T37.1X6
Sulfur, sulfurated, sulfuric, sulfurous, sulfuryl (compounds NEC) (medicinal)	T49.4X1	T49.4X2	T49.4X3	T49.4X4	T49.4X5	T49.4X6
acid	T54.2X1	T54.2X2	T54.2X3	T54.2X4	—	—
dioxide (gas)	T59.1X1	T59.1X2	T59.1X3	T59.1X4	—	—
ether—*see* Ether(s)						
hydrogen	T59.6X1	T59.6X2	T59.6X3	T59.6X4	—	—
medicinal (keratolytic) (ointment) NEC	T49.4X1	T49.4X2	T49.4X3	T49.4X4	T49.4X5	T49.4X6
ointment	T49.ØX1	T49.ØX2	T49.ØX3	T49.ØX4	T49.ØX5	T49.ØX6
pesticide (vapor)	T6Ø.91	T6Ø.92	T6Ø.93	T6Ø.94	—	—
vapor NEC	T59.891	T59.892	T59.893	T59.894	—	—
Sulfuric acid	T54.2X1	T54.2X2	T54.2X3	T54.2X4	—	—
Sulglicotide	T47.1X1	T47.1X2	T47.1X3	T47.1X4	T47.1X5	T47.1X6
Sulindac	T39.391	T39.392	T39.393	T39.394	T39.395	T39.396
Sulisatin	T47.2X1	T47.2X2	T47.2X3	T47.2X4	T47.2X5	T47.2X6
Sulisobenzone	T49.3X1	T49.3X2	T49.3X3	T49.3X4	T49.3X5	T49.3X6
Sulkowitch's reagent	T5Ø.8X1	T5Ø.8X2	T5Ø.8X3	T5Ø.8X4	T5Ø.8X5	T5Ø.8X6
Sulmetozine	T44.3X1	T44.3X2	T44.3X3	T44.3X4	T44.3X5	T44.3X6
Suloctidil	T46.7X1	T46.7X2	T46.7X3	T46.7X4	T46.7X5	T46.7X6
Sulph —*see also* Sulf-						
Sulphadiazine	T37.ØX1	T37.ØX2	T37.ØX3	T37.ØX4	T37.ØX5	T37.ØX6
Sulphadimethoxine	T37.ØX1	T37.ØX2	T37.ØX3	T37.ØX4	T37.ØX5	T37.ØX6
Sulphadimidine	T37.ØX1	T37.ØX2	T37.ØX3	T37.ØX4	T37.ØX5	T37.ØX6
Sulphadione	T37.1X1	T37.1X2	T37.1X3	T37.1X4	T37.1X5	T37.1X6
Sulphafurazole	T37.ØX1	T37.ØX2	T37.ØX3	T37.ØX4	T37.ØX5	T37.ØX6
Sulphamethizole	T37.ØX1	T37.ØX2	T37.ØX3	T37.ØX4	T37.ØX5	T37.ØX6
Sulphamethoxazole	T37.ØX1	T37.ØX2	T37.ØX3	T37.ØX4	T37.ØX5	T37.ØX6
Sulphan blue	T5Ø.8X1	T5Ø.8X2	T5Ø.8X3	T5Ø.8X4	T5Ø.8X5	T5Ø.8X6
Sulphaphenazole	T37.ØX1	T37.ØX2	T37.ØX3	T37.ØX4	T37.ØX5	T37.ØX6
Sulphapyridine	T37.ØX1	T37.ØX2	T37.ØX3	T37.ØX4	T37.ØX5	T37.ØX6
Sulphasalazine	T37.ØX1	T37.ØX2	T37.ØX3	T37.ØX4	T37.ØX5	T37.ØX6
Sulphinpyrazone	T5Ø.4X1	T5Ø.4X2	T5Ø.4X3	T5Ø.4X4	T5Ø.4X5	T5Ø.4X6
Sulpiride	T43.591	T43.592	T43.593	T43.594	T43.595	T43.596
Sulprostone	T48.ØX1	T48.ØX2	T48.ØX3	T48.ØX4	T48.ØX5	T48.ØX6
Sulpyrine	T39.2X1	T39.2X2	T39.2X3	T39.2X4	T39.2X5	T39.2X6
Sultamicillin	T36.ØX1	T36.ØX2	T36.ØX3	T36.ØX4	T36.ØX5	T36.ØX6
Sulthiame	T42.6X1	T42.6X2	T42.6X3	T42.6X4	T42.6X5	T42.6X6
Sultiame	T42.6X1	T42.6X2	T42.6X3	T42.6X4	T42.6X5	T42.6X6
Sultopride	T43.591	T43.592	T43.593	T43.594	T43.595	T43.596
Sumatriptan	T39.8X1	T39.8X2	T39.8X3	T39.8X4	T39.8X5	T39.8X6
Sunflower seed oil	T46.6X1	T46.6X2	T46.6X3	T46.6X4	T46.6X5	T46.6X6
Superinone	T48.4X1	T48.4X2	T48.4X3	T48.4X4	T48.4X5	T48.4X6
Suprofen	T39.311	T39.312	T39.313	T39.314	T39.315	T39.316
Suramin (sodium)	T37.4X1	T37.4X2	T37.4X3	T37.4X4	T37.4X5	T37.4X6
Surfacaine	T41.3X1	T41.3X2	T41.3X3	T41.3X4	T41.3X5	T41.3X6
Surital	T41.1X1	T41.1X2	T41.1X3	T41.1X4	T41.1X5	T41.1X6
Sutilains	T45.3X1	T45.3X2	T45.3X3	T45.3X4	T45.3X5	T45.3X6
Suxamethonium (chloride)	T48.1X1	T48.1X2	T48.1X3	T48.1X4	T48.1X5	T48.1X6
Suxethonium (chloride)	T48.1X1	T48.1X2	T48.1X3	T48.1X4	T48.1X5	T48.1X6
Suxibuzone	T39.2X1	T39.2X2	T39.2X3	T39.2X4	T39.2X5	T39.2X6
Sweet oil (birch)	T49.3X1	T49.3X2	T49.3X3	T49.3X4	T49.3X5	T49.3X6
Sweet niter spirit	T46.3X1	T46.3X2	T46.3X3	T46.3X4	T46.3X5	T46.3X6
Sweetener	T5Ø.9Ø1	T5Ø.9Ø2	T5Ø.9Ø3	T5Ø.9Ø4	T5Ø.9Ø5	T5Ø.9Ø6
Sym-dichloroethyl ether	T53.6X1	T53.6X2	T53.6X3	T53.6X4	—	—
Sympatholytic NEC	T44.8X1	T44.8X2	T44.8X3	T44.8X4	T44.8X5	T44.8X6
haloalkylamine	T44.8X1	T44.8X2	T44.8X3	T44.8X4	T44.8X5	T44.8X6
Sympathomimetic NEC	T44.9Ø1	T44.9Ø2	T44.9Ø3	T44.9Ø4	T44.9Ø5	T44.9Ø6
anti-common-cold	T48.5X1	T48.5X2	T48.5X3	T48.5X4	T48.5X5	T48.5X6
bronchodilator	T48.6X1	T48.6X2	T48.6X3	T48.6X4	T48.6X5	T48.6X6
specified NEC	T44.991	T44.992	T44.993	T44.994	T44.995	T44.996
Synagis	T5Ø.B91	T5Ø.B92	T5Ø.B93	T5Ø.B94	T5Ø.B95	T5Ø.B96
Synalar	T49.ØX1	T49.ØX2	T49.ØX3	T49.ØX4	T49.ØX5	T49.ØX6
Synthroid	T38.1X1	T38.1X2	T38.1X3	T38.1X4	T38.1X5	T38.1X6
Syntocinon	T48.ØX1	T48.ØX2	T48.ØX3	T48.ØX4	T48.ØX5	T48.ØX6
Syrosingopine	T46.5X1	T46.5X2	T46.5X3	T46.5X4	T46.5X5	T46.5X6
Systemic drug	T45.91	T45.92	T45.93	T45.94	T45.95	T45.96
specified NEC	T45.8X1	T45.8X2	T45.8X3	T45.8X4	T45.8X5	T45.8X6
T						
2,4,5-T	T6Ø.3X1	T6Ø.3X2	T6Ø.3X3	T6Ø.3X4	—	—
2,4,5-T (trichloro-phenoxyacetic acid)	T6Ø.1X1	T6Ø.1X2	T6Ø.1X3	T6Ø.1X4	—	—
Tablets (*see also* specified substance)	T5Ø.9Ø1	T5Ø.9Ø2	T5Ø.9Ø3	T5Ø.9Ø4	T5Ø.9Ø5	T5Ø.9Ø6
Tace	T38.5X1	T38.5X2	T38.5X3	T38.5X4	T38.5X5	T38.5X6
Tacrine	T44.ØX1	T44.ØX2	T44.ØX3	T44.ØX4	T44.ØX5	T44.ØX6
Tadalafil	T46.7X1	T46.7X2	T46.7X3	T46.7X4	T46.7X5	T46.7X6
Talampicillin	T36.ØX1	T36.ØX2	T36.ØX3	T36.ØX4	T36.ØX5	T36.ØX6
Talbutal	T42.3X1	T42.3X2	T42.3X3	T42.3X4	T42.3X5	T42.3X6
Talc powder	T49.3X1	T49.3X2	T49.3X3	T49.3X4	T49.3X5	T49.3X6
Talcum	T49.3X1	T49.3X2	T49.3X3	T49.3X4	T49.3X5	T49.3X6
Taleranol	T38.6X1	T38.6X2	T38.6X3	T38.6X4	T38.6X5	T38.6X6
Tamoxifen	T38.6X1	T38.6X2	T38.6X3	T38.6X4	T38.6X5	T38.6X6
Tamsulosin	T44.6X1	T44.6X2	T44.6X3	T44.6X4	T44.6X5	T44.6X6
Tandearil, tanderil	T39.2X1	T39.2X2	T39.2X3	T39.2X4	T39.2X5	T39.2X6
Tannic acid	T49.2X1	T49.2X2	T49.2X3	T49.2X4	T49.2X5	T49.2X6
medicinal (astringent)	T49.2X1	T49.2X2	T49.2X3	T49.2X4	T49.2X5	T49.2X6
Tannin—*see* Tannic acid						
Tansy	T62.2X1	T62.2X2	T62.2X3	T62.2X4	—	—
TAO	T36.3X1	T36.3X2	T36.3X3	T36.3X4	T36.3X5	T36.3X6
Tapazole	T38.2X1	T38.2X2	T38.2X3	T38.2X4	T38.2X5	T38.2X6
Tar NEC	T52.ØX1	T52.ØX2	T52.ØX3	T52.ØX4	—	—
camphor	T6Ø.1X1	T6Ø.1X2	T6Ø.1X3	T6Ø.1X4	—	—
distillate	T49.1X1	T49.1X2	T49.1X3	T49.1X4	T49.1X5	T49.1X6
fumes	T59.891	T59.892	T59.893	T59.894	—	—
medicinal	T49.1X1	T49.1X2	T49.1X3	T49.1X4	T49.1X5	T49.1X6
ointment	T49.1X1	T49.1X2	T49.1X3	T49.1X4	T49.1X5	T49.1X6
Taractan	T43.591	T43.592	T43.593	T43.594	T43.595	T43.596
Tarantula (venomous)	T63.321	T63.322	T63.323	T63.324	—	—
Tartar emetic	T37.8X1	T37.8X2	T37.8X3	T37.8X4	T37.8X5	T37.8X6
Tartaric acid	T65.891	T65.892	T65.893	T65.894	—	—
Tartrated antimony (anti-infective)	T37.8X1	T37.8X2	T37.8X3	T37.8X4	T37.8X5	T37.8X6
Tartrate, laxative	T47.4X1	T47.4X2	T47.4X3	T47.4X4	T47.4X5	T47.4X6
Tauromustine	T45.1X1	T45.1X2	T45.1X3	T45.1X4	T45.1X5	T45.1X6
TCA—*see* Trichloroacetic acid						
TCDD	T53.7X1	T53.7X2	T53.7X3	T53.7X4	—	—
TDI (vapor)	T65.ØX1	T65.ØX2	T65.ØX3	T65.ØX4	—	—
Tear						
gas	T59.3X1	T59.3X2	T59.3X3	T59.3X4	—	—
solution	T49.5X1	T49.5X2	T49.5X3	T49.5X4	T49.5X5	T49.5X6
Teclothiazide	T5Ø.2X1	T5Ø.2X2	T5Ø.2X3	T5Ø.2X4	T5Ø.2X5	T5Ø.2X6
Teclozan	T37.3X1	T37.3X2	T37.3X3	T37.3X4	T37.3X5	T37.3X6
Tegafur	T45.1X1	T45.1X2	T45.1X3	T45.1X4	T45.1X5	T45.1X6
Tegretol	T42.1X1	T42.1X2	T42.1X3	T42.1X4	T42.1X5	T42.1X6
Teicoplanin	T36.8X1	T36.8X2	T36.8X3	T36.8X4	T36.8X5	T36.8X6
Telepaque	T5Ø.8X1	T5Ø.8X2	T5Ø.8X3	T5Ø.8X4	T5Ø.8X5	T5Ø.8X6
Tellurium	T56.891	T56.892	T56.893	T56.894	—	—
fumes	T56.891	T56.892	T56.893	T56.894	—	—
TEM	T45.1X1	T45.1X2	T45.1X3	T45.1X4	T45.1X5	T45.1X6
Temazepam	T42.4X1	T42.4X2	T42.4X3	T42.4X4	T42.4X5	T42.4X6
Temocillin	T36.ØX1	T36.ØX2	T36.ØX3	T36.ØX4	T36.ØX5	T36.ØX6
Tenamfetamine	T43.621	T43.622	T43.623	T43.624	T43.625	T43.626
Teniposide	T45.1X1	T45.1X2	T45.1X3	T45.1X4	T45.1X5	T45.1X6
Tenitramine	T46.3X1	T46.3X2	T46.3X3	T46.3X4	T46.3X5	T46.3X6
Tenoglicin	T48.4X1	T48.4X2	T48.4X3	T48.4X4	T48.4X5	T48.4X6
Tenonitrozole	T37.3X1	T37.3X2	T37.3X3	T37.3X4	T37.3X5	T37.3X6
Tenoxicam	T39.391	T39.392	T39.393	T39.394	T39.395	T39.396
TEPA	T45.1X1	T45.1X2	T45.1X3	T45.1X4	T45.1X5	T45.1X6
TEPP	T6Ø.ØX1	T6Ø.ØX2	T6Ø.ØX3	T6Ø.ØX4	—	—
Teprotide	T46.5X1	T46.5X2	T46.5X3	T46.5X4	T46.5X5	T46.5X6
Terazosin	T44.6X1	T44.6X2	T44.6X3	T44.6X4	T44.6X5	T44.6X6
Terbufos	T6Ø.ØX1	T6Ø.ØX2	T6Ø.ØX3	T6Ø.ØX4	—	—
Terbutaline	T48.6X1	T48.6X2	T48.6X3	T48.6X4	T48.6X5	T48.6X6
Terconazole	T49.ØX1	T49.ØX2	T49.ØX3	T49.ØX4	T49.ØX5	T49.ØX6
Terfenadine	T45.ØX1	T45.ØX2	T45.ØX3	T45.ØX4	T45.ØX5	T45.ØX6
Teriparatide (acetate)	T5Ø.991	T5Ø.992	T5Ø.993	T5Ø.994	T5Ø.995	T5Ø.996

Substance	Poisoning, Accidental (unintentional)	Poisoning, Intentional Self-harm	Poisoning, Assault	Poisoning, Undetermined	Adverse Effect	Under-dosing
Terizidone	T37.1X1	T37.1X2	T37.1X3	T37.1X4	T37.1X5	T37.1X6
Terlipressin	T38.891	T38.892	T38.893	T38.894	T38.895	T38.896
Terodiline	T46.3X1	T46.3X2	T46.3X3	T46.3X4	T46.3X5	T46.3X6
Teroxalene	T37.4X1	T37.4X2	T37.4X3	T37.4X4	T37.4X5	T37.4X6
Terpin(cis) hydrate	T48.4X1	T48.4X2	T48.4X3	T48.4X4	T48.4X5	T48.4X6
Terramycin	T36.4X1	T36.4X2	T36.4X3	T36.4X4	T36.4X5	T36.4X6
Tertatolol	T44.7X1	T44.7X2	T44.7X3	T44.7X4	T44.7X5	T44.7X6
Tessalon	T48.3X1	T48.3X2	T48.3X3	T48.3X4	T48.3X5	T48.3X6
Testolactone	T38.7X1	T38.7X2	T38.7X3	T38.7X4	T38.7X5	T38.7X6
Testosterone	T38.7X1	T38.7X2	T38.7X3	T38.7X4	T38.7X5	T38.7X6
Tetanus toxoid or vaccine	T5Ø.A91	T5Ø.A92	T5Ø.A93	T5Ø.A94	T5Ø.A95	T5Ø.A96
antitoxin	T5Ø.Z11	T5Ø.Z12	T5Ø.Z13	T5Ø.Z14	T5Ø.Z15	T5Ø.Z16
immune globulin (human)	T5Ø.Z11	T5Ø.Z12	T5Ø.Z13	T5Ø.Z14	T5Ø.Z15	T5Ø.Z16
toxoid	T5Ø.A91	T5Ø.A92	T5Ø.A93	T5Ø.A94	T5Ø.A95	T5Ø.A96
with diphtheria toxoid	T5Ø.A21	T5Ø.A22	T5Ø.A23	T5Ø.A24	T5Ø.A25	T5Ø.A26
with pertussis	T5Ø.A11	T5Ø.A12	T5Ø.A13	T5Ø.A14	T5Ø.A15	T5Ø.A16
Tetrabenazine	T43.591	T43.592	T43.593	T43.594	T43.595	T43.596
Tetracaine	T41.3X1	T41.3X2	T41.3X3	T41.3X4	T41.3X5	T41.3X6
nerve block (peripheral) (plexus)	T41.3X1	T41.3X2	T41.3X3	T41.3X4	T41.3X5	T41.3X6
regional	T41.3X1	T41.3X2	T41.3X3	T41.3X4	T41.3X5	T41.3X6
spinal	T41.3X1	T41.3X2	T41.3X3	T41.3X4	T41.3X5	T41.3X6
Tetrachlorethylene—*see* Tetrachloroethylene						
Tetrachlormethiazide	T5Ø.2X1	T5Ø.2X2	T5Ø.2X3	T5Ø.2X4	T5Ø.2X5	T5Ø.2X6
2,3,7,8-Tetrachlorodibenzo-p-dioxin	T53.7X1	T53.7X2	T53.7X3	T53.7X4	—	—
Tetrachloroethane	T53.6X1	T53.6X2	T53.6X3	T53.6X4	—	—
vapor	T53.6X1	T53.6X2	T53.6X3	T53.6X4	—	—
paint or varnish	T53.6X1	T53.6X2	T53.6X3	T53.6X4	—	—
Tetrachloroethylene (liquid)	T53.3X1	T53.3X2	T53.3X3	T53.3X4	—	—
medicinal	T37.4X1	T37.4X2	T37.4X3	T37.4X4	T37.4X5	T37.4X6
vapor	T53.3X1	T53.3X2	T53.3X3	T53.3X4	—	—
Tetrachloromethane—*see* Carbon tetrachloride						
Tetracosactide	T38.811	T38.812	T38.813	T38.814	T38.815	T38.816
Tetracosactrin	T38.811	T38.812	T38.813	T38.814	T38.815	T38.816
Tetracycline	T36.4X1	T36.4X2	T36.4X3	T36.4X4	T36.4X5	T36.4X6
ophthalmic preparation	T49.5X1	T49.5X2	T49.5X3	T49.5X4	T49.5X5	T49.5X6
topical NEC	T49.ØX1	T49.ØX2	T49.ØX3	T49.ØX4	T49.ØX5	T49.ØX6
Tetradifon	T6Ø.8X1	T6Ø.8X2	T6Ø.8X3	T6Ø.8X4	—	—
Tetradotoxin	T61.771	T61.772	T61.773	T61.774	—	—
Tetraethyl						
lead	T56.ØX1	T56.ØX2	T56.ØX3	T56.ØX4	—	—
pyrophosphate	T6Ø.ØX1	T6Ø.ØX2	T6Ø.ØX3	T6Ø.ØX4	—	—
Tetraethylammonium chloride	T44.2X1	T44.2X2	T44.2X3	T44.2X4	T44.2X5	T44.2X6
Tetraethylthiuram disulfide	T5Ø.6X1	T5Ø.6X2	T5Ø.6X3	T5Ø.6X4	T5Ø.6X5	T5Ø.6X6
Tetrahydroaminoacridine	T44.ØX1	T44.ØX2	T44.ØX3	T44.ØX4	T44.ØX5	T44.ØX6
Tetrahydrocannabinol	T4Ø.7X1	T4Ø.7X2	T4Ø.7X3	T4Ø.7X4	T4Ø.7X5	T4Ø.7X6
Tetrahydrofuran	T52.8X1	T52.8X2	T52.8X3	T52.8X4	—	—
Tetrahydronaphthalene	T52.8X1	T52.8X2	T52.8X3	T52.8X4	—	—
Tetrahydrozoline	T49.5X1	T49.5X2	T49.5X3	T49.5X4	T49.5X5	T49.5X6
Tetralin	T52.8X1	T52.8X2	T52.8X3	T52.8X4	—	—
Tetramethrin	T6Ø.2X1	T6Ø.2X2	T6Ø.2X3	T6Ø.2X4	—	—
Tetramethylthiuram (disulfide) **NEC**	T6Ø.3X1	T6Ø.3X2	T6Ø.3X3	T6Ø.3X4	—	—
medicinal	T49.ØX1	T49.ØX2	T49.ØX3	T49.ØX4	T49.ØX5	T49.ØX6
Tetramisole	T37.4X1	T37.4X2	T37.4X3	T37.4X4	T37.4X5	T37.4X6
Tetranicotinoyl fructose	T46.7X1	T46.7X2	T46.7X3	T46.7X4	T46.7X5	T46.7X6
Tetronal	T42.6X1	T42.6X2	T42.6X3	T42.6X4	T42.6X5	T42.6X6
Tetrazepam	T42.4X1	T42.4X2	T42.4X3	T42.4X4	T42.4X5	T42.4X6
Tetryl	T65.3X1	T65.3X2	T65.3X3	T65.3X4	—	—
Tetrylammonium chloride	T44.2X1	T44.2X2	T44.2X3	T44.2X4	T44.2X5	T44.2X6
Tetryzoline	T49.5X1	T49.5X2	T49.5X3	T49.5X4	T49.5X5	T49.5X6
Thalidomide	T45.1X1	T45.1X2	T45.1X3	T45.1X4	T45.1X5	T45.1X6
Thallium (compounds) (dust) **NEC**	T56.811	T56.812	T56.813	T56.814	—	—
pesticide	T6Ø.4X1	T6Ø.4X2	T6Ø.4X3	T6Ø.4X4	—	—
THC	T4Ø.7X1	T4Ø.7X2	T4Ø.7X3	T4Ø.7X4	T4Ø.7X5	T4Ø.7X6
Thebacon	T48.3X1	T48.3X2	T48.3X3	T48.3X4	T48.3X5	T48.3X6
Thebaine	T4Ø.2X1	T4Ø.2X2	T4Ø.2X3	T4Ø.2X4	T4Ø.2X5	T4Ø.2X6
Thenoic acid	T49.6X1	T49.6X2	T49.6X3	T49.6X4	T49.6X5	T49.6X6
Thenyldiamine	T45.ØX1	T45.ØX2	T45.ØX3	T45.ØX4	T45.ØX5	T45.ØX6
Theobromine (calcium salicylate)	T48.6X1	T48.6X2	T48.6X3	T48.6X4	T48.6X5	T48.6X6
sodium salicylate	T48.6X1	T48.6X2	T48.6X3	T48.6X4	T48.6X5	T48.6X6
Theophyllamine	T48.6X1	T48.6X2	T48.6X3	T48.6X4	T48.6X5	T48.6X6
Theophylline	T48.6X1	T48.6X2	T48.6X3	T48.6X4	T48.6X5	T48.6X6
aminobenzoic acid	T48.6X1	T48.6X2	T48.6X3	T48.6X4	T48.6X5	T48.6X6
ethylenediamine	T48.6X1	T48.6X2	T48.6X3	T48.6X4	T48.6X5	T48.6X6
piperazine p-aminobenzoate	T48.6X1	T48.6X2	T48.6X3	T48.6X4	T48.6X5	T48.6X6
Thiabendazole	T37.4X1	T37.4X2	T37.4X3	T37.4X4	T37.4X5	T37.4X6
Thialbarbital	T41.1X1	T41.1X2	T41.1X3	T41.1X4	T41.1X5	T41.1X6
Thiamazole	T38.2X1	T38.2X2	T38.2X3	T38.2X4	T38.2X5	T38.2X6
Thiambutosine	T37.1X1	T37.1X2	T37.1X3	T37.1X4	T37.1X5	T37.1X6
Thiamine	T45.2X1	T45.2X2	T45.2X3	T45.2X4	T45.2X5	T45.2X6
Thiamphenicol	T36.2X1	T36.2X2	T36.2X3	T36.2X4	T36.2X5	T36.2X6
Thiamylal	T41.1X1	T41.1X2	T41.1X3	T41.1X4	T41.1X5	T41.1X6
sodium	T41.1X1	T41.1X2	T41.1X3	T41.1X4	T41.1X5	T41.1X6
Thiazesim	T43.291	T43.292	T43.293	T43.294	T43.295	T43.296
Thiazides (diuretics)	T5Ø.2X1	T5Ø.2X2	T5Ø.2X3	T5Ø.2X4	T5Ø.2X5	T5Ø.2X6
Thiazinamium metilsulfate	T43.3X1	T43.3X2	T43.3X3	T43.3X4	T43.3X5	T43.3X6
Thiethylperazine	T43.3X1	T43.3X2	T43.3X3	T43.3X4	T43.3X5	T43.3X6
Thimerosal	T49.ØX1	T49.ØX2	T49.ØX3	T49.ØX4	T49.ØX5	T49.ØX6
ophthalmic preparation	T49.5X1	T49.5X2	T49.5X3	T49.5X4	T49.5X5	T49.5X6
Thioacetazone	T37.1X1	T37.1X2	T37.1X3	T37.1X4	T37.1X5	T37.1X6
with isoniazid	T37.1X1	T37.1X2	T37.1X3	T37.1X4	T37.1X5	T37.1X6
Thiobarbital sodium	T41.1X1	T41.1X2	T41.1X3	T41.1X4	T41.1X5	T41.1X6
Thiobarbiturate anesthetic	T41.1X1	T41.1X2	T41.1X3	T41.1X4	T41.1X5	T41.1X6
Thiobismol	T37.8X1	T37.8X2	T37.8X3	T37.8X4	T37.8X5	T37.8X6
Thiobutabarbital sodium	T41.1X1	T41.1X2	T41.1X3	T41.1X4	T41.1X5	T41.1X6
Thiocarbamate (insecticide)	T6Ø.ØX1	T6Ø.ØX2	T6Ø.ØX3	T6Ø.ØX4	—	—
Thiocarbamide	T38.2X1	T38.2X2	T38.2X3	T38.2X4	T38.2X5	T38.2X6
Thiocarbarsone	T37.8X1	T37.8X2	T37.8X3	T37.8X4	T37.8X5	T37.8X6
Thiocarlide	T37.1X1	T37.1X2	T37.1X3	T37.1X4	T37.1X5	T37.1X6
Thioctamide	T5Ø.991	T5Ø.992	T5Ø.993	T5Ø.994	T5Ø.995	T5Ø.996
Thioctic acid	T5Ø.991	T5Ø.992	T5Ø.993	T5Ø.994	T5Ø.995	T5Ø.996
Thiofos	T6Ø.ØX1	T6Ø.ØX2	T6Ø.ØX3	T6Ø.ØX4	—	—
Thioglycolate	T49.4X1	T49.4X2	T49.4X3	T49.4X4	T49.4X5	T49.4X6
Thioglycolic acid	T65.891	T65.892	T65.893	T65.894	—	—
Thioguanine	T45.1X1	T45.1X2	T45.1X3	T45.1X4	T45.1X5	T45.1X6
Thiomercaptomerin	T5Ø.2X1	T5Ø.2X2	T5Ø.2X3	T5Ø.2X4	T5Ø.2X5	T5Ø.2X6
Thiomerin	T5Ø.2X1	T5Ø.2X2	T5Ø.2X3	T5Ø.2X4	T5Ø.2X5	T5Ø.2X6
Thiomersal	T49.ØX1	T49.ØX2	T49.ØX3	T49.ØX4	T49.ØX5	T49.ØX6
Thionazin	T6Ø.ØX1	T6Ø.ØX2	T6Ø.ØX3	T6Ø.ØX4	—	—
Thiopental (sodium)	T41.1X1	T41.1X2	T41.1X3	T41.1X4	T41.1X5	T41.1X6
Thiopentone (sodium)	T41.1X1	T41.1X2	T41.1X3	T41.1X4	T41.1X5	T41.1X6
Thiopropazate	T43.3X1	T43.3X2	T43.3X3	T43.3X4	T43.3X5	T43.3X6
Thioproperazine	T43.3X1	T43.3X2	T43.3X3	T43.3X4	T43.3X5	T43.3X6
Thioridazine	T43.3X1	T43.3X2	T43.3X3	T43.3X4	T43.3X5	T43.3X6
Thiosinamine	T49.3X1	T49.3X2	T49.3X3	T49.3X4	T49.3X5	T49.3X6
Thiotepa	T45.1X1	T45.1X2	T45.1X3	T45.1X4	T45.1X5	T45.1X6
Thiothixene	T43.4X1	T43.4X2	T43.4X3	T43.4X4	T43.4X5	T43.4X6
Thiouracil (benzyl) (methyl) (propyl)	T38.2X1	T38.2X2	T38.2X3	T38.2X4	T38.2X5	T38.2X6
Thiourea	T38.2X1	T38.2X2	T38.2X3	T38.2X4	T38.2X5	T38.2X6
Thiphenamil	T44.3X1	T44.3X2	T44.3X3	T44.3X4	T44.3X5	T44.3X6
Thiram	T6Ø.3X1	T6Ø.3X2	T6Ø.3X3	T6Ø.3X4	—	—
medicinal	T49.2X1	T49.2X2	T49.2X3	T49.2X4	T49.2X5	T49.2X6
Thonzylamine (systemic)	T45.ØX1	T45.ØX2	T45.ØX3	T45.ØX4	T45.ØX5	T45.ØX6
mucosal decongestant	T48.5X1	T48.5X2	T48.5X3	T48.5X4	T48.5X5	T48.5X6
Thorazine	T43.3X1	T43.3X2	T43.3X3	T43.3X4	T43.3X5	T43.3X6
Thorium dioxide suspension	T5Ø.8X1	T5Ø.8X2	T5Ø.8X3	T5Ø.8X4	T5Ø.8X5	T5Ø.8X6
Thornapple	T62.2X1	T62.2X2	T62.2X3	T62.2X4	—	—
Throat drug NEC	T49.6X1	T49.6X2	T49.6X3	T49.6X4	T49.6X5	T49.6X6
Thrombin	T45.7X1	T45.7X2	T45.7X3	T45.7X4	T45.7X5	T45.7X6
Thrombolysin	T45.611	T45.612	T45.613	T45.614	T45.615	T45.616
Thromboplastin	T45.7X1	T45.7X2	T45.7X3	T45.7X4	T45.7X5	T45.7X6
Thurfyl nicotinate	T46.7X1	T46.7X2	T46.7X3	T46.7X4	T46.7X5	T46.7X6
Thymol	T49.ØX1	T49.ØX2	T49.ØX3	T49.ØX4	T49.ØX5	T49.ØX6
Thymopentin	T37.5X1	T37.5X2	T37.5X3	T37.5X4	T37.5X5	T37.5X6
Thymoxamine	T46.7X1	T46.7X2	T46.7X3	T46.7X4	T46.7X5	T46.7X6
Thymus extract	T38.891	T38.892	T38.893	T38.894	T38.895	T38.896
Thyreotrophic hormone	T38.811	T38.812	T38.813	T38.814	T38.815	T38.816
Thyroglobulin	T38.1X1	T38.1X2	T38.1X3	T38.1X4	T38.1X5	T38.1X6

Substance	Poisoning, Accidental (unintentional)	Poisoning, Intentional Self-harm	Poisoning, Assault	Poisoning, Undetermined	Adverse Effect	Under-dosing
Thyroid (hormone)	T38.1X1	T38.1X2	T38.1X3	T38.1X4	T38.1X5	T38.1X6
Thyrolar	T38.1X1	T38.1X2	T38.1X3	T38.1X4	T38.1X5	T38.1X6
Thyrotrophin	T38.811	T38.812	T38.813	T38.814	T38.815	T38.816
Thyrotropic hormone	T38.811	T38.812	T38.813	T38.814	T38.815	T38.816
Thyroxine	T38.1X1	T38.1X2	T38.1X3	T38.1X4	T38.1X5	T38.1X6
Tiabendazole	T37.4X1	T37.4X2	T37.4X3	T37.4X4	T37.4X5	T37.4X6
Tiamizide	T50.2X1	T50.2X2	T50.2X3	T50.2X4	T50.2X5	T50.2X6
Tianeptine	T43.291	T43.292	T43.293	T43.294	T43.295	T43.296
Tiapamil	T46.1X1	T46.1X2	T46.1X3	T46.1X4	T46.1X5	T46.1X6
Tiapride	T43.591	T43.592	T43.593	T43.594	T43.595	T43.596
Tiaprofenic acid	T39.311	T39.312	T39.313	T39.314	T39.315	T39.316
Tiaramide	T39.8X1	T39.8X2	T39.8X3	T39.8X4	T39.8X5	T39.8X6
Ticarcillin	T36.0X1	T36.0X2	T36.0X3	T36.0X4	T36.0X5	T36.0X6
Ticlatone	T49.0X1	T49.0X2	T49.0X3	T49.0X4	T49.0X5	T49.0X6
Ticlopidine	T45.521	T45.522	T45.523	T45.524	T45.525	T45.526
Ticrynafen	T50.1X1	T50.1X2	T50.1X3	T50.1X4	T50.1X5	T50.1X6
Tidiacic	T50.991	T50.992	T50.993	T50.994	T50.995	T50.996
Tiemonium	T44.3X1	T44.3X2	T44.3X3	T44.3X4	T44.3X5	T44.3X6
iodide	T44.3X1	T44.3X2	T44.3X3	T44.3X4	T44.3X5	T44.3X6
Tienilic acid	T50.1X1	T50.1X2	T50.1X3	T50.1X4	T50.1X5	T50.1X6
Tifenamil	T44.3X1	T44.3X2	T44.3X3	T44.3X4	T44.3X5	T44.3X6
Tigan	T45.0X1	T45.0X2	T45.0X3	T45.0X4	T45.0X5	T45.0X6
Tigloidine	T44.3X1	T44.3X2	T44.3X3	T44.3X4	T44.3X5	T44.3X6
Tilactase	T47.5X1	T47.5X2	T47.5X3	T47.5X4	T47.5X5	T47.5X6
Tiletamine	T41.291	T41.292	T41.293	T41.294	T41.295	T41.296
Tilidine	T40.4X1	T40.4X2	T40.4X3	T40.4X4	—	—
Timepidium bromide	T44.3X1	T44.3X2	T44.3X3	T44.3X4	T44.3X5	T44.3X6
Timiperone	T43.4X1	T43.4X2	T43.4X3	T43.4X4	T43.4X5	T43.4X6
Timolol	T44.7X1	T44.7X2	T44.7X3	T44.7X4	T44.7X5	T44.7X6
Tin (chloride) (dust) (oxide) **NEC**	T56.6X1	T56.6X2	T56.6X3	T56.6X4	—	—
anti-infectives	T37.8X1	T37.8X2	T37.8X3	T37.8X4	T37.8X5	T37.8X6
Tincture, iodine—*see* Iodine						
Tindal	T43.3X1	T43.3X2	T43.3X3	T43.3X4	T43.3X5	T43.3X6
Tinidazole	T37.3X1	T37.3X2	T37.3X3	T37.3X4	T37.3X5	T37.3X6
Tinoridine	T39.8X1	T39.8X2	T39.8X3	T39.8X4	T39.8X5	T39.8X6
Tiocarlide	T37.1X1	T37.1X2	T37.1X3	T37.1X4	T37.1X5	T37.1X6
Tioclomarol	T45.511	T45.512	T45.513	T45.514	T45.515	T45.516
Tioconazole	T49.0X1	T49.0X2	T49.0X3	T49.0X4	T49.0X5	T49.0X6
Tioguanine	T45.1X1	T45.1X2	T45.1X3	T45.1X4	T45.1X5	T45.1X6
Tiopronin	T50.991	T50.992	T50.993	T50.994	T50.995	T50.996
Tiotixene	T43.4X1	T43.4X2	T43.4X3	T43.4X4	T43.4X5	T43.4X6
Tioxolone	T49.4X1	T49.4X2	T49.4X3	T49.4X4	T49.4X5	T49.4X6
Tipepidine	T48.3X1	T48.3X2	T48.3X3	T48.3X4	T48.3X5	T48.3X6
Tiquizium bromide	T44.3X1	T44.3X2	T44.3X3	T44.3X4	T44.3X5	T44.3X6
Tiratricol	T38.1X1	T38.1X2	T38.1X3	T38.1X4	T38.1X5	T38.1X6
Tisopurine	T50.4X1	T50.4X2	T50.4X3	T50.4X4	T50.4X5	T50.4X6
Titanium (compounds) (vapor)	T56.891	T56.892	T56.893	T56.894	—	—
dioxide	T49.3X1	T49.3X2	T49.3X3	T49.3X4	T49.3X5	T49.3X6
ointment	T49.3X1	T49.3X2	T49.3X3	T49.3X4	T49.3X5	T49.3X6
oxide	T49.3X1	T49.3X2	T49.3X3	T49.3X4	T49.3X5	T49.3X6
tetrachloride	T56.891	T56.892	T56.893	T56.894	—	—
Titanocene	T56.891	T56.892	T56.893	T56.894	—	—
Titroid	T38.1X1	T38.1X2	T38.1X3	T38.1X4	T38.1X5	T38.1X6
Tizanidine	T42.8X1	T42.8X2	T42.8X3	T42.8X4	T42.8X5	T42.8X6
TMTD	T60.3X1	T60.3X2	T60.3X3	T60.3X4	—	—
TNT (fumes)	T65.3X1	T65.3X2	T65.3X3	T65.3X4	—	—
Toadstool	T62.0X1	T62.0X2	T62.0X3	T62.0X4	—	—
Tobacco NEC	T65.291	T65.292	T65.293	T65.294	—	—
cigarettes	T65.221	T65.222	T65.223	T65.224	—	—
Indian	T62.291	T62.292	T62.293	T62.294	—	—
smoke, second-hand	T65.221	T65.222	T65.223	T65.224	—	—
Tobramycin	T36.5X1	T36.5X2	T36.5X3	T36.5X4	T36.5X5	T36.5X6
Tocainide	T46.2X1	T46.2X2	T46.2X3	T46.2X4	T46.2X5	T46.2X6
Tocoferol	T45.2X1	T45.2X2	T45.2X3	T45.2X4	T45.2X5	T45.2X6
Tocopherol	T45.2X1	T45.2X2	T45.2X3	T45.2X4	T45.2X5	T45.2X6
acetate	T45.2X1	T45.2X2	T45.2X3	T45.2X4	T45.2X5	T45.2X6
Tocosamine	T48.0X1	T48.0X2	T48.0X3	T48.0X4	T48.0X5	T48.0X6
Todralazine	T46.5X1	T46.5X2	T46.5X3	T46.5X4	T46.5X5	T46.5X6
Tofisopam	T42.4X1	T42.4X2	T42.4X3	T42.4X4	T42.4X5	T42.4X6
Tofranil	T43.011	T43.012	T43.013	T43.014	T43.015	T43.016
Toilet deodorizer	T65.891	T65.892	T65.893	T65.894	—	—

Substance	Poisoning, Accidental (unintentional)	Poisoning, Intentional Self-harm	Poisoning, Assault	Poisoning, Undetermined	Adverse Effect	Under-dosing
Tolamolol	T44.7X1	T44.7X2	T44.7X3	T44.7X4	T44.7X5	T44.7X6
Tolazamide	T38.3X1	T38.3X2	T38.3X3	T38.3X4	T38.3X5	T38.3X6
Tolazoline	T46.7X1	T46.7X2	T46.7X3	T46.7X4	T46.7X5	T46.7X6
Tolbutamide (sodium)	T38.3X1	T38.3X2	T38.3X3	T38.3X4	T38.3X5	T38.3X6
Tolciclate	T49.0X1	T49.0X2	T49.0X3	T49.0X4	T49.0X5	T49.0X6
Tolmetin	T39.391	T39.392	T39.393	T39.394	T39.395	T39.396
Tolnaftate	T49.0X1	T49.0X2	T49.0X3	T49.0X4	T49.0X5	T49.0X6
Tolonidine	T46.5X1	T46.5X2	T46.5X3	T46.5X4	T46.5X5	T46.5X6
Toloxatone	T42.6X1	T42.6X2	T42.6X3	T42.6X4	T42.6X5	T42.6X6
Tolperisone	T44.3X1	T44.3X2	T44.3X3	T44.3X4	T44.3X5	T44.3X6
Tolserol	T42.8X1	T42.8X2	T42.8X3	T42.8X4	T42.8X5	T42.8X6
Toluene (liquid)	T52.2X1	T52.2X2	T52.2X3	T52.2X4	—	—
diisocyanate	T65.0X1	T65.0X2	T65.0X3	T65.0X4	—	—
Toluidine	T65.891	T65.892	T65.893	T65.894	—	—
vapor	T59.891	T59.892	T59.893	T59.894	—	—
Toluol (liquid)	T52.2X1	T52.2X2	T52.2X3	T52.2X4	—	—
vapor	T52.2X1	T52.2X2	T52.2X3	T52.2X4	—	—
Toluylenediamine	T65.3X1	T65.3X2	T65.3X3	T65.3X4	—	—
Tolylene-2,4-diisocyanate	T65.0X1	T65.0X2	T65.0X3	T65.0X4	—	—
Tonic NEC	T50.901	T50.902	T50.903	T50.904	T50.905	T50.906
Topical action drug NEC	T49.91	T49.92	T49.93	T49.94	T49.95	T49.96
ear, nose or throat	T49.6X1	T49.6X2	T49.6X3	T49.6X4	T49.6X5	T49.6X6
eye	T49.5X1	T49.5X2	T49.5X3	T49.5X4	T49.5X5	T49.5X6
skin	T49.91	T49.92	T49.93	T49.94	T49.95	T49.96
specified NEC	T49.8X1	T49.8X2	T49.8X3	T49.8X4	T49.8X5	T49.8X6
Toquizine	T44.3X1	T44.3X2	T44.3X3	T44.3X4	T44.3X5	T44.3X6
Toremifene	T38.6X1	T38.6X2	T38.6X3	T38.6X4	T38.6X5	T38.6X6
Tosylchloramide sodium	T49.8X1	T49.8X2	T49.8X3	T49.8X4	T49.8X5	T49.8X6
Toxaphene (dust) (spray)	T60.1X1	T60.1X2	T60.1X3	T60.1X4	—	—
Toxin, diphtheria (Schick Test)	T50.8X1	T50.8X2	T50.8X3	T50.8X4	T50.8X5	T50.8X6
Toxoid						
combined	T50.A21	T50.A22	T50.A23	T50.A24	T50.A25	T50.A26
diphtheria	T50.A91	T50.A92	T50.A93	T50.A94	T50.A95	T50.A96
tetanus	T50.A91	T50.A92	T50.A93	T50.A94	T50.A95	T50.A96
Trace element NEC	T45.8X1	T45.8X2	T45.8X3	T45.8X4	T45.8X5	T45.8X6
Tractor fuel NEC	T52.0X1	T52.0X2	T52.0X3	T52.0X4	—	—
Tragacanth	T50.991	T50.992	T50.993	T50.994	T50.995	T50.996
Tramadol	T40.4X1	T40.4X2	T40.4X3	T40.4X4	T40.4X5	T40.4X6
Tramazoline	T48.5X1	T48.5X2	T48.5X3	T48.5X4	T48.5X5	T48.5X6
Tranexamic acid	T45.621	T45.622	T45.623	T45.624	T45.625	T45.626
Tranilast	T45.0X1	T45.0X2	T45.0X3	T45.0X4	T45.0X5	T45.0X6
Tranquilizer NEC	T43.501	T43.502	T43.503	T43.504	T43.505	T43.506
with hypnotic or sedative	T42.6X1	T42.6X2	T42.6X3	T42.6X4	T42.6X5	T42.6X6
benzodiazepine NEC	T42.4X1	T42.4X2	T42.4X3	T42.4X4	T42.4X5	T42.4X6
butyrophenone NEC	T43.4X1	T43.4X2	T43.4X3	T43.4X4	T43.4X5	T43.4X6
carbamate	T43.591	T43.592	T43.593	T43.594	T43.595	T43.596
dimethylamine	T43.3X1	T43.3X2	T43.3X3	T43.3X4	T43.3X5	T43.3X6
ethylamine	T43.3X1	T43.3X2	T43.3X3	T43.3X4	T43.3X5	T43.3X6
hydroxyzine	T43.591	T43.592	T43.593	T43.594	T43.595	T43.596
major NEC	T43.501	T43.502	T43.503	T43.504	T43.505	T43.506
penothiazine NEC	T43.3X1	T43.3X2	T43.3X3	T43.3X4	T43.3X5	T43.3X6
phenothiazine-based	T43.3X1	T43.3X2	T43.3X3	T43.3X4	T43.3X5	T43.3X6
piperazine NEC	T43.3X1	T43.3X2	T43.3X3	T43.3X4	T43.3X5	T43.3X6
piperidine	T43.3X1	T43.3X2	T43.3X3	T43.3X4	T43.3X5	T43.3X6
propylamine	T43.3X1	T43.3X2	T43.3X3	T43.3X4	T43.3X5	T43.3X6
specified NEC	T43.591	T43.592	T43.593	T43.594	T43.595	T43.596
thioxanthene NEC	T43.591	T43.592	T43.593	T43.594	T43.595	T43.596
Tranxene	T42.4X1	T42.4X2	T42.4X3	T42.4X4	T42.4X5	T42.4X6
Tranylcypromine	T43.1X1	T43.1X2	T43.1X3	T43.1X4	T43.1X5	T43.1X6
Trapidil	T46.3X1	T46.3X2	T46.3X3	T46.3X4	T46.3X5	T46.3X6
Trasentine	T44.3X1	T44.3X2	T44.3X3	T44.3X4	T44.3X5	T44.3X6
Travert	T50.3X1	T50.3X2	T50.3X3	T50.3X4	T50.3X5	T50.3X6
Trazodone	T43.211	T43.212	T43.213	T43.214	T43.215	T43.216
Trecator	T37.1X1	T37.1X2	T37.1X3	T37.1X4	T37.1X5	T37.1X6
Treosulfan	T45.1X1	T45.1X2	T45.1X3	T45.1X4	T45.1X5	T45.1X6
Tretamine	T45.1X1	T45.1X2	T45.1X3	T45.1X4	T45.1X5	T45.1X6
Tretinoin	T49.0X1	T49.0X2	T49.0X3	T49.0X4	T49.0X5	T49.0X6
Tretoquinol	T48.6X1	T48.6X2	T48.6X3	T48.6X4	T48.6X5	T48.6X6
Triacetin	T49.0X1	T49.0X2	T49.0X3	T49.0X4	T49.0X5	T49.0X6
Triacetoxyanthracene	T49.4X1	T49.4X2	T49.4X3	T49.4X4	T49.4X5	T49.4X6
Triacetyloleandomycin	T36.3X1	T36.3X2	T36.3X3	T36.3X4	T36.3X5	T36.3X6

Substance	Poisoning, Accidental (unintentional)	Poisoning, Intentional Self-harm	Poisoning, Assault	Poisoning, Undetermined	Adverse Effect	Under-dosing
Triamcinolone	T49.ØX1	T49.ØX2	T49.ØX3	T49.ØX4	T49.ØX5	T49.ØX6
ENT agent	T49.6X1	T49.6X2	T49.6X3	T49.6X4	T49.6X5	T49.6X6
hexacetonide	T49.ØX1	T49.ØX2	T49.ØX3	T49.ØX4	T49.ØX5	T49.ØX6
ophthalmic preparation	T49.5X1	T49.5X2	T49.5X3	T49.5X4	T49.5X5	T49.5X6
topical NEC	T49.ØX1	T49.ØX2	T49.ØX3	T49.ØX4	T49.ØX5	T49.ØX6
Triampyzine	T44.3X1	T44.3X2	T44.3X3	T44.3X4	T44.3X5	T44.3X6
Triamterene	T5Ø.2X1	T5Ø.2X2	T5Ø.2X3	T5Ø.2X4	T5Ø.2X5	T5Ø.2X6
Triazine (herbicide)	T6Ø.3X1	T6Ø.3X2	T6Ø.3X3	T6Ø.3X4	—	—
Triaziquone	T45.1X1	T45.1X2	T45.1X3	T45.1X4	T45.1X5	T45.1X6
Triazolam	T42.4X1	T42.4X2	T42.4X3	T42.4X4	T42.4X5	T42.4X6
Triazole (herbicide)	T6Ø.3X1	T6Ø.3X2	T6Ø.3X3	T6Ø.3X4	—	—
Tribenoside	T46.991	T46.992	T46.993	T46.994	T46.995	T46.996
Tribromacetaldehyde	T42.6X1	T42.6X2	T42.6X3	T42.6X4	T42.6X5	T42.6X6
Tribromoethanol, rectal	T41.291	T41.292	T41.293	T41.294	T41.295	T41.296
Tribromomethane	T42.6X1	T42.6X2	T42.6X3	T42.6X4	T42.6X5	T42.6X6
Trichlorethane	T53.2X1	T53.2X2	T53.2X3	T53.2X4	—	—
Trichlorethylene	T53.2X1	T53.2X2	T53.2X3	T53.2X4	—	—
Trichlorfon	T6Ø.ØX1	T6Ø.ØX2	T6Ø.ØX3	T6Ø.ØX4	—	—
Trichlormethiazide	T5Ø.2X1	T5Ø.2X2	T5Ø.2X3	T5Ø.2X4	T5Ø.2X5	T5Ø.2X6
Trichlormethine	T45.1X1	T45.1X2	T45.1X3	T45.1X4	T45.1X5	T45.1X6
Trichloroacetic acid, Trichloracetic acid	T54.2X1	T54.2X2	T54.2X3	T54.2X4	—	—
medicinal	T49.4X1	T49.4X2	T49.4X3	T49.4X4	T49.4X5	T49.4X6
Trichloroethane	T53.2X1	T53.2X2	T53.2X3	T53.2X4	—	—
Trichloroethanol	T42.6X1	T42.6X2	T42.6X3	T42.6X4	T42.6X5	T42.6X6
Trichloroethylene (liquid) (vapor)	T53.2X1	T53.2X2	T53.2X3	T53.2X4	—	—
anesthetic (gas)	T41.ØX1	T41.ØX2	T41.ØX3	T41.ØX4	T41.ØX5	T41.ØX6
vapor NEC	T53.2X1	T53.2X2	T53.2X3	T53.2X4	—	—
Trichloroethyl phosphate	T42.6X1	T42.6X2	T42.6X3	T42.6X4	T42.6X5	T42.6X6
Trichlorofluoromethane NEC	T53.5X1	T53.5X2	T53.5X3	T53.5X4	—	—
Trichloronate	T6Ø.ØX1	T6Ø.ØX2	T6Ø.ØX3	T6Ø.ØX4	—	—
Trichloropropane	T53.6X1	T53.6X2	T53.6X3	T53.6X4	—	—
2,4,5-Trichlorophen-oxyacetic acid	T6Ø.3X1	T6Ø.3X2	T6Ø.3X3	T6Ø.3X4	—	—
Trichlorotriethylamine	T45.1X1	T45.1X2	T45.1X3	T45.1X4	T45.1X5	T45.1X6
Trichomonacides NEC	T37.3X1	T37.3X2	T37.3X3	T37.3X4	T37.3X5	T37.3X6
Trichomycin	T36.7X1	T36.7X2	T36.7X3	T36.7X4	T36.7X5	T36.7X6
Triclobisonium chloride	T49.ØX1	T49.ØX2	T49.ØX3	T49.ØX4	T49.ØX5	T49.ØX6
Triclocarban	T49.ØX1	T49.ØX2	T49.ØX3	T49.ØX4	T49.ØX5	T49.ØX6
Triclofos	T42.6X1	T42.6X2	T42.6X3	T42.6X4	T42.6X5	T42.6X6
Triclosan	T49.ØX1	T49.ØX2	T49.ØX3	T49.ØX4	T49.ØX5	T49.ØX6
Tricresyl phosphate	T65.891	T65.892	T65.893	T65.894	—	—
solvent	T52.91	T52.92	T52.93	T52.94	—	—
Tricyclamol chloride	T44.3X1	T44.3X2	T44.3X3	T44.3X4	T44.3X5	T44.3X6
Tridesilon	T49.ØX1	T49.ØX2	T49.ØX3	T49.ØX4	T49.ØX5	T49.ØX6
Tridihexethyl iodide	T44.3X1	T44.3X2	T44.3X3	T44.3X4	T44.3X5	T44.3X6
Tridione	T42.2X1	T42.2X2	T42.2X3	T42.2X4	T42.2X5	T42.2X6
Trientine	T45.8X1	T45.8X2	T45.8X3	T45.8X4	T45.8X5	T45.8X6
Triethanolamine NEC	T54.3X1	T54.3X2	T54.3X3	T54.3X4	—	—
detergent	T54.3X1	T54.3X2	T54.3X3	T54.3X4	—	—
trinitrate (biphosphate)	T46.3X1	T46.3X2	T46.3X3	T46.3X4	T46.3X5	T46.3X6
Triethanomelamine	T45.1X1	T45.1X2	T45.1X3	T45.1X4	T45.1X5	T45.1X6
Triethylenemelamine	T45.1X1	T45.1X2	T45.1X3	T45.1X4	T45.1X5	T45.1X6
Triethylenephosphoramide	T45.1X1	T45.1X2	T45.1X3	T45.1X4	T45.1X5	T45.1X6
Triethylenethiophosphoramide	T45.1X1	T45.1X2	T45.1X3	T45.1X4	T45.1X5	T45.1X6
Trifluoperazine	T43.3X1	T43.3X2	T43.3X3	T43.3X4	T43.3X5	T43.3X6
Trifluoroethyl vinyl ether	T41.ØX1	T41.ØX2	T41.ØX3	T41.ØX4	T41.ØX5	T41.ØX6
Trifluperidol	T43.4X1	T43.4X2	T43.4X3	T43.4X4	T43.4X5	T43.4X6
Triflupromazine	T43.3X1	T43.3X2	T43.3X3	T43.3X4	T43.3X5	T43.3X6
Trifluridine	T37.5X1	T37.5X2	T37.5X3	T37.5X4	T37.5X5	T37.5X6
Triflusal	T45.521	T45.522	T45.523	T45.524	T45.525	T45.526
Trihexyphenidyl	T44.3X1	T44.3X2	T44.3X3	T44.3X4	T44.3X5	T44.3X6
Triiodothyronine	T38.1X1	T38.1X2	T38.1X3	T38.1X4	T38.1X5	T38.1X6
Trilene	T41.ØX1	T41.ØX2	T41.ØX3	T41.ØX4	T41.ØX5	T41.ØX6
Trilostane	T38.991	T38.992	T38.993	T38.994	T38.995	T38.996
Trimebutine	T44.3X1	T44.3X2	T44.3X3	T44.3X4	T44.3X5	T44.3X6
Trimecaine	T41.3X1	T41.3X2	T41.3X3	T41.3X4	T41.3X5	T41.3X6
Trimeprazine (tartrate)	T44.3X1	T44.3X2	T44.3X3	T44.3X4	T44.3X5	T44.3X6
Trimetaphan camsilate	T44.2X1	T44.2X2	T44.2X3	T44.2X4	T44.2X5	T44.2X6
Trimetazidine	T46.7X1	T46.7X2	T46.7X3	T46.7X4	T46.7X5	T46.7X6
Trimethadione	T42.2X1	T42.2X2	T42.2X3	T42.2X4	T42.2X5	T42.2X6
Trimethaphan	T44.2X1	T44.2X2	T44.2X3	T44.2X4	T44.2X5	T44.2X6
Trimethidinium	T44.2X1	T44.2X2	T44.2X3	T44.2X4	T44.2X5	T44.2X6
Trimethobenzamide	T45.ØX1	T45.ØX2	T45.ØX3	T45.ØX4	T45.ØX5	T45.ØX6
Trimethoprim	T37.8X1	T37.8X2	T37.8X3	T37.8X4	T37.8X5	T37.8X6
with sulfamethoxazole	T36.8X1	T36.8X2	T36.8X3	T36.8X4	T36.8X5	T36.8X6
Trimethylcarbinol	T51.3X1	T51.3X2	T51.3X3	T51.3X4	—	—
Trimethylpsoralen	T49.3X1	T49.3X2	T49.3X3	T49.3X4	T49.3X5	T49.3X6
Trimeton	T45.ØX1	T45.ØX2	T45.ØX3	T45.ØX4	T45.ØX5	T45.ØX6
Trimetrexate	T45.1X1	T45.1X2	T45.1X3	T45.1X4	T45.1X5	T45.1X6
Trimipramine	T43.Ø11	T43.Ø12	T43.Ø13	T43.Ø14	T43.Ø15	T43.Ø16
Trimustine	T45.1X1	T45.1X2	T45.1X3	T45.1X4	T45.1X5	T45.1X6
Trinitrine	T46.3X1	T46.3X2	T46.3X3	T46.3X4	T46.3X5	T46.3X6
Trinitrobenzol	T65.3X1	T65.3X2	T65.3X3	T65.3X4	—	—
Trinitrophenol	T65.3X1	T65.3X2	T65.3X3	T65.3X4	—	—
Trinitrotoluene (fumes)	T65.3X1	T65.3X2	T65.3X3	T65.3X4	—	—
Trional	T42.6X1	T42.6X2	T42.6X3	T42.6X4	T42.6X5	T42.6X6
Triorthocresyl phosphate	T65.891	T65.892	T65.893	T65.894	—	—
Trioxide of arsenic	T57.ØX1	T57.ØX2	T57.ØX3	T57.ØX4	—	—
Trioxysalen	T49.4X1	T49.4X2	T49.4X3	T49.4X4	T49.4X5	T49.4X6
Tripamide	T5Ø.2X1	T5Ø.2X2	T5Ø.2X3	T5Ø.2X4	T5Ø.2X5	T5Ø.2X6
Triparanol	T46.6X1	T46.6X2	T46.6X3	T46.6X4	T46.6X5	T46.6X6
Tripelennamine	T45.ØX1	T45.ØX2	T45.ØX3	T45.ØX4	T45.ØX5	T45.ØX6
Triperiden	T44.3X1	T44.3X2	T44.3X3	T44.3X4	T44.3X5	T44.3X6
Triperidol	T43.4X1	T43.4X2	T43.4X3	T43.4X4	T43.4X5	T43.4X6
Triphenylphosphate	T65.891	T65.892	T65.893	T65.894	—	—
Triple						
bromides	T42.6X1	T42.6X2	T42.6X3	T42.6X4	T42.6X5	T42.6X6
carbonate	T47.1X1	T47.1X2	T47.1X3	T47.1X4	T47.1X5	T47.1X6
vaccine						
DPT	T5Ø.A11	T5Ø.A12	T5Ø.A13	T5Ø.A14	T5Ø.A15	T5Ø.A16
including pertussis	T5Ø.A11	T5Ø.A12	T5Ø.A13	T5Ø.A14	T5Ø.A15	T5Ø.A16
MMR	T5Ø.B91	T5Ø.B92	T5Ø.B93	T5Ø.B94	T5Ø.B95	T5Ø.B96
Triprolidine	T45.ØX1	T45.ØX2	T45.ØX3	T45.ØX4	T45.ØX5	T45.ØX6
Trisodium hydrogen edetate	T5Ø.6X1	T5Ø.6X2	T5Ø.6X3	T5Ø.6X4	T5Ø.6X5	T5Ø.6X6
Trisoralen	T49.3X1	T49.3X2	T49.3X3	T49.3X4	T49.3X5	T49.3X6
Trisulfapyrimidines	T37.ØX1	T37.ØX2	T37.ØX3	T37.ØX4	T37.ØX5	T37.ØX6
Trithiozine	T44.3X1	T44.3X2	T44.3X3	T44.3X4	T44.3X5	T44.3X6
Tritiozine	T44.3X1	T44.3X2	T44.3X3	T44.3X4	T44.3X5	T44.3X6
Tritoqualine	T45.ØX1	T45.ØX2	T45.ØX3	T45.ØX4	T45.ØX5	T45.ØX6
Trofosfamide	T45.1X1	T45.1X2	T45.1X3	T45.1X4	T45.1X5	T45.1X6
Troleandomycin	T36.3X1	T36.3X2	T36.3X3	T36.3X4	T36.3X5	T36.3X6
Trolnitrate (phosphate)	T46.3X1	T46.3X2	T46.3X3	T46.3X4	T46.3X5	T46.3X6
Tromantadine	T37.5X1	T37.5X2	T37.5X3	T37.5X4	T37.5X5	T37.5X6
Trometamol	T5Ø.2X1	T5Ø.2X2	T5Ø.2X3	T5Ø.2X4	T5Ø.2X5	T5Ø.2X6
Tromethamine	T5Ø.2X1	T5Ø.2X2	T5Ø.2X3	T5Ø.2X4	T5Ø.2X5	T5Ø.2X6
Tronothane	T41.3X1	T41.3X2	T41.3X3	T41.3X4	T41.3X5	T41.3X6
Tropacine	T44.3X1	T44.3X2	T44.3X3	T44.3X4	T44.3X5	T44.3X6
Tropatepine	T44.3X1	T44.3X2	T44.3X3	T44.3X4	T44.3X5	T44.3X6
Tropicamide	T44.3X1	T44.3X2	T44.3X3	T44.3X4	T44.3X5	T44.3X6
Trospium chloride	T44.3X1	T44.3X2	T44.3X3	T44.3X4	T44.3X5	T44.3X6
Troxerutin	T46.991	T46.992	T46.993	T46.994	T46.995	T46.996
Troxidone	T42.2X1	T42.2X2	T42.2X3	T42.2X4	T42.2X5	T42.2X6
Tryparsamide	T37.3X1	T37.3X2	T37.3X3	T37.3X4	T37.3X5	T37.3X6
Trypsin	T45.3X1	T45.3X2	T45.3X3	T45.3X4	T45.3X5	T45.3X6
Tryptizol	T43.Ø11	T43.Ø12	T43.Ø13	T43.Ø14	T43.Ø15	T43.Ø16
TSH	T38.811	T38.812	T38.813	T38.814	T38.815	T38.816
Tuaminoheptane	T48.5X1	T48.5X2	T48.5X3	T48.5X4	T48.5X5	T48.5X6
Tuberculin, purified protein derivative (PPD)	T5Ø.8X1	T5Ø.8X2	T5Ø.8X3	T5Ø.8X4	T5Ø.8X5	T5Ø.8X6
Tubocurare	T48.1X1	T48.1X2	T48.1X3	T48.1X4	T48.1X5	T48.1X6
Tubocurarine (chloride)	T48.1X1	T48.1X2	T48.1X3	T48.1X4	T48.1X5	T48.1X6
Tulobuterol	T48.6X1	T48.6X2	T48.6X3	T48.6X4	T48.6X5	T48.6X6
Turpentine (spirits of)	T52.8X1	T52.8X2	T52.8X3	T52.8X4	—	—
vapor	T52.8X1	T52.8X2	T52.8X3	T52.8X4	—	—
Tybamate	T43.591	T43.592	T43.593	T43.594	T43.595	T43.596
Tyloxapol	T48.4X1	T48.4X2	T48.4X3	T48.4X4	T48.4X5	T48.4X6
Tymazoline	T48.5X1	T48.5X2	T48.5X3	T48.5X4	T48.5X5	T48.5X6
Typhoid-paratyphoid vaccine	T5Ø.A91	T5Ø.A92	T5Ø.A93	T5Ø.A94	T5Ø.A95	T5Ø.A96
Typhus vaccine	T5Ø.A91	T5Ø.A92	T5Ø.A93	T5Ø.A94	T5Ø.A95	T5Ø.A96
Tyropanoate	T5Ø.8X1	T5Ø.8X2	T5Ø.8X3	T5Ø.8X4	T5Ø.8X5	T5Ø.8X6

Substance	Poisoning, Accidental (unintentional)	Poisoning, Intentional Self-harm	Poisoning, Assault	Poisoning, Undetermined	Adverse Effect	Under-dosing
Tyrothricin	T49.6X1	T49.6X2	T49.6X3	T49.6X4	T49.6X5	T49.6X6
ENT agent	T49.6X1	T49.6X2	T49.6X3	T49.6X4	T49.6X5	T49.6X6
ophthalmic preparation	T49.5X1	T49.5X2	T49.5X3	T49.5X4	T49.5X5	T49.5X6
U						
Ufenamate	T39.391	T39.392	T39.393	T39.394	T39.395	T39.396
Ultraviolet light protectant	T49.3X1	T49.3X2	T49.3X3	T49.3X4	T49.3X5	T49.3X6
Undecenoic acid	T49.ØX1	T49.ØX2	T49.ØX3	T49.ØX4	T49.ØX5	T49.ØX6
Undecoylium	T49.ØX1	T49.ØX2	T49.ØX3	T49.ØX4	T49.ØX5	T49.ØX6
Undecylenic acid (derivatives)	T49.ØX1	T49.ØX2	T49.ØX3	T49.ØX4	T49.ØX5	T49.ØX6
Unna's boot	T49.3X1	T49.3X2	T49.3X3	T49.3X4	T49.3X5	T49.3X6
Unsaturated fatty acid	T46.6X1	T46.6X2	T46.6X3	T46.6X4	T46.6X5	T46.6X6
Uracil mustard	T45.1X1	T45.1X2	T45.1X3	T45.1X4	T45.1X5	T45.1X6
Uramustine	T45.1X1	T45.1X2	T45.1X3	T45.1X4	T45.1X5	T45.1X6
Urapidil	T46.5X1	T46.5X2	T46.5X3	T46.5X4	T46.5X5	T46.5X6
Urari	T48.1X1	T48.1X2	T48.1X3	T48.1X4	T48.1X5	T48.1X6
Urate oxidase	T5Ø.4X1	T5Ø.4X2	T5Ø.4X3	T5Ø.4X4	T5Ø.4X5	T5Ø.4X6
Urea	T47.3X1	T47.3X2	T47.3X3	T47.3X4	T47.3X5	T47.3X6
peroxide	T49.ØX1	T49.ØX2	T49.ØX3	T49.ØX4	T49.ØX5	T49.ØX6
stibamine	T37.4X1	T37.4X2	T37.4X3	T37.4X4	T37.4X5	T37.4X6
topical	T49.8X1	T49.8X2	T49.8X3	T49.8X4	T49.8X5	T49.8X6
Urethane	T45.1X1	T45.1X2	T45.1X3	T45.1X4	T45.1X5	T45.1X6
Urginea (maritima) (scilla)—*see* Squill						
Uric acid metabolism drug NEC	T5Ø.4X1	T5Ø.4X2	T5Ø.4X3	T5Ø.4X4	T5Ø.4X5	T5Ø.4X6
Uricosuric agent	T5Ø.4X1	T5Ø.4X2	T5Ø.4X3	T5Ø.4X4	T5Ø.4X5	T5Ø.4X6
Urinary anti-infective	T37.8X1	T37.8X2	T37.8X3	T37.8X4	T37.8X5	T37.8X6
Urofollitropin	T38.811	T38.812	T38.813	T38.814	T38.815	T38.816
Urokinase	T45.611	T45.612	T45.613	T45.614	T45.615	T45.616
Urokon	T5Ø.8X1	T5Ø.8X2	T5Ø.8X3	T5Ø.8X4	T5Ø.8X5	T5Ø.8X6
Ursodeoxycholic acid	T5Ø.991	T5Ø.992	T5Ø.993	T5Ø.994	T5Ø.995	T5Ø.996
Ursodiol	T5Ø.991	T5Ø.992	T5Ø.993	T5Ø.994	T5Ø.995	T5Ø.996
Urtica	T62.2X1	T62.2X2	T62.2X3	T62.2X4	—	—
Utility gas—*see* Gas, utility						
V						
Vaccine NEC	T5Ø.Z91	T5Ø.Z92	T5Ø.Z93	T5Ø.Z94	T5Ø.Z95	T5Ø.Z96
antineoplastic	T5Ø.Z91	T5Ø.Z92	T5Ø.Z93	T5Ø.Z94	T5Ø.Z95	T5Ø.Z96
bacterial NEC	T5Ø.A91	T5Ø.A92	T5Ø.A93	T5Ø.A94	T5Ø.A95	T5Ø.A96
with						
other bacterial component	T5Ø.A21	T5Ø.A22	T5Ø.A23	T5Ø.A24	T5Ø.A25	T5Ø.A26
pertussis component	T5Ø.A11	T5Ø.A12	T5Ø.A13	T5Ø.A14	T5Ø.A15	T5Ø.A16
viral-rickettsial component	T5Ø.A21	T5Ø.A22	T5Ø.A23	T5Ø.A24	T5Ø.A25	T5Ø.A26
mixed NEC	T5Ø.A21	T5Ø.A22	T5Ø.A23	T5Ø.A24	T5Ø.A25	T5Ø.A26
BCG	T5Ø.A91	T5Ø.A92	T5Ø.A93	T5Ø.A94	T5Ø.A95	T5Ø.A96
cholera	T5Ø.A91	T5Ø.A92	T5Ø.A93	T5Ø.A94	T5Ø.A95	T5Ø.A96
diphtheria	T5Ø.A91	T5Ø.A92	T5Ø.A93	T5Ø.A94	T5Ø.A95	T5Ø.A96
with tetanus	T5Ø.A21	T5Ø.A22	T5Ø.A23	T5Ø.A24	T5Ø.A25	T5Ø.A26
and pertussis	T5Ø.A11	T5Ø.A12	T5Ø.A13	T5Ø.A14	T5Ø.A15	T5Ø.A16
influenza	T5Ø.B91	T5Ø.B92	T5Ø.B93	T5Ø.B94	T5Ø.B95	T5Ø.B96
measles	T5Ø.B91	T5Ø.B92	T5Ø.B93	T5Ø.B94	T5Ø.B95	T5Ø.B96
with mumps and rubella	T5Ø.B91	T5Ø.B92	T5Ø.B93	T5Ø.B94	T5Ø.B95	T5Ø.B96
meningococcal	T5Ø.A91	T5Ø.A92	T5Ø.A93	T5Ø.A94	T5Ø.A95	T5Ø.A96
mumps	T5Ø.B91	T5Ø.B92	T5Ø.B93	T5Ø.B94	T5Ø.B95	T5Ø.B96
paratyphoid	T5Ø.A91	T5Ø.A92	T5Ø.A93	T5Ø.A94	T5Ø.A95	T5Ø.A96
pertussis	T5Ø.A11	T5Ø.A12	T5Ø.A13	T5Ø.A14	T5Ø.A15	T5Ø.A16
with diphtheria	T5Ø.A11	T5Ø.A12	T5Ø.A13	T5Ø.A14	T5Ø.A15	T5Ø.A16
and tetanus	T5Ø.A11	T5Ø.A12	T5Ø.A13	T5Ø.A14	T5Ø.A15	T5Ø.A16
with other component	T5Ø.A11	T5Ø.A12	T5Ø.A13	T5Ø.A14	T5Ø.A15	T5Ø.A16
plague	T5Ø.A91	T5Ø.A92	T5Ø.A93	T5Ø.A94	T5Ø.A95	T5Ø.A96
poliomyelitis	T5Ø.B91	T5Ø.B92	T5Ø.B93	T5Ø.B94	T5Ø.B95	T5Ø.B96
poliovirus	T5Ø.B91	T5Ø.B92	T5Ø.B93	T5Ø.B94	T5Ø.B95	T5Ø.B96
rabies	T5Ø.B91	T5Ø.B92	T5Ø.B93	T5Ø.B94	T5Ø.B95	T5Ø.B96
respiratory syncytial virus	T5Ø.B91	T5Ø.B92	T5Ø.B93	T5Ø.B94	T5Ø.B95	T5Ø.B96
rickettsial NEC	T5Ø.A91	T5Ø.A92	T5Ø.A93	T5Ø.A94	T5Ø.A95	T5Ø.A96
with						
bacterial component	T5Ø.A21	T5Ø.A22	T5Ø.A23	T5Ø.A24	T5Ø.A25	T5Ø.A26
Rocky Mountain spotted fever	T5Ø.A91	T5Ø.A92	T5Ø.A93	T5Ø.A94	T5Ø.A95	T5Ø.A96
rubella	T5Ø.B91	T5Ø.B92	T5Ø.B93	T5Ø.B94	T5Ø.B95	T5Ø.B96
sabin oral	T5Ø.B91	T5Ø.B92	T5Ø.B93	T5Ø.B94	T5Ø.B95	T5Ø.B96
smallpox	T5Ø.B11	T5Ø.B12	T5Ø.B13	T5Ø.B14	T5Ø.B15	T5Ø.B16
TAB	T5Ø.A91	T5Ø.A92	T5Ø.A93	T5Ø.A94	T5Ø.A95	T5Ø.A96

Substance	Poisoning, Accidental (unintentional)	Poisoning, Intentional Self-harm	Poisoning, Assault	Poisoning, Undetermined	Adverse Effect	Under-dosing
Vaccine NEC—*continued*						
tetanus	T5Ø.A91	T5Ø.A92	T5Ø.A93	T5Ø.A94	T5Ø.A95	T5Ø.A96
typhoid	T5Ø.A91	T5Ø.A92	T5Ø.A93	T5Ø.A94	T5Ø.A95	T5Ø.A96
typhus	T5Ø.A91	T5Ø.A92	T5Ø.A93	T5Ø.A94	T5Ø.A95	T5Ø.A96
viral NEC	T5Ø.B91	T5Ø.B92	T5Ø.B93	T5Ø.B94	T5Ø.B95	T5Ø.B96
yellow fever	T5Ø.B91	T5Ø.B92	T5Ø.B93	T5Ø.B94	T5Ø.B95	T5Ø.B96
Vaccinia immune globulin	T5Ø.Z11	T5Ø.Z12	T5Ø.Z13	T5Ø.Z14	T5Ø.Z15	T5Ø.Z16
Vaginal contraceptives	T49.8X1	T49.8X2	T49.8X3	T49.8X4	T49.8X5	T49.8X6
Valerian						
root	T42.6X1	T42.6X2	T42.6X3	T42.6X4	T42.6X5	T42.6X6
tincture	T42.6X1	T42.6X2	T42.6X3	T42.6X4	T42.6X5	T42.6X6
Valethamate bromide	T44.3X1	T44.3X2	T44.3X3	T44.3X4	T44.3X5	T44.3X6
Valisone	T49.ØX1	T49.ØX2	T49.ØX3	T49.ØX4	T49.ØX5	T49.ØX6
Valium	T42.4X1	T42.4X2	T42.4X3	T42.4X4	T42.4X5	T42.4X6
Valmid	T42.6X1	T42.6X2	T42.6X3	T42.6X4	T42.6X5	T42.6X6
Valnoctamide	T42.6X1	T42.6X2	T42.6X3	T42.6X4	T42.6X5	T42.6X6
Valproate (sodium)	T42.6X1	T42.6X2	T42.6X3	T42.6X4	T42.6X5	T42.6X6
Valproic acid	T42.6X1	T42.6X2	T42.6X3	T42.6X4	T42.6X5	T42.6X6
Valpromide	T42.6X1	T42.6X2	T42.6X3	T42.6X4	T42.6X5	T42.6X6
Vanadium	T56.891	T56.892	T56.893	T56.894	—	—
Vancomycin	T36.8X1	T36.8X2	T36.8X3	T36.8X4	T36.8X5	T36.8X6
Vapor—*see also* Gas	T59.91	T59.92	T59.93	T59.94	—	—
kiln (carbon monoxide)	T58.8X1	T58.8X2	T58.8X3	T58.8X4	—	—
lead—*see* lead						
specified source NEC	T59.891	T59.892	T59.893	T59.894	—	—
Vardenafil	T46.7X1	T46.7X2	T46.7X3	T46.7X4	T46.7X5	T46.7X6
Varicose reduction drug	T46.8X1	T46.8X2	T46.8X3	T46.8X4	T46.8X5	T46.8X6
Varnish	T65.4X1	T65.4X2	T65.4X3	T65.4X4	—	—
cleaner	T52.91	T52.92	T52.93	T52.94	—	—
Vaseline	T49.3X1	T49.3X2	T49.3X3	T49.3X4	T49.3X5	T49.3X6
Vasodilan	T46.7X1	T46.7X2	T46.7X3	T46.7X4	T46.7X5	T46.7X6
Vasodilator						
coronary NEC	T46.3X1	T46.3X2	T46.3X3	T46.3X4	T46.3X5	T46.3X6
peripheral NEC	T46.7X1	T46.7X2	T46.7X3	T46.7X4	T46.7X5	T46.7X6
Vasopressin	T38.891	T38.892	T38.893	T38.894	T38.895	T38.896
Vasopressor drugs	T38.891	T38.892	T38.893	T38.894	T38.895	T38.896
Vecuronium bromide	T48.1X1	T48.1X2	T48.1X3	T48.1X4	T48.1X5	T48.1X6
Vegetable extract, astringent	T49.2X1	T49.2X2	T49.2X3	T49.2X4	T49.2X5	T49.2X6
Venlafaxine	T43.211	T43.212	T43.213	T43.214	T43.215	T43.216
Venom, venomous (bite) (sting)	T63.91	T63.92	T63.93	T63.94	—	—
ant	T63.421	T63.422	T63.423	T63.424	—	—
amphibian NEC	T63.831	T63.832	T63.833	T63.834	—	—
animal NEC	T63.891	T63.892	T63.893	T63.894	—	—
arthropod NEC	T63.481	T63.482	T63.483	T63.484	—	—
bee	T63.441	T63.442	T63.443	T63.444	—	—
centipede	T63.411	T63.412	T63.413	T63.414	—	—
fish	T63.591	T63.592	T63.593	T63.594	—	—
frog	T63.811	T63.812	T63.813	T63.814	—	—
hornet	T63.451	T63.452	T63.453	T63.454	—	—
insect NEC	T63.481	T63.482	T63.483	T63.484	—	—
lizard	T63.121	T63.122	T63.123	T63.124	—	—
marine						
animals	T63.691	T63.692	T63.693	T63.694	—	—
bluebottle	T63.611	T63.612	T63.613	T63.614	—	—
jellyfish NEC	T63.621	T63.622	T63.623	T63.624	—	—
Portuguese Man-o-war	T63.611	T63.612	T63.613	T63.614	—	—
sea anemone	T63.631	T63.632	T63.633	T63.634	—	—
specified NEC	T63.691	T63.692	T63.693	T63.694	—	—
plants	T63.711	T63.712	T63.713	T63.714	—	—
millipede (tropical)	T63.411	T63.412	T63.413	T63.414	—	—
plant NEC	T63.791	T63.792	T63.793	T63.794	—	—
marine	T63.711	T63.712	T63.713	T63.714	—	—
reptile	T63.191	T63.192	T63.193	T63.194	—	—
gila monster	T63.111	T63.112	T63.113	T63.114	—	—
lizard NEC	T63.121	T63.122	T63.123	T63.124	—	—
scorpion	T63.2X1	T63.2X2	T63.2X3	T63.2X4	—	—
snake	T63.ØØ1	T63.ØØ2	T63.ØØ3	T63.ØØ4	—	—
African NEC	T63.Ø81	T63.Ø82	T63.Ø83	T63.Ø84	—	—
American (North) (South) NEC	T63.Ø61	T63.Ø62	T63.Ø63	T63.Ø64	—	—
Asian	T63.Ø81	T63.Ø82	T63.Ø83	T63.Ø84	—	—
Australian	T63.Ø71	T63.Ø72	T63.Ø73	T63.Ø74	—	—

Substance	Poisoning, Accidental (unintentional)	Poisoning, Intentional Self-harm	Poisoning, Assault	Poisoning, Undetermined	Adverse Effect	Under-dosing
Venom, venomous (bite) (sting) *— continued*						
snake						
cobra	T63.041	T63.042	T63.043	T63.044	—	—
coral snake	T63.021	T63.022	T63.023	T63.024	—	—
rattlesnake	T63.011	T63.012	T63.013	T63.014	—	—
specified NEC	T63.091	T63.092	T63.093	T63.094	—	—
taipan	T63.031	T63.032	T63.033	T63.034	—	—
specified NEC	T63.891	T63.892	T63.893	T63.894	—	—
spider	T63.301	T63.302	T63.303	T63.304	—	—
black widow	T63.311	T63.312	T63.313	T63.314	—	—
brown recluse	T63.331	T63.332	T63.333	T63.334	—	—
specified NEC	T63.391	T63.392	T63.393	T63.394	—	—
tarantula	T63.321	T63.322	T63.323	T63.324	—	—
sting ray	T63.511	T63.512	T63.513	T63.514	—	—
toad	T63.821	T63.822	T63.823	T63.824	—	—
wasp	T63.461	T63.462	T63.463	T63.464	—	—
Venous sclerosing drug NEC	T46.8X1	T46.8X2	T46.8X3	T46.8X4	T46.8X5	T46.8X6
Ventolin—*see* Albuterol						
Verapamil	T46.1X1	T46.1X2	T46.1X3	T46.1X4	T46.1X5	T46.1X6
Veramon	T42.3X1	T42.3X2	T42.3X3	T42.3X4	T42.3X5	T42.3X6
Veratrine	T46.5X1	T46.5X2	T46.5X3	T46.5X4	T46.5X5	T46.5X6
Veratrum						
album	T62.2X1	T62.2X2	T62.2X3	T62.2X4	—	—
alkaloids	T46.5X1	T46.5X2	T46.5X3	T46.5X4	T46.5X5	T46.5X6
viride	T62.2X1	T62.2X2	T62.2X3	T62.2X4	—	—
Verdigris	T60.3X1	T60.3X2	T60.3X3	T60.3X4	—	—
Veronal	T42.3X1	T42.3X2	T42.3X3	T42.3X4	T42.3X5	T42.3X6
Veroxil	T37.4X1	T37.4X2	T37.4X3	T37.4X4	T37.4X5	T37.4X6
Versenate	T50.6X1	T50.6X2	T50.6X3	T50.6X4	T50.6X5	T50.6X6
Versidyne	T39.8X1	T39.8X2	T39.8X3	T39.8X4	T39.8X5	T39.8X6
Vetrabutine	T48.0X1	T48.0X2	T48.0X3	T48.0X4	T48.0X5	T48.0X6
Vidarabine	T37.5X1	T37.5X2	T37.5X3	T37.5X4	T37.5X5	T37.5X6
Vienna						
green	T57.0X1	T57.0X2	T57.0X3	T57.0X4	—	—
insecticide	T60.2X1	T60.2X2	T60.2X3	T60.2X4	—	—
red	T57.0X1	T57.0X2	T57.0X3	T57.0X4	—	—
pharmaceutical dye	T50.991	T50.992	T50.993	T50.994	T50.995	T50.996
Vigabatrin	T42.6X1	T42.6X2	T42.6X3	T42.6X4	T42.6X5	T42.6X6
Viloxazine	T43.291	T43.292	T43.293	T43.294	T43.295	T43.296
Viminol	T39.8X1	T39.8X2	T39.8X3	T39.8X4	T39.8X5	T39.8X6
Vinbarbital, vinbarbitone	T42.3X1	T42.3X2	T42.3X3	T42.3X4	T42.3X5	T42.3X6
Vinblastine	T45.1X1	T45.1X2	T45.1X3	T45.1X4	T45.1X5	T45.1X6
Vinburnine	T46.7X1	T46.7X2	T46.7X3	T46.7X4	T46.7X5	T46.7X6
Vincamine	T45.1X1	T45.1X2	T45.1X3	T45.1X4	T45.1X5	T45.1X6
Vincristine	T45.1X1	T45.1X2	T45.1X3	T45.1X4	T45.1X5	T45.1X6
Vindesine	T45.1X1	T45.1X2	T45.1X3	T45.1X4	T45.1X5	T45.1X6
Vinesthene, vinethene	T41.0X1	T41.0X2	T41.0X3	T41.0X4	T41.0X5	T41.0X6
Vinorelbine tartrate	T45.1X1	T45.1X2	T45.1X3	T45.1X4	T45.1X5	T45.1X6
Vinpocetine	T46.7X1	T46.7X2	T46.7X3	T46.7X4	T46.7X5	T46.7X6
Vinyl						
acetate	T65.891	T65.892	T65.893	T65.894	—	—
bital	T42.3X1	T42.3X2	T42.3X3	T42.3X4	T42.3X5	T42.3X6
bromide	T65.891	T65.892	T65.893	T65.894	—	—
chloride	T59.891	T59.892	T59.893	T59.894	—	—
ether	T41.0X1	T41.0X2	T41.0X3	T41.0X4	T41.0X5	T41.0X6
Vinylbital	T42.3X1	T42.3X2	T42.3X3	T42.3X4	T42.3X5	T42.3X6
Vinylidene chloride	T65.891	T65.892	T65.893	T65.894	—	—
Vioform	T37.8X1	T37.8X2	T37.8X3	T37.8X4	T37.8X5	T37.8X6
topical	T49.0X1	T49.0X2	T49.0X3	T49.0X4	T49.0X5	T49.0X6
Viomycin	T36.8X1	T36.8X2	T36.8X3	T36.8X4	T36.8X5	T36.8X6
Viosterol	T45.2X1	T45.2X2	T45.2X3	T45.2X4	T45.2X5	T45.2X6
Viper (venom)	T63.091	T63.092	T63.093	T63.094	—	—
Viprynium	T37.4X1	T37.4X2	T37.4X3	T37.4X4	T37.4X5	T37.4X6
Viquidil	T46.7X1	T46.7X2	T46.7X3	T46.7X4	T46.7X5	T46.7X6
Viral vaccine NEC	T50.B91	T50.B92	T50.B93	T50.B94	T50.B95	T50.B96
Virginiamycin	T36.8X1	T36.8X2	T36.8X3	T36.8X4	T36.8X5	T36.8X6
Virugon	T37.5X1	T37.5X2	T37.5X3	T37.5X4	T37.5X5	T37.5X6
Viscous agent	T50.901	T50.902	T50.903	T50.904	T50.905	T50.906
Visine	T49.5X1	T49.5X2	T49.5X3	T49.5X4	T49.5X5	T49.5X6
Visnadine	T46.3X1	T46.3X2	T46.3X3	T46.3X4	T46.3X5	T46.3X6

Substance	Poisoning, Accidental (unintentional)	Poisoning, Intentional Self-harm	Poisoning, Assault	Poisoning, Undetermined	Adverse Effect	Under-dosing
Vitamin NEC	T45.2X1	T45.2X2	T45.2X3	T45.2X4	T45.2X5	T45.2X6
A	T45.2X1	T45.2X2	T45.2X3	T45.2X4	T45.2X5	T45.2X6
B NEC	T45.2X1	T45.2X2	T45.2X3	T45.2X4	T45.2X5	T45.2X6
nicotinic acid	T46.7X1	T46.7X2	T46.7X3	T46.7X4	T46.7X5	T46.7X6
B1	T45.2X1	T45.2X2	T45.2X3	T45.2X4	T45.2X5	T45.2X6
B2	T45.2X1	T45.2X2	T45.2X3	T45.2X4	T45.2X5	T45.2X6
B6	T45.2X1	T45.2X2	T45.2X3	T45.2X4	T45.2X5	T45.2X6
B12	T45.2X1	T45.2X2	T45.2X3	T45.2X4	T45.2X5	T45.2X6
B15	T45.2X1	T45.2X2	T45.2X3	T45.2X4	T45.2X5	T45.2X6
C	T45.2X1	T45.2X2	T45.2X3	T45.2X4	T45.2X5	T45.2X6
D	T45.2X1	T45.2X2	T45.2X3	T45.2X4	T45.2X5	T45.2X6
D2	T45.2X1	T45.2X2	T45.2X3	T45.2X4	T45.2X5	T45.2X6
D3	T45.2X1	T45.2X2	T45.2X3	T45.2X4	T45.2X5	T45.2X6
E	T45.2X1	T45.2X2	T45.2X3	T45.2X4	T45.2X5	T45.2X6
E acetate	T45.2X1	T45.2X2	T45.2X3	T45.2X4	T45.2X5	T45.2X6
hematopoietic	T45.8X1	T45.8X2	T45.8X3	T45.8X4	T45.8X5	T45.8X6
K NEC	T45.7X1	T45.7X2	T45.7X3	T45.7X4	T45.7X5	T45.7X6
K1	T45.7X1	T45.7X2	T45.7X3	T45.7X4	T45.7X5	T45.7X6
K2	T45.7X1	T45.7X2	T45.7X3	T45.7X4	T45.7X5	T45.7X6
PP	T45.2X1	T45.2X2	T45.2X3	T45.2X4	T45.2X5	T45.2X6
ulceroprotectant	T47.1X1	T47.1X2	T47.1X3	T47.1X4	T47.1X5	T47.1X6
Vleminckx's solution	T49.4X1	T49.4X2	T49.4X3	T49.4X4	T49.4X5	T49.4X6
Voltaren—*see* Diclofenac sodium						
W						
Warfarin	T45.511	T45.512	T45.513	T45.514	T45.515	T45.516
rodenticide	T60.4X1	T60.4X2	T60.4X3	T60.4X4	—	—
sodium	T60.4X1	T60.4X2	T60.4X3	T60.4X4	—	—
Wasp (sting)	T63.461	T63.462	T63.463	T63.464	—	—
Water						
balance drug	T50.3X1	T50.3X2	T50.3X3	T50.3X4	T50.3X5	T50.3X6
distilled	T50.3X1	T50.3X2	T50.3X3	T50.3X4	T50.3X5	T50.3X6
gas—*see* Gas, water						
incomplete combustion of—*see* Carbon, monoxide, fuel, utility						
hemlock	T62.2X1	T62.2X2	T62.2X3	T62.2X4	—	—
moccasin (venom)	T63.061	T63.062	T63.063	T63.064	—	—
purified	T50.3X1	T50.3X2	T50.3X3	T50.3X4	T50.3X5	T50.3X6
Wax (paraffin) (petroleum)	T52.0X1	T52.0X2	T52.0X3	T52.0X4	—	—
automobile	T65.891	T65.892	T65.893	T65.894	—	—
floor	T52.0X1	T52.0X2	T52.0X3	T52.0X4	—	—
Weed killers NEC	T60.3X1	T60.3X2	T60.3X3	T60.3X4	—	—
Welldorm	T42.6X1	T42.6X2	T42.6X3	T42.6X4	T42.6X5	T42.6X6
White						
arsenic	T57.0X1	T57.0X2	T57.0X3	T57.0X4	—	—
hellebore	T62.2X1	T62.2X2	T62.2X3	T62.2X4	—	—
lotion (keratolytic)	T49.4X1	T49.4X2	T49.4X3	T49.4X4	T49.4X5	T49.4X6
spirit	T52.0X1	T52.0X2	T52.0X3	T52.0X4	—	—
Whitewash	T65.891	T65.892	T65.893	T65.894	—	—
Whole Blood (human)	T45.8X1	T45.8X2	T45.8X3	T45.8X4	T45.8X5	T45.8X6
Wild						
black cherry	T62.2X1	T62.2X2	T62.2X3	T62.2X4	—	—
poisonous plants NEC	T62.2X1	T62.2X2	T62.2X3	T62.2X4	—	—
Window cleaning fluid	T65.891	T65.892	T65.893	T65.894	—	—
Wintergreen (oil)	T49.3X1	T49.3X2	T49.3X3	T49.3X4	T49.3X5	T49.3X6
Witch hazel	T49.2X1	T49.2X2	T49.2X3	T49.2X4	T49.2X5	T49.2X6
Wisterine	T62.2X1	T62.2X2	T62.2X3	T62.2X4	—	—
Witch hazel	T49.2X1	T49.2X2	T49.2X3	T49.2X4	T49.2X5	T49.2X6
Wood alcohol or spirit	T51.1X1	T51.1X2	T51.1X3	T51.1X4	—	—
Wool fat (hydrous)	T49.3X1	T49.3X2	T49.3X3	T49.3X4	T49.3X5	T49.3X6
Woorali	T48.1X1	T48.1X2	T48.1X3	T48.1X4	T48.1X5	T48.1X6
Wormseed, American	T37.4X1	T37.4X2	T37.4X3	T37.4X4	T37.4X5	T37.4X6
X						
Xamoterol	T44.5X1	T44.5X2	T44.5X3	T44.5X4	T44.5X5	T44.5X6
Xanthine diuretics	T50.2X1	T50.2X2	T50.2X3	T50.2X4	T50.2X5	T50.2X6
Xanthinol nicotinate	T46.7X1	T46.7X2	T46.7X3	T46.7X4	T46.7X5	T46.7X6
Xanthotoxin	T49.3X1	T49.3X2	T49.3X3	T49.3X4	T49.3X5	T49.3X6
Xantinol nicotinate	T46.7X1	T46.7X2	T46.7X3	T46.7X4	T46.7X5	T46.7X6
Xantocillin	T36.0X1	T36.0X2	T36.0X3	T36.0X4	T36.0X5	T36.0X6
Xenon (127Xe) (133Xe)	T50.8X1	T50.8X2	T50.8X3	T50.8X4	T50.8X5	T50.8X6

Substance	Poisoning, Accidental (unintentional)	Poisoning, Intentional Self-harm	Poisoning, Assault	Poisoning, Undetermined	Adverse Effect	Under-dosing
Xenysalate	T49.4X1	T49.4X2	T49.4X3	T49.4X4	T49.4X5	T49.4X6
Xibornol	T37.8X1	T37.8X2	T37.8X3	T37.8X4	T37.8X5	T37.8X6
Xigris	T45.511	T45.512	T45.513	T45.514	T45.515	T45.516
Xipamide	T5Ø.2X1	T5Ø.2X2	T5Ø.2X3	T5Ø.2X4	T5Ø.2X5	T5Ø.2X6
Xylene (vapor)	T52.2X1	T52.2X2	T52.2X3	T52.2X4	—	—
Xylocaine (infiltration) (topical)	T41.3X1	T41.3X2	T41.3X3	T41.3X4	T41.3X5	T41.3X6
nerve block (peripheral) (plexus)	T41.3X1	T41.3X2	T41.3X3	T41.3X4	T41.3X5	T41.3X6
spinal	T41.3X1	T41.3X2	T41.3X3	T41.3X4	T41.3X5	T41.3X6
Xylol (vapor)	T52.2X1	T52.2X2	T52.2X3	T52.2X4	—	—
Xylometazoline	T48.5X1	T48.5X2	T48.5X3	T48.5X4	T48.5X5	T48.5X6
Y						
Yeast	T45.2X1	T45.2X2	T45.2X3	T45.2X4	T45.2X5	T45.2X6
dried	T45.2X1	T45.2X2	T45.2X3	T45.2X4	T45.2X5	T45.2X6
Yellow						
fever vaccine	T5Ø.B91	T5Ø.B92	T5Ø.B93	T5Ø.B94	T5Ø.B95	T5Ø.B96
jasmine	T62.2X1	T62.2X2	T62.2X3	T62.2X4	—	—
phenolphthalein	T47.2X1	T47.2X2	T47.2X3	T47.2X4	T47.2X5	T47.2X6
Yew	T62.2X1	T62.2X2	T62.2X3	T62.2X4	—	—
Yohimbic acid	T4Ø.991	T4Ø.992	T4Ø.993	T4Ø.994	T4Ø.995	T4Ø.996
Z						
Zactane	T39.8X1	T39.8X2	T39.8X3	T39.8X4	T39.8X5	T39.8X6
Zalcitabine	T37.5X1	T37.5X2	T37.5X3	T37.5X4	T37.5X5	T37.5X6
Zaroxolyn	T5Ø.2X1	T5Ø.2X2	T5Ø.2X3	T5Ø.2X4	T5Ø.2X5	T5Ø.2X6
Zephiran (topical)	T49.ØX1	T49.ØX2	T49.ØX3	T49.ØX4	T49.ØX5	T49.ØX6
ophthalmic preparation	T49.5X1	T49.5X2	T49.5X3	T49.5X4	T49.5X5	T49.5X6
Zeranol	T38.7X1	T38.7X2	T38.7X3	T38.7X4	T38.7X5	T38.7X6
Zerone	T51.1X1	T51.1X2	T51.1X3	T51.1X4	—	—
Zidovudine	T37.5X1	T37.5X2	T37.5X3	T37.5X4	T37.5X5	T37.5X6
Zimeldine	T43.221	T43.222	T43.223	T43.224	T43.225	T43.226
Zinc (compounds) (fumes) (vapor) **NEC**	T56.5X1	T56.5X2	T56.5X3	T56.5X4	—	—
anti-infectives	T49.ØX1	T49.ØX2	T49.ØX3	T49.ØX4	T49.ØX5	T49.ØX6
antivaricose	T46.8X1	T46.8X2	T46.8X3	T46.8X4	T46.8X5	T46.8X6
Zinc NEC — *continued*						
bacitracin	T49.ØX1	T49.ØX2	T49.ØX3	T49.ØX4	T49.ØX5	T49.ØX6
chloride (mouthwash)	T49.6X1	T49.6X2	T49.6X3	T49.6X4	T49.6X5	T49.6X6
chromate	T56.5X1	T56.5X2	T56.5X3	T56.5X4	—	—
gelatin	T49.3X1	T49.3X2	T49.3X3	T49.3X4	T49.3X5	T49.3X6
oxide	T49.3X1	T49.3X2	T49.3X3	T49.3X4	T49.3X5	T49.3X6
plaster	T49.3X1	T49.3X2	T49.3X3	T49.3X4	T49.3X5	T49.3X6
peroxide	T49.ØX1	T49.ØX2	T49.ØX3	T49.ØX4	T49.ØX5	T49.ØX6
pesticides	T56.5X1	T56.5X2	T56.5X3	T56.5X4	—	—
phosphide	T6Ø.4X1	T6Ø.4X2	T6Ø.4X3	T6Ø.4X4	—	—
pyrithionate	T49.4X1	T49.4X2	T49.4X3	T49.4X4	T49.4X5	T49.4X6
stearate	T49.3X1	T49.3X2	T49.3X3	T49.3X4	T49.3X5	T49.3X6
sulfate	T49.5X1	T49.5X2	T49.5X3	T49.5X4	T49.5X5	T49.5X6
ENT agent	T49.6X1	T49.6X2	T49.6X3	T49.6X4	T49.6X5	T49.6X6
ophthalmic solution	T49.5X1	T49.5X2	T49.5X3	T49.5X4	T49.5X5	T49.5X6
topical NEC	T49.ØX1	T49.ØX2	T49.ØX3	T49.ØX4	T49.ØX5	T49.ØX6
undecylenate	T49.ØX1	T49.ØX2	T49.ØX3	T49.ØX4	T49.ØX5	T49.ØX6
Zineb	T6Ø.ØX1	T6Ø.ØX2	T6Ø.ØX3	T6Ø.ØX4	—	—
Zinostatin	T45.1X1	T45.1X2	T45.1X3	T45.1X4	T45.1X5	T45.1X6
Zipeprol	T48.3X1	T48.3X2	T48.3X3	T48.3X4	T48.3X5	T48.3X6
Zofenopril	T46.4X1	T46.4X2	T46.4X3	T46.4X4	T46.4X5	T46.4X6
Zolpidem	T42.6X1	T42.6X2	T42.6X3	T42.6X4	T42.6X5	T42.6X6
Zomepirac	T39.391	T39.392	T39.393	T39.394	T39.395	T39.396
Zopiclone	T42.6X1	T42.6X2	T42.6X3	T42.6X4	T42.6X5	T42.6X6
Zorubicin	T45.1X1	T45.1X2	T45.1X3	T45.1X4	T45.1X5	T45.1X6
Zotepine	T43.591	T43.592	T43.593	T43.594	T43.595	T43.596
Zovant	T45.511	T45.512	T45.513	T45.514	T45.515	T45.516
Zoxazolamine	T42.8X1	T42.8X2	T42.8X3	T42.8X4	T42.8X5	T42.8X6
Zuclopenthixol	T43.4X1	T43.4X2	T43.4X3	T43.4X4	T43.4X5	T43.4X6
Zygadenus (venenosus)	T62.2X1	T62.2X2	T62.2X3	T62.2X4	—	—
Zyprexa	T43.591	T43.592	T43.593	T43.594	T43.595	T43.596

ICD-1Ø-CM Index to External Causes

A

- **Abandonment** (causing exposure to weather conditions) (with intent to injure or kill) NEC X58
- **Abuse** (adult) (child) (mental) (physical) (sexual) X58
- **Accident** (to) X58
  - aircraft (in transit) (powered) (*see also* Accident, transport, aircraft)
    - due to, caused by cataclysm — *see* Forces of nature, by type
  - animal-rider — *see* Accident, transport, animal-rider
  - animal-drawn vehicle — *see* Accident, transport, animal-drawn vehicle occupant
  - automobile — *see* Accident, transport, car occupant
  - bare foot water skiier V94.4
  - boat, boating (*see also* Accident, watercraft)
    - striking swimmer
      - powered V94.11
      - unpowered V94.12
  - bus — *see* Accident, transport, bus occupant
  - cable car, not on rails V98.Ø
    - on rails — *see* Accident, transport, streetcar occupant
  - car — *see* Accident, transport, car occupant
  - caused by, due to
    - animal NEC W64
    - chain hoist W24.Ø
    - cold (excessive) — *see* Exposure, cold
    - corrosive liquid, substance — *see* Table of Drugs and Chemicals
    - cutting or piercing instrument — *see* Contact, with, by type of instrument
    - drive belt W24.Ø
    - electric
      - current — *see* Exposure, electric current
      - motor (*see also* Contact, with, by type of machine) W31.3
        - current (of) W86.8
    - environmental factor NEC X58
    - explosive material — *see* Explosion
    - fire, flames — *see* Exposure, fire
    - firearm missile — *see* Discharge, firearm by type
    - heat (excessive) — *see* Heat
    - hot — *see* Contact, with, hot
    - ignition — *see* Ignition
    - lifting device W24.Ø
    - lightning — *see* subcategory T75.Ø
      - causing fire — *see* Exposure, fire
    - machine, machinery — *see* Contact, with, by type of machine
    - natural factor NEC X58
    - pulley (block) W24.Ø
    - radiation — *see* Radiation
    - steam X13.1
      - inhalation X13.Ø
      - pipe X16
    - thunderbolt — *see* subcategory T75.Ø
      - causing fire — *see* Exposure, fire
    - transmission device W24.1
  - coach — *see* Accident, transport, bus occupant
  - coal car — *see* Accident, transport, industrial vehicle occupant
  - diving (*see also* Fall, into, water)
    - with
      - drowning or submersion — *see* Drowning
  - forklift — *see* Accident, transport, industrial vehicle occupant
  - heavy transport vehicle NOS — *see* Accident, transport, truck occupant
  - ice yacht V98.2
  - in
    - medical, surgical procedure
      - as, or due to misadventure — *see* Misadventure

Accident— *continued*

- in— *continued*
  - medical, surgical procedure— *continued*
    - causing an abnormal reaction or later complication without mention of misadventure (*see also* Complication of or following, by type of procedure) Y84.9
- land yacht V98.1
- late effect of — *see* WØØ-X58 with 7th character S
- logging car — *see* Accident, transport, industrial vehicle occupant
- machine, machinery (*see also* Contact, with, by type of machine)
  - on board watercraft V93.69
    - explosion — *see* Explosion, in, watercraft
    - fire — *see* Burn, on board watercraft
    - powered craft V93.63
      - ferry boat V93.61
      - fishing boat V93.62
      - jetskis V93.63
      - liner V93.61
      - merchant ship V93.6Ø
      - passenger ship V93.61
      - sailboat V93.64
- mine tram — *see* Accident, transport, industrial vehicle occupant
- mobility scooter (motorized) — *see* Accident, transport, pedestrian, conveyance, specified type NEC
- motor scooter — *see* Accident, transport, motorcyclist
- motor vehicle NOS (traffic) (*see also* Accident, transport) V89.2
  - nontraffic V89.Ø
  - three-wheeled NOS — *see* Accident, transport, three-wheeled motor vehicle occupant
- motorcycle NOS — *see* Accident, transport, motorcyclist
- nonmotor vehicle NOS (nontraffic) (*see also* Accident, transport) V89.1
  - traffic NOS V89.3
- nontraffic (victim's mode of transport NOS) V88.9
  - collision (between) V88.7
    - bus and truck V88.5
    - car and:
      - bus V88.3
      - pickup V88.2
      - three-wheeled motor vehicle V88.Ø
      - train V88.6
      - truck V88.4
      - two-wheeled motor vehicle V88.Ø
      - van V88.2
    - specified vehicle NEC and:
      - three-wheeled motor vehicle V88.1
      - two-wheeled motor vehicle V88.1
  - known mode of transport — *see* Accident, transport, by type of vehicle
  - noncollision V88.8
- on board watercraft V93.89
  - powered craft V93.83
    - ferry boat V93.81
    - fishing boat V93.82
    - jetskis V93.83
    - liner V93.81
    - merchant ship V93.8Ø
    - passenger ship V93.81
  - unpowered craft V93.88
    - canoe V93.85
    - inflatable V93.86
      - in tow
        - recreational V94.31
        - specified NEC V94.32
    - kayak V93.85
    - sailboat V93.84
    - surf-board V93.88
    - water skis V93.87

Accident— *continued*

- on board watercraft— *continued*
  - unpowered craft— *continued*
    - windsurfer V93.88
- parachutist V97.29
  - entangled in object V97.21
  - injured on landing V97.22
- pedal cycle — *see* Accident, transport, pedal cyclist
- pedestrian (on foot)
  - with
    - another pedestrian W51
      - with fall WØ3
        - due to ice or snow WØØ.Ø
        - on pedestrian conveyance NEC VØØ.Ø9
    - roller skater (in-line) VØØ.Ø1
    - skate boarder VØØ.Ø2
    - transport vehicle — *see* Accident, transport
  - on pedestrian conveyance — *see* Accident, transport, pedestrian, conveyance
- pick-up truck or van — *see* Accident, transport, pickup truck occupant
- quarry truck — *see* Accident, transport, industrial vehicle occupant
- railway vehicle (any) (in motion) — *see* Accident, transport, railway vehicle occupant
  - due to cataclysm — *see* Forces of nature, by type
- scooter (non-motorized) — *see* Accident, transport, pedestrian, conveyance, scooter
- sequelae of — *see* categories WØØ-X58 with 7th character S
- skateboard — *see* Accident, transport, pedestrian, conveyance, skateboard
- ski(ing) — *see* Accident, transport, pedestrian, conveyance
  - lift V98.3
- specified cause NEC X58
- streetcar — *see* Accident, transport, streetcar occupant
- traffic (victim's mode of transport NOS) V87.9
  - collision (between) V87.7
    - bus and truck V87.5
    - car and:
      - bus V87.3
      - pickup V87.2
      - three-wheeled motor vehicle V87.Ø
      - train V87.6
      - truck V87.4
      - two-wheeled motor vehicle V87.Ø
      - van V87.2
    - specified vehicle NEC and:
      - three-wheeled motor vehicle V87.1
      - two-wheeled motor vehicle V87.1
  - known mode of transport — *see* Accident, transport, by type of vehicle
  - noncollision V87.8
- transport (involving injury to) V99
  - 18 wheeler — *see* Accident, transport, truck occupant
  - agricultural vehicle occupant (nontraffic) V84.9
    - driver V84.5
    - hanger-on V84.7
    - passenger V84.6
    - traffic V84.3
      - driver V84.Ø
    - while boarding or alighting V84.4
  - aircraft NEC V97.89
    - military NEC V97.818
      - with civlian aircraft V97.81Ø
      - civilian injured by V97.811
    - occupant injured (in)
      - nonpowered craft accident V96.9
        - balloon V96.ØØ
          - collision V96.Ø3
          - crash V96.Ø1
          - explosion V96.Ø5
          - fire V96.Ø4

- **Accident**— *continued*
  - transport— *continued*
    - aircraft— *continued*
      - occupant injured— *continued*
        - nonpowered craft accident— *continued*
          - balloon— *continued*
            - forced landing V96.Ø2
            - specified type NEC V96.Ø9
          - glider V96.2Ø
            - collision V96.23
            - crash V96.21
            - explosion V96.25
            - fire V96.24
            - forced landing V96.22
            - specified type NEC V96.29
          - hang glider V96.1Ø
            - collision V96.13
            - crash V96.11
            - explosion V96.15
            - fire V96.14
            - forced landing V96.12
            - specified type NEC V96.19
          - specified craft NEC V96.8
        - powered craft accident V95.9
          - fixed wing NEC
            - commercial V95.3Ø
              - collision V95.33
              - crash V95.31
              - explosion V95.35
              - fire V95.34
              - forced landing V95.32
              - specified type NEC V95.39
            - private V95.2Ø
              - collision V95.23
              - crash V95.21
              - explosion V95.25
              - fire V95.24
              - forced landing V95.22
              - specified type NEC V95.29
          - glider V95.1Ø
            - collision V95.13
            - crash V95.11
            - explosion V95.15
            - fire V95.14
            - forced landing V95.12
            - specified type NEC V95.19
          - helicopter V95.ØØ
            - collision V95.Ø3
            - crash V95.Ø1
            - explosion V95.Ø5
            - fire V95.Ø4
            - forced landing V95.Ø2
            - specified type NEC V95.Ø9
          - spacecraft V95.4Ø
            - collision V95.43
            - crash V95.41
            - explosion V95.45
            - fire V95.44
            - forced landing V95.42
            - specified type NEC V95.49
          - specified craft NEC V95.8
          - ultralight V95.1Ø
            - collision V95.13
            - crash V95.11
            - explosion V95.15
            - fire V95.14
            - forced landing V95.12
            - specified type NEC V95.19
        - specified accident NEC V97.Ø
        - while boarding or alighting V97.1
      - person (injured by)
        - falling from, in or on aircraft V97.Ø
        - machinery on aircraft V97.89
        - on ground with aircraft involvement V97.39
        - rotating propeller V97.32
        - struck by object falling from aircraft V97.31
        - sucked into aircraft jet V97.33
        - while boarding or alighting aircraft V97.1
    - airport (battery-powered) passenger vehicle — *see* Accident, transport, industrial vehicle occupant

- **Accident**— *continued*
  - transport— *continued*
    - all-terrain vehicle occupant (nontraffic) V86.99
      - driver V86.59
      - dune buggy — *see* Accident, transport, dune buggy occupant
      - hanger-on V86.79
      - passenger V86.69
      - snowmobile — *see* Accident, transport, snowmobile occupant
      - traffic V86.39
        - driver V86.Ø9
        - hanger-on V86.29
        - passenger V86.19
      - while boarding or alighting V86.49
    - ambulance occupant (traffic) V86.31
      - driver V86.Ø1
      - hanger-on V86.21
      - nontraffic V86.91
        - driver V86.51
        - hanger-on V86.71
        - passenger V86.61
      - passenger V86.11
      - while boarding or alighting V86.41
    - animal-drawn vehicle occupant (in) V8Ø.929
      - collision (with)
        - animal V8Ø.12
          - being ridden V8Ø.711
        - animal-drawn vehicle V8Ø.721
        - bus V8Ø.42
        - car V8Ø.42
        - fixed or stationary object V8Ø.82
        - military vehicle V8Ø.92Ø
        - nonmotor vehicle V8Ø.791
        - pedal cycle V8Ø.22
        - pedestrian V8Ø.12
        - pickup V8Ø.42
        - railway train or vehicle V8Ø.62
        - specified motor vehicle NEC V8Ø.52
        - streetcar V8Ø.731
        - truck V8Ø.42
        - two or three-wheeled motor vehicle V8Ø.32
        - van V8Ø.42
      - noncollision V8Ø.Ø2
      - specified circumstance NEC V8Ø.928
    - animal-rider V8Ø.919
      - collision (with)
        - animal V8Ø.11
          - being ridden V8Ø.71Ø
        - animal-drawn vehicle V8Ø.72Ø
        - bus V8Ø.41
        - car V8Ø.41
        - fixed or stationary object V8Ø.81
        - military vehicle V8Ø.91Ø
        - nonmotor vehicle V8Ø.79Ø
        - pedal cycle V8Ø.21
        - pedestrian V8Ø.11
        - pickup V8Ø.41
        - railway train or vehicle V8Ø.61
        - specified motor vehicle NEC V8Ø.51
        - streetcar V8Ø.73Ø
        - truck V8Ø.41
        - two or three-wheeled motor vehicle V8Ø.31
        - van V8Ø.41
      - noncollision V8Ø.Ø18
        - specified as horse rider V8Ø.Ø1Ø
      - specified circumstance NEC V8Ø.918
    - armored car — *see* Accident, transport, truck occupant
    - battery-powered truck (baggage) (mail) — *see* Accident, transport, industrial vehicle occupant
    - bus occupant V79.9
      - collision (with)
        - animal (traffic) V7Ø.9
          - being ridden (traffic) V76.9
            - nontraffic V76.3
            - while boarding or alighting V76.4
          - nontraffic V7Ø.3

- **Accident**— *continued*
  - transport— *continued*
    - bus occupant— *continued*
      - collision— *continued*
        - animal— *continued*
          - while boarding or alighting V7Ø.4
        - animal-drawn vehicle (traffic) V76.9
          - nontraffic V76.3
          - while boarding or alighting V76.4
        - bus (traffic) V74.9
          - nontraffic V74.3
          - while boarding or alighting V74.4
        - car (traffic) V73.9
          - nontraffic V73.3
          - while boarding or alighting V73.4
        - motor vehicle NOS (traffic) V79.6Ø
          - nontraffic V79.2Ø
          - specified type NEC (traffic) V79.69
            - nontraffic V79.29
        - pedal cycle (traffic) V71.9
          - nontraffic V71.3
          - while boarding or alighting V71.4
        - pickup truck (traffic) V73.9
          - nontraffic V73.3
          - while boarding or alighting V73.4
        - railway vehicle (traffic) V75.9
          - nontraffic V75.3
          - while boarding or alighting V75.4
        - specified vehicle NEC (traffic) V76.9
          - nontraffic V76.3
          - while boarding or alighting V76.4
        - stationary object (traffic) V77.9
          - nontraffic V77.3
          - while boarding or alighting V77.4
        - streetcar (traffic) V76.9
          - nontraffic V76.3
          - while boarding or alighting V76.4
        - three wheeled motor vehicle (traffic) V72.9
          - nontraffic V72.3
          - while boarding or alighting V72.4
        - truck (traffic) V74.9
          - nontraffic V74.3
          - while boarding or alighting V74.4
        - two wheeled motor vehicle (traffic) V72.9
          - nontraffic V72.3
          - while boarding or alighting V72.4
        - van (traffic) V73.9
          - nontraffic V73.3
          - while boarding or alighting V73.4
      - driver
        - collision (with)
          - animal (traffic) V7Ø.5
            - being ridden (traffic) V76.5
              - nontraffic V76.Ø
            - nontraffic V7Ø.Ø
          - animal-drawn vehicle (traffic) V76.5
            - nontraffic V76.Ø
          - bus (traffic) V74.5
            - nontraffic V74.Ø
          - car (traffic) V73.5
            - nontraffic V73.Ø
          - motor vehicle NOS (traffic) V79.4Ø
            - nontraffic V79.ØØ
            - specified type NEC (traffic) V79.49
              - nontraffic V79.Ø9
          - pedal cycle (traffic) V71.5
            - nontraffic V71.Ø
          - pickup truck (traffic) V73.5
            - nontraffic V73.Ø
          - railway vehicle (traffic) V75.5
            - nontraffic V75.Ø
          - specified vehicle NEC (traffic) V76.5
            - nontraffic V76.Ø
          - stationary object (traffic) V77.5
            - nontraffic V77.Ø
          - streetcar (traffic) V76.5
            - nontraffic V76.Ø
          - three wheeled motor vehicle (traffic) V72.5
            - nontraffic V72.Ø
          - truck (traffic) V74.5
            - nontraffic V74.Ø

- **Accident**— *continued*
  - transport— *continued*
    - bus occupant— *continued*
      - driver— *continued*
        - collision— *continued*
          - two wheeled motor vehicle (traffic) V72.5
            - nontraffic V72.Ø
          - van (traffic) V73.5
            - nontraffic V73.Ø
        - noncollision accident (traffic) V78.5
          - nontraffic V78.Ø
      - noncollision accident (traffic) V78.9
        - nontraffic V78.3
        - while boarding or alighting V78.4
      - nontraffic V79.3
      - hanger-on
        - collision (with)
          - animal (traffic) V7Ø.7
            - being ridden (traffic) V76.7
              - nontraffic V76.2
            - nontraffic V7Ø.2
          - animal-drawn vehicle (traffic) V76.7
            - nontraffic V76.2
          - bus (traffic) V74.7
            - nontraffic V74.2
          - car (traffic) V73.7
            - nontraffic V73.2
          - pedal cycle (traffic) V71.7
            - nontraffic V71.2
          - pickup truck (traffic) V73.7
            - nontraffic V73.2
          - railway vehicle (traffic) V75.7
            - nontraffic V75.2
          - specified vehicle NEC (traffic) V76.7
            - nontraffic V76.2
          - stationary object (traffic) V77.7
            - nontraffic V77.2
          - streetcar (traffic) V76.7
            - nontraffic V76.2
          - three wheeled motor vehicle (traffic) V72.7
            - nontraffic V72.2
          - truck (traffic) V74.7
            - nontraffic V74.2
          - two wheeled motor vehicle (traffic) V72.7
            - nontraffic V72.2
          - van (traffic) V73.7
            - nontraffic V73.2
        - noncollision accident (traffic) V78.7
          - nontraffic V78.2
      - passenger
        - collision (with)
          - animal (traffic) V7Ø.6
            - being ridden (traffic) V76.6
              - nontraffic V76.1
            - nontraffic V7Ø.1
          - animal-drawn vehicle (traffic) V76.6
            - nontraffic V76.1
          - bus (traffic) V74.6
            - nontraffic V74.1
          - car (traffic) V73.6
            - nontraffic V73.1
          - motor vehicle NOS (traffic) V79.5Ø
            - nontraffic V79.1Ø
            - specified type NEC (traffic) V79.59
              - nontraffic V79.19
          - pedal cycle (traffic) V71.6
            - nontraffic V71.1
          - pickup truck (traffic) V73.6
            - nontraffic V73.1
          - railway vehicle (traffic) V75.6
            - nontraffic V75.1
          - specified vehicle NEC (traffic) V76.6
            - nontraffic V76.1
          - stationary object (traffic) V77.6
            - nontraffic V77.1
          - streetcar (traffic) V76.6
            - nontraffic V76.1
          - three wheeled motor vehicle (traffic) V72.6
            - nontraffic V72.1

- **Accident**— *continued*
  - transport— *continued*
    - bus occupant— *continued*
      - passenger— *continued*
        - collision— *continued*
          - truck (traffic) V74.6
            - nontraffic V74.1
          - two wheeled motor vehicle (traffic) V72.6
            - nontraffic V72.1
          - van (traffic) V73.6
            - nontraffic V73.1
        - noncollision accident (traffic) V78.6
          - nontraffic V78.1
      - specified type NEC V79.88
        - military vehicle V79.81
    - cable car, not on rails V98.Ø
      - on rails — *see* Accident, transport, streetcar occupant
    - car occupant V49.9
      - ambulance occupant — *see* Accident, transport, ambulance occupant
      - collision (with)
        - animal (traffic) V4Ø.9
          - being ridden (traffic) V46.9
            - nontraffic V46.3
            - while boarding or alighting V46.4
          - nontraffic V4Ø.3
          - while boarding or alighting V4Ø.4
        - animal-drawn vehicle (traffic) V46.9
          - nontraffic V46.3
          - while boarding or alighting V46.4
        - bus (traffic) V44.9
          - nontraffic V44.3
          - while boarding or alighting V44.4
        - car (traffic) V43.92
          - nontraffic V43.32
          - while boarding or alighting V43.42
        - motor vehicle NOS (traffic) V49.6Ø
          - nontraffic V49.2Ø
          - specified type NEC (traffic) V49.69
            - nontraffic V49.29
        - pedal cycle (traffic) V41.9
          - nontraffic V41.3
          - while boarding or alighting V41.4
        - pickup truck (traffic) V43.93
          - nontraffic V43.33
          - while boarding or alighting V43.43
        - railway vehicle (traffic) V45.9
          - nontraffic V45.3
          - while boarding or alighting V45.4
        - specified vehicle NEC (traffic) V46.9
          - nontraffic V46.3
          - while boarding or alighting V46.4
        - sport utility vehicle (traffic) V43.91
          - nontraffic V43.31
          - while boarding or alighting V43.41
        - stationary object (traffic) V47.92
          - nontraffic V47.32
          - while boarding or alighting V47.4
        - streetcar (traffic) V46.9
          - nontraffic V46.3
          - while boarding or alighting V46.4
        - three wheeled motor vehicle (traffic) V42.9
          - nontraffic V42.3
          - while boarding or alighting V42.4
        - truck (traffic) V44.9
          - nontraffic V44.3
          - while boarding or alighting V44.4
        - two wheeled motor vehicle (traffic) V42.9
          - nontraffic V42.3
          - while boarding or alighting V42.4
        - van (traffic) V43.94
          - nontraffic V43.34
          - while boarding or alighting V43.44
      - driver
        - collision (with)
          - animal (traffic) V4Ø.5
            - being ridden (traffic) V46.5
              - nontraffic V46.Ø
            - nontraffic V4Ø.Ø
          - animal-drawn vehicle (traffic) V46.5

- **Accident**— *continued*
  - transport— *continued*
    - car occupant— *continued*
      - driver— *continued*
        - collision— *continued*
          - animal-drawn vehicle— *continued*
            - nontraffic V46.Ø
          - bus (traffic) V44.5
            - nontraffic V44.Ø
          - car (traffic) V43.52
            - nontraffic V43.Ø2
          - motor vehicle NOS (traffic) V49.4Ø
            - nontraffic V49.ØØ
            - specified type NEC (traffic) V49.49
              - nontraffic V49.Ø9
          - pedal cycle (traffic) V41.5
            - nontraffic V41.Ø
          - pickup truck (traffic) V43.53
            - nontraffic V43.Ø3
          - railway vehicle (traffic) V45.5
            - nontraffic V45.Ø
          - specified vehicle NEC (traffic) V46.5
            - nontraffic V46.Ø
          - sport utility vehicle (traffic) V43.51
            - nontraffic V43.Ø1
          - stationary object (traffic) V47.52
            - nontraffic V47.Ø2
          - streetcar (traffic) V46.5
            - nontraffic V46.Ø
          - three wheeled motor vehicle (traffic) V42.5
            - nontraffic V42.Ø
          - truck (traffic) V44.5
            - nontraffic V44.Ø
          - two wheeled motor vehicle (traffic) V42.5
            - nontraffic V42.Ø
          - van (traffic) V43.54
            - nontraffic V43.Ø4
        - noncollision accident (traffic) V48.5
          - nontraffic V48.Ø
      - noncollision accident (traffic) V48.9
        - nontraffic V48.3
        - while boarding or alighting V48.4
      - nontraffic V49.3
      - hanger-on
        - collision (with)
          - animal (traffic) V4Ø.7
            - being ridden (traffic) V46.7
              - nontraffic V46.2
            - nontraffic V4Ø.2
          - animal-drawn vehicle (traffic) V46.7
            - nontraffic V46.2
          - bus (traffic) V44.7
            - nontraffic V44.2
          - car (traffic) V43.72
            - nontraffic V43.22
          - pedal cycle (traffic) V41.7
            - nontraffic V41.2
          - pickup truck (traffic) V43.73
            - nontraffic V43.23
          - railway vehicle (traffic) V45.7
            - nontraffic V45.2
          - specified vehicle NEC (traffic) V46.7
            - nontraffic V46.2
          - sport utility vehicle (traffic) V43.71
            - nontraffic V43.21
          - stationary object (traffic) V47.7
            - nontraffic V47.2
          - streetcar (traffic) V46.7
            - nontraffic V46.2
          - three wheeled motor vehicle (traffic) V42.7
            - nontraffic V42.2
          - truck (traffic) V44.7
            - nontraffic V44.2
          - two wheeled motor vehicle (traffic) V42.7
            - nontraffic V42.2
          - van (traffic) V43.74
            - nontraffic V43.24
        - noncollision accident (traffic) V48.7
          - nontraffic V48.2

- **Accident**— *continued*
  - transport— *continued*
    - car occupant— *continued*
      - passenger
        - collision (with)
          - animal (traffic) V4Ø.6
            - being ridden (traffic) V46.6
              - nontraffic V46.1
            - nontraffic V4Ø.1
          - animal-drawn vehicle (traffic) V46.6
            - nontraffic V46.1
          - bus (traffic) V44.6
            - nontraffic V44.1
          - car (traffic) V43.62
            - nontraffic V43.12
          - motor vehicle NOS (traffic) V49.5Ø
            - nontraffic V49.1Ø
            - specified type NEC (traffic) V49.59
              - nontraffic V49.19
          - pedal cycle (traffic) V41.6
            - nontraffic V41.1
          - pickup truck (traffic) V43.63
            - nontraffic V43.13
          - railway vehicle (traffic) V45.6
            - nontraffic V45.1
          - specified vehicle NEC (traffic) V46.6
            - nontraffic V46.1
          - sport utility vehicle (traffic) V43.61
            - nontraffic V43.11
          - stationary object (traffic) V47.62
            - nontraffic V47.12
          - streetcar (traffic) V46.6
            - nontraffic V46.1
          - three wheeled motor vehicle (traffic) V42.6
            - nontraffic V42.1
          - truck (traffic) V44.6
            - nontraffic V44.1
          - two wheeled motor vehicle (traffic) V42.6
            - nontraffic V42.1
          - van (traffic) V43.64
            - nontraffic V43.14
        - noncollision accident (traffic) V48.6
          - nontraffic V48.1
      - specified type NEC V49.88
        - military vehicle V49.81
    - coal car — *see* Accident, transport, industrial vehicle occupant
    - construction vehicle occupant (nontraffic) V85.9
      - driver V85.5
      - hanger-on V85.7
      - passenger V85.6
      - traffic V85.3
        - driver V85.Ø
        - hanger-on V85.2
        - passenger V85.1
      - while boarding or alighting V85.4
    - dirt bike rider — *see* Accident, transport, all-terrain vehicle occupant
    - due to cataclysm — *see* Forces of nature, by type
    - dune buggy occupant (nontraffic) V86.93
      - driver V86.53
      - hanger-on V86.73
      - passenger V86.63
      - traffic V86.33
        - driver V86.Ø3
        - hanger-on V86.23
        - passenger V86.13
      - while boarding or alighting V86.43
    - forklift — *see* Accident, transport, industrial vehicle occupant
    - go cart — *see* Accident, transport, all-terrain vehicle occupant
    - golf cart — *see* Accident, transport, all-terrain vehicle occupant
    - heavy transport vehicle occupant — *see* Accident, transport, truck occupant
    - ice yacht V98.2
    - industrial vehicle occupant (nontraffic) V83.9
      - driver V83.5
      - hanger-on V83.7
      - passenger V83.6

- **Accident**— *continued*
  - transport— *continued*
    - industrial vehicle occupant— *continued*
      - traffic V83.3
        - driver V83.Ø
        - hanger-on V83.2
        - passenger V83.1
      - while boarding or alighting V83.4
    - interurban electric car — *see* Accident, transport, streetcar
    - land yacht V98.1
    - logging car — *see* Accident, transport, industrial vehicle occupant
    - military vehicle occupant (traffic) V86.34
      - driver V86.Ø4
      - hanger-on V86.24
      - nontraffic V86.94
        - driver V86.54
        - hanger-on V86.74
        - passenger V86.64
      - passenger V86.14
      - while boarding or alighting V86.44
    - mine tram — *see* Accident, transport, industrial vehicle occupant
    - motorcoach — *see* Accident, transport, bus occupant
    - motorcyclist V29.9
      - collision (with)
        - animal (traffic) V2Ø.9
          - being ridden (traffic) V26.9
            - nontraffic V26.2
            - while boarding or alighting V26.3
          - nontraffic V2Ø.2
          - while boarding or alighting V2Ø.3
        - animal-drawn vehicle (traffic) V26.9
          - nontraffic V26.2
          - while boarding or alighting V26.3
        - bus (traffic) V24.9
          - nontraffic V24.2
          - while boarding or alighting V24.3
        - car (traffic) V23.9
          - nontraffic V23.2
          - while boarding or alighting V23.3
        - motor vehicle NOS (traffic) V29.6Ø
          - nontraffic V29.2Ø
          - specified type NEC (traffic) V29.69
            - nontraffic V29.29
        - pedal cycle (traffic) V21.9
          - nontraffic V21.2
          - while boarding or alighting V21.3
        - pickup truck (traffic) V23.9
          - nontraffic V23.2
          - while boarding or alighting V23.3
        - railway vehicle (traffic) V25.9
          - nontraffic V25.2
          - while boarding or alighting V25.3
        - specified vehicle NEC (traffic) V26.9
          - nontraffic V26.2
          - while boarding or alighting V26.3
        - stationary object (traffic) V27.9
          - nontraffic V27.2
          - while boarding or alighting V27.3
        - streetcar (traffic) V26.9
          - nontraffic V26.2
          - while boarding or alighting V26.3
        - three wheeled motor vehicle (traffic) V22.9
          - nontraffic V22.2
          - while boarding or alighting V22.3
        - truck (traffic) V24.9
          - nontraffic V24.2
          - while boarding or alighting V24.3
        - two wheeled motor vehicle (traffic) V22.9
          - nontraffic V22.2
          - while boarding or alighting V22.3
        - van (traffic) V23.9
          - nontraffic V23.2
          - while boarding or alighting V23.3
      - driver
        - collision (with)
          - animal (traffic) V2Ø.4
            - being ridden (traffic) V26.4
              - nontraffic V26.Ø

- **Accident**— *continued*
  - transport— *continued*
    - motorcyclist— *continued*
      - driver— *continued*
        - collision— *continued*
          - animal— *continued*
            - nontraffic V2Ø.Ø
          - animal-drawn vehicle (traffic) V26.4
            - nontraffic V26.Ø
          - bus (traffic) V24.4
            - nontraffic V24.Ø
          - car (traffic) V23.4
            - nontraffic V23.Ø
          - motor vehicle NOS (traffic) V29.4Ø
            - nontraffic V29.ØØ
            - specified type NEC (traffic) V29.49
              - nontraffic V29.Ø9
          - pedal cycle (traffic) V21.4
            - nontraffic V21.Ø
          - pickup truck (traffic) V23.4
            - nontraffic V23.Ø
          - railway vehicle (traffic) V25.4
            - nontraffic V25.Ø
          - specified vehicle NEC (traffic) V26.4
            - nontraffic V26.Ø
          - stationary object (traffic) V27.4
            - nontraffic V27.Ø
          - streetcar (traffic) V26.4
            - nontraffic V26.Ø
          - three wheeled motor vehicle (traffic) V22.4
            - nontraffic V22.Ø
          - truck (traffic) V24.4
            - nontraffic V24.Ø
          - two wheeled motor vehicle (traffic) V22.4
            - nontraffic V22.Ø
          - van (traffic) V23.4
            - nontraffic V23.Ø
        - noncollision accident (traffic) V28.4
          - nontraffic V28.Ø
      - noncollision accident (traffic) V28.9
        - nontraffic V28.2
        - while boarding or alighting V28.3
      - nontraffic V29.3
      - passenger
        - collision (with)
          - animal (traffic) V2Ø.5
            - being ridden (traffic) V26.5
              - nontraffic V26.1
            - nontraffic V2Ø.1
          - animal-drawn vehicle (traffic) V26.5
            - nontraffic V26.1
          - bus (traffic) V24.5
            - nontraffic V24.1
          - car (traffic) V23.5
            - nontraffic V23.1
          - motor vehicle NOS (traffic) V29.5Ø
            - nontraffic V29.1Ø
            - specified type NEC (traffic) V29.59
              - nontraffic V29.19
          - pedal cycle (traffic) V21.5
            - nontraffic V21.1
          - pickup truck (traffic) V23.5
            - nontraffic V23.1
          - railway vehicle (traffic) V25.5
            - nontraffic V25.1
          - specified vehicle NEC (traffic) V26.5
            - nontraffic V26.1
          - stationary object (traffic) V27.5
            - nontraffic V27.1
          - streetcar (traffic) V26.5
            - nontraffic V26.1
          - three wheeled motor vehicle (traffic) V22.5
            - nontraffic V22.1
          - truck (traffic) V24.5
            - nontraffic V24.1
          - two wheeled motor vehicle (traffic) V22.5
            - nontraffic V22.1
          - van (traffic) V23.5
            - nontraffic V23.1

- **Accident**— *continued*
  - transport— *continued*
    - motorcyclist— *continued*
      - passenger— *continued*
        - noncollision accident (traffic) V28.5
          - nontraffic V28.1
      - specified type NEC V29.88
        - military vehicle V29.81
    - motor vehicle NEC occupant (traffic) V86.39
      - driver V86.Ø9
      - hanger-on V86.29
      - nontraffic V86.99
        - driver V86.59
        - hanger-on V86.79
        - passenger V86.69
      - passenger V86.19
      - while boarding or alighting V86.49
    - occupant (of)
      - aircraft (powered) V95.9
        - fixed wing
          - commercial — *see* Accident, transport, aircraft, occupant, powered, fixed wing, commercial
          - private — *see* Accident, transport, aircraft, occupant, powered, fixed wing, private
        - nonpowered V96.9
        - specified NEC V95.8
      - airport battery-powered vehicle — *see* Accident, transport, industrial vehicle occupant
      - all-terrain vehicle (ATV) — *see* Accident, transport, all-terrain vehicle occupant
      - animal-drawn vehicle — *see* Accident, transport, animal-drawn vehicle occupant
      - automobile — *see* Accident, transport, car occupant
      - balloon V96.ØØ
      - battery-powered vehicle — *see* Accident, transport, industrial vehicle occupant
      - bicycle — *see* Accident, transport, pedal cyclist
        - motorized — *see* Accident, transport, motorcycle rider
      - boat NEC — *see* Accident, watercraft
      - bulldozer — *see* Accident, transport, construction vehicle occupant
      - bus — *see* Accident, transport, bus occupant
      - cable car (on rails) (*see also* Accident, transport, streetcar occupant)
        - not on rails V98.Ø
      - car (*see also* Accident, transport, car occupant)
        - cable (on rails) (*see also* Accident, transport, streetcar occupant)
          - not on rails V98.Ø
      - coach — *see* Accident, transport, bus occupant
      - coal-car — *see* Accident, transport, industrial vehicle occupant
      - digger — *see* Accident, transport, construction vehicle occupant
      - dump truck — *see* Accident, transport, construction vehicle occupant
      - earth-leveler — *see* Accident, transport, construction vehicle occupant
      - farm machinery (self-propelled) — *see* Accident, transport, agricultural vehicle occupant
      - forklift — *see* Accident, transport, industrial vehicle occupant
      - glider (unpowered) V96.2Ø
        - hang V96.1Ø
        - powered (microlight) (ultralight) — *see* Accident, transport, aircraft, occupant, powered, glider
      - glider (unpowered) NEC V96.2Ø
      - hang-glider V96.1Ø
      - harvester — *see* Accident, transport, agricultural vehicle occupant
      - heavy (transport) vehicle — *see* Accident, transport, truck occupant

- **Accident**— *continued*
  - transport— *continued*
    - occupant— *continued*
      - helicopter — *see* Accident, transport, aircraft, occupant, helicopter
      - ice-yacht V98.2
      - kite (carrying person) V96.8
      - land-yacht V98.1
      - logging car — *see* Accident, transport, industrial vehicle occupant
      - mechanical shovel — *see* Accident, transport, construction vehicle occupant
      - microlight — *see* Accident, transport, aircraft, occupant, powered, glider
      - minibus — *see* Accident, transport, car occupant
      - minivan — *see* Accident, transport, car occupant
      - moped — *see* Accident, transport, motorcycle
      - motor scooter — *see* Accident, transport, motorcycle
      - motorcycle (with sidecar) — *see* Accident, transport, motorcycle
      - pedal cycle (*see also* Accident, transport, pedal cyclist)
      - pick-up (truck) — *see* Accident, transport, pickup truck occupant
      - railway (train) (vehicle) (subterranean) (elevated) — *see* Accident, transport, railway vehicle occupant
      - rickshaw — *see* Accident, transport, pedal cycle
        - pedal driven — *see* Accident, transport, pedal cyclist
      - road-roller — *see* Accident, transport, construction vehicle occupant
      - ship NOS V94.9
      - ski-lift (chair) (gondola) V98.3
      - snowmobile — *see* Accident, transport, snowmobile occupant
      - spacecraft, spaceship — *see* Accident, transport, aircraft, occupant, spacecraft
      - sport utility vehicle — *see* Accident, transport, car occupant
      - streetcar (interurban) (operating on public street or highway) — *see* Accident, transport, streetcar occupant
      - SUV — *see* Accident, transport, car occupant
      - téléférique V98.Ø
      - three-wheeled vehicle (motorized) (*see also* Accident, transport, three-wheeled motor vehicle occupant)
        - nonmotorized — *see* Accident, transport, pedal cycle
      - tractor (farm) (and trailer) — *see* Accident, transport, agricultural vehicle occupant
      - train — *see* Accident, transport, railway vehicle occupant
      - tram — *see* Accident, transport, streetcar occupant
        - in mine or quarry — *see* Accident, transport, industrial vehicle occupant
      - tricycle — *see* Accident, transport, pedal cycle
        - motorized — *see* Accident, transport, three-wheeled motor vehicle
      - trolley — *see* Accident, transport, streetcar occupant
        - in mine or quarry — *see* Accident, transport, industrial vehicle occupant
      - tub, in mine or quarry — *see* Accident, transport, industrial vehicle occupant
      - ultralight — *see* Accident, transport, aircraft, occupant, powered, glider
      - van — *see* Accident, transport, van occupant
      - vehicle NEC V89.9
        - heavy transport — *see* Accident, transport, truck occupant
        - motor (traffic) NEC V89.2
          - nontraffic NEC V89.Ø

- **Accident**— *continued*
  - transport— *continued*
    - occupant— *continued*
      - watercraft NOS V94.9
        - causing drowning — *see* Drowning, resulting from accident to boat
    - parachutist V97.29
      - after accident to aircraft — *see* Accident, transport, aircraft
      - entangled in object V97.21
      - injured on landing V97.22
    - pedal cyclist V19.9
      - collision (with)
        - animal (traffic) V1Ø.9
          - being ridden (traffic) V16.9
            - nontraffic V16.2
              - while boarding or alighting V16.3
          - nontraffic V1Ø.2
          - while boarding or alighting V1Ø.3
        - animal-drawn vehicle (traffic) V16.9
          - nontraffic V16.2
          - while boarding or alighting V16.3
        - bus (traffic) V14.9
          - nontraffic V14.2
          - while boarding or alighting V14.3
        - car (traffic) V13.9
          - nontraffic V13.2
          - while boarding or alighting V13.3
        - motor vehicle NOS (traffic) V19.6Ø
          - nontraffic V19.2Ø
          - specified type NEC (traffic) V19.69
            - nontraffic V19.29
        - pedal cycle (traffic) V11.9
          - nontraffic V11.2
          - while boarding or alighting V11.3
        - pickup truck (traffic) V13.9
          - nontraffic V13.2
          - while boarding or alighting V13.3
        - railway vehicle (traffic) V15.9
          - nontraffic V15.2
          - while boarding or alighting V15.3
        - specified vehicle NEC (traffic) V16.9
          - nontraffic V16.2
          - while boarding or alighting V16.3
        - stationary object (traffic) V17.9
          - nontraffic V17.2
          - while boarding or alighting V17.3
        - streetcar (traffic) V16.9
          - nontraffic V16.2
          - while boarding or alighting V16.3
        - three wheeled motor vehicle (traffic) V12.9
          - nontraffic V12.2
          - while boarding or alighting V12.3
        - truck (traffic) V14.9
          - nontraffic V14.2
          - while boarding or alighting V14.3
        - two wheeled motor vehicle (traffic) V12.9
          - nontraffic V12.2
          - while boarding or alighting V12.3
        - van (traffic) V13.9
          - nontraffic V13.2
          - while boarding or alighting V13.3
      - driver
        - collision (with)
          - animal (traffic) V1Ø.4
            - being ridden (traffic) V16.4
              - nontraffic V16.Ø
            - nontraffic V1Ø.Ø
          - animal-drawn vehicle (traffic) V16.4
            - nontraffic V16.Ø
          - bus (traffic) V14.4
            - nontraffic V14.Ø
          - car (traffic) V13.4
            - nontraffic V13.Ø
          - motor vehicle NOS (traffic) V19.4Ø
            - nontraffic V19.ØØ
            - specified type NEC (traffic) V19.49
              - nontraffic V19.Ø9
          - pedal cycle (traffic) V11.4
            - nontraffic V11.Ø
          - pickup truck (traffic) V13.4
            - nontraffic V13.Ø

- **Accident**— *continued*
  - transport— *continued*
    - pedal cyclist— *continued*
      - driver— *continued*
        - collision— *continued*
          - railway vehicle (traffic) V15.4
            - nontraffic V15.Ø
          - specified vehicle NEC (traffic) V16.4
            - nontraffic V16.Ø
          - stationary object (traffic) V17.4
            - nontraffic V17.Ø
          - streetcar (traffic) V16.4
            - nontraffic V16.Ø
          - three wheeled motor vehicle (traffic) V12.4
            - nontraffic V12.Ø
          - truck (traffic) V14.4
            - nontraffic V14.Ø
          - two wheeled motor vehicle (traffic) V12.4
            - nontraffic V12.Ø
          - van (traffic) V13.4
            - nontraffic V13.Ø
        - noncollision accident (traffic) V18.4
          - nontraffic V18.Ø
      - noncollision accident (traffic) V18.9
        - nontraffic V18.2
        - while boarding or alighting V18.3
      - nontraffic V19.3
      - passenger
        - collision (with)
          - animal (traffic) V1Ø.5
            - being ridden (traffic) V16.5
              - nontraffic V16.1
            - nontraffic V1Ø.1
          - animal-drawn vehicle (traffic) V16.5
            - nontraffic V16.1
          - bus (traffic) V14.5
            - nontraffic V14.1
          - car (traffic) V13.5
            - nontraffic V13.1
          - motor vehicle NOS (traffic) V19.5Ø
            - nontraffic V19.1Ø
            - specified type NEC (traffic) V19.59
              - nontraffic V19.19
          - pedal cycle (traffic) V11.5
            - nontraffic V11.1
          - pickup truck (traffic) V13.5
            - nontraffic V13.1
          - railway vehicle (traffic) V15.5
            - nontraffic V15.1
          - specified vehicle NEC (traffic) V16.5
            - nontraffic V16.1
          - stationary object (traffic) V17.5
            - nontraffic V17.1
          - streetcar (traffic) V16.5
            - nontraffic V16.1
          - three wheeled motor vehicle (traffic) V12.5
            - nontraffic V12.1
          - truck (traffic) V14.5
            - nontraffic V14.1
          - two wheeled motor vehicle (traffic) V12.5
            - nontraffic V12.1
          - van (traffic) V13.5
            - nontraffic V13.1
        - noncollision accident (traffic) V18.5
          - nontraffic V18.1
      - specified type NEC V19.88
        - military vehicle V19.81
    - pedestrian
      - conveyance (occupant) VØ9.9
        - babystroller VØØ.828
          - collision (with) VØ9.9
            - animal being ridden or animal drawn vehicle VØ6.99
              - nontraffic VØ6.Ø9
              - traffic VØ6.19
            - bus or heavy transport VØ4.99
              - nontraffic VØ4.Ø9
              - traffic VØ4.19

- **Accident**— *continued*
  - transport— *continued*
    - pedestrian— *continued*
      - conveyance— *continued*
        - babystroller— *continued*
          - collision— *continued*
            - car VØ3.99
              - nontraffic VØ3.Ø9
              - traffic VØ3.19
            - pedal cycle VØ1.99
              - nontraffic VØ1.Ø9
              - traffic VØ1.19
            - pick-up truck or van VØ3.99
              - nontraffic VØ3.Ø9
              - traffic VØ3.19
            - railway (train) (vehicle) VØ5.99
              - nontraffic VØ5.Ø9
              - traffic VØ5.19
            - streetcar VØ6.99
              - nontraffic VØ6.Ø9
              - traffic VØ6.19
            - stationary object VØØ.822
            - two or three-wheeled motor vehicle VØ2.99
              - nontraffic VØ2.Ø9
              - traffic VØ2.19
            - vehicle VØ9.9
              - animal-drawn VØ6.99
                - nontraffic VØ6.Ø9
                - traffic VØ6.19
              - motor
                - nontraffic VØ9.ØØ
                - traffic VØ9.2Ø
          - fall VØØ.821
          - nontraffic VØ9.1
            - involving motor vehicle NEC VØ9.ØØ
          - traffic VØ9.3
            - involving motor vehicle NEC VØ9.2Ø
        - flat-bottomed NEC VØØ.388
          - collision (with) VØ9.9
            - animal being ridden or animal drawn vehicle VØ6.99
              - nontraffic VØ6.Ø9
              - traffic VØ6.19
            - bus or heavy transport VØ4.99
              - nontraffic VØ4.Ø9
              - traffic VØ4.19
            - car VØ3.99
              - nontraffic VØ3.Ø9
              - traffic VØ3.19
            - pedal cycle VØ1.99
              - nontraffic VØ1.Ø9
              - traffic VØ1.19
            - pick-up truck or van VØ3.99
              - nontraffic VØ3.Ø9
              - traffic VØ3.19
            - railway (train) (vehicle) VØ5.99
              - nontraffic VØ5.Ø9
              - traffic VØ5.19
            - stationary object VØØ.382
            - streetcar VØ6.99
              - nontraffic VØ6.Ø9
              - traffic VØ6.19
              - two or three-wheeled motor vehicle VØ2.99
                - nontraffic VØ2.Ø9
                - traffic VØ2.19
            - vehicle VØ9.9
              - animal-drawn VØ6.99
                - nontraffic VØ6.Ø9
                - traffic VØ6.19
              - motor
                - nontraffic VØ9.ØØ
                - traffic VØ9.2Ø
          - fall VØØ.381
          - nontraffic VØ9.1
            - involving motor vehicle NEC VØ9.ØØ

- **Accident**— *continued*
  - transport— *continued*
    - pedestrian— *continued*
      - conveyance— *continued*
        - flat-bottomed— *continued*
          - snow
            - board — *see* Accident, transport, pedestrian, conveyance, snow board
            - ski — *see* Accident, transport, pedestrian, conveyance, skis (snow)
          - traffic VØ9.3
            - involving motor vehicle NEC VØ9.2Ø
        - gliding type NEC VØØ.288
          - collision (with) VØ9.9
            - animal being ridden or animal drawn vehicle VØ6.99
              - nontraffic VØ6.Ø9
              - traffic VØ6.19
            - bus or heavy transport VØ4.99
              - nontraffic VØ4.Ø9
              - traffic VØ4.19
            - car VØ3.99
              - nontraffic VØ3.Ø9
              - traffic VØ3.19
            - pedal cycle VØ1.99
              - nontraffic VØ1.Ø9
              - traffic VØ1.19
            - pick-up truck or van VØ3.99
              - nontraffic VØ3.Ø9
              - traffic VØ3.19
            - railway (train) (vehicle) VØ5.99
              - nontraffic VØ5.Ø9
              - traffic VØ5.19
            - stationary object VØØ.282
            - streetcar VØ6.99
              - nontraffic VØ6.Ø9
              - traffic VØ6.19
            - two or three-wheeled motor vehicle VØ2.99
              - nontraffic VØ2.Ø9
              - traffic VØ2.19
            - vehicle VØ9.9
              - animal-drawn VØ6.99
                - nontraffic VØ6.Ø9
                - traffic VØ6.19
              - motor
                - nontraffic VØ9.ØØ
                - traffic VØ9.2Ø
          - fall VØØ.281
          - heelies — *see* Accident, transport, pedestrian, conveyance, heelies
          - ice skate — *see* Accident, transport, pedestrian, conveyance, ice skate
          - nontraffic VØ9.1
            - involving motor vehicle NEC VØ9.ØØ
          - sled — *see* Accident, transport, pedestrian, conveyance, sled
          - traffic VØ9.3
            - involving motor vehicle NEC VØ9.2Ø
          - wheelies — *see* Accident, transport, pedestrian, conveyance, heelies
        - heelies VØØ.158
          - colliding with stationary object VØØ.152
          - fall VØØ.151
        - ice skates VØØ.218
          - collision (with) VØ9.9
            - animal being ridden or animal drawn vehicle VØ6.99
              - nontraffic VØ6.Ø9
              - traffic VØ6.19
            - bus or heavy transport VØ4.99
              - nontraffic VØ4.Ø9
              - traffic VØ4.19
            - car VØ3.99
              - nontraffic VØ3.Ø9

Accident— *continued*
transport— *continued*
pedestrian— *continued*
conveyance— *continued*
ice skates — *continued*
collision— *continued*
car— *continued*
traffic V03.19
pedal cycle V01.99
nontraffic V01.09
traffic V01.19
pick-up truck or van V03.99
nontraffic V03.09
traffic V03.19
railway (train) (vehicle) V05.99
nontraffic V05.09
traffic V05.19
streetcar V06.99
nontraffic V06.09
traffic V06.19
stationary object V00.212
two or three-wheeled motor vehicle V02.99
nontraffic V02.09
traffic V02.19
vehicle V09.9
animal-drawn V06.99
nontraffic V06.09
traffic V06.19
motor
nontraffic V09.00
traffic V09.20
fall V00.211
nontraffic V09.1
involving motor vehicle NEC V09.00
traffic V09.3
involving motor vehicle NEC V09.20
motorized mobility scooter V00.838
collision with stationary object V00.832
fall from V00.831
nontraffic V09.1
involving motor vehicle V09.00
military V09.01
specified type NEC V09.09
rolling shoes V00.158
roller skates (non in-line) V00.128
collision (with) V09.9
animal being ridden or animal drawn vehicle V06.91
nontraffic V06.01
traffic V06.11
bus or heavy transport V04.91
nontraffic V04.01
traffic V04.11
car V03.91
nontraffic V03.01
traffic V03.11
pedal cycle V01.91
nontraffic V01.01
traffic V01.11
pick-up truck or van V03.91
nontraffic V03.01
traffic V03.11
railway (train) (vehicle) V05.91
nontraffic V05.01
traffic V05.11
streetcar V06.91
nontraffic V06.01
traffic V06.11
stationary object V00.122
two or three-wheeled motor vehicle V02.91
nontraffic V02.01
traffic V02.11
vehicle V09.9
animal-drawn V06.91
nontraffic V06.01
traffic V06.11
motor
nontraffic V09.00

Accident— *continued*
transport— *continued*
pedestrian— *continued*
conveyance— *continued*
roller skates— *continued*
collision— *continued*
vehicle— *continued*
motor— *continued*
traffic V09.20
fall V00.121
in-line V00.118
collision (*see also* Accident, transport, pedestrian, conveyance occupant, roller skates, collision)
with stationary object V00.112
fall V00.111
nontraffic V09.1
involving motor vehicle NEC V09.00
traffic V09.3
involving motor vehicle NEC V09.20
rolling type NEC V00.188
collision (with) V09.9
animal being ridden or animal drawn vehicle V06.99
nontraffic V06.09
traffic V06.19
bus or heavy transport V04.99
nontraffic V04.09
traffic V04.19
car V03.99
nontraffic V03.09
traffic V03.19
pedal cycle V01.99
nontraffic V01.09
traffic V01.19
pick-up truck or van V03.99
nontraffic V03.09
traffic V03.19
railway (train) (vehicle) V05.99
nontraffic V05.09
traffic V05.19
stationary object V00.182
streetcar V06.99
nontraffic V06.09
traffic V06.19
two or three-wheeled motor vehicle V02.99
nontraffic V02.09
traffic V02.19
vehicle V09.9
animal-drawn V06.99
nontraffic V06.09
traffic V06.19
motor
nontraffic V09.00
traffic V09.20
fall V00.181
in-line roller skate — *see* Accident, transport, pedestrian, conveyance, roller skate, in-line
nontraffic V09.1
involving motor vehicle NEC V09.00
roller skate — *see* Accident, transport, pedestrian, conveyance, roller skate
scooter (non-motorized) — *see* Accident, transport, pedestrian, conveyance, scooter
skateboard — *see* Accident, transport, pedestrian, conveyance, skateboard
traffic V09.3
involving motor vehicle NEC V09.20
scooter (non-motorized) V00.148
collision (with) V09.9
animal being ridden or animal drawn vehicle V06.99
nontraffic V06.09

Accident— *continued*
transport— *continued*
pedestrian— *continued*
conveyance— *continued*
scooter— *continued*
collision— *continued*
animal being ridden or animal drawn vehicle— *continued*
traffic V06.19
bus or heavy transport V04.99
nontraffic V04.09
traffic V04.19
car V03.99
nontraffic V03.09
traffic V03.19
pedal cycle V01.99
nontraffic V01.09
traffic V01.19
pick-up truck or van V03.99
nontraffic V03.09
traffic V03.19
railway (train) (vehicle) V05.99
nontraffic V05.09
traffic V05.19
streetcar V06.99
nontraffic V06.09
traffic V06.19
stationary object V00.142
two or three-wheeled motor vehicle V02.99
nontraffic V02.09
traffic V02.19
vehicle V09.9
animal-drawn V06.99
nontraffic V06.09
traffic V06.19
motor
nontraffic V09.00
traffic V09.20
fall V00.141
nontraffic V09.1
involving motor vehicle NEC V09.00
traffic V09.3
involving motor vehicle NEC V09.20
skate board V00.138
collision (with) V09.9
animal being ridden or animal drawn vehicle V06.92
nontraffic V06.02
traffic V06.12
bus or heavy transport V04.92
nontraffic V04.02
traffic V04.12
car V03.92
nontraffic V03.02
traffic V03.12
pedal cycle V01.92
nontraffic V01.02
traffic V01.12
pick-up truck or van V03.92
nontraffic V03.02
traffic V03.12
railway (train) (vehicle) V05.92
nontraffic V05.02
traffic V05.12
streetcar V06.92
nontraffic V06.02
traffic V06.12
stationary object V00.132
two or three-wheeled motor vehicle V02.92
nontraffic V02.02
traffic V02.12
vehicle V09.9
animal-drawn V06.92
nontraffic V06.02
traffic V06.12
motor
nontraffic V09.00
traffic V09.20
fall V00.131

- **Accident**—*continued*
  - transport—*continued*
    - pedestrian—*continued*
      - conveyance—*continued*
        - skate board—*continued*
          - nontraffic VØ9.1
            - involving motor vehicle NEC VØ9.ØØ
          - traffic VØ9.3
            - involving motor vehicle NEC VØ9.2Ø
        - sled VØØ.228
          - collision (with) VØ9.9
            - animal being ridden or animal drawn vehicle VØ6.99
              - nontraffic VØ6.Ø9
              - traffic VØ6.19
            - bus or heavy transport VØ4.99
              - nontraffic VØ4.Ø9
              - traffic VØ4.19
            - car VØ3.99
              - nontraffic VØ3.Ø9
              - traffic VØ3.19
            - pedal cycle VØ1.99
              - nontraffic VØ1.Ø9
              - traffic VØ1.19
            - pick-up truck or van VØ3.99
              - nontraffic VØ3.Ø9
              - traffic VØ3.19
            - railway (train) (vehicle) VØ5.99
              - nontraffic VØ5.Ø9
              - traffic VØ5.19
            - streetcar VØ6.99
              - nontraffic VØ6.Ø9
              - traffic VØ6.19
            - stationary object VØØ.222
            - two or three-wheeled motor vehicle VØ2.99
              - nontraffic VØ2.Ø9
              - traffic VØ2.19
            - vehicle VØ9.9
              - animal-drawn VØ6.99
                - nontraffic VØ6.Ø9
                - traffic VØ6.19
              - motor
                - nontraffic VØ9.ØØ
                - traffic VØ9.2Ø
          - fall VØØ.221
          - nontraffic VØ9.1
            - involving motor vehicle NEC VØ9.ØØ
          - traffic VØ9.3
            - involving motor vehicle NEC VØ9.2Ø
        - skis (snow) VØØ.328
          - collision (with) VØ9.9
            - animal being ridden or animal drawn vehicle VØ6.99
              - nontraffic VØ6.Ø9
              - traffic VØ6.19
            - bus or heavy transport VØ4.99
              - nontraffic VØ4.Ø9
              - traffic VØ4.19
            - car VØ3.99
              - nontraffic VØ3.Ø9
              - traffic VØ3.19
            - pedal cycle VØ1.99
              - nontraffic VØ1.Ø9
              - traffic VØ1.19
            - pick-up truck or van VØ3.99
              - nontraffic VØ3.Ø9
              - traffic VØ3.19
            - railway (train) (vehicle) VØ5.99
              - nontraffic VØ5.Ø9
              - traffic VØ5.19
            - streetcar VØ6.99
              - nontraffic VØ6.Ø9
              - traffic VØ6.19
            - stationary object VØØ.322
            - two or three-wheeled motor vehicle VØ2.99
              - nontraffic VØ2.Ø9
              - traffic VØ2.19

- **Accident**—*continued*
  - transport—*continued*
    - pedestrian—*continued*
      - conveyance—*continued*
        - skis—*continued*
          - collision—*continued*
            - vehicle VØ9.9
              - animal-drawn VØ6.99
                - nontraffic VØ6.Ø9
                - traffic VØ6.19
              - motor
                - nontraffic VØ9.ØØ
                - traffic VØ9.2Ø
          - fall VØØ.321
          - nontraffic VØ9.1
            - involving motor vehicle NEC VØ9.ØØ
          - traffic VØ9.3
            - involving motor vehicle NEC VØ9.2Ø
        - snow board VØØ.318
          - collision (with) VØ9.9
            - animal being ridden or animal drawn vehicle VØ6.99
              - nontraffic VØ6.Ø9
              - traffic VØ6.19
            - bus or heavy transport VØ4.99
              - nontraffic VØ4.Ø9
              - traffic VØ4.19
            - car VØ3.99
              - nontraffic VØ3.Ø9
              - traffic VØ3.19
            - pedal cycle VØ1.99
              - nontraffic VØ1.Ø9
              - traffic VØ1.19
            - pick-up truck or van VØ3.99
              - nontraffic VØ3.Ø9
              - traffic VØ3.19
            - railway (train) (vehicle) VØ5.99
              - nontraffic VØ5.Ø9
              - traffic VØ5.19
            - streetcar VØ6.99
              - nontraffic VØ6.Ø9
              - traffic VØ6.19
            - stationary object VØØ.312
            - two or three-wheeled motor vehicle VØ2.99
              - nontraffic VØ2.Ø9
              - traffic VØ2.19
            - vehicle VØ9.9
              - animal-drawn VØ6.99
                - nontraffic VØ6.Ø9
                - traffic VØ6.19
              - motor
                - nontraffic VØ9.ØØ
                - traffic VØ9.2Ø
          - fall VØØ.311
          - nontraffic VØ9.1
            - involving motor vehicle NEC VØ9.ØØ
          - traffic VØ9.3
            - involving motor vehicle NEC VØ9.2Ø
        - specified type NEC VØØ.898
          - collision (with) VØ9.9
            - animal being ridden or animal drawn vehicle VØ6.99
              - nontraffic VØ6.Ø9
              - traffic VØ6.19
            - bus or heavy transport VØ4.99
              - nontraffic VØ4.Ø9
              - traffic VØ4.19
            - car VØ3.99
              - nontraffic VØ3.Ø9
              - traffic VØ3.19
            - pedal cycle VØ1.99
              - nontraffic VØ1.Ø9
              - traffic VØ1.19
            - pick-up truck or van VØ3.99
              - nontraffic VØ3.Ø9
              - traffic VØ3.19
            - railway (train) (vehicle) VØ5.99
              - nontraffic VØ5.Ø9

- **Accident**—*continued*
  - transport—*continued*
    - pedestrian—*continued*
      - conveyance—*continued*
        - specified type—*continued*
          - collision—*continued*
            - railway—*continued*
              - traffic VØ5.19
            - streetcar VØ6.99
              - nontraffic VØ6.Ø9
              - traffic VØ6.19
            - stationary object VØØ.892
            - two or three-wheeled motor vehicle VØ2.99
              - nontraffic VØ2.Ø9
              - traffic VØ2.19
            - vehicle VØ9.9
              - animal-drawn VØ6.99
                - nontraffic VØ6.Ø9
                - traffic VØ6.19
              - motor
                - nontraffic VØ9.ØØ
                - traffic VØ9.2Ø
          - fall VØØ.891
          - nontraffic VØ9.1
            - involving motor vehicle NEC VØ9.ØØ
          - traffic VØ9.3
            - involving motor vehicle NEC VØ9.2Ø
        - traffic VØ9.3
          - involving motor vehicle VØ9.2Ø
            - military VØ9.21
            - specified type NEC VØ9.29
        - wheelchair (powered) VØØ.818
          - collision (with) VØ9.9
            - animal being ridden or animal drawn vehicle VØ6.99
              - nontraffic VØ6.Ø9
              - traffic VØ6.19
            - bus or heavy transport VØ4.99
              - nontraffic VØ4.Ø9
              - traffic VØ4.19
            - car VØ3.99
              - nontraffic VØ3.Ø9
              - traffic VØ3.19
            - pedal cycle VØ1.99
              - nontraffic VØ1.Ø9
              - traffic VØ1.19
            - pick-up truck or van VØ3.99
              - nontraffic VØ3.Ø9
              - traffic VØ3.19
            - railway (train) (vehicle) VØ5.99
              - nontraffic VØ5.Ø9
              - traffic VØ5.19
            - streetcar VØ6.99
              - nontraffic VØ6.Ø9
              - traffic VØ6.19
            - stationary object VØØ.812
            - two or three-wheeled motor vehicle VØ2.99
              - nontraffic VØ2.Ø9
              - traffic VØ2.19
            - vehicle VØ9.9
              - animal-drawn VØ6.99
                - nontraffic VØ6.Ø9
                - traffic VØ6.19
              - motor
                - nontraffic VØ9.ØØ
                - traffic VØ9.2Ø
          - fall VØØ.811
          - nontraffic VØ9.1
            - involving motor vehicle NEC VØ9.ØØ
          - traffic VØ9.3
            - involving motor vehicle NEC VØ9.2Ø
        - wheeled shoe VØØ.158
      - on foot (*see also* Accident, pedestrian)
        - collision (with)
          - animal being ridden or animal drawn vehicle VØ6.9Ø
            - nontraffic VØ6.ØØ

- **Accident**— *continued*
  - transport— *continued*
    - pedestrian— *continued*
      - on foot— *continued*
        - collision— *continued*
          - animal being ridden or animal drawn vehicle— *continued*
            - traffic VØ6.1Ø
          - bus or heavy transport VØ4.9Ø
            - nontraffic VØ4.ØØ
            - traffic VØ4.1Ø
          - car VØ3.9Ø
            - nontraffic VØ3.ØØ
            - traffic VØ3.1Ø
          - pedal cycle VØ1.9Ø
            - nontraffic VØ1.ØØ
            - traffic VØ1.1Ø
          - pick-up truck or van VØ3.9Ø
            - nontraffic VØ3.ØØ
            - traffic VØ3.1Ø
          - railway (train) (vehicle) VØ5.9Ø
            - nontraffic VØ5.ØØ
            - traffic VØ5.1Ø
          - streetcar VØ6.9Ø
            - nontraffic VØ6.ØØ
            - traffic VØ6.1Ø
          - two or three-wheeled motor vehicle VØ2.9Ø
            - nontraffic VØ2.ØØ
            - traffic VØ2.1Ø
          - vehicle VØ9.9
            - animal-drawn VØ6.9Ø
              - nontraffic VØ6.ØØ
              - traffic VØ6.1Ø
            - motor
              - nontraffic VØ9.ØØ
              - traffic VØ9.2Ø
        - nontraffic VØ9.1
          - involving motor vehicle VØ9.ØØ
            - military VØ9.Ø1
            - specified type NEC VØ9.Ø9
        - traffic VØ9.3
          - involving motor vehicle VØ9.2Ø
            - military VØ9.21
            - specified type NEC VØ9.29
    - person NEC (unknown way or transportation) V99
      - collision (between)
        - bus (with)
          - heavy transport vehicle (traffic) V87.5
            - nontraffic V88.5
        - car (with)
          - bus (traffic) V87.3
            - nontraffic V88.3
          - heavy transport vehicle (traffic) V87.4
            - nontraffic V88.4
          - nontraffic V88.5
          - pick-up truck or van (traffic) V87.2
            - nontraffic V88.2
          - train or railway vehicle (traffic) V87.6
            - nontraffic V88.6
          - two-or three-wheeled motor vehicle (traffic) V87.Ø
            - nontraffic V88.Ø
        - motor vehicle (traffic) NEC V87.7
          - nontraffic V88.7
        - two-or three-wheeled vehicle (with) (traffic)
          - motor vehicle NEC V87.1
            - nontraffic V88.1
      - nonmotor vehicle (collision) (noncollision) (traffic) V87.9
        - nontraffic V88.9
    - pickup truck occupant V59.9
      - collision (with)
        - animal (traffic) V5Ø.9
          - being ridden (traffic) V56.9
            - nontraffic V56.3
            - while boarding or alighting V56.4
          - nontraffic V5Ø.3
          - while boarding or alighting V5Ø.4
        - animal-drawn vehicle (traffic) V56.9
          - nontraffic V56.3
          - while boarding or alighting V56.4

- **Accident**— *continued*
  - transport— *continued*
    - pickup truck occupant— *continued*
      - collision— *continued*
        - bus (traffic) V54.9
          - nontraffic V54.3
          - while boarding or alighting V54.4
        - car (traffic) V53.9
          - nontraffic V53.3
          - while boarding or alighting V53.4
        - motor vehicle NOS (traffic) V59.6Ø
          - nontraffic V59.2Ø
          - specified type NEC (traffic) V59.69
            - nontraffic V59.29
        - pedal cycle (traffic) V51.9
          - nontraffic V51.3
          - while boarding or alighting V51.4
        - pickup truck (traffic) V53.9
          - nontraffic V53.3
          - while boarding or alighting V53.4
        - railway vehicle (traffic) V55.9
          - nontraffic V55.3
          - while boarding or alighting V55.4
        - specified vehicle NEC (traffic) V56.9
          - nontraffic V56.3
          - while boarding or alighting V56.4
        - stationary object (traffic) V57.9
          - nontraffic V57.3
          - while boarding or alighting V57.4
        - streetcar (traffic) V56.9
          - nontraffic V56.3
          - while boarding or alighting V56.4
        - three wheeled motor vehicle (traffic) V52.9
          - nontraffic V52.3
          - while boarding or alighting V52.4
        - truck (traffic) V54.9
          - nontraffic V54.3
          - while boarding or alighting V54.4
        - two wheeled motor vehicle (traffic) V52.9
          - nontraffic V52.3
          - while boarding or alighting V52.4
        - van (traffic) V53.9
          - nontraffic V53.3
          - while boarding or alighting V53.4
      - driver
        - collision (with)
          - animal (traffic) V5Ø.5
            - being ridden (traffic) V56.5
              - nontraffic V56.Ø
            - nontraffic V5Ø.Ø
          - animal-drawn vehicle (traffic) V56.5
            - nontraffic V56.Ø
          - bus (traffic) V54.5
            - nontraffic V54.Ø
          - car (traffic) V53.5
            - nontraffic V53.Ø
          - motor vehicle NOS (traffic) V59.4Ø
            - nontraffic V59.ØØ
            - specified type NEC (traffic) V59.49
              - nontraffic V59.Ø9
          - pedal cycle (traffic) V51.5
            - nontraffic V51.Ø
          - pickup truck (traffic) V53.5
            - nontraffic V53.Ø
          - railway vehicle (traffic) V55.5
            - nontraffic V55.Ø
          - specified vehicle NEC (traffic) V56.5
            - nontraffic V56.Ø
          - stationary object (traffic) V57.5
            - nontraffic V57.Ø
          - streetcar (traffic) V56.5
            - nontraffic V56.Ø
          - three wheeled motor vehicle (traffic) V52.5
            - nontraffic V52.Ø
          - truck (traffic) V54.5
            - nontraffic V54.Ø
          - two wheeled motor vehicle (traffic) V52.5
            - nontraffic V52.Ø
          - van (traffic) V53.5
            - nontraffic V53.Ø

- **Accident**— *continued*
  - transport— *continued*
    - pickup truck occupant— *continued*
      - driver— *continued*
        - noncollision accident (traffic) V58.5
          - nontraffic V58.Ø
      - noncollision accident (traffic) V58.9
        - nontraffic V58.3
        - while boarding or alighting V58.4
      - nontraffic V59.3
      - hanger-on
        - collision (with)
          - animal (traffic) V5Ø.7
            - being ridden (traffic) V56.7
              - nontraffic V56.2
            - nontraffic V5Ø.2
          - animal-drawn vehicle (traffic) V56.7
            - nontraffic V56.2
          - bus (traffic) V54.7
            - nontraffic V54.2
          - car (traffic) V53.7
            - nontraffic V53.2
          - pedal cycle (traffic) V51.7
            - nontraffic V51.2
          - pickup truck (traffic) V53.7
            - nontraffic V53.2
          - railway vehicle (traffic) V55.7
            - nontraffic V55.2
          - specified vehicle NEC (traffic) V56.7
            - nontraffic V56.2
          - stationary object (traffic) V57.7
            - nontraffic V57.2
          - streetcar (traffic) V56.7
            - nontraffic V56.2
          - three wheeled motor vehicle (traffic) V52.7
            - nontraffic V52.2
          - truck (traffic) V54.7
            - nontraffic V54.2
          - two wheeled motor vehicle (traffic) V52.7
            - nontraffic V52.2
          - van (traffic) V53.7
            - nontraffic V53.2
        - noncollision accident (traffic) V58.7
          - nontraffic V58.2
      - passenger
        - collision (with)
          - animal (traffic) V5Ø.6
            - being ridden (traffic) V56.6
              - nontraffic V56.1
            - nontraffic V5Ø.1
          - animal-drawn vehicle (traffic) V56.6
            - nontraffic V56.1
          - bus (traffic) V54.6
            - nontraffic V54.1
          - car (traffic) V53.6
            - nontraffic V53.1
          - motor vehicle NOS (traffic) V59.5Ø
            - nontraffic V59.1Ø
            - specified type NEC (traffic) V59.59
              - nontraffic V59.19
          - pedal cycle (traffic) V51.6
            - nontraffic V51.1
          - pickup truck (traffic) V53.6
            - nontraffic V53.1
          - railway vehicle (traffic) V55.6
            - nontraffic V55.1
          - specified vehicle NEC (traffic) V56.6
            - nontraffic V56.1
          - stationary object (traffic) V57.6
            - nontraffic V57.1
          - streetcar (traffic) V56.6
            - nontraffic V56.1
          - three wheeled motor vehicle (traffic) V52.6
            - nontraffic V52.1
          - truck (traffic) V54.6
            - nontraffic V54.1
          - two wheeled motor vehicle (traffic) V52.6
            - nontraffic V52.1
          - van (traffic) V53.6

Accident— *continued*
- watercraft— *continued*
  - causing— *continued*
    - injury— *continued*
      - specified type— *continued*
        - powered craft— *continued*
          - jetskis V91.83
          - liner V91.81
          - merchant ship V91.8Ø
          - passenger ship V91.81
        - unpowered craft V91.88
          - canoe V91.85
          - inflatable V91.86
          - kayak V91.85
          - sailboat V91.84
          - surf-board V91.88
          - water skis V91.87
          - windsurfer V91.88
  - due to, caused by cataclysm — *see* Forces of nature, by type
  - military NEC V94.818
    - with civilian watercraft V94.81Ø
    - civilian in water injured by V94.811
  - nonpowered, struck by
    - nonpowered vessel V94.22
    - powered vessel V94.21
  - specified type NEC V94.89
  - striking swimmer
    - powered V94.11
    - unpowered V94.12

Acid throwing (assault) YØ8.89

Activity (involving) (of victim at time of event) Y93.9
- aerobic and step exercise (class) Y93.A3
- alpine skiing Y93.23
- animal care NEC Y93.K9
- arts and handcrafts NEC Y93.D9
- athletics NEC Y93.79
- athletics played as a team or group NEC Y93.69
- athletics played individually NEC Y93.59
- baking Y93.G3
- ballet Y93.41
- barbells Y93.B3
- BASE (Building, Antenna, Span, Earth) jumping Y93.33
- baseball Y93.64
- basketball Y93.67
- bathing (personal) Y93.E1
- beach volleyball Y93.68
- bike riding Y93.55
- boogie boarding Y93.18
- bowling Y93.54
- boxing Y93.71
- brass instrument playing Y93.J4
- building construction Y93.H3
- bungee jumping Y93.34
- calisthenics Y93.A2
- canoeing (in calm and turbulent water) Y93.16
- capture the flag Y93.6A
- cardiorespiratory exercise NEC Y93.A9
- caregiving (providing) NEC Y93.F9
  - bathing Y93.F1
  - lifting Y93.F2
- cellular
  - communication device Y93.C2
  - telephone Y93.C2
- challenge course Y93.A5
- cheerleading Y93.45
- circuit training Y93.A4
- cleaning
  - floor Y93.E5
- climbing NEC Y93.39
  - mountain Y93.31
  - rock Y93.31
  - wall Y93.31
- clothing care and maintenance NEC Y93.E9
- cool down exercises Y93.A2
- combatives Y93.75
- computer
  - keyboarding Y93.C1
  - technology NEC Y93.C9
- confidence course Y93.A5

Activity— *continued*
- construction (building) Y93.H3
- cooking and baking Y93.G3
- cricket Y93.69
- crocheting Y93.D1
- cross country skiing Y93.24
- dancing (all types) Y93.41
- digging
  - dirt Y93.H1
- dirt digging Y93.H1
- dishwashing Y93.G1
- diving (platform) (springboard) Y93.12
  - underwater Y93.15
- dodge ball Y93.6A
- downhill skiing Y93.23
- drum playing Y93.J2
- dumbbells Y93.B3
- electronic
  - devices NEC Y93.C9
    - hand held interactive Y93.C2
  - game playing (using) (with)
    - keyboard or other stationary device Y93.C1
    - interactive device Y93.C2
- elliptical machine Y93.A1
- exercise(s)
  - machines ((primarily) for)
    - cardiorespiratory conditioning Y93.A1
    - muscle strengthening Y93.B1
  - muscle strengthening (non-machine) NEC Y93.B9
- external motion NEC Y93.I9
  - rollercoaster Y93.I1
- field hockey Y93.65
- figure skating (pairs) (singles) Y93.21
- flag football Y93.62
- floor mopping and cleaning Y93.E5
- food preparation and clean up Y93.G1
- football (American) NOS Y93.61
  - flag Y93.62
  - tackle Y93.61
  - touch Y93.62
- four square Y93..6A
- free weights Y93.B3
- frisbee (ultimate) Y93.74
- furniture
  - building Y93.D3
  - finishing Y93.D3
  - repair Y93.D3
- game playing (electronic)
  - using keyboard or other stationary device Y93.C1
  - using interactive device Y93.C2
- gardening Y93.H2
- golf Y93.53
- grass drills Y93.A6
- grilling and smoking food Y93.G2
- grooming and shearing an animal Y93.K3
- guerilla drills Y93.A6
- gymnastics (rhythmic) Y93.43
- handball Y93.73
- handcrafts NEC Y93.D9
- hand held interactive electronic device Y93.C2
- hang gliding Y93.35
- hiking (on level or elevated terrain) Y93.Ø1
- hockey (ice) Y93.22
  - field Y93.65
- horseback riding Y93.52
- household (interior) maintenance NEC Y93.E9
- ice NEC Y93.29
  - dancing Y93.21
  - hockey Y93.22
  - skating Y93.21
- inline roller skating Y93.51
- ironing Y93.E4
- judo Y93.75
- jumping (off) NEC Y93.39
  - BASE (Building, Antenna, Span, Earth) Y93.33
  - bungee Y93.34
  - jacks Y93.A2
  - rope Y93.56
- jumping jacks Y93.A2
- jumping rope Y93.56
- karate Y93.75
- kayaking (in calm and turbulent water) Y93.16

Activity— *continued*
- keyboarding (computer) Y93.C1
- kickball Y93.6A
- knitting Y93.D1
- lacrosse Y93.65
- land maintenance NEC Y93.H9
- landscaping Y93.H2
- laundry Y93.E2
- machines (exercise)
  - primarily for cardiorespiratory conditioning Y93.A1
  - primarily for muscle strengthening Y93.B1
- maintenance
  - exterior building NEC Y93.H9
  - household (interior) NEC Y93.E9
  - land Y93.H9
  - property Y93.H9
- marching (on level or elevated terrain) Y93.Ø1
- martial arts Y93.75
- microwave oven Y93.G3
- mopping (floor) Y93.E5
- mountain climbing Y93.31
- milking an animal Y93.K2
- muscle strengthening
  - exercises (non-machine) NEC Y93.B9
  - machines Y93.B1
- musical keyboard (electronic) playing Y93.J1
- nordic skiing Y93.24
- obstacle course Y93.A5
- oven (microwave) Y93.G3
- packing up and unpacking in moving to a new residence Y93.E6
- parasailing Y93.19
- percussion instrument playing NEC Y93.J2
- personal
  - bathing and showering Y93.E1
  - hygiene NEC Y93.E8
  - showering Y93.E1
- physical games generally associated with school recess, summer camp and children Y93.6A
- physical training NEC Y93.A9
- piano playing Y93.J1
- pilates Y93.B4
- platform diving Y93.12
- playing musical instrument
  - brass instrument Y93.J4
  - drum Y93.J2
  - musical keyboard (electronic) Y93.J1
  - percussion instrument NEC Y93.J2
  - piano Y93.J1
  - string instrument Y93.J3
  - winds instrument Y93.J4
- property maintenance
  - exterior NEC Y93.H9
  - interior NEC Y93.E9
- pruning (garden and lawn) Y93.H2
- pull-ups Y93.B2
- push-ups Y93.B2
- racquetball Y93.73
- rafting (in calm and turbulent water) Y93.16
- raking (leaves) Y93.H1
- rappelling Y93.32
- refereeing a sports activity Y93.81
- residential relocation Y93.E6
- rhythmic gymnastics Y93.43
- rhythmic movement NEC Y93.49
- riding
  - horseback Y93.52
  - rollercoaster Y93.I1
- rock climbing Y93.31
- rollercoaster riding Y93.I1
- roller skating (inline) Y93.51
- rough housing and horseplay Y93.83
- rowing (in calm and turbulent water) Y93.16
- rugby Y93.63
- SCUBA diving Y93.15
- sewing Y93.D2
- shoveling Y93.H1
  - dirt Y93.H1
  - snow Y93.H1
- showering (personal) Y93.E1
- sit-ups Y93.B2

- **Activity**— *continued*
  - skateboarding Y93.51
  - skating (ice) Y93.21
    - roller Y93.51
  - skiing (alpine) (downhill) Y93.23
    - cross country Y93.24
    - nordic Y93.24
    - water Y93.17
  - sledding (snow) Y93.23
  - sleeping (sleep) Y93.84
  - smoking and grilling food Y93.G2
  - snorkeling Y93.15
  - snow NEC Y93.29
    - boarding Y93.23
    - shoveling Y93.H1
    - sledding Y93.23
    - tubing Y93.23
  - soccer Y93.66
  - softball Y93.64
  - specified NEC Y93.89
  - spectator at an event Y93.82
  - sports NEC Y93.79
    - sports played as a team or group NEC Y93.69
    - sports played individually NEC Y93.59
  - springboard diving Y93.12
  - squash Y93.73
  - stationary bike Y93.A1
  - step (stepping) exercise (class) Y93.A3
  - stepper machine Y93.A1
  - stove Y93.G3
  - string instrument playing Y93.J3
  - surfing Y93.18
    - wind Y93.18
  - swimming Y93.11
  - tackle football Y93.61
  - tap dancing Y93.41
  - tennis Y93.73
  - tobogganing Y93.23
  - touch football Y93.62
  - track and field events (non-running) Y93.57
    - running Y93.Ø2
  - trampoline Y93.44
  - treadmill Y93.A1
  - trimming shrubs Y93.H2
  - tubing (in calm and turbulent water) Y93.16
    - snow Y93.23
  - ultimate frisbee Y93.74
  - underwater diving Y93.15
  - unpacking in moving to a new residence Y93.E6
  - use of stove, oven and microwave oven Y93.G3
    - vacuuming Y93.E3
  - volleyball (beach) (court) Y93.68
  - wake boarding Y93.17
  - walking an animal Y93.K1
  - walking (on level or elevated terrain) Y93.Ø1
    - an animal Y93.K1
  - wall climbing Y93.31
  - warm up and cool down exercises Y93.A2
  - water NEC Y93.19
    - aerobics Y93.14
    - craft NEC Y93.19
    - exercise Y93.14
    - polo Y93.13
    - skiing Y93.17
    - sliding Y93.18
    - survival training and testing Y93.19
  - weeding (garden and lawn) Y93.H2
  - wind instrument playing Y93.J4
  - windsurfing Y93.18
  - wrestling Y93.72
  - yoga Y93.42
- **Adverse effect of drugs** - *see* Table of Drugs and Chemicals
- **Aerosinusitis** — *see* Air, pressure
- **After-effect, late** — *see* Sequelae
- **Air**
  - blast in war operations — *see* War operations, air blast
  - pressure
    - change, rapid
      - during
        - ascent W94.29
- **Air**— *continued*
  - pressure— *continued*
    - change, rapid— *continued*
      - during— *continued*
        - ascent— *continued*
          - while (in) (surfacing from)
            - aircraft W94.23
            - deep water diving W94.21
            - underground W94.22
        - descent W94.39
          - in
            - aircraft W94.31
            - water W94.32
    - high, prolonged W94.Ø
    - low, prolonged W94.12
      - due to residence or long visit at high altitude W94.11
- **Alpine sickness** W94.11
- **Altitude sickness** W94.11
- **Anaphylactic shock, anaphylaxis** — *see* Table of Drugs and Chemicals
- **Andes disease** W94.11
- **Arachnidism, arachnoidism** X58
- **Arson** (with intent to injure or kill) X97
- **Asphyxia, asphyxiation**
  - by
    - food (bone) (seed) — *see* categories T17 and T18
    - gas (*see also* Table of Drugs and Chemicals)
      - legal
        - execution — *see* Legal, intervention, gas
        - intervention — *see* Legal, intervention, gas
  - from
    - fire (*see also* Exposure, fire)
      - in war operations — *see* War operations, fire
    - ignition — *see* Ignition
    - vomitus T17.81
  - in war operations — *see* War operations, restriction of airway
- **Aspiration**
  - food (any type) (into respiratory tract) (with asphyxia, obstruction respiratory tract, suffocation) — *see* categories T17 and T18
  - foreign body — *see* Foreign body, aspiration
  - vomitus (with asphyxia, obstruction respiratory tract, suffocation) T17.81
- **Assassination** (attempt) — *see* Assault
- **Assault** (homicidal) (by) (in) YØ9
  - arson X97
  - bite (of human being) YØ4.1
  - bodily force YØ4.8
    - bite YØ4.1
    - bumping into YØ4.2
    - sexual — *see* subcategories T74.Ø, T76.Ø
    - unarmed fight YØ4.Ø
  - bomb X96.9
    - antipersonnel X96.Ø
    - fertilizer X96.3
    - gasoline X96.1
    - letter X96.2
    - petrol X96.1
    - pipe X96.3
    - specified NEC X96.8
  - brawl (hand) (fists) (foot) (unarmed) YØ4.Ø
  - burning, burns (by fire) NEC X97
    - acid YØ8.89
    - caustic, corrosive substance YØ8.89
    - chemical from swallowing caustic, corrosive substance — *see* Table of Drugs and Chemicals
    - cigarette(s) X97
    - hot object X98.9
      - fluid NEC X98.2
      - household appliance X98.3
      - specified NEC X98.8
      - steam X98.Ø
      - tap water X98.1
      - vapors X98.Ø
    - scalding — *see* Assault, burning
    - steam X98.Ø
    - vitriol YØ8.89
  - caustic, corrosive substance (gas) YØ8.89
- **Assault**— *continued*
  - crashing of
    - aircraft YØ8.81
    - motor vehicle YØ3.8
      - pushed in front of YØ2.Ø
      - run over YØ3.Ø
      - specified NEC YØ3.8
  - cutting or piercing instrument X99.9
    - dagger X99.2
    - glass X99.Ø
    - knife X99.1
    - specified NEC X99.8
    - sword X99.2
  - dagger X99.2
  - drowning (in) X92.9
    - bathtub X92.Ø
    - natural water X92.3
    - specified NEC X92.8
    - swimming pool X92.1
      - following fall X92.2
  - dynamite X96.8
  - explosive(s) (material) X96.9
  - fight (hand) (fists) (foot) (unarmed) YØ4.Ø
    - with weapon — *see* Assault, by type of weapon
  - fire X97
  - firearm X95.9
    - airgun X95.Ø1
    - handgun X93
    - hunting rifle X94.1
    - larger X94.9
      - specified NEC X94.8
    - machine gun X94.2
    - shotgun X94.Ø
    - specified NEC X95.8
  - from high place YØ1
  - gunshot (wound) NEC — *see* Assault, firearm, by type
  - incendiary device X97
  - injury YØ9
    - to child due to criminal abortion attempt NEC YØ8.89
  - knife X99.1
  - late effect of — *see* categories X92-YØ8 with 7th character S
  - placing before moving object NEC YØ2.8
    - motor vehicle YØ2.Ø
  - poisoning — *see* categories T36-T65 with 7th character S
  - puncture, any part of body — *see* Assault, cutting or piercing instrument
  - pushing
    - before moving object NEC YØ2.8
      - motor vehicle YØ2.Ø
      - subway train YØ2.1
      - train YØ2.1
    - from high place YØ1.-
  - rape T74.2-
  - scalding — *see* Assault, burning
  - sequelae of — *see* categories X92-YØ8 with 7th character S
  - sexual (by bodily force) T74.2-
  - shooting — *see* Assault, firearm
  - specified means NEC YØ8.89
  - stab, any part of body — *see* Assault, cutting or piercing instrument
  - steam X98.Ø
  - striking against
    - other person YØ4.2
    - sports equipment YØ8.Ø9
      - baseball bat YØ8.Ø2
      - hockey stick YØ8.Ø1
  - struck by
    - sports equipment YØ8.Ø9
      - baseball bat YØ8.Ø2
      - hockey stick YØ8.Ø1
  - submersion — *see* Assault, drowning
  - violence YØ9
  - weapon YØ9
    - blunt YØØ
    - cutting or piercing — *see* Assault, cutting or piercing instrument
    - firearm — *see* Assault, firearm

Assault— *continued*
- wound YØ9
  - cutting — *see* Assault, cutting or piercing instrument
  - gunshot — *see* Assault, firearm
  - knife X99.1
  - piercing — *see* Assault, cutting or piercing instrument
  - puncture — *see* Assault, cutting or piercing instrument
  - stab — *see* Assault, cutting or piercing instrument

Attack by mammals NEC W55.89
Avalanche — *see* Landslide
Aviator's disease — *see* Air, pressure

B

Barotitis, barodontalgia, barosinusitis, barotrauma (otitic) (sinus) — *see* Air, pressure
Battered (baby) (child) (person) (syndrome) X58
Bayonet wound W26.1
- in
  - legal intervention — *see* Legal, intervention, sharp object, bayonet
  - war operations — *see* War operations, combat
- stated as undetermined whether accidental or intentional Y28.8
- suicide (attempt) X78.2

Bean in nose - *see* categories T17 and T18
Bed set on fire NEC — *see* Exposure, fire, uncontrolled, building, bed
Beheading (by guillotine)
- homicide X99.9
- legal execution — *see* Legal, intervention

Bending, injury in — *see* Overexertion
Bends — *see* Air, pressure, change
Bite, bitten by
- alligator W58.Ø1
- arthropod (nonvenomous) NEC W57
- bull W55.21
- cat W55.Ø1
- cow W55.21
- crocodile W58.11
- dog W54.Ø
- goat W55.31
- hoof stock NEC W55.31
- horse W55.11
- human being (accidentally) W5Ø.3
  - with intent to injure or kill YØ4.1
  - as, or caused by, a crowd or human stampede (with fall) W52
  - assault YØ4.1
  - homicide (attempt) YØ4.1
  - in
    - fight YØ4.1
- insect (nonvenomous) W57
- lizard (nonvenomous) W59.Ø1
- millipede W57
- mammal NEC W55.81
  - marine W56.31
- marine animal (nonvenomous) W56.81
- moray eel W56.51
- mouse W53.Ø1
- person(s) (accidentally) W5Ø.3
  - with intent to injure or kill YØ4.1
  - as, or caused by, a crowd or human stampede (with fall) W52
  - assault YØ4.1
  - homicide (attempt) YØ4.1
  - in
    - fight YØ4.1
- pig W55.41
- raccoon W55.51
- rat W53.11
- reptile W59.81
  - lizard W59.Ø1
  - snake W59.11
  - turtle W59.21
    - terrestrial W59.81
- rodent W53.81
  - mouse W53.Ø1

Bite, bitten by— *continued*
- rodent— *continued*
  - rat W53.11
  - specified NEC W53.81
  - squirrel W53.21
- shark W56.41
- sheep W55.31
- snake (nonvenomous) W59.11
- spider (nonvenomous) W57
- squirrel W53.21

Blast (air) **in war operations** - *see* War operations, blast
Blizzard X37.2
Blood alcohol level Y9Ø.9
- less than 2Ømg/1ØØml Y9Ø.Ø
- presence in blood, level not specified Y9Ø.9
- 2Ø-39mg/1ØØml Y9Ø.1
- 4Ø-59mg/1ØØml Y9Ø.2
- 6Ø-79mg/1ØØml Y9Ø.3
- 8Ø-99mg/1ØØml Y9Ø.4
- 1ØØ-119mg/1ØØml Y9Ø.5
- 12Ø-199mg/1ØØml Y9Ø.6
- 2ØØ-239mg/1ØØml Y9Ø.7

Blow X58
- by law-enforcing agent, police (on duty) — *see* Legal, intervention, manhandling
  - blunt object — *see* Legal, intervention, blunt object

Blowing up — *see* Explosion
Brawl (hand) (fists) (foot) YØ4.Ø
Breakage (accidental) (part of)
- ladder (causing fall) W11
- scaffolding (causing fall) W12

Broken
- glass, contact with — *see* Contact, with, glass
- power line (causing electric shock) W85

Bumping against, into (accidentally)
- object NEC W22.8
  - with fall — *see* Fall, due to, bumping against, object
  - caused by crowd or human stampede (with fall) W52
  - sports equipment W21.9
- person(s) W51
  - with fall WØ3
    - due to ice or snow WØØ.Ø
  - assault YØ4.2
  - caused by, a crowd or human stampede (with fall) W52
  - homicide (attempt) YØ4.2
- sports equipment W21.9

Burn, burned, burning (accidental) (by) (from) (on)
- acid NEC — *see* Table of Drugs and Chemicals
- bed linen — *see* Exposure, fire, uncontrolled, in building, bed
- blowtorch XØ8.8
  - with ignition of clothing NEC XØ6.2
    - nightwear XØ5
- bonfire, campfire (controlled) (*see also* Exposure, fire, controlled, not in building)
  - uncontrolled — *see* Exposure, fire, uncontrolled, not in building
- candle XØ8.8
  - with ignition of clothing NEC XØ6.2
    - nightwear XØ5
- caustic liquid, substance (external) (internal) NEC — *see* Table of Drugs and Chemicals
- chemical (external) (internal) (*see also* Table of Drugs and Chemicals)
  - in war operations — *see* War operations. fire
- cigar(s) or cigarette(s) XØ8.8
  - with ignition of clothing NEC XØ6.2
    - nightwear XØ5
- clothes, clothing NEC (from controlled fire) XØ6.2
  - with conflagration — *see* Exposure, fire, uncontrolled, building
    - not in building or structure — *see* Exposure, fire, uncontrolled, not in building
- cooker (hot) X15.8
  - stated as undetermined whether accidental or intentional Y27.3
  - suicide (attempt) X77.3

Burn, burned, burning— *continued*
- electric blanket X16
- engine (hot) X17
- fire, flames — *see* Exposure, fire
- flare, Very pistol — *see* Discharge, firearm NEC
- heat
  - from appliance (electrical) (household) X15.8
    - cooker X15.8
    - hotplate X15.2
    - kettle X15.8
    - light bulb X15.8
    - saucepan X15.3
    - skillet X15.3
    - stove X15.Ø
    - stated as undetermined whether accidental or intentional Y27.3
    - suicide (attempt) X77.3
    - toaster X15.1
  - in local application or packing during medical or surgical procedure Y63.5
- heating
  - appliance, radiator or pipe X16
- homicide (attempt) — *see* Assault, burning
- hot
  - air X14.1
  - cooker X15.8
  - drink X1Ø.Ø
  - engine X17
  - fat X1Ø.2
  - fluid NEC X12
  - food X1Ø.1
  - gases X14.1
  - heating appliance X16
  - household appliance NEC X15.8
  - kettle X15.8
  - liquid NEC X12
  - machinery X17
  - metal (molten) (liquid) NEC X18
  - object (not producing fire or flames) NEC X19
  - oil (cooking) X1Ø.2
  - pipe(s) X16
  - radiator X16
  - saucepan (glass) (metal) X15.3
  - stove (kitchen) X15.Ø
  - substance NEC X19
    - caustic or corrosive NEC — *see* Table of Drugs and Chemicals
  - toaster X15.1
  - tool X17
  - vapor X13.1
  - water (tap) — *see* Contact, with, hot, tap water
- hotplate X15.2
  - suicide (attempt) X77.3
- ignition — *see* Ignition
- in war operations — *see* War operations, fire
- inflicted by other person X97
  - by hot objects, hot vapor, and steam — *see* Assault, burning, hot object
- internal, from swallowed caustic, corrosive liquid, substance — *see* Table of Drugs and Chemicals
- iron (hot) X15.8
  - stated as undetermined whether accidental or intentional Y27.3
  - suicide (attempt) X77.3
- kettle (hot) X15.8
  - stated as undetermined whether accidental or intentional Y27.3
  - suicide (attempt) X77.3
- lamp (flame) XØ8.8
  - with ignition of clothing NEC XØ6.2
    - nightwear XØ5
- lighter (cigar) (cigarette) XØ8.8
  - with ignition of clothing NEC XØ6.2
    - nightwear XØ5
- lightning — *see* subcategory T75.Ø
  - causing fire — *see* Exposure, fire
- liquid (boiling) (hot) NEC X12
  - stated as undetermined whether accidental or intentional Y27.2
  - suicide (attempt) X77.2
- local application of externally applied substance in medical or surgical care Y63.5

- **Burn, burned, burning**— *continued*
  - machinery (hot) X17
  - matches X08.8
    - with ignition of clothing NEC X06.2
      - nightwear X05
  - mattress — *see* Exposure, fire, uncontrolled, building, bed
  - medicament, externally applied Y63.5
  - metal (hot) (liquid) (molten) NEC X18
  - nightwear (nightclothes, nightdress, gown, pajamas, robe) X05
  - object (hot) NEC X19
  - on board watercraft
    - due to
      - accident to watercraft V91.09
        - powered craft V91.03
          - ferry boat V91.01
          - fishing boat V91.02
          - jetskis V91.03
          - liner V91.01
          - merchant ship V91.00
          - passenger ship V91.01
        - unpowered craft V91.08
          - canoe V91.05
          - inflatable V91.06
          - kayak V91.05
          - sailboat V91.04
          - surf-board V91.08
          - water skis V91.07
          - windsurfer V91.08
      - fire on board V93.09
        - ferry boat V93.01
        - fishing boat V93.02
        - jetskis V93.03
        - liner V93.01
        - merchant ship V93.00
        - passenger ship V93.01
        - powered craft NEC V93.03
        - sailboat V93.04
      - specified heat source NEC on board V93.19
        - ferry boat V93.11
        - fishing boat V93.12
        - jetskis V93.13
        - liner V93.11
        - merchant ship V93.10
        - passenger ship V93.11
        - powered craft NEC V93.13
        - sailboat V93.14
  - pipe (hot) X16
    - smoking X08.8
      - with ignition of clothing NEC X06.2
        - nightwear X05
  - powder — *see* Powder burn
  - radiator (hot) X16
  - saucepan (hot) (glass) (metal) X15.3
    - stated as undetermined whether accidental or intentional Y27.3
    - suicide (attempt) X77.3
  - self-inflicted X76
    - stated as undetermined whether accidental or intentional Y26
  - steam X13.1
    - pipe X16
      - stated as undetermined whether accidental or intentional Y27.8
    - stated as undetermined whether accidental or intentional Y27.0
    - suicide (attempt) X77.0
  - stove (hot) (kitchen) X15.0
    - stated as undetermined whether accidental or intentional Y27.3
    - suicide (attempt) X77.3
  - substance (hot) NEC X19
    - boiling X12
      - stated as undetermined whether accidental or intentional Y27.2
      - suicide (attempt) X77.2
    - molten (metal) X18
  - suicide (attempt) NEC X76
    - hot
      - household appliance X77.3
      - object X77.9

- **Burn, burned, burning**— *continued*
  - therapeutic misadventure
    - heat in local application or packing during medical or surgical procedure Y63.5
    - overdose of radiation Y63.2
  - toaster (hot) X15.1
    - stated as undetermined whether accidental or intentional Y27.3
    - suicide (attempt) X77.3
  - tool (hot) X17
  - torch, welding X08.8
    - with ignition of clothing NEC X06.2
      - nightwear X05
  - trash fire (controlled) — *see* Exposure, fire, controlled, not in building
    - uncontrolled — *see* Exposure, fire, uncontrolled, not in building
  - vapor (hot) X13.1
    - stated as undetermined whether accidental or intentional Y27.0
    - suicide (attempt) X77.0
  - Very pistol — *see* Discharge, firearm NEC
- **Butted by animal** W55.82
  - bull W55.22
  - cow W55.22
  - goat W55.32
  - horse W55.12
  - pig W55.42
  - sheep W55.32

C

- **Caisson disease** — *see* Air, pressure, change
- **Campfire** (exposure to) (controlled) (*see also* Exposure, fire, controlled, not in building)
  - uncontrolled — *see* Exposure, fire, uncontrolled, not in building
- **Capital punishment** (any means) — *see* Legal, intervention
- **Car sickness** T75.3
- **Casualty** (not due to war) NEC X58
  - war — *see* War operations
- **Cat**
  - bite W55.01
  - scratch W55.03
- **Cataclysm, cataclysmic** (any injury) NEC — *see* Forces of nature
- **Catching fire** — *see* Exposure, fire
- **Caught**
  - between
    - folding object W23.0
    - objects (moving) (stationary and moving) W23.0
      - and machinery — *see* Contact, with, by type of machine
      - stationary W23.1
    - sliding door and door frame W23.0
  - by, in
    - machinery (moving parts of) — *see* Contact, with, by type of machine
    - washing-machine wringer W23.0
  - under packing crate (due to losing grip) W23.1
- **Cave-in** caused by cataclysmic earth surface movement or eruption — *see* Landslide
- **Change(s) in air pressure** — *see* Air, pressure, change
- **Choked, choking** (on) (any object except food or vomitus)
  - food (bone) (seed) — *see* categories T17 and T18
  - vomitus T17.81-
- **Civil insurrection** — *see* War operations
- **Cloudburst** (any injury) X37.8
- **Cold, exposure to (accidental) (excessive)** (extreme) (natural) (place) **NEC** — see Exposure, cold
- **Collapse**
  - building W20.1
    - burning (uncontrolled fire) X00.2
  - dam or man-made structure (causing earth movement) X36.0
  - machinery — *see* Contact, with, by type of machine
  - structure W20.1
    - burning (uncontrolled fire) X00.2

- **Collision** (accidental) NEC (*see also* Accident, transport) V89.9
  - pedestrian W51
    - with fall W03
      - due to ice or snow W00.0
      - involving pedestrian conveyance — *see* Accident, transport, pedestrian, conveyance
    - and
      - crowd or human stampede (with fall) W52
      - object W22.8
        - with fall — *see* Fall, due to, bumping against, object
  - person(s) — *see* Collision, pedestrian
  - transport vehicle NEC V89.9
    - and
      - avalanche, fallen or not moving — *see* Accident, transport
        - falling or moving — *see* Landslide
      - landslide, fallen or not moving — *see* Accident, transport
        - falling or moving — *see* Landslide
    - due to cataclysm — *see* Forces of nature, by type
    - intentional, purposeful suicide (attempt) — *see* Suicide, collision
- **Combustion, spontaneous** — *see* Ignition
- **Complication** (delayed) **of or following** medical or surgical procedure Y84.9
  - with misadventure — *see* Misadventure
  - amputation of limb(s) Y83.5
  - anastomosis (arteriovenous) (blood vessel) (gastrojejunal) (tendon) (natural or artificial material) Y83.2
  - aspiration (of fluid) Y84.4
    - tissue Y84.8
  - biopsy Y84.8
  - blood
    - sampling Y84.7
    - transfusion
      - procedure Y84.8
  - bypass Y83.2
  - catheterization (urinary) Y84.6
    - cardiac Y84.0
  - colostomy Y83.3
  - cystostomy Y83.3
  - dialysis (kidney) Y84.1
  - drug — *see* Table of Drugs and Chemicals
    - due to misadventure — *see* Misadventure
  - duodenostomy Y83.3
  - electroshock therapy Y84.3
  - external stoma, creation of Y83.3
  - formation of external stoma Y83.3
  - gastrostomy Y83.3
  - graft Y83.2
  - hypothermia (medically-induced) Y84.8
  - implant, implantation (of)
    - artificial
      - internal device (cardiac pacemaker) (electrodes in brain) (heart valve prosthesis) (orthopedic) Y83.1
      - material or tissue (for anastomosis or bypass) Y83.2
        - with creation of external stoma Y83.3
    - natural tissues (for anastomosis or bypass) Y83.2
      - with creation of external stoma Y83.3
  - infusion
    - procedure Y84.8
  - injection — *see* Table of Drugs and Chemicals
    - procedure Y84.8
  - insertion of gastric or duodenal sound Y84.5
  - insulin-shock therapy Y84.3
  - paracentesis (abdominal) (thoracic) (aspirative) Y84.4
  - procedures other than surgical operation — *see* Complication of or following, by type of procedure
  - radiological procedure or therapy Y84.2
  - removal of organ (partial) (total) NEC Y83.6
  - sampling
    - blood Y84.7
    - fluid NEC Y84.4
    - tissue Y84.8

- **Complication of or following**— *continued*
  - shock therapy Y84.3
  - surgical operation NEC (*see also* Complication of or following, by type of operation) Y83.9
    - reconstructive NEC Y83.4
      - with
        - anastomosis, bypass or graft Y83.2
        - formation of external stoma Y83.3
    - specified NEC Y83.8
  - transfusion (*see also* Table of Drugs and Chemicals)
    - procedure Y84.8
  - transplant, transplantation (heart) (kidney) (liver) (whole organ, any) Y83.Ø
    - partial organ Y83.4
  - ureterostomy Y83.3
  - vaccination (*see also* Table of Drugs and Chemicals)
    - procedure Y84.8
- **Compression**
  - divers' squeeze — *see* Air, pressure, change
  - trachea by
    - food (lodged in esophagus) — *see* categories T17 and T18
    - vomitus (lodged in esophagus) T17.81-
- **Conflagration** — *see* Exposure, fire, uncontrolled
- **Constriction** (external)
  - hair W49.Ø1
  - jewelry W49.Ø4
  - ring W49.Ø4
  - rubber band W49.Ø3
  - specified item NEC W49.Ø9
  - string W49.Ø2
  - thread W49.Ø2
- **Contact** (accidental)
  - with
    - abrasive wheel (metalworking) W31.1
    - alligator W58.Ø9
      - bite W58.Ø1
      - crushing W58.Ø3
      - strike W58.Ø2
    - amphibian W62.9
      - frog W62.Ø
      - toad W62.1
    - animal (nonvenomous) NEC W64
      - marine W56.89
        - bite W56.81
        - dolphin — *see* Contact, with, dolphin
        - fish NEC — *see* Contact, with, fish
        - mammal — *see* Contact, with, mammal, marine
        - orca — *see* Contact, with, orca
        - sea lion — *see* Contact, with, sea lion
        - shark — *see* Contact, with, shark
        - strike W56.82
    - animate mechanical force NEC W64
    - arrow W21.89
      - not thrown, projected or falling W45.8
    - arthropods (nonvenomous) W57
    - axe W27.Ø
    - band-saw (industrial) W31.2
    - bayonet — *see* Bayonet wound
    - bee(s) X58
    - bench-saw (industrial) W31.2
    - bird W61.99
      - bite W61.91
      - chicken — *see* Contact, with, chicken
      - duck — *see* Contact, with, duck
      - goose — *see* Contact, with, goose
      - macaw — *see* Contact, with, macaw
      - parrot — *see* Contact, with, parrot
      - psittacine — *see* Contact, with, psittacine
      - strike W61.92
      - turkey — *see* Contact, with, turkey
    - blender W29.Ø
    - boiling water X12
      - stated as undetermined whether accidental or intentional Y27.2
      - suicide (attempt) X77.2
    - bore, earth-drilling or mining (land) (seabed) W31.Ø
    - buffalo — *see* Contact, with, hoof stock NEC
    - bull W55.29

- **Contact**— *continued*
  - with— *continued*
    - bull— *continued*
      - bite W55.21
      - gored W55.22
      - strike W55.22
    - bumper cars W31.81
    - camel — *see* Contact, with, hoof stock NEC
    - can
      - lid W45.2
      - opener W27.4
        - powered W29.Ø
    - cat W55.Ø9
      - bite W55.Ø1
      - scratch W55.Ø3
    - caterpillar (venomous) X58
    - centipede (venomous) X58
    - chain
      - hoist W24.Ø
        - agricultural operations W3Ø.89
      - saw W29.3
    - chicken W61.39
      - peck W61.33
      - strike W61.32
    - chisel W27.Ø
    - circular saw W31.2
    - cobra X58
    - combine (harvester) W3Ø.Ø
    - conveyer belt W24.1
    - cooker (hot) X15.8
      - stated as undetermined whether accidental or intentional Y27.3
      - suicide (attempt) X77.3
    - coral X58
    - cotton gin W31.82
    - cow W55.29
      - bite W55.21
      - strike W55.22
    - crane W24.Ø
      - agricultural operations W3Ø.89
    - crocodile W58.19
      - bite W58.11
      - crushing W58.13
      - strike W58.12
    - dagger W26.1
      - stated as undetermined whether accidental or intentional Y28.2
      - suicide (attempt) X78.2
    - dairy equipment W31.82
    - dart W21.89
      - not thrown, projected or falling W45.8
    - deer — *see* Contact, with, hoof stock NEC
    - derrick W24.Ø
      - agricultural operations W3Ø.89
        - hay W3Ø.2
    - dog W54.8
      - bite W54.Ø
      - strike W54.1
    - dolphin W56.Ø9
      - bite W56.Ø1
      - strike W56.Ø2
    - donkey — *see* Contact, with, hoof stock NEC
    - drill (powered) W29.8
      - earth (land) (seabed) W31.Ø
      - nonpowered W27.8
    - drive belt W24.Ø
      - agricultural operations W3Ø.89
    - dry ice — *see* Exposure, cold, man-made
    - dryer (clothes) (powered) (spin) W29.2
    - duck W61.69
      - bite W61.61
      - strike W61.62
    - earth(-)
      - drilling machine (industrial) W31.Ø
      - scraping machine in stationary use W31.83
    - edge of stiff paper W45.1
    - electric
      - beater W29.Ø
      - blanket X16
      - fan W29.2
        - commercial W31.82
      - knife W29.1
      - mixer W29.Ø

- **Contact**— *continued*
  - with— *continued*
    - elevator (building) W24.Ø
      - agricultural operations W3Ø.89
        - grain W3Ø.3
    - engine(s), hot NEC X17
    - excavating machine W31.Ø
    - farm machine W3Ø.9
    - feces — *see* Contact, with, by type of animal
    - fer de lance X58
    - fish W56.59
      - bite W56.51
      - shark — *see* Contact, with, shark
      - strike W56.52
    - flying horses W31.81
    - forging (metalworking) machine W31.1
    - fork W27.4
    - forklift (truck) W24.Ø
      - agricultural operations W3Ø.89
    - frog W62.Ø
    - garden
      - cultivator (powered) W29.3
        - riding W3Ø.89
      - fork W27.1
    - gas turbine W31.3
    - Gila monster X58
    - giraffe — *see* Contact, with, hoof stock NEC
    - glass (sharp) (broken) W25
      - with subsequent fall W18.Ø2
      - assault X99.Ø
      - due to fall — *see* Fall, by type
      - stated as undetermined whether accidental or intentional Y28.Ø
      - suicide (attempt) X78.Ø
    - goat W55.39
      - bite W55.31
      - strike W55.32
    - goose W61.59
      - bite W61.51
      - strike W61.52
    - hand
      - saw W27.Ø
      - tool (not powered) NEC W27.8
        - powered W29.8
    - harvester W3Ø.Ø
    - hay-derrick W3Ø.2
    - heat NEC X19
      - from appliance (electrical) (household) — *see* Contact, with, hot, household appliance
        - heating appliance X16
    - heating
      - appliance (hot) X16
      - pad (electric) X16
    - hedge-trimmer (powered) W29.3
    - hoe W27.1
    - hoist (chain) (shaft) NEC W24.Ø
      - agricultural W3Ø.89
    - hoof stock NEC W55.39
      - bite W55.31
      - strike W55.32
    - hornet(s) X58
    - horse W55.19
      - bite W55.11
      - strike W55.12
    - hot
      - air X14.1
        - inhalation X14.Ø
      - cooker X15.8
      - drinks X1Ø.Ø
      - engine X17
      - fats X1Ø.2
      - fluids NEC X12
        - assault X98.2
        - suicide (attempt) X77.2
        - undetermined whether accidental or intentional Y27.2
      - food X1Ø.1
      - gases X14.1
        - inhalation X14.Ø
      - heating appliance X16
      - household appliance X15.8
        - assault X98.3
        - cooker X15.8

- **Contact**— *continued*
  - with— *continued*
    - hot— *continued*
      - household appliance— *continued*
        - hotplate X15.2
        - kettle X15.8
        - light bulb X15.8
        - object NEC X19
          - assault X98.8
          - stated as undetermined whether accidental or intentional Y27.9
          - suicide (attempt) X77.8
        - saucepan X15.3
        - skillet X15.3
        - stove X15.Ø
        - stated as undetermined whether accidental or intentional Y27.3
        - suicide (attempt) X77.3
        - toaster X15.1
      - kettle X15.8
      - light bulb X15.8
      - liquid NEC (*see also* Burning) X12
        - drinks X1Ø.Ø
        - stated as undetermined whether accidental or intentional Y27.2
        - suicide (attempt) X77.2
        - tap water X11.8
          - stated as undetermined whether accidental or intentional Y27.1
          - suicide (attempt) X77.1
      - machinery X17
      - metal (molten) (liquid) NEC X18
      - object (not producing fire or flames) NEC X19
      - oil (cooking) X1Ø.2
      - pipe X16
      - plate X15.2
      - radiator X16
      - saucepan (glass) (metal) X15.3
      - skillet X15.3
      - stove (kitchen) X15.Ø
      - substance NEC X19
      - tap-water X11.8
        - assault X98.1
        - heated on stove X12
          - stated as undetermined whether accidental or intentional Y27.2
          - suicide (attempt) X77.2
        - in bathtub X11.Ø
        - running X11.1
        - stated as undetermined whether accidental or intentional Y27.1
        - suicide (attempt) X77.1
      - toaster X15.1
      - tool X17
      - vapors X13.1
        - inhalation X13.Ø
      - water (tap) X11.8
        - boiling X12
          - stated as undetermined whether accidental or intentional Y27.2
          - suicide (attempt) X77.2
        - heated on stove X12
          - stated as undetermined whether accidental or intentional Y27.2
          - suicide (attempt) X77.2
        - in bathtub X11.Ø
        - running X11.1
        - stated as undetermined whether accidental or intentional Y27.1
        - suicide (attempt) X77.1
    - hotplate X15.2
    - ice-pick W27.4
    - insect (nonvenomous) NEC W57
    - kettle (hot) X15.8
    - knife W26.Ø
      - assault X99.1
      - electric W29.1
      - stated as undetermined whether accidental or intentional Y28.1
      - suicide (attempt) X78.1
    - lathe (metalworking) W31.1
      - turnings W45.8
      - woodworking W31.2

- **Contact**— *continued*
  - with— *continued*
    - lawnmower (powered) (ridden) W28
      - causing electrocution W86.8
        - suicide (attempt) X83.1
      - unpowered W27.1
    - lift, lifting (devices) W24.Ø
      - agricultural operations W3Ø.89
      - shaft W24.Ø
    - liquefied gas — *see* Exposure, cold, man-made
    - liquid air, hydrogen, nitrogen — *see* Exposure, cold, man-made
    - lizard (nonvenomous) W59.Ø9
      - bite W59.Ø1
      - strike W59.Ø2
    - llama — *see* Contact, with, hoof stock NEC
    - macaw W61.19
      - bite W61.11
      - strike W61.12
    - machine, machinery W31.9
      - abrasive wheel W31.1
      - agricultural including animal-powered W3Ø.9
        - combine harvester W3Ø.Ø
        - grain storage elevator W3Ø.3
        - hay derrick W3Ø.2
        - power take-off device W3Ø.1
        - reaper W3Ø.Ø
        - specified NEC W3Ø.89
        - thresher W3Ø.Ø
        - transport vehicle, stationary W3Ø.81
      - band saw W31.2
      - bench saw W31.2
      - circular saw W31.2
      - commercial NEC W31.82
      - drilling, metal (industrial) W31.1
      - earth-drilling W31.Ø
      - earthmoving or scraping W31.89
      - excavating W31.89
      - forging machine W31.1
      - gas turbine W31.3
      - hot X17
      - internal combustion engine W31.3
      - land drill W31.Ø
      - lathe W31.1
      - lifting (devices) W24.Ø
      - metal drill W31.1
      - metalworking (industrial) W31.1
      - milling, metal W31.1
      - mining W31.Ø
      - molding W31.2
      - overhead plane W31.2
      - power press, metal W31.1
      - prime mover W31.3
      - printing W31.89
      - radial saw W31.2
      - recreational W31.81
      - roller-coaster W31.81
      - rolling mill, metal W31.1
      - sander W31.2
      - seabed drill W31.Ø
      - shaft
        - hoist W31.Ø
        - lift W31.Ø
      - specified NEC W31.89
      - spinning W31.89
      - steam engine W31.3
      - transmission W24.1
      - undercutter W31.Ø
      - water driven turbine W31.3
      - weaving W31.89
      - woodworking or forming (industrial) W31.2
    - mammal (feces) (urine) W55.89
      - bull — *see* Contact, with, bull
      - cat — *see* Contact, with, cat
      - cow — *see* Contact, with, cow
      - goat — *see* Contact, with, goat
      - hoof stock — *see* Contact, with, hoof stock
      - horse — *see* Contact, with, horse
      - marine W56.39
        - dolphin — *see* Contact, with, dolphin
        - orca — *see* Contact, with, orca
        - sea lion — *see* Contact, with, sea lion
        - specified NEC W56.39

- **Contact**— *continued*
  - with— *continued*
    - mammal— *continued*
      - marine— *continued*
        - specified— *continued*
          - bite W56.31
          - strike W56.32
      - pig — *see* Contact, with, pig
      - raccoon — *see* Contact, with, raccoon
      - rodent — *see* Contact, with, rodent
      - sheep — *see* Contact, with, sheep
      - specified NEC W55.89
        - bite W55.81
        - strike W55.82
    - marine
      - animal W56.89
        - bite W56.81
        - dolphin — *see* Contact, with, dolphin
        - fish NEC — *see* Contact, with, fish
        - mammal — *see* Contact, with, mammal, marine
        - orca — *see* Contact, with, orca
        - sea lion — *see* Contact, with, sea lion
        - shark — *see* Contact, with, shark
        - strike W56.82
    - meat
      - grinder (domestic) W29.Ø
        - industrial W31.82
        - nonpowered W27.4
      - slicer (domestic) W29.Ø
        - industrial W31.82
    - merry go round W31.81
    - metal, hot (liquid) (molten) NEC X18
    - millipede W57
    - nail W45.Ø
      - gun W29.4
    - needle (sewing) W27.3
      - hypodermic W46.Ø
        - contaminated W46.1
    - object (blunt) NEC
      - hot NEC X19
      - legal intervention — *see* Legal, intervention, blunt object
      - sharp NEC W45.8
        - inflicted by other person NEC W45.8
          - stated as
            - intentional homicide (attempt) — *see* Assault, cutting or piercing instrument
        - legal intervention — *see* Legal, intervention, sharp object
        - self-inflicted X78.9
    - orca W56.29
      - bite W56.21
      - strike W56.22
    - overhead plane W31.2
    - paper (as sharp object) W45.1
    - paper-cutter W27.5
    - parrot W61.Ø9
      - bite W61.Ø1
      - strike W61.Ø2
    - pig W55.49
      - bite W55.41
      - strike W55.42
    - pipe, hot X16
    - pitchfork W27.1
    - plane (metal) (wood) W27.Ø
      - overhead W31.2
    - plant thorns, spines, sharp leaves or other mechanisms W6Ø
    - powered
      - garden cultivator W29.3
      - household appliance, implement, or machine W29.8
      - saw (industrial) W31.2
        - hand W29.8
    - printing machine W31.89
    - psittacine bird W61.29
      - bite W61.21
      - macaw — *see* Contace, with, macaw
      - parrot — *see* Contact, with, parrot
      - strike W61.22

Contact— *continued*
- with— *continued*
  - pulley (block) (transmission) W24.Ø
    - agricultural operations W3Ø.89
  - raccoon W55.59
    - bite W55.51
    - strike W55.52
  - radial-saw (industrial) W31.2
  - radiator (hot) X16
  - rake W27.1
  - rattlesnake X58
  - reaper W3Ø.Ø
  - reptile W59.89
    - lizard — *see* Contact, with, lizard
    - snake — *see* Contact, with, snake
    - specified NEC W59.89
      - bite W59.81
      - crushing W59.83
      - strike W59.82
    - turtle — *see* Contact, with, turtle
  - rivet gun (powered) W29.4
  - road scraper — *see* Accident, transport, construction vehicle
  - rodent (feces) (urine) W53.89
    - bite W53.81
    - mouse W53.Ø9
      - bite W53.Ø1
    - rat W53.19
      - bite W53.11
    - specified NEC W53.89
      - bite W53.81
    - squirrel W53.29
      - bite W53.21
  - roller coaster W31.81
  - rope NEC W24.Ø
    - agricultural operations W3Ø.89
  - saliva — *see* Contact, with, by type of animal
  - sander W29.8
    - industrial W31.2
  - saucepan (hot) (glass) (metal) X15.3
  - saw W27.Ø
    - band (industrial) W31.2
    - bench (industrial) W31.2
    - chain W29.3
    - hand W27.Ø
  - sawing machine, metal W31.1
  - scissors W27.2
  - scorpion X58
  - screwdriver W27.Ø
    - powered W29.8
  - sea
    - anemone, cucumber or urchin (spine) X58
    - lion W56.19
      - bite W56.11
      - strike W56.12
  - serpent — *see* Contact, with, snake, by type
  - sewing-machine (electric) (powered) W29.2
    - not powered W27.8
  - shaft (hoist) (lift) (transmission) NEC W24.Ø
    - agricultural W3Ø.89
  - shark W56.49
    - bite W56.41
    - strike W56.42
  - shears (hand) W27.2
    - powered (industrial) W31.1
      - domestic W29.2
  - sheep W55.39
    - bite W55.31
    - strike W55.32
  - shovel W27.8
    - steam — *see* Accident, transport, construction vehicle
  - snake (nonvenomous) W59.19
    - bite W59.11
    - crushing W59.13
    - strike W59.12
  - spade W27.1
  - spider (venomous) X58
  - spin-drier W29.2
  - spinning machine W31.89
  - splinter W45.8
  - sports equipment W21.9
  - staple gun (powered) W29.8
  - steam X13.1
    - engine W31.3
    - inhalation X13.Ø
    - pipe X16
    - shovel W31.89
  - stove (hot) (kitchen) X15.Ø
  - substance, hot NEC X19
    - molten (metal) X18
  - sword W26.1
    - assault X99.2
    - stated as undetermined whether accidental or intentional Y28.2
    - suicide (attempt) X78.2
  - tarantula X58
  - thresher W3Ø.Ø
  - tin can lid W45.2
  - toad W62.1
  - toaster (hot) X15.1
  - tool W27.8
    - hand (not powered) W27.8
      - auger W27.Ø
      - axe W27.Ø
      - can opener W27.4
      - chisel W27.Ø
      - fork W27.4
      - garden W27.1
      - handsaw W27.Ø
      - hoe W27.1
      - ice-pick W27.4
      - kitchen utensil W27.4
      - manual
        - lawn mower W27.1
        - sewing machine W27.8
      - meat grinder W27.4
      - needle (sewing) W27.3
        - hypodermic W46.Ø
          - contaminated W46.1
      - paper cutter W27.5
      - pitchfork W27.1
      - rake W27.1
      - scissors W27.2
      - screwdriver W27.Ø
      - specified NEC W27.8
      - workbench W27.Ø
    - hot X17
    - powered W29.8
      - blender W29.Ø
        - commercial W31.82
      - can opener W29.Ø
        - commercial W31.82
      - chainsaw W29.3
      - clothes dryer W29.2
        - commercial W31.82
      - dishwasher W29.2
        - commercial W31.82
      - edger W29.3
      - electric fan W29.2
        - commercial W31.82
      - electric knife W29.1
      - food processor W29.Ø
        - commercial W31.82
      - garbage disposal W29.Ø
        - commercial W31.82
      - garden tool W29.3
      - hedge trimmer W29.3
      - ice maker W29.Ø
        - commercial W31.82
      - kitchen appliance W29.Ø
        - commercial W31.82
      - lawn mower W28
      - meat grinder W29.Ø
        - commercial W31.82
      - mixer W29.Ø
        - commercial W31.82
      - rototiller W29.3
      - sewing machine W29.2
        - commercial W31.82
      - washing machine W29.2
        - commercial W31.82
  - transmission device (belt, cable, chain, gear, pinion, shaft) W24.1
    - agricultural operations W3Ø.89
  - turbine (gas) (water-driven) W31.3
  - turkey W61.49
    - peck W61.43
    - strike W61.42
  - turtle (nonvenomous) W59.29
    - bite W59.21
    - strike W59.22
    - terrestrial W59.89
      - bite W59.81
      - crushing W59.83
      - strike W59.82
  - under-cutter W31.Ø
  - urine — *see* Contact, with, by type of animal
  - vehicle
    - agricultural use (transport) — *see* Accident, transport, agricultural vehicle
      - not on public highway W3Ø.81
    - industrial use (transport) — *see* Accident, transport, industrial vehicle
      - not on public highway W31.83
    - off-road use (transport) — *see* Accident, transport, all-terrain or off-road vehicle
      - not on public highway W31.83
    - special construction use (transport) — *see* Accident, transport, construction vehicle
      - not on public highway W31.83
  - venomous
    - animal X58
    - arthropods X58
    - lizard X58
    - marine animal NEC X58
    - marine plant NEC X58
    - millipedes (tropical) X58
    - plant(s) X58
    - snake X58
    - spider X58
  - viper X58
  - washing-machine (powered) W29.2
  - wasp X58
  - weaving-machine W31.89
  - winch W24.Ø
    - agricultural operations W3Ø.89
  - wire NEC W24.Ø
    - agricultural operations W3Ø.89
  - wood slivers W45.8
  - yellow jacket X58
  - zebra — *see* Contact, with, hoof stock NEC

Coup de soleil X32

Crash
- aircraft (in transit) (powered) V95.9
  - balloon V96.Ø1
  - fixed wing NEC (private) V95.21
    - commercial V95.31
  - glider V96.21
    - hang V96.11
    - powered V95.11
  - helicopter V95.Ø1
  - in war operations — *see* War operations, destruction of aircraft
  - microlight V95.11
  - nonpowered V96.9
    - specified NEC V96.8
  - powered NEC V95.8
  - stated as
    - homicide (attempt) YØ8.81
    - suicide (attempt) X83.Ø
  - ultralight V95.11
- spacecraft V95.41
- transport vehicle NEC (*see also* Accident, transport) V89.9
  - homicide (attempt) YØ3.8
  - motor NEC (traffic) V89.2
    - homicide (attempt) YØ3.8
    - suicide (attempt) — *see* Suicide, collision

Cruelty (mental) (physical) (sexual) X58

Crushed (accidentally) X58
- between objects (moving) (stationary and moving) W23.Ø

- **Crushed**— *continued*
  - between objects— *continued*
    - stationary W23.1
  - by
    - alligator W58.Ø3
    - avalanche NEC — *see* Landslide
    - cave-in W2Ø.Ø
      - caused by cataclysmic earth surface movement — *see* Landslide
    - crocodile W58.13
    - crowd or human stampede W52
    - falling
      - aircraft V97.39
        - in war operations — *see* War operations, destruction of aircraft
      - earth, material W2Ø.Ø
        - caused by cataclysmic earth surface movement — *see* Landslide
      - object NEC W2Ø.8
    - landslide NEC — *see* Landslide
    - lizard (nonvenomous) W59.Ø9
    - machinery — *see* Contact, with, by type of machine
    - reptile NEC W59.89
    - snake (nonvenomous) W59.13
  - in
    - machinery — *see* Contact, with, by type of machine
- **Cut, cutting** (any part of body) (accidental) (*see also* Contact, with, by object or machine)
  - during medical or surgical treatment as misadventure — *see* Misadventure, cut, by type of procedure
  - homicide (attempt) — *see* Assault, cutting or piercing instrument
  - inflicted by other person — *see* Assault, cutting or piercing instrument
  - legal
    - execution — *see* Legal, intervention
    - intervention — *see* Legal, intervention, sharp object
  - machine NEC (*see also* Contact, with, by type of machine) W31.9
  - self-inflicted — *see* Suicide, cutting or piercing instrument
  - suicide (attempt) — *see* Suicide, cutting or piercing instrument
- **Cyclone** (any injury) X37.1

D

- **Decapitation** (accidental circumstances) NEC X58
  - homicide X99.9
  - legal execution — *see* Legal, intervention
- **Dehydration from lack of water** X58
- **Deprivation** X58
- **Derailment** (accidental)
  - railway (rolling stock) (train) (vehicle) (without antecedent collision) V81.7
    - with antecedent collision — *see* Accident, transport, railway vehicle occupant
  - streetcar (without antecedent collision) V82.7
    - with antecedent collision — *see* Accident, transport, streetcar occupant
- **Descent**
  - parachute (voluntary) (without accident to aircraft) V97.29
    - due to accident to aircraft — *see* Accident, transport, aircraft
- **Desertion** X58
- **Destitution** X58
- **Disability, late effect or sequela of injury** — *see* Sequelae
- **Discharge** (accidental)
  - airgun W34.Ø1Ø
    - assault X95.Ø1
    - homicide (attempt) X95.Ø1
    - stated as undetermined whether accidental or intentional Y24.Ø
    - suicide (attempt) X74.Ø1
  - BB gun — *see* Discharge, airgun

- **Discharge**— *continued*
  - firearm (accidental) W34.ØØ
    - assault X95.9
    - handgun (pistol) (revolver) W32.Ø
      - assault X93
      - homicide (attempt) X93
      - legal intervention — *see* Legal, intervention, firearm, handgun
      - stated as undetermined whether accidental or intentional Y22
      - suicide (attempt) X72
    - homicide (attempt) X95.9
    - hunting rifle W33.Ø2
      - assault X94.1
      - homicide (attempt) X94.1
      - legal intervention
        - injuring
          - bystander Y35.Ø32
          - law enforcement personnel Y35.Ø31
          - suspect Y35.Ø33
      - stated as undetermined whether accidental or intentional Y23.1
      - suicide (attempt) X73.1
    - larger W33.ØØ
      - assault X94.9
      - homicide (attempt) X94.9
      - hunting rifle — *see* Discharge, firearm, hunting rifle
      - legal intervention — *see* Legal, intervention, firearm by type of firearm
      - machine gun — *see* Discharge, firearm, machine gun
      - shotgun — *see* Discharge, firearm, shotgun
      - specified NEC W33.Ø9
        - assault X94.8
        - homicide (attempt) X94.8
        - legal intervention
          - injuring
            - bystander Y35.Ø92
            - law enforcement personnel Y35.Ø91
            - suspect Y35.Ø93
        - stated as undetermined whether accidental or intentional Y23.8
        - suicide (attempt) X73.8
      - stated as undetermined whether accidental or intentional Y23.9
      - suicide (attempt) X73.9
    - legal intervention
      - injuring
        - bystander Y35.ØØ2
        - law enforcement personnel Y35.ØØ1
        - suspect Y35.ØØ3
      - using rubber bullet
        - injuring
          - bystander Y35.Ø42
          - law enforcement personnel Y35.Ø41
          - suspect Y35.Ø43
    - machine gun W33.Ø3
      - assault X94.2
      - homicide (attempt) X94.2
      - legal intervention — *see* Legal, intervention, firearm, machine gun
      - stated as undetermined whether accidental or intentional Y23.3
      - suicide (attempt) X73.2
    - pellet gun — *see* Discharge, airgun
    - shotgun W33.Ø1
      - assault X94.Ø
      - homicide (attempt) X94.Ø
      - legal intervention — *see* Legal, intervention, firearm, specified NEC
      - stated as undetermined whether accidental or intentional Y23.Ø
      - suicide (attempt) X73.Ø
    - specified NEC W34.Ø9
      - assault X95.8
      - homicide (attempt) X95.8
      - legal intervention — *see* Legal, intervention, firearm, specified NEC
      - stated as undetermined whether accidental or intentional Y24.8
      - suicide (attempt) X74.8

- **Discharge**— *continued*
  - firearm— *continued*
    - stated as undetermined whether accidental or intentional Y24.9
    - suicide (attempt) X74.9
    - Very pistol W34.Ø9
      - assault X95.8
      - homicide (attempt) X95.8
      - stated as undetermined whether accidental or intentional Y24.8
      - suicide (attempt) X74.8
  - firework(s) W39
    - stated as undetermined whether accidental or intentional Y25
  - gas-operated gun NEC W34.Ø18
    - airgun — *see* Discharge, airgun
    - assault X95.Ø9
    - homicide (attempt) X95.Ø9
    - paintball gun — *see* Discharge, paintball gun
    - stated as undetermined whether accidental or intentional Y24.8
    - suicide (attempt) X74.Ø9
  - gun NEC (*see also* Discharge, firearm NEC)
    - air — *see* Discharge, airgun
    - B— *see* Discharge, airgun
    - for single hand use — *see* Discharge, firearm, handgun
    - hand — *see* Discharge, firearm, handgun
    - machine — *see* Discharge, firearm, machine gun
    - other specified — *see* Discharge, firearm NEC
    - paintball — *see* Discharge, paintball gun
    - pellet — *see* Discharge, airgun
  - handgun — *see* Discharge, firearm, handgun
  - machine gun — *see* Discharge, firearm, machine gun
  - paintball gun W34.Ø11
    - assault X95.Ø2
    - homicide (attempt) X95.Ø2
    - stated as undetermined whether accidental or intentional Y24.8
    - suicide (attempt) X74.Ø2
  - pistol — *see* Discharge, firearm, handgun
    - flare — *see* Discharge, firearm, Very pistol
    - pellet — *see* Discharge, airgun
    - Very — *see* Discharge, firearm, Very pistol
  - revolver — *see* Discharge, firearm, handgun
  - rifle (hunting) — *see* Discharge, firearm, hunting rifle
  - shotgun — *see* Discharge, firearm, shotgun
  - spring-operated gun NEC W34.Ø18
    - assault X95.Ø9
    - homicide (attempt) X95.Ø9
    - stated as undetermined whether accidental or intentional Y24.8
    - suicide (attempt) X74.Ø9
- **Disease**
  - Andes W94.11
  - aviator's — *see* Air, pressure
  - range W94.11
- **Diver's disease, palsy, paralysis, squeeze** — *see* Air, pressure
- **Diving** (into water) — *see* Accident, diving
- **Dog bite** W54.Ø
- **Dragged by transport vehicle NEC** (*see also* Accident, transport) VØ9.9
- **Drinking poison** (accidental) — *see* Table of Drugs and Chemicals
- **Dropped** (accidentally) **while being carried or supported by other person** WØ4
- **Drowning** (accidental) W74
  - assault X92.9
  - due to
    - accident (to)
      - machinery — *see* Contact, with, by type of machine
      - watercraft V9Ø.89
        - burning V9Ø.29
          - powered V9Ø.23
            - merchant ship V9Ø.2Ø
            - passenger ship V9Ø.21
            - fishing boat V9Ø.22
            - jetskis V9Ø.23
          - unpowered V9Ø.28

- **Drowning** — *continued*
  - in— *continued*
    - war operations — *see* War operations, restriction of airway
  - resulting from accident to watercraft — *see* Drowning, due to, accident, watercraft
  - self-inflicted X71.9
  - stated as undetermined whether accidental or intentional Y21.9
  - suicide (attempt) X71.9

E

- **Earth** (surface) **movement NEC** — *see* Forces of nature, earth movement
- **Earth falling** (on) W2Ø.Ø
  - caused by cataclysmic earth surface movement or eruption — *see* Landslide
- **Earthquake** (any injury) X34
- **Effect**(s) (adverse) **of**
  - air pressure (any) — *see* Air, pressure
  - cold, excessive (exposure to) — *see* Exposure, cold
  - heat (excessive) — *see* Heat
  - hot place (weather) — *see* Heat
  - insolation X3Ø
  - late — *see* Sequelae
  - motion — *see* Motion
  - nuclear explosion or weapon in war operations — *see* War operations, nuclear weapon
  - radiation — *see* Radiation
  - travel — *see* Travel
- **Electric shock** (accidental) (by) (in) — *see* Exposure, electric current
- **Electrocution** (accidental) — *see* Exposure, electric current
- **Endotracheal tube wrongly placed during anesthetic procedure**
- **Entanglement**
  - in
    - bed linen, causing suffocation — *see* category T71
    - wheel of pedal cycle V19.88
- **Entry of foreign body or material** - *see* Foreign body
- **Environmental pollution related condition**- *see* Z57
- **Execution, legal** (any method)— *see* Legal, intervention
- **Exhaustion**
  - cold — *see* Exposure, cold
  - due to excessive exertion — *see* Overexertion
  - heat — *see* Heat
- **Explosion** (accidental) (of) (with secondary fire) W4Ø.9
  - acetylene W4Ø.1
  - aerosol can W36.1
  - air tank (compressed) (in machinery) W36.2
  - aircraft (in transit) (powered) NEC V95.9
    - balloon V96.Ø5
    - fixed wing NEC (private) V95.25
      - commercial V95.35
    - glider V96.25
      - hang V96.15
      - powered V95.15
    - helicopter V95.Ø5
    - in war operations — *see* War operations, destruction of aircraft
    - microlight V95.15
    - nonpowered V96.9
      - specified NEC V96.8
    - powered NEC V95.8
    - stated as
      - homicide (attempt) YØ3.8
      - suicide (attempt) X83.Ø
    - ultralight V95.15
  - anesthetic gas in operating room W4Ø.1
  - antipersonnel bomb W4Ø.8
    - assault X96.Ø
    - homicide (attempt) X96.Ø
    - suicide (attempt) X75
  - assault X96.9
  - bicycle tire W37.Ø
  - blasting (cap) (materials) W4Ø.Ø
  - boiler (machinery), not on transport vehicle W35
    - on watercraft — *see* Explosion, in, watercraft

- **Explosion** — *continued*
  - butane W4Ø.1
  - caused by other person X96.9
  - coal gas W4Ø.1
  - detonator W4Ø.Ø
  - dump (munitions) W4Ø.8
  - dynamite W4Ø.Ø
    - in
      - assault X96.8
      - homicide (attempt) X96.8
      - legal intervention
        - injuring
          - bystander Y35.112
          - law enforcement personnel Y35.111
          - suspect Y35.113
      - suicide (attempt) X75
  - explosive (material) W4Ø.9
    - gas W4Ø.1
    - in blasting operation W4Ø.Ø
    - specified NEC W4Ø.8
      - in
        - assault X96.8
        - homicide (attempt) X96.8
        - legal intervention
          - injuring
            - bystander Y35.192
            - law enforcement personnel Y35.191
            - suspect Y35.193
        - suicide (attempt) X75
  - factory (munitions) W4Ø.8
  - fertilizer bomb W4Ø.8
    - assault X96.3
    - homicide (attempt) X96.3
    - suicide (attempt) X75
  - firearm (parts) NEC W34.19
    - airgun W34.11Ø
    - BB gun W34.11Ø
    - gas, air or spring-operated gun NEC W34.118
    - hangun W32.1
    - hunting rifle W33.12
    - larger firearm W33.1Ø
      - specified NEC W33.19
    - machine gun W33.13
    - paintball gun W34.111
    - pellet gun W34.11Ø
    - shotgun W33.11
    - Very pistol [flare] W34.19
  - fire-damp W4Ø.1
  - fireworks W39
  - gas (coal) (explosive) W4Ø.1
    - cylinder W36.9
      - aerosol can W36.1
      - air tank W36.2
      - pressurized W36.3
      - specified NEC W36.8
  - gasoline (fumes) (tank) not in moving motor vehicle W4Ø.1
    - bomb W4Ø.8
      - assault X96.1
      - homicide (attempt) X96.1
      - suicide (attempt) X75
    - in motor vehicle — *see* Accident, transport, by type of vehicle
  - grain store W4Ø.8
  - grenade W4Ø.8
    - in
      - assault X96.8
      - homicide (attempt) X96.8
      - legal intervention
        - injuring
          - bystander Y35.192
          - law enforcement personnel Y35.191
          - suspect Y35.193
      - suicide (attempt) X75
  - handgun (parts) — *see* Explosion, firearm, hangun (parts)
  - homicide (attempt) X96.9
    - antipersonnel bomb — *see* Explosion, antipersonnel bomb
    - fertilizer bomb — *see* Explosion, fertilizer bomb
    - gasoline bomb — *see* Explosion, gasoline bomb
    - letter bomb — *see* Explosion, letter bomb

- **Explosion** — *continued*
  - homicide— *continued*
    - pipe bomb — *see* Explosion, pipe bomb
    - specified NEC X96.8
  - hose, pressurized W37.8
  - hot water heater, tank (in machinery) W35
    - on watercraft — *see* Explosion, in, watercraft
  - in, on
    - dump W4Ø.8
    - factory W4Ø.8
    - mine (of explosive gases) NEC W4Ø.1
    - watercraft V93.59
      - powered craft V93.53
        - ferry boat V93.51
        - fishing boat V93.52
        - jetskis V93.53
        - liner V93.51
        - merchant ship V93.5Ø
        - passenger ship V93.51
        - sailboat V93.54
  - letter bomb W4Ø.8
    - assault X96.2
    - homicide (attempt) X96.2
    - suicide (attempt) X75
  - machinery (*see also* Contact, with, by type of machine)
    - on board watercraft — *see* Explosion, in, watercraft
    - pressure vessel — *see* Explosion, by type of vessel
  - methane W4Ø.1
  - mine W4Ø.1
  - missile NEC W4Ø.8
  - mortar bomb W4Ø.8
    - in
      - assault X96.8
      - homicide (attempt) X96.8
      - legal intervention
        - injuring
          - bystander Y35.192
          - law enforcement personnel Y35.191
          - suspect Y35.193
      - suicide (attempt) X75
  - munitions (dump) (factory) W4Ø.8
  - pipe, pressurized W37.8
    - bomb W4Ø.8
      - assault X96.4
      - homicide (attempt) X96.4
      - suicide (attempt) X75
  - pressure, pressurized
    - cooker W38
    - gas tank (in machinery) W36.3
    - hose W37.8
    - pipe W37.8
    - specified device NEC W38
    - tire W37.8
      - bicycle W37.Ø
    - vessel (in machinery) W38
  - propane W4Ø.1
  - self-inflicted X75
  - shell (artillery) NEC W4Ø.8
    - during war operations — *see* War operations, explosion
    - in
      - legal intervention
        - injuring
          - bystander Y35.122
          - law enforcement personnel Y35.121
          - suspect Y35.123
      - war — *see* War operations, explosion
  - spacecraft V95.45
  - steam or water lines (in machinery) W37.8
  - stove W4Ø.9
  - stated as undetermined whether accidental or intentional Y25
  - suicide (attempt) X75
  - tire, pressurized W37.8
    - bicycle W37.Ø
  - undetermined whether accidental or intentional Y25
  - vehicle tire NEC W37.8
    - bicycle W37.Ø
  - war operations — *see* War operations, explosion

- **Exposure** (to) X58
  - air pressure change — *see* Air, pressure
  - cold (accidental) (excessive) (extreme) (natural) (place) X31
    - assault YØ8.89
    - due to
      - man-made conditions W93.8
        - dry ice (contact) W93.Ø1
          - inhalation W93.Ø2
        - liquid air (contact) (hydrogen) (nitrogen) W93.11
          - inhalation W93.12
        - refrigeration unit (deep freeze) W93.2
        - suicide (attempt) X83.2
      - weather (conditions) X31
    - homicide (attempt) YØ8.89
    - self-inflicted X83.2
  - due to abandonment or neglect X58
  - electric current W86.8
    - appliance (faulty) W86.8
      - domestic W86.Ø
    - caused by other person YØ8.89
    - conductor (faulty) W86.1
    - control apparatus (faulty) W86.1
    - electric power generating plant, distribution station W86.1
    - electroshock gun — *see* Exposure, electric current, taser
    - high-voltage cable W85
    - homicide (attempt) YØ8.89
    - legal execution — *see* Legal, intervention, specified means NEC
    - lightning — *see* subcategory T75.Ø
    - live rail W86.8
    - misadventure in medical or surgical procedure in electroshock therapy Y63.4
    - motor (electric) (faulty) W86.8
      - domestic W86.Ø
    - self-inflicted X83.1
    - specified NEC W86.8
      - domestic W86.Ø
    - stun gun — *see* Exposure, electric current, taser
    - suicide (attempt) X83.1
    - taser W86.8
      - assault YØ8.89
      - legal intervention — *see* category Y35
      - self-harm (intentional) X83.8
      - undeternined intent Y33
    - third rail W86.8
    - transformer (faulty) W86.1
    - transmission lines W85
  - environmental tobacco smoke X58
  - excessive
    - cold — *see* Exposure, cold
    - heat (natural) NEC X3Ø
      - man-made W92
  - factor(s) NOS X58
    - environmental NEC X58
      - man-made NEC W99
      - natural NEC — *see* Forces of nature
    - specified NEC X58
  - fire, flames (accidental) XØ8.8
    - assault X97
    - campfire — *see* Exposure, fire, controlled, not in building
    - controlled (in)
      - with ignition (of) clothing (*see also* Ignition, clothes) XØ6.2
        - nightwear XØ5
      - bonfire — *see* Exposure, fire, controlled, not in building
      - brazier (in building or structure) (*see also* Exposure, fire, controlled, building)
        - not in building or structure — *see* Exposure, fire, controlled, not in building
      - building or structure XØ2.Ø
        - with
          - fall from building XØ2.3
          - injury due to building collapse XØ2.2
          - from building XØ2.5
          - smoke inhalation XØ2.1
        - hit by object from building XØ2.4

- **Exposure**— *continued*
  - fire, flames— *continued*
    - controlled— *continued*
      - building or structure— *continued*
        - specified mode of injury NEC XØ2.8
      - fireplace, furnace or stove — *see* Exposure, fire, controlled, building
      - not in building or structure XØ3.Ø
        - with
          - fall XØ3.3
          - smoke inhalation XØ3.1
        - hit by object XØ3.4
        - specified mode of injury NEC XØ3.8
      - trash — *see* Exposure, fire, controlled, not in building
    - fireplace — *see* Exposure, fire, controlled, building
    - fittings or furniture (in building or structure) (uncontrolled) — *see* Exposure, fire, uncontrolled, building
    - forest (uncontrolled) — *see* Exposure, fire, uncontrolled, not in building
    - grass (uncontrolled) — *see* Exposure, fire, uncontrolled, not in building
    - hay (uncontrolled) — *see* Exposure, fire, uncontrolled, not in building
    - homicide (attempt) X97
    - ignition of highly flammable material XØ4
    - in, of, on, starting in
      - machinery — *see* Contact, with, by type of machine
      - motor vehicle (in motion) (*see also* Accident, transport, occupant by type of vehicle) V87.8
        - with collision — *see* Collision
      - railway rolling stock, train, vehicle V81.81
        - with collision — *see* Accident, transport, railway vehicle occupant
      - street car (in motion) V82.8
        - with collision — *see* Accident, transport, streetcar occupant
      - transport vehicle NEC (*see also* Accident, transport)
        - with collision — *see* Collision
      - war operations (*see also* War operations, fire)
        - from nuclear explosion — *see* War operations, nuclear weapons
      - watercraft (in transit) (not in transit) V91.Ø9
        - localized — *see* Burn, on board watercraft, due to, fire on board
        - powered craft V91.Ø3
          - ferry boat V91.Ø1
          - fishing boat V91.Ø2
          - jet skis V91.Ø3
          - liner V91.Ø1
          - merchant ship V91.ØØ
          - passenger ship V91.Ø1
        - unpowered craft V91.Ø8
          - canoe V91.Ø5
          - inflatable V91.Ø6
          - kayak V91.Ø5
          - sailboat V91.Ø4
          - surf-board V91.Ø8
          - waterskis V91.Ø7
          - windsurfer V91.Ø8
    - lumber (uncontrolled) — *see* Exposure, fire, uncontrolled, not in building
    - mine (uncontrolled) — *see* Exposure, fire, uncontrolled, not in building
    - prairie (uncontrolled) — *see* Exposure, fire, uncontrolled, not in building
    - resulting from
      - explosion — *see* Explosion
      - lightning XØ8.8
    - self-inflicted X76
    - specified NEC XØ8.8
    - started by other person X97
    - stove — *see* Exposure, fire, controlled, building
    - stated as undetermined whether accidental or intentional Y26
    - suicide (attempt) X76
    - tunnel (uncontrolled) — *see* Exposure, fire, uncontrolled, not in building

- **Exposure**— *continued*
  - fire, flames— *continued*
    - uncontrolled
      - in building or structure XØØ.Ø
        - with
          - fall from building XØØ.3
          - injury due to building collapse XØØ.2
          - jump from building XØØ.5
          - smoke inhalation XØØ.1
        - bed XØ8.ØØ
          - due to
            - cigarette XØ8.Ø1
            - specified material NEC XØ8.Ø9
        - furniture NEC XØ8.2Ø
          - due to
            - cigarette XØ8.21
            - specified material NEC XØ8.29
        - hit by object from building XØØ.4
        - sofa XØ8.1Ø
          - due to
            - cigarette XØ8.11
            - specified material NEC XØ8.19
        - specified mode of injury NEC XØØ.8
      - not in building or structure (any) XØ1.Ø
        - with
          - fall XØ1.3
          - smoke inhalation XØ1.1
        - hit by object XØ1.4
        - specified mode of injury NEC XØ1.8
    - undetermined whether accidental or intentional Y26
  - forces of nature NEC — *see* Forces of nature
  - G-forces (abnormal) W49.9
  - gravitational forces (abnormal) W49.9
  - heat (natural) NEC — *see* Heat
  - high-pressure jet (hydraulic) (pneumatic) W49.9
  - hydraulic jet W49.9
  - inanimate mechanical force W49.9
  - jet, high-pressure (hydraulic) (pneumatic) W49.9
  - lightning — *see* subcategory T75.Ø
    - causing fire — *see* Exposure, fire
  - mechanical forces NEC W49.9
    - animate NEC W64
    - inanimate NEC W49.9
  - noise W42.9
    - supersonic W42.Ø
  - noxious substance — *see* Table of Drugs and Chemicals
  - pneumatic jet W49.9
  - prolonged in deep-freeze unit or refrigerator W93.2
  - radiation — *see* Radiation
  - smoke (*see also* Exposure, fire)
    - tobacco, second hand Z77.22
  - specified factors NEC X58
  - sunlight X32
    - man-made (sun lamp) W89.8
      - tanning bed W89.1
  - supersonic waves W42.Ø
  - transmission line(s), electric W85
  - vibration W49.9
  - waves
    - infrasound W49.9
    - sound W42.9
    - supersonic W42.Ø
  - weather NEC — *see* Forces of nature
- **External cause status** Y99.9
  - child assisting in compensated work for family Y99.8
  - civilian activity done for financial or other compensation Y99.Ø
  - civilian activity done for income or pay Y99.Ø
  - family member assisting in compensated work for other family member Y99.8
  - hobby not done for income Y99.8
  - leisure activity Y99.8
  - military activity Y99.1
  - off-duty activity of military personnel Y99.8
  - recreation or sport not for income or while a student Y99.8
  - specified NEC Y99.8
  - student activity Y99.8
  - volunteer activity Y99.2

F

- **Factors, supplemental**
  - alcohol
    - blood level
      - less than 20mg/100ml Y90.0
      - presence in blood, level not specified Y90.9
      - 20-39mg/100ml Y90.1
      - 40-59mg/100ml Y90.2
      - 60-79mg/100ml Y90.3
      - 80-99mg/100ml Y90.4
      - 100-119mg/100ml Y90.5
      - 120-199mg/100ml Y90.6
      - 200-239mg/100ml Y90.7
      - 240 mg/100ml or more Y90.8
    - presence in blood, but level not specified Y90.9
  - environmental-pollution-related condition — *see* Z57
  - nosocomial condition Y95
  - work-related condition Y99.0
- **Failure**
  - in suture or ligature during surgical procedure Y65.2
  - mechanical, of instrument or apparatus (any) (during any medical or surgical procedure) Y65.8
  - sterile precautions (during medical and surgical care) — *see* Misadventure, failure, sterile precautions, by type of procedure
  - to
    - introduce tube or instrument Y65.4
      - endotracheal tube during anesthesia Y65.3
    - make curve (transport vehicle) NEC — *see* Accident, transport
    - remove tube or instrument Y65.4
- **Fall, falling** (accidental) W19
  - building W20.1
    - burning (uncontrolled fire) X00.3
  - down
    - embankment W17.81
    - escalator W10.0
    - hill W17.81
    - ladder W11
    - ramp W10.2
    - stairs, steps W10.9
  - due to
    - bumping against
      - object W18.00
        - sharp glass W18.02
        - specified NEC W18.09
        - sports equipment W18.01
      - person W03
        - due to ice or snow W00.0
        - on pedestrian conveyance — *see* Accident, transport, pedestrian, conveyance
    - collision with another person W03
      - due to ice or snow W00.0
      - involving pedestrian conveyance — *see* Accident, transport, pedestrian, conveyance
    - grocery cart tipping over W17.82
    - ice or snow W00.9
      - from one level to another W00.2
        - on stairs or steps W00.1
      - involving pedestrian conveyance — *see* Accident, transport, pedestrian, conveyance
      - on same level W00.0
    - slipping (on moving sidewalk) W01.0
      - with subsequent striking against object W01.10
        - furniture W01.190
        - sharp object W01.119
          - glass W01.110
          - power tool or machine W01.111
          - specified NEC W01.118
        - specified NEC W01.198
    - striking against
      - object W18.00
        - sharp glass W18.02
        - specified NEC W18.09
        - sports equipment W18.01
      - person W03

- **Fall, falling**— *continued*
  - due to— *continued*
    - striking against— *continued*
      - person— *continued*
        - due to ice or snow W00.0
        - on pedestrian conveyance — *see* Accident, transport, pedestrian, conveyance
  - earth (with asphyxia or suffocation (by pressure)) — *see* Earth, falling
  - from, off, out of
    - aircraft NEC (with accident to aircraft NEC) V97.0
      - while boarding or alighting V97.1
    - balcony W13.0
    - bed W06
    - boat, ship, watercraft NEC (with drowning or submersion) — *see* Drowning, due to, fall overboard
      - with hitting bottom or object V94.0
    - bridge W13.1
    - building W13.9
      - burning (uncontrolled fire) X00.3
    - cavity W17.2
    - cherry picker W17.89
    - chair W07
    - cliff W15
    - dock W17.4
    - embankment W17.81
    - escalator W10.0
    - flagpole W13.8
    - furniture NEC W08
    - grocery cart W17.82
    - haystack W17.89
    - high place NEC W17.89
      - stated as undetermined whether accidental or intentional Y30
    - hole W17.2
    - incline W10.2
    - ladder W11
    - lifting device W17.89
    - machine, machinery (*see also* Contact, with, by type of machine)
      - not in operation W17.89
    - manhole W17.1
    - mobile elevated work platform [MEWP] W17.89
    - motorized mobility scooter W05.2
    - one level to another NEC W17.89
      - intentional, purposeful, suicide (attempt) X80
      - stated as undetermined whether accidental or intentional Y30
    - pit W17.2
    - playground equipment W09.8
      - jungle gym W09.2
      - slide W09.0
      - swing W09.1
    - quarry W17.89
    - railing W13.9
    - ramp W10.2
    - roof W13.2
    - scaffolding W12
    - scooter (nonmotorized) W05.1
      - motorized mobility W05.2
    - sky lift W17.89
    - stairs, steps W10.9
      - curb W10.1
      - due to ice or snow W00.1
      - escalator W10.0
      - incline W10.2
      - ramp W10.2
      - sidewalk curb W10.1
      - specified NEC W10.8
    - stepladder W11
    - storm drain W17.1
    - streetcar NEC V82.6
      - with antecedent collision — *see* Accident, transport, streetcar occupant
      - while boarding or alighting V82.4
    - structure NEC W13.8
      - burning (uncontrolled fire) X00.3
    - table W08
    - toilet W18.11
      - with subsequent striking against object W18.12

- **Fall, falling**— *continued*
  - from, off, out of — *continued*
    - train NEC V81.6
      - during derailment (without antecedent collision) V81.7
        - with antecedent collision — *see* Accident, transport, railway vehicle occupant
      - while boarding or alighting V81.4
    - transport vehicle after collision — *see* Accident, transport, by type of vehicle, collision
    - tree W14
    - vehicle (in motion) NEC (*see also* Accident, transport) V89.9
      - motor NEC (*see also* Accident, transport, occupant, by type of vehicle) V87.8
      - stationary W17.89
        - while boarding or alighting — *see* Accident, transport, by type of vehicle, while boarding or alighting
    - viaduct W13.8
    - wall W13.8
    - watercraft (*see also* Drowning, due to, fall overboard)
      - with hitting bottom or object V94.0
    - well W17.0
    - wheelchair, non-moving W05.0
      - powered — *see* Accident, transport, pedestrian, conveyance occupant, specified type NEC
    - window W13.4
  - in, on
    - aircraft NEC V97.0
      - with accident to aircraft V97.0
      - while boarding or alighting V97.1
    - bathtub (empty) W18.2
      - filled W16.212
        - causing drowning W16.211
    - escalator W10.0
    - incline W10.2
    - ladder W11
    - machine, machinery — *see* Contact, with, by type of machine
    - object, edged, pointed or sharp (with cut) — *see* Fall, by type
    - playground equipment W09.8
      - jungle gym W09.2
      - slide W09.0
      - swing W09.1
    - ramp W10.2
    - scaffolding W12
    - shower W18.2
      - causing drowning W16.211
    - staircase, stairs, steps W10.9
      - curb W10.1
      - due to ice or snow W00.1
      - escalator W10.0
      - incline W10.2
      - specified NEC W10.8
    - streetcar (without antecedent collision) V82.5
      - with antecedent collision — *see* Accident, transport, streetcar occupant
      - while boarding or alighting V82.4
    - train (without antecedent collision) V81.5
      - with antecedent collision — *see* Accident, transport, railway vehicle occupant
      - during derailment (without antecedent collision) V81.7
        - with antecedent collision — *see* Accident, transport, railway vehicle occupant
      - while boarding or alighting V81.4
    - transport vehicle after collision — *see* Accident, transport, by type of vehicle, collision
    - watercraft V93.39
      - due to
        - accident to craft V91.29
          - powered craft V91.23
            - ferry boat V91.21
            - fishing boat V91.22
            - jetskis V91.23
            - liner V91.21
            - merchant ship V91.20
            - passenger ship V91.21
          - unpowered craft

- **Fall, falling**— *continued*
  - in on— *continued*
    - watercraft— *continued*
      - due to— *continued*
        - accident to craft— *continued*
          - unpowered craft— *continued*
            - canoe V91.25
            - inflatable V91.26
            - kayak V91.25
            - sailboat V91.24
      - powered craft V93.33
        - ferry boat V93.31
        - fishing boat V93.32
        - jetskis V93.33
        - liner V93.31
        - merchant ship V93.3Ø
        - passenger ship V93.31
      - unpowered craft V93.38
        - canoe V93.35
        - inflatable V93.36
        - kayak V93.35
        - sailboat V93.34
        - surf-board V93.38
        - windsurfer V93.38
  - into
    - cavity W17.2
    - dock W17.4
    - fire — *see* Exposure, fire, by type
    - haystack W17.89
    - hole W17.2
    - lake — *see* Fall, into, water
    - manhole W17.1
    - moving part of machinery — *see* Contact, with, by type of machine
    - ocean — *see* Fall, into, water
    - opening in surface NEC W17.89
    - pit W17.2
    - pond — *see* Fall, into, water
    - quarry W17.89
    - river — *see* Fall, into, water
    - shaft W17.89
    - storm drain W17.1
    - stream — *see* Fall, into, water
    - swimming pool (*see also* Fall, into, water, in, swimming pool
      - empty W17.3
    - tank W17.89
    - water W16.42
      - causing drowning W16.41
      - from watercraft — *see* Drowning, due to, fall overboard
      - hitting diving board W21.4
      - in
        - bathtub W16.212
          - causing drowning W16.211
        - bucket W16.222
          - causing drowning W16.221
        - natural body of water W16.112
          - causing drowning W16.111
          - striking
            - bottom W16.122
              - causing drowning W16.121
            - side W16.132
              - causing drowning W16.131
        - specified water NEC W16.312
          - causing drowning W16.311
          - striking
            - bottom W16.322
              - causing drowning W16.321
            - wall W16.332
              - causing drowning W16.331
        - swimming pool W16.Ø12
          - causing drowning W16.Ø11
          - striking
            - bottom W16.Ø22
              - causing drowning W16.Ø21
            - wall W16.Ø32
              - causing drowning W16.Ø31
        - utility bucket W16.222
          - causing drowning W16.221
    - well W17.Ø
  - involving
    - bed WØ6

- **Fall, falling**— *continued*
  - involving— *continued*
    - chair WØ7
    - furniture NEC WØ8
    - glass — *see* Fall, by type
    - playground equipment WØ9.8
      - jungle gym WØ9.2
      - slide WØ9.Ø
      - swing WØ9.1
    - roller blades — *see* Accident, transport, pedestrian, conveyance
    - skateboard(s) — *see* Accident, transport, pedestrian, conveyance
    - skates (ice) (in line) (roller) — *see* Accident, transport, pedestrian, conveyance
    - skis — *see* Accident, transport, pedestrian, conveyance
    - table WØ8
    - wheelchair, non-moving WØ5.Ø
      - powered — *see* Accident, transport, pedestrian, conveyance, specified type NEC
  - object — *see* Struck by, object, falling
  - off
    - toilet W18.11
      - with subsequent striking against object W18.12
  - on same level W18.3Ø
    - due to
      - specified NEC W18.39
      - stepping on an object W18.31
  - out of
    - bed WØ6
    - building NEC W13.8
    - chair WØ7
    - furniture NEC WØ8
    - wheelchair, non-moving WØ5.Ø
      - powered — *see* Accident, transport, pedestrian, conveyance, specified type NEC
    - window W13.4
  - over
    - animal WØ1.Ø
    - cliff W15
    - embankment W17.81
    - small object WØ1.Ø
  - rock W2Ø.8
  - same level W18.3Ø
    - from
      - being crushed, pushed, or stepped on by a crowd or human stampede W52
      - collision, pushing, shoving, by or with other person WØ3
      - slipping, stumbling, tripping WØ1.Ø
    - involving ice or snow WØØ.Ø
      - involving skates (ice) (roller), skateboard, skis — *see* Accident, transport, pedestrian, conveyance
  - snowslide (avalanche) — *see* Landslide
  - stone W2Ø.8
  - structure W2Ø.1
    - burning (uncontrolled fire) XØØ.3
  - through
    - bridge W13.1
    - floor W13.3
    - roof W13.2
    - wall W13.8
    - window W13.4
  - timber W2Ø.8
  - tree (caused by lightning) W2Ø.8
  - while being carried or supported by other person(s) WØ4
- **Fallen on by**
  - animal (not being ridden) NEC W55.89
- **Felo-de-se** — *see* Suicide
- **Fight** (hand) (fists) (foot) — *see* Assault, fight
- **Fire** (accidental) — *see* Exposure, fire
- **Firearm discharge** — *see* Discharge, firearm
- **Fireball effects from nuclear explosion in war operations** — *see* War operations, nuclear weapons
- **Fireworks** (explosion) W39
- **Flash burns from explosion** — *see* Explosion

- **Flood** (any injury) (caused by) X38
  - collapse of man-made structure causing earth movement X36.Ø
  - tidal wave — *see* Forces of nature, tidal wave
- **Food** (any type) **in**
  - air passages (with asphyxia, obstruction, or suffocation) — *see* categories T17 and T18
  - alimentary tract causing asphyxia (due to compression of trachea) — *see* categories T17 and T18
- **Forces of nature** X39.8
  - avalanche X36.1
    - causing transport accident — *see* Accident, transport, by type of vehicle
  - blizzard X37.2
  - cataclysmic storm X37.9
    - with flood X38
    - blizzard X37.2
    - cloudburst X37.8
    - cyclone X37.1
    - dust storm X37.3
    - hurricane X37.Ø
    - specified storm NEC X37.8
    - storm surge X37.Ø
    - tornado X37.1
    - twister X37.1
    - typhoon X37.Ø
  - cloudburst X37.8
  - cold (natural) X31
  - cyclone X37.1
  - dam collapse causing earth movement X36.Ø
  - dust storm X37.3
  - earth movement X36.1
    - earthquake X34
    - caused by dam or structure collapse X36.Ø
  - earthquake X34
  - flood (caused by) X38
    - dam collapse X36.Ø
    - tidal wave — *see* Forces of nature, tidal wave
  - heat (natural) X3Ø
  - hurricane X37.Ø
  - landslide X36.1
    - causing transport accident — *see* Accident, transport, by type of vehicle
  - lightning — *see* subcategory T75.Ø
    - causing fire — *see* Exposure, fire
  - mudslide X36.1
    - causing transport accident — *see* Accident, transport, by type of vehicle
  - radiation (natural) X39.Ø8
    - radon X39.Ø1
  - radon X39.Ø1
  - specified force NEC X39.8
  - storm surge X37.Ø
  - structure collapse causing earth movement X36.Ø
  - sunlight X32
  - tidal wave X37.41
    - due to
      - earthquake X37.41
      - landslide X37.43
      - storm X37.42
      - volcanic eruption X37.41
  - tornado X37.1
  - tsunami X37.41
  - twister X37.1
  - typhoon X37.Ø
  - volcanic eruption X35
- **Foreign body entering through skin** W45.8
  - can lid W45.2
  - nail W45.Ø
  - paper W45.1
  - specified NEC W45.8
  - splinter W45.8
- **Forest fire** (exposure to) — *see* Exposure, fire, uncontrolled, not in building
- **Found injured** X58
  - from exposure (to) — *see* Exposure
  - on
    - highway, road(way), street V89.9
    - railway right of way V81.9
- **Fracture** (circumstances unknown or unspecified) X58
  - due to specified cause NEC X58
- **Freezing** — *see* Exposure, cold

- **Frostbite** X31
  - due to man-made conditions — *see* Exposure, cold, man-made
- **Frozen** — *see* Exposure, cold

G

- **Gored by bull** W55.22
- **Gunshot wound** W34.00

H

- **Hailstones, injured by** X39.8
- **Hanged herself or himself** — *see* Hanging, self-inflicted
- **Hanging** (accidental) (*see also* category T71)
  - legal execution — *see* Legal, intervention, specified means NEC
- **Heat** (effects of) (excessive) X3Ø
  - due to
    - man-made conditions W92
      - on board watercraft V93.29
        - fishing boat V93.22
        - merchant ship V93.2Ø
        - passenger ship V93.21
        - sailboat V93.24
        - specified powered craft NEC V93.23
    - weather (conditions) X3Ø
  - from
    - electric heating apparatus causing burning X16
    - nuclear explosion in war operations — *see* War operations, nuclear weapons
  - inappropriate in local application or packing in medical or surgical procedure Y63.5
- **Hemorrhage**
  - delayed following medical or surgical treatment without mention of misadventure — *see* Complication of or following, by type of procedure
  - during medical or surgical treatment as misadventure — *see* Misadventure, cut, by type of procedure
- **High**
  - altitude (effects) — *see* Air, pressure, low
  - level of radioactivity, effects — *see* Radiation
  - pressure (effects) — *see* Air, pressure, high
  - temperature, effects *see* Heat
- **Hit, hitting** (accidental) **by** — *see* Struck by
- **Hitting against** - *see* Striking against
- **Homicide** (attempt) (justifiable) — *see* Assault
- **Hot**
  - place, effects (*see also* Heat)
  - weather, effects X3Ø
- **House fire** (uncontrolled) — *see* Exposure, fire, uncontrolled, building
- **Humidity, causing problem** X39.8
- **Hunger** X58
- **Hurricane** (any injury) X37.Ø
- **Hypobarism, hypobaropathy** — *see* Air, pressure, low

I

- **Ictus**
  - caloris (*see also* Heat)
  - solaris X3Ø
- **Ignition** (accidental) (*see also* Exposure, fire) XØ8.8
  - anesthetic gas in operating room W4Ø.1
  - apparel XØ6.2
    - from highly flammable material XØ4
    - nightwear XØ5
  - bed linen (sheets) (spreads) (pillows) (mattress) — *see* Exposure, fire, uncontrolled, building, bed
  - benzine XØ4
  - clothes, clothing NEC (from controlled fire) XØ6.2
    - from
      - highly flammable material XØ4
  - ether XØ4
    - in operating room W4Ø.1
  - explosive material — *see* Explosion
- **Ignition** — *continued*
  - gasoline XØ4
  - jewelry (plastic) (any) XØ6.Ø
  - kerosene XØ4
  - material
    - explosive — *see* Explosion
    - highly flammable with secondary explosion XØ4
  - nightwear XØ5
  - paraffin XØ4
  - petrol XØ4
- **Immersion** (accidental) (*see also* Drowning)
  - hand or foot due to cold (excessive) X31
- **Implantation of quills of porcupine** W55.89
- **Inanition** (from) (hunger) X58
  - thirst X58
- **Inappropriate operation performed**
  - correct operation on wrong side of body part (wrong side) (wrong site) Y65.53
  - operation intended for another patient done on wrong patient Y65.52
  - wrong operation performed on correct patient Y65.51
- **Inattention after, at birth** (homicidal intent) (infanticidal intent) X58
- **Incident, adverse**
  - device
    - anesthesiology Y7Ø.8
      - accessory Y7Ø.2
      - diagnostic Y7Ø.Ø
      - miscellaneous Y7Ø.8
      - monitoring Y7Ø.Ø
      - prosthetic Y7Ø.2
      - rehabilitative Y7Ø.1
      - surgical Y7Ø.3
      - therapeutic Y7Ø.1
    - cardiovascular Y71.8
      - accessory Y71.2
      - diagnostic Y71.Ø
      - miscellaneous Y71.8
      - monitoring Y71.Ø
      - prosthetic Y71.2
      - rehabilitative Y71.1
      - surgical Y71.3
      - therapeutic Y71.1
    - gastroenterology Y73.8
      - accessory Y73.2
      - diagnostic Y73.Ø
      - miscellaneous Y73.8
      - monitoring Y73.Ø
      - prosthetic Y73.2
      - rehabilitative Y73.1
      - surgical Y73.3
      - therapeutic Y73.1
    - general
      - hospital Y74.8
        - accessory Y74.2
        - diagnostic Y74.Ø
        - miscellaneous Y74.8
        - monitoring Y74.Ø
        - prosthetic Y74.2
        - rehabilitative Y74.1
        - surgical Y74.3
        - therapeutic Y74.1
      - surgical Y81.8
        - accessory Y81.2
        - diagnostic Y81.Ø
        - miscellaneous Y81.8
        - monitoring Y81.Ø
        - prosthetic Y81.2
        - rehabilitative Y81.1
        - surgical Y81.3
        - therapeutic Y81.1
    - gynecological Y76.8
      - accessory Y76.2
      - diagnostic Y76.Ø
      - miscellaneous Y76.8
      - monitoring Y76.Ø
      - prosthetic Y76.2
      - rehabilitative Y76.1
      - surgical Y76.3
      - therapeutic Y76.1
    - medical Y82.9
      - specified type NEC Y82.8
- **Incident, adverse**— *continued*
  - device— *continued*
    - neurological Y75.8
      - accessory Y75.2
      - diagnostic Y75.Ø
      - miscellaneous Y75.8
      - monitoring Y75.Ø
      - prosthetic Y75.2
      - rehabilitative Y75.1
      - surgical Y75.3
      - therapeutic Y75.1
    - obstetrical Y76.8
      - accessory Y76.2
      - diagnostic Y76.Ø
      - miscellaneous Y76.8
      - monitoring Y76.Ø
      - prosthetic Y76.2
      - rehabilitative Y76.1
      - surgical Y76.3
      - therapeutic Y76.1
    - ophthalmic Y77.8
      - accessory Y77.2
      - diagnostic Y77.Ø
      - miscellaneous Y77.8
      - monitoring Y77.Ø
      - prosthetic Y77.2
      - rehabilitative Y77.1
      - surgical Y77.3
      - therapeutic Y77.1
    - orthopedic Y79.8
      - accessory Y79.2
      - diagnostic Y79.Ø
      - miscellaneous Y79.8
      - monitoring Y79.Ø
      - prosthetic Y79.2
      - rehabilitative Y79.1
      - surgical Y79.3
      - therapeutic Y79.1
    - otorhinolaryngological Y72.8
      - accessory Y72.2
      - diagnostic Y72.Ø
      - miscellaneous Y72.8
      - monitoring Y72.Ø
      - prosthetic Y72.2
      - rehabilitative Y72.1
      - surgical Y72.3
      - therapeutic Y72.1
    - personal use Y74.8
      - accessory Y74.2
      - diagnostic Y74.Ø
      - miscellaneous Y74.8
      - monitoring Y74.Ø
      - prosthetic Y74.2
      - rehabilitative Y74.1
      - surgical Y74.3
      - therapeutic Y74.1
    - physical medicine Y8Ø.8
      - accessory Y8Ø.2
      - diagnostic Y8Ø.Ø
      - miscellaneous Y8Ø.8
      - monitoring Y8Ø.Ø
      - prosthetic Y8Ø.2
      - rehabilitative Y8Ø.1
      - surgical Y8Ø.3
      - therapeutic Y8Ø.1
    - plastic surgical Y81.8
      - accessory Y81.2
      - diagnostic Y81.Ø
      - miscellaneous Y81.8
      - monitoring Y81.Ø
      - prosthetic Y81.2
      - rehabilitative Y81.1
      - surgical Y81.3
      - therapeutic Y81.1
    - radiological Y78.8
      - accessory Y78.2
      - diagnostic Y78.Ø
      - miscellaneous Y78.8
      - monitoring Y78.Ø
      - prosthetic Y78.2
      - rehabilitative Y78.1
      - surgical Y78.3
      - therapeutic Y78.1

Incident, adverse— *continued*
- device— *continued*
  - urology Y73.8
    - accessory Y73.2
    - diagnostic Y73.Ø
    - miscellaneous Y73.8
    - monitoring Y73.Ø
    - prosthetic Y73.2
    - rehabilitative Y73.1
    - surgical Y73.3
    - therapeutic Y73.1

Incineration (accidental) — *see* Exposure, fire

Infanticide — *see* Assault

Infrasound waves (causing injury) W49.9

Ingestion
- foreign body (causing injury) (with obstruction) — *see* Foreign body, alimentary canal
- poisonous
  - plant(s) X58
  - substance NEC — *see* Table of Drugs and Chemicals

Inhalation
- excessively cold substance, man-made — *see* Exposure, cold, man-made
- food (any type) (into respiratory tract) (with asphyxia, obstruction respiratory tract, suffocation) — *see* categories T17 and T18
- foreign body — *see* Foreign body, aspiration
- gastric contents (with asphyxia, obstruction respiratory passage, suffocation) T17.81-
- hot air or gases X14.Ø
- liquid air, hydrogen, nitrogen W93.12
  - suicide (attempt) X83.2
- steam X13.Ø
  - assault X98.Ø
  - stated as undetermined whether accidental or intentional Y27.Ø
  - suicide (attempt) X77.Ø
- toxic gas — *see* Table of Drugs and Chemicals
- vomitus (with asphyxia, obstruction respiratory passage, suffocation) T17.81-

Injury, injured (accidental(ly)) NOS X58
- by, caused by, from
  - assault — *see* Assault
  - law-enforcing agent, police, in course of legal intervention — *see* Legal intervention
  - suicide (attempt) X83.8
- due to, in
  - civil insurrection — *see* War operations
  - fight (*see also* Assault, fight) YØ4.Ø
  - war operations — *see* War operations
- homicide (*see also* Assault) YØ9
- inflicted (by)
  - in course of arrest (attempted), suppression of disturbance, maintenance of order, by law-enforcing agents — *see* Legal intervention
  - other person
    - stated as
      - accidental X58
      - intentional, homicide (attempt) — *see* Assault
      - undetermined whether accidental or intentional Y33
- purposely (inflicted) by other person(s) — *see* Assault
- self-inflicted X83.8
  - stated as accidental X58
- specified cause NEC X58
- undetermined whether accidental or intentional Y33

Insolation, effects X3Ø

Insufficient nourishment X58

Interruption of respiration (by)
- food (lodged in esophagus) — *see* categories T17 and T18
- vomitus (lodged in esophagus) T17.81-

Intervention, legal — *see* Legal intervention

Intoxication
- drug — *see* Table of Drugs and Chemicals
- poison — *see* Table of Drugs and Chemicals

J

Jammed (accidentally)
- between objects (moving) (stationary and moving) W23.Ø
  - stationary W23.1

Jumped, jumping
- before moving object NEC X81.8
  - motor vehicle X81.Ø
  - subway train X81.1
  - train X81.1
  - undetermined whether accidental or intentional Y31
- from
  - boat (into water) voluntarily, without accident (to or on boat) W16.712
    - with
      - accident to or on boat — *see* Accident, watercraft
      - drowning or submersion W16.711
        - suicide (attempt) X71.3
    - striking bottom W16.722
      - causing drowning W16.721
  - building (*see also* Jumped, from, high place) W13.9
    - burning (uncontrolled fire) XØØ.5
  - high place NEC W17.89
    - suicide (attempt) X8Ø
    - undetermined whether accidental or intentional Y3Ø
  - structure (*see also* Jumped, from, high place) W13.9
    - burning (uncontrolled fire) XØØ.5
- into water W16.92
  - causing drowning W16.91
  - from, off watercraft — *see* Jumped, from, boat
  - in
    - natural body W16.612
      - causing drowning W16.611
      - striking bottom W16.622
        - causing drowning W16.621
    - specified place NEC W16.812
      - causing drowning W16.811
      - striking
        - bottom W16.822
          - causing drowning W16.821
        - wall W16.832
          - causing drowning W16.831
    - swimming pool W16.512
      - causing drowning W16.511
      - striking
        - bottom W16.522
          - causing drowning W16.521
        - wall W16.532
          - causing drowning W16.531
  - suicide (attempt) X71.3

K

Kicked by
- animal NEC W55.82
- person(s) (accidentally) W5Ø.1
  - with intent to injure or kill YØ4.Ø
  - as, or caused by, a crowd or human stampede (with fall) W52
  - assault YØ4.Ø
  - homicide (attempt) YØ4.Ø
  - in
    - fight YØ4.Ø
    - legal intervention
      - injuring
        - bystander Y35.812
        - law enforcement personnel Y35.811
        - suspect Y35.813

Kicking against
- object W22.8
  - sports equipment W21.9
  - stationary W22.Ø9
    - sports equipment W21.89
- person — *see* Striking against, person
- sports equipment W21.9

Killed, killing (accidentally) **NOS** (*see also* Injury) X58
- in
  - action — *see* War operations
  - brawl, fight (hand) (fists) (foot) YØ4.Ø
    - by weapon (*see also* Assault)
      - cutting, piercing — *see* Assault, cutting or piercing instrument
      - firearm — *see* Discharge, firearm, by type, homicide
- self
  - stated as
    - accident NOS X58
    - suicide — *see* Suicide
    - undetermined whether accidental or intentional Y33

Knocked down (accidentally) (by) NOS X58
- animal (not being ridden) NEC (*see also* Struck by, by type of animal)
- crowd or human stampede W52
- person W51
  - in brawl, fight YØ4.Ø
- transport vehicle NEC (*see also* Accident, transport) VØ9.9

L

Laceration NEC — *see* Injury

Lack of
- care (helpless person) (infant) (newborn) X58
- food except as result of abandonment or neglect X58
  - due to abandonment or neglect X58
- water except as result of transport accident X58
  - due to transport accident — *see* Accident, transport, by type
  - helpless person, infant, newborn X58

Landslide (falling on transport vehicle) X36.1
- caused by collapse of man-made structure X36.Ø

Late effect — *see* Sequelae

Legal
- execution (any method) — *see* Legal, intervention
- intervention (by)
  - baton — *see* Legal, intervention, blunt object, baton
  - bayonet — *see* Legal, intervention, sharp object, bayonet
  - blow — *see* Legal, intervention, manhandling
  - blunt object
    - baton
      - injuring
        - bystander Y35.312
        - law enforcement personnel Y35.311
        - suspect Y35.313
    - injuring
      - bystander Y35.3Ø2
      - law enforcement personnel Y35.3Ø1
      - suspect Y35.3Ø3
    - specified NEC
      - injuring
        - bystander Y35.392
        - law enforcement personnel Y35.391
        - suspect Y35.393
    - stave
      - injuring
        - bystander Y35.392
        - law enforcement personnel Y35.391
        - suspect Y35.393
  - bomb — *see* Legal, intervention, explosive
  - cutting or piercing instrument — *see* Legal, intervention, sharp object
  - dynamite — *see* Legal, intervention, explosive, dynamite
  - explosive(s)
    - dynamite
      - injuring
        - bystander Y35.112
        - law enforcement personnel Y35.111
        - suspect Y35.113

- **Legal**— *continued*
  - intervention— *continued*
    - explosive(s)— *continued*
      - grenade
        - injuring
          - bystander Y35.192
          - law enforcement personnel Y35.191
          - suspect Y35.193
      - injuring
        - bystander Y35.1Ø2
        - law enforcement personnel Y35.1Ø1
        - suspect Y35.1Ø3
      - mortar bomb
        - injuring
          - bystander Y35.192
          - law enforcement personnel Y35.191
          - suspect Y35.193
      - shell
        - injuring
          - bystander Y35.122
          - law enforcement personnel Y35.121
          - suspect Y35.123
      - specified NEC
        - injuring
          - bystander Y35.192
          - law enforcement personnel Y35.191
          - suspect Y35.193
    - firearm(s) (discharge)
      - handgun
        - injuring
          - bystander Y35.Ø22
          - law enforcement personnel Y35.Ø21
          - suspect Y35.Ø23
      - injuring
        - bystander Y35.ØØ2
        - law enforcement personnel Y35.ØØ1
        - suspect Y35.ØØ3
      - machine gun
        - injuring
          - bystander Y35.Ø12
          - law enforcement personnel Y35.Ø11
          - suspect Y35.Ø13
      - rifle pellet
        - injuring
          - bystander Y35.Ø32
          - law enforcement personnel Y35.Ø31
          - suspect Y35.Ø33
      - rubber bullet
        - injuring
          - bystander Y35.Ø42
          - law enforcement personnel Y35.Ø41
          - suspect Y35.Ø43
      - shotgun — *see* Legal, intervention, firearm, specified NEC
      - specified NEC
        - injuring
          - bystander Y35.Ø92
          - law enforcement personnel Y35.Ø91
          - suspect Y35.Ø93
    - gas (asphyxiation) (poisoning)
      - injuring
        - bystander Y35.2Ø2
        - law enforcement personnel Y35.2Ø1
        - suspect Y35.2Ø3
      - specified NEC
        - injuring
          - bystander Y35.292
          - law enforcement personnel Y35.291
          - suspect Y35.293
      - tear gas
        - injuring
          - bystander Y35.212
          - law enforcement personnel Y35.211
          - suspect Y35.213
    - grenade — *see* Legal, intervention, explosive, grenade
    - injuring
      - bystander Y35.92
      - law enforcement personnel Y35.91
      - suspect Y35.93

- **Legal**— *continued*
  - intervention— *continued*
    - late effect (of) — *see* category Y35 with 7th character S
    - manhandling
      - injuring
        - bystander Y35.812
        - law enforcement personnel Y35.811
        - suspect Y35.813
    - sequelae (of) — *see* category Y35 with 7th character S
    - sharp objects
      - bayonet
        - injuring
          - bystander Y35.412
          - law enforcement personnel Y35.411
          - suspect Y35.413
      - injuring
        - bystander Y35.4Ø2
        - law enforcement personnel Y35.4Ø1
        - suspect Y35.4Ø3
      - specified NEC
        - injuring
          - bystander Y35.492
          - law enforcement personnel Y35.491
          - suspect Y35.493
    - specified means NEC
      - injuring
        - bystander Y35.892
        - law enforcement personnel Y35.891
        - suspect Y35.893
    - stabbing — *see* Legal, intervention, sharp object
    - stave — *see* Legal, intervention, blunt object, stave
    - tear gas — *see* Legal, intervention, gas, tear gas
    - truncheon — *see* Legal, intervention, blunt object, stave
- **Lightning** (shock) (stroke) (struck by) — *see* subcategory T75.Ø
  - causing fire — *see* Exposure, fire
- **Loss of control** (transport vehicle) **NEC** — *see* Accident, transport
- **Lost at sea NOS** — *see* Drowning, due to, fall overboard
- **Low**
  - pressure (effects) — *see* Air, pressure, low
  - temperature (effects) — *see* Exposure, cold
- **Lying before train, vehicle or other moving object** X81.8
  - subway train X81.1
  - train X81.1
  - undetermined whether accidental or intentional Y31
- **Lynching** — *see* Assault

M

- **Malfunction** (mechanism or component) (of)
  - firearm W34.1Ø
    - airgun W34.11Ø
    - BB gun W34.11Ø
    - gas, air or spring-operated gun NEC W34.118
    - handgun W32.1
    - hunting rifle W33.12
    - larger firearm W33.1Ø
      - specified NEC W33.19
    - machine gun W33.13
    - paintball gun W34.111
    - pellet gun W34.11Ø
    - shotgun W33.11
    - specified NEC W34.19
    - Very pistol [flare] W34.19
  - handgun — *see* Malfunction, firearm, handgun
- **Maltreatment** — *see* Perpetrator
- **Mangled** (accidentally) NOS X58
- **Manhandling** (in brawl, fight) YØ4.Ø
  - legal intervention — *see* Legal, intervention, manhandling
- **Manslaughter** (nonaccidental) — *see* Assault
- **Mauled by animal NEC** W55.89

- **Medical procedure, complication of** (delayed or as an abnormal reaction without mention of misadventure) — *see* Complication of or following, by specified type of procedure
  - due to or as a result of misadventure — *see* Misadventure
- **Melting** (due to fire) (*see also* Exposure, fire)
  - apparel NEC XØ6.3
  - clothes, clothing NEC XØ6.3
    - nightwear XØ5
  - fittings or furniture (burning building) (uncontrolled fire) XØØ.8
  - nightwear XØ5
  - plastic jewelry XØ6.1
- **Mental cruelty** X58
- **Military operations** (injuries to military and civilians occuring during peacetime on military property and during routine military exercises and operations) (by) (from) (involving) Y37.9Ø-
  - air blast Y37.2Ø-
  - aircraft
    - destruction — *see* Military operations, destruction of aircraft
  - airway restriction — *see* Military operations, restriction of airways
  - asphyxiation — *see* Military operations, restriction of airways
  - biological weapons Y37.6X-
  - blast Y37.2Ø-
  - blast fragments Y37.2Ø-
  - blast wave Y37.2Ø-
  - blast wind Y37.2Ø-
  - bomb Y37.2Ø-
    - dirty Y37.5Ø-
    - gasoline Y37.31-
    - incendiary Y37.31-
    - petrol Y37.31-
  - bullet Y37.43-
    - incendiary Y37.32-
    - rubber Y37.41-
  - chemical weapons Y37.7X-
  - combat
    - hand to hand (unarmed) combat Y37.44-
    - using blunt or piercing object Y37.45-
  - conflagration — *see* Military operations, fire
  - conventional warfare NEC Y37.49-
  - depth-charge Y37.Ø1-
  - destruction of aircraft Y37.1Ø-
    - due to
      - air to air missile Y37.11-
      - collision with other aircraft Y37.12-
      - detonation (accidental) of onboard munitions and explosives Y37.14-
      - enemy fire or explosives Y37.11-
      - explosive placed on aircraft Y37.11-
      - onboard fire Y37.13-
      - rocket propelled grenade [RPG] Y37.11-
      - small arms fire Y37.11-
      - surface to air missile Y37.11-
    - specified NEC Y37.19-
  - detonation (accidental) of
    - onboard marine weapons Y37.Ø5-
    - own munitions or munitions launch device Y37.24-
  - dirty bomb Y37.5Ø-
  - explosion (of) Y37.2Ø-
    - aerial bomb Y37.21-
    - bomb NOS Y37.2Ø*see also* Military operations, bomb(s)
    - own munitions or munitions launch device (accidental) Y37.24-
    - fragments Y37.2Ø-
    - grenade Y37.29-
    - guided missile Y37.22-
    - improvised explosive device [IED] (person-borne) (roadside) (vehicle-borne) Y37.23-
    - land mine Y37.29-
    - marine mine (at sea) (in harbor) Y37.Ø2-
    - marine weapon Y37.ØØ-
      - specified NEC Y37.Ø9-
    - sea-based artillery shell Y37.Ø3-
    - specified NEC Y37.29-
    - torpedo Y37.Ø4-

- **Military operations**— *continued*
  - fire Y37.3Ø-
    - specified NEC Y37.39-
  - firearms
    - discharge Y37.43-
    - pellets Y37.42-
  - flamethrower Y37.33-
  - fragments (from) (of)
    - improvised explosive device [IED] (person-borne) (roadside) (vehicle-borne) Y37.26-
    - munitions Y37.25-
    - specified NEC Y37.29-
    - weapons Y37.27-
  - friendly fire Y37.92-
  - hand to hand (unarmed) combat Y37.44-
  - hot substances — *see* Military operations, fire
  - incendiary bullet Y37.32-
  - nuclear weapon (effects of) Y37.5Ø-
    - acute radiation exposure Y37.54-
    - blast pressure Y37.51-
    - direct blast Y37.51-
    - direct heat Y37.53-
    - fallout exposure Y37.54-
    - fireball Y37.53-
    - indirect blast (struck or crushed by blast debris) (being thrown by blast) Y37.52-
    - ionizing radiation (immediate exposure) Y37.54-
    - nuclear radiation Y37.54-
    - radiation
      - ionizing (immediate exposure) Y37.54-
      - nuclear Y37.54-
      - thermal Y37.53-
    - specified NEC Y37.59-
    - secondary effects Y37.54-
    - thermal radiation Y37.53-
  - restriction of air (airway)
    - intentional Y37.46-
    - unintentional Y37.47-
  - rubber bullets Y37.41-
  - shrapnel NOS Y37.29-
  - suffocation — *see* Military operations, restriction of airways
  - unconventional warfare NEC Y37.7X-
  - underwater blast NOS Y37.ØØ-
  - warfare
    - conventional NEC Y37.49-
    - unconventional NEC Y37.7X-
  - weapons
    - biological weapons Y37.6X-
    - chemical Y37.7X-
    - nuclear (effects of) Y37.5Ø-
      - acute radiation exposure Y37.54-
      - blast pressure Y37.51-
      - direct blast Y37.51-
      - direct heat Y37.53-
      - fallout exposure Y37.54-
      - fireball Y37.53-
      - radiation
        - ionizing (immediate exposure) Y37.54-
        - nuclear Y37.54-
        - thermal Y37.53-
      - secondary effects Y37.54-
      - specified NEC Y37.59-
    - of mass destruction [WMD] Y37.91-
  - weapon of mass destruction [WMD] Y37.91-
- **Misadventure**(s) **to patient**(s) **during surgical or medical care** Y69
  - contaminated medical or biological substance (blood, drug, fluid) Y64.9
    - administered (by) NEC Y64.9
      - immunization Y64.1
      - infusion Y64.Ø
      - injection Y64.1
      - specified means NEC Y64.8
      - transfusion Y64.Ø
      - vaccination Y64.1
  - excessive amount of blood or other fluid during transfusion or infusion Y63.Ø

- **Misadventure**(s) **to patient**(s) **during surgical or medical care** — *continued*
  - failure
    - in dosage Y63.9
      - electroshock therapy Y63.4
      - inappropriate temperature (too hot or too cold) in local application and packing Y63.5
      - infusion
        - excessive amount of fluid Y63.Ø
        - incorrect dilution of fluid Y63.1
      - insulin-shock therapy Y63.4
      - nonadministration of necessary drug or biological substance Y63.62
      - overdose — *see* Table of Drugs and Chemicals
        - radiation, in therapy Y63.2
      - radiation
        - overdose Y63.2
      - specified procedure NEC Y63.8
      - transfusion
        - excessive amount of blood Y63.Ø
    - mechanical, of instrument or apparatus (any) (during any procedure) Y65.8
    - sterile precautions (during procedure) Y62.9
      - aspiration of fluid or tissue (by puncture or catheterization, except heart) Y62.6
      - biopsy (except needle aspiration) Y62.8
        - needle (aspirating) Y62.6
      - blood sampling Y62.6
      - catheterization Y62.6
        - heart Y62.5
      - dialysis (kidney) Y62.2
      - endoscopic examination Y62.4
      - enema Y62.8
      - immunization Y62.3
      - infusion Y62.1
      - injection Y62.3
      - needle biopsy Y62.6
      - paracentesis (abdominal) (thoracic) Y62.6
      - perfusion Y62.2
      - puncture (lumbar) Y62.6
      - removal of catheter or packing Y62.8
      - specified procedure NEC Y62.8
      - surgical operation Y62.Ø
      - transfusion Y62.1
      - vaccination Y62.3
    - suture or ligature during surgical procedure Y65.2
    - to introduce or to remove tube or instrument — *see* Failure, to
  - hemorrhage — *see* Misadventure, cut, by type of procedure
  - inadvertent exposure of patient to radiation Y63.3
  - inappropriate
    - operation performed — *see* Inappropriate operation performed
    - temperature (too hot or too cold) in local application or packing Y63.5
  - infusion (*see also* Misadventure, by type, infusion) Y69
    - excessive amount of fluid Y63.Ø
    - incorrect dilution of fluid Y63.1
    - wrong fluid Y65.1
  - mismatched blood in transfusion Y65.Ø
  - nonadministration of necessary drug or biological substance Y63.62
  - overdose — *see* Table of Drugs and Chemicals
    - radiation (in therapy) Y63.2
  - perforation — *see* Misadventure, cut, by type of procedure
  - performance of inappropriate operation — *see* Inappropriate operation performed
  - puncture — *see* Misadventure, cut, by type of procedure
  - specified type NEC Y65.8
    - failure
      - suture or ligature during surgical operation Y65.2
      - to introduce or to remove tube or instrument — *see* Failure, to

- **Misadventure**(s) **to patient**(s) **during surgical or medical care** — *continued*
  - specified type— *continued*
    - infusion of wrong fluid Y65.1
    - performance of inappropriate operation — *see* Inappropriate operation performed
    - transfusion of mismatched blood Y65.Ø
    - wrong
      - fluid in infusion Y65.1
      - placement of endotracheal tube during anesthetic procedure Y65.3
  - transfusion — *see* Misadventure, by type, transfusion
    - excessive amount of blood Y63.Ø
    - mismatched blood Y65.Ø
  - wrong
    - drug given in error — *see* Table of Drugs and Chemicals
    - fluid in infusion Y65.1
    - placement of endotracheal tube during anesthetic procedure Y65.3
- **Mismatched blood in transfusion** Y65.Ø
- **Motion sickness** T75.3
- **Mountain sickness** W94.11
- **Mudslide** (of cataclysmic nature) — *see* Landslide
- **Murder** (attempt) — *see* Assault

N

- **Nail, contact with** W45.Ø
  - gun W29.4
- **Neglect** (criminal) (homicidal intent) X58
- **Noise** (causing injury) (pollution) W42.9
  - supersonic W42.Ø
- **Nonadministration** (of)
  - drug or biological substance (necessary) Y63.62
  - surgical and medical care Y66
- **Nosocomial condition** Y95

O

- **Object**
  - falling
    - from, in, on, hitting
      - machinery — *see* Contact, with, by type of machine
  - set in motion by
    - accidental explosion or rupture of pressure vessel W38
    - firearm — *see* Discharge, firearm, by type
    - machine(ry) — *see* Contact, with, by type of machine
- **Overdose** (drug) — *see* Table of Drugs and Chemicals
  - radiation Y63.2
- **Overexertion** — *see* category Y93
- **Overexposure** (accidental) (to)
  - cold (*see also* Exposure, cold) X31
    - due to man-made conditions — *see* Exposure, cold, man-made
  - heat (*see also* Heat) X3Ø
  - radiation — *see* Radiation
  - radioactivity W88.Ø
  - sun (sunburn) X32
  - weather NEC — *see* Forces of nature
  - wind NEC — *see* Forces of nature
- **Overheated** — *see* Heat
- **Overturning** (accidental)
  - machinery — *see* Contact, with, by type of machine
  - transport vehicle NEC (*see also* Accident, transport) V89.9
  - watercraft (causing drowning, submersion) (*see also* Drowning, due to, accident to, watercraft, overturning)
    - causing injury except drowning or submersion — *see* Accident, watercraft, causing, injury NEC

P

- **Parachute descent** (voluntary) (without accident to aircraft) V97.29
  - due to accident to aircraft — *see* Accident, transport, aircraft
- **Pecked by bird** W61.99
- **Perforation during medical or surgical treatment as misadventure** — *see* Misadventure, cut, by type of procedure
- **Perpetrator, perpetration, of assault, maltreatment and neglect (by)** YØ7.9
  - boyfriend YØ7.Ø3
  - brother YØ7.41Ø
    - stepbrother YØ7.435
  - coach YØ7.53
  - cousin
    - female YØ7.491
    - male YØ7.49Ø
  - daycare provider YØ7.519
    - at-home
      - adult care YØ7.512
      - childcare YØ7.51Ø
    - care center
      - adult care YØ7.513
      - childcare YØ7.511
  - family member NEC YØ7.499
  - father YØ7.11
    - adoptive YØ7.13
    - foster YØ7.42Ø
    - stepfather YØ7.43Ø
  - foster father YØ7.42Ø
  - foster mother YØ7.421
  - girl friend YØ7.Ø4
  - healthcare provider YØ7.529
    - mental health YØ7.521
    - specified NEC YØ7.528
  - husband YØ7.Ø1
  - instructor YØ7.53
  - mother YØ7.12
    - adoptive YØ7.14
    - foster YØ7.421
    - stepmother YØ7.433
  - nonfamily member YØ7.5Ø
    - specifed NEC YØ7.59
  - nurse YØ7.528
  - occupational therapist YØ7.528
  - partner of parent
    - female YØ7.434
    - male YØ7.432
  - physical therapist YØ7.528
  - sister YØ7.411
  - speech therapist YØ7.528
  - stepbrother YØ7.435
  - stepfather YØ7.43Ø
  - stepmother YØ7.433
  - stepsister YØ7.436
  - teacher YØ7.53
  - wife YØ7.Ø2
- **Piercing** — *see* Contact, with, by type of object or machine
- **Pinched**
  - between objects (moving) (stationary and moving) W23.Ø
    - stationary W23.1
- **Pinned under machine(ry)** — *see* Contact, with, by type of machine
- **Place of occurrence** Y92.9
  - abandoned house Y92.89
  - airplane Y92.813
  - airport Y92.52Ø
  - ambulatory health services establishment NEC Y92.538
  - ambulatory surgery center Y92.53Ø
  - amusement park Y92.831
  - apartment (co-op) — *see* Place of occurrence, residence, apartment
  - assembly hall Y92.29
  - bank Y92.51Ø
  - barn Y92.71
  - baseball field Y92.32Ø
  - basketball court Y92.31Ø

- **Place of occurrence** — *continued*
  - beach Y92.832
  - boarding house — *see* Place of occurrence, residence, boarding house
  - boat Y92.814
  - bowling alley Y92.39
  - bridge Y92.89
  - building under construction Y92.61
  - bus Y92.811
    - station Y92.521
  - cafe Y92.511
  - campsite Y92.833
  - campus — *see* Place of occurrence, school
  - canal Y92.89
  - car Y92.81Ø
  - casino Y92.59
  - children's home — *see* Place of occurrence, residence, institutional, orphanage
  - church Y92.22
  - cinema Y92.26
  - clubhouse Y92.29
  - coal pit Y92.64
  - college (community) Y92.214
  - condominium — *see* Place of occurrence, residence, apartment
  - construction area — *see* Place of occurrence, industrial and construction area
  - convalescent home — *see* Place of occurrence, residence, institutional, nursing home
  - court-house Y92.24Ø
  - cricket ground Y92.328
  - cultural building Y92.258
    - art gallery Y92.25Ø
    - museum Y92.251
    - music hall Y92.252
    - opera house Y92.253
    - specified NEC Y92.258
    - theater Y92.254
  - dancehall Y92.252
  - day nursery Y92.21Ø
  - dentist office Y92.531
  - derelict house Y92.89
  - desert Y92.82Ø
  - dock NOS Y92.89
  - dockyard Y92.62
  - doctor's office Y92.531
  - dormitory — *see* Place of occurrence, residence, institutional, school dormitory
  - dry dock Y92.62
  - factory (building) (premises) Y92.63
  - farm (land under cultivation) (outbuildings) Y92.79
    - barn Y92.71
    - chicken coop Y92.72
    - field Y92.73
    - hen house Y92.72
    - house — *see* Place of occurrence, residence, house
    - orchard Y92.74
    - specified NEC Y92.79
  - football field Y92.321
  - forest Y92.821
  - freeway Y92.411
  - gallery Y92.25Ø
  - garage (commercial) Y92.59
    - boarding house Y92.Ø44
    - military base Y92.135
    - mobile home Y92.Ø25
    - nursing home Y92.124
    - orphanage Y92.114
    - private house Y92.Ø15
    - reform school Y92.155
  - gas station Y92.524
  - gasworks Y92.69
  - golf course Y92.39
  - gravel pit Y92.64
  - grocery Y92.512
  - gymnasium Y92.39
  - handball court Y92.318
  - harbor Y92.89
  - harness racing course Y92.39
  - healthcare provider office Y92.531
  - highway (interstate) Y92.411
  - hill Y92.828

- **Place of occurrence** — *continued*
  - hockey rink Y92.33Ø
  - home — *see* Place of occurrence, residence
  - hospice — *see* Place of occurrence, residence, institutional, nursing home
  - hospital Y92.239
    - cafeteria Y92.233
    - corridor Y92.232
    - operating room Y92.234
    - patient
      - bathroom Y92.231
      - room Y92.23Ø
    - specified NEC Y92.238
  - hotel Y92.59
  - house (*see also* Place of occurrence, residence)
    - abandoned Y92.89
    - under construction Y92.61
  - industrial and construction area (yard) Y92.69
    - building under construction Y92.61
    - dock Y92.62
    - dry dock Y92.62
    - factory Y92.63
    - gasworks Y92.69
    - mine Y92.64
    - oil rig Y92.65
    - pit Y92.64
    - power station Y92.69
    - shipyard Y92.62
    - specified NEC Y92.69
    - tunnel under construction Y92.69
    - workshop Y92.69
  - kindergarten Y92.211
  - lacrosse field Y92.328
  - lake Y92.828
  - library Y92.241
  - mall Y92.59
  - market Y92.512
  - marsh Y92.828
  - military
    - base — *see* Place of occurrence, residence, institutional, military base
    - training ground Y92.84
  - mine Y92.64
  - mosque Y92.22
  - motel Y92.59
  - motorway (interstate) Y92.411
  - mountain Y92.828
  - movie-house Y92.26
  - museum Y92.251
  - music-hall Y92.252
  - not applicable Y92.9
  - nuclear power station Y92.69
  - nursing home — *see* Place of occurrence, residence, institutional, nursing home
  - office building Y92.59
  - offshore installation Y92.65
  - oil rig Y92.65
  - old people's home — *see* Place of occurrence, residence, institutional, specified NEC
  - opera-house Y92.253
  - orphanage — *see* Place of occurrence, residence, institutional, orphanage
  - outpatient surgery center Y92.53Ø
  - park (public) Y92.83Ø
    - amusement Y92.831
  - parking garage Y92.89
    - lot Y92.481
  - pavement Y92.48Ø
  - physician office Y92.531
  - polo field Y92.328
  - pond Y92.828
  - post office Y92.242
  - power station Y92.69
  - prairie Y92.828
  - prison — *see* Place of occurrence, residence, institutional, prison
  - public
    - administration building Y92.248
      - city hall Y92.243
      - courthouse Y92.24Ø
      - library Y92.241
      - post office Y92.242
      - specified NEC Y92.248

- **Place of occurrence** — *continued*
  - trade area— *continued*
    - radio station Y92.59
    - restaurant Y92.511
    - shop Y92.513
    - shopping mall Y92.59
    - store Y92.512
    - supermarket Y92.512
    - television station Y92.59
    - warehouse Y92.59
  - trailer park, residential — *see* Place of occurrence, residence, mobile home
  - trailer site NOS Y92.89
  - train Y92.815
    - station Y92.522
  - truck Y92.812
  - tunnel under construction Y92.69
  - university Y92.214
  - urgent (health) care center Y92.532
  - vehicle (transport) Y92.818
    - airplane Y92.813
    - boat Y92.814
    - bus Y92.811
    - car Y92.810
    - specified NEC Y92.818
    - subway car Y92.816
    - train Y92.815
    - truck Y92.812
  - warehouse Y92.59
  - water reservoir Y92.89
  - wilderness area Y92.828
    - desert Y92.820
    - forest Y92.821
    - marsh Y92.828
    - mountain Y92.828
    - prairie Y92.828
    - specified NEC Y92.828
    - swamp Y92.828
  - workshop Y92.69
  - yard, private Y92.096
    - boarding house Y92.046
    - single family house Y92.017
    - mobile home Y92.027
  - youth center Y92.29
  - zoo (zoological garden) Y92.834
- **Plumbism** — *see* Table of Drugs and Chemicals, lead
- **Poisoning** (accidental) (by) (*see also* Table of Drugs and Chemicals)
  - by plant, thorns, spines, sharp leaves or other mechanisms NEC X58
  - carbon monoxide
    - generated by
      - motor vehicle — *see* Accident, transport
      - watercraft (in transit) (not in transit) V93.89
        - ferry boat V93.81
        - fishing boat V93.82
        - jet skis V93.83
        - liner V93.81
        - merchant ship V93.80
        - passenger ship V93.81
        - powered craft NEC V93.83
  - caused by injection of poisons into skin by plant thorns, spines, sharp leaves X58
    - marine or sea plants (venomous) X58
  - execution— *see* Legal, intervention, gas
    - intervention
      - by gas — *see* Legal, intervention, gas
      - other specified means — *see* Legal, intervention, specified means NEC
  - exhaust gas
    - generated by
      - motor vehicle — *see* Accident, transport
      - watercraft (in transit) (not in transit) V93.89
        - ferry boat V93.81
        - fishing boat V93.82
        - jet skis V93.83
        - liner V93.81
        - merchant ship V93.80
        - passenger ship V93.81
        - powered craft NEC V93.83
  - fumes or smoke due to
    - explosion (*see also* Explosion) W40.9
    - fire — *see* Exposure, fire
- **Poisoning** — *continued*
  - fumes or smoke due to— *continued*
    - ignition — *see* Ignition
  - gas
    - in legal intervention — *see* Legal, intervention, gas
    - legal execution — *see* Legal, intervention, gas
  - in war operations — *see* War operations
- **Powder burn** (by) (from)
  - airgun W34.110
  - BB gun W34.110
  - firearn NEC W34.19
  - gas, air or spring-operated gun NEC W34.118
  - handgun W32.1
  - hunting rifle W33.12
  - larger firearm W33.10
    - specified NEC W33.19
  - machine gun W33.13
  - paintball gun W34.111
  - pellet gun W34.110
  - shotgun W33.11
  - Very pistol [flare] W34.19
- **Premature cessation** (of) **surgical and medical care** Y66
- **Privation** (food) (water) X58
- **Procedure** (operation)
  - correct, on wrong side or body part (wrong side) (wrong site) Y65.53
  - intended for another patient done on wrong patient Y65.52
  - performed on patient not scheduled for surgery Y65.52
  - performed on wrong patient Y65.52
  - wrong, performed on correct patient Y65.51
- **Prolonged**
  - sitting in transport vehicle — *see* Travel, by type of vehicle
  - stay in
    - high altitude as cause of anoxia, barodontalgia, barotitis or hypoxia W94.11
    - weightless environment X52
- **Pulling, excessive** — *see* Overexertion
- **Puncture, puncturing** (*see also* Contact, with, by type of object or machine)
  - by
    - plant thorns, spines, sharp leaves or other mechanisms NEC W60
  - during medical or surgical treatment as misadventure — *see* Misadventure, cut, by type of procedure
- **Pushed, pushing** (accidental) (injury in) (overexertion) (*see also* Overexertion)
  - by other person(s) (accidental) W51
    - with fall W03
      - due to ice or snow W00.0
    - as, or caused by, a crowd or human stampede (with fall) W52
    - before moving object NEC Y02.8
      - motor vehicle Y02.0
      - subway train Y02.1
      - train Y02.1
    - from
      - high place NEC
        - in accidental circumstances W17.89
        - stated as
          - intentional, homicide (attempt) Y01
          - undetermined whether accidental or intentional Y30
      - transport vehicle NEC (*see also* Accident, transport) V89.9
        - stated as
          - intentional, homicide (attempt) Y08.89

R

- **Radiation** (exposure to)
  - arc lamps W89.0
  - atomic power plant (malfunction) NEC W88.1
  - complication of or abnormal reaction to medical radiotherapy Y84.2
- **Radiation** — *continued*
  - electromagnetic, ionizing W88.0
  - gamma rays W88.1
  - in
    - war operations (from or following nuclear explosion) — *see* War operations
  - inadvertent exposure of patient (receiving test or therapy) Y63.3
  - infrared (heaters and lamps) W90.1
    - excessive heat from W92
  - ionized, ionizing (particles, artificially accelerated)
    - radioisotopes W88.1
    - specified NEC W88.8
    - x-rays W88.0
  - isotopes, radioactive — *see* Radiation, radioactive isotopes
  - laser(s) W90.2
    - in war operations — *see* War operations
    - misadventure in medical care Y63.2
  - light sources (man-made visible and ultraviolet) W89.9
    - natural X32
    - specified NEC W89.8
    - tanning bed W89.1
    - welding light W89.0
  - man-made visible light W89.9
    - specified NEC W89.8
    - tanning bed W89.1
    - welding light W89.0
  - microwave W90.8
  - misadventure in medical or surgical procedure Y63.2
  - natural NEC X39.08
    - radon X39.01
  - overdose (in medical or surgical procedure) Y63.2
  - radar W90.0
  - radioactive isotopes (any) W88.1
    - atomic power plant malfunction W88.1
    - misadventure in medical or surgical treatment Y63.2
  - radiofrequency W90.0
  - radium NEC W88.1
  - sun X32
  - ultraviolet (light) (man-made) W89.9
    - natural X32
    - specified NEC W89.8
    - tanning bed W89.1
    - welding light W89.0
  - welding arc, torch, or light W89.0
    - excessive heat from W92
  - x-rays (hard) (soft) W88.0
- **Range disease** W94.11
- **Rape** (attempted) T74.2-
- **Rat bite** W53.11
- **Reaction, abnormal to medical procedure** (*see also* Complication of or following, by type of procedure) Y84.9
  - with misadventure — *see* Misadventure
  - biologicals — *see* Table of Drugs and Chemicals
  - drugs — *see* Table of Drugs and Chemicals
  - vaccine — *see* Table of Drugs and Chemicals
- **Recoil**
  - airgun W34.110
  - BB gun W34.110
  - firearn NEC W34.19
  - gas, air or spring-operated gun NEC W34.118
  - handgun W32.1
  - hunting rifle W33.12
  - larger firearm W33.10
    - specified NEC W33.19
  - machine gun W33.13
  - paintball gun W34.111
  - pellet W34.110
  - shotgun W33.11
  - Very pistol [flare] W34.19
- **Reduction in**
  - atmospheric pressure — *see* Air, pressure, change
- **Rock falling on or hitting** (accidentally) (person) W20.8
  - in cave-in W20.0
- **Run over** (accidentally) (by)
  - animal (not being ridden) NEC W55.89
  - machinery — *see* Contact, with, by specified type of machine

Run over — *continued*
- transport vehicle NEC (*see also* Accident, transport) V09.9
  - intentional homicide (attempt) Y03.0
  - motor NEC V09.20
    - intentional homicide (attempt) Y03.0

Running
- before moving object X81.8
  - motor vehicle X81.0

Running off, away
- animal (being ridden) (*see also* Accident, transport) V80.918
  - not being ridden W55.89
- animal-drawn vehicle NEC (*see also* Accident, transport) V80.928
- highway, road(way), street
  - transport vehicle NEC (*see also* Accident, transport) V89.9

Rupture pressurized devices — *see* Explosion, by type of device

S

Saturnism — *see* Table of Drugs and Chemicals, lead

Scald, scalding (accidental) (by) (from) (in) X19
- air (hot) X14.1
- gases (hot) X14.1
- homicide (attempt) — *see* Assault, burning, hot object
- inflicted by other person
  - stated as intentional, homicide (attempt) — *see* Assault, burning, hot object
- liquid (boiling) (hot) NEC X12
  - stated as undetermined whether accidental or intentional Y27.2
  - suicide (attempt) X77.2
- local application of externally applied substance in medical or surgical care Y63.5
- metal (molten) (liquid) (hot) NEC X18
- self-inflicted X77.9
- stated as undetermined whether accidental or intentional Y27.8
- steam X13.1
  - assault X98.0
  - stated as undetermined whether accidental or intentional Y27.0
  - suicide (attempt) X77.0
- suicide (attempt) X77.9
- vapor (hot) X13.1
  - assault X98.0
  - stated as undetermined whether accidental or intentional Y27.0
  - suicide (attempt) X77.0

Scratched by
- cat W55.03
- person(s) (accidentally) W50.4
  - with intent to injure or kill Y04.0
  - as, or caused by, a crowd or human stampede (with fall) W52
  - assault Y04.0
  - homicide (attempt) Y04.0
  - in
    - fight Y04.0
    - legal intervention
      - injuring
        - bystander Y35.892
        - law enforcement personnel Y35.891
        - suspect Y35.893

Seasickness T75.3

Self-harm NEC (*see also* External cause by type, undetermined whether accidental or intentional)
- intentional — *see* Suicide
- poisoning NEC — *see* Table of drugs and biologicals, accident

Self-inflicted (injury) **NEC** (*see also* External cause by type, undetermined whether accidental or intentional)
- intentional — *see* Suicide
- poisoning NEC — *see* Table of drugs and biologicals, accident

Sequelae (of)
- accident NEC — *see* categories W00-X58 with 7th character S
- assault (homicidal) (any means) — *see* categories X92-Y08 with 7th character S
- homicide, attempt (any means) — *see* categories X92-Y08 with 7th character S
- injury undetermined whether accidentally or purposely inflicted —*see* categories Y21-Y33 with 7th character S
- intentional self-harm (classifiable to X71-X83) — *see* categories X71-X83 with 7th character S
- legal intervention — *see* category Y35 with 7th character S
- motor vehicle accident — *see* categories V00-V99 with 7th character S
- suicide, attempt (any means) — *see* categories X71-X83 with 7th character S
- transport accident — *see* categories V00-V99 with 7th character S
- war operations — *see* War operations

Shock
- electric — *see* Exposure, electric current
- from electric appliance (any) (faulty) W86.8
  - domestic W86.0
  - suicide (attempt) X83.1

Shooting, shot (accidental(ly)) (*see also* Discharge, firearm, by type)
- herself or himself — *see* Discharge, firearm by type, self-inflicted
- homicide (attempt) — *see* Discharge, firearm by type, homicide
- in war operations — *see* War operations
- inflicted by other person — *see* Discharge, firearm by type, homicide
  - accidental — *see* Discharge, firearm, by type of firearm
- legal
  - execution — *see* Legal, intervention, firearm
  - intervention — *see* Legal, intervention, firearm
- self-inflicted — *see* Discharge, firearm by type, suicide
  - accidental — *see* Discharge, firearm, by type of firearm
- suicide (attempt) — *see* Discharge, firearm by type, suicide

Shoving (accidentally) **by other person** — *see* Pushing, by other person

Sickness
- alpine W94.11
- motion — *see* Motion
- mountain W94.11

Sinking (accidental)
- watercraft (causing drowning, submersion) (*see also* Drowning, due to, accident to, watercraft, sinking)
  - causing injury except drowning or submersion — *see* Accident, watercraft, causing, injury NEC

Siriasis X32

Slashed wrists — *see* Cut, self-inflicted

Slipping (accidental) (on same level) (with fall) W01.0
- on
  - ice W00.0
    - with skates — *see* Accident, transport, pedestrian, conveyance
  - mud W01.0
  - oil W01.0
  - snow W00.0
    - with skis — *see* Accident, transport, pedestrian, conveyance
  - surface (slippery) (wet) NEC W01.0
- without fall W18.40
  - due to
    - specified NEC W18.49
    - stepping from one level to another W18.43
    - stepping into hole or opening W18.42
    - stepping on object W18.41

Sliver, wood, contact with W45.8

Smoldering (due to fire) — *see* Exposure, fire

Sodomy (attempted) **by force** T74.2-

Sound waves (causing injury) W42.9
- supersonic W42.0

Splinter, contact with W45.8

Stab, stabbing B *see* Cut

Starvation X58

Status of external cause Y99.9
- child assisting in compensated work for family Y99.8
- civilian activity done for financial or other compensation Y99.0
- civilian activity done for income or pay Y99.0
- family member assisting in compensated work for other family member Y99.8
- hobby not done for income Y99.8
- leisure activity Y99.8
- military activity Y99.1
- off-duty activity of military personnel Y99.8
- recreation or sport not for income or while a student Y99.8
- specified NEC Y99.8
- student activity Y99.8
- volunteer activity Y99.2

Stepped on
- by
  - animal (not being ridden) NEC W55.89
  - crowd or human stampede W52
  - person W50.0

Stepping on
- object W22.8
  - with fall W18.31
  - sports equipment W21.9
  - stationary W22.09
    - sports equipment W21.89
- person W51
  - by crowd or human stampede W52
- sports equipment W21.9

Sting
- arthropod, nonvenomous W57
- insect, nonvenomous W57

Storm (cataclysmic) — *see* Forces of nature, cataclysmic storm

Straining, excessive — *see* Overexertion

Strangling — *see* Strangulation

Strangulation (accidental) — *see* category T71

Strenuous movements — *see* Repetitive movements

Striking against
- airbag (automobile) W22.10
  - driver side W22.11
  - front passenger side W22.12
  - specified NEC W22.19
- bottom when
  - diving or jumping into water (in) W16.822
    - causing drowning W16.821
    - from boat W16.722
      - causing drowning W16.721
    - natural body W16.622
      - causing drowning W16.821
    - swimming pool W16.522
      - causing drowning W16.521
  - falling into water (in) W16.322
    - causing drowning W16.321
    - fountain — *see* Striking against, bottom when, falling into water, specified NEC
    - natural body W16.122
      - causing drowning W16.121
    - reservoir — *see* Striking against, bottom when, falling into water, specified NEC
    - specified NEC W16.322
      - causing drowning W16.321
    - swimming pool W16.022
      - causing drowning W16.021
- diving board (swimming-pool) W21.4
- object W22.8
  - with
    - drowning or submersion — *see* Drowning
    - fall — *see* Fall, due to, bumping against, object
  - caused by crowd or human stampede (with fall) W52
  - furniture W22.03
  - lamppost W22.02
  - sports equipment W21.9
  - stationary W22.09
    - sports equipment W21.89
  - wall W22.01

Struck by— *continued*
- sports equipment— *continued*
  - foot wear NEC W21.39
  - football helmet W21.81
  - hockey (ice)
    - field
      - puck W21.221
      - stick W21.211
    - puck W21.22Ø
    - stick W21.21Ø
      - assault YØ8.Ø1
  - skate blades W21.32
  - specified NEC W21.89
    - assault YØ8.Ø9
- thunderbolt — *see* subcategory T75.Ø
  - causing fire — *see* Exposure, fire
- transport vehicle NEC (*see also* Accident, transport) VØ9.9
  - intentional, homicide (attempt) YØ3.Ø
  - motor NEC (*see also* Accident, transport) VØ9.2Ø
    - homicide YØ3.Ø
- vehicle (transport) NEC — *see* Accident, transport, by type of vehicle
  - stationary (falling from jack, hydraulic lift, ramp) W2Ø.8

Stumbling
- over
  - animal NEC WØ1.Ø
    - with fall WØ1.Ø
  - carpet, rug or (small) object W22.8
    - with fall W18.Ø9
  - person W51
    - with fall WØ3
      - due to ice or snow WØØ.Ø
- without fall W18.49
  - due to
    - specifed NEC W18.49
    - stepping from one level to another W18.43
    - stepping into hole or opening W18.42
    - stepping on object W18.41

Submersion (accidental) — *see* Drowning

Suffocation (accidental) (by external means) (by pressure) (mechanical) (*see also* category T71)
- due to, by
  - avalanche — *see* Landslide
  - explosion — *see* Explosion
  - fire — *see* Exposure, fire
  - food, any type (aspiration) (ingestion) (inhalation) — *see* categories T17 and T18
  - ignition — *see* Ignition
  - landslide — *see* Landslide
  - machine(ry) — *see* Contact, with, by type of machine
  - vomitus (aspiration) (inhalation) T17.81-
- in
  - burning building XØØ.8

Suicide, suicidal (attempted) (by) X83.8
- blunt object X79
- burning, burns X76
  - hot object X77.9
    - fluid NEC X77.2
    - household appliance X77.3
    - specified NEC X77.8
    - steam X77.Ø
    - tap water X77.1
    - vapors X77.Ø
- caustic substance — *see* Table of Drugs and Chemicals
- cold, extreme X83.2
- collision of motor vehicle with
  - motor vehicle X82.Ø
  - specified NEC X82.8
  - train X82.1
  - tree X82.2
- crashing of aircraft X83.Ø
- cut (any part of body) X78.9
- cutting or piercing instrument X78.9
  - dagger X78.2
  - glass X78.Ø
  - knife X78.1
  - specified NEC X78.8
  - sword X78.2

Suicide, suicidal — *continued*
- drowning (in) X71.9
  - bathtub X71.Ø
  - natural water X71.3
  - specified NEC X71.8
  - swimming pool X71.1
    - following fall X71.2
- electrocution X83.1
- explosive(s) (material) X75
- fire, flames X76
- firearm X74.9
  - airgun X74.Ø1
  - handgun X72
  - hunting rifle X73.1
  - larger X73.9
    - specified NEC X73.8
  - machine gun X73.2
  - shotgun X73.Ø
  - specified NEC X74.8
- hanging X83.8
- hot object — *see* Suicide, burning, hot object
- jumping
  - before moving object X81.8
    - motor vehicle X81.Ø
    - subway train X81.1
    - train X81.1
  - from high place X8Ø
- late effect of attempt — *see* categories X71-X83 with 7th character S
- lying before moving object, train, vehicle X81.8
- poisoning — *see* Table of Drugs and Chemicals
- puncture (any part of body) — *see* Suicide, cutting or piercing instrument
- scald — *see* Suicide, burning, hot object
- sequelae of attempt — *see* categories X71-X83 with 7th character S
- sharp object (any) — *see* Suicide, cutting or piercing instrument
- shooting — *see* Suicide, firearm
- specified means NEC X83.8
- stab (any part of body) — *see* Suicide, cutting or piercing instrument
- steam, hot vapors X77.Ø
- strangulation X83.8
- submersion — *see* Suicide, drowning
- suffocation X83.8
- wound NEC X83.8

Sunstroke X32

Supersonic waves (causing injury) W42.Ø

Surgical procedure, complication of (delayed or as an abnormal reaction without mention of misadventure) (*see also* Complication of or following, by type of procedure)
- due to or as a result of misadventure — *see* Misadventure

Swallowed, swallowing
- foreign body — *see* Foreign body, alimentary canal
- poison — *see* Table of Drugs and Chemicals
- substance
  - caustic or corrosive — *see* Table of Drugs and Chemicals
  - poisonous — *see* Table of Drugs and Chemicals

T

Tackle in sport WØ3

Terrorism (involving) Y38.8Ø
- biological weapons Y38.6X-
- chemical weapons Y38.7X-
- conflagration Y38.3X-
- explosion Y38.2X-
  - destruction of aircraft Y38.1X-
  - marine weapons Y38.Ø X-
- fire Y38.3X-
- firearms Y38.4X-
- hot substances Y38.5X-
- nuclear weapons Y38.5X-
- specified method NEC Y38.8X-

Thirst X58

Threat to breathing aspiration — *see* Aspiration
- due to cave-in, falling earth or substance NEC — *see* category T71

Thrown (accidentally)
- against part (any) of or object in transport vehicle (in motion) NEC (*see also* Accident, transport)
- from
  - high place, homicide (attempt) YØ1
  - machinery — *see* Contact, with, by type of machine
  - transport vehicle NEC (*see also* Accident, transport) V89.9
- off — *see* Thrown, from

Thunderbolt — *see* subcategory T75.Ø
- causing fire — *see* Exposure, fire

Tidal wave (any injury) NEC — *see* Forces of nature, tidal wave

Took
- overdose (drug) — *see* Table of Drugs and Chemicals
- poison — *see* Table of Drugs and Chemicals

Tornado (any injury) X37.1

Torrential rain (any injury) X37.8

Torture X58

Trampled by animal NEC W55.89

Trapped (accidentally)
- between objects (moving) (stationary and moving) — *see* Caught
- by part (any) of
  - motorcycle V29.88
  - pedal cycle V19.88
  - transport vehicle NEC (*see also* Accident, transport) V89.9

Travel (effects) (sickness) T75.3

Tree falling on or hitting (accidentally) (person) W2Ø.8

Tripping
- over
  - animal WØ1.Ø
    - with fall WØ1.Ø
  - carpet, rug or (small) object W22.8
    - with fall W18.Ø9
  - person W51
    - with fall WØ3
      - due to ice or snow WØØ.Ø
- without fall W18.4Ø
  - due to
    - specified NEC W18.49
    - stepping from one level to another W18.43
    - stepping into hole or opening W18.42
    - stepping on object W18.41

Twisted by person(s) (accidentally) W5Ø.2
- with intent to injure or kill YØ4.Ø
- as, or caused by, a crowd or human stampede (with fall) W52
- assault YØ4.Ø
- homicide (attempt) YØ4.Ø
- in
  - fight YØ4.Ø
  - legal intervention — *see* Legal, intervention, manhandling

Twisting, excessive — *see* Overexertion

U

Underdosing of necessary drugs, medicaments or biological substances Y63.61

Undetermined intent (contact) (exposure)
- automobile collision Y32
- blunt object Y29
- drowning (submersion) (in) Y21.9
  - bathtub Y21.Ø
    - after fall Y21.1
  - natural water (lake) (ocean) (pond) (river) (stream) Y21.4
  - specified place NEC Y21.8
  - swimming pool Y21.2
    - after fall Y21.3
- explosive material Y25
- fall, jump or push from high place Y3Ø
- falling, lying or running before moving object Y31
- fire Y26

Undetermined intent — *continued*
- firearm discharge Y24.9
  - airgun (BB) (pellet) Y24.Ø
  - handgun (pistol) (revolver) Y22
  - hunting rifle Y23.1
  - larger Y23.9
    - hunting rifle Y23.1
    - machine gun Y23.3
    - military Y23.2
    - shotgun Y23.Ø
    - specified type NEC Y23.8
  - machine gun Y23.3
  - military Y23.2
  - shotgun Y23.Ø
  - specified type NEC Y24.8
  - Very pistol Y24.8
- hot object Y27.9
  - fluid NEC Y27.2
  - household appliance Y27.3
  - specified object NEC Y27.8
  - steam Y27.Ø
  - tap water Y27.1
  - vapor Y27.Ø
- jump, fall or push from high place Y3Ø
- lying, falling or running before moving object Y31
- motor vehicle crash Y32
- push, fall or jump from high place Y3Ø
- running, falling or lying before moving object Y31
- sharp object Y28.9
  - dagger Y28.2
  - glass Y28.Ø
  - knife Y28.1
  - specified object NEC Y28.8
  - sword Y28.2
- smoke Y26
- specified event NEC Y33

V

Vibration (causing injury) W49.9

Victim (of)
- avalanche — *see* Landslide
- earth movements NEC — *see* Forces of nature, earth movement
- earthquake X34
- flood — *see* Flood
- landslide — *see* Landslide
- lightning — *see* subcategory T75.Ø
  - causing fire — *see* Exposure, fire
- storm (cataclysmic) NEC — *see* Forces of nature, cataclysmic storm
- volcanic eruption X35-

Volcanic eruption (any injury) X35

Vomitus, gastric contents in air passages (with asphyxia, obstruction or suffocation) T17.81-

W

Walked into stationary object (any) W22.Ø9
- furniture W22.Ø3
- lamppost W22.Ø2
- wall W22.Ø1

War operations (injuries to military personnel and civilians during war, civil insurrection and peacekeeping missions) (by) (from) (involving) Y36.9Ø-
- after cessation of hostilities Y36.89-
  - explosion (of)
    - bomb placed during war operations Y36.82
    - mine placed during war operations Y36.81-
  - specified NEC Y36.88-
- air blast Y36.2Ø-
- aircraft
  - destruction- *see* War operations, destruction of aircraft
- airway restriction — *see* War operations, restriction of airways
- asphyxiation — *see* War operations, restriction of airways
- biological weapons Y36.6X-

War operations — *continued*
- blast Y36.2Ø-
- blast fragments Y36.2Ø-
- blast wave Y36.2Ø-
- blast wind Y36.2Ø-
- bomb Y36.2Ø-
  - dirty Y36.5Ø-
  - gasoline Y36.31-
  - incendiary Y36.31-
  - petrol Y36.31-
- bullet Y36.43-
  - incendiary Y36.32-
  - rubber Y36.41-
- chemical weapons Y36.7X-
- combat
  - hand to hand (unarmed) combat Y36.44-
  - using blunt or piercing object Y36.45-
- conflagration — *see* War operations, fire
- conventional warfare NEC Y36.49-
- depth-charge Y36.Ø1-
- destruction of aircraft Y36.1Ø-
  - due to
    - air to air missile Y36.11-
    - collision with other aircraft Y36.12-
    - detonation (accidental) of onboard munitions and explosives Y36.14-
    - enemy fire or explosives Y36.11-
    - explosive placed on aircraft Y36.11-
    - onboard fire Y36.13-
    - rocket propelled grenade [RPG] Y36.11-
    - small arms fire Y36.11-
    - surface to air missile Y36.11-
  - specified NEC Y36.19-
- detonation (accidental) of
  - onboard marine weapons Y36.Ø5-
  - own munitions or munitions launch device Y36.24-
- dirty bomb Y36.5Ø-
- explosion (of) Y36.2Ø-
  - after cessation of hostilities
    - bomb placed during war operations Y36.82
    - mine placed during war operations Y36.81-
  - aerial bomb Y36.21-
  - bomb NOS Y36.2Ø (*see also* War operations, bomb(s))
  - own munitions or munitions launch device (accidental) Y36.24-
- fragments Y36.2Ø-
- grenade Y36.29-
- guided missile Y36.22-
- improvised explosive device [IED] (person-borne) (roadside) (vehicle-borne) Y36.23-
- land mine Y36.29-
- marine mine (at sea) (in harbor) Y36.Ø2-
- marine weapon Y36.ØØ-
  - specified NEC Y36.Ø9-
- sea-based artillery shell Y36.Ø3-
- specified NEC Y36.29-
- torpedo Y36.Ø4-
- fire Y36.3Ø-
  - specified NEC Y36.39-
- firearms
  - discharge Y36.43-
  - pellets Y36.42-
- flamethrower Y36.33-
- fragments (from) (of)
  - improvised explosive device [IED] (person-borne) (roadside) (vehicle-borne) Y36.26-
  - munitions Y36.25-
  - specified NEC Y36.29-
  - weapons Y36.27-
- friendly fire Y36.92-
- hand to hand (unarmed) combat Y36.44-
- hot substances — *see* War operations, fire
- incendiary bullet Y36.32-
- nuclear weapon (effects of) Y36.5Ø-
  - acute radiation exposure Y36.54-
  - blast pressure Y36.51-
  - direct blast Y36.51-
  - direct heat Y36.53-
  - fallout exposure Y36.54-
  - fireball Y36.53-
  - ionizing radiation (immediate exposure) Y36.54-

War operations — *continued*
- nuclear weapon — *continued*
  - nuclear radiation Y36.54-
  - radiation
    - ionizing (immediate exposure) Y36.54-
    - nuclear Y36.54-
    - thermal Y36.53-
  - specified NEC Y36.59-
  - secondary effects Y36.54-
  - thermal radiation Y36.53-
- restriction of air (airway)
  - intentional Y36.46-
  - unintentional Y36.47-
- rubber bullets Y36.41-
- shrapnel NOS Y36.29-
- suffocation — *see* War operations, restriction of airways
- unconventional warfare NEC Y36.7X-
- underwater blast NOS Y36.ØØ-
- warfare
  - conventional NEC Y36.49-
  - unconventional NEC Y36.7X-
- weapons
  - biological weapons Y36.6X-
  - chemical Y36.7X-
  - nuclear (effects of) Y36.5Ø-
    - acute radiation exposure Y36.54-
    - blast pressure Y36.51-
    - direct blast Y36.51-
    - direct heat Y36.53-
    - fallout exposure Y36.54-
    - fireball Y36.53-
    - indirect blast (struck or crushed by blast debris) (being thrown by blast) Y36.52-
    - radiation
      - ionizing (immediate exposure) Y36.54-
      - nuclear Y36.54-
      - thermal Y36.53-
    - secondary effects Y36.54-
    - specified NEC Y36.59-
  - of mass destruction [WMD] Y36.91-
- weapon of mass destruction [WMD] Y36.91-

Washed
- away by flood — *see* Flood
- off road by storm (transport vehicle) — *see* Forces of nature, cataclysmic storm

Weather exposure NEC - *see* Forces of nature

Weightlessness (causing injury) (effects of) (in spacecraft, real or simulated) X52

Work related condition Y99.Ø

Wound (accidental) **NEC** (*see also* Injury) X58
- battle (*see also* War operations) Y36.9Ø
- gunshot — *see* Discharge, firearm by type

Wreck transport vehicle NEC (*see also* Accident, transport) V89.9

Wrong
- device implanted into correct surgical site Y65.51
- fluid in infusion Y65.1
- procedure (operation) on correct patient Y65.51
- patient, procedure performed on Y65.52

ICD-10-CM Tabular List of Diseases and Injuries

Chapter 1. Certain Infectious and Parasitic Diseases (A00-B99)

INCLUDES diseases generally recognized as communicable or transmissible

Use additional code to identify resistance to antimicrobial drugs (Z16.-)

EXCLUDES 1 *certain localized infections—see body system-related chapters*
infectious and parasitic diseases complicating pregnancy, childbirth and the puerperium (O98.-)
influenza and other acute respiratory infections (J00-J22)

EXCLUDES 2 *carrier or suspected carrier of infectious disease (Z22.-)*
infectious and parasitic diseases specific to the perinatal period (P35-P39)

This chapter contains the following blocks:

A00-A09	Intestinal infectious diseases
A15-A19	Tuberculosis
A20-A28	Certain zoonotic bacterial diseases
A30-A49	Other bacterial diseases
A50-A64	Infections with a predominantly sexual mode of transmission
A65-A69	Other spirochetal diseases
A70-A74	Other diseases caused by chlamydiae
A75-A79	Rickettsioses
A80-A89	Viral infections of the central nervous system
A90-A99	Arthropod-borne viral fevers and viral hemorrhagic fevers
B00-B09	Viral infections characterized by skin and mucous membrane lesions
B10	Other human herpesviruses
B15-B19	Viral hepatitis
B20	Human immunodeficiency virus [HIV] disease
B25-B34	Other viral diseases
B35-B49	Mycoses
B50-B64	Protozoal diseases
B65-B83	Helminthiases
B85-B89	Pediculosis, acariasis and other infestations
B90-B94	Sequelae of infectious and parasitic diseases
B95-B97	Bacterial and viral infectious agents
B99	Other infectious diseases

Intestinal Infectious Diseases (A00-A09)

✓4th **A00 Cholera**

A00.0 Cholera due to Vibrio cholerae 01, biovar cholerae
Classical cholera

A00.1 Cholera due to Vibrio cholerae 01, biovar eltor
Cholera eltor

A00.9 Cholera, unspecified

✓4th **A01 Typhoid and paratyphoid fevers**

✓5th **A01.0 Typhoid fever**
Infection due to Salmonella typhi

A01.00 Typhoid fever, unspecified

A01.01 Typhoid meningitis

A01.02 Typhoid fever with heart involvement
Typhoid endocarditis
Typhoid myocarditis

A01.03 Typhoid pneumonia

A01.04 Typhoid arthritis

A01.05 Typhoid osteomyelitis

A01.09 Typhoid fever with other complications

A01.1 Paratyphoid fever A

A01.2 Paratyphoid fever B

A01.3 Paratyphoid fever C

A01.4 Paratyphoid fever, unspecified
Infection due to Salmonella paratyphi NOS

✓4th **A02 Other salmonella infections**

INCLUDES infection or foodborne intoxication due to any Salmonella species other than S. typhi and S. paratyphi

A02.0 Salmonella enteritis
Salmonellosis

A02.1 Salmonella sepsis

✓5th **A02.2 Localized salmonella infections**

A02.20 Localized salmonella infection, unspecified

A02.21 Salmonella meningitis

A02.22 Salmonella pneumonia

A02.23 Salmonella arthritis

A02.24 Salmonella osteomyelitis

A02.25 Salmonella pyelonephritis
Salmonella tubulo-interstitial nephropathy

A02.29 Salmonella with other localized infection

A02.8 Other specified salmonella infections

A02.9 Salmonella infection, unspecified

✓4th **A03 Shigellosis**

A03.0 Shigellosis due to Shigella dysenteriae
Group A shigellosis [Shiga-Kruse dysentery]

A03.1 Shigellosis due to Shigella flexneri
Group B shigellosis

A03.2 Shigellosis due to Shigella boydii
Group C shigellosis

A03.3 Shigellosis due to Shigella sonnei
Group D shigellosis

A03.8 Other shigellosis

A03.9 Shigellosis, unspecified
Bacillary dysentery NOS

✓4th **A04 Other bacterial intestinal infections**

EXCLUDES 1 *bacterial foodborne intoxications, NEC (A05.-)*
tuberculous enteritis (A18.32)

A04.0 Enteropathogenic Escherichia coli infection

A04.1 Enterotoxigenic Escherichia coli infection

A04.2 Enteroinvasive Escherichia coli infection

A04.3 Enterohemorrhagic Escherichia coli infection

A04.4 Other intestinal Escherichia coli infections
Escherichia coli enteritis NOS

A04.5 Campylobacter enteritis

A04.6 Enteritis due to Yersinia enterocolitica
EXCLUDES 1 *extraintestinal yersiniosis (A28.2)*

A04.7 Enterocolitis due to Clostridium difficile
Foodborne intoxication by Clostridium difficile
Pseudomembraneous colitis

A04.8 Other specified bacterial intestinal infections

A04.9 Bacterial intestinal infection, unspecified
Bacterial enteritis NOS

✓4th **A05 Other bacterial foodborne intoxications, not elsewhere classified**

EXCLUDES 1 *Clostridium difficile foodborne intoxication and infection (A04.7)*
Escherichia coli infection (A04.0-A04.4)
listeriosis (A32.-)
salmonella foodborne intoxication and infection (A02.-)
toxic effect of noxious foodstuffs (T61-T62)

A05.0 Foodborne staphylococcal intoxication

A05.1 Botulism food poisoning
Botulism NOS
Classical foodborne intoxication due to Clostridium botulinum
EXCLUDES 1 *infant botulism (A48.51)*
wound botulism (A48.52)

A05.2 Foodborne Clostridium perfringens [Clostridium welchii] intoxication
Enteritis necroticans
Pig-bel

A05.3 Foodborne Vibrio parahaemolyticus intoxication

A05.4 Foodborne Bacillus cereus intoxication

A05.5 Foodborne Vibrio vulnificus intoxication

A05.8 Other specified bacterial foodborne intoxications

A05.9 Bacterial foodborne intoxication, unspecified

✓4th **A06 Amebiasis**

INCLUDES infection due to Entamoeba histolytica

EXCLUDES 1 *other protozoal intestinal diseases (A07.-)*

EXCLUDES 2 *acanthamebiasis (B60.1-)*
Naegleriasis (B60.2)

A06.0 Acute amebic dysentery
Acute amebiasis
Intestinal amebiasis NOS

A06.1 Chronic intestinal amebiasis

A06.2 Amebic nondysenteric colitis

A06.3 Ameboma of intestine
Ameboma NOS

A06.4 Amebic liver abscess
Hepatic amebiasis

A06.5 Amebic lung abscess
Amebic abscess of lung (and liver)

A06.6 Amebic brain abscess
Amebic abscess of brain (and liver) (and lung)

A06.7 Cutaneous amebiasis

✓5th **A06.8 Amebic infection of other sites**

A06.81 Amebic cystitis

A06.82 Other amebic genitourinary infections
Amebic balanitis
Amebic vesiculitis
Amebic vulvovaginitis

A06.89 Other amebic infections
Amebic appendicitis
Amebic splenic abscess

A06.9 Amebiasis, unspecified

✓4th **A07 Other protozoal intestinal diseases**

A07.0 Balantidiasis
Balantidial dysentery

A07.1 Giardiasis [lambliasis]

A07.2 Cryptosporidiosis

A07.3 Isosporiasis
Infection due to Isospora belli and Isospora hominis
Intestinal coccidiosis
Isosporosis

A07.4 Cyclosporiasis

A07.8 Other specified protozoal intestinal diseases
Intestinal microsporidiosis
Intestinal trichomoniasis
Sarcocystosis
Sarcosporidiosis

A07.9 Protozoal intestinal disease, unspecified
Flagellate diarrhea
Protozoal colitis
Protozoal diarrhea
Protozoal dysentery

✓4th **A08 Viral and other specified intestinal infections**

EXCLUDES 1 *influenza with involvement of gastrointestinal tract (J09.X3, J10.2, J11.2)*

A08.0 Rotaviral enteritis

✓5th **A08.1 Acute gastroenteropathy due to Norwalk agent and other small round viruses**

A08.11 Acute gastroenteropathy due to Norwalk agent
Acute gastroenteropathy due to Norovirus
Acute gastroenteropathy due to Norwalk-like agent

A08.19 Acute gastroenteropathy due to other small round viruses
Acute gastroenteropathy due to small round virus [SRV] NOS

A08.2 Adenoviral enteritis

✓5th **A08.3 Other viral enteritis**

A08.31 Calicivirus enteritis

A08.32 Astrovirus enteritis

A08.39 Other viral enteritis
Coxsackie virus enteritis
Echovirus enteritis
Enterovirus enteritis NEC
Torovirus enteritis

A08.4 Viral intestinal infection, unspecified
Viral enteritis NOS
Viral gastroenteritis NOS
Viral gastroenteropathy NOS

A08.8 Other specified intestinal infections

A09 Infectious gastroenteritis and colitis, unspecified
Infectious colitis NOS
Infectious enteritis NOS
Infectious gastroenteritis NOS

EXCLUDES 1 *colitis NOS (K52.9)*
diarrhea NOS (R19.7)
enteritis NOS (K52.9)
gastroenteritis NOS (K52.9)
noninfective gastroenteritis and colitis, unspecified (K52.9)

Tuberculosis (A15-A19)

INCLUDES infections due to Mycobacterium tuberculosis and Mycobacterium bovis

EXCLUDES 1 *congenital tuberculosis (P37.0)*
nonspecific reaction to test for tuberculosis without active tuberculosis (R76.1-)
pneumoconiosis associated with tuberculosis, any type in A15 (J65)
positive PPD (R76.11)
positive tuberculin skin test without active tuberculosis (R76.11)
sequelae of tuberculosis (B90.-)
silicotuberculosis (J65)

✓4th **A15 Respiratory tuberculosis**

A15.0 Tuberculosis of lung
Tuberculous bronchiectasis
Tuberculous fibrosis of lung
Tuberculous pneumonia
Tuberculous pneumothorax

A15.4 Tuberculosis of intrathoracic lymph nodes
Tuberculosis of hilar lymph nodes
Tuberculosis of mediastinal lymph nodes
Tuberculosis of tracheobronchial lymph nodes

EXCLUDES 1 *tuberculosis specified as primary (A15.7)*

A15.5 Tuberculosis of larynx, trachea and bronchus
Tuberculosis of bronchus
Tuberculosis of glottis
Tuberculosis of larynx
Tuberculosis of trachea

A15.6 Tuberculous pleurisy
Tuberculosis of pleura Tuberculous empyema

EXCLUDES 1 *primary respiratory tuberculosis (A15.7)*

A15.7 Primary respiratory tuberculosis

A15.8 Other respiratory tuberculosis
Mediastinal tuberculosis
Nasopharyngeal tuberculosis
Tuberculosis of nose
Tuberculosis of sinus [any nasal]

A15.9 Respiratory tuberculosis unspecified

✓4th **A17 Tuberculosis of nervous system**

A17.0 Tuberculous meningitis
Tuberculosis of meninges (cerebral)(spinal)
Tuberculous leptomeningitis

EXCLUDES 1 *tuberculous meningoencephalitis (A17.82)*

A17.1 Meningeal tuberculoma
Tuberculoma of meninges (cerebral) (spinal)

EXCLUDES 2 *tuberculoma of brain and spinal cord (A17.81)*

✓5th **A17.8 Other tuberculosis of nervous system**

A17.81 Tuberculoma of brain and spinal cord
Tuberculous abscess of brain and spinal cord

A17.82 Tuberculous meningoencephalitis
Tuberculous myelitis

A17.83 Tuberculous neuritis
Tuberculous mononeuropathy

A17.89 Other tuberculosis of nervous system
Tuberculous polyneuropathy

A17.9 Tuberculosis of nervous system, unspecified

✓4th **A18 Tuberculosis of other organs**

✓5th **A18.0 Tuberculosis of bones and joints**

A18.01 Tuberculosis of spine
Pott's disease or curvature of spine
Tuberculous arthritis
Tuberculous osteomyelitis of spine
Tuberculous spondylitis

A18.02 Tuberculous arthritis of other joints
Tuberculosis of hip (joint)
Tuberculosis of knee (joint)

A18.03 Tuberculosis of other bones
Tuberculous mastoiditis
Tuberculous osteomyelitis

A18.09 Other musculoskeletal tuberculosis
Tuberculous myositis
Tuberculous synovitis
Tuberculous tenosynovitis

✓5th **A18.1 Tuberculosis of genitourinary system**

A18.10 Tuberculosis of genitourinary system, unspecified

A18.11 Tuberculosis of kidney and ureter

A18.12 Tuberculosis of bladder

A18.13 Tuberculosis of other urinary organs
Tuberculous urethritis

A18.14 Tuberculosis of prostate
A18.15 Tuberculosis of other male genital organs
A18.16 Tuberculosis of cervix
A18.17 Tuberculous female pelvic inflammatory disease
Tuberculous endometritis
Tuberculous oophoritis and salpingitis
A18.18 Tuberculosis of other female genital organs
Tuberculous ulceration of vulva

A18.2 Tuberculous peripheral lymphadenopathy
Tuberculous adenitis
EXCLUDES 2 *tuberculosis of bronchial and mediastinal lymph nodes (A15.4)*
tuberculosis of mesenteric and retroperitoneal lymph nodes (A18.39)
tuberculous tracheobronchial adenopathy (A15.4)

✓5th **A18.3 Tuberculosis of intestines, peritoneum and mesenteric glands**
A18.31 Tuberculous peritonitis
Tuberculous ascites
A18.32 Tuberculous enteritis
Tuberculosis of anus and rectum
Tuberculosis of intestine (large) (small)
A18.39 Retroperitoneal tuberculosis
Tuberculosis of mesenteric glands
Tuberculosis of retroperitoneal (lymph glands)

A18.4 Tuberculosis of skin and subcutaneous tissue
Erythema induratum, tuberculous
Lupus excedens
Lupus vulgaris NOS
Lupus vulgaris of eyelid
Scrofuloderma
Tuberculosis of external ear
EXCLUDES 2 *lupus erythematosus (L93.-)*
lupus NOS (M32.9)
systemic (M32.-)

✓5th **A18.5 Tuberculosis of eye**
EXCLUDES 2 *lupus vulgaris of eyelid (A18.4)*
A18.50 Tuberculosis of eye, unspecified
A18.51 Tuberculous episcleritis
A18.52 Tuberculous keratitis
Tuberculous interstitial keratitis
Tuberculous keratoconjunctivitis (interstitial) (phlyctenular)
A18.53 Tuberculous chorioretinitis
A18.54 Tuberculous iridocyclitis
A18.59 Other tuberculosis of eye
Tuberculous conjunctivitis

A18.6 Tuberculosis of (inner) (middle) ear
Tuberculous otitis media
EXCLUDES 2 *tuberculosis of external ear (A18.4)*
tuberculous mastoiditis (A18.03)

A18.7 Tuberculosis of adrenal glands
Tuberculous Addison's disease

✓5th **A18.8 Tuberculosis of other specified organs**
A18.81 Tuberculosis of thyroid gland
A18.82 Tuberculosis of other endocrine glands
Tuberculosis of pituitary gland
Tuberculosis of thymus gland
A18.83 Tuberculosis of digestive tract organs, not elsewhere classified
EXCLUDES 1 *tuberculosis of intestine (A18.32)*
A18.84 Tuberculosis of heart
Tuberculous cardiomyopathy
Tuberculous endocarditis
Tuberculous myocarditis
Tuberculous pericarditis
A18.85 Tuberculosis of spleen
A18.89 Tuberculosis of other sites
Tuberculosis of muscle
Tuberculous cerebral arteritis

✓4th **A19 Miliary tuberculosis**
INCLUDES disseminated tuberculosis
generalized tuberculosis
tuberculous polyserositis
A19.0 Acute miliary tuberculosis of a single specified site
A19.1 Acute miliary tuberculosis of multiple sites
A19.2 Acute miliary tuberculosis, unspecified
A19.8 Other miliary tuberculosis
A19.9 Miliary tuberculosis, unspecified

Certain zoonotic bacterial diseases (A20-A28)

✓4th **A20 Plague**
INCLUDES infection due to Yersinia pestis
A20.0 Bubonic plague
A20.1 Cellulocutaneous plague
A20.2 Pneumonic plague
A20.3 Plague meningitis
A20.7 Septicemic plague
A20.8 Other forms of plague
Abortive plague
Asymptomatic plague
Pestis minor
A20.9 Plague, unspecified

✓4th **A21 Tularemia**
INCLUDES deer-fly fever
infection due to Francisella tularensis
rabbit fever
A21.0 Ulceroglandular tularemia
A21.1 Oculoglandular tularemia
Ophthalmic tularemia
A21.2 Pulmonary tularemia
A21.3 Gastrointestinal tularemia
Abdominal tularemia
A21.7 Generalized tularemia
A21.8 Other forms of tularemia
A21.9 Tularemia, unspecified

✓4th **A22 Anthrax**
INCLUDES infection due to Bacillus anthracis
A22.0 Cutaneous anthrax
Malignant carbuncle
Malignant pustule
A22.1 Pulmonary anthrax
Inhalation anthrax
Ragpicker's disease
Woolsorter's disease
A22.2 Gastrointestinal anthrax
A22.7 Anthrax sepsis
A22.8 Other forms of anthrax
Anthrax meningitis
A22.9 Anthrax, unspecified

✓4th **A23 Brucellosis**
Malta fever
Mediterranean fever
Undulant fever
A23.0 Brucellosis due to Brucella melitensis
A23.1 Brucellosis due to Brucella abortus
A23.2 Brucellosis due to Brucella suis
A23.3 Brucellosis due to Brucella canis
A23.8 Other brucellosis
A23.9 Brucellosis, unspecified

✓4th **A24 Glanders and melioidosis**
A24.0 Glanders
Infection due to Pseudomonas mallei
Malleus
A24.1 Acute and fulminating melioidosis
Melioidosis pneumonia
Melioidosis sepsis
A24.2 Subacute and chronic melioidosis
A24.3 Other melioidosis
A24.9 Melioidosis, unspecified
Infection due to Pseudomonas pseudomallei NOS
Whitmore's disease

✓4th **A25 Rat-bite fevers**
A25.0 Spirillosis
Sodoku
A25.1 Streptobacillosis
Epidemic arthritic erythema
Haverhill fever
Streptobacillary rat-bite fever
A25.9 Rat-bite fever, unspecified

A26 Erysipeloid
- **A26.0 Cutaneous erysipeloid**
  - Erythema migrans
- **A26.7 Erysipelothrix sepsis**
- **A26.8 Other forms of erysipeloid**
- **A26.9 Erysipeloid, unspecified**

A27 Leptospirosis
- **A27.0 Leptospirosis icterohemorrhagica**
  - Leptospiral or spirochetal jaundice (hemorrhagic)
  - Weil's disease
- **A27.8 Other forms of leptospirosis**
  - **A27.81 Aseptic meningitis in leptospirosis**
  - **A27.89 Other forms of leptospirosis**
- **A27.9 Leptospirosis, unspecified**

A28 Other zoonotic bacterial diseases, not elsewhere classified
- **A28.0 Pasteurellosis**
- **A28.1 Cat-scratch disease**
  - Cat-scratch fever
- **A28.2 Extraintestinal yersiniosis**
  - EXCLUDES 1 *enteritis due to Yersinia enterocolitica (A04.6)*
  - *plague (A20.-)*
- **A28.8 Other specified zoonotic bacterial diseases, not elsewhere classified**
- **A28.9 Zoonotic bacterial disease, unspecified**

Other bacterial diseases (A30-A49)

A30 Leprosy [Hansen's disease]
- INCLUDES infection due to Mycobacterium leprae
- EXCLUDES 1 *sequelae of leprosy (B92)*
- **A30.0 Indeterminate leprosy**
  - I leprosy
- **A30.1 Tuberculoid leprosy**
  - TT leprosy
- **A30.2 Borderline tuberculoid leprosy**
  - BT leprosy
- **A30.3 Borderline leprosy**
  - BB leprosy
- **A30.4 Borderline lepromatous leprosy**
  - BL leprosy
- **A30.5 Lepromatous leprosy**
  - LL leprosy
- **A30.8 Other forms of leprosy**
- **A30.9 Leprosy, unspecified**

A31 Infection due to other mycobacteria
- EXCLUDES 2 *leprosy (A30.-)*
  - *tuberculosis (A15-A19)*
- **A31.0 Pulmonary mycobacterial infection**
  - Infection due to Mycobacterium avium
  - Infection due to Mycobacterium intracellulare [Battey bacillus]
  - Infection due to Mycobacterium kansasii
- **A31.1 Cutaneous mycobacterial infection**
  - Buruli ulcer
  - Infection due to Mycobacterium marinum
  - Infection due to Mycobacterium ulcerans
- **A31.2 Disseminated mycobacterium avium-intracellulare complex (DMAC)**
  - MAC sepsis
- **A31.8 Other mycobacterial infections**
- **A31.9 Mycobacterial infection, unspecified**
  - Atypical mycobacterial infection NOS
  - Mycobacteriosis NOS

A32 Listeriosis
- INCLUDES listerial foodborne infection
- EXCLUDES 1 *neonatal (disseminated) listeriosis (P37.2)*
- **A32.0 Cutaneous listeriosis**
- **A32.1 Listerial meningitis and meningoencephalitis**
  - **A32.11 Listerial meningitis**
  - **A32.12 Listerial meningoencephalitis**
- **A32.7 Listerial sepsis**
- **A32.8 Other forms of listeriosis**
  - **A32.81 Oculoglandular listeriosis**
  - **A32.82 Listerial endocarditis**
  - **A32.89 Other forms of listeriosis**
    - Listerial cerebral arteritis
- **A32.9 Listeriosis, unspecified**

A33 Tetanus neonatorum

A34 Obstetrical tetanus

A35 Other tetanus
- Tetanus NOS
- EXCLUDES 1 *obstetrical tetanus (A34)*
  - *tetanus neonatorum (A33)*

A36 Diphtheria
- **A36.0 Pharyngeal diphtheria**
  - Diphtheritic membranous angina
  - Tonsillar diphtheria
- **A36.1 Nasopharyngeal diphtheria**
- **A36.2 Laryngeal diphtheria**
  - Diphtheritic laryngotracheitis
- **A36.3 Cutaneous diphtheria**
  - EXCLUDES 2 *erythrasma (L08.1)*
- **A36.8 Other diphtheria**
  - **A36.81 Diphtheritic cardiomyopathy**
    - Diphtheritic myocarditis
  - **A36.82 Diphtheritic radiculomyelitis**
  - **A36.83 Diphtheritic polyneuritis**
  - **A36.84 Diphtheritic tubulo-interstitial nephropathy**
  - **A36.85 Diphtheritic cystitis**
  - **A36.86 Diphtheritic conjunctivitis**
  - **A36.89 Other diphtheritic complications**
    - Diphtheritic peritonitis
- **A36.9 Diphtheria, unspecified**

A37 Whooping cough
- **A37.0 Whooping cough due to Bordetella pertussis**
  - **A37.00 Whooping cough due to Bordetella pertussis without pneumonia**
  - **A37.01 Whooping cough due to Bordetella pertussis with pneumonia**
- **A37.1 Whooping cough due to Bordetella parapertussis**
  - **A37.10 Whooping cough due to Bordetella parapertussis without pneumonia**
  - **A37.11 Whooping cough due to Bordetella parapertussis with pneumonia**
- **A37.8 Whooping cough due to other Bordetella species**
  - **A37.80 Whooping cough due to other Bordetella species without pneumonia**
  - **A37.81 Whooping cough due to other Bordetella species with pneumonia**
- **A37.9 Whooping cough, unspecified species**
  - **A37.90 Whooping cough, unspecified species without pneumonia**
  - **A37.91 Whooping cough, unspecified species with pneumonia**

A38 Scarlet fever
- INCLUDES scarlatina
- EXCLUDES 2 *streptococcal sore throat (J02.0)*
- **A38.0 Scarlet fever with otitis media**
- **A38.1 Scarlet fever with myocarditis**
- **A38.8 Scarlet fever with other complications**
- **A38.9 Scarlet fever, uncomplicated**
  - Scarlet fever, NOS

A39 Meningococcal infection
- **A39.0 Meningococcal meningitis**
- **A39.1 Waterhouse-Friderichsen syndrome**
  - Meningococcal hemorrhagic adrenalitis
  - Meningococcic adrenal syndrome
- **A39.2 Acute meningococcemia**
- **A39.3 Chronic meningococcemia**
- **A39.4 Meningococcemia, unspecified**
- **A39.5 Meningococcal heart disease**
  - **A39.50 Meningococcal carditis, unspecified**
  - **A39.51 Meningococcal endocarditis**
  - **A39.52 Meningococcal myocarditis**
  - **A39.53 Meningococcal pericarditis**
- **A39.8 Other meningococcal infections**
  - **A39.81 Meningococcal encephalitis**
  - **A39.82 Meningococcal retrobulbar neuritis**
  - **A39.83 Meningococcal arthritis**
  - **A39.84 Postmeningococcal arthritis**

A39.89 Other meningococcal infections
Meningococcal conjunctivitis

A39.9 Meningococcal infection, unspecified
Meningococcal disease NOS

A40 Streptococcal sepsis
Code first: postprocedural streptococcal sepsis (T81.4)
streptococcal sepsis during labor (O75.3)
streptococcal sepsis following abortion or ectopic or molar pregnancy (O03-O07, O08.0)
streptococcal sepsis following immunization (T88.0)
streptococcal sepsis following infusion, transfusion or therapeutic injection (T80.2-)

EXCLUDES 1 *neonatal (P36.0-P36.1)*
puerperal sepsis (O85)
sepsis due to Streptococcus, group D (A41.81)

A40.0 Sepsis due to streptococcus, group A
A40.1 Sepsis due to streptococcus, group B
A40.3 Sepsis due to Streptococcus pneumoniae
Pneumococcal sepsis
A40.8 Other streptococcal sepsis
A40.9 Streptococcal sepsis, unspecified

A41 Other sepsis
Code first: postprocedural sepsis (T81.4)
sepsis during labor (O75.3)
sepsis following abortion, ectopic or molar pregnancy (O03-O07, O08.0)
sepsis following immunization (T88.0)
sepsis following infusion, transfusion or therapeutic injection (T80.2-)

EXCLUDES 1 *bacteremia NOS (R78.81)*
neonatal (P36.-)
puerperal sepsis (O85)
sepsis NOS (A41.9)
streptococcal sepsis (A40.-)

EXCLUDES 2 *sepsis (due to) (in) actinomycotic (A42.7)*
sepsis (due to) (in) anthrax (A22.7)
sepsis (due to) (in) candidal (B37.7)
sepsis (due to) (in) Erysipelothrix (A26.7)
sepsis (due to) (in) extraintestinal yersiniosis (A28.2)
sepsis (due to) (in) gonococcal (A54.86)
sepsis (due to) (in) herpesviral (B00.7)
sepsis (due to) (in) listerial (A32.7)
sepsis (due to) (in) melioidosis (A24.1)
sepsis (due to) (in) meningococcal (A39.2-A39.4)
sepsis (due to) (in) plague (A20.7)
sepsis (due to) (in) tularemia (A21.7)
toxic shock syndrome (A48.3)

A41.0 Sepsis due to Staphylococcus aureus
A41.01 Sepsis due to methicillin susceptible Staphylococcus aureus
MSSA sepsis
Staphylococcus aureus sepsis NOS
A41.02 Sepsis due to methicillin resistant Staphylococcus aureus
A41.1 Sepsis due to other specified staphylococcus
Coagulase negative staphylococcus sepsis
A41.2 Sepsis due to unspecified staphylococcus
A41.3 Sepsis due to Hemophilus influenzae
A41.4 Sepsis due to anaerobes
EXCLUDES 1 *gas gangrene (A48.0)*
A41.5 Sepsis due to other Gram-negative organisms
A41.50 Gram-negative sepsis, unspecified
Gram-negative sepsis NOS
A41.51 Sepsis due to Escherichia coli [E. coli]
A41.52 Sepsis due to Pseudomonas
Pseudomonas aeroginosa
A41.53 Sepsis due to Serratia
A41.59 Other Gram-negative sepsis
A41.8 Other specified sepsis
A41.81 Sepsis due to Enterococcus
A41.89 Other specified sepsis
A41.9 Sepsis, unspecified organism
Septicemia NOS

A42 Actinomycosis
EXCLUDES 1 *actinomycetoma (B47.1)*
A42.0 Pulmonary actinomycosis
A42.1 Abdominal actinomycosis
A42.2 Cervicofacial actinomycosis
A42.7 Actinomycotic sepsis
A42.8 Other forms of actinomycosis
A42.81 Actinomycotic meningitis
A42.82 Actinomycotic encephalitis
A42.89 Other forms of actinomycosis
A42.9 Actinomycosis, unspecified

A43 Nocardiosis
A43.0 Pulmonary nocardiosis
A43.1 Cutaneous nocardiosis
A43.8 Other forms of nocardiosis
A43.9 Nocardiosis, unspecified

A44 Bartonellosis
A44.0 Systemic bartonellosis
Oroya fever
A44.1 Cutaneous and mucocutaneous bartonellosis
Verruga peruana
A44.8 Other forms of bartonellosis
A44.9 Bartonellosis, unspecified

A46 Erysipelas
EXCLUDES 1 *postpartum or puerperal erysipelas (O86.89)*

A48 Other bacterial diseases, not elsewhere classified
EXCLUDES 1 *actinomycetoma (B47.1)*
A48.0 Gas gangrene
Clostridial cellulitis
Clostridial myonecrosis
A48.1 Legionnaires' disease
A48.2 Nonpneumonic Legionnaires' disease [Pontiac fever]
A48.3 Toxic shock syndrome
Use additional code to identify the organism (B95, B96)
EXCLUDES 1 *endotoxic shock NOS (R57.8)*
sepsis NOS (A41.9)
A48.4 Brazilian purpuric fever
Systemic Hemophilus aegyptius infection
A48.5 Other specified botulism
Non-foodborne intoxication due to toxins of Clostridium botulinum [C. botulinum]
EXCLUDES 1 *food poisoning due to toxins of Clostridium botulinum (A05.1)*
A48.51 Infant botulism
A48.52 Wound botulism
Non-foodborne botulism NOS
Use additional code for associated wound
A48.8 Other specified bacterial diseases

A49 Bacterial infection of unspecified site
EXCLUDES 1 *bacterial agents as the cause of diseases classified elsewhere (B95-B96)*
chlamydial infection NOS (A74.9)
meningococcal infection NOS (A39.9)
rickettsial infection NOS (A79.9)
spirochetal infection NOS (A69.9)
A49.0 Staphylococcal infection, unspecified site
A49.01 Methicillin susceptible Staphylococcus aureus infection, unspecified site
Methicillin susceptible Staphylococcus aureus (MSSA) infection
Staphylococcus aureus infection NOS
A49.02 Methicillin resistant Staphylococcus aureus infection, unspecified site
Methicillin resistant Staphylococcus aureus (MRSA) infection
A49.1 Streptococcal infection, unspecified site
A49.2 Hemophilus influenzae infection, unspecified site
A49.3 Mycoplasma infection, unspecified site
A49.8 Other bacterial infections of unspecified site
A49.9 Bacterial infection, unspecified
EXCLUDES 1 *bacteremia NOS (R78.81)*

Infections with a predominantly sexual mode of transmission (A50-A64)

EXCLUDES 1 *human immunodeficiency virus [HIV] disease (B20)*
nonspecific and nongonococcal urethritis (N34.1)
Reiter's disease (M02.3-)

A50 Congenital syphilis

A50.0 Early congenital syphilis, symptomatic
Any congenital syphilitic condition specified as early or manifest less than two years after birth.
A50.01 Early congenital syphilitic oculopathy
A50.02 Early congenital syphilitic osteochondropathy
A50.03 Early congenital syphilitic pharyngitis
Early congenital syphilitic laryngitis
A50.04 Early congenital syphilitic pneumonia
A50.05 Early congenital syphilitic rhinitis
A50.06 Early cutaneous congenital syphilis
A50.07 Early mucocutaneous congenital syphilis
A50.08 Early visceral congenital syphilis
A50.09 Other early congenital syphilis, symptomatic

A50.1 Early congenital syphilis, latent
Congenital syphilis without clinical manifestations, with positive serological reaction and negative spinal fluid test, less than two years after birth.

A50.2 Early congenital syphilis, unspecified
Congenital syphilis NOS less than two years after birth.

A50.3 Late congenital syphilitic oculopathy
EXCLUDES 1 *Hutchinson's triad (A50.53)*
A50.30 Late congenital syphilitic oculopathy, unspecified
A50.31 Late congenital syphilitic interstitial keratitis
A50.32 Late congenital syphilitic chorioretinitis
A50.39 Other late congenital syphilitic oculopathy

A50.4 Late congenital neurosyphilis [juvenile neurosyphilis]
Use additional code to identify any associated mental disorder
EXCLUDES 1 *Hutchinson's triad (A50.53)*
A50.40 Late congenital neurosyphilis, unspecified
Juvenile neurosyphilis NOS
A50.41 Late congenital syphilitic meningitis
A50.42 Late congenital syphilitic encephalitis
A50.43 Late congenital syphilitic polyneuropathy
A50.44 Late congenital syphilitic optic nerve atrophy
A50.45 Juvenile general paresis
Dementia paralytica juvenilis
Juvenile tabetoparetic neurosyphilis
A50.49 Other late congenital neurosyphilis
Juvenile tabes dorsalis

A50.5 Other late congenital syphilis, symptomatic
Any congenital syphilitic condition specified as late or manifest two years or more after birth.
A50.51 Clutton's joints
A50.52 Hutchinson's teeth
A50.53 Hutchinson's triad
A50.54 Late congenital cardiovascular syphilis
A50.55 Late congenital syphilitic arthropathy
A50.56 Late congenital syphilitic osteochondropathy
A50.57 Syphilitic saddle nose
A50.59 Other late congenital syphilis, symptomatic

A50.6 Late congenital syphilis, latent
Congenital syphilis without clinical manifestations, with positive serological reaction and negative spinal fluid test, two years or more after birth.

A50.7 Late congenital syphilis, unspecified
Congenital syphilis NOS two years or more after birth.

A50.9 Congenital syphilis, unspecified

A51 Early syphilis

A51.0 Primary genital syphilis
Syphilitic chancre NOS

A51.1 Primary anal syphilis

A51.2 Primary syphilis of other sites

A51.3 Secondary syphilis of skin and mucous membranes
A51.31 Condyloma latum
A51.32 Syphilitic alopecia
A51.39 Other secondary syphilis of skin
Syphilitic leukoderma
Syphilitic mucous patch
EXCLUDES 1 *late syphilitic leukoderma (A52.79)*

A51.4 Other secondary syphilis
A51.41 Secondary syphilitic meningitis
A51.42 Secondary syphilitic female pelvic disease
A51.43 Secondary syphilitic oculopathy
Secondary syphilitic chorioretinitis
Secondary syphilitic iridocyclitis, iritis
Secondary syphilitic uveitis
A51.44 Secondary syphilitic nephritis
A51.45 Secondary syphilitic hepatitis
A51.46 Secondary syphilitic osteopathy
A51.49 Other secondary syphilitic conditions
Secondary syphilitic lymphadenopathy
Secondary syphilitic myositis

A51.5 Early syphilis, latent
Syphilis (acquired) without clinical manifestations, with positive serological reaction and negative spinal fluid test, less than two years after infection.

A51.9 Early syphilis, unspecified

A52 Late syphilis

A52.0 Cardiovascular and cerebrovascular syphilis
A52.00 Cardiovascular syphilis, unspecified
A52.01 Syphilitic aneurysm of aorta
A52.02 Syphilitic aortitis
A52.03 Syphilitic endocarditis
Syphilitic aortic valve incompetence or stenosis
Syphilitic mitral valve stenosis
Syphilitic pulmonary valve regurgitation
A52.04 Syphilitic cerebral arteritis
A52.05 Other cerebrovascular syphilis
Syphilitic cerebral aneurysm (ruptured) (non-ruptured)
Syphilitic cerebral thrombosis
A52.06 Other syphilitic heart involvement
Syphilitic coronary artery disease
Syphilitic myocarditis
Syphilitic pericarditis
A52.09 Other cardiovascular syphilis

A52.1 Symptomatic neurosyphilis
A52.10 Symptomatic neurosyphilis, unspecified
A52.11 Tabes dorsalis
Locomotor ataxia (progressive)
Tabetic neurosyphilis
A52.12 Other cerebrospinal syphilis
A52.13 Late syphilitic meningitis
A52.14 Late syphilitic encephalitis
A52.15 Late syphilitic neuropathy
Late syphilitic acoustic neuritis
Late syphilitic optic (nerve) atrophy
Late syphilitic polyneuropathy
Late syphilitic retrobulbar neuritis
A52.16 Charcôt's arthropathy (tabetic)
A52.17 General paresis
Dementia paralytica
A52.19 Other symptomatic neurosyphilis
Syphilitic parkinsonism

A52.2 Asymptomatic neurosyphilis

A52.3 Neurosyphilis, unspecified
Gumma (syphilitic)
Syphilis (late)
Syphiloma

A52.7 Other symptomatic late syphilis
A52.71 Late syphilitic oculopathy
Late syphilitic chorioretinitis
Late syphilitic episcleritis
A52.72 Syphilis of lung and bronchus
A52.73 Symptomatic late syphilis of other respiratory organs
A52.74 Syphilis of liver and other viscera
Late syphilitic peritonitis
A52.75 Syphilis of kidney and ureter
Syphilitic glomerular disease
A52.76 Other genitourinary symptomatic late syphilis
Late syphilitic female pelvic inflammatory disease
A52.77 Syphilis of bone and joint

DRAFT

A52.78 **Syphilis of other musculoskeletal tissue**
Late syphilitic bursitis
Syphilis [stage unspecified] of bursa
Syphilis [stage unspecified] of muscle
Syphilis [stage unspecified] of synovium
Syphilis [stage unspecified] of tendon

A52.79 **Other symptomatic late syphilis**
Late syphilitic leukoderma
Syphilis of adrenal gland
Syphilis of pituitary gland
Syphilis of thyroid gland
Syphilitic splenomegaly
EXCLUDES 1 *syphilitic leukoderma (secondary) (A51.39)*

A52.8 **Late syphilis, latent**
Syphilis (acquired) without clinical manifestations, with positive serological reaction and negative spinal fluid test, two years or more after infection

A52.9 **Late syphilis, unspecified**

✓4th **A53 Other and unspecified syphilis**

A53.0 **Latent syphilis, unspecified as early or late**
Latent syphilis NOS
Positive serological reaction for syphilis

A53.9 **Syphilis, unspecified**
Infection due to Treponema pallidum NOS
Syphilis (acquired) NOS
EXCLUDES 1 *syphilis NOS under two years of age (A50.2)*

✓4th **A54 Gonococcal infection**

✓5th A54.0 **Gonococcal infection of lower genitourinary tract without periurethral or accessory gland abscess**
EXCLUDES 1 *gonococcal infection with genitourinary gland abscess (A54.1)*
gonococcal infection with periurethral abscess (A54.1)

A54.00 **Gonococcal infection of lower genitourinary tract, unspecified**
A54.01 **Gonococcal cystitis and urethritis, unspecified**
A54.02 **Gonococcal vulvovaginitis, unspecified**
A54.03 **Gonococcal cervicitis, unspecified**
A54.09 **Other gonococcal infection of lower genitourinary tract**

A54.1 **Gonococcal infection of lower genitourinary tract with periurethral and accessory gland abscess**
Gonococcal Bartholin's gland abscess

✓5th A54.2 **Gonococcal pelviperitonitis and other gonococcal genitourinary infection**
A54.21 **Gonococcal infection of kidney and ureter**
A54.22 **Gonococcal prostatitis**
A54.23 **Gonococcal infection of other male genital organs**
Gonococcal epididymitis
Gonococcal orchitis
A54.24 **Gonococcal female pelvic inflammatory disease**
Gonococcal pelviperitonitis
EXCLUDES 1 *gonococcal peritonitis (A54.85)*
A54.29 **Other gonococcal genitourinary infections**

✓5th A54.3 **Gonococcal infection of eye**
A54.30 **Gonococcal infection of eye, unspecified**
A54.31 **Gonococcal conjunctivitis**
Ophthalmia neonatorum due to gonococcus
A54.32 **Gonococcal iridocyclitis**
A54.33 **Gonococcal keratitis**
A54.39 **Other gonococcal eye infection**
Gonococcal endophthalmia

✓5th A54.4 **Gonococcal infection of musculoskeletal system**
A54.40 **Gonococcal infection of musculoskeletal system, unspecified**
A54.41 **Gonococcal spondylopathy**
A54.42 **Gonococcal arthritis**
EXCLUDES 2 *gonococcal infection of spine (A54.41)*
A54.43 **Gonococcal osteomyelitis**
EXCLUDES 2 *gonococcal infection of spine (A54.41)*
A54.49 **Gonococcal infection of other musculoskeletal tissue**
Gonococcal bursitis
Gonococcal myositis
Gonococcal synovitis
Gonococcal tenosynovitis

A54.5 **Gonococcal pharyngitis**

A54.6 **Gonococcal infection of anus and rectum**

✓5th A54.8 **Other gonococcal infections**
A54.81 **Gonococcal meningitis**
A54.82 **Gonococcal brain abscess**
A54.83 **Gonococcal heart infection**
Gonococcal endocarditis
Gonococcal myocarditis
Gonococcal pericarditis
A54.84 **Gonococcal pneumonia**
A54.85 **Gonococcal peritonitis**
EXCLUDES 1 *gonococcal pelviperitonitis (A54.24)*
A54.86 **Gonococcal sepsis**
A54.89 **Other gonococcal infections**
Gonococcal keratoderma
Gonococcal lymphadenitis

A54.9 **Gonococcal infection, unspecified**

A55 Chlamydial lymphogranuloma (venereum)
Climatic or tropical bubo
Durand-Nicolas-Favre disease
Esthiomene
Lymphogranuloma inguinale

✓4th **A56 Other sexually transmitted chlamydial diseases**
INCLUDES sexually transmitted diseases due to Chlamydia trachomatis
EXCLUDES 1 *neonatal chlamydial conjunctivitis (P39.1)*
neonatal chlamydial pneumonia (P23.1)
EXCLUDES 2 *chlamydial lymphogranuloma (A55)*
conditions classified to A74-

✓5th A56.0 **Chlamydial infection of lower genitourinary tract**
A56.00 **Chlamydial infection of lower genitourinary tract, unspecified**
A56.01 **Chlamydial cystitis and urethritis**
A56.02 **Chlamydial vulvovaginitis**
A56.09 **Other chlamydial infection of lower genitourinary tract**
Chlamydial cervicitis

✓5th A56.1 **Chlamydial infection of pelviperitoneum and other genitourinary organs**
A56.11 **Chlamydial female pelvic inflammatory disease**
A56.19 **Other chlamydial genitourinary infection**
Chlamydial epididymitis
Chlamydial orchitis

A56.2 **Chlamydial infection of genitourinary tract, unspecified**
A56.3 **Chlamydial infection of anus and rectum**
A56.4 **Chlamydial infection of pharynx**
A56.8 **Sexually transmitted chlamydial infection of other sites**

A57 Chancroid
Ulcus molle

A58 Granuloma inguinale
Donovanosis

✓4th **A59 Trichomoniasis**
EXCLUDES 2 *intestinal trichomoniasis (A07.8)*

✓5th A59.0 **Urogenital trichomoniasis**
A59.00 **Urogenital trichomoniasis, unspecified**
Fluor (vaginalis) due to Trichomonas
Leukorrhea (vaginalis) due to Trichomonas
A59.01 **Trichomonal vulvovaginitis**
A59.02 **Trichomonal prostatitis**
A59.03 **Trichomonal cystitis and urethritis**
A59.09 **Other urogenital trichomoniasis**
Trichomonas cervicitis

A59.8 **Trichomoniasis of other sites**
A59.9 **Trichomoniasis, unspecified**

✓4th **A60 Anogenital herpesviral [herpes simplex] infections**

✓5th A60.0 **Herpesviral infection of genitalia and urogenital tract**
A60.00 **Herpesviral infection of urogenital system, unspecified**
A60.01 **Herpesviral infection of penis**
A60.02 **Herpesviral infection of other male genital organs**
A60.03 **Herpesviral cervicitis**
A60.04 **Herpesviral vulvovaginitis**
Herpesviral [herpes simplex] ulceration
Herpesviral [herpes simplex] vaginitis
Herpesviral [herpes simplex] vulvitis
A60.09 **Herpesviral infection of other urogenital tract**

A60.1 Herpesviral infection of perianal skin and rectum

A60.9 Anogenital herpesviral infection, unspecified

✓4th **A63 Other predominantly sexually transmitted diseases, not elsewhere classified**

EXCLUDES 2 *molluscum contagiosum (B08.1)*
papilloma of cervix (D26.0)

A63.0 Anogenital (venereal) warts
Anogenital warts due to (human) papillomavirus [HPV]
Condyloma acuminatum

A63.8 Other specified predominantly sexually transmitted diseases

A64 Unspecified sexually transmitted disease

Other spirochetal diseases (A65-A69)

EXCLUDES 2 *leptospirosis (A27.-)*
syphilis (A50-A53)

A65 Nonvenereal syphilis
Bejel
Endemic syphilis
Njovera

✓4th **A66 Yaws**

INCLUDES bouba
frambesia (tropica)
pian

A66.0 Initial lesions of yaws
Chancre of yaws
Frambesia, initial or primary
Initial frambesial ulcer
Mother yaw

A66.1 Multiple papillomata and wet crab yaws
Frambesioma
Pianoma
Plantar or palmar papilloma of yaws

A66.2 Other early skin lesions of yaws
Cutaneous yaws, less than five years after infection
Early yaws (cutaneous) (macular) (maculopapular) (micropapular) (papular)
Frambeside of early yaws

A66.3 Hyperkeratosis of yaws
Ghoul hand
Hyperkeratosis, palmar or plantar (early) (late) due to yaws
Worm-eaten soles

A66.4 Gummata and ulcers of yaws
Gummatous frambeside
Nodular late yaws (ulcerated)

A66.5 Gangosa
Rhinopharyngitis mutilans

A66.6 Bone and joint lesions of yaws
Yaws ganglion
Yaws goundou
Yaws gumma, bone
Yaws gummatous osteitis or periostitis
Yaws hydrarthrosis
Yaws osteitis
Yaws periostitis (hypertrophic)

A66.7 Other manifestations of yaws
Juxta-articular nodules of yaws
Mucosal yaws

A66.8 Latent yaws
Yaws without clinical manifestations, with positive serology

A66.9 Yaws, unspecified

✓4th **A67 Pinta [carate]**

A67.0 Primary lesions of pinta
Chancre (primary) of pinta
Papule (primary) of pinta

A67.1 Intermediate lesions of pinta
Erythematous plaques of pinta
Hyperchromic lesions of pinta
Hyperkeratosis of pinta
Pintids

A67.2 Late lesions of pinta
Achromic skin lesions of pinta
Cicatricial skin lesions of pinta
Dyschromic skin lesions of pinta

A67.3 Mixed lesions of pinta
Achromic with hyperchromic skin lesions of pinta [carate]

A67.9 Pinta, unspecified

✓4th **A68 Relapsing fevers**

INCLUDES recurrent fever

EXCLUDES 2 *Lyme disease (A69.2-)*

A68.0 Louse-borne relapsing fever
Relapsing fever due to Borrelia recurrentis

A68.1 Tick-borne relapsing fever
Relapsing fever due to any Borrelia species other than Borrelia recurrentis

A68.9 Relapsing fever, unspecified

✓4th **A69 Other spirochetal infections**

A69.0 Necrotizing ulcerative stomatitis
Cancrum oris
Fusospirochetal gangrene
Noma
Stomatitis gangrenosa

A69.1 Other Vincent's infections
Fusospirochetal pharyngitis
Necrotizing ulcerative (acute) gingivitis
Necrotizing ulcerative (acute) gingivostomatitis
Spirochetal stomatitis
Trench mouth
Vincent's angina
Vincent's gingivitis

✓5th **A69.2 Lyme disease**
Erythema chronicum migrans due to Borrelia burgdorferi

A69.20 Lyme disease, unspecified

A69.21 Meningitis due to Lyme disease

A69.22 Other neurologic disorders in Lyme disease
Cranial neuritis
Meningoencephalitis
Polyneuropathy

A69.23 Arthritis due to Lyme disease

A69.29 Other conditions associated with Lyme disease
Myopericarditis due to Lyme disease

A69.8 Other specified spirochetal infections

A69.9 Spirochetal infection, unspecified

Other diseases caused by chlamydiae (A70-A74)

EXCLUDES 1 *sexually transmitted chlamydial diseases (A55-A56)*

A70 Chlamydia psittaci infections
Ornithosis
Parrot fever
Psittacosis

✓4th **A71 Trachoma**

EXCLUDES 1 *sequelae of trachoma (B94.0)*

A71.0 Initial stage of trachoma
Trachoma dubium

A71.1 Active stage of trachoma
Granular conjunctivitis (trachomatous)
Trachomatous follicular conjunctivitis
Trachomatous pannus

A71.9 Trachoma, unspecified

✓4th **A74 Other diseases caused by chlamydiae**

EXCLUDES 1 *neonatal chlamydial conjunctivitis (P39.1)*
neonatal chlamydial pneumonia (P23.1)
Reiter's disease (M02.3-)
sexually transmitted chlamydial diseases (A55-A56)

EXCLUDES 2 *chlamydial pneumonia (J16.0)*

A74.0 Chlamydial conjunctivitis
Paratrachoma

✓5th **A74.8 Other chlamydial diseases**

A74.81 Chlamydial peritonitis

A74.89 Other chlamydial diseases

A74.9 Chlamydial infection, unspecified
Chlamydiosis NOS

Rickettsioses (A75-A79)

✓4th **A75 Typhus fever**

EXCLUDES 1 *rickettsiosis due to Ehrlichia sennetsu (A79.81)*

A75.0 Epidemic louse-borne typhus fever due to Rickettsia prowazekii
Classical typhus (fever)
Epidemic (louse-borne) typhus

A75.1 Recrudescent typhus [Brill's disease]
Brill-Zinsser disease

A75.2 Typhus fever due to Rickettsia typhi
Murine (flea-borne) typhus

A75.3 Typhus fever due to Rickettsia tsutsugamushi
Scrub (mite-borne) typhus
Tsutsugamushi fever

A75.9 Typhus fever, unspecified
Typhus (fever) NOS

√4th **A77 Spotted fever [tick-borne rickettsioses]**

A77.0 Spotted fever due to Rickettsia rickettsii
Rocky Mountain spotted fever
Sao Paulo fever

A77.1 Spotted fever due to Rickettsia conorii
African tick typhus
Boutonneuse fever
India tick typhus
Kenya tick typhus
Marseilles fever
Mediterranean tick fever

A77.2 Spotted fever due to Rickettsia siberica
North Asian tick fever
Siberian tick typhus

A77.3 Spotted fever due to Rickettsia australis
Queensland tick typhus

√5th **A77.4 Ehrlichiosis**
EXCLUDES 1 *Rickettsiosis due to Ehrlichia sennetsu (A79.81)*

A77.40 Ehrlichiosis, unspecified
A77.41 Ehrlichiosis chafeensis [E. chafeensis]
A77.49 Other ehrlichiosis

A77.8 Other spotted fevers

A77.9 Spotted fever, unspecified
Tick-borne typhus NOS

A78 Q fever
Infection due to Coxiella burnetii
Nine Mile fever
Quadrilateral fever

√4th **A79 Other rickettsioses**

A79.0 Trench fever
Quintan fever
Wolhynian fever

A79.1 Rickettsialpox due to Rickettsia akari
Kew Garden fever
Vesicular rickettsiosis

√5th **A79.8 Other specified rickettsioses**

A79.81 Rickettsiosis due to Ehrlichia sennetsu
A79.89 Other specified rickettsioses

A79.9 Rickettsiosis, unspecified
Rickettsial infection NOS

Viral and prion infections of the central nervous system (A80-A89)

EXCLUDES 1 *postpolio syndrome (G14)*
sequelae of poliomyelitis (B91)
sequelae of viral encephalitis (B94.1)

√4th **A80 Acute poliomyelitis**

A80.0 Acute paralytic poliomyelitis, vaccine-associated
A80.1 Acute paralytic poliomyelitis, wild virus, imported
A80.2 Acute paralytic poliomyelitis, wild virus, indigenous

√5th **A80.3 Acute paralytic poliomyelitis, other and unspecified**

A80.30 Acute paralytic poliomyelitis, unspecified
A80.39 Other acute paralytic poliomyelitis

A80.4 Acute nonparalytic poliomyelitis
A80.9 Acute poliomyelitis, unspecified

√4th **A81 Atypical virus infections of central nervous system**
INCLUDES diseases of the central nervous system caused by prions
Use additional code to identify:
dementia with behavioral disturbance (F02.81)
dementia without behavioral disturbance (F02.80)

√5th **A81.0 Creutzfeldt-Jakob disease**

A81.00 Creutzfeldt-Jakob disease, unspecified
Jakob-Creutzfeldt disease, unspecified

A81.01 Variant Creutzfeldt-Jakob disease
vCJD

A81.09 Other Creutzfeldt-Jakob disease
CJD
Familial Creutzfeldt-Jakob disease
Iatrogenic Creutzfeldt-Jakob disease
Sporadic Creutzfeldt-Jakob disease
Subacute spongiform encephalopathy (with dementia)

A81.1 Subacute sclerosing panencephalitis
Dawson's inclusion body encephalitis
Van Bogaert's sclerosing leukoencephalopathy

A81.2 Progressive multifocal leukoencephalopathy
Multifocal leukoencephalopathy NOS

√5th **A81.8 Other atypical virus infections of central nervous system**

A81.81 Kuru

A81.82 Gerstmann-Sträussler-Scheinker syndrome
GSS syndrome

A81.83 Fatal familial insomnia
FFI

A81.89 Other atypical virus infections of central nervous system

A81.9 Atypical virus infection of central nervous system, unspecified
Prion diseases of the central nervous system NOS

√4th **A82 Rabies**

A82.0 Sylvatic rabies
A82.1 Urban rabies
A82.9 Rabies, unspecified

√4th **A83 Mosquito-borne viral encephalitis**
INCLUDES mosquito-borne viral meningoencephalitis
EXCLUDES 2 *Venezuelan equine encephalitis (A92.2)*
West Nile fever (A92.3-)
West Nile virus (A92.3-)

A83.0 Japanese encephalitis
A83.1 Western equine encephalitis
A83.2 Eastern equine encephalitis
A83.3 St Louis encephalitis

A83.4 Australian encephalitis
Kunjin virus disease

A83.5 California encephalitis
California meningoencephalitis
La Crosse encephalitis

A83.6 Rocio virus disease
A83.8 Other mosquito-borne viral encephalitis
A83.9 Mosquito-borne viral encephalitis, unspecified

√4th **A84 Tick-borne viral encephalitis**
INCLUDES tick-borne viral meningoencephalitis

A84.0 Far Eastern tick-borne encephalitis [Russian spring-summer encephalitis]
A84.1 Central European tick-borne encephalitis

A84.8 Other tick-borne viral encephalitis
Louping ill
Powassan virus disease

A84.9 Tick-borne viral encephalitis, unspecified

√4th **A85 Other viral encephalitis, not elsewhere classified**
INCLUDES specified viral encephalomyelitis NEC
specified viral meningoencephalitis NEC
EXCLUDES 1 *benign myalgic encephalomyelitis (G93.3)*
encephalitis due to:
cytomegalovirus (B25.8)
herpesvirus NEC (B10.0-)
herpesvirus [herpes simplex] (B00.4)
measles virus (B05.0)
mumps virus (B26.2)
poliomyelitis virus (A80.-)
zoster (B02.0)
lymphocytic choriomeningitis (A87.2)

A85.0 Enteroviral encephalitis
Enteroviral encephalomyelitis

A85.1 Adenoviral encephalitis
Adenoviral meningoencephalitis

A85.2 Arthropod-borne viral encephalitis, unspecified
EXCLUDES 1 *West nile virus with encephalitis (A92.31)*

A85.8 Other specified viral encephalitis
Encephalitis lethargica
Von Economo-Cruchet disease

A86 Unspecified viral encephalitis
Viral encephalomyelitis NOS
Viral meningoencephalitis NOS

✓4th **A87 Viral meningitis**
EXCLUDES 1 *meningitis due to herpesvirus [herpes simplex] (B00.3)*
meningitis due to measles virus (B05.1)
meningitis due to mumps virus (B26.1)
meningitis due to poliomyelitis virus (A80.-)
meningitis due to zoster (B02.1)

A87.0 Enteroviral meningitis
Coxsackievirus meningitis
Echovirus meningitis

A87.1 Adenoviral meningitis

A87.2 Lymphocytic choriomeningitis
Lymphocytic meningoencephalitis

A87.8 Other viral meningitis

A87.9 Viral meningitis, unspecified

✓4th **A88 Other viral infections of central nervous system, not elsewhere classified**
EXCLUDES 1 *viral encephalitis NOS (A86)*
viral meningitis NOS (A87.9)

A88.0 Enteroviral exanthematous fever [Boston exanthem]

A88.1 Epidemic vertigo

A88.8 Other specified viral infections of central nervous system

A89 Unspecified viral infection of central nervous system

Arthropod-borne viral fevers and viral hemorrhagic fevers (A90-A99)

A90 Dengue fever [classical dengue]
EXCLUDES 1 *dengue hemorrhagic fever (A91)*

A91 Dengue hemorrhagic fever

✓4th **A92 Other mosquito-borne viral fevers**
EXCLUDES 1 *Ross River disease (B33.1)*

A92.0 Chikungunya virus disease
Chikungunya (hemorrhagic) fever

A92.1 O'nyong-nyong fever

A92.2 Venezuelan equine fever
Venezuelan equine encephalitis
Venezuelan equine encephalomyelitis virus disease

✓5th **A92.3 West Nile virus infection**
West Nile fever

A92.30 West Nile virus infection, unspecified
West Nile fever NOS
West Nile fever without complications
West Nile virus NOS

A92.31 West Nile virus infection with encephalitis
West Nile encephalitis
West Nile encephalomyelitis

A92.32 West Nile virus infection with other neurologic manifestation
Use additional code to specify the neurologic manifestation

A92.39 West Nile virus infection with other complications
Use additional code to specify the other conditions

A92.4 Rift Valley fever

A92.8 Other specified mosquito-borne viral fevers

A92.9 Mosquito-borne viral fever, unspecified

✓4th **A93 Other arthropod-borne viral fevers, not elsewhere classified**

A93.0 Oropouche virus disease
Oropouche fever

A93.1 Sandfly fever
Pappataci fever
Phlebotomus fever

A93.2 Colorado tick fever

A93.8 Other specified arthropod-borne viral fevers
Piry virus disease
Vesicular stomatitis virus disease [Indiana fever]

A94 Unspecified arthropod-borne viral fever
Arboviral fever NOS
Arbovirus infection NOS

✓4th **A95 Yellow fever**

A95.0 Sylvatic yellow fever
Jungle yellow fever

A95.1 Urban yellow fever

A95.9 Yellow fever, unspecified

✓4th **A96 Arenaviral hemorrhagic fever**

A96.0 Junin hemorrhagic fever
Argentinian hemorrhagic fever

A96.1 Machupo hemorrhagic fever
Bolivian hemorrhagic fever

A96.2 Lassa fever

A96.8 Other arenaviral hemorrhagic fevers

A96.9 Arenaviral hemorrhagic fever, unspecified

✓4th **A98 Other viral hemorrhagic fevers, not elsewhere classified**
EXCLUDES 1 *chikungunya hemorrhagic fever (A92.0)*
dengue hemorrhagic fever (A91)

A98.0 Crimean-Congo hemorrhagic fever
Central Asian hemorrhagic fever

A98.1 Omsk hemorrhagic fever

A98.2 Kyasanur Forest disease

A98.3 Marburg virus disease

A98.4 Ebola virus disease

A98.5 Hemorrhagic fever with renal syndrome
Epidemic hemorrhagic fever
Korean hemorrhagic fever
Russian hemorrhagic fever
Hantaan virus disease
Hantavirus disease with renal manifestations
Nephropathia epidemica
Songo fever
EXCLUDES 1 *hantavirus (cardio)-pulmonary syndrome (B33.4)*

A98.8 Other specified viral hemorrhagic fevers

A99 Unspecified viral hemorrhagic fever

Viral infections characterized by skin and mucous membrane lesions (B00-B09)

✓4th **B00 Herpesviral [herpes simplex] infections**
EXCLUDES 1 *congenital herpesviral infections (P35.2)*
EXCLUDES 2 *anogenital herpesviral infection (A60.-)*
gammaherpesviral mononucleosis (B27.0-)
herpangina (B08.5)

B00.0 Eczema herpeticum
Kaposi's varicelliform eruption

B00.1 Herpesviral vesicular dermatitis
Herpes simplex facialis
Herpes simplex labialis
Herpes simplex otitis externa
Vesicular dermatitis of ear
Vesicular dermatitis of lip

B00.2 Herpesviral gingivostomatitis and pharyngotonsillitis
Herpesviral pharyngitis

B00.3 Herpesviral meningitis

B00.4 Herpesviral encephalitis
Herpesviral meningoencephalitis
Simian B disease
EXCLUDES 1 *herpesviral encephalitis due to herpesvirus 6 and 7 (B10.01, B10.09)*
non-simplex herpesviral encephalitis (B10.0-)

✓5th **B00.5 Herpesviral ocular disease**

B00.50 Herpesviral ocular disease, unspecified

B00.51 Herpesviral iridocyclitis
Herpesviral iritis
Herpesviral uveitis, anterior

B00.52 Herpesviral keratitis
Herpesviral keratoconjunctivitis

B00.53 Herpesviral conjunctivitis

B00.59 Other herpesviral disease of eye
Herpesviral dermatitis of eyelid

B00.7 Disseminated herpesviral disease
Herpesviral sepsis

✓5th **B00.8 Other forms of herpesviral infections**

B00.81 Herpesviral hepatitis

B00.82 Herpes simplex myelitis

B00.89 Other herpesviral infection
Herpesviral whitlow

B00.9 Herpesviral infection, unspecified
Herpes simplex infection NOS

✓4th **B01 Varicella [chickenpox]**

B01.0 Varicella meningitis

✓5th **B01.1 Varicella encephalitis, myelitis and encephalomyelitis**
Postchickenpox encephalitis, myelitis and encephalomyelitis
B01.11 Varicella encephalitis and encephalomyelitis
Postchickenpox encephalitis and encephalomyelitis
B01.12 Varicella myelitis
Postchickenpox myelitis
B01.2 Varicella pneumonia
✓5th **B01.8 Varicella with other complications**
B01.81 Varicella keratitis
B01.89 Other varicella complications
B01.9 Varicella without complication
Varicella NOS

✓4th **B02 Zoster [herpes zoster]**
INCLUDES shingles
zona
B02.0 Zoster encephalitis
Zoster meningoencephalitis
B02.1 Zoster meningitis
✓5th **B02.2 Zoster with other nervous system involvement**
B02.21 Postherpetic geniculate ganglionitis
B02.22 Postherpetic trigeminal neuralgia
B02.23 Postherpetic polyneuropathy
B02.24 Postherpetic myelitis
Herpes zoster myelitis
B02.29 Other postherpetic nervous system involvement
Postherpetic radiculopathy
✓5th **B02.3 Zoster ocular disease**
B02.30 Zoster ocular disease, unspecified
B02.31 Zoster conjunctivitis
B02.32 Zoster iridocyclitis
B02.33 Zoster keratitis
Herpes zoster keratoconjunctivitis
B02.34 Zoster scleritis
B02.39 Other herpes zoster eye disease
Zoster blepharitis
B02.7 Disseminated zoster
B02.8 Zoster with other complications
Herpes zoster otitis externa
B02.9 Zoster without complications
Zoster NOS

B03 Smallpox
NOTE In 1980 the 33rd World Health Assembly declared that smallpox had been eradicated.
The classification is maintained for surveillance purposes.

B04 Monkeypox

✓4th **B05 Measles**
INCLUDES morbilli
EXCLUDES 1 *subacute sclerosing panencephalitis (A81.1)*
B05.0 Measles complicated by encephalitis
Postmeasles encephalitis
B05.1 Measles complicated by meningitis
Postmeasles meningitis
B05.2 Measles complicated by pneumonia
Postmeasles pneumonia
B05.3 Measles complicated by otitis media
Postmeasles otitis media
B05.4 Measles with intestinal complications
✓5th **B05.8 Measles with other complications**
B05.81 Measles keratitis and keratoconjunctivitis
B05.89 Other measles complications
B05.9 Measles without complication
Measles NOS

✓4th **B06 Rubella [German measles]**
EXCLUDES 1 *congenital rubella (P35.0)*
✓5th **B06.0 Rubella with neurological complications**
B06.00 Rubella with neurological complication, unspecified
B06.01 Rubella encephalitis
Rubella meningoencephalitis
B06.02 Rubella meningitis
B06.09 Other neurological complications of rubella
✓5th **B06.8 Rubella with other complications**
B06.81 Rubella pneumonia
B06.82 Rubella arthritis
B06.89 Other rubella complications
B06.9 Rubella without complication
Rubella NOS

✓4th **B07 Viral warts**
INCLUDES verruca simplex
verruca vulgaris
viral warts due to human papillomavirus
EXCLUDES 2 *anogenital (venereal) warts (A63.0)*
papilloma of bladder (D41.4)
papilloma of cervix (D26.0)
papilloma larynx (D14.1)
B07.0 Plantar wart
Verruca plantaris
B07.8 Other viral warts
Common wart
Flat wart
Verruca plana
B07.9 Viral wart, unspecified

✓4th **B08 Other viral infections characterized by skin and mucous membrane lesions, not elsewhere classified**
EXCLUDES 1 *vesicular stomatitis virus disease (A93.8)*
✓5th **B08.0 Other orthopoxvirus infections**
EXCLUDES 2 *monkeypox (B04)*
✓6th **B08.01 Cowpox and vaccinia not from vaccine**
B08.010 Cowpox
B08.011 Vaccinia not from vaccine
EXCLUDES 1 *vaccinia (from vaccination) (generalized) (T88.1)*
B08.02 Orf virus disease
Contagious pustular dermatitis
Ecthyma contagiosum
B08.03 Pseudocowpox [milker's node]
B08.04 Paravaccinia, unspecified
B08.09 Other orthopoxvirus infections
Orthopoxvirus infection NOS
B08.1 Molluscum contagiosum
✓5th **B08.2 Exanthema subitum [sixth disease]**
Roseola infantum
B08.20 Exanthema subitum [sixth disease], unspecified
Roseola infantum, unspecified
B08.21 Exanthema subitum [sixth disease] due to human herpesvirus 6
Roseola infantum due to human herpesvirus 6
B08.22 Exanthema subitum [sixth disease] due to human herpesvirus 7
Roseola infantum due to human herpesvirus 7
B08.3 Erythema infectiosum [fifth disease]
B08.4 Enteroviral vesicular stomatitis with exanthem
Hand, foot and mouth disease
B08.5 Enteroviral vesicular pharyngitis
Herpangina
✓5th **B08.6 Parapoxvirus infections**
B08.60 Parapoxvirus infection, unspecified
B08.61 Bovine stomatitis
B08.62 Sealpox
B08.69 Other parapoxvirus infections
✓5th **B08.7 Yatapoxvirus infections**
B08.70 Yatapoxvirus infection, unspecified
B08.71 Tanapox virus disease
B08.72 Yaba pox virus disease
Yaba monkey tumor disease
B08.79 Other yatapoxvirus infections
B08.8 Other specified viral infections characterized by skin and mucous membrane lesions
Enteroviral lymphonodular pharyngitis
Foot-and-mouth disease
Poxvirus NEC

B09 Unspecified viral infection characterized by skin and mucous membrane lesions
Viral enanthema NOS
Viral exanthema NOS

DRAFT

Other human herpesviruses (B10)

✓4th B10 Other human herpesviruses

EXCLUDES 2 *cytomegalovirus (B25.9)*
Epstein-Barr virus (B27.0-)
herpes NOS (B00.9)
herpes simplex (B00.-)
herpes zoster (B02.-)
human herpesvirus NOS (B00.-)
human herpesvirus 1 and 2 (B00.-)
human herpesvirus 3 (B01.-, B02.-)
human herpesvirus 4 (B27.0-)
human herpesvirus 5 (B25.-)
varicella (B01.-)
zoster (B02.-)

✓5th **B10.0 Other human herpesvirus encephalitis**

EXCLUDES 2 *herpes encephalitis NOS (B00.4)*
herpes simplex encephalitis (B00.4)
human herpesvirus encephalitis (B00.4)
simian B herpes virus encephalitis (B00.4)

B10.01 Human herpesvirus 6 encephalitis
B10.09 Other human herpesvirus encephalitis
Human herpesvirus 7 encephalitis

✓5th **B10.8 Other human herpesvirus infection**
B10.81 Human herpesvirus 6 infection
B10.82 Human herpesvirus 7 infection
B10.89 Other human herpesvirus infection
Human herpesvirus 8 infection
Kaposi's sarcoma-associated herpesvirus infection

Viral hepatitis (B15-B19)

EXCLUDES 1 *sequelae of viral hepatitis (B94.2)*
EXCLUDES 2 *cytomegaloviral hepatitis (B25.1)*
herpesviral [herpes simplex] hepatitis (B00.81)

✓4th B15 Acute hepatitis A
B15.0 Hepatitis A with hepatic coma
B15.9 Hepatitis A without hepatic coma
Hepatitis A (acute)(viral) NOS

✓4th B16 Acute hepatitis B
B16.0 Acute hepatitis B with delta-agent with hepatic coma
B16.1 Acute hepatitis B with delta-agent without hepatic coma
B16.2 Acute hepatitis B without delta-agent with hepatic coma
B16.9 Acute hepatitis B without delta-agent and without hepatic coma
Hepatitis B (acute) (viral) NOS

✓4th B17 Other acute viral hepatitis
B17.0 Acute delta-(super) infection of hepatitis B carrier
✓5th **B17.1 Acute hepatitis C**
B17.10 Acute hepatitis C without hepatic coma
Acute hepatitis C NOS
B17.11 Acute hepatitis C with hepatic coma
B17.2 Acute hepatitis E
B17.8 Other specified acute viral hepatitis
Hepatitis non-A non-B (acute) (viral) NEC
B17.9 Acute viral hepatitis, unspecified
Acute hepatitis NOS

✓4th B18 Chronic viral hepatitis
B18.0 Chronic viral hepatitis B with delta-agent
B18.1 Chronic viral hepatitis B without delta-agent
Chronic (viral) hepatitis B
B18.2 Chronic viral hepatitis C
B18.8 Other chronic viral hepatitis
B18.9 Chronic viral hepatitis, unspecified

✓4th B19 Unspecified viral hepatitis
B19.0 Unspecified viral hepatitis with hepatic coma
✓5th **B19.1 Unspecified viral hepatitis B**
B19.10 Unspecified viral hepatitis B without hepatic coma
Unspecified viral hepatitis B NOS
B19.11 Unspecified viral hepatitis B with hepatic coma
✓5th **B19.2 Unspecified viral hepatitis C**
B19.20 Unspecified viral hepatitis C without hepatic coma
Viral hepatitis C NOS
B19.21 Unspecified viral hepatitis C with hepatic coma
B19.9 Unspecified viral hepatitis without hepatic coma
Viral hepatitis NOS

Human immunodeficiency virus [HIV] disease (B20)

B20 Human immunodeficiency virus [HIV] disease

INCLUDES acquired immune deficiency syndrome [AIDS]
AIDS-related complex [ARC]
HIV infection, symptomatic

Code first human immunodeficiency virus [HIV] disease complicating pregnancy, childbirth and the puerperium, if applicable (O98.7-)
Use additional code(s) to identify all manifestations of HIV infection

EXCLUDES 1 *asymptomatic human immunodeficiency virus [HIV] infection status (Z21)*
exposure to HIV virus (Z20.6)
inconclusive serologic evidence of HIV (R75)

Other viral diseases (B25-B34)

✓4th B25 Cytomegaloviral disease

EXCLUDES 1 *congenital cytomegalovirus infection (P35.1)*
cytomegaloviral mononucleosis (B27.1-)

B25.0 Cytomegaloviral pneumonitis
B25.1 Cytomegaloviral hepatitis
B25.2 Cytomegaloviral pancreatitis
B25.8 Other cytomegaloviral diseases
Cytomegaloviral encephalitis
B25.9 Cytomegaloviral disease, unspecified

✓4th B26 Mumps

INCLUDES epidemic parotitis
infectious parotitis

B26.0 Mumps orchitis
B26.1 Mumps meningitis
B26.2 Mumps encephalitis
B26.3 Mumps pancreatitis
✓5th **B26.8 Mumps with other complications**
B26.81 Mumps hepatitis
B26.82 Mumps myocarditis
B26.83 Mumps nephritis
B26.84 Mumps polyneuropathy
B26.85 Mumps arthritis
B26.89 Other mumps complications
B26.9 Mumps without complication
Mumps NOS
Mumps parotitis NOS

✓4th B27 Infectious mononucleosis

INCLUDES glandular fever
monocytic angina
Pfeiffer's disease

✓5th **B27.0 Gammaherpesviral mononucleosis**
Mononucleosis due to Epstein-Barr virus
B27.00 Gammaherpesviral mononucleosis without complication
B27.01 Gammaherpesviral mononucleosis with polyneuropathy
B27.02 Gammaherpesviral mononucleosis with meningitis
B27.09 Gammaherpesviral mononucleosis with other complications
Hepatomegaly in gammaherpesviral mononucleosis
✓5th **B27.1 Cytomegaloviral mononucleosis**
B27.10 Cytomegaloviral mononucleosis without complications
B27.11 Cytomegaloviral mononucleosis with polyneuropathy
B27.12 Cytomegaloviral mononucleosis with meningitis
B27.19 Cytomegaloviral mononucleosis with other complication
Hepatomegaly in cytomegaloviral mononucleosis
✓5th **B27.8 Other infectious mononucleosis**
B27.80 Other infectious mononucleosis without complication
B27.81 Other infectious mononucleosis with polyneuropathy
B27.82 Other infectious mononucleosis with meningitis
B27.89 Other infectious mononucleosis with other complication
Hepatomegaly in other infectious mononucleosis
✓5th **B27.9 Infectious mononucleosis, unspecified**
B27.90 Infectious mononucleosis, unspecified without complication

B27.91 Infectious mononucleosis, unspecified with polyneuropathy

B27.92 Infectious mononucleosis, unspecified with meningitis

B27.99 Infectious mononucleosis, unspecified with other complication
Hepatomegaly in unspecified infectious mononucleosis

✓4th B30 Viral conjunctivitis
EXCLUDES 1 *herpesviral [herpes simplex] ocular disease (B00.5)*
ocular zoster (B02.3)

B30.0 Keratoconjunctivitis due to adenovirus
Epidemic keratoconjunctivitis
Shipyard eye

B30.1 Conjunctivitis due to adenovirus
Acute adenoviral follicular conjunctivitis
Swimming-pool conjunctivitis

B30.2 Viral pharyngoconjunctivitis

B30.3 Acute epidemic hemorrhagic conjunctivitis (enteroviral)
Conjunctivitis due to coxsackievirus 24
Conjunctivitis due to enterovirus 70
Hemorrhagic conjunctivitis (acute)(epidemic)

B30.8 Other viral conjunctivitis
Newcastle conjunctivitis

B30.9 Viral conjunctivitis, unspecified

✓4th B33 Other viral diseases, not elsewhere classified

B33.0 Epidemic myalgia
Bornholm disease

B33.1 Ross River disease
Epidemic polyarthritis and exanthema
Ross River fever

✓5th **B33.2 Viral carditis**
Coxsackie (virus) carditis

B33.20 Viral carditis, unspecified

B33.21 Viral endocarditis

B33.22 Viral myocarditis

B33.23 Viral pericarditis

B33.24 Viral cardiomyopathy

B33.3 Retrovirus infections, not elsewhere classified
Retrovirus infection NOS

B33.4 Hantavirus (cardio)-pulmonary syndrome [HPS] [HCPS]
Hantavirus disease with pulmonary manifestations
Sin nombre virus disease
Use additional code to identify any associated acute kidney failure (N17.9)
EXCLUDES 1 *hantavirus disease with renal manifestations (A98.5)*
hemorrhagic fever with renal manifestations (A98.5)

B33.8 Other specified viral diseases
EXCLUDES 1 *anogenital human papillomavirus infection (A63.0)*
viral warts due to human papillomavirus infection (B07)

✓4th B34 Viral infection of unspecified site
EXCLUDES 1 *anogenital human papillomavirus infection (A63.0)*
cytomegaloviral disease NOS (B25.9)
herpesvirus [herpes simplex] infection NOS (B00.9)
retrovirus infection NOS (B33.3)
viral agents as the cause of diseases classified elsewhere (B97.-)
viral warts due to human papillomavirus infection (B07)

B34.0 Adenovirus infection, unspecified

B34.1 Enterovirus infection, unspecified
Coxsackievirus infection NOS
Echovirus infection NOS

B34.2 Coronavirus infection, unspecified
EXCLUDES 1 *pneumonia due to SARS-associated coronavirus (J12.81)*

B34.3 Parvovirus infection, unspecified

B34.4 Papovavirus infection, unspecified

B34.8 Other viral infections of unspecified site

B34.9 Viral infection, unspecified
Viremia NOS

Mycoses (B35-B49)

EXCLUDES 2 *hypersensitivity pneumonitis due to organic dust (J67.-)*
mycosis fungoides (C84.0-)

✓4th B35 Dermatophytosis
INCLUDES favus
infections due to species of Epidermophyton, Micro-sporum and Trichophyton
tinea, any type except those in B36-

B35.0 Tinea barbae and tinea capitis
Beard ringworm
Kerion
Scalp ringworm
Sycosis, mycotic

B35.1 Tinea unguium
Dermatophytic onychia
Dermatophytosis of nail
Onychomycosis
Ringworm of nails

B35.2 Tinea manuum
Dermatophytosis of hand
Hand ringworm

B35.3 Tinea pedis
Athlete's foot
Dermatophytosis of foot
Foot ringworm

B35.4 Tinea corporis
Ringworm of the body

B35.5 Tinea imbricata
Tokelau

B35.6 Tinea cruris
Dhobi itch
Groin ringworm
Jock itch

B35.8 Other dermatophytoses
Disseminated dermatophytosis
Granulomatous dermatophytosis

B35.9 Dermatophytosis, unspecified
Ringworm NOS

✓4th B36 Other superficial mycoses

B36.0 Pityriasis versicolor
Tinea flava
Tinea versicolor

B36.1 Tinea nigra
Keratomycosis nigricans palmaris
Microsporosis nigra
Pityriasis nigra

B36.2 White piedra
Tinea blanca

B36.3 Black piedra

B36.8 Other specified superficial mycoses

B36.9 Superficial mycosis, unspecified

✓4th B37 Candidiasis
INCLUDES candidosis
moniliasis
EXCLUDES 1 *neonatal candidiasis (P37.5)*

B37.0 Candidal stomatitis
Oral thrush

B37.1 Pulmonary candidiasis
Candidal bronchitis
Candidal pneumonia

B37.2 Candidiasis of skin and nail
Candidal onychia
Candidal paronychia
EXCLUDES 2 *diaper dermatitis (L22)*

B37.3 Candidiasis of vulva and vagina
Candidal vulvovaginitis
Monilial vulvovaginitis
Vaginal thrush

✓5th **B37.4 Candidiasis of other urogenital sites**

B37.41 Candidal cystitis and urethritis

B37.42 Candidal balanitis

B37.49 Other urogenital candidiasis
Candidal pyelonephritis

B37.5 Candidal meningitis

B37.6 Candidal endocarditis

B37.7 Candidal sepsis
Disseminated candidiasis
Systemic candidiasis

DRAFT

✓ Appropriate additional character required
✓x7th Requires 7th character, placeholder x must fill empty characters

√5th **B37.8 Candidiasis of other sites**
- **B37.81 Candidal esophagitis**
- **B37.82 Candidal enteritis**
  - Candidal proctitis
- **B37.83 Candidal cheilitis**
- **B37.84 Candidal otitis externa**
- **B37.89 Other sites of candidiasis**
  - Candidal osteomyelitis

B37.9 Candidiasis, unspecified
- Thrush NOS

√4th **B38 Coccidioidomycosis**
- **B38.0 Acute pulmonary coccidioidomycosis**
- **B38.1 Chronic pulmonary coccidioidomycosis**
- **B38.2 Pulmonary coccidioidomycosis, unspecified**
- **B38.3 Cutaneous coccidioidomycosis**
- **B38.4 Coccidioidomycosis meningitis**
- **B38.7 Disseminated coccidioidomycosis**
  - Generalized coccidioidomycosis
- √5th **B38.8 Other forms of coccidioidomycosis**
  - **B38.81 Prostatic coccidioidomycosis**
  - **B38.89 Other forms of coccidioidomycosis**
- **B38.9 Coccidioidomycosis, unspecified**

√4th **B39 Histoplasmosis**

Code first associated AIDS (B20)

Use additional code for any associated manifestations, such as:
- endocarditis (I39)
- meningitis (G02)
- pericarditis (I32)
- retinitis (H32)

- **B39.0 Acute pulmonary histoplasmosis capsulati**
- **B39.1 Chronic pulmonary histoplasmosis capsulati**
- **B39.2 Pulmonary histoplasmosis capsulati, unspecified**
- **B39.3 Disseminated histoplasmosis capsulati**
  - Generalized histoplasmosis capsulati
- **B39.4 Histoplasmosis capsulati, unspecified**
  - American histoplasmosis
- **B39.5 Histoplasmosis duboisii**
  - African histoplasmosis
- **B39.9 Histoplasmosis, unspecified**

√4th **B40 Blastomycosis**

EXCLUDES 1 *Brazilian blastomycosis (B41.-)*
keloidal blastomycosis (B48.0)

- **B40.0 Acute pulmonary blastomycosis**
- **B40.1 Chronic pulmonary blastomycosis**
- **B40.2 Pulmonary blastomycosis, unspecified**
- **B40.3 Cutaneous blastomycosis**
- **B40.7 Disseminated blastomycosis**
  - Generalized blastomycosis
- √5th **B40.8 Other forms of blastomycosis**
  - **B40.81 Blastomycotic meningoencephalitis**
    - Meningomyelitis due to blastomycosis
  - **B40.89 Other forms of blastomycosis**
- **B40.9 Blastomycosis, unspecified**

√4th **B41 Paracoccidioidomycosis**

INCLUDES Brazilian blastomycosis
Lutz' disease

- **B41.0 Pulmonary paracoccidioidomycosis**
- **B41.7 Disseminated paracoccidioidomycosis**
  - Generalized paracoccidioidomycosis
- **B41.8 Other forms of paracoccidioidomycosis**
- **B41.9 Paracoccidioidomycosis, unspecified**

√4th **B42 Sporotrichosis**
- **B42.0 Pulmonary sporotrichosis**
- **B42.1 Lymphocutaneous sporotrichosis**
- **B42.7 Disseminated sporotrichosis**
  - Generalized sporotrichosis
- √5th **B42.8 Other forms of sporotrichosis**
  - **B42.81 Cerebral sporotrichosis**
    - Meningitis due to sporotrichosis
  - **B42.82 Sporotrichosis arthritis**
  - **B42.89 Other forms of sporotrichosis**
- **B42.9 Sporotrichosis, unspecified**

√4th **B43 Chromomycosis and pheomycotic abscess**
- **B43.0 Cutaneous chromomycosis**
  - Dermatitis verrucosa
- **B43.1 Pheomycotic brain abscess**
  - Cerebral chromomycosis
- **B43.2 Subcutaneous pheomycotic abscess and cyst**
- **B43.8 Other forms of chromomycosis**
- **B43.9 Chromomycosis, unspecified**

√4th **B44 Aspergillosis**

INCLUDES aspergilloma

- **B44.0 Invasive pulmonary aspergillosis**
- **B44.1 Other pulmonary aspergillosis**
- **B44.2 Tonsillar aspergillosis**
- **B44.7 Disseminated aspergillosis**
  - Generalized aspergillosis
- √5th **B44.8 Other forms of aspergillosis**
  - **B44.81 Allergic bronchopulmonary aspergillosis**
  - **B44.89 Other forms of aspergillosis**
- **B44.9 Aspergillosis, unspecified**

√4th **B45 Cryptococcosis**
- **B45.0 Pulmonary cryptococcosis**
- **B45.1 Cerebral cryptococcosis**
  - Cryptococcal meningitis
  - Cryptococcosis meningocerebralis
- **B45.2 Cutaneous cryptococcosis**
- **B45.3 Osseous cryptococcosis**
- **B45.7 Disseminated cryptococcosis**
  - Generalized cryptococcosis
- **B45.8 Other forms of cryptococcosis**
- **B45.9 Cryptococcosis, unspecified**

√4th **B46 Zygomycosis**
- **B46.0 Pulmonary mucormycosis**
- **B46.1 Rhinocerebral mucormycosis**
- **B46.2 Gastrointestinal mucormycosis**
- **B46.3 Cutaneous mucormycosis**
  - Subcutaneous mucormycosis
- **B46.4 Disseminated mucormycosis**
  - Generalized mucormycosis
- **B46.5 Mucormycosis, unspecified**
- **B46.8 Other zygomycoses**
  - Entomophthoromycosis
- **B46.9 Zygomycosis, unspecified**
  - Phycomycosis NOS

√4th **B47 Mycetoma**
- **B47.0 Eumycetoma**
  - Madura foot, mycotic
  - Maduromycosis
- **B47.1 Actinomycetoma**
- **B47.9 Mycetoma, unspecified**
  - Madura foot NOS

√4th **B48 Other mycoses, not elsewhere classified**
- **B48.0 Lobomycosis**
  - Keloidal blastomycosis
  - Lobo's disease
- **B48.1 Rhinosporidiosis**
- **B48.2 Allescheriasis**
  - Infection due to Pseudallescheria boydii
  - EXCLUDES 1 *eumycetoma (B47.0)*
- **B48.3 Geotrichosis**
  - Geotrichum stomatitis
- **B48.4 Penicillosis**
- **B48.8 Other specified mycoses**
  - Adiaspiromycosis
  - Infection of tissue and organs by Alternaria
  - Infection of tissue and organs by Drechslera
  - Infection of tissue and organs by Fusarium
  - Infection of tissue and organs by saprophytic fungi NEC

B49 Unspecified mycosis
- Fungemia NOS

Protozoal diseases (B50-B64)

EXCLUDES 1 *amebiasis (A06.-)*
other protozoal intestinal diseases (A07.-)

✓4th **B50 Plasmodium falciparum malaria**
INCLUDES mixed infections of Plasmodium falciparum with any other Plasmodium species

B50.0 Plasmodium falciparum malaria with cerebral complications
Cerebral malaria NOS

B50.8 Other severe and complicated Plasmodium falciparum malaria
Severe or complicated Plasmodium falciparum malaria NOS

B50.9 Plasmodium falciparum malaria, unspecified

✓4th **B51 Plasmodium vivax malaria**
INCLUDES mixed infections of Plasmodium vivax with other Plasmodium species, except Plasmodium falciparum
EXCLUDES 1 *plasmodium vivax with Plasmodium falciparum (B50.-)*

B51.0 Plasmodium vivax malaria with rupture of spleen
B51.8 Plasmodium vivax malaria with other complications
B51.9 Plasmodium vivax malaria without complication
Plasmodium vivax malaria NOS

✓4th **B52 Plasmodium malariae malaria**
INCLUDES mixed infections of Plasmodium malariae with other Plasmodium species, except Plasmodium falciparum and Plasmodium vivax
EXCLUDES 1 *Plasmodium falciparum (B50.-)*
Plasmodium vivax (B51.-)

B52.0 Plasmodium malariae malaria with nephropathy
B52.8 Plasmodium malariae malaria with other complications
B52.9 Plasmodium malariae malaria without complication
Plasmodium malariae malaria NOS

✓4th **B53 Other specified malaria**

B53.0 Plasmodium ovale malaria
EXCLUDES 1 *Plasmodium ovale with Plasmodium falciparum (B50.-)*
Plasmodium ovale with Plasmodium malariae (B52.-)
Plasmodium ovale with Plasmodium vivax (B51.-)

B53.1 Malaria due to simian plasmodia
EXCLUDES 1 *Malaria due to simian plasmodia with Plasmodium falciparum (B50.-)*
Malaria due to simian plasmodia with Plasmodium malariae (B52.-)
Malaria due to simian plasmodia with Plasmodium ovale (B53.0)
Malaria due to simian plasmodia with Plasmodium vivax (B51.-)

B53.8 Other malaria, not elsewhere classified

B54 Unspecified malaria

✓4th **B55 Leishmaniasis**

B55.0 Visceral leishmaniasis
Kala-azar
Post-kala-azar dermal leishmaniasis

B55.1 Cutaneous leishmaniasis
B55.2 Mucocutaneous leishmaniasis
B55.9 Leishmaniasis, unspecified

✓4th **B56 African trypanosomiasis**

B56.0 Gambiense trypanosomiasis
Infection due to Trypanosoma brucei gambiense
West African sleeping sickness

B56.1 Rhodesiense trypanosomiasis
East African sleeping sickness
Infection due to Trypanosoma brucei rhodesiense

B56.9 African trypanosomiasis, unspecified
Sleeping sickness NOS

✓4th **B57 Chagas' disease**
INCLUDES American trypanosomiasis
infection due to Trypanosoma cruzi

B57.0 Acute Chagas' disease with heart involvement
Acute Chagas' disease with myocarditis

B57.1 Acute Chagas' disease without heart involvement
Acute Chagas' disease NOS

B57.2 Chagas' disease (chronic) with heart involvement
American trypanosomiasis NOS
Chagas' disease (chronic) NOS
Chagas' disease (chronic) with myocarditis
Trypanosomiasis NOS

✓5th **B57.3 Chagas' disease (chronic) with digestive system involvement**

B57.30 Chagas' disease with digestive system involvement, unspecified
B57.31 Megaesophagus in Chagas' disease
B57.32 Megacolon in Chagas' disease
B57.39 Other digestive system involvement in Chagas' disease

✓5th **B57.4 Chagas' disease (chronic) with nervous system involvement**

B57.40 Chagas' disease with nervous system involvement, unspecified
B57.41 Meningitis in Chagas' disease
B57.42 Meningoencephalitis in Chagas' disease
B57.49 Other nervous system involvement in Chagas' disease

B57.5 Chagas' disease (chronic) with other organ involvement

✓4th **B58 Toxoplasmosis**
INCLUDES infection due to Toxoplasma gondii
EXCLUDES 1 *congenital toxoplasmosis (P37.1)*

✓5th **B58.0 Toxoplasma oculopathy**

B58.00 Toxoplasma oculopathy, unspecified
B58.01 Toxoplasma chorioretinitis
B58.09 Other toxoplasma oculopathy
Toxoplasma uveitis

B58.1 Toxoplasma hepatitis
B58.2 Toxoplasma meningoencephalitis
B58.3 Pulmonary toxoplasmosis

✓5th **B58.8 Toxoplasmosis with other organ involvement**

B58.81 Toxoplasma myocarditis
B58.82 Toxoplasma myositis
B58.83 Toxoplasma tubulo-interstitial nephropathy
Toxoplasma pyelonephritis
B58.89 Toxoplasmosis with other organ involvement

B58.9 Toxoplasmosis, unspecified

B59 Pneumocystosis
Pneumonia due to Pneumocystis carinii
Pneumonia due to Pneumocystis jiroveci

✓4th **B60 Other protozoal diseases, not elsewhere classified**
EXCLUDES 1 *cryptosporidiosis (A07.2)*
intestinal microsporidiosis (A07.8)
isosporiasis (A07.3)

B60.0 Babesiosis
Piroplasmosis

✓5th **B60.1 Acanthamebiasis**

B60.10 Acanthamebiasis, unspecified
B60.11 Meningoencephalitis due to Acanthamoeba (culbertsoni)
B60.12 Conjunctivitis due to Acanthamoeba
B60.13 Keratoconjunctivitis due to Acanthamoeba
B60.19 Other acanthamebic disease

B60.2 Naegleriasis
Primary amebic meningoencephalitis

B60.8 Other specified protozoal diseases
Microsporidiosis

B64 Unspecified protozoal disease

Helminthiases (B65-B83)

✓4th **B65 Schistosomiasis [bilharziasis]**
INCLUDES snail fever

B65.0 Schistosomiasis due to Schistosoma haematobium [urinary schistosomiasis]
B65.1 Schistosomiasis due to Schistosoma mansoni [intestinal schistosomiasis]
B65.2 Schistosomiasis due to Schistosoma japonicum
Asiatic schistosomiasis
B65.3 Cercarial dermatitis
Swimmer's itch

✓ Appropriate additional character required
✓x7th Requires 7th character, placeholder x must fill empty characters

B65.8 Other schistosomiasis
Infection due to Schistosoma intercalatum
Infection due to Schistosoma mattheei
Infection due to Schistosoma mekongi

B65.9 Schistosomiasis, unspecified

4th B66 Other fluke infections

B66.Ø Opisthorchiasis
Infection due to cat liver fluke
Infection due to Opisthorchis (felineus)(viverrini)

B66.1 Clonorchiasis
Chinese liver fluke disease
Infection due to Clonorchis sinensis
Oriental liver fluke disease

B66.2 Dicroceliasis
Infection due to Dicrocoelium dendriticum
Lancet fluke infection

B66.3 Fascioliasis
Infection due to Fasciola gigantica
Infection due to Fasciola hepatica
Infection due to Fasciola indica
Sheep liver fluke disease

B66.4 Paragonimiasis
Infection due to Paragonimus species
Lung fluke disease
Pulmonary distomiasis

B66.5 Fasciolopsiasis
Infection due to Fasciolopsis buski
Intestinal distomiasis

B66.8 Other specified fluke infections
Echinostomiasis
Heterophyiasis
Metagonimiasis
Nanophyetiasis
Watsoniasis

B66.9 Fluke infection, unspecified

4th B67 Echinococcosis
INCLUDES hydatidosis

B67.Ø Echinococcus granulosus infection of liver

B67.1 Echinococcus granulosus infection of lung

B67.2 Echinococcus granulosus infection of bone

5th B67.3 Echinococcus granulosus infection, other and multiple sites

B67.31 Echinococcus granulosus infection, thyroid gland

B67.32 Echinococcus granulosus infection, multiple sites

B67.39 Echinococcus granulosus infection, other sites

B67.4 Echinococcus granulosus infection, unspecified
Dog tapeworm (infection)

B67.5 Echinococcus multilocularis infection of liver

5th B67.6 Echinococcus multilocularis infection, other and multiple sites

B67.61 Echinococcus multilocularis infection, multiple sites

B67.69 Echinococcus multilocularis infection, other sites

B67.7 Echinococcus multilocularis infection, unspecified

B67.8 Echinococcosis, unspecified, of liver

5th B67.9 Echinococcosis, other and unspecified

B67.9Ø Echinococcosis, unspecified
Echinococcosis NOS

B67.99 Other echinococcosis

4th B68 Taeniasis
EXCLUDES1 *cysticercosis (B69.-)*

B68.Ø Taenia solium taeniasis
Pork tapeworm (infection)

B68.1 Taenia saginata taeniasis
Beef tapeworm (infection)
Infection due to adult tapeworm Taenia saginata

B68.9 Taeniasis, unspecified

4th B69 Cysticercosis
INCLUDES cysticerciasis infection due to larval form of Taenia solium

B69.Ø Cysticercosis of central nervous system

B69.1 Cysticercosis of eye

5th B69.8 Cysticercosis of other sites

B69.81 Myositis in cysticercosis

B69.89 Cysticercosis of other sites

B69.9 Cysticercosis, unspecified

4th B7Ø Diphyllobothriasis and sparganosis

B7Ø.Ø Diphyllobothriasis
Diphyllobothrium (adult) (latum) (pacificum) infection
Fish tapeworm (infection)
EXCLUDES2 *larval diphyllobothriasis (B7Ø.1)*

B7Ø.1 Sparganosis
Infection due to Sparganum (mansoni) (proliferum)
Infection due to Spirometra larva
Larval diphyllobothriasis
Spirometrosis

4th B71 Other cestode infections

B71.Ø Hymenolepiasis
Dwarf tapeworm infection
Rat tapeworm (infection)

B71.1 Dipylidiasis

B71.8 Other specified cestode infections
Coenurosis

B71.9 Cestode infection, unspecified
Tapeworm (infection) NOS

B72 Dracunculiasis
INCLUDES guinea worm infection
infection due to Dracunculus medinensis

4th B73 Onchocerciasis
INCLUDES onchocerca volvulus infection
onchocercosis
river blindness

5th B73.Ø Onchocerciasis with eye disease

B73.ØØ Onchocerciasis with eye involvement, unspecified

B73.Ø1 Onchocerciasis with endophthalmitis

B73.Ø2 Onchocerciasis with glaucoma

B73.Ø9 Onchocerciasis with other eye involvement
Infestation of eyelid due to onchocerciasis

B73.1 Onchocerciasis without eye disease

4th B74 Filariasis
EXCLUDES2 *onchocerciasis (B73)*
tropical (pulmonary) eosinophilia NOS (J82)

B74.Ø Filariasis due to Wuchereria bancrofti
Bancroftian elephantiasis
Bancroftian filariasis

B74.1 Filariasis due to Brugia malayi

B74.2 Filariasis due to Brugia timori

B74.3 Loiasis
Calabar swelling
Eyeworm disease of Africa
Loa loa infection

B74.4 Mansonelliasis
Infection due to Mansonella ozzardi
Infection due to Mansonella perstans
Infection due to Mansonella streptocerca

B74.8 Other filariases
Dirofilariasis

B74.9 Filariasis, unspecified

B75 Trichinellosis
INCLUDES infection due to Trichinella species
trichiniasis

4th B76 Hookworm diseases
INCLUDES uncinariasis

B76.Ø Ancylostomiasis
Infection due to Ancylostoma species

B76.1 Necatoriasis
Infection due to Necator americanus

B76.8 Other hookworm diseases

B76.9 Hookworm disease, unspecified
Cutaneous larva migrans NOS

4th B77 Ascariasis
INCLUDES ascaridiasis
roundworm infection

B77.Ø Ascariasis with intestinal complications

5th B77.8 Ascariasis with other complications

B77.81 Ascariasis pneumonia

B77.89 Ascariasis with other complications

B77.9 Ascariasis, unspecified

4th B78 Strongyloidiasis
EXCLUDES1 *trichostrongyliasis (B81.2)*

B78.Ø Intestinal strongyloidiasis

B78.1 **Cutaneous strongyloidiasis**
B78.7 **Disseminated strongyloidiasis**
B78.9 **Strongyloidiasis, unspecified**

B79 Trichuriasis
INCLUDES trichocephaliasis
whipworm (disease)(infection)

B80 Enterobiasis
INCLUDES oxyuriasis
pinworm infection
threadworm infection

✓4th **B81 Other intestinal helminthiases, not elsewhere classified**
EXCLUDES 1 *angiostrongyliasis due to Parastrongylus cantonensis (B83.2)*
B81.0 **Anisakiasis**
Infection due to Anisakis larva
B81.1 **Intestinal capillariasis**
Capillariasis NOS
Infection due to Capillaria philippinensis
EXCLUDES 2 *hepatic capillariasis (B83.8)*
B81.2 **Trichostrongyliasis**
B81.3 **Intestinal angiostrongyliasis**
Angiostrongyliasis due to Parastrongylus costaricensis
B81.4 **Mixed intestinal helminthiases**
Infection due to intestinal helminths classified to more than one of the categories B65.0-B81.3 and B81.8
Mixed helminthiasis NOS
B81.8 **Other specified intestinal helminthiases**
Infection due to Oesophagostomum species [esophagostomiasis]
Infection due to Ternidens diminutus [ternidensiasis]

✓4th **B82 Unspecified intestinal parasitism**
B82.0 **Intestinal helminthiasis, unspecified**
B82.9 **Intestinal parasitism, unspecified**

✓4th **B83 Other helminthiases**
EXCLUDES 1 *capillariasis NOS (B81.1)*
EXCLUDES 2 *intestinal capillariasis (B81.1)*
B83.0 **Visceral larva migrans**
Toxocariasis
B83.1 **Gnathostomiasis**
Wandering swelling
B83.2 **Angiostrongyliasis due to Parastrongylus cantonensis**
Eosinophilic meningoencephalitis due to Parastrongylus cantonensis
EXCLUDES 2 *intestinal angiostrongyliasis (B81.3)*
B83.3 **Syngamiasis**
Syngamosis
B83.4 **Internal hirudiniasis**
EXCLUDES 2 *external hirudiniasis (B88.3)*
B83.8 **Other specified helminthiases**
Acanthocephaliasis
Gongylonemiasis
Hepatic capillariasis
Metastrongyliasis
Thelaziasis
B83.9 **Helminthiasis, unspecified**
Worms NOS
EXCLUDES 1 *intestinal helminthiasis NOS (B82.0)*

Pediculosis, acariasis and other infestations (B85-B89)

✓4th **B85 Pediculosis and phthiriasis**
B85.0 **Pediculosis due to Pediculus humanus capitis**
Head-louse infestation
B85.1 **Pediculosis due to Pediculus humanus corporis**
Body-louse infestation
B85.2 **Pediculosis, unspecified**
B85.3 **Phthiriasis**
Infestation by crab-louse
Infestation by Phthirus pubis
B85.4 **Mixed pediculosis and phthiriasis**
Infestation classifiable to more than one of the categories B85.0- B85.3

B86 Scabies
Sarcoptic itch

✓4th **B87 Myiasis**
INCLUDES infestation by larva of flies
B87.0 **Cutaneous myiasis**
Creeping myiasis
B87.1 **Wound myiasis**
Traumatic myiasis
B87.2 **Ocular myiasis**
B87.3 **Nasopharyngeal myiasis**
Laryngeal myiasis
B87.4 **Aural myiasis**
✓5th B87.8 **Myiasis of other sites**
B87.81 **Genitourinary myiasis**
B87.82 **Intestinal myiasis**
B87.89 **Myiasis of other sites**
B87.9 **Myiasis, unspecified**

✓4th **B88 Other infestations**
B88.0 **Other acariasis**
Acarine dermatitis
Dermatitis due to Demodex species
Dermatitis due to Dermanyssus gallinae
Dermatitis due to Liponyssoides sanguineus
Trombiculosis
EXCLUDES 2 *scabies (B86)*
B88.1 **Tungiasis [sandflea infestation]**
B88.2 **Other arthropod infestations**
Scarabiasis
B88.3 **External hirudiniasis**
Leech infestation NOS
EXCLUDES 2 *internal hirudiniasis (B83.4)*
B88.8 **Other specified infestations**
Ichthyoparasitism due to Vandellia cirrhosa
Linguatulosis
Porocephaliasis
B88.9 **Infestation, unspecified**
Infestation (skin) NOS
Infestation by mites NOS
Skin parasites NOS

B89 Unspecified parasitic disease

Sequelae of infectious and parasitic diseases (B90-B94)

NOTE Categories B90-B94 are to be used to indicate conditions in categories A00-B89 as the cause of sequelae, which are themselves classified elsewhere. The "sequelae" include conditions specified as such; they also include residuals of diseases classifiable to the above categories if there is evidence that the disease itself is no longer present. Codes from these categories are not to be used for chronic infections. Code chronic current infections to active infectious disease as appropriate.

Code first condition resulting from (sequela) the infectious or parasitic disease

✓4th **B90 Sequelae of tuberculosis**
B90.0 **Sequelae of central nervous system tuberculosis**
B90.1 **Sequelae of genitourinary tuberculosis**
B90.2 **Sequelae of tuberculosis of bones and joints**
B90.8 **Sequelae of tuberculosis of other organs**
EXCLUDES 2 *sequelae of respiratory tuberculosis (B90.9)*
B90.9 **Sequelae of respiratory and unspecified tuberculosis**
Sequelae of tuberculosis NOS

B91 Sequelae of poliomyelitis
EXCLUDES 1 *postpolio syndrome (G14)*

B92 Sequelae of leprosy

✓4th **B94 Sequelae of other and unspecified infectious and parasitic diseases**
B94.0 **Sequelae of trachoma**
B94.1 **Sequelae of viral encephalitis**
B94.2 **Sequelae of viral hepatitis**
B94.8 **Sequelae of other specified infectious and parasitic diseases**
B94.9 **Sequelae of unspecified infectious and parasitic disease**

Bacterial and viral infectious agents (B95-B97)

NOTE These categories are provided for use as supplementary or additional codes to identify the infectious agent(s) in diseases classified elsewhere.

✓4th **B95 Streptococcus, Staphylococcus, and Enterococcus as the cause of diseases classified elsewhere**

B95.0 Streptococcus, group A, as the cause of diseases classified elsewhere

B95.1 Streptococcus, group B, as the cause of diseases classified elsewhere

B95.2 Enterococcus as the cause of diseases classified elsewhere

B95.3 Streptococcus pneumoniae as the cause of diseases classified elsewhere

B95.4 Other streptococcus as the cause of diseases classified elsewhere

B95.5 Unspecified streptococcus as the cause of diseases classified elsewhere

✓5th **B95.6 Staphylococcus aureus as the cause of diseases classified elsewhere**

B95.61 Methicillin susceptible Staphylococcus aureus infection as the cause of diseases classified elsewhere

Methicillin susceptible Staphylococcus aureus (MSSA) infection as the cause of diseases classified elsewhere

Staphylococcus aureus infection NOS as the cause of diseases classified elsewhere

B95.62 Methicillin resistant Staphylococcus aureus infection as the cause of diseases classified elsewhere

Methicillin resistant Staphylococcus aureus (MRSA) infection as the cause of diseases classified elsewhere

B95.7 Other staphylococcus as the cause of diseases classified elsewhere

B95.8 Unspecified staphylococcus as the cause of diseases classified elsewhere

✓4th **B96 Other bacterial agents as the cause of diseases classified elsewhere**

B96.0 Mycoplasma pneumoniae [M. pneumoniae] as the cause of diseases classified elsewhere

Pleuro-pneumonia-like-organism [PPLO]

B96.1 Klebsiella pneumoniae [K. pneumoniae] as the cause of diseases classified elsewhere

✓5th **B96.2 Escherichia coli [E. coli] as the cause of diseases classified elsewhere**

B96.20 Unspecified Escherichia coli [E. coli] as the cause of diseases classified elsewhere

Escherichia coli [E. coli] NOS

B96.21 Shiga toxin-producing Escherichia coli [E. coli] (STEC) O157 as the cause of diseases classified elsewhere

E. coli O157:H- (nonmotile) with confirmation of Shiga toxin

E. coli O157 with confirmation of Shiga toxin when H antigen is unknown, or is not H7

O157:H7 Escherichia coli [E.coli] with or without confirmation of Shiga toxin-production

Shiga toxin-producing Escherichia coli [E.coli] O157:H7 with or without confirmation of Shiga toxin-production

STEC O157:H7 with or without confirmation of Shiga toxin-production

B96.22 Other specified Shiga toxin-producing Escherichia coli [E. coli] (STEC) as the cause of diseases classified elsewhere

Non-O157 Shiga toxin-producing Escherichia coli [E.coli]

Non-O157 Shiga toxin-producing Escherichia coli [E.coli] with known O group

B96.23 Unspecified Shiga toxin-producing Escherichia coli [E. coli] (STEC) as the cause of diseases classified elsewhere

Shiga toxin-producing Escherichia coli [E. coli] with unspecified O group

STEC NOS

B96.29 Other Escherichia coli [E. coli] as the cause of diseases classified elsewhere

Non-Shiga toxin-producing E. coli

B96.3 Hemophilus influenzae [H. influenzae] as the cause of diseases classified elsewhere

B96.4 Proteus (mirabilis) (morganii) as the cause of diseases classified elsewhere

B96.5 Pseudomonas (aeruginosa) (mallei) (pseudomallei) as the cause of diseases classified elsewhere

B96.6 Bacteroides fragilis [B. fragilis] as the cause of diseases classified elsewhere

B96.7 Clostridium perfringens [C. perfringens] as the cause of diseases classified elsewhere

✓5th **B96.8 Other specified bacterial agents as the cause of diseases classified elsewhere**

B96.81 Helicobacter pylori [H. pylori] as the cause of diseases classified elsewhere

B96.82 Vibrio vulnificus as the cause of diseases classified elsewhere

B96.89 Other specified bacterial agents as the cause of diseases classified elsewhere

✓4th **B97 Viral agents as the cause of diseases classified elsewhere**

B97.0 Adenovirus as the cause of diseases classified elsewhere

✓5th **B97.1 Enterovirus as the cause of diseases classified elsewhere**

B97.10 Unspecified enterovirus as the cause of diseases classified elsewhere

B97.11 Coxsackievirus as the cause of diseases classified elsewhere

B97.12 Echovirus as the cause of diseases classified elsewhere

B97.19 Other enterovirus as the cause of diseases classified elsewhere

✓5th **B97.2 Coronavirus as the cause of diseases classified elsewhere**

B97.21 SARS-associated coronavirus as the cause of diseases classified elsewhere

EXCLUDES 1 *pneumonia due to SARS-associated coronavirus (J12.81)*

B97.29 Other coronavirus as the cause of diseases classified elsewhere

✓5th **B97.3 Retrovirus as the cause of diseases classified elsewhere**

EXCLUDES 1 *human immunodeficiency virus [HIV} disease (B20)*

B97.30 Unspecified retrovirus as the cause of diseases classified elsewhere

B97.31 Lentivirus as the cause of diseases classified elsewhere

B97.32 Oncovirus as the cause of diseases classified elsewhere

B97.33 Human T-cell lymphotrophic virus, type I [HTLV-I] as the cause of diseases classified elsewhere

B97.34 Human T-cell lymphotrophic virus, type II [HTLV-II] as the cause of diseases classified elsewhere

B97.35 Human immunodeficiency virus, type 2 [HIV 2] as the cause of diseases classified elsewhere

B97.39 Other retrovirus as the cause of diseases classified elsewhere

B97.4 Respiratory syncytial virus as the cause of diseases classified elsewhere

B97.5 Reovirus as the cause of diseases classified elsewhere

B97.6 Parvovirus as the cause of diseases classified elsewhere

B97.7 Papillomavirus as the cause of diseases classified elsewhere

✓5th **B97.8 Other viral agents as the cause of diseases classified elsewhere**

B97.81 Human metapneumovirus as the cause of diseases classified elsewhere

B97.89 Other viral agents as the cause of diseases classified elsewhere

Other infectious diseases (B99)

✓4th **B99 Other and unspecified infectious diseases**

B99.8 Other infectious disease

B99.9 Unspecified infectious disease

Chapter 2. Neoplasms (C00-D49)

This chapter contains the following broad groups of neoplasms:

C00-C14	Malignant neoplasms of lip, oral cavity and pharynx
C15-C26	Malignant neoplasms of digestive organs
C30-C39	Malignant neoplasms of respiratory and intrathoracic organs
C40-C41	Malignant neoplasms of bone and articular cartilage
C43-C44	Melanoma and other malignant neoplasms of skin
C45-C49	Malignant neoplasms of mesothelial and soft tissue
C50	Malignant neoplasms of breast
C51-C58	Malignant neoplasms of female genital organs
C60-C63	Malignant neoplasms of male genital organs
C64-C68	Malignant neoplasms of urinary tract
C69-C72	Malignant neoplasms of eye, brain and other parts of central nervous system
C73-C75	Malignant neoplasms of thyroid and other endocrine glands
C7A	Malignant neuroendocrine tumors
C7B	Secondary neuroendocrine tumors
C76-C80	Malignant neoplasms of ill-defined, other secondary and unspecified sites
C81-C96	Malignant neoplasms of lymphoid, hematopoietic and related tissue
D00-D09	In situ neoplasms
D10-D36	Benign neoplasms, except benign neuroendocrine tumors
D3A	Benign neuroendocrine tumors
D37-D48	Neoplasms of uncertain behavior, polycythemia vera and myelodysplastic syndromes
D49	Neoplasms of unspecified behavior

NOTE

Functional activity

All neoplasms are classified in this chapter, whether they are functionally active or not. An additional code from Chapter 4 may be used, to identify functional activity associated with any neoplasm.

Morphology [Histology]

Chapter 2 classifies neoplasms primarily by site (topography), with broad groupings for behavior, malignant, in situ, benign, etc. The Table of Neoplasms should be used to identify the correct topography code. In a few cases, such as for malignant melanoma and certain neuroendocrine tumors, the morphology (histologic type) is included in the category and codes.

Primary malignant neoplasms overlapping site boundaries

A primary malignant neoplasm that overlaps two or more contiguous (next to each other) sites should be classified to the subcategory/code .8 ("overlapping lesion"), unless the combination is specifically indexed elsewhere. For multiple neoplasms of the same site that are not contiguous, such as tumors in different quadrants of the same breast, codes for each site should be assigned.

Malignant neoplasm of ectopic tissue

Malignant neoplasms of ectopic tissue are to be coded to the site mentioned, e.g., ectopic pancreatic malignant neoplasms are coded to pancreas, unspecified (C25.9).

MALIGNANT NEOPLASMS (C00-C96)

NOTE Malignant neoplasms, stated or presumed to be primary (of specified sites), and certain specified histologies, except neuroendocrine, and of lymphoid, hematopoietic and related tissue (C00-C75)

Malignant neoplasms of lip, oral cavity and pharynx (C00-C14)

✓4th C00 Malignant neoplasm of lip

EXCLUDES 1 *malignant melanoma of lip (C43.0)*
Merkel cell carcinoma of lip (C4A.0)
other and unspecified malignant neoplasm of skin of lip (C44.0-)

Use additional code to identify:
alcohol abuse and dependence (F10.-)
history of tobacco use (Z87.891)
tobacco dependence (F17.-)
tobacco use (Z72.0)

C00.0 Malignant neoplasm of external upper lip
Malignant neoplasm of lipstick area of upper lip
Malignant neoplasm of upper lip NOS
Malignant neoplasm of vermilion border of upper lip

C00.1 Malignant neoplasm of external lower lip
Malignant neoplasm of lower lip NOS
Malignant neoplasm of lipstick area of lower lip
Malignant neoplasm of vermilion border of lower lip

C00.2 Malignant neoplasm of external lip, unspecified
Malignant neoplasm of vermilion border of lip NOS

C00.3 Malignant neoplasm of upper lip, inner aspect
Malignant neoplasm of buccal aspect of upper lip
Malignant neoplasm of frenulum of upper lip
Malignant neoplasm of mucosa of upper lip
Malignant neoplasm of oral aspect of upper lip

C00.4 Malignant neoplasm of lower lip, inner aspect
Malignant neoplasm of buccal aspect of lower lip
Malignant neoplasm of frenulum of lower lip
Malignant neoplasm of mucosa of lower lip
Malignant neoplasm of oral aspect of lower lip

C00.5 Malignant neoplasm of lip, unspecified, inner aspect
Malignant neoplasm of buccal aspect of lip, unspecified
Malignant neoplasm of frenulum of lip, unspecified
Malignant neoplasm of mucosa of lip, unspecified
Malignant neoplasm of oral aspect of lip, unspecified

C00.6 Malignant neoplasm of commissure of lip, unspecified

C00.8 Malignant neoplasm of overlapping sites of lip

C00.9 Malignant neoplasm of lip, unspecified

C01 Malignant neoplasm of base of tongue
Malignant neoplasm of dorsal surface of base of tongue
Malignant neoplasm of fixed part of tongue NOS
Malignant neoplasm of posterior third of tongue

Use additional code to identify:
alcohol abuse and dependence (F10.-)
history of tobacco use (Z87.891)
tobacco dependence (F17.-)
tobacco use (Z72.0)

✓4th C02 Malignant neoplasm of other and unspecified parts of tongue

Use additional code to identify:
alcohol abuse and dependence (F10.-)
history of tobacco use (Z87.891)
tobacco dependence (F17.-)
tobacco use (Z72.0)

C02.0 Malignant neoplasm of dorsal surface of tongue
Malignant neoplasm of anterior two-thirds of tongue, dorsal surface

EXCLUDES 2 *malignant neoplasm of dorsal surface of base of tongue (C01)*

C02.1 Malignant neoplasm of border of tongue
Malignant neoplasm of tip of tongue

C02.2 Malignant neoplasm of ventral surface of tongue
Malignant neoplasm of anterior two-thirds of tongue, ventral surface
Malignant neoplasm of frenulum linguae

C02.3 Malignant neoplasm of anterior two-thirds of tongue, part unspecified
Malignant neoplasm of middle third of tongue NOS
Malignant neoplasm of mobile part of tongue NOS

C02.4 Malignant neoplasm of lingual tonsil

EXCLUDES 2 *malignant neoplasm of tonsil NOS (C09.9)*

C02.8 Malignant neoplasm of overlapping sites of tongue
Malignant neoplasm of two or more contiguous sites of tongue

C02.9 Malignant neoplasm of tongue, unspecified

✓4th C03 Malignant neoplasm of gum

INCLUDES malignant neoplasm of alveolar (ridge) mucosa
malignant neoplasm of gingiva

EXCLUDES 2 *malignant odontogenic neoplasms (C41.0-C41.1)*

Use additional code to identify:
alcohol abuse and dependence (F10.-)
history of tobacco use (Z87.891)
tobacco dependence (F17.-)
tobacco use (Z72.0)

C03.0 Malignant neoplasm of upper gum

C03.1 Malignant neoplasm of lower gum

C03.9 Malignant neoplasm of gum, unspecified

✓4th C04 Malignant neoplasm of floor of mouth

Use additional code to identify:
alcohol abuse and dependence (F10.-)
history of tobacco use (Z87.891)
tobacco dependence (F17.-)
tobacco use (Z72.0)

C04.0 Malignant neoplasm of anterior floor of mouth
Malignant neoplasm of anterior to the premolar-canine junction

C04.1 Malignant neoplasm of lateral floor of mouth

C04.8 Malignant neoplasm of overlapping sites of floor of mouth

C04.9 Malignant neoplasm of floor of mouth, unspecified

CØ5 Malignant neoplasm of palate

EXCLUDES 1 Kaposi's sarcoma of palate (C46.2)

Use additional code to identify:
- alcohol abuse and dependence (F1Ø.-)
- history of tobacco use (Z87.891)
- tobacco dependence (F17.-)
- tobacco use (Z72.Ø)

CØ5.Ø Malignant neoplasm of hard palate

CØ5.1 Malignant neoplasm of soft palate

EXCLUDES 2 malignant neoplasm of nasopharyngeal surface of soft palate (C11.3)

CØ5.2 Malignant neoplasm of uvula

CØ5.8 Malignant neoplasm of overlapping sites of palate

CØ5.9 Malignant neoplasm of palate, unspecified

Malignant neoplasm of roof of mouth

CØ6 Malignant neoplasm of other and unspecified parts of mouth

Use additional code to identify:
- alcohol abuse and dependence (F1Ø.-)
- history of tobacco use (Z87.891)
- tobacco dependence (F17.-)
- tobacco use (Z72.Ø)

CØ6.Ø Malignant neoplasm of cheek mucosa

Malignant neoplasm of buccal mucosa NOS
Malignant neoplasm of internal cheek

CØ6.1 Malignant neoplasm of vestibule of mouth

Malignant neoplasm of buccal sulcus (upper) (lower)
Malignant neoplasm of labial sulcus (upper) (lower)

CØ6.2 Malignant neoplasm of retromolar area

CØ6.8 Malignant neoplasm of overlapping sites of other and unspecified parts of mouth

CØ6.8Ø Malignant neoplasm of overlapping sites of unspecified parts of mouth

CØ6.89 Malignant neoplasm of overlapping sites of other parts of mouth

"book leaf" neoplasm [ventral surface of tongue and floor of mouth]

CØ6.9 Malignant neoplasm of mouth, unspecified

Malignant neoplasm of minor salivary gland, unspecified site
Malignant neoplasm of oral cavity NOS

CØ7 Malignant neoplasm of parotid gland

Use additional code to identify:
- alcohol abuse and dependence (F1Ø.-)
- exposure to environmental tobacco smoke (Z77.22)
- exposure to tobacco smoke in the perinatal period (P96.81)
- history of tobacco use (Z87.891)
- occupational exposure to environmental tobacco smoke (Z57.31)
- tobacco dependence (F17.-)
- tobacco use (Z72.Ø)

CØ8 Malignant neoplasm of other and unspecified major salivary glands

INCLUDES malignant neoplasm of salivary ducts

EXCLUDES 1 malignant neoplasms of specified minor salivary glands which are classified according to their anatomical location

EXCLUDES 2 malignant neoplasms of minor salivary glands NOS (CØ6.9)
malignant neoplasm of parotid gland (CØ7)

Use additional code to identify:
- alcohol abuse and dependence (F1Ø.-)
- exposure to environmental tobacco smoke (Z77.22)
- exposure to tobacco smoke in the perinatal period (P96.81)
- history of tobacco use (Z87.891)
- occupational exposure to environmental tobacco smoke (Z57.31)
- tobacco dependence (F17.-)
- tobacco use (Z72.Ø)

CØ8.Ø Malignant neoplasm of submandibular gland

Malignant neoplasm of submaxillary gland

CØ8.1 Malignant neoplasm of sublingual gland

CØ8.9 Malignant neoplasm of major salivary gland, unspecified

Malignant neoplasm of salivary gland (major) NOS

CØ9 Malignant neoplasm of tonsil

EXCLUDES 2 malignant neoplasm of lingual tonsil (CØ2.4)
malignant neoplasm of pharyngeal tonsil (C11.1)

Use additional code to identify:
- alcohol abuse and dependence (F1Ø.-)
- exposure to environmental tobacco smoke (Z77.22)
- exposure to tobacco smoke in the perinatal period (P96.81)
- history of tobacco use (Z87.891)
- occupational exposure to environmental tobacco smoke (Z57.31)
- tobacco dependence (F17.-)
- tobacco use (Z72.Ø)

CØ9.Ø Malignant neoplasm of tonsillar fossa

CØ9.1 Malignant neoplasm of tonsillar pillar (anterior) (posterior)

CØ9.8 Malignant neoplasm of overlapping sites of tonsil

CØ9.9 Malignant neoplasm of tonsil, unspecified

Malignant neoplasm of tonsil NOS
Malignant neoplasm of faucial tonsils
Malignant neoplasm of palatine tonsils

C1Ø Malignant neoplasm of oropharynx

EXCLUDES 2 malignant neoplasm of tonsil (CØ9.-)

Use additional code to identify:
- alcohol abuse and dependence (F1Ø.-)
- exposure to environmental tobacco smoke (Z77.22)
- exposure to tobacco smoke in the perinatal period (P96.81)
- history of tobacco use (Z87.891)
- occupational exposure to environmental tobacco smoke (Z57.31)
- tobacco dependence (F17.-)
- tobacco use (Z72.Ø)

C1Ø.Ø Malignant neoplasm of vallecula

C1Ø.1 Malignant neoplasm of anterior surface of epiglottis

Malignant neoplasm of epiglottis, free border [margin]
Malignant neoplasm of glossoepiglottic fold(s)

EXCLUDES 2 malignant neoplasm of epiglottis (suprahyoid portion) NOS (C32.1)

C1Ø.2 Malignant neoplasm of lateral wall of oropharynx

C1Ø.3 Malignant neoplasm of posterior wall of oropharynx

C1Ø.4 Malignant neoplasm of branchial cleft

Malignant neoplasm of branchial cyst [site of neoplasm]

C1Ø.8 Malignant neoplasm of overlapping sites of oropharynx

Malignant neoplasm of junctional region of oropharynx

C1Ø.9 Malignant neoplasm of oropharynx, unspecified

C11 Malignant neoplasm of nasopharynx

Use additional code to identify:
- exposure to environmental tobacco smoke (Z77.22)
- exposure to tobacco smoke in the perinatal period (P96.81)
- history of tobacco use (Z87.891)
- occupational exposure to environmental tobacco smoke (Z57.31)
- tobacco dependence (F17.-)
- tobacco use (Z72.Ø)

C11.Ø Malignant neoplasm of superior wall of nasopharynx

Malignant neoplasm of roof of nasopharynx

C11.1 Malignant neoplasm of posterior wall of nasopharynx

Malignant neoplasm of adenoid
Malignant neoplasm of pharyngeal tonsil

C11.2 Malignant neoplasm of lateral wall of nasopharynx

Malignant neoplasm of fossa of Rosenmüller
Malignant neoplasm of opening of auditory tube
Malignant neoplasm of pharyngeal recess

C11.3 Malignant neoplasm of anterior wall of nasopharynx

Malignant neoplasm of floor of nasopharynx
Malignant neoplasm of nasopharyngeal (anterior) (posterior) surface of soft palate
Malignant neoplasm of posterior margin of nasal choana
Malignant neoplasm of posterior margin of nasal septum

C11.8 Malignant neoplasm of overlapping sites of nasopharynx

C11.9 Malignant neoplasm of nasopharynx, unspecified

Malignant neoplasm of nasopharyngeal wall NOS

C12 Malignant neoplasm of pyriform sinus

Malignant neoplasm of pyriform fossa

Use additional code to identify:
- exposure to environmental tobacco smoke (Z77.22)
- exposure to tobacco smoke in the perinatal period (P96.81)
- history of tobacco use (Z87.891)
- occupational exposure to environmental tobacco smoke (Z57.31)
- tobacco dependence (F17.-)
- tobacco use (Z72.Ø)

C13 Malignant neoplasm of hypopharynx
EXCLUDES 2 *malignant neoplasm of pyriform sinus (C12)*
Use additional code to identify:
exposure to environmental tobacco smoke (Z77.22)
exposure to tobacco smoke in the perinatal period (P96.81)
history of tobacco use (Z87.891)
occupational exposure to environmental tobacco smoke (Z57.31)
tobacco dependence (F17.-)
tobacco use (Z72.0)

C13.0 Malignant neoplasm of postcricoid region

C13.1 Malignant neoplasm of aryepiglottic fold, hypopharyngeal aspect
Malignant neoplasm of aryepiglottic fold NOS
Malignant neoplasm of interarytenoid fold NOS
Malignant neoplasm of aryepiglottic fold marginal zone
Malignant neoplasm of interarytenoid fold marginal zone
EXCLUDES 2 *malignant neoplasm of aryepiglottic fold or interarytenoid fold, laryngeal aspect (C32.1)*

C13.2 Malignant neoplasm of posterior wall of hypopharynx

C13.8 Malignant neoplasm of overlapping sites of hypopharynx

C13.9 Malignant neoplasm of hypopharynx, unspecified
Malignant neoplasm of hypopharyngeal wall NOS

C14 Malignant neoplasm of other and ill-defined sites in the lip, oral cavity and pharynx
EXCLUDES 1 *malignant neoplasm of oral cavity NOS (C06.9)*
Use additional code to identify:
alcohol abuse and dependence (F10.-)
exposure to environmental tobacco smoke (Z77.22)
exposure to tobacco smoke in the perinatal period (P96.81)
history of tobacco use (Z87.891)
occupational exposure to environmental tobacco smoke (Z57.31)
tobacco dependence (F17.-)
tobacco use (Z72.0)

C14.0 Malignant neoplasm of pharynx, unspecified

C14.2 Malignant neoplasm of Waldeyer's ring

C14.8 Malignant neoplasm of overlapping sites of lip, oral cavity and pharynx
Primary malignant neoplasm of two or more contiguous sites of lip, oral cavity and pharynx
EXCLUDES 1 *"book leaf" neoplasm [ventral surface of tongue and floor of mouth] (C06.89)*

Malignant neoplasms of digestive organs (C15-C26)

EXCLUDES 1 *Kaposi's sarcoma of gastrointestinal sites (C46.4)*

C15 Malignant neoplasm of esophagus
Use additional code to identify:
alcohol abuse and dependence (F10.-)

C15.3 Malignant neoplasm of upper third of esophagus

C15.4 Malignant neoplasm of middle third of esophagus

C15.5 Malignant neoplasm of lower third of esophagus
EXCLUDES 1 *malignant neoplasm of cardio-esophageal junction (C16.0)*

C15.8 Malignant neoplasm of overlapping sites of esophagus

C15.9 Malignant neoplasm of esophagus, unspecified

C16 Malignant neoplasm of stomach
Use additional code to identify:
alcohol abuse and dependence (F10.-)
EXCLUDES 2 *malignant carcinoid tumor of the stomach (C7A.092)*

C16.0 Malignant neoplasm of cardia
Malignant neoplasm of cardiac orifice
Malignant neoplasm of cardio-esophageal junction
Malignant neoplasm of esophagus and stomach
Malignant neoplasm of gastro-esophageal junction

C16.1 Malignant neoplasm of fundus of stomach

C16.2 Malignant neoplasm of body of stomach

C16.3 Malignant neoplasm of pyloric antrum
Malignant neoplasm of gastric antrum

C16.4 Malignant neoplasm of pylorus
Malignant neoplasm of prepylorus
Malignant neoplasm of pyloric canal

C16.5 Malignant neoplasm of lesser curvature of stomach, unspecified
Malignant neoplasm of lesser curvature of stomach, not classifiable to C16.1-C16.4

C16.6 Malignant neoplasm of greater curvature of stomach, unspecified
Malignant neoplasm of greater curvature of stomach, not classifiable to C16.0-C16.4

C16.8 Malignant neoplasm of overlapping sites of stomach

C16.9 Malignant neoplasm of stomach, unspecified
Gastric cancer NOS

C17 Malignant neoplasm of small intestine
EXCLUDES 1 *malignant carcinoid tumors of the small intestine (C7A.01)*

C17.0 Malignant neoplasm of duodenum

C17.1 Malignant neoplasm of jejunum

C17.2 Malignant neoplasm of ileum
EXCLUDES 1 *malignant neoplasm of ileocecal valve (C18.0)*

C17.3 Meckel's diverticulum, malignant
EXCLUDES 1 *Meckel's diverticulum, congenital (Q43.0)*

C17.8 Malignant neoplasm of overlapping sites of small intestine

C17.9 Malignant neoplasm of small intestine, unspecified

C18 Malignant neoplasm of colon
EXCLUDES 1 *malignant carcinoid tumors of the colon (C7A.02-)*

C18.0 Malignant neoplasm of cecum
Malignant neoplasm of ileocecal valve

C18.1 Malignant neoplasm of appendix

C18.2 Malignant neoplasm of ascending colon

C18.3 Malignant neoplasm of hepatic flexure

C18.4 Malignant neoplasm of transverse colon

C18.5 Malignant neoplasm of splenic flexure

C18.6 Malignant neoplasm of descending colon

C18.7 Malignant neoplasm of sigmoid colon
Malignant neoplasm of sigmoid (flexure)
EXCLUDES 1 *malignant neoplasm of rectosigmoid junction (C19)*

C18.8 Malignant neoplasm of overlapping sites of colon

C18.9 Malignant neoplasm of colon, unspecified
Malignant neoplasm of large intestine NOS

C19 Malignant neoplasm of rectosigmoid junction
Malignant neoplasm of colon with rectum
Malignant neoplasm of rectosigmoid (colon)
EXCLUDES 1 *malignant carcinoid tumors of the colon (C7A.02-)*

C20 Malignant neoplasm of rectum
Malignant neoplasm of rectal ampulla
EXCLUDES 1 *malignant carcinoid tumor of the rectum (C7A.026)*

C21 Malignant neoplasm of anus and anal canal
EXCLUDES 2 *malignant carcinoid tumors of the colon (C7A.02-)*
other and unspecified malignant neoplasm of anal margin (C44.500, C44.510, C44.520, C44.590)
other and unspecified malignant neoplasm of anal skin (C44.500, C44.510, C44.520, C44.590)
other and unspecified malignant neoplasm of perianal skin (C44.500, C44.510, C44.520, C44.590)

C21.0 Malignant neoplasm of anus, unspecified

C21.1 Malignant neoplasm of anal canal
Malignant neoplasm of anal sphincter

C21.2 Malignant neoplasm of cloacogenic zone

C21.8 Malignant neoplasm of overlapping sites of rectum, anus and anal canal
Malignant neoplasm of anorectal junction
Malignant neoplasm of anorectum
Primary malignant neoplasm of two or more contiguous sites of rectum, anus and anal canal

C22 Malignant neoplasm of liver and intrahepatic bile ducts
EXCLUDES 1 *malignant neoplasm of biliary tract NOS (C24.9)*
secondary malignant neoplasm of liver and intrahepatic bile duct (C78.7)
Use additional code to identify:
alcohol abuse and dependence (F10.-)
hepatitis B (B16.-, B18.0-B18.1)
hepatitis C (B17.1-, B18.2)

C22.0 Liver cell carcinoma
Hepatocellular carcinoma
Hepatoma

C22.1 Intrahepatic bile duct carcinoma
Cholangiocarcinoma
EXCLUDES 1 *malignant neoplasm of hepatic duct (C24.0)*

C22.2 Hepatoblastoma

C22.3 Angiosarcoma of liver
Kupffer cell sarcoma

C22.4 Other sarcomas of liver
C22.7 Other specified carcinomas of liver
C22.8 Malignant neoplasm of liver, primary, unspecified as to type
C22.9 Malignant neoplasm of liver, not specified as primary or secondary

C23 Malignant neoplasm of gallbladder

✓4th **C24 Malignant neoplasm of other and unspecified parts of biliary tract**
EXCLUDES 1 *malignant neoplasm of intrahepatic bile duct (C22.1)*
C24.0 Malignant neoplasm of extrahepatic bile duct
Malignant neoplasm of biliary duct or passage NOS
Malignant neoplasm of common bile duct
Malignant neoplasm of cystic duct
Malignant neoplasm of hepatic duct
C24.1 Malignant neoplasm of ampulla of Vater
C24.8 Malignant neoplasm of overlapping sites of biliary tract
Malignant neoplasm involving both intrahepatic and extrahepatic bile ducts
Primary malignant neoplasm of two or more contiguous sites of biliary tract
C24.9 Malignant neoplasm of biliary tract, unspecified

✓4th **C25 Malignant neoplasm of pancreas**
Use additional code to identify:
alcohol abuse and dependence (F10.-)
C25.0 Malignant neoplasm of head of pancreas
C25.1 Malignant neoplasm of body of pancreas
C25.2 Malignant neoplasm of tail of pancreas
C25.3 Malignant neoplasm of pancreatic duct
C25.4 Malignant neoplasm of endocrine pancreas
Malignant neoplasm of islets of Langerhans
Use additional code to identify any functional activity
C25.7 Malignant neoplasm of other parts of pancreas
Malignant neoplasm of neck of pancreas
C25.8 Malignant neoplasm of overlapping sites of pancreas
C25.9 Malignant neoplasm of pancreas, unspecified

✓4th **C26 Malignant neoplasm of other and ill-defined digestive organs**
EXCLUDES 1 *malignant neoplasm of peritoneum and retroperitoneum (C48.-)*
C26.0 Malignant neoplasm of intestinal tract, part unspecified
Malignant neoplasm of intestine NOS
C26.1 Malignant neoplasm of spleen
EXCLUDES 1 *Hodgkin lymphoma (C81.-)*
non-Hodgkin lymphoma (C82-C85)
C26.9 Malignant neoplasm of ill-defined sites within the digestive system
Malignant neoplasm of alimentary canal or tract NOS
Malignant neoplasm of gastrointestinal tract NOS
EXCLUDES 1 *malignant neoplasm of abdominal NOS (C76.2)*
malignant neoplasm of intra-abdominal NOS (C76.2)

Malignant neoplasms of respiratory and intrathoracic organs (C30-C39)

INCLUDES malignant neoplasm of middle ear
EXCLUDES 1 *mesothelioma (C45.-)*

✓4th **C30 Malignant neoplasm of nasal cavity and middle ear**
C30.0 Malignant neoplasm of nasal cavity
Malignant neoplasm of cartilage of nose
Malignant neoplasm of nasal concha
Malignant neoplasm of internal nose
Malignant neoplasm of septum of nose
Malignant neoplasm of vestibule of nose
EXCLUDES 1 *malignant melanoma of skin of nose (C43.31)*
malignant neoplasm of nasal bone (C41.0)
malignant neoplasm of nose NOS (C76.0)
malignant neoplasm of olfactory bulb (C72.2-)
malignant neoplasm of posterior margin of nasal septum and choana (C11.3)
malignant neoplasm of turbinates (C41.0)
other and unspecified malignant neoplasm of skin of nose (C44.301, C44.311, C44.321, C44.391)
C30.1 Malignant neoplasm of middle ear
Malignant neoplasm of antrum tympanicum
Malignant neoplasm of auditory tube
Malignant neoplasm of eustachian tube
Malignant neoplasm of inner ear
Malignant neoplasm of mastoid air cells
Malignant neoplasm of tympanic cavity
EXCLUDES 1 *malignant melanoma of skin of (external) ear (C43.2-)*
malignant neoplasm of auricular canal (external) (C43.2-, C44.2-)
malignant neoplasm of bone of ear (meatus) (C41.0)
malignant neoplasm of cartilage of ear (C49.0)
other and unspecified malignant neoplasm of skin of (external) ear (C44.2-)

✓4th **C31 Malignant neoplasm of accessory sinuses**
C31.0 Malignant neoplasm of maxillary sinus
Malignant neoplasm of antrum (Highmore) (maxillary)
C31.1 Malignant neoplasm of ethmoidal sinus
C31.2 Malignant neoplasm of frontal sinus
C31.3 Malignant neoplasm of sphenoid sinus
C31.8 Malignant neoplasm of overlapping sites of accessory sinuses
C31.9 Malignant neoplasm of accessory sinus, unspecified

✓4th **C32 Malignant neoplasm of larynx**
Use additional code to identify:
alcohol abuse and dependence (F10.-)
exposure to environmental tobacco smoke (Z77.22)
exposure to tobacco smoke in the perinatal period (P96.81)
history of tobacco use (Z87.891)
occupational exposure to environmental tobacco smoke (Z57.31)
tobacco dependence (F17.-)
tobacco use (Z72.0)
C32.0 Malignant neoplasm of glottis
Malignant neoplasm of intrinsic larynx
Malignant neoplasm of laryngeal commissure (anterior)(posterior)
Malignant neoplasm of vocal cord (true) NOS
C32.1 Malignant neoplasm of supraglottis
Malignant neoplasm of aryepiglottic fold or interarytenoid fold, laryngeal aspect
Malignant neoplasm of epiglottis (suprahyoid portion) NOS
Malignant neoplasm of extrinsic larynx
Malignant neoplasm of false vocal cord
Malignant neoplasm of posterior (laryngeal) surface of epiglottis
Malignant neoplasm of ventricular bands
EXCLUDES 2 *malignant neoplasm of anterior surface of epiglottis (C10.1)*
malignant neoplasm of aryepiglottic fold or interarytenoid fold:
NOS (C13.1)
hypopharyngeal aspect (C13.1)
marginal zone (C13.1)
C32.2 Malignant neoplasm of subglottis
C32.3 Malignant neoplasm of laryngeal cartilage
C32.8 Malignant neoplasm of overlapping sites of larynx
C32.9 Malignant neoplasm of larynx, unspecified

C33 Malignant neoplasm of trachea
Use additional code to identify:
exposure to environmental tobacco smoke (Z77.22)
exposure to tobacco smoke in the perinatal period (P96.81)
history of tobacco use (Z87.891)
occupational exposure to environmental tobacco smoke (Z57.31)
tobacco dependence (F17.-)
tobacco use (Z72.0)

C34 Malignant neoplasm of bronchus and lung

EXCLUDES 1 *Kaposi's sarcoma of lung (C46.5-)*
malignant carcinoid tumor of the bronchus and lung (C7A.090)

Use additional code to identify:
exposure to environmental tobacco smoke (Z77.22)
exposure to tobacco smoke in the perinatal period (P96.81)
history of tobacco use (Z87.891)
occupational exposure to environmental tobacco smoke (Z57.31)
tobacco dependence (F17.-)
tobacco use (Z72.0)

C34.0 Malignant neoplasm of main bronchus
Malignant neoplasm of carina
Malignant neoplasm of hilus (of lung)

C34.00 Malignant neoplasm of unspecified main bronchus
C34.01 Malignant neoplasm of right main bronchus
C34.02 Malignant neoplasm of left main bronchus

C34.1 Malignant neoplasm of upper lobe, bronchus or lung

C34.10 Malignant neoplasm of upper lobe, unspecified bronchus or lung
C34.11 Malignant neoplasm of upper lobe, right bronchus or lung
C34.12 Malignant neoplasm of upper lobe, left bronchus or lung

C34.2 Malignant neoplasm of middle lobe, bronchus or lung

C34.3 Malignant neoplasm of lower lobe, bronchus or lung

C34.30 Malignant neoplasm of lower lobe, unspecified bronchus or lung
C34.31 Malignant neoplasm of lower lobe, right bronchus or lung
C34.32 Malignant neoplasm of lower lobe, left bronchus or lung

C34.8 Malignant neoplasm of overlapping sites of bronchus and lung

C34.80 Malignant neoplasm of overlapping sites of unspecified bronchus and lung
C34.81 Malignant neoplasm of overlapping sites of right bronchus and lung
C34.82 Malignant neoplasm of overlapping sites of left bronchus and lung

C34.9 Malignant neoplasm of unspecified part of bronchus or lung

C34.90 Malignant neoplasm of unspecified part of unspecified bronchus or lung
Lung cancer NOS
C34.91 Malignant neoplasm of unspecified part of right bronchus or lung
C34.92 Malignant neoplasm of unspecified part of left bronchus or lung

C37 Malignant neoplasm of thymus

EXCLUDES 1 *malignant carcinoid tumor of the thymus (C7A.091)*

C38 Malignant neoplasm of heart, mediastinum and pleura

EXCLUDES 1 *mesothelioma (C45.-)*

C38.0 Malignant neoplasm of heart
Malignant neoplasm of pericardium
EXCLUDES 1 *malignant neoplasm of great vessels (C49.3)*
C38.1 Malignant neoplasm of anterior mediastinum
C38.2 Malignant neoplasm of posterior mediastinum
C38.3 Malignant neoplasm of mediastinum, part unspecified
C38.4 Malignant neoplasm of pleura
C38.8 Malignant neoplasm of overlapping sites of heart, mediastinum and pleura

C39 Malignant neoplasm of other and ill-defined sites in the respiratory system and intrathoracic organs

EXCLUDES 1 *intrathoracic malignant neoplasm NOS (C76.1)*
thoracic malignant neoplasm NOS (C76.1)

Use additional code to identify:
exposure to environmental tobacco smoke (Z77.22)
exposure to tobacco smoke in the perinatal period (P96.81)
history of tobacco use (Z87.891)
occupational exposure to environmental tobacco smoke (Z57.31)
tobacco dependence (F17.-)
tobacco use (Z72.0)

C39.0 Malignant neoplasm of upper respiratory tract, part unspecified
C39.9 Malignant neoplasm of lower respiratory tract, part unspecified
Malignant neoplasm of respiratory tract NOS

Malignant neoplasms of bone and articular cartilage (C40-C41)

INCLUDES malignant neoplasm of cartilage (articular) (joint)
malignant neoplasm of periosteum

EXCLUDES 1 *malignant neoplasm of bone marrow NOS (C96.9)*
malignant neoplasm of synovia (C49.-)

C40 Malignant neoplasm of bone and articular cartilage of limbs

Use additional code to identify major osseous defect, if applicable (M89.7-)

C40.0 Malignant neoplasm of scapula and long bones of upper limb

C40.00 Malignant neoplasm of scapula and long bones of unspecified upper limb
C40.01 Malignant neoplasm of scapula and long bones of right upper limb
C40.02 Malignant neoplasm of scapula and long bones of left upper limb

C40.1 Malignant neoplasm of short bones of upper limb

C40.10 Malignant neoplasm of short bones of unspecified upper limb
C40.11 Malignant neoplasm of short bones of right upper limb
C40.12 Malignant neoplasm of short bones of left upper limb

C40.2 Malignant neoplasm of long bones of lower limb

C40.20 Malignant neoplasm of long bones of unspecified lower limb
C40.21 Malignant neoplasm of long bones of right lower limb
C40.22 Malignant neoplasm of long bones of left lower limb

C40.3 Malignant neoplasm of short bones of lower limb

C40.30 Malignant neoplasm of short bones of unspecified lower limb
C40.31 Malignant neoplasm of short bones of right lower limb
C40.32 Malignant neoplasm of short bones of left lower limb

C40.8 Malignant neoplasm of overlapping sites of bone and articular cartilage of limb

C40.80 Malignant neoplasm of overlapping sites of bone and articular cartilage of unspecified limb
C40.81 Malignant neoplasm of overlapping sites of bone and articular cartilage of right limb
C40.82 Malignant neoplasm of overlapping sites of bone and articular cartilage of left limb

C40.9 Malignant neoplasm of unspecified bones and articular cartilage of limb

C40.90 Malignant neoplasm of unspecified bones and articular cartilage of unspecified limb
C40.91 Malignant neoplasm of unspecified bones and articular cartilage of right limb
C40.92 Malignant neoplasm of unspecified bones and articular cartilage of left limb

C41 Malignant neoplasm of bone and articular cartilage of other and unspecified sites

EXCLUDES 1 *malignant neoplasm of bones of limbs (C40.-)*
malignant neoplasm of cartilage of:
ear (C49.0)
eyelid (C49.0)
larynx (C32.3)
limbs (C40.-)
nose (C30.0)

C41.0 Malignant neoplasm of bones of skull and face
Malignant neoplasm of maxilla (superior)
Malignant neoplasm of orbital bone
EXCLUDES 2 *carcinoma, any type except intraosseous or odontogenic of:*
maxillary sinus (C31.0)
upper jaw (C03.0)
malignant neoplasm of jaw bone (lower) (C41.1)

C41.1 Malignant neoplasm of mandible
Malignant neoplasm of inferior maxilla
Malignant neoplasm of lower jaw bone
EXCLUDES 2 *carcinoma, any type except intraosseous or odontogenic of:*
jaw NOS (C03.9)
lower (C03.1)
malignant neoplasm of upper jaw bone (C41.0)

C41.2 Malignant neoplasm of vertebral column
EXCLUDES 1 *malignant neoplasm of sacrum and coccyx (C41.4)*

C41.3 Malignant neoplasm of ribs, sternum and clavicle

C41.4 Malignant neoplasm of pelvic bones, sacrum and coccyx

C41.9 Malignant neoplasm of bone and articular cartilage, unspecified

Melanoma and other malignant neoplasms of skin (C43-C44)

✓4th **C43 Malignant melanoma of skin**
EXCLUDES 1 *melanoma in situ (D03.-)*
EXCLUDES 2 *malignant melanoma of skin of genital organs (C51-C52, C60.-, C63.-)*
Merkel cell carcinoma (C4A.-)
sites other than skin—code to malignant neoplasm of the site

C43.0 Malignant melanoma of lip
EXCLUDES 1 *malignant neoplasm of vermilion border of lip (C00.0-C00.2)*

✓5th **C43.1 Malignant melanoma of eyelid, including canthus**
C43.10 Malignant melanoma of unspecified eyelid, including canthus
C43.11 Malignant melanoma of right eyelid, including canthus
C43.12 Malignant melanoma of left eyelid, including canthus

✓5th **C43.2 Malignant melanoma of ear and external auricular canal**
C43.20 Malignant melanoma of unspecified ear and external auricular canal
C43.21 Malignant melanoma of right ear and external auricular canal
C43.22 Malignant melanoma of left ear and external auricular canal

✓5th **C43.3 Malignant melanoma of other and unspecified parts of face**
C43.30 Malignant melanoma of unspecified part of face
C43.31 Malignant melanoma of nose
C43.39 Malignant melanoma of other parts of face

C43.4 Malignant melanoma of scalp and neck

✓5th **C43.5 Malignant melanoma of trunk**
EXCLUDES 2 *malignant neoplasm of anus NOS (C21.0)*
malignant neoplasm of scrotum (C63.2)
C43.51 Malignant melanoma of anal skin
Malignant melanoma of anal margin
Malignant melanoma of perianal skin
C43.52 Malignant melanoma of skin of breast
C43.59 Malignant melanoma of other part of trunk

✓5th **C43.6 Malignant melanoma of upper limb, including shoulder**
C43.60 Malignant melanoma of unspecified upper limb, including shoulder
C43.61 Malignant melanoma of right upper limb, including shoulder
C43.62 Malignant melanoma of left upper limb, including shoulder

✓5th **C43.7 Malignant melanoma of lower limb, including hip**
C43.70 Malignant melanoma of unspecified lower limb, including hip
C43.71 Malignant melanoma of right lower limb, including hip
C43.72 Malignant melanoma of left lower limb, including hip

C43.8 Malignant melanoma of overlapping sites of skin

C43.9 Malignant melanoma of skin, unspecified
Malignant melanoma of unspecified site of skin

✓4th **C4A Merkel cell carcinoma**

C4A.0 Merkel cell carcinoma of lip
EXCLUDES 1 *malignant neoplasm of vermilion border of lip (C00.0-C00.2)*

✓5th **C4A.1 Merkel cell carcinoma of eyelid, including canthus**
C4A.10 Merkel cell carcinoma of unspecified eyelid, including canthus
C4A.11 Merkel cell carcinoma of right eyelid, including canthus
C4A.12 Merkel cell carcinoma of left eyelid, including canthus

✓5th **C4A.2 Merkel cell carcinoma of ear and external auricular canal**
C4A.20 Merkel cell carcinoma of unspecified ear and external auricular canal
C4A.21 Merkel cell carcinoma of right ear and external auricular canal
C4A.22 Merkel cell carcinoma of left ear and external auricular canal

✓5th **C4A.3 Merkel cell carcinoma of other and unspecified parts of face**
C4A.30 Merkel cell carcinoma of unspecified part of face
C4A.31 Merkel cell carcinoma of nose
C4A.39 Merkel cell carcinoma of other parts of face

C4A.4 Merkel cell carcinoma of scalp and neck

✓5th **C4A.5 Merkel cell carcinoma of trunk**
EXCLUDES 2 *malignant neoplasm of anus NOS (C21.0)*
malignant neoplasm of scrotum (C63.2)
C4A.51 Merkel cell carcinoma of anal skin
Merkel cell carcinoma of anal margin
Merkel cell carcinoma of perianal skin
C4A.52 Merkel cell carcinoma of skin of breast
C4A.59 Merkel cell carcinoma of other part of trunk

✓5th **C4A.6 Merkel cell carcinoma of upper limb, including shoulder**
C4A.60 Merkel cell carcinoma of unspecified upper limb, including shoulder
C4A.61 Merkel cell carcinoma of right upper limb, including shoulder
C4A.62 Merkel cell carcinoma of left upper limb, including shoulder

✓5th **C4A.7 Merkel cell carcinoma of lower limb, including hip**
C4A.70 Merkel cell carcinoma of unspecified lower limb, including hip
C4A.71 Merkel cell carcinoma of right lower limb, including hip
C4A.72 Merkel cell carcinoma of left lower limb, including hip

C4A.8 Merkel cell carcinoma of overlapping sites

C4A.9 Merkel cell carcinoma, unspecified
Merkel cell carcinoma of unspecified site

✓4th **C44 Other and unspecified malignant neoplasm of skin**
INCLUDES malignant neoplasm of sebaceous glands
malignant neoplasm of sweat glands
EXCLUDES 1 *Kaposi's sarcoma of skin (C46.0)*
malignant melanoma of skin (C43.-)
malignant neoplasm of skin of genital organs (C51-C52, C60-, C63.2)
Merkel cell carcinoma (C4A.-)

✓5th **C44.0 Other and unspecified malignant neoplasm of skin of lip**
EXCLUDES 1 *malignant neoplasm of lip (C00.-)*
C44.00 Unspecified malignant neoplasm of skin of lip
C44.01 Basal cell carcinoma of skin of lip
C44.02 Squamous cell carcinoma of skin of lip
C44.09 Other specified malignant neoplasm of skin of lip

✓5th **C44.1 Other and unspecified malignant neoplasm of skin of eyelid, including canthus**
EXCLUDES 1 *connective tissue of eyelid (C49.0)*

✓6th **C44.10 Unspecified malignant neoplasm of skin of eyelid, including canthus**
C44.101 Unspecified malignant neoplasm of skin of unspecified eyelid, including canthus
C44.102 Unspecified malignant neoplasm of skin of right eyelid, including canthus
C44.109 Unspecified malignant neoplasm of skin of left eyelid, including canthus

✓6th **C44.11 Basal cell carcinoma of skin of eyelid, including canthus**
C44.111 Basal cell carcinoma of skin of unspecified eyelid, including canthus
C44.112 Basal cell carcinoma of skin of right eyelid, including canthus
C44.119 Basal cell carcinoma of skin of left eyelid, including canthus

C44.12 Squamous cell carcinoma of skin of eyelid, including canthus
- **C44.121 Squamous cell carcinoma of skin of unspecified eyelid, including canthus**
- **C44.122 Squamous cell carcinoma of skin of right eyelid, including canthus**
- **C44.129 Squamous cell carcinoma of skin of left eyelid, including canthus**

C44.19 Other specified malignant neoplasm of skin of eyelid, including canthus
- **C44.191 Other specified malignant neoplasm of skin of unspecified eyelid, including canthus**
- **C44.192 Other specified malignant neoplasm of skin of right eyelid, including canthus**
- **C44.199 Other specified malignant neoplasm of skin of left eyelid, including canthus**

C44.2 Other and unspecified malignant neoplasm of skin of ear and external auricular canal

EXCLUDES 1 *connective tissue of ear (C49.0)*

C44.20 Unspecified malignant neoplasm of skin of ear and external auricular canal
- **C44.201 Unspecified malignant neoplasm of skin of unspecified ear and external auricular canal**
- **C44.202 Unspecified malignant neoplasm of skin of right ear and external auricular canal**
- **C44.209 Unspecified malignant neoplasm of skin of left ear and external auricular canal**

C44.21 Basal cell carcinoma of skin of ear and external auricular canal
- **C44.211 Basal cell carcinoma of skin of unspecified ear and external auricular canal**
- **C44.212 Basal cell carcinoma of skin of right ear and external auricular canal**
- **C44.219 Basal cell carcinoma of skin of left ear and external auricular canal**

C44.22 Squamous cell carcinoma of skin of ear and external auricular canal
- **C44.221 Squamous cell carcinoma of skin of unspecified ear and external auricular canal**
- **C44.222 Squamous cell carcinoma of skin of right ear and external auricular canal**
- **C44.229 Squamous cell carcinoma of skin of left ear and external auricular canal**

C44.29 Other specified malignant neoplasm of skin of ear and external auricular canal
- **C44.291 Other specified malignant neoplasm of skin of unspecified ear and external auricular canal**
- **C44.292 Other specified malignant neoplasm of skin of right ear and external auricular canal**
- **C44.299 Other specified malignant neoplasm of skin of left ear and external auricular canal**

C44.3 Other and unspecified malignant neoplasm of skin of other and unspecified parts of face

C44.30 Unspecified malignant neoplasm of skin of other and unspecified parts of face
- **C44.300 Unspecified malignant neoplasm of skin of unspecified part of face**
- **C44.301 Unspecified malignant neoplasm of skin of nose**
- **C44.309 Unspecified malignant neoplasm of skin of other parts of face**

C44.31 Basal cell carcinoma of skin of other and unspecified parts of face
- **C44.310 Basal cell carcinoma of skin of unspecified parts of face**
- **C44.311 Basal cell carcinoma of skin of nose**
- **C44.319 Basal cell carcinoma of skin of other parts of face**

C44.32 Squamous cell carcinoma of skin of other and unspecified parts of face
- **C44.320 Squamous cell carcinoma of skin of unspecified parts of face**
- **C44.321 Squamous cell carcinoma of skin of nose**
- **C44.329 Squamous cell carcinoma of skin of other parts of face**

C44.39 Other specified malignant neoplasm of skin of other and unspecified parts of face
- **C44.390 Other specified malignant neoplasm of skin of unspecified parts of face**
- **C44.391 Other specified malignant neoplasm of skin of nose**
- **C44.399 Other specified malignant neoplasm of skin of other parts of face**

C44.4 Other and unspecified malignant neoplasm of skin of scalp and neck
- **C44.40 Unspecified malignant neoplasm of skin of scalp and neck**
- **C44.41 Basal cell carcinoma of skin of scalp and neck**
- **C44.42 Squamous cell carcinoma of skin of scalp and neck**
- **C44.49 Other specified malignant neoplasm of skin of scalp and neck**

C44.5 Other and unspecified malignant neoplasm of skin of trunk

EXCLUDES 1 *anus NOS (C21.0)*
scrotum (C63.2)

C44.50 Unspecified malignant neoplasm of skin of trunk
- **C44.500 Unspecified malignant neoplasm of anal skin**
  - Unspecified malignant neoplasm of anal margin
  - Unspecified malignant neoplasm of perianal skin
- **C44.501 Unspecified malignant neoplasm of skin of breast**
- **C44.509 Unspecified malignant neoplasm of skin of other part of trunk**

C44.51 Basal cell carcinoma of skin of trunk
- **C44.510 Basal cell carcinoma of anal skin**
  - Basal cell carcinoma of anal margin
  - Basal cell carcinoma of perianal skin
- **C44.511 Basal cell carcinoma of skin of breast**
- **C44.519 Basal cell carcinoma of skin of other part of trunk**

C44.52 Squamous cell carcinoma of skin of trunk
- **C44.520 Squamous cell carcinoma of anal skin**
  - Squamous cell carcinoma of anal margin
  - Squamous cell carcinoma of perianal skin
- **C44.521 Squamous cell carcinoma of skin of breast**
- **C44.529 Squamous cell carcinoma of skin of other part of trunk**

C44.59 Other specified malignant neoplasm of skin of trunk
- **C44.590 Other specified malignant neoplasm of anal skin**
  - Other specified malignant neoplasm of anal margin
  - Other specified malignant neoplasm of perianal skin
- **C44.591 Other specified malignant neoplasm of skin of breast**
- **C44.599 Other specified malignant neoplasm of skin of other part of trunk**

C44.6 Other and unspecified malignant neoplasm of skin of upper limb, including shoulder

C44.60 Unspecified malignant neoplasm of skin of upper limb, including shoulder
- **C44.601 Unspecified malignant neoplasm of skin of unspecified upper limb, including shoulder**
- **C44.602 Unspecified malignant neoplasm of skin of right upper limb, including shoulder**
- **C44.609 Unspecified malignant neoplasm of skin of left upper limb, including shoulder**

√6th **C44.61 Basal cell carcinoma of skin of upper limb, including shoulder**
C44.611 Basal cell carcinoma of skin of unspecified upper limb, including shoulder
C44.612 Basal cell carcinoma of skin of right upper limb, including shoulder
C44.619 Basal cell carcinoma of skin of left upper limb, including shoulder

√6th **C44.62 Squamous cell carcinoma of skin of upper limb, including shoulder**
C44.621 Squamous cell carcinoma of skin of unspecified upper limb, including shoulder
C44.622 Squamous cell carcinoma of skin of right upper limb, including shoulder
C44.629 Squamous cell carcinoma of skin of left upper limb, including shoulder

√6th **C44.69 Other specified malignant neoplasm of skin of upper limb, including shoulder**
C44.691 Other specified malignant neoplasm of skin of unspecified upper limb, including shoulder
C44.692 Other specified malignant neoplasm of skin of right upper limb, including shoulder
C44.699 Other specified malignant neoplasm of skin of left upper limb, including shoulder

√5th **C44.7 Other and unspecified malignant neoplasm of skin of lower limb, including hip**

√6th **C44.70 Unspecified malignant neoplasm of skin of lower limb, including hip**
C44.701 Unspecified malignant neoplasm of skin of unspecified lower limb, including hip
C44.702 Unspecified malignant neoplasm of skin of right lower limb, including hip
C44.709 Unspecified malignant neoplasm of skin of left lower limb, including hip

√6th **C44.71 Basal cell carcinoma of skin of lower limb, including hip**
C44.711 Basal cell carcinoma of skin of unspecified lower limb, including hip
C44.712 Basal cell carcinoma of skin of right lower limb, including hip
C44.719 Basal cell carcinoma of skin of left lower limb, including hip

√6th **C44.72 Squamous cell carcinoma of skin of lower limb, including hip**
C44.721 Squamous cell carcinoma of skin of unspecified lower limb, including hip
C44.722 Squamous cell carcinoma of skin of right lower limb, including hip
C44.729 Squamous cell carcinoma of skin of left lower limb, including hip

√6th **C44.79 Other specified malignant neoplasm of skin of lower limb, including hip**
C44.791 Other specified malignant neoplasm of skin of unspecified lower limb, including hip
C44.792 Other specified malignant neoplasm of skin of right lower limb, including hip
C44.799 Other specified malignant neoplasm of skin of left lower limb, including hip

√5th **C44.8 Other and unspecified malignant neoplasm of overlapping sites of skin**
C44.80 Unspecified malignant neoplasm of overlapping sites of skin
C44.81 Basal cell carcinoma of overlapping sites of skin
C44.82 Squamous cell carcinoma of overlapping sites of skin
C44.89 Other specified malignant neoplasm of overlapping sites of skin

√5th **C44.9 Other and unspecified malignant neoplasm of skin, unspecified**
C44.90 Unspecified malignant neoplasm of skin, unspecified
Malignant neoplasm of unspecified site of skin
C44.91 Basal cell carcinoma of skin, unspecified
C44.92 Squamous cell carcinoma of skin, unspecified
C44.99 Other specified malignant neoplasm of skin, unspecified

Malignant neoplasms of mesothelial and soft tissue (C45-C49)

√4th **C45 Mesothelioma**
C45.0 Mesothelioma of pleura
EXCLUDES1 *other malignant neoplasm of pleura (C38.4)*
C45.1 Mesothelioma of peritoneum
Mesothelioma of cul-de-sac
Mesothelioma of mesentery
Mesothelioma of mesocolon
Mesothelioma of omentum
Mesothelioma of peritoneum (parietal) (pelvic)
EXCLUDES1 *other malignant neoplasm of soft tissue of peritoneum (C48.-)*
C45.2 Mesothelioma of pericardium
EXCLUDES1 *other malignant neoplasm of pericardium (C38.0)*
C45.7 Mesothelioma of other sites
C45.9 Mesothelioma, unspecified

√4th **C46 Kaposi's sarcoma**
Code first any human immunodeficiency virus [HIV] disease (B20)
C46.0 Kaposi's sarcoma of skin
C46.1 Kaposi's sarcoma of soft tissue
Kaposi's sarcoma of blood vessel
Kaposi's sarcoma of connective tissue
Kaposi's sarcoma of fascia
Kaposi's sarcoma of ligament
Kaposi's sarcoma of lymphatic(s) NEC
Kaposi's sarcoma of muscle
EXCLUDES2 *Kaposi's sarcoma of lymph glands and nodes (C46.3)*
C46.2 Kaposi's sarcoma of palate
C46.3 Kaposi's sarcoma of lymph nodes
C46.4 Kaposi's sarcoma of gastrointestinal sites
√5th **C46.5 Kaposi's sarcoma of lung**
C46.50 Kaposi's sarcoma of unspecified lung
C46.51 Kaposi's sarcoma of right lung
C46.52 Kaposi's sarcoma of left lung
C46.7 Kaposi's sarcoma of other sites
C46.9 Kaposi's sarcoma, unspecified
Kaposi's sarcoma of unspecified site

√4th **C47 Malignant neoplasm of peripheral nerves and autonomic nervous system**
INCLUDES malignant neoplasm of sympathetic and parasympathetic nerves and ganglia
EXCLUDES1 *Kaposi's sarcoma of soft tissue (C46.1)*
C47.0 Malignant neoplasm of peripheral nerves of head, face and neck
EXCLUDES1 *malignant neoplasm of peripheral nerves of orbit (C69.6-)*
√5th **C47.1 Malignant neoplasm of peripheral nerves of upper limb, including shoulder**
C47.10 Malignant neoplasm of peripheral nerves of unspecified upper limb, including shoulder
C47.11 Malignant neoplasm of peripheral nerves of right upper limb, including shoulder
C47.12 Malignant neoplasm of peripheral nerves of left upper limb, including shoulder
√5th **C47.2 Malignant neoplasm of peripheral nerves of lower limb, including hip**
C47.20 Malignant neoplasm of peripheral nerves of unspecified lower limb, including hip
C47.21 Malignant neoplasm of peripheral nerves of right lower limb, including hip
C47.22 Malignant neoplasm of peripheral nerves of left lower limb, including hip
C47.3 Malignant neoplasm of peripheral nerves of thorax
C47.4 Malignant neoplasm of peripheral nerves of abdomen
C47.5 Malignant neoplasm of peripheral nerves of pelvis
C47.6 Malignant neoplasm of peripheral nerves of trunk, unspecified
Malignant neoplasm of peripheral nerves of unspecified part of trunk
C47.8 Malignant neoplasm of overlapping sites of peripheral nerves and autonomic nervous system

C47.9 Malignant neoplasm of peripheral nerves and autonomic nervous system, unspecified
Malignant neoplasm of unspecified site of peripheral nerves and autonomic nervous system

C48 Malignant neoplasm of retroperitoneum and peritoneum
EXCLUDES 1 *Kaposi's sarcoma of connective tissue (C46.1)*
mesothelioma (C45.-)

C48.0 Malignant neoplasm of retroperitoneum

C48.1 Malignant neoplasm of specified parts of peritoneum
Malignant neoplasm of cul-de-sac
Malignant neoplasm of mesentery
Malignant neoplasm of mesocolon
Malignant neoplasm of omentum
Malignant neoplasm of parietal peritoneum
Malignant neoplasm of pelvic peritoneum

C48.2 Malignant neoplasm of peritoneum, unspecified

C48.8 Malignant neoplasm of overlapping sites of retroperitoneum and peritoneum

C49 Malignant neoplasm of other connective and soft tissue
INCLUDES malignant neoplasm of blood vessel
malignant neoplasm of bursa
malignant neoplasm of cartilage
malignant neoplasm of fascia
malignant neoplasm of fat
malignant neoplasm of ligament, except uterine
malignant neoplasm of lymphatic vessel
malignant neoplasm of muscle
malignant neoplasm of synovia
malignant neoplasm of tendon (sheath)
EXCLUDES 1 *malignant neoplasm of cartilage (of):*
articular (C40-C41)
larynx (C32.3)
nose (C30.0)
malignant neoplasm of connective tissue of breast (C50.-)
EXCLUDES 2 *Kaposi's sarcoma of soft tissue (C46.1)*
malignant neoplasm of heart (C38.0)
malignant neoplasm of peripheral nerves and autonomic nervous system (C47.-)
malignant neoplasm of peritoneum (C48.2)
malignant neoplasm of retroperitoneum (C48.0)
malignant neoplasm of uterine ligament (C57.3)
mesothelioma (C45.-)

C49.0 Malignant neoplasm of connective and soft tissue of head, face and neck
Malignant neoplasm of connective tissue of ear
Malignant neoplasm of connective tissue of eyelid
EXCLUDES 1 *connective tissue of orbit (C69.6-)*

C49.1 Malignant neoplasm of connective and soft tissue of upper limb, including shoulder

C49.10 Malignant neoplasm of connective and soft tissue of unspecified upper limb, including shoulder

C49.11 Malignant neoplasm of connective and soft tissue of right upper limb, including shoulder

C49.12 Malignant neoplasm of connective and soft tissue of left upper limb, including shoulder

C49.2 Malignant neoplasm of connective and soft tissue of lower limb, including hip

C49.20 Malignant neoplasm of connective and soft tissue of unspecified lower limb, including hip

C49.21 Malignant neoplasm of connective and soft tissue of right lower limb, including hip

C49.22 Malignant neoplasm of connective and soft tissue of left lower limb, including hip

C49.3 Malignant neoplasm of connective and soft tissue of thorax
Malignant neoplasm of axilla
Malignant neoplasm of diaphragm
Malignant neoplasm of great vessels
EXCLUDES 1 *malignant neoplasm of breast (C50.-)*
malignant neoplasm of heart (C38.0)
malignant neoplasm of mediastinum (C38.1-C38.3)
malignant neoplasm of thymus (C37)

C49.4 Malignant neoplasm of connective and soft tissue of abdomen
Malignant neoplasm of abdominal wall
Malignant neoplasm of hypochondrium

C49.5 Malignant neoplasm of connective and soft tissue of pelvis
Malignant neoplasm of buttock
Malignant neoplasm of groin
Malignant neoplasm of perineum

C49.6 Malignant neoplasm of connective and soft tissue of trunk, unspecified
Malignant neoplasm of back NOS

C49.8 Malignant neoplasm of overlapping sites of connective and soft tissue
Primary malignant neoplasm of two or more contiguous sites of connective and soft tissue

C49.9 Malignant neoplasm of connective and soft tissue, unspecified

Malignant neoplasms of breast (C50)

C50 Malignant neoplasm of breast
INCLUDES connective tissue of breast
Paget's disease of breast
Paget's disease of nipple
Use additional code to identify estrogen receptor status (Z17.0, Z17.1)
EXCLUDES 1 *skin of breast (C44.501, C44.511, C44.521, C44.591)*

C50.0 Malignant neoplasm of nipple and areola

C50.01 Malignant neoplasm of nipple and areola, female

C50.011 Malignant neoplasm of nipple and areola, right female breast

C50.012 Malignant neoplasm of nipple and areola, left female breast

C50.019 Malignant neoplasm of nipple and areola, unspecified female breast

C50.02 Malignant neoplasm of nipple and areola, male

C50.021 Malignant neoplasm of nipple and areola, right male breast

C50.022 Malignant neoplasm of nipple and areola, left male breast

C50.029 Malignant neoplasm of nipple and areola, unspecified male breast

C50.1 Malignant neoplasm of central portion of breast

C50.11 Malignant neoplasm of central portion of breast, female

C50.111 Malignant neoplasm of central portion of right female breast

C50.112 Malignant neoplasm of central portion of left female breast

C50.119 Malignant neoplasm of central portion of unspecified female breast

C50.12 Malignant neoplasm of central portion of breast, male

C50.121 Malignant neoplasm of central portion of right male breast

C50.122 Malignant neoplasm of central portion of left male breast

C50.129 Malignant neoplasm of central portion of unspecified male breast

C50.2 Malignant neoplasm of upper-inner quadrant of breast

C50.21 Malignant neoplasm of upper-inner quadrant of breast, female

C50.211 Malignant neoplasm of upper-inner quadrant of right female breast

C50.212 Malignant neoplasm of upper-inner quadrant of left female breast

C50.219 Malignant neoplasm of upper-inner quadrant of unspecified female breast

C50.22 Malignant neoplasm of upper-inner quadrant of breast, male

C50.221 Malignant neoplasm of upper-inner quadrant of right male breast

C50.222 Malignant neoplasm of upper-inner quadrant of left male breast

C50.229 Malignant neoplasm of upper-inner quadrant of unspecified male breast

C50.3 Malignant neoplasm of lower-inner quadrant of breast

C50.31 Malignant neoplasm of lower-inner quadrant of breast, female

C50.311 Malignant neoplasm of lower-inner quadrant of right female breast

C50.312 Malignant neoplasm of lower-inner quadrant of left female breast

C50.319 Malignant neoplasm of lower-inner quadrant of unspecified female breast

✓6th **C50.32 Malignant neoplasm of lower-inner quadrant of breast, male**
- **C50.321 Malignant neoplasm of lower-inner quadrant of right male breast**
- **C50.322 Malignant neoplasm of lower-inner quadrant of left male breast**
- **C50.329 Malignant neoplasm of lower-inner quadrant of unspecified male breast**

✓5th **C50.4 Malignant neoplasm of upper-outer quadrant of breast**

✓6th **C50.41 Malignant neoplasm of upper-outer quadrant of breast, female**
- **C50.411 Malignant neoplasm of upper-outer quadrant of right female breast**
- **C50.412 Malignant neoplasm of upper-outer quadrant of left female breast**
- **C50.419 Malignant neoplasm of upper-outer quadrant of unspecified female breast**

✓6th **C50.42 Malignant neoplasm of upper-outer quadrant of breast, male**
- **C50.421 Malignant neoplasm of upper-outer quadrant of right male breast**
- **C50.422 Malignant neoplasm of upper-outer quadrant of left male breast**
- **C50.429 Malignant neoplasm of upper-outer quadrant of unspecified male breast**

✓5th **C50.5 Malignant neoplasm of lower-outer quadrant of breast**

✓6th **C50.51 Malignant neoplasm of lower-outer quadrant of breast, female**
- **C50.511 Malignant neoplasm of lower-outer quadrant of right female breast**
- **C50.512 Malignant neoplasm of lower-outer quadrant of left female breast**
- **C50.519 Malignant neoplasm of lower-outer quadrant of unspecified female breast**

✓6th **C50.52 Malignant neoplasm of lower-outer quadrant of breast, male**
- **C50.521 Malignant neoplasm of lower-outer quadrant of right male breast**
- **C50.522 Malignant neoplasm of lower-outer quadrant of left male breast**
- **C50.529 Malignant neoplasm of lower-outer quadrant of unspecified male breast**

✓5th **C50.6 Malignant neoplasm of axillary tail of breast**

✓6th **C50.61 Malignant neoplasm of axillary tail of breast, female**
- **C50.611 Malignant neoplasm of axillary tail of right female breast**
- **C50.612 Malignant neoplasm of axillary tail of left female breast**
- **C50.619 Malignant neoplasm of axillary tail of unspecified female breast**

✓6th **C50.62 Malignant neoplasm of axillary tail of breast, male**
- **C50.621 Malignant neoplasm of axillary tail of right male breast**
- **C50.622 Malignant neoplasm of axillary tail of left male breast**
- **C50.629 Malignant neoplasm of axillary tail of unspecified male breast**

✓5th **C50.8 Malignant neoplasm of overlapping sites of breast**

✓6th **C50.81 Malignant neoplasm of overlapping sites of breast, female**
- **C50.811 Malignant neoplasm of overlapping sites of right female breast**
- **C50.812 Malignant neoplasm of overlapping sites of left female breast**
- **C50.819 Malignant neoplasm of overlapping sites of unspecified female breast**

✓6th **C50.82 Malignant neoplasm of overlapping sites of breast, male**
- **C50.821 Malignant neoplasm of overlapping sites of right male breast**
- **C50.822 Malignant neoplasm of overlapping sites of left male breast**
- **C50.829 Malignant neoplasm of overlapping sites of unspecified male breast**

✓5th **C50.9 Malignant neoplasm of breast of unspecified site**

✓6th **C50.91 Malignant neoplasm of breast of unspecified site, female**
- **C50.911 Malignant neoplasm of unspecified site of right female breast**
- **C50.912 Malignant neoplasm of unspecified site of left female breast**
- **C50.919 Malignant neoplasm of unspecified site of unspecified female breast**

✓6th **C50.92 Malignant neoplasm of breast of unspecified site, male**
- **C50.921 Malignant neoplasm of unspecified site of right male breast**
- **C50.922 Malignant neoplasm of unspecified site of left male breast**
- **C50.929 Malignant neoplasm of unspecified site of unspecified male breast**

Malignant neoplasms of female genital organs (C51-C58)

INCLUDES malignant neoplasm of skin of female genital organs

✓4th **C51 Malignant neoplasm of vulva**

EXCLUDES1 *carcinoma in situ of vulva (D07.1)*

- **C51.0 Malignant neoplasm of labium majus**
  Malignant neoplasm of Bartholin's [greater vestibular] gland
- **C51.1 Malignant neoplasm of labium minus**
- **C51.2 Malignant neoplasm of clitoris**
- **C51.8 Malignant neoplasm of overlapping sites of vulva**
- **C51.9 Malignant neoplasm of vulva, unspecified**
  Malignant neoplasm of external female genitalia NOS
  Malignant neoplasm of pudendum

C52 Malignant neoplasm of vagina

EXCLUDES1 *carcinoma in situ of vagina (D07.2)*

✓4th **C53 Malignant neoplasm of cervix uteri**

EXCLUDES1 *carcinoma in situ of cervix uteri (D06.-)*

- **C53.0 Malignant neoplasm of endocervix**
- **C53.1 Malignant neoplasm of exocervix**
- **C53.8 Malignant neoplasm of overlapping sites of cervix uteri**
- **C53.9 Malignant neoplasm of cervix uteri, unspecified**

✓4th **C54 Malignant neoplasm of corpus uteri**
- **C54.0 Malignant neoplasm of isthmus uteri**
  Malignant neoplasm of lower uterine segment
- **C54.1 Malignant neoplasm of endometrium**
- **C54.2 Malignant neoplasm of myometrium**
- **C54.3 Malignant neoplasm of fundus uteri**
- **C54.8 Malignant neoplasm of overlapping sites of corpus uteri**
- **C54.9 Malignant neoplasm of corpus uteri, unspecified**

C55 Malignant neoplasm of uterus, part unspecified

✓4th **C56 Malignant neoplasm of ovary**

Use additional code to identify any functional activity

- **C56.1 Malignant neoplasm of right ovary**
- **C56.2 Malignant neoplasm of left ovary**
- **C56.9 Malignant neoplasm of unspecified ovary**

✓4th **C57 Malignant neoplasm of other and unspecified female genital organs**

✓5th **C57.0 Malignant neoplasm of fallopian tube**

Malignant neoplasm of oviduct
Malignant neoplasm of uterine tube

- **C57.00 Malignant neoplasm of unspecified fallopian tube**
- **C57.01 Malignant neoplasm of right fallopian tube**
- **C57.02 Malignant neoplasm of left fallopian tube**

✓5th **C57.1 Malignant neoplasm of broad ligament**
- **C57.10 Malignant neoplasm of unspecified broad ligament**
- **C57.11 Malignant neoplasm of right broad ligament**
- **C57.12 Malignant neoplasm of left broad ligament**

✓5th **C57.2 Malignant neoplasm of round ligament**
- **C57.20 Malignant neoplasm of unspecified round ligament**
- **C57.21 Malignant neoplasm of right round ligament**
- **C57.22 Malignant neoplasm of left round ligament**

C57.3 Malignant neoplasm of parametrium

Malignant neoplasm of uterine ligament NOS

C57.4 Malignant neoplasm of uterine adnexa, unspecified

C57.7 Malignant neoplasm of other specified female genital organs
Malignant neoplasm of wolffian body or duct

C57.8 Malignant neoplasm of overlapping sites of female genital organs
Primary malignant neoplasm of two or more contiguous sites of the female genital organs whose point of origin cannot be determined
Primary tubo-ovarian malignant neoplasm whose point of origin cannot be determined
Primary utero-ovarian malignant neoplasm whose point of origin cannot be determined

C57.9 Malignant neoplasm of female genital organ, unspecified
Malignant neoplasm of female genitourinary tract NOS

C58 Malignant neoplasm of placenta
INCLUDES choriocarcinoma NOS
chorionepithelioma NOS
EXCLUDES 1 *chorioadenoma (destruens) (D39.2)*
hydatidiform mole NOS (O01.9)
invasive hydatidiform mole (D39.2)
male choriocarcinoma NOS (C62.9-)
malignant hydatidiform mole (D39.2)

Malignant neoplasms of male genital organs (C60-C63)

INCLUDES malignant neoplasm of skin of male genital organs

✓4th **C60 Malignant neoplasm of penis**
C60.0 Malignant neoplasm of prepuce
Malignant neoplasm of foreskin
C60.1 Malignant neoplasm of glans penis
C60.2 Malignant neoplasm of body of penis
Malignant neoplasm of corpus cavernosum
C60.8 Malignant neoplasm of overlapping sites of penis
C60.9 Malignant neoplasm of penis, unspecified
Malignant neoplasm of skin of penis NOS

C61 Malignant neoplasm of prostate
EXCLUDES 1 *malignant neoplasm of seminal vesicle (C63.7)*

✓4th **C62 Malignant neoplasm of testis**
Use additional code to identify any functional activity
✓5th **C62.0 Malignant neoplasm of undescended testis**
Malignant neoplasm of ectopic testis
Malignant neoplasm of retained testis
C62.00 Malignant neoplasm of unspecified undescended testis
C62.01 Malignant neoplasm of undescended right testis
C62.02 Malignant neoplasm of undescended left testis
✓5th **C62.1 Malignant neoplasm of descended testis**
Malignant neoplasm of scrotal testis
C62.10 Malignant neoplasm of unspecified descended testis
C62.11 Malignant neoplasm of descended right testis
C62.12 Malignant neoplasm of descended left testis
✓5th **C62.9 Malignant neoplasm of testis, unspecified whether descended or undescended**
C62.90 Malignant neoplasm of unspecified testis, unspecified whether descended or undescended
Malignant neoplasm of testis NOS
C62.91 Malignant neoplasm of right testis, unspecified whether descended or undescended
C62.92 Malignant neoplasm of left testis, unspecified whether descended or undescended

✓4th **C63 Malignant neoplasm of other and unspecified male genital organs**
✓5th **C63.0 Malignant neoplasm of epididymis**
C63.00 Malignant neoplasm of unspecified epididymis
C63.01 Malignant neoplasm of right epididymis
C63.02 Malignant neoplasm of left epididymis
✓5th **C63.1 Malignant neoplasm of spermatic cord**
C63.10 Malignant neoplasm of unspecified spermatic cord
C63.11 Malignant neoplasm of right spermatic cord
C63.12 Malignant neoplasm of left spermatic cord
C63.2 Malignant neoplasm of scrotum
Malignant neoplasm of skin of scrotum
C63.7 Malignant neoplasm of other specified male genital organs
Malignant neoplasm of seminal vesicle
Malignant neoplasm of tunica vaginalis
C63.8 Malignant neoplasm of overlapping sites of male genital organs
Primary malignant neoplasm of two or more contiguous sites of male genital organs whose point of origin cannot be determined
C63.9 Malignant neoplasm of male genital organ, unspecified
Malignant neoplasm of male genitourinary tract NOS

Malignant neoplasms of urinary tract (C64-C68)

✓4th **C64 Malignant neoplasm of kidney, except renal pelvis**
EXCLUDES 1 *malignant carcinoid tumor of the kidney (C7A.093)*
malignant neoplasm of renal calyces (C65.-)
malignant neoplasm of renal pelvis (C65.-)
C64.1 Malignant neoplasm of right kidney, except renal pelvis
C64.2 Malignant neoplasm of left kidney, except renal pelvis
C64.9 Malignant neoplasm of unspecified kidney, except renal pelvis

✓4th **C65 Malignant neoplasm of renal pelvis**
INCLUDES malignant neoplasm of pelviureteric junction
malignant neoplasm of renal calyces
C65.1 Malignant neoplasm of right renal pelvis
C65.2 Malignant neoplasm of left renal pelvis
C65.9 Malignant neoplasm of unspecified renal pelvis

✓4th **C66 Malignant neoplasm of ureter**
EXCLUDES 1 *malignant neoplasm of ureteric orifice of bladder (C67.6)*
C66.1 Malignant neoplasm of right ureter
C66.2 Malignant neoplasm of left ureter
C66.9 Malignant neoplasm of unspecified ureter

✓4th **C67 Malignant neoplasm of bladder**
C67.0 Malignant neoplasm of trigone of bladder
C67.1 Malignant neoplasm of dome of bladder
C67.2 Malignant neoplasm of lateral wall of bladder
C67.3 Malignant neoplasm of anterior wall of bladder
C67.4 Malignant neoplasm of posterior wall of bladder
C67.5 Malignant neoplasm of bladder neck
Malignant neoplasm of internal urethral orifice
C67.6 Malignant neoplasm of ureteric orifice
C67.7 Malignant neoplasm of urachus
C67.8 Malignant neoplasm of overlapping sites of bladder
C67.9 Malignant neoplasm of bladder, unspecified

✓4th **C68 Malignant neoplasm of other and unspecified urinary organs**
EXCLUDES 1 *malignant neoplasm of female genitourinary tract NOS (C57.9)*
malignant neoplasm of male genitourinary tract NOS (C63.9)
C68.0 Malignant neoplasm of urethra
EXCLUDES 1 *malignant neoplasm of urethral orifice of bladder (C67.5)*
C68.1 Malignant neoplasm of paraurethral glands
C68.8 Malignant neoplasm of overlapping sites of urinary organs
Primary malignant neoplasm of two or more contiguous sites of urinary organs whose point of origin cannot be determined
C68.9 Malignant neoplasm of urinary organ, unspecified
Malignant neoplasm of urinary system NOS

Malignant neoplasms of eye, brain and other parts of central nervous system (C69-C72)

✓4th **C69 Malignant neoplasm of eye and adnexa**
EXCLUDES 1 *malignant neoplasm of connective tissue of eyelid (C49.0)*
malignant neoplasm of eyelid (skin) (C43.1-, C44.1-)
malignant neoplasm of optic nerve (C72.3-)
✓5th **C69.0 Malignant neoplasm of conjunctiva**
C69.00 Malignant neoplasm of unspecified conjunctiva
C69.01 Malignant neoplasm of right conjunctiva
C69.02 Malignant neoplasm of left conjunctiva
✓5th **C69.1 Malignant neoplasm of cornea**
C69.10 Malignant neoplasm of unspecified cornea
C69.11 Malignant neoplasm of right cornea
C69.12 Malignant neoplasm of left cornea

DRAFT

✓5th **C69.2 Malignant neoplasm of retina**
EXCLUDES 1 *dark area on retina (D49.81)*
neoplasm of unspecified behavior of retina and choroid (D49.81)
retinal freckle (D49.81)
C69.20 Malignant neoplasm of unspecified retina
C69.21 Malignant neoplasm of right retina
C69.22 Malignant neoplasm of left retina

✓5th **C69.3 Malignant neoplasm of choroid**
C69.30 Malignant neoplasm of unspecified choroid
C69.31 Malignant neoplasm of right choroid
C69.32 Malignant neoplasm of left choroid

✓5th **C69.4 Malignant neoplasm of ciliary body**
Malignant neoplasm of eyeball
C69.40 Malignant neoplasm of unspecified ciliary body
C69.41 Malignant neoplasm of right ciliary body
C69.42 Malignant neoplasm of left ciliary body

✓5th **C69.5 Malignant neoplasm of lacrimal gland and duct**
Malignant neoplasm of lacrimal sac
Malignant neoplasm of nasolacrimal duct
C69.50 Malignant neoplasm of unspecified lacrimal gland and duct
C69.51 Malignant neoplasm of right lacrimal gland and duct
C69.52 Malignant neoplasm of left lacrimal gland and duct

✓5th **C69.6 Malignant neoplasm of orbit**
Malignant neoplasm of connective tissue of orbit
Malignant neoplasm of extraocular muscle
Malignant neoplasm of peripheral nerves of orbit
Malignant neoplasm of retrobulbar tissue
Malignant neoplasm of retro-ocular tissue
EXCLUDES 1 *malignant neoplasm of orbital bone (C41.0)*
C69.60 Malignant neoplasm of unspecified orbit
C69.61 Malignant neoplasm of right orbit
C69.62 Malignant neoplasm of left orbit

✓5th **C69.8 Malignant neoplasm of overlapping sites of eye and adnexa**
C69.80 Malignant neoplasm of overlapping sites of unspecified eye and adnexa
C69.81 Malignant neoplasm of overlapping sites of right eye and adnexa
C69.82 Malignant neoplasm of overlapping sites of left eye and adnexa

✓5th **C69.9 Malignant neoplasm of unspecified site of eye**
C69.90 Malignant neoplasm of unspecified site of unspecified eye
C69.91 Malignant neoplasm of unspecified site of right eye
C69.92 Malignant neoplasm of unspecified site of left eye

✓4th **C70 Malignant neoplasm of meninges**
C70.0 Malignant neoplasm of cerebral meninges
C70.1 Malignant neoplasm of spinal meninges
C70.9 Malignant neoplasm of meninges, unspecified

✓4th **C71 Malignant neoplasm of brain**
EXCLUDES 1 *malignant neoplasm of cranial nerves (C72.2-C72.5)*
retrobulbar malignant neoplasm (C69.6-)
C71.0 Malignant neoplasm of cerebrum, except lobes and ventricles
Malignant neoplasm of supratentorial NOS
C71.1 Malignant neoplasm of frontal lobe
C71.2 Malignant neoplasm of temporal lobe
C71.3 Malignant neoplasm of parietal lobe
C71.4 Malignant neoplasm of occipital lobe
C71.5 Malignant neoplasm of cerebral ventricle
EXCLUDES 1 *malignant neoplasm of fourth cerebral ventricle (C71.7)*
C71.6 Malignant neoplasm of cerebellum
C71.7 Malignant neoplasm of brain stem
Malignant neoplasm of fourth cerebral ventricle
Infratentorial malignant neoplasm NOS
C71.8 Malignant neoplasm of overlapping sites of brain
C71.9 Malignant neoplasm of brain, unspecified

✓4th **C72 Malignant neoplasm of spinal cord, cranial nerves and other parts of central nervous system**
EXCLUDES 1 *malignant neoplasm of meninges (C70.-)*
malignant neoplasm of peripheral nerves and autonomic nervous system (C47.-)
C72.0 Malignant neoplasm of spinal cord
C72.1 Malignant neoplasm of cauda equina

✓5th **C72.2 Malignant neoplasm of olfactory nerve**
Malignant neoplasm of olfactory bulb
C72.20 Malignant neoplasm of unspecified olfactory nerve
C72.21 Malignant neoplasm of right olfactory nerve
C72.22 Malignant neoplasm of left olfactory nerve

✓5th **C72.3 Malignant neoplasm of optic nerve**
C72.30 Malignant neoplasm of unspecified optic nerve
C72.31 Malignant neoplasm of right optic nerve
C72.32 Malignant neoplasm of left optic nerve

✓5th **C72.4 Malignant neoplasm of acoustic nerve**
C72.40 Malignant neoplasm of unspecified acoustic nerve
C72.41 Malignant neoplasm of right acoustic nerve
C72.42 Malignant neoplasm of left acoustic nerve

✓5th **C72.5 Malignant neoplasm of other and unspecified cranial nerves**
C72.50 Malignant neoplasm of unspecified cranial nerve
Malignant neoplasm of cranial nerve NOS
C72.59 Malignant neoplasm of other cranial nerves
C72.9 Malignant neoplasm of central nervous system, unspecified
Malignant neoplasm of unspecified site of central nervous system
Malignant neoplasm of nervous system NOS

Malignant neoplasms of thyroid and other endocrine glands (C73-C75)

C73 Malignant neoplasm of thyroid gland
Use additional code to identify any functional activity

✓4th **C74 Malignant neoplasm of adrenal gland**

✓5th **C74.0 Malignant neoplasm of cortex of adrenal gland**
C74.00 Malignant neoplasm of cortex of unspecified adrenal gland
C74.01 Malignant neoplasm of cortex of right adrenal gland
C74.02 Malignant neoplasm of cortex of left adrenal gland

✓5th **C74.1 Malignant neoplasm of medulla of adrenal gland**
C74.10 Malignant neoplasm of medulla of unspecified adrenal gland
C74.11 Malignant neoplasm of medulla of right adrenal gland
C74.12 Malignant neoplasm of medulla of left adrenal gland

✓5th **C74.9 Malignant neoplasm of unspecified part of adrenal gland**
C74.90 Malignant neoplasm of unspecified part of unspecified adrenal gland
C74.91 Malignant neoplasm of unspecified part of right adrenal gland
C74.92 Malignant neoplasm of unspecified part of left adrenal gland

✓4th **C75 Malignant neoplasm of other endocrine glands and related structures**
EXCLUDES 1 *malignant carcinoid tumors (C7A.0-)*
malignant neoplasm of adrenal gland (C74.-)
malignant neoplasm of endocrine pancreas (C25.4)
malignant neoplasm of islets of Langerhans (C25.4)
malignant neoplasm of ovary (C56.-)
malignant neoplasm of testis (C62.-)
malignant neoplasm of thymus (C37)
malignant neoplasm of thyroid gland (C73)
malignant neuroendocrine tumors (C7A.-)
C75.0 Malignant neoplasm of parathyroid gland
C75.1 Malignant neoplasm of pituitary gland
C75.2 Malignant neoplasm of craniopharyngeal duct
C75.3 Malignant neoplasm of pineal gland
C75.4 Malignant neoplasm of carotid body
C75.5 Malignant neoplasm of aortic body and other paraganglia
C75.8 Malignant neoplasm with pluriglandular involvement, unspecified
C75.9 Malignant neoplasm of endocrine gland, unspecified

Malignant neuroendocrine tumors (C7A)

C7A Malignant neuroendocrine tumors
Code also any associated multiple endocrine neoplasia [MEN] syndromes (E31.2-)
Use additional code to identify any associated endocrine syndrome, such as:
carcinoid syndrome (E34.0)
EXCLUDES 2 *malignant pancreatic islet cell tumors (C25.4)*
Merkel cell carcinoma (C4A.-)

C7A.0 Malignant carcinoid tumors
C7A.00 Malignant carcinoid tumor of unspecified site
C7A.01 Malignant carcinoid tumors of the small intestine
C7A.010 Malignant carcinoid tumor of the duodenum
C7A.011 Malignant carcinoid tumor of the jejunum
C7A.012 Malignant carcinoid tumor of the ileum
C7A.019 Malignant carcinoid tumor of the small intestine, unspecified portion
C7A.02 Malignant carcinoid tumors of the appendix, large intestine, and rectum
C7A.020 Malignant carcinoid tumor of the appendix
C7A.021 Malignant carcinoid tumor of the cecum
C7A.022 Malignant carcinoid tumor of the ascending colon
C7A.023 Malignant carcinoid tumor of the transverse colon
C7A.024 Malignant carcinoid tumor of the descending colon
C7A.025 Malignant carcinoid tumor of the sigmoid colon
C7A.026 Malignant carcinoid tumor of the rectum
C7A.029 Malignant carcinoid tumor of the large intestine, unspecified portion
Malignant carcinoid tumor of the colon NOS
C7A.09 Malignant carcinoid tumors of other sites
C7A.090 Malignant carcinoid tumor of the bronchus and lung
C7A.091 Malignant carcinoid tumor of the thymus
C7A.092 Malignant carcinoid tumor of the stomach
C7A.093 Malignant carcinoid tumor of the kidney
C7A.094 Malignant carcinoid tumor of the foregut NOS
C7A.095 Malignant carcinoid tumor of the midgut NOS
C7A.096 Malignant carcinoid tumor of the hindgut NOS
C7A.098 Malignant carcinoid tumors of other sites
C7A.1 Malignant poorly differentiated neuroendocrine tumors
High grade neuroendocrine carcinoma, any site
Malignant poorly differentiated neuroendocrine tumor NOS
Malignant poorly differentiated neuroendocrine carcinoma, any site
C7A.8 Other malignant neuroendocrine tumors

Secondary neuroendocrine tumors (C7B)

C7B Secondary neuroendocrine tumors
Use additional code to identify any functional activity
C7B.0 Secondary carcinoid tumors
C7B.00 Secondary carcinoid tumors, unspecified site
C7B.01 Secondary carcinoid tumors of distant lymph nodes
C7B.02 Secondary carcinoid tumors of liver
C7B.03 Secondary carcinoid tumors of bone
C7B.04 Secondary carcinoid tumors of peritoneum
Mesentery metastasis of carcinoid tumor
C7B.09 Secondary carcinoid tumors of other sites
C7B.1 Secondary Merkel cell carcinoma
Merkel cell carcinoma nodal presentation
Merkel cell carcinoma visceral metastatic presentation
C7B.8 Other secondary neuroendocrine tumors

Malignant neoplasms of ill-defined, other secondary and unspecified sites (C76-C80)

C76 Malignant neoplasm of other and ill-defined sites
EXCLUDES 1 *malignant neoplasm of female genitourinary tract NOS (C57.9)*
malignant neoplasm of male genitourinary tract NOS (C63.9)
malignant neoplasm of lymphoid, hematopoietic and related tissue (C81-C96)
malignant neoplasm of skin (C44.-)
malignant neoplasm of unspecified site NOS (C80.1)
C76.0 Malignant neoplasm of head, face and neck
Malignant neoplasm of cheek NOS
Malignant neoplasm of nose NOS
C76.1 Malignant neoplasm of thorax
Intrathoracic malignant neoplasm NOS
Malignant neoplasm of axilla NOS
Thoracic malignant neoplasm NOS
C76.2 Malignant neoplasm of abdomen
C76.3 Malignant neoplasm of pelvis
Malignant neoplasm of groin NOS
Malignant neoplasm of sites overlapping systems within the pelvis
Rectovaginal (septum) malignant neoplasm
Rectovesical (septum) malignant neoplasm
C76.4 Malignant neoplasm of upper limb
C76.40 Malignant neoplasm of unspecified upper limb
C76.41 Malignant neoplasm of right upper limb
C76.42 Malignant neoplasm of left upper limb
C76.5 Malignant neoplasm of lower limb
C76.50 Malignant neoplasm of unspecified lower limb
C76.51 Malignant neoplasm of right lower limb
C76.52 Malignant neoplasm of left lower limb
C76.8 Malignant neoplasm of other specified ill-defined sites
Malignant neoplasm of overlapping ill-defined sites

C77 Secondary and unspecified malignant neoplasm of lymph nodes
EXCLUDES 1 *malignant neoplasm of lymph nodes, specified as primary (C81-C88, C96.-)*
mesentery metastasis of carcinoid tumor (C7B.04)
secondary carcinoid tumors of distant lymph nodes (C7B.01)
C77.0 Secondary and unspecified malignant neoplasm of lymph nodes of head, face and neck
Secondary and unspecified malignant neoplasm of supraclavicular lymph nodes
C77.1 Secondary and unspecified malignant neoplasm of intrathoracic lymph nodes
C77.2 Secondary and unspecified malignant neoplasm of intra-abdominal lymph nodes
C77.3 Secondary and unspecified malignant neoplasm of axilla and upper limb lymph nodes
Secondary and unspecified malignant neoplasm of pectoral lymph nodes
C77.4 Secondary and unspecified malignant neoplasm of inguinal and lower limb lymph nodes
C77.5 Secondary and unspecified malignant neoplasm of intrapelvic lymph nodes
C77.8 Secondary and unspecified malignant neoplasm of lymph nodes of multiple regions
C77.9 Secondary and unspecified malignant neoplasm of lymph node, unspecified

C78 Secondary malignant neoplasm of respiratory and digestive organs
EXCLUDES 1 *lymph node metastases (C77.0)*
secondary carcinoid tumors of liver (C7B.02)
secondary carcinoid tumors of peritoneum (C7B.04)
C78.0 Secondary malignant neoplasm of lung
C78.00 Secondary malignant neoplasm of unspecified lung
C78.01 Secondary malignant neoplasm of right lung
C78.02 Secondary malignant neoplasm of left lung
C78.1 Secondary malignant neoplasm of mediastinum
C78.2 Secondary malignant neoplasm of pleura

✓5th **C78.3 Secondary malignant neoplasm of other and unspecified respiratory organs**
C78.30 Secondary malignant neoplasm of unspecified respiratory organ
C78.39 Secondary malignant neoplasm of other respiratory organs
C78.4 Secondary malignant neoplasm of small intestine
C78.5 Secondary malignant neoplasm of large intestine and rectum
C78.6 Secondary malignant neoplasm of retroperitoneum and peritoneum
C78.7 Secondary malignant neoplasm of liver and intrahepatic bile duct
✓5th **C78.8 Secondary malignant neoplasm of other and unspecified digestive organs**
C78.80 Secondary malignant neoplasm of unspecified digestive organ
C78.89 Secondary malignant neoplasm of other digestive organs

✓4th **C79 Secondary malignant neoplasm of other and unspecified sites**
EXCLUDES 1 *lymph node metastases (C77.0)*
secondary carcinoid tumors (C7B.-)
secondary neuroendocrine tumors (C7B.-)
✓5th **C79.0 Secondary malignant neoplasm of kidney and renal pelvis**
C79.00 Secondary malignant neoplasm of unspecified kidney and renal pelvis
C79.01 Secondary malignant neoplasm of right kidney and renal pelvis
C79.02 Secondary malignant neoplasm of left kidney and renal pelvis
✓5th **C79.1 Secondary malignant neoplasm of bladder and other and unspecified urinary organs**
C79.10 Secondary malignant neoplasm of unspecified urinary organs
C79.11 Secondary malignant neoplasm of bladder
C79.19 Secondary malignant neoplasm of other urinary organs
C79.2 Secondary malignant neoplasm of skin
EXCLUDES 1 *secondary Merkel cell carcinoma (C7B.1)*
✓5th **C79.3 Secondary malignant neoplasm of brain and cerebral meninges**
C79.31 Secondary malignant neoplasm of brain
C79.32 Secondary malignant neoplasm of cerebral meninges
✓5th **C79.4 Secondary malignant neoplasm of other and unspecified parts of nervous system**
C79.40 Secondary malignant neoplasm of unspecified part of nervous system
C79.49 Secondary malignant neoplasm of other parts of nervous system
✓5th **C79.5 Secondary malignant neoplasm of bone and bone marrow**
EXCLUDES 1 *secondary carcinoid tumors of bone (C7B.03)*
C79.51 Secondary malignant neoplasm of bone
C79.52 Secondary malignant neoplasm of bone marrow
✓5th **C79.6 Secondary malignant neoplasm of ovary**
C79.60 Secondary malignant neoplasm of unspecified ovary
C79.61 Secondary malignant neoplasm of right ovary
C79.62 Secondary malignant neoplasm of left ovary
✓5th **C79.7 Secondary malignant neoplasm of adrenal gland**
C79.70 Secondary malignant neoplasm of unspecified adrenal gland
C79.71 Secondary malignant neoplasm of right adrenal gland
C79.72 Secondary malignant neoplasm of left adrenal gland
✓5th **C79.8 Secondary malignant neoplasm of other specified sites**
C79.81 Secondary malignant neoplasm of breast
C79.82 Secondary malignant neoplasm of genital organs
C79.89 Secondary malignant neoplasm of other specified sites
C79.9 Secondary malignant neoplasm of unspecified site
Metastatic cancer NOS
Metastatic disease NOS
EXCLUDES 1 *carcinomatosis NOS (C80.0)*
generalized cancer NOS (C80.0)
malignant (primary) neoplasm of unspecified site (C80.1)

✓4th **C80 Malignant neoplasm without specification of site**
EXCLUDES 1 *malignant carcinoid tumor of unspecified site (C7A.00)*
malignant neoplasm of specified multiple sites—code to each site
C80.0 Disseminated malignant neoplasm, unspecified
Carcinomatosis NOS
Generalized cancer, unspecified site (primary) (secondary)
Generalized malignancy, unspecified site (primary) (secondary)
C80.1 Malignant (primary) neoplasm, unspecified
Cancer NOS
Cancer unspecified site (primary)
Carcinoma unspecified site (primary)
Malignancy unspecified site (primary)
EXCLUDES 1 *secondary malignant neoplasm of unspecified site (C79.9)*
C80.2 Malignant neoplasm associated with transplanted organ
Code first complication of transplanted organ (T86.-)
Use additional code to identify the specific malignancy

Malignant neoplasms of lymphoid, hematopoietic and related tissue (C81-C96)

EXCLUDES 2 *Kaposi's sarcoma of lymph nodes (C46.3)*
secondary and unspecified neoplasm of lymph nodes (C77.-)
secondary neoplasm of bone marrow (C79.52)
secondary neoplasm of spleen (C78.89)

✓4th **C81 Hodgkin lymphoma**
EXCLUDES 1 *personal history of Hodgkin lymphoma (Z85.71)*
✓5th **C81.0 Nodular lymphocyte predominant Hodgkin lymphoma**
C81.00 Nodular lymphocyte predominant Hodgkin lymphoma, unspecified site
C81.01 Nodular lymphocyte predominant Hodgkin lymphoma, lymph nodes of head, face, and neck
C81.02 Nodular lymphocyte predominant Hodgkin lymphoma, intrathoracic lymph nodes
C81.03 Nodular lymphocyte predominant Hodgkin lymphoma, intra-abdominal lymph nodes
C81.04 Nodular lymphocyte predominant Hodgkin lymphoma, lymph nodes of axilla and upper limb
C81.05 Nodular lymphocyte predominant Hodgkin lymphoma, lymph nodes of inguinal region and lower limb
C81.06 Nodular lymphocyte predominant Hodgkin lymphoma, intrapelvic lymph nodes
C81.07 Nodular lymphocyte predominant Hodgkin lymphoma, spleen
C81.08 Nodular lymphocyte predominant Hodgkin lymphoma, lymph nodes of multiple sites
C81.09 Nodular lymphocyte predominant Hodgkin lymphoma, extranodal and solid organ sites
✓5th **C81.1 Nodular sclerosis classical Hodgkin lymphoma**
C81.10 Nodular sclerosis classical Hodgkin lymphoma, unspecified site
C81.11 Nodular sclerosis classical Hodgkin lymphoma, lymph nodes of head, face, and neck
C81.12 Nodular sclerosis classical Hodgkin lymphoma, intrathoracic lymph nodes
C81.13 Nodular sclerosis classical Hodgkin lymphoma, intra-abdominal lymph nodes
C81.14 Nodular sclerosis classical Hodgkin lymphoma, lymph nodes of axilla and upper limb
C81.15 Nodular sclerosis classical Hodgkin lymphoma, lymph nodes of inguinal region and lower limb
C81.16 Nodular sclerosis classical Hodgkin lymphoma, intrapelvic lymph nodes
C81.17 Nodular sclerosis classical Hodgkin lymphoma, spleen
C81.18 Nodular sclerosis classical Hodgkin lymphoma, lymph nodes of multiple sites

C81.19 Nodular sclerosis classical Hodgkin lymphoma, extranodal and solid organ sites

✓5th C81.2 Mixed cellularity classical Hodgkin lymphoma
C81.20 Mixed cellularity classical Hodgkin lymphoma, unspecified site
C81.21 Mixed cellularity classical Hodgkin lymphoma, lymph nodes of head, face, and neck
C81.22 Mixed cellularity classical Hodgkin lymphoma, intrathoracic lymph nodes
C81.23 Mixed cellularity classical Hodgkin lymphoma, intra-abdominal lymph nodes
C81.24 Mixed cellularity classical Hodgkin lymphoma, lymph nodes of axilla and upper limb
C81.25 Mixed cellularity classical Hodgkin lymphoma, lymph nodes of inguinal region and lower limb
C81.26 Mixed cellularity classical Hodgkin lymphoma, intrapelvic lymph nodes
C81.27 Mixed cellularity classical Hodgkin lymphoma, spleen
C81.28 Mixed cellularity classical Hodgkin lymphoma, lymph nodes of multiple sites
C81.29 Mixed cellularity classical Hodgkin lymphoma, extranodal and solid organ sites

✓5th C81.3 Lymphocyte-depleted classical Hodgkin lymphoma
C81.30 Lymphocyte-depleted classical Hodgkin lymphoma, unspecified site
C81.31 Lymphocyte-depleted classical Hodgkin lymphoma, lymph nodes of head, face, and neck
C81.32 Lymphocyte-depleted classical Hodgkin lymphoma, intrathoracic lymph nodes
C81.33 Lymphocyte-depleted classical Hodgkin lymphoma, intra-abdominal lymph nodes
C81.34 Lymphocyte-depleted classical Hodgkin lymphoma, lymph nodes of axilla and upper limb
C81.35 Lymphocyte-depleted classical Hodgkin lymphoma, lymph nodes of inguinal region and lower limb
C81.36 Lymphocyte-depleted classical Hodgkin lymphoma, intrapelvic lymph nodes
C81.37 Lymphocyte-depleted classical Hodgkin lymphoma, spleen
C81.38 Lymphocyte-depleted classical Hodgkin lymphoma, lymph nodes of multiple sites
C81.39 Lymphocyte-depleted classical Hodgkin lymphoma, extranodal and solid organ sites

✓5th C81.4 Lymphocyte-rich classical Hodgkin lymphoma
EXCLUDES 1 *nodular lymphocyte predominant Hodgkin lymphoma (C81.0-)*
C81.40 Lymphocyte-rich classical Hodgkin lymphoma, unspecified site
C81.41 Lymphocyte-rich classical Hodgkin lymphoma, lymph nodes of head, face, and neck
C81.42 Lymphocyte-rich classical Hodgkin lymphoma, intrathoracic lymph nodes
C81.43 Lymphocyte-rich classical Hodgkin lymphoma, intra-abdominal lymph nodes
C81.44 Lymphocyte-rich classical Hodgkin lymphoma, lymph nodes of axilla and upper limb
C81.45 Lymphocyte-rich classical Hodgkin lymphoma, lymph nodes of inguinal region and lower limb
C81.46 Lymphocyte-rich classical Hodgkin lymphoma, intrapelvic lymph nodes
C81.47 Lymphocyte-rich classical Hodgkin lymphoma, spleen
C81.48 Lymphocyte-rich classical Hodgkin lymphoma, lymph nodes of multiple sites
C81.49 Lymphocyte-rich classical Hodgkin lymphoma, extranodal and solid organ sites

✓5th C81.7 Other classical Hodgkin lymphoma
Classical Hodgkin lymphoma NOS
C81.70 Other classical Hodgkin lymphoma, unspecified site
C81.71 Other classical Hodgkin lymphoma, lymph nodes of head, face, and neck
C81.72 Other classical Hodgkin lymphoma, intrathoracic lymph nodes
C81.73 Other classical Hodgkin lymphoma, intra-abdominal lymph nodes
C81.74 Other classical Hodgkin lymphoma, lymph nodes of axilla and upper limb
C81.75 Other classical Hodgkin lymphoma, lymph nodes of inguinal region and lower limb
C81.76 Other classical Hodgkin lymphoma, intrapelvic lymph nodes
C81.77 Other classical Hodgkin lymphoma, spleen
C81.78 Other classical Hodgkin lymphoma, lymph nodes of multiple sites
C81.79 Other classical Hodgkin lymphoma, extranodal and solid organ sites

✓5th C81.9 Hodgkin lymphoma, unspecified
C81.90 Hodgkin lymphoma, unspecified, unspecified site
C81.91 Hodgkin lymphoma, unspecified, lymph nodes of head, face, and neck
C81.92 Hodgkin lymphoma, unspecified, intrathoracic lymph nodes
C81.93 Hodgkin lymphoma, unspecified, intra-abdominal lymph nodes
C81.94 Hodgkin lymphoma, unspecified, lymph nodes of axilla and upper limb
C81.95 Hodgkin lymphoma, unspecified, lymph nodes of inguinal region and lower limb
C81.96 Hodgkin lymphoma, unspecified, intrapelvic lymph nodes
C81.97 Hodgkin lymphoma, unspecified, spleen
C81.98 Hodgkin lymphoma, unspecified, lymph nodes of multiple sites
C81.99 Hodgkin lymphoma, unspecified, extranodal and solid organ sites

✓4th C82 Follicular lymphoma

INCLUDES follicular lymphoma with or without diffuse areas
EXCLUDES 1 *mature T/NK-cell lymphomas (C84.-)*
personal history of non-Hodgkin lymphoma (Z85.72)

✓5th C82.0 Follicular lymphoma grade I
C82.00 Follicular lymphoma grade I, unspecified site
C82.01 Follicular lymphoma grade I, lymph nodes of head, face, and neck
C82.02 Follicular lymphoma grade I, intrathoracic lymph nodes
C82.03 Follicular lymphoma grade I, intra-abdominal lymph nodes
C82.04 Follicular lymphoma grade I, lymph nodes of axilla and upper limb
C82.05 Follicular lymphoma grade I, lymph nodes of inguinal region and lower limb
C82.06 Follicular lymphoma grade I, intrapelvic lymph nodes
C82.07 Follicular lymphoma grade I, spleen
C82.08 Follicular lymphoma grade I, lymph nodes of multiple sites
C82.09 Follicular lymphoma grade I, extranodal and solid organ sites

✓5th C82.1 Follicular lymphoma grade II
C82.10 Follicular lymphoma grade II, unspecified site
C82.11 Follicular lymphoma grade II, lymph nodes of head, face, and neck
C82.12 Follicular lymphoma grade II, intrathoracic lymph nodes
C82.13 Follicular lymphoma grade II, intra-abdominal lymph nodes
C82.14 Follicular lymphoma grade II, lymph nodes of axilla and upper limb
C82.15 Follicular lymphoma grade II, lymph nodes of inguinal region and lower limb
C82.16 Follicular lymphoma grade II, intrapelvic lymph nodes
C82.17 Follicular lymphoma grade II, spleen
C82.18 Follicular lymphoma grade II, lymph nodes of multiple sites
C82.19 Follicular lymphoma grade II, extranodal and solid organ sites

✓5th C82.2 Follicular lymphoma grade III, unspecified
C82.20 Follicular lymphoma grade III, unspecified, unspecified site
C82.21 Follicular lymphoma grade III, unspecified, lymph nodes of head, face, and neck

C82.22 Follicular lymphoma grade III, unspecified, intrathoracic lymph nodes
C82.23 Follicular lymphoma grade III, unspecified, intra-abdominal lymph nodes
C82.24 Follicular lymphoma grade III, unspecified, lymph nodes of axilla and upper limb
C82.25 Follicular lymphoma grade III, unspecified, lymph nodes of inguinal region and lower limb
C82.26 Follicular lymphoma grade III, unspecified, intrapelvic lymph nodes
C82.27 Follicular lymphoma grade III, unspecified, spleen
C82.28 Follicular lymphoma grade III, unspecified, lymph nodes of multiple sites
C82.29 Follicular lymphoma grade III, unspecified, extranodal and solid organ sites

✓5th **C82.3 Follicular lymphoma grade IIIa**
C82.3Ø Follicular lymphoma grade IIIa, unspecified site
C82.31 Follicular lymphoma grade IIIa, lymph nodes of head, face, and neck
C82.32 Follicular lymphoma grade IIIa, intrathoracic lymph nodes
C82.33 Follicular lymphoma grade IIIa, intra-abdominal lymph nodes
C82.34 Follicular lymphoma grade IIIa, lymph nodes of axilla and upper limb
C82.35 Follicular lymphoma grade IIIa, lymph nodes of inguinal region and lower limb
C82.36 Follicular lymphoma grade IIIa, intrapelvic lymph nodes
C82.37 Follicular lymphoma grade IIIa, spleen
C82.38 Follicular lymphoma grade IIIa, lymph nodes of multiple sites
C82.39 Follicular lymphoma grade IIIa, extranodal and solid organ sites

✓5th **C82.4 Follicular lymphoma grade IIIb**
C82.4Ø Follicular lymphoma grade IIIb, unspecified site
C82.41 Follicular lymphoma grade IIIb, lymph nodes of head, face, and neck
C82.42 Follicular lymphoma grade IIIb, intrathoracic lymph nodes
C82.43 Follicular lymphoma grade IIIb, intra-abdominal lymph nodes
C82.44 Follicular lymphoma grade IIIb, lymph nodes of axilla and upper limb
C82.45 Follicular lymphoma grade IIIb, lymph nodes of inguinal region and lower limb
C82.46 Follicular lymphoma grade IIIb, intrapelvic lymph nodes
C82.47 Follicular lymphoma grade IIIb, spleen
C82.48 Follicular lymphoma grade IIIb, lymph nodes of multiple sites
C82.49 Follicular lymphoma grade IIIb, extranodal and solid organ sites

✓5th **C82.5 Diffuse follicle center lymphoma**
C82.5Ø Diffuse follicle center lymphoma, unspecified site
C82.51 Diffuse follicle center lymphoma, lymph nodes of head, face, and neck
C82.52 Diffuse follicle center lymphoma, intrathoracic lymph nodes
C82.53 Diffuse follicle center lymphoma, intra-abdominal lymph nodes
C82.54 Diffuse follicle center lymphoma, lymph nodes of axilla and upper limb
C82.55 Diffuse follicle center lymphoma, lymph nodes of inguinal region and lower limb
C82.56 Diffuse follicle center lymphoma, intrapelvic lymph nodes
C82.57 Diffuse follicle center lymphoma, spleen
C82.58 Diffuse follicle center lymphoma, lymph nodes of multiple sites
C82.59 Diffuse follicle center lymphoma, extranodal and solid organ sites

✓5th **C82.6 Cutaneous follicle center lymphoma**
C82.6Ø Cutaneous follicle center lymphoma, unspecified site
C82.61 Cutaneous follicle center lymphoma, lymph nodes of head, face, and neck
C82.62 Cutaneous follicle center lymphoma, intrathoracic lymph nodes
C82.63 Cutaneous follicle center lymphoma, intra-abdominal lymph nodes
C82.64 Cutaneous follicle center lymphoma, lymph nodes of axilla and upper limb
C82.65 Cutaneous follicle center lymphoma, lymph nodes of inguinal region and lower limb
C82.66 Cutaneous follicle center lymphoma, intrapelvic lymph nodes
C82.67 Cutaneous follicle center lymphoma, spleen
C82.68 Cutaneous follicle center lymphoma, lymph nodes of multiple sites
C82.69 Cutaneous follicle center lymphoma, extranodal and solid organ sites

✓5th **C82.8 Other types of follicular lymphoma**
C82.8Ø Other types of follicular lymphoma, unspecified site
C82.81 Other types of follicular lymphoma, lymph nodes of head, face, and neck
C82.82 Other types of follicular lymphoma, intrathoracic lymph nodes
C82.83 Other types of follicular lymphoma, intra-abdominal lymph nodes
C82.84 Other types of follicular lymphoma, lymph nodes of axilla and upper limb
C82.85 Other types of follicular lymphoma, lymph nodes of inguinal region and lower limb
C82.86 Other types of follicular lymphoma, intrapelvic lymph nodes
C82.87 Other types of follicular lymphoma, spleen
C82.88 Other types of follicular lymphoma, lymph nodes of multiple sites
C82.89 Other types of follicular lymphoma, extranodal and solid organ sites

✓5th **C82.9 Follicular lymphoma, unspecified**
C82.9Ø Follicular lymphoma, unspecified, unspecified site
C82.91 Follicular lymphoma, unspecified, lymph nodes of head, face, and neck
C82.92 Follicular lymphoma, unspecified, intrathoracic lymph nodes
C82.93 Follicular lymphoma, unspecified, intra-abdominal lymph nodes
C82.94 Follicular lymphoma, unspecified, lymph nodes of axilla and upper limb
C82.95 Follicular lymphoma, unspecified, lymph nodes of inguinal region and lower limb
C82.96 Follicular lymphoma, unspecified, intrapelvic lymph nodes
C82.97 Follicular lymphoma, unspecified, spleen
C82.98 Follicular lymphoma, unspecified, lymph nodes of multiple sites
C82.99 Follicular lymphoma, unspecified, extranodal and solid organ sites

✓4th **C83 Non-follicular lymphoma**
EXCLUDES 1 *personal history of non-Hodgkin lymphoma (Z85.72)*

✓5th **C83.Ø Small cell B-cell lymphoma**
Lymphoplasmacytic lymphoma
Nodal marginal zone lymphoma
Non-leukemic variant of B-CLL
Splenic marginal zone lymphoma
EXCLUDES 1 *chronic lymphocytic leukemia (C91.1)*
mature T/NK-cell lymphomas (C84.-)
Waldenström macroglobulinemia (C88.Ø)
C83.ØØ Small cell B-cell lymphoma, unspecified site
C83.Ø1 Small cell B-cell lymphoma, lymph nodes of head, face, and neck
C83.Ø2 Small cell B-cell lymphoma, intrathoracic lymph nodes
C83.Ø3 Small cell B-cell lymphoma, intra-abdominal lymph nodes
C83.Ø4 Small cell B-cell lymphoma, lymph nodes of axilla and upper limb
C83.Ø5 Small cell B-cell lymphoma, lymph nodes of inguinal region and lower limb
C83.Ø6 Small cell B-cell lymphoma, intrapelvic lymph nodes
C83.Ø7 Small cell B-cell lymphoma, spleen

C83.08 Small cell B-cell lymphoma, lymph nodes of multiple sites
C83.09 Small cell B-cell lymphoma, extranodal and solid organ sites

C83.1 Mantle cell lymphoma
Centrocytic lymphoma
Malignant lymphomatous polyposis
C83.10 Mantle cell lymphoma, unspecified site
C83.11 Mantle cell lymphoma, lymph nodes of head, face, and neck
C83.12 Mantle cell lymphoma, intrathoracic lymph nodes
C83.13 Mantle cell lymphoma, intra-abdominal lymph nodes
C83.14 Mantle cell lymphoma, lymph nodes of axilla and upper limb
C83.15 Mantle cell lymphoma, lymph nodes of inguinal region and lower limb
C83.16 Mantle cell lymphoma, intrapelvic lymph nodes
C83.17 Mantle cell lymphoma, spleen
C83.18 Mantle cell lymphoma, lymph nodes of multiple sites
C83.19 Mantle cell lymphoma, extranodal and solid organ sites

C83.3 Diffuse large B-cell lymphoma
Anaplastic diffuse large B-cell lymphoma
CD30-positive diffuse large B-cell lymphoma
Centroblastic diffuse large B-cell lymphoma
Diffuse large B-cell lymphoma, subtype not specified
Immunoblastic diffuse large B-cell lymphoma
Plasmablastic diffuse large B-cell lymphoma
T-cell rich diffuse large B-cell lymphoma
EXCLUDES 1 *mediastinal (thymic) large B-cell lymphoma (C85.2-)*
mature T/NK-cell lymphomas (C84.-)
C83.30 Diffuse large B-cell lymphoma, unspecified site
C83.31 Diffuse large B-cell lymphoma, lymph nodes of head, face, and neck
C83.32 Diffuse large B-cell lymphoma, intrathoracic lymph nodes
C83.33 Diffuse large B-cell lymphoma, intra-abdominal lymph nodes
C83.34 Diffuse large B-cell lymphoma, lymph nodes of axilla and upper limb
C83.35 Diffuse large B-cell lymphoma, lymph nodes of inguinal region and lower limb
C83.36 Diffuse large B-cell lymphoma, intrapelvic lymph nodes
C83.37 Diffuse large B-cell lymphoma, spleen
C83.38 Diffuse large B-cell lymphoma, lymph nodes of multiple sites
C83.39 Diffuse large B-cell lymphoma, extranodal and solid organ sites

C83.5 Lymphoblastic (diffuse) lymphoma
B-precursor lymphoma
Lymphoblastic B-cell lymphoma
Lymphoblastic lymphoma NOS
Lymphoblastic T-cell lymphoma
T-precursor lymphoma
C83.50 Lymphoblastic (diffuse) lymphoma, unspecified site
C83.51 Lymphoblastic (diffuse) lymphoma, lymph nodes of head, face, and neck
C83.52 Lymphoblastic (diffuse) lymphoma, intrathoracic lymph nodes
C83.53 Lymphoblastic (diffuse) lymphoma, intra-abdominal lymph nodes
C83.54 Lymphoblastic (diffuse) lymphoma, lymph nodes of axilla and upper limb
C83.55 Lymphoblastic (diffuse) lymphoma, lymph nodes of inguinal region and lower limb
C83.56 Lymphoblastic (diffuse) lymphoma, intrapelvic lymph nodes
C83.57 Lymphoblastic (diffuse) lymphoma, spleen
C83.58 Lymphoblastic (diffuse) lymphoma, lymph nodes of multiple sites
C83.59 Lymphoblastic (diffuse) lymphoma, extranodal and solid organ sites

C83.7 Burkitt lymphoma
Atypical Burkitt lymphoma
Burkitt-like lymphoma
EXCLUDES 1 *mature B-cell leukemia Burkitt type (C91.A-)*
C83.70 Burkitt lymphoma, unspecified site
C83.71 Burkitt lymphoma, lymph nodes of head, face, and neck
C83.72 Burkitt lymphoma, intrathoracic lymph nodes
C83.73 Burkitt lymphoma, intra-abdominal lymph nodes
C83.74 Burkitt lymphoma, lymph nodes of axilla and upper limb
C83.75 Burkitt lymphoma, lymph nodes of inguinal region and lower limb
C83.76 Burkitt lymphoma, intrapelvic lymph nodes
C83.77 Burkitt lymphoma, spleen
C83.78 Burkitt lymphoma, lymph nodes of multiple sites
C83.79 Burkitt lymphoma, extranodal and solid organ sites

C83.8 Other non-follicular lymphoma
Intravascular large B-cell lymphoma
Lymphoid granulomatosis
Primary effusion B-cell lymphoma
EXCLUDES 1 *mediastinal (thymic) large B-cell lymphoma (C85.2-)*
T-cell rich B-cell lymphoma (C83.3-)
C83.80 Other non-follicular lymphoma, unspecified site
C83.81 Other non-follicular lymphoma, lymph nodes of head, face, and neck
C83.82 Other non-follicular lymphoma, intrathoracic lymph nodes
C83.83 Other non-follicular lymphoma, intra-abdominal lymph nodes
C83.84 Other non-follicular lymphoma, lymph nodes of axilla and upper limb
C83.85 Other non-follicular lymphoma, lymph nodes of inguinal region and lower limb
C83.86 Other non-follicular lymphoma, intrapelvic lymph nodes
C83.87 Other non-follicular lymphoma, spleen
C83.88 Other non-follicular lymphoma, lymph nodes of multiple sites
C83.89 Other non-follicular lymphoma, extranodal and solid organ sites

C83.9 Non-follicular (diffuse) lymphoma, unspecified
C83.90 Non-follicular (diffuse) lymphoma, unspecified, unspecified site
C83.91 Non-follicular (diffuse) lymphoma, unspecified, lymph nodes of head, face, and neck
C83.92 Non-follicular (diffuse) lymphoma, unspecified, intrathoracic lymph nodes
C83.93 Non-follicular (diffuse) lymphoma, unspecified, intra-abdominal lymph nodes
C83.94 Non-follicular (diffuse) lymphoma, unspecified, lymph nodes of axilla and upper limb
C83.95 Non-follicular (diffuse) lymphoma, unspecified, lymph nodes of inguinal region and lower limb
C83.96 Non-follicular (diffuse) lymphoma, unspecified, intrapelvic lymph nodes
C83.97 Non-follicular (diffuse) lymphoma, unspecified, spleen
C83.98 Non-follicular (diffuse) lymphoma, unspecified, lymph nodes of multiple sites
C83.99 Non-follicular (diffuse) lymphoma, unspecified, extranodal and solid organ sites

C84 Mature T/NK-cell lymphomas
EXCLUDES 1 *personal history of non-Hodgkin lymphoma (Z85.72)*

C84.0 Mycosis fungoides
EXCLUDES 1 *peripheral T-cell lymphoma, not classified (C84.4-)*
C84.00 Mycosis fungoides, unspecified site
C84.01 Mycosis fungoides, lymph nodes of head, face, and neck
C84.02 Mycosis fungoides, intrathoracic lymph nodes
C84.03 Mycosis fungoides, intra-abdominal lymph nodes
C84.04 Mycosis fungoides, lymph nodes of axilla and upper limb
C84.05 Mycosis fungoides, lymph nodes of inguinal region and lower limb
C84.06 Mycosis fungoides, intrapelvic lymph nodes

Appropriate additional character required
Requires 7th character, placeholder x must fill empty characters

C84.07 Mycosis fungoides, spleen
C84.08 Mycosis fungoides, lymph nodes of multiple sites
C84.09 Mycosis fungoides, extranodal and solid organ sites

✓5th **C84.1 Sézary disease**
C84.10 Sézary disease, unspecified site
C84.11 Sézary disease, lymph nodes of head, face, and neck
C84.12 Sézary disease, intrathoracic lymph nodes
C84.13 Sézary disease, intra-abdominal lymph nodes
C84.14 Sézary disease, lymph nodes of axilla and upper limb
C84.15 Sézary disease, lymph nodes of inguinal region and lower limb
C84.16 Sézary disease, intrapelvic lymph nodes
C84.17 Sézary disease, spleen
C84.18 Sézary disease, lymph nodes of multiple sites
C84.19 Sézary disease, extranodal and solid organ sites

✓5th **C84.4 Peripheral T-cell lymphoma, not classified**
Lennert's lymphoma
Lymphoepithelioid lymphoma
Mature T-cell lymphoma, not elsewhere classified
C84.40 Peripheral T-cell lymphoma, not classified, unspecified site
C84.41 Peripheral T-cell lymphoma, not classified, lymph nodes of head, face, and neck
C84.42 Peripheral T-cell lymphoma, not classified, intrathoracic lymph nodes
C84.43 Peripheral T-cell lymphoma, not classified, intra-abdominal lymph nodes
C84.44 Peripheral T-cell lymphoma, not classified, lymph nodes of axilla and upper limb
C84.45 Peripheral T-cell lymphoma, not classified, lymph nodes of inguinal region and lower limb
C84.46 Peripheral T-cell lymphoma, not classified, intrapelvic lymph nodes
C84.47 Peripheral T-cell lymphoma, not classified, spleen
C84.48 Peripheral T-cell lymphoma, not classified, lymph nodes of multiple sites
C84.49 Peripheral T-cell lymphoma, not classified, extranodal and solid organ sites

✓5th **C84.6 Anaplastic large cell lymphoma, ALK-positive**
Anaplastic large cell lymphoma, CD30-positive
C84.60 Anaplastic large cell lymphoma, ALK-positive, unspecified site
C84.61 Anaplastic large cell lymphoma, ALK-positive, lymph nodes of head, face, and neck
C84.62 Anaplastic large cell lymphoma, ALK-positive, intrathoracic lymph nodes
C84.63 Anaplastic large cell lymphoma, ALK-positive, intra-abdominal lymph nodes
C84.64 Anaplastic large cell lymphoma, ALK-positive, lymph nodes of axilla and upper limb
C84.65 Anaplastic large cell lymphoma, ALK-positive, lymph nodes of inguinal region and lower limb
C84.66 Anaplastic large cell lymphoma, ALK-positive, intrapelvic lymph nodes
C84.67 Anaplastic large cell lymphoma, ALK-positive, spleen
C84.68 Anaplastic large cell lymphoma, ALK-positive, lymph nodes of multiple sites
C84.69 Anaplastic large cell lymphoma, ALK-positive, extranodal and solid organ sites

✓5th **C84.7 Anaplastic large cell lymphoma, ALK-negative**
EXCLUDES 1 *primary cutaneous CD30-positive T-cell proliferations (C86.6-)*
C84.70 Anaplastic large cell lymphoma, ALK-negative, unspecified site
C84.71 Anaplastic large cell lymphoma, ALK-negative, lymph nodes of head, face, and neck
C84.72 Anaplastic large cell lymphoma, ALK-negative, intrathoracic lymph nodes
C84.73 Anaplastic large cell lymphoma, ALK-negative, intra-abdominal lymph nodes
C84.74 Anaplastic large cell lymphoma, ALK-negative, lymph nodes of axilla and upper limb
C84.75 Anaplastic large cell lymphoma, ALK-negative, lymph nodes of inguinal region and lower limb
C84.76 Anaplastic large cell lymphoma, ALK-negative, intrapelvic lymph nodes
C84.77 Anaplastic large cell lymphoma, ALK-negative, spleen
C84.78 Anaplastic large cell lymphoma, ALK-negative, lymph nodes of multiple sites
C84.79 Anaplastic large cell lymphoma, ALK-negative, extranodal and solid organ sites

✓5th **C84.A Cutaneous T-cell lymphoma, unspecified**
C84.A0 Cutaneous T-cell lymphoma, unspecified, unspecified site
C84.A1 Cutaneous T-cell lymphoma, unspecified lymph nodes of head, face, and neck
C84.A2 Cutaneous T-cell lymphoma, unspecified, intrathoracic lymph nodes
C84.A3 Cutaneous T-cell lymphoma, unspecified, intra-abdominal lymph nodes
C84.A4 Cutaneous T-cell lymphoma, unspecified, lymph nodes of axilla and upper limb
C84.A5 Cutaneous T-cell lymphoma, unspecified, lymph nodes of inguinal region and lower limb
C84.A6 Cutaneous T-cell lymphoma, unspecified, intrapelvic lymph nodes
C84.A7 Cutaneous T-cell lymphoma, unspecified, spleen
C84.A8 Cutaneous T-cell lymphoma, unspecified, lymph nodes of multiple sites
C84.A9 Cutaneous T-cell lymphoma, unspecified, extranodal and solid organ sites

✓5th **C84.Z Other mature T/NK-cell lymphomas**
NOTE If T-cell lineage or involvement is mentioned in conjunction with a specific lymphoma, code to the more specific description.
EXCLUDES 1 *angioimmunoblastic T-cell lymphoma (C86.5)*
blastic NK-cell lymphoma (C86.4)
enteropathy-type T-cell lymphoma (C86.2)
extranodal NK-cell lymphoma, nasal type (C86.0)
hepatosplenic T-cell lymphoma (C86.1)
primary cutaneous CD30-positive T-cell proliferations (C86.6)
subcutaneous panniculitis-like T-cell lymphoma (C86.3)
T-cell leukemia (C91.1-)
C84.Z0 Other mature T/NK-cell lymphomas, unspecified site
C84.Z1 Other mature T/NK-cell lymphomas, lymph nodes of head, face, and neck
C84.Z2 Other mature T/NK-cell lymphomas, intrathoracic lymph nodes
C84.Z3 Other mature T/NK-cell lymphomas, intra-abdominal lymph nodes
C84.Z4 Other mature T/NK-cell lymphomas, lymph nodes of axilla and upper limb
C84.Z5 Other mature T/NK-cell lymphomas, lymph nodes of inguinal region and lower limb
C84.Z6 Other mature T/NK-cell lymphomas, intrapelvic lymph nodes
C84.Z7 Other mature T/NK-cell lymphomas, spleen
C84.Z8 Other mature T/NK-cell lymphomas, lymph nodes of multiple sites
C84.Z9 Other mature T/NK-cell lymphomas, extranodal and solid organ sites

✓5th **C84.9 Mature T/NK-cell lymphomas, unspecified**
NK/T cell lymphoma NOS
EXCLUDES 1 *mature T-cell lymphoma, not elsewhere classified (C84.4-)*
C84.90 Mature T/NK-cell lymphomas, unspecified, unspecified site
C84.91 Mature T/NK-cell lymphomas, unspecified, lymph nodes of head, face, and neck
C84.92 Mature T/NK-cell lymphomas, unspecified, intrathoracic lymph nodes
C84.93 Mature T/NK-cell lymphomas, unspecified, intra-abdominal lymph nodes
C84.94 Mature T/NK-cell lymphomas, unspecified, lymph nodes of axilla and upper limb
C84.95 Mature T/NK-cell lymphomas, unspecified, lymph nodes of inguinal region and lower limb
C84.96 Mature T/NK-cell lymphomas, unspecified, intrapelvic lymph nodes

C84.97 Mature T/NK-cell lymphomas, unspecified, spleen
C84.98 Mature T/NK-cell lymphomas, unspecified, lymph nodes of multiple sites
C84.99 Mature T/NK-cell lymphomas, unspecified, extranodal and solid organ sites

✓4th C85 Other specified and unspecified types of non-Hodgkin lymphoma
EXCLUDES 1 *other specified types of T/NK-cell lymphoma (C86.-)*
personal history of non-Hodgkin lymphoma (Z85.72)

✓5th C85.1 Unspecified B-cell lymphoma
NOTE If B-cell lineage or involvement is mentioned in conjunction with a specific lymphoma, code to the more specific description.
C85.10 Unspecified B-cell lymphoma, unspecified site
C85.11 Unspecified B-cell lymphoma, lymph nodes of head, face, and neck
C85.12 Unspecified B-cell lymphoma, intrathoracic lymph nodes
C85.13 Unspecified B-cell lymphoma, intra-abdominal lymph nodes
C85.14 Unspecified B-cell lymphoma, lymph nodes of axilla and upper limb
C85.15 Unspecified B-cell lymphoma, lymph nodes of inguinal region and lower limb
C85.16 Unspecified B-cell lymphoma, intrapelvic lymph nodes
C85.17 Unspecified B-cell lymphoma, spleen
C85.18 Unspecified B-cell lymphoma, lymph nodes of multiple sites
C85.19 Unspecified B-cell lymphoma, extranodal and solid organ sites

✓5th C85.2 Mediastinal (thymic) large B-cell lymphoma
C85.20 Mediastinal (thymic) large B-cell lymphoma, unspecified site
C85.21 Mediastinal (thymic) large B-cell lymphoma, lymph nodes of head, face, and neck
C85.22 Mediastinal (thymic) large B-cell lymphoma, intrathoracic lymph nodes
C85.23 Mediastinal (thymic) large B-cell lymphoma, intra-abdominal lymph nodes
C85.24 Mediastinal (thymic) large B-cell lymphoma, lymph nodes of axilla and upper limb
C85.25 Mediastinal (thymic) large B-cell lymphoma, lymph nodes of inguinal region and lower limb
C85.26 Mediastinal (thymic) large B-cell lymphoma, intrapelvic lymph nodes
C85.27 Mediastinal (thymic) large B-cell lymphoma, spleen
C85.28 Mediastinal (thymic) large B-cell lymphoma, lymph nodes of multiple sites
C85.29 Mediastinal (thymic) large B-cell lymphoma, extranodal and solid organ sites

✓5th C85.8 Other specified types of non-Hodgkin lymphoma
C85.80 Other specified types of non-Hodgkin lymphoma, unspecified site
C85.81 Other specified types of non-Hodgkin lymphoma, lymph nodes of head, face, and neck
C85.82 Other specified types of non-Hodgkin lymphoma, intrathoracic lymph nodes
C85.83 Other specified types of non-Hodgkin lymphoma, intra-abdominal lymph nodes
C85.84 Other specified types of non-Hodgkin lymphoma, lymph nodes of axilla and upper limb
C85.85 Other specified types of non-Hodgkin lymphoma, lymph nodes of inguinal region and lower limb
C85.86 Other specified types of non-Hodgkin lymphoma, intrapelvic lymph nodes
C85.87 Other specified types of non-Hodgkin lymphoma, spleen
C85.88 Other specified types of non-Hodgkin lymphoma, lymph nodes of multiple sites
C85.89 Other specified types of non-Hodgkin lymphoma, extranodal and solid organ sites

✓5th C85.9 Non-Hodgkin lymphoma, unspecified
Lymphoma NOS
Malignant lymphoma NOS
Non-Hodgkin lymphoma NOS
C85.90 Non-Hodgkin lymphoma, unspecified, unspecified site
C85.91 Non-Hodgkin lymphoma, unspecified, lymph nodes of head, face, and neck
C85.92 Non-Hodgkin lymphoma, unspecified, intrathoracic lymph nodes
C85.93 Non-Hodgkin lymphoma, unspecified, intra-abdominal lymph nodes
C85.94 Non-Hodgkin lymphoma, unspecified, lymph nodes of axilla and upper limb
C85.95 Non-Hodgkin lymphoma, unspecified, lymph nodes of inguinal region and lower limb
C85.96 Non-Hodgkin lymphoma, unspecified, intrapelvic lymph nodes
C85.97 Non-Hodgkin lymphoma, unspecified, spleen
C85.98 Non-Hodgkin lymphoma, unspecified, lymph nodes of multiple sites
C85.99 Non-Hodgkin lymphoma, unspecified, extranodal and solid organ sites

✓4th C86 Other specified types of T/NK-cell lymphoma
EXCLUDES 1 *anaplastic large cell lymphoma, ALK negative (C84.7-)*
anaplastic large cell lymphoma, ALK positive (C84.6-)
mature T/NK-cell lymphomas (C84.-)
other specified types of non-Hodgkin lymphoma (C85.8-)
C86.0 Extranodal NK/T-cell lymphoma, nasal type
C86.1 Hepatosplenic T-cell lymphoma
Alpha-beta and gamma delta types
C86.2 Enteropathy-type (intestinal) T-cell lymphoma
Enteropathy associated T-cell lymphoma
C86.3 Subcutaneous panniculitis-like T-cell lymphoma
C86.4 Blastic NK-cell lymphoma
C86.5 Angioimmunoblastic T-cell lymphoma
Angioimmunoblastic lymphadenopathy with dysproteinemia [AILD]
C86.6 Primary cutaneous CD30-positive T-cell proliferations
Lymphomatoid papulosis
Primary cutaneous anaplastic large cell lymphoma
Primary cutaneous CD30-positive large T-cell lymphoma

✓4th C88 Malignant immunoproliferative diseases and certain other B-cell lymphomas
EXCLUDES 1 *B-cell lymphoma, unspecified C85.1-*
personal history of other malignant neoplasms of lymphoid, hematopoietic and related tissues (Z85.79)
C88.0 Waldenström macroglobulinemia
Lymphoplasmacytic lymphoma with IgM-production
Macroglobulinemia (idiopathic) (primary)
EXCLUDES 1 *small cell B-cell lymphoma (C83.0)*
C88.2 Heavy chain disease
Franklin disease
Gamma heavy chain disease
Mu heavy chain disease
C88.3 Immunoproliferative small intestinal disease
Alpha heavy chain disease
Mediterranean lymphoma
C88.4 Extranodal marginal zone B-cell lymphoma of mucosa-associated lymphoid tissue [MALT-lymphoma]
Lymphoma of skin-associated lymphoid tissue [SALT-lymphoma]
Lymphoma of bronchial-associated lymphoid tissue [BALT-lymphoma]
EXCLUDES 1 *high malignant (diffuse large B-cell) lymphoma (C83.3-)*
C88.8 Other malignant immunoproliferative diseases
C88.9 Malignant immunoproliferative disease, unspecified
Immunoproliferative disease NOS

✓4th C90 Multiple myeloma and malignant plasma cell neoplasms
EXCLUDES 1 *personal history of other malignant neoplasms of lymphoid, hematopoietic and related tissues (Z85.79)*
✓5th C90.0 Multiple myeloma
Kahler's disease
Medullary plasmacytoma
Myelomatosis
Plasma cell myeloma
EXCLUDES 1 *solitary myeloma (C90.3-)*
solitary plasmactyoma (C90.3-)
C90.00 Multiple myeloma not having achieved remission
Multiple myeloma with failed remission
Multiple myeloma NOS

C90.01 Multiple myeloma in remission
C90.02 Multiple myeloma in relapse

✓5th **C90.1 Plasma cell leukemia**
Plasmacytic leukemia
C90.10 Plasma cell leukemia not having achieved remission
Plasma cell leukemia with failed remission
Plasma cell leukemia NOS
C90.11 Plasma cell leukemia in remission
C90.12 Plasma cell leukemia in relapse

✓5th **C90.2 Extramedullary plasmacytoma**
C90.20 Extramedullary plasmacytoma not having achieved remission
Extramedullary plasmacytoma with failed remission
Extramedullary plasmacytoma NOS
C90.21 Extramedullary plasmacytoma in remission
C90.22 Extramedullary plasmacytoma in relapse

✓5th **C90.3 Solitary plasmacytoma**
Localized malignant plasma cell tumor NOS
Plasmacytoma NOS
Solitary myeloma
C90.30 Solitary plasmacytoma not having achieved remission
Solitary plasmacytoma with failed remission
Solitary plasmacytoma NOS
C90.31 Solitary plasmacytoma in remission
C90.32 Solitary plasmacytoma in relapse

✓4th **C91 Lymphoid leukemia**
EXCLUDES 1 *personal history of leukemia (Z85.6)*

✓5th **C91.0 Acute lymphoblastic leukemia [ALL]**
NOTE Code C91.0 should only be used for T-cell and B-cell precursor leukemia
C91.00 Acute lymphoblastic leukemia not having achieved remission
Acute lymphoblastic leukemia with failed remission
Acute lymphoblastic leukemia NOS
C91.01 Acute lymphoblastic leukemia, in remission
C91.02 Acute lymphoblastic leukemia, in relapse

✓5th **C91.1 Chronic lymphocytic leukemia of B-cell type**
Lymphoplasmacytic leukemia
Richter syndrome
EXCLUDES 1 *lymphoplasmacytic lymphoma (C83.0-)*
C91.10 Chronic lymphocytic leukemia of B-cell type not having achieved remission
Chronic lymphocytic leukemia of B-cell type with failed remission
Chronic lymphocytic leukemia of B-cell type NOS
C91.11 Chronic lymphocytic leukemia of B-cell type in remission
C91.12 Chronic lymphocytic leukemia of B-cell type in relapse

✓5th **C91.3 Prolymphocytic leukemia of B-cell type**
C91.30 Prolymphocytic leukemia of B-cell type not having achieved remission
Prolymphocytic leukemia of B-cell type with failed remission
Prolymphocytic leukemia of B-cell type NOS
C91.31 Prolymphocytic leukemia of B-cell type, in remission
C91.32 Prolymphocytic leukemia of B-cell type, in relapse

✓5th **C91.4 Hairy cell leukemia**
Leukemic reticuloendotheliosis
C91.40 Hairy cell leukemia not having achieved remission
Hairy cell leukemia with failed remission
Hairy cell leukemia NOS
C91.41 Hairy cell leukemia, in remission
C91.42 Hairy cell leukemia, in relapse

✓5th **C91.5 Adult T-cell lymphoma/leukemia (HTLV-1-associated)**
Acute variant of adult T-cell lymphoma/leukemia (HTLV-1-associated)
Chronic variant of adult T-cell lymphoma/leukemia (HTLV-1-associated)
Lymphomatoid variant of adult T-cell lymphoma/leukemia (HTLV-1-associated)
Smouldering variant of adult T-cell lymphoma/leukemia (HTLV-1-associated)
C91.50 Adult T-cell lymphoma/leukemia (HTLV-1-associated) not having achieved remission
Adult T-cell lymphoma/leukemia (HTLV-1-associated) with failed remission
Adult T-cell lymphoma/leukemia (HTLV-1-associated) NOS
C91.51 Adult T-cell lymphoma/leukemia (HTLV-1-associated), in remission
C91.52 Adult T-cell lymphoma/leukemia (HTLV-1-associated), in relapse

✓5th **C91.6 Prolymphocytic leukemia of T-cell type**
C91.60 Prolymphocytic leukemia of T-cell type not having achieved remission
Prolymphocytic leukemia of T-cell type with failed remission
Prolymphocytic leukemia of T-cell type NOS
C91.61 Prolymphocytic leukemia of T-cell type, in remission
C91.62 Prolymphocytic leukemia of T-cell type, in relapse

✓5th **C91.A Mature B-cell leukemia Burkitt-type**
EXCLUDES 1 *Burkitt lymphoma (C83.7-)*
C91.A0 Mature B-cell leukemia Burkitt-type not having achieved remission
Mature B-cell leukemia Burkitt-type with failed remission
Mature B-cell leukemia Burkitt-type NOS
C91.A1 Mature B-cell leukemia Burkitt-type, in remission
C91.A2 Mature B-cell leukemia Burkitt-type, in relapse

✓5th **C91.Z Other lymphoid leukemia**
T-cell large granular lymphocytic leukemia (associated with rheumatoid arthritis)
C91.Z0 Other lymphoid leukemia not having achieved remission
Other lymphoid leukemia with failed remission
Other lymphoid leukemia NOS
C91.Z1 Other lymphoid leukemia, in remission
C91.Z2 Other lymphoid leukemia, in relapse

✓5th **C91.9 Lymphoid leukemia, unspecified**
C91.90 Lymphoid leukemia, unspecified not having achieved remission
Lymphoid leukemia with failed remission
Lymphoid leukemia NOS
C91.91 Lymphoid leukemia, unspecified, in remission
C91.92 Lymphoid leukemia, unspecified, in relapse

✓4th **C92 Myeloid leukemia**
INCLUDES granulocytic leukemia
myelogenous leukemia
EXCLUDES 1 *personal history of leukemia (Z85.6)*

✓5th **C92.0 Acute myeloblastic leukemia**
Acute myeloblastic leukemia, minimal differentiation
Acute myeloblastic leukemia (with maturation)
Acute myeloblastic leukemia 1/ETO
Acute myeloblastic leukemia M0
Acute myeloblastic leukemia M1
Acute myeloblastic leukemia M2
Acute myeloblastic leukemia with t(8;21)
Acute myeloblastic leukemia (without a FAB classification) NOS
Refractory anemia with excess blasts in transformation [RAEB T]
EXCLUDES 1 *acute exacerbation of chronic myeloid leukemia (C92.10)*
refractory anemia with excess of blasts not in transformation (D46.2-)
C92.00 Acute myeloblastic leukemia, not having achieved remission
Acute myeloblastic leukemia with failed remission
Acute myeloblastic leukemia NOS
C92.01 Acute myeloblastic leukemia, in remission
C92.02 Acute myeloblastic leukemia, in relapse

C92.1 Chronic myeloid leukemia, BCR/ABL-positive
Chronic myelogenous leukemia, Philadelphia chromosome (Ph1) positive
Chronic myelogenous leukemia, t(9;22) (q34;q11)
Chronic myelogenous leukemia with crisis of blast cells
EXCLUDES 1 *atypical chronic myeloid leukemia BCR/ABL-negative (C92.2-)*
chronic myelomonocytic leukemia (C93.1-)
chronic myeloproliferative disease (D47.1)

C92.10 Chronic myeloid leukemia, BCR/ABL-positive, not having achieved remission
Chronic myeloid leukemia, BCR/ABL-positive with failed remission
Chronic myeloid leukemia, BCR/ABL-positive NOS

C92.11 Chronic myeloid leukemia, BCR/ABL-positive, in remission

C92.12 Chronic myeloid leukemia, BCR/ABL-positive, in relapse

C92.2 Atypical chronic myeloid leukemia, BCR/ABL-negative

C92.20 Atypical chronic myeloid leukemia, BCR/ABL-negative, not having achieved remission
Atypical chronic myeloid leukemia, BCR/ABL-negative with failed remission
Atypical chronic myeloid leukemia, BCR/ABL-negative NOS

C92.21 Atypical chronic myeloid leukemia, BCR/ABL-negative, in remission

C92.22 Atypical chronic myeloid leukemia, BCR/ABL-negative, in relapse

C92.3 Myeloid sarcoma
A malignant tumor of immature myeloid cells
Chloroma
Granulocytic sarcoma

C92.30 Myeloid sarcoma, not having achieved remission
Myeloid sarcoma with failed remission
Myeloid sarcoma NOS

C92.31 Myeloid sarcoma, in remission

C92.32 Myeloid sarcoma, in relapse

C92.4 Acute promyelocytic leukemia
AML M3
AML Me with t(15;17) and variants

C92.40 Acute promyelocytic leukemia, not having achieved remission
Acute promyelocytic leukemia with failed remission
Acute promyelocytic leukemia NOS

C92.41 Acute promyelocytic leukemia, in remission

C92.42 Acute promyelocytic leukemia, in relapse

C92.5 Acute myelomonocytic leukemia
AML M4
AML M4 Eo with inv(16) or t(16;16)

C92.50 Acute myelomonocytic leukemia, not having achieved remission
Acute myelomonocytic leukemia with failed remission
Acute myelomonocytic leukemia NOS

C92.51 Acute myelomonocytic leukemia, in remission

C92.52 Acute myelomonocytic leukemia, in relapse

C92.6 Acute myeloid leukemia with 11q23-abnormality
Acute myeloid leukemia with variation of MLL-gene

C92.60 Acute myeloid leukemia with 11q23-abnormality not having achieved remission
Acute myeloid leukemia with 11q23-abnormality with failed remission
Acute myeloid leukemia with 11q23-abnormality NOS

C92.61 Acute myeloid leukemia with 11q23-abnormality in remission

C92.62 Acute myeloid leukemia with 11q23-abnormality in relapse

C92.A Acute myeloid leukemia with multilineage dysplasia
Acute myeloid leukemia with dysplasia of remaining hematopoesis and/or myelodysplastic disease in its history

C92.A0 Acute myeloid leukemia with multilineage dysplasia, not having achieved remission
Acute myeloid leukemia with multilineage dysplasia with failed remission
Acute myeloid leukemia with multilineage dysplasia NOS

C92.A1 Acute myeloid leukemia with multilineage dysplasia, in remission

C92.A2 Acute myeloid leukemia with multilineage dysplasia, in relapse

C92.Z Other myeloid leukemia

C92.Z0 Other myeloid leukemia not having achieved remission
Myeloid leukemia NEC with failed remission
Myeloid leukemia NEC

C92.Z1 Other myeloid leukemia, in remission

C92.Z2 Other myeloid leukemia, in relapse

C92.9 Myeloid leukemia, unspecified

C92.90 Myeloid leukemia, unspecified, not having achieved remission
Myeloid leukemia, unspecified with failed remission
Myeloid leukemia, unspecified NOS

C92.91 Myeloid leukemia, unspecified in remission

C92.92 Myeloid leukemia, unspecified in relapse

C93 Monocytic leukemia
INCLUDES monocytoid leukemia
EXCLUDES 1 *personal history of leukemia (Z85.6)*

C93.0 Acute monoblastic/monocytic leukemia
AML M5
AML M5a
AML M5b

C93.00 Acute monoblastic/monocytic leukemia, not having achieved remission
Acute monoblastic/monocytic leukemia with failed remission
Acute monoblastic/monocytic leukemia NOS

C93.01 Acute monoblastic/monocytic leukemia, in remission

C93.02 Acute monoblastic/monocytic leukemia, in relapse

C93.1 Chronic myelomonocytic leukemia
Chronic monocytic leukemia
CMML-1
CMML-2
CMML with eosinophilia

C93.10 Chronic myelomonocytic leukemia not having achieved remission
Chronic myelomonocytic leukemia with failed remission
Chronic myelomonocytic leukemia NOS

C93.11 Chronic myelomonocytic leukemia, in remission

C93.12 Chronic myelomonocytic leukemia, in relapse

C93.3 Juvenile myelomonocytic leukemia

C93.30 Juvenile myelomonocytic leukemia, not having achieved remission
Juvenile myelomonocytic leukemia with failed remission
Juvenile myelomonocytic leukemia NOS

C93.31 Juvenile myelomonocytic leukemia, in remission

C93.32 Juvenile myelomonocytic leukemia, in relapse

C93.Z Other monocytic leukemia

C93.Z0 Other monocytic leukemia, not having achieved remission
Other monocytic leukemia NOS

C93.Z1 Other monocytic leukemia, in remission

C93.Z2 Other monocytic leukemia, in relapse

C93.9 Monocytic leukemia, unspecified

C93.90 Monocytic leukemia, unspecified, not having achieved remission
Monocytic leukemia, unspecified with failed remission
Monocytic leukemia, unspecified NOS

C93.91 Monocytic leukemia, unspecified in remission

C93.92 Monocytic leukemia, unspecified in relapse

C94 Other leukemias of specified cell type
EXCLUDES 1 *leukemic reticuloendotheliosis (C91.4-)*
myelodysplastic syndromes (D46.-)
personal history of leukemia (Z85.6)
plasma cell leukemia (C90.1-)

C94.0 Acute erythroid leukemia
Acute myeloid leukemia M6(a)(b)
Erythroleukemia

C94.00 Acute erythroid leukemia, not having achieved remission
Acute erythroid leukemia with failed remission
Acute erythroid leukemia NOS

Appropriate additional character required
Requires 7th character, placeholder x must fill empty characters

C94.Ø1 Acute erythroid leukemia, in remission
C94.Ø2 Acute erythroid leukemia, in relapse

√5th **C94.2 Acute megakaryoblastic leukemia**
Acute myeloid leukemia M7
Acute megakaryocytic leukemia
C94.2Ø Acute megakaryoblastic leukemia not having achieved remission
Acute megakaryoblastic leukemia with failied remission
Acute megakaryoblastic leukemia NOS
C94.21 Acute megakaryoblastic leukemia, in remission
C94.22 Acute megakaryoblastic leukemia, in relapse

√5th **C94.3 Mast cell leukemia**
C94.3Ø Mast cell leukemia not having achieved remission
Mast cell leukemia with failed remission
Mast cell leukemia NOS
C94.31 Mast cell leukemia, in remission
C94.32 Mast cell leukemia, in relapse

√5th **C94.4 Acute panmyelosis with myelofibrosis**
Acute myelofibrosis
EXCLUDES 1 *myelofibrosis NOS (D75.81)*
secondary myelofibrosis NOS (D75.81)
C94.4Ø Acute panmyelosis with myelofibrosis not having achieved remission
Acute myelofibrosis NOS
Acute panmyelosis with myelofibrosis with failed remission
Acute panmyelosis NOS
C94.41 Acute panmyelosis with myelofibrosis, in remission
C94.42 Acute panmyelosis with myelofibrosis, in relapse

C94.6 Myelodysplastic disease, not classified
Myeloproliferative disease, not classified

√5th **C94.8 Other specified leukemias**
Aggressive NK-cell leukemia
Acute basophilic leukemia
C94.8Ø Other specified leukemias not having achieved remission
Other specified leukemia with failed remission
Other specified leukemias NOS
C94.81 Other specified leukemias, in remission
C94.82 Other specified leukemias, in relapse

√4th **C95 Leukemia of unspecified cell type**
EXCLUDES 1 *personal history of leukemia (Z85.6)*

√5th **C95.Ø Acute leukemia of unspecified cell type**
Acute bilineal leukemia
Acute mixed lineage leukemia
Biphenotypic acute leukemia
Stem cell leukemia of unclear lineage
EXCLUDES 1 *acute exacerbation of unspecified chronic leukemia (C95.1Ø)*
C95.ØØ Acute leukemia of unspecified cell type not having achieved remission
Acute leukemia of unspecified cell type with failed remission
Acute leukemia NOS
C95.Ø1 Acute leukemia of unspecified cell type, in remission
C95.Ø2 Acute leukemia of unspecified cell type, in relapse

√5th **C95.1 Chronic leukemia of unspecified cell type**
C95.1Ø Chronic leukemia of unspecified cell type not having achieved remission
Chronic leukemia of unspecified cell type with failed remission
Chronic leukemia NOS
C95.11 Chronic leukemia of unspecified cell type, in remission
C95.12 Chronic leukemia of unspecified cell type, in relapse

√5th **C95.9 Leukemia, unspecified**
C95.9Ø Leukemia, unspecified not having achieved remission
Leukemia, unspecified with failed remission
Leukemia NOS
C95.91 Leukemia, unspecified, in remission
C95.92 Leukemia, unspecified, in relapse

√4th **C96 Other and unspecified malignant neoplasms of lymphoid, hematopoietic and related tissue**
EXCLUDES 1 *personal history of other malignant neoplasms of lymphoid, hematopoietic and related tissues (Z85.79)*

C96.Ø Multifocal and multisystemic (disseminated) Langerhans-cell histiocytosis
Histiocytosis X, multisystemic
Letterer-Siwe disease
EXCLUDES 1 *adult pulmonary Langerhans cell histiocytosis (J84.82)*
multifocal and unisystemic Langerhans-cell histiocytosis (C96.5)
unifocal Langerhans-cell histiocytosis (C96.6)

C96.2 Malignant mast cell tumor
Aggressive systemic mastocytosis
Mast cell sarcoma
EXCLUDES 1 *indolent mastocytosis (D47.Ø)*
mast cell leukemia (C94.3Ø)
mastocytosis (congenital) (cutaneous) (Q82.2)

C96.4 Sarcoma of dendritic cells (accessory cells)
Follicular dendritic cell sarcoma
Interdigitating dendritic cell sarcoma
Langerhans cell sarcoma

C96.5 Multifocal and unisystemic Langerhans-cell histiocytosis
Hand-Schüller-Christian disease
Histiocytosis X, multifocal
EXCLUDES 1 *multifocal and multisystemic (disseminated) Langerhans-cell histiocytosis (C96.Ø)*
unifocal Langerhans-cell histiocytosis (C96.6)

C96.6 Unifocal Langerhans-cell histiocytosis
Eosinophilic granuloma
Histiocytosis X, unifocal
Histiocytosis X NOS
Langerhans-cell histiocytosis NOS
EXCLUDES 1 *multifocal and multisysemic (disseminated) Langerhans-cell histiocytosis (C96.Ø)*
multifocal and unisystemic Langerhans-cell histiocytosis (C96.5)

C96.A Histiocytic sarcoma
Malignant histiocytosis

C96.Z Other specified malignant neoplasms of lymphoid, hematopoietic and related tissue

C96.9 Malignant neoplasm of lymphoid, hematopoietic and related tissue, unspecified

In situ neoplasms (DØØ-DØ9)

INCLUDES Bowen's disease
erythroplasia
grade III intraepithelial neoplasia
Queyrat's erythroplasia

√4th **DØØ Carcinoma in situ of oral cavity, esophagus and stomach**
EXCLUDES 1 *melanoma in situ (DØ3.-)*

√5th **DØØ.Ø Carcinoma in situ of lip, oral cavity and pharynx**
EXCLUDES 1 *carcinoma in situ of aryepiglottic fold or interarytenoid fold, laryngeal aspect (DØ2.Ø)*
carcinoma in situ of epiglottis NOS (DØ2.Ø)
carcinoma in situ of epiglottis suprahyoid portion (DØ2.Ø)
carcinoma in situ of skin of lip (DØ3.Ø, DØ4.Ø)
Use additional code to identify:
exposure to environmental tobacco smoke (Z77.22)
exposure to tobacco smoke in the perinatal period (P96.81)
history of tobacco use (Z87.891)
occupational exposure to environmental tobacco smoke (Z57.31)
tobacco dependence (F17.-)
tobacco use (Z72.Ø)
DØØ.ØØ Carcinoma in situ of oral cavity, unspecified site
DØØ.Ø1 Carcinoma in situ of labial mucosa and vermilion border
DØØ.Ø2 Carcinoma in situ of buccal mucosa
DØØ.Ø3 Carcinoma in situ of gingiva and edentulous alveolar ridge
DØØ.Ø4 Carcinoma in situ of soft palate
DØØ.Ø5 Carcinoma in situ of hard palate
DØØ.Ø6 Carcinoma in situ of floor of mouth
DØØ.Ø7 Carcinoma in situ of tongue

D00.08 Carcinoma in situ of pharynx
Carcinoma in situ of aryepiglottic fold NOS
Carcinoma in situ of hypopharyngeal aspect of aryepiglottic fold
Carcinoma in situ of marginal zone of aryepiglottic fold

D00.1 Carcinoma in situ of esophagus

D00.2 Carcinoma in situ of stomach

✓4th **D01 Carcinoma in situ of other and unspecified digestive organs**
EXCLUDES 1 *melanoma in situ (D03.-)*

D01.0 Carcinoma in situ of colon
EXCLUDES 1 *carcinoma in situ of rectosigmoid junction (D01.1)*

D01.1 Carcinoma in situ of rectosigmoid junction

D01.2 Carcinoma in situ of rectum

D01.3 Carcinoma in situ of anus and anal canal
EXCLUDES 1 *carcinoma in situ of anal margin (D04.5)*
carcinoma in situ of anal skin (D04.5)
carcinoma in situ of perianal skin (D04.5)

✓5th **D01.4 Carcinoma in situ of other and unspecified parts of intestine**
EXCLUDES 1 *carcinoma in situ of ampulla of Vater (D01.5)*

D01.40 Carcinoma in situ of unspecified part of intestine

D01.49 Carcinoma in situ of other parts of intestine

D01.5 Carcinoma in situ of liver, gallbladder and bile ducts
Carcinoma in situ of ampulla of Vater

D01.7 Carcinoma in situ of other specified digestive organs
Carcinoma in situ of pancreas

D01.9 Carcinoma in situ of digestive organ, unspecified

✓4th **D02 Carcinoma in situ of middle ear and respiratory system**
EXCLUDES 1 *melanoma in situ (D03.-)*
Use additional code to identify:
exposure to environmental tobacco smoke (Z77.22)
exposure to tobacco smoke in the perinatal period (P96.81)
history of tobacco use (Z87.891)
occupational exposure to environmental tobacco smoke (Z57.31)
tobacco dependence (F17.-)
tobacco use (Z72.0)

D02.0 Carcinoma in situ of larynx
Carcinoma in situ of aryepiglottic fold or interarytenoid fold, laryngeal aspect
Carcinoma in situ of epiglottis (suprahyoid portion)
EXCLUDES 1 *carcinoma in situ of aryepiglottic fold or interarytenoid fold NOS (D00.08)*
carcinoma in situ of hypopharyngeal aspect (D00.08)
carcinoma in situ of marginal zone (D00.08)

D02.1 Carcinoma in situ of trachea

✓5th **D02.2 Carcinoma in situ of bronchus and lung**

D02.20 Carcinoma in situ of unspecified bronchus and lung

D02.21 Carcinoma in situ of right bronchus and lung

D02.22 Carcinoma in situ of left bronchus and lung

D02.3 Carcinoma in situ of other parts of respiratory system
Carcinoma in situ of accessory sinuses
Carcinoma in situ of middle ear
Carcinoma in situ of nasal cavities
EXCLUDES 1 *carcinoma in situ of ear (external) (skin) (D04.2-)*
carcinoma in situ of nose NOS (D09.8)
carcinoma in situ of skin of nose (D04.3)

D02.4 Carcinoma in situ of respiratory system, unspecified

✓4th **D03 Melanoma in situ**

D03.0 Melanoma in situ of lip

✓5th **D03.1 Melanoma in situ of eyelid, including canthus**

D03.10 Melanoma in situ of unspecified eyelid, including canthus

D03.11 Melanoma in situ of right eyelid, including canthus

D03.12 Melanoma in situ of left eyelid, including canthus

✓5th **D03.2 Melanoma in situ of ear and external auricular canal**

D03.20 Melanoma in situ of unspecified ear and external auricular canal

D03.21 Melanoma in situ of right ear and external auricular canal

D03.22 Melanoma in situ of left ear and external auricular canal

✓5th **D03.3 Melanoma in situ of other and unspecified parts of face**

D03.30 Melanoma in situ of unspecified part of face

D03.39 Melanoma in situ of other parts of face

D03.4 Melanoma in situ of scalp and neck

✓5th **D03.5 Melanoma in situ of trunk**

D03.51 Melanoma in situ of anal skin
Melanoma in situ of anal margin
Melanoma in situ of perianal skin

D03.52 Melanoma in situ of breast (skin) (soft tissue)

D03.59 Melanoma in situ of other part of trunk

✓5th **D03.6 Melanoma in situ of upper limb, including shoulder**

D03.60 Melanoma in situ of unspecified upper limb, including shoulder

D03.61 Melanoma in situ of right upper limb, including shoulder

D03.62 Melanoma in situ of left upper limb, including shoulder

✓5th **D03.7 Melanoma in situ of lower limb, including hip**

D03.70 Melanoma in situ of unspecified lower limb, including hip

D03.71 Melanoma in situ of right lower limb, including hip

D03.72 Melanoma in situ of left lower limb, including hip

D03.8 Melanoma in situ of other sites
Melanoma in situ of scrotum
EXCLUDES 1 *carcinoma in situ of scrotum (D07.61)*

D03.9 Melanoma in situ, unspecified

✓4th **D04 Carcinoma in situ of skin**
EXCLUDES 1 *erythroplasia of Queyrat (penis) NOS (D07.4)*
melanoma in situ (D03.-)

D04.0 Carcinoma in situ of skin of lip
EXCLUDES 1 *carcinoma in situ of vermilion border of lip (D00.01)*

✓5th **D04.1 Carcinoma in situ of skin of eyelid, including canthus**

D04.10 Carcinoma in situ of skin of unspecified eyelid, including canthus

D04.11 Carcinoma in situ of skin of right eyelid, including canthus

D04.12 Carcinoma in situ of skin of left eyelid, including canthus

✓5th **D04.2 Carcinoma in situ of skin of ear and external auricular canal**

D04.20 Carcinoma in situ of skin of unspecified ear and external auricular canal

D04.21 Carcinoma in situ of skin of right ear and external auricular canal

D04.22 Carcinoma in situ of skin of left ear and external auricular canal

✓5th **D04.3 Carcinoma in situ of skin of other and unspecified parts of face**

D04.30 Carcinoma in situ of skin of unspecified part of face

D04.39 Carcinoma in situ of skin of other parts of face

D04.4 Carcinoma in situ of skin of scalp and neck

D04.5 Carcinoma in situ of skin of trunk
Carcinoma in situ of anal margin
Carcinoma in situ of anal skin
Carcinoma in situ of perianal skin
Carcinoma in situ of skin of breast
EXCLUDES 1 *carcinoma in situ of anus NOS (D01.3)*
carcinoma in situ of scrotum (D07.61)
carcinoma in situ of skin of genital organs (D07.-)

✓5th **D04.6 Carcinoma in situ of skin of upper limb, including shoulder**

D04.60 Carcinoma in situ of skin of unspecified upper limb, including shoulder

D04.61 Carcinoma in situ of skin of right upper limb, including shoulder

D04.62 Carcinoma in situ of skin of left upper limb, including shoulder

✓5th **D04.7 Carcinoma in situ of skin of lower limb, including hip**

D04.70 Carcinoma in situ of skin of unspecified lower limb, including hip

D04.71 Carcinoma in situ of skin of right lower limb, including hip

D04.72 Carcinoma in situ of skin of left lower limb, including hip

D04.8 Carcinoma in situ of skin of other sites

D04.9 Carcinoma in situ of skin, unspecified

✓4th **D05 Carcinoma in situ of breast**
EXCLUDES 1 *carcinoma in situ of skin of breast (D04.5)*
melanoma in situ of breast (skin) (D03.5)
Paget's disease of breast or nipple (C50.-)

✓5th **D05.0 Lobular carcinoma in situ of breast**

D05.00 Lobular carcinoma in situ of unspecified breast

D05.01 Lobular carcinoma in situ of right breast
D05.02 Lobular carcinoma in situ of left breast
✓5th **D05.1 Intraductal carcinoma in situ of breast**
D05.10 Intraductal carcinoma in situ of unspecified breast
D05.11 Intraductal carcinoma in situ of right breast
D05.12 Intraductal carcinoma in situ of left breast
✓5th **D05.8 Other specified type of carcinoma in situ of breast**
D05.80 Other specified type of carcinoma in situ of unspecified breast
D05.81 Other specified type of carcinoma in situ of right breast
D05.82 Other specified type of carcinoma in situ of left breast
✓5th **D05.9 Unspecified type of carcinoma in situ of breast**
D05.90 Unspecified type of carcinoma in situ of unspecified breast
D05.91 Unspecified type of carcinoma in situ of right breast
D05.92 Unspecified type of carcinoma in situ of left breast

✓4th **D06 Carcinoma in situ of cervix uteri**
INCLUDES cervical adenocarcinoma in situ
cervical intraepithelial glandular neoplasia
cervical intraepithelial neoplasia III [CIN III]
severe dysplasia of cervix uteri
EXCLUDES 1 *cervical intraepithelial neoplasia II [CIN II] (N87.1)*
cytologic evidence of malignancy of cervix without histologic confirmation (R87.614)
high grade squamous intraepithelial lesion (HGSIL) of cervix (R87.613)
melanoma in situ of cervix (D03.5)
moderate cervical dysplasia (N87.1)
D06.0 Carcinoma in situ of endocervix
D06.1 Carcinoma in situ of exocervix
D06.7 Carcinoma in situ of other parts of cervix
D06.9 Carcinoma in situ of cervix, unspecified

✓4th **D07 Carcinoma in situ of other and unspecified genital organs**
EXCLUDES 1 *melanoma in situ of trunk (D03.5)*
D07.0 Carcinoma in situ of endometrium
D07.1 Carcinoma in situ of vulva
Severe dysplasia of vulva
Vulvar intraepithelial neoplasia III [VIN III]
EXCLUDES 1 *moderate dysplasia of vulva (N90.1)*
vulvar intraepithelial neoplasia II [VIN II] (N90.1)
D07.2 Carcinoma in situ of vagina
Severe dysplasia of vagina
Vaginal intraepithelial neoplasia III [VAIN III]
EXCLUDES 1 *moderate dysplasia of vagina (N89.1)*
vaginal intraepithelial neoplasia II [VIN II] (N89.1)
✓5th **D07.3 Carcinoma in situ of other and unspecified female genital organs**
D07.30 Carcinoma in situ of unspecified female genital organs
D07.39 Carcinoma in situ of other female genital organs
D07.4 Carcinoma in situ of penis
Erythroplasia of Queyrat NOS
D07.5 Carcinoma in situ of prostate
Prostatic intraepithelial neoplasia III (PIN III)
Severe dysplasia of prostate
EXCLUDES 1 *dysplasia (mild) (moderate) of prostate (N42.3)*
✓5th **D07.6 Carcinoma in situ of other and unspecified male genital organs**
D07.60 Carcinoma in situ of unspecified male genital organs
D07.61 Carcinoma in situ of scrotum
D07.69 Carcinoma in situ of other male genital organs

✓4th **D09 Carcinoma in situ of other and unspecified sites**
EXCLUDES 1 *melanoma in situ (D03.-)*
D09.0 Carcinoma in situ of bladder
✓5th **D09.1 Carcinoma in situ of other and unspecified urinary organs**
D09.10 Carcinoma in situ of unspecified urinary organ
D09.19 Carcinoma in situ of other urinary organs
✓5th **D09.2 Carcinoma in situ of eye**
EXCLUDES 1 *carcinoma in situ of skin of eyelid (D04.1-)*
D09.20 Carcinoma in situ of unspecified eye
D09.21 Carcinoma in situ of right eye
D09.22 Carcinoma in situ of left eye
D09.3 Carcinoma in situ of thyroid and other endocrine glands
EXCLUDES 1 *carcinoma in situ of endocrine pancreas (D01.7)*
carcinoma in situ of ovary (D07.39)
carcinoma in situ of testis (D07.69)
D09.8 Carcinoma in situ of other specified sites
D09.9 Carcinoma in situ, unspecified

Benign neoplasms, except benign neuroendocrine tumors (D10-D36)

✓4th **D10 Benign neoplasm of mouth and pharynx**
D10.0 Benign neoplasm of lip
Benign neoplasm of lip (frenulum) (inner aspect) (mucosa) (vermilion border)
EXCLUDES 1 *benign neoplasm of skin of lip (D22.0, D23.0)*
D10.1 Benign neoplasm of tongue
Benign neoplasm of lingual tonsil
D10.2 Benign neoplasm of floor of mouth
✓5th **D10.3 Other and unspecified parts of mouth**
D10.30 Benign neoplasm of unspecified part of mouth
D10.39 Benign neoplasm of other parts of mouth
Benign neoplasm of minor salivary gland NOS
EXCLUDES 1 *benign odontogenic neoplasms (D16.4-D16.5)*
benign neoplasm of mucosa of lip (D10.0)
benign neoplasm of nasopharyngeal surface of soft palate (D10.6)
D10.4 Benign neoplasm of tonsil
Benign neoplasm of tonsil (faucial) (palatine)
EXCLUDES 1 *benign neoplasm of lingual tonsil (D10.1)*
benign neoplasm of pharyngeal tonsil (D10.6)
benign neoplasm of tonsillar fossa (D10.5)
benign neoplasm of tonsillar pillars (D10.5)
D10.5 Benign neoplasm of other parts of oropharynx
Benign neoplasm of epiglottis, anterior aspect
Benign neoplasm of tonsillar fossa
Benign neoplasm of tonsillar pillars
Benign neoplasm of vallecula
EXCLUDES 1 *benign neoplasm of epiglottis NOS (D14.1)*
benign neoplasm of epiglottis, suprahyoid portion (D14.1)
D10.6 Benign neoplasm of nasopharynx
Benign neoplasm of pharyngeal tonsil
Benign neoplasm of posterior margin of septum and choanae
D10.7 Benign neoplasm of hypopharynx
D10.9 Benign neoplasm of pharynx, unspecified

✓4th **D11 Benign neoplasm of major salivary glands**
EXCLUDES 1 *benign neoplasms of specified minor salivary glands which are classified according to their anatomical location*
benign neoplasms of minor salivary glands NOS (D10.39)
D11.0 Benign neoplasm of parotid gland
D11.7 Benign neoplasm of other major salivary glands
Benign neoplasm of sublingual salivary gland
Benign neoplasm of submandibular salivary gland
D11.9 Benign neoplasm of major salivary gland, unspecified

✓4th **D12 Benign neoplasm of colon, rectum, anus and anal canal**
EXCLUDES 1 *benign carcinoid tumors of the large intestine, and rectum (D3A.02-)*
D12.0 Benign neoplasm of cecum
Benign neoplasm of ileocecal valve
D12.1 Benign neoplasm of appendix
EXCLUDES 1 *benign carcinoid tumor of the appendix (D3A.020)*
D12.2 Benign neoplasm of ascending colon
D12.3 Benign neoplasm of transverse colon
Benign neoplasm of hepatic flexure
Benign neoplasm of splenic flexure
D12.4 Benign neoplasm of descending colon
D12.5 Benign neoplasm of sigmoid colon
D12.6 Benign neoplasm of colon, unspecified
Adenomatosis of colon
Benign neoplasm of large intestine NOS
Polyposis (hereditary) of colon
EXCLUDES 1 *inflammatory polyp of colon (K51.4-)*
polyp of colon NOS (K63.5)
D12.7 Benign neoplasm of rectosigmoid junction
D12.8 Benign neoplasm of rectum
EXCLUDES 1 *benign carcinoid tumor of the rectum (D3A.026)*

D12.9 Benign neoplasm of anus and anal canal
Benign neoplasm of anus NOS
EXCLUDES 1 *benign neoplasm of anal margin (D22.5, D23.5)*
benign neoplasm of anal skin (D22.5, D23.5)
benign neoplasm of perianal skin (D22.5, D23.5)

D13 Benign neoplasm of other and ill-defined parts of digestive system
EXCLUDES 1 *benign stromal tumors of digestive system (D21.4)*
D13.0 Benign neoplasm of esophagus
D13.1 Benign neoplasm of stomach
EXCLUDES 1 *benign carcinoid tumor of the stomach (D3A.092)*
D13.2 Benign neoplasm of duodenum
EXCLUDES 1 *benign carcinoid tumor of the duodenum (D3A.010)*
D13.3 Benign neoplasm of other and unspecified parts of small intestine
EXCLUDES 1 *benign carcinoid tumors of the small intestine (D3A.01-)*
benign neoplasm of ileocecal valve (D12.0)
D13.30 Benign neoplasm of unspecified part of small intestine
D13.39 Benign neoplasm of other parts of small intestine
D13.4 Benign neoplasm of liver
Benign neoplasm of intrahepatic bile ducts
D13.5 Benign neoplasm of extrahepatic bile ducts
D13.6 Benign neoplasm of pancreas
EXCLUDES 1 *benign neoplasm of endocrine pancreas (D13.7)*
D13.7 Benign neoplasm of endocrine pancreas
Islet cell tumor
Benign neoplasm of islets of Langerhans
Use additional code to identify any functional activity
D13.9 Benign neoplasm of ill-defined sites within the digestive system
Benign neoplasm of digestive system NOS
Benign neoplasm of intestine NOS
Benign neoplasm of spleen

D14 Benign neoplasm of middle ear and respiratory system
D14.0 Benign neoplasm of middle ear, nasal cavity and accessory sinuses
Benign neoplasm of cartilage of nose
EXCLUDES 1 *benign neoplasm of auricular canal (external) (D22.2-, D23.2-)*
benign neoplasm of bone of ear (D16.4)
benign neoplasm of bone of nose (D16.4)
benign neoplasm of cartilage of ear (D21.0)
benign neoplasm of ear (external)(skin) (D22.2-, D23.2-)
benign neoplasm of nose NOS (D36.7)
benign neoplasm of skin of nose (D22.39, D23.39)
benign neoplasm of olfactory bulb (D33.3)
benign neoplasm of posterior margin of septum and choanae (D10.6)
polyp of accessory sinus (J33.8)
polyp of ear (middle) (H74.4)
polyp of nasal (cavity) (J33.-)
D14.1 Benign neoplasm of larynx
Adenomatous polyp of larynx
Benign neoplasm of epiglottis (suprahyoid portion)
EXCLUDES 1 *benign neoplasm of epiglottis, anterior aspect (D10.5)*
polyp (nonadenomatous) of vocal cord or larynx (J38.1)
D14.2 Benign neoplasm of trachea
D14.3 Benign neoplasm of bronchus and lung
EXCLUDES 1 *benign carcinoid tumor of the bronchus and lung (D3A.090)*
D14.30 Benign neoplasm of unspecified bronchus and lung
D14.31 Benign neoplasm of right bronchus and lung
D14.32 Benign neoplasm of left bronchus and lung
D14.4 Benign neoplasm of respiratory system, unspecified

D15 Benign neoplasm of other and unspecified intrathoracic organs
EXCLUDES 1 *benign neoplasm of mesothelial tissue (D19.-)*
D15.0 Benign neoplasm of thymus
EXCLUDES 1 *benign carcinoid tumor of the thymus (D3A.091)*
D15.1 Benign neoplasm of heart
EXCLUDES 1 *benign neoplasm of great vessels (D21.3)*
D15.2 Benign neoplasm of mediastinum
D15.7 Benign neoplasm of other specified intrathoracic organs
D15.9 Benign neoplasm of intrathoracic organ, unspecified

D16 Benign neoplasm of bone and articular cartilage
EXCLUDES 1 *benign neoplasm of connective tissue of ear (D21.0)*
benign neoplasm of connective tissue of eyelid (D21.0)
benign neoplasm of connective tissue of larynx (D14.1)
benign neoplasm of connective tissue of nose (D14.0)
benign neoplasm of synovia (D21.-)
D16.0 Benign neoplasm of scapula and long bones of upper limb
D16.00 Benign neoplasm of scapula and long bones of unspecified upper limb
D16.01 Benign neoplasm of scapula and long bones of right upper limb
D16.02 Benign neoplasm of scapula and long bones of left upper limb
D16.1 Benign neoplasm of short bones of upper limb
D16.10 Benign neoplasm of short bones of unspecified upper limb
D16.11 Benign neoplasm of short bones of right upper limb
D16.12 Benign neoplasm of short bones of left upper limb
D16.2 Benign neoplasm of long bones of lower limb
D16.20 Benign neoplasm of long bones of unspecified lower limb
D16.21 Benign neoplasm of long bones of right lower limb
D16.22 Benign neoplasm of long bones of left lower limb
D16.3 Benign neoplasm of short bones of lower limb
D16.30 Benign neoplasm of short bones of unspecified lower limb
D16.31 Benign neoplasm of short bones of right lower limb
D16.32 Benign neoplasm of short bones of left lower limb
D16.4 Benign neoplasm of bones of skull and face
Benign neoplasm of maxilla (superior)
Benign neoplasm of orbital bone
Keratocyst of maxilla
Keratocystic odontogenic tumor of maxilla
EXCLUDES 1 *benign neoplasm of lower jaw bone (D16.5)*
D16.5 Benign neoplasm of lower jaw bone
Keratocyst of mandible
Keratocystic odontogenic tumor of mandible
D16.6 Benign neoplasm of vertebral column
EXCLUDES 1 *benign neoplasm of sacrum and coccyx (D16.8)*
D16.7 Benign neoplasm of ribs, sternum and clavicle
D16.8 Benign neoplasm of pelvic bones, sacrum and coccyx
D16.9 Benign neoplasm of bone and articular cartilage, unspecified

D17 Benign lipomatous neoplasm
D17.0 Benign lipomatous neoplasm of skin and subcutaneous tissue of head, face and neck
D17.1 Benign lipomatous neoplasm of skin and subcutaneous tissue of trunk
D17.2 Benign lipomatous neoplasm of skin and subcutaneous tissue of limb
D17.20 Benign lipomatous neoplasm of skin and subcutaneous tissue of unspecified limb
D17.21 Benign lipomatous neoplasm of skin and subcutaneous tissue of right arm
D17.22 Benign lipomatous neoplasm of skin and subcutaneous tissue of left arm
D17.23 Benign lipomatous neoplasm of skin and subcutaneous tissue of right leg
D17.24 Benign lipomatous neoplasm of skin and subcutaneous tissue of left leg
D17.3 Benign lipomatous neoplasm of skin and subcutaneous tissue of other and unspecified sites
D17.30 Benign lipomatous neoplasm of skin and subcutaneous tissue of unspecified sites
D17.39 Benign lipomatous neoplasm of skin and subcutaneous tissue of other sites
D17.4 Benign lipomatous neoplasm of intrathoracic organs
D17.5 Benign lipomatous neoplasm of intra-abdominal organs
EXCLUDES 1 *benign lipomatous neoplasm of peritoneum and retroperitoneum (D17.79)*
D17.6 Benign lipomatous neoplasm of spermatic cord

✓5th **D17.7 Benign lipomatous neoplasm of other sites**

D17.71 Benign lipomatous neoplasm of kidney

D17.72 Benign lipomatous neoplasm of other genitourinary organ

D17.79 Benign lipomatous neoplasm of other sites

Benign lipomatous neoplasm of peritoneum

Benign lipomatous neoplasm of retroperitoneum

D17.9 Benign lipomatous neoplasm, unspecified

Lipoma NOS

✓4th **D18 Hemangioma and lymphangioma, any site**

EXCLUDES 1 *benign neoplasm of glomus jugulare (D35.6)*
blue or pigmented nevus (D22.-)
nevus NOS (D22.-)
vascular nevus (Q82.5)

✓5th **D18.Ø Hemangioma**

Angioma NOS

Cavernous nevus

D18.ØØ Hemangioma unspecified site

D18.Ø1 Hemangioma of skin and subcutaneous tissue

D18.Ø2 Hemangioma of intracranial structures

D18.Ø3 Hemangioma of intra-abdominal structures

D18.Ø9 Hemangioma of other sites

D18.1 Lymphangioma, any site

✓4th **D19 Benign neoplasm of mesothelial tissue**

D19.Ø Benign neoplasm of mesothelial tissue of pleura

D19.1 Benign neoplasm of mesothelial tissue of peritoneum

D19.7 Benign neoplasm of mesothelial tissue of other sites

D19.9 Benign neoplasm of mesothelial tissue, unspecified

Benign mesothelioma NOS

✓4th **D2Ø Benign neoplasm of soft tissue of retroperitoneum and peritoneum**

EXCLUDES 1 *benign lipomatous neoplasm of peritoneum and retroperitoneum (D17.79)*
benign neoplasm of mesothelial tissue (D19.-)

D2Ø.Ø Benign neoplasm of soft tissue of retroperitoneum

D2Ø.1 Benign neoplasm of soft tissue of peritoneum

✓4th **D21 Other benign neoplasms of connective and other soft tissue**

INCLUDES benign neoplasm of blood vessel
benign neoplasm of bursa
benign neoplasm of cartilage
benign neoplasm of fascia
benign neoplasm of fat
benign neoplasm of ligament, except uterine
benign neoplasm of lymphatic channel
benign neoplasm of muscle
benign neoplasm of synovia
benign neoplasm of tendon (sheath)
benign stromal tumors

EXCLUDES 1 *benign neoplasm of articular cartilage (D16.-)*
benign neoplasm of cartilage of larynx (D14.1)
benign neoplasm of cartilage of nose (D14.Ø)
benign neoplasm of connective tissue of breast (D24.-)
benign neoplasm of peripheral nerves and autonomic nervous system (D36.1-)
benign neoplasm of peritoneum (D2Ø.1)
benign neoplasm of retroperitoneum (D2Ø.Ø)
benign neoplasm of uterine ligament, any (D28.2)
benign neoplasm of vascular tissue (D18.-)
hemangioma (D18.Ø-)
lipomatous neoplasm (D17.-)
lymphangioma (D18.1)
uterine leiomyoma (D25.-)

D21.Ø Benign neoplasm of connective and other soft tissue of head, face and neck

Benign neoplasm of connective tissue of ear

Benign neoplasm of connective tissue of eyelid

EXCLUDES 1 *benign neoplasm of connective tissue of orbit (D31.6-)*

✓5th **D21.1 Benign neoplasm of connective and other soft tissue of upper limb, including shoulder**

D21.1Ø Benign neoplasm of connective and other soft tissue of unspecified upper limb, including shoulder

D21.11 Benign neoplasm of connective and other soft tissue of right upper limb, including shoulder

D21.12 Benign neoplasm of connective and other soft tissue of left upper limb, including shoulder

✓5th **D21.2 Benign neoplasm of connective and other soft tissue of lower limb, including hip**

D21.2Ø Benign neoplasm of connective and other soft tissue of unspecified lower limb, including hip

D21.21 Benign neoplasm of connective and other soft tissue of right lower limb, including hip

D21.22 Benign neoplasm of connective and other soft tissue of left lower limb, including hip

D21.3 Benign neoplasm of connective and other soft tissue of thorax

Benign neoplasm of axilla

Benign neoplasm of diaphragm

Benign neoplasm of great vessels

EXCLUDES 1 *benign neoplasm of heart (D15.1)*
benign neoplasm of mediastinum (D15.2)
benign neoplasm of thymus (D15.Ø)

D21.4 Benign neoplasm of connective and other soft tissue of abdomen

Benign stromal tumors of abdomen

D21.5 Benign neoplasm of connective and other soft tissue of pelvis

EXCLUDES 1 *benign neoplasm of any uterine ligament (D28.2)*
uterine leiomyoma (D25.-)

D21.6 Benign neoplasm of connective and other soft tissue of trunk, unspecified

Benign neoplasm of back NOS

D21.9 Benign neoplasm of connective and other soft tissue, unspecified

✓4th **D22 Melanocytic nevi**

INCLUDES atypical nevus
blue hairy pigmented nevus
nevus NOS

D22.Ø Melanocytic nevi of lip

✓5th **D22.1 Melanocytic nevi of eyelid, including canthus**

D22.1Ø Melanocytic nevi of unspecified eyelid, including canthus

D22.11 Melanocytic nevi of right eyelid, including canthus

D22.12 Melanocytic nevi of left eyelid, including canthus

✓5th **D22.2 Melanocytic nevi of ear and external auricular canal**

D22.2Ø Melanocytic nevi of unspecified ear and external auricular canal

D22.21 Melanocytic nevi of right ear and external auricular canal

D22.22 Melanocytic nevi of left ear and external auricular canal

✓5th **D22.3 Melanocytic nevi of other and unspecified parts of face**

D22.3Ø Melanocytic nevi of unspecified part of face

D22.39 Melanocytic nevi of other parts of face

D22.4 Melanocytic nevi of scalp and neck

D22.5 Melanocytic nevi of trunk

Melanocytic nevi of anal margin

Melanocytic nevi of anal skin

Melanocytic nevi of perianal skin

Melanocytic nevi of skin of breast

✓5th **D22.6 Melanocytic nevi of upper limb, including shoulder**

D22.6Ø Melanocytic nevi of unspecified upper limb, including shoulder

D22.61 Melanocytic nevi of right upper limb, including shoulder

D22.62 Melanocytic nevi of left upper limb, including shoulder

✓5th **D22.7 Melanocytic nevi of lower limb, including hip**

D22.7Ø Melanocytic nevi of unspecified lower limb, including hip

D22.71 Melanocytic nevi of right lower limb, including hip

D22.72 Melanocytic nevi of left lower limb, including hip

D22.9 Melanocytic nevi, unspecified

✓4th **D23 Other benign neoplasms of skin**

INCLUDES benign neoplasm of hair follicles
benign neoplasm of sebaceous glands
benign neoplasm of sweat glands

EXCLUDES 1 *benign lipomatous neoplasms of skin (D17.Ø-D17.3)*
melanocytic nevi (D22.-)

D23.Ø Other benign neoplasm of skin of lip

EXCLUDES 1 *benign neoplasm of vermilion border of lip (D1Ø.Ø)*

✓5th **D23.1 Other benign neoplasm of skin of eyelid, including canthus**
D23.10 Other benign neoplasm of skin of unspecified eyelid, including canthus
D23.11 Other benign neoplasm of skin of right eyelid, including canthus
D23.12 Other benign neoplasm of skin of left eyelid, including canthus

✓5th **D23.2 Other benign neoplasm of skin of ear and external auricular canal**
D23.20 Other benign neoplasm of skin of unspecified ear and external auricular canal
D23.21 Other benign neoplasm of skin of right ear and external auricular canal
D23.22 Other benign neoplasm of skin of left ear and external auricular canal

✓5th **D23.3 Other benign neoplasm of skin of other and unspecified parts of face**
D23.30 Other benign neoplasm of skin of unspecified part of face
D23.39 Other benign neoplasm of skin of other parts of face

D23.4 Other benign neoplasm of skin of scalp and neck

D23.5 Other benign neoplasm of skin of trunk
Other benign neoplasm of anal margin
Other benign neoplasm of anal skin
Other benign neoplasm of perianal skin
Other benign neoplasm of skin of breast
EXCLUDES 1 *benign neoplasm of anus NOS (D12.9)*

✓5th **D23.6 Other benign neoplasm of skin of upper limb, including shoulder**
D23.60 Other benign neoplasm of skin of unspecified upper limb, including shoulder
D23.61 Other benign neoplasm of skin of right upper limb, including shoulder
D23.62 Other benign neoplasm of skin of left upper limb, including shoulder

✓5th **D23.7 Other benign neoplasm of skin of lower limb, including hip**
D23.70 Other benign neoplasm of skin of unspecified lower limb, including hip
D23.71 Other benign neoplasm of skin of right lower limb, including hip
D23.72 Other benign neoplasm of skin of left lower limb, including hip

D23.9 Other benign neoplasm of skin, unspecified

✓4th **D24 Benign neoplasm of breast**
INCLUDES benign neoplasm of connective tissue of breast
benign neoplasm of soft parts of breast
fibroadenoma of breast
EXCLUDES 2 *adenofibrosis of breast (N60.2)*
benign cyst of breast (N60.-)
benign mammary dysplasia (N60.-)
benign neoplasm of skin of breast (D22.5, D23.5)
fibrocystic disease of breast (N60.-)

D24.1 Benign neoplasm of right breast
D24.2 Benign neoplasm of left breast
D24.9 Benign neoplasm of unspecified breast

✓4th **D25 Leiomyoma of uterus**
INCLUDES uterine fibroid
uterine fibromyoma
uterine myoma

D25.0 Submucous leiomyoma of uterus
D25.1 Intramural leiomyoma of uterus
Interstitial leiomyoma of uterus
D25.2 Subserosal leiomyoma of uterus
Subperitoneal leiomyoma of uterus
D25.9 Leiomyoma of uterus, unspecified

✓4th **D26 Other benign neoplasms of uterus**
D26.0 Other benign neoplasm of cervix uteri
D26.1 Other benign neoplasm of corpus uteri
D26.7 Other benign neoplasm of other parts of uterus
D26.9 Other benign neoplasm of uterus, unspecified

✓4th **D27 Benign neoplasm of ovary**
Use additional code to identify any functional activity
EXCLUDES 2 *corpus albicans cyst (N83.2)*
corpus luteum cyst (N83.1)
endometrial cyst (N80.1)
follicular (atretic) cyst (N83.0)
graafian follicle cyst (N83.0)
ovarian cyst NEC (N83.2)
ovarian retention cyst (N83.2)

D27.0 Benign neoplasm of right ovary
D27.1 Benign neoplasm of left ovary
D27.9 Benign neoplasm of unspecified ovary

✓4th **D28 Benign neoplasm of other and unspecified female genital organs**
INCLUDES adenomatous polyp
benign neoplasm of skin of female genital organs
benign teratoma
EXCLUDES 1 *epoophoron cyst (Q50.5)*
fimbrial cyst (Q50.4)
Gartner's duct cyst (Q52.4)
parovarian cyst (Q50.5)

D28.0 Benign neoplasm of vulva
D28.1 Benign neoplasm of vagina
D28.2 Benign neoplasm of uterine tubes and ligaments
Benign neoplasm of fallopian tube
Benign neoplasm of uterine ligament (broad) (round)
D28.7 Benign neoplasm of other specified female genital organs
D28.9 Benign neoplasm of female genital organ, unspecified

✓4th **D29 Benign neoplasm of male genital organs**
INCLUDES benign neoplasm of skin of male genital organs

D29.0 Benign neoplasm of penis
D29.1 Benign neoplasm of prostate
EXCLUDES 1 *enlarged prostate (N40.-)*

✓5th **D29.2 Benign neoplasm of testis**
Use additional code to identify any functional activity
D29.20 Benign neoplasm of unspecified testis
D29.21 Benign neoplasm of right testis
D29.22 Benign neoplasm of left testis

✓5th **D29.3 Benign neoplasm of epididymis**
D29.30 Benign neoplasm of unspecified epididymis
D29.31 Benign neoplasm of right epididymis
D29.32 Benign neoplasm of left epididymis

D29.4 Benign neoplasm of scrotum
Benign neoplasm of skin of scrotum
D29.8 Benign neoplasm of other specified male genital organs
Benign neoplasm of seminal vesicle
Benign neoplasm of spermatic cord
Benign neoplasm of tunica vaginalis
D29.9 Benign neoplasm of male genital organ, unspecified

✓4th **D30 Benign neoplasm of urinary organs**

✓5th **D30.0 Benign neoplasm of kidney**
EXCLUDES 1 *benign carcinoid tumor of the kidney (D3A.093)*
benign neoplasm of renal calyces (D30.1-)
benign neoplasm of renal pelvis (D30.1-)
D30.00 Benign neoplasm of unspecified kidney
D30.01 Benign neoplasm of right kidney
D30.02 Benign neoplasm of left kidney

✓5th **D30.1 Benign neoplasm of renal pelvis**
D30.10 Benign neoplasm of unspecified renal pelvis
D30.11 Benign neoplasm of right renal pelvis
D30.12 Benign neoplasm of left renal pelvis

✓5th **D30.2 Benign neoplasm of ureter**
EXCLUDES 1 *benign neoplasm of ureteric orifice of bladder (D30.3)*
D30.20 Benign neoplasm of unspecified ureter
D30.21 Benign neoplasm of right ureter
D30.22 Benign neoplasm of left ureter

D30.3 Benign neoplasm of bladder
Benign neoplasm of ureteric orifice of bladder
Benign neoplasm of urethral orifice of bladder
D30.4 Benign neoplasm of urethra
EXCLUDES 1 *benign neoplasm of urethral orifice of bladder (D30.3)*
D30.8 Benign neoplasm of other specified urinary organs
Benign neoplasm of paraurethral glands
D30.9 Benign neoplasm of urinary organ, unspecified
Benign neoplasm of urinary system NOS

D31 Benign neoplasm of eye and adnexa
EXCLUDES 1 *benign neoplasm of connective tissue of eyelid (D21.Ø)*
benign neoplasm of optic nerve (D33.3)
benign neoplasm of skin of eyelid (D22.1-, D23.1-)

D31.Ø Benign neoplasm of conjunctiva
D31.ØØ Benign neoplasm of unspecified conjunctiva
D31.Ø1 Benign neoplasm of right conjunctiva
D31.Ø2 Benign neoplasm of left conjunctiva

D31.1 Benign neoplasm of cornea
D31.1Ø Benign neoplasm of unspecified cornea
D31.11 Benign neoplasm of right cornea
D31.12 Benign neoplasm of left cornea

D31.2 Benign neoplasm of retina
EXCLUDES 1 *dark area on retina (D49.81)*
hemangioma of retina (D49.81)
neoplasm of unspecified behavior of retina and choroid (D49.81)
retinal freckle (D49.81)
D31.2Ø Benign neoplasm of unspecified retina
D31.21 Benign neoplasm of right retina
D31.22 Benign neoplasm of left retina

D31.3 Benign neoplasm of choroid
D31.3Ø Benign neoplasm of unspecified choroid
D31.31 Benign neoplasm of right choroid
D31.32 Benign neoplasm of left choroid

D31.4 Benign neoplasm of ciliary body
D31.4Ø Benign neoplasm of unspecified ciliary body
D31.41 Benign neoplasm of right ciliary body
D31.42 Benign neoplasm of left ciliary body

D31.5 Benign neoplasm of lacrimal gland and duct
Benign neoplasm of lacrimal sac
Benign neoplasm of nasolacrimal duct
D31.5Ø Benign neoplasm of unspecified lacrimal gland and duct
D31.51 Benign neoplasm of right lacrimal gland and duct
D31.52 Benign neoplasm of left lacrimal gland and duct

D31.6 Benign neoplasm of unspecified site of orbit
Benign neoplasm of connective tissue of orbit
Benign neoplasm of extraocular muscle
Benign neoplasm of peripheral nerves of orbit
Benign neoplasm of retrobulbar tissue
Benign neoplasm of retro-ocular tissue
EXCLUDES 1 *benign neoplasm of orbital bone (D16.4)*
D31.6Ø Benign neoplasm of unspecified site of unspecified orbit
D31.61 Benign neoplasm of unspecified site of right orbit
D31.62 Benign neoplasm of unspecified site of left orbit

D31.9 Benign neoplasm of unspecified part of eye
D31.9Ø Benign neoplasm of unspecified part of unspecified eye
D31.91 Benign neoplasm of unspecified part of right eye
D31.92 Benign neoplasm of unspecified part of left eye

D32 Benign neoplasm of meninges
D32.Ø Benign neoplasm of cerebral meninges
D32.1 Benign neoplasm of spinal meninges
D32.9 Benign neoplasm of meninges, unspecified
Meningioma NOS

D33 Benign neoplasm of brain and other parts of central nervous system
EXCLUDES 1 *angioma (D18.Ø-)*
benign neoplasm of meninges (D32.-)
benign neoplasm of peripheral nerves and autonomic nervous system (D36.1-)
hemangioma (D18.Ø-)
neurofibromatosis (Q85.Ø-)
retro-ocular benign neoplasm (D31.6-)

D33.Ø Benign neoplasm of brain, supratentorial
Benign neoplasm of cerebral ventricle
Benign neoplasm of cerebrum
Benign neoplasm of frontal lobe
Benign neoplasm of occipital lobe
Benign neoplasm of parietal lobe
Benign neoplasm of temporal lobe
EXCLUDES 1 *benign neoplasm of fourth ventricle (D33.1)*

D33.1 Benign neoplasm of brain, infratentorial
Benign neoplasm of brain stem
Benign neoplasm of cerebellum
Benign neoplasm of fourth ventricle
D33.2 Benign neoplasm of brain, unspecified
D33.3 Benign neoplasm of cranial nerves
Benign neoplasm of olfactory bulb
D33.4 Benign neoplasm of spinal cord
D33.7 Benign neoplasm of other specified parts of central nervous system
D33.9 Benign neoplasm of central nervous system, unspecified
Benign neoplasm of nervous system (central) NOS

D34 Benign neoplasm of thyroid gland
Use additional code to identify any functional activity

D35 Benign neoplasm of other and unspecified endocrine glands
Use additional code to identify any functional activity
EXCLUDES 1 *benign neoplasm of endocrine pancreas (D13.7)*
benign neoplasm of ovary (D27.-)
benign neoplasm of testis (D29.2-)
benign neoplasm of thymus (D15.Ø)

D35.Ø Benign neoplasm of adrenal gland
D35.ØØ Benign neoplasm of unspecified adrenal gland
D35.Ø1 Benign neoplasm of right adrenal gland
D35.Ø2 Benign neoplasm of left adrenal gland
D35.1 Benign neoplasm of parathyroid gland
D35.2 Benign neoplasm of pituitary gland
D35.3 Benign neoplasm of craniopharyngeal duct
D35.4 Benign neoplasm of pineal gland
D35.5 Benign neoplasm of carotid body
D35.6 Benign neoplasm of aortic body and other paraganglia
Benign tumor of glomus jugulare
D35.7 Benign neoplasm of other specified endocrine glands
D35.9 Benign neoplasm of endocrine gland, unspecified
Benign neoplasm of unspecified endocrine gland

D36 Benign neoplasm of other and unspecified sites
D36.Ø Benign neoplasm of lymph nodes
EXCLUDES 1 *lymphangioma (D18.1)*
D36.1 Benign neoplasm of peripheral nerves and autonomic nervous system
EXCLUDES 1 *benign neoplasm of peripheral nerves of orbit (D31.6-)*
neurofibromatosis (Q85.Ø-)
D36.1Ø Benign neoplasm of peripheral nerves and autonomic nervous system, unspecified
D36.11 Benign neoplasm of peripheral nerves and autonomic nervous system of face, head, and neck
D36.12 Benign neoplasm of peripheral nerves and autonomic nervous system, upper limb, including shoulder
D36.13 Benign neoplasm of peripheral nerves and autonomic nervous system of lower limb, including hip
D36.14 Benign neoplasm of peripheral nerves and autonomic nervous system of thorax
D36.15 Benign neoplasm of peripheral nerves and autonomic nervous system of abdomen
D36.16 Benign neoplasm of peripheral nerves and autonomic nervous system of pelvis
D36.17 Benign neoplasm of peripheral nerves and autonomic nervous system of trunk, unspecified
D36.7 Benign neoplasm of other specified sites
Benign neoplasm of nose NOS
D36.9 Benign neoplasm, unspecified site

Benign neuroendocrine tumors (D3A)

D3A Benign neuroendocrine tumors
Code also any associated multiple endocrine neoplasia [MEN] syndromes (E31.2-)
Use additional code to identify any associated endocrine syndrome, such as:
carcinoid syndrome (E34.Ø)
EXCLUDES 2 *benign pancreatic islet cell tumors (D13.7)*
D3A.Ø Benign carcinoid tumors
D3A.ØØ Benign carcinoid tumor of unspecified site
Carcinoid tumor NOS

EXCLUDES 1 Not coded here EXCLUDES 2 Not included here ***Manifestation Code***

D3A.01 Benign carcinoid tumors of the small intestine
D3A.010 Benign carcinoid tumor of the duodenum
D3A.011 Benign carcinoid tumor of the jejunum
D3A.012 Benign carcinoid tumor of the ileum
D3A.019 Benign carcinoid tumor of the small intestine, unspecified portion
D3A.02 Benign carcinoid tumors of the appendix, large intestine, and rectum
D3A.020 Benign carcinoid tumor of the appendix
D3A.021 Benign carcinoid tumor of the cecum
D3A.022 Benign carcinoid tumor of the ascending colon
D3A.023 Benign carcinoid tumor of the transverse colon
D3A.024 Benign carcinoid tumor of the descending colon
D3A.025 Benign carcinoid tumor of the sigmoid colon
D3A.026 Benign carcinoid tumor of the rectum
D3A.029 Benign carcinoid tumor of the large intestine, unspecified portion
Benign carcinoid tumor of the colon NOS
D3A.09 Benign carcinoid tumors of other sites
D3A.090 Benign carcinoid tumor of the bronchus and lung
D3A.091 Benign carcinoid tumor of the thymus
D3A.092 Benign carcinoid tumor of the stomach
D3A.093 Benign carcinoid tumor of the kidney
D3A.094 Benign carcinoid tumor of the foregut NOS
D3A.095 Benign carcinoid tumor of the midgut NOS
D3A.096 Benign carcinoid tumor of the hindgut NOS
D3A.098 Benign carcinoid tumors of other sites
D3A.8 Other benign neuroendocrine tumors
Neuroendocrine tumor NOS

Neoplasms of uncertain behavior, polycythemia vera and myelodysplastic syndromes (D37-D48)

NOTE Categories D37-D44, and D48 classify by site neoplasms of uncertain behavior, i.e., histologic confirmation whether the neoplasm is malignant or benign cannot be made.

EXCLUDES 1 *neoplasms of unspecified behavior (D49.-)*

D37 Neoplasm of uncertain behavior of oral cavity and digestive organs
EXCLUDES 1 *stromal tumors of uncertain behavior of digestive system (D48.1)*
D37.0 Neoplasm of uncertain behavior of lip, oral cavity and pharynx
EXCLUDES 1 *neoplasm of uncertain behavior of aryepiglottic fold or interarytenoid fold, laryngeal aspect (D38.0)*
neoplasm of uncertain behavior of epiglottis NOS (D38.0)
neoplasm of uncertain behavior of skin of lip (D48.5)
neoplasm of uncertain behavior of suprahyoid portion of epiglottis (D38.0)
D37.01 Neoplasm of uncertain behavior of lip
Neoplasm of uncertain behavior of vermilion border of lip
D37.02 Neoplasm of uncertain behavior of tongue
D37.03 Neoplasm of uncertain behavior of the major salivary glands
D37.030 Neoplasm of uncertain behavior of the parotid salivary glands
D37.031 Neoplasm of uncertain behavior of the sublingual salivary glands
D37.032 Neoplasm of uncertain behavior of the submandibular salivary glands
D37.039 Neoplasm of uncertain behavior of the major salivary glands, unspecified
D37.04 Neoplasm of uncertain behavior of the minor salivary glands
Neoplasm of uncertain behavior of submucosal salivary glands of lip
Neoplasm of uncertain behavior of submucosal salivary glands of cheek
Neoplasm of uncertain behavior of submucosal salivary glands of hard palate
Neoplasm of uncertain behavior of submucosal salivary glands of soft palate
D37.05 Neoplasm of uncertain behavior of pharynx
Neoplasm of uncertain behavior of aryepiglottic fold of pharynx NOS
Neoplasm of uncertain behavior of hypopharyngeal aspect of aryepiglottic fold of pharynx
Neoplasm of uncertain behavior of marginal zone of aryepiglottic fold of pharynx
D37.09 Neoplasm of uncertain behavior of other specified sites of the oral cavity
D37.1 Neoplasm of uncertain behavior of stomach
D37.2 Neoplasm of uncertain behavior of small intestine
D37.3 Neoplasm of uncertain behavior of appendix
D37.4 Neoplasm of uncertain behavior of colon
D37.5 Neoplasm of uncertain behavior of rectum
Neoplasm of uncertain behavior of rectosigmoid junction
D37.6 Neoplasm of uncertain behavior of liver, gallbladder and bile ducts
Neoplasm of uncertain behavior of ampulla of Vater
D37.8 Neoplasm of uncertain behavior of other specified digestive organs
Neoplasm of uncertain behavior of anal canal
Neoplasm of uncertain behavior of anal sphincter
Neoplasm of uncertain behavior of anus NOS
Neoplasm of uncertain behavior of esophagus
Neoplasm of uncertain behavior of intestine NOS
Neoplasm of uncertain behavior of pancreas
EXCLUDES 1 *neoplasm of uncertain behavior of anal margin (D48.5)*
neoplasm of uncertain behavior of anal skin (D48.5)
neoplasm of uncertain behavior of perianal skin (D48.5)
D37.9 Neoplasm of uncertain behavior of digestive organ, unspecified
D38 Neoplasm of uncertain behavior of middle ear and respiratory and intrathoracic organs
EXCLUDES 1 *neoplasm of uncertain behavior of heart (D48.7)*
D38.0 Neoplasm of uncertain behavior of larynx
Neoplasm of uncertain behavior of aryepiglottic fold or interarytenoid fold, laryngeal aspect
Neoplasm of uncertain behavior of epiglottis (suprahyoid portion)
EXCLUDES 1 *neoplasm of uncertain behavior of aryepiglottic fold or interarytenoid fold NOS (D37.05)*
neoplasm of uncertain behavior of hypopharyngeal aspect of aryepiglottic fold (D37.05)
neoplasm of uncertain behavior of marginal zone of aryepiglottic fold (D37.05)
D38.1 Neoplasm of uncertain behavior of trachea, bronchus and lung
D38.2 Neoplasm of uncertain behavior of pleura
D38.3 Neoplasm of uncertain behavior of mediastinum
D38.4 Neoplasm of uncertain behavior of thymus
D38.5 Neoplasm of uncertain behavior of other respiratory organs
Neoplasm of uncertain behavior of accessory sinuses
Neoplasm of uncertain behavior of cartilage of nose
Neoplasm of uncertain behavior of middle ear
Neoplasm of uncertain behavior of nasal cavities
EXCLUDES 1 *neoplasm of uncertain behavior of ear (external) (skin) (D48.5)*
neoplasm of uncertain behavior of nose NOS (D48.7)
neoplasm of uncertain behavior of skin of nose (D48.5)
D38.6 Neoplasm of uncertain behavior of respiratory organ, unspecified
D39 Neoplasm of uncertain behavior of female genital organs
D39.0 Neoplasm of uncertain behavior of uterus

5th **D39.1 Neoplasm of uncertain behavior of ovary**
Use additional code to identify any functional activity
D39.1Ø Neoplasm of uncertain behavior of unspecified ovary
D39.11 Neoplasm of uncertain behavior of right ovary
D39.12 Neoplasm of uncertain behavior of left ovary
D39.2 Neoplasm of uncertain behavior of placenta
Chorioadenoma destruens
Invasive hydatidiform mole
Malignant hydatidiform mole
EXCLUDES1 *hydatidiform mole NOS (OØ1.9)*
D39.8 Neoplasm of uncertain behavior of other specified female genital organs
Neoplasm of uncertain behavior of skin of female genital organs
D39.9 Neoplasm of uncertain behavior of female genital organ, unspecified

4th **D4Ø Neoplasm of uncertain behavior of male genital organs**
D4Ø.Ø Neoplasm of uncertain behavior of prostate
5th **D4Ø.1 Neoplasm of uncertain behavior of testis**
D4Ø.1Ø Neoplasm of uncertain behavior of unspecified testis
D4Ø.11 Neoplasm of uncertain behavior of right testis
D4Ø.12 Neoplasm of uncertain behavior of left testis
D4Ø.8 Neoplasm of uncertain behavior of other specified male genital organs
Neoplasm of uncertain behavior of skin of male genital organs
D4Ø.9 Neoplasm of uncertain behavior of male genital organ, unspecified

4th **D41 Neoplasm of uncertain behavior of urinary organs**
5th **D41.Ø Neoplasm of uncertain behavior of kidney**
EXCLUDES1 *neoplasm of uncertain behavior of renal pelvis (D41.1-)*
D41.ØØ Neoplasm of uncertain behavior of unspecified kidney
D41.Ø1 Neoplasm of uncertain behavior of right kidney
D41.Ø2 Neoplasm of uncertain behavior of left kidney
5th **D41.1 Neoplasm of uncertain behavior of renal pelvis**
D41.1Ø Neoplasm of uncertain behavior of unspecified renal pelvis
D41.11 Neoplasm of uncertain behavior of right renal pelvis
D41.12 Neoplasm of uncertain behavior of left renal pelvis
5th **D41.2 Neoplasm of uncertain behavior of ureter**
D41.2Ø Neoplasm of uncertain behavior of unspecified ureter
D41.21 Neoplasm of uncertain behavior of right ureter
D41.22 Neoplasm of uncertain behavior of left ureter
D41.3 Neoplasm of uncertain behavior of urethra
D41.4 Neoplasm of uncertain behavior of bladder
D41.8 Neoplasm of uncertain behavior of other specified urinary organs
D41.9 Neoplasm of uncertain behavior of unspecified urinary organ

4th **D42 Neoplasm of uncertain behavior of meninges**
D42.Ø Neoplasm of uncertain behavior of cerebral meninges
D42.1 Neoplasm of uncertain behavior of spinal meninges
D42.9 Neoplasm of uncertain behavior of meninges, unspecified

4th **D43 Neoplasm of uncertain behavior of brain and central nervous system**
EXCLUDES1 *neoplasm of uncertain behavior of peripheral nerves and autonomic nervous system (D48.2)*
D43.Ø Neoplasm of uncertain behavior of brain, supratentorial
Neoplasm of uncertain behavior of cerebral ventricle
Neoplasm of uncertain behavior of cerebrum
Neoplasm of uncertain behavior of frontal lobe
Neoplasm of uncertain behavior of occipital lobe
Neoplasm of uncertain behavior of parietal lobe
Neoplasm of uncertain behavior of temporal lobe
EXCLUDES1 *neoplasm of uncertain behavior of fourth ventricle (D43.1)*
D43.1 Neoplasm of uncertain behavior of brain, infratentorial
Neoplasm of uncertain behavior of brain stem
Neoplasm of uncertain behavior of cerebellum
Neoplasm of uncertain behavior of fourth ventricle
D43.2 Neoplasm of uncertain behavior of brain, unspecified
D43.3 Neoplasm of uncertain behavior of cranial nerves
D43.4 Neoplasm of uncertain behavior of spinal cord
D43.8 Neoplasm of uncertain behavior of other specified parts of central nervous system
D43.9 Neoplasm of uncertain behavior of central nervous system, unspecified
Neoplasm of uncertain behavior of nervous system (central) NOS

4th **D44 Neoplasm of uncertain behavior of endocrine glands**
EXCLUDES1 *multiple endocrine adenomatosis (E31.2-)*
multiple endocrine neoplasia (E31.2-)
neoplasm of uncertain behavior of endocrine pancreas (D37.8)
neoplasm of uncertain behavior of ovary (D39.1-)
neoplasm of uncertain behavior of testis (D4Ø.1-)
neoplasm of uncertain behavior of thymus (D38.4)
D44.Ø Neoplasm of uncertain behavior of thyroid gland
5th **D44.1 Neoplasm of uncertain behavior of adrenal gland**
Use additional code to identify any functional activity
D44.1Ø Neoplasm of uncertain behavior of unspecified adrenal gland
D44.11 Neoplasm of uncertain behavior of right adrenal gland
D44.12 Neoplasm of uncertain behavior of left adrenal gland
D44.2 Neoplasm of uncertain behavior of parathyroid gland
D44.3 Neoplasm of uncertain behavior of pituitary gland
Use additional code to identify any functional activity
D44.4 Neoplasm of uncertain behavior of craniopharyngeal duct
D44.5 Neoplasm of uncertain behavior of pineal gland
D44.6 Neoplasm of uncertain behavior of carotid body
D44.7 Neoplasm of uncertain behavior of aortic body and other paraganglia
D44.9 Neoplasm of uncertain behavior of unspecified endocrine gland

D45 Polycythemia vera
EXCLUDES1 *familial polycythemia (D75.Ø)*
secondary polycythemia (D75.1)

4th **D46 Myelodysplastic syndromes**
Use additional code for adverse effect, if applicable, to identify drug (T36-T5Ø with fifth or sixth character 5)
EXCLUDES2 *drug-induced aplastic anemia (D61.1)*
D46.Ø Refractory anemia without ring sideroblasts, so stated
Refractory anemia without sideroblasts, without excess of blasts
D46.1 Refractory anemia with ring sideroblasts
RARS
5th **D46.2 Refractory anemia with excess of blasts**
D46.2Ø Refractory anemia with excess of blasts, unspecified
RAEB NOS
D46.21 Refractory anemia with excess of blasts 1
RAEB 1
D46.22 Refractory anemia with excess of blasts 2
RAEB 2
D46.A Refractory cytopenia with multilineage dysplasia
D46.B Refractory cytopenia with multilineage dysplasia and ring sideroblasts
RCMD RS
D46.C Myelodysplastic syndrome with isolated del(5q) chromosomal abnormality
Myelodysplastic syndrome with 5q deletion
5q minus syndrome NOS
D46.4 Refractory anemia, unspecified
D46.Z Other myelodysplastic syndromes
EXCLUDES1 *chronic myelomonocytic leukemia (C93.1-)*
D46.9 Myelodysplastic syndrome, unspecified
Myelodysplasia NOS

4th **D47 Other neoplasms of uncertain behavior of lymphoid, hematopoietic and related tissue**
D47.Ø Histiocytic and mast cell tumors of uncertain behavior
Indolent systemic mastocytosis
Mast cell tumor NOS
Mastocytoma NOS
EXCLUDES1 *malignant mast cell tumor (C96.2)*
mastocytosis (congenital) (cutaneous) (Q82.2)

D47.1 Chronic myeloproliferative disease
Chronic neutrophilic leukemia
Myeloproliferative disease, unspecified
EXCLUDES 1 *atypical chronic myeloid leukemia BCR/ABL-negative (C92.2-)*
chronic myeloid leukemia BCR/ABL-positive (C92.1-)
myelofibrosis NOS (D75.81)
myelophthisic anemia (D61.82)
myelophthisis (D61.82)
secondary myelofibrosis NOS (D75.81)

D47.2 Monoclonal gammopathy
Monoclonal gammopathy of undetermined significance [MGUS]

D47.3 Essential (hemorrhagic) thrombocythemia
Essential thrombocytosis
Idiopathic hemorrhagic thrombocythemia

D47.4 Osteomyelofibrosis
Chronic idiopathic myelofibrosis
Myelofibrosis (idiopathic) (with myeloid metaplasia)
Myelosclerosis (megakaryocytic) with myeloid metaplasia
Secondary myelofibrosis in myeloproliferative disease
EXCLUDES 1 *acute myelofibrosis (C94.4-)*

✓5th **D47.Z Other specified neoplasms of uncertain behavior of lymphoid, hematopoietic and related tissue**

D47.Z1 Post-transplant lymphoproliferative disorder (PTLD)
Code first complications of transplanted organs and tissue (T86.-)

D47.Z9 Other specified neoplasms of uncertain behavior of lymphoid, hematopoietic and related tissue
Histiocytic tumors of uncertain behavior

D47.9 Neoplasm of uncertain behavior of lymphoid, hematopoietic and related tissue, unspecified
Lymphoproliferative disease NOS

✓4th **D48 Neoplasm of uncertain behavior of other and unspecified sites**
EXCLUDES 1 *neurofibromatosis (nonmalignant) (Q85.0-)*

D48.0 Neoplasm of uncertain behavior of bone and articular cartilage
EXCLUDES 1 *neoplasm of uncertain behavior of cartilage of ear (D48.1)*
neoplasm of uncertain behavior of cartilage of larynx (D38.0)
neoplasm of uncertain behavior of cartilage of nose (D38.5)
neoplasm of uncertain behavior of connective tissue of eyelid (D48.1)
neoplasm of uncertain behavior of synovia (D48.1)

D48.1 Neoplasm of uncertain behavior of connective and other soft tissue
Neoplasm of uncertain behavior of connective tissue of ear
Neoplasm of uncertain behavior of connective tissue of eyelid
Stromal tumors of uncertain behavior of digestive system
EXCLUDES 1 *neoplasm of uncertain behavior of articular cartilage (D48.0)*
neoplasm of uncertain behavior of cartilage of larynx (D38.0)
neoplasm of uncertain behavior of cartilage of nose (D38.5)
neoplasm of uncertain behavior of connective tissue of breast (D48.6-)

D48.2 Neoplasm of uncertain behavior of peripheral nerves and autonomic nervous system
EXCLUDES 1 *neoplasm of uncertain behavior of peripheral nerves of orbit (D48.7)*

D48.3 Neoplasm of uncertain behavior of retroperitoneum

D48.4 Neoplasm of uncertain behavior of peritoneum

D48.5 Neoplasm of uncertain behavior of skin
Neoplasm of uncertain behavior of anal margin
Neoplasm of uncertain behavior of anal skin
Neoplasm of uncertain behavior of perianal skin
Neoplasm of uncertain behavior of skin of breast
EXCLUDES 1 *neoplasm of uncertain behavior of anus NOS (D37.8)*
neoplasm of uncertain behavior of skin of genital organs (D39.8, D40.7)
neoplasm of uncertain behavior of vermilion border of lip (D37.0)

✓5th **D48.6 Neoplasm of uncertain behavior of breast**
Neoplasm of uncertain behavior of connective tissue of breast
Cystosarcoma phyllodes
EXCLUDES 1 *neoplasm of uncertain behavior of skin of breast (D48.5)*

D48.60 Neoplasm of uncertain behavior of unspecified breast

D48.61 Neoplasm of uncertain behavior of right breast

D48.62 Neoplasm of uncertain behavior of left breast

D48.7 Neoplasm of uncertain behavior of other specified sites
Neoplasm of uncertain behavior of eye
Neoplasm of uncertain behavior of heart
Neoplasm of uncertain behavior of peripheral nerves of orbit
EXCLUDES 1 *neoplasm of uncertain behavior of connective tissue (D48.1)*
neoplasm of uncertain behavior of skin of eyelid (D48.5)

D48.9 Neoplasm of uncertain behavior, unspecified

Neoplasms of uncertain behavior (D49)

✓4th **D49 Neoplasms of unspecified behavior**
NOTE Category D49 classifies by site neoplasms of unspecified morphology and behavior. The term "mass", unless otherwise stated, is not to be regarded as a neoplastic growth.
INCLUDES "growth" NOS
neoplasm NOS
new growth NOS
tumor NOS
EXCLUDES 1 *neoplasms of uncertain behavior (D37-D44, D48)*

D49.0 Neoplasm of unspecified behavior of digestive system
EXCLUDES 1 *neoplasm of unspecified behavior of margin of anus (D49.2)*
neoplasm of unspecified behavior of perianal skin (D49.2)
neoplasm of unspecified behavior of skin of anus (D49.2)

D49.1 Neoplasm of unspecified behavior of respiratory system

D49.2 Neoplasm of unspecified behavior of bone, soft tissue, and skin
EXCLUDES 1 *neoplasm of unspecified behavior of anal canal (D49.0)*
neoplasm of unspecified behavior of anus NOS (D49.0)
neoplasm of unspecified behavior of bone marrow (D49.9)
neoplasm of unspecified behavior of cartilage of larynx (D49.1)
neoplasm of unspecified behavior of cartilage of nose (D49.1)
neoplasm of unspecified behavior of connective tissue of breast (D49.3)
neoplasm of unspecified behavior of skin of genital organs (D49.5)
neoplasm of unspecified behavior of vermilion border of lip (D49.0)

D49.3 Neoplasm of unspecified behavior of breast
EXCLUDES 1 *neoplasm of unspecified behavior of skin of breast (D49.2)*

D49.4 Neoplasm of unspecified behavior of bladder

D49.5 Neoplasm of unspecified behavior of other genitourinary organs

D49.6 Neoplasm of unspecified behavior of brain
EXCLUDES 1 *neoplasm of unspecified behavior of cerebral meninges (D49.7)*
neoplasm of unspecified behavior of cranial nerves (D49.7)

D49.7 Neoplasm of unspecified behavior of endocrine glands and other parts of nervous system
EXCLUDES 1 *neoplasm of unspecified behavior of peripheral, sympathetic, and parasympathetic nerves and ganglia (D49.2)*

✓5th **D49.8 Neoplasm of unspecified behavior of other specified sites**

EXCLUDES 1 *neoplasm of unspecified behavior of eyelid (skin) (D49.2)*
neoplasm of unspecified behavior of eyelid cartilage (D49.2)
neoplasm of unspecified behavior of great vessels (D49.2)
neoplasm of unspecified behavior of optic nerve (D49.7)

D49.81 Neoplasm of unspecified behavior of retina and choroid

Dark area on retina
Retinal freckle

D49.89 Neoplasm of unspecified behavior of other specified sites

D49.9 Neoplasm of unspecified behavior of unspecified site

Chapter 3. Diseases of the Blood and Blood-forming Organs and Certain Disorders Involving the Immune Mechanism (D50-D89)

EXCLUDES 2 *autoimmune disease (systemic) NOS (M35.9)*
certain conditions originating in the perinatal period (P00-P96)
complications of pregnancy, childbirth and the puerperium (O00-O9A)
congenital malformations, deformations and chromosomal abnormalities (Q00-Q99)
endocrine, nutritional and metabolic diseases (E00-E88)
human immunodeficiency virus [HIV] disease (B20)
injury, poisoning and certain other consequences of external causes (S00-T88)
neoplasms (C00-D49)
symptoms, signs and abnormal clinical and laboratory findings, not elsewhere classified (R00-R94)

This chapter contains the following blocks:

D50-D53	Nutritional anemias
D55-D59	Hemolytic anemias
D60-D64	Aplastic and other anemias and other bone marrow failure syndromes
D65-D69	Coagulation defects, purpura and other hemorrhagic conditions
D70-D77	Other disorders of blood and blood-forming organs
D78	Intraoperative and postprocedural complications of the spleen
D80-D89	Certain disorders involving the immune mechanism

Nutritional anemias (D50-D53)

✓4th **D50 Iron deficiency anemia**
INCLUDES asiderotic anemia
hypochromic anemia

D50.0 Iron deficiency anemia secondary to blood loss (chronic)
Posthemorrhagic anemia (chronic)
EXCLUDES 1 *acute posthemorrhagic anemia (D62)*
congenital anemia from fetal blood loss (P61.3)

D50.1 Sideropenic dysphagia
Kelly-Paterson syndrome
Plummer-Vinson syndrome

D50.8 Other iron deficiency anemias
Iron deficiency anemia due to inadequate dietary iron intake

D50.9 Iron deficiency anemia, unspecified

✓4th **D51 Vitamin B12 deficiency anemia**
EXCLUDES 1 *vitamin B12 deficiency (E53.8)*

D51.0 Vitamin B12 deficiency anemia due to intrinsic factor deficiency
Addison anemia
Biermer anemia
Pernicious (congenital) anemia
Congenital intrinsic factor deficiency

D51.1 Vitamin B12 deficiency anemia due to selective vitamin B12 malabsorption with proteinuria
Imerslund (Gräsbeck) syndrome
Megaloblastic hereditary anemia

D51.2 Transcobalamin II deficiency

D51.3 Other dietary vitamin B12 deficiency anemia
Vegan anemia

D51.8 Other vitamin B12 deficiency anemias

D51.9 Vitamin B12 deficiency anemia, unspecified

✓4th **D52 Folate deficiency anemia**
EXCLUDES 1 *folate deficiency without anemia (E53.8)*

D52.0 Dietary folate deficiency anemia
Nutritional megaloblastic anemia

D52.1 Drug-induced folate deficiency anemia
Use additional code for adverse effect, if applicable, to identify drug (T36-T50 with fifth or sixth character 5)

D52.8 Other folate deficiency anemias

D52.9 Folate deficiency anemia, unspecified
Folic acid deficiency anemia NOS

✓4th **D53 Other nutritional anemias**
INCLUDES megaloblastic anemia unresponsive to vitamin B12 or folate therapy

D53.0 Protein deficiency anemia
Amino-acid deficiency anemia
Orotaciduric anemia
EXCLUDES 1 *Lesch-Nyhan syndrome (E79.1)*

D53.1 Other megaloblastic anemias, not elsewhere classified
Megaloblastic anemia NOS
EXCLUDES 1 *Di Guglielmo's disease (C94.0)*

D53.2 Scorbutic anemia
EXCLUDES 1 *scurvy (E54)*

D53.8 Other specified nutritional anemias
Anemia associated with deficiency of copper
Anemia associated with deficiency of molybdenum
Anemia associated with deficiency of zinc
EXCLUDES 1 *nutritional deficiencies without anemia, such as:*
copper deficiency NOS (E61.0)
molybdenum deficiency NOS (E61.5)
zinc deficiency NOS (E60)

D53.9 Nutritional anemia, unspecified
Simple chronic anemia
EXCLUDES 1 *anemia NOS (D64.9)*

Hemolytic anemias (D55-D59)

✓4th **D55 Anemia due to enzyme disorders**
EXCLUDES 1 *drug-induced enzyme deficiency anemia (D59.2)*

D55.0 Anemia due to glucose-6-phosphate dehydrogenase [G6PD] deficiency
Favism
G6PD deficiency anemia

D55.1 Anemia due to other disorders of glutathione metabolism
Anemia (due to) enzyme deficiencies, except G6PD, related to the hexose monophosphate [HMP] shunt pathway
Anemia (due to) hemolytic nonspherocytic (hereditary), type I

D55.2 Anemia due to disorders of glycolytic enzymes
Hemolytic nonspherocytic (hereditary) anemia, type II
Hexokinase deficiency anemia
Pyruvate kinase [PK] deficiency anemia
Triose-phosphate isomerase deficiency anemia
EXCLUDES 1 *disorders of glycolysis not associated with anemia (E74.8)*

D55.3 Anemia due to disorders of nucleotide metabolism

D55.8 Other anemias due to enzyme disorders

D55.9 Anemia due to enzyme disorder, unspecified

✓4th **D56 Thalassemia**
EXCLUDES 1 *sickle-cell thalassemia (D57.4-)*

D56.0 Alpha thalassemia
Alpha thalassemia major
Hemoglobin H Constant Spring
Hemoglobin H disease
Hydrops fetalis due to alpha thalassemia
Severe alpha thalassemia
Triple gene defect alpha thalassemia
Use additional code, if applicable, for hydrops fetalis due to alpha thalassemia (P56.99)
EXCLUDES 1 *alpha thalassemia trait or minor (D56.3)*
asymptomatic alpha thalassemia (D56.3)
hydrops fetalis due to isoimmunization (P56.0)
hydrops fetalis not due to immune hemolysis (P83.2)

D56.1 Beta thalassemia
Beta thalassemia major
Cooley's anemia
Homozygous beta thalassemia
Severe beta thalassemia
Thalassemia intermedia
Thalassemia major
EXCLUDES 1 *beta thalassemia minor (D56.3)*
beta thalassemia trait (D56.3)
delta-beta thalassemia (D56.2)
hemoglobin E-beta thalassemia (D56.5)
sickle-cell beta thalassemia (D57.4-)

D56.2 Delta-beta thalassemia
Homozygous delta-beta thalassemia
EXCLUDES 1 *delta-beta thalassemia minor (D56.3)*
delta-beta thalassemia trait (D56.3)

DRAFT

D56.3 Thalassemia minor
Alpha thalassemia minor
Alpha thalassemia silent carrier
Alpha thalassemia trait
Beta thalassemia minor
Beta thalassemia trait
Delta-beta thalassemia minor
Delta-beta thalassemia trait
Thalassemia trait NOS
EXCLUDES 1 *alpha thalassemia (D56.0)*
beta thalassemia (D56.1)
delta-beta thalassemia (D56.2)
hemoglobin E-beta thalassemia (D56.5)
sickle-cell trait (D57.3)

D56.4 Hereditary persistence of fetal hemoglobin [HPFH]

D56.5 Hemoglobin E-beta thalassemia
EXCLUDES 1 *beta thalassemia (D56.1)*
beta thalassemia minor (D56.3)
beta thalassemia trait (D56.3)
delta-beta thalassemia (D56.2)
delta-beta thalassemia trait (D56.3)
hemoglobin E disease (D58.2)
other hemoglobinopathies (D58.2)
sickle-cell beta thalassemia (D57.4-)

D56.8 Other thalassemias
Dominant thalassemia
Hemoglobin C thalassemia
Mixed thalassemia
Thalassemia with other hemoglobinopathy
EXCLUDES 1 *hemoglobin C disease (D58.2)*
hemoglobin E disease (D58.2)
other hemoglobinopathies (D58.2)
sickle-cell anemia (D57.-)
sickle-cell thalassemia (D57.4)

D56.9 Thalassemia, unspecified
Mediterranean anemia (with other hemoglobinopathy)

✓4th **D57 Sickle-cell disorders**
Use additional code for any associated fever (R50.81)
EXCLUDES 1 *other hemoglobinopathies (D58.-)*

✓5th **D57.0 Hb-SS disease with crisis**
Sickle-cell disease NOS with crisis
Hb-SS disease with vasoocclusive pain
D57.00 Hb-SS disease with crisis, unspecified
D57.01 Hb-SS disease with acute chest syndrome
D57.02 Hb-SS disease with splenic sequestration

D57.1 Sickle-cell disease without crisis
Hb-SS disease without crisis
Sickle-cell anemia NOS
Sickle-cell disease NOS
Sickle-cell disorder NOS

✓5th **D57.2 Sickle-cell/Hb-C disease**
Hb-SC disease
Hb-S/Hb-C disease
D57.20 Sickle-cell/Hb-C disease without crisis
✓6th **D57.21 Sickle-cell/Hb-C disease with crisis**
D57.211 Sickle-cell/Hb-C disease with acute chest syndrome
D57.212 Sickle-cell/Hb-C disease with splenic sequestration
D57.219 Sickle-cell/Hb-C disease with crisis, unspecified
Sickle-cell/Hb-C disease with crisis NOS

D57.3 Sickle-cell trait
Hb-S trait
Heterozygous hemoglobin S

✓5th **D57.4 Sickle-cell thalassemia**
Sickle-cell beta thalassemia
Thalassemia Hb-S disease
D57.40 Sickle-cell thalassemia without crisis
Microdrepanocytosis
Sickle-cell thalassemia NOS
✓6th **D57.41 Sickle-cell thalassemia with crisis**
Sickle-cell thalassemia with vasoocclusive pain
D57.411 Sickle-cell thalassemia with acute chest syndrome
D57.412 Sickle-cell thalassemia with splenic sequestration
D57.419 Sickle-cell thalassemia with crisis, unspecified
Sickle-cell thalassemia with crisis NOS

✓5th **D57.8 Other sickle-cell disorders**
Hb-SD disease
Hb-SE disease
D57.80 Other sickle-cell disorders without crisis
✓6th **D57.81 Other sickle-cell disorders with crisis**
D57.811 Other sickle-cell disorders with acute chest syndrome
D57.812 Other sickle-cell disorders with splenic sequestration
D57.819 Other sickle-cell disorders with crisis, unspecified
Other sickle-cell disorders with crisis NOS

✓4th **D58 Other hereditary hemolytic anemias**
EXCLUDES 1 *hemolytic anemia of the newborn (P55.-)*

D58.0 Hereditary spherocytosis
Acholuric (familial) jaundice
Congenital (spherocytic) hemolytic icterus
Minkowski-Chauffard syndrome

D58.1 Hereditary elliptocytosis
Elliptocytosis (congenital)
Ovalocytosis (congenital) (hereditary)

D58.2 Other hemoglobinopathies
Abnormal hemoglobin NOS
Congenital Heinz body anemia
Hb-C disease
Hb-D disease
Hb-E disease
Hemoglobinopathy NOS
Unstable hemoglobin hemolytic disease
EXCLUDES 1 *familial polycythemia (D75.0)*
Hb-M disease (D74.0)
hemoglobin E-beta thalassemia (D56.5)
hereditary persistence of fetal hemoglobin [HPFH] (D56.4)
high-altitude polycythemia (D75.1)
methemoglobinemia (D74.-)
other hemoglobinopathies with thalassemia (D56.8)

D58.8 Other specified hereditary hemolytic anemias
Stomatocytosis

D58.9 Hereditary hemolytic anemia, unspecified

✓4th **D59 Acquired hemolytic anemia**

D59.0 Drug-induced autoimmune hemolytic anemia
Use additional code for adverse effect, if applicable, to identify drug (T36-T50 with fifth or sixth character 5)

D59.1 Other autoimmune hemolytic anemias
Autoimmune hemolytic disease (cold type) (warm type)
Chronic cold hemagglutinin disease
Cold agglutinin disease
Cold agglutinin hemoglobinuria
Cold type (secondary) (symptomatic) hemolytic anemia
Warm type (secondary) (symptomatic) hemolytic anemia
EXCLUDES 1 *Evans syndrome (D69.41)*
hemolytic disease of newborn (P55.-)
paroxysmal cold hemoglobinuria (D59.6)

D59.2 Drug-induced nonautoimmune hemolytic anemia
Drug-induced enzyme deficiency anemia
Use additional code for adverse effect, if applicable, to identify drug (T36-T50 with fifth or sixth character 5)

D59.3 Hemolytic-uremic syndrome
Use additional code to identify associated:
E. coli infection (B96.2-)
Pneumococcal pneumonia (J13)
Shigella dysenteriae (A03.9)

D59.4 Other nonautoimmune hemolytic anemias
Mechanical hemolytic anemia
Microangiopathic hemolytic anemia
Toxic hemolytic anemia

D59.5 Paroxysmal nocturnal hemoglobinuria [Marchiafava-Micheli]
EXCLUDES 1 *hemoglobinuria NOS (R82.3)*

D59.6 Hemoglobinuria due to hemolysis from other external causes
Hemoglobinuria from exertion
March hemoglobinuria
Paroxysmal cold hemoglobinuria
Use additional code (Chapter 20) to identify external cause
EXCLUDES 1 *hemoglobinuria NOS (R82.3)*

D59.8 Other acquired hemolytic anemias

D59.9 Acquired hemolytic anemia, unspecified
Idiopathic hemolytic anemia, chronic

Aplastic and other anemias and other bone marrow failure syndromes (D60-D64)

✓4th D60 Acquired pure red cell aplasia [erythroblastopenia]
INCLUDES red cell aplasia (acquired) (adult) (with thymoma)
EXCLUDES 1 *congenital red cell aplasia (D61.01)*

D60.0 Chronic acquired pure red cell aplasia

D60.1 Transient acquired pure red cell aplasia

D60.8 Other acquired pure red cell aplasias

D60.9 Acquired pure red cell aplasia, unspecified

✓4th D61 Other aplastic anemias and other bone marrow failure syndromes
EXCLUDES 1 *neutropenia (D70.-)*

✓5th D61.0 Constitutional aplastic anemia

D61.01 Constitutional (pure) red blood cell aplasia
Blackfan-Diamond syndrome
Congenital (pure) red cell aplasia
Familial hypoplastic anemia
Primary (pure) red cell aplasia
Red cell (pure) aplasia of infants
EXCLUDES 1 *acquired red cell aplasia (D60.9)*

D61.09 Other constitutional aplastic anemia
Fanconi's anemia
Pancytopenia with malformations

D61.1 Drug-induced aplastic anemia
Use additional code for adverse effect, if applicable, to identify drug (T36-T50 with fifth or sixth character 5)

D61.2 Aplastic anemia due to other external agents
Code first, if applicable, toxic effects of substances chiefly nonmedicinal as to source (T51-T65)

D61.3 Idiopathic aplastic anemia

✓5th D61.8 Other specified aplastic anemias and other bone marrow failure syndromes

✓6th D61.81 Pancytopenia
EXCLUDES 1 *pancytopenia (due to) (with) aplastic anemia (D61.9)*
pancytopenia (due to) (with) bone marrow infiltration (D61.82)
pancytopenia (due to) (with) congenital (pure) red cell aplasia (D61.01)
pancytopenia (due to) (with) hairy cell leukemia (C91.4-)
pancytopenia (due to) (with) human immunodeficiency virus disease (B20)
pancytopenia (due to) (with) leukoerythroblastic anemia (D61.82)
pancytopenia (due to) (with) myelodysplastic syndromes (D46.-)
pancytopenia (due to) (with) myeloproliferative disease (D47.1)

D61.810 Antineoplastic chemotherapy induced pancytopenia
EXCLUDES 2 *aplastic anemia due to antineoplastic chemotherapy (D61.1)*

D61.811 Other drug-induced pancytopenia
EXCLUDES 2 *aplastic anemia due to drugs (D61.1)*

D61.818 Other pancytopenia

D61.82 Myelophthisis
Leukoerythroblastic anemia
Myelophthisic anemia
Panmyelophthisis
Code also the underlying disorder, such as:
malignant neoplasm of breast (C50.-)
tuberculosis (A15.-)
EXCLUDES 1 *idiopathic myelofibrosis (D47.1)*
myelofibrosis NOS (D75.81)
myelofibrosis with myeloid metaplasia (D47.4)
primary myelofibrosis (D47.1)
secondary myelofibrosis (D75.81)

D61.89 Other specified aplastic anemias and other bone marrow failure syndromes

D61.9 Aplastic anemia, unspecified
Hypoplastic anemia NOS
Medullary hypoplasia

D62 Acute posthemorrhagic anemia
EXCLUDES 1 *anemia due to chronic blood loss (D50.0)*
blood loss anemia NOS (D50.0)
congenital anemia from fetal blood loss (P61.3)

✓4th D63 Anemia in chronic diseases classified elsewhere

D63.0 Anemia in neoplastic disease
Code first neoplasm (C00-D49)
EXCLUDES 1 *anemia due to antineoplastic chemotherapy (D64.81)*
aplastic anemia due to antineoplastic chemotherapy (D61.1)

D63.1 Anemia in chronic kidney disease
Erythropoietin resistant anemia (EPO resistant anemia)
Code first underlying chronic kidney disease (CKD) (N18.-)

D63.8 Anemia in other chronic diseases classified elsewhere
Code first underlying disease, such as:
diphyllobothriasis (B70.0)
hookworm disease (B76.0-B76.9)
hypothyroidism (E00.0-E03.9)
malaria (B50.0-B54)
symptomatic late syphilis (A52.79)
tuberculosis (A18.89)

✓4th D64 Other anemias
EXCLUDES 1 *refractory anemia (D46.-)*
refractory anemia with excess blasts in transformation [RAEB T] (C92.0-)

D64.0 Hereditary sideroblastic anemia
Sex-linked hypochromic sideroblastic anemia

D64.1 Secondary sideroblastic anemia due to disease
Code first underlying disease

D64.2 Secondary sideroblastic anemia due to drugs and toxins
Code first poisoning due to drug or toxin, if applicable (T36-T65 with fifth or sixth character 1-4 or 6)
Use additional code for adverse effect, if applicable, to identify drug (T36-T50 with fifth or sixth character 5)

D64.3 Other sideroblastic anemias
Sideroblastic anemia NOS
Pyridoxine-responsive sideroblastic anemia NEC

D64.4 Congenital dyserythropoietic anemia
Dyshematopoietic anemia (congenital)
EXCLUDES 1 *Blackfan-Diamond syndrome (D61.01)*
Di Guglielmo's disease (C94.0)

✓5th D64.8 Other specified anemias

D64.81 Anemia due to antineoplastic chemotherapy
Antineoplastic chemotherapy induced anemia
EXCLUDES 1 *anemia in neoplastic disease (D63.0)*
aplastic anemia due to antineoplastic chemotherapy (D61.1)

D64.89 Other specified anemias
Infantile pseudoleukemia

D64.9 Anemia, unspecified

Coagulation defects, purpura and other hemorrhagic conditions (D65-D69)

D65 Disseminated intravascular coagulation [defibrination syndrome]
Afibrinogenemia, acquired
Consumption coagulopathy
Diffuse or disseminated intravascular coagulation [DIC]
Fibrinolytic hemorrhage, acquired
Fibrinolytic purpura
Purpura fulminans
EXCLUDES 1 *disseminated intravascular coagulation (complicating):*
abortion or ectopic or molar pregnancy (O00-O07, O08.1)
in newborn (P60)
pregnancy, childbirth and the puerperium (O45.0, O46.0, O67.0, O72.3)

D66 Hereditary factor VIII deficiency
Classical hemophilia
Deficiency factor VIII (with functional defect)
Hemophilia NOS
Hemophilia A
EXCLUDES 1 *factor VIII deficiency with vascular defect (D68.0)*

D67 Hereditary factor IX deficiency
Christmas disease
Factor IX deficiency (with functional defect)
Hemophilia B
Plasma thromboplastin component [PTC] deficiency

✓4th **D68 Other coagulation defects**
EXCLUDES 1 *abnormal coagulation profile (R79.1)*
coagulation defects complicating:
abortion or ectopic or molar pregnancy (O00-O07, O08.1)
pregnancy, childbirth and the puerperium (O45.0, O46.0, O67.0, O72.3)

D68.0 Von Willebrand's disease
Angiohemophilia
Factor VIII deficiency with vascular defect
Vascular hemophilia
EXCLUDES 1 *capillary fragility (hereditary) (D69.8)*
factor VIII deficiency NOS (D66)
factor VIII deficiency with functional defect (D66)

D68.1 Hereditary factor XI deficiency
Hemophilia C
Plasma thromboplastin antecedent [PTA] deficiency
Rosenthal's disease

D68.2 Hereditary deficiency of other clotting factors
AC globulin deficiency
Congenital afibrinogenemia
Deficiency of factor I [fibrinogen]
Deficiency of factor II [prothrombin]
Deficiency of factor V [labile]
Deficiency of factor VII [stable]
Deficiency of factor X [Stuart-Prower]
Deficiency of factor XII [Hageman]
Deficiency of factor XIII [fibrin stabilizing]
Dysfibrinogenemia (congenital)
Hypoproconvertinemia
Owren's disease
Proaccelerin deficiency

✓5th **D68.3 Hemorrhagic disorder due to circulating anticoagulants**

✓6th **D68.31 Hemorrhagic disorder due to intrinsic circulating anticoagulants, antibodies, or inhibitors**

D68.311 Acquired hemophilia
Autoimmune hemophilia
Autoimmune inhibitors to clotting factors
Secondary hemophilia

D68.312 Antiphospholipid antibody with hemorrhagic disorder
Lupus anticoagulant (LAC) with hemorrhagic disorder
Systemic lupus erythematosus [SLE] inhibitor with hemorrhagic disorder
EXCLUDES 1 *antiphospholipid antibody, finding without diagnosis (R76.0)*
antiphospholipid antibody syndrome (D68.61)
antiphospholipid antibody with hypercoagulable state (D68.61)
lupus anticoagulant (LAC) finding without diagnosis (R76.0)
lupus anticoagulant (LAC) with hypercoagulable state (D68.62)
systemic lupus erythematosus [SLE] inhibitor finding without diagnosis (R76.0)
systemic lupus erythematosus [SLE] inhibitor with hypercoagulable state (D68.62)

D68.318 Other hemorrhagic disorder due to intrinsic circulating anticoagulants, antibodies, or inhibitors
Antithromboplastinemia
Antithromboplastinogenemia
Hemorrhagic disorder due to intrinsic increase in antithrombin
Hemorrhagic disorder due to intrinsic increase in anti-VIIIa
Hemorrhagic disorder due to intrinsic increase in anti-IXa
Hemorrhagic disorder due to intrinsic increase in anti-XIa

D68.32 Hemorrhagic disorder due to extrinsic circulating anticoagulants
Drug-induced hemorrhagic disorder
Hemorrhagic disorder due to increase in anti-IIa
Hemorrhagic disorder due to increase in anti-Xa
Hyperheparinemia
Use additional code for adverse effect, if applicable, to identify drug (T45.515, T45.525)

D68.4 Acquired coagulation factor deficiency
Deficiency of coagulation factor due to liver disease
Deficiency of coagulation factor due to vitamin K deficiency
EXCLUDES 1 *vitamin K deficiency of newborn (P53)*

✓5th **D68.5 Primary thrombophilia**
Primary hypercoagulable states
EXCLUDES 1 *antiphospholipid syndrome (D68.61)*
lupus anticoagulant (D68.62)
secondary activated protein C resistance (D68.69)
secondary antiphospholipid antibody syndrome (D68.69)
secondary lupus anticoagulant with hypercoagulable state (D68.69)
secondary systemic lupus erythematosus [SLE] inhibitor with hypercoagulable state (D68.69)
systemic lupus erythematosus [SLE] inhibitor finding without diagnosis (R76.0)
systemic lupus erythematosus [SLE] inhibitor with hemorrhagic disorder (D68.312)
thrombotic thrombocytopenic purpura (M31.1)

D68.51 Activated protein C resistance
Factor V Leiden mutation

D68.52 Prothrombin gene mutation

D68.59 Other primary thrombophilia
Antithrombin III deficiency
Hypercoagulable state NOS
Primary hypercoagulable state NEC
Primary thrombophilia NEC
Protein C deficiency
Protein S deficiency
Thrombophilia NOS

√5th **D68.6 Other thrombophilia**
Other hypercoagulable states
EXCLUDES 1 *diffuse or disseminated intravascular coagulation [DIC] (D65)*
heparin induced thrombocytopenia (HIT) (D75.82)
hyperhomocysteinemia (E72.11)

D68.61 Antiphospholipid syndrome
Anticardiolipin syndrome
Antiphospholipid antibody syndrome
EXCLUDES 1 *antiphospholipid antibody, finding without diagnosis (R76.0)*
antiphospholipid antibody with hemorrhagic disorder (D68.312)
lupus anticoagulant syndrome (D68.62)

D68.62 Lupus anticoagulant syndrome
Lupus anticoagulant
Presence of systemic lupus erythematosus [SLE] inhibitor
EXCLUDES 1 *anticardiolipin syndrome (D68.61)*
antiphospholipid syndrome (D68.61)
lupus anticoagulant (LAC) finding without diagnosis (R79.0)
lupus anticoagulant (LAC) with hemorrhagic disorder (D68.312)

D68.69 Other thrombophilia
Hypercoagulable states NEC
Secondary hypercoagulable state NOS

D68.8 Other specified coagulation defects
EXCLUDES 1 *hemorrhagic disease of newborn (P53)*

D68.9 Coagulation defect, unspecified

√4th **D69 Purpura and other hemorrhagic conditions**
EXCLUDES 1 *benign hypergammaglobulinemic purpura (D89.0)*
cryoglobulinemic purpura (D89.1)
essential (hemorrhagic) thrombocythemia (D47.3)
hemorrhagic thrombocythemia (D47.3)
purpura fulminans (D65)
thrombotic thrombocytopenic purpura (M31.1)
Waldenström hypergammaglobulinemic purpura (D89.0)

D69.0 Allergic purpura
Allergic vasculitis
Nonthrombocytopenic hemorrhagic purpura
Nonthrombocytopenic idiopathic purpura
Purpura anaphylactoid
Purpura Henoch(-Schönlein)
Purpura rheumatica
Vascular purpura
EXCLUDES 1 *thrombocytopenic hemorrhagic purpura (D69.3)*

D69.1 Qualitative platelet defects
Bernard-Soulier [giant platelet] syndrome
Glanzmann's disease
Grey platelet syndrome
Thromboasthenia (hemorrhagic) (hereditary)
Thrombocytopathy
EXCLUDES 1 *von Willebrand's disease (D68.0)*

D69.2 Other nonthrombocytopenic purpura
Purpura NOS
Purpura simplex
Senile purpura

D69.3 Immune thrombocytopenic purpura
Hemorrhagic (thrombocytopenic) purpura
Idiopathic thrombocytopenic purpura
Tidal platelet dysgenesis

√5th **D69.4 Other primary thrombocytopenia**
EXCLUDES 1 *transient neonatal thrombocytopenia (P61.0)*
Wiskott-Aldrich syndrome (D82.0)

D69.41 Evans syndrome

D69.42 Congenital and hereditary thrombocytopenia purpura
Congenital thrombocytopenia
Hereditary thrombocytopenia
Code first congenital or hereditary disorder, such as:
thrombocytopenia with absent radius (TAR syndrome) (Q87.2)

D69.49 Other primary thrombocytopenia
Megakaryocytic hypoplasia
Primary thrombocytopenia NOS

√5th **D69.5 Secondary thrombocytopenia**
EXCLUDES 1 *heparin induced thrombocytopenia (HIT) (D75.82)*
transient thrombocytopenia of newborn (P61.0)

D69.51 Posttransfusion purpura
Posttransfusion purpura from whole blood (fresh) or blood products
PTP

D69.59 Other secondary thrombocytopenia

D69.6 Thrombocytopenia, unspecified

D69.8 Other specified hemorrhagic conditions
Capillary fragility (hereditary)
Vascular pseudohemophilia

D69.9 Hemorrhagic condition, unspecified

Other disorders of blood and blood-forming organs (D70-D77)

√4th **D70 Neutropenia**
INCLUDES agranulocytosis
decreased absolute neurophile count (ANC)
Use additional code for any associated:
fever (R50.81)
mucositis (J34.81, K12.3-, K92.81, N76.81)
EXCLUDES 1 *neutropenic splenomegaly (D73.81)*
transient neonatal neutropenia (P61.5)

D70.0 Congenital agranulocytosis
Congenital neutropenia
Infantile genetic agranulocytosis
Kostmann's disease

D70.1 Agranulocytosis secondary to cancer chemotherapy
Use additional code for adverse effect, if applicable, to identify drug (T45.1X5)
Code also underlying neoplasm

D70.2 Other drug-induced agranulocytosis
Use additional code for adverse effect, if applicable, to identify drug (T36-T50 with fifth or sixth character 5)

D70.3 Neutropenia due to infection

D70.4 Cyclic neutropenia
Cyclic hematopoiesis
Periodic neutropenia

D70.8 Other neutropenia

D70.9 Neutropenia, unspecified

D71 Functional disorders of polymorphonuclear neutrophils
Cell membrane receptor complex [CR3] defect
Chronic (childhood) granulomatous disease
Congenital dysphagocytosis
Progressive septic granulomatosis

√4th **D72 Other disorders of white blood cells**
EXCLUDES 1 *basophilia (D72.824)*
immunity disorders (D80-D89)
neutropenia (D70)
preleukemia (syndrome) (D46.9)

D72.0 Genetic anomalies of leukocytes
Alder (granulation) (granulocyte) anomaly
Alder syndrome
Hereditary leukocytic hypersegmentation
Hereditary leukocytic hyposegmentation
Hereditary leukomelanopathy
May-Hegglin (granulation) (granulocyte) anomaly
May-Hegglin syndrome
Pelger-Huët (granulation) (granulocyte) anomaly
Pelger-Huët syndrome
EXCLUDES 1 *Chédiak (-Steinbrinck)-Higashi syndrome (E70.330)*

D72.1 Eosinophilia
Allergic eosinophilia
Hereditary eosinophilia
EXCLUDES 1 *Löffler's syndrome (J82)*
pulmonary eosinophilia (J82)

√5th **D72.8 Other specified disorders of white blood cells**
EXCLUDES 1 *leukemia (C91-C95)*

√6th **D72.81 Decreased white blood cell count**
EXCLUDES 1 *neutropenia (D70.-)*

D72.810 Lymphocytopenia
Decreased lymphocytes

D72.818 Other decreased white blood cell count
Basophilic leukopenia
Eosinophilic leukopenia
Monocytopenia
Other decreased leukocytes
Plasmacytopenia

D72.819 Decreased white blood cell count, unspecified
Decreased leukocytes, unspecified
Leukocytopenia, unspecified
Leukopenia
EXCLUDES 1 *malignant leukopenia (D70.9)*

✓6th **D72.82 Elevated white blood cell count**
EXCLUDES 1 *eosinophilia (D72.1)*

D72.820 Lymphocytosis (symptomatic)
Elevated lymphocytes

D72.821 Monocytosis (symptomatic)
EXCLUDES 1 *infectious mononucleosis (B27.-)*

D72.822 Plasmacytosis

D72.823 Leukemoid reaction
Basophilic leukemoid reaction
Leukemoid reaction NOS
Lymphocytic leukemoid reaction
Monocytic leukemoid reaction
Myelocytic leukemoid reaction
Neutrophilic leukemoid reaction

D72.824 Basophilia

D72.825 Bandemia
Bandemia without diagnosis of specific infection
EXCLUDES 1 *confirmed infection—code to infection*
leukemia (C91.-, C92.-, C93.-, C94.-, C95.-)

D72.828 Other elevated white blood cell count

D72.829 Elevated white blood cell count, unspecified
Elevated leukocytes, unspecified
Leukocytosis, unspecified

D72.89 Other specified disorders of white blood cells
Abnormality of white blood cells NEC

D72.9 Disorder of white blood cells, unspecified
Abnormal leukocyte differential NOS

✓4th **D73 Diseases of spleen**

D73.0 Hyposplenism
Atrophy of spleen
EXCLUDES 1 *asplenia (congenital) (Q89.01)*
postsurgical absence of spleen (Z90.81)

D73.1 Hypersplenism
EXCLUDES 1 *neutropenic splenomegaly (D73.81)*
primary splenic neutropenia (D73.81)
splenitis, splenomegaly in late syphilis (A52.79)
splenitis, splenomegaly in tuberculosis (A18.85)
splenomegaly NOS (R16.1)
splenomegaly congenital (Q89.0)

D73.2 Chronic congestive splenomegaly

D73.3 Abscess of spleen

D73.4 Cyst of spleen

D73.5 Infarction of spleen
Splenic rupture, nontraumatic
Torsion of spleen
EXCLUDES 1 *rupture of spleen due to Plasmodium vivax malaria (B51.0)*
traumatic rupture of spleen (S36.03-)

✓5th **D73.8 Other diseases of spleen**

D73.81 Neutropenic splenomegaly
Werner-Schultz disease

D73.89 Other diseases of spleen
Fibrosis of spleen NOS
Perisplenitis
Splenitis NOS

D73.9 Disease of spleen, unspecified

✓4th **D74 Methemoglobinemia**

D74.0 Congenital methemoglobinemia
Congenital NADH-methemoglobin reductase deficiency
Hemoglobin-M [Hb-M] disease
Methemoglobinemia, hereditary

D74.8 Other methemoglobinemias
Acquired methemoglobinemia (with sulfhemoglobinemia)
Toxic methemoglobinemia

D74.9 Methemoglobinemia, unspecified

✓4th **D75 Other and unspecified diseases of blood and blood-forming organs**
EXCLUDES 2 *acute lymphadenitis (L04.-)*
chronic lymphadenitis (I88.1)
enlarged lymph nodes (R59.-)
hypergammaglobulinemia NOS (D89.2)
lymphadenitis NOS (I88.9)
mesenteric lymphadenitis (acute) (chronic) (I88.0)

D75.0 Familial erythrocytosis
Benign polycythemia
Familial polycythemia
EXCLUDES 1 *hereditary ovalocytosis (D58.1)*

D75.1 Secondary polycythemia
Acquired polycythemia
Emotional polycythemia
Erythrocytosis NOS
Hypoxemic polycythemia
Nephrogenous polycythemia
Polycythemia due to erythropoietin
Polycythemia due to fall in plasma volume
Polycythemia due to high altitude
Polycythemia due to stress
Polycythemia NOS
Relative polycythemia
EXCLUDES 1 *polycythemia neonatorum (P61.1)*
polycythemia vera (D45)

✓5th **D75.8 Other specified diseases of blood and blood-forming organs**

D75.81 Myelofibrosis
Myelofibrosis NOS
Secondary myelofibrosis NOS
Code first the underlying disorder, such as:
malignant neoplasm of breast (C50.-)
Use additional code, if applicable, for associated therapy-related myelodysplastic syndrome (D46.-)
Use additional code for adverse effect, if applicable, to identify drug (T45.1X5)
EXCLUDES 1 *acute myelofibrosis (C94.4-)*
idiopathic myelofibrosis (D47.1)
leukoerythroblastic anemia (D61.82)
myelofibrosis with myeloid metaplasia (D47.4)
myelophthisic anemia (D61.82)
myelophthisis (D61.82)
primary myelofibrosis (D47.1)

D75.82 Heparin induced thrombocytopenia (HIT)

D75.89 Other specified diseases of blood and blood-forming organs

D75.9 Disease of blood and blood-forming organs, unspecified

✓4th **D76 Other specified diseases with participation of lymphoreticular and reticulohistiocytic tissue**
EXCLUDES 1 *(Abt-) Letterer-Siwe disease (C96.0)*
eosinophilic granuloma (C96.6)
Hand-Schüller-Christian disease (C96.5)
histiocytic sarcoma (C96.A)
histiocytosis X, multifocal (C96.5)
histiocytosis X, unifocal (C96.6)
malignant histiocytosis (C96.A)
Langerhans-cell histiocytosis, multifocal (C96.5)
Langerhans-cell histiocytosis NOS (C96.6)
Langerhans-cell histiocytosis, unifocal (C96.6)
leukemic reticuloendotheliosis or reticulosis (C91.4-)
lipomelanotic reticuloendotheliosis or reticulosis (I89.8)

D76.1 Hemophagocytic lymphohistiocytosis
Familial hemophagocytic reticulosis
Histiocytoses of mononuclear phagocytes

D76.2 Hemophagocytic syndrome, infection-associated
Use additional code to identify infectious agent or disease

D76.3 Other histiocytosis syndromes
Reticulohistiocytoma (giant-cell)
Sinus histiocytosis with massive lymphadenopathy
Xanthogranuloma

D77 ***Other disorders of blood and blood-forming organs in diseases classified elsewhere***

Code first underlying disease, such as:
amyloidosis (E85.-)
congenital early syphilis (A50.0)
echinococcosis (B67.0-B67.9)
malaria (B50.0-B54)
schistosomiasis [bilharziasis] (B65.0-B65.9)
vitamin C deficiency (E54)

EXCLUDES 1 *rupture of spleen due to Plasmodium vivax malaria (B51.0)*
splenitis, splenomegaly in:
late syphilis (A52.79)
tuberculosis (A18.85)

Intraoperative and postprocedural complications of the spleen (D78)

✓4th **D78 Intraoperative and postprocedural complications of the spleen**

✓5th **D78.0 Intraoperative hemorrhage and hematoma of the spleen complicating a procedure**

EXCLUDES 1 *intraoperative hemorrhage and hematoma of the spleen due to accidental puncture or laceration during a procedure (D78.1-)*

D78.01 Intraoperative hemorrhage and hematoma of the spleen complicating a procedure on the spleen
D78.02 Intraoperative hemorrhage and hematoma of the spleen complicating other procedure

✓5th **D78.1 Accidental puncture and laceration of the spleen during a procedure**

D78.11 Accidental puncture and laceration of the spleen during a procedure on the spleen
D78.12 Accidental puncture and laceration of the spleen during other procedure

✓5th **D78.2 Postprocedural hemorrhage and hematoma of the spleen following a procedure**

D78.21 Postprocedural hemorrhage and hematoma of the spleen following a procedure on the spleen
D78.22 Postprocedural hemorrhage and hematoma of the spleen following other procedure

✓5th **D78.8 Other intraoperative and postprocedural complications of the spleen**

Use additional code, if applicable, to further specify disorder

D78.81 Other intraoperative complications of the spleen
D78.89 Other postprocedural complications of the spleen

Certain disorders involving the immune mechanism (D80-D89)

INCLUDES defects in the complement system
immunodeficiency disorders, except human immunodeficiency virus [HIV] disease
sarcoidosis

EXCLUDES 1 *autoimmune disease (systemic) NOS (M35.9)*
functional disorders of polymorphonuclear neutrophils (D71)
human immunodeficiency virus [HIV] disease (B20)

✓4th **D80 Immunodeficiency with predominantly antibody defects**

D80.0 Hereditary hypogammaglobulinemia
Autosomal recessive agammaglobulinemia (Swiss type)
X-linked agammaglobulinemia [Bruton] (with growth hormone deficiency)

D80.1 Nonfamilial hypogammaglobulinemia
Agammaglobulinemia with immunoglobulin-bearing B-lymphocytes
Common variable agammaglobulinemia [CVAgamma]
Hypogammaglobulinemia NOS

D80.2 Selective deficiency of immunoglobulin A [IgA]
D80.3 Selective deficiency of immunoglobulin G [IgG] subclasses
D80.4 Selective deficiency of immunoglobulin M [IgM]
D80.5 Immunodeficiency with increased immunoglobulin M [IgM]
D80.6 Antibody deficiency with near-normal immunoglobulins or with hyperimmunoglobulinemia
D80.7 Transient hypogammaglobulinemia of infancy
D80.8 Other immunodeficiencies with predominantly antibody defects
Kappa light chain deficiency
D80.9 Immunodeficiency with predominantly antibody defects, unspecified

✓4th **D81 Combined immunodeficiencies**

EXCLUDES 1 *autosomal recessive agammaglobulinemia (Swiss type) (D80.0)*

D81.0 Severe combined immunodeficiency [SCID] with reticular dysgenesis
D81.1 Severe combined immunodeficiency [SCID] with low T- and B-cell numbers
D81.2 Severe combined immunodeficiency [SCID] with low or normal B-cell numbers
D81.3 Adenosine deaminase [ADA] deficiency
D81.4 Nezelof's syndrome
D81.5 Purine nucleoside phosphorylase [PNP] deficiency
D81.6 Major histocompatibility complex class I deficiency
Bare lymphocyte syndrome
D81.7 Major histocompatibility complex class II deficiency

✓5th **D81.8 Other combined immunodeficiencies**

✓6th **D81.81 Biotin-dependent carboxylase deficiency**
Multiple carboxylase deficiency

EXCLUDES 1 *biotin-dependent carboxylase deficiency due to dietary deficiency of biotin (E53.8)*

D81.810 Biotinidase deficiency
D81.818 Other biotin-dependent carboxylase deficiency
Holocarboxylase synthetase deficiency
Other multiple carboxylase deficiency
D81.819 Biotin-dependent carboxylase deficiency, unspecified
Multiple carboxylase deficiency, unspecified

D81.89 Other combined immunodeficiencies

D81.9 Combined immunodeficiency, unspecified
Severe combined immunodeficiency disorder [SCID] NOS

✓4th **D82 Immunodeficiency associated with other major defects**

EXCLUDES 1 *ataxia telangiectasia [Louis-Bar] (G11.3)*

D82.0 Wiskott-Aldrich syndrome
Immunodeficiency with thrombocytopenia and eczema
D82.1 Di George's syndrome
Pharyngeal pouch syndrome
Thymic alymphoplasia
Thymic aplasia or hypoplasia with immunodeficiency
D82.2 Immunodeficiency with short-limbed stature
D82.3 Immunodeficiency following hereditary defective response to Epstein-Barr virus
X-linked lymphoproliferative disease
D82.4 Hyperimmunoglobulin E [IgE] syndrome
D82.8 Immunodeficiency associated with other specified major defects
D82.9 Immunodeficiency associated with major defect, unspecified

✓4th **D83 Common variable immunodeficiency**

D83.0 Common variable immunodeficiency with predominant abnormalities of B-cell numbers and function
D83.1 Common variable immunodeficiency with predominant immunoregulatory T-cell disorders
D83.2 Common variable immunodeficiency with autoantibodies to B- or T-cells
D83.8 Other common variable immunodeficiencies
D83.9 Common variable immunodeficiency, unspecified

✓4th **D84 Other immunodeficiencies**

D84.0 Lymphocyte function antigen-1 [LFA-1] defect
D84.1 Defects in the complement system
C1 esterase inhibitor [C1-INH] deficiency
D84.8 Other specified immunodeficiencies
D84.9 Immunodeficiency, unspecified

✓4th **D86 Sarcoidosis**

D86.0 Sarcoidosis of lung
D86.1 Sarcoidosis of lymph nodes
D86.2 Sarcoidosis of lung with sarcoidosis of lymph nodes
D86.3 Sarcoidosis of skin

✓5th **D86.8 Sarcoidosis of other sites**

D86.81 Sarcoid meningitis
D86.82 Multiple cranial nerve palsies in sarcoidosis
D86.83 Sarcoid iridocyclitis
D86.84 Sarcoid pyelonephritis
Tubulo-interstitial nephropathy in sarcoidosis

Diseases of the Blood and Blood-forming Organs D77–D86.84

D86.85 Sarcoid myocarditis

D86.86 Sarcoid arthropathy
Polyarthritis in sarcoidosis

D86.87 Sarcoid myositis

D86.89 Sarcoidosis of other sites
Hepatic granuloma
Uveoparotid fever [Heerfordt]

D86.9 Sarcoidosis, unspecified

✓4th **D89 Other disorders involving the immune mechanism, not elsewhere classified**

EXCLUDES 1 *hyperglobulinemia NOS (R77.1)*
monoclonal gammopathy (of undetermined significance) (D47.2)

EXCLUDES 2 *transplant failure and rejection (T86.-)*

D89.0 Polyclonal hypergammaglobulinemia
Benign hypergammaglobulinemic purpura
Polyclonal gammopathy NOS

D89.1 Cryoglobulinemia
Cryoglobulinemic purpura
Cryoglobulinemic vasculitis
Essential cryoglobulinemia
Idiopathic cryoglobulinemia
Mixed cryoglobulinemia
Primary cryoglobulinemia
Secondary cryoglobulinemia

D89.2 Hypergammaglobulinemia, unspecified

D89.3 Immune reconstitution syndrome
Immune reconstitution inflammatory syndrome [IRIS]
Use additional code for adverse effect, if applicable, to identify drug (T36-T50 with fifth or sixth character 5)

✓5th **D89.8 Other specified disorders involving the immune mechanism, not elsewhere classified**

✓6th **D89.81 Graft-versus-host disease**
Code first underlying cause, such as:
complications of transplanted organs and tissue (T86.-)
complications of blood transfusion (T80.89)
Use additional code to identify associated manifestations, such as:
desquamative dermatitis (L30.8)
diarrhea (R19.7)
elevated bilirubin (R17)
hair loss (L65.9)

D89.810 Acute graft-versus-host disease

D89.811 Chronic graft-versus-host disease

D89.812 Acute on chronic graft-versus-host disease

D89.813 Graft-versus-host disease, unspecified

D89.82 Autoimmune lymphoproliferative syndrome [ALPS]

D89.89 Other specified disorders involving the immune mechanism, not elsewhere classified

EXCLUDES 1 *human immunodeficiency virus disease (B20)*

D89.9 Disorder involving the immune mechanism, unspecified
Immune disease NOS

Chapter 4. Endocrine, Nutritional and Metabolic Diseases (EØØ-E89)

NOTE All neoplasms, whether functionally active or not, are classified in Chapter 2. Appropriate codes in this chapter (i.e. EØ5.8, EØ7.Ø, E16-E31, E34-) may be used as additional codes to indicate either functional activity by neoplasms and ectopic endocrine tissue or hyperfunction and hypofunction of endocrine glands associated with neoplasms and other conditions classified elsewhere.

EXCLUDES 1 *transitory endocrine and metabolic disorders specific to newborn (P7Ø-P74)*

This chapter contains the following blocks:

EØØ-EØ7 Disorders of thyroid gland
EØ8-E13 Diabetes mellitus
E15-E16 Other disorders of glucose regulation and pancreatic internal secretion
E2Ø-E35 Disorders of other endocrine glands
E36 Intraoperative complications of endocrine system
E4Ø-E46 Malnutrition
E5Ø-E64 Other nutritional deficiencies
E65-E68 Overweight, obesity and other hyperalimentation
E7Ø-E88 Metabolic disorders
E89 Postprocedural endocrine and metabolic complications and disorders, not elsewhere classified

Disorders of thyroid gland (EØØ-EØ7)

✓4th **EØØ Congenital iodine-deficiency syndrome**
Use additional code (F7Ø-F79) to identify associated intellectual disabilities
EXCLUDES 1 *subclinical iodine-deficiency hypothyroidism (EØ2)*

EØØ.Ø Congenital iodine-deficiency syndrome, neurological type
Endemic cretinism, neurological type

EØØ.1 Congenital iodine-deficiency syndrome, myxedematous type
Endemic hypothyroid cretinism
Endemic cretinism, myxedematous type

EØØ.2 Congenital iodine-deficiency syndrome, mixed type
Endemic cretinism, mixed type

EØØ.9 Congenital iodine-deficiency syndrome, unspecified
Congenital iodine-deficiency hypothyroidism NOS
Endemic cretinism NOS

✓4th **EØ1 Iodine-deficiency related thyroid disorders and allied conditions**
EXCLUDES 1 *congenital iodine-deficiency syndrome (EØØ.-)*
subclinical iodine-deficiency hypothyroidism (EØ2)

EØ1.Ø Iodine-deficiency related diffuse (endemic) goiter

EØ1.1 Iodine-deficiency related multinodular (endemic) goiter
Iodine-deficiency related nodular goiter

EØ1.2 Iodine-deficiency related (endemic) goiter, unspecified
Endemic goiter NOS

EØ1.8 Other iodine-deficiency related thyroid disorders and allied conditions
Acquired iodine-deficiency hypothyroidism NOS

EØ2 Subclinical iodine-deficiency hypothyroidism

✓4th **EØ3 Other hypothyroidism**
EXCLUDES 1 *iodine-deficiency related hypothyroidism (EØØ-EØ2)*
postprocedural hypothyroidism (E89.Ø)

EØ3.Ø Congenital hypothyroidism with diffuse goiter
Congenital parenchymatous goiter (nontoxic)
Congenital goiter (nontoxic) NOS
EXCLUDES 1 *transitory congenital goiter with normal function (P72.Ø)*

EØ3.1 Congenital hypothyroidism without goiter
Aplasia of thyroid (with myxedema)
Congenital atrophy of thyroid
Congenital hypothyroidism NOS

EØ3.2 Hypothyroidism due to medicaments and other exogenous substances
Code first poisoning due to drug or toxin, if applicable (T36-T65 with fifth or sixth character 1-4 or 6)
Use additional code for adverse effect, if applicable, to identify drug (T36-T5Ø with fifth or sixth character 5)

EØ3.3 Postinfectious hypothyroidism

EØ3.4 Atrophy of thyroid (acquired)
EXCLUDES 1 *congenital atrophy of thyroid (EØ3.1)*

EØ3.5 Myxedema coma

EØ3.8 Other specified hypothyroidism

EØ3.9 Hypothyroidism, unspecified
Myxedema NOS

✓4th **EØ4 Other nontoxic goiter**
EXCLUDES 1 *congenital goiter (NOS) (diffuse) (parenchymatous) (EØ3.Ø)*
iodine-deficiency related goiter (EØØ-EØ2)

EØ4.Ø Nontoxic diffuse goiter
Diffuse (colloid) nontoxic goiter
Simple nontoxic goiter

EØ4.1 Nontoxic single thyroid nodule
Colloid nodule (cystic) (thyroid)
Nontoxic uninodular goiter
Thyroid (cystic) nodule NOS

EØ4.2 Nontoxic multinodular goiter
Cystic goiter NOS
Multinodular (cystic) goiter NOS

EØ4.8 Other specified nontoxic goiter

EØ4.9 Nontoxic goiter, unspecified
Goiter NOS
Nodular goiter (nontoxic) NOS

✓4th **EØ5 Thyrotoxicosis [hyperthyroidism]**
EXCLUDES 1 *chronic thyroiditis with transient thyrotoxicosis (EØ6.2)*
neonatal thyrotoxicosis (P72.1)

✓5th **EØ5.Ø Thyrotoxicosis with diffuse goiter**
Exophthalmic or toxic goiter NOS
Graves' disease
Toxic diffuse goiter

EØ5.ØØ Thyrotoxicosis with diffuse goiter without thyrotoxic crisis or storm

EØ5.Ø1 Thyrotoxicosis with diffuse goiter with thyrotoxic crisis or storm

✓5th **EØ5.1 Thyrotoxicosis with toxic single thyroid nodule**
Thyrotoxicosis with toxic uninodular goiter

EØ5.1Ø Thyrotoxicosis with toxic single thyroid nodule without thyrotoxic crisis or storm

EØ5.11 Thyrotoxicosis with toxic single thyroid nodule with thyrotoxic crisis or storm

✓5th **EØ5.2 Thyrotoxicosis with toxic multinodular goiter**
Toxic nodular goiter NOS

EØ5.2Ø Thyrotoxicosis with toxic multinodular goiter without thyrotoxic crisis or storm

EØ5.21 Thyrotoxicosis with toxic multinodular goiter with thyrotoxic crisis or storm

✓5th **EØ5.3 Thyrotoxicosis from ectopic thyroid tissue**

EØ5.3Ø Thyrotoxicosis from ectopic thyroid tissue without thyrotoxic crisis or storm

EØ5.31 Thyrotoxicosis from ectopic thyroid tissue with thyrotoxic crisis or storm

✓5th **EØ5.4 Thyrotoxicosis factitia**

EØ5.4Ø Thyrotoxicosis factitia without thyrotoxic crisis or storm

EØ5.41 Thyrotoxicosis factitia with thyrotoxic crisis or storm

✓5th **EØ5.8 Other thyrotoxicosis**
Overproduction of thyroid-stimulating hormone

EØ5.8Ø Other thyrotoxicosis without thyrotoxic crisis or storm

EØ5.81 Other thyrotoxicosis with thyrotoxic crisis or storm

✓5th **EØ5.9 Thyrotoxicosis, unspecified**
Hyperthyroidism NOS

EØ5.9Ø Thyrotoxicosis, unspecified without thyrotoxic crisis or storm

EØ5.91 Thyrotoxicosis, unspecified with thyrotoxic crisis or storm

✓4th **EØ6 Thyroiditis**
EXCLUDES 1 *postpartum thyroiditis (O9Ø.5)*

EØ6.Ø Acute thyroiditis
Abscess of thyroid
Pyogenic thyroiditis
Suppurative thyroiditis
Use additional code (B95-B97) to identify infectious agent

EØ6.1 Subacute thyroiditis
de Quervain thyroiditis
Giant-cell thyroiditis
Granulomatous thyroiditis
Nonsuppurative thyroiditis
Viral thyroiditis
EXCLUDES 1 *autoimmune thyroiditis (EØ6.3)*

E06.2 Chronic thyroiditis with transient thyrotoxicosis
EXCLUDES 1 *autoimmune thyroiditis (E06.3)*

E06.3 Autoimmune thyroiditis
Hashimoto's thyroiditis
Hashitoxicosis (transient)
Lymphadenoid goiter
Lymphocytic thyroiditis
Struma lymphomatosa

E06.4 Drug-induced thyroiditis
Use additional code for adverse effect, if applicable, to identify drug (T36-T50 with fifth or sixth character 5)

E06.5 Other chronic thyroiditis
Chronic fibrous thyroiditis
Chronic thyroiditis NOS
Ligneous thyroiditis
Riedel thyroiditis

E06.9 Thyroiditis, unspecified

✓4th **E07 Other disorders of thyroid**

E07.0 Hypersecretion of calcitonin
C-cell hyperplasia of thyroid
Hypersecretion of thyrocalcitonin

E07.1 Dyshormogenetic goiter
Familial dyshormogenetic goiter
Pendred's syndrome
EXCLUDES 1 *transitory congenital goiter with normal function (P72.0)*

✓5th **E07.8 Other specified disorders of thyroid**

E07.81 Sick-euthyroid syndrome
Euthyroid sick-syndrome

E07.89 Other specified disorders of thyroid
Abnormality of thyroid-binding globulin
Hemorrhage of thyroid
Infarction of thyroid

E07.9 Disorder of thyroid, unspecified

Diabetes mellitus (E08-E13)

✓4th **E08 Diabetes mellitus due to underlying condition**
Code first the underlying condition, such as:
congenital rubella (P35.0)
cushing's syndrome (E24.-)
cystic fibrosis (E84.-)
malignant neoplasm (C00-C96)
malnutrition (E40-E46)
pancreatitis and other diseases of the pancreas (K85.-, K86.-)
Use additional code to identify any insulin use (Z79.4)
EXCLUDES 1 *drug or chemical induced diabetes mellitus (E09.-)*
gestational diabetes (O24.4-)
neonatal diabetes mellitus (P70.2)
postpancreatectomy diabetes mellitus (E13.-)
postprocedural diabetes mellitus (E13.-)
secondary diabetes mellitus NEC (E13.-)
type 1 diabetes mellitus (E10.-)
type 2 diabetes mellitus (E11.-)

✓5th **E08.0 Diabetes mellitus due to underlying condition with hyperosmolarity**

E08.00 Diabetes mellitus due to underlying condition with hyperosmolarity without nonketotic hyperglycemic-hyperosmolar coma (NKHHC)

E08.01 Diabetes mellitus due to underlying condition with hyperosmolarity with coma

✓5th **E08.1 Diabetes mellitus due to underlying condition with ketoacidosis**

E08.10 Diabetes mellitus due to underlying condition with ketoacidosis without coma

E08.11 Diabetes mellitus due to underlying condition with ketoacidosis with coma

✓5th **E08.2 Diabetes mellitus due to underlying condition with kidney complications**

E08.21 Diabetes mellitus due to underlying condition with diabetic nephropathy
Diabetes mellitus due to underlying condition with intercapillary glomerulosclerosis
Diabetes mellitus due to underlying condition with intracapillary glomerulonephrosis
Diabetes mellitus due to underlying condition with Kimmelstiel-Wilson disease

E08.22 Diabetes mellitus due to underlying condition with diabetic chronic kidney disease
Diabetes mellitus due to underlying condition with chronic kidney disease due to conditions classified to .21 and .22
Use additional code to identify stage of chronic kidney disease (N18.1-N18.6)

E08.29 Diabetes mellitus due to underlying condition with other diabetic kidney complication
Renal tubular degeneration in diabetes mellitus due to underlying condition

✓5th **E08.3 Diabetes mellitus due to underlying condition with ophthalmic complications**

✓6th **E08.31 Diabetes mellitus due to underlying condition with unspecified diabetic retinopathy**

E08.311 Diabetes mellitus due to underlying condition with unspecified diabetic retinopathy with macular edema

E08.319 Diabetes mellitus due to underlying condition with unspecified diabetic retinopathy without macular edema

✓6th **E08.32 Diabetes mellitus due to underlying condition with mild nonproliferative diabetic retinopathy**
Diabetes mellitus due to underlying condition with nonproliferative diabetic retinopathy NOS

E08.321 Diabetes mellitus due to underlying condition with mild nonproliferative diabetic retinopathy with macular edema

E08.329 Diabetes mellitus due to underlying condition with mild nonproliferative diabetic retinopathy without macular edema

✓6th **E08.33 Diabetes mellitus due to underlying condition with moderate nonproliferative diabetic retinopathy**

E08.331 Diabetes mellitus due to underlying condition with moderate nonproliferative diabetic retinopathy with macular edema

E08.339 Diabetes mellitus due to underlying condition with moderate nonproliferative diabetic retinopathy without macular edema

✓6th **E08.34 Diabetes mellitus due to underlying condition with severe nonproliferative diabetic retinopathy**

E08.341 Diabetes mellitus due to underlying condition with severe nonproliferative diabetic retinopathy with macular edema

E08.349 Diabetes mellitus due to underlying condition with severe nonproliferative diabetic retinopathy without macular edema

✓6th **E08.35 Diabetes mellitus due to underlying condition with proliferative diabetic retinopathy**

E08.351 Diabetes mellitus due to underlying condition with proliferative diabetic retinopathy with macular edema

E08.359 Diabetes mellitus due to underlying condition with proliferative diabetic retinopathy without macular edema

E08.36 Diabetes mellitus due to underlying condition with diabetic cataract

E08.39 Diabetes mellitus due to underlying condition with other diabetic ophthalmic complication

✓5th **E08.4 Diabetes mellitus due to underlying condition with neurological complications**

E08.40 Diabetes mellitus due to underlying condition with diabetic neuropathy, unspecified

E08.41 Diabetes mellitus due to underlying condition with diabetic mononeuropathy

E08.42 Diabetes mellitus due to underlying condition with diabetic polyneuropathy
Diabetes mellitus due to underlying condition with diabetic neuralgia

E08.43 Diabetes mellitus due to underlying condition with diabetic autonomic (poly)neuropathy
Diabetes mellitus due to underlying condition with diabetic gastroparesis

E08.44 Diabetes mellitus due to underlying condition with diabetic amyotrophy

E08.49 Diabetes mellitus due to underlying condition with other diabetic neurological complication

E08.5 Diabetes mellitus due to underlying condition with circulatory complications

E08.51 Diabetes mellitus due to underlying condition with diabetic peripheral angiopathy without gangrene

E08.52 Diabetes mellitus due to underlying condition with diabetic peripheral angiopathy with gangrene

Diabetes mellitus due to underlying condition with diabetic gangrene

E08.59 Diabetes mellitus due to underlying condition with other circulatory complications

E08.6 Diabetes mellitus due to underlying condition with other specified complications

E08.61 Diabetes mellitus due to underlying condition with diabetic arthropathy

E08.610 Diabetes mellitus due to underlying condition with diabetic neuropathic arthropathy

Diabetes mellitus due to underlying condition with Charcôt's joints

E08.618 Diabetes mellitus due to underlying condition with other diabetic arthropathy

E08.62 Diabetes mellitus due to underlying condition with skin complications

E08.620 Diabetes mellitus due to underlying condition with diabetic dermatitis

Diabetes mellitus due to underlying condition with diabetic necrobiosis lipoidica

E08.621 Diabetes mellitus due to underlying condition with foot ulcer

Use additional code to identify site of ulcer (L97.4-, L97.5-)

E08.622 Diabetes mellitus due to underlying condition with other skin ulcer

Use additional code to identify site of ulcer (L97.1-L97.9, L98.41-L98.49)

E08.628 Diabetes mellitus due to underlying condition with other skin complications

E08.63 Diabetes mellitus due to underlying condition with oral complications

E08.630 Diabetes mellitus due to underlying condition with periodontal disease

E08.638 Diabetes mellitus due to underlying condition with other oral complications

E08.64 Diabetes mellitus due to underlying condition with hypoglycemia

E08.641 Diabetes mellitus due to underlying condition with hypoglycemia with coma

E08.649 Diabetes mellitus due to underlying condition with hypoglycemia without coma

E08.65 Diabetes mellitus due to underlying condition with hyperglycemia

E08.69 Diabetes mellitus due to underlying condition with other specified complication

Use additional code to identify complication

E08.8 Diabetes mellitus due to underlying condition with unspecified complications

E08.9 Diabetes mellitus due to underlying condition without complications

E09 Drug or chemical induced diabetes mellitus

Code first poisoning due to drug or toxin, if applicable (T36-T65 with fifth or sixth character 1-4 or 6)

Use additional code for adverse effect, if applicable, to identify drug (T36-T50 with fifth or sixth character 5)

Use additional code to identify any insulin use (Z79.4)

EXCLUDES 1 *diabetes mellitus due to underlying condition (E08.-)*
gestational diabetes (O24.4-)
neonatal diabetes mellitus (P70.2)
postpancreatectomy diabetes mellitus (E13.-)
postprocedural diabetes mellitus (E13.-)
secondary diabetes mellitus NEC (E13.-)
type 1 diabetes mellitus (E10.-)
type 2 diabetes mellitus (E11.-)

E09.0 Drug or chemical induced diabetes mellitus with hyperosmolarity

E09.00 Drug or chemical induced diabetes mellitus with hyperosmolarity without nonketotic hyperglycemic-hyperosmolar coma (NKHHC)

E09.01 Drug or chemical induced diabetes mellitus with hyperosmolarity with coma

E09.1 Drug or chemical induced diabetes mellitus with ketoacidosis

E09.10 Drug or chemical induced diabetes mellitus with ketoacidosis without coma

E09.11 Drug or chemical induced diabetes mellitus with ketoacidosis with coma

E09.2 Drug or chemical induced diabetes mellitus with kidney complications

E09.21 Drug or chemical induced diabetes mellitus with diabetic nephropathy

Drug or chemical induced diabetes mellitus with intercapillary glomerulosclerosis

Drug or chemical induced diabetes mellitus with intracapillary glomerulonephrosis

Drug or chemical induced diabetes mellitus with Kimmelstiel-Wilson disease

E09.22 Drug or chemical induced diabetes mellitus with diabetic chronic kidney disease

Drug or chemical induced diabetes mellitus with chronic kidney disease due to conditions classified to .21 and .22

Use additional code to identify stage of chronic kidney disease (N18.1-N18.6)

E09.29 Drug or chemical induced diabetes mellitus with other diabetic kidney complication

Drug or chemical induced diabetes mellitus with renal tubular degeneration

E09.3 Drug or chemical induced diabetes mellitus with ophthalmic complications

E09.31 Drug or chemical induced diabetes mellitus with unspecified diabetic retinopathy

E09.311 Drug or chemical induced diabetes mellitus with unspecified diabetic retinopathy with macular edema

E09.319 Drug or chemical induced diabetes mellitus with unspecified diabetic retinopathy without macular edema

E09.32 Drug or chemical induced diabetes mellitus with mild nonproliferative diabetic retinopathy

Drug or chemical induced diabetes mellitus with nonproliferative diabetic retinopathy NOS

E09.321 Drug or chemical induced diabetes mellitus with mild nonproliferative diabetic retinopathy with macular edema

E09.329 Drug or chemical induced diabetes mellitus with mild nonproliferative diabetic retinopathy without macular edema

E09.33 Drug or chemical induced diabetes mellitus with moderate nonproliferative diabetic retinopathy

E09.331 Drug or chemical induced diabetes mellitus with moderate nonproliferative diabetic retinopathy with macular edema

E09.339 Drug or chemical induced diabetes mellitus with moderate nonproliferative diabetic retinopathy without macular edema

✓6th **E09.34 Drug or chemical induced diabetes mellitus with severe nonproliferative diabetic retinopathy**

E09.341 Drug or chemical induced diabetes mellitus with severe nonproliferative diabetic retinopathy with macular edema

E09.349 Drug or chemical induced diabetes mellitus with severe nonproliferative diabetic retinopathy without macular edema

✓6th **E09.35 Drug or chemical induced diabetes mellitus with proliferative diabetic retinopathy**

E09.351 Drug or chemical induced diabetes mellitus with proliferative diabetic retinopathy with macular edema

E09.359 Drug or chemical induced diabetes mellitus with proliferative diabetic retinopathy without macular edema

E09.36 Drug or chemical induced diabetes mellitus with diabetic cataract

E09.39 Drug or chemical induced diabetes mellitus with other diabetic ophthalmic complication

✓5th **E09.4 Drug or chemical induced diabetes mellitus with neurological complications**

E09.40 Drug or chemical induced diabetes mellitus with neurological complications with diabetic neuropathy, unspecified

E09.41 Drug or chemical induced diabetes mellitus with neurological complications with diabetic mononeuropathy

E09.42 Drug or chemical induced diabetes mellitus with neurological complications with diabetic polyneuropathy

Drug or chemical induced diabetes mellitus with diabetic neuralgia

E09.43 Drug or chemical induced diabetes mellitus with neurological complications with diabetic autonomic (poly)neuropathy

Drug or chemical induced diabetes mellitus with diabetic gastroparesis

E09.44 Drug or chemical induced diabetes mellitus with neurological complications with diabetic amyotrophy

E09.49 Drug or chemical induced diabetes mellitus with neurological complications with other diabetic neurological complication

✓5th **E09.5 Drug or chemical induced diabetes mellitus with circulatory complications**

E09.51 Drug or chemical induced diabetes mellitus with diabetic peripheral angiopathy without gangrene

E09.52 Drug or chemical induced diabetes mellitus with diabetic peripheral angiopathy with gangrene

Drug or chemical induced diabetes mellitus with diabetic gangrene

E09.59 Drug or chemical induced diabetes mellitus with other circulatory complications

✓5th **E09.6 Drug or chemical induced diabetes mellitus with other specified complications**

✓6th **E09.61 Drug or chemical induced diabetes mellitus with diabetic arthropathy**

E09.610 Drug or chemical induced diabetes mellitus with diabetic neuropathic arthropathy

Drug or chemical induced diabetes mellitus with Charcôt's joints

E09.618 Drug or chemical induced diabetes mellitus with other diabetic arthropathy

✓6th **E09.62 Drug or chemical induced diabetes mellitus with skin complications**

E09.620 Drug or chemical induced diabetes mellitus with diabetic dermatitis

Drug or chemical induced diabetes mellitus with diabetic necrobiosis lipoidica

E09.621 Drug or chemical induced diabetes mellitus with foot ulcer

Use additional code to identify site of ulcer (L97.4-, L97.5-)

E09.622 Drug or chemical induced diabetes mellitus with other skin ulcer

Use additional code to identify site of ulcer (L97.1-L97.9, L98.41-L98.49)

E09.628 Drug or chemical induced diabetes mellitus with other skin complications

✓6th **E09.63 Drug or chemical induced diabetes mellitus with oral complications**

E09.630 Drug or chemical induced diabetes mellitus with periodontal disease

E09.638 Drug or chemical induced diabetes mellitus with other oral complications

✓6th **E09.64 Drug or chemical induced diabetes mellitus with hypoglycemia**

E09.641 Drug or chemical induced diabetes mellitus with hypoglycemia with coma

E09.649 Drug or chemical induced diabetes mellitus with hypoglycemia without coma

E09.65 Drug or chemical induced diabetes mellitus with hyperglycemia

E09.69 Drug or chemical induced diabetes mellitus with other specified complication

Use additional code to identify complication

E09.8 Drug or chemical induced diabetes mellitus with unspecified complications

E09.9 Drug or chemical induced diabetes mellitus without complications

✓4th **E10 Type 1 diabetes mellitus**

INCLUDES brittle diabetes (mellitus)
diabetes (mellitus) due to autoimmune process
diabetes (mellitus) due to immune mediated pancreatic islet beta-cell destruction
idiopathic diabetes (mellitus)
juvenile onset diabetes (mellitus)
ketosis-prone diabetes (mellitus)

EXCLUDES 1 *diabetes mellitus due to underlying condition (E08.-)*
drug or chemical induced diabetes mellitus (E09.-)
gestational diabetes (O24.4-)
hyperglycemia NOS (R73.9)
neonatal diabetes mellitus (P70.2)
postpancreatectomy diabetes mellitus (E13.-)
postprocedural diabetes mellitus (E13.-)
secondary diabetes mellitus NEC (E13.-)
type 2 diabetes mellitus (E11.-)

✓5th **E10.1 Type 1 diabetes mellitus with ketoacidosis**

E10.10 Type 1 diabetes mellitus with ketoacidosis without coma

E10.11 Type 1 diabetes mellitus with ketoacidosis with coma

✓5th **E10.2 Type 1 diabetes mellitus with kidney complications**

E10.21 Type 1 diabetes mellitus with diabetic nephropathy

Type 1 diabetes mellitus with intercapillary glomerulosclerosis
Type 1 diabetes mellitus with intracapillary glomerulonephrosis
Type 1 diabetes mellitus with Kimmelstiel-Wilson disease

E10.22 Type 1 diabetes mellitus with diabetic chronic kidney disease

Type 1 diabetes mellitus with chronic kidney disease due to conditions classified to .21 and .22
Use additional code to identify stage of chronic kidney disease (N18.1-N18.6)

E10.29 Type 1 diabetes mellitus with other diabetic kidney complication

Type 1 diabetes mellitus with renal tubular degeneration

✓5th **E10.3 Type 1 diabetes mellitus with ophthalmic complications**

✓6th **E10.31 Type 1 diabetes mellitus with unspecified diabetic retinopathy**

E10.311 Type 1 diabetes mellitus with unspecified diabetic retinopathy with macular edema

E10.319 Type 1 diabetes mellitus with unspecified diabetic retinopathy without macular edema

✓6th **E10.32 Type 1 diabetes mellitus with mild nonproliferative diabetic retinopathy**
Type 1 diabetes mellitus with nonproliferative diabetic retinopathy NOS

E10.321 Type 1 diabetes mellitus with mild nonproliferative diabetic retinopathy with macular edema

E10.329 Type 1 diabetes mellitus with mild nonproliferative diabetic retinopathy without macular edema

✓6th **E10.33 Type 1 diabetes mellitus with moderate nonproliferative diabetic retinopathy**

E10.331 Type 1 diabetes mellitus with moderate nonproliferative diabetic retinopathy with macular edema

E10.339 Type 1 diabetes mellitus with moderate nonproliferative diabetic retinopathy without macular edema

✓6th **E10.34 Type 1 diabetes mellitus with severe nonproliferative diabetic retinopathy**

E10.341 Type 1 diabetes mellitus with severe nonproliferative diabetic retinopathy with macular edema

E10.349 Type 1 diabetes mellitus with severe nonproliferative diabetic retinopathy without macular edema

✓6th **E10.35 Type 1 diabetes mellitus with proliferative diabetic retinopathy**

E10.351 Type 1 diabetes mellitus with proliferative diabetic retinopathy with macular edema

E10.359 Type 1 diabetes mellitus with proliferative diabetic retinopathy without macular edema

E10.36 Type 1 diabetes mellitus with diabetic cataract

E10.39 Type 1 diabetes mellitus with other diabetic ophthalmic complication

✓5th **E10.4 Type 1 diabetes mellitus with neurological complications**

E10.40 Type 1 diabetes mellitus with diabetic neuropathy, unspecified

E10.41 Type 1 diabetes mellitus with diabetic mononeuropathy

E10.42 Type 1 diabetes mellitus with diabetic polyneuropathy
Type 1 diabetes mellitus with diabetic neuralgia

E10.43 Type 1 diabetes mellitus with diabetic autonomic (poly)neuropathy
Type 1 diabetes mellitus with diabetic gastroparesis

E10.44 Type 1 diabetes mellitus with diabetic amyotrophy

E10.49 Type 1 diabetes mellitus with other diabetic neurological complication

✓5th **E10.5 Type 1 diabetes mellitus with circulatory complications**

E10.51 Type 1 diabetes mellitus with diabetic peripheral angiopathy without gangrene

E10.52 Type 1 diabetes mellitus with diabetic peripheral angiopathy with gangrene
Type 1 diabetes mellitus with diabetic gangrene

E10.59 Type 1 diabetes mellitus with other circulatory complications

✓5th **E10.6 Type 1 diabetes mellitus with other specified complications**

✓6th **E10.61 Type 1 diabetes mellitus with diabetic arthropathy**

E10.610 Type 1 diabetes mellitus with diabetic neuropathic arthropathy
Type 1 diabetes mellitus with Charcôt's joints

E10.618 Type 1 diabetes mellitus with other diabetic arthropathy

✓6th **E10.62 Type 1 diabetes mellitus with skin complications**

E10.620 Type 1 diabetes mellitus with diabetic dermatitis
Type 1 diabetes mellitus with diabetic necrobiosis lipoidica

E10.621 Type 1 diabetes mellitus with foot ulcer
Use additional code to identify site of ulcer (L97.4-, L97.5-)

E10.622 Type 1 diabetes mellitus with other skin ulcer
Use additional code to identify site of ulcer (L97.1-L97.9, L98.41-L98.49)

E10.628 Type 1 diabetes mellitus with other skin complications

✓6th **E10.63 Type 1 diabetes mellitus with oral complications**

E10.630 Type 1 diabetes mellitus with periodontal disease

E10.638 Type 1 diabetes mellitus with other oral complications

✓6th **E10.64 Type 1 diabetes mellitus with hypoglycemia**

E10.641 Type 1 diabetes mellitus with hypoglycemia with coma

E10.649 Type 1 diabetes mellitus with hypoglycemia without coma

E10.65 Type 1 diabetes mellitus with hyperglycemia

E10.69 Type 1 diabetes mellitus with other specified complication
Use additional code to identify complication

E10.8 Type 1 diabetes mellitus with unspecified complications

E10.9 Type 1 diabetes mellitus without complications

✓4th **E11 Type 2 diabetes mellitus**

INCLUDES diabetes (mellitus) due to insulin secretory defect
diabetes NOS
insulin resistant diabetes (mellitus)

Use additional code to identify any insulin use (Z79.4)

EXCLUDES 1 *diabetes mellitus due to underlying condition (E08.-)*
drug or chemical induced diabetes mellitus (E09.-)
gestational diabetes (O24.4-)
neonatal diabetes mellitus (P70.2)
postpancreatectomy diabetes mellitus (E13.-)
postprocedural diabetes mellitus (E13.-)
secondary diabetes mellitus NEC (E13.-)
type 1 diabetes mellitus (E10.-)

✓5th **E11.0 Type 2 diabetes mellitus with hyperosmolarity**

E11.00 Type 2 diabetes mellitus with hyperosmolarity without nonketotic hyperglycemic-hyperosmolar coma (NKHHC)

E11.01 Type 2 diabetes mellitus with hyperosmolarity with coma

✓5th **E11.2 Type 2 diabetes mellitus with kidney complications**

E11.21 Type 2 diabetes mellitus with diabetic nephropathy
Type 2 diabetes mellitus with intercapillary glomerulosclerosis
Type 2 diabetes mellitus with intracapillary glomerulonephrosis
Type 2 diabetes mellitus with Kimmelstiel-Wilson disease

E11.22 Type 2 diabetes mellitus with diabetic chronic kidney disease
Type 2 diabetes mellitus with chronic kidney disease due to conditions classified to .21 and .22
Use additional code to identify stage of chronic kidney disease (N18.1-N18.6)

E11.29 Type 2 diabetes mellitus with other diabetic kidney complication
Type 2 diabetes mellitus with renal tubular degeneration

✓5th **E11.3 Type 2 diabetes mellitus with ophthalmic complications**

✓6th **E11.31 Type 2 diabetes mellitus with unspecified diabetic retinopathy**

E11.311 Type 2 diabetes mellitus with unspecified diabetic retinopathy with macular edema

E11.319 Type 2 diabetes mellitus with unspecified diabetic retinopathy without macular edema

✓6th **E11.32 Type 2 diabetes mellitus with mild nonproliferative diabetic retinopathy**
Type 2 diabetes mellitus with nonproliferative diabetic retinopathy NOS

E11.321 Type 2 diabetes mellitus with mild nonproliferative diabetic retinopathy with macular edema

E11.329 Type 2 diabetes mellitus with mild nonproliferative diabetic retinopathy without macular edema

☑ Appropriate additional character required   x7th Requires 7th character, placeholder x must fill empty characters

E11.33 Type 2 diabetes mellitus with moderate nonproliferative diabetic retinopathy
- **E11.331 Type 2 diabetes mellitus with moderate nonproliferative diabetic retinopathy with macular edema**
- **E11.339 Type 2 diabetes mellitus with moderate nonproliferative diabetic retinopathy without macular edema**

E11.34 Type 2 diabetes mellitus with severe nonproliferative diabetic retinopathy
- **E11.341 Type 2 diabetes mellitus with severe nonproliferative diabetic retinopathy with macular edema**
- **E11.349 Type 2 diabetes mellitus with severe nonproliferative diabetic retinopathy without macular edema**

E11.35 Type 2 diabetes mellitus with proliferative diabetic retinopathy
- **E11.351 Type 2 diabetes mellitus with proliferative diabetic retinopathy with macular edema**
- **E11.359 Type 2 diabetes mellitus with proliferative diabetic retinopathy without macular edema**

E11.36 Type 2 diabetes mellitus with diabetic cataract

E11.39 Type 2 diabetes mellitus with other diabetic ophthalmic complication

E11.4 Type 2 diabetes mellitus with neurological complications
- **E11.40 Type 2 diabetes mellitus with diabetic neuropathy, unspecified**
- **E11.41 Type 2 diabetes mellitus with diabetic mononeuropathy**
- **E11.42 Type 2 diabetes mellitus with diabetic polyneuropathy**
  - Type 2 diabetes mellitus with diabetic neuralgia
- **E11.43 Type 2 diabetes mellitus with diabetic autonomic (poly)neuropathy**
  - Type 2 diabetes mellitus with diabetic gastroparesis
- **E11.44 Type 2 diabetes mellitus with diabetic amyotrophy**
- **E11.49 Type 2 diabetes mellitus with other diabetic neurological complication**

E11.5 Type 2 diabetes mellitus with circulatory complications
- **E11.51 Type 2 diabetes mellitus with diabetic peripheral angiopathy without gangrene**
- **E11.52 Type 2 diabetes mellitus with diabetic peripheral angiopathy with gangrene**
  - Type 2 diabetes mellitus with diabetic gangrene
- **E11.59 Type 2 diabetes mellitus with other circulatory complications**

E11.6 Type 2 diabetes mellitus with other specified complications
- **E11.61 Type 2 diabetes mellitus with diabetic arthropathy**
  - **E11.610 Type 2 diabetes mellitus with diabetic neuropathic arthropathy**
    - Type 2 diabetes mellitus with Charcôt's joints
  - **E11.618 Type 2 diabetes mellitus with other diabetic arthropathy**
- **E11.62 Type 2 diabetes mellitus with skin complications**
  - **E11.620 Type 2 diabetes mellitus with diabetic dermatitis**
    - Type 2 diabetes mellitus with diabetic necrobiosis lipoidica
  - **E11.621 Type 2 diabetes mellitus with foot ulcer**
    - Use additional code to identify site of ulcer (L97.4-, L97.5-)
  - **E11.622 Type 2 diabetes mellitus with other skin ulcer**
    - Use additional code to identify site of ulcer (L97.1-L97.9, L98.41-L98.49)
  - **E11.628 Type 2 diabetes mellitus with other skin complications**
- **E11.63 Type 2 diabetes mellitus with oral complications**
  - **E11.630 Type 2 diabetes mellitus with periodontal disease**
  - **E11.638 Type 2 diabetes mellitus with other oral complications**
- **E11.64 Type 2 diabetes mellitus with hypoglycemia**
  - **E11.641 Type 2 diabetes mellitus with hypoglycemia with coma**
  - **E11.649 Type 2 diabetes mellitus with hypoglycemia without coma**
- **E11.65 Type 2 diabetes mellitus with hyperglycemia**
- **E11.69 Type 2 diabetes mellitus with other specified complication**
  - Use additional code to identify complication

E11.8 Type 2 diabetes mellitus with unspecified complications

E11.9 Type 2 diabetes mellitus without complications

E13 Other specified diabetes mellitus

Diabetes mellitus due to genetic defects of beta-cell function
Diabetes mellitus due to genetic defects in insulin action
Postpancreatectomy diabetes mellitus
Postprocedural diabetes mellitus
Secondary diabetes mellitus NEC
Use additional code to identify any insulin use (Z79.4)

EXCLUDES 1 *diabetes (mellitus) due to autoimmune process (E10.-)*
diabetes (mellitus) due to immune mediated pancreatic islet beta-cell destruction (E10.-)
diabetes mellitus due to underlying condition (E08.-)
drug or chemical induced diabetes mellitus (E09.-)
gestational diabetes (O24.4-)
neonatal diabetes mellitus (P70.2)
type 2 diabetes mellitus (E11.-)

E13.0 Other specified diabetes mellitus with hyperosmolarity
- **E13.00 Other specified diabetes mellitus with hyperosmolarity without nonketotic hyperglycemic-hyperosmolar coma (NKHHC)**
- **E13.01 Other specified diabetes mellitus with hyperosmolarity with coma**

E13.1 Other specified diabetes mellitus with ketoacidosis
- **E13.10 Other specified diabetes mellitus with ketoacidosis without coma**
- **E13.11 Other specified diabetes mellitus with ketoacidosis with coma**

E13.2 Other specified diabetes mellitus with kidney complications
- **E13.21 Other specified diabetes mellitus with diabetic nephropathy**
  - Other specified diabetes mellitus with intercapillary glomerulosclerosis
  - Other specified diabetes mellitus with intracapillary glomerulonephrosis
  - Other specified diabetes mellitus with Kimmelstiel-Wilson disease
- **E13.22 Other specified diabetes mellitus with diabetic chronic kidney disease**
  - Other specified diabetes mellitus with chronic kidney disease due to conditions classified to .21 and .22
  - Use additional code to identify stage of chronic kidney disease (N18.1-N18.6)
- **E13.29 Other specified diabetes mellitus with other diabetic kidney complication**
  - Other specified diabetes mellitus with renal tubular degeneration

E13.3 Other specified diabetes mellitus with ophthalmic complications
- **E13.31 Other specified diabetes mellitus with unspecified diabetic retinopathy**
  - **E13.311 Other specified diabetes mellitus with unspecified diabetic retinopathy with macular edema**
  - **E13.319 Other specified diabetes mellitus with unspecified diabetic retinopathy without macular edema**
- **E13.32 Other specified diabetes mellitus with mild nonproliferative diabetic retinopathy**
  - Other specified diabetes mellitus with nonproliferative diabetic retinopathy NOS
  - **E13.321 Other specified diabetes mellitus with mild nonproliferative diabetic retinopathy with macular edema**
  - **E13.329 Other specified diabetes mellitus with mild nonproliferative diabetic retinopathy without macular edema**

√6th **E13.33 Other specified diabetes mellitus with moderate nonproliferative diabetic retinopathy**
E13.331 Other specified diabetes mellitus with moderate nonproliferative diabetic retinopathy with macular edema
E13.339 Other specified diabetes mellitus with moderate nonproliferative diabetic retinopathy without macular edema

√6th **E13.34 Other specified diabetes mellitus with severe nonproliferative diabetic retinopathy**
E13.341 Other specified diabetes mellitus with severe nonproliferative diabetic retinopathy with macular edema
E13.349 Other specified diabetes mellitus with severe nonproliferative diabetic retinopathy without macular edema

√6th **E13.35 Other specified diabetes mellitus with proliferative diabetic retinopathy**
E13.351 Other specified diabetes mellitus with proliferative diabetic retinopathy with macular edema
E13.359 Other specified diabetes mellitus with proliferative diabetic retinopathy without macular edema

E13.36 Other specified diabetes mellitus with diabetic cataract

E13.39 Other specified diabetes mellitus with other diabetic ophthalmic complication

√5th **E13.4 Other specified diabetes mellitus with neurological complications**
E13.40 Other specified diabetes mellitus with diabetic neuropathy, unspecified
E13.41 Other specified diabetes mellitus with diabetic mononeuropathy
E13.42 Other specified diabetes mellitus with diabetic polyneuropathy
Other specified diabetes mellitus with diabetic neuralgia
E13.43 Other specified diabetes mellitus with diabetic autonomic (poly)neuropathy
Other specified diabetes mellitus with diabetic gastroparesis
E13.44 Other specified diabetes mellitus with diabetic amyotrophy
E13.49 Other specified diabetes mellitus with other diabetic neurological complication

√5th **E13.5 Other specified diabetes mellitus with circulatory complications**
E13.51 Other specified diabetes mellitus with diabetic peripheral angiopathy without gangrene
E13.52 Other specified diabetes mellitus with diabetic peripheral angiopathy with gangrene
Other specified diabetes mellitus with diabetic gangrene
E13.59 Other specified diabetes mellitus with other circulatory complications

√5th **E13.6 Other specified diabetes mellitus with other specified complications**

√6th **E13.61 Other specified diabetes mellitus with diabetic arthropathy**
E13.610 Other specified diabetes mellitus with diabetic neuropathic arthropathy
Other specified diabetes mellitus with Charcôt's joints
E13.618 Other specified diabetes mellitus with other diabetic arthropathy

√6th **E13.62 Other specified diabetes mellitus with skin complications**
E13.620 Other specified diabetes mellitus with diabetic dermatitis
Other specified diabetes mellitus with diabetic necrobiosis lipoidica
E13.621 Other specified diabetes mellitus with foot ulcer
Use additional code to identify site of ulcer (L97.4-, L97.5-)
E13.622 Other specified diabetes mellitus with other skin ulcer
Use additional code to identify site of ulcer (L97.1-L97.9, L98.41-L98.49)
E13.628 Other specified diabetes mellitus with other skin complications

√6th **E13.63 Other specified diabetes mellitus with oral complications**
E13.630 Other specified diabetes mellitus with periodontal disease
E13.638 Other specified diabetes mellitus with other oral complications

√6th **E13.64 Other specified diabetes mellitus with hypoglycemia**
E13.641 Other specified diabetes mellitus with hypoglycemia with coma
E13.649 Other specified diabetes mellitus with hypoglycemia without coma

E13.65 Other specified diabetes mellitus with hyperglycemia

E13.69 Other specified diabetes mellitus with other specified complication
Use additional code to identify complication

E13.8 Other specified diabetes mellitus with unspecified complications

E13.9 Other specified diabetes mellitus without complications

Other disorders of glucose regulation and pancreatic internal secretion (E15-E16)

E15 Nondiabetic hypoglycemic coma
INCLUDES drug-induced insulin coma in nondiabetic
hyperinsulinism with hypoglycemic coma
hypoglycemic coma NOS

√4th **E16 Other disorders of pancreatic internal secretion**

E16.0 Drug-induced hypoglycemia without coma
Use additional code for adverse effect, if applicable, to identify drug (T36-T50 with fifth or sixth character 5)

E16.1 Other hypoglycemia
Functional hyperinsulinism
Functional nonhyperinsulinemic hypoglycemia
Hyperinsulinism NOS
Hyperplasia of pancreatic islet beta cells NOS
EXCLUDES 1 *hypoglycemia in infant of diabetic mother (P70.1)*
neonatal hypoglycemia (P70.4)

E16.2 Hypoglycemia, unspecified

E16.3 Increased secretion of glucagon
Hyperplasia of pancreatic endocrine cells with glucagon excess

E16.4 Increased secretion of gastrin
Hypergastrinemia
Hyperplasia of pancreatic endocrine cells with gastrin excess
Zollinger-Ellison syndrome

E16.8 Other specified disorders of pancreatic internal secretion
Increased secretion from endocrine pancreas of growth hormone-releasing hormone
Increased secretion from endocrine pancreas of pancreatic polypeptide
Increased secretion from endocrine pancreas of somatostatin
Increased secretion from endocrine pancreas of vasoactive-intestinal polypeptide

E16.9 Disorder of pancreatic internal secretion, unspecified
Islet-cell hyperplasia NOS
Pancreatic endocrine cell hyperplasia NOS

Disorders of other endocrine glands (E20-E35)

EXCLUDES 1 *galactorrhea (N64.3)*
gynecomastia (N62)

√4th **E20 Hypoparathyroidism**
EXCLUDES 1 *Di George's syndrome (D82.1)*
postprocedural hypoparathyroidism (E89.2)
tetany NOS (R29.0)
transitory neonatal hypoparathyroidism (P71.4)

E20.0 Idiopathic hypoparathyroidism

E20.1 Pseudohypoparathyroidism

E20.8 Other hypoparathyroidism

E20.9 Hypoparathyroidism, unspecified
Parathyroid tetany

✓4th E21 Hyperparathyroidism and other disorders of parathyroid gland
EXCLUDES 1 *adult osteomalacia (M83.-)*
ectopic hyperparathyroidism (E34.2)
familial hypocalciuric hypercalcemia (E83.52)
hungry bone syndrome (E83.81)
infantile and juvenile osteomalacia (E55.0)

E21.0 Primary hyperparathyroidism
Hyperplasia of parathyroid
Osteitis fibrosa cystica generalisata [von Recklinghausen's disease of bone]

E21.1 Secondary hyperparathyroidism, not elsewhere classified
EXCLUDES 1 *secondary hyperparathyroidism of renal origin (N25.81)*

E21.2 Other hyperparathyroidism
Tertiary hyperparathyroidism
EXCLUDES 1 *familial hypocalciuric hypercalcemia (E83.52)*

E21.3 Hyperparathyroidism, unspecified

E21.4 Other specified disorders of parathyroid gland

E21.5 Disorder of parathyroid gland, unspecified

✓4th E22 Hyperfunction of pituitary gland
EXCLUDES 1 *Cushing's syndrome (E24.-)*
Nelson's syndrome (E24.1)
overproduction of ACTH not associated with Cushing's disease (E27.0)
overproduction of pituitary ACTH (E24.0)
overproduction of thyroid-stimulating hormone (E05.8-)

E22.0 Acromegaly and pituitary gigantism
Overproduction of growth hormone
EXCLUDES 1 *constitutional gigantism (E34.4)*
constitutional tall stature (E34.4)
increased secretion from endocrine pancreas of growth hormone-releasing hormone (E16.8)

E22.1 Hyperprolactinemia
Use additional code for adverse effect, if applicable, to identify drug (T36-T50 with fifth or sixth character 5)

E22.2 Syndrome of inappropriate secretion of antidiuretic hormone

E22.8 Other hyperfunction of pituitary gland
Central precocious puberty

E22.9 Hyperfunction of pituitary gland, unspecified

✓4th E23 Hypofunction and other disorders of the pituitary gland
INCLUDES the listed conditions whether the disorder is in the pituitary or the hypothalamus
EXCLUDES 1 *postprocedural hypopituitarism (E89.3)*

E23.0 Hypopituitarism
Fertile eunuch syndrome
Hypogonadotropic hypogonadism
Idiopathic growth hormone deficiency
Isolated deficiency of gonadotropin
Isolated deficiency of growth hormone
Isolated deficiency of pituitary hormone
Kallmann's syndrome
Lorain-Levi short stature
Necrosis of pituitary gland (postpartum)
Panhypopituitarism
Pituitary cachexia
Pituitary insufficiency NOS
Pituitary short stature
Sheehan's syndrome
Simmonds' disease

E23.1 Drug-induced hypopituitarism
Use additional code for adverse effect, if applicable, to identify drug (T36-T50 with fifth or sixth character 5)

E23.2 Diabetes insipidus
EXCLUDES 1 *nephrogenic diabetes insipidus (N25.1)*

E23.3 Hypothalamic dysfunction, not elsewhere classified
EXCLUDES 1 *Prader-Willi syndrome (Q87.1)*
Russell-Silver syndrome (Q87.1)

E23.6 Other disorders of pituitary gland
Abscess of pituitary
Adiposogenital dystrophy

E23.7 Disorder of pituitary gland, unspecified

✓4th E24 Cushing's syndrome
EXCLUDES 1 *congenital adrenal hyperplasia (E25.0)*

E24.0 Pituitary-dependent Cushing's disease
Overproduction of pituitary ACTH
Pituitary-dependent hypercorticalism

E24.1 Nelson's syndrome

E24.2 Drug-induced Cushing's syndrome
Use additional code for adverse effect, if applicable, to identify drug (T36-T50 with fifth or sixth character 5)

E24.3 Ectopic ACTH syndrome

E24.4 Alcohol-induced pseudo-Cushing's syndrome

E24.8 Other Cushing's syndrome

E24.9 Cushing's syndrome, unspecified

✓4th E25 Adrenogenital disorders
Adrenogenital syndromes, virilizing or feminizing, whether acquired or due to adrenal hyperplasia
Consequent on inborn enzyme defects in hormone synthesis
Female adrenal pseudohermaphroditism
Female heterosexual precocious pseudopuberty
Male isosexual precocious pseudopuberty
Male macrogenitosomia praecox
Male sexual precocity with adrenal hyperplasia
Male virilization (female)
EXCLUDES 1 *indeterminate sex and pseudohermaphroditism (Q56)*
chromosomal abnormalities (Q90-Q99)

E25.0 Congenital adrenogenital disorders associated with enzyme deficiency
Congenital adrenal hyperplasia
21-Hydroxylase deficiency
Salt-losing congenital adrenal hyperplasia

E25.8 Other adrenogenital disorders
Idiopathic adrenogenital disorder
Use additional code for adverse effect, if applicable, to identify drug (T36-T50 with fifth or sixth character 5)

E25.9 Adrenogenital disorder, unspecified
Adrenogenital syndrome NOS

✓4th E26 Hyperaldosteronism

✓5th E26.0 Primary hyperaldosteronism

E26.01 Conn's syndrome
Code also adrenal adenoma (D35.0)

E26.02 Glucocorticoid-remediable aldosteronism
Familial aldosteronism type I

E26.09 Other primary hyperaldosteronism
Primary aldosteronism due to adrenal hyperplasia (bilateral)

E26.1 Secondary hyperaldosteronism

✓5th E26.8 Other hyperaldosteronism

E26.81 Bartter's syndrome

E26.89 Other hyperaldosteronism

E26.9 Hyperaldosteronism, unspecified
Aldosteronism NOS
Hyperaldosteronism NOS

✓4th E27 Other disorders of adrenal gland

E27.0 Other adrenocortical overactivity
Overproduction of ACTH, not associated with Cushing's disease
Premature adrenarche
EXCLUDES 1 *Cushing's syndrome (E24.-)*

E27.1 Primary adrenocortical insufficiency
Addison's disease
Autoimmune adrenalitis
EXCLUDES 1 *Addison only phenotype adrenoleukodystrophy (E71.528)*
amyloidosis (E85.-)
tuberculous Addison's disease (A18.7)
Waterhouse-Friderichsen syndrome (A39.1)

E27.2 Addisonian crisis
Adrenal crisis
Adrenocortical crisis

E27.3 Drug-induced adrenocortical insufficiency
Use additional code for adverse effect, if applicable, to identify drug (T36-T50 with fifth or sixth character 5)

✓5th E27.4 Other and unspecified adrenocortical insufficiency
EXCLUDES 1 *adrenoleukodystrophy [Addison-Schilder] (E71.528)*
Waterhouse-Friderichsen syndrome (A39.1)

E27.40 Unspecified adrenocortical insufficiency
Adrenocortical insufficiency NOS
Hypoaldosteronism

E27.49 Other adrenocortical insufficiency
Adrenal hemorrhage
Adrenal infarction

E27.5 Adrenomedullary hyperfunction
Adrenomedullary hyperplasia
Catecholamine hypersecretion

E27.8 Other specified disorders of adrenal gland
Abnormality of cortisol-binding globulin

E27.9 Disorder of adrenal gland, unspecified

✓4th **E28 Ovarian dysfunction**
EXCLUDES 1 *isolated gonadotropin deficiency (E23.0)*
postprocedural ovarian failure (E89.4-)

E28.0 Estrogen excess
Use additional code for adverse effect, if applicable, to identify drug (T36-T50 with fifth or sixth character 5)

E28.1 Androgen excess
Hypersecretion of ovarian androgens
Use additional code for adverse effect, if applicable, to identify drug (T36-T50 with fifth or sixth character 5)

E28.2 Polycystic ovarian syndrome
Sclerocystic ovary syndrome
Stein-Leventhal syndrome

✓5th **E28.3 Primary ovarian failure**
EXCLUDES 1 *pure gonadal dysgenesis (Q99.1)*
Turner's syndrome (Q96.-)

✓6th **E28.31 Premature menopause**

E28.310 Symptomatic premature menopause
Symptoms such as flushing, sleeplessness, headache, lack of concentration, associated with premature menopause

E28.319 Asymptomatic premature menopause
Premature menopause NOS

E28.39 Other primary ovarian failure
Decreased estrogen
Resistant ovary syndrome

E28.8 Other ovarian dysfunction
Ovarian hyperfunction NOS
EXCLUDES 1 *postprocedural ovarian failure (E89.4-)*

E28.9 Ovarian dysfunction, unspecified

✓4th **E29 Testicular dysfunction**
EXCLUDES 1 *androgen insensitivity syndrome (E34.5-)*
azoospermia or oligospermia NOS (N46.0-N46.1)
isolated gonadotropin deficiency (E23.0)
Klinefelter's syndrome (Q98.0-Q98.2, Q98.4)

E29.0 Testicular hyperfunction
Hypersecretion of testicular hormones

E29.1 Testicular hypofunction
Defective biosynthesis of testicular androgen NOS
5-delta-Reductase deficiency (with male pseudohermaphroditism)
Testicular hypogonadism NOS
Use additional code for adverse effect, if applicable, to identify drug (T36-T50 with fifth or sixth character 5)
EXCLUDES 1 *postprocedural testicular hypofunction (E89.5)*

E29.8 Other testicular dysfunction

E29.9 Testicular dysfunction, unspecified

✓4th **E30 Disorders of puberty, not elsewhere classified**

E30.0 Delayed puberty
Constitutional delay of puberty
Delayed sexual development

E30.1 Precocious puberty
Precocious menstruation
EXCLUDES 1 *Albright (-McCune) (-Sternberg) syndrome (Q78.1)*
central precocious puberty (E22.8)
congenital adrenal hyperplasia (E25.0)
female heterosexual precocious pseudopuberty (E25.-)
male isosexual precocious pseudopuberty (E25.-)

E30.8 Other disorders of puberty
Premature thelarche

E30.9 Disorder of puberty, unspecified

✓4th **E31 Polyglandular dysfunction**
EXCLUDES 1 *ataxia telangiectasia [Louis-Bar] (G11.3)*
dystrophia myotonica [Steinert] (G71.11)
pseudohypoparathyroidism (E20.1)

E31.0 Autoimmune polyglandular failure
Schmidt's syndrome

E31.1 Polyglandular hyperfunction
EXCLUDES 1 *multiple endocrine adenomatosis (E31.2-)*
multiple endocrine neoplasia (E31.2-)

✓5th **E31.2 Multiple endocrine neoplasia [MEN] syndromes**
Multiple endocrine adenomatosis
Code also any associated malignancies and other conditions associated with the syndromes

E31.20 Multiple endocrine neoplasia [MEN] syndrome, unspecified
Multiple endocrine adenomatosis NOS
Multiple endocrine neoplasia [MEN] syndrome NOS

E31.21 Multiple endocrine neoplasia [MEN] type I
Wermer's syndrome

E31.22 Multiple endocrine neoplasia [MEN] type IIA
Sipple's syndrome

E31.23 Multiple endocrine neoplasia [MEN] type IIB

E31.8 Other polyglandular dysfunction

E31.9 Polyglandular dysfunction, unspecified

✓4th **E32 Diseases of thymus**
EXCLUDES 1 *aplasia or hypoplasia of thymus with immunodeficiency (D82.1)*
myasthenia gravis (G70.0)

E32.0 Persistent hyperplasia of thymus
Hypertrophy of thymus

E32.1 Abscess of thymus

E32.8 Other diseases of thymus
EXCLUDES 1 *aplasia or hypoplasia with immunodeficiency (D82.1)*
thymoma (D15.0)

E32.9 Disease of thymus, unspecified

✓4th **E34 Other endocrine disorders**
EXCLUDES 1 *pseudohypoparathyroidism (E20.1)*

E34.0 Carcinoid syndrome
NOTE May be used as an additional code to identify functional activity associated with a carcinoid tumor.

E34.1 Other hypersecretion of intestinal hormones

E34.2 Ectopic hormone secretion, not elsewhere classified
EXCLUDES 1 *ectopic ACTH syndrome (E24.3)*

E34.3 Short stature due to endocrine disorder
Constitutional short stature
Laron-type short stature
EXCLUDES 1 *achondroplastic short stature (Q77.4)*
hypochondroplastic short stature (Q77.4)
nutritional short stature (E45)
pituitary short stature (E23.0)
progeria (E34.8)
renal short stature (N25.0)
Russell-Silver syndrome (Q87.1)
short-limbed stature with immunodeficiency (D82.2)
short stature in specific dysmorphic syndromes—code to syndrome—see Alphabetical Index
short stature NOS (R62.52)

E34.4 Constitutional tall stature
Constitutional gigantism

✓5th **E34.5 Androgen insensitivity syndrome**

E34.50 Androgen insensitivity syndrome, unspecified
Androgen insensitivity NOS

E34.51 Complete androgen insensitivity syndrome
Complete androgen insensitivity
de Quervain syndrome
Goldberg-Maxwell syndrome

E34.52 Partial androgen insensitivity syndrome
Partial androgen insensitivity
Reifenstein syndrome

E34.8 Other specified endocrine disorders
Pineal gland dysfunction
Progeria
EXCLUDES 2 *pseudohypoparathyroidism (E20.1)*

E34.9 Endocrine disorder, unspecified
Endocrine disturbance NOS
Hormone disturbance NOS

E35 *Disorders of endocrine glands in diseases classified elsewhere*
Code first underlying disease, such as:
late congenital syphilis of thymus gland [Dubois disease] (A50.5)
tuberculous calcification of adrenal gland (B90.8)
EXCLUDES 1 *Echinococcus granulosus infection of thyroid gland (B67.3)*
meningococcal hemorrhagic adrenalitis (A39.1)
syphilis of endocrine gland (A52.79)
tuberculosis of adrenal gland, except calcification (A18.7)
tuberculosis of endocrine gland NEC (A18.82)
tuberculosis of thyroid gland (A18.81)
Waterhouse-Friderichsen syndrome (A39.1)

✓4th **E36 Intraoperative complications of endocrine system**
EXCLUDES 2 *postprocedural endocrine and metabolic complications and disorders, not elsewhere classified (E89.-)*

✓5th **E36.0 Intraoperative hemorrhage and hematoma of an endocrine system organ or structure complicating a procedure**
EXCLUDES 1 *intraoperative hemorrhage and hematoma of an endocrine system organ or structure due to accidental puncture or laceration during a procedure (E36.1-)*
E36.01 Intraoperative hemorrhage and hematoma of an endocrine system organ or structure complicating an endocrine system procedure
E36.02 Intraoperative hemorrhage and hematoma of an endocrine system organ or structure complicating other procedure

✓5th **E36.1 Accidental puncture and laceration of an endocrine system organ or structure during a procedure**
E36.11 Accidental puncture and laceration of an endocrine system organ or structure during an endocrine system procedure
E36.12 Accidental puncture and laceration of an endocrine system organ or structure during other procedure

E36.8 Other intraoperative complications of endocrine system
Use additional code, if applicable, to further specify disorder

Malnutrition (E40-E46)

EXCLUDES 1 *intestinal malabsorption (K90.-)*
sequelae of protein-calorie malnutrition (E64.0)
EXCLUDES 2 *nutritional anemias (D50-D53)*
starvation (T73.0)

E40 Kwashiorkor
Severe malnutrition with nutritional edema with dyspigmentation of skin and hair
EXCLUDES 1 *marasmic kwashiorkor (E42)*

E41 Nutritional marasmus
Severe malnutrition with marasmus
EXCLUDES 1 *marasmic kwashiorkor (E42)*

E42 Marasmic kwashiorkor
Intermediate form severe protein-calorie malnutrition
Severe protein-calorie malnutrition with signs of both kwashiorkor and marasmus

E43 Unspecified severe protein-calorie malnutrition
Starvation edema

✓4th **E44 Protein-calorie malnutrition of moderate and mild degree**
E44.0 Moderate protein-calorie malnutrition
E44.1 Mild protein-calorie malnutrition

E45 Retarded development following protein-calorie malnutrition
Nutritional short stature
Nutritional stunting
Physical retardation due to malnutrition

E46 Unspecified protein-calorie malnutrition
Malnutrition NOS
Protein-calorie imbalance NOS
EXCLUDES 1 *nutritional deficiency NOS (E63.9)*

Other nutritional deficiencies (E50-E64)

EXCLUDES 2 *nutritional anemias (D50-D53)*

✓4th **E50 Vitamin A deficiency**
EXCLUDES 1 *sequelae of vitamin A deficiency (E64.1)*
E50.0 Vitamin A deficiency with conjunctival xerosis
E50.1 Vitamin A deficiency with Bitot's spot and conjunctival xerosis
Bitot's spot in the young child
E50.2 Vitamin A deficiency with corneal xerosis
E50.3 Vitamin A deficiency with corneal ulceration and xerosis
E50.4 Vitamin A deficiency with keratomalacia
E50.5 Vitamin A deficiency with night blindness
E50.6 Vitamin A deficiency with xerophthalmic scars of cornea
E50.7 Other ocular manifestations of vitamin A deficiency
Xerophthalmia NOS
E50.8 Other manifestations of vitamin A deficiency
Follicular keratosis
Xeroderma
E50.9 Vitamin A deficiency, unspecified
Hypovitaminosis A NOS

✓4th **E51 Thiamine deficiency**
EXCLUDES 1 *sequelae of thiamine deficiency (E64.8)*
✓5th **E51.1 Beriberi**
E51.11 Dry beriberi
Beriberi NOS
Beriberi with polyneuropathy
E51.12 Wet beriberi
Beriberi with cardiovascular manifestations
Cardiovascular beriberi
Shoshin disease
E51.2 Wernicke's encephalopathy
E51.8 Other manifestations of thiamine deficiency
E51.9 Thiamine deficiency, unspecified

E52 Niacin deficiency [pellagra]
Niacin (-tryptophan) deficiency
Nicotinamide deficiency
Pellagra (alcoholic)
EXCLUDES 1 *sequelae of niacin deficiency (E64.8)*

✓4th **E53 Deficiency of other B group vitamins**
EXCLUDES 1 *sequelae of vitamin B deficiency (E64.8)*
E53.0 Riboflavin deficiency
Ariboflavinosis
Vitamin B2 deficiency
E53.1 Pyridoxine deficiency
Vitamin B6 deficiency
EXCLUDES 1 *pyridoxine-responsive sideroblastic anemia (D64.3)*
E53.8 Deficiency of other specified B group vitamins
Biotin deficiency
Cyanocobalamin deficiency
Folate deficiency
Folic acid deficiency
Pantothenic acid deficiency
Vitamin B12 deficiency
EXCLUDES 1 *folate deficiency anemia (D52.-)*
vitamin B12 deficiency anemia (D51.-)
E53.9 Vitamin B deficiency, unspecified

E54 Ascorbic acid deficiency
Deficiency of vitamin C
Scurvy
EXCLUDES 1 *scorbutic anemia (D53.2)*
sequelae of vitamin C deficiency (E64.2)

✓4th **E55 Vitamin D deficiency**
EXCLUDES 1 *adult osteomalacia (M83.-)*
osteoporosis (M80.-)
sequelae of rickets (E64.3)
E55.0 Rickets, active
Infantile Osteomalacia
Juvenile Osteomalacia
EXCLUDES 1 *celiac rickets (K90.0)*
Crohn's rickets (K50.-)
hereditary vitamin D-dependent rickets (E83.32)
inactive rickets (E64.3)
renal rickets (N25.0)
sequelae of rickets (E64.3)
vitamin D-resistant rickets (E83.31)
E55.9 Vitamin D deficiency, unspecified
Avitaminosis D

✓4th **E56 Other vitamin deficiencies**
EXCLUDES 1 *sequelae of other vitamin deficiencies (E64.8)*
E56.0 Deficiency of vitamin E

E56.1 Deficiency of vitamin K
EXCLUDES 1 *deficiency of coagulation factor due to vitamin K deficiency (D68.4)*
vitamin K deficiency of newborn (P53)
E56.8 Deficiency of other vitamins
E56.9 Vitamin deficiency, unspecified

E58 Dietary calcium deficiency
EXCLUDES 1 *disorders of calcium metabolism (E83.5-)*
sequelae of calcium deficiency (E64.8)

E59 Dietary selenium deficiency
Keshan disease
EXCLUDES 1 *sequelae of selenium deficiency (E64.8)*

E60 Dietary zinc deficiency

✓4th **E61 Deficiency of other nutrient elements**
Use additional code for adverse effect, if applicable, to identify drug (T36-T50 with fifth or sixth character 5)
EXCLUDES 1 *disorders of mineral metabolism (E83.-)*
iodine deficiency related thyroid disorders (E00-E02)
sequelae of malnutrition and other nutritional deficiencies (E64.-)
E61.0 Copper deficiency
E61.1 Iron deficiency
EXCLUDES 1 *iron deficiency anemia (D50.-)*
E61.2 Magnesium deficiency
E61.3 Manganese deficiency
E61.4 Chromium deficiency
E61.5 Molybdenum deficiency
E61.6 Vanadium deficiency
E61.7 Deficiency of multiple nutrient elements
E61.8 Deficiency of other specified nutrient elements
E61.9 Deficiency of nutrient element, unspecified

✓4th **E63 Other nutritional deficiencies**
EXCLUDES 1 *dehydration (E86.0)*
failure to thrive, adult (R62.7)
failure to thrive, child (R62.51)
feeding problems in newborn (P92.-)
sequelae of malnutrition and other nutritional deficiencies (E64.-)
E63.0 Essential fatty acid [EFA] deficiency
E63.1 Imbalance of constituents of food intake
E63.8 Other specified nutritional deficiencies
E63.9 Nutritional deficiency, unspecified

✓4th **E64 Sequelae of malnutrition and other nutritional deficiencies**
NOTE This category is to be used to indicate conditions in categories E43, E44, E46, E50-E63 as the cause of sequelae, which are themselves classified elsewhere. The 'sequelae' include conditions specified as such; they also include the late effects of diseases classifiable to the above categories if the disease itself is no longer present
Code first condition resulting from (sequela) of malnutrition and other nutritional deficiencies
E64.0 Sequelae of protein-calorie malnutrition
EXCLUDES 2 *retarded development following protein-calorie malnutrition (E45)*
E64.1 Sequelae of vitamin A deficiency
E64.2 Sequelae of vitamin C deficiency
E64.3 Sequelae of rickets
E64.8 Sequelae of other nutritional deficiencies
E64.9 Sequelae of unspecified nutritional deficiency

Overweight, obesity and other hyperalimentation (E65-E68)

E65 Localized adiposity
Fat pad

✓4th **E66 Overweight and obesity**
Code first obesity complicating pregnancy, childbirth and the puerperium, if applicable (O99.21-)
Use additional code to identify body mass index (BMI), if known (Z68.-)
EXCLUDES 1 *adiposogenital dystrophy (E23.6)*
lipomatosis NOS (E88.2)
lipomatosis dolorosa [Dercum] (E88.2)
Prader-Willi syndrome (Q87.1)
✓5th **E66.0 Obesity due to excess calories**
E66.01 Morbid (severe) obesity due to excess calories
EXCLUDES 1 *morbid (severe) obesity with alveolar hypoventilation (E66.2)*
E66.09 Other obesity due to excess calories
E66.1 Drug-induced obesity
Use additional code for adverse effect, if applicable, to identify drug (T36-T50 with fifth or sixth character 5)
E66.2 Morbid (severe) obesity with alveolar hypoventilation
Pickwickian syndrome
E66.3 Overweight
E66.8 Other obesity
E66.9 Obesity, unspecified
Obesity NOS

✓4th **E67 Other hyperalimentation**
EXCLUDES 1 *hyperalimentation NOS (R63.2)*
sequelae of hyperalimentation (E68)
E67.0 Hypervitaminosis A
E67.1 Hypercarotinemia
E67.2 Megavitamin-B6 syndrome
E67.3 Hypervitaminosis D
E67.8 Other specified hyperalimentation

E68 Sequelae of hyperalimentation
Code first condition resulting from (sequela) of hyperalimentation

Metabolic disorders (E70-E88)

EXCLUDES 1 *androgen insensitivity syndrome (E34.5-)*
congenital adrenal hyperplasia (E25.0)
Ehlers-Danlos syndrome (Q79.6)
hemolytic anemias attributable to enzyme disorders (D55.-)
Marfan's syndrome (Q87.4)
5-alpha-reductase deficiency (E29.1)

✓4th **E70 Disorders of aromatic amino-acid metabolism**
E70.0 Classical phenylketonuria
E70.1 Other hyperphenylalaninemias
✓5th **E70.2 Disorders of tyrosine metabolism**
EXCLUDES 1 *transitory tyrosinemia of newborn (P74.5)*
E70.20 Disorder of tyrosine metabolism, unspecified
E70.21 Tyrosinemia
Hypertyrosinemia
E70.29 Other disorders of tyrosine metabolism
Alkaptonuria
Ochronosis
✓5th **E70.3 Albinism**
E70.30 Albinism, unspecified
✓6th **E70.31 Ocular albinism**
E70.310 X-linked ocular albinism
E70.311 Autosomal recessive ocular albinism
E70.318 Other ocular albinism
E70.319 Ocular albinism, unspecified
✓6th **E70.32 Oculocutaneous albinism**
EXCLUDES 1 *Chediak-Higashi syndrome (E70.330)*
Hermansky-Pudlak syndrome (E70.331)
E70.320 Tyrosinase negative oculocutaneous albinism
Albinism I
Oculocutaneous albinism ty-neg
E70.321 Tyrosinase positive oculocutaneous albinism
Albinism II
Oculocutaneous albinism ty-pos
E70.328 Other oculocutaneous albinism
Cross syndrome
E70.329 Oculocutaneous albinism, unspecified
✓6th **E70.33 Albinism with hematologic abnormality**
E70.330 Chediak-Higashi syndrome
E70.331 Hermansky-Pudlak syndrome
E70.338 Other albinism with hematologic abnormality
E70.339 Albinism with hematologic abnormality, unspecified
E70.39 Other specified albinism
Piebaldism
✓5th **E70.4 Disorders of histidine metabolism**
E70.40 Disorders of histidine metabolism, unspecified
E70.41 Histidinemia
E70.49 Other disorders of histidine metabolism
E70.5 Disorders of tryptophan metabolism

E70.8 **Other disorders of aromatic amino-acid metabolism**
E70.9 **Disorder of aromatic amino-acid metabolism, unspecified**

4th **E71 Disorders of branched-chain amino-acid metabolism and fatty-acid metabolism**
E71.0 **Maple-syrup-urine disease**
5th E71.1 **Other disorders of branched-chain amino-acid metabolism**
6th E71.11 **Branched-chain organic acidurias**
E71.110 **Isovaleric acidemia**
E71.111 **3-methylglutaconic aciduria**
E71.118 **Other branched-chain organic acidurias**
6th E71.12 **Disorders of propionate metabolism**
E71.120 **Methylmalonic acidemia**
E71.121 **Propionic acidemia**
E71.128 **Other disorders of propionate metabolism**
E71.19 **Other disorders of branched-chain amino-acid metabolism**
Hyperleucine-isoleucinemia
Hypervalinemia
E71.2 **Disorder of branched-chain amino-acid metabolism, unspecified**
5th E71.3 **Disorders of fatty-acid metabolism**
EXCLUDES 1 *peroxisomal disorders (E71.5)*
Refsum's disease (G60.1)
Schilder's disease (G37.0)
EXCLUDES 2 *carnitine deficiency due to inborn error of metabolism (E71.42)*
E71.30 **Disorder of fatty-acid metabolism, unspecified**
6th E71.31 **Disorders of fatty-acid oxidation**
E71.310 **Long chain/very long chain acyl CoA dehydrogenase deficiency**
LCAD
VLCAD
E71.311 **Medium chain acyl CoA dehydrogenase deficiency**
MCAD
E71.312 **Short chain acyl CoA dehydrogenase deficiency**
SCAD
E71.313 **Glutaric aciduria type II**
Glutaric aciduria type II A
Glutaric aciduria type II B
Glutaric aciduria type II C
EXCLUDES 1 *glutaric aciduria (type 1) NOS (E72.3)*
E71.314 **Muscle carnitine palmitoyltransferase deficiency**
E71.318 **Other disorders of fatty-acid oxidation**
E71.32 **Disorders of ketone metabolism**
E71.39 **Other disorders of fatty-acid metabolism**
5th E71.4 **Disorders of carnitine metabolism**
EXCLUDES 1 *muscle carnitine palmitoyltransferase deficiency (E71.314)*
E71.40 **Disorder of carnitine metabolism, unspecified**
E71.41 **Primary carnitine deficiency**
E71.42 **Carnitine deficiency due to inborn errors of metabolism**
Code also associated inborn error or metabolism
E71.43 **Iatrogenic carnitine deficiency**
Carnitine deficiency due to:
hemodialysis
valproic acid therapy
6th E71.44 **Other secondary carnitine deficiency**
E71.440 **Ruvalcaba-Myhre-Smith syndrome**
E71.448 **Other secondary carnitine deficiency**
5th E71.5 **Peroxisomal disorders**
EXCLUDES 1 *Schilder's disease (G37.0)*
E71.50 **Peroxisomal disorder, unspecified**
6th E71.51 **Disorders of peroxisome biogenesis**
Group 1 peroxisomal disorders
EXCLUDES 1 *Refsum's disease (G60.1)*
E71.510 **Zellweger syndrome**
E71.511 **Neonatal adrenoleukodystrophy**
EXCLUDES 1 *X-linked adrenoleukodystrophy (E71.52-)*
E71.518 **Other disorders of peroxisome biogenesis**
6th E71.52 **X-linked adrenoleukodystrophy**
E71.520 **Childhood cerebral X-linked adrenoleukodystrophy**
E71.521 **Adolescent X-linked adrenoleukodystrophy**
E71.522 **Adrenomyeloneuropathy**
E71.528 **Other X-linked adrenoleukodystrophy**
Addison only phenotype adrenoleukodystrophy
Addison-Schilder adrenoleukodystrophy
E71.529 **X-linked adrenoleukodystrophy, unspecified type**
E71.53 **Other group 2 peroxisomal disorders**
6th E71.54 **Other peroxisomal disorders**
E71.540 **Rhizomelic chondrodysplasia punctata**
EXCLUDES 1 *chondrodysplasia punctata NOS (Q77.3)*
E71.541 **Zellweger-like syndrome**
E71.542 **Other group 3 peroxisomal disorders**
E71.548 **Other peroxisomal disorders**

4th **E72 Other disorders of amino-acid metabolism**
EXCLUDES 1 *disorders of:*
aromatic amino-acid metabolism (E70.-)
branched-chain amino-acid metabolism (E71.0-E71.2)
fatty-acid metabolism (E71.3)
purine and pyrimidine metabolism (E79.-)
gout (M1A.-, M10.-)
5th E72.0 **Disorders of amino-acid transport**
EXCLUDES 1 *disorders of tryptophan metabolism (E70.5)*
E72.00 **Disorders of amino-acid transport, unspecified**
E72.01 **Cystinuria**
E72.02 **Hartnup's disease**
E72.03 **Lowe's syndrome**
Use additional code for associated glaucoma (H42)
E72.04 **Cystinosis**
Fanconi (-de Toni) (-Debré) syndrome with cystinosis
EXCLUDES 1 *Fanconi (-de Toni) (-Debré) syndrome without cystinosis (E72.09)*
E72.09 **Other disorders of amino-acid transport**
Fanconi (-de Toni) (-Debré) syndrome, unspecified
5th E72.1 **Disorders of sulfur-bearing amino-acid metabolism**
EXCLUDES 1 *cystinosis (E72.04)*
cystinuria (E72.01)
transcobalamin II deficiency (D51.2)
E72.10 **Disorders of sulfur-bearing amino-acid metabolism, unspecified**
E72.11 **Homocystinuria**
Cystathionine synthase deficiency
E72.12 **Methylenetetrahydrofolate reductase deficiency**
E72.19 **Other disorders of sulfur-bearing amino-acid metabolism**
Cystathioninuria
Methioninemia
Sulfite oxidase deficiency
5th E72.2 **Disorders of urea cycle metabolism**
EXCLUDES 1 *disorders of ornithine metabolism (E72.4)*
E72.20 **Disorder of urea cycle metabolism, unspecified**
Hyperammonemia
EXCLUDES 1 *hyperammonemia- hyperornithinemia-homocitrullinemia syndrome (E72.4)*
transient hyperammonemia of newborn (P74.6)
E72.21 **Argininemia**
E72.22 **Arginosuccinic aciduria**
E72.23 **Citrullinemia**
E72.29 **Other disorders of urea cycle metabolism**
E72.3 **Disorders of lysine and hydroxylysine metabolism**
Glutaric aciduria NOS
Glutaric aciduria (type I)
Hydroxylysinemia
Hyperlysinemia
EXCLUDES 1 *glutaric aciduria type II (E71.313)*
Refsum's disease (G60.1)
Zellweger syndrome (E71.510)

E72.4 Disorders of ornithine metabolism
Hyperammonemia-hyperornithinemia-homocitrullinemia syndrome
Ornithinemia (types I, II)
Ornithine transcarbamylase deficiency
EXCLUDES 1 *hereditary choroidal dystrophy (H31.2-)*

✓5th **E72.5 Disorders of glycine metabolism**
E72.50 Disorder of glycine metabolism, unspecified
E72.51 Non-ketotic hyperglycinemia
E72.52 Trimethylaminuria
E72.53 Hyperoxaluria
Oxalosis
Oxaluria
E72.59 Other disorders of glycine metabolism
D-glycericacidemia
Hyperhydroxyprolinemia
Hyperprolinemia (types I, II)
Sarcosinemia

E72.8 Other specified disorders of amino-acid metabolism
Disorders of beta-amino-acid metabolism
Disorders of gamma-glutamyl cycle

E72.9 Disorder of amino-acid metabolism, unspecified

✓4th **E73 Lactose intolerance**
E73.0 Congenital lactase deficiency
E73.1 Secondary lactase deficiency
E73.8 Other lactose intolerance
E73.9 Lactose intolerance, unspecified

✓4th **E74 Other disorders of carbohydrate metabolism**
EXCLUDES 1 *diabetes mellitus (E08-E13)*
hypoglycemia NOS (E16.2)
increased secretion of glucagon (E16.3)
mucopolysaccharidosis (E76.0-E76.3)

✓5th **E74.0 Glycogen storage disease**
E74.00 Glycogen storage disease, unspecified
E74.01 von Gierke disease
Type I glycogen storage disease
E74.02 Pompe disease
Cardiac glycogenosis
Type II glycogen storage disease
E74.03 Cori disease
Forbes disease
Type III glycogen storage disease
E74.04 McArdle disease
Type V glycogen storage disease
E74.09 Other glycogen storage disease
Andersen disease
Hers disease
Tauri disease
Glycogen storage disease, types 0, IV, VI-XI
Liver phosphorylase deficiency
Muscle phosphofructokinase deficiency

✓5th **E74.1 Disorders of fructose metabolism**
EXCLUDES 1 *muscle phosphofructokinase deficiency (E74.09)*
E74.10 Disorder of fructose metabolism, unspecified
E74.11 Essential fructosuria
Fructokinase deficiency
E74.12 Hereditary fructose intolerance
Fructosemia
E74.19 Other disorders of fructose metabolism
Fructose-1, 6-diphosphatase deficiency

✓5th **E74.2 Disorders of galactose metabolism**
E74.20 Disorders of galactose metabolism, unspecified
E74.21 Galactosemia
E74.29 Other disorders of galactose metabolism
Galactokinase deficiency

✓5th **E74.3 Other disorders of intestinal carbohydrate absorption**
EXCLUDES 2 *lactose intolerance (E73.-)*
E74.31 Sucrase-isomaltase deficiency
E74.39 Other disorders of intestinal carbohydrate absorption
Disorder of intestinal carbohydrate absorption NOS
Glucose-galactose malabsorption
Sucrase deficiency

E74.4 Disorders of pyruvate metabolism and gluconeogenesis
Deficiency of phosphoenolpyruvate carboxykinase
Deficiency of pyruvate carboxylase
Deficiency of pyruvate dehydrogenase
EXCLUDES 1 *disorders of pyruvate metabolism and gluconeogenesis with anemia (D55.-)*
Leigh's syndrome (G31.82)

E74.8 Other specified disorders of carbohydrate metabolism
Essential pentosuria
Renal glycosuria

E74.9 Disorder of carbohydrate metabolism, unspecified

✓4th **E75 Disorders of sphingolipid metabolism and other lipid storage disorders**
EXCLUDES 1 *mucolipidosis, types I-III (E77.0-E77.1)*
Refsum's disease (G60.1)

✓5th **E75.0 GM2 gangliosidosis**
E75.00 GM2 gangliosidosis, unspecified
E75.01 Sandhoff disease
E75.02 Tay-Sachs disease
E75.09 Other GM2 gangliosidosis
Adult GM2 gangliosidosis
Juvenile GM2 gangliosidosis

✓5th **E75.1 Other and unspecified gangliosidosis**
E75.10 Unspecified gangliosidosis
Gangliosidosis NOS
E75.11 Mucolipidosis IV
E75.19 Other gangliosidosis
GM1 gangliosidosis
GM3 gangliosidosis

✓5th **E75.2 Other sphingolipidosis**
EXCLUDES 1 *adrenoleukodystrophy [Addison-Schilder] (E71.528)*
E75.21 Fabry (-Anderson) disease
E75.22 Gaucher disease
E75.23 Krabbe disease
✓6th **E75.24 Niemann-Pick disease**
E75.240 Niemann-Pick disease type A
E75.241 Niemann-Pick disease type B
E75.242 Niemann-Pick disease type C
E75.243 Niemann-Pick disease type D
E75.248 Other Niemann-Pick disease
E75.249 Niemann-Pick disease, unspecified
E75.25 Metachromatic leukodystrophy
E75.29 Other sphingolipidosis
Farber's syndrome
Sulfatase deficiency
Sulfatide lipidosis

E75.3 Sphingolipidosis, unspecified
E75.4 Neuronal ceroid lipofuscinosis
Batten disease
Bielschowsky-Jansky disease
Kufs disease
Spielmeyer-Vogt disease
E75.5 Other lipid storage disorders
Cerebrotendinous cholesterosis [van Bogaert-Scherer-Epstein]
Wolman's disease
E75.6 Lipid storage disorder, unspecified

✓4th **E76 Disorders of glycosaminoglycan metabolism**
✓5th **E76.0 Mucopolysaccharidosis, type I**
E76.01 Hurler's syndrome
E76.02 Hurler-Scheie syndrome
E76.03 Scheie's syndrome
E76.1 Mucopolysaccharidosis, type II
Hunter's syndrome
✓5th **E76.2 Other mucopolysaccharidoses**
✓6th **E76.21 Morquio mucopolysaccharidoses**
E76.210 Morquio A mucopolysaccharidoses
Classic Morquio syndrome
Morquio syndrome A
Mucopolysaccharidosis, type IVA
E76.211 Morquio B mucopolysaccharidoses
Morquio-like mucopolysaccharidoses
Morquio-like syndrome
Morquio syndrome B
Mucopolysaccharidosis, type IVB

E76.219 **Morquio mucopolysaccharidoses, unspecified**
Morquio syndrome
Mucopolysaccharidosis, type IV

E76.22 **Sanfilippo mucopolysaccharidoses**
Mucopolysaccharidosis, type III (A) (B) (C) (D)
Sanfilippo A syndrome
Sanfilippo B syndrome
Sanfilippo C syndrome
Sanfilippo D syndrome

E76.29 **Other mucopolysaccharidoses**
beta-Glucuronidase deficiency
Maroteaux-Lamy (mild) (severe) syndrome
Mucopolysaccharidosis, types VI, VII

E76.3 **Mucopolysaccharidosis, unspecified**

E76.8 **Other disorders of glucosaminoglycan metabolism**

E76.9 **Glucosaminoglycan metabolism disorder, unspecified**

✓4th **E77 Disorders of glycoprotein metabolism**

E77.Ø **Defects in post-translational modification of lysosomal enzymes**
Mucolipidosis II [I-cell disease]
Mucolipidosis III [pseudo-Hurler polydystrophy]

E77.1 **Defects in glycoprotein degradation**
Aspartylglucosaminuria
Fucosidosis
Mannosidosis
Sialidosis [mucolipidosis I]

E77.8 **Other disorders of glycoprotein metabolism**

E77.9 **Disorder of glycoprotein metabolism, unspecified**

✓4th **E78 Disorders of lipoprotein metabolism and other lipidemias**

EXCLUDES 1 *sphingolipidosis (E75.Ø-E75.3)*

E78.Ø **Pure hypercholesterolemia**
Familial hypercholesterolemia
Fredrickson's hyperlipoproteinemia, type IIa
Hyperbetalipoproteinemia
Hyperlipidemia, Group A
Low-density-lipoprotein-type [LDL] hyperlipoproteinemia

E78.1 **Pure hyperglyceridemia**
Elevated fasting triglycerides
Endogenous hyperglyceridemia
Fredrickson's hyperlipoproteinemia, type IV
Hyperlipidemia, group B
Hyperprebetalipoproteinemia
Very-low-density-lipoprotein-type [VLDL] hyperlipoproteinemia

E78.2 **Mixed hyperlipidemia**
Broad- or floating-betalipoproteinemia
Combined hyperlipidemia NOS
Elevated cholesterol with elevated triglycerides NEC
Fredrickson's hyperlipoproteinemia, type IIb or III
Hyperbetalipoproteinemia with prebetalipoproteinemia
Hypercholesteremia with endogenous hyperglyceridemia
Hyperlipidemia, group C
Tubo-eruptive xanthoma
Xanthoma tuberosum

EXCLUDES 1 *cerebrotendinous cholesterosis [van Bogaert-Scherer- Epstein] (E75.5)*
familial combined hyperlipidemia (E78.4)

E78.3 **Hyperchylomicronemia**
Chylomicron retention disease
Fredrickson's hyperlipoproteinemia, type I or V
Hyperlipidemia, group D
Mixed hyperglyceridemia

E78.4 **Other hyperlipidemia**
Familial combined hyperlipidemia

E78.5 **Hyperlipidemia, unspecified**

E78.6 **Lipoprotein deficiency**
Abetalipoproteinemia
Depressed HDL cholesterol
High-density lipoprotein deficiency
Hypoalphalipoproteinemia
Hypobetalipoproteinemia (familial)
Lecithin cholesterol acyltransferase deficiency
Tangier disease

✓5th E78.7 **Disorders of bile acid and cholesterol metabolism**

EXCLUDES 1 *Niemann-Pick disease type C (E75.242)*

E78.7Ø **Disorder of bile acid and cholesterol metabolism, unspecified**

E78.71 **Barth syndrome**

E78.72 **Smith-Lemli-Opitz syndrome**

E78.79 **Other disorders of bile acid and cholesterol metabolism**

✓5th E78.8 **Other disorders of lipoprotein metabolism**

E78.81 **Lipoid dermatoarthritis**

E78.89 **Other lipoprotein metabolism disorders**

E78.9 **Disorder of lipoprotein metabolism, unspecified**

✓4th **E79 Disorders of purine and pyrimidine metabolism**

EXCLUDES 1 *Ataxia-telangiectasia (G11.3)*
Bloom's syndrome (Q82.8)
Cockayne's syndrome (Q87.1)
calculus of kidney (N2Ø.Ø)
combined immunodeficiency disorders (D81.-)
Fanconi's anemia (D61.Ø9)
gout (M1A.-, M1Ø.-)
orotaciduric anemia (D53.Ø)
progeria (E34.8)
Werner's syndrome (E34.8)
xeroderma pigmentosum (Q82.1)

E79.Ø **Hyperuricemia without signs of inflammatory arthritis and tophaceous disease**
Asymptomatic hyperuricemia

E79.1 **Lesch-Nyhan syndrome**
HGPRT deficiency

E79.2 **Myoadenylate deaminase deficiency**

E79.8 **Other disorders of purine and pyrimidine metabolism**
Hereditary xanthinuria

E79.9 **Disorder of purine and pyrimidine metabolism, unspecified**

✓4th **E8Ø Disorders of porphyrin and bilirubin metabolism**

INCLUDES defects of catalase and peroxidase

E8Ø.Ø **Hereditary erythropoietic porphyria**
Congenital erythropoietic porphyria
Erythropoietic protoporphyria

E8Ø.1 **Porphyria cutanea tarda**

✓5th E8Ø.2 **Other and unspecified porphyria**

E8Ø.2Ø **Unspecified porphyria**
Porphyria NOS

E8Ø.21 **Acute intermittent (hepatic) porphyria**

E8Ø.29 **Other porphyria**
Hereditary coproporphyria

E8Ø.3 **Defects of catalase and peroxidase**
Acatalasia [Takahara]

E8Ø.4 **Gilbert syndrome**

E8Ø.5 **Crigler-Najjar syndrome**

E8Ø.6 **Other disorders of bilirubin metabolism**
Dubin-Johnson syndrome
Rotor's syndrome

E8Ø.7 **Disorder of bilirubin metabolism, unspecified**

✓4th **E83 Disorders of mineral metabolism**

EXCLUDES 1 *dietary mineral deficiency (E58-E61)*
parathyroid disorders (E2Ø-E21)
vitamin D deficiency (E55.-)

✓5th E83.Ø **Disorders of copper metabolism**

E83.ØØ **Disorder of copper metabolism, unspecified**

E83.Ø1 **Wilson's disease**
Code also associated Kayser Fleischer ring (H18.Ø4-)

E83.Ø9 **Other disorders of copper metabolism**
Menkes' (kinky hair) (steely hair) disease

✓5th E83.1 **Disorders of iron metabolism**

EXCLUDES 1 *iron deficiency anemia (D5Ø.-)*
sideroblastic anemia (D64.Ø-D64.3)

E83.1Ø **Disorder of iron metabolism, unspecified**

✓6th E83.11 **Hemochromatosis**

E83.11Ø **Hereditary hemochromatosis**
Bronzed diabetes
Pigmentary cirrhosis (of liver)
Primary (hereditary) hemochromatosis

E83.111 **Hemochromatosis due to repeated red blood cell transfusions**
Iron overload due to repeated red blood cell transfusions
Transfusion (red blood cell) associated hemochromatosis

E83.118 **Other hemochromatosis**

E83.119 **Hemochromatosis, unspecified**

E83.19 Other disorders of iron metabolism
Use additional code, if applicable, for idiopathic pulmonary hemosiderosis (J84.03)

E83.2 Disorders of zinc metabolism
Acrodermatitis enteropathica

✓5th **E83.3 Disorders of phosphorus metabolism and phosphatases**
EXCLUDES 1 *adult osteomalacia (M83.-)*
osteoporosis (M80.-)

E83.30 Disorder of phosphorus metabolism, unspecified

E83.31 Familial hypophosphatemia
Vitamin D-resistant osteomalacia
Vitamin D-resistant rickets
EXCLUDES 1 *vitamin D-deficiency rickets (E55.0)*

E83.32 Hereditary vitamin D-dependent rickets (type 1) (type 2)
25-hydroxyvitamin D 1-alpha-hydroxylase deficiency
Pseudovitamin D deficiency
Vitamin D receptor defect

E83.39 Other disorders of phosphorus metabolism
Acid phosphatase deficiency
Hypophosphatasia

✓5th **E83.4 Disorders of magnesium metabolism**

E83.40 Disorders of magnesium metabolism, unspecified

E83.41 Hypermagnesemia

E83.42 Hypomagnesemia

E83.49 Other disorders of magnesium metabolism

✓5th **E83.5 Disorders of calcium metabolism**
EXCLUDES 1 *chondrocalcinosis (M11.1-M11.2)*
hungry bone syndrome (E83.81)
hyperparathyroidism (E21.0-E21.3)

E83.50 Unspecified disorder of calcium metabolism

E83.51 Hypocalcemia

E83.52 Hypercalcemia
Familial hypocalciuric hypercalcemia

E83.59 Other disorders of calcium metabolism
Idiopathic hypercalciuria

✓5th **E83.8 Other disorders of mineral metabolism**

E83.81 Hungry bone syndrome

E83.89 Other disorders of mineral metabolism

E83.9 Disorder of mineral metabolism, unspecified

✓4th **E84 Cystic fibrosis**
INCLUDES mucoviscidosis

E84.0 Cystic fibrosis with pulmonary manifestations
Use additional code to identify any infectious organism present, such as:
Pseudomonas (B96.5)

✓5th **E84.1 Cystic fibrosis with intestinal manifestations**

E84.11 Meconium ileus in cystic fibrosis
EXCLUDES 1 *meconium ileus not due to cystic fibrosis (P76.0)*

E84.19 Cystic fibrosis with other intestinal manifestations
Distal intestinal obstruction syndrome

E84.8 Cystic fibrosis with other manifestations

E84.9 Cystic fibrosis, unspecified

✓4th **E85 Amyloidosis**
EXCLUDES 1 *Alzheimer's disease (G30.0-)*

E85.0 Non-neuropathic heredofamilial amyloidosis
Familial Mediterranean fever
Hereditary amyloid nephropathy

E85.1 Neuropathic heredofamilial amyloidosis
Amyloid polyneuropathy (Portuguese)

E85.2 Heredofamilial amyloidosis, unspecified

E85.3 Secondary systemic amyloidosis
Hemodialysis-associated amyloidosis

E85.4 Organ-limited amyloidosis
Localized amyloidosis

E85.8 Other amyloidosis

E85.9 Amyloidosis, unspecified

✓4th **E86 Volume depletion**
EXCLUDES 1 *dehydration of newborn (P74.1)*
hypovolemic shock NOS (R57.1)
postprocedural hypovolemic shock (T81.11)
traumatic hypovolemic shock (T79.4)

E86.0 Dehydration

E86.1 Hypovolemia
Depletion of volume of plasma

E86.9 Volume depletion, unspecified

✓4th **E87 Other disorders of fluid, electrolyte and acid-base balance**
EXCLUDES 1 *diabetes insipidus (E23.2)*
electrolyte imbalance associated with hyperemesis gravidarum (O21.1)
electrolyte imbalance following ectopic or molar pregnancy (O08.5)
familial periodic paralysis (G72.3)

E87.0 Hyperosmolality and hypernatremia
Sodium [Na] excess
Sodium [Na] overload

E87.1 Hypo-osmolality and hyponatremia
Sodium [Na] deficiency
EXCLUDES 1 *syndrome of inappropriate secretion of antidiuretic hormone (E22.2)*

E87.2 Acidosis
Acidosis NOS
Lactic acidosis
Metabolic acidosis
Respiratory acidosis
EXCLUDES 1 *diabetic acidosis—see categories E08-E13 with ketoacidosis*

E87.3 Alkalosis
Alkalosis NOS
Metabolic alkalosis
Respiratory alkalosis

E87.4 Mixed disorder of acid-base balance

E87.5 Hyperkalemia
Potassium [K] excess
Potassium [K] overload

E87.6 Hypokalemia
Potassium [K] deficiency

✓5th **E87.7 Fluid overload**
EXCLUDES 1 *edema NOS (R60.9)*
fluid retention (R60.9)

E87.70 Fluid overload, unspecified

E87.71 Transfusion associated circulatory overload
Fluid overload due to transfusion (blood) (blood components)
TACO

E87.79 Other fluid overload

E87.8 Other disorders of electrolyte and fluid balance, not elsewhere classified
Electrolyte imbalance NOS
Hyperchloremia
Hypochloremia

✓4th **E88 Other and unspecified metabolic disorders**
Use additional codes for associated conditions
EXCLUDES 1 *histiocytosis X (chronic) (C96.6)*

✓5th **E88.0 Disorders of plasma-protein metabolism, not elsewhere classified**
EXCLUDES 1 *disorder of lipoprotein metabolism (E78.-)*
monoclonal gammopathy (of undetermined significance) (D47.2)
polyclonal hypergammaglobulinemia (D89.0)
Waldenström's macroglobulinemia (C88.0)

E88.01 Alpha-1-antitrypsin deficiency
AAT deficiency

E88.09 Other disorders of plasma-protein metabolism, not elsewhere classified
Bisalbuminemia

E88.1 Lipodystrophy, not elsewhere classified
Lipodystrophy NOS
EXCLUDES 1 *Whipple's disease (K90.81)*

E88.2 Lipomatosis, not elsewhere classified
Lipomatosis NOS
Lipomatosis (Check) dolorosa [Dercum]

E88.3 Tumor lysis syndrome
Tumor lysis syndrome (spontaneous)
Tumor lysis syndrome following antineoplastic drug chemotherapy
Use additional code for adverse effect, if applicable, to identify drug (T45.1X5)

✓5th **E88.4 Mitochondrial metabolism disorders**

EXCLUDES 1 *disorders of pyruvate metabolism (E74.4)*
Kearns-Sayre syndrome (H49.81)
Leber's disease (H47.22)
Leigh's encephalopathy (G31.82)
Mitochondrial myopathy, NEC (G71.3)
Reye's syndrome (G93.7)

E88.40 Mitochondrial metabolism disorder, unspecified

E88.41 MELAS syndrome
Mitochondrial myopathy, encephalopathy, lactic acidosis and stroke-like episodes

E88.42 MERRF syndrome
Myoclonic epilepsy associated with ragged-red fibers
Code also myoclonic epilepsy (G40.3-)

E88.49 Other mitochondrial metabolism disorders

✓5th **E88.8 Other specified metabolic disorders**

E88.81 Metabolic syndrome
Dysmetabolic syndrome X
Use additional codes for associated manifestations, such as:
obesity (E66.-)

E88.89 Other specified metabolic disorders
Launois-Bensaude adenolipomatosis
EXCLUDES 1 *adult pulmonary Langerhans cell histiocytosis (J84.82)*

E88.9 Metabolic disorder, unspecified

✓4th **E89 Postprocedural endocrine and metabolic complications and disorders, not elsewhere classified**

EXCLUDES 2 *intraoperative complications of endocrine system organ or structure (E36.0-, E36.1-, E36.8)*

E89.0 Postprocedural hypothyroidism
Postirradiation hypothyroidism
Postsurgical hypothyroidism

E89.1 Postprocedural hypoinsulinemia
Postpancreatectomy hyperglycemia
Postsurgical hypoinsulinemia
Use additional code, if applicable, to identify:
acquired absence of pancreas (Z90.41-)
diabetes mellitus (postpancreatectomy) (postprocedural) (E13.-)
insulin use (Z79.4)
EXCLUDES 1 *transient postprocedural hyperglycemia (R73.9)*
transient postprocedural hypoglycemia (E16.2)

E89.2 Postprocedural hypoparathyroidism
Parathyroprival tetany

E89.3 Postprocedural hypopituitarism
Postirradiation hypopituitarism

✓5th **E89.4 Postprocedural ovarian failure**

E89.40 Asymptomatic postprocedural ovarian failure
Postprocedural ovarian failure NOS

E89.41 Symptomatic postprocedural ovarian failure
Symptoms such as flushing, sleeplessness, headache, lack of concentration, associated with postprocedural menopause

E89.5 Postprocedural testicular hypofunction

E89.6 Postprocedural adrenocortical (-medullary) hypofunction

✓5th **E89.8 Other postprocedural endocrine and metabolic complications and disorders**

✓6th **E89.81 Postprocedural hemorrhage and hematoma of an endocrine system organ or structure following a procedure**

E89.810 Postprocedural hemorrhage and hematoma of an endocrine system organ or structure following an endocrine system procedure

E89.811 Postprocedural hemorrhage and hematoma of an endocrine system organ or structure following other procedure

E89.89 Other postprocedural endocrine and metabolic complications and disorders
Use additional code, if applicable, to further specify disorder

Chapter 5. Mental, Behavioral, and Neurodevelopmental Disorders (FØ1-F99)

INCLUDES disorders of psychological development

EXCLUDES 2 *symptoms, signs and abnormal clinical laboratory findings, not elsewhere classified (RØØ-R99)*

This chapter contains the following blocks:

FØ1-FØ9	Mental disorders due to known physiological conditions
F1Ø-F19	Mental and behavioral disorders due to psychoactive substance use
F2Ø-F29	Schizophrenia, schizotypal, delusional, and other non-mood psychotic disorders
F3Ø-F39	Mood [affective] disorders
F4Ø-F48	Anxiety, dissociative, stress-related, somatoform and other nonpsychotic mental disorders
F5Ø-F59	Behavioral syndromes associated with physiological disturbances and physical factors
F6Ø-F69	Disorders of adult personality and behavior
F7Ø-F79	Intellectual disabilities
F8Ø-F89	Pervasive and specific developmental disorders
F9Ø-F98	Behavioral and emotional disorders with onset usually occurring in childhood and adolescence
F99	Unspecified mental disorder

Mental disorders due to known physiological conditions (FØ1-FØ9)

NOTE This block comprises a range of mental disorders grouped together on the basis of their having in common a demonstrable etiology in cerebral disease, brain injury, or other insult leading to cerebral dysfunction. The dysfunction may be primary, as in diseases, injuries, and insults that affect the brain directly and selectively; or secondary, as in systemic diseases and disorders that attack the brain only as one of the multiple organs or systems of the body that are involved.

✓4th **FØ1 Vascular dementia**

Vascular dementia as a result of infarction of the brain due to vascular disease, including hypertensive cerebrovascular disease.

INCLUDES arteriosclerotic dementia

Code first the underlying physiological condition or sequelae of cerebrovascular disease.

✓5th **FØ1.5 Vascular dementia**

FØ1.5Ø Vascular dementia without behavioral disturbance

FØ1.51 Vascular dementia with behavioral disturbance

Vascular dementia with aggressive behavior
Vascular dementia with combative behavior
Vascular dementia with violent behavior
Use additional code, if applicable, to identify wandering in vascular dementia (Z91.83)

✓4th **FØ2 Dementia in other diseases classified elsewhere**

Code first the underlying physiological condition, such as:
Alzheimer's (G3Ø.-)
cerebral lipidosis (E75.4)
Creutzfeldt-Jakob disease (A81.Ø-)
dementia with Lewy bodies (G31.83)
epilepsy and recurrent seizures (G4Ø.-)
frontotemporal dementia (G31.Ø9)
hepatolenticular degeneration (E83.Ø)
human immunodeficiency virus [HIV] disease (B2Ø)
hypercalcemia (E83.52)
hypothyroidism, acquired (EØØ-EØ3.-)
intoxications (T36-T65)
Jakob-Creutzfeldt disease (A81.Ø-)
multiple sclerosis (G35)
neurosyphilis (A52.17)
niacin deficiency [pellagra] (E52)
Parkinson's disease (G2Ø)
Pick's disease (G31.Ø1)
polyarteritis nodosa (M3Ø.Ø)
systemic lupus erythematosus (M32.-)
trypanosomiasis (B56.-, B57.-)
vitamin B deficiency (E53.8)

EXCLUDES 1 *dementia with Parkinsonism (G31.83)*

EXCLUDES 2 *dementia in alcohol and psychoactive substance disorders (F1Ø-F19, with .17, .27, .97)*
vascular dementia (FØ1.5-)

✓5th **FØ2.8 Dementia in other diseases classified elsewhere**

FØ2.8Ø Dementia in other diseases classified elsewhere without behavioral disturbance

Dementia in other diseases classified elsewhere NOS

FØ2.81 Dementia in other diseases classified elsewhere with behavioral disturbance

Dementia in other diseases classified elsewhere with aggressive behavior
Dementia in other diseases classified elsewhere with combative behavior
Dementia in other diseases classified elsewhere with violent behavior
Use additional code, if applicable, to identify wandering in dementia in conditions classified elsewhere (Z91.83)

✓4th **FØ3 Unspecified dementia**

Presenile dementia NOS
Presenile psychosis NOS
Primary degenerative dementia NOS
Senile dementia NOS
Senile dementia depressed or paranoid type
Senile psychosis NOS

EXCLUDES 1 *senility NOS (R41.81)*

EXCLUDES 2 *mild memory disturbance due to known physiological condition (FØ6.8)*
senile dementia with delirium or acute confusional state (FØ5)

✓5th **FØ3.9 Unspecified dementia**

FØ3.9Ø Unspecified dementia without behavioral disturbance

Dementia NOS

FØ3.91 Unspecified dementia with behavioral disturbance

Unspecified dementia with aggressive behavior
Unspecified dementia with combative behavior
Unspecified dementia with violent behavior
Use additional code, if applicable, to identify wandering in unspecified dementia (Z91.83)

FØ4 Amnestic disorder due to known physiological condition

Korsakov's psychosis or syndrome, nonalcoholic
Code first the underlying physiological condition

EXCLUDES 1 *amnesia NOS (R41.3)*
anterograde amnesia (R41.1)
dissociative amnesia (F44.Ø)
retrograde amnesia (R41.2)

EXCLUDES 2 *alcohol-induced or unspecified Korsakov's syndrome (F1Ø.26, F1Ø.96)*
Korsakov's syndrome induced by other psychoactive substances (F13.26, F13.96, F19.16, F19.26, F19.96)

FØ5 Delirium due to known physiological condition

Acute or subacute brain syndrome
Acute or subacute confusional state (nonalcoholic)
Acute or subacute infective psychosis
Acute or subacute organic reaction
Acute or subacute psycho-organic syndrome
Delirium of mixed etiology
Delirium superimposed on dementia
Sundowning
Code first the underlying physiological condition

EXCLUDES 1 *delirium NOS (R41.Ø)*

EXCLUDES 2 *delirium tremens alcohol-induced or unspecified (F1Ø.231, F1Ø.921)*

✓4th F06 Other mental disorders due to known physiological condition
INCLUDES mental disorders due to endocrine disorder
mental disorders due to exogenous hormone
mental disorders due to exogenous toxic substance
mental disorders due to primary cerebral disease
mental disorders due to somatic illness
mental disorders due to systemic disease affecting the brain
Code first the underlying physiological condition
EXCLUDES 1 *unspecified dementia (F03)*
EXCLUDES 2 *delirium due to known physiological condition (F05)*
dementia as classified in F01-F02
other mental disorders associated with alcohol and other psychoactive substances (F10-F19)

F06.0 Psychotic disorder with hallucinations due to known physiological condition
Organic hallucinatory state (nonalcoholic)
EXCLUDES 2 *hallucinations and perceptual disturbance induced by alcohol and other psychoactive substances (F10-F19 with .151, .251, .951)*
schizophrenia (F20.-)

F06.1 Catatonic disorder due to known physiological condition
EXCLUDES 1 *catatonic stupor (R40.1)*
stupor NOS (R40.1)
EXCLUDES 2 *catatonic schizophrenia (F20.2)*
dissociative stupor (F44.2)

F06.2 Psychotic disorder with delusions due to known physiological condition
Paranoid and paranoid-hallucinatory organic states
Schizophrenia-like psychosis in epilepsy
EXCLUDES 2 *alcohol and drug-induced psychotic disorder (F10-F19 with .150, .250, .950)*
brief psychotic disorder (F23)
delusional disorder (F22)
schizophrenia (F20.-)

✓5th F06.3 Mood disorder due to known physiological condition
EXCLUDES 2 *mood disorders due to alcohol and other psychoactive substances (F10-F19 with .14, .24, .94)*
mood disorders, not due to known physiological condition or unspecified (F30-F39)

F06.30 Mood disorder due to known physiological condition, unspecified
F06.31 Mood disorder due to known physiological condition with depressive features
F06.32 Mood disorder due to known physiological condition with major depressive-like episode
F06.33 Mood disorder due to known physiological condition with manic features
F06.34 Mood disorder due to known physiological condition with mixed features

F06.4 Anxiety disorder due to known physiological condition
EXCLUDES 2 *anxiety disorders due to alcohol and other psychoactive substances (F10-F19 with .180, .280, .980)*
anxiety disorders, not due to known physiological condition or unspecified (F40.-, F41.-)

F06.8 Other specified mental disorders due to known physiological condition
Epileptic psychosis NOS
Organic dissociative disorder
Organic emotionally labile [asthenic] disorder

✓4th F07 Personality and behavioral disorders due to known physiological condition
Code first the underlying physiological condition

F07.0 Personality change due to known physiological condition
Frontal lobe syndrome
Limbic epilepsy personality syndrome
Lobotomy syndrome
Organic personality disorder
Organic pseudopsychopathic personality
Organic pseudoretarded personality
Postleucotomy syndrome
Code first underlying physiological condition
EXCLUDES 1 *mild cognitive impairment (G31.84)*
postconcussional syndrome (F07.81)
postencephalitic syndrome (F07.89)
signs and symptoms involving emotional state (R45.-)
EXCLUDES 2 *specific personality disorder (F60.-)*

✓5th F07.8 Other personality and behavioral disorders due to known physiological condition

F07.81 Postconcussional syndrome
Postcontusional syndrome (encephalopathy)
Post-traumatic brain syndrome, nonpsychotic
Use additional code to identify associated post-traumatic headache, if applicable (G44.3-)
EXCLUDES 1 *current concussion (brain) (S06.0-)*
postencephalitic syndrome (F07.89)

F07.89 Other personality and behavioral disorders due to known physiological condition
Postencephalitic syndrome
Right hemispheric organic affective disorder

F07.9 Unspecified personality and behavioral disorder due to known physiological condition
Organic psychosyndrome

F09 Unspecified mental disorder due to known physiological condition
Mental disorder NOS due to known physiological condition
Organic brain syndrome NOS
Organic mental disorder NOS
Organic psychosis NOS
Symptomatic psychosis NOS
Code first the underlying physiological condition
EXCLUDES 1 *psychosis NOS (F29)*

Mental and behavioral disorders due to psychoactive substance use (F10-F19)

✓4th F10 Alcohol related disorders
Use additional code for blood alcohol level, if applicable (Y90.-)

✓5th F10.1 Alcohol abuse
EXCLUDES 1 *alcohol dependence (F10.2-)*
alcohol use, unspecified (F10.9-)

F10.10 Alcohol abuse, uncomplicated
✓6th F10.12 Alcohol abuse with intoxication
F10.120 Alcohol abuse with intoxication, uncomplicated
F10.121 Alcohol abuse with intoxication delirium
F10.129 Alcohol abuse with intoxication, unspecified
F10.14 Alcohol abuse with alcohol-induced mood disorder
✓6th F10.15 Alcohol abuse with alcohol-induced psychotic disorder
F10.150 Alcohol abuse with alcohol-induced psychotic disorder with delusions
F10.151 Alcohol abuse with alcohol-induced psychotic disorder with hallucinations
F10.159 Alcohol abuse with alcohol-induced psychotic disorder, unspecified
✓6th F10.18 Alcohol abuse with other alcohol-induced disorders
F10.180 Alcohol abuse with alcohol-induced anxiety disorder
F10.181 Alcohol abuse with alcohol-induced sexual dysfunction
F10.182 Alcohol abuse with alcohol-induced sleep disorder
F10.188 Alcohol abuse with other alcohol-induced disorder
F10.19 Alcohol abuse with unspecified alcohol-induced disorder

✓5th F10.2 Alcohol dependence
EXCLUDES 1 *alcohol abuse (F10.1-)*
alcohol use, unspecified (F10.9-)
EXCLUDES 2 *toxic effect of alcohol (T51.0-)*

F10.20 Alcohol dependence, uncomplicated
F10.21 Alcohol dependence, in remission
✓6th F10.22 Alcohol dependence with intoxication
Acute drunkenness (in alcoholism)
EXCLUDES 1 *alcohol dependence with withdrawal (F10.23-)*
F10.220 Alcohol dependence with intoxication, uncomplicated
F10.221 Alcohol dependence with intoxication delirium

F10.229 **Alcohol dependence with intoxication, unspecified**

✓6th F10.23 **Alcohol dependence with withdrawal**

EXCLUDES 1 *Alcohol dependence with intoxication (F10.22-)*

F10.230 **Alcohol dependence with withdrawal, uncomplicated**

F10.231 **Alcohol dependence with withdrawal delirium**

F10.232 **Alcohol dependence with withdrawal with perceptual disturbance**

F10.239 **Alcohol dependence with withdrawal, unspecified**

F10.24 **Alcohol dependence with alcohol-induced mood disorder**

✓6th F10.25 **Alcohol dependence with alcohol-induced psychotic disorder**

F10.250 **Alcohol dependence with alcohol-induced psychotic disorder with delusions**

F10.251 **Alcohol dependence with alcohol-induced psychotic disorder with hallucinations**

F10.259 **Alcohol dependence with alcohol-induced psychotic disorder, unspecified**

F10.26 **Alcohol dependence with alcohol-induced persisting amnestic disorder**

F10.27 **Alcohol dependence with alcohol-induced persisting dementia**

✓6th F10.28 **Alcohol dependence with other alcohol-induced disorders**

F10.280 **Alcohol dependence with alcohol-induced anxiety disorder**

F10.281 **Alcohol dependence with alcohol-induced sexual dysfunction**

F10.282 **Alcohol dependence with alcohol-induced sleep disorder**

F10.288 **Alcohol dependence with other alcohol-induced disorder**

F10.29 **Alcohol dependence with unspecified alcohol-induced disorder**

✓5th F10.9 **Alcohol use, unspecified**

EXCLUDES 1 *alcohol abuse (F10.1-)*
alcohol dependence (F10.2-)

✓6th F10.92 **Alcohol use, unspecified with intoxication**

F10.920 **Alcohol use, unspecified with intoxication, uncomplicated**

F10.921 **Alcohol use, unspecified with intoxication delirium**

F10.929 **Alcohol use, unspecified with intoxication, unspecified**

F10.94 **Alcohol use, unspecified with alcohol-induced mood disorder**

✓6th F10.95 **Alcohol use, unspecified with alcohol-induced psychotic disorder**

F10.950 **Alcohol use, unspecified with alcohol-induced psychotic disorder with delusions**

F10.951 **Alcohol use, unspecified with alcohol-induced psychotic disorder with hallucinations**

F10.959 **Alcohol use, unspecified with alcohol-induced psychotic disorder, unspecified**

F10.96 **Alcohol use, unspecified with alcohol-induced persisting amnestic disorder**

F10.97 **Alcohol use, unspecified with alcohol-induced persisting dementia**

✓6th F10.98 **Alcohol use, unspecified with other alcohol-induced disorders**

F10.980 **Alcohol use, unspecified with alcohol-induced anxiety disorder**

F10.981 **Alcohol use, unspecified with alcohol-induced sexual dysfunction**

F10.982 **Alcohol use, unspecified with alcohol-induced sleep disorder**

F10.988 **Alcohol use, unspecified with other alcohol-induced disorder**

F10.99 **Alcohol use, unspecified with unspecified alcohol-induced disorder**

✓4th **F11 Opioid related disorders**

✓5th F11.1 **Opioid abuse**

EXCLUDES 1 *opioid dependence (F11.2-)*
opioid use, unspecified (F11.9-)

F11.10 **Opioid abuse, uncomplicated**

✓6th F11.12 **Opioid abuse with intoxication**

F11.120 **Opioid abuse with intoxication, uncomplicated**

F11.121 **Opioid abuse with intoxication delirium**

F11.122 **Opioid abuse with intoxication with perceptual disturbance**

F11.129 **Opioid abuse with intoxication, unspecified**

F11.14 **Opioid abuse with opioid-induced mood disorder**

✓6th F11.15 **Opioid abuse with opioid-induced psychotic disorder**

F11.150 **Opioid abuse with opioid-induced psychotic disorder with delusions**

F11.151 **Opioid abuse with opioid-induced psychotic disorder with hallucinations**

F11.159 **Opioid abuse with opioid-induced psychotic disorder, unspecified**

✓6th F11.18 **Opioid abuse with other opioid-induced disorder**

F11.181 **Opioid abuse with opioid-induced sexual dysfunction**

F11.182 **Opioid abuse with opioid-induced sleep disorder**

F11.188 **Opioid abuse with other opioid-induced disorder**

F11.19 **Opioid abuse with unspecified opioid-induced disorder**

✓5th F11.2 **Opioid dependence**

EXCLUDES 1 *opioid abuse (F11.1-)*
opioid use, unspecified (F11.9-)

EXCLUDES 2 *opioid poisoning (T40.0-T40.2-)*

F11.20 **Opioid dependence, uncomplicated**

F11.21 **Opioid dependence, in remission**

✓6th F11.22 **Opioid dependence with intoxication**

EXCLUDES 1 *opioid dependence with withdrawal (F11.23)*

F11.220 **Opioid dependence with intoxication, uncomplicated**

F11.221 **Opioid dependence with intoxication delirium**

F11.222 **Opioid dependence with intoxication with perceptual disturbance**

F11.229 **Opioid dependence with intoxication, unspecified**

F11.23 **Opioid dependence with withdrawal**

EXCLUDES 1 *opioid dependence with intoxication (F11.22-)*

F11.24 **Opioid dependence with opioid-induced mood disorder**

✓6th F11.25 **Opioid dependence with opioid-induced psychotic disorder**

F11.250 **Opioid dependence with opioid-induced psychotic disorder with delusions**

F11.251 **Opioid dependence with opioid-induced psychotic disorder with hallucinations**

F11.259 **Opioid dependence with opioid-induced psychotic disorder, unspecified**

✓6th F11.28 **Opioid dependence with other opioid-induced disorder**

F11.281 **Opioid dependence with opioid-induced sexual dysfunction**

F11.282 **Opioid dependence with opioid-induced sleep disorder**

F11.288 **Opioid dependence with other opioid-induced disorder**

F11.29 **Opioid dependence with unspecified opioid-induced disorder**

✓5th **F11.9 Opioid use, unspecified**
EXCLUDES 1 *opioid abuse (F11.1-)*
opioid dependence (F11.2-)
F11.90 Opioid use, unspecified, uncomplicated
✓6th **F11.92 Opioid use, unspecified with intoxication**
EXCLUDES 1 *opioid use, unspecified with withdrawal (F11.93)*
F11.920 Opioid use, unspecified with intoxication, uncomplicated
F11.921 Opioid use, unspecified with intoxication delirium
F11.922 Opioid use, unspecified with intoxication with perceptual disturbance
F11.929 Opioid use, unspecified with intoxication, unspecified
F11.93 Opioid use, unspecified with withdrawal
EXCLUDES 1 *opioid use, unspecified with intoxication (F11.92-)*
F11.94 Opioid use, unspecified with opioid-induced mood disorder
✓6th **F11.95 Opioid use, unspecified with opioid-induced psychotic disorder**
F11.950 Opioid use, unspecified with opioid-induced psychotic disorder with delusions
F11.951 Opioid use, unspecified with opioid-induced psychotic disorder with hallucinations
F11.959 Opioid use, unspecified with opioid-induced psychotic disorder, unspecified
✓6th **F11.98 Opioid use, unspecified with other specified opioid-induced disorder**
F11.981 Opioid use, unspecified with opioid-induced sexual dysfunction
F11.982 Opioid use, unspecified with opioid-induced sleep disorder
F11.988 Opioid use, unspecified with other opioid-induced disorder
F11.99 Opioid use, unspecified with unspecified opioid-induced disorder

✓4th **F12 Cannabis related disorders**
INCLUDES marijuana
✓5th **F12.1 Cannabis abuse**
EXCLUDES 1 *cannabis dependence (F12.2-)*
cannabis use, unspecified (F12.9-)
F12.10 Cannabis abuse, uncomplicated
✓6th **F12.12 Cannabis abuse with intoxication**
F12.120 Cannabis abuse with intoxication, uncomplicated
F12.121 Cannabis abuse with intoxication delirium
F12.122 Cannabis abuse with intoxication with perceptual disturbance
F12.129 Cannabis abuse with intoxication, unspecified
✓6th **F12.15 Cannabis abuse with psychotic disorder**
F12.150 Cannabis abuse with psychotic disorder with delusions
F12.151 Cannabis abuse with psychotic disorder with hallucinations
F12.159 Cannabis abuse with psychotic disorder, unspecified
✓6th **F12.18 Cannabis abuse with other cannabis-induced disorder**
F12.180 Cannabis abuse with cannabis-induced anxiety disorder
F12.188 Cannabis abuse with other cannabis-induced disorder
F12.19 Cannabis abuse with unspecified cannabis-induced disorder
✓5th **F12.2 Cannabis dependence**
EXCLUDES 1 *cannabis abuse (F12.1-)*
cannabis use, unspecified (F12.9-)
EXCLUDES 2 *cannabis poisoning (T40.7-)*
F12.20 Cannabis dependence, uncomplicated
F12.21 Cannabis dependence, in remission
✓6th **F12.22 Cannabis dependence with intoxication**
F12.220 Cannabis dependence with intoxication, uncomplicated
F12.221 Cannabis dependence with intoxication delirium
F12.222 Cannabis dependence with intoxication with perceptual disturbance
F12.229 Cannabis dependence with intoxication, unspecified
✓6th **F12.25 Cannabis dependence with psychotic disorder**
F12.250 Cannabis dependence with psychotic disorder with delusions
F12.251 Cannabis dependence with psychotic disorder with hallucinations
F12.259 Cannabis dependence with psychotic disorder, unspecified
✓6th **F12.28 Cannabis dependence with other cannabis-induced disorder**
F12.280 Cannabis dependence with cannabis-induced anxiety disorder
F12.288 Cannabis dependence with other cannabis-induced disorder
F12.29 Cannabis dependence with unspecified cannabis-induced disorder
✓5th **F12.9 Cannabis use, unspecified**
EXCLUDES 1 *cannabis abuse (F12.1-)*
cannabis dependence (F12.2-)
F12.90 Cannabis use, unspecified, uncomplicated
✓6th **F12.92 Cannabis use, unspecified with intoxication**
F12.920 Cannabis use, unspecified with intoxication, uncomplicated
F12.921 Cannabis use, unspecified with intoxication delirium
F12.922 Cannabis use, unspecified with intoxication with perceptual disturbance
F12.929 Cannabis use, unspecified with intoxication, unspecified
✓6th **F12.95 Cannabis use, unspecified with psychotic disorder**
F12.950 Cannabis use, unspecified with psychotic disorder with delusions
F12.951 Cannabis use, unspecified with psychotic disorder with hallucinations
F12.959 Cannabis use, unspecified with psychotic disorder, unspecified
✓6th **F12.98 Cannabis use, unspecified with other cannabis-induced disorder**
F12.980 Cannabis use, unspecified with anxiety disorder
F12.988 Cannabis use, unspecified with other cannabis-induced disorder
F12.99 Cannabis use, unspecified with unspecified cannabis-induced disorder

✓4th **F13 Sedative, hypnotic, or anxiolytic related disorders**
✓5th **F13.1 Sedative, hypnotic or anxiolytic-related abuse**
EXCLUDES 1 *sedative, hypnotic or anxiolytic-related dependence (F13.2-)*
sedative, hypnotic, or anxiolytic use, unspecified (F13.9-)
F13.10 Sedative, hypnotic or anxiolytic abuse, uncomplicated
✓6th **F13.12 Sedative, hypnotic or anxiolytic abuse with intoxication**
F13.120 Sedative, hypnotic or anxiolytic abuse with intoxication, uncomplicated
F13.121 Sedative, hypnotic or anxiolytic abuse with intoxication delirium
F13.129 Sedative, hypnotic or anxiolytic abuse with intoxication, unspecified
F13.14 Sedative, hypnotic or anxiolytic abuse with sedative, hypnotic or anxiolytic-induced mood disorder
✓6th **F13.15 Sedative, hypnotic or anxiolytic abuse with sedative, hypnotic or anxiolytic-induced psychotic disorder**

EXCLUDES 1 Not coded here EXCLUDES 2 Not included here *Manifestation Code*

F13.150 Sedative, hypnotic or anxiolytic abuse with sedative, hypnotic or anxiolytic-induced psychotic disorder with delusions

F13.151 Sedative, hypnotic or anxiolytic abuse with sedative, hypnotic or anxiolytic-induced psychotic disorder with hallucinations

F13.159 Sedative, hypnotic or anxiolytic abuse with sedative, hypnotic or anxiolytic-induced psychotic disorder, unspecified

✓6th F13.18 Sedative, hypnotic or anxiolytic abuse with other sedative, hypnotic or anxiolytic-induced disorders

F13.180 Sedative, hypnotic or anxiolytic abuse with sedative, hypnotic or anxiolytic-induced anxiety disorder

F13.181 Sedative, hypnotic or anxiolytic abuse with sedative, hypnotic or anxiolytic-induced sexual dysfunction

F13.182 Sedative, hypnotic or anxiolytic abuse with sedative, hypnotic or anxiolytic-induced sleep disorder

F13.188 Sedative, hypnotic or anxiolytic abuse with other sedative, hypnotic or anxiolytic-induced disorder

F13.19 Sedative, hypnotic or anxiolytic abuse with unspecified sedative, hypnotic or anxiolytic-induced disorder

✓5th F13.2 Sedative, hypnotic or anxiolytic-related dependence

EXCLUDES 1 *sedative, hypnotic or anxiolytic-related abuse (F13.1-)*
sedative, hypnotic, or anxiolytic use, unspecified (F13.9-)

EXCLUDES 2 *sedative, hypnotic, or anxiolytic poisoning (T42.-)*

F13.20 Sedative, hypnotic or anxiolytic dependence, uncomplicated

F13.21 Sedative, hypnotic or anxiolytic dependence, in remission

✓6th F13.22 Sedative, hypnotic or anxiolytic dependence with intoxication

EXCLUDES 1 *sedative, hypnotic or anxiolytic dependence with withdrawal (F13.23-)*

F13.220 Sedative, hypnotic or anxiolytic dependence with intoxication, uncomplicated

F13.221 Sedative, hypnotic or anxiolytic dependence with intoxication delirium

F13.229 Sedative, hypnotic or anxiolytic dependence with intoxication, unspecified

✓6th F13.23 Sedative, hypnotic or anxiolytic dependence with withdrawal

EXCLUDES 1 *sedative, hypnotic or anxiolytic dependence with intoxication (F13.22-)*

F13.230 Sedative, hypnotic or anxiolytic dependence with withdrawal, uncomplicated

F13.231 Sedative, hypnotic or anxiolytic dependence with withdrawal delirium

F13.232 Sedative, hypnotic or anxiolytic dependence with withdrawal with perceptual disturbance

F13.239 Sedative, hypnotic or anxiolytic dependence with withdrawal, unspecified

F13.24 Sedative, hypnotic or anxiolytic dependence with sedative, hypnotic or anxiolytic-induced mood disorder

✓6th F13.25 Sedative, hypnotic or anxiolytic dependence with sedative, hypnotic or anxiolytic-induced psychotic disorder

F13.250 Sedative, hypnotic or anxiolytic dependence with sedative, hypnotic or anxiolytic-induced psychotic disorder with delusions

F13.251 Sedative, hypnotic or anxiolytic dependence with sedative, hypnotic or anxiolytic-induced psychotic disorder with hallucinations

F13.259 Sedative, hypnotic or anxiolytic dependence with sedative, hypnotic or anxiolytic-induced psychotic disorder, unspecified

F13.26 Sedative, hypnotic or anxiolytic dependence with sedative, hypnotic or anxiolytic-induced persisting amnestic disorder

F13.27 Sedative, hypnotic or anxiolytic dependence with sedative, hypnotic or anxiolytic-induced persisting dementia

✓6th F13.28 Sedative, hypnotic or anxiolytic dependence with other sedative, hypnotic or anxiolytic-induced disorders

F13.280 Sedative, hypnotic or anxiolytic dependence with sedative, hypnotic or anxiolytic-induced anxiety disorder

F13.281 Sedative, hypnotic or anxiolytic dependence with sedative, hypnotic or anxiolytic-induced sexual dysfunction

F13.282 Sedative, hypnotic or anxiolytic dependence with sedative, hypnotic or anxiolytic-induced sleep disorder

F13.288 Sedative, hypnotic or anxiolytic dependence with other sedative, hypnotic or anxiolytic-induced disorder

F13.29 Sedative, hypnotic or anxiolytic dependence with unspecified sedative, hypnotic or anxiolytic-induced disorder

✓5th F13.9 Sedative, hypnotic or anxiolytic-related use, unspecified

EXCLUDES 1 *sedative, hypnotic or anxiolytic-related abuse (F13.1-)*
sedative, hypnotic or anxiolytic-related dependence (F13.2-)

F13.90 Sedative, hypnotic, or anxiolytic use, unspecified, uncomplicated

✓6th F13.92 Sedative, hypnotic or anxiolytic use, unspecified with intoxication

EXCLUDES 1 *sedative, hypnotic or anxiolytic use, unspecified with withdrawal (F13.93-)*

F13.920 Sedative, hypnotic or anxiolytic use, unspecified with intoxication, uncomplicated

F13.921 Sedative, hypnotic or anxiolytic use, unspecified with intoxication delirium

F13.929 Sedative, hypnotic or anxiolytic use, unspecified with intoxication, unspecified

✓6th F13.93 Sedative, hypnotic or anxiolytic use, unspecified with withdrawal

EXCLUDES 1 *sedative, hypnotic or anxiolytic use, unspecified with intoxication (F13.92-)*

F13.930 Sedative, hypnotic or anxiolytic use, unspecified with withdrawal, uncomplicated

F13.931 Sedative, hypnotic or anxiolytic use, unspecified with withdrawal delirium

F13.932 Sedative, hypnotic or anxiolytic use, unspecified with withdrawal with perceptual disturbances

F13.939 Sedative, hypnotic or anxiolytic use, unspecified with withdrawal, unspecified

F13.94 Sedative, hypnotic or anxiolytic use, unspecified with sedative, hypnotic or anxiolytic-induced mood disorder

✓6th F13.95 Sedative, hypnotic or anxiolytic use, unspecified with sedative, hypnotic or anxiolytic-induced psychotic disorder

F13.950 Sedative, hypnotic or anxiolytic use, unspecified with sedative, hypnotic or anxiolytic-induced psychotic disorder with delusions

F13.951 Sedative, hypnotic or anxiolytic use, unspecified with sedative, hypnotic or anxiolytic-induced psychotic disorder with hallucinations

F13.959 Sedative, hypnotic or anxiolytic use, unspecified with sedative, hypnotic or anxiolytic-induced psychotic disorder, unspecified

F13.96 Sedative, hypnotic or anxiolytic use, unspecified with sedative, hypnotic or anxiolytic-induced persisting amnestic disorder

F13.97 Sedative, hypnotic or anxiolytic use, unspecified with sedative, hypnotic or anxiolytic-induced persisting dementia

✓6th **F13.98 Sedative, hypnotic or anxiolytic use, unspecified with other sedative, hypnotic or anxiolytic-induced disorders**

F13.980 Sedative, hypnotic or anxiolytic use, unspecified with sedative, hypnotic or anxiolytic-induced anxiety disorder

F13.981 Sedative, hypnotic or anxiolytic use, unspecified with sedative, hypnotic or anxiolytic-induced sexual dysfunction

F13.982 Sedative, hypnotic or anxiolytic use, unspecified with sedative, hypnotic or anxiolytic-induced sleep disorder

F13.988 Sedative, hypnotic or anxiolytic use, unspecified with other sedative, hypnotic or anxiolytic-induced disorder

F13.99 Sedative, hypnotic or anxiolytic use, unspecified with unspecified sedative, hypnotic or anxiolytic-induced disorder

✓4th **F14 Cocaine related disorders**

EXCLUDES 2 *other stimulant-related disorders (F15.-)*

✓5th **F14.1 Cocaine abuse**

EXCLUDES 1 *cocaine dependence (F14.2-)*
cocaine use, unspecified (F14.9-)

F14.10 Cocaine abuse, uncomplicated

✓6th **F14.12 Cocaine abuse with intoxication**

F14.120 Cocaine abuse with intoxication, uncomplicated

F14.121 Cocaine abuse with intoxication with delirium

F14.122 Cocaine abuse with intoxication with perceptual disturbance

F14.129 Cocaine abuse with intoxication, unspecified

F14.14 Cocaine abuse with cocaine-induced mood disorder

✓6th **F14.15 Cocaine abuse with cocaine-induced psychotic disorder**

F14.150 Cocaine abuse with cocaine-induced psychotic disorder with delusions

F14.151 Cocaine abuse with cocaine-induced psychotic disorder with hallucinations

F14.159 Cocaine abuse with cocaine-induced psychotic disorder, unspecified

✓6th **F14.18 Cocaine abuse with other cocaine-induced disorder**

F14.180 Cocaine abuse with cocaine-induced anxiety disorder

F14.181 Cocaine abuse with cocaine-induced sexual dysfunction

F14.182 Cocaine abuse with cocaine-induced sleep disorder

F14.188 Cocaine abuse with other cocaine-induced disorder

F14.19 Cocaine abuse with unspecified cocaine-induced disorder

✓5th **F14.2 Cocaine dependence**

EXCLUDES 1 *cocaine abuse (F14.1-)*
cocaine use, unspecified (F14.9-)

EXCLUDES 2 *cocaine poisoning (T40.5-)*

F14.20 Cocaine dependence, uncomplicated

F14.21 Cocaine dependence, in remission

✓6th **F14.22 Cocaine dependence with intoxication**

EXCLUDES 1 *cocaine dependence with withdrawal (F14.23)*

F14.220 Cocaine dependence with intoxication, uncomplicated

F14.221 Cocaine dependence with intoxication delirium

F14.222 Cocaine dependence with intoxication with perceptual disturbance

F14.229 Cocaine dependence with intoxication, unspecified

F14.23 Cocaine dependence with withdrawal

EXCLUDES 1 *cocaine dependence with intoxication (F14.22-)*

F14.24 Cocaine dependence with cocaine-induced mood disorder

✓6th **F14.25 Cocaine dependence with cocaine-induced psychotic disorder**

F14.250 Cocaine dependence with cocaine-induced psychotic disorder with delusions

F14.251 Cocaine dependence with cocaine-induced psychotic disorder with hallucinations

F14.259 Cocaine dependence with cocaine-induced psychotic disorder, unspecified

✓6th **F14.28 Cocaine dependence with other cocaine-induced disorder**

F14.280 Cocaine dependence with cocaine-induced anxiety disorder

F14.281 Cocaine dependence with cocaine-induced sexual dysfunction

F14.282 Cocaine dependence with cocaine-induced sleep disorder

F14.288 Cocaine dependence with other cocaine-induced disorder

F14.29 Cocaine dependence with unspecified cocaine-induced disorder

✓5th **F14.9 Cocaine use, unspecified**

EXCLUDES 1 *cocaine abuse (F14.1-)*
cocaine dependence (F14.2-)

F14.90 Cocaine use, unspecified, uncomplicated

✓6th **F14.92 Cocaine use, unspecified with intoxication**

F14.920 Cocaine use, unspecified with intoxication, uncomplicated

F14.921 Cocaine use, unspecified with intoxication delirium

F14.922 Cocaine use, unspecified with intoxication with perceptual disturbance

F14.929 Cocaine use, unspecified with intoxication, unspecified

F14.94 Cocaine use, unspecified with cocaine-induced mood disorder

✓6th **F14.95 Cocaine use, unspecified with cocaine-induced psychotic disorder**

F14.950 Cocaine use, unspecified with cocaine-induced psychotic disorder with delusions

F14.951 Cocaine use, unspecified with cocaine-induced psychotic disorder with hallucinations

F14.959 Cocaine use, unspecified with cocaine-induced psychotic disorder, unspecified

✓6th **F14.98 Cocaine use, unspecified with other specified cocaine-induced disorder**

F14.980 Cocaine use, unspecified with cocaine-induced anxiety disorder

F14.981 Cocaine use, unspecified with cocaine-induced sexual dysfunction

F14.982 Cocaine use, unspecified with cocaine-induced sleep disorder

F14.988 Cocaine use, unspecified with other cocaine-induced disorder

F14.99 Cocaine use, unspecified with unspecified cocaine-induced disorder

✓4th F15 Other stimulant related disorders
Amphetamine-related disorders
Caffeine
EXCLUDES 2 *cocaine-related disorders (F14.-)*

✓5th F15.1 Other stimulant abuse
EXCLUDES 1 *other stimulant dependence (F15.2-)*
other stimulant use, unspecified (F15.9-)

F15.10 Other stimulant abuse, uncomplicated

✓6th F15.12 Other stimulant abuse with intoxication

F15.120 Other stimulant abuse with intoxication, uncomplicated

F15.121 Other stimulant abuse with intoxication delirium

F15.122 Other stimulant abuse with intoxication with perceptual disturbance

F15.129 Other stimulant abuse with intoxication, unspecified

F15.14 Other stimulant abuse with stimulant-induced mood disorder

✓6th F15.15 Other stimulant abuse with stimulant-induced psychotic disorder

F15.150 Other stimulant abuse with stimulant-induced psychotic disorder with delusions

F15.151 Other stimulant abuse with stimulant-induced psychotic disorder with hallucinations

F15.159 Other stimulant abuse with stimulant-induced psychotic disorder, unspecified

✓6th F15.18 Other stimulant abuse with other stimulant-induced disorder

F15.180 Other stimulant abuse with stimulant-induced anxiety disorder

F15.181 Other stimulant abuse with stimulant-induced sexual dysfunction

F15.182 Other stimulant abuse with stimulant-induced sleep disorder

F15.188 Other stimulant abuse with other stimulant-induced disorder

F15.19 Other stimulant abuse with unspecified stimulant-induced disorder

✓5th F15.2 Other stimulant dependence
EXCLUDES 1 *other stimulant abuse (F15.1-)*
other stimulant use, unspecified (F15.9-)

F15.20 Other stimulant dependence, uncomplicated

F15.21 Other stimulant dependence, in remission

✓6th F15.22 Other stimulant dependence with intoxication
EXCLUDES 1 *other stimulant dependence with withdrawal (F15.23)*

F15.220 Other stimulant dependence with intoxication, uncomplicated

F15.221 Other stimulant dependence with intoxication delirium

F15.222 Other stimulant dependence with intoxication with perceptual disturbance

F15.229 Other stimulant dependence with intoxication, unspecified

F15.23 Other stimulant dependence with withdrawal
EXCLUDES 1 *other stimulant dependence with intoxication (F15.22-)*

F15.24 Other stimulant dependence with stimulant-induced mood disorder

✓6th F15.25 Other stimulant dependence with stimulant-induced psychotic disorder

F15.250 Other stimulant dependence with stimulant-induced psychotic disorder with delusions

F15.251 Other stimulant dependence with stimulant-induced psychotic disorder with hallucinations

F15.259 Other stimulant dependence with stimulant-induced psychotic disorder, unspecified

✓6th F15.28 Other stimulant dependence with other stimulant-induced disorder

F15.280 Other stimulant dependence with stimulant-induced anxiety disorder

F15.281 Other stimulant dependence with stimulant-induced sexual dysfunction

F15.282 Other stimulant dependence with stimulant-induced sleep disorder

F15.288 Other stimulant dependence with other stimulant-induced disorder

F15.29 Other stimulant dependence with unspecified stimulant-induced disorder

✓5th F15.9 Other stimulant use, unspecified
EXCLUDES 1 *other stimulant abuse (F15.1-)*
other stimulant dependence (F15.2-)

F15.90 Other stimulant use, unspecified, uncomplicated

✓6th F15.92 Other stimulant use, unspecified with intoxication
EXCLUDES 1 *other stimulant use, unspecified with withdrawal (F15.93)*

F15.920 Other stimulant use, unspecified with intoxication, uncomplicated

F15.921 Other stimulant use, unspecified with intoxication delirium

F15.922 Other stimulant use, unspecified with intoxication with perceptual disturbance

F15.929 Other stimulant use, unspecified with intoxication, unspecified

F15.93 Other stimulant use, unspecified with withdrawal
EXCLUDES 1 *other stimulant use, unspecified with intoxication (F15.92-)*

F15.94 Other stimulant use, unspecified with stimulant-induced mood disorder

✓6th F15.95 Other stimulant use, unspecified with stimulant-induced psychotic disorder

F15.950 Other stimulant use, unspecified with stimulant-induced psychotic disorder with delusions

F15.951 Other stimulant use, unspecified with stimulant-induced psychotic disorder with hallucinations

F15.959 Other stimulant use, unspecified with stimulant-induced psychotic disorder, unspecified

✓6th F15.98 Other stimulant use, unspecified with other stimulant-induced disorder

F15.980 Other stimulant use, unspecified with stimulant-induced anxiety disorder

F15.981 Other stimulant use, unspecified with stimulant-induced sexual dysfunction

F15.982 Other stimulant use, unspecified with stimulant-induced sleep disorder

F15.988 Other stimulant use, unspecified with other stimulant-induced disorder

F15.99 Other stimulant use, unspecified with unspecified stimulant-induced disorder

✓4th F16 Hallucinogen related disorders
INCLUDES ecstasy
PCP
phencyclidine

✓5th F16.1 Hallucinogen abuse
EXCLUDES 1 *hallucinogen dependence (F16.2-)*
hallucinogen use, unspecified (F16.9-)

F16.10 Hallucinogen abuse, uncomplicated

✓6th F16.12 Hallucinogen abuse with intoxication

F16.120 Hallucinogen abuse with intoxication, uncomplicated

F16.121 Hallucinogen abuse with intoxication with delirium

F16.122 Hallucinogen abuse with intoxication with perceptual disturbance

F16.129 Hallucinogen abuse with intoxication, unspecified

F16.14 Hallucinogen abuse with hallucinogen-induced mood disorder

✓6th F16.15 Hallucinogen abuse with hallucinogen-induced psychotic disorder

F16.150 Hallucinogen abuse with hallucinogen-induced psychotic disorder with delusions

✓ Appropriate additional character required   ✓x7th Requires 7th character, placeholder x must fill empty characters

F16.151 Hallucinogen abuse with hallucinogen-induced psychotic disorder with hallucinations
F16.159 Hallucinogen abuse with hallucinogen-induced psychotic disorder, unspecified
6th **F16.18** Hallucinogen abuse with other hallucinogen-induced disorder
F16.180 Hallucinogen abuse with hallucinogen-induced anxiety disorder
F16.183 Hallucinogen abuse with hallucinogen persisting perception disorder (flashbacks)
F16.188 Hallucinogen abuse with other hallucinogen-induced disorder
F16.19 Hallucinogen abuse with unspecified hallucinogen-induced disorder

5th **F16.2 Hallucinogen dependence**
EXCLUDES 1 *hallucinogen abuse (F16.1-)*
hallucinogen use, unspecified (F16.9-)
F16.20 Hallucinogen dependence, uncomplicated
F16.21 Hallucinogen dependence, in remission
6th **F16.22** Hallucinogen dependence with intoxication
F16.220 Hallucinogen dependence with intoxication, uncomplicated
F16.221 Hallucinogen dependence with intoxication with delirium
F16.229 Hallucinogen dependence with intoxication, unspecified
F16.24 Hallucinogen dependence with hallucinogen-induced mood disorder
6th **F16.25** Hallucinogen dependence with hallucinogen-induced psychotic disorder
F16.250 Hallucinogen dependence with hallucinogen-induced psychotic disorder with delusions
F16.251 Hallucinogen dependence with hallucinogen-induced psychotic disorder with hallucinations
F16.259 Hallucinogen dependence with hallucinogen-induced psychotic disorder, unspecified
6th **F16.28** Hallucinogen dependence with other hallucinogen-induced disorder
F16.280 Hallucinogen dependence with hallucinogen-induced anxiety disorder
F16.283 Hallucinogen dependence with hallucinogen persisting perception disorder (flashbacks)
F16.288 Hallucinogen dependence with other hallucinogen-induced disorder
F16.29 Hallucinogen dependence with unspecified hallucinogen-induced disorder

5th **F16.9 Hallucinogen use, unspecified**
EXCLUDES 1 *hallucinogen abuse (F16.1-)*
hallucinogen dependence (F16.2-)
F16.90 Hallucinogen use, unspecified, uncomplicated
6th **F16.92** Hallucinogen use, unspecified with intoxication
F16.920 Hallucinogen use, unspecified with intoxication, uncomplicated
F16.921 Hallucinogen use, unspecified with intoxication with delirium
F16.929 Hallucinogen use, unspecified with intoxication, unspecified
F16.94 Hallucinogen use, unspecified with hallucinogen-induced mood disorder
6th **F16.95** Hallucinogen use, unspecified with hallucinogen-induced psychotic disorder
F16.950 Hallucinogen use, unspecified with hallucinogen-induced psychotic disorder with delusions
F16.951 Hallucinogen use, unspecified with hallucinogen-induced psychotic disorder with hallucinations
F16.959 Hallucinogen use, unspecified with hallucinogen-induced psychotic disorder, unspecified
6th **F16.98** Hallucinogen use, unspecified with other specified hallucinogen-induced disorder
F16.980 Hallucinogen use, unspecified with hallucinogen-induced anxiety disorder
F16.983 Hallucinogen use, unspecified with hallucinogen persisting perception disorder (flashbacks)
F16.988 Hallucinogen use, unspecified with other hallucinogen-induced disorder
F16.99 Hallucinogen use, unspecified with unspecified hallucinogen-induced disorder

4th F17 Nicotine dependence
EXCLUDES 1 *history of tobacco dependence (Z87.891)*
tobacco use NOS (Z72.0)
EXCLUDES 2 *tobacco use (smoking) during pregnancy, childbirth and the puerperium (O99.33-)*
toxic effect of nicotine (T65.2-)

5th **F17.2 Nicotine dependence**
6th **F17.20** Nicotine dependence, unspecified
F17.200 Nicotine dependence, unspecified, uncomplicated
F17.201 Nicotine dependence, unspecified, in remission
F17.203 Nicotine dependence unspecified, with withdrawal
F17.208 Nicotine dependence, unspecified, with other nicotine-induced disorders
F17.209 Nicotine dependence, unspecified, with unspecified nicotine-induced disorders
6th **F17.21** Nicotine dependence, cigarettes
F17.210 Nicotine dependence, cigarettes, uncomplicated
F17.211 Nicotine dependence, cigarettes, in remission
F17.213 Nicotine dependence, cigarettes, with withdrawal
F17.218 Nicotine dependence, cigarettes, with other nicotine-induced disorders
F17.219 Nicotine dependence, cigarettes, with unspecified nicotine-induced disorders
6th **F17.22** Nicotine dependence, chewing tobacco
F17.220 Nicotine dependence, chewing tobacco, uncomplicated
F17.221 Nicotine dependence, chewing tobacco, in remission
F17.223 Nicotine dependence, chewing tobacco, with withdrawal
F17.228 Nicotine dependence, chewing tobacco, with other nicotine-induced disorders
F17.229 Nicotine dependence, chewing tobacco, with unspecified nicotine-induced disorders
6th **F17.29** Nicotine dependence, other tobacco product
F17.290 Nicotine dependence, other tobacco product, uncomplicated
F17.291 Nicotine dependence, other tobacco product, in remission
F17.293 Nicotine dependence, other tobacco product, with withdrawal
F17.298 Nicotine dependence, other tobacco product, with other nicotine-induced disorders
F17.299 Nicotine dependence, other tobacco product, with unspecified nicotine-induced disorders

4th F18 Inhalant related disorders
INCLUDES volatile solvents

5th **F18.1 Inhalant abuse**
EXCLUDES 1 *inhalant dependence (F18.2-)*
inhalant use, unspecified (F18.9-)
F18.10 Inhalant abuse, uncomplicated
6th **F18.12** Inhalant abuse with intoxication
F18.120 Inhalant abuse with intoxication, uncomplicated
F18.121 Inhalant abuse with intoxication delirium

F18.129 Inhalant abuse with intoxication, unspecified

F18.14 Inhalant abuse with inhalant-induced mood disorder

√6th **F18.15 Inhalant abuse with inhalant-induced psychotic disorder**

F18.150 Inhalant abuse with inhalant-induced psychotic disorder with delusions

F18.151 Inhalant abuse with inhalant-induced psychotic disorder with hallucinations

F18.159 Inhalant abuse with inhalant-induced psychotic disorder, unspecified

F18.17 Inhalant abuse with inhalant-induced dementia

√6th **F18.18 Inhalant abuse with other inhalant-induced disorders**

F18.180 Inhalant abuse with inhalant-induced anxiety disorder

F18.188 Inhalant abuse with other inhalant-induced disorder

F18.19 Inhalant abuse with unspecified inhalant-induced disorder

√5th **F18.2 Inhalant dependence**

EXCLUDES 1 *inhalant abuse (F18.1-)*
inhalant use, unspecified (F18.9-)

F18.20 Inhalant dependence, uncomplicated

F18.21 Inhalant dependence, in remission

√6th **F18.22 Inhalant dependence with intoxication**

F18.220 Inhalant dependence with intoxication, uncomplicated

F18.221 Inhalant dependence with intoxication delirium

F18.229 Inhalant dependence with intoxication, unspecified

F18.24 Inhalant dependence with inhalant-induced mood disorder

√6th **F18.25 Inhalant dependence with inhalant-induced psychotic disorder**

F18.250 Inhalant dependence with inhalant-induced psychotic disorder with delusions

F18.251 Inhalant dependence with inhalant-induced psychotic disorder with hallucinations

F18.259 Inhalant dependence with inhalant-induced psychotic disorder, unspecified

F18.27 Inhalant dependence with inhalant-induced dementia

√6th **F18.28 Inhalant dependence with other inhalant-induced disorders**

F18.280 Inhalant dependence with inhalant-induced anxiety disorder

F18.288 Inhalant dependence with other inhalant-induced disorder

F18.29 Inhalant dependence with unspecified inhalant-induced disorder

√5th **F18.9 Inhalant use, unspecified**

EXCLUDES 1 *inhalant abuse (F18.1-)*
inhalant dependence (F18.2-)

F18.90 Inhalant use, unspecified, uncomplicated

√6th **F18.92 Inhalant use, unspecified with intoxication**

F18.920 Inhalant use, unspecified with intoxication, uncomplicated

F18.921 Inhalant use, unspecified with intoxication with delirium

F18.929 Inhalant use, unspecified with intoxication, unspecified

F18.94 Inhalant use, unspecified with inhalant-induced mood disorder

√6th **F18.95 Inhalant use, unspecified with inhalant-induced psychotic disorder**

F18.950 Inhalant use, unspecified with inhalant-induced psychotic disorder with delusions

F18.951 Inhalant use, unspecified with inhalant-induced psychotic disorder with hallucinations

F18.959 Inhalant use, unspecified with inhalant-induced psychotic disorder, unspecified

F18.97 Inhalant use, unspecified with inhalant-induced persisting dementia

√6th **F18.98 Inhalant use, unspecified with other inhalant-induced disorders**

F18.980 Inhalant use, unspecified with inhalant-induced anxiety disorder

F18.988 Inhalant use, unspecified with other inhalant-induced disorder

F18.99 Inhalant use, unspecified with unspecified inhalant-induced disorder

√4th **F19 Other psychoactive substance related disorders**

INCLUDES polysubstance drug use (indiscriminate drug use)

√5th **F19.1 Other psychoactive substance abuse**

EXCLUDES 1 *other psychoactive substance dependence (F19.2-)*
other psychoactive substance use, unspecified (F19.9-)

F19.10 Other psychoactive substance abuse, uncomplicated

√6th **F19.12 Other psychoactive substance abuse with intoxication**

F19.120 Other psychoactive substance abuse with intoxication, uncomplicated

F19.121 Other psychoactive substance abuse with intoxication delirium

F19.122 Other psychoactive substance abuse with intoxication with perceptual disturbances

F19.129 Other psychoactive substance abuse with intoxication, unspecified

F19.14 Other psychoactive substance abuse with psychoactive substance-induced mood disorder

√6th **F19.15 Other psychoactive substance abuse with psychoactive substance-induced psychotic disorder**

F19.150 Other psychoactive substance abuse with psychoactive substance-induced psychotic disorder with delusions

F19.151 Other psychoactive substance abuse with psychoactive substance-induced psychotic disorder with hallucinations

F19.159 Other psychoactive substance abuse with psychoactive substance-induced psychotic disorder, unspecified

F19.16 Other psychoactive substance abuse with psychoactive substance-induced persisting amnestic disorder

F19.17 Other psychoactive substance abuse with psychoactive substance-induced persisting dementia

√6th **F19.18 Other psychoactive substance abuse with other psychoactive substance-induced disorders**

F19.180 Other psychoactive substance abuse with psychoactive substance-induced anxiety disorder

F19.181 Other psychoactive substance abuse with psychoactive substance-induced sexual dysfunction

F19.182 Other psychoactive substance abuse with psychoactive substance-induced sleep disorder

F19.188 Other psychoactive substance abuse with other psychoactive substance-induced disorder

F19.19 Other psychoactive substance abuse with unspecified psychoactive substance-induced disorder

√5th **F19.2 Other psychoactive substance dependence**

EXCLUDES 1 *other psychoactive substance abuse (F19.1-)*
other psychoactive substance use, unspecified (F19.9-)

F19.20 Other psychoactive substance dependence, uncomplicated

F19.21 Other psychoactive substance dependence, in remission

6th **F19.22 Other psychoactive substance dependence with intoxication**
EXCLUDES 1 *other psychoactive substance dependence with withdrawal (F19.23-)*
F19.220 Other psychoactive substance dependence with intoxication, uncomplicated
F19.221 Other psychoactive substance dependence with intoxication delirium
F19.222 Other psychoactive substance dependence with intoxication with perceptual disturbance
F19.229 Other psychoactive substance dependence with intoxication, unspecified

6th **F19.23 Other psychoactive substance dependence with withdrawal**
EXCLUDES 1 *other psychoactive substance dependence with intoxication (F19.22-)*
F19.230 Other psychoactive substance dependence with withdrawal, uncomplicated
F19.231 Other psychoactive substance dependence with withdrawal delirium
F19.232 Other psychoactive substance dependence with withdrawal with perceptual disturbance
F19.239 Other psychoactive substance dependence with withdrawal, unspecified

F19.24 Other psychoactive substance dependence with psychoactive substance-induced mood disorder

6th **F19.25 Other psychoactive substance dependence with psychoactive substance-induced psychotic disorder**
F19.250 Other psychoactive substance dependence with psychoactive substance-induced psychotic disorder with delusions
F19.251 Other psychoactive substance dependence with psychoactive substance-induced psychotic disorder with hallucinations
F19.259 Other psychoactive substance dependence with psychoactive substance-induced psychotic disorder, unspecified

F19.26 Other psychoactive substance dependence with psychoactive substance-induced persisting amnestic disorder

F19.27 Other psychoactive substance dependence with psychoactive substance-induced persisting dementia

6th **F19.28 Other psychoactive substance dependence with other psychoactive substance-induced disorders**
F19.280 Other psychoactive substance dependence with psychoactive substance-induced anxiety disorder
F19.281 Other psychoactive substance dependence with psychoactive substance-induced sexual dysfunction
F19.282 Other psychoactive substance dependence with psychoactive substance-induced sleep disorder
F19.288 Other psychoactive substance dependence with other psychoactive substance-induced disorder

F19.29 Other psychoactive substance dependence with unspecified psychoactive substance-induced disorder

5th **F19.9 Other psychoactive substance use, unspecified**
EXCLUDES 1 *other psychoactive substance abuse (F19.1-)*
other psychoactive substance dependence (F19.2-)

F19.90 Other psychoactive substance use, unspecified, uncomplicated

6th **F19.92 Other psychoactive substance use, unspecified with intoxication**
EXCLUDES 1 *other psychoactive substance use, unspecified with withdrawal (F19.93)*
F19.920 Other psychoactive substance use, unspecified with intoxication, uncomplicated
F19.921 Other psychoactive substance use, unspecified with intoxication with delirium
F19.922 Other psychoactive substance use, unspecified with intoxication with perceptual disturbance
F19.929 Other psychoactive substance use, unspecified with intoxication, unspecified

6th **F19.93 Other psychoactive substance use, unspecified with withdrawal**
EXCLUDES 1 *other psychoactive substance use, unspecified with intoxication (F19.92-)*
F19.930 Other psychoactive substance use, unspecified with withdrawal, uncomplicated
F19.931 Other psychoactive substance use, unspecified with withdrawal delirium
F19.932 Other psychoactive substance use, unspecified with withdrawal with perceptual disturbance
F19.939 Other psychoactive substance use, unspecified with withdrawal, unspecified

F19.94 Other psychoactive substance use, unspecified with psychoactive substance-induced mood disorder

6th **F19.95 Other psychoactive substance use, unspecified with psychoactive substance-induced psychotic disorder**
F19.950 Other psychoactive substance use, unspecified with psychoactive substance-induced psychotic disorder with delusions
F19.951 Other psychoactive substance use, unspecified with psychoactive substance-induced psychotic disorder with hallucinations
F19.959 Other psychoactive substance use, unspecified with psychoactive substance-induced psychotic disorder, unspecified

F19.96 Other psychoactive substance use, unspecified with psychoactive substance-induced persisting amnestic disorder

F19.97 Other psychoactive substance use, unspecified with psychoactive substance-induced persisting dementia

6th **F19.98 Other psychoactive substance use, unspecified with other psychoactive substance-induced disorders**
F19.980 Other psychoactive substance use, unspecified with psychoactive substance-induced anxiety disorder
F19.981 Other psychoactive substance use, unspecified with psychoactive substance-induced sexual dysfunction
F19.982 Other psychoactive substance use, unspecified with psychoactive substance-induced sleep disorder
F19.988 Other psychoactive substance use, unspecified with other psychoactive substance-induced disorder

F19.99 Other psychoactive substance use, unspecified with unspecified psychoactive substance-induced disorder

Schizophrenia, schizotypal, delusional, and other non-mood psychotic disorders (F20-F29)

4th F20 Schizophrenia

EXCLUDES 1 *brief psychotic disorder (F23)*
cyclic schizophrenia (F25.0)
mood [affective] disorders with psychotic symptoms (F30.2, F31.2, F31.5, F31.64, F32.3, F33.3)
schizoaffective disorder (F25.-)
schizophrenic reaction NOS (F23)

EXCLUDES 2 *schizophrenic reaction in:*
alcoholism (F10.15-, F10.25-, F10.95-)
brain disease (F06.2)
epilepsy (F06.2)
psychoactive drug use (F11-F19 with .15. .25, .95)
schizotypal disorder (F21)

F20.0 Paranoid schizophrenia
Paraphrenic schizophrenia
EXCLUDES 1 *involutional paranoid state (F22)*
paranoia (F22)

F20.1 Disorganized schizophrenia
Hebephrenic schizophrenia
Hebephrenia

F20.2 Catatonic schizophrenia
Schizophrenic catalepsy
Schizophrenic catatonia
Schizophrenic flexibilitas cerea
EXCLUDES 1 *catatonic stupor (R40.1)*

F20.3 Undifferentiated schizophrenia
Atypical schizophrenia
EXCLUDES 1 *acute schizophrenia-like psychotic disorder (F23)*
EXCLUDES 2 *post-schizophrenic depression (F32.8)*

F20.5 Residual schizophrenia
Restzustand (schizophrenic)
Schizophrenic residual state

5th F20.8 Other schizophrenia

F20.81 Schizophreniform disorder
Schizophreniform psychosis NOS

F20.89 Other schizophrenia
Cenesthopathic schizophrenia
Simple schizophrenia

F20.9 Schizophrenia, unspecified

F21 Schizotypal disorder
Borderline schizophrenia
Latent schizophrenia
Latent schizophrenic reaction
Prepsychotic schizophrenia
Prodromal schizophrenia
Pseudoneurotic schizophrenia
Pseudopsychopathic schizophrenia
Schizotypal personality disorder
EXCLUDES 2 *Asperger's syndrome (F84.5)*
schizoid personality disorder (F60.1)

F22 Delusional disorders
Delusional dysmorphophobia
Involutional paranoid state
Paranoia
Paranoia querulans
Paranoid psychosis
Paranoid state
Paraphrenia (late)
Sensitiver Beziehungswahn
EXCLUDES 1 *mood [affective] disorders with psychotic symptoms (F30.2, F31.2, F31.5, F31.64, F32.3, F33.3)*
paranoid schizophrenia (F20.0)
EXCLUDES 2 *paranoid personality disorder (F60.0)*
paranoid psychosis, psychogenic (F23)
paranoid reaction (F23)

F23 Brief psychotic disorder
Paranoid reaction
Psychogenic paranoid psychosis
EXCLUDES 2 *mood [affective] disorders with psychotic symptoms (F30.2, F31.2, F31.5, F31.64, F32.3, F33.3)*

F24 Shared psychotic disorder
Folie à deux
Induced paranoid disorder
Induced psychotic disorder

4th F25 Schizoaffective disorders
EXCLUDES 1 *mood [affective] disorders with psychotic symptoms (F30.2, F31.2, F31.5, F31.64, F32.3, F33.3)*
schizophrenia (F20.-)

F25.0 Schizoaffective disorder, bipolar type
Cyclic schizophrenia
Schizoaffective disorder, manic type
Schizoaffective disorder, mixed type
Schizoaffective psychosis, bipolar type
Schizophreniform psychosis, manic type

F25.1 Schizoaffective disorder, depressive type
Schizoaffective psychosis, depressive type
Schizophreniform psychosis, depressive type

F25.8 Other schizoaffective disorders

F25.9 Schizoaffective disorder, unspecified
Schizoaffective psychosis NOS

F28 Other psychotic disorder not due to a substance or known physiological condition
Chronic hallucinatory psychosis

F29 Unspecified psychosis not due to a substance or known physiological condition
Psychosis NOS
EXCLUDES 1 *mental disorder NOS (F99)*
unspecified mental disorder due to known physiological condition (F09)

Mood [affective] disorders (F30-F39)

4th F30 Manic episode
INCLUDES bipolar disorder, single manic episode
mixed affective episode
EXCLUDES 1 *bipolar disorder (F31.-)*
major depressive disorder, single episode (F32.-)
major depressive disorder, recurrent (F33.-)

5th F30.1 Manic episode without psychotic symptoms

F30.10 Manic episode without psychotic symptoms, unspecified

F30.11 Manic episode without psychotic symptoms, mild

F30.12 Manic episode without psychotic symptoms, moderate

F30.13 Manic episode, severe, without psychotic symptoms

F30.2 Manic episode, severe with psychotic symptoms
Manic stupor
Mania with mood-congruent psychotic symptoms
Mania with mood-incongruent psychotic symptoms

F30.3 Manic episode in partial remission

F30.4 Manic episode in full remission

F30.8 Other manic episodes
Hypomania

F30.9 Manic episode, unspecified
Mania NOS

4th F31 Bipolar disorder
INCLUDES manic-depressive illness
manic-depressive psychosis
manic-depressive reaction
EXCLUDES 1 *bipolar disorder, single manic episode (F30.-)*
major depressive disorder, single episode (F32.-)
major depressive disorder, recurrent (F33.-)
EXCLUDES 2 *cyclothymia (F34.0)*

F31.0 Bipolar disorder, current episode hypomanic

5th F31.1 Bipolar disorder, current episode manic without psychotic features

F31.10 Bipolar disorder, current episode manic without psychotic features, unspecified

F31.11 Bipolar disorder, current episode manic without psychotic features, mild

F31.12 Bipolar disorder, current episode manic without psychotic features, moderate

F31.13 Bipolar disorder, current episode manic without psychotic features, severe

F31.2 Bipolar disorder, current episode manic severe with psychotic features
Bipolar disorder, current episode manic with mood-congruent psychotic symptoms
Bipolar disorder, current episode manic with mood-incongruent psychotic symptoms

√5th **F31.3 Bipolar disorder, current episode depressed, mild or moderate severity**

F31.30 Bipolar disorder, current episode depressed, mild or moderate severity, unspecified

F31.31 Bipolar disorder, current episode depressed, mild

F31.32 Bipolar disorder, current episode depressed, moderate

F31.4 Bipolar disorder, current episode depressed, severe, without psychotic features

F31.5 Bipolar disorder, current episode depressed, severe, with psychotic features

Bipolar disorder, current episode depressed with mood-incongruent psychotic symptoms

Bipolar disorder, current episode depressed with mood-congruent psychotic symptoms

√5th **F31.6 Bipolar disorder, current episode mixed**

F31.60 Bipolar disorder, current episode mixed, unspecified

F31.61 Bipolar disorder, current episode mixed, mild

F31.62 Bipolar disorder, current episode mixed, moderate

F31.63 Bipolar disorder, current episode mixed, severe, without psychotic features

F31.64 Bipolar disorder, current episode mixed, severe, with psychotic features

Bipolar disorder, current episode mixed with mood-congruent psychotic symptoms

Bipolar disorder, current episode mixed with mood-incongruent psychotic symptoms

√5th **F31.7 Bipolar disorder, currently in remission**

F31.70 Bipolar disorder, currently in remission, most recent episode unspecified

F31.71 Bipolar disorder, in partial remission, most recent episode hypomanic

F31.72 Bipolar disorder, in full remission, most recent episode hypomanic

F31.73 Bipolar disorder, in partial remission, most recent episode manic

F31.74 Bipolar disorder, in full remission, most recent episode manic

F31.75 Bipolar disorder, in partial remission, most recent episode depressed

F31.76 Bipolar disorder, in full remission, most recent episode depressed

F31.77 Bipolar disorder, in partial remission, most recent episode mixed

F31.78 Bipolar disorder, in full remission, most recent episode mixed

√5th **F31.8 Other bipolar disorders**

F31.81 Bipolar II disorder

F31.89 Other bipolar disorder

Recurrent manic episodes NOS

F31.9 Bipolar disorder, unspecified

√4th **F32 Major depressive disorder, single episode**

INCLUDES single episode of agitated depression
single episode of depressive reaction
single episode of major depression
single episode of psychogenic depression
single episode of reactive depression
single episode of vital depression

EXCLUDES 1 *bipolar disorder (F31.-)*
manic episode (F30.-)
recurrent depressive disorder (F33.-)

EXCLUDES 2 *adjustment disorder (F43.2)*

F32.0 Major depressive disorder, single episode, mild

F32.1 Major depressive disorder, single episode, moderate

F32.2 Major depressive disorder, single episode, severe without psychotic features

F32.3 Major depressive disorder, single episode, severe with psychotic features

Single episode of major depression with mood-congruent psychotic symptoms

Single episode of major depression with mood-incongruent psychotic symptoms

Single episode of major depression with psychotic symptoms

Single episode of psychogenic depressive psychosis

Single episode of psychotic depression

Single episode of reactive depressive psychosis

F32.4 Major depressive disorder, single episode, in partial remission

F32.5 Major depressive disorder, single episode, in full remission

F32.8 Other depressive episodes

Atypical depression

Post-schizophrenic depression

Single episode of 'masked' depression NOS

F32.9 Major depressive disorder, single episode, unspecified

Depression NOS

Depressive disorder NOS

Major depression NOS

√4th **F33 Major depressive disorder, recurrent**

Recurrent episodes of depressive reaction
Recurrent episodes of endogenous depression
Recurrent episodes of major depression
Recurrent episodes of psychogenic depression
Recurrent episodes of reactive depression
Recurrent episodes of seasonal depressive disorder
Recurrent episodes of vital depression

EXCLUDES 1 *bipolar disorder (F31.-)*
manic episode (F30.-)

F33.0 Major depressive disorder, recurrent, mild

F33.1 Major depressive disorder, recurrent, moderate

F33.2 Major depressive disorder, recurrent severe without psychotic features

F33.3 Major depressive disorder, recurrent, severe with psychotic symptoms

Endogenous depression with psychotic symptoms

Recurrent severe episodes of major depression with mood-congruent psychotic symptoms

Recurrent severe episodes of major depression with mood-incongruent psychotic symptoms

Recurrent severe episodes of major depression with psychotic symptoms

Recurrent severe episodes of psychogenic depressive psychosis

Recurrent severe episodes of psychotic depression

Recurrent severe episodes of reactive depressive psychosis

√5th **F33.4 Major depressive disorder, recurrent, in remission**

F33.40 Major depressive disorder, recurrent, in remission, unspecified

F33.41 Major depressive disorder, recurrent, in partial remission

F33.42 Major depressive disorder, recurrent, in full remission

F33.8 Other recurrent depressive disorders

Recurrent brief depressive episodes

F33.9 Major depressive disorder, recurrent, unspecified

Monopolar depression NOS

√4th **F34 Persistent mood [affective] disorders**

F34.0 Cyclothymic disorder

Affective personality disorder

Cycloid personality

Cyclothymia

Cyclothymic personality

F34.1 Dysthymic disorder

Depressive neurosis

Depressive personality disorder

Dysthymia

Neurotic depression

Persistent anxiety depression

EXCLUDES 2 *anxiety depression (mild or not persistent) (F41.8)*

F34.8 Other persistent mood [affective] disorders

F34.9 Persistent mood [affective] disorder, unspecified

F39 Unspecified mood [affective] disorder

Affective psychosis NOS

Anxiety, dissociative, stress-related, somatoform and other nonpsychotic mental disorders (F40-F48)

√4th **F40 Phobic anxiety disorders**

√5th **F40.0 Agoraphobia**

F40.00 Agoraphobia, unspecified

F40.01 Agoraphobia with panic disorder

Panic disorder with agoraphobia

EXCLUDES 1 *panic disorder without agoraphobia (F41.0)*

F40.02 Agoraphobia without panic disorder

✓5th **F40.1 Social phobias**
Anthropophobia
Social anxiety disorder of childhood
Social neurosis
F40.10 Social phobia, unspecified
F40.11 Social phobia, generalized

✓5th **F40.2 Specific (isolated) phobias**
EXCLUDES 2 *dysmorphophobia (nondelusional) (F45.22)*
nosophobia (F45.22)

✓6th **F40.21 Animal type phobia**
F40.210 Arachnophobia
Fear of spiders
F40.218 Other animal type phobia

✓6th **F40.22 Natural environment type phobia**
F40.220 Fear of thunderstorms
F40.228 Other natural environment type phobia

✓6th **F40.23 Blood, injection, injury type phobia**
F40.230 Fear of blood
F40.231 Fear of injections and transfusions
F40.232 Fear of other medical care
F40.233 Fear of injury

✓6th **F40.24 Situational type phobia**
F40.240 Claustrophobia
F40.241 Acrophobia
F40.242 Fear of bridges
F40.243 Fear of flying
F40.248 Other situational type phobia

✓6th **F40.29 Other specified phobia**
F40.290 Androphobia
Fear of men
F40.291 Gynephobia
Fear of women
F40.298 Other specified phobia

F40.8 Other phobic anxiety disorders
Phobic anxiety disorder of childhood

F40.9 Phobic anxiety disorder, unspecified
Phobia NOS
Phobic state NOS

✓4th **F41 Other anxiety disorders**
EXCLUDES 2 *anxiety in:*
acute stress reaction (F43.0)
transient adjustment reaction (F43.2)
neurasthenia (F48.8)
psychophysiologic disorders (F45.-)
separation anxiety (F93.0)

F41.0 Panic disorder [episodic paroxysmal anxiety] without agoraphobia
Panic attack
Panic state
EXCLUDES 1 *panic disorder with agoraphobia (F40.01)*

F41.1 Generalized anxiety disorder
Anxiety neurosis
Anxiety reaction
Anxiety state
Overanxious disorder
EXCLUDES 2 *neurasthenia (F48.8)*

F41.3 Other mixed anxiety disorders

F41.8 Other specified anxiety disorders
Anxiety depression (mild or not persistent)
Anxiety hysteria
Mixed anxiety and depressive disorder

F41.9 Anxiety disorder, unspecified
Anxiety NOS

F42 Obsessive-compulsive disorder
Anancastic neurosis
Obsessive-compulsive neurosis
EXCLUDES 2 *obsessive-compulsive personality (disorder) (F60.5)*
obsessive-compulsive symptoms occurring in:
depression (F32-F33)
schizophrenia (F20.-)

✓4th **F43 Reaction to severe stress, and adjustment disorders**

F43.0 Acute stress reaction
Acute crisis reaction
Acute reaction to stress
Combat and operational stress reaction
Combat fatigue
Crisis state
Psychic shock

✓5th **F43.1 Post-traumatic stress disorder (PTSD)**
Traumatic neurosis
F43.10 Post-traumatic stress disorder, unspecified
F43.11 Post-traumatic stress disorder, acute
F43.12 Post-traumatic stress disorder, chronic

✓5th **F43.2 Adjustment disorders**
Culture shock
Grief reaction
Hospitalism in children
EXCLUDES 2 *separation anxiety disorder of childhood (F93.0)*
F43.20 Adjustment disorder, unspecified
F43.21 Adjustment disorder with depressed mood
F43.22 Adjustment disorder with anxiety
F43.23 Adjustment disorder with mixed anxiety and depressed mood
F43.24 Adjustment disorder with disturbance of conduct
F43.25 Adjustment disorder with mixed disturbance of emotions and conduct
F43.29 Adjustment disorder with other symptoms

F43.8 Other reactions to severe stress

F43.9 Reaction to severe stress, unspecified

✓4th **F44 Dissociative and conversion disorders**
INCLUDES conversion hysteria
conversion reaction
hysteria
hysterical psychosis
EXCLUDES 2 *malingering [conscious simulation] (Z76.5)*

F44.0 Dissociative amnesia
EXCLUDES 1 *amnesia NOS (R41.3)*
anterograde amnesia (R41.1)
retrograde amnesia (R41.2)
EXCLUDES 2 *alcohol-or other psychoactive substance-induced amnestic disorder (F10, F13, F19 with .26, .96)*
amnestic disorder due to known physiological condition (F04)
postictal amnesia in epilepsy (G40.-)

F44.1 Dissociative fugue
EXCLUDES 2 *postictal fugue in epilepsy (G40.-)*

F44.2 Dissociative stupor
EXCLUDES 1 *catatonic stupor (R40.1)*
stupor NOS (R40.1)
EXCLUDES 2 *catatonic disorder due to known physiological condition (F06.1)*
depressive stupor (F32, F33)
manic stupor (F30, F31)

F44.4 Conversion disorder with motor symptom or deficit
Dissociative motor disorders
Psychogenic aphonia
Psychogenic dysphonia

F44.5 Conversion disorder with seizures or convulsions
Dissociative convulsions

F44.6 Conversion disorder with sensory symptom or deficit
Dissociative anesthesia and sensory loss
Psychogenic deafness

F44.7 Conversion disorder with mixed symptom presentation

✓5th **F44.8 Other dissociative and conversion disorders**
F44.81 Dissociative identity disorder
Multiple personality disorder
F44.89 Other dissociative and conversion disorders
Ganser's syndrome
Psychogenic confusion
Psychogenic twilight state
Trance and possession disorders

F44.9 Dissociative and conversion disorder, unspecified
Dissociative disorder NOS

✓4th F45 Somatoform disorders
EXCLUDES 2 *dissociative and conversion disorders (F44.-)*
factitious disorders (F68.1-)
hair-plucking (F63.3)
lalling (F80.0)
lisping (F80.0)
malingering [conscious simulation] (Z76.5)
nail-biting (F98.8)
psychological or behavioral factors associated with disorders or diseases classified elsewhere (F54)
sexual dysfunction, not due to a substance or known physiological condition (F52.-)
thumb-sucking (F98.8)
tic disorders (in childhood and adolescence) (F95.-)
Tourette's syndrome (F95.2)
trichotillomania (F63.3)

F45.0 Somatization disorder
Briquet's disorder
Multiple psychosomatic disorder

F45.1 Undifferentiated somatoform disorder
Undifferentiated psychosomatic disorder

✓5th F45.2 Hypochondriacal disorders
EXCLUDES 2 *delusional dysmorphophobia (F22)*
fixed delusions about bodily functions or shape (F22)

F45.20 Hypochondriacal disorder, unspecified

F45.21 Hypochondriasis
Hypochondriacal neurosis

F45.22 Body dysmorphic disorder
Dysmorphophobia (nondelusional)
Nosophobia

F45.29 Other hypochondriacal disorders

✓5th F45.4 Pain disorders related to psychological factors
EXCLUDES 1 *pain NOS (R52)*

F45.41 Pain disorder exclusively related to psychological factors
Somatoform pain disorder (persistent)

F45.42 Pain disorder with related psychological factors
Code also associated acute or chronic pain (G89.-)

F45.8 Other somatoform disorders
Psychogenic dysmenorrhea
Psychogenic dysphagia, including "globus hystericus"
Psychogenic pruritus
Psychogenic torticollis
Somatoform autonomic dysfunction
Teeth grinding
EXCLUDES 1 *sleep related teeth grinding (G47.63)*

F45.9 Somatoform disorder, unspecified
Psychosomatic disorder NOS

✓4th F48 Other nonpsychotic mental disorders

F48.1 Depersonalization-derealization syndrome

F48.2 Pseudobulbar affect
Involuntary emotional expression disorder
Code first underlying cause, if known, such as:
amyotrophic lateral sclerosis (G12.21)
multiple sclerosis (G35)
sequelae of cerebrovascular disease (I69.-)
sequelae of traumatic intracranial injury (S06.-)

F48.8 Other specified nonpsychotic mental disorders
Dhat syndrome
Neurasthenia
Occupational neurosis, including writer's cramp
Psychasthenia
Psychasthenic neurosis
Psychogenic syncope

F48.9 Nonpsychotic mental disorder, unspecified
Neurosis NOS

Behavioral syndromes associated with physiological disturbances and physical factors (F50-F59)

✓4th F50 Eating disorders
EXCLUDES 1 *anorexia NOS (R63.0)*
feeding difficulties (R63.3)
polyphagia (R63.2)
EXCLUDES 2 *feeding disorder in infancy or childhood (F98.2-)*

✓5th F50.0 Anorexia nervosa
EXCLUDES 1 *loss of appetite (R63.0)*
psychogenic loss of appetite (F50.8)

F50.00 Anorexia nervosa, unspecified

F50.01 Anorexia nervosa, restricting type

F50.02 Anorexia nervosa, binge eating/purging type
EXCLUDES 1 *bulimia nervosa (F50.2)*

F50.2 Bulimia nervosa
Bulimia NOS
Hyperorexia nervosa
EXCLUDES 1 *anorexia nervosa, binge eating/purging type (F50.02)*

F50.8 Other eating disorders
Pica in adults
Psychogenic loss of appetite
EXCLUDES 2 *pica of infancy and childhood (F98.3)*

F50.9 Eating disorder, unspecified
Atypical anorexia nervosa
Atypical bulimia nervosa

✓4th F51 Sleep disorders not due to a substance or known physiological condition
EXCLUDES 2 *organic sleep disorders (G47.-)*

✓5th F51.0 Insomnia not due to a substance or known physiological condition
EXCLUDES 2 *alcohol related insomnia (F10.182, F10.282, F10.982)*
drug related insomnia (F11.182, F11.282, F11.982, F13.182, F13.282, F13.982, F14.182, F14.282, F14.982, F15.182, F15.282, F15.982, F19.182, F19.282, F19.982)
insomnia NOS (G47.0-)
insomnia due to known physiological condition (G47.0-)
organic insomnia (G47.0-)
sleep deprivation (Z72.820)

F51.01 Primary insomnia
Idiopathic insomnia

F51.02 Adjustment insomnia

F51.03 Paradoxical insomnia

F51.04 Psychophysiologic insomnia

F51.05 Insomnia due to other mental disorder
Code also associated mental disorder

F51.09 Other insomnia not due to a substance or known physiological condition

✓5th F51.1 Hypersomnia not due to a substance or known physiological condition
EXCLUDES 2 *alcohol related hypersomnia (F10.182, F10.282, F10.982)*
drug related hypersomnia (F11.182, F11.282, F11.982, F13.182, F13.282, F13.982, F14.182, F14.282, F14.982, F15.182, F15.282, F15.982, F19.182, F19.282, F19.982)
hypersomnia NOS (G47.10)
hypersomnia due to known physiological condition (G47.10)
idiopathic hypersomnia (G47.11, G47.12)
narcolepsy (G47.4-)

F51.11 Primary hypersomnia

F51.12 Insufficient sleep syndrome
EXCLUDES 1 *sleep deprivation (Z72.820)*

F51.13 Hypersomnia due to other mental disorder
Code also associated mental disorder

F51.19 Other hypersomnia not due to a substance or known physiological condition

F51.3 Sleepwalking [somnambulism]

F51.4 Sleep terrors [night terrors]

F51.5 Nightmare disorder
Dream anxiety disorder

F51.8 Other sleep disorders not due to a substance or known physiological condition

F51.9 Sleep disorder not due to a substance or known physiological condition, unspecified
Emotional sleep disorder NOS

✓4th F52 Sexual dysfunction not due to a substance or known physiological condition
EXCLUDES 2 *Dhat syndrome (F48.8)*

F52.0 Hypoactive sexual desire disorder
Anhedonia (sexual)
Lack or loss of sexual desire
EXCLUDES 1 *decreased libido (R68.82)*

F52.1 Sexual aversion disorder
Sexual aversion and lack of sexual enjoyment

✓5th **F52.2 Sexual arousal disorders**
Failure of genital response
F52.21 Male erectile disorder
Psychogenic impotence
EXCLUDES 1 *impotence of organic origin (N52.-)*
impotence NOS (N52.-)
F52.22 Female sexual arousal disorder
Frigidity
✓5th **F52.3 Orgasmic disorder**
Inhibited orgasm
Psychogenic anorgasmy
F52.31 Female orgasmic disorder
F52.32 Male orgasmic disorder
F52.4 Premature ejaculation
F52.5 Vaginismus not due to a substance or known physiological condition
Psychogenic vaginismus
EXCLUDES 2 *vaginismus (due to a known physiological condition) (N94.2)*
F52.6 Dyspareunia not due to a substance or known physiological condition
Psychogenic dyspareunia
EXCLUDES 2 *dyspareunia (due to a known physiological condition) (N94.1)*
F52.8 Other sexual dysfunction not due to a substance or known physiological condition
Excessive sexual drive
Nymphomania
Satyriasis
F52.9 Unspecified sexual dysfunction not due to a substance or known physiological condition
Sexual dysfunction NOS

F53 Puerperal psychosis
Postpartum depression
EXCLUDES 1 *mood disorders with psychotic features (F30.2, F31.2, F31.5, F31.64, F32.3, F33.3)*
postpartum dysphoria (O90.6)
psychosis in schizophrenia, schizotypal, delusional, and other psychotic disorders (F20-F29)

F54 Psychological and behavioral factors associated with disorders or diseases classified elsewhere
Psychological factors affecting physical conditions
Code first the associated physical disorder, such as:
asthma (J45.-)
dermatitis (L23-L25)
gastric ulcer (K25.-)
mucous colitis (K58.-)
ulcerative colitis (K51.-)
urticaria (L50.-)
EXCLUDES 2 *tension-type headache (G44.2)*

✓4th **F55 Abuse of non-psychoactive substances**
EXCLUDES 2 *abuse of psychoactive substances (F10-F19)*
F55.0 Abuse of antacids
F55.1 Abuse of herbal or folk remedies
F55.2 Abuse of laxatives
F55.3 Abuse of steroids or hormones
F55.4 Abuse of vitamins
F55.8 Abuse of other non-psychoactive substances

F59 Unspecified behavioral syndromes associated with physiological disturbances and physical factors
Psychogenic physiological dysfunction NOS

Disorders of adult personality and behavior (F60-F69)

✓4th **F60 Specific personality disorders**
F60.0 Paranoid personality disorder
Expansive paranoid personality (disorder)
Fanatic personality (disorder)
Querulant personality (disorder)
Paranoid personality (disorder)
Sensitive paranoid personality (disorder)
EXCLUDES 2 *paranoia (F22)*
paranoia querulans (F22)
paranoid psychosis (F22)
paranoid schizophrenia (F20.0)
paranoid state (F22)
F60.1 Schizoid personality disorder
EXCLUDES 2 *Asperger's syndrome (F84.5)*
delusional disorder (F22)
schizoid disorder of childhood (F84.5)
schizophrenia (F20.-)
schizotypal disorder (F21)
F60.2 Antisocial personality disorder
Amoral personality (disorder)
Asocial personality (disorder)
Dissocial personality disorder
Psychopathic personality (disorder)
Sociopathic personality (disorder)
EXCLUDES 1 *conduct disorders (F91.-)*
EXCLUDES 2 *borderline personality disorder (F60.3)*
F60.3 Borderline personality disorder
Aggressive personality (disorder)
Emotionally unstable personality disorder
Explosive personality (disorder)
EXCLUDES 2 *antisocial personality disorder (F60.2)*
F60.4 Histrionic personality disorder
Hysterical personality (disorder)
Psychoinfantile personality (disorder)
F60.5 Obsessive-compulsive personality disorder
Anankastic personality (disorder)
Compulsive personality (disorder)
Obsessional personality (disorder)
EXCLUDES 2 *obsessive-compulsive disorder (F42)*
F60.6 Avoidant personality disorder
Anxious personality disorder
F60.7 Dependent personality disorder
Asthenic personality (disorder)
Inadequate personality (disorder)
Passive personality (disorder)
✓5th **F60.8 Other specific personality disorders**
F60.81 Narcissistic personality disorder
F60.89 Other specific personality disorders
Eccentric personality disorder
"Haltlose" type personality disorder
Immature personality disorder
Passive-aggressive personality disorder
Psychoneurotic personality disorder
Self-defeating personality disorder
F60.9 Personality disorder, unspecified
Character disorder NOS
Character neurosis NOS
Pathological personality NOS

✓4th **F63 Impulse disorders**
EXCLUDES 2 *habitual excessive use of alcohol or psychoactive substances (F10-F19)*
impulse disorders involving sexual behavior (F65.-)
F63.0 Pathological gambling
Compulsive gambling
EXCLUDES 1 *gambling and betting NOS (Z72.6)*
EXCLUDES 2 *excessive gambling by manic patients (F30, F31)*
gambling in antisocial personality disorder (F60.2)
F63.1 Pyromania
Pathological fire-setting
EXCLUDES 2 *fire-setting (by) (in):*
adult with antisocial personality disorder (F60.2)
alcohol or psychoactive substance intoxication (F10-F19)
conduct disorders (F91.-)
mental disorders due to known physiological condition (F01-F09)
schizophrenia (F20.-)
F63.2 Kleptomania
Pathological stealing
EXCLUDES 1 *shoplifting as the reason for observation for suspected mental disorder (Z03.8)*
EXCLUDES 2 *depressive disorder with stealing (F31-F33)*
stealing due to underlying mental condition—code to mental condition
stealing in mental disorders due to known physiological condition (F01-F09)
F63.3 Trichotillomania
Hair plucking
EXCLUDES 2 *other stereotyped movement disorder (F98.4)*
✓5th **F63.8 Other impulse disorders**
F63.81 Intermittent explosive disorder

F63.89 Other impulse disorders
F63.9 Impulse disorder, unspecified
Impulse control disorder NOS

✓4th **F64 Gender identity disorders**
F64.1 Gender identity disorder in adolescence and adulthood
Dual role transvestism
Transsexualism
Use additional code to identify sex reassignment status (Z87.890)
EXCLUDES 1 *gender identity disorder in childhood (F64.2)*
EXCLUDES 2 *fetishistic transvestism (F65.1)*
F64.2 Gender identity disorder of childhood
EXCLUDES 1 *gender identity disorder in adolescence and adulthood (F64.1)*
EXCLUDES 2 *sexual maturation disorder (F66)*
F64.8 Other gender identity disorders
F64.9 Gender identity disorder, unspecified
Gender-role disorder NOS

✓4th **F65 Paraphilias**
F65.Ø Fetishism
F65.1 Transvestic fetishism
Fetishistic transvestism
F65.2 Exhibitionism
F65.3 Voyeurism
F65.4 Pedophilia
✓5th **F65.5 Sadomasochism**
F65.5Ø Sadomasochism, unspecified
F65.51 Sexual masochism
F65.52 Sexual sadism
✓5th **F65.8 Other paraphilias**
F65.81 Frotteurism
F65.89 Other paraphilias
Necrophilia
F65.9 Paraphilia, unspecified
Sexual deviation NOS

F66 Other sexual disorders
Sexual maturation disorder
Sexual relationship disorder

✓4th **F68 Other disorders of adult personality and behavior**
✓5th **F68.1 Factitious disorder**
Compensation neurosis
Elaboration of physical symptoms for psychological reasons
Hospital hopper syndrome
Münchhausen's syndrome
Peregrinating patient
EXCLUDES 2 *factitial dermatitis (L98.1)*
person feigning illness (with obvious motivation) (Z76.5)
F68.1Ø Factitious disorder, unspecified
F68.11 Factitious disorder with predominantly psychological signs and symptoms
F68.12 Factitious disorder with predominantly physical signs and symptoms
F68.13 Factitious disorder with combined psychological and physical signs and symptoms
F68.8 Other specified disorders of adult personality and behavior
F69 Unspecified disorder of adult personality and behavior

Intellectual Disabilities (F7Ø-F79)

Code first any associated physical or developmental disorders
EXCLUDES 1 *borderline intellectual functioning, IQ above 7Ø to 84 (R41.83)*

F7Ø Mild intellectual disabilities
IQ level 5Ø-55 to approximately 7Ø
Mild mental subnormality

F71 Moderate intellectual disabilities
IQ level 35-4Ø to 5Ø-55
Moderate mental subnormality

F72 Severe intellectual disabilities
IQ 2Ø-25 to 35-4Ø
Severe mental subnormality

F73 Profound intellectual disabilities
IQ level below 2Ø-25
Profound mental subnormality

F78 Other intellectual disabilities

F79 Unspecified intellectual disabilities
Mental deficiency NOS
Mental subnormality NOS

Pervasive and specific developmental disorders (F8Ø-F89)

✓4th **F8Ø Specific developmental disorders of speech and language**
F8Ø.Ø Phonological disorder
Dyslalia
Functional speech articulation disorder
Lalling
Lisping
Phonological developmental disorder
Speech articulation developmental disorder
EXCLUDES 1 *speech articulation impairment due to aphasia NOS (R47.Ø1)*
speech articulation impairment due to apraxia (R48.2)
EXCLUDES 2 *speech articulation impairment due to hearing loss (F8Ø.4)*
speech articulation impairment due to intellectual disabilities (F7Ø-F79)
speech articulation impairment with expressive language developmental disorder (F8Ø.1)
speech articulation impairment with mixed receptive expressive language developmental disorder (F8Ø.2)
F8Ø.1 Expressive language disorder
Developmental dysphasia or aphasia, expressive type
EXCLUDES 1 *dysphasia and aphasia NOS (R47.-)*
mixed receptive-expressive language disorder (F8Ø.2)
EXCLUDES 2 *acquired aphasia with epilepsy [Landau-Kleffner] (G4Ø.8Ø-)*
intellectual disabilities (F7Ø-F79)
pervasive developmental disorders (F84.-)
selective mutism (F94.Ø)
F8Ø.2 Mixed receptive-expressive language disorder
Developmental dysphasia or aphasia, receptive type
Developmental Wernicke's aphasia
EXCLUDES 1 *central auditory processing disorder (H93.25)*
dysphasia or aphasia NOS (R47.-)
expressive language disorder (F8Ø.1)
expressive type dysphasia or aphasia (F8Ø.1)
word deafness (H93.25)
EXCLUDES 2 *acquired aphasia with epilepsy [Landau-Kleffner] (G4Ø.8Ø-)*
intellectual disabilities (F7Ø-F79)
pervasive developmental disorders (F84.-)
selective mutism (F94.Ø)
F8Ø.4 Speech and language development delay due to hearing loss
Code also type of hearing loss (H9Ø.-, H91.-)
✓5th **F8Ø.8 Other developmental disorders of speech and language**
F8Ø.81 Childhood onset fluency disorder
Cluttering NOS
Stuttering NOS
EXCLUDES 1 *adult onset fluency disorder (F98.5)*
fluency disorder in conditions classified elsewhere (R47.82)
fluency disorder (stuttering) following cerebrovascular disease (I69. with final characters-23)
F8Ø.89 Other developmental disorders of speech and language
F8Ø.9 Developmental disorder of speech and language, unspecified
Communication disorder NOS
Language disorder NOS

✓4th **F81 Specific developmental disorders of scholastic skills**
F81.Ø Specific reading disorder
"Backward reading"
Developmental dyslexia
Specific reading retardation
EXCLUDES 1 *alexia NOS (R48.Ø)*
dyslexia NOS (R48.Ø)

F81.2 Mathematics disorder
Developmental acalculia
Developmental arithmetical disorder
Developmental Gerstmann's syndrome
EXCLUDES 1 *acalculia NOS (R48.8)*
EXCLUDES 2 *arithmetical difficulties associated with a reading disorder (F81.0)*
arithmetical difficulties associated with a spelling disorder (F81.81)
arithmetical difficulties due to inadequate teaching (Z55.8)

✓5th **F81.8 Other developmental disorders of scholastic skills**
F81.81 Disorder of written expression
Specific spelling disorder
F81.89 Other developmental disorders of scholastic skills

F81.9 Developmental disorder of scholastic skills, unspecified
Knowledge acquisition disability NOS
Learning disability NOS
Learning disorder NOS

F82 Specific developmental disorder of motor function
Clumsy child syndrome
Developmental coordination disorder
Developmental dyspraxia
EXCLUDES 1 *abnormalities of gait and mobility (R26.-)*
lack of coordination (R27.-)
EXCLUDES 2 *lack of coordination secondary to intellectual disabilities (F70-F79)*

✓4th **F84 Pervasive developmental disorders**
Use additional code to identify any associated medical condition and intellectual disabilities

F84.0 Autistic disorder
Infantile autism
Infantile psychosis
Kanner's syndrome
EXCLUDES 1 *Asperger's syndrome (F84.5)*

F84.2 Rett's syndrome
EXCLUDES 1 *Asperger's syndrome (F84.5)*
Autistic disorder (F84.0)
Other childhood disintegrative disorder (F84.3)

F84.3 Other childhood disintegrative disorder
Dementia infantilis
Disintegrative psychosis
Heller's syndrome
Symbiotic psychosis
Use additional code to identify any associated neurological condition
EXCLUDES 1 *Asperger's syndrome (F84.5)*
Autistic disorder (F84.0)
Rett's syndrome (F84.2)

F84.5 Asperger's syndrome
Asperger's disorder
Autistic psychopathy
Schizoid disorder of childhood

F84.8 Other pervasive developmental disorders
Overactive disorder associated with intellectual disabilities and stereotyped movements

F84.9 Pervasive developmental disorder, unspecified
Atypical autism

F88 Other disorders of psychological development
Developmental agnosia

F89 Unspecified disorder of psychological development
Developmental disorder NOS

Behavioral and emotional disorders with onset usually occurring in childhood and adolescence (F90-F98)

NOTE Codes within categories F90-F98may be used regardless of the age of a patient. These disorders generally have onset within the childhood or adolescent years, but may continue throughout life or not be diagnosed until adulthood

✓4th **F90 Attention-deficit hyperactivity disorders**
INCLUDES attention deficit disorder with hyperactivity
attention deficit syndrome with hyperactivity
EXCLUDES 2 *anxiety disorders (F40.-, F41.-)*
mood [affective] disorders (F30-F39)
pervasive developmental disorders (F84.-)
schizophrenia (F20.-)

F90.0 Attention-deficit hyperactivity disorder, predominantly inattentive type
F90.1 Attention-deficit hyperactivity disorder, predominantly hyperactive type
F90.2 Attention-deficit hyperactivity disorder, combined type
F90.8 Attention-deficit hyperactivity disorder, other type
F90.9 Attention-deficit hyperactivity disorder, unspecified type
Attention-deficit hyperactivity disorder of childhood or adolescence NOS
Attention-deficit hyperactivity disorder NOS

✓4th **F91 Conduct disorders**
EXCLUDES 1 *antisocial behavior (Z72.81-)*
antisocial personality disorder (F60.2)
EXCLUDES 2 *conduct problems associated with attention-deficit hyperactivity disorder (F90.-)*
mood [affective] disorders (F30-F39)
pervasive developmental disorders (F84.-)
schizophrenia (F20.-)

F91.0 Conduct disorder confined to family context
F91.1 Conduct disorder, childhood-onset type
Unsocialized conduct disorder
Conduct disorder, solitary aggressive type
Unsocialized aggressive disorder
F91.2 Conduct disorder, adolescent-onset type
Socialized conduct disorder
Conduct disorder, group type
F91.3 Oppositional defiant disorder
F91.8 Other conduct disorders
F91.9 Conduct disorder, unspecified
Behavioral disorder NOS
Conduct disorder NOS
Disruptive behavior disorder NOS

✓4th **F93 Emotional disorders with onset specific to childhood**
F93.0 Separation anxiety disorder of childhood
EXCLUDES 2 *mood [affective] disorders (F30-F39)*
nonpsychotic mental disorders (F40-F48)
phobic anxiety disorder of childhood (F40.8)
social phobia (F40.1)
F93.8 Other childhood emotional disorders
Identity disorder
EXCLUDES 2 *gender identity disorder of childhood (F64.2)*
F93.9 Childhood emotional disorder, unspecified

✓4th **F94 Disorders of social functioning with onset specific to childhood and adolescence**
F94.0 Selective mutism
Elective mutism
EXCLUDES 2 *pervasive developmental disorders (F84.-)*
schizophrenia (F20.-)
specific developmental disorders of speech and language (F80.-)
transient mutism as part of separation anxiety in young children (F93.0)
F94.1 Reactive attachment disorder of childhood
Use additional code to identify any associated failure to thrive or growth retardation
EXCLUDES 1 *disinhibited attachment disorder of childhood (F94.2)*
normal variation in pattern of selective attachment
EXCLUDES 2 *Asperger's syndrome (F84.5)*
maltreatment syndromes (T74.-)
sexual or physical abuse in childhood, resulting in psychosocial problems (Z62.81-)
F94.2 Disinhibited attachment disorder of childhood
Affectionless psychopathy
Institutional syndrome
EXCLUDES 1 *reactive attachment disorder of childhood (F94.l)*
EXCLUDES 2 *Asperger's syndrome (F84.5)*
attention-deficit hyperactivity disorders (F90.-)
hospitalism in children (F43.2-)
F94.8 Other childhood disorders of social functioning
F94.9 Childhood disorder of social functioning, unspecified

✓4th **F95 Tic disorder**
F95.0 Transient tic disorder
F95.1 Chronic motor or vocal tic disorder
F95.2 Tourette's disorder
Combined vocal and multiple motor tic disorder [de la Tourette]
Tourette's syndrome

F95.8 Other tic disorders

F95.9 Tic disorder, unspecified
Tic NOS

✓4th **F98 Other behavioral and emotional disorders with onset usually occurring in childhood and adolescence**
EXCLUDES 2 *breath-holding spells (R06.89)*
gender identity disorder of childhood (F64.2)
Kleine-Levin syndrome (G47.13)
obsessive-compulsive disorder (F42)
sleep disorders not due to a substance or known physiological condition (F51.-)

F98.0 Enuresis not due to a substance or known physiological condition
Enuresis (primary) (secondary) of nonorganic origin
Functional enuresis
Psychogenic enuresis
Urinary incontinence of nonorganic origin
EXCLUDES 1 *enuresis NOS (R32)*

F98.1 Encopresis not due to a substance or known physiological condition
Functional encopresis
Incontinence of feces of nonorganic origin
Psychogenic encopresis
Use additional code to identify the cause of any coexisting constipation
EXCLUDES 1 *encopresis NOS (R15.-)*

✓5th **F98.2 Other feeding disorders of infancy and childhood**
EXCLUDES 1 *feeding difficulties (R63.3)*
EXCLUDES 2 *anorexia nervosa and other eating disorders (F50.-)*
feeding problems of newborn (P92.-)
pica of infancy or childhood (F98.3)

F98.21 Rumination disorder of infancy

F98.29 Other feeding disorders of infancy and early childhood

F98.3 Pica of infancy and childhood

F98.4 Stereotyped movement disorders
Stereotype/habit disorder
EXCLUDES 1 *abnormal involuntary movements (R25.-)*
EXCLUDES 2 *compulsions in obsessive-compulsive disorder (F42)*
hair plucking (F63.3)
movement disorders of organic origin (G20-G25)
nail-biting (F98.8)
nose-picking (F98.8)
stereotypies that are part of a broader psychiatric condition (F01-F95)
thumb-sucking (F98.8)
tic disorders (F95.-)
trichotillomania (F63.3)

F98.5 Adult onset fluency disorder
EXCLUDES 1 *childhood onset fluency disorder (F80.81)*
dysphasia (R47.02)
fluency disorder in conditions classified elsewhere (R47.82)
fluency disorder (stuttering) following cerebrovascular disease (I69. with final characters -23)
tic disorders (F95.-)

F98.8 Other specified behavioral and emotional disorders with onset usually occurring in childhood and adolescence
Excessive masturbation
Nail-biting
Nose-picking
Thumb-sucking

F98.9 Unspecified behavioral and emotional disorders with onset usually occurring in childhood and adolescence

Unspecified mental disorder (F99)

F99 Mental disorder, not otherwise specified
Mental illness NOS
EXCLUDES 1 *unspecified mental disorder due to known physiological condition (F09)*

Chapter 6. Diseases of the Nervous System (G00-G99)

EXCLUDES 2 *certain conditions originating in the perinatal period (P04-P96)*
certain infectious and parasitic diseases (A00-B99)
complications of pregnancy, childbirth and the puerperium (O00-O99A)
congenital malformations, deformations, and chromosomal abnormalities (Q00-Q99)
endocrine, nutritional and metabolic diseases (E00-E88)
injury, poisoning and certain other consequences of external causes (S00-T88)
neoplasms (C00-D49)
symptoms, signs and abnormal clinical and laboratory findings, not elsewhere classified (R00-R94)

This chapter contains the following blocks:

G00-G09	Inflammatory diseases of the central nervous system
G10-G14	Systemic atrophies primarily affecting the central nervous system
G20-G26	Extrapyramidal and movement disorders
G30-G32	Other degenerative diseases of the nervous system
G35-G37	Demyelinating diseases of the central nervous system
G40-G47	Episodic and paroxysmal disorders
G50-G59	Nerve, nerve root and plexus disorders
G60-G65	Polyneuropathies and other disorders of the peripheral nervous system
G70-G73	Diseases of myoneural junction and muscle
G80-G83	Cerebral palsy and other paralytic syndromes
G89-G99	Other disorders of the nervous system

Inflammatory diseases of the central nervous system (G00-G09)

✓4th **G00 Bacterial meningitis, not elsewhere classified**
INCLUDES bacterial arachnoiditis
bacterial leptomeningitis
bacterial meningitis
bacterial pachymeningitis
EXCLUDES 1 *bacterial:*
meningoencephalitis (G04.2)
meningomyelitis (G04.2)

G00.0 Hemophilus meningitis
Meningitis due to Hemophilus influenzae

G00.1 Pneumococcal meningitis

G00.2 Streptococcal meningitis
Use additional code to further identify organism (B95.0-B95.5)

G00.3 Staphylococcal meningitis
Use additional code to further identify organism (B95.61-B95.8)

G00.8 Other bacterial meningitis
Meningitis due to Escherichia coli
Meningitis due to Friedländer's bacillus
Meningitis due to Klebsiella
Use additional code to further identify organism (B96.-)

G00.9 Bacterial meningitis, unspecified
Meningitis due to gram-negative bacteria, unspecified
Purulent meningitis NOS
Pyogenic meningitis NOS
Suppurative meningitis NOS

G01 Meningitis in bacterial diseases classified elsewhere
Code first underlying disease
EXCLUDES 1 *meningitis (in):*
gonococcal (A54.81)
leptospirosis (A27.81)
listeriosis (A32.11)
Lyme disease (A69.21)
meningococcal (A39.0)
neurosyphilis (A52.13)
tuberculosis (A17.0)
meningoencephalitis and meningomyelitis in bacterial diseases classified elsewhere (G05)

G02 Meningitis in other infectious and parasitic diseases classified elsewhere
Code first underlying disease, such as:
African trypanosomiasis (B56.-)
poliovirus infection (A80.-)
EXCLUDES 1 *candidal meningitis (B37.5)*
coccidioidomycosis meningitis (B38.4)
cryptococcal meningitis (B45.1)
herpesviral [herpes simplex] meningitis (B00.3)
infectious mononucleosis complicated by meningitis (B27.- with fourth character 2)
measles complicated by meningitis (B05.1)
meningoencephalitis and meningomyelitis in other infectious and parasitic diseases classified elsewhere (G05)
mumps meningitis (B26.1)
rubella meningitis (B06.02)
varicella [chickenpox] meningitis (B01.0)
zoster meningitis (B02.1)

✓4th **G03 Meningitis due to other and unspecified causes**
INCLUDES arachnoiditis NOS
leptomeningitis NOS
meningitis NOS
pachymeningitis NOS
EXCLUDES 1 *meningoencephalitis (G04.-)*
meningomyelitis (G04.-)

G03.0 Nonpyogenic meningitis
Aseptic meningitis
Nonbacterial meningitis

G03.1 Chronic meningitis

G03.2 Benign recurrent meningitis [Mollaret]

G03.8 Meningitis due to other specified causes

G03.9 Meningitis, unspecified
Arachnoiditis (spinal) NOS

✓4th **G04 Encephalitis, myelitis and encephalomyelitis**
INCLUDES acute ascending myelitis
meningoencephalitis
meningomyelitis
EXCLUDES 1 *encephalopathy NOS (G93.40)*
EXCLUDES 2 *acute transverse myelitis (G37.3-)*
alcoholic encephalopathy (G31.2)
benign myalgic encephalomyelitis (G93.3)
multiple sclerosis (G35)
subacute necrotizing myelitis (G37.4)
toxic encephalitis (G92)
toxic encephalopathy (G92)

✓5th **G04.0 Acute disseminated encephalitis and encephalomyelitis (ADEM)**
EXCLUDES 1 *acute necrotizing hemorrhagic encephalopathy (G04.3-)*
other noninfectious acute disseminated encephalomyelitis (noninfectious ADEM) (G04.81)

G04.00 Acute disseminated encephalitis and encephalomyelitis, unspecified

G04.01 Postinfectious acute disseminated encephalitis and encephalomyelitis (postinfectious ADEM)
EXCLUDES 1 *post chickenpox encephalitis (B01.1)*
post measles encephalitis (B05.0)
post measles myelitis (B05.1)

G04.02 Postimmunization acute disseminated encephalitis, myelitis and encephalomyelitis
Encephalitis, postimmunization
Encephalomyelitis, postimmunization

G04.1 Tropical spastic paraplegia

G04.2 Bacterial meningoencephalitis and meningomyelitis, not elsewhere classified

✓5th **G04.3 Acute necrotizing hemorrhagic encephalopathy**
EXCLUDES 1 *acute disseminated encephalitis and encephalomyelitis (G04.0-)*

G04.30 Acute necrotizing hemorrhagic encephalopathy, unspecified

G04.31 Postinfectious acute necrotizing hemorrhagic encephalopathy

G04.32 Postimmunization acute necrotizing hemorrhagic encephalopathy

G04.39 Other acute necrotizing hemorrhagic encephalopathy
Code also underlying etiology, if applicable

√5th **G04.8 Other encephalitis, myelitis and encephalomyelitis**
Code also any associated seizure (G40.-, R56.9)
G04.81 Other encephalitis and encephalomyelitis
Noninfectious acute disseminated encephalomyelitis (noninfectious ADEM)
G04.89 Other myelitis

√5th **G04.9 Encephalitis, myelitis and encephalomyelitis, unspecified**
G04.90 Encephalitis and encephalomyelitis, unspecified
Ventriculitis (cerebral) NOS
G04.91 Myelitis, unspecified

√4th **G05 Encephalitis, myelitis and encephalomyelitis in diseases classified elsewhere**
Code first underlying disease, such as:
human immunodeficiency virus [HIV] disease (B20)
poliovirus (A80.-)
suppurative otitis media (H66.01-H66.4)
trichinellosis (B75)
EXCLUDES 1 *adenoviral encephalitis, myelitis and encephalomyelitis (A85.1)*
congenital toxoplasmosis encephalitis, myelitis and encephalomyelitis (P37.1)
cytomegaloviral encephalitis, myelitis and encephalomyelitis (B25.8)
encephalitis, myelitis and encephalomyelitis (in) measles (B05.0)
encephalitis, myelitis and encephalomyelitis (in) systemic lupus erythematosus (M32.19)
enteroviral encephalitis, myelitis and encephalomyelitis (A85.0)
eosinophilic meningoencephalitis (B83.2)
herpesviral [herpes simplex] encephalitis, myelitis and encephalomyelitis (B00.4)
listerial encephalitis, myelitis and encephalomyelitis (A32.12)
meningococcal encephalitis, myelitis and encephalomyelitis (A39.81)
mumps encephalitis, myelitis and encephalomyelitis (B26.2)
postchickenpox encephalitis, myelitis and encephalomyelitis (B01.1-)
rubella encephalitis, myelitis and encephalomyelitis (B06.01)
toxoplasmosis encephalitis, myelitis and encephalomyelitis (B58.2)
zoster encephalitis, myelitis and encephalomyelitis (B02.0)

G05.3 Encephalitis and encephalomyelitis in diseases classified elsewhere
Meningoencephalitis in diseases classified elsewhere
G05.4 Myelitis in diseases classified elsewhere
Meningomyelitis in diseases classified elsewhere

√4th **G06 Intracranial and intraspinal abscess and granuloma**
Use additional code (B95-B97) to identify infectious agent
G06.0 Intracranial abscess and granuloma
Brain [any part] abscess (embolic)
Cerebellar abscess (embolic)
Cerebral abscess (embolic)
Intracranial epidural abscess or granuloma
Intracranial extradural abscess or granuloma
Intracranial subdural abscess or granuloma
Otogenic abscess (embolic)
EXCLUDES 1 *tuberculous intracranial abscess and granuloma (A17.81)*
G06.1 Intraspinal abscess and granuloma
Abscess (embolic) of spinal cord [any part]
Intraspinal epidural abscess or granuloma
Intraspinal extradural abscess or granuloma
Intraspinal subdural abscess or granuloma
EXCLUDES 1 *tuberculous intraspinal abscess and granuloma (A17.81)*
G06.2 Extradural and subdural abscess, unspecified

G07 Intracranial and intraspinal abscess and granuloma in diseases classified elsewhere
Code first, underlying disease, such as:
schistosomiasis granuloma of brain (B65.-)
EXCLUDES 1 *abscess of brain:*
amebic (A06.6)
chromomycotic (B43.1)
gonococcal (A54.82)
tuberculous (A17.81)
tuberculoma of meninges (A17.1)

G08 Intracranial and intraspinal phlebitis and thrombophlebitis
Septic embolism of intracranial or intraspinal venous sinuses and veins
Septic endophlebitis of intracranial or intraspinal venous sinuses and veins
Septic phlebitis of intracranial or intraspinal venous sinuses and veins
Septic thrombophlebitis of intracranial or intraspinal venous sinuses and veins
Septic thrombosis of intracranial or intraspinal venous sinuses and veins
EXCLUDES 1 *intracranial phlebitis and thrombophlebitis complicating:*
abortion, ectopic or molar pregnancy (O00-O07, O08.7)
pregnancy, childbirth and the puerperium (O22.5, O87.3)
nonpyogenic intracranial phlebitis and thrombophlebitis (I67.6)
nonpyogenic intraspinal phlebitis and thrombophlebitis (G95.1)

G09 Sequelae of inflammatory diseases of central nervous system
NOTE Category G09 is to be used to indicate conditions whose primary classification is to G00-G08 as the cause of sequelae, themselves classifiable elsewhere. The "sequelae" include conditions specified as residuals.
Code first condition resulting from (sequela) of inflammatory diseases of central nervous system

Systemic atrophies primarily affecting the central nervous system (G10-G14)

G10 Huntington's disease
Huntington's chorea
Huntington's dementia

√4th **G11 Hereditary ataxia**
EXCLUDES 2 *cerebral palsy (G80.-)*
hereditary and idiopathic neuropathy (G60.-)
metabolic disorders (E70-E88)
G11.0 Congenital nonprogressive ataxia
G11.1 Early-onset cerebellar ataxia
Early-onset cerebellar ataxia with essential tremor
Early-onset cerebellar ataxia with myoclonus [Hunt's ataxia]
Early-onset cerebellar ataxia with retained tendon reflexes
Friedreich's ataxia (autosomal recessive)
X-linked recessive spinocerebellar ataxia
G11.2 Late-onset cerebellar ataxia
G11.3 Cerebellar ataxia with defective DNA repair
Ataxia telangiectasia [Louis-Bar]
EXCLUDES 2 *Cockayne's syndrome (Q87.1)*
other disorders of purine and pyrimidine metabolism (E79.-)
xeroderma pigmentosum (Q82.1)
G11.4 Hereditary spastic paraplegia
G11.8 Other hereditary ataxias
G11.9 Hereditary ataxia, unspecified
Hereditary cerebellar ataxia NOS
Hereditary cerebellar degeneration
Hereditary cerebellar disease
Hereditary cerebellar syndrome

√4th **G12 Spinal muscular atrophy and related syndromes**
G12.0 Infantile spinal muscular atrophy, type I [Werdnig-Hoffman]
G12.1 Other inherited spinal muscular atrophy
Adult form spinal muscular atrophy
Childhood form, type II spinal muscular atrophy
Distal spinal muscular atrophy
Juvenile form, type III spinal muscular atrophy [Kugelberg-Welander]
Progressive bulbar palsy of childhood [Fazio-Londe]
Scapuloperoneal form spinal muscular atrophy

√5th **G12.2 Motor neuron disease**
G12.20 Motor neuron disease, unspecified
G12.21 Amyotrophic lateral sclerosis
Progressive spinal muscle atrophy
G12.22 Progressive bulbar palsy
G12.29 Other motor neuron disease
Familial motor neuron disease
Primary lateral sclerosis
G12.8 Other spinal muscular atrophies and related syndromes
G12.9 Spinal muscular atrophy, unspecified

G13 Systemic atrophies primarily affecting central nervous system in diseases classified elsewhere

G13.0 ***Paraneoplastic neuromyopathy and neuropathy***
Carcinomatous neuromyopathy
Sensorial paraneoplastic neuropathy [Denny Brown]
Code first underlying neoplasm (C00-D49)

G13.1 ***Other systemic atrophy primarily affecting central nervous system in neoplastic disease***
Paraneoplastic limbic encephalopathy
Code first underlying neoplasm (C00-D49)

G13.2 Systemic atrophy primarily affecting the central nervous system in myxedema
Code first underlying disease, such as:
hypothyroidism (E03.-)
myxedematous congenital iodine deficiency (E00.1)

G13.8 ***Systemic atrophy primarily affecting central nervous system in other diseases classified elsewhere***
Code first underlying disease

G14 Postpolio syndrome
Postpolio myelitic syndrome
EXCLUDES 1 *sequelae of poliomyelitis (B91)*

Extrapyramidal and movement disorders (G20-G26)

G20 Parkinson's disease
Hemiparkinsonism
Idiopathic Parkinsonism or Parkinson's disease
Paralysis agitans
Parkinsonism or Parkinson's disease NOS
Primary Parkinsonism or Parkinson's disease
EXCLUDES 1 *dementia with Parkinsonism (G31.83)*

G21 Secondary parkinsonism
EXCLUDES 1 *dementia with Parkinsonism (G31.83)*
Huntington's disease (G10)
Shy-Drager syndrome (G90.3)
syphilitic Parkinsonism (A52.19)

G21.0 Malignant neuroleptic syndrome
Use additional code for adverse effect, if applicable, to identify drug (T43.3X5, T43.4X5, T43.505, T43.595)
EXCLUDES 1 *neuroleptic induced parkinsonism (G21.11)*

G21.1 Other drug-induced secondary parkinsonism

G21.11 Neuroleptic induced parkinsonism
Use additional code for adverse effect, if applicable, to identify drug (T43.3X5, T43.4X5, T43.505, T43.595)
EXCLUDES 1 *malignant neuroleptic syndrome (G21.0)*

G21.19 Other drug induced secondary parkinsonism
Use additional code for adverse effect, if applicable, to identify drug (T36-T50 with fifth or sixth character 5)

G21.2 Secondary parkinsonism due to other external agents
Code first (T51-T65) to identify external agent

G21.3 Postencephalitic parkinsonism
G21.4 Vascular parkinsonism
G21.8 Other secondary parkinsonism
G21.9 Secondary parkinsonism, unspecified

G23 Other degenerative diseases of basal ganglia
EXCLUDES 2 *multi-system degeneration of the autonomic nervous system (G90.3)*

G23.0 Hallervorden-Spatz disease
Pigmentary pallidal degeneration

G23.1 Progressive supranuclear ophthalmoplegia [Steele-Richardson-Olszewski]
Progressive supranuclear palsy

G23.2 Striatonigral degeneration

G23.8 Other specified degenerative diseases of basal ganglia
Calcification of basal ganglia

G23.9 Degenerative disease of basal ganglia, unspecified

G24 Dystonia
INCLUDES dyskinesia
EXCLUDES 2 *athetoid cerebral palsy (G80.3)*

G24.0 Drug induced dystonia
Use additional code code for adverse effect, if applicable, to identify drug (T36-T50 with fifth or sixth character5)

G24.01 Drug induced subacute dyskinesia
Drug induced blepharospasm
Drug induced orofacial dyskinesia
Neuroleptic induced tardive dyskinesia
Tardive dyskinesia

G24.02 Drug induced acute dystonia
Acute dystonic reaction to drugs
Neuroleptic induced acute dystonia

G24.09 Other drug induced dystonia

G24.1 Genetic torsion dystonia
Dystonia deformans progressiva
Dystonia musculorum deformans
Familial torsion dystonia
Idiopathic familial dystonia
Idiopathic (torsion) dystonia NOS
(Schwalbe-) Ziehen-Oppenheim disease

G24.2 Idiopathic nonfamilial dystonia

G24.3 Spasmodic torticollis
EXCLUDES 1 *congenital torticollis (Q68.0)*
hysterical torticollis (F44.4)
ocular torticollis (R29.891)
psychogenic torticollis (F45.8)
torticollis NOS (M43.6)
traumatic recurrent torticollis (S13.4)

G24.4 Idiopathic orofacial dystonia
Orofacial dyskinesia
EXCLUDES 1 *drug induced orofacial dyskinesia (G24.01)*

G24.5 Blepharospasm
EXCLUDES 1 *drug induced blepharospasm (G24.01)*

G24.8 Other dystonia
Acquired torsion dystonia NOS

G24.9 Dystonia, unspecified
Dyskinesia NOS

G25 Other extrapyramidal and movement disorders
EXCLUDES 2 *sleep related movement disorders (G47.6-)*

G25.0 Essential tremor
Familial tremor
EXCLUDES 1 *tremor NOS (R25.1)*

G25.1 Drug-induced tremor
Use additional code for adverse effect, if applicable, to identify drug (T36-T50 with fifth or sixth character 5)

G25.2 Other specified forms of tremor
Intention tremor

G25.3 Myoclonus
Drug-induced myoclonus
Palatal myoclonus
Use additional code for adverse effect, if applicable, to identify drug (T36-T50 with fifth or sixth character 5)
EXCLUDES 1 *facial myokymia (G51.4)*
myoclonic epilepsy (G40.-)

G25.4 Drug-induced chorea
Use additional code for adverse effect, if applicable, to identify drug (T36-T50 with fifth or sixth character 5)

G25.5 Other chorea
Chorea NOS
EXCLUDES 1 *chorea NOS with heart involvement (I02.0)*
Huntington's chorea (G10)
rheumatic chorea (I02.-)
Sydenham's chorea (I02.-)

G25.6 Drug induced tics and other tics of organic origin

G25.61 Drug induced tics
Use additional code for adverse effect, if applicable, to identify drug (T36-T50 with fifth or sixth character 5)

G25.69 Other tics of organic origin
EXCLUDES 1 *habit spasm (F95.9)*
tic NOS (F95.9)
Tourette's syndrome (F95.2)

G25.7 Other and unspecified drug induced movement disorders
Use additional code for adverse effect, if applicable, to identify drug (T36-T50 with fifth or sixth character 5)

G25.70 Drug induced movement disorder, unspecified

G25.71 **Drug induced akathisia**
Drug induced acathisia
Neuroleptic induced acute akathisia

G25.79 **Other drug induced movement disorders**

√5th G25.8 **Other specified extrapyramidal and movement disorders**

G25.81 **Restless legs syndrome**

G25.82 **Stiff-man syndrome**

G25.83 **Benign shuddering attacks**

G25.89 **Other specified extrapyramidal and movement disorders**

G25.9 **Extrapyramidal and movement disorder, unspecified**

G26 Extrapyramidal and movement disorders in diseases classified elsewhere
Code first underlying disease

Other degenerative diseases of the nervous system (G30-G32)

√4th **G30 Alzheimer's disease**
INCLUDES Alzheimer's dementia senile and presenile forms
Use additional code to identify:
delirium, if applicable (F05)
dementia with behavioral disturbance (F02.81)
dementia without behavioral disturbance (F02.80)
EXCLUDES 1 *senile degeneration of brain NEC (G31.1)*
senile dementia NOS (F03)
senility NOS (R41.81)

G30.0 **Alzheimer's disease with early onset**

G30.1 **Alzheimer's disease with late onset**

G30.8 **Other Alzheimer's disease**

G30.9 **Alzheimer's disease, unspecified**

√4th **G31 Other degenerative diseases of nervous system, not elsewhere classified**
Use additional code to identify:
dementia with behavioral disturbance (F02.81)
dementia without behavioral disturbance (F02.80)
EXCLUDES 2 *Reye's syndrome (G93.7)*

√5th G31.0 **Frontotemporal dementia**

G31.01 **Pick's disease**
Primary progressive aphasia
Progressive isolated aphasia

G31.09 **Other frontotemporal dementia**
Frontal dementia

G31.1 **Senile degeneration of brain, not elsewhere classified**
EXCLUDES 1 *Alzheimer's disease (G30.-)*
senility NOS (R41.81)

G31.2 **Degeneration of nervous system due to alcohol**
Alcoholic cerebellar ataxia
Alcoholic cerebellar degeneration
Alcoholic cerebral degeneration
Alcoholic encephalopathy
Dysfunction of the autonomic nervous system due to alcohol
Code also associated alcoholism (F10.-)

√5th G31.8 **Other specified degenerative diseases of nervous system**

G31.81 **Alpers disease**
Grey-matter degeneration

G31.82 **Leigh's disease**
Subacute necrotizing encephalopathy

G31.83 **Dementia with Lewy bodies**
Dementia with Parkinsonism
Lewy body dementia
Lewy body disease

G31.84 **Mild cognitive impairment, so stated**
EXCLUDES 1 *age related cognitive decline (R41.81)*
altered mental status (R41.82)
cerebral degeneration (G31.9)
change in mental status (R41.82)
cognitive deficits following (sequelae of) cerebral hemorrhage or infarction (I69.01, I69.11, I69.21, I69.31, I69.81, I69.91)
cognitive impairment due to intracranial or head injury (S06.-)
dementia (F01.-, F02.-, F03)
mild memory disturbance (F06.8)
neurologic neglect syndrome (R41.4)
personality change, nonpsychotic (F68.8)

G31.85 **Corticobasal degeneration**

G31.89 **Other specified degenerative diseases of nervous system**

G31.9 **Degenerative disease of nervous system, unspecified**

√4th **G32 Other degenerative disorders of nervous system in diseases classified elsewhere**

G32.0 Subacute combined degeneration of spinal cord in diseases classified elsewhere
Dana-Putnam syndrome
Sclerosis of spinal cord (combined) (dorsolateral) (posterolateral)
Code first underlying disease, such as:
vitamin B12 deficiency (E53.8)
vitamin B12 deficiency:
anemia (D51.9)
dietary (D51.3)
pernicious (D51.0)
EXCLUDES 1 *syphilitic combined degeneration of spinal cord (A52.11)*

√5th G32.8 **Other specified degenerative disorders of nervous system in diseases classified elsewhere**
Code first underlying disease, such as:
amyloidosis cerebral degeneration (E85.-)
cerebral degeneration (due to) hypothyroidism (E00.0-E03.9)
cerebral degeneration (due to) neoplasm (C00-D49)
cerebral degeneration (due to) vitamin B deficiency, except thiamine (E52-E53.-)
EXCLUDES 1 *superior hemorrhagic polioencephalitis [Wernicke's encephalopathy] (E51.2)*

G32.81 Cerebellar ataxia in diseases classified elsewhere
Code first underlying disease, such as:
cerebellar ataxia (in) neoplastic disease (paraneoplastic cerebellar degeneration) (C00-D49)
EXCLUDES 1 *systemic atrophy primarily affecting the central nervous system in alcoholic cerebellar ataxia (G31.2)*
systemic atrophy primarily affecting the central nervous system in myxedema (G13.2)

G32.89 Other specified degenerative disorders of nervous system in diseases classified elsewhere
Degenerative encephalopathy in diseases classified elsewhere

Demyelinating diseases of the central nervous system (G35-G37)

G35 Multiple sclerosis
Disseminated multiple sclerosis
Generalized multiple sclerosis
Multiple sclerosis NOS
Multiple sclerosis of brain stem
Multiple sclerosis of cord

√4th **G36 Other acute disseminated demyelination**
EXCLUDES 1 *postinfectious encephalitis and encephalomyelitis NOS (G04.01)*

G36.0 **Neuromyelitis optica [Devic]**
Demyelination in optic neuritis
EXCLUDES 1 *optic neuritis NOS (H46)*

G36.1 **Acute and subacute hemorrhagic leukoencephalitis [Hurst]**

G36.8 **Other specified acute disseminated demyelination**

G36.9 **Acute disseminated demyelination, unspecified**

√4th **G37 Other demyelinating diseases of central nervous system**

G37.0 **Diffuse sclerosis of central nervous system**
Periaxial encephalitis
Schilder's disease
EXCLUDES 1 *X linked adrenoleukodystrophy (E71.52-)*

G37.1 **Central demyelination of corpus callosum**

G37.2 **Central pontine myelinolysis**

G37.3 **Acute transverse myelitis in demyelinating disease of central nervous system**
Acute transverse myelitis NOS
Acute transverse myelopathy
EXCLUDES 1 *multiple sclerosis (G35)*
neuromyelitis optica [Devic] (G36.0)

G37.4 **Subacute necrotizing myelitis of central nervous system**

G37.5 **Concentric sclerosis [Balo] of central nervous system**

G37.8 **Other specified demyelinating diseases of central nervous system**

G37.9 Demyelinating disease of central nervous system, unspecified

Episodic and paroxysmal disorders (G40-G47)

✓4th G40 Epilepsy and recurrent seizures

NOTE The following terms are to be considered equivalent to intractable: pharmacoresistant (pharmacologically resistant), treatment resistant, refractory (medically) and poorly controlled

EXCLUDES 1 *conversion disorder with seizures (F44.5)*
convulsions NOS (R56.9)
hippocampal sclerosis (G93.81)
mesial temporal sclerosis (G93.81)
post traumatic seizures (R56.1)
seizure (convulsive) NOS (R56.9)
seizure of newborn (P90)
temporal sclerosis (G93.81)
Todd's paralysis (G83.8)

✓5th G40.0 Localization-related (focal) (partial) idiopathic epilepsy and epileptic syndromes with seizures of localized onset
Benign childhood epilepsy with centrotemporal EEG spikes
Childhood epilepsy with occipital EEG paroxysms
EXCLUDES 1 *adult onset localization-related epilepsy (G40.1-, G40.2-)*

✓6th G40.00 Localization-related (focal) (partial) idiopathic epilepsy and epileptic syndromes with seizures of localized onset, not intractable
Localization-related (focal) (partial) idiopathic epilepsy and epileptic syndromes with seizures of localized onset without intractability

G40.001 Localization-related (focal) (partial) idiopathic epilepsy and epileptic syndromes with seizures of localized onset, not intractable, with status epilepticus

G40.009 Localization-related (focal) (partial) idiopathic epilepsy and epileptic syndromes with seizures of localized onset, not intractable, without status epilepticus
Localization-related (focal) (partial) idiopathic epilepsy and epileptic syndromes with seizures of localized onset NOS

✓6th G40.01 Localization-related (focal) (partial) idiopathic epilepsy and epileptic syndromes with seizures of localized onset, intractable

G40.011 Localization-related (focal) (partial) idiopathic epilepsy and epileptic syndromes with seizures of localized onset, intractable, with status epilepticus

G40.019 Localization-related (focal) (partial) idiopathic epilepsy and epileptic syndromes with seizures of localized onset, intractable, without status epilepticus

✓5th G40.1 Localization-related (focal) (partial) symptomatic epilepsy and epileptic syndromes with simple partial seizures
Attacks without alteration of consciousness
Epilepsia partialis continua [Kozhevnikof]
Simple partial seizures developing into secondarily generalized seizures

✓6th G40.10 Localization-related (focal) (partial) symptomatic epilepsy and epileptic syndromes with simple partial seizures, not intractable
Localization-related (focal) (partial) symptomatic epilepsy and epileptic syndromes with simple partial seizures without intractability

G40.101 Localization-related (focal) (partial) symptomatic epilepsy and epileptic syndromes with simple partial seizures, not intractable, with status epilepticus

G40.109 Localization-related (focal) (partial) symptomatic epilepsy and epileptic syndromes with simple partial seizures, not intractable, without status epilepticus
Localization-related (focal) (partial) symptomatic epilepsy and epileptic syndromes with simple partial seizures NOS

✓6th G40.11 Localization-related (focal) (partial) symptomatic epilepsy and epileptic syndromes with simple partial seizures, intractable

G40.111 Localization-related (focal) (partial) symptomatic epilepsy and epileptic syndromes with simple partial seizures, intractable, with status epilepticus

G40.119 Localization-related (focal) (partial) symptomatic epilepsy and epileptic syndromes with simple partial seizures, intractable, without status epilepticus

✓5th G40.2 Localization-related (focal) (partial) symptomatic epilepsy and epileptic syndromes with complex partial seizures
Attacks with alteration of consciousness, often with automatisms
Complex partial seizures developing into secondarily generalized seizures

✓6th G40.20 Localization-related (focal) (partial) symptomatic epilepsy and epileptic syndromes with complex partial seizures, not intractable
Localization-related (focal) (partial) symptomatic epilepsy and epileptic syndromes with complex partial seizures without intractability

G40.201 Localization-related (focal) (partial) symptomatic epilepsy and epileptic syndromes with complex partial seizures, not intractable, with status epilepticus

G40.209 Localization-related (focal) (partial) symptomatic epilepsy and epileptic syndromes with complex partial seizures, not intractable, without status epilepticus
Localization-related (focal) (partial) symptomatic epilepsy and epileptic syndromes with complex partial seizures NOS

✓6th G40.21 Localization-related (focal) (partial) symptomatic epilepsy and epileptic syndromes with complex partial seizures, intractable

G40.211 Localization-related (focal) (partial) symptomatic epilepsy and epileptic syndromes with complex partial seizures, intractable, with status epilepticus

G40.219 Localization-related (focal) (partial) symptomatic epilepsy and epileptic syndromes with complex partial seizures, intractable, without status epilepticus

✓5th G40.3 Generalized idiopathic epilepsy and epileptic syndromes
Code also MERRF syndrome, if applicable (E88.42)

✓6th G40.30 Generalized idiopathic epilepsy and epileptic syndromes, not intractable
Generalized idiopathic epilepsy and epileptic syndromes without intractability

G40.301 Generalized idiopathic epilepsy and epileptic syndromes, not intractable, with status epilepticus

G40.309 Generalized idiopathic epilepsy and epileptic syndromes, not intractable, without status epilepticus
Generalized idiopathic epilepsy and epileptic syndromes NOS

✓6th G40.31 Generalized idiopathic epilepsy and epileptic syndromes, intractable

G40.311 Generalized idiopathic epilepsy and epileptic syndromes, intractable, with status epilepticus

G40.319 Generalized idiopathic epilepsy and epileptic syndromes, intractable, without status epilepticus

G40.A Absence epileptic syndrome
Childhood absence epilepsy [pyknolepsy]
Juvenile absence epilepsy
Absence epileptic syndrome, NOS

G40.A0 Absence epileptic syndrome, not intractable

G40.A01 Absence epileptic syndrome, not intractable, with status epilepticus

G40.A09 Absence epileptic syndrome, not intractable, without status epilepticus

G40.A1 Absence epileptic syndrome, intractable

G40.A11 Absence epileptic syndrome, intractable, with status epilepticus

G40.A19 Absence epileptic syndrome, intractable, without status epilepticus

G40.B Juvenile myoclonic epilepsy [impulsive petit mal]

G40.B0 Juvenile myoclonic epilepsy, not intractable

G40.B01 Juvenile myoclonic epilepsy, not intractable, with status epilepticus

G40.B09 Juvenile myoclonic epilepsy, not intractable, without status epilepticus

G40.B1 Juvenile myoclonic epilepsy, intractable

G40.B11 Juvenile myoclonic epilepsy, intractable, with status epilepticus

G40.B19 Juvenile myoclonic epilepsy, intractable, without status epilepticus

G40.4 Other generalized epilepsy and epileptic syndromes
Epilepsy with grand mal seizures on awakening
Epilepsy with myoclonic absences
Epilepsy with myoclonic-astatic seizures
Grand mal seizure NOS
Nonspecific atonic epileptic seizures
Nonspecific clonic epileptic seizures
Nonspecific myoclonic epileptic seizures
Nonspecific tonic epileptic seizures
Nonspecific tonic-clonic epileptic seizures
Symptomatic early myoclonic encephalopathy

G40.40 Other generalized epilepsy and epileptic syndromes, not intractable
Other generalized epilepsy and epileptic syndromes without intractability
Other generalized epilepsy and epileptic syndromes NOS

G40.401 Other generalized epilepsy and epileptic syndromes, not intractable, with status epilepticus

G40.409 Other generalized epilepsy and epileptic syndromes, not intractable, without status epilepticus

G40.41 Other generalized epilepsy and epileptic syndromes, intractable

G40.411 Other generalized epilepsy and epileptic syndromes, intractable, with status epilepticus

G40.419 Other generalized epilepsy and epileptic syndromes, intractable, without status epilepticus

G40.5 Epileptic seizures related to external causes
Epileptic seizures related to alcohol
Epileptic seizures related to drugs
Epileptic seizures related to hormonal changes
Epileptic seizures related to sleep deprivation
Epileptic seizures related to stress
Use additional code for adverse effect, if applicable, to identify drug (T36-T50 with fifth or sixth character 5)
Code also, if applicable, associated epilepsy and recurrent seizures (G40.-)

G40.50 Epileptic seizures related to external causes, not intractable

G40.501 Epileptic seizures related to external causes, not intractable, with status epilepticus

G40.509 Epileptic seizures related to external causes, not intractable, without status epilepticus
Epileptic seizures related to external causes, NOS

G40.8 Other epilepsy and recurrent seizures
Epilepsies and epileptic syndromes undetermined as to whether they are focal or generalized
Landau-Kleffner syndrome

G40.80 Other epilepsy

G40.801 Other epilepsy, not intractable, with status epilepticus
Other epilepsy without intractability with status epilepticus

G40.802 Other epilepsy, not intractable, without status epilepticus
Other epilepsy without intractability without status epilepticus

G40.803 Other epilepsy, intractable, with status epilepticus

G40.804 Other epilepsy, intractable, without status epilepticus

G40.81 Lennox-Gastaut syndrome

G40.811 Lennox-Gastaut syndrome, not intractable, with status epilepticus

G40.812 Lennox-Gastaut syndrome, not intractable, without status epilepticus

G40.813 Lennox-Gastaut syndrome, intractable, with status epilepticus

G40.814 Lennox-Gastaut syndrome, intractable, without status epilepticus

G40.82 Epileptic spasms
Infantile spasms
Salaam attacks
West's syndrome

G40.821 Epileptic spasms, not intractable, with status epilepticus

G40.822 Epileptic spasms, not intractable, without status epilepticus

G40.823 Epileptic spasms, intractable, with status epilepticus

G40.824 Epileptic spasms, intractable, without status epilepticus

G40.89 Other seizures
EXCLUDES 1 *post traumatic seizures (R56.1)*
recurrent seizures NOS (G40.909)
seizure NOS (R56.9)

G40.9 Epilepsy, unspecified

G40.90 Epilepsy, unspecified, not intractable
Epilepsy, unspecified, without intractability

G40.901 Epilepsy, unspecified, not intractable, with status epilepticus

G40.909 Epilepsy, unspecified, not intractable, without status epilepticus
Epilepsy NOS
Epileptic convulsions NOS
Epileptic fits NOS
Epileptic seizures NOS
Recurrent seizures NOS
Seizure disorder NOS

G40.91 Epilepsy, unspecified, intractable
Intractable seizure disorder NOS

G40.911 Epilepsy, unspecified, intractable, with status epilepticus

G40.919 Epilepsy, unspecified, intractable, without status epilepticus

G43 Migraine
NOTE The following terms are to be considered equivalent to intractable: pharmacoresistant (pharmacologically resistant), treatment resistant, refractory (medically) and poorly controlled
Use additional code for adverse effect, if applicable, to identify drug (T36-T50 with fifth or sixth character 5)
EXCLUDES 1 *headache NOS (R51)*
headache syndromes (G44.-)
lower half migraine (G44.00)

G43.0 Migraine without aura
Common migraine
EXCLUDES 1 *chronic migraine without aura (G43.7-)*

G43.00 Migraine without aura, not intractable
Migraine without aura without mention of refractory migraine

G43.001 Migraine without aura, not intractable, with status migrainosus

G43.009 Migraine without aura, not intractable, without status migrainosus
Migraine without aura NOS

√6th **G43.01 Migraine without aura, intractable**
Migraine without aura with refractory migraine

G43.011 Migraine without aura, intractable, with status migrainosus

G43.019 Migraine without aura, intractable, without status migrainosus

√5th **G43.1 Migraine with aura**
Basilar migraine
Classical migraine
Migraine equivalents
Migraine preceded or accompanied by transient focal neurological phenomena
Migraine triggered seizures
Migraine with acute-onset aura
Migraine with aura without headache (migraine equivalents)
Migraine with prolonged aura
Migraine with typical aura
Retinal migraine
Code also any associated seizure (G40.-, R56.9)
EXCLUDES 1 *persistent migraine aura (G43.5-, G43.6-)*

√6th **G43.10 Migraine with aura, not intractable**
Migraine with aura without mention of refractory migraine

G43.101 Migraine with aura, not intractable, with status migrainosus

G43.109 Migraine with aura, not intractable, without status migrainosus
Migraine with aura NOS

√6th **G43.11 Migraine with aura, intractable**
Migraine with aura with refractory migraine

G43.111 Migraine with aura, intractable, with status migrainosus

G43.119 Migraine with aura, intractable, without status migrainosus

√5th **G43.4 Hemiplegic migraine**
Familial migraine
Sporadic migraine

√6th **G43.40 Hemiplegic migraine, not intractable**
Hemiplegic migraine without refractory migraine

G43.401 Hemiplegic migraine, not intractable, with status migrainosus

G43.409 Hemiplegic migraine, not intractable, without status migrainosus
Hemiplegic migraine NOS

√6th **G43.41 Hemiplegic migraine, intractable**
Hemiplegic migraine with refractory migraine

G43.411 Hemiplegic migraine, intractable, with status migrainosus

G43.419 Hemiplegic migraine, intractable, without status migrainosus

√5th **G43.5 Persistent migraine aura without cerebral infarction**

√6th **G43.50 Persistent migraine aura without cerebral infarction, not intractable**
Persistent migraine aura without cerebral infarction, without refractory migraine

G43.501 Persistent migraine aura without cerebral infarction, not intractable, with status migrainosus

G43.509 Persistent migraine aura without cerebral infarction, not intractable, without status migrainosus
Persistent migraine aura NOS

√6th **G43.51 Persistent migraine aura without cerebral infarction, intractable**
Persistent migraine aura without cerebral infarction, with refractory migraine

G43.511 Persistent migraine aura without cerebral infarction, intractable, with status migrainosus

G43.519 Persistent migraine aura without cerebral infarction, intractable, without status migrainosus

√5th **G43.6 Persistent migraine aura with cerebral infarction**
Code also the type of cerebral infarction (I63.-)

√6th **G43.60 Persistent migraine aura with cerebral infarction, not intractable**
Persistent migraine aura with cerebral infarction, without refractory migraine

G43.601 Persistent migraine aura with cerebral infarction, not intractable, with status migrainosus

G43.609 Persistent migraine aura with cerebral infarction, not intractable, without status migrainosus

√6th **G43.61 Persistent migraine aura with cerebral infarction, intractable**
Persistent migraine aura with cerebral infarction, with refractory migraine

G43.611 Persistent migraine aura with cerebral infarction, intractable, with status migrainosus

G43.619 Persistent migraine aura with cerebral infarction, intractable, without status migrainosus

√5th **G43.7 Chronic migraine without aura**
Transformed migraine
EXCLUDES 1 *migraine without aura (G43.0-)*

√6th **G43.70 Chronic migraine without aura, not intractable**
Chronic migraine without aura, without refractory migraine

G43.701 Chronic migraine without aura, not intractable, with status migrainosus

G43.709 Chronic migraine without aura, not intractable, without status migrainosus
Chronic migraine without aura NOS

√6th **G43.71 Chronic migraine without aura, intractable**
Chronic migraine without aura, with refractory migraine

G43.711 Chronic migraine without aura, intractable, with status migrainosus

G43.719 Chronic migraine without aura, intractable, without status migrainosus

√5th **G43.A Cyclical vomiting**

G43.A0 Cyclical vomiting, not intractable
Cyclical vomiting, without refractory migraine

G43.A1 Cyclical vomiting, intractable
Cyclical vomiting, with refractory migraine

√5th **G43.B Ophthalmoplegic migraine**

G43.B0 Ophthalmoplegic migraine, not intractable
Ophthalmoplegic migraine, without refractory migraine

G43.B1 Ophthalmoplegic migraine, intractable
Ophthalmoplegic migraine, with refractory migraine

√5th **G43.C Periodic headache syndromes in child or adult**

G43.C0 Periodic headache syndromes in child or adult, not intractable
Periodic headache syndromes in child or adult, without refractory migraine

G43.C1 Periodic headache syndromes in child or adult, intractable
Periodic headache syndromes in child or adult, with refractory migraine

√5th **G43.D Abdominal migraine**

G43.D0 Abdominal migraine, not intractable
Abdominal migraine, without refractory migraine

G43.D1 Abdominal migraine, intractable
Abdominal migraine, with refractory migraine

√5th **G43.8 Other migraine**

√6th **G43.80 Other migraine, not intractable**
Other migraine, without refractory migraine

G43.801 Other migraine, not intractable, with status migrainosus

G43.809 Other migraine, not intractable, without status migrainosus

√6th **G43.81 Other migraine, intractable**
Other migraine, with refractory migraine

G43.811 Other migraine, intractable, with status migrainosus

G43.819 Other migraine, intractable, without status migrainosus

✓6th **G43.82 Menstrual migraine, not intractable**
Menstrual headache, not intractable
Menstrual migraine, without refractory migraine
Menstrually related migraine, not intractable
Pre-menstrual headache, not intractable
Pre-menstrual migraine, not intractable
Pure menstrual migraine, not intractable
Code also associated premenstrual tension syndrome (N94.3)

G43.821 Menstrual migraine, not intractable, with status migrainosus

G43.829 Menstrual migraine, not intractable, without status migrainosus
Menstrual migraine NOS

✓6th **G43.83 Menstrual migraine, intractable**
Menstrual headache, intractable
Menstrual migraine, with refractory migraine
Menstrually related migraine, intractable
Pre-menstrual headache, intractable
Pre-menstrual migraine, intractable
Pure menstrual migraine, intractable
Code also associated premenstrual tension syndrome (N94.3)

G43.831 Menstrual migraine, intractable, with status migrainosus

G43.839 Menstrual migraine, intractable, without status migrainosus

✓5th **G43.9 Migraine, unspecified**

✓6th **G43.90 Migraine, unspecified, not intractable**
Migraine, unspecified, without refractory migraine

G43.901 Migraine, unspecified, not intractable, with status migrainosus
Status migrainosus NOS

G43.909 Migraine, unspecified, not intractable, without status migrainosus
Migraine NOS

✓6th **G43.91 Migraine, unspecified, intractable**
Migraine, unspecified, with refractory migraine

G43.911 Migraine, unspecified, intractable, with status migrainosus

G43.919 Migraine, unspecified, intractable, without status migrainosus

✓4th **G44 Other headache syndromes**
EXCLUDES 1 *headache NOS (R51)*
EXCLUDES 2 *atypical facial pain (G50.1)*
headache due to lumbar puncture (G97.1)
migraines (G43.-)
trigeminal neuralgia (G50.0)

✓5th **G44.0 Cluster headaches and other trigeminal autonomic cephalgias (TAC)**

✓6th **G44.00 Cluster headache syndrome, unspecified**
Ciliary neuralgia
Cluster headache NOS
Histamine cephalgia
Lower half migraine
Migrainous neuralgia

G44.001 Cluster headache syndrome, unspecified, intractable

G44.009 Cluster headache syndrome, unspecified, not intractable
Cluster headache syndrome NOS

✓6th **G44.01 Episodic cluster headache**

G44.011 Episodic cluster headache, intractable

G44.019 Episodic cluster headache, not intractable
Episodic cluster headache NOS

✓6th **G44.02 Chronic cluster headache**

G44.021 Chronic cluster headache, intractable

G44.029 Chronic cluster headache, not intractable
Chronic cluster headache NOS

✓6th **G44.03 Episodic paroxysmal hemicrania**
Paroxysmal hemicrania NOS

G44.031 Episodic paroxysmal hemicrania, intractable

G44.039 Episodic paroxysmal hemicrania, not intractable
Episodic paroxysmal hemicrania NOS

✓6th **G44.04 Chronic paroxysmal hemicrania**

G44.041 Chronic paroxysmal hemicrania, intractable

G44.049 Chronic paroxysmal hemicrania, not intractable
Chronic paroxysmal hemicrania NOS

✓6th **G44.05 Short lasting unilateral neuralgiform headache with conjunctival injection and tearing (SUNCT)**

G44.051 Short lasting unilateral neuralgiform headache with conjunctival injection and tearing (SUNCT), intractable

G44.059 Short lasting unilateral neuralgiform headache with conjunctival injection and tearing (SUNCT), not intractable
Short lasting unilateral neuralgiform headache with conjunctival injection and tearing (SUNCT) NOS

✓6th **G44.09 Other trigeminal autonomic cephalgias (TAC)**

G44.091 Other trigeminal autonomic cephalgias (TAC), intractable

G44.099 Other trigeminal autonomic cephalgias (TAC), not intractable

G44.1 Vascular headache, not elsewhere classified
EXCLUDES 2 *cluster headache (G44.0)*
complicated headache syndromes (G44.5-)
drug-induced headache (G44.4-)
migraine (G43.-)
other specified headache syndromes (G44.8-)
post-traumatic headache (G44.3-)
tension-type headache (G44.2-)

✓5th **G44.2 Tension-type headache**

✓6th **G44.20 Tension-type headache, unspecified**

G44.201 Tension-type headache, unspecified, intractable

G44.209 Tension-type headache, unspecified, not intractable
Tension headache NOS

✓6th **G44.21 Episodic tension-type headache**

G44.211 Episodic tension-type headache, intractable

G44.219 Episodic tension-type headache, not intractable
Episodic tension-type headache NOS

✓6th **G44.22 Chronic tension-type headache**

G44.221 Chronic tension-type headache, intractable

G44.229 Chronic tension-type headache, not intractable
Chronic tension-type headache NOS

✓5th **G44.3 Post-traumatic headache**

✓6th **G44.30 Post-traumatic headache, unspecified**

G44.301 Post-traumatic headache, unspecified, intractable

G44.309 Post-traumatic headache, unspecified, not intractable
Post-traumatic headache NOS

✓6th **G44.31 Acute post-traumatic headache**

G44.311 Acute post-traumatic headache, intractable

G44.319 Acute post-traumatic headache, not intractable
Acute post-traumatic headache NOS

✓6th **G44.32 Chronic post-traumatic headache**

G44.321 Chronic post-traumatic headache, intractable

G44.329 Chronic post-traumatic headache, not intractable
Chronic post-traumatic headache NOS

✓5th **G44.4 Drug-induced headache, not elsewhere classified**
Medication overuse headache
Use additional code for adverse effect, if applicable, to identify drug (T36-T50 with fifth or sixth character 5)

G44.40 Drug-induced headache, not elsewhere classified, not intractable

G44.41 Drug-induced headache, not elsewhere classified, intractable

✓5th **G44.5 Complicated headache syndromes**

G44.51 Hemicrania continua

G44.52 New daily persistent headache (NDPH)

G44.53 **Primary thunderclap headache**
G44.59 **Other complicated headache syndrome**

✓5th **G44.8 Other specified headache syndromes**
G44.81 **Hypnic headache**
G44.82 **Headache associated with sexual activity**
Orgasmic headache
Preorgasmic headache
G44.83 **Primary cough headache**
G44.84 **Primary exertional headache**
G44.85 **Primary stabbing headache**
G44.89 **Other headache syndrome**

✓4th **G45 Transient cerebral ischemic attacks and related syndromes**
EXCLUDES 1 *neonatal cerebral ischemia (P91.0)*
transient retinal artery occlusion (H34.0-)
G45.0 **Vertebro-basilar artery syndrome**
G45.1 **Carotid artery syndrome (hemispheric)**
G45.2 **Multiple and bilateral precerebral artery syndromes**
G45.3 **Amaurosis fugax**
G45.4 **Transient global amnesia**
EXCLUDES 1 *amnesia NOS (R41.3)*
G45.8 **Other transient cerebral ischemic attacks and related syndromes**
G45.9 **Transient cerebral ischemic attack, unspecified**
Spasm of cerebral artery
TIA
Transient cerebral ischemia NOS

✓4th **G46 Vascular syndromes of brain in cerebrovascular diseases**
Code first underlying cerebrovascular disease (I60-I69)
G46.0 **Middle cerebral artery syndrome**
G46.1 **Anterior cerebral artery syndrome**
G46.2 **Posterior cerebral artery syndrome**
G46.3 **Brain stem stroke syndrome**
Benedikt syndrome
Claude syndrome
Foville syndrome
Millard-Gubler syndrome
Wallenberg syndrome
Weber syndrome
G46.4 **Cerebellar stroke syndrome**
G46.5 **Pure motor lacunar syndrome**
G46.6 **Pure sensory lacunar syndrome**
G46.7 **Other lacunar syndromes**
G46.8 **Other vascular syndromes of brain in cerebrovascular diseases**

✓4th **G47 Sleep disorders**
EXCLUDES 2 *nightmares (F51.5)*
nonorganic sleep disorders (F51.-)
sleep terrors (F51.4)
sleepwalking (F51.3)

✓5th **G47.0 Insomnia**
EXCLUDES 2 *alcohol related insomnia (F10.182, F10.282, F10.982)*
drug related insomnia (F11.182, F11.282, F11.982, F13.182, F13.282, F13.982, F14.182, F14.282, F14.982, F15.182, F15.282, F15.982, F19.182, F19.282, F19.982)
idiopathic insomnia (F51.01)
insomnia due to a mental disorder (F51.05)
insomnia not due to a substance or known physiological condition (F51.0-)
nonorganic insomnia (F51.0-)
primary insomnia (F51.01)
sleep apnea (G47.3-)
G47.00 **Insomnia, unspecified**
Insomnia NOS
G47.01 **Insomnia due to medical condition**
Code also associated medical condition
G47.09 **Other insomnia**

✓5th **G47.1 Hypersomnia**
EXCLUDES 2 *alcohol-related hypersomnia (F10.182, F10.282, F10.982)*
drug-related hypersomnia (F11.182, F11.282, F11.982, F13.182, F13.282, F13.982, F14.182, F14.282, F14.982, F15.182, F15.282, F15.982, F19.182, F19.282, F19.982)
hypersomnia due to a mental disorder (F51.13)
hypersomnia not due to a substance or known physiological condition (F51.1-)
primary hypersomnia (F51.11)
sleep apnea (G47.3-)
G47.10 **Hypersomnia, unspecified**
Hypersomnia NOS
G47.11 **Idiopathic hypersomnia with long sleep time**
Idiopathic hypersomnia NOS
G47.12 **Idiopathic hypersomnia without long sleep time**
G47.13 **Recurrent hypersomnia**
Kleine-Levin syndrome
Menstrual related hypersomnia
G47.14 **Hypersomnia due to medical condition**
Code also associated medical condition
G47.19 **Other hypersomnia**

✓5th **G47.2 Circadian rhythm sleep disorders**
Disorders of the sleep wake schedule
Inversion of nyctohemeral rhythm
Inversion of sleep rhythm
G47.20 **Circadian rhythm sleep disorder, unspecified type**
Sleep wake schedule disorder NOS
G47.21 **Circadian rhythm sleep disorder, delayed sleep phase type**
Delayed sleep phase syndrome
G47.22 **Circadian rhythm sleep disorder, advanced sleep phase type**
G47.23 **Circadian rhythm sleep disorder, irregular sleep wake type**
Irregular sleep-wake pattern
G47.24 **Circadian rhythm sleep disorder, free running type**
G47.25 **Circadian rhythm sleep disorder, jet lag type**
G47.26 **Circadian rhythm sleep disorder, shift work type**
G47.27 ***Circadian rhythm sleep disorder in conditions classified elsewhere***
Code first underlying condition
G47.29 **Other circadian rhythm sleep disorder**

✓5th **G47.3 Sleep apnea**
Code also any associated underlying condition
EXCLUDES 1 *apnea NOS R06.81*
Cheyne-Stokes breathing (R06.3)
pickwickian syndrome (E66.2)
sleep apnea of newborn (P28.3)
G47.30 **Sleep apnea, unspecified**
Sleep apnea NOS
G47.31 **Primary central sleep apnea**
G47.32 **High altitude periodic breathing**
G47.33 **Obstructive sleep apnea (adult) (pediatric)**
EXCLUDES 1 *obstructive sleep apnea of newborn (P28.3)*
G47.34 **Idiopathic sleep related nonobstructive alveolar hypoventilation**
Sleep related hypoxia
G47.35 **Congenital central alveolar hypoventilation syndrome**
G47.36 ***Sleep related hypoventilation in conditions classified elsewhere***
Sleep related hypoxemia in conditions classified elsewhere
Code first underlying condition
G47.37 ***Central sleep apnea in conditions classified elsewhere***
Code first underlying condition
G47.39 **Other sleep apnea**

✓5th **G47.4 Narcolepsy and cataplexy**
✓6th G47.41 **Narcolepsy**
G47.411 **Narcolepsy with cataplexy**
G47.419 **Narcolepsy without cataplexy**
Narcolepsy NOS
✓6th G47.42 **Narcolepsy in conditions classified elsewhere**
G47.421 ***Narcolepsy in conditions classified elsewhere with cataplexy***

G47.429 Narcolepsy in conditions classified elsewhere without cataplexy

G47.5 Parasomnia

EXCLUDES 1 *alcohol induced parasomnia (F10.182, F10.282, F10.982)*
drug induced parasomnia (F11.182, F11.282, F11.982, F13.182, F13.282, F13.982, F14.182, F14.282, F14.982, F15.182, F15.282, F15.982, F19.182, F19.282, F19.982)
parasomnia not due to a substance or known physiological condition (F51.8)

G47.50 Parasomnia, unspecified
Parasomnia NOS
G47.51 Confusional arousals
G47.52 REM sleep behavior disorder
G47.53 Recurrent isolated sleep paralysis
G47.54 Parasomnia in conditions classified elsewhere
Code first underlying condition
G47.59 Other parasomnia

G47.6 Sleep related movement disorders
EXCLUDES 2 *restless legs syndrome (G25.81)*
G47.61 Periodic limb movement disorder
G47.62 Sleep related leg cramps
G47.63 Sleep related bruxism
EXCLUDES 1 *psychogenic bruxism (F45.8)*
G47.69 Other sleep related movement disorders

G47.8 Other sleep disorders
G47.9 Sleep disorder, unspecified
Sleep disorder NOS

Nerve, nerve root and plexus disorders (G50-G59)

EXCLUDES 1 *current traumatic nerve, nerve root and plexus disorders—see Injury, nerve by body region*
neuralgia NOS (M79.2)
neuritis NOS (M79.2)
peripheral neuritis in pregnancy (O26.82-)
radiculitis NOS (M54.1-)

G50 Disorders of trigeminal nerve
INCLUDES disorders of 5th cranial nerve
G50.0 Trigeminal neuralgia
Syndrome of paroxysmal facial pain
Tic douloureux
G50.1 Atypical facial pain
G50.8 Other disorders of trigeminal nerve
G50.9 Disorder of trigeminal nerve, unspecified

G51 Facial nerve disorders
INCLUDES disorders of 7th cranial nerve
G51.0 Bell's palsy
Facial palsy
G51.1 Geniculate ganglionitis
EXCLUDES 1 *postherpetic geniculate ganglionitis (B02.21)*
G51.2 Melkersson's syndrome
Melkersson-Rosenthal syndrome
G51.3 Clonic hemifacial spasm
G51.4 Facial myokymia
G51.8 Other disorders of facial nerve
G51.9 Disorder of facial nerve, unspecified

G52 Disorders of other cranial nerves
EXCLUDES 2 *disorders of acoustic [8th] nerve (H93.3)*
disorders of optic [2nd] nerve (H46, H47.0)
paralytic strabismus due to nerve palsy (H49.0-H49.2)
G52.0 Disorders of olfactory nerve
Disorders of 1st cranial nerve
G52.1 Disorders of glossopharyngeal nerve
Disorder of 9th cranial nerve
Glossopharyngeal neuralgia
G52.2 Disorders of vagus nerve
Disorders of pneumogastric [10th] nerve
G52.3 Disorders of hypoglossal nerve
Disorders of 12th cranial nerve
G52.7 Disorders of multiple cranial nerves
Polyneuritis cranialis
G52.8 Disorders of other specified cranial nerves
G52.9 Cranial nerve disorder, unspecified

G53 Cranial nerve disorders in diseases classified elsewhere
Code first underlying disease, such as:
neoplasm (C00-D49)
EXCLUDES 1 *multiple cranial nerve palsy in sarcoidosis (D86.82)*
multiple cranial nerve palsy in syphilis (A52.15)
postherpetic geniculate ganglionitis (B02.21)
postherpetic trigeminal neuralgia (B02.22)

G54 Nerve root and plexus disorders
EXCLUDES 1 *current traumatic nerve root and plexus disorders—see nerve injury by body region*
intervertebral disc disorders (M50-M51)
neuralgia or neuritis NOS (M79.2)
neuritis or radiculitis:
brachial NOS (M54.13)
lumbar NOS (M54.16)
lumbosacral NOS (M54.17)
thoracic NOS (M54.14)
radiculitis NOS (M54.10)
radiculopathy NOS (M54.10)
spondylosis (M47.-)
G54.0 Brachial plexus disorders
Thoracic outlet syndrome
G54.1 Lumbosacral plexus disorders
G54.2 Cervical root disorders, not elsewhere classified
G54.3 Thoracic root disorders, not elsewhere classified
G54.4 Lumbosacral root disorders, not elsewhere classified
G54.5 Neuralgic amyotrophy
Parsonage-Aldren-Turner syndrome
Shoulder-girdle neuritis
EXCLUDES 1 *neuralgic amyotrophy in diabetes mellitus (E08-E13 with .44)*
G54.6 Phantom limb syndrome with pain
G54.7 Phantom limb syndrome without pain
Phantom limb syndrome NOS
G54.8 Other nerve root and plexus disorders
G54.9 Nerve root and plexus disorder, unspecified

G55 Nerve root and plexus compressions in diseases classified elsewhere
Code first underlying disease, such as:
neoplasm (C00-D49)
EXCLUDES 1 *nerve root compression (due to) (in) ankylosing spondylitis (M45.-)*
nerve root compression (due to) (in) dorsopathies (M53.-, M54.-)
nerve root compression (due to) (in) intervertebral disc disorders (M50.1-, M51.1-)
nerve root compression (due to) (in) spondylopathies (M46.-, M48.-)
nerve root compression (due to) (in) spondylosis (M47.0-M47.2-)

G56 Mononeuropathies of upper limb
EXCLUDES 1 *current traumatic nerve disorder—see nerve injury by body region*
G56.0 Carpal tunnel syndrome
G56.00 Carpal tunnel syndrome, unspecified upper limb
G56.01 Carpal tunnel syndrome, right upper limb
G56.02 Carpal tunnel syndrome, left upper limb
G56.1 Other lesions of median nerve
G56.10 Other lesions of median nerve, unspecified upper limb
G56.11 Other lesions of median nerve, right upper limb
G56.12 Other lesions of median nerve, left upper limb
G56.2 Lesion of ulnar nerve
Tardy ulnar nerve palsy
G56.20 Lesion of ulnar nerve, unspecified upper limb
G56.21 Lesion of ulnar nerve, right upper limb
G56.22 Lesion of ulnar nerve, left upper limb
G56.3 Lesion of radial nerve
G56.30 Lesion of radial nerve, unspecified upper limb
G56.31 Lesion of radial nerve, right upper limb
G56.32 Lesion of radial nerve, left upper limb

- ✓5th **G56.4 Causalgia of upper limb**
  - Complex regional pain syndrome II of upper limb
  - EXCLUDES 1 *complex regional pain syndrome I of lower limb (G90.52-)*
    complex regional pain syndrome I of upper limb (G90.51-)
    complex regional pain syndrome II of lower limb (G57.7-)
    reflex sympathetic dystrophy of lower limb (G90.52-)
    reflex sympathetic dystrophy of upper limb (G90.51-)
  - **G56.40 Causalgia of unspecified upper limb**
  - **G56.41 Causalgia of right upper limb**
  - **G56.42 Causalgia of left upper limb**
- ✓5th **G56.8 Other specified mononeuropathies of upper limb**
  - Interdigital neuroma of upper limb
  - **G56.80 Other specified mononeuropathies of unspecified upper limb**
  - **G56.81 Other specified mononeuropathies of right upper limb**
  - **G56.82 Other specified mononeuropathies of left upper limb**
- ✓5th **G56.9 Unspecified mononeuropathy of upper limb**
  - **G56.90 Unspecified mononeuropathy of unspecified upper limb**
  - **G56.91 Unspecified mononeuropathy of right upper limb**
  - **G56.92 Unspecified mononeuropathy of left upper limb**

✓4th **G57 Mononeuropathies of lower limb**

EXCLUDES 1 *current traumatic nerve disorder—see nerve injury by body region*

- ✓5th **G57.0 Lesion of sciatic nerve**
  - EXCLUDES 1 *sciatica NOS (M54.3-)*
  - EXCLUDES 2 *sciatica attributed to intervertebral disc disorder (M51.1-)*
  - **G57.00 Lesion of sciatic nerve, unspecified lower limb**
  - **G57.01 Lesion of sciatic nerve, right lower limb**
  - **G57.02 Lesion of sciatic nerve, left lower limb**
- ✓5th **G57.1 Meralgia paresthetica**
  - Lateral cutaneous nerve of thigh syndrome
  - **G57.10 Meralgia paresthetica, unspecified lower limb**
  - **G57.11 Meralgia paresthetica, right lower limb**
  - **G57.12 Meralgia paresthetica, left lower limb**
- ✓5th **G57.2 Lesion of femoral nerve**
  - **G57.20 Lesion of femoral nerve, unspecified lower limb**
  - **G57.21 Lesion of femoral nerve, right lower limb**
  - **G57.22 Lesion of femoral nerve, left lower limb**
- ✓5th **G57.3 Lesion of lateral popliteal nerve**
  - Peroneal nerve palsy
  - **G57.30 Lesion of lateral popliteal nerve, unspecified lower limb**
  - **G57.31 Lesion of lateral popliteal nerve, right lower limb**
  - **G57.32 Lesion of lateral popliteal nerve, left lower limb**
- ✓5th **G57.4 Lesion of medial popliteal nerve**
  - **G57.40 Lesion of medial popliteal nerve, unspecified lower limb**
  - **G57.41 Lesion of medial popliteal nerve, right lower limb**
  - **G57.42 Lesion of medial popliteal nerve, left lower limb**
- ✓5th **G57.5 Tarsal tunnel syndrome**
  - **G57.50 Tarsal tunnel syndrome, unspecified lower limb**
  - **G57.51 Tarsal tunnel syndrome, right lower limb**
  - **G57.52 Tarsal tunnel syndrome, left lower limb**
- ✓5th **G57.6 Lesion of plantar nerve**
  - Morton's metatarsalgia
  - **G57.60 Lesion of plantar nerve, unspecified lower limb**
  - **G57.61 Lesion of plantar nerve, right lower limb**
  - **G57.62 Lesion of plantar nerve, left lower limb**
- ✓5th **G57.7 Causalgia of lower limb**
  - Complex regional pain syndrome II of lower limb
  - EXCLUDES 1 *complex regional pain syndrome I of lower limb (G90.52-)*
    complex regional pain syndrome I of upper limb (G90.51-)
    complex regional pain syndrome II of upper limb (G56.4-)
    reflex sympathetic dystrophy of lower limb (G90.52-)
    reflex sympathetic dystrophy of upper limb (G90.51-)
  - **G57.70 Causalgia of unspecified lower limb**
  - **G57.71 Causalgia of right lower limb**
  - **G57.72 Causalgia of left lower limb**
- ✓5th **G57.8 Other specified mononeuropathies of lower limb**
  - Interdigital neuroma of lower limb
  - **G57.80 Other specified mononeuropathies of unspecified lower limb**
  - **G57.81 Other specified mononeuropathies of right lower limb**
  - **G57.82 Other specified mononeuropathies of left lower limb**
- ✓5th **G57.9 Unspecified mononeuropathy of lower limb**
  - **G57.90 Unspecified mononeuropathy of unspecified lower limb**
  - **G57.91 Unspecified mononeuropathy of right lower limb**
  - **G57.92 Unspecified mononeuropathy of left lower limb**

✓4th **G58 Other mononeuropathies**

- **G58.0 Intercostal neuropathy**
- **G58.7 Mononeuritis multiplex**
- **G58.8 Other specified mononeuropathies**
- **G58.9 Mononeuropathy, unspecified**

G59 Mononeuropathy in diseases classified elsewhere

Code first underlying disease

EXCLUDES 1 *diabetic mononeuropathy (E09-E14 with .41)*
syphilitic nerve paralysis (A52.19)
syphilitic neuritis (A52.15)
tuberculous mononeuropathy (A17.83)

Polyneuropathies and other disorders of the peripheral nervous system (G60-G65)

EXCLUDES 1 *neuralgia NOS (M79.2)*
neuritis NOS (M79.2)
peripheral neuritis in pregnancy (O26.82-)
radiculitis NOS (M54.10)

✓4th **G60 Hereditary and idiopathic neuropathy**

- **G60.0 Hereditary motor and sensory neuropathy**
  - Charcôt-Marie-Tooth disease
  - Déjérine-Sottas disease
  - Hereditary motor and sensory neuropathy, types I-IV
  - Hypertrophic neuropathy of infancy
  - Peroneal muscular atrophy (axonal type) (hypertrophic type)
  - Roussy-Levy syndrome
- **G60.1 Refsum's disease**
  - Infantile Refsum disease
- **G60.2 Neuropathy in association with hereditary ataxia**
- **G60.3 Idiopathic progressive neuropathy**
- **G60.8 Other hereditary and idiopathic neuropathies**
  - Dominantly inherited sensory neuropathy
  - Morvan's disease
  - Nelaton's syndrome
  - Recessively inherited sensory neuropathy
- **G60.9 Hereditary and idiopathic neuropathy, unspecified**

✓4th **G61 Inflammatory polyneuropathy**

- **G61.0 Guillain-Barre syndrome**
  - Acute (post-)infective polyneuritis
  - Miller Fisher syndrome
- **G61.1 Serum neuropathy**
  - Use additional code for adverse effect, if applicable, to identify serum (T50.-)
- ✓5th **G61.8 Other inflammatory polyneuropathies**
  - **G61.81 Chronic inflammatory demyelinating polyneuritis**
  - **G61.89 Other inflammatory polyneuropathies**
- **G61.9 Inflammatory polyneuropathy, unspecified**

✓4th **G62 Other and unspecified polyneuropathies**

- **G62.0 Drug-induced polyneuropathy**
  - Use additional code for adverse effect, if applicable, to identify drug (T36-T50 with fifth or sixth character 5)
- **G62.1 Alcoholic polyneuropathy**
- **G62.2 Polyneuropathy due to other toxic agents**
  - Code first (T51-T65) to identify toxic agent
- ✓5th **G62.8 Other specified polyneuropathies**
  - **G62.81 Critical illness polyneuropathy**
    - Acute motor neuropathy
  - **G62.82 Radiation-induced polyneuropathy**
    - Use additional external cause code (W88-W90, X39.0-) to identify cause
  - **G62.89 Other specified polyneuropathies**

G62.9 Polyneuropathy, unspecified
Neuropathy NOS

G63 Polyneuropathy in diseases classified elsewhere
Code first underlying disease, such as:
amyloidosis (E85.-)
endocrine disease, except diabetes (E00-E07, E15-E16, E20-E34)
metabolic diseases (E70-E88)
neoplasm (C00-D49)
nutritional deficiency (E40-E64)

EXCLUDES 1 *polyneuropathy (in):*
diabetes mellitus (E08-E13 with .42)
diphtheria (A36.83)
infectious mononucleosis (B27.0-B27.9 with 1)
Lyme disease (A69.22)
mumps (B26.84)
postherpetic (B02.23)
rheumatoid arthritis (M05.33)
scleroderma (M34.83)
systemic lupus erythematosus (M32.19)

G64 Other disorders of peripheral nervous system
Disorder of peripheral nervous system NOS

✓4th **G65 Sequelae of inflammatory and toxic polyneuropathies**
Code first condition resulting from (sequela) of inflammatory and toxic polyneuropathies

G65.0 Sequelae of Guillain-Barré syndrome
G65.1 Sequelae of other inflammatory polyneuropathy
G65.2 Sequelae of toxic polyneuropathy

Diseases of myoneural junction and muscle (G70-G73)

✓4th **G70 Myasthenia gravis and other myoneural disorders**
EXCLUDES 1 *botulism (A05.1, A48.51-A48.52)*
transient neonatal myasthenia gravis (P94.0)

✓5th **G70.0 Myasthenia gravis**
G70.00 Myasthenia gravis without (acute) exacerbation
Myasthenia gravis NOS
G70.01 Myasthenia gravis with (acute) exacerbation
Myasthenia gravis in crisis

G70.1 Toxic myoneural disorders
Code first (T51-T65) to identify toxic agent

G70.2 Congenital and developmental myasthenia

✓5th **G70.8 Other specified myoneural disorders**
G70.80 Lambert-Eaton syndrome, unspecified
Lambert-Eaton syndrome NOS
G70.81 Lambert-Eaton syndrome in disease classified elsewhere
Code first underlying disease
EXCLUDES 1 *Lambert-Eaton syndrome in neoplastic disease (G73.1)*
G70.89 Other specified myoneural disorders

G70.9 Myoneural disorder, unspecified

✓4th **G71 Primary disorders of muscles**
EXCLUDES 2 *arthrogryposis multiplex congenita (Q74.3)*
metabolic disorders (E70-E88)
myositis (M60.-)

G71.0 Muscular dystrophy
Autosomal recessive, childhood type, muscular dystrophy resembling Duchenne or Becker muscular dystrophy
Benign [Becker] muscular dystrophy
Benign scapuloperoneal muscular dystrophy with early contractures [Emery-Dreifuss]
Congenital muscular dystrophy NOS
Congenital muscular dystrophy with specific morphological abnormalities of the muscle fiber
Distal muscular dystrophy
Facioscapulohumeral muscular dystrophy
Limb-girdle muscular dystrophy
Ocular muscular dystrophy
Oculopharyngeal muscular dystrophy
Scapuloperoneal muscular dystrophy
Severe [Duchenne] muscular dystrophy

✓5th **G71.1 Myotonic disorders**
G71.11 Myotonic muscular dystrophy
Dystrophia myotonica [Steinert]
Myotonia atrophica
Myotonic dystrophy
Proximal myotonic myopathy (PROMM)
Steinert disease

G71.12 Myotonia congenita
Acetazolamide responsive myotonia congenita
Dominant myotonia congenita [Thomsen disease]
Myotonia levior
Recessive myotonia congenita [Becker disease]

G71.13 Myotonic chondrodystrophy
Chondrodystrophic myotonia
Congenital myotonic chondrodystrophy
Schwartz-Jampel disease

G71.14 Drug induced myotonia
Use additional code for adverse effect, if applicable, to identify drug (T36-T50 with fifth or sixth character 5)

G71.19 Other specified myotonic disorders
Myotonia fluctuans
Myotonia permanens
Neuromyotonia [Isaacs]
Paramyotonia congenita (of von Eulenburg)
Pseudomyotonia
Symptomatic myotonia

G71.2 Congenital myopathies
Central core disease
Fiber-type disproportion
Minicore disease
Multicore disease
Myotubular (centronuclear) myopathy
Nemaline myopathy
EXCLUDES 1 *arthrogryposis multiplex congenita (Q74.3)*

G71.3 Mitochondrial myopathy, not elsewhere classified
EXCLUDES 1 *Kearns-Sayre syndrome (H49.81)*
Leber's disease (H47.21)
Leigh's encephalopathy (G31.82)
mitochondrial metabolism disorders (E88.4-)
Reye's syndrome (G93.7)

G71.8 Other primary disorders of muscles
G71.9 Primary disorder of muscle, unspecified
Hereditary myopathy NOS

✓4th **G72 Other and unspecified myopathies**
EXCLUDES 1 *arthrogryposis multiplex congenita (Q74.3)*
dermatopolymyositis (M33.-)
ischemic infarction of muscle (M62.2-)
myositis (M60.-)
polymyositis (M33.2-)

G72.0 Drug-induced myopathy
Use additional code for adverse effect, if applicable, to identify drug (T36-T50 with fifth or sixth character 5)

G72.1 Alcoholic myopathy
Use additional code to identify alcoholism (F10.-)

G72.2 Myopathy due to other toxic agents
Code first (T51-T65) to identify toxic agent

G72.3 Periodic paralysis
Familial periodic paralysis
Hyperkalemic periodic paralysis (familial)
Hypokalemic periodic paralysis (familial)
Myotonic periodic paralysis (familial)
Normokalemic paralysis (familial)
Potassium sensitive periodic paralysis
EXCLUDES 1 *paramyotonia congenita (of von Eulenburg) (G71.19)*

✓5th **G72.4 Inflammatory and immune myopathies, not elsewhere classified**
G72.41 Inclusion body myositis [IBM]
G72.49 Other inflammatory and immune myopathies, not elsewhere classified
Inflammatory myopathy NOS

✓5th **G72.8 Other specified myopathies**
G72.81 Critical illness myopathy
Acute necrotizing myopathy
Acute quadriplegic myopathy
Intensive care (ICU) myopathy
Myopathy of critical illness
G72.89 Other specified myopathies

G72.9 Myopathy, unspecified

✓4th **G73 Disorders of myoneural junction and muscle in diseases classified elsewhere**
G73.1 Lambert-Eaton syndrome in neoplastic disease
Code first underlying neoplasm (C00-D49)
EXCLUDES 1 *Lambert-Eaton syndrome not associated with neoplasm (G70.80-G70.81)*

G73.3 Myasthenic syndromes in other diseases classified elsewhere
Code first underlying disease, such as:
neoplasm (C00-D49)
thyrotoxicosis (E05.-)

G73.7 Myopathy in diseases classified elsewhere
Code first underlying disease, such as:
hyperparathyroidism (E21.0, E21.3)
hypoparathyroidism (E20.-)
glycogen storage disease (E74.0)
lipid storage disorders (E75.-)
EXCLUDES 1 *myopathy in:*
rheumatoid arthritis (M05.4-)
sarcoidosis (D86.87)
scleroderma (M34.82)
sicca syndrome [Sjögren] (M35.03)
systemic lupus erythematosus (M32.19)

Cerebral palsy and other paralytic syndromes (G80-G83)

✓4th G80 Cerebral palsy
EXCLUDES 1 *hereditary spastic paraplegia (G11.4)*
G80.0 Spastic quadriplegic cerebral palsy
Congenital spastic paralysis (cerebral)
G80.1 Spastic diplegic cerebral palsy
Spastic cerebral palsy NOS
G80.2 Spastic hemiplegic cerebral palsy
G80.3 Athetoid cerebral palsy
Double athetosis (syndrome)
Dyskinetic cerebral palsy
Dystonic cerebral palsy
Vogt disease
G80.4 Ataxic cerebral palsy
G80.8 Other cerebral palsy
Mixed cerebral palsy syndromes
G80.9 Cerebral palsy, unspecified
Cerebral palsy NOS

✓4th G81 Hemiplegia and hemiparesis
NOTE This category is to be used only when hemiplegia (complete)(incomplete) is reported without further specification, or is stated to be old or longstanding but of unspecified cause. The category is also for use in multiple coding to identify these types of hemiplegia resulting from any cause.
EXCLUDES 1 *congenital cerebral palsy (G80.-)*
hemiplegia and hemiparesis due to sequela of cerebrovascular disease (I69.05-, I69.15-, I69.25-, I69.35-, I69.85-, I69.95-)

✓5th G81.0 Flaccid hemiplegia
G81.00 Flaccid hemiplegia affecting unspecified side
G81.01 Flaccid hemiplegia affecting right dominant side
G81.02 Flaccid hemiplegia affecting left dominant side
G81.03 Flaccid hemiplegia affecting right nondominant side
G81.04 Flaccid hemiplegia affecting left nondominant side

✓5th G81.1 Spastic hemiplegia
G81.10 Spastic hemiplegia affecting unspecified side
G81.11 Spastic hemiplegia affecting right dominant side
G81.12 Spastic hemiplegia affecting left dominant side
G81.13 Spastic hemiplegia affecting right nondominant side
G81.14 Spastic hemiplegia affecting left nondominant side

✓5th G81.9 Hemiplegia, unspecified
G81.90 Hemiplegia, unspecified affecting unspecified side
G81.91 Hemiplegia, unspecified affecting right dominant side
G81.92 Hemiplegia, unspecified affecting left dominant side
G81.93 Hemiplegia, unspecified affecting right nondominant side
G81.94 Hemiplegia, unspecified affecting left nondominant side

✓4th G82 Paraplegia (paraparesis) and quadriplegia (quadriparesis)
NOTE This category is to be used only when the listed conditions are reported without further specification, or are stated to be old or longstanding but of unspecified cause. The category is also for use in multiple coding to identify these conditions resulting from any cause
EXCLUDES 1 *congenital cerebral palsy (G80.-)*
functional quadriplegia (R53.2)
hysterical paralysis (F44.4)

✓5th G82.2 Paraplegia
Paralysis of both lower limbs NOS
Paraparesis (lower) NOS
Paraplegia (lower) NOS
G82.20 Paraplegia, unspecified
G82.21 Paraplegia, complete
G82.22 Paraplegia, incomplete

✓5th G82.5 Quadriplegia
G82.50 Quadriplegia, unspecified
G82.51 Quadriplegia, C1-C4 complete
G82.52 Quadriplegia, C1-C4 incomplete
G82.53 Quadriplegia, C5-C7 complete
G82.54 Quadriplegia, C5-C7 incomplete

✓4th G83 Other paralytic syndromes
NOTE This category is to be used only when the listed conditions are reported without further specification, or are stated to be old or longstanding but of unspecified cause. The category is also for use in multiple coding to identify these conditions resulting from any cause.
INCLUDES paralysis (complete) (incomplete), except as in G80-G82
G83.0 Diplegia of upper limbs
Diplegia (upper)
Paralysis of both upper limbs

✓5th G83.1 Monoplegia of lower limb
Paralysis of lower limb
EXCLUDES 1 *monoplegia of lower limbs due to sequela of cerebrovascular disease (I69.04-, I69.14-, I69.24-, I69.34-, I69.84-, I69.94-)*
G83.10 Monoplegia of lower limb affecting unspecified side
G83.11 Monoplegia of lower limb affecting right dominant side
G83.12 Monoplegia of lower limb affecting left dominant side
G83.13 Monoplegia of lower limb affecting right nondominant side
G83.14 Monoplegia of lower limb affecting left nondominant side

✓5th G83.2 Monoplegia of upper limb
Paralysis of upper limb
EXCLUDES 1 *monoplegia of upper limbs due to sequela of cerebrovascular disease (I69.03-, I69.13-, I69.23-, I69.33-, I69.83-, I69.93-)*
G83.20 Monoplegia of upper limb affecting unspecified side
G83.21 Monoplegia of upper limb affecting right dominant side
G83.22 Monoplegia of upper limb affecting left dominant side
G83.23 Monoplegia of upper limb affecting right nondominant side
G83.24 Monoplegia of upper limb affecting left nondominant side

✓5th G83.3 Monoplegia, unspecified
G83.30 Monoplegia, unspecified affecting unspecified side
G83.31 Monoplegia, unspecified affecting right dominant side
G83.32 Monoplegia, unspecified affecting left dominant side
G83.33 Monoplegia, unspecified affecting right nondominant side
G83.34 Monoplegia, unspecified affecting left nondominant side

G83.4 Cauda equina syndrome
Neurogenic bladder due to cauda equina syndrome
EXCLUDES 1 *cord bladder NOS (G95.89)*
neurogenic bladder NOS (N31.9)

G83.5 Locked-in state

✓5th **G83.8 Other specified paralytic syndromes**
EXCLUDES 1 *paralytic syndromes due to current spinal cord injury—code to spinal cord injury (S14, S24, S34)*
G83.81 Brown-Séquard syndrome
G83.82 Anterior cord syndrome
G83.83 Posterior cord syndrome
G83.84 Todd's paralysis (postepileptic)
G83.89 Other specified paralytic syndromes
G83.9 Paralytic syndrome, unspecified

Other disorders of the nervous system (G89-G99)

✓4th **G89 Pain, not elsewhere classified**
Code also related psychological factors associated with pain (F45.42)
EXCLUDES 1 *generalized pain NOS (R52)*
pain disorders exclusively related to psychological factors (F45.41)
pain NOS (R52)
EXCLUDES 2 *atypical face pain (G50.1)*
headache syndromes (G44.-)
localized pain, unspecified type—code to pain by site, such as:
abdomen pain (R10.-)
back pain (M54.9)
breast pain (N64.4)
chest pain (R07.1-R07.9)
ear pain (H92.0-)
eye pain (H57.1)
headache (R51)
joint pain (M25.5-)
limb pain (M79.6-)
lumbar region pain (M54.5)
painful urination (R30.9)
pelvic and perineal pain (R10.2)
renal colic (N23)
shoulder pain (M25.51-)
spine pain (M54.-)
throat pain (R07.0)
tongue pain (K14.6)
tooth pain (K08.8)
migraines (G43.-)
myalgia (M79.1)
pain from prosthetic devices, implants, and grafts (T82.84, T83.84, T84.84, T85.84)
phantom limb syndrome with pain (G54.6)
vulvar vestibulitis (N94.810)
vulvodynia (N94.81-)
G89.0 Central pain syndrome
Déjérine-Roussy syndrome
Myelopathic pain syndrome
Thalamic pain syndrome (hyperesthetic)
✓5th **G89.1 Acute pain, not elsewhere classified**
G89.11 Acute pain due to trauma
G89.12 Acute post-thoracotomy pain
Post-thoracotomy pain NOS
G89.18 Other acute postprocedural pain
Postoperative pain NOS
Postprocedural pain NOS
✓5th **G89.2 Chronic pain, not elsewhere classified**
EXCLUDES 1 *causalgia, lower limb (G57.7-)*
causalgia, upper limb (G56.4-)
central pain syndrome (G89.0)
chronic pain syndrome (G89.4)
complex regional pain syndrome II, lower limb (G57.7-)
complex regional pain syndrome II, upper limb (G56.4-)
neoplasm related chronic pain (G89.3)
reflex sympathetic dystrophy (G90.5-)
G89.21 Chronic pain due to trauma
G89.22 Chronic post-thoracotomy pain
G89.28 Other chronic postprocedural pain
Other chronic postoperative pain
G89.29 Other chronic pain
G89.3 Neoplasm related pain (acute) (chronic)
Cancer associated pain
Pain due to malignancy (primary) (secondary)
Tumor associated pain
G89.4 Chronic pain syndrome
Chronic pain associated with significant psychosocial dysfunction

✓4th **G90 Disorders of autonomic nervous system**
EXCLUDES 1 *dysfunction of the autonomic nervous system due to alcohol (G31.2)*
✓5th **G90.0 Idiopathic peripheral autonomic neuropathy**
G90.01 Carotid sinus syncope
Carotid sinus syndrome
G90.09 Other idiopathic peripheral autonomic neuropathy
Idiopathic peripheral autonomic neuropathy NOS
G90.1 Familial dysautonomia [Riley-Day]
G90.2 Horner's syndrome
Bernard(-Horner) syndrome
Cervical sympathetic dystrophy or paralysis
G90.3 Multi-system degeneration of the autonomic nervous system
Neurogenic orthostatic hypotension [Shy-Drager]
EXCLUDES 1 *orthostatic hypotension NOS (I95.1)*
G90.4 Autonomic dysreflexia
Use additional code to identify the cause, such as:
fecal impaction (K56.41)
pressure ulcer (pressure area) (L89.-)
urinary tract infection (N39.0)
✓5th **G90.5 Complex regional pain syndrome I (CRPS I)**
Reflex sympathetic dystrophy
EXCLUDES 1 *causalgia of lower limb (G57.7-)*
causalgia of upper limb (G56.4-)
complex regional pain syndrome II of lower limb (G57.7-)
complex regional pain syndrome II of upper limb (G56.4-)
G90.50 Complex regional pain syndrome I, unspecified
✓6th **G90.51 Complex regional pain syndrome I of upper limb**
G90.511 Complex regional pain syndrome I of right upper limb
G90.512 Complex regional pain syndrome I of left upper limb
G90.513 Complex regional pain syndrome I of upper limb, bilateral
G90.519 Complex regional pain syndrome I of unspecified upper limb
✓6th **G90.52 Complex regional pain syndrome I of lower limb**
G90.521 Complex regional pain syndrome I of right lower limb
G90.522 Complex regional pain syndrome I of left lower limb
G90.523 Complex regional pain syndrome I of lower limb, bilateral
G90.529 Complex regional pain syndrome I of unspecified lower limb
G90.59 Complex regional pain syndrome I of other specified site
G90.8 Other disorders of autonomic nervous system
G90.9 Disorder of the autonomic nervous system, unspecified

✓4th **G91 Hydrocephalus**
INCLUDES acquired hydrocephalus
EXCLUDES 1 *Arnold-Chiari syndrome with hydrocephalus (Q07.-)*
congenital hydrocephalus (Q03.-)
spina bifida with hydrocephalus (Q05.-)
G91.0 Communicating hydrocephalus
Secondary normal pressure hydrocephalus
G91.1 Obstructive hydrocephalus
G91.2 (Idiopathic) normal pressure hydrocephalus
Normal pressure hydrocephalus NOS
G91.3 Post-traumatic hydrocephalus, unspecified
G91.4 ***Hydrocephalus in diseases classified elsewhere***
Code first underlying condition, such as:
congenital syphilis (A50.4-)
neoplasm (C00-D49)
EXCLUDES 1 *hydrocephalus due to congenital toxoplasmosis (P37.1)*
G91.8 Other hydrocephalus
G91.9 Hydrocephalus, unspecified

G92 Toxic encephalopathy
Toxic encephalitis
Toxic metabolic encephalopathy
Code first (T51-T65) to identify toxic agent

✓4th **G93 Other disorders of brain**

G93.0 Cerebral cysts
Arachnoid cyst
Porencephalic cyst, acquired
EXCLUDES 1 *acquired periventricular cysts of newborn (P91.1)*
congenital cerebral cysts (Q04.6)

G93.1 Anoxic brain damage, not elsewhere classified
EXCLUDES 1 *cerebral anoxia due to anesthesia during labor and delivery (O74.3)*
cerebral anoxia due to anesthesia during the puerperium (O89.2)
neonatal anoxia (P84)

G93.2 Benign intracranial hypertension
EXCLUDES 1 *hypertensive encephalopathy (I67.4)*

G93.3 Postviral fatigue syndrome
Benign myalgic encephalomyelitis
EXCLUDES 1 *chronic fatigue syndrome NOS (R53.82)*

✓5th **G93.4 Other and unspecified encephalopathy**
EXCLUDES 1 *alcoholic encephalopathy (G31.2)*
encephalopathy in diseases classified elsewhere (G94)
hypertensive encephalopathy (I67.4)
toxic (metabolic) encephalopathy (G92)

G93.40 Encephalopathy, unspecified

G93.41 Metabolic encephalopathy
Septic encephalopathy

G93.49 Other encephalopathy
Encephalopathy NEC

G93.5 Compression of brain
Arnold-Chiari type 1 compression of brain
Compression of brain (stem)
Herniation of brain (stem)
EXCLUDES 1 *diffuse traumatic compression of brain (S06.2-)*
focal traumatic compression of brain (S06.3-)

G93.6 Cerebral edema
EXCLUDES 1 *cerebral edema due to birth injury (P11.0)*
traumatic cerebral edema (S06.1-)

G93.7 Reye's syndrome
Code first (T39.0-), if salicylates-induced

✓5th **G93.8 Other specified disorders of brain**

G93.81 Temporal sclerosis
Hippocampal sclerosis
Mesial temporal sclerosis

G93.82 Brain death

G93.89 Other specified disorders of brain
Postradiation encephalopathy

G93.9 Disorder of brain, unspecified

G94 Other disorders of brain in diseases classified elsewhere
Code first underlying disease
EXCLUDES 1 *encephalopathy in congenital syphilis (A50.49)*
encephalopathy in influenza (J09.X9, J10.81, J11.81)
encephalopathy in syphilis (A52.19)
hydrocephalus in diseases classified elsewhere (G91.4)

✓4th **G95 Other and unspecified diseases of spinal cord**
EXCLUDES 2 *myelitis (G04.-)*

G95.0 Syringomyelia and syringobulbia

✓5th **G95.1 Vascular myelopathies**
EXCLUDES 2 *intraspinal phlebitis and thrombophlebitis, except non-pyogenic (G08)*

G95.11 Acute infarction of spinal cord (embolic) (nonembolic)
Anoxia of spinal cord
Arterial thrombosis of spinal cord

G95.19 Other vascular myelopathies
Edema of spinal cord
Hematomyelia
Nonpyogenic intraspinal phlebitis and thrombophlebitis
Subacute necrotic myelopathy

✓5th **G95.2 Other and unspecified cord compression**

G95.20 Unspecified cord compression

G95.29 Other cord compression

✓5th **G95.8 Other specified diseases of spinal cord**
EXCLUDES 1 *neurogenic bladder NOS (N31.9)*
neurogenic bladder due to cauda equina syndrome (G83.4)
neuromuscular dysfunction of bladder without spinal cord lesion (N31.-)

G95.81 Conus medullaris syndrome

G95.89 Other specified diseases of spinal cord
Cord bladder NOS
Drug-induced myelopathy
Radiation-induced myelopathy
EXCLUDES 1 *myelopathy NOS (G95.9)*

G95.9 Disease of spinal cord, unspecified
Myelopathy NOS

✓4th **G96 Other disorders of central nervous system**

G96.0 Cerebrospinal fluid leak
EXCLUDES 1 *cerebrospinal fluid leak from spinal puncture (G97.0)*

✓5th **G96.1 Disorders of meninges, not elsewhere classified**

G96.11 Dural tear
EXCLUDES 1 *accidental puncture or laceration of dura during a procedure (G97.41)*

G96.12 Meningeal adhesions (cerebral) (spinal)

G96.19 Other disorders of meninges, not elsewhere classified

G96.8 Other specified disorders of central nervous system

G96.9 Disorder of central nervous system, unspecified

✓4th **G97 Intraoperative and postprocedural complications and disorders of nervous system, not elsewhere classified**
EXCLUDES 2 *intraoperative and postprocedural cerebrovascular infarction (I97.81-, I97.82-)*

G97.0 Cerebrospinal fluid leak from spinal puncture

G97.1 Other reaction to spinal and lumbar puncture
Headache due to lumbar puncture

G97.2 Intracranial hypotension following ventricular shunting

✓5th **G97.3 Intraoperative hemorrhage and hematoma of a nervous system organ or structure complicating a procedure**
EXCLUDES 1 *intraoperative hemorrhage and hematoma of a nervous system organ or structure due to accidental puncture and laceration during a procedure (G97.4-)*

G97.31 Intraoperative hemorrhage and hematoma of a nervous system organ or structure complicating a nervous system procedure

G97.32 Intraoperative hemorrhage and hematoma of a nervous system organ or structure complicating other procedure

✓5th **G97.4 Accidental puncture and laceration of a nervous system organ or structure during a procedure**

G97.41 Accidental puncture or laceration of dura during a procedure
Incidental (inadvertent) durotomy

G97.48 Accidental puncture and laceration of other nervous system organ or structure during a nervous system procedure

G97.49 Accidental puncture and laceration of other nervous system organ or structure during other procedure

✓5th **G97.5 Postprocedural hemorrhage and hematoma of a nervous system organ or structure following a procedure**

G97.51 Postprocedural hemorrhage and hematoma of a nervous system organ or structure following a nervous system procedure

G97.52 Postprocedural hemorrhage and hematoma of a nervous system organ or structure following other procedure

✓5th **G97.8 Other intraoperative and postprocedural complications and disorders of nervous system**
Use additional code to further specify disorder

G97.81 Other intraoperative complications of nervous system

G97.82 Other postprocedural complications and disorders of nervous system

✓4th G98 Other disorders of nervous system not elsewhere classified

INCLUDES nervous system disorder NOS

G98.0 Neurogenic arthritis, not elsewhere classified

Nonsyphilitic neurogenic arthropathy NEC

Nonsyphilitic neurogenic spondylopathy NEC

EXCLUDES 1 *spondylopathy (in):*

syringomyelia and syringobulbia (G95.0)

tabes dorsalis (A52.11)

G98.8 Other disorders of nervous system

Nervous system disorder NOS

✓4th G99 Other disorders of nervous system in diseases classified elsewhere

G99.0 Autonomic neuropathy in diseases classified elsewhere

Code first underlying disease, such as:

amyloidosis (E85.-)

gout (M1A.-, M10.-)

hyperthyroidism (E05.-)

EXCLUDES 1 *diabetic autonomic neuropathy (E09-14 with .43)*

G99.2 Myelopathy in diseases classified elsewhere

Code first underlying disease, such as:

neoplasm (C00-D49)

EXCLUDES 1 *myelopathy in:*

intervertebral disease (M50.0-, M51.0-)

spondylosis (M47.0-, M47.1-)

G99.8 Other specified disorders of nervous system in diseases classified elsewhere

Code first underlying disorder, such as:

amyloidosis (E85.-)

avitaminosis (E56.9)

EXCLUDES 1 *nervous system involvement in:*

cysticercosis (B69.0)

rubella (B06.0-)

syphilis (A52.1-)

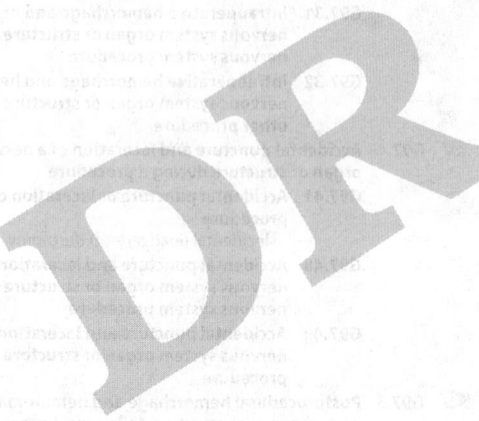

Chapter 7. Diseases of the Eye and Adnexa (H00-H59)

NOTE Use an external cause code following the code for the eye condition, if applicable, to identify the cause of the eye condition

EXCLUDES 2 *certain conditions originating in the perinatal period (P04-P96)*
certain infectious and parasitic diseases (A00-B99)
complications of pregnancy, childbirth and the puerperium (O00-O9A)
congenital malformations, deformations, and chromosomal abnormalities (Q00-Q99)
diabetes mellitus related eye conditions (E09.3-, E10.3-, E11.3-, E13.3-)
endocrine, nutritional and metabolic diseases (E00-E88)
injury (trauma) of eye and orbit (S05.-)
injury, poisoning and certain other consequences of external causes (S00-T88)
neoplasms (C00-D49)
symptoms, signs and abnormal clinical and laboratory findings, not elsewhere classified (R00-R94)
syphilis related eye disorders (A50.01, A50.3-, A51.43, A52.71)

This chapter contains the following blocks:

H00-H05	Disorders of eyelid, lacrimal system and orbit
H10-H11	Disorders of conjunctiva
H15-H22	Disorders of sclera, cornea, iris and ciliary body
H25-H28	Disorders of lens
H30-H36	Disorders of choroid and retina
H40-H42	Glaucoma
H43-H44	Disorders of vitreous body and globe
H46-H47	Disorders of optic nerve and visual pathways
H49-H52	Disorders of ocular muscles, binocular movement, accommodation and refraction
H53-H54	Visual disturbances and blindness
H55-H57	Other disorders of eye and adnexa
H59	Intraoperative and postprocedural complications and disorders of eye and adnexa, not elsewhere classified

Disorders of eyelid, lacrimal system and orbit (H00-H05)

EXCLUDES 2 *open wound of eyelid (S01.1-)*
superficial injury of eyelid (S00.1-, S00.2-)

✓4th **H00 Hordeolum and chalazion**

✓5th **H00.0 Hordeolum (externum) (internum) of eyelid**

✓6th **H00.01 Hordeolum externum**
Hordeolum NOS
Stye

H00.011 Hordeolum externum right upper eyelid
H00.012 Hordeolum externum right lower eyelid
H00.013 Hordeolum externum right eye, unspecified eyelid
H00.014 Hordeolum externum left upper eyelid
H00.015 Hordeolum externum left lower eyelid
H00.016 Hordeolum externum left eye, unspecified eyelid
H00.019 Hordeolum externum unspecified eye, unspecified eyelid

✓6th **H00.02 Hordeolum internum**
Infection of meibomian gland

H00.021 Hordeolum internum right upper eyelid
H00.022 Hordeolum internum right lower eyelid
H00.023 Hordeolum internum right eye, unspecified eyelid
H00.024 Hordeolum internum left upper eyelid
H00.025 Hordeolum internum left lower eyelid
H00.026 Hordeolum internum left eye, unspecified eyelid
H00.029 Hordeolum internum unspecified eye, unspecified eyelid

✓6th **H00.03 Abscess of eyelid**
Furuncle of eyelid

H00.031 Abscess of right upper eyelid
H00.032 Abscess of right lower eyelid
H00.033 Abscess of eyelid right eye, unspecified eyelid
H00.034 Abscess of left upper eyelid
H00.035 Abscess of left lower eyelid
H00.036 Abscess of eyelid left eye, unspecified eyelid
H00.039 Abscess of eyelid unspecified eye, unspecified eyelid

✓5th **H00.1 Chalazion**
Meibomian (gland) cyst
EXCLUDES 2 *infected meibomian gland (H00.02-)*

H00.11 Chalazion right upper eyelid
H00.12 Chalazion right lower eyelid
H00.13 Chalazion right eye, unspecified eyelid
H00.14 Chalazion left upper eyelid
H00.15 Chalazion left lower eyelid
H00.16 Chalazion left eye, unspecified eyelid
H00.19 Chalazion unspecified eye, unspecified eyelid

✓4th **H01 Other inflammation of eyelid**

✓5th **H01.0 Blepharitis**
EXCLUDES 1 *blepharoconjunctivitis (H10.5-)*

✓6th **H01.00 Unspecified blepharitis**

H01.001 Unspecified blepharitis right upper eyelid
H01.002 Unspecified blepharitis right lower eyelid
H01.003 Unspecified blepharitis right eye, unspecified eyelid
H01.004 Unspecified blepharitis left upper eyelid
H01.005 Unspecified blepharitis left lower eyelid
H01.006 Unspecified blepharitis left eye, unspecified eyelid
H01.009 Unspecified blepharitis unspecified eye, unspecified eyelid

✓6th **H01.01 Ulcerative blepharitis**

H01.011 Ulcerative blepharitis right upper eyelid
H01.012 Ulcerative blepharitis right lower eyelid
H01.013 Ulcerative blepharitis right eye, unspecified eyelid
H01.014 Ulcerative blepharitis left upper eyelid
H01.015 Ulcerative blepharitis left lower eyelid
H01.016 Ulcerative blepharitis left eye, unspecified eyelid
H01.019 Ulcerative blepharitis unspecified eye, unspecified eyelid

✓6th **H01.02 Squamous blepharitis**

H01.021 Squamous blepharitis right upper eyelid
H01.022 Squamous blepharitis right lower eyelid
H01.023 Squamous blepharitis right eye, unspecified eyelid
H01.024 Squamous blepharitis left upper eyelid
H01.025 Squamous blepharitis left lower eyelid
H01.026 Squamous blepharitis left eye, unspecified eyelid
H01.029 Squamous blepharitis unspecified eye, unspecified eyelid

✓5th **H01.1 Noninfectious dermatoses of eyelid**

✓6th **H01.11 Allergic dermatitis of eyelid**
Contact dermatitis of eyelid

H01.111 Allergic dermatitis of right upper eyelid
H01.112 Allergic dermatitis of right lower eyelid
H01.113 Allergic dermatitis of right eye, unspecified eyelid
H01.114 Allergic dermatitis of left upper eyelid
H01.115 Allergic dermatitis of left lower eyelid
H01.116 Allergic dermatitis of left eye, unspecified eyelid
H01.119 Allergic dermatitis of unspecified eye, unspecified eyelid

✓6th **H01.12 Discoid lupus erythematosus of eyelid**

H01.121 Discoid lupus erythematosus of right upper eyelid
H01.122 Discoid lupus erythematosus of right lower eyelid
H01.123 Discoid lupus erythematosus of right eye, unspecified eyelid
H01.124 Discoid lupus erythematosus of left upper eyelid
H01.125 Discoid lupus erythematosus of left lower eyelid
H01.126 Discoid lupus erythematosus of left eye, unspecified eyelid
H01.129 Discoid lupus erythematosus of unspecified eye, unspecified eyelid

✓6th **HØ1.13 Eczematous dermatitis of eyelid**
- **HØ1.131 Eczematous dermatitis of right upper eyelid**
- **HØ1.132 Eczematous dermatitis of right lower eyelid**
- **HØ1.133 Eczematous dermatitis of right eye, unspecified eyelid**
- **HØ1.134 Eczematous dermatitis of left upper eyelid**
- **HØ1.135 Eczematous dermatitis of left lower eyelid**
- **HØ1.136 Eczematous dermatitis of left eye, unspecified eyelid**
- **HØ1.139 Eczematous dermatitis of unspecified eye, unspecified eyelid**

✓6th **HØ1.14 Xeroderma of eyelid**
- **HØ1.141 Xeroderma of right upper eyelid**
- **HØ1.142 Xeroderma of right lower eyelid**
- **HØ1.143 Xeroderma of right eye, unspecified eyelid**
- **HØ1.144 Xeroderma of left upper eyelid**
- **HØ1.145 Xeroderma of left lower eyelid**
- **HØ1.146 Xeroderma of left eye, unspecified eyelid**
- **HØ1.149 Xeroderma of unspecified eye, unspecified eyelid**

HØ1.8 Other specified inflammations of eyelid

HØ1.9 Unspecified inflammation of eyelid
Inflammation of eyelid NOS

✓4th **HØ2 Other disorders of eyelid**
EXCLUDES 1 *congenital malformations of eyelid (Q1Ø.Ø-Q1Ø.3)*

✓5th **HØ2.Ø Entropion and trichiasis of eyelid**

✓6th **HØ2.ØØ Unspecified entropion of eyelid**
- **HØ2.ØØ1 Unspecified entropion of right upper eyelid**
- **HØ2.ØØ2 Unspecified entropion of right lower eyelid**
- **HØ2.ØØ3 Unspecified entropion of right eye, unspecified eyelid**
- **HØ2.ØØ4 Unspecified entropion of left upper eyelid**
- **HØ2.ØØ5 Unspecified entropion of left lower eyelid**
- **HØ2.ØØ6 Unspecified entropion of left eye, unspecified eyelid**
- **HØ2.ØØ9 Unspecified entropion of unspecified eye, unspecified eyelid**

✓6th **HØ2.Ø1 Cicatricial entropion of eyelid**
- **HØ2.Ø11 Cicatricial entropion of right upper eyelid**
- **HØ2.Ø12 Cicatricial entropion of right lower eyelid**
- **HØ2.Ø13 Cicatricial entropion of right eye, unspecified eyelid**
- **HØ2.Ø14 Cicatricial entropion of left upper eyelid**
- **HØ2.Ø15 Cicatricial entropion of left lower eyelid**
- **HØ2.Ø16 Cicatricial entropion of left eye, unspecified eyelid**
- **HØ2.Ø19 Cicatricial entropion of unspecified eye, unspecified eyelid**

✓6th **HØ2.Ø2 Mechanical entropion of eyelid**
- **HØ2.Ø21 Mechanical entropion of right upper eyelid**
- **HØ2.Ø22 Mechanical entropion of right lower eyelid**
- **HØ2.Ø23 Mechanical entropion of right eye, unspecified eyelid**
- **HØ2.Ø24 Mechanical entropion of left upper eyelid**
- **HØ2.Ø25 Mechanical entropion of left lower eyelid**
- **HØ2.Ø26 Mechanical entropion of left eye, unspecified eyelid**
- **HØ2.Ø29 Mechanical entropion of unspecified eye, unspecified eyelid**

✓6th **HØ2.Ø3 Senile entropion of eyelid**
- **HØ2.Ø31 Senile entropion of right upper eyelid**
- **HØ2.Ø32 Senile entropion of right lower eyelid**
- **HØ2.Ø33 Senile entropion of right eye, unspecified eyelid**
- **HØ2.Ø34 Senile entropion of left upper eyelid**
- **HØ2.Ø35 Senile entropion of left lower eyelid**
- **HØ2.Ø36 Senile entropion of left eye, unspecified eyelid**
- **HØ2.Ø39 Senile entropion of unspecified eye, unspecified eyelid**

✓6th **HØ2.Ø4 Spastic entropion of eyelid**
- **HØ2.Ø41 Spastic entropion of right upper eyelid**
- **HØ2.Ø42 Spastic entropion of right lower eyelid**
- **HØ2.Ø43 Spastic entropion of right eye, unspecified eyelid**
- **HØ2.Ø44 Spastic entropion of left upper eyelid**
- **HØ2.Ø45 Spastic entropion of left lower eyelid**
- **HØ2.Ø46 Spastic entropion of left eye, unspecified eyelid**
- **HØ2.Ø49 Spastic entropion of unspecified eye, unspecified eyelid**

✓6th **HØ2.Ø5 Trichiasis without entropian**
- **HØ2.Ø51 Trichiasis without entropian right upper eyelid**
- **HØ2.Ø52 Trichiasis without entropian right lower eyelid**
- **HØ2.Ø53 Trichiasis without entropian right eye, unspecified eyelid**
- **HØ2.Ø54 Trichiasis without entropian left upper eyelid**
- **HØ2.Ø55 Trichiasis without entropian left lower eyelid**
- **HØ2.Ø56 Trichiasis without entropian left eye, unspecified eyelid**
- **HØ2.Ø59 Trichiasis without entropian unspecified eye, unspecified eyelid**

✓5th **HØ2.1 Ectropion of eyelid**

✓6th **HØ2.1Ø Unspecified ectropion of eyelid**
- **HØ2.1Ø1 Unspecified ectropion of right upper eyelid**
- **HØ2.1Ø2 Unspecified ectropion of right lower eyelid**
- **HØ2.1Ø3 Unspecified ectropion of right eye, unspecified eyelid**
- **HØ2.1Ø4 Unspecified ectropion of left upper eyelid**
- **HØ2.1Ø5 Unspecified ectropion of left lower eyelid**
- **HØ2.1Ø6 Unspecified ectropion of left eye, unspecified eyelid**
- **HØ2.1Ø9 Unspecified ectropion of unspecified eye, unspecified eyelid**

✓6th **HØ2.11 Cicatricial ectropion of eyelid**
- **HØ2.111 Cicatricial ectropion of right upper eyelid**
- **HØ2.112 Cicatricial ectropion of right lower eyelid**
- **HØ2.113 Cicatricial ectropion of right eye, unspecified eyelid**
- **HØ2.114 Cicatricial ectropion of left upper eyelid**
- **HØ2.115 Cicatricial ectropion of left lower eyelid**
- **HØ2.116 Cicatricial ectropion of left eye, unspecified eyelid**
- **HØ2.119 Cicatricial ectropion of unspecified eye, unspecified eyelid**

✓6th **HØ2.12 Mechanical ectropion of eyelid**
- **HØ2.121 Mechanical ectropion of right upper eyelid**
- **HØ2.122 Mechanical ectropion of right lower eyelid**
- **HØ2.123 Mechanical ectropion of right eye, unspecified eyelid**
- **HØ2.124 Mechanical ectropion of left upper eyelid**
- **HØ2.125 Mechanical ectropion of left lower eyelid**
- **HØ2.126 Mechanical ectropion of left eye, unspecified eyelid**

H02.129 **Mechanical ectropion of unspecified eye, unspecified eyelid**

✓6th **H02.13 Senile ectropion of eyelid**

H02.131 **Senile ectropion of right upper eyelid**
H02.132 **Senile ectropion of right lower eyelid**
H02.133 **Senile ectropion of right eye, unspecified eyelid**
H02.134 **Senile ectropion of left upper eyelid**
H02.135 **Senile ectropion of left lower eyelid**
H02.136 **Senile ectropion of left eye, unspecified eyelid**
H02.139 **Senile ectropion of unspecified eye, unspecified eyelid**

✓6th **H02.14 Spastic ectropion of eyelid**

H02.141 **Spastic ectropion of right upper eyelid**
H02.142 **Spastic ectropion of right lower eyelid**
H02.143 **Spastic ectropion of right eye, unspecified eyelid**
H02.144 **Spastic ectropion of left upper eyelid**
H02.145 **Spastic ectropion of left lower eyelid**
H02.146 **Spastic ectropion of left eye, unspecified eyelid**
H02.149 **Spastic ectropion of unspecified eye, unspecified eyelid**

✓5th **H02.2 Lagophthalmos**

✓6th **H02.20 Unspecified lagophthalmos**

H02.201 **Unspecified lagophthalmos right upper eyelid**
H02.202 **Unspecified lagophthalmos right lower eyelid**
H02.203 **Unspecified lagophthalmos right eye, unspecified eyelid**
H02.204 **Unspecified lagophthalmos left upper eyelid**
H02.205 **Unspecified lagophthalmos left lower eyelid**
H02.206 **Unspecified lagophthalmos left eye, unspecified eyelid**
H02.209 **Unspecified lagophthalmos unspecified eye, unspecified eyelid**

✓6th **H02.21 Cicatricial lagophthalmos**

H02.211 **Cicatricial lagophthalmos right upper eyelid**
H02.212 **Cicatricial lagophthalmos right lower eyelid**
H02.213 **Cicatricial lagophthalmos right eye, unspecified eyelid**
H02.214 **Cicatricial lagophthalmos left upper eyelid**
H02.215 **Cicatricial lagophthalmos left lower eyelid**
H02.216 **Cicatricial lagophthalmos left eye, unspecified eyelid**
H02.219 **Cicatricial lagophthalmos unspecified eye, unspecified eyelid**

✓6th **H02.22 Mechanical lagophthalmos**

H02.221 **Mechanical lagophthalmos right upper eyelid**
H02.222 **Mechanical lagophthalmos right lower eyelid**
H02.223 **Mechanical lagophthalmos right eye, unspecified eyelid**
H02.224 **Mechanical lagophthalmos left upper eyelid**
H02.225 **Mechanical lagophthalmos left lower eyelid**
H02.226 **Mechanical lagophthalmos left eye, unspecified eyelid**
H02.229 **Mechanical lagophthalmos unspecified eye, unspecified eyelid**

✓6th **H02.23 Paralytic lagophthalmos**

H02.231 **Paralytic lagophthalmos right upper eyelid**
H02.232 **Paralytic lagophthalmos right lower eyelid**
H02.233 **Paralytic lagophthalmos right eye, unspecified eyelid**
H02.234 **Paralytic lagophthalmos left upper eyelid**
H02.235 **Paralytic lagophthalmos left lower eyelid**
H02.236 **Paralytic lagophthalmos left eye, unspecified eyelid**
H02.239 **Paralytic lagophthalmos unspecified eye, unspecified eyelid**

✓5th **H02.3 Blepharochalasis**

Pseudoptosis

H02.30 **Blepharochalasis unspecified eye, unspecified eyelid**
H02.31 **Blepharochalasis right upper eyelid**
H02.32 **Blepharochalasis right lower eyelid**
H02.33 **Blepharochalasis right eye, unspecified eyelid**
H02.34 **Blepharochalasis left upper eyelid**
H02.35 **Blepharochalasis left lower eyelid**
H02.36 **Blepharochalasis left eye, unspecified eyelid**

✓5th **H02.4 Ptosis of eyelid**

✓6th **H02.40 Unspecified ptosis of eyelid**

H02.401 **Unspecified ptosis of right eyelid**
H02.402 **Unspecified ptosis of left eyelid**
H02.403 **Unspecified ptosis of bilateral eyelids**
H02.409 **Unspecified ptosis of unspecified eyelid**

✓6th **H02.41 Mechanical ptosis of eyelid**

H02.411 **Mechanical ptosis of right eyelid**
H02.412 **Mechanical ptosis of left eyelid**
H02.413 **Mechanical ptosis of bilateral eyelids**
H02.419 **Mechanical ptosis of unspecified eyelid**

✓6th **H02.42 Myogenic ptosis of eyelid**

H02.421 **Myogenic ptosis of right eyelid**
H02.422 **Myogenic ptosis of left eyelid**
H02.423 **Myogenic ptosis of bilateral eyelids**
H02.429 **Myogenic ptosis of unspecified eyelid**

✓6th **H02.43 Paralytic ptosis of eyelid**

Neurogenic ptosis of eyelid

H02.431 **Paralytic ptosis of right eyelid**
H02.432 **Paralytic ptosis of left eyelid**
H02.433 **Paralytic ptosis of bilateral eyelids**
H02.439 **Paralytic ptosis unspecified eyelid**

✓5th **H02.5 Other disorders affecting eyelid function**

EXCLUDES 2 *blepharospasm (G24.5)*
organic tic (G25.69)
psychogenic tic (F95.-)

✓6th **H02.51 Abnormal innervation syndrome**

H02.511 **Abnormal innervation syndrome right upper eyelid**
H02.512 **Abnormal innervation syndrome right lower eyelid**
H02.513 **Abnormal innervation syndrome right eye, unspecified eyelid**
H02.514 **Abnormal innervation syndrome left upper eyelid**
H02.515 **Abnormal innervation syndrome left lower eyelid**
H02.516 **Abnormal innervation syndrome left eye, unspecified eyelid**
H02.519 **Abnormal innervation syndrome unspecified eye, unspecified eyelid**

✓6th **H02.52 Blepharophimosis**

Ankyloblepharon

H02.521 **Blepharophimosis right upper eyelid**
H02.522 **Blepharophimosis right lower eyelid**
H02.523 **Blepharophimosis right eye, unspecified eyelid**
H02.524 **Blepharophimosis left upper eyelid**
H02.525 **Blepharophimosis left lower eyelid**
H02.526 **Blepharophimosis left eye, unspecified eyelid**
H02.529 **Blepharophimosis unspecified eye, unspecified lid**

✓6th **H02.53 Eyelid retraction**

Eyelid lag

H02.531 **Eyelid retraction right upper eyelid**
H02.532 **Eyelid retraction right lower eyelid**

✓ Appropriate additional character required ✓x7th Requires 7th character, placeholder x must fill empty characters

H02.533 Eyelid retraction right eye, unspecified eyelid
H02.534 Eyelid retraction left upper eyelid
H02.535 Eyelid retraction left lower eyelid
H02.536 Eyelid retraction left eye, unspecified eyelid
H02.539 Eyelid retraction unspecified eye, unspecified lid

H02.59 Other disorders affecting eyelid function
Deficient blink reflex
Sensory disorders

✓5th H02.6 Xanthelasma of eyelid
H02.60 Xanthelasma of unspecified eye, unspecified eyelid
H02.61 Xanthelasma of right upper eyelid
H02.62 Xanthelasma of right lower eyelid
H02.63 Xanthelasma of right eye, unspecified eyelid
H02.64 Xanthelasma of left upper eyelid
H02.65 Xanthelasma of left lower eyelid
H02.66 Xanthelasma of left eye, unspecified eyelid

✓5th H02.7 Other and unspecified degenerative disorders of eyelid and periocular area
H02.70 Unspecified degenerative disorders of eyelid and periocular area
✓6th H02.71 Chloasma of eyelid and periocular area
Dyspigmentation of eyelid
Hyperpigmentation of eyelid
H02.711 Chloasma of right upper eyelid and periocular area
H02.712 Chloasma of right lower eyelid and periocular area
H02.713 Chloasma of right eye, unspecified eyelid and periocular area
H02.714 Chloasma of left upper eyelid and periocular area
H02.715 Chloasma of left lower eyelid and periocular area
H02.716 Chloasma of left eye, unspecified eyelid and periocular area
H02.719 Chloasma of unspecified eye, unspecified eyelid and periocular area
✓6th H02.72 Madarosis of eyelid and periocular area
Hypotrichosis of eyelid
H02.721 Madarosis of right upper eyelid and periocular area
H02.722 Madarosis of right lower eyelid and periocular area
H02.723 Madarosis of right eye, unspecified eyelid and periocular area
H02.724 Madarosis of left upper eyelid and periocular area
H02.725 Madarosis of left lower eyelid and periocular area
H02.726 Madarosis of left eye, unspecified eyelid and periocular area
H02.729 Madarosis of unspecified eye, unspecified eyelid and periocular area
✓6th H02.73 Vitiligo of eyelid and periocular area
Hypopigmentation of eyelid
H02.731 Vitiligo of right upper eyelid and periocular area
H02.732 Vitiligo of right lower eyelid and periocular area
H02.733 Vitiligo of right eye, unspecified eyelid and periocular area
H02.734 Vitiligo of left upper eyelid and periocular area
H02.735 Vitiligo of left lower eyelid and periocular area
H02.736 Vitiligo of left eye, unspecified eyelid and periocular area
H02.739 Vitiligo of unspecified eye, unspecified eyelid and periocular area
H02.79 Other degenerative disorders of eyelid and periocular area

✓5th H02.8 Other specified disorders of eyelid
✓6th H02.81 Retained foreign body in eyelid
Use additional code to identify the type of retained foreign body (Z18.-)
EXCLUDES 1 *laceration of eyelid with foreign body (S01.12-)*
retained intraocular foreign body (H44.6-, H44.7-)
superficial foreign body of eyelid and periocular area (S00.25-)
H02.811 Retained foreign body in right upper eyelid
H02.812 Retained foreign body in right lower eyelid
H02.813 Retained foreign body in right eye, unspecified eyelid
H02.814 Retained foreign body in left upper eyelid
H02.815 Retained foreign body in left lower eyelid
H02.816 Retained foreign body in left eye, unspecified eyelid
H02.819 Retained foreign body in unspecified eye, unspecified eyelid
✓6th H02.82 Cysts of eyelid
Sebaceous cyst of eyelid
H02.821 Cysts of right upper eyelid
H02.822 Cysts of right lower eyelid
H02.823 Cysts of right eye, unspecified eyelid
H02.824 Cysts of left upper eyelid
H02.825 Cysts of left lower eyelid
H02.826 Cysts of left eye, unspecified eyelid
H02.829 Cysts of unspecified eye, unspecified eyelid
✓6th H02.83 Dermatochalasis of eyelid
H02.831 Dermatochalasis of right upper eyelid
H02.832 Dermatochalasis of right lower eyelid
H02.833 Dermatochalasis of right eye, unspecified eyelid
H02.834 Dermatochalasis of left upper eyelid
H02.835 Dermatochalasis of left lower eyelid
H02.836 Dermatochalasis of left eye, unspecified eyelid
H02.839 Dermatochalasis of unspecified eye, unspecified eyelid
✓6th H02.84 Edema of eyelid
Hyperemia of eyelid
H02.841 Edema of right upper eyelid
H02.842 Edema of right lower eyelid
H02.843 Edema of right eye, unspecified eyelid
H02.844 Edema of left upper eyelid
H02.845 Edema of left lower eyelid
H02.846 Edema of left eye, unspecified eyelid
H02.849 Edema of unspecified eye, unspecified eyelid
✓6th H02.85 Elephantiasis of eyelid
H02.851 Elephantiasis of right upper eyelid
H02.852 Elephantiasis of right lower eyelid
H02.853 Elephantiasis of right eye, unspecified eyelid
H02.854 Elephantiasis of left upper eyelid
H02.855 Elephantiasis of left lower eyelid
H02.856 Elephantiasis of left eye, unspecified eyelid
H02.859 Elephantiasis of unspecified eye, unspecified eyelid
✓6th H02.86 Hypertrichosis of eyelid
H02.861 Hypertrichosis of right upper eyelid
H02.862 Hypertrichosis of right lower eyelid
H02.863 Hypertrichosis of right eye, unspecified eyelid
H02.864 Hypertrichosis of left upper eyelid
H02.865 Hypertrichosis of left lower eyelid
H02.866 Hypertrichosis of left eye, unspecified eyelid
H02.869 Hypertrichosis of unspecified eye, unspecified eyelid

H02.87 Vascular anomalies of eyelid
- **H02.871 Vascular anomalies of right upper eyelid**
- **H02.872 Vascular anomalies of right lower eyelid**
- **H02.873 Vascular anomalies of right eye, unspecified eyelid**
- **H02.874 Vascular anomalies of left upper eyelid**
- **H02.875 Vascular anomalies of left lower eyelid**
- **H02.876 Vascular anomalies of left eye, unspecified eyelid**
- **H02.879 Vascular anomalies of unspecified eye, unspecified eyelid**

H02.89 Other specified disorders of eyelid
Hemorrhage of eyelid

H02.9 Unspecified disorder of eyelid
Disorder of eyelid NOS

H04 Disorders of lacrimal system
EXCLUDES 1 *congenital malformations of lacrimal system (Q10.4-Q10.6)*

H04.0 Dacryoadenitis
H04.00 Unspecified dacryoadenitis
- **H04.001 Unspecified dacryoadenitis, right lacrimal gland**
- **H04.002 Unspecified dacryoadenitis, left lacrimal gland**
- **H04.003 Unspecified dacryoadenitis, bilateral lacrimal glands**
- **H04.009 Unspecified dacryoadenitis, unspecified lacrimal gland**

H04.01 Acute dacryoadenitis
- **H04.011 Acute dacryoadenitis, right lacrimal gland**
- **H04.012 Acute dacryoadenitis, left lacrimal gland**
- **H04.013 Acute dacryoadenitis, bilateral lacrimal glands**
- **H04.019 Acute dacryoadenitis, unspecified lacrimal gland**

H04.02 Chronic dacryoadenitis
- **H04.021 Chronic dacryoadenitis, right lacrimal gland**
- **H04.022 Chronic dacryoadenitis, left lacrimal gland**
- **H04.023 Chronic dacryoadenitis, bilateral lacrimal glands**
- **H04.029 Chronic dacryoadenitis, unspecified lacrimal gland**

H04.03 Chronic enlargement of lacrimal gland
- **H04.031 Chronic enlargement of right lacrimal gland**
- **H04.032 Chronic enlargement of left lacrimal gland**
- **H04.033 Chronic enlargement of bilateral lacrimal glands**
- **H04.039 Chronic enlargement of unspecified lacrimal gland**

H04.1 Other disorders of lacrimal gland
H04.11 Dacryops
- **H04.111 Dacryops of right lacrimal gland**
- **H04.112 Dacryops of left lacrimal gland**
- **H04.113 Dacryops of bilateral lacrimal glands**
- **H04.119 Dacryops of unspecified lacrimal gland**

H04.12 Dry eye syndrome
Tear film insufficiency, NOS
- **H04.121 Dry eye syndrome of right lacrimal gland**
- **H04.122 Dry eye syndrome of left lacrimal gland**
- **H04.123 Dry eye syndrome of bilateral lacrimal glands**
- **H04.129 Dry eye syndrome of unspecified lacrimal gland**

H04.13 Lacrimal cyst
Lacrimal cystic degeneration
- **H04.131 Lacrimal cyst, right lacrimal gland**
- **H04.132 Lacrimal cyst, left lacrimal gland**
- **H04.133 Lacrimal cyst, bilateral lacrimal glands**
- **H04.139 Lacrimal cyst, unspecified lacrimal gland**

H04.14 Primary lacrimal gland atrophy
- **H04.141 Primary lacrimal gland atrophy, right lacrimal gland**
- **H04.142 Primary lacrimal gland atrophy, left lacrimal gland**
- **H04.143 Primary lacrimal gland atrophy, bilateral lacrimal glands**
- **H04.149 Primary lacrimal gland atrophy, unspecified lacrimal gland**

H04.15 Secondary lacrimal gland atrophy
- **H04.151 Secondary lacrimal gland atrophy, right lacrimal gland**
- **H04.152 Secondary lacrimal gland atrophy, left lacrimal gland**
- **H04.153 Secondary lacrimal gland atrophy, bilateral lacrimal glands**
- **H04.159 Secondary lacrimal gland atrophy, unspecified lacrimal gland**

H04.16 Lacrimal gland dislocation
- **H04.161 Lacrimal gland dislocation, right lacrimal gland**
- **H04.162 Lacrimal gland dislocation, left lacrimal gland**
- **H04.163 Lacrimal gland dislocation, bilateral lacrimal glands**
- **H04.169 Lacrimal gland dislocation, unspecified lacrimal gland**

H04.19 Other specified disorders of lacrimal gland

H04.2 Epiphora
H04.20 Unspecified epiphora
- **H04.201 Unspecified epiphora, right lacrimal gland**
- **H04.202 Unspecified epiphora, left lacrimal gland**
- **H04.203 Unspecified epiphora, bilateral lacrimal glands**
- **H04.209 Unspecified epiphora, unspecified lacrimal gland**

H04.21 Epiphora due to excess lacrimation
- **H04.211 Epiphora due to excess lacrimation, right lacrimal gland**
- **H04.212 Epiphora due to excess lacrimation, left lacrimal gland**
- **H04.213 Epiphora due to excess lacrimation, bilateral lacrimal glands**
- **H04.219 Epiphora due to excess lacrimation, unspecified lacrimal gland**

H04.22 Epiphora due to insufficient drainage
- **H04.221 Epiphora due to insufficient drainage, right lacrimal gland**
- **H04.222 Epiphora due to insufficient drainage, left lacrimal gland**
- **H04.223 Epiphora due to insufficient drainage, bilateral lacrimal glands**
- **H04.229 Epiphora due to insufficient drainage, unspecified lacrimal gland**

H04.3 Acute and unspecified inflammation of lacrimal passages
EXCLUDES 1 *neonatal dacryocystitis (P39.1)*

H04.30 Unspecified dacryocystitis
- **H04.301 Unspecified dacryocystitis of right lacrimal passage**
- **H04.302 Unspecified dacryocystitis of left lacrimal passage**
- **H04.303 Unspecified dacryocystitis of bilateral lacrimal passages**
- **H04.309 Unspecified dacryocystitis of unspecified lacrimal passage**

H04.31 Phlegmonous dacryocystitis
- **H04.311 Phlegmonous dacryocystitis of right lacrimal passage**
- **H04.312 Phlegmonous dacryocystitis of left lacrimal passage**
- **H04.313 Phlegmonous dacryocystitis of bilateral lacrimal passages**
- **H04.319 Phlegmonous dacryocystitis of unspecified lacrimal passage**

6th H04.32 Acute dacryocystitis
Acute dacryopericystitis
H04.321 Acute dacryocystitis of right lacrimal passage
H04.322 Acute dacryocystitis of left lacrimal passage
H04.323 Acute dacryocystitis of bilateral lacrimal passages
H04.329 Acute dacryocystitis of unspecified lacrimal passage
6th H04.33 Acute lacrimal canaliculitis
H04.331 Acute lacrimal canaliculitis of right lacrimal passage
H04.332 Acute lacrimal canaliculitis of left lacrimal passage
H04.333 Acute lacrimal canaliculitis of bilateral lacrimal passages
H04.339 Acute lacrimal canaliculitis of unspecified lacrimal passage
5th H04.4 Chronic inflammation of lacrimal passages
6th H04.41 Chronic dacryocystitis
H04.411 Chronic dacryocystitis of right lacrimal passage
H04.412 Chronic dacryocystitis of left lacrimal passage
H04.413 Chronic dacryocystitis of bilateral lacrimal passages
H04.419 Chronic dacryocystitis of unspecified lacrimal passage
6th H04.42 Chronic lacrimal canaliculitis
H04.421 Chronic lacrimal canaliculitis of right lacrimal passage
H04.422 Chronic lacrimal canaliculitis of left lacrimal passage
H04.423 Chronic lacrimal canaliculitis of bilateral lacrimal passages
H04.429 Chronic lacrimal canaliculitis of unspecified lacrimal passage
6th H04.43 Chronic lacrimal mucocele
H04.431 Chronic lacrimal mucocele of right lacrimal passage
H04.432 Chronic lacrimal mucocele of left lacrimal passage
H04.433 Chronic lacrimal mucocele of bilateral lacrimal passages
H04.439 Chronic lacrimal mucocele of unspecified lacrimal passage
5th H04.5 Stenosis and insufficiency of lacrimal passages
6th H04.51 Dacryolith
H04.511 Dacryolith of right lacrimal passage
H04.512 Dacryolith of left lacrimal passage
H04.513 Dacryolith of bilateral lacrimal passages
H04.519 Dacryolith of unspecified lacrimal passage
6th H04.52 Eversion of lacrimal punctum
H04.521 Eversion of right lacrimal punctum
H04.522 Eversion of left lacrimal punctum
H04.523 Eversion of bilateral lacrimal punctum
H04.529 Eversion of unspecified lacrimal punctum
6th H04.53 Neonatal obstruction of nasolacrimal duct
EXCLUDES1 *congenital stenosis and stricture of lacrimal duct (Q10.5)*
H04.531 Neonatal obstruction of right nasolacrimal duct
H04.532 Neonatal obstruction of left nasolacrimal duct
H04.533 Neonatal obstruction of bilateral nasolacrimal duct
H04.539 Neonatal obstruction of unspecified nasolacrimal duct
6th H04.54 Stenosis of lacrimal canaliculi
H04.541 Stenosis of right lacrimal canaliculi
H04.542 Stenosis of left lacrimal canaliculi
H04.543 Stenosis of bilateral lacrimal canaliculi
H04.549 Stenosis of unspecified lacrimal canaliculi
6th H04.55 Acquired stenosis of nasolacrimal duct
H04.551 Acquired stenosis of right nasolacrimal duct
H04.552 Acquired stenosis of left nasolacrimal duct
H04.553 Acquired stenosis of bilateral nasolacrimal duct
H04.559 Acquired stenosis of unspecified nasolacrimal duct
6th H04.56 Stenosis of lacrimal punctum
H04.561 Stenosis of right lacrimal punctum
H04.562 Stenosis of left lacrimal punctum
H04.563 Stenosis of bilateral lacrimal punctum
H04.569 Stenosis of unspecified lacrimal punctum
6th H04.57 Stenosis of lacrimal sac
H04.571 Stenosis of right lacrimal sac
H04.572 Stenosis of left lacrimal sac
H04.573 Stenosis of bilateral lacrimal sac
H04.579 Stenosis of unspecified lacrimal sac
5th H04.6 Other changes of lacrimal passages
6th H04.61 Lacrimal fistula
H04.611 Lacrimal fistula right lacrimal passage
H04.612 Lacrimal fistula left lacrimal passage
H04.613 Lacrimal fistula bilateral lacrimal passages
H04.619 Lacrimal fistula unspecified lacrimal passage
H04.69 Other changes of lacrimal passages
5th H04.8 Other disorders of lacrimal system
6th H04.81 Granuloma of lacrimal passages
H04.811 Granuloma of right lacrimal passage
H04.812 Granuloma of left lacrimal passage
H04.813 Granuloma of bilateral lacrimal passages
H04.819 Granuloma of unspecified lacrimal passage
H04.89 Other disorders of lacrimal system
H04.9 Disorder of lacrimal system, unspecified
4th H05 Disorders of orbit
EXCLUDES1 *congenital malformation of orbit (Q10.7)*
5th H05.0 Acute inflammation of orbit
H05.00 Unspecified acute inflammation of orbit
6th H05.01 Cellulitis of orbit
Abscess of orbit
H05.011 Cellulitis of right orbit
H05.012 Cellulitis of left orbit
H05.013 Cellulitis of bilateral orbits
H05.019 Cellulitis of unspecified orbit
6th H05.02 Osteomyelitis of orbit
H05.021 Osteomyelitis of right orbit
H05.022 Osteomyelitis of left orbit
H05.023 Osteomyelitis of bilateral orbits
H05.029 Osteomyelitis of unspecified orbit
6th H05.03 Periostitis of orbit
H05.031 Periostitis of right orbit
H05.032 Periostitis of left orbit
H05.033 Periostitis of bilateral orbits
H05.039 Periostitis of unspecified orbit
6th H05.04 Tenonitis of orbit
H05.041 Tenonitis of right orbit
H05.042 Tenonitis of left orbit
H05.043 Tenonitis of bilateral orbits
H05.049 Tenonitis of unspecified orbit
5th H05.1 Chronic inflammatory disorders of orbit
H05.10 Unspecified chronic inflammatory disorders of orbit
6th H05.11 Granuloma of orbit
Pseudotumor (inflammatory) of orbit
H05.111 Granuloma of right orbit
H05.112 Granuloma of left orbit
H05.113 Granuloma of bilateral orbits
H05.119 Granuloma of unspecified orbit
6th H05.12 Orbital myositis
H05.121 Orbital myositis, right orbit

H05.122 Orbital myositis, left orbit
H05.123 Orbital myositis, bilateral
H05.129 Orbital myositis, unspecified orbit

✓5th H05.2 Exophthalmic conditions
H05.20 Unspecified exophthalmos
✓6th H05.21 Displacement (lateral) of globe
H05.211 Displacement (lateral) of globe, right eye
H05.212 Displacement (lateral) of globe, left eye
H05.213 Displacement (lateral) of globe, bilateral
H05.219 Displacement (lateral) of globe, unspecified eye
✓6th H05.22 Edema of orbit
Orbital congestion
H05.221 Edema of right orbit
H05.222 Edema of left orbit
H05.223 Edema of bilateral orbit
H05.229 Edema of unspecified orbit
✓6th H05.23 Hemorrhage of orbit
H05.231 Hemorrhage of right orbit
H05.232 Hemorrhage of left orbit
H05.233 Hemorrhage of bilateral orbit
H05.239 Hemorrhage of unspecified orbit
✓6th H05.24 Constant exophthalmos
H05.241 Constant exophthalmos, right eye
H05.242 Constant exophthalmos, left eye
H05.243 Constant exophthalmos, bilateral
H05.249 Constant exophthalmos, unspecified eye
✓6th H05.25 Intermittent exophthalmos
H05.251 Intermittent exophthalmos, right eye
H05.252 Intermittent exophthalmos, left eye
H05.253 Intermittent exophthalmos, bilateral
H05.259 Intermittent exophthalmos, unspecified eye
✓6th H05.26 Pulsating exophthalmos
H05.261 Pulsating exophthalmos, right eye
H05.262 Pulsating exophthalmos, left eye
H05.263 Pulsating exophthalmos, bilateral
H05.269 Pulsating exophthalmos, unspecified eye

✓5th H05.3 Deformity of orbit
EXCLUDES 1 *congenital deformity of orbit (Q10.7)*
hypertelorism (Q75.2)
H05.30 Unspecified deformity of orbit
✓6th H05.31 Atrophy of orbit
H05.311 Atrophy of right orbit
H05.312 Atrophy of left orbit
H05.313 Atrophy of bilateral orbit
H05.319 Atrophy of unspecified orbit
✓6th H05.32 Deformity of orbit due to bone disease
Code also associated bone disease
H05.321 Deformity of right orbit due to bone disease
H05.322 Deformity of left orbit due to bone disease
H05.323 Deformity of bilateral orbits due to bone disease
H05.329 Deformity of unspecified orbit due to bone disease
✓6th H05.33 Deformity of orbit due to trauma or surgery
H05.331 Deformity of right orbit due to trauma or surgery
H05.332 Deformity of left orbit due to trauma or surgery
H05.333 Deformity of bilateral orbits due to trauma or surgery
H05.339 Deformity of unspecified orbit due to trauma or surgery
✓6th H05.34 Enlargement of orbit
H05.341 Enlargement of right orbit
H05.342 Enlargement of left orbit
H05.343 Enlargement of bilateral orbits
H05.349 Enlargement of unspecified orbit
✓6th H05.35 Exostosis of orbit
H05.351 Exostosis of right orbit
H05.352 Exostosis of left orbit
H05.353 Exostosis of bilateral orbits
H05.359 Exostosis of unspecified orbit

✓5th H05.4 Enophthalmos
✓6th H05.40 Unspecified enophthalmos
H05.401 Unspecified enophthalmos, right eye
H05.402 Unspecified enophthalmos, left eye
H05.403 Unspecified enophthalmos, bilateral
H05.409 Unspecified enophthalmos, unspecified eye
✓6th H05.41 Enophthalmos due to atrophy of orbital tissue
H05.411 Enophthalmos due to atrophy of orbital tissue, right eye
H05.412 Enophthalmos due to atrophy of orbital tissue, left eye
H05.413 Enophthalmos due to atrophy of orbital tissue, bilateral
H05.419 Enophthalmos due to atrophy of orbital tissue, unspecified eye
✓6th H05.42 Enophthalmos due to trauma or surgery
H05.421 Enophthalmos due to trauma or surgery, right eye
H05.422 Enophthalmos due to trauma or surgery, left eye
H05.423 Enophthalmos due to trauma or surgery, bilateral
H05.429 Enophthalmos due to trauma or surgery, unspecified eye

✓5th H05.5 Retained (old) foreign body following penetrating wound of orbit
Use additional code to identify the type of retained foreign body (Z18.-)
Retrobulbar foreign body
EXCLUDES 1 *current penetrating wound of orbit (S05.4-)*
EXCLUDES 2 *retained foreign body of eyelid (H02.81-)*
retained intraocular foreign body (H44.6-, H44.7-)
H05.50 Retained (old) foreign body following penetrating wound of unspecified orbit
H05.51 Retained (old) foreign body following penetrating wound of right orbit
H05.52 Retained (old) foreign body following penetrating wound of left orbit
H05.53 Retained (old) foreign body following penetrating wound of bilateral orbits

✓5th H05.8 Other disorders of orbit
✓6th H05.81 Cyst of orbit
Encephalocele of orbit
H05.811 Cyst of right orbit
H05.812 Cyst of left orbit
H05.813 Cyst of bilateral orbits
H05.819 Cyst of unspecified orbit
✓6th H05.82 Myopathy of extraocular muscles
H05.821 Myopathy of extraocular muscles, right orbit
H05.822 Myopathy of extraocular muscles, left orbit
H05.823 Myopathy of extraocular muscles, bilateral
H05.829 Myopathy of extraocular muscles, unspecified orbit
H05.89 Other disorders of orbit
H05.9 Unspecified disorder of orbit

Disorders of conjunctiva (H10-H11)

✓4th **H10 Conjunctivitis**
EXCLUDES 1 *keratoconjunctivitis (H16.2-)*
✓5th H10.0 Mucopurulent conjunctivitis
✓6th H10.01 Acute follicular conjunctivitis
H10.011 Acute follicular conjunctivitis, right eye
H10.012 Acute follicular conjunctivitis, left eye
H10.013 Acute follicular conjunctivitis, bilateral
H10.019 Acute follicular conjunctivitis, unspecified eye
✓6th H10.02 Other mucopurulent conjunctivitis
H10.021 Other mucopurulent conjunctivitis, right eye

H10.022 Other mucopurulent conjunctivitis, left eye
H10.023 Other mucopurulent conjunctivitis, bilateral
H10.029 Other mucopurulent conjunctivitis, unspecified eye

✓5th **H10.1 Acute atopic conjunctivitis**
Acute papillary conjunctivitis
H10.10 Acute atopic conjunctivitis, unspecified eye
H10.11 Acute atopic conjunctivitis, right eye
H10.12 Acute atopic conjunctivitis, left eye
H10.13 Acute atopic conjunctivitis, bilateral

✓5th **H10.2 Other acute conjunctivitis**
✓6th **H10.21 Acute toxic conjunctivitis**
Acute chemical conjunctivitis
Code first (T51-T65) to identify chemical and intent
EXCLUDES 1 *burn and corrosion of eye and adnexa (T26.-)*
H10.211 Acute toxic conjunctivitis, right eye
H10.212 Acute toxic conjunctivitis, left eye
H10.213 Acute toxic conjunctivitis, bilateral
H10.219 Acute toxic conjunctivitis, unspecified eye

✓6th **H10.22 Pseudomembranous conjunctivitis**
H10.221 Pseudomembranous conjunctivitis, right eye
H10.222 Pseudomembranous conjunctivitis, left eye
H10.223 Pseudomembranous conjunctivitis, bilateral
H10.229 Pseudomembranous conjunctivitis, unspecified eye

✓6th **H10.23 Serous conjunctivitis, except viral**
EXCLUDES 1 *viral conjunctivitis (B30.-)*
H10.231 Serous conjunctivitis, except viral, right eye
H10.232 Serous conjunctivitis, except viral, left eye
H10.233 Serous conjunctivitis, except viral, bilateral
H10.239 Serous conjunctivitis, except viral, unspecified eye

✓5th **H10.3 Unspecified acute conjunctivitis**
EXCLUDES 1 *ophthalmia neonatorum NOS (P39.1)*
H10.30 Unspecified acute conjunctivitis, unspecified eye
H10.31 Unspecified acute conjunctivitis, right eye
H10.32 Unspecified acute conjunctivitis, left eye
H10.33 Unspecified acute conjunctivitis, bilateral

✓5th **H10.4 Chronic conjunctivitis**
✓6th **H10.40 Unspecified chronic conjunctivitis**
H10.401 Unspecified chronic conjunctivitis, right eye
H10.402 Unspecified chronic conjunctivitis, left eye
H10.403 Unspecified chronic conjunctivitis, bilateral
H10.409 Unspecified chronic conjunctivitis, unspecified eye

✓6th **H10.41 Chronic giant papillary conjunctivitis**
H10.411 Chronic giant papillary conjunctivitis, right eye
H10.412 Chronic giant papillary conjunctivitis, left eye
H10.413 Chronic giant papillary conjunctivitis, bilateral
H10.419 Chronic giant papillary conjunctivitis, unspecified eye

✓6th **H10.42 Simple chronic conjunctivitis**
H10.421 Simple chronic conjunctivitis, right eye
H10.422 Simple chronic conjunctivitis, left eye
H10.423 Simple chronic conjunctivitis, bilateral
H10.429 Simple chronic conjunctivitis, unspecified eye

✓6th **H10.43 Chronic follicular conjunctivitis**
H10.431 Chronic follicular conjunctivitis, right eye
H10.432 Chronic follicular conjunctivitis, left eye
H10.433 Chronic follicular conjunctivitis, bilateral
H10.439 Chronic follicular conjunctivitis, unspecified eye

H10.44 Vernal conjunctivitis
EXCLUDES 1 *vernal keratoconjunctivitis with limbar and corneal involvement (H16.26-)*

H10.45 Other chronic allergic conjunctivitis

✓5th **H10.5 Blepharoconjunctivitis**
✓6th **H10.50 Unspecified blepharoconjunctivitis**
H10.501 Unspecified blepharoconjunctivitis, right eye
H10.502 Unspecified blepharoconjunctivitis, left eye
H10.503 Unspecified blepharoconjunctivitis, bilateral
H10.509 Unspecified blepharoconjunctivitis, unspecified eye

✓6th **H10.51 Ligneous conjunctivitis**
H10.511 Ligneous conjunctivitis, right eye
H10.512 Ligneous conjunctivitis, left eye
H10.513 Ligneous conjunctivitis, bilateral
H10.519 Ligneous conjunctivitis, unspecified eye

✓6th **H10.52 Angular blepharoconjunctivitis**
H10.521 Angular blepharoconjunctivitis, right eye
H10.522 Angular blepharoconjunctivitis, left eye
H10.523 Angular blepharoconjunctivitis, bilateral
H10.529 Angular blepharoconjunctivitis, unspecified eye

✓6th **H10.53 Contact blepharoconjunctivitis**
H10.531 Contact blepharoconjunctivitis, right eye
H10.532 Contact blepharoconjunctivitis, left eye
H10.533 Contact blepharoconjunctivitis, bilateral
H10.539 Contact blepharoconjunctivitis, unspecified eye

✓5th **H10.8 Other conjunctivitis**
✓6th **H10.81 Pingueculitis**
EXCLUDES 1 *pinguecula (H11.15-)*
H10.811 Pingueculitis, right eye
H10.812 Pingueculitis, left eye
H10.813 Pingueculitis, bilateral
H10.819 Pingueculitis, unspecified eye

H10.89 Other conjunctivitis

H10.9 Unspecified conjunctivitis

✓4th H11 Other disorders of conjunctiva
EXCLUDES 1 *keratoconjunctivitis (H16.2-)*

✓5th **H11.0 Pterygium of eye**
EXCLUDES 1 *pseudopterygium (H11.81-)*
✓6th **H11.00 Unspecified pterygium of eye**
H11.001 Unspecified pterygium of right eye
H11.002 Unspecified pterygium of left eye
H11.003 Unspecified pterygium of eye, bilateral
H11.009 Unspecified pterygium of unspecified eye

✓6th **H11.01 Amyloid pterygium**
H11.011 Amyloid pterygium of right eye
H11.012 Amyloid pterygium of left eye
H11.013 Amyloid pterygium of eye, bilateral
H11.019 Amyloid pterygium of unspecified eye

✓6th **H11.02 Central pterygium of eye**
H11.021 Central pterygium of right eye
H11.022 Central pterygium of left eye
H11.023 Central pterygium of eye, bilateral
H11.029 Central pterygium of unspecified eye

✓6th **H11.03 Double pterygium of eye**
H11.031 Double pterygium of right eye
H11.032 Double pterygium of left eye
H11.033 Double pterygium of eye, bilateral
H11.039 Double pterygium of unspecified eye

H10.022–H11.039

✓6th **H11.04 Peripheral pterygium of eye, stationary**
H11.041 Peripheral pterygium, stationary, right eye
H11.042 Peripheral pterygium, stationary, left eye
H11.043 Peripheral pterygium, stationary, bilateral
H11.049 Peripheral pterygium, stationary, unspecified eye

✓6th **H11.05 Peripheral pterygium of eye, progressive**
H11.051 Peripheral pterygium, progressive, right eye
H11.052 Peripheral pterygium, progressive, left eye
H11.053 Peripheral pterygium, progressive, bilateral
H11.059 Peripheral pterygium, progressive, unspecified eye

✓6th **H11.06 Recurrent pterygium of eye**
H11.061 Recurrent pterygium of right eye
H11.062 Recurrent pterygium of left eye
H11.063 Recurrent pterygium of eye, bilateral
H11.069 Recurrent pterygium of unspecified eye

✓5th **H11.1 Conjunctival degenerations and deposits**
EXCLUDES 2 *pseudopterygium (H11.81)*
H11.10 Unspecified conjunctival degenerations

✓6th **H11.11 Conjunctival deposits**
H11.111 Conjunctival deposits, right eye
H11.112 Conjunctival deposits, left eye
H11.113 Conjunctival deposits, bilateral
H11.119 Conjunctival deposits, unspecified eye

✓6th **H11.12 Conjunctival concretions**
H11.121 Conjunctival concretions, right eye
H11.122 Conjunctival concretions, left eye
H11.123 Conjunctival concretions, bilateral
H11.129 Conjunctival concretions, unspecified eye

✓6th **H11.13 Conjunctival pigmentations**
Conjunctival argyrosis [argyria]
H11.131 Conjunctival pigmentations, right eye
H11.132 Conjunctival pigmentations, left eye
H11.133 Conjunctival pigmentations, bilateral
H11.139 Conjunctival pigmentations, unspecified eye

✓6th **H11.14 Conjunctival xerosis, unspecified**
EXCLUDES 1 *xerosis of conjunctiva due to vitamin A deficiency (E50.0, E50.1)*
H11.141 Conjunctival xerosis, unspecified, right eye
H11.142 Conjunctival xerosis , unspecified, left eye
H11.143 Conjunctival xerosis, unspecified, bilateral
H11.149 Conjunctival xerosis, unspecified, unspecified eye

✓6th **H11.15 Pinguecula**
EXCLUDES 1 *pingueculitis (H10.81-)*
H11.151 Pinguecula, right eye
H11.152 Pinguecula, left eye
H11.153 Pinguecula, bilateral
H11.159 Pinguecula, unspecified eye

✓5th **H11.2 Conjunctival scars**

✓6th **H11.21 Conjunctival adhesions and strands (localized)**
H11.211 Conjunctival adhesions and strands (localized), right eye
H11.212 Conjunctival adhesions and strands (localized), left eye
H11.213 Conjunctival adhesions and strands (localized), bilateral
H11.219 Conjunctival adhesions and strands (localized), unspecified eye

✓6th **H11.22 Conjunctival granuloma**
H11.221 Conjunctival granuloma, right eye
H11.222 Conjunctival granuloma, left eye
H11.223 Conjunctival granuloma, bilateral
H11.229 Conjunctival granuloma, unspecified

✓6th **H11.23 Symblepharon**
H11.231 Symblepharon, right eye
H11.232 Symblepharon, left eye
H11.233 Symblepharon, bilateral
H11.239 Symblepharon, unspecified eye

✓6th **H11.24 Scarring of conjunctiva**
H11.241 Scarring of conjunctiva, right eye
H11.242 Scarring of conjunctiva, left eye
H11.243 Scarring of conjunctiva, bilateral
H11.249 Scarring of conjunctiva, unspecified eye

✓5th **H11.3 Conjunctival hemorrhage**
Subconjunctival hemorrhage
H11.30 Conjunctival hemorrhage, unspecified eye
H11.31 Conjunctival hemorrhage, right eye
H11.32 Conjunctival hemorrhage, left eye
H11.33 Conjunctival hemorrhage, bilateral

✓5th **H11.4 Other conjunctival vascular disorders and cysts**

✓6th **H11.41 Vascular abnormalities of conjunctiva**
Conjunctival aneurysm
H11.411 Vascular abnormalities of conjunctiva, right eye
H11.412 Vascular abnormalities of conjunctiva, left eye
H11.413 Vascular abnormalities of conjunctiva, bilateral
H11.419 Vascular abnormalities of conjunctiva, unspecified eye

✓6th **H11.42 Conjunctival edema**
H11.421 Conjunctival edema, right eye
H11.422 Conjunctival edema, left eye
H11.423 Conjunctival edema, bilateral
H11.429 Conjunctival edema, unspecified eye

✓6th **H11.43 Conjunctival hyperemia**
H11.431 Conjunctival hyperemia, right eye
H11.432 Conjunctival hyperemia, left eye
H11.433 Conjunctival hyperemia, bilateral
H11.439 Conjunctival hyperemia, unspecified eye

✓6th **H11.44 Conjunctival cysts**
H11.441 Conjunctival cysts, right eye
H11.442 Conjunctival cysts, left eye
H11.443 Conjunctival cysts, bilateral
H11.449 Conjunctival cysts, unspecified eye

✓5th **H11.8 Other specified disorders of conjunctiva**

✓6th **H11.81 Pseudopterygium of conjunctiva**
H11.811 Pseudopterygium of conjunctiva, right eye
H11.812 Pseudopterygium of conjunctiva, left eye
H11.813 Pseudopterygium of conjunctiva, bilateral
H11.819 Pseudopterygium of conjunctiva, unspecified eye

✓6th **H11.82 Conjunctivochalasis**
H11.821 Conjunctivochalasis, right eye
H11.822 Conjunctivochalasis, left eye
H11.823 Conjunctivochalasis, bilateral
H11.829 Conjunctivochalasis, unspecified eye
H11.89 Other specified disorders of conjunctiva
H11.9 Unspecified disorder of conjunctiva

Disorders of sclera, cornea, iris and ciliary body (H15-H22)

✓4th **H15 Disorders of sclera**

✓5th **H15.0 Scleritis**

✓6th **H15.00 Unspecified scleritis**
H15.001 Unspecified scleritis, right eye
H15.002 Unspecified scleritis, left eye
H15.003 Unspecified scleritis, bilateral
H15.009 Unspecified scleritis, unspecified eye

✓6th **H15.01 Anterior scleritis**
H15.011 Anterior scleritis, right eye
H15.012 Anterior scleritis, left eye
H15.013 Anterior scleritis, bilateral
H15.019 Anterior scleritis, unspecified eye

√6th H15.02 Brawny scleritis
H15.021 Brawny scleritis, right eye
H15.022 Brawny scleritis, left eye
H15.023 Brawny scleritis, bilateral
H15.029 Brawny scleritis, unspecified eye
√6th H15.03 Posterior scleritis
Sclerotenonitis
H15.031 Posterior scleritis, right eye
H15.032 Posterior scleritis, left eye
H15.033 Posterior scleritis, bilateral
H15.039 Posterior scleritis, unspecified eye
√6th H15.04 Scleritis with corneal involvement
H15.041 Scleritis with corneal involvement, right eye
H15.042 Scleritis with corneal involvement, left eye
H15.043 Scleritis with corneal involvement, bilateral
H15.049 Scleritis with corneal involvement, unspecified eye
√6th H15.05 Scleromalacia perforans
H15.051 Scleromalacia perforans, right eye
H15.052 Scleromalacia perforans, left eye
H15.053 Scleromalacia perforans, bilateral
H15.059 Scleromalacia perforans, unspecified eye
√6th H15.09 Other scleritis
Scleral abscess
H15.091 Other scleritis, right eye
H15.092 Other scleritis, left eye
H15.093 Other scleritis, bilateral
H15.099 Other scleritis, unspecified eye
√5th H15.1 Episcleritis
√6th H15.10 Unspecified episcleritis
H15.101 Unspecified episcleritis, right eye
H15.102 Unspecified episcleritis, left eye
H15.103 Unspecified episcleritis, bilateral
H15.109 Unspecified episcleritis, unspecified eye
√6th H15.11 Episcleritis periodica fugax
H15.111 Episcleritis periodica fugax, right eye
H15.112 Episcleritis periodica fugax, left eye
H15.113 Episcleritis periodica fugax, bilateral
H15.119 Episcleritis periodica fugax, unspecified eye
√6th H15.12 Nodular episcleritis
H15.121 Nodular episcleritis, right eye
H15.122 Nodular episcleritis, left eye
H15.123 Nodular episcleritis, bilateral
H15.129 Nodular episcleritis, unspecified eye
√5th H15.8 Other disorders of sclera
EXCLUDES 2 *blue sclera (Q13.5)*
degenerative myopia (H44.2-)
√6th H15.81 Equatorial staphyloma
H15.811 Equatorial staphyloma, right eye
H15.812 Equatorial staphyloma, left eye
H15.813 Equatorial staphyloma, bilateral
H15.819 Equatorial staphyloma, unspecified eye
√6th H15.82 Localized anterior staphyloma
H15.821 Localized anterior staphyloma, right eye
H15.822 Localized anterior staphyloma, left eye
H15.823 Localized anterior staphyloma, bilateral
H15.829 Localized anterior staphyloma, unspecified eye
√6th H15.83 Staphyloma posticum
H15.831 Staphyloma posticum, right eye
H15.832 Staphyloma posticum, left eye
H15.833 Staphyloma posticum, bilateral
H15.839 Staphyloma posticum, unspecified eye
√6th H15.84 Scleral ectasia
H15.841 Scleral ectasia, right eye
H15.842 Scleral ectasia, left eye
H15.843 Scleral ectasia, bilateral
H15.849 Scleral ectasia, unspecified eye
√6th H15.85 Ring staphyloma
H15.851 Ring staphyloma, right eye
H15.852 Ring staphyloma, left eye
H15.853 Ring staphyloma, bilateral
H15.859 Ring staphyloma, unspecified eye
H15.89 Other disorders of sclera
H15.9 Unspecified disorder of sclera

√4th **H16 Keratitis**
√5th H16.0 Corneal ulcer
√6th H16.00 Unspecified corneal ulcer
H16.001 Unspecified corneal ulcer, right eye
H16.002 Unspecified corneal ulcer, left eye
H16.003 Unspecified corneal ulcer, bilateral
H16.009 Unspecified corneal ulcer, unspecified eye
√6th H16.01 Central corneal ulcer
H16.011 Central corneal ulcer, right eye
H16.012 Central corneal ulcer, left eye
H16.013 Central corneal ulcer, bilateral
H16.019 Central corneal ulcer, unspecified eye
√6th H16.02 Ring corneal ulcer
H16.021 Ring corneal ulcer, right eye
H16.022 Ring corneal ulcer, left eye
H16.023 Ring corneal ulcer, bilateral
H16.029 Ring corneal ulcer, unspecified eye
√6th H16.03 Corneal ulcer with hypopyon
H16.031 Corneal ulcer with hypopyon, right eye
H16.032 Corneal ulcer with hypopyon, left eye
H16.033 Corneal ulcer with hypopyon, bilateral
H16.039 Corneal ulcer with hypopyon, unspecified eye
√6th H16.04 Marginal corneal ulcer
H16.041 Marginal corneal ulcer, right eye
H16.042 Marginal corneal ulcer, left eye
H16.043 Marginal corneal ulcer, bilateral
H16.049 Marginal corneal ulcer, unspecified eye
√6th H16.05 Mooren's corneal ulcer
H16.051 Mooren's corneal ulcer, right eye
H16.052 Mooren's corneal ulcer, left eye
H16.053 Mooren's corneal ulcer, bilateral
H16.059 Mooren's corneal ulcer, unspecified eye
√6th H16.06 Mycotic corneal ulcer
H16.061 Mycotic corneal ulcer, right eye
H16.062 Mycotic corneal ulcer, left eye
H16.063 Mycotic corneal ulcer, bilateral
H16.069 Mycotic corneal ulcer, unspecified eye
√6th H16.07 Perforated corneal ulcer
H16.071 Perforated corneal ulcer, right eye
H16.072 Perforated corneal ulcer, left eye
H16.073 Perforated corneal ulcer, bilateral
H16.079 Perforated corneal ulcer, unspecified eye
√5th H16.1 Other and unspecified superficial keratitis without conjunctivitis
√6th H16.10 Unspecified superficial keratitis
H16.101 Unspecified superficial keratitis, right eye
H16.102 Unspecified superficial keratitis, left eye
H16.103 Unspecified superficial keratitis, bilateral
H16.109 Unspecified superficial keratitis, unspecified eye
√6th H16.11 Macular keratitis
Areolar keratitis
Nummular keratitis
Stellate keratitis
Striate keratitis
H16.111 Macular keratitis, right eye
H16.112 Macular keratitis, left eye
H16.113 Macular keratitis, bilateral
H16.119 Macular keratitis, unspecified eye
√6th H16.12 Filamentary keratitis
H16.121 Filamentary keratitis, right eye
H16.122 Filamentary keratitis, left eye
H16.123 Filamentary keratitis, bilateral
H16.129 Filamentary keratitis, unspecified eye

√6th H16.13 Photokeratitis
Snow blindness
Welders keratitis
H16.131 Photokeratitis, right eye
H16.132 Photokeratitis, left eye
H16.133 Photokeratitis, bilateral
H16.139 Photokeratitis, unspecified eye
√6th H16.14 Punctate keratitis
H16.141 Punctate keratitis, right eye
H16.142 Punctate keratitis, left eye
H16.143 Punctate keratitis, bilateral
H16.149 Punctate keratitis, unspecified eye
√5th H16.2 Keratoconjunctivitis
√6th H16.20 Unspecified keratoconjunctivitis
Superficial keratitis with conjunctivitis NOS
H16.201 Unspecified keratoconjunctivitis, right eye
H16.202 Unspecified keratoconjunctivitis, left eye
H16.203 Unspecified keratoconjunctivitis, bilateral
H16.209 Unspecified keratoconjunctivitis, unspecified eye
√6th H16.21 Exposure keratoconjunctivitis
H16.211 Exposure keratoconjunctivitis, right eye
H16.212 Exposure keratoconjunctivitis, left eye
H16.213 Exposure keratoconjunctivitis, bilateral
H16.219 Exposure keratoconjunctivitis, unspecified eye
√6th H16.22 Keratoconjunctivitis sicca, not specified as Sjögren's
EXCLUDES1 *Sjögren's syndrome (M35.01)*
H16.221 Keratoconjunctivitis sicca, not specified as Sjögren's, right eye
H16.222 Keratoconjunctivitis sicca, not specified as Sjögren's, left eye
H16.223 Keratoconjunctivitis sicca, not specified as Sjögren's, bilateral
H16.229 Keratoconjunctivitis sicca, not specified as Sjögren's, unspecified eye
√6th H16.23 Neurotrophic keratoconjunctivitis
H16.231 Neurotrophic keratoconjunctivitis, right eye
H16.232 Neurotrophic keratoconjunctivitis, left eye
H16.233 Neurotrophic keratoconjunctivitis, bilateral
H16.239 Neurotrophic keratoconjunctivitis, unspecified eye
√6th H16.24 Ophthalmia nodosa
H16.241 Ophthalmia nodosa, right eye
H16.242 Ophthalmia nodosa, left eye
H16.243 Ophthalmia nodosa, bilateral
H16.249 Ophthalmia nodosa, unspecified eye
√6th H16.25 Phlyctenular keratoconjunctivitis
H16.251 Phlyctenular keratoconjunctivitis, right eye
H16.252 Phlyctenular keratoconjunctivitis, left eye
H16.253 Phlyctenular keratoconjunctivitis, bilateral
H16.259 Phlyctenular keratoconjunctivitis, unspecified eye
√6th H16.26 Vernal keratoconjunctivitis, with limbar and corneal involvement
EXCLUDES1 *vernal conjunctivitis without limbar and corneal involvement (H10.44)*
H16.261 Vernal keratoconjunctivitis, with limbar and corneal involvement, right eye
H16.262 Vernal keratoconjunctivitis, with limbar and corneal involvement, left eye
H16.263 Vernal keratoconjunctivitis, with limbar and corneal involvement, bilateral
H16.269 Vernal keratoconjunctivitis, with limbar and corneal involvement, unspecified eye
√6th H16.29 Other keratoconjunctivitis
H16.291 Other keratoconjunctivitis, right eye
H16.292 Other keratoconjunctivitis, left eye
H16.293 Other keratoconjunctivitis, bilateral
H16.299 Other keratoconjunctivitis, unspecified eye
√5th H16.3 Interstitial and deep keratitis
√6th H16.30 Unspecified interstitial keratitis
H16.301 Unspecified interstitial keratitis, right eye
H16.302 Unspecified interstitial keratitis, left eye
H16.303 Unspecified interstitial keratitis, bilateral
H16.309 Unspecified interstitial keratitis, unspecified eye
√6th H16.31 Corneal abscess
H16.311 Corneal abscess, right eye
H16.312 Corneal abscess, left eye
H16.313 Corneal abscess, bilateral
H16.319 Corneal abscess, unspecified eye
√6th H16.32 Diffuse interstitial keratitis
Cogan's syndrome
H16.321 Diffuse interstitial keratitis, right eye
H16.322 Diffuse interstitial keratitis, left eye
H16.323 Diffuse interstitial keratitis, bilateral
H16.329 Diffuse interstitial keratitis, unspecified eye
√6th H16.33 Sclerosing keratitis
H16.331 Sclerosing keratitis, right eye
H16.332 Sclerosing keratitis, left eye
H16.333 Sclerosing keratitis, bilateral
H16.339 Sclerosing keratitis, unspecified eye
√6th H16.39 Other interstitial and deep keratitis
H16.391 Other interstitial and deep keratitis, right eye
H16.392 Other interstitial and deep keratitis, left eye
H16.393 Other interstitial and deep keratitis, bilateral
H16.399 Other interstitial and deep keratitis, unspecified eye
√5th H16.4 Corneal neovascularization
√6th H16.40 Unspecified corneal neovascularization
H16.401 Unspecified corneal neovascularization, right eye
H16.402 Unspecified corneal neovascularization, left eye
H16.403 Unspecified corneal neovascularization, bilateral
H16.409 Unspecified corneal neovascularization, unspecified eye
√6th H16.41 Ghost vessels (corneal)
H16.411 Ghost vessels (corneal), right eye
H16.412 Ghost vessels (corneal), left eye
H16.413 Ghost vessels (corneal), bilateral
H16.419 Ghost vessels (corneal), unspecified eye
√6th H16.42 Pannus (corneal)
H16.421 Pannus (corneal), right eye
H16.422 Pannus (corneal), left eye
H16.423 Pannus (corneal), bilateral
H16.429 Pannus (corneal), unspecified eye
√6th H16.43 Localized vascularization of cornea
H16.431 Localized vascularization of cornea, right eye
H16.432 Localized vascularization of cornea, left eye
H16.433 Localized vascularization of cornea, bilateral
H16.439 Localized vascularization of cornea, unspecified eye
√6th H16.44 Deep vascularization of cornea
H16.441 Deep vascularization of cornea, right eye
H16.442 Deep vascularization of cornea, left eye
H16.443 Deep vascularization of cornea, bilateral

H16.449 Deep vascularization of cornea, unspecified eye

H16.8 Other keratitis

H16.9 Unspecified keratitis

✓4th **H17 Corneal scars and opacities**

✓5th H17.0 Adherent leukoma

H17.00 Adherent leukoma, unspecified eye

H17.01 Adherent leukoma, right eye

H17.02 Adherent leukoma, left eye

H17.03 Adherent leukoma, bilateral

✓5th H17.1 Central corneal opacity

H17.10 Central corneal opacity, unspecified eye

H17.11 Central corneal opacity, right eye

H17.12 Central corneal opacity, left eye

H17.13 Central corneal opacity, bilateral

✓5th H17.8 Other corneal scars and opacities

✓6th H17.81 Minor opacity of cornea

Corneal nebula

H17.811 Minor opacity of cornea, right eye

H17.812 Minor opacity of cornea, left eye

H17.813 Minor opacity of cornea, bilateral

H17.819 Minor opacity of cornea, unspecified eye

✓6th H17.82 Peripheral opacity of cornea

H17.821 Peripheral opacity of cornea, right eye

H17.822 Peripheral opacity of cornea, left eye

H17.823 Peripheral opacity of cornea, bilateral

H17.829 Peripheral opacity of cornea, unspecified eye

H17.89 Other corneal scars and opacities

H17.9 Unspecified corneal scar and opacity

✓4th **H18 Other disorders of cornea**

✓5th H18.0 Corneal pigmentations and deposits

✓6th H18.00 Unspecified corneal deposit

H18.001 Unspecified corneal deposit, right eye

H18.002 Unspecified corneal deposit, left eye

H18.003 Unspecified corneal deposit, bilateral

H18.009 Unspecified corneal deposit, unspecified eye

✓6th H18.01 Anterior corneal pigmentations

Staehli's line

H18.011 Anterior corneal pigmentations, right eye

H18.012 Anterior corneal pigmentations, left eye

H18.013 Anterior corneal pigmentations, bilateral

H18.019 Anterior corneal pigmentations, unspecified eye

✓6th H18.02 Argentous corneal deposits

H18.021 Argentous corneal deposits, right eye

H18.022 Argentous corneal deposits, left eye

H18.023 Argentous corneal deposits, bilateral

H18.029 Argentous corneal deposits, unspecified eye

✓6th H18.03 Corneal deposits in metabolic disorders

Code also associated metabolic disorder

H18.031 Corneal deposits in metabolic disorders, right eye

H18.032 Corneal deposits in metabolic disorders, left eye

H18.033 Corneal deposits in metabolic disorders, bilateral

H18.039 Corneal deposits in metabolic disorders, unspecified eye

✓6th H18.04 Kayser-Fleischer ring

Code also associated Wilson's disease (E83.01)

H18.041 Kayser-Fleischer ring, right eye

H18.042 Kayser-Fleischer ring, left eye

H18.043 Kayser-Fleischer ring, bilateral

H18.049 Kayser-Fleischer ring, unspecified eye

✓6th H18.05 Posterior corneal pigmentations

Krukenberg's spindle

H18.051 Posterior corneal pigmentations, right eye

H18.052 Posterior corneal pigmentations, left eye

H18.053 Posterior corneal pigmentations, bilateral

H18.059 Posterior corneal pigmentations, unspecified eye

✓6th H18.06 Stromal corneal pigmentations

Hematocornea

H18.061 Stromal corneal pigmentations, right eye

H18.062 Stromal corneal pigmentations, left eye

H18.063 Stromal corneal pigmentations, bilateral

H18.069 Stromal corneal pigmentations, unspecified eye

✓5th H18.1 Bullous keratopathy

H18.10 Bullous keratopathy, unspecified eye

H18.11 Bullous keratopathy, right eye

H18.12 Bullous keratopathy, left eye

H18.13 Bullous keratopathy, bilateral

✓5th H18.2 Other and unspecified corneal edema

H18.20 Unspecified corneal edema

✓6th H18.21 Corneal edema secondary to contact lens

EXCLUDES 2 *other corneal disorders due to contact lens (H18.82-)*

H18.211 Corneal edema secondary to contact lens, right eye

H18.212 Corneal edema secondary to contact lens, left eye

H18.213 Corneal edema secondary to contact lens, bilateral

H18.219 Corneal edema secondary to contact lens, unspecified eye

✓6th H18.22 Idiopathic corneal edema

H18.221 Idiopathic corneal edema, right eye

H18.222 Idiopathic corneal edema, left eye

H18.223 Idiopathic corneal edema, bilateral

H18.229 Idiopathic corneal edema, unspecified eye

✓6th H18.23 Secondary corneal edema

H18.231 Secondary corneal edema, right eye

H18.232 Secondary corneal edema, left eye

H18.233 Secondary corneal edema, bilateral

H18.239 Secondary corneal edema, unspecified eye

✓5th H18.3 Changes of corneal membranes

H18.30 Unspecified corneal membrane change

✓6th H18.31 Folds and rupture in Bowman's membrane

H18.311 Folds and rupture in Bowman's membrane, right eye

H18.312 Folds and rupture in Bowman's membrane, left eye

H18.313 Folds and rupture in Bowman's membrane, bilateral

H18.319 Folds and rupture in Bowman's membrane, unspecified eye

✓6th H18.32 Folds in Descemet's membrane

H18.321 Folds in Descemet's membrane, right eye

H18.322 Folds in Descemet's membrane, left eye

H18.323 Folds in Descemet's membrane, bilateral

H18.329 Folds in Descemet's membrane, unspecified eye

✓6th H18.33 Rupture in Descemet's membrane

H18.331 Rupture in Descemet's membrane, right eye

H18.332 Rupture in Descemet's membrane, left eye

H18.333 Rupture in Descemet's membrane, bilateral

H18.339 Rupture in Descemet's membrane, unspecified eye

✓5th H18.4 Corneal degeneration

EXCLUDES 1 *Mooren's ulcer (H16.0-)*
recurrent erosion of cornea (H18.83-)

H18.40 Unspecified corneal degeneration

✓6th **H18.41 Arcus senilis**
Senile corneal changes
H18.411 Arcus senilis, right eye
H18.412 Arcus senilis, left eye
H18.413 Arcus senilis, bilateral
H18.419 Arcus senilis, unspecified eye

✓6th **H18.42 Band keratopathy**
H18.421 Band keratopathy, right eye
H18.422 Band keratopathy, left eye
H18.423 Band keratopathy, bilateral
H18.429 Band keratopathy, unspecified eye

H18.43 Other calcerous corneal degeneration

✓6th **H18.44 Keratomalacia**
EXCLUDES 1 *keratomalacia due to vitamin A deficiency (E50.4)*
H18.441 Keratomalacia, right eye
H18.442 Keratomalacia, left eye
H18.443 Keratomalacia, bilateral
H18.449 Keratomalacia, unspecified eye

✓6th **H18.45 Nodular corneal degeneration**
H18.451 Nodular corneal degeneration, right eye
H18.452 Nodular corneal degeneration, left eye
H18.453 Nodular corneal degeneration, bilateral
H18.459 Nodular corneal degeneration, unspecified eye

✓6th **H18.46 Peripheral corneal degeneration**
H18.461 Peripheral corneal degeneration, right eye
H18.462 Peripheral corneal degeneration, left eye
H18.463 Peripheral corneal degeneration, bilateral
H18.469 Peripheral corneal degeneration, unspecified eye

H18.49 Other corneal degeneration

✓5th **H18.5 Hereditary corneal dystrophies**
H18.50 Unspecified hereditary corneal dystrophies
H18.51 Endothelial corneal dystrophy
Fuchs' dystrophy
H18.52 Epithelial (juvenile) corneal dystrophy
H18.53 Granular corneal dystrophy
H18.54 Lattice corneal dystrophy
H18.55 Macular corneal dystrophy
H18.59 Other hereditary corneal dystrophies

✓5th **H18.6 Keratoconus**
✓6th **H18.60 Keratoconus, unspecified**
H18.601 Keratoconus, unspecified, right eye
H18.602 Keratoconus, unspecified, left eye
H18.603 Keratoconus, unspecified, bilateral
H18.609 Keratoconus, unspecified, unspecified eye

✓6th **H18.61 Keratoconus, stable**
H18.611 Keratoconus, stable, right eye
H18.612 Keratoconus, stable, left eye
H18.613 Keratoconus, stable, bilateral
H18.619 Keratoconus, stable, unspecified eye

✓6th **H18.62 Keratoconus, unstable**
Acute hydrops
H18.621 Keratoconus, unstable, right eye
H18.622 Keratoconus, unstable, left eye
H18.623 Keratoconus, unstable, bilateral
H18.629 Keratoconus, unstable, unspecified eye

✓5th **H18.7 Other and unspecified corneal deformities**
EXCLUDES 1 *congenital malformations of cornea (Q13.3-Q13.4)*
H18.70 Unspecified corneal deformity

✓6th **H18.71 Corneal ectasia**
H18.711 Corneal ectasia, right eye
H18.712 Corneal ectasia, left eye
H18.713 Corneal ectasia, bilateral
H18.719 Corneal ectasia, unspecified eye

✓6th **H18.72 Corneal staphyloma**
H18.721 Corneal staphyloma, right eye
H18.722 Corneal staphyloma, left eye
H18.723 Corneal staphyloma, bilateral
H18.729 Corneal staphyloma, unspecified eye

✓6th **H18.73 Descemetocele**
H18.731 Descemetocele, right eye
H18.732 Descemetocele, left eye
H18.733 Descemetocele, bilateral
H18.739 Descemetocele, unspecified eye

✓6th **H18.79 Other corneal deformities**
H18.791 Other corneal deformities, right eye
H18.792 Other corneal deformities, left eye
H18.793 Other corneal deformities, bilateral
H18.799 Other corneal deformities, unspecified eye

✓5th **H18.8 Other specified disorders of cornea**
✓6th **H18.81 Anesthesia and hypoesthesia of cornea**
H18.811 Anesthesia and hypoesthesia of cornea, right eye
H18.812 Anesthesia and hypoesthesia of cornea, left eye
H18.813 Anesthesia and hypoesthesia of cornea, bilateral
H18.819 Anesthesia and hypoesthesia of cornea, unspecified eye

✓6th **H18.82 Corneal disorder due to contact lens**
EXCLUDES 2 *corneal edema due to contact lens (H18.21-)*
H18.821 Corneal disorder due to contact lens, right eye
H18.822 Corneal disorder due to contact lens, left eye
H18.823 Corneal disorder due to contact lens, bilateral
H18.829 Corneal disorder due to contact lens, unspecified eye

✓6th **H18.83 Recurrent erosion of cornea**
H18.831 Recurrent erosion of cornea, right eye
H18.832 Recurrent erosion of cornea, left eye
H18.833 Recurrent erosion of cornea, bilateral
H18.839 Recurrent erosion of cornea, unspecified eye

✓6th **H18.89 Other specified disorders of cornea**
H18.891 Other specified disorders of cornea, right eye
H18.892 Other specified disorders of cornea, left eye
H18.893 Other specified disorders of cornea, bilateral
H18.899 Other specified disorders of cornea, unspecified eye

H18.9 Unspecified disorder of cornea

✓4th H20 Iridocyclitis

✓5th **H20.0 Acute and subacute iridocyclitis**
Acute anterior uveitis
Acute cyclitis
Acute iritis
Subacute anterior uveitis
Subacute cyclitis
Subacute iritis
EXCLUDES 1 *iridocyclitis, iritis, uveitis (due to) (in) diabetes mellitus (E08-E13 with .39)*
iridocyclitis, iritis, uveitis (due to) (in) diphtheria (A36.89)
iridocyclitis, iritis, uveitis (due to) (in) gonococcal (A54.32)
iridocyclitis, iritis, uveitis (due to) (in) herpes (simplex) (B00.51)
iridocyclitis, iritis, uveitis (due to) (in) herpes zoster (B02.32)
iridocyclitis, iritis, uveitis (due to) (in) late congenital syphilis (A50.39)
iridocyclitis, iritis, uveitis (due to) (in) late syphilis (A52.71)
iridocyclitis, iritis, uveitis (due to) (in) sarcoidosis (D86.83)
iridocyclitis, iritis, uveitis (due to) (in) syphilis (A51.43)
iridocyclitis, iritis, uveitis (due to) (in) toxoplasmosis (B58.09)
iridocyclitis, iritis, uveitis (due to) (in) tuberculosis (A18.54)

H20.00 Unspecified acute and subacute iridocyclitis

✓6th **H20.01 Primary iridocyclitis**
- **H20.011 Primary iridocyclitis, right eye**
- **H20.012 Primary iridocyclitis, left eye**
- **H20.013 Primary iridocyclitis, bilateral**
- **H20.019 Primary iridocyclitis, unspecified eye**

✓6th **H20.02 Recurrent acute iridocyclitis**
- **H20.021 Recurrent acute iridocyclitis, right eye**
- **H20.022 Recurrent acute iridocyclitis, left eye**
- **H20.023 Recurrent acute iridocyclitis, bilateral**
- **H20.029 Recurrent acute iridocyclitis, unspecified eye**

✓6th **H20.03 Secondary infectious iridocyclitis**
- **H20.031 Secondary infectious iridocyclitis, right eye**
- **H20.032 Secondary infectious iridocyclitis, left eye**
- **H20.033 Secondary infectious iridocyclitis, bilateral**
- **H20.039 Secondary infectious iridocyclitis, unspecified eye**

✓6th **H20.04 Secondary noninfectious iridocyclitis**
- **H20.041 Secondary noninfectious iridocyclitis, right eye**
- **H20.042 Secondary noninfectious iridocyclitis, left eye**
- **H20.043 Secondary noninfectious iridocyclitis, bilateral**
- **H20.049 Secondary noninfectious iridocyclitis, unspecified eye**

✓6th **H20.05 Hypopyon**
- **H20.051 Hypopyon, right eye**
- **H20.052 Hypopyon, left eye**
- **H20.053 Hypopyon, bilateral**
- **H20.059 Hypopyon, unspecified eye**

✓5th **H20.1 Chronic iridocyclitis**

Use additional code for any associated cataract (H26.21-)

EXCLUDES 2 *posterior cyclitis (H30.2-)*

- **H20.10 Chronic iridocyclitis, unspecified eye**
- **H20.11 Chronic iridocyclitis, right eye**
- **H20.12 Chronic iridocyclitis, left eye**
- **H20.13 Chronic iridocyclitis, bilateral**

✓5th **H20.2 Lens-induced iridocyclitis**
- **H20.20 Lens-induced iridocyclitis, unspecified eye**
- **H20.21 Lens-induced iridocyclitis, right eye**
- **H20.22 Lens-induced iridocyclitis, left eye**
- **H20.23 Lens-induced iridocyclitis, bilateral**

✓5th **H20.8 Other iridocyclitis**

EXCLUDES 2 *glaucomatocyclitis crises (H40.4-)*
posterior cyclitis (H30.2-)
sympathetic uveitis (H44.13-)

✓6th **H20.81 Fuchs' heterochromic cyclitis**
- **H20.811 Fuchs' heterochromic cyclitis, right eye**
- **H20.812 Fuchs' heterochromic cyclitis, left eye**
- **H20.813 Fuchs' heterochromic cyclitis, bilateral**
- **H20.819 Fuchs' heterochromic cyclitis, unspecified eye**

✓6th **H20.82 Vogt-Koyanagi syndrome**
- **H20.821 Vogt-Koyanagi syndrome, right eye**
- **H20.822 Vogt-Koyanagi syndrome, left eye**
- **H20.823 Vogt-Koyanagi syndrome, bilateral**
- **H20.829 Vogt-Koyanagi syndrome, unspecified eye**

H20.9 Unspecified iridocyclitis

Uveitis NOS

✓4th H21 Other disorders of iris and ciliary body

EXCLUDES 2 *sympathetic uveitis (H44.1-)*

✓5th **H21.0 Hyphema**

EXCLUDES 1 *traumatic hyphema (S05.1-)*

- **H21.00 Hyphema, unspecified eye**
- **H21.01 Hyphema, right eye**
- **H21.02 Hyphema, left eye**
- **H21.03 Hyphema, bilateral**

✓5th **H21.1 Other vascular disorders of iris and ciliary body**

Neovascularization of iris or ciliary body
Rubeosis iridis
Rubeosis of iris

✓6th **H21.1X Other vascular disorders of iris and ciliary body**
- **H21.1X1 Other vascular disorders of iris and ciliary body, right eye**
- **H21.1X2 Other vascular disorders of iris and ciliary body, left eye**
- **H21.1X3 Other vascular disorders of iris and ciliary body, bilateral**
- **H21.1X9 Other vascular disorders of iris and ciliary body, unspecified eye**

✓5th **H21.2 Degeneration of iris and ciliary body**

✓6th **H21.21 Degeneration of chamber angle**
- **H21.211 Degeneration of chamber angle, right eye**
- **H21.212 Degeneration of chamber angle, left eye**
- **H21.213 Degeneration of chamber angle, bilateral**
- **H21.219 Degeneration of chamber angle, unspecified eye**

✓6th **H21.22 Degeneration of ciliary body**
- **H21.221 Degeneration of ciliary body, right eye**
- **H21.222 Degeneration of ciliary body, left eye**
- **H21.223 Degeneration of ciliary body, bilateral**
- **H21.229 Degeneration of ciliary body, unspecified eye**

✓6th **H21.23 Degeneration of iris (pigmentary)**

Translucency of iris

- **H21.231 Degeneration of iris (pigmentary), right eye**
- **H21.232 Degeneration of iris (pigmentary), left eye**
- **H21.233 Degeneration of iris (pigmentary), bilateral**
- **H21.239 Degeneration of iris (pigmentary), unspecified eye**

✓6th **H21.24 Degeneration of pupillary margin**
- **H21.241 Degeneration of pupillary margin, right eye**
- **H21.242 Degeneration of pupillary margin, left eye**
- **H21.243 Degeneration of pupillary margin, bilateral**
- **H21.249 Degeneration of pupillary margin, unspecified eye**

✓6th **H21.25 Iridoschisis**
- **H21.251 Iridoschisis, right eye**
- **H21.252 Iridoschisis, left eye**
- **H21.253 Iridoschisis, bilateral**
- **H21.259 Iridoschisis, unspecified eye**

✓6th **H21.26 Iris atrophy (essential) (progressive)**
- **H21.261 Iris atrophy (essential) (progressive), right eye**
- **H21.262 Iris atrophy (essential) (progressive), left eye**
- **H21.263 Iris atrophy (essential) (progressive), bilateral**
- **H21.269 Iris atrophy (essential) (progressive), unspecified eye**

✓6th **H21.27 Miotic pupillary cyst**
- **H21.271 Miotic pupillary cyst, right eye**
- **H21.272 Miotic pupillary cyst, left eye**
- **H21.273 Miotic pupillary cyst, bilateral**
- **H21.279 Miotic pupillary cyst, unspecified eye**

H21.29 Other iris atrophy

✓5th **H21.3 Cyst of iris, ciliary body and anterior chamber**

EXCLUDES 2 *miotic pupillary cyst (H21.27-)*

✓6th **H21.30 Idiopathic cysts of iris, ciliary body or anterior chamber**

Cyst of iris, ciliary body or anterior chamber NOS

- **H21.301 Idiopathic cysts of iris, ciliary body or anterior chamber, right eye**
- **H21.302 Idiopathic cysts of iris, ciliary body or anterior chamber, left eye**

H21.303 **Idiopathic cysts of iris, ciliary body or anterior chamber, bilateral**
H21.309 **Idiopathic cysts of iris, ciliary body or anterior chamber, unspecified eye**

✓6th **H21.31 Exudative cysts of iris or anterior chamber**
H21.311 **Exudative cysts of iris or anterior chamber, right eye**
H21.312 **Exudative cysts of iris or anterior chamber, left eye**
H21.313 **Exudative cysts of iris or anterior chamber, bilateral**
H21.319 **Exudative cysts of iris or anterior chamber, unspecified eye**

✓6th **H21.32 Implantation cysts of iris, ciliary body or anterior chamber**
H21.321 **Implantation cysts of iris, ciliary body or anterior chamber, right eye**
H21.322 **Implantation cysts of iris, ciliary body or anterior chamber, left eye**
H21.323 **Implantation cysts of iris, ciliary body or anterior chamber, bilateral**
H21.329 **Implantation cysts of iris, ciliary body or anterior chamber, unspecified eye**

✓6th **H21.33 Parasitic cyst of iris, ciliary body or anterior chamber**
H21.331 **Parasitic cyst of iris, ciliary body or anterior chamber, right eye**
H21.332 **Parasitic cyst of iris, ciliary body or anterior chamber, left eye**
H21.333 **Parasitic cyst of iris, ciliary body or anterior chamber, bilateral**
H21.339 **Parasitic cyst of iris, ciliary body or anterior chamber, unspecified eye**

✓6th **H21.34 Primary cyst of pars plana**
H21.341 **Primary cyst of pars plana, right eye**
H21.342 **Primary cyst of pars plana, left eye**
H21.343 **Primary cyst of pars plana, bilateral**
H21.349 **Primary cyst of pars plana, unspecified eye**

✓6th **H21.35 Exudative cyst of pars plana**
H21.351 **Exudative cyst of pars plana, right eye**
H21.352 **Exudative cyst of pars plana, left eye**
H21.353 **Exudative cyst of pars plana, bilateral**
H21.359 **Exudative cyst of pars plana, unspecified eye**

✓5th **H21.4 Pupillary membranes**
Iris bombé
Pupillary occlusion
Pupillary seclusion
EXCLUDES 1 *congenital pupillary membranes (Q13.8)*
H21.40 **Pupillary membranes, unspecified eye**
H21.41 **Pupillary membranes, right eye**
H21.42 **Pupillary membranes, left eye**
H21.43 **Pupillary membranes, bilateral**

✓5th **H21.5 Other and unspecified adhesions and disruptions of iris and ciliary body**
EXCLUDES 1 *corectopia (Q13.2)*

✓6th **H21.50 Unspecified adhesions of iris**
Synechia (iris) NOS
H21.501 **Unspecified adhesions of iris, right eye**
H21.502 **Unspecified adhesions of iris, left eye**
H21.503 **Unspecified adhesions of iris, bilateral**
H21.509 **Unspecified adhesions of iris and ciliary body, unspecified eye**

✓6th **H21.51 Anterior synechiae (iris)**
H21.511 **Anterior synechiae (iris), right eye**
H21.512 **Anterior synechiae (iris), left eye**
H21.513 **Anterior synechiae (iris), bilateral**
H21.519 **Anterior synechiae (iris), unspecified eye**

✓6th **H21.52 Goniosynechiae**
H21.521 **Goniosynechiae, right eye**
H21.522 **Goniosynechiae, left eye**
H21.523 **Goniosynechiae, bilateral**
H21.529 **Goniosynechiae, unspecified eye**

✓6th **H21.53 Iridodialysis**
H21.531 **Iridodialysis, right eye**
H21.532 **Iridodialysis, left eye**
H21.533 **Iridodialysis, bilateral**
H21.539 **Iridodialysis, unspecified eye**

✓6th **H21.54 Posterior synechiae (iris)**
H21.541 **Posterior synechiae (iris), right eye**
H21.542 **Posterior synechiae (iris), left eye**
H21.543 **Posterior synechiae (iris), bilateral**
H21.549 **Posterior synechiae (iris), unspecified eye**

✓6th **H21.55 Recession of chamber angle**
H21.551 **Recession of chamber angle, right eye**
H21.552 **Recession of chamber angle, left eye**
H21.553 **Recession of chamber angle, bilateral**
H21.559 **Recession of chamber angle, unspecified eye**

✓6th **H21.56 Pupillary abnormalities**
Deformed pupil
Ectopic pupil
Rupture of sphincter, pupil
EXCLUDES 1 *congenital deformity of pupil (Q13.2-)*
H21.561 **Pupillary abnormality, right eye**
H21.562 **Pupillary abnormality, left eye**
H21.563 **Pupillary abnormality, bilateral**
H21.569 **Pupillary abnormality, unspecified eye**

✓5th **H21.8 Other specified disorders of iris and ciliary body**
H21.81 **Floppy iris syndrome**
Intraoperative floppy iris syndrome (IFIS)
Use additional code for adverse effect, if applicable, to identify drug (T36-T50 with fifth or sixth character 5)
H21.82 **Plateau iris syndrome (post-iridectomy) (postprocedural)**
H21.89 **Other specified disorders of iris and ciliary body**

H21.9 Unspecified disorder of iris and ciliary body

H22 Disorders of iris and ciliary body in diseases classified elsewhere
Code first underlying disease, such as:
gout (M1A.-, M10.-)

Disorders of lens (H25-H28)

✓4th **H25 Age-related cataract**
Senile cataract
EXCLUDES 2 *capsular glaucoma with pseudoexfoliation of lens (H40.1-)*

✓5th **H25.0 Age-related incipient cataract**

✓6th **H25.01 Cortical age-related cataract**
H25.011 **Cortical age-related cataract, right eye**
H25.012 **Cortical age-related cataract, left eye**
H25.013 **Cortical age-related cataract, bilateral**
H25.019 **Cortical age-related cataract, unspecified eye**

✓6th **H25.03 Anterior subcapsular polar age-related cataract**
H25.031 **Anterior subcapsular polar age-related cataract, right eye**
H25.032 **Anterior subcapsular polar age-related cataract, left eye**
H25.033 **Anterior subcapsular polar age-related cataract, bilateral**
H25.039 **Anterior subcapsular polar age-related cataract, unspecified eye**

✓6th **H25.04 Posterior subcapsular polar age-related cataract**
H25.041 **Posterior subcapsular polar age-related cataract, right eye**
H25.042 **Posterior subcapsular polar age-related cataract, left eye**
H25.043 **Posterior subcapsular polar age-related cataract, bilateral**
H25.049 **Posterior subcapsular polar age-related cataract, unspecified eye**

✓6th **H25.09 Other age-related incipient cataract**
Coronary age-related cataract
Punctate age-related cataract
Water clefts
H25.091 **Other age-related incipient cataract, right eye**
H25.092 **Other age-related incipient cataract, left eye**

H25.093 **Other age-related incipient cataract, bilateral**

H25.099 **Other age-related incipient cataract, unspecified eye**

✓5th **H25.1** **Age-related nuclear cataract**
Cataracta brunescens
Nuclear sclerosis cataract

H25.10 **Age-related nuclear cataract, unspecified eye**

H25.11 **Age-related nuclear cataract, right eye**

H25.12 **Age-related nuclear cataract, left eye**

H25.13 **Age-related nuclear cataract, bilateral**

✓5th **H25.2** **Age-related cataract, morgagnian type**
Age-related hypermature cataract

H25.20 **Age-related cataract, morgagnian type, unspecified eye**

H25.21 **Age-related cataract, morgagnian type, right eye**

H25.22 **Age-related cataract, morgagnian type, left eye**

H25.23 **Age-related cataract, morgagnian type, bilateral**

✓5th **H25.8** **Other age-related cataract**

✓6th **H25.81** **Combined forms of age-related cataract**

H25.811 **Combined forms of age-related cataract, right eye**

H25.812 **Combined forms of age-related cataract, left eye**

H25.813 **Combined forms of age-related cataract, bilateral**

H25.819 **Combined forms of age-related cataract, unspecified eye**

H25.89 **Other age-related cataract**

H25.9 **Unspecified age-related cataract**

✓4th **H26** **Other cataract**

EXCLUDES 1 *congenital cataract (Q12.0)*

✓5th **H26.0** **Infantile and juvenile cataract**

✓6th **H26.00** **Unspecified infantile and juvenile cataract**

H26.001 **Unspecified infantile and juvenile cataract, right eye**

H26.002 **Unspecified infantile and juvenile cataract, left eye**

H26.003 **Unspecified infantile and juvenile cataract, bilateral**

H26.009 **Unspecified infantile and juvenile cataract, unspecified eye**

✓6th **H26.01** **Infantile and juvenile cortical, lamellar, or zonular cataract**

H26.011 **Infantile and juvenile cortical, lamellar, or zonular cataract, right eye**

H26.012 **Infantile and juvenile cortical, lamellar, or zonular cataract, left eye**

H26.013 **Infantile and juvenile cortical, lamellar, or zonular cataract, bilateral**

H26.019 **Infantile and juvenile cortical, lamellar, or zonular cataract, unspecified eye**

✓6th **H26.03** **Infantile and juvenile nuclear cataract**

H26.031 **Infantile and juvenile nuclear cataract, right eye**

H26.032 **Infantile and juvenile nuclear cataract, left eye**

H26.033 **Infantile and juvenile nuclear cataract, bilateral**

H26.039 **Infantile and juvenile nuclear cataract, unspecified eye**

✓6th **H26.04** **Anterior subcapsular polar infantile and juvenile cataract**

H26.041 **Anterior subcapsular polar infantile and juvenile cataract, right eye**

H26.042 **Anterior subcapsular polar infantile and juvenile cataract, left eye**

H26.043 **Anterior subcapsular polar infantile and juvenile cataract, bilateral**

H26.049 **Anterior subcapsular polar infantile and juvenile cataract, unspecified eye**

✓6th **H26.05** **Posterior subcapsular polar infantile and juvenile cataract**

H26.051 **Posterior subcapsular polar infantile and juvenile cataract, right eye**

H26.052 **Posterior subcapsular polar infantile and juvenile cataract, left eye**

H26.053 **Posterior subcapsular polar infantile and juvenile cataract, bilateral**

H26.059 **Posterior subcapsular polar infantile and juvenile cataract, unspecified eye**

✓6th **H26.06** **Combined forms of infantile and juvenile cataract**

H26.061 **Combined forms of infantile and juvenile cataract, right eye**

H26.062 **Combined forms of infantile and juvenile cataract, left eye**

H26.063 **Combined forms of infantile and juvenile cataract, bilateral**

H26.069 **Combined forms of infantile and juvenile cataract, unspecified eye**

H26.09 **Other infantile and juvenile cataract**

✓5th **H26.1** **Traumatic cataract**
Use additional code (Chapter 20) to identify external cause

✓6th **H26.10** **Unspecified traumatic cataract**

H26.101 **Unspecified traumatic cataract, right eye**

H26.102 **Unspecified traumatic cataract, left eye**

H26.103 **Unspecified traumatic cataract, bilateral**

H26.109 **Unspecified traumatic cataract, unspecified eye**

✓6th **H26.11** **Localized traumatic opacities**

H26.111 **Localized traumatic opacities, right eye**

H26.112 **Localized traumatic opacities, left eye**

H26.113 **Localized traumatic opacities, bilateral**

H26.119 **Localized traumatic opacities, unspecified eye**

✓6th **H26.12** **Partially resolved traumatic cataract**

H26.121 **Partially resolved traumatic cataract, right eye**

H26.122 **Partially resolved traumatic cataract, left eye**

H26.123 **Partially resolved traumatic cataract, bilateral**

H26.129 **Partially resolved traumatic cataract, unspecified eye**

✓6th **H26.13** **Total traumatic cataract**

H26.131 **Total traumatic cataract, right eye**

H26.132 **Total traumatic cataract, left eye**

H26.133 **Total traumatic cataract, bilateral**

H26.139 **Total traumatic cataract, unspecified eye**

✓5th **H26.2** **Complicated cataract**

H26.20 **Unspecified complicated cataract**
Cataracta complicata NOS

✓6th **H26.21** **Cataract with neovascularization**
Code also associated condition, such as:
chronic iridocyclitis (H20.1-)

H26.211 **Cataract with neovascularization, right eye**

H26.212 **Cataract with neovascularization, left eye**

H26.213 **Cataract with neovascularization, bilateral**

H26.219 **Cataract with neovascularization, unspecified eye**

✓6th **H26.22** **Cataract secondary to ocular disorders (degenerative) (inflammatory)**
Code also associated ocular disorder

H26.221 **Cataract secondary to ocular disorders (degenerative) (inflammatory), right eye**

H26.222 **Cataract secondary to ocular disorders (degenerative) (inflammatory), left eye**

H26.223 **Cataract secondary to ocular disorders (degenerative) (inflammatory), bilateral**

H26.229 **Cataract secondary to ocular disorders (degenerative) (inflammatory), unspecified eye**

✓6th **H26.23** **Glaucomatous flecks (subcapsular)**
Code first underlying glaucoma (H40-H42)

H26.231 **Glaucomatous flecks (subcapsular), right eye**

H26.232 **Glaucomatous flecks (subcapsular), left eye**

H26.233 **Glaucomatous flecks (subcapsular), bilateral**
H26.239 **Glaucomatous flecks (subcapsular), unspecified eye**

✓5th **H26.3 Drug-induced cataract**
Toxic cataract
Use additional code for adverse effect, if applicable, to identify drug (T36-T50 with fifth or sixth character 5)
H26.30 **Drug-induced cataract, unspecified eye**
H26.31 **Drug-induced cataract, right eye**
H26.32 **Drug-induced cataract, left eye**
H26.33 **Drug-induced cataract, bilateral**

✓5th **H26.4 Secondary cataract**
H26.40 **Unspecified secondary cataract**
✓6th **H26.41 Soemmering's ring**
H26.411 **Soemmering's ring, right eye**
H26.412 **Soemmering's ring, left eye**
H26.413 **Soemmering's ring, bilateral**
H26.419 **Soemmering's ring, unspecified eye**
✓6th **H26.49 Other secondary cataract**
H26.491 **Other secondary cataract, right eye**
H26.492 **Other secondary cataract, left eye**
H26.493 **Other secondary cataract, bilateral**
H26.499 **Other secondary cataract, unspecified eye**

H26.8 Other specified cataract
H26.9 Unspecified cataract

✓4th **H27 Other disorders of lens**
EXCLUDES 1 *congenital lens malformations (Q12.-)*
mechanical complications of intraocular lens implant (T85.2)
pseudophakia (Z96.1)

✓5th **H27.0 Aphakia**
Acquired absence of lens
Acquired aphakia
Aphakia due to trauma
EXCLUDES 1 *cataract extraction status (Z98.4-)*
congenital absence of lens (Q12.3)
congenital aphakia (Q12.3)
H27.00 **Aphakia, unspecified eye**
H27.01 **Aphakia, right eye**
H27.02 **Aphakia, left eye**
H27.03 **Aphakia, bilateral**

✓5th **H27.1 Dislocation of lens**
H27.10 **Unspecified dislocation of lens**
✓6th **H27.11 Subluxation of lens**
H27.111 **Subluxation of lens, right eye**
H27.112 **Subluxation of lens, left eye**
H27.113 **Subluxation of lens, bilateral**
H27.119 **Subluxation of lens, unspecified eye**
✓6th **H27.12 Anterior dislocation of lens**
H27.121 **Anterior dislocation of lens, right eye**
H27.122 **Anterior dislocation of lens, left eye**
H27.123 **Anterior dislocation of lens, bilateral**
H27.129 **Anterior dislocation of lens, unspecified eye**
✓6th **H27.13 Posterior dislocation of lens**
H27.131 **Posterior dislocation of lens, right eye**
H27.132 **Posterior dislocation of lens, left eye**
H27.133 **Posterior dislocation of lens, bilateral**
H27.139 **Posterior dislocation of lens, unspecified eye**

H27.8 Other specified disorders of lens
H27.9 Unspecified disorder of lens

H28 Cataract in diseases classified elsewhere
Code first underlying disease, such as:
hypoparathyroidism (E20.-)
myotonia (G71.1-)
myxedema (E03.-)
protein-calorie malnutrition (E40-E46)
EXCLUDES 1 *cataract in diabetes mellitus (E08.33, E09.33, E10.33, E11.33, E13.33)*

Disorders of choroid and retina (H30-H36)

✓4th **H30 Chorioretinal inflammation**

✓5th **H30.0 Focal chorioretinal inflammation**
Focal chorioretinitis
Focal choroiditis
Focal retinitis
Focal retinochoroiditis
✓6th **H30.00 Unspecified focal chorioretinal inflammation**
Focal chorioretinitis NOS
Focal choroiditis NOS
Focal retinitis NOS
Focal retinochoroiditis NOS
H30.001 **Unspecified focal chorioretinal inflammation, right eye**
H30.002 **Unspecified focal chorioretinal inflammation, left eye**
H30.003 **Unspecified focal chorioretinal inflammation, bilateral**
H30.009 **Unspecified focal chorioretinal inflammation, unspecified eye**
✓6th **H30.01 Focal chorioretinal inflammation, juxtapapillary**
H30.011 **Focal chorioretinal inflammation, juxtapapillary, right eye**
H30.012 **Focal chorioretinal inflammation, juxtapapillary, left eye**
H30.013 **Focal chorioretinal inflammation, juxtapapillary, bilateral**
H30.019 **Focal chorioretinal inflammation, juxtapapillary, unspecified eye**
✓6th **H30.02 Focal chorioretinal inflammation of posterior pole**
H30.021 **Focal chorioretinal inflammation of posterior pole, right eye**
H30.022 **Focal chorioretinal inflammation of posterior pole, left eye**
H30.023 **Focal chorioretinal inflammation of posterior pole, bilateral**
H30.029 **Focal chorioretinal inflammation of posterior pole, unspecified eye**
✓6th **H30.03 Focal chorioretinal inflammation, peripheral**
H30.031 **Focal chorioretinal inflammation, peripheral, right eye**
H30.032 **Focal chorioretinal inflammation, peripheral, left eye**
H30.033 **Focal chorioretinal inflammation, peripheral, bilateral**
H30.039 **Focal chorioretinal inflammation, peripheral, unspecified eye**
✓6th **H30.04 Focal chorioretinal inflammation, macular or paramacular**
H30.041 **Focal chorioretinal inflammation, macular or paramacular, right eye**
H30.042 **Focal chorioretinal inflammation, macular or paramacular, left eye**
H30.043 **Focal chorioretinal inflammation, macular or paramacular, bilateral**
H30.049 **Focal chorioretinal inflammation, macular or paramacular, unspecified eye**

✓5th **H30.1 Disseminated chorioretinal inflammation**
Disseminated chorioretinitis
Disseminated choroiditis
Disseminated retinitis
Disseminated retinochoroiditis
EXCLUDES 2 *exudative retinopathy (H35.02-)*
✓6th **H30.10 Unspecified disseminated chorioretinal inflammation**
Disseminated chorioretinitis NOS
Disseminated choroiditis NOS
Disseminated retinitis NOS
Disseminated retinochoroiditis NOS
H30.101 **Unspecified disseminated chorioretinal inflammation, right eye**
H30.102 **Unspecified disseminated chorioretinal inflammation, left eye**
H30.103 **Unspecified disseminated chorioretinal inflammation, bilateral**
H30.109 **Unspecified disseminated chorioretinal inflammation, unspecified eye**

√6th **H30.11 Disseminated chorioretinal inflammation of posterior pole**
- **H30.111 Disseminated chorioretinal inflammation of posterior pole, right eye**
- **H30.112 Disseminated chorioretinal inflammation of posterior pole, left eye**
- **H30.113 Disseminated chorioretinal inflammation of posterior pole, bilateral**
- **H30.119 Disseminated chorioretinal inflammation of posterior pole, unspecified eye**

√6th **H30.12 Disseminated chorioretinal inflammation, peripheral**
- **H30.121 Disseminated chorioretinal inflammation, peripheral right eye**
- **H30.122 Disseminated chorioretinal inflammation, peripheral, left eye**
- **H30.123 Disseminated chorioretinal inflammation, peripheral, bilateral**
- **H30.129 Disseminated chorioretinal inflammation, peripheral, unspecified eye**

√6th **H30.13 Disseminated chorioretinal inflammation, generalized**
- **H30.131 Disseminated chorioretinal inflammation, generalized, right eye**
- **H30.132 Disseminated chorioretinal inflammation, generalized, left eye**
- **H30.133 Disseminated chorioretinal inflammation, generalized, bilateral**
- **H30.139 Disseminated chorioretinal inflammation, generalized, unspecified eye**

√6th **H30.14 Acute posterior multifocal placoid pigment epitheliopathy**
- **H30.141 Acute posterior multifocal placoid pigment epitheliopathy, right eye**
- **H30.142 Acute posterior multifocal placoid pigment epitheliopathy, left eye**
- **H30.143 Acute posterior multifocal placoid pigment epitheliopathy, bilateral**
- **H30.149 Acute posterior multifocal placoid pigment epitheliopathy, unspecified eye**

√5th **H30.2 Posterior cyclitis**

Pars planitis
- **H30.20 Posterior cyclitis, unspecified eye**
- **H30.21 Posterior cyclitis, right eye**
- **H30.22 Posterior cyclitis, left eye**
- **H30.23 Posterior cyclitis, bilateral**

√5th **H30.8 Other chorioretinal inflammations**

√6th **H30.81 Harada's disease**
- **H30.811 Harada's disease, right eye**
- **H30.812 Harada's disease, left eye**
- **H30.813 Harada's disease, bilateral**
- **H30.819 Harada's disease, unspecified eye**

√6th **H30.89 Other chorioretinal inflammations**
- **H30.891 Other chorioretinal inflammations, right eye**
- **H30.892 Other chorioretinal inflammations, left eye**
- **H30.893 Other chorioretinal inflammations, bilateral**
- **H30.899 Other chorioretinal inflammations, unspecified eye**

√5th **H30.9 Unspecified chorioretinal inflammation**

Chorioretinitis NOS
Choroiditis NOS
Neuroretinitis NOS
Retinitis NOS
Retinochoroiditis NOS
- **H30.90 Unspecified chorioretinal inflammation, unspecified eye**
- **H30.91 Unspecified chorioretinal inflammation, right eye**
- **H30.92 Unspecified chorioretinal inflammation, left eye**
- **H30.93 Unspecified chorioretinal inflammation, bilateral**

√4th **H31 Other disorders of choroid**

√5th **H31.0 Chorioretinal scars**

EXCLUDES 2 *postsurgical chorioretinal scars (H59.81-)*

√6th **H31.00 Unspecified chorioretinal scars**
- **H31.001 Unspecified chorioretinal scars, right eye**
- **H31.002 Unspecified chorioretinal scars, left eye**
- **H31.003 Unspecified chorioretinal scars, bilateral**
- **H31.009 Unspecified chorioretinal scars, unspecified eye**

√6th **H31.01 Macula scars of posterior pole (postinflammatory) (post-traumatic)**

EXCLUDES 1 *postprocedural chorioretinal scar (H59.81-)*
- **H31.011 Macula scars of posterior pole (postinflammatory) (post-traumatic), right eye**
- **H31.012 Macula scars of posterior pole (postinflammatory) (post-traumatic), left eye**
- **H31.013 Macula scars of posterior pole (postinflammatory) (post-traumatic), bilateral**
- **H31.019 Macula scars of posterior pole (postinflammatory) (post-traumatic), unspecified eye**

√6th **H31.02 Solar retinopathy**
- **H31.021 Solar retinopathy, right eye**
- **H31.022 Solar retinopathy, left eye**
- **H31.023 Solar retinopathy, bilateral**
- **H31.029 Solar retinopathy, unspecified eye**

√6th **H31.09 Other chorioretinal scars**
- **H31.091 Other chorioretinal scars, right eye**
- **H31.092 Other chorioretinal scars, left eye**
- **H31.093 Other chorioretinal scars, bilateral**
- **H31.099 Other chorioretinal scars, unspecified eye**

√5th **H31.1 Choroidal degeneration**

EXCLUDES 2 *angioid streaks of macula (H35.33)*

√6th **H31.10 Unspecified choroidal degeneration**

Choroidal sclerosis NOS
- **H31.101 Choroidal degeneration, unspecified, right eye**
- **H31.102 Choroidal degeneration, unspecified, left eye**
- **H31.103 Choroidal degeneration, unspecified, bilateral**
- **H31.109 Choroidal degeneration, unspecified, unspecified eye**

√6th **H31.11 Age-related choroidal atrophy**
- **H31.111 Age-related choroidal atrophy, right eye**
- **H31.112 Age-related choroidal atrophy, left eye**
- **H31.113 Age-related choroidal atrophy, bilateral**
- **H31.119 Age-related choroidal atrophy, unspecified eye**

√6th **H31.12 Diffuse secondary atrophy of choroid**
- **H31.121 Diffuse secondary atrophy of choroid, right eye**
- **H31.122 Diffuse secondary atrophy of choroid, left eye**
- **H31.123 Diffuse secondary atrophy of choroid, bilateral**
- **H31.129 Diffuse secondary atrophy of choroid, unspecified eye**

√5th **H31.2 Hereditary choroidal dystrophy**

EXCLUDES 2 *hyperornithinemia (E72.4)*
ornithinemia (E72.4)
- **H31.20 Hereditary choroidal dystrophy, unspecified**
- **H31.21 Choroideremia**
- **H31.22 Choroidal dystrophy (central areolar) (generalized) (peripapillary)**
- **H31.23 Gyrate atrophy, choroid**
- **H31.29 Other hereditary choroidal dystrophy**

√5th **H31.3 Choroidal hemorrhage and rupture**

√6th **H31.30 Unspecified choroidal hemorrhage**
- **H31.301 Unspecified choroidal hemorrhage, right eye**

H31.302 Unspecified choroidal hemorrhage, left eye
H31.303 Unspecified choroidal hemorrhage, bilateral
H31.309 Unspecified choroidal hemorrhage, unspecified eye

✓6th H31.31 Expulsive choroidal hemorrhage
H31.311 Expulsive choroidal hemorrhage, right eye
H31.312 Expulsive choroidal hemorrhage, left eye
H31.313 Expulsive choroidal hemorrhage, bilateral
H31.319 Expulsive choroidal hemorrhage, unspecified eye

✓6th H31.32 Choroidal rupture
H31.321 Choroidal rupture, right eye
H31.322 Choroidal rupture, left eye
H31.323 Choroidal rupture, bilateral
H31.329 Choroidal rupture, unspecified eye

✓5th H31.4 Choroidal detachment

✓6th H31.40 Unspecified choroidal detachment
H31.401 Unspecified choroidal detachment, right eye
H31.402 Unspecified choroidal detachment, left eye
H31.403 Unspecified choroidal detachment, bilateral
H31.409 Unspecified choroidal detachment, unspecified eye

✓6th H31.41 Hemorrhagic choroidal detachment
H31.411 Hemorrhagic choroidal detachment, right eye
H31.412 Hemorrhagic choroidal detachment, left eye
H31.413 Hemorrhagic choroidal detachment, bilateral
H31.419 Hemorrhagic choroidal detachment, unspecified eye

✓6th H31.42 Serous choroidal detachment
H31.421 Serous choroidal detachment, right eye
H31.422 Serous choroidal detachment, left eye
H31.423 Serous choroidal detachment, bilateral
H31.429 Serous choroidal detachment, unspecified eye

H31.8 Other specified disorders of choroid
H31.9 Unspecified disorder of choroid

H32 *Chorioretinal disorders in diseases classified elsewhere*

Code first underlying disease, such as:
congenital toxoplasmosis (P37.1)
histoplasmosis (B39.-)
leprosy (A30.-)

EXCLUDES 1 *chorioretinitis (in):*
toxoplasmosis (acquired) (B58.01)
tuberculosis (A18.53)

✓4th **H33 Retinal detachments and breaks**

EXCLUDES 1 *detachment of retinal pigment epithelium (H35.72-, H35.73-)*

✓5th H33.0 Retinal detachment with retinal break
Rhegmatogenous retinal detachment
EXCLUDES 1 *serous retinal detachment (without retinal break) (H33.2-)*

✓6th H33.00 Unspecified retinal detachment with retinal break
H33.001 Unspecified retinal detachment with retinal break, right eye
H33.002 Unspecified retinal detachment with retinal break, left eye
H33.003 Unspecified retinal detachment with retinal break, bilateral
H33.009 Unspecified retinal detachment with retinal break, unspecified eye

✓6th H33.01 Retinal detachment with single break
H33.011 Retinal detachment with single break, right eye
H33.012 Retinal detachment with single break, left eye
H33.013 Retinal detachment with single break, bilateral
H33.019 Retinal detachment with single break, unspecified eye

✓6th H33.02 Retinal detachment with multiple breaks
H33.021 Retinal detachment with multiple breaks, right eye
H33.022 Retinal detachment with multiple breaks, left eye
H33.023 Retinal detachment with multiple breaks, bilateral
H33.029 Retinal detachment with multiple breaks, unspecified eye

✓6th H33.03 Retinal detachment with giant retinal tear
H33.031 Retinal detachment with giant retinal tear, right eye
H33.032 Retinal detachment with giant retinal tear, left eye
H33.033 Retinal detachment with giant retinal tear, bilateral
H33.039 Retinal detachment with giant retinal tear, unspecified eye

✓6th H33.04 Retinal detachment with retinal dialysis
H33.041 Retinal detachment with retinal dialysis, right eye
H33.042 Retinal detachment with retinal dialysis, left eye
H33.043 Retinal detachment with retinal dialysis, bilateral
H33.049 Retinal detachment with retinal dialysis, unspecified eye

✓6th H33.05 Total retinal detachment
H33.051 Total retinal detachment, right eye
H33.052 Total retinal detachment, left eye
H33.053 Total retinal detachment, bilateral
H33.059 Total retinal detachment, unspecified eye

✓5th H33.1 Retinoschisis and retinal cysts
EXCLUDES 1 *congenital retinoschisis (Q14.1)*
microcystoid degeneration of retina (H35.42-)

✓6th H33.10 Unspecified retinoschisis
H33.101 Unspecified retinoschisis, right eye
H33.102 Unspecified retinoschisis, left eye
H33.103 Unspecified retinoschisis, bilateral
H33.109 Unspecified retinoschisis, unspecified eye

✓6th H33.11 Cyst of ora serrata
H33.111 Cyst of ora serrata, right eye
H33.112 Cyst of ora serrata, left eye
H33.113 Cyst of ora serrata, bilateral
H33.119 Cyst of ora serrata, unspecified eye

✓6th H33.12 Parasitic cyst of retina
H33.121 Parasitic cyst of retina, right eye
H33.122 Parasitic cyst of retina, left eye
H33.123 Parasitic cyst of retina, bilateral
H33.129 Parasitic cyst of retina, unspecified eye

✓6th H33.19 Other retinoschisis and retinal cysts
Pseudocyst of retina
H33.191 Other retinoschisis and retinal cysts, right eye
H33.192 Other retinoschisis and retinal cysts, left eye
H33.193 Other retinoschisis and retinal cysts, bilateral
H33.199 Other retinoschisis and retinal cysts, unspecified eye

✓5th H33.2 Serous retinal detachment
Retinal detachment NOS
Retinal detachment without retinal break
EXCLUDES 1 *central serous chorioretinopathy (H35.71-)*
H33.20 Serous retinal detachment, unspecified eye
H33.21 Serous retinal detachment, right eye
H33.22 Serous retinal detachment, left eye
H33.23 Serous retinal detachment, bilateral

✓5th **H33.3 Retinal breaks without detachment**
EXCLUDES1 *chorioretinal scars after surgery for detachment (H59.81-)*
peripheral retinal degeneration without break (H35.4-)
✓6th **H33.30 Unspecified retinal break**
H33.301 Unspecified retinal break, right eye
H33.302 Unspecified retinal break, left eye
H33.303 Unspecified retinal break, bilateral
H33.309 Unspecified retinal break, unspecified eye
✓6th **H33.31 Horseshoe tear of retina without detachment**
Operculum of retina without detachment
H33.311 Horseshoe tear of retina without detachment, right eye
H33.312 Horseshoe tear of retina without detachment, left eye
H33.313 Horseshoe tear of retina without detachment, bilateral
H33.319 Horseshoe tear of retina without detachment, unspecified eye
✓6th **H33.32 Round hole of retina without detachment**
H33.321 Round hole, right eye
H33.322 Round hole, left eye
H33.323 Round hole, bilateral
H33.329 Round hole, unspecified eye
✓6th **H33.33 Multiple defects of retina without detachment**
H33.331 Multiple defects of retina without detachment, right eye
H33.332 Multiple defects of retina without detachment, left eye
H33.333 Multiple defects of retina without detachment, bilateral
H33.339 Multiple defects of retina without detachment, unspecified eye
✓5th **H33.4 Traction detachment of retina**
Proliferative vitreo-retinopathy with retinal detachment
H33.40 Traction detachment of retina, unspecified eye
H33.41 Traction detachment of retina, right eye
H33.42 Traction detachment of retina, left eye
H33.43 Traction detachment of retina, bilateral
H33.8 Other retinal detachments

✓4th **H34 Retinal vascular occlusions**
EXCLUDES1 *amaurosis fugax (G45.3)*
✓5th **H34.0 Transient retinal artery occlusion**
H34.00 Transient retinal artery occlusion, unspecified eye
H34.01 Transient retinal artery occlusion, right eye
H34.02 Transient retinal artery occlusion, left eye
H34.03 Transient retinal artery occlusion, bilateral
✓5th **H34.1 Central retinal artery occlusion**
H34.10 Central retinal artery occlusion, unspecified eye
H34.11 Central retinal artery occlusion, right eye
H34.12 Central retinal artery occlusion, left eye
H34.13 Central retinal artery occlusion, bilateral
✓5th **H34.2 Other retinal artery occlusions**
✓6th **H34.21 Partial retinal artery occlusion**
Hollenhorst's plaque
Retinal microembolism
H34.211 Partial retinal artery occlusion, right eye
H34.212 Partial retinal artery occlusion, left eye
H34.213 Partial retinal artery occlusion, bilateral
H34.219 Partial retinal artery occlusion, unspecified eye
✓6th **H34.23 Retinal artery branch occlusion**
H34.231 Retinal artery branch occlusion, right eye
H34.232 Retinal artery branch occlusion, left eye
H34.233 Retinal artery branch occlusion, bilateral
H34.239 Retinal artery branch occlusion, unspecified eye
✓5th **H34.8 Other retinal vascular occlusions**
✓6th **H34.81 Central retinal vein occlusion**
H34.811 Central retinal vein occlusion, right eye
H34.812 Central retinal vein occlusion, left eye
H34.813 Central retinal vein occlusion, bilateral
H34.819 Central retinal vein occlusion, unspecified eye
✓6th **H34.82 Venous engorgement**
Incipient retinal vein occlusion
Partial retinal vein occlusion
H34.821 Venous engorgement, right eye
H34.822 Venous engorgement, left eye
H34.823 Venous engorgement, bilateral
H34.829 Venous engorgement, unspecified eye
✓6th **H34.83 Tributary (branch) retinal vein occlusion**
H34.831 Tributary (branch) retinal vein occlusion, right eye
H34.832 Tributary (branch) retinal vein occlusion, left eye
H34.833 Tributary (branch) retinal vein occlusion, bilateral
H34.839 Tributary (branch) retinal vein occlusion, unspecified eye
H34.9 Unspecified retinal vascular occlusion

✓4th **H35 Other retinal disorders**
EXCLUDES2 *diabetic retinal disorders (E08.311-E08.359, E09.311-E09.359, E10.311-E10.359, E11.311-E11.359, E13.311-E13.359)*
✓5th **H35.0 Background retinopathy and retinal vascular changes**
Code also any associated hypertension (I10)
H35.00 Unspecified background retinopathy
✓6th **H35.01 Changes in retinal vascular appearance**
Retinal vascular sheathing
H35.011 Changes in retinal vascular appearance, right eye
H35.012 Changes in retinal vascular appearance, left eye
H35.013 Changes in retinal vascular appearance, bilateral
H35.019 Changes in retinal vascular appearance, unspecified eye
✓6th **H35.02 Exudative retinopathy**
Coats retinopathy
H35.021 Exudative retinopathy, right eye
H35.022 Exudative retinopathy, left eye
H35.023 Exudative retinopathy, bilateral
H35.029 Exudative retinopathy, unspecified eye
✓6th **H35.03 Hypertensive retinopathy**
H35.031 Hypertensive retinopathy, right eye
H35.032 Hypertensive retinopathy, left eye
H35.033 Hypertensive retinopathy, bilateral
H35.039 Hypertensive retinopathy, unspecified eye
✓6th **H35.04 Retinal micro-aneurysms, unspecified**
H35.041 Retinal micro-aneurysms, unspecified, right eye
H35.042 Retinal micro-aneurysms, unspecified, left eye
H35.043 Retinal micro-aneurysms, unspecified, bilateral
H35.049 Retinal micro-aneurysms, unspecified, unspecified eye
✓6th **H35.05 Retinal neovascularization, unspecified**
H35.051 Retinal neovascularization, unspecified, right eye
H35.052 Retinal neovascularization, unspecified, left eye
H35.053 Retinal neovascularization, unspecified, bilateral
H35.059 Retinal neovascularization, unspecified, unspecified eye
✓6th **H35.06 Retinal vasculitis**
Eales disease
Retinal perivasculitis
H35.061 Retinal vasculitis, right eye
H35.062 Retinal vasculitis, left eye
H35.063 Retinal vasculitis, bilateral
H35.069 Retinal vasculitis, unspecified eye
✓6th **H35.07 Retinal telangiectasis**
H35.071 Retinal telangiectasis, right eye
H35.072 Retinal telangiectasis, left eye
H35.073 Retinal telangiectasis, bilateral

EXCLUDES1 Not coded here EXCLUDES2 Not included here *Manifestation Code*

H35.079 Retinal telangiectasis, unspecified eye

H35.09 Other intraretinal microvascular abnormalities
Retinal varices

✓5th H35.1 Retinopathy of prematurity

✓6th H35.10 Retinopathy of prematurity, unspecified
Retinopathy of prematurity NOS

H35.101 Retinopathy of prematurity, unspecified, right eye
H35.102 Retinopathy of prematurity, unspecified, left eye
H35.103 Retinopathy of prematurity, unspecified, bilateral
H35.109 Retinopathy of prematurity, unspecified, unspecified eye

✓6th H35.11 Retinopathy of prematurity, stage 0
H35.111 Retinopathy of prematurity, stage 0, right eye
H35.112 Retinopathy of prematurity, stage 0, left eye
H35.113 Retinopathy of prematurity, stage 0, bilateral
H35.119 Retinopathy of prematurity, stage 0, unspecified eye

✓6th H35.12 Retinopathy of prematurity, stage 1
H35.121 Retinopathy of prematurity, stage 1, right eye
H35.122 Retinopathy of prematurity, stage 1, left eye
H35.123 Retinopathy of prematurity, stage 1, bilateral
H35.129 Retinopathy of prematurity, stage 1, unspecified eye

✓6th H35.13 Retinopathy of prematurity, stage 2
H35.131 Retinopathy of prematurity, stage 2, right eye
H35.132 Retinopathy of prematurity, stage 2, left eye
H35.133 Retinopathy of prematurity, stage 2, bilateral
H35.139 Retinopathy of prematurity, stage 2, unspecified eye

✓6th H35.14 Retinopathy of prematurity, stage 3
H35.141 Retinopathy of prematurity, stage 3, right eye
H35.142 Retinopathy of prematurity, stage 3, left eye
H35.143 Retinopathy of prematurity, stage 3, bilateral
H35.149 Retinopathy of prematurity, stage 3, unspecified eye

✓6th H35.15 Retinopathy of prematurity, stage 4
H35.151 Retinopathy of prematurity, stage 4, right eye
H35.152 Retinopathy of prematurity, stage 4, left eye
H35.153 Retinopathy of prematurity, stage 4, bilateral
H35.159 Retinopathy of prematurity, stage 4, unspecified eye

✓6th H35.16 Retinopathy of prematurity, stage 5
H35.161 Retinopathy of prematurity, stage 5, right eye
H35.162 Retinopathy of prematurity, stage 5, left eye
H35.163 Retinopathy of prematurity, stage 5, bilateral
H35.169 Retinopathy of prematurity, stage 5, unspecified eye

✓6th H35.17 Retrolental fibroplasia
H35.171 Retrolental fibroplasia, right eye
H35.172 Retrolental fibroplasia, left eye
H35.173 Retrolental fibroplasia, bilateral
H35.179 Retrolental fibroplasia, unspecified eye

✓5th H35.2 Other non-diabetic proliferative retinopathy
Proliferative vitreo-retinopathy
EXCLUDES 1 *proliferative vitreo-retinopathy with retinal detachment (H33.4-)*

H35.20 Other non-diabetic proliferative retinopathy, unspecified eye
H35.21 Other non-diabetic proliferative retinopathy, right eye
H35.22 Other non-diabetic proliferative retinopathy, left eye
H35.23 Other non-diabetic proliferative retinopathy, bilateral

✓5th H35.3 Degeneration of macula and posterior pole

H35.30 Unspecified macular degeneration
Age-related macular degeneration

H35.31 Nonexudative age-related macular degeneration
Atrophic age-related macular degeneration

H35.32 Exudative age-related macular degeneration

H35.33 Angioid streaks of macula

✓6th H35.34 Macular cyst, hole, or pseudohole
H35.341 Macular cyst, hole, or pseudohole, right eye
H35.342 Macular cyst, hole, or pseudohole, left eye
H35.343 Macular cyst, hole, or pseudohole, bilateral
H35.349 Macular cyst, hole, or pseudohole, unspecified eye

✓6th H35.35 Cystoid macular degeneration
EXCLUDES 1 *cystoid macular edema following cataract surgery (H59.03-)*
H35.351 Cystoid macular degeneration, right eye
H35.352 Cystoid macular degeneration, left eye
H35.353 Cystoid macular degeneration, bilateral
H35.359 Cystoid macular degeneration, unspecified eye

✓6th H35.36 Drusen (degenerative) of macula
H35.361 Drusen (degenerative) of macula, right eye
H35.362 Drusen (degenerative) of macula, left eye
H35.363 Drusen (degenerative) of macula, bilateral
H35.369 Drusen (degenerative) of macula, unspecified eye

✓6th H35.37 Puckering of macula
H35.371 Puckering of macula, right eye
H35.372 Puckering of macula, left eye
H35.373 Puckering of macula, bilateral
H35.379 Puckering of macula, unspecified eye

✓6th H35.38 Toxic maculopathy
Code first poisoning due to drug or toxin, if applicable (T36-T65 with fifth or sixth character 1-4 or 6)
Use additional code for adverse effect, if applicable, to identify drug (T36-T50 with fifth or sixth character 5)
H35.381 Toxic maculopathy, right eye
H35.382 Toxic maculopathy, left eye
H35.383 Toxic maculopathy, bilateral
H35.389 Toxic maculopathy, unspecified eye

✓5th H35.4 Peripheral retinal degeneration
EXCLUDES 1 *hereditary retinal degeneration (dystrophy) (H35.5-)*
peripheral retinal degeneration with retinal break (H33.3-)

H35.40 Unspecified peripheral retinal degeneration

✓6th H35.41 Lattice degeneration of retina
Palisade degeneration of retina
H35.411 Lattice degeneration of retina, right eye
H35.412 Lattice degeneration of retina, left eye
H35.413 Lattice degeneration of retina, bilateral
H35.419 Lattice degeneration of retina, unspecified eye

✓6th H35.42 Microcystoid degeneration of retina
H35.421 Microcystoid degeneration of retina, right eye

✓ Appropriate additional character required ✓x7th Requires 7th character, placeholder x must fill empty characters

H35.422 **Microcystoid degeneration of retina, left eye**

H35.423 **Microcystoid degeneration of retina, bilateral**

H35.429 **Microcystoid degeneration of retina, unspecified eye**

✓6th **H35.43** **Paving stone degeneration of retina**

H35.431 **Paving stone degeneration of retina, right eye**

H35.432 **Paving stone degeneration of retina, left eye**

H35.433 **Paving stone degeneration of retina, bilateral**

H35.439 **Paving stone degeneration of retina, unspecified eye**

✓6th **H35.44** **Age-related reticular degeneration of retina**

H35.441 **Age-related reticular degeneration of retina, right eye**

H35.442 **Age-related reticular degeneration of retina, left eye**

H35.443 **Age-related reticular degeneration of retina, bilateral**

H35.449 **Age-related reticular degeneration of retina, unspecified eye**

✓6th **H35.45** **Secondary pigmentary degeneration**

H35.451 **Secondary pigmentary degeneration, right eye**

H35.452 **Secondary pigmentary degeneration, left eye**

H35.453 **Secondary pigmentary degeneration, bilateral**

H35.459 **Secondary pigmentary degeneration, unspecified eye**

✓6th **H35.46** **Secondary vitreoretinal degeneration**

H35.461 **Secondary vitreoretinal degeneration, right eye**

H35.462 **Secondary vitreoretinal degeneration, left eye**

H35.463 **Secondary vitreoretinal degeneration, bilateral**

H35.469 **Secondary vitreoretinal degeneration, unspecified eye**

✓5th **H35.5** **Hereditary retinal dystrophy**

EXCLUDES 1 *dystrophies primarily involving Bruch's membrane (H31.1-)*

H35.5Ø **Unspecified hereditary retinal dystrophy**

H35.51 **Vitreoretinal dystrophy**

H35.52 **Pigmentary retinal dystrophy**

Albipunctate retinal dystrophy
Retinitis pigmentosa
Tapetoretinal dystrophy

H35.53 **Other dystrophies primarily involving the sensory retina**

Stargardt's disease

H35.54 **Dystrophies primarily involving the retinal pigment epithelium**

Vitelliform retinal dystrophy

✓5th **H35.6** **Retinal hemorrhage**

H35.6Ø **Retinal hemorrhage, unspecified eye**

H35.61 **Retinal hemorrhage, right eye**

H35.62 **Retinal hemorrhage, left eye**

H35.63 **Retinal hemorrhage, bilateral**

✓5th **H35.7** **Separation of retinal layers**

EXCLUDES 1 *retinal detachment (serous) (H33.2-)*
rhegmatogenous retinal detachment (H33.Ø-)

H35.7Ø **Unspecified separation of retinal layers**

✓6th **H35.71** **Central serous chorioretinopathy**

H35.711 **Central serous chorioretinopathy, right eye**

H35.712 **Central serous chorioretinopathy, left eye**

H35.713 **Central serous chorioretinopathy, bilateral**

H35.719 **Central serous chorioretinopathy, unspecified eye**

✓6th **H35.72** **Serous detachment of retinal pigment epithelium**

H35.721 **Serous detachment of retinal pigment epithelium, right eye**

H35.722 **Serous detachment of retinal pigment epithelium, left eye**

H35.723 **Serous detachment of retinal pigment epithelium, bilateral**

H35.729 **Serous detachment of retinal pigment epithelium, unspecified eye**

✓6th **H35.73** **Hemorrhagic detachment of retinal pigment epithelium**

H35.731 **Hemorrhagic detachment of retinal pigment epithelium, right eye**

H35.732 **Hemorrhagic detachment of retinal pigment epithelium, left eye**

H35.733 **Hemorrhagic detachment of retinal pigment epithelium, bilateral**

H35.739 **Hemorrhagic detachment of retinal pigment epithelium, unspecified eye**

✓5th **H35.8** **Other specified retinal disorders**

EXCLUDES 2 *retinal hemorrhage (H35.6-)*

H35.81 **Retinal edema**

Retinal cotton wool spots

H35.82 **Retinal ischemia**

H35.89 **Other specified retinal disorders**

H35.9 **Unspecified retinal disorder**

H36 ***Retinal disorders in diseases classified elsewhere***

Code first underlying disease, such as:
lipid storage disorders (E75.-)
sickle-cell disorders (D57.-)

EXCLUDES 1 *arteriosclerotic retinopathy (H35.Ø-)*
diabetic retinopathy (EØ8.3-, EØ9.3-, E1Ø.3-, E11.3-, E13.3-)

Glaucoma (H4Ø-H42)

✓4th **H4Ø** **Glaucoma**

EXCLUDES 1 *absolute glaucoma (H44.51-)*
congenital glaucoma (Q15.Ø)
traumatic glaucoma due to birth injury (P15.3)

✓5th **H4Ø.Ø** **Glaucoma suspect**

✓6th **H4Ø.ØØ** **Preglaucoma, unspecified**

H4Ø.ØØ1 **Preglaucoma, unspecified, right eye**

H4Ø.ØØ2 **Preglaucoma, unspecified, left eye**

H4Ø.ØØ3 **Preglaucoma, unspecified, bilateral**

H4Ø.ØØ9 **Preglaucoma, unspecified, unspecified eye**

✓6th **H4Ø.Ø1** **Open angle with borderline findings, low risk**

Open angle, low risk

H4Ø.Ø11 **Open angle with borderline findings, low risk, right eye**

H4Ø.Ø12 **Open angle with borderline findings, low risk, left eye**

H4Ø.Ø13 **Open angle with borderline findings, low risk, bilateral**

H4Ø.Ø19 **Open angle with borderline findings, low risk, unspecified eye**

✓6th **H4Ø.Ø2** **Open angle with borderline findings, high risk**

Open angle, high risk

H4Ø.Ø21 **Open angle with borderline findings, high risk, right eye**

H4Ø.Ø22 **Open angle with borderline findings, high risk, left eye**

H4Ø.Ø23 **Open angle with borderline findings, high risk, bilateral**

H4Ø.Ø29 **Open angle with borderline findings, high risk, unspecified eye**

✓6th **H4Ø.Ø3** **Anatomical narrow angle**

Primary angle closure suspect

H4Ø.Ø31 **Anatomical narrow angle, right eye**

H4Ø.Ø32 **Anatomical narrow angle, left eye**

H4Ø.Ø33 **Anatomical narrow angle, bilateral**

H4Ø.Ø39 **Anatomical narrow angle, unspecified eye**

✓6th **H4Ø.Ø4** **Steroid responder**

H4Ø.Ø41 **Steroid responder, right eye**

H4Ø.Ø42 **Steroid responder, left eye**

H4Ø.Ø43 **Steroid responder, bilateral**

H4Ø.Ø49 **Steroid responder, unspecified eye**

✓6th **H4Ø.Ø5** **Ocular hypertension**

H4Ø.Ø51 **Ocular hypertension, right eye**

H40.052 Ocular hypertension, left eye
H40.053 Ocular hypertension, bilateral
H40.059 Ocular hypertension, unspecified eye

✓6th **H40.06 Primary angle closure without glaucoma damage**
H40.061 Primary angle closure without glaucoma damage, right eye
H40.062 Primary angle closure without glaucoma damage, left eye
H40.063 Primary angle closure without glaucoma damage, bilateral
H40.069 Primary angle closure without glaucoma damage, unspecified eye

✓5th **H40.1 Open-angle glaucoma**

One of the following 7th characters is to be assigned to each code in subcategories H40.10, H40.11, H40.12-, H40.13-, and H40.15- to designate the stage of glaucoma.
0 stage unspecified
1 mild stage
2 moderate stage
3 severe stage
4 indeterminate stage

✓x7th **H40.10 Unspecified open-angle glaucoma**
✓x7th **H40.11 Primary open-angle glaucoma**
Chronic simple glaucoma
✓6th **H40.12 Low-tension glaucoma**
✓7th H40.121 Low-tension glaucoma, right eye
✓7th H40.122 Low-tension glaucoma, left eye
✓7th H40.123 Low-tension glaucoma, bilateral
✓7th H40.129 Low-tension glaucoma, unspecified eye
✓6th **H40.13 Pigmentary glaucoma**
✓7th H40.131 Pigmentary glaucoma, right eye
✓7th H40.132 Pigmentary glaucoma, left eye
✓7th H40.133 Pigmentary glaucoma, bilateral
✓7th H40.139 Pigmentary glaucoma, unspecified eye
✓6th **H40.14 Capsular glaucoma with pseudoexfoliation of lens**
H40.141 Capsular glaucoma with pseudoexfoliation of lens, right eye
H40.142 Capsular glaucoma with pseudoexfoliation of lens, left eye
H40.143 Capsular glaucoma with pseudoexfoliation of lens, bilateral
H40.149 Capsular glaucoma with pseudoexfoliation of lens, unspecified eye
✓6th **H40.15 Residual stage of open-angle glaucoma**
✓7th H40.151 Residual stage of open-angle glaucoma, right eye
✓7th H40.152 Residual stage of open-angle glaucoma, left eye
✓7th H40.153 Residual stage of open-angle glaucoma, bilateral
✓7th H40.159 Residual stage of open-angle glaucoma, unspecified eye

✓5th **H40.2 Primary angle-closure glaucoma**

One of the following 7th characters is to be assigned to each code in subcategories H40.20 and H40.22- to designate the stage of glaucoma.
0 stage unspecified
1 mild stage
2 moderate stage
3 severe stage
4 indeterminate stage

EXCLUDES 1 *aqueous misdirection (H40.83-)*
malignant glaucoma (H40.83-)

✓x7th **H40.20 Unspecified primary angle-closure glaucoma**
✓6th **H40.21 Acute angle-closure glaucoma**
Acute angle-closure glaucoma attack
Acute angle-closure glaucoma crisis
H40.211 Acute angle-closure glaucoma, right eye
H40.212 Acute angle-closure glaucoma, left eye
H40.213 Acute angle-closure glaucoma, bilateral
H40.219 Acute angle-closure glaucoma, unspecified eye
✓6th **H40.22 Chronic angle-closure glaucoma**
Chronic primary angle-closure glaucoma
✓7th H40.221 Chronic angle-closure glaucoma, right eye
✓7th H40.222 Chronic angle-closure glaucoma, left eye
✓7th H40.223 Chronic angle-closure glaucoma, bilateral
✓7th H40.229 Chronic angle-closure glaucoma, unspecified eye
✓6th **H40.23 Intermittent angle-closure glaucoma**
H40.231 Intermittent angle-closure glaucoma, right eye
H40.232 Intermittent angle-closure glaucoma, left eye
H40.233 Intermittent angle-closure glaucoma, bilateral
H40.239 Intermittent angle-closure glaucoma, unspecified eye
✓6th **H40.24 Residual stage of angle-closure glaucoma**
H40.241 Residual stage of angle-closure glaucoma, right eye
H40.242 Residual stage of angle-closure glaucoma, left eye
H40.243 Residual stage of angle-closure glaucoma, bilateral
H40.249 Residual stage of angle-closure glaucoma, unspecified eye

✓5th **H40.3 Glaucoma secondary to eye trauma**
Code also underlying condition

One of the following 7th characters is to be assigned to each code in subcategory H40.3- to designate the stage of glaucoma.
0 stage unspecified
1 mild stage
2 moderate stage
3 severe stage
4 indeterminate stage

✓x7th **H40.30 Glaucoma secondary to eye trauma, unspecified eye**
✓x7th **H40.31 Glaucoma secondary to eye trauma, right eye**
✓x7th **H40.32 Glaucoma secondary to eye trauma, left eye**
✓x7th **H40.33 Glaucoma secondary to eye trauma, bilateral**

✓5th **H40.4 Glaucoma secondary to eye inflammation**
Code also underlying condition

One of the following 7th characters is to be assigned to each code in subcategory H40.4- to designate the stage of glaucoma.
0 stage unspecified
1 mild stage
2 moderate stage
3 severe stage
4 indeterminate stage

✓x7th **H40.40 Glaucoma secondary to eye inflammation, unspecified eye**
✓x7th **H40.41 Glaucoma secondary to eye inflammation, right eye**
✓x7th **H40.42 Glaucoma secondary to eye inflammation, left eye**
✓x7th **H40.43 Glaucoma secondary to eye inflammation, bilateral**

✓5th **H40.5 Glaucoma secondary to other eye disorders**
Code also underlying eye disorder

One of the following 7th characters is to be assigned to each code in subcategory H40.5- to designate the stage of glaucoma.
0 stage unspecified
1 mild stage
2 moderate stage
3 severe stage
4 indeterminate stage

✓x7th **H40.50 Glaucoma secondary to other eye disorders, unspecified eye**
✓x7th **H40.51 Glaucoma secondary to other eye disorders, right eye**

✓ Appropriate additional character required
✓x7th Requires 7th character, placeholder x must fill empty characters

√x7th **H40.52 Glaucoma secondary to other eye disorders, left eye**
√x7th **H40.53 Glaucoma secondary to other eye disorders, bilateral**

√5th **H40.6 Glaucoma secondary to drugs**
Use additional code for adverse effect, if applicable, to identify drug (T36-T50 with fifth or sixth character 5)

One of the following 7th characters is to be assigned to each code in subcategory H40.6- to designate the stage of glaucoma.
0 stage unspecified
1 mild stage
2 moderate stage
3 severe stage
4 indeterminate stage

√x7th **H40.60 Glaucoma secondary to drugs, unspecified eye**
√x7th **H40.61 Glaucoma secondary to drugs, right eye**
√x7th **H40.62 Glaucoma secondary to drugs, left eye**
√x7th **H40.63 Glaucoma secondary to drugs, bilateral**

√5th **H40.8 Other glaucoma**
√6th **H40.81 Glaucoma with increased episcleral venous pressure**
H40.811 Glaucoma with increased episcleral venous pressure, right eye
H40.812 Glaucoma with increased episcleral venous pressure, left eye
H40.813 Glaucoma with increased episcleral venous pressure, bilateral
H40.819 Glaucoma with increased episcleral venous pressure, unspecified eye
√6th **H40.82 Hypersecretion glaucoma**
H40.821 Hypersecretion glaucoma, right eye
H40.822 Hypersecretion glaucoma, left eye
H40.823 Hypersecretion glaucoma, bilateral
H40.829 Hypersecretion glaucoma, unspecified eye
√6th **H40.83 Aqueous misdirection**
Malignant glaucoma
H40.831 Aqueous misdirection, right eye
H40.832 Aqueous misdirection, left eye
H40.833 Aqueous misdirection, bilateral
H40.839 Aqueous misdirection, unspecified eye
H40.89 Other specified glaucoma
H40.9 Unspecified glaucoma

H42 Glaucoma in diseases classified elsewhere
Code first underlying condition, such as:
amyloidosis (E85.-)
aniridia (Q13.1)
Lowe's syndrome (E72.03)
Reiger's anomaly (Q13.81)
specified metabolic disorder (E70-E88)
EXCLUDES 1 *glaucoma (in):*
diabetes mellitus (E08.39, E09.39, E10.39, E11.39, E13.39)
onchocerciasis (B73.02)
syphilis (A52.71)
tuberculous (A18.59)

Disorders of vitreous body and globe (H43-H44)

√4th **H43 Disorders of vitreous body**
√5th **H43.0 Vitreous prolapse**
EXCLUDES 1 *vitreous syndrome following cataract surgery (H59.0-)*
traumatic vitreous prolapse (S05.2-)
H43.00 Vitreous prolapse, unspecified eye
H43.01 Vitreous prolapse, right eye
H43.02 Vitreous prolapse, left eye
H43.03 Vitreous prolapse, bilateral
√5th **H43.1 Vitreous hemorrhage**
H43.10 Vitreous hemorrhage, unspecified eye
H43.11 Vitreous hemorrhage, right eye
H43.12 Vitreous hemorrhage, left eye
H43.13 Vitreous hemorrhage, bilateral
√5th **H43.2 Crystalline deposits in vitreous body**
H43.20 Crystalline deposits in vitreous body, unspecified eye
H43.21 Crystalline deposits in vitreous body, right eye
H43.22 Crystalline deposits in vitreous body, left eye
H43.23 Crystalline deposits in vitreous body, bilateral
√5th **H43.3 Other vitreous opacities**
√6th **H43.31 Vitreous membranes and strands**
H43.311 Vitreous membranes and strands, right eye
H43.312 Vitreous membranes and strands, left eye
H43.313 Vitreous membranes and strands, bilateral
H43.319 Vitreous membranes and strands, unspecified eye
√6th **H43.39 Other vitreous opacities**
Vitreous floaters
H43.391 Other vitreous opacities, right eye
H43.392 Other vitreous opacities, left eye
H43.393 Other vitreous opacities, bilateral
H43.399 Other vitreous opacities, unspecified eye
√5th **H43.8 Other disorders of vitreous body**
EXCLUDES 1 *proliferative vitreo-retinopathy with retinal detachment (H33.4-)*
EXCLUDES 2 *vitreous abscess (H44.02-)*
√6th **H43.81 Vitreous degeneration**
Vitreous detachment
H43.811 Vitreous degeneration, right eye
H43.812 Vitreous degeneration, left eye
H43.813 Vitreous degeneration, bilateral
H43.819 Vitreous degeneration, unspecified eye
√6th **H43.82 Vitreomacular adhesion**
Vitreomacular traction
H43.821 Vitreomacular adhesion, right eye
H43.822 Vitreomacular adhesion, left eye
H43.823 Vitreomacular adhesion, bilateral
H43.829 Vitreomacular adhesion, unspecified eye
H43.89 Other disorders of vitreous body
H43.9 Unspecified disorder of vitreous body

√4th **H44 Disorders of globe**
INCLUDES disorders affecting multiple structures of eye
√5th **H44.0 Purulent endophthalmitis**
Use additional code to identify organism
EXCLUDES 1 *bleb associated endophthalmitis (H59.4-)*
√6th **H44.00 Unspecified purulent endophthalmitis**
H44.001 Unspecified purulent endophthalmitis, right eye
H44.002 Unspecified purulent endophthalmitis, left eye
H44.003 Unspecified purulent endophthalmitis, bilateral
H44.009 Unspecified purulent endophthalmitis, unspecified eye
√6th **H44.01 Panophthalmitis (acute)**
H44.011 Panophthalmitis (acute), right eye
H44.012 Panophthalmitis (acute), left eye
H44.013 Panophthalmitis (acute), bilateral
H44.019 Panophthalmitis (acute), unspecified eye
√6th **H44.02 Vitreous abscess (chronic)**
H44.021 Vitreous abscess (chronic), right eye
H44.022 Vitreous abscess (chronic), left eye
H44.023 Vitreous abscess (chronic), bilateral
H44.029 Vitreous abscess (chronic), unspecified eye
√5th **H44.1 Other endophthalmitis**
EXCLUDES 1 *bleb associated endophthalmitis (H59.4-)*
EXCLUDES 2 *ophthalmia nodosa (H16.2-)*
√6th **H44.11 Panuveitis**
H44.111 Panuveitis, right eye
H44.112 Panuveitis, left eye
H44.113 Panuveitis, bilateral
H44.119 Panuveitis, unspecified eye
√6th **H44.12 Parasitic endophthalmitis, unspecified**
H44.121 Parasitic endophthalmitis, unspecified, right eye

H44.122 Parasitic endophthalmitis, unspecified, left eye
H44.123 Parasitic endophthalmitis, unspecified, bilateral
H44.129 Parasitic endophthalmitis, unspecified, unspecified eye

✓6th H44.13 Sympathetic uveitis
H44.131 Sympathetic uveitis, right eye
H44.132 Sympathetic uveitis, left eye
H44.133 Sympathetic uveitis, bilateral
H44.139 Sympathetic uveitis, unspecified eye

H44.19 Other endophthalmitis

✓5th H44.2 Degenerative myopia
Malignant myopia
H44.20 Degenerative myopia, unspecified eye
H44.21 Degenerative myopia, right eye
H44.22 Degenerative myopia, left eye
H44.23 Degenerative myopia, bilateral

✓5th H44.3 Other and unspecified degenerative disorders of globe
H44.30 Unspecified degenerative disorder of globe
✓6th H44.31 Chalcosis
H44.311 Chalcosis, right eye
H44.312 Chalcosis, left eye
H44.313 Chalcosis, bilateral
H44.319 Chalcosis, unspecified eye
✓6th H44.32 Siderosis of eye
H44.321 Siderosis of eye, right eye
H44.322 Siderosis of eye, left eye
H44.323 Siderosis of eye, bilateral
H44.329 Siderosis of eye, unspecified eye
✓6th H44.39 Other degenerative disorders of globe
H44.391 Other degenerative disorders of globe, right eye
H44.392 Other degenerative disorders of globe, left eye
H44.393 Other degenerative disorders of globe, bilateral
H44.399 Other degenerative disorders of globe, unspecified eye

✓5th H44.4 Hypotony of eye
H44.40 Unspecified hypotony of eye
✓6th H44.41 Flat anterior chamber hypotony of eye
H44.411 Flat anterior chamber hypotony of right eye
H44.412 Flat anterior chamber hypotony of left eye
H44.413 Flat anterior chamber hypotony of eye, bilateral
H44.419 Flat anterior chamber hypotony of unspecified eye
✓6th H44.42 Hypotony of eye due to ocular fistula
H44.421 Hypotony of right eye due to ocular fistula
H44.422 Hypotony of left eye due to ocular fistula
H44.423 Hypotony of eye due to ocular fistula, bilateral
H44.429 Hypotony of unspecified eye due to ocular fistula
✓6th H44.43 Hypotony of eye due to other ocular disorders
H44.431 Hypotony of eye due to other ocular disorders, right eye
H44.432 Hypotony of eye due to other ocular disorders, left eye
H44.433 Hypotony of eye due to other ocular disorders, bilateral
H44.439 Hypotony of eye due to other ocular disorders, unspecified eye
✓6th H44.44 Primary hypotony of eye
H44.441 Primary hypotony of right eye
H44.442 Primary hypotony of left eye
H44.443 Primary hypotony of eye, bilateral
H44.449 Primary hypotony of unspecified eye

✓5th H44.5 Degenerated conditions of globe
H44.50 Unspecified degenerated conditions of globe
✓6th H44.51 Absolute glaucoma
H44.511 Absolute glaucoma, right eye
H44.512 Absolute glaucoma, left eye
H44.513 Absolute glaucoma, bilateral
H44.519 Absolute glaucoma, unspecified eye
✓6th H44.52 Atrophy of globe
Phthisis bulbi
H44.521 Atrophy of globe, right eye
H44.522 Atrophy of globe, left eye
H44.523 Atrophy of globe, bilateral
H44.529 Atrophy of globe, unspecified eye
✓6th H44.53 Leucocoria
H44.531 Leucocoria, right eye
H44.532 Leucocoria, left eye
H44.533 Leucocoria, bilateral
H44.539 Leucocoria, unspecified eye

✓5th H44.6 Retained (old) intraocular foreign body, magnetic
Use additional code to identify magnetic foreign body (Z18.11)
EXCLUDES 1 *current intraocular foreign body (S05.-)*
EXCLUDES 2 *retained foreign body in eyelid (H02.81-)*
retained (old) foreign body following penetrating wound of orbit (H05.5-)
retained (old) intraocular foreign body, nonmagnetic (H44.7-)
✓6th H44.60 Unspecified retained (old) intraocular foreign body, magnetic
H44.601 Unspecified retained (old) intraocular foreign body, magnetic, right eye
H44.602 Unspecified retained (old) intraocular foreign body, magnetic, left eye
H44.603 Unspecified retained (old) intraocular foreign body, magnetic, bilateral
H44.609 Unspecified retained (old) intraocular foreign body, magnetic, unspecified eye
✓6th H44.61 Retained (old) magnetic foreign body in anterior chamber
H44.611 Retained (old) magnetic foreign body in anterior chamber, right eye
H44.612 Retained (old) magnetic foreign body in anterior chamber, left eye
H44.613 Retained (old) magnetic foreign body in anterior chamber, bilateral
H44.619 Retained (old) magnetic foreign body in anterior chamber, unspecified eye
✓6th H44.62 Retained (old) magnetic foreign body in iris or ciliary body
H44.621 Retained (old) magnetic foreign body in iris or ciliary body, right eye
H44.622 Retained (old) magnetic foreign body in iris or ciliary body, left eye
H44.623 Retained (old) magnetic foreign body in iris or ciliary body, bilateral
H44.629 Retained (old) magnetic foreign body in iris or ciliary body, unspecified eye
✓6th H44.63 Retained (old) magnetic foreign body in lens
H44.631 Retained (old) magnetic foreign body in lens, right eye
H44.632 Retained (old) magnetic foreign body in lens, left eye
H44.633 Retained (old) magnetic foreign body in lens, bilateral
H44.639 Retained (old) magnetic foreign body in lens, unspecified eye
✓6th H44.64 Retained (old) magnetic foreign body in posterior wall of globe
H44.641 Retained (old) magnetic foreign body in posterior wall of globe, right eye
H44.642 Retained (old) magnetic foreign body in posterior wall of globe, left eye
H44.643 Retained (old) magnetic foreign body in posterior wall of globe, bilateral
H44.649 Retained (old) magnetic foreign body in posterior wall of globe, unspecified eye
✓6th H44.65 Retained (old) magnetic foreign body in vitreous body
H44.651 Retained (old) magnetic foreign body in vitreous body, right eye

H44.652 Retained (old) magnetic foreign body in vitreous body, left eye
H44.653 Retained (old) magnetic foreign body in vitreous body, bilateral
H44.659 Retained (old) magnetic foreign body in vitreous body, unspecified eye

✓6th **H44.69** Retained (old) intraocular foreign body, magnetic, in other or multiple sites
H44.691 Retained (old) intraocular foreign body, magnetic, in other or multiple sites, right eye
H44.692 Retained (old) intraocular foreign body, magnetic, in other or multiple sites, left eye
H44.693 Retained (old) intraocular foreign body, magnetic, in other or multiple sites, bilateral
H44.699 Retained (old) intraocular foreign body, magnetic, in other or multiple sites, unspecified eye

✓5th **H44.7** Retained (old) intraocular foreign body, nonmagnetic
Use additional code to identify nonmagnetic foreign body (Z18.01-Z18.10, Z18.12, Z18.2-Z18.9)
EXCLUDES 1 *current intraocular foreign body (S05.-)*
EXCLUDES 2 *retained foreign body in eyelid (H02.81-)*
retained (old) foreign body following penetrating wound of orbit (H05.5-)
retained (old) intraocular foreign body, magnetic (H44.6-)

✓6th **H44.70** Unspecified retained (old) intraocular foreign body, nonmagnetic
H44.701 Unspecified retained (old) intraocular foreign body, nonmagnetic, right eye
H44.702 Unspecified retained (old) intraocular foreign body, nonmagnetic, left eye
H44.703 Unspecified retained (old) intraocular foreign body, nonmagnetic, bilateral
H44.709 Unspecified retained (old) intraocular foreign body, nonmagnetic, unspecified eye
Retained (old) intraocular foreign body NOS

✓6th **H44.71** Retained (nonmagnetic) (old) foreign body in anterior chamber
H44.711 Retained (nonmagnetic) (old) foreign body in anterior chamber, right eye
H44.712 Retained (nonmagnetic) (old) foreign body in anterior chamber, left eye
H44.713 Retained (nonmagnetic) (old) foreign body in anterior chamber, bilateral
H44.719 Retained (nonmagnetic) (old) foreign body in anterior chamber, unspecified eye

✓6th **H44.72** Retained (nonmagnetic) (old) foreign body in iris or ciliary body
H44.721 Retained (nonmagnetic) (old) foreign body in iris or ciliary body, right eye
H44.722 Retained (nonmagnetic) (old) foreign body in iris or ciliary body, left eye
H44.723 Retained (nonmagnetic) (old) foreign body in iris or ciliary body, bilateral
H44.729 Retained (nonmagnetic) (old) foreign body in iris or ciliary body, unspecified eye

✓6th **H44.73** Retained (nonmagnetic) (old) foreign body in lens
H44.731 Retained (nonmagnetic) (old) foreign body in lens, right eye
H44.732 Retained (nonmagnetic) (old) foreign body in lens, left eye
H44.733 Retained (nonmagnetic) (old) foreign body in lens, bilateral
H44.739 Retained (nonmagnetic) (old) foreign body in lens, unspecified eye

✓6th **H44.74** Retained (nonmagnetic) (old) foreign body in posterior wall of globe
H44.741 Retained (nonmagnetic) (old) foreign body in posterior wall of globe, right eye
H44.742 Retained (nonmagnetic) (old) foreign body in posterior wall of globe, left eye
H44.743 Retained (nonmagnetic) (old) foreign body in posterior wall of globe, bilateral
H44.749 Retained (nonmagnetic) (old) foreign body in posterior wall of globe, unspecified eye

✓6th **H44.75** Retained (nonmagnetic) (old) foreign body in vitreous body
H44.751 Retained (nonmagnetic) (old) foreign body in vitreous body, right eye
H44.752 Retained (nonmagnetic) (old) foreign body in vitreous body, left eye
H44.753 Retained (nonmagnetic) (old) foreign body in vitreous body, bilateral
H44.759 Retained (nonmagnetic) (old) foreign body in vitreous body, unspecified eye

✓6th **H44.79** Retained (old) intraocular foreign body, nonmagnetic, in other or multiple sites
H44.791 Retained (old) intraocular foreign body, nonmagnetic, in other or multiple sites, right eye
H44.792 Retained (old) intraocular foreign body, nonmagnetic, in other or multiple sites, left eye
H44.793 Retained (old) intraocular foreign body, nonmagnetic, in other or multiple sites, bilateral
H44.799 Retained (old) intraocular foreign body, nonmagnetic, in other or multiple sites, unspecified eye

✓5th **H44.8** Other disorders of globe
✓6th **H44.81** Hemophthalmos
H44.811 Hemophthalmos, right eye
H44.812 Hemophthalmos, left eye
H44.813 Hemophthalmos, bilateral
H44.819 Hemophthalmos, unspecified eye

✓6th **H44.82** Luxation of globe
H44.821 Luxation of globe, right eye
H44.822 Luxation of globe, left eye
H44.823 Luxation of globe, bilateral
H44.829 Luxation of globe, unspecified eye

H44.89 Other disorders of globe
H44.9 Unspecified disorder of globe

Disorders of optic nerve and visual pathways (H46-H47)

✓4th **H46 Optic neuritis**
EXCLUDES 2 *ischemic optic neuropathy (H47.01-)*
neuromyelitis optica [Devic] (G36.0)

✓5th **H46.0** Optic papillitis
H46.00 Optic papillitis, unspecified eye
H46.01 Optic papillitis, right eye
H46.02 Optic papillitis, left eye
H46.03 Optic papillitis, bilateral

✓5th **H46.1** Retrobulbar neuritis
Retrobulbar neuritis NOS
EXCLUDES 1 *syphilitic retrobulbar neuritis (A52.15)*
H46.10 Retrobulbar neuritis, unspecified eye
H46.11 Retrobulbar neuritis, right eye
H46.12 Retrobulbar neuritis, left eye
H46.13 Retrobulbar neuritis, bilateral

H46.2 Nutritional optic neuropathy
H46.3 Toxic optic neuropathy
Code first (T51-T65) to identify cause
H46.8 Other optic neuritis
H46.9 Unspecified optic neuritis

✓4th **H47 Other disorders of optic [2nd] nerve and visual pathways**
✓5th **H47.0** Disorders of optic nerve, not elsewhere classified
✓6th **H47.01** Ischemic optic neuropathy
H47.011 Ischemic optic neuropathy, right eye
H47.012 Ischemic optic neuropathy, left eye
H47.013 Ischemic optic neuropathy, bilateral
H47.019 Ischemic optic neuropathy, unspecified eye

✓6th **H47.02** Hemorrhage in optic nerve sheath
H47.021 Hemorrhage in optic nerve sheath, right eye

H47.022 Hemorrhage in optic nerve sheath, left eye
H47.023 Hemorrhage in optic nerve sheath, bilateral
H47.029 Hemorrhage in optic nerve sheath, unspecified eye

✓6th H47.03 Optic nerve hypoplasia
H47.031 Optic nerve hypoplasia, right eye
H47.032 Optic nerve hypoplasia, left eye
H47.033 Optic nerve hypoplasia, bilateral
H47.039 Optic nerve hypoplasia, unspecified eye

✓6th H47.09 Other disorders of optic nerve, not elsewhere classified
Compression of optic nerve
H47.091 Other disorders of optic nerve, not elsewhere classified, right eye
H47.092 Other disorders of optic nerve, not elsewhere classified, left eye
H47.093 Other disorders of optic nerve, not elsewhere classified, bilateral
H47.099 Other disorders of optic nerve, not elsewhere classified, unspecified eye

✓5th H47.1 Papilledema
H47.10 Unspecified papilledema
H47.11 Papilledema associated with increased intracranial pressure
H47.12 Papilledema associated with decreased ocular pressure
H47.13 Papilledema associated with retinal disorder

✓6th H47.14 Foster-Kennedy syndrome
H47.141 Foster-Kennedy syndrome, right eye
H47.142 Foster-Kennedy syndrome, left eye
H47.143 Foster-Kennedy syndrome, bilateral
H47.149 Foster-Kennedy syndrome, unspecified eye

✓5th H47.2 Optic atrophy
H47.20 Unspecified optic atrophy

✓6th H47.21 Primary optic atrophy
H47.211 Primary optic atrophy, right eye
H47.212 Primary optic atrophy, left eye
H47.213 Primary optic atrophy, bilateral
H47.219 Primary optic atrophy, unspecified eye

H47.22 Hereditary optic atrophy
Leber's optic atrophy

✓6th H47.23 Glaucomatous optic atrophy
H47.231 Glaucomatous optic atrophy, right eye
H47.232 Glaucomatous optic atrophy, left eye
H47.233 Glaucomatous optic atrophy, bilateral
H47.239 Glaucomatous optic atrophy, unspecified eye

✓6th H47.29 Other optic atrophy
Temporal pallor of optic disc
H47.291 Other optic atrophy, right eye
H47.292 Other optic atrophy, left eye
H47.293 Other optic atrophy, bilateral
H47.299 Other optic atrophy, unspecified eye

✓5th H47.3 Other disorders of optic disc

✓6th H47.31 Coloboma of optic disc
H47.311 Coloboma of optic disc, right eye
H47.312 Coloboma of optic disc, left eye
H47.313 Coloboma of optic disc, bilateral
H47.319 Coloboma of optic disc, unspecified eye

✓6th H47.32 Drusen of optic disc
H47.321 Drusen of optic disc, right eye
H47.322 Drusen of optic disc, left eye
H47.323 Drusen of optic disc, bilateral
H47.329 Drusen of optic disc, unspecified eye

✓6th H47.33 Pseudopapilledema of optic disc
H47.331 Pseudopapilledema of optic disc, right eye
H47.332 Pseudopapilledema of optic disc, left eye
H47.333 Pseudopapilledema of optic disc, bilateral
H47.339 Pseudopapilledema of optic disc, unspecified eye

✓6th H47.39 Other disorders of optic disc
H47.391 Other disorders of optic disc, right eye
H47.392 Other disorders of optic disc, left eye
H47.393 Other disorders of optic disc, bilateral
H47.399 Other disorders of optic disc, unspecified eye

✓5th H47.4 Disorders of optic chiasm
Code also underlying condition
H47.41 Disorders of optic chiasm in (due to) inflammatory disorders
H47.42 Disorders of optic chiasm in (due to) neoplasm
H47.43 Disorders of optic chiasm in (due to) vascular disorders
H47.49 Disorders of optic chiasm in (due to) other disorders

✓5th H47.5 Disorders of other visual pathways
Disorders of optic tracts, geniculate nuclei and optic radiations
Code also underlying condition

✓6th H47.51 Disorders of visual pathways in (due to) inflammatory disorders
H47.511 Disorders of visual pathways in (due to) inflammatory disorders, right side
H47.512 Disorders of visual pathways in (due to) inflammatory disorders, left side
H47.519 Disorders of visual pathways in (due to) inflammatory disorders, unspecified side

✓6th H47.52 Disorders of visual pathways in (due to) neoplasm
H47.521 Disorders of visual pathways in (due to) neoplasm, right side
H47.522 Disorders of visual pathways in (due to) neoplasm, left side
H47.529 Disorders of visual pathways in (due to) neoplasm, unspecified side

✓6th H47.53 Disorders of visual pathways in (due to) vascular disorders
H47.531 Disorders of visual pathways in (due to) vascular disorders, right side
H47.532 Disorders of visual pathways in (due to) vascular disorders, left side
H47.539 Disorders of visual pathways in (due to) vascular disorders, unspecified side

✓5th H47.6 Disorders of visual cortex
Code also underlying condition
EXCLUDES 1 *injury to visual cortex S04.04*

✓6th H47.61 Cortical blindness
H47.611 Cortical blindness, right side of brain
H47.612 Cortical blindness, left side of brain
H47.619 Cortical blindness, unspecified side of brain

✓6th H47.62 Disorders of visual cortex in (due to) inflammatory disorders
H47.621 Disorders of visual cortex in (due to) inflammatory disorders, right side of brain
H47.622 Disorders of visual cortex in (due to) inflammatory disorders, left side of brain
H47.629 Disorders of visual cortex in (due to) inflammatory disorders, unspecified side of brain

✓6th H47.63 Disorders of visual cortex in (due to) neoplasm
H47.631 Disorders of visual cortex in (due to) neoplasm, right side of brain
H47.632 Disorders of visual cortex in (due to) neoplasm, left side of brain
H47.639 Disorders of visual cortex in (due to) neoplasm, unspecified side of brain

✓6th H47.64 Disorders of visual cortex in (due to) vascular disorders
H47.641 Disorders of visual cortex in (due to) vascular disorders, right side of brain
H47.642 Disorders of visual cortex in (due to) vascular disorders, left side of brain
H47.649 Disorders of visual cortex in (due to) vascular disorders, unspecified side of brain

H47.9 Unspecified disorder of visual pathways

Disorders of ocular muscles, binocular movement, accommodation and refraction (H49-H52)

EXCLUDES 2 *nystagmus and other irregular eye movements (H55)*

✓4th **H49 Paralytic strabismus**

EXCLUDES 2 *internal ophthalmoplegia (H52.51-)*
internuclear ophthalmoplegia (H51.2-)
progressive supranuclear ophthalmoplegia (G23.1)

✓5th **H49.Ø Third [oculomotor] nerve palsy**
H49.ØØ Third [oculomotor] nerve palsy, unspecified eye
H49.Ø1 Third [oculomotor] nerve palsy, right eye
H49.Ø2 Third [oculomotor] nerve palsy, left eye
H49.Ø3 Third [oculomotor] nerve palsy, bilateral

✓5th **H49.1 Fourth [trochlear] nerve palsy**
H49.1Ø Fourth [trochlear] nerve palsy, unspecified eye
H49.11 Fourth [trochlear] nerve palsy, right eye
H49.12 Fourth [trochlear] nerve palsy, left eye
H49.13 Fourth [trochlear] nerve palsy, bilateral

✓5th **H49.2 Sixth [abducent] nerve palsy**
H49.2Ø Sixth [abducent] nerve palsy, unspecified eye
H49.21 Sixth [abducent] nerve palsy, right eye
H49.22 Sixth [abducent] nerve palsy, left eye
H49.23 Sixth [abducent] nerve palsy, bilateral

✓5th **H49.3 Total (external) ophthalmoplegia**
H49.3Ø Total (external) ophthalmoplegia, unspecified eye
H49.31 Total (external) ophthalmoplegia, right eye
H49.32 Total (external) ophthalmoplegia, left eye
H49.33 Total (external) ophthalmoplegia, bilateral

✓5th **H49.4 Progressive external ophthalmoplegia**

EXCLUDES 1 *Kearns-Sayre syndrome (H49.81-)*

H49.4Ø Progressive external ophthalmoplegia, unspecified eye
H49.41 Progressive external ophthalmoplegia, right eye
H49.42 Progressive external ophthalmoplegia, left eye
H49.43 Progressive external ophthalmoplegia, bilateral

✓5th **H49.8 Other paralytic strabismus**

✓6th **H49.81 Kearns-Sayre syndrome**
Progressive external ophthalmoplegia with pigmentary retinopathy
Use additional code for other manifestation, such as: heart block (I45.9)
H49.811 Kearns-Sayre syndrome, right eye
H49.812 Kearns-Sayre syndrome, left eye
H49.813 Kearns-Sayre syndrome, bilateral
H49.819 Kearns-Sayre syndrome, unspecified eye

✓6th **H49.88 Other paralytic strabismus**
External ophthalmoplegia NOS
H49.881 Other paralytic strabismus, right eye
H49.882 Other paralytic strabismus, left eye
H49.883 Other paralytic strabismus, bilateral
H49.889 Other paralytic strabismus, unspecified eye

H49.9 Unspecified paralytic strabismus

✓4th **H5Ø Other strabismus**

✓5th **H5Ø.Ø Esotropia**
Convergent concomitant strabismus

EXCLUDES 1 *intermittent esotropia (H5Ø.31-, H5Ø.32)*

H5Ø.ØØ Unspecified esotropia

✓6th **H5Ø.Ø1 Monocular esotropia**
H5Ø.Ø11 Monocular esotropia, right eye
H5Ø.Ø12 Monocular esotropia, left eye

✓6th **H5Ø.Ø2 Monocular esotropia with A pattern**
H5Ø.Ø21 Monocular esotropia with A pattern, right eye
H5Ø.Ø22 Monocular esotropia with A pattern, left eye

✓6th **H5Ø.Ø3 Monocular esotropia with V pattern**
H5Ø.Ø31 Monocular esotropia with V pattern, right eye
H5Ø.Ø32 Monocular esotropia with V pattern, left eye

✓6th **H5Ø.Ø4 Monocular esotropia with other noncomitancies**
H5Ø.Ø41 Monocular esotropia with other noncomitancies, right eye
H5Ø.Ø42 Monocular esotropia with other noncomitancies, left eye

H5Ø.Ø5 Alternating esotropia
H5Ø.Ø6 Alternating esotropia with A pattern
H5Ø.Ø7 Alternating esotropia with V pattern
H5Ø.Ø8 Alternating esotropia with other noncomitancies

✓5th **H5Ø.1 Exotropia**
Divergent concomitant strabismus

EXCLUDES 1 *intermittent exotropia (H5Ø.33-, H5Ø.34)*

H5Ø.1Ø Unspecified exotropia

✓6th **H5Ø.11 Monocular exotropia**
H5Ø.111 Monocular exotropia, right eye
H5Ø.112 Monocular exotropia, left eye

✓6th **H5Ø.12 Monocular exotropia with A pattern**
H5Ø.121 Monocular exotropia with A pattern, right eye
H5Ø.122 Monocular exotropia with A pattern, left eye

✓6th **H5Ø.13 Monocular exotropia with V pattern**
H5Ø.131 Monocular exotropia with V pattern, right eye
H5Ø.132 Monocular exotropia with V pattern, left eye

✓6th **H5Ø.14 Monocular exotropia with other noncomitancies**
H5Ø.141 Monocular exotropia with other noncomitancies, right eye
H5Ø.142 Monocular exotropia with other noncomitancies, left eye

H5Ø.15 Alternating exotropia
H5Ø.16 Alternating exotropia with A pattern
H5Ø.17 Alternating exotropia with V pattern
H5Ø.18 Alternating exotropia with other noncomitancies

✓5th **H5Ø.2 Vertical strabismus**
Hypertropia
H5Ø.21 Vertical strabismus, right eye
H5Ø.22 Vertical strabismus, left eye

✓5th **H5Ø.3 Intermittent heterotropia**
H5Ø.3Ø Unspecified intermittent heterotropia

✓6th **H5Ø.31 Intermittent monocular esotropia**
H5Ø.311 Intermittent monocular esotropia, right eye
H5Ø.312 Intermittent monocular esotropia, left eye

H5Ø.32 Intermittent alternating esotropia

✓6th **H5Ø.33 Intermittent monocular exotropia**
H5Ø.331 Intermittent monocular exotropia, right eye
H5Ø.332 Intermittent monocular exotropia, left eye

H5Ø.34 Intermittent alternating exotropia

✓5th **H5Ø.4 Other and unspecified heterotropia**
H5Ø.4Ø Unspecified heterotropia

✓6th **H5Ø.41 Cyclotropia**
H5Ø.411 Cyclotropia, right eye
H5Ø.412 Cyclotropia, left eye

H5Ø.42 Monofixation syndrome
H5Ø.43 Accommodative component in esotropia

✓5th **H5Ø.5 Heterophoria**
H5Ø.5Ø Unspecified heterophoria
H5Ø.51 Esophoria
H5Ø.52 Exophoria
H5Ø.53 Vertical heterophoria
H5Ø.54 Cyclophoria
H5Ø.55 Alternating heterophoria

✓5th **H5Ø.6 Mechanical strabismus**
H5Ø.6Ø Mechanical strabismus, unspecified

✓6th **H5Ø.61 Brown's sheath syndrome**
H5Ø.611 Brown's sheath syndrome, right eye
H5Ø.612 Brown's sheath syndrome, left eye

H5Ø.69 Other mechanical strabismus
Strabismus due to adhesions
Traumatic limitation of duction of eye muscle

✓5th **H5Ø.8 Other specified strabismus**

✓6th **H5Ø.81 Duane's syndrome**
H5Ø.811 Duane's syndrome, right eye
H5Ø.812 Duane's syndrome, left eye

H50.89 Other specified strabismus
H50.9 Unspecified strabismus

✓4th **H51 Other disorders of binocular movement**
H51.0 Palsy (spasm) of conjugate gaze
✓5th H51.1 Convergence insufficiency and excess
H51.11 Convergence insufficiency
H51.12 Convergence excess
✓5th H51.2 Internuclear ophthalmoplegia
H51.20 Internuclear ophthalmoplegia, unspecified eye
H51.21 Internuclear ophthalmoplegia, right eye
H51.22 Internuclear ophthalmoplegia, left eye
H51.23 Internuclear ophthalmoplegia, bilateral
H51.8 Other specified disorders of binocular movement
H51.9 Unspecified disorder of binocular movement

✓4th **H52 Disorders of refraction and accommodation**
✓5th H52.0 Hypermetropia
H52.00 Hypermetropia, unspecified eye
H52.01 Hypermetropia, right eye
H52.02 Hypermetropia, left eye
H52.03 Hypermetropia, bilateral
✓5th H52.1 Myopia
EXCLUDES 1 *degenerative myopia (H44.2-)*
H52.10 Myopia, unspecified eye
H52.11 Myopia, right eye
H52.12 Myopia, left eye
H52.13 Myopia, bilateral
✓5th H52.2 Astigmatism
✓6th H52.20 Unspecified astigmatism
H52.201 Unspecified astigmatism, right eye
H52.202 Unspecified astigmatism, left eye
H52.203 Unspecified astigmatism, bilateral
H52.209 Unspecified astigmatism, unspecified eye
✓6th H52.21 Irregular astigmatism
H52.211 Irregular astigmatism, right eye
H52.212 Irregular astigmatism, left eye
H52.213 Irregular astigmatism, bilateral
H52.219 Irregular astigmatism, unspecified eye
✓6th H52.22 Regular astigmatism
H52.221 Regular astigmatism, right eye
H52.222 Regular astigmatism, left eye
H52.223 Regular astigmatism, bilateral
H52.229 Regular astigmatism, unspecified eye
✓5th H52.3 Anisometropia and aniseikonia
H52.31 Anisometropia
H52.32 Aniseikonia
H52.4 Presbyopia
✓5th H52.5 Disorders of accommodation
✓6th H52.51 Internal ophthalmoplegia (complete) (total)
H52.511 Internal ophthalmoplegia (complete) (total), right eye
H52.512 Internal ophthalmoplegia (complete) (total), left eye
H52.513 Internal ophthalmoplegia (complete) (total), bilateral
H52.519 Internal ophthalmoplegia (complete) (total), unspecified eye
✓6th H52.52 Paresis of accommodation
H52.521 Paresis of accommodation, right eye
H52.522 Paresis of accommodation, left eye
H52.523 Paresis of accommodation, bilateral
H52.529 Paresis of accommodation, unspecified eye
✓6th H52.53 Spasm of accommodation
H52.531 Spasm of accommodation, right eye
H52.532 Spasm of accommodation, left eye
H52.533 Spasm of accommodation, bilateral
H52.539 Spasm of accommodation, unspecified eye
H52.6 Other disorders of refraction
H52.7 Unspecified disorder of refraction

Visual disturbances and blindness (H53-H54)

✓4th **H53 Visual disturbances**
✓5th H53.0 Amblyopia ex anopsia
EXCLUDES 1 *amblyopia due to vitamin A deficiency (E50.5)*
✓6th H53.00 Unspecified amblyopia
H53.001 Unspecified amblyopia, right eye
H53.002 Unspecified amblyopia, left eye
H53.003 Unspecified amblyopia, bilateral
H53.009 Unspecified amblyopia, unspecified eye
✓6th H53.01 Deprivation amblyopia
H53.011 Deprivation amblyopia, right eye
H53.012 Deprivation amblyopia, left eye
H53.013 Deprivation amblyopia, bilateral
H53.019 Deprivation amblyopia, unspecified eye
✓6th H53.02 Refractive amblyopia
H53.021 Refractive amblyopia, right eye
H53.022 Refractive amblyopia, left eye
H53.023 Refractive amblyopia, bilateral
H53.029 Refractive amblyopia, unspecified eye
✓6th H53.03 Strabismic amblyopia
EXCLUDES 1 *strabismus (H50.-)*
H53.031 Strabismic amblyopia, right eye
H53.032 Strabismic amblyopia, left eye
H53.033 Strabismic amblyopia, bilateral
H53.039 Strabismic amblyopia, unspecified eye
✓5th H53.1 Subjective visual disturbances
EXCLUDES 1 *subjective visual disturbances due to vitamin A deficiency (E50.5)*
visual hallucinations (R44.1)
H53.10 Unspecified subjective visual disturbances
H53.11 Day blindness
Hemeralopia
✓6th H53.12 Transient visual loss
Scintillating scotoma
EXCLUDES 1 *amaurosis fugax (G45.3-)*
transient retinal artery occlusion (H34.0-)
H53.121 Transient visual loss, right eye
H53.122 Transient visual loss, left eye
H53.123 Transient visual loss, bilateral
H53.129 Transient visual loss, unspecified eye
✓6th H53.13 Sudden visual loss
H53.131 Sudden visual loss, right eye
H53.132 Sudden visual loss, left eye
H53.133 Sudden visual loss, bilateral
H53.139 Sudden visual loss, unspecified eye
✓6th H53.14 Visual discomfort
Asthenopia
Photophobia
H53.141 Visual discomfort, right eye
H53.142 Visual discomfort, left eye
H53.143 Visual discomfort, bilateral
H53.149 Visual discomfort, unspecified
H53.15 Visual distortions of shape and size
Metamorphopsia
H53.16 Psychophysical visual disturbances
H53.19 Other subjective visual disturbances
Visual halos
H53.2 Diplopia
Double vision
✓5th H53.3 Other and unspecified disorders of binocular vision
H53.30 Unspecified disorder of binocular vision
H53.31 Abnormal retinal correspondence
H53.32 Fusion with defective stereopsis
H53.33 Simultaneous visual perception without fusion
H53.34 Suppression of binocular vision
✓5th H53.4 Visual field defects
H53.40 Unspecified visual field defects
✓6th H53.41 Scotoma involving central area
Central scotoma
H53.411 Scotoma involving central area, right eye
H53.412 Scotoma involving central area, left eye
H53.413 Scotoma involving central area, bilateral

H53.419 Scotoma involving central area, unspecified eye

✓6th **H53.42 Scotoma of blind spot area**
Enlarged blind spot
H53.421 Scotoma of blind spot area, right eye
H53.422 Scotoma of blind spot area, left eye
H53.423 Scotoma of blind spot area, bilateral
H53.429 Scotoma of blind spot area, unspecified eye

✓6th **H53.43 Sector or arcuate defects**
Arcuate scotoma
Bjerrum scotoma
H53.431 Sector or arcuate defects, right eye
H53.432 Sector or arcuate defects, left eye
H53.433 Sector or arcuate defects, bilateral
H53.439 Sector or arcuate defects, unspecified eye

✓6th **H53.45 Other localized visual field defect**
Peripheral visual field defect
Ring scotoma NOS
Scotoma NOS
H53.451 Other localized visual field defect, right eye
H53.452 Other localized visual field defect, left eye
H53.453 Other localized visual field defect, bilateral
H53.459 Other localized visual field defect, unspecified eye

✓6th **H53.46 Homonymous bilateral field defects**
Homonymous hemianop(s)ia
Quadrant anop(s)ia
H53.461 Homonymous bilateral field defects, right side
H53.462 Homonymous bilateral field defects, left side
H53.469 Homonymous bilateral field defects, unspecified side
Homonymous bilateral field defects NOS

H53.47 Heteronymous bilateral field defects
Heteronymous hemianop(s)ia

✓6th **H53.48 Generalized contraction of visual field**
H53.481 Generalized contraction of visual field, right eye
H53.482 Generalized contraction of visual field, left eye
H53.483 Generalized contraction of visual field, bilateral
H53.489 Generalized contraction of visual field, unspecified eye

✓5th **H53.5 Color vision deficiencies**
Color blindness
EXCLUDES 2 *day blindness (H53.11)*
H53.50 Unspecified color vision deficiencies
Color blindness NOS
H53.51 Achromatopsia
H53.52 Acquired color vision deficiency
H53.53 Deuteranomaly
Deuteranopia
H53.54 Protanomaly
Protanopia
H53.55 Tritanomaly
Tritanopia
H53.59 Other color vision deficiencies

✓5th **H53.6 Night blindness**
EXCLUDES 1 *night blindness due to vitamin A deficiency (E50.5)*
H53.60 Unspecified night blindness
H53.61 Abnormal dark adaptation curve
H53.62 Acquired night blindness
H53.63 Congenital night blindness
H53.69 Other night blindness

✓5th **H53.7 Vision sensitivity deficiencies**
H53.71 Glare sensitivity
H53.72 Impaired contrast sensitivity

H53.8 Other visual disturbances

H53.9 Unspecified visual disturbance

✓4th **H54 Blindness and low vision**
NOTE For definition of visual impairment categories see table below
Code first any associated underlying cause of the blindness
EXCLUDES 1 *amaurosis fugax (G45.3)*

H54.0 Blindness, both eyes
Visual impairment categories 3, 4, 5 in both eyes.

✓5th **H54.1 Blindness, one eye, low vision other eye**
Visual impairment categories 3, 4, 5 in one eye, with categories 1 or 2 in the other eye.
H54.10 Blindness, one eye, low vision other eye, unspecified eyes
H54.11 Blindness, right eye, low vision left eye
H54.12 Blindness, left eye, low vision right eye

H54.2 Low vision, both eyes
Visual impairment categories 1 or 2 in both eyes.

H54.3 Unqualified visual loss, both eyes
Visual impairment category 9 in both eyes.

✓5th **H54.4 Blindness, one eye**
Visual impairment categories 3, 4, 5 in one eye [normal vision in other eye]
H54.40 Blindness, one eye, unspecified eye
H54.41 Blindness, right eye, normal vision left eye
H54.42 Blindness, left eye, normal vision right eye

✓5th **H54.5 Low vision, one eye**
Visual impairment categories 1 or 2 in one eye [normal vision in other eye].
H54.50 Low vision, one eye, unspecified eye
H54.51 Low vision, right eye, normal vision left eye
H54.52 Low vision, left eye, normal vision right eye

✓5th **H54.6 Unqualified visual loss, one eye**
Visual impairment category 9 in one eye [normal vision in other eye].
H54.60 Unqualified visual loss, one eye, unspecified
H54.61 Unqualified visual loss, right eye, normal vision left eye
H54.62 Unqualified visual loss, left eye, normal vision right eye

H54.7 Unspecified visual loss
Visual impairment category 9 NOS

H54.8 Legal blindness, as defined in USA
Blindness NOS according to USA definition
EXCLUDES 1 *legal blindness with specification of impairment level (H54.0-H54.7)*

NOTE The following table gives a classification of severity of visual impairment recommended by a WHO Study Group on the Prevention of Blindness, Geneva, 6-10 November I972.

The term "low vision" in category H54 comprises categories 1 and 2 of the table, the term "blindness" categories 3, 4 and 5, and the term "unqualified visual loss" category 9.

If the extent of the visual field is taken into account, patients with a field no greater than 10 but greater than 5 around central fixation should be placed in category 3 and patients with a field no greater than 5 around central fixation should be placed in category 4, even if the central acuity is not impaired.

Category of visual impairment	Visual acuity with best possible correction	
	Maximum less than:	Minimum equal to or better than:
1	6/18 3/10 (0.3) 20/70	6/60 1/10 (0.1) 20/200
2	6/60 1/10 (0.1) 20/200	3/60 1/20 (0.5) 20/400
3	3/60 1/20 (0.05) 20/400	1/60 (finger counting at one meter) 1/50 (0.02) 5/300 (20/1200)
4	1/60 (finger counting at one meter) 1/50 (0.02) 5/300	Light perception
5	No light perception	
9	Undetermined or unspecified	

Other disorders of eye and adnexa (H55-H59)

✓4th H55 Nystagmus and other irregular eye movements

- ✓5th **H55.0 Nystagmus**
  - **H55.00 Unspecified nystagmus**
  - **H55.01 Congenital nystagmus**
  - **H55.02 Latent nystagmus**
  - **H55.03 Visual deprivation nystagmus**
  - **H55.04 Dissociated nystagmus**
  - **H55.09 Other forms of nystagmus**
- ✓5th **H55.8 Other irregular eye movements**
  - **H55.81 Saccadic eye movements**
  - **H55.89 Other irregular eye movements**

✓4th H57 Other disorders of eye and adnexa

- ✓5th **H57.0 Anomalies of pupillary function**
  - **H57.00 Unspecified anomaly of pupillary function**
  - **H57.01 Argyll Robertson pupil, atypical**
    - EXCLUDES 1 *syphilitic Argyll Robertson pupil (A52.19)*
  - **H57.02 Anisocoria**
  - **H57.03 Miosis**
  - **H57.04 Mydriasis**
  - ✓6th **H57.05 Tonic pupil**
    - **H57.051 Tonic pupil, right eye**
    - **H57.052 Tonic pupil, left eye**
    - **H57.053 Tonic pupil, bilateral**
    - **H57.059 Tonic pupil, unspecified eye**
  - **H57.09 Other anomalies of pupillary function**
- ✓5th **H57.1 Ocular pain**
  - **H57.10 Ocular pain, unspecified eye**
  - **H57.11 Ocular pain, right eye**
  - **H57.12 Ocular pain, left eye**
  - **H57.13 Ocular pain, bilateral**
- **H57.8 Other specified disorders of eye and adnexa**
- **H57.9 Unspecified disorder of eye and adnexa**

✓4th H59 Intraoperative and postprocedural complications and disorders of eye and adnexa, not elsewhere classified

EXCLUDES 1 *mechanical complication of intraocular lens (T85.2)*
mechanical complication of other ocular prosthetic devices, implants and grafts (T85.3)
pseudophakia (Z96.1)
secondary cataracts (H26.4-)

- ✓5th **H59.0 Disorders of the eye following cataract surgery**
  - ✓6th **H59.01 Keratopathy (bullous aphakic) following cataract surgery**
    - Vitreal corneal syndrome
    - Vitreous (touch) syndrome
    - **H59.011 Keratopathy (bullous aphakic) following cataract surgery, right eye**
    - **H59.012 Keratopathy (bullous aphakic) following cataract surgery, left eye**
    - **H59.013 Keratopathy (bullous aphakic) following cataract surgery, bilateral**
    - **H59.019 Keratopathy (bullous aphakic) following cataract surgery, unspecified eye**
  - ✓6th **H59.02 Cataract (lens) fragments in eye following cataract surgery**
    - **H59.021 Cataract (lens) fragments in eye following cataract surgery, right eye**
    - **H59.022 Cataract (lens) fragments in eye following cataract surgery, left eye**
    - **H59.023 Cataract (lens) fragments in eye following cataract surgery, bilateral**
    - **H59.029 Cataract (lens) fragments in eye following cataract surgery, unspecified eye**
  - ✓6th **H59.03 Cystoid macular edema following cataract surgery**
    - **H59.031 Cystoid macular edema following cataract surgery, right eye**
    - **H59.032 Cystoid macular edema following cataract surgery, left eye**
    - **H59.033 Cystoid macular edema following cataract surgery, bilateral**
    - **H59.039 Cystoid macular edema following cataract surgery, unspecified eye**
  - ✓6th **H59.09 Other disorders of the eye following cataract surgery**
    - **H59.091 Other disorders of the right eye following cataract surgery**
    - **H59.092 Other disorders of the left eye following cataract surgery**
    - **H59.093 Other disorders of the eye following cataract surgery, bilateral**
    - **H59.099 Other disorders of unspecified eye following cataract surgery**
- ✓5th **H59.1 Intraoperative hemorrhage and hematoma of eye and adnexa complicating a procedure**
  - EXCLUDES 1 *intraoperative hemorrhage and hematoma of eye and adnexa due to accidental puncture or laceration during a procedure (H59.2-)*
  - ✓6th **H59.11 Intraoperative hemorrhage and hematoma of eye and adnexa complicating an ophthalmic procedure**
    - **H59.111 Intraoperative hemorrhage and hematoma of right eye and adnexa complicating an ophthalmic procedure**
    - **H59.112 Intraoperative hemorrhage and hematoma of left eye and adnexa complicating an ophthalmic procedure**
    - **H59.113 Intraoperative hemorrhage and hematoma of eye and adnexa complicating an ophthalmic procedure, bilateral**
    - **H59.119 Intraoperative hemorrhage and hematoma of unspecified eye and adnexa complicating an ophthalmic procedure**
  - ✓6th **H59.12 Intraoperative hemorrhage and hematoma of eye and adnexa complicating other procedure**
    - **H59.121 Intraoperative hemorrhage and hematoma of right eye and adnexa complicating other procedure**
    - **H59.122 Intraoperative hemorrhage and hematoma of left eye and adnexa complicating other procedure**
    - **H59.123 Intraoperative hemorrhage and hematoma of eye and adnexa complicating other procedure, bilateral**
    - **H59.129 Intraoperative hemorrhage and hematoma of unspecified eye and adnexa complicating other procedure**
- ✓5th **H59.2 Accidental puncture and laceration of eye and adnexa during a procedure**
  - ✓6th **H59.21 Accidental puncture and laceration of eye and adnexa during an ophthalmic procedure**
    - **H59.211 Accidental puncture and laceration of right eye and adnexa during an ophthalmic procedure**
    - **H59.212 Accidental puncture and laceration of left eye and adnexa during an ophthalmic procedure**
    - **H59.213 Accidental puncture and laceration of eye and adnexa during an ophthalmic procedure, bilateral**
    - **H59.219 Accidental puncture and laceration of unspecified eye and adnexa during an ophthalmic procedure**
  - ✓6th **H59.22 Accidental puncture and laceration of eye and adnexa during other procedure**
    - **H59.221 Accidental puncture and laceration of right eye and adnexa during other procedure**
    - **H59.222 Accidental puncture and laceration of left eye and adnexa during other procedure**
    - **H59.223 Accidental puncture and laceration of eye and adnexa during other procedure, bilateral**
    - **H59.229 Accidental puncture and laceration of unspecified eye and adnexa during other procedure**

H59.3 Postprocedural hemorrhage and hematoma of eye and adnexa following a procedure

H59.31 Postprocedural hemorrhage and hematoma of eye and adnexa following an ophthalmic procedure

H59.311 Postprocedural hemorrhage and hematoma of right eye and adnexa following an ophthalmic procedure

H59.312 Postprocedural hemorrhage and hematoma of left eye and adnexa following an ophthalmic procedure

H59.313 Postprocedural hemorrhage and hematoma of eye and adnexa following an ophthalmic procedure, bilateral

H59.319 Postprocedural hemorrhage and hematoma of unspecified eye and adnexa following an ophthalmic procedure

H59.32 Postprocedural hemorrhage and hematoma of eye and adnexa following other procedure

H59.321 Postprocedural hemorrhage and hematoma of right eye and adnexa following other procedure

H59.322 Postprocedural hemorrhage and hematoma of left eye and adnexa following other procedure

H59.323 Postprocedural hemorrhage and hematoma of eye and adnexa following other procedure, bilateral

H59.329 Postprocedural hemorrhage and hematoma of unspecified eye and adnexa following other procedure

H59.4 Inflammation (infection) of postprocedural bleb

Postprocedural blebitis

EXCLUDES1 *filtering (vitreous) bleb after glaucoma surgery status (Z98.83)*

H59.40 Inflammation (infection) of postprocedural bleb, unspecified

H59.41 Inflammation (infection) of postprocedural bleb, stage 1

H59.42 Inflammation (infection) of postprocedural bleb, stage 2

H59.43 Inflammation (infection) of postprocedural bleb, stage 3

Bleb endophthalmitis

H59.8 Other intraoperative and postprocedural complications and disorders of eye and adnexa, not elsewhere classified

H59.81 Chorioretinal scars after surgery for detachment

H59.811 Chorioretinal scars after surgery for detachment, right eye

H59.812 Chorioretinal scars after surgery for detachment, left eye

H59.813 Chorioretinal scars after surgery for detachment, bilateral

H59.819 Chorioretinal scars after surgery for detachment, unspecified eye

H59.88 Other intraoperative complications of eye and adnexa, not elsewhere classified

H59.89 Other postprocedural complications and disorders of eye and adnexa, not elsewhere classified

Chapter 8. Diseases of the Ear and Mastoid Process (H60-H95)

NOTE Use an external cause code following the code for the ear condition, if applicable, to identify the cause of the ear condition

EXCLUDES 2 *certain conditions originating in the perinatal period (P04-P96)*
certain infectious and parasitic diseases (A00-B99)
complications of pregnancy, childbirth and the puerperium (O00-O9A)
congenital malformations, deformations and chromosomal abnormalities (Q00-Q99)
endocrine, nutritional and metabolic diseases (E00-E88)
injury, poisoning and certain other consequences of external causes (S00-T88)
neoplasms (C00-D49)
symptoms, signs and abnormal clinical and laboratory findings, not elsewhere classified (R00-R94)

This chapter contains the following blocks:

H60-H62 Diseases of external ear
H65-H75 Diseases of middle ear and mastoid
H80-H83 Diseases of inner ear
H90-H94 Other disorders of ear
H95 Intraoperative and postprocedural complications and disorders of ear and mastoid process, not elsewhere classified

Diseases of external ear (H60-H62)

✓4th **H60 Otitis externa**

✓5th **H60.0 Abscess of external ear**
Boil of external ear
Carbuncle of auricle or external auditory canal
Furuncle of external ear
H60.00 Abscess of external ear, unspecified ear
H60.01 Abscess of right external ear
H60.02 Abscess of left external ear
H60.03 Abscess of external ear, bilateral

✓5th **H60.1 Cellulitis of external ear**
Cellulitis of auricle
Cellulitis of external auditory canal
H60.10 Cellulitis of external ear, unspecified ear
H60.11 Cellulitis of right external ear
H60.12 Cellulitis of left external ear
H60.13 Cellulitis of external ear, bilateral

✓5th **H60.2 Malignant otitis externa**
H60.20 Malignant otitis externa, unspecified ear
H60.21 Malignant otitis externa, right ear
H60.22 Malignant otitis externa, left ear
H60.23 Malignant otitis externa, bilateral

✓5th **H60.3 Other infective otitis externa**
✓6th **H60.31 Diffuse otitis externa**
H60.311 Diffuse otitis externa, right ear
H60.312 Diffuse otitis externa, left ear
H60.313 Diffuse otitis externa, bilateral
H60.319 Diffuse otitis externa, unspecified ear
✓6th **H60.32 Hemorrhagic otitis externa**
H60.321 Hemorrhagic otitis externa, right ear
H60.322 Hemorrhagic otitis externa, left ear
H60.323 Hemorrhagic otitis externa, bilateral
H60.329 Hemorrhagic otitis externa, unspecified ear
✓6th **H60.33 Swimmer's ear**
H60.331 Swimmer's ear, right ear
H60.332 Swimmer's ear, left ear
H60.333 Swimmer's ear, bilateral
H60.339 Swimmer's ear, unspecified ear
✓6th **H60.39 Other infective otitis externa**
H60.391 Other infective otitis externa, right ear
H60.392 Other infective otitis externa, left ear
H60.393 Other infective otitis externa, bilateral
H60.399 Other infective otitis externa, unspecified ear

✓5th **H60.4 Cholesteatoma of external ear**
Keratosis obturans of external ear (canal)
EXCLUDES 2 *cholesteatoma of middle ear (H71.-)*
recurrent cholesteatoma of postmastoidectomy cavity (H95.0-)
H60.40 Cholesteatoma of external ear, unspecified ear
H60.41 Cholesteatoma of right external ear
H60.42 Cholesteatoma of left external ear
H60.43 Cholesteatoma of external ear, bilateral

✓5th **H60.5 Acute noninfective otitis externa**
✓6th **H60.50 Unspecified acute noninfective otitis externa**
Acute otitis externa NOS
H60.501 Unspecified acute noninfective otitis externa, right ear
H60.502 Unspecified acute noninfective otitis externa, left ear
H60.503 Unspecified acute noninfective otitis externa, bilateral
H60.509 Unspecified acute noninfective otitis externa, unspecified ear
✓6th **H60.51 Acute actinic otitis externa**
H60.511 Acute actinic otitis externa, right ear
H60.512 Acute actinic otitis externa, left ear
H60.513 Acute actinic otitis externa, bilateral
H60.519 Acute actinic otitis externa, unspecified ear
✓6th **H60.52 Acute chemical otitis externa**
H60.521 Acute chemical otitis externa, right ear
H60.522 Acute chemical otitis externa, left ear
H60.523 Acute chemical otitis externa, bilateral
H60.529 Acute chemical otitis externa, unspecified ear
✓6th **H60.53 Acute contact otitis externa**
H60.531 Acute contact otitis externa, right ear
H60.532 Acute contact otitis externa, left ear
H60.533 Acute contact otitis externa, bilateral
H60.539 Acute contact otitis externa, unspecified ear
✓6th **H60.54 Acute eczematoid otitis externa**
H60.541 Acute eczematoid otitis externa, right ear
H60.542 Acute eczematoid otitis externa, left ear
H60.543 Acute eczematoid otitis externa, bilateral
H60.549 Acute eczematoid otitis externa, unspecified ear
✓6th **H60.55 Acute reactive otitis externa**
H60.551 Acute reactive otitis externa, right ear
H60.552 Acute reactive otitis externa, left ear
H60.553 Acute reactive otitis externa, bilateral
H60.559 Acute reactive otitis externa, unspecified ear
✓6th **H60.59 Other noninfective acute otitis externa**
H60.591 Other noninfective acute otitis externa, right ear
H60.592 Other noninfective acute otitis externa, left ear
H60.593 Other noninfective acute otitis externa, bilateral
H60.599 Other noninfective acute otitis externa, unspecified ear

✓5th **H60.6 Unspecified chronic otitis externa**
H60.60 Unspecified chronic otitis externa, unspecified ear
H60.61 Unspecified chronic otitis externa, right ear
H60.62 Unspecified chronic otitis externa, left ear
H60.63 Unspecified chronic otitis externa, bilateral

✓5th **H60.8 Other otitis externa**
✓6th **H60.8X Other otitis externa**
H60.8X1 Other otitis externa, right ear
H60.8X2 Other otitis externa, left ear
H60.8X3 Other otitis externa, bilateral
H60.8X9 Other otitis externa, unspecified ear

✓5th **H60.9 Unspecified otitis externa**
H60.90 Unspecified otitis externa, unspecified ear
H60.91 Unspecified otitis externa, right ear
H60.92 Unspecified otitis externa, left ear
H60.93 Unspecified otitis externa, bilateral

4th H61 Other disorders of external ear

5th H61.0 Chondritis and perichondritis of external ear
Chondrodermatitis nodularis chronica helicis
Perichondritis of auricle
Perichondritis of pinna

6th H61.00 Unspecified perichondritis of external ear
- **H61.001 Unspecified perichondritis of right external ear**
- **H61.002 Unspecified perichondritis of left external ear**
- **H61.003 Unspecified perichondritis of external ear, bilateral**
- **H61.009 Unspecified perichondritis of external ear, unspecified ear**

6th H61.01 Acute perichondritis of external ear
- **H61.011 Acute perichondritis of right external ear**
- **H61.012 Acute perichondritis of left external ear**
- **H61.013 Acute perichondritis of external ear, bilateral**
- **H61.019 Acute perichondritis of external ear, unspecified ear**

6th H61.02 Chronic perichondritis of external ear
- **H61.021 Chronic perichondritis of right external ear**
- **H61.022 Chronic perichondritis of left external ear**
- **H61.023 Chronic perichondritis of external ear, bilateral**
- **H61.029 Chronic perichondritis of external ear, unspecified ear**

6th H61.03 Chondritis of external ear
Chondritis of auricle
Chondritis of pinna
- **H61.031 Chondritis of right external ear**
- **H61.032 Chondritis of left external ear**
- **H61.033 Chondritis of external ear, bilateral**
- **H61.039 Chondritis of external ear, unspecified ear**

5th H61.1 Noninfective disorders of pinna
EXCLUDES 2 *cauliflower ear (M95.1-)*
gouty tophi of ear (M1A.-, M10.-)

6th H61.10 Unspecified noninfective disorders of pinna
Disorder of pinna NOS
- **H61.101 Unspecified noninfective disorders of pinna, right ear**
- **H61.102 Unspecified noninfective disorders of pinna, left ear**
- **H61.103 Unspecified noninfective disorders of pinna, bilateral**
- **H61.109 Unspecified noninfective disorders of pinna, unspecified ear**

6th H61.11 Acquired deformity of pinna
Acquired deformity of auricle
EXCLUDES 2 *cauliflower ear (M95.1-)*
- **H61.111 Acquired deformity of pinna, right ear**
- **H61.112 Acquired deformity of pinna, left ear**
- **H61.113 Acquired deformity of pinna, bilateral**
- **H61.119 Acquired deformity of pinna, unspecified ear**

6th H61.12 Hematoma of pinna
Hematoma of auricle
- **H61.121 Hematoma of pinna, right ear**
- **H61.122 Hematoma of pinna, left ear**
- **H61.123 Hematoma of pinna, bilateral**
- **H61.129 Hematoma of pinna, unspecified ear**

6th H61.19 Other noninfective disorders of pinna
- **H61.191 Noninfective disorders of pinna, right ear**
- **H61.192 Noninfective disorders of pinna, left ear**
- **H61.193 Noninfective disorders of pinna, bilateral**
- **H61.199 Noninfective disorders of pinna, unspecified ear**

5th H61.2 Impacted cerumen
Wax in ear
- **H61.20 Impacted cerumen, unspecified ear**
- **H61.21 Impacted cerumen, right ear**
- **H61.22 Impacted cerumen, left ear**
- **H61.23 Impacted cerumen, bilateral**

5th H61.3 Acquired stenosis of external ear canal
Collapse of external ear canal
EXCLUDES 1 *postprocedural stenosis of external ear canal (H95.81-)*

6th H61.30 Acquired stenosis of external ear canal, unspecified
- **H61.301 Acquired stenosis of right external ear canal, unspecified**
- **H61.302 Acquired stenosis of left external ear canal, unspecified**
- **H61.303 Acquired stenosis of external ear canal, unspecified, bilateral**
- **H61.309 Acquired stenosis of external ear canal, unspecified, unspecified ear**

6th H61.31 Acquired stenosis of external ear canal secondary to trauma
- **H61.311 Acquired stenosis of right external ear canal secondary to trauma**
- **H61.312 Acquired stenosis of left external ear canal secondary to trauma**
- **H61.313 Acquired stenosis of external ear canal secondary to trauma, bilateral**
- **H61.319 Acquired stenosis of external ear canal secondary to trauma, unspecified ear**

6th H61.32 Acquired stenosis of external ear canal secondary to inflammation and infection
- **H61.321 Acquired stenosis of right external ear canal secondary to inflammation and infection**
- **H61.322 Acquired stenosis of left external ear canal secondary to inflammation and infection**
- **H61.323 Acquired stenosis of external ear canal secondary to inflammation and infection, bilateral**
- **H61.329 Acquired stenosis of external ear canal secondary to inflammation and infection, unspecified ear**

6th H61.39 Other acquired stenosis of external ear canal
- **H61.391 Other acquired stenosis of right external ear canal**
- **H61.392 Other acquired stenosis of left external ear canal**
- **H61.393 Other acquired stenosis of external ear canal, bilateral**
- **H61.399 Other acquired stenosis of external ear canal, unspecified ear**

5th H61.8 Other specified disorders of external ear

6th H61.81 Exostosis of external canal
- **H61.811 Exostosis of right external canal**
- **H61.812 Exostosis of left external canal**
- **H61.813 Exostosis of external canal, bilateral**
- **H61.819 Exostosis of external canal, unspecified ear**

6th H61.89 Other specified disorders of external ear
- **H61.891 Other specified disorders of right external ear**
- **H61.892 Other specified disorders of left external ear**
- **H61.893 Other specified disorders of external ear, bilateral**
- **H61.899 Other specified disorders of external ear, unspecified ear**

5th H61.9 Disorder of external ear, unspecified
- **H61.90 Disorder of external ear, unspecified, unspecified ear**
- **H61.91 Disorder of right external ear, unspecified**
- **H61.92 Disorder of left external ear, unspecified**
- **H61.93 Disorder of external ear, unspecified, bilateral**

H62 Disorders of external ear in diseases classified elsewhere

H62.4 Otitis externa in other diseases classified elsewhere

Code first underlying disease, such as:
erysipelas (A46)
impetigo (L01.0)

EXCLUDES1 *otitis externa (in):*
candidiasis (B37.84)
herpes viral [herpes simplex] (B00.1)
herpes zoster (B02.8)

H62.40 Otitis externa in other diseases classified elsewhere, unspecified ear
H62.41 Otitis externa in other diseases classified elsewhere, right ear
H62.42 Otitis externa in other diseases classified elsewhere, left ear
H62.43 Otitis externa in other diseases classified elsewhere, bilateral

H62.8 Other disorders of external ear in diseases classified elsewhere

Code first underlying disease, such as:
gout (M1A-, M10.-)

H62.8X Other disorders of external ear in diseases classified elsewhere

H62.8X1 Other disorders of right external ear in diseases classified elsewhere
H62.8X2 Other disorders of left external ear in diseases classified elsewhere
H62.8X3 Other disorders of external ear in diseases classified elsewhere, bilateral
H62.8X9 Other disorders of external ear in diseases classified elsewhere, unspecified ear

Diseases of middle ear and mastoid (H65-H75)

H65 Nonsuppurative otitis media

INCLUDES nonsuppurative otitis media with myringitis

Use additional code for any associated perforated tympanic membrane (H72.-)

Use additional code to identify:
exposure to environmental tobacco smoke (Z77.22)
exposure to tobacco smoke in the perinatal period (P96.81)
history of tobacco use (Z87.891)
occupational exposure to environmental tobacco smoke (Z57.31)
tobacco dependence (F17.-)
tobacco use (Z72.0)

H65.0 Acute serous otitis media

Acute and subacute secretory otitis

H65.00 Acute serous otitis media, unspecified ear
H65.01 Acute serous otitis media, right ear
H65.02 Acute serous otitis media, left ear
H65.03 Acute serous otitis media, bilateral
H65.04 Acute serous otitis media, recurrent, right ear
H65.05 Acute serous otitis media, recurrent, left ear
H65.06 Acute serous otitis media, recurrent, bilateral
H65.07 Acute serous otitis media, recurrent, unspecified ear

H65.1 Other acute nonsuppurative otitis media

EXCLUDES1 *otitic barotrauma (T70.0)*
otitis media (acute) NOS (H66.9)

H65.11 Acute and subacute allergic otitis media (mucoid) (sanguinous) (serous)

H65.111 Acute and subacute allergic otitis media (mucoid) (sanguinous) (serous), right ear
H65.112 Acute and subacute allergic otitis media (mucoid) (sanguinous) (serous), left ear
H65.113 Acute and subacute allergic otitis media (mucoid) (sanguinous) (serous), bilateral
H65.114 Acute and subacute allergic otitis media (mucoid) (sanguinous) (serous), recurrent, right ear
H65.115 Acute and subacute allergic otitis media (mucoid) (sanguinous) (serous), recurrent, left ear
H65.116 Acute and subacute allergic otitis media (mucoid) (sanguinous) (serous), recurrent, bilateral
H65.117 Acute and subacute allergic otitis media (mucoid) (sanguinous) (serous), recurrent, unspecified ear
H65.119 Acute and subacute allergic otitis media (mucoid) (sanguinous) (serous), unspecified ear

H65.19 Other acute nonsuppurative otitis media

Acute and subacute mucoid otitis media
Acute and subacute nonsuppurative otitis media NOS
Acute and subacute sanguinous otitis media
Acute and subacute seromucinous otitis media

H65.191 Other acute nonsuppurative otitis media, right ear
H65.192 Other acute nonsuppurative otitis media, left ear
H65.193 Other acute nonsuppurative otitis media, bilateral
H65.194 Other acute nonsuppurative otitis media, recurrent, right ear
H65.195 Other acute nonsuppurative otitis media, recurrent, left ear
H65.196 Other acute nonsuppurative otitis media, recurrent, bilateral
H65.197 Other acute nonsuppurative otitis media recurrent, unspecified ear
H65.199 Other acute nonsuppurative otitis media, unspecified ear

H65.2 Chronic serous otitis media

Chronic tubotympanal catarrh

H65.20 Chronic serous otitis media, unspecified ear
H65.21 Chronic serous otitis media, right ear
H65.22 Chronic serous otitis media, left ear
H65.23 Chronic serous otitis media, bilateral

H65.3 Chronic mucoid otitis media

Chronic mucinous otitis media
Chronic secretory otitis media
Chronic transudative otitis media
Glue ear

EXCLUDES1 *adhesive middle ear disease (H74.1)*

H65.30 Chronic mucoid otitis media, unspecified ear
H65.31 Chronic mucoid otitis media, right ear
H65.32 Chronic mucoid otitis media, left ear
H65.33 Chronic mucoid otitis media, bilateral

H65.4 Other chronic nonsuppurative otitis media

H65.41 Chronic allergic otitis media

H65.411 Chronic allergic otitis media, right ear
H65.412 Chronic allergic otitis media, left ear
H65.413 Chronic allergic otitis media, bilateral
H65.419 Chronic allergic otitis media, unspecified ear

H65.49 Other chronic nonsuppurative otitis media

Chronic exudative otitis media
Chronic nonsuppurative otitis media NOS
Chronic otitis media with effusion (nonpurulent)
Chronic seromucinous otitis media

H65.491 Other chronic nonsuppurative otitis media, right ear
H65.492 Other chronic nonsuppurative otitis media, left ear
H65.493 Other chronic nonsuppurative otitis media, bilateral
H65.499 Other chronic nonsuppurative otitis media, unspecified ear

H65.9 Unspecified nonsuppurative otitis media

Allergic otitis media NOS
Catarrhal otitis media NOS
Exudative otitis media NOS
Mucoid otitis media NOS
Otitis media with effusion (nonpurulent) NOS
Secretory otitis media NOS
Seromucinous otitis media NOS
Serous otitis media NOS
Transudative otitis media NOS

H65.90 Unspecified nonsuppurative otitis media, unspecified ear
H65.91 Unspecified nonsuppurative otitis media, right ear
H65.92 Unspecified nonsuppurative otitis media, left ear

Appropriate additional character required
Requires 7th character, placeholder x must fill empty characters

H65.93 Unspecified nonsuppurative otitis media, bilateral

✓4th **H66 Suppurative and unspecified otitis media**

INCLUDES suppurative and unspecified otitis media with myringitis

Use additional code for any associated perforated tympanic membrane (H72.-)

Use additional code to identify:
exposure to environmental tobacco smoke (Z77.22)
exposure to tobacco smoke in the perinatal period (P96.81)
history of tobacco use (Z87.891)
occupational exposure to environmental tobacco smoke (Z57.31)
tobacco dependence (F17.-)
tobacco use (Z72.0)

✓5th **H66.0 Acute suppurative otitis media**

✓6th **H66.00 Acute suppurative otitis media without spontaneous rupture of ear drum**

H66.001 Acute suppurative otitis media without spontaneous rupture of ear drum, right ear

H66.002 Acute suppurative otitis media without spontaneous rupture of ear drum, left ear

H66.003 Acute suppurative otitis media without spontaneous rupture of ear drum, bilateral

H66.004 Acute suppurative otitis media without spontaneous rupture of ear drum, recurrent, right ear

H66.005 Acute suppurative otitis media without spontaneous rupture of ear drum, recurrent, left ear

H66.006 Acute suppurative otitis media without spontaneous rupture of ear drum, recurrent, bilateral

H66.007 Acute suppurative otitis media without spontaneous rupture of ear drum, recurrent, unspecified ear

H66.009 Acute suppurative otitis media without spontaneous rupture of ear drum, unspecified ear

✓6th **H66.01 Acute suppurative otitis media with spontaneous rupture of ear drum**

H66.011 Acute suppurative otitis media with spontaneous rupture of ear drum, right ear

H66.012 Acute suppurative otitis media with spontaneous rupture of ear drum, left ear

H66.013 Acute suppurative otitis media with spontaneous rupture of ear drum, bilateral

H66.014 Acute suppurative otitis media with spontaneous rupture of ear drum, recurrent, right ear

H66.015 Acute suppurative otitis media with spontaneous rupture of ear drum, recurrent, left ear

H66.016 Acute suppurative otitis media with spontaneous rupture of ear drum, recurrent, bilateral

H66.017 Acute suppurative otitis media with spontaneous rupture of ear drum, recurrent, unspecified ear

H66.019 Acute suppurative otitis media with spontaneous rupture of ear drum, unspecified ear

✓5th **H66.1 Chronic tubotympanic suppurative otitis media**

Benign chronic suppurative otitis media
Chronic tubotympanic disease

H66.10 Chronic tubotympanic suppurative otitis media, unspecified

H66.11 Chronic tubotympanic suppurative otitis media, right ear

H66.12 Chronic tubotympanic suppurative otitis media, left ear

H66.13 Chronic tubotympanic suppurative otitis media, bilateral

✓5th **H66.2 Chronic atticoantral suppurative otitis media**

Chronic atticoantral disease

H66.20 Chronic atticoantral suppurative otitis media, unspecified ear

H66.21 Chronic atticoantral suppurative otitis media, right ear

H66.22 Chronic atticoantral suppurative otitis media, left ear

H66.23 Chronic atticoantral suppurative otitis media, bilateral

✓5th **H66.3 Other chronic suppurative otitis media**

Chronic suppurative otitis media NOS

EXCLUDES1 *tuberculous otitis media (A18.6)*

✓6th **H66.3X Other chronic suppurative otitis media**

H66.3X1 Other chronic suppurative otitis media, right ear

H66.3X2 Other chronic suppurative otitis media, left ear

H66.3X3 Other chronic suppurative otitis media, bilateral

H66.3X9 Other chronic suppurative otitis media, unspecified ear

✓5th **H66.4 Suppurative otitis media, unspecified**

Purulent otitis media NOS

H66.40 Suppurative otitis media, unspecified, unspecified ear

H66.41 Suppurative otitis media, unspecified, right ear

H66.42 Suppurative otitis media, unspecified, left ear

H66.43 Suppurative otitis media, unspecified, bilateral

✓5th **H66.9 Otitis media, unspecified**

Otitis media NOS
Acute otitis media NOS
Chronic otitis media NOS

H66.90 Otitis media, unspecified, unspecified ear

H66.91 Otitis media, unspecified. right ear

H66.92 Otitis media, unspecified, left ear

H66.93 Otitis media, unspecified, bilateral

✓4th **H67 Otitis media in diseases classified elsewhere**

Code first underlying disease, such as:
viral disease NEC (B00-B34)

Use additional code for any associated perforated tympanic membrane (H72.-)

EXCLUDES1 *otitis media in:*
influenza (J09.X9, J10.83, J11.83)
measles (B05.3)
scarlet fever (A38.0)
tuberculosis (A18.6)

H67.1 ***Otitis media in diseases classified elsewhere, right ear***

H67.2 ***Otitis media in diseases classified elsewhere, left ear***

H67.3 ***Otitis media in diseases classified elsewhere, bilateral***

H67.9 ***Otitis media in diseases classified elsewhere, unspecified ear***

✓4th **H68 Eustachian salpingitis and obstruction**

✓5th **H68.0 Eustachian salpingitis**

✓6th **H68.00 Unspecified Eustachian salpingitis**

H68.001 Unspecified Eustachian salpingitis, right ear

H68.002 Unspecified Eustachian salpingitis, left ear

H68.003 Unspecified Eustachian salpingitis, bilateral

H68.009 Unspecified Eustachian salpingitis, unspecified ear

✓6th **H68.01 Acute Eustachian salpingitis**

H68.011 Acute Eustachian salpingitis, right ear

H68.012 Acute Eustachian salpingitis, left ear

H68.013 Acute Eustachian salpingitis, bilateral

H68.019 Acute Eustachian salpingitis, unspecified ear

✓6th **H68.02 Chronic Eustachian salpingitis**

H68.021 Chronic Eustachian salpingitis, right ear

H68.022 Chronic Eustachian salpingitis, left ear

H68.023 Chronic Eustachian salpingitis, bilateral

H68.029 Chronic Eustachian salpingitis, unspecified ear

H68.1 Obstruction of Eustachian tube
Stenosis of Eustachian tube
Stricture of Eustachian tube
H68.10 Unspecified obstruction of Eustachian tube
H68.101 Unspecified obstruction of Eustachian tube, right ear
H68.102 Unspecified obstruction of Eustachian tube, left ear
H68.103 Unspecified obstruction of Eustachian tube, bilateral
H68.109 Unspecified obstruction of Eustachian tube, unspecified ear
H68.11 Osseous obstruction of Eustachian tube
H68.111 Osseous obstruction of Eustachian tube, right ear
H68.112 Osseous obstruction of Eustachian tube, left ear
H68.113 Osseous obstruction of Eustachian tube, bilateral
H68.119 Osseous obstruction of Eustachian tube, unspecified ear
H68.12 Intrinsic cartilagenous obstruction of Eustachian tube
H68.121 Intrinsic cartilagenous obstruction of Eustachian tube, right ear
H68.122 Intrinsic cartilagenous obstruction of Eustachian tube, left ear
H68.123 Intrinsic cartilagenous obstruction of Eustachian tube, bilateral
H68.129 Intrinsic cartilagenous obstruction of Eustachian tube, unspecified ear
H68.13 Extrinsic cartilagenous obstruction of Eustachian tube
Compression of Eustachian tube
H68.131 Extrinsic cartilagenous obstruction of Eustachian tube, right ear
H68.132 Extrinsic cartilagenous obstruction of Eustachian tube, left ear
H68.133 Extrinsic cartilagenous obstruction of Eustachian tube, bilateral
H68.139 Extrinsic cartilagenous obstruction of Eustachian tube, unspecified ear

H69 Other and unspecified disorders of Eustachian tube

H69.0 Patulous Eustachian tube
H69.00 Patulous Eustachian tube, unspecified ear
H69.01 Patulous Eustachian tube, right ear
H69.02 Patulous Eustachian tube, left ear
H69.03 Patulous Eustachian tube, bilateral
H69.8 Other specified disorders of Eustachian tube
H69.80 Other specified disorders of Eustachian tube, unspecified ear
H69.81 Other specified disorders of Eustachian tube, right ear
H69.82 Other specified disorders of Eustachian tube, left ear
H69.83 Other specified disorders of Eustachian tube, bilateral
H69.9 Unspecified Eustachian tube disorder
H69.90 Unspecified Eustachian tube disorder, unspecified ear
H69.91 Unspecified Eustachian tube disorder, right ear
H69.92 Unspecified Eustachian tube disorder, left ear
H69.93 Unspecified Eustachian tube disorder, bilateral

H70 Mastoiditis and related conditions

H70.0 Acute mastoiditis
Abscess of mastoid
Empyema of mastoid
H70.00 Acute mastoiditis without complications
H70.001 Acute mastoiditis without complications, right ear
H70.002 Acute mastoiditis without complications, left ear
H70.003 Acute mastoiditis without complications, bilateral
H70.009 Acute mastoiditis without complications, unspecified ear
H70.01 Subperiosteal abscess of mastoid
H70.011 Subperiosteal abscess of mastoid, right ear
H70.012 Subperiosteal abscess of mastoid, left ear
H70.013 Subperiosteal abscess of mastoid, bilateral
H70.019 Subperiosteal abscess of mastoid, unspecified ear
H70.09 Acute mastoiditis with other complications
H70.091 Acute mastoiditis with other complications, right ear
H70.092 Acute mastoiditis with other complications, left ear
H70.093 Acute mastoiditis with other complications, bilateral
H70.099 Acute mastoiditis with other complications, unspecified ear
H70.1 Chronic mastoiditis
Caries of mastoid
Fistula of mastoid
EXCLUDES 1 *tuberculous mastoiditis (A18.03)*
H70.10 Chronic mastoiditis, unspecified ear
H70.11 Chronic mastoiditis, right ear
H70.12 Chronic mastoiditis, left ear
H70.13 Chronic mastoiditis, bilateral
H70.2 Petrositis
Inflammation of petrous bone
H70.20 Unspecified petrositis
H70.201 Unspecified petrositis, right ear
H70.202 Unspecified petrositis, left ear
H70.203 Unspecified petrositis, bilateral
H70.209 Unspecified petrositis, unspecified ear
H70.21 Acute petrositis
H70.211 Acute petrositis, right ear
H70.212 Acute petrositis, left ear
H70.213 Acute petrositis, bilateral
H70.219 Acute petrositis, unspecified ear
H70.22 Chronic petrositis
H70.221 Chronic petrositis, right ear
H70.222 Chronic petrositis, left ear
H70.223 Chronic petrositis, bilateral
H70.229 Chronic petrositis, unspecified ear
H70.8 Other mastoiditis and related conditions
EXCLUDES 1 *preauricular sinus and cyst (Q18.1)*
sinus, fistula, and cyst of branchial cleft (Q18.0)
H70.81 Postauricular fistula
H70.811 Postauricular fistula, right ear
H70.812 Postauricular fistula, left ear
H70.813 Postauricular fistula, bilateral
H70.819 Postauricular fistula, unspecified ear
H70.89 Other mastoiditis and related conditions
H70.891 Other mastoiditis and related conditions, right ear
H70.892 Other mastoiditis and related conditions, left ear
H70.893 Other mastoiditis and related conditions, bilateral
H70.899 Other mastoiditis and related conditions, unspecified ear
H70.9 Unspecified mastoiditis
H70.90 Unspecified mastoiditis, unspecified ear
H70.91 Unspecified mastoiditis, right ear
H70.92 Unspecified mastoiditis, left ear
H70.93 Unspecified mastoiditis, bilateral

H71 Cholesteatoma of middle ear

EXCLUDES 2 *cholesteatoma of external ear (H60.4-)*
recurrent cholesteatoma of postmastoidectomy cavity (H95.0-)
H71.0 Cholesteatoma of attic
H71.00 Cholesteatoma of attic, unspecified ear
H71.01 Cholesteatoma of attic, right ear
H71.02 Cholesteatoma of attic, left ear
H71.03 Cholesteatoma of attic, bilateral

√5th **H71.1 Cholesteatoma of tympanum**
- **H71.10 Cholesteatoma of tympanum, unspecified ear**
- **H71.11 Cholesteatoma of tympanum, right ear**
- **H71.12 Cholesteatoma of tympanum, left ear**
- **H71.13 Cholesteatoma of tympanum, bilateral**

√5th **H71.2 Cholesteatoma of mastoid**
- **H71.20 Cholesteatoma of mastoid, unspecified ear**
- **H71.21 Cholesteatoma of mastoid, right ear**
- **H71.22 Cholesteatoma of mastoid, left ear**
- **H71.23 Cholesteatoma of mastoid, bilateral**

√5th **H71.3 Diffuse cholesteatosis**
- **H71.30 Diffuse cholesteatosis, unspecified ear**
- **H71.31 Diffuse cholesteatosis, right ear**
- **H71.32 Diffuse cholesteatosis, left ear**
- **H71.33 Diffuse cholesteatosis, bilateral**

√5th **H71.9 Unspecified cholesteatoma**
- **H71.90 Unspecified cholesteatoma, unspecified ear**
- **H71.91 Unspecified cholesteatoma, right ear**
- **H71.92 Unspecified cholesteatoma, left ear**
- **H71.93 Unspecified cholesteatoma, bilateral**

√4th H72 Perforation of tympanic membrane

INCLUDES persistent post-traumatic perforation of ear drum
postinflammatory perforation of ear drum

Code first any associated otitis media (H65.-, H66.1-, H66.2-, H66.3-, H66.4-, H66.9-, H67.-)

EXCLUDES 1 *acute suppurative otitis media with rupture of the tympanic membrane (H66.01-)*
traumatic rupture of ear drum (S09.2-)

√5th **H72.0 Central perforation of tympanic membrane**
- **H72.00 Central perforation of tympanic membrane, unspecified ear**
- **H72.01 Central perforation of tympanic membrane, right ear**
- **H72.02 Central perforation of tympanic membrane, left ear**
- **H72.03 Central perforation of tympanic membrane, bilateral**

√5th **H72.1 Attic perforation of tympanic membrane**
Perforation of pars flaccida
- **H72.10 Attic perforation of tympanic membrane, unspecified ear**
- **H72.11 Attic perforation of tympanic membrane, right ear**
- **H72.12 Attic perforation of tympanic membrane, left ear**
- **H72.13 Attic perforation of tympanic membrane, bilateral**

√5th **H72.2 Other marginal perforations of tympanic membrane**
- √6th **H72.2X Other marginal perforations of tympanic membrane**
  - **H72.2X1 Other marginal perforations of tympanic membrane, right ear**
  - **H72.2X2 Other marginal perforations of tympanic membrane, left ear**
  - **H72.2X3 Other marginal perforations of tympanic membrane, bilateral**
  - **H72.2X9 Other marginal perforations of tympanic membrane, unspecified ear**

√5th **H72.8 Other perforations of tympanic membrane**
- √6th **H72.81 Multiple perforations of tympanic membrane**
  - **H72.811 Multiple perforations of tympanic membrane, right ear**
  - **H72.812 Multiple perforations of tympanic membrane, left ear**
  - **H72.813 Multiple perforations of tympanic membrane, bilateral**
  - **H72.819 Multiple perforations of tympanic membrane, unspecified ear**
- √6th **H72.82 Total perforations of tympanic membrane**
  - **H72.821 Total perforations of tympanic membrane, right ear**
  - **H72.822 Total perforations of tympanic membrane, left ear**
  - **H72.823 Total perforations of tympanic membrane, bilateral**
  - **H72.829 Total perforations of tympanic membrane, unspecified ear**

√5th **H72.9 Unspecified perforation of tympanic membrane**
- **H72.90 Unspecified perforation of tympanic membrane, unspecified ear**
- **H72.91 Unspecified perforation of tympanic membrane, right ear**
- **H72.92 Unspecified perforation of tympanic membrane, left ear**
- **H72.93 Unspecified perforation of tympanic membrane, bilateral**

√4th H73 Other disorders of tympanic membrane

√5th **H73.0 Acute myringitis**
EXCLUDES 1 *acute myringitis with otitis media (H65, H66)*
- √6th **H73.00 Unspecified acute myringitis**
  Acute tympanitis NOS
  - **H73.001 Acute myringitis, right ear**
  - **H73.002 Acute myringitis, left ear**
  - **H73.003 Acute myringitis, bilateral**
  - **H73.009 Acute myringitis, unspecified ear**
- √6th **H73.01 Bullous myringitis**
  - **H73.011 Bullous myringitis, right ear**
  - **H73.012 Bullous myringitis, left ear**
  - **H73.013 Bullous myringitis, bilateral**
  - **H73.019 Bullous myringitis, unspecified ear**
- √6th **H73.09 Other acute myringitis**
  - **H73.091 Other acute myringitis, right ear**
  - **H73.092 Other acute myringitis, left ear**
  - **H73.093 Other acute myringitis, bilateral**
  - **H73.099 Other acute myringitis, unspecified ear**

√5th **H73.1 Chronic myringitis**
Chronic tympanitis
EXCLUDES 1 *chronic myringitis with otitis media (H65, H66)*
- **H73.10 Chronic myringitis, unspecified ear**
- **H73.11 Chronic myringitis, right ear**
- **H73.12 Chronic myringitis, left ear**
- **H73.13 Chronic myringitis, bilateral**

√5th **H73.2 Unspecified myringitis**
- **H73.20 Unspecified myringitis, unspecified ear**
- **H73.21 Unspecified myringitis, right ear**
- **H73.22 Unspecified myringitis, left ear**
- **H73.23 Unspecified myringitis, bilateral**

√5th **H73.8 Other specified disorders of tympanic membrane**
- √6th **H73.81 Atrophic flaccid tympanic membrane**
  - **H73.811 Atrophic flaccid tympanic membrane, right ear**
  - **H73.812 Atrophic flaccid tympanic membrane, left ear**
  - **H73.813 Atrophic flaccid tympanic membrane, bilateral**
  - **H73.819 Atrophic flaccid tympanic membrane, unspecified ear**
- √6th **H73.82 Atrophic nonflaccid tympanic membrane**
  - **H73.821 Atrophic nonflaccid tympanic membrane, right ear**
  - **H73.822 Atrophic nonflaccid tympanic membrane, left ear**
  - **H73.823 Atrophic nonflaccid tympanic membrane, bilateral**
  - **H73.829 Atrophic nonflaccid tympanic membrane, unspecified ear**
- √6th **H73.89 Other specified disorders of tympanic membrane**
  - **H73.891 Other specified disorders of tympanic membrane, right ear**
  - **H73.892 Other specified disorders of tympanic membrane, left ear**
  - **H73.893 Other specified disorders of tympanic membrane, bilateral**
  - **H73.899 Other specified disorders of tympanic membrane, unspecified ear**

√5th **H73.9 Unspecified disorder of tympanic membrane**
- **H73.90 Unspecified disorder of tympanic membrane, unspecified ear**
- **H73.91 Unspecified disorder of tympanic membrane, right ear**
- **H73.92 Unspecified disorder of tympanic membrane, left ear**

H73.93 **Unspecified disorder of tympanic membrane, bilateral**

✓4th H74 Other disorders of middle ear mastoid

EXCLUDES 2 *mastoiditis (H70.-)*

✓5th **H74.0 Tympanosclerosis**

- **H74.01 Tympanosclerosis, right ear**
- **H74.02 Tympanosclerosis, left ear**
- **H74.03 Tympanosclerosis, bilateral**
- **H74.09 Tympanosclerosis, unspecified ear**

✓5th **H74.1 Adhesive middle ear disease**

Adhesive otitis

EXCLUDES 1 *glue ear (H65.3-)*

- **H74.11 Adhesive right middle ear disease**
- **H74.12 Adhesive left middle ear disease**
- **H74.13 Adhesive middle ear disease, bilateral**
- **H74.19 Adhesive middle ear disease, unspecified ear**

✓5th **H74.2 Discontinuity and dislocation of ear ossicles**

- **H74.20 Discontinuity and dislocation of ear ossicles, unspecified ear**
- **H74.21 Discontinuity and dislocation of right ear ossicles**
- **H74.22 Discontinuity and dislocation of left ear ossicles**
- **H74.23 Discontinuity and dislocation of ear ossicles, bilateral**

✓5th **H74.3 Other acquired abnormalities of ear ossicles**

✓6th **H74.31 Ankylosis of ear ossicles**

- **H74.311 Ankylosis of ear ossicles, right ear**
- **H74.312 Ankylosis of ear ossicles, left ear**
- **H74.313 Ankylosis of ear ossicles, bilateral**
- **H74.319 Ankylosis of ear ossicles, unspecified ear**

✓6th **H74.32 Partial loss of ear ossicles**

- **H74.321 Partial loss of ear ossicles, right ear**
- **H74.322 Partial loss of ear ossicles, left ear**
- **H74.323 Partial loss of ear ossicles, bilateral**
- **H74.329 Partial loss of ear ossicles, unspecified ear**

✓6th **H74.39 Other acquired abnormalities of ear ossicles**

- **H74.391 Other acquired abnormalities of right ear ossicles**
- **H74.392 Other acquired abnormalities of left ear ossicles**
- **H74.393 Other acquired abnormalities of ear ossicles, bilateral**
- **H74.399 Other acquired abnormalities of ear ossicles, unspecified ear**

✓5th **H74.4 Polyp of middle ear**

- **H74.40 Polyp of middle ear, unspecified ear**
- **H74.41 Polyp of right middle ear**
- **H74.42 Polyp of left middle ear**
- **H74.43 Polyp of middle ear, bilateral**

✓5th **H74.8 Other specified disorders of middle ear and mastoid**

✓6th **H74.8X Other specified disorders of middle ear and mastoid**

- **H74.8X1 Other specified disorders of right middle ear and mastoid**
- **H74.8X2 Other specified disorders of left middle ear and mastoid**
- **H74.8X3 Other specified disorders of middle ear and mastoid, bilateral**
- **H74.8X9 Other specified disorders of middle ear and mastoid, unspecified ear**

✓5th **H74.9 Unspecified disorder of middle ear and mastoid**

- **H74.90 Unspecified disorder of middle ear and mastoid, unspecified ear**
- **H74.91 Unspecified disorder of right middle ear and mastoid**
- **H74.92 Unspecified disorder of left middle ear and mastoid**
- **H74.93 Unspecified disorder of middle ear and mastoid, bilateral**

✓4th H75 Other disorders of middle ear and mastoid in diseases classified elsewhere

Code first underlying disease

✓5th **H75.0 Mastoiditis in infectious and parasitic diseases classified elsewhere**

EXCLUDES 1 *mastoiditis (in):*
syphilis (A52.77)
tuberculosis (A18.03)

- **H75.00** ***Mastoiditis in infectious and parasitic diseases classified elsewhere, unspecified ear***
- **H75.01** ***Mastoiditis in infectious and parasitic diseases classified elsewhere, right ear***
- **H75.02** ***Mastoiditis in infectious and parasitic diseases classified elsewhere, left ear***
- **H75.03** ***Mastoiditis in infectious and parasitic diseases classified elsewhere, bilateral***

✓5th **H75.8 Other specified disorders of middle ear and mastoid in diseases classified elsewhere**

- **H75.80** ***Other specified disorders of middle ear and mastoid in diseases classified elsewhere, unspecified ear***
- **H75.81** ***Other specified disorders of right middle ear and mastoid in diseases classified elsewhere***
- **H75.82** ***Other specified disorders of left middle ear and mastoid in diseases classified elsewhere***
- **H75.83** ***Other specified disorders of middle ear and mastoid in diseases classified elsewhere, bilateral***

Diseases of inner ear (H80-H83)

✓4th H80 Otosclerosis

INCLUDES Otospongiosis

✓5th **H80.0 Otosclerosis involving oval window, nonobliterative**

- **H80.00 Otosclerosis involving oval window, nonobliterative, unspecified ear**
- **H80.01 Otosclerosis involving oval window, nonobliterative, right ear**
- **H80.02 Otosclerosis involving oval window, nonobliterative, left ear**
- **H80.03 Otosclerosis involving oval window, nonobliterative, bilateral**

✓5th **H80.1 Otosclerosis involving oval window, obliterative**

- **H80.10 Otosclerosis involving oval window, obliterative, unspecified ear**
- **H80.11 Otosclerosis involving oval window, obliterative, right ear**
- **H80.12 Otosclerosis involving oval window, obliterative, left ear**
- **H80.13 Otosclerosis involving oval window, obliterative, bilateral**

✓5th **H80.2 Cochlear otosclerosis**

Otosclerosis involving otic capsule
Otosclerosis involving round window

- **H80.20 Cochlear otosclerosis, unspecified ear**
- **H80.21 Cochlear otosclerosis, right ear**
- **H80.22 Cochlear otosclerosis, left ear**
- **H80.23 Cochlear otosclerosis, bilateral**

✓5th **H80.8 Other otosclerosis**

- **H80.80 Other otosclerosis, unspecified ear**
- **H80.81 Other otosclerosis, right ear**
- **H80.82 Other otosclerosis, left ear**
- **H80.83 Other otosclerosis, bilateral**

✓5th **H80.9 Unspecified otosclerosis**

- **H80.90 Unspecified otosclerosis, unspecified ear**
- **H80.91 Unspecified otosclerosis, right ear**
- **H80.92 Unspecified otosclerosis, left ear**
- **H80.93 Unspecified otosclerosis, bilateral**

✓4th H81 Disorders of vestibular function

EXCLUDES 1 *epidemic vertigo (A88.1)*
vertigo NOS (R42)

✓5th **H81.0 Ménière's disease**

Labyrinthine hydrops
Ménière's syndrome or vertigo

- **H81.01 Ménière's disease, right ear**
- **H81.02 Ménière's disease, left ear**
- **H81.03 Ménière's disease, bilateral**
- **H81.09 Ménière's disease, unspecified ear**

5th **H81.1 Benign paroxysmal vertigo**
- **H81.10 Benign paroxysmal vertigo, unspecified ear**
- **H81.11 Benign paroxysmal vertigo, right ear**
- **H81.12 Benign paroxysmal vertigo, left ear**
- **H81.13 Benign paroxysmal vertigo, bilateral**

5th **H81.2 Vestibular neuronitis**
- **H81.20 Vestibular neuronitis, unspecified ear**
- **H81.21 Vestibular neuronitis, right ear**
- **H81.22 Vestibular neuronitis, left ear**
- **H81.23 Vestibular neuronitis, bilateral**

5th **H81.3 Other peripheral vertigo**

6th **H81.31 Aural vertigo**
- **H81.311 Aural vertigo, right ear**
- **H81.312 Aural vertigo, left ear**
- **H81.313 Aural vertigo, bilateral**
- **H81.319 Aural vertigo, unspecified ear**

6th **H81.39 Other peripheral vertigo**
Lermoyez' syndrome
Otogenic vertigo
Peripheral vertigo NOS
- **H81.391 Other peripheral vertigo, right ear**
- **H81.392 Other peripheral vertigo, left ear**
- **H81.393 Other peripheral vertigo, bilateral**
- **H81.399 Other peripheral vertigo, unspecified ear**

5th **H81.4 Vertigo of central origin**
Central positional nystagmus
- **H81.41 Vertigo of central origin, right ear**
- **H81.42 Vertigo of central origin, left ear**
- **H81.43 Vertigo of central origin, bilateral**
- **H81.49 Vertigo of central origin, unspecified ear**

5th **H81.8 Other disorders of vestibular function**

6th **H81.8X Other disorders of vestibular function**
- **H81.8X1 Other disorders of vestibular function, right ear**
- **H81.8X2 Other disorders of vestibular function, left ear**
- **H81.8X3 Other disorders of vestibular function, bilateral**
- **H81.8X9 Other disorders of vestibular function, unspecified ear**

5th **H81.9 Unspecified disorder of vestibular function**
Vertiginous syndrome NOS
- **H81.90 Unspecified disorder of vestibular function, unspecified ear**
- **H81.91 Unspecified disorder of vestibular function, right ear**
- **H81.92 Unspecified disorder of vestibular function, left ear**
- **H81.93 Unspecified disorder of vestibular function, bilateral**

4th **H82 Vertiginous syndromes in diseases classified elsewhere**
Code first underlying disease
EXCLUDES1 *epidemic vertigo (A88.1)*
- **H82.1 *Vertiginous syndromes in diseases classified elsewhere, right ear***
- **H82.2 *Vertiginous syndromes in diseases classified elsewhere, left ear***
- **H82.3 *Vertiginous syndromes in diseases classified elsewhere, bilateral***
- **H82.9 *Vertiginous syndromes in diseases classified elsewhere, unspecified ear***

4th **H83 Other diseases of inner ear**

5th **H83.0 Labyrinthitis**
- **H83.01 Labyrinthitis, right ear**
- **H83.02 Labyrinthitis, left ear**
- **H83.03 Labyrinthitis, bilateral**
- **H83.09 Labyrinthitis, unspecified ear**

5th **H83.1 Labyrinthine fistula**
- **H83.11 Labyrinthine fistula, right ear**
- **H83.12 Labyrinthine fistula, left ear**
- **H83.13 Labyrinthine fistula, bilateral**
- **H83.19 Labyrinthine fistula, unspecified ear**

5th **H83.2 Labyrinthine dysfunction**
Labyrinthine hypersensitivity
Labyrinthine hypofunction
Labyrinthine loss of function

6th **H83.2X Labyrinthine dysfunction**
- **H83.2X1 Labyrinthine dysfunction, right ear**
- **H83.2X2 Labyrinthine dysfunction, left ear**
- **H83.2X3 Labyrinthine dysfunction, bilateral**
- **H83.2X9 Labyrinthine dysfunction, unspecified ear**

5th **H83.3 Noise effects on inner ear**
Acoustic trauma of inner ear
Noise-induced hearing loss of inner ear

6th **H83.3X Noise effects on inner ear**
- **H83.3X1 Noise effects on right inner ear**
- **H83.3X2 Noise effects on left inner ear**
- **H83.3X3 Noise effects on inner ear, bilateral**
- **H83.3X9 Noise effects on inner ear, unspecified ear**

5th **H83.8 Other specified diseases of inner ear**

6th **H83.8X Other specified diseases of inner ear**
- **H83.8X1 Other specified diseases of right inner ear**
- **H83.8X2 Other specified diseases of left inner ear**
- **H83.8X3 Other specified diseases of inner ear, bilateral**
- **H83.8X9 Other specified diseases of inner ear, unspecified ear**

5th **H83.9 Unspecified disease of inner ear**
- **H83.90 Unspecified disease of inner ear, unspecified ear**
- **H83.91 Unspecified disease of right inner ear**
- **H83.92 Unspecified disease of left inner ear**
- **H83.93 Unspecified disease of inner ear, bilateral**

Other disorders of ear (H90-H94)

4th **H90 Conductive and sensorineural hearing loss**
EXCLUDES1 *deaf nonspeaking NEC (H91.3)*
deafness NOS (H91.9-)
hearing loss NOS (H91.9-)
noise-induced hearing loss (H83.3-)
ototoxic hearing loss (H91.0-)
sudden (idiopathic) hearing loss (H91.2-)

H90.0 Conductive hearing loss, bilateral

5th **H90.1 Conductive hearing loss, unilateral with unrestricted hearing on the contralateral side**
- **H90.11 Conductive hearing loss, unilateral, right ear, with unrestricted hearing on the contralateral side**
- **H90.12 Conductive hearing loss, unilateral, left ear, with unrestricted hearing on the contralateral side**

H90.2 Conductive hearing loss, unspecified
Conductive deafness NOS

H90.3 Sensorineural hearing loss, bilateral

5th **H90.4 Sensorineural hearing loss, unilateral with unrestricted hearing on the contralateral side**
- **H90.41 Sensorineural hearing loss, unilateral, right ear, with unrestricted hearing on the contralateral side**
- **H90.42 Sensorineural hearing loss, unilateral, left ear, with unrestricted hearing on the contralateral side**

H90.5 Unspecified sensorineural hearing loss
Central hearing loss NOS
Congenital deafness NOS
Neural hearing loss NOS
Perceptive hearing loss NOS
Sensorineural deafness NOS
Sensory hearing loss NOS
EXCLUDES1 *abnormal auditory perception (H93.2-)*
psychogenic deafness (F44.6)

H90.6 Mixed conductive and sensorineural hearing loss, bilateral

5th **H90.7 Mixed conductive and sensorineural hearing loss, unilateral with unrestricted hearing on the contralateral side**
- **H90.71 Mixed conductive and sensorineural hearing loss, unilateral, right ear, with unrestricted hearing on the contralateral side**
- **H90.72 Mixed conductive and sensorineural hearing loss, unilateral, left ear, with unrestricted hearing on the contralateral side**

H9Ø.8 Mixed conductive and sensorineural hearing loss, unspecified

✓4th **H91 Other and unspecified hearing loss**

EXCLUDES 1 *abnormal auditory perception (H93.2-)*
hearing loss as classified in H9Ø-
impacted cerumen (H61.2-)
noise-induced hearing loss (H83.3-)
psychogenic deafness (F44.6)
transient ischemic deafness (H93.Ø1-)

✓5th **H91.Ø Ototoxic hearing loss**
Code first poisoning due to drug or toxin, if applicable (T36-T65 with fifth or sixth character 1-4 or 6)
Use additional code for adverse effect, if applicable, to identify drug (T36-T5Ø with fifth or sixth character 5)
H91.Ø1 Ototoxic hearing loss, right ear
H91.Ø2 Ototoxic hearing loss, left ear
H91.Ø3 Ototoxic hearing loss, bilateral
H91.Ø9 Ototoxic hearing loss, unspecified ear

✓5th **H91.1 Presbycusis**
Presbyacusia
H91.1Ø Presbycusis, unspecified ear
H91.11 Presbycusis, right ear
H91.12 Presbycusis, left ear
H91.13 Presbycusis, bilateral

✓5th **H91.2 Sudden idiopathic hearing loss**
Sudden hearing loss NOS
H91.2Ø Sudden idiopathic hearing loss, unspecified ear
H91.21 Sudden idiopathic hearing loss, right ear
H91.22 Sudden idiopathic hearing loss, left ear
H91.23 Sudden idiopathic hearing loss, bilateral

H91.3 Deaf nonspeaking, not elsewhere classified

✓5th **H91.8 Other specified hearing loss**
✓6th **H91.8X Other specified hearing loss**
H91.8X1 Other specified hearing loss, right ear
H91.8X2 Other specified hearing loss, left ear
H91.8X3 Other specified hearing loss, bilateral
H91.8X9 Other specified hearing loss, unspecified ear

✓5th **H91.9 Unspecified hearing loss**
Deafness NOS
High frequency deafness
Low frequency deafness
H91.9Ø Unspecified hearing loss, unspecified ear
H91.91 Unspecified hearing loss, right ear
H91.92 Unspecified hearing loss, left ear
H91.93 Unspecified hearing loss, bilateral

✓4th **H92 Otalgia and effusion of ear**

✓5th **H92.Ø Otalgia**
H92.Ø1 Otalgia, right ear
H92.Ø2 Otalgia, left ear
H92.Ø3 Otalgia, bilateral
H92.Ø9 Otalgia, unspecified ear

✓5th **H92.1 Otorrhea**
EXCLUDES 1 *leakage of cerebrospinal fluid through ear (G96.Ø)*
H92.1Ø Otorrhea, unspecified ear
H92.11 Otorrhea, right ear
H92.12 Otorrhea, left ear
H92.13 Otorrhea, bilateral

✓5th **H92.2 Otorrhagia**
EXCLUDES 1 *traumatic otorrhagia—code to injury*
H92.2Ø Otorrhagia, unspecified ear
H92.21 Otorrhagia, right ear
H92.22 Otorrhagia, left ear
H92.23 Otorrhagia, bilateral

✓4th **H93 Other disorders of ear, not elsewhere classified**

✓5th **H93.Ø Degenerative and vascular disorders of ear**
EXCLUDES 1 *presbycusis (H91.1)*
✓6th **H93.Ø1 Transient ischemic deafness**
H93.Ø11 Transient ischemic deafness, right ear
H93.Ø12 Transient ischemic deafness, left ear
H93.Ø13 Transient ischemic deafness, bilateral
H93.Ø19 Transient ischemic deafness, unspecified ear
✓6th **H93.Ø9 Unspecified degenerative and vascular disorders of ear**
H93.Ø91 Unspecified degenerative and vascular disorders of right ear
H93.Ø92 Unspecified degenerative and vascular disorders of left ear
H93.Ø93 Unspecified degenerative and vascular disorders of ear, bilateral
H93.Ø99 Unspecified degenerative and vascular disorders of unspecified ear

✓5th **H93.1 Tinnitus**
H93.11 Tinnitus, right ear
H93.12 Tinnitus, left ear
H93.13 Tinnitus, bilateral
H93.19 Tinnitus, unspecified ear

✓5th **H93.2 Other abnormal auditory perceptions**
EXCLUDES 2 *auditory hallucinations (R44.Ø)*
✓6th **H93.21 Auditory recruitment**
H93.211 Auditory recruitment, right ear
H93.212 Auditory recruitment, left ear
H93.213 Auditory recruitment, bilateral
H93.219 Auditory recruitment, unspecified ear
✓6th **H93.22 Diplacusis**
H93.221 Diplacusis, right ear
H93.222 Diplacusis, left ear
H93.223 Diplacusis, bilateral
H93.229 Diplacusis, unspecified ear
✓6th **H93.23 Hyperacusis**
H93.231 Hyperacusis, right ear
H93.232 Hyperacusis, left ear
H93.233 Hyperacusis, bilateral
H93.239 Hyperacusis, unspecified ear
✓6th **H93.24 Temporary auditory threshold shift**
H93.241 Temporary auditory threshold shift, right ear
H93.242 Temporary auditory threshold shift, left ear
H93.243 Temporary auditory threshold shift, bilateral
H93.249 Temporary auditory threshold shift, unspecified ear
H93.25 Central auditory processing disorder
Congenital auditory imperception
Word deafness
EXCLUDES 1 *mixed receptive-expressive language disorder (F8Ø.2)*
✓6th **H93.29 Other abnormal auditory perceptions**
H93.291 Other abnormal auditory perceptions, right ear
H93.292 Other abnormal auditory perceptions, left ear
H93.293 Other abnormal auditory perceptions, bilateral
H93.299 Other abnormal auditory perceptions, unspecified ear

✓5th **H93.3 Disorders of acoustic nerve**
Disorder of 8th cranial nerve
EXCLUDES 1 *acoustic neuroma (D33.3)*
syphilitic acoustic neuritis (A52.15)
✓6th **H93.3X Disorders of acoustic nerve**
H93.3X1 Disorders of right acoustic nerve
H93.3X2 Disorders of left acoustic nerve
H93.3X3 Disorders of bilateral acoustic nerves
H93.3X9 Disorders of unspecified acoustic nerve

✓5th **H93.8 Other specified disorders of ear**
✓6th **H93.8X Other specified disorders of ear**
H93.8X1 Other specified disorders of right ear
H93.8X2 Other specified disorders of left ear
H93.8X3 Other specified disorders of ear, bilateral
H93.8X9 Other specified disorders of ear, unspecified ear

✓5th **H93.9 Unspecified disorder of ear**
H93.9Ø Unspecified disorder of ear, unspecified ear
H93.91 Unspecified disorder of right ear
H93.92 Unspecified disorder of left ear

H93.93 **Unspecified disorder of ear, bilateral**

✓4th **H94 Other disorders of ear in diseases classified elsewhere**

✓5th **H94.0 Acoustic neuritis in infectious and parasitic diseases classified elsewhere**

Code first underlying disease, such as:
parasitic disease (B65-B89)

EXCLUDES 1 *acoustic neuritis (in):*
herpes zoster (B02.29)
syphilis (A52.15)

H94.00 ***Acoustic neuritis in infectious and parasitic diseases classified elsewhere, unspecified ear***

H94.01 ***Acoustic neuritis in infectious and parasitic diseases classified elsewhere, right ear***

H94.02 ***Acoustic neuritis in infectious and parasitic diseases classified elsewhere, left ear***

H94.03 ***Acoustic neuritis in infectious and parasitic diseases classified elsewhere, bilateral***

✓5th **H94.8 Other specified disorders of ear in diseases classified elsewhere**

Code first underlying disease, such as:
congenital syphilis (A50.0)

EXCLUDES 1 *aural myiasis (B87.4)*
syphilitic labyrinthitis (A52.79)

H94.80 ***Other specified disorders of ear in diseases classified elsewhere, unspecified ear***

H94.81 ***Other specified disorders of right ear in diseases classified elsewhere***

H94.82 ***Other specified disorders of left ear in diseases classified elsewhere***

H94.83 ***Other specified disorders of ear in diseases classified elsewhere, bilateral***

Intraoperative and postprocedural complications and disorders of ear and mastoid process, not elsewhere classified (H95)

✓4th **H95 Intraoperative and postprocedural complications and disorders of ear and mastoid process, not elsewhere classified**

✓5th **H95.0 Recurrent cholesteatoma of postmastoidectomy cavity**

H95.00 Recurrent cholesteatoma of postmastoidectomy cavity, unspecified ear

H95.01 Recurrent cholesteatoma of postmastoidectomy cavity, right ear

H95.02 Recurrent cholesteatoma of postmastoidectomy cavity, left ear

H95.03 Recurrent cholesteatoma of postmastoidectomy cavity, bilateral ears

✓5th **H95.1 Other disorders of ear and mastoid process following mastoidectomy**

✓6th **H95.11 Chronic inflammation of postmastoidectomy cavity**

H95.111 Chronic inflammation of postmastoidectomy cavity, right ear

H95.112 Chronic inflammation of postmastoidectomy cavity, left ear

H95.113 Chronic inflammation of postmastoidectomy cavity, bilateral ears

H95.119 Chronic inflammation of postmastoidectomy cavity, unspecified ear

✓6th **H95.12 Granulation of postmastoidectomy cavity**

H95.121 Granulation of postmastoidectomy cavity, right ear

H95.122 Granulation of postmastoidectomy cavity, left ear

H95.123 Granulation of postmastoidectomy cavity, bilateral ears

H95.129 Granulation of postmastoidectomy cavity, unspecified ear

✓6th **H95.13 Mucosal cyst of postmastoidectomy cavity**

H95.131 Mucosal cyst of postmastoidectomy cavity, right ear

H95.132 Mucosal cyst of postmastoidectomy cavity, left ear

H95.133 Mucosal cyst of postmastoidectomy cavity, bilateral ears

H95.139 Mucosal cyst of postmastoidectomy cavity, unspecified ear

✓6th **H95.19 Other disorders following mastoidectomy**

H95.191 Other disorders following mastoidectomy, right ear

H95.192 Other disorders following mastoidectomy, left ear

H95.193 Other disorders following mastoidectomy, bilateral ears

H95.199 Other disorders following mastoidectomy, unspecified ear

✓5th **H95.2 Intraoperative hemorrhage and hematoma of ear and mastoid process complicating a procedure**

EXCLUDES 1 *intraoperative hemorrhage and hematoma of ear and mastoid process due to accidental puncture or laceration during a procedure (H95.3-)*

H95.21 Intraoperative hemorrhage and hematoma of ear and mastoid process complicating a procedure on the ear and mastoid process

H95.22 Intraoperative hemorrhage and hematoma of ear and mastoid process complicating other procedure

✓5th **H95.3 Accidental puncture and laceration of ear and mastoid process during a procedure**

H95.31 Accidental puncture and laceration of the ear and mastoid process during a procedure on the ear and mastoid process

H95.32 Accidental puncture and laceration of the ear and mastoid process during other procedure

✓5th **H95.4 Postprocedural hemorrhage and hematoma of ear and mastoid process following a procedure**

H95.41 Postprocedural hemorrhage and hematoma of ear and mastoid process following a procedure on the ear and mastoid process

H95.42 Postprocedural hemorrhage and hematoma of ear and mastoid process following other procedure

✓5th **H95.8 Other intraoperative and postprocedural complications and disorders of the ear and mastoid process, not elsewhere classified**

EXCLUDES 2 *postprocedural complications and disorders following mastoidectomy (H95.0-, H95.1-)*

✓6th **H95.81 Postprocedural stenosis of external ear canal**

H95.811 Postprocedural stenosis of right external ear canal

H95.812 Postprocedural stenosis of left external ear canal

H95.813 Postprocedural stenosis of external ear canal, bilateral

H95.819 Postprocedural stenosis of unspecified external ear canal

H95.88 Other intraoperative complications and disorders of the ear and mastoid process, not elsewhere classified

Use additional code, if applicable, to further specify disorder

H95.89 Other postprocedural complications and disorders of the ear and mastoid process, not elsewhere classified

Use additional code, if applicable, to further specify disorder

Chapter 9. Diseases of the Circulatory System (IØØ-I99)

EXCLUDES 2 *certain conditions originating in the perinatal period (PØ4-P96)*
certain infectious and parasitic diseases (AØØ-B99)
complications of pregnancy, childbirth and the puerperium (OØØ-O9A)
congenital malformations, deformations, and chromosomal abnormalities (QØØ-Q99)
endocrine, nutritional and metabolic diseases (EØØ-E88)
injury, poisoning and certain other consequences of external causes (SØØ-T88)
neoplasms (CØØ-D49)
symptoms, signs and abnormal clinical and laboratory findings, not elsewhere classified (RØØ-R94)
systemic connective tissue disorders (M3Ø-M36)
transient cerebral ischemic attacks and related syndromes (G45.-)

This chapter contains the following blocks:

IØØ-IØ2	Acute rheumatic fever
IØ5-IØ9	Chronic rheumatic heart diseases
I1Ø-I15	Hypertensive diseases
I2Ø-I25	Ischemic heart diseases
I26-I28	Pulmonary heart disease and diseases of pulmonary circulation
I3Ø-I52	Other forms of heart disease
I6Ø-I69	Cerebrovascular diseases
I7Ø-I79	Diseases of arteries, arterioles and capillaries
I8Ø-I89	Diseases of veins, lymphatic vessels and lymph nodes, not elsewhere classified
I95-I99	Other and unspecified disorders of the circulatory system

Acute rheumatic fever (IØØ-IØ2)

IØØ Rheumatic fever without heart involvement
INCLUDES arthritis, rheumatic, acute or subacute
EXCLUDES 1 *rheumatic fever with heart involvement (IØ1.Ø–IØ1.9)*

✓4th **IØ1 Rheumatic fever with heart involvement**
EXCLUDES 1 *chronic diseases of rheumatic origin (IØ5-IØ9) unless rheumatic fever is also present or there is evidence of reactivation or activity of the rheumatic process.*

IØ1.Ø Acute rheumatic pericarditis
Any condition in IØØ with pericarditis
Rheumatic pericarditis (acute)
EXCLUDES 1 *acute pericarditis not specified as rheumatic (I3Ø.-)*

IØ1.1 Acute rheumatic endocarditis
Any condition in IØØ with endocarditis or valvulitis
Acute rheumatic valvulitis

IØ1.2 Acute rheumatic myocarditis
Any condition in IØØ with myocarditis

IØ1.8 Other acute rheumatic heart disease
Any condition in IØØ with other or multiple types of heart involvement
Acute rheumatic pancarditis

IØ1.9 Acute rheumatic heart disease, unspecified
Any condition in IØØ with unspecified type of heart involvement
Rheumatic carditis, acute
Rheumatic heart disease, active or acute

✓4th **IØ2 Rheumatic chorea**
INCLUDES Sydenham's chorea
EXCLUDES 1 *chorea NOS (G25.5)*
Huntington's chorea (G1Ø)

IØ2.Ø Rheumatic chorea with heart involvement
Chorea NOS with heart involvement
Rheumatic chorea with heart involvement of any type classifiable under IØ1-

IØ2.9 Rheumatic chorea without heart involvement
Rheumatic chorea NOS

Chronic rheumatic heart diseases (IØ5-IØ9)

✓4th **IØ5 Rheumatic mitral valve diseases**
INCLUDES conditions classifiable to both IØ5.Ø and IØ5.2-IØ5.9, whether specified as rheumatic or not
EXCLUDES 1 *mitral valve disease specified as nonrheumatic (I34.-)*
mitral valve disease with aortic and/or tricuspid valve involvement (IØ8.-)

IØ5.Ø Rheumatic mitral stenosis
Mitral (valve) obstruction (rheumatic)

IØ5.1 Rheumatic mitral insufficiency
Rheumatic mitral incompetence
Rheumatic mitral regurgitation
EXCLUDES 1 *mitral insufficiency not specified as rheumatic (I34.Ø)*

IØ5.2 Rheumatic mitral stenosis with insufficiency
Rheumatic mitral stenosis with incompetence or regurgitation

IØ5.8 Other rheumatic mitral valve diseases
Rheumatic mitral (valve) failure

IØ5.9 Rheumatic mitral valve disease, unspecified
Rheumatic mitral (valve) disorder (chronic) NOS

✓4th **IØ6 Rheumatic aortic valve diseases**
EXCLUDES 1 *aortic valve disease not specified as rheumatic (I35.-)*
aortic valve disease with mitral and/or tricuspid valve involvement (IØ8.-)

IØ6.Ø Rheumatic aortic stenosis
Rheumatic aortic (valve) obstruction

IØ6.1 Rheumatic aortic insufficiency
Rheumatic aortic incompetence
Rheumatic aortic regurgitation

IØ6.2 Rheumatic aortic stenosis with insufficiency
Rheumatic aortic stenosis with incompetence or regurgitation

IØ6.8 Other rheumatic aortic valve diseases

IØ6.9 Rheumatic aortic valve disease, unspecified
Rheumatic aortic (valve) disease NOS

✓4th **IØ7 Rheumatic tricuspid valve diseases**
INCLUDES rheumatic tricuspid valve diseases specified as rheumatic or unspecified
EXCLUDES 1 *tricuspid valve disease specified as nonrheumatic (I36.-)*
tricuspid valve disease with aortic and/or mitral valve involvement (IØ8.-)

IØ7.Ø Rheumatic tricuspid stenosis
Tricuspid (valve) stenosis (rheumatic)

IØ7.1 Rheumatic tricuspid insufficiency
Tricuspid (valve) insufficiency (rheumatic)

IØ7.2 Rheumatic tricuspid stenosis and insufficiency

IØ7.8 Other rheumatic tricuspid valve diseases

IØ7.9 Rheumatic tricuspid valve disease, unspecified
Rheumatic tricuspid valve disorder NOS

✓4th **IØ8 Multiple valve diseases**
INCLUDES multiple valve diseases specified as rheumatic or unspecified
EXCLUDES 1 *endocarditis, valve unspecified (I38)*
multiple valve disease specified a nonrheumatic (I34.-, I35.-, I36.-, I37.-, I38.-, Q22.-, Q23.-, Q24.8-)
rheumatic valve disease NOS (IØ9.1)

IØ8.Ø Rheumatic disorders of both mitral and aortic valves
Involvement of both mitral and aortic valves specified as rheumatic or unspecified

IØ8.1 Rheumatic disorders of both mitral and tricuspid valves

IØ8.2 Rheumatic disorders of both aortic and tricuspid valves

IØ8.3 Combined rheumatic disorders of mitral, aortic and tricuspid valves

IØ8.8 Other rheumatic multiple valve diseases

IØ8.9 Rheumatic multiple valve disease, unspecified

✓4th **IØ9 Other rheumatic heart diseases**

IØ9.Ø Rheumatic myocarditis
EXCLUDES 1 *myocarditis not specified as rheumatic (I51.4)*

IØ9.1 Rheumatic diseases of endocardium, valve unspecified
Rheumatic endocarditis (chronic)
Rheumatic valvulitis (chronic)
EXCLUDES 1 *endocarditis, valve unspecified (I38)*

IØ9.2 Chronic rheumatic pericarditis
Adherent pericardium, rheumatic
Chronic rheumatic mediastinopericarditis
Chronic rheumatic myopericarditis
EXCLUDES 1 *chronic pericarditis not specified as rheumatic (I31.-)*

✓5th **IØ9.8 Other specified rheumatic heart diseases**

IØ9.81 Rheumatic heart failure
Use additional code to identify type of heart failure (I5Ø.-)

IØ9.89 Other specified rheumatic heart diseases
Rheumatic disease of pulmonary valve

IØ9.9 Rheumatic heart disease, unspecified
Rheumatic carditis
EXCLUDES 1 *rheumatoid carditis (MØ5.31)*

Hypertensive diseases (I1Ø-I15)

Use additional code to identify:
exposure to environmental tobacco smoke (Z77.22)
history of tobacco use (Z87.891)
occupational exposure to environmental tobacco smoke (Z57.31)
tobacco dependence (F17.-)
tobacco use (Z72.Ø)

EXCLUDES 1 *hypertensive disease complicating pregnancy, childbirth and the puerperium (O1Ø-O11, O13-O16)*
neonatal hypertension (P29.2)
primary pulmonary hypertension (I27.Ø)

I1Ø Essential (primary) hypertension
INCLUDES high blood pressure
hypertension (arterial) (benign) (essential) (malignant) (primary) (systemic)
EXCLUDES 1 *hypertensive disease complicating pregnancy, childbirth and the puerperium (O1Ø-O11, O13-O16)*
EXCLUDES 2 *essential (primary) hypertension involving vessels of brain (I6Ø-I69)*
essential (primary) hypertension involving vessels of eye (H35.Ø-)

✓4th **I11 Hypertensive heart disease**
INCLUDES any condition in I51.4-I51.9 due to hypertension

I11.Ø Hypertensive heart disease with heart failure
Hypertensive heart failure
Use additional code to identify type of heart failure (I5Ø.-)

I11.9 Hypertensive heart disease without heart failure
Hypertensive heart disease NOS

✓4th **I12 Hypertensive chronic kidney disease**
INCLUDES any condition in N18- and N26- due to hypertension
arteriosclerosis of kidney
arteriosclerotic nephritis (chronic) (interstitial)
hypertensive nephropathy
nephrosclerosis
EXCLUDES 1 *hypertension due to kidney disease (I15.Ø, I15.1)*
renovascular hypertension (I15.Ø)
secondary hypertension (I15.-)
EXCLUDES 2 *acute kidney failure (N17.-)*

I12.Ø Hypertensive chronic kidney disease with stage 5 chronic kidney disease or end stage renal disease
Use additional code to identify the stage of chronic kidney disease (N18.5, N18.6)

I12.9 Hypertensive chronic kidney disease with stage 1 through stage 4 chronic kidney disease, or unspecified chronic kidney disease
Hypertensive chronic kidney disease NOS
Hypertensive renal disease NOS
Use additional code to identify the stage of chronic kidney disease (N18.1-N18.4, N18.9)

✓4th **I13 Hypertensive heart and chronic kidney disease**
INCLUDES any condition in I11- with any condition in I12-
cardiorenal disease
cardiovascular renal disease

I13.Ø Hypertensive heart and chronic kidney disease with heart failure and stage 1 through stage 4 chronic kidney disease, or unspecified chronic kidney disease
Use additional code to identify type of heart failure (I5Ø.-)
Use additional code to identify stage of chronic kidney disease (N18.1-N18.4, N18.9)

✓5th **I13.1 Hypertensive heart and chronic kidney disease without heart failure**

I13.1Ø Hypertensive heart and chronic kidney disease without heart failure, with stage 1 through stage 4 chronic kidney disease, or unspecified chronic kidney disease
Hypertensive heart disease and hypertensive chronic kidney disease NOS
Use additional code to identify the stage of chronic kidney disease (N18.1-N18.4, N18.9)

I13.11 Hypertensive heart and chronic kidney disease without heart failure, with stage 5 chronic kidney disease, or end stage renal disease
Use additional code to identify the stage of chronic kidney disease (N18.5, N18.6)

I13.2 Hypertensive heart and chronic kidney disease with heart failure and with stage 5 chronic kidney disease, or end stage renal disease
Use additional code to identify type of heart failure (I5Ø.-)
Use additional code to identify the stage of chronic kidney disease (N18.5, N18.6)

✓4th **I15 Secondary hypertension**
Code also underlying condition
EXCLUDES 1 *postprocedural hypertension (I97.3)*
EXCLUDES 2 *secondary hypertension involving vessels of brain (I6Ø-I69)*
secondary hypertension involving vessels of eye (H35.Ø-)

I15.Ø Renovascular hypertension
I15.1 Hypertension secondary to other renal disorders
I15.2 Hypertension secondary to endocrine disorders
I15.8 Other secondary hypertension
I15.9 Secondary hypertension, unspecified

Ischemic heart diseases (I2Ø-I25)

Use additional code to identify presence of hypertension (I1Ø-I15)

✓4th **I2Ø Angina pectoris**
Use additional code to identify:
exposure to environmental tobacco smoke (Z77.22)
history of tobacco use (Z87.891)
occupational exposure to environmental tobacco smoke (Z57.31)
tobacco dependence (F17.-)
tobacco use (Z72.Ø)
EXCLUDES 1 *angina pectoris with atherosclerotic heart disease of native coronary arteries (I25.1-)*
atherosclerosis of coronary artery bypass graft(s) and coronary artery of transplanted heart with angina pectoris (I25.7-)
postinfarction angina (I23.7)

I2Ø.Ø Unstable angina
Accelerated angina
Crescendo angina
De novo effort angina
Intermediate coronary syndrome
Preinfarction syndrome
Worsening effort angina

I2Ø.1 Angina pectoris with documented spasm
Angiospastic angina
Prinzmetal angina
Spasm-induced angina
Variant angina

I2Ø.8 Other forms of angina pectoris
Angina equivalent
Angina of effort
Coronary slow flow syndrome
Stenocardia
Use additional code(s) for symptoms associated with angina equivalent

I2Ø.9 Angina pectoris, unspecified
Angina NOS
Anginal syndrome
Cardiac angina
Ischemic chest pain

I21 ST elevation (STEMI) and non-ST elevation (NSTEMI) myocardial infarction

INCLUDES cardiac infarction
coronary (artery) embolism
coronary (artery) occlusion
coronary (artery) rupture
coronary (artery) thrombosis
infarction of heart, myocardium, or ventricle
myocardial infarction specified as acute or with a stated duration of 4 weeks (28 days) or less from onset

Use additional code, if applicable, to identify:
exposure to environmental tobacco smoke (Z77.22)
history of tobacco use (Z87.891)
occupational exposure to environmental tobacco smoke (Z57.31)
status post administration of tPA (rtPA) in a different facility within the last 24 hours prior to admission to current facility (Z92.82)
tobacco dependence (F17.-)
tobacco use (Z72.0)

EXCLUDES 2 *old myocardial infarction (I25.2)*
postmyocardial infarction syndrome (I24.1)
subsequent myocardial infarction (I22.-)

I21.0 ST elevation (STEMI) myocardial infarction of anterior wall

I21.01 ST elevation (STEMI) myocardial infarction involving left main coronary artery

I21.02 ST elevation (STEMI) myocardial infarction involving left anterior descending coronary artery
ST elevation (STEMI) myocardial infarction involving diagonal coronary artery

I21.09 ST elevation (STEMI) myocardial infarction involving other coronary artery of anterior wall
Acute transmural myocardial infarction of anterior wall
Anteroapical transmural (Q wave) infarction (acute)
Anterolateral transmural (Q wave) infarction (acute)
Anteroseptal transmural (Q wave) infarction (acute)
Transmural (Q wave) infarction (acute) (of) anterior (wall) NOS

I21.1 ST elevation (STEMI) myocardial infarction of inferior wall

I21.11 ST elevation (STEMI) myocardial infarction involving right coronary artery
Inferoposterior transmural (Q wave) infarction (acute)

I21.19 ST elevation (STEMI) myocardial infarction involving other coronary artery of inferior wall
Acute transmural myocardial infarction of inferior wall
Inferolateral transmural (Q wave) infarction (acute)
Transmural (Q wave) infarction (acute) (of) diaphragmatic wall
Transmural (Q wave) infarction (acute) (of) inferior (wall) NOS

EXCLUDES 2 *ST elevation (STEMI) myocardial infarction involving left circumflex coronary artery (I21.21)*

I21.2 ST elevation (STEMI) myocardial infarction of other sites

I21.21 ST elevation (STEMI) myocardial infarction involving left circumflex coronary artery
ST elevation (STEMI) myocardial infarction involving oblique marginal coronary artery

I21.29 ST elevation (STEMI) myocardial infarction involving other sites
Acute transmural myocardial infarction of other sites
Apical-lateral transmural (Q wave) infarction (acute)
Basal-lateral transmural (Q wave) infarction (acute)
High lateral transmural (Q wave) infarction (acute)
Lateral (wall) NOS transmural (Q wave) infarction (acute)
Posterior (true) transmural (Q wave) infarction (acute)
Posterobasal transmural (Q wave) infarction (acute)
Posterolateral transmural (Q wave) infarction (acute)
Posteroseptal transmural (Q wave) infarction (acute)
Septal transmural (Q wave) infarction (acute) NOS

I21.3 ST elevation (STEMI) myocardial infarction of unspecified site
Acute transmural myocardial infarction of unspecified site
Myocardial infarction (acute) NOS
Transmural (Q wave) myocardial infarction NOS

I21.4 Non-ST elevation (NSTEMI) myocardial infarction
Acute subendocardial myocardial infarction
Non-Q wave myocardial infarction NOS
Nontransmural myocardial infarction NOS

I22 Subsequent ST elevation (STEMI) and non-ST elevation (NSTEMI) myocardial infarction

INCLUDES acute myocardial infarction occurring within four weeks (28 days) of a previous acute myocardial infarction, regardless of site
cardiac infarction
coronary (artery) embolism
coronary (artery) occlusion
coronary (artery) rupture
coronary (artery) thrombosis
infarction of heart, myocardium, or ventricle
recurrent myocardial infarction
reinfarction of myocardium
rupture of heart, myocardium, or ventricle

Use additional code, if applicable, to identify:
exposure to environmental tobacco smoke (Z77.22)
history of tobacco use (Z87.891)
occupational exposure to environmental tobacco smoke (Z57.31)
status post administration of tPA (rtPA) in a different facility within the last 24 hours prior to admission to current facility (Z92.82)
tobacco dependence (F17.-)
tobacco use (Z72.0)

I22.0 Subsequent ST elevation (STEMI) myocardial infarction of anterior wall
Subsequent acute transmural myocardial infarction of anterior wall
Subsequent transmural (Q wave) infarction (acute)(of) anterior (wall) NOS
Subsequent anteroapical transmural (Q wave) infarction (acute)
Subsequent anterolateral transmural (Q wave) infarction (acute)
Subsequent anteroseptal transmural (Q wave) infarction (acute)

I22.1 Subsequent ST elevation (STEMI) myocardial infarction of inferior wall
Subsequent acute transmural myocardial infarction of inferior wall
Subsequent transmural (Q wave) infarction (acute)(of) diaphragmatic wall
Subsequent transmural (Q wave) infarction (acute)(of) inferior (wall) NOS
Subsequent inferolateral transmural (Q wave) infarction (acute)
Subsequent inferoposterior transmural (Q wave) infarction (acute)

I22.2 Subsequent non-ST elevation (NSTEMI) myocardial infarction
Subsequent acute subendocardial myocardial infarction
Subsequent non-Q wave myocardial infarction NOS
Subsequent nontransmural myocardial infarction NOS

I22.8 Subsequent ST elevation (STEMI) myocardial infarction of other sites
Subsequent acute transmural myocardial infarction of other sites
Subsequent apical-lateral transmural (Q wave) myocardial infarction (acute)
Subsequent basal-lateral transmural (Q wave) myocardial infarction (acute)
Subsequent high lateral transmural (Q wave) myocardial infarction (acute)
Subsequent transmural (Q wave) myocardial infarction (acute)(of) lateral (wall) NOS
Subsequent posterior (true)transmural (Q wave) myocardial infarction (acute)
Subsequent posterobasal transmural (Q wave) myocardial infarction (acute)
Subsequent posterolateral transmural (Q wave) myocardial infarction (acute)
Subsequent posteroseptal transmural (Q wave) myocardial infarction (acute)
Subsequent septal NOS transmural (Q wave) myocardial infarction (acute)

I22.9 Subsequent ST elevation (STEMI) myocardial infarction of unspecified site
Subsequent acute myocardial infarction of unspecified site
Subsequent myocardial infarction (acute) NOS

I23 Certain current complications following ST elevation (STEMI) and non-ST elevation (NSTEMI) myocardial infarction (within the 28 day period)

NOTE A code from category I23 must be used in conjunction with a code from category I21 or category I22. The I23 code should be sequenced first, if it is the reason for encounter, or, it should be sequenced after the I21 or I22 code if the complication of the MI occurs during the encounter for the MI.

I23.0 Hemopericardium as current complication following acute myocardial infarction

EXCLUDES 1 *hemopericardium not specified as current complication following acute myocardial infarction (I31.2)*

I23.1 Atrial septal defect as current complication following acute myocardial infarction

EXCLUDES 1 *acquired atrial septal defect not specified as current complication following acute myocardial infarction (I51.0)*

I23.2 Ventricular septal defect as current complication following acute myocardial infarction

EXCLUDES 1 *acquired ventricular septal defect not specified as current complication following acute myocardial infarction (I51.0)*

I23.3 Rupture of cardiac wall without hemopericardium as current complication following acute myocardial infarction

I23.4 Rupture of chordae tendineae as current complication following acute myocardial infarction

EXCLUDES 1 *rupture of chordae tendineae not specified as current complication following acute myocardial infarction (I51.1)*

I23.5 Rupture of papillary muscle as current complication following acute myocardial infarction

EXCLUDES 1 *rupture of papillary muscle not specified as current complication following acute myocardial infarction (I51.2)*

I23.6 Thrombosis of atrium, auricular appendage, and ventricle as current complications following acute myocardial infarction

EXCLUDES 1 *thrombosis of atrium, auricular appendage, and ventricle not specified as current complication following acute myocardial infarction (I51.3)*

I23.7 Postinfarction angina

I23.8 Other current complications following acute myocardial infarction

I24 Other acute ischemic heart diseases

EXCLUDES 1 *angina pectoris (I20.-)*
transient myocardial ischemia in newborn (P29.4)

I24.0 Acute coronary thrombosis not resulting in myocardial infarction

Acute coronary (artery) (vein) embolism not resulting in myocardial infarction
Acute coronary (artery) (vein) occlusion not resulting in myocardial infarction
Acute coronary (artery) (vein) thromboembolism not resulting in myocardial infarction

EXCLUDES 1 *atherosclerotic heart disease (I25.1-)*

I24.1 Dressler's syndrome

Postmyocardial infarction syndrome

EXCLUDES 1 *postinfarction angina (I23.7)*

I24.8 Other forms of acute ischemic heart disease

I24.9 Acute ischemic heart disease, unspecified

EXCLUDES 1 *ischemic heart disease (chronic) NOS (I25.9)*

I25 Chronic ischemic heart disease

Use additional code to identify:
chronic total occlusion of coronary artery (I25.82)
exposure to environmental tobacco smoke (Z77.22)
history of tobacco use (Z87.891)
occupational exposure to environmental tobacco smoke (Z57.31)
tobacco dependence (F17.-)
tobacco use (Z72.0)

I25.1 Atherosclerotic heart disease of native coronary artery

Atherosclerotic cardiovascular disease
Coronary (artery) atheroma
Coronary (artery) atherosclerosis
Coronary (artery) disease
Coronary (artery) sclerosis

Use additional code, if applicable, to identify:
coronary atherosclerosis due to calcified coronary lesion (I25.84)
coronary atherosclerosis due to lipid rich plaque (I25.83)

EXCLUDES 2 *atheroembolism (I75.-)*
atherosclerosis of coronary artery bypass graft(s) and transplanted heart (I25.7-)

I25.10 Atherosclerotic heart disease of native coronary artery without angina pectoris

Atherosclerotic heart disease NOS

I25.11 Atherosclerotic heart disease of native coronary artery with angina pectoris

I25.110 Atherosclerotic heart disease of native coronary artery with unstable angina pectoris

EXCLUDES 1 *unstable angina without atherosclerotic heart disease (I20.0)*

I25.111 Atherosclerotic heart disease of native coronary artery with angina pectoris with documented spasm

EXCLUDES 1 *angina pectoris with documented spasm without atherosclerotic heart disease (I20.1)*

I25.118 Atherosclerotic heart disease of native coronary artery with other forms of angina pectoris

EXCLUDES 1 *other forms of angina pectoris without atherosclerotic heart disease (I20.8)*

I25.119 Atherosclerotic heart disease of native coronary artery with unspecified angina pectoris

Atherosclerotic heart disease with angina NOS
Atherosclerotic heart disease with ischemic chest pain

EXCLUDES 1 *unspecified angina pectoris without atherosclerotic heart disease (I20.9)*

I25.2 Old myocardial infarction

Healed myocardial infarction
Past myocardial infarction diagnosed by ECG or other investigation, but currently presenting no symptoms

I25.3 Aneurysm of heart

Mural aneurysm
Ventricular aneurysm

I25.4 Coronary artery aneurysm and dissection

I25.41 Coronary artery aneurysm

Coronary arteriovenous fistula, acquired

EXCLUDES 1 *congenital coronary (artery) aneurysm (Q24.5)*

I25.42 Coronary artery dissection

I25.5 Ischemic cardiomyopathy

EXCLUDES 2 *coronary atherosclerosis (I25.1-, I25.7-)*

I25.6 Silent myocardial ischemia

I25.7 Atherosclerosis of coronary artery bypass graft(s) and coronary artery of transplanted heart with angina pectoris
Use additional code, if applicable, to identify:
coronary atherosclerosis due to calcified coronary lesion (I25.84)
coronary atherosclerosis due to lipid rich plaque (I25.83)
EXCLUDES 1 *atherosclerosis of bypass graft(s) of transplanted heart without angina pectoris (I25.812)*
atherosclerosis of coronary artery bypass graft(s) without angina pectoris (I25.810)
atherosclerosis of native coronary artery of transplanted heart without angina pectoris (I25.811)
embolism or thrombus of coronary artery bypass graft(s) (T82.8-)

I25.70 Atherosclerosis of coronary artery bypass graft(s), unspecified, with angina pectoris

I25.700 Atherosclerosis of coronary artery bypass graft(s), unspecified, with unstable angina pectoris
EXCLUDES 1 *unstable angina pectoris without atherosclerosis of coronary artery bypass graft (I20.0)*

I25.701 Atherosclerosis of coronary artery bypass graft(s), unspecified, with angina pectoris with documented spasm
EXCLUDES 1 *angina pectoris with documented spasm without atherosclerosis of coronary artery bypass graft (I20.1)*

I25.708 Atherosclerosis of coronary artery bypass graft(s), unspecified, with other forms of angina pectoris
EXCLUDES 1 *other forms of angina pectoris without atherosclerosis of coronary artery bypass graft (I20.8)*

I25.709 Atherosclerosis of coronary artery bypass graft(s), unspecified, with unspecified angina pectoris
EXCLUDES 1 *unspecified angina pectoris without atherosclerosis of coronary artery bypass graft (I20.9)*

I25.71 Atherosclerosis of autologous vein coronary artery bypass graft(s) with angina pectoris

I25.710 Atherosclerosis of autologous vein coronary artery bypass graft(s) with unstable angina pectoris
EXCLUDES 1 *unstable angina without atherosclerosis of autologous vein coronary artery bypass graft(s) (I20.0)*

I25.711 Atherosclerosis of autologous vein coronary artery bypass graft(s) with angina pectoris with documented spasm
EXCLUDES 1 *angina pectoris with documented spasm without atherosclerosis of autologous vein coronary artery bypass graft(s) (I20.1)*

I25.718 Atherosclerosis of autologous vein coronary artery bypass graft(s) with other forms of angina pectoris
EXCLUDES 1 *other forms of angina pectoris without atherosclerosis of autologous vein coronary artery bypass graft(s) (I20.8)*

I25.719 Atherosclerosis of autologous vein coronary artery bypass graft(s) with unspecified angina pectoris
EXCLUDES 1 *unspecified angina pectoris without atherosclerosis of autologous vein coronary artery bypass graft(s) (I20.9)*

I25.72 Atherosclerosis of autologous artery coronary artery bypass graft(s) with angina pectoris
Atherosclerosis of internal mammary artery graft with angina pectoris

I25.720 Atherosclerosis of autologous artery coronary artery bypass graft(s) with unstable angina pectoris
EXCLUDES 1 *unstable angina without atherosclerosis of autologous artery coronary artery bypass graft(s) (I20.0)*

I25.721 Atherosclerosis of autologous artery coronary artery bypass graft(s) with angina pectoris with documented spasm
EXCLUDES 1 *angina pectoris with documented spasm without atherosclerosis of autologous artery coronary artery bypass graft(s) (I20.1)*

I25.728 Atherosclerosis of autologous artery coronary artery bypass graft(s) with other forms of angina pectoris
EXCLUDES 1 *other forms of angina pectoris without atherosclerosis of autologous artery coronary artery bypass graft(s) (I20.8)*

I25.729 Atherosclerosis of autologous artery coronary artery bypass graft(s) with unspecified angina pectoris
EXCLUDES 1 *unspecified angina pectoris without atherosclerosis of autologous artery coronary artery bypass graft(s) (I20.9)*

I25.73 Atherosclerosis of nonautologous biological coronary artery bypass graft(s) with angina pectoris

I25.730 Atherosclerosis of nonautologous biological coronary artery bypass graft(s) with unstable angina pectoris
EXCLUDES 1 *unstable angina without atherosclerosis of nonautologous biological coronary artery bypass graft(s) (I20.0)*

I25.731 Atherosclerosis of nonautologous biological coronary artery bypass graft(s) with angina pectoris with documented spasm
EXCLUDES 1 *angina pectoris with documented spasm without atherosclerosis of nonautologous biological coronary artery bypass graft(s) (I20.1)*

I25.738 Atherosclerosis of nonautologous biological coronary artery bypass graft(s) with other forms of angina pectoris
EXCLUDES 1 *other forms of angina pectoris without atherosclerosis of nonautologous biological coronary artery bypass graft(s) (I20.8)*

I25.739 Atherosclerosis of nonautologous biological coronary artery bypass graft(s) with unspecified angina pectoris
EXCLUDES 1 *unspecified angina pectoris without atherosclerosis of nonautologous biological coronary artery bypass graft(s) (I20.9)*

I25.75 Atherosclerosis of native coronary artery of transplanted heart with angina pectoris

EXCLUDES 1 *atherosclerosis of native coronary artery of transplanted heart without angina pectoris (I25.811)*

I25.750 Atherosclerosis of native coronary artery of transplanted heart with unstable angina

I25.751 Atherosclerosis of native coronary artery of transplanted heart with angina pectoris with documented spasm

I25.758 Atherosclerosis of native coronary artery of transplanted heart with other forms of angina pectoris

I25.759 Atherosclerosis of native coronary artery of transplanted heart with unspecified angina pectoris

I25.76 Atherosclerosis of bypass graft of coronary artery of transplanted heart with angina pectoris

EXCLUDES 1 *atherosclerosis of bypass graft of coronary artery of transplanted heart without angina pectoris (I25.812)*

I25.760 Atherosclerosis of bypass graft of coronary artery of transplanted heart with unstable angina

I25.761 Atherosclerosis of bypass graft of coronary artery of transplanted heart with angina pectoris with documented spasm

I25.768 Atherosclerosis of bypass graft of coronary artery of transplanted heart with other forms of angina pectoris

I25.769 Atherosclerosis of bypass graft of coronary artery of transplanted heart with unspecified angina pectoris

I25.79 Atherosclerosis of other coronary artery bypass graft(s) with angina pectoris

I25.790 Atherosclerosis of other coronary artery bypass graft(s) with unstable angina pectoris

EXCLUDES 1 *unstable angina without atherosclerosis of other coronary artery bypass graft(s) (I20.0)*

I25.791 Atherosclerosis of other coronary artery bypass graft(s) with angina pectoris with documented spasm

EXCLUDES 1 *angina pectoris with documented spasm without atherosclerosis of other coronary artery bypass graft(s) (I20.1)*

I25.798 Atherosclerosis of other coronary artery bypass graft(s) with other forms of angina pectoris

EXCLUDES 1 *other forms of angina pectoris without atherosclerosis of other coronary artery bypass graft(s)(I20.8)*

I25.799 Atherosclerosis of other coronary artery bypass graft(s) with unspecified angina pectoris

EXCLUDES 1 *unspecified angina pectoris without atherosclerosis of other coronary artery bypass graft(s) (I20.9)*

I25.8 Other forms of chronic ischemic heart disease

I25.81 Atherosclerosis of other coronary vessels without angina pectoris

Use additional code, if applicable, to identify:
coronary atherosclerosis due to calcified coronary lesion (I25.84)
coronary atherosclerosis due to lipid rich plaque (I25.83)

EXCLUDES 1 *atherosclerotic heart disease of native coronary artery without angina pectoris (I25.10)*

I25.810 Atherosclerosis of coronary artery bypass graft(s) without angina pectoris

Atherosclerosis of coronary artery bypass graft NOS

EXCLUDES 1 *atherosclerosis of coronary bypass graft(s) with angina pectoris (I25.70–I25.73-, I25.79-)*

I25.811 Atherosclerosis of native coronary artery of transplanted heart without angina pectoris

Atherosclerosis of native coronary artery of transplanted heart NOS

EXCLUDES 1 *atherosclerosis of native coronary artery of transplanted heart with angina pectoris (I25.75-)*

I25.812 Atherosclerosis of bypass graft of coronary artery of transplanted heart without angina pectoris

Atherosclerosis of bypass graft of transplanted heart NOS

EXCLUDES 1 *atherosclerosis of bypass graft of transplanted heart with angina pectoris (I25.76)*

I25.82 Chronic total occlusion of coronary artery

Complete occlusion of coronary artery
Total occlusion of coronary artery
Code first coronary atherosclerosis (I25.1-, I25.7-, I25.81-)

EXCLUDES 1 *acute coronary occulsion with myocardial infarction (I21.-, I22.-)*
acute coronary occulsion without myocardial infarction (I24.0)

I25.83 Coronary atherosclerosis due to lipid rich plaque

Code first coronary atherosclerosis (I25.1-, I25.7-, I25.81-)

I25.84 Coronary atherosclerosis due to calcified coronary lesion

Coronary atherosclerosis due to severely calcified coronary lesion
Code first coronary atherosclerosis (I25.1-, I25.7-, I25.81-)

I25.89 Other forms of chronic ischemic heart disease

I25.9 Chronic ischemic heart disease, unspecified

Ischemic heart disease (chronic) NOS

Pulmonary heart disease and diseases of pulmonary circulation (I26-I28)

I26 Pulmonary embolism

Pulmonary (acute) (artery)(vein) infarction
Pulmonary (acute) (artery)(vein) thromboembolism
Pulmonary (acute) (artery)(vein) thrombosis

EXCLUDES 2 *chronic pulmonary embolism (I27.82)*
personal history of pulmonary embolism (Z86.711)
pulmonary embolism due to trauma (T79.0, T79.1)
pulmonary embolism due to complications of surgical and medical care (T80.0, T81.7-, T82.8-)
pulmonary embolism complicating:
abortion, ectopic or molar pregnancy (O00-O07, O08.2)
pregnancy, childbirth and the puerperium (O88.-)
septic (non-pulmonary) arterial embolism (I76)

I26.0 Pulmonary embolism with acute cor pulmonale

I26.01 Septic pulmonary embolism with acute cor pulmonale

Code first underlying infection

I26.02 Saddle embolus of pulmonary artery with acute cor pulmonale

I26.09 Other pulmonary embolism with acute cor pulmonale
Acute cor pulmonale NOS

✓5th **I26.9 Pulmonary embolism without acute cor pulmonale**

I26.90 Septic pulmonary embolism without acute cor pulmonale
Code first underlying infection

I26.92 Saddle embolus of pulmonary artery without acute cor pulmonale

I26.99 Other pulmonary embolism without acute cor pulmonale
Acute pulmonary embolism NOS
Pulmonary embolism NOS

✓4th **I27 Other pulmonary heart diseases**

I27.0 Primary pulmonary hypertension
EXCLUDES 1 *pulmonary hypertension NOS (I27.2)*
secondary pulmonary hypertension (I27.2)

I27.1 Kyphoscoliotic heart disease

I27.2 Other secondary pulmonary hypertension
Pulmonary hypertension NOS
Code also associated underlying condition

✓5th **I27.8 Other specified pulmonary heart diseases**

I27.81 Cor pulmonale (chronic)
Cor pulmonale NOS
EXCLUDES 1 *acute cor pulmonale (I26.0-)*

I27.82 Chronic pulmonary embolism
Use additional code, if applicable, for associated long-term (current) use of anticoagulants (Z79.01)
EXCLUDES 1 *personal history of pulmonary embolism (Z86.711)*

I27.89 Other specified pulmonary heart diseases
Eisenmenger's complex
Eisenmenger's syndrome
EXCLUDES 1 *Eisenmenger's defect (Q21.8)*

I27.9 Pulmonary heart disease, unspecified
Chronic cardiopulmonary disease

✓4th **I28 Other diseases of pulmonary vessels**

I28.0 Arteriovenous fistula of pulmonary vessels
EXCLUDES 1 *congenital arteriovenous fistula (Q25.72)*

I28.1 Aneurysm of pulmonary artery
EXCLUDES 1 *congenital aneurysm (Q25.79)*
congenital arteriovenous aneurysm (Q25.72)

I28.8 Other diseases of pulmonary vessels
Pulmonary arteritis
Pulmonary endarteritis
Rupture of pulmonary vessels
Stenosis of pulmonary vessels
Stricture of pulmonary vessels

I28.9 Disease of pulmonary vessels, unspecified

Other forms of heart disease (I30-I52)

✓4th **I30 Acute pericarditis**
INCLUDES acute mediastinopericarditis
acute myopericarditis
acute pericardial effusion
acute pleuropericarditis
acute pneumopericarditis
EXCLUDES 1 *Dressler's syndrome (I24.1)*
rheumatic pericarditis (acute) (I01.0)

I30.0 Acute nonspecific idiopathic pericarditis

I30.1 Infective pericarditis
Pneumococcal pericarditis
Pneumopyopericardium
Purulent pericarditis
Pyopericarditis
Pyopericardium
Pyopneumopericardium
Staphylococcal pericarditis
Streptococcal pericarditis
Suppurative pericarditis
Viral pericarditis
Use additional code (B95-B97) to identify infectious agent

I30.8 Other forms of acute pericarditis

I30.9 Acute pericarditis, unspecified

✓4th **I31 Other diseases of pericardium**
EXCLUDES 1 *diseases of pericardium specified as rheumatic (I09.2)*
postcardiotomy syndrome (I97.0)
traumatic injury to pericardium (S26.-)

I31.0 Chronic adhesive pericarditis
Accretio cordis
Adherent pericardium
Adhesive mediastinopericarditis

I31.1 Chronic constrictive pericarditis
Concretio cordis
Pericardial calcification

I31.2 Hemopericardium, not elsewhere classified
EXCLUDES 1 *hemopericardium as current complication following acute myocardial infarction (I23.0)*

I31.3 Pericardial effusion (noninflammatory)
Chylopericardium
EXCLUDES 1 *acute pericardial effusion (I30.9)*

I31.4 Cardiac tamponade
Code first underlying cause

I31.8 Other specified diseases of pericardium
Epicardial plaques
Focal pericardial adhesions

I31.9 Disease of pericardium, unspecified
Pericarditis (chronic) NOS

I32 Pericarditis in diseases classified elsewhere
Code first underlying disease
EXCLUDES 1 *pericarditis (in):*
coxsackie (virus) (B33.23)
gonococcal (A54.83)
meningococcal (A39.53)
rheumatoid (arthritis) (M05.31)
syphilitic (A52.06)
systemic lupus erythematosus (M32.12)
tuberculosis (A18.84)

✓4th **I33 Acute and subacute endocarditis**
EXCLUDES 1 *acute rheumatic endocarditis (I01.1)*
endocarditis NOS (I38)

I33.0 Acute and subacute infective endocarditis
Bacterial endocarditis (acute) (subacute)
Infective endocarditis (acute) (subacute) NOS
Endocarditis lenta (acute) (subacute)
Malignant endocarditis (acute) (subacute)
Purulent endocarditis (acute) (subacute)
Septic endocarditis (acute) (subacute)
Ulcerative endocarditis (acute) (subacute)
Vegetative endocarditis (acute) (subacute)
Use additional code (B95-B97) to identify infectious agent

I33.9 Acute and subacute endocarditis, unspecified
Acute endocarditis NOS
Acute myoendocarditis NOS
Acute periendocarditis NOS
Subacute endocarditis NOS
Subacute myoendocarditis NOS
Subacute periendocarditis NOS

✓4th **I34 Nonrheumatic mitral valve disorders**
EXCLUDES 1 *mitral valve disease (I05.9)*
mitral valve failure (I05.8)
mitral valve stenosis (I05.0)
mitral valve disorder of unspecified cause with diseases of aortic and/or tricuspid valve(s) (I08.-)
mitral valve disorder of unspecified cause with mitral stenosis or obstruction (I05.0)
mitral valve disorder specified as congenital (Q23.2, Q23.3)
mitral valve disorder specified as rheumatic (I05.-)

I34.0 Nonrheumatic mitral (valve) insufficiency
Nonrheumatic mitral (valve) incompetence NOS
Nonrheumatic mitral (valve) regurgitation NOS

I34.1 Nonrheumatic mitral (valve) prolapse
Floppy nonrheumatic mitral valve syndrome
EXCLUDES 1 *Marfan's syndrome (Q87.4-)*

I34.2 Nonrheumatic mitral (valve) stenosis

I34.8 Other nonrheumatic mitral valve disorders

I34.9 Nonrheumatic mitral valve disorder, unspecified

I35 Nonrheumatic aortic valve disorders

EXCLUDES 1 *aortic valve disorder of unspecified cause but with diseases of mitral and/or tricuspid valve(s) (I08.-)*
aortic valve disorder specified as congenital (Q23.0, Q23.1)
aortic valve disorder specified as rheumatic (I06.-)
hypertrophic subaortic stenosis (I42.1)

I35.0 Nonrheumatic aortic (valve) stenosis

I35.1 Nonrheumatic aortic (valve) insufficiency
Nonrheumatic aortic (valve) incompetence NOS
Nonrheumatic aortic (valve) regurgitation NOS

I35.2 Nonrheumatic aortic (valve) stenosis with insufficiency

I35.8 Other nonrheumatic aortic valve disorders

I35.9 Nonrheumatic aortic valve disorder, unspecified

I36 Nonrheumatic tricuspid valve disorders

EXCLUDES 1 *tricuspid valve disorders of unspecified cause (I07.-)*
tricuspid valve disorders specified as congenital (Q22.4, Q22.8, Q22.9)
tricuspid valve disorders specified as rheumatic (I07.-)
tricuspid valve disorders with aortic and/or mitral valve involvement (I08.-)

I36.0 Nonrheumatic tricuspid (valve) stenosis

I36.1 Nonrheumatic tricuspid (valve) insufficiency
Nonrheumatic tricuspid (valve) incompetence
Nonrheumatic tricuspid (valve) regurgitation

I36.2 Nonrheumatic tricuspid (valve) stenosis with insufficiency

I36.8 Other nonrheumatic tricuspid valve disorders

I36.9 Nonrheumatic tricuspid valve disorder, unspecified

I37 Nonrheumatic pulmonary valve disorders

EXCLUDES 1 *pulmonary valve disorder specified as congenital (Q22.1, Q22.2, Q22.3)*
pulmonary valve disorder specified as rheumatic (I09.89)

I37.0 Nonrheumatic pulmonary valve stenosis

I37.1 Nonrheumatic pulmonary valve insufficiency
Nonrheumatic pulmonary valve incompetence
Nonrheumatic pulmonary valve regurgitation

I37.2 Nonrheumatic pulmonary valve stenosis with insufficiency

I37.8 Other nonrheumatic pulmonary valve disorders

I37.9 Nonrheumatic pulmonary valve disorder, unspecified

I38 Endocarditis, valve unspecified

INCLUDES endocarditis (chronic) NOS
valvular incompetence NOS
valvular insufficiency NOS
valvular regurgitation NOS
valvular stenosis NOS
valvulitis (chronic) NOS

EXCLUDES 1 *congenital insufficiency of cardiac valve NOS (Q24.8)*
congenital stenosis of cardiac valve NOS (Q24.8)
endocardial fibroelastosis (I42.4)
endocarditis specified as rheumatic (I09.1)

I39 Endocarditis and heart valve disorders in diseases classified elsewhere

Code first underlying disease, such as:
Q fever (A78)

EXCLUDES 1 *endocardial involvement in:*
candidiasis (B37.6)
gonococcal infection (A54.83)
Libman-Sacks disease (M32.11)
listerosis (A32.82)
meningococcal infection (A39.51)
rheumatoid arthritis (M05.31)
syphilis (A52.03)
tuberculosis (A18.84)
typhoid fever (A01.02)

I40 Acute myocarditis

INCLUDES subacute myocarditis

EXCLUDES 1 *acute rheumatic myocarditis (I01.2)*

I40.0 Infective myocarditis
Septic myocarditis
Use additional code (B95-B97) to identify infectious agent

I40.1 Isolated myocarditis
Fiedler's myocarditis
Giant cell myocarditis
Idiopathic myocarditis

I40.8 Other acute myocarditis

I40.9 Acute myocarditis, unspecified

I41 Myocarditis in diseases classified elsewhere

Code first underlying disease, such as:
typhus (A75.0-A75.9)

EXCLUDES 1 *myocarditis (in):*
Chagas' disease (chronic) (B57.2)
acute (B57.0)
coxsackie (virus) infection (B33.22)
diphtheritic (A36.81)
gonococcal (A54.83)
influenzal (J09.X9, J10.82, J11.82)
meningococcal (A39.52)
mumps (B26.82)
rheumatoid arthritis (M05.31)
sarcoid (D86.85)
syphilis (A52.06)
toxoplasmosis (B58.81)
tuberculous (A18.84)

I42 Cardiomyopathy

INCLUDES myocardiopathy

Code first cardiomyopathy complicating pregnancy and puerperium (O99.4)

EXCLUDES 1 *ischemic cardiomyopathy (I25.5)*
peripartum cardiomyopathy (O90.3)

EXCLUDES 2 *ventricular hypertrophy (I51.7)*

I42.0 Dilated cardiomyopathy
Congestive cardiomyopathy

I42.1 Obstructive hypertrophic cardiomyopathy
Hypertrophic subaortic stenosis (idiopathic)

I42.2 Other hypertrophic cardiomyopathy
Nonobstructive hypertrophic cardiomyopathy

I42.3 Endomyocardial (eosinophilic) disease
Endomyocardial (tropical) fibrosis
Löffler's endocarditis

I42.4 Endocardial fibroelastosis
Congenital cardiomyopathy
Elastomyofibrosis

I42.5 Other restrictive cardiomyopathy
Constrictive cardiomyopathy NOS

I42.6 Alcoholic cardiomyopathy
Code also presence of alcoholism (F10.-)

I42.7 Cardiomyopathy due to drug and external agent
Code first poisoning due to drug or toxin, if applicable (T36-T65 with fifth or sixth character 1-4 or 6)
Use additional code for adverse effect, if applicable, to identify drug (T36-T50 with fifth or sixth character 5)

I42.8 Other cardiomyopathies

I42.9 Cardiomyopathy, unspecified
Cardiomyopathy (primary) (secondary) NOS

I43 Cardiomyopathy in diseases classified elsewhere

Code first underlying disease, such as:
amyloidosis (E85.-)
glycogen storage disease (E74.0)
gout (M10.0-)
thyrotoxicosis (E05.0-E05.9-)

EXCLUDES 1 *cardiomyopathy (in):*
coxsackie (virus) (B33.24)
diphtheria (A36.81)
sarcoidosis (D86.85)
tuberculosis (A18.84)

I44 Atrioventricular and left bundle-branch block

I44.0 Atrioventricular block, first degree

I44.1 Atrioventricular block, second degree
Atrioventricular block, type I and II
Möbitz block, type I and II
Second degree block, type I and II
Wenckebach's block

I44.2 Atrioventricular block, complete
Complete heart block NOS
Third degree block

I44.3 Other and unspecified atrioventricular block
Atrioventricular block NOS

I44.30 Unspecified atrioventricular block

I44.39 Other atrioventricular block

I44.4 Left anterior fascicular block

I44.5 Left posterior fascicular block

I44.6 Other and unspecified fascicular block

I44.60 Unspecified fascicular block
Left bundle-branch hemiblock NOS

I44.69 **Other fascicular block**
I44.7 **Left bundle-branch block, unspecified**

✓4th I45 Other conduction disorders
I45.0 **Right fascicular block**
✓5th I45.1 **Other and unspecified right bundle-branch block**
I45.10 **Unspecified right bundle-branch block**
Right bundle-branch block NOS
I45.19 **Other right bundle-branch block**
I45.2 **Bifascicular block**
I45.3 **Trifascicular block**
I45.4 **Nonspecific intraventricular block**
Bundle-branch block NOS
I45.5 **Other specified heart block**
Sinoatrial block
Sinoauricular block
EXCLUDES 1 *heart block NOS (I45.9)*
I45.6 **Pre-excitation syndrome**
Accelerated atrioventricular conduction
Accessory atrioventricular conduction
Anomalous atrioventricular excitation
Lown-Ganong-Levine syndrome
Pre-excitation atrioventricular conduction
Wolff-Parkinson-White syndrome
✓5th I45.8 **Other specified conduction disorders**
I45.81 **Long QT syndrome**
I45.89 **Other specified conduction disorders**
Atrioventricular [AV] dissociation
Interference dissociation
Isorhythmic dissociation
Nonparoxysmal AV nodal tachycardia
I45.9 **Conduction disorder, unspecified**
Heart block NOS
Stokes-Adams syndrome

✓4th I46 Cardiac arrest
EXCLUDES 1 *cardiogenic shock (R57.0)*
I46.2 **Cardiac arrest due to underlying cardiac condition**
Code first underlying cardiac condition
I46.8 **Cardiac arrest due to other underlying condition**
Code first underlying condition
I46.9 **Cardiac arrest, cause unspecified**

✓4th I47 Paroxysmal tachycardia
Code first tachycardia complicating:
abortion or ectopic or molar pregnancy (O00-O07, O08.8)
obstetric surgery and procedures (O75.4)
EXCLUDES 1 *tachycardia:*
NOS (R00.0)
sinoauricular NOS (R00.0)
sinus [sinusal] NOS (R00.0)
I47.0 **Re-entry ventricular arrhythmia**
I47.1 **Supraventricular tachycardia**
Atrial (paroxysmal) tachycardia
Atrioventricular [AV] (paroxysmal) tachycardia
Atrioventricular re-entrant (nodal) tachycardia [AVNRT] [AVRT]
Junctional (paroxysmal) tachycardia
Nodal (paroxysmal) tachycardia
I47.2 **Ventricular tachycardia**
I47.9 **Paroxysmal tachycardia, unspecified**
Bouveret (-Hoffman) syndrome

✓4th I48 Atrial fibrillation and flutter
I48.0 **Paroxysmal atrial fibrillation**
I48.1 **Persistent atrial fibrillation**
I48.2 **Chronic atrial fibrillation**
Permanent atrial fibrillation
I48.3 **Typical atrial flutter**
Type I atrial flutter
I48.4 **Atypical atrial flutter**
Type II atrial flutter
✓5th I48.9 **Unspecified atrial fibrillation and atrial flutter**
I48.91 **Unspecified atrial fibrillation**
I48.92 **Unspecified atrial flutter**

✓4th I49 Other cardiac arrhythmias
Code first cardiac arrhythmia complicating:
abortion or ectopic or molar pregnancy (O00-O07, O08.8)
obstetric surgery and procedures (O75.4)
EXCLUDES 1 *bradycardia:*
NOS (R00.1)
sinoatrial (R00.1)
sinus (R00.1)
vagal (R00.1)
neonatal dysrhythmia (P29.1-)
✓5th I49.0 **Ventricular fibrillation and flutter**
I49.01 **Ventricular fibrillation**
I49.02 **Ventricular flutter**
I49.1 **Atrial premature depolarization**
Atrial premature beats
I49.2 **Junctional premature depolarization**
I49.3 **Ventricular premature depolarization**
✓5th I49.4 **Other and unspecified premature depolarization**
I49.40 **Unspecified premature depolarization**
Premature beats NOS
I49.49 **Other premature depolarization**
Ectopic beats
Extrasystoles
Extrasystolic arrhythmias
Premature contractions
I49.5 **Sick sinus syndrome**
Tachycardia-bradycardia syndrome
I49.8 **Other specified cardiac arrhythmias**
Coronary sinus rhythm disorder
Ectopic rhythm disorder
Nodal rhythm disorder
I49.9 **Cardiac arrhythmia, unspecified**
Arrhythmia (cardiac) NOS

✓4th I50 Heart failure
Code first:
heart failure complicating abortion or ectopic or molar pregnancy (O00-O07, O08.8)
heart failure following surgery (I97.13-)
heart failure due to hypertension (I11.0)
heart failure due to hypertension with chronic kidney disease (I13.-)
obstetric surgery and procedures (O75.4)
rheumatic heart failure (I09.81)
EXCLUDES 1 *cardiac arrest (I46.-)*
neonatal cardiac failure (P29.0)
I50.1 **Left ventricular failure**
Cardiac asthma
Edema of lung with heart disease NOS
Edema of lung with heart failure
Left heart failure
Pulmonary edema with heart disease NOS
Pulmonary edema with heart failure
EXCLUDES 1 *edema of lung without heart disease or heart failure (J81.-)*
pulmonary edema without heart disease or failure (J81.-)
✓5th I50.2 **Systolic (congestive) heart failure**
EXCLUDES 1 *combined systolic (congestive) and diastolic (congestive) heart failure (I50.4-)*
I50.20 **Unspecified systolic (congestive) heart failure**
I50.21 **Acute systolic (congestive) heart failure**
I50.22 **Chronic systolic (congestive) heart failure**
I50.23 **Acute on chronic systolic (congestive) heart failure**
✓5th I50.3 **Diastolic (congestive) heart failure**
EXCLUDES 1 *combined systolic (congestive) and diastolic (congestive) heart failure (I50.4-)*
I50.30 **Unspecified diastolic (congestive) heart failure**
I50.31 **Acute diastolic (congestive) heart failure**
I50.32 **Chronic diastolic (congestive) heart failure**
I50.33 **Acute on chronic diastolic (congestive) heart failure**
✓5th I50.4 **Combined systolic (congestive) and diastolic (congestive) heart failure**
I50.40 **Unspecified combined systolic (congestive) and diastolic (congestive) heart failure**
I50.41 **Acute combined systolic (congestive) and diastolic (congestive) heart failure**

I50.42 Chronic combined systolic (congestive) and diastolic (congestive) heart failure

I50.43 Acute on chronic combined systolic (congestive) and diastolic (congestive) heart failure

I50.9 Heart failure, unspecified
Biventricular (heart) failure NOS
Cardiac, heart or myocardial failure NOS
Congestive heart disease
Congestive heart failure NOS
Right ventricular failure (secondary to left heart failure)
EXCLUDES 1 *fluid overload (E87.70)*

✓4th **I51 Complications and ill-defined descriptions of heart disease**
EXCLUDES 1 *any condition in I51.4-I51.9 due to hypertension (I11.-)*
any condition in I51.4-I51.9 due to hypertension and chronic kidney disease (I13.-)
heart disease specified as rheumatic (I00-I09)

I51.0 Cardiac septal defect, acquired
Acquired septal atrial defect (old)
Acquired septal auricular defect (old)
Acquired septal ventricular defect (old)
EXCLUDES 1 *cardiac septal defect as current complication following acute myocardial infarction (I23.1, I23.2)*

I51.1 Rupture of chordae tendineae, not elsewhere classified
EXCLUDES 1 *rupture of chordae tendineae as current complication following acute myocardial infarction (I23.4)*

I51.2 Rupture of papillary muscle, not elsewhere classified
EXCLUDES 1 *rupture of papillary muscle as current complication following acute myocardial infarction (I23.5)*

I51.3 Intracardiac thrombosis, not elsewhere classified
Apical thrombosis (old)
Atrial thrombosis (old)
Auricular thrombosis (old)
Mural thrombosis (old)
Ventricular thrombosis (old)
EXCLUDES 1 *intracardiac thrombosis as current complication following acute myocardial infarction (I23.6)*

I51.4 Myocarditis, unspecified
Chronic (interstitial) myocarditis
Myocardial fibrosis
Myocarditis NOS
EXCLUDES 1 *acute or subacute myocarditis (I40.-)*

I51.5 Myocardial degeneration
Fatty degeneration of heart or myocardium
Myocardial disease
Senile degeneration of heart or myocardium

I51.7 Cardiomegaly
Cardiac dilatation
Cardiac hypertrophy
Ventricular dilatation

✓5th **I51.8 Other ill-defined heart diseases**

I51.81 Takotsubo syndrome
Reversible left ventricular dysfunction following sudden emotional stress
Stress induced cardiomyopathy
Takotsubo cardiomyopathy
Transient left ventricular apical ballooning syndrome

I51.89 Other ill-defined heart diseases
Carditis (acute)(chronic)
Pancarditis (acute)(chronic)

I51.9 Heart disease, unspecified

I52 Other heart disorders in diseases classified elsewhere
Code first underlying disease, such as:
congenital syphilis (A50.5)
mucopolysaccharidosis (E76.3)
schistosomiasis (B65.0-B65.9)
EXCLUDES 1 *heart disease (in):*
gonococcal infection (A54.83)
meningococcal infection (A39.50)
rheumatoid arthritis (M05.31)
syphilis (A52.06)

Cerebrovascular diseases (I60-I69)

Use additional code to identify presence of:
alcohol abuse and dependence (F10.-)
exposure to environmental tobacco smoke (Z77.22)
history of tobacco use (Z87.891)
hypertension (I10-I15)
occupational exposure to environmental tobacco smoke (Z57.31)
tobacco dependence (F17.-)
tobacco use (Z72.0)
EXCLUDES 1 *transient cerebral ischemic attacks and related syndromes (G45.-)*
traumatic intracranial hemorrhage (S06.-)

✓4th **I60 Nontraumatic subarachnoid hemorrhage**
INCLUDES ruptured cerebral aneurysm
EXCLUDES 1 *sequelae of subarachnoid hemorrhage (I69.0-)*
syphilitic ruptured cerebral aneurysm (A52.05)

✓5th **I60.0 Nontraumatic subarachnoid hemorrhage from carotid siphon and bifurcation**

I60.00 Nontraumatic subarachnoid hemorrhage from unspecified carotid siphon and bifurcation

I60.01 Nontraumatic subarachnoid hemorrhage from right carotid siphon and bifurcation

I60.02 Nontraumatic subarachnoid hemorrhage from left carotid siphon and bifurcation

✓5th **I60.1 Nontraumatic subarachnoid hemorrhage from middle cerebral artery**

I60.10 Nontraumatic subarachnoid hemorrhage from unspecified middle cerebral artery

I60.11 Nontraumatic subarachnoid hemorrhage from right middle cerebral artery

I60.12 Nontraumatic subarachnoid hemorrhage from left middle cerebral artery

✓5th **I60.2 Nontraumatic subarachnoid hemorrhage from anterior communicating artery**

I60.20 Nontraumatic subarachnoid hemorrhage from unspecified anterior communicating artery

I60.21 Nontraumatic subarachnoid hemorrhage from right anterior communicating artery

I60.22 Nontraumatic subarachnoid hemorrhage from left anterior communicating artery

✓5th **I60.3 Nontraumatic subarachnoid hemorrhage from posterior communicating artery**

I60.30 Nontraumatic subarachnoid hemorrhage from unspecified posterior communicating artery

I60.31 Nontraumatic subarachnoid hemorrhage from right posterior communicating artery

I60.32 Nontraumatic subarachnoid hemorrhage from left posterior communicating artery

I60.4 Nontraumatic subarachnoid hemorrhage from basilar artery

✓5th **I60.5 Nontraumatic subarachnoid hemorrhage from vertebral artery**

I60.50 Nontraumatic subarachnoid hemorrhage from unspecified vertebral artery

I60.51 Nontraumatic subarachnoid hemorrhage from right vertebral artery

I60.52 Nontraumatic subarachnoid hemorrhage from left vertebral artery

I60.6 Nontraumatic subarachnoid hemorrhage from other intracranial arteries

I60.7 Nontraumatic subarachnoid hemorrhage from unspecified intracranial artery
Ruptured (congenital) berry aneurysm
Ruptured (congenital) cerebral aneurysm
Subarachnoid hemorrhage (nontraumatic) from cerebral artery NOS
Subarachnoid hemorrhage (nontraumatic) from communicating artery NOS
EXCLUDES 1 *berry aneurysm, nonruptured (I67.1)*

I60.8 Other nontraumatic subarachnoid hemorrhage
Meningeal hemorrhage
Rupture of cerebral arteriovenous malformation

I60.9 Nontraumatic subarachnoid hemorrhage, unspecified

✓4th **I61 Nontraumatic intracerebral hemorrhage**
EXCLUDES 1 *sequelae of intracerebral hemorrhage (I69.1-)*

I61.0 Nontraumatic intracerebral hemorrhage in hemisphere, subcortical
Deep intracerebral hemorrhage (nontraumatic)

I61.1 **Nontraumatic intracerebral hemorrhage in hemisphere, cortical**
Cerebral lobe hemorrhage (nontraumatic)
Superficial intracerebral hemorrhage (nontraumatic)
I61.2 **Nontraumatic intracerebral hemorrhage in hemisphere, unspecified**
I61.3 **Nontraumatic intracerebral hemorrhage in brain stem**
I61.4 **Nontraumatic intracerebral hemorrhage in cerebellum**
I61.5 **Nontraumatic intracerebral hemorrhage, intraventricular**
I61.6 **Nontraumatic intracerebral hemorrhage, multiple localized**
I61.8 **Other nontraumatic intracerebral hemorrhage**
I61.9 **Nontraumatic intracerebral hemorrhage, unspecified**

✓4th **I62 Other and unspecified nontraumatic intracranial hemorrhage**
EXCLUDES 1 *sequelae of intracranial hemorrhage (I69.2)*
✓5th I62.0 **Nontraumatic subdural hemorrhage**
I62.00 **Nontraumatic subdural hemorrhage, unspecified**
I62.01 **Nontraumatic acute subdural hemorrhage**
I62.02 **Nontraumatic subacute subdural hemorrhage**
I62.03 **Nontraumatic chronic subdural hemorrhage**
I62.1 **Nontraumatic extradural hemorrhage**
Nontraumatic epidural hemorrhage
I62.9 **Nontraumatic intracranial hemorrhage, unspecified**

✓4th **I63 Cerebral infarction**
INCLUDES occlusion and stenosis of cerebral and precerebral arteries, resulting in cerebral infarction
Use additional code, if applicable, to identify status post administration of tPA (rtPA) in a different facility within the last 24 hours prior to admission to current facility (Z92.82)
EXCLUDES 1 *sequelae of cerebral infarction (I69.3-)*
✓5th I63.0 **Cerebral infarction due to thrombosis of precerebral arteries**
I63.00 **Cerebral infarction due to thrombosis of unspecified precerebral artery**
✓6th I63.01 **Cerebral infarction due to thrombosis of vertebral artery**
I63.011 **Cerebral infarction due to thrombosis of right vertebral artery**
I63.012 **Cerebral infarction due to thrombosis of left vertebral artery**
I63.019 **Cerebral infarction due to thrombosis of unspecified vertebral artery**
I63.02 **Cerebral infarction due to thrombosis of basilar artery**
✓6th I63.03 **Cerebral infarction due to thrombosis of carotid artery**
I63.031 **Cerebral infarction due to thrombosis of right carotid artery**
I63.032 **Cerebral infarction due to thrombosis of left carotid artery**
I63.039 **Cerebral infarction due to thrombosis of unspecified carotid artery**
I63.09 **Cerebral infarction due to thrombosis of other precerebral artery**
✓5th I63.1 **Cerebral infarction due to embolism of precerebral arteries**
I63.10 **Cerebral infarction due to embolism of unspecified precerebral artery**
✓6th I63.11 **Cerebral infarction due to embolism of vertebral artery**
I63.111 **Cerebral infarction due to embolism of right vertebral artery**
I63.112 **Cerebral infarction due to embolism of left vertebral artery**
I63.119 **Cerebral infarction due to embolism of unspecified vertebral artery**
I63.12 **Cerebral infarction due to embolism of basilar artery**
✓6th I63.13 **Cerebral infarction due to embolism of carotid artery**
I63.131 **Cerebral infarction due to embolism of right carotid artery**
I63.132 **Cerebral infarction due to embolism of left carotid artery**
I63.139 **Cerebral infarction due to embolism of unspecified carotid artery**
I63.19 **Cerebral infarction due to embolism of other precerebral artery**
✓5th I63.2 **Cerebral infarction due to unspecified occlusion or stenosis of precerebral arteries**
I63.20 **Cerebral infarction due to unspecified occlusion or stenosis of unspecified precerebral arteries**
✓6th I63.21 **Cerebral infarction due to unspecified occlusion or stenosis of vertebral arteries**
I63.211 **Cerebral infarction due to unspecified occlusion or stenosis of right vertebral arteries**
I63.212 **Cerebral infarction due to unspecified occlusion or stenosis of left vertebral arteries**
I63.219 **Cerebral infarction due to unspecified occlusion or stenosis of unspecified vertebral arteries**
I63.22 **Cerebral infarction due to unspecified occlusion or stenosis of basilar arteries**
✓6th I63.23 **Cerebral infarction due to unspecified occlusion or stenosis of carotid arteries**
I63.231 **Cerebral infarction due to unspecified occlusion or stenosis of right carotid arteries**
I63.232 **Cerebral infarction due to unspecified occlusion or stenosis of left carotid arteries**
I63.239 **Cerebral infarction due to unspecified occlusion or stenosis of unspecified carotid arteries**
I63.29 **Cerebral infarction due to unspecified occlusion or stenosis of other precerebral arteries**
✓5th I63.3 **Cerebral infarction due to thrombosis of cerebral arteries**
I63.30 **Cerebral infarction due to thrombosis of unspecified cerebral artery**
✓6th I63.31 **Cerebral infarction due to thrombosis of middle cerebral artery**
I63.311 **Cerebral infarction due to thrombosis of right middle cerebral artery**
I63.312 **Cerebral infarction due to thrombosis of left middle cerebral artery**
I63.319 **Cerebral infarction due to thrombosis of unspecified middle cerebral artery**
✓6th I63.32 **Cerebral infarction due to thrombosis of anterior cerebral artery**
I63.321 **Cerebral infarction due to thrombosis of right anterior cerebral artery**
I63.322 **Cerebral infarction due to thrombosis of left anterior cerebral artery**
I63.329 **Cerebral infarction due to thrombosis of unspecified anterior cerebral artery**
✓6th I63.33 **Cerebral infarction due to thrombosis of posterior cerebral artery**
I63.331 **Cerebral infarction due to thrombosis of right posterior cerebral artery**
I63.332 **Cerebral infarction due to thrombosis of left posterior cerebral artery**
I63.339 **Cerebral infarction due to thrombosis of unspecified posterior cerebral artery**
✓6th I63.34 **Cerebral infarction due to thrombosis of cerebellar artery**
I63.341 **Cerebral infarction due to thrombosis of right cerebellar artery**
I63.342 **Cerebral infarction due to thrombosis of left cerebellar artery**
I63.349 **Cerebral infarction due to thrombosis of unspecified cerebellar artery**
I63.39 **Cerebral infarction due to thrombosis of other cerebral artery**
✓5th I63.4 **Cerebral infarction due to embolism of cerebral arteries**
I63.40 **Cerebral infarction due to embolism of unspecified cerebral artery**
✓6th I63.41 **Cerebral infarction due to embolism of middle cerebral artery**
I63.411 **Cerebral infarction due to embolism of right middle cerebral artery**
I63.412 **Cerebral infarction due to embolism of left middle cerebral artery**
I63.419 **Cerebral infarction due to embolism of unspecified middle cerebral artery**

✓6th **I63.42 Cerebral infarction due to embolism of anterior cerebral artery**

I63.421 Cerebral infarction due to embolism of right anterior cerebral artery

I63.422 Cerebral infarction due to embolism of left anterior cerebral artery

I63.429 Cerebral infarction due to embolism of unspecified anterior cerebral artery

✓6th **I63.43 Cerebral infarction due to embolism of posterior cerebral artery**

I63.431 Cerebral infarction due to embolism of right posterior cerebral artery

I63.432 Cerebral infarction due to embolism of left posterior cerebral artery

I63.439 Cerebral infarction due to embolism of unspecified posterior cerebral artery

✓6th **I63.44 Cerebral infarction due to embolism of cerebellar artery**

I63.441 Cerebral infarction due to embolism of right cerebellar artery

I63.442 Cerebral infarction due to embolism of left cerebellar artery

I63.449 Cerebral infarction due to embolism of unspecified cerebellar artery

I63.49 Cerebral infarction due to embolism of other cerebral artery

✓5th **I63.5 Cerebral infarction due to unspecified occlusion or stenosis of cerebral arteries**

I63.5Ø Cerebral infarction due to unspecified occlusion or stenosis of unspecified cerebral artery

✓6th **I63.51 Cerebral infarction due to unspecified occlusion or stenosis of middle cerebral artery**

I63.511 Cerebral infarction due to unspecified occlusion or stenosis of right middle cerebral artery

I63.512 Cerebral infarction due to unspecified occlusion or stenosis of left middle cerebral artery

I63.519 Cerebral infarction due to unspecified occlusion or stenosis of unspecified middle cerebral artery

✓6th **I63.52 Cerebral infarction due to unspecified occlusion or stenosis of anterior cerebral artery**

I63.521 Cerebral infarction due to unspecified occlusion or stenosis of right anterior cerebral artery

I63.522 Cerebral infarction due to unspecified occlusion or stenosis of left anterior cerebral artery

I63.529 Cerebral infarction due to unspecified occlusion or stenosis of unspecified anterior cerebral artery

✓6th **I63.53 Cerebral infarction due to unspecified occlusion or stenosis of posterior cerebral artery**

I63.531 Cerebral infarction due to unspecified occlusion or stenosis of right posterior cerebral artery

I63.532 Cerebral infarction due to unspecified occlusion or stenosis of left posterior cerebral artery

I63.539 Cerebral infarction due to unspecified occlusion or stenosis of unspecified posterior cerebral artery

✓6th **I63.54 Cerebral infarction due to unspecified occlusion or stenosis of cerebellar artery**

I63.541 Cerebral infarction due to unspecified occlusion or stenosis of right cerebellar artery

I63.542 Cerebral infarction due to unspecified occlusion or stenosis of left cerebellar artery

I63.549 Cerebral infarction due to unspecified occlusion or stenosis of unspecified cerebellar artery

I63.59 Cerebral infarction due to unspecified occlusion or stenosis of other cerebral artery

I63.6 Cerebral infarction due to cerebral venous thrombosis, nonpyogenic

I63.8 Other cerebral infarction

I63.9 Cerebral infarction, unspecified
Stroke NOS

✓4th **I65 Occlusion and stenosis of precerebral arteries, not resulting in cerebral infarction**

INCLUDES embolism of precerebral artery
narrowing of precerebral artery
obstruction (complete) (partial) of precerebral artery
thrombosis of precerebral artery

EXCLUDES 1 *insufficiency, NOS, of precerebral artery (G45.-)*
insufficiency of precerebral arteries causing cerebral infarction (I63.Ø-I63.2)

✓5th **I65.Ø Occlusion and stenosis of vertebral artery**

I65.Ø1 Occlusion and stenosis of right vertebral artery

I65.Ø2 Occlusion and stenosis of left vertebral artery

I65.Ø3 Occlusion and stenosis of bilateral vertebral arteries

I65.Ø9 Occlusion and stenosis of unspecified vertebral artery

I65.1 Occlusion and stenosis of basilar artery

✓5th **I65.2 Occlusion and stenosis of carotid artery**

I65.21 Occlusion and stenosis of right carotid artery

I65.22 Occlusion and stenosis of left carotid artery

I65.23 Occlusion and stenosis of bilateral carotid arteries

I65.29 Occlusion and stenosis of unspecified carotid artery

I65.8 Occlusion and stenosis of other precerebral arteries

I65.9 Occlusion and stenosis of unspecified precerebral artery
Occlusion and stenosis of precerebral artery NOS

✓4th **I66 Occlusion and stenosis of cerebral arteries, not resulting in cerebral infarction**

INCLUDES embolism of cerebral artery
narrowing of cerebral artery
obstruction (complete) (partial) of cerebral artery
thrombosis of cerebral artery

EXCLUDES 1 *occlusion and stenosis of cerebral artery causing cerebral infarction (I63.3-I63.5)*

✓5th **I66.Ø Occlusion and stenosis of middle cerebral artery**

I66.Ø1 Occlusion and stenosis of right middle cerebral artery

I66.Ø2 Occlusion and stenosis of left middle cerebral artery

I66.Ø3 Occlusion and stenosis of bilateral middle cerebral arteries

I66.Ø9 Occlusion and stenosis of unspecified middle cerebral artery

✓5th **I66.1 Occlusion and stenosis of anterior cerebral artery**

I66.11 Occlusion and stenosis of right anterior cerebral artery

I66.12 Occlusion and stenosis of left anterior cerebral artery

I66.13 Occlusion and stenosis of bilateral anterior cerebral arteries

I66.19 Occlusion and stenosis of unspecified anterior cerebral artery

✓5th **I66.2 Occlusion and stenosis of posterior cerebral artery**

I66.21 Occlusion and stenosis of right posterior cerebral artery

I66.22 Occlusion and stenosis of left posterior cerebral artery

I66.23 Occlusion and stenosis of bilateral posterior cerebral arteries

I66.29 Occlusion and stenosis of unspecified posterior cerebral artery

I66.3 Occlusion and stenosis of cerebellar arteries

I66.8 Occlusion and stenosis of other cerebral arteries
Occlusion and stenosis of perforating arteries

I66.9 Occlusion and stenosis of unspecified cerebral artery

✓4th **I67 Other cerebrovascular diseases**

EXCLUDES 1 *sequelae of the listed conditions (I69.8)*

I67.Ø Dissection of cerebral arteries, nonruptured

EXCLUDES 1 *ruptured cerebral arteries (I6Ø.7)*

I67.1 Cerebral aneurysm, nonruptured
Cerebral aneurysm NOS
Cerebral arteriovenous fistula, acquired
Internal carotid artery aneurysm, intracranial portion
Internal carotid artery aneurysm, NOS
EXCLUDES 1 *congenital cerebral aneurysm, nonruptured (Q28.-)*
ruptured cerebral aneurysm (I60.7)

I67.2 Cerebral atherosclerosis
Atheroma of cerebral and precerebral arteries

I67.3 Progressive vascular leukoencephalopathy
Binswanger's disease

I67.4 Hypertensive encephalopathy

I67.5 Moyamoya disease

I67.6 Nonpyogenic thrombosis of intracranial venous system
Nonpyogenic thrombosis of cerebral vein
Nonpyogenic thrombosis of intracranial venous sinus
EXCLUDES 1 *nonpyogenic thrombosis of intracranial venous system causing infarction (I63.6)*

I67.7 Cerebral arteritis, not elsewhere classified
Granulomatous angiitis of the nervous system
EXCLUDES 1 *allergic granulomatous angiitis (M30.1)*

✓5th **I67.8 Other specified cerebrovascular diseases**

I67.81 Acute cerebrovascular insufficiency
Acute cerebrovascular insufficiency unspecified as to location or reversibility

I67.82 Cerebral ischemia
Chronic cerebral ischemia

I67.83 Posterior reversible encephalopathy syndrome
PRES

✓6th **I67.84 Cerebral vasospasm and vasoconstriction**

I67.841 Reversible cerebrovascular vasoconstriction syndrome
Call-Fleming syndrome
Code first underlying condition, if applicable, such as eclampsia (O15.00-O15.9)

I67.848 Other cerebrovascular vasospasm and vasoconstriction

I67.89 Other cerebrovascular disease

I67.9 Cerebrovascular disease, unspecified

✓4th **I68 Cerebrovascular disorders in diseases classified elsewhere**

I68.0 Cerebral amyloid angiopathy
Code first underlying amyloidosis (E85.-)

I68.2 Cerebral arteritis in other diseases classified elsewhere
Code first underlying disease
EXCLUDES 1 *cerebral arteritis (in):*
listerosis (A32.89)
systemic lupus erythematosus (M32.19)
syphilis (A52.04)
tuberculosis (A18.89)

I68.8 Other cerebrovascular disorders in diseases classified elsewhere
Code first underlying disease
EXCLUDES 1 *syphilitic cerebral aneurysm (A52.05)*

✓4th **I69 Sequelae of cerebrovascular disease**
NOTE Category I69 is to be used to indicate conditions in I60-I67 as the cause of sequelae. The "sequelae" include conditions specified as such or as residuals which may occur at any time after the onset of the causal condition
EXCLUDES 1 *personal history of cerebral infarction without residual deficit (Z86.73)*
personal history of prolonged reversible ischemic neurologic deficit (PRIND) (Z86.73)
personal history of reversible ischemic neurologcial deficit (RIND) (Z86.73)
sequelae of traumatic intracranial injury (S06.-)
transient ischemic attack (TIA) (G45.9)

✓5th **I69.0 Sequelae of nontraumatic subarachnoid hemorrhage**

I69.00 Unspecified sequelae of nontraumatic subarachnoid hemorrhage

I69.01 Cognitive deficits following nontraumatic subarachnoid hemorrhage

✓6th **I69.02 Speech and language deficits following nontraumatic subarachnoid hemorrhage**

I69.020 Aphasia following nontraumatic subarachnoid hemorrhage

I69.021 Dysphasia following nontraumatic subarachnoid hemorrhage

I69.022 Dysarthria following nontraumatic subarachnoid hemorrhage

I69.023 Fluency disorder following nontraumatic subarachnoid hemorrhage
Stuttering following nontraumatic subarachnoid hemorrhage

I69.028 Other speech and language deficits following nontraumatic subarachnoid hemorrhage

✓6th **I69.03 Monoplegia of upper limb following nontraumatic subarachnoid hemorrhage**

I69.031 Monoplegia of upper limb following nontraumatic subarachnoid hemorrhage affecting right dominant side

I69.032 Monoplegia of upper limb following nontraumatic subarachnoid hemorrhage affecting left dominant side

I69.033 Monoplegia of upper limb following nontraumatic subarachnoid hemorrhage affecting right non-dominant side

I69.034 Monoplegia of upper limb following nontraumatic subarachnoid hemorrhage affecting left non-dominant side

I69.039 Monoplegia of upper limb following nontraumatic subarachnoid hemorrhage affecting unspecified side

✓6th **I69.04 Monoplegia of lower limb following nontraumatic subarachnoid hemorrhage**

I69.041 Monoplegia of lower limb following nontraumatic subarachnoid hemorrhage affecting right dominant side

I69.042 Monoplegia of lower limb following nontraumatic subarachnoid hemorrhage affecting left dominant side

I69.043 Monoplegia of lower limb following nontraumatic subarachnoid hemorrhage affecting right non-dominant side

I69.044 Monoplegia of lower limb following nontraumatic subarachnoid hemorrhage affecting left non-dominant side

I69.049 Monoplegia of lower limb following nontraumatic subarachnoid hemorrhage affecting unspecified side

✓6th **I69.05 Hemiplegia and hemiparesis following nontraumatic subarachnoid hemorrhage**

I69.051 Hemiplegia and hemiparesis following nontraumatic subarachnoid hemorrhage affecting right dominant side

I69.052 Hemiplegia and hemiparesis following nontraumatic subarachnoid hemorrhage affecting left dominant side

I69.053 Hemiplegia and hemiparesis following nontraumatic subarachnoid hemorrhage affecting right non-dominant side

I69.054 Hemiplegia and hemiparesis following nontraumatic subarachnoid hemorrhage affecting left non-dominant side

I69.059 Hemiplegia and hemiparesis following nontraumatic subarachnoid hemorrhage affecting unspecified side

✓6th **I69.06 Other paralytic syndrome following nontraumatic subarachnoid hemorrhage**
Use additional code to identify type of paralytic syndrome, such as:
locked-in state (G83.5)
quadriplegia (G82.5-)
EXCLUDES 1 *hemiplegia/hemiparesis following nontraumatic subarachnoid hemorrhage (I69.05-)*
monoplegia of lower limb following nontraumatic subarachnoid hemorrhage (I69.04-)
monoplegia of upper limb following nontraumatic subarachnoid hemorrhage (I69.03-)

I69.061 Other paralytic syndrome following nontraumatic subarachnoid hemorrhage affecting right dominant side
I69.062 Other paralytic syndrome following nontraumatic subarachnoid hemorrhage affecting left dominant side
I69.063 Other paralytic syndrome following nontraumatic subarachnoid hemorrhage affecting right non-dominant side
I69.064 Other paralytic syndrome following nontraumatic subarachnoid hemorrhage affecting left non-dominant side
I69.065 Other paralytic syndrome following nontraumatic subarachnoid hemorrhage, bilateral
I69.069 Other paralytic syndrome following nontraumatic subarachnoid hemorrhage affecting unspecified side

✓6th **I69.09 Other sequelae of nontraumatic subarachnoid hemorrhage**
I69.090 Apraxia following nontraumatic subarachnoid hemorrhage
I69.091 Dysphagia following nontraumatic subarachnoid hemorrhage
Use additional code to identify the type of dysphagia, if known (R13.1-)
I69.092 Facial weakness following nontraumatic subarachnoid hemorrhage
Facial droop following nontraumatic subarachnoid hemorrhage
I69.093 Ataxia following nontraumatic subarachnoid hemorrhage
I69.098 Other sequelae following nontraumatic subarachnoid hemorrhage
Alterations of sensation following nontraumatic subarachnoid hemorrhage
Disturbance of vision following nontraumatic subarachnoid hemorrhage
Use additional code to identify the sequelae

✓5th **I69.1 Sequelae of nontraumatic intracerebral hemorrhage**
I69.10 Unspecified sequelae of nontraumatic intracerebral hemorrhage
I69.11 Cognitive deficits following nontraumatic intracerebral hemorrhage

✓6th **I69.12 Speech and language deficits following nontraumatic intracerebral hemorrhage**
I69.120 Aphasia following nontraumatic intracerebral hemorrhage
I69.121 Dysphasia following nontraumatic intracerebral hemorrhage
I69.122 Dysarthria following nontraumatic intracerebral hemorrhage
I69.123 Fluency disorder following nontraumatic intracerebral hemorrhage
Stuttering following nontraumatic subarachnoid hemorrhage
I69.128 Other speech and language deficits following nontraumatic intracerebral hemorrhage

✓6th **I69.13 Monoplegia of upper limb following nontraumatic intracerebral hemorrhage**
I69.131 Monoplegia of upper limb following nontraumatic intracerebral hemorrhage affecting right dominant side
I69.132 Monoplegia of upper limb following nontraumatic intracerebral hemorrhage affecting left dominant side
I69.133 Monoplegia of upper limb following nontraumatic intracerebral hemorrhage affecting right non-dominant side
I69.134 Monoplegia of upper limb following nontraumatic intracerebral hemorrhage affecting left non-dominant side
I69.139 Monoplegia of upper limb following nontraumatic intracerebral hemorrhage affecting unspecified side

✓6th **I69.14 Monoplegia of lower limb following nontraumatic intracerebral hemorrhage**
I69.141 Monoplegia of lower limb following nontraumatic intracerebral hemorrhage affecting right dominant side
I69.142 Monoplegia of lower limb following nontraumatic intracerebral hemorrhage affecting left dominant side
I69.143 Monoplegia of lower limb following nontraumatic intracerebral hemorrhage affecting right non-dominant side
I69.144 Monoplegia of lower limb following nontraumatic intracerebral hemorrhage affecting left non-dominant side
I69.149 Monoplegia of lower limb following nontraumatic intracerebral hemorrhage affecting unspecified side

✓6th **I69.15 Hemiplegia and hemiparesis following nontraumatic intracerebral hemorrhage**
I69.151 Hemiplegia and hemiparesis following nontraumatic intracerebral hemorrhage affecting right dominant side
I69.152 Hemiplegia and hemiparesis following nontraumatic intracerebral hemorrhage affecting left dominant side
I69.153 Hemiplegia and hemiparesis following nontraumatic intracerebral hemorrhage affecting right non-dominant side
I69.154 Hemiplegia and hemiparesis following nontraumatic intracerebral hemorrhage affecting left non-dominant side
I69.159 Hemiplegia and hemiparesis following nontraumatic intracerebral hemorrhage affecting unspecified side

✓6th **I69.16 Other paralytic syndrome following nontraumatic intracerebral hemorrhage**
Use additional code to identify type of paralytic syndrome, such as:
locked-in state (G83.5)
quadriplegia (G82.5-)
EXCLUDES 1 *hemiplegia/hemiparesis following nontraumatic intracerebral hemorrhage (I69.15-)*
monoplegia of lower limb following nontraumatic intracerebral hemorrhage (I69.14-)
monoplegia of upper limb following nontraumatic intracerebral hemorrhage (I69.13-)

I69.161 Other paralytic syndrome following nontraumatic intracerebral hemorrhage affecting right dominant side
I69.162 Other paralytic syndrome following nontraumatic intracerebral hemorrhage affecting left dominant side
I69.163 Other paralytic syndrome following nontraumatic intracerebral hemorrhage affecting right non-dominant side

I69.164 **Other paralytic syndrome following nontraumatic intracerebral hemorrhage affecting left non-dominant side**

I69.165 **Other paralytic syndrome following nontraumatic intracerebral hemorrhage, bilateral**

I69.169 **Other paralytic syndrome following nontraumatic intracerebral hemorrhage affecting unspecified side**

✓6th **I69.19 Other sequelae of nontraumatic intracerebral hemorrhage**

I69.190 **Apraxia following nontraumatic intracerebral hemorrhage**

I69.191 **Dysphagia following nontraumatic intracerebral hemorrhage**

Use additional code to identify the type of dysphagia, if known (R13.1-)

I69.192 **Facial weakness following nontraumatic intracerebral hemorrhage**

Facial droop following nontraumatic intracerebral hemorrhage

I69.193 **Ataxia following nontraumatic intracerebral hemorrhage**

I69.198 **Other sequelae of nontraumatic intracerebral hemorrhage**

Alteration of sensations following nontraumatic intracerebral hemorrhage

Disturbance of vision following nontraumatic intracerebral hemorrhage

Use additional code to identify the sequelae

✓5th **I69.2 Sequelae of other nontraumatic intracranial hemorrhage**

I69.20 **Unspecified sequelae of other nontraumatic intracranial hemorrhage**

I69.21 **Cognitive deficits following other nontraumatic intracranial hemorrhage**

✓6th **I69.22 Speech and language deficits following other nontraumatic intracranial hemorrhage**

I69.220 **Aphasia following other nontraumatic intracranial hemorrhage**

I69.221 **Dysphasia following other nontraumatic intracranial hemorrhage**

I69.222 **Dysarthria following other nontraumatic intracranial hemorrhage**

I69.223 **Fluency disorder following other nontraumatic intracranial hemorrhage**

Stuttering following nontraumatic subarachnoid hemorrhage

I69.228 **Other speech and language deficits following other nontraumatic intracranial hemorrhage**

✓6th **I69.23 Monoplegia of upper limb following other nontraumatic intracranial hemorrhage**

I69.231 **Monoplegia of upper limb following other nontraumatic intracranial hemorrhage affecting right dominant side**

I69.232 **Monoplegia of upper limb following other nontraumatic intracranial hemorrhage affecting left dominant side**

I69.233 **Monoplegia of upper limb following other nontraumatic intracranial hemorrhage affecting right non-dominant side**

I69.234 **Monoplegia of upper limb following other nontraumatic intracranial hemorrhage affecting left non-dominant side**

I69.239 **Monoplegia of upper limb following other nontraumatic intracranial hemorrhage affecting unspecified side**

✓6th **I69.24 Monoplegia of lower limb following other nontraumatic intracranial hemorrhage**

I69.241 **Monoplegia of lower limb following other nontraumatic intracranial hemorrhage affecting right dominant side**

I69.242 **Monoplegia of lower limb following other nontraumatic intracranial hemorrhage affecting left dominant side**

I69.243 **Monoplegia of lower limb following other nontraumatic intracranial hemorrhage affecting right non-dominant side**

I69.244 **Monoplegia of lower limb following other nontraumatic intracranial hemorrhage affecting left non-dominant side**

I69.249 **Monoplegia of lower limb following other nontraumatic intracranial hemorrhage affecting unspecified side**

✓6th **I69.25 Hemiplegia and hemiparesis following other nontraumatic intracranial hemorrhage**

I69.251 **Hemiplegia and hemiparesis following other nontraumatic intracranial hemorrhage affecting right dominant side**

I69.252 **Hemiplegia and hemiparesis following other nontraumatic intracranial hemorrhage affecting left dominant side**

I69.253 **Hemiplegia and hemiparesis following other nontraumatic intracranial hemorrhage affecting right non-dominant side**

I69.254 **Hemiplegia and hemiparesis following other nontraumatic intracranial hemorrhage affecting left non-dominant side**

I69.259 **Hemiplegia and hemiparesis following other nontraumatic intracranial hemorrhage affecting unspecified side**

✓6th **I69.26 Other paralytic syndrome following other nontraumatic intracranial hemorrhage**

Use additional code to identify type of paralytic syndrome, such as:
locked-in state (G83.5)
quadriplegia (G82.5-)

EXCLUDES 1 *hemiplegia/hemiparesis following other nontraumatic intracranial hemorrhage (I69.25-)*
monoplegia of lower limb following other nontraumatic intracranial hemorrhage (I69.24-)
monoplegia of upper limb following other nontraumatic intracranial hemorrhage (I69.23-)

I69.261 **Other paralytic syndrome following other nontraumatic intracranial hemorrhage affecting right dominant side**

I69.262 **Other paralytic syndrome following other nontraumatic intracranial hemorrhage affecting left dominant side**

I69.263 **Other paralytic syndrome following other nontraumatic intracranial hemorrhage affecting right non-dominant side**

I69.264 **Other paralytic syndrome following other nontraumatic intracranial hemorrhage affecting left non-dominant side**

I69.265 **Other paralytic syndrome following other nontraumatic intracranial hemorrhage, bilateral**

I69.269 **Other paralytic syndrome following other nontraumatic intracranial hemorrhage affecting unspecified side**

✓6th **I69.29 Other sequelae of other nontraumatic intracranial hemorrhage**

I69.290 **Apraxia following other nontraumatic intracranial hemorrhage**

I69.291 Dysphagia following other nontraumatic intracranial hemorrhage
Use additional code to identify the type of dysphagia, if known (R13.1-)

I69.292 Facial weakness following other nontraumatic intracranial hemorrhage
Facial droop following other nontraumatic intracranial hemorrhage

I69.293 Ataxia following other nontraumatic intracranial hemorrhage

I69.298 Other sequelae of other nontraumatic intracranial hemorrhage
Alteration of sensation following other nontraumatic intracranial hemorrhage
Disturbance of vision following other nontraumatic intracranial hemorrhage
Use additional code to identify the sequelae

✓5th **I69.3 Sequelae of cerebral infarction**
Sequelae of stroke NOS

I69.30 Unspecified sequelae of cerebral infarction

I69.31 Cognitive deficits following cerebral infarction

✓6th **I69.32 Speech and language deficits following cerebral infarction**

I69.320 Aphasia following cerebral infarction

I69.321 Dysphasia following cerebral infarction

I69.322 Dysarthria following cerebral infarction

I69.323 Fluency disorder following cerebral infarction
Stuttering following nontraumatic subarachnoid hemorrhage

I69.328 Other speech and language deficits following cerebral infarction

✓6th **I69.33 Monoplegia of upper limb following cerebral infarction**

I69.331 Monoplegia of upper limb following cerebral infarction affecting right dominant side

I69.332 Monoplegia of upper limb following cerebral infarction affecting left dominant side

I69.333 Monoplegia of upper limb following cerebral infarction affecting right non-dominant side

I69.334 Monoplegia of upper limb following cerebral infarction affecting left non-dominant side

I69.339 Monoplegia of upper limb following cerebral infarction affecting unspecified side

✓6th **I69.34 Monoplegia of lower limb following cerebral infarction**

I69.341 Monoplegia of lower limb following cerebral infarction affecting right dominant side

I69.342 Monoplegia of lower limb following cerebral infarction affecting left dominant side

I69.343 Monoplegia of lower limb following cerebral infarction affecting right non-dominant side

I69.344 Monoplegia of lower limb following cerebral infarction affecting left non-dominant side

I69.349 Monoplegia of lower limb following cerebral infarction affecting unspecified side

✓6th **I69.35 Hemiplegia and hemiparesis following cerebral infarction**

I69.351 Hemiplegia and hemiparesis following cerebral infarction affecting right dominant side

I69.352 Hemiplegia and hemiparesis following cerebral infarction affecting left dominant side

I69.353 Hemiplegia and hemiparesis following cerebral infarction affecting right non-dominant side

I69.354 Hemiplegia and hemiparesis following cerebral infarction affecting left non-dominant side

I69.359 Hemiplegia and hemiparesis following cerebral infarction affecting unspecified side

✓6th **I69.36 Other paralytic syndrome following cerebral infarction**
Use additional code to identify type of paralytic syndrome, such as:
locked-in state (G83.5)
quadriplegia (G82.5-)

EXCLUDES 1 *hemiplegia/hemiparesis following cerebral infarction (I69.35-)*
monoplegia of lower limb following cerebral infarction (I69.34-)
monoplegia of upper limb following cerebral infarction (I69.33-)

I69.361 Other paralytic syndrome following cerebral infarction affecting right dominant side

I69.362 Other paralytic syndrome following cerebral infarction affecting left dominant side

I69.363 Other paralytic syndrome following cerebral infarction affecting right non-dominant side

I69.364 Other paralytic syndrome following cerebral infarction affecting left non-dominant side

I69.365 Other paralytic syndrome following cerebral infarction, bilateral

I69.369 Other paralytic syndrome following cerebral infarction affecting unspecified side

✓6th **I69.39 Other sequelae of cerebral infarction**

I69.390 Apraxia following cerebral infarction

I69.391 Dysphagia following cerebral infarction
Use additional code to identify the type of dysphagia, if known (R13.1-)

I69.392 Facial weakness following cerebral infarction
Facial droop following cerebral infarction

I69.393 Ataxia following cerebral infarction

I69.398 Other sequelae of cerebral infarction
Alteration of sensation following cerebral infarction
Disturbance of vision following cerebral infarction
Use additional code to identify the sequelae

✓5th **I69.8 Sequelae of other cerebrovascular diseases**
EXCLUDES 1 *sequelae of traumatic intracranial injury (S06.-)*

I69.80 Unspecified sequelae of other cerebrovascular disease

I69.81 Cognitive deficits following other cerebrovascular disease

✓6th **I69.82 Speech and language deficits following other cerebrovascular disease**

I69.820 Aphasia following other cerebrovascular disease

I69.821 Dysphasia following other cerebrovascular disease

I69.822 Dysarthria following other cerebrovascular disease

I69.823 Fluency disorder following other cerebrovascular disease
Stuttering following nontraumatic subarachnoid hemorrhage

I69.828 Other speech and language deficits following other cerebrovascular disease

✓6th **I69.83 Monoplegia of upper limb following other cerebrovascular disease**

I69.831 Monoplegia of upper limb following other cerebrovascular disease affecting right dominant side

I69.832 **Monoplegia of upper limb following other cerebrovascular disease affecting left dominant side**

I69.833 **Monoplegia of upper limb following other cerebrovascular disease affecting right non-dominant side**

I69.834 **Monoplegia of upper limb following other cerebrovascular disease affecting left non-dominant side**

I69.839 **Monoplegia of upper limb following other cerebrovascular disease affecting unspecified side**

✓6th I69.84 **Monoplegia of lower limb following other cerebrovascular disease**

I69.841 **Monoplegia of lower limb following other cerebrovascular disease affecting right dominant side**

I69.842 **Monoplegia of lower limb following other cerebrovascular disease affecting left dominant side**

I69.843 **Monoplegia of lower limb following other cerebrovascular disease affecting right non-dominant side**

I69.844 **Monoplegia of lower limb following other cerebrovascular disease affecting left non-dominant side**

I69.849 **Monoplegia of lower limb following other cerebrovascular disease affecting unspecified side**

✓6th I69.85 **Hemiplegia and hemiparesis following other cerebrovascular disease**

I69.851 **Hemiplegia and hemiparesis following other cerebrovascular disease affecting right dominant side**

I69.852 **Hemiplegia and hemiparesis following other cerebrovascular disease affecting left dominant side**

I69.853 **Hemiplegia and hemiparesis following other cerebrovascular disease affecting right non-dominant side**

I69.854 **Hemiplegia and hemiparesis following other cerebrovascular disease affecting left non-dominant side**

I69.859 **Hemiplegia and hemiparesis following other cerebrovascular disease affecting unspecified side**

✓6th I69.86 **Other paralytic syndrome following other cerebrovascular disease**

Use additional code to identify type of paralytic syndrome, such as:
locked-in state (G83.5)
quadriplegia (G82.5-)

EXCLUDES 1 *hemiplegia/hemiparesis following other cerebrovascular disease (I69.85-)*
monoplegia of lower limb following other cerebrovascular disease (I69.84-)
monoplegia of upper limb following other cerebrovascular disease (I69.83-)

I69.861 **Other paralytic syndrome following other cerebrovascular disease affecting right dominant side**

I69.862 **Other paralytic syndrome following other cerebrovascular disease affecting left dominant side**

I69.863 **Other paralytic syndrome following other cerebrovascular disease affecting right non-dominant side**

I69.864 **Other paralytic syndrome following other cerebrovascular disease affecting left non-dominant side**

I69.865 **Other paralytic syndrome following other cerebrovascular disease, bilateral**

I69.869 **Other paralytic syndrome following other cerebrovascular disease affecting unspecified side**

✓6th I69.89 **Other sequelae of other cerebrovascular disease**

I69.890 **Apraxia following other cerebrovascular disease**

I69.891 **Dysphagia following other cerebrovascular disease**

Use additional code to identify the type of dysphagia, if known (R13.1-)

I69.892 **Facial weakness following other cerebrovascular disease**

Facial droop following other cerebrovascular disease

I69.893 **Ataxia following other cerebrovascular disease**

I69.898 **Other sequelae of other cerebrovascular disease**

Alteration of sensation following other cerebrovascular disease
Disturbance of vision following other cerebrovascular disease
Use additional code to identify the sequelae

✓5th I69.9 **Sequelae of unspecified cerebrovascular diseases**

EXCLUDES 1 *sequelae of stroke (I69.3)*
sequelae of traumatic intracranial injury (S06.-)

I69.90 **Unspecified sequelae of unspecified cerebrovascular disease**

I69.91 **Cognitive deficits following unspecified cerebrovascular disease**

✓6th I69.92 **Speech and language deficits following unspecified cerebrovascular disease**

I69.920 **Aphasia following unspecified cerebrovascular disease**

I69.921 **Dysphasia following unspecified cerebrovascular disease**

I69.922 **Dysarthria following unspecified cerebrovascular disease**

I69.923 **Fluency disorder following unspecified cerebrovascular disease**

Stuttering following nontraumatic subarachnoid hemorrhage

I69.928 **Other speech and language deficits following unspecified cerebrovascular disease**

✓6th I69.93 **Monoplegia of upper limb following unspecified cerebrovascular disease**

I69.931 **Monoplegia of upper limb following unspecified cerebrovascular disease affecting right dominant side**

I69.932 **Monoplegia of upper limb following unspecified cerebrovascular disease affecting left dominant side**

I69.933 **Monoplegia of upper limb following unspecified cerebrovascular disease affecting right non-dominant side**

I69.934 **Monoplegia of upper limb following unspecified cerebrovascular disease affecting left non-dominant side**

I69.939 **Monoplegia of upper limb following unspecified cerebrovascular disease affecting unspecified side**

✓6th I69.94 **Monoplegia of lower limb following unspecified cerebrovascular disease**

I69.941 **Monoplegia of lower limb following unspecified cerebrovascular disease affecting right dominant side**

I69.942 **Monoplegia of lower limb following unspecified cerebrovascular disease affecting left dominant side**

I69.943 **Monoplegia of lower limb following unspecified cerebrovascular disease affecting right non-dominant side**

I69.944 **Monoplegia of lower limb following unspecified cerebrovascular disease affecting left non-dominant side**

I69.949 **Monoplegia of lower limb following unspecified cerebrovascular disease affecting unspecified side**

✓6th I69.95 **Hemiplegia and hemiparesis following unspecified cerebrovascular disease**

I69.951 **Hemiplegia and hemiparesis following unspecified cerebrovascular disease affecting right dominant side**

I69.952 Hemiplegia and hemiparesis following unspecified cerebrovascular disease affecting left dominant side

I69.953 Hemiplegia and hemiparesis following unspecified cerebrovascular disease affecting right non-dominant side

I69.954 Hemiplegia and hemiparesis following unspecified cerebrovascular disease affecting left non-dominant side

I69.959 Hemiplegia and hemiparesis following unspecified cerebrovascular disease affecting unspecified side

✓6th **I69.96 Other paralytic syndrome following unspecified cerebrovascular disease**

Use additional code to identify type of paralytic syndrome, such as:
locked-in state (G83.5)
quadriplegia (G82.5-)

EXCLUDES 1 *hemiplegia/hemiparesis following unspecified cerebrovascular disease (I69.95-)*
monoplegia of lower limb following unspecified cerebrovascular disease (I69.94-)
monoplegia of upper limb following unspecified cerebrovascular disease (I69.93-)

I69.961 Other paralytic syndrome following unspecified cerebrovascular disease affecting right dominant side

I69.962 Other paralytic syndrome following unspecified cerebrovascular disease affecting left dominant side

I69.963 Other paralytic syndrome following unspecified cerebrovascular disease affecting right non-dominant side

I69.964 Other paralytic syndrome following unspecified cerebrovascular disease affecting left non-dominant side

I69.965 Other paralytic syndrome following unspecified cerebrovascular disease, bilateral

I69.969 Other paralytic syndrome following unspecified cerebrovascular disease affecting unspecified side

✓6th **I69.99 Other sequelae of unspecified cerebrovascular disease**

I69.990 Apraxia following unspecified cerebrovascular disease

I69.991 Dysphagia following unspecified cerebrovascular disease

Use additional code to identify the type of dysphagia, if known (R13.1-)

I69.992 Facial weakness following unspecified cerebrovascular disease

Facial droop following unspecified cerebrovascular disease

I69.993 Ataxia following unspecified cerebrovascular disease

I69.998 Other sequelae following unspecified cerebrovascular disease

Alteration in sensation following unspecified cerebrovascular disease
Disturbance of vision following unspecified cerebrovascular disease
Use additional code to identify the sequelae

Diseases of arteries, arterioles and capillaries (I70-I79)

✓4th **I70 Atherosclerosis**

INCLUDES arteriolosclerosis
arterial degeneration
arteriosclerosis
arteriosclerotic vascular disease
arteriovascular degeneration
atheroma
endarteritis deformans or obliterans
senile arteritis
senile endarteritis
vascular degeneration

Use additional code to identify:
exposure to environmental tobacco smoke (Z77.22)
history of tobacco use (Z87.891)
occupational exposure to environmental tobacco smoke (Z57.31)
tobacco dependence (F17.-)
tobacco use (Z72.0)

EXCLUDES 2 *arteriosclerotic cardiovascular disease (I25.1-)*
arteriosclerotic heart disease (I25.1-)
atheroembolism (I75.-)
cerebral atherosclerosis (I67.2)
coronary atherosclerosis (I25.1-)
mesenteric atherosclerosis (K55.1)
precerebral atherosclerosis (I67.2)
primary pulmonary atherosclerosis (I27.0)

I70.0 Atherosclerosis of aorta

I70.1 Atherosclerosis of renal artery

Goldblatt's kidney

EXCLUDES 2 *atherosclerosis of renal arterioles (I12.-)*

✓5th **I70.2 Atherosclerosis of native arteries of the extremities**

Mönckeberg's (medial) sclerosis
Use additional code, if applicable, to identify chronic total occlusion of artery of extremity (I70.92)

EXCLUDES 2 *atherosclerosis of bypass graft of extremities (I70.30-I70.79)*

✓6th **I70.20 Unspecified atherosclerosis of native arteries of extremities**

I70.201 Unspecified atherosclerosis of native arteries of extremities, right leg

I70.202 Unspecified atherosclerosis of native arteries of extremities, left leg

I70.203 Unspecified atherosclerosis of native arteries of extremities, bilateral legs

I70.208 Unspecified atherosclerosis of native arteries of extremities, other extremity

I70.209 Unspecified atherosclerosis of native arteries of extremities, unspecified extremity

✓6th **I70.21 Atherosclerosis of native arteries of extremities with intermittent claudication**

I70.211 Atherosclerosis of native arteries of extremities with intermittent claudication, right leg

I70.212 Atherosclerosis of native arteries of extremities with intermittent claudication, left leg

I70.213 Atherosclerosis of native arteries of extremities with intermittent claudication, bilateral legs

I70.218 Atherosclerosis of native arteries of extremities with intermittent claudication, other extremity

I70.219 Atherosclerosis of native arteries of extremities with intermittent claudication, unspecified extremity

✓6th **I70.22 Atherosclerosis of native arteries of extremities with rest pain**

Includes any condition classifiable to I70.21-

I70.221 Atherosclerosis of native arteries of extremities with rest pain, right leg

I70.222 Atherosclerosis of native arteries of extremities with rest pain, left leg

I70.223 Atherosclerosis of native arteries of extremities with rest pain, bilateral legs

I70.228 Atherosclerosis of native arteries of extremities with rest pain, other extremity

I70.229 Atherosclerosis of native arteries of extremities with rest pain, unspecified extremity

I70.23 Atherosclerosis of native arteries of right leg with ulceration
Includes any condition classifiable to I70.211 and I70.221
Use additional code to identify severity of ulcer (L97.- with fifth character 1)

I70.231 Atherosclerosis of native arteries of right leg with ulceration of thigh

I70.232 Atherosclerosis of native arteries of right leg with ulceration of calf

I70.233 Atherosclerosis of native arteries of right leg with ulceration of ankle

I70.234 Atherosclerosis of native arteries of right leg with ulceration of heel and midfoot
Atherosclerosis of native arteries of right leg with ulceration of plantar surface of midfoot

I70.235 Atherosclerosis of native arteries of right leg with ulceration of other part of foot
Atherosclerosis of native arteries of right leg extremities with ulceration of toe

I70.238 Atherosclerosis of native arteries of right leg with ulceration of other part of lower right leg

I70.239 Atherosclerosis of native arteries of right leg with ulceration of unspecified site

I70.24 Atherosclerosis of native arteries of left leg with ulceration
Includes any condition classifiable to I70.212 and I70.222
Use additional code to identify severity of ulcer (L97.- with fifth character 2)

I70.241 Atherosclerosis of native arteries of left leg with ulceration of thigh

I70.242 Atherosclerosis of native arteries of left leg with ulceration of calf

I70.243 Atherosclerosis of native arteries of left leg with ulceration of ankle

I70.244 Atherosclerosis of native arteries of left leg with ulceration of heel and midfoot
Atherosclerosis of native arteries of left leg with ulceration of plantar surface of midfoot

I70.245 Atherosclerosis of native arteries of left leg with ulceration of other part of foot
Atherosclerosis of native arteries of left leg extremities with ulceration of toe

I70.248 Atherosclerosis of native arteries of left leg with ulceration of other part of lower left leg

I70.249 Atherosclerosis of native arteries of left leg with ulceration of unspecified site

I70.25 Atherosclerosis of native arteries of other extremities with ulceration
Includes any condition classifiable to I70.218 and I70.228
Use additional code to identify the severity of the ulcer (L98.49-)

I70.26 Atherosclerosis of native arteries of extremities with gangrene
Includes any condition classifiable to I70.21-, I70.22-, I70.23-, I70.24-, and I70.25-
Use additional code to identify the severity of any ulcer (L98.49-), if applicable

I70.261 Atherosclerosis of native arteries of extremities with gangrene, right leg

I70.262 Atherosclerosis of native arteries of extremities with gangrene, left leg

I70.263 Atherosclerosis of native arteries of extremities with gangrene, bilateral legs

I70.268 Atherosclerosis of native arteries of extremities with gangrene, other extremity

I70.269 Atherosclerosis of native arteries of extremities with gangrene, unspecified extremity

I70.29 Other atherosclerosis of native arteries of extremities

I70.291 Other atherosclerosis of native arteries of extremities, right leg

I70.292 Other atherosclerosis of native arteries of extremities, left leg

I70.293 Other atherosclerosis of native arteries of extremities, bilateral legs

I70.298 Other atherosclerosis of native arteries of extremities, other extremity

I70.299 Other atherosclerosis of native arteries of extremities, unspecified extremity

I70.3 Atherosclerosis of unspecified type of bypass graft(s) of the extremities
Use additional code, if applicable, to identify chronic total occlusion of artery of extremity (I70.92)
EXCLUDES 1 *embolism or thrombus of bypass graft(s) of extremities (T82.8-)*

I70.30 Unspecified atherosclerosis of unspecified type of bypass graft(s) of the extremities

I70.301 Unspecified atherosclerosis of unspecified type of bypass graft(s) of the extremities, right leg

I70.302 Unspecified atherosclerosis of unspecified type of bypass graft(s) of the extremities, left leg

I70.303 Unspecified atherosclerosis of unspecified type of bypass graft(s) of the extremities, bilateral legs

I70.308 Unspecified atherosclerosis of unspecified type of bypass graft(s) of the extremities, other extremity

I70.309 Unspecified atherosclerosis of unspecified type of bypass graft(s) of the extremities, unspecified extremity

I70.31 Atherosclerosis of unspecified type of bypass graft(s) of the extremities with intermittent claudication

I70.311 Atherosclerosis of unspecified type of bypass graft(s) of the extremities with intermittent claudication, right leg

I70.312 Atherosclerosis of unspecified type of bypass graft(s) of the extremities with intermittent claudication, left leg

I70.313 Atherosclerosis of unspecified type of bypass graft(s) of the extremities with intermittent claudication, bilateral legs

I70.318 Atherosclerosis of unspecified type of bypass graft(s) of the extremities with intermittent claudication, other extremity

I70.319 Atherosclerosis of unspecified type of bypass graft(s) of the extremities with intermittent claudication, unspecified extremity

I70.32 Atherosclerosis of unspecified type of bypass graft(s) of the extremities with rest pain
Includes any condition classifiable to I70.31-

I70.321 Atherosclerosis of unspecified type of bypass graft(s) of the extremities with rest pain, right leg

I70.322 Atherosclerosis of unspecified type of bypass graft(s) of the extremities with rest pain, left leg

I70.323 Atherosclerosis of unspecified type of bypass graft(s) of the extremities with rest pain, bilateral legs

I70.328 Atherosclerosis of unspecified type of bypass graft(s) of the extremities with rest pain, other extremity

I70.329 Atherosclerosis of unspecified type of bypass graft(s) of the extremities with rest pain, unspecified extremity

Appropriate additional character required
Requires 7th character, placeholder x must fill empty characters

✓6th **I70.33 Atherosclerosis of unspecified type of bypass graft(s) of the right leg with ulceration**
Includes any condition classifiable to I70.311 and I70.321
Use additional code to identify severity of ulcer (L97.- with fifth character 1)

I70.331 Atherosclerosis of unspecified type of bypass graft(s) of the right leg with ulceration of thigh

I70.332 Atherosclerosis of unspecified type of bypass graft(s) of the right leg with ulceration of calf

I70.333 Atherosclerosis of unspecified type of bypass graft(s) of the right leg with ulceration of ankle

I70.334 Atherosclerosis of unspecified type of bypass graft(s) of the right leg with ulceration of heel and midfoot
Atherosclerosis of unspecified type of bypass graft(s) of right leg with ulceration of plantar surface of midfoot

I70.335 Atherosclerosis of unspecified type of bypass graft(s) of the right leg with ulceration of other part of foot
Atherosclerosis of unspecified type of bypass graft(s) of the right leg with ulceration of toe

I70.338 Atherosclerosis of unspecified type of bypass graft(s) of the right leg with ulceration of other part of lower leg

I70.339 Atherosclerosis of unspecified type of bypass graft(s) of the right leg with ulceration of unspecified site

✓6th **I70.34 Atherosclerosis of unspecified type of bypass graft(s) of the left leg with ulceration**
Includes any condition classifiable to I70.312 and I70.322
Use additional code to identify severity of ulcer (L97.- with fifth character 2)

I70.341 Atherosclerosis of unspecified type of bypass graft(s) of the left leg with ulceration of thigh

I70.342 Atherosclerosis of unspecified type of bypass graft(s) of the left leg with ulceration of calf

I70.343 Atherosclerosis of unspecified type of bypass graft(s) of the left leg with ulceration of ankle

I70.344 Atherosclerosis of unspecified type of bypass graft(s) of the left leg with ulceration of heel and midfoot
Atherosclerosis of unspecified type of bypass graft(s) of left leg with ulceration of plantar surface of midfoot

I70.345 Atherosclerosis of unspecified type of bypass graft(s) of the left leg with ulceration of other part of foot
Atherosclerosis of unspecified type of bypass graft(s) of the left leg with ulceration of toe

I70.348 Atherosclerosis of unspecified type of bypass graft(s) of the left leg with ulceration of other part of lower leg

I70.349 Atherosclerosis of unspecified type of bypass graft(s) of the left leg with ulceration of unspecified site

I70.35 Atherosclerosis of unspecified type of bypass graft(s) of other extremity with ulceration
Includes any condition classifiable to I70.318 and I70.328
Use additional code to identify severity of ulcer (L98.49-)

✓6th **I70.36 Atherosclerosis of unspecified type of bypass graft(s) of the extremities with gangrene**
Includes any condition classifiable to I70.31-, I70.32-, I70.33-, I70.34-, I70.35
Use additional code to identify the severity of any ulcer (L98.49-), if applicable

I70.361 Atherosclerosis of unspecified type of bypass graft(s) of the extremities with gangrene, right leg

I70.362 Atherosclerosis of unspecified type of bypass graft(s) of the extremities with gangrene, left leg

I70.363 Atherosclerosis of unspecified type of bypass graft(s) of the extremities with gangrene, bilateral legs

I70.368 Atherosclerosis of unspecified type of bypass graft(s) of the extremities with gangrene, other extremity

I70.369 Atherosclerosis of unspecified type of bypass graft(s) of the extremities with gangrene, unspecified extremity

✓6th **I70.39 Other atherosclerosis of unspecified type of bypass graft(s) of the extremities**

I70.391 Other atherosclerosis of unspecified type of bypass graft(s) of the extremities, right leg

I70.392 Other atherosclerosis of unspecified type of bypass graft(s) of the extremities, left leg

I70.393 Other atherosclerosis of unspecified type of bypass graft(s) of the extremities, bilateral legs

I70.398 Other atherosclerosis of unspecified type of bypass graft(s) of the extremities, other extremity

I70.399 Other atherosclerosis of unspecified type of bypass graft(s) of the extremities, unspecified extremity

✓5th **I70.4 Atherosclerosis of autologous vein bypass graft(s) of the extremities**
Use additional code, if applicable, to identify chronic total occlusion of artery of extremity (I70.92)

✓6th **I70.40 Unspecified atherosclerosis of autologous vein bypass graft(s) of the extremities**

I70.401 Unspecified atherosclerosis of autologous vein bypass graft(s) of the extremities, right leg

I70.402 Unspecified atherosclerosis of autologous vein bypass graft(s) of the extremities, left leg

I70.403 Unspecified atherosclerosis of autologous vein bypass graft(s) of the extremities, bilateral legs

I70.408 Unspecified atherosclerosis of autologous vein bypass graft(s) of the extremities, other extremity

I70.409 Unspecified atherosclerosis of autologous vein bypass graft(s) of the extremities, unspecified extremity

✓6th **I70.41 Atherosclerosis of autologous vein bypass graft(s) of the extremities with intermittent claudication**

I70.411 Atherosclerosis of autologous vein bypass graft(s) of the extremities with intermittent claudication, right leg

I70.412 Atherosclerosis of autologous vein bypass graft(s) of the extremities with intermittent claudication, left leg

I70.413 Atherosclerosis of autologous vein bypass graft(s) of the extremities with intermittent claudication, bilateral legs

I70.418 Atherosclerosis of autologous vein bypass graft(s) of the extremities with intermittent claudication, other extremity

I70.419 Atherosclerosis of autologous vein bypass graft(s) of the extremities with intermittent claudication, unspecified extremity

✓6th I70.42 Atherosclerosis of autologous vein bypass graft(s) of the extremities with rest pain
Includes any condition classifiable to I70.41-

I70.421 Atherosclerosis of autologous vein bypass graft(s) of the extremities with rest pain, right leg

I70.422 Atherosclerosis of autologous vein bypass graft(s) of the extremities with rest pain, left leg

I70.423 Atherosclerosis of autologous vein bypass graft(s) of the extremities with rest pain, bilateral legs

I70.428 Atherosclerosis of autologous vein bypass graft(s) of the extremities with rest pain, other extremity

I70.429 Atherosclerosis of autologous vein bypass graft(s) of the extremities with rest pain, unspecified extremity

✓6th I70.43 Atherosclerosis of autologous vein bypass graft(s) of the right leg with ulceration
Includes any condition classifiable to I70.411 and I70.421
Use additional code to identify severity of ulcer (L97.- with fifth character 1)

I70.431 Atherosclerosis of autologous vein bypass graft(s) of the right leg with ulceration of thigh

I70.432 Atherosclerosis of autologous vein bypass graft(s) of the right leg with ulceration of calf

I70.433 Atherosclerosis of autologous vein bypass graft(s) of the right leg with ulceration of ankle

I70.434 Atherosclerosis of autologous vein bypass graft(s) of the right leg with ulceration of heel and midfoot
Atherosclerosis of autologous vein bypass graft(s) of right leg with ulceration of plantar surface of midfoot

I70.435 Atherosclerosis of autologous vein bypass graft(s) of the right leg with ulceration of other part of foot
Atherosclerosis of autologous vein bypass graft(s) of right leg with ulceration of toe

I70.438 Atherosclerosis of autologous vein bypass graft(s) of the right leg with ulceration of other part of lower leg

I70.439 Atherosclerosis of autologous vein bypass graft(s) of the right leg with ulceration of unspecified site

✓6th I70.44 Atherosclerosis of autologous vein bypass graft(s) of the left leg with ulceration
Includes any condition classifiable to I70.412 and I70.422
Use additional code to identify severity of ulcer (L97.- with fifth character 2)

I70.441 Atherosclerosis of autologous vein bypass graft(s) of the left leg with ulceration of thigh

I70.442 Atherosclerosis of autologous vein bypass graft(s) of the left leg with ulceration of calf

I70.443 Atherosclerosis of autologous vein bypass graft(s) of the left leg with ulceration of ankle

I70.444 Atherosclerosis of autologous vein bypass graft(s) of the left leg with ulceration of heel and midfoot
Atherosclerosis of autologous vein bypass graft(s) of left leg with ulceration of plantar surface of midfoot

I70.445 Atherosclerosis of autologous vein bypass graft(s) of the left leg with ulceration of other part of foot
Atherosclerosis of autologous vein bypass graft(s) of left leg with ulceration of toe

I70.448 Atherosclerosis of autologous vein bypass graft(s) of the left leg with ulceration of other part of lower leg

I70.449 Atherosclerosis of autologous vein bypass graft(s) of the left leg with ulceration of unspecified site

I70.45 Atherosclerosis of autologous vein bypass graft(s) of other extremity with ulceration
Includes any condition classifiable to I70.418, I70.428, and I70.438
Use additional code to identify severity of ulcer (L98.49)

✓6th I70.46 Atherosclerosis of autologous vein bypass graft(s) of the extremities with gangrene
Includes any condition classifiable to I70.41-, I70.42-, and I70.43-, I70.44-, I70.45
Use additional code to identify the severity of any ulcer (L98.49-), if applicable

I70.461 Atherosclerosis of autologous vein bypass graft(s) of the extremities with gangrene, right leg

I70.462 Atherosclerosis of autologous vein bypass graft(s) of the extremities with gangrene, left leg

I70.463 Atherosclerosis of autologous vein bypass graft(s) of the extremities with gangrene, bilateral legs

I70.468 Atherosclerosis of autologous vein bypass graft(s) of the extremities with gangrene, other extremity

I70.469 Atherosclerosis of autologous vein bypass graft(s) of the extremities with gangrene, unspecified extremity

✓6th I70.49 Other atherosclerosis of autologous vein bypass graft(s) of the extremities

I70.491 Other atherosclerosis of autologous vein bypass graft(s) of the extremities, right leg

I70.492 Other atherosclerosis of autologous vein bypass graft(s) of the extremities, left leg

I70.493 Other atherosclerosis of autologous vein bypass graft(s) of the extremities, bilateral legs

I70.498 Other atherosclerosis of autologous vein bypass graft(s) of the extremities, other extremity

I70.499 Other atherosclerosis of autologous vein bypass graft(s) of the extremities, unspecified extremity

✓5th I70.5 Atherosclerosis of nonautologous biological bypass graft(s) of the extremities
Use additional code, if applicable, to identify chronic total occlusion of artery of extremity (I70.92)

✓6th I70.50 Unspecified atherosclerosis of nonautologous biological bypass graft(s) of the extremities

I70.501 Unspecified atherosclerosis of nonautologous biological bypass graft(s) of the extremities, right leg

I70.502 Unspecified atherosclerosis of nonautologous biological bypass graft(s) of the extremities, left leg

I70.503 Unspecified atherosclerosis of nonautologous biological bypass graft(s) of the extremities, bilateral legs

I70.508 Unspecified atherosclerosis of nonautologous biological bypass graft(s) of the extremities, other extremity

I70.509 Unspecified atherosclerosis of nonautologous biological bypass graft(s) of the extremities, unspecified extremity

✓6th I70.51 Atherosclerosis of nonautologous biological bypass graft(s) of the extremities with intermittent claudication

I70.511 Atherosclerosis of nonautologous biological bypass graft(s) of the extremities with intermittent claudication, right leg

I7Ø.512 Atherosclerosis of nonautologous biological bypass graft(s) of the extremities with intermittent claudication, left leg

I7Ø.513 Atherosclerosis of nonautologous biological bypass graft(s) of the extremities with intermittent claudication, bilateral legs

I7Ø.518 Atherosclerosis of nonautologous biological bypass graft(s) of the extremities with intermittent claudication, other extremity

I7Ø.519 Atherosclerosis of nonautologous biological bypass graft(s) of the extremities with intermittent claudication, unspecified extremity

✓6th **I7Ø.52 Atherosclerosis of nonautologous biological bypass graft(s) of the extremities with rest pain**

Includes any condition classifiable to I7Ø.51-

I7Ø.521 Atherosclerosis of nonautologous biological bypass graft(s) of the extremities with rest pain, right leg

I7Ø.522 Atherosclerosis of nonautologous biological bypass graft(s) of the extremities with rest pain, left leg

I7Ø.523 Atherosclerosis of nonautologous biological bypass graft(s) of the extremities with rest pain, bilateral legs

I7Ø.528 Atherosclerosis of nonautologous biological bypass graft(s) of the extremities with rest pain, other extremity

I7Ø.529 Atherosclerosis of nonautologous biological bypass graft(s) of the extremities with rest pain, unspecified extremity

✓6th **I7Ø.53 Atherosclerosis of nonautologous biological bypass graft(s) of the right leg with ulceration**

Includes any condition classifiable to I7Ø.511 and I7Ø.521

Use additional code to identify severity of ulcer (L97.- with fifth character 1)

I7Ø.531 Atherosclerosis of nonautologous biological bypass graft(s) of the right leg with ulceration of thigh

I7Ø.532 Atherosclerosis of nonautologous biological bypass graft(s) of the right leg with ulceration of calf

I7Ø.533 Atherosclerosis of nonautologous biological bypass graft(s) of the right leg with ulceration of ankle

I7Ø.534 Atherosclerosis of nonautologous biological bypass graft(s) of the right leg with ulceration of heel and midfoot

Atherosclerosis of nonautologous biological bypass graft(s) of right leg with ulceration of plantar surface of midfoot

I7Ø.535 Atherosclerosis of nonautologous biological bypass graft(s) of the right leg with ulceration of other part of foot

Atherosclerosis of nonautologous biological bypass graft(s) of the right leg with ulceration of toe

I7Ø.538 Atherosclerosis of nonautologous biological bypass graft(s) of the right leg with ulceration of other part of lower leg

I7Ø.539 Atherosclerosis of nonautologous biological bypass graft(s) of the right leg with ulceration of unspecified site

✓6th **I7Ø.54 Atherosclerosis of nonautologous biological bypass graft(s) of the left leg with ulceration**

Includes any condition classifiable to I7Ø.512 and I7Ø.522

Use additional code to identify severity of ulcer (L97.- with fifth character 2)

I7Ø.541 Atherosclerosis of nonautologous biological bypass graft(s) of the left leg with ulceration of thigh

I7Ø.542 Atherosclerosis of nonautologous biological bypass graft(s) of the left leg with ulceration of calf

I7Ø.543 Atherosclerosis of nonautologous biological bypass graft(s) of the left leg with ulceration of ankle

I7Ø.544 Atherosclerosis of nonautologous biological bypass graft(s) of the left leg with ulceration of heel and midfoot

Atherosclerosis of nonautologous biological bypass graft(s) of left leg with ulceration of plantar surface of midfoot

I7Ø.545 Atherosclerosis of nonautologous biological bypass graft(s) of the left leg with ulceration of other part of foot

Atherosclerosis of nonautologous biological bypass graft(s) of the left leg with ulceration of toe

I7Ø.548 Atherosclerosis of nonautologous biological bypass graft(s) of the left leg with ulceration of other part of lower leg

I7Ø.549 Atherosclerosis of nonautologous biological bypass graft(s) of the left leg with ulceration of unspecified site

I7Ø.55 Atherosclerosis of nonautologous biological bypass graft(s) of other extremity with ulceration

Includes any condition classifiable to I7Ø.518, I7Ø.528, and I7Ø.538

Use additional code to identify severity of ulcer (L98.49)

✓6th **I7Ø.56 Atherosclerosis of nonautologous biological bypass graft(s) of the extremities with gangrene**

Includes any condition classifiable to I7Ø.51-, I7Ø.52-, and I7Ø.53-, I7Ø.54-, I7Ø.55

Use additional code to identify the severity of any ulcer (L98.49-), if applicable

I7Ø.561 Atherosclerosis of nonautologous biological bypass graft(s) of the extremities with gangrene, right leg

I7Ø.562 Atherosclerosis of nonautologous biological bypass graft(s) of the extremities with gangrene, left leg

I7Ø.563 Atherosclerosis of nonautologous biological bypass graft(s) of the extremities with gangrene, bilateral legs

I7Ø.568 Atherosclerosis of nonautologous biological bypass graft(s) of the extremities with gangrene, other extremity

I7Ø.569 Atherosclerosis of nonautologous biological bypass graft(s) of the extremities with gangrene, unspecified extremity

✓6th **I7Ø.59 Other atherosclerosis of nonautologous biological bypass graft(s) of the extremities**

I7Ø.591 Other atherosclerosis of nonautologous biological bypass graft(s) of the extremities, right leg

I7Ø.592 Other atherosclerosis of nonautologous biological bypass graft(s) of the extremities, left leg

I7Ø.593 Other atherosclerosis of nonautologous biological bypass graft(s) of the extremities, bilateral legs

I7Ø.598 Other atherosclerosis of nonautologous biological bypass graft(s) of the extremities, other extremity

I7Ø.599 Other atherosclerosis of nonautologous biological bypass graft(s) of the extremities, unspecified extremity

✓5th I70.6 Atherosclerosis of nonbiological bypass graft(s) of the extremities

Use additional code, if applicable, to identify chronic total occlusion of artery of extremity (I70.92)

✓6th I70.60 Unspecified atherosclerosis of nonbiological bypass graft(s) of the extremities

I70.601 Unspecified atherosclerosis of nonbiological bypass graft(s) of the extremities, right leg

I70.602 Unspecified atherosclerosis of nonbiological bypass graft(s) of the extremities, left leg

I70.603 Unspecified atherosclerosis of nonbiological bypass graft(s) of the extremities, bilateral legs

I70.608 Unspecified atherosclerosis of nonbiological bypass graft(s) of the extremities, other extremity

I70.609 Unspecified atherosclerosis of nonbiological bypass graft(s) of the extremities, unspecified extremity

✓6th I70.61 Atherosclerosis of nonbiological bypass graft(s) of the extremities with intermittent claudication

I70.611 Atherosclerosis of nonbiological bypass graft(s) of the extremities with intermittent claudication, right leg

I70.612 Atherosclerosis of nonbiological bypass graft(s) of the extremities with intermittent claudication, left leg

I70.613 Atherosclerosis of nonbiological bypass graft(s) of the extremities with intermittent claudication, bilateral legs

I70.618 Atherosclerosis of nonbiological bypass graft(s) of the extremities with intermittent claudication, other extremity

I70.619 Atherosclerosis of nonbiological bypass graft(s) of the extremities with intermittent claudication, unspecified extremity

✓6th I70.62 Atherosclerosis of nonbiological bypass graft(s) of the extremities with rest pain

Includes any condition classifiable to I70.61-

I70.621 Atherosclerosis of nonbiological bypass graft(s) of the extremities with rest pain, right leg

I70.622 Atherosclerosis of nonbiological bypass graft(s) of the extremities with rest pain, left leg

I70.623 Atherosclerosis of nonbiological bypass graft(s) of the extremities with rest pain, bilateral legs

I70.628 Atherosclerosis of nonbiological bypass graft(s) of the extremities with rest pain, other extremity

I70.629 Atherosclerosis of nonbiological bypass graft(s) of the extremities with rest pain, unspecified extremity

✓6th I70.63 Atherosclerosis of nonbiological bypass graft(s) of the right leg with ulceration

Includes any condition classifiable to I70.611 and I70.621

Use additional code to identify severity of ulcer (L97.- with fifth character 1)

I70.631 Atherosclerosis of nonbiological bypass graft(s) of the right leg with ulceration of thigh

I70.632 Atherosclerosis of nonbiological bypass graft(s) of the right leg with ulceration of calf

I70.633 Atherosclerosis of nonbiological bypass graft(s) of the right leg with ulceration of ankle

I70.634 Atherosclerosis of nonbiological bypass graft(s) of the right leg with ulceration of heel and midfoot

Atherosclerosis of nonbiological bypass graft(s) of right leg with ulceration of plantar surface of midfoot

I70.635 Atherosclerosis of nonbiological bypass graft(s) of the right leg with ulceration of other part of foot

Atherosclerosis of nonbiological bypass graft(s) of the right leg with ulceration of toe

I70.638 Atherosclerosis of nonbiological bypass graft(s) of the right leg with ulceration of other part of lower leg

I70.639 Atherosclerosis of nonbiological bypass graft(s) of the right leg with ulceration of unspecified site

✓6th I70.64 Atherosclerosis of nonbiological bypass graft(s) of the left leg with ulceration

Includes any condition classifiable to I70.612 and I70.622

Use additional code to identify severity of ulcer (L97.- with fifth character 2)

I70.641 Atherosclerosis of nonbiological bypass graft(s) of the left leg with ulceration of thigh

I70.642 Atherosclerosis of nonbiological bypass graft(s) of the left leg with ulceration of calf

I70.643 Atherosclerosis of nonbiological bypass graft(s) of the left leg with ulceration of ankle

I70.644 Atherosclerosis of nonbiological bypass graft(s) of the left leg with ulceration of heel and midfoot

Atherosclerosis of nonbiological bypass graft(s) of left leg with ulceration of plantar surface of midfoot

I70.645 Atherosclerosis of nonbiological bypass graft(s) of the left leg with ulceration of other part of foot

Atherosclerosis of nonbiological bypass graft(s) of the left leg with ulceration of toe

I70.648 Atherosclerosis of nonbiological bypass graft(s) of the left leg with ulceration of other part of lower leg

I70.649 Atherosclerosis of nonbiological bypass graft(s) of the left leg with ulceration of unspecified site

I70.65 Atherosclerosis of nonbiological bypass graft(s) of other extremity with ulceration

Includes any condition classifiable to I70.618 and I70.628

Use additional code to identify severity of ulcer (L98.49)

✓6th I70.66 Atherosclerosis of nonbiological bypass graft(s) of the extremities with gangrene

Includes any condition classifiable to I70.61-, I70.62-, I70.63-, I70.64-, I70.65

Use additional code to identify the severity of any ulcer (L98.49-), if applicable

I70.661 Atherosclerosis of nonbiological bypass graft(s) of the extremities with gangrene, right leg

I70.662 Atherosclerosis of nonbiological bypass graft(s) of the extremities with gangrene, left leg

I70.663 Atherosclerosis of nonbiological bypass graft(s) of the extremities with gangrene, bilateral legs

I70.668 Atherosclerosis of nonbiological bypass graft(s) of the extremities with gangrene, other extremity

I70.669 Atherosclerosis of nonbiological bypass graft(s) of the extremities with gangrene, unspecified extremity

✓6th I70.69 Other atherosclerosis of nonbiological bypass graft(s) of the extremities

I70.691 Other atherosclerosis of nonbiological bypass graft(s) of the extremities, right leg

I70.692 Other atherosclerosis of nonbiological bypass graft(s) of the extremities, left leg

✓ Appropriate additional character required ✓x7th Requires 7th character, placeholder x must fill empty characters

I7Ø.693 Other atherosclerosis of nonbiological bypass graft(s) of the extremities, bilateral legs

I7Ø.698 Other atherosclerosis of nonbiological bypass graft(s) of the extremities, other extremity

I7Ø.699 Other atherosclerosis of nonbiological bypass graft(s) of the extremities, unspecified extremity

5th I7Ø.7 Atherosclerosis of other type of bypass graft(s) of the extremities

Use additional code, if applicable, to identify chronic total occlusion of artery of extremity (I7Ø.92)

6th I7Ø.7Ø Unspecified atherosclerosis of other type of bypass graft(s) of the extremities

I7Ø.7Ø1 Unspecified atherosclerosis of other type of bypass graft(s) of the extremities, right leg

I7Ø.7Ø2 Unspecified atherosclerosis of other type of bypass graft(s) of the extremities, left leg

I7Ø.7Ø3 Unspecified atherosclerosis of other type of bypass graft(s) of the extremities, bilateral legs

I7Ø.7Ø8 Unspecified atherosclerosis of other type of bypass graft(s) of the extremities, other extremity

I7Ø.7Ø9 Unspecified atherosclerosis of other type of bypass graft(s) of the extremities, unspecified extremity

6th I7Ø.71 Atherosclerosis of other type of bypass graft(s) of the extremities with intermittent claudication

I7Ø.711 Atherosclerosis of other type of bypass graft(s) of the extremities with intermittent claudication, right leg

I7Ø.712 Atherosclerosis of other type of bypass graft(s) of the extremities with intermittent claudication, left leg

I7Ø.713 Atherosclerosis of other type of bypass graft(s) of the extremities with intermittent claudication, bilateral legs

I7Ø.718 Atherosclerosis of other type of bypass graft(s) of the extremities with intermittent claudication, other extremity

I7Ø.719 Atherosclerosis of other type of bypass graft(s) of the extremities with intermittent claudication, unspecified extremity

6th I7Ø.72 Atherosclerosis of other type of bypass graft(s) of the extremities with rest pain

Includes any condition classifiable to I7Ø.71-

I7Ø.721 Atherosclerosis of other type of bypass graft(s) of the extremities with rest pain, right leg

I7Ø.722 Atherosclerosis of other type of bypass graft(s) of the extremities with rest pain, left leg

I7Ø.723 Atherosclerosis of other type of bypass graft(s) of the extremities with rest pain, bilateral legs

I7Ø.728 Atherosclerosis of other type of bypass graft(s) of the extremities with rest pain, other extremity

I7Ø.729 Atherosclerosis of other type of bypass graft(s) of the extremities with rest pain, unspecified extremity

6th I7Ø.73 Atherosclerosis of other type of bypass graft(s) of the right leg with ulceration

Includes any condition classifiable to I7Ø.711 and I7Ø.721

Use additional code to identify severity of ulcer (L97.- with fifth character 1)

I7Ø.731 Atherosclerosis of other type of bypass graft(s) of the right leg with ulceration of thigh

I7Ø.732 Atherosclerosis of other type of bypass graft(s) of the right leg with ulceration of calf

I7Ø.733 Atherosclerosis of other type of bypass graft(s) of the right leg with ulceration of ankle

I7Ø.734 Atherosclerosis of other type of bypass graft(s) of the right leg with ulceration of heel and midfoot

Atherosclerosis of other type of bypass graft(s) of right leg with ulceration of plantar surface of midfoot

I7Ø.735 Atherosclerosis of other type of bypass graft(s) of the right leg with ulceration of other part of foot

Atherosclerosis of other type of bypass graft(s) of right leg with ulceration of toe

I7Ø.738 Atherosclerosis of other type of bypass graft(s) of the right leg with ulceration of other part of lower leg

I7Ø.739 Atherosclerosis of other type of bypass graft(s) of the right leg with ulceration of unspecified site

6th I7Ø.74 Atherosclerosis of other type of bypass graft(s) of the left leg with ulceration

Includes any condition classifiable to I7Ø.712 and I7Ø.722

Use additional code to identify severity of ulcer (L97.- with fifth character 2)

I7Ø.741 Atherosclerosis of other type of bypass graft(s) of the left leg with ulceration of thigh

I7Ø.742 Atherosclerosis of other type of bypass graft(s) of the left leg with ulceration of calf

I7Ø.743 Atherosclerosis of other type of bypass graft(s) of the left leg with ulceration of ankle

I7Ø.744 Atherosclerosis of other type of bypass graft(s) of the left leg with ulceration of heel and midfoot

Atherosclerosis of other type of bypass graft(s) of left leg with ulceration of plantar surface of midfoot

I7Ø.745 Atherosclerosis of other type of bypass graft(s) of the left leg with ulceration of other part of foot

Atherosclerosis of other type of bypass graft(s) of left leg with ulceration of toe

I7Ø.748 Atherosclerosis of other type of bypass graft(s) of the left leg with ulceration of other part of lower leg

I7Ø.749 Atherosclerosis of other type of bypass graft(s) of the left leg with ulceration of unspecified site

I7Ø.75 Atherosclerosis of other type of bypass graft(s) of other extremity with ulceration

Includes any condition classifiable to I7Ø.718 and I7Ø.728

Use additional code to identify severity of ulcer (L98.49)

6th I7Ø.76 Atherosclerosis of other type of bypass graft(s) of the extremities with gangrene

Includes any condition classifiable to I7Ø.71-, I7Ø.72-, I7Ø.73-, I7Ø.74-, I7Ø.75

Use additional code to identify the severity of any ulcer (L98.49-), if applicable

I7Ø.761 Atherosclerosis of other type of bypass graft(s) of the extremities with gangrene, right leg

I7Ø.762 Atherosclerosis of other type of bypass graft(s) of the extremities with gangrene, left leg

I7Ø.763 Atherosclerosis of other type of bypass graft(s) of the extremities with gangrene, bilateral legs

I7Ø.768 Atherosclerosis of other type of bypass graft(s) of the extremities with gangrene, other extremity

I7Ø.769 Atherosclerosis of other type of bypass graft(s) of the extremities with gangrene, unspecified extremity

✓6th **I70.79 Other atherosclerosis of other type of bypass graft(s) of the extremities**
I70.791 Other atherosclerosis of other type of bypass graft(s) of the extremities, right leg
I70.792 Other atherosclerosis of other type of bypass graft(s) of the extremities, left leg
I70.793 Other atherosclerosis of other type of bypass graft(s) of the extremities, bilateral legs
I70.798 Other atherosclerosis of other type of bypass graft(s) of the extremities, other extremity
I70.799 Other atherosclerosis of other type of bypass graft(s) of the extremities, unspecified extremity

I70.8 Atherosclerosis of other arteries

✓5th **I70.9 Other and unspecified atherosclerosis**
I70.90 Unspecified atherosclerosis
I70.91 Generalized atherosclerosis
I70.92 Chronic total occlusion of artery of the extremities
Complete occlusion of artery of the extremities
Total occlusion of artery of the extremities
Code first atherosclerosis of arteries of the extremities (I70.2-, I70.3-, I70.4-, I70.5-, I70.6-, I70.7-)
EXCLUDES 1 *acute occlusion of artery of the extremity (I70.2-, I70.3-, I70.4-)*

✓4th **I71 Aortic aneurysm and dissection**
EXCLUDES 1 *aortic ectasia (I77.81-)*
syphilitic aortic aneurysm (A52.01)
traumatic aortic aneurysm (S25.09, S35.09)

✓5th **I71.0 Dissection of aorta**
I71.00 Dissection of unspecified site of aorta
I71.01 Dissection of thoracic aorta
I71.02 Dissection of abdominal aorta
I71.03 Dissection of thoracoabdominal aorta

I71.1 Thoracic aortic aneurysm, ruptured
I71.2 Thoracic aortic aneurysm, without rupture
I71.3 Abdominal aortic aneurysm, ruptured
I71.4 Abdominal aortic aneurysm, without rupture
I71.5 Thoracoabdominal aortic aneurysm, ruptured
I71.6 Thoracoabdominal aortic aneurysm, without rupture
I71.8 Aortic aneurysm of unspecified site, ruptured
Rupture of aorta NOS
I71.9 Aortic aneurysm of unspecified site, without rupture
Aneurysm of aorta
Dilatation of aorta
Hyaline necrosis of aorta

✓4th **I72 Other aneurysm**
INCLUDES aneurysm (cirsoid) (false) (ruptured)
EXCLUDES 2 *acquired aneurysm (I77.0)*
aneurysm (of) aorta (I71.-)
aneurysm (of) arteriovenous NOS (Q27.3-)
carotid artery dissection (I77.71)
cerebral (nonruptured) aneurysm (I67.1)
coronary aneurysm (I25.4)
coronary artery dissection (I25.42)
dissection of artery NEC (I77.79)
heart aneurysm (I25.3)
iliac artery dissection (I77.72)
pulmonary artery aneurysm (I28.1)
renal artery dissection (I77.73)
retinal aneurysm (H35.0)
ruptured cerebral aneurysm (I60.7)
varicose aneurysm (I77.0)
vertebral artery dissection (I77.74)

I72.0 Aneurysm of carotid artery
Aneurysm of common carotid artery
Aneurysm of external carotid artery
Aneurysm of internal carotid artery, extracranial portion
EXCLUDES 1 *aneurysm of internal carotid artery, intracranial portion (I67.1)*
aneurysm of internal carotid artery NOS (I67.1)
I72.1 Aneurysm of artery of upper extremity
I72.2 Aneurysm of renal artery
I72.3 Aneurysm of iliac artery
I72.4 Aneurysm of artery of lower extremity
I72.8 Aneurysm of other specified arteries
I72.9 Aneurysm of unspecified site

✓4th **I73 Other peripheral vascular diseases**
EXCLUDES 2 *chilblains (T69.1)*
frostbite (T33-T34)
immersion hand or foot (T69.0-)
spasm of cerebral artery (G45.9)

✓5th **I73.0 Raynaud's syndrome**
Raynaud's disease
Raynaud's phenomenon (secondary)
I73.00 Raynaud's syndrome without gangrene
I73.01 Raynaud's syndrome with gangrene

I73.1 Thromboangiitis obliterans [Buerger's disease]

✓5th **I73.8 Other specified peripheral vascular diseases**
EXCLUDES 1 *diabetic (peripheral) angiopathy (E08-E13 with .51-.52)*
I73.81 Erythromelalgia
I73.89 Other specified peripheral vascular diseases
Acrocyanosis
Erythrocyanosis
Simple acroparesthesia [Schultze's type]
Vasomotor acroparesthesia [Nothnagel's type]

I73.9 Peripheral vascular disease, unspecified
Intermittent claudication
Peripheral angiopathy NOS
Spasm of artery
EXCLUDES 1 *atherosclerosis of the extremities (I70.2--I70.7-)*

✓4th **I74 Arterial embolism and thrombosis**
Embolic infarction
Embolic occlusion
Thrombotic infarction
Thrombotic occlusion
Code first:
embolism and thrombosis complicating abortion or ectopic or molar pregnancy (O00-O07, O08.2)
embolism and thrombosis complicating pregnancy, childbirth and the puerperium (O88.-)
EXCLUDES 2 *atheroembolism (I75.-)*
basilar embolism and thrombosis (I63.0-I63.2, I65.1)
carotid embolism and thrombosis (I63.0-I63.2, I65.2)
cerebral embolism and thrombosis (I63.3-I63.5, I66-)
coronary embolism and thrombosis (I21-I25)
mesenteric embolism and thrombosis (K55.0)
ophthalmic embolism and thrombosis (H34.-)
precerebral embolism and thrombosis NOS (I63.0-I63.2, I65.9)
pulmonary embolism and thrombosis (I26.-)
renal embolism and thrombosis (N28.0)
retinal embolism and thrombosis (H34.-)
septic embolism and thrombosis (I76)
vertebral embolism and thrombosis (I63.0-I63.2, I65.0)

✓5th **I74.0 Embolism and thrombosis of abdominal aorta**
I74.01 Saddle embolus of abdominal aorta
I74.09 Other arterial embolism and thrombosis of abdominal aorta
Aortic bifurcation syndrome
Aortoiliac obstruction
Leriche's syndrome

✓5th **I74.1 Embolism and thrombosis of other and unspecified parts of aorta**
I74.10 Embolism and thrombosis of unspecified parts of aorta
I74.11 Embolism and thrombosis of thoracic aorta
I74.19 Embolism and thrombosis of other parts of aorta

I74.2 Embolism and thrombosis of arteries of the upper extremities
I74.3 Embolism and thrombosis of arteries of the lower extremities
I74.4 Embolism and thrombosis of arteries of extremities, unspecified
Peripheral arterial embolism NOS
I74.5 Embolism and thrombosis of iliac artery
I74.8 Embolism and thrombosis of other arteries
I74.9 Embolism and thrombosis of unspecified artery

√4th **I75 Atheroembolism**
Atherothrombotic microembolism
Cholesterol embolism

√5th **I75.Ø Atheroembolism of extremities**

√6th **I75.Ø1 Atheroembolism of upper extremity**

I75.Ø11 Atheroembolism of right upper extremity

I75.Ø12 Atheroembolism of left upper extremity

I75.Ø13 Atheroembolism of bilateral upper extremities

I75.Ø19 Atheroembolism of unspecified upper extremity

√6th **I75.Ø2 Atheroembolism of lower extremity**

I75.Ø21 Atheroembolism of right lower extremity

I75.Ø22 Atheroembolism of left lower extremity

I75.Ø23 Atheroembolism of bilateral lower extremities

I75.Ø29 Atheroembolism of unspecified lower extremity

√5th **I75.8 Atheroembolism of other sites**

I75.81 Atheroembolism of kidney
Use additional code for any associated acute kidney failure and chronic kidney disease (N17.-, N18.-)

I75.89 Atheroembolism of other site

I76 Septic arterial embolism
Code first underlying infection, such as:
infective endocarditis (I33.Ø)
lung abscess (J85.-)
Use additional code to identify the site of the embolism (I74.-)
EXCLUDES 2 *septic pulmonary embolism (I26.Ø1, I26.9Ø)*

√4th **I77 Other disorders of arteries and arterioles**
EXCLUDES 2 *collagen (vascular) diseases (M3Ø-M36)*
hypersensitivity angiitis (M31.Ø)
pulmonary artery (I28.-)

I77.Ø Arteriovenous fistula, acquired
Aneurysmal varix
Arteriovenous aneurysm, acquired
EXCLUDES 1 *arteriovenous aneurysm NOS (Q27.3-)*
presence of arteriovenous shunt (fistula) for dialysis (Z99.2)
traumatic—see injury of blood vessel by body region
EXCLUDES 2 *cerebral (I67.1)*
coronary (I25.4)

I77.1 Stricture of artery
Narrowing of artery

I77.2 Rupture of artery
Erosion of artery
Fistula of artery
Ulcer of artery
EXCLUDES 1 *traumatic rupture of artery—see injury of blood vessel by body region*

I77.3 Arterial fibromuscular dysplasia
Fibromuscular hyperplasia (of) carotid artery
Fibromuscular hyperplasia (of) renal artery

I77.4 Celiac artery compression syndrome

I77.5 Necrosis of artery

I77.6 Arteritis, unspecified
Aortitis NOS
Endarteritis NOS
EXCLUDES 1 *arteritis or endarteritis:*
aortic arch (M31.4)
cerebral NEC (I67.7)
coronary (I25.89)
deformans (I7Ø.-)
giant cell (M31.5., M31.6)
obliterans (I7Ø.-)
senile (I7Ø.-)

√5th **I77.7 Other arterial dissection**
EXCLUDES 2 *dissection of aorta (I71.Ø-)*
dissection of coronary artery (I25.42)

I77.71 Dissection of carotid artery

I77.72 Dissection of iliac artery

I77.73 Dissection of renal artery

I77.74 Dissection of vertebral artery

I77.79 Dissection of other artery

√5th **I77.8 Other specified disorders of arteries and arterioles**

√6th **I77.81 Aortic ectasia**
Ectasis aorta
EXCLUDES 1 *aortic aneurysm and dissection (I71.Ø-)*

I77.81Ø Thoracic aortic ectasia

I77.811 Abdominal aortic ectasia

I77.812 Thoracoabdominal aortic ectasia

I77.819 Aortic ectasia, unspecified site

I77.89 Other specified disorders of arteries and arterioles

I77.9 Disorder of arteries and arterioles, unspecified

√4th **I78 Diseases of capillaries**

I78.Ø Hereditary hemorrhagic telangiectasia
Rendu-Osler-Weber disease

I78.1 Nevus, non-neoplastic
Araneus nevus
Senile nevus
Spider nevus
Stellar nevus
EXCLUDES 1 *nevus NOS (D22.-)*
vascular NOS (Q82.5)
EXCLUDES 2 *blue nevus (D22.-)*
flammeus nevus (Q82.5)
hairy nevus (D22.-)
melanocytic nevus (D22.-)
pigmented nevus (D22.-)
portwine nevus (Q82.5)
sanguineous nevus (Q82.5)
strawberry nevus (Q82.5)
verrucous nevus (Q82.5)

I78.8 Other diseases of capillaries

I78.9 Disease of capillaries, unspecified

√4th **I79 Disorders of arteries, arterioles and capillaries in diseases classified elsewhere**

I79.Ø Aneurysm of aorta in diseases classified elsewhere
Code first underlying disease
EXCLUDES 1 *syphilitic aneurysm (A52.Ø1)*

I79.1 Aortitis in diseases classified elsewhere
Code first underlying disease
EXCLUDES 1 *syphilitic aortitis (A52.Ø2)*

I79.8 Other disorders of arteries, arterioles and capillaries in diseases classified elsewhere
Code first underlying disease, such as:
amyloidosis (E85.-)
EXCLUDES 1 *diabetic (peripheral) angiopathy (EØ8-E13 with .51-.52)*
endarteritis:
syphilitic (A52.Ø9)
tuberculous (A18.89)

Diseases of veins, lymphatic vessels and lymph nodes, not elsewhere classified. (I8Ø-I89)

√4th **I8Ø Phlebitis and thrombophlebitis**
INCLUDES endophlebitis
inflammation, vein
periphlebitis
suppurative phlebitis
Code first:
phlebitis and thrombophlebitis complicating abortion, ectopic or molar pregnancy (OØØ-OØ7, OØ8.7)
phlebitis and thrombophlebitis complicating pregnancy, childbirth and the puerperium (O22.-, O87.-)
EXCLUDES 1 *venous embolism and thrombosis of lower extremities ((I82.4-, I82.5-, I82.81-)*

√5th **I8Ø.Ø Phlebitis and thrombophlebitis of superficial vessels of lower extremities**
Phlebitis and thrombophlebitis of femoropopliteal vein

I8Ø.ØØ Phlebitis and thrombophlebitis of superficial vessels of unspecified lower extremity

I8Ø.Ø1 Phlebitis and thrombophlebitis of superficial vessels of right lower extremity

I8Ø.Ø2 Phlebitis and thrombophlebitis of superficial vessels of left lower extremity

I8Ø.Ø3 Phlebitis and thrombophlebitis of superficial vessels of lower extremities, bilateral

√5th **I8Ø.1 Phlebitis and thrombophlebitis of femoral vein**

I8Ø.1Ø Phlebitis and thrombophlebitis of unspecified femoral vein

I80.11 Phlebitis and thrombophlebitis of right femoral vein

I80.12 Phlebitis and thrombophlebitis of left femoral vein

I80.13 Phlebitis and thrombophlebitis of femoral vein, bilateral

✓5th **I80.2 Phlebitis and thrombophlebitis of other and unspecified deep vessels of lower extremities**

✓6th **I80.20 Phlebitis and thrombophlebitis of unspecified deep vessels of lower extremities**

I80.201 Phlebitis and thrombophlebitis of unspecified deep vessels of right lower extremity

I80.202 Phlebitis and thrombophlebitis of unspecified deep vessels of left lower extremity

I80.203 Phlebitis and thrombophlebitis of unspecified deep vessels of lower extremities, bilateral

I80.209 Phlebitis and thrombophlebitis of unspecified deep vessels of unspecified lower extremity

✓6th **I80.21 Phlebitis and thrombophlebitis of iliac vein**

I80.211 Phlebitis and thrombophlebitis of right iliac vein

I80.212 Phlebitis and thrombophlebitis of left iliac vein

I80.213 Phlebitis and thrombophlebitis of iliac vein, bilateral

I80.219 Phlebitis and thrombophlebitis of unspecified iliac vein

✓6th **I80.22 Phlebitis and thrombophlebitis of popliteal vein**

I80.221 Phlebitis and thrombophlebitis of right popliteal vein

I80.222 Phlebitis and thrombophlebitis of left popliteal vein

I80.223 Phlebitis and thrombophlebitis of popliteal vein, bilateral

I80.229 Phlebitis and thrombophlebitis of unspecified popliteal vein

✓6th **I80.23 Phlebitis and thrombophlebitis of tibial vein**

I80.231 Phlebitis and thrombophlebitis of right tibial vein

I80.232 Phlebitis and thrombophlebitis of left tibial vein

I80.233 Phlebitis and thrombophlebitis of tibial vein, bilateral

I80.239 Phlebitis and thrombophlebitis of unspecified tibial vein

✓6th **I80.29 Phlebitis and thrombophlebitis of other deep vessels of lower extremities**

I80.291 Phlebitis and thrombophlebitis of other deep vessels of right lower extremity

I80.292 Phlebitis and thrombophlebitis of other deep vessels of left lower extremity

I80.293 Phlebitis and thrombophlebitis of other deep vessels of lower extremity, bilateral

I80.299 Phlebitis and thrombophlebitis of other deep vessels of unspecified lower extremity

I80.3 Phlebitis and thrombophlebitis of lower extremities, unspecified

I80.8 Phlebitis and thrombophlebitis of other sites

I80.9 Phlebitis and thrombophlebitis of unspecified site

I81 Portal vein thrombosis

Portal (vein) obstruction

EXCLUDES 2 *hepatic vein thrombosis (I82.0)*
phlebitis of portal vein (K75.1)

✓4th I82 Other venous embolism and thrombosis

Code first venous embolism and thrombosis complicating:
abortion, ectopic or molar pregnancy (O00-O07, O08.7)
pregnancy, childbirth and the puerperium (O22.-, O87.-)

EXCLUDES 2 *venous embolism and thrombosis (of):*
cerebral (I63.6, I67.6)
coronary (I21-I25)
intracranial and intraspinal, septic or NOS (G08)
intracranial, nonpyogenic (I67.6)
intraspinal, nonpyogenic (G95.1)
mesenteric (K55.0)
portal (I81)
pulmonary (I26.-)

I82.0 Budd-Chiari syndrome
Hepatic vein thrombosis

I82.1 Thrombophlebitis migrans

✓5th **I82.2 Embolism and thrombosis of vena cava and other thoracic veins**

✓6th **I82.21 Embolism and thrombosis of superior vena cava**

I82.210 Acute embolism and thrombosis of superior vena cava
Embolism and thrombosis of superior vena cava NOS

I82.211 Chronic embolism and thrombosis of superior vena cava

✓6th **I82.22 Embolism and thrombosis of inferior vena cava**

I82.220 Acute embolism and thrombosis of inferior vena cava
Embolism and thrombosis of inferior vena cava NOS

I82.221 Chronic embolism and thrombosis of inferior vena cava

✓6th **I82.29 Embolism and thrombosis of other thoracic veins**
Embolism and thrombosis of brachiocephalic (innominate) vein

I82.290 Acute embolism and thrombosis of other thoracic veins

I82.291 Chronic embolism and thrombosis of other thoracic veins

I82.3 Embolism and thrombosis of renal vein

✓5th **I82.4 Acute embolism and thrombosis of deep veins of lower extremity**

✓6th **I82.40 Acute embolism and thrombosis of unspecified deep veins of lower extremity**
Deep vein thrombosis NOS
DVT NOS

EXCLUDES 1 *acute embolism and thrombosis of unspecified deep veins of distal lower extremity (I82.4b-)*
acute embolism and thrombosis of unspecified deep veins of proximal lower extremity (I82.4a-)

I82.401 Acute embolism and thrombosis of unspecified deep veins of right lower extremity

I82.402 Acute embolism and thrombosis of unspecified deep veins of left lower extremity

I82.403 Acute embolism and thrombosis of unspecified deep veins of lower extremity, bilateral

I82.409 Acute embolism and thrombosis of unspecified deep veins of unspecified lower extremity

✓6th **I82.41 Acute embolism and thrombosis of femoral vein**

I82.411 Acute embolism and thrombosis of right femoral vein

I82.412 Acute embolism and thrombosis of left femoral vein

I82.413 Acute embolism and thrombosis of femoral vein, bilateral

I82.419 Acute embolism and thrombosis of unspecified femoral vein

✓6th **I82.42 Acute embolism and thrombosis of iliac vein**

I82.421 Acute embolism and thrombosis of right iliac vein

I82.422 Acute embolism and thrombosis of left iliac vein

I82.423 Acute embolism and thrombosis of iliac vein, bilateral

I82.429 Acute embolism and thrombosis of unspecified iliac vein

√6ᵗʰ **I82.43** Acute embolism and thrombosis of popliteal vein

I82.431 Acute embolism and thrombosis of right popliteal vein

I82.432 Acute embolism and thrombosis of left popliteal vein

I82.433 Acute embolism and thrombosis of popliteal vein, bilateral

I82.439 Acute embolism and thrombosis of unspecified popliteal vein

√6ᵗʰ **I82.44** Acute embolism and thrombosis of tibial vein

I82.441 Acute embolism and thrombosis of right tibial vein

I82.442 Acute embolism and thrombosis of left tibial vein

I82.443 Acute embolism and thrombosis of tibial vein, bilateral

I82.449 Acute embolism and thrombosis of unspecified tibial vein

√6ᵗʰ **I82.49** Acute embolism and thrombosis of other specified deep vein of lower extremity

I82.491 Acute embolism and thrombosis of other specified deep vein of right lower extremity

I82.492 Acute embolism and thrombosis of other specified deep vein of left lower extremity

I82.493 Acute embolism and thrombosis of other specified deep vein of lower extremity, bilateral

I82.499 Acute embolism and thrombosis of other specified deep vein of unspecified lower extremity

√6ᵗʰ **I82.4Y** Acute embolism and thrombosis of unspecified deep veins of proximal lower extremity

Acute embolism and thrombosis of deep vein of thigh NOS

Acute embolism and thrombosis of deep vein of upper leg NOS

I82.4Y1 Acute embolism and thrombosis of unspecified deep veins of right proximal lower extremity

I82.4Y2 Acute embolism and thrombosis of unspecified deep veins of left proximal lower extremity

I82.4Y3 Acute embolism and thrombosis of unspecified deep veins of proximal lower extremity, bilateral

I82.4Y9 Acute embolism and thrombosis of unspecified deep veins of unspecified proximal lower extremity

√6ᵗʰ **I82.4Z** Acute embolism and thrombosis of unspecified deep veins of distal lower extremity

Acute embolism and thrombosis of deep vein of calf NOS

Acute embolism and thrombosis of deep vein of lower leg NOS

I82.4Z1 Acute embolism and thrombosis of unspecified deep veins of right distal lower extremity

I82.4Z2 Acute embolism and thrombosis of unspecified deep veins of left distal lower extremity

I82.4Z3 Acute embolism and thrombosis of unspecified deep veins of distal lower extremity, bilateral

I82.4Z9 Acute embolism and thrombosis of unspecified deep veins of unspecified distal lower extremity

√5ᵗʰ **I82.5** Chronic embolism and thrombosis of deep veins of lower extremity

Use additional code, if applicable, for associated long-term (current) use of anticoagulants (Z79.01)

EXCLUDES 1 personal history of venous embolism and thrombosis (Z86.718)

√6ᵗʰ **I82.50** Chronic embolism and thrombosis of unspecified deep veins of lower extremity

EXCLUDES 1 chronic embolism and thrombosis of unspecified deep veins of distal lower extremity (I82.5b-)
chronic embolism and thrombosis of unspecified deep veins of proximal lower extremity (I82.5a-)

I82.501 Chronic embolism and thrombosis of unspecified deep veins of right lower extremity

I82.502 Chronic embolism and thrombosis of unspecified deep veins of left lower extremity

I82.503 Chronic embolism and thrombosis of unspecified deep veins of lower extremity, bilateral

I82.509 Chronic embolism and thrombosis of unspecified deep veins of unspecified lower extremity

√6ᵗʰ **I82.51** Chronic embolism and thrombosis of femoral vein

I82.511 Chronic embolism and thrombosis of right femoral vein

I82.512 Chronic embolism and thrombosis of left femoral vein

I82.513 Chronic embolism and thrombosis of femoral vein, bilateral

I82.519 Chronic embolism and thrombosis of unspecified femoral vein

√6ᵗʰ **I82.52** Chronic embolism and thrombosis of iliac vein

I82.521 Chronic embolism and thrombosis of right iliac vein

I82.522 Chronic embolism and thrombosis of left iliac vein

I82.523 Chronic embolism and thrombosis of iliac vein, bilateral

I82.529 Chronic embolism and thrombosis of unspecified iliac vein

√6ᵗʰ **I82.53** Chronic embolism and thrombosis of popliteal vein

I82.531 Chronic embolism and thrombosis of right popliteal vein

I82.532 Chronic embolism and thrombosis of left popliteal vein

I82.533 Chronic embolism and thrombosis of popliteal vein, bilateral

I82.539 Chronic embolism and thrombosis of unspecified popliteal vein

√6ᵗʰ **I82.54** Chronic embolism and thrombosis of tibial vein

I82.541 Chronic embolism and thrombosis of right tibial vein

I82.542 Chronic embolism and thrombosis of left tibial vein

I82.543 Chronic embolism and thrombosis of tibial vein, bilateral

I82.549 Chronic embolism and thrombosis of unspecified tibial vein

√6ᵗʰ **I82.59** Chronic embolism and thrombosis of other specified deep vein of lower extremity

I82.591 Chronic embolism and thrombosis of other specified deep vein of right lower extremity

I82.592 Chronic embolism and thrombosis of other specified deep vein of left lower extremity

I82.593 Chronic embolism and thrombosis of other specified deep vein of lower extremity, bilateral

I82.599 Chronic embolism and thrombosis of other specified deep vein of unspecified lower extremity

I82.5Y Chronic embolism and thrombosis of unspecified deep veins of proximal lower extremity
Chronic embolism and thrombosis of deep veins of thigh NOS
Chronic embolism and thrombosis of deep veins of upper leg NOS
- **I82.5Y1 Chronic embolism and thrombosis of unspecified deep veins of right proximal lower extremity**
- **I82.5Y2 Chronic embolism and thrombosis of unspecified deep veins of left proximal lower extremity**
- **I82.5Y3 Chronic embolism and thrombosis of unspecified deep veins of proximal lower extremity, bilateral**
- **I82.5Y9 Chronic embolism and thrombosis of unspecified deep veins of unspecified proximal lower extremity**

I82.5Z Chronic embolism and thrombosis of unspecified deep veins of distal lower extremity
Chronic embolism and thrombosis of deep veins of calf NOS
Chronic embolism and thrombosis of deep veins of lower leg NOS
- **I82.5Z1 Chronic embolism and thrombosis of unspecified deep veins of right distal lower extremity**
- **I82.5Z2 Chronic embolism and thrombosis of unspecified deep veins of left distal lower extremity**
- **I82.5Z3 Chronic embolism and thrombosis of unspecified deep veins of distal lower extremity, bilateral**
- **I82.5Z9 Chronic embolism and thrombosis of unspecified deep veins of unspecified distal lower extremity**

I82.6 Acute embolism and thrombosis of veins of upper extremity

I82.60 Acute embolism and thrombosis of unspecified veins of upper extremity
- **I82.601 Acute embolism and thrombosis of unspecified veins of right upper extremity**
- **I82.602 Acute embolism and thrombosis of unspecified veins of left upper extremity**
- **I82.603 Acute embolism and thrombosis of unspecified veins of upper extremity, bilateral**
- **I82.609 Acute embolism and thrombosis of unspecified veins of unspecified upper extremity**

I82.61 Acute embolism and thrombosis of superficial veins of upper extremity
Acute embolism and thrombosis of antecubital vein
Acute embolism and thrombosis of basilic vein
Acute embolism and thrombosis of cephalic vein
- **I82.611 Acute embolism and thrombosis of superficial veins of right upper extremity**
- **I82.612 Acute embolism and thrombosis of superficial veins of left upper extremity**
- **I82.613 Acute embolism and thrombosis of superficial veins of upper extremity, bilateral**
- **I82.619 Acute embolism and thrombosis of superficial veins of unspecified upper extremity**

I82.62 Acute embolism and thrombosis of deep veins of upper extremity
Acute embolism and thrombosis of brachial vein
Acute embolism and thrombosis of radial vein
Acute embolism and thrombosis of ulnar vein
- **I82.621 Acute embolism and thrombosis of deep veins of right upper extremity**
- **I82.622 Acute embolism and thrombosis of deep veins of left upper extremity**
- **I82.623 Acute embolism and thrombosis of deep veins of upper extremity, bilateral**
- **I82.629 Acute embolism and thrombosis of deep veins of unspecified upper extremity**

I82.7 Chronic embolism and thrombosis of veins of upper extremity
Use additional code, if applicable, for associated long-term (current) use of anticoagulants (Z79.01)
EXCLUDES 1 *personal history of venous embolism and thrombosis (Z86.718)*

I82.70 Chronic embolism and thrombosis of unspecified veins of upper extremity
- **I82.701 Chronic embolism and thrombosis of unspecified veins of right upper extremity**
- **I82.702 Chronic embolism and thrombosis of unspecified veins of left upper extremity**
- **I82.703 Chronic embolism and thrombosis of unspecified veins of upper extremity, bilateral**
- **I82.709 Chronic embolism and thrombosis of unspecified veins of unspecified upper extremity**

I82.71 Chronic embolism and thrombosis of superficial veins of upper extremity
Chronic embolism and thrombosis of antecubital vein
Chronic embolism and thrombosis of basilic vein
Chronic embolism and thrombosis of cephalic vein
- **I82.711 Chronic embolism and thrombosis of superficial veins of right upper extremity**
- **I82.712 Chronic embolism and thrombosis of superficial veins of left upper extremity**
- **I82.713 Chronic embolism and thrombosis of superficial veins of upper extremity, bilateral**
- **I82.719 Chronic embolism and thrombosis of superficial veins of unspecified upper extremity**

I82.72 Chronic embolism and thrombosis of deep veins of upper extremity
Chronic embolism and thrombosis of brachial vein
Chronic embolism and thrombosis of radial vein
Chronic embolism and thrombosis of ulnar vein
- **I82.721 Chronic embolism and thrombosis of deep veins of right upper extremity**
- **I82.722 Chronic embolism and thrombosis of deep veins of left upper extremity**
- **I82.723 Chronic embolism and thrombosis of deep veins of upper extremity, bilateral**
- **I82.729 Chronic embolism and thrombosis of deep veins of unspecified upper extremity**

I82.A Embolism and thrombosis of axillary vein

I82.A1 Acute embolism and thrombosis of axillary vein
- **I82.A11 Acute embolism and thrombosis of right axillary vein**
- **I82.A12 Acute embolism and thrombosis of left axillary vein**
- **I82.A13 Acute embolism and thrombosis of axillary vein, bilateral**
- **I82.A19 Acute embolism and thrombosis of unspecified axillary vein**

I82.A2 Chronic embolism and thrombosis of axillary vein
- **I82.A21 Chronic embolism and thrombosis of right axillary vein**
- **I82.A22 Chronic embolism and thrombosis of left axillary vein**
- **I82.A23 Chronic embolism and thrombosis of axillary vein, bilateral**
- **I82.A29 Chronic embolism and thrombosis of unspecified axillary vein**

I82.B Embolism and thrombosis of subclavian vein

I82.B1 Acute embolism and thrombosis of subclavian vein
- **I82.B11 Acute embolism and thrombosis of right subclavian vein**
- **I82.B12 Acute embolism and thrombosis of left subclavian vein**
- **I82.B13 Acute embolism and thrombosis of subclavian vein, bilateral**

I82.B19 Acute embolism and thrombosis of unspecified subclavian vein

✓6th **I82.B2 Chronic embolism and thrombosis of subclavian vein**

I82.B21 Chronic embolism and thrombosis of right subclavian vein

I82.B22 Chronic embolism and thrombosis of left subclavian vein

I82.B23 Chronic embolism and thrombosis of subclavian vein, bilateral

I82.B29 Chronic embolism and thrombosis of unspecified subclavian vein

✓5th **I82.C Embolism and thrombosis of internal jugular vein**

✓6th **I82.C1 Acute embolism and thrombosis of internal jugular vein**

I82.C11 Acute embolism and thrombosis of right internal jugular vein

I82.C12 Acute embolism and thrombosis of left internal jugular vein

I82.C13 Acute embolism and thrombosis of internal jugular vein, bilateral

I82.C19 Acute embolism and thrombosis of unspecified internal jugular vein

✓6th **I82.C2 Chronic embolism and thrombosis of internal jugular vein**

I82.C21 Chronic embolism and thrombosis of right internal jugular vein

I82.C22 Chronic embolism and thrombosis of left internal jugular vein

I82.C23 Chronic embolism and thrombosis of internal jugular vein, bilateral

I82.C29 Chronic embolism and thrombosis of unspecified internal jugular vein

✓5th **I82.8 Embolism and thrombosis of other specified veins**

Use additional code, if applicable, for associated long-term (current) use of anticoagulants (Z79.01)

✓6th **I82.81 Embolism and thrombosis of superficial veins of lower extremities**

Embolism and thrombosis of saphenous vein (greater) (lesser)

I82.811 Embolism and thrombosis of superficial veins of right lower extremities

I82.812 Embolism and thrombosis of superficial veins of left lower extremities

I82.813 Embolism and thrombosis of superficial veins of lower extremities, bilateral

I82.819 Embolism and thrombosis of superficial veins of unspecified lower extremities

✓6th **I82.89 Embolism and thrombosis of other specified veins**

I82.890 Acute embolism and thrombosis of other specified veins

I82.891 Chronic embolism and thrombosis of other specified veins

✓5th **I82.9 Embolism and thrombosis of unspecified vein**

I82.90 Acute embolism and thrombosis of unspecified vein

Embolism of vein NOS

Thrombosis (vein) NOS

I82.91 Chronic embolism and thrombosis of unspecified vein

✓4th **I83 Varicose veins of lower extremities**

EXCLUDES 1 *varicose veins complicating pregnancy (O22.0-)*

varicose veins complicating the puerperium (O87.4)

✓5th **I83.0 Varicose veins of lower extremities with ulcer**

Use additional code to identify severity of ulcer (L97.-)

✓6th **I83.00 Varicose veins of unspecified lower extremity with ulcer**

I83.001 Varicose veins of unspecified lower extremity with ulcer of thigh

I83.002 Varicose veins of unspecified lower extremity with ulcer of calf

I83.003 Varicose veins of unspecified lower extremity with ulcer of ankle

I83.004 Varicose veins of unspecified lower extremity with ulcer of heel and midfoot

Varicose veins of unspecified lower extremity with ulcer of plantar surface of midfoot

I83.005 Varicose veins of unspecified lower extremity with ulcer other part of foot

Varicose veins of unspecified lower extremity with ulcer of toe

I83.008 Varicose veins of unspecified lower extremity with ulcer other part of lower leg

I83.009 Varicose veins of unspecified lower extremity with ulcer of unspecified site

✓6th **I83.01 Varicose veins of right lower extremity with ulcer**

I83.011 Varicose veins of right lower extremity with ulcer of thigh

I83.012 Varicose veins of right lower extremity with ulcer of calf

I83.013 Varicose veins of right lower extremity with ulcer of ankle

I83.014 Varicose veins of right lower extremity with ulcer of heel and midfoot

Varicose veins of right lower extremity with ulcer of plantar surface of midfoot

I83.015 Varicose veins of right lower extremity with ulcer other part of foot

Varicose veins of right lower extremity with ulcer of toe

I83.018 Varicose veins of right lower extremity with ulcer other part of lower leg

I83.019 Varicose veins of right lower extremity with ulcer of unspecified site

✓6th **I83.02 Varicose veins of left lower extremity with ulcer**

I83.021 Varicose veins of left lower extremity with ulcer of thigh

I83.022 Varicose veins of left lower extremity with ulcer of calf

I83.023 Varicose veins of left lower extremity with ulcer of ankle

I83.024 Varicose veins of left lower extremity with ulcer of heel and midfoot

Varicose veins of left lower extremity with ulcer of plantar surface of midfoot

I83.025 Varicose veins of left lower extremity with ulcer other part of foot

Varicose veins of left lower extremity with ulcer of toe

I83.028 Varicose veins of left lower extremity with ulcer other part of lower leg

I83.029 Varicose veins of left lower extremity with ulcer of unspecified site

✓5th **I83.1 Varicose veins of lower extremities with inflammation**

Stasis dermatitis

I83.10 Varicose veins of unspecified lower extremity with inflammation

I83.11 Varicose veins of right lower extremity with inflammation

I83.12 Varicose veins of left lower extremity with inflammation

✓5th **I83.2 Varicose veins of lower extremities with both ulcer and inflammation**

Use additional code to identify severity of ulcer (L97.-)

✓6th **I83.20 Varicose veins of unspecified lower extremity with both ulcer and inflammation**

I83.201 Varicose veins of unspecified lower extremity with both ulcer of thigh and inflammation

I83.202 Varicose veins of unspecified lower extremity with both ulcer of calf and inflammation

I83.203 Varicose veins of unspecified lower extremity with both ulcer of ankle and inflammation

I83.204 Varicose veins of unspecified lower extremity with both ulcer of heel and midfoot and inflammation

Varicose veins of unspecified lower extremity with both ulcer of plantar surface of midfoot and inflammation

I83.205 Varicose veins of unspecified lower extremity with both ulcer other part of foot and inflammation
Varicose veins of unspecified lower extremity with both ulcer of toe and inflammation

I83.208 Varicose veins of unspecified lower extremity with both ulcer of other part of lower extremity and inflammation

I83.209 Varicose veins of unspecified lower extremity with both ulcer of unspecified site and inflammation

✓6th **I83.21 Varicose veins of right lower extremity with both ulcer and inflammation**

I83.211 Varicose veins of right lower extremity with both ulcer of thigh and inflammation

I83.212 Varicose veins of right lower extremity with both ulcer of calf and inflammation

I83.213 Varicose veins of right lower extremity with both ulcer of ankle and inflammation

I83.214 Varicose veins of right lower extremity with both ulcer of heel and midfoot and inflammation
Varicose veins of right lower extremity with both ulcer of plantar surface of midfoot and inflammation

I83.215 Varicose veins of right lower extremity with both ulcer other part of foot and inflammation
Varicose veins of right lower extremity with both ulcer of toe and inflammation

I83.218 Varicose veins of right lower extremity with both ulcer of other part of lower extremity and inflammation

I83.219 Varicose veins of right lower extremity with both ulcer of unspecified site and inflammation

✓6th **I83.22 Varicose veins of left lower extremity with both ulcer and inflammation**

I83.221 Varicose veins of left lower extremity with both ulcer of thigh and inflammation

I83.222 Varicose veins of left lower extremity with both ulcer of calf and inflammation

I83.223 Varicose veins of left lower extremity with both ulcer of ankle and inflammation

I83.224 Varicose veins of left lower extremity with both ulcer of heel and midfoot and inflammation
Varicose veins of left lower extremity with both ulcer of plantar surface of midfoot and inflammation

I83.225 Varicose veins of left lower extremity with both ulcer other part of foot and inflammation
Varicose veins of left lower extremity with both ulcer of toe and inflammation

I83.228 Varicose veins of left lower extremity with both ulcer of other part of lower extremity and inflammation

I83.229 Varicose veins of left lower extremity with both ulcer of unspecified site and inflammation

✓5th **I83.8 Varicose veins of lower extremities with other complications**

✓6th **I83.81 Varicose veins of lower extremities with pain**

I83.811 Varicose veins of right lower extremities with pain

I83.812 Varicose veins of left lower extremities with pain

I83.813 Varicose veins of bilateral lower extremities with pain

I83.819 Varicose veins of unspecified lower extremities with pain

✓6th **I83.89 Varicose veins of lower extremities with other complications**
Varicose veins of lower extremities with edema
Varicose veins of lower extremities with swelling

I83.891 Varicose veins of right lower extremities with other complications

I83.892 Varicose veins of left lower extremities with other complications

I83.893 Varicose veins of bilateral lower extremities with other complications

I83.899 Varicose veins of unspecified lower extremities with other complications

✓5th **I83.9 Asymptomatic varicose veins of lower extremities**
Phlebectasia of lower extremities
Varicose veins of lower extremities
Varix of lower extremities

I83.90 Asymptomatic varicose veins of unspecified lower extremity
Varicose veins NOS

I83.91 Asymptomatic varicose veins of right lower extremity

I83.92 Asymptomatic varicose veins of left lower extremity

I83.93 Asymptomatic varicose veins of bilateral lower extremities

✓4th **I85 Esophageal varices**
Use additional code to identify:
alcohol abuse and dependence (F10.-)

✓5th **I85.0 Esophageal varices**
Idiopathic esophageal varices
Primary esophageal varices

I85.00 Esophageal varices without bleeding
Esophageal varices NOS

I85.01 Esophageal varices with bleeding

✓5th **I85.1 Secondary esophageal varices**
Esophageal varices secondary to alcoholic liver disease
Esophageal varices secondary to cirrhosis of liver
Esophageal varices secondary to schistosomiasis
Esophageal varices secondary to toxic liver disease
Code first underlying disease

I85.10 Secondary esophageal varices without bleeding

I85.11 Secondary esophageal varices with bleeding

✓4th **I86 Varicose veins of other sites**
EXCLUDES 1 *varicose veins of unspecified site (I83.9-)*
EXCLUDES 2 *retinal varices (H35.0-)*

I86.0 Sublingual varices

I86.1 Scrotal varices
Varicocele

I86.2 Pelvic varices

I86.3 Vulval varices
EXCLUDES 1 *vulval varices complicating childbirth and the puerperium (O87.8)*
vulval varices complicating pregnancy (O22.1-)

I86.4 Gastric varices

I86.8 Varicose veins of other specified sites
Varicose ulcer of nasal septum

✓4th **I87 Other disorders of veins**

✓5th **I87.0 Postthrombotic syndrome**
Chronic venous hypertension due to deep vein thrombosis
Postphlebitic syndrome
EXCLUDES 1 *chronic venous hypertension without deep vein thrombosis (I87.3-)*

✓6th **I87.00 Postthrombotic syndrome without complications**
Asymptomatic postthrombotic syndrome

I87.001 Postthrombotic syndrome without complications of right lower extremity

I87.002 Postthrombotic syndrome without complications of left lower extremity

I87.003 Postthrombotic syndrome without complications of bilateral lower extremity

I87.009 Postthrombotic syndrome without complications of unspecified extremity
Postthrombotic syndrome NOS

DRAFT

√6th **I87.Ø1 Postthrombotic syndrome with ulcer**
Use additional code to specify site and severity of ulcer (L97.-)
I87.Ø11 Postthrombotic syndrome with ulcer of right lower extremity
I87.Ø12 Postthrombotic syndrome with ulcer of left lower extremity
I87.Ø13 Postthrombotic syndrome with ulcer of bilateral lower extremity
I87.Ø19 Postthrombotic syndrome with ulcer of unspecified lower extremity

√6th **I87.Ø2 Postthrombotic syndrome with inflammation**
I87.Ø21 Postthrombotic syndrome with inflammation of right lower extremity
I87.Ø22 Postthrombotic syndrome with inflammation of left lower extremity
I87.Ø23 Postthrombotic syndrome with inflammation of bilateral lower extremity
I87.Ø29 Postthrombotic syndrome with inflammation of unspecified lower extremity

√6th **I87.Ø3 Postthrombotic syndrome with ulcer and inflammation**
Use additional code to specify site and severity of ulcer (L97.-)
I87.Ø31 Postthrombotic syndrome with ulcer and inflammation of right lower extremity
I87.Ø32 Postthrombotic syndrome with ulcer and inflammation of left lower extremity
I87.Ø33 Postthrombotic syndrome with ulcer and inflammation of bilateral lower extremity
I87.Ø39 Postthrombotic syndrome with ulcer and inflammation of unspecified lower extremity

√6th **I87.Ø9 Postthrombotic syndrome with other complications**
I87.Ø91 Postthrombotic syndrome with other complications of right lower extremity
I87.Ø92 Postthrombotic syndrome with other complications of left lower extremity
I87.Ø93 Postthrombotic syndrome with other complications of bilateral lower extremity
I87.Ø99 Postthrombotic syndrome with other complications of unspecified lower extremity

I87.1 Compression of vein
Stricture of vein
Vena cava syndrome (inferior) (superior)
EXCLUDES 2 *compression of pulmonary vein (I28.8)*

I87.2 Venous insufficiency (chronic) (peripheral)

√5th **I87.3 Chronic venous hypertension (idiopathic)**
Stasis edema
EXCLUDES 1 *chronic venous hypertension due to deep vein thrombosis (I87.Ø-)*
varicose veins of lower extremities (I83.-)

√6th **I87.3Ø Chronic venous hypertension (idiopathic) without complications**
Asymptomatic chronic venous hypertension (idiopathic)
I87.3Ø1 Chronic venous hypertension (idiopathic) without complications of right lower extremity
I87.3Ø2 Chronic venous hypertension (idiopathic) without complications of left lower extremity
I87.3Ø3 Chronic venous hypertension (idiopathic) without complications of bilateral lower extremity
I87.3Ø9 Chronic venous hypertension (idiopathic) without complications of unspecified lower extremity
Chronic venous hypertension NOS

√6th **I87.31 Chronic venous hypertension (idiopathic) with ulcer**
Use additional code to specify site and severity of ulcer (L97.-)
I87.311 Chronic venous hypertension (idiopathic) with ulcer of right lower extremity
I87.312 Chronic venous hypertension (idiopathic) with ulcer of left lower extremity
I87.313 Chronic venous hypertension (idiopathic) with ulcer of bilateral lower extremity
I87.319 Chronic venous hypertension (idiopathic) with ulcer of unspecified lower extremity

√6th **I87.32 Chronic venous hypertension (idiopathic) with inflammation**
I87.321 Chronic venous hypertension (idiopathic) with inflammation of right lower extremity
I87.322 Chronic venous hypertension (idiopathic) with inflammation of left lower extremity
I87.323 Chronic venous hypertension (idiopathic) with inflammation of bilateral lower extremity
I87.329 Chronic venous hypertension (idiopathic) with inflammation of unspecified lower extremity

√6th **I87.33 Chronic venous hypertension (idiopathic) with ulcer and inflammation**
Use additional code to specify site and severity of ulcer (L97.-)
I87.331 Chronic venous hypertension (idiopathic) with ulcer and inflammation of right lower extremity
I87.332 Chronic venous hypertension (idiopathic) with ulcer and inflammation of left lower extremity
I87.333 Chronic venous hypertension (idiopathic) with ulcer and inflammation of bilateral lower extremity
I87.339 Chronic venous hypertension (idiopathic) with ulcer and inflammation of unspecified lower extremity

√6th **I87.39 Chronic venous hypertension (idiopathic) with other complications**
I87.391 Chronic venous hypertension (idiopathic) with other complications of right lower extremity
I87.392 Chronic venous hypertension (idiopathic) with other complications of left lower extremity
I87.393 Chronic venous hypertension (idiopathic) with other complications of bilateral lower extremity
I87.399 Chronic venous hypertension (idiopathic) with other complications of unspecified lower extremity

I87.8 Other specified disorders of veins
Phlebosclerosis
Venofibrosis

I87.9 Disorder of vein, unspecified

√4th **I88 Nonspecific lymphadenitis**
EXCLUDES 1 *acute lymphadenitis, except mesenteric (LØ4.-)*
enlarged lymph nodes NOS (R59.-)
human immunodeficiency virus [HIV] disease resulting in generalized lymphadenopathy (B2Ø)

I88.Ø Nonspecific mesenteric lymphadenitis
Mesenteric lymphadenitis (acute)(chronic)

I88.1 Chronic lymphadenitis, except mesenteric
Adenitis
Lymphadenitis

I88.8 Other nonspecific lymphadenitis

I88.9 Nonspecific lymphadenitis, unspecified
Lymphadenitis NOS

I89 Other noninfective disorders of lymphatic vessels and lymph nodes

EXCLUDES 1 *chylocele, tunica vaginalis (nonfilarial) NOS (N50.8)*
enlarged lymph nodes NOS (R59.-)
filarial chylocele (B74.-)
hereditary lymphedema (Q82.0)

I89.0 Lymphedema, not elsewhere classified
Elephantiasis (nonfilarial) NOS
Lymphangiectasis
Obliteration, lymphatic vessel
Praecox lymphedema
Secondary lymphedema
EXCLUDES 1 *postmastectomy lymphedema (I97.2)*

I89.1 Lymphangitis
Chronic lymphangitis
Lymphangitis NOS
Subacute lymphangitis
EXCLUDES 1 *acute lymphangitis (L03.-)*

I89.8 Other specified noninfective disorders of lymphatic vessels and lymph nodes
Chylocele (nonfilarial)
Chylous ascites
Chylous cyst
Lipomelanotic reticulosis
Lymph node or vessel fistula
Lymph node or vessel infarction
Lymph node or vessel rupture

I89.9 Noninfective disorder of lymphatic vessels and lymph nodes, unspecified
Disease of lymphatic vessels NOS

Other and unspecified disorders of the circulatory system (I95-I99)

I95 Hypotension

EXCLUDES 1 *cardiovascular collapse (R57.9)*
maternal hypotension syndrome (O26.5-)
nonspecific low blood pressure reading NOS (R03.1)

I95.0 Idiopathic hypotension

I95.1 Orthostatic hypotension
Hypotension, postural
EXCLUDES 1 *neurogenic orthostatic hypotension [Shy-Drager] (G90.3)*
orthostatic hypotension due to drugs (I95.2)

I95.2 Hypotension due to drugs
Orthostatic hypotension due to drugs
Use additional code for adverse effect, if applicable, to identify drug (T36-T50 with fifth or sixth character 5)

I95.3 Hypotension of hemodialysis
Intra-dialytic hypotension

I95.8 Other hypotension
I95.81 Postprocedural hypotension
I95.89 Other hypotension
Chronic hypotension

I95.9 Hypotension, unspecified

I96 Gangrene, not elsewhere classified
Gangrenous cellulitis
EXCLUDES 1 *gangrene in atherosclerosis of native arteries of the extremities (I70.26)*
gangrene in diabetes mellitus (E08-E13)
gangrene in hernia (K40.1, K40.4, K41.1, K41.4, K42.1, K43.1-, K44.1, K45.1, K46.1)
gangrene in other peripheral vascular diseases (I73.-)
gangrene of certain specified sites—see Alphabetical Index
gas gangrene (A48.0)
pyoderma gangrenosum (L88)

I97 Intraoperative and postprocedural complications and disorders of circulatory system, not elsewhere classified

EXCLUDES 2 *postprocedural shock (T81.1-)*

I97.0 Postcardiotomy syndrome

I97.1 Other postprocedural cardiac functional disturbances
EXCLUDES 2 *acute pulmonary insufficiency following thoracic surgery (J95.1)*
intraoperative cardiac functional disturbances (I97.7-)

I97.11 Postprocedural cardiac insufficiency
I97.110 Postprocedural cardiac insufficiency following cardiac surgery
I97.111 Postprocedural cardiac insufficiency following other surgery

I97.12 Postprocedural cardiac arrest
I97.120 Postprocedural cardiac arrest following cardiac surgery
I97.121 Postprocedural cardiac arrest following other surgery

I97.13 Postprocedural heart failure
Use additional code to identify the heart failure (I50.-)
I97.130 Postprocedural heart failure following cardiac surgery
I97.131 Postprocedural heart failure following other surgery

I97.19 Other postprocedural cardiac functional disturbances
Use additional code, if applicable, to further specify disorder
I97.190 Other postprocedural cardiac functional disturbances following cardiac surgery
I97.191 Other postprocedural cardiac functional disturbances following other surgery

I97.2 Postmastectomy lymphedema syndrome
Elephantiasis due to mastectomy
Obliteration of lymphatic vessels

I97.3 Postprocedural hypertension

I97.4 Intraoperative hemorrhage and hematoma of a circulatory system organ or structure complicating a procedure
EXCLUDES 1 *intraoperative hemorrhage and hematoma of a circulatory system organ or structure due to accidental puncture and laceration during a procedure (I97.5-)*
EXCLUDES 2 *intraoperative cerebrovascular hemorrhage complicating a procedure (G97.3-)*

I97.41 Intraoperative hemorrhage and hematoma of a circulatory system organ or structure complicating a circulatory system procedure
I97.410 Intraoperative hemorrhage and hematoma of a circulatory system organ or structure complicating a cardiac catheterization
I97.411 Intraoperative hemorrhage and hematoma of a circulatory system organ or structure complicating a cardiac bypass
I97.418 Intraoperative hemorrhage and hematoma of a circulatory system organ or structure complicating other circulatory system procedure

I97.42 Intraoperative hemorrhage and hematoma of a circulatory system organ or structure complicating other procedure

I97.5 Accidental puncture and laceration of a circulatory system organ or structure during a procedure
EXCLUDES 2 *accidental puncture and laceration of brain during a procedure (G97.4-)*
I97.51 Accidental puncture and laceration of a circulatory system organ or structure during a circulatory system procedure
I97.52 Accidental puncture and laceration of a circulatory system organ or structure during other procedure

I97.6 Postprocedural hemorrhage and hematoma of a circulatory system organ or structure following a procedure
EXCLUDES 2 *postprocedural cerebrovascular hemorrhage complicating a procedure (G97.5-)*

I97.61 Postprocedural hemorrhage and hematoma of a circulatory system organ or structure following a circulatory system procedure
I97.610 Postprocedural hemorrhage and hematoma of a circulatory system organ or structure following a cardiac catheterization
I97.611 Postprocedural hemorrhage and hematoma of a circulatory system organ or structure following cardiac bypass
I97.618 Postprocedural hemorrhage and hematoma of a circulatory system organ or structure following other circulatory system procedure

I97.62 Postprocedural hemorrhage and hematoma of a circulatory system organ or structure following other procedure

✓5th **I97.7 Intraoperative cardiac functional disturbances**

EXCLUDES 2 *acute pulmonary insufficiency following thoracic surgery (J95.1)*

postprocedural cardiac functional disturbances (I97.1-)

✓6th **I97.71 Intraoperative cardiac arrest**

I97.71Ø Intraoperative cardiac arrest during cardiac surgery

I97.711 Intraoperative cardiac arrest during other surgery

✓6th **I97.79 Other intraoperative cardiac functional disturbances**

Use additional code, if applicable, to further specify disorder

I97.79Ø Other intraoperative cardiac functional disturbances during cardiac surgery

I97.791 Other intraoperative cardiac functional disturbances during other surgery

✓5th **I97.8 Other intraoperative and postprocedural complications and disorders of the circulatory system, not elsewhere classified**

Use additional code, if applicable, to further specify disorder

✓6th **I97.81 Intraoperative cerebrovascular infarction**

I97.81Ø Intraoperative cerebrovascular infarction during cardiac surgery

I97.811 Intraoperative cerebrovascular infarction during other surgery

✓6th **I97.82 Postprocedural cerebrovascular infarction**

I97.82Ø Postprocedural cerebrovascular infarction during cardiac surgery

I97.821 Postprocedural cerebrovascular infarction during other surgery

I97.88 Other intraoperative complications of the circulatory system, not elsewhere classified

I97.89 Other postprocedural complications and disorders of the circulatory system, not elsewhere classified

✓4th **I99 Other and unspecified disorders of circulatory system**

I99.8 Other disorder of circulatory system

I99.9 Unspecified disorder of circulatory system

Chapter 10. Diseases of the Respiratory System (J00-J99)

NOTE When a respiratory condition is described as occurring in more than one site and is not specifically indexed, it should be classified to the lower anatomic site (e.g. tracheobronchitis to bronchitis in J40).

Use additional code, where applicable, to identify:
- exposure to environmental tobacco smoke (Z77.22)
- exposure to tobacco smoke in the perinatal period (P96.81)
- history of tobacco use (Z87.891)
- occupational exposure to environmental tobacco smoke (Z57.31)
- tobacco dependence (F17.-)
- tobacco use (Z72.0)

EXCLUDES 2 *certain conditions originating in the perinatal period (P04-P96)*
certain infectious and parasitic diseases (A00-B99)
complications of pregnancy, childbirth and the puerperium (O00-O9A)
congenital malformations, deformations and chromosomal abnormalities (Q00-Q99)
endocrine, nutritional and metabolic diseases (E00-E88)
injury, poisoning and certain other consequences of external causes (S00-T88)
neoplasms (C00-D49)
smoke inhalation (T59.81-)
symptoms, signs and abnormal clinical and laboratory findings, not elsewhere classified (R00-R94)

This chapter contains the following blocks:

J00-J06	Acute upper respiratory infections
J09-J18	Influenza and pneumonia
J20-J22	Other acute lower respiratory infections
J30-J39	Other diseases of upper respiratory tract
J40-J47	Chronic lower respiratory diseases
J60-J70	Lung diseases due to external agents
J80-J84	Other respiratory diseases principally affecting the interstitium
J85-J86	Suppurative and necrotic conditions of the lower respiratory tract
J90-J94	Other diseases of the pleura
J95	Intraoperative and postprocedural complications and disorders of respiratory system, not elsewhere classified
J96-J99	Other diseases of the respiratory system

Acute upper respiratory infections (J00-J06)

EXCLUDES 1 *chronic obstructive pulmonary disease with acute lower respiratory infection (J44.0)*
influenza virus with other respiratory manifestations (J09.X2, J10.1, J11.1)

J00 Acute nasopharyngitis (common cold)
Acute rhinitis
Coryza (acute)
Infective nasopharyngitis NOS
Infective rhinitis
Nasal catarrh, acute
Nasopharyngitis NOS
EXCLUDES 1 *acute pharyngitis (J02.-)*
acute sore throat NOS (J02.9)
pharyngitis NOS (J02.9)
rhinitis NOS (J31.0)
sore throat NOS (J02.9)
EXCLUDES 2 *allergic rhinitis (J30.1-J30.9)*
chronic pharyngitis (J31.2)
chronic rhinitis (J31.0)
chronic sore throat (J31.2)
nasopharyngitis, chronic (J31.1)
vasomotor rhinitis (J30.0)

4th **J01 Acute sinusitis**
INCLUDES acute abscess of sinus
acute empyema of sinus
acute infection of sinus
acute inflammation of sinus
acute suppuration of sinus
Use additional code (B95-B97) to identify infectious agent
EXCLUDES 1 *sinusitis NOS (J32.9)*
EXCLUDES 2 *chronic sinusitis (J32.0-J32.8)*

5th **J01.0 Acute maxillary sinusitis**
Acute antritis
J01.00 Acute maxillary sinusitis, unspecified
J01.01 Acute recurrent maxillary sinusitis

5th **J01.1 Acute frontal sinusitis**
J01.10 Acute frontal sinusitis, unspecified
J01.11 Acute recurrent frontal sinusitis

5th **J01.2 Acute ethmoidal sinusitis**
J01.20 Acute ethmoidal sinusitis, unspecified
J01.21 Acute recurrent ethmoidal sinusitis

5th **J01.3 Acute sphenoidal sinusitis**
J01.30 Acute sphenoidal sinusitis, unspecified
J01.31 Acute recurrent sphenoidal sinusitis

5th **J01.4 Acute pansinusitis**
J01.40 Acute pansinusitis, unspecified
J01.41 Acute recurrent pansinusitis

5th **J01.8 Other acute sinusitis**
J01.80 Other acute sinusitis
Acute sinusitis involving more than one sinus but not pansinusitis
J01.81 Other acute recurrent sinusitis
Acute recurrent sinusitis involving more than one sinus but not pansinusitis

5th **J01.9 Acute sinusitis, unspecified**
J01.90 Acute sinusitis, unspecified
J01.91 Acute recurrent sinusitis, unspecified

4th **J02 Acute pharyngitis**
INCLUDES acute sore throat
EXCLUDES 1 *acute laryngopharyngitis (J06.0)*
peritonsillar abscess (J36)
pharyngeal abscess (J39.1)
retropharyngeal abscess (J39.0)
EXCLUDES 2 *chronic pharyngitis (J31.2)*

J02.0 Streptococcal pharyngitis
Septic pharyngitis
Streptococcal sore throat
EXCLUDES 2 *scarlet fever (A38.-)*

J02.8 Acute pharyngitis due to other specified organisms
Use additional code (B95-B97) to identify infectious agent
EXCLUDES 1 *acute pharyngitis due to coxsackie virus (B08.5)*
acute pharyngitis due to gonococcus (A54.5)
acute pharyngitis due to herpes [simplex] virus (B00.2)
acute pharyngitis due to infectious mononucleosis (B27.-)
enteroviral vesicular pharyngitis (B08.5)

J02.9 Acute pharyngitis, unspecified
Gangrenous pharyngitis (acute)
Infective pharyngitis (acute) NOS
Pharyngitis (acute) NOS
Sore throat (acute) NOS
Suppurative pharyngitis (acute)
Ulcerative pharyngitis (acute)

4th **J03 Acute tonsillitis**
EXCLUDES 1 *acute sore throat (J02.-)*
hypertrophy of tonsils (J35.1)
peritonsillar abscess (J36)
sore throat NOS (J02.9)
streptococcal sore throat (J02.0)
EXCLUDES 2 *chronic tonsillitis (J35.0)*

5th **J03.0 Streptococcal tonsillitis**
J03.00 Acute streptococcal tonsillitis, unspecified
J03.01 Acute recurrent streptococcal tonsillitis

5th **J03.8 Acute tonsillitis due to other specified organisms**
Use additional code (B95-B97) to identify infectious agent
EXCLUDES 1 *diphtheritic tonsillitis (A36.0)*
herpesviral pharyngotonsillitis (B00.2)
streptococcal tonsillitis (J03.0)
tuberculous tonsillitis (A15.8)
Vincent's tonsillitis (A69.1)
J03.80 Acute tonsillitis due to other specified organisms
J03.81 Acute recurrent tonsillitis due to other specified organisms

5th **J03.9 Acute tonsillitis, unspecified**
Follicular tonsillitis (acute)
Gangrenous tonsillitis (acute)
Infective tonsillitis (acute)
Tonsillitis (acute) NOS
Ulcerative tonsillitis (acute)
J03.90 Acute tonsillitis, unspecified
J03.91 Acute recurrent tonsillitis, unspecified

√4th **J04 Acute laryngitis and tracheitis**
Use additional code (B95-B97) to identify infectious agent
EXCLUDES 1 *acute obstructive laryngitis [croup] and epiglottitis (J05.-)*
EXCLUDES 2 *laryngismus (stridulus) (J38.5)*

J04.0 Acute laryngitis
Edematous laryngitis (acute)
Laryngitis (acute) NOS
Subglottic laryngitis (acute)
Suppurative laryngitis (acute)
Ulcerative laryngitis (acute)
EXCLUDES 1 *acute obstructive laryngitis (J05.0)*
EXCLUDES 2 *chronic laryngitis (J37.0)*

√5th **J04.1 Acute tracheitis**
Acute viral tracheitis
Catarrhal tracheitis (acute)
Tracheitis (acute) NOS
EXCLUDES 2 *chronic tracheitis (J42)*

J04.10 Acute tracheitis without obstruction
J04.11 Acute tracheitis with obstruction

J04.2 Acute laryngotracheitis
Laryngotracheitis NOS
Tracheitis (acute) with laryngitis (acute)
EXCLUDES 1 *acute obstructive laryngotracheitis (J05.0)*
EXCLUDES 2 *chronic laryngotracheitis (J37.1)*

√5th **J04.3 Supraglottitis, unspecified**
J04.30 Supraglottitis, unspecified, without obstruction
J04.31 Supraglottitis, unspecified, with obstruction

√4th **J05 Acute obstructive laryngitis [croup] and epiglottitis**
Use additional code (B95-B97) to identify infectious agent

J05.0 Acute obstructive laryngitis [croup]
Obstructive laryngitis (acute) NOS
Obstructive laryngotracheitis NOS

√5th **J05.1 Acute epiglottitis**
EXCLUDES 2 *epiglottitis, chronic (J37.0)*

J05.10 Acute epiglottitis without obstruction
Epiglottitis NOS
J05.11 Acute epiglottitis with obstruction

√4th **J06 Acute upper respiratory infections of multiple and unspecified sites**
EXCLUDES 1 *acute respiratory infection NOS (J22)*
streptococcal pharyngitis (J02.0)

J06.0 Acute laryngopharyngitis
J06.9 Acute upper respiratory infection, unspecified
Upper respiratory disease, acute
Upper respiratory infection NOS

Influenza and pneumonia (J09-J18)

EXCLUDES 2 *allergic or eosinophilic pneumonia (J82)*
aspiration pneumonia NOS (J69.0)
congenital pneumonia (P23.9)
lipid pneumonia (J69.1)
meconium pneumonia (P24.01)
neonatal aspiration pneumonia (P24.-)
pneumonia due to solids and liquids (J69.-)
rheumatic pneumonia (I00)
ventilator associated pneumonia (J95.851)

√4th **J09 Influenza due to certain identified influenza viruses**
EXCLUDES 1 *seasonal influenza due to other identified influenza virus (J10.-)*
seasonal influenza due to unidentified influenza virus (J11.-)

√5th **J09.X Influenza due to identified novel influenza A virus**
Avian influenza
Bird influenza
Influenza A/H5N1
Influenza of other animal origin, not bird or swine
Swine influenza virus (viruses that normally cause infections in pigs)

J09.X1 Influenza due to identified novel influenza A virus with pneumonia
Code also, if applicable, associated:
lung abscess (J85.1)
other specified type of pneumonia

J09.X2 Influenza due to identified novel influenza A virus with other respiratory manifestations
Influenza due to identified novel influenza A virus NOS
Influenza due to identified novel influenza A virus with laryngitis
Influenza due to identified novel influenza A virus with pharyngitis
Influenza due to identified novel influenza A virus with upper respiratory symptoms
Use additional code, if applicable, for associated:
pleural effusion (J91.8)
sinusitis (J01.-)

J09.X3 Influenza due to identified novel influenza A virus with gastrointestinal manifestations
Influenza due to identified novel influenza A virus gastroenteritis
EXCLUDES 1 *'intestinal flu' [viral gastroenteritis] (A08.-)*

J09.X9 Influenza due to identified novel influenza A virus with other manifestations
Influenza due to identified novel influenza A virus with encephalopathy
Influenza due to identified novel influenza A virus with myocarditis
Influenza due to identified novel influenza A virus with otitis media
Use additional code to identify manifestation

√4th **J10 Influenza due to other identified influenza virus**
Use additional code to identify the virus (B97.-)
EXCLUDES 1 *influenza due to avian influenza virus (J09.X-)*
influenza due to swine flu (J09.X-)
influenza due to unidentifed influenza virus (J11.-)

√5th **J10.0 Influenza due to other identified influenza virus with pneumonia**
Code also associated lung abscess, if applicable (J85.1)

J10.00 Influenza due to other identified influenza virus with unspecified type of pneumonia
J10.01 Influenza due to other identified influenza virus with the same other identified influenza virus pneumonia
J10.08 Influenza due to other identified influenza virus with other specified pneumonia
Code also other specified type of pneumonia

J10.1 Influenza due to other identified influenza virus with other respiratory manifestations
Influenza due to other identified influenza virus NOS
Influenza due to other identified influenza virus with laryngitis
Influenza due to other identified influenza virus with pharyngitis
Influenza due to other identified influenza virus with upper respiratory symptoms
Use additional code for associated pleural effusion, if applicable (J91.8)
Use additional code for associated sinusitis, if applicable (J01.-)

J10.2 Influenza due to other identified influenza virus with gastrointestinal manifestations
Influenza due to other identified influenza virus gastroenteritis
EXCLUDES 1 *'intestinal flu' [viral gastroenteritis] (A08.-)*

√5th **J10.8 Influenza due to other identified influenza virus with other manifestations**
J10.81 Influenza due to other identified influenza virus with encephalopathy
J10.82 Influenza due to other identified influenza virus with myocarditis
J10.83 Influenza due to other identified influenza virus with otitis media
Use additional code for any associated perforated tympanic membrane (H72.-)
J10.89 Influenza due to other identified influenza virus with other manifestations
Use additional codes to identify the manifestations

J11 Influenza due to unidentified influenza virus

J11.0 Influenza due to unidentified influenza virus with pneumonia

Code also associated lung abscess, if applicable (J85.1)

J11.00 Influenza due to unidentified influenza virus with unspecified type of pneumonia

Influenza with pneumonia NOS

J11.08 Influenza due to unidentified influenza virus with specified pneumonia

Code also other specified type of pneumonia

J11.1 Influenza due to unidentified influenza virus with other respiratory manifestations

Influenza NOS
Influenzal laryngitis NOS
Influenzal pharyngitis NOS
Influenza with upper respiratory symptoms NOS

Use additional code for associated pleural effusion, if applicable (J91.8)

Use additional code for associated sinusitis, if applicable (J01.-)

J11.2 Influenza due to unidentified influenza virus with gastrointestinal manifestations

Influenza gastroenteritis NOS

EXCLUDES 1 *'intestinal flu' [viral gastroenteritis] (A08.-)*

J11.8 Influenza due to unidentified influenza virus with other manifestations

J11.81 Influenza due to unidentified influenza virus with encephalopathy

Influenzal encephalopathy NOS

J11.82 Influenza due to unidentified influenza virus with myocarditis

Influenzal myocarditis NOS

J11.83 Influenza due to unidentified influenza virus with otitis media

Influenzal otitis media NOS

Use additional code for any associated perforated tympanic membrane (H72.-)

J11.89 Influenza due to unidentified influenza virus with other manifestations

Use additional codes to identify the manifestations

J12 Viral pneumonia, not elsewhere classified

INCLUDES bronchopneumonia due to viruses other than influenza viruses

Code first associated influenza, if applicable (J09.X1, J10.0-, J11.0-)

Code also associated abscess, if applicable (J85.1)

EXCLUDES 1 *aspiration pneumonia due to anesthesia during labor and delivery (O74.0)*
aspiration pneumonia due to anesthesia during pregnancy (O29)
aspiration pneumonia due to anesthesia during puerperium (O89.0)
aspiration pneumonia due to solids and liquids (J69.-)
aspiration pneumonia NOS (J69.0)
congenital pneumonia (P23.0)
congenital rubella pneumonitis (P35.0)
interstitial pneumonia NOS (J84.9)
lipid pneumonia (J69.1)
neonatal aspiration pneumonia (P24.-)

J12.0 Adenoviral pneumonia

J12.1 Respiratory syncytial virus pneumonia

J12.2 Parainfluenza virus pneumonia

J12.3 Human metapneumovirus pneumonia

J12.8 Other viral pneumonia

J12.81 Pneumonia due to SARS-associated coronavirus

Severe acute respiratory syndrome NOS

J12.89 Other viral pneumonia

J12.9 Viral pneumonia, unspecified

J13 Pneumonia due to Streptococcus pneumoniae

Bronchopneumonia due to S. pneumoniae

Code first associated influenza, if applicable (J09.X1, J10.0-, -J11.0-)

Code also associated lung abscess, if applicable (J85.1)

EXCLUDES 1 *congenital pneumonia due to S. pneumoniae (P23.6)*
lobar pneumonia, unspecified organism (J18.1)
pneumonia due to other streptococci (J15.3-J15.4)

J14 Pneumonia due to Hemophilus influenzae

Bronchopneumonia due to H. influenzae

Code first associated influenza, if applicable (J09.X1, J10.0-, -J11.0-)

Code also associated lung abscess, if applicable (J85.1)

EXCLUDES 1 *congenital pneumonia due to H. influenzae (P23.6)*

J15 Bacterial pneumonia, not elsewhere classified

Bronchopneumonia due to bacteria other than S. pneumoniae and H. influenzae

Code first associated influenza, if applicable (J09.X1, J10.0-, -J11.0-)

Code also associated lung abscess, if applicable (J85.1)

EXCLUDES 1 *chlamydial pneumonia (J16.0)*
congenital pneumonia (P23.-)
Legionnaires' disease (A48.1)
spirochetal pneumonia (A69.8)

J15.0 Pneumonia due to Klebsiella pneumoniae

J15.1 Pneumonia due to Pseudomonas

J15.2 Pneumonia due to staphylococcus

J15.20 Pneumonia due to staphylococcus, unspecified

J15.21 Pneumonia due to Staphylococcus aureus

J15.211 Pneumonia due to methicillin susceptible Staphylococcus aureus

MSSA pneumonia
Pneumonia due to Staphylococcus aureus NOS

J15.212 Pneumonia due to methicillin resistant Staphylococcus aureus

J15.29 Pneumonia due to other staphylococcus

J15.3 Pneumonia due to streptococcus, group B

J15.4 Pneumonia due to other streptococci

EXCLUDES 1 *pneumonia due to streptococcus, group B (J15.3)*
pneumonia due to Streptococcus pneumoniae (J13)

J15.5 Pneumonia due to Escherichia coli

J15.6 Pneumonia due to other aerobic Gram-negative bacteria

Pneumonia due to Serratia marcescens

J15.7 Pneumonia due to Mycoplasma pneumoniae

J15.8 Pneumonia due to other specified bacteria

J15.9 Unspecified bacterial pneumonia

Pneumonia due to gram-positive bacteria

J16 Pneumonia due to other infectious organisms, not elsewhere classified

Code first associated influenza, if applicable (J09.X1, J10.0-, -J11.0-)

Code also associated lung abscess, if applicable (J85.1)

EXCLUDES 1 *congenital pneumonia (P23.-)*
ornithosis (A70)
pneumocystosis (B59)
pneumonia NOS (J18.9)

J16.0 Chlamydial pneumonia

J16.8 Pneumonia due to other specified infectious organisms

J17 Pneumonia in diseases classified elsewhere

Code first underlying disease, such as:
Q fever (A78)
rheumatic fever (I00)
schistosomiasis (B65.0-B65.9)

EXCLUDES 1 *candidial pneumonia (B37.1)*
chlamydial pneumonia (J16.0)
gonorrheal pneumonia (A54.84)
histoplasmosis pneumonia (B39.0-B39.2)
measles pneumonia (B05.2)
nocardiosis pneumonia (A43.0)
pneumocystosis (B59)
pneumonia due to Pneumocystis carinii (B59)
pneumonia due to Pneumocystis jiroveci (B59)
pneumonia in actinomycosis (A42.0)
pneumonia in anthrax (A22.1)
pneumonia in ascariasis (B77.81)
pneumonia in aspergillosis (B44.0-B44.1)
pneumonia in coccidioidomycosis (B38.0-B38.2)
pneumonia in cytomegalovirus disease (B25.0)
pneumonia in toxoplasmosis (B58.3)
rubella pneumonia (B06.81)
salmonella pneumonia (A02.22)
spirochetal infection NEC with pneumonia (A69.8)
tularemia pneumonia (A21.2)
typhoid fever with pneumonia (A01.03)
varicella pneumonia (B01.2)
whooping cough with pneumonia (A37 with fifth-character 1)

✓4th J18 Pneumonia, unspecified organism
Code first associated influenza, if applicable (J09.X1, J10.0-, -J11.0-)
EXCLUDES 1 *abscess of lung with pneumonia (J85.1)*
aspiration pneumonia due to anesthesia during labor and delivery (O74.0)
aspiration pneumonia due to anesthesia during pregnancy (O29)
aspiration pneumonia due to anesthesia during puerperium (O89.0)
aspiration pneumonia due to solids and liquids (J69.-)
aspiration pneumonia NOS (J69.0)
congenital pneumonia (P23.0)
drug-induced interstitial lung disorder (J70.2-J70.4)
interstitial pneumonia NOS (J84.9)
lipid pneumonia (J69.1)
neonatal aspiration pneumonia (P24.-)
pneumonitis due to external agents (J67-J70)
pneumonitis due to fumes and vapors (J68.0)
usual interstitial pneumonia (J84.17)

J18.0 Bronchopneumonia, unspecified organism
EXCLUDES 1 *hypostatic bronchopneumonia (J18.2)*
lipid pneumonia (J69.1)
EXCLUDES 2 *acute bronchiolitis (J21.-)*
chronic bronchiolitis (J44.9)

J18.1 Lobar pneumonia, unspecified organism

J18.2 Hypostatic pneumonia, unspecified organism
Hypostatic bronchopneumonia
Passive pneumonia

J18.8 Other pneumonia, unspecified organism

J18.9 Pneumonia, unspecified organism

Other acute lower respiratory infections (J20-J22)

EXCLUDES 1 *chronic obstructive pulmonary disease with acute lower respiratory infection (J44.0)*

✓4th J20 Acute bronchitis
INCLUDES acute and subacute bronchitis (with) bronchospasm
acute and subacute bronchitis (with) tracheitis
acute and subacute bronchitis (with) tracheobronchitis, acute
acute and subacute fibrinous bronchitis
acute and subacute membranous bronchitis
acute and subacute purulent bronchitis
acute and subacute septic bronchitis
EXCLUDES 2 *acute bronchitis with bronchiectasis (J47.0)*
acute bronchitis with chronic obstructive asthma (J44.0)
acute bronchitis with chronic obstructive pulmonary disease (J44.0)
allergic bronchitis NOS (J45.909)
bronchitis due to chemicals, fumes and vapors (J68.0)
bronchitis NOS (J40)
chronic bronchitis NOS (J42)
chronic mucopurulent bronchitis (J41.1)
chronic obstructive bronchitis (J44.-)
chronic obstructive tracheobronchitis (J44.-)
chronic simple bronchitis (J41.0)
chronic tracheobronchitis (J42)
tracheobronchitis NOS (J40)

J20.0 Acute bronchitis due to Mycoplasma pneumoniae
J20.1 Acute bronchitis due to Hemophilus influenzae
J20.2 Acute bronchitis due to streptococcus
J20.3 Acute bronchitis due to coxsackievirus
J20.4 Acute bronchitis due to parainfluenza virus
J20.5 Acute bronchitis due to respiratory syncytial virus
J20.6 Acute bronchitis due to rhinovirus
J20.7 Acute bronchitis due to echovirus
J20.8 Acute bronchitis due to other specified organisms
J20.9 Acute bronchitis, unspecified

✓4th J21 Acute bronchiolitis
Acute bronchiolitis with bronchospasm
EXCLUDES 2 *respiratory bronchiolitis interstitial lung disease (J84.115)*

J21.0 Acute bronchiolitis due to respiratory syncytial virus
J21.1 Acute bronchiolitis due to human metapneumovirus
J21.8 Acute bronchiolitis due to other specified organisms
J21.9 Acute bronchiolitis, unspecified
Bronchiolitis (acute)
EXCLUDES 1 *chronic bronchiolitis (J44.-)*

J22 Unspecified acute lower respiratory infection
Acute (lower) respiratory (tract) infection NOS
EXCLUDES 1 *upper respiratory infection (acute) (J06.9)*

Other diseases of upper respiratory tract (J30-J39)

✓4th J30 Vasomotor and allergic rhinitis
INCLUDES spasmodic rhinorrhea
EXCLUDES 1 *allergic rhinitis with asthma (bronchial) (J45.909)*
rhinitis NOS (J31.0)

J30.0 Vasomotor rhinitis
J30.1 Allergic rhinitis due to pollen
Allergy NOS due to pollen
Hay fever
Pollinosis
J30.2 Other seasonal allergic rhinitis
J30.5 Allergic rhinitis due to food
✓5th J30.8 Other allergic rhinitis
J30.81 Allergic rhinitis due to animal (cat) (dog) hair and dander
J30.89 Other allergic rhinitis
Perennial allergic rhinitis
J30.9 Allergic rhinitis, unspecified

✓4th J31 Chronic rhinitis, nasopharyngitis and pharyngitis
Use additional code to identify:
exposure to environmental tobacco smoke (Z77.22)
exposure to tobacco smoke in the perinatal period (P96.81)
history of tobacco use (Z87.891)
occupational exposure to environmental tobacco smoke (Z57.31)
tobacco dependence (F17.-)
tobacco use (Z72.0)

J31.0 Chronic rhinitis
Atrophic rhinitis (chronic)
Granulomatous rhinitis (chronic)
Hypertrophic rhinitis (chronic)
Obstructive rhinitis (chronic)
Ozena
Purulent rhinitis (chronic)
Rhinitis (chronic) NOS
Ulcerative rhinitis (chronic)
EXCLUDES 1 *allergic rhinitis (J30.1-J30.9)*
vasomotor rhinitis (J30.0)

J31.1 Chronic nasopharyngitis
EXCLUDES 2 *acute nasopharyngitis (J00)*

J31.2 Chronic pharyngitis
Atrophic pharyngitis (chronic)
Chronic sore throat
Granular pharyngitis (chronic)
Hypertrophic pharyngitis (chronic)
EXCLUDES 2 *acute pharyngitis (J02.9)*

✓4th J32 Chronic sinusitis
INCLUDES sinus abscess
sinus empyema
sinus infection
sinus suppuration
Use additional code to identify:
exposure to environmental tobacco smoke (Z77.22)
exposure to tobacco smoke in the perinatal period (P96.81)
history of tobacco use (Z87.891)
infectious agent (B95-B97)
occupational exposure to environmental tobacco smoke (Z57.31)
tobacco dependence (F17.-)
tobacco use (Z72.0)
EXCLUDES 2 *acute sinusitis (J01.-)*

J32.0 Chronic maxillary sinusitis
Antritis (chronic)
Maxillary sinusitis NOS
J32.1 Chronic frontal sinusitis
Frontal sinusitis NOS
J32.2 Chronic ethmoidal sinusitis
Ethmoidal sinusitis NOS
EXCLUDES 1 *Woakes' ethmoiditis (J33.1)*
J32.3 Chronic sphenoidal sinusitis
Sphenoidal sinusitis NOS
J32.4 Chronic pansinusitis
Pansinusitis NOS
J32.8 Other chronic sinusitis
Sinusitis (chronic) involving more than one sinus but not pansinusitis

J32.9 Chronic sinusitis, unspecified
Sinusitis (chronic) NOS

✓4th J33 Nasal polyp
Use additional code to identify:
exposure to environmental tobacco smoke (Z77.22)
exposure to tobacco smoke in the perinatal period (P96.81)
history of tobacco use (Z87.891)
occupational exposure to environmental tobacco smoke (Z57.31)
tobacco dependence (F17.-)
tobacco use (Z72.0)
EXCLUDES 1 *adenomatous polyps (D14.0)*

J33.0 Polyp of nasal cavity
Choanal polyp
Nasopharyngeal polyp

J33.1 Polypoid sinus degeneration
Woakes' syndrome or ethmoiditis

J33.8 Other polyp of sinus
Accessory polyp of sinus
Ethmoidal polyp of sinus
Maxillary polyp of sinus
Sphenoidal polyp of sinus

J33.9 Nasal polyp, unspecified

✓4th J34 Other and unspecified disorders of nose and nasal sinuses
EXCLUDES 2 *varicose ulcer of nasal septum (I86.8)*

J34.0 Abscess, furuncle and carbuncle of nose
Cellulitis of nose
Necrosis of nose
Ulceration of nose

J34.1 Cyst and mucocele of nose and nasal sinus

J34.2 Deviated nasal septum
Deflection or deviation of septum (nasal) (acquired)
EXCLUDES 1 *congenital deviated nasal septum (Q67.4)*

J34.3 Hypertrophy of nasal turbinates

✓5th J34.8 Other specified disorders of nose and nasal sinuses

J34.81 Nasal mucositis (ulcerative)
Code also type of associated therapy, such as:
antineoplastic and immunosuppressive drugs (T45.1X-)
radiological procedure and radiotherapy (Y84.2)
EXCLUDES 2 *gastrointestinal mucositis (ulcerative) (K92.81)*
mucositis (ulcerative) of vagina and vulva (N76.81)
oral mucositis (ulcerative) (K12.3-)

J34.89 Other specified disorders of nose and nasal sinuses
Perforation of nasal septum NOS
Rhinolith

J34.9 Unspecified disorder of nose and nasal sinuses

✓4th J35 Chronic diseases of tonsils and adenoids
Use additional code to identify:
exposure to environmental tobacco smoke (Z77.22)
exposure to tobacco smoke in the perinatal period (P96.81)
history of tobacco use (Z87.891)
occupational exposure to environmental tobacco smoke (Z57.31)
tobacco dependence (F17.-)
tobacco use (Z72.0)

✓5th J35.0 Chronic tonsillitis and adenoiditis
EXCLUDES 2 *acute tonsillitis (J03.-)*

J35.01 Chronic tonsillitis

J35.02 Chronic adenoiditis

J35.03 Chronic tonsillitis and adenoiditis

J35.1 Hypertrophy of tonsils
Enlargement of tonsils
EXCLUDES 1 *hypertrophy of tonsils with tonsillitis (J35.0-)*

J35.2 Hypertrophy of adenoids
Enlargement of adenoids
EXCLUDES 1 *hypertrophy of adenoids with adenoiditis (J35.0-)*

J35.3 Hypertrophy of tonsils with hypertrophy of adenoids
EXCLUDES 1 *hypertrophy of tonsils and adenoids with tonsillitis and adenoiditis (J35.03)*

J35.8 Other chronic diseases of tonsils and adenoids
Adenoid vegetations
Amygdalolith
Calculus, tonsil
Cicatrix of tonsil (and adenoid)
Tonsillar tag
Ulcer of tonsil

J35.9 Chronic disease of tonsils and adenoids, unspecified
Disease (chronic) of tonsils and adenoids NOS

J36 Peritonsillar abscess
INCLUDES abscess of tonsil
peritonsillar cellulitis
quinsy
Use additional code (B95-B97) to identify infectious agent
EXCLUDES 1 *acute tonsillitis (J03.-)*
chronic tonsillitis (J35.0)
retropharyngeal abscess (J39.0)
tonsillitis NOS (J03.9-)

✓4th J37 Chronic laryngitis and laryngotracheitis
Use additional code to identify:
exposure to environmental tobacco smoke (Z77.22)
exposure to tobacco smoke in the perinatal period (P96.81)
history of tobacco use (Z87.891)
infectious agent (B95-B97)
occupational exposure to environmental tobacco smoke (Z57.31)
tobacco dependence (F17.-)
tobacco use (Z72.0)

J37.0 Chronic laryngitis
Catarrhal laryngitis
Hypertrophic laryngitis
Sicca laryngitis
EXCLUDES 2 *acute laryngitis (J04.0)*
obstructive (acute) laryngitis (J05.0)

J37.1 Chronic laryngotracheitis
Laryngitis, chronic, with tracheitis (chronic)
Tracheitis, chronic, with laryngitis
EXCLUDES 1 *chronic tracheitis (J42)*
EXCLUDES 2 *acute laryngotracheitis (J04.2)*
acute tracheitis (J04.1)

✓4th J38 Diseases of vocal cords and larynx, not elsewhere classified
Use additional code to identify:
exposure to environmental tobacco smoke (Z77.22)
exposure to tobacco smoke in the perinatal period (P96.81)
history of tobacco use (Z87.891)
occupational exposure to environmental tobacco smoke (Z57.31)
tobacco dependence (F17.-)
tobacco use (Z72.0)
EXCLUDES 1 *congenital laryngeal stridor (P28.89)*
obstructive laryngitis (acute) (J05.0)
postprocedural subglottic stenosis (J95.5)
stridor (R06.1)
ulcerative laryngitis (J04.0)

✓5th J38.0 Paralysis of vocal cords and larynx
Laryngoplegia
Paralysis of glottis

J38.00 Paralysis of vocal cords and larynx, unspecified

J38.01 Paralysis of vocal cords and larynx, unilateral

J38.02 Paralysis of vocal cords and larynx, bilateral

J38.1 Polyp of vocal cord and larynx
EXCLUDES 1 *adenomatous polyps (D14.1)*

J38.2 Nodules of vocal cords
Chorditis (fibrinous)(nodosa)(tuberosa)
Singer's nodes
Teacher's nodes

J38.3 Other diseases of vocal cords
Abscess of vocal cords
Cellulitis of vocal cords
Granuloma of vocal cords
Leukokeratosis of vocal cords
Leukoplakia of vocal cords

J38.4 Edema of larynx
Edema (of) glottis
Subglottic edema
Supraglottic edema
EXCLUDES 1 *acute obstructive laryngitis [croup] (J05.0)*
edematous laryngitis (J04.0)

J38.5 Laryngeal spasm
Laryngismus (stridulus)

J38.6 Stenosis of larynx

J38.7 Other diseases of larynx
Abscess of larynx
Cellulitis of larynx
Disease of larynx NOS
Necrosis of larynx
Pachyderma of larynx
Perichondritis of larynx
Ulcer of larynx

✓4th J39 Other diseases of upper respiratory tract
EXCLUDES 1 *acute respiratory infection NOS (J22)*
acute upper respiratory infection (J06.9)
upper respiratory inflammation due to chemicals, gases, fumes or vapors (J68.2)

J39.0 Retropharyngeal and parapharyngeal abscess
Peripharyngeal abscess
EXCLUDES 1 *peritonsillar abscess (J36)*

J39.1 Other abscess of pharynx
Cellulitis of pharynx
Nasopharyngeal abscess

J39.2 Other diseases of pharynx
Cyst of pharynx
Edema of pharynx
EXCLUDES 2 *chronic pharyngitis (J31.2)*
ulcerative pharyngitis (J02.9)

J39.3 Upper respiratory tract hypersensitivity reaction, site unspecified
EXCLUDES 1 *hypersensitivity reaction of upper respiratory tract, such as:*
extrinsic allergic alveolitis (J67.9)
pneumoconiosis (J60-J67.9)

J39.8 Other specified diseases of upper respiratory tract

J39.9 Disease of upper respiratory tract, unspecified

Chronic lower respiratory diseases (J40-J47)

EXCLUDES 1 *bronchitis due to chemicals, gases, fumes and vapors (J68.0)*
EXCLUDES 2 *cystic fibrosis (E84.-)*

J40 Bronchitis, not specified as acute or chronic
Bronchitis NOS
Bronchitis with tracheitis NOS
Catarrhal bronchitis
Tracheobronchitis NOS
Use additional code to identify:
exposure to environmental tobacco smoke (Z77.22)
exposure to tobacco smoke in the perinatal period (P96.81)
history of tobacco use (Z87.891)
occupational exposure to environmental tobacco smoke (Z57.31)
tobacco dependence (F17.-)
tobacco use (Z72.0)
EXCLUDES 1 *allergic bronchitis NOS (J45.909)*
asthmatic bronchitis NOS (J45.9-)
bronchitis due to chemicals, gases, fumes and vapors (J68.0)

✓4th J41 Simple and mucopurulent chronic bronchitis
Use additional code to identify:
exposure to environmental tobacco smoke (Z77.22)
exposure to tobacco smoke in the perinatal period (P96.81)
history of tobacco use (Z87.891)
occupational exposure to environmental tobacco smoke (Z57.31)
tobacco dependence (F17.-)
tobacco use (Z72.0)
EXCLUDES 1 *chronic bronchitis NOS (J42)*
chronic obstructive bronchitis (J44.-)

J41.0 Simple chronic bronchitis

J41.1 Mucopurulent chronic bronchitis

J41.8 Mixed simple and mucopurulent chronic bronchitis

J42 Unspecified chronic bronchitis
Chronic bronchitis NOS
Chronic tracheitis
Chronic tracheobronchitis
Use additional code to identify:
exposure to environmental tobacco smoke (Z77.22)
exposure to tobacco smoke in the perinatal period (P96.81)
history of tobacco use (Z87.891)
occupational exposure to environmental tobacco smoke (Z57.31)
tobacco dependence (F17.-)
tobacco use (Z72.0)
EXCLUDES 1 *chronic asthmatic bronchitis (J44.-)*
chronic bronchitis with airways obstruction (J44.-)
chronic emphysematous bronchitis (J44.-)
chronic obstructive pulmonary disease NOS (J44.9)
simple and mucopurulent chronic bronchitis (J41.-)

✓4th J43 Emphysema
Use additional code to identify:
exposure to environmental tobacco smoke (Z77.22)
history of tobacco use (Z87.891)
occupational exposure to environmental tobacco smoke (Z57.31)
tobacco dependence (F17.-)
tobacco use (Z72.0)
EXCLUDES 1 *compensatory emphysema (J98.3)*
emphysema due to inhalation of chemicals, gases, fumes or vapors (J68.4)
emphysema with chronic (obstructive) bronchitis (J44.-)
emphysematous (obstructive) bronchitis (J44.-)
interstitial emphysema (J98.2)
mediastinal emphysema (J98.2)
neonatal interstitial emphysema (P25.0)
surgical (subcutaneous) emphysema (T81.82)
traumatic subcutaneous emphysema (T79.7)

J43.0 Unilateral pulmonary emphysema [MacLeod's syndrome]
Swyer-James syndrome
Unilateral emphysema
Unilateral hyperlucent lung
Unilateral pulmonary artery functional hypoplasia
Unilateral transparency of lung

J43.1 Panlobular emphysema
Panacinar emphysema

J43.2 Centrilobular emphysema

J43.8 Other emphysema

J43.9 Emphysema, unspecified
Bullous emphysema (lung)(pulmonary)
Emphysema (lung)(pulmonary) NOS
Emphysematous bleb
Vesicular emphysema (lung)(pulmonary)

✓4th J44 Other chronic obstructive pulmonary disease
INCLUDES asthma with chronic obstructive pulmonary disease
chronic asthmatic (obstructive) bronchitis
chronic bronchitis with airways obstruction
chronic bronchitis with emphysema
chronic emphysematous bronchitis
chronic obstructive asthma
chronic obstructive bronchitis
chronic obstructive tracheobronchitis
Code also type of asthma, if applicable (J45.-)
Use additional code to identify:
exposure to environmental tobacco smoke (Z77.22)
history of tobacco use (Z87.891)
occupational exposure to environmental tobacco smoke (Z57.31)
tobacco dependence (F17.-)
tobacco use (Z72.0)
EXCLUDES 1 *bronchiectasis (J47.-)*
chronic bronchitis NOS (J42)
chronic simple and mucopurulent bronchitis (J41.-)
chronic tracheitis (J42)
chronic tracheobronchitis (J42)
emphysema without chronic bronchitis (J43.-)
lung diseases due to external agents (J60-J70)

J44.0 Chronic obstructive pulmonary disease with acute lower respiratory infection
Use additional code to identify the infection

J44.1 Chronic obstructive pulmonary disease with (acute) exacerbation
Decompensated COPD
Decompensated COPD with (acute) exacerbation
EXCLUDES 2 *chronic obstructive pulmonary disease [COPD] with acute bronchitis (J44.0)*

J44.9 Chronic obstructive pulmonary disease, unspecified
Chronic obstructive airway disease NOS
Chronic obstructive lung disease NOS

J45 Asthma
Allergic (predominantly) asthma
Allergic bronchitis NOS
Allergic rhinitis with asthma
Atopic asthma
Extrinsic allergic asthma
Hay fever with asthma
Idiosyncratic asthma
Intrinsic nonallergic asthma
Nonallergic asthma
Use additional code to identify:
exposure to environmental tobacco smoke (Z77.22)
exposure to tobacco smoke in the perinatal period (P96.81)
history of tobacco use (Z87.891)
occupational exposure to environmental tobacco smoke (Z57.31)
tobacco dependence (F17.-)
tobacco use (Z72.0)
EXCLUDES 1 *detergent asthma (J69.8)*
eosinophilic asthma (J82)
lung diseases due to external agents (J60-J70)
miner's asthma (J60)
wheezing NOS (R06.2)
wood asthma (J67.8)
EXCLUDES 2 *asthma with chronic obstructive pulmonary disease (J44.9)*
chronic asthmatic (obstructive) bronchitis (J44.9)
chronic obstructive asthma (J44.9)

J45.2 Mild intermittent asthma
J45.20 Mild intermittent asthma, uncomplicated
Mild intermittent asthma NOS
J45.21 Mild intermittent asthma with (acute) exacerbation
J45.22 Mild intermittent asthma with status asthmaticus

J45.3 Mild persistent asthma
J45.30 Mild persistent asthma, uncomplicated
Mild persistent asthma NOS
J45.31 Mild persistent asthma with (acute) exacerbation
J45.32 Mild persistent asthma with status asthmaticus

J45.4 Moderate persistent asthma
J45.40 Moderate persistent asthma, uncomplicated
Moderate persistent asthma NOS
J45.41 Moderate persistent asthma with (acute) exacerbation
J45.42 Moderate persistent asthma with status asthmaticus

J45.5 Severe persistent asthma
J45.50 Severe persistent asthma, uncomplicated
Severe persistent asthma NOS
J45.51 Severe persistent asthma with (acute) exacerbation
J45.52 Severe persistent asthma with status asthmaticus

J45.9 Other and unspecified asthma
J45.90 Unspecified asthma
Asthmatic bronchitis NOS
Childhood asthma NOS
Late onset asthma
J45.901 Unspecified asthma with (acute) exacerbation
J45.902 Unspecified asthma with status asthmaticus
J45.909 Unspecified asthma, uncomplicated
Asthma NOS
J45.99 Other asthma
J45.990 Exercise induced bronchospasm
J45.991 Cough variant asthma
J45.998 Other asthma

J47 Bronchiectasis
INCLUDES bronchiolectasis
Use additional code to identify:
exposure to environmental tobacco smoke (Z77.22)
exposure to tobacco smoke in the perinatal period (P96.81)
history of tobacco use (Z87.891)
occupational exposure to environmental tobacco smoke (Z57.31)
tobacco dependence (F17.-)
tobacco use (Z72.0)
EXCLUDES 1 *congenital bronchiectasis (Q33.4)*
tuberculous bronchiectasis (current disease) (A15.0)
J47.0 Bronchiectasis with acute lower respiratory infection
Bronchiectasis with acute bronchitis
J47.1 Bronchiectasis with (acute) exacerbation
J47.9 Bronchiectasis, uncomplicated
Bronchiectasis NOS

Lung diseases due to external agents (J60-J70)

EXCLUDES 2 *asthma (J45.-)*
malignant neoplasm of bronchus and lung (C34.-)

J60 Coalworker's pneumoconiosis
Anthracosilicosis
Anthracosis
Black lung disease
Coalworker's lung
EXCLUDES 1 *coalworker pneumoconiosis with tuberculosis, any type in A15 (J65)*

J61 Pneumoconiosis due to asbestos and other mineral fibers
Asbestosis
EXCLUDES 1 *pleural plaque with asbestosis (J92.0)*
pneumoconiosis with tuberculosis, any type in A15 (J65)

J62 Pneumoconiosis due to dust containing silica
INCLUDES silicotic fibrosis (massive) of lung
EXCLUDES 1 *pneumoconiosis with tuberculosis, any type in A15 (J65)*
J62.0 Pneumoconiosis due to talc dust
J62.8 Pneumoconiosis due to other dust containing silica
Silicosis NOS

J63 Pneumoconiosis due to other inorganic dusts
EXCLUDES 1 *pneumoconiosis with tuberculosis, any type in A15 (J65)*
J63.0 Aluminosis (of lung)
J63.1 Bauxite fibrosis (of lung)
J63.2 Berylliosis
J63.3 Graphite fibrosis (of lung)
J63.4 Siderosis
J63.5 Stannosis
J63.6 Pneumoconiosis due to other specified inorganic dusts

J64 Unspecified pneumoconiosis
EXCLUDES 1 *pneumonoconiosis with tuberculosis, any type in A15 (J65)*

J65 Pneumoconiosis associated with tuberculosis
Any condition in J60-J64 with tuberculosis, any type in A15
silicotuberculosis

J66 Airway disease due to specific organic dust
EXCLUDES 2 *allergic alveolitis (J67.-)*
asbestosis (J61)
bagassosis (J67.1)
farmer's lung (J67.0)
hypersensitivity pneumonitis due to organic dust (J67.-)
reactive airways dysfunction syndrome (J68.3)
J66.0 Byssinosis
Airway disease due to cotton dust
J66.1 Flax-dressers' disease
J66.2 Cannabinosis
J66.8 Airway disease due to other specific organic dusts

J67 Hypersensitivity pneumonitis due to organic dust
INCLUDES allergic alveolitis and pneumonitis due to inhaled organic dust and particles of fungal, actinomycetic or other origin
EXCLUDES 1 *pneumonitis due to inhalation of chemicals, gases, fumes or vapors (J68.0)*
J67.0 Farmer's lung
Harvester's lung
Haymaker's lung
Moldy hay disease
J67.1 Bagassosis
Bagasse disease
Bagasse pneumonitis
J67.2 Bird fancier's lung
Budgerigar fancier's disease or lung
Pigeon fancier's disease or lung
J67.3 Suberosis
Corkhandler's disease or lung
Corkworker's disease or lung
J67.4 Maltworker's lung
Alveolitis due to Aspergillus clavatus
J67.5 Mushroom-worker's lung
J67.6 Maple-bark-stripper's lung
Alveolitis due to Cryptostroma corticale
Cryptostromosis

J67.7 Air conditioner and humidifier lung
Allergic alveolitis due to fungal, thermophilic actinomycetes and other organisms growing in ventilation [air conditioning] systems

J67.8 Hypersensitivity pneumonitis due to other organic dusts
Cheese-washer's lung
Coffee-worker's lung
Fish-meal worker's lung
Furrier's lung
Sequoiosis

J67.9 Hypersensitivity pneumonitis due to unspecified organic dust
Allergic alveolitis (extrinsic) NOS
Hypersensitivity pneumonitis NOS

4th J68 Respiratory conditions due to inhalation of chemicals, gases, fumes and vapors
Code first (T51-T65) to identify cause
Use additional code to identify associated respiratory conditions, such as:
acute respiratory failure (J96.0-)

J68.0 Bronchitis and pneumonitis due to chemicals, gases, fumes and vapors
Chemical bronchitis (acute)

J68.1 Pulmonary edema due to chemicals, gases, fumes and vapors
Chemical pulmonary edema (acute) (chronic)
EXCLUDES 1 *pulmonary edema (acute) (chronic) NOS (J81.-)*

J68.2 Upper respiratory inflammation due to chemicals, gases, fumes and vapors, not elsewhere classified

J68.3 Other acute and subacute respiratory conditions due to chemicals, gases, fumes and vapors
Reactive airways dysfunction syndrome

J68.4 Chronic respiratory conditions due to chemicals, gases, fumes and vapors
Emphysema (diffuse) (chronic) due to inhalation of chemicals, gases, fumes and vapors
Obliterative bronchiolitis (chronic) (subacute) due to inhalation of chemicals, gases, fumes and vapors
Pulmonary fibrosis (chronic) due to inhalation of chemicals, gases, fumes and vapors
EXCLUDES 1 *chronic pulmonary edema due to chemicals, gases, fumes and vapors (J68.1)*

J68.8 Other respiratory conditions due to chemicals, gases, fumes and vapors

J68.9 Unspecified respiratory condition due to chemicals, gases, fumes and vapors

4th J69 Pneumonitis due to solids and liquids
EXCLUDES 1 *neonatal aspiration syndromes (P24.-)*
postprocedural pneumonitis (J95.4)

J69.0 Pneumonitis due to inhalation of food and vomit
Aspiration pneumonia NOS
Aspiration pneumonia (due to) food (regurgitated)
Aspiration pneumonia (due to) gastric secretions
Aspiration pneumonia (due to) milk
Aspiration pneumonia (due to) vomit
Code also any associated foreign body in respiratory tract (T17.-)
EXCLUDES 1 *chemical pneumonitis due to anesthesia (J95.4)*
obstetric aspiration pneumonitis (O74.0)

J69.1 Pneumonitis due to inhalation of oils and essences
Exogenous lipoid pneumonia
Lipid pneumonia NOS
Code first (T51-T65) to identify substance
EXCLUDES 1 *endogenous lipoid pneumonia (J84.89)*

J69.8 Pneumonitis due to inhalation of other solids and liquids
Pneumonitis due to aspiration of blood
Pneumonitis due to aspiration of detergent
Code first (T51-T65) to identify substance

4th J70 Respiratory conditions due to other external agents

J70.0 Acute pulmonary manifestations due to radiation
Radiation pneumonitis
Use additional code (W88-W90, X39.0-) to identify the external cause

J70.1 Chronic and other pulmonary manifestations due to radiation
Fibrosis of lung following radiation
Use additional code (W88-W90, X39.0-) to identify the external cause

J70.2 Acute drug-induced interstitial lung disorders
Use additional code for adverse effect, if applicable, to identify drug (T36-T50 with fifth or sixth character 5)
EXCLUDES 1 *interstitial pneumonia NOS (J84.9)*
lymphoid interstitial pneumonia (J84.2)

J70.3 Chronic drug-induced interstitial lung disorders
Use additional code for adverse effect, if applicable, to identify drug (T36-T50 with fifth or sixth character 5)
EXCLUDES 1 *interstitial pneumonia NOS (J84.9)*
lymphoid interstitial pneumonia (J84.2)

J70.4 Drug-induced interstitial lung disorders, unspecified
Use additional code for adverse effect, if applicable, to identify drug (T36-T50 with fifth or sixth character 5)
EXCLUDES 1 *interstitial pneumonia NOS (J84.9)*
lymphoid interstitial pneumonia (J84.2)

J70.5 Respiratory conditions due to smoke inhalation
Smoke inhalation NOS
EXCLUDES 1 *smoke inhalation due to chemicals, gases, fumes and vapors (J68.9)*

J70.8 Respiratory conditions due to other specified external agents
Code first (T51-T65) to identify the external agent

J70.9 Respiratory conditions due to unspecified external agent
Code first (T51-T65) to identify the external agent

Other respiratory diseases principally affecting the interstitium (J80-J84)

J80 Acute respiratory distress syndrome
Acute respiratory distress syndrome in adult or child
Adult hyaline membrane disease
EXCLUDES 1 *respiratory distress syndrome in newborn (perinatal) (P22.0)*

4th J81 Pulmonary edema
Use additional code to identify:
exposure to environmental tobacco smoke (Z77.22)
history of tobacco use (Z87.891)
occupational exposure to environmental tobacco smoke (Z57.31)
tobacco dependence (F17.-)
tobacco use (Z72.0)
EXCLUDES 1 *chemical (acute) pulmonary edema (J68.1)*
hypostatic pneumonia (J18.2)
passive pneumonia (J18.2)
pulmonary edema due to external agents (J60-J70)
pulmonary edema with heart disease NOS (I50.1)
pulmonary edema with heart failure (I50.1)

J81.0 Acute pulmonary edema
Acute edema of lung

J81.1 Chronic pulmonary edema
Pulmonary congestion (chronic) (passive)
Pulmonary edema NOS

J82 Pulmonary eosinophilia, not elsewhere classified
Allergic pneumonia
Eosinophilic asthma
Eosinophilic pneumonia
Löffler's pneumonia
Tropical (pulmonary) eosinophilia NOS
EXCLUDES 1 *pulmonary eosinophilia due to aspergillosis (B44.-)*
pulmonary eosinophilia due to drugs (J70.2-J70.4)
pulmonary eosinophilia due to specified parasitic infection (B50-B83)
pulmonary eosinophilia due to systemic connective tissue disorders (M30-M36)
pulmonary infiltrate NOS (R91.8)

4th J84 Other interstitial pulmonary diseases
EXCLUDES 1 *drug-induced interstitial lung disorders (J70.2-J70.4)*
interstitial emphysema (J98.2)
lung diseases due to external agents (J60-J70)

5th J84.0 Alveolar and parieto-alveolar conditions

J84.01 Alveolar proteinosis

J84.02 Pulmonary alveolar microlithiasis

J84.03 Idiopathic pulmonary hemosiderosis
Essential brown induration of lung
Code first underlying disease, such as:
disorders of iron metabolism (E83.1-)
EXCLUDES 1 *acute idiopathic pulmonary hemorrhage in infants [AIPHI] (R04.81)*

J84.09 Other alveolar and parieto-alveolar conditions

J84.1 Other interstitial pulmonary diseases with fibrosis

EXCLUDES 1 *pulmonary fibrosis (chronic) due to inhalation of chemicals, gases, fumes or vapors (J68.4)*
pulmonary fibrosis (chronic) following radiation (J70.1)

J84.10 Pulmonary fibrosis, unspecified

Capillary fibrosis of lung
Cirrhosis of lung (chronic) NOS
Fibrosis of lung (atrophic) (chronic) (confluent) (massive) (perialveolar) (peribronchial) NOS
Induration of lung (chronic) NOS
Postinflammatory pulmonary fibrosis

J84.11 Idiopathic interstitial pneumonia

EXCLUDES 1 *lymphoid interstitial pneumonia (J84.2)*
pneumocystis pneumonia (B59)

J84.111 Idiopathic interstitial pneumonia, not otherwise specified

J84.112 Idiopathic pulmonary fibrosis

Cryptogenic fibrosing alveolitis
Idiopathic fibrosing alveolitis

J84.113 Idiopathic non-specific interstitial pneumonitis

EXCLUDES 1 *non-specific interstitial pneumonia NOS, or due to known underlying cause (J84.89)*

J84.114 Acute interstitial pneumonitis

Hamman-Rich syndrome
EXCLUDES 1 *pneumocystis pneumonia (B59)*

J84.115 Respiratory bronchiolitis interstitial lung disease

J84.116 Cryptogenic organizing pneumonia

EXCLUDES 1 *organizing pneumonia NOS, or due to known underlying cause (J84.89)*

J84.117 Desquamative interstitial pneumonia

J84.17 Other interstitial pulmonary diseases with fibrosis in diseases classified elsewhere

Interstitial pneumonia (nonspecific) (usual) due to collagen vascular disease
Interstitial pneumonia (nonspecific) (usual) in diseases classified elsewhere
Organizing pneumonia due to collagen vascular disease
Organizing pneumonia in diseases classified elsewhere
Code first underlying disease, such as:
progressive systemic sclerosis (M34.0)
rheumatoid arthritis (M05.00-M06.9)
systemic lupus erythematosis (M32.0-M32.9)

J84.2 Lymphoid interstitial pneumonia

Lymphoid interstitial pneumonitis

J84.8 Other specified interstitial pulmonary diseases

EXCLUDES 1 *exogenous lipoid pneumonia (J69.1)*
unspecified lipoid pneumonia (J69.1)

J84.81 Lymphangioleiomyomatosis

Lymphangiomyomatosis

J84.82 Adult pulmonary Langerhans cell histiocytosis

Adult PLCH

J84.83 Surfactant mutations of the lung

J84.84 Other interstitial lung diseases of childhood

J84.841 Neuroendocrine cell hyperplasia of infancy

J84.842 Pulmonary interstitial glycogenosis

J84.843 Alveolar capillary dysplasia with vein misalignment

J84.848 Other interstitial lung diseases of childhood

J84.89 Other specified interstitial pulmonary diseases

Endogenous lipoid pneumonia
Interstitial pneumonitis
Non-specific interstitial pneumonitis NOS
Organizing pneumonia due to known underlying cause
Organizing pneumonia NOS
Code first, if applicable:
poisoning due to drug or toxin (T51-T65 with fifth or sixth character to indicate intent), for toxic pneumonopathy
underlying cause of pneumonopathy, if known
Use additional code, for adverse effect, to identify drug (T36-T50 with fifth or sixth character 5), if drug-induced
EXCLUDES 1 *cryptogenic organizing pneumonia (J84.846)*
idiopathic non-specific interstitial pneumonitis (J84.843)
lipoid pneumonia, exogenous or unspecified (J69.1)
lymphoid interstitial pneumonia (J84.2)

J84.9 Interstitial pulmonary disease, unspecified

Interstitial pneumonia NOS

Suppurative and necrotic conditions of the lower respiratory tract (J85-J86)

J85 Abscess of lung and mediastinum

Use additional code (B95-B97) to identify infectious agent.

J85.0 Gangrene and necrosis of lung

J85.1 Abscess of lung with pneumonia

Code also the type of pneumonia

J85.2 Abscess of lung without pneumonia

Abscess of lung NOS

J85.3 Abscess of mediastinum

J86 Pyothorax

Use additional code (B95-B97) to identify infectious agent
EXCLUDES 1 *abscess of lung (J85.-)*
pyothorax due to tuberculosis (A15.6)

J86.0 Pyothorax with fistula

Bronchocutaneous fistula
Bronchopleural fistula
Hepatopleural fistula
Mediastinal fistula
Pleural fistula
Thoracic fistula
Any condition classifiable to J86.9 with fistula

J86.9 Pyothorax without fistula

Abscess of pleura
Abscess of thorax
Empyema (chest) (lung) (pleura)
Fibrinopurulent pleurisy
Purulent pleurisy
Pyopneumothorax
Septic pleurisy
Seropurulent pleurisy
Suppurative pleurisy

Other diseases of the pleura (J90-J94)

J90 Pleural effusion, not elsewhere classified

Encysted pleurisy
Pleural effusion NOS
Pleurisy with effusion (exudative) (serous)
EXCLUDES 1 *chylous (pleural) effusion (J94.0)*
malignant pleural effusion (J91.0))
pleurisy NOS (R09.1)
tuberculous pleural effusion (A15.6)

J91 Pleural effusion in conditions classified elsewhere

EXCLUDES 2 *pleural effusion in heart failure (I50.-)*
pleural effusion in systemic lupus erythematosus (M32.13)

J91.0 Malignant pleural effusion

Code first underlying neoplasm

J91.8 Pleural effusion in other conditions classified elsewhere

Code first underlying disease, such as:
filariasis (B74.0-B74.9)
influenza (J09.X2, J10.1, J11.1)

DRAFT

Appropriate additional character required
Requires 7th character, placeholder x must fill empty characters

J92 Pleural plaque
INCLUDES pleural thickening
J92.Ø Pleural plaque with presence of asbestos
J92.9 Pleural plaque without asbestos
Pleural plaque NOS

J93 Pneumothorax and air leak
EXCLUDES 1 *congenital or perinatal pneumothorax (P25.1)*
postprocedural air leak (J95.812)
postprocedural pneumothorax (J95.811)
traumatic pneumothorax (S27.Ø)
tuberculous (current disease) pneumothorax (A15.-)
pyopneumothorax (J86.-)
J93.Ø Spontaneous tension pneumothorax
J93.1 Other spontaneous pneumothorax
J93.11 Primary spontaneous pneumothorax
J93.12 Secondary spontaneous pneumothorax
Code first underlying condition, such as:
catamenial pneumothorax due to endometriosis (N8Ø.8)
cystic fibrosis (E84.-)
eosinophilic pneumonia (J82)
lymphangioleiomyomatosis (J84.81)
malignant neoplasm of bronchus and lung (C34.-)
Marfan's syndrome (Q87.4)
pneumonia due to Pneumocystis carinii (B59)
secondary malignant neoplasm of lung (C78.Ø-)
spontaneous rupture of the esophagus (K22.3)
J93.8 Other pneumothorax and air leak
J93.81 Chronic pneumothorax
J93.82 Other air leak
Persistent air leak
J93.83 Other pneumothorax
Acute pneumothorax
Spontaneous pneumothorax NOS
J93.9 Pneumothorax, unspecified
Pneumothorax NOS

J94 Other pleural conditions
EXCLUDES 1 *pleurisy NOS (RØ9.1)*
traumatic hemopneumothorax (S27.2)
traumatic hemothorax (S27.1)
tuberculous pleural conditions (current disease) (A15.-)
J94.Ø Chylous effusion
Chyliform effusion
J94.1 Fibrothorax
J94.2 Hemothorax
Hemopneumothorax
J94.8 Other specified pleural conditions
Hydropneumothorax
Hydrothorax
J94.9 Pleural condition, unspecified

Intraoperative and postprocedural complications and disorders of respiratory system, not elsewhere classified (J95)

J95 Intraoperative and postprocedural complications and disorders of respiratory system, not elsewhere classified
EXCLUDES 2 *aspiration pneumonia (J69.-)*
emphysema (subcutaneous) resulting from a procedure (T81.82)
hypostatic pneumonia (J18.2)
pulmonary manifestations due to radiation (J7Ø.Ø- J7Ø.1)
J95.Ø Tracheostomy complications
J95.ØØ Unspecified tracheostomy complication
J95.Ø1 Hemorrhage from tracheostomy stoma
J95.Ø2 Infection of tracheostomy stoma
Use additional code to identify type of infection, such as:
cellulitis of neck (LØ3.8)
sepsis (A4Ø, A41-)
J95.Ø3 Malfunction of tracheostomy stoma
Mechanical complication of tracheostomy stoma
Obstruction of tracheostomy airway
Tracheal stenosis due to tracheostomy
J95.Ø4 Tracheo-esophageal fistula following tracheostomy
J95.Ø9 Other tracheostomy complication
J95.1 Acute pulmonary insufficiency following thoracic surgery
EXCLUDES 2 *functional disturbances following cardiac surgery (I97.Ø, I97.1-)*
J95.2 Acute pulmonary insufficiency following nonthoracic surgery
EXCLUDES 2 *functional disturbances following cardiac surgery (I97.Ø, I97.1-)*
J95.3 Chronic pulmonary insufficiency following surgery
EXCLUDES 2 *functional disturbances following cardiac surgery (I97.Ø, I97.1-)*
J95.4 Chemical pneumonitis due to anesthesia
Code first:
Mendelson's syndrome
Postprocedural aspiration pneumonia
Use additional code for adverse effect, if applicable, to identify drug (T41.- with fifth or sixth character 5)
EXCLUDES 1 *aspiration pneumonitis due to anesthesia complicating labor and delivery (O74.Ø)*
aspiration pneumonitis due to anesthesia complicating pregnancy (O29)
aspiration pneumonitis due to anesthesia complicating the puerperium (O89.Ø1)
J95.5 Postprocedural subglottic stenosis
J95.6 Intraoperative hemorrhage and hematoma of a respiratory system organ or structure complicating a procedure
EXCLUDES 1 *intraoperative hemorrhage and hematoma of a respiratory system organ or structure due to accidental puncture and laceration during procedure (J95.7-)*
J95.61 Intraoperative hemorrhage and hematoma of a respiratory system organ or structure complicating a respiratory system procedure
J95.62 Intraoperative hemorrhage and hematoma of a respiratory system organ or structure complicating other procedure
J95.7 Accidental puncture and laceration of a respiratory system organ or structure during a procedure
EXCLUDES 2 *postprocedural pneumothorax (J95.8)*
J95.71 Accidental puncture and laceration of a respiratory system organ or structure during a respiratory system procedure
J95.72 Accidental puncture and laceration of a respiratory system organ or structure during other procedure
J95.8 Other intraoperative and postprocedural complications and disorders of respiratory system, not elsewhere classified
J95.81 Postprocedural pneumothorax and air leak
J95.811 Postprocedural pneumothorax
J95.812 Postprocedural air leak
J95.82 Postprocedural respiratory failure
EXCLUDES 1 *respiratory failure in other conditions (J96.-)*
J95.821 Acute postprocedural respiratory failure
Postprocedural respiratory failure NOS
J95.822 Acute and chronic postprocedural respiratory failure
J95.83 Postprocedural hemorrhage and hematoma of a respiratory system organ or structure following a procedure
J95.83Ø Postprocedural hemorrhage and hematoma of a respiratory system organ or structure following a respiratory system procedure
J95.831 Postprocedural hemorrhage and hematoma of a respiratory system organ or structure following other procedure
J95.84 Transfusion-related acute lung injury (TRALI)
J95.85 Complication of respirator [ventilator]
J95.85Ø Mechanical complication of respirator
EXCLUDES 1 *encounter for respirator [ventilator] dependence during power failure (Z99.12)*

J95.851 Ventilator associated pneumonia
Ventilator associated pneumonitis
Use additional code to identify the organism, if known (B95.-, B96.-, B97.-)
EXCLUDES 1 *ventilator lung in newborn (P27.8)*

J95.859 Other complication of respirator [ventilator]

J95.88 Other intraoperative complications of respiratory system, not elsewhere classified

J95.89 Other postprocedural complications and disorders of respiratory system, not elsewhere classified
Use additional code to identify disorder, such as:
aspiration pneumonia (J69.-)
bacterial or viral pneumonia (J12-J18)
EXCLUDES 2 *acute pulmonary insufficiency following thoracic surgery (J95.1)*
postprocedural subglottic stenosis (J95.5)

Other diseases of the respiratory system (J96-J99)

✓4th **J96 Respiratory failure, not elsewhere classified**
EXCLUDES 1 *acute respiratory distress syndrome (J80)*
cardiorespiratory failure (R09.2)
newborn respiratory distress syndrome (P22.0)
postprocedural respiratory failure (J95.82-)
respiratory arrest (R09.2)
respiratory arrest of newborn (P28.81)
respiratory failure of newborn (P28.5)

✓5th **J96.0 Acute respiratory failure**
J96.00 Acute respiratory failure, unspecified whether with hypoxia or hypercapnia
J96.01 Acute respiratory failure with hypoxia
J96.02 Acute respiratory failure with hypercapnia

✓5th **J96.1 Chronic respiratory failure**
J96.10 Chronic respiratory failure, unspecified whether with hypoxia or hypercapnia
J96.11 Chronic respiratory failure with hypoxia
J96.12 Chronic respiratory failure with hypercapnia

✓5th **J96.2 Acute and chronic respiratory failure**
Acute on chronic respiratory failure
J96.20 Acute and chronic respiratory failure, unspecified whether with hypoxia or hypercapnia
J96.21 Acute and chronic respiratory failure with hypoxia
J96.22 Acute and chronic respiratory failure with hypercapnia

✓5th **J96.9 Respiratory failure, unspecified**
J96.90 Respiratory failure, unspecified, unspecified whether with hypoxia or hypercapnia
J96.91 Respiratory failure, unspecified with hypoxia
J96.92 Respiratory failure, unspecified with hypercapnia

✓4th **J98 Other respiratory disorders**
Use additional code to identify:
exposure to environmental tobacco smoke (Z77.22)
exposure to tobacco smoke in the perinatal period (P96.81)
history of tobacco use (Z87.891)
occupational exposure to environmental tobacco smoke (Z57.31)
tobacco dependence (F17.-)
tobacco use (Z72.0)
EXCLUDES 1 *newborn apnea (P28.4)*
newborn sleep apnea (P28.3)
EXCLUDES 2 *apnea NOS (R06.81)*
sleep apnea (G47.3-)

✓5th **J98.0 Diseases of bronchus, not elsewhere classified**
J98.01 Acute bronchospasm
EXCLUDES 1 *acute bronchiolitis with bronchospasm (J21.-)*
acute bronchitis with bronchospasm (J20.-)
asthma (J45.-)
exercise induced bronchospasm (J45.990)

J98.09 Other diseases of bronchus, not elsewhere classified
Broncholithiasis
Calcification of bronchus
Stenosis of bronchus
Tracheobronchial collapse
Tracheobronchial dyskinesia
Ulcer of bronchus

✓5th **J98.1 Pulmonary collapse**
EXCLUDES 1 *therapeutic collapse of lung status (Z98.3)*
J98.11 Atelectasis
EXCLUDES 1 *newborn atelectasis*
tuberculous atelectasis (current disease) (A15)
J98.19 Other pulmonary collapse

J98.2 Interstitial emphysema
Mediastinal emphysema
EXCLUDES 1 *emphysema NOS (J43.9)*
emphysema in newborn (P25.0)
surgical emphysema (subcutaneous) (T81.82)
traumatic subcutaneous emphysema (T79.7)

J98.3 Compensatory emphysema

J98.4 Other disorders of lung
Calcification of lung
Cystic lung disease (acquired)
Lung disease NOS
Pulmolithiasis
EXCLUDES 1 *acute interstitial pneumonitis (J84.114)*
pulmonary insufficiency following surgery (J95.1-J95.2)

J98.5 Diseases of mediastinum, not elsewhere classified
Fibrosis of mediastinum
Hernia of mediastinum
Retraction of mediastinum
Mediastinitis
EXCLUDES 2 *abscess of mediastinum (J85.3)*

J98.6 Disorders of diaphragm
Diaphragmatitis
Paralysis of diaphragm
Relaxation of diaphragm
EXCLUDES 1 *congenital malformation of diaphragm NEC (Q79.1)*
congenital diaphragmatic hernia (Q79.0)
EXCLUDES 2 *diaphragmatic hernia (K44.-)*

J98.8 Other specified respiratory disorders

J98.9 Respiratory disorder, unspecified
Respiratory disease (chronic) NOS

J99 Respiratory disorders in diseases classified elsewhere
Code first underlying disease, such as:
amyloidosis (E85.-)
ankylosing spondylitis (M45)
congenital syphilis (A50.5)
cryoglobulinemia (D89.1)
early congenital syphilis (A50.0)
schistosomiasis (B65.0-B65.9)
EXCLUDES 1 *respiratory disorders in:*
amebiasis (A06.5)
blastomycosis (B40.0-B40.2)
candidiasis (B37.1)
coccidioidomycosis (B38.0-B38.2)
cystic fibrosis with pulmonary manifestations (E84.0)
dermatomyositis (M33.01, M33.11)
histoplasmosis (B39.0-B39.2)
late syphilis (A52.72, A52.73)
polymyositis (M33.21)
sicca syndrome (M35.02)
systemic lupus erythematosus (M32.13)
systemic sclerosis (M34.81)
Wegener's granulomatosis (M31.30-M31.31)

Chapter 11. Diseases of the Digestive System (KØØ-K95)

EXCLUDES 2 *certain conditions originating in the perinatal period (PØ4-P96)*
certain infectious and parasitic diseases (AØØ-B99)
complications of pregnancy, childbirth and the puerperium (OØØ-O9A)
congenital malformations, deformations and chromosomal abnormalities (QØØ-Q99)
endocrine, nutritional and metabolic diseases (EØØ-E88)
injury, poisoning and certain other consequences of external causes (SØØ-T88)
neoplasms (CØØ-D49)
symptoms, signs and abnormal clinical and laboratory findings, not elsewhere classified (RØØ-R94)

This chapter contains the following blocks:

KØØ-K14 Diseases of oral cavity and salivary glands
K2Ø-K31 Diseases of esophagus, stomach and duodenum
K35-K38 Diseases of appendix
K4Ø-K46 Hernia
K5Ø-K52 Noninfective enteritis and colitis
K55-K64 Other diseases of intestines
K65-K68 Diseases of peritoneum and retroperitoneum
K7Ø-K77 Diseases of liver
K8Ø-K87 Disorders of gallbladder, biliary tract and pancreas
K9Ø-K95 Other diseases of the digestive system

Diseases of oral cavity and salivary glands (KØØ-K14)

✓4th KØØ Disorders of tooth development and eruption
EXCLUDES 2 *embedded and impacted teeth (KØ1.-)*

KØØ.Ø Anodontia
Hypodontia
Oligodontia
EXCLUDES 1 *acquired absence of teeth (KØ8.1-)*

KØØ.1 Supernumerary teeth
Distomolar
Fourth molar
Mesiodens
Paramolar
Supplementary teeth
EXCLUDES 2 *supernumerary roots (KØØ.2)*

KØØ.2 Abnormalities of size and form of teeth
Concrescence of teeth
Dens evaginatus
Dens in dente
Dens invaginatus
Enamel pearls
Fusion of teeth
Gemination of teeth
Macrodontia
Microdontia
Peg-shaped [conical] teeth
Supernumerary roots
Taurodontism
Tuberculum paramolare
EXCLUDES 1 *abnormalities of teeth due to congenital syphilis (A5Ø.5)*
tuberculum Carabelli, which is regarded as a normal variation and should not be coded

KØØ.3 Mottled teeth
Dental fluorosis
Mottling of enamel
Nonfluoride enamel opacities
EXCLUDES 2 *deposits [accretions] on teeth (KØ3.6)*

KØØ.4 Disturbances in tooth formation
Aplasia and hypoplasia of cementum
Dilaceration of tooth
Enamel hypoplasia (neonatal) (postnatal) (prenatal)
Regional odontodysplasia
Turner's tooth
EXCLUDES 1 *Hutchinson's teeth and mulberry molars in congenital syphilis (A5Ø.5)*
EXCLUDES 2 *mottled teeth (KØØ.3)*

KØØ.5 Hereditary disturbances in tooth structure, not elsewhere classified
Amelogenesis imperfecta
Dentinogenesis imperfecta
Odontogenesis imperfecta
Dentinal dysplasia
Shell teeth

KØØ.6 Disturbances in tooth eruption
Dentia praecox
Natal tooth
Neonatal tooth
Premature eruption of tooth
Premature shedding of primary [deciduous] tooth
Prenatal teeth
Retained [persistent] primary tooth
EXCLUDES 2 *embedded and impacted teeth (KØ1.-)*

KØØ.7 Teething syndrome

KØØ.8 Other disorders of tooth development
Color changes during tooth formation
Intrinsic staining of teeth NOS
EXCLUDES 2 *posteruptive color changes (KØ3.7)*

KØØ.9 Disorder of tooth development, unspecified
Disorder of odontogenesis NOS

✓4th KØ1 Embedded and impacted teeth
EXCLUDES 1 *abnormal position of fully erupted teeth (M26.3-)*

KØ1.Ø Embedded teeth

KØ1.1 Impacted teeth

✓4th KØ2 Dental caries
Dental cavities
Tooth decay

KØ2.3 Arrested dental caries
Arrested coronal and root caries

✓5th KØ2.5 Dental caries on pit and fissure surface
Dental caries on chewing surface of tooth

KØ2.51 Dental caries on pit and fissure surface limited to enamel
White spot lesions [initial caries] on pit and fissure surface of tooth

KØ2.52 Dental caries on pit and fissure surface penetrating into dentin

KØ2.53 Dental caries on pit and fissure surface penetrating into pulp

✓5th KØ2.6 Dental caries on smooth surface

KØ2.61 Dental caries on smooth surface limited to enamel
White spot lesions [initial caries] on smooth surface of tooth

KØ2.62 Dental caries on smooth surface penetrating into dentin

KØ2.63 Dental caries on smooth surface penetrating into pulp

KØ2.7 Dental root caries

KØ2.9 Dental caries, unspecified

✓4th KØ3 Other diseases of hard tissues of teeth
EXCLUDES 2 *bruxism (F45.8)*
dental caries (KØ2.-)
teeth-grinding NOS (F45.8)

KØ3.Ø Excessive attrition of teeth
Approximal wear of teeth
Occlusal wear of teeth

KØ3.1 Abrasion of teeth
Dentifrice abrasion of teeth
Habitual abrasion of teeth
Occupational abrasion of teeth
Ritual abrasion of teeth
Traditional abrasion of teeth
Wedge defect NOS

KØ3.2 Erosion of teeth
Erosion of teeth due to diet
Erosion of teeth due to drugs and medicaments
Erosion of teeth due to persistent vomiting
Erosion of teeth NOS
Idiopathic erosion of teeth
Occupational erosion of teeth

KØ3.3 Pathological resorption of teeth
Internal granuloma of pulp
Resorption of teeth (external)

KØ3.4 Hypercementosis
Cementation hyperplasia

KØ3.5 Ankylosis of teeth

K03.6 **Deposits [accretions] on teeth**
Betel deposits [accretions] on teeth
Black deposits [accretions] on teeth
Extrinsic staining of teeth NOS
Green deposits [accretions] on teeth
Materia alba deposits [accretions] on teeth
Orange deposits [accretions] on teeth
Staining of teeth NOS
Subgingival dental calculus
Supragingival dental calculus
Tobacco deposits [accretions] on teeth

K03.7 **Posteruptive color changes of dental hard tissues**
EXCLUDES 2 *deposits [accretions] on teeth (K03.6)*

✓5th K03.8 **Other specified diseases of hard tissues of teeth**

K03.81 **Cracked tooth**
EXCLUDES 1 *asymptomatic craze lines in enamel—omit code*
broken or fractured tooth due to trauma (S02.5)

K03.89 **Other specified diseases of hard tissues of teeth**

K03.9 **Disease of hard tissues of teeth, unspecified**

✓4th **K04 Diseases of pulp and periapical tissues**

K04.0 **Pulpitis**
Acute pulpitis
Chronic (hyperplastic) (ulcerative) pulpitis
Irreversible pulpitis
Reversible pulpitis

K04.1 **Necrosis of pulp**
Pulpal gangrene

K04.2 **Pulp degeneration**
Denticles
Pulpal calcifications
Pulpal stones

K04.3 **Abnormal hard tissue formation in pulp**
Secondary or irregular dentine

K04.4 **Acute apical periodontitis of pulpal origin**
Acute apical periodontitis NOS
EXCLUDES 1 *acute periodontitis (K05.2-)*

K04.5 **Chronic apical periodontitis**
Apical or periapical granuloma
Apical periodontitis NOS
EXCLUDES 1 *chronic periodontitis (K05.3-)*

K04.6 **Periapical abscess with sinus**
Dental abscess with sinus
Dentoalveolar abscess with sinus

K04.7 **Periapical abscess without sinus**
Dental abscess without sinus
Dentoalveolar abscess without sinus
Periapical abscess without sinus

K04.8 **Radicular cyst**
Apical (periodontal) cyst
Periapical cyst
Residual radicular cyst
EXCLUDES 2 *lateral periodontal cyst (K09.0)*

✓5th K04.9 **Other and unspecified diseases of pulp and periapical tissues**

K04.90 **Unspecified diseases of pulp and periapical tissues**

K04.99 **Other diseases of pulp and periapical tissues**

✓4th **K05 Gingivitis and periodontal diseases**

Use additional code to identify:
alcohol abuse and dependence (F10.-)
exposure to environmental tobacco smoke (Z77.22)
exposure to tobacco smoke in the perinatal period (P96.81)
history of tobacco use (Z87.891)
occupational exposure to environmental tobacco smoke (Z57.31)
tobacco dependence (F17.-)
tobacco use (Z72.0)

✓5th K05.0 **Acute gingivitis**
EXCLUDES 1 *acute necrotizing ulcerative gingivitis (A69.1)*
herpesviral [herpes simplex] gingivostomatitis (B00.2)

K05.00 **Acute gingivitis, plaque induced**
Acute gingivitis NOS

K05.01 **Acute gingivitis, non-plaque induced**

✓5th K05.1 **Chronic gingivitis**
Desquamative gingivitis (chronic)
Gingivitis (chronic) NOS
Hyperplastic gingivitis (chronic)
Simple marginal gingivitis (chronic)
Ulcerative gingivitis (chronic)

K05.10 **Chronic gingivitis, plaque induced**
Chronic gingivitis NOS
Gingivitis NOS

K05.11 **Chronic gingivitis, non-plaque induced**

✓5th K05.2 **Aggressive periodontitis**
Acute pericoronitis
EXCLUDES 1 *acute apical periodontitis (K04.4)*
periapical abscess (K04.7)
periapical abscess with sinus (K04.6)

K05.20 **Aggressive periodontitis, unspecified**

K05.21 **Aggressive periodontitis, localized**
Periodontal abscess

K05.22 **Aggressive periodontitis, generalized**

✓5th K05.3 **Chronic periodontitis**
Chronic pericoronitis
Complex periodontitis
Periodontitis NOS
Simplex periodontitis
EXCLUDES 1 *chronic apical periodontitis (K04.5)*

K05.30 **Chronic periodontitis, unspecified**

K05.31 **Chronic periodontitis, localized**

K05.32 **Chronic periodontitis, generalized**

K05.4 **Periodontosis**
Juvenile periodontosis

K05.5 **Other periodontal diseases**
EXCLUDES 2 *leukoplakia of gingiva (K13.21)*

K05.6 **Periodontal disease, unspecified**

✓4th **K06 Other disorders of gingiva and edentulous alveolar ridge**
EXCLUDES 2 *acute gingivitis (K05.0)*
atrophy of edentulous alveolar ridge (K08.2)
chronic gingivitis (K05.1)
gingivitis NOS (K05.1)

K06.0 **Gingival recession**
Gingival recession (generalized) (localized) (postinfective) (postprocedural)

K06.1 **Gingival enlargement**
Gingival fibromatosis

K06.2 **Gingival and edentulous alveolar ridge lesions associated with trauma**
Irritative hyperplasia of edentulous ridge [denture hyperplasia]
Use additional code (Chapter 20) to identify external cause or denture status (Z97.2)

K06.8 **Other specified disorders of gingiva and edentulous alveolar ridge**
Fibrous epulis
Flabby alveolar ridge
Giant cell epulis
Peripheral giant cell granuloma of gingiva
Pyogenic granuloma of gingiva
EXCLUDES 2 *gingival cyst (K09.0)*

K06.9 **Disorder of gingiva and edentulous alveolar ridge, unspecified**

✓4th **K08 Other disorders of teeth and supporting structures**
EXCLUDES 2 *dentofacial anomalies [including malocclusion] (M26.-)*
disorders of jaw (M27.-)

K08.0 **Exfoliation of teeth due to systemic causes**
Code also underlying systemic condition

✓5th K08.1 **Complete loss of teeth**
Acquired loss of teeth, complete
EXCLUDES 1 *congenital absence of teeth (K00.0)*
exfoliation of teeth due to systemic causes (K08.0)
partial loss of teeth (K08.4-)

✓6th K08.10 **Complete loss of teeth, unspecified cause**

K08.101 **Complete loss of teeth, unspecified cause, class I**

K08.102 **Complete loss of teeth, unspecified cause, class II**

K08.103 **Complete loss of teeth, unspecified cause, class III**

K08.104 **Complete loss of teeth, unspecified cause, class IV**

K08.109 Complete loss of teeth, unspecified cause, unspecified class
Edentulism NOS

√6th **K08.11 Complete loss of teeth due to trauma**

K08.111 Complete loss of teeth due to trauma, class I

K08.112 Complete loss of teeth due to trauma, class II

K08.113 Complete loss of teeth due to trauma, class III

K08.114 Complete loss of teeth due to trauma, class IV

K08.119 Complete loss of teeth due to trauma, unspecified class

√6th **K08.12 Complete loss of teeth due to periodontal diseases**

K08.121 Complete loss of teeth due to periodontal diseases, class I

K08.122 Complete loss of teeth due to periodontal diseases, class II

K08.123 Complete loss of teeth due to periodontal diseases, class III

K08.124 Complete loss of teeth due to periodontal diseases, class IV

K08.129 Complete loss of teeth due to periodontal diseases, unspecified class

√6th **K08.13 Complete loss of teeth due to caries**

K08.131 Complete loss of teeth due to caries, class I

K08.132 Complete loss of teeth due to caries, class II

K08.133 Complete loss of teeth due to caries, class III

K08.134 Complete loss of teeth due to caries, class IV

K08.139 Complete loss of teeth due to caries, unspecified class

√6th **K08.19 Complete loss of teeth due to other specified cause**

K08.191 Complete loss of teeth due to other specified cause, class I

K08.192 Complete loss of teeth due to other specified cause, class II

K08.193 Complete loss of teeth due to other specified cause, class III

K08.194 Complete loss of teeth due to other specified cause, class IV

K08.199 Complete loss of teeth due to other specified cause, unspecified class

√5th **K08.2 Atrophy of edentulous alveolar ridge**

K08.20 Unspecified atrophy of edentulous alveolar ridge
Atrophy of the mandible NOS
Atrophy of the maxilla NOS

K08.21 Minimal atrophy of the mandible
Minimal atrophy of the edentulous mandible

K08.22 Moderate atrophy of the mandible
Moderate atrophy of the edentulous mandible

K08.23 Severe atrophy of the mandible
Severe atrophy of the edentulous mandible

K08.24 Minimal atrophy of maxilla
Minimal atrophy of the edentulous maxilla

K08.25 Moderate atrophy of the maxilla
Moderate atrophy of the edentulous maxilla

K08.26 Severe atrophy of the maxilla
Severe atrophy of the edentulous maxilla

K08.3 Retained dental root

√5th **K08.4 Partial loss of teeth**
Acquired loss of teeth, partial
EXCLUDES 1 *complete loss of teeth (K08.1-)*
congenital absence of teeth (K00.0)
EXCLUDES 2 *exfoliation of teeth due to systemic causes (K08.0)*

√6th **K08.40 Partial loss of teeth, unspecified cause**

K08.401 Partial loss of teeth, unspecified cause, class I

K08.402 Partial loss of teeth, unspecified cause, class II

K08.403 Partial loss of teeth, unspecified cause, class III

K08.404 Partial loss of teeth, unspecified cause, class IV

K08.409 Partial loss of teeth, unspecified cause, unspecified class
Tooth extraction status NOS

√6th **K08.41 Partial loss of teeth due to trauma**

K08.411 Partial loss of teeth due to trauma, class I

K08.412 Partial loss of teeth due to trauma, class II

K08.413 Partial loss of teeth due to trauma, class III

K08.414 Partial loss of teeth due to trauma, class IV

K08.419 Partial loss of teeth due to trauma, unspecified class

√6th **K08.42 Partial loss of teeth due to periodontal diseases**

K08.421 Partial loss of teeth due to periodontal diseases, class I

K08.422 Partial loss of teeth due to periodontal diseases, class II

K08.423 Partial loss of teeth due to periodontal diseases, class III

K08.424 Partial loss of teeth due to periodontal diseases, class IV

K08.429 Partial loss of teeth due to periodontal diseases, unspecified class

√6th **K08.43 Partial loss of teeth due to caries**

K08.431 Partial loss of teeth due to caries, class I

K08.432 Partial loss of teeth due to caries, class II

K08.433 Partial loss of teeth due to caries, class III

K08.434 Partial loss of teeth due to caries, class IV

K08.439 Partial loss of teeth due to caries, unspecified class

√6th **K08.49 Partial loss of teeth due to other specified cause**

K08.491 Partial loss of teeth due to other specified cause, class I

K08.492 Partial loss of teeth due to other specified cause, class II

K08.493 Partial loss of teeth due to other specified cause, class III

K08.494 Partial loss of teeth due to other specified cause, class IV

K08.499 Partial loss of teeth due to other specified cause, unspecified class

√5th **K08.5 Unsatisfactory restoration of tooth**
Defective bridge, crown, filling
Defective dental restoration
EXCLUDES 1 *dental restoration status (Z98.811)*
EXCLUDES 2 *endosseous dental implant failure (M27.6-)*
unsatisfactory endodontic treatment (M27.5-)

K08.50 Unsatisfactory restoration of tooth, unspecified
Defective dental restoration NOS

K08.51 Open restoration margins of tooth
Dental restoration failure of marginal integrity
Open margin on tooth restoration
Poor gingival margin to tooth restoration

K08.52 Unrepairable overhanging of dental restorative materials
Overhanging of tooth restoration

√6th **K08.53 Fractured dental restorative material**
EXCLUDES 1 *cracked tooth (K03.81)*
traumatic fracture of tooth (S02.5)

K08.530 Fractured dental restorative material without loss of material

K08.531 Fractured dental restorative material with loss of material

K08.539 Fractured dental restorative material, unspecified

K08.54 Contour of existing restoration of tooth biologically incompatible with oral health
Dental restoration failure of periodontal anatomical integrity
Unacceptable contours of existing restoration of tooth
Unacceptable morphology of existing restoration of tooth

K08.55 Allergy to existing dental restorative material
Use additional code to identify the specific type of allergy

K08.56 Poor aesthetic of existing restoration of tooth
Dental restoration aesthetically inadequate or displeasing

K08.59 Other unsatisfactory restoration of tooth
Other defective dental restoration

K08.8 Other specified disorders of teeth and supporting structures
Enlargement of alveolar ridge NOS
Irregular alveolar process
Toothache NOS

K08.9 Disorder of teeth and supporting structures, unspecified

K09 Cysts of oral region, not elsewhere classified
INCLUDES lesions showing histological features both of aneurysmal cyst and of another fibro-osseous lesion
EXCLUDES 2 *cysts of jaw (M27.0-, M27.4-)*
radicular cyst (K04.8)

K09.0 Developmental odontogenic cysts
Dentigerous cyst
Eruption cyst
Follicular cyst
Gingival cyst
Lateral periodontal cyst
Primordial cyst
EXCLUDES 2 *keratocysts (D16.4, D16.5)*
odontogenic keratocystic tumors (D16.4, D16.5)

K09.1 Developmental (nonodontogenic) cysts of oral region
Cyst (of) incisive canal
Cyst (of) palatine of papilla
Globulomaxillary cyst
Median palatal cyst
Nasoalveolar cyst
Nasolabial cyst
Nasopalatine duct cyst

K09.8 Other cysts of oral region, not elsewhere classified
Dermoid cyst
Epidermoid cyst
Lymphoepithelial cyst
Epstein's pearl

K09.9 Cyst of oral region, unspecified

K11 Diseases of salivary glands
Use additional code to identify:
alcohol abuse and dependence (F10.-)
exposure to environmental tobacco smoke (Z77.22)
exposure to tobacco smoke in the perinatal period (P96.81)
history of tobacco use (Z87.891)
occupational exposure to environmental tobacco smoke (Z57.31)
tobacco dependence (F17.-)
tobacco use (Z72.0)

K11.0 Atrophy of salivary gland

K11.1 Hypertrophy of salivary gland

K11.2 Sialoadenitis
Parotitis
EXCLUDES 1 *epidemic parotitis (B26.-)*
mumps (B26.-)
uveoparotid fever [Heerfordt] (D86.89)

K11.20 Sialoadenitis, unspecified

K11.21 Acute sialoadenitis
EXCLUDES 1 *acute recurrent sialoadenitis (K11.22)*

K11.22 Acute recurrent sialoadenitis

K11.23 Chronic sialoadenitis

K11.3 Abscess of salivary gland

K11.4 Fistula of salivary gland
EXCLUDES 1 *congenital fistula of salivary gland (Q38.4)*

K11.5 Sialolithiasis
Calculus of salivary gland or duct
Stone of salivary gland or duct

K11.6 Mucocele of salivary gland
Mucous extravasation cyst of salivary gland
Mucous retention cyst of salivary gland
Ranula

K11.7 Disturbances of salivary secretion
Hypoptyalism
Ptyalism
Xerostomia
EXCLUDES 2 *dry mouth NOS (R68.2)*

K11.8 Other diseases of salivary glands
Benign lymphoepithelial lesion of salivary gland
Mikulicz' disease
Necrotizing sialometaplasia
Sialectasia
Stenosis of salivary duct
Stricture of salivary duct
EXCLUDES 1 *sicca syndrome [Sjögren] (M35.0-)*

K11.9 Disease of salivary gland, unspecified
Sialoadenopathy NOS

K12 Stomatitis and related lesions
Use additional code to identify:
alcohol abuse and dependence (F10.-)
exposure to environmental tobacco smoke (Z77.22)
exposure to tobacco smoke in the perinatal period (P96.81)
history of tobacco use (Z87.891)
occupational exposure to environmental tobacco smoke (Z57.31)
tobacco dependence (F17.-)
tobacco use (Z72.0)
EXCLUDES 1 *cancrum oris (A69.0)*
cheilitis (K13.0)
gangrenous stomatitis (A69.0)
herpesviral [herpes simplex] gingivostomatitis (B00.2)
noma (A69.0)

K12.0 Recurrent oral aphthae
Aphthous stomatitis (major) (minor)
Bednar's aphthae
Periadenitis mucosa necrotica recurrens
Recurrent aphthous ulcer
Stomatitis herpetiformis

K12.1 Other forms of stomatitis
Stomatitis NOS
Denture stomatitis
Ulcerative stomatitis
Vesicular stomatitis
EXCLUDES 1 *acute necrotizing ulcerative stomatitis (A69.1)*
Vincent's stomatitis (A69.1)

K12.2 Cellulitis and abscess of mouth
Cellulitis of mouth (floor)
Submandibular abscess
EXCLUDES 2 *abscess of salivary gland (K11.3)*
abscess of tongue (K14.0)
periapical abscess (K04.6-K04.7)
periodontal abscess (K05.21)
peritonsillar abscess (J36)

K12.3 Oral mucositis (ulcerative)
Mucositis (oral) (oropharyneal)
EXCLUDES 2 *gastrointestinal mucositis (ulcerative) (K92.81)*
mucositis (ulcerative) of vagina and vulva (N76.81)
nasal mucositis (ulcerative) (J34.81)

K12.30 Oral mucositis (ulcerative), unspecified

K12.31 Oral mucositis (ulcerative) due to antineoplastic therapy
Use additional code for adverse effect, if applicable, to identify antineoplastic and immunosuppressive drugs (T45.1X5)
Use additional code for other antineoplastic therapy, such as:
radiological procedure and radiotherapy (Y84.2)

K12.32 Oral mucositis (ulcerative) due to other drugs
Use additional code for adverse effect, if applicable, to identify drug (T36-T50 with fifth or sixth character 5)

K12.33 Oral mucositis (ulcerative) due to radiation
Use additional external cause code (W88-W90, X39.0-) to identify cause

K12.39 Other oral mucositis (ulcerative)
Viral oral mucositis (ulcerative)

✓4th K13 Other diseases of lip and oral mucosa

INCLUDES epithelial disturbances of tongue

Use additional code to identify:
- alcohol abuse and dependence (F1Ø.-)
- exposure to environmental tobacco smoke (Z77.22)
- exposure to tobacco smoke in the perinatal period (P96.81)
- history of tobacco use (Z87.891)
- occupational exposure to environmental tobacco smoke (Z57.31)
- tobacco dependence (F17.-)
- tobacco use (Z72.Ø)

EXCLUDES 2 *certain disorders of gingiva and edentulous alveolar ridge (KØ5-KØ6)*
cysts of oral region (KØ9.-)
diseases of tongue (K14.-)
stomatitis and related lesions (K12.-)

K13.Ø Diseases of lips
- Abscess of lips
- Angular cheilitis
- Cellulitis of lips
- Cheilitis NOS
- Cheilodynia
- Cheilosis
- Exfoliative cheilitis
- Fistula of lips
- Glandular cheilitis
- Hypertrophy of lips
- Perlèche NEC

EXCLUDES 1 *ariboflavinosis (E53.Ø)*
cheilitis due to radiation-related disorders (L55-L59)
congenital fistula of lips (Q38.Ø)
congenital hypertrophy of lips (Q18.6)
Perlèche due to candidiasis (B37.83)
Perlèche due to riboflavin deficiency (E53.Ø)

K13.1 Cheek and lip biting

✓5th K13.2 Leukoplakia and other disturbances of oral epithelium, including tongue

EXCLUDES 1 *carcinoma in situ of oral epithelium (DØØ.Ø-)*
hairy leukoplakia (K13.3)

K13.21 Leukoplakia of oral mucosa, including tongue
- Leukokeratosis of oral mucosa
- Leukoplakia of gingiva, lips, tongue

EXCLUDES 1 *hairy leukoplakia (K13.3)*
leukokeratosis nicotina palati (K13.24)

K13.22 Minimal keratinized residual ridge mucosa
- Minimal keratinization of alveolar ridge mucosa

K13.23 Excessive keratinized residual ridge mucosa
- Excessive keratinization of alveolar ridge mucosa

K13.24 Leukokeratosis nicotina palati
- Smoker's palate

K13.29 Other disturbances of oral epithelium, including tongue
- Erythroplakia of mouth or tongue
- Focal epithelial hyperplasia of mouth or tongue
- Leukoedema of mouth or tongue
- Other oral epithelium disturbances

K13.3 Hairy leukoplakia

K13.4 Granuloma and granuloma-like lesions of oral mucosa
- Eosinophilic granuloma
- Granuloma pyogenicum
- Verrucous xanthoma

K13.5 Oral submucous fibrosis
- Submucous fibrosis of tongue

K13.6 Irritative hyperplasia of oral mucosa

EXCLUDES 2 *irritative hyperplasia of edentulous ridge [denture hyperplasia] (KØ6.2)*

✓5th K13.7 Other and unspecified lesions of oral mucosa

K13.7Ø Unspecified lesions of oral mucosa

K13.79 Other lesions of oral mucosa
- Focal oral mucinosis

✓4th K14 Diseases of tongue

Use additional code to identify:
- alcohol abuse and dependence (F1Ø.-)
- exposure to environmental tobacco smoke (Z77.22)
- history of tobacco use (Z87.891)
- occupational exposure to environmental tobacco smoke (Z57.31)
- tobacco dependence (F17.-)
- tobacco use (Z72.Ø)

EXCLUDES 2 *erythroplakia (K13.29)*
focal epithelial hyperplasia (K13.29)
leukedema of tongue (K13.29)
leukoplakia of tongue (K13.21)
hairy leukoplakia (K13.3)
macroglossia (congenital) (Q38.2)
submucous fibrosis of tongue (K13.5)

K14.Ø Glossitis
- Abscess of tongue
- Ulceration (traumatic) of tongue

EXCLUDES 1 *atrophic glossitis (K14.4)*

K14.1 Geographic tongue
- Benign migratory glossitis
- Glossitis areata exfoliativa

K14.2 Median rhomboid glossitis

K14.3 Hypertrophy of tongue papillae
- Black hairy tongue
- Coated tongue
- Hypertrophy of foliate papillae
- Lingua villosa nigra

K14.4 Atrophy of tongue papillae
- Atrophic glossitis

K14.5 Plicated tongue
- Fissured tongue
- Furrowed tongue
- Scrotal tongue

EXCLUDES 1 *fissured tongue, congenital (Q38.3)*

K14.6 Glossodynia
- Glossopyrosis
- Painful tongue

K14.8 Other diseases of tongue
- Atrophy of tongue
- Crenated tongue
- Enlargement of tongue
- Glossocele
- Glossoptosis
- Hypertrophy of tongue

K14.9 Disease of tongue, unspecified
- Glossopathy NOS

Diseases of esophagus, stomach and duodenum (K2Ø-K31)

EXCLUDES 2 *hiatus hernia (K44.-)*

✓4th K2Ø Esophagitis

Use additional code to identify:
- alcohol abuse and dependence (F1Ø.-)

EXCLUDES 1 *erosion of esophagus (K22.1-)*
esophagitis with gastro-esophageal reflux disease (K21.Ø)
reflux esophagitis (K21.Ø)
ulcerative esophagitis (K22.1-)

EXCLUDES 2 *eosinophilic gastritis or gastroenteritis (K52.81)*

K2Ø.Ø Eosinophilic esophagitis

K2Ø.8 Other esophagitis
- Abscess of esophagus

K2Ø.9 Esophagitis, unspecified
- Esophagitis NOS

✓4th K21 Gastro-esophageal reflux disease

EXCLUDES 1 *newborn esophageal reflux (P78.83)*

K21.Ø Gastro-esophageal reflux disease with esophagitis
- Reflux esophagitis

K21.9 Gastro-esophageal reflux disease without esophagitis
- Esophageal reflux NOS

✓4th K22 Other diseases of esophagus

EXCLUDES 2 *esophageal varices (I85.-)*

K22.Ø Achalasia of cardia
- Achalasia NOS
- Cardiospasm

EXCLUDES 1 *congenital cardiospasm (Q39.5)*

✓5th **K22.1 Ulcer of esophagus**
Barrett's ulcer
Erosion of esophagus
Fungal ulcer of esophagus
Peptic ulcer of esophagus
Ulcer of esophagus due to ingestion of chemicals
Ulcer of esophagus due to ingestion of drugs and medicaments
Ulcerative esophagitis
Code first poisoning due to drug or toxin, if applicable (T36-T65 with fifth or sixth character 1-4 or 6)
Use additional code for adverse effect, if applicable, to identify drug (T36-T50 with fifth or sixth character 5)
EXCLUDES 1 *Barrett's esophagus (K22.7-)*

K22.10 Ulcer of esophagus without bleeding
Ulcer of esophagus NOS

K22.11 Ulcer of esophagus with bleeding
EXCLUDES 2 *bleeding esophageal varices (I85.01, I85.11)*

K22.2 Esophageal obstruction
Compression of esophagus
Constriction of esophagus
Stenosis of esophagus
Stricture of esophagus
EXCLUDES 1 *congenital stenosis or stricture of esophagus (Q39.3)*

K22.3 Perforation of esophagus
Rupture of esophagus
EXCLUDES 1 *traumatic perforation of (thoracic) esophagus (S27.8-)*

K22.4 Dyskinesia of esophagus
Corkscrew esophagus
Diffuse esophageal spasm
Spasm of esophagus
EXCLUDES 1 *cardiospasm (K22.0)*

K22.5 Diverticulum of esophagus, acquired
Esophageal pouch, acquired
EXCLUDES 1 *diverticulum of esophagus (congenital) (Q39.6)*

K22.6 Gastro-esophageal laceration-hemorrhage syndrome
Mallory-Weiss syndrome

✓5th **K22.7 Barrett's esophagus**
Barrett's disease
Barrett's syndrome
EXCLUDES 1 *Barrett's ulcer (K22.1)*
malignant neoplasm of esophagus (C15.-)

K22.70 Barrett's esophagus without dysplasia
Barrett's esophagus NOS

✓6th **K22.71 Barrett's esophagus with dysplasia**
K22.710 Barrett's esophagus with low grade dysplasia
K22.711 Barrett's esophagus with high grade dysplasia
K22.719 Barrett's esophagus with dysplasia, unspecified

K22.8 Other specified diseases of esophagus
Hemorrhage of esophagus NOS
EXCLUDES 2 *esophageal varices (I85.-)*
Paterson-Kelly syndrome (D50.1)

K22.9 Disease of esophagus, unspecified

K23 Disorders of esophagus in diseases classified elsewhere
Code first underlying disease, such as:
congenital syphilis (A50.5)
EXCLUDES 1 *late syphilis (A52.79)*
megaesophagus due to Chagas' disease (B57.31)
tuberculosis (A18.83)

✓4th **K25 Gastric ulcer**
INCLUDES erosion (acute) of stomach
pylorus ulcer (peptic)
stomach ulcer (peptic)
Use additional code to identify:
alcohol abuse and dependence (F10.-)
EXCLUDES 1 *acute gastritis (K29.0-)*
peptic ulcer NOS (K27.-)

K25.0 Acute gastric ulcer with hemorrhage
K25.1 Acute gastric ulcer with perforation
K25.2 Acute gastric ulcer with both hemorrhage and perforation
K25.3 Acute gastric ulcer without hemorrhage or perforation
K25.4 Chronic or unspecified gastric ulcer with hemorrhage
K25.5 Chronic or unspecified gastric ulcer with perforation
K25.6 Chronic or unspecified gastric ulcer with both hemorrhage and perforation
K25.7 Chronic gastric ulcer without hemorrhage or perforation
K25.9 Gastric ulcer, unspecified as acute or chronic, without hemorrhage or perforation

✓4th **K26 Duodenal ulcer**
INCLUDES erosion (acute) of duodenum
duodenum ulcer (peptic)
postpyloric ulcer (peptic)
Use additional code to identify:
alcohol abuse and dependence (F10.-)
EXCLUDES 1 *peptic ulcer NOS (K27.-)*

K26.0 Acute duodenal ulcer with hemorrhage
K26.1 Acute duodenal ulcer with perforation
K26.2 Acute duodenal ulcer with both hemorrhage and perforation
K26.3 Acute duodenal ulcer without hemorrhage or perforation
K26.4 Chronic or unspecified duodenal ulcer with hemorrhage
K26.5 Chronic or unspecified duodenal ulcer with perforation
K26.6 Chronic or unspecified duodenal ulcer with both hemorrhage and perforation
K26.7 Chronic duodenal ulcer without hemorrhage or perforation
K26.9 Duodenal ulcer, unspecified as acute or chronic, without hemorrhage or perforation

✓4th **K27 Peptic ulcer, site unspecified**
INCLUDES gastroduodenal ulcer NOS
peptic ulcer NOS
Use additional code to identify:
alcohol abuse and dependence (F10.-)
EXCLUDES 1 *peptic ulcer of newborn (P78.82)*

K27.0 Acute peptic ulcer, site unspecified, with hemorrhage
K27.1 Acute peptic ulcer, site unspecified, with perforation
K27.2 Acute peptic ulcer, site unspecified, with both hemorrhage and perforation
K27.3 Acute peptic ulcer, site unspecified, without hemorrhage or perforation
K27.4 Chronic or unspecified peptic ulcer, site unspecified, with hemorrhage
K27.5 Chronic or unspecified peptic ulcer, site unspecified, with perforation
K27.6 Chronic or unspecified peptic ulcer, site unspecified, with both hemorrhage and perforation
K27.7 Chronic peptic ulcer, site unspecified, without hemorrhage or perforation
K27.9 Peptic ulcer, site unspecified, unspecified as acute or chronic, without hemorrhage or perforation

✓4th **K28 Gastrojejunal ulcer**
INCLUDES anastomotic ulcer (peptic) or erosion
gastrocolic ulcer (peptic) or erosion
gastrointestinal ulcer (peptic) or erosion
gastrojejunal ulcer (peptic) or erosion
jejunal ulcer (peptic) or erosion
marginal ulcer (peptic) or erosion
stomal ulcer (peptic) or erosion
Use additional code to identify:
alcohol abuse and dependence (F10.-)
EXCLUDES 1 *primary ulcer of small intestine (K63.3)*

K28.0 Acute gastrojejunal ulcer with hemorrhage
K28.1 Acute gastrojejunal ulcer with perforation
K28.2 Acute gastrojejunal ulcer with both hemorrhage and perforation
K28.3 Acute gastrojejunal ulcer without hemorrhage or perforation
K28.4 Chronic or unspecified gastrojejunal ulcer with hemorrhage
K28.5 Chronic or unspecified gastrojejunal ulcer with perforation
K28.6 Chronic or unspecified gastrojejunal ulcer with both hemorrhage and perforation
K28.7 Chronic gastrojejunal ulcer without hemorrhage or perforation
K28.9 Gastrojejunal ulcer, unspecified as acute or chronic, without hemorrhage or perforation

✓4th **K29 Gastritis and duodenitis**
EXCLUDES 1 *eosinophilic gastritis or gastroenteritis (K52.81)*
Zollinger-Ellison syndrome (E16.4)

✓5th **K29.Ø Acute gastritis**
Use additional code to identify:
alcohol abuse and dependence (F1Ø.-)
EXCLUDES 1 *erosion (acute) of stomach (K25.-)*
K29.ØØ Acute gastritis without bleeding
K29.Ø1 Acute gastritis with bleeding

✓5th **K29.2 Alcoholic gastritis**
Use additional code to identify:
alcohol abuse and dependence (F1Ø.-)
K29.2Ø Alcoholic gastritis without bleeding
K29.21 Alcoholic gastritis with bleeding

✓5th **K29.3 Chronic superficial gastritis**
K29.3Ø Chronic superficial gastritis without bleeding
K29.31 Chronic superficial gastritis with bleeding

✓5th **K29.4 Chronic atrophic gastritis**
Gastric atrophy
K29.4Ø Chronic atrophic gastritis without bleeding
K29.41 Chronic atrophic gastritis with bleeding

✓5th **K29.5 Unspecified chronic gastritis**
Chronic antral gastritis
Chronic fundal gastritis
K29.5Ø Unspecified chronic gastritis without bleeding
K29.51 Unspecified chronic gastritis with bleeding

✓5th **K29.6 Other gastritis**
Giant hypertrophic gastritis
Granulomatous gastritis
Ménétrier's disease
K29.6Ø Other gastritis without bleeding
K29.61 Other gastritis with bleeding

✓5th **K29.7 Gastritis, unspecified**
K29.7Ø Gastritis, unspecified, without bleeding
K29.71 Gastritis, unspecified, with bleeding

✓5th **K29.8 Duodenitis**
K29.8Ø Duodenitis without bleeding
K29.81 Duodenitis with bleeding

✓5th **K29.9 Gastroduodenitis, unspecified**
K29.9Ø Gastroduodenitis, unspecified, without bleeding
K29.91 Gastroduodenitis, unspecified, with bleeding

K3Ø Functional dyspepsia
Indigestion
EXCLUDES 1 *dyspepsia NOS (R1Ø.13)*
heartburn (R12)
nervous dyspepsia (F45.8)
neurotic dyspepsia (F45.8)
psychogenic dyspepsia (F45.8)

✓4th **K31 Other diseases of stomach and duodenum**
INCLUDES functional disorders of stomach
EXCLUDES 2 *diabetic gastroparesis (EØ8.43, EØ9.43, E1Ø.43, E11.43, E13.43)*
diverticulum of duodenum (K57.ØØ-K57.13)

K31.Ø Acute dilatation of stomach
Acute distention of stomach

K31.1 Adult hypertrophic pyloric stenosis
Pyloric stenosis NOS
EXCLUDES 1 *congenital or infantile pyloric stenosis (Q4Ø.Ø)*

K31.2 Hourglass stricture and stenosis of stomach
EXCLUDES 1 *congenital hourglass stomach (Q4Ø.2)*
hourglass contraction of stomach (K31.89)

K31.3 Pylorospasm, not elsewhere classified
EXCLUDES 1 *congenital or infantile pylorospasm (Q4Ø.Ø)*
neurotic pylorospasm (F45.8)
psychogenic pylorospasm (F45.8)

K31.4 Gastric diverticulum
EXCLUDES 1 *congenital diverticulum of stomach (Q4Ø.2)*

K31.5 Obstruction of duodenum
Constriction of duodenum
Duodenal ileus (chronic)
Stenosis of duodenum
Stricture of duodenum
Volvulus of duodenum
EXCLUDES 1 *congenital stenosis of duodenum (Q41.Ø)*

K31.6 Fistula of stomach and duodenum
Gastrocolic fistula
Gastrojejunocolic fistula

K31.7 Polyp of stomach and duodenum
EXCLUDES 1 *adenomatous polyp of stomach (D13.1)*

✓5th **K31.8 Other specified diseases of stomach and duodenum**
✓6th **K31.81 Angiodysplasia of stomach and duodenum**
K31.811 Angiodysplasia of stomach and duodenum with bleeding
K31.819 Angiodysplasia of stomach and duodenum without bleeding
Angiodysplasia of stomach and duodenum NOS
K31.82 Dieulafoy lesion (hemorrhagic) of stomach and duodenum
EXCLUDES 2 *Dieulafoy lesion of intestine (K63.81)*
K31.83 Achlorhydria
K31.84 Gastroparesis
Gastroparalysis
Code first underlying disease, if known, such as:
anorexia nervosa (F5Ø.Ø-)
diabetes mellitus (EØ8.43, EØ9.43, E1Ø.43, E11.43, E13.43)
scleroderma (M34.-)
K31.89 Other diseases of stomach and duodenum

K31.9 Disease of stomach and duodenum, unspecified

Diseases of appendix (K35-K38)

✓4th **K35 Acute appendicitis**

K35.2 Acute appendicitis with generalized peritonitis
Appendicitis (acute) with generalized (diffuse) peritonitis following rupture or perforation of appendix
Appendicitis with peritonitis NOS
Perforated appendix NOS
Ruptured appendix NOS

K35.3 Acute appendicitis with localized peritonitis
Acute appendicitis with localized peritonitis with or without rupture or perforation of appendix
Acute appendicitis with peritoneal abscess

✓5th **K35.8 Other and unspecified acute appendicitis**
K35.8Ø Unspecified acute appendicitis
Acute appendicitis NOS
Acute appendicitis without (localized) (generalized) peritonitis
K35.89 Other acute appendicitis

K36 Other appendicitis
Chronic appendicitis
Recurrent appendicitis

K37 Unspecified appendicitis
EXCLUDES 1 *unspecified appendicitis with peritonitis (K35.2-K35.3)*

✓4th **K38 Other diseases of appendix**
K38.Ø Hyperplasia of appendix
K38.1 Appendicular concretions
Fecalith of appendix
Stercolith of appendix
K38.2 Diverticulum of appendix
K38.3 Fistula of appendix
K38.8 Other specified diseases of appendix
Intussusception of appendix
K38.9 Disease of appendix, unspecified

Hernia (K40-K46)

NOTE Hernia with both gangrene and obstruction is classified to hernia with gangrene.

INCLUDES acquired hernia
congenital [except diaphragmatic or hiatus] hernia
recurrent hernia

K40 Inguinal hernia

INCLUDES bubonocele
direct inguinal hernia
double inguinal hernia
indirect inguinal hernia
inguinal hernia NOS
oblique inguinal hernia
scrotal hernia

K40.0 Bilateral inguinal hernia, with obstruction, without gangrene
Inguinal hernia (bilateral) causing obstruction without gangrene
Incarcerated inguinal hernia (bilateral) without gangrene
Irreducible inguinal hernia (bilateral) without gangrene
Strangulated inguinal hernia (bilateral) without gangrene

K40.00 Bilateral inguinal hernia, with obstruction, without gangrene, not specified as recurrent
Bilateral inguinal hernia, with obstruction, without gangrene NOS

K40.01 Bilateral inguinal hernia, with obstruction, without gangrene, recurrent

K40.1 Bilateral inguinal hernia, with gangrene

K40.10 Bilateral inguinal hernia, with gangrene, not specified as recurrent
Bilateral inguinal hernia, with gangrene NOS

K40.11 Bilateral inguinal hernia, with gangrene, recurrent

K40.2 Bilateral inguinal hernia, without obstruction or gangrene

K40.20 Bilateral inguinal hernia, without obstruction or gangrene, not specified as recurrent
Bilateral inguinal hernia NOS

K40.21 Bilateral inguinal hernia, without obstruction or gangrene, recurrent

K40.3 Unilateral inguinal hernia, with obstruction, without gangrene
Inguinal hernia (unilateral) causing obstruction without gangrene
Incarcerated inguinal hernia (unilateral) without gangrene
Irreducible inguinal hernia (unilateral) without gangrene
Strangulated inguinal hernia (unilateral) without gangrene

K40.30 Unilateral inguinal hernia, with obstruction, without gangrene, not specified as recurrent
Inguinal hernia, with obstruction NOS
Unilateral inguinal hernia, with obstruction, without gangrene NOS

K40.31 Unilateral inguinal hernia, with obstruction, without gangrene, recurrent

K40.4 Unilateral inguinal hernia, with gangrene

K40.40 Unilateral inguinal hernia, with gangrene, not specified as recurrent
Inguinal hernia with gangrene NOS
Unilateral inguinal hernia with gangrene NOS

K40.41 Unilateral inguinal hernia, with gangrene, recurrent

K40.9 Unilateral inguinal hernia, without obstruction or gangrene

K40.90 Unilateral inguinal hernia, without obstruction or gangrene, not specified as recurrent
Inguinal hernia NOS
Unilateral inguinal hernia NOS

K40.91 Unilateral inguinal hernia, without obstruction or gangrene, recurrent

K41 Femoral hernia

K41.0 Bilateral femoral hernia, with obstruction, without gangrene
Femoral hernia (bilateral) causing obstruction, without gangrene
Incarcerated femoral hernia (bilateral), without gangrene
Irreducible femoral hernia (bilateral), without gangrene
Strangulated femoral hernia (bilateral), without gangrene

K41.00 Bilateral femoral hernia, with obstruction, without gangrene, not specified as recurrent
Bilateral femoral hernia, with obstruction, without gangrene NOS

K41.01 Bilateral femoral hernia, with obstruction, without gangrene, recurrent

K41.1 Bilateral femoral hernia, with gangrene

K41.10 Bilateral femoral hernia, with gangrene, not specified as recurrent
Bilateral femoral hernia, with gangrene NOS

K41.11 Bilateral femoral hernia, with gangrene, recurrent

K41.2 Bilateral femoral hernia, without obstruction or gangrene

K41.20 Bilateral femoral hernia, without obstruction or gangrene, not specified as recurrent
Bilateral femoral hernia NOS

K41.21 Bilateral femoral hernia, without obstruction or gangrene, recurrent

K41.3 Unilateral femoral hernia, with obstruction, without gangrene
Femoral hernia (unilateral) causing obstruction, without gangrene
Incarcerated femoral hernia (unilateral), without gangrene
Irreducible femoral hernia (unilateral), without gangrene
Strangulated femoral hernia (unilateral), without gangrene

K41.30 Unilateral femoral hernia, with obstruction, without gangrene, not specified as recurrent
Femoral hernia, with obstruction NOS
Unilateral femoral hernia, with obstruction NOS

K41.31 Unilateral femoral hernia, with obstruction, without gangrene, recurrent

K41.4 Unilateral femoral hernia, with gangrene

K41.40 Unilateral femoral hernia, with gangrene, not specified as recurrent
Femoral hernia, with gangrene NOS
Unilateral femoral hernia, with gangrene NOS

K41.41 Unilateral femoral hernia, with gangrene, recurrent

K41.9 Unilateral femoral hernia, without obstruction or gangrene

K41.90 Unilateral femoral hernia, without obstruction or gangrene, not specified as recurrent
Femoral hernia NOS
Unilateral femoral hernia NOS

K41.91 Unilateral femoral hernia, without obstruction or gangrene, recurrent

K42 Umbilical hernia

INCLUDES paraumbilical hernia
EXCLUDES 1 *omphalocele (Q79.2)*

K42.0 Umbilical hernia with obstruction, without gangrene
Umbilical hernia causing obstruction, without gangrene
Incarcerated umbilical hernia, without gangrene
Irreducible umbilical hernia, without gangrene
Strangulated umbilical hernia, without gangrene

K42.1 Umbilical hernia with gangrene
Gangrenous umbilical hernia

K42.9 Umbilical hernia without obstruction or gangrene
Umbilical hernia NOS

K43 Ventral hernia

K43.0 Incisional hernia with obstruction, without gangrene
Incisional hernia causing obstruction, without gangrene
Incarcerated incisional hernia, without gangrene
Irreducible incisional hernia, without gangrene
Strangulated incisional hernia, without gangrene

K43.1 Incisional hernia with gangrene
Gangrenous incisional hernia

K43.2 Incisional hernia without obstruction or gangrene
Incisional hernia NOS

K43.3 Parastomal hernia with obstruction, without gangrene
Incarcerated parastomal hernia, without gangrene
Irreducible parastomal hernia, without gangrene
Parastomal hernia causing obstruction, without gangrene
Strangulated parastomal hernia, without gangrene

K43.4 Parastomal hernia with gangrene
Gangrenous parastomal hernia

K43.5 Parastomal hernia without obstruction or gangrene
Parastomal hernia NOS

K43.6 Other and unspecified ventral hernia with obstruction, without gangrene
Epigastric hernia causing obstruction, without gangrene
Hypogastric hernia causing obstruction, without gangrene
Incarcerated epigastric hernia without gangrene
Incarcerated hypogastric hernia without gangrene
Incarcerated midline hernia without gangrene
Incarcerated spigelian hernia without gangrene
Incarcerated subxiphoid hernia without gangrene
Irreducible epigastric hernia without gangrene
Irreducible hypogastric hernia without gangrene
Irreducible midline hernia without gangrene
Irreducible spigelian hernia without gangrene
Irreducible subxiphoid hernia without gangrene
Midline hernia causing obstruction, without gangrene
Spigelian hernia causing obstruction, without gangrene
Strangulated epigastric hernia without gangrene
Strangulated hypogastric hernia without gangrene
Strangulated midline hernia without gangrene
Strangulated spigelian hernia without gangrene
Strangulated subxiphoid hernia without gangrene
Subxiphoid hernia causing obstruction, without gangrene

K43.7 Other and unspecified ventral hernia with gangrene
Any condition listed under K43.6 specified as gangrenous

K43.9 Ventral hernia without obstruction or gangrene
Epigastric hernia
Ventral hernia NOS

✓4th K44 Diaphragmatic hernia
INCLUDES hiatus hernia (esophageal) (sliding)
paraesophageal hernia
EXCLUDES 1 *congenital diaphragmatic hernia (Q79.Ø)*
congenital hiatus hernia (Q4Ø.1)

K44.Ø Diaphragmatic hernia with obstruction, without gangrene
Diaphragmatic hernia causing obstruction
Incarcerated diaphragmatic hernia
Irreducible diaphragmatic hernia
Strangulated diaphragmatic hernia

K44.1 Diaphragmatic hernia with gangrene
Gangrenous diaphragmatic hernia

K44.9 Diaphragmatic hernia without obstruction or gangrene
Diaphragmatic hernia NOS

✓4th K45 Other abdominal hernia
INCLUDES abdominal hernia, specified site NEC
lumbar hernia
obturator hernia
pudendal hernia
retroperitoneal hernia
sciatic hernia

K45.Ø Other specified abdominal hernia with obstruction, without gangrene
Other specified abdominal hernia causing obstruction
Other specified incarcerated abdominal hernia
Other specified irreducible abdominal hernia
Other specified strangulated abdominal hernia

K45.1 Other specified abdominal hernia with gangrene
Any condition listed under K4 specified as gangrenous

K45.8 Other specified abdominal hernia without obstruction or gangrene

✓4th K46 Unspecified abdominal hernia
INCLUDES enterocele
epiplocele
hernia NOS
interstitial hernia
intestinal hernia
intra-abdominal hernia
EXCLUDES 1 *vaginal enterocele (N81.5)*

K46.Ø Unspecified abdominal hernia with obstruction, without gangrene
Unspecified abdominal hernia causing obstruction
Unspecified incarcerated abdominal hernia
Unspecified irreducible abdominal hernia
Unspecified strangulated abdominal hernia

K46.1 Unspecified abdominal hernia with gangrene
Any condition listed under K46 specified as gangrenous

K46.9 Unspecified abdominal hernia without obstruction or gangrene
Abdominal hernia NOS

Noninfective enteritis and colitis (K5Ø-K52)

INCLUDES noninfective inflammatory bowel disease
EXCLUDES 1 *irritable bowel syndrome (K58.-)*
megacolon (K59.3)

✓4th K5Ø Crohn's disease [regional enteritis]
INCLUDES granulomatous enteritis
EXCLUDES 1 *ulcerative colitis (K51.-)*
Use additional code to identify manifestations, such as:
pyoderma gangrenosum (L88)

✓5th K5Ø.Ø Crohn's disease of small intestine
Crohn's disease [regional enteritis] of duodenum
Crohn's disease [regional enteritis] of ileum
Crohn's disease [regional enteritis] of jejunum
Regional ileitis
Terminal ileitis
EXCLUDES 1 *Crohn's disease of both small and large intestine (K5Ø.8-)*

K5Ø.ØØ Crohn's disease of small intestine without complications

✓6th K5Ø.Ø1 Crohn's disease of small intestine with complications

K5Ø.Ø11 Crohn's disease of small intestine with rectal bleeding

K5Ø.Ø12 Crohn's disease of small intestine with intestinal obstruction

K5Ø.Ø13 Crohn's disease of small intestine with fistula

K5Ø.Ø14 Crohn's disease of small intestine with abscess

K5Ø.Ø18 Crohn's disease of small intestine with other complication

K5Ø.Ø19 Crohn's disease of small intestine with unspecified complications

✓5th K5Ø.1 Crohn's disease of large intestine
Crohn's disease [regional enteritis] of colon
Crohn's disease [regional enteritis] of large bowel
Crohn's disease [regional enteritis] of rectum
Granulomatous colitis
Regional colitis
EXCLUDES 1 *Crohn's disease of both small and large intestine (K5Ø.8)*

K5Ø.1Ø Crohn's disease of large intestine without complications

✓6th K5Ø.11 Crohn's disease of large intestine with complications

K5Ø.111 Crohn's disease of large intestine with rectal bleeding

K5Ø.112 Crohn's disease of large intestine with intestinal obstruction

K5Ø.113 Crohn's disease of large intestine with fistula

K5Ø.114 Crohn's disease of large intestine with abscess

K5Ø.118 Crohn's disease of large intestine with other complication

K5Ø.119 Crohn's disease of large intestine with unspecified complications

✓5th K5Ø.8 Crohn's disease of both small and large intestine

K5Ø.8Ø Crohn's disease of both small and large intestine without complications

✓6th K5Ø.81 Crohn's disease of both small and large intestine with complications

K5Ø.811 Crohn's disease of both small and large intestine with rectal bleeding

K5Ø.812 Crohn's disease of both small and large intestine with intestinal obstruction

K5Ø.813 Crohn's disease of both small and large intestine with fistula

K5Ø.814 Crohn's disease of both small and large intestine with abscess

K5Ø.818 Crohn's disease of both small and large intestine with other complication

K5Ø.819 Crohn's disease of both small and large intestine with unspecified complications

☑5th **K50.9 Crohn's disease, unspecified**

K50.90 Crohn's disease, unspecified, without complications
Crohn's disease NOS
Regional enteritis NOS

☑6th **K50.91 Crohn's disease, unspecified, with complications**

K50.911 Crohn's disease, unspecified, with rectal bleeding

K50.912 Crohn's disease, unspecified, with intestinal obstruction

K50.913 Crohn's disease, unspecified, with fistula

K50.914 Crohn's disease, unspecified, with abscess

K50.918 Crohn's disease, unspecified, with other complication

K50.919 Crohn's disease, unspecified, with unspecified complications

☑4th **K51 Ulcerative colitis**

Use additional code to identify manifestations, such as:
pyoderma gangrenosum (L88)

EXCLUDES 1 *Crohn's disease [regional enteritis] (K50.-)*

☑5th **K51.0 Ulcerative (chronic) pancolitis**
Backwash ileitis

K51.00 Ulcerative (chronic) pancolitis without complications
Ulcerative (chronic) pancolitis NOS

☑6th **K51.01 Ulcerative (chronic) pancolitis with complications**

K51.011 Ulcerative (chronic) pancolitis with rectal bleeding

K51.012 Ulcerative (chronic) pancolitis with intestinal obstruction

K51.013 Ulcerative (chronic) pancolitis with fistula

K51.014 Ulcerative (chronic) pancolitis with abscess

K51.018 Ulcerative (chronic) pancolitis with other complication

K51.019 Ulcerative (chronic) pancolitis with unspecified complications

☑5th **K51.2 Ulcerative (chronic) proctitis**

K51.20 Ulcerative (chronic) proctitis without complications
Ulcerative (chronic) proctitis NOS

☑6th **K51.21 Ulcerative (chronic) proctitis with complications**

K51.211 Ulcerative (chronic) proctitis with rectal bleeding

K51.212 Ulcerative (chronic) proctitis with intestinal obstruction

K51.213 Ulcerative (chronic) proctitis with fistula

K51.214 Ulcerative (chronic) proctitis with abscess

K51.218 Ulcerative (chronic) proctitis with other complication

K51.219 Ulcerative (chronic) proctitis with unspecified complications

☑5th **K51.3 Ulcerative (chronic) rectosigmoiditis**

K51.30 Ulcerative (chronic) rectosigmoiditis without complications
Ulcerative (chronic) rectosigmoiditis NOS

☑6th **K51.31 Ulcerative (chronic) rectosigmoiditis with complications**

K51.311 Ulcerative (chronic) rectosigmoiditis with rectal bleeding

K51.312 Ulcerative (chronic) rectosigmoiditis with intestinal obstruction

K51.313 Ulcerative (chronic) rectosigmoiditis with fistula

K51.314 Ulcerative (chronic) rectosigmoiditis with abscess

K51.318 Ulcerative (chronic) rectosigmoiditis with other complication

K51.319 Ulcerative (chronic) rectosigmoiditis with unspecified complications

☑5th **K51.4 Inflammatory polyps of colon**

EXCLUDES 1 *adenomatous polyp of colon (D12.6)*
polyposis of colon (D12.6)
polyps of colon NOS (K63.5)

K51.40 Inflammatory polyps of colon without complications
Inflammatory polyps of colon NOS

☑6th **K51.41 Inflammatory polyps of colon with complications**

K51.411 Inflammatory polyps of colon with rectal bleeding

K51.412 Inflammatory polyps of colon with intestinal obstruction

K51.413 Inflammatory polyps of colon with fistula

K51.414 Inflammatory polyps of colon with abscess

K51.418 Inflammatory polyps of colon with other complication

K51.419 Inflammatory polyps of colon with unspecified complications

☑5th **K51.5 Left sided colitis**
Left hemicolitis

K51.50 Left sided colitis without complications
Left sided colitis NOS

☑6th **K51.51 Left sided colitis with complications**

K51.511 Left sided colitis with rectal bleeding

K51.512 Left sided colitis with intestinal obstruction

K51.513 Left sided colitis with fistula

K51.514 Left sided colitis with abscess

K51.518 Left sided colitis with other complication

K51.519 Left sided colitis with unspecified complications

☑5th **K51.8 Other ulcerative colitis**

K51.80 Other ulcerative colitis without complications

☑6th **K51.81 Other ulcerative colitis with complications**

K51.811 Other ulcerative colitis with rectal bleeding

K51.812 Other ulcerative colitis with intestinal obstruction

K51.813 Other ulcerative colitis with fistula

K51.814 Other ulcerative colitis with abscess

K51.818 Other ulcerative colitis with other complication

K51.819 Other ulcerative colitis with unspecified complications

☑5th **K51.9 Ulcerative colitis, unspecified**

K51.90 Ulcerative colitis, unspecified, without complications

☑6th **K51.91 Ulcerative colitis, unspecified, with complications**

K51.911 Ulcerative colitis, unspecified with rectal bleeding

K51.912 Ulcerative colitis, unspecified with intestinal obstruction

K51.913 Ulcerative colitis, unspecified with fistula

K51.914 Ulcerative colitis, unspecified with abscess

K51.918 Ulcerative colitis, unspecified with other complication

K51.919 Ulcerative colitis, unspecified with unspecified complications

☑4th **K52 Other and unspecified noninfective gastroenteritis and colitis**

K52.0 Gastroenteritis and colitis due to radiation

K52.1 Toxic gastroenteritis and colitis
Drug-induced gastroenteritis and colitis
Code first (T51-T65) to identify toxic agent
Use additional code for adverse effect, if applicable, to identify drug (T36-T50 with fifth or sixth character 5)

K52.2 Allergic and dietetic gastroenteritis and colitis
Food hypersensitivity gastroenteritis or colitis
Use additional code to identify type of food allergy (Z91.01-, Z91.02-)

✓5th **K52.8 Other specified noninfective gastroenteritis and colitis**
K52.81 Eosinophilic gastritis or gastroenteritis
Eosinophilic enteritis
EXCLUDES 1 *eosinophilic esophagitis (K20.0)*
K52.82 Eosinophilic colitis
K52.89 Other specified noninfective gastroenteritis and colitis
Collagenous colitis
Lymphocytic colitis
Microscopic colitis (collagenous or lymphocytic)
K52.9 Noninfective gastroenteritis and colitis, unspecified
Colitis NOS
Enteritis NOS
Gastroenteritis NOS
Ileitis NOS
Jejunitis NOS
Sigmoiditis NOS
EXCLUDES 1 *diarrhea NOS (R19.7)*
functional diarrhea (K59.1)
infectious gastroenteritis and colitis NOS (A09)
neonatal diarrhea (noninfective) (P78.3)
psychogenic diarrhea (F45.8)

Other diseases of intestines (K55-K64)

✓4th **K55 Vascular disorders of intestine**
EXCLUDES 1 *necrotizing enterocolitis of newborn (P77.-)*
K55.0 Acute vascular disorders of intestine
Acute fulminant ischemic colitis
Acute intestinal infarction
Acute small intestine ischemia
Infarction of appendices epiploicae
Mesenteric (artery) (vein) embolism
Mesenteric (artery) (vein) infarction
Mesenteric (artery) (vein) thrombosis
Necrosis of intestine
Subacute ischemic colitis
K55.1 Chronic vascular disorders of intestine
Chronic ischemic colitis
Chronic ischemic enteritis
Chronic ischemic enterocolitis
Ischemic stricture of intestine
Mesenteric atherosclerosis
Mesenteric vascular insufficiency
✓5th **K55.2 Angiodysplasia of colon**
K55.20 Angiodysplasia of colon without hemorrhage
K55.21 Angiodysplasia of colon with hemorrhage
K55.8 Other vascular disorders of intestine
K55.9 Vascular disorder of intestine, unspecified
Ischemic colitis
Ischemic enteritis
Ischemic enterocolitis

✓4th **K56 Paralytic ileus and intestinal obstruction without hernia**
EXCLUDES 1 *congenital stricture or stenosis of intestine (Q41-Q42)*
cystic fibrosis with meconium ileus (E84.11)
intestinal obstruction with hernia (K40-K46)
ischemic stricture of intestine (K55.1)
meconium ileus NOS (P76.0)
neonatal intestinal obstructions classifiable to P76-
obstruction of duodenum (K31.5)
postprocedural intestinal obstruction (K91.3)
stenosis of anus or rectum (K62.4)
K56.0 Paralytic ileus
Paralysis of bowel
Paralysis of colon
Paralysis of intestine
EXCLUDES 1 *gallstone ileus (K56.3)*
ileus NOS (K56.7)
obstructive ileus NOS (K56.69)
K56.1 Intussusception
Intussusception or invagination of bowel
Intussusception or invagination of colon
Intussusception or invagination of intestine
Intussusception or invagination of rectum
EXCLUDES 2 *intussusception of appendix (K38.8)*
K56.2 Volvulus
Strangulation of colon or intestine
Torsion of colon or intestine
Twist of colon or intestine
EXCLUDES 2 *volvulus of duodenum (K31.5)*
K56.3 Gallstone ileus
Obstruction of intestine by gallstone
✓5th **K56.4 Other impaction of intestine**
K56.41 Fecal impaction
EXCLUDES 1 *constipation (K59.0-)*
incomplete defecation (R15.0)
K56.49 Other impaction of intestine
K56.5 Intestinal adhesions [bands] with obstruction (postprocedural) (postinfection)
Abdominal hernia due to adhesions with obstruction
Peritoneal adhesions [bands] with intestinal obstruction (postprocedural) (postinfection)
✓5th **K56.6 Other and unspecified intestinal obstruction**
K56.60 Unspecified intestinal obstruction
Intestinal obstruction NOS
EXCLUDES 1 *intestinal obstruction due to specified condition—code to condition*
K56.69 Other intestinal obstruction
Enterostenosis NOS
Obstructive ileus NOS
Occlusion of colon or intestine NOS
Stenosis of colon or intestine NOS
Stricture of colon or intestine NOS
EXCLUDES 1 *intestinal obstruction due to specified condition—code to condition*
K56.7 Ileus, unspecified
EXCLUDES 1 *obstructive ileus (K56.69)*

✓4th **K57 Diverticular disease of intestine**
EXCLUDES 1 *congenital diverticulum of intestine (Q43.8)*
Meckel's diverticulum (Q43.0)
EXCLUDES 2 *diverticulum of appendix (K38.2)*
✓5th **K57.0 Diverticulitis of small intestine with perforation and abscess**
Diverticulitis of small intestine with peritonitis
EXCLUDES 1 *diverticulitis of both small and large intestine with perforation and abscess (K57.4-)*
K57.00 Diverticulitis of small intestine with perforation and abscess without bleeding
K57.01 Diverticulitis of small intestine with perforation and abscess with bleeding
✓5th **K57.1 Diverticular disease of small intestine without perforation or abscess**
EXCLUDES 1 *diverticular disease of both small and large intestine without perforation or abscess (K57.5-)*
K57.10 Diverticulosis of small intestine without perforation or abscess without bleeding
Diverticular disease of small intestine NOS
K57.11 Diverticulosis of small intestine without perforation or abscess with bleeding
K57.12 Diverticulitis of small intestine without perforation or abscess without bleeding
K57.13 Diverticulitis of small intestine without perforation or abscess with bleeding
✓5th **K57.2 Diverticulitis of large intestine with perforation and abscess**
Diverticulitis of colon with peritonitis
EXCLUDES 1 *diverticulitis of both small and large intestine with perforation and abscess (K57.4-)*
K57.20 Diverticulitis of large intestine with perforation and abscess without bleeding
K57.21 Diverticulitis of large intestine with perforation and abscess with bleeding
✓5th **K57.3 Diverticular disease of large intestine without perforation or abscess**
EXCLUDES 1 *diverticular disease of both small and large intestine without perforation or abscess (K57.5-)*
K57.30 Diverticulosis of large intestine without perforation or abscess without bleeding
Diverticular disease of colon NOS
K57.31 Diverticulosis of large intestine without perforation or abscess with bleeding
K57.32 Diverticulitis of large intestine without perforation or abscess without bleeding
K57.33 Diverticulitis of large intestine without perforation or abscess with bleeding

✓5th **K57.4 Diverticulitis of both small and large intestine with perforation and abscess**
Diverticulitis of both small and large intestine with peritonitis
K57.40 Diverticulitis of both small and large intestine with perforation and abscess without bleeding
K57.41 Diverticulitis of both small and large intestine with perforation and abscess with bleeding

✓5th **K57.5 Diverticular disease of both small and large intestine without perforation or abscess**
K57.50 Diverticulosis of both small and large intestine without perforation or abscess without bleeding
Diverticular disease of both small and large intestine NOS
K57.51 Diverticulosis of both small and large intestine without perforation or abscess with bleeding
K57.52 Diverticulitis of both small and large intestine without perforation or abscess without bleeding
K57.53 Diverticulitis of both small and large intestine without perforation or abscess with bleeding

✓5th **K57.8 Diverticulitis of intestine, part unspecified, with perforation and abscess**
Diverticulitis of intestine NOS with peritonitis
K57.80 Diverticulitis of intestine, part unspecified, with perforation and abscess without bleeding
K57.81 Diverticulitis of intestine, part unspecified, with perforation and abscess with bleeding

✓5th **K57.9 Diverticular disease of intestine, part unspecified, without perforation or abscess**
K57.90 Diverticulosis of intestine, part unspecified, without perforation or abscess without bleeding
Diverticular disease of intestine NOS
K57.91 Diverticulosis of intestine, part unspecified, without perforation or abscess with bleeding
K57.92 Diverticulitis of intestine, part unspecified, without perforation or abscess without bleeding
K57.93 Diverticulitis of intestine, part unspecified, without perforation or abscess with bleeding

✓4th **K58 Irritable bowel syndrome**
INCLUDES irritable colon
spastic colon
K58.0 Irritable bowel syndrome with diarrhea
K58.9 Irritable bowel syndrome without diarrhea
Irritable bowel syndrome NOS

✓4th **K59 Other functional intestinal disorders**
EXCLUDES 1 *change in bowel habit NOS (R19.4)*
intestinal malabsorption (K90.-)
psychogenic intestinal disorders (F45.8)
EXCLUDES 2 *functional disorders of stomach (K31.-)*

✓5th **K59.0 Constipation**
EXCLUDES 1 *fecal impaction (K56.41)*
incomplete defecation (R15.0)
K59.00 Constipation, unspecified
K59.01 Slow transit constipation
K59.02 Outlet dysfunction constipation
K59.09 Other constipation

K59.1 Functional diarrhea
EXCLUDES 1 *diarrhea NOS (R19.7)*
irritable bowel syndrome with diarrhea (K58.0)

K59.2 Neurogenic bowel, not elsewhere classified

K59.3 Megacolon, not elsewhere classified
Dilatation of colon
Toxic megacolon
Code first (T51-T65) to identify toxic agent
EXCLUDES 1 *congenital megacolon (aganglionic) (Q43.1)*
megacolon (due to) (in) Chagas' disease (B57.32)
megacolon (due to) (in) Clostridium difficile (A04.7)
megacolon (due to) (in) Hirschsprung's disease (Q43.1)

K59.4 Anal spasm
Proctalgia fugax

K59.8 Other specified functional intestinal disorders
Atony of colon
Pseudo-obstruction (acute) (chronic) of intestine

K59.9 Functional intestinal disorder, unspecified

✓4th **K60 Fissure and fistula of anal and rectal regions**
EXCLUDES 1 *fissure and fistula of anal and rectal regions with abscess or cellulitis (K61.-)*
EXCLUDES 2 *anal sphincter tear (healed) (nontraumatic) (old) (K62.81)*
K60.0 Acute anal fissure
K60.1 Chronic anal fissure
K60.2 Anal fissure, unspecified
K60.3 Anal fistula
K60.4 Rectal fistula
Fistula of rectum to skin
EXCLUDES 1 *rectovaginal fistula (N82.3)*
vesicorectal fistual (N32.1)
K60.5 Anorectal fistula

✓4th **K61 Abscess of anal and rectal regions**
INCLUDES abscess of anal and rectal regions
cellulitis of anal and rectal regions
K61.0 Anal abscess
Perianal abscess
EXCLUDES 1 *intrasphincteric abscess (K61.4)*
K61.1 Rectal abscess
Perirectal abscess
EXCLUDES 1 *ischiorectal abscess (K61.3)*
K61.2 Anorectal abscess
K61.3 Ischiorectal abscess
Abscess of ischiorectal fossa
K61.4 Intrasphincteric abscess

✓4th **K62 Other diseases of anus and rectum**
INCLUDES anal canal
EXCLUDES 2 *colostomy and enterostomy malfunction (K94.0-, K94.1-)*
fecal incontinence (R15)
hemorrhoids (K64.-)
K62.0 Anal polyp
K62.1 Rectal polyp
EXCLUDES 1 *adenomatous polyp (D12.8)*
K62.2 Anal prolapse
Prolapse of anal canal
K62.3 Rectal prolapse
Prolapse of rectal mucosa
K62.4 Stenosis of anus and rectum
Stricture of anus (sphincter)
K62.5 Hemorrhage of anus and rectum
EXCLUDES 1 *gastrointestinal bleeding NOS (K92.2)*
melena (K92.1)
neonatal rectal hemorrhage (P54.2)
K62.6 Ulcer of anus and rectum
Solitary ulcer of anus and rectum
Stercoral ulcer of anus and rectum
EXCLUDES 1 *fissure and fistula of anus and rectum (K60.-)*
ulcerative colitis (K51.-)
K62.7 Radiation proctitis
Use additional code to identify the type of radiation (W90.-)

✓5th **K62.8 Other specified diseases of anus and rectum**
EXCLUDES 2 *ulcerative proctitis (K51.2)*
K62.81 Anal sphincter tear (healed) (nontraumatic) (old)
Tear of anus, nontraumatic
Use additional code for any associated fecal incontinence (R15.-)
EXCLUDES 2 *anal fissure (K60.-)*
anal sphincter tear (healed) (old) complicating delivery (O34.7-)
traumatic tear of anal sphincter (S31.831)
K62.82 Dysplasia of anus
Anal intraepithelial neoplasia I and II (AIN I and II) (histologically confirmed)
Dysplasia of anus NOS
Mild and moderate dysplasia of anus (histologically confirmed)
EXCLUDES 1 *abnormal results from anal cytologic examination without histologic confirmation (R85.61-)*
anal intraepithelial neoplasia III (D01.3)
carcinoma in situ of anus (D01.3)
HGSIL of anus (R85.613)
severe dysplasia of anus (D01.3)

K62.89 Other specified diseases of anus and rectum
Proctitis NOS
Use additional code for any associated fecal incontinence (R15.-)

K62.9 Disease of anus and rectum, unspecified

✓4th K63 Other diseases of intestine

K63.0 Abscess of intestine
EXCLUDES 1 *abscess of intestine with Crohn's disease (K50.014, K50.114, K50.814, K50.914)*
abscess of intestine with diverticular disease (K57.0, K57.2, K57.4, K57.8)
abscess of intestine with ulcerative colitis (K51.014, K51.114, K51.214, K51.314, K51.414, K51.514, K51.814, K51.914)
EXCLUDES 2 *abscess of anal and rectal regions (K61.-)*
abscess of appendix (K35.3)

K63.1 Perforation of intestine (nontraumatic)
Perforation (nontraumatic) of rectum
EXCLUDES 1 *perforation (nontraumatic) of duodenum (K26.-)*
perforation (nontraumatic) of intestine with diverticular disease (K57.0, K57.2, K57.4, K57.8)
EXCLUDES 2 *perforation (nontraumatic) of appendix (K35.2, K35.3)*

K63.2 Fistula of intestine
EXCLUDES 1 *fistula of duodenum (K31.6)*
fistula of intestine with Crohn's disease (K50.013, K50.113, K50.813, K50.913)
fistula of intestine with ulcerative colitis (K51.013, K51.113, K51.213, K51.313, K51.413, K51.513, K51.813, K51.913)
EXCLUDES 2 *fistula of anal and rectal regions (K60.-)*
fistula of appendix (K38.3)
intestinal-genital fistula, female (N82.2-N82.4)
vesicointestinal fistula (N32.1)

K63.3 Ulcer of intestine
Primary ulcer of small intestine
EXCLUDES 1 *duodenal ulcer (K26.-)*
gastrointestinal ulcer (K28.-)
gastrojejunal ulcer (K28.-)
jejunal ulcer (K28.-)
peptic ulcer, site unspecified (K27.-)
ulcer of intestine with perforation (K63.1)
ulcer of anus or rectum (K62.6)
ulcerative colitis (K51.-)

K63.4 Enteroptosis

K63.5 Polyp of colon
EXCLUDES 1 *adenomatous polyp of colon (D12.6)*
inflammatory polyp of colon (K51.4-)
polyposis of colon (D12.6)

✓5th K63.8 Other specified diseases of intestine

K63.81 Dieulafoy lesion of intestine
EXCLUDES 2 *Dieulafoy lesion of stomach and duodenum (K31.82)*

K63.89 Other specified diseases of intestine

K63.9 Disease of intestine, unspecified

✓4th K64 Hemorrhoids and perianal venous thrombosis
INCLUDES piles
EXCLUDES 1 *hemorrhoids complicating childbirth and the puerperium (O87.2)*
hemorrhoids complicating pregnancy (O22.4)

K64.0 First degree hemorrhoids
Grade/stage I hemorrhoids
Hemorrhoids (bleeding) without prolapse outside of anal canal

K64.1 Second degree hemorrhoids
Grade/stage II hemorrhoids
Hemorrhoids (bleeding) that prolapse with straining, but retract spontaneously

K64.2 Third degree hemorrhoids
Grade/stage III hemorrhoids
Hemorrhoids (bleeding) that prolapse with straining and require manual replacement back inside anal canal

K64.3 Fourth degree hemorrhoids
Grade/stage IV hemorrhoids
Hemorrhoids (bleeding) with prolapsed tissue that cannot be manually replaced

K64.4 Residual hemorrhoidal skin tags
External hemorrhoids, NOS
Skin tags of anus

K64.5 Perianal venous thrombosis
External hemorrhoids with thrombosis
Perianal hematoma
Thrombosed hemorrhoids NOS

K64.8 Other hemorrhoids
Internal hemorrhoids, without mention of degree
Prolapsed hemorrhoids, degree not specified

K64.9 Unspecified hemorrhoids
Hemorrhoids (bleeding) NOS
Hemorrhoids (bleeding) without mention of degree

Diseases of peritoneum and retroperitoneum (K65-K68)

✓4th K65 Peritonitis
Use additional code (B95-B97), to identify infectious agent
EXCLUDES 1 *acute appendicitis with generalized peritonitis (K35.2)*
aseptic peritonitis (T81.6)
benign paroxysmal peritonitis (E85.0)
chemical peritonitis (T81.6)
diverticulitis of both small and large intestine with peritonitis (K57.4-)
diverticulitis of colon with peritonitis (K57.2-)
diverticulitis of intestine, NOS, with peritonitis (K57.8-)
diverticulitis of small intestine with peritonitis (K57.0-)
gonococcal peritonitis (A54.85)
neonatal peritonitis (P78.0-P78.1)
pelvic peritonitis, female (N73.3-N73.5)
periodic familial peritonitis (E85.0)
peritonitis due to talc or other foreign substance (T81.6)
peritonitis in chlamydia (A74.81)
peritonitis in diphtheria (A36.89)
peritonitis in syphilis (late) (A52.74)
peritonitis in tuberculosis (A18.31)
peritonitis with or following abortion or ectopic or molar pregnancy (O00-O07, O08.0)
peritonitis with or following appendicitis (K35.-)
peritonitis with or following diverticular disease of intestine (K57.-)
puerperal peritonitis (O85)
retroperitoneal infections (K68.-)

K65.0 Generalized (acute) peritonitis
Pelvic peritonitis (acute), male
Subphrenic peritonitis (acute)
Suppurative peritonitis (acute)

K65.1 Peritoneal abscess
Abdominopelvic abscess
Abscess (of) omentum
Abscess (of) peritoneum
Mesenteric abscess
Retrocecal abscess
Subdiaphragmatic abscess
Subhepatic abscess
Subphrenic abscess

K65.2 Spontaneous bacterial peritonitis
EXCLUDES 1 *bacterial peritonitis NOS K65.9*

K65.3 Choleperitonitis
Peritonitis due to bile

K65.4 Sclerosing mesenteritis
Fat necrosis of peritoneum
(Idiopathic) sclerosing mesenteric fibrosis
Mesenteric lipodystrophy
Mesenteric panniculitis
Retractile mesenteritis

K65.8 Other peritonitis
Chronic proliferative peritonitis
Peritonitis due to urine

K65.9 Peritonitis, unspecified
Bacterial peritonitis NOS

✓4th K66 Other disorders of peritoneum
EXCLUDES 2 *ascites (R18.-)*
peritoneal effusion (chronic) (R18.8)

K66.0 Peritoneal adhesions (postprocedural) (postinfection)
Adhesions (of) abdominal (wall)
Adhesions (of) diaphragm
Adhesions (of) intestine
Adhesions (of) male pelvis
Adhesions (of) omentum
Adhesions (of) stomach
Adhesive bands
Mesenteric adhesions
EXCLUDES 1 *female pelvic adhesions [bands] (N73.6)*
peritoneal adhesions with intestinal obstruction (K56.5)

K66.1 Hemoperitoneum
EXCLUDES 1 *traumatic hemoperitoneum (S36.8-)*

K66.8 Other specified disorders of peritoneum

K66.9 Disorder of peritoneum, unspecified

K67 Disorders of peritoneum in infectious diseases classified elsewhere

Code first underlying disease, such as:
congenital syphilis (A50.0)
helminthiasis (B65.0–B83.9)

EXCLUDES 1 *peritonitis in chlamydia (A74.81)*
peritonitis in diphtheria (A36.89)
peritonitis in gonococcal (A54.85)
peritonitis in syphilis (late) (A52.74)
peritonitis in tuberculosis (A18.31)

√4th **K68 Disorders of retroperitoneum**

√5th **K68.1 Retroperitoneal abscess**
K68.11 Postprocedural retroperitoneal abscess
K68.12 Psoas muscle abscess
K68.19 Other retroperitoneal abscess

K68.9 Other disorders of retroperitoneum

Diseases of liver (K70-K77)

EXCLUDES 1 *jaundice NOS (R17)*
EXCLUDES 2 *hemochromatosis (E83.11-)*
Reye's syndrome (G93.7)
vira lhepatitis (B15-B19)
Wilson's disease (E83.0)

√4th **K70 Alcoholic liver disease**

Use additional code to identify:
alcohol abuse and dependence (F10.-)

K70.0 Alcoholic fatty liver

√5th **K70.1 Alcoholic hepatitis**
K70.10 Alcoholic hepatitis without ascites
K70.11 Alcoholic hepatitis with ascites

K70.2 Alcoholic fibrosis and sclerosis of liver

√5th **K70.3 Alcoholic cirrhosis of liver**
Alcoholic cirrhosis NOS
K70.30 Alcoholic cirrhosis of liver without ascites
K70.31 Alcoholic cirrhosis of liver with ascites

√5th **K70.4 Alcoholic hepatic failure**
Acute alcoholic hepatic failure
Alcoholic hepatic failure NOS
Chronic alcoholic hepatic failure
Subacute alcoholic hepatic failure
K70.40 Alcoholic hepatic failure without coma
K70.41 Alcoholic hepatic failure with coma

K70.9 Alcoholic liver disease, unspecified

√4th **K71 Toxic liver disease**

INCLUDES drug-induced idiosyncratic (unpredictable) liver disease
drug-induced toxic (predictable) liver disease

Code first poisoning due to drug or toxin, if applicable (T36-T65 with fifth or sixth character 1-4 or 6)

Use additional code for adverse effect, if applicable, to identify drug (T36-T50 with fifth or sixth character 5)

EXCLUDES 2 *alcoholic liver disease (K70.-)*
Budd-Chiari syndrome (I82.0)

K71.0 Toxic liver disease with cholestasis
Cholestasis with hepatocyte injury
"Pure" cholestasis

√5th **K71.1 Toxic liver disease with hepatic necrosis**
Hepatic failure (acute) (chronic) due to drugs
K71.10 Toxic liver disease with hepatic necrosis, without coma
K71.11 Toxic liver disease with hepatic necrosis, with coma

K71.2 Toxic liver disease with acute hepatitis
K71.3 Toxic liver disease with chronic persistent hepatitis
K71.4 Toxic liver disease with chronic lobular hepatitis

√5th **K71.5 Toxic liver disease with chronic active hepatitis**
Toxic liver disease with lupoid hepatitis
K71.50 Toxic liver disease with chronic active hepatitis without ascites
K71.51 Toxic liver disease with chronic active hepatitis with ascites

K71.6 Toxic liver disease with hepatitis, not elsewhere classified
K71.7 Toxic liver disease with fibrosis and cirrhosis of liver
K71.8 Toxic liver disease with other disorders of liver
Toxic liver disease with focal nodular hyperplasia
Toxic liver disease with hepatic granulomas
Toxic liver disease with peliosis hepatis
Toxic liver disease with veno-occlusive disease of liver
K71.9 Toxic liver disease, unspecified

√4th **K72 Hepatic failure, not elsewhere classified**

INCLUDES acute hepatitis NEC, with hepatic failure
fulminant hepatitis NEC, with hepatic failure
hepatic encephalopathy NOS
liver (cell) necrosis with hepatic failure
malignant hepatitis NEC, with hepatic failure
yellow liver atrophy or dystrophy

EXCLUDES 1 *alcoholic hepatic failure (K70.4)*
hepatic failure complicating abortion or ectopic or molar pregnancy (O00-O07, O08.8)
hepatic failure complicating pregnancy, childbirth and the puerperium (O26.6-)
hepatic failure with toxic liver disease (K71.1-)
icterus of newborn (P55-P59)
postprocedural hepatic failure (K91.82)
viral hepatitis with hepatic coma (B15-B19)

√5th **K72.0 Acute and subacute hepatic failure**
K72.00 Acute and subacute hepatic failure without coma
K72.01 Acute and subacute hepatic failure with coma

√5th **K72.1 Chronic hepatic failure**
K72.10 Chronic hepatic failure without coma
K72.11 Chronic hepatic failure with coma

√5th **K72.9 Hepatic failure, unspecified**
K72.90 Hepatic failure, unspecified without coma
K72.91 Hepatic failure, unspecified with coma
Hepatic coma NOS

√4th **K73 Chronic hepatitis, not elsewhere classified**

EXCLUDES 1 *alcoholic hepatitis (chronic) (K70.1-)*
drug-induced hepatitis (chronic) (K71.-)
granulomatous hepatitis (chronic) NEC (K75.3)
reactive, nonspecific hepatitis (chronic) (K75.2)
viral hepatitis (chronic) (B15-B19)

K73.0 Chronic persistent hepatitis, not elsewhere classified
K73.1 Chronic lobular hepatitis, not elsewhere classified
K73.2 Chronic active hepatitis, not elsewhere classified
K73.8 Other chronic hepatitis, not elsewhere classified
K73.9 Chronic hepatitis, unspecified

√4th **K74 Fibrosis and cirrhosis of liver**

Code also, if applicable, viral hepatitis (acute) (chronic) (B15-B19)

EXCLUDES 1 *alcoholic cirrhosis (of liver) (K70.3)*
alcoholic fibrosis of liver (K70.2)
cardiac sclerosis of liver (K76.1)
cirrhosis (of liver) with toxic liver disease (K71.7)
congenital cirrhosis (of liver) (P78.81)
pigmentary cirrhosis (of liver) (E83.110)

K74.0 Hepatic fibrosis
K74.1 Hepatic sclerosis
K74.2 Hepatic fibrosis with hepatic sclerosis
K74.3 Primary biliary cirrhosis
Chronic nonsuppurative destructive cholangitis
K74.4 Secondary biliary cirrhosis
K74.5 Biliary cirrhosis, unspecified

√5th **K74.6 Other and unspecified cirrhosis of liver**
K74.60 Unspecified cirrhosis of liver
Cirrhosis (of liver) NOS
K74.69 Other cirrhosis of liver
Cryptogenic cirrhosis (of liver)
Macronodular cirrhosis (of liver)
Micronodular cirrhosis (of liver)
Mixed type cirrhosis (of liver)
Portal cirrhosis (of liver)
Postnecrotic cirrhosis (of liver)

K75 Other inflammatory liver diseases (4th)
EXCLUDES 2 *toxic liver disease (K71.-)*

K75.0 Abscess of liver
Cholangitic hepatic abscess
Hematogenic hepatic abscess
Hepatic abscess NOS
Lymphogenic hepatic abscess
Pylephlebitic hepatic abscess
EXCLUDES 1 *amebic liver abscess (A06.4)*
cholangitis without liver abscess (K83.0)
pylephlebitis without liver abscess (K75.1)

K75.1 Phlebitis of portal vein
Pylephlebitis
EXCLUDES 1 *pylephlebitic liver abscess (K75.0)*

K75.2 Nonspecific reactive hepatitis
EXCLUDES 1 *acute or subacute hepatitis (K72.0-)*
chronic hepatitis NEC (K73.-)
viral hepatitis (B15-B19)

K75.3 Granulomatous hepatitis, not elsewhere classified
EXCLUDES 1 *acute or subacute hepatitis (K72.0-)*
chronic hepatitis NEC (K73.-)
viral hepatitis (B15-B19)

K75.4 Autoimmune hepatitis
Lupoid hepatitis NEC

K75.8 Other specified inflammatory liver diseases (5th)
K75.81 Nonalcoholic steatohepatitis (NASH)
K75.89 Other specified inflammatory liver diseases

K75.9 Inflammatory liver disease, unspecified
Hepatitis NOS
EXCLUDES 1 *acute or subacute hepatitis (K72.0-)*
chronic hepatitis NEC (K73.-)
viral hepatitis (B15-B19)

K76 Other diseases of liver (4th)
EXCLUDES 2 *alcoholic liver disease (K70.-)*
amyloid degeneration of liver (E85.-)
cystic disease of liver (congenital) (Q44.6)
hepatic vein thrombosis (I82.0)
hepatomegaly NOS (R16.0)
pigmentary cirrhosis (of liver) (E83.110)
portal vein thrombosis (I81)
toxic liver disease (K71.-)

K76.0 Fatty (change of) liver, not elsewhere classified
Nonalcoholic fatty liver disease (NAFLD)
EXCLUDES 1 *nonalcoholic steatohepatitis (NASH) (K75.81)*

K76.1 Chronic passive congestion of liver
Cardiac cirrhosis
Cardiac sclerosis

K76.2 Central hemorrhagic necrosis of liver
EXCLUDES 1 *liver necrosis with hepatic failure (K72.-)*

K76.3 Infarction of liver

K76.4 Peliosis hepatis
Hepatic angiomatosis

K76.5 Hepatic veno-occlusive disease
EXCLUDES 1 *Budd-Chiari syndrome (I82.0)*

K76.6 Portal hypertension
Use additional code for any associated complications, such as:
portal hypertensive gastropathy (K31.89)

K76.7 Hepatorenal syndrome
EXCLUDES 1 *hepatorenal syndrome following labor and delivery (O90.4)*
postprocedural hepatorenal syndrome (K91.82)

K76.8 Other specified diseases of liver (5th)
K76.81 Hepatopulmonary syndrome
Code first underlying liver disease, such as:
alcoholic cirrhosis of liver (K70.3-)
cirrhosis of liver without mention of alcohol (K74.6-)
K76.89 Other specified diseases of liver
Cyst (simple) of liver
Focal nodular hyperplasia of liver
Hepatoptosis

K76.9 Liver disease, unspecified

K77 Liver disorders in diseases classified elsewhere
Code first underlying disease, such as:
amyloidosis (E85.-)
congenital syphilis (A50.0, A50.5)
congenital toxoplasmosis (P37.1)
schistosomiasis (B65.0-B65.9)
EXCLUDES 1 *alcoholic hepatitis (K70.1-)*
alcoholic liver disease (K70-.)
cytomegaloviral hepatitis (B25.1)
herpesviral [herpes simplex] hepatitis (B00.81)
infectious mononucleosis with liver disease (B27.0-B27.9 with .9)
mumps hepatitis (B26.81)
sarcoidosis with liver disease (D86.89)
secondary syphilis with liver disease (A51.45)
syphilis (late) with liver disease (A52.74)
toxoplasmosis (acquired) hepatitis (B58.1)
tuberculosis with liver disease (A18.83)

Disorders of gallbladder, biliary tract and pancreas (K80-K87)

K80 Cholelithiasis (4th)
EXCLUDES 1 *retained cholelithiasis following cholecystectomy (K91.86)*

K80.0 Calculus of gallbladder with acute cholecystitis (5th)
Any condition listed in K80.2 with acute cholecystitis
K80.00 Calculus of gallbladder with acute cholecystitis without obstruction
K80.01 Calculus of gallbladder with acute cholecystitis with obstruction

K80.1 Calculus of gallbladder with other cholecystitis (5th)
K80.10 Calculus of gallbladder with chronic cholecystitis without obstruction
Cholelithiasis with cholecystitis NOS
K80.11 Calculus of gallbladder with chronic cholecystitis with obstruction
K80.12 Calculus of gallbladder with acute and chronic cholecystitis without obstruction
K80.13 Calculus of gallbladder with acute and chronic cholecystitis with obstruction
K80.18 Calculus of gallbladder with other cholecystitis without obstruction
K80.19 Calculus of gallbladder with other cholecystitis with obstruction

K80.2 Calculus of gallbladder without cholecystitis (5th)
Cholecystolithiasis without cholecystitis
Cholelithiasis (without cholecystitis)
Colic (recurrent) of gallbladder (without cholecystitis)
Gallstone (impacted) of cystic duct (without cholecystitis)
Gallstone (impacted) of gallbladder (without cholecystitis)
K80.20 Calculus of gallbladder without cholecystitis without obstruction
K80.21 Calculus of gallbladder without cholecystitis with obstruction

K80.3 Calculus of bile duct with cholangitis (5th)
Any condition listed in K80.5 with cholangitis
K80.30 Calculus of bile duct with cholangitis, unspecified, without obstruction
K80.31 Calculus of bile duct with cholangitis, unspecified, with obstruction
K80.32 Calculus of bile duct with acute cholangitis without obstruction
K80.33 Calculus of bile duct with acute cholangitis with obstruction
K80.34 Calculus of bile duct with chronic cholangitis without obstruction
K80.35 Calculus of bile duct with chronic cholangitis with obstruction
K80.36 Calculus of bile duct with acute and chronic cholangitis without obstruction
K80.37 Calculus of bile duct with acute and chronic cholangitis with obstruction

K80.4 Calculus of bile duct with cholecystitis (5th)
Any condition listed in K80.5 with cholecystitis (with cholangitis)
K80.40 Calculus of bile duct with cholecystitis, unspecified, without obstruction
K80.41 Calculus of bile duct with cholecystitis, unspecified, with obstruction

K80.42 **Calculus of bile duct with acute cholecystitis without obstruction**

K80.43 **Calculus of bile duct with acute cholecystitis with obstruction**

K80.44 **Calculus of bile duct with chronic cholecystitis without obstruction**

K80.45 **Calculus of bile duct with chronic cholecystitis with obstruction**

K80.46 **Calculus of bile duct with acute and chronic cholecystitis without obstruction**

K80.47 **Calculus of bile duct with acute and chronic cholecystitis with obstruction**

✓5th **K80.5 Calculus of bile duct without cholangitis or cholecystitis**

Choledocholithiasis (without cholangitis or cholecystitis)
Gallstone (impacted) of bile duct NOS (without cholangitis or cholecystitis)
Gallstone (impacted) of common duct (without cholangitis or cholecystitis)
Gallstone (impacted) of hepatic duct (without cholangitis or cholecystitis)
Hepatic cholelithiasis (without cholangitis or cholecystitis)
Hepatic colic (recurrent) (without cholangitis or cholecystitis)

K80.50 **Calculus of bile duct without cholangitis or cholecystitis without obstruction**

K80.51 **Calculus of bile duct without cholangitis or cholecystitis with obstruction**

✓5th **K80.6 Calculus of gallbladder and bile duct with cholecystitis**

K80.60 **Calculus of gallbladder and bile duct with cholecystitis, unspecified, without obstruction**

K80.61 **Calculus of gallbladder and bile duct with cholecystitis, unspecified, with obstruction**

K80.62 **Calculus of gallbladder and bile duct with acute cholecystitis without obstruction**

K80.63 **Calculus of gallbladder and bile duct with acute cholecystitis with obstruction**

K80.64 **Calculus of gallbladder and bile duct with chronic cholecystitis without obstruction**

K80.65 **Calculus of gallbladder and bile duct with chronic cholecystitis with obstruction**

K80.66 **Calculus of gallbladder and bile duct with acute and chronic cholecystitis without obstruction**

K80.67 **Calculus of gallbladder and bile duct with acute and chronic cholecystitis with obstruction**

✓5th **K80.7 Calculus of gallbladder and bile duct without cholecystitis**

K80.70 **Calculus of gallbladder and bile duct without cholecystitis without obstruction**

K80.71 **Calculus of gallbladder and bile duct without cholecystitis with obstruction**

✓5th **K80.8 Other cholelithiasis**

K80.80 **Other cholelithiasis without obstruction**

K80.81 **Other cholelithiasis with obstruction**

✓4th K81 Cholecystitis

EXCLUDES 1 *cholecystitis with cholelithiasis (K80.-)*

K81.0 Acute cholecystitis

Abscess of gallbladder
Angiocholecystitis
Emphysematous (acute) cholecystitis
Empyema of gallbladder
Gangrene of gallbladder
Gangrenous cholecystitis
Suppurative cholecystitis

K81.1 Chronic cholecystitis

K81.2 Acute cholecystitis with chronic cholecystitis

K81.9 Cholecystitis, unspecified

✓4th K82 Other diseases of gallbladder

EXCLUDES 1 *nonvisualization of gallbladder (R93.2)*
postcholecystectomy syndrome (K91.5)

K82.0 Obstruction of gallbladder

Occlusion of cystic duct or gallbladder without cholelithiasis
Stenosis of cystic duct or gallbladder without cholelithiasis
Stricture of cystic duct or gallbladder without cholelithiasis
EXCLUDES 1 *obstruction of gallbladder with cholelithiasis (K80.-)*

K82.1 Hydrops of gallbladder

Mucocele of gallbladder

K82.2 Perforation of gallbladder

Rupture of cystic duct or gallbladder

K82.3 Fistula of gallbladder

Cholecystocolic fistula
Cholecystoduodenal fistula

K82.4 Cholesterolosis of gallbladder

Strawberry gallbladder
EXCLUDES 1 *cholesterolosis of gallbladder with cholecystitis (K81.-)*
cholesterolosis of gallbladder with cholelithiasis (K80.-)

K82.8 Other specified diseases of gallbladder

Adhesions of cystic duct or gallbladder
Atrophy of cystic duct or gallbladder
Cyst of cystic duct or gallbladder
Dyskinesia of cystic duct or gallbladder
Hypertrophy of cystic duct or gallbladder
Nonfunctioning of cystic duct or gallbladder
Ulcer of cystic duct or gallbladder

K82.9 Disease of gallbladder, unspecified

✓4th K83 Other diseases of biliary tract

EXCLUDES 1 *postcholecystectomy syndrome (K91.5)*
EXCLUDES 2 *conditions involving the gallbladder (K81-K82)*
conditions involving the cystic duct (K81-K82)

K83.0 Cholangitis

Ascending cholangitis
Cholangitis NOS
Primary cholangitis
Recurrent cholangitis
Sclerosing cholangitis
Secondary cholangitis
Stenosing cholangitis
Suppurative cholangitis
EXCLUDES 1 *cholangitic liver abscess (K75.0)*
cholangitis with choledocholithiasis (K80.3-, K80.4-)
chronic nonsuppurative destructive cholangitis (K74.3)

K83.1 Obstruction of bile duct

Occlusion of bile duct without cholelithiasis
Stenosis of bile duct without cholelithiasis
Stricture of bile duct without cholelithiasis
EXCLUDES 1 *congenital obstruction of bile duct (Q44.3)*
obstruction of bile duct with cholelithiasis (K80.-)

K83.2 Perforation of bile duct

Rupture of bile duct

K83.3 Fistula of bile duct

Choledochoduodenal fistula

K83.4 Spasm of sphincter of Oddi

K83.5 Biliary cyst

K83.8 Other specified diseases of biliary tract

Adhesions of biliary tract
Atrophy of biliary tract
Hypertrophy of biliary tract
Ulcer of biliary tract

K83.9 Disease of biliary tract, unspecified

✓4th K85 Acute pancreatitis

Abscess of pancreas
Acute necrosis of pancreas
Acute (recurrent) pancreatitis
Gangrene of (gangrenous) pancreas
Hemorrhagic pancreatitis
Infective necrosis of pancreas
Subacute pancreatitis
Suppurative pancreatitis

K85.0 Idiopathic acute pancreatitis

K85.1 Biliary acute pancreatitis

Gallstone pancreatitis

K85.2 Alcohol induced acute pancreatitis

EXCLUDES 2 *alcohol induced chronic pancreatitis (K86.0)*

K85.3 Drug induced acute pancreatitis

Use additional code for adverse effect, if applicable, to identify drug (T36-T50 with fifth or sixth character 5)
Use additional code to identify drug abuse and dependence (F11.- F17.-)

K85.8 Other acute pancreatitis

K85.9 Acute pancreatitis, unspecified

Pancreatitis NOS

✓4th K86 Other diseases of pancreas

EXCLUDES 2 *fibrocystic disease of pancreas (E84.-)*
islet cell tumor (of pancreas) (D13.7)
pancreatic steatorrhea (K9Ø.3)

K86.Ø Alcohol-induced chronic pancreatitis
Use additional code to identify:
alcohol abuse and dependence (F1Ø.-)
EXCLUDES 2 *alcohol induced acute pancreatitis (K85.2)*

K86.1 Other chronic pancreatitis
Chronic pancreatitis NOS
Infectious chronic pancreatitis
Recurrent chronic pancreatitis
Relapsing chronic pancreatitis

K86.2 Cyst of pancreas

K86.3 Pseudocyst of pancreas

K86.8 Other specified diseases of pancreas
Aseptic pancreatic necrosis
Atrophy of pancreas
Calculus of pancreas
Cirrhosis of pancreas
Fibrosis of pancreas
Pancreatic fat necrosis
Pancreatic infantilism
Pancreatic necrosis NOS

K86.9 Disease of pancreas, unspecified

K87 Disorders of gallbladder, biliary tract and pancreas in diseases classified elsewhere

Code first underlying disease
EXCLUDES 1 *cytomegaloviral pancreatitis (B25.2)*
mumps pancreatitis (B26.3)
syphilitic gallbladder (A52.74)
syphilitic pancreas (A52.74)
tuberculosis of gallbladder (A18.83)
tuberculosis of pancreas (A18.83)

Other diseases of the digestive system (K9Ø-K95)

✓4th K9Ø Intestinal malabsorption

EXCLUDES 1 *intestinal malabsorption following gastrointestinal surgery (K91.2)*

K9Ø.Ø Celiac disease
Gluten-sensitive enteropathy
Idiopathic steatorrhea
Nontropical sprue

K9Ø.1 Tropical sprue
Sprue NOS
Tropical steatorrhea

K9Ø.2 Blind loop syndrome, not elsewhere classified
Blind loop syndrome NOS
EXCLUDES 1 *congenital blind loop syndrome (Q43.8)*
postsurgical blind loop syndrome (K91.2)

K9Ø.3 Pancreatic steatorrhea

K9Ø.4 Malabsorption due to intolerance, not elsewhere classified
Malabsorption due to intolerance to carbohydrate
Malabsorption due to intolerance to fat
Malabsorption due to intolerance to protein
Malabsorption due to intolerance to starch
EXCLUDES 2 *gluten-sensitive enteropathy (K9Ø.Ø)*
lactose intolerance (E73.-)

✓5th K9Ø.8 Other intestinal malabsorption

K9Ø.81 Whipple's disease

K9Ø.89 Other intestinal malabsorption

K9Ø.9 Intestinal malabsorption, unspecified

✓4th K91 Intraoperative and postprocedural complications and disorders of digestive system, not elsewhere classified

EXCLUDES 2 *complications of artificial opening of digestive system (K94.-)*
complications of bariatric procedures (K95.-)
gastrojejunal ulcer (K28.-)
postprocedural (radiation) retroperitoneal abscess (K68.11)
radiation colitis (K52.Ø)
radiation gastroenteritis (K52.Ø)
radiation proctitis (K62.7)

K91.Ø Vomiting following gastrointestinal surgery

K91.1 Postgastric surgery syndromes
Dumping syndrome
Postgastrectomy syndrome
Postvagotomy syndrome

K91.2 Postsurgical malabsorption, not elsewhere classified
Postsurgical blind loop syndrome
EXCLUDES 1 *malabsorption osteomalacia in adults (M83.2)*
malabsorption osteoporosis, postsurgical (M8Ø.8-, M81.8)

K91.3 Postprocedural intestinal obstruction

K91.5 Postcholecystectomy syndrome

✓5th K91.6 Intraoperative hemorrhage and hematoma of a digestive system organ or structure complicating a procedure

EXCLUDES 1 *intraoperative hemorrhage and hematoma of a digestive system organ or structure due to accidental puncture and laceration during a procedure (K91.7-)*

K91.61 Intraoperative hemorrhage and hematoma of a digestive system organ or structure complicating a digestive sytem procedure

K91.62 Intraoperative hemorrhage and hematoma of a digestive system organ or structure complicating other procedure

✓5th K91.7 Accidental puncture and laceration of a digestive system organ or structure during a procedure

K91.71 Accidental puncture and laceration of a digestive system organ or structure during a digestive system procedure

K91.72 Accidental puncture and laceration of a digestive system organ or structure during other procedure

✓5th K91.8 Other intraoperative and postprocedural complications and disorders of digestive system

K91.81 Other intraoperative complications of digestive system

K91.82 Postprocedural hepatic failure

K91.83 Postprocedural hepatorenal syndrome

✓6th K91.84 Postprocedural hemorrhage and hematoma of a digestive system organ or structure following a procedure

K91.84Ø Postprocedural hemorrhage and hematoma of a digestive system organ or structure following a digestive system procedure

K91.841 Postprocedural hemorrhage and hematoma of a digestive system organ or structure following other procedure

✓6th K91.85 Complications of intestinal pouch

K91.85Ø Pouchitis
Inflammation of internal ileoanal pouch

K91.858 Other complications of intestinal pouch

K91.86 Retained cholelithiasis following cholecystectomy

K91.89 Other postprocedural complications and disorders of digestive system
Use additional code, if applicable, to further specify disorder
EXCLUDES 2 *postprocedural retroperitoneal abscess (K68.11)*

✓4th K92 Other diseases of digestive system

EXCLUDES 1 *neonatal gastrointestinal hemorrhage (P54.Ø-P54.3)*

K92.Ø Hematemesis

K92.1 Melena
EXCLUDES 1 *occult blood in feces (R19.5)*

K92.2 Gastrointestinal hemorrhage, unspecified
Gastric hemorrhage NOS
Intestinal hemorrhage NOS
EXCLUDES 1 *acute hemorrhagic gastritis (K29.Ø1)*
hemorrhage of anus and rectum (K62.5)
angiodysplasia of stomach with hemorrhage (K31.811)
diverticular disease with hemorrhage (K57.-)
gastritis and duodenitis with hemorrhage (K29.-)
peptic ulcer with hemorrhage (K25-K28)

✓5th K92.8 Other specified diseases of the digestive system

K92.81 Gastrointestinal mucositis (ulcerative)
Code also type of associated therapy, such as:
antineoplastic and immunosuppressive drugs (T45.1X-)
radiological procedure and radiotherapy (Y84.2)
EXCLUDES 2 *mucositis (ulcerative) of vagina and vulva (N76.81)*
nasal mucositis (ulcerative) (J34.81)
oral mucositis (ulcerative) (K12.3-)

K92.89 Other specified diseases of the digestive system

K92.9 Disease of digestive system, unspecified

K94 Complications of artificial openings of the digestive system

K94.0 Colostomy complications

K94.00 Colostomy complication, unspecified

K94.01 Colostomy hemorrhage

K94.02 Colostomy infection

Use additional code to specify type of infection, such as:
- cellulitis of abdominal wall (L03.311)
- sepsis (A40-, A41-)

K94.03 Colostomy malfunction

Mechanical complication of colostomy

K94.09 Other complications of colostomy

K94.1 Enterostomy complications

K94.10 Enterostomy complication, unspecified

K94.11 Enterostomy hemorrhage

K94.12 Enterostomy infection

Use additional code to specify type of infection, such as:
- cellulitis of abdominal wall (L03.311)
- sepsis (A40-, A41-)

K94.13 Enterostomy malfunction

Mechanical complication of enterostomy

K94.19 Other complications of enterostomy

K94.2 Gastrostomy complications

K94.20 Gastrostomy complication, unspecified

K94.21 Gastrostomy hemorrhage

K94.22 Gastrostomy infection

Use additional code to specify type of infection, such as:
- cellulitis of abdominal wall (L03.311)
- sepsis (A40-, A41-)

K94.23 Gastrostomy malfunction

Mechanical complication of gastrostomy

K94.29 Other complications of gastrostomy

K94.3 Esophagostomy complications

K94.30 Esophagostomy complications, unspecified

K94.31 Esophagostomy hemorrhage

K94.32 Esophagostomy infection

Use additional code to identify the infection

K94.33 Esophagostomy malfunction

Mechanical complication of esophagostomy

K94.39 Other complications of esophagostomy

K95 Complications of bariatric procedures

K95.0 Complications of gastric band procedure

K95.01 Infection due to gastric band procedure

Use additional code to specify type of infection or organism, such as:
- bacterial and viral infectious agents (B95.-, B96.-)
- cellulitis of abdominal wall (L03.311)
- sepsis (A40.-, A41.-)

K95.09 Other complications of gastric band procedure

Use additional code, if applicable, to further specify complication

K95.8 Complications of other bariatric procedure

EXCLUDES 1 *complications of gastric band surgery (K95.0-)*

K95.81 Infection due to other bariatric procedure

Use additional code to specify type of infection or organism, such as:
- bacterial and viral infectious agents (B95.-, B96.-)
- cellulitis of abdominal wall (L03.311)
- sepsis (A40.-, A41.-)

K95.89 Other complications of other bariatric procedure

Use additional code, if applicable, to further specify complication

Chapter 12. Diseases of the Skin and Subcutaneous Tissue (LØØ-L99)

EXCLUDES 2 *certain conditions originating in the perinatal period (PØ4-P96)*
certain infectious and parasitic diseases (AØØ-B99)
complications of pregnancy, childbirth and the puerperium (OØØ-O9A)
congenital malformations, deformations, and chromosomal abnormalities (QØØ-Q99)
endocrine, nutritional and metabolic diseases (EØØ-E88)
lipomelanotic reticulosis (I89.8)
neoplasms (CØØ-D49)
symptoms, signs and abnormal clinical and laboratory findings, not elsewhere classified (RØØ-R94)
systemic connective tissue disorders (M3Ø-M36)
viral warts (BØ7.-)

This chapter contains the following blocks:

LØØ-LØ8	Infections of the skin and subcutaneous tissue
L1Ø-L14	Bullous disorders
L2Ø-L3Ø	Dermatitis and eczema
L4Ø-L45	Papulosquamous disorders
L49-L54	Urticaria and erythema
L55-L59	Radiation-related disorders of the skin and subcutaneous tissue
L6Ø-L75	Disorders of skin appendages
L76	Intraoperative and postprocedural complications of skin and subcutaneous tissue
L8Ø-L99	Other disorders of the skin and subcutaneous tissue

Infections of the skin and subcutaneous tissue (LØØ-LØ8)

Use additional code (B95-B97) to identify infectious agent

EXCLUDES 2 *hordeolum (HØØ.Ø)*
infective dermatitis (L3Ø.3)
local infections of skin classified in Chapter 1
lupus panniculitis (L93.2)
panniculitis NOS (M79.3)
panniculitis of neck and back (M54.Ø-)
Perlèche NOS (K13.Ø)
Perlèche due to candidiasis (B37.Ø)
Perlèche due to riboflavin deficiency (E53.Ø)
pyogenic granuloma (L98.Ø)
relapsing panniculitis [Weber-Christian] (M35.6)
viral warts (BØ7.-)
zoster (BØ2.-)

LØØ Staphylococcal scalded skin syndrome
Ritter's disease
Use additional code to identify percentage of skin exfoliation (L49.-)
EXCLUDES 1 *bullous impetigo (LØ1.Ø3)*
pemphigus neonatorum (LØ1.Ø3)
toxic epidermal necrolysis [Lyell] (L51.2)

✓4th **LØ1 Impetigo**
EXCLUDES 1 *impetigo herpetiformis (L4Ø.1)*

✓5th **LØ1.Ø Impetigo**
Impetigo contagiosa
Impetigo vulgaris

LØ1.ØØ Impetigo, unspecified
Impetigo NOS

LØ1.Ø1 Non-bullous impetigo

LØ1.Ø2 Bockhart's impetigo
Impetigo follicularis
Perifolliculitis NOS
Superficial pustular perifolliculitis

LØ1.Ø3 Bullous impetigo
Impetigo neonatorum
Pemphigus neonatorum

LØ1.Ø9 Other impetigo
Ulcerative impetigo

LØ1.1 Impetiginization of other dermatoses

✓4th **LØ2 Cutaneous abscess, furuncle and carbuncle**
Use additional code to identify organism (B95-B96)
EXCLUDES 2 *abscess of anus and rectal regions (K61.-)*
abscess of female genital organs (external) (N76.4)
abscess of male genital organs (external) (N48.2, N49-)

✓5th **LØ2.Ø Cutaneous abscess, furuncle and carbuncle of face**
EXCLUDES 2 *abscess of ear, external (H6Ø.Ø)*
abscess of eyelid (HØØ.Ø)
abscess of head [any part, except face] (LØ2.8)
abscess of lacrimal gland (HØ4.Ø)
abscess of lacrimal passages (HØ4.3)
abscess of mouth (K12.2)
abscess of nose (J34.Ø)
abscess of orbit (HØ5.Ø)
submandibular abscess (K12.2)

LØ2.Ø1 Cutaneous abscess of face

LØ2.Ø2 Furuncle of face
Boil of face
Folliculitis of face

LØ2.Ø3 Carbuncle of face

✓5th **LØ2.1 Cutaneous abscess, furuncle and carbuncle of neck**

LØ2.11 Cutaneous abscess of neck

LØ2.12 Furuncle of neck
Boil of neck
Folliculitis of neck

LØ2.13 Carbuncle of neck

✓5th **LØ2.2 Cutaneous abscess, furuncle and carbuncle of trunk**
EXCLUDES 1 *non-newborn omphalitis (LØ8.82)*
omphalitis of newborn (P38.-)
EXCLUDES 2 *abscess of breast (N61)*
abscess of buttocks (LØ2.3)
abscess of female external genital organs (N76.4)
abscess of hip (LØ2.4)
abscess of male external genital organs (N48.2, N49-)

✓6th **LØ2.21 Cutaneous abscess of trunk**

LØ2.211 Cutaneous abscess of abdominal wall
LØ2.212 Cutaneous abscess of back [any part, except buttock]
LØ2.213 Cutaneous abscess of chest wall
LØ2.214 Cutaneous abscess of groin
LØ2.215 Cutaneous abscess of perineum
LØ2.216 Cutaneous abscess of umbilicus
LØ2.219 Cutaneous abscess of trunk, unspecified

✓6th **LØ2.22 Furuncle of trunk**
Boil of trunk
Folliculitis of trunk

LØ2.221 Furuncle of abdominal wall
LØ2.222 Furuncle of back [any part, except buttock]
LØ2.223 Furuncle of chest wall
LØ2.224 Furuncle of groin
LØ2.225 Furuncle of perineum
LØ2.226 Furuncle of umbilicus
LØ2.229 Furuncle of trunk, unspecified

✓6th **LØ2.23 Carbuncle of trunk**

LØ2.231 Carbuncle of abdominal wall
LØ2.232 Carbuncle of back [any part, except buttock]
LØ2.233 Carbuncle of chest wall
LØ2.234 Carbuncle of groin
LØ2.235 Carbuncle of perineum
LØ2.236 Carbuncle of umbilicus
LØ2.239 Carbuncle of trunk, unspecified

✓5th **LØ2.3 Cutaneous abscess, furuncle and carbuncle of buttock**
EXCLUDES 1 *pilonidal cyst with abscess (LØ5.Ø1)*

LØ2.31 Cutaneous abscess of buttock
Cutaneous abscess of gluteal region

LØ2.32 Furuncle of buttock
Boil of buttock
Folliculitis of buttock
Furuncle of gluteal region

LØ2.33 Carbuncle of buttock
Carbuncle of gluteal region

✓5th **L02.4 Cutaneous abscess, furuncle and carbuncle of limb**
EXCLUDES 2 *cutaneous abscess, furuncle and carbuncle of groin (L02.214, L02.224, L02.234)*
cutaneous abscess, furuncle and carbuncle of hand (L02.5-)
cutaneous abscess, furuncle and carbuncle of foot (L02.6-)

✓6th **L02.41 Cutaneous abscess of limb**
L02.411 Cutaneous abscess of right axilla
L02.412 Cutaneous abscess of left axilla
L02.413 Cutaneous abscess of right upper limb
L02.414 Cutaneous abscess of left upper limb
L02.415 Cutaneous abscess of right lower limb
L02.416 Cutaneous abscess of left lower limb
L02.419 Cutaneous abscess of limb, unspecified

✓6th **L02.42 Furuncle of limb**
Boil of limb
Folliculitis of limb
L02.421 Furuncle of right axilla
L02.422 Furuncle of left axilla
L02.423 Furuncle of right upper limb
L02.424 Furuncle of left upper limb
L02.425 Furuncle of right lower limb
L02.426 Furuncle of left lower limb
L02.429 Furuncle of limb, unspecified

✓6th **L02.43 Carbuncle of limb**
L02.431 Carbuncle of right axilla
L02.432 Carbuncle of left axilla
L02.433 Carbuncle of right upper limb
L02.434 Carbuncle of left upper limb
L02.435 Carbuncle of right lower limb
L02.436 Carbuncle of left lower limb
L02.439 Carbuncle of limb, unspecified

✓5th **L02.5 Cutaneous abscess, furuncle and carbuncle of hand**
✓6th **L02.51 Cutaneous abscess of hand**
L02.511 Cutaneous abscess of right hand
L02.512 Cutaneous abscess of left hand
L02.519 Cutaneous abscess of unspecified hand

✓6th **L02.52 Furuncle hand**
Boil of hand
Folliculitis of hand
L02.521 Furuncle right hand
L02.522 Furuncle left hand
L02.529 Furuncle unspecified hand

✓6th **L02.53 Carbuncle of hand**
L02.531 Carbuncle of right hand
L02.532 Carbuncle of left hand
L02.539 Carbuncle of unspecified hand

✓5th **L02.6 Cutaneous abscess, furuncle and carbuncle of foot**
✓6th **L02.61 Cutaneous abscess of foot**
L02.611 Cutaneous abscess of right foot
L02.612 Cutaneous abscess of left foot
L02.619 Cutaneous abscess of unspecified foot

✓6th **L02.62 Furuncle of foot**
Boil of foot
Folliculitis of foot
L02.621 Furuncle of right foot
L02.622 Furuncle of left foot
L02.629 Furuncle of unspecified foot

✓6th **L02.63 Carbuncle of foot**
L02.631 Carbuncle of right foot
L02.632 Carbuncle of left foot
L02.639 Carbuncle of unspecified foot

✓5th **L02.8 Cutaneous abscess, furuncle and carbuncle of other sites**
✓6th **L02.81 Cutaneous abscess of other sites**
L02.811 Cutaneous abscess of head [any part, except face]
L02.818 Cutaneous abscess of other sites

✓6th **L02.82 Furuncle of other sites**
Boil of other sites
Folliculitis of other sites
L02.821 Furuncle of head [any part, except face]
L02.828 Furuncle of other sites

✓6th **L02.83 Carbuncle of other sites**
L02.831 Carbuncle of head [any part, except face]
L02.838 Carbuncle of other sites

✓5th **L02.9 Cutaneous abscess, furuncle and carbuncle, unspecified**
L02.91 Cutaneous abscess, unspecified
L02.92 Furuncle, unspecified
Boil NOS
Furunculosis NOS
L02.93 Carbuncle, unspecified

✓4th **L03 Cellulitis and acute lymphangitis**
EXCLUDES 2 *cellulitis of anal and rectal region (K61.-)*
cellulitis of external auditory canal (H60.1)
cellulitis of eyelid (H00.03-)
cellulitis of female external genital organs (N76.4)
cellulitis of lacrimal apparatus (H04.3)
cellulitis of male external genital organs (N48.2, N49-)
cellulitis of mouth (K12.2)
cellulitis of nose (J34.0)
eosinophilic cellulitis [Wells] (L98.3)
febrile neutrophilic dermatosis [Sweet] (L98.2)
lymphangitis (chronic) (subacute) (I89.1)

✓5th **L03.0 Cellulitis and acute lymphangitis of finger and toe**
Infection of nail
Onychia
Paronychia
Perionychia

✓6th **L03.01 Cellulitis of finger**
Felon
Whitlow
EXCLUDES 1 *herpetic whitlow (B00.89)*
L03.011 Cellulitis of right finger
L03.012 Cellulitis of left finger
L03.019 Cellulitis of unspecified finger

✓6th **L03.02 Acute lymphangitis of finger**
Hangnail with lymphangitis of finger
L03.021 Acute lymphangitis of right finger
L03.022 Acute lymphangitis of left finger
L03.029 Acute lymphangitis of unspecified finger

✓6th **L03.03 Cellulitis of toe**
L03.031 Cellulitis of right toe
L03.032 Cellulitis of left toe
L03.039 Cellulitis of unspecified toe

✓6th **L03.04 Acute lymphangitis of toe**
Hangnail with lymphangitis of toe
L03.041 Acute lymphangitis of right toe
L03.042 Acute lymphangitis of left toe
L03.049 Acute lymphangitis of unspecified toe

✓5th **L03.1 Cellulitis and acute lymphangitis of other parts of limb**
✓6th **L03.11 Cellulitis of other parts of limb**
EXCLUDES 2 *cellulitis of fingers (L03.01-)*
cellulitis of toes (L03.03-)
groin (L03.314)
L03.111 Cellulitis of right axilla
L03.112 Cellulitis of left axilla
L03.113 Cellulitis of right upper limb
L03.114 Cellulitis of left upper limb
L03.115 Cellulitis of right lower limb
L03.116 Cellulitis of left lower limb
L03.119 Cellulitis of unspecified part of limb

✓6th **L03.12 Acute lymphangitis of other parts of limb**
EXCLUDES 2 *acute lymphangitis of fingers (L03.02-)*
acute lymphangitis of groin (L03.324)
acute lymphangitis of toes (L03.04-)
L03.121 Acute lymphangitis of right axilla
L03.122 Acute lymphangitis of left axilla
L03.123 Acute lymphangitis of right upper limb
L03.124 Acute lymphangitis of left upper limb
L03.125 Acute lymphangitis of right lower limb
L03.126 Acute lymphangitis of left lower limb
L03.129 Acute lymphangitis of unspecified part of limb

✓5th **LØ3.2 Cellulitis and acute lymphangitis of face and neck**
✓6th **LØ3.21 Cellulitis and acute lymphangitis of face**
LØ3.211 Cellulitis of face
EXCLUDES 2 *cellulitis of ear (H6Ø.1-)*
cellulitis of eyelid (HØØ.Ø3-)
cellulitis of head (LØ3.811)
cellulitis of lacrimal apparatus (HØ4.3)
cellulitis of lip (K13.Ø)
cellulitis of mouth (K12.2)
cellulitis of nose (internal) (J34.Ø)
cellulitis of orbit (HØ5.Ø)
cellulitis of scalp (LØ3.811)
LØ3.212 Acute lymphangitis of face
✓6th **LØ3.22 Cellulitis and acute lymphangitis of neck**
LØ3.221 Cellulitis of neck
LØ3.222 Acute lymphangitis of neck
✓5th **LØ3.3 Cellulitis and acute lymphangitis of trunk**
✓6th **LØ3.31 Cellulitis of trunk**
EXCLUDES 2 *cellulitis of anal and rectal regions (K61.-)*
cellulitis of breast NOS (N61)
cellulitis of female external genital organs (N76.4)
cellulitis of male external genital organs (N48.2, N49-)
omphalitis of newborn (P38.-)
puerperal cellulitis of breast (O91.2)
LØ3.311 Cellulitis of abdominal wall
EXCLUDES 2 *cellulitis of umbilicus (LØ3.316)*
cellulitis of groin (LØ3.314)
LØ3.312 Cellulitis of back [any part except buttock]
LØ3.313 Cellulitis of chest wall
LØ3.314 Cellulitis of groin
LØ3.315 Cellulitis of perineum
LØ3.316 Cellulitis of umbilicus
LØ3.317 Cellulitis of buttock
LØ3.319 Cellulitis of trunk, unspecified
✓6th **LØ3.32 Acute lymphangitis of trunk**
LØ3.321 Acute lymphangitis of abdominal wall
LØ3.322 Acute lymphangitis of back [any part except buttock]
LØ3.323 Acute lymphangitis of chest wall
LØ3.324 Acute lymphangitis of groin
LØ3.325 Acute lymphangitis of perineum
LØ3.326 Acute lymphangitis of umbilicus
LØ3.327 Acute lymphangitis of buttock
LØ3.329 Acute lymphangitis of trunk, unspecified
✓5th **LØ3.8 Cellulitis and acute lymphangitis of other sites**
✓6th **LØ3.81 Cellulitis of other sites**
LØ3.811 Cellulitis of head [any part, except face]
Cellulitis of scalp
EXCLUDES 2 *cellulitis of face (LØ3.211)*
LØ3.818 Cellulitis of other sites
✓6th **LØ3.89 Acute lymphangitis of other sites**
LØ3.891 Acute lymphangitis of head [any part, except face]
LØ3.898 Acute lymphangitis of other sites
✓5th **LØ3.9 Cellulitis and acute lymphangitis, unspecified**
LØ3.9Ø Cellulitis, unspecified
LØ3.91 Acute lymphangitis, unspecified
EXCLUDES 1 *lymphangitis NOS (I89.1)*

✓4th **LØ4 Acute lymphadenitis**
INCLUDES abscess (acute) of lymph nodes, except mesenteric
acute lymphadenitis, except mesenteric
EXCLUDES 1 *chronic or subacute lymphadenitis, except mesenteric (I88.1)*
enlarged lymph nodes (R59.-)
human immunodeficiency virus [HIV] disease resulting in generalized lymphadenopathy (B2Ø)
lymphadenitis NOS (I88.9)
nonspecific mesenteric lymphadenitis (I88.Ø)
LØ4.Ø Acute lymphadenitis of face, head and neck
LØ4.1 Acute lymphadenitis of trunk
LØ4.2 Acute lymphadenitis of upper limb
Acute lymphadenitis of axilla
Acute lymphadenitis of shoulder
LØ4.3 Acute lymphadenitis of lower limb
Acute lymphadenitis of hip
EXCLUDES 2 *acute lymphadenitis of groin (LØ4.1)*
LØ4.8 Acute lymphadenitis of other sites
LØ4.9 Acute lymphadenitis, unspecified

✓4th **LØ5 Pilonidal cyst and sinus**
✓5th **LØ5.Ø Pilonidal cyst and sinus with abscess**
LØ5.Ø1 Pilonidal cyst with abscess
Parasacral dimple with abscess
Pilonidal abscess
Pilonidal dimple with abscess
Postanal dimple with abscess
LØ5.Ø2 Pilonidal sinus with abscess
Coccygeal fistula with abscess
Coccygeal sinus with abscess
Pilonidal fistula with abscess
✓5th **LØ5.9 Pilonidal cyst and sinus without abscess**
LØ5.91 Pilonidal cyst without abscess
Parasacral dimple
Pilonidal dimple
Postanal dimple
Pilonidal cyst NOS
LØ5.92 Pilonidal sinus without abscess
Coccygeal fistula
Coccygeal sinus without abscess
Pilonidal fistula

✓4th **LØ8 Other local infections of skin and subcutaneous tissue**
LØ8.Ø Pyoderma
Dermatitis gangrenosa
Purulent dermatitis
Septic dermatitis
Suppurative dermatitis
EXCLUDES 1 *pyoderma gangrenosum (L88)*
pyoderma vegetans (LØ8.81)
LØ8.1 Erythrasma
✓5th **LØ8.8 Other specified local infections of the skin and subcutaneous tissue**
LØ8.81 Pyoderma vegetans
EXCLUDES 1 *pyoderma gangrenosum (L88)*
pyoderma NOS (LØ8.Ø)
LØ8.82 Omphalitis not of newborn
EXCLUDES 1 *omphalitis of newborn (P38.-)*
LØ8.89 Other specified local infections of the skin and subcutaneous tissue
LØ8.9 Local infection of the skin and subcutaneous tissue, unspecified

Bullous disorders (L1Ø-L14)

EXCLUDES 1 *benign familial pemphigus [Hailey-Hailey] (Q82.8)*
staphylococcal scalded skin syndrome (LØØ)
toxic epidermal necrolysis [Lyell] (L51.2)

✓4th **L1Ø Pemphigus**
EXCLUDES 1 *pemphigus neonatorum (LØ1.Ø3)*
L1Ø.Ø Pemphigus vulgaris
L1Ø.1 Pemphigus vegetans
L1Ø.2 Pemphigus foliaceous
L1Ø.3 Brazilian pemphigus [fogo selvagem]
L1Ø.4 Pemphigus erythematosus
Senear-Usher syndrome
L1Ø.5 Drug-induced pemphigus
Use additional code for adverse effect, if applicable, to identify drug (T36-T5Ø with fifth or sixth character 5)
✓5th **L1Ø.8 Other pemphigus**
L1Ø.81 Paraneoplastic pemphigus
L1Ø.89 Other pemphigus
L1Ø.9 Pemphigus, unspecified

✓4th **L11 Other acantholytic disorders**
L11.Ø Acquired keratosis follicularis
EXCLUDES 1 *keratosis follicularis (congenital) [Darier-White] (Q82.8)*
L11.1 Transient acantholytic dermatosis [Grover]
L11.8 Other specified acantholytic disorders
L11.9 Acantholytic disorder, unspecified

√4th **L12 Pemphigoid**
EXCLUDES 1 *herpes gestationis (O26.4-)*
impetigo herpetiformis (L40.1)
L12.0 Bullous pemphigoid
L12.1 Cicatricial pemphigoid
Benign mucous membrane pemphigoid
L12.2 Chronic bullous disease of childhood
Juvenile dermatitis herpetiformis
√5th **L12.3 Acquired epidermolysis bullosa**
EXCLUDES 1 *epidermolysis bullosa (congenital) (Q81.-)*
L12.30 Acquired epidermolysis bullosa, unspecified
L12.31 Epidermolysis bullosa due to drug
Use additional code for adverse effect, if applicable, to identify drug (T36-T50 with fifth or sixth character 5)
L12.35 Other acquired epidermolysis bullosa
L12.8 Other pemphigoid
L12.9 Pemphigoid, unspecified

√4th **L13 Other bullous disorders**
L13.0 Dermatitis herpetiformis
Duhring's disease
Hydroa herpetiformis
EXCLUDES 1 *juvenile dermatitis herpetiformis (L12.2)*
senile dermatitis herpetiformis (L12.0)
L13.1 Subcorneal pustular dermatitis
Sneddon-Wilkinson disease
L13.8 Other specified bullous disorders
L13.9 Bullous disorder, unspecified

L14 Bullous disorders in diseases classified elsewhere
Code first underlying disease

Dermatitis and eczema (L20-L30)

NOTE In this block the terms dermatitis and eczema are used synonymously and interchangeably.

EXCLUDES 2 *chronic (childhood) granulomatous disease (D71)*
dermatitis gangrenosa (L08.0)
dermatitis herpetiformis (L13.0)
dry skin dermatitis (L85.3)
factitial dermatitis (L98.1)
perioral dermatitis (L71.0)
radiation-related disorders of the skin and subcutaneous tissue (L55-L59)
stasis dermatitis (I83.1-I83.2)

√4th **L20 Atopic dermatitis**
L20.0 Besnier's prurigo
√5th **L20.8 Other atopic dermatitis**
EXCLUDES 2 *circumscribed neurodermatitis (L28.0)*
L20.81 Atopic neurodermatitis
Diffuse neurodermatitis
L20.82 Flexural eczema
L20.83 Infantile (acute) (chronic) eczema
L20.84 Intrinsic (allergic) eczema
L20.89 Other atopic dermatitis
L20.9 Atopic dermatitis, unspecified

√4th **L21 Seborrheic dermatitis**
EXCLUDES 2 *infective dermatitis (L30.3)*
seborrheic keratosis (L82.-)
L21.0 Seborrhea capitis
Cradle cap
L21.1 Seborrheic infantile dermatitis
L21.8 Other seborrheic dermatitis
L21.9 Seborrheic dermatitis, unspecified
Seborrhea NOS

L22 Diaper dermatitis
Diaper erythema
Diaper rash
Psoriasiform diaper rash

√4th **L23 Allergic contact dermatitis**
EXCLUDES 1 *allergy NOS (T78.40)*
contact dermatitis NOS (L25.9)
dermatitis NOS (L30.9)
EXCLUDES 2 *dermatitis due to substances taken internally (L27.-)*
dermatitis of eyelid (H01.1-)
diaper dermatitis (L22)
eczema of external ear (H60.5-)
irritant contact dermatitis (L24.-)
perioral dermatitis (L71.0)
radiation-related disorders of the skin and subcutaneous tissue (L55-L59)
L23.0 Allergic contact dermatitis due to metals
Allergic contact dermatitis due to chromium
Allergic contact dermatitis due to nickel
L23.1 Allergic contact dermatitis due to adhesives
L23.2 Allergic contact dermatitis due to cosmetics
L23.3 Allergic contact dermatitis due to drugs in contact with skin
Use additional code for adverse effect, if applicable, to identify drug (T36-T50 with fifth or sixth character 5)
EXCLUDES 2 *dermatitis due to ingested drugs and medicaments (L27.0-L27.1)*
L23.4 Allergic contact dermatitis due to dyes
L23.5 Allergic contact dermatitis due to other chemical products
Allergic contact dermatitis due to cement
Allergic contact dermatitis due to insecticide
Allergic contact dermatitis due to plastic
Allergic contact dermatitis due to rubber
L23.6 Allergic contact dermatitis due to food in contact with the skin
EXCLUDES 2 *dermatitis due to ingested food (L27.2)*
L23.7 Allergic contact dermatitis due to plants, except food
EXCLUDES 2 *allergy NOS due to pollen (J30.1)*
√5th **L23.8 Allergic contact dermatitis due to other agents**
L23.81 Allergic contact dermatitis due to animal (cat) (dog) dander
Allergic contact dermatitis due to animal (cat) (dog) hair
L23.89 Allergic contact dermatitis due to other agents
L23.9 Allergic contact dermatitis, unspecified cause
Allergic contact eczema NOS

√4th **L24 Irritant contact dermatitis**
EXCLUDES 1 *allergy NOS (T78.40)*
contact dermatitis NOS (L25.9)
dermatitis NOS (L30.9)
EXCLUDES 2 *allergic contact dermatitis (L23.-)*
dermatitis due to substances taken internally (L27.-)
dermatitis of eyelid (H01.1-)
diaper dermatitis (L22)
eczema of external ear (H60.5-)
perioral dermatitis (L71.0)
radiation-related disorders of the skin and subcutaneous tissue (L55-L59)
L24.0 Irritant contact dermatitis due to detergents
L24.1 Irritant contact dermatitis due to oils and greases
L24.2 Irritant contact dermatitis due to solvents
Irritant contact dermatitis due to chlorocompound
Irritant contact dermatitis due to cyclohexane
Irritant contact dermatitis due to ester
Irritant contact dermatitis due to glycol
Irritant contact dermatitis due to hydrocarbon
Irritant contact dermatitis due to ketone
L24.3 Irritant contact dermatitis due to cosmetics
L24.4 Irritant contact dermatitis due to drugs in contact with skin
Use additional code for adverse effect, if applicable, to identify drug (T36-T50 with fifth or sixth character 5)
L24.5 Irritant contact dermatitis due to other chemical products
Irritant contact dermatitis due to cement
Irritant contact dermatitis due to insecticide
Irritant contact dermatitis due to plastic
Irritant contact dermatitis due to rubber
L24.6 Irritant contact dermatitis due to food in contact with skin
EXCLUDES 2 *dermatitis due to ingested food (L27.2)*
L24.7 Irritant contact dermatitis due to plants, except food
EXCLUDES 2 *allergy NOS to pollen (J30.1)*

✓5th **L24.8 Irritant contact dermatitis due to other agents**
L24.81 Irritant contact dermatitis due to metals
Irritant contact dermatitis due to chromium
Irritant contact dermatitis due to nickel
L24.89 Irritant contact dermatitis due to other agents
Irritant contact dermatitis due to dyes
L24.9 Irritant contact dermatitis, unspecified cause
Irritant contact eczema NOS

✓4th **L25 Unspecified contact dermatitis**
EXCLUDES 1 *allergic contact dermatitis (L23.-)*
allergy NOS (T78.40)
dermatitis NOS (L30.9)
irritant contact dermatitis (L24.-)
EXCLUDES 2 *dermatitis due to ingested substances (L27.-)*
dermatitis of eyelid (H01.1-)
eczema of external ear (H60.5-)
perioral dermatitis (L71.0)
radiation-related disorders of the skin and subcutaneous tissue (L55-L59)
L25.0 Unspecified contact dermatitis due to cosmetics
L25.1 Unspecified contact dermatitis due to drugs in contact with skin
Use additional code for adverse effect, if applicable, to identify drug (T36-T50 with fifth or sixth character 5)
EXCLUDES 2 *dermatitis due to ingested drugs and medicaments (L27.0-L27.1)*
L25.2 Unspecified contact dermatitis due to dyes
L25.3 Unspecified contact dermatitis due to other chemical products
Unspecified contact dermatitis due to cement
Unspecified contact dermatitis due to insecticide
L25.4 Unspecified contact dermatitis due to food in contact with skin
EXCLUDES 2 *dermatitis due to ingested food (L27.2)*
L25.5 Unspecified contact dermatitis due to plants, except food
EXCLUDES 1 *nettle rash (L50.9)*
EXCLUDES 2 *allergy NOS due to pollen (J30.1)*
L25.8 Unspecified contact dermatitis due to other agents
L25.9 Unspecified contact dermatitis, unspecified cause
Contact dermatitis (occupational) NOS
Contact eczema (occupational) NOS

L26 Exfoliative dermatitis
Hebra's pityriasis
EXCLUDES 1 *Ritter's disease (L00)*

✓4th **L27 Dermatitis due to substances taken internally**
EXCLUDES 1 *allergy NOS (T78.40)*
EXCLUDES 2 *adverse food reaction, except dermatitis (T78.0-T78.1)*
contact dermatitis (L23-L25)
drug photoallergic response (L56.1)
drug phototoxic response (L56.0)
urticaria (L50.-)
L27.0 Generalized skin eruption due to drugs and medicaments taken internally
Use additional code for adverse effect, if applicable, to identify drug (T36-T50 with fifth or sixth character 5)
L27.1 Localized skin eruption due to drugs and medicaments taken internally
Use additional code for adverse effect, if applicable, to identify drug (T36-T50 with fifth or sixth character 5)
L27.2 Dermatitis due to ingested food
EXCLUDES 2 *dermatitis due to food in contact with skin (L23.6, L24.6, L25.4)*
L27.8 Dermatitis due to other substances taken internally
L27.9 Dermatitis due to unspecified substance taken internally

✓4th **L28 Lichen simplex chronicus and prurigo**
L28.0 Lichen simplex chronicus
Circumscribed neurodermatitis
Lichen NOS
L28.1 Prurigo nodularis
L28.2 Other prurigo
Prurigo NOS
Prurigo Hebra
Prurigo mitis
Urticaria papulosa

✓4th **L29 Pruritus**
EXCLUDES 1 *neurotic excoriation (L98.1)*
psychogenic pruritus (F45.8)
L29.0 Pruritus ani
L29.1 Pruritus scroti
L29.2 Pruritus vulvae
L29.3 Anogenital pruritus, unspecified
L29.8 Other pruritus
L29.9 Pruritus, unspecified
Itch NOS

✓4th **L30 Other and unspecified dermatitis**
EXCLUDES 2 *contact dermatitis (L23-L25)*
dry skin dermatitis (L85.3)
small plaque parapsoriasis (L41.3)
stasis dermatitis (I83.1-.2)
L30.0 Nummular dermatitis
L30.1 Dyshidrosis [pompholyx]
L30.2 Cutaneous autosensitization
Candidid [levurid]
Dermatophytid
Eczematid
L30.3 Infective dermatitis
Infectious eczematoid dermatitis
L30.4 Erythema intertrigo
L30.5 Pityriasis alba
L30.8 Other specified dermatitis
L30.9 Dermatitis, unspecified
Eczema NOS

Papulosquamous disorders (L40-L45)

✓4th **L40 Psoriasis**
L40.0 Psoriasis vulgaris
Nummular psoriasis
Plaque psoriasis
L40.1 Generalized pustular psoriasis
Impetigo herpetiformis
Von Zumbusch's disease
L40.2 Acrodermatitis continua
L40.3 Pustulosis palmaris et plantaris
L40.4 Guttate psoriasis
✓5th **L40.5 Arthropathic psoriasis**
L40.50 Arthropathic psoriasis, unspecified
L40.51 Distal interphalangeal psoriatic arthropathy
L40.52 Psoriatic arthritis mutilans
L40.53 Psoriatic spondylitis
L40.54 Psoriatic juvenile arthropathy
L40.59 Other psoriatic arthropathy
L40.8 Other psoriasis
Flexural psoriasis
L40.9 Psoriasis, unspecified

✓4th **L41 Parapsoriasis**
EXCLUDES 1 *poikiloderma vasculare atrophicans (L94.5)*
L41.0 Pityriasis lichenoides et varioliformis acuta
Mucha-Habermann disease
L41.1 Pityriasis lichenoides chronica
L41.2 Lymphomatoid papulosis
L41.3 Small plaque parapsoriasis
L41.4 Large plaque parapsoriasis
L41.5 Retiform parapsoriasis
L41.8 Other parapsoriasis
L41.9 Parapsoriasis, unspecified

L42 Pityriasis rosea

✓4th **L43 Lichen planus**
EXCLUDES 1 *lichen planopilaris (L66.1)*
L43.0 Hypertrophic lichen planus
L43.1 Bullous lichen planus
L43.2 Lichenoid drug reaction
Use additional code for adverse effect, if applicable, to identify drug (T36-T50 with fifth or sixth character 5)
L43.3 Subacute (active) lichen planus
Lichen planus tropicus
L43.8 Other lichen planus
L43.9 Lichen planus, unspecified

✓4th **L44 Other papulosquamous disorders**
L44.0 Pityriasis rubra pilaris
L44.1 Lichen nitidus
L44.2 Lichen striatus
L44.3 Lichen ruber moniliformis
L44.4 Infantile papular acrodermatitis [Gianotti-Crosti]
L44.8 Other specified papulosquamous disorders
L44.9 Papulosquamous disorder, unspecified

L45 Papulosquamous disorders in diseases classified elsewhere
Code first underlying disease

Urticaria and erythema (L49-L54)

EXCLUDES 1 *Lyme disease (A69.2-)*
rosacea (L71.-)

✓4th **L49 Exfoliation due to erythematous conditions according to extent of body surface involved**
Code first erythematous condition causing exfoliation, such as:
Ritter's disease (L00)
(Staphylococcal) scalded skin syndrom (L00)
Stevens-Johnson syndrome (L51.1)
Stevens-Johnson syndrome-toxic epidermal necrolysis overlap syndrome (L51.3)
toxic epidermal necrolysis (L51.2)
L49.0 Exfoliation due to erythematous condition involving less than 10 percent of body surface
Exfoliation due to erythematous condition NOS
L49.1 Exfoliation due to erythematous condition involving 10-19 percent of body surface
L49.2 Exfoliation due to erythematous condition involving 20-29 percent of body surface
L49.3 Exfoliation due to erythematous condition involving 30-39 percent of body surface
L49.4 Exfoliation due to erythematous condition involving 40-49 percent of body surface
L49.5 Exfoliation due to erythematous condition involving 50-59 percent of body surface
L49.6 Exfoliation due to erythematous condition involving 60-69 percent of body surface
L49.7 Exfoliation due to erythematous condition involving 70-79 percent of body surface
L49.8 Exfoliation due to erythematous condition involving 80-89 percent of body surface
L49.9 Exfoliation due to erythematous condition involving 90 or more percent of body surface

✓4th **L50 Urticaria**
EXCLUDES 1 *allergic contact dermatitis (L23.-)*
angioneurotic edema (T78.3)
giant urticaria (T78.3)
hereditary angio-edema (D84.1)
Quincke's edema (T78.3)
serum urticaria (T80.6-)
solar urticaria (L56.3)
urticaria neonatorum (P83.8)
urticaria papulosa (L28.2)
urticaria pigmentosa (Q82.2)
L50.0 Allergic urticaria
L50.1 Idiopathic urticaria
L50.2 Urticaria due to cold and heat
L50.3 Dermatographic urticaria
L50.4 Vibratory urticaria
L50.5 Cholinergic urticaria
L50.6 Contact urticaria
L50.8 Other urticaria
Chronic urticaria
Recurrent periodic urticaria
L50.9 Urticaria, unspecified

✓4th **L51 Erythema multiforme**
Use additional code for adverse effect, if applicable, to identify drug (T36-T50 with fifth or sixth character 5)
Use additional code to identify associated manifestations, such as:
arthropathy associated with dermatological disorders (M14.8-)
conjunctival edema (H11.42)
conjunctivitis (H10.22-)
corneal scars and opacities (H17.-)
corneal ulcer (H16.0-)
edema of eyelid (H02.84)
inflammation of eyelid (H01.8)
keratoconjunctivitis sicca (H16.22-)
mechanical lagophthalmos (H02.22-)
stomatitis (K12.-)
symblepharon (H11.23-)
Use additional code to identify percentage of skin exfoliation (L49.-)
EXCLUDES 1 *staphylococcal scalded skin syndrome (L00)*
Ritter's disease (L00)
L51.0 Nonbullous erythema multiforme
L51.1 Stevens-Johnson syndrome
L51.2 Toxic epidermal necrolysis [Lyell]
L51.3 Stevens-Johnson syndrome-toxic epidermal necrolysis overlap syndrome
SJS-TEN overlap syndrome
L51.8 Other erythema multiforme
L51.9 Erythema multiforme, unspecified
Erythema iris
Erythema multiforme major NOS
Erythema multiforme minor NOS
Herpes iris

L52 Erythema nodosum
EXCLUDES 1 *tuberculous erythema nodosum (A18.4)*

✓4th **L53 Other erythematous conditions**
EXCLUDES 1 *erythema ab igne (L59.0)*
erythema due to external agents in contact with skin (L23-L25)
erythema intertrigo (L30.4)
L53.0 Toxic erythema
Code first poisoning due to drug or toxin, if applicable (T36-T65 with fifth or sixth character 1-4 or 6)
Use additional code for adverse effect, if applicable, to identify drug (T36-T50 with fifth or sixth character 5)
EXCLUDES 1 *neonatal erythema toxicum (P83.1)*
L53.1 Erythema annulare centrifugum
L53.2 Erythema marginatum
L53.3 Other chronic figurate erythema
L53.8 Other specified erythematous conditions
L53.9 Erythematous condition, unspecified
Erythema NOS
Erythroderma NOS

L54 Erythema in diseases classified elsewhere
Code first underlying disease

Radiation-related disorders of the skin and subcutaneous tissue (L55-L59)

✓4th **L55 Sunburn**
L55.0 Sunburn of first degree
L55.1 Sunburn of second degree
L55.2 Sunburn of third degree
L55.9 Sunburn, unspecified

✓4th **L56 Other acute skin changes due to ultraviolet radiation**
Use additional code to identify the source of the ultraviolet radiation (W89, X32)
L56.0 Drug phototoxic response
Use additional code for adverse effect, if applicable, to identify drug (T36-T50 with fifth or sixth character 5)
L56.1 Drug photoallergic response
Use additional code for adverse effect, if applicable, to identify drug (T36-T50 with fifth or sixth character 5)
L56.2 Photocontact dermatitis [berloque dermatitis]
L56.3 Solar urticaria
L56.4 Polymorphous light eruption
L56.5 Disseminated superficial actinic porokeratosis (DSAP)
L56.8 Other specified acute skin changes due to ultraviolet radiation
L56.9 Acute skin change due to ultraviolet radiation, unspecified

4th L57 Skin changes due to chronic exposure to nonionizing radiation
Use additional code to identify the source of the ultraviolet radiation (W89, X32)

L57.0 Actinic keratosis
Keratosis NOS
Senile keratosis
Solar keratosis

L57.1 Actinic reticuloid

L57.2 Cutis rhomboidalis nuchae

L57.3 Poikiloderma of Civatte

L57.4 Cutis laxa senilis
Elastosis senilis

L57.5 Actinic granuloma

L57.8 Other skin changes due to chronic exposure to nonionizing radiation
Farmer's skin
Sailor's skin
Solar dermatitis

L57.9 Skin changes due to chronic exposure to nonionizing radiation, unspecified

4th L58 Radiodermatitis
Use additional code to identify the source of the radiation (W88, W90)

L58.0 Acute radiodermatitis

L58.1 Chronic radiodermatitis

L58.9 Radiodermatitis, unspecified

4th L59 Other disorders of skin and subcutaneous tissue related to radiation

L59.0 Erythema ab igne [dermatitis ab igne]

L59.8 Other specified disorders of the skin and subcutaneous tissue related to radiation

L59.9 Disorder of the skin and subcutaneous tissue related to radiation, unspecified

Disorders of skin appendages (L60-L75)

EXCLUDES 1 *congenital malformations of integument (Q84.-)*

4th L60 Nail disorders
EXCLUDES 2 *clubbing of nails (R68.3)*
onychia and paronychia (L03.0-)

L60.0 Ingrowing nail

L60.1 Onycholysis

L60.2 Onychogryphosis

L60.3 Nail dystrophy

L60.4 Beau's lines

L60.5 Yellow nail syndrome

L60.8 Other nail disorders

L60.9 Nail disorder, unspecified

L62 Nail disorders in diseases classified elsewhere
Code first underlying disease, such as:
pachydermoperiostosis (M89.4-)

4th L63 Alopecia areata

L63.0 Alopecia (capitis) totalis

L63.1 Alopecia universalis

L63.2 Ophiasis

L63.8 Other alopecia areata

L63.9 Alopecia areata, unspecified

4th L64 Androgenic alopecia
INCLUDES male-pattern baldness

L64.0 Drug-induced androgenic alopecia
Use additional code for adverse effect, if applicable, to identify drug (T36-T50 with fifth or sixth character 5)

L64.8 Other androgenic alopecia

L64.9 Androgenic alopecia, unspecified

4th L65 Other nonscarring hair loss
Use additional code for adverse effect, if applicable, to identify drug (T36-T50 with fifth or sixth character 5)
EXCLUDES 1 *trichotillomania (F63.3)*

L65.0 Telogen effluvium

L65.1 Anagen effluvium

L65.2 Alopecia mucinosa

L65.8 Other specified nonscarring hair loss

L65.9 Nonscarring hair loss, unspecified
Alopecia NOS

4th L66 Cicatricial alopecia [scarring hair loss]

L66.0 Pseudopelade

L66.1 Lichen planopilaris
Follicular lichen planus

L66.2 Folliculitis decalvans

L66.3 Perifolliculitis capitis abscedens

L66.4 Folliculitis ulerythematosa reticulata

L66.8 Other cicatricial alopecia

L66.9 Cicatricial alopecia, unspecified

4th L67 Hair color and hair shaft abnormalities
EXCLUDES 1 *monilethrix (Q84.1)*
pili annulati (Q84.1)
telogen effluvium (L65.0)

L67.0 Trichorrhexis nodosa

L67.1 Variations in hair color
Canities
Greyness, hair (premature)
Heterochromia of hair
Poliosis circumscripta, acquired
Poliosis NOS

L67.8 Other hair color and hair shaft abnormalities
Fragilitas crinium

L67.9 Hair color and hair shaft abnormality, unspecified

4th L68 Hypertrichosis
INCLUDES excess hair
EXCLUDES 1 *congenital hypertrichosis (Q84.2)*
persistent lanugo (Q84.2)

L68.0 Hirsutism

L68.1 Acquired hypertrichosis lanuginosa

L68.2 Localized hypertrichosis

L68.3 Polytrichia

L68.8 Other hypertrichosis

L68.9 Hypertrichosis, unspecified

4th L70 Acne
EXCLUDES 2 *acne keloid (L73.0)*

L70.0 Acne vulgaris

L70.1 Acne conglobata

L70.2 Acne varioliformis
Acne necrotica miliaris

L70.3 Acne tropica

L70.4 Infantile acne

L70.5 Acné excoriée des jeunes filles
Picker's acne

L70.8 Other acne

L70.9 Acne, unspecified

4th L71 Rosacea
Use additional code for adverse effect, if applicable, to identify drug (T36-T50 with fifth or sixth character 5)

L71.0 Perioral dermatitis

L71.1 Rhinophyma

L71.8 Other rosacea

L71.9 Rosacea, unspecified

4th L72 Follicular cysts of skin and subcutaneous tissue

L72.0 Epidermal cyst

5th L72.1 Pilar and trichodermal cyst

L72.11 Pilar cyst

L72.12 Trichodermal cyst
Trichilemmal (proliferating) cyst

L72.2 Steatocystoma multiplex

L72.3 Sebaceous cyst
EXCLUDES 2 *pilar cyst (L72.11)*
trichilemmal (proliferating) cyst (L72.12)

L72.8 Other follicular cysts of the skin and subcutaneous tissue

L72.9 Follicular cyst of the skin and subcutaneous tissue, unspecified

4th L73 Other follicular disorders

L73.0 Acne keloid

L73.1 Pseudofolliculitis barbae

L73.2 Hidradenitis suppurativa

L73.8 Other specified follicular disorders
Sycosis barbae

L73.9 Follicular disorder, unspecified

L74 Eccrine sweat disorders
EXCLUDES 2 *generalized hyperhidrosis (R61)*
L74.0 Miliaria rubra
L74.1 Miliaria crystallina
L74.2 Miliaria profunda
Miliaria tropicalis
L74.3 Miliaria, unspecified
L74.4 Anhidrosis
Hypohidrosis
L74.5 Focal hyperhidrosis
L74.51 Primary focal hyperhidrosis
L74.510 Primary focal hyperhidrosis, axilla
L74.511 Primary focal hyperhidrosis, face
L74.512 Primary focal hyperhidrosis, palms
L74.513 Primary focal hyperhidrosis, soles
L74.519 Primary focal hyperhidrosis, unspecified
L74.52 Secondary focal hyperhidrosis
Frey's syndrome
L74.8 Other eccrine sweat disorders
L74.9 Eccrine sweat disorder, unspecified
Sweat gland disorder NOS

L75 Apocrine sweat disorders
EXCLUDES 1 *dyshidrosis (L30.1)*
hidradenitis suppurativa (L73.2)
L75.0 Bromhidrosis
L75.1 Chromhidrosis
L75.2 Apocrine miliaria
Fox-Fordyce disease
L75.8 Other apocrine sweat disorders
L75.9 Apocrine sweat disorder, unspecified

Intraoperative and postprocedural complications of skin and subcutaneous tissue (L76)

L76 Intraoperative and postprocedural complications of skin and subcutaneous tissue
L76.0 Intraoperative hemorrhage and hematoma of skin and subcutaneous tissue complicating a procedure
EXCLUDES 1 *intraoperative hemorrhage and hematoma of skin and subcutaneous tissue due to accidental puncture and laceration during a procedure (L76.1-)*
L76.01 Intraoperative hemorrhage and hematoma of skin and subcutaneous tissue complicating a dermatologic procedure
L76.02 Intraoperative hemorrhage and hematoma of skin and subcutaneous tissue complicating other procedure
L76.1 Accidental puncture and laceration of skin and subcutaneous tissue during a procedure
L76.11 Accidental puncture and laceration of skin and subcutaneous tissue during a dermatologic procedure
L76.12 Accidental puncture and laceration of skin and subcutaneous tissue during other procedure
L76.2 Postprocedural hemorrhage and hematoma of skin and subcutaneous tissue following a procedure
L76.21 Postprocedural hemorrhage and hematoma of skin and subcutaneous tissue following a dermatologic procedure
L76.22 Postprocedural hemorrhage and hematoma of skin and subcutaneous tissue following other procedure
L76.8 Other intraoperative and postprocedural complications of skin and subcutaneous tissue
Use additional code, if applicable, to further specify disorder
L76.81 Other intraoperative complications of skin and subcutaneous tissue
L76.82 Other postprocedural complications of skin and subcutaneous tissue

Other disorders of the skin and subcutaneous tissue (L80-L99)

L80 Vitiligo
EXCLUDES 2 *vitiligo of eyelids (H02.73-)*
vitiligo of vulva (N90.89)

L81 Other disorders of pigmentation
EXCLUDES 1 *birthmark NOS (Q82.5)*
Peutz-Jeghers syndrome (Q85.8)
EXCLUDES 2 *nevus—see Alphabetical Index*
L81.0 Postinflammatory hyperpigmentation
L81.1 Chloasma
L81.2 Freckles
L81.3 Café au lait spots
L81.4 Other melanin hyperpigmentation
Lentigo
L81.5 Leukoderma, not elsewhere classified
L81.6 Other disorders of diminished melanin formation
L81.7 Pigmented purpuric dermatosis
Angioma serpiginosum
L81.8 Other specified disorders of pigmentation
Iron pigmentation
Tattoo pigmentation
L81.9 Disorder of pigmentation, unspecified

L82 Seborrheic keratosis
INCLUDES dermatosis papulosa nigra
Leser-Trélat disease
EXCLUDES 2 *seborrheic dermatitis (L21.-)*
L82.0 Inflamed seborrheic keratosis
L82.1 Other seborrheic keratosis
Seborrheic keratosis NOS

L83 Acanthosis nigricans
Confluent and reticulated papillomatosis

L84 Corns and callosities
Callus
Clavus

L85 Other epidermal thickening
EXCLUDES 2 *hypertrophic disorders of the skin (L91.-)*
L85.0 Acquired ichthyosis
EXCLUDES 1 *congenital ichthyosis (Q80.-)*
L85.1 Acquired keratosis [keratoderma] palmaris et plantaris
EXCLUDES 1 *inherited keratosis palmaris et plantaris (Q82.8)*
L85.2 Keratosis punctata (palmaris et plantaris)
L85.3 Xerosis cutis
Dry skin dermatitis
L85.8 Other specified epidermal thickening
Cutaneous horn
L85.9 Epidermal thickening, unspecified

L86 Keratoderma in diseases classified elsewhere
Code first underlying disease, such as:
Reiter's disease (M02.3-)
EXCLUDES 1 *gonococcal keratoderma (A54.89)*
gonococcal keratosis (A54.89)
keratoderma due to vitamin A deficiency (E50.8)
keratosis due to vitamin A deficiency (E50.8)
xeroderma due to vitamin A deficiency (E50.8)

L87 Transepidermal elimination disorders
EXCLUDES 1 *granuloma annulare (perforating) (L92.0)*
L87.0 Keratosis follicularis et parafollicularis in cutem penetrans
Kyrle disease
Hyperkeratosis follicularis penetrans
L87.1 Reactive perforating collagenosis
L87.2 Elastosis perforans serpiginosa
L87.8 Other transepidermal elimination disorders
L87.9 Transepidermal elimination disorder, unspecified

L88 Pyoderma gangrenosum
Phagedenic pyoderma
EXCLUDES 1 *dermatitis gangrenosa (L08.0)*

L89 Pressure ulcer
Bed sore
Decubitus ulcer
Plaster ulcer
Pressure area
Pressure sore
Code first any associated gangrene (I96)
EXCLUDES 2 *decubitus (trophic) ulcer of cervix (uteri) (N86)*
diabetic ulcers (E08.621, E08.622, E09.621, E09.622, E10.621, E10.622, E11.621, E11.622, E13.621, E13.622)
non-pressure chronic ulcer of skin (L97.-)
skin infections (L00-L08)
varicose ulcer (I83.0, I83.2)

✓5th **L89.0 Pressure ulcer of elbow**

✓6th **L89.00 Pressure ulcer of unspecified elbow**

L89.000 Pressure ulcer of unspecified elbow, unstageable

L89.001 Pressure ulcer of unspecified elbow, stage 1
Healing pressure ulcer of unspecified elbow, stage 1
Pressure pre-ulcer skin changes limited to persistent focal edema, unspecified elbow

L89.002 Pressure ulcer of unspecified elbow, stage 2
Healing pressure ulcer of unspecified elbow, stage 2
Pressure ulcer with abrasion, blister, partial thickness skin loss involving epidermis and/or dermis, unspecified elbow

L89.003 Pressure ulcer of unspecified elbow, stage 3
Healing pressure ulcer of unspecified elbow, stage 3
Pressure ulcer with full thickness skin loss involving damage or necrosis of subcutaneous tissue, unspecified elbow

L89.004 Pressure ulcer of unspecified elbow, stage 4
Healing pressure ulcer of unspecified elbow, stage 4
Pressure ulcer with necrosis of soft tissues through to underlying muscle, tendon, or bone, unspecified elbow

L89.009 Pressure ulcer of unspecified elbow, unspecified stage
Healing pressure ulcer of elbow NOS
Healing pressure ulcer of unspecified elbow, unspecified stage

✓6th **L89.01 Pressure ulcer of right elbow**

L89.010 Pressure ulcer of right elbow, unstageable

L89.011 Pressure ulcer of right elbow, stage 1
Healing pressure ulcer of right elbow, stage 1
Pressure pre-ulcer skin changes limited to persistent focal edema, right elbow

L89.012 Pressure ulcer of right elbow, stage 2
Healing pressure ulcer of right elbow, stage 2
Pressure ulcer with abrasion, blister, partial thickness skin loss involving epidermis and/or dermis, right elbow

L89.013 Pressure ulcer of right elbow, stage 3
Healing pressure ulcer of right elbow, stage 3
Pressure ulcer with full thickness skin loss involving damage or necrosis of subcutaneous tissue, right elbow

L89.014 Pressure ulcer of right elbow, stage 4
Healing pressure ulcer of right elbow, stage 4
Pressure ulcer with necrosis of soft tissues through to underlying muscle, tendon, or bone, right elbow

L89.019 Pressure ulcer of right elbow, unspecified stage
Healing pressure right of elbow NOS
Healing pressure ulcer of unspecified elbow, unspecified stage

✓6th **L89.02 Pressure ulcer of left elbow**

L89.020 Pressure ulcer of left elbow, unstageable

L89.021 Pressure ulcer of left elbow, stage 1
Healing pressure ulcer of left elbow, stage 1
Pressure pre-ulcer skin changes limited to persistent focal edema, left elbow

L89.022 Pressure ulcer of left elbow, stage 2
Healing pressure ulcer of left elbow, stage 2
Pressure ulcer with abrasion, blister, partial thickness skin loss involving epidermis and/or dermis, left elbow

L89.023 Pressure ulcer of left elbow, stage 3
Healing pressure ulcer of left elbow, stage 3
Pressure ulcer with full thickness skin loss involving damage or necrosis of subcutaneous tissue, left elbow

L89.024 Pressure ulcer of left elbow, stage 4
Healing pressure ulcer of left elbow, stage 4
Pressure ulcer with necrosis of soft tissues through to underlying muscle, tendon, or bone, left elbow

L89.029 Pressure ulcer of left elbow, unspecified stage
Healing pressure ulcer of left of elbow NOS
Healing pressure ulcer of unspecified elbow, unspecified stage

✓5th **L89.1 Pressure ulcer of back**

✓6th **L89.10 Pressure ulcer of unspecified part of back**

L89.100 Pressure ulcer of unspecified part of back, unstageable

L89.101 Pressure ulcer of unspecified part of back, stage 1
Healing pressure ulcer of unspecified part of back, stage 1
Pressure pre-ulcer skin changes limited to persistent focal edema, unspecified part of back

L89.102 Pressure ulcer of unspecified part of back, stage 2
Healing pressure ulcer of unspecified part of back, stage 2
Pressure ulcer with abrasion, blister, partial thickness skin loss involving epidermis and/or dermis, unspecified part of back

L89.103 Pressure ulcer of unspecified part of back, stage 3
Healing pressure ulcer of unspecified part of back, stage 3
Pressure ulcer with full thickness skin loss involving damage or necrosis of subcutaneous tissue, unspecified part of back

L89.104 Pressure ulcer of unspecified part of back, stage 4
Healing pressure ulcer of unspecified part of back, stage 4
Pressure ulcer with necrosis of soft tissues through to underlying muscle, tendon, or bone, unspecified part of back

L89.109 Pressure ulcer of unspecified part of back, unspecified stage
Healing pressure ulcer of unspecified part of back NOS
Healing pressure ulcer of unspecified part of back, unspecified stage

L89.11 Pressure ulcer of right upper back (6th)
Pressure ulcer of right shoulder blade

L89.110 Pressure ulcer of right upper back, unstageable

L89.111 Pressure ulcer of right upper back, stage 1
Healing pressure ulcer of right upper back, stage 1
Pressure pre-ulcer skin changes limited to persistent focal edema, right upper back

L89.112 Pressure ulcer of right upper back, stage 2
Healing pressure ulcer of right upper back, stage 2
Pressure ulcer with abrasion, blister, partial thickness skin loss involving epidermis and/or dermis, right upper back

L89.113 Pressure ulcer of right upper back, stage 3
Healing pressure ulcer of right upper back, stage 3
Pressure ulcer with full thickness skin loss involving damage or necrosis of subcutaneous tissue, right upper back

L89.114 Pressure ulcer of right upper back, stage 4
Healing pressure ulcer of right upper back, stage 4
Pressure ulcer with necrosis of soft tissues through to underlying muscle, tendon, or bone, right upper back

L89.119 Pressure ulcer of right upper back, unspecified stage
Healing pressure ulcer of right upper back NOS
Healing pressure ulcer of right upper back, unspecified stage

L89.12 Pressure ulcer of left upper back (6th)
Pressure ulcer of left shoulder blade

L89.120 Pressure ulcer of left upper back, unstageable

L89.121 Pressure ulcer of left upper back, stage 1
Healing pressure ulcer of left upper back, stage 1
Pressure pre-ulcer skin changes limited to persistent focal edema, left upper back

L89.122 Pressure ulcer of left upper back, stage 2
Healing pressure ulcer of left upper back, stage 2
Pressure ulcer with abrasion, blister, partial thickness skin loss involving epidermis and/or dermis, left upper back

L89.123 Pressure ulcer of left upper back, stage 3
Healing pressure ulcer of left upper back, stage 3
Pressure ulcer with full thickness skin loss involving damage or necrosis of subcutaneous tissue, left upper back

L89.124 Pressure ulcer of left upper back, stage 4
Healing pressure ulcer of left upper back, stage 4
Pressure ulcer with necrosis of soft tissues through to underlying muscle, tendon, or bone, left upper back

L89.129 Pressure ulcer of left upper back, unspecified stage
Healing pressure ulcer of left upper back NOS
Healing pressure ulcer of left upper back, unspecified stage

L89.13 Pressure ulcer of right lower back (6th)

L89.130 Pressure ulcer of right lower back, unstageable

L89.131 Pressure ulcer of right lower back, stage 1
Healing pressure ulcer of right lower back, stage 1
Pressure pre-ulcer skin changes limited to persistent focal edema, right lower back

L89.132 Pressure ulcer of right lower back, stage 2
Healing pressure ulcer of right lower back, stage 2
Pressure ulcer with abrasion, blister, partial thickness skin loss involving epidermis and/or dermis, right lower back

L89.133 Pressure ulcer of right lower back, stage 3
Healing pressure ulcer of right lower back, stage 3
Pressure ulcer with full thickness skin loss involving damage or necrosis of subcutaneous tissue, right lower back

L89.134 Pressure ulcer of right lower back, stage 4
Healing pressure ulcer of right lower back, stage 4
Pressure ulcer with necrosis of soft tissues through to underlying muscle, tendon, or bone, right lower back

L89.139 Pressure ulcer of right lower back, unspecified stage
Healing pressure ulcer of right lower back NOS
Healing pressure ulcer of right lower back, unspecified stage

L89.14 Pressure ulcer of left lower back (6th)

L89.140 Pressure ulcer of left lower back, unstageable

L89.141 Pressure ulcer of left lower back, stage 1
Healing pressure ulcer of left lower back, stage 1
Pressure pre-ulcer skin changes limited to persistent focal edema, left lower back

L89.142 Pressure ulcer of left lower back, stage 2
Healing pressure ulcer of left lower back, stage 2
Pressure ulcer with abrasion, blister, partial thickness skin loss involving epidermis and/or dermis, left lower back

L89.143 Pressure ulcer of left lower back, stage 3
Healing pressure ulcer of left lower back, stage 3
Pressure ulcer with full thickness skin loss involving damage or necrosis of subcutaneous tissue, left lower back

L89.144 Pressure ulcer of left lower back, stage 4
Healing pressure ulcer of left lower back, stage 4
Pressure ulcer with necrosis of soft tissues through to underlying muscle, tendon, or bone, left lower back

L89.149 Pressure ulcer of left lower back, unspecified stage
Healing pressure ulcer of left lower back NOS
Healing pressure ulcer of left lower back, unspecified stage

6th **L89.15 Pressure ulcer of sacral region**
Pressure ulcer of coccyx
Pressure ulcer of tailbone

L89.150 Pressure ulcer of sacral region, unstageable

L89.151 Pressure ulcer of sacral region, stage 1
Healing pressure ulcer of sacral region, stage 1
Pressure pre-ulcer skin changes limited to persistent focal edema, sacral region

L89.152 Pressure ulcer of sacral region, stage 2
Healing pressure ulcer of sacral region, stage 2
Pressure ulcer with abrasion, blister, partial thickness skin loss involving epidermis and/or dermis, sacral region

L89.153 Pressure ulcer of sacral region, stage 3
Healing pressure ulcer of sacral region, stage 3
Pressure ulcer with full thickness skin loss involving damage or necrosis of subcutaneous tissue, sacral region

L89.154 Pressure ulcer of sacral region, stage 4
Healing pressure ulcer of sacral region, stage 4
Pressure ulcer with necrosis of soft tissues through to underlying muscle, tendon, or bone, sacral region

L89.159 Pressure ulcer of sacral region, unspecified stage
Healing pressure ulcer of sacral region NOS
Healing pressure ulcer of sacral region, unspecified stage

5th **L89.2 Pressure ulcer of hip**

6th **L89.20 Pressure ulcer of unspecified hip**

L89.200 Pressure ulcer of unspecified hip, unstageable

L89.201 Pressure ulcer of unspecified hip, stage 1
Healing pressure ulcer of unspecified hip back, stage 1
Pressure pre-ulcer skin changes limited to persistent focal edema, unspecified hip

L89.202 Pressure ulcer of unspecified hip, stage 2
Healing pressure ulcer of unspecified hip, stage 2
Pressure ulcer with abrasion, blister, partial thickness skin loss involving epidermis and/or dermis, unspecified hip

L89.203 Pressure ulcer of unspecified hip, stage 3
Healing pressure ulcer of unspecified hip, stage 3
Pressure ulcer with full thickness skin loss involving damage or necrosis of subcutaneous tissue, unspecified hip

L89.204 Pressure ulcer of unspecified hip, stage 4
Healing pressure ulcer of unspecified hip, stage 4
Pressure ulcer with necrosis of soft tissues through to underlying muscle, tendon, or bone, unspecified hip

L89.209 Pressure ulcer of unspecified hip, unspecified stage
Healing pressure ulcer of unspecified hip NOS
Healing pressure ulcer of unspecified hip, unspecified stage

6th **L89.21 Pressure ulcer of right hip**

L89.210 Pressure ulcer of right hip, unstageable

L89.211 Pressure ulcer of right hip, stage 1
Healing pressure ulcer of right hip back, stage 1
Pressure pre-ulcer skin changes limited to persistent focal edema, right hip

L89.212 Pressure ulcer of right hip, stage 2
Healing pressure ulcer of right hip, stage 2
Pressure ulcer with abrasion, blister, partial thickness skin loss involving epidermis and/or dermis, right hip

L89.213 Pressure ulcer of right hip, stage 3
Healing pressure ulcer of right hip, stage 3
Pressure ulcer with full thickness skin loss involving damage or necrosis of subcutaneous tissue, right hip

L89.214 Pressure ulcer of right hip, stage 4
Healing pressure ulcer of right hip, stage 4
Pressure ulcer with necrosis of soft tissues through to underlying muscle, tendon, or bone, right hip

L89.219 Pressure ulcer of right hip, unspecified stage
Healing pressure ulcer of right hip NOS
Healing pressure ulcer of right hip, unspecified stage

6th **L89.22 Pressure ulcer of left hip**

L89.220 Pressure ulcer of left hip, unstageable

L89.221 Pressure ulcer of left hip, stage 1
Healing pressure ulcer of left hip back, stage 1
Pressure pre-ulcer skin changes limited to persistent focal edema, left hip

L89.222 Pressure ulcer of left hip, stage 2
Healing pressure ulcer of left hip, stage 2
Pressure ulcer with abrasion, blister, partial thickness skin loss involving epidermis and/or dermis, left hip

L89.223 Pressure ulcer of left hip, stage 3
Healing pressure ulcer of left hip, stage 3
Pressure ulcer with full thickness skin loss involving damage or necrosis of subcutaneous tissue, left hip

L89.224 Pressure ulcer of left hip, stage 4
Healing pressure ulcer of left hip, stage 4
Pressure ulcer with necrosis of soft tissues through to underlying muscle, tendon, or bone, left hip

L89.229 Pressure ulcer of left hip, unspecified stage
Healing pressure ulcer of left hip NOS
Healing pressure ulcer of left hip, unspecified stage

5th **L89.3 Pressure ulcer of buttock**

6th **L89.30 Pressure ulcer of unspecified buttock**

L89.300 Pressure ulcer of unspecified buttock, unstageable

L89.301 Pressure ulcer of unspecified buttock, stage 1
Healing pressure ulcer of unspecified buttock, stage 1
Pressure pre-ulcer skin changes limited to persistent focal edema, unspecified buttock

L89.302 Pressure ulcer of unspecified buttock, stage 2
Healing pressure ulcer of unspecified buttock, stage 2
Pressure ulcer with abrasion, blister, partial thickness skin loss involving epidermis and/or dermis, unspecified buttock

L89.303 Pressure ulcer of unspecified buttock, stage 3
Healing pressure ulcer of unspecified buttock, stage 3
Pressure ulcer with full thickness skin loss involving damage or necrosis of subcutaneous tissue, unspecified buttock

L89.304 Pressure ulcer of unspecified buttock, stage 4
Healing pressure ulcer of unspecified buttock, stage 4
Pressure ulcer with necrosis of soft tissues through to underlying muscle, tendon, or bone, unspecified buttock

L89.309 Pressure ulcer of unspecified buttock, unspecified stage
Healing pressure ulcer of unspecified buttock NOS
Healing pressure ulcer of unspecified buttock, unspecified stage

✓6th **L89.31 Pressure ulcer of right buttock**

L89.310 Pressure ulcer of right buttock, unstageable

L89.311 Pressure ulcer of right buttock, stage 1
Healing pressure ulcer of right buttock, stage 1
Pressure pre-ulcer skin changes limited to persistent focal edema, right buttock

L89.312 Pressure ulcer of right buttock, stage 2
Healing pressure ulcer of right buttock, stage 2
Pressure ulcer with abrasion, blister, partial thickness skin loss involving epidermis and/or dermis, right buttock

L89.313 Pressure ulcer of right buttock, stage 3
Healing pressure ulcer of right buttock, stage 3
Pressure ulcer with full thickness skin loss involving damage or necrosis of subcutaneous tissue, right buttock

L89.314 Pressure ulcer of right buttock, stage 4
Healing pressure ulcer of right buttock, stage 4
Pressure ulcer with necrosis of soft tissues through to underlying muscle, tendon, or bone, right buttock

L89.319 Pressure ulcer of right buttock, unspecified stage
Healing pressure ulcer of right buttock NOS
Healing pressure ulcer of right buttock, unspecified stage

✓6th **L89.32 Pressure ulcer of left buttock**

L89.320 Pressure ulcer of left buttock, unstageable

L89.321 Pressure ulcer of left buttock, stage 1
Healing pressure ulcer of left buttock, stage 1
Pressure pre-ulcer skin changes limited to persistent focal edema, left buttock

L89.322 Pressure ulcer of left buttock, stage 2
Healing pressure ulcer of left buttock, stage 2
Pressure ulcer with abrasion, blister, partial thickness skin loss involving epidermis and/or dermis, left buttock

L89.323 Pressure ulcer of left buttock, stage 3
Healing pressure ulcer of left buttock, stage 3
Pressure ulcer with full thickness skin loss involving damage or necrosis of subcutaneous tissue, left buttock

L89.324 Pressure ulcer of left buttock, stage 4
Healing pressure ulcer of left buttock, stage 4
Pressure ulcer with necrosis of soft tissues through to underlying muscle, tendon, or bone, left buttock

L89.329 Pressure ulcer of left buttock, unspecified stage
Healing pressure ulcer of left buttock NOS
Healing pressure ulcer of left buttock, unspecified stage

✓5th **L89.4 Pressure ulcer of contiguous site of back, buttock and hip**

L89.40 Pressure ulcer of contiguous site of back, buttock and hip, unspecified stage
Healing pressure ulcer of contiguous site of back, buttock and hip NOS
Healing pressure ulcer of contiguous site of back, buttock and hip, unspecified stage

L89.41 Pressure ulcer of contiguous site of back, buttock and hip, stage 1
Healing pressure ulcer of contiguous site of back, buttock and hip, stage 1
Pressure pre-ulcer skin changes limited to persistent focal edema, contiguous site of back, buttock and hip

L89.42 Pressure ulcer of contiguous site of back, buttock and hip, stage 2
Healing pressure ulcer of contiguous site of back, buttock and hip, stage 2
Pressure ulcer with abrasion, blister, partial thickness skin loss involving epidermis and/or dermis, contiguous site of back, buttock and hip

L89.43 Pressure ulcer of contiguous site of back, buttock and hip, stage 3
Healing pressure ulcer of contiguous site of back, buttock and hip, stage 3
Pressure ulcer with full thickness skin loss involving damage or necrosis of subcutaneous tissue, contiguous site of back, buttock and hip

L89.44 Pressure ulcer of contiguous site of back, buttock and hip, stage 4
Healing pressure ulcer of contiguous site of back, buttock and hip, stage 4
Pressure ulcer with necrosis of soft tissues through to underlying muscle, tendon, or bone, contiguous site of back, buttock and hip

L89.45 Pressure ulcer of contiguous site of back, buttock and hip, unstageable

✓5th **L89.5 Pressure ulcer of ankle**

✓6th **L89.50 Pressure ulcer of unspecified ankle**

L89.500 Pressure ulcer of unspecified ankle, unstageable

L89.501 Pressure ulcer of unspecified ankle, stage 1
Healing pressure ulcer of unspecified ankle, stage 1
Pressure pre-ulcer skin changes limited to persistent focal edema, unspecified ankle

L89.502 Pressure ulcer of unspecified ankle, stage 2
Healing pressure ulcer of unspecified ankle, stage 2
Pressure ulcer with abrasion, blister, partial thickness skin loss involving epidermis and/or dermis, unspecified ankle

L89.503 Pressure ulcer of unspecified ankle, stage 3
Healing pressure ulcer of unspecified ankle, stage 3
Pressure ulcer with full thickness skin loss involving damage or necrosis of subcutaneous tissue, unspecified ankle

L89.504 Pressure ulcer of unspecified ankle, stage 4
Healing pressure ulcer of unspecified ankle, stage 4
Pressure ulcer with necrosis of soft tissues through to underlying muscle, tendon, or bone, unspecified ankle

L89.509 Pressure ulcer of unspecified ankle, unspecified stage
Healing pressure ulcer of unspecified ankle NOS
Healing pressure ulcer of unspecified ankle, unspecified stage

✓6th **L89.51 Pressure ulcer of right ankle**

L89.510 Pressure ulcer of right ankle, unstageable

L89.511 Pressure ulcer of right ankle, stage 1
Healing pressure ulcer of right ankle, stage 1
Pressure pre-ulcer skin changes limited to persistent focal edema, right ankle

L89.512 Pressure ulcer of right ankle, stage 2
Healing pressure ulcer of right ankle, stage 2
Pressure ulcer with abrasion, blister, partial thickness skin loss involving epidermis and/or dermis, right ankle

L89.513 Pressure ulcer of right ankle, stage 3
Healing pressure ulcer of right ankle, stage 3
Pressure ulcer with full thickness skin loss involving damage or necrosis of subcutaneous tissue, right ankle

L89.514 Pressure ulcer of right ankle, stage 4
Healing pressure ulcer of right ankle, stage 4
Pressure ulcer with necrosis of soft tissues through to underlying muscle, tendon, or bone, right ankle

L89.519 Pressure ulcer of right ankle, unspecified stage
Healing pressure ulcer of right ankle NOS
Healing pressure ulcer of right ankle, unspecified stage

✓6th **L89.52 Pressure ulcer of left ankle**

L89.520 Pressure ulcer of left ankle, unstageable

L89.521 Pressure ulcer of left ankle, stage 1
Healing pressure ulcer of left ankle, stage 1
Pressure pre-ulcer skin changes limited to persistnt focal edema, left ankle

L89.522 Pressure ulcer of left ankle, stage 2
Healing pressure ulcer of left ankle, stage 2
Pressure ulcer with abrasion, blister, partial thickness skin loss involving epidermis and/or dermis, left ankle

L89.523 Pressure ulcer of left ankle, stage 3
Healing pressure ulcer of left ankle, stage 3
Pressure ulcer with full thickness skin loss involving damage or necrosis of subcutaneous tissue, left ankle

L89.524 Pressure ulcer of left ankle, stage 4
Healing pressure ulcer of left ankle, stage 4
Pressure ulcer with necrosis of soft tissues through to underlying muscle, tendon, or bone, left ankle

L89.529 Pressure ulcer of left ankle, unspecified stage
Healing pressure ulcer of left ankle NOS
Healing pressure ulcer of left ankle, unspecified stage

✓5th **L89.6 Pressure ulcer of heel**

✓6th **L89.60 Pressure ulcer of unspecified heel**

L89.600 Pressure ulcer of unspecified heel, unstageable

L89.601 Pressure ulcer of unspecified heel, stage 1
Healing pressure ulcer of unspecified heel, stage 1
Pressure pre-ulcer skin changes limited to persistent focal edema, unspecified heel

L89.602 Pressure ulcer of unspecified heel, stage 2
Healing pressure ulcer of unspecified heel, stage 2
Pressure ulcer with abrasion, blister, partial thickness skin loss involving epidermis and/or dermis, unspecified heel

L89.603 Pressure ulcer of unspecified heel, stage 3
Healing pressure ulcer of unspecified heel, stage 3
Pressure ulcer with full thickness skin loss involving damage or necrosis of subcutaneous tissue, unspecified heel

L89.604 Pressure ulcer of unspecified heel, stage 4
Healing pressure ulcer of unspecified heel, stage 4
Pressure ulcer with necrosis of soft tissues through to underlying muscle, tendon, or bone, unspecified heel

L89.609 Pressure ulcer of unspecified heel, unspecified stage
Healing pressure ulcer of unspecified heel NOS
Healing pressure ulcer of unspecified heel, unspecified stage

✓6th **L89.61 Pressure ulcer of right heel**

L89.610 Pressure ulcer of right heel, unstageable

L89.611 Pressure ulcer of right heel, stage 1
Healing pressure ulcer of right heel, stage 1
Pressure pre-ulcer skin changes limited to persistent focal edema, right heel

L89.612 Pressure ulcer of right heel, stage 2
Healing pressure ulcer of right heel, stage 2
Pressure ulcer with abrasion, blister, partial thickness skin loss involving epidermis and/or dermis, right heel

L89.613 Pressure ulcer of right heel, stage 3
Healing pressure ulcer of right heel, stage 3
Pressure ulcer with full thickness skin loss involving damage or necrosis of subcutaneous tissue, right heel

L89.614 Pressure ulcer of right heel, stage 4
Healing pressure ulcer of right heel, stage 4
Pressure ulcer with necrosis of soft tissues through to underlying muscle, tendon, or bone, right heel

L89.619 Pressure ulcer of right heel, unspecified stage
Healing pressure ulcer of right heel NOS
Healing pressure ulcer of unspecified heel, right stage

✓6th **L89.62 Pressure ulcer of left heel**

L89.620 Pressure ulcer of left heel, unstageable

L89.621 Pressure ulcer of left heel, stage 1
Healing pressure ulcer of left heel, stage 1
Pressure pre-ulcer skin changes limited to persistent focal edema, left heel

L89.622 Pressure ulcer of left heel, stage 2
Healing pressure ulcer of left heel, stage 2
Pressure ulcer with abrasion, blister, partial thickness skin loss involving epidermis and/or dermis, left heel

L89.623 Pressure ulcer of left heel, stage 3
Healing pressure ulcer of left heel, stage 3
Pressure ulcer with full thickness skin loss involving damage or necrosis of subcutaneous tissue, left heel

L89.624 Pressure ulcer of left heel, stage 4
Healing pressure ulcer of left heel, stage 4
Pressure ulcer with necrosis of soft tissues through to underlying muscle, tendon, or bone, left heel

L89.629 Pressure ulcer of left heel, unspecified stage
Healing pressure ulcer of left heel NOS
Healing pressure ulcer of left heel, unspecified stage

5th **L89.8 Pressure ulcer of other site**

6th **L89.81 Pressure ulcer of head**
Pressure ulcer of face

L89.810 Pressure ulcer of head, unstageable

L89.811 Pressure ulcer of head, stage 1
Healing pressure ulcer of head, stage 1
Pressure pre-ulcer skin changes limited to persistent focal edema, head

L89.812 Pressure ulcer of head, stage 2
Healing pressure ulcer of head, stage 2
Pressure ulcer with abrasion, blister, partial thickness skin loss involving epidermis and/or dermis, head

L89.813 Pressure ulcer of head, stage 3
Healing pressure ulcer of head, stage 3
Pressure ulcer with full thickness skin loss involving damage or necrosis of subcutaneous tissue, head

L89.814 Pressure ulcer of head, stage 4
Healing pressure ulcer of head, stage 4
Pressure ulcer with necrosis of soft tissues through to underlying muscle, tendon, or bone, head

L89.819 Pressure ulcer of head, unspecified stage
Healing pressure ulcer of head NOS
Healing pressure ulcer of head, unspecified stage

6th **L89.89 Pressure ulcer of other site**

L89.890 Pressure ulcer of other site, unstageable

L89.891 Pressure ulcer of other site, stage 1
Healing pressure ulcer of other site, stage 1
Pressure pre-ulcer skin changes limited to persistent focal edema, other site

L89.892 Pressure ulcer of other site, stage 2
Healing pressure ulcer of other site, stage 2
Pressure ulcer with abrasion, blister, partial thickness skin loss involving epidermis and/or dermis, other site

L89.893 Pressure ulcer of other site, stage 3
Healing pressure ulcer of other site, stage 3
Pressure ulcer with full thickness skin loss involving damage or necrosis of subcutaneous tissue, other site

L89.894 Pressure ulcer of other site, stage 4
Healing pressure ulcer of other site, stage 4
Pressure ulcer with necrosis of soft tissues through to underlying muscle, tendon, or bone, other site

L89.899 Pressure ulcer of other site, unspecified stage
Healing pressure ulcer of other site NOS
Healing pressure ulcer of other site, unspecified stage

5th **L89.9 Pressure ulcer of unspecified site**

L89.90 Pressure ulcer of unspecified site, unspecified stage
Healing pressure ulcer of unspecified site NOS
Healing pressure ulcer of unspecified site, unspecified stage

L89.91 Pressure ulcer of unspecified site, stage 1
Healing pressure ulcer of unspecified site, stage 1
Pressure pre-ulcer skin changes limited to persistent focal edema, unspecified site

L89.92 Pressure ulcer of unspecified site, stage 2
Healing pressure ulcer of unspecified site, stage 2
Pressure ulcer with abrasion, blister, partial thickness skin loss involving epidermis and/or dermis, unspecified site

L89.93 Pressure ulcer of unspecified site, stage 3
Healing pressure ulcer of unspecified site, stage 3
Pressure ulcer with full thickness skin loss involving damage or necrosis of subcutaneous tissue, unspecified site

L89.94 Pressure ulcer of unspecified site, stage 4
Healing pressure ulcer of unspecified site, stage 4
Pressure ulcer with necrosis of soft tissues through to underlying muscle, tendon, or bone, unspecified site

L89.95 Pressure ulcer of unspecified site, unstageable

4th **L90 Atrophic disorders of skin**

L90.0 Lichen sclerosus et atrophicus
EXCLUDES 2 *lichen sclerosus of external female genital organs (N90.4)*
lichen sclerosus of external male genital organs (N48.0)

L90.1 Anetoderma of Schweninger-Buzzi

L90.2 Anetoderma of Jadassohn-Pellizzari

L90.3 Atrophoderma of Pasini and Pierini

L90.4 Acrodermatitis chronica atrophicans

L90.5 Scar conditions and fibrosis of skin
Adherent scar (skin)
Cicatrix
Disfigurement of skin due to scar
Fibrosis of skin NOS
Scar NOS
EXCLUDES 2 *hypertrophic scar (L91.0)*
keloid scar (L91.0)

L90.6 Striae atrophicae

L90.8 Other atrophic disorders of skin

L90.9 Atrophic disorder of skin, unspecified

4th **L91 Hypertrophic disorders of skin**

L91.0 Hypertrophic scar
Keloid
Keloid scar
EXCLUDES 2 *acne keloid (L73.0)*
scar NOS (L90.5)

L91.8 Other hypertrophic disorders of the skin

L91.9 Hypertrophic disorder of the skin, unspecified

4th **L92 Granulomatous disorders of skin and subcutaneous tissue**
EXCLUDES 2 *actinic granuloma (L57.5)*

L92.0 Granuloma annulare
Perforating granuloma annulare

L92.1 Necrobiosis lipoidica, not elsewhere classified
EXCLUDES 1 *necrobiosis lipoidica associated with diabetes mellitus (E08-E13 with .620)*

L92.2 Granuloma faciale [eosinophilic granuloma of skin]

L92.3 Foreign body granuloma of the skin and subcutaneous tissue
Use additional code to identify the type of retained foreign body (Z18.-)

L92.8 Other granulomatous disorders of the skin and subcutaneous tissue

L92.9 Granulomatous disorder of the skin and subcutaneous tissue, unspecified

√4th **L93 Lupus erythematosus**

Use additional code for adverse effect, if applicable, to identify drug (T36-T50 with fifth or sixth character 5)

EXCLUDES 1 *lupus exedens (A18.4)*
lupus vulgaris (A18.4)
scleroderma (M34.-)
systemic lupus erythematosus (M32.-)

L93.0 Discoid lupus erythematosus
Lupus erythematosus NOS

L93.1 Subacute cutaneous lupus erythematosus

L93.2 Other local lupus erythematosus
Lupus erythematosus profundus
Lupus panniculitis

√4th **L94 Other localized connective tissue disorders**

EXCLUDES 1 *systemic connective tissue disorders (M30-M36)*

L94.0 Localized scleroderma [morphea]
Circumscribed scleroderma

L94.1 Linear scleroderma
En coup de sabre lesion

L94.2 Calcinosis cutis

L94.3 Sclerodactyly

L94.4 Gottron's papules

L94.5 Poikiloderma vasculare atrophicans

L94.6 Ainhum

L94.8 Other specified localized connective tissue disorders

L94.9 Localized connective tissue disorder, unspecified

√4th **L95 Vasculitis limited to skin, not elsewhere classified**

EXCLUDES 1 *angioma serpiginosum (L81.7)*
Henoch(-Schönlein) purpura (D69.0)
hypersensitivity angiitis (M31.0)
lupus panniculitis (L93.2)
panniculitis NOS (M79.3)
panniculitis of neck and back (M54.0-)
polyarteritis nodosa (M30.0)
relapsing panniculitis (M35.6)
rheumatoid vasculitis (M05.2)
serum sickness (T80.6-)
urticaria (L50.-)
Wegener's granulomatosis (M31.3-)

L95.0 Livedoid vasculitis
Atrophie blanche (en plaque)

L95.1 Erythema elevatum diutinum

L95.8 Other vasculitis limited to the skin

L95.9 Vasculitis limited to the skin, unspecified

√4th **L97 Non-pressure chronic ulcer of lower limb, not elsewhere classified**

INCLUDES chronic ulcer of skin of lower limb NOS
non-healing ulcer of skin
non-infected sinus of skin
trophic ulcer NOS
tropical ulcer NOS
ulcer of skin of lower limb NOS

Code first any associated underlying condition, such as:
atherosclerosis of the lower extremities (I70.23-, I70.24-, I70.33-, I70.34-, I70.43-, I70.44-, I70.53-, I70.54-, I70.63-, I70.64-, I70.73-, I70.74-)
chronic venous hypertension (I87.31-, I87.33-)
diabetic ulcers (E08.621, E08.622, E09.621, E09.622, E10.621, E10.622, E11.621, E11.622, E13.621, E13.622)
postphlebitic syndrome (I87.01-, I87.03-)
postthrombotic syndrome (I87.01-, I87.03-)
varicose ulcer (I83.0-, I83.2-)

Code first any associated gangrene (I96)

EXCLUDES 2 *pressure ulcer (pressure area) (L89.-)*
skin infections (L00-L08)
specific infections classified to A00-B99

√5th **L97.1 Non-pressure chronic ulcer of thigh**

√6th **L97.10 Non-pressure chronic ulcer of unspecified thigh**

L97.101 Non-pressure chronic ulcer of unspecified thigh limited to breakdown of skin

L97.102 Non-pressure chronic ulcer of unspecified thigh with fat layer exposed

L97.103 Non-pressure chronic ulcer of unspecified thigh with necrosis of muscle

L97.104 Non-pressure chronic ulcer of unspecified thigh with necrosis of bone

L97.109 Non-pressure chronic ulcer of unspecified thigh with unspecified severity

√6th **L97.11 Non-pressure chronic ulcer of right thigh**

L97.111 Non-pressure chronic ulcer of right thigh limited to breakdown of skin

L97.112 Non-pressure chronic ulcer of right thigh with fat layer exposed

L97.113 Non-pressure chronic ulcer of right thigh with necrosis of muscle

L97.114 Non-pressure chronic ulcer of right thigh with necrosis of bone

L97.119 Non-pressure chronic ulcer of right thigh with unspecified severity

√6th **L97.12 Non-pressure chronic ulcer of left thigh**

L97.121 Non-pressure chronic ulcer of left thigh limited to breakdown of skin

L97.122 Non-pressure chronic ulcer of left thigh with fat layer exposed

L97.123 Non-pressure chronic ulcer of left thigh with necrosis of muscle

L97.124 Non-pressure chronic ulcer of left thigh with necrosis of bone

L97.129 Non-pressure chronic ulcer of left thigh with unspecified severity

√5th **L97.2 Non-pressure chronic ulcer of calf**

√6th **L97.20 Non-pressure chronic ulcer of unspecified calf**

L97.201 Non-pressure chronic ulcer of unspecified calf limited to breakdown of skin

L97.202 Non-pressure chronic ulcer of unspecified calf with fat layer exposed

L97.203 Non-pressure chronic ulcer of unspecified calf with necrosis of muscle

L97.204 Non-pressure chronic ulcer of unspecified calf with necrosis of bone

L97.209 Non-pressure chronic ulcer of unspecified calf with unspecified severity

√6th **L97.21 Non-pressure chronic ulcer of right calf**

L97.211 Non-pressure chronic ulcer of right calf limited to breakdown of skin

L97.212 Non-pressure chronic ulcer of right calf with fat layer exposed

L97.213 Non-pressure chronic ulcer of right calf with necrosis of muscle

L97.214 Non-pressure chronic ulcer of right calf with necrosis of bone

L97.219 Non-pressure chronic ulcer of right calf with unspecified severity

√6th **L97.22 Non-pressure chronic ulcer of left calf**

L97.221 Non-pressure chronic ulcer of left calf limited to breakdown of skin

L97.222 Non-pressure chronic ulcer of left calf with fat layer exposed

L97.223 Non-pressure chronic ulcer of left calf with necrosis of muscle

L97.224 Non-pressure chronic ulcer of left calf with necrosis of bone

L97.229 Non-pressure chronic ulcer of left calf with unspecified severity

√5th **L97.3 Non-pressure chronic ulcer of ankle**

√6th **L97.30 Non-pressure chronic ulcer of unspecified ankle**

L97.301 Non-pressure chronic ulcer of unspecified ankle limited to breakdown of skin

L97.302 Non-pressure chronic ulcer of unspecified ankle with fat layer exposed

L97.303 Non-pressure chronic ulcer of unspecified ankle with necrosis of muscle

L97.304 Non-pressure chronic ulcer of unspecified ankle with necrosis of bone

L97.309 Non-pressure chronic ulcer of unspecified ankle with unspecified severity

✓6th L97.31 Non-pressure chronic ulcer of right ankle
- **L97.311 Non-pressure chronic ulcer of right ankle limited to breakdown of skin**
- **L97.312 Non-pressure chronic ulcer of right ankle with fat layer exposed**
- **L97.313 Non-pressure chronic ulcer of right ankle with necrosis of muscle**
- **L97.314 Non-pressure chronic ulcer of right ankle with necrosis of bone**
- **L97.319 Non-pressure chronic ulcer of right ankle with unspecified severity**

✓6th L97.32 Non-pressure chronic ulcer of left ankle
- **L97.321 Non-pressure chronic ulcer of left ankle limited to breakdown of skin**
- **L97.322 Non-pressure chronic ulcer of left ankle with fat layer exposed**
- **L97.323 Non-pressure chronic ulcer of left ankle with necrosis of muscle**
- **L97.324 Non-pressure chronic ulcer of left ankle with necrosis of bone**
- **L97.329 Non-pressure chronic ulcer of left ankle with unspecified severity**

✓5th L97.4 Non-pressure chronic ulcer of heel and midfoot
Non-pressure chronic ulcer of plantar surface of midfoot

✓6th L97.40 Non-pressure chronic ulcer of unspecified heel and midfoot
- **L97.401 Non-pressure chronic ulcer of unspecified heel and midfoot limited to breakdown of skin**
- **L97.402 Non-pressure chronic ulcer of unspecified heel and midfoot with fat layer exposed**
- **L97.403 Non-pressure chronic ulcer of unspecified heel and midfoot with necrosis of muscle**
- **L97.404 Non-pressure chronic ulcer of unspecified heel and midfoot with necrosis of bone**
- **L97.409 Non-pressure chronic ulcer of unspecified heel and midfoot with unspecified severity**

✓6th L97.41 Non-pressure chronic ulcer of right heel and midfoot
- **L97.411 Non-pressure chronic ulcer of right heel and midfoot limited to breakdown of skin**
- **L97.412 Non-pressure chronic ulcer of right heel and midfoot with fat layer exposed**
- **L97.413 Non-pressure chronic ulcer of right heel and midfoot with necrosis of muscle**
- **L97.414 Non-pressure chronic ulcer of right heel and midfoot with necrosis of bone**
- **L97.419 Non-pressure chronic ulcer of right heel and midfoot with unspecified severity**

✓6th L97.42 Non-pressure chronic ulcer of left heel and midfoot
- **L97.421 Non-pressure chronic ulcer of left heel and midfoot limited to breakdown of skin**
- **L97.422 Non-pressure chronic ulcer of left heel and midfoot with fat layer exposed**
- **L97.423 Non-pressure chronic ulcer of left heel and midfoot with necrosis of muscle**
- **L97.424 Non-pressure chronic ulcer of left heel and midfoot with necrosis of bone**
- **L97.429 Non-pressure chronic ulcer of left heel and midfoot with unspecified severity**

✓5th L97.5 Non-pressure chronic ulcer of other part of foot
Non-pressure chronic ulcer of toe

✓6th L97.50 Non-pressure chronic ulcer of other part of unspecified foot
- **L97.501 Non-pressure chronic ulcer of other part of unspecified foot limited to breakdown of skin**
- **L97.502 Non-pressure chronic ulcer of other part of unspecified foot with fat layer exposed**
- **L97.503 Non-pressure chronic ulcer of other part of unspecified foot with necrosis of muscle**
- **L97.504 Non-pressure chronic ulcer of other part of unspecified foot with necrosis of bone**
- **L97.509 Non-pressure chronic ulcer of other part of unspecified foot with unspecified severity**

✓6th L97.51 Non-pressure chronic ulcer of other part of right foot
- **L97.511 Non-pressure chronic ulcer of other part of right foot limited to breakdown of skin**
- **L97.512 Non-pressure chronic ulcer of other part of right foot with fat layer exposed**
- **L97.513 Non-pressure chronic ulcer of other part of right foot with necrosis of muscle**
- **L97.514 Non-pressure chronic ulcer of other part of right foot with necrosis of bone**
- **L97.519 Non-pressure chronic ulcer of other part of right foot with unspecified severity**

✓6th L97.52 Non-pressure chronic ulcer of other part of left foot
- **L97.521 Non-pressure chronic ulcer of other part of left foot limited to breakdown of skin**
- **L97.522 Non-pressure chronic ulcer of other part of left foot with fat layer exposed**
- **L97.523 Non-pressure chronic ulcer of other part of left foot with necrosis of muscle**
- **L97.524 Non-pressure chronic ulcer of other part of left foot with necrosis of bone**
- **L97.529 Non-pressure chronic ulcer of other part of left foot with unspecified severity**

✓5th L97.8 Non-pressure chronic ulcer of other part of lower leg

✓6th L97.80 Non-pressure chronic ulcer of other part of unspecified lower leg
- **L97.801 Non-pressure chronic ulcer of other part of unspecified lower leg limited to breakdown of skin**
- **L97.802 Non-pressure chronic ulcer of other part of unspecified lower leg with fat layer exposed**
- **L97.803 Non-pressure chronic ulcer of other part of unspecified lower leg with necrosis of muscle**
- **L97.804 Non-pressure chronic ulcer of other part of unspecified lower leg with necrosis of bone**
- **L97.809 Non-pressure chronic ulcer of other part of unspecified lower leg with unspecified severity**

✓6th L97.81 Non-pressure chronic ulcer of other part of right lower leg
- **L97.811 Non-pressure chronic ulcer of other part of right lower leg limited to breakdown of skin**
- **L97.812 Non-pressure chronic ulcer of other part of right lower leg with fat layer exposed**
- **L97.813 Non-pressure chronic ulcer of other part of right lower leg with necrosis of muscle**
- **L97.814 Non-pressure chronic ulcer of other part of right lower leg with necrosis of bone**
- **L97.819 Non-pressure chronic ulcer of other part of right lower leg with unspecified severity**

✓6th L97.82 Non-pressure chronic ulcer of other part of left lower leg
- **L97.821 Non-pressure chronic ulcer of other part of left lower leg limited to breakdown of skin**
- **L97.822 Non-pressure chronic ulcer of other part of left lower leg with fat layer exposed**
- **L97.823 Non-pressure chronic ulcer of other part of left lower leg with necrosis of muscle**
- **L97.824 Non-pressure chronic ulcer of other part of left lower leg with necrosis of bone**

L97.829 Non-pressure chronic ulcer of other part of left lower leg with unspecified severity

✓5th **L97.9 Non-pressure chronic ulcer of unspecified part of lower leg**

✓6th **L97.90 Non-pressure chronic ulcer of unspecified part of unspecified lower leg**

L97.901 Non-pressure chronic ulcer of unspecified part of unspecified lower leg limited to breakdown of skin

L97.902 Non-pressure chronic ulcer of unspecified part of unspecified lower leg with fat layer exposed

L97.903 Non-pressure chronic ulcer of unspecified part of unspecified lower leg with necrosis of muscle

L97.904 Non-pressure chronic ulcer of unspecified part of unspecified lower leg with necrosis of bone

L97.909 Non-pressure chronic ulcer of unspecified part of unspecified lower leg with unspecified severity

✓6th **L97.91 Non-pressure chronic ulcer of unspecified part of right lower leg**

L97.911 Non-pressure chronic ulcer of unspecified part of right lower leg limited to breakdown of skin

L97.912 Non-pressure chronic ulcer of unspecified part of right lower leg with fat layer exposed

L97.913 Non-pressure chronic ulcer of unspecified part of right lower leg with necrosis of muscle

L97.914 Non-pressure chronic ulcer of unspecified part of right lower leg with necrosis of bone

L97.919 Non-pressure chronic ulcer of unspecified part of right lower leg with unspecified severity

✓6th **L97.92 Non-pressure chronic ulcer of unspecified part of left lower leg**

L97.921 Non-pressure chronic ulcer of unspecified part of left lower leg limited to breakdown of skin

L97.922 Non-pressure chronic ulcer of unspecified part of left lower leg with fat layer exposed

L97.923 Non-pressure chronic ulcer of unspecified part of left lower leg with necrosis of muscle

L97.924 Non-pressure chronic ulcer of unspecified part of left lower leg with necrosis of bone

L97.929 Non-pressure chronic ulcer of unspecified part of left lower leg with unspecified severity

✓4th **L98 Other disorders of skin and subcutaneous tissue, not elsewhere classified**

L98.0 Pyogenic granuloma

EXCLUDES 2 *pyogenic granuloma of gingiva (K06.8)*
pyogenic granuloma of maxillary alveolar ridge (K04.5)
pyogenic granuloma of oral mucosa (K13.4)

L98.1 Factitial dermatitis

Neurotic excoriation

L98.2 Febrile neutrophilic dermatosis [Sweet]

L98.3 Eosinophilic cellulitis [Wells]

✓5th **L98.4 Non-pressure chronic ulcer of skin, not elsewhere classified**

Chronic ulcer of skin NOS
Tropical ulcer NOS
Ulcer of skin NOS

EXCLUDES 2 *pressure ulcer (pressure area) (L89.-)*
gangrene (I96)
skin infections (L00-L08)
specific infections classified to A00-B99
ulcer of lower limb NEC (L97.-)
varicose ulcer (I83.0-I82.2)

✓6th **L98.41 Non-pressure chronic ulcer of buttock**

L98.411 Non-pressure chronic ulcer of buttock limited to breakdown of skin

L98.412 Non-pressure chronic ulcer of buttock with fat layer exposed

L98.413 Non-pressure chronic ulcer of buttock with necrosis of muscle

L98.414 Non-pressure chronic ulcer of buttock with necrosis of bone

L98.419 Non-pressure chronic ulcer of buttock with unspecified severity

✓6th **L98.42 Non-pressure chronic ulcer of back**

L98.421 Non-pressure chronic ulcer of back limited to breakdown of skin

L98.422 Non-pressure chronic ulcer of back with fat layer exposed

L98.423 Non-pressure chronic ulcer of back with necrosis of muscle

L98.424 Non-pressure chronic ulcer of back with necrosis of bone

L98.429 Non-pressure chronic ulcer of back with unspecified severity

✓6th **L98.49 Non-pressure chronic ulcer of skin of other sites**

Non-pressure chronic ulcer of skin NOS

L98.491 Non-pressure chronic ulcer of skin of other sites limited to breakdown of skin

L98.492 Non-pressure chronic ulcer of skin of other sites with fat layer exposed

L98.493 Non-pressure chronic ulcer of skin of other sites with necrosis of muscle

L98.494 Non-pressure chronic ulcer of skin of other sites with necrosis of bone

L98.499 Non-pressure chronic ulcer of skin of other sites with unspecified severity

L98.5 Mucinosis of the skin

Focal mucinosis
Lichen myxedematosus

EXCLUDES 1 *focal oral mucinosis (K13.79)*
myxedema (E03.9)

L98.6 Other infiltrative disorders of the skin and subcutaneous tissue

EXCLUDES 1 *hyalinosis cutis et mucosae (E78.89)*

L98.8 Other specified disorders of the skin and subcutaneous tissue

L98.9 Disorder of the skin and subcutaneous tissue, unspecified

L99 Other disorders of skin and subcutaneous tissue in diseases classified elsewhere

Code first underlying disease, such as:
amyloidosis (E85.-)

EXCLUDES 1 *skin disorders in diabetes (E08-E13 with .62)*
skin disorders in gonorrhea (A54.89)
skin disorders in syphilis (A51.31, A52.79)

Chapter 13. Diseases of the Musculoskeletal System and Connective Tissue (M00-M99)

NOTE Use an external cause code following the code for the musculoskeletal condition, if applicable, to identify the cause of the musculoskeletal condition

EXCLUDES 2 *arthropathic psoriasis (L40.5-)*
certain conditions originating in the perinatal period (P04-P96)
certain infectious and parasitic diseases (A00-B99)
compartment syndrome (traumatic) (T79.A-)
complications of pregnancy, childbirth and the puerperium (O00-O9A)
congenital malformations, deformations, and chromosomal abnormalities (Q00-Q99)
endocrine, nutritional and metabolic diseases (E00-E88)
injury, poisoning and certain other consequences of external causes (S00-T88)
neoplasms (C00-D49)
symptoms, signs and abnormal clinical and laboratory findings, not elsewhere classified (R00-R94)

This chapter contains the following blocks:

M00-M02 Infectious arthropathies
M05-M14 Inflammatory polyarthropathies
M15-M19 Osteoarthritis
M20-M25 Other joint disorders
M26-M27 Dentofacial anomalies [including malocclusion] and other disorders of jaw
M30-M36 Systemic connective tissue disorders
M40-M43 Deforming dorsopathies
M45-M49 Spondylopathies
M50-M54 Other dorsopathies
M60-M63 Disorders of muscles
M65-M67 Disorders of synovium and tendon
M70-M79 Other soft tissue disorders
M80-M85 Disorders of bone density and structure
M86-M90 Other osteopathies
M91-M94 Chondropathies
M95 Other disorders of the musculoskeletal system and connective tissue
M96 Intraoperative and postprocedural complications and disorders of musculoskeletal system, not elsewhere classified
M99 Biomechanical lesions, not elsewhere classified

ARTHROPATHIES (M00-M25)

INCLUDES disorders affecting predominantly peripheral (limb) joints

Infectious arthropathies (M00-M02)

This block comprises arthropathies due to microbiological agents. Distinction is made between the following types of etiological relationship:

a) direct infection of joint, where organisms invade synovial tissue and microbial antigen is present in the joint;
b) indirect infection, which may be of two types: a reactive arthropathy, where microbial infection of the body is established but neither organisms nor antigens can be identified in the joint, and a postinfective arthropathy, where microbial antigen is present but recovery of an organism is inconstant and evidence of local multiplication is lacking.

✓4th **M00 Pyogenic arthritis**
✓5th **M00.0 Staphylococcal arthritis and polyarthritis**
Use additional code (B95.61-B95.8) to identify bacterial agent
EXCLUDES 2 *infection and inflammatory reaction due to internal joint prosthesis (T84.5-)*
M00.00 Staphylococcal arthritis, unspecified joint
✓6th **M00.01 Staphylococcal arthritis, shoulder**
M00.011 Staphylococcal arthritis, right shoulder
M00.012 Staphylococcal arthritis, left shoulder
M00.019 Staphylococcal arthritis, unspecified shoulder
✓6th **M00.02 Staphylococcal arthritis, elbow**
M00.021 Staphylococcal arthritis, right elbow
M00.022 Staphylococcal arthritis, left elbow
M00.029 Staphylococcal arthritis, unspecified elbow
✓6th **M00.03 Staphylococcal arthritis, wrist**
Staphylococcal arthritis of carpal bones
M00.031 Staphylococcal arthritis, right wrist
M00.032 Staphylococcal arthritis, left wrist
M00.039 Staphylococcal arthritis, unspecified wrist
✓6th **M00.04 Staphylococcal arthritis, hand**
Staphylococcal arthritis of metacarpus and phalanges
M00.041 Staphylococcal arthritis, right hand
M00.042 Staphylococcal arthritis, left hand
M00.049 Staphylococcal arthritis, unspecified hand
✓6th **M00.05 Staphylococcal arthritis, hip**
M00.051 Staphylococcal arthritis, right hip
M00.052 Staphylococcal arthritis, left hip
M00.059 Staphylococcal arthritis, unspecified hip
✓6th **M00.06 Staphylococcal arthritis, knee**
M00.061 Staphylococcal arthritis, right knee
M00.062 Staphylococcal arthritis, left knee
M00.069 Staphylococcal arthritis, unspecified knee
✓6th **M00.07 Staphylococcal arthritis, ankle and foot**
Staphylococcal arthritis, tarsus, metatarsus and phalanges
M00.071 Staphylococcal arthritis, right ankle and foot
M00.072 Staphylococcal arthritis, left ankle and foot
M00.079 Staphylococcal arthritis, unspecified ankle and foot
M00.08 Staphylococcal arthritis, vertebrae
M00.09 Staphylococcal polyarthritis
✓5th **M00.1 Pneumococcal arthritis and polyarthritis**
M00.10 Pneumococcal arthritis, unspecified joint
✓6th **M00.11 Pneumococcal arthritis, shoulder**
M00.111 Pneumococcal arthritis, right shoulder
M00.112 Pneumococcal arthritis, left shoulder
M00.119 Pneumococcal arthritis, unspecified shoulder
✓6th **M00.12 Pneumococcal arthritis, elbow**
M00.121 Pneumococcal arthritis, right elbow
M00.122 Pneumococcal arthritis, left elbow
M00.129 Pneumococcal arthritis, unspecified elbow
✓6th **M00.13 Pneumococcal arthritis, wrist**
Pneumococcal arthritis of carpal bones
M00.131 Pneumococcal arthritis, right wrist
M00.132 Pneumococcal arthritis, left wrist
M00.139 Pneumococcal arthritis, unspecified wrist
✓6th **M00.14 Pneumococcal arthritis, hand**
Pneumococcal arthritis of metacarpus and phalanges
M00.141 Pneumococcal arthritis, right hand
M00.142 Pneumococcal arthritis, left hand
M00.149 Pneumococcal arthritis, unspecified hand
✓6th **M00.15 Pneumococcal arthritis, hip**
M00.151 Pneumococcal arthritis, right hip
M00.152 Pneumococcal arthritis, left hip
M00.159 Pneumococcal arthritis, unspecified hip
✓6th **M00.16 Pneumococcal arthritis, knee**
M00.161 Pneumococcal arthritis, right knee
M00.162 Pneumococcal arthritis, left knee
M00.169 Pneumococcal arthritis, unspecified knee
✓6th **M00.17 Pneumococcal arthritis, ankle and foot**
Pneumococcal arthritis, tarsus, metatarsus and phalanges
M00.171 Pneumococcal arthritis, right ankle and foot
M00.172 Pneumococcal arthritis, left ankle and foot
M00.179 Pneumococcal arthritis, unspecified ankle and foot
M00.18 Pneumococcal arthritis, vertebrae
M00.19 Pneumococcal polyarthritis

√5th **M00.2 Other streptococcal arthritis and polyarthritis**
Use additional code (B95.0-B95.2, B95.4-B95.5) to identify bacterial agent
M00.20 Other streptococcal arthritis, unspecified joint
√6th **M00.21 Other streptococcal arthritis, shoulder**
M00.211 Other streptococcal arthritis, right shoulder
M00.212 Other streptococcal arthritis, left shoulder
M00.219 Other streptococcal arthritis, unspecified shoulder
√6th **M00.22 Other streptococcal arthritis, elbow**
M00.221 Other streptococcal arthritis, right elbow
M00.222 Other streptococcal arthritis, left elbow
M00.229 Other streptococcal arthritis, unspecified elbow
√6th **M00.23 Other streptococcal arthritis, wrist**
Other streptococcal arthritis of carpal bones
M00.231 Other streptococcal arthritis, right wrist
M00.232 Other streptococcal arthritis, left wrist
M00.239 Other streptococcal arthritis, unspecified wrist
√6th **M00.24 Other streptococcal arthritis, hand**
Other streptococcal arthritis metacarpus and phalanges
M00.241 Other streptococcal arthritis, right hand
M00.242 Other streptococcal arthritis, left hand
M00.249 Other streptococcal arthritis, unspecified hand
√6th **M00.25 Other streptococcal arthritis, hip**
M00.251 Other streptococcal arthritis, right hip
M00.252 Other streptococcal arthritis, left hip
M00.259 Other streptococcal arthritis, unspecified hip
√6th **M00.26 Other streptococcal arthritis, knee**
M00.261 Other streptococcal arthritis, right knee
M00.262 Other streptococcal arthritis, left knee
M00.269 Other streptococcal arthritis, unspecified knee
√6th **M00.27 Other streptococcal arthritis, ankle and foot**
Other streptococcal arthritis, tarsus, metatarsus and phalanges
M00.271 Other streptococcal arthritis, right ankle and foot
M00.272 Other streptococcal arthritis, left ankle and foot
M00.279 Other streptococcal arthritis, unspecified ankle and foot
M00.28 Other streptococcal arthritis, vertebrae
M00.29 Other streptococcal polyarthritis
√5th **M00.8 Arthritis and polyarthritis due to other bacteria**
Use additional code (B96) to identify bacteria
M00.80 Arthritis due to other bacteria, unspecified joint
√6th **M00.81 Arthritis due to other bacteria, shoulder**
M00.811 Arthritis due to other bacteria, right shoulder
M00.812 Arthritis due to other bacteria, left shoulder
M00.819 Arthritis due to other bacteria, unspecified shoulder
√6th **M00.82 Arthritis due to other bacteria, elbow**
M00.821 Arthritis due to other bacteria, right elbow
M00.822 Arthritis due to other bacteria, left elbow
M00.829 Arthritis due to other bacteria, unspecified elbow
√6th **M00.83 Arthritis due to other bacteria, wrist**
Arthritis due to other bacteria, carpal bones
M00.831 Arthritis due to other bacteria, right wrist
M00.832 Arthritis due to other bacteria, left wrist
M00.839 Arthritis due to other bacteria, unspecified wrist
√6th **M00.84 Arthritis due to other bacteria, hand**
Arthritis due to other bacteria, metacarpus and phalanges
M00.841 Arthritis due to other bacteria, right hand
M00.842 Arthritis due to other bacteria, left hand
M00.849 Arthritis due to other bacteria, unspecified hand
√6th **M00.85 Arthritis due to other bacteria, hip**
M00.851 Arthritis due to other bacteria, right hip
M00.852 Arthritis due to other bacteria, left hip
M00.859 Arthritis due to other bacteria, unspecified hip
√6th **M00.86 Arthritis due to other bacteria, knee**
M00.861 Arthritis due to other bacteria, right knee
M00.862 Arthritis due to other bacteria, left knee
M00.869 Arthritis due to other bacteria, unspecified knee
√6th **M00.87 Arthritis due to other bacteria, ankle and foot**
Arthritis due to other bacteria, tarsus, metatarsus, and phalanges
M00.871 Arthritis due to other bacteria, right ankle and foot
M00.872 Arthritis due to other bacteria, left ankle and foot
M00.879 Arthritis due to other bacteria, unspecified ankle and foot
M00.88 Arthritis due to other bacteria, vertebrae
M00.89 Polyarthritis due to other bacteria
M00.9 Pyogenic arthritis, unspecified
Infective arthritis NOS

√4th **M01 Direct infections of joint in infectious and parasitic diseases classified elsewhere**
Code first underlying disease, such as:
leprosy [Hansen's disease] (A30.-)
mycoses (B35-B49)
O'nyong-nyong fever (A92.1)
paratyphoid fever (A01.1-A01.4)
EXCLUDES 1 *arthritis, arthropathy (in):*
gonococcal (A54.42)
Lyme disease (A69.23)
meningococcal (A39.83)
mumps (B26.85)
postinfective (M02.-)
postmeningococcal (A39.84)
reactive (M04.0-)
rubella (B06.82)
sarcoidosis (D86.86)
spine (A18.01)
typhoid fever (A01.04)
tuberculosis (A18.02)
√5th **M01.X Direct infection of joint in infectious and parasitic diseases classified elsewhere**
M01.X0 Direct infection of unspecified joint in infectious and parasitic diseases classified elsewhere
√6th **M01.X1 Direct infection of shoulder joint in infectious and parasitic diseases classified elsewhere**
M01.X11 Direct infection of right shoulder in infectious and parasitic diseases classified elsewhere
M01.X12 Direct infection of left shoulder in infectious and parasitic diseases classified elsewhere
M01.X19 Direct infection of unspecified shoulder in infectious and parasitic diseases classified elsewhere
√6th **M01.X2 Direct infection of elbow in infectious and parasitic diseases classified elsewhere**
M01.X21 Direct infection of right elbow in infectious and parasitic diseases classified elsewhere
M01.X22 Direct infection of left elbow in infectious and parasitic diseases classified elsewhere
M01.X29 Direct infection of unspecified elbow in infectious and parasitic diseases classified elsewhere

6th **M01.X3 Direct infection of wrist in infectious and parasitic diseases classified elsewhere**
Direct infection of carpal bones in infectious and parasitic diseases classified elsewhere
M01.X31 Direct infection of right wrist in infectious and parasitic diseases classified elsewhere
M01.X32 Direct infection of left wrist in infectious and parasitic diseases classified elsewhere
M01.X39 Direct infection of unspecified wrist in infectious and parasitic diseases classified elsewhere

6th **M01.X4 Direct infection of hand in infectious and parasitic diseases classified elsewhere**
Direct infection of metacarpus and phalanges in infectious and parasitic diseases classified elsewhere
M01.X41 Direct infection of right hand in infectious and parasitic diseases classified elsewhere
M01.X42 Direct infection of left hand in infectious and parasitic diseases classified elsewhere
M01.X49 Direct infection of unspecified hand in infectious and parasitic diseases classified elsewhere

6th **M01.X5 Direct infection of hip in infectious and parasitic diseases classified elsewhere**
M01.X51 Direct infection of right hip in infectious and parasitic diseases classified elsewhere
M01.X52 Direct infection of left hip in infectious and parasitic diseases classified elsewhere
M01.X59 Direct infection of unspecified hip in infectious and parasitic diseases classified elsewhere

6th **M01.X6 Direct infection of knee in infectious and parasitic diseases classified elsewhere**
M01.X61 Direct infection of right knee in infectious and parasitic diseases classified elsewhere
M01.X62 Direct infection of left knee in infectious and parasitic diseases classified elsewhere
M01.X69 Direct infection of unspecified knee in infectious and parasitic diseases classified elsewhere

6th **M01.X7 Direct infection of ankle and foot in infectious and parasitic diseases classified elsewhere**
Direct infection of tarsus, metatarsus and phalanges in infectious and parasitic diseases classified elsewhere
M01.X71 Direct infection of right ankle and foot in infectious and parasitic diseases classified elsewhere
M01.X72 Direct infection of left ankle and foot in infectious and parasitic diseases classified elsewhere
M01.X79 Direct infection of unspecified ankle and foot in infectious and parasitic diseases classified elsewhere

M01.X8 Direct infection of vertebrae in infectious and parasitic diseases classified elsewhere
M01.X9 Direct infection of multiple joints in infectious and parasitic diseases classified elsewhere

4th **M02 Postinfective and reactive arthropathies**
Code first underlying disease, such as:
congenital syphilis [Clutton's joints] (A50.5)
enteritis due to Yersinia enterocolitica (A04.6)
infective endocarditis (I33.0)
viral hepatitis (B15-B19)

EXCLUDES 1 *Behçet's disease (M35.2)*
direct infections of joint in infectious and parasitic diseases classified elsewhere (M01.-)
postinfectious arthritis (in):
meningococcal (A39.84)
mumps (B26.85)
rheumatic fever (I00)
rubella (B06.82)
syphilis (late) (A52.77)
tabetic arthropathy [Charcôt's] (A52.16)

5th **M02.0 Arthropathy following intestinal bypass**
M02.00 Arthropathy following intestinal bypass, unspecified site

6th **M02.01 Arthropathy following intestinal bypass, shoulder**
M02.011 Arthropathy following intestinal bypass, right shoulder
M02.012 Arthropathy following intestinal bypass, left shoulder
M02.019 Arthropathy following intestinal bypass, unspecified shoulder

6th **M02.02 Arthropathy following intestinal bypass, elbow**
M02.021 Arthropathy following intestinal bypass, right elbow
M02.022 Arthropathy following intestinal bypass, left elbow
M02.029 Arthropathy following intestinal bypass, unspecified elbow

6th **M02.03 Arthropathy following intestinal bypass, wrist**
Arthropathy following intestinal bypass, carpal bones
M02.031 Arthropathy following intestinal bypass, right wrist
M02.032 Arthropathy following intestinal bypass, left wrist
M02.039 Arthropathy following intestinal bypass, unspecified wrist

6th **M02.04 Arthropathy following intestinal bypass, hand**
Arthropathy following intestinal bypass, metacarpals and phalanges
M02.041 Arthropathy following intestinal bypass, right hand
M02.042 Arthropathy following intestinal bypass, left hand
M02.049 Arthropathy following intestinal bypass, unspecified hand

6th **M02.05 Arthropathy following intestinal bypass, hip**
M02.051 Arthropathy following intestinal bypass, right hip
M02.052 Arthropathy following intestinal bypass, left hip
M02.059 Arthropathy following intestinal bypass, unspecified hip

6th **M02.06 Arthropathy following intestinal bypass, knee**
M02.061 Arthropathy following intestinal bypass, right knee
M02.062 Arthropathy following intestinal bypass, left knee
M02.069 Arthropathy following intestinal bypass, unspecified knee

6th **M02.07 Arthropathy following intestinal bypass, ankle and foot**
Arthropathy following intestinal bypass, tarsus, metatarsus and phalanges
M02.071 Arthropathy following intestinal bypass, right ankle and foot
M02.072 Arthropathy following intestinal bypass, left ankle and foot
M02.079 Arthropathy following intestinal bypass, unspecified ankle and foot

M02.08 Arthropathy following intestinal bypass, vertebrae
M02.09 Arthropathy following intestinal bypass, multiple sites

✓5th **MØ2.1 Postdysenteric arthropathy**

MØ2.1Ø Postdysenteric arthropathy, unspecified site

✓6th **MØ2.11 Postdysenteric arthropathy, shoulder**

MØ2.111 Postdysenteric arthropathy, right shoulder

MØ2.112 Postdysenteric arthropathy, left shoulder

MØ2.119 Postdysenteric arthropathy, unspecified shoulder

✓6th **MØ2.12 Postdysenteric arthropathy, elbow**

MØ2.121 Postdysenteric arthropathy, right elbow

MØ2.122 Postdysenteric arthropathy, left elbow

MØ2.129 Postdysenteric arthropathy, unspecified elbow

✓6th **MØ2.13 Postdysenteric arthropathy, wrist**

Postdysenteric arthropathy, carpal bones

MØ2.131 Postdysenteric arthropathy, right wrist

MØ2.132 Postdysenteric arthropathy, left wrist

MØ2.139 Postdysenteric arthropathy, unspecified wrist

✓6th **MØ2.14 Postdysenteric arthropathy, hand**

Postdysenteric arthropathy, metacarpus and phalanges

MØ2.141 Postdysenteric arthropathy, right hand

MØ2.142 Postdysenteric arthropathy, left hand

MØ2.149 Postdysenteric arthropathy, unspecified hand

✓6th **MØ2.15 Postdysenteric arthropathy, hip**

MØ2.151 Postdysenteric arthropathy, right hip

MØ2.152 Postdysenteric arthropathy, left hip

MØ2.159 Postdysenteric arthropathy, unspecified hip

✓6th **MØ2.16 Postdysenteric arthropathy, knee**

MØ2.161 Postdysenteric arthropathy, right knee

MØ2.162 Postdysenteric arthropathy, left knee

MØ2.169 Postdysenteric arthropathy, unspecified knee

✓6th **MØ2.17 Postdysenteric arthropathy, ankle and foot**

Postdysenteric arthropathy, tarsus, metatarsus and phalanges

MØ2.171 Postdysenteric arthropathy, right ankle and foot

MØ2.172 Postdysenteric arthropathy, left ankle and foot

MØ2.179 Postdysenteric arthropathy, unspecified ankle and foot

MØ2.18 Postdysenteric arthropathy, vertebrae

MØ2.19 Postdysenteric arthropathy, multiple sites

✓5th **MØ2.2 Postimmunization arthropathy**

MØ2.2Ø Postimmunization arthropathy, unspecified site

✓6th **MØ2.21 Postimmunization arthropathy, shoulder**

MØ2.211 Postimmunization arthropathy, right shoulder

MØ2.212 Postimmunization arthropathy, left shoulder

MØ2.219 Postimmunization arthropathy, unspecified shoulder

✓6th **MØ2.22 Postimmunization arthropathy, elbow**

MØ2.221 Postimmunization arthropathy, right elbow

MØ2.222 Postimmunization arthropathy, left elbow

MØ2.229 Postimmunization arthropathy, unspecified elbow

✓6th **MØ2.23 Postimmunization arthropathy, wrist**

Postimmunization arthropathy, carpal bones

MØ2.231 Postimmunization arthropathy, right wrist

MØ2.232 Postimmunization arthropathy, left wrist

MØ2.239 Postimmunization arthropathy, unspecified wrist

✓6th **MØ2.24 Postimmunization arthropathy, hand**

Postimmunization arthropathy, metacarpus and phalanges

MØ2.241 Postimmunization arthropathy, right hand

MØ2.242 Postimmunization arthropathy, left hand

MØ2.249 Postimmunization arthropathy, unspecified hand

✓6th **MØ2.25 Postimmunization arthropathy, hip**

MØ2.251 Postimmunization arthropathy, right hip

MØ2.252 Postimmunization arthropathy, left hip

MØ2.259 Postimmunization arthropathy, unspecified hip

✓6th **MØ2.26 Postimmunization arthropathy, knee**

MØ2.261 Postimmunization arthropathy, right knee

MØ2.262 Postimmunization arthropathy, left knee

MØ2.269 Postimmunization arthropathy, unspecified knee

✓6th **MØ2.27 Postimmunization arthropathy, ankle and foot**

Postimmunization arthropathy, tarsus, metatarsus and phalanges

MØ2.271 Postimmunization arthropathy, right ankle and foot

MØ2.272 Postimmunization arthropathy, left ankle and foot

MØ2.279 Postimmunization arthropathy, unspecified ankle and foot

MØ2.28 Postimmunization arthropathy, vertebrae

MØ2.29 Postimmunization arthropathy, multiple sites

✓5th **MØ2.3 Reiter's disease**

Reactive arthritis

MØ2.3Ø Reiter's disease, unspecified site

✓6th **MØ2.31 Reiter's disease, shoulder**

MØ2.311 Reiter's disease, right shoulder

MØ2.312 Reiter's disease, left shoulder

MØ2.319 Reiter's disease, unspecified shoulder

✓6th **MØ2.32 Reiter's disease, elbow**

MØ2.321 Reiter's disease, right elbow

MØ2.322 Reiter's disease, left elbow

MØ2.329 Reiter's disease, unspecified elbow

✓6th **MØ2.33 Reiter's disease, wrist**

Reiter's disease, carpal bones

MØ2.331 Reiter's disease, right wrist

MØ2.332 Reiter's disease, left wrist

MØ2.339 Reiter's disease, unspecified wrist

✓6th **MØ2.34 Reiter's disease, hand**

Reiter's disease, metacarpus and phalanges

MØ2.341 Reiter's disease, right hand

MØ2.342 Reiter's disease, left hand

MØ2.349 Reiter's disease, unspecified hand

✓6th **MØ2.35 Reiter's disease, hip**

MØ2.351 Reiter's disease, right hip

MØ2.352 Reiter's disease, left hip

MØ2.359 Reiter's disease, unspecified hip

✓6th **MØ2.36 Reiter's disease, knee**

MØ2.361 Reiter's disease, right knee

MØ2.362 Reiter's disease, left knee

MØ2.369 Reiter's disease, unspecified knee

✓6th **MØ2.37 Reiter's disease, ankle and foot**

Reiter's disease, tarsus, metatarsus and phalanges

MØ2.371 Reiter's disease, right ankle and foot

MØ2.372 Reiter's disease, left ankle and foot

MØ2.379 Reiter's disease, unspecified ankle and foot

MØ2.38 Reiter's disease, vertebrae

MØ2.39 Reiter's disease, multiple sites

✓5th **MØ2.8 Other reactive arthropathies**

MØ2.8Ø Other reactive arthropathies, unspecified site

✓6th **MØ2.81 Other reactive arthropathies, shoulder**

MØ2.811 Other reactive arthropathies, right shoulder

MØ2.812 Other reactive arthropathies, left shoulder

MØ2.819 Other reactive arthropathies, unspecified shoulder

6th **M02.82 Other reactive arthropathies, elbow**
M02.821 Other reactive arthropathies, right elbow
M02.822 Other reactive arthropathies, left elbow
M02.829 Other reactive arthropathies, unspecified elbow

6th **M02.83 Other reactive arthropathies, wrist**
Other reactive arthropathies, carpal bones
M02.831 Other reactive arthropathies, right wrist
M02.832 Other reactive arthropathies, left wrist
M02.839 Other reactive arthropathies, unspecified wrist

6th **M02.84 Other reactive arthropathies, hand**
Other reactive arthropathies, metacarpus and phalanges
M02.841 Other reactive arthropathies, right hand
M02.842 Other reactive arthropathies, left hand
M02.849 Other reactive arthropathies, unspecified hand

6th **M02.85 Other reactive arthropathies, hip**
M02.851 Other reactive arthropathies, right hip
M02.852 Other reactive arthropathies, left hip
M02.859 Other reactive arthropathies, unspecified hip

6th **M02.86 Other reactive arthropathies, knee**
M02.861 Other reactive arthropathies, right knee
M02.862 Other reactive arthropathies, left knee
M02.869 Other reactive arthropathies, unspecified knee

6th **M02.87 Other reactive arthropathies, ankle and foot**
Other reactive arthropathies, tarsus, metatarsus and phalanges
M02.871 Other reactive arthropathies, right ankle and foot
M02.872 Other reactive arthropathies, left ankle and foot
M02.879 Other reactive arthropathies, unspecified ankle and foot

M02.88 Other reactive arthropathies, vertebrae

M02.89 Other reactive arthropathies, multiple sites

M02.9 Reactive arthropathy, unspecified

Inflammatory polyarthropathies (M05-M14)

4th **M05 Rheumatoid arthritis with rheumatoid factor**
EXCLUDES 1 *rheumatic fever (I00)*
juvenile rheumatoid arthritis (M08.-)
rheumatoid arthritis of spine (M45.-)

5th **M05.0 Felty's syndrome**
Rheumatoid arthritis with splenoadenomegaly and leukopenia
M05.00 Felty's syndrome, unspecified site

6th **M05.01 Felty's syndrome, shoulder**
M05.011 Felty's syndrome, right shoulder
M05.012 Felty's syndrome, left shoulder
M05.019 Felty's syndrome, unspecified shoulder

6th **M05.02 Felty's syndrome, elbow**
M05.021 Felty's syndrome, right elbow
M05.022 Felty's syndrome, left elbow
M05.029 Felty's syndrome, unspecified elbow

6th **M05.03 Felty's syndrome, wrist**
Felty's syndrome, carpal bones
M05.031 Felty's syndrome, right wrist
M05.032 Felty's syndrome, left wrist
M05.039 Felty's syndrome, unspecified wrist

6th **M05.04 Felty's syndrome, hand**
Felty's syndrome, metacarpus and phalanges
M05.041 Felty's syndrome, right hand
M05.042 Felty's syndrome, left hand
M05.049 Felty's syndrome, unspecified hand

6th **M05.05 Felty's syndrome, hip**
M05.051 Felty's syndrome, right hip
M05.052 Felty's syndrome, left hip
M05.059 Felty's syndrome, unspecified hip

6th **M05.06 Felty's syndrome, knee**
M05.061 Felty's syndrome, right knee
M05.062 Felty's syndrome, left knee
M05.069 Felty's syndrome, unspecified knee

6th **M05.07 Felty's syndrome, ankle and foot**
Felty's syndrome, tarsus, metatarsus and phalanges
M05.071 Felty's syndrome, right ankle and foot
M05.072 Felty's syndrome, left ankle and foot
M05.079 Felty's syndrome, unspecified ankle and foot

M05.09 Felty's syndrome, multiple sites

5th **M05.1 Rheumatoid lung disease with rheumatoid arthritis**
M05.10 Rheumatoid lung disease with rheumatoid arthritis of unspecified site

6th **M05.11 Rheumatoid lung disease with rheumatoid arthritis of shoulder**
M05.111 Rheumatoid lung disease with rheumatoid arthritis of right shoulder
M05.112 Rheumatoid lung disease with rheumatoid arthritis of left shoulder
M05.119 Rheumatoid lung disease with rheumatoid arthritis of unspecified shoulder

6th **M05.12 Rheumatoid lung disease with rheumatoid arthritis of elbow**
M05.121 Rheumatoid lung disease with rheumatoid arthritis of right elbow
M05.122 Rheumatoid lung disease with rheumatoid arthritis of left elbow
M05.129 Rheumatoid lung disease with rheumatoid arthritis of unspecified elbow

6th **M05.13 Rheumatoid lung disease with rheumatoid arthritis of wrist**
Rheumatoid lung disease with rheumatoid arthritis, carpal bones
M05.131 Rheumatoid lung disease with rheumatoid arthritis of right wrist
M05.132 Rheumatoid lung disease with rheumatoid arthritis of left wrist
M05.139 Rheumatoid lung disease with rheumatoid arthritis of unspecified wrist

6th **M05.14 Rheumatoid lung disease with rheumatoid arthritis of hand**
Rheumatoid lung disease with rheumatoid arthritis, metacarpus and phalanges
M05.141 Rheumatoid lung disease with rheumatoid arthritis of right hand
M05.142 Rheumatoid lung disease with rheumatoid arthritis of left hand
M05.149 Rheumatoid lung disease with rheumatoid arthritis of unspecified hand

6th **M05.15 Rheumatoid lung disease with rheumatoid arthritis of hip**
M05.151 Rheumatoid lung disease with rheumatoid arthritis of right hip
M05.152 Rheumatoid lung disease with rheumatoid arthritis of left hip
M05.159 Rheumatoid lung disease with rheumatoid arthritis of unspecified hip

6th **M05.16 Rheumatoid lung disease with rheumatoid arthritis of knee**
M05.161 Rheumatoid lung disease with rheumatoid arthritis of right knee
M05.162 Rheumatoid lung disease with rheumatoid arthritis of left knee
M05.169 Rheumatoid lung disease with rheumatoid arthritis of unspecified knee

6th **M05.17 Rheumatoid lung disease with rheumatoid arthritis of ankle and foot**
Rheumatoid lung disease with rheumatoid arthritis, tarsus, metatarsus and phalanges
M05.171 Rheumatoid lung disease with rheumatoid arthritis of right ankle and foot

MØ5.172 Rheumatoid lung disease with rheumatoid arthritis of left ankle and foot

MØ5.179 Rheumatoid lung disease with rheumatoid arthritis of unspecified ankle and foot

MØ5.19 Rheumatoid lung disease with rheumatoid arthritis of multiple sites

5th **MØ5.2 Rheumatoid vasculitis with rheumatoid arthritis**

MØ5.2Ø Rheumatoid vasculitis with rheumatoid arthritis of unspecified site

6th **MØ5.21 Rheumatoid vasculitis with rheumatoid arthritis of shoulder**

MØ5.211 Rheumatoid vasculitis with rheumatoid arthritis of right shoulder

MØ5.212 Rheumatoid vasculitis with rheumatoid arthritis of left shoulder

MØ5.219 Rheumatoid vasculitis with rheumatoid arthritis of unspecified shoulder

6th **MØ5.22 Rheumatoid vasculitis with rheumatoid arthritis of elbow**

MØ5.221 Rheumatoid vasculitis with rheumatoid arthritis of right elbow

MØ5.222 Rheumatoid vasculitis with rheumatoid arthritis of left elbow

MØ5.229 Rheumatoid vasculitis with rheumatoid arthritis of unspecified elbow

6th **MØ5.23 Rheumatoid vasculitis with rheumatoid arthritis of wrist**

Rheumatoid vasculitis with rheumatoid arthritis, carpal bones

MØ5.231 Rheumatoid vasculitis with rheumatoid arthritis of right wrist

MØ5.232 Rheumatoid vasculitis with rheumatoid arthritis of left wrist

MØ5.239 Rheumatoid vasculitis with rheumatoid arthritis of unspecified wrist

6th **MØ5.24 Rheumatoid vasculitis with rheumatoid arthritis of hand**

Rheumatoid vasculitis with rheumatoid arthritis, metacarpus and phalanges

MØ5.241 Rheumatoid vasculitis with rheumatoid arthritis of right hand

MØ5.242 Rheumatoid vasculitis with rheumatoid arthritis of left hand

MØ5.249 Rheumatoid vasculitis with rheumatoid arthritis of unspecified hand

6th **MØ5.25 Rheumatoid vasculitis with rheumatoid arthritis of hip**

MØ5.251 Rheumatoid vasculitis with rheumatoid arthritis of right hip

MØ5.252 Rheumatoid vasculitis with rheumatoid arthritis of left hip

MØ5.259 Rheumatoid vasculitis with rheumatoid arthritis of unspecified hip

6th **MØ5.26 Rheumatoid vasculitis with rheumatoid arthritis of knee**

MØ5.261 Rheumatoid vasculitis with rheumatoid arthritis of right knee

MØ5.262 Rheumatoid vasculitis with rheumatoid arthritis of left knee

MØ5.269 Rheumatoid vasculitis with rheumatoid arthritis of unspecified knee

6th **MØ5.27 Rheumatoid vasculitis with rheumatoid arthritis of ankle and foot**

Rheumatoid vasculitis with rheumatoid arthritis, tarsus, metatarsus and phalanges

MØ5.271 Rheumatoid vasculitis with rheumatoid arthritis of right ankle and foot

MØ5.272 Rheumatoid vasculitis with rheumatoid arthritis of left ankle and foot

MØ5.279 Rheumatoid vasculitis with rheumatoid arthritis of unspecified ankle and foot

MØ5.29 Rheumatoid vasculitis with rheumatoid arthritis of multiple sites

5th **MØ5.3 Rheumatoid heart disease with rheumatoid arthritis**

Rheumatoid carditis
Rheumatoid endocarditis
Rheumatoid myocarditis
Rheumatoid pericarditis

MØ5.3Ø Rheumatoid heart disease with rheumatoid arthritis of unspecified site

6th **MØ5.31 Rheumatoid heart disease with rheumatoid arthritis of shoulder**

MØ5.311 Rheumatoid heart disease with rheumatoid arthritis of right shoulder

MØ5.312 Rheumatoid heart disease with rheumatoid arthritis of left shoulder

MØ5.319 Rheumatoid heart disease with rheumatoid arthritis of unspecified shoulder

6th **MØ5.32 Rheumatoid heart disease with rheumatoid arthritis of elbow**

MØ5.321 Rheumatoid heart disease with rheumatoid arthritis of right elbow

MØ5.322 Rheumatoid heart disease with rheumatoid arthritis of left elbow

MØ5.329 Rheumatoid heart disease with rheumatoid arthritis of unspecified elbow

6th **MØ5.33 Rheumatoid heart disease with rheumatoid arthritis of wrist**

Rheumatoid heart disease with rheumatoid arthritis, carpal bones

MØ5.331 Rheumatoid heart disease with rheumatoid arthritis of right wrist

MØ5.332 Rheumatoid heart disease with rheumatoid arthritis of left wrist

MØ5.339 Rheumatoid heart disease with rheumatoid arthritis of unspecified wrist

6th **MØ5.34 Rheumatoid heart disease with rheumatoid arthritis of hand**

Rheumatoid heart disease with rheumatoid arthritis, metacarpus and phalanges

MØ5.341 Rheumatoid heart disease with rheumatoid arthritis of right hand

MØ5.342 Rheumatoid heart disease with rheumatoid arthritis of left hand

MØ5.349 Rheumatoid heart disease with rheumatoid arthritis of unspecified hand

6th **MØ5.35 Rheumatoid heart disease with rheumatoid arthritis of hip**

MØ5.351 Rheumatoid heart disease with rheumatoid arthritis of right hip

MØ5.352 Rheumatoid heart disease with rheumatoid arthritis of left hip

MØ5.359 Rheumatoid heart disease with rheumatoid arthritis of unspecified hip

6th **MØ5.36 Rheumatoid heart disease with rheumatoid arthritis of knee**

MØ5.361 Rheumatoid heart disease with rheumatoid arthritis of right knee

MØ5.362 Rheumatoid heart disease with rheumatoid arthritis of left knee

MØ5.369 Rheumatoid heart disease with rheumatoid arthritis of unspecified knee

6th **MØ5.37 Rheumatoid heart disease with rheumatoid arthritis of ankle and foot**

Rheumatoid heart disease with rheumatoid arthritis, tarsus, metatarsus and phalanges

MØ5.371 Rheumatoid heart disease with rheumatoid arthritis of right ankle and foot

MØ5.372 Rheumatoid heart disease with rheumatoid arthritis of left ankle and foot

MØ5.379 Rheumatoid heart disease with rheumatoid arthritis of unspecified ankle and foot

MØ5.39 Rheumatoid heart disease with rheumatoid arthritis of multiple sites

5th **MØ5.4 Rheumatoid myopathy with rheumatoid arthritis**

MØ5.4Ø Rheumatoid myopathy with rheumatoid arthritis of unspecified site

M05.41 Rheumatoid myopathy with rheumatoid arthritis of shoulder
- **M05.411 Rheumatoid myopathy with rheumatoid arthritis of right shoulder**
- **M05.412 Rheumatoid myopathy with rheumatoid arthritis of left shoulder**
- **M05.419 Rheumatoid myopathy with rheumatoid arthritis of unspecified shoulder**

M05.42 Rheumatoid myopathy with rheumatoid arthritis of elbow
- **M05.421 Rheumatoid myopathy with rheumatoid arthritis of right elbow**
- **M05.422 Rheumatoid myopathy with rheumatoid arthritis of left elbow**
- **M05.429 Rheumatoid myopathy with rheumatoid arthritis of unspecified elbow**

M05.43 Rheumatoid myopathy with rheumatoid arthritis of wrist
Rheumatoid myopathy with rheumatoid arthritis, carpal bones
- **M05.431 Rheumatoid myopathy with rheumatoid arthritis of right wrist**
- **M05.432 Rheumatoid myopathy with rheumatoid arthritis of left wrist**
- **M05.439 Rheumatoid myopathy with rheumatoid arthritis of unspecified wrist**

M05.44 Rheumatoid myopathy with rheumatoid arthritis of hand
Rheumatoid myopathy with rheumatoid arthritis, metacarpus and phalanges
- **M05.441 Rheumatoid myopathy with rheumatoid arthritis of right hand**
- **M05.442 Rheumatoid myopathy with rheumatoid arthritis of left hand**
- **M05.449 Rheumatoid myopathy with rheumatoid arthritis of unspecified hand**

M05.45 Rheumatoid myopathy with rheumatoid arthritis of hip
- **M05.451 Rheumatoid myopathy with rheumatoid arthritis of right hip**
- **M05.452 Rheumatoid myopathy with rheumatoid arthritis of left hip**
- **M05.459 Rheumatoid myopathy with rheumatoid arthritis of unspecified hip**

M05.46 Rheumatoid myopathy with rheumatoid arthritis of knee
- **M05.461 Rheumatoid myopathy with rheumatoid arthritis of right knee**
- **M05.462 Rheumatoid myopathy with rheumatoid arthritis of left knee**
- **M05.469 Rheumatoid myopathy with rheumatoid arthritis of unspecified knee**

M05.47 Rheumatoid myopathy with rheumatoid arthritis of ankle and foot
Rheumatoid myopathy with rheumatoid arthritis, tarsus, metatarsus and phalanges
- **M05.471 Rheumatoid myopathy with rheumatoid arthritis of right ankle and foot**
- **M05.472 Rheumatoid myopathy with rheumatoid arthritis of left ankle and foot**
- **M05.479 Rheumatoid myopathy with rheumatoid arthritis of unspecified ankle and foot**

M05.49 Rheumatoid myopathy with rheumatoid arthritis of multiple sites

M05.5 Rheumatoid polyneuropathy with rheumatoid arthritis

M05.50 Rheumatoid polyneuropathy with rheumatoid arthritis of unspecified site

M05.51 Rheumatoid polyneuropathy with rheumatoid arthritis of shoulder
- **M05.511 Rheumatoid polyneuropathy with rheumatoid arthritis of right shoulder**
- **M05.512 Rheumatoid polyneuropathy with rheumatoid arthritis of left shoulder**
- **M05.519 Rheumatoid polyneuropathy with rheumatoid arthritis of unspecified shoulder**

M05.52 Rheumatoid polyneuropathy with rheumatoid arthritis of elbow
- **M05.521 Rheumatoid polyneuropathy with rheumatoid arthritis of right elbow**
- **M05.522 Rheumatoid polyneuropathy with rheumatoid arthritis of left elbow**
- **M05.529 Rheumatoid polyneuropathy with rheumatoid arthritis of unspecified elbow**

M05.53 Rheumatoid polyneuropathy with rheumatoid arthritis of wrist
Rheumatoid polyneuropathy with rheumatoid arthritis, carpal bones
- **M05.531 Rheumatoid polyneuropathy with rheumatoid arthritis of right wrist**
- **M05.532 Rheumatoid polyneuropathy with rheumatoid arthritis of left wrist**
- **M05.539 Rheumatoid polyneuropathy with rheumatoid arthritis of unspecified wrist**

M05.54 Rheumatoid polyneuropathy with rheumatoid arthritis of hand
Rheumatoid polyneuropathy with rheumatoid arthritis, metacarpus and phalanges
- **M05.541 Rheumatoid polyneuropathy with rheumatoid arthritis of right hand**
- **M05.542 Rheumatoid polyneuropathy with rheumatoid arthritis of left hand**
- **M05.549 Rheumatoid polyneuropathy with rheumatoid arthritis of unspecified hand**

M05.55 Rheumatoid polyneuropathy with rheumatoid arthritis of hip
- **M05.551 Rheumatoid polyneuropathy with rheumatoid arthritis of right hip**
- **M05.552 Rheumatoid polyneuropathy with rheumatoid arthritis of left hip**
- **M05.559 Rheumatoid polyneuropathy with rheumatoid arthritis of unspecified hip**

M05.56 Rheumatoid polyneuropathy with rheumatoid arthritis of knee
- **M05.561 Rheumatoid polyneuropathy with rheumatoid arthritis of right knee**
- **M05.562 Rheumatoid polyneuropathy with rheumatoid arthritis of left knee**
- **M05.569 Rheumatoid polyneuropathy with rheumatoid arthritis of unspecified knee**

M05.57 Rheumatoid polyneuropathy with rheumatoid arthritis of ankle and foot
Rheumatoid polyneuropathy with rheumatoid arthritis, tarsus, metatarsus and phalanges
- **M05.571 Rheumatoid polyneuropathy with rheumatoid arthritis of right ankle and foot**
- **M05.572 Rheumatoid polyneuropathy with rheumatoid arthritis of left ankle and foot**
- **M05.579 Rheumatoid polyneuropathy with rheumatoid arthritis of unspecified ankle and foot**

M05.59 Rheumatoid polyneuropathy with rheumatoid arthritis of multiple sites

M05.6 Rheumatoid arthritis with involvement of other organs and systems

M05.60 Rheumatoid arthritis of unspecified site with involvement of other organs and systems

M05.61 Rheumatoid arthritis of shoulder with involvement of other organs and systems
- **M05.611 Rheumatoid arthritis of right shoulder with involvement of other organs and systems**
- **M05.612 Rheumatoid arthritis of left shoulder with involvement of other organs and systems**
- **M05.619 Rheumatoid arthritis of unspecified shoulder with involvement of other organs and systems**

Appropriate additional character required | x7th Requires 7th character, placeholder x must fill empty characters

6th **MØ5.62 Rheumatoid arthritis of elbow with involvement of other organs and systems**
- **MØ5.621 Rheumatoid arthritis of right elbow with involvement of other organs and systems**
- **MØ5.622 Rheumatoid arthritis of left elbow with involvement of other organs and systems**
- **MØ5.629 Rheumatoid arthritis of unspecified elbow with involvement of other organs and systems**

6th **MØ5.63 Rheumatoid arthritis of wrist with involvement of other organs and systems**

Rheumatoid arthritis of carpal bones with involvement of other organs and systems

- **MØ5.631 Rheumatoid arthritis of right wrist with involvement of other organs and systems**
- **MØ5.632 Rheumatoid arthritis of left wrist with involvement of other organs and systems**
- **MØ5.639 Rheumatoid arthritis of unspecified wrist with involvement of other organs and systems**

6th **MØ5.64 Rheumatoid arthritis of hand with involvement of other organs and systems**

Rheumatoid arthritis of metacarpus and phalanges with involvement of other organs and systems

- **MØ5.641 Rheumatoid arthritis of right hand with involvement of other organs and systems**
- **MØ5.642 Rheumatoid arthritis of left hand with involvement of other organs and systems**
- **MØ5.649 Rheumatoid arthritis of unspecified hand with involvement of other organs and systems**

6th **MØ5.65 Rheumatoid arthritis of hip with involvement of other organs and systems**
- **MØ5.651 Rheumatoid arthritis of right hip with involvement of other organs and systems**
- **MØ5.652 Rheumatoid arthritis of left hip with involvement of other organs and systems**
- **MØ5.659 Rheumatoid arthritis of unspecified hip with involvement of other organs and systems**

6th **MØ5.66 Rheumatoid arthritis of knee with involvement of other organs and systems**
- **MØ5.661 Rheumatoid arthritis of right knee with involvement of other organs and systems**
- **MØ5.662 Rheumatoid arthritis of left knee with involvement of other organs and systems**
- **MØ5.669 Rheumatoid arthritis of unspecified knee with involvement of other organs and systems**

6th **MØ5.67 Rheumatoid arthritis of ankle and foot with involvement of other organs and systems**

Rheumatoid arthritis of tarsus, metatarsus and phalanges with involvement of other organs and systems

- **MØ5.671 Rheumatoid arthritis of right ankle and foot with involvement of other organs and systems**
- **MØ5.672 Rheumatoid arthritis of left ankle and foot with involvement of other organs and systems**
- **MØ5.679 Rheumatoid arthritis of unspecified ankle and foot with involvement of other organs and systems**

MØ5.69 Rheumatoid arthritis of multiple sites with involvement of other organs and systems

5th **MØ5.7 Rheumatoid arthritis with rheumatoid factor without organ or systems involvement**

MØ5.7Ø Rheumatoid arthritis with rheumatoid factor of unspecified site without organ or systems involvement

6th **MØ5.71 Rheumatoid arthritis with rheumatoid factor of shoulder without organ or systems involvement**
- **MØ5.711 Rheumatoid arthritis with rheumatoid factor of right shoulder without organ or systems involvement**
- **MØ5.712 Rheumatoid arthritis with rheumatoid factor of left shoulder without organ or systems involvement**
- **MØ5.719 Rheumatoid arthritis with rheumatoid factor of unspecified shoulder without organ or systems involvement**

6th **MØ5.72 Rheumatoid arthritis with rheumatoid factor of elbow without organ or systems involvement**
- **MØ5.721 Rheumatoid arthritis with rheumatoid factor of right elbow without organ or systems involvement**
- **MØ5.722 Rheumatoid arthritis with rheumatoid factor of left elbow without organ or systems involvement**
- **MØ5.729 Rheumatoid arthritis with rheumatoid factor of unspecified elbow without organ or systems involvement**

6th **MØ5.73 Rheumatoid arthritis with rheumatoid factor of wrist without organ or systems involvement**
- **MØ5.731 Rheumatoid arthritis with rheumatoid factor of right wrist without organ or systems involvement**
- **MØ5.732 Rheumatoid arthritis with rheumatoid factor of left wrist without organ or systems involvement**
- **MØ5.739 Rheumatoid arthritis with rheumatoid factor of unspecified wrist without organ or systems involvement**

6th **MØ5.74 Rheumatoid arthritis with rheumatoid factor of hand without organ or systems involvement**
- **MØ5.741 Rheumatoid arthritis with rheumatoid factor of right hand without organ or systems involvement**
- **MØ5.742 Rheumatoid arthritis with rheumatoid factor of left hand without organ or systems involvement**
- **MØ5.749 Rheumatoid arthritis with rheumatoid factor of unspecified hand without organ or systems involvement**

6th **MØ5.75 Rheumatoid arthritis with rheumatoid factor of hip without organ or systems involvement**
- **MØ5.751 Rheumatoid arthritis with rheumatoid factor of right hip without organ or systems involvement**
- **MØ5.752 Rheumatoid arthritis with rheumatoid factor of left hip without organ or systems involvement**
- **MØ5.759 Rheumatoid arthritis with rheumatoid factor of unspecified hip without organ or systems involvement**

6th **MØ5.76 Rheumatoid arthritis with rheumatoid factor of knee without organ or systems involvement**
- **MØ5.761 Rheumatoid arthritis with rheumatoid factor of right knee without organ or systems involvement**
- **MØ5.762 Rheumatoid arthritis with rheumatoid factor of left knee without organ or systems involvement**
- **MØ5.769 Rheumatoid arthritis with rheumatoid factor of unspecified knee without organ or systems involvement**

6th **MØ5.77 Rheumatoid arthritis with rheumatoid factor of ankle and foot without organ or systems involvement**
- **MØ5.771 Rheumatoid arthritis with rheumatoid factor of right ankle and foot without organ or systems involvement**
- **MØ5.772 Rheumatoid arthritis with rheumatoid factor of left ankle and foot without organ or systems involvement**
- **MØ5.779 Rheumatoid arthritis with rheumatoid factor of unspecified ankle and foot without organ or systems involvement**

M05.79 Rheumatoid arthritis with rheumatoid factor of multiple sites without organ or systems involvement

✓5th M05.8 Other rheumatoid arthritis with rheumatoid factor

M05.80 Other rheumatoid arthritis with rheumatoid factor of unspecified site

✓6th M05.81 Other rheumatoid arthritis with rheumatoid factor of shoulder

M05.811 Other rheumatoid arthritis with rheumatoid factor of right shoulder

M05.812 Other rheumatoid arthritis with rheumatoid factor of left shoulder

M05.819 Other rheumatoid arthritis with rheumatoid factor of unspecified shoulder

✓6th M05.82 Other rheumatoid arthritis with rheumatoid factor of elbow

M05.821 Other rheumatoid arthritis with rheumatoid factor of right elbow

M05.822 Other rheumatoid arthritis with rheumatoid factor of left elbow

M05.829 Other rheumatoid arthritis with rheumatoid factor of unspecified elbow

✓6th M05.83 Other rheumatoid arthritis with rheumatoid factor of wrist

M05.831 Other rheumatoid arthritis with rheumatoid factor of right wrist

M05.832 Other rheumatoid arthritis with rheumatoid factor of left wrist

M05.839 Other rheumatoid arthritis with rheumatoid factor of unspecified wrist

✓6th M05.84 Other rheumatoid arthritis with rheumatoid factor of hand

M05.841 Other rheumatoid arthritis with rheumatoid factor of right hand

M05.842 Other rheumatoid arthritis with rheumatoid factor of left hand

M05.849 Other rheumatoid arthritis with rheumatoid factor of unspecified hand

✓6th M05.85 Other rheumatoid arthritis with rheumatoid factor of hip

M05.851 Other rheumatoid arthritis with rheumatoid factor of right hip

M05.852 Other rheumatoid arthritis with rheumatoid factor of left hip

M05.859 Other rheumatoid arthritis with rheumatoid factor of unspecified hip

✓6th M05.86 Other rheumatoid arthritis with rheumatoid factor of knee

M05.861 Other rheumatoid arthritis with rheumatoid factor of right knee

M05.862 Other rheumatoid arthritis with rheumatoid factor of left knee

M05.869 Other rheumatoid arthritis with rheumatoid factor of unspecified knee

✓6th M05.87 Other rheumatoid arthritis with rheumatoid factor of ankle and foot

M05.871 Other rheumatoid arthritis with rheumatoid factor of right ankle and foot

M05.872 Other rheumatoid arthritis with rheumatoid factor of left ankle and foot

M05.879 Other rheumatoid arthritis with rheumatoid factor of unspecified ankle and foot

M05.89 Other rheumatoid arthritis with rheumatoid factor of multiple sites

M05.9 Rheumatoid arthritis with rheumatoid factor, unspecified

✓4th M06 Other rheumatoid arthritis

✓5th M06.0 Rheumatoid arthritis without rheumatoid factor

M06.00 Rheumatoid arthritis without rheumatoid factor, unspecified site

✓6th M06.01 Rheumatoid arthritis without rheumatoid factor, shoulder

M06.011 Rheumatoid arthritis without rheumatoid factor, right shoulder

M06.012 Rheumatoid arthritis without rheumatoid factor, left shoulder

M06.019 Rheumatoid arthritis without rheumatoid factor, unspecified shoulder

✓6th M06.02 Rheumatoid arthritis without rheumatoid factor, elbow

M06.021 Rheumatoid arthritis without rheumatoid factor, right elbow

M06.022 Rheumatoid arthritis without rheumatoid factor, left elbow

M06.029 Rheumatoid arthritis without rheumatoid factor, unspecified elbow

✓6th M06.03 Rheumatoid arthritis without rheumatoid factor, wrist

M06.031 Rheumatoid arthritis without rheumatoid factor, right wrist

M06.032 Rheumatoid arthritis without rheumatoid factor, left wrist

M06.039 Rheumatoid arthritis without rheumatoid factor, unspecified wrist

✓6th M06.04 Rheumatoid arthritis without rheumatoid factor, hand

M06.041 Rheumatoid arthritis without rheumatoid factor, right hand

M06.042 Rheumatoid arthritis without rheumatoid factor, left hand

M06.049 Rheumatoid arthritis without rheumatoid factor, unspecified hand

✓6th M06.05 Rheumatoid arthritis without rheumatoid factor, hip

M06.051 Rheumatoid arthritis without rheumatoid factor, right hip

M06.052 Rheumatoid arthritis without rheumatoid factor, left hip

M06.059 Rheumatoid arthritis without rheumatoid factor, unspecified hip

✓6th M06.06 Rheumatoid arthritis without rheumatoid factor, knee

M06.061 Rheumatoid arthritis without rheumatoid factor, right knee

M06.062 Rheumatoid arthritis without rheumatoid factor, left knee

M06.069 Rheumatoid arthritis without rheumatoid factor, unspecified knee

✓6th M06.07 Rheumatoid arthritis without rheumatoid factor, ankle and foot

M06.071 Rheumatoid arthritis without rheumatoid factor, right ankle and foot

M06.072 Rheumatoid arthritis without rheumatoid factor, left ankle and foot

M06.079 Rheumatoid arthritis without rheumatoid factor, unspecified ankle and foot

M06.08 Rheumatoid arthritis without rheumatoid factor, vertebrae

M06.09 Rheumatoid arthritis without rheumatoid factor, multiple sites

M06.1 Adult-onset Still's disease

EXCLUDES1 *Still's disease NOS (M08.2-)*

✓5th M06.2 Rheumatoid bursitis

M06.20 Rheumatoid bursitis, unspecified site

✓6th M06.21 Rheumatoid bursitis, shoulder

M06.211 Rheumatoid bursitis, right shoulder

M06.212 Rheumatoid bursitis, left shoulder

M06.219 Rheumatoid bursitis, unspecified shoulder

✓6th M06.22 Rheumatoid bursitis, elbow

M06.221 Rheumatoid bursitis, right elbow

M06.222 Rheumatoid bursitis, left elbow

M06.229 Rheumatoid bursitis, unspecified elbow

✓6th M06.23 Rheumatoid bursitis, wrist

M06.231 Rheumatoid bursitis, right wrist

M06.232 Rheumatoid bursitis, left wrist

M06.239 Rheumatoid bursitis, unspecified wrist

✓6th M06.24 Rheumatoid bursitis, hand

M06.241 Rheumatoid bursitis, right hand

M06.242 Rheumatoid bursitis, left hand

M06.249 Rheumatoid bursitis, unspecified hand

✓6th **MØ6.25 Rheumatoid bursitis, hip**
MØ6.251 Rheumatoid bursitis, right hip
MØ6.252 Rheumatoid bursitis, left hip
MØ6.259 Rheumatoid bursitis, unspecified hip

✓6th **MØ6.26 Rheumatoid bursitis, knee**
MØ6.261 Rheumatoid bursitis, right knee
MØ6.262 Rheumatoid bursitis, left knee
MØ6.269 Rheumatoid bursitis, unspecified knee

✓6th **MØ6.27 Rheumatoid bursitis, ankle and foot**
MØ6.271 Rheumatoid bursitis, right ankle and foot
MØ6.272 Rheumatoid bursitis, left ankle and foot
MØ6.279 Rheumatoid bursitis, unspecified ankle and foot

MØ6.28 Rheumatoid bursitis, vertebrae
MØ6.29 Rheumatoid bursitis, multiple sites

✓5th **MØ6.3 Rheumatoid nodule**
MØ6.3Ø Rheumatoid nodule, unspecified site

✓6th **MØ6.31 Rheumatoid nodule, shoulder**
MØ6.311 Rheumatoid nodule, right shoulder
MØ6.312 Rheumatoid nodule, left shoulder
MØ6.319 Rheumatoid nodule, unspecified shoulder

✓6th **MØ6.32 Rheumatoid nodule, elbow**
MØ6.321 Rheumatoid nodule, right elbow
MØ6.322 Rheumatoid nodule, left elbow
MØ6.329 Rheumatoid nodule, unspecified elbow

✓6th **MØ6.33 Rheumatoid nodule, wrist**
MØ6.331 Rheumatoid nodule, right wrist
MØ6.332 Rheumatoid nodule, left wrist
MØ6.339 Rheumatoid nodule, unspecified wrist

✓6th **MØ6.34 Rheumatoid nodule, hand**
MØ6.341 Rheumatoid nodule, right hand
MØ6.342 Rheumatoid nodule, left hand
MØ6.349 Rheumatoid nodule, unspecified hand

✓6th **MØ6.35 Rheumatoid nodule, hip**
MØ6.351 Rheumatoid nodule, right hip
MØ6.352 Rheumatoid nodule, left hip
MØ6.359 Rheumatoid nodule, unspecified hip

✓6th **MØ6.36 Rheumatoid nodule, knee**
MØ6.361 Rheumatoid nodule, right knee
MØ6.362 Rheumatoid nodule, left knee
MØ6.369 Rheumatoid nodule, unspecified knee

✓6th **MØ6.37 Rheumatoid nodule, ankle and foot**
MØ6.371 Rheumatoid nodule, right ankle and foot
MØ6.372 Rheumatoid nodule, left ankle and foot
MØ6.379 Rheumatoid nodule, unspecified ankle and foot

MØ6.38 Rheumatoid nodule, vertebrae
MØ6.39 Rheumatoid nodule, multiple sites

MØ6.4 Inflammatory polyarthropathy
EXCLUDES 1 *polyarthritis NOS (M13.Ø)*

✓5th **MØ6.8 Other specified rheumatoid arthritis**
MØ6.8Ø Other specified rheumatoid arthritis, unspecified site

✓6th **MØ6.81 Other specified rheumatoid arthritis, shoulder**
MØ6.811 Other specified rheumatoid arthritis, right shoulder
MØ6.812 Other specified rheumatoid arthritis, left shoulder
MØ6.819 Other specified rheumatoid arthritis, unspecified shoulder

✓6th **MØ6.82 Other specified rheumatoid arthritis, elbow**
MØ6.821 Other specified rheumatoid arthritis, right elbow
MØ6.822 Other specified rheumatoid arthritis, left elbow
MØ6.829 Other specified rheumatoid arthritis, unspecified elbow

✓6th **MØ6.83 Other specified rheumatoid arthritis, wrist**
MØ6.831 Other specified rheumatoid arthritis, right wrist
MØ6.832 Other specified rheumatoid arthritis, left wrist
MØ6.839 Other specified rheumatoid arthritis, unspecified wrist

✓6th **MØ6.84 Other specified rheumatoid arthritis, hand**
MØ6.841 Other specified rheumatoid arthritis, right hand
MØ6.842 Other specified rheumatoid arthritis, left hand
MØ6.849 Other specified rheumatoid arthritis, unspecified hand

✓6th **MØ6.85 Other specified rheumatoid arthritis, hip**
MØ6.851 Other specified rheumatoid arthritis, right hip
MØ6.852 Other specified rheumatoid arthritis, left hip
MØ6.859 Other specified rheumatoid arthritis, unspecified hip

✓6th **MØ6.86 Other specified rheumatoid arthritis, knee**
MØ6.861 Other specified rheumatoid arthritis, right knee
MØ6.862 Other specified rheumatoid arthritis, left knee
MØ6.869 Other specified rheumatoid arthritis, unspecified knee

✓6th **MØ6.87 Other specified rheumatoid arthritis, ankle and foot**
MØ6.871 Other specified rheumatoid arthritis, right ankle and foot
MØ6.872 Other specified rheumatoid arthritis, left ankle and foot
MØ6.879 Other specified rheumatoid arthritis, unspecified ankle and foot

MØ6.88 Other specified rheumatoid arthritis, vertebrae
MØ6.89 Other specified rheumatoid arthritis, multiple sites

MØ6.9 Rheumatoid arthritis, unspecified

✓4th **MØ7 Enteropathic arthropathies**
Code also associated enteropathy, such as:
regional enteritis [Crohn's disease] (K5Ø.-)
ulcerative colitis (K51.-)
EXCLUDES 1 *psoriatic arthropathies (L4Ø.5-)*

✓5th **MØ7.6 Enteropathic arthropathies**
MØ7.6Ø Enteropathic arthropathies, unspecified site

✓6th **MØ7.61 Enteropathic arthropathies, shoulder**
MØ7.611 Enteropathic arthropathies, right shoulder
MØ7.612 Enteropathic arthropathies, left shoulder
MØ7.619 Enteropathic arthropathies, unspecified shoulder

✓6th **MØ7.62 Enteropathic arthropathies, elbow**
MØ7.621 Enteropathic arthropathies, right elbow
MØ7.622 Enteropathic arthropathies, left elbow
MØ7.629 Enteropathic arthropathies, unspecified elbow

✓6th **MØ7.63 Enteropathic arthropathies, wrist**
MØ7.631 Enteropathic arthropathies, right wrist
MØ7.632 Enteropathic arthropathies, left wrist
MØ7.639 Enteropathic arthropathies, unspecified wrist

✓6th **MØ7.64 Enteropathic arthropathies, hand**
MØ7.641 Enteropathic arthropathies, right hand
MØ7.642 Enteropathic arthropathies, left hand
MØ7.649 Enteropathic arthropathies, unspecified hand

✓6th **MØ7.65 Enteropathic arthropathies, hip**
MØ7.651 Enteropathic arthropathies, right hip
MØ7.652 Enteropathic arthropathies, left hip
MØ7.659 Enteropathic arthropathies, unspecified hip

✓6th **MØ7.66 Enteropathic arthropathies, knee**
MØ7.661 Enteropathic arthropathies, right knee
MØ7.662 Enteropathic arthropathies, left knee
MØ7.669 Enteropathic arthropathies, unspecified knee

✓6th **MØ7.67 Enteropathic arthropathies, ankle and foot**
MØ7.671 Enteropathic arthropathies, right ankle and foot

M07.672 Enteropathic arthropathies, left ankle and foot
M07.679 Enteropathic arthropathies, unspecified ankle and foot
M07.68 Enteropathic arthropathies, vertebrae
M07.69 Enteropathic arthropathies, multiple sites

✓4th M08 Juvenile arthritis
Code also any associated underlying condition, such as:
regional enteritis [Crohn's disease] (K50.-)
ulcerative colitis (K51.-)
EXCLUDES 1 *arthropathy in Whipple's disease (M14.8)*
Felty's syndrome (M05.0)
juvenile dermatomyositis (M33.0-)
psoriatic juvenile arthropathy (L40.54)

✓5th M08.0 Unspecified juvenile rheumatoid arthritis
Juvenile rheumatoid arthritis with or without rheumatoid factor
M08.00 Unspecified juvenile rheumatoid arthritis of unspecified site
✓6th M08.01 Unspecified juvenile rheumatoid arthritis, shoulder
M08.011 Unspecified juvenile rheumatoid arthritis, right shoulder
M08.012 Unspecified juvenile rheumatoid arthritis, left shoulder
M08.019 Unspecified juvenile rheumatoid arthritis, unspecified shoulder
✓6th M08.02 Unspecified juvenile rheumatoid arthritis of elbow
M08.021 Unspecified juvenile rheumatoid arthritis, right elbow
M08.022 Unspecified juvenile rheumatoid arthritis, left elbow
M08.029 Unspecified juvenile rheumatoid arthritis, unspecified elbow
✓6th M08.03 Unspecified juvenile rheumatoid arthritis, wrist
M08.031 Unspecified juvenile rheumatoid arthritis, right wrist
M08.032 Unspecified juvenile rheumatoid arthritis, left wrist
M08.039 Unspecified juvenile rheumatoid arthritis, unspecified wrist
✓6th M08.04 Unspecified juvenile rheumatoid arthritis, hand
M08.041 Unspecified juvenile rheumatoid arthritis, right hand
M08.042 Unspecified juvenile rheumatoid arthritis, left hand
M08.049 Unspecified juvenile rheumatoid arthritis, unspecified hand
✓6th M08.05 Unspecified juvenile rheumatoid arthritis, hip
M08.051 Unspecified juvenile rheumatoid arthritis, right hip
M08.052 Unspecified juvenile rheumatoid arthritis, left hip
M08.059 Unspecified juvenile rheumatoid arthritis, unspecified hip
✓6th M08.06 Unspecified juvenile rheumatoid arthritis, knee
M08.061 Unspecified juvenile rheumatoid arthritis, right knee
M08.062 Unspecified juvenile rheumatoid arthritis, left knee
M08.069 Unspecified juvenile rheumatoid arthritis, unspecified knee
✓6th M08.07 Unspecified juvenile rheumatoid arthritis, ankle and foot
M08.071 Unspecified juvenile rheumatoid arthritis, right ankle and foot
M08.072 Unspecified juvenile rheumatoid arthritis, left ankle and foot
M08.079 Unspecified juvenile rheumatoid arthritis, unspecified ankle and foot
M08.08 Unspecified juvenile rheumatoid arthritis, vertebrae
M08.09 Unspecified juvenile rheumatoid arthritis, multiple sites

M08.1 Juvenile ankylosing spondylitis
EXCLUDES 1 *ankylosing spondylitis in adults (M45.0-)*

✓5th M08.2 Juvenile rheumatoid arthritis with systemic onset
Still's disease NOS
EXCLUDES 1 *adult-onset Still's disease (M06.1-)*
M08.20 Juvenile rheumatoid arthritis with systemic onset, unspecified site
✓6th M08.21 Juvenile rheumatoid arthritis with systemic onset, shoulder
M08.211 Juvenile rheumatoid arthritis with systemic onset, right shoulder
M08.212 Juvenile rheumatoid arthritis with systemic onset, left shoulder
M08.219 Juvenile rheumatoid arthritis with systemic onset, unspecified shoulder
✓6th M08.22 Juvenile rheumatoid arthritis with systemic onset, elbow
M08.221 Juvenile rheumatoid arthritis with systemic onset, right elbow
M08.222 Juvenile rheumatoid arthritis with systemic onset, left elbow
M08.229 Juvenile rheumatoid arthritis with systemic onset, unspecified elbow
✓6th M08.23 Juvenile rheumatoid arthritis with systemic onset, wrist
M08.231 Juvenile rheumatoid arthritis with systemic onset, right wrist
M08.232 Juvenile rheumatoid arthritis with systemic onset, left wrist
M08.239 Juvenile rheumatoid arthritis with systemic onset, unspecified wrist
✓6th M08.24 Juvenile rheumatoid arthritis with systemic onset, hand
M08.241 Juvenile rheumatoid arthritis with systemic onset, right hand
M08.242 Juvenile rheumatoid arthritis with systemic onset, left hand
M08.249 Juvenile rheumatoid arthritis with systemic onset, unspecified hand
✓6th M08.25 Juvenile rheumatoid arthritis with systemic onset, hip
M08.251 Juvenile rheumatoid arthritis with systemic onset, right hip
M08.252 Juvenile rheumatoid arthritis with systemic onset, left hip
M08.259 Juvenile rheumatoid arthritis with systemic onset, unspecified hip
✓6th M08.26 Juvenile rheumatoid arthritis with systemic onset, knee
M08.261 Juvenile rheumatoid arthritis with systemic onset, right knee
M08.262 Juvenile rheumatoid arthritis with systemic onset, left knee
M08.269 Juvenile rheumatoid arthritis with systemic onset, unspecified knee
✓6th M08.27 Juvenile rheumatoid arthritis with systemic onset, ankle and foot
M08.271 Juvenile rheumatoid arthritis with systemic onset, right ankle and foot
M08.272 Juvenile rheumatoid arthritis with systemic onset, left ankle and foot
M08.279 Juvenile rheumatoid arthritis with systemic onset, unspecified ankle and foot
M08.28 Juvenile rheumatoid arthritis with systemic onset, vertebrae
M08.29 Juvenile rheumatoid arthritis with systemic onset, multiple sites

M08.3 Juvenile rheumatoid polyarthritis (seronegative)

✓5th M08.4 Pauciarticular juvenile rheumatoid arthritis
M08.40 Pauciarticular juvenile rheumatoid arthritis, unspecified site
✓6th M08.41 Pauciarticular juvenile rheumatoid arthritis, shoulder
M08.411 Pauciarticular juvenile rheumatoid arthritis, right shoulder
M08.412 Pauciarticular juvenile rheumatoid arthritis, left shoulder
M08.419 Pauciarticular juvenile rheumatoid arthritis, unspecified shoulder

✓6th **MØ8.42 Pauciarticular juvenile rheumatoid arthritis, elbow**
MØ8.421 Pauciarticular juvenile rheumatoid arthritis, right elbow
MØ8.422 Pauciarticular juvenile rheumatoid arthritis, left elbow
MØ8.429 Pauciarticular juvenile rheumatoid arthritis, unspecified elbow

✓6th **MØ8.43 Pauciarticular juvenile rheumatoid arthritis, wrist**
MØ8.431 Pauciarticular juvenile rheumatoid arthritis, right wrist
MØ8.432 Pauciarticular juvenile rheumatoid arthritis, left wrist
MØ8.439 Pauciarticular juvenile rheumatoid arthritis, unspecified wrist

✓6th **MØ8.44 Pauciarticular juvenile rheumatoid arthritis, hand**
MØ8.441 Pauciarticular juvenile rheumatoid arthritis, right hand
MØ8.442 Pauciarticular juvenile rheumatoid arthritis, left hand
MØ8.449 Pauciarticular juvenile rheumatoid arthritis, unspecified hand

✓6th **MØ8.45 Pauciarticular juvenile rheumatoid arthritis, hip**
MØ8.451 Pauciarticular juvenile rheumatoid arthritis, right hip
MØ8.452 Pauciarticular juvenile rheumatoid arthritis, left hip
MØ8.459 Pauciarticular juvenile rheumatoid arthritis, unspecified hip

✓6th **MØ8.46 Pauciarticular juvenile rheumatoid arthritis, knee**
MØ8.461 Pauciarticular juvenile rheumatoid arthritis, right knee
MØ8.462 Pauciarticular juvenile rheumatoid arthritis, left knee
MØ8.469 Pauciarticular juvenile rheumatoid arthritis, unspecified knee

✓6th **MØ8.47 Pauciarticular juvenile rheumatoid arthritis, ankle and foot**
MØ8.471 Pauciarticular juvenile rheumatoid arthritis, right ankle and foot
MØ8.472 Pauciarticular juvenile rheumatoid arthritis, left ankle and foot
MØ8.479 Pauciarticular juvenile rheumatoid arthritis, unspecified ankle and foot

MØ8.48 Pauciarticular juvenile rheumatoid arthritis, vertebrae

✓5th **MØ8.8 Other juvenile arthritis**
MØ8.8Ø Other juvenile arthritis, unspecified site

✓6th **MØ8.81 Other juvenile arthritis, shoulder**
MØ8.811 Other juvenile arthritis, right shoulder
MØ8.812 Other juvenile arthritis, left shoulder
MØ8.819 Other juvenile arthritis, unspecified shoulder

✓6th **MØ8.82 Other juvenile arthritis, elbow**
MØ8.821 Other juvenile arthritis, right elbow
MØ8.822 Other juvenile arthritis, left elbow
MØ8.829 Other juvenile arthritis, unspecified elbow

✓6th **MØ8.83 Other juvenile arthritis, wrist**
MØ8.831 Other juvenile arthritis, right wrist
MØ8.832 Other juvenile arthritis, left wrist
MØ8.839 Other juvenile arthritis, unspecified wrist

✓6th **MØ8.84 Other juvenile arthritis, hand**
MØ8.841 Other juvenile arthritis, right hand
MØ8.842 Other juvenile arthritis, left hand
MØ8.849 Other juvenile arthritis, unspecified hand

✓6th **MØ8.85 Other juvenile arthritis, hip**
MØ8.851 Other juvenile arthritis, right hip
MØ8.852 Other juvenile arthritis, left hip
MØ8.859 Other juvenile arthritis, unspecified hip

✓6th **MØ8.86 Other juvenile arthritis, knee**
MØ8.861 Other juvenile arthritis, right knee
MØ8.862 Other juvenile arthritis, left knee
MØ8.869 Other juvenile arthritis, unspecified knee

✓6th **MØ8.87 Other juvenile arthritis, ankle and foot**
MØ8.871 Other juvenile arthritis, right ankle and foot
MØ8.872 Other juvenile arthritis, left ankle and foot
MØ8.879 Other juvenile arthritis, unspecified ankle and foot

MØ8.88 Other juvenile arthritis, vertebrae
MØ8.89 Other juvenile arthritis, multiple sites

✓5th **MØ8.9 Juvenile arthritis, unspecified**

EXCLUDES 1 *juvenile rheumatoid arthritis, unspecified (MØ8.Ø-)*

MØ8.9Ø Juvenile arthritis, unspecified, unspecified site

✓6th **MØ8.91 Juvenile arthritis, unspecified, shoulder**
MØ8.911 Juvenile arthritis, unspecified, right shoulder
MØ8.912 Juvenile arthritis, unspecified, left shoulder
MØ8.919 Juvenile arthritis, unspecified, unspecified shoulder

✓6th **MØ8.92 Juvenile arthritis, unspecified, elbow**
MØ8.921 Juvenile arthritis, unspecified, right elbow
MØ8.922 Juvenile arthritis, unspecified, left elbow
MØ8.929 Juvenile arthritis, unspecified, unspecified elbow

✓6th **MØ8.93 Juvenile arthritis, unspecified, wrist**
MØ8.931 Juvenile arthritis, unspecified, right wrist
MØ8.932 Juvenile arthritis, unspecified, left wrist
MØ8.939 Juvenile arthritis, unspecified, unspecified wrist

✓6th **MØ8.94 Juvenile arthritis, unspecified, hand**
MØ8.941 Juvenile arthritis, unspecified, right hand
MØ8.942 Juvenile arthritis, unspecified, left hand
MØ8.949 Juvenile arthritis, unspecified, unspecified hand

✓6th **MØ8.95 Juvenile arthritis, unspecified, hip**
MØ8.951 Juvenile arthritis, unspecified, right hip
MØ8.952 Juvenile arthritis, unspecified, left hip
MØ8.959 Juvenile arthritis, unspecified, unspecified hip

✓6th **MØ8.96 Juvenile arthritis, unspecified, knee**
MØ8.961 Juvenile arthritis, unspecified, right knee
MØ8.962 Juvenile arthritis, unspecified, left knee
MØ8.969 Juvenile arthritis, unspecified, unspecified knee

✓6th **MØ8.97 Juvenile arthritis, unspecified, ankle and foot**
MØ8.971 Juvenile arthritis, unspecified, right ankle and foot
MØ8.972 Juvenile arthritis, unspecified, left ankle and foot
MØ8.979 Juvenile arthritis, unspecified, unspecified ankle and foot

MØ8.98 Juvenile arthritis, unspecified, vertebrae
MØ8.99 Juvenile arthritis, unspecified, multiple sites

✓4th **M1A Chronic gout**

Use additional code to identify:
- autonomic neuropathy in diseases classified elsewhere (G99.Ø)
- calculus of urinary tract in diseases classified elsewhere (N22)
- cardiomyopathy in diseases classified elsewhere (I43)
- disorders of external ear in diseases classified elsewhere (H61.1-, H62.8-)
- disorders of iris and ciliary body in diseases classified elsewhere (H22)
- glomerular disorders in diseases classified elsewhere (NØ8)

The appropriate 7th character is to be added to each code from category M1A.
Ø without tophus (tophi)
1 with tophus (tophi)

EXCLUDES 1 *acute gout (M1Ø.-)*
gout NOS (M1Ø.-)

- ✓5th **M1A.0 Idiopathic chronic gout**
  Chronic gouty bursitis
  Primary chronic gout
  - ✓x7th **M1A.00 Idiopathic chronic gout, unspecified site**
  - ✓6th **M1A.01 Idiopathic chronic gout, shoulder**
    - ✓7th **M1A.011 Idiopathic chronic gout, right shoulder**
    - ✓7th **M1A.012 Idiopathic chronic gout, left shoulder**
    - ✓7th **M1A.019 Idiopathic chronic gout, unspecified shoulder**
  - ✓6th **M1A.02 Idiopathic chronic gout, elbow**
    - ✓7th **M1A.021 Idiopathic chronic gout, right elbow**
    - ✓7th **M1A.022 Idiopathic chronic gout, left elbow**
    - ✓7th **M1A.029 Idiopathic chronic gout, unspecified elbow**
  - ✓6th **M1A.03 Idiopathic chronic gout, wrist**
    - ✓7th **M1A.031 Idiopathic chronic gout, right wrist**
    - ✓7th **M1A.032 Idiopathic chronic gout, left wrist**
    - ✓7th **M1A.039 Idiopathic chronic gout, unspecified wrist**
  - ✓6th **M1A.04 Idiopathic chronic gout, hand**
    - ✓7th **M1A.041 Idiopathic chronic gout, right hand**
    - ✓7th **M1A.042 Idiopathic chronic gout, left hand**
    - ✓7th **M1A.049 Idiopathic chronic gout, unspecified hand**
  - ✓6th **M1A.05 Idiopathic chronic gout, hip**
    - ✓7th **M1A.051 Idiopathic chronic gout, right hip**
    - ✓7th **M1A.052 Idiopathic chronic gout, left hip**
    - ✓7th **M1A.059 Idiopathic chronic gout, unspecified hip**
  - ✓6th **M1A.06 Idiopathic chronic gout, knee**
    - ✓7th **M1A.061 Idiopathic chronic gout, right knee**
    - ✓7th **M1A.062 Idiopathic chronic gout, left knee**
    - ✓7th **M1A.069 Idiopathic chronic gout, unspecified knee**
  - ✓6th **M1A.07 Idiopathic chronic gout, ankle and foot**
    - ✓7th **M1A.071 Idiopathic chronic gout, right ankle and foot**
    - ✓7th **M1A.072 Idiopathic chronic gout, left ankle and foot**
    - ✓7th **M1A.079 Idiopathic chronic gout, unspecified ankle and foot**
  - ✓x7th **M1A.08 Idiopathic chronic gout, vertebrae**
  - ✓x7th **M1A.09 Idiopathic chronic gout, multiple sites**
- ✓5th **M1A.1 Lead-induced chronic gout**
  Code first: toxic effects of lead and its compounds (T56.0-)
  - ✓x7th **M1A.10 Lead-induced chronic gout, unspecified site**
  - ✓6th **M1A.11 Lead-induced chronic gout, shoulder**
    - ✓7th **M1A.111 Lead-induced chronic gout, right shoulder**
    - ✓7th **M1A.112 Lead-induced chronic gout, left shoulder**
    - ✓7th **M1A.119 Lead-induced chronic gout, unspecified shoulder**
  - ✓6th **M1A.12 Lead-induced chronic gout, elbow**
    - ✓7th **M1A.121 Lead-induced chronic gout, right elbow**
    - ✓7th **M1A.122 Lead-induced chronic gout, left elbow**
    - ✓7th **M1A.129 Lead-induced chronic gout, unspecified elbow**
  - ✓6th **M1A.13 Lead-induced chronic gout, wrist**
    - ✓7th **M1A.131 Lead-induced chronic gout, right wrist**
    - ✓7th **M1A.132 Lead-induced chronic gout, left wrist**
    - ✓7th **M1A.139 Lead-induced chronic gout, unspecified wrist**
  - ✓6th **M1A.14 Lead-induced chronic gout, hand**
    - ✓7th **M1A.141 Lead-induced chronic gout, right hand**
    - ✓7th **M1A.142 Lead-induced chronic gout, left hand**
    - ✓7th **M1A.149 Lead-induced chronic gout, unspecified hand**
  - ✓6th **M1A.15 Lead-induced chronic gout, hip**
    - ✓7th **M1A.151 Lead-induced chronic gout, right hip**
    - ✓7th **M1A.152 Lead-induced chronic gout, left hip**
    - ✓7th **M1A.159 Lead-induced chronic gout, unspecified hip**
  - ✓6th **M1A.16 Lead-induced chronic gout, knee**
    - ✓7th **M1A.161 Lead-induced chronic gout, right knee**
    - ✓7th **M1A.162 Lead-induced chronic gout, left knee**
    - ✓7th **M1A.169 Lead-induced chronic gout, unspecified knee**
  - ✓6th **M1A.17 Lead-induced chronic gout, ankle and foot**
    - ✓7th **M1A.171 Lead-induced chronic gout, right ankle and foot**
    - ✓7th **M1A.172 Lead-induced chronic gout, left ankle and foot**
    - ✓7th **M1A.179 Lead-induced chronic gout, unspecified ankle and foot**
  - ✓x7th **M1A.18 Lead-induced chronic gout, vertebrae**
  - ✓x7th **M1A.19 Lead-induced chronic gout, multiple sites**
- ✓5th **M1A.2 Drug-induced chronic gout**
  Use additional code for adverse effect, if applicable, to identify drug (T36-T50 with fifth or sixth character 5)
  - ✓x7th **M1A.20 Drug-induced chronic gout, unspecified site**
  - ✓6th **M1A.21 Drug-induced chronic gout, shoulder**
    - ✓7th **M1A.211 Drug-induced chronic gout, right shoulder**
    - ✓7th **M1A.212 Drug-induced chronic gout, left shoulder**
    - ✓7th **M1A.219 Drug-induced chronic gout, unspecified shoulder**
  - ✓6th **M1A.22 Drug-induced chronic gout, elbow**
    - ✓7th **M1A.221 Drug-induced chronic gout, right elbow**
    - ✓7th **M1A.222 Drug-induced chronic gout, left elbow**
    - ✓7th **M1A.229 Drug-induced chronic gout, unspecified elbow**
  - ✓6th **M1A.23 Drug-induced chronic gout, wrist**
    - ✓7th **M1A.231 Drug-induced chronic gout, right wrist**
    - ✓7th **M1A.232 Drug-induced chronic gout, left wrist**
    - ✓7th **M1A.239 Drug-induced chronic gout, unspecified wrist**
  - ✓6th **M1A.24 Drug-induced chronic gout, hand**
    - ✓7th **M1A.241 Drug-induced chronic gout, right hand**
    - ✓7th **M1A.242 Drug-induced chronic gout, left hand**
    - ✓7th **M1A.249 Drug-induced chronic gout, unspecified hand**
  - ✓6th **M1A.25 Drug-induced chronic gout, hip**
    - ✓7th **M1A.251 Drug-induced chronic gout, right hip**
    - ✓7th **M1A.252 Drug-induced chronic gout, left hip**
    - ✓7th **M1A.259 Drug-induced chronic gout, unspecified hip**
  - ✓6th **M1A.26 Drug-induced chronic gout, knee**
    - ✓7th **M1A.261 Drug-induced chronic gout, right knee**
    - ✓7th **M1A.262 Drug-induced chronic gout, left knee**
    - ✓7th **M1A.269 Drug-induced chronic gout, unspecified knee**
  - ✓6th **M1A.27 Drug-induced chronic gout, ankle and foot**
    - ✓7th **M1A.271 Drug-induced chronic gout, right ankle and foot**
    - ✓7th **M1A.272 Drug-induced chronic gout, left ankle and foot**
    - ✓7th **M1A.279 Drug-induced chronic gout, unspecified ankle and foot**
  - ✓x7th **M1A.28 Drug-induced chronic gout, vertebrae**
  - ✓x7th **M1A.29 Drug-induced chronic gout, multiple sites**
- ✓5th **M1A.3 Chronic gout due to renal impairment**
  Code first associated renal disease
  - ✓x7th **M1A.30 Chronic gout due to renal impairment, unspecified site**
  - ✓6th **M1A.31 Chronic gout due to renal impairment, shoulder**
    - ✓7th **M1A.311 Chronic gout due to renal impairment, right shoulder**
    - ✓7th **M1A.312 Chronic gout due to renal impairment, left shoulder**
    - ✓7th **M1A.319 Chronic gout due to renal impairment, unspecified shoulder**
  - ✓6th **M1A.32 Chronic gout due to renal impairment, elbow**
    - ✓7th **M1A.321 Chronic gout due to renal impairment, right elbow**
    - ✓7th **M1A.322 Chronic gout due to renal impairment, left elbow**
    - ✓7th **M1A.329 Chronic gout due to renal impairment, unspecified elbow**

✓ Appropriate additional character required
✓x7th Requires 7th character, placeholder x must fill empty characters

✓6th **M1A.33 Chronic gout due to renal impairment, wrist**

✓7th **M1A.331 Chronic gout due to renal impairment, right wrist**

✓7th **M1A.332 Chronic gout due to renal impairment, left wrist**

✓7th **M1A.339 Chronic gout due to renal impairment, unspecified wrist**

✓6th **M1A.34 Chronic gout due to renal impairment, hand**

✓7th **M1A.341 Chronic gout due to renal impairment, right hand**

✓7th **M1A.342 Chronic gout due to renal impairment, left hand**

✓7th **M1A.349 Chronic gout due to renal impairment, unspecified hand**

✓6th **M1A.35 Chronic gout due to renal impairment, hip**

✓7th **M1A.351 Chronic gout due to renal impairment, right hip**

✓7th **M1A.352 Chronic gout due to renal impairment, left hip**

✓7th **M1A.359 Chronic gout due to renal impairment, unspecified hip**

✓6th **M1A.36 Chronic gout due to renal impairment, knee**

✓7th **M1A.361 Chronic gout due to renal impairment, right knee**

✓7th **M1A.362 Chronic gout due to renal impairment, left knee**

✓7th **M1A.369 Chronic gout due to renal impairment, unspecified knee**

✓6th **M1A.37 Chronic gout due to renal impairment, ankle and foot**

✓7th **M1A.371 Chronic gout due to renal impairment, right ankle and foot**

✓7th **M1A.372 Chronic gout due to renal impairment, left ankle and foot**

✓7th **M1A.379 Chronic gout due to renal impairment, unspecified ankle and foot**

✓x7th **M1A.38 Chronic gout due to renal impairment, vertebrae**

✓x7th **M1A.39 Chronic gout due to renal impairment, multiple sites**

✓5th **M1A.4 Other secondary chronic gout**

Code first associated condition

✓x7th **M1A.4Ø Other secondary chronic gout, unspecified site**

✓6th **M1A.41 Other secondary chronic gout, shoulder**

✓7th **M1A.411 Other secondary chronic gout, right shoulder**

✓7th **M1A.412 Other secondary chronic gout, left shoulder**

✓7th **M1A.419 Other secondary chronic gout, unspecified shoulder**

✓6th **M1A.42 Other secondary chronic gout, elbow**

✓7th **M1A.421 Other secondary chronic gout, right elbow**

✓7th **M1A.422 Other secondary chronic gout, left elbow**

✓7th **M1A.429 Other secondary chronic gout, unspecified elbow**

✓6th **M1A.43 Other secondary chronic gout, wrist**

✓7th **M1A.431 Other secondary chronic gout, right wrist**

✓7th **M1A.432 Other secondary chronic gout, left wrist**

✓7th **M1A.439 Other secondary chronic gout, unspecified wrist**

✓6th **M1A.44 Other secondary chronic gout, hand**

✓7th **M1A.441 Other secondary chronic gout, right hand**

✓7th **M1A.442 Other secondary chronic gout, left hand**

✓7th **M1A.449 Other secondary chronic gout, unspecified hand**

✓6th **M1A.45 Other secondary chronic gout, hip**

✓7th **M1A.451 Other secondary chronic gout, right hip**

✓7th **M1A.452 Other secondary chronic gout, left hip**

✓7th **M1A.459 Other secondary chronic gout, unspecified hip**

✓6th **M1A.46 Other secondary chronic gout, knee**

✓7th **M1A.461 Other secondary chronic gout, right knee**

✓7th **M1A.462 Other secondary chronic gout, left knee**

✓7th **M1A.469 Other secondary chronic gout, unspecified knee**

✓6th **M1A.47 Other secondary chronic gout, ankle and foot**

✓7th **M1A.471 Other secondary chronic gout, right ankle and foot**

✓7th **M1A.472 Other secondary chronic gout, left ankle and foot**

✓7th **M1A.479 Other secondary chronic gout, unspecified ankle and foot**

✓x7th **M1A.48 Other secondary chronic gout, vertebrae**

✓x7th **M1A.49 Other secondary chronic gout, multiple sites**

✓x7th **M1A.9 Chronic gout, unspecified**

✓4th **M1Ø Gout**

Acute gout
Gout attack
Gout flare
Gout NOS
Podagra

Use additional code to identify:
- autonomic neuropathy in diseases classified elsewhere (G99.Ø)
- calculus of urinary tract in diseases classified elsewhere (N22)
- cardiomyopathy in diseases classified elsewhere (I43)
- disorders of external ear in diseases classified elsewhere (H61.1-, H62.8-)
- disorders of iris and ciliary body in diseases classified elsewhere (H22)
- glomerular disorders in diseases classified elsewhere (NØ8)

EXCLUDES 1 *chronic gout (M1A.-)*

✓5th **M1Ø.Ø Idiopathic gout**

Gouty bursitis
Primary gout

M1Ø.ØØ Idiopathic gout, unspecified site

✓6th **M1Ø.Ø1 Idiopathic gout, shoulder**

M1Ø.Ø11 Idiopathic gout, right shoulder

M1Ø.Ø12 Idiopathic gout, left shoulder

M1Ø.Ø19 Idiopathic gout, unspecified shoulder

✓6th **M1Ø.Ø2 Idiopathic gout, elbow**

M1Ø.Ø21 Idiopathic gout, right elbow

M1Ø.Ø22 Idiopathic gout, left elbow

M1Ø.Ø29 Idiopathic gout, unspecified elbow

✓6th **M1Ø.Ø3 Idiopathic gout, wrist**

M1Ø.Ø31 Idiopathic gout, right wrist

M1Ø.Ø32 Idiopathic gout, left wrist

M1Ø.Ø39 Idiopathic gout, unspecified wrist

✓6th **M1Ø.Ø4 Idiopathic gout, hand**

M1Ø.Ø41 Idiopathic gout, right hand

M1Ø.Ø42 Idiopathic gout, left hand

M1Ø.Ø49 Idiopathic gout, unspecified hand

✓6th **M1Ø.Ø5 Idiopathic gout, hip**

M1Ø.Ø51 Idiopathic gout, right hip

M1Ø.Ø52 Idiopathic gout, left hip

M1Ø.Ø59 Idiopathic gout, unspecified hip

✓6th **M1Ø.Ø6 Idiopathic gout, knee**

M1Ø.Ø61 Idiopathic gout, right knee

M1Ø.Ø62 Idiopathic gout, left knee

M1Ø.Ø69 Idiopathic gout, unspecified knee

✓6th **M1Ø.Ø7 Idiopathic gout, ankle and foot**

M1Ø.Ø71 Idiopathic gout, right ankle and foot

M1Ø.Ø72 Idiopathic gout, left ankle and foot

M1Ø.Ø79 Idiopathic gout, unspecified ankle and foot

M1Ø.Ø8 Idiopathic gout, vertebrae

M1Ø.Ø9 Idiopathic gout, multiple sites

✓5th **M1Ø.1 Lead-induced gout**

Code first: toxic effects of lead and its compounds (T56.Ø-)

M1Ø.1Ø Lead-induced gout, unspecified site

✓6th **M1Ø.11 Lead-induced gout, shoulder**

M1Ø.111 Lead-induced gout, right shoulder

M1Ø.112 Lead-induced gout, left shoulder

M1Ø.119 Lead-induced gout, unspecified shoulder

✓6th **M1Ø.12 Lead-induced gout, elbow**

M1Ø.121 Lead-induced gout, right elbow

M1Ø.122 Lead-induced gout, left elbow

M10.129 **Lead-induced gout, unspecified elbow**
✓6th **M10.13 Lead-induced gout, wrist**
M10.131 **Lead-induced gout, right wrist**
M10.132 **Lead-induced gout, left wrist**
M10.139 **Lead-induced gout, unspecified wrist**
✓6th **M10.14 Lead-induced gout, hand**
M10.141 **Lead-induced gout, right hand**
M10.142 **Lead-induced gout, left hand**
M10.149 **Lead-induced gout, unspecified hand**
✓6th **M10.15 Lead-induced gout, hip**
M10.151 **Lead-induced gout, right hip**
M10.152 **Lead-induced gout, left hip**
M10.159 **Lead-induced gout, unspecified hip**
✓6th **M10.16 Lead-induced gout, knee**
M10.161 **Lead-induced gout, right knee**
M10.162 **Lead-induced gout, left knee**
M10.169 **Lead-induced gout, unspecified knee**
✓6th **M10.17 Lead-induced gout, ankle and foot**
M10.171 **Lead-induced gout, right ankle and foot**
M10.172 **Lead-induced gout, left ankle and foot**
M10.179 **Lead-induced gout, unspecified ankle and foot**
M10.18 Lead-induced gout, vertebrae
M10.19 Lead-induced gout, multiple sites

✓5th **M10.2 Drug-induced gout**
Use additional code for adverse effect, if applicable, to identify drug (T36-T50 with fifth or sixth character 5)
M10.20 Drug-induced gout, unspecified site
✓6th **M10.21 Drug-induced gout, shoulder**
M10.211 **Drug-induced gout, right shoulder**
M10.212 **Drug-induced gout, left shoulder**
M10.219 **Drug-induced gout, unspecified shoulder**
✓6th **M10.22 Drug-induced gout, elbow**
M10.221 **Drug-induced gout, right elbow**
M10.222 **Drug-induced gout, left elbow**
M10.229 **Drug-induced gout, unspecified elbow**
✓6th **M10.23 Drug-induced gout, wrist**
M10.231 **Drug-induced gout, right wrist**
M10.232 **Drug-induced gout, left wrist**
M10.239 **Drug-induced gout, unspecified wrist**
✓6th **M10.24 Drug-induced gout, hand**
M10.241 **Drug-induced gout, right hand**
M10.242 **Drug-induced gout, left hand**
M10.249 **Drug-induced gout, unspecified hand**
✓6th **M10.25 Drug-induced gout, hip**
M10.251 **Drug-induced gout, right hip**
M10.252 **Drug-induced gout, left hip**
M10.259 **Drug-induced gout, unspecified hip**
✓6th **M10.26 Drug-induced gout, knee**
M10.261 **Drug-induced gout, right knee**
M10.262 **Drug-induced gout, left knee**
M10.269 **Drug-induced gout, unspecified knee**
✓6th **M10.27 Drug-induced gout, ankle and foot**
M10.271 **Drug-induced gout, right ankle and foot**
M10.272 **Drug-induced gout, left ankle and foot**
M10.279 **Drug-induced gout, unspecified ankle and foot**
M10.28 Drug-induced gout, vertebrae
M10.29 Drug-induced gout, multiple sites

✓5th **M10.3 Gout due to renal impairment**
Code first associated renal disease
M10.30 Gout due to renal impairment, unspecified site
✓6th **M10.31 Gout due to renal impairment, shoulder**
M10.311 **Gout due to renal impairment, right shoulder**
M10.312 **Gout due to renal impairment, left shoulder**
M10.319 **Gout due to renal impairment, unspecified shoulder**
✓6th **M10.32 Gout due to renal impairment, elbow**
M10.321 **Gout due to renal impairment, right elbow**
M10.322 **Gout due to renal impairment, left elbow**
M10.329 **Gout due to renal impairment, unspecified elbow**
✓6th **M10.33 Gout due to renal impairment, wrist**
M10.331 **Gout due to renal impairment, right wrist**
M10.332 **Gout due to renal impairment, left wrist**
M10.339 **Gout due to renal impairment, unspecified wrist**
✓6th **M10.34 Gout due to renal impairment, hand**
M10.341 **Gout due to renal impairment, right hand**
M10.342 **Gout due to renal impairment, left hand**
M10.349 **Gout due to renal impairment, unspecified hand**
✓6th **M10.35 Gout due to renal impairment, hip**
M10.351 **Gout due to renal impairment, right hip**
M10.352 **Gout due to renal impairment, left hip**
M10.359 **Gout due to renal impairment, unspecified hip**
✓6th **M10.36 Gout due to renal impairment, knee**
M10.361 **Gout due to renal impairment, right knee**
M10.362 **Gout due to renal impairment, left knee**
M10.369 **Gout due to renal impairment, unspecified knee**
✓6th **M10.37 Gout due to renal impairment, ankle and foot**
M10.371 **Gout due to renal impairment, right ankle and foot**
M10.372 **Gout due to renal impairment, left ankle and foot**
M10.379 **Gout due to renal impairment, unspecified ankle and foot**
M10.38 Gout due to renal impairment, vertebrae
M10.39 Gout due to renal impairment, multiple sites

✓5th **M10.4 Other secondary gout**
Code first associated condition
M10.40 Other secondary gout, unspecified site
✓6th **M10.41 Other secondary gout, shoulder**
M10.411 **Other secondary gout, right shoulder**
M10.412 **Other secondary gout, left shoulder**
M10.419 **Other secondary gout, unspecified shoulder**
✓6th **M10.42 Other secondary gout, elbow**
M10.421 **Other secondary gout, right elbow**
M10.422 **Other secondary gout, left elbow**
M10.429 **Other secondary gout, unspecified elbow**
✓6th **M10.43 Other secondary gout, wrist**
M10.431 **Other secondary gout, right wrist**
M10.432 **Other secondary gout, left wrist**
M10.439 **Other secondary gout, unspecified wrist**
✓6th **M10.44 Other secondary gout, hand**
M10.441 **Other secondary gout, right hand**
M10.442 **Other secondary gout, left hand**
M10.449 **Other secondary gout, unspecified hand**
✓6th **M10.45 Other secondary gout, hip**
M10.451 **Other secondary gout, right hip**
M10.452 **Other secondary gout, left hip**
M10.459 **Other secondary gout, unspecified hip**
✓6th **M10.46 Other secondary gout, knee**
M10.461 **Other secondary gout, right knee**
M10.462 **Other secondary gout, left knee**
M10.469 **Other secondary gout, unspecified knee**
✓6th **M10.47 Other secondary gout, ankle and foot**
M10.471 **Other secondary gout, right ankle and foot**
M10.472 **Other secondary gout, left ankle and foot**
M10.479 **Other secondary gout, unspecified ankle and foot**
M10.48 Other secondary gout, vertebrae
M10.49 Other secondary gout, multiple sites

M10.9 Gout, unspecified
Gout NOS

✓ Appropriate additional character required
✓x7th Requires 7th character, placeholder x must fill empty characters

M11 Other crystal arthropathies
- **M11.0 Hydroxyapatite deposition disease**
  - **M11.00 Hydroxyapatite deposition disease, unspecified site**
  - **M11.01 Hydroxyapatite deposition disease, shoulder**
    - **M11.011 Hydroxyapatite deposition disease, right shoulder**
    - **M11.012 Hydroxyapatite deposition disease, left shoulder**
    - **M11.019 Hydroxyapatite deposition disease, unspecified shoulder**
  - **M11.02 Hydroxyapatite deposition disease, elbow**
    - **M11.021 Hydroxyapatite deposition disease, right elbow**
    - **M11.022 Hydroxyapatite deposition disease, left elbow**
    - **M11.029 Hydroxyapatite deposition disease, unspecified elbow**
  - **M11.03 Hydroxyapatite deposition disease, wrist**
    - **M11.031 Hydroxyapatite deposition disease, right wrist**
    - **M11.032 Hydroxyapatite deposition disease, left wrist**
    - **M11.039 Hydroxyapatite deposition disease, unspecified wrist**
  - **M11.04 Hydroxyapatite deposition disease, hand**
    - **M11.041 Hydroxyapatite deposition disease, right hand**
    - **M11.042 Hydroxyapatite deposition disease, left hand**
    - **M11.049 Hydroxyapatite deposition disease, unspecified hand**
  - **M11.05 Hydroxyapatite deposition disease, hip**
    - **M11.051 Hydroxyapatite deposition disease, right hip**
    - **M11.052 Hydroxyapatite deposition disease, left hip**
    - **M11.059 Hydroxyapatite deposition disease, unspecified hip**
  - **M11.06 Hydroxyapatite deposition disease, knee**
    - **M11.061 Hydroxyapatite deposition disease, right knee**
    - **M11.062 Hydroxyapatite deposition disease, left knee**
    - **M11.069 Hydroxyapatite deposition disease, unspecified knee**
  - **M11.07 Hydroxyapatite deposition disease, ankle and foot**
    - **M11.071 Hydroxyapatite deposition disease, right ankle and foot**
    - **M11.072 Hydroxyapatite deposition disease, left ankle and foot**
    - **M11.079 Hydroxyapatite deposition disease, unspecified ankle and foot**
  - **M11.08 Hydroxyapatite deposition disease, vertebrae**
  - **M11.09 Hydroxyapatite deposition disease, multiple sites**
- **M11.1 Familial chondrocalcinosis**
  - **M11.10 Familial chondrocalcinosis, unspecified site**
  - **M11.11 Familial chondrocalcinosis, shoulder**
    - **M11.111 Familial chondrocalcinosis, right shoulder**
    - **M11.112 Familial chondrocalcinosis, left shoulder**
    - **M11.119 Familial chondrocalcinosis, unspecified shoulder**
  - **M11.12 Familial chondrocalcinosis, elbow**
    - **M11.121 Familial chondrocalcinosis, right elbow**
    - **M11.122 Familial chondrocalcinosis, left elbow**
    - **M11.129 Familial chondrocalcinosis, unspecified elbow**
  - **M11.13 Familial chondrocalcinosis, wrist**
    - **M11.131 Familial chondrocalcinosis, right wrist**
    - **M11.132 Familial chondrocalcinosis, left wrist**
    - **M11.139 Familial chondrocalcinosis, unspecified wrist**
  - **M11.14 Familial chondrocalcinosis, hand**
    - **M11.141 Familial chondrocalcinosis, right hand**
    - **M11.142 Familial chondrocalcinosis, left hand**
    - **M11.149 Familial chondrocalcinosis, unspecified hand**
  - **M11.15 Familial chondrocalcinosis, hip**
    - **M11.151 Familial chondrocalcinosis, right hip**
    - **M11.152 Familial chondrocalcinosis, left hip**
    - **M11.159 Familial chondrocalcinosis, unspecified hip**
  - **M11.16 Familial chondrocalcinosis, knee**
    - **M11.161 Familial chondrocalcinosis, right knee**
    - **M11.162 Familial chondrocalcinosis, left knee**
    - **M11.169 Familial chondrocalcinosis, unspecified knee**
  - **M11.17 Familial chondrocalcinosis, ankle and foot**
    - **M11.171 Familial chondrocalcinosis, right ankle and foot**
    - **M11.172 Familial chondrocalcinosis, left ankle and foot**
    - **M11.179 Familial chondrocalcinosis, unspecified ankle and foot**
  - **M11.18 Familial chondrocalcinosis, vertebrae**
  - **M11.19 Familial chondrocalcinosis, multiple sites**
- **M11.2 Other chondrocalcinosis**
  Chondrocalcinosis NOS
  - **M11.20 Other chondrocalcinosis, unspecified site**
  - **M11.21 Other chondrocalcinosis, shoulder**
    - **M11.211 Other chondrocalcinosis, right shoulder**
    - **M11.212 Other chondrocalcinosis, left shoulder**
    - **M11.219 Other chondrocalcinosis, unspecified shoulder**
  - **M11.22 Other chondrocalcinosis, elbow**
    - **M11.221 Other chondrocalcinosis, right elbow**
    - **M11.222 Other chondrocalcinosis, left elbow**
    - **M11.229 Other chondrocalcinosis, unspecified elbow**
  - **M11.23 Other chondrocalcinosis, wrist**
    - **M11.231 Other chondrocalcinosis, right wrist**
    - **M11.232 Other chondrocalcinosis, left wrist**
    - **M11.239 Other chondrocalcinosis, unspecified wrist**
  - **M11.24 Other chondrocalcinosis, hand**
    - **M11.241 Other chondrocalcinosis, right hand**
    - **M11.242 Other chondrocalcinosis, left hand**
    - **M11.249 Other chondrocalcinosis, unspecified hand**
  - **M11.25 Other chondrocalcinosis, hip**
    - **M11.251 Other chondrocalcinosis, right hip**
    - **M11.252 Other chondrocalcinosis, left hip**
    - **M11.259 Other chondrocalcinosis, unspecified hip**
  - **M11.26 Other chondrocalcinosis, knee**
    - **M11.261 Other chondrocalcinosis, right knee**
    - **M11.262 Other chondrocalcinosis, left knee**
    - **M11.269 Other chondrocalcinosis, unspecified knee**
  - **M11.27 Other chondrocalcinosis, ankle and foot**
    - **M11.271 Other chondrocalcinosis, right ankle and foot**
    - **M11.272 Other chondrocalcinosis, left ankle and foot**
    - **M11.279 Other chondrocalcinosis, unspecified ankle and foot**
  - **M11.28 Other chondrocalcinosis, vertebrae**
  - **M11.29 Other chondrocalcinosis, multiple sites**
- **M11.8 Other specified crystal arthropathies**
  - **M11.80 Other specified crystal arthropathies, unspecified site**
  - **M11.81 Other specified crystal arthropathies, shoulder**
    - **M11.811 Other specified crystal arthropathies, right shoulder**
    - **M11.812 Other specified crystal arthropathies, left shoulder**
    - **M11.819 Other specified crystal arthropathies, unspecified shoulder**
  - **M11.82 Other specified crystal arthropathies, elbow**
    - **M11.821 Other specified crystal arthropathies, right elbow**

M11.822 Other specified crystal arthropathies, left elbow
M11.829 Other specified crystal arthropathies, unspecified elbow
✓6th M11.83 Other specified crystal arthropathies, wrist
M11.831 Other specified crystal arthropathies, right wrist
M11.832 Other specified crystal arthropathies, left wrist
M11.839 Other specified crystal arthropathies, unspecified wrist
✓6th M11.84 Other specified crystal arthropathies, hand
M11.841 Other specified crystal arthropathies, right hand
M11.842 Other specified crystal arthropathies, left hand
M11.849 Other specified crystal arthropathies, unspecified hand
✓6th M11.85 Other specified crystal arthropathies, hip
M11.851 Other specified crystal arthropathies, right hip
M11.852 Other specified crystal arthropathies, left hip
M11.859 Other specified crystal arthropathies, unspecified hip
✓6th M11.86 Other specified crystal arthropathies, knee
M11.861 Other specified crystal arthropathies, right knee
M11.862 Other specified crystal arthropathies, left knee
M11.869 Other specified crystal arthropathies, unspecified knee
✓6th M11.87 Other specified crystal arthropathies, ankle and foot
M11.871 Other specified crystal arthropathies, right ankle and foot
M11.872 Other specified crystal arthropathies, left ankle and foot
M11.879 Other specified crystal arthropathies, unspecified ankle and foot
M11.88 Other specified crystal arthropathies, vertebrae
M11.89 Other specified crystal arthropathies, multiple sites
M11.9 Crystal arthropathy, unspecified

✓4th **M12 Other and unspecified arthropathy**
EXCLUDES 1 *arthrosis (M15-M19)*
cricoarytenoid arthropathy (J38.7)

✓5th M12.0 Chronic postrheumatic arthropathy [Jaccoud]
M12.00 Chronic postrheumatic arthropathy [Jaccoud], unspecified site
✓6th M12.01 Chronic postrheumatic arthropathy [Jaccoud], shoulder
M12.011 Chronic postrheumatic arthropathy [Jaccoud], right shoulder
M12.012 Chronic postrheumatic arthropathy [Jaccoud], left shoulder
M12.019 Chronic postrheumatic arthropathy [Jaccoud], unspecified shoulder
✓6th M12.02 Chronic postrheumatic arthropathy [Jaccoud], elbow
M12.021 Chronic postrheumatic arthropathy [Jaccoud], right elbow
M12.022 Chronic postrheumatic arthropathy [Jaccoud], left elbow
M12.029 Chronic postrheumatic arthropathy [Jaccoud], unspecified elbow
✓6th M12.03 Chronic postrheumatic arthropathy [Jaccoud], wrist
M12.031 Chronic postrheumatic arthropathy [Jaccoud], right wrist
M12.032 Chronic postrheumatic arthropathy [Jaccoud], left wrist
M12.039 Chronic postrheumatic arthropathy [Jaccoud], unspecified wrist
✓6th M12.04 Chronic postrheumatic arthropathy [Jaccoud], hand
M12.041 Chronic postrheumatic arthropathy [Jaccoud], right hand
M12.042 Chronic postrheumatic arthropathy [Jaccoud], left hand
M12.049 Chronic postrheumatic arthropathy [Jaccoud], unspecified hand
✓6th M12.05 Chronic postrheumatic arthropathy [Jaccoud], hip
M12.051 Chronic postrheumatic arthropathy [Jaccoud], right hip
M12.052 Chronic postrheumatic arthropathy [Jaccoud], left hip
M12.059 Chronic postrheumatic arthropathy [Jaccoud], unspecified hip
✓6th M12.06 Chronic postrheumatic arthropathy [Jaccoud], knee
M12.061 Chronic postrheumatic arthropathy [Jaccoud], right knee
M12.062 Chronic postrheumatic arthropathy [Jaccoud], left knee
M12.069 Chronic postrheumatic arthropathy [Jaccoud], unspecified knee
✓6th M12.07 Chronic postrheumatic arthropathy [Jaccoud], ankle and foot
M12.071 Chronic postrheumatic arthropathy [Jaccoud], right ankle and foot
M12.072 Chronic postrheumatic arthropathy [Jaccoud], left ankle and foot
M12.079 Chronic postrheumatic arthropathy [Jaccoud], unspecified ankle and foot
M12.08 Chronic postrheumatic arthropathy [Jaccoud], vertebrae
M12.09 Chronic postrheumatic arthropathy [Jaccoud], multiple sites
✓5th M12.1 Kaschin-Beck disease
Osteochondroarthrosis deformans endemica
M12.10 Kaschin-Beck disease, unspecified site
✓6th M12.11 Kaschin-Beck disease, shoulder
M12.111 Kaschin-Beck disease, right shoulder
M12.112 Kaschin-Beck disease, left shoulder
M12.119 Kaschin-Beck disease, unspecified shoulder
✓6th M12.12 Kaschin-Beck disease, elbow
M12.121 Kaschin-Beck disease, right elbow
M12.122 Kaschin-Beck disease, left elbow
M12.129 Kaschin-Beck disease, unspecified elbow
✓6th M12.13 Kaschin-Beck disease, wrist
M12.131 Kaschin-Beck disease, right wrist
M12.132 Kaschin-Beck disease, left wrist
M12.139 Kaschin-Beck disease, unspecified wrist
✓6th M12.14 Kaschin-Beck disease, hand
M12.141 Kaschin-Beck disease, right hand
M12.142 Kaschin-Beck disease, left hand
M12.149 Kaschin-Beck disease, unspecified hand
✓6th M12.15 Kaschin-Beck disease, hip
M12.151 Kaschin-Beck disease, right hip
M12.152 Kaschin-Beck disease, left hip
M12.159 Kaschin-Beck disease, unspecified hip
✓6th M12.16 Kaschin-Beck disease, knee
M12.161 Kaschin-Beck disease, right knee
M12.162 Kaschin-Beck disease, left knee
M12.169 Kaschin-Beck disease, unspecified knee
✓6th M12.17 Kaschin-Beck disease, ankle and foot
M12.171 Kaschin-Beck disease, right ankle and foot
M12.172 Kaschin-Beck disease, left ankle and foot
M12.179 Kaschin-Beck disease, unspecified ankle and foot
M12.18 Kaschin-Beck disease, vertebrae
M12.19 Kaschin-Beck disease, multiple sites
✓5th M12.2 Villonodular synovitis (pigmented)
M12.20 Villonodular synovitis (pigmented), unspecified site

✓6th **M12.21 Villonodular synovitis (pigmented), shoulder**
- **M12.211 Villonodular synovitis (pigmented), right shoulder**
- **M12.212 Villonodular synovitis (pigmented), left shoulder**
- **M12.219 Villonodular synovitis (pigmented), unspecified shoulder**

✓6th **M12.22 Villonodular synovitis (pigmented), elbow**
- **M12.221 Villonodular synovitis (pigmented), right elbow**
- **M12.222 Villonodular synovitis (pigmented), left elbow**
- **M12.229 Villonodular synovitis (pigmented), unspecified elbow**

✓6th **M12.23 Villonodular synovitis (pigmented), wrist**
- **M12.231 Villonodular synovitis (pigmented), right wrist**
- **M12.232 Villonodular synovitis (pigmented), left wrist**
- **M12.239 Villonodular synovitis (pigmented), unspecified wrist**

✓6th **M12.24 Villonodular synovitis (pigmented), hand**
- **M12.241 Villonodular synovitis (pigmented), right hand**
- **M12.242 Villonodular synovitis (pigmented), left hand**
- **M12.249 Villonodular synovitis (pigmented), unspecified hand**

✓6th **M12.25 Villonodular synovitis (pigmented), hip**
- **M12.251 Villonodular synovitis (pigmented), right hip**
- **M12.252 Villonodular synovitis (pigmented), left hip**
- **M12.259 Villonodular synovitis (pigmented), unspecified hip**

✓6th **M12.26 Villonodular synovitis (pigmented), knee**
- **M12.261 Villonodular synovitis (pigmented), right knee**
- **M12.262 Villonodular synovitis (pigmented), left knee**
- **M12.269 Villonodular synovitis (pigmented), unspecified knee**

✓6th **M12.27 Villonodular synovitis (pigmented), ankle and foot**
- **M12.271 Villonodular synovitis (pigmented), right ankle and foot**
- **M12.272 Villonodular synovitis (pigmented), left ankle and foot**
- **M12.279 Villonodular synovitis (pigmented), unspecified ankle and foot**

M12.28 Villonodular synovitis (pigmented), vertebrae

M12.29 Villonodular synovitis (pigmented), multiple sites

✓5th **M12.3 Palindromic rheumatism**

M12.30 Palindromic rheumatism, unspecified site

✓6th **M12.31 Palindromic rheumatism, shoulder**
- **M12.311 Palindromic rheumatism, right shoulder**
- **M12.312 Palindromic rheumatism, left shoulder**
- **M12.319 Palindromic rheumatism, unspecified shoulder**

✓6th **M12.32 Palindromic rheumatism, elbow**
- **M12.321 Palindromic rheumatism, right elbow**
- **M12.322 Palindromic rheumatism, left elbow**
- **M12.329 Palindromic rheumatism, unspecified elbow**

✓6th **M12.33 Palindromic rheumatism, wrist**
- **M12.331 Palindromic rheumatism, right wrist**
- **M12.332 Palindromic rheumatism, left wrist**
- **M12.339 Palindromic rheumatism, unspecified wrist**

✓6th **M12.34 Palindromic rheumatism, hand**
- **M12.341 Palindromic rheumatism, right hand**
- **M12.342 Palindromic rheumatism, left hand**
- **M12.349 Palindromic rheumatism, unspecified hand**

✓6th **M12.35 Palindromic rheumatism, hip**
- **M12.351 Palindromic rheumatism, right hip**
- **M12.352 Palindromic rheumatism, left hip**
- **M12.359 Palindromic rheumatism, unspecified hip**

✓6th **M12.36 Palindromic rheumatism, knee**
- **M12.361 Palindromic rheumatism, right knee**
- **M12.362 Palindromic rheumatism, left knee**
- **M12.369 Palindromic rheumatism, unspecified knee**

✓6th **M12.37 Palindromic rheumatism, ankle and foot**
- **M12.371 Palindromic rheumatism, right ankle and foot**
- **M12.372 Palindromic rheumatism, left ankle and foot**
- **M12.379 Palindromic rheumatism, unspecified ankle and foot**

M12.38 Palindromic rheumatism, vertebrae

M12.39 Palindromic rheumatism, multiple sites

✓5th **M12.4 Intermittent hydrarthrosis**

M12.40 Intermittent hydrarthrosis, unspecified site

✓6th **M12.41 Intermittent hydrarthrosis, shoulder**
- **M12.411 Intermittent hydrarthrosis, right shoulder**
- **M12.412 Intermittent hydrarthrosis, left shoulder**
- **M12.419 Intermittent hydrarthrosis, unspecified shoulder**

✓6th **M12.42 Intermittent hydrarthrosis, elbow**
- **M12.421 Intermittent hydrarthrosis, right elbow**
- **M12.422 Intermittent hydrarthrosis, left elbow**
- **M12.429 Intermittent hydrarthrosis, unspecified elbow**

✓6th **M12.43 Intermittent hydrarthrosis, wrist**
- **M12.431 Intermittent hydrarthrosis, right wrist**
- **M12.432 Intermittent hydrarthrosis, left wrist**
- **M12.439 Intermittent hydrarthrosis, unspecified wrist**

✓6th **M12.44 Intermittent hydrarthrosis, hand**
- **M12.441 Intermittent hydrarthrosis, right hand**
- **M12.442 Intermittent hydrarthrosis, left hand**
- **M12.449 Intermittent hydrarthrosis, unspecified hand**

✓6th **M12.45 Intermittent hydrarthrosis, hip**
- **M12.451 Intermittent hydrarthrosis, right hip**
- **M12.452 Intermittent hydrarthrosis, left hip**
- **M12.459 Intermittent hydrarthrosis, unspecified hip**

✓6th **M12.46 Intermittent hydrarthrosis, knee**
- **M12.461 Intermittent hydrarthrosis, right knee**
- **M12.462 Intermittent hydrarthrosis, left knee**
- **M12.469 Intermittent hydrarthrosis, unspecified knee**

✓6th **M12.47 Intermittent hydrarthrosis, ankle and foot**
- **M12.471 Intermittent hydrarthrosis, right ankle and foot**
- **M12.472 Intermittent hydrarthrosis, left ankle and foot**
- **M12.479 Intermittent hydrarthrosis, unspecified ankle and foot**

M12.48 Intermittent hydrarthrosis, other site

M12.49 Intermittent hydrarthrosis, multiple sites

✓5th **M12.5 Traumatic arthropathy**

EXCLUDES1 *current injury-see Alphabetic Index*
post-traumatic osteoarthritis (of):
NOS (M19.1-)
first carpometacarpal joint (M18.2-M18.3)
hip (M16.4-M16.5)
knee (M17.2-M17.3)
other single joints (M19.1-)

M12.50 Traumatic arthropathy, unspecified site

✓6th **M12.51 Traumatic arthropathy, shoulder**
- **M12.511 Traumatic arthropathy, right shoulder**
- **M12.512 Traumatic arthropathy, left shoulder**
- **M12.519 Traumatic arthropathy, unspecified shoulder**

✓6th **M12.52 Traumatic arthropathy, elbow**
- **M12.521 Traumatic arthropathy, right elbow**
- **M12.522 Traumatic arthropathy, left elbow**
- **M12.529 Traumatic arthropathy, unspecified elbow**

✓6th **M12.53 Traumatic arthropathy, wrist**
M12.531 Traumatic arthropathy, right wrist
M12.532 Traumatic arthropathy, left wrist
M12.539 Traumatic arthropathy, unspecified wrist

✓6th **M12.54 Traumatic arthropathy, hand**
M12.541 Traumatic arthropathy, right hand
M12.542 Traumatic arthropathy, left hand
M12.549 Traumatic arthropathy, unspecified hand

✓6th **M12.55 Traumatic arthropathy, hip**
M12.551 Traumatic arthropathy, right hip
M12.552 Traumatic arthropathy, left hip
M12.559 Traumatic arthropathy, unspecified hip

✓6th **M12.56 Traumatic arthropathy, knee**
M12.561 Traumatic arthropathy, right knee
M12.562 Traumatic arthropathy, left knee
M12.569 Traumatic arthropathy, unspecified knee

✓6th **M12.57 Traumatic arthropathy, ankle and foot**
M12.571 Traumatic arthropathy, right ankle and foot
M12.572 Traumatic arthropathy, left ankle and foot
M12.579 Traumatic arthropathy, unspecified ankle and foot

M12.58 Traumatic arthropathy, vertebrae
M12.59 Traumatic arthropathy, multiple sites

✓5th **M12.8 Other specific arthropathies, not elsewhere classified**
Transient arthropathy

M12.80 Other specific arthropathies, not elsewhere classified, unspecified site

✓6th **M12.81 Other specific arthropathies, not elsewhere classified, shoulder**
M12.811 Other specific arthropathies, not elsewhere classified, right shoulder
M12.812 Other specific arthropathies, not elsewhere classified, left shoulder
M12.819 Other specific arthropathies, not elsewhere classified, unspecified shoulder

✓6th **M12.82 Other specific arthropathies, not elsewhere classified, elbow**
M12.821 Other specific arthropathies, not elsewhere classified, right elbow
M12.822 Other specific arthropathies, not elsewhere classified, left elbow
M12.829 Other specific arthropathies, not elsewhere classified, unspecified elbow

✓6th **M12.83 Other specific arthropathies, not elsewhere classified, wrist**
M12.831 Other specific arthropathies, not elsewhere classified, right wrist
M12.832 Other specific arthropathies, not elsewhere classified, left wrist
M12.839 Other specific arthropathies, not elsewhere classified, unspecified wrist

✓6th **M12.84 Other specific arthropathies, not elsewhere classified, hand**
M12.841 Other specific arthropathies, not elsewhere classified, right hand
M12.842 Other specific arthropathies, not elsewhere classified, left hand
M12.849 Other specific arthropathies, not elsewhere classified, unspecified hand

✓6th **M12.85 Other specific arthropathies, not elsewhere classified, hip**
M12.851 Other specific arthropathies, not elsewhere classified, right hip
M12.852 Other specific arthropathies, not elsewhere classified, left hip
M12.859 Other specific arthropathies, not elsewhere classified, unspecified hip

✓6th **M12.86 Other specific arthropathies, not elsewhere classified, knee**
M12.861 Other specific arthropathies, not elsewhere classified, right knee
M12.862 Other specific arthropathies, not elsewhere classified, left knee
M12.869 Other specific arthropathies, not elsewhere classified, unspecified knee

✓6th **M12.87 Other specific arthropathies, not elsewhere classified, ankle and foot**
M12.871 Other specific arthropathies, not elsewhere classified, right ankle and foot
M12.872 Other specific arthropathies, not elsewhere classified, left ankle and foot
M12.879 Other specific arthropathies, not elsewhere classified, unspecified ankle and foot

M12.88 Other specific arthropathies, not elsewhere classified, vertebrae
M12.89 Other specific arthropathies, not elsewhere classified, multiple sites

M12.9 Arthropathy, unspecified

✓4th M13 Other arthritis

EXCLUDES 1 *arthrosis (M15-M19)*
osteoarthritis (M15-M19)

M13.0 Polyarthritis, unspecified

✓5th **M13.1 Monoarthritis, not elsewhere classified**

M13.10 Monoarthritis, not elsewhere classified, unspecified site

✓6th **M13.11 Monoarthritis, not elsewhere classified, shoulder**
M13.111 Monoarthritis, not elsewhere classified, right shoulder
M13.112 Monoarthritis, not elsewhere classified, left shoulder
M13.119 Monoarthritis, not elsewhere classified, unspecified shoulder

✓6th **M13.12 Monoarthritis, not elsewhere classified, elbow**
M13.121 Monoarthritis, not elsewhere classified, right elbow
M13.122 Monoarthritis, not elsewhere classified, left elbow
M13.129 Monoarthritis, not elsewhere classified, unspecified elbow

✓6th **M13.13 Monoarthritis, not elsewhere classified, wrist**
M13.131 Monoarthritis, not elsewhere classified, right wrist
M13.132 Monoarthritis, not elsewhere classified, left wrist
M13.139 Monoarthritis, not elsewhere classified, unspecified wrist

✓6th **M13.14 Monoarthritis, not elsewhere classified, hand**
M13.141 Monoarthritis, not elsewhere classified, right hand
M13.142 Monoarthritis, not elsewhere classified, left hand
M13.149 Monoarthritis, not elsewhere classified, unspecified hand

✓6th **M13.15 Monoarthritis, not elsewhere classified, hip**
M13.151 Monoarthritis, not elsewhere classified, right hip
M13.152 Monoarthritis, not elsewhere classified, left hip
M13.159 Monoarthritis, not elsewhere classified, unspecified hip

✓6th **M13.16 Monoarthritis, not elsewhere classified, knee**
M13.161 Monoarthritis, not elsewhere classified, right knee
M13.162 Monoarthritis, not elsewhere classified, left knee
M13.169 Monoarthritis, not elsewhere classified, unspecified knee

✓6th **M13.17 Monoarthritis, not elsewhere classified, ankle and foot**
M13.171 Monoarthritis, not elsewhere classified, right ankle and foot
M13.172 Monoarthritis, not elsewhere classified, left ankle and foot
M13.179 Monoarthritis, not elsewhere classified, unspecified ankle and foot

5th **M13.8 Other specified arthritis**
Allergic arthritis
EXCLUDES1 *osteoarthritis (M15-M19)*

M13.80 Other specified arthritis, unspecified site

6th **M13.81 Other specified arthritis, shoulder**
- **M13.811 Other specified arthritis, right shoulder**
- **M13.812 Other specified arthritis, left shoulder**
- **M13.819 Other specified arthritis, unspecified shoulder**

6th **M13.82 Other specified arthritis, elbow**
- **M13.821 Other specified arthritis, right elbow**
- **M13.822 Other specified arthritis, left elbow**
- **M13.829 Other specified arthritis, unspecified elbow**

6th **M13.83 Other specified arthritis, wrist**
- **M13.831 Other specified arthritis, right wrist**
- **M13.832 Other specified arthritis, left wrist**
- **M13.839 Other specified arthritis, unspecified wrist**

6th **M13.84 Other specified arthritis, hand**
- **M13.841 Other specified arthritis, right hand**
- **M13.842 Other specified arthritis, left hand**
- **M13.849 Other specified arthritis, unspecified hand**

6th **M13.85 Other specified arthritis, hip**
- **M13.851 Other specified arthritis, right hip**
- **M13.852 Other specified arthritis, left hip**
- **M13.859 Other specified arthritis, unspecified hip**

6th **M13.86 Other specified arthritis, knee**
- **M13.861 Other specified arthritis, right knee**
- **M13.862 Other specified arthritis, left knee**
- **M13.869 Other specified arthritis, unspecified knee**

6th **M13.87 Other specified arthritis, ankle and foot**
- **M13.871 Other specified arthritis, right ankle and foot**
- **M13.872 Other specified arthritis, left ankle and foot**
- **M13.879 Other specified arthritis, unspecified ankle and foot**

M13.88 Other specified arthritis, other site

M13.89 Other specified arthritis, multiple sites

4th **M14 Arthropathies in other diseases classified elsewhere**

EXCLUDES1 *arthropathy in:*
- *diabetes mellitus (E08-E13 with 4th and 5th characters 61)*
- *hematological disorders (M36.2-M36.3)*
- *hypersensitivity reactions (M36.4)*
- *neoplastic disease (M36.1)*
- *neurosyphillis (A52.16)*
- *sarcoidosis (D86.86)*

enteropathic arthropathies (M07.-)
juvenile psoriatic arthropathy (L40.54)
lipoid dermatoarthritis (E78.81)

5th **M14.6 Charcôt's joint**
Neuropathic arthropathy
EXCLUDES1 *Charcôt's joint in diabetes mellitus (E08-E13 with final characters 610)*
Charcôt's joint in tabes dorsalis (A52.16)

M14.60 Charcôt's joint, unspecified site

6th **M14.61 Charcôt's joint, shoulder**
- **M14.611 Charcôt's joint, right shoulder**
- **M14.612 Charcôt's joint, left shoulder**
- **M14.619 Charcôt's joint, unspecified shoulder**

6th **M14.62 Charcôt's joint, elbow**
- **M14.621 Charcôt's joint, right elbow**
- **M14.622 Charcôt's joint, left elbow**
- **M14.629 Charcôt's joint, unspecified elbow**

6th **M14.63 Charcôt's joint, wrist**
- **M14.631 Charcôt's joint, right wrist**
- **M14.632 Charcôt's joint, left wrist**
- **M14.639 Charcôt's joint, unspecified wrist**

6th **M14.64 Charcôt's joint, hand**
- **M14.641 Charcôt's joint, right hand**
- **M14.642 Charcôt's joint, left hand**
- **M14.649 Charcôt's joint, unspecified hand**

6th **M14.65 Charcôt's joint, hip**
- **M14.651 Charcôt's joint, right hip**
- **M14.652 Charcôt's joint, left hip**
- **M14.659 Charcôt's joint, unspecified hip**

6th **M14.66 Charcôt's joint, knee**
- **M14.661 Charcôt's joint, right knee**
- **M14.662 Charcôt's joint, left knee**
- **M14.669 Charcôt's joint, unspecified knee**

6th **M14.67 Charcôt's joint, ankle and foot**
- **M14.671 Charcôt's joint, right ankle and foot**
- **M14.672 Charcôt's joint, left ankle and foot**
- **M14.679 Charcôt's joint, unspecified ankle and foot**

M14.68 Charcôt's joint, vertebrae

M14.69 Charcôt's joint, multiple sites

5th **M14.8 Arthropathies in other specified diseases classified elsewhere**
Code first underlying disease, such as:
- *amyloidosis (E85.-)*
- *erythema multiforme (L51.-)*
- *erythema nodosum (L52)*
- *hemochromatosis (E83.11-)*
- *hyperparathyroidism (E21.-)*
- *hypothyroidism (E00-E03)*
- *sickle-cell disorders (D57.-)*
- *thyrotoxicosis [hyperthyroidism] (E05.-)*
- *Whipple's disease (K90.81)*

M14.80 Arthropathies in other specified diseases classified elsewhere, unspecified site

6th **M14.81 Arthropathies in other specified diseases classified elsewhere, shoulder**
- ***M14.811 Arthropathies in other specified diseases classified elsewhere, right shoulder***
- ***M14.812 Arthropathies in other specified diseases classified elsewhere, left shoulder***
- ***M14.819 Arthropathies in other specified diseases classified elsewhere, unspecified shoulder***

6th **M14.82 Arthropathies in other specified diseases classified elsewhere, elbow**
- ***M14.821 Arthropathies in other specified diseases classified elsewhere, right elbow***
- ***M14.822 Arthropathies in other specified diseases classified elsewhere, left elbow***
- ***M14.829 Arthropathies in other specified diseases classified elsewhere, unspecified elbow***

6th **M14.83 Arthropathies in other specified diseases classified elsewhere, wrist**
- ***M14.831 Arthropathies in other specified diseases classified elsewhere, right wrist***
- ***M14.832 Arthropathies in other specified diseases classified elsewhere, left wrist***
- ***M14.839 Arthropathies in other specified diseases classified elsewhere, unspecified wrist***

6th **M14.84 Arthropathies in other specified diseases classified elsewhere, hand**
- ***M14.841 Arthropathies in other specified diseases classified elsewhere, right hand***
- ***M14.842 Arthropathies in other specified diseases classified elsewhere, left hand***
- ***M14.849 Arthropathies in other specified diseases classified elsewhere, unspecified hand***

6th **M14.85 Arthropathies in other specified diseases classified elsewhere, hip**
- ***M14.851 Arthropathies in other specified diseases classified elsewhere, right hip***
- ***M14.852 Arthropathies in other specified diseases classified elsewhere, left hip***
- ***M14.859 Arthropathies in other specified diseases classified elsewhere, unspecified hip***

6th **M14.86 Arthropathies in other specified diseases classified elsewhere, knee**
- ***M14.861 Arthropathies in other specified diseases classified elsewhere, right knee***
- ***M14.862 Arthropathies in other specified diseases classified elsewhere, left knee***
- ***M14.869 Arthropathies in other specified diseases classified elsewhere, unspecified knee***

✓6th **M14.87 Arthropathies in other specified diseases classified elsewhere, ankle and foot**
- *M14.871 Arthropathies in other specified diseases classified elsewhere, right ankle and foot*
- *M14.872 Arthropathies in other specified diseases classified elsewhere, left ankle and foot*
- *M14.879 Arthropathies in other specified diseases classified elsewhere, unspecified ankle and foot*

M14.88 Arthropathies in other specified diseases classified elsewhere, vertebrae

M14.89 Arthropathies in other specified diseases classified elsewhere, multiple sites

Osteoarthritis (M15-M19)

EXCLUDES 2 *osteoarthritis of spine (M47.-)*

✓4th **M15 Polyosteoarthritis**

INCLUDES arthritis of multiple sites

EXCLUDES 1 *bilateral involvement of single joint (M16-M19)*

- **M15.0 Primary generalized (osteo)arthritis**
- **M15.1 Heberden's nodes (with arthropathy)**
  Interphalangeal distal osteoarthritis
- **M15.2 Bouchard's nodes (with arthropathy)**
  Juxtaphalangeal distal osteoarthritis
- **M15.3 Secondary multiple arthritis**
  Post-traumatic polyosteoarthritis
- **M15.4 Erosive (osteo)arthritis**
- **M15.8 Other polyosteoarthritis**
- **M15.9 Polyosteoarthritis, unspecified**
  Generalized osteoarthritis NOS

✓4th **M16 Osteoarthritis of hip**
- **M16.0 Bilateral primary osteoarthritis of hip**
- ✓5th **M16.1 Unilateral primary osteoarthritis of hip**
  Primary osteoarthritis of hip NOS
  - **M16.10 Unilateral primary osteoarthritis, unspecified hip**
  - **M16.11 Unilateral primary osteoarthritis, right hip**
  - **M16.12 Unilateral primary osteoarthritis, left hip**
- **M16.2 Bilateral osteoarthritis resulting from hip dysplasia**
- ✓5th **M16.3 Unilateral osteoarthritis resulting from hip dysplasia**
  Dysplastic osteoarthritis of hip NOS
  - **M16.30 Unilateral osteoarthritis resulting from hip dysplasia, unspecified hip**
  - **M16.31 Unilateral osteoarthritis resulting from hip dysplasia, right hip**
  - **M16.32 Unilateral osteoarthritis resulting from hip dysplasia, left hip**
- **M16.4 Bilateral post-traumatic osteoarthritis of hip**
- ✓5th **M16.5 Unilateral post-traumatic osteoarthritis of hip**
  Post-traumatic osteoarthritis of hip NOS
  - **M16.50 Unilateral post-traumatic osteoarthritis, unspecified hip**
  - **M16.51 Unilateral post-traumatic osteoarthritis, right hip**
  - **M16.52 Unilateral post-traumatic osteoarthritis, left hip**
- **M16.6 Other bilateral secondary osteoarthritis of hip**
- **M16.7 Other unilateral secondary osteoarthritis of hip**
  Secondary osteoarthritis of hip NOS
- **M16.9 Osteoarthritis of hip, unspecified**

✓4th **M17 Osteoarthritis of knee**
- **M17.0 Bilateral primary osteoarthritis of knee**
- ✓5th **M17.1 Unilateral primary osteoarthritis of knee**
  Primary osteoarthritis of knee NOS
  - **M17.10 Unilateral primary osteoarthritis, unspecified knee**
  - **M17.11 Unilateral primary osteoarthritis, right knee**
  - **M17.12 Unilateral primary osteoarthritis, left knee**
- **M17.2 Bilateral post-traumatic osteoarthritis of knee**
- ✓5th **M17.3 Unilateral post-traumatic osteoarthritis of knee**
  Post-traumatic osteoarthritis of knee NOS
  - **M17.30 Unilateral post-traumatic osteoarthritis, unspecified knee**
  - **M17.31 Unilateral post-traumatic osteoarthritis, right knee**
  - **M17.32 Unilateral post-traumatic osteoarthritis, left knee**
- **M17.4 Other bilateral secondary osteoarthritis of knee**
- **M17.5 Other unilateral secondary osteoarthritis of knee**
  Secondary osteoarthritis of knee NOS
- **M17.9 Osteoarthritis of knee, unspecified**

✓4th **M18 Osteoarthritis of first carpometacarpal joint**
- **M18.0 Bilateral primary osteoarthritis of first carpometacarpal joints**
- ✓5th **M18.1 Unilateral primary osteoarthritis of first carpometacarpal joint**
  Primary osteoarthritis of first carpometacarpal joint NOS
  - **M18.10 Unilateral primary osteoarthritis of first carpometacarpal joint, unspecified hand**
  - **M18.11 Unilateral primary osteoarthritis of first carpometacarpal joint, right hand**
  - **M18.12 Unilateral primary osteoarthritis of first carpometacarpal joint, left hand**
- **M18.2 Bilateral post-traumatic osteoarthritis of first carpometacarpal joints**
- ✓5th **M18.3 Unilateral post-traumatic osteoarthritis of first carpometacarpal joint**
  Post-traumatic osteoarthritis of first carpometacarpal joint NOS
  - **M18.30 Unilateral post-traumatic osteoarthritis of first carpometacarpal joint, unspecified hand**
  - **M18.31 Unilateral post-traumatic osteoarthritis of first carpometacarpal joint, right hand**
  - **M18.32 Unilateral post-traumatic osteoarthritis of first carpometacarpal joint, left hand**
- **M18.4 Other bilateral secondary osteoarthritis of first carpometacarpal joints**
- ✓5th **M18.5 Other unilateral secondary osteoarthritis of first carpometacarpal joint**
  Secondary osteoarthritis of first carpometacarpal joint NOS
  - **M18.50 Other unilateral secondary osteoarthritis of first carpometacarpal joint, unspecified hand**
  - **M18.51 Other unilateral secondary osteoarthritis of first carpometacarpal joint, right hand**
  - **M18.52 Other unilateral secondary osteoarthritis of first carpometacarpal joint, left hand**
- **M18.9 Osteoarthritis of first carpometacarpal joint, unspecified**

✓4th **M19 Other and unspecified osteoarthritis**

EXCLUDES 1 *polyarthritis (M15.-)*

EXCLUDES 2 *arthrosis of spine (M47.-)*
hallux rigidus (M20.2)
osteoarthritis of spine (M47.-)

- ✓5th **M19.0 Primary osteoarthritis of other joints**
  - ✓6th **M19.01 Primary osteoarthritis, shoulder**
    - **M19.011 Primary osteoarthritis, right shoulder**
    - **M19.012 Primary osteoarthritis, left shoulder**
    - **M19.019 Primary osteoarthritis, unspecified shoulder**
  - ✓6th **M19.02 Primary osteoarthritis, elbow**
    - **M19.021 Primary osteoarthritis, right elbow**
    - **M19.022 Primary osteoarthritis, left elbow**
    - **M19.029 Primary osteoarthritis, unspecified elbow**
  - ✓6th **M19.03 Primary osteoarthritis, wrist**
    - **M19.031 Primary osteoarthritis, right wrist**
    - **M19.032 Primary osteoarthritis, left wrist**
    - **M19.039 Primary osteoarthritis, unspecified wrist**
  - ✓6th **M19.04 Primary osteoarthritis, hand**
    EXCLUDES 2 *primary osteoarthritis of first carpometacarpal joint (M18.0-, M18.1-)*
    - **M19.041 Primary osteoarthritis, right hand**
    - **M19.042 Primary osteoarthritis, left hand**
    - **M19.049 Primary osteoarthritis, unspecified hand**
  - ✓6th **M19.07 Primary osteoarthritis ankle and foot**
    - **M19.071 Primary osteoarthritis, right ankle and foot**
    - **M19.072 Primary osteoarthritis, left ankle and foot**
    - **M19.079 Primary osteoarthritis, unspecified ankle and foot**

✓ Appropriate additional character required   ✓x7th Requires 7th character, placeholder x must fill empty characters

√5th **M19.1 Post-traumatic osteoarthritis of other joints**
√6th **M19.11 Post-traumatic osteoarthritis, shoulder**
M19.111 Post-traumatic osteoarthritis, right shoulder
M19.112 Post-traumatic osteoarthritis, left shoulder
M19.119 Post-traumatic osteoarthritis, unspecified shoulder
√6th **M19.12 Post-traumatic osteoarthritis, elbow**
M19.121 Post-traumatic osteoarthritis, right elbow
M19.122 Post-traumatic osteoarthritis, left elbow
M19.129 Post-traumatic osteoarthritis, unspecified elbow
√6th **M19.13 Post-traumatic osteoarthritis, wrist**
M19.131 Post-traumatic osteoarthritis, right wrist
M19.132 Post-traumatic osteoarthritis, left wrist
M19.139 Post-traumatic osteoarthritis, unspecified wrist
√6th **M19.14 Post-traumatic osteoarthritis, hand**
EXCLUDES 2 *post-traumatic osteoarthritis of first carpometacarpal joint (M18.2-, M18.3-)*
M19.141 Post-traumatic osteoarthritis, right hand
M19.142 Post-traumatic osteoarthritis, left hand
M19.149 Post-traumatic osteoarthritis, unspecified hand
√6th **M19.17 Post-traumatic osteoarthritis, ankle and foot**
M19.171 Post-traumatic osteoarthritis, right ankle and foot
M19.172 Post-traumatic osteoarthritis, left ankle and foot
M19.179 Post-traumatic osteoarthritis, unspecified ankle and foot
√5th **M19.2 Secondary osteoarthritis of other joints**
√6th **M19.21 Secondary osteoarthritis, shoulder**
M19.211 Secondary osteoarthritis, right shoulder
M19.212 Secondary osteoarthritis, left shoulder
M19.219 Secondary osteoarthritis, unspecified shoulder
√6th **M19.22 Secondary osteoarthritis, elbow**
M19.221 Secondary osteoarthritis, right elbow
M19.222 Secondary osteoarthritis, left elbow
M19.229 Secondary osteoarthritis, unspecified elbow
√6th **M19.23 Secondary osteoarthritis, wrist**
M19.231 Secondary osteoarthritis, right wrist
M19.232 Secondary osteoarthritis, left wrist
M19.239 Secondary osteoarthritis, unspecified wrist
√6th **M19.24 Secondary osteoarthritis, hand**
M19.241 Secondary osteoarthritis, right hand
M19.242 Secondary osteoarthritis, left hand
M19.249 Secondary osteoarthritis, unspecified hand
√6th **M19.27 Secondary osteoarthritis, ankle and foot**
M19.271 Secondary osteoarthritis, right ankle and foot
M19.272 Secondary osteoarthritis, left ankle and foot
M19.279 Secondary osteoarthritis, unspecified ankle and foot
√5th **M19.9 Osteoarthritis, unspecified site**
M19.90 Unspecified osteoarthritis, unspecified site
Arthrosis NOS
Arthritis NOS
Osteoarthritis NOS
M19.91 Primary osteoarthritis, unspecified site
Primary osteoarthritis NOS
M19.92 Post-traumatic osteoarthritis, unspecified site
Post-traumatic osteoarthritis NOS
M19.93 Secondary osteoarthritis, unspecified site
Secondary osteoarthritis NOS

Other joint disorders (M20-M25)

EXCLUDES 2 *joints of the spine (M40-M54)*

√4th **M20 Acquired deformities of fingers and toes**
EXCLUDES 1 *acquired absence of fingers and toes (Z89.-)*
congenital absence of fingers and toes (Q71.3-, Q72.3-)
congenital deformities and malformations of fingers and toes (Q66-, Q68-Q70, Q74-)
√5th **M20.0 Deformity of finger(s)**
EXCLUDES 1 *clubbing of fingers (R68.3)*
palmar fascial fibromatosis [Dupuytren] (M72.0)
trigger finger (M65.3)
√6th **M20.00 Unspecified deformity of finger(s)**
M20.001 Unspecified deformity of right finger(s)
M20.002 Unspecified deformity of left finger(s)
M20.009 Unspecified deformity of unspecified finger(s)
√6th **M20.01 Mallet finger**
M20.011 Mallet finger of right finger(s)
M20.012 Mallet finger of left finger(s)
M20.019 Mallet finger of unspecified finger(s)
√6th **M20.02 Boutonnière deformity**
M20.021 Boutonnière deformity of right finger(s)
M20.022 Boutonnière deformity of left finger(s)
M20.029 Boutonnière deformity of unspecified finger(s)
√6th **M20.03 Swan-neck deformity**
M20.031 Swan-neck deformity of right finger(s)
M20.032 Swan-neck deformity of left finger(s)
M20.039 Swan-neck deformity of unspecified finger(s)
√6th **M20.09 Other deformity of finger(s)**
M20.091 Other deformity of right finger(s)
M20.092 Other deformity of left finger(s)
M20.099 Other deformity of finger(s), unspecified finger(s)
√5th **M20.1 Hallux valgus (acquired)**
Bunion
M20.10 Hallux valgus (acquired), unspecified foot
M20.11 Hallux valgus (acquired), right foot
M20.12 Hallux valgus (acquired), left foot
√5th **M20.2 Hallux rigidus**
M20.20 Hallux rigidus, unspecified foot
M20.21 Hallux rigidus, right foot
M20.22 Hallux rigidus, left foot
√5th **M20.3 Hallux varus (acquired)**
M20.30 Hallux varus (acquired), unspecified foot
M20.31 Hallux varus (acquired), right foot
M20.32 Hallux varus (acquired), left foot
√5th **M20.4 Other hammer toe(s) (acquired)**
M20.40 Other hammer toe(s) (acquired), unspecified foot
M20.41 Other hammer toe(s) (acquired), right foot
M20.42 Other hammer toe(s) (acquired), left foot
√5th **M20.5 Other deformities of toe(s) (acquired)**
√6th **M20.5X Other deformities of toe(s) (acquired)**
M20.5X1 Other deformities of toe(s) (acquired), right foot
M20.5X2 Other deformities of toe(s) (acquired), left foot
M20.5X9 Other deformities of toe(s) (acquired), unspecified foot
√5th **M20.6 Acquired deformities of toe(s), unspecified**
M20.60 Acquired deformities of toe(s), unspecified, unspecified foot
M20.61 Acquired deformities of toe(s), unspecified, right foot
M20.62 Acquired deformities of toe(s), unspecified, left foot

M21 Other acquired deformities of limbs

EXCLUDES 1 *acquired absence of limb (Z89.-)*
congenital absence of limbs (Q71-Q73)
congenital deformities and malformations of limbs (Q65-Q66, Q68-Q74)

EXCLUDES 2 *acquired deformities of fingers or toes (M20.-)*
coxa plana (M91.2)

M21.0 Valgus deformity, not elsewhere classified

EXCLUDES 1 *metatarsus valgus (Q66.6)*
talipes calcaneovalgus (Q66.4)

M21.00 Valgus deformity, not elsewhere classified, unspecified site

M21.02 Valgus deformity, not elsewhere classified, elbow

Cubitus valgus

M21.021 Valgus deformity, not elsewhere classified, right elbow

M21.022 Valgus deformity, not elsewhere classified, left elbow

M21.029 Valgus deformity, not elsewhere classified, unspecified elbow

M21.05 Valgus deformity, not elsewhere classified, hip

M21.051 Valgus deformity, not elsewhere classified, right hip

M21.052 Valgus deformity, not elsewhere classified, left hip

M21.059 Valgus deformity, not elsewhere classified, unspecified hip

M21.06 Valgus deformity, not elsewhere classified, knee

Genu valgum
Knock knee

M21.061 Valgus deformity, not elsewhere classified, right knee

M21.062 Valgus deformity, not elsewhere classified, left knee

M21.069 Valgus deformity, not elsewhere classified, unspecified knee

M21.07 Valgus deformity, not elsewhere classified, ankle

M21.071 Valgus deformity, not elsewhere classified, right ankle

M21.072 Valgus deformity, not elsewhere classified, left ankle

M21.079 Valgus deformity, not elsewhere classified, unspecified ankle

M21.1 Varus deformity, not elsewhere classified

EXCLUDES 1 *metatarsus varus (Q66.2)*
tibia vara (M92.5)

M21.10 Varus deformity, not elsewhere classified, unspecified site

M21.12 Varus deformity, not elsewhere classified, elbow

Cubitus varus, elbow

M21.121 Varus deformity, not elsewhere classified, right elbow

M21.122 Varus deformity, not elsewhere classified, left elbow

M21.129 Varus deformity, not elsewhere classified, unspecified elbow

M21.15 Varus deformity, not elsewhere classified, hip

M21.151 Varus deformity, not elsewhere classified, right hip

M21.152 Varus deformity, not elsewhere classified, left hip

M21.159 Varus deformity, not elsewhere classified, unspecified

M21.16 Varus deformity, not elsewhere classified, knee

Bow leg
Genu varum

M21.161 Varus deformity, not elsewhere classified, right knee

M21.162 Varus deformity, not elsewhere classified, left knee

M21.169 Varus deformity, not elsewhere classified, unspecified knee

M21.17 Varus deformity, not elsewhere classified, ankle

M21.171 Varus deformity, not elsewhere classified, right ankle

M21.172 Varus deformity, not elsewhere classified, left ankle

M21.179 Varus deformity, not elsewhere classified, unspecified ankle

M21.2 Flexion deformity

M21.20 Flexion deformity, unspecified site

M21.21 Flexion deformity, shoulder

M21.211 Flexion deformity, right shoulder

M21.212 Flexion deformity, left shoulder

M21.219 Flexion deformity, unspecified shoulder

M21.22 Flexion deformity, elbow

M21.221 Flexion deformity, right elbow

M21.222 Flexion deformity, left elbow

M21.229 Flexion deformity, unspecified elbow

M21.23 Flexion deformity, wrist

M21.231 Flexion deformity, right wrist

M21.232 Flexion deformity, left wrist

M21.239 Flexion deformity, unspecified wrist

M21.24 Flexion deformity, finger joints

M21.241 Flexion deformity, right finger joints

M21.242 Flexion deformity, left finger joints

M21.249 Flexion deformity, unspecified finger joints

M21.25 Flexion deformity, hip

M21.251 Flexion deformity, right hip

M21.252 Flexion deformity, left hip

M21.259 Flexion deformity, unspecified hip

M21.26 Flexion deformity, knee

M21.261 Flexion deformity, right knee

M21.262 Flexion deformity, left knee

M21.269 Flexion deformity, unspecified knee

M21.27 Flexion deformity, ankle and toes

M21.271 Flexion deformity, right ankle and toes

M21.272 Flexion deformity, left ankle and toes

M21.279 Flexion deformity, unspecified ankle and toes

M21.3 Wrist or foot drop (acquired)

M21.33 Wrist drop (acquired)

M21.331 Wrist drop, right wrist

M21.332 Wrist drop, left wrist

M21.339 Wrist drop, unspecified wrist

M21.37 Foot drop (acquired)

M21.371 Foot drop, right foot

M21.372 Foot drop, left foot

M21.379 Foot drop, unspecified foot

M21.4 Flat foot [pes planus] (acquired)

EXCLUDES 1 *congenital pes planus (Q66.5-)*

M21.40 Flat foot [pes planus] (acquired), unspecified foot

M21.41 Flat foot [pes planus] (acquired), right foot

M21.42 Flat foot [pes planus] (acquired), left foot

M21.5 Acquired clawhand, clubhand, clawfoot and clubfoot

EXCLUDES 1 *clubfoot, not specified as acquired (Q66.89)*

M21.51 Acquired clawhand

M21.511 Acquired clawhand, right hand

M21.512 Acquired clawhand, left hand

M21.519 Acquired clawhand, unspecified hand

M21.52 Acquired clubhand

M21.521 Acquired clubhand, right hand

M21.522 Acquired clubhand, left hand

M21.529 Acquired clubhand, unspecified hand

M21.53 Acquired clawfoot

M21.531 Acquired clawfoot, right foot

M21.532 Acquired clawfoot, left foot

M21.539 Acquired clawfoot, unspecified foot

M21.54 Acquired clubfoot

M21.541 Acquired clubfoot, right foot

M21.542 Acquired clubfoot, left foot

M21.549 Acquired clubfoot, unspecified foot

M21.6 Other acquired deformities of foot

EXCLUDES 2 *deformities of toe (acquired) (M20.1-M20.6)*

M21.6X Other acquired deformities of foot

M21.6X1 Other acquired deformities of right foot

M21.6X2 Other acquired deformities of left foot

M21.6X9 Other acquired deformities of unspecified foot

5th **M21.7 Unequal limb length (acquired)**
NOTE The site used should correspond to the shorter limb
M21.70 Unequal limb length (acquired), unspecified site
6th **M21.72 Unequal limb length (acquired), humerus**
M21.721 Unequal limb length (acquired), right humerus
M21.722 Unequal limb length (acquired), left humerus
M21.729 Unequal limb length (acquired), unspecified humerus
6th **M21.73 Unequal limb length (acquired), ulna and radius**
M21.731 Unequal limb length (acquired), right ulna
M21.732 Unequal limb length (acquired), left ulna
M21.733 Unequal limb length (acquired), right radius
M21.734 Unequal limb length (acquired), left radius
M21.739 Unequal limb length (acquired), unspecified ulna and radius
6th **M21.75 Unequal limb length (acquired), femur**
M21.751 Unequal limb length (acquired), right femur
M21.752 Unequal limb length (acquired), left femur
M21.759 Unequal limb length (acquired), unspecified femur
6th **M21.76 Unequal limb length (acquired), tibia and fibula**
M21.761 Unequal limb length (acquired), right tibia
M21.762 Unequal limb length (acquired), left tibia
M21.763 Unequal limb length (acquired), right fibula
M21.764 Unequal limb length (acquired), left fibula
M21.769 Unequal limb length (acquired), unspecified tibia and fibula
5th **M21.8 Other specified acquired deformities of limbs**
EXCLUDES 2 *coxa plana (M91.2)*
M21.80 Other specified acquired deformities of unspecified limb
6th **M21.82 Other specified acquired deformities of upper arm**
M21.821 Other specified acquired deformities of right upper arm
M21.822 Other specified acquired deformities of left upper arm
M21.829 Other specified acquired deformities of unspecified upper arm
6th **M21.83 Other specified acquired deformities of forearm**
M21.831 Other specified acquired deformities of right forearm
M21.832 Other specified acquired deformities of left forearm
M21.839 Other specified acquired deformities of unspecified forearm
6th **M21.85 Other specified acquired deformities of thigh**
M21.851 Other specified acquired deformities of right thigh
M21.852 Other specified acquired deformities of left thigh
M21.859 Other specified acquired deformities of unspecified thigh
6th **M21.86 Other specified acquired deformities of lower leg**
M21.861 Other specified acquired deformities of right lower leg
M21.862 Other specified acquired deformities of left lower leg
M21.869 Other specified acquired deformities of unspecified lower leg
5th **M21.9 Unspecified acquired deformity of limb and hand**
M21.90 Unspecified acquired deformity of unspecified limb
6th **M21.92 Unspecified acquired deformity of upper arm**
M21.921 Unspecified acquired deformity of right upper arm
M21.922 Unspecified acquired deformity of left upper arm
M21.929 Unspecified acquired deformity of unspecified upper arm
6th **M21.93 Unspecified acquired deformity of forearm**
M21.931 Unspecified acquired deformity of right forearm
M21.932 Unspecified acquired deformity of left forearm
M21.939 Unspecified acquired deformity of unspecified forearm
6th **M21.94 Unspecified acquired deformity of hand**
M21.941 Unspecified acquired deformity of hand, right hand
M21.942 Unspecified acquired deformity of hand, left hand
M21.949 Unspecified acquired deformity of hand, unspecified hand
6th **M21.95 Unspecified acquired deformity of thigh**
M21.951 Unspecified acquired deformity of right thigh
M21.952 Unspecified acquired deformity of left thigh
M21.959 Unspecified acquired deformity of unspecified thigh
6th **M21.96 Unspecified acquired deformity of lower leg**
M21.961 Unspecified acquired deformity of right lower leg
M21.962 Unspecified acquired deformity of left lower leg
M21.969 Unspecified acquired deformity of unspecified lower leg

4th **M22 Disorder of patella**
EXCLUDES 1 *traumatic dislocation of patella (S83.0-)*
5th **M22.0 Recurrent dislocation of patella**
M22.00 Recurrent dislocation of patella, unspecified knee
M22.01 Recurrent dislocation of patella, right knee
M22.02 Recurrent dislocation of patella, left knee
5th **M22.1 Recurrent subluxation of patella**
Incomplete dislocation of patella
M22.10 Recurrent subluxation of patella, unspecified knee
M22.11 Recurrent subluxation of patella, right knee
M22.12 Recurrent subluxation of patella, left knee
5th **M22.2 Patellofemoral disorders**
6th **M22.2X Patellofemoral disorders**
M22.2X1 Patellofemoral disorders, right knee
M22.2X2 Patellofemoral disorders, left knee
M22.2X9 Patellofemoral disorders, unspecified knee
5th **M22.3 Other derangements of patella**
6th **M22.3X Other derangements of patella**
M22.3X1 Other derangements of patella, right knee
M22.3X2 Other derangements of patella, left knee
M22.3X9 Other derangements of patella, unspecified knee
5th **M22.4 Chondromalacia patellae**
M22.40 Chondromalacia patellae, unspecified knee
M22.41 Chondromalacia patellae, right knee
M22.42 Chondromalacia patellae, left knee
5th **M22.8 Other disorders of patella**
6th **M22.8X Other disorders of patella**
M22.8X1 Other disorders of patella, right knee
M22.8X2 Other disorders of patella, left knee
M22.8X9 Other disorders of patella, unspecified knee
5th **M22.9 Unspecified disorder of patella**
M22.90 Unspecified disorder of patella, unspecified knee
M22.91 Unspecified disorder of patella, right knee
M22.92 Unspecified disorder of patella, left knee

M23 Internal derangement of knee

EXCLUDES 1 *ankylosis (M24.66)*
current injury—see injury of knee and lower leg (S80-S89)
deformity of knee (M21.-)
osteochondritis dissecans (M93.2)
recurrent dislocation or subluxation of joints (M24.4)
recurrent dislocation or subluxation of patella (M22.0-M22.1)

M23.0 Cystic meniscus

M23.00 Cystic meniscus, unspecified meniscus
Cystic meniscus, unspecified lateral meniscus
Cystic meniscus, unspecified medial meniscus

M23.000 Cystic meniscus, unspecified lateral meniscus, right knee
M23.001 Cystic meniscus, unspecified lateral meniscus, left knee
M23.002 Cystic meniscus, unspecified lateral meniscus, unspecified knee
M23.003 Cystic meniscus, unspecified medial meniscus, right knee
M23.004 Cystic meniscus, unspecified medial meniscus, left knee
M23.005 Cystic meniscus, unspecified medial meniscus, unspecified knee
M23.006 Cystic meniscus, unspecified meniscus, right knee
M23.007 Cystic meniscus, unspecified meniscus, left knee
M23.009 Cystic meniscus, unspecified meniscus, unspecified knee

M23.01 Cystic meniscus, anterior horn of medial meniscus
M23.011 Cystic meniscus, anterior horn of medial meniscus, right knee
M23.012 Cystic meniscus, anterior horn of medial meniscus, left knee
M23.019 Cystic meniscus, anterior horn of medial meniscus, unspecified knee

M23.02 Cystic meniscus, posterior horn of medial meniscus
M23.021 Cystic meniscus, posterior horn of medial meniscus, right knee
M23.022 Cystic meniscus, posterior horn of medial meniscus, left knee
M23.029 Cystic meniscus, posterior horn of medial meniscus, unspecified knee

M23.03 Cystic meniscus, other medial meniscus
M23.031 Cystic meniscus, other medial meniscus, right knee
M23.032 Cystic meniscus, other medial meniscus, left knee
M23.039 Cystic meniscus, other medial meniscus, unspecified knee

M23.04 Cystic meniscus, anterior horn of lateral meniscus
M23.041 Cystic meniscus, anterior horn of lateral meniscus, right knee
M23.042 Cystic meniscus, anterior horn of lateral meniscus, left knee
M23.049 Cystic meniscus, anterior horn of lateral meniscus, unspecified knee

M23.05 Cystic meniscus, posterior horn of lateral meniscus
M23.051 Cystic meniscus, posterior horn of lateral meniscus, right knee
M23.052 Cystic meniscus, posterior horn of lateral meniscus, left knee
M23.059 Cystic meniscus, posterior horn of lateral meniscus, unspecified knee

M23.06 Cystic meniscus, other lateral meniscus
M23.061 Cystic meniscus, other lateral meniscus, right knee
M23.062 Cystic meniscus, other lateral meniscus, left knee
M23.069 Cystic meniscus, other lateral meniscus, unspecified knee

M23.2 Derangement of meniscus due to old tear or injury
Old bucket-handle tear

M23.20 Derangement of unspecified meniscus due to old tear or injury
Derangement of unspecified lateral meniscus due to old tear or injury
Derangement of unspecified medial meniscus due to old tear or injury

M23.200 Derangement of unspecified lateral meniscus due to old tear or injury, right knee
M23.201 Derangement of unspecified lateral meniscus due to old tear or injury, left knee
M23.202 Derangement of unspecified lateral meniscus due to old tear or injury, unspecified knee
M23.203 Derangement of unspecified medial meniscus due to old tear or injury, right knee
M23.204 Derangement of unspecified medial meniscus due to old tear or injury, left knee
M23.205 Derangement of unspecified medial meniscus due to old tear or injury, unspecified knee
M23.206 Derangement of unspecified meniscus due to old tear or injury, right knee
M23.207 Derangement of unspecified meniscus due to old tear or injury, left knee
M23.209 Derangement of unspecified meniscus due to old tear or injury, unspecified knee

M23.21 Derangement of anterior horn of medial meniscus due to old tear or injury
M23.211 Derangement of anterior horn of medial meniscus due to old tear or injury, right knee
M23.212 Derangement of anterior horn of medial meniscus due to old tear or injury, left knee
M23.219 Derangement of anterior horn of medial meniscus due to old tear or injury, unspecified knee

M23.22 Derangement of posterior horn of medial meniscus due to old tear or injury
M23.221 Derangement of posterior horn of medial meniscus due to old tear or injury, right knee
M23.222 Derangement of posterior horn of medial meniscus due to old tear or injury, left knee
M23.229 Derangement of posterior horn of medial meniscus due to old tear or injury, unspecified knee

M23.23 Derangement of other medial meniscus due to old tear or injury
M23.231 Derangement of other medial meniscus due to old tear or injury, right knee
M23.232 Derangement of other medial meniscus due to old tear or injury, left knee
M23.239 Derangement of other medial meniscus due to old tear or injury, unspecified knee

M23.24 Derangement of anterior horn of lateral meniscus due to old tear or injury
M23.241 Derangement of anterior horn of lateral meniscus due to old tear or injury, right knee
M23.242 Derangement of anterior horn of lateral meniscus due to old tear or injury, left knee
M23.249 Derangement of anterior horn of lateral meniscus due to old tear or injury, unspecified knee

6th **M23.25 Derangement of posterior horn of lateral meniscus due to old tear or injury**
- **M23.251 Derangement of posterior horn of lateral meniscus due to old tear or injury, right knee**
- **M23.252 Derangement of posterior horn of lateral meniscus due to old tear or injury, left knee**
- **M23.259 Derangement of posterior horn of lateral meniscus due to old tear or injury, unspecified knee**

6th **M23.26 Derangement of other lateral meniscus due to old tear or injury**
- **M23.261 Derangement of other lateral meniscus due to old tear or injury, right knee**
- **M23.262 Derangement of other lateral meniscus due to old tear or injury, left knee**
- **M23.269 Derangement of other lateral meniscus due to old tear or injury, unspecified knee**

5th **M23.3 Other meniscus derangements**

Degenerate meniscus
Detached meniscus
Retained meniscus

6th **M23.30 Other meniscus derangements, unspecified meniscus**

Other meniscus derangements, unspecified lateral meniscus
Other meniscus derangements, unspecified medial meniscus

- **M23.300 Other meniscus derangements, unspecified lateral meniscus, right knee**
- **M23.301 Other meniscus derangements, unspecified lateral meniscus, left knee**
- **M23.302 Other meniscus derangements, unspecified lateral meniscus, unspecified knee**
- **M23.303 Other meniscus derangements, unspecified medial meniscus, right knee**
- **M23.304 Other meniscus derangements, unspecified medial meniscus, left knee**
- **M23.305 Other meniscus derangements, unspecified medial meniscus, unspecified knee**
- **M23.306 Other meniscus derangements, unspecified meniscus, right knee**
- **M23.307 Other meniscus derangements, unspecified meniscus, left knee**
- **M23.309 Other meniscus derangements, unspecified meniscus, unspecified knee**

6th **M23.31 Other meniscus derangements, anterior horn of medial meniscus**
- **M23.311 Other meniscus derangements, anterior horn of medial meniscus, right knee**
- **M23.312 Other meniscus derangements, anterior horn of medial meniscus, left knee**
- **M23.319 Other meniscus derangements, anterior horn of medial meniscus, unspecified knee**

6th **M23.32 Other meniscus derangements, posterior horn of medial meniscus**
- **M23.321 Other meniscus derangements, posterior horn of medial meniscus, right knee**
- **M23.322 Other meniscus derangements, posterior horn of medial meniscus, left knee**
- **M23.329 Other meniscus derangements, posterior horn of medial meniscus, unspecified knee**

6th **M23.33 Other meniscus derangements, other medial meniscus**
- **M23.331 Other meniscus derangements, other medial meniscus, right knee**
- **M23.332 Other meniscus derangements, other medial meniscus, left knee**
- **M23.339 Other meniscus derangements, other medial meniscus, unspecified knee**

6th **M23.34 Other meniscus derangements, anterior horn of lateral meniscus**
- **M23.341 Other meniscus derangements, anterior horn of lateral meniscus, right knee**
- **M23.342 Other meniscus derangements, anterior horn of lateral meniscus, left knee**
- **M23.349 Other meniscus derangements, anterior horn of lateral meniscus, unspecified knee**

6th **M23.35 Other meniscus derangements, posterior horn of lateral meniscus**
- **M23.351 Other meniscus derangements, posterior horn of lateral meniscus, right knee**
- **M23.352 Other meniscus derangements, posterior horn of lateral meniscus, left knee**
- **M23.359 Other meniscus derangements, posterior horn of lateral meniscus, unspecified knee**

6th **M23.36 Other meniscus derangements, other lateral meniscus**
- **M23.361 Other meniscus derangements, other lateral meniscus, right knee**
- **M23.362 Other meniscus derangements, other lateral meniscus, left knee**
- **M23.369 Other meniscus derangements, other lateral meniscus, unspecified knee**

5th **M23.4 Loose body in knee**
- **M23.40 Loose body in knee, unspecified knee**
- **M23.41 Loose body in knee, right knee**
- **M23.42 Loose body in knee, left knee**

5th **M23.5 Chronic instability of knee**
- **M23.50 Chronic instability of knee, unspecified knee**
- **M23.51 Chronic instability of knee, right knee**
- **M23.52 Chronic instability of knee, left knee**

5th **M23.6 Other spontaneous disruption of ligament(s) of knee**

6th **M23.60 Other spontaneous disruption of unspecified ligament of knee**
- **M23.601 Other spontaneous disruption of unspecified ligament of right knee**
- **M23.602 Other spontaneous disruption of unspecified ligament of left knee**
- **M23.609 Other spontaneous disruption of unspecified ligament of unspecified knee**

6th **M23.61 Other spontaneous disruption of anterior cruciate ligament of knee**
- **M23.611 Other spontaneous disruption of anterior cruciate ligament of right knee**
- **M23.612 Other spontaneous disruption of anterior cruciate ligament of left knee**
- **M23.619 Other spontaneous disruption of anterior cruciate ligament of unspecified knee**

6th **M23.62 Other spontaneous disruption of posterior cruciate ligament of knee**
- **M23.621 Other spontaneous disruption of posterior cruciate ligament of right knee**
- **M23.622 Other spontaneous disruption of posterior cruciate ligament of left knee**
- **M23.629 Other spontaneous disruption of posterior cruciate ligament of unspecified knee**

6th **M23.63 Other spontaneous disruption of medial collateral ligament of knee**
- **M23.631 Other spontaneous disruption of medial collateral ligament of right knee**
- **M23.632 Other spontaneous disruption of medial collateral ligament of left knee**
- **M23.639 Other spontaneous disruption of medial collateral ligament of unspecified knee**

6th **M23.64 Other spontaneous disruption of lateral collateral ligament of knee**
- **M23.641 Other spontaneous disruption of lateral collateral ligament of right knee**
- **M23.642 Other spontaneous disruption of lateral collateral ligament of left knee**

M23.649 Other spontaneous disruption of lateral collateral ligament of unspecified knee

✓6th **M23.67 Other spontaneous disruption of capsular ligament of knee**

M23.671 Other spontaneous disruption of capsular ligament of right knee

M23.672 Other spontaneous disruption of capsular ligament of left knee

M23.679 Other spontaneous disruption of capsular ligament of unspecified knee

✓5th **M23.8 Other internal derangements of knee**

Laxity of ligament of knee

Snapping knee

✓6th **M23.8X Other internal derangements of knee**

M23.8X1 Other internal derangements of right knee

M23.8X2 Other internal derangements of left knee

M23.8X9 Other internal derangements of unspecified knee

✓5th **M23.9 Unspecified internal derangement of knee**

M23.90 Unspecified internal derangement of unspecified knee

M23.91 Unspecified internal derangement of right knee

M23.92 Unspecified internal derangement of left knee

✓4th **M24 Other specific joint derangements**

EXCLUDES 1 *current injury—see injury of joint by body region*

EXCLUDES 2 *ganglion (M67.4)*

snapping knee (M23.8-)

temporomandibular joint disorders (M26.6-)

✓5th **M24.0 Loose body in joint**

EXCLUDES 2 *loose body in knee (M23.4)*

M24.00 Loose body in unspecified joint

✓6th **M24.01 Loose body in shoulder**

M24.011 Loose body in right shoulder

M24.012 Loose body in left shoulder

M24.019 Loose body in unspecified shoulder

✓6th **M24.02 Loose body in elbow**

M24.021 Loose body in right elbow

M24.022 Loose body in left elbow

M24.029 Loose body in unspecified elbow

✓6th **M24.03 Loose body in wrist**

M24.031 Loose body in right wrist

M24.032 Loose body in left wrist

M24.039 Loose body in unspecified wrist

✓6th **M24.04 Loose body in finger joints**

M24.041 Loose body in right finger joint(s)

M24.042 Loose body in left finger joint(s)

M24.049 Loose body in unspecified finger joint(s)

✓6th **M24.05 Loose body in hip**

M24.051 Loose body in right hip

M24.052 Loose body in left hip

M24.059 Loose body in unspecified hip

✓6th **M24.07 Loose body in ankle and toe joints**

M24.071 Loose body in right ankle

M24.072 Loose body in left ankle

M24.073 Loose body in unspecified ankle

M24.074 Loose body in right toe joint(s)

M24.075 Loose body in left toe joint(s)

M24.076 Loose body in unspecified toe joints

M24.08 Loose body, other site

✓5th **M24.1 Other articular cartilage disorders**

EXCLUDES 2 *chondrocalcinosis (M11.1, M11.2-)*

internal derangement of knee (M23.-)

metastatic calcification (E83.5)

ochronosis (E70.2)

M24.10 Other articular cartilage disorders, unspecified site

✓6th **M24.11 Other articular cartilage disorders, shoulder**

M24.111 Other articular cartilage disorders, right shoulder

M24.112 Other articular cartilage disorders, left shoulder

M24.119 Other articular cartilage disorders, unspecified shoulder

✓6th **M24.12 Other articular cartilage disorders, elbow**

M24.121 Other articular cartilage disorders, right elbow

M24.122 Other articular cartilage disorders, left elbow

M24.129 Other articular cartilage disorders, unspecified elbow

✓6th **M24.13 Other articular cartilage disorders, wrist**

M24.131 Other articular cartilage disorders, right wrist

M24.132 Other articular cartilage disorders, left wrist

M24.139 Other articular cartilage disorders, unspecified wrist

✓6th **M24.14 Other articular cartilage disorders, hand**

M24.141 Other articular cartilage disorders, right hand

M24.142 Other articular cartilage disorders, left hand

M24.149 Other articular cartilage disorders, unspecified hand

✓6th **M24.15 Other articular cartilage disorders, hip**

M24.151 Other articular cartilage disorders, right hip

M24.152 Other articular cartilage disorders, left hip

M24.159 Other articular cartilage disorders, unspecified hip

✓6th **M24.17 Other articular cartilage disorders, ankle and foot**

M24.171 Other articular cartilage disorders, right ankle

M24.172 Other articular cartilage disorders, left ankle

M24.173 Other articular cartilage disorders, unspecified ankle

M24.174 Other articular cartilage disorders, right foot

M24.175 Other articular cartilage disorders, left foot

M24.176 Other articular cartilage disorders, unspecified foot

✓5th **M24.2 Disorder of ligament**

Instability secondary to old ligament injury

Ligamentous laxity NOS

EXCLUDES 1 *familial ligamentous laxity (M35.7)*

EXCLUDES 2 *internal derangement of knee (M23.5-M23.89)*

M24.20 Disorder of ligament, unspecified site

✓6th **M24.21 Disorder of ligament, shoulder**

M24.211 Disorder of ligament, right shoulder

M24.212 Disorder of ligament, left shoulder

M24.219 Disorder of ligament, unspecified shoulder

✓6th **M24.22 Disorder of ligament, elbow**

M24.221 Disorder of ligament, right elbow

M24.222 Disorder of ligament, left elbow

M24.229 Disorder of ligament, unspecified elbow

✓6th **M24.23 Disorder of ligament, wrist**

M24.231 Disorder of ligament, right wrist

M24.232 Disorder of ligament, left wrist

M24.239 Disorder of ligament, unspecified wrist

✓6th **M24.24 Disorder of ligament, hand**

M24.241 Disorder of ligament, right hand

M24.242 Disorder of ligament, left hand

M24.249 Disorder of ligament, unspecified hand

✓6th **M24.25 Disorder of ligament, hip**

M24.251 Disorder of ligament, right hip

M24.252 Disorder of ligament, left hip

M24.259 Disorder of ligament, unspecified hip

✓6th **M24.27 Disorder of ligament, ankle and foot**

M24.271 Disorder of ligament, right ankle

M24.272 Disorder of ligament, left ankle

M24.273 Disorder of ligament, unspecified ankle

M24.274 Disorder of ligament, right foot

M24.275 Disorder of ligament, left foot

M24.276 Disorder of ligament, unspecified foot

M24.28 Disorder of ligament, vertebrae

✓ Appropriate additional character required ✓x7th Requires 7th character, placeholder x must fill empty characters

M24.3 Pathological dislocation of joint, not elsewhere classified
EXCLUDES 1 *congenital dislocation or displacement of joint—see congenital malformations and deformations of the musculoskeletal system (Q65-Q79)*
current injury—see injury of joints and ligaments by body region
recurrent dislocation of joint (M24.4-)
M24.30 Pathological dislocation of unspecified joint, not elsewhere classified
M24.31 Pathological dislocation of shoulder, not elsewhere classified
M24.311 Pathological dislocation of right shoulder, not elsewhere classified
M24.312 Pathological dislocation of left shoulder, not elsewhere classified
M24.319 Pathological dislocation of unspecified shoulder, not elsewhere classified
M24.32 Pathological dislocation of elbow, not elsewhere classified
M24.321 Pathological dislocation of right elbow, not elsewhere classified
M24.322 Pathological dislocation of left elbow, not elsewhere classified
M24.329 Pathological dislocation of unspecified elbow, not elsewhere classified
M24.33 Pathological dislocation of wrist, not elsewhere classified
M24.331 Pathological dislocation of right wrist, not elsewhere classified
M24.332 Pathological dislocation of left wrist, not elsewhere classified
M24.339 Pathological dislocation of unspecified wrist, not elsewhere classified
M24.34 Pathological dislocation of hand, not elsewhere classified
M24.341 Pathological dislocation of right hand, not elsewhere classified
M24.342 Pathological dislocation of left hand, not elsewhere classified
M24.349 Pathological dislocation of unspecified hand, not elsewhere classified
M24.35 Pathological dislocation of hip, not elsewhere classified
M24.351 Pathological dislocation of right hip, not elsewhere classified
M24.352 Pathological dislocation of left hip, not elsewhere classified
M24.359 Pathological dislocation of unspecified hip, not elsewhere classified
M24.36 Pathological dislocation of knee, not elsewhere classified
M24.361 Pathological dislocation of right knee, not elsewhere classified
M24.362 Pathological dislocation of left knee, not elsewhere classified
M24.369 Pathological dislocation of unspecified knee, not elsewhere classified
M24.37 Pathological dislocation of ankle and foot, not elsewhere classified
M24.371 Pathological dislocation of right ankle, not elsewhere classified
M24.372 Pathological dislocation of left ankle, not elsewhere classified
M24.373 Pathological dislocation of unspecified ankle, not elsewhere classified
M24.374 Pathological dislocation of right foot, not elsewhere classified
M24.375 Pathological dislocation of left foot, not elsewhere classified
M24.376 Pathological dislocation of unspecified foot, not elsewhere classified

M24.4 Recurrent dislocation of joint
Recurrent subluxation of joint
EXCLUDES 2 *recurrent dislocation of patella (M22.0-M22.1)*
recurrent vertebral dislocation (M43.3-, M43.4, M43.5-)
M24.40 Recurrent dislocation, unspecified joint
M24.41 Recurrent dislocation, shoulder
M24.411 Recurrent dislocation, right shoulder
M24.412 Recurrent dislocation, left shoulder
M24.419 Recurrent dislocation, unspecified shoulder
M24.42 Recurrent dislocation, elbow
M24.421 Recurrent dislocation, right elbow
M24.422 Recurrent dislocation, left elbow
M24.429 Recurrent dislocation, unspecified elbow
M24.43 Recurrent dislocation, wrist
M24.431 Recurrent dislocation, right wrist
M24.432 Recurrent dislocation, left wrist
M24.439 Recurrent dislocation, unspecified wrist
M24.44 Recurrent dislocation, hand and finger(s)
M24.441 Recurrent dislocation, right hand
M24.442 Recurrent dislocation, left hand
M24.443 Recurrent dislocation, unspecified hand
M24.444 Recurrent dislocation, right finger
M24.445 Recurrent dislocation, left finger
M24.446 Recurrent dislocation, unspecified finger
M24.45 Recurrent dislocation, hip
M24.451 Recurrent dislocation, right hip
M24.452 Recurrent dislocation, left hip
M24.459 Recurrent dislocation, unspecified hip
M24.46 Recurrent dislocation, knee
M24.461 Recurrent dislocation, right knee
M24.462 Recurrent dislocation, left knee
M24.469 Recurrent dislocation, unspecified knee
M24.47 Recurrent dislocation, ankle, foot and toes
M24.471 Recurrent dislocation, right ankle
M24.472 Recurrent dislocation, left ankle
M24.473 Recurrent dislocation, unspecified ankle
M24.474 Recurrent dislocation, right foot
M24.475 Recurrent dislocation, left foot
M24.476 Recurrent dislocation, unspecified foot
M24.477 Recurrent dislocation, right toe(s)
M24.478 Recurrent dislocation, left toe(s)
M24.479 Recurrent dislocation, unspecified toe(s)

M24.5 Contracture of joint
EXCLUDES 1 *contracture of muscle without contracture of joint (M62.4-)*
contracture of tendon (sheath) without contracture of joint (M62.4-)
Dupuytren's contracture (M72.0)
EXCLUDES 2 *acquired deformities of limbs (M20-M21)*
M24.50 Contracture, unspecified joint
M24.51 Contracture, shoulder
M24.511 Contracture, right shoulder
M24.512 Contracture, left shoulder
M24.519 Contracture, unspecified shoulder
M24.52 Contracture, elbow
M24.521 Contracture, right elbow
M24.522 Contracture, left elbow
M24.529 Contracture, unspecified elbow
M24.53 Contracture, wrist
M24.531 Contracture, right wrist
M24.532 Contracture, left wrist
M24.539 Contracture, unspecified wrist
M24.54 Contracture, hand
M24.541 Contracture, right hand
M24.542 Contracture, left hand
M24.549 Contracture, unspecified hand
M24.55 Contracture, hip
M24.551 Contracture, right hip
M24.552 Contracture, left hip
M24.559 Contracture, unspecified hip
M24.56 Contracture, knee
M24.561 Contracture, right knee
M24.562 Contracture, left knee
M24.569 Contracture, unspecified knee
M24.57 Contracture, ankle and foot
M24.571 Contracture, right ankle
M24.572 Contracture, left ankle

EXCLUDES 1 Not coded here EXCLUDES 2 Not included here *Manifestation Code*

M24.573 Contracture, unspecified ankle
M24.574 Contracture, right foot
M24.575 Contracture, left foot
M24.576 Contracture, unspecified foot

✓5th M24.6 Ankylosis of joint
EXCLUDES 1 *stiffness of joint without ankylosis (M25.6-)*
EXCLUDES 2 *spine (M43.2-)*
M24.60 Ankylosis, unspecified joint
✓6th M24.61 Ankylosis, shoulder
M24.611 Ankylosis, right shoulder
M24.612 Ankylosis, left shoulder
M24.619 Ankylosis, unspecified shoulder
✓6th M24.62 Ankylosis, elbow
M24.621 Ankylosis, right elbow
M24.622 Ankylosis, left elbow
M24.629 Ankylosis, unspecified elbow
✓6th M24.63 Ankylosis, wrist
M24.631 Ankylosis, right wrist
M24.632 Ankylosis, left wrist
M24.639 Ankylosis, unspecified wrist
✓6th M24.64 Ankylosis, hand
M24.641 Ankylosis, right hand
M24.642 Ankylosis, left hand
M24.649 Ankylosis, unspecified hand
✓6th M24.65 Ankylosis, hip
M24.651 Ankylosis, right hip
M24.652 Ankylosis, left hip
M24.659 Ankylosis, unspecified hip
✓6th M24.66 Ankylosis, knee
M24.661 Ankylosis, right knee
M24.662 Ankylosis, left knee
M24.669 Ankylosis, unspecified knee
✓6th M24.67 Ankylosis, ankle and foot
M24.671 Ankylosis, right ankle
M24.672 Ankylosis, left ankle
M24.673 Ankylosis, unspecified ankle
M24.674 Ankylosis, right foot
M24.675 Ankylosis, left foot
M24.676 Ankylosis, unspecified foot

M24.7 Protrusio acetabuli

✓5th M24.8 Other specific joint derangements, not elsewhere classified
EXCLUDES 2 *iliotibial band syndrome (M76.3)*
M24.80 Other specific joint derangements of unspecified joint, not elsewhere classified
✓6th M24.81 Other specific joint derangements of shoulder, not elsewhere classified
M24.811 Other specific joint derangements of right shoulder, not elsewhere classified
M24.812 Other specific joint derangements of left shoulder, not elsewhere classified
M24.819 Other specific joint derangements of unspecified shoulder, not elsewhere classified
✓6th M24.82 Other specific joint derangements of elbow, not elsewhere classified
M24.821 Other specific joint derangements of right elbow, not elsewhere classified
M24.822 Other specific joint derangements of left elbow, not elsewhere classified
M24.829 Other specific joint derangements of unspecified elbow, not elsewhere classified
✓6th M24.83 Other specific joint derangements of wrist, not elsewhere classified
M24.831 Other specific joint derangements of right wrist, not elsewhere classified
M24.832 Other specific joint derangements of left wrist, not elsewhere classified
M24.839 Other specific joint derangements of unspecified wrist, not elsewhere classified
✓6th M24.84 Other specific joint derangements of hand, not elsewhere classified
M24.841 Other specific joint derangements of right hand, not elsewhere classified
M24.842 Other specific joint derangements of left hand, not elsewhere classified
M24.849 Other specific joint derangements of unspecified hand, not elsewhere classified
✓6th M24.85 Other specific joint derangements of hip, not elsewhere classified
Irritable hip
M24.851 Other specific joint derangements of right hip, not elsewhere classified
M24.852 Other specific joint derangements of left hip, not elsewhere classified
M24.859 Other specific joint derangements of unspecified hip, not elsewhere classified
✓6th M24.87 Other specific joint derangements of ankle and foot, not elsewhere classified
M24.871 Other specific joint derangements of right ankle, not elsewhere classified
M24.872 Other specific joint derangements of left ankle, not elsewhere classified
M24.873 Other specific joint derangements of unspecified ankle, not elsewhere classified
M24.874 Other specific joint derangements of right foot, not elsewhere classified
M24.875 Other specific joint derangements left foot, not elsewhere classified
M24.876 Other specific joint derangements of unspecified foot, not elsewhere classified

M24.9 Joint derangement, unspecified

M25 Other joint disorder, not elsewhere classified

EXCLUDES 2 *abnormality of gait and mobility (R26.-)*
acquired deformities of limb (M20-M21)
calcification of bursa (M71.4-)
calcification of shoulder (joint) (M75.3)
calcification of tendon (M65.2-)
difficulty in walking (R26.2)
temporomandibular joint disorder (M26.6-)

✓5th M25.0 Hemarthrosis
EXCLUDES 1 *current injury—see injury of joint by body region*
hemophilic arthropathy (M36.2)
M25.00 Hemarthrosis, unspecified joint
✓6th M25.01 Hemarthrosis, shoulder
M25.011 Hemarthrosis, right shoulder
M25.012 Hemarthrosis, left shoulder
M25.019 Hemarthrosis, unspecified shoulder
✓6th M25.02 Hemarthrosis, elbow
M25.021 Hemarthrosis, right elbow
M25.022 Hemarthrosis, left elbow
M25.029 Hemarthrosis, unspecified elbow
✓6th M25.03 Hemarthrosis, wrist
M25.031 Hemarthrosis, right wrist
M25.032 Hemarthrosis, left wrist
M25.039 Hemarthrosis, unspecified wrist
✓6th M25.04 Hemarthrosis, hand
M25.041 Hemarthrosis, right hand
M25.042 Hemarthrosis, left hand
M25.049 Hemarthrosis, unspecified hand
✓6th M25.05 Hemarthrosis, hip
M25.051 Hemarthrosis, right hip
M25.052 Hemarthrosis, left hip
M25.059 Hemarthrosis, unspecified hip
✓6th M25.06 Hemarthrosis, knee
M25.061 Hemarthrosis, right knee
M25.062 Hemarthrosis, left knee
M25.069 Hemarthrosis, unspecified knee
✓6th M25.07 Hemarthrosis, ankle and foot
M25.071 Hemarthrosis, right ankle
M25.072 Hemarthrosis, left ankle
M25.073 Hemarthrosis, unspecified ankle
M25.074 Hemarthrosis, right foot
M25.075 Hemarthrosis, left foot
M25.076 Hemarthrosis, unspecified foot
M25.08 Hemarthrosis, vertebrae

✓5th **M25.1 Fistula of joint**
- **M25.10 Fistula, unspecified joint**
- ✓6th **M25.11 Fistula, shoulder**
  - **M25.111 Fistula, right shoulder**
  - **M25.112 Fistula, left shoulder**
  - **M25.119 Fistula, unspecified shoulder**
- ✓6th **M25.12 Fistula, elbow**
  - **M25.121 Fistula, right elbow**
  - **M25.122 Fistula, left elbow**
  - **M25.129 Fistula, unspecified elbow**
- ✓6th **M25.13 Fistula, wrist**
  - **M25.131 Fistula, right wrist**
  - **M25.132 Fistula, left wrist**
  - **M25.139 Fistula, unspecified wrist**
- ✓6th **M25.14 Fistula, hand**
  - **M25.141 Fistula, right hand**
  - **M25.142 Fistula, left hand**
  - **M25.149 Fistula, unspecified hand**
- ✓6th **M25.15 Fistula, hip**
  - **M25.151 Fistula, right hip**
  - **M25.152 Fistula, left hip**
  - **M25.159 Fistula, unspecified hip**
- ✓6th **M25.16 Fistula, knee**
  - **M25.161 Fistula, right knee**
  - **M25.162 Fistula, left knee**
  - **M25.169 Fistula, unspecified knee**
- ✓6th **M25.17 Fistula, ankle and foot**
  - **M25.171 Fistula, right ankle**
  - **M25.172 Fistula, left ankle**
  - **M25.173 Fistula, unspecified ankle**
  - **M25.174 Fistula, right foot**
  - **M25.175 Fistula, left foot**
  - **M25.176 Fistula, unspecified foot**
- **M25.18 Fistula, vertebrae**

✓5th **M25.2 Flail joint**
- **M25.20 Flail joint, unspecified joint**
- ✓6th **M25.21 Flail joint, shoulder**
  - **M25.211 Flail joint, right shoulder**
  - **M25.212 Flail joint, left shoulder**
  - **M25.219 Flail joint, unspecified shoulder**
- ✓6th **M25.22 Flail joint, elbow**
  - **M25.221 Flail joint, right elbow**
  - **M25.222 Flail joint, left elbow**
  - **M25.229 Flail joint, unspecified elbow**
- ✓6th **M25.23 Flail joint, wrist**
  - **M25.231 Flail joint, right wrist**
  - **M25.232 Flail joint, left wrist**
  - **M25.239 Flail joint, unspecified wrist**
- ✓6th **M25.24 Flail joint, hand**
  - **M25.241 Flail joint, right hand**
  - **M25.242 Flail joint, left hand**
  - **M25.249 Flail joint, unspecified hand**
- ✓6th **M25.25 Flail joint, hip**
  - **M25.251 Flail joint, right hip**
  - **M25.252 Flail joint, left hip**
  - **M25.259 Flail joint, unspecified hip**
- ✓6th **M25.26 Flail joint, knee**
  - **M25.261 Flail joint, right knee**
  - **M25.262 Flail joint, left knee**
  - **M25.269 Flail joint, unspecified knee**
- ✓6th **M25.27 Flail joint, ankle and foot**
  - **M25.271 Flail joint, right ankle and foot**
  - **M25.272 Flail joint, left ankle and foot**
  - **M25.279 Flail joint, unspecified ankle and foot**
- **M25.28 Flail joint, other site**

✓5th **M25.3 Other instability of joint**

EXCLUDES 1 *instability of joint secondary to old ligament injury (M24.2-)*
instability of joint secondary to removal of joint prosthesis (M96.8-)

EXCLUDES 2 *spinal instabilities (M53.2-)*

- **M25.30 Other instability, unspecified joint**
- ✓6th **M25.31 Other instability, shoulder**
  - **M25.311 Other instability, right shoulder**
  - **M25.312 Other instability, left shoulder**
  - **M25.319 Other instability, unspecified shoulder**
- ✓6th **M25.32 Other instability, elbow**
  - **M25.321 Other instability, right elbow**
  - **M25.322 Other instability, left elbow**
  - **M25.329 Other instability, unspecified elbow**
- ✓6th **M25.33 Other instability, wrist**
  - **M25.331 Other instability, right wrist**
  - **M25.332 Other instability, left wrist**
  - **M25.339 Other instability, unspecified wrist**
- ✓6th **M25.34 Other instability, hand**
  - **M25.341 Other instability, right hand**
  - **M25.342 Other instability, left hand**
  - **M25.349 Other instability, unspecified hand**
- ✓6th **M25.35 Other instability, hip**
  - **M25.351 Other instability, right hip**
  - **M25.352 Other instability, left hip**
  - **M25.359 Other instability, unspecified hip**
- ✓6th **M25.36 Other instability, knee**
  - **M25.361 Other instability, right knee**
  - **M25.362 Other instability, left knee**
  - **M25.369 Other instability, unspecified knee**
- ✓6th **M25.37 Other instability, ankle and foot**
  - **M25.371 Other instability, right ankle**
  - **M25.372 Other instability, left ankle**
  - **M25.373 Other instability, unspecified ankle**
  - **M25.374 Other instability, right foot**
  - **M25.375 Other instability, left foot**
  - **M25.376 Other instability, unspecified foot**

✓5th **M25.4 Effusion of joint**

EXCLUDES 1 *hydrarthrosis in yaws (A66.6)*
intermittent hydrarthrosis (M12.4-)
other infective (teno)synovitis (M65.1-)

- **M25.40 Effusion, unspecified joint**
- ✓6th **M25.41 Effusion, shoulder**
  - **M25.411 Effusion, right shoulder**
  - **M25.412 Effusion, left shoulder**
  - **M25.419 Effusion, unspecified shoulder**
- ✓6th **M25.42 Effusion, elbow**
  - **M25.421 Effusion, right elbow**
  - **M25.422 Effusion, left elbow**
  - **M25.429 Effusion, unspecified elbow**
- ✓6th **M25.43 Effusion, wrist**
  - **M25.431 Effusion, right wrist**
  - **M25.432 Effusion, left wrist**
  - **M25.439 Effusion, unspecified wrist**
- ✓6th **M25.44 Effusion, hand**
  - **M25.441 Effusion, right hand**
  - **M25.442 Effusion, left hand**
  - **M25.449 Effusion, unspecified hand**
- ✓6th **M25.45 Effusion, hip**
  - **M25.451 Effusion, right hip**
  - **M25.452 Effusion, left hip**
  - **M25.459 Effusion, unspecified hip**
- ✓6th **M25.46 Effusion, knee**
  - **M25.461 Effusion, right knee**
  - **M25.462 Effusion, left knee**
  - **M25.469 Effusion, unspecified knee**
- ✓6th **M25.47 Effusion, ankle and foot**
  - **M25.471 Effusion, right ankle**
  - **M25.472 Effusion, left ankle**
  - **M25.473 Effusion, unspecified ankle**
  - **M25.474 Effusion, right foot**
  - **M25.475 Effusion, left foot**
  - **M25.476 Effusion, unspecified foot**
- **M25.48 Effusion, other site**

✓5th **M25.5 Pain in joint**

EXCLUDES 2 *pain in hand (M79.64-)*
pain in fingers (M79.64-)
pain in foot (M79.67-)
pain in limb (M79.6-)
pain in toes (M79.67-)

- **M25.50 Pain in unspecified joint**
- ✓6th **M25.51 Pain in shoulder**
  - **M25.511 Pain in right shoulder**

M25.512 Pain in left shoulder
M25.519 Pain in unspecified shoulder
✓6th M25.52 Pain in elbow
M25.521 Pain in right elbow
M25.522 Pain in left elbow
M25.529 Pain in unspecified elbow
✓6th M25.53 Pain in wrist
M25.531 Pain in right wrist
M25.532 Pain in left wrist
M25.539 Pain in unspecified wrist
✓6th M25.55 Pain in hip
M25.551 Pain in right hip
M25.552 Pain in left hip
M25.559 Pain in unspecified hip
✓6th M25.56 Pain in knee
M25.561 Pain in right knee
M25.562 Pain in left knee
M25.569 Pain in unspecified knee
✓6th M25.57 Pain in ankle
M25.571 Pain in right ankle
M25.572 Pain in left ankle
M25.579 Pain in unspecified ankle
✓5th M25.6 Stiffness of joint, not elsewhere classified
EXCLUDES 1 *ankylosis of joint (M24.6-)*
contracture of joint (M24.5-)
M25.60 Stiffness of unspecified joint, not elsewhere classified
✓6th M25.61 Stiffness of shoulder, not elsewhere classified
M25.611 Stiffness of right shoulder, not elsewhere classified
M25.612 Stiffness of left shoulder, not elsewhere classified
M25.619 Stiffness of unspecified shoulder, not elsewhere classified
✓6th M25.62 Stiffness of elbow, not elsewhere classified
M25.621 Stiffness of right elbow, not elsewhere classified
M25.622 Stiffness of left elbow, not elsewhere classified
M25.629 Stiffness of unspecified elbow, not elsewhere classified
✓6th M25.63 Stiffness of wrist, not elsewhere classified
M25.631 Stiffness of right wrist, not elsewhere classified
M25.632 Stiffness of left wrist, not elsewhere classified
M25.639 Stiffness of unspecified wrist, not elsewhere classified
✓6th M25.64 Stiffness of hand, not elsewhere classified
M25.641 Stiffness of right hand, not elsewhere classified
M25.642 Stiffness of left hand, not elsewhere classified
M25.649 Stiffness of unspecified hand, not elsewhere classified
✓6th M25.65 Stiffness of hip, not elsewhere classified
M25.651 Stiffness of right hip, not elsewhere classified
M25.652 Stiffness of left hip, not elsewhere classified
M25.659 Stiffness of unspecified hip, not elsewhere classified
✓6th M25.66 Stiffness of knee, not elsewhere classified
M25.661 Stiffness of right knee, not elsewhere classified
M25.662 Stiffness of left knee, not elsewhere classified
M25.669 Stiffness of unspecified knee, not elsewhere classified
✓6th M25.67 Stiffness of ankle and foot, not elsewhere classified
M25.671 Stiffness of right ankle, not elsewhere classified
M25.672 Stiffness of left ankle, not elsewhere classified
M25.673 Stiffness of unspecified ankle, not elsewhere classified
M25.674 Stiffness of right foot, not elsewhere classified
M25.675 Stiffness of left foot, not elsewhere classified
M25.676 Stiffness of unspecified foot, not elsewhere classified
✓5th M25.7 Osteophyte
M25.70 Osteophyte, unspecified joint
✓6th M25.71 Osteophyte, shoulder
M25.711 Osteophyte, right shoulder
M25.712 Osteophyte, left shoulder
M25.719 Osteophyte, unspecified shoulder
✓6th M25.72 Osteophyte, elbow
M25.721 Osteophyte, right elbow
M25.722 Osteophyte, left elbow
M25.729 Osteophyte, unspecified elbow
✓6th M25.73 Osteophyte, wrist
M25.731 Osteophyte, right wrist
M25.732 Osteophyte, left wrist
M25.739 Osteophyte, unspecified wrist
✓6th M25.74 Osteophyte, hand
M25.741 Osteophyte, right hand
M25.742 Osteophyte, left hand
M25.749 Osteophyte, unspecified hand
✓6th M25.75 Osteophyte, hip
M25.751 Osteophyte, right hip
M25.752 Osteophyte, left hip
M25.759 Osteophyte, unspecified hip
✓6th M25.76 Osteophyte, knee
M25.761 Osteophyte, right knee
M25.762 Osteophyte, left knee
M25.769 Osteophyte, unspecified knee
✓6th M25.77 Osteophyte, ankle and foot
M25.771 Osteophyte, right ankle
M25.772 Osteophyte, left ankle
M25.773 Osteophyte, unspecified ankle
M25.774 Osteophyte, right foot
M25.775 Osteophyte, left foot
M25.776 Osteophyte, unspecified foot
M25.78 Osteophyte, vertebrae
✓5th M25.8 Other specified joint disorders
M25.80 Other specified joint disorders, unspecified joint
✓6th M25.81 Other specified joint disorders, shoulder
M25.811 Other specified joint disorders, right shoulder
M25.812 Other specified joint disorders, left shoulder
M25.819 Other specified joint disorders, unspecified shoulder
✓6th M25.82 Other specified joint disorders, elbow
M25.821 Other specified joint disorders, right elbow
M25.822 Other specified joint disorders, left elbow
M25.829 Other specified joint disorders, unspecified elbow
✓6th M25.83 Other specified joint disorders, wrist
M25.831 Other specified joint disorders, right wrist
M25.832 Other specified joint disorders, left wrist
M25.839 Other specified joint disorders, unspecified wrist
✓6th M25.84 Other specified joint disorders, hand
M25.841 Other specified joint disorders, right hand
M25.842 Other specified joint disorders, left hand
M25.849 Other specified joint disorders, unspecified hand
✓6th M25.85 Other specified joint disorders, hip
M25.851 Other specified joint disorders, right hip
M25.852 Other specified joint disorders, left hip
M25.859 Other specified joint disorders, unspecified hip
✓6th M25.86 Other specified joint disorders, knee
M25.861 Other specified joint disorders, right knee

M25.862 Other specified joint disorders, left knee
M25.869 Other specified joint disorders, unspecified knee
✓6th **M25.87 Other specified joint disorders, ankle and foot**
M25.871 Other specified joint disorders, right ankle and foot
M25.872 Other specified joint disorders, left ankle and foot
M25.879 Other specified joint disorders, unspecified ankle and foot
M25.9 Joint disorder, unspecified

Dentofacial anomalies [including malocclusion] and other disorders of jaw (M26-M27)

EXCLUDES 1 *hemifacial atrophy or hypertrophy (Q67.4)*
unilateral condylar hyperplasia or hypoplasia (M27.8)

✓4th **M26 Dentofacial anomalies [including malocclusion]**
✓5th **M26.0 Major anomalies of jaw size**
EXCLUDES 1 *acromegaly (E22.0)*
Robin's syndrome (Q87.0)
M26.00 Unspecified anomaly of jaw size
M26.01 Maxillary hyperplasia
M26.02 Maxillary hypoplasia
M26.03 Mandibular hyperplasia
M26.04 Mandibular hypoplasia
M26.05 Macrogenia
M26.06 Microgenia
M26.07 Excessive tuberosity of jaw
Entire maxillary tuberosity
M26.09 Other specified anomalies of jaw size
✓5th **M26.1 Anomalies of jaw-cranial base relationship**
M26.10 Unspecified anomaly of jaw-cranial base relationship
M26.11 Maxillary asymmetry
M26.12 Other jaw asymmetry
M26.19 Other specified anomalies of jaw-cranial base relationship
✓5th **M26.2 Anomalies of dental arch relationship**
M26.20 Unspecified anomaly of dental arch relationship
✓6th **M26.21 Malocclusion, Angle's class**
M26.211 Malocclusion, Angle's class I
Neutro-occlusion
M26.212 Malocclusion, Angle's class II
Disto-occlusion Division I
Disto-occlusion Division II
M26.213 Malocclusion, Angle's class III
Mesio-occlusion
M26.219 Malocclusion, Angle's class, unspecified
✓6th **M26.22 Open occlusal relationship**
M26.220 Open anterior occlusal relationship
Anterior openbite
M26.221 Open posterior occlusal relationship
Posterior openbite
M26.23 Excessive horizontal overlap
Excessive horizontal overjet
M26.24 Reverse articulation
Crossbite (anterior) (posterior)
M26.25 Anomalies of interarch distance
M26.29 Other anomalies of dental arch relationship
Midline deviation of dental arch
Overbite (excessive) deep
Overbite (excessive) horizontal
Overbite (excessive) vertical
Posterior lingual occlusion of mandibular teeth
✓5th **M26.3 Anomalies of tooth position of fully erupted tooth or teeth**
EXCLUDES 2 *embedded and impacted teeth (K01.-)*
M26.30 Unspecified anomaly of tooth position of fully erupted tooth or teeth
Abnormal spacing of fully erupted tooth or teeth NOS
Displacement of fully erupted tooth or teeth NOS
Transposition of fully erupted tooth or teeth NOS
M26.31 Crowding of fully erupted teeth
M26.32 Excessive spacing of fully erupted teeth
Diastema of fully erupted tooth or teeth NOS
M26.33 Horizontal displacement of fully erupted tooth or teeth
Tipped tooth or teeth
Tipping of fully erupted tooth
M26.34 Vertical displacement of fully erupted tooth or teeth
Extruded tooth
Infraeruption of tooth or teeth
Supraeruption of tooth or teeth
M26.35 Rotation of fully erupted tooth or teeth
M26.36 Insufficient interocclusal distance of fully erupted teeth (ridge)
Lack of adequate intermaxillary vertical dimension of fully erupted teeth
M26.37 Excessive interocclusal distance of fully erupted teeth
Excessive intermaxillary vertical dimension of fully erupted teeth
Loss of occlusal vertical dimension of fully erupted teeth
M26.39 Other anomalies of tooth position of fully erupted tooth or teeth
M26.4 Malocclusion, unspecified
✓5th **M26.5 Dentofacial functional abnormalities**
EXCLUDES 1 *bruxism (F45.8)*
teeth-grinding NOS (F45.8)
M26.50 Dentofacial functional abnormalities, unspecified
M26.51 Abnormal jaw closure
M26.52 Limited mandibular range of motion
M26.53 Deviation in opening and closing of the mandible
M26.54 Insufficient anterior guidance
Insufficient anterior occlusal guidance
M26.55 Centric occlusion maximum intercuspation discrepancy
EXCLUDES 1 *centric occlusion NOS (M26.59)*
M26.56 Non-working side interference
Balancing side interference
M26.57 Lack of posterior occlusal support
M26.59 Other dentofacial functional abnormalities
Centric occlusion (of teeth) NOS
Malocclusion due to abnormal swallowing
Malocclusion due to mouth breathing
Malocclusion due to tongue, lip or finger habits
✓5th **M26.6 Temporomandibular joint disorders**
EXCLUDES 2 *current temporomandibular joint dislocation (S03.0)*
current temporomandibular joint sprain (S03.4)
M26.60 Temporomandibular joint disorder, unspecified
M26.61 Adhesions and ankylosis of temporomandibular joint
M26.62 Arthralgia of temporomandibular joint
M26.63 Articular disc disorder of temporomandibular joint
M26.69 Other specified disorders of temporomandibular joint
✓5th **M26.7 Dental alveolar anomalies**
M26.70 Unspecified alveolar anomaly
M26.71 Alveolar maxillary hyperplasia
M26.72 Alveolar mandibular hyperplasia
M26.73 Alveolar maxillary hypoplasia
M26.74 Alveolar mandibular hypoplasia
M26.79 Other specified alveolar anomalies
✓5th **M26.8 Other dentofacial anomalies**
M26.81 Anterior soft tissue impingement
Anterior soft tissue impingement on teeth
M26.82 Posterior soft tissue impingement
Posterior soft tissue impingement on teeth
M26.89 Other dentofacial anomalies
M26.9 Dentofacial anomaly, unspecified
✓4th **M27 Other diseases of jaws**
M27.0 Developmental disorders of jaws
Latent bone cyst of jaw
Stafne's cyst
Torus mandibularis
Torus palatinus
M27.1 Giant cell granuloma, central
Giant cell granuloma NOS
EXCLUDES 1 *peripheral giant cell granuloma (K06.8)*

M27.2 Inflammatory conditions of jaws
Osteitis of jaw(s)
Osteomyelitis (neonatal) jaw(s)
Osteoradionecrosis jaw(s)
Periostitis jaw(s)
Sequestrum of jaw bone
Use additional code (W88-W90, X39.0) to identify radiation, if radiation-induced
EXCLUDES 2 *osteonecrosis of jaw due to drug (M87.180)*

M27.3 Alveolitis of jaws
Alveolar osteitis
Dry socket

✓5th **M27.4 Other and unspecified cysts of jaw**
EXCLUDES 1 *cysts of oral region (K09.-)*
latent bone cyst of jaw (M27.0)
Stafne's cyst (M27.0)

M27.40 Unspecified cyst of jaw
Cyst of jaw NOS

M27.49 Other cysts of jaw
Aneurysmal cyst of jaw
Hemorrhagic cyst of jaw
Traumatic cyst of jaw

✓5th **M27.5 Periradicular pathology associated with previous endodontic treatment**

M27.51 Perforation of root canal space due to endodontic treatment

M27.52 Endodontic overfill

M27.53 Endodontic underfill

M27.59 Other periradicular pathology associated with previous endodontic treatment

✓5th **M27.6 Endosseous dental implant failure**

M27.61 Osseointegration failure of dental implant
Hemorrhagic complications of dental implant placement
Iatrogenic osseointegration failure of dental implant
Osseointegration failure of dental implant due to complications of systemic disease
Osseointegration failure of dental implant due to poor bone quality
Pre-integration failure of dental implant NOS
Pre-osseointegration failure of dental implant

M27.62 Post-osseointegration biological failure of dental implant
Failure of dental implant due to lack of attached gingiva
Failure of dental implant due to occlusal trauma (caused by poor prosthetic design)
Failure of dental implant due to parafunctional habits
Failure of dental implant due to periodontal infection (peri-implantitis)
Failure of dental implant due to poor oral hygiene
Iatrogenic post-osseointegration failure of dental implant
Post-osseointegration failure of dental implant due to complications of systemic disease

M27.63 Post-osseointegration mechanical failure of dental implant
Failure of dental prosthesis causing loss of dental implant
Fracture of dental implant
EXCLUDES 2 *cracked tooth (K03.81)*
fractured dental restorative material with loss of material (K08.531)
fractured dental restorative material without loss of material (K08.530)
fractured tooth (S02.5)

M27.69 Other endosseous dental implant failure
Dental implant failure NOS

M27.8 Other specified diseases of jaws
Cherubism
Exostosis
Fibrous dysplasia
Unilateral condylar hyperplasia
Unilateral condylar hypoplasia
EXCLUDES 1 *jaw pain (R68.84)*

M27.9 Disease of jaws, unspecified

Systemic connective tissue disorders (M30-M36)

INCLUDES autoimmune disease NOS
collagen (vascular) disease NOS
systemic autoimmune disease
systemic collagen (vascular) disease

EXCLUDES 1 *autoimmune disease, single organ or single cell-type—code to relevant condition category*

✓4th **M30 Polyarteritis nodosa and related conditions**
EXCLUDES 1 *microscopic polyarteritis (M31.7)*

M30.0 Polyarteritis nodosa

M30.1 Polyarteritis with lung involvement [Churg-Strauss]
Allergic granulomatous angiitis

M30.2 Juvenile polyarteritis

M30.3 Mucocutaneous lymph node syndrome [Kawasaki]

M30.8 Other conditions related to polyarteritis nodosa
Polyangiitis overlap syndrome

✓4th **M31 Other necrotizing vasculopathies**

M31.0 Hypersensitivity angiitis
Goodpasture's syndrome

M31.1 Thrombotic microangiopathy
Thrombotic thrombocytopenic purpura

M31.2 Lethal midline granuloma

✓5th **M31.3 Wegener's granulomatosis**
Necrotizing respiratory granulomatosis

M31.30 Wegener's granulomatosis without renal involvement
Wegener's granulomatosis NOS

M31.31 Wegener's granulomatosis with renal involvement

M31.4 Aortic arch syndrome [Takayasu]

M31.5 Giant cell arteritis with polymyalgia rheumatica

M31.6 Other giant cell arteritis

M31.7 Microscopic polyangiitis
Microscopic polyarteritis
EXCLUDES 1 *polyarteritis nodosa (M30.0)*

M31.8 Other specified necrotizing vasculopathies
Hypocomplementemic vasculitis
Septic vasculitis

M31.9 Necrotizing vasculopathy, unspecified

✓4th **M32 Systemic lupus erythematosus (SLE)**
EXCLUDES 1 *lupus erythematosus (discoid) (NOS) (L93.0)*

M32.0 Drug-induced systemic lupus erythematosus
Use additional code for adverse effect, if applicable, to identify drug (T36-T50 with fifth or sixth character 5)

✓5th **M32.1 Systemic lupus erythematosus with organ or system involvement**

M32.10 Systemic lupus erythematosus, organ or system involvement unspecified

M32.11 Endocarditis in systemic lupus erythematosus
Libman-Sacks disease

M32.12 Pericarditis in systemic lupus erythematosus
Lupus pericarditis

M32.13 Lung involvement in systemic lupus erythematosus
Pleural effusion due to systemic lupus erythematosus

M32.14 Glomerular disease in systemic lupus erythematosus
Lupus renal disease NOS

M32.15 Tubulo-interstitial nephropathy in systemic lupus erythematosus

M32.19 Other organ or system involvement in systemic lupus erythematosus

M32.8 Other forms of systemic lupus erythematosus

M32.9 Systemic lupus erythematosus, unspecified
SLE NOS
Systemic lupus erythematosus NOS
Systemic lupus erythematosus without organ involvement

✓4th **M33 Dermatopolymyositis**

✓5th **M33.0 Juvenile dermatopolymyositis**

M33.00 Juvenile dermatopolymyositis, organ involvement unspecified

M33.01 Juvenile dermatopolymyositis with respiratory involvement

M33.02 Juvenile dermatopolymyositis with myopathy

M33.09 Juvenile dermatopolymyositis with other organ involvement

M33.1 Other dermatopolymyositis
- **M33.10 Other dermatopolymyositis, organ involvement unspecified**
- **M33.11 Other dermatopolymyositis with respiratory involvement**
- **M33.12 Other dermatopolymyositis with myopathy**
- **M33.19 Other dermatopolymyositis with other organ involvement**

M33.2 Polymyositis
- **M33.20 Polymyositis, organ involvement unspecified**
- **M33.21 Polymyositis with respiratory involvement**
- **M33.22 Polymyositis with myopathy**
- **M33.29 Polymyositis with other organ involvement**

M33.9 Dermatopolymyositis, unspecified
- **M33.90 Dermatopolymyositis, unspecified, organ involvement unspecified**
- **M33.91 Dermatopolymyositis, unspecified with respiratory involvement**
- **M33.92 Dermatopolymyositis, unspecified with myopathy**
- **M33.99 Dermatopolymyositis, unspecified with other organ involvement**

M34 Systemic sclerosis [scleroderma]

EXCLUDES 1 *circumscribed scleroderma (L94.0)*
neonatal scleroderma (P83.8)

M34.0 Progressive systemic sclerosis

M34.1 CR(E)ST syndrome
Combination of calcinosis, Raynaud's phenomenon, esophageal dysfunction, sclerodactyly, telangiectasia

M34.2 Systemic sclerosis induced by drug and chemical
Code first poisoning due to drug or toxin, if applicable (T36-T65 with fifth or sixth character 1-4 or 6)
Use additional code for adverse effect, if applicable, to identify drug (T36-T50 with fifth or sixth character 5)

M34.8 Other forms of systemic sclerosis
- **M34.81 Systemic sclerosis with lung involvement**
- **M34.82 Systemic sclerosis with myopathy**
- **M34.83 Systemic sclerosis with polyneuropathy**
- **M34.89 Other systemic sclerosis**

M34.9 Systemic sclerosis, unspecified

M35 Other systemic involvement of connective tissue

EXCLUDES 1 *reactive perforating collagenosis (L87.1)*

M35.0 Sicca syndrome [Sjögren]
- **M35.00 Sicca syndrome, unspecified**
- **M35.01 Sicca syndrome with keratoconjunctivitis**
- **M35.02 Sicca syndrome with lung involvement**
- **M35.03 Sicca syndrome with myopathy**
- **M35.04 Sicca syndrome with tubulo-interstitial nephropathy**
  Renal tubular acidosis in sicca syndrome
- **M35.09 Sicca syndrome with other organ involvement**

M35.1 Other overlap syndromes
Mixed connective tissue disease
EXCLUDES 1 *polyangiitis overlap syndrome (M30.8)*

M35.2 Behçet's disease

M35.3 Polymyalgia rheumatica
EXCLUDES 1 *polymyalgia rheumatica with giant cell arteritis (M31.5)*

M35.4 Diffuse (eosinophilic) fasciitis

M35.5 Multifocal fibrosclerosis

M35.6 Relapsing panniculitis [Weber-Christian]
EXCLUDES 1 *lupus panniculitis (L93.2)*
panniculitis NOS (M79.3-)

M35.7 Hypermobility syndrome
Familial ligamentous laxity
EXCLUDES 1 *Ehlers-Danlos syndrome (Q79.6)*
ligamentous laxity, NOS (M24.2-)

M35.8 Other specified systemic involvement of connective tissue

M35.9 Systemic involvement of connective tissue, unspecified
Autoimmune disease (systemic) NOS
Collagen (vascular) disease NOS

M36 Systemic disorders of connective tissue in diseases classified elsewhere

EXCLUDES 2 *arthropathies in diseases classified elsewhere (M14.-)*

M36.0 Dermato(poly)myositis in neoplastic disease
Code first underlying neoplasm (C00-D49)

M36.1 Arthropathy in neoplastic disease
Code first underlying neoplasm, such as:
leukemia (C91-C95)
malignant histiocytosis (C96.A)
multiple myeloma (C90.0)

M36.2 Hemophilic arthropathy
Hemarthrosis in hemophilic arthropathy
Code first underlying disease, such as:
factor VIII deficiency (D66)
with vascular defect (D68.0)
factor IX deficiency (D67)
hemophilia (classical) (D66)
hemophilia B (D67)
hemophilia C (D68.1)

M36.3 Arthropathy in other blood disorders

M36.4 Arthropathy in hypersensitivity reactions classified elsewhere
Code first underlying disease, such as:
Henoch (-Schönlein) purpura (D69.0)
serum sickness (T80.6-)

M36.8 Systemic disorders of connective tissue in other diseases classified elsewhere
Code first underlying disease, such as:
alkaptonuria (E70.2)
hypogammaglobulinemia (D80.-)
ochronosis (E70.2)

DORSOPATHIES (M40-M54)

Deforming dorsopathies (M40-M43)

M40 Kyphosis and lordosis

EXCLUDES 1 *congenital kyphosis and lordosis (Q76.4)*
kyphoscoliosis (M41.-)
postprocedural kyphosis and lordosis (M96.-)

M40.0 Postural kyphosis
EXCLUDES 1 *osteochondrosis of spine (M42.-)*
- **M40.00 Postural kyphosis, site unspecified**
- **M40.03 Postural kyphosis, cervicothoracic region**
- **M40.04 Postural kyphosis, thoracic region**
- **M40.05 Postural kyphosis, thoracolumbar region**

M40.1 Other secondary kyphosis
- **M40.10 Other secondary kyphosis, site unspecified**
- **M40.12 Other secondary kyphosis, cervical region**
- **M40.13 Other secondary kyphosis, cervicothoracic region**
- **M40.14 Other secondary kyphosis, thoracic region**
- **M40.15 Other secondary kyphosis, thoracolumbar region**

M40.2 Other and unspecified kyphosis
- **M40.20 Unspecified kyphosis**
  - **M40.202 Unspecified kyphosis, cervical region**
  - **M40.203 Unspecified kyphosis, cervicothoracic region**
  - **M40.204 Unspecified kyphosis, thoracic region**
  - **M40.205 Unspecified kyphosis, thoracolumbar region**
  - **M40.209 Unspecified kyphosis, site unspecified**
- **M40.29 Other kyphosis**
  - **M40.292 Other kyphosis, cervical region**
  - **M40.293 Other kyphosis, cervicothoracic region**
  - **M40.294 Other kyphosis, thoracic region**
  - **M40.295 Other kyphosis, thoracolumbar region**
  - **M40.299 Other kyphosis, site unspecified**

M40.3 Flatback syndrome
- **M40.30 Flatback syndrome, site unspecified**
- **M40.35 Flatback syndrome, thoracolumbar region**
- **M40.36 Flatback syndrome, lumbar region**
- **M40.37 Flatback syndrome, lumbosacral region**

M40.4 Postural lordosis
Acquired lordosis
- **M40.40 Postural lordosis, site unspecified**
- **M40.45 Postural lordosis, thoracolumbar region**
- **M40.46 Postural lordosis, lumbar region**
- **M40.47 Postural lordosis, lumbosacral region**

M40.5 Lordosis, unspecified
- **M40.50 Lordosis, unspecified, site unspecified**
- **M40.55 Lordosis, unspecified, thoracolumbar region**

M40.56 Lordosis, unspecified, lumbar region
M40.57 Lordosis, unspecified, lumbosacral region

√4th M41 Scoliosis
INCLUDES kyphoscoliosis
EXCLUDES 1 *congenital scoliosis NOS (Q67.5)*
congenital scoliosis due to bony malformation (Q76.3)
kyphoscoliotic heart disease (I27.1)
postprocedural scoliosis (M96.-)
postural congenital scoliosis (Q67.5)

√5th M41.0 Infantile idiopathic scoliosis
M41.00 Infantile idiopathic scoliosis, site unspecified
M41.02 Infantile idiopathic scoliosis, cervical region
M41.03 Infantile idiopathic scoliosis, cervicothoracic region
M41.04 Infantile idiopathic scoliosis, thoracic region
M41.05 Infantile idiopathic scoliosis, thoracolumbar region
M41.06 Infantile idiopathic scoliosis, lumbar region
M41.07 Infantile idiopathic scoliosis, lumbosacral region
M41.08 Infantile idiopathic scoliosis, sacral and sacrococcygeal region

√5th M41.1 Juvenile and adolescent idiopathic scoliosis
√6th M41.11 Juvenile idiopathic scoliosis
M41.112 Juvenile idiopathic scoliosis, cervical region
M41.113 Juvenile idiopathic scoliosis, cervicothoracic region
M41.114 Juvenile idiopathic scoliosis, thoracic region
M41.115 Juvenile idiopathic scoliosis, thoracolumbar region
M41.116 Juvenile idiopathic scoliosis, lumbar region
M41.117 Juvenile idiopathic scoliosis, lumbosacral region
M41.119 Juvenile idiopathic scoliosis, site unspecified
√6th M41.12 Adolescent scoliosis
M41.122 Adolescent idiopathic scoliosis, cervical region
M41.123 Adolescent idiopathic scoliosis, cervicothoracic region
M41.124 Adolescent idiopathic scoliosis, thoracic region
M41.125 Adolescent idiopathic scoliosis, thoracolumbar region
M41.126 Adolescent idiopathic scoliosis, lumbar region
M41.127 Adolescent idiopathic scoliosis, lumbosacral region
M41.129 Adolescent idiopathic scoliosis, site unspecified

√5th M41.2 Other idiopathic scoliosis
M41.20 Other idiopathic scoliosis, site unspecified
M41.22 Other idiopathic scoliosis, cervical region
M41.23 Other idiopathic scoliosis, cervicothoracic region
M41.24 Other idiopathic scoliosis, thoracic region
M41.25 Other idiopathic scoliosis, thoracolumbar region
M41.26 Other idiopathic scoliosis, lumbar region
M41.27 Other idiopathic scoliosis, lumbosacral region

√5th M41.3 Thoracogenic scoliosis
M41.30 Thoracogenic scoliosis, site unspecified
M41.34 Thoracogenic scoliosis, thoracic region
M41.35 Thoracogenic scoliosis, thoracolumbar region

√5th M41.4 Neuromuscular scoliosis
Scoliosis secondary to cerebral palsy, Friedreich's ataxia, poliomyelitis and other neuromuscular disorders
Code also underlying condition
M41.40 Neuromuscular scoliosis, site unspecified
M41.41 Neuromuscular scoliosis, occipito-atlanto-axial region
M41.42 Neuromuscular scoliosis, cervical region
M41.43 Neuromuscular scoliosis, cervicothoracic region
M41.44 Neuromuscular scoliosis, thoracic region
M41.45 Neuromuscular scoliosis, thoracolumbar region
M41.46 Neuromuscular scoliosis, lumbar region
M41.47 Neuromuscular scoliosis, lumbosacral region

√5th M41.5 Other secondary scoliosis
M41.50 Other secondary scoliosis, site unspecified
M41.52 Other secondary scoliosis, cervical region
M41.53 Other secondary scoliosis, cervicothoracic region
M41.54 Other secondary scoliosis, thoracic region
M41.55 Other secondary scoliosis, thoracolumbar region
M41.56 Other secondary scoliosis, lumbar region
M41.57 Other secondary scoliosis, lumbosacral region

√5th M41.8 Other forms of scoliosis
M41.80 Other forms of scoliosis, site unspecified
M41.82 Other forms of scoliosis, cervical region
M41.83 Other forms of scoliosis, cervicothoracic region
M41.84 Other forms of scoliosis, thoracic region
M41.85 Other forms of scoliosis, thoracolumbar region
M41.86 Other forms of scoliosis, lumbar region
M41.87 Other forms of scoliosis, lumbosacral region
M41.9 Scoliosis, unspecified

√4th M42 Spinal osteochondrosis
√5th M42.0 Juvenile osteochondrosis of spine
Calvé's disease
Scheuermann's disease
EXCLUDES 1 *postural kyphosis (M40.0)*
M42.00 Juvenile osteochondrosis of spine, site unspecified
M42.01 Juvenile osteochondrosis of spine, occipito-atlanto-axial region
M42.02 Juvenile osteochondrosis of spine, cervical region
M42.03 Juvenile osteochondrosis of spine, cervicothoracic region
M42.04 Juvenile osteochondrosis of spine, thoracic region
M42.05 Juvenile osteochondrosis of spine, thoracolumbar region
M42.06 Juvenile osteochondrosis of spine, lumbar region
M42.07 Juvenile osteochondrosis of spine, lumbosacral region
M42.08 Juvenile osteochondrosis of spine, sacral and sacrococcygeal region
M42.09 Juvenile osteochondrosis of spine, multiple sites in spine

√5th M42.1 Adult osteochondrosis of spine
M42.10 Adult osteochondrosis of spine, site unspecified
M42.11 Adult osteochondrosis of spine, occipito-atlanto-axial region
M42.12 Adult osteochondrosis of spine, cervical region
M42.13 Adult osteochondrosis of spine, cervicothoracic region
M42.14 Adult osteochondrosis of spine, thoracic region
M42.15 Adult osteochondrosis of spine, thoracolumbar region
M42.16 Adult osteochondrosis of spine, lumbar region
M42.17 Adult osteochondrosis of spine, lumbosacral region
M42.18 Adult osteochondrosis of spine, sacral and sacrococcygeal region
M42.19 Adult osteochondrosis of spine, multiple sites in spine
M42.9 Spinal osteochondrosis, unspecified

√4th M43 Other deforming dorsopathies
EXCLUDES 1 *congenital spondylolysis and spondylolisthesis (Q76.2)*
hemivertebra (Q76.3-Q76.4)
Klippel-Feil syndrome (Q76.1)
lumbarization and sacralization (Q76.4)
platyspondylisis (Q76.4)
spina bifida occulta (Q76.0)
spinal curvature in osteoporosis (M80.-)
spinal curvature in Paget's disease of bone [osteitis deformans] (M88.-)

√5th M43.0 Spondylolysis
EXCLUDES 1 *congenital spondylolysis (Q76.2)*
spondylolisthesis (M43.1)
M43.00 Spondylolysis, site unspecified
M43.01 Spondylolysis, occipito-atlanto-axial region
M43.02 Spondylolysis, cervical region
M43.03 Spondylolysis, cervicothoracic region
M43.04 Spondylolysis, thoracic region
M43.05 Spondylolysis, thoracolumbar region

M43.06 Spondylolysis, lumbar region
M43.07 Spondylolysis, lumbosacral region
M43.08 Spondylolysis, sacral and sacrococcygeal region
M43.09 Spondylolysis, multiple sites in spine

✓5th **M43.1 Spondylolisthesis**
EXCLUDES 1 *acute traumatic of lumbosacral region (S33.1)*
acute traumatic of sites other than lumbosacral—code to Fracture, vertebra, by region
congenital spondylolisthesis (Q76.2)

M43.10 Spondylolisthesis, site unspecified
M43.11 Spondylolisthesis, occipito-atlanto-axial region
M43.12 Spondylolisthesis, cervical region
M43.13 Spondylolisthesis, cervicothoracic region
M43.14 Spondylolisthesis, thoracic region
M43.15 Spondylolisthesis, thoracolumbar region
M43.16 Spondylolisthesis, lumbar region
M43.17 Spondylolisthesis, lumbosacral region
M43.18 Spondylolisthesis, sacral and sacrococcygeal region
M43.19 Spondylolisthesis, multiple sites in spine

✓5th **M43.2 Fusion of spine**
Ankylosis of spinal joint
EXCLUDES 1 *ankylosing spondylitis (M45.0-)*
congenital fusion of spine (Q76.4)
EXCLUDES 2 *arthrodesis status (Z98.1)*
pseudoarthrosis after fusion or arthrodesis (M96.0)

M43.20 Fusion of spine, site unspecified
M43.21 Fusion of spine, occipito-atlanto-axial region
M43.22 Fusion of spine, cervical region
M43.23 Fusion of spine, cervicothoracic region
M43.24 Fusion of spine, thoracic region
M43.25 Fusion of spine, thoracolumbar region
M43.26 Fusion of spine, lumbar region
M43.27 Fusion of spine, lumbosacral region
M43.28 Fusion of spine, sacral and sacrococcygeal region

M43.3 Recurrent atlantoaxial dislocation with myelopathy
M43.4 Other recurrent atlantoaxial dislocation

✓5th **M43.5 Other recurrent vertebral dislocation**
EXCLUDES 1 *biomechanical lesions NEC (M99.-)*

✓6th **M43.5X Other recurrent vertebral dislocation**
M43.5X2 Other recurrent vertebral dislocation, cervical region
M43.5X3 Other recurrent vertebral dislocation, cervicothoracic region
M43.5X4 Other recurrent vertebral dislocation, thoracic region
M43.5X5 Other recurrent vertebral dislocation, thoracolumbar region
M43.5X6 Other recurrent vertebral dislocation, lumbar region
M43.5X7 Other recurrent vertebral dislocation, lumbosacral region
M43.5X8 Other recurrent vertebral dislocation, sacral and sacrococcygeal region
M43.5X9 Other recurrent vertebral dislocation, site unspecified

M43.6 Torticollis
EXCLUDES 1 *congenital (sternomastoid) torticollis (Q68.0)*
current injury—see Injury, of spine, by body region
ocular torticollis (R29.891)
psychogenic torticollis (F45.8)
spasmodic torticollis (G24.3)
torticollis due to birth injury (P15.2)

✓5th **M43.8 Other specified deforming dorsopathies**
EXCLUDES 2 *kyphosis and lordosis (M40.-)*
scoliosis (M41.-)

✓6th **M43.8X Other specified deforming dorsopathies**
M43.8X1 Other specified deforming dorsopathies, occipito-atlanto-axial region
M43.8X2 Other specified deforming dorsopathies, cervical region
M43.8X3 Other specified deforming dorsopathies, cervicothoracic region
M43.8X4 Other specified deforming dorsopathies, thoracic region
M43.8X5 Other specified deforming dorsopathies, thoracolumbar region
M43.8X6 Other specified deforming dorsopathies, lumbar region
M43.8X7 Other specified deforming dorsopathies, lumbosacral region
M43.8X8 Other specified deforming dorsopathies, sacral and sacrococcygeal region
M43.8X9 Other specified deforming dorsopathies, site unspecified

M43.9 Deforming dorsopathy, unspecified
Curvature of spine NOS

Spondylopathies (M45-M49)

✓4th **M45 Ankylosing spondylitis**
Rheumatoid arthritis of spine
EXCLUDES 1 *arthropathy in Reiter's disease (M02.3-)*
juvenile (ankylosing) spondylitis (M08.1)
EXCLUDES 2 *Behçet's disease (M35.2)*

M45.0 Ankylosing spondylitis of multiple sites in spine
M45.1 Ankylosing spondylitis of occipito-atlanto-axial region
M45.2 Ankylosing spondylitis of cervical region
M45.3 Ankylosing spondylitis of cervicothoracic region
M45.4 Ankylosing spondylitis of thoracic region
M45.5 Ankylosing spondylitis of thoracolumbar region
M45.6 Ankylosing spondylitis lumbar region
M45.7 Ankylosing spondylitis of lumbosacral region
M45.8 Ankylosing spondylitis sacral and sacrococcygeal region
M45.9 Ankylosing spondylitis of unspecified sites in spine

✓4th **M46 Other inflammatory spondylopathies**

✓5th **M46.0 Spinal enthesopathy**
Disorder of ligamentous or muscular attachments of spine

M46.00 Spinal enthesopathy, site unspecified
M46.01 Spinal enthesopathy, occipito-atlanto-axial region
M46.02 Spinal enthesopathy, cervical region
M46.03 Spinal enthesopathy, cervicothoracic region
M46.04 Spinal enthesopathy, thoracic region
M46.05 Spinal enthesopathy, thoracolumbar region
M46.06 Spinal enthesopathy, lumbar region
M46.07 Spinal enthesopathy, lumbosacral region
M46.08 Spinal enthesopathy, sacral and sacrococcygeal region
M46.09 Spinal enthesopathy, multiple sites in spine

M46.1 Sacroiliitis, not elsewhere classified

✓5th **M46.2 Osteomyelitis of vertebra**
M46.20 Osteomyelitis of vertebra, site unspecified
M46.21 Osteomyelitis of vertebra, occipito-atlanto-axial region
M46.22 Osteomyelitis of vertebra, cervical region
M46.23 Osteomyelitis of vertebra, cervicothoracic region
M46.24 Osteomyelitis of vertebra, thoracic region
M46.25 Osteomyelitis of vertebra, thoracolumbar region
M46.26 Osteomyelitis of vertebra, lumbar region
M46.27 Osteomyelitis of vertebra, lumbosacral region
M46.28 Osteomyelitis of vertebra, sacral and sacrococcygeal region

✓5th **M46.3 Infection of intervertebral disc (pyogenic)**
Use additional code (B95-B97) to identify infectious agent

M46.30 Infection of intervertebral disc (pyogenic), site unspecified
M46.31 Infection of intervertebral disc (pyogenic), occipito-atlanto-axial region
M46.32 Infection of intervertebral disc (pyogenic), cervical region
M46.33 Infection of intervertebral disc (pyogenic), cervicothoracic region
M46.34 Infection of intervertebral disc (pyogenic), thoracic region
M46.35 Infection of intervertebral disc (pyogenic), thoracolumbar region
M46.36 Infection of intervertebral disc (pyogenic), lumbar region
M46.37 Infection of intervertebral disc (pyogenic), lumbosacral region

M46.38 Infection of intervertebral disc (pyogenic), sacral and sacrococcygeal region
M46.39 Infection of intervertebral disc (pyogenic), multiple sites in spine

✓5th M46.4 Discitis, unspecified
M46.40 Discitis, unspecified, site unspecified
M46.41 Discitis, unspecified, occipito-atlanto-axial region
M46.42 Discitis, unspecified, cervical region
M46.43 Discitis, unspecified, cervicothoracic region
M46.44 Discitis, unspecified, thoracic region
M46.45 Discitis, unspecified, thoracolumbar region
M46.46 Discitis, unspecified, lumbar region
M46.47 Discitis, unspecified, lumbosacral region
M46.48 Discitis, unspecified, sacral and sacrococcygeal region
M46.49 Discitis, unspecified, multiple sites in spine

✓5th M46.5 Other infective spondylopathies
M46.50 Other infective spondylopathies, site unspecified
M46.51 Other infective spondylopathies, occipito-atlanto-axial region
M46.52 Other infective spondylopathies, cervical region
M46.53 Other infective spondylopathies, cervicothoracic region
M46.54 Other infective spondylopathies, thoracic region
M46.55 Other infective spondylopathies, thoracolumbar region
M46.56 Other infective spondylopathies, lumbar region
M46.57 Other infective spondylopathies, lumbosacral region
M46.58 Other infective spondylopathies, sacral and sacrococcygeal region
M46.59 Other infective spondylopathies, multiple sites in spine

✓5th M46.8 Other specified inflammatory spondylopathies
M46.80 Other specified inflammatory spondylopathies, site unspecified
M46.81 Other specified inflammatory spondylopathies, occipito-atlanto-axial region
M46.82 Other specified inflammatory spondylopathies, cervical region
M46.83 Other specified inflammatory spondylopathies, cervicothoracic region
M46.84 Other specified inflammatory spondylopathies, thoracic region
M46.85 Other specified inflammatory spondylopathies, thoracolumbar region
M46.86 Other specified inflammatory spondylopathies, lumbar region
M46.87 Other specified inflammatory spondylopathies, lumbosacral region
M46.88 Other specified inflammatory spondylopathies, sacral and sacrococcygeal region
M46.89 Other specified inflammatory spondylopathies, multiple sites in spine

✓5th M46.9 Unspecified inflammatory spondylopathy
M46.90 Unspecified inflammatory spondylopathy, site unspecified
M46.91 Unspecified inflammatory spondylopathy, occipito-atlanto-axial region
M46.92 Unspecified inflammatory spondylopathy, cervical region
M46.93 Unspecified inflammatory spondylopathy, cervicothoracic region
M46.94 Unspecified inflammatory spondylopathy, thoracic region
M46.95 Unspecified inflammatory spondylopathy, thoracolumbar region
M46.96 Unspecified inflammatory spondylopathy, lumbar region
M46.97 Unspecified inflammatory spondylopathy, lumbosacral region
M46.98 Unspecified inflammatory spondylopathy, sacral and sacrococcygeal region
M46.99 Unspecified inflammatory spondylopathy, multiple sites in spine

✓4th **M47 Spondylosis**
INCLUDES arthrosis or osteoarthritis of spine
degeneration of facet joints

✓5th M47.0 Anterior spinal and vertebral artery compression syndromes
✓6th M47.01 Anterior spinal artery compression syndromes
M47.011 Anterior spinal artery compression syndromes, occipito-atlanto-axial region
M47.012 Anterior spinal artery compression syndromes, cervical region
M47.013 Anterior spinal artery compression syndromes, cervicothoracic region
M47.014 Anterior spinal artery compression syndromes, thoracic region
M47.015 Anterior spinal artery compression syndromes, thoracolumbar region
M47.016 Anterior spinal artery compression syndromes, lumbar region
M47.019 Anterior spinal artery compression syndromes, site unspecified
✓6th M47.02 Vertebral artery compression syndromes
M47.021 Vertebral artery compression syndromes, occipito-atlanto-axial region
M47.022 Vertebral artery compression syndromes, cervical region
M47.029 Vertebral artery compression syndromes, site unspecified

✓5th M47.1 Other spondylosis with myelopathy
Spondylogenic compression of spinal cord
EXCLUDES 1 *vertebral subluxation (M43.3-M43.5X9)*
M47.10 Other spondylosis with myelopathy, site unspecified
M47.11 Other spondylosis with myelopathy, occipito-atlanto-axial region
M47.12 Other spondylosis with myelopathy, cervical region
M47.13 Other spondylosis with myelopathy, cervicothoracic region
M47.14 Other spondylosis with myelopathy, thoracic region
M47.15 Other spondylosis with myelopathy, thoracolumbar region
M47.16 Other spondylosis with myelopathy, lumbar region
M47.17 Other spondylosis with myelopathy, lumbosacral region
M47.18 Other spondylosis with myelopathy, sacral and sacrococcygeal region

✓5th M47.2 Other spondylosis with radiculopathy
M47.20 Other spondylosis with radiculopathy, site unspecified
M47.21 Other spondylosis with radiculopathy, occipito-atlanto-axial region
M47.22 Other spondylosis with radiculopathy, cervical region
M47.23 Other spondylosis with radiculopathy, cervicothoracic region
M47.24 Other spondylosis with radiculopathy, thoracic region
M47.25 Other spondylosis with radiculopathy, thoracolumbar region
M47.26 Other spondylosis with radiculopathy, lumbar region
M47.27 Other spondylosis with radiculopathy, lumbosacral region
M47.28 Other spondylosis with radiculopathy, sacral and sacrococcygeal region

✓5th M47.8 Other spondylosis
✓6th M47.81 Spondylosis without myelopathy or radiculopathy
M47.811 Spondylosis without myelopathy or radiculopathy, occipito-atlanto-axial region
M47.812 Spondylosis without myelopathy or radiculopathy, cervical region
M47.813 Spondylosis without myelopathy or radiculopathy, cervicothoracic region

M47.814 Spondylosis without myelopathy or radiculopathy, thoracic region

M47.815 Spondylosis without myelopathy or radiculopathy, thoracolumbar region

M47.816 Spondylosis without myelopathy or radiculopathy, lumbar region

M47.817 Spondylosis without myelopathy or radiculopathy, lumbosacral region

M47.818 Spondylosis without myelopathy or radiculopathy, sacral and sacrococcygeal region

M47.819 Spondylosis without myelopathy or radiculopathy, site unspecified

✓6th **M47.89 Other spondylosis**

M47.891 Other spondylosis, occipito-atlanto-axial region

M47.892 Other spondylosis, cervical region

M47.893 Other spondylosis, cervicothoracic region

M47.894 Other spondylosis, thoracic region

M47.895 Other spondylosis, thoracolumbar region

M47.896 Other spondylosis, lumbar region

M47.897 Other spondylosis, lumbosacral region

M47.898 Other spondylosis, sacral and sacrococcygeal region

M47.899 Other spondylosis, site unspecified

M47.9 Spondylosis, unspecified

✓4th **M48 Other spondylopathies**

✓5th **M48.0 Spinal stenosis**

Caudal stenosis

M48.00 Spinal stenosis, site unspecified

M48.01 Spinal stenosis, occipito-atlanto-axial region

M48.02 Spinal stenosis, cervical region

M48.03 Spinal stenosis, cervicothoracic region

M48.04 Spinal stenosis, thoracic region

M48.05 Spinal stenosis, thoracolumbar region

M48.06 Spinal stenosis, lumbar region

M48.07 Spinal stenosis, lumbosacral region

M48.08 Spinal stenosis, sacral and sacrococcygeal region

✓5th **M48.1 Ankylosing hyperostosis [Forestier]**

Diffuse idiopathic skeletal hyperostosis [DISH]

M48.10 Ankylosing hyperostosis [Forestier], site unspecified

M48.11 Ankylosing hyperostosis [Forestier], occipito-atlanto-axial region

M48.12 Ankylosing hyperostosis [Forestier], cervical region

M48.13 Ankylosing hyperostosis [Forestier], cervicothoracic region

M48.14 Ankylosing hyperostosis [Forestier], thoracic region

M48.15 Ankylosing hyperostosis [Forestier], thoracolumbar region

M48.16 Ankylosing hyperostosis [Forestier], lumbar region

M48.17 Ankylosing hyperostosis [Forestier], lumbosacral region

M48.18 Ankylosing hyperostosis [Forestier], sacral and sacrococcygeal region

M48.19 Ankylosing hyperostosis [Forestier], multiple sites in spine

✓5th **M48.2 Kissing spine**

M48.20 Kissing spine, site unspecified

M48.21 Kissing spine, occipito-atlanto-axial region

M48.22 Kissing spine, cervical region

M48.23 Kissing spine, cervicothoracic region

M48.24 Kissing spine, thoracic region

M48.25 Kissing spine, thoracolumbar region

M48.26 Kissing spine, lumbar region

M48.27 Kissing spine, lumbosacral region

✓5th **M48.3 Traumatic spondylopathy**

M48.30 Traumatic spondylopathy, site unspecified

M48.31 Traumatic spondylopathy, occipito-atlanto-axial region

M48.32 Traumatic spondylopathy, cervical region

M48.33 Traumatic spondylopathy, cervicothoracic region

M48.34 Traumatic spondylopathy, thoracic region

M48.35 Traumatic spondylopathy, thoracolumbar region

M48.36 Traumatic spondylopathy, lumbar region

M48.37 Traumatic spondylopathy, lumbosacral region

M48.38 Traumatic spondylopathy, sacral and sacrococcygeal region

✓5th **M48.4 Fatigue fracture of vertebra**

Stress fracture of vertebra

EXCLUDES 1 *pathological fracture NOS (M84.4-)*
pathological fracture of vertebra due to neoplasm (M84.58)
pathological fracture of vertebra due to other diagnosis (M84.68)
pathological fracture of vertebra due to osteoporosis (M80.-)
traumatic fracture of vertebrae (S12.0-S12.3-, S22.0-, S32.0-)

The appropriate 7th character is to be added to each code from subcategory M48.4.

- A initial encounter for fracture
- D subsequent encounter for fracture with routine healing
- G subsequent encounter for fracture with delayed healing
- S sequela of fracture

✓x7th **M48.40 Fatigue fracture of vertebra, site unspecified**

✓x7th **M48.41 Fatigue fracture of vertebra, occipito-atlanto-axial region**

✓x7th **M48.42 Fatigue fracture of vertebra, cervical region**

✓x7th **M48.43 Fatigue fracture of vertebra, cervicothoracic region**

✓x7th **M48.44 Fatigue fracture of vertebra, thoracic region**

✓x7th **M48.45 Fatigue fracture of vertebra, thoracolumbar region**

✓x7th **M48.46 Fatigue fracture of vertebra, lumbar region**

✓x7th **M48.47 Fatigue fracture of vertebra, lumbosacral region**

✓x7th **M48.48 Fatigue fracture of vertebra, sacral and sacrococcygeal region**

✓5th **M48.5 Collapsed vertebra, not elsewhere classified**

Collapsed vertebra NOS
Wedging of vertebra NOS

EXCLUDES 1 *current injury—see Injury of spine, by body region*
fatigue fracture of vertebra (M48.4)
pathological fracture of vertebra due to neoplasm (M84.58)
pathological fracture of vertebra due to other diagnosis (M84.68)
pathological fracture of vertebra due to osteoporosis (M80.-)
pathological fracture NOS (M84.4-)
stress fracture of vertebra (M48.4-)
traumatic fracture of vertebra (S12-, S22-, S32-)

The appropriate 7th character is to be added to each code from subcategory M48.5.

- A initial encounter for fracture
- D subsequent encounter for fracture with routine healing
- G subsequent encounter for fracture with delayed healing
- S sequela of fracture

✓x7th **M48.50 Collapsed vertebra, not elsewhere classified, site unspecified**

✓x7th **M48.51 Collapsed vertebra, not elsewhere classified, occipito-atlanto-axial region**

✓x7th **M48.52 Collapsed vertebra, not elsewhere classified, cervical region**

✓x7th **M48.53 Collapsed vertebra, not elsewhere classified, cervicothoracic region**

✓x7th **M48.54 Collapsed vertebra, not elsewhere classified, thoracic region**

✓x7th **M48.55 Collapsed vertebra, not elsewhere classified, thoracolumbar region**

✓x7th **M48.56 Collapsed vertebra, not elsewhere classified, lumbar region**

✓x7th **M48.57 Collapsed vertebra, not elsewhere classified, lumbosacral region**

M48.58 Collapsed vertebra, not elsewhere classified, sacral and sacrococcygeal region

M48.8 Other specified spondylopathies
Ossification of posterior longitudinal ligament

M48.8X Other specified spondylopathies
M48.8X1 Other specified spondylopathies, occipito-atlanto-axial region
M48.8X2 Other specified spondylopathies, cervical region
M48.8X3 Other specified spondylopathies, cervicothoracic region
M48.8X4 Other specified spondylopathies, thoracic region
M48.8X5 Other specified spondylopathies, thoracolumbar region
M48.8X6 Other specified spondylopathies, lumbar region
M48.8X7 Other specified spondylopathies, lumbosacral region
M48.8X8 Other specified spondylopathies, sacral and sacrococcygeal region
M48.8X9 Other specified spondylopathies, site unspecified

M48.9 Spondylopathy, unspecified

M49 Spondylopathies in diseases classified elsewhere
Curvature of spine in diseases classified elsewhere
Deformity of spine in diseases classified elsewhere
Kyphosis in diseases classified elsewhere
Scoliosis in diseases classified elsewhere
Spondylopathy in diseases classified elsewhere

EXCLUDES 1 *curvature of spine in tuberculosis [Pott's] (A18.Ø1)*
enteropathic arthropathies (MØ7.-)
neuropathic spondylopathy (in):
nonsyphilitic NEC (G98.Ø)
syringomyelia (G95.Ø)
tabes dorsalis (A52.11)
spondylitis (in):
gonococcal (A54.41)
syphilis (acquired) (A52.77)
neuropathic [tabes dorsalis] (A52.11)
tuberculosis (A18.Ø1)
typhoid fever (AØ1.Ø5)

Code first underlying disease, such as:
brucellosis (A23.-)
Charcôt-Marie-Tooth disease (G6Ø.Ø)
enterobacterial infections (AØ1-AØ4)
osteitis fibrosa cystica (E21.Ø)

M49.8 Spondylopathy in diseases classified elsewhere
M49.8Ø Spondylopathy in diseases classified elsewhere, site unspecified
M49.81 Spondylopathy in diseases classified elsewhere, occipito-atlanto-axial region
M49.82 Spondylopathy in diseases classified elsewhere, cervical region
M49.83 Spondylopathy in diseases classified elsewhere, cervicothoracic region
M49.84 Spondylopathy in diseases classified elsewhere, thoracic region
M49.85 Spondylopathy in diseases classified elsewhere, thoracolumbar region
M49.86 Spondylopathy in diseases classified elsewhere, lumbar region
M49.87 Spondylopathy in diseases classified elsewhere, lumbosacral region
M49.88 Spondylopathy in diseases classified elsewhere, sacral and sacrococcygeal region
M49.89 Spondylopathy in diseases classified elsewhere, multiple sites in spine

Other dorsopathies (M5Ø-M54)

EXCLUDES 1 *current injury—see injury of spine by body region*
discitis NOS (M46.4-)

M5Ø Cervical disc disorders
INCLUDES cervicothoracic disc disorders with cervicalgia
cervicothoracic disc disorders
NOTE Code to the most superior level of disorder

M5Ø.Ø Cervical disc disorder with myelopathy
M5Ø.ØØ Cervical disc disorder with myelopathy, unspecified cervical region
M5Ø.Ø1 Cervical disc disorder with myelopathy, occipito-atlanto-axial region
M5Ø.Ø2 Cervical disc disorder with myelopathy, mid-cervical region
M5Ø.Ø3 Cervical disc disorder with myelopathy, cervicothoracic region

M5Ø.1 Cervical disc disorder with radiculopathy
EXCLUDES 2 *brachial radiculitis NOS (M54.13)*
M5Ø.1Ø Cervical disc disorder with radiculopathy, unspecified cervical region
M5Ø.11 Cervical disc disorder with radiculopathy, occipito-atlanto-axial region
M5Ø.12 Cervical disc disorder with radiculopathy, mid-cervical region
M5Ø.13 Cervical disc disorder with radiculopathy, cervicothoracic region

M5Ø.2 Other cervical disc displacement
M5Ø.2Ø Other cervical disc displacement, unspecified cervical region
M5Ø.21 Other cervical disc displacement, occipito-atlanto-axial region
M5Ø.22 Other cervical disc displacement, mid-cervical region
M5Ø.23 Other cervical disc displacement, cervicothoracic region

M5Ø.3 Other cervical disc degeneration
M5Ø.3Ø Other cervical disc degeneration, unspecified cervical region
M5Ø.31 Other cervical disc degeneration, occipito-atlanto-axial region
M5Ø.32 Other cervical disc degeneration, mid-cervical region
M5Ø.33 Other cervical disc degeneration, cervicothoracic region

M5Ø.8 Other cervical disc disorders
M5Ø.8Ø Other cervical disc disorders, unspecified cervical region
M5Ø.81 Other cervical disc disorders, occipito-atlanto-axial region
M5Ø.82 Other cervical disc disorders, mid-cervical region
M5Ø.83 Other cervical disc disorders, cervicothoracic region

M5Ø.9 Cervical disc disorder, unspecified
M5Ø.9Ø Cervical disc disorder, unspecified, unspecified cervical region
M5Ø.91 Cervical disc disorder, unspecified, occipito-atlanto-axial region
M5Ø.92 Cervical disc disorder, unspecified, mid-cervical region
M5Ø.93 Cervical disc disorder, unspecified, cervicothoracic region

M51 Thoracic, thoracolumbar, and lumbosacral intervertebral disc disorders
EXCLUDES 2 *cervical and cervicothoracic disc disorders (M5Ø.-)*
sacral and sacrococcygeal disorders (M53.3)

M51.Ø Thoracic, thoracolumbar and lumbosacral intervertebral disc disorders with myelopathy
M51.Ø4 Intervertebral disc disorders with myelopathy, thoracic region
M51.Ø5 Intervertebral disc disorders with myelopathy, thoracolumbar region
M51.Ø6 Intervertebral disc disorders with myelopathy, lumbar region
M51.Ø7 Intervertebral disc disorders with myelopathy, lumbosacral region

✓5th **M51.1 Thoracic, thoracolumbar and lumbosacral intervertebral disc disorders with radiculopathy**
Sciatica due to intervertebral disc disorder
EXCLUDES 1 *lumbar radiculitis NOS (M54.16)*
sciatica NOS (M54.3)
M51.14 Intervertebral disc disorders with radiculopathy, thoracic region
M51.15 Intervertebral disc disorders with radiculopathy, thoracolumbar region
M51.16 Intervertebral disc disorders with radiculopathy, lumbar region
M51.17 Intervertebral disc disorders with radiculopathy, lumbosacral region

✓5th **M51.2 Other thoracic, thoracolumbar and lumbosacral intervertebral disc displacement**
Lumbago due to displacement of intervertebral disc
M51.24 Other intervertebral disc displacement, thoracic region
M51.25 Other intervertebral disc displacement, thoracolumbar region
M51.26 Other intervertebral disc displacement, lumbar region
M51.27 Other intervertebral disc displacement, lumbosacral region

✓5th **M51.3 Other thoracic, thoracolumbar and lumbosacral intervertebral disc degeneration**
M51.34 Other intervertebral disc degeneration, thoracic region
M51.35 Other intervertebral disc degeneration, thoracolumbar region
M51.36 Other intervertebral disc degeneration, lumbar region
M51.37 Other intervertebral disc degeneration, lumbosacral region

✓5th **M51.4 Schmorl's nodes**
M51.44 Schmorl's nodes, thoracic region
M51.45 Schmorl's nodes, thoracolumbar region
M51.46 Schmorl's nodes, lumbar region
M51.47 Schmorl's nodes, lumbosacral region

✓5th **M51.8 Other thoracic, thoracolumbar and lumbosacral intervertebral disc disorders**
M51.84 Other intervertebral disc disorders, thoracic region
M51.85 Other intervertebral disc disorders, thoracolumbar region
M51.86 Other intervertebral disc disorders, lumbar region
M51.87 Other intervertebral disc disorders, lumbosacral region

M51.9 Unspecified thoracic, thoracolumbar and lumbosacral intervertebral disc disorder

✓4th **M53 Other and unspecified dorsopathies, not elsewhere classified**

M53.Ø Cervicocranial syndrome
Posterior cervical sympathetic syndrome

M53.1 Cervicobrachial syndrome
EXCLUDES 2 *cervical disc disorder (M5Ø.-)*
thoracic outlet syndrome (G54.Ø)

✓5th **M53.2 Spinal instabilities**
✓6th **M53.2X Spinal instabilities**
M53.2X1 Spinal instabilities, occipito-atlanto-axial region
M53.2X2 Spinal instabilities, cervical region
M53.2X3 Spinal instabilities, cervicothoracic region
M53.2X4 Spinal instabilities, thoracic region
M53.2X5 Spinal instabilities, thoracolumbar region
M53.2X6 Spinal instabilities, lumbar region
M53.2X7 Spinal instabilities, lumbosacral region
M53.2X8 Spinal instabilities, sacral and sacrococcygeal region
M53.2X9 Spinal instabilities, site unspecified

M53.3 Sacrococcygeal disorders, not elsewhere classified
Coccygodynia

✓5th **M53.8 Other specified dorsopathies**
M53.8Ø Other specified dorsopathies, site unspecified
M53.81 Other specified dorsopathies, occipito-atlanto-axial region
M53.82 Other specified dorsopathies, cervical region
M53.83 Other specified dorsopathies, cervicothoracic region
M53.84 Other specified dorsopathies, thoracic region
M53.85 Other specified dorsopathies, thoracolumbar region
M53.86 Other specified dorsopathies, lumbar region
M53.87 Other specified dorsopathies, lumbosacral region
M53.88 Other specified dorsopathies, sacral and sacrococcygeal region

M53.9 Dorsopathy, unspecified

✓4th **M54 Dorsalgia**
EXCLUDES 1 *psychogenic dorsalgia (F45.41)*

✓5th **M54.Ø Panniculitis affecting regions of neck and back**
EXCLUDES 1 *lupus panniculitis (L93.2)*
panniculitis NOS (M79.3)
relapsing [Weber-Christian] panniculitis (M35.6)
M54.ØØ Panniculitis affecting regions of neck and back, site unspecified
M54.Ø1 Panniculitis affecting regions of neck and back, occipito-atlanto-axial region
M54.Ø2 Panniculitis affecting regions of neck and back, cervical region
M54.Ø3 Panniculitis affecting regions of neck and back, cervicothoracic region
M54.Ø4 Panniculitis affecting regions of neck and back, thoracic region
M54.Ø5 Panniculitis affecting regions of neck and back, thoracolumbar region
M54.Ø6 Panniculitis affecting regions of neck and back, lumbar region
M54.Ø7 Panniculitis affecting regions of neck and back, lumbosacral region
M54.Ø8 Panniculitis affecting regions of neck and back, sacral and sacrococcygeal region
M54.Ø9 Panniculitis affecting regions, neck and back, multiple sites in spine

✓5th **M54.1 Radiculopathy**
Brachial neuritis or radiculitis NOS
Lumbar neuritis or radiculitis NOS
Lumbosacral neuritis or radiculitis NOS
Thoracic neuritis or radiculitis NOS
Radiculitis NOS
EXCLUDES 1 *neuralgia and neuritis NOS (M79.2)*
radiculopathy with cervical disc disorder (M5Ø.1)
radiculopathy with lumbar and other intervertebral disc disorder (M51.1-)
radiculopathy with spondylosis (M47.2-)
M54.1Ø Radiculopathy, site unspecified
M54.11 Radiculopathy, occipito-atlanto-axial region
M54.12 Radiculopathy, cervical region
M54.13 Radiculopathy, cervicothoracic region
M54.14 Radiculopathy, thoracic region
M54.15 Radiculopathy, thoracolumbar region
M54.16 Radiculopathy, lumbar region
M54.17 Radiculopathy, lumbosacral region
M54.18 Radiculopathy, sacral and sacrococcygeal region

M54.2 Cervicalgia
EXCLUDES 1 *cervicalgia due to intervertebral cervical disc disorder (M5Ø.-)*

✓5th **M54.3 Sciatica**
EXCLUDES 1 *lesion of sciatic nerve (G57.Ø)*
sciatica due to intervertebral disc disorder (M51.1-)
sciatica with lumbago (M54.4-)
M54.3Ø Sciatica, unspecified side
M54.31 Sciatica, right side
M54.32 Sciatica, left side

✓5th **M54.4 Lumbago with sciatica**
EXCLUDES 1 *lumbago with sciatica due to intervertebral disc disorder (M51.1-)*
M54.4Ø Lumbago with sciatica, unspecified side
M54.41 Lumbago with sciatica, right side
M54.42 Lumbago with sciatica, left side

M54.5 Low back pain
Loin pain
Lumbago NOS
EXCLUDES 1 *low back strain S39.012*
lumbago due to intervertebral disc displacement (M51.2-)
lumbago with sciatica (M54.4-)

M54.6 Pain in thoracic spine
EXCLUDES 1 *pain in thoracic spine due to intervertebral disc disorder (M51.-)*

✓5th **M54.8 Other dorsalgia**
EXCLUDES 1 *dorsalgia in thoracic region (M54.6)*
low back pain (M54.5)
M54.81 Occipital neuralgia
M54.89 Other dorsalgia

M54.9 Dorsalgia, unspecified
Backache NOS
Back pain NOS

SOFT TISSUE DISORDERS (M60-M79)

Disorders of muscles (M60-M63)

EXCLUDES 1 *dermatopolymyositis (M33.-)*
muscular dystrophies and myopathies (G71-G72)
myopathy in:
amyloidosis (E85.-)
polyarteritis nodosa (M30.0)
rheumatoid arthritis (M05.32)
scleroderma (M34.-)
Sjögren's syndrome (M35.03)
systemic lupus erythematosus (M32.-)

✓4th **M60 Myositis**
EXCLUDES 2 *inclusion body myositis [IBM] (G72.41)*

✓5th **M60.0 Infective myositis**
Tropical pyomyositis
Use additional code (B95-B97) to identify infectious agent
✓6th **M60.00 Infective myositis, unspecified site**
M60.000 Infective myositis, unspecified right arm
Infective myositis, right upper limb NOS
M60.001 Infective myositis, unspecified left arm
Infective myositis, left upper limb NOS
M60.002 Infective myositis, unspecified arm
Infective myositis, upper limb NOS
M60.003 Infective myositis, unspecified right leg
Infective myositis, right lower limb NOS
M60.004 Infective myositis, unspecified left leg
Infective myositis, left lower limb NOS
M60.005 Infective myositis, unspecified leg
Infective myositis, lower limb NOS
M60.009 Infective myositis, unspecified site
✓6th **M60.01 Infective myositis, shoulder**
M60.011 Infective myositis, right shoulder
M60.012 Infective myositis, left shoulder
M60.019 Infective myositis, unspecified shoulder
✓6th **M60.02 Infective myositis, upper arm**
M60.021 Infective myositis, right upper arm
M60.022 Infective myositis, left upper arm
M60.029 Infective myositis, unspecified upper arm
✓6th **M60.03 Infective myositis, forearm**
M60.031 Infective myositis, right forearm
M60.032 Infective myositis, left forearm
M60.039 Infective myositis, unspecified forearm
✓6th **M60.04 Infective myositis, hand and fingers**
M60.041 Infective myositis, right hand
M60.042 Infective myositis, left hand
M60.043 Infective myositis, unspecified hand
M60.044 Infective myositis, right finger(s)
M60.045 Infective myositis, left finger(s)
M60.046 Infective myositis, unspecified finger(s)
✓6th **M60.05 Infective myositis, thigh**
M60.051 Infective myositis, right thigh
M60.052 Infective myositis, left thigh
M60.059 Infective myositis, unspecified thigh
✓6th **M60.06 Infective myositis, lower leg**
M60.061 Infective myositis, right lower leg
M60.062 Infective myositis, left lower leg
M60.069 Infective myositis, unspecified lower leg
✓6th **M60.07 Infective myositis, ankle, foot and toes**
M60.070 Infective myositis, right ankle
M60.071 Infective myositis, left ankle
M60.072 Infective myositis, unspecified ankle
M60.073 Infective myositis, right foot
M60.074 Infective myositis, left foot
M60.075 Infective myositis, unspecified foot
M60.076 Infective myositis, right toe(s)
M60.077 Infective myositis, left toe(s)
M60.078 Infective myositis, unspecified toe(s)
M60.08 Infective myositis, other site
M60.09 Infective myositis, multiple sites

✓5th **M60.1 Interstitial myositis**
M60.10 Interstitial myositis of unspecified site
✓6th **M60.11 Interstitial myositis, shoulder**
M60.111 Interstitial myositis, right shoulder
M60.112 Interstitial myositis, left shoulder
M60.119 Interstitial myositis, unspecified shoulder
✓6th **M60.12 Interstitial myositis, upper arm**
M60.121 Interstitial myositis, right upper arm
M60.122 Interstitial myositis, left upper arm
M60.129 Interstitial myositis, unspecified upper arm
✓6th **M60.13 Interstitial myositis, forearm**
M60.131 Interstitial myositis, right forearm
M60.132 Interstitial myositis, left forearm
M60.139 Interstitial myositis, unspecified forearm
✓6th **M60.14 Interstitial myositis, hand**
M60.141 Interstitial myositis, right hand
M60.142 Interstitial myositis, left hand
M60.149 Interstitial myositis, unspecified hand
✓6th **M60.15 Interstitial myositis, thigh**
M60.151 Interstitial myositis, right thigh
M60.152 Interstitial myositis, left thigh
M60.159 Interstitial myositis, unspecified thigh
✓6th **M60.16 Interstitial myositis, lower leg**
M60.161 Interstitial myositis, right lower leg
M60.162 Interstitial myositis, left lower leg
M60.169 Interstitial myositis, unspecified lower leg
✓6th **M60.17 Interstitial myositis, ankle and foot**
M60.171 Interstitial myositis, right ankle and foot
M60.172 Interstitial myositis, left ankle and foot
M60.179 Interstitial myositis, unspecified ankle and foot
M60.18 Interstitial myositis, other site
M60.19 Interstitial myositis, multiple sites

✓5th **M60.2 Foreign body granuloma of soft tissue, not elsewhere classified**
Use additional code to identify the type of retained foreign body (Z18.-)
EXCLUDES 1 *foreign body granuloma of skin and subcutaneous tissue (L92.3)*
M60.20 Foreign body granuloma of soft tissue, not elsewhere classified, unspecified site
✓6th **M60.21 Foreign body granuloma of soft tissue, not elsewhere classified, shoulder**
M60.211 Foreign body granuloma of soft tissue, not elsewhere classified, right shoulder
M60.212 Foreign body granuloma of soft tissue, not elsewhere classified, left shoulder
M60.219 Foreign body granuloma of soft tissue, not elsewhere classified, unspecified shoulder
✓6th **M60.22 Foreign body granuloma of soft tissue, not elsewhere classified, upper arm**
M60.221 Foreign body granuloma of soft tissue, not elsewhere classified, right upper arm
M60.222 Foreign body granuloma of soft tissue, not elsewhere classified, left upper arm

M6Ø.229 Foreign body granuloma of soft tissue, not elsewhere classified, unspecified upper arm

✓6th **M6Ø.23** Foreign body granuloma of soft tissue, not elsewhere classified, forearm

M6Ø.231 Foreign body granuloma of soft tissue, not elsewhere classified, right forearm

M6Ø.232 Foreign body granuloma of soft tissue, not elsewhere classified, left forearm

M6Ø.239 Foreign body granuloma of soft tissue, not elsewhere classified, unspecified forearm

✓6th **M6Ø.24** Foreign body granuloma of soft tissue, not elsewhere classified, hand

M6Ø.241 Foreign body granuloma of soft tissue, not elsewhere classified, right hand

M6Ø.242 Foreign body granuloma of soft tissue, not elsewhere classified, left hand

M6Ø.249 Foreign body granuloma of soft tissue, not elsewhere classified, unspecified hand

✓6th **M6Ø.25** Foreign body granuloma of soft tissue, not elsewhere classified, thigh

M6Ø.251 Foreign body granuloma of soft tissue, not elsewhere classified, right thigh

M6Ø.252 Foreign body granuloma of soft tissue, not elsewhere classified, left thigh

M6Ø.259 Foreign body granuloma of soft tissue, not elsewhere classified, unspecified thigh

✓6th **M6Ø.26** Foreign body granuloma of soft tissue, not elsewhere classified, lower leg

M6Ø.261 Foreign body granuloma of soft tissue, not elsewhere classified, right lower leg

M6Ø.262 Foreign body granuloma of soft tissue, not elsewhere classified, left lower leg

M6Ø.269 Foreign body granuloma of soft tissue, not elsewhere classified, unspecified lower leg

✓6th **M6Ø.27** Foreign body granuloma of soft tissue, not elsewhere classified, ankle and foot

M6Ø.271 Foreign body granuloma of soft tissue, not elsewhere classified, right ankle and foot

M6Ø.272 Foreign body granuloma of soft tissue, not elsewhere classified, left ankle and foot

M6Ø.279 Foreign body granuloma of soft tissue, not elsewhere classified, unspecified ankle and foot

M6Ø.28 Foreign body granuloma of soft tissue, not elsewhere classified, other site

✓5th **M6Ø.8** Other myositis

M6Ø.8Ø Other myositis, unspecified site

✓6th **M6Ø.81** Other myositis shoulder

M6Ø.811 Other myositis, right shoulder

M6Ø.812 Other myositis, left shoulder

M6Ø.819 Other myositis, unspecified shoulder

✓6th **M6Ø.82** Other myositis, upper arm

M6Ø.821 Other myositis, right upper arm

M6Ø.822 Other myositis, left upper arm

M6Ø.829 Other myositis, unspecified upper arm

✓6th **M6Ø.83** Other myositis, forearm

M6Ø.831 Other myositis, right forearm

M6Ø.832 Other myositis, left forearm

M6Ø.839 Other myositis, unspecified forearm

✓6th **M6Ø.84** Other myositis, hand

M6Ø.841 Other myositis, right hand

M6Ø.842 Other myositis, left hand

M6Ø.849 Other myositis, unspecified hand

✓6th **M6Ø.85** Other myositis, thigh

M6Ø.851 Other myositis, right thigh

M6Ø.852 Other myositis, left thigh

M6Ø.859 Other myositis, unspecified thigh

✓6th **M6Ø.86** Other myositis, lower leg

M6Ø.861 Other myositis, right lower leg

M6Ø.862 Other myositis, left lower leg

M6Ø.869 Other myositis, unspecified lower leg

✓6th **M6Ø.87** Other myositis, ankle and foot

M6Ø.871 Other myositis, right ankle and foot

M6Ø.872 Other myositis, left ankle and foot

M6Ø.879 Other myositis, unspecified ankle and foot

M6Ø.88 Other myositis, other site

M6Ø.89 Other myositis, multiple sites

M6Ø.9 Myositis, unspecified

✓4th **M61 Calcification and ossification of muscle**

✓5th **M61.Ø** Myositis ossificans traumatica

M61.ØØ Myositis ossificans traumatica, unspecified site

✓6th **M61.Ø1** Myositis ossificans traumatica, shoulder

M61.Ø11 Myositis ossificans traumatica, right shoulder

M61.Ø12 Myositis ossificans traumatica, left shoulder

M61.Ø19 Myositis ossificans traumatica, unspecified shoulder

✓6th **M61.Ø2** Myositis ossificans traumatica, upper arm

M61.Ø21 Myositis ossificans traumatica, right upper arm

M61.Ø22 Myositis ossificans traumatica, left upper arm

M61.Ø29 Myositis ossificans traumatica, unspecified upper arm

✓6th **M61.Ø3** Myositis ossificans traumatica, forearm

M61.Ø31 Myositis ossificans traumatica, right forearm

M61.Ø32 Myositis ossificans traumatica, left forearm

M61.Ø39 Myositis ossificans traumatica, unspecified forearm

✓6th **M61.Ø4** Myositis ossificans traumatica, hand

M61.Ø41 Myositis ossificans traumatica, right hand

M61.Ø42 Myositis ossificans traumatica, left hand

M61.Ø49 Myositis ossificans traumatica, unspecified hand

✓6th **M61.Ø5** Myositis ossificans traumatica, thigh

M61.Ø51 Myositis ossificans traumatica, right thigh

M61.Ø52 Myositis ossificans traumatica, left thigh

M61.Ø59 Myositis ossificans traumatica, unspecified thigh

✓6th **M61.Ø6** Myositis ossificans traumatica, lower leg

M61.Ø61 Myositis ossificans traumatica, right lower leg

M61.Ø62 Myositis ossificans traumatica, left lower leg

M61.Ø69 Myositis ossificans traumatica, unspecified lower leg

✓6th **M61.Ø7** Myositis ossificans traumatica, ankle and foot

M61.Ø71 Myositis ossificans traumatica, right ankle and foot

M61.Ø72 Myositis ossificans traumatica, left ankle and foot

M61.Ø79 Myositis ossificans traumatica, unspecified ankle and foot

M61.Ø8 Myositis ossificans traumatica, other site

M61.Ø9 Myositis ossificans traumatica, multiple sites

✓5th **M61.1** Myositis ossificans progressiva

Fibrodysplasia ossificans progressiva

M61.1Ø Myositis ossificans progressiva, unspecified site

✓6th **M61.11** Myositis ossificans progressiva, shoulder

M61.111 Myositis ossificans progressiva, right shoulder

M61.112 Myositis ossificans progressiva, left shoulder

M61.119 Myositis ossificans progressiva, unspecified shoulder

✓6th **M61.12** Myositis ossificans progressiva, upper arm

M61.121 Myositis ossificans progressiva, right upper arm

M61.122 Myositis ossificans progressiva, left upper arm

M61.129 **Myositis ossificans progressiva, unspecified arm**

✓6th M61.13 **Myositis ossificans progressiva, forearm**

M61.131 **Myositis ossificans progressiva, right forearm**

M61.132 **Myositis ossificans progressiva, left forearm**

M61.139 **Myositis ossificans progressiva, unspecified forearm**

✓6th M61.14 **Myositis ossificans progressiva, hand and finger(s)**

M61.141 **Myositis ossificans progressiva, right hand**

M61.142 **Myositis ossificans progressiva, left hand**

M61.143 **Myositis ossificans progressiva, unspecified hand**

M61.144 **Myositis ossificans progressiva, right finger(s)**

M61.145 **Myositis ossificans progressiva, left finger(s)**

M61.146 **Myositis ossificans progressiva, unspecified finger(s)**

✓6th M61.15 **Myositis ossificans progressiva, thigh**

M61.151 **Myositis ossificans progressiva, right thigh**

M61.152 **Myositis ossificans progressiva, left thigh**

M61.159 **Myositis ossificans progressiva, unspecified thigh**

✓6th M61.16 **Myositis ossificans progressiva, lower leg**

M61.161 **Myositis ossificans progressiva, right lower leg**

M61.162 **Myositis ossificans progressiva, left lower leg**

M61.169 **Myositis ossificans progressiva, unspecified lower leg**

✓6th M61.17 **Myositis ossificans progressiva, ankle, foot and toe(s)**

M61.171 **Myositis ossificans progressiva, right ankle**

M61.172 **Myositis ossificans progressiva, left ankle**

M61.173 **Myositis ossificans progressiva, unspecified ankle**

M61.174 **Myositis ossificans progressiva, right foot**

M61.175 **Myositis ossificans progressiva, left foot**

M61.176 **Myositis ossificans progressiva, unspecified foot**

M61.177 **Myositis ossificans progressiva, right toe(s)**

M61.178 **Myositis ossificans progressiva, left toe(s)**

M61.179 **Myositis ossificans progressiva, unspecified toe(s)**

M61.18 **Myositis ossificans progressiva, other site**

M61.19 **Myositis ossificans progressiva, multiple sites**

✓5th M61.2 **Paralytic calcification and ossification of muscle**

Myositis ossificans associated with quadriplegia or paraplegia

M61.20 **Paralytic calcification and ossification of muscle, unspecified site**

✓6th M61.21 **Paralytic calcification and ossification of muscle, shoulder**

M61.211 **Paralytic calcification and ossification of muscle, right shoulder**

M61.212 **Paralytic calcification and ossification of muscle, left shoulder**

M61.219 **Paralytic calcification and ossification of muscle, unspecified shoulder**

✓6th M61.22 **Paralytic calcification and ossification of muscle, upper arm**

M61.221 **Paralytic calcification and ossification of muscle, right upper arm**

M61.222 **Paralytic calcification and ossification of muscle, left upper arm**

M61.229 **Paralytic calcification and ossification of muscle, unspecified upper arm**

✓6th M61.23 **Paralytic calcification and ossification of muscle, forearm**

M61.231 **Paralytic calcification and ossification of muscle, right forearm**

M61.232 **Paralytic calcification and ossification of muscle, left forearm**

M61.239 **Paralytic calcification and ossification of muscle, unspecified forearm**

✓6th M61.24 **Paralytic calcification and ossification of muscle, hand**

M61.241 **Paralytic calcification and ossification of muscle, right hand**

M61.242 **Paralytic calcification and ossification of muscle, left hand**

M61.249 **Paralytic calcification and ossification of muscle, unspecified hand**

✓6th M61.25 **Paralytic calcification and ossification of muscle, thigh**

M61.251 **Paralytic calcification and ossification of muscle, right thigh**

M61.252 **Paralytic calcification and ossification of muscle, left thigh**

M61.259 **Paralytic calcification and ossification of muscle, unspecified thigh**

✓6th M61.26 **Paralytic calcification and ossification of muscle, lower leg**

M61.261 **Paralytic calcification and ossification of muscle, right lower leg**

M61.262 **Paralytic calcification and ossification of muscle, left lower leg**

M61.269 **Paralytic calcification and ossification of muscle, unspecified lower leg**

✓6th M61.27 **Paralytic calcification and ossification of muscle, ankle and foot**

M61.271 **Paralytic calcification and ossification of muscle, right ankle and foot**

M61.272 **Paralytic calcification and ossification of muscle, left ankle and foot**

M61.279 **Paralytic calcification and ossification of muscle, unspecified ankle and foot**

M61.28 **Paralytic calcification and ossification of muscle, other site**

M61.29 **Paralytic calcification and ossification of muscle, multiple sites**

✓5th M61.3 **Calcification and ossification of muscles associated with burns**

Myositis ossificans associated with burns

M61.30 **Calcification and ossification of muscles associated with burns, unspecified site**

✓6th M61.31 **Calcification and ossification of muscles associated with burns, shoulder**

M61.311 **Calcification and ossification of muscles associated with burns, right shoulder**

M61.312 **Calcification and ossification of muscles associated with burns, left shoulder**

M61.319 **Calcification and ossification of muscles associated with burns, unspecified shoulder**

✓6th M61.32 **Calcification and ossification of muscles associated with burns, upper arm**

M61.321 **Calcification and ossification of muscles associated with burns, right upper arm**

M61.322 **Calcification and ossification of muscles associated with burns, left upper arm**

M61.329 **Calcification and ossification of muscles associated with burns, unspecified upper arm**

✓6th M61.33 **Calcification and ossification of muscles associated with burns, forearm**

M61.331 **Calcification and ossification of muscles associated with burns, right forearm**

M61.332 **Calcification and ossification of muscles associated with burns, left forearm**

M61.339 **Calcification and ossification of muscles associated with burns, unspecified forearm**

√6th **M61.34 Calcification and ossification of muscles associated with burns, hand**
M61.341 Calcification and ossification of muscles associated with burns, right hand
M61.342 Calcification and ossification of muscles associated with burns, left hand
M61.349 Calcification and ossification of muscles associated with burns, unspecified hand
√6th **M61.35 Calcification and ossification of muscles associated with burns, thigh**
M61.351 Calcification and ossification of muscles associated with burns, right thigh
M61.352 Calcification and ossification of muscles associated with burns, left thigh
M61.359 Calcification and ossification of muscles associated with burns, unspecified thigh
√6th **M61.36 Calcification and ossification of muscles associated with burns, lower leg**
M61.361 Calcification and ossification of muscles associated with burns, right lower leg
M61.362 Calcification and ossification of muscles associated with burns, left lower leg
M61.369 Calcification and ossification of muscles associated with burns, unspecified lower leg
√6th **M61.37 Calcification and ossification of muscles associated with burns, ankle and foot**
M61.371 Calcification and ossification of muscles associated with burns, right ankle and foot
M61.372 Calcification and ossification of muscles associated with burns, left ankle and foot
M61.379 Calcification and ossification of muscles associated with burns, unspecified ankle and foot
M61.38 Calcification and ossification of muscles associated with burns, other site
M61.39 Calcification and ossification of muscles associated with burns, multiple sites
√5th **M61.4 Other calcification of muscle**
EXCLUDES 1 *calcific tendinitis NOS (M65.2-)*
calcific tendinitis of shoulder (M75.3)
M61.40 Other calcification of muscle, unspecified site
√6th **M61.41 Other calcification of muscle, shoulder**
M61.411 Other calcification of muscle, right shoulder
M61.412 Other calcification of muscle, left shoulder
M61.419 Other calcification of muscle, unspecified shoulder
√6th **M61.42 Other calcification of muscle, upper arm**
M61.421 Other calcification of muscle, right upper arm
M61.422 Other calcification of muscle, left upper arm
M61.429 Other calcification of muscle, unspecified upper arm
√6th **M61.43 Other calcification of muscle, forearm**
M61.431 Other calcification of muscle, right forearm
M61.432 Other calcification of muscle, left forearm
M61.439 Other calcification of muscle, unspecified forearm
√6th **M61.44 Other calcification of muscle, hand**
M61.441 Other calcification of muscle, right hand
M61.442 Other calcification of muscle, left hand
M61.449 Other calcification of muscle, unspecified hand
√6th **M61.45 Other calcification of muscle, thigh**
M61.451 Other calcification of muscle, right thigh
M61.452 Other calcification of muscle, left thigh
M61.459 Other calcification of muscle, unspecified thigh
√6th **M61.46 Other calcification of muscle, lower leg**
M61.461 Other calcification of muscle, right lower leg
M61.462 Other calcification of muscle, left lower leg
M61.469 Other calcification of muscle, unspecified lower leg
√6th **M61.47 Other calcification of muscle, ankle and foot**
M61.471 Other calcification of muscle, right ankle and foot
M61.472 Other calcification of muscle, left ankle and foot
M61.479 Other calcification of muscle, unspecified ankle and foot
M61.48 Other calcification of muscle, other site
M61.49 Other calcification of muscle, multiple sites
√5th **M61.5 Other ossification of muscle**
M61.50 Other ossification of muscle, unspecified site
√6th **M61.51 Other ossification of muscle, shoulder**
M61.511 Other ossification of muscle, right shoulder
M61.512 Other ossification of muscle, left shoulder
M61.519 Other ossification of muscle, unspecified shoulder
√6th **M61.52 Other ossification of muscle, upper arm**
M61.521 Other ossification of muscle, right upper arm
M61.522 Other ossification of muscle, left upper arm
M61.529 Other ossification of muscle, unspecified upper arm
√6th **M61.53 Other ossification of muscle, forearm**
M61.531 Other ossification of muscle, right forearm
M61.532 Other ossification of muscle, left forearm
M61.539 Other ossification of muscle, unspecified forearm
√6th **M61.54 Other ossification of muscle, hand**
M61.541 Other ossification of muscle, right hand
M61.542 Other ossification of muscle, left hand
M61.549 Other ossification of muscle, unspecified hand
√6th **M61.55 Other ossification of muscle, thigh**
M61.551 Other ossification of muscle, right thigh
M61.552 Other ossification of muscle, left thigh
M61.559 Other ossification of muscle, unspecified thigh
√6th **M61.56 Other ossification of muscle, lower leg**
M61.561 Other ossification of muscle, right lower leg
M61.562 Other ossification of muscle, left lower leg
M61.569 Other ossification of muscle, unspecified lower leg
√6th **M61.57 Other ossification of muscle, ankle and foot**
M61.571 Other ossification of muscle, right ankle and foot
M61.572 Other ossification of muscle, left ankle and foot
M61.579 Other ossification of muscle, unspecified ankle and foot
M61.58 Other ossification of muscle, other site
M61.59 Other ossification of muscle, multiple sites
M61.9 Calcification and ossification of muscle, unspecified

DRAFT

✓4th M62 Other disorders of muscle

EXCLUDES 1 *alcoholic myopathy (G72.1)*
cramp and spasm (R25.2)
drug-induced myopathy (G72.Ø)
myalgia (M79.1)
stiff-man syndrome (G25.82)

EXCLUDES 2 *nontraumatic hematoma of muscle (M79.81)*

✓5th M62.Ø Separation of muscle (nontraumatic)

Diastasis of muscle

EXCLUDES 1 *diastasis recti complicating pregnancy, labor and delivery (O71.8)*
traumatic separation of muscle—see strain of muscle by body region

M62.ØØ Separation of muscle (nontraumatic), unspecified site

✓6th M62.Ø1 Separation of muscle (nontraumatic), shoulder
- **M62.Ø11 Separation of muscle (nontraumatic), right shoulder**
- **M62.Ø12 Separation of muscle (nontraumatic), left shoulder**
- **M62.Ø19 Separation of muscle (nontraumatic), unspecified shoulder**

✓6th M62.Ø2 Separation of muscle (nontraumatic), upper arm
- **M62.Ø21 Separation of muscle (nontraumatic), right upper arm**
- **M62.Ø22 Separation of muscle (nontraumatic), left upper arm**
- **M62.Ø29 Separation of muscle (nontraumatic), unspecified upper arm**

✓6th M62.Ø3 Separation of muscle (nontraumatic), forearm
- **M62.Ø31 Separation of muscle (nontraumatic), right forearm**
- **M62.Ø32 Separation of muscle (nontraumatic), left forearm**
- **M62.Ø39 Separation of muscle (nontraumatic), unspecified forearm**

✓6th M62.Ø4 Separation of muscle (nontraumatic), hand
- **M62.Ø41 Separation of muscle (nontraumatic), right hand**
- **M62.Ø42 Separation of muscle (nontraumatic), left hand**
- **M62.Ø49 Separation of muscle (nontraumatic), unspecified hand**

✓6th M62.Ø5 Separation of muscle (nontraumatic), thigh
- **M62.Ø51 Separation of muscle (nontraumatic), right thigh**
- **M62.Ø52 Separation of muscle (nontraumatic), left thigh**
- **M62.Ø59 Separation of muscle (nontraumatic), unspecified thigh**

✓6th M62.Ø6 Separation of muscle (nontraumatic), lower leg
- **M62.Ø61 Separation of muscle (nontraumatic), right lower leg**
- **M62.Ø62 Separation of muscle (nontraumatic), left lower leg**
- **M62.Ø69 Separation of muscle (nontraumatic), unspecified lower leg**

✓6th M62.Ø7 Separation of muscle (nontraumatic), ankle and foot
- **M62.Ø71 Separation of muscle (nontraumatic), right ankle and foot**
- **M62.Ø72 Separation of muscle (nontraumatic), left ankle and foot**
- **M62.Ø79 Separation of muscle (nontraumatic), unspecified ankle and foot**

M62.Ø8 Separation of muscle (nontraumatic), other site

✓5th M62.1 Other rupture of muscle (nontraumatic)

EXCLUDES 1 *traumatic rupture of muscle—see strain of muscle by body region*

EXCLUDES 2 *rupture of tendon (M66.-)*

M62.1Ø Other rupture of muscle (nontraumatic), unspecified site

✓6th M62.11 Other rupture of muscle (nontraumatic), shoulder
- **M62.111 Other rupture of muscle (nontraumatic), right shoulder**
- **M62.112 Other rupture of muscle (nontraumatic), left shoulder**
- **M62.119 Other rupture of muscle (nontraumatic), unspecified shoulder**

✓6th M62.12 Other rupture of muscle (nontraumatic), upper arm
- **M62.121 Other rupture of muscle (nontraumatic), right upper arm**
- **M62.122 Other rupture of muscle (nontraumatic), left upper arm**
- **M62.129 Other rupture of muscle (nontraumatic), unspecified upper arm**

✓6th M62.13 Other rupture of muscle (nontraumatic), forearm
- **M62.131 Other rupture of muscle (nontraumatic), right forearm**
- **M62.132 Other rupture of muscle (nontraumatic), left forearm**
- **M62.139 Other rupture of muscle (nontraumatic), unspecified forearm**

✓6th M62.14 Other rupture of muscle (nontraumatic), hand
- **M62.141 Other rupture of muscle (nontraumatic), right hand**
- **M62.142 Other rupture of muscle (nontraumatic), left hand**
- **M62.149 Other rupture of muscle (nontraumatic), unspecified hand**

✓6th M62.15 Other rupture of muscle (nontraumatic), thigh
- **M62.151 Other rupture of muscle (nontraumatic), right thigh**
- **M62.152 Other rupture of muscle (nontraumatic), left thigh**
- **M62.159 Other rupture of muscle (nontraumatic), unspecified thigh**

✓6th M62.16 Other rupture of muscle (nontraumatic), lower leg
- **M62.161 Other rupture of muscle (nontraumatic), right lower leg**
- **M62.162 Other rupture of muscle (nontraumatic), left lower leg**
- **M62.169 Other rupture of muscle (nontraumatic), unspecified lower leg**

✓6th M62.17 Other rupture of muscle (nontraumatic), ankle and foot
- **M62.171 Other rupture of muscle (nontraumatic), right ankle and foot**
- **M62.172 Other rupture of muscle (nontraumatic), left ankle and foot**
- **M62.179 Other rupture of muscle (nontraumatic), unspecified ankle and foot**

M62.18 Other rupture of muscle (nontraumatic), other site

✓5th M62.2 Nontraumatic ischemic infarction of muscle

EXCLUDES 1 *compartment syndrome (traumatic) (T79.A-)*
nontraumatic compartment syndrome (M79.A-)
rhabdomyolysis (M62.82)
traumatic ischemia of muscle (T79.6)
Volkmann's ischemic contracture (T79.6)

M62.2Ø Nontraumatic ischemic infarction of muscle, unspecified site

✓6th M62.21 Nontraumatic ischemic infarction of muscle, shoulder
- **M62.211 Nontraumatic ischemic infarction of muscle, right shoulder**
- **M62.212 Nontraumatic ischemic infarction of muscle, left shoulder**
- **M62.219 Nontraumatic ischemic infarction of muscle, unspecified shoulder**

✓6th M62.22 Nontraumatic ischemic infarction of muscle, upper arm
- **M62.221 Nontraumatic ischemic infarction of muscle, right upper arm**
- **M62.222 Nontraumatic ischemic infarction of muscle, left upper arm**
- **M62.229 Nontraumatic ischemic infarction of muscle, unspecified upper arm**

✓6th M62.23 Nontraumatic ischemic infarction of muscle, forearm
- **M62.231 Nontraumatic ischemic infarction of muscle, right forearm**
- **M62.232 Nontraumatic ischemic infarction of muscle, left forearm**

Diseases of the Musculoskeletal System and Connective Tissue
M62–M62.232

M62.239 Nontraumatic ischemic infarction of muscle, unspecified forearm

✓6th **M62.24 Nontraumatic ischemic infarction of muscle, hand**

M62.241 Nontraumatic ischemic infarction of muscle, right hand

M62.242 Nontraumatic ischemic infarction of muscle, left hand

M62.249 Nontraumatic ischemic infarction of muscle, unspecified hand

✓6th **M62.25 Nontraumatic ischemic infarction of muscle, thigh**

M62.251 Nontraumatic ischemic infarction of muscle, right thigh

M62.252 Nontraumatic ischemic infarction of muscle, left thigh

M62.259 Nontraumatic ischemic infarction of muscle, unspecified thigh

✓6th **M62.26 Nontraumatic ischemic infarction of muscle, lower leg**

M62.261 Nontraumatic ischemic infarction of muscle, right lower leg

M62.262 Nontraumatic ischemic infarction of muscle, left lower leg

M62.269 Nontraumatic ischemic infarction of muscle, unspecified lower leg

✓6th **M62.27 Nontraumatic ischemic infarction of muscle, ankle and foot**

M62.271 Nontraumatic ischemic infarction of muscle, right ankle and foot

M62.272 Nontraumatic ischemic infarction of muscle, left ankle and foot

M62.279 Nontraumatic ischemic infarction of muscle, unspecified ankle and foot

M62.28 Nontraumatic ischemic infarction of muscle, other site

M62.3 Immobility syndrome (paraplegic)

✓5th **M62.4 Contracture of muscle**

Contracture of tendon (sheath)

EXCLUDES 1 *contracture of joint (M24.5-)*

M62.40 Contracture of muscle, unspecified site

✓6th **M62.41 Contracture of muscle, shoulder**

M62.411 Contracture of muscle, right shoulder

M62.412 Contracture of muscle, left shoulder

M62.419 Contracture of muscle, unspecified shoulder

✓6th **M62.42 Contracture of muscle, upper arm**

M62.421 Contracture of muscle, right upper arm

M62.422 Contracture of muscle, left upper arm

M62.429 Contracture of muscle, unspecified upper arm

✓6th **M62.43 Contracture of muscle, forearm**

M62.431 Contracture of muscle, right forearm

M62.432 Contracture of muscle, left forearm

M62.439 Contracture of muscle, unspecified forearm

✓6th **M62.44 Contracture of muscle, hand**

M62.441 Contracture of muscle, right hand

M62.442 Contracture of muscle, left hand

M62.449 Contracture of muscle, unspecified hand

✓6th **M62.45 Contracture of muscle, thigh**

M62.451 Contracture of muscle, right thigh

M62.452 Contracture of muscle, left thigh

M62.459 Contracture of muscle, unspecified thigh

✓6th **M62.46 Contracture of muscle, lower leg**

M62.461 Contracture of muscle, right lower leg

M62.462 Contracture of muscle, left lower leg

M62.469 Contracture of muscle, unspecified lower leg

✓6th **M62.47 Contracture of muscle, ankle and foot**

M62.471 Contracture of muscle, right ankle and foot

M62.472 Contracture of muscle, left ankle and foot

M62.479 Contracture of muscle, unspecified ankle and foot

M62.48 Contracture of muscle, other site

M62.49 Contracture of muscle, multiple sites

✓5th **M62.5 Muscle wasting and atrophy, not elsewhere classified**

Disuse atrophy NEC

EXCLUDES 1 *neuralgic amyotrophy (G54.5)*
progressive muscular atrophy (G12.29)

EXCLUDES 2 *pelvic muscle wasting (N81.84)*

M62.50 Muscle wasting and atrophy, not elsewhere classified, unspecified site

✓6th **M62.51 Muscle wasting and atrophy, not elsewhere classified, shoulder**

M62.511 Muscle wasting and atrophy, not elsewhere classified, right shoulder

M62.512 Muscle wasting and atrophy, not elsewhere classified, left shoulder

M62.519 Muscle wasting and atrophy, not elsewhere classified, unspecified shoulder

✓6th **M62.52 Muscle wasting and atrophy, not elsewhere classified, upper arm**

M62.521 Muscle wasting and atrophy, not elsewhere classified, right upper arm

M62.522 Muscle wasting and atrophy, not elsewhere classified, left upper arm

M62.529 Muscle wasting and atrophy, not elsewhere classified, unspecified upper arm

✓6th **M62.53 Muscle wasting and atrophy, not elsewhere classified, forearm**

M62.531 Muscle wasting and atrophy, not elsewhere classified, right forearm

M62.532 Muscle wasting and atrophy, not elsewhere classified, left forearm

M62.539 Muscle wasting and atrophy, not elsewhere classified, unspecified forearm

✓6th **M62.54 Muscle wasting and atrophy, not elsewhere classified, hand**

M62.541 Muscle wasting and atrophy, not elsewhere classified, right hand

M62.542 Muscle wasting and atrophy, not elsewhere classified, left hand

M62.549 Muscle wasting and atrophy, not elsewhere classified, unspecified hand

✓6th **M62.55 Muscle wasting and atrophy, not elsewhere classified, thigh**

M62.551 Muscle wasting and atrophy, not elsewhere classified, right thigh

M62.552 Muscle wasting and atrophy, not elsewhere classified, left thigh

M62.559 Muscle wasting and atrophy, not elsewhere classified, unspecified thigh

✓6th **M62.56 Muscle wasting and atrophy, not elsewhere classified, lower leg**

M62.561 Muscle wasting and atrophy, not elsewhere classified, right lower leg

M62.562 Muscle wasting and atrophy, not elsewhere classified, left lower leg

M62.569 Muscle wasting and atrophy, not elsewhere classified, unspecified lower leg

✓6th **M62.57 Muscle wasting and atrophy, not elsewhere classified, ankle and foot**

M62.571 Muscle wasting and atrophy, not elsewhere classified, right ankle and foot

M62.572 Muscle wasting and atrophy, not elsewhere classified, left ankle and foot

M62.579 Muscle wasting and atrophy, not elsewhere classified, unspecified ankle and foot

M62.58 Muscle wasting and atrophy, not elsewhere classified, other site

M62.59 Muscle wasting and atrophy, not elsewhere classified, multiple sites

✓5th **M62.8 Other specified disorders of muscle**

EXCLUDES 2 *nontraumatic hematoma of muscle (M79.81)*

M62.81 Muscle weakness (generalized)

M62.82 Rhabdomyolysis

EXCLUDES 1 *traumatic rhabdomyolysis (T79.6)*

M62.83 Muscle spasm
M62.830 Muscle spasm of back
M62.831 Muscle spasm of calf
Charley-horse
M62.838 Other muscle spasm
M62.89 Other specified disorders of muscle
Muscle (sheath) hernia
M62.9 Disorder of muscle, unspecified

M63 Disorders of muscle in diseases classified elsewhere
EXCLUDES 1 *myopathy in cysticercosis (B69.81)*
myopathy in endocrine diseases (G73.7)
myopathy in metabolic diseases (G73.7)
myopathy in sarcoidosis (D86.87)
myopathy in secondary syphilis (A51.49)
myopathy in syphilis (late) (A52.78)
myopathy in toxoplasmosis (B58.82)
myopathy in tuberculosis (A18.09)
Code first underlying disease, such as:
leprosy (A30.-)
neoplasm (C49-, C79.89, D21-, D48.1)
schistosomiasis (B65.-)
trichinellosis (B75)

M63.8 Disorders of muscle in diseases classified elsewhere
M63.80 Disorders of muscle in diseases classified elsewhere, unspecified site
M63.81 Disorders of muscle in diseases classified elsewhere, shoulder
M63.811 Disorders of muscle in diseases classified elsewhere, right shoulder
M63.812 Disorders of muscle in diseases classified elsewhere, left shoulder
M63.819 Disorders of muscle in diseases classified elsewhere, unspecified shoulder
M63.82 Disorders of muscle in diseases classified elsewhere, upper arm
M63.821 Disorders of muscle in diseases classified elsewhere, right upper arm
M63.822 Disorders of muscle in diseases classified elsewhere, left upper arm
M63.829 Disorders of muscle in diseases classified elsewhere, unspecified upper arm
M63.83 Disorders of muscle in diseases classified elsewhere, forearm
M63.831 Disorders of muscle in diseases classified elsewhere, right forearm
M63.832 Disorders of muscle in diseases classified elsewhere, left forearm
M63.839 Disorders of muscle in diseases classified elsewhere, unspecified forearm
M63.84 Disorders of muscle in diseases classified elsewhere, hand
M63.841 Disorders of muscle in diseases classified elsewhere, right hand
M63.842 Disorders of muscle in diseases classified elsewhere, left hand
M63.849 Disorders of muscle in diseases classified elsewhere, unspecified hand
M63.85 Disorders of muscle in diseases classified elsewhere, thigh
M63.851 Disorders of muscle in diseases classified elsewhere, right thigh
M63.852 Disorders of muscle in diseases classified elsewhere, left thigh
M63.859 Disorders of muscle in diseases classified elsewhere, unspecified thigh
M63.86 Disorders of muscle in diseases classified elsewhere, lower leg
M63.861 Disorders of muscle in diseases classified elsewhere, right lower leg
M63.862 Disorders of muscle in diseases classified elsewhere, left lower leg
M63.869 Disorders of muscle in diseases classified elsewhere, unspecified lower leg
M63.87 Disorders of muscle in diseases classified elsewhere, ankle and foot
M63.871 Disorders of muscle in diseases classified elsewhere, right ankle and foot
M63.872 Disorders of muscle in diseases classified elsewhere, left ankle and foot
M63.879 Disorders of muscle in diseases classified elsewhere, unspecified ankle and foot
M63.88 Disorders of muscle in diseases classified elsewhere, other site
M63.89 Disorders of muscle in diseases classified elsewhere, multiple sites

Disorders of synovium and tendon (M65-M67)

M65 Synovitis and tenosynovitis
EXCLUDES 1 *chronic crepitant synovitis of hand and wrist (M70.0-)*
current injury—see injury of ligament or tendon by body region
soft tissue disorders related to use, overuse and pressure (M70.-)

M65.0 Abscess of tendon sheath
Use additional code (B95-B96) to identify bacterial agent.
M65.00 Abscess of tendon sheath, unspecified site
M65.01 Abscess of tendon sheath, shoulder
M65.011 Abscess of tendon sheath, right shoulder
M65.012 Abscess of tendon sheath, left shoulder
M65.019 Abscess of tendon sheath, unspecified shoulder
M65.02 Abscess of tendon sheath, upper arm
M65.021 Abscess of tendon sheath, right upper arm
M65.022 Abscess of tendon sheath, left upper arm
M65.029 Abscess of tendon sheath, unspecified upper arm
M65.03 Abscess of tendon sheath, forearm
M65.031 Abscess of tendon sheath, right forearm
M65.032 Abscess of tendon sheath, left forearm
M65.039 Abscess of tendon sheath, unspecified forearm
M65.04 Abscess of tendon sheath, hand
M65.041 Abscess of tendon sheath, right hand
M65.042 Abscess of tendon sheath, left hand
M65.049 Abscess of tendon sheath, unspecified hand
M65.05 Abscess of tendon sheath, thigh
M65.051 Abscess of tendon sheath, right thigh
M65.052 Abscess of tendon sheath, left thigh
M65.059 Abscess of tendon sheath, unspecified thigh
M65.06 Abscess of tendon sheath, lower leg
M65.061 Abscess of tendon sheath, right lower leg
M65.062 Abscess of tendon sheath, left lower leg
M65.069 Abscess of tendon sheath, unspecified lower leg
M65.07 Abscess of tendon sheath, ankle and foot
M65.071 Abscess of tendon sheath, right ankle and foot
M65.072 Abscess of tendon sheath, left ankle and foot
M65.079 Abscess of tendon sheath, unspecified ankle and foot
M65.08 Abscess of tendon sheath, other site
M65.1 Other infective (teno)synovitis
M65.10 Other infective (teno)synovitis, unspecified site
M65.11 Other infective (teno)synovitis, shoulder
M65.111 Other infective (teno)synovitis, right shoulder
M65.112 Other infective (teno)synovitis, left shoulder

M65.119 Other infective (teno)synovitis, unspecified shoulder

✓6th M65.12 Other infective (teno)synovitis, elbow
M65.121 Other infective (teno)synovitis, right elbow
M65.122 Other infective (teno)synovitis, left elbow
M65.129 Other infective (teno)synovitis, unspecified elbow

✓6th M65.13 Other infective (teno)synovitis, wrist
M65.131 Other infective (teno)synovitis, right wrist
M65.132 Other infective (teno)synovitis, left wrist
M65.139 Other infective (teno)synovitis, unspecified wrist

✓6th M65.14 Other infective (teno)synovitis, hand
M65.141 Other infective (teno)synovitis, right hand
M65.142 Other infective (teno)synovitis, left hand
M65.149 Other infective (teno)synovitis, unspecified hand

✓6th M65.15 Other infective (teno)synovitis, hip
M65.151 Other infective (teno)synovitis, right hip
M65.152 Other infective (teno)synovitis, left hip
M65.159 Other infective (teno)synovitis, unspecified hip

✓6th M65.16 Other infective (teno)synovitis, knee
M65.161 Other infective (teno)synovitis, right knee
M65.162 Other infective (teno)synovitis, left knee
M65.169 Other infective (teno)synovitis, unspecified knee

✓6th M65.17 Other infective (teno)synovitis, ankle and foot
M65.171 Other infective (teno)synovitis, right ankle and foot
M65.172 Other infective (teno)synovitis, left ankle and foot
M65.179 Other infective (teno)synovitis, unspecified ankle and foot

M65.18 Other infective (teno)synovitis, other site
M65.19 Other infective (teno)synovitis, multiple sites

✓5th M65.2 Calcific tendinitis
EXCLUDES1 *tendinitis as classified in M75-M77*
calcified tendinitis of shoulder (M75.3)

M65.20 Calcific tendinitis, unspecified site

✓6th M65.22 Calcific tendinitis, upper arm
M65.221 Calcific tendinitis, right upper arm
M65.222 Calcific tendinitis, left upper arm
M65.229 Calcific tendinitis, unspecified upper arm

✓6th M65.23 Calcific tendinitis, forearm
M65.231 Calcific tendinitis, right forearm
M65.232 Calcific tendinitis, left forearm
M65.239 Calcific tendinitis, unspecified forearm

✓6th M65.24 Calcific tendinitis, hand
M65.241 Calcific tendinitis, right hand
M65.242 Calcific tendinitis, left hand
M65.249 Calcific tendinitis, unspecified hand

✓6th M65.25 Calcific tendinitis, thigh
M65.251 Calcific tendinitis, right thigh
M65.252 Calcific tendinitis, left thigh
M65.259 Calcific tendinitis, unspecified thigh

✓6th M65.26 Calcific tendinitis, lower leg
M65.261 Calcific tendinitis, right lower leg
M65.262 Calcific tendinitis, left lower leg
M65.269 Calcific tendinitis, unspecified lower leg

✓6th M65.27 Calcific tendinitis, ankle and foot
M65.271 Calcific tendinitis, right ankle and foot
M65.272 Calcific tendinitis, left ankle and foot
M65.279 Calcific tendinitis, unspecified ankle and foot

M65.28 Calcific tendinitis, other site
M65.29 Calcific tendinitis, multiple sites

✓5th M65.3 Trigger finger
Nodular tendinous disease

M65.30 Trigger finger, unspecified finger

✓6th M65.31 Trigger thumb
M65.311 Trigger thumb, right thumb
M65.312 Trigger thumb, left thumb
M65.319 Trigger thumb, unspecified thumb

✓6th M65.32 Trigger finger, index finger
M65.321 Trigger finger, right index finger
M65.322 Trigger finger, left index finger
M65.329 Trigger finger, unspecified index finger

✓6th M65.33 Trigger finger, middle finger
M65.331 Trigger finger, right middle finger
M65.332 Trigger finger, left middle finger
M65.339 Trigger finger, unspecified middle finger

✓6th M65.34 Trigger finger, ring finger
M65.341 Trigger finger, right ring finger
M65.342 Trigger finger, left ring finger
M65.349 Trigger finger, unspecified ring finger

✓6th M65.35 Trigger finger, little finger
M65.351 Trigger finger, right little finger
M65.352 Trigger finger, left little finger
M65.359 Trigger finger, unspecified little finger

M65.4 Radial styloid tenosynovitis [de Quervain]

✓5th M65.8 Other synovitis and tenosynovitis

M65.80 Other synovitis and tenosynovitis, unspecified site

✓6th M65.81 Other synovitis and tenosynovitis, shoulder
M65.811 Other synovitis and tenosynovitis, right shoulder
M65.812 Other synovitis and tenosynovitis, left shoulder
M65.819 Other synovitis and tenosynovitis, unspecified shoulder

✓6th M65.82 Other synovitis and tenosynovitis, upper arm
M65.821 Other synovitis and tenosynovitis, right upper arm
M65.822 Other synovitis and tenosynovitis, left upper arm
M65.829 Other synovitis and tenosynovitis, unspecified upper arm

✓6th M65.83 Other synovitis and tenosynovitis, forearm
M65.831 Other synovitis and tenosynovitis, right forearm
M65.832 Other synovitis and tenosynovitis, left forearm
M65.839 Other synovitis and tenosynovitis, unspecified forearm

✓6th M65.84 Other synovitis and tenosynovitis, hand
M65.841 Other synovitis and tenosynovitis, right hand
M65.842 Other synovitis and tenosynovitis, left hand
M65.849 Other synovitis and tenosynovitis, unspecified hand

✓6th M65.85 Other synovitis and tenosynovitis, thigh
M65.851 Other synovitis and tenosynovitis, right thigh
M65.852 Other synovitis and tenosynovitis, left thigh
M65.859 Other synovitis and tenosynovitis, unspecified thigh

✓6th M65.86 Other synovitis and tenosynovitis, lower leg
M65.861 Other synovitis and tenosynovitis, right lower leg
M65.862 Other synovitis and tenosynovitis, left lower leg
M65.869 Other synovitis and tenosynovitis, unspecified lower leg

✓6th M65.87 Other synovitis and tenosynovitis, ankle and foot
M65.871 Other synovitis and tenosynovitis, right ankle and foot
M65.872 Other synovitis and tenosynovitis, left ankle and foot
M65.879 Other synovitis and tenosynovitis, unspecified ankle and foot

M65.88 Other synovitis and tenosynovitis, other site
M65.89 Other synovitis and tenosynovitis, multiple sites
M65.9 Synovitis and tenosynovitis, unspecified

M66 Spontaneous rupture of synovium and tendon

INCLUDES rupture that occurs when a normal force is applied to tissues that are inferred to have less than normal strength

EXCLUDES 2 *rotator cuff syndrome (M75.1-)*
rupture where an abnormal force is applied to normal tissue—see injury of tendon by body region

M66.0 Rupture of popliteal cyst

M66.1 Rupture of synovium
Rupture of synovial cyst
EXCLUDES 2 *rupture of popliteal cyst (M66.0)*

M66.10 Rupture of synovium, unspecified joint
M66.11 Rupture of synovium, shoulder
M66.111 Rupture of synovium, right shoulder
M66.112 Rupture of synovium, left shoulder
M66.119 Rupture of synovium, unspecified shoulder
M66.12 Rupture of synovium, elbow
M66.121 Rupture of synovium, right elbow
M66.122 Rupture of synovium, left elbow
M66.129 Rupture of synovium, unspecified elbow
M66.13 Rupture of synovium, wrist
M66.131 Rupture of synovium, right wrist
M66.132 Rupture of synovium, left wrist
M66.139 Rupture of synovium, unspecified wrist
M66.14 Rupture of synovium, hand and fingers
M66.141 Rupture of synovium, right hand
M66.142 Rupture of synovium, left hand
M66.143 Rupture of synovium, unspecified hand
M66.144 Rupture of synovium, right finger(s)
M66.145 Rupture of synovium, left finger(s)
M66.146 Rupture of synovium, unspecified finger(s)
M66.15 Rupture of synovium, hip
M66.151 Rupture of synovium, right hip
M66.152 Rupture of synovium, left hip
M66.159 Rupture of synovium, unspecified hip
M66.17 Rupture of synovium, ankle, foot and toes
M66.171 Rupture of synovium, right ankle
M66.172 Rupture of synovium, left ankle
M66.173 Rupture of synovium, unspecified ankle
M66.174 Rupture of synovium, right foot
M66.175 Rupture of synovium, left foot
M66.176 Rupture of synovium, unspecified foot
M66.177 Rupture of synovium, right toe(s)
M66.178 Rupture of synovium, left toe(s)
M66.179 Rupture of synovium, unspecified toe(s)
M66.18 Rupture of synovium, other site

M66.2 Spontaneous rupture of extensor tendons
M66.20 Spontaneous rupture of extensor tendons, unspecified site
M66.21 Spontaneous rupture of extensor tendons, shoulder
M66.211 Spontaneous rupture of extensor tendons, right shoulder
M66.212 Spontaneous rupture of extensor tendons, left shoulder
M66.219 Spontaneous rupture of extensor tendons, unspecified shoulder
M66.22 Spontaneous rupture of extensor tendons, upper arm
M66.221 Spontaneous rupture of extensor tendons, right upper arm
M66.222 Spontaneous rupture of extensor tendons, left upper arm
M66.229 Spontaneous rupture of extensor tendons, unspecified upper arm
M66.23 Spontaneous rupture of extensor tendons, forearm
M66.231 Spontaneous rupture of extensor tendons, right forearm
M66.232 Spontaneous rupture of extensor tendons, left forearm
M66.239 Spontaneous rupture of extensor tendons, unspecified forearm
M66.24 Spontaneous rupture of extensor tendons, hand
M66.241 Spontaneous rupture of extensor tendons, right hand
M66.242 Spontaneous rupture of extensor tendons, left hand
M66.249 Spontaneous rupture of extensor tendons, unspecified hand
M66.25 Spontaneous rupture of extensor tendons, thigh
M66.251 Spontaneous rupture of extensor tendons, right thigh
M66.252 Spontaneous rupture of extensor tendons, left thigh
M66.259 Spontaneous rupture of extensor tendons, unspecified thigh
M66.26 Spontaneous rupture of extensor tendons, lower leg
M66.261 Spontaneous rupture of extensor tendons, right lower leg
M66.262 Spontaneous rupture of extensor tendons, left lower leg
M66.269 Spontaneous rupture of extensor tendons, unspecified lower leg
M66.27 Spontaneous rupture of extensor tendons, ankle and foot
M66.271 Spontaneous rupture of extensor tendons, right ankle and foot
M66.272 Spontaneous rupture of extensor tendons, left ankle and foot
M66.279 Spontaneous rupture of extensor tendons, unspecified ankle and foot
M66.28 Spontaneous rupture of extensor tendons, other site
M66.29 Spontaneous rupture of extensor tendons, multiple sites

M66.3 Spontaneous rupture of flexor tendons
M66.30 Spontaneous rupture of flexor tendons, unspecified site
M66.31 Spontaneous rupture of flexor tendons, shoulder
M66.311 Spontaneous rupture of flexor tendons, right shoulder
M66.312 Spontaneous rupture of flexor tendons, left shoulder
M66.319 Spontaneous rupture of flexor tendons, unspecified shoulder
M66.32 Spontaneous rupture of flexor tendons, upper arm
M66.321 Spontaneous rupture of flexor tendons, right upper arm
M66.322 Spontaneous rupture of flexor tendons, left upper arm
M66.329 Spontaneous rupture of flexor tendons, unspecified upper arm
M66.33 Spontaneous rupture of flexor tendons, forearm
M66.331 Spontaneous rupture of flexor tendons, right forearm
M66.332 Spontaneous rupture of flexor tendons, left forearm
M66.339 Spontaneous rupture of flexor tendons, unspecified forearm
M66.34 Spontaneous rupture of flexor tendons, hand
M66.341 Spontaneous rupture of flexor tendons, right hand
M66.342 Spontaneous rupture of flexor tendons, left hand
M66.349 Spontaneous rupture of flexor tendons, unspecified hand
M66.35 Spontaneous rupture of flexor tendons, thigh
M66.351 Spontaneous rupture of flexor tendons, right thigh
M66.352 Spontaneous rupture of flexor tendons, left thigh
M66.359 Spontaneous rupture of flexor tendons, unspecified thigh
M66.36 Spontaneous rupture of flexor tendons, lower leg
M66.361 Spontaneous rupture of flexor tendons, right lower leg

M66.362 Spontaneous rupture of flexor tendons, left lower leg
M66.369 Spontaneous rupture of flexor tendons, unspecified lower leg
✓6th M66.37 Spontaneous rupture of flexor tendons, ankle and foot
M66.371 Spontaneous rupture of flexor tendons, right ankle and foot
M66.372 Spontaneous rupture of flexor tendons, left ankle and foot
M66.379 Spontaneous rupture of flexor tendons, unspecified ankle and foot
M66.38 Spontaneous rupture of flexor tendons, other site
M66.39 Spontaneous rupture of flexor tendons, multiple sites
✓5th M66.8 Spontaneous rupture of other tendons
M66.80 Spontaneous rupture of other tendons, unspecified site
✓6th M66.81 Spontaneous rupture of other tendons, shoulder
M66.811 Spontaneous rupture of other tendons, right shoulder
M66.812 Spontaneous rupture of other tendons, left shoulder
M66.819 Spontaneous rupture of other tendons, unspecified shoulder
✓6th M66.82 Spontaneous rupture of other tendons, upper arm
M66.821 Spontaneous rupture of other tendons, right upper arm
M66.822 Spontaneous rupture of other tendons, left upper arm
M66.829 Spontaneous rupture of other tendons, unspecified upper arm
✓6th M66.83 Spontaneous rupture of other tendons, forearm
M66.831 Spontaneous rupture of other tendons, right forearm
M66.832 Spontaneous rupture of other tendons, left forearm
M66.839 Spontaneous rupture of other tendons, unspecified forearm
✓6th M66.84 Spontaneous rupture of other tendons, hand
M66.841 Spontaneous rupture of other tendons, right hand
M66.842 Spontaneous rupture of other tendons, left hand
M66.849 Spontaneous rupture of other tendons, unspecified hand
✓6th M66.85 Spontaneous rupture of other tendons, thigh
M66.851 Spontaneous rupture of other tendons, right thigh
M66.852 Spontaneous rupture of other tendons, left thigh
M66.859 Spontaneous rupture of other tendons, unspecified thigh
✓6th M66.86 Spontaneous rupture of other tendons, lower leg
M66.861 Spontaneous rupture of other tendons, right lower leg
M66.862 Spontaneous rupture of other tendons, left lower leg
M66.869 Spontaneous rupture of other tendons, unspecified lower leg
✓6th M66.87 Spontaneous rupture of other tendons, ankle and foot
M66.871 Spontaneous rupture of other tendons, right ankle and foot
M66.872 Spontaneous rupture of other tendons, left ankle and foot
M66.879 Spontaneous rupture of other tendons, unspecified ankle and foot
M66.88 Spontaneous rupture of other tendons, other
M66.89 Spontaneous rupture of other tendons, multiple sites
M66.9 Spontaneous rupture of unspecified tendon
Rupture at musculotendinous junction, nontraumatic

✓4th **M67 Other disorders of synovium and tendon**
EXCLUDES 1 *palmar fascial fibromatosis [Dupuytren] (M72.0)*
tendinitis NOS (M77.9-)
xanthomatosis localized to tendons (E78.2)
✓5th M67.0 Short Achilles tendon (acquired)
M67.00 Short Achilles tendon (acquired), unspecified ankle
M67.01 Short Achilles tendon (acquired), right ankle
M67.02 Short Achilles tendon (acquired), left ankle
✓5th M67.2 Synovial hypertrophy, not elsewhere classified
EXCLUDES 1 *villonodular synovitis (pigmented) (M12.2-)*
M67.20 Synovial hypertrophy, not elsewhere classified, unspecified site
✓6th M67.21 Synovial hypertrophy, not elsewhere classified, shoulder
M67.211 Synovial hypertrophy, not elsewhere classified, right shoulder
M67.212 Synovial hypertrophy, not elsewhere classified, left shoulder
M67.219 Synovial hypertrophy, not elsewhere classified, unspecified shoulder
✓6th M67.22 Synovial hypertrophy, not elsewhere classified, upper arm
M67.221 Synovial hypertrophy, not elsewhere classified, right upper arm
M67.222 Synovial hypertrophy, not elsewhere classified, left upper arm
M67.229 Synovial hypertrophy, not elsewhere classified, unspecified upper arm
✓6th M67.23 Synovial hypertrophy, not elsewhere classified, forearm
M67.231 Synovial hypertrophy, not elsewhere classified, right forearm
M67.232 Synovial hypertrophy, not elsewhere classified, left forearm
M67.239 Synovial hypertrophy, not elsewhere classified, unspecified forearm
✓6th M67.24 Synovial hypertrophy, not elsewhere classified, hand
M67.241 Synovial hypertrophy, not elsewhere classified, right hand
M67.242 Synovial hypertrophy, not elsewhere classified, left hand
M67.249 Synovial hypertrophy, not elsewhere classified, unspecified hand
✓6th M67.25 Synovial hypertrophy, not elsewhere classified, thigh
M67.251 Synovial hypertrophy, not elsewhere classified, right thigh
M67.252 Synovial hypertrophy, not elsewhere classified, left thigh
M67.259 Synovial hypertrophy, not elsewhere classified, unspecified thigh
✓6th M67.26 Synovial hypertrophy, not elsewhere classified, lower leg
M67.261 Synovial hypertrophy, not elsewhere classified, right lower leg
M67.262 Synovial hypertrophy, not elsewhere classified, left lower leg
M67.269 Synovial hypertrophy, not elsewhere classified, unspecified lower leg
✓6th M67.27 Synovial hypertrophy, not elsewhere classified, ankle and foot
M67.271 Synovial hypertrophy, not elsewhere classified, right ankle and foot
M67.272 Synovial hypertrophy, not elsewhere classified, left ankle and foot
M67.279 Synovial hypertrophy, not elsewhere classified, unspecified ankle and foot
M67.28 Synovial hypertrophy, not elsewhere classified, other site
M67.29 Synovial hypertrophy, not elsewhere classified, multiple sites
✓5th M67.3 Transient synovitis
Toxic synovitis
EXCLUDES 1 *palindromic rheumatism (M12.3-)*
M67.30 Transient synovitis, unspecified site

✓6th M67.31 Transient synovitis, shoulder
M67.311 Transient synovitis, right shoulder
M67.312 Transient synovitis, left shoulder
M67.319 Transient synovitis, unspecified shoulder
✓6th M67.32 Transient synovitis, elbow
M67.321 Transient synovitis, right elbow
M67.322 Transient synovitis, left elbow
M67.329 Transient synovitis, unspecified elbow
✓6th M67.33 Transient synovitis, wrist
M67.331 Transient synovitis, right wrist
M67.332 Transient synovitis, left wrist
M67.339 Transient synovitis, unspecified wrist
✓6th M67.34 Transient synovitis, hand
M67.341 Transient synovitis, right hand
M67.342 Transient synovitis, left hand
M67.349 Transient synovitis, unspecified hand
✓6th M67.35 Transient synovitis, hip
M67.351 Transient synovitis, right hip
M67.352 Transient synovitis, left hip
M67.359 Transient synovitis, unspecified hip
✓6th M67.36 Transient synovitis, knee
M67.361 Transient synovitis, right knee
M67.362 Transient synovitis, left knee
M67.369 Transient synovitis, unspecified knee
✓6th M67.37 Transient synovitis, ankle and foot
M67.371 Transient synovitis, right ankle and foot
M67.372 Transient synovitis, left ankle and foot
M67.379 Transient synovitis, unspecified ankle and foot
M67.38 Transient synovitis, other site
M67.39 Transient synovitis, multiple sites
✓5th M67.4 Ganglion
Ganglion of joint or tendon (sheath)
EXCLUDES 1 *ganglion in yaws (A66.6)*
EXCLUDES 2 *cyst of bursa (M71.2-M71.3)*
cyst of synovium (M71.2-M71.3)
M67.40 Ganglion, unspecified site
✓6th M67.41 Ganglion, shoulder
M67.411 Ganglion, right shoulder
M67.412 Ganglion, left shoulder
M67.419 Ganglion, unspecified shoulder
✓6th M67.42 Ganglion, elbow
M67.421 Ganglion, right elbow
M67.422 Ganglion, left elbow
M67.429 Ganglion, unspecified elbow
✓6th M67.43 Ganglion, wrist
M67.431 Ganglion, right wrist
M67.432 Ganglion, left wrist
M67.439 Ganglion, unspecified wrist
✓6th M67.44 Ganglion, hand
M67.441 Ganglion, right hand
M67.442 Ganglion, left hand
M67.449 Ganglion, unspecified hand
✓6th M67.45 Ganglion, hip
M67.451 Ganglion, right hip
M67.452 Ganglion, left hip
M67.459 Ganglion, unspecified hip
✓6th M67.46 Ganglion, knee
M67.461 Ganglion, right knee
M67.462 Ganglion, left knee
M67.469 Ganglion, unspecified knee
✓6th M67.47 Ganglion, ankle and foot
M67.471 Ganglion, right ankle and foot
M67.472 Ganglion, left ankle and foot
M67.479 Ganglion, unspecified ankle and foot
M67.48 Ganglion, other site
M67.49 Ganglion, multiple sites
✓5th M67.5 Plica syndrome
Plica knee
M67.50 Plica syndrome, unspecified knee
M67.51 Plica syndrome, right knee
M67.52 Plica syndrome, left knee

✓5th M67.8 Other specified disorders of synovium and tendon
M67.80 Other specified disorders of synovium and tendon, unspecified site
✓6th M67.81 Other specified disorders of synovium and tendon, shoulder
M67.811 Other specified disorders of synovium, right shoulder
M67.812 Other specified disorders of synovium, left shoulder
M67.813 Other specified disorders of tendon, right shoulder
M67.814 Other specified disorders of tendon, left shoulder
M67.819 Other specified disorders of synovium and tendon, unspecified shoulder
✓6th M67.82 Other specified disorders of synovium and tendon, elbow
M67.821 Other specified disorders of synovium, right elbow
M67.822 Other specified disorders of synovium, left elbow
M67.823 Other specified disorders of tendon, right elbow
M67.824 Other specified disorders of tendon, left elbow
M67.829 Other specified disorders of synovium and tendon, unspecified elbow
✓6th M67.83 Other specified disorders of synovium and tendon, wrist
M67.831 Other specified disorders of synovium, right wrist
M67.832 Other specified disorders of synovium, left wrist
M67.833 Other specified disorders of tendon, right wrist
M67.834 Other specified disorders of tendon, left wrist
M67.839 Other specified disorders of synovium and tendon, unspecified forearm
✓6th M67.84 Other specified disorders of synovium and tendon, hand
M67.841 Other specified disorders of synovium, right hand
M67.842 Other specified disorders of synovium, left hand
M67.843 Other specified disorders of tendon, right hand
M67.844 Other specified disorders of tendon, left hand
M67.849 Other specified disorders of synovium and tendon, unspecified hand
✓6th M67.85 Other specified disorders of synovium and tendon, hip
M67.851 Other specified disorders of synovium, right hip
M67.852 Other specified disorders of synovium, left hip
M67.853 Other specified disorders of tendon, right hip
M67.854 Other specified disorders of tendon, left hip
M67.859 Other specified disorders of synovium and tendon, unspecified hip
✓6th M67.86 Other specified disorders of synovium and tendon, knee
M67.861 Other specified disorders of synovium, right knee
M67.862 Other specified disorders of synovium, left knee
M67.863 Other specified disorders of tendon, right knee
M67.864 Other specified disorders of tendon, left knee
M67.869 Other specified disorders of synovium and tendon, unspecified knee

✓6th **M67.87 Other specified disorders of synovium and tendon, ankle and foot**
M67.871 Other specified disorders of synovium, right ankle and foot
M67.872 Other specified disorders of synovium, left ankle and foot
M67.873 Other specified disorders of tendon, right ankle and foot
M67.874 Other specified disorders of tendon, left ankle and foot
M67.879 Other specified disorders of synovium and tendon, unspecified ankle and foot
M67.88 Other specified disorders of synovium and tendon, other site
M67.89 Other specified disorders of synovium and tendon, multiple sites

✓5th **M67.9 Unspecified disorder of synovium and tendon**
M67.90 Unspecified disorder of synovium and tendon, unspecified site

✓6th **M67.91 Unspecified disorder of synovium and tendon, shoulder**
M67.911 Unspecified disorder of synovium and tendon, right shoulder
M67.912 Unspecified disorder of synovium and tendon, left shoulder
M67.919 Unspecified disorder of synovium and tendon, unspecified shoulder

✓6th **M67.92 Unspecified disorder of synovium and tendon, upper arm**
M67.921 Unspecified disorder of synovium and tendon, right upper arm
M67.922 Unspecified disorder of synovium and tendon, left upper arm
M67.929 Unspecified disorder of synovium and tendon, unspecified upper arm

✓6th **M67.93 Unspecified disorder of synovium and tendon, forearm**
M67.931 Unspecified disorder of synovium and tendon, right forearm
M67.932 Unspecified disorder of synovium and tendon, left forearm
M67.939 Unspecified disorder of synovium and tendon, unspecified forearm

✓6th **M67.94 Unspecified disorder of synovium and tendon, hand**
M67.941 Unspecified disorder of synovium and tendon, right hand
M67.942 Unspecified disorder of synovium and tendon, left hand
M67.949 Unspecified disorder of synovium and tendon, unspecified hand

✓6th **M67.95 Unspecified disorder of synovium and tendon, thigh**
M67.951 Unspecified disorder of synovium and tendon, right thigh
M67.952 Unspecified disorder of synovium and tendon, left thigh
M67.959 Unspecified disorder of synovium and tendon, unspecified thigh

✓6th **M67.96 Unspecified disorder of synovium and tendon, lower leg**
M67.961 Unspecified disorder of synovium and tendon, right lower leg
M67.962 Unspecified disorder of synovium and tendon, left lower leg
M67.969 Unspecified disorder of synovium and tendon, unspecified lower leg

✓6th **M67.97 Unspecified disorder of synovium and tendon, ankle and foot**
M67.971 Unspecified disorder of synovium and tendon, right ankle and foot
M67.972 Unspecified disorder of synovium and tendon, left ankle and foot
M67.979 Unspecified disorder of synovium and tendon, unspecified ankle and foot
M67.98 Unspecified disorder of synovium and tendon, other site
M67.99 Unspecified disorder of synovium and tendon, multiple sites

Other soft tissue disorders (M70-M79)

✓4th **M70 Soft tissue disorders related to use, overuse and pressure**

INCLUDES soft tissue disorders of occupational origin

EXCLUDES 1 *bursitis NOS (M71.9-)*

EXCLUDES 2 *bursitis of shoulder (M75.5)*
enthesopathies (M76-M77)
pressure ulcer (pressure area) (L89.-)

Use additional external cause code to identify activity causing disorder (Y93.-)

✓5th **M70.0 Crepitant synovitis (acute) (chronic) of hand and wrist**

✓6th **M70.03 Crepitant synovitis (acute) (chronic), wrist**
M70.031 Crepitant synovitis (acute) (chronic), right wrist
M70.032 Crepitant synovitis (acute) (chronic), left wrist
M70.039 Crepitant synovitis (acute) (chronic), unspecified wrist

✓6th **M70.04 Crepitant synovitis (acute) (chronic), hand**
M70.041 Crepitant synovitis (acute) (chronic), right hand
M70.042 Crepitant synovitis (acute) (chronic), left hand
M70.049 Crepitant synovitis (acute) (chronic), unspecified hand

✓5th **M70.1 Bursitis of hand**
M70.10 Bursitis, unspecified hand
M70.11 Bursitis, right hand
M70.12 Bursitis, left hand

✓5th **M70.2 Olecranon bursitis**
M70.20 Olecranon bursitis, unspecified elbow
M70.21 Olecranon bursitis, right elbow
M70.22 Olecranon bursitis, left elbow

✓5th **M70.3 Other bursitis of elbow**
M70.30 Other bursitis of elbow, unspecified elbow
M70.31 Other bursitis of elbow, right elbow
M70.32 Other bursitis of elbow, left elbow

✓5th **M70.4 Prepatellar bursitis**
M70.40 Prepatellar bursitis, unspecified knee
M70.41 Prepatellar bursitis, right knee
M70.42 Prepatellar bursitis, left knee

✓5th **M70.5 Other bursitis of knee**
M70.50 Other bursitis of knee, unspecified knee
M70.51 Other bursitis of knee, right knee
M70.52 Other bursitis of knee, left knee

✓5th **M70.6 Trochanteric bursitis**
Trochanteric tendinitis
M70.60 Trochanteric bursitis, unspecified hip
M70.61 Trochanteric bursitis, right hip
M70.62 Trochanteric bursitis, left hip

✓5th **M70.7 Other bursitis of hip**
Ischial bursitis
M70.70 Other bursitis of hip, unspecified hip
M70.71 Other bursitis of hip, right hip
M70.72 Other bursitis of hip, left hip

✓5th **M70.8 Other soft tissue disorders related to use, overuse and pressure**
M70.80 Other soft tissue disorders related to use, overuse and pressure of unspecified site

✓6th **M70.81 Other soft tissue disorders related to use, overuse and pressure of shoulder**
M70.811 Other soft tissue disorders related to use, overuse and pressure, right shoulder
M70.812 Other soft tissue disorders related to use, overuse and pressure, left shoulder
M70.819 Other soft tissue disorders related to use, overuse and pressure, unspecified shoulder

✓6th **M70.82 Other soft tissue disorders related to use, overuse and pressure of upper arm**
M70.821 Other soft tissue disorders related to use, overuse and pressure, right upper arm

M70.822 Other soft tissue disorders related to use, overuse and pressure, left upper arm
M70.829 Other soft tissue disorders related to use, overuse and pressure, unspecified upper arms
✓6th **M70.83 Other soft tissue disorders related to use, overuse and pressure of forearm**
M70.831 Other soft tissue disorders related to use, overuse and pressure, right forearm
M70.832 Other soft tissue disorders related to use, overuse and pressure, left forearm
M70.839 Other soft tissue disorders related to use, overuse and pressure, unspecified forearm
✓6th **M70.84 Other soft tissue disorders related to use, overuse and pressure of hand**
M70.841 Other soft tissue disorders related to use, overuse and pressure, right hand
M70.842 Other soft tissue disorders related to use, overuse and pressure, left hand
M70.849 Other soft tissue disorders related to use, overuse and pressure, unspecified hand
✓6th **M70.85 Other soft tissue disorders related to use, overuse and pressure of thigh**
M70.851 Other soft tissue disorders related to use, overuse and pressure, right thigh
M70.852 Other soft tissue disorders related to use, overuse and pressure, left thigh
M70.859 Other soft tissue disorders related to use, overuse and pressure, unspecified thigh
✓6th **M70.86 Other soft tissue disorders related to use, overuse and pressure lower leg**
M70.861 Other soft tissue disorders related to use, overuse and pressure, right lower leg
M70.862 Other soft tissue disorders related to use, overuse and pressure, left lower leg
M70.869 Other soft tissue disorders related to use, overuse and pressure, unspecified leg
✓6th **M70.87 Other soft tissue disorders related to use, overuse and pressure of ankle and foot**
M70.871 Other soft tissue disorders related to use, overuse and pressure, right ankle and foot
M70.872 Other soft tissue disorders related to use, overuse and pressure, left ankle and foot
M70.879 Other soft tissue disorders related to use, overuse and pressure, unspecified ankle and foot
M70.88 Other soft tissue disorders related to use, overuse and pressure other site
M70.89 Other soft tissue disorders related to use, overuse and pressure multiple sites
✓5th **M70.9 Unspecified soft tissue disorder related to use, overuse and pressure**
M70.90 Unspecified soft tissue disorder related to use, overuse and pressure of unspecified site
✓6th **M70.91 Unspecified soft tissue disorder related to use, overuse and pressure of shoulder**
M70.911 Unspecified soft tissue disorder related to use, overuse and pressure, right shoulder
M70.912 Unspecified soft tissue disorder related to use, overuse and pressure, left shoulder
M70.919 Unspecified soft tissue disorder related to use, overuse and pressure, unspecified shoulder
✓6th **M70.92 Unspecified soft tissue disorder related to use, overuse and pressure of upper arm**
M70.921 Unspecified soft tissue disorder related to use, overuse and pressure, right upper arm
M70.922 Unspecified soft tissue disorder related to use, overuse and pressure, left upper arm
M70.929 Unspecified soft tissue disorder related to use, overuse and pressure, unspecified upper arm
✓6th **M70.93 Unspecified soft tissue disorder related to use, overuse and pressure of forearm**
M70.931 Unspecified soft tissue disorder related to use, overuse and pressure, right forearm
M70.932 Unspecified soft tissue disorder related to use, overuse and pressure, left forearm
M70.939 Unspecified soft tissue disorder related to use, overuse and pressure, unspecified forearm
✓6th **M70.94 Unspecified soft tissue disorder related to use, overuse and pressure of hand**
M70.941 Unspecified soft tissue disorder related to use, overuse and pressure, right hand
M70.942 Unspecified soft tissue disorder related to use, overuse and pressure, left hand
M70.949 Unspecified soft tissue disorder related to use, overuse and pressure, unspecified hand
✓6th **M70.95 Unspecified soft tissue disorder related to use, overuse and pressure of thigh**
M70.951 Unspecified soft tissue disorder related to use, overuse and pressure, right thigh
M70.952 Unspecified soft tissue disorder related to use, overuse and pressure, left thigh
M70.959 Unspecified soft tissue disorder related to use, overuse and pressure, unspecified thigh
✓6th **M70.96 Unspecified soft tissue disorder related to use, overuse and pressure lower leg**
M70.961 Unspecified soft tissue disorder related to use, overuse and pressure, right lower leg
M70.962 Unspecified soft tissue disorder related to use, overuse and pressure, left lower leg
M70.969 Unspecified soft tissue disorder related to use, overuse and pressure, unspecified lower leg
✓6th **M70.97 Unspecified soft tissue disorder related to use, overuse and pressure of ankle and foot**
M70.971 Unspecified soft tissue disorder related to use, overuse and pressure, right ankle and foot
M70.972 Unspecified soft tissue disorder related to use, overuse and pressure, left ankle and foot
M70.979 Unspecified soft tissue disorder related to use, overuse and pressure, unspecified ankle and foot
M70.98 Unspecified soft tissue disorder related to use, overuse and pressure other
M70.99 Unspecified soft tissue disorder related to use, overuse and pressure multiple sites

✓4th **M71 Other bursopathies**
EXCLUDES 1 *bunion (M20.1)*
bursitis related to use, overuse or pressure (M70.-)
enthesopathies (M76-M77)
✓5th **M71.0 Abscess of bursa**
Use additional code (B95.-, B96.-) to identify causative organism
M71.00 Abscess of bursa, unspecified site
✓6th **M71.01 Abscess of bursa, shoulder**
M71.011 Abscess of bursa, right shoulder
M71.012 Abscess of bursa, left shoulder
M71.019 Abscess of bursa, unspecified shoulder
✓6th **M71.02 Abscess of bursa, elbow**
M71.021 Abscess of bursa, right elbow
M71.022 Abscess of bursa, left elbow
M71.029 Abscess of bursa, unspecified elbow

✓6th **M71.03 Abscess of bursa, wrist**
M71.031 Abscess of bursa, right wrist
M71.032 Abscess of bursa, left wrist
M71.039 Abscess of bursa, unspecified wrist

✓6th **M71.04 Abscess of bursa, hand**
M71.041 Abscess of bursa, right hand
M71.042 Abscess of bursa, left hand
M71.049 Abscess of bursa, unspecified hand

✓6th **M71.05 Abscess of bursa, hip**
M71.051 Abscess of bursa, right hip
M71.052 Abscess of bursa, left hip
M71.059 Abscess of bursa, unspecified hip

✓6th **M71.06 Abscess of bursa, knee**
M71.061 Abscess of bursa, right knee
M71.062 Abscess of bursa, left knee
M71.069 Abscess of bursa, unspecified knee

✓6th **M71.07 Abscess of bursa, ankle and foot**
M71.071 Abscess of bursa, right ankle and foot
M71.072 Abscess of bursa, left ankle and foot
M71.079 Abscess of bursa, unspecified ankle and foot

M71.08 Abscess of bursa, other site
M71.09 Abscess of bursa, multiple sites

✓5th **M71.1 Other infective bursitis**
Use additional code (B95.-, B96.-) to identify causative organism

M71.10 Other infective bursitis, unspecified site

✓6th **M71.11 Other infective bursitis, shoulder**
M71.111 Other infective bursitis, right shoulder
M71.112 Other infective bursitis, left shoulder
M71.119 Other infective bursitis, unspecified shoulder

✓6th **M71.12 Other infective bursitis, elbow**
M71.121 Other infective bursitis, right elbow
M71.122 Other infective bursitis, left elbow
M71.129 Other infective bursitis, unspecified elbow

✓6th **M71.13 Other infective bursitis, wrist**
M71.131 Other infective bursitis, right wrist
M71.132 Other infective bursitis, left wrist
M71.139 Other infective bursitis, unspecified wrist

✓6th **M71.14 Other infective bursitis, hand**
M71.141 Other infective bursitis, right hand
M71.142 Other infective bursitis, left hand
M71.149 Other infective bursitis, unspecified hand

✓6th **M71.15 Other infective bursitis, hip**
M71.151 Other infective bursitis, right hip
M71.152 Other infective bursitis, left hip
M71.159 Other infective bursitis, unspecified hip

✓6th **M71.16 Other infective bursitis, knee**
M71.161 Other infective bursitis, right knee
M71.162 Other infective bursitis, left knee
M71.169 Other infective bursitis, unspecified knee

✓6th **M71.17 Other infective bursitis, ankle and foot**
M71.171 Other infective bursitis, right ankle and foot
M71.172 Other infective bursitis, left ankle and foot
M71.179 Other infective bursitis, unspecified ankle and foot

M71.18 Other infective bursitis, other site
M71.19 Other infective bursitis, multiple sites

✓5th **M71.2 Synovial cyst of popliteal space [Baker]**
EXCLUDES 1 *synovial cyst of popliteal space with rupture (M66.0)*

M71.20 Synovial cyst of popliteal space [Baker], unspecified knee
M71.21 Synovial cyst of popliteal space [Baker], right knee
M71.22 Synovial cyst of popliteal space [Baker], left knee

✓5th **M71.3 Other bursal cyst**
Synovial cyst NOS
EXCLUDES 1 *synovial cyst with rupture (M66.1-)*

M71.30 Other bursal cyst, unspecified site

✓6th **M71.31 Other bursal cyst, shoulder**
M71.311 Other bursal cyst, right shoulder
M71.312 Other bursal cyst, left shoulder
M71.319 Other bursal cyst, unspecified shoulder

✓6th **M71.32 Other bursal cyst, elbow**
M71.321 Other bursal cyst, right elbow
M71.322 Other bursal cyst, left elbow
M71.329 Other bursal cyst, unspecified elbow

✓6th **M71.33 Other bursal cyst, wrist**
M71.331 Other bursal cyst, right wrist
M71.332 Other bursal cyst, left wrist
M71.339 Other bursal cyst, unspecified wrist

✓6th **M71.34 Other bursal cyst, hand**
M71.341 Other bursal cyst, right hand
M71.342 Other bursal cyst, left hand
M71.349 Other bursal cyst, unspecified hand

✓6th **M71.35 Other bursal cyst, hip**
M71.351 Other bursal cyst, right hip
M71.352 Other bursal cyst, left hip
M71.359 Other bursal cyst, unspecified hip

✓6th **M71.37 Other bursal cyst, ankle and foot**
M71.371 Other bursal cyst, right ankle and foot
M71.372 Other bursal cyst, left ankle and foot
M71.379 Other bursal cyst, unspecified ankle and foot

M71.38 Other bursal cyst, other site
M71.39 Other bursal cyst, multiple sites

✓5th **M71.4 Calcium deposit in bursa**
EXCLUDES 2 *calcium deposit in bursa of shoulder (M75.3)*

M71.40 Calcium deposit in bursa, unspecified site

✓6th **M71.42 Calcium deposit in bursa, elbow**
M71.421 Calcium deposit in bursa, right elbow
M71.422 Calcium deposit in bursa, left elbow
M71.429 Calcium deposit in bursa, unspecified elbow

✓6th **M71.43 Calcium deposit in bursa, wrist**
M71.431 Calcium deposit in bursa, right wrist
M71.432 Calcium deposit in bursa, left wrist
M71.439 Calcium deposit in bursa, unspecified wrist

✓6th **M71.44 Calcium deposit in bursa, hand**
M71.441 Calcium deposit in bursa, right hand
M71.442 Calcium deposit in bursa, left hand
M71.449 Calcium deposit in bursa, unspecified hand

✓6th **M71.45 Calcium deposit in bursa, hip**
M71.451 Calcium deposit in bursa, right hip
M71.452 Calcium deposit in bursa, left hip
M71.459 Calcium deposit in bursa, unspecified hip

✓6th **M71.46 Calcium deposit in bursa, knee**
M71.461 Calcium deposit in bursa, right knee
M71.462 Calcium deposit in bursa, left knee
M71.469 Calcium deposit in bursa, unspecified knee

✓6th **M71.47 Calcium deposit in bursa, ankle and foot**
M71.471 Calcium deposit in bursa, right ankle and foot
M71.472 Calcium deposit in bursa, left ankle and foot
M71.479 Calcium deposit in bursa, unspecified ankle and foot

M71.48 Calcium deposit in bursa, other site
M71.49 Calcium deposit in bursa, multiple sites

✓5th **M71.5 Other bursitis, not elsewhere classified**
EXCLUDES 1 *bursitis NOS (M71.9-)*
EXCLUDES 2 *bursitis of shoulder (M75.5)*
bursitis of tibial collateral [Pellegrini-Stieda] (M76.4)

M71.50 Other bursitis, not elsewhere classified, unspecified site

✓6th **M71.52 Other bursitis, not elsewhere classified, elbow**
M71.521 Other bursitis, not elsewhere classified, right elbow
M71.522 Other bursitis, not elsewhere classified, left elbow

EXCLUDES 1 Not coded here EXCLUDES 2 Not included here *Manifestation Code*

M71.529 Other bursitis, not elsewhere classified, unspecified elbow

✓6th M71.53 Other bursitis, not elsewhere classified, wrist
M71.531 Other bursitis, not elsewhere classified, right wrist
M71.532 Other bursitis, not elsewhere classified, left wrist
M71.539 Other bursitis, not elsewhere classified, unspecified wrist

✓6th M71.54 Other bursitis, not elsewhere classified, hand
M71.541 Other bursitis, not elsewhere classified, right hand
M71.542 Other bursitis, not elsewhere classified, left hand
M71.549 Other bursitis, not elsewhere classified, unspecified hand

✓6th M71.55 Other bursitis, not elsewhere classified, hip
M71.551 Other bursitis, not elsewhere classified, right hip
M71.552 Other bursitis, not elsewhere classified, left hip
M71.559 Other bursitis, not elsewhere classified, unspecified hip

✓6th M71.56 Other bursitis, not elsewhere classified, knee
M71.561 Other bursitis, not elsewhere classified, right knee
M71.562 Other bursitis, not elsewhere classified, left knee
M71.569 Other bursitis, not elsewhere classified, unspecified knee

✓6th M71.57 Other bursitis, not elsewhere classified, ankle and foot
M71.571 Other bursitis, not elsewhere classified, right ankle and foot
M71.572 Other bursitis, not elsewhere classified, left ankle and foot
M71.579 Other bursitis, not elsewhere classified, unspecified ankle and foot

M71.58 Other bursitis, not elsewhere classified, other site

✓5th M71.8 Other specified bursopathies
M71.80 Other specified bursopathies, unspecified site

✓6th M71.81 Other specified bursopathies, shoulder
M71.811 Other specified bursopathies, right shoulder
M71.812 Other specified bursopathies, left shoulder
M71.819 Other specified bursopathies, unspecified shoulder

✓6th M71.82 Other specified bursopathies, elbow
M71.821 Other specified bursopathies, right elbow
M71.822 Other specified bursopathies, left elbow
M71.829 Other specified bursopathies, unspecified elbow

✓6th M71.83 Other specified bursopathies, wrist
M71.831 Other specified bursopathies, right wrist
M71.832 Other specified bursopathies, left wrist
M71.839 Other specified bursopathies, unspecified wrist

✓6th M71.84 Other specified bursopathies, hand
M71.841 Other specified bursopathies, right hand
M71.842 Other specified bursopathies, left hand
M71.849 Other specified bursopathies, unspecified hand

✓6th M71.85 Other specified bursopathies, hip
M71.851 Other specified bursopathies, right hip
M71.852 Other specified bursopathies, left hip
M71.859 Other specified bursopathies, unspecified hip

✓6th M71.86 Other specified bursopathies, knee
M71.861 Other specified bursopathies, right knee
M71.862 Other specified bursopathies, left knee
M71.869 Other specified bursopathies, unspecified knee

✓6th M71.87 Other specified bursopathies, ankle and foot
M71.871 Other specified bursopathies, right ankle and foot
M71.872 Other specified bursopathies, left ankle and foot
M71.879 Other specified bursopathies, unspecified ankle and foot

M71.88 Other specified bursopathies, other site
M71.89 Other specified bursopathies, multiple sites
M71.9 Bursopathy, unspecified
Bursitis NOS

✓4th **M72 Fibroblastic disorders**
EXCLUDES 2 *retroperitoneal fibromatosis (D48.3)*

M72.0 Palmar fascial fibromatosis [Dupuytren]
M72.1 Knuckle pads
M72.2 Plantar fascial fibromatosis
Plantar fasciitis
M72.4 Pseudosarcomatous fibromatosis
Nodular fasciitis
M72.6 Necrotizing fasciitis
Use additional code (B95.-, B96.-) to identify causative organism
M72.8 Other fibroblastic disorders
Abscess of fascia
Fasciitis NEC
Other infective fasciitis
Use additional code to (B95.-, B96.-) identify causative organism
EXCLUDES 1 *diffuse (eosinophilic) fasciitis (M35.4)*
necrotizing fasciitis (M72.6)
nodular fasciitis (M72.4)
perirenal fasciitis NOS (N13.5)
perirenal fasciitis with infection (N13.6)
plantar fasciitis (M72.2)
M72.9 Fibroblastic disorder, unspecified
Fasciitis NOS
Fibromatosis NOS

✓4th **M75 Shoulder lesions**
EXCLUDES 2 *shoulder-hand syndrome (M89.0-)*

✓5th M75.0 Adhesive capsulitis of shoulder
Frozen shoulder
Periarthritis of shoulder
M75.00 Adhesive capsulitis of unspecified shoulder
M75.01 Adhesive capsulitis of right shoulder
M75.02 Adhesive capsulitis of left shoulder

✓5th M75.1 Rotator cuff tear or rupture, not specified as traumatic
Rotator cuff syndrome
Supraspinatus syndrome
Supraspinatus tear or rupture, not specified as traumatic
EXCLUDES 1 *tear of rotator cuff, traumatic (S46.01-)*

✓6th M75.10 Unspecified rotator cuff tear or rupture, not specified as traumatic
M75.100 Unspecified rotator cuff tear or rupture of unspecified shoulder, not specified as traumatic
M75.101 Unspecified rotator cuff tear or rupture of right shoulder, not specified as traumatic
M75.102 Unspecified rotator cuff tear or rupture of left shoulder, not specified as traumatic

✓6th M75.11 Incomplete rotator cuff tear or rupture not specified as traumatic
M75.110 Incomplete rotator cuff tear or rupture of unspecified shoulder, not specified as traumatic
M75.111 Incomplete rotator cuff tear or rupture of right shoulder, not specified as traumatic
M75.112 Incomplete rotator cuff tear or rupture of left shoulder, not specified as traumatic

✓6th M75.12 Complete rotator cuff tear or rupture not specified astraumatic
M75.120 Complete rotator cuff tear or rupture of unspecified shoulder, not specified as traumatic
M75.121 Complete rotator cuff tear or rupture of right shoulder, not specified as traumatic

M75.122 Complete rotator cuff tear or rupture of left shoulder, not specified as traumatic

5th **M75.2 Bicipital tendinitis**
- **M75.20 Bicipital tendinitis, unspecified shoulder**
- **M75.21 Bicipital tendinitis, right shoulder**
- **M75.22 Bicipital tendinitis, left shoulder**

5th **M75.3 Calcific tendinitis of shoulder**
Calcified bursa of shoulder
- **M75.30 Calcific tendinitis of unspecified shoulder**
- **M75.31 Calcific tendinitis of right shoulder**
- **M75.32 Calcific tendinitis of left shoulder**

5th **M75.4 Impingement syndrome of shoulder**
- **M75.40 Impingement syndrome of unspecified shoulder**
- **M75.41 Impingement syndrome of right shoulder**
- **M75.42 Impingement syndrome of left shoulder**

5th **M75.5 Bursitis of shoulder**
- **M75.50 Bursitis of unspecified shoulder**
- **M75.51 Bursitis of right shoulder**
- **M75.52 Bursitis of left shoulder**

5th **M75.8 Other shoulder lesions**
- **M75.80 Other shoulder lesions, unspecified shoulder**
- **M75.81 Other shoulder lesions, right shoulder**
- **M75.82 Other shoulder lesions, left shoulder**

5th **M75.9 Shoulder lesion, unspecified**
- **M75.90 Shoulder lesion, unspecified, unspecified shoulder**
- **M75.91 Shoulder lesion, unspecified, right shoulder**
- **M75.92 Shoulder lesion, unspecified, left shoulder**

4th M76 Enthesopathies, lower limb, excluding foot

EXCLUDES 2 *bursitis due to use, overuse and pressure (M70.-)*
enthesopathies of ankle and foot (M77.5-)

5th **M76.0 Gluteal tendinitis**
- **M76.00 Gluteal tendinitis, unspecified hip**
- **M76.01 Gluteal tendinitis, right hip**
- **M76.02 Gluteal tendinitis, left hip**

5th **M76.1 Psoas tendinitis**
- **M76.10 Psoas tendinitis, unspecified hip**
- **M76.11 Psoas tendinitis, right hip**
- **M76.12 Psoas tendinitis, left hip**

5th **M76.2 Iliac crest spur**
- **M76.20 Iliac crest spur, unspecified hip**
- **M76.21 Iliac crest spur, right hip**
- **M76.22 Iliac crest spur, left hip**

5th **M76.3 Iliotibial band syndrome**
- **M76.30 Iliotibial band syndrome, unspecified leg**
- **M76.31 Iliotibial band syndrome, right leg**
- **M76.32 Iliotibial band syndrome, left leg**

5th **M76.4 Tibial collateral bursitis [Pellegrini-Stieda]**
- **M76.40 Tibial collateral bursitis [Pellegrini-Stieda], unspecified leg**
- **M76.41 Tibial collateral bursitis [Pellegrini-Stieda], right leg**
- **M76.42 Tibial collateral bursitis [Pellegrini-Stieda], left leg**

5th **M76.5 Patellar tendinitis**
- **M76.50 Patellar tendinitis, unspecified knee**
- **M76.51 Patellar tendinitis, right knee**
- **M76.52 Patellar tendinitis, left knee**

5th **M76.6 Achilles tendinitis**
Achilles bursitis
- **M76.60 Achilles tendinitis, unspecified leg**
- **M76.61 Achilles tendinitis, right leg**
- **M76.62 Achilles tendinitis, left leg**

5th **M76.7 Peroneal tendinitis**
- **M76.70 Peroneal tendinitis, unspecified leg**
- **M76.71 Peroneal tendinitis, right leg**
- **M76.72 Peroneal tendinitis, left leg**

5th **M76.8 Other specified enthesopathies of lower limb, excluding foot**

6th **M76.81 Anterior tibial syndrome**
- **M76.811 Anterior tibial syndrome, right leg**
- **M76.812 Anterior tibial syndrome, left leg**
- **M76.819 Anterior tibial syndrome, unspecified leg**

6th **M76.82 Posterior tibial tendinitis**
- **M76.821 Posterior tibial tendinitis, right leg**
- **M76.822 Posterior tibial tendinitis, left leg**
- **M76.829 Posterior tibial tendinitis, unspecified leg**

6th **M76.89 Other specified enthesopathies of lower limb, excluding foot**
- **M76.891 Other specified enthesopathies of right lower limb, excluding foot**
- **M76.892 Other specified enthesopathies of left lower limb, excluding foot**
- **M76.899 Other specified enthesopathies of unspecified lower limb, excluding foot**

M76.9 Unspecified enthesopathy, lower limb, excluding foot

4th M77 Other enthesopathies

EXCLUDES 1 *bursitis NOS (M71.9-)*

EXCLUDES 2 *bursitis due to use, overuse and pressure (M70.-)*
osteophyte (M25.7)
spinal enthesopathy (M46.0-)

5th **M77.0 Medial epicondylitis**
- **M77.00 Medial epicondylitis, unspecified elbow**
- **M77.01 Medial epicondylitis, right elbow**
- **M77.02 Medial epicondylitis, left elbow**

5th **M77.1 Lateral epicondylitis**
Tennis elbow
- **M77.10 Lateral epicondylitis, unspecified elbow**
- **M77.11 Lateral epicondylitis, right elbow**
- **M77.12 Lateral epicondylitis, left elbow**

5th **M77.2 Periarthritis of wrist**
- **M77.20 Periarthritis, unspecified wrist**
- **M77.21 Periarthritis, right wrist**
- **M77.22 Periarthritis, left wrist**

5th **M77.3 Calcaneal spur**
- **M77.30 Calcaneal spur, unspecified foot**
- **M77.31 Calcaneal spur, right foot**
- **M77.32 Calcaneal spur, left foot**

5th **M77.4 Metatarsalgia**

EXCLUDES 1 *Morton's metatarsalgia (G57.6)*
- **M77.40 Metatarsalgia, unspecified foot**
- **M77.41 Metatarsalgia, right foot**
- **M77.42 Metatarsalgia, left foot**

5th **M77.5 Other enthesopathy of foot**
- **M77.50 Other enthesopathy of unspecified foot**
- **M77.51 Other enthesopathy of right foot**
- **M77.52 Other enthesopathy of left foot**

M77.8 Other enthesopathies, not elsewhere classified

M77.9 Enthesopathy, unspecified
Bone spur NOS
Capsulitis NOS
Periarthritis NOS
Tendinitis NOS

4th M79 Other and unspecified soft tissue disorders, not elsewhere classified

EXCLUDES 1 *psychogenic rheumatism (F45.8)*
soft tissue pain, psychogenic (F45.41)

M79.0 Rheumatism, unspecified

EXCLUDES 1 *fibromyalgia (M79.7)*
palindromic rheumatism (M12.3-)

M79.1 Myalgia
Myofascial pain syndrome

EXCLUDES 1 *fibromyalgia (M79.7)*
myositis (M60.-)

M79.2 Neuralgia and neuritis, unspecified

EXCLUDES 1 *brachial radiculitis NOS (M54.1)*
lumbosacral radiculitis NOS (M54.1)
mononeuropathies (G56-G58)
radiculitis NOS (M54.1)
sciatica (M54.3-M54.4)

M79.3 Panniculitis, unspecified

EXCLUDES 1 *lupus panniculitis (L93.2)*
neck and back panniculitis (M54.0-)
relapsing [Weber-Christian] panniculitis (M35.6)

M79.4 Hypertrophy of (infrapatellar) fat pad

M79.5 Residual foreign body in soft tissue

EXCLUDES 1 *foreign body granuloma of skin and subcutaneous tissue (L92.3)*
foreign body granuloma of soft tissue (M60.2-)

M79.6 Pain in limb, hand, foot, fingers and toes
EXCLUDES 2 *pain in joint (M25.5-)*

M79.60 Pain in limb, unspecified
M79.601 Pain in right arm
Pain in right upper limb NOS
M79.602 Pain in left arm
Pain in left upper limb NOS
M79.603 Pain in arm, unspecified
Pain in upper limb NOS
M79.604 Pain in right leg
Pain in right lower limb NOS
M79.605 Pain in left leg
Pain in left lower limb NOS
M79.606 Pain in leg, unspecified
Pain in lower limb NOS
M79.609 Pain in unspecified limb
Pain in limb NOS

M79.62 Pain in upper arm
Pain in axillary region
M79.621 Pain in right upper arm
M79.622 Pain in left upper arm
M79.629 Pain in unspecified upper arm

M79.63 Pain in forearm
M79.631 Pain in right forearm
M79.632 Pain in left forearm
M79.639 Pain in unspecified forearm

M79.64 Pain in hand and fingers
M79.641 Pain in right hand
M79.642 Pain in left hand
M79.643 Pain in unspecified hand
M79.644 Pain in right finger(s)
M79.645 Pain in left finger(s)
M79.646 Pain in unspecified finger(s)

M79.65 Pain in thigh
M79.651 Pain in right thigh
M79.652 Pain in left thigh
M79.659 Pain in unspecified thigh

M79.66 Pain in lower leg
M79.661 Pain in right lower leg
M79.662 Pain in left lower leg
M79.669 Pain in unspecified lower leg

M79.67 Pain in foot and toes
M79.671 Pain in right foot
M79.672 Pain in left foot
M79.673 Pain in unspecified foot
M79.674 Pain in right toe(s)
M79.675 Pain in left toe(s)
M79.676 Pain in unspecified toe(s)

M79.7 Fibromyalgia
Fibromyositis
Fibrositis
Myofibrositis

M79.A Nontraumatic compartment syndrome
Code first, if applicable, associated postprocedural complication
EXCLUDES 1 *compartment syndrome NOS (T79.A-)*
fibromyalgia (M79.7)
nontraumatic ischemic infarction of muscle (M62.2-)
traumatic compartment syndrome (T79.A-)

M79.A1 Nontraumatic compartment syndrome of upper extremity
Nontraumatic compartment syndrome of shoulder, arm, forearm, wrist, hand, and fingers
M79.A11 Nontraumatic compartment syndrome of right upper extremity
M79.A12 Nontraumatic compartment syndrome of left upper extremity
M79.A19 Nontraumatic compartment syndrome of unspecified upper extremity

M79.A2 Nontraumatic compartment syndrome of lower extremity
Nontraumatic compartment syndrome of hip, buttock, thigh, leg, foot, and toes
M79.A21 Nontraumatic compartment syndrome of right lower extremity
M79.A22 Nontraumatic compartment syndrome of left lower extremity
M79.A29 Nontraumatic compartment syndrome of unspecified lower extremity

M79.A3 Nontraumatic compartment syndrome of abdomen
M79.A9 Nontraumatic compartment syndrome of other sites

M79.8 Other specified soft tissue disorders
M79.81 Nontraumatic hematoma of soft tissue
Nontraumatic hematoma of muscle
Nontraumatic seroma of muscle and soft tissue
M79.89 Other specified soft tissue disorders
Polyalgia
M79.9 Soft tissue disorder, unspecified

OSTEOPATHIES AND CHONDROPATHIES (M80-M94)

Disorders of bone density and structure (M80-M85)

M80 Osteoporosis with current pathological fracture
INCLUDES osteoporosis with current fragility fracture
Use additional code to identify major osseous defect, if applicable (M89.7-)
EXCLUDES 1 *collapsed vertebra NOS (M48.5)*
pathological fracture NOS (M84.4)
wedging of vertebra NOS (M48.5)
EXCLUDES 2 *personal history of (healed) osteoporosis fracture (Z87.310)*

The appropriate 7th character is to be added to each code from category M80.
A initial encounter for fracture
D subsequent encounter for fracture with routine healing
G subsequent encounter for fracture with delayed healing
K subsequent encounter for fracture with nonunion
P subsequent encounter for fracture with malunion
S sequela

M80.0 Age-related osteoporosis with current pathological fracture
Involutional osteoporosis with current pathological fracture
Osteoporosis NOS with current pathological fracture
Postmenopausal osteoporosis with current pathological fracture
Senile osteoporosis with current pathological fracture

M80.00 Age-related osteoporosis with current pathological fracture, unspecified site

M80.01 Age-related osteoporosis with current pathological fracture, shoulder
M80.011 Age-related osteoporosis with current pathological fracture, right shoulder
M80.012 Age-related osteoporosis with current pathological fracture, left shoulder
M80.019 Age-related osteoporosis with current pathological fracture, unspecified shoulder

M80.02 Age-related osteoporosis with current pathological fracture, humerus
M80.021 Age-related osteoporosis with current pathological fracture, right humerus
M80.022 Age-related osteoporosis with current pathological fracture, left humerus
M80.029 Age-related osteoporosis with current pathological fracture, unspecified humerus

M80.03 Age-related osteoporosis with current pathological fracture, forearm
Age-related osteoporosis with current pathological fracture of wrist
M80.031 Age-related osteoporosis with current pathological fracture, right forearm
M80.032 Age-related osteoporosis with current pathological fracture, left forearm
M80.039 Age-related osteoporosis with current pathological fracture, unspecified forearm

M80.04 Age-related osteoporosis with current pathological fracture, hand
M80.041 Age-related osteoporosis with current pathological fracture, right hand
M80.042 Age-related osteoporosis with current pathological fracture, left hand

Appropriate additional character required
Requires 7th character, placeholder x must fill empty characters

✓7th **M8Ø.Ø49 Age-related osteoporosis with current pathological fracture, unspecified hand**

✓6th **M8Ø.Ø5 Age-related osteoporosis with current pathological fracture, femur**
Age-related osteoporosis with current pathological fracture of hip

✓7th **M8Ø.Ø51 Age-related osteoporosis with current pathological fracture, right femur**

✓7th **M8Ø.Ø52 Age-related osteoporosis with current pathological fracture, left femur**

✓7th **M8Ø.Ø59 Age-related osteoporosis with current pathological fracture, unspecified femur**

✓6th **M8Ø.Ø6 Age-related osteoporosis with current pathological fracture, lower leg**

✓7th **M8Ø.Ø61 Age-related osteoporosis with current pathological fracture, right lower leg**

✓7th **M8Ø.Ø62 Age-related osteoporosis with current pathological fracture, left lower leg**

✓7th **M8Ø.Ø69 Age-related osteoporosis with current pathological fracture, unspecified lower leg**

✓6th **M8Ø.Ø7 Age-related osteoporosis with current pathological fracture, ankle and foot**

✓7th **M8Ø.Ø71 Age-related osteoporosis with current pathological fracture, right ankle and foot**

✓7th **M8Ø.Ø72 Age-related osteoporosis with current pathological fracture, left ankle and foot**

✓7th **M8Ø.Ø79 Age-related osteoporosis with current pathological fracture, unspecified ankle and foot**

✓x7th **M8Ø.Ø8 Age-related osteoporosis with current pathological fracture, vertebra(e)**

✓5th **M8Ø.8 Other osteoporosis with current pathological fracture**
Drug-induced osteoporosis with current pathological fracture
Idiopathic osteoporosis with current pathological fracture
Osteoporosis of disuse with current pathological fracture
Postoophorectomy osteoporosis with current pathological fracture
Postsurgical malabsorption osteoporosis with current pathological fracture
Post-traumatic osteoporosis with current pathological fracture
Use additional code for adverse effect, if applicable, to identify drug (T36-T5Ø with fifth or sixth character 5)

✓x7th **M8Ø.8Ø Other osteoporosis with current pathological fracture, unspecified site**

✓6th **M8Ø.81 Other osteoporosis with pathological fracture, shoulder**

✓7th **M8Ø.811 Other osteoporosis with current pathological fracture, right shoulder**

✓7th **M8Ø.812 Other osteoporosis with current pathological fracture, left shoulder**

✓7th **M8Ø.819 Other osteoporosis with current pathological fracture, unspecified shoulder**

✓6th **M8Ø.82 Other osteoporosis with current pathological fracture, humerus**

✓7th **M8Ø.821 Other osteoporosis with current pathological fracture, right humerus**

✓7th **M8Ø.822 Other osteoporosis with current pathological fracture, left humerus**

✓7th **M8Ø.829 Other osteoporosis with current pathological fracture, unspecified humerus**

✓6th **M8Ø.83 Other osteoporosis with current pathological fracture, forearm**
Other osteoporosis with current pathological fracture of wrist

✓7th **M8Ø.831 Other osteoporosis with current pathological fracture, right forearm**

✓7th **M8Ø.832 Other osteoporosis with current pathological fracture, left forearm**

✓7th **M8Ø.839 Other osteoporosis with current pathological fracture, unspecified forearm**

✓6th **M8Ø.84 Other osteoporosis with current pathological fracture, hand**

✓7th **M8Ø.841 Other osteoporosis with current pathological fracture, right hand**

✓7th **M8Ø.842 Other osteoporosis with current pathological fracture, left hand**

✓7th **M8Ø.849 Other osteoporosis with current pathological fracture, unspecified hand**

✓6th **M8Ø.85 Other osteoporosis with current pathological fracture, femur**
Other osteoporosis with current pathological fracture of hip

✓7th **M8Ø.851 Other osteoporosis with current pathological fracture, right femur**

✓7th **M8Ø.852 Other osteoporosis with current pathological fracture, left femur**

✓7th **M8Ø.859 Other osteoporosis with current pathological fracture, unspecified femur**

✓6th **M8Ø.86 Other osteoporosis with current pathological fracture, lower leg**

✓7th **M8Ø.861 Other osteoporosis with current pathological fracture, right lower leg**

✓7th **M8Ø.862 Other osteoporosis with current pathological fracture, left lower leg**

✓7th **M8Ø.869 Other osteoporosis with current pathological fracture, unspecified lower leg**

✓6th **M8Ø.87 Other osteoporosis with current pathological fracture, ankle and foot**

✓7th **M8Ø.871 Other osteoporosis with current pathological fracture, right ankle and foot**

✓7th **M8Ø.872 Other osteoporosis with current pathological fracture, left ankle and foot**

✓7th **M8Ø.879 Other osteoporosis with current pathological fracture, unspecified ankle and foot**

✓x7th **M8Ø.88 Other osteoporosis with current pathological fracture, vertebra(e)**

✓4th **M81 Osteoporosis without current pathological fracture**
Use additional code to identify:
major osseous defect, if applicable (M89.7-)
personal history of (healed) osteoporosis fracture, if applicable (Z87.31Ø)
EXCLUDES 1 *osteoporosis with current pathological fracture (M8Ø.-)*
Sudeck's atrophy (M89.Ø)

M81.Ø Age-related osteoporosis without current pathological fracture
Involutional osteoporosis without current pathological fracture
Osteoporosis NOS
Postmenopausal osteoporosis without current pathological fracture
Senile osteoporosis without current pathological fracture

M81.6 Localized osteoporosis [Lequesne]
EXCLUDES 1 *Sudeck's atrophy (M89.Ø)*

M81.8 Other osteoporosis without current pathological fracture
Drug-induced osteoporosis without current pathological fracture
Idiopathic osteoporosis without current pathological fracture
Osteoporosis of disuse without current pathological fracture
Postoophorectomy osteoporosis without current pathological fracture
Postsurgical malabsorption osteoporosis without current pathological fracture
Post-traumatic osteoporosis without current pathological fracture
Use additional code for adverse effect, if applicable, to identify drug (T36-T5Ø with fifth or sixth character 5)

✓4th **M83 Adult osteomalacia**
EXCLUDES 1 *infantile and juvenile osteomalacia (E55.Ø)*
renal osteodystrophy (N25.Ø)
rickets (active) (E55.Ø)
rickets (active) sequelae (E64.3)
vitamin D-resistant osteomalacia (E83.3)
vitamin D-resistant rickets (active) (E83.3)

M83.Ø Puerperal osteomalacia

M83.1 Senile osteomalacia

M83.2 Adult osteomalacia due to malabsorption
Postsurgical malabsorption osteomalacia in adults

M83.3 Adult osteomalacia due to malnutrition

M83.4 Aluminum bone disease

M83.5 Other drug-induced osteomalacia in adults
Use additional code for adverse effect, if applicable, to identify drug (T36-T50 with fifth or sixth character 5)

M83.8 Other adult osteomalacia

M83.9 Adult osteomalacia, unspecified

✓4th **M84 Disorder of continuity of bone**
EXCLUDES 2 *traumatic fracture of bone-see fracture, by site*

✓5th **M84.3 Stress fracture**
Fatigue fracture
March fracture
Stress fracture NOS
Stress reaction
Use additional external cause code(s) to identify the cause of the stress fracture
EXCLUDES 1 *pathological fracture NOS (M84.4-)*
pathological fracture due to osteoporosis (M80.-)
traumatic fracture (S12-, S22-, S32-, S42-, S52-, S62-, S72-, S82-, S92-)
EXCLUDES 2 *personal history of (healed) stress (fatigue) fracture (Z87.312)*
stress fracture of vertebra (M48.4-)

The appropriate 7th character is to be added to each code from subcategory M84.3.
A initial encounter for fracture
D subsequent encounter for fracture with routine healing
G subsequent encounter for fracture with delayed healing
K subsequent encounter for fracture with nonunion
P subsequent encounter for fracture with malunion
S sequela

✓x7th **M84.30 Stress fracture, unspecified site**
✓6th **M84.31 Stress fracture, shoulder**
✓7th **M84.311 Stress fracture, right shoulder**
✓7th **M84.312 Stress fracture, left shoulder**
✓7th **M84.319 Stress fracture, unspecified shoulder**
✓6th **M84.32 Stress fracture, humerus**
✓7th **M84.321 Stress fracture, right humerus**
✓7th **M84.322 Stress fracture, left humerus**
✓7th **M84.329 Stress fracture, unspecified humerus**
✓6th **M84.33 Stress fracture, ulna and radius**
✓7th **M84.331 Stress fracture, right ulna**
✓7th **M84.332 Stress fracture, left ulna**
✓7th **M84.333 Stress fracture, right radius**
✓7th **M84.334 Stress fracture, left radius**
✓7th **M84.339 Stress fracture, unspecified ulna and radius**
✓6th **M84.34 Stress fracture, hand and fingers**
✓7th **M84.341 Stress fracture, right hand**
✓7th **M84.342 Stress fracture, left hand**
✓7th **M84.343 Stress fracture, unspecified hand**
✓7th **M84.344 Stress fracture, right finger(s)**
✓7th **M84.345 Stress fracture, left finger(s)**
✓7th **M84.346 Stress fracture, unspecified finger(s)**
✓6th **M84.35 Stress fracture, pelvis and femur**
Stress fracture, hip
✓7th **M84.350 Stress fracture, pelvis**
✓7th **M84.351 Stress fracture, right femur**
✓7th **M84.352 Stress fracture, left femur**
✓7th **M84.353 Stress fracture, unspecified femur**
✓7th **M84.359 Stress fracture, hip, unspecified**
✓6th **M84.36 Stress fracture, tibia and fibula**
✓7th **M84.361 Stress fracture, right tibia**
✓7th **M84.362 Stress fracture, left tibia**
✓7th **M84.363 Stress fracture, right fibula**
✓7th **M84.364 Stress fracture, left fibula**
✓7th **M84.369 Stress fracture, unspecified tibia and fibula**
✓6th **M84.37 Stress fracture, ankle, foot and toes**
✓7th **M84.371 Stress fracture, right ankle**
✓7th **M84.372 Stress fracture, left ankle**
✓7th **M84.373 Stress fracture, unspecified ankle**
✓7th **M84.374 Stress fracture, right foot**
✓7th **M84.375 Stress fracture, left foot**
✓7th **M84.376 Stress fracture, unspecified foot**
✓7th **M84.377 Stress fracture, right toe(s)**
✓7th **M84.378 Stress fracture, left toe(s)**
✓7th **M84.379 Stress fracture, unspecified toe(s)**
✓x7th **M84.38 Stress fracture, other site**
EXCLUDES 2 *stress fracture of vertebra (M48.4-)*

✓5th **M84.4 Pathological fracture, not elsewhere classified**
Chronic fracture
Pathological fracture NOS
EXCLUDES 1 *collapsed vertebra NEC (M48.5)*
pathological fracture in neoplastic disease (M84.5-)
pathological fracture in osteoporosis (M80.-)
pathological fracture in other disease (M84.6-)
stress fracture (M84.3-)
traumatic fracture (S12.-, S22.-, S32.-, S42.-, S52.-, S62.-, S72.-, S82.-, S92.-)
EXCLUDES 2 *personal history of (healed) pathological fracture (Z87.311)*

The appropriate 7th character is to be added to each code from subcategory M84.4.
A initial encounter for fracture
D subsequent encounter for fracture with routine healing
G subsequent encounter for fracture with delayed healing
K subsequent encounter for fracture with nonunion
P subsequent encounter for fracture with malunion
S sequela

✓x7th **M84.40 Pathological fracture, unspecified site**
✓6th **M84.41 Pathological fracture, shoulder**
✓7th **M84.411 Pathological fracture, right shoulder**
✓7th **M84.412 Pathological fracture, left shoulder**
✓7th **M84.419 Pathological fracture, unspecified shoulder**
✓6th **M84.42 Pathological fracture, humerus**
✓7th **M84.421 Pathological fracture, right humerus**
✓7th **M84.422 Pathological fracture, left humerus**
✓7th **M84.429 Pathological fracture, unspecified humerus**
✓6th **M84.43 Pathological fracture, ulna and radius**
✓7th **M84.431 Pathological fracture, right ulna**
✓7th **M84.432 Pathological fracture, left ulna**
✓7th **M84.433 Pathological fracture, right radius**
✓7th **M84.434 Pathological fracture, left radius**
✓7th **M84.439 Pathological fracture, unspecified ulna and radius**
✓6th **M84.44 Pathological fracture, hand and fingers**
✓7th **M84.441 Pathological fracture, right hand**
✓7th **M84.442 Pathological fracture, left hand**
✓7th **M84.443 Pathological fracture, unspecified hand**
✓7th **M84.444 Pathological fracture, right finger(s)**
✓7th **M84.445 Pathological fracture, left finger(s)**
✓7th **M84.446 Pathological fracture, unspecified finger(s)**
✓6th **M84.45 Pathological fracture, femur and pelvis**
✓7th **M84.451 Pathological fracture, right femur**
✓7th **M84.452 Pathological fracture, left femur**
✓7th **M84.453 Pathological fracture, unspecified femur**
✓7th **M84.454 Pathological fracture, pelvis**
✓7th **M84.459 Pathological fracture, hip, unspecified**
✓6th **M84.46 Pathological fracture, tibia and fibula**
✓7th **M84.461 Pathological fracture, right tibia**
✓7th **M84.462 Pathological fracture, left tibia**
✓7th **M84.463 Pathological fracture, right fibula**
✓7th **M84.464 Pathological fracture, left fibula**
✓7th **M84.469 Pathological fracture, unspecified tibia and fibula**
✓6th **M84.47 Pathological fracture, ankle, foot and toes**
✓7th **M84.471 Pathological fracture, right ankle**
✓7th **M84.472 Pathological fracture, left ankle**

√7th M84.473 **Pathological fracture, unspecified ankle**
√7th M84.474 **Pathological fracture, right foot**
√7th M84.475 **Pathological fracture, left foot**
√7th M84.476 **Pathological fracture, unspecified foot**
√7th M84.477 **Pathological fracture, right toe(s)**
√7th M84.478 **Pathological fracture, left toe(s)**
√7th M84.479 **Pathological fracture, unspecified toe(s)**

√x7th M84.48 **Pathological fracture, other site**

√5th M84.5 **Pathological fracture in neoplastic disease**

Code also underlying neoplasm

The appropriate 7th character is to be added to each code from subcategory M84.5.
- A initial encounter for fracture
- D subsequent encounter for fracture with routine healing
- G subsequent encounter for fracture with delayed healing
- K subsequent encounter for fracture with nonunion
- P subsequent encounter for fracture with malunion
- S sequela

√x7th M84.50 **Pathological fracture in neoplastic disease, unspecified site**

√6th M84.51 **Pathological fracture in neoplastic disease, shoulder**
√7th M84.511 **Pathological fracture in neoplastic disease, right shoulder**
√7th M84.512 **Pathological fracture in neoplastic disease, left shoulder**
√7th M84.519 **Pathological fracture in neoplastic disease, unspecified shoulder**

√6th M84.52 **Pathological fracture in neoplastic disease, humerus**
√7th M84.521 **Pathological fracture in neoplastic disease, right humerus**
√7th M84.522 **Pathological fracture in neoplastic disease, left humerus**
√7th M84.529 **Pathological fracture in neoplastic disease, unspecified humerus**

√6th M84.53 **Pathological fracture in neoplastic disease, ulna and radius**
√7th M84.531 **Pathological fracture in neoplastic disease, right ulna**
√7th M84.532 **Pathological fracture in neoplastic disease, left ulna**
√7th M84.533 **Pathological fracture in neoplastic disease, right radius**
√7th M84.534 **Pathological fracture in neoplastic disease, left radius**
√7th M84.539 **Pathological fracture in neoplastic disease, unspecified ulna and radius**

√6th M84.54 **Pathological fracture in neoplastic disease, hand**
√7th M84.541 **Pathological fracture in neoplastic disease, right hand**
√7th M84.542 **Pathological fracture in neoplastic disease, left hand**
√7th M84.549 **Pathological fracture in neoplastic disease, unspecified hand**

√6th M84.55 **Pathological fracture in neoplastic disease, pelvis and femur**
√7th M84.550 **Pathological fracture in neoplastic disease, pelvis**
√7th M84.551 **Pathological fracture in neoplastic disease, right femur**
√7th M84.552 **Pathological fracture in neoplastic disease, left femur**
√7th M84.553 **Pathological fracture in neoplastic disease, unspecified femur**
√7th M84.559 **Pathological fracture in neoplastic disease, hip, unspecified**

√6th M84.56 **Pathological fracture in neoplastic disease, tibia and fibula**
√7th M84.561 **Pathological fracture in neoplastic disease, right tibia**
√7th M84.562 **Pathological fracture in neoplastic disease, left tibia**
√7th M84.563 **Pathological fracture in neoplastic disease, right fibula**
√7th M84.564 **Pathological fracture in neoplastic disease, left fibula**
√7th M84.569 **Pathological fracture in neoplastic disease, unspecified tibia and fibula**

√6th M84.57 **Pathological fracture in neoplastic disease, ankle and foot**
√7th M84.571 **Pathological fracture in neoplastic disease, right ankle**
√7th M84.572 **Pathological fracture in neoplastic disease, left ankle**
√7th M84.573 **Pathological fracture in neoplastic disease, unspecified ankle**
√7th M84.574 **Pathological fracture in neoplastic disease, right foot**
√7th M84.575 **Pathological fracture in neoplastic disease, left foot**
√7th M84.576 **Pathological fracture in neoplastic disease, unspecified foot**

√x7th M84.58 **Pathological fracture in neoplastic disease, vertebrae**

√5th M84.6 **Pathological fracture in other disease**

Code also underlying condition

EXCLUDES 1 *pathological fracture in osteoporosis (M80.-)*

The appropriate 7th character is to be added to each code from subcategory M84.6.
- A initial encounter for fracture
- D subsequent encounter for fracture with routine healing
- G subsequent encounter for fracture with delayed healing
- K subsequent encounter for fracture with nonunion
- P subsequent encounter for fracture with malunion
- S sequela

√x7th M84.60 **Pathological fracture in other disease, unspecified site**

√6th M84.61 **Pathological fracture in other disease, shoulder**
√7th M84.611 **Pathological fracture in other disease, right shoulder**
√7th M84.612 **Pathological fracture in other disease, left shoulder**
√7th M84.619 **Pathological fracture in other disease, unspecified shoulder**

√6th M84.62 **Pathological fracture in other disease, humerus**
√7th M84.621 **Pathological fracture in other disease, right humerus**
√7th M84.622 **Pathological fracture in other disease, left humerus**
√7th M84.629 **Pathological fracture in other disease, unspecified humerus**

√6th M84.63 **Pathological fracture in other disease, ulna and radius**
√7th M84.631 **Pathological fracture in other disease, right ulna**
√7th M84.632 **Pathological fracture in other disease, left ulna**
√7th M84.633 **Pathological fracture in other disease, right radius**
√7th M84.634 **Pathological fracture in other disease, left radius**
√7th M84.639 **Pathological fracture in other disease, unspecified ulna and radius**

√6th M84.64 **Pathological fracture in other disease, hand**
√7th M84.641 **Pathological fracture in other disease, right hand**
√7th M84.642 **Pathological fracture in other disease, left hand**
√7th M84.649 **Pathological fracture in other disease, unspecified hand**

√6th M84.65 **Pathological fracture in other disease, pelvis and femur**
√7th M84.650 **Pathological fracture in other disease, pelvis**
√7th M84.651 **Pathological fracture in other disease, right femur**

M84.652 Pathological fracture in other disease, left femur
M84.653 Pathological fracture in other disease, unspecified femur
M84.659 Pathological fracture in other disease, hip, unspecified
M84.66 Pathological fracture in other disease, tibia and fibula
M84.661 Pathological fracture in other disease, right tibia
M84.662 Pathological fracture in other disease, left tibia
M84.663 Pathological fracture in other disease, right fibula
M84.664 Pathological fracture in other disease, left fibula
M84.669 Pathological fracture in other disease, unspecified tibia and fibula
M84.67 Pathological fracture in other disease, ankle and foot
M84.671 Pathological fracture in other disease, right ankle
M84.672 Pathological fracture in other disease, left ankle
M84.673 Pathological fracture in other disease, unspecified ankle
M84.674 Pathological fracture in other disease, right foot
M84.675 Pathological fracture in other disease, left foot
M84.676 Pathological fracture in other disease, unspecified foot
M84.68 Pathological fracture in other disease, other site
M84.8 Other disorders of continuity of bone
M84.80 Other disorders of continuity of bone, unspecified site
M84.81 Other disorders of continuity of bone, shoulder
M84.811 Other disorders of continuity of bone, right shoulder
M84.812 Other disorders of continuity of bone, left shoulder
M84.819 Other disorders of continuity of bone, unspecified shoulder
M84.82 Other disorders of continuity of bone, humerus
M84.821 Other disorders of continuity of bone, right humerus
M84.822 Other disorders of continuity of bone, left humerus
M84.829 Other disorders of continuity of bone, unspecified humerus
M84.83 Other disorders of continuity of bone, ulna and radius
M84.831 Other disorders of continuity of bone, right ulna
M84.832 Other disorders of continuity of bone, left ulna
M84.833 Other disorders of continuity of bone, right radius
M84.834 Other disorders of continuity of bone, left radius
M84.839 Other disorders of continuity of bone, unspecified ulna and radius
M84.84 Other disorders of continuity of bone, hand
M84.841 Other disorders of continuity of bone, right hand
M84.842 Other disorders of continuity of bone, left hand
M84.849 Other disorders of continuity of bone, unspecified hand
M84.85 Other disorders of continuity of bone, pelvic region and thigh
M84.851 Other disorders of continuity of bone, right pelvic region and thigh
M84.852 Other disorders of continuity of bone, left pelvic region and thigh
M84.859 Other disorders of continuity of bone, unspecified pelvic region and thigh
M84.86 Other disorders of continuity of bone, tibia and fibula
M84.861 Other disorders of continuity of bone, right tibia
M84.862 Other disorders of continuity of bone, left tibia
M84.863 Other disorders of continuity of bone, right fibula
M84.864 Other disorders of continuity of bone, left fibula
M84.869 Other disorders of continuity of bone, unspecified tibia and fibula
M84.87 Other disorders of continuity of bone, ankle and foot
M84.871 Other disorders of continuity of bone, right ankle and foot
M84.872 Other disorders of continuity of bone, left ankle and foot
M84.879 Other disorders of continuity of bone, unspecified ankle and foot
M84.88 Other disorders of continuity of bone, other site
M84.9 Disorder of continuity of bone, unspecified

M85 Other disorders of bone density and structure

EXCLUDES 1 *osteogenesis imperfecta (Q78.0)*
osteopetrosis (Q78.2)
osteopoikilosis (Q78.8)
polyostotic fibrous dysplasia (Q78.1)

M85.0 Fibrous dysplasia (monostotic)
EXCLUDES 2 *fibrous dysplasia of jaw (M27.8)*
M85.00 Fibrous dysplasia (monostotic), unspecified site
M85.01 Fibrous dysplasia (monostotic), shoulder
M85.011 Fibrous dysplasia (monostotic), right shoulder
M85.012 Fibrous dysplasia (monostotic), left shoulder
M85.019 Fibrous dysplasia (monostotic), unspecified shoulder
M85.02 Fibrous dysplasia (monostotic), upper arm
M85.021 Fibrous dysplasia (monostotic), right upper arm
M85.022 Fibrous dysplasia (monostotic), left upper arm
M85.029 Fibrous dysplasia (monostotic), unspecified upper arm
M85.03 Fibrous dysplasia (monostotic), forearm
M85.031 Fibrous dysplasia (monostotic), right forearm
M85.032 Fibrous dysplasia (monostotic), left forearm
M85.039 Fibrous dysplasia (monostotic), unspecified forearm
M85.04 Fibrous dysplasia (monostotic), hand
M85.041 Fibrous dysplasia (monostotic), right hand
M85.042 Fibrous dysplasia (monostotic), left hand
M85.049 Fibrous dysplasia (monostotic), unspecified hand
M85.05 Fibrous dysplasia (monostotic), thigh
M85.051 Fibrous dysplasia (monostotic), right thigh
M85.052 Fibrous dysplasia (monostotic), left thigh
M85.059 Fibrous dysplasia (monostotic), unspecified thigh
M85.06 Fibrous dysplasia (monostotic), lower leg
M85.061 Fibrous dysplasia (monostotic), right lower leg
M85.062 Fibrous dysplasia (monostotic), left lower leg
M85.069 Fibrous dysplasia (monostotic), unspecified lower leg
M85.07 Fibrous dysplasia (monostotic), ankle and foot
M85.071 Fibrous dysplasia (monostotic), right ankle and foot
M85.072 Fibrous dysplasia (monostotic), left ankle and foot

M85.079 Fibrous dysplasia (monostotic), unspecified ankle and foot
M85.08 Fibrous dysplasia (monostotic), other site
M85.09 Fibrous dysplasia (monostotic), multiple sites
✓5th M85.1 Skeletal fluorosis
M85.10 Skeletal fluorosis, unspecified site
✓6th M85.11 Skeletal fluorosis, shoulder
M85.111 Skeletal fluorosis, right shoulder
M85.112 Skeletal fluorosis, left shoulder
M85.119 Skeletal fluorosis, unspecified shoulder
✓6th M85.12 Skeletal fluorosis, upper arm
M85.121 Skeletal fluorosis, right upper arm
M85.122 Skeletal fluorosis, left upper arm
M85.129 Skeletal fluorosis, unspecified upper arm
✓6th M85.13 Skeletal fluorosis, forearm
M85.131 Skeletal fluorosis, right forearm
M85.132 Skeletal fluorosis, left forearm
M85.139 Skeletal fluorosis, unspecified forearm
✓6th M85.14 Skeletal fluorosis, hand
M85.141 Skeletal fluorosis, right hand
M85.142 Skeletal fluorosis, left hand
M85.149 Skeletal fluorosis, unspecified hand
✓6th M85.15 Skeletal fluorosis, thigh
M85.151 Skeletal fluorosis, right thigh
M85.152 Skeletal fluorosis, left thigh
M85.159 Skeletal fluorosis, unspecified thigh
✓6th M85.16 Skeletal fluorosis, lower leg
M85.161 Skeletal fluorosis, right lower leg
M85.162 Skeletal fluorosis, left lower leg
M85.169 Skeletal fluorosis, unspecified lower leg
✓6th M85.17 Skeletal fluorosis, ankle and foot
M85.171 Skeletal fluorosis, right ankle and foot
M85.172 Skeletal fluorosis, left ankle and foot
M85.179 Skeletal fluorosis, unspecified ankle and foot
M85.18 Skeletal fluorosis, other site
M85.19 Skeletal fluorosis, multiple sites
M85.2 Hyperostosis of skull
✓5th M85.3 Osteitis condensans
M85.30 Osteitis condensans, unspecified site
✓6th M85.31 Osteitis condensans, shoulder
M85.311 Osteitis condensans, right shoulder
M85.312 Osteitis condensans, left shoulder
M85.319 Osteitis condensans, unspecified shoulder
✓6th M85.32 Osteitis condensans, upper arm
M85.321 Osteitis condensans, right upper arm
M85.322 Osteitis condensans, left upper arm
M85.329 Osteitis condensans, unspecified upper arm
✓6th M85.33 Osteitis condensans, forearm
M85.331 Osteitis condensans, right forearm
M85.332 Osteitis condensans, left forearm
M85.339 Osteitis condensans, unspecified forearm
✓6th M85.34 Osteitis condensans, hand
M85.341 Osteitis condensans, right hand
M85.342 Osteitis condensans, left hand
M85.349 Osteitis condensans, unspecified hand
✓6th M85.35 Osteitis condensans, thigh
M85.351 Osteitis condensans, right thigh
M85.352 Osteitis condensans, left thigh
M85.359 Osteitis condensans, unspecified thigh
✓6th M85.36 Osteitis condensans, lower leg
M85.361 Osteitis condensans, right lower leg
M85.362 Osteitis condensans, left lower leg
M85.369 Osteitis condensans, unspecified lower leg
✓6th M85.37 Osteitis condensans, ankle and foot
M85.371 Osteitis condensans, right ankle and foot
M85.372 Osteitis condensans, left ankle and foot
M85.379 Osteitis condensans, unspecified ankle and foot

M85.38 Osteitis condensans, other site
M85.39 Osteitis condensans, multiple sites
✓5th M85.4 Solitary bone cyst
EXCLUDES 2 *solitary cyst of jaw (M27.4)*
M85.40 Solitary bone cyst, unspecified site
✓6th M85.41 Solitary bone cyst, shoulder
M85.411 Solitary bone cyst, right shoulder
M85.412 Solitary bone cyst, left shoulder
M85.419 Solitary bone cyst, unspecified shoulder
✓6th M85.42 Solitary bone cyst, humerus
M85.421 Solitary bone cyst, right humerus
M85.422 Solitary bone cyst, left humerus
M85.429 Solitary bone cyst, unspecified humerus
✓6th M85.43 Solitary bone cyst, ulna and radius
M85.431 Solitary bone cyst, right ulna and radius
M85.432 Solitary bone cyst, left ulna and radius
M85.439 Solitary bone cyst, unspecified ulna and radius
✓6th M85.44 Solitary bone cyst, hand
M85.441 Solitary bone cyst, right hand
M85.442 Solitary bone cyst, left hand
M85.449 Solitary bone cyst, unspecified hand
✓6th M85.45 Solitary bone cyst, pelvis
M85.451 Solitary bone cyst, right pelvis
M85.452 Solitary bone cyst, left pelvis
M85.459 Solitary bone cyst, unspecified pelvis
✓6th M85.46 Solitary bone cyst, tibia and fibula
M85.461 Solitary bone cyst, right tibia and fibula
M85.462 Solitary bone cyst, left tibia and fibula
M85.469 Solitary bone cyst, unspecified tibia and fibula
✓6th M85.47 Solitary bone cyst, ankle and foot
M85.471 Solitary bone cyst, right ankle and foot
M85.472 Solitary bone cyst, left ankle and foot
M85.479 Solitary bone cyst, unspecified ankle and foot
M85.48 Solitary bone cyst, other site
✓5th M85.5 Aneurysmal bone cyst
EXCLUDES 2 *aneurysmal cyst of jaw (M27.4)*
M85.50 Aneurysmal bone cyst, unspecified site
✓6th M85.51 Aneurysmal bone cyst, shoulder
M85.511 Aneurysmal bone cyst, right shoulder
M85.512 Aneurysmal bone cyst, left shoulder
M85.519 Aneurysmal bone cyst, unspecified shoulder
✓6th M85.52 Aneurysmal bone cyst, upper arm
M85.521 Aneurysmal bone cyst, right upper arm
M85.522 Aneurysmal bone cyst, left upper arm
M85.529 Aneurysmal bone cyst, unspecified upper arm
✓6th M85.53 Aneurysmal bone cyst, forearm
M85.531 Aneurysmal bone cyst, right forearm
M85.532 Aneurysmal bone cyst, left forearm
M85.539 Aneurysmal bone cyst, unspecified forearm
✓6th M85.54 Aneurysmal bone cyst, hand
M85.541 Aneurysmal bone cyst, right hand
M85.542 Aneurysmal bone cyst, left hand
M85.549 Aneurysmal bone cyst, unspecified hand
✓6th M85.55 Aneurysmal bone cyst, thigh
M85.551 Aneurysmal bone cyst, right thigh
M85.552 Aneurysmal bone cyst, left thigh
M85.559 Aneurysmal bone cyst, unspecified thigh
✓6th M85.56 Aneurysmal bone cyst, lower leg
M85.561 Aneurysmal bone cyst, right lower leg
M85.562 Aneurysmal bone cyst, left lower leg
M85.569 Aneurysmal bone cyst, unspecified lower leg
✓6th M85.57 Aneurysmal bone cyst, ankle and foot
M85.571 Aneurysmal bone cyst, right ankle and foot
M85.572 Aneurysmal bone cyst, left ankle and foot

M85.579 **Aneurysmal bone cyst, unspecified ankle and foot**
M85.58 **Aneurysmal bone cyst, other site**
M85.59 **Aneurysmal bone cyst, multiple sites**
✓5th M85.6 **Other cyst of bone**
EXCLUDES 1 *cyst of jaw NEC (M27.4)*
osteitis fibrosa cystica generalisata [von Recklinghausen's disease of bone] (E21.0)
M85.60 **Other cyst of bone, unspecified site**
✓6th M85.61 **Other cyst of bone, shoulder**
M85.611 **Other cyst of bone, right shoulder**
M85.612 **Other cyst of bone, left shoulder**
M85.619 **Other cyst of bone, unspecified shoulder**
✓6th M85.62 **Other cyst of bone, upper arm**
M85.621 **Other cyst of bone, right upper arm**
M85.622 **Other cyst of bone, left upper arm**
M85.629 **Other cyst of bone, unspecified upper arm**
✓6th M85.63 **Other cyst of bone, forearm**
M85.631 **Other cyst of bone, right forearm**
M85.632 **Other cyst of bone, left forearm**
M85.639 **Other cyst of bone, unspecified forearm**
✓6th M85.64 **Other cyst of bone, hand**
M85.641 **Other cyst of bone, right hand**
M85.642 **Other cyst of bone, left hand**
M85.649 **Other cyst of bone, unspecified hand**
✓6th M85.65 **Other cyst of bone, thigh**
M85.651 **Other cyst of bone, right thigh**
M85.652 **Other cyst of bone, left thigh**
M85.659 **Other cyst of bone, unspecified thigh**
✓6th M85.66 **Other cyst of bone, lower leg**
M85.661 **Other cyst of bone, right lower leg**
M85.662 **Other cyst of bone, left lower leg**
M85.669 **Other cyst of bone, unspecified lower leg**
✓6th M85.67 **Other cyst of bone, ankle and foot**
M85.671 **Other cyst of bone, right ankle and foot**
M85.672 **Other cyst of bone, left ankle and foot**
M85.679 **Other cyst of bone, unspecified ankle and foot**
M85.68 **Other cyst of bone, other site**
M85.69 **Other cyst of bone, multiple sites**
✓5th M85.8 **Other specified disorders of bone density and structure**
Hyperostosis of bones, except skull
Osteosclerosis, acquired
EXCLUDES 1 *diffuse idiopathic skeletal hyperostosis [DISH] (M48.1)*
osteosclerosis congenita (Q77.4)
osteosclerosis fragilitas (generalista) (Q78.2)
osteosclerosis myelofibrosis (D75.81)
M85.80 **Other specified disorders of bone density and structure, unspecified site**
✓6th M85.81 **Other specified disorders of bone density and structure, shoulder**
M85.811 **Other specified disorders of bone density and structure, right shoulder**
M85.812 **Other specified disorders of bone density and structure, left shoulder**
M85.819 **Other specified disorders of bone density and structure, unspecified shoulder**
✓6th M85.82 **Other specified disorders of bone density and structure, upper arm**
M85.821 **Other specified disorders of bone density and structure, right upper arm**
M85.822 **Other specified disorders of bone density and structure, left upper arm**
M85.829 **Other specified disorders of bone density and structure, unspecified upper arm**
✓6th M85.83 **Other specified disorders of bone density and structure, forearm**
M85.831 **Other specified disorders of bone density and structure, right forearm**
M85.832 **Other specified disorders of bone density and structure, left forearm**
M85.839 **Other specified disorders of bone density and structure, unspecified forearm**
✓6th M85.84 **Other specified disorders of bone density and structure, hand**
M85.841 **Other specified disorders of bone density and structure, right hand**
M85.842 **Other specified disorders of bone density and structure, left hand**
M85.849 **Other specified disorders of bone density and structure, unspecified hand**
✓6th M85.85 **Other specified disorders of bone density and structure, thigh**
M85.851 **Other specified disorders of bone density and structure, right thigh**
M85.852 **Other specified disorders of bone density and structure, left thigh**
M85.859 **Other specified disorders of bone density and structure, unspecified thigh**
✓6th M85.86 **Other specified disorders of bone density and structure, lower leg**
M85.861 **Other specified disorders of bone density and structure, right lower leg**
M85.862 **Other specified disorders of bone density and structure, left lower leg**
M85.869 **Other specified disorders of bone density and structure, unspecified lower leg**
✓6th M85.87 **Other specified disorders of bone density and structure, ankle and foot**
M85.871 **Other specified disorders of bone density and structure, right ankle and foot**
M85.872 **Other specified disorders of bone density and structure, left ankle and foot**
M85.879 **Other specified disorders of bone density and structure, unspecified ankle and foot**
M85.88 **Other specified disorders of bone density and structure, other site**
M85.89 **Other specified disorders of bone density and structure, multiple sites**
M85.9 **Disorder of bone density and structure, unspecified**

Other osteopathies (M86-M90)

EXCLUDES 1 *postprocedural osteopathies (M96.-)*

✓4th **M86 Osteomyelitis**
Use additional code (B95-B97) to identify infectious agent
Use additional code to identify major osseous defect, if applicable (M89.7-)
EXCLUDES 1 *osteomyelitis due to:*
echinococcus (B67.2)
gonococcus (A54.43)
salmonella (A02.24)
EXCLUDES 2 *ostemyelitis of:*
orbit (H05.0-)
petrous bone (H70.2-)
vertebra (M46.2-)
✓5th M86.0 **Acute hematogenous osteomyelitis**
M86.00 **Acute hematogenous osteomyelitis, unspecified site**
✓6th M86.01 **Acute hematogenous osteomyelitis, shoulder**
M86.011 **Acute hematogenous osteomyelitis, right shoulder**
M86.012 **Acute hematogenous osteomyelitis, left shoulder**
M86.019 **Acute hematogenous osteomyelitis, unspecified shoulder**
✓6th M86.02 **Acute hematogenous osteomyelitis, humerus**
M86.021 **Acute hematogenous osteomyelitis, right humerus**
M86.022 **Acute hematogenous osteomyelitis, left humerus**
M86.029 **Acute hematogenous osteomyelitis, unspecified humerus**

√6th M86.03 Acute hematogenous osteomyelitis, radius and ulna
M86.031 Acute hematogenous osteomyelitis, right radius and ulna
M86.032 Acute hematogenous osteomyelitis, left radius and ulna
M86.039 Acute hematogenous osteomyelitis, unspecified radius and ulna
√6th M86.04 Acute hematogenous osteomyelitis, hand
M86.041 Acute hematogenous osteomyelitis, right hand
M86.042 Acute hematogenous osteomyelitis, left hand
M86.049 Acute hematogenous osteomyelitis, unspecified hand
√6th M86.05 Acute hematogenous osteomyelitis, femur
M86.051 Acute hematogenous osteomyelitis, right femur
M86.052 Acute hematogenous osteomyelitis, left femur
M86.059 Acute hematogenous osteomyelitis, unspecified femur
√6th M86.06 Acute hematogenous osteomyelitis, tibia and fibula
M86.061 Acute hematogenous osteomyelitis, right tibia and fibula
M86.062 Acute hematogenous osteomyelitis, left tibia and fibula
M86.069 Acute hematogenous osteomyelitis, unspecified tibia and fibula
√6th M86.07 Acute hematogenous osteomyelitis, ankle and foot
M86.071 Acute hematogenous osteomyelitis, right ankle and foot
M86.072 Acute hematogenous osteomyelitis, left ankle and foot
M86.079 Acute hematogenous osteomyelitis, unspecified ankle and foot
M86.08 Acute hematogenous osteomyelitis, other sites
M86.09 Acute hematogenous osteomyelitis, multiple sites
√5th M86.1 Other acute osteomyelitis
M86.10 Other acute osteomyelitis, unspecified site
√6th M86.11 Other acute osteomyelitis, shoulder
M86.111 Other acute osteomyelitis, right shoulder
M86.112 Other acute osteomyelitis, left shoulder
M86.119 Other acute osteomyelitis, unspecified shoulder
√6th M86.12 Other acute osteomyelitis, humerus
M86.121 Other acute osteomyelitis, right humerus
M86.122 Other acute osteomyelitis, left humerus
M86.129 Other acute osteomyelitis, unspecified humerus
√6th M86.13 Other acute osteomyelitis, radius and ulna
M86.131 Other acute osteomyelitis, right radius and ulna
M86.132 Other acute osteomyelitis, left radius and ulna
M86.139 Other acute osteomyelitis, unspecified radius and ulna
√6th M86.14 Other acute osteomyelitis, hand
M86.141 Other acute osteomyelitis, right hand
M86.142 Other acute osteomyelitis, left hand
M86.149 Other acute osteomyelitis, unspecified hand
√6th M86.15 Other acute osteomyelitis, femur
M86.151 Other acute osteomyelitis, right femur
M86.152 Other acute osteomyelitis, left femur
M86.159 Other acute osteomyelitis, unspecified femur
√6th M86.16 Other acute osteomyelitis, tibia and fibula
M86.161 Other acute osteomyelitis, right tibia and fibula
M86.162 Other acute osteomyelitis, left tibia and fibula
M86.169 Other acute osteomyelitis, unspecified tibia and fibula
√6th M86.17 Other acute osteomyelitis, ankle and foot
M86.171 Other acute osteomyelitis, right ankle and foot
M86.172 Other acute osteomyelitis, left ankle and foot
M86.179 Other acute osteomyelitis, unspecified ankle and foot
M86.18 Other acute osteomyelitis, other site
M86.19 Other acute osteomyelitis, multiple sites
√5th M86.2 Subacute osteomyelitis
M86.20 Subacute osteomyelitis, unspecified site
√6th M86.21 Subacute osteomyelitis, shoulder
M86.211 Subacute osteomyelitis, right shoulder
M86.212 Subacute osteomyelitis, left shoulder
M86.219 Subacute osteomyelitis, unspecified shoulder
√6th M86.22 Subacute osteomyelitis, humerus
M86.221 Subacute osteomyelitis, right humerus
M86.222 Subacute osteomyelitis, left humerus
M86.229 Subacute osteomyelitis, unspecified humerus
√6th M86.23 Subacute osteomyelitis, radius and ulna
M86.231 Subacute osteomyelitis, right radius and ulna
M86.232 Subacute osteomyelitis, left radius and ulna
M86.239 Subacute osteomyelitis, unspecified radius and ulna
√6th M86.24 Subacute osteomyelitis, hand
M86.241 Subacute osteomyelitis, right hand
M86.242 Subacute osteomyelitis, left hand
M86.249 Subacute osteomyelitis, unspecified hand
√6th M86.25 Subacute osteomyelitis, femur
M86.251 Subacute osteomyelitis, right femur
M86.252 Subacute osteomyelitis, left femur
M86.259 Subacute osteomyelitis, unspecified femur
√6th M86.26 Subacute osteomyelitis, tibia and fibula
M86.261 Subacute osteomyelitis, right tibia and fibula
M86.262 Subacute osteomyelitis, left tibia and fibula
M86.269 Subacute osteomyelitis, unspecified tibia and fibula
√6th M86.27 Subacute osteomyelitis, ankle and foot
M86.271 Subacute osteomyelitis, right ankle and foot
M86.272 Subacute osteomyelitis, left ankle and foot
M86.279 Subacute osteomyelitis, unspecified ankle and foot
M86.28 Subacute osteomyelitis, other site
M86.29 Subacute osteomyelitis, multiple sites
√5th M86.3 Chronic multifocal osteomyelitis
M86.30 Chronic multifocal osteomyelitis, unspecified site
√6th M86.31 Chronic multifocal osteomyelitis, shoulder
M86.311 Chronic multifocal osteomyelitis, right shoulder
M86.312 Chronic multifocal osteomyelitis, left shoulder
M86.319 Chronic multifocal osteomyelitis, unspecified shoulder
√6th M86.32 Chronic multifocal osteomyelitis, humerus
M86.321 Chronic multifocal osteomyelitis, right humerus
M86.322 Chronic multifocal osteomyelitis, left humerus
M86.329 Chronic multifocal osteomyelitis, unspecified humerus
√6th M86.33 Chronic multifocal osteomyelitis, radius and ulna
M86.331 Chronic multifocal osteomyelitis, right radius and ulna
M86.332 Chronic multifocal osteomyelitis, left radius and ulna

M86.339 Chronic multifocal osteomyelitis, unspecified radius and ulna
✓6th M86.34 Chronic multifocal osteomyelitis, hand
M86.341 Chronic multifocal osteomyelitis, right hand
M86.342 Chronic multifocal osteomyelitis, left hand
M86.349 Chronic multifocal osteomyelitis, unspecified hand
✓6th M86.35 Chronic multifocal osteomyelitis, femur
M86.351 Chronic multifocal osteomyelitis, right femur
M86.352 Chronic multifocal osteomyelitis, left femur
M86.359 Chronic multifocal osteomyelitis, unspecified femur
✓6th M86.36 Chronic multifocal osteomyelitis, tibia and fibula
M86.361 Chronic multifocal osteomyelitis, right tibia and fibula
M86.362 Chronic multifocal osteomyelitis, left tibia and fibula
M86.369 Chronic multifocal osteomyelitis, unspecified tibia and fibula
✓6th M86.37 Chronic multifocal osteomyelitis, ankle and foot
M86.371 Chronic multifocal osteomyelitis, right ankle and foot
M86.372 Chronic multifocal osteomyelitis, left ankle and foot
M86.379 Chronic multifocal osteomyelitis, unspecified ankle and foot
M86.38 Chronic multifocal osteomyelitis, other site
M86.39 Chronic multifocal osteomyelitis, multiple sites
✓5th M86.4 Chronic osteomyelitis with draining sinus
M86.40 Chronic osteomyelitis with draining sinus, unspecified site
✓6th M86.41 Chronic osteomyelitis with draining sinus, shoulder
M86.411 Chronic osteomyelitis with draining sinus, right shoulder
M86.412 Chronic osteomyelitis with draining sinus, left shoulder
M86.419 Chronic osteomyelitis with draining sinus, unspecified shoulder
✓6th M86.42 Chronic osteomyelitis with draining sinus, humerus
M86.421 Chronic osteomyelitis with draining sinus, right humerus
M86.422 Chronic osteomyelitis with draining sinus, left humerus
M86.429 Chronic osteomyelitis with draining sinus, unspecified humerus
✓6th M86.43 Chronic osteomyelitis with draining sinus, radius and ulna
M86.431 Chronic osteomyelitis with draining sinus, right radius and ulna
M86.432 Chronic osteomyelitis with draining sinus, left radius and ulna
M86.439 Chronic osteomyelitis with draining sinus, unspecified radius and ulna
✓6th M86.44 Chronic osteomyelitis with draining sinus, hand
M86.441 Chronic osteomyelitis with draining sinus, right hand
M86.442 Chronic osteomyelitis with draining sinus, left hand
M86.449 Chronic osteomyelitis with draining sinus, unspecified hand
✓6th M86.45 Chronic osteomyelitis with draining sinus, femur
M86.451 Chronic osteomyelitis with draining sinus, right femur
M86.452 Chronic osteomyelitis with draining sinus, left femur
M86.459 Chronic osteomyelitis with draining sinus, unspecified femur
✓6th M86.46 Chronic osteomyelitis with draining sinus, tibia and fibula
M86.461 Chronic osteomyelitis with draining sinus, right tibia and fibula
M86.462 Chronic osteomyelitis with draining sinus, left tibia and fibula
M86.469 Chronic osteomyelitis with draining sinus, unspecified tibia and fibula
✓6th M86.47 Chronic osteomyelitis with draining sinus, ankle and foot
M86.471 Chronic osteomyelitis with draining sinus, right ankle and foot
M86.472 Chronic osteomyelitis with draining sinus, left ankle and foot
M86.479 Chronic osteomyelitis with draining sinus, unspecified ankle and foot
M86.48 Chronic osteomyelitis with draining sinus, other site
M86.49 Chronic osteomyelitis with draining sinus, multiple sites
✓5th M86.5 Other chronic hematogenous osteomyelitis
M86.50 Other chronic hematogenous osteomyelitis, unspecified site
✓6th M86.51 Other chronic hematogenous osteomyelitis, shoulder
M86.511 Other chronic hematogenous osteomyelitis, right shoulder
M86.512 Other chronic hematogenous osteomyelitis, left shoulder
M86.519 Other chronic hematogenous osteomyelitis, unspecified shoulder
✓6th M86.52 Other chronic hematogenous osteomyelitis, humerus
M86.521 Other chronic hematogenous osteomyelitis, right humerus
M86.522 Other chronic hematogenous osteomyelitis, left humerus
M86.529 Other chronic hematogenous osteomyelitis, unspecified humerus
✓6th M86.53 Other chronic hematogenous osteomyelitis, radius and ulna
M86.531 Other chronic hematogenous osteomyelitis, right radius and ulna
M86.532 Other chronic hematogenous osteomyelitis, left radius and ulna
M86.539 Other chronic hematogenous osteomyelitis, unspecified radius and ulna
✓6th M86.54 Other chronic hematogenous osteomyelitis, hand
M86.541 Other chronic hematogenous osteomyelitis, right hand
M86.542 Other chronic hematogenous osteomyelitis, left hand
M86.549 Other chronic hematogenous osteomyelitis, unspecified hand
✓6th M86.55 Other chronic hematogenous osteomyelitis, femur
M86.551 Other chronic hematogenous osteomyelitis, right femur
M86.552 Other chronic hematogenous osteomyelitis, left femur
M86.559 Other chronic hematogenous osteomyelitis, unspecified femur
✓6th M86.56 Other chronic hematogenous osteomyelitis, tibia and fibula
M86.561 Other chronic hematogenous osteomyelitis, right tibia and fibula
M86.562 Other chronic hematogenous osteomyelitis, left tibia and fibula
M86.569 Other chronic hematogenous osteomyelitis, unspecified tibia and fibula
✓6th M86.57 Other chronic hematogenous osteomyelitis, ankle and foot
M86.571 Other chronic hematogenous osteomyelitis, right ankle and foot
M86.572 Other chronic hematogenous osteomyelitis, left ankle and foot
M86.579 Other chronic hematogenous osteomyelitis, unspecified ankle and foot
M86.58 Other chronic hematogenous osteomyelitis, other site

M86.59 Other chronic hematogenous osteomyelitis, multiple sites

✓5th **M86.6 Other chronic osteomyelitis**

M86.6Ø Other chronic osteomyelitis, unspecified site

✓6th **M86.61 Other chronic osteomyelitis, shoulder**

M86.611 Other chronic osteomyelitis, right shoulder

M86.612 Other chronic osteomyelitis, left shoulder

M86.619 Other chronic osteomyelitis, unspecified shoulder

✓6th **M86.62 Other chronic osteomyelitis, humerus**

M86.621 Other chronic osteomyelitis, right humerus

M86.622 Other chronic osteomyelitis, left humerus

M86.629 Other chronic osteomyelitis, unspecified humerus

✓6th **M86.63 Other chronic osteomyelitis, radius and ulna**

M86.631 Other chronic osteomyelitis, right radius and ulna

M86.632 Other chronic osteomyelitis, left radius and ulna

M86.639 Other chronic osteomyelitis, unspecified radius and ulna

✓6th **M86.64 Other chronic osteomyelitis, hand**

M86.641 Other chronic osteomyelitis, right hand

M86.642 Other chronic osteomyelitis, left hand

M86.649 Other chronic osteomyelitis, unspecified hand

✓6th **M86.65 Other chronic osteomyelitis, thigh**

M86.651 Other chronic osteomyelitis, right thigh

M86.652 Other chronic osteomyelitis, left thigh

M86.659 Other chronic osteomyelitis, unspecified thigh

✓6th **M86.66 Other chronic osteomyelitis, tibia and fibula**

M86.661 Other chronic osteomyelitis, right tibia and fibula

M86.662 Other chronic osteomyelitis, left tibia and fibula

M86.669 Other chronic osteomyelitis, unspecified tibia and fibula

✓6th **M86.67 Other chronic osteomyelitis, ankle and foot**

M86.671 Other chronic osteomyelitis, right ankle and foot

M86.672 Other chronic osteomyelitis, left ankle and foot

M86.679 Other chronic osteomyelitis, unspecified ankle and foot

M86.68 Other chronic osteomyelitis, other site

M86.69 Other chronic osteomyelitis, multiple sites

✓5th **M86.8 Other osteomyelitis**

Brodie's abscess

✓6th **M86.8X Other osteomyelitis**

M86.8XØ Other osteomyelitis, multiple sites

M86.8X1 Other osteomyelitis, shoulder

M86.8X2 Other osteomyelitis, upper arm

M86.8X3 Other osteomyelitis, forearm

M86.8X4 Other osteomyelitis, hand

M86.8X5 Other osteomyelitis, thigh

M86.8X6 Other osteomyelitis, lower leg

M86.8X7 Other osteomyelitis, ankle and foot

M86.8X8 Other osteomyelitis, other site

M86.8X9 Other osteomyelitis, unspecified sites

M86.9 Osteomyelitis, unspecified

Infection of bone NOS

Periostitis without osteomyelitis

✓4th **M87 Osteonecrosis**

INCLUDES avascular necrosis of bone

Use additional code to identify major osseous defect, if applicable (M89.7-)

EXCLUDES 1 *juvenile osteonecrosis (M91-M92)*

osteochondropathies (M9Ø-M93)

✓5th **M87.Ø Idiopathic aseptic necrosis of bone**

M87.ØØ Idiopathic aseptic necrosis of unspecified bone

✓6th **M87.Ø1 Idiopathic aseptic necrosis of shoulder**

Idiopathic aseptic necrosis of clavicle and scapula

M87.Ø11 Idiopathic aseptic necrosis of right shoulder

M87.Ø12 Idiopathic aseptic necrosis of left shoulder

M87.Ø19 Idiopathic aseptic necrosis of unspecified shoulder

✓6th **M87.Ø2 Idiopathic aseptic necrosis of humerus**

M87.Ø21 Idiopathic aseptic necrosis of right humerus

M87.Ø22 Idiopathic aseptic necrosis of left humerus

M87.Ø29 Idiopathic aseptic necrosis of unspecified humerus

✓6th **M87.Ø3 Idiopathic aseptic necrosis of radius, ulna and carpus**

M87.Ø31 Idiopathic aseptic necrosis of right radius

M87.Ø32 Idiopathic aseptic necrosis of left radius

M87.Ø33 Idiopathic aseptic necrosis of unspecified radius

M87.Ø34 Idiopathic aseptic necrosis of right ulna

M87.Ø35 Idiopathic aseptic necrosis of left ulna

M87.Ø36 Idiopathic aseptic necrosis of unspecified ulna

M87.Ø37 Idiopathic aseptic necrosis of right carpus

M87.Ø38 Idiopathic aseptic necrosis of left carpus

M87.Ø39 Idiopathic aseptic necrosis of unspecified carpus

✓6th **M87.Ø4 Idiopathic aseptic necrosis of hand and fingers**

Idiopathic aseptic necrosis of metacarpals and phalanges of hands

M87.Ø41 Idiopathic aseptic necrosis of right hand

M87.Ø42 Idiopathic aseptic necrosis of left hand

M87.Ø43 Idiopathic aseptic necrosis of unspecified hand

M87.Ø44 Idiopathic aseptic necrosis of right finger(s)

M87.Ø45 Idiopathic aseptic necrosis of left finger(s)

M87.Ø46 Idiopathic aseptic necrosis of unspecified finger(s)

✓6th **M87.Ø5 Idiopathic aseptic necrosis of pelvis and femur**

M87.Ø5Ø Idiopathic aseptic necrosis of pelvis

M87.Ø51 Idiopathic aseptic necrosis of right femur

M87.Ø52 Idiopathic aseptic necrosis of left femur

M87.Ø59 Idiopathic aseptic necrosis of unspecified femur

Idiopathic aseptic necrosis of hip NOS

✓6th **M87.Ø6 Idiopathic aseptic necrosis of tibia and fibula**

M87.Ø61 Idiopathic aseptic necrosis of right tibia

M87.Ø62 Idiopathic aseptic necrosis of left tibia

M87.Ø63 Idiopathic aseptic necrosis of unspecified tibia

M87.Ø64 Idiopathic aseptic necrosis of right fibula

M87.Ø65 Idiopathic aseptic necrosis of left fibula

M87.Ø66 Idiopathic aseptic necrosis of unspecified fibula

✓6th **M87.Ø7 Idiopathic aseptic necrosis of ankle, foot and toes**

Idiopathic aseptic necrosis of metatarsus, tarsus, and phalanges of toes

M87.Ø71 Idiopathic aseptic necrosis of right ankle

M87.Ø72 Idiopathic aseptic necrosis of left ankle

M87.Ø73 Idiopathic aseptic necrosis of unspecified ankle

M87.Ø74 Idiopathic aseptic necrosis of right foot

M87.Ø75 Idiopathic aseptic necrosis of left foot

M87.Ø76 Idiopathic aseptic necrosis of unspecified foot

M87.Ø77 Idiopathic aseptic necrosis of right toe(s)

M87.Ø78 Idiopathic aseptic necrosis of left toe(s)

M87.Ø79 Idiopathic aseptic necrosis of unspecified toe(s)

M87.08 Idiopathic aseptic necrosis of bone, other site
M87.09 Idiopathic aseptic necrosis of bone, multiple sites
✓5th M87.1 Osteonecrosis due to drugs
Use additional code for adverse effect, if applicable, to identify drug (T36-T50 with fifth or sixth character 5)
M87.10 Osteonecrosis due to drugs, unspecified bone
✓6th M87.11 Osteonecrosis due to drugs, shoulder
M87.111 Osteonecrosis due to drugs, right shoulder
M87.112 Osteonecrosis due to drugs, left shoulder
M87.119 Osteonecrosis due to drugs, unspecified shoulder
✓6th M87.12 Osteonecrosis due to drugs, humerus
M87.121 Osteonecrosis due to drugs, right humerus
M87.122 Osteonecrosis due to drugs, left humerus
M87.129 Osteonecrosis due to drugs, unspecified humerus
✓6th M87.13 Osteonecrosis due to drugs of radius, ulna and carpus
M87.131 Osteonecrosis due to drugs of right radius
M87.132 Osteonecrosis due to drugs of left radius
M87.133 Osteonecrosis due to drugs of unspecified radius
M87.134 Osteonecrosis due to drugs of right ulna
M87.135 Osteonecrosis due to drugs of left ulna
M87.136 Osteonecrosis due to drugs of unspecified ulna
M87.137 Osteonecrosis due to drugs of right carpus
M87.138 Osteonecrosis due to drugs of left carpus
M87.139 Osteonecrosis due to drugs of unspecified carpus
✓6th M87.14 Osteonecrosis due to drugs, hand and fingers
M87.141 Osteonecrosis due to drugs, right hand
M87.142 Osteonecrosis due to drugs, left hand
M87.143 Osteonecrosis due to drugs, unspecified hand
M87.144 Osteonecrosis due to drugs, right finger(s)
M87.145 Osteonecrosis due to drugs, left finger(s)
M87.146 Osteonecrosis due to drugs, unspecified finger(s)
✓6th M87.15 Osteonecrosis due to drugs, pelvis and femur
M87.150 Osteonecrosis due to drugs, pelvis
M87.151 Osteonecrosis due to drugs, right femur
M87.152 Osteonecrosis due to drugs, left femur
M87.159 Osteonecrosis due to drugs, unspecified femur
✓6th M87.16 Osteonecrosis due to drugs, tibia and fibula
M87.161 Osteonecrosis due to drugs, right tibia
M87.162 Osteonecrosis due to drugs, left tibia
M87.163 Osteonecrosis due to drugs, unspecified tibia
M87.164 Osteonecrosis due to drugs, right fibula
M87.165 Osteonecrosis due to drugs, left fibula
M87.166 Osteonecrosis due to drugs, unspecified fibula
✓6th M87.17 Osteonecrosis due to drugs, ankle, foot and toes
M87.171 Osteonecrosis due to drugs, right ankle
M87.172 Osteonecrosis due to drugs, left ankle
M87.173 Osteonecrosis due to drugs, unspecified ankle
M87.174 Osteonecrosis due to drugs, right foot
M87.175 Osteonecrosis due to drugs, left foot
M87.176 Osteonecrosis due to drugs, unspecified foot
M87.177 Osteonecrosis due to drugs, right toe(s)
M87.178 Osteonecrosis due to drugs, left toe(s)
M87.179 Osteonecrosis due to drugs, unspecified toe(s)
✓6th M87.18 Osteonecrosis due to drugs, other site
M87.180 Osteonecrosis due to drugs, jaw
M87.188 Osteonecrosis due to drugs, other site
M87.19 Osteonecrosis due to drugs, multiple sites
✓5th M87.2 Osteonecrosis due to previous trauma
M87.20 Osteonecrosis due to previous trauma, unspecified bone
✓6th M87.21 Osteonecrosis due to previous trauma, shoulder
M87.211 Osteonecrosis due to previous trauma, right shoulder
M87.212 Osteonecrosis due to previous trauma, left shoulder
M87.219 Osteonecrosis due to previous trauma, unspecified shoulder
✓6th M87.22 Osteonecrosis due to previous trauma, humerus
M87.221 Osteonecrosis due to previous trauma, right humerus
M87.222 Osteonecrosis due to previous trauma, left humerus
M87.229 Osteonecrosis due to previous trauma, unspecified humerus
✓6th M87.23 Osteonecrosis due to previous trauma of radius, ulna and carpus
M87.231 Osteonecrosis due to previous trauma of right radius
M87.232 Osteonecrosis due to previous trauma of left radius
M87.233 Osteonecrosis due to previous trauma of unspecified radius
M87.234 Osteonecrosis due to previous trauma of right ulna
M87.235 Osteonecrosis due to previous trauma of left ulna
M87.236 Osteonecrosis due to previous trauma of unspecified ulna
M87.237 Osteonecrosis due to previous trauma of right carpus
M87.238 Osteonecrosis due to previous trauma of left carpus
M87.239 Osteonecrosis due to previous trauma of unspecified carpus
✓6th M87.24 Osteonecrosis due to previous trauma, hand and fingers
M87.241 Osteonecrosis due to previous trauma, right hand
M87.242 Osteonecrosis due to previous trauma, left hand
M87.243 Osteonecrosis due to previous trauma, unspecified hand
M87.244 Osteonecrosis due to previous trauma, right finger(s)
M87.245 Osteonecrosis due to previous trauma, left finger(s)
M87.246 Osteonecrosis due to previous trauma, unspecified finger(s)
✓6th M87.25 Osteonecrosis due to previous trauma, pelvis and femur
M87.250 Osteonecrosis due to previous trauma, pelvis
M87.251 Osteonecrosis due to previous trauma, right femur
M87.252 Osteonecrosis due to previous trauma, left femur
M87.256 Osteonecrosis due to previous trauma, unspecified femur
✓6th M87.26 Osteonecrosis due to previous trauma, tibia and fibula
M87.261 Osteonecrosis due to previous trauma, right tibia
M87.262 Osteonecrosis due to previous trauma, left tibia
M87.263 Osteonecrosis due to previous trauma, unspecified tibia
M87.264 Osteonecrosis due to previous trauma, right fibula
M87.265 Osteonecrosis due to previous trauma, left fibula

- M87.266 Osteonecrosis due to previous trauma, unspecified fibula
- ✓6th M87.27 Osteonecrosis due to previous trauma, ankle, foot and toes
  - M87.271 Osteonecrosis due to previous trauma, right ankle
  - M87.272 Osteonecrosis due to previous trauma, left ankle
  - M87.273 Osteonecrosis due to previous trauma, unspecified ankle
  - M87.274 Osteonecrosis due to previous trauma, right foot
  - M87.275 Osteonecrosis due to previous trauma, left foot
  - M87.276 Osteonecrosis due to previous trauma, unspecified foot
  - M87.277 Osteonecrosis due to previous trauma, right toe(s)
  - M87.278 Osteonecrosis due to previous trauma, left toe(s)
  - M87.279 Osteonecrosis due to previous trauma, unspecified toe(s)
- M87.28 Osteonecrosis due to previous trauma, other site
- M87.29 Osteonecrosis due to previous trauma, multiple sites

✓5th M87.3 Other secondary osteonecrosis
- M87.30 Other secondary osteonecrosis, unspecified bone
- ✓6th M87.31 Other secondary osteonecrosis, shoulder
  - M87.311 Other secondary osteonecrosis, right shoulder
  - M87.312 Other secondary osteonecrosis, left shoulder
  - M87.319 Other secondary osteonecrosis, unspecified shoulder
- ✓6th M87.32 Other secondary osteonecrosis, humerus
  - M87.321 Other secondary osteonecrosis, right humerus
  - M87.322 Other secondary osteonecrosis, left humerus
  - M87.329 Other secondary osteonecrosis, unspecified humerus
- ✓6th M87.33 Other secondary osteonecrosis of radius, ulna and carpus
  - M87.331 Other secondary osteonecrosis of right radius
  - M87.332 Other secondary osteonecrosis of left radius
  - M87.333 Other secondary osteonecrosis of unspecified radius
  - M87.334 Other secondary osteonecrosis of right ulna
  - M87.335 Other secondary osteonecrosis of left ulna
  - M87.336 Other secondary osteonecrosis of unspecified ulna
  - M87.337 Other secondary osteonecrosis of right carpus
  - M87.338 Other secondary osteonecrosis of left carpus
  - M87.339 Other secondary osteonecrosis of unspecified carpus
- ✓6th M87.34 Other secondary osteonecrosis, hand and fingers
  - M87.341 Other secondary osteonecrosis, right hand
  - M87.342 Other secondary osteonecrosis, left hand
  - M87.343 Other secondary osteonecrosis, unspecified hand
  - M87.344 Other secondary osteonecrosis, right finger(s)
  - M87.345 Other secondary osteonecrosis, left finger(s)
  - M87.346 Other secondary osteonecrosis, unspecified finger(s)
- ✓6th M87.35 Other secondary osteonecrosis, pelvis and femur
  - M87.350 Other secondary osteonecrosis, pelvis
  - M87.351 Other secondary osteonecrosis, right femur
  - M87.352 Other secondary osteonecrosis, left femur
  - M87.353 Other secondary osteonecrosis, unspecified femur
- ✓6th M87.36 Other secondary osteonecrosis, tibia and fibula
  - M87.361 Other secondary osteonecrosis, right tibia
  - M87.362 Other secondary osteonecrosis, left tibia
  - M87.363 Other secondary osteonecrosis, unspecified tibia
  - M87.364 Other secondary osteonecrosis, right fibula
  - M87.365 Other secondary osteonecrosis, left fibula
  - M87.366 Other secondary osteonecrosis, unspecified fibula
- ✓6th M87.37 Other secondary osteonecrosis, ankle and foot
  - M87.371 Other secondary osteonecrosis, right ankle
  - M87.372 Other secondary osteonecrosis, left ankle
  - M87.373 Other secondary osteonecrosis, unspecified ankle
  - M87.374 Other secondary osteonecrosis, right foot
  - M87.375 Other secondary osteonecrosis, left foot
  - M87.376 Other secondary osteonecrosis, unspecified foot
  - M87.377 Other secondary osteonecrosis, right toe(s)
  - M87.378 Other secondary osteonecrosis, left toe(s)
  - M87.379 Other secondary osteonecrosis, unspecified toe(s)
- M87.38 Other secondary osteonecrosis, other site
- M87.39 Other secondary osteonecrosis, multiple sites

✓5th M87.8 Other osteonecrosis
- M87.80 Other osteonecrosis, unspecified bone
- ✓6th M87.81 Other osteonecrosis, shoulder
  - M87.811 Other osteonecrosis, right shoulder
  - M87.812 Other osteonecrosis, left shoulder
  - M87.819 Other osteonecrosis, unspecified shoulder
- ✓6th M87.82 Other osteonecrosis, humerus
  - M87.821 Other osteonecrosis, right humerus
  - M87.822 Other osteonecrosis, left humerus
  - M87.829 Other osteonecrosis, unspecified humerus
- ✓6th M87.83 Other osteonecrosis of radius, ulna and carpus
  - M87.831 Other osteonecrosis of right radius
  - M87.832 Other osteonecrosis of left radius
  - M87.833 Other osteonecrosis of unspecified radius
  - M87.834 Other osteonecrosis of right ulna
  - M87.835 Other osteonecrosis of left ulna
  - M87.836 Other osteonecrosis of unspecified ulna
  - M87.837 Other osteonecrosis of right carpus
  - M87.838 Other osteonecrosis of left carpus
  - M87.839 Other osteonecrosis of unspecified carpus
- ✓6th M87.84 Other osteonecrosis, hand and fingers
  - M87.841 Other osteonecrosis, right hand
  - M87.842 Other osteonecrosis, left hand
  - M87.843 Other osteonecrosis, unspecified hand
  - M87.844 Other osteonecrosis, right finger(s)
  - M87.845 Other osteonecrosis, left finger(s)
  - M87.849 Other osteonecrosis, unspecified finger(s)
- ✓6th M87.85 Other osteonecrosis, pelvis and femur
  - M87.850 Other osteonecrosis, pelvis
  - M87.851 Other osteonecrosis, right femur
  - M87.852 Other osteonecrosis, left femur
  - M87.859 Other osteonecrosis, unspecified femur
- ✓6th M87.86 Other osteonecrosis, tibia and fibula
  - M87.861 Other osteonecrosis, right tibia
  - M87.862 Other osteonecrosis, left tibia

EXCLUDES1 Not coded here EXCLUDES2 Not included here *Manifestation Code*

M87.863 Other osteonecrosis, unspecified tibia
M87.864 Other osteonecrosis, right fibula
M87.865 Other osteonecrosis, left fibula
M87.869 Other osteonecrosis, unspecified fibula
✓6th M87.87 Other osteonecrosis, ankle, foot and toes
M87.871 Other osteonecrosis, right ankle
M87.872 Other osteonecrosis, left ankle
M87.873 Other osteonecrosis, unspecified ankle
M87.874 Other osteonecrosis, right foot
M87.875 Other osteonecrosis, left foot
M87.876 Other osteonecrosis, unspecified foot
M87.877 Other osteonecrosis, right toe(s)
M87.878 Other osteonecrosis, left toe(s)
M87.879 Other osteonecrosis, unspecified toe(s)
M87.88 Other osteonecrosis, other site
M87.89 Other osteonecrosis, multiple sites
M87.9 Osteonecrosis, unspecified
Necrosis of bone NOS

✓4th **M88 Osteitis deformans [Paget's disease of bone]**
EXCLUDES 1 *osteitis deformans in neoplastic disease (M9Ø.6)*
M88.Ø Osteitis deformans of skull
M88.1 Osteitis deformans of vertebrae
✓5th M88.8 Osteitis deformans of other bones
✓6th M88.81 Osteitis deformans of shoulder
M88.811 Osteitis deformans of right shoulder
M88.812 Osteitis deformans of left shoulder
M88.819 Osteitis deformans of unspecified shoulder
✓6th M88.82 Osteitis deformans of upper arm
M88.821 Osteitis deformans of right upper arm
M88.822 Osteitis deformans of left upper arm
M88.829 Osteitis deformans of unspecified upper arm
✓6th M88.83 Osteitis deformans of forearm
M88.831 Osteitis deformans of right forearm
M88.832 Osteitis deformans of left forearm
M88.839 Osteitis deformans of unspecified forearm
✓6th M88.84 Osteitis deformans of hand
M88.841 Osteitis deformans of right hand
M88.842 Osteitis deformans of left hand
M88.849 Osteitis deformans of unspecified hand
✓6th M88.85 Osteitis deformans of thigh
M88.851 Osteitis deformans of right thigh
M88.852 Osteitis deformans of left thigh
M88.859 Osteitis deformans of unspecified thigh
✓6th M88.86 Osteitis deformans of lower leg
M88.861 Osteitis deformans of right lower leg
M88.862 Osteitis deformans of left lower leg
M88.869 Osteitis deformans of unspecified lower leg
✓6th M88.87 Osteitis deformans of ankle and foot
M88.871 Osteitis deformans of right ankle and foot
M88.872 Osteitis deformans of left ankle and foot
M88.879 Osteitis deformans of unspecified ankle and foot
M88.88 Osteitis deformans of other bones
EXCLUDES 2 *osteitis deformans of skull (M88.Ø)*
osteitis deformans of vertebrae (M88.1)
M88.89 Osteitis deformans of multiple sites
M88.9 Osteitis deformans of unspecified bone

✓4th **M89 Other disorders of bone**
✓5th M89.Ø Algoneurodystrophy
Shoulder-hand syndrome
Sudeck's atrophy
EXCLUDES 1 *causalgia, lower limb (G57.7-)*
causalgia, upper limb (G56.4-)
complex regional pain syndrome II, lower limb (G57.7-)
complex regional pain syndrome II, upper limb (G56.4-)
reflex sympathetic dystrophy (G9Ø.5-)
M89.ØØ Algoneurodystrophy, unspecified site
✓6th M89.Ø1 Algoneurodystrophy, shoulder
M89.Ø11 Algoneurodystrophy, right shoulder
M89.Ø12 Algoneurodystrophy, left shoulder
M89.Ø19 Algoneurodystrophy, unspecified shoulder
✓6th M89.Ø2 Algoneurodystrophy, upper arm
M89.Ø21 Algoneurodystrophy, right upper arm
M89.Ø22 Algoneurodystrophy, left upper arm
M89.Ø29 Algoneurodystrophy, unspecified upper arm
✓6th M89.Ø3 Algoneurodystrophy, forearm
M89.Ø31 Algoneurodystrophy, right forearm
M89.Ø32 Algoneurodystrophy, left forearm
M89.Ø39 Algoneurodystrophy, unspecified forearm
✓6th M89.Ø4 Algoneurodystrophy, hand
M89.Ø41 Algoneurodystrophy, right hand
M89.Ø42 Algoneurodystrophy, left hand
M89.Ø49 Algoneurodystrophy, unspecified hand
✓6th M89.Ø5 Algoneurodystrophy, thigh
M89.Ø51 Algoneurodystrophy, right thigh
M89.Ø52 Algoneurodystrophy, left thigh
M89.Ø59 Algoneurodystrophy, unspecified thigh
✓6th M89.Ø6 Algoneurodystrophy, lower leg
M89.Ø61 Algoneurodystrophy, right lower leg
M89.Ø62 Algoneurodystrophy, left lower leg
M89.Ø69 Algoneurodystrophy, unspecified lower leg
✓6th M89.Ø7 Algoneurodystrophy, ankle and foot
M89.Ø71 Algoneurodystrophy, right ankle and foot
M89.Ø72 Algoneurodystrophy, left ankle and foot
M89.Ø79 Algoneurodystrophy, unspecified ankle and foot
M89.Ø8 Algoneurodystrophy, other site
M89.Ø9 Algoneurodystrophy, multiple sites
✓5th M89.1 Physeal arrest
Arrest of growth plate
Epiphyseal arrest
Growth plate arrest
✓6th M89.12 Physeal arrest, humerus
M89.121 Complete physeal arrest, right proximal humerus
M89.122 Complete physeal arrest, left proximal humerus
M89.123 Partial physeal arrest, right proximal humerus
M89.124 Partial physeal arrest, left proximal humerus
M89.125 Complete physeal arrest, right distal humerus
M89.126 Complete physeal arrest, left distal humerus
M89.127 Partial physeal arrest, right distal humerus
M89.128 Partial physeal arrest, left distal humerus
M89.129 Physeal arrest, humerus, unspecified
✓6th M89.13 Physeal arrest, forearm
M89.131 Complete physeal arrest, right distal radius
M89.132 Complete physeal arrest, left distal radius
M89.133 Partial physeal arrest, right distal radius
M89.134 Partial physeal arrest, left distal radius
M89.138 Other physeal arrest of forearm
M89.139 Physeal arrest, forearm, unspecified
✓6th M89.15 Physeal arrest, femur
M89.151 Complete physeal arrest, right proximal femur
M89.152 Complete physeal arrest, left proximal femur
M89.153 Partial physeal arrest, right proximal femur
M89.154 Partial physeal arrest, left proximal femur

M89.155 Complete physeal arrest, right distal femur
M89.156 Complete physeal arrest, left distal femur
M89.157 Partial physeal arrest, right distal femur
M89.158 Partial physeal arrest, left distal femur
M89.159 Physeal arrest, femur, unspecified
✓6th M89.16 Physeal arrest, lower leg
M89.160 Complete physeal arrest, right proximal tibia
M89.161 Complete physeal arrest, left proximal tibia
M89.162 Partial physeal arrest, right proximal tibia
M89.163 Partial physeal arrest, left proximal tibia
M89.164 Complete physeal arrest, right distal tibia
M89.165 Complete physeal arrest, left distal tibia
M89.166 Partial physeal arrest, right distal tibia
M89.167 Partial physeal arrest, left distal tibia
M89.168 Other physeal arrest of lower leg
M89.169 Physeal arrest, lower leg, unspecified
M89.18 Physeal arrest, other site
✓5th M89.2 Other disorders of bone development and growth
M89.20 Other disorders of bone development and growth, unspecified site
✓6th M89.21 Other disorders of bone development and growth, shoulder
M89.211 Other disorders of bone development and growth, right shoulder
M89.212 Other disorders of bone development and growth, left shoulder
M89.219 Other disorders of bone development and growth, unspecified shoulder
✓6th M89.22 Other disorders of bone development and growth, humerus
M89.221 Other disorders of bone development and growth, right humerus
M89.222 Other disorders of bone development and growth, left humerus
M89.229 Other disorders of bone development and growth, unspecified humerus
✓6th M89.23 Other disorders of bone development and growth, ulna and radius
M89.231 Other disorders of bone development and growth, right ulna
M89.232 Other disorders of bone development and growth, left ulna
M89.233 Other disorders of bone development and growth, right radius
M89.234 Other disorders of bone development and growth, left radius
M89.239 Other disorders of bone development and growth, unspecified ulna and radius
✓6th M89.24 Other disorders of bone development and growth, hand
M89.241 Other disorders of bone development and growth, right hand
M89.242 Other disorders of bone development and growth, left hand
M89.249 Other disorders of bone development and growth, unspecified hand
✓6th M89.25 Other disorders of bone development and growth, femur
M89.251 Other disorders of bone development and growth, right femur
M89.252 Other disorders of bone development and growth, left femur
M89.259 Other disorders of bone development and growth, unspecified femur
✓6th M89.26 Other disorders of bone development and growth, tibia and fibula
M89.261 Other disorders of bone development and growth, right tibia
M89.262 Other disorders of bone development and growth, left tibia
M89.263 Other disorders of bone development and growth, right fibula
M89.264 Other disorders of bone development and growth, left fibula
M89.269 Other disorders of bone development and growth, unspecified lower leg
✓6th M89.27 Other disorders of bone development and growth, ankle and foot
M89.271 Other disorders of bone development and growth, right ankle and foot
M89.272 Other disorders of bone development and growth, left ankle and foot
M89.279 Other disorders of bone development and growth, unspecified ankle and foot
M89.28 Other disorders of bone development and growth, other site
M89.29 Other disorders of bone development and growth, multiple sites
✓5th M89.3 Hypertrophy of bone
M89.30 Hypertrophy of bone, unspecified site
✓6th M89.31 Hypertrophy of bone, shoulder
M89.311 Hypertrophy of bone, right shoulder
M89.312 Hypertrophy of bone, left shoulder
M89.319 Hypertrophy of bone, unspecified shoulder
✓6th M89.32 Hypertrophy of bone, humerus
M89.321 Hypertrophy of bone, right humerus
M89.322 Hypertrophy of bone, left humerus
M89.329 Hypertrophy of bone, unspecified humerus
✓6th M89.33 Hypertrophy of bone, ulna and radius
M89.331 Hypertrophy of bone, right ulna
M89.332 Hypertrophy of bone, left ulna
M89.333 Hypertrophy of bone, right radius
M89.334 Hypertrophy of bone, left radius
M89.339 Hypertrophy of bone, unspecified ulna and radius
✓6th M89.34 Hypertrophy of bone, hand
M89.341 Hypertrophy of bone, right hand
M89.342 Hypertrophy of bone, left hand
M89.349 Hypertrophy of bone, unspecified hand
✓6th M89.35 Hypertrophy of bone, femur
M89.351 Hypertrophy of bone, right femur
M89.352 Hypertrophy of bone, left femur
M89.359 Hypertrophy of bone, unspecified femur
✓6th M89.36 Hypertrophy of bone, tibia and fibula
M89.361 Hypertrophy of bone, right tibia
M89.362 Hypertrophy of bone, left tibia
M89.363 Hypertrophy of bone, right fibula
M89.364 Hypertrophy of bone, left fibula
M89.369 Hypertrophy of bone, unspecified tibia and fibula
✓6th M89.37 Hypertrophy of bone, ankle and foot
M89.371 Hypertrophy of bone, right ankle and foot
M89.372 Hypertrophy of bone, left ankle and foot
M89.379 Hypertrophy of bone, unspecified ankle and foot
M89.38 Hypertrophy of bone, other site
M89.39 Hypertrophy of bone, multiple sites
✓5th M89.4 Other hypertrophic osteoarthropathy
Marie-Bamberger disease
Pachydermoperiostosis
M89.40 Other hypertrophic osteoarthropathy, unspecified site
✓6th M89.41 Other hypertrophic osteoarthropathy, shoulder
M89.411 Other hypertrophic osteoarthropathy, right shoulder
M89.412 Other hypertrophic osteoarthropathy, left shoulder
M89.419 Other hypertrophic osteoarthropathy, unspecified shoulder
✓6th M89.42 Other hypertrophic osteoarthropathy, upper arm
M89.421 Other hypertrophic osteoarthropathy, right upper arm
M89.422 Other hypertrophic osteoarthropathy, left upper arm
M89.429 Other hypertrophic osteoarthropathy, unspecified upper arm

✓6th **M89.43 Other hypertrophic osteoarthropathy, forearm**
- **M89.431 Other hypertrophic osteoarthropathy, right forearm**
- **M89.432 Other hypertrophic osteoarthropathy, left forearm**
- **M89.439 Other hypertrophic osteoarthropathy, unspecified forearm**

✓6th **M89.44 Other hypertrophic osteoarthropathy, hand**
- **M89.441 Other hypertrophic osteoarthropathy, right hand**
- **M89.442 Other hypertrophic osteoarthropathy, left hand**
- **M89.449 Other hypertrophic osteoarthropathy, unspecified hand**

✓6th **M89.45 Other hypertrophic osteoarthropathy, thigh**
- **M89.451 Other hypertrophic osteoarthropathy, right thigh**
- **M89.452 Other hypertrophic osteoarthropathy, left thigh**
- **M89.459 Other hypertrophic osteoarthropathy, unspecified thigh**

✓6th **M89.46 Other hypertrophic osteoarthropathy, lower leg**
- **M89.461 Other hypertrophic osteoarthropathy, right lower leg**
- **M89.462 Other hypertrophic osteoarthropathy, left lower leg**
- **M89.469 Other hypertrophic osteoarthropathy, unspecified lower leg**

✓6th **M89.47 Other hypertrophic osteoarthropathy, ankle and foot**
- **M89.471 Other hypertrophic osteoarthropathy, right ankle and foot**
- **M89.472 Other hypertrophic osteoarthropathy, left ankle and foot**
- **M89.479 Other hypertrophic osteoarthropathy, unspecified ankle and foot**

M89.48 Other hypertrophic osteoarthropathy, other site

M89.49 Other hypertrophic osteoarthropathy, multiple sites

✓5th **M89.5 Osteolysis**

Use additional code to identify major osseous defect, if applicable (M89.7-)

EXCLUDES 2 *periprosthetic osteolysis of internal prosthetic joint (T84.05-)*

M89.50 Osteolysis, unspecified site

✓6th **M89.51 Osteolysis, shoulder**
- **M89.511 Osteolysis, right shoulder**
- **M89.512 Osteolysis, left shoulder**
- **M89.519 Osteolysis, unspecified shoulder**

✓6th **M89.52 Osteolysis, upper arm**
- **M89.521 Osteolysis, right upper arm**
- **M89.522 Osteolysis, left upper arm**
- **M89.529 Osteolysis, unspecified upper arm**

✓6th **M89.53 Osteolysis, forearm**
- **M89.531 Osteolysis, right forearm**
- **M89.532 Osteolysis, left forearm**
- **M89.539 Osteolysis, unspecified forearm**

✓6th **M89.54 Osteolysis, hand**
- **M89.541 Osteolysis, right hand**
- **M89.542 Osteolysis, left hand**
- **M89.549 Osteolysis, unspecified hand**

✓6th **M89.55 Osteolysis, thigh**
- **M89.551 Osteolysis, right thigh**
- **M89.552 Osteolysis, left thigh**
- **M89.559 Osteolysis, unspecified thigh**

✓6th **M89.56 Osteolysis, lower leg**
- **M89.561 Osteolysis, right lower leg**
- **M89.562 Osteolysis, left lower leg**
- **M89.569 Osteolysis, unspecified lower leg**

✓6th **M89.57 Osteolysis, ankle and foot**
- **M89.571 Osteolysis, right ankle and foot**
- **M89.572 Osteolysis, left ankle and foot**
- **M89.579 Osteolysis, unspecified ankle and foot**

M89.58 Osteolysis, other site

M89.59 Osteolysis, multiple sites

✓5th **M89.6 Osteopathy after poliomyelitis**

Use additional code (B91) to identify previous poliomyelitis

EXCLUDES 1 *postpolio syndrome (G14)*

M89.60 Osteopathy after poliomyelitis, unspecified site

✓6th **M89.61 Osteopathy after poliomyelitis, shoulder**
- **M89.611 Osteopathy after poliomyelitis, right shoulder**
- **M89.612 Osteopathy after poliomyelitis, left shoulder**
- **M89.619 Osteopathy after poliomyelitis, unspecified shoulder**

✓6th **M89.62 Osteopathy after poliomyelitis, upper arm**
- **M89.621 Osteopathy after poliomyelitis, right upper arm**
- **M89.622 Osteopathy after poliomyelitis, left upper arm**
- **M89.629 Osteopathy after poliomyelitis, unspecified upper arm**

✓6th **M89.63 Osteopathy after poliomyelitis, forearm**
- **M89.631 Osteopathy after poliomyelitis, right forearm**
- **M89.632 Osteopathy after poliomyelitis, left forearm**
- **M89.639 Osteopathy after poliomyelitis, unspecified forearm**

✓6th **M89.64 Osteopathy after poliomyelitis, hand**
- **M89.641 Osteopathy after poliomyelitis, right hand**
- **M89.642 Osteopathy after poliomyelitis, left hand**
- **M89.649 Osteopathy after poliomyelitis, unspecified hand**

✓6th **M89.65 Osteopathy after poliomyelitis, thigh**
- **M89.651 Osteopathy after poliomyelitis, right thigh**
- **M89.652 Osteopathy after poliomyelitis, left thigh**
- **M89.659 Osteopathy after poliomyelitis, unspecified thigh**

✓6th **M89.66 Osteopathy after poliomyelitis, lower leg**
- **M89.661 Osteopathy after poliomyelitis, right lower leg**
- **M89.662 Osteopathy after poliomyelitis, left lower leg**
- **M89.669 Osteopathy after poliomyelitis, unspecified lower leg**

✓6th **M89.67 Osteopathy after poliomyelitis, ankle and foot**
- **M89.671 Osteopathy after poliomyelitis, right ankle and foot**
- **M89.672 Osteopathy after poliomyelitis, left ankle and foot**
- **M89.679 Osteopathy after poliomyelitis, unspecified ankle and foot**

M89.68 Osteopathy after poliomyelitis, other site

M89.69 Osteopathy after poliomyelitis, multiple sites

✓5th **M89.7 Major osseous defect**

Code first underlying disease, if known, such as:
- aseptic necrosis of bone (M87.-)
- malignant neoplasm of bone (C40.-)
- osteolysis (M89.5)
- osteomyelitis (M86.-)
- osteonecrosis (M87.-)
- osteoporosis (M80.-, M81.-)
- periprosthetic osteolysis (T84.05-)

M89.70 Major osseous defect, unspecified site

✓6th **M89.71 Major osseous defect, shoulder region**

Major osseous defect clavicle or scapula
- **M89.711 Major osseous defect, right shoulder region**
- **M89.712 Major osseous defect, left shoulder region**
- **M89.719 Major osseous defect, unspecified shoulder region**

✓6th **M89.72 Major osseous defect, humerus**
- **M89.721 Major osseous defect, right humerus**
- **M89.722 Major osseous defect, left humerus**

M89.729 **Major osseous defect, unspecified humerus**

✓6th M89.73 **Major osseous defect, forearm**

Major osseous defect of radius and ulna

M89.731 **Major osseous defect, right forearm**

M89.732 **Major osseous defect, left forearm**

M89.739 **Major osseous defect, unspecified forearm**

✓6th M89.74 **Major osseous defect, hand**

Major osseous defect of carpus, fingers, metacarpus

M89.741 **Major osseous defect, right hand**

M89.742 **Major osseous defect, left hand**

M89.749 **Major osseous defect, unspecified hand**

✓6th M89.75 **Major osseous defect, pelvic region and thigh**

Major osseous defect of femur and pelvis

M89.751 **Major osseous defect, right pelvic region and thigh**

M89.752 **Major osseous defect, left pelvic region and thigh**

M89.759 **Major osseous defect, unspecified pelvic region and thigh**

✓6th M89.76 **Major osseous defect, lower leg**

Major osseous defect of fibula and tibia

M89.761 **Major osseous defect, right lower leg**

M89.762 **Major osseous defect, left lower leg**

M89.769 **Major osseous defect, unspecified lower leg**

✓6th M89.77 **Major osseous defect, ankle and foot**

Major osseous defect of metatarsus, tarsus, toes

M89.771 **Major osseous defect, right ankle and foot**

M89.772 **Major osseous defect, left ankle and foot**

M89.779 **Major osseous defect, unspecified ankle and foot**

M89.78 **Major osseous defect, other site**

M89.79 **Major osseous defect, multiple sites**

✓5th M89.8 **Other specified disorders of bone**

Infantile cortical hyperostoses

Post-traumatic subperiosteal ossification

✓6th M89.8X **Other specified disorders of bone**

M89.8X0 **Other specified disorders of bone, multiple sites**

M89.8X1 **Other specified disorders of bone, shoulder**

M89.8X2 **Other specified disorders of bone, upper arm**

M89.8X3 **Other specified disorders of bone, forearm**

M89.8X4 **Other specified disorders of bone, hand**

M89.8X5 **Other specified disorders of bone, thigh**

M89.8X6 **Other specified disorders of bone, lower leg**

M89.8X7 **Other specified disorders of bone, ankle and foot**

M89.8X8 **Other specified disorders of bone, other site**

M89.8X9 **Other specified disorders of bone, unspecified site**

M89.9 **Disorder of bone, unspecified**

✓4th **M90 Osteopathies in diseases classified elsewhere**

EXCLUDES 1 *osteochondritis, osteomyelitis, and osteopathy (in):*
- *cryptococcosis (B45.3)*
- *diabetes mellitus (E08-E13 with 4th character .61-)*
- *gonococcal (A54.43)*
- *neurogenic syphilis (A52.11)*
- *renal osteodystrophy (N25.0)*
- *salmonellosis (A02.24)*
- *secondary syphilis (A51.46)*
- *syphilis (late) (A52.77)*

✓5th M90.5 **Osteonecrosis in diseases classified elsewhere**

Code first underlying disease, such as:
- *caisson disease (T70.3)*
- *hemoglobinopathy (D50-D64)*

M90.50 ***Osteonecrosis in diseases classified elsewhere, unspecified site***

✓6th M90.51 **Osteonecrosis in diseases classified elsewhere, shoulder**

M90.511 ***Osteonecrosis in diseases classified elsewhere, right shoulder***

M90.512 ***Osteonecrosis in diseases classified elsewhere, left shoulder***

M90.519 ***Osteonecrosis in diseases classified elsewhere, unspecified shoulder***

✓6th M90.52 **Osteonecrosis in diseases classified elsewhere, upper arm**

M90.521 ***Osteonecrosis in diseases classified elsewhere, right upper arm***

M90.522 ***Osteonecrosis in diseases classified elsewhere, left upper arm***

M90.529 ***Osteonecrosis in diseases classified elsewhere, unspecified upper arm***

✓6th M90.53 **Osteonecrosis in diseases classified elsewhere, forearm**

M90.531 ***Osteonecrosis in diseases classified elsewhere, right forearm***

M90.532 ***Osteonecrosis in diseases classified elsewhere, left forearm***

M90.539 ***Osteonecrosis in diseases classified elsewhere, unspecified forearm***

✓6th M90.54 **Osteonecrosis in diseases classified elsewhere, hand**

M90.541 ***Osteonecrosis in diseases classified elsewhere, right hand***

M90.542 ***Osteonecrosis in diseases classified elsewhere, left hand***

M90.549 ***Osteonecrosis in diseases classified elsewhere, unspecified hand***

✓6th M90.55 **Osteonecrosis in diseases classified elsewhere, thigh**

M90.551 ***Osteonecrosis in diseases classified elsewhere, right thigh***

M90.552 ***Osteonecrosis in diseases classified elsewhere, left thigh***

M90.559 ***Osteonecrosis in diseases classified elsewhere, unspecified thigh***

✓6th M90.56 **Osteonecrosis in diseases classified elsewhere, lower leg**

M90.561 ***Osteonecrosis in diseases classified elsewhere, right lower leg***

M90.562 ***Osteonecrosis in diseases classified elsewhere, left lower leg***

M90.569 ***Osteonecrosis in diseases classified elsewhere, unspecified lower leg***

✓6th M90.57 **Osteonecrosis in diseases classified elsewhere, ankle and foot**

M90.571 ***Osteonecrosis in diseases classified elsewhere, right ankle and foot***

M90.572 ***Osteonecrosis in diseases classified elsewhere, left ankle and foot***

M90.579 ***Osteonecrosis in diseases classified elsewhere, unspecified ankle and foot***

M90.58 ***Osteonecrosis in diseases classified elsewhere, other site***

M90.59 ***Osteonecrosis in diseases classified elsewhere, multiple sites***

✓5th M90.6 **Osteitis deformans in neoplastic diseases**

Osteitis deformans in malignant neoplasm of bone

Code first the neoplasm (C40-, C41-)

EXCLUDES 1 *osteitis deformans [Paget's disease of bone] (M88.-)*

M90.60 ***Osteitis deformans in neoplastic diseases, unspecified site***

✓6th M90.61 **Osteitis deformans in neoplastic diseases, shoulder**

M90.611 ***Osteitis deformans in neoplastic diseases, right shoulder***

M90.612 ***Osteitis deformans in neoplastic diseases, left shoulder***

M90.619 ***Osteitis deformans in neoplastic diseases, unspecified shoulder***

✓6th M90.62 **Osteitis deformans in neoplastic diseases, upper arm**

M90.621 ***Osteitis deformans in neoplastic diseases, right upper arm***

M90.622 *Osteitis deformans in neoplastic diseases, left upper arm*
M90.629 *Osteitis deformans in neoplastic diseases, unspecified upper arm*

M90.63 Osteitis deformans in neoplastic diseases, forearm (6th)
M90.631 *Osteitis deformans in neoplastic diseases, right forearm*
M90.632 *Osteitis deformans in neoplastic diseases, left forearm*
M90.639 *Osteitis deformans in neoplastic diseases, unspecified forearm*

M90.64 Osteitis deformans in neoplastic diseases, hand (6th)
M90.641 *Osteitis deformans in neoplastic diseases, right hand*
M90.642 *Osteitis deformans in neoplastic diseases, left hand*
M90.649 *Osteitis deformans in neoplastic diseases, unspecified hand*

M90.65 Osteitis deformans in neoplastic diseases, thigh (6th)
M90.651 *Osteitis deformans in neoplastic diseases, right thigh*
M90.652 *Osteitis deformans in neoplastic diseases, left thigh*
M90.659 *Osteitis deformans in neoplastic diseases, unspecified thigh*

M90.66 Osteitis deformans in neoplastic diseases, lower leg (6th)
M90.661 *Osteitis deformans in neoplastic diseases, right lower leg*
M90.662 *Osteitis deformans in neoplastic diseases, left lower leg*
M90.669 *Osteitis deformans in neoplastic diseases, unspecified lower leg*

M90.67 Osteitis deformans in neoplastic diseases, ankle and foot (6th)
M90.671 *Osteitis deformans in neoplastic diseases, right ankle and foot*
M90.672 *Osteitis deformans in neoplastic diseases, left ankle and foot*
M90.679 *Osteitis deformans in neoplastic diseases, unspecified ankle and foot*

M90.68 *Osteitis deformans in neoplastic diseases, other site*
M90.69 *Osteitis deformans in neoplastic diseases, multiple sites*

M90.8 Osteopathy in diseases classified elsewhere (5th)
Code first underlying disease, such as:
rickets (E55.0)
vitamin-D-resistant rickets (E83.3)

M90.80 *Osteopathy in diseases classified elsewhere, unspecified site*

M90.81 Osteopathy in diseases classified elsewhere, shoulder (6th)
M90.811 *Osteopathy in diseases classified elsewhere, right shoulder*
M90.812 *Osteopathy in diseases classified elsewhere, left shoulder*
M90.819 *Osteopathy in diseases classified elsewhere, unspecified shoulder*

M90.82 Osteopathy in diseases classified elsewhere, upper arm (6th)
M90.821 *Osteopathy in diseases classified elsewhere, right upper arm*
M90.822 *Osteopathy in diseases classified elsewhere, left upper arm*
M90.829 *Osteopathy in diseases classified elsewhere, unspecified upper arm*

M90.83 Osteopathy in diseases classified elsewhere, forearm (6th)
M90.831 *Osteopathy in diseases classified elsewhere, right forearm*
M90.832 *Osteopathy in diseases classified elsewhere, left forearm*
M90.839 *Osteopathy in diseases classified elsewhere, unspecified forearm*

M90.84 Osteopathy in diseases classified elsewhere, hand (6th)
M90.841 *Osteopathy in diseases classified elsewhere, right hand*
M90.842 *Osteopathy in diseases classified elsewhere, left hand*
M90.849 *Osteopathy in diseases classified elsewhere, unspecified hand*

M90.85 Osteopathy in diseases classified elsewhere, thigh (6th)
M90.851 *Osteopathy in diseases classified elsewhere, right thigh*
M90.852 *Osteopathy in diseases classified elsewhere, left thigh*
M90.859 *Osteopathy in diseases classified elsewhere, unspecified thigh*

M90.86 Osteopathy in diseases classified elsewhere, lower leg (6th)
M90.861 *Osteopathy in diseases classified elsewhere, right lower leg*
M90.862 *Osteopathy in diseases classified elsewhere, left lower leg*
M90.869 *Osteopathy in diseases classified elsewhere, unspecified lower leg*

M90.87 Osteopathy in diseases classified elsewhere, ankle and foot (6th)
M90.871 *Osteopathy in diseases classified elsewhere, right ankle and foot*
M90.872 *Osteopathy in diseases classified elsewhere, left ankle and foot*
M90.879 *Osteopathy in diseases classified elsewhere, unspecified ankle and foot*

M90.88 *Osteopathy in diseases classified elsewhere, other site*
M90.89 *Osteopathy in diseases classified elsewhere, multiple sites*

Chondropathies (M91-M94)

EXCLUDES 1 *postprocedural chondropathies (M96.-)*

M91 Juvenile osteochondrosis of hip and pelvis (4th)
EXCLUDES 1 *slipped upper femoral epiphysis (nontraumatic) (M93.0)*

M91.0 Juvenile osteochondrosis of pelvis
Osteochondrosis (juvenile) of:
- acetabulum
- iliac crest [Buchanan]
- ischiopubic synchondrosis [van Neck]
- symphysis pubis [Pierson]

M91.1 Juvenile osteochondrosis of head of femur [Legg-Calvé-Perthes] (5th)
M91.10 Juvenile osteochondrosis of head of femur [Legg-Calvé-Perthes], unspecified leg
M91.11 Juvenile osteochondrosis of head of femur [Legg-Calvé-Perthes], right leg
M91.12 Juvenile osteochondrosis of head of femur [Legg-Calvé-Perthes], left leg

M91.2 Coxa plana (5th)
Hip deformity due to previous juvenile osteochondrosis
M91.20 Coxa plana, unspecified hip
M91.21 Coxa plana, right hip
M91.22 Coxa plana, left hip

M91.3 Pseudocoxalgia (5th)
M91.30 Pseudocoxalgia, unspecified hip
M91.31 Pseudocoxalgia, right hip
M91.32 Pseudocoxalgia, left hip

M91.4 Coxa magna (5th)
M91.40 Coxa magna, unspecified hip
M91.41 Coxa magna, right hip
M91.42 Coxa magna, left hip

M91.8 Other juvenile osteochondrosis of hip and pelvis (5th)
Juvenile osteochondrosis after reduction of congenital dislocation of hip
M91.80 Other juvenile osteochondrosis of hip and pelvis, unspecified leg
M91.81 Other juvenile osteochondrosis of hip and pelvis, right leg
M91.82 Other juvenile osteochondrosis of hip and pelvis, left leg

M91.9 Juvenile osteochondrosis of hip and pelvis, unspecified (5th)
M91.90 Juvenile osteochondrosis of hip and pelvis, unspecified, unspecified leg

M91.91 Juvenile osteochondrosis of hip and pelvis, unspecified, right leg

M91.92 Juvenile osteochondrosis of hip and pelvis, unspecified, left leg

✓4th **M92 Other juvenile osteochondrosis**

✓5th **M92.0 Juvenile osteochondrosis of humerus**
Osteochondrosis (juvenile) of capitulum of humerus [Panner]
Osteochondrosis (juvenile) of head of humerus [Haas]

M92.00 Juvenile osteochondrosis of humerus, unspecified arm

M92.01 Juvenile osteochondrosis of humerus, right arm

M92.02 Juvenile osteochondrosis of humerus, left arm

✓5th **M92.1 Juvenile osteochondrosis of radius and ulna**
Osteochondrosis (juvenile) of lower ulna [Burns]
Osteochondrosis (juvenile) of radial head [Brailsford]

M92.10 Juvenile osteochondrosis of radius and ulna, unspecified arm

M92.11 Juvenile osteochondrosis of radius and ulna, right arm

M92.12 Juvenile osteochondrosis of radius and ulna, left arm

✓5th **M92.2 Juvenile osteochondrosis, hand**

✓6th **M92.20 Unspecified juvenile osteochondrosis, hand**

M92.201 Unspecified juvenile osteochondrosis, right hand

M92.202 Unspecified juvenile osteochondrosis, left hand

M92.209 Unspecified juvenile osteochondrosis, unspecified hand

✓6th **M92.21 Osteochondrosis (juvenile) of carpal lunate [Kienböck]**

M92.211 Osteochondrosis (juvenile) of carpal lunate [Kienböck], right hand

M92.212 Osteochondrosis (juvenile) of carpal lunate [Kienböck], left hand

M92.219 Osteochondrosis (juvenile) of carpal lunate [Kienböck], unspecified hand

✓6th **M92.22 Osteochondrosis (juvenile) of metacarpal heads [Mauclaire]**

M92.221 Osteochondrosis (juvenile) of metacarpal heads [Mauclaire], right hand

M92.222 Osteochondrosis (juvenile) of metacarpal heads [Mauclaire], left hand

M92.229 Osteochondrosis (juvenile) of metacarpal heads [Mauclaire], unspecified hand

✓6th **M92.29 Other juvenile osteochondrosis, hand**

M92.291 Other juvenile osteochondrosis, right hand

M92.292 Other juvenile osteochondrosis, left hand

M92.299 Other juvenile osteochondrosis, unspecified hand

✓5th **M92.3 Other juvenile osteochondrosis, upper limb**

M92.30 Other juvenile osteochondrosis, unspecified upper limb

M92.31 Other juvenile osteochondrosis, right upper limb

M92.32 Other juvenile osteochondrosis, left upper limb

✓5th **M92.4 Juvenile osteochondrosis of patella**
Osteochondrosis (juvenile) of primary patellar center [Köhler]
Osteochondrosis (juvenile) of secondary patellar centre [Sinding Larsen]

M92.40 Juvenile osteochondrosis of patella, unspecified knee

M92.41 Juvenile osteochondrosis of patella, right knee

M92.42 Juvenile osteochondrosis of patella, left knee

✓5th **M92.5 Juvenile osteochondrosis of tibia and fibula**
Osteochondrosis (juvenile) of proximal tibia [Blount]
Osteochondrosis (juvenile) of tibial tubercle [Osgood-Schlatter]
Tibia vara

M92.50 Juvenile osteochondrosis of tibia and fibula, unspecified leg

M92.51 Juvenile osteochondrosis of tibia and fibula, right leg

M92.52 Juvenile osteochondrosis of tibia and fibula, left leg

✓5th **M92.6 Juvenile osteochondrosis of tarsus**
Osteochondrosis (juvenile) of calcaneum [Sever]
Osteochondrosis (juvenile) of os tibiale externum [Haglund]
Osteochondrosis (juvenile) of talus [Diaz]
Osteochondrosis (juvenile) of tarsal navicular [Köhler]

M92.60 Juvenile osteochondrosis of tarsus, unspecified ankle

M92.61 Juvenile osteochondrosis of tarsus, right ankle

M92.62 Juvenile osteochondrosis of tarsus, left ankle

✓5th **M92.7 Juvenile osteochondrosis of metatarsus**
Osteochondrosis (juvenile) of fifth metatarsus [Iselin]
Osteochondrosis (juvenile) of second metatarsus [Freiberg]

M92.70 Juvenile osteochondrosis of metatarsus, unspecified foot

M92.71 Juvenile osteochondrosis of metatarsus, right foot

M92.72 Juvenile osteochondrosis of metatarsus, left foot

M92.8 Other specified juvenile osteochondrosis
Calcaneal apophysitis

M92.9 Juvenile osteochondrosis, unspecified
Juvenile apophysitis NOS
Juvenile epiphysitis NOS
Juvenile osteochondritis NOS
Juvenile osteochondrosis NOS

✓4th **M93 Other osteochondropathies**
EXCLUDES 2 *osteochondrosis of spine (M42.-)*

✓5th **M93.0 Slipped upper femoral epiphysis (nontraumatic)**
Use additional code for associated chondrolysis (M94.3)

✓6th **M93.00 Unspecified slipped upper femoral epiphysis (nontraumatic)**

M93.001 Unspecified slipped upper femoral epiphysis (nontraumatic), right hip

M93.002 Unspecified slipped upper femoral epiphysis (nontraumatic), left hip

M93.003 Unspecified slipped upper femoral epiphysis (nontraumatic), unspecified hip

✓6th **M93.01 Acute slipped upper femoral epiphysis (nontraumatic)**

M93.011 Acute slipped upper femoral epiphysis (nontraumatic), right hip

M93.012 Acute slipped upper femoral epiphysis (nontraumatic), left hip

M93.013 Acute slipped upper femoral epiphysis (nontraumatic), unspecified hip

✓6th **M93.02 Chronic slipped upper femoral epiphysis (nontraumatic)**

M93.021 Chronic slipped upper femoral epiphysis (nontraumatic), right hip

M93.022 Chronic slipped upper femoral epiphysis (nontraumatic), left hip

M93.023 Chronic slipped upper femoral epiphysis (nontraumatic), unspecified hip

✓6th **M93.03 Acute on chronic slipped upper femoral epiphysis (nontraumatic)**

M93.031 Acute on chronic slipped upper femoral epiphysis (nontraumatic), right hip

M93.032 Acute on chronic slipped upper femoral epiphysis (nontraumatic), left hip

M93.033 Acute on chronic slipped upper femoral epiphysis (nontraumatic), unspecified hip

M93.1 Kienböck's disease of adults
Adult osteochondrosis of carpal lunates

✓5th **M93.2 Osteochondritis dissecans**

M93.20 Osteochondritis dissecans of unspecified site

✓6th **M93.21 Osteochondritis dissecans of shoulder**

M93.211 Osteochondritis dissecans, right shoulder

M93.212 Osteochondritis dissecans, left shoulder

M93.219 Osteochondritis dissecans, unspecified shoulder

✓6th **M93.22 Osteochondritis dissecans of elbow**

M93.221 Osteochondritis dissecans, right elbow

M93.222 Osteochondritis dissecans, left elbow

M93.229 Osteochondritis dissecans, unspecified elbow

√6th M93.23 Osteochondritis dissecans of wrist
M93.231 Osteochondritis dissecans, right wrist
M93.232 Osteochondritis dissecans, left wrist
M93.239 Osteochondritis dissecans, unspecified wrist
√6th M93.24 Osteochondritis dissecans of joints of hand
M93.241 Osteochondritis dissecans, joints of right hand
M93.242 Osteochondritis dissecans, joints of left hand
M93.249 Osteochondritis dissecans, joints of unspecified hand
√6th M93.25 Osteochondritis dissecans of hip
M93.251 Osteochondritis dissecans, right hip
M93.252 Osteochondritis dissecans, left hip
M93.259 Osteochondritis dissecans, unspecified hip
√6th M93.26 Osteochondritis dissecans knee
M93.261 Osteochondritis dissecans, right knee
M93.262 Osteochondritis dissecans, left knee
M93.269 Osteochondritis dissecans, unspecified knee
√6th M93.27 Osteochondritis dissecans of ankle and joints of foot
M93.271 Osteochondritis dissecans, right ankle and joints of right foot
M93.272 Osteochondritis dissecans, left ankle and joints of left foot
M93.279 Osteochondritis dissecans, unspecified ankle and joints of foot
M93.28 Osteochondritis dissecans other site
M93.29 Osteochondritis dissecans multiple sites
√5th M93.8 Other specified osteochondropathies
M93.80 Other specified osteochondropathies of unspecified site
√6th M93.81 Other specified osteochondropathies of shoulder
M93.811 Other specified osteochondropathies, right shoulder
M93.812 Other specified osteochondropathies, left shoulder
M93.819 Other specified osteochondropathies, unspecified shoulder
√6th M93.82 Other specified osteochondropathies of upper arm
M93.821 Other specified osteochondropathies, right upper arm
M93.822 Other specified osteochondropathies, left upper arm
M93.829 Other specified osteochondropathies, unspecified upper arm
√6th M93.83 Other specified osteochondropathies of forearm
M93.831 Other specified osteochondropathies, right forearm
M93.832 Other specified osteochondropathies, left forearm
M93.839 Other specified osteochondropathies, unspecified forearm
√6th M93.84 Other specified osteochondropathies of hand
M93.841 Other specified osteochondropathies, right hand
M93.842 Other specified osteochondropathies, left hand
M93.849 Other specified osteochondropathies, unspecified hand
√6th M93.85 Other specified osteochondropathies of thigh
M93.851 Other specified osteochondropathies, right thigh
M93.852 Other specified osteochondropathies, left thigh
M93.859 Other specified osteochondropathies, unspecified thigh
√6th M93.86 Other specified osteochondropathies lower leg
M93.861 Other specified osteochondropathies, right lower leg
M93.862 Other specified osteochondropathies, left lower leg
M93.869 Other specified osteochondropathies, unspecified lower leg
√6th M93.87 Other specified osteochondropathies of ankle and foot
M93.871 Other specified osteochondropathies, right ankle and foot
M93.872 Other specified osteochondropathies, left ankle and foot
M93.879 Other specified osteochondropathies, unspecified ankle and foot
M93.88 Other specified osteochondropathies other
M93.89 Other specified osteochondropathies multiple sites
√5th M93.9 Osteochondropathy, unspecified
Apophysitis NOS
Epiphysitis NOS
Osteochondritis NOS
Osteochondrosis NOS
M93.90 Osteochondropathy, unspecified of unspecified site
√6th M93.91 Osteochondropathy, unspecified of shoulder
M93.911 Osteochondropathy, unspecified, right shoulder
M93.912 Osteochondropathy, unspecified, left shoulder
M93.919 Osteochondropathy, unspecified, unspecified shoulder
√6th M93.92 Osteochondropathy, unspecified of upper arm
M93.921 Osteochondropathy, unspecified, right upper arm
M93.922 Osteochondropathy, unspecified, left upper arm
M93.929 Osteochondropathy, unspecified, unspecified upper arm
√6th M93.93 Osteochondropathy, unspecified of forearm
M93.931 Osteochondropathy, unspecified, right forearm
M93.932 Osteochondropathy, unspecified, left forearm
M93.939 Osteochondropathy, unspecified, unspecified forearm
√6th M93.94 Osteochondropathy, unspecified of hand
M93.941 Osteochondropathy, unspecified, right hand
M93.942 Osteochondropathy, unspecified, left hand
M93.949 Osteochondropathy, unspecified, unspecified hand
√6th M93.95 Osteochondropathy, unspecified of thigh
M93.951 Osteochondropathy, unspecified, right thigh
M93.952 Osteochondropathy, unspecified, left thigh
M93.959 Osteochondropathy, unspecified, unspecified thigh
√6th M93.96 Osteochondropathy, unspecified lower leg
M93.961 Osteochondropathy, unspecified, right lower leg
M93.962 Osteochondropathy, unspecified, left lower leg
M93.969 Osteochondropathy, unspecified, unspecified lower leg
√6th M93.97 Osteochondropathy, unspecified of ankle and foot
M93.971 Osteochondropathy, unspecified, right ankle and foot
M93.972 Osteochondropathy, unspecified, left ankle and foot
M93.979 Osteochondropathy, unspecified, unspecified ankle and foot
M93.98 Osteochondropathy, unspecified other
M93.99 Osteochondropathy, unspecified multiple sites

√4th **M94 Other disorders of cartilage**
M94.0 Chondrocostal junction syndrome [Tietze]
Costochondritis
M94.1 Relapsing polychondritis
√5th M94.2 Chondromalacia
EXCLUDES 1 *chondromalacia patellae (M22.4)*
M94.20 Chondromalacia, unspecified site

✓6th **M94.21 Chondromalacia, shoulder**
M94.211 Chondromalacia, right shoulder
M94.212 Chondromalacia, left shoulder
M94.219 Chondromalacia, unspecified shoulder

✓6th **M94.22 Chondromalacia, elbow**
M94.221 Chondromalacia, right elbow
M94.222 Chondromalacia, left elbow
M94.229 Chondromalacia, unspecified elbow

✓6th **M94.23 Chondromalacia, wrist**
M94.231 Chondromalacia, right wrist
M94.232 Chondromalacia, left wrist
M94.239 Chondromalacia, unspecified wrist

✓6th **M94.24 Chondromalacia, joints of hand**
M94.241 Chondromalacia, joints of right hand
M94.242 Chondromalacia, joints of left hand
M94.249 Chondromalacia, joints of unspecified hand

✓6th **M94.25 Chondromalacia, hip**
M94.251 Chondromalacia, right hip
M94.252 Chondromalacia, left hip
M94.259 Chondromalacia, unspecified hip

✓6th **M94.26 Chondromalacia, knee**
M94.261 Chondromalacia, right knee
M94.262 Chondromalacia, left knee
M94.269 Chondromalacia, unspecified knee

✓6th **M94.27 Chondromalacia, ankle and joints of foot**
M94.271 Chondromalacia, right ankle and joints of right foot
M94.272 Chondromalacia, left ankle and joints of left foot
M94.279 Chondromalacia, unspecified ankle and joints of foot

M94.28 Chondromalacia, other site
M94.29 Chondromalacia, multiple sites

✓5th **M94.3 Chondrolysis**
Code first any associated slipped upper femoral epiphysis (nontraumatic) (M93.0-)

✓6th **M94.35 Chondrolysis, hip**
M94.351 Chondrolysis, right hip
M94.352 Chondrolysis, left hip
M94.359 Chondrolysis, unspecified hip

✓5th **M94.8 Other specified disorders of cartilage**
✓6th **M94.8X Other specified disorders of cartilage**
M94.8X0 Other specified disorders of cartilage, multiple sites
M94.8X1 Other specified disorders of cartilage, shoulder
M94.8X2 Other specified disorders of cartilage, upper arm
M94.8X3 Other specified disorders of cartilage, forearm
M94.8X4 Other specified disorders of cartilage, hand
M94.8X5 Other specified disorders of cartilage, thigh
M94.8X6 Other specified disorders of cartilage, lower leg
M94.8X7 Other specified disorders of cartilage, ankle and foot
M94.8X8 Other specified disorders of cartilage, other site
M94.8X9 Other specified disorders of cartilage, unspecified sites

M94.9 Disorder of cartilage, unspecified

Other disorders of the musculoskeletal system and connective tissue (M95)

✓4th **M95 Other acquired deformities of musculoskeletal system and connective tissue**
EXCLUDES 2 *acquired absence of limbs and organs (Z89-Z90)*
acquired deformities of limbs (M20-M21)
congenital malformations and deformations of the musculoskeletal system (Q65-Q79)
deforming dorsopathies (M40-M43)
dentofacial anomalies [including malocclusion] (M26.-)
postprocedural musculoskeletal disorders (M96.-)

M95.0 Acquired deformity of nose
EXCLUDES 2 *deviated nasal septum (J34.2)*

✓5th **M95.1 Cauliflower ear**
EXCLUDES 2 *other acquired deformities of ear (H61.1)*
M95.10 Cauliflower ear, unspecified ear
M95.11 Cauliflower ear, right ear
M95.12 Cauliflower ear, left ear

M95.2 Other acquired deformity of head
M95.3 Acquired deformity of neck
M95.4 Acquired deformity of chest and rib
M95.5 Acquired deformity of pelvis
EXCLUDES 1 *maternal care for known or suspected disproportion (O33.-)*
M95.8 Other specified acquired deformities of musculoskeletal system
M95.9 Acquired deformity of musculoskeletal system, unspecified

Intraoperative and postprocedural complications and disorders of musculoskeletal system, not elsewhere classified (M96)

✓4th **M96 Intraoperative and postprocedural complications and disorders of musculoskeletal system, not elsewhere classified**
EXCLUDES 2 *arthropathy following intestinal bypass (M02.0-)*
complications of internal orthopedic prosthetic devices, implants and grafts (T84.-)
disorders associated with osteoporosis (M80)
presence of functional implants and other devices (Z96-Z97)

M96.0 Pseudarthrosis after fusion or arthrodesis
M96.1 Postlaminectomy syndrome, not elsewhere classified
M96.2 Postradiation kyphosis
M96.3 Postlaminectomy kyphosis
M96.4 Postsurgical lordosis
M96.5 Postradiation scoliosis

✓5th **M96.6 Fracture of bone following insertion of orthopedic implant, joint prosthesis, or bone plate**
Intraoperative fracture of bone during insertion of orthopedic implant, joint prosthesis, or bone plate
EXCLUDES 2 *complication of internal orthopedic devices, implants or grafts (T84.-)*

✓6th **M96.62 Fracture of humerus following insertion of orthopedic implant, joint prosthesis, or bone plate**
M96.621 Fracture of humerus following insertion of orthopedic implant, joint prosthesis, or bone plate, right arm
M96.622 Fracture of humerus following insertion of orthopedic implant, joint prosthesis, or bone plate, left arm
M96.629 Fracture of humerus following insertion of orthopedic implant, joint prosthesis, or bone plate, unspecified arm

✓6th **M96.63 Fracture of radius or ulna following insertion of orthopedic implant, joint prosthesis, or bone plate**
M96.631 Fracture of radius or ulna following insertion of orthopedic implant, joint prosthesis, or bone plate, right arm
M96.632 Fracture of radius or ulna following insertion of orthopedic implant, joint prosthesis, or bone plate, left arm
M96.639 Fracture of radius or ulna following insertion of orthopedic implant, joint prosthesis, or bone plate, unspecified arm

M96.65 Fracture of pelvis following insertion of orthopedic implant, joint prosthesis, or bone plate

✓6th **M96.66 Fracture of femur following insertion of orthopedic implant, joint prosthesis, or bone plate**
M96.661 Fracture of femur following insertion of orthopedic implant, joint prosthesis, or bone plate, right leg
M96.662 Fracture of femur following insertion of orthopedic implant, joint prosthesis, or bone plate, left leg
M96.669 Fracture of femur following insertion of orthopedic implant, joint prosthesis, or bone plate, unspecified leg
✓6th **M96.67 Fracture of tibia or fibula following insertion of orthopedic implant, joint prosthesis, or bone plate**
M96.671 Fracture of tibia or fibula following insertion of orthopedic implant, joint prosthesis, or bone plate, right leg
M96.672 Fracture of tibia or fibula following insertion of orthopedic implant, joint prosthesis, or bone plate, left leg
M96.679 Fracture of tibia or fibula following insertion of orthopedic implant, joint prosthesis, or bone plate, unspecified leg
M96.69 Fracture of other bone following insertion of orthopedic implant, joint prosthesis, or bone plate
✓5th **M96.8 Other intraoperative and postprocedural complications and disorders of musculoskeletal system, not elsewhere classified**
✓6th **M96.81 Intraoperative hemorrhage and hematoma of a musculoskeletal structure complicating a procedure**
EXCLUDES 1 *intraoperative hemorrhage and hematoma of a musculoskeletal structure due to accidental puncture and laceration during a procedure (M98.82-)*
M96.810 Intraoperative hemorrhage and hematoma of a musculoskeletal structure complicating a musculoskeletal system procedure
M96.811 Intraoperative hemorrhage and hematoma of a musculoskeletal structure complicating other procedure
✓6th **M96.82 Accidental puncture and laceration of a musculoskeletal structure during a procedure**
M96.820 Accidental puncture and laceration of a musculoskeletal structure during a musculoskeletal system procedure
M96.821 Accidental puncture and laceration of a musculoskeletal structure during other procedure
✓6th **M96.83 Postprocedural hemorrhage and hematoma of a musculoskeletal structure following a procedure**
M96.830 Postprocedural hemorrhage and hematoma of a musculoskeletal structure following a musculoskeletal system procedure
M96.831 Postprocedural hemorrhage and hematoma of a musculoskeletal structure following other procedure
M96.89 Other intraoperative and postprocedural complications and disorders of the musculoskeletal system
Instability of joint secondary to removal of joint prosthesis
Use additional code, if applicable, to further specify disorder

Biomechanical lesions, not elsewhere classified (M99)

✓4th **M99 Biomechanical lesions, not elsewhere classified**
NOTE This category should not be used if the condition can be classified elsewhere.
✓5th **M99.0 Segmental and somatic dysfunction**
M99.00 Segmental and somatic dysfunction of head region
M99.01 Segmental and somatic dysfunction of cervical region
M99.02 Segmental and somatic dysfunction of thoracic region
M99.03 Segmental and somatic dysfunction of lumbar region
M99.04 Segmental and somatic dysfunction of sacral region
M99.05 Segmental and somatic dysfunction of pelvic region
M99.06 Segmental and somatic dysfunction of lower extremity
M99.07 Segmental and somatic dysfunction of upper extremity
M99.08 Segmental and somatic dysfunction of rib cage
M99.09 Segmental and somatic dysfunction of abdomen and other regions
✓5th **M99.1 Subluxation complex (vertebral)**
M99.10 Subluxation complex (vertebral) of head region
M99.11 Subluxation complex (vertebral) of cervical region
M99.12 Subluxation complex (vertebral) of thoracic region
M99.13 Subluxation complex (vertebral) of lumbar region
M99.14 Subluxation complex (vertebral) of sacral region
M99.15 Subluxation complex (vertebral) of pelvic region
M99.16 Subluxation complex (vertebral) of lower extremity
M99.17 Subluxation complex (vertebral) of upper extremity
M99.18 Subluxation complex (vertebral) of rib cage
M99.19 Subluxation complex (vertebral) of abdomen and other regions
✓5th **M99.2 Subluxation stenosis of neural canal**
M99.20 Subluxation stenosis of neural canal of head region
M99.21 Subluxation stenosis of neural canal of cervical region
M99.22 Subluxation stenosis of neural canal of thoracic region
M99.23 Subluxation stenosis of neural canal of lumbar region
M99.24 Subluxation stenosis of neural canal of sacral region
M99.25 Subluxation stenosis of neural canal of pelvic region
M99.26 Subluxation stenosis of neural canal of lower extremity
M99.27 Subluxation stenosis of neural canal of upper extremity
M99.28 Subluxation stenosis of neural canal of rib cage
M99.29 Subluxation stenosis of neural canal of abdomen and other regions
✓5th **M99.3 Osseous stenosis of neural canal**
M99.30 Osseous stenosis of neural canal of head region
M99.31 Osseous stenosis of neural canal of cervical region
M99.32 Osseous stenosis of neural canal of thoracic region
M99.33 Osseous stenosis of neural canal of lumbar region
M99.34 Osseous stenosis of neural canal of sacral region
M99.35 Osseous stenosis of neural canal of pelvic region
M99.36 Osseous stenosis of neural canal of lower extremity
M99.37 Osseous stenosis of neural canal of upper extremity
M99.38 Osseous stenosis of neural canal of rib cage
M99.39 Osseous stenosis of neural canal of abdomen and other regions
✓5th **M99.4 Connective tissue stenosis of neural canal**
M99.40 Connective tissue stenosis of neural canal of head region
M99.41 Connective tissue stenosis of neural canal of cervical region
M99.42 Connective tissue stenosis of neural canal of thoracic region
M99.43 Connective tissue stenosis of neural canal of lumbar region
M99.44 Connective tissue stenosis of neural canal of sacral region
M99.45 Connective tissue stenosis of neural canal of pelvic region
M99.46 Connective tissue stenosis of neural canal of lower extremity

M99.47 Connective tissue stenosis of neural canal of upper extremity
M99.48 Connective tissue stenosis of neural canal of rib cage
M99.49 Connective tissue stenosis of neural canal of abdomen and other regions

✓5th M99.5 Intervertebral disc stenosis of neural canal
M99.50 Intervertebral disc stenosis of neural canal of head region
M99.51 Intervertebral disc stenosis of neural canal of cervical region
M99.52 Intervertebral disc stenosis of neural canal of thoracic region
M99.53 Intervertebral disc stenosis of neural canal of lumbar region
M99.54 Intervertebral disc stenosis of neural canal of sacral region
M99.55 Intervertebral disc stenosis of neural canal of pelvic region
M99.56 Intervertebral disc stenosis of neural canal of lower extremity
M99.57 Intervertebral disc stenosis of neural canal of upper extremity
M99.58 Intervertebral disc stenosis of neural canal of rib cage
M99.59 Intervertebral disc stenosis of neural canal of abdomen and other regions

✓5th M99.6 Osseous and subluxation stenosis of intervertebral foramina
M99.60 Osseous and subluxation stenosis of intervertebral foramina of head region
M99.61 Osseous and subluxation stenosis of intervertebral foramina of cervical region
M99.62 Osseous and subluxation stenosis of intervertebral foramina of thoracic region
M99.63 Osseous and subluxation stenosis of intervertebral foramina of lumbar region
M99.64 Osseous and subluxation stenosis of intervertebral foramina of sacral region
M99.65 Osseous and subluxation stenosis of intervertebral foramina of pelvic region
M99.66 Osseous and subluxation stenosis of intervertebral foramina of lower extremity
M99.67 Osseous and subluxation stenosis of intervertebral foramina of upper extremity
M99.68 Osseous and subluxation stenosis of intervertebral foramina of rib cage
M99.69 Osseous and subluxation stenosis of intervertebral foramina of abdomen and other regions

✓5th M99.7 Connective tissue and disc stenosis of intervertebral foramina
M99.70 Connective tissue and disc stenosis of intervertebral foramina of head region
M99.71 Connective tissue and disc stenosis of intervertebral foramina of cervical region
M99.72 Connective tissue and disc stenosis of intervertebral foramina of thoracic region
M99.73 Connective tissue and disc stenosis of intervertebral foramina of lumbar region
M99.74 Connective tissue and disc stenosis of intervertebral foramina of sacral region
M99.75 Connective tissue and disc stenosis of intervertebral foramina of pelvic region
M99.76 Connective tissue and disc stenosis of intervertebral foramina of lower extremity
M99.77 Connective tissue and disc stenosis of intervertebral foramina of upper extremity
M99.78 Connective tissue and disc stenosis of intervertebral foramina of rib cage
M99.79 Connective tissue and disc stenosis of intervertebral foramina of abdomen and other regions

✓5th M99.8 Other biomechanical lesions
M99.80 Other biomechanical lesions of head region
M99.81 Other biomechanical lesions of cervical region
M99.82 Other biomechanical lesions of thoracic region
M99.83 Other biomechanical lesions of lumbar region
M99.84 Other biomechanical lesions of sacral region
M99.85 Other biomechanical lesions of pelvic region
M99.86 Other biomechanical lesions of lower extremity
M99.87 Other biomechanical lesions of upper extremity
M99.88 Other biomechanical lesions of rib cage
M99.89 Other biomechanical lesions of abdomen and other regions

M99.9 Biomechanical lesion, unspecified

Chapter 14. Diseases of the Genitourinary System (N00-N99)

EXCLUDES 2 *certain conditions originating in the perinatal period (P04-P96)*
certain infectious and parasitic diseases (A00-B99)
complications of pregnancy, childbirth and the puerperium (O00-O9A)
congenital malformations, deformations and chromosomal abnormalities (Q00-Q99)
endocrine, nutritional and metabolic diseases (E00-E88)
injury, poisoning and certain other consequences of external causes (S00-T88)
neoplasms (C00-D49)
symptoms, signs and abnormal clinical and laboratory findings, not elsewhere classified (R00-R94)

This chapter contains the following blocks:

N00-N08	Glomerular diseases
N10-N16	Renal tubulo-interstitial diseases
N17-N19	Acute kidney failure and chronic kidney disease
N20-N23	Urolithiasis
N25-N29	Other disorders of kidney and ureter
N30-N39	Other diseases of the urinary system
N40-N53	Diseases of male genital organs
N60-N65	Disorders of breast
N70-N77	Inflammatory diseases of female pelvic organs
N80-N98	Noninflammatory disorders of female genital tract
N99	Intraoperative and postprocedural complications and disorders of genitourinary system, not elsewhere classified

Glomerular diseases (N00-N08)

Code also any associated kidney failure (N17-N19).

EXCLUDES 1 *hypertensive chronic kidney disease (I12.-)*

✓4th N00 Acute nephritic syndrome

INCLUDES acute glomerular disease
acute glomerulonephritis
acute nephritis

EXCLUDES 1 *acute tubulo-interstitial nephritis (N10)*
nephritic syndrome NOS (N05.-)

N00.0 Acute nephritic syndrome with minor glomerular abnormality
Acute nephritic syndrome with minimal change lesion

N00.1 Acute nephritic syndrome with focal and segmental glomerular lesions
Acute nephritic syndrome with focal and segmental hyalinosis
Acute nephritic syndrome with focal and segmental sclerosis
Acute nephritic syndrome with focal glomerulonephritis

N00.2 Acute nephritic syndrome with diffuse membranous glomerulonephritis

N00.3 Acute nephritic syndrome with diffuse mesangial proliferative glomerulonephritis

N00.4 Acute nephritic syndrome with diffuse endocapillary proliferative glomerulonephritis

N00.5 Acute nephritic syndrome with diffuse mesangiocapillary glomerulonephritis
Acute nephritic syndrome with membranoproliferative glomerulonephritis, types 1 and 3, or NOS

N00.6 Acute nephritic syndrome with dense deposit disease
Acute nephritic syndrome with membranoproliferative glomerulonephritis, type 2

N00.7 Acute nephritic syndrome with diffuse crescentic glomerulonephritis
Acute nephritic syndrome with extracapillary glomerulonephritis

N00.8 Acute nephritic syndrome with other morphologic changes
Acute nephritic syndrome with proliferative glomerulonephritis NOS

N00.9 Acute nephritic syndrome with unspecified morphologic changes

✓4th N01 Rapidly progressive nephritic syndrome

INCLUDES rapidly progressive glomerular disease
rapidly progressive glomerulonephritis
rapidly progressive nephritis

EXCLUDES 1 *nephritic syndrome NOS (N05.-)*

N01.0 Rapidly progressive nephritic syndrome with minor glomerular abnormality
Rapidly progressive nephritic syndrome with minimal change lesion

N01.1 Rapidly progressive nephritic syndrome with focal and segmental glomerular lesions
Rapidly progressive nephritic syndrome with focal and segmental hyalinosis
Rapidly progressive nephritic syndrome with focal and segmental sclerosis
Rapidly progressive nephritic syndrome with focal glomerulonephritis

N01.2 Rapidly progressive nephritic syndrome with diffuse membranous glomerulonephritis

N01.3 Rapidly progressive nephritic syndrome with diffuse mesangial proliferative glomerulonephritis

N01.4 Rapidly progressive nephritic syndrome with diffuse endocapillary proliferative glomerulonephritis

N01.5 Rapidly progressive nephritic syndrome with diffuse mesangiocapillary glomerulonephritis
Rapidly progressive nephritic syndrome with membranoproliferative glomerulonephritis, types 1 and 3, or NOS

N01.6 Rapidly progressive nephritic syndrome with dense deposit disease
Rapidly progressive nephritic syndrome with membranoproliferative glomerulonephritis, type 2

N01.7 Rapidly progressive nephritic syndrome with diffuse crescentic glomerulonephritis
Rapidly progressive nephritic syndrome with extracapillary glomerulonephritis

N01.8 Rapidly progressive nephritic syndrome with other morphologic changes
Rapidly progressive nephritic syndrome with proliferative glomerulonephritis NOS

N01.9 Rapidly progressive nephritic syndrome with unspecified morphologic changes

✓4th N02 Recurrent and persistent hematuria

EXCLUDES 1 *acute cystitis with hematuria (N30.01)*
acute prostatitis with hematuria (N41.01)
chronic prostatitis with hematuria (N41.11)
hematuria NOS (R31.9)
hematuria not associated with specified morphologic lesions (R31.-)

N02.0 Recurrent and persistent hematuria with minor glomerular abnormality
Recurrent and persistent hematuria with minimal change lesion

N02.1 Recurrent and persistent hematuria with focal and segmental glomerular lesions
Recurrent and persistent hematuria with focal and segmental hyalinosis
Recurrent and persistent hematuria with focal and segmental sclerosis
Recurrent and persistent hematuria with focal glomerulonephritis

N02.2 Recurrent and persistent hematuria with diffuse membranous glomerulonephritis

N02.3 Recurrent and persistent hematuria with diffuse mesangial proliferative glomerulonephritis

N02.4 Recurrent and persistent hematuria with diffuse endocapillary proliferative glomerulonephritis

N02.5 Recurrent and persistent hematuria with diffuse mesangiocapillary glomerulonephritis
Recurrent and persistent hematuria with membranoproliferative glomerulonephritis, types 1 and 3, or NOS

N02.6 Recurrent and persistent hematuria with dense deposit disease
Recurrent and persistent hematuria with membranoproliferative glomerulonephritis, type 2

N02.7 Recurrent and persistent hematuria with diffuse crescentic glomerulonephritis
Recurrent and persistent hematuria with extracapillary glomerulonephritis

N02.8 Recurrent and persistent hematuria with other morphologic changes
Recurrent and persistent hematuria with proliferative glomerulonephritis NOS

N02.9 Recurrent and persistent hematuria with unspecified morphologic changes

NØ3 Chronic nephritic syndrome

INCLUDES chronic glomerular disease
chronic glomerulonephritis
chronic nephritis

EXCLUDES 1 *chronic tubulo-interstitial nephritis (N11.-)*
diffuse sclerosing glomerulonephritis (NØ5.8-)
nephritic syndrome NOS (NØ5.-)

NØ3.Ø Chronic nephritic syndrome with minor glomerular abnormality
Chronic nephritic syndrome with minimal change lesion

NØ3.1 Chronic nephritic syndrome with focal and segmental glomerular lesions
Chronic nephritic syndrome with focal and segmental hyalinosis
Chronic nephritic syndrome with focal and segmental sclerosis
Chronic nephritic syndrome with focal glomerulonephritis

NØ3.2 Chronic nephritic syndrome with diffuse membranous glomerulonephritis

NØ3.3 Chronic nephritic syndrome with diffuse mesangial proliferative glomerulonephritis

NØ3.4 Chronic nephritic syndrome with diffuse endocapillary proliferative glomerulonephritis

NØ3.5 Chronic nephritic syndrome with diffuse mesangiocapillary glomerulonephritis
Chronic nephritic syndrome with membranoproliferative glomerulonephritis, types 1 and 3, or NOS

NØ3.6 Chronic nephritic syndrome with dense deposit disease
Chronic nephritic syndrome with membranoproliferative glomerulonephritis, type 2

NØ3.7 Chronic nephritic syndrome with diffuse crescentic glomerulonephritis
Chronic nephritic syndrome with extracapillary glomerulonephritis

NØ3.8 Chronic nephritic syndrome with other morphologic changes
Chronic nephritic syndrome with proliferative glomerulonephritis NOS

NØ3.9 Chronic nephritic syndrome with unspecified morphologic changes

NØ4 Nephrotic syndrome

INCLUDES congenital nephrotic syndrome
lipoid nephrosis

NØ4.Ø Nephrotic syndrome with minor glomerular abnormality
Nephrotic syndrome with minimal change lesion

NØ4.1 Nephrotic syndrome with focal and segmental glomerular lesions
Nephrotic syndrome with focal and segmental hyalinosis
Nephrotic syndrome with focal and segmental sclerosis
Nephrotic syndrome with focal glomerulonephritis

NØ4.2 Nephrotic syndrome with diffuse membranous glomerulonephritis

NØ4.3 Nephrotic syndrome with diffuse mesangial proliferative glomerulonephritis

NØ4.4 Nephrotic syndrome with diffuse endocapillary proliferative glomerulonephritis

NØ4.5 Nephrotic syndrome with diffuse mesangiocapillary glomerulonephritis
Nephrotic syndrome with membranoproliferative glomerulonephritis, types 1 and 3, or NOS

NØ4.6 Nephrotic syndrome with dense deposit disease
Nephrotic syndrome with membranoproliferative glomerulonephritis, type 2

NØ4.7 Nephrotic syndrome with diffuse crescentic glomerulonephritis
Nephrotic syndrome with extracapillary glomerulonephritis

NØ4.8 Nephrotic syndrome with other morphologic changes
Nephrotic syndrome with proliferative glomerulonephritis NOS

NØ4.9 Nephrotic syndrome with unspecified morphologic changes

NØ5 Unspecified nephritic syndrome

INCLUDES glomerular disease NOS
glomerulonephritis NOS
nephritis NOS
nephropathy NOS and renal disease NOS with morphological lesion specified in .Ø-.8

EXCLUDES 1 *nephropathy NOS with no stated morphological lesion (N28.9)*
renal disease NOS with no stated morphological lesion (N28.9)
tubulo-interstitial nephritis NOS (N12)

NØ5.Ø Unspecified nephritic syndrome with minor glomerular abnormality
Unspecified nephritic syndrome with minimal change lesion

NØ5.1 Unspecified nephritic syndrome with focal and segmental glomerular lesions
Unspecified nephritic syndrome with focal and segmental hyalinosis
Unspecified nephritic syndrome with focal and segmental sclerosis
Unspecified nephritic syndrome with focal glomerulonephritis

NØ5.2 Unspecified nephritic syndrome with diffuse membranous glomerulonephritis

NØ5.3 Unspecified nephritic syndrome with diffuse mesangial proliferative glomerulonephritis

NØ5.4 Unspecified nephritic syndrome with diffuse endocapillary proliferative glomerulonephritis

NØ5.5 Unspecified nephritic syndrome with diffuse mesangiocapillary glomerulonephritis
Unspecified nephritic syndrome with membranoproliferative glomerulonephritis, types 1 and 3, or NOS

NØ5.6 Unspecified nephritic syndrome with dense deposit disease
Unspecified nephritic syndrome with membranoproliferative glomerulonephritis, type 2

NØ5.7 Unspecified nephritic syndrome with diffuse crescentic glomerulonephritis
Unspecified nephritic syndrome with extracapillary glomerulonephritis

NØ5.8 Unspecified nephritic syndrome with other morphologic changes
Unspecified nephritic syndrome with proliferative glomerulonephritis NOS

NØ5.9 Unspecified nephritic syndrome with unspecified morphologic changes

NØ6 Isolated proteinuria with specified morphological lesion

EXCLUDES 1 *proteinuria not associated with specific morphologic lesions (R8Ø.Ø)*

NØ6.Ø Isolated proteinuria with minor glomerular abnormality
Isolated proteinuria with minimal change lesion

NØ6.1 Isolated proteinuria with focal and segmental glomerular lesions
Isolated proteinuria with focal and segmental hyalinosis
Isolated proteinuria with focal and segmental sclerosis
Isolated proteinuria with focal glomerulonephritis

NØ6.2 Isolated proteinuria with diffuse membranous glomerulonephritis

NØ6.3 Isolated proteinuria with diffuse mesangial proliferative glomerulonephritis

NØ6.4 Isolated proteinuria with diffuse endocapillary proliferative glomerulonephritis

NØ6.5 Isolated proteinuria with diffuse mesangiocapillary glomerulonephritis
Isolated proteinuria with membranoproliferative glomerulonephritis, types 1 and 3, or NOS

NØ6.6 Isolated proteinuria with dense deposit disease
Isolated proteinuria with membranoproliferative glomerulonephritis, type 2

NØ6.7 Isolated proteinuria with diffuse crescentic glomerulonephritis
Isolated proteinuria with extracapillary glomerulonephritis

NØ6.8 Isolated proteinuria with other morphologic lesion
Isolated proteinuria with proliferative glomerulonephritis NOS

NØ6.9 Isolated proteinuria with unspecified morphologic lesion

✓4th N07 Hereditary nephropathy, not elsewhere classified

EXCLUDES 2 *Alport's syndrome (Q87.81-)*
hereditary amyloid nephropathy (E85.-)
nail patella syndrome (Q87.2)
non-neuropathic heredofamilial amyloidosis (E85.-)

N07.0 Hereditary nephropathy, not elsewhere classified with minor glomerular abnormality
Hereditary nephropathy, not elsewhere classified with minimal change lesion

N07.1 Hereditary nephropathy, not elsewhere classified with focal and segmental glomerular lesions
Hereditary nephropathy, not elsewhere classified with focal and segmental hyalinosis
Hereditary nephropathy, not elsewhere classified with focal and segmental sclerosis
Hereditary nephropathy, not elsewhere classified with focal glomerulonephritis

N07.2 Hereditary nephropathy, not elsewhere classified with diffuse membranous glomerulonephritis

N07.3 Hereditary nephropathy, not elsewhere classified with diffuse mesangial proliferative glomerulonephritis

N07.4 Hereditary nephropathy, not elsewhere classified with diffuse endocapillary proliferative glomerulonephritis

N07.5 Hereditary nephropathy, not elsewhere classified with diffuse mesangiocapillary glomerulonephritis
Hereditary nephropathy, not elsewhere classified with membranoproliferative glomerulonephritis, types 1 and 3, or NOS

N07.6 Hereditary nephropathy, not elsewhere classified with dense deposit disease
Hereditary nephropathy, not elsewhere classified with membranoproliferative glomerulonephritis, type 2

N07.7 Hereditary nephropathy, not elsewhere classified with diffuse crescentic glomerulonephritis
Hereditary nephropathy, not elsewhere classified with extracapillary glomerulonephritis

N07.8 Hereditary nephropathy, not elsewhere classified with other morphologic lesions
Hereditary nephropathy, not elsewhere classified with proliferative glomerulonephritis NOS

N07.9 Hereditary nephropathy, not elsewhere classified with unspecified morphologic lesions

N08 Glomerular disorders in diseases classified elsewhere
Glomerulonephritis
Nephritis
Nephropathy
Code first underlying disease, such as:
amyloidosis (E85.-)
congenital syphilis (A50.5)
cryoglobulinemia (D89.1)
disseminated intravascular coagulation (D65)
gout (M1A.-, M10.-)
microscopic polyangiitis (M31.7)
multiple myeloma (C90.0-)
sepsis (A40.0-A41.9)
sickle-cell disease (D57.0-D57.8)

EXCLUDES 1 *glomerulonephritis, nephritis and nephropathy (in):*
antiglomerular basement membrane disease (M31.0)
diabetes (E08-E13 with .21)
gonococcal (A54.21)
Goodpasture's syndrome (M31.0)
hemolytic-uremic syndrome (D59.3)
lupus (M32.14)
mumps (B26.83)
syphilis (A52.75)
systemic lupus erythematosus (M32.14)
Wegener's granulomatosis (M31.31)
pyelonephritis in diseases classified elsewhere (N16)
renal tubulo-interstitial disorders classified elsewhere (N16)

Renal tubulo-interstitial diseases (N10-N16)

INCLUDES pyelonephritis
EXCLUDES 1 *pyeloureteritis cystica (N28.85)*

N10 Acute tubulo-interstitial nephritis
Acute infectious interstitial nephritis
Acute pyelitis
Acute pyelonephritis
Hemoglobin nephrosis
Myoglobin nephrosis
Use additional code (B95-B97), to identify infectious agent

✓4th N11 Chronic tubulo-interstitial nephritis

INCLUDES chronic infectious interstitial nephritis
chronic pyelitis
chronic pyelonephritis

Use additional code (B95-B97), to identify infectious agent

N11.0 Nonobstructive reflux-associated chronic pyelonephritis
Pyelonephritis (chronic) associated with (vesicoureteral) reflux
EXCLUDES 1 *vesicoureteral reflux NOS (N13.70)*

N11.1 Chronic obstructive pyelonephritis
Pyelonephritis (chronic) associated with anomaly of pelviureteric junction
Pyelonephritis (chronic) associated with anomaly of pyeloureteric junction
Pyelonephritis (chronic) associated with crossing of vessel
Pyelonephritis (chronic) associated with kinking of ureter
Pyelonephritis (chronic) associated with obstruction of ureter
Pyelonephritis (chronic) associated with stricture of pelviureteric junction
Pyelonephritis (chronic) associated with stricture of ureter
EXCLUDES 1 *calculous pyelonephritis (N20.9)*
obstructive uropathy (N13.-)

N11.8 Other chronic tubulo-interstitial nephritis
Nonobstructive chronic pyelonephritis NOS

N11.9 Chronic tubulo-interstitial nephritis, unspecified
Chronic interstitial nephritis NOS
Chronic pyelitis NOS
Chronic pyelonephritis NOS

N12 Tubulo-interstitial nephritis, not specified as acute or chronic
Interstitial nephritis NOS
Pyelitis NOS
Pyelonephritis NOS
EXCLUDES 1 *calculous pyelonephritis (N20.9)*

✓4th N13 Obstructive and reflux uropathy

EXCLUDES 2 *calculus of kidney and ureter without hydronephrosis (N20.-)*
congenital obstructive defects of renal pelvis and ureter (Q62.0-Q62.3)
hydronephrosis with ureteropelvic junction obstruction (Q62.1)
obstructive pyelonephritis (N11.1)

N13.1 Hydronephrosis with ureteral stricture, not elsewhere classified
EXCLUDES 1 *hydronephrosis with ureteral stricture with infection (N13.6)*

N13.2 Hydronephrosis with renal and ureteral calculous obstruction
EXCLUDES 1 *hydronephrosis with renal and ureteral calculous obstruction with infection (N13.6)*

✓5th N13.3 Other and unspecified hydronephrosis
EXCLUDES 1 *hydronephrosis with infection (N13.6)*

N13.30 Unspecified hydronephrosis

N13.39 Other hydronephrosis

N13.4 Hydroureter
EXCLUDES 1 *congenital hydroureter (Q62.3-)*
hydroureter with infection (N13.6)
vesicoureteral-reflux with hydroureter (N13.73-)

N13.5 Crossing vessel and stricture of ureter without hydronephrosis
Kinking and stricture of ureter without hydronephrosis
EXCLUDES 1 *crossing vessel and stricture of ureter without hydronephrosis with infection (N13.6)*

N13.6 Pyonephrosis
Conditions in N13.1-N13.5 with infection
Obstructive uropathy with infection
Use additional code (B95-B97), to identify infectious agent

✓5th **N13.7 Vesicoureteral-reflux**
EXCLUDES 1 *reflux-associated pyelonephritis (N11.Ø)*

N13.7Ø Vesicoureteral-reflux, unspecified
Vesicoureteral-reflux NOS

N13.71 Vesicoureteral-reflux without reflux nephropathy

✓6th **N13.72 Vesicoureteral-reflux with reflux nephropathy without hydroureter**

N13.721 Vesicoureteral-reflux with reflux nephropathy without hydroureter, unilateral

N13.722 Vesicoureteral-reflux with reflux nephropathy without hydroureter, bilateral

N13.729 Vesicoureteral-reflux with reflux nephropathy without hydroureter, unspecified

✓6th **N13.73 Vesicoureteral-reflux with reflux nephropathy with hydroureter**

N13.731 Vesicoureteral-reflux with reflux nephropathy with hydroureter, unilateral

N13.732 Vesicoureteral-reflux with reflux nephropathy with hydroureter, bilateral

N13.739 Vesicoureteral-reflux with reflux nephropathy with hydroureter, unspecified

N13.8 Other obstructive and reflux uropathy
Urinary tract obstruction due to specified cause
Code first, if applicable, any causal condition, such as:
enlarged prostate (N4Ø.1)

N13.9 Obstructive and reflux uropathy, unspecified
Urinary tract obstruction NOS

✓4th **N14 Drug- and heavy-metal-induced tubulo-interstitial and tubular conditions**
Code first poisoning due to drug or toxin, if applicable (T36-T65 with fifth or sixth character 1-4 or 6)
Use additional code for adverse effect, if applicable, to identify drug (T36-T5Ø with fifth or sixth character 5)

N14.Ø Analgesic nephropathy

N14.1 Nephropathy induced by other drugs, medicaments and biological substances

N14.2 Nephropathy induced by unspecified drug, medicament or biological substance

N14.3 Nephropathy induced by heavy metals

N14.4 Toxic nephropathy, not elsewhere classified

✓4th **N15 Other renal tubulo-interstitial diseases**

N15.Ø Balkan nephropathy
Balkan endemic nephropathy

N15.1 Renal and perinephric abscess

N15.8 Other specified renal tubulo-interstitial diseases

N15.9 Renal tubulo-interstitial disease, unspecified
Infection of kidney NOS
EXCLUDES 1 *urinary tract infection NOS (N39.Ø)*

N16 Renal tubulo-interstitial disorders in diseases classified elsewhere
Pyelonephritis
Tubulo-interstitial nephritis
Code first underlying disease, such as:
brucellosis (A23.Ø-A23.9)
cryoglobulinemia (D89.1)
glycogen storage disease (E74.Ø)
leukemia (C91-C95)
lymphoma (C81.Ø-C85.9, C96.Ø-C96.9)
multiple myeloma (C9Ø.Ø-)
sepsis (A4Ø.Ø-A41.9)
Wilson's disease (E83.Ø)
EXCLUDES 1 *diphtheritic pyelonephritis and tubulo-interstitial nephritis (A36.84)*
pyelonephritis and tubulo-interstitial nephritis in candidiasis (B37.49)
pyelonephritis and tubulo-interstitial nephritis in cystinosis (E72.Ø4)
pyelonephritis and tubulo-interstitial nephritis in salmonella infection (AØ2.25)
pyelonephritis and tubulo-interstitial nephritis in sarcoidosis (D86.84)
pyelonephritis and tubulo-interstitial nephritis in sicca syndrome [Sjogren's] (M35.Ø4)
pyelonephritis and tubulo-interstitial nephritis in systemic lupus erythematosus (M32.15)
pyelonephritis and tubulo-interstitial nephritis in toxoplasmosis (B58.83)
renal tubular degeneration in diabetes (EØ8-E13 with .29)
syphilitic pyelonephritis and tubulo-interstitial nephritis (A52.75)

Acute kidney failure and chronic kidney disease (N17-N19)

EXCLUDES 2 *congenital renal failure (P96.Ø)*
drug- and heavy-metal-induced tubulo-interstitial and tubular conditions (N14.-)
extrarenal uremia (R39.2)
hemolytic-uremic syndrome (D59.3)
hepatorenal syndrome (K76.7)
postpartum hepatorenal syndrome (O9Ø.4)
posttraumatic renal failure (T79.5)
prerenal uremia (R39.2)
renal failure:
complicating abortion or ectopic or molar pregnancy (OØØ-OØ7, OØ8.4)
following labor and delivery (O9Ø.4)
postprocedural (N99.Ø)

✓4th **N17 Acute kidney failure**
Code also associated underlying condition
EXCLUDES 1 *posttraumatic renal failure (T79.5)*

N17.Ø Acute kidney failure with tubular necrosis
Acute tubular necrosis
Renal tubular necrosis
Tubular necrosis NOS

N17.1 Acute kidney failure with acute cortical necrosis
Acute cortical necrosis
Cortical necrosis NOS
Renal cortical necrosis

N17.2 Acute kidney failure with medullary necrosis
Medullary [papillary] necrosis NOS
Acute medullary [papillary] necrosis
Renal medullary [papillary] necrosis

N17.8 Other acute kidney failure

N17.9 Acute kidney failure, unspecified
Acute kidney injury (nontraumatic)
EXCLUDES 2 *traumatic kidney injury (S37.Ø-)*

✓4th **N18 Chronic kidney disease (CKD)**
Code first any associated:
diabetic chronic kidney disease (EØ8.22, EØ9.22, E1Ø.22, E11.22, E13.22)
hypertensive chronic kidney disease (I12-, I13-)
Use additional code to identify kidney transplant status, if applicable, (Z94.Ø)

N18.1 Chronic kidney disease, stage 1

N18.2 Chronic kidney disease, stage 2 (mild)

N18.3 Chronic kidney disease, stage 3 (moderate)

N18.4 Chronic kidney disease, stage 4 (severe)

N18.5 Chronic kidney disease, stage 5
EXCLUDES 1 *chronic kidney disease, stage 5 requiring chronic dialysis (N18.6)*

N18.6 End stage renal disease
Chronic kidney disease requiring chronic dialysis
Use additional code to identify dialysis status (Z99.2)

N18.9 Chronic kidney disease, unspecified
Chronic renal disease
Chronic renal failure NOS
Chronic renal insufficiency
Chronic uremia
Renal disease NOS

N19 Unspecified kidney failure
Uremia NOS
EXCLUDES 1 *acute kidney failure (N17.-)*
chronic kidney disease (N18.-)
chronic uremia (N18.9)
extrarenal uremia (R39.2)
prerenal uremia (R39.2)
renal insufficiency (acute) (N28.9)
uremia of newborn (P96.0)

Urolithiasis (N20-N23)

✓4th N20 Calculus of kidney and ureter
Calculous pyelonephritis
EXCLUDES 1 *nephrocalcinosis (E83.5)*
that with hydronephrosis (N13.2)

N20.0 Calculus of kidney
Nephrolithiasis NOS
Renal calculus
Renal stone
Staghorn calculus
Stone in kidney

N20.1 Calculus of ureter
Ureteric stone

N20.2 Calculus of kidney with calculus of ureter

N20.9 Urinary calculus, unspecified

✓4th N21 Calculus of lower urinary tract
Calculus of lower urinary tract with cystitis and urethritis

N21.0 Calculus in bladder
Calculus in diverticulum of bladder
Urinary bladder stone
EXCLUDES 2 *staghorn calculus (N20.0)*

N21.1 Calculus in urethra
EXCLUDES 2 *calculus of prostate (N42.0)*

N21.8 Other lower urinary tract calculus

N21.9 Calculus of lower urinary tract, unspecified
EXCLUDES 1 *calculus of urinary tract NOS (N20.9)*

N22 Calculus of urinary tract in diseases classified elsewhere
Code first underlying disease, such as:
gout (M1A.-, M10.-)
schistosomiasis (B65.0-B65.9)

N23 Unspecified renal colic

Other disorders of kidney and ureter (N25-N29)

EXCLUDES 2 *disorders of kidney and ureter with urolithiasis (N20-N23)*

✓4th N25 Disorders resulting from impaired renal tubular function
EXCLUDES 1 *metabolic disorders classifiable to E70-E88*

N25.0 Renal osteodystrophy
Azotemic osteodystrophy
Phosphate-losing tubular disorders
Renal rickets
Renal short stature

N25.1 Nephrogenic diabetes insipidus
EXCLUDES 1 *diabetes insipidus NOS (E23.2)*

✓5th N25.8 Other disorders resulting from impaired renal tubular function

N25.81 Secondary hyperparathyroidism of renal origin
EXCLUDES 1 *secondary hyperparathyroidism, non-renal (E21.1)*

N25.89 Other disorders resulting from impaired renal tubular function
Hypokalemic nephropathy
Lightwood-Albright syndrome
Renal tubular acidosis NOS

N25.9 Disorder resulting from impaired renal tubular function, unspecified

✓4th N26 Unspecified contracted kidney
EXCLUDES 1 *contracted kidney due to hypertension (I12.-)*
diffuse sclerosing glomerulonephritis (N05.8-)
hypertensive nephrosclerosis (arteriolar) (arteriosclerotic) (I12.-)
small kidney of unknown cause (N27.-)

N26.1 Atrophy of kidney (terminal)

N26.2 Page kidney

N26.9 Renal sclerosis, unspecified

✓4th N27 Small kidney of unknown cause
INCLUDES oligonephronia

N27.0 Small kidney, unilateral

N27.1 Small kidney, bilateral

N27.9 Small kidney, unspecified

✓4th N28 Other disorders of kidney and ureter, not elsewhere classified

N28.0 Ischemia and infarction of kidney
Renal artery embolism
Renal artery obstruction
Renal artery occlusion
Renal artery thrombosis
Renal infarct
EXCLUDES 1 *atherosclerosis of renal artery (extrarenal part) (I70.1)*
congenital stenosis of renal artery (Q27.1)
Goldblatt's kidney (I70.1)

N28.1 Cyst of kidney, acquired
Cyst (multiple)(solitary) of kidney, acquired
EXCLUDES 1 *cystic kidney disease (congenital) (Q61.-)*

✓5th N28.8 Other specified disorders of kidney and ureter
EXCLUDES 1 *hydroureter (N13.4)*
ureteric stricture with hydronephrosis (N13.1)
ureteric stricture without hydronephrosis (N13.5)

N28.81 Hypertrophy of kidney

N28.82 Megaloureter

N28.83 Nephroptosis

N28.84 Pyelitis cystica

N28.85 Pyeloureteritis cystica

N28.86 Ureteritis cystica

N28.89 Other specified disorders of kidney and ureter

N28.9 Disorder of kidney and ureter, unspecified
Nephropathy NOS
Renal disease (acute) NOS
Renal insufficiency (acute)
EXCLUDES 1 *chronic renal insufficiency (N18.9)*
unspecified nephritic syndrome (N05.-)

N29 Other disorders of kidney and ureter in diseases classified elsewhere
Code first underlying disease, such as:
amyloidosis (E85.-)
nephrocalcinosis (E83.5)
schistosomiasis (B65.0-B65.9)
EXCLUDES 1 *disorders of kidney and ureter in:*
cystinosis (E72.0)
gonorrhea (A54.21)
syphilis (A52.75)
tuberculosis (A18.11)

Other diseases of the urinary system (N30-N39)

EXCLUDES 1 *urinary infection (complicating):*
abortion or ectopic or molar pregnancy (O00-O07, O08.8)
pregnancy, childbirth and the puerperium (O23-, O75.3, O86.2-)

✓4th N30 Cystitis
Use additional code to identify infectious agent (B95-B97)
EXCLUDES 1 *prostatocystitis (N41.3)*

✓5th N30.0 Acute cystitis
EXCLUDES 1 *irradiation cystitis (N30.4-)*
trigonitis (N30.3-)

N30.00 Acute cystitis without hematuria

N30.01 Acute cystitis with hematuria

✓5th N30.1 Interstitial cystitis (chronic)

N30.10 Interstitial cystitis (chronic) without hematuria

N30.11 Interstitial cystitis (chronic) with hematuria

✓5th N30.2 Other chronic cystitis

N30.20 Other chronic cystitis without hematuria

N3Ø.21 **Other chronic cystitis with hematuria**

✓5th **N3Ø.3 Trigonitis**
Urethrotrigonitis
N3Ø.3Ø Trigonitis without hematuria
N3Ø.31 Trigonitis with hematuria

✓5th **N3Ø.4 Irradiation cystitis**
N3Ø.4Ø Irradiation cystitis without hematuria
N3Ø.41 Irradiation cystitis with hematuria

✓5th **N3Ø.8 Other cystitis**
Abscess of bladder
N3Ø.8Ø Other cystitis without hematuria
N3Ø.81 Other cystitis with hematuria

✓5th **N3Ø.9 Cystitis, unspecified**
N3Ø.9Ø Cystitis, unspecified without hematuria
N3Ø.91 Cystitis, unspecified with hematuria

✓4th **N31 Neuromuscular dysfunction of bladder, not elsewhere classified**
Use additional code to identify any associated urinary incontinence (N39.3-N39.4-)
EXCLUDES 1 *cord bladder NOS (G95.89)*
neurogenic bladder due to cauda equina syndrome (G83.4)
neuromuscular dysfunction due to spinal cord lesion (G95.89)
N31.Ø Uninhibited neuropathic bladder, not elsewhere classified
N31.1 Reflex neuropathic bladder, not elsewhere classified
N31.2 Flaccid neuropathic bladder, not elsewhere classified
Atonic (motor) (sensory) neuropathic bladder
Autonomous neuropathic bladder
Nonreflex neuropathic bladder
N31.8 Other neuromuscular dysfunction of bladder
N31.9 Neuromuscular dysfunction of bladder, unspecified
Neurogenic bladder dysfunction NOS

✓4th **N32 Other disorders of bladder**
EXCLUDES 2 *calculus of bladder (N21.Ø)*
cystocele (N81.1-)
hernia or prolapse of bladder, female (N81.1-)
N32.Ø Bladder-neck obstruction
Bladder-neck stenosis (acquired)
EXCLUDES 1 *congenital bladder-neck obstruction (Q64.3-)*
N32.1 Vesicointestinal fistula
Vesicorectal fistula
N32.2 Vesical fistula, not elsewhere classified
EXCLUDES 1 *fistula between bladder and female genital tract (N82.Ø-N82.1)*
N32.3 Diverticulum of bladder
EXCLUDES 1 *congenital diverticulum of bladder (Q64.6)*
diverticulitis of bladder (N3Ø.8-)
✓5th **N32.8 Other specified disorders of bladder**
N32.81 Overactive bladder
Detrusor muscle hyperactivity
EXCLUDES 1 *frequent urination due to specified bladder condition—code to condition*
N32.89 Other specified disorders of bladder
Bladder hemorrhage
Bladder hypertrophy
Calcified bladder
Contracted bladder
N32.9 Bladder disorder, unspecified

N33 Bladder disorders in diseases classified elsewhere
Code first underlying disease, such as:
schistosomiasis (B65.Ø-B65.9)
EXCLUDES 1 *bladder disorder in:*
syphilis (A52.76)
tuberculosis (A18.12)
cystitis (in):
candidal infection (B37.41)
chlamydial (A56.Ø1)
diphtheritic (A36.85)
gonorrhea (A54.Ø1)
syphilitic (A52.76)
trichomonal infection (A59.Ø3)
neurogenic bladder (N31.-)

✓4th **N34 Urethritis and urethral syndrome**
Use additional code (B95-B97), to identify infectious agent
EXCLUDES 2 *Reiter's disease (MØ2.3-)*
urethritis in diseases with a predominantly sexual mode of transmission (A5Ø-A64)
urethrotrigonitis (N3Ø.3-)
N34.Ø Urethral abscess
Abscess (of) Cowper's gland
Abscess (of) Littrés gland
Abscess (of) urethral (gland)
Periurethral abscess
EXCLUDES 1 *urethral caruncle (N36.2)*
N34.1 Nonspecific urethritis
Nongonococcal urethritis
Nonvenereal urethritis
N34.2 Other urethritis
Meatitis, urethral
Postmenopausal urethritis
Ulcer of urethra (meatus)
Urethritis NOS
N34.3 Urethral syndrome, unspecified

✓4th **N35 Urethral stricture**
EXCLUDES 1 *congenital urethral stricture (Q64.3-)*
postprocedural urethral stricture (N99.1-)
✓5th **N35.Ø Post-traumatic urethral stricture**
Urethral stricture due to injury
EXCLUDES 1 *postprocedural urethral stricture (N99.1-)*
✓6th **N35.Ø1 Post-traumatic urethral stricture, male**
N35.Ø1Ø Post-traumatic urethral stricture, male, meatal
N35.Ø11 Post-traumatic bulbous urethral stricture
N35.Ø12 Post-traumatic membranous urethral stricture
N35.Ø13 Post-traumatic anterior urethral stricture
N35.Ø14 Post-traumatic urethral stricture, male, unspecified
✓6th **N35.Ø2 Post-traumatic urethral stricture, female**
N35.Ø21 Urethral stricture due to childbirth
N35.Ø28 Other post-traumatic urethral stricture, female
✓5th **N35.1 Postinfective urethral stricture, not elsewhere classified**
EXCLUDES 1 *urethral stricture associated with schistosomiasis (B65-, N29)*
gonococcal urethral stricture (A54.Ø1)
syphilitic urethral stricture (A52.76)
✓6th **N35.11 Postinfective urethral stricture, not elsewhere classified, male**
N35.111 Postinfective urethral stricture, not elsewhere classified, male, meatal
N35.112 Postinfective bulbous urethral stricture, not elsewhere classified
N35.113 Postinfective membranous urethral stricture, not elsewhere classified
N35.114 Postinfective anterior urethral stricture, not elsewhere classified
N35.119 Postinfective urethral stricture, not elsewhere classified, male, unspecified
N35.12 Postinfective urethral stricture, not elsewhere classified, female
N35.8 Other urethral stricture
EXCLUDES 1 *postprocedural urethral stricture (N99.1-)*
N35.9 Urethral stricture, unspecified

✓4th **N36 Other disorders of urethra**
N36.Ø Urethral fistula
Urethroperineal fistula
Urethrorectal fistula
Urinary fistula NOS
EXCLUDES 1 *urethroscrotal fistula (N5Ø.8)*
urethrovaginal fistula (N82.1)
urethrovesicovaginal fistula (N82.1)
N36.1 Urethral diverticulum
N36.2 Urethral caruncle

√5th **N36.4 Urethral functional and muscular disorders**
Use additional code to identify associated urinary stress incontinence (N39.3)
N36.41 Hypermobility of urethra
N36.42 Intrinsic sphincter deficiency (ISD)
N36.43 Combined hypermobility of urethra and intrinsic sphincter deficiency
N36.44 Muscular disorders of urethra
Bladder sphincter dyssynergy
N36.5 Urethral false passage
N36.8 Other specified disorders of urethra
N36.9 Urethral disorder, unspecified

N37 Urethral disorders in diseases classified elsewhere
Code first underlying disease
EXCLUDES 1 *urethritis (in):*
candidal infection (B37.41)
chlamydial (A56.01)
gonorrhea (A54.01)
syphilis (A52.76)
trichomonal infection (A59.03)
tuberculosis (A18.13)

√4th **N39 Other disorders of urinary system**
EXCLUDES 2 *hematuria NOS (R31.-)*
recurrent or persistent hematuria (N02.-)
recurrent or persistent hematuria with specified morphological lesion (N02.-)
proteinuria NOS (R80.-)
N39.0 Urinary tract infection, site not specified
Use additional code (B95-B97), to identify infectious agent
EXCLUDES 1 *candidiasis of urinary tract (B37.4-)*
neonatal urinary tract infection (P39.3)
urinary tract infection of specified site, such as:
cystitis (N30.-)
urethritis (N34.-)
N39.3 Stress incontinence (female) (male)
Code also any associated overactive bladder (N32.81)
EXCLUDES 1 *mixed incontinence (N39.46)*
√5th **N39.4 Other specified urinary incontinence**
Code also any associated overactive bladder (N32.81)
EXCLUDES 1 *enuresis NOS (R32)*
functional urinary incontinence (R39.81)
urinary incontinence associated with cognitive impairment (R39.81)
urinary incontinence NOS (R32)
urinary incontinence of nonorganic origin (F98.0)
N39.41 Urge incontinence
EXCLUDES 1 *mixed incontinence (N39.46)*
N39.42 Incontinence without sensory awareness
N39.43 Post-void dribbling
N39.44 Nocturnal enuresis
N39.45 Continuous leakage
N39.46 Mixed incontinence
Urge and stress incontinence
√6th **N39.49 Other specified urinary incontinence**
N39.490 Overflow incontinence
N39.498 Other specified urinary incontinence
Reflex incontinence
Total incontinence
N39.8 Other specified disorders of urinary system
N39.9 Disorder of urinary system, unspecified

Diseases of male genital organs (N40-N53)

√4th **N40 Enlarged prostate**
Adenofibromatous hypertrophy of prostate
Benign hypertrophy of the prostate
Benign prostatic hyperplasia
Benign prostatic hypertrophy
BPH
Nodular prostate
Polyp of prostate
EXCLUDES 1 *benign neoplasms of prostate (adenoma, benign) (fibroadenoma) (fibroma) (myoma) (D29.1)*
EXCLUDES 2 *malignant neoplasm of prostate (C61)*
N40.0 Enlarged prostate without lower urinary tract symptoms
Enlarged prostate NOS
Enlarged prostate without LUTS
N40.1 Enlarged prostate with lower urinary tract symptoms
Enlarged prostate with LUTS
Use additional code for associated symptoms, when specified:
incomplete bladder emptying (R39.14)
nocturia (R35.1)
straining on urination (R39.16)
urinary frequency (R35.0)
urinary hesitancy (R39.11)
urinary incontinence (N39.4-)
urinary obstruction (N13.8)
urinary retention (R33.8)
urinary urgency (R39.15)
weak urinary stream (R39.12)
N40.2 Nodular prostate without lower urinary tract symptoms
Nodular prostate without LUTS
N40.3 Nodular prostate with lower urinary tract symptoms
Use additional code for associated symptoms, when specified:
incomplete bladder emptying (R39.14)
nocturia (R35.1)
straining on urination (R39.16)
urinary frequency (R35.0)
urinary hesitancy (R39.11)
urinary incontinence (N39.4-)
urinary obstruction (N13.8)
urinary retention (R33.8)
urinary urgency (R39.15)
weak urinary stream (R39.12)

√4th **N41 Inflammatory diseases of prostate**
Use additional code (B95-B97), to identify infectious agent
N41.0 Acute prostatitis
N41.1 Chronic prostatitis
N41.2 Abscess of prostate
N41.3 Prostatocystitis
N41.4 Granulomatous prostatitis
N41.8 Other inflammatory diseases of prostate
N41.9 Inflammatory disease of prostate, unspecified
Prostatitis NOS

√4th **N42 Other and unspecified disorders of prostate**
N42.0 Calculus of prostate
Prostatic stone
N42.1 Congestion and hemorrhage of prostate
EXCLUDES 1 *enlarged prostate (N40.-)*
hematuria (R31.-)
hyperplasia of prostate (N40.-)
inflammatory diseases of prostate (N41.-)
N42.3 Dysplasia of prostate
Prostatic intraepithelial neoplasia I (PIN I)
Prostatic intraepithelial neoplasia II (PIN II)
EXCLUDES 1 *prostatic intraepithelial neoplasia III (PIN III) (D07.5)*
√5th **N42.8 Other specified disorders of prostate**
N42.81 Prostatodynia syndrome
Painful prostate syndrome
N42.82 Prostatosis syndrome
N42.83 Cyst of prostate
N42.89 Other specified disorders of prostate
N42.9 Disorder of prostate, unspecified

N43 Hydrocele and spermatocele
INCLUDES hydrocele of spermatic cord, testis or tunica vaginalis
EXCLUDES 1 *congenital hydrocele (P83.5)*
N43.Ø Encysted hydrocele
N43.1 Infected hydrocele
Use additional code (B95-B97), to identify infectious agent
N43.2 Other hydrocele
N43.3 Hydrocele, unspecified
N43.4 Spermatocele of epididymis
Spermatic cyst
N43.4Ø Spermatocele of epididymis, unspecified
N43.41 Spermatocele of epididymis, single
N43.42 Spermatocele of epididymis, multiple

N44 Noninflammatory disorders of testis
N44.Ø Torsion of testis
N44.ØØ Torsion of testis, unspecified
N44.Ø1 Extravaginal torsion of spermatic cord
N44.Ø2 Intravaginal torsion of spermatic cord
Torsion of spermatic cord NOS
N44.Ø3 Torsion of appendix testis
N44.Ø4 Torsion of appendix epididymis
N44.1 Cyst of tunica albuginea testis
N44.2 Benign cyst of testis
N44.8 Other noninflammatory disorders of the testis

N45 Orchitis and epididymitis
Use additional code (B95-B97), to identify infectious agent
N45.1 Epididymitis
N45.2 Orchitis
N45.3 Epididymo-orchitis
N45.4 Abscess of epididymis or testis

N46 Male infertility
EXCLUDES 1 *vasectomy status (Z98.52)*
N46.Ø Azoospermia
Absolute male infertility
Male infertility due to germinal (cell) aplasia
Male infertility due to spermatogenic arrest (complete)
N46.Ø1 Organic azoospermia
Azoospermia NOS
N46.Ø2 Azoospermia due to extratesticular causes
Code also associated cause
N46.Ø21 Azoospermia due to drug therapy
N46.Ø22 Azoospermia due to infection
N46.Ø23 Azoospermia due to obstruction of efferent ducts
N46.Ø24 Azoospermia due to radiation
N46.Ø25 Azoospermia due to systemic disease
N46.Ø29 Azoospermia due to other extratesticular causes
N46.1 Oligospermia
Male infertility due to germinal cell desquamation
Male infertility due to hypospermatogenesis
Male infertility due to incomplete spermatogenic arrest
N46.11 Organic oligospermia
Oligospermia NOS
N46.12 Oligospermia due to extratesticular causes
Code also associated cause
N46.121 Oligospermia due to drug therapy
N46.122 Oligospermia due to infection
N46.123 Oligospermia due to obstruction of efferent ducts
N46.124 Oligospermia due to radiation
N46.125 Oligospermia due to systemic disease
N46.129 Oligospermia due to other extratesticular causes
N46.8 Other male infertility
N46.9 Male infertility, unspecified

N47 Disorders of prepuce
N47.Ø Adherent prepuce, newborn
N47.1 Phimosis
N47.2 Paraphimosis
N47.3 Deficient foreskin
N47.4 Benign cyst of prepuce
N47.5 Adhesions of prepuce and glans penis
N47.6 Balanoposthitis
EXCLUDES 1 *balanitis (N48.1)*
Use additional code (B95-B97), to identify infectious agent
N47.7 Other inflammatory diseases of prepuce
Use additional code (B95-B97), to identify infectious agent
N47.8 Other disorders of prepuce

N48 Other disorders of penis
N48.Ø Leukoplakia of penis
Balanitis xerotica obliterans
Kraurosis of penis
Lichen sclerosus of external male genital organs
EXCLUDES 1 *carcinoma in situ of penis (DØ7.4)*
N48.1 Balanitis
EXCLUDES 1 *amebic balanitis (AØ6.8)*
balanitis xerotica obliterans (N48.Ø)
candidal balanitis (B37.42)
gonococcal balanitis (A54.23)
herpesviral [herpes simplex] balanitis (A6Ø.Ø1)
Use additional code (B95-B97), to identify infectious agent
N48.2 Other inflammatory disorders of penis
Use additional code (B95-B97), to identify infectious agent
EXCLUDES 1 *balanitis (N48.1)*
balanitis xerotica obliterans (N48.Ø)
balanoposthitis (N47.6)
N48.21 Abscess of corpus cavernosum and penis
N48.22 Cellulitis of corpus cavernosum and penis
N48.29 Other inflammatory disorders of penis
N48.3 Priapism
Painful erection
Code first underlying cause
N48.3Ø Priapism, unspecified
N48.31 Priapism due to trauma
N48.32 Priapism due to disease classified elsewhere
N48.33 Priapism, drug-induced
N48.39 Other priapism
N48.5 Ulcer of penis
N48.6 Induration penis plastica
Peyronie's disease
Plastic induration of penis
N48.8 Other specified disorders of penis
N48.81 Thrombosis of superficial vein of penis
N48.82 Acquired torsion of penis
Acquired torsion of penis NOS
EXCLUDES 1 *congenital torsion of penis (Q55.63)*
N48.83 Acquired buried penis
EXCLUDES 1 *congenital hidden penis (Q55.64)*
N48.89 Other specified disorders of penis
N48.9 Disorder of penis, unspecified

N49 Inflammatory disorders of male genital organs, not elsewhere classified
Use additional code (B95-B97), to identify infectious agent
EXCLUDES 1 *inflammation of penis (N48.1, N48.2-)*
orchitis and epididymitis (N45.-)
N49.Ø Inflammatory disorders of seminal vesicle
Vesiculitis NOS
N49.1 Inflammatory disorders of spermatic cord, tunica vaginalis and vas deferens
Vasitis
N49.2 Inflammatory disorders of scrotum
N49.3 Fournier gangrene
N49.8 Inflammatory disorders of other specified male genital organs
Inflammation of multiple sites in male genital organs
N49.9 Inflammatory disorder of unspecified male genital organ
Abscess of unspecified male genital organ
Boil of unspecified male genital organ
Carbuncle of unspecified male genital organ
Cellulitis of unspecified male genital organ

N5Ø Other and unspecified disorders of male genital organs
EXCLUDES 2 *torsion of testis (N44.Ø-)*
N5Ø.Ø Atrophy of testis
N5Ø.1 Vascular disorders of male genital organs
Hematocele, NOS, of male genital organs
Hemorrhage of male genital organs
Thrombosis of male genital organs
N5Ø.3 Cyst of epididymis

N50.8 Other specified disorders of male genital organs
Atrophy of scrotum, seminal vesicle, spermatic cord, tunica vaginalis and vas deferens
Chylocele, tunica vaginalis (nonfilarial) NOS
Edema of scrotum, seminal vesicle, spermatic cord, testis, tunica vaginalis and vas deferens
Hypertrophy of scrotum, seminal vesicle, spermatic cord, testis, tunica vaginalis and vas deferens
Stricture of spermatic cord, tunica vaginalis, and vas deferens
Ulcer of scrotum, seminal vesicle, spermatic cord, testis, tunica vaginalis and vas deferens
Urethroscrotal fistula

N50.9 Disorder of male genital organs, unspecified

N51 Disorders of male genital organs in diseases classified elsewhere
Code first underlying disease, such as:
filariasis (B74.0-B74.9)
EXCLUDES 1 *amebic balanitis (A06.8)*
candidal balanitis (B37.42)
gonococcal balanitis (A54.23)
gonococcal prostatitis (A54.22)
herpesviral [herpes simplex] balanitis (A60.01)
trichomonal prostatitis (A59.02)
tuberculous prostatitis (A18.14)

✓4th **N52 Male erectile dysfunction**
EXCLUDES 1 *psychogenic impotence (F52.21)*

✓5th **N52.0 Vasculogenic erectile dysfunction**
N52.01 Erectile dysfunction due to arterial insufficiency
N52.02 Corporo-venous occlusive erectile dysfunction
N52.03 Combined arterial insufficiency and corporo-venous occlusive erectile dysfunction

N52.1 Erectile dysfunction due to diseases classified elsewhere
Code first underlying disease

N52.2 Drug-induced erectile dysfunction

✓5th **N52.3 Post-surgical erectile dysfunction**
N52.31 Erectile dysfunction following radical prostatectomy
N52.32 Erectile dysfunction following radical cystectomy
N52.33 Erectile dysfunction following urethral surgery
N52.34 Erectile dysfunction following simple prostatectomy
N52.39 Other post-surgical erectile dysfunction

N52.8 Other male erectile dysfunction
N52.9 Male erectile dysfunction, unspecified
Impotence NOS

✓4th **N53 Other male sexual dysfunction**
EXCLUDES 1 *psychogenic sexual dysfunction (F52.-)*

✓5th **N53.1 Ejaculatory dysfunction**
EXCLUDES 1 *premature ejaculation (F52.4)*
N53.11 Retarded ejaculation
N53.12 Painful ejaculation
N53.13 Anejaculatory orgasm
N53.14 Retrograde ejaculation
N53.19 Other ejaculatory dysfunction
Ejaculatory dysfunction NOS

N53.8 Other male sexual dysfunction
N53.9 Unspecified male sexual dysfunction

Disorders of breast (N60-N65)

EXCLUDES 1 *disorders of breast associated with childbirth (O91-O92)*

✓4th **N60 Benign mammary dysplasia**
INCLUDES fibrocystic mastopathy

✓5th **N60.0 Solitary cyst of breast**
Cyst of breast
N60.01 Solitary cyst of right breast
N60.02 Solitary cyst of left breast
N60.09 Solitary cyst of unspecified breast

✓5th **N60.1 Diffuse cystic mastopathy**
Cystic breast
Fibrocystic disease of breast
EXCLUDES 1 *diffuse cystic mastopathy with epithelial proliferation (N60.3-)*
N60.11 Diffuse cystic mastopathy of right breast
N60.12 Diffuse cystic mastopathy of left breast
N60.19 Diffuse cystic mastopathy of unspecified breast

✓5th **N60.2 Fibroadenosis of breast**
Adenofibrosis of breast
EXCLUDES 2 *fibroadenoma of breast (D24.-)*
N60.21 Fibroadenosis of right breast
N60.22 Fibroadenosis of left breast
N60.29 Fibroadenosis of unspecified breast

✓5th **N60.3 Fibrosclerosis of breast**
Cystic mastopathy with epithelial proliferation
N60.31 Fibrosclerosis of right breast
N60.32 Fibrosclerosis of left breast
N60.39 Fibrosclerosis of unspecified breast

✓5th **N60.4 Mammary duct ectasia**
N60.41 Mammary duct ectasia of right breast
N60.42 Mammary duct ectasia of left breast
N60.49 Mammary duct ectasia of unspecified breast

✓5th **N60.8 Other benign mammary dysplasias**
N60.81 Other benign mammary dysplasias of right breast
N60.82 Other benign mammary dysplasias of left breast
N60.89 Other benign mammary dysplasias of unspecified breast

✓5th **N60.9 Unspecified benign mammary dysplasia**
N60.91 Unspecified benign mammary dysplasia of right breast
N60.92 Unspecified benign mammary dysplasia of left breast
N60.99 Unspecified benign mammary dysplasia of unspecified breast

N61 Inflammatory disorders of breast
Abscess (acute) (chronic) (nonpuerperal) of areola
Abscess (acute) (chronic) (nonpuerperal) of breast
Carbuncle of breast
Infective mastitis (acute) (subacute) (nonpuerperal)
Mastitis (acute) (subacute) (nonpuerperal) NOS
EXCLUDES 1 *inflammatory carcinoma of breast (C50.9)*
inflammatory disorder of breast associated with childbirth (O91.-)
neonatal infective mastitis (P39.0)
thrombophlebitis of breast [Mondor's disease] (I80.8)

N62 Hypertrophy of breast
Gynecomastia
Hypertrophy of breast NOS
Massive pubertal hypertrophy of breast
EXCLUDES 1 *breast engorgement of newborn (P83.4)*
disproportion of reconstructed breast (N65.1)

N63 Unspecified lump in breast
Nodule(s) NOS in breast

✓4th **N64 Other disorders of breast**
EXCLUDES 2 *mechanical complication of breast prosthesis and implant (T85.4-)*

N64.0 Fissure and fistula of nipple
N64.1 Fat necrosis of breast
Fat necrosis (segmental) of breast
Code first breast necrosis due to breast graft (T85.89)
N64.2 Atrophy of breast
N64.3 Galactorrhea not associated with childbirth
N64.4 Mastodynia

✓5th **N64.5 Other signs and symptoms in breast**
EXCLUDES 2 *abnormal findings on diagnostic imaging of breast (R92.-)*
N64.51 Induration of breast
N64.52 Nipple discharge
EXCLUDES 1 *abnormal findings in nipple discharge (R89.-)*
N64.53 Retraction of nipple
N64.59 Other signs and symptoms in breast

✓5th **N64.8 Other specified disorders of breast**
N64.81 Ptosis of breast
EXCLUDES 1 *ptosis of native breast in relation to reconstructed breast (N65.1)*
N64.82 Hypoplasia of breast
Micromastia
EXCLUDES 1 *congenital absence of breast (Q83.0)*
hypoplasia of native breast in relation to reconstructed breast (N65.1)

N64.89 Other specified disorders of breast
Galactocele
Subinvolution of breast (postlactational)

N64.9 Disorder of breast, unspecified

✓4th **N65 Deformity and disproportion of reconstructed breast**

N65.0 Deformity of reconstructed breast
Contour irregularity in reconstructed breast
Excess tissue in reconstructed breast
Misshapen reconstructed breast

N65.1 Disproportion of reconstructed breast
Breast asymmetry between native breast and reconstructed breast
Disproportion between native breast and reconstructed breast

Inflammatory diseases of female pelvic organs (N70-N77)

EXCLUDES 1 *inflammatory diseases of female pelvic organs complicating:*
abortion or ectopic or molar pregnancy (O00-O07, O08.0)
pregnancy, childbirth and the puerperium (O23-, O75.3, O85, O86-)

✓4th **N70 Salpingitis and oophoritis**
INCLUDES abscess (of) fallopian tube
abscess (of) ovary
pyosalpinx
salpingo-oophoritis
tubo-ovarian abscess
tubo-ovarian inflammatory disease
Use additional code (B95-B97), to identify infectious agent
EXCLUDES 1 *gonococcal infection (A54.24)*
tuberculous infection (A18.17)

✓5th **N70.0 Acute salpingitis and oophoritis**
N70.01 Acute salpingitis
N70.02 Acute oophoritis
N70.03 Acute salpingitis and oophoritis

✓5th **N70.1 Chronic salpingitis and oophoritis**
Hydrosalpinx
N70.11 Chronic salpingitis
N70.12 Chronic oophoritis
N70.13 Chronic salpingitis and oophoritis

✓5th **N70.9 Salpingitis and oophoritis, unspecified**
N70.91 Salpingitis, unspecified
N70.92 Oophoritis, unspecified
N70.93 Salpingitis and oophoritis, unspecified

✓4th **N71 Inflammatory disease of uterus, except cervix**
Endo (myo) metritis
Metritis
Myometritis
Pyometra
Uterine abscess
Use additional code (B95-B97), to identify infectious agent
EXCLUDES 1 *hyperplastic endometritis (N85.0-)*
infection of uterus following delivery (O85, O86-)

N71.0 Acute inflammatory disease of uterus
N71.1 Chronic inflammatory disease of uterus
N71.9 Inflammatory disease of uterus, unspecified

N72 Inflammatory disease of cervix uteri
Cervicitis (with or without erosion or ectropion)
Endocervicitis (with or without erosion or ectropion)
Exocervicitis (with or without erosion or ectropion)
Use additional code (B95-B97), to identify infectious agent
EXCLUDES 1 *erosion and ectropion of cervix without cervicitis (N86)*

✓4th **N73 Other female pelvic inflammatory diseases**
Use additional code (B95-B97), to identify infectious agent

N73.0 Acute parametritis and pelvic cellulitis
Abscess of broad ligament
Abscess of parametrium
Pelvic cellulitis, female

N73.1 Chronic parametritis and pelvic cellulitis
Any condition in N73.0 specified as chronic
EXCLUDES 1 *tuberculous parametritis and pelvic cellultis (A18.17)*

N73.2 Unspecified parametritis and pelvic cellulitis
Any condition in N73.0 unspecified whether acute or chronic

N73.3 Female acute pelvic peritonitis

N73.4 Female chronic pelvic peritonitis
EXCLUDES 1 *tuberculous pelvic (female) peritonitis (A18.17)*

N73.5 Female pelvic peritonitis, unspecified

N73.6 Female pelvic peritoneal adhesions (postinfective)
EXCLUDES 2 *postprocedural pelvic peritoneal adhesions (N99.4)*

N73.8 Other specified female pelvic inflammatory diseases

N73.9 Female pelvic inflammatory disease, unspecified
Female pelvic infection or inflammation NOS

N74 Female pelvic inflammatory disorders in diseases classified elsewhere
Code first underlying disease
EXCLUDES 1 *cervicitis:*
chlamydial (A56.02)
gonococcal (A54.03)
herpesviral [herpes simplex] (A60.03)
syphilitic (A52.76)
trichomonal (A59.09)
tuberculous (A18.16)
pelvic inflammatory disease:
chlamydial (A56.11)
gonococcal (A54.24)
herpesviral [herpes simplex] (A60.09)
syphilitic (A52.76)
tuberculous (A18.17)

✓4th **N75 Diseases of Bartholin's gland**
N75.0 Cyst of Bartholin's gland
N75.1 Abscess of Bartholin's gland
N75.8 Other diseases of Bartholin's gland
Bartholinitis
N75.9 Disease of Bartholin's gland, unspecified

✓4th **N76 Other inflammation of vagina and vulva**
Use additional code (B95-B97), to identify infectious agent
EXCLUDES 2 *senile (atrophic) vaginitis (N95.2)*
vulvar vestibulitis (N94.810)

N76.0 Acute vaginitis
Acute vulvovaginitis
Vaginitis NOS
Vulvovaginitis NOS

N76.1 Subacute and chronic vaginitis
Chronic vulvovaginitis
Subacute vulvovaginitis

N76.2 Acute vulvitis
Vulvitis NOS

N76.3 Subacute and chronic vulvitis

N76.4 Abscess of vulva
Furuncle of vulva

N76.5 Ulceration of vagina

N76.6 Ulceration of vulva

✓5th **N76.8 Other specified inflammation of vagina and vulva**
N76.81 Mucositis (ulcerative) of vagina and vulva
Code also type of associated therapy, such as:
antineoplastic and immunosuppressive drugs (T45.1X-)
radiological procedure and radiotherapy (Y84.2)
EXCLUDES 2 *gastrointestinal mucositis (ulcerative) (K92.81)*
nasal mucositis (ulcerative) (J34.81)
oral mucositis (ulcerative) (K12.3-)
N76.89 Other specified inflammation of vagina and vulva

✓4th **N77 Vulvovaginal ulceration and inflammation in diseases classified elsewhere**

N77.0 Ulceration of vulva in diseases classified elsewhere
Code first underlying disease, such as:
Behçet's disease (M35.2)
EXCLUDES 1 *ulceration of vulva in gonococcal infection (A54.02)*
ulceration of vulva in herpesviral [herpes simplex] infection (A60.04)
ulceration of vulva in syphilis (A51.0)
ulceration of vulva in tuberculosis (A18.18)

N77.1 Vaginitis, vulvitis and vulvovaginitis in diseases classified elsewhere
Code first underlying disease, such as:
pinworm (B80)
EXCLUDES 1 *vaginitis, vulvitis and vulvovaginitis (in):*
candidiasis (B37.3)
chlamydial (A56.02)
gonococcal infection (A54.02)
herpesviral [herpes simplex] infection (A60.04)
syphilitic, early (A51.0)
syphilitic, late (A52.76)
trichomonal (A59.01)
tuberculous (A18.18)

Noninflammatory disorders of female genital tract (N80-N98)

N80 Endometriosis
- **N80.0 Endometriosis of uterus**
  Adenomyosis
  EXCLUDES 1 *stromal endometriosis (D39.0)*
- **N80.1 Endometriosis of ovary**
- **N80.2 Endometriosis of fallopian tube**
- **N80.3 Endometriosis of pelvic peritoneum**
- **N80.4 Endometriosis of rectovaginal septum and vagina**
- **N80.5 Endometriosis of intestine**
- **N80.6 Endometriosis in cutaneous scar**
- **N80.8 Other endometriosis**
- **N80.9 Endometriosis, unspecified**

N81 Female genital prolapse
EXCLUDES 1 *genital prolapse complicating pregnancy, labor or delivery (O34.5-)*
prolapse and hernia of ovary and fallopian tube (N83.4)
prolapse of vaginal vault after hysterectomy (N99.3)
- **N81.0 Urethrocele**
  EXCLUDES 1 *urethrocele with cystocele (N81.1-)*
  urethrocele with prolapse of uterus (N81.2-N81.4)
- **N81.1 Cystocele**
  Cystocele with urethrocele
  Cystourethrocele
  EXCLUDES 1 *cystocele with prolapse of uterus (N81.2-N81.4)*
  - **N81.10 Cystocele, unspecified**
    Prolapse of (anterior) vaginal wall NOS
  - **N81.11 Cystocele, midline**
  - **N81.12 Cystocele, lateral**
    Paravaginal cystocele
- **N81.2 Incomplete uterovaginal prolapse**
  First degree uterine prolapse
  Prolapse of cervix NOS
  Second degree uterine prolapse
  EXCLUDES 1 *cervical stump prolaspe (N81.85)*
- **N81.3 Complete uterovaginal prolapse**
  Procidentia (uteri) NOS
  Third degree uterine prolapse
- **N81.4 Uterovaginal prolapse, unspecified**
  Prolapse of uterus NOS
- **N81.5 Vaginal enterocele**
  EXCLUDES 1 *enterocele with prolapse of uterus (N81.2-N81.4)*
- **N81.6 Rectocele**
  Prolapse of posterior vaginal wall
  Use additional code for any associated fecal incontinence, if applicable (R15.-)
  EXCLUDES 2 *perineocele N81.81*
  rectal prolapse (K62.3)
  rectocele with prolapse of uterus (N81.2-N81.4)
- **N81.8 Other female genital prolapse**
  - **N81.81 Perineocele**
  - **N81.82 Incompetence or weakening of pubocervical tissue**
  - **N81.83 Incompetence or weakening of rectovaginal tissue**
  - **N81.84 Pelvic muscle wasting**
    Disuse atrophy of pelvic muscles and anal sphincter
  - **N81.85 Cervical stump prolapse**
  - **N81.89 Other female genital prolapse**
    Deficient perineum
    Old laceration of muscles of pelvic floor
- **N81.9 Female genital prolapse, unspecified**

N82 Fistulae involving female genital tract
EXCLUDES 1 *vesicointestinal fistulae (N32.1)*
- **N82.0 Vesicovaginal fistula**
- **N82.1 Other female urinary-genital tract fistulae**
  Cervicovesical fistula
  Ureterovaginal fistula
  Urethrovaginal fistula
  Uteroureteric fistula
  Uterovesical fistula
- **N82.2 Fistula of vagina to small intestine**
- **N82.3 Fistula of vagina to large intestine**
  Rectovaginal fistula
- **N82.4 Other female intestinal-genital tract fistulae**
  Intestinouterine fistula
- **N82.5 Female genital tract-skin fistulae**
  Uterus to abdominal wall fistula
  Vaginoperineal fistula
- **N82.8 Other female genital tract fistulae**
- **N82.9 Female genital tract fistula, unspecified**

N83 Noninflammatory disorders of ovary, fallopian tube and broad ligament
EXCLUDES 2 *hydrosalpinx (N70.1-)*
- **N83.0 Follicular cyst of ovary**
  Cyst of graafian follicle
  Hemorrhagic follicular cyst (of ovary)
- **N83.1 Corpus luteum cyst**
  Hemorrhagic corpus luteum cyst
- **N83.2 Other and unspecified ovarian cysts**
  EXCLUDES 1 *developmental ovarian cyst (Q50.1)*
  neoplastic ovarian cyst (D27.-)
  polycystic ovarian syndrome (E28.2)
  Stein-Leventhal syndrome (E28.2)
  - **N83.20 Unspecified ovarian cysts**
  - **N83.29 Other ovarian cysts**
    Retention cyst of ovary
    Simple cyst of ovary
- **N83.3 Acquired atrophy of ovary and fallopian tube**
  - **N83.31 Acquired atrophy of ovary**
  - **N83.32 Acquired atrophy of fallopian tube**
  - **N83.33 Acquired atrophy of ovary and fallopian tube**
- **N83.4 Prolapse and hernia of ovary and fallopian tube**
- **N83.5 Torsion of ovary, ovarian pedicle and fallopian tube**
  Torsion of accessory tube
  - **N83.51 Torsion of ovary and ovarian pedicle**
  - **N83.52 Torsion of fallopian tube**
    Torsion of hydatid of Morgagni
  - **N83.53 Torsion of ovary, ovarian pedicle and fallopian tube**
- **N83.6 Hematosalpinx**
  EXCLUDES 1 *hematosalpinx (with) (in):*
  hematocolpos (N89.7)
  hematometra (N85.7)
  tubal pregnancy (O00.1)
- **N83.7 Hematoma of broad ligament**
- **N83.8 Other noninflammatory disorders of ovary, fallopian tube and broad ligament**
  Broad ligament laceration syndrome [Allen-Masters]
- **N83.9 Noninflammatory disorder of ovary, fallopian tube and broad ligament, unspecified**

N84 Polyp of female genital tract
EXCLUDES 1 *adenomatous polyp (D28.-)*
placental polyp (O90.89)
- **N84.0 Polyp of corpus uteri**
  Polyp of endometrium
  Polyp of uterus NOS
  EXCLUDES 1 *polypoid endometrial hyperplasia (N85.0-)*
- **N84.1 Polyp of cervix uteri**
  Mucous polyp of cervix
- **N84.2 Polyp of vagina**
- **N84.3 Polyp of vulva**
  Polyp of labia
- **N84.8 Polyp of other parts of female genital tract**
- **N84.9 Polyp of female genital tract, unspecified**

N85 Other noninflammatory disorders of uterus, except cervix
EXCLUDES 1 *endometriosis (N80.-)*
inflammatory diseases of uterus (N71.-)
noninflammatory disorders of cervix, except malposition (N86-N88)
polyp of corpus uteri (N84.0)
uterine prolapse (N81.-)
- **N85.0 Endometrial hyperplasia**
  - **N85.00 Endometrial hyperplasia, unspecified**
    Hyperplasia (adenomatous) (cystic) (glandular) of endometrium
    Hyperplastic endometritis
  - **N85.01 Benign endometrial hyperplasia**
    Endometrial hyperplasia (complex) (simple) without atypia

N85.02 Endometrial intraepithelial neoplasia [EIN]
Endometrial hyperplasia with atypia
EXCLUDES 1 *malignant neoplasm of endometrium (with endometrial intraepithelial neoplasia [EIN]) (C54.1)*

N85.2 Hypertrophy of uterus
Bulky or enlarged uterus
EXCLUDES 1 *puerperal hypertrophy of uterus (O90.89)*

N85.3 Subinvolution of uterus
EXCLUDES 1 *puerperal subinvolution of uterus (O90.89)*

N85.4 Malposition of uterus
Anteversion of uterus
Retroflexion of uterus
Retroversion of uterus
EXCLUDES 1 *malposition of uterus complicating pregnancy, labor or delivery (O34.5-, O65.5)*

N85.5 Inversion of uterus
EXCLUDES 1 *current obstetric trauma (O71.2)*
postpartum inversion of uterus (O71.2)

N85.6 Intrauterine synechiae

N85.7 Hematometra
Hematosalpinx with hematometra
EXCLUDES 1 *hematometra with hematocolpos (N89.7)*

N85.8 Other specified noninflammatory disorders of uterus
Atrophy of uterus, acquired
Fibrosis of uterus NOS

N85.9 Noninflammatory disorder of uterus, unspecified
Disorder of uterus NOS

N86 Erosion and ectropion of cervix uteri
Decubitus (trophic) ulcer of cervix
Eversion of cervix
EXCLUDES 1 *erosion and ectropion of cervix with cervicitis (N72)*

✓4th **N87 Dysplasia of cervix uteri**
EXCLUDES 1 *abnormal results from cervical cytologic examination without histologic confirmation (R87.61-)*
carcinoma in situ of cervix uteri (D06.-)
cervical intraepithelial neoplasia III [CIN III] (D06.-)
HGSIL of cervix (R87.613)
severe dysplasia of cervix uteri (D06.-)

N87.0 Mild cervical dysplasia
Cervical intraepithelial neoplasia I [CIN I]

N87.1 Moderate cervical dysplasia
Cervical intraepithelial neoplasia II [CIN II]

N87.9 Dysplasia of cervix uteri, unspecified
Anaplasia of cervix
Cervical atypism
Cervical dysplasia NOS

✓4th **N88 Other noninflammatory disorders of cervix uteri**
EXCLUDES 2 *inflammatory disease of cervix (N72)*
polyp of cervix (N84.1)

N88.0 Leukoplakia of cervix uteri

N88.1 Old laceration of cervix uteri
Adhesions of cervix
EXCLUDES 1 *current obstetric trauma (O71.3)*

N88.2 Stricture and stenosis of cervix uteri
EXCLUDES 1 *stricture and stenosis of cervix uteri complicating labor (O65.5)*

N88.3 Incompetence of cervix uteri
Investigation and management of (suspected) cervical incompetence in a nonpregnant woman
EXCLUDES 1 *cervical incompetence complicating pregnancy (O34.3-)*

N88.4 Hypertrophic elongation of cervix uteri

N88.8 Other specified noninflammatory disorders of cervix uteri
EXCLUDES 1 *current obstetric trauma (O71.3)*

N88.9 Noninflammatory disorder of cervix uteri, unspecified

✓4th **N89 Other noninflammatory disorders of vagina**
EXCLUDES 1 *abnormal results from vaginal cytologic examination without histologic confirmation (R87.62-)*
carcinoma in situ of vagina (D07.2)
HGSIL of vagina (R87.623)
inflammation of vagina (N76.-)
senile (atrophic) vaginitis (N95.2)
severe dysplasia of vagina (D07.2)
trichomonal leukorrhea (A59.00)
vaginal intraepithelial neoplasia [VAIN], grade III (D07.2)

N89.0 Mild vaginal dysplasia
Vaginal intraepithelial neoplasia [VAIN], grade I

N89.1 Moderate vaginal dysplasia
Vaginal intraepithelial neoplasia [VAIN], grade II

N89.3 Dysplasia of vagina, unspecified

N89.4 Leukoplakia of vagina

N89.5 Stricture and atresia of vagina
Vaginal adhesions
Vaginal stenosis
EXCLUDES 1 *congenital atresia or stricture (Q52.4)*
postprocedural adhesions of vagina (N99.2)

N89.6 Tight hymenal ring
Rigid hymen
Tight introitus
EXCLUDES 1 *imperforate hymen (Q52.3)*

N89.7 Hematocolpos
Hematocolpos with hematometra or hematosalpinx

N89.8 Other specified noninflammatory disorders of vagina
Leukorrhea NOS
Old vaginal laceration
Pessary ulcer of vagina
EXCLUDES 1 *current obstetric trauma (O70-, O71.4, O71.7-O71.8)*
old laceration involving muscles of pelvic floor (N81.8)

N89.9 Noninflammatory disorder of vagina, unspecified

✓4th **N90 Other noninflammatory disorders of vulva and perineum**
EXCLUDES 1 *anogenital (venereal) warts (A63.0)*
carcinoma in situ of vulva (D07.1)
condyloma acuminatum (A63.0)
current obstetric trauma (O70-, O71.7-O71.8)
inflammation of vulva (N76.-)
severe dysplasia of vulva (D07.1)
vulvar intraepithelial neoplasm III [VIN III] (D07.1)

N90.0 Mild vulvar dysplasia
Vulvar intraepithelial neoplasia [VIN], grade I

N90.1 Moderate vulvar dysplasia
Vulvar intraepithelial neoplasia [VIN], grade II

N90.3 Dysplasia of vulva, unspecified

N90.4 Leukoplakia of vulva
Dystrophy of vulva
Kraurosis of vulva
Lichen sclerosus of external female genital organs

N90.5 Atrophy of vulva
Stenosis of vulva

N90.6 Hypertrophy of vulva
Hypertrophy of labia

N90.7 Vulvar cyst

✓5th **N90.8 Other specified noninflammatory disorders of vulva and perineum**

✓6th **N90.81 Female genital mutilation status**
Female genital cutting status

N90.810 Female genital mutilation status, unspecified
Female genital cutting status, unspecified
Female genital mutilation status NOS

N90.811 Female genital mutilation Type I status
Clitorectomy status
Female genital cutting Type I status

N90.812 Female genital mutilation Type II status
Clitorectomy with excision of labia minora status
Female genital cutting Type II status

N90.813 Female genital mutilation Type III status
Female genital cutting Type III status
Infibulation status

N90.818 **Other female genital mutilation status**
Female genital cutting Type IV status
Female genital mutilation Type IV status
Other female genital cutting status

N90.89 **Other specified noninflammatory disorders of vulva and perineum**
Adhesions of vulva
Hypertrophy of clitoris

N90.9 **Noninflammatory disorder of vulva and perineum, unspecified**

N91 Absent, scanty and rare menstruation
EXCLUDES 1 *ovarian dysfunction (E28.-)*

N91.0 **Primary amenorrhea**
N91.1 **Secondary amenorrhea**
N91.2 **Amenorrhea, unspecified**
N91.3 **Primary oligomenorrhea**
N91.4 **Secondary oligomenorrhea**
N91.5 **Oligomenorrhea, unspecified**
Hypomenorrhea NOS

N92 Excessive, frequent and irregular menstruation
EXCLUDES 1 *postmenopausal bleeding (N95.0)*
precocious puberty (menstruation) (E30.1)

N92.0 **Excessive and frequent menstruation with regular cycle**
Heavy periods NOS
Menorrhagia NOS
Polymenorrhea

N92.1 **Excessive and frequent menstruation with irregular cycle**
Irregular intermenstrual bleeding
Irregular, shortened intervals between menstrual bleeding
Menometrorrhagia
Metrorrhagia

N92.2 **Excessive menstruation at puberty**
Excessive bleeding associated with onset of menstrual periods
Pubertal menorrhagia
Puberty bleeding

N92.3 **Ovulation bleeding**
Regular intermenstrual bleeding

N92.4 **Excessive bleeding in the premenopausal period**
Climacteric menorrhagia or metrorrhagia
Menopausal menorrhagia or metrorrhagia
Preclimacteric menorrhagia or metrorrhagia
Premenopausal menorrhagia or metrorrhagia

N92.5 **Other specified irregular menstruation**

N92.6 **Irregular menstruation, unspecified**
Irregular bleeding NOS
Irregular periods NOS
EXCLUDES 1 *irregular menstruation with:*
lengthened intervals or scanty bleeding (N91.3-N91.5)
shortened intervals or excessive bleeding (N92.1)

N93 Other abnormal uterine and vaginal bleeding
EXCLUDES 1 *neonatal vaginal hemorrhage (P54.6)*
precocious puberty (menstruation) (E30.1)
pseudomenses (P54.6)

N93.0 **Postcoital and contact bleeding**
N93.8 **Other specified abnormal uterine and vaginal bleeding**
Dysfunctional or functional uterine or vaginal bleeding NOS
N93.9 **Abnormal uterine and vaginal bleeding, unspecified**

N94 Pain and other conditions associated with female genital organs and menstrual cycle

N94.0 **Mittelschmerz**
N94.1 **Dyspareunia**
EXCLUDES 1 *psychogenic dyspareunia (F52.6)*
N94.2 **Vaginismus**
EXCLUDES 1 *psychogenic vaginismus (F52.5)*
N94.3 **Premenstrual tension syndrome**
Premenstrual dysphoric disorder
Code also associated menstrual migraine (G43.82-, G43.83-)
N94.4 **Primary dysmenorrhea**
N94.5 **Secondary dysmenorrhea**
N94.6 **Dysmenorrhea, unspecified**
EXCLUDES 1 *psychogenic dysmenorrhea (F45.8)*

N94.8 **Other specified conditions associated with female genital organs and menstrual cycle**
N94.81 **Vulvodynia**
N94.810 **Vulvar vestibulitis**
N94.818 **Other vulvodynia**
N94.819 **Vulvodynia, unspecified**
Vulvodynia NOS
N94.89 **Other specified conditions associated with female genital organs and menstrual cycle**
N94.9 **Unspecified condition associated with female genital organs and menstrual cycle**

N95 Menopausal and other perimenopausal disorders
Menopausal and other perimenopausal disorders due to naturally occurring (age-related) menopause and perimenopause
EXCLUDES 1 *excessive bleeding in the premenopausal period (N92.4)*
menopausal and perimenopausal disorders due to artificial or premature menopause (E89.4-, E28.31-)
premature menopause (E28.31-)
EXCLUDES 2 *postmenopausal osteoporosis (M81.0-)*
postmenopausal osteoporosis with current pathological fracture (M80.0-)
postmenopausal urethritis (N34.2)

N95.0 **Postmenopausal bleeding**
N95.1 **Menopausal and female climacteric states**
Symptoms such as flushing, sleeplessness, headache, lack of concentration, associated with natural (age-related) menopause
Use additional code for associated symptoms
EXCLUDES 1 *asymptomatic menopausal state (Z78.0)*
symptoms associated with artificial menopause (E89.41)
symptoms associated with premature menopause (E28.310)
N95.2 **Postmenopausal atrophic vaginitis**
Senile (atrophic) vaginitis
N95.8 **Other specified menopausal and perimenopausal disorders**
N95.9 **Unspecified menopausal and perimenopausal disorder**

N96 Recurrent pregnancy loss
Investigation or care in a nonpregnant woman with history of recurrent pregnancy loss
EXCLUDES 1 *recurrent pregnancy loss with current pregnancy (O26.2-)*

N97 Female infertility
INCLUDES inability to achieve a pregnancy
sterility, female NOS
EXCLUDES 1 *female infertility associated with:*
hypopituitarism (E23.0)
Stein-Leventhal syndrome (E28.2)
EXCLUDES 2 *incompetence of cervix uteri (N88.3)*

N97.0 **Female infertility associated with anovulation**
N97.1 **Female infertility of tubal origin**
Female infertility associated with congenital anomaly of tube
Female infertility due to tubal block
Female infertility due to tubal occlusion
Female infertility due to tubal stenosis
N97.2 **Female infertility of uterine origin**
Female infertility associated with congenital anomaly of uterus
Female infertility due to nonimplantation of ovum
N97.8 **Female infertility of other origin**
N97.9 **Female infertility, unspecified**

N98 Complications associated with artificial fertilization

N98.0 **Infection associated with artificial insemination**
N98.1 **Hyperstimulation of ovaries**
Hyperstimulation of ovaries NOS
Hyperstimulation of ovaries associated with induced ovulation
N98.2 **Complications of attempted introduction of fertilized ovum following in vitro fertilization**
N98.3 **Complications of attempted introduction of embryo in embryo transfer**
N98.8 **Other complications associated with artificial fertilization**
N98.9 **Complication associated with artificial fertilization, unspecified**

Intraoperative and postprocedural complications and disorders of genitourinary system, not elsewhere classified (N99)

✓4th **N99 Intraoperative and postprocedural complications and disorders of genitourinary system, not elsewhere classified**

EXCLUDES 2 *irradiation cystitis (N30.4-)*
postoophorectomy osteoporosis with current pathological fracture (M80.8-)
postoophorectomy osteoporosis without current pathological fracture (M81.8)

N99.0 Postprocedural (acute) (chronic) kidney failure
Use additional code to type of kidney disease

✓5th **N99.1 Postprocedural urethral stricture**
Postcatheterization urethral stricture

✓6th **N99.11 Postprocedural urethral stricture, male**
N99.110 Postprocedural urethral stricture, male, meatal
N99.111 Postprocedural bulbous urethral stricture
N99.112 Postprocedural membranous urethral stricture
N99.113 Postprocedural anterior urethral stricture
N99.114 Postprocedural urethral stricture, male, unspecified

N99.12 Postprocedural urethral stricture, female

N99.2 Postprocedural adhesions of vagina

N99.3 Prolapse of vaginal vault after hysterectomy

N99.4 Postprocedural pelvic peritoneal adhesions
EXCLUDES 2 *pelvic peritoneal adhesions NOS (N73.6)*
postinfective pelvic peritoneal adhesions (N73.6)

✓5th **N99.5 Complications of stoma of urinary tract**
EXCLUDES 2 *mechanical complication of urinary (indwelling) catheter (T83.0-)*

✓6th **N99.51 Complication of cystostomy**
N99.510 Cystostomy hemorrhage
N99.511 Cystostomy infection
N99.512 Cystostomy malfunction
N99.518 Other cystostomy complication

✓6th **N99.52 Complication of other external stoma of urinary tract**
N99.520 Hemorrhage of other external stoma of urinary tract
N99.521 Infection of other external stoma of urinary tract
N99.522 Malfunction of other external stoma of urinary tract
N99.528 Other complication of other external stoma of urinary tract

✓6th **N99.53 Complication of other stoma of urinary tract**
N99.530 Hemorrhage of other stoma of urinary tract
N99.531 Infection of other stoma of urinary tract
N99.532 Malfunction of other stoma of urinary tract
N99.538 Other complication of other stoma of urinary tract

✓5th **N99.6 Intraoperative hemorrhage and hematoma of a genitourinary system organ or structure complicating a procedure**
EXCLUDES 1 *intraoperative hemorrhage and hematoma of a genitourinary system organ or structure due to accidental puncture or laceration during a procedure (N99.7-)*

N99.61 Intraoperative hemorrhage and hematoma of a genitourinary system organ or structure complicating a genitourinary system procedure

N99.62 Intraoperative hemorrhage and hematoma of a genitourinary system organ or structure complicating other procedure

✓5th **N99.7 Accidental puncture and laceration of a genitourinary system organ or structure during a procedure**

N99.71 Accidental puncture and laceration of a genitourinary system organ or structure during a genitourinary system procedure

N99.72 Accidental puncture and laceration of a genitourinary system organ or structure during other procedure

✓5th **N99.8 Other intraoperative and postprocedural complications and disorders of genitourinary system**

N99.81 Other intraoperative complications of genitourinary system

✓6th **N99.82 Postprocedural hemorrhage and hematoma of a genitourinary system organ or structure following a procedure**
N99.820 Postprocedural hemorrhage and hematoma of a genitourinary system organ or structure following a genitourinary system procedure
N99.821 Postprocedural hemorrhage and hematoma of a genitourinary system organ or structure following other procedure

N99.83 Residual ovary syndrome

N99.89 Other postprocedural complications and disorders of genitourinary system

Chapter 15. Pregnancy, Childbirth and the Puerperium (O00-O9A)

NOTE CODES FROM THIS CHAPTER ARE FOR USE ONLY ON MATERNAL RECORDS, NEVER ON NEWBORN RECORDS.

Codes from this chapter are for use for conditions related to or aggravated by the pregnancy, childbirth, or by the puerperium (maternal causes or obstetric causes).

NOTE Trimesters are counted from the first day of the last menstrual period. They are defined as follows:

1st trimester- less than 14 weeks 0 days
2nd trimester- 14 weeks 0 days to less than 28 weeks 0 days
3rd trimester- 28 weeks 0 days until delivery

Use additional code from category Z3A, Weeks of gestation, to identify the specific week of the pregnancy

EXCLUDES 1 *supervision of normal pregnancy (Z34.-)*

EXCLUDES 2 *mental and behavioral disorders associated with the puerperium (F53)*
obstetrical tetanus (A34)
postpartum necrosis of pituitary gland (E23.0)
puerperal osteomalacia (M83.0)

This chapter contains the following blocks:

O00-O08	Pregnancy with abortive outcome
O09	Supervision of high risk pregnancy
O10-O16	Edema, proteinuria and hypertensive disorders in pregnancy, childbirth and the puerperium
O20-O29	Other maternal disorders predominantly related to pregnancy
O30-O48	Maternal care related to the fetus and amniotic cavity and possible delivery problems
O60-O77	Complications of labor and delivery
O80, O82	Encounter for delivery
O85-O92	Complications predominantly related to the puerperium
O94-O9A	Other obstetric conditions, not elsewhere classified

Pregnancy with abortive outcome (O00-O08)

EXCLUDES 1 *continuing pregnancy in multiple gestation after abortion of one fetus or more (O31.1-, O31.3-)*

✓4th O00 Ectopic pregnancy

INCLUDES ruptured ectopic pregnancy

Use additional code from category O08 to identify any associated complication

O00.0 Abdominal pregnancy

EXCLUDES 1 *maternal care for viable fetus in abdominal pregnancy (O36.7-)*

O00.1 Tubal pregnancy

Fallopian pregnancy
Rupture of (fallopian) tube due to pregnancy
Tubal abortion

O00.2 Ovarian pregnancy

O00.8 Other ectopic pregnancy

Cervical pregnancy
Cornual pregnancy
Intraligamentous pregnancy
Mural pregnancy

O00.9 Ectopic pregnancy, unspecified

✓4th O01 Hydatidiform mole

Use additional code from category O08 to identify any associated complication

EXCLUDES 1 *chorioadenoma (destruens) (D39.2)*
malignant hydatidiform mole (D39.2)

O01.0 Classical hydatidiform mole

Complete hydatidiform mole

O01.1 Incomplete and partial hydatidiform mole

O01.9 Hydatidiform mole, unspecified

Trophoblastic disease NOS
Vesicular mole NOS

✓4th O02 Other abnormal products of conception

Use additional code from category O08 to identify any associated complication

EXCLUDES 1 *papyraceous fetus (O31.0-)*

O02.0 Blighted ovum and nonhydatidiform mole

Carneous mole
Fleshy mole
Intrauterine mole NOS
Molar pregnancy NEC
Pathological ovum

O02.1 Missed abortion

Early fetal death, before completion of 20 weeks of gestation, with retention of dead fetus

EXCLUDES 1 *failed induced abortion (O07.-)*
fetal death (intrauterine) (late) (O36.4)
missed abortion with blighted ovum (O02.0)
missed abortion with hydatidiform mole (O01.-)
missed abortion with nonhydatidiform (O02.0)
missed abortion with other abnormal products of conception (O02.8-)
missed delivery (O36.4)
stillbirth (P95)

✓5th O02.8 Other specified abnormal products of conception

EXCLUDES 1 *abnormal products of conception with blighted ovum (O02.0)*
abnormal products of conception with hydatidiform mole (O01.-)
abnormal products of conception with nonhydatidiform mole (O02.0)

O02.81 Inappropriate change in quantitative human chorionic gonadotropin (hCG) in early pregnancy

Biochemical pregnancy
Chemical pregnancy
Inappropriate level of quantitative human chorionic gonadotropin (hCG) for gestational age in early pregnancy

O02.89 Other abnormal products of conception

O02.9 Abnormal product of conception, unspecified

✓4th O03 Spontaneous abortion

NOTE Incomplete abortion includes retained products of conception following spontaneous abortion

INCLUDES miscarriage

O03.0 Genital tract and pelvic infection following incomplete spontaneous abortion

Endometritis following incomplete spontaneous abortion
Oophoritis following incomplete spontaneous abortion
Parametritis following incomplete spontaneous abortion
Pelvic peritonitis following incomplete spontaneous abortion
Salpingitis following incomplete spontaneous abortion
Salpingo-oophoritis following incomplete spontaneous abortion

EXCLUDES 1 *sepsis following incomplete spontaneous abortion (O03.37)*
urinary tract infection following incomplete spontaneous abortion (O03.38)

O03.1 Delayed or excessive hemorrhage following incomplete spontaneous abortion

Afibrinogenemia following incomplete spontaneous abortion
Defibrination syndrome following incomplete spontaneous abortion
Hemolysis following incomplete spontaneous abortion
Intravascular coagulation following incomplete spontaneous abortion

O03.2 Embolism following incomplete spontaneous abortion

Air embolism following incomplete spontaneous abortion
Amniotic fluid embolism following incomplete spontaneous abortion
Blood-clot embolism following incomplete spontaneous abortion
Embolism NOS following incomplete spontaneous abortion
Fat embolism following incomplete spontaneous abortion
Pulmonary embolism following incomplete spontaneous abortion
Pyemic embolism following incomplete spontaneous abortion
Septic or septicopyemic embolism following incomplete spontaneous abortion
Soap embolism following incomplete spontaneous abortion

✓5th O03.3 Other and unspecified complications following incomplete spontaneous abortion

O03.30 Unspecified complication following incomplete spontaneous abortion

O03.31 Shock following incomplete spontaneous abortion

Circulatory collapse following incomplete spontaneous abortion
Shock (postprocedural) following incomplete spontaneous abortion

EXCLUDES 1 *shock due to infection following incomplete spontaneous abortion (O03.37)*

OØ3.32 Renal failure following incomplete spontaneous abortion
Kidney failure (acute) following incomplete spontaneous abortion
Oliguria following incomplete spontaneous abortion
Renal shutdown following incomplete spontaneous abortion
Renal tubular necrosis following incomplete spontaneous abortion
Uremia following incomplete spontaneous abortion

OØ3.33 Metabolic disorder following incomplete spontaneous abortion

OØ3.34 Damage to pelvic organs following incomplete spontaneous abortion
Laceration, perforation, tear or chemical damage of bladder following incomplete spontaneous abortion
Laceration, perforation, tear or chemical damage of bowel following incomplete spontaneous abortion
Laceration, perforation, tear or chemical damage of broad ligament following incomplete spontaneous abortion
Laceration, perforation, tear or chemical damage of cervix following incomplete spontaneous abortion
Laceration, perforation, tear or chemical damage of periurethral tissue following incomplete spontaneous abortion
Laceration, perforation, tear or chemical damage of uterus following incomplete spontaneous abortion
Laceration, perforation, tear or chemical damage of vagina following incomplete spontaneous abortion

OØ3.35 Other venous complications following incomplete spontaneous abortion

OØ3.36 Cardiac arrest following incomplete spontaneous abortion

OØ3.37 Sepsis following incomplete spontaneous abortion
Use additional code to identify infectious agent (B95-B97)
Use additional code to identify severe sepsis, if applicable (R65.2-)
EXCLUDES 1 *septic or septicopyemic embolism following incomplete spontaneous abortion (OØ3.2)*

OØ3.38 Urinary tract infection following incomplete spontaneous abortion
Cystitis following incomplete spontaneous abortion

OØ3.39 Incomplete spontaneous abortion with other complications

OØ3.4 Incomplete spontaneous abortion without complication

OØ3.5 Genital tract and pelvic infection following complete or unspecified spontaneous abortion
Endometritis following complete or unspecified spontaneous abortion
Oophoritis following complete or unspecified spontaneous abortion
Parametritis following complete or unspecified spontaneous abortion
Pelvic peritonitis following complete or unspecified spontaneous abortion
Salpingitis following complete or unspecified spontaneous abortion
Salpingo-oophoritis following complete or unspecified spontaneous abortion
EXCLUDES 1 *sepsis following complete or unspecified spontaneous abortion (OØ3.87)*
urinary tract infection following complete or unspecified spontaneous abortion (OØ3.88)

OØ3.6 Delayed or excessive hemorrhage following complete or unspecified spontaneous abortion
Afibrinogenemia following complete or unspecified spontaneous abortion
Defibrination syndrome following complete or unspecified spontaneous abortion
Hemolysis following complete or unspecified spontaneous abortion
Intravascular coagulation following complete or unspecified spontaneous abortion

OØ3.7 Embolism following complete or unspecified spontaneous abortion
Air embolism following complete or unspecified spontaneous abortion
Amniotic fluid embolism following complete or unspecified spontaneous abortion
Blood-clot embolism following complete or unspecified spontaneous abortion
Embolism NOS following complete or unspecified spontaneous abortion
Fat embolism following complete or unspecified spontaneous abortion
Pulmonary embolism following complete or unspecified spontaneous abortion
Pyemic embolism following complete or unspecified spontaneous abortion
Septic or septicopyemic embolism following complete or unspecified spontaneous abortion
Soap embolism following complete or unspecified spontaneous abortion

✓5th **OØ3.8 Other and unspecified complications following complete or unspecified spontaneous abortion**

OØ3.8Ø Unspecified complication following complete or unspecified spontaneous abortion

OØ3.81 Shock following complete or unspecified spontaneous abortion
Circulatory collapse following complete or unspecified spontaneous abortion
Shock (postprocedural) following complete or unspecified spontaneous abortion
EXCLUDES 1 *shock due to infection following complete or unspecified spontaneous abortion (OØ3.87)*

OØ3.82 Renal failure following complete or unspecified spontaneous abortion
Kidney failure (acute) following complete or unspecified spontaneous abortion
Oliguria following complete or unspecified spontaneous abortion
Renal shutdown following complete or unspecified spontaneous abortion
Renal tubular necrosis following complete or unspecified spontaneous abortion
Uremia following complete or unspecified spontaneous abortion

OØ3.83 Metabolic disorder following complete or unspecified spontaneous abortion

OØ3.84 Damage to pelvic organs following complete or unspecified spontaneous abortion
Laceration, perforation, tear or chemical damage of bladder following complete or unspecified spontaneous abortion
Laceration, perforation, tear or chemical damage of bowel following complete or unspecified spontaneous abortion
Laceration, perforation, tear or chemical damage of broad ligament following complete or unspecified spontaneous abortion
Laceration, perforation, tear or chemical damage of cervix following complete or unspecified spontaneous abortion
Laceration, perforation, tear or chemical damage of periurethral tissue following complete or unspecified spontaneous abortion
Laceration, perforation, tear or chemical damage of uterus following complete or unspecified spontaneous abortion
Laceration, perforation, tear or chemical damage of vagina following complete or unspecified spontaneous abortion

OØ3.85 Other venous complications following complete or unspecified spontaneous abortion

O03.86 Cardiac arrest following complete or unspecified spontaneous abortion

O03.87 Sepsis following complete or unspecified spontaneous abortion
Use additional code to identify infectious agent (B95-B97)
Use additional code to identify severe sepsis, if applicable (R65.2-)
EXCLUDES 1 *septic or septicopyemic embolism following complete or unspecified spontaneous abortion (O03.7)*

O03.88 Urinary tract infection following complete or unspecified spontaneous abortion
Cystitis following complete or unspecified spontaneous abortion

O03.89 Complete or unspecified spontaneous abortion with other complications

O03.9 Complete or unspecified spontaneous abortion without complication
Miscarriage NOS
Spontaneous abortion NOS

✓4th O04 Complications following (induced) termination of pregnancy
INCLUDES complications following (induced) termination of pregnancy
EXCLUDES 1 *encounter for elective termination of pregnancy, uncomplicated (Z33.2)*
failed attempted termination of pregnancy (O07.-)

O04.5 Genital tract and pelvic infection following (induced) termination of pregnancy
Endometritis following (induced) termination of pregnancy
Oophoritis following (induced) termination of pregnancy
Parametritis following (induced) termination of pregnancy
Pelvic peritonitis following (induced) termination of pregnancy
Salpingitis following (induced) termination of pregnancy
Salpingo-oophoritis following (induced) termination of pregnancy
EXCLUDES 1 *sepsis following (induced) termination of pregnancy (O04.87)*
urinary tract infection following (induced) termination of pregnancy (O04.88)

O04.6 Delayed or excessive hemorrhage following (induced) termination of pregnancy
Afibrinogenemia following (induced) termination of pregnancy
Defibrination syndrome following (induced) termination of pregnancy
Hemolysis following (induced) termination of pregnancy
Intravascular coagulation following (induced) termination of pregnancy

O04.7 Embolism following (induced) termination of pregnancy
Air embolism following (induced) termination of pregnancy
Amniotic fluid embolism following (induced) termination of pregnancy
Blood-clot embolism following (induced) termination of pregnancy
Embolism NOS following (induced) termination of pregnancy
Fat embolism following (induced) termination of pregnancy
Pulmonary embolism following (induced) termination of pregnancy
Pyemic embolism following (induced) termination of pregnancy
Septic or septicopyemic embolism following (induced) termination of pregnancy
Soap embolism following (induced) termination of pregnancy

✓5th O04.8 (Induced) termination of pregnancy with other and unspecified complications

O04.80 (Induced) termination of pregnancy with unspecified complications

O04.81 Shock following (induced) termination of pregnancy
Circulatory collapse following (induced) termination of pregnancy
Shock (postprocedural) following (induced) termination of pregnancy
EXCLUDES 1 *shock due to infection following (induced) termination of pregnancy (O04.87)*

O04.82 Renal failure following (induced) termination of pregnancy
Kidney failure (acute) following (induced) termination of pregnancy
Oliguria following (induced) termination of pregnancy
Renal shutdown following (induced) termination of pregnancy
Renal tubular necrosis following (induced) termination of pregnancy
Uremia following (induced) termination of pregnancy

O04.83 Metabolic disorder following (induced) termination of pregnancy

O04.84 Damage to pelvic organs following (induced) termination of pregnancy
Laceration, perforation, tear or chemical damage of bladder following (induced) termination of pregnancy
Laceration, perforation, tear or chemical damage of bowel following (induced) termination of pregnancy
Laceration, perforation, tear or chemical damage of broad ligament following (induced) termination of pregnancy
Laceration, perforation, tear or chemical damage of cervix following (induced) termination of pregnancy
Laceration, perforation, tear or chemical damage of periurethral tissue following (induced) termination of pregnancy
Laceration, perforation, tear or chemical damage of uterus following (induced) termination of pregnancy
Laceration, perforation, tear or chemical damage of vagina following (induced) termination of pregnancy

O04.85 Other venous complications following (induced) termination of pregnancy

O04.86 Cardiac arrest following (induced) termination of pregnancy

O04.87 Sepsis following (induced) termination of pregnancy
Use additional code to identify infectious agent (B95-B97)
Use additional code to identify severe sepsis, if applicable (R65.2-)
EXCLUDES 1 *septic or septicopyemic embolism following (induced) termination of pregnancy (O04.7)*

O04.88 Urinary tract infection following (induced) termination of pregnancy
Cystitis following (induced) termination of pregnancy

O04.89 (Induced) termination of pregnancy with other complications

✓4th O07 Failed attempted termination of pregnancy
INCLUDES failure of attempted induction of termination of pregnancy
incomplete elective abortion
EXCLUDES 1 *incomplete spontaneous abortion (O03.0-)*

O07.0 Genital tract and pelvic infection following failed attempted termination of pregnancy
Endometritis following failed attempted termination of pregnancy
Oophoritis following failed attempted termination of pregnancy
Parametritis following failed attempted termination of pregnancy
Pelvic peritonitis following failed attempted termination of pregnancy
Salpingitis following failed attempted termination of pregnancy
Salpingo-oophoritis following failed attempted termination of pregnancy
EXCLUDES 1 *sepsis following failed attempted termination of pregnancy (O07.37)*
urinary tract infection following failed attempted termination of pregnancy (O07.38)

O07.1 Delayed or excessive hemorrhage following failed attempted termination of pregnancy
Afibrinogenemia following failed attempted termination of pregnancy
Defibrination syndrome following failed attempted termination of pregnancy
Hemolysis following failed attempted termination of pregnancy
Intravascular coagulation following failed attempted termination of pregnancy

O07.2 Embolism following failed attempted termination of pregnancy
Air embolism following failed attempted termination of pregnancy
Amniotic fluid embolism following failed attempted termination of pregnancy
Blood-clot embolism following failed attempted termination of pregnancy
Embolism NOS following failed attempted termination of pregnancy
Fat embolism following failed attempted termination of pregnancy
Pulmonary embolism following failed attempted termination of pregnancy
Pyemic embolism following failed attempted termination of pregnancy
Septic or septicopyemic embolism following failed attempted termination of pregnancy
Soap embolism following failed attempted termination of pregnancy

✓5th **O07.3 Failed attempted termination of pregnancy with other and unspecified complications**

O07.30 Failed attempted termination of pregnancy with unspecified complications

O07.31 Shock following failed attempted termination of pregnancy
Circulatory collapse following failed attempted termination of pregnancy
Shock (postprocedural) following failed attempted termination of pregnancy
EXCLUDES 1 *shock due to infection following failed attempted termination of pregnancy (O07.37)*

O07.32 Renal failure following failed attempted termination of pregnancy
Kidney failure (acute) following failed attempted termination of pregnancy
Oliguria following failed attempted termination of pregnancy
Renal shutdown following failed attempted termination of pregnancy
Renal tubular necrosis following failed attempted termination of pregnancy
Uremia following failed attempted termination of pregnancy

O07.33 Metabolic disorder following failed attempted termination of pregnancy

O07.34 Damage to pelvic organs following failed attempted termination of pregnancy
Laceration, perforation, tear or chemical damage of bladder following failed attempted termination of pregnancy
Laceration, perforation, tear or chemical damage of bowel following failed attempted termination of pregnancy
Laceration, perforation, tear or chemical damage of broad ligament following failed attempted termination of pregnancy
Laceration, perforation, tear or chemical damage of cervix following failed attempted termination of pregnancy
Laceration, perforation, tear or chemical damage of periurethral tissue following failed attempted termination of pregnancy
Laceration, perforation, tear or chemical damage of uterus following failed attempted termination of pregnancy
Laceration, perforation, tear or chemical damage of vagina following failed attempted termination of pregnancy

O07.35 Other venous complications following failed attempted termination of pregnancy

O07.36 Cardiac arrest following failed attempted termination of pregnancy

O07.37 Sepsis following failed attempted termination of pregnancy
Use additional code to identify infectious agent (B95-B97)
Use additional code to identify severe sepsis, if applicable (R65.2-)
EXCLUDES 1 *septic or septicopyemic embolism following failed attempted termination of pregnancy (O07.2)*

O07.38 Urinary tract infection following failed attempted termination of pregnancy
Cystitis following failed attempted termination of pregnancy

O07.39 Failed attempted termination of pregnancy with other complications

O07.4 Failed attempted termination of pregnancy without complication

✓4th **O08 Complications following ectopic and molar pregnancy**
This category is for use with categories O00-O02 to identify any associated complications

O08.0 Genital tract and pelvic infection following ectopic and molar pregnancy
Endometritis following ectopic and molar pregnancy
Oophoritis following ectopic and molar pregnancy
Parametritis following ectopic and molar pregnancy
Pelvic peritonitis following ectopic and molar pregnancy
Salpingitis following ectopic and molar pregnancy
Salpingo-oophoritis following ectopic and molar pregnancy
EXCLUDES 1 *sepsis following ectopic and molar pregnancy (O08.82)*
urinary tract infection (O08.83)

O08.1 Delayed or excessive hemorrhage following ectopic and molar pregnancy
Afibrinogenemia following ectopic and molar pregnancy
Defibrination syndrome following ectopic and molar pregnancy
Hemolysis following ectopic and molar pregnancy
Intravascular coagulation following ectopic and molar pregnancy
EXCLUDES 1 *delayed or excessive hemorrhage due to incomplete abortion (O03.1)*

O08.2 Embolism following ectopic and molar pregnancy
Air embolism following ectopic and molar pregnancy
Amniotic fluid embolism following ectopic and molar pregnancy
Blood-clot embolism following ectopic and molar pregnancy
Embolism NOS following ectopic and molar pregnancy
Fat embolism following ectopic and molar pregnancy
Pulmonary embolism following ectopic and molar pregnancy
Pyemic embolism following ectopic and molar pregnancy
Septic or septicopyemic embolism following ectopic and molar pregnancy
Soap embolism following ectopic and molar pregnancy

O08.3 Shock following ectopic and molar pregnancy
Circulatory collapse following ectopic and molar pregnancy
Shock (postprocedural) following ectopic and molar pregnancy
EXCLUDES 1 *shock due to infection following ectopic and molar pregnancy (O08.82)*

O08.4 Renal failure following ectopic and molar pregnancy
Kidney failure (acute) following ectopic and molar pregnancy
Oliguria following ectopic and molar pregnancy
Renal shutdown following ectopic and molar pregnancy
Renal tubular necrosis following ectopic and molar pregnancy
Uremia following ectopic and molar pregnancy

O08.5 Metabolic disorders following an ectopic and molar pregnancy

O08.6 Damage to pelvic organs and tissues following an ectopic and molar pregnancy
Laceration, perforation, tear or chemical damage of bladder following an ectopic and molar pregnancy
Laceration, perforation, tear or chemical damage of bowel following an ectopic and molar pregnancy
Laceration, perforation, tear or chemical damage of broad ligament following an ectopic and molar pregnancy
Laceration, perforation, tear or chemical damage of cervix following an ectopic and molar pregnancy
Laceration, perforation, tear or chemical damage of periurethral tissue following an ectopic and molar pregnancy
Laceration, perforation, tear or chemical damage of uterus following an ectopic and molar pregnancy
Laceration, perforation, tear or chemical damage of vagina following an ectopic and molar pregnancy

O08.7 Other venous complications following an ectopic and molar pregnancy

✓5th **O08.8 Other complications following an ectopic and molar pregnancy**

O08.81 Cardiac arrest following an ectopic and molar pregnancy

O08.82 Sepsis following ectopic and molar pregnancy
Use additional code to identify infectious agent (B95-B97)
Use additional code to identify severe sepsis, if applicable (R65.2-)
EXCLUDES 1 *septic or septicopyemic embolism following ectopic and molar pregnancy (O08.2)*

O08.83 Urinary tract infection following an ectopic and molar pregnancy
Cystitis following an ectopic and molar pregnancy

O08.89 Other complications following an ectopic and molar pregnancy

O08.9 Unspecified complication following an ectopic and molar pregnancy

Supervision of high risk pregnancy (O09)

✓4th **O09 Supervision of high risk pregnancy**

✓5th **O09.0 Supervision of pregnancy with history of infertility**

O09.00 Supervision of pregnancy with history of infertility, unspecified trimester

O09.01 Supervision of pregnancy with history of infertility, first trimester

O09.02 Supervision of pregnancy with history of infertility, second trimester

O09.03 Supervision of pregnancy with history of infertility, third trimester

✓5th **O09.1 Supervision of pregnancy with history of ectopic or molar pregnancy**

O09.10 Supervision of pregnancy with history of ectopic or molar pregnancy, unspecified trimester

O09.11 Supervision of pregnancy with history of ectopic or molar pregnancy, first trimester

O09.12 Supervision of pregnancy with history of ectopic or molar pregnancy, second trimester

O09.13 Supervision of pregnancy with history of ectopic or molar pregnancy, third trimester

✓5th **O09.2 Supervision of pregnancy with other poor reproductive or obstetric history**
EXCLUDES 2 *pregnancy care for patient with history of recurrent pregnancy loss (O26.2-)*

✓6th **O09.21 Supervision of pregnancy with history of pre-term labor**

O09.211 Supervision of pregnancy with history of pre-term labor, first trimester

O09.212 Supervision of pregnancy with history of pre-term labor, second trimester

O09.213 Supervision of pregnancy with history of pre-term labor, third trimester

O09.219 Supervision of pregnancy with history of pre-term labor, unspecified trimester

✓6th **O09.29 Supervision of pregnancy with other poor reproductive or obstetric history**
Supervision of pregnancy with history of neonatal death
Supervision of pregnancy with history of stillbirth

O09.291 Supervision of pregnancy with other poor reproductive or obstetric history, first trimester

O09.292 Supervision of pregnancy with other poor reproductive or obstetric history, second trimester

O09.293 Supervision of pregnancy with other poor reproductive or obstetric history, third trimester

O09.299 Supervision of pregnancy with other poor reproductive or obstetric history, unspecified trimester

✓5th **O09.3 Supervision of pregnancy with insufficient antenatal care**
Supervision of concealed pregnancy
Supervision of hidden pregnancy

O09.30 Supervision of pregnancy with insufficient antenatal care, unspecified trimester

O09.31 Supervision of pregnancy with insufficient antenatal care, first trimester

O09.32 Supervision of pregnancy with insufficient antenatal care, second trimester

O09.33 Supervision of pregnancy with insufficient antenatal care, third trimester

✓5th **O09.4 Supervision of pregnancy with grand multiparity**

O09.40 Supervision of pregnancy with grand multiparity, unspecified trimester

O09.41 Supervision of pregnancy with grand multiparity, first trimester

O09.42 Supervision of pregnancy with grand multiparity, second trimester

O09.43 Supervision of pregnancy with grand multiparity, third trimester

✓5th **O09.5 Supervision of elderly primigravida and multigravida**
Pregnancy for a female 35 years and older at expected date of delivery

✓6th **O09.51 Supervision of elderly primigravida**

O09.511 Supervision of elderly primigravida, first trimester

O09.512 Supervision of elderly primigravida, second trimester

O09.513 Supervision of elderly primigravida, third trimester

O09.519 Supervision of elderly primigravida, unspecified trimester

✓6th **O09.52 Supervision of elderly multigravida**

O09.521 Supervision of elderly multigravida, first trimester

O09.522 Supervision of elderly multigravida, second trimester

O09.523 Supervision of elderly multigravida, third trimester

O09.529 Supervision of elderly multigravida, unspecified trimester

✓5th **O09.6 Supervision of young primigravida and multigravida**
Supervision of pregnancy for a female less than 16 years old at expected date of delivery

✓6th **O09.61 Supervision of young primigravida**

O09.611 Supervision of young primigravida, first trimester

O09.612 Supervision of young primigravida, second trimester

O09.613 Supervision of young primigravida, third trimester

O09.619 Supervision of young primigravida, unspecified trimester

✓6th **O09.62 Supervision of young multigravida**

O09.621 Supervision of young multigravida, first trimester

O09.622 Supervision of young multigravida, second trimester

O09.623 Supervision of young multigravida, third trimester

O09.629 Supervision of young multigravida, unspecified trimester

✓5th **O09.7 Supervision of high risk pregnancy due to social problems**

O09.70 Supervision of high risk pregnancy due to social problems, unspecified trimester

O09.71 Supervision of high risk pregnancy due to social problems, first trimester

O09.72 Supervision of high risk pregnancy due to social problems, second trimester

O09.73 Supervision of high risk pregnancy due to social problems, third trimester

✓5th **O09.8 Supervision of other high risk pregnancies**

✓6th **O09.81 Supervision of pregnancy resulting from assisted reproductive technology**

Supervision of pregnancy resulting from in-vitro fertilization

O09.811 Supervision of pregnancy resulting from assisted reproductive technology, first trimester

O09.812 Supervision of pregnancy resulting from assisted reproductive technology, second trimester

O09.813 Supervision of pregnancy resulting from assisted reproductive technology, third trimester

O09.819 Supervision of pregnancy resulting from assisted reproductive technology, unspecified trimester

✓6th **O09.82 Supervision of pregnancy with history of in utero procedure during previous pregnancy**

O09.821 Supervision of pregnancy with history of in utero procedure during previous pregnancy, first trimester

O09.822 Supervision of pregnancy with history of in utero procedure during previous pregnancy, second trimester

O09.823 Supervision of pregnancy with history of in utero procedure during previous pregnancy, third trimester

O09.829 Supervision of pregnancy with history of in utero procedure during previous pregnancy, unspecified trimester

EXCLUDES 1 *supervision of pregnancy affected by in utero procedure during current pregnancy (O35.7)*

✓6th **O09.89 Supervision of other high risk pregnancies**

O09.891 Supervision of other high risk pregnancies, first trimester

O09.892 Supervision of other high risk pregnancies, second trimester

O09.893 Supervision of other high risk pregnancies, third trimester

O09.899 Supervision of other high risk pregnancies, unspecified trimester

✓5th **O09.9 Supervision of high risk pregnancy, unspecified**

O09.90 Supervision of high risk pregnancy, unspecified, unspecified trimester

O09.91 Supervision of high risk pregnancy, unspecified, first trimester

O09.92 Supervision of high risk pregnancy, unspecified, second trimester

O09.93 Supervision of high risk pregnancy, unspecified, third trimester

Edema, proteinuria and hypertensive disorders in pregnancy, childbirth and the puerperium (O10-O16)

✓4th **O10 Pre-existing hypertension complicating pregnancy, childbirth and the puerperium**

Pre-existing hypertension with pre-existing proteinuria complicating pregnancy, childbirth and the puerperium

EXCLUDES 2 *pre-existing hypertension with superimposed pre-eclampsia complicating pregnancy, childbirth and the puerperium (O11.-)*

✓5th **O10.0 Pre-existing essential hypertension complicating pregnancy, childbirth and the puerperium**

Any condition in I10 specified as a reason for obstetric care during pregnancy, childbirth or the puerperium

✓6th **O10.01 Pre-existing essential hypertension complicating pregnancy,**

O10.011 Pre-existing essential hypertension complicating pregnancy, first trimester

O10.012 Pre-existing essential hypertension complicating pregnancy, second trimester

O10.013 Pre-existing essential hypertension complicating pregnancy, third trimester

O10.019 Pre-existing essential hypertension complicating pregnancy, unspecified trimester

O10.02 Pre-existing essential hypertension complicating childbirth

O10.03 Pre-existing essential hypertension complicating the puerperium

✓5th **O10.1 Pre-existing hypertensive heart disease complicating pregnancy, childbirth and the puerperium**

Any condition in I11 specified as a reason for obstetric care during pregnancy, childbirth or the puerperium

Use additional code from I11 to identify the type of hypertensive heart disease

✓6th **O10.11 Pre-existing hypertensive heart disease complicating pregnancy**

O10.111 Pre-existing hypertensive heart disease complicating pregnancy, first trimester

O10.112 Pre-existing hypertensive heart disease complicating pregnancy, second trimester

O10.113 Pre-existing hypertensive heart disease complicating pregnancy, third trimester

O10.119 Pre-existing hypertensive heart disease complicating pregnancy, unspecified trimester

O10.12 Pre-existing hypertensive heart disease complicating childbirth

O10.13 Pre-existing hypertensive heart disease complicating the puerperium

✓5th **O10.2 Pre-existing hypertensive chronic kidney disease complicating pregnancy, childbirth and the puerperium**

Any condition in I12 specified as a reason for obstetric care during pregnancy, childbirth or the puerperium

Use additional code from I12 to identify the type of hypertensive chronic kidney disease

✓6th **O10.21 Pre-existing hypertensive chronic kidney disease complicating pregnancy**

O10.211 Pre-existing hypertensive chronic kidney disease complicating pregnancy, first trimester

O10.212 Pre-existing hypertensive chronic kidney disease complicating pregnancy, second trimester

O10.213 Pre-existing hypertensive chronic kidney disease complicating pregnancy, third trimester

O10.219 Pre-existing hypertensive chronic kidney disease complicating pregnancy, unspecified trimester

O10.22 Pre-existing hypertensive chronic kidney disease complicating childbirth

O10.23 Pre-existing hypertensive chronic kidney disease complicating the puerperium

EXCLUDES 1 Not coded here EXCLUDES 2 Not included here **Manifestation Code**

O10.3 Pre-existing hypertensive heart and chronic kidney disease complicating pregnancy, childbirth and the puerperium
Any condition in I13 specified as a reason for obstetric care during pregnancy, childbirth or the puerperium
Use additional code from I13 to identify the type of hypertensive heart and chronic kidney disease

O10.31 Pre-existing hypertensive heart and chronic kidney disease complicating pregnancy
O10.311 Pre-existing hypertensive heart and chronic kidney disease complicating pregnancy, first trimester
O10.312 Pre-existing hypertensive heart and chronic kidney disease complicating pregnancy, second trimester
O10.313 Pre-existing hypertensive heart and chronic kidney disease complicating pregnancy, third trimester
O10.319 Pre-existing hypertensive heart and chronic kidney disease complicating pregnancy, unspecified trimester
O10.32 Pre-existing hypertensive heart and chronic kidney disease complicating childbirth
O10.33 Pre-existing hypertensive heart and chronic kidney disease complicating the puerperium

O10.4 Pre-existing secondary hypertension complicating pregnancy, childbirth and the puerperium
Any condition in I15 specified as a reason for obstetric care during pregnancy, childbirth or the puerperium
Use additional code from I15 to identify the type of secondary hypertension

O10.41 Pre-existing secondary hypertension complicating pregnancy
O10.411 Pre-existing secondary hypertension complicating pregnancy, first trimester
O10.412 Pre-existing secondary hypertension complicating pregnancy, second trimester
O10.413 Pre-existing secondary hypertension complicating pregnancy, third trimester
O10.419 Pre-existing secondary hypertension complicating pregnancy, unspecified trimester
O10.42 Pre-existing secondary hypertension complicating childbirth
O10.43 Pre-existing secondary hypertension complicating the puerperium

O10.9 Unspecified pre-existing hypertension complicating pregnancy, childbirth and the puerperium
O10.91 Unspecified pre-existing hypertension complicating pregnancy
O10.911 Unspecified pre-existing hypertension complicating pregnancy, first trimester
O10.912 Unspecified pre-existing hypertension complicating pregnancy, second trimester
O10.913 Unspecified pre-existing hypertension complicating pregnancy, third trimester
O10.919 Unspecified pre-existing hypertension complicating pregnancy, unspecified trimester
O10.92 Unspecified pre-existing hypertension complicating childbirth
O10.93 Unspecified pre-existing hypertension complicating the puerperium

O11 Pre-existing hypertension with pre-eclampsia
Conditions in O10 complicated by pre-eclampsia
Pre-eclampsia superimposed pre-existing hypertension
Use additional code from O10 to identify the type of hypertension
O11.1 Pre-existing hypertension with pre-eclampsia, first trimester
O11.2 Pre-existing hypertension with pre-eclampsia, second trimester
O11.3 Pre-existing hypertension with pre-eclampsia, third trimester
O11.9 Pre-existing hypertension with pre-eclampsia, unspecified trimester

O12 Gestational [pregnancy-induced] edema and proteinuria without hypertension
O12.0 Gestational edema
O12.00 Gestational edema, unspecified trimester
O12.01 Gestational edema, first trimester
O12.02 Gestational edema, second trimester
O12.03 Gestational edema, third trimester
O12.1 Gestational proteinuria
O12.10 Gestational proteinuria, unspecified trimester
O12.11 Gestational proteinuria, first trimester
O12.12 Gestational proteinuria, second trimester
O12.13 Gestational proteinuria, third trimester
O12.2 Gestational edema with proteinuria
O12.20 Gestational edema with proteinuria, unspecified trimester
O12.21 Gestational edema with proteinuria, first trimester
O12.22 Gestational edema with proteinuria, second trimester
O12.23 Gestational edema with proteinuria, third trimester

O13 Gestational [pregnancy-induced] hypertension without significant proteinuria
INCLUDES gestational hypertension NOS
O13.1 Gestational [pregnancy-induced] hypertension without significant proteinuria, first trimester
O13.2 Gestational [pregnancy-induced] hypertension without significant proteinuria, second trimester
O13.3 Gestational [pregnancy-induced] hypertension without significant proteinuria, third trimester
O13.9 Gestational [pregnancy-induced] hypertension without significant proteinuria, unspecified trimester

O14 Pre-eclampsia
EXCLUDES 1 *pre-existing hypertension with pre-eclampsia (O11)*
O14.0 Mild to moderate pre-eclampsia
O14.00 Mild to moderate pre-eclampsia, unspecified trimester
O14.02 Mild to moderate pre-eclampsia, second trimester
O14.03 Mild to moderate pre-eclampsia, third trimester
O14.1 Severe pre-eclampsia
EXCLUDES 1 *HELLP syndrome (O14.2-)*
O14.10 Severe pre-eclampsia, unspecified trimester
O14.12 Severe pre-eclampsia, second trimester
O14.13 Severe pre-eclampsia, third trimester
O14.2 HELLP syndrome
Severe pre-eclampsia with hemolysis, elevated liver enzymes and low platelet count (HELLP)
O14.20 HELLP syndrome (HELLP), unspecified trimester
O14.22 HELLP syndrome (HELLP), second trimester
O14.23 HELLP syndrome (HELLP), third trimester
O14.9 Unspecified pre-eclampsia
O14.90 Unspecified pre-eclampsia, unspecified trimester
O14.92 Unspecified pre-eclampsia, second trimester
O14.93 Unspecified pre-eclampsia, third trimester

O15 Eclampsia
INCLUDES convulsions following conditions in O10-O14 and O16
O15.0 Eclampsia in pregnancy
O15.00 Eclampsia in pregnancy, unspecified trimester
O15.02 Eclampsia in pregnancy, second trimester
O15.03 Eclampsia in pregnancy, third trimester
O15.1 Eclampsia in labor
O15.2 Eclampsia in the puerperium
O15.9 Eclampsia, unspecified as to time period
Eclampsia NOS

O16 Unspecified maternal hypertension
O16.1 Unspecified maternal hypertension, first trimester
O16.2 Unspecified maternal hypertension, second trimester
O16.3 Unspecified maternal hypertension, third trimester
O16.9 Unspecified maternal hypertension, unspecified trimester

Other maternal disorders predominantly related to pregnancy (O20-O29)

EXCLUDES 2 *maternal care related to the fetus and amniotic cavity and possible delivery problems (O30-O48)*
maternal diseases classifiable elsewhere but complicating pregnancy, labor and delivery, and the puerperium (O98-O99)

✓4th **O20 Hemorrhage in early pregnancy**
Hemorrhage before completion of 20 weeks gestation
EXCLUDES 1 *pregnancy with abortive outcome (O00-O08)*

O20.0 Threatened abortion
Hemorrhage specified as due to threatened abortion

O20.8 Other hemorrhage in early pregnancy

O20.9 Hemorrhage in early pregnancy, unspecified

✓4th **O21 Excessive vomiting in pregnancy**

O21.0 Mild hyperemesis gravidarum
Hyperemesis gravidarum, mild or unspecified, starting before the end of the 20th week of gestation

O21.1 Hyperemesis gravidarum with metabolic disturbance
Hyperemesis gravidarum, starting before the end of the 20th week of gestation, with metabolic disturbance such as carbohydrate depletion
Hyperemesis gravidarum, starting before the end of the 20th week of gestation, with metabolic disturbance such as dehydration
Hyperemesis gravidarum, starting before the end of the 20th week of gestation, with metabolic disturbance such as electrolyte imbalance

O21.2 Late vomiting of pregnancy
Excessive vomiting starting after 20 completed weeks of gestation

O21.8 Other vomiting complicating pregnancy
Vomiting due to diseases classified elsewhere, complicating pregnancy
Use additional code, to identify cause

O21.9 Vomiting of pregnancy, unspecified

✓4th **O22 Venous complications and hemorrhoids in pregnancy**
EXCLUDES 1 *venous complications of:*
abortion NOS (O03.9)
ectopic or molar pregnancy (O08.7)
failed attempted abortion (O07.35)
induced abortion (O04.85)
spontaneous abortion (O03.89)
EXCLUDES 2 *obstetric pulmonary embolism (O88.-)*
venous complications and hemorrhoids of childbirth and the puerperium (O87.-)

✓5th **O22.0 Varicose veins of lower extremity in pregnancy**
Varicose veins NOS in pregnancy

O22.00 Varicose veins of lower extremity in pregnancy, unspecified trimester

O22.01 Varicose veins of lower extremity in pregnancy, first trimester

O22.02 Varicose veins of lower extremity in pregnancy, second trimester

O22.03 Varicose veins of lower extremity in pregnancy, third trimester

✓5th **O22.1 Genital varices in pregnancy**
Perineal varices in pregnancy
Vaginal varices in pregnancy
Vulval varices in pregnancy

O22.10 Genital varices in pregnancy, unspecified trimester

O22.11 Genital varices in pregnancy, first trimester

O22.12 Genital varices in pregnancy, second trimester

O22.13 Genital varices in pregnancy, third trimester

✓5th **O22.2 Superficial thrombophlebitis in pregnancy**
Phlebitis in pregnancy NOS
Thrombophlebitis of legs in pregnancy
Thrombosis in pregnancy NOS
Use additional code to identify the superficial thrombophlebitis (I80.0-)

O22.20 Superficial thrombophlebitis in pregnancy, unspecified trimester

O22.21 Superficial thrombophlebitis in pregnancy, first trimester

O22.22 Superficial thrombophlebitis in pregnancy, second trimester

O22.23 Superficial thrombophlebitis in pregnancy, third trimester

✓5th **O22.3 Deep phlebothrombosis in pregnancy**
Deep vein thrombosis, antepartum
Use additional code to identify the deep vein thrombosis (I82.4-, I82.5-, I82.62-, I82.72-)
Use additional code, if applicable, for associated long-term (current) use of anticoagulants (Z79.01)

O22.30 Deep phlebothrombosis in pregnancy, unspecified trimester

O22.31 Deep phlebothrombosis in pregnancy, first trimester

O22.32 Deep phlebothrombosis in pregnancy, second trimester

O22.33 Deep phlebothrombosis in pregnancy, third trimester

✓5th **O22.4 Hemorrhoids in pregnancy**

O22.40 Hemorrhoids in pregnancy, unspecified trimester

O22.41 Hemorrhoids in pregnancy, first trimester

O22.42 Hemorrhoids in pregnancy, second trimester

O22.43 Hemorrhoids in pregnancy, third trimester

✓5th **O22.5 Cerebral venous thrombosis in pregnancy**
Cerebrovenous sinus thrombosis in pregnancy

O22.50 Cerebral venous thrombosis in pregnancy, unspecified trimester

O22.51 Cerebral venous thrombosis in pregnancy, first trimester

O22.52 Cerebral venous thrombosis in pregnancy, second trimester

O22.53 Cerebral venous thrombosis in pregnancy, third trimester

✓5th **O22.8 Other venous complications in pregnancy**

✓6th **O22.8X Other venous complications in pregnancy**

O22.8X1 Other venous complications in pregnancy, first trimester

O22.8X2 Other venous complications in pregnancy, second trimester

O22.8X3 Other venous complications in pregnancy, third trimester

O22.8X9 Other venous complications in pregnancy, unspecified trimester

✓5th **O22.9 Venous complication in pregnancy, unspecified**
Gestational phlebitis NOS
Gestational phlebopathy NOS
Gestational thrombosis NOS

O22.90 Venous complication in pregnancy, unspecified, unspecified trimester

O22.91 Venous complication in pregnancy, unspecified, first trimester

O22.92 Venous complication in pregnancy, unspecified, second trimester

O22.93 Venous complication in pregnancy, unspecified, third trimester

✓4th **O23 Infections of genitourinary tract in pregnancy**
Use additional code to identify organism (B95.-, B96.-)
EXCLUDES 2 *gonococcal infections complicating pregnancy, childbirth and the puerperium (O98.2)*
infections with a predominantly sexual mode of transmission NOS complicating pregnancy, childbirth and the puerperium (O98.3)
syphilis complicating pregnancy, childbirth and the puerperium (O98.1)
tuberculosis of genitourinary system complicating pregnancy, childbirth and the puerperium (O98.0)
venereal disease NOS complicating pregnancy, childbirth and the puerperium (O98.3)

✓5th **O23.0 Infections of kidney in pregnancy**
Pyelonephritis in pregnancy

O23.00 Infections of kidney in pregnancy, unspecified trimester

O23.01 Infections of kidney in pregnancy, first trimester

O23.02 Infections of kidney in pregnancy, second trimester

O23.03 Infections of kidney in pregnancy, third trimester

✓5th **O23.1 Infections of bladder in pregnancy**

O23.10 Infections of bladder in pregnancy, unspecified trimester

O23.11 Infections of bladder in pregnancy, first trimester

O23.12 Infections of bladder in pregnancy, second trimester

O23.13 Infections of bladder in pregnancy, third trimester

✓5th O23.2 Infections of urethra in pregnancy

O23.20 Infections of urethra in pregnancy, unspecified trimester

O23.21 Infections of urethra in pregnancy, first trimester

O23.22 Infections of urethra in pregnancy, second trimester

O23.23 Infections of urethra in pregnancy, third trimester

✓5th O23.3 Infections of other parts of urinary tract in pregnancy

O23.30 Infections of other parts of urinary tract in pregnancy, unspecified trimester

O23.31 Infections of other parts of urinary tract in pregnancy, first trimester

O23.32 Infections of other parts of urinary tract in pregnancy, second trimester

O23.33 Infections of other parts of urinary tract in pregnancy, third trimester

✓5th O23.4 Unspecified infection of urinary tract in pregnancy

O23.40 Unspecified infection of urinary tract in pregnancy, unspecified trimester

O23.41 Unspecified infection of urinary tract in pregnancy, first trimester

O23.42 Unspecified infection of urinary tract in pregnancy, second trimester

O23.43 Unspecified infection of urinary tract in pregnancy, third trimester

✓5th O23.5 Infections of the genital tract in pregnancy

✓6th O23.51 Infection of cervix in pregnancy

O23.511 Infections of cervix in pregnancy, first trimester

O23.512 Infections of cervix in pregnancy, second trimester

O23.513 Infections of cervix in pregnancy, third trimester

O23.519 Infections of cervix in pregnancy, unspecified trimester

✓6th O23.52 Salpingo-oophoritis in pregnancy

Oophoritis in pregnancy

Salpingitis in pregnancy

O23.521 Salpingo-oophoritis in pregnancy, first trimester

O23.522 Salpingo-oophoritis in pregnancy, second trimester

O23.523 Salpingo-oophoritis in pregnancy, third trimester

O23.529 Salpingo-oophoritis in pregnancy, unspecified trimester

✓6th O23.59 Infection of other part of genital tract in pregnancy

O23.591 Infection of other part of genital tract in pregnancy, first trimester

O23.592 Infection of other part of genital tract in pregnancy, second trimester

O23.593 Infection of other part of genital tract in pregnancy, third trimester

O23.599 Infection of other part of genital tract in pregnancy, unspecified trimester

✓5th O23.9 Unspecified genitourinary tract infection in pregnancy

Genitourinary tract infection in pregnancy NOS

O23.90 Unspecified genitourinary tract infection in pregnancy, unspecified trimester

O23.91 Unspecified genitourinary tract infection in pregnancy, first trimester

O23.92 Unspecified genitourinary tract infection in pregnancy, second trimester

O23.93 Unspecified genitourinary tract infection in pregnancy, third trimester

✓4th O24 Diabetes mellitus in pregnancy, childbirth, and the puerperium

✓5th O24.0 Pre-existing diabetes mellitus, type 1, in pregnancy, childbirth and the puerperium

Juvenile onset diabetes mellitus, in pregnancy, childbirth and the puerperium

Ketosis-prone diabetes mellitus in pregnancy, childbirth and the puerperium

Use additional code from category E10 to further identify any manifestations

✓6th O24.01 Pre-existing diabetes mellitus, type 1, in pregnancy

O24.011 Pre-existing diabetes mellitus, type 1, in pregnancy, first trimester

O24.012 Pre-existing diabetes mellitus, type 1, in pregnancy, second trimester

O24.013 Pre-existing diabetes mellitus, type 1, in pregnancy, third trimester

O24.019 Pre-existing diabetes mellitus, type 1, in pregnancy, unspecified trimester

O24.02 Pre-existing diabetes mellitus, type 1, in childbirth

O24.03 Pre-existing diabetes mellitus, type 1, in the puerperium

✓5th O24.1 Pre-existing diabetes mellitus, type 2, in pregnancy, childbirth and the puerperium

Insulin-resistant diabetes mellitus in pregnancy, childbirth and the puerperium

Use additional code (for):

from category E11 to further identify any manifestations

long-term (current) use of insulin (Z79.4)

✓6th O24.11 Pre-existing diabetes mellitus, type 2, in pregnancy

O24.111 Pre-existing diabetes mellitus, type 2, in pregnancy, first trimester

O24.112 Pre-existing diabetes mellitus, type 2, in pregnancy, second trimester

O24.113 Pre-existing diabetes mellitus, type 2, in pregnancy, third trimester

O24.119 Pre-existing diabetes mellitus, type 2, in pregnancy, unspecified trimester

O24.12 Pre-existing diabetes mellitus, type 2, in childbirth

O24.13 Pre-existing diabetes mellitus, type 2, in the puerperium

✓5th O24.3 Unspecified pre-existing diabetes mellitus in pregnancy, childbirth and the puerperium

Use additional code (for):

from category E11 to further identify any manifestation

long-term (current) use of insulin (Z79.4)

✓6th O24.31 Unspecified pre-existing diabetes mellitus in pregnancy

O24.311 Unspecified pre-existing diabetes mellitus in pregnancy, first trimester

O24.312 Unspecified pre-existing diabetes mellitus in pregnancy, second trimester

O24.313 Unspecified pre-existing diabetes mellitus in pregnancy, third trimester

O24.319 Unspecified pre-existing diabetes mellitus in pregnancy, unspecified trimester

O24.32 Unspecified pre-existing diabetes mellitus in childbirth

O24.33 Unspecified pre-existing diabetes mellitus in the puerperium

✓5th O24.4 Gestational diabetes mellitus

Diabetes mellitus arising in pregnancy

Gestational diabetes mellitus NOS

✓6th O24.41 Gestational diabetes mellitus in pregnancy

O24.410 Gestational diabetes mellitus in pregnancy, diet controlled

O24.414 Gestational diabetes mellitus in pregnancy, insulin controlled

O24.419 Gestational diabetes mellitus in pregnancy, unspecified control

✓6th O24.42 Gestational diabetes mellitus in childbirth

O24.420 Gestational diabetes mellitus in childbirth, diet controlled

O24.424 Gestational diabetes mellitus in childbirth, insulin controlled

O24.429 Gestational diabetes mellitus in childbirth, unspecified control

✓6th **O24.43 Gestational diabetes mellitus in the puerperium**

O24.430 Gestational diabetes mellitus in the puerperium, diet controlled

O24.434 Gestational diabetes mellitus in the puerperium, insulin controlled

O24.439 Gestational diabetes mellitus in the puerperium, unspecified control

✓5th **O24.8 Other pre-existing diabetes mellitus in pregnancy, childbirth, and the puerperium**

Use additional code (for):

from categories E08, E09 and E13 to further identify any manifestation

long-term (current) use of insulin (Z79.4)

✓6th **O24.81 Other pre-existing diabetes mellitus in pregnancy**

O24.811 Other pre-existing diabetes mellitus in pregnancy, first trimester

O24.812 Other pre-existing diabetes mellitus in pregnancy, second trimester

O24.813 Other pre-existing diabetes mellitus in pregnancy, third trimester

O24.819 Other pre-existing diabetes mellitus in pregnancy, unspecified trimester

O24.82 Other pre-existing diabetes mellitus in childbirth

O24.83 Other pre-existing diabetes mellitus in the puerperium

✓5th **O24.9 Unspecified diabetes mellitus in pregnancy, childbirth and the puerperium**

Use additional code for long-term (current) use of insulin (Z79.4)

✓6th **O24.91 Unspecified diabetes mellitus in pregnancy**

O24.911 Unspecified diabetes mellitus in pregnancy, first trimester

O24.912 Unspecified diabetes mellitus in pregnancy, second trimester

O24.913 Unspecified diabetes mellitus in pregnancy, third trimester

O24.919 Unspecified diabetes mellitus in pregnancy, unspecified trimester

O24.92 Unspecified diabetes mellitus in childbirth

O24.93 Unspecified diabetes mellitus in the puerperium

✓4th **O25 Malnutrition in pregnancy, childbirth and the puerperium**

✓5th **O25.1 Malnutrition in pregnancy**

O25.10 Malnutrition in pregnancy, unspecified trimester

O25.11 Malnutrition in pregnancy, first trimester

O25.12 Malnutrition in pregnancy, second trimester

O25.13 Malnutrition in pregnancy, third trimester

O25.2 Malnutrition in childbirth

O25.3 Malnutrition in the puerperium

✓4th **O26 Maternal care for other conditions predominantly related to pregnancy**

✓5th **O26.0 Excessive weight gain in pregnancy**

EXCLUDES 2 *gestational edema (O12.0, O12.2)*

O26.00 Excessive weight gain in pregnancy, unspecified trimester

O26.01 Excessive weight gain in pregnancy, first trimester

O26.02 Excessive weight gain in pregnancy, second trimester

O26.03 Excessive weight gain in pregnancy, third trimester

✓5th **O26.1 Low weight gain in pregnancy**

O26.10 Low weight gain in pregnancy, unspecified trimester

O26.11 Low weight gain in pregnancy, first trimester

O26.12 Low weight gain in pregnancy, second trimester

O26.13 Low weight gain in pregnancy, third trimester

✓5th **O26.2 Pregnancy care for patient with recurrent pregnancy loss**

O26.20 Pregnancy care for patient with recurrent pregnancy loss, unspecified trimester

O26.21 Pregnancy care for patient with recurrent pregnancy loss, first trimester

O26.22 Pregnancy care for patient with recurrent pregnancy loss, second trimester

O26.23 Pregnancy care for patient with recurrent pregnancy loss, third trimester

✓5th **O26.3 Retained intrauterine contraceptive device in pregnancy**

O26.30 Retained intrauterine contraceptive device in pregnancy, unspecified trimester

O26.31 Retained intrauterine contraceptive device in pregnancy, first trimester

O26.32 Retained intrauterine contraceptive device in pregnancy, second trimester

O26.33 Retained intrauterine contraceptive device in pregnancy, third trimester

✓5th **O26.4 Herpes gestationis**

O26.40 Herpes gestationis, unspecified trimester

O26.41 Herpes gestationis, first trimester

O26.42 Herpes gestationis, second trimester

O26.43 Herpes gestationis, third trimester

✓5th **O26.5 Maternal hypotension syndrome**

Supine hypotensive syndrome

O26.50 Maternal hypotension syndrome, unspecified trimester

O26.51 Maternal hypotension syndrome, first trimester

O26.52 Maternal hypotension syndrome, second trimester

O26.53 Maternal hypotension syndrome, third trimester

✓5th **O26.6 Liver and biliary tract disorders in pregnancy, childbirth and the puerperium**

Use additional code to identify the specific disorder

EXCLUDES 2 *hepatorenal syndrome following labor and delivery (O90.4)*

✓6th **O26.61 Liver and biliary tract disorders in pregnancy**

O26.611 Liver and biliary tract disorders in pregnancy, first trimester

O26.612 Liver and biliary tract disorders in pregnancy, second trimester

O26.613 Liver and biliary tract disorders in pregnancy, third trimester

O26.619 Liver and biliary tract disorders in pregnancy, unspecified trimester

O26.62 Liver and biliary tract disorders in childbirth

O26.63 Liver and biliary tract disorders in the puerperium

✓5th **O26.7 Subluxation of symphysis (pubis) in pregnancy, childbirth and the puerperium**

EXCLUDES 1 *traumatic separation of symphysis (pubis) during childbirth (O71.6)*

✓6th **O26.71 Subluxation of symphysis (pubis) in pregnancy**

O26.711 Subluxation of symphysis (pubis) in pregnancy, first trimester

O26.712 Subluxation of symphysis (pubis) in pregnancy, second trimester

O26.713 Subluxation of symphysis (pubis) in pregnancy, third trimester

O26.719 Subluxation of symphysis (pubis) in pregnancy, unspecified trimester

O26.72 Subluxation of symphysis (pubis) in childbirth

O26.73 Subluxation of symphysis (pubis) in the puerperium

✓5th **O26.8 Other specified pregnancy related conditions**

✓6th **O26.81 Pregnancy related exhaustion and fatigue**

O26.811 Pregnancy related exhaustion and fatigue, first trimester

O26.812 Pregnancy related exhaustion and fatigue, second trimester

O26.813 Pregnancy related exhaustion and fatigue, third trimester

O26.819 Pregnancy related exhaustion and fatigue, unspecified trimester

✓6th **O26.82 Pregnancy related peripheral neuritis**

O26.821 Pregnancy related peripheral neuritis, first trimester

O26.822 Pregnancy related peripheral neuritis, second trimester

O26.823 Pregnancy related peripheral neuritis, third trimester

O26.829 Pregnancy related peripheral neuritis, unspecified trimester

✓6th **O26.83 Pregnancy related renal disease**

Use additional code to identify the specific disorder

O26.831 Pregnancy related renal disease, first trimester

O26.832 Pregnancy related renal disease, second trimester

O26.833 Pregnancy related renal disease, third trimester

O26.839 Pregnancy related renal disease, unspecified trimester

√6th **O26.84 Uterine size-date discrepancy complicating pregnancy**

EXCLUDES 1 *encounter for suspected problem with fetal growth ruled out (Z03.74)*

O26.841 Uterine size-date discrepancy, first trimester

O26.842 Uterine size-date discrepancy, second trimester

O26.843 Uterine size-date discrepancy, third trimester

O26.849 Uterine size-date discrepancy, unspecified trimester

√6th **O26.85 Spotting complicating pregnancy**

O26.851 Spotting complicating pregnancy, first trimester

O26.852 Spotting complicating pregnancy, second trimester

O26.853 Spotting complicating pregnancy, third trimester

O26.859 Spotting complicating pregnancy, unspecified trimester

O26.86 Pruritic urticarial papules and plaques of pregnancy (PUPPP)

Polymorphic eruption of pregnancy

√6th **O26.87 Cervical shortening**

EXCLUDES 1 *encounter for suspected cervical shortening ruled out (Z03.75)*

O26.872 Cervical shortening, second trimester

O26.873 Cervical shortening, third trimester

O26.879 Cervical shortening, unspecified trimester

√6th **O26.89 Other specified pregnancy related conditions**

O26.891 Other specified pregnancy related conditions, first trimester

O26.892 Other specified pregnancy related conditions, second trimester

O26.893 Other specified pregnancy related conditions, third trimester

O26.899 Other specified pregnancy related conditions, unspecified trimester

√5th **O26.9 Pregnancy related conditions, unspecified**

O26.90 Pregnancy related conditions, unspecified, unspecified trimester

O26.91 Pregnancy related conditions, unspecified, first trimester

O26.92 Pregnancy related conditions, unspecified, second trimester

O26.93 Pregnancy related conditions, unspecified, third trimester

√4th **O28 Abnormal findings on antenatal screening of mother**

EXCLUDES 1 *diagnostic findings classified elsewhere—see Alphabetical Index*

O28.0 Abnormal hematological finding on antenatal screening of mother

O28.1 Abnormal biochemical finding on antenatal screening of mother

O28.2 Abnormal cytological finding on antenatal screening of mother

O28.3 Abnormal ultrasonic finding on antenatal screening of mother

O28.4 Abnormal radiological finding on antenatal screening of mother

O28.5 Abnormal chromosomal and genetic finding on antenatal screening of mother

O28.8 Other abnormal findings on antenatal screening of mother

O28.9 Unspecified abnormal findings on antenatal screening of mother

√4th **O29 Complications of anesthesia during pregnancy**

INCLUDES maternal complications arising from the administration of a general, regional or local anesthetic, analgesic or other sedation during pregnancy

Use additional code, if necessary, to identify the complication

EXCLUDES 2 *complications of anesthesia during labor and delivery (O74.-)*
complications of anesthesia during the puerperium (O89.-)

√5th **O29.0 Pulmonary complications of anesthesia during pregnancy**

√6th **O29.01 Aspiration pneumonitis due to anesthesia during pregnancy**

Inhalation of stomach contents or secretions NOS due to anesthesia during pregnancy

Mendelson's syndrome due to anesthesia during pregnancy

O29.011 Aspiration pneumonitis due to anesthesia during pregnancy, first trimester

O29.012 Aspiration pneumonitis due to anesthesia during pregnancy, second trimester

O29.013 Aspiration pneumonitis due to anesthesia during pregnancy, third trimester

O29.019 Aspiration pneumonitis due to anesthesia during pregnancy, unspecified trimester

√6th **O29.02 Pressure collapse of lung due to anesthesia during pregnancy**

O29.021 Pressure collapse of lung due to anesthesia during pregnancy, first trimester

O29.022 Pressure collapse of lung due to anesthesia during pregnancy, second trimester

O29.023 Pressure collapse of lung due to anesthesia during pregnancy, third trimester

O29.029 Pressure collapse of lung due to anesthesia during pregnancy, unspecified trimester

√6th **O29.09 Other pulmonary complications of anesthesia during pregnancy**

O29.091 Other pulmonary complications of anesthesia during pregnancy, first trimester

O29.092 Other pulmonary complications of anesthesia during pregnancy, second trimester

O29.093 Other pulmonary complications of anesthesia during pregnancy, third trimester

O29.099 Other pulmonary complications of anesthesia during pregnancy, unspecified trimester

√5th **O29.1 Cardiac complications of anesthesia during pregnancy**

√6th **O29.11 Cardiac arrest due to anesthesia during pregnancy**

O29.111 Cardiac arrest due to anesthesia during pregnancy, first trimester

O29.112 Cardiac arrest due to anesthesia during pregnancy, second trimester

O29.113 Cardiac arrest due to anesthesia during pregnancy, third trimester

O29.119 Cardiac arrest due to anesthesia during pregnancy, unspecified trimester

√6th **O29.12 Cardiac failure due to anesthesia during pregnancy**

O29.121 Cardiac failure due to anesthesia during pregnancy, first trimester

O29.122 Cardiac failure due to anesthesia during pregnancy, second trimester

O29.123 Cardiac failure due to anesthesia during pregnancy, third trimester

O29.129 Cardiac failure due to anesthesia during pregnancy, unspecified trimester

√6th **O29.19 Other cardiac complications of anesthesia during pregnancy**

O29.191 Other cardiac complications of anesthesia during pregnancy, first trimester

O29.192 **Other cardiac complications of anesthesia during pregnancy, second trimester**

O29.193 **Other cardiac complications of anesthesia during pregnancy, third trimester**

O29.199 **Other cardiac complications of anesthesia during pregnancy, unspecified trimester**

5th **O29.2** **Central nervous system complications of anesthesia during pregnancy**

6th **O29.21** **Cerebral anoxia due to anesthesia during pregnancy**

O29.211 **Cerebral anoxia due to anesthesia during pregnancy, first trimester**

O29.212 **Cerebral anoxia due to anesthesia during pregnancy, second trimester**

O29.213 **Cerebral anoxia due to anesthesia during pregnancy, third trimester**

O29.219 **Cerebral anoxia due to anesthesia during pregnancy, unspecified trimester**

6th **O29.29** **Other central nervous system complications of anesthesia during pregnancy**

O29.291 **Other central nervous system complications of anesthesia during pregnancy, first trimester**

O29.292 **Other central nervous system complications of anesthesia during pregnancy, second trimester**

O29.293 **Other central nervous system complications of anesthesia during pregnancy, third trimester**

O29.299 **Other central nervous system complications of anesthesia during pregnancy, unspecified trimester**

5th **O29.3** **Toxic reaction to local anesthesia during pregnancy**

6th **O29.3X** **Toxic reaction to local anesthesia during pregnancy**

O29.3X1 **Toxic reaction to local anesthesia during pregnancy, first trimester**

O29.3X2 **Toxic reaction to local anesthesia during pregnancy, second trimester**

O29.3X3 **Toxic reaction to local anesthesia during pregnancy, third trimester**

O29.3X9 **Toxic reaction to local anesthesia during pregnancy, unspecified trimester**

5th **O29.4** **Spinal and epidural anesthesia induced headache during pregnancy**

O29.4Ø **Spinal and epidural anesthesia induced headache during pregnancy, unspecified trimester**

O29.41 **Spinal and epidural anesthesia induced headache during pregnancy, first trimester**

O29.42 **Spinal and epidural anesthesia induced headache during pregnancy, second trimester**

O29.43 **Spinal and epidural anesthesia induced headache during pregnancy, third trimester**

5th **O29.5** **Other complications of spinal and epidural anesthesia during pregnancy**

6th **O29.5X** **Other complications of spinal and epidural anesthesia during pregnancy**

O29.5X1 **Other complications of spinal and epidural anesthesia during pregnancy, first trimester**

O29.5X2 **Other complications of spinal and epidural anesthesia during pregnancy, second trimester**

O29.5X3 **Other complications of spinal and epidural anesthesia during pregnancy, third trimester**

O29.5X9 **Other complications of spinal and epidural anesthesia during pregnancy, unspecified trimester**

5th **O29.6** **Failed or difficult intubation for anesthesia during pregnancy**

O29.6Ø **Failed or difficult intubation for anesthesia during pregnancy, unspecified trimester**

O29.61 **Failed or difficult intubation for anesthesia during pregnancy, first trimester**

O29.62 **Failed or difficult intubation for anesthesia during pregnancy, second trimester**

O29.63 **Failed or difficult intubation for anesthesia during pregnancy, third trimester**

5th **O29.8** **Other complications of anesthesia during pregnancy**

6th **O29.8X** **Other complications of anesthesia during pregnancy**

O29.8X1 **Other complications of anesthesia during pregnancy, first trimester**

O29.8X2 **Other complications of anesthesia during pregnancy, second trimester**

O29.8X3 **Other complications of anesthesia during pregnancy, third trimester**

O29.8X9 **Other complications of anesthesia during pregnancy, unspecified trimester**

5th **O29.9** **Unspecified complication of anesthesia during pregnancy**

O29.9Ø **Unspecified complication of anesthesia during pregnancy, unspecified trimester**

O29.91 **Unspecified complication of anesthesia during pregnancy, first trimester**

O29.92 **Unspecified complication of anesthesia during pregnancy, second trimester**

O29.93 **Unspecified complication of anesthesia during pregnancy, third trimester**

Maternal care related to the fetus and amniotic cavity and possible delivery problems (O3Ø-O48)

4th **O3Ø** **Multiple gestation**

Code also any complications specific to multiple gestation

5th **O3Ø.Ø** **Twin pregnancy**

6th **O3Ø.ØØ** **Twin pregnancy, unspecified number of placenta and unspecified number of amniotic sacs**

O3Ø.ØØ1 **Twin pregnancy, unspecified number of placenta and unspecified number of amniotic sacs, first trimester**

O3Ø.ØØ2 **Twin pregnancy, unspecified number of placenta and unspecified number of amniotic sacs, second trimester**

O3Ø.ØØ3 **Twin pregnancy, unspecified number of placenta and unspecified number of amniotic sacs, third trimester**

O3Ø.ØØ9 **Twin pregnancy, unspecified number of placenta and unspecified number of amniotic sacs, unspecified trimester**

6th **O3Ø.Ø1** **Twin pregnancy, monochorionic/monoamniotic**

Twin pregnancy, one placenta, one amniotic sac

EXCLUDES 1 *conjoined twins (O3Ø.Ø2-)*

O3Ø.Ø11 **Twin pregnancy, monochorionic/monoamniotic, first trimester**

O3Ø.Ø12 **Twin pregnancy, monochorionic/monoamniotic, second trimester**

O3Ø.Ø13 **Twin pregnancy, monochorionic/monoamniotic, third trimester**

O3Ø.Ø19 **Twin pregnancy, monochorionic/monoamniotic, unspecified trimester**

6th **O3Ø.Ø2** **Conjoined twin pregnancy**

O3Ø.Ø21 **Conjoined twin pregnancy, first trimester**

O3Ø.Ø22 **Conjoined twin pregnancy, second trimester**

O3Ø.Ø23 **Conjoined twin pregnancy, third trimester**

O3Ø.Ø29 **Conjoined twin pregnancy, unspecified trimester**

6th **O3Ø.Ø3** **Twin pregnancy, monochorionic/diamniotic**

Twin pregnancy, one placenta, two amniotic sacs

O3Ø.Ø31 **Twin pregnancy, monochorionic/diamniotic, first trimester**

O3Ø.Ø32 **Twin pregnancy, monochorionic/diamniotic, second trimester**

O3Ø.Ø33 **Twin pregnancy, monochorionic/diamniotic, third trimester**

O3Ø.Ø39 **Twin pregnancy, monochorionic/diamniotic, unspecified trimester**

✓6th O3Ø.Ø4 Twin pregnancy, dichorionic/diamniotic
Twin pregnancy, two placentae, two amniotic sacs
O3Ø.Ø41 Twin pregnancy, dichorionic/diamniotic, first trimester
O3Ø.Ø42 Twin pregnancy, dichorionic/diamniotic, second trimester
O3Ø.Ø43 Twin pregnancy, dichorionic/diamniotic, third trimester
O3Ø.Ø49 Twin pregnancy, dichorionic/diamniotic, unspecified trimester

✓6th O3Ø.Ø9 Twin pregnancy, unable to determine number of placenta and number of amniotic sacs
O3Ø.Ø91 Twin pregnancy, unable to determine number of placenta and number of amniotic sacs, first trimester
O3Ø.Ø92 Twin pregnancy, unable to determine number of placenta and number of amniotic sacs, second trimester
O3Ø.Ø93 Twin pregnancy, unable to determine number of placenta and number of amniotic sacs, third trimester
O3Ø.Ø99 Twin pregnancy, unable to determine number of placenta and number of amniotic sacs, unspecified trimester

✓5th O3Ø.1 Triplet pregnancy, unspecified number of placenta and unspecified number of amniotic sacs

✓6th O3Ø.1Ø Triplet pregnancy, unspecified number of placenta and unspecified number of amniotic sacs
O3Ø.1Ø1 Triplet pregnancy, unspecified number of placenta and unspecified number of amniotic sacs, first trimester
O3Ø.1Ø2 Triplet pregnancy, unspecified number of placenta and unspecified number of amniotic sacs, second trimester
O3Ø.1Ø3 Triplet pregnancy, unspecified number of placenta and unspecified number of amniotic sacs, third trimester
O3Ø.1Ø9 Triplet pregnancy, unspecified number of placenta and unspecified number of amniotic sacs, unspecified trimester

✓6th O3Ø.11 Triplet pregnancy with two or more monochorionic fetuses
O3Ø.111 Triplet pregnancy with two or more monochorionic fetuses, first trimester
O3Ø.112 Triplet pregnancy with two or more monochorionic fetuses, second trimester
O3Ø.113 Triplet pregnancy with two or more monochorionic fetuses, third trimester
O3Ø.119 Triplet pregnancy with two or more monochorionic fetuses, unspecified trimester

✓6th O3Ø.12 Triplet pregnancy with two or more monoamniotic fetuses
O3Ø.121 Triplet pregnancy with two or more monoamniotic fetuses, first trimester
O3Ø.122 Triplet pregnancy with two or more monoamniotic fetuses, second trimester
O3Ø.123 Triplet pregnancy with two or more monoamniotic fetuses, third trimester
O3Ø.129 Triplet pregnancy with two or more monoamniotic fetuses, unspecified trimester

✓6th O3Ø.19 Triplet pregnancy, unable to determine number of placenta and number of amniotic sacs
O3Ø.191 Triplet pregnancy, unable to determine number of placenta and number of amniotic sacs, first trimester
O3Ø.192 Triplet pregnancy, unable to determine number of placenta and number of amniotic sacs, second trimester
O3Ø.193 Triplet pregnancy, unable to determine number of placenta and number of amniotic sacs, third trimester
O3Ø.199 Triplet pregnancy, unable to determine number of placenta and number of amniotic sacs, unspecified trimester

✓6th O3Ø.2 Quadruplet pregnancy

✓6th O3Ø.2Ø Quadruplet pregnancy, unspecified number of placenta and unspecified number of amniotic sacs
O3Ø.2Ø1 Quadruplet pregnancy, unspecified number of placenta and unspecified number of amniotic sacs, first trimester
O3Ø.2Ø2 Quadruplet pregnancy, unspecified number of placenta and unspecified number of amniotic sacs, second trimester
O3Ø.2Ø3 Quadruplet pregnancy, unspecified number of placenta and unspecified number of amniotic sacs, third trimester
O3Ø.2Ø9 Quadruplet pregnancy, unspecified number of placenta and unspecified number of amniotic sacs, unspecified trimester

✓6th O3Ø.21 Quadruplet pregnancy with two or more monochorionic fetuses
O3Ø.211 Quadruplet pregnancy with two or more monochorionic fetuses, first trimester
O3Ø.212 Quadruplet pregnancy with two or more monochorionic fetuses, second trimester
O3Ø.213 Quadruplet pregnancy with two or more monochorionic fetuses, third trimester
O3Ø.219 Quadruplet pregnancy with two or more monochorionic fetuses, unspecified trimester

✓6th O3Ø.22 Quadruplet pregnancy with two or more monoamniotic fetuses
O3Ø.221 Quadruplet pregnancy with two or more monoamniotic fetuses, first trimester
O3Ø.222 Quadruplet pregnancy with two or more monoamniotic fetuses, second trimester
O3Ø.223 Quadruplet pregnancy with two or more monoamniotic fetuses, third trimester
O3Ø.229 Quadruplet pregnancy with two or more monoamniotic fetuses, unspecified trimester

✓6th O3Ø.29 Quadruplet pregnancy, unable to determine number of placenta and number of amniotic sacs
O3Ø.291 Quadruplet pregnancy, unable to determine number of placenta and number of amniotic sacs, first trimester
O3Ø.292 Quadruplet pregnancy, unable to determine number of placenta and number of amniotic sacs, second trimester
O3Ø.293 Quadruplet pregnancy, unable to determine number of placenta and number of amniotic sacs, third trimester
O3Ø.299 Quadruplet pregnancy, unable to determine number of placenta and number of amniotic sacs, unspecified trimester

✓5th O3Ø.8 Other specified multiple gestation
Multiple gestation pregnancy greater than quadruplets

✓6th O3Ø.8Ø Other specified multiple gestation, unspecified number of placenta and unspecified number of amniotic sacs
O3Ø.8Ø1 Other specified multiple gestation, unspecified number of placenta and unspecified number of amniotic sacs, first trimester
O3Ø.8Ø2 Other specified multiple gestation, unspecified number of placenta and unspecified number of amniotic sacs, second trimester
O3Ø.8Ø3 Other specified multiple gestation, unspecified number of placenta and unspecified number of amniotic sacs, third trimester
O3Ø.8Ø9 Other specified multiple gestation, unspecified number of placenta and unspecified number of amniotic sacs, unspecified trimester

√6th **O3Ø.81 Other specified multiple gestation with two or more monochorionic fetuses**

O3Ø.811 Other specified multiple gestation with two or more monochorionic fetuses, first trimester

O3Ø.812 Other specified multiple gestation with two or more monochorionic fetuses, second trimester

O3Ø.813 Other specified multiple gestation with two or more monochorionic fetuses, third trimester

O3Ø.819 Other specified multiple gestation with two or more monochorionic fetuses, unspecified trimester

√6th **O3Ø.82 Other specified multiple gestation with two or more monoamniotic fetuses**

O3Ø.821 Other specified multiple gestation with two or more monoamniotic fetuses, first trimester

O3Ø.822 Other specified multiple gestation with two or more monoamniotic fetuses, second trimester

O3Ø.823 Other specified multiple gestation with two or more monoamniotic fetuses, third trimester

O3Ø.829 Other specified multiple gestation with two or more monoamniotic fetuses, unspecified trimester

√6th **O3Ø.89 Other specified multiple gestation, unable to determine number of placenta and number of amniotic sacs**

O3Ø.891 Other specified multiple gestation, unable to determine number of placenta and number of amniotic sacs, first trimester

O3Ø.892 Other specified multiple gestation, unable to determine number of placenta and number of amniotic sacs, second trimester

O3Ø.893 Other specified multiple gestation, unable to determine number of placenta and number of amniotic sacs, third trimester

O3Ø.899 Other specified multiple gestation, unable to determine number of placenta and number of amniotic sacs, unspecified trimester

√5th **O3Ø.9 Multiple gestation, unspecified**

Multiple pregnancy NOS

O3Ø.9Ø Multiple gestation, unspecified, unspecified trimester

O3Ø.91 Multiple gestation, unspecified, first trimester

O3Ø.92 Multiple gestation, unspecified, second trimester

O3Ø.93 Multiple gestation, unspecified, third trimester

√4th **O31 Complications specific to multiple gestation**

EXCLUDES 2 *delayed delivery of second twin, triplet, etc. (O63.2)*
malpresentation of one fetus or more (O32.5)
placental transfusion syndromes (O43.Ø-)

One of the following 7th characters is to be assigned to each code under category O31. 7th character Ø is for single gestations and multiple gestations where the fetus is unspecified. 7th characters 1 through 9 are for cases of multiple gestations to identify the fetus for which the code applies. The appropriate code from category O3Ø, Multiple gestation, must also be assigned when assigning a code from category O31 that has a 7th character of 1 through 9.

Ø not applicable or unspecified
1 fetus 1
2 fetus 2
3 fetus 3
4 fetus 4
5 fetus 5
9 other fetus

√5th **O31.Ø Papyraceous fetus**

Fetus compressus

√x7th **O31.ØØ Papyraceous fetus, unspecified trimester**

√x7th **O31.Ø1 Papyraceous fetus, first trimester**

√x7th **O31.Ø2 Papyraceous fetus, second trimester**

√x7th **O31.Ø3 Papyraceous fetus, third trimester**

√5th **O31.1 Continuing pregnancy after spontaneous abortion of one fetus or more**

√x7th **O31.1Ø Continuing pregnancy after spontaneous abortion of one fetus or more, unspecified trimester**

√x7th **O31.11 Continuing pregnancy after spontaneous abortion of one fetus or more, first trimester**

√x7th **O31.12 Continuing pregnancy after spontaneous abortion of one fetus or more, second trimester**

√x7th **O31.13 Continuing pregnancy after spontaneous abortion of one fetus or more, third trimester**

√5th **O31.2 Continuing pregnancy after intrauterine death of one fetus or more**

√x7th **O31.2Ø Continuing pregnancy after intrauterine death of one fetus or more, unspecified trimester**

√x7th **O31.21 Continuing pregnancy after intrauterine death of one fetus or more, first trimester**

√x7th **O31.22 Continuing pregnancy after intrauterine death of one fetus or more, second trimester**

√x7th **O31.23 Continuing pregnancy after intrauterine death of one fetus or more, third trimester**

√5th **O31.3 Continuing pregnancy after elective fetal reduction of one fetus or more**

Continuing pregnancy after selective termination of one fetus or more

√x7th **O31.3Ø Continuing pregnancy after elective fetal reduction of one fetus or more, unspecified trimester**

√x7th **O31.31 Continuing pregnancy after elective fetal reduction of one fetus or more, first trimester**

√x7th **O31.32 Continuing pregnancy after elective fetal reduction of one fetus or more, second trimester**

√x7th **O31.33 Continuing pregnancy after elective fetal reduction of one fetus or more, third trimester**

√5th **O31.8 Other complications specific to multiple gestation**

√6th **O31.8X Other complications specific to multiple gestation**

√7th **O31.8X1 Other complications specific to multiple gestation, first trimester**

√7th **O31.8X2 Other complications specific to multiple gestation, second trimester**

√7th **O31.8X3 Other complications specific to multiple gestation, third trimester**

√7th **O31.8X9 Other complications specific to multiple gestation, unspecified trimester**

√4th **O32 Maternal care for malpresentation of fetus**

INCLUDES the listed conditions as a reason for observation, hospitalization or other obstetric care of the mother, or for cesarean delivery before onset of labor

EXCLUDES 1 *malpresentation of fetus with obstructed labor (O64.-)*

One of the following 7th characters is to be assigned to each code under category O32. 7th character Ø is for single gestations and multiple gestations where the fetus is unspecified. 7th characters 1 through 9 are for cases of multiple gestations to identify the fetus for which the code applies. The appropriate code from category O3Ø, Multiple gestation, must also be assigned when assigning a code from category O32 that has a 7th character of 1 through 9.

Ø not applicable or unspecified
1 fetus 1
2 fetus 2
3 fetus 3
4 fetus 4
5 fetus 5
9 other fetus

√x7th **O32.Ø Maternal care for unstable lie**

√x7th **O32.1 Maternal care for breech presentation**

Maternal care for buttocks presentation
Maternal care for complete breech
Maternal care for frank breech

EXCLUDES 1 *footling presentation (O32.8)*
incomplete breech (O32.8)

√x7th **O32.2 Maternal care for transverse and oblique lie**

Maternal care for oblique presentation
Maternal care for transverse presentation

√x7th **O32.3 Maternal care for face, brow and chin presentation**

√x7th **O32.4 Maternal care for high head at term**

Maternal care for failure of head to enter pelvic brim

√x7th **O32.6 Maternal care for compound presentation**

✓x7th O32.8 Maternal care for other malpresentation of fetus
Maternal care for footling presentation
Maternal care for incomplete breech

✓x7th O32.9 Maternal care for malpresentation of fetus, unspecified

✓4th O33 Maternal care for disproportion
INCLUDES the listed conditions as a reason for observation, hospitalization or other obstetric care of the mother, or for cesarean delivery before onset of labor
EXCLUDES 1 *disproportion with obstructed labor (O65- O66)*

O33.Ø Maternal care for disproportion due to deformity of maternal pelvic bones
Maternal care for disproportion due to pelvic deformity causing disproportion NOS

O33.1 Maternal care for disproportion due to generally contracted pelvis
Maternal care for disproportion due to contracted pelvis NOS causing disproportion

O33.2 Maternal care for disproportion due to inlet contraction of pelvis
Maternal care for disproportion due to inlet contraction (pelvis) causing disproportion

✓x7th O33.3 Maternal care for disproportion due to outlet contraction of pelvis
Maternal care for disproportion due to mid-cavity contraction (pelvis)
Maternal care for disproportion due to outlet contraction (pelvis)

One of the following 7th characters is to be assigned to code O33.3. 7th character Ø is for single gestations and multiple gestations where the fetus is unspecified. 7th characters 1 through 9 are for cases of multiple gestations to identify the fetus for which the code applies. The appropriate code from category O3Ø, Multiple gestation, must also be assigned when assigning code O33.3 with a 7th character of 1 through 9.
Ø not applicable or unspecified
1 fetus 1
2 fetus 2
3 fetus 3
4 fetus 4
5 fetus 5
9 other fetus

✓x7th O33.4 Maternal care for disproportion of mixed maternal and fetal origin

One of the following 7th characters is to be assigned to code O33.4. 7th character Ø is for single gestations and multiple gestations where the fetus is unspecified. 7th characters 1 through 9 are for cases of multiple gestations to identify the fetus for which the code applies. The appropriate code from category O3Ø, Multiple gestation, must also be assigned when assigning code O33.4 with a 7th character of 1 through 9.
Ø not applicable or unspecified
1 fetus 1
2 fetus 2
3 fetus 3
4 fetus 4
5 fetus 5
9 other fetus

✓x7th O33.5 Maternal care for disproportion due to unusually large fetus
Maternal care for disproportion due to disproportion of fetal origin with normally formed fetus
Maternal care for disproportion due to fetal disproportion NOS

One of the following 7th characters is to be assigned to code O33.5. 7th character Ø is for single gestations and multiple gestations where the fetus is unspecified. 7th characters 1 through 9 are for cases of multiple gestations to identify the fetus for which the code applies. The appropriate code from category O3Ø, Multiple gestation, must also be assigned when assigning code O33.5 with a 7th character of 1 through 9.
Ø not applicable or unspecified
1 fetus 1
2 fetus 2
3 fetus 3
4 fetus 4
5 fetus 5
9 other fetus

✓x7th O33.6 Maternal care for disproportion due to hydrocephalic fetus

One of the following 7th characters is to be assigned to code O33.6. 7th character Ø is for single gestations and multiple gestations where the fetus is unspecified. 7th characters 1 through 9 are for cases of multiple gestations to identify the fetus for which the code applies. The appropriate code from category O3Ø, Multiple gestation, must also be assigned when assigning code O33.6 with a 7th character of 1 through 9.
Ø not applicable or unspecified
1 fetus 1
2 fetus 2
3 fetus 3
4 fetus 4
5 fetus 5
9 other fetus

✓x7th O33.7 Maternal care for disproportion due to other fetal deformities

One of the following 7th characters is to be assigned to code O33.7. 7th character Ø is for single gestations and multiple gestations where the fetus is unspecified. 7th characters 1 through 9 are for cases of multiple gestations to identify the fetus for which the code applies. The appropriate code from category O3Ø, Multiple gestation, must also be assigned when assigning code O33.7 with a 7th character of 1 through 9.
Ø not applicable or unspecified
1 fetus 1
2 fetus 2
3 fetus 3
4 fetus 4
5 fetus 5
9 other fetus

Maternal care for disproportion due to fetal ascites
Maternal care for disproportion due to fetal hydrops
Maternal care for disproportion due to fetal meningomyelocele
Maternal care for disproportion due to fetal sacral teratoma
Maternal care for disproportion due to fetal tumor
EXCLUDES 1 *obstructed labor due to other fetal deformities (O66.3)*

O33.8 Maternal care for disproportion of other origin

O33.9 Maternal care for disproportion, unspecified
Maternal care for disproportion due to cephalopelvic disproportion NOS
Maternal care for disproportion due to fetopelvic disproportion NOS

✓4th O34 Maternal care for abnormality of pelvic organs
INCLUDES the listed conditions as a reason for hospitalization or other obstetric care of the mother, or for cesarean delivery before onset of labor
Code first any associated obstructed labor (O65.5)
Use additional code for specific condition

✓5th O34.Ø Maternal care for congenital malformation of uterus
O34.ØØ Maternal care for unspecified congenital malformation of uterus, unspecified trimester
O34.Ø1 Maternal care for unspecified congenital malformation of uterus, first trimester
O34.Ø2 Maternal care for unspecified congenital malformation of uterus, second trimester
O34.Ø3 Maternal care for unspecified congenital malformation of uterus, third trimester

✓5th O34.1 Maternal care for benign tumor of corpus uteri
EXCLUDES 2 *maternal care for benign tumor of cervix (O34.4-)*
maternal care for malignant neoplasm of uterus (O9A.1-)
O34.1Ø Maternal care for benign tumor of corpus uteri, unspecified trimester
O34.11 Maternal care for benign tumor of corpus uteri, first trimester
O34.12 Maternal care for benign tumor of corpus uteri, second trimester
O34.13 Maternal care for benign tumor of corpus uteri, third trimester

✓5th O34.2 Maternal care due to uterine scar from previous surgery
O34.21 Maternal care for scar from previous cesarean delivery

O34.29 Maternal care due to uterine scar from other previous surgery

✓5th **O34.3 Maternal care for cervical incompetence**
Maternal care for cerclage with or without cervical incompetence
Maternal care for Shirodkar suture with or without cervical incompetence

O34.30 Maternal care for cervical incompetence, unspecified trimester
O34.31 Maternal care for cervical incompetence, first trimester
O34.32 Maternal care for cervical incompetence, second trimester
O34.33 Maternal care for cervical incompetence, third trimester

✓5th **O34.4 Maternal care for other abnormalities of cervix**
O34.40 Maternal care for other abnormalities of cervix, unspecified trimester
O34.41 Maternal care for other abnormalities of cervix, first trimester
O34.42 Maternal care for other abnormalities of cervix, second trimester
O34.43 Maternal care for other abnormalities of cervix, third trimester

✓5th **O34.5 Maternal care for other abnormalities of gravid uterus**
✓6th **O34.51 Maternal care for incarceration of gravid uterus**
O34.511 Maternal care for incarceration of gravid uterus, first trimester
O34.512 Maternal care for incarceration of gravid uterus, second trimester
O34.513 Maternal care for incarceration of gravid uterus, third trimester
O34.519 Maternal care for incarceration of gravid uterus, unspecified trimester
✓6th **O34.52 Maternal care for prolapse of gravid uterus**
O34.521 Maternal care for prolapse of gravid uterus, first trimester
O34.522 Maternal care for prolapse of gravid uterus, second trimester
O34.523 Maternal care for prolapse of gravid uterus, third trimester
O34.529 Maternal care for prolapse of gravid uterus, unspecified trimester
✓6th **O34.53 Maternal care for retroversion of gravid uterus**
O34.531 Maternal care for retroversion of gravid uterus, first trimester
O34.532 Maternal care for retroversion of gravid uterus, second trimester
O34.533 Maternal care for retroversion of gravid uterus, third trimester
O34.539 Maternal care for retroversion of gravid uterus, unspecified trimester
✓6th **O34.59 Maternal care for other abnormalities of gravid uterus**
O34.591 Maternal care for other abnormalities of gravid uterus, first trimester
O34.592 Maternal care for other abnormalities of gravid uterus, second trimester
O34.593 Maternal care for other abnormalities of gravid uterus, third trimester
O34.599 Maternal care for other abnormalities of gravid uterus, unspecified trimester

✓5th **O34.6 Maternal care for abnormality of vagina**
EXCLUDES 2 *maternal care for vaginal varices in pregnancy (O22.1-)*

O34.60 Maternal care for abnormality of vagina, unspecified trimester
O34.61 Maternal care for abnormality of vagina, first trimester
O34.62 Maternal care for abnormality of vagina, second trimester
O34.63 Maternal care for abnormality of vagina, third trimester

✓5th **O34.7 Maternal care for abnormality of vulva and perineum**
EXCLUDES 2 *maternal care for perineal and vulval varices in pregnancy (O22.1-)*

O34.70 Maternal care for abnormality of vulva and perineum, unspecified trimester
O34.71 Maternal care for abnormality of vulva and perineum, first trimester
O34.72 Maternal care for abnormality of vulva and perineum, second trimester
O34.73 Maternal care for abnormality of vulva and perineum, third trimester

✓5th **O34.8 Maternal care for other abnormalities of pelvic organs**
O34.80 Maternal care for other abnormalities of pelvic organs, unspecified trimester
O34.81 Maternal care for other abnormalities of pelvic organs, first trimester
O34.82 Maternal care for other abnormalities of pelvic organs, second trimester
O34.83 Maternal care for other abnormalities of pelvic organs, third trimester

✓5th **O34.9 Maternal care for abnormality of pelvic organ, unspecified**
O34.90 Maternal care for abnormality of pelvic organ, unspecified, unspecified trimester
O34.91 Maternal care for abnormality of pelvic organ, unspecified, first trimester
O34.92 Maternal care for abnormality of pelvic organ, unspecified, second trimester
O34.93 Maternal care for abnormality of pelvic organ, unspecified, third trimester

✓4th **O35 Maternal care for known or suspected fetal abnormality and damage**
INCLUDES the listed conditions in the fetus as a reason for hospitalization or other obstetric care to the mother, or for termination of pregnancy
Code also any associated maternal condition
EXCLUDES 1 *encounter for suspected maternal and fetal conditions ruled out (Z03.7-)*

One of the following 7th characters is to be assigned to each code under category O35. 7th character 0 is for single gestations and multiple gestations where the fetus is unspecified. 7th characters 1 through 9 are for cases of multiple gestations to identify the fetus for which the code applies. The appropriate code from category O30, Multiple gestation, must also be assigned when assigning a code from category O35 that has a 7th character of 1 through 9.

0 not applicable or unspecified
1 fetus 1
2 fetus 2
3 fetus 3
4 fetus 4
5 fetus 5
9 other fetus

✓x7th **O35.0 Maternal care for (suspected) central nervous system malformation in fetus**
Maternal care for fetal anencephaly
Maternal care for fetal hydrocephalus
Maternal care for fetal spina bifida
EXCLUDES 2 *chromosomal abnormality in fetus (O35.1)*

✓x7th **O35.1 Maternal care for (suspected) chromosomal abnormality in fetus**

✓x7th **O35.2 Maternal care for (suspected) hereditary disease in fetus**
EXCLUDES 2 *chromosomal abnormality in fetus (O35.1)*

✓x7th **O35.3 Maternal care for (suspected) damage to fetus from viral disease in mother**
Maternal care for damage to fetus from maternal cytomegalovirus infection
Maternal care for damage to fetus from maternal rubella

✓x7th **O35.4 Maternal care for (suspected) damage to fetus from alcohol**

✓x7th **O35.5 Maternal care for (suspected) damage to fetus by drugs**
Maternal care for damage to fetus from drug addiction

✓x7th **O35.6 Maternal care for (suspected) damage to fetus by radiation**

✓x7th **O35.7 Maternal care for (suspected) damage to fetus by other medical procedures**
Maternal care for damage to fetus by amniocentesis
Maternal care for damage to fetus by biopsy procedures
Maternal care for damage to fetus by hematological investigation
Maternal care for damage to fetus by intrauterine contraceptive device
Maternal care for damage to fetus by intrauterine surgery

√x7th **O35.8 Maternal care for other (suspected) fetal abnormality and damage**
Maternal care for damage to fetus from maternal listeriosis
Maternal care for damage to fetus from maternal toxoplasmosis

√x7th **O35.9 Maternal care for (suspected) fetal abnormality and damage, unspecified**

√4th **O36 Maternal care for other fetal problems**
INCLUDES the listed conditions in the fetus as a reason for hospitalization or other obstetric care of the mother, or for termination of pregnancy
EXCLUDES 1 *encounter for suspected maternal and fetal conditions ruled out (Z03.7-)*
placental transfusion syndromes (O43.0-)
EXCLUDES 2 *labor and delivery complicated by fetal stress (O77.-)*

One of the following 7th characters is to be assigned to each code under category O36. 7th character 0 is for single gestations and multiple gestations where the fetus is unspecified. 7th characters 1 through 9 are for cases of multiple gestations to identify the fetus for which the code applies. The appropriate code from category O30, Multiple gestation, must also be assigned when assigning a code from category O36 that has a 7th character of 1 through 9.
0 not applicable or unspecified
1 fetus 1
2 fetus 2
3 fetus 3
4 fetus 4
5 fetus 5
9 other fetus

√5th **O36.0 Maternal care for rhesus isoimmunization**
Maternal care for Rh incompatibility (with hydrops fetalis)

√6th **O36.01 Maternal care for anti-D [Rh] antibodies**
√7th **O36.011 Maternal care for anti-D [Rh] antibodies, first trimester**
√7th **O36.012 Maternal care for anti-D [Rh] antibodies, second trimester**
√7th **O36.013 Maternal care for anti-D [Rh] antibodies, third trimester**
√7th **O36.019 Maternal care for anti-D [Rh] antibodies, unspecified trimester**

√6th **O36.09 Maternal care for other rhesus isoimmunization**
√7th **O36.091 Maternal care for other rhesus isoimmunization, first trimester**
√7th **O36.092 Maternal care for other rhesus isoimmunization, second trimester**
√7th **O36.093 Maternal care for other rhesus isoimmunization, third trimester**
√7th **O36.099 Maternal care for other rhesus isoimmunization, unspecified trimester**

√5th **O36.1 Maternal care for other isoimmunization**
Maternal care for ABO isoimmunization

√6th **O36.11 Maternal care for Anti-A sensitization**
Maternal care for isoimmunization NOS (with hydrops fetalis)
√7th **O36.111 Maternal care for Anti-A sensitization, first trimester**
√7th **O36.112 Maternal care for Anti-A sensitization, second trimester**
√7th **O36.113 Maternal care for Anti-A sensitization, third trimester**
√7th **O36.119 Maternal care for Anti-A sensitization, unspecified trimester**

√6th **O36.19 Maternal care for other isoimmunization**
Maternal care for Anti-B sensitization
√7th **O36.191 Maternal care for other isoimmunization, first trimester**
√7th **O36.192 Maternal care for other isoimmunization, second trimester**
√7th **O36.193 Maternal care for other isoimmunization, third trimester**
√7th **O36.199 Maternal care for other isoimmunization, unspecified trimester**

√5th **O36.2 Maternal care for hydrops fetalis**
Maternal care for hydrops fetalis NOS
Maternal care for hydrops fetalis not associated with isoimmunization
EXCLUDES 1 *hydrops fetalis associated with ABO isoimmunization (O36.1-)*
hydrops fetalis associated with rhesus isoimmunization (O36.0-)

√x7th **O36.20 Maternal care for hydrops fetalis, unspecified trimester**
√x7th **O36.21 Maternal care for hydrops fetalis, first trimester**
√x7th **O36.22 Maternal care for hydrops fetalis, second trimester**
√x7th **O36.23 Maternal care for hydrops fetalis, third trimester**

√x7th **O36.4 Maternal care for intrauterine death**
Maternal care for intrauterine fetal death NOS
Maternal care for intrauterine fetal death after completion of 20 weeks of gestation
Maternal care for late fetal death
Maternal care for missed delivery
EXCLUDES 1 *missed abortion (O02.1)*
stillbirth (P95)

√5th **O36.5 Maternal care for known or suspected poor fetal growth**
√6th **O36.51 Maternal care for known or suspected placental insufficiency**
√7th **O36.511 Maternal care for known or suspected placental insufficiency, first trimester**
√7th **O36.512 Maternal care for known or suspected placental insufficiency, second trimester**
√7th **O36.513 Maternal care for known or suspected placental insufficiency, third trimester**
√7th **O36.519 Maternal care for known or suspected placental insufficiency, unspecified trimester**

√6th **O36.59 Maternal care for other known or suspected poor fetal growth**
Maternal care for known or suspected light-for-dates NOS
Maternal care for known or suspected small-for-dates NOS
√7th **O36.591 Maternal care for other known or suspected poor fetal growth, first trimester**
√7th **O36.592 Maternal care for other known or suspected poor fetal growth, second trimester**
√7th **O36.593 Maternal care for other known or suspected poor fetal growth, third trimester**
√7th **O36.599 Maternal care for other known or suspected poor fetal growth, unspecified trimester**

√5th **O36.6 Maternal care for excessive fetal growth**
Maternal care for known or suspected large-for-dates
√x7th **O36.60 Maternal care for excessive fetal growth, unspecified trimester**
√x7th **O36.61 Maternal care for excessive fetal growth, first trimester**
√x7th **O36.62 Maternal care for excessive fetal growth, second trimester**
√x7th **O36.63 Maternal care for excessive fetal growth, third trimester**

√5th **O36.7 Maternal care for viable fetus in abdominal pregnancy**
√x7th **O36.70 Maternal care for viable fetus in abdominal pregnancy, unspecified trimester**
√x7th **O36.71 Maternal care for viable fetus in abdominal pregnancy, first trimester**
√x7th **O36.72 Maternal care for viable fetus in abdominal pregnancy, second trimester**
√x7th **O36.73 Maternal care for viable fetus in abdominal pregnancy, third trimester**

√5th **O36.8 Maternal care for other specified fetal problems**
O36.80 Pregnancy with inconclusive fetal viability
Encounter to determine fetal viability of pregnancy

√6th **O36.81 Decreased fetal movements**
√7th **O36.812 Decreased fetal movements, second trimester**
√7th **O36.813 Decreased fetal movements, third trimester**

√7th **O36.819 Decreased fetal movements, unspecified trimester**

√6th **O36.82 Fetal anemia and thrombocytopenia**

√7th **O36.821 Fetal anemia and thrombocytopenia, first trimester**

√7th **O36.822 Fetal anemia and thrombocytopenia, second trimester**

√7th **O36.823 Fetal anemia and thrombocytopenia, third trimester**

√7th **O36.829 Fetal anemia and thrombocytopenia, unspecified trimester**

√6th **O36.89 Maternal care for other specified fetal problems**

√7th **O36.891 Maternal care for other specified fetal problems, first trimester**

√7th **O36.892 Maternal care for other specified fetal problems, second trimester**

√7th **O36.893 Maternal care for other specified fetal problems, third trimester**

√7th **O36.899 Maternal care for other specified fetal problems, unspecified trimester**

√5th **O36.9 Maternal care for fetal problem, unspecified**

√x7th **O36.9Ø Maternal care for fetal problem, unspecified, unspecified trimester**

√x7th **O36.91 Maternal care for fetal problem, unspecified, first trimester**

√x7th **O36.92 Maternal care for fetal problem, unspecified, second trimester**

√x7th **O36.93 Maternal care for fetal problem, unspecified, third trimester**

√4th **O4Ø Polyhydramnios**

Hydramnios

EXCLUDES 1 *encounter for suspected maternal and fetal conditions ruled out (ZØ3.7-)*

One of the following 7th characters is to be assigned to each code under category O4Ø. 7th character Ø is for single gestations and multiple gestations where the fetus is unspecified. 7th characters 1 through 9 are for cases of multiple gestations to identify the fetus for which the code applies. The appropriate code from category O3Ø, Multiple gestation, must also be assigned when assigning a code from category O4Ø that has a 7th character of 1 through 9.

Ø not applicable or unspecified
1 fetus 1
2 fetus 2
3 fetus 3
4 fetus 4
5 fetus 5
9 other fetus

√x7th **O4Ø.1 Polyhydramnios, first trimester**

√x7th **O4Ø.2 Polyhydramnios, second trimester**

√x7th **O4Ø.3 Polyhydramnios, third trimester**

√x7th **O4Ø.9 Polyhydramnios, unspecified trimester**

√4th **O41 Other disorders of amniotic fluid and membranes**

EXCLUDES 1 *encounter for suspected maternal and fetal conditions ruled out (ZØ3.7-)*

One of the following 7th characters is to be assigned to each code under category O41. 7th character Ø is for single gestations and multiple gestations where the fetus is unspecified. 7th characters 1 through 9 are for cases of multiple gestations to identify the fetus for which the code applies. The appropriate code from category O3Ø, Multiple gestation, must also be assigned when assigning a code from category O41 that has a 7th character of 1 through 9.

Ø not applicable or unspecified
1 fetus 1
2 fetus 2
3 fetus 3
4 fetus 4
5 fetus 5
9 other fetus

√5th **O41.Ø Oligohydramnios**

Oligohydramnios without rupture of membranes

√x7th **O41.ØØ Oligohydramnios, unspecified trimester**

√x7th **O41.Ø1 Oligohydramnios, first trimester**

√x7th **O41.Ø2 Oligohydramnios, second trimester**

√x7th **O41.Ø3 Oligohydramnios, third trimester**

√5th **O41.1 Infection of amniotic sac and membranes**

√6th **O41.1Ø Infection of amniotic sac and membranes, unspecified**

√7th **O41.1Ø1 Infection of amniotic sac and membranes, unspecified, first trimester**

√7th **O41.1Ø2 Infection of amniotic sac and membranes, unspecified, second trimester**

√7th **O41.1Ø3 Infection of amniotic sac and membranes, unspecified, third trimester**

√7th **O41.1Ø9 Infection of amniotic sac and membranes, unspecified, unspecified trimester**

√6th **O41.12 Chorioamnionitis**

√7th **O41.121 Chorioamnionitis, first trimester**

√7th **O41.122 Chorioamnionitis, second trimester**

√7th **O41.123 Chorioamnionitis, third trimester**

√7th **O41.129 Chorioamnionitis, unspecified trimester**

√6th **O41.14 Placentitis**

√7th **O41.141 Placentitis, first trimester**

√7th **O41.142 Placentitis, second trimester**

√7th **O41.143 Placentitis, third trimester**

√7th **O41.149 Placentitis, unspecified trimester**

√5th **O41.8 Other specified disorders of amniotic fluid and membranes**

√6th **O41.8X Other specified disorders of amniotic fluid and membranes**

√7th **O41.8X1 Other specified disorders of amniotic fluid and membranes, first trimester**

√7th **O41.8X2 Other specified disorders of amniotic fluid and membranes, second trimester**

√7th **O41.8X3 Other specified disorders of amniotic fluid and membranes, third trimester**

√7th **O41.8X9 Other specified disorders of amniotic fluid and membranes, unspecified trimester**

√5th **O41.9 Disorder of amniotic fluid and membranes, unspecified**

√x7th **O41.9Ø Disorder of amniotic fluid and membranes, unspecified, unspecified trimester**

√x7th **O41.91 Disorder of amniotic fluid and membranes, unspecified, first trimester**

√x7th **O41.92 Disorder of amniotic fluid and membranes, unspecified, second trimester**

√x7th **O41.93 Disorder of amniotic fluid and membranes, unspecified, third trimester**

√4th **O42 Premature rupture of membranes**

√5th **O42.Ø Premature rupture of membranes, onset of labor within 24 hours of rupture**

O42.ØØ Premature rupture of membranes, onset of labor within 24 hours of rupture, unspecified weeks of gestation

√6th **O42.Ø1 Preterm premature rupture of membranes, onset of labor within 24 hours of rupture**

Premature rupture of membranes before 37 completed weeks of gestation

O42.Ø11 Preterm premature rupture of membranes, onset of labor within 24 hours of rupture, first trimester

O42.Ø12 Preterm premature rupture of membranes, onset of labor within 24 hours of rupture, second trimester

O42.Ø13 Preterm premature rupture of membranes, onset of labor within 24 hours of rupture, third trimester

O42.Ø19 Preterm premature rupture of membranes, onset of labor within 24 hours of rupture, unspecified trimester

O42.Ø2 Full-term premature rupture of membranes, onset of labor within 24 hours of rupture

Premature rupture of membranes after 37 completed weeks of gestation

√5th **O42.1 Premature rupture of membranes, onset of labor more than 24 hours following rupture**

O42.1Ø Premature rupture of membranes, onset of labor more than 24 hours following rupture, unspecified weeks of gestation

√6th **O42.11 Preterm premature rupture of membranes, onset of labor more than 24 hours following rupture**
Premature rupture of membranes before 37 completed weeks of gestation
O42.111 Preterm premature rupture of membranes, onset of labor more than 24 hours following rupture, first trimester
O42.112 Preterm premature rupture of membranes, onset of labor more than 24 hours following rupture, second trimester
O42.113 Preterm premature rupture of membranes, onset of labor more than 24 hours following rupture, third trimester
O42.119 Preterm premature rupture of membranes, onset of labor more than 24 hours following rupture, unspecified trimester
O42.12 Full-term premature rupture of membranes, onset of labor more than 24 hours following rupture
Premature rupture of membranes after 37 completed weeks of gestation

√5th **O42.9 Premature rupture of membranes, unspecified as to length of time between rupture and onset of labor**
O42.90 Premature rupture of membranes, unspecified as to length of time between rupture and onset of labor, unspecified weeks of gestation
√6th **O42.91 Preterm premature rupture of membranes, unspecified as to length of time between rupture and onset of labor**
Premature rupture of membranes before 37 completed weeks of gestation
O42.911 Preterm premature rupture of membranes, unspecified as to length of time between rupture and onset of labor, first trimester
O42.912 Preterm premature rupture of membranes, unspecified as to length of time between rupture and onset of labor, second trimester
O42.913 Preterm premature rupture of membranes, unspecified as to length of time between rupture and onset of labor, third trimester
O42.919 Preterm premature rupture of membranes, unspecified as to length of time between rupture and onset of labor, unspecified trimester
O42.92 Full-term premature rupture of membranes, unspecified as to length of time between rupture and onset of labor
Premature rupture of membranes after 37 completed weeks of gestation

√4th **O43 Placental disorders**
EXCLUDES 2 *maternal care for poor fetal growth due to placental insufficiency (O36.5-)*
placenta previa (O44.-)
placental polyp (O90.89)
placentitis (O41.14-)
premature separation of placenta [abruptio placentae] (O45.-)

√5th **O43.0 Placental transfusion syndromes**
√6th **O43.01 Fetomaternal placental transfusion syndrome**
Maternofetal placental transfusion syndrome
O43.011 Fetomaternal placental transfusion syndrome, first trimester
O43.012 Fetomaternal placental transfusion syndrome, second trimester
O43.013 Fetomaternal placental transfusion syndrome, third trimester
O43.019 Fetomaternal placental transfusion syndrome, unspecified trimester
√6th **O43.02 Fetus-to-fetus placental transfusion syndrome**
O43.021 Fetus-to-fetus placental transfusion syndrome, first trimester
O43.022 Fetus-to-fetus placental transfusion syndrome, second trimester
O43.023 Fetus-to-fetus placental transfusion syndrome, third trimester
O43.029 Fetus-to-fetus placental transfusion syndrome, unspecified trimester

√5th **O43.1 Malformation of placenta**
√6th **O43.10 Malformation of placenta, unspecified**
Abnormal placenta NOS
O43.101 Malformation of placenta, unspecified, first trimester
O43.102 Malformation of placenta, unspecified, second trimester
O43.103 Malformation of placenta, unspecified, third trimester
O43.109 Malformation of placenta, unspecified, unspecified trimester
√6th **O43.11 Circumvallate placenta**
O43.111 Circumvallate placenta, first trimester
O43.112 Circumvallate placenta, second trimester
O43.113 Circumvallate placenta, third trimester
O43.119 Circumvallate placenta, unspecified trimester
√6th **O43.12 Velamentous insertion of umbilical cord**
O43.121 Velamentous insertion of umbilical cord, first trimester
O43.122 Velamentous insertion of umbilical cord, second trimester
O43.123 Velamentous insertion of umbilical cord, third trimester
O43.129 Velamentous insertion of umbilical cord, unspecified trimester
√6th **O43.19 Other malformation of placenta**
O43.191 Other malformation of placenta, first trimester
O43.192 Other malformation of placenta, second trimester
O43.193 Other malformation of placenta, third trimester
O43.199 Other malformation of placenta, unspecified trimester

√5th **O43.2 Morbidly adherent placenta**
Code also associated third stage postpartum hemorrhage, if applicable (O72.0)
EXCLUDES 1 *retained placenta (O73.-)*
√6th **O43.21 Placenta accreta**
O43.211 Placenta accreta, first trimester
O43.212 Placenta accreta, second trimester
O43.213 Placenta accreta, third trimester
O43.219 Placenta accreta, unspecified trimester
√6th **O43.22 Placenta increta**
O43.221 Placenta increta, first trimester
O43.222 Placenta increta, second trimester
O43.223 Placenta increta, third trimester
O43.229 Placenta increta, unspecified trimester
√6th **O43.23 Placenta percreta**
O43.231 Placenta percreta, first trimester
O43.232 Placenta percreta, second trimester
O43.233 Placenta percreta, third trimester
O43.239 Placenta percreta, unspecified trimester

√5th **O43.8 Other placental disorders**
√6th **O43.81 Placental infarction**
O43.811 Placental infarction, first trimester
O43.812 Placental infarction, second trimester
O43.813 Placental infarction, third trimester
O43.819 Placental infarction, unspecified trimester
√6th **O43.89 Other placental disorders**
Placental dysfunction
O43.891 Other placental disorders, first trimester
O43.892 Other placental disorders, second trimester
O43.893 Other placental disorders, third trimester
O43.899 Other placental disorders, unspecified trimester

O43.9 Unspecified placental disorder

O43.90 Unspecified placental disorder, unspecified trimester

O43.91 Unspecified placental disorder, first trimester

O43.92 Unspecified placental disorder, second trimester

O43.93 Unspecified placental disorder, third trimester

O44 Placenta previa

O44.0 Placenta previa specified as without hemorrhage

Low implantation of placenta specified as without hemorrhage

O44.00 Placenta previa specified as without hemorrhage, unspecified trimester

O44.01 Placenta previa specified as without hemorrhage, first trimester

O44.02 Placenta previa specified as without hemorrhage, second trimester

O44.03 Placenta previa specified as without hemorrhage, third trimester

O44.1 Placenta previa with hemorrhage

Low implantation of placenta, NOS or with hemorrhage
Marginal placenta previa, NOS or with hemorrhage
Partial placenta previa, NOS or with hemorrhage
Total placenta previa, NOS or with hemorrhage

EXCLUDES 1 *labor and delivery complicated by hemorrhage from vasa previa (O69.4)*

O44.10 Placenta previa with hemorrhage, unspecified trimester

O44.11 Placenta previa with hemorrhage, first trimester

O44.12 Placenta previa with hemorrhage, second trimester

O44.13 Placenta previa with hemorrhage, third trimester

O45 Premature separation of placenta [abruptio placentae]

O45.0 Premature separation of placenta with coagulation defect

O45.00 Premature separation of placenta with coagulation defect, unspecified

O45.001 Premature separation of placenta with coagulation defect, unspecified, first trimester

O45.002 Premature separation of placenta with coagulation defect, unspecified, second trimester

O45.003 Premature separation of placenta with coagulation defect, unspecified, third trimester

O45.009 Premature separation of placenta with coagulation defect, unspecified, unspecified trimester

O45.01 Premature separation of placenta with afibrinogenemia

Premature separation of placenta with hypofibrinogenemia

O45.011 Premature separation of placenta with afibrinogenemia, first trimester

O45.012 Premature separation of placenta with afibrinogenemia, second trimester

O45.013 Premature separation of placenta with afibrinogenemia, third trimester

O45.019 Premature separation of placenta with afibrinogenemia, unspecified trimester

O45.02 Premature separation of placenta with disseminated intravascular coagulation

O45.021 Premature separation of placenta with disseminated intravascular coagulation, first trimester

O45.022 Premature separation of placenta with disseminated intravascular coagulation, second trimester

O45.023 Premature separation of placenta with disseminated intravascular coagulation, third trimester

O45.029 Premature separation of placenta with disseminated intravascular coagulation, unspecified trimester

O45.09 Premature separation of placenta with other coagulation defect

O45.091 Premature separation of placenta with other coagulation defect, first trimester

O45.092 Premature separation of placenta with other coagulation defect, second trimester

O45.093 Premature separation of placenta with other coagulation defect, third trimester

O45.099 Premature separation of placenta with other coagulation defect, unspecified trimester

O45.8 Other premature separation of placenta

O45.8X Other premature separation of placenta

O45.8X1 Other premature separation of placenta, first trimester

O45.8X2 Other premature separation of placenta, second trimester

O45.8X3 Other premature separation of placenta, third trimester

O45.8X9 Other premature separation of placenta, unspecified trimester

O45.9 Premature separation of placenta, unspecified

Abruptio placentae NOS

O45.90 Premature separation of placenta, unspecified, unspecified trimester

O45.91 Premature separation of placenta, unspecified, first trimester

O45.92 Premature separation of placenta, unspecified, second trimester

O45.93 Premature separation of placenta, unspecified, third trimester

O46 Antepartum hemorrhage, not elsewhere classified

EXCLUDES 1 *hemorrhage in early pregnancy (O20.-)*
intrapartum hemorrhage NEC (O67.-)
placenta previa (O44.-)
premature separation of placenta [abruptio placentae] (O45.-)

O46.0 Antepartum hemorrhage with coagulation defect

O46.00 Antepartum hemorrhage with coagulation defect, unspecified

O46.001 Antepartum hemorrhage with coagulation defect, unspecified, first trimester

O46.002 Antepartum hemorrhage with coagulation defect, unspecified, second trimester

O46.003 Antepartum hemorrhage with coagulation defect, unspecified, third trimester

O46.009 Antepartum hemorrhage with coagulation defect, unspecified, unspecified trimester

O46.01 Antepartum hemorrhage with afibrinogenemia

Antepartum hemorrhage with hypofibrinogenemia

O46.011 Antepartum hemorrhage with afibrinogenemia, first trimester

O46.012 Antepartum hemorrhage with afibrinogenemia, second trimester

O46.013 Antepartum hemorrhage with afibrinogenemia, third trimester

O46.019 Antepartum hemorrhage with afibrinogenemia, unspecified trimester

O46.02 Antepartum hemorrhage with disseminated intravascular coagulation

O46.021 Antepartum hemorrhage with disseminated intravascular coagulation, first trimester

O46.022 Antepartum hemorrhage with disseminated intravascular coagulation, second trimester

O46.023 Antepartum hemorrhage with disseminated intravascular coagulation, third trimester

O46.029 Antepartum hemorrhage with disseminated intravascular coagulation, unspecified trimester

O46.09 Antepartum hemorrhage with other coagulation defect

O46.091 Antepartum hemorrhage with other coagulation defect, first trimester

O46.092 Antepartum hemorrhage with other coagulation defect, second trimester

O46.093 Antepartum hemorrhage with other coagulation defect, third trimester

O46.099 Antepartum hemorrhage with other coagulation defect, unspecified trimester

5th **O46.8 Other antepartum hemorrhage**

6th **O46.8X Other antepartum hemorrhage**

O46.8X1 Other antepartum hemorrhage, first trimester

O46.8X2 Other antepartum hemorrhage, second trimester

O46.8X3 Other antepartum hemorrhage, third trimester

O46.8X9 Other antepartum hemorrhage, unspecified trimester

5th **O46.9 Antepartum hemorrhage, unspecified**

O46.90 Antepartum hemorrhage, unspecified, unspecified trimester

O46.91 Antepartum hemorrhage, unspecified, first trimester

O46.92 Antepartum hemorrhage, unspecified, second trimester

O46.93 Antepartum hemorrhage, unspecified, third trimester

4th **O47 False labor**

Braxton Hicks contractions

Threatened labor

EXCLUDES 1 *preterm labor (O60.-)*

5th **O47.0 False labor before 37 completed weeks of gestation**

O47.00 False labor before 37 completed weeks of gestation, unspecified trimester

O47.02 False labor before 37 completed weeks of gestation, second trimester

O47.03 False labor before 37 completed weeks of gestation, third trimester

O47.1 False labor at or after 37 completed weeks of gestation

O47.9 False labor, unspecified

4th **O48 Late pregnancy**

O48.0 Post-term pregnancy

Pregnancy over 40 completed weeks to 42 completed weeks gestation

O48.1 Prolonged pregnancy

Pregnancy which has advanced beyond 42 completed weeks gestation

Complications of labor and delivery (O60-O77)

4th **O60 Preterm labor**

INCLUDES onset (spontaneous) of labor before 37 completed weeks of gestation

EXCLUDES 1 *false labor (O47.0-)*

threatened labor NOS (O47.0-)

5th **O60.0 Preterm labor without delivery**

O60.00 Preterm labor without delivery, unspecified trimester

O60.02 Preterm labor without delivery, second trimester

O60.03 Preterm labor without delivery, third trimester

5th **O60.1 Preterm labor with preterm delivery**

One of the following 7th characters is to be assigned to each code under subcategory O60.1. 7th character 0 is for single gestations and multiple gestations where the fetus is unspecified. 7th characters 1 through 9 are for cases of multiple gestations to identify the fetus for which the code applies. The appropriate code from category O30, Multiple gestation, must also be assigned when assigning a code from subcategory O60.1 that has a 7th character of 1 through 9.

0	not applicable or unspecified
1	fetus 1
2	fetus 2
3	fetus 3
4	fetus 4
5	fetus 5
9	other fetus

x7th **O60.10 Preterm labor with preterm delivery, unspecified trimester**

Preterm labor with delivery NOS

x7th **O60.12 Preterm labor second trimester with preterm delivery second trimester**

x7th **O60.13 Preterm labor second trimester with preterm delivery third trimester**

x7th **O60.14 Preterm labor third trimester with preterm delivery third trimester**

5th **O60.2 Term delivery with preterm labor**

One of the following 7th characters is to be assigned to each code under subcategory O60.2. 7th character 0 is for single gestations and multiple gestations where the fetus is unspecified. 7th characters 1 through 9 are for cases of multiple gestations to identify the fetus for which the code applies. The appropriate code from category O30, Multiple gestation, must also be assigned when assigning a code from subcategory O60.2 that has a 7th character of 1 through 9.

0	not applicable or unspecified
1	fetus 1
2	fetus 2
3	fetus 3
4	fetus 4
5	fetus 5
9	other fetus

x7th **O60.20 Term delivery with preterm labor, unspecified trimester**

x7th **O60.22 Term delivery with preterm labor, second trimester**

x7th **O60.23 Term delivery with preterm labor, third trimester**

4th **O61 Failed induction of labor**

O61.0 Failed medical induction of labor

Failed induction (of labor) by oxytocin

Failed induction (of labor) by prostaglandins

O61.1 Failed instrumental induction of labor

Failed mechanical induction (of labor)

Failed surgical induction (of labor)

O61.8 Other failed induction of labor

O61.9 Failed induction of labor, unspecified

4th **O62 Abnormalities of forces of labor**

O62.0 Primary inadequate contractions

Failure of cervical dilatation

Primary hypotonic uterine dysfunction

Uterine inertia during latent phase of labor

O62.1 Secondary uterine inertia

Arrested active phase of labor

Secondary hypotonic uterine dysfunction

O62.2 Other uterine inertia

Atony of uterus without hemorrhage

Atony of uterus NOS

Desultory labor

Hypotonic uterine dysfunction NOS

Irregular labor

Poor contractions

Slow slope active phase of labor

Uterine inertia NOS

EXCLUDES 1 *atony of uterus with hemorrhage (postpartum) (O72.1)*

postpartum atony of uterus without hemorrhage (O75.89)

O62.3 Precipitate labor

O62.4 Hypertonic, incoordinate, and prolonged uterine contractions

Cervical spasm

Contraction ring dystocia

Dyscoordinate labor

Hour-glass contraction of uterus

Hypertonic uterine dysfunction

Incoordinate uterine action

Tetanic contractions

Uterine dystocia NOS

Uterine spasm

EXCLUDES 1 *dystocia (fetal) (maternal) NOS (O66.9)*

O62.8 Other abnormalities of forces of labor

O62.9 Abnormality of forces of labor, unspecified

4th **O63 Long labor**

O63.0 Prolonged first stage (of labor)

O63.1 Prolonged second stage (of labor)

O63.2 Delayed delivery of second twin, triplet, etc.

DRAFT

O63.9 Long labor, unspecified
Prolonged labor NOS

✓4th **O64 Obstructed labor due to malposition and malpresentation of fetus**

One of the following 7th characters is to be assigned to each code under category O64. 7th character Ø is for single gestations and multiple gestations where the fetus is unspecified. 7th characters 1 through 9 are for cases of multiple gestations to identify the fetus for which the code applies. The appropriate code from category O3Ø, Multiple gestation, must also be assigned when assigning a code from category O64 that has a 7th character of 1 through 9.
Ø not applicable or unspecified
1 fetus 1
2 fetus 2
3 fetus 3
4 fetus 4
5 fetus 5
9 other fetus

✓x7th **O64.Ø Obstructed labor due to incomplete rotation of fetal head**
Deep transverse arrest
Obstructed labor due to persistent occipitoiliac (position)
Obstructed labor due to persistent occipitoposterior (position)
Obstructed labor due to persistent occipitosacral (position)
Obstructed labor due to persistent occipitotransverse (position)

✓x7th **O64.1 Obstructed labor due to breech presentation**
Obstructed labor due to buttocks presentation
Obstructed labor due to complete breech presentation
Obstructed labor due to frank breech presentation

✓x7th **O64.2 Obstructed labor due to face presentation**
Obstructed labor due to chin presentation

✓x7th **O64.3 Obstructed labor due to brow presentation**

✓x7th **O64.4 Obstructed labor due to shoulder presentation**
Prolapsed arm
EXCLUDES1 *impacted shoulders (O66.Ø)*
shoulder dystocia (O66.Ø)

✓x7th **O64.5 Obstructed labor due to compound presentation**

✓x7th **O64.8 Obstructed labor due to other malposition and malpresentation**
Obstructed labor due to footling presentation
Obstructed labor due to incomplete breech presentation

✓x7th **O64.9 Obstructed labor due to malposition and malpresentation, unspecified**

✓4th **O65 Obstructed labor due to maternal pelvic abnormality**

O65.Ø Obstructed labor due to deformed pelvis

O65.1 Obstructed labor due to generally contracted pelvis

O65.2 Obstructed labor due to pelvic inlet contraction

O65.3 Obstructed labor due to pelvic outlet and mid-cavity contraction

O65.4 Obstructed labor due to fetopelvic disproportion, unspecified
EXCLUDES1 *dystocia due to abnormality of fetus (O66.2-O66.3)*

O65.5 Obstructed labor due to abnormality of maternal pelvic organs
Obstructed labor due to conditions listed in O34-
Use additional code to identify abnormality of pelvic organs (O34.-)

O65.8 Obstructed labor due to other maternal pelvic abnormalities

O65.9 Obstructed labor due to maternal pelvic abnormality, unspecified

✓4th **O66 Other obstructed labor**

O66.Ø Obstructed labor due to shoulder dystocia
Impacted shoulders

O66.1 Obstructed labor due to locked twins

O66.2 Obstructed labor due to unusually large fetus

O66.3 Obstructed labor due to other abnormalities of fetus
Dystocia due to fetal ascites
Dystocia due to fetal hydrops
Dystocia due to fetal meningomyelocele
Dystocia due to fetal sacral teratoma
Dystocia due to fetal tumor
Dystocia due to hydrocephalic fetus
Use additional code to identify cause of obstruction

✓5th **O66.4 Failed trial of labor**

O66.4Ø Failed trial of labor, unspecified

O66.41 Failed attempted vaginal birth after previous cesarean delivery
Code first rupture of uterus, if applicable (O71.Ø-, O71.1)

O66.5 Attempted application of vacuum extractor and forceps
Attempted application of vacuum or forceps, with subsequent delivery by forceps or cesarean delivery

O66.6 Obstructed labor due to other multiple fetuses

O66.8 Other specified obstructed labor
Use additional code to identify cause of obstruction

O66.9 Obstructed labor, unspecified
Dystocia NOS
Fetal dystocia NOS
Maternal dystocia NOS

✓4th **O67 Labor and delivery complicated by intrapartum hemorrhage, not elsewhere classified**
EXCLUDES1 *antepartum hemorrhage NEC (O46.-)*
placenta previa (O44.-)
premature separation of placenta [abruptio placentae] (O45.-)
EXCLUDES2 *postpartum hemorrhage (O72.-)*

O67.Ø Intrapartum hemorrhage with coagulation defect
Intrapartum hemorrhage (excessive) associated with afibrinogenemia
Intrapartum hemorrhage (excessive) associated with disseminated intravascular coagulation
Intrapartum hemorrhage (excessive) associated with hyperfibrinolysis
Intrapartum hemorrhage (excessive) associated with hypofibrinogenemia

O67.8 Other intrapartum hemorrhage
Excessive intrapartum hemorrhage

O67.9 Intrapartum hemorrhage, unspecified

O68 Labor and delivery complicated by abnormality of fetal acid-base balance
Fetal acidemia complicating labor and delivery
Fetal acidosis complicating labor and delivery
Fetal alkalosis complicating labor and delivery
Fetal metabolic acidemia complicating labor and delivery
EXCLUDES1 *fetal stress NOS (O77.9)*
labor and delivery complicated by electrocardiographic evidence of fetal stress (O77.8)
labor and delivery complicated by ultrasonic evidence of fetal stress (O77.8)
EXCLUDES2 *abnormality in fetal heart rate or rhythm (O76)*
labor and delivery complicated by meconium in amniotic fluid (O77.Ø)

✓4th **O69 Labor and delivery complicated by umbilical cord complications**

One of the following 7th characters is to be assigned to each code under category O69. 7th character Ø is for single gestations and multiple gestations where the fetus is unspecified. 7th characters 1 through 9 are for cases of multiple gestations to identify the fetus for which the code applies. The appropriate code from category O3Ø, Multiple gestation, must also be assigned when assigning a code from category O69 that has a 7th character of 1 through 9.
Ø not applicable or unspecified
1 fetus 1
2 fetus 2
3 fetus 3
4 fetus 4
5 fetus 5
9 other fetus

✓x7th **O69.Ø Labor and delivery complicated by prolapse of cord**

✓x7th **O69.1 Labor and delivery complicated by cord around neck, with compression**
EXCLUDES1 *labor and delivery complicated by cord around neck, without compression (O69.81)*

✓x7th **O69.2 Labor and delivery complicated by other cord entanglement, with compression**
Labor and delivery complicated by compression of cord NOS
Labor and delivery complicated by entanglement of cords of twins in monoamniotic sac
Labor and delivery complicated by knot in cord
EXCLUDES1 *labor and delivery complicated by other cord entanglement, without compression (O69.82)*

✓x7th **O69.3 Labor and delivery complicated by short cord**

√x7th **O69.4 Labor and delivery complicated by vasa previa**
Labor and delivery complicated by hemorrhage from vasa previa

√x7th **O69.5 Labor and delivery complicated by vascular lesion of cord**
Labor and delivery complicated by cord bruising
Labor and delivery complicated by cord hematoma
Labor and delivery complicated by thrombosis of umbilical vessels

√5th **O69.8 Labor and delivery complicated by other cord complications**

√x7th **O69.81 Labor and delivery complicated by cord around neck, without compression**

√x7th **O69.82 Labor and delivery complicated by other cord entanglement, without compression**

√x7th **O69.89 Labor and delivery complicated by other cord complications**

√x7th **O69.9 Labor and delivery complicated by cord complication, unspecified**

√4th **O70 Perineal laceration during delivery**
Episiotomy extended by laceration
EXCLUDES 1 *obstetric high vaginal laceration alone (O71.4)*

O70.0 First degree perineal laceration during delivery
Perineal laceration, rupture or tear involving fourchette during delivery
Perineal laceration, rupture or tear involving labia during delivery
Perineal laceration, rupture or tear involving skin during delivery
Perineal laceration, rupture or tear involving vagina during delivery
Perineal laceration, rupture or tear involving vulva during delivery
Slight perineal laceration, rupture or tear during delivery

O70.1 Second degree perineal laceration during delivery
Perineal laceration, rupture or tear during delivery as in O70.0, also involving pelvic floor
Perineal laceration, rupture or tear during delivery as in O70.0, also involving perineal muscles
Perineal laceration, rupture or tear during delivery as in O70.0, also involving vaginal muscles
EXCLUDES 1 *perineal laceration involving anal sphincter (O70.2)*

O70.2 Third degree perineal laceration during delivery
Perineal laceration, rupture or tear during delivery as in O70.1, also involving anal sphincter
Perineal laceration, rupture or tear during delivery as in O70.1, also involving rectovaginal septum
Perineal laceration, rupture or tear during delivery as in O70.1, also involving sphincter NOS
EXCLUDES 1 *anal sphincter tear during delivery without third degree perineal laceration (O70.4)*
perineal laceration involving anal or rectal mucosa (O70.3)

O70.3 Fourth degree perineal laceration during delivery
Perineal laceration, rupture or tear during delivery as in O70.2, also involving anal mucosa
Perineal laceration, rupture or tear during delivery as in O70.2, also involving rectal mucosa

O70.4 Anal sphincter tear complicating delivery, not associated with third degree laceration
EXCLUDES 1 *anal sphincter tear with third degree perineal laceration (O70.2)*

O70.9 Perineal laceration during delivery, unspecified

√4th **O71 Other obstetric trauma**
Obstetric damage from instruments

√5th **O71.0 Rupture of uterus (spontaneous) before onset of labor**
EXCLUDES 1 *disruption of (current) cesarean delivery wound (O90.0)*
laceration of uterus, NEC (O71.81)

O71.00 Rupture of uterus before onset of labor, unspecified trimester

O71.02 Rupture of uterus before onset of labor, second trimester

O71.03 Rupture of uterus before onset of labor, third trimester

O71.1 Rupture of uterus during labor
Rupture of uterus not stated as occurring before onset of labor
EXCLUDES 1 *disruption of cesarean delivery wound (O90.0)*
laceration of uterus, NEC (O71.81)

O71.2 Postpartum inversion of uterus

O71.3 Obstetric laceration of cervix
Annular detachment of cervix

O71.4 Obstetric high vaginal laceration alone
Laceration of vaginal wall without perineal laceration
EXCLUDES 1 *obstetric high vaginal laceration with perineal laceration (O70.-)*

O71.5 Other obstetric injury to pelvic organs
Obstetric injury to bladder
Obstetric injury to urethra
EXCLUDES 2 *obstetric periurethral trauma (O71.82)*

O71.6 Obstetric damage to pelvic joints and ligaments
Obstetric avulsion of inner symphyseal cartilage
Obstetric damage to coccyx
Obstetric traumatic separation of symphysis (pubis)

O71.7 Obstetric hematoma of pelvis
Obstetric hematoma of perineum
Obstetric hematoma of vagina
Obstetric hematoma of vulva

√5th **O71.8 Other specified obstetric trauma**

O71.81 Laceration of uterus, not elsewhere classified

O71.82 Other specified trauma to perineum and vulva
Obstetric periurethral trauma

O71.89 Other specified obstetric trauma

O71.9 Obstetric trauma, unspecified

√4th **O72 Postpartum hemorrhage**
INCLUDES hemorrhage after delivery of fetus or infant

O72.0 Third-stage hemorrhage
Hemorrhage associated with retained, trapped or adherent placenta
Retained placenta NOS
Code also type of adherent placenta (O43.2-)

O72.1 Other immediate postpartum hemorrhage
Hemorrhage following delivery of placenta
Postpartum hemorrhage (atonic) NOS
Uterine atony with hemorrhage
EXCLUDES 1 *uterine atony NOS (O62.2)*
uterine atony without hemorrhage (O62.2)
postpartum atony of uterus without hemorrhage (O75.89)

O72.2 Delayed and secondary postpartum hemorrhage
Hemorrhage associated with retained portions of placenta or membranes after the first 24 hours following delivery of placenta
Retained products of conception NOS, following delivery

O72.3 Postpartum coagulation defects
Postpartum afibrinogenemia
Postpartum fibrinolysis

√4th **O73 Retained placenta and membranes, without hemorrhage**
EXCLUDES 1 *placenta accreta (O43.21-)*
placenta increta (O43.22-)
placenta percreta (O43.23-)

O73.0 Retained placenta without hemorrhage
Adherent placenta, without hemorrhage
Trapped placenta without hemorrhage

O73.1 Retained portions of placenta and membranes, without hemorrhage
Retained products of conception following delivery, without hemorrhage

√4th **O74 Complications of anesthesia during labor and delivery**
INCLUDES maternal complications arising from the administration of a general, regional or local anesthetic, analgesic or other sedation during labor and delivery
Use additional code, if applicable, to identify specific complication

O74.0 Aspiration pneumonitis due to anesthesia during labor and delivery
Inhalation of stomach contents or secretions NOS due to anesthesia during labor and delivery
Mendelson's syndrome due to anesthesia during labor and delivery

O74.1 Other pulmonary complications of anesthesia during labor and delivery

O74.2 Cardiac complications of anesthesia during labor and delivery

O74.3 Central nervous system complications of anesthesia during labor and delivery

O74.4 Toxic reaction to local anesthesia during labor and delivery

O74.5 Spinal and epidural anesthesia-induced headache during labor and delivery

O74.6 Other complications of spinal and epidural anesthesia during labor and delivery

O74.7 Failed or difficult intubation for anesthesia during labor and delivery

O74.8 Other complications of anesthesia during labor and delivery

O74.9 Complication of anesthesia during labor and delivery, unspecified

√4th **O75 Other complications of labor and delivery, not elsewhere classified**

EXCLUDES 2 *puerperal (postpartum) infection (O86.-)*
puerperal (postpartum) sepsis (O85)

O75.0 Maternal distress during labor and delivery

O75.1 Shock during or following labor and delivery
Obstetric shock following labor and delivery

O75.2 Pyrexia during labor, not elsewhere classified

O75.3 Other infection during labor
Sepsis during labor
Use additional code (B95-B97), to identify infectious agent

O75.4 Other complications of obstetric surgery and procedures
Cardiac arrest following obstetric surgery or procedures
Cardiac failure following obstetric surgery or procedures
Cerebral anoxia following obstetric surgery or procedures
Pulmonary edema following obstetric surgery or procedures
Use additional code to identify specific complication
EXCLUDES 2 *complications of anesthesia during labor and delivery (O74.-)*
disruption of obstetrical (surgical) wound (O90.0-O90.1)
hematoma of obstetrical (surgical) wound (O90.2)
infection of obstetrical (surgical) wound (O86.0)

O75.5 Delayed delivery after artificial rupture of membranes

√5th **O75.8 Other specified complications of labor and delivery**

O75.81 Maternal exhaustion complicating labor and delivery

O75.82 Onset (spontaneous) of labor after 37 completed weeks of gestation but before 39 completed weeks gestation, with delivery by (planned) cesarean section
Delivery by (planned) cesarean section occurring after 37 completed weeks of gestation but before 39 completed weeks gestation due to (spontaneous) onset of labor
Use additional code to specify reason for planned cesarean section such as:
cephalopelvic disproportion (normally formed fetus) (O33.9)
previous cesarean delivery (O34.21)

O75.89 Other specified complications of labor and delivery

O75.9 Complication of labor and delivery, unspecified

O76 Abnormality in fetal heart rate and rhythm complicating labor and delivery
Depressed fetal heart rate tones complicating labor and delivery
Fetal bradycardia complicating labor and delivery
Fetal heart rate decelerations complicating labor and delivery
Fetal heart rate irregularity complicating labor and delivery
Fetal heart rate abnormal variability complicating labor and delivery
Fetal tachycardia complicating labor and delivery
Non-reassuring fetal heart rate or rhythm complicating labor and delivery
EXCLUDES 1 *fetal stress NOS (O77.9)*
labor and delivery complicated by electrocardiographic evidence of fetal stress (O77.8)
labor and delivery complicated by ultrasonic evidence of fetal stress (O77.8)
EXCLUDES 2 *fetal metabolic acidemia (O68)*
other fetal stress (O77.0-O77.1)

√4th **O77 Other fetal stress complicating labor and delivery**

O77.0 Labor and delivery complicated by meconium in amniotic fluid

O77.1 Fetal stress in labor or delivery due to drug administration

O77.8 Labor and delivery complicated by other evidence of fetal stress
Labor and delivery complicated by electrocardiographic evidence of fetal stress
Labor and delivery complicated by ultrasonic evidence of fetal stress
EXCLUDES 1 *abnormality of fetal acid-base balance (O68)*
abnormality in fetal heart rate or rhythm (O76)
fetal metabolic acidemia (O68)

O77.9 Labor and delivery complicated by fetal stress, unspecified
EXCLUDES 1 *abnormality of fetal acid-base balance (O68)*
abnormality in fetal heart rate or rhythm (O76)
fetal metabolic acidemia (O68)

Encounter for delivery (O80, O82)

O80 Encounter for full-term uncomplicated delivery
NOTE Delivery requiring minimal or no assistance, with or without episiotomy, without fetal manipulation [e.g., rotation version] or instrumentation [forceps] of a spontaneous, cephalic, vaginal, full-term, single, live-born infant. This code is for use as a single diagnosis code and is not to be used with any other code from chapter 15. This code must be accompanied by a delivery code from the appropriate procedure classification.
Use additional code to indicate outcome of delivery (Z37.0)

O82 Encounter for cesarean delivery without indication
NOTE This code must be accompanied by a delivery code from the appropriate procedure classification.
Use additional code to indicate outcome of delivery (Z37.0)

Complications predominantly related to the puerperium (O85-O92)

EXCLUDES 2 *mental and behavioral disorders associated with the puerperium (F53)*
obstetrical tetanus (A34)
puerperal osteomalacia (M83.0)

O85 Puerperal sepsis
Postpartum sepsis
Puerperal peritonitis
Puerperal pyemia
Use additional code (B95-B97), to identify infectious agent
Use additional code (R65.2-) to identify severe sepsis, if applicable
EXCLUDES 1 *fever of unknown origin following delivery (O86.4)*
genital tract infection following delivery (O86.1-)
obstetric pyemic and septic embolism (O88.3-)
puerperal septic thrombophlebitis (O86.81)
urinary tract infection following delivery (O86.2-)
EXCLUDES 2 *sepsis during labor (O75.3)*

√4th **O86 Other puerperal infections**
Use additional code (B95-B97), to identify infectious agent
EXCLUDES 2 *infection during labor (O75.3)*
obstetrical tetanus (A34)

O86.0 Infection of obstetric surgical wound
Infected cesarean delivery wound following delivery
Infected perineal repair following delivery

√5th **O86.1 Other infection of genital tract following delivery**

O86.11 Cervicitis following delivery

O86.12 Endometritis following delivery

O86.13 Vaginitis following delivery

O86.19 Other infection of genital tract following delivery

√5th **O86.2 Urinary tract infection following delivery**

O86.20 Urinary tract infection following delivery, unspecified
Puerperal urinary tract infection NOS

O86.21 Infection of kidney following delivery

O86.22 Infection of bladder following delivery
Infection of urethra following delivery

O86.29 Other urinary tract infection following delivery

O86.4 Pyrexia of unknown origin following delivery
Puerperal infection NOS following delivery
Puerperal pyrexia NOS following delivery
EXCLUDES 2 *pyrexia during labor (O75.2)*

√5th **O86.8 Other specified puerperal infections**

O86.81 Puerperal septic thrombophlebitis

O86.89 Other specified puerperal infections

O87 Venous complications and hemorrhoids in the puerperium
Venous complications in labor, delivery and the puerperium
EXCLUDES 2 *obstetric embolism (O88.-)*
puerperal septic thrombophlebitis (O86.81)
venous complications in pregnancy (O22.-)

O87.0 Superficial thrombophlebitis in the puerperium
Puerperal phlebitis NOS
Puerperal thrombosis NOS

O87.1 Deep phlebothrombosis in the puerperium
Deep vein thrombosis, postpartum
Pelvic thrombophlebitis, postpartum
Use additional code to identify the deep vein thrombosis (I82.4-, I82.5-, I82.62-. I82.72-)
Use additional code, if applicable, for associated long-term (current) use of anticoagulants (Z79.01)

O87.2 Hemorrhoids in the puerperium

O87.3 Cerebral venous thrombosis in the puerperium
Cerebrovenous sinus thrombosis in the puerperium

O87.4 Varicose veins of lower extremity in the puerperium

O87.8 Other venous complications in the puerperium
Genital varices in the puerperium

O87.9 Venous complication in the puerperium, unspecified
Puerperal phlebopathy NOS

O88 Obstetric embolism
EXCLUDES 1 *embolism complicating abortion NOS (O03.2)*
embolism complicating ectopic or molar pregnancy (O08.2)
embolism complicating failed attempted abortion (O07.2, O07.7)
embolism complicating induced abortion (O04.7)
embolism complicating spontaneous abortion (O03.2, O03.7)

O88.0 Obstetric air embolism
O88.01 Obstetric air embolism in pregnancy
O88.011 Air embolism in pregnancy, first trimester
O88.012 Air embolism in pregnancy, second trimester
O88.013 Air embolism in pregnancy, third trimester
O88.019 Air embolism in pregnancy, unspecified trimester
O88.02 Air embolism in childbirth
O88.03 Air embolism in the puerperium

O88.1 Amniotic fluid embolism
Anaphylactoid syndrome in pregnancy
O88.11 Amniotic fluid embolism in pregnancy
O88.111 Amniotic fluid embolism in pregnancy, first trimester
O88.112 Amniotic fluid embolism in pregnancy, second trimester
O88.113 Amniotic fluid embolism in pregnancy, third trimester
O88.119 Amniotic fluid embolism in pregnancy, unspecified trimester
O88.12 Amniotic fluid embolism in childbirth
O88.13 Amniotic fluid embolism in the puerperium

O88.2 Obstetric thromboembolism
O88.21 Thromboembolism in pregnancy
Obstetric (pulmonary) embolism NOS
O88.211 Thromboembolism in pregnancy, first trimester
O88.212 Thromboembolism in pregnancy, second trimester
O88.213 Thromboembolism in pregnancy, third trimester
O88.219 Thromboembolism in pregnancy, unspecified trimester
O88.22 Thromboembolism in childbirth
O88.23 Thromboembolism in the puerperium
Puerperal (pulmonary) embolism NOS

O88.3 Obstetric pyemic and septic embolism
O88.31 Pyemic and septic embolism in pregnancy
O88.311 Pyemic and septic embolism in pregnancy, first trimester
O88.312 Pyemic and septic embolism in pregnancy, second trimester
O88.313 Pyemic and septic embolism in pregnancy, third trimester
O88.319 Pyemic and septic embolism in pregnancy, unspecified trimester
O88.32 Pyemic and septic embolism in childbirth
O88.33 Pyemic and septic embolism in the puerperium

O88.8 Other obstetric embolism
Obstetric fat embolism
O88.81 Other embolism in pregnancy
O88.811 Other embolism in pregnancy, first trimester
O88.812 Other embolism in pregnancy, second trimester
O88.813 Other embolism in pregnancy, third trimester
O88.819 Other embolism in pregnancy, unspecified trimester
O88.82 Other embolism in childbirth
O88.83 Other embolism in the puerperium

O89 Complications of anesthesia during the puerperium
INCLUDES maternal complications arising from the administration of a general, regional or local anesthetic, analgesic or other sedation during the puerperium
Use additional code, if applicable, to identify specific complication

O89.0 Pulmonary complications of anesthesia during the puerperium
O89.01 Aspiration pneumonitis due to anesthesia during the puerperium
Inhalation of stomach contents or secretions NOS due to anesthesia during the puerperium
Mendelson's syndrome due to anesthesia during the puerperium
O89.09 Other pulmonary complications of anesthesia during the puerperium

O89.1 Cardiac complications of anesthesia during the puerperium

O89.2 Central nervous system complications of anesthesia during the puerperium

O89.3 Toxic reaction to local anesthesia during the puerperium

O89.4 Spinal and epidural anesthesia-induced headache during the puerperium

O89.5 Other complications of spinal and epidural anesthesia during the puerperium

O89.6 Failed or difficult intubation for anesthesia during the puerperium

O89.8 Other complications of anesthesia during the puerperium

O89.9 Complication of anesthesia during the puerperium, unspecified

O90 Complications of the puerperium, not elsewhere classified

O90.0 Disruption of cesarean delivery wound
Dehiscence of cesarean delivery wound
EXCLUDES 1 *rupture of uterus (spontaneous) before onset of labor (O71.0-)*
rupture of uterus during labor (O71.1)

O90.1 Disruption of perineal obstetric wound
Disruption of wound of episiotomy
Disruption of wound of perineal laceration
Secondary perineal tear

O90.2 Hematoma of obstetric wound

O90.3 Peripartum cardiomyopathy
Conditions in I42- arising during pregnancy and the puerperium
EXCLUDES 1 *pre-existing heart disease complicating pregnancy and the puerperium (O99.4-)*

O90.4 Postpartum acute kidney failure
Hepatorenal syndrome following labor and delivery

O90.5 Postpartum thyroiditis

O90.6 Postpartum mood disturbance
Postpartum blues
Postpartum dysphoria
Postpartum sadness
EXCLUDES 1 *postpartum depression (F53)*
puerperal psychosis (F53)

O90.8 Other complications of the puerperium, not elsewhere classified
O90.81 Anemia of the puerperium
Postpartum anemia NOS
EXCLUDES 1 *pre-existing anemia complicating the puerperium (O99.03)*

O9Ø.89 Other complications of the puerperium, not elsewhere classified
Placental polyp

O9Ø.9 Complication of the puerperium, unspecified

O91 Infections of breast associated with pregnancy, the puerperium and lactation
Use additional code to identify infection

O91.Ø Infection of nipple associated with pregnancy, the puerperium and lactation

O91.Ø1 Infection of nipple associated with pregnancy
Gestational abscess of nipple

O91.Ø11 Infection of nipple associated with pregnancy, first trimester

O91.Ø12 Infection of nipple associated with pregnancy, second trimester

O91.Ø13 Infection of nipple associated with pregnancy, third trimester

O91.Ø19 Infection of nipple associated with pregnancy, unspecified trimester

O91.Ø2 Infection of nipple associated with the puerperium
Puerperal abscess of nipple

O91.Ø3 Infection of nipple associated with lactation
Abscess of nipple associated with lactation

O91.1 Abscess of breast associated with pregnancy, the puerperium and lactation

O91.11 Abscess of breast associated with pregnancy
Gestational mammary abscess
Gestational purulent mastitis
Gestational subareolar abscess

O91.111 Abscess of breast associated with pregnancy, first trimester

O91.112 Abscess of breast associated with pregnancy, second trimester

O91.113 Abscess of breast associated with pregnancy, third trimester

O91.119 Abscess of breast associated with pregnancy, unspecified trimester

O91.12 Abscess of breast associated with the puerperium
Puerperal mammary abscess
Puerperal purulent mastitis
Puerperal subareolar abscess

O91.13 Abscess of breast associated with lactation
Mammary abscess associated with lactation
Purulent mastitis associated with lactation
Subareolar abscess associated with lactation

O91.2 Nonpurulent mastitis associated with pregnancy, the puerperium and lactation

O91.21 Nonpurulent mastitis associated with pregnancy
Gestational interstitial mastitis
Gestational lymphangitis of breast
Gestational mastitis NOS
Gestational parenchymatous mastitis

O91.211 Nonpurulent mastitis associated with pregnancy, first trimester

O91.212 Nonpurulent mastitis associated with pregnancy, second trimester

O91.213 Nonpurulent mastitis associated with pregnancy, third trimester

O91.219 Nonpurulent mastitis associated with pregnancy, unspecified trimester

O91.22 Nonpurulent mastitis associated with the puerperium
Puerperal interstitial mastitis
Puerperal lymphangitis of breast
Puerperal mastitis NOS
Puerperal parenchymatous mastitis

O91.23 Nonpurulent mastitis associated with lactation
Interstitial mastitis associated with lactation
Lymphangitis of breast associated with lactation
Mastitis NOS associated with lactation
Parenchymatous mastitis associated with lactation

O92 Other disorders of breast and disorders of lactation associated with pregnancy and the puerperium

O92.Ø Retracted nipple associated with pregnancy, the puerperium, and lactation

O92.Ø1 Retracted nipple associated with pregnancy

O92.Ø11 Retracted nipple associated with pregnancy, first trimester

O92.Ø12 Retracted nipple associated with pregnancy, second trimester

O92.Ø13 Retracted nipple associated with pregnancy, third trimester

O92.Ø19 Retracted nipple associated with pregnancy, unspecified trimester

O92.Ø2 Retracted nipple associated with the puerperium

O92.Ø3 Retracted nipple associated with lactation

O92.1 Cracked nipple associated with pregnancy, the puerperium, and lactation
Fissure of nipple, gestational or puerperal

O92.11 Cracked nipple associated with pregnancy

O92.111 Cracked nipple associated with pregnancy, first trimester

O92.112 Cracked nipple associated with pregnancy, second trimester

O92.113 Cracked nipple associated with pregnancy, third trimester

O92.119 Cracked nipple associated with pregnancy, unspecified trimester

O92.12 Cracked nipple associated with the puerperium

O92.13 Cracked nipple associated with lactation

O92.2 Other and unspecified disorders of breast associated with pregnancy and the puerperium

O92.2Ø Unspecified disorder of breast associated with pregnancy and the puerperium

O92.29 Other disorders of breast associated with pregnancy and the puerperium

O92.3 Agalactia
Primary agalactia
EXCLUDES 1 *elective agalactia (O92.5)*
secondary agalactia (O92.5)
therapeutic agalactia (O92.5)

O92.4 Hypogalactia

O92.5 Suppressed lactation
Elective agalactia
Secondary agalactia
Therapeutic agalactia
EXCLUDES 1 *primary agalactia (O92.3)*

O92.6 Galactorrhea

O92.7 Other and unspecified disorders of lactation

O92.7Ø Unspecified disorders of lactation

O92.79 Other disorders of lactation
Puerperal galactocele

Other obstetric conditions, not elsewhere classified (O94-O9A)

O94 Sequelae of complication of pregnancy, childbirth, and the puerperium
NOTE This category is to be used to indicate conditions in OØØ-O77.-, O85-O94 and O98-O9A.- as the cause of late effects. The sequelae include conditions specified as such, or as late effects, which may occur at any time after the puerperium
Code first condition resulting from (sequela) of complication of pregnancy, childbirth, and the puerperium

O98 Maternal infectious and parasitic diseases classifiable elsewhere but complicating pregnancy, childbirth and the puerperium
INCLUDES the listed conditions when complicating the pregnant state, when aggravated by the pregnancy, or as a reason for obstetric care
Use additional code (Chapter 1), to identify specific infectious or parasitic disease
EXCLUDES 2 *herpes gestationis (O26.4-)*
infectious carrier state (O99.82-, O99.83-)
obstetrical tetanus (A34)
puerperal infection (O86.-)
puerperal sepsis (O85)
when the reason for maternal care is that the disease is known or suspected to have affected the fetus (O35-O36)

O98.Ø Tuberculosis complicating pregnancy, childbirth and the puerperium
Conditions in A15-A19

O98.Ø1 Tuberculosis complicating pregnancy

O98.Ø11 Tuberculosis complicating pregnancy, first trimester

O98.012 Tuberculosis complicating pregnancy, second trimester

O98.013 Tuberculosis complicating pregnancy, third trimester

O98.019 Tuberculosis complicating pregnancy, unspecified trimester

O98.02 Tuberculosis complicating childbirth

O98.03 Tuberculosis complicating the puerperium

√5th **O98.1 Syphilis complicating pregnancy, childbirth and the puerperium**

Conditions in A50-A53

√6th **O98.11 Syphilis complicating pregnancy**

O98.111 Syphilis complicating pregnancy, first trimester

O98.112 Syphilis complicating pregnancy, second trimester

O98.113 Syphilis complicating pregnancy, third trimester

O98.119 Syphilis complicating pregnancy, unspecified trimester

O98.12 Syphilis complicating childbirth

O98.13 Syphilis complicating the puerperium

√5th **O98.2 Gonorrhea complicating pregnancy, childbirth and the puerperium**

Conditions in A54-

√6th **O98.21 Gonorrhea complicating pregnancy**

O98.211 Gonorrhea complicating pregnancy, first trimester

O98.212 Gonorrhea complicating pregnancy, second trimester

O98.213 Gonorrhea complicating pregnancy, third trimester

O98.219 Gonorrhea complicating pregnancy, unspecified trimester

O98.22 Gonorrhea complicating childbirth

O98.23 Gonorrhea complicating the puerperium

√5th **O98.3 Other infections with a predominantly sexual mode of transmission complicating pregnancy, childbirth and the puerperium**

Conditions in A55-A64

√6th **O98.31 Other infections with a predominantly sexual mode of transmission complicating pregnancy**

O98.311 Other infections with a predominantly sexual mode of transmission complicating pregnancy, first trimester

O98.312 Other infections with a predominantly sexual mode of transmission complicating pregnancy, second trimester

O98.313 Other infections with a predominantly sexual mode of transmission complicating pregnancy, third trimester

O98.319 Other infections with a predominantly sexual mode of transmission complicating pregnancy, unspecified trimester

O98.32 Other infections with a predominantly sexual mode of transmission complicating childbirth

O98.33 Other infections with a predominantly sexual mode of transmission complicating the puerperium

√5th **O98.4 Viral hepatitis complicating pregnancy, childbirth and the puerperium**

Conditions in B15-B19

√6th **O98.41 Viral hepatitis complicating pregnancy**

O98.411 Viral hepatitis complicating pregnancy, first trimester

O98.412 Viral hepatitis complicating pregnancy, second trimester

O98.413 Viral hepatitis complicating pregnancy, third trimester

O98.419 Viral hepatitis complicating pregnancy, unspecified trimester

O98.42 Viral hepatitis complicating childbirth

O98.43 Viral hepatitis complicating the puerperium

√5th **O98.5 Other viral diseases complicating pregnancy, childbirth and the puerperium**

Conditions in A80-B09, B25-B34, R87.81-, R87.82-

EXCLUDES 1 *human immunodeficiency virus [HIV] disease complicating pregnancy, childbirth and the puerperium (O98.7-)*

√6th **O98.51 Other viral diseases complicating pregnancy**

O98.511 Other viral diseases complicating pregnancy, first trimester

O98.512 Other viral diseases complicating pregnancy, second trimester

O98.513 Other viral diseases complicating pregnancy, third trimester

O98.519 Other viral diseases complicating pregnancy, unspecified trimester

O98.52 Other viral diseases complicating childbirth

O98.53 Other viral diseases complicating the puerperium

√5th **O98.6 Protozoal diseases complicating pregnancy, childbirth and the puerperium**

Conditions in B50-B64

√6th **O98.61 Protozoal diseases complicating pregnancy**

O98.611 Protozoal diseases complicating pregnancy, first trimester

O98.612 Protozoal diseases complicating pregnancy, second trimester

O98.613 Protozoal diseases complicating pregnancy, third trimester

O98.619 Protozoal diseases complicating pregnancy, unspecified trimester

O98.62 Protozoal diseases complicating childbirth

O98.63 Protozoal diseases complicating the puerperium

√5th **O98.7 Human immunodeficiency virus [HIV] disease complicating pregnancy, childbirth and the puerperium**

Use additional code to identify the type of HIV disease:
- acquired immune deficiency syndrome (AIDS) (B20)
- asymptomatic HIV status (Z21)
- HIV positive NOS (Z21)
- symptomatic HIV disease (B20)

√6th **O98.71 Human immunodeficiency virus [HIV] disease complicating pregnancy**

O98.711 Human immunodeficiency virus [HIV] disease complicating pregnancy, first trimester

O98.712 Human immunodeficiency virus [HIV] disease complicating pregnancy, second trimester

O98.713 Human immunodeficiency virus [HIV] disease complicating pregnancy, third trimester

O98.719 Human immunodeficiency virus [HIV] disease complicating pregnancy, unspecified trimester

O98.72 Human immunodeficiency virus [HIV] disease complicating childbirth

O98.73 Human immunodeficiency virus [HIV] disease complicating the puerperium

√5th **O98.8 Other maternal infectious and parasitic diseases complicating pregnancy, childbirth and the puerperium**

√6th **O98.81 Other maternal infectious and parasitic diseases complicating pregnancy**

O98.811 Other maternal infectious and parasitic diseases complicating pregnancy, first trimester

O98.812 Other maternal infectious and parasitic diseases complicating pregnancy, second trimester

O98.813 Other maternal infectious and parasitic diseases complicating pregnancy, third trimester

O98.819 Other maternal infectious and parasitic diseases complicating pregnancy, unspecified trimester

O98.82 Other maternal infectious and parasitic diseases complicating childbirth

O98.83 Other maternal infectious and parasitic diseases complicating the puerperium

5th **O98.9 Unspecified maternal infectious and parasitic disease complicating pregnancy, childbirth and the puerperium**

6th **O98.91 Unspecified maternal infectious and parasitic disease complicating pregnancy**

O98.911 Unspecified maternal infectious and parasitic disease complicating pregnancy, first trimester

O98.912 Unspecified maternal infectious and parasitic disease complicating pregnancy, second trimester

O98.913 Unspecified maternal infectious and parasitic disease complicating pregnancy, third trimester

O98.919 Unspecified maternal infectious and parasitic disease complicating pregnancy, unspecified trimester

O98.92 Unspecified maternal infectious and parasitic disease complicating childbirth

O98.93 Unspecified maternal infectious and parasitic disease complicating the puerperium

4th **O99 Other maternal diseases classifiable elsewhere but complicating pregnancy, childbirth and the puerperium**

Conditions which complicate the pregnant state, are aggravated by the pregnancy or are a main reason for obstetric care

Use additional code to identify specific condition

EXCLUDES 2 *when the reason for maternal care is that the condition is known or suspected to have affected the fetus (O35-O36)*

5th **O99.Ø Anemia complicating pregnancy, childbirth and the puerperium**

Conditions in D5Ø-D64

EXCLUDES 1 *anemia arising in the puerperium (O9Ø.81)*
postpartum anemia NOS (O9Ø.81)

6th **O99.Ø1 Anemia complicating pregnancy**

O99.Ø11 Anemia complicating pregnancy, first trimester

O99.Ø12 Anemia complicating pregnancy, second trimester

O99.Ø13 Anemia complicating pregnancy, third trimester

O99.Ø19 Anemia complicating pregnancy, unspecified trimester

O99.Ø2 Anemia complicating childbirth

O99.Ø3 Anemia complicating the puerperium

EXCLUDES 1 *postpartum anemia not pre-existing prior to delivery (O9Ø-.81)*

5th **O99.1 Other diseases of the blood and blood-forming organs and certain disorders involving the immune mechanism complicating pregnancy, childbirth and the puerperium**

Conditions in D65-D89

EXCLUDES 2 *hemorrhage with coagulation defects (O45.-, O46.Ø-, O67.Ø, O72.3)*

6th **O99.11 Other diseases of the blood and blood-forming organs and certain disorders involving the immune mechanism complicating pregnancy**

O99.111 Other diseases of the blood and blood-forming organs and certain disorders involving the immune mechanism complicating pregnancy, first trimester

O99.112 Other diseases of the blood and blood-forming organs and certain disorders involving the immune mechanism complicating pregnancy, second trimester

O99.113 Other diseases of the blood and blood-forming organs and certain disorders involving the immune mechanism complicating pregnancy, third trimester

O99.119 Other diseases of the blood and blood-forming organs and certain disorders involving the immune mechanism complicating pregnancy, unspecified trimester

O99.12 Other diseases of the blood and blood-forming organs and certain disorders involving the immune mechanism complicating childbirth

O99.13 Other diseases of the blood and blood-forming organs and certain disorders involving the immune mechanism complicating the puerperium

5th **O99.2 Endocrine, nutritional and metabolic diseases complicating pregnancy, childbirth and the puerperium**

Conditions in EØØ-E88

EXCLUDES 2 *diabetes mellitus (O24.-)*
malnutrition (O25.-)
postpartum thyroiditis (O9Ø.5)

6th **O99.21 Obesity complicating pregnancy, childbirth, and the puerperium**

Use additional code to identify the type of obesity (E66.-)

O99.21Ø Obesity complicating pregnancy, unspecified trimester

O99.211 Obesity complicating pregnancy, first trimester

O99.212 Obesity complicating pregnancy, second trimester

O99.213 Obesity complicating pregnancy, third trimester

O99.214 Obesity complicating childbirth

O99.215 Obesity complicating the puerperium

6th **O99.28 Other endocrine, nutritional and metabolic diseases complicating pregnancy, childbirth and the puerperium**

O99.28Ø Endocrine, nutritional and metabolic diseases complicating pregnancy, unspecified trimester

O99.281 Endocrine, nutritional and metabolic diseases complicating pregnancy, first trimester

O99.282 Endocrine, nutritional and metabolic diseases complicating pregnancy, second trimester

O99.283 Endocrine, nutritional and metabolic diseases complicating pregnancy, third trimester

O99.284 Endocrine, nutritional and metabolic diseases complicating childbirth

O99.285 Endocrine, nutritional and metabolic diseases complicating the puerperium

5th **O99.3 Mental disorders and diseases of the nervous system complicating pregnancy, childbirth and the puerperium**

6th **O99.31 Alcohol use complicating pregnancy, childbirth, and the puerperium**

Use additional code(s) from F1Ø to identify manifestations of the alcohol use

O99.31Ø Alcohol use complicating pregnancy, unspecified trimester

O99.311 Alcohol use complicating pregnancy, first trimester

O99.312 Alcohol use complicating pregnancy, second trimester

O99.313 Alcohol use complicating pregnancy, third trimester

O99.314 Alcohol use complicating childbirth

O99.315 Alcohol use complicating the puerperium

6th **O99.32 Drug use complicating pregnancy, childbirth, and the puerperium**

Use additional code(s) from F11-F16 and F18-F19 to identify manifestations of the drug use

O99.32Ø Drug use complicating pregnancy, unspecified trimester

O99.321 Drug use complicating pregnancy, first trimester

O99.322 Drug use complicating pregnancy, second trimester

O99.323 Drug use complicating pregnancy, third trimester

O99.324 Drug use complicating childbirth

O99.325 Drug use complicating the puerperium

6th **O99.33 Smoking (tobacco) complicating pregnancy, childbirth, and the puerperium**

Use additional code from F17 to identify type of tobacco

O99.33Ø Smoking (tobacco) complicating pregnancy, unspecified trimester

O99.331 **Smoking (tobacco) complicating pregnancy, first trimester**
O99.332 **Smoking (tobacco) complicating pregnancy, second trimester**
O99.333 **Smoking (tobacco) complicating pregnancy, third trimester**
O99.334 **Smoking (tobacco) complicating childbirth**
O99.335 **Smoking (tobacco) complicating the puerperium**

6th O99.34 **Other mental disorders complicating pregnancy, childbirth, and the puerperium**
Conditions in F01-F09 and F20-F99
EXCLUDES 2 *postpartum mood disturbance (O90.6)*
postnatal psychosis (F53)
puerperal psychosis (F53)
O99.340 **Other mental disorders complicating pregnancy, unspecified trimester**
O99.341 **Other mental disorders complicating pregnancy, first trimester**
O99.342 **Other mental disorders complicating pregnancy, second trimester**
O99.343 **Other mental disorders complicating pregnancy, third trimester**
O99.344 **Other mental disorders complicating childbirth**
O99.345 **Other mental disorders complicating the puerperium**

6th O99.35 **Diseases of the nervous system complicating pregnancy, childbirth, and the puerperium**
Conditions in G00-G99
EXCLUDES 2 *pregnancy related peripheral neuritis (O26.8-)*
O99.350 **Diseases of the nervous system complicating pregnancy, unspecified trimester**
O99.351 **Diseases of the nervous system complicating pregnancy, first trimester**
O99.352 **Diseases of the nervous system complicating pregnancy, second trimester**
O99.353 **Diseases of the nervous system complicating pregnancy, third trimester**
O99.354 **Diseases of the nervous system complicating childbirth**
O99.355 **Diseases of the nervous system complicating the puerperium**

5th O99.4 **Diseases of the circulatory system complicating pregnancy, childbirth and the puerperium**
Conditions in I00-I99
EXCLUDES 1 *peripartum cardiomyopathy (O90.3)*
EXCLUDES 2 *hypertensive disorders (O10-O16)*
obstetric embolism (O88.-)
venous complications and cerebrovenous sinus thrombosis in labor, childbirth and the puerperium (O87.-)
venous complications and cerebrovenous sinus thrombosis in pregnancy (O22.-)

6th O99.41 **Diseases of the circulatory system complicating pregnancy**
O99.411 **Diseases of the circulatory system complicating pregnancy, first trimester**
O99.412 **Diseases of the circulatory system complicating pregnancy, second trimester**
O99.413 **Diseases of the circulatory system complicating pregnancy, third trimester**
O99.419 **Diseases of the circulatory system complicating pregnancy, unspecified trimester**
O99.42 **Diseases of the circulatory system complicating childbirth**
O99.43 **Diseases of the circulatory system complicating the puerperium**

5th O99.5 **Diseases of the respiratory system complicating pregnancy, childbirth and the puerperium**
Conditions in J00-J99
6th O99.51 **Diseases of the respiratory system complicating pregnancy**
O99.511 **Diseases of the respiratory system complicating pregnancy, first trimester**
O99.512 **Diseases of the respiratory system complicating pregnancy, second trimester**
O99.513 **Diseases of the respiratory system complicating pregnancy, third trimester**
O99.519 **Diseases of the respiratory system complicating pregnancy, unspecified trimester**
O99.52 **Diseases of the respiratory system complicating childbirth**
O99.53 **Diseases of the respiratory system complicating the puerperium**

5th O99.6 **Diseases of the digestive system complicating pregnancy, childbirth and the puerperium**
Conditions in K00-K93
EXCLUDES 2 *liver and biliary tract disorders in pregnancy, childbirth and the puerperium (O26.6-)*
6th O99.61 **Diseases of the digestive system complicating pregnancy**
O99.611 **Diseases of the digestive system complicating pregnancy, first trimester**
O99.612 **Diseases of the digestive system complicating pregnancy, second trimester**
O99.613 **Diseases of the digestive system complicating pregnancy, third trimester**
O99.619 **Diseases of the digestive system complicating pregnancy, unspecified trimester**
O99.62 **Diseases of the digestive system complicating childbirth**
O99.63 **Diseases of the digestive system complicating the puerperium**

5th O99.7 **Diseases of the skin and subcutaneous tissue complicating pregnancy, childbirth and the puerperium**
Conditions in L00-L99
EXCLUDES 2 *herpes gestationis (O26.4)*
pruritic urticarial papules and plaques of pregnancy (PUPPP) (O26.86)
6th O99.71 **Diseases of the skin and subcutaneous tissue complicating pregnancy**
O99.711 **Diseases of the skin and subcutaneous tissue complicating pregnancy, first trimester**
O99.712 **Diseases of the skin and subcutaneous tissue complicating pregnancy, second trimester**
O99.713 **Diseases of the skin and subcutaneous tissue complicating pregnancy, third trimester**
O99.719 **Diseases of the skin and subcutaneous tissue complicating pregnancy, unspecified trimester**
O99.72 **Diseases of the skin and subcutaneous tissue complicating childbirth**
O99.73 **Diseases of the skin and subcutaneous tissue complicating the puerperium**

5th O99.8 **Other specified diseases and conditions complicating pregnancy, childbirth and the puerperium**
Conditions in D00-D48, H00-H95, M00-N99, and Q00-Q99
Use additional code to identify condition
EXCLUDES 2 *genitourinary infections in pregnancy (O23.-)*
infection of genitourinary tract following delivery (O86.1-O86.3)
malignant neoplasm complicating pregnancy, childbirth and the puerperium (O9A.1-)
maternal care for known or suspected abnormality of maternal pelvic organs (O34.-)
postpartum acute kidney failure (O90.4)
traumatic injuries in pregnancy (O9A.2)
6th O99.81 **Abnormal glucose complicating pregnancy, childbirth and the puerperium**
EXCLUDES 1 *gestational diabetes (O24.4-)*
O99.810 **Abnormal glucose complicating pregnancy**
O99.814 **Abnormal glucose complicating childbirth**

O99.815 **Abnormal glucose complicating the puerperium**

✓6th O99.82 **Streptococcus B carrier state complicating pregnancy, childbirth and the puerperium**

O99.820 **Streptococcus B carrier state complicating pregnancy**

O99.824 **Streptococcus B carrier state complicating childbirth**

O99.825 **Streptococcus B carrier state complicating the puerperium**

✓6th O99.83 **Other infection carrier state complicating pregnancy, childbirth and the puerperium**

Use additional code to identify the carrier state (Z22.-)

O99.830 **Other infection carrier state complicating pregnancy**

O99.834 **Other infection carrier state complicating childbirth**

O99.835 **Other infection carrier state complicating the puerperium**

✓6th O99.84 **Bariatric surgery status complicating pregnancy, childbirth and the puerperium**

Gastric banding status complicating pregnancy, childbirth and the puerperium

Gastric bypass status for obesity complicating pregnancy, childbirth and the puerperium

Obesity surgery status complicating pregnancy, childbirth and the puerperium

O99.840 **Bariatric surgery status complicating pregnancy, unspecified trimester**

O99.841 **Bariatric surgery status complicating pregnancy, first trimester**

O99.842 **Bariatric surgery status complicating pregnancy, second trimester**

O99.843 **Bariatric surgery status complicating pregnancy, third trimester**

O99.844 **Bariatric surgery status complicating childbirth**

O99.845 **Bariatric surgery status complicating the puerperium**

O99.89 **Other specified diseases and conditions complicating pregnancy, childbirth and the puerperium**

✓4th **O9A Maternal malignant neoplasms, traumatic injuries and abuse classifiable elsewhere but complicating pregnancy, childbirth and the puerperium**

✓5th O9A.1 **Malignant neoplasm complicating pregnancy, childbirth and the puerperium**

Conditions in CØØ-C96

Use additional code to identify neoplasm

EXCLUDES 2 *maternal care for benign tumor of corpus uteri (O34.1-)*

maternal care for benign tumor of cervix (O34.4-)

✓6th O9A.11 **Malignant neoplasm complicating pregnancy**

O9A.111 **Malignant neoplasm complicating pregnancy, first trimester**

O9A.112 **Malignant neoplasm complicating pregnancy, second trimester**

O9A.113 **Malignant neoplasm complicating pregnancy, third trimester**

O9A.119 **Malignant neoplasm complicating pregnancy, unspecified trimester**

O9A.12 **Malignant neoplasm complicating childbirth**

O9A.13 **Malignant neoplasm complicating the puerperium**

✓5th O9A.2 **Injury, poisoning and certain other consequences of external causes complicating pregnancy, childbirth and the puerperium**

Conditions in SØØ-T88, except T74 and T76

Use additional code(s) to identify the injury or poisoning

EXCLUDES 2 *physical, sexual and psychological abuse complicating pregnancy, childbirth and the puerperium (O9A.3-, O9A.4-, O9A.5-)*

✓6th O9A.21 **Injury, poisoning and certain other consequences of external causes complicating pregnancy**

O9A.211 **Injury, poisoning and certain other consequences of external causes complicating pregnancy, first trimester**

O9A.212 **Injury, poisoning and certain other consequences of external causes complicating pregnancy, second trimester**

O9A.213 **Injury, poisoning and certain other consequences of external causes complicating pregnancy, third trimester**

O9A.219 **Injury, poisoning and certain other consequences of external causes complicating pregnancy, unspecified trimester**

O9A.22 **Injury, poisoning and certain other consequences of external causes complicating childbirth**

O9A.23 **Injury, poisoning and certain other consequences of external causes complicating the puerperium**

✓5th O9A.3 **Physical abuse complicating pregnancy, childbirth and the puerperium**

Conditions in T74.11 or T76.11

Use additional code (if applicable):

to identify any associated current injury due to physical abuse

to identify the perpetrator of abuse (YØ7.-)

EXCLUDES 2 *sexual abuse complicating pregnancy, childbirth and the puerperium (O9A.4)*

✓6th O9A.31 **Physical abuse complicating pregnancy**

O9A.311 **Physical abuse complicating pregnancy, first trimester**

O9A.312 **Physical abuse complicating pregnancy, second trimester**

O9A.313 **Physical abuse complicating pregnancy, third trimester**

O9A.319 **Physical abuse complicating pregnancy, unspecified trimester**

O9A.32 **Physical abuse complicating childbirth**

O9A.33 **Physical abuse complicating the puerperium**

✓5th O9A.4 **Sexual abuse complicating pregnancy, childbirth and the puerperium**

Conditions in T74.21 or T76.21

Use additional code (if applicable):

to identify any associated current injury due to sexual abuse

to identify the perpetrator of abuse (YØ7.-)

✓6th O9A.41 **Sexual abuse complicating pregnancy**

O9A.411 **Sexual abuse complicating pregnancy, first trimester**

O9A.412 **Sexual abuse complicating pregnancy, second trimester**

O9A.413 **Sexual abuse complicating pregnancy, third trimester**

O9A.419 **Sexual abuse complicating pregnancy, unspecified trimester**

O9A.42 **Sexual abuse complicating childbirth**

O9A.43 **Sexual abuse complicating the puerperium**

✓5th O9A.5 **Psychological abuse complicating pregnancy, childbirth and the puerperium**

Conditions in T74.31 or T76.31

Use additional code to identify the perpetrator of abuse (YØ7.-)

✓6th O9A.51 **Psychological abuse complicating pregnancy**

O9A.511 **Psychological abuse complicating pregnancy, first trimester**

O9A.512 **Psychological abuse complicating pregnancy, second trimester**

O9A.513 **Psychological abuse complicating pregnancy, third trimester**

O9A.519 **Psychological abuse complicating pregnancy, unspecified trimester**

O9A.52 **Psychological abuse complicating childbirth**

O9A.53 **Psychological abuse complicating the puerperium**

Chapter 16. Certain Conditions Originating in the Perinatal Period (PØØ-P96)

NOTE Codes from this chapter are for use on newborn records only, never on maternal records

INCLUDES conditions that have their origin in the fetal or perinatal period (before birth through the first 28 days after birth) even if morbidity occurs later

EXCLUDES 2 *congenital malformations, deformations and chromosomal abnormalities (QØØ-Q99)*
endocrine, nutritional and metabolic diseases (EØØ-E88)
injury, poisoning and certain other consequences of external causes (SØØ-T88)
neoplasms (CØØ-D49)
tetanus neonatorum (A33)

This chapter contains the following blocks:

PØØ-PØ4	Newborn affected by maternal factors and by complications of pregnancy, labor, and delivery
PØ5-PØ8	Disorders of newborn related to length of gestation and fetal growth
PØ9	Abnormal findings on neonatal screening
P1Ø-P15	Birth trauma
P19-P29	Respiratory and cardiovascular disorders specific to the perinatal period
P35-P39	Infections specific to the perinatal period
P5Ø-P61	Hemorrhagic and hematological disorders of newborn
P7Ø-P74	Transitory endocrine and metabolic disorders specific to newborn
P76-P78	Digestive system disorders of newborn
P8Ø-P83	Conditions involving the integument and temperature regulation of newborn
P84	Other problems with newborn
P9Ø-P96	Other disorders originating in the perinatal period

Newborn affected by maternal factors and by complications of pregnancy, labor, and delivery (PØØ-PØ4)

NOTE These codes are for use when the listed maternal conditions are specified as the cause of confirmed morbidity or potential morbidity which have their origin in the perinatal period (before birth through the first 28 days after birth). Codes from these categories are also for use for newborns who are suspected of having an abnormal condition resulting from exposure from the mother or the birth process, but without signs or symptoms, and, which after examination and observation, is found not to exist. These codes may be used even if treatment is begun for a suspected condition that is ruled out.

✓4th **PØØ Newborn (suspected to be) affected by maternal conditions that may be unrelated to present pregnancy**
Code first any current condition in newborn
EXCLUDES 2 *newborn (suspected to be) affected by maternal complications of pregnancy (PØ1.-)*
newborn affected by maternal endocrine and metabolic disorders (P7Ø-P74)
newborn affected by noxious substances transmitted via placenta or breast milk (PØ4.-)

PØØ.Ø Newborn (suspected to be) affected by maternal hypertensive disorders
Newborn (suspected to be) affected by maternal conditions classifiable to O1Ø-O11, O13-O16

PØØ.1 Newborn (suspected to be) affected by maternal renal and urinary tract diseases
Newborn (suspected to be) affected by maternal conditions classifiable to NØØ-N39

PØØ.2 Newborn (suspected to be) affected by maternal infectious and parasitic diseases
Newborn (suspected to be) affected by maternal infectious disease classifiable to AØØ-B99, JØ9 and J1Ø
EXCLUDES 1 *infections specific to the perinatal period (P35-P39)*
maternal genital tract or other localized infections (PØØ.8)

PØØ.3 Newborn (suspected to be) affected by other maternal circulatory and respiratory diseases
Newborn (suspected to be) affected by maternal conditions classifiable to IØØ-I99, JØØ-J99, Q2Ø-Q34 and not included in PØØ.Ø, PØØ.2

PØØ.4 Newborn (suspected to be) affected by maternal nutritional disorders
Newborn (suspected to be) affected by maternal disorders classifiable to E4Ø-E64
Maternal malnutrition NOS

PØØ.5 Newborn (suspected to be) affected by maternal injury
Newborn (suspected to be) affected by maternal conditions classifiable to O9A.2-

PØØ.6 Newborn (suspected to be) affected by surgical procedure on mother
Newborn (suspected to be) affected by amniocentesis
EXCLUDES 1 *Cesarean delivery for present delivery (PØ3.4)*
damage to placenta from amniocentesis, Cesarean delivery or surgical induction (PØ2.1)
previous surgery to uterus or pelvic organs (PØ3.89)
EXCLUDES 2 *newborn affected by complication of (fetal) intrauterine procedure (P96.5)*

PØØ.7 Newborn (suspected to be) affected by other medical procedures on mother, not elsewhere classified
Newborn (suspected to be) affected by radiation to mother
EXCLUDES 1 *damage to placenta from amniocentesis, cesarean delivery or surgical induction (PØ2.1)*
newborn affected by other complications of labor and delivery (PØ3.-)

✓5th **PØØ.8 Newborn (suspected to be) affected by other maternal conditions**

PØØ.81 Newborn (suspected to be) affected by periodontal disease in mother

PØØ.89 Newborn (suspected to be) affected by other maternal conditions
Newborn (suspected to be) affected by conditions classifiable to T8Ø-T88
Newborn (suspected to be) affected by maternal genital tract or other localized infections
Newborn (suspected to be) affected by maternal systemic lupus erythematosus

PØØ.9 Newborn (suspected to be) affected by unspecified maternal condition

✓4th **PØ1 Newborn (suspected to be) affected by maternal complications of pregnancy**
Code first any current condition in newborn

PØ1.Ø Newborn (suspected to be) affected by incompetent cervix

PØ1.1 Newborn (suspected to be) affected by premature rupture of membranes

PØ1.2 Newborn (suspected to be) affected by oligohydramnios
EXCLUDES 1 *oligohydramnios due to premature rupture of membranes (PØ1.1)*

PØ1.3 Newborn (suspected to be) affected by polyhydramnios
Newborn (suspected to be) affected by hydramnios

PØ1.4 Newborn (suspected to be) affected by ectopic pregnancy
Newborn (suspected to be) affected by abdominal pregnancy

PØ1.5 Newborn (suspected to be) affected by multiple pregnancy
Newborn (suspected to be) affected by triplet (pregnancy)
Newborn (suspected to be) affected by twin (pregnancy)

PØ1.6 Newborn (suspected to be) affected by maternal death

PØ1.7 Newborn (suspected to be) affected by malpresentation before labor
Newborn (suspected to be) affected by breech presentation before labor
Newborn (suspected to be) affected by external version before labor
Newborn (suspected to be) affected by face presentation before labor
Newborn (suspected to be) affected by transverse lie before labor
Newborn (suspected to be) affected by unstable lie before labor

PØ1.8 Newborn (suspected to be) affected by other maternal complications of pregnancy

PØ1.9 Newborn (suspected to be) affected by maternal complication of pregnancy, unspecified

✓4th **PØ2 Newborn (suspected to be) affected by complications of placenta, cord and membranes**
Code first any current condition in newborn

PØ2.Ø Newborn (suspected to be) affected by placenta previa

P02.1 Newborn (suspected to be) affected by other forms of placental separation and hemorrhage
Newborn (suspected to be) affected by abruptio placenta
Newborn (suspected to be) affected by accidental hemorrhage
Newborn (suspected to be) affected by antepartum hemorrhage
Newborn (suspected to be) affected by damage to placenta from amniocentesis, cesarean delivery or surgical induction
Newborn (suspected to be) affected by maternal blood loss
Newborn (suspected to be) affected by premature separation of placenta

✓5th **P02.2 Newborn (suspected to be) affected by other and unspecified morphological and functional abnormalities of placenta**

P02.20 Newborn (suspected to be) affected by unspecified morphological and functional abnormalities of placenta

P02.29 Newborn (suspected to be) affected by other morphological and functional abnormalities of placenta
Newborn (suspected to be) affected by placental dysfunction
Newborn (suspected to be) affected by placental infarction
Newborn (suspected to be) affected by placental insufficiency

P02.3 Newborn (suspected to be) affected by placental transfusion syndromes
Newborn (suspected to be) affected by placental and cord abnormalities resulting in twin-to-twin or other transplacental transfusion

P02.4 Newborn (suspected to be) affected by prolapsed cord

P02.5 Newborn (suspected to be) affected by other compression of umbilical cord
Newborn (suspected to be) affected by umbilical cord (tightly) around neck
Newborn (suspected to be) affected by entanglement of umbilical cord
Newborn (suspected to be) affected by knot in umbilical cord

✓5th **P02.6 Newborn (suspected to be) affected by other and unspecified conditions of umbilical cord**

P02.60 Newborn (suspected to be) affected by unspecified conditions of umbilical cord

P02.69 Newborn (suspected to be) affected by other conditions of umbilical cord
Newborn (suspected to be) affected by short umbilical cord
Newborn (suspected to be) affected by vasa previa
EXCLUDES 1 *newborn affected by single umbilical artery (Q27.0)*

P02.7 Newborn (suspected to be) affected by chorioamnionitis
Newborn (suspected to be) affected by amnionitis
Newborn (suspected to be) affected by membranitis
Newborn (suspected to be) affected by placentitis

P02.8 Newborn (suspected to be) affected by other abnormalities of membranes

P02.9 Newborn (suspected to be) affected by abnormality of membranes, unspecified

✓4th **P03 Newborn (suspected to be) affected by other complications of labor and delivery**
Code first any current condition in newborn

P03.0 Newborn (suspected to be) affected by breech delivery and extraction

P03.1 Newborn (suspected to be) affected by other malpresentation, malposition and disproportion during labor and delivery
Newborn (suspected to be) affected by contracted pelvis
Newborn (suspected to be) affected by conditions classifiable to O64-O66
Newborn (suspected to be) affected by persistent occipitoposterior
Newborn (suspected to be) affected by transverse lie

P03.2 Newborn (suspected to be) affected by forceps delivery

P03.3 Newborn (suspected to be) affected by delivery by vacuum extractor [ventouse]

P03.4 Newborn (suspected to be) affected by Cesarean delivery

P03.5 Newborn (suspected to be) affected by precipitate delivery
Newborn (suspected to be) affected by rapid second stage

P03.6 Newborn (suspected to be) affected by abnormal uterine contractions
Newborn (suspected to be) affected by conditions classifiable to O62-, except O62.3
Newborn (suspected to be) affected by hypertonic labor
Newborn (suspected to be) affected by uterine inertia

✓5th **P03.8 Newborn (suspected to be) affected by other specified complications of labor and delivery**

✓6th **P03.81 Newborn (suspected to be) affected by abnormality in fetal (intrauterine) heart rate or rhythm**
EXCLUDES 1 *neonatal cardiac dysrhythmia (P29.1-)*

P03.810 Newborn (suspected to be) affected by abnormality in fetal (intrauterine) heart rate or rhythm before the onset of labor

P03.811 Newborn (suspected to be) affected by abnormality in fetal (intrauterine) heart rate or rhythm during labor

P03.819 Newborn (suspected to be) affected by abnormality in fetal (intrauterine) heart rate or rhythm, unspecified as to time of onset

P03.82 Meconium passage during delivery
EXCLUDES 1 *meconium aspiration (P24.00, P24.01)*
meconium staining (P96.83)

P03.89 Newborn (suspected to be) affected by other specified complications of labor and delivery
Newborn (suspected to be) affected by abnormality of maternal soft tissues
Newborn (suspected to be) affected by conditions classifiable to O60-O75 and by procedures used in labor and delivery not included in P02- and P03.0-P03.6
Newborn (suspected to be) affected by induction of labor

P03.9 Newborn (suspected to be) affected by complication of labor and delivery, unspecified

✓4th **P04 Newborn (suspected to be) affected by noxious substances transmitted via placenta or breast milk**
INCLUDES nonteratogenic effects of substances transmitted via placenta
EXCLUDES 2 *congenital malformations (Q00-Q99)*
neonatal jaundice from excessive hemolysis due to drugs or toxins transmitted from mother (P58.4)
newborn in contact with and (suspected) exposures hazardous to health not transmitted via placenta or breast milk (Z77.-)

P04.0 Newborn (suspected to be) affected by maternal anesthesia and analgesia in pregnancy, labor and delivery
Newborn (suspected to be) affected by reactions and intoxications from maternal opiates and tranquilizers administered during labor and delivery

P04.1 Newborn (suspected to be) affected by other maternal medication
Newborn (suspected to be) affected by cancer chemotherapy
Newborn (suspected to be) affected by cytotoxic drugs
EXCLUDES 1 *dysmorphism due to warfarin (Q86.2)*
fetal hydantoin syndrome (Q86.1)
maternal use of drugs of addiction (P04.4-)

P04.2 Newborn (suspected to be) affected by maternal use of tobacco
Newborn (suspected to be) affected by exposure in utero to tobacco smoke
EXCLUDES 2 *newborn exposure to environmental tobacco smoke (P96.81)*

P04.3 Newborn (suspected to be) affected by maternal use of alcohol
EXCLUDES 1 *fetal alcohol syndrome (Q86.0)*

✓5th **P04.4 Newborn (suspected to be) affected by maternal use of drugs of addiction**

P04.41 Newborn (suspected to be) affected by maternal use of cocaine
"Crack baby"

P04.49 Newborn (suspected to be) affected by maternal use of other drugs of addiction
EXCLUDES 2 *newborn (suspected to be) affected by maternal anesthesia and analgesia (P04.0)*
withdrawal symptoms from maternal use of drugs of addiction (P96.1)

PØ4.5 Newborn (suspected to be) affected by maternal use of nutritional chemical substances

PØ4.6 Newborn (suspected to be) affected by maternal exposure to environmental chemical substances

PØ4.8 Newborn (suspected to be) affected by other maternal noxious substances

PØ4.9 Newborn (suspected to be) affected by maternal noxious substance, unspecified

Disorders of newborn related to length of gestation and fetal growth (PØ5-PØ8)

✓4th **PØ5 Disorders of newborn related to slow fetal growth and fetal malnutrition**

✓5th **PØ5.Ø Newborn light for gestational age**
Newborn light-for-dates

PØ5.ØØ Newborn light for gestational age, unspecified weight

PØ5.Ø1 Newborn light for gestational age, less than 5ØØ grams

PØ5.Ø2 Newborn light for gestational age, 5ØØ-749 grams

PØ5.Ø3 Newborn light for gestational age, 75Ø-999 grams

PØ5.Ø4 Newborn light for gestational age, 1ØØØ-1249 grams

PØ5.Ø5 Newborn light for gestational age, 125Ø-1499 grams

PØ5.Ø6 Newborn light for gestational age, 15ØØ-1749 grams

PØ5.Ø7 Newborn light for gestational age, 175Ø-1999 grams

PØ5.Ø8 Newborn light for gestational age, 2ØØØ-2499 grams

✓5th **PØ5.1 Newborn small for gestational age**
Newborn small-and-light-for-dates
Newborn small-for-dates

PØ5.1Ø Newborn small for gestational age, unspecified weight

PØ5.11 Newborn small for gestational age, less than 5ØØ grams

PØ5.12 Newborn small for gestational age, 5ØØ-749 grams

PØ5.13 Newborn small for gestational age, 75Ø-999 grams

PØ5.14 Newborn small for gestational age, 1ØØØ-1249 grams

PØ5.15 Newborn small for gestational age, 125Ø-1499 grams

PØ5.16 Newborn small for gestational age, 15ØØ-1749 grams

PØ5.17 Newborn small for gestational age, 175Ø-1999 grams

PØ5.18 Newborn small for gestational age, 2ØØØ-2499 grams

PØ5.2 Newborn affected by fetal (intrauterine) malnutrition not light or small for gestational age
Infant, not light or small for gestational age, showing signs of fetal malnutrition, such as dry, peeling skin and loss of subcutaneous tissue

EXCLUDES 1 *newborn affected by fetal malnutrition with light for gestational age (PØ5.Ø-)*
newborn affected by fetal malnutrition with small for gestational age (PØ5.1-)

PØ5.9 Newborn affected by slow intrauterine growth, unspecified
Newborn affected by fetal growth retardation NOS

✓4th **PØ7 Disorders of newborn related to short gestation and low birth weight, not elsewhere classified**

NOTE When both birth weight and gestational age of the newborn are available, both should be coded with birth weight sequenced before gestational age

The listed conditions, without further specification, as the cause of morbidity or additional care, in newborn

EXCLUDES 1 *low birth weight due to slow fetal growth and fetal malnutrition (PØ5.-)*

✓5th **PØ7.Ø Extremely low birth weight newborn**
Newborn birth weight 999 g. or less

PØ7.ØØ Extremely low birth weight newborn, unspecified weight

PØ7.Ø1 Extremely low birth weight newborn, less than 5ØØ grams

PØ7.Ø2 Extremely low birth weight newborn, 5ØØ-749 grams

PØ7.Ø3 Extremely low birth weight newborn, 75Ø-999 grams

✓5th **PØ7.1 Other low birth weight newborn**
Newborn birth weight 1ØØØ-2499 g.

PØ7.1Ø Other low birth weight newborn, unspecified weight

PØ7.14 Other low birth weight newborn, 1ØØØ-1249 grams

PØ7.15 Other low birth weight newborn, 125Ø-1499 grams

PØ7.16 Other low birth weight newborn, 15ØØ-1749 grams

PØ7.17 Other low birth weight newborn, 175Ø-1999 grams

PØ7.18 Other low birth weight newborn, 2ØØØ-2499 grams

✓5th **PØ7.2 Extreme immaturity of newborn**
Less than 28 completed weeks (less than 196 completed days) of gestation.

PØ7.2Ø Extreme immaturity of newborn, unspecified weeks of gestation
Gestational age less than 28 completed weeks NOS

PØ7.21 Extreme immaturity of newborn, gestational age less than 23 completed weeks
Extreme immaturity of newborn, gestational age less than 23 weeks, Ø days

PØ7.22 Extreme immaturity of newborn, gestational age 23 completed weeks
Extreme immaturity of newborn, gestational age 23 weeks, Ø days through 23 weeks, 6 days

PØ7.23 Extreme immaturity of newborn, gestational age 24 completed weeks
Extreme immaturity of newborn, gestational age 24 weeks, Ø days through 24 weeks, 6 days

PØ7.24 Extreme immaturity of newborn, gestational age 25 completed weeks
Extreme immaturity of newborn, gestational age 25 weeks, Ø days through 25 weeks, 6 days

PØ7.25 Extreme immaturity of newborn, gestational age 26 completed weeks
Extreme immaturity of newborn, gestational age 26 weeks, Ø days through 26 weeks, 6 days

PØ7.26 Extreme immaturity of newborn, gestational age 27 completed weeks
Extreme immaturity of newborn, gestational age 27 weeks, Ø days through 27 weeks, 6 days

✓5th **PØ7.3 Preterm [premature] newborn [other]**
28 completed weeks or more but less than 37 completed weeks (196 completed days but less than 259 completed days) of gestation
Prematurity NOS

PØ7.3Ø Preterm newborn, unspecified weeks of gestation

PØ7.31 Preterm newborn, gestational age 28 completed weeks
Preterm newborn, gestational age 28 weeks, Ø days through 28 weeks, 6 days

PØ7.32 Preterm newborn, gestational age 29 completed weeks
Preterm newborn, gestational age 29 weeks, Ø days through 29 weeks, 6 days

PØ7.33 Preterm newborn, gestational age 3Ø completed weeks
Preterm newborn, gestational age 3Ø weeks, Ø days through 3Ø weeks, 6 days

PØ7.34 Preterm newborn, gestational age 31 completed weeks
Preterm newborn, gestational age 31 weeks, Ø days through 31 weeks, 6 days

PØ7.35 Preterm newborn, gestational age 32 completed weeks
Preterm newborn, gestational age 32 weeks, Ø days through 32 weeks, 6 days

PØ7.36 Preterm newborn, gestational age 33 completed weeks
Preterm newborn, gestational age 33 weeks, Ø days through 33 weeks, 6 days

PØ7.37 Preterm newborn, gestational age 34 completed weeks
Preterm newborn, gestational age 34 weeks, Ø days through 34 weeks, 6 days

PØ7.38 Preterm newborn, gestational age 35 completed weeks
Preterm newborn, gestational age 35 weeks, Ø days through 35 weeks, 6 days

PØ7.39 Preterm newborn, gestational age 36 completed weeks
Preterm newborn, gestational age 36 weeks, Ø days through 36 weeks, 6 days

√4th **PØ8 Disorders of newborn related to long gestation and high birth weight**

NOTE When both birth weight and gestational age of the newborn are available, priority of assignment should be given to birth weight

INCLUDES the listed conditions, without further specification, as causes of morbidity or additional care, in newborn

PØ8.Ø Exceptionally large newborn baby
Usually implies a birth weight of 45ØØ g. or more
EXCLUDES 1 *syndrome of infant of diabetic mother (P7Ø.1)*
syndrome of infant of mother with gestational diabetes (P7Ø.Ø)

PØ8.1 Other heavy for gestational age newborn
Other newborn heavy- or large-for-dates regardless of period of gestation
Usually implies a birth weight of 4ØØØ g. to 4499 g.
EXCLUDES 1 *newborn with a birth weight of 45ØØ or more (PØ8.Ø)*
syndrome of infant of diabetic mother (P7Ø.1)
syndrome of infant of mother with gestational diabetes (P7Ø.Ø).

√5th **PØ8.2 Late newborn, not heavy for gestational age**

PØ8.21 Post-term newborn
Newborn with gestation period over 4Ø completed weeks to 42 completed weeks

PØ8.22 Prolonged gestation of newborn
Newborn with gestation period over 42 completed weeks (294 days or more), not heavy- or large-for-dates.
Postmaturity NOS

Abnormal findings on neonatal screening (PØ9)

PØ9 Abnormal findings on neonatal screening
Use additional code to identify signs, symptoms and conditions associated with the screening
EXCLUDES 2 *nonspecific serologic evidence of human immunodeficiency virus [HIV] (R75)*

Birth trauma (P1Ø-P15)

√4th **P1Ø Intracranial laceration and hemorrhage due to birth injury**
EXCLUDES 1 *intracranial hemorrhage of newborn NOS (P52.9)*
intracranial hemorrhage of newborn due to anoxia or hypoxia (P52.-)
nontraumatic intracranial hemorrhage of newborn (P52.-)

P1Ø.Ø Subdural hemorrhage due to birth injury
Subdural hematoma (localized) due to birth injury
EXCLUDES 1 *subdural hemorrhage accompanying tentorial tear (P1Ø.4)*

P1Ø.1 Cerebral hemorrhage due to birth injury

P1Ø.2 Intraventricular hemorrhage due to birth injury

P1Ø.3 Subarachnoid hemorrhage due to birth injury

P1Ø.4 Tentorial tear due to birth injury

P1Ø.8 Other intracranial lacerations and hemorrhages due to birth injury

P1Ø.9 Unspecified intracranial laceration and hemorrhage due to birth injury

√4th **P11 Other birth injuries to central nervous system**

P11.Ø Cerebral edema due to birth injury

P11.1 Other specified brain damage due to birth injury

P11.2 Unspecified brain damage due to birth injury

P11.3 Birth injury to facial nerve
Facial palsy due to birth injury

P11.4 Birth injury to other cranial nerves

P11.5 Birth injury to spine and spinal cord
Fracture of spine due to birth injury

P11.9 Birth injury to central nervous system, unspecified

√4th **P12 Birth injury to scalp**

P12.Ø Cephalhematoma due to birth injury

P12.1 Chignon (from vacuum extraction) due to birth injury

P12.2 Epicranial subaponeurotic hemorrhage due to birth injury
Subgaleal hemorrhage

P12.3 Bruising of scalp due to birth injury

P12.4 Injury of scalp of newborn due to monitoring equipment
Sampling incision of scalp of newborn
Scalp clip (electrode) injury of newborn

√5th **P12.8 Other birth injuries to scalp**

P12.81 Caput succedaneum

P12.89 Other birth injuries to scalp

P12.9 Birth injury to scalp, unspecified

√4th **P13 Birth injury to skeleton**
EXCLUDES 2 *birth injury to spine (P11.5)*

P13.Ø Fracture of skull due to birth injury

P13.1 Other birth injuries to skull
EXCLUDES 1 *cephalhematoma (P12.Ø)*

P13.2 Birth injury to femur

P13.3 Birth injury to other long bones

P13.4 Fracture of clavicle due to birth injury

P13.8 Birth injuries to other parts of skeleton

P13.9 Birth injury to skeleton, unspecified

√4th **P14 Birth injury to peripheral nervous system**

P14.Ø Erb's paralysis due to birth injury

P14.1 Klumpke's paralysis due to birth injury

P14.2 Phrenic nerve paralysis due to birth injury

P14.3 Other brachial plexus birth injuries

P14.8 Birth injuries to other parts of peripheral nervous system

P14.9 Birth injury to peripheral nervous system, unspecified

√4th **P15 Other birth injuries**

P15.Ø Birth injury to liver
Rupture of liver due to birth injury

P15.1 Birth injury to spleen
Rupture of spleen due to birth injury

P15.2 Sternomastoid injury due to birth injury

P15.3 Birth injury to eye
Subconjunctival hemorrhage due to birth injury
Traumatic glaucoma due to birth injury

P15.4 Birth injury to face
Facial congestion due to birth injury

P15.5 Birth injury to external genitalia

P15.6 Subcutaneous fat necrosis due to birth injury

P15.8 Other specified birth injuries

P15.9 Birth injury, unspecified

Respiratory and cardiovascular disorders specific to the perinatal period (P19-P29)

√4th **P19 Metabolic acidemia in newborn**
Metabolic acidemia in newborn

P19.Ø Metabolic acidemia in newborn first noted before onset of labor

P19.1 Metabolic acidemia in newborn first noted during labor

P19.2 Metabolic acidemia noted at birth

P19.9 Metabolic acidemia, unspecified

√4th **P22 Respiratory distress of newborn**
EXCLUDES 1 *respiratory arrest of newborn (P28.81)*
respiratory failure of newborn NOS (P28.5)

P22.0 Respiratory distress syndrome of newborn
Cardiorespiratory distress syndrome of newborn
Hyaline membrane disease
Idiopathic respiratory distress syndrome [IRDS or RDS] of newborn
Pulmonary hypoperfusion syndrome
Respiratory distress syndrome, type I

P22.1 Transient tachypnea of newborn
Idiopathic tachypnea of newborn
Respiratory distress syndrome, type II
Wet lung syndrome

P22.8 Other respiratory distress of newborn

P22.9 Respiratory distress of newborn, unspecified

✓4th P23 Congenital pneumonia
INCLUDES infective pneumonia acquired in utero or during birth
EXCLUDES 1 *neonatal pneumonia resulting from aspiration (P24.-)*

P23.0 Congenital pneumonia due to viral agent
Use additional code (B97) to identify organism
EXCLUDES 1 *congenital rubella pneumonitis (P35.0)*

P23.1 Congenital pneumonia due to Chlamydia

P23.2 Congenital pneumonia due to staphylococcus

P23.3 Congenital pneumonia due to streptococcus, group B

P23.4 Congenital pneumonia due to Escherichia coli

P23.5 Congenital pneumonia due to Pseudomonas

P23.6 Congenital pneumonia due to other bacterial agents
Congenital pneumonia due to Hemophilus influenzae
Congenital pneumonia due to Klebsiella pneumoniae
Congenital pneumonia due to Mycoplasma
Congenital pneumonia due to Streptococcus, except group B
Use additional code (B95-B96) to identify organism

P23.8 Congenital pneumonia due to other organisms

P23.9 Congenital pneumonia, unspecified

✓4th P24 Neonatal aspiration
INCLUDES aspiration in utero and during delivery

✓5th P24.0 Meconium aspiration
EXCLUDES 1 *meconium passage (without aspiration) during delivery (P03.82)*
meconium staining (P96.83)

P24.00 Meconium aspiration without respiratory symptoms
Meconium aspiration NOS

P24.01 Meconium aspiration with respiratory symptoms
Meconium aspiration pneumonia
Meconium aspiration pneumonitis
Meconium aspiration syndrome NOS
Use additional code to identify any secondary pulmonary hypertension, if applicable (I27.2)

✓5th P24.1 Neonatal aspiration of (clear) amniotic fluid and mucus
Neonatal aspiration of liquor (amnii)

P24.10 Neonatal aspiration of (clear) amniotic fluid and mucus without respiratory symptoms
Neonatal aspiration of amniotic fluid and mucus NOS

P24.11 Neonatal aspiration of (clear) amniotic fluid and mucus with respiratory symptoms
Neonatal aspiration of amniotic fluid and mucus with pneumonia
Neonatal aspiration of amniotic fluid and mucus with pneumonitis
Use additional code to identify any secondary pulmonary hypertension, if applicable (I27.2)

✓5th P24.2 Neonatal aspiration of blood

P24.20 Neonatal aspiration of blood without respiratory symptoms
Neonatal aspiration of blood NOS

P24.21 Neonatal aspiration of blood with respiratory symptoms
Neonatal aspiration of blood with pneumonia
Neonatal aspiration of blood with pneumonitis
Use additional code to identify any secondary pulmonary hypertension, if applicable (I27.2)

✓5th P24.3 Neonatal aspiration of milk and regurgitated food
Neonatal aspiration of stomach contents

P24.30 Neonatal aspiration of milk and regurgitated food without respiratory symptoms
Neonatal aspiration of milk and regurgitated food NOS

P24.31 Neonatal aspiration of milk and regurgitated food with respiratory symptoms
Neonatal aspiration of milk and regurgitated food with pneumonia
Neonatal aspiration of milk and regurgitated food with pneumonitis
Use additional code to identify any secondary pulmonary hypertension, if applicable (I27.2)

✓5th P24.8 Other neonatal aspiration

P24.80 Other neonatal aspiration without respiratory symptoms
Neonatal aspiration NEC

P24.81 Other neonatal aspiration with respiratory symptoms
Neonatal aspiration pneumonia NEC
Neonatal aspiration with pneumonitis NEC
Neonatal aspiration with pneumonia NOS
Neonatal aspiration with pneumonitis NOS
Use additional code to identify any secondary pulmonary hypertension, if applicable (I27.2)

P24.9 Neonatal aspiration, unspecified

✓4th P25 Interstitial emphysema and related conditions originating in the perinatal period

P25.0 Interstitial emphysema originating in the perinatal period

P25.1 Pneumothorax originating in the perinatal period

P25.2 Pneumomediastinum originating in the perinatal period

P25.3 Pneumopericardium originating in the perinatal period

P25.8 Other conditions related to interstitial emphysema originating in the perinatal period

✓4th P26 Pulmonary hemorrhage originating in the perinatal period
EXCLUDES 1 *acute idiopathic hemorrhage in infants over 28 days old (R04.81)*

P26.0 Tracheobronchial hemorrhage originating in the perinatal period

P26.1 Massive pulmonary hemorrhage originating in the perinatal period

P26.8 Other pulmonary hemorrhages originating in the perinatal period

P26.9 Unspecified pulmonary hemorrhage originating in the perinatal period

✓4th P27 Chronic respiratory disease originating in the perinatal period
EXCLUDES 1 *respiratory distress of newborn (P22.0-P22.9)*

P27.0 Wilson-Mikity syndrome
Pulmonary dysmaturity

P27.1 Bronchopulmonary dysplasia originating in the perinatal period

P27.8 Other chronic respiratory diseases originating in the perinatal period
Congenital pulmonary fibrosis
Ventilator lung in newborn

P27.9 Unspecified chronic respiratory disease originating in the perinatal period

✓4th P28 Other respiratory conditions originating in the perinatal period
EXCLUDES 1 *congenital malformations of the respiratory system (Q30-Q34)*

P28.0 Primary atelectasis of newborn
Primary failure to expand terminal respiratory units
Pulmonary hypoplasia associated with short gestation
Pulmonary immaturity NOS

✓5th P28.1 Other and unspecified atelectasis of newborn

P28.10 Unspecified atelectasis of newborn
Atelectasis of newborn NOS

P28.11 Resorption atelectasis without respiratory distress syndrome
EXCLUDES 1 *resorption atelectasis with respiratory distress syndrome (P22.0)*

P28.19 Other atelectasis of newborn
Partial atelectasis of newborn
Secondary atelectasis of newborn

P28.2 Cyanotic attacks of newborn
EXCLUDES 1 *apnea of newborn (P28.3-P28.4)*

P28.3 Primary sleep apnea of newborn
Central sleep apnea of newborn
Obstructive sleep apnea of newborn
Sleep apnea of newborn NOS

P28.4 Other apnea of newborn
Apnea of prematurity
Obstructive apnea of newborn
EXCLUDES 1 *obstructive sleep apnea of newborn (P28.3)*

P28.5 Respiratory failure of newborn
EXCLUDES 1 *respiratory arrest of newborn (P28.81)*
respiratory distress of newborn (P22.Ø-)

5th **P28.8 Other specified respiratory conditions of newborn**
P28.81 Respiratory arrest of newborn
P28.89 Other specified respiratory conditions of newborn
Congenital laryngeal stridor
Sniffles in newborn
Snuffles in newborn
EXCLUDES 1 *early congenital syphilitic rhinitis (A5Ø.Ø)*

P28.9 Respiratory condition of newborn, unspecified
Respiratory depression in newborn

4th **P29 Cardiovascular disorders originating in the perinatal period**
EXCLUDES 1 *congenital malformations of the circulatory system (Q2Ø-Q28)*

P29.Ø Neonatal cardiac failure
5th **P29.1 Neonatal cardiac dysrhythmia**
P29.11 Neonatal tachycardia
P29.12 Neonatal bradycardia
P29.2 Neonatal hypertension
P29.3 Persistent fetal circulation
Delayed closure of ductus arteriosus
(Persistent) pulmonary hypertension of newborn
P29.4 Transient myocardial ischemia in newborn
5th **P29.8 Other cardiovascular disorders originating in the perinatal period**
P29.81 Cardiac arrest of newborn
P29.89 Other cardiovascular disorders originating in the perinatal period
P29.9 Cardiovascular disorder originating in the perinatal period, unspecified

Infections specific to the perinatal period (P35-P39)

Infections acquired in utero, during birth via the umbilicus, or during the first 28 days after birth
EXCLUDES 2 *asymptomatic human immunodeficiency virus [HIV] infection status (Z21)*
congenital gonococcal infection (A54.-)
congenital pneumonia (P23.-)
congenital syphilis (A5Ø.-)
human immunodeficiency virus [HIV] disease (B2Ø)
infant botulism (A48.51)
infectious diseases not specific to the perinatal period (AØØ-B99, JØ9, J1Ø-)
intestinal infectious disease (AØØ-AØ9)
laboratory evidence of human immunodeficiency virus [HIV] (R75)
tetanus neonatorum (A33)

4th **P35 Congenital viral diseases**
INCLUDES infections acquired in utero or during birth
P35.Ø Congenital rubella syndrome
Congenital rubella pneumonitis
P35.1 Congenital cytomegalovirus infection
P35.2 Congenital herpesviral [herpes simplex] infection
P35.3 Congenital viral hepatitis
P35.8 Other congenital viral diseases
Congenital varicella [chickenpox]
P35.9 Congenital viral disease, unspecified

4th **P36 Bacterial sepsis of newborn**
INCLUDES congenital sepsis
Use additional code(s), if applicable, to identify severe sepsis (R65.2-) and associated acute organ dysfunction(s)
P36.Ø Sepsis of newborn due to streptococcus, group B
5th **P36.1 Sepsis of newborn due to other and unspecified streptococci**
P36.1Ø Sepsis of newborn due to unspecified streptococci
P36.19 Sepsis of newborn due to other streptococci
P36.2 Sepsis of newborn due to Staphylococcus aureus
5th **P36.3 Sepsis of newborn due to other and unspecified staphylococci**
P36.3Ø Sepsis of newborn due to unspecified staphylococci
P36.39 Sepsis of newborn due to other staphylococci
P36.4 Sepsis of newborn due to Escherichia coli
P36.5 Sepsis of newborn due to anaerobes
P36.8 Other bacterial sepsis of newborn
Use additional code from category B96 to identify organism
P36.9 Bacterial sepsis of newborn, unspecified

4th **P37 Other congenital infectious and parasitic diseases**
EXCLUDES 2 *congenital syphilis (A5Ø.-)*
infectious neonatal diarrhea (AØØ-AØ9)
necrotizing enterocolitis in newborn (P77.-)
noninfectious neonatal diarrhea (P78.3)
ophthalmia neonatorum due to gonococcus (A54.31)
tetanus neonatorum (A33)
P37.Ø Congenital tuberculosis
P37.1 Congenital toxoplasmosis
Hydrocephalus due to congenital toxoplasmosis
P37.2 Neonatal (disseminated) listeriosis
P37.3 Congenital falciparum malaria
P37.4 Other congenital malaria
P37.5 Neonatal candidiasis
P37.8 Other specified congenital infectious and parasitic diseases
P37.9 Congenital infectious or parasitic disease, unspecified

4th **P38 Omphalitis of newborn**
EXCLUDES 1 *omphalitis not of newborn (LØ8.82)*
tetanus omphalitis (A33)
umbilical hemorrhage of newborn (P51.-)
P38.1 Omphalitis with mild hemorrhage
P38.9 Omphalitis without hemorrhage
Omphalitis of newborn NOS

4th **P39 Other infections specific to the perinatal period**
Use additional code to identify organism or specific infection
P39.Ø Neonatal infective mastitis
EXCLUDES 1 *breast engorgement of newborn (P83.4)*
noninfective mastitis of newborn (P83.4)
P39.1 Neonatal conjunctivitis and dacryocystitis
Neonatal chlamydial conjunctivitis
Ophthalmia neonatorum NOS
EXCLUDES 1 *gonococcal conjunctivitis (A54.31)*
P39.2 Intra-amniotic infection affecting newborn, not elsewhere classified
P39.3 Neonatal urinary tract infection
P39.4 Neonatal skin infection
Neonatal pyoderma
EXCLUDES 1 *pemphigus neonatorum (LØØ)*
staphylococcal scalded skin syndrome (LØØ)
P39.8 Other specified infections specific to the perinatal period
P39.9 Infection specific to the perinatal period, unspecified

Hemorrhagic and hematological disorders of newborn (P5Ø-P61)

EXCLUDES 1 *congenital stenosis and stricture of bile ducts (Q44.3)*
Crigler-Najjar syndrome (E8Ø.5)
Dubin-Johnson syndrome (E8Ø.6)
Gilbert syndrome (E8Ø.4)
hereditary hemolytic anemias (D55-D58)

4th **P5Ø Newborn affected by intrauterine (fetal) blood loss**
EXCLUDES 1 *congenital anemia from intrauterine (fetal) blood loss (P61.3)*
P5Ø.Ø Newborn affected by intrauterine (fetal) blood loss from vasa previa
P5Ø.1 Newborn affected by intrauterine (fetal) blood loss from ruptured cord
P5Ø.2 Newborn affected by intrauterine (fetal) blood loss from placenta
P5Ø.3 Newborn affected by hemorrhage into co-twin
P5Ø.4 Newborn affected by hemorrhage into maternal circulation
P5Ø.5 Newborn affected by intrauterine (fetal) blood loss from cut end of co-twin's cord
P5Ø.8 Newborn affected by other intrauterine (fetal) blood loss
P5Ø.9 Newborn affected by intrauterine (fetal) blood loss, unspecified
Newborn affected by fetal hemorrhage NOS

4th **P51 Umbilical hemorrhage of newborn**
EXCLUDES 1 *omphalitis with mild hemorrhage (P38.1)*
umbilical hemorrhage from cut end of co-twins cord (P5Ø.5)
P51.Ø Massive umbilical hemorrhage of newborn

P51.8 Other umbilical hemorrhages of newborn
Slipped umbilical ligature NOS

P51.9 Umbilical hemorrhage of newborn, unspecified

✓4th **P52 Intracranial nontraumatic hemorrhage of newborn**
Intracranial hemorrhage due to anoxia or hypoxia
EXCLUDES 1 *intracranial hemorrhage due to birth injury (P10.-)*
intracranial hemorrhage due to other injury (S06.-)

P52.0 Intraventricular (nontraumatic) hemorrhage, grade 1, of newborn
Subependymal hemorrhage (without intraventricular extension)
Bleeding into germinal matrix

P52.1 Intraventricular (nontraumatic) hemorrhage, grade 2, of newborn
Subependymal hemorrhage with intraventricular extension
Bleeding into ventricle

✓5th **P52.2 Intraventricular (nontraumatic) hemorrhage, grade 3 and grade 4, of newborn**

P52.21 Intraventricular (nontraumatic) hemorrhage, grade 3, of newborn
Subependymal hemorrhage with intraventricular extension with enlargement of ventricle

P52.22 Intraventricular (nontraumatic) hemorrhage, grade 4, of newborn
Bleeding into cerebral cortex
Subependymal hemorrhage with intracerebral extension

P52.3 Unspecified intraventricular (nontraumatic) hemorrhage of newborn

P52.4 Intracerebral (nontraumatic) hemorrhage of newborn

P52.5 Subarachnoid (nontraumatic) hemorrhage of newborn

P52.6 Cerebellar (nontraumatic) and posterior fossa hemorrhage of newborn

P52.8 Other intracranial (nontraumatic) hemorrhages of newborn

P52.9 Intracranial (nontraumatic) hemorrhage of newborn, unspecified

P53 Hemorrhagic disease of newborn
Vitamin K deficiency of newborn

✓4th **P54 Other neonatal hemorrhages**
EXCLUDES 1 *newborn affected by (intrauterine) blood loss (P50.-)*
pulmonary hemorrhage originating in the perinatal period (P26.-)

P54.0 Neonatal hematemesis
EXCLUDES 1 *neonatal hematemesis due to swallowed maternal blood (P78.2)*

P54.1 Neonatal melena
EXCLUDES 1 *neonatal melena due to swallowed maternal blood (P78.2)*

P54.2 Neonatal rectal hemorrhage

P54.3 Other neonatal gastrointestinal hemorrhage

P54.4 Neonatal adrenal hemorrhage

P54.5 Neonatal cutaneous hemorrhage
Neonatal bruising
Neonatal ecchymoses
Neonatal petechiae
Neonatal superficial hematomata
EXCLUDES 2 *bruising of scalp due to birth injury (P12.3)*
cephalhematoma due to birth injury (P12.0)

P54.6 Neonatal vaginal hemorrhage
Neonatal pseudomenses

P54.8 Other specified neonatal hemorrhages

P54.9 Neonatal hemorrhage, unspecified

✓4th **P55 Hemolytic disease of newborn**

P55.0 Rh isoimmunization of newborn

P55.1 ABO isoimmunization of newborn

P55.8 Other hemolytic diseases of newborn

P55.9 Hemolytic disease of newborn, unspecified

✓4th **P56 Hydrops fetalis due to hemolytic disease**
EXCLUDES 1 *hydrops fetalis NOS (P83.2)*

P56.0 Hydrops fetalis due to isoimmunization

✓5th **P56.9 Hydrops fetalis due to other and unspecified hemolytic disease**

P56.90 Hydrops fetalis due to unspecified hemolytic disease

P56.99 Hydrops fetalis due to other hemolytic disease

✓4th **P57 Kernicterus**

P57.0 Kernicterus due to isoimmunization

P57.8 Other specified kernicterus
EXCLUDES 1 *Crigler-Najjar syndrome (E80.5)*

P57.9 Kernicterus, unspecified

✓4th **P58 Neonatal jaundice due to other excessive hemolysis**
EXCLUDES 1 *jaundice due to isoimmunization (P55-P57)*

P58.0 Neonatal jaundice due to bruising

P58.1 Neonatal jaundice due to bleeding

P58.2 Neonatal jaundice due to infection

P58.3 Neonatal jaundice due to polycythemia

✓5th **P58.4 Neonatal jaundice due to drugs or toxins transmitted from mother or given to newborn**
Code first poisoning due to drug or toxin, if applicable (T36-T65 with fifth or sixth character 1-4 or 6)
Use additional code for adverse effect, if applicable, to identify drug (T36-T50 with fifth or sixth character 5)

P58.41 Neonatal jaundice due to drugs or toxins transmitted from mother

P58.42 Neonatal jaundice due to drugs or toxins given to newborn

P58.5 Neonatal jaundice due to swallowed maternal blood

P58.8 Neonatal jaundice due to other specified excessive hemolysis

P58.9 Neonatal jaundice due to excessive hemolysis, unspecified

✓4th **P59 Neonatal jaundice from other and unspecified causes**
EXCLUDES 1 *jaundice due to inborn errors of metabolism (E70-E88)*
kernicterus (P57.-)

P59.0 Neonatal jaundice associated with preterm delivery
Hyperbilirubinemia of prematurity
Jaundice due to delayed conjugation associated with preterm delivery

P59.1 Inspissated bile syndrome

✓5th **P59.2 Neonatal jaundice from other and unspecified hepatocellular damage**
EXCLUDES 1 *congenital viral hepatitis (P35.3)*

P59.20 Neonatal jaundice from unspecified hepatocellular damage

P59.29 Neonatal jaundice from other hepatocellular damage
Neonatal giant cell hepatitis
Neonatal (idiopathic) hepatitis

P59.3 Neonatal jaundice from breast milk inhibitor

P59.8 Neonatal jaundice from other specified causes

P59.9 Neonatal jaundice, unspecified
Neonatal physiological jaundice (intense)(prolonged) NOS

P60 Disseminated intravascular coagulation of newborn
Defibrination syndrome of newborn

✓4th **P61 Other perinatal hematological disorders**
EXCLUDES 1 *transient hypogammaglobulinemia of infancy (D80.7)*

P61.0 Transient neonatal thrombocytopenia
Neonatal thrombocytopenia due to exchange transfusion
Neonatal thrombocytopenia due to idiopathic maternal thrombocytopenia
Neonatal thrombocytopenia due to isoimmunization

P61.1 Polycythemia neonatorum

P61.2 Anemia of prematurity

P61.3 Congenital anemia from fetal blood loss

P61.4 Other congenital anemias, not elsewhere classified
Congenital anemia NOS

P61.5 Transient neonatal neutropenia
EXCLUDES 1 *congenital neutropenia (nontransient) (D70.0)*

P61.6 Other transient neonatal disorders of coagulation

P61.8 Other specified perinatal hematological disorders

P61.9 Perinatal hematological disorder, unspecified

Transitory endocrine and metabolic disorders specific to newborn (P70-P74)

INCLUDES transitory endocrine and metabolic disturbances caused by the infant's response to maternal endocrine and metabolic factors, or its adjustment to extrauterine environment

P70 Transitory disorders of carbohydrate metabolism specific to newborn

P70.0 Syndrome of infant of mother with gestational diabetes
Newborn (with hypoglycemia) affected by maternal gestational diabetes
EXCLUDES 1 *newborn (with hypoglycemia) affected by maternal (pre-existing) diabetes mellitus (P70.1)*
syndrome of infant of a diabetic mother (P70.1)

P70.1 Syndrome of infant of a diabetic mother
Newborn (with hypoglycemia) affected by maternal (pre-existing) diabetes mellitus
EXCLUDES 1 *newborn (with hypoglycemia) affected by maternal gestational diabetes (P70.0)*
syndrome of infant of mother with gestational diabetes (P70.0)

P70.2 Neonatal diabetes mellitus

P70.3 Iatrogenic neonatal hypoglycemia

P70.4 Other neonatal hypoglycemia
Transitory neonatal hypoglycemia

P70.8 Other transitory disorders of carbohydrate metabolism of newborn

P70.9 Transitory disorder of carbohydrate metabolism of newborn, unspecified

P71 Transitory neonatal disorders of calcium and magnesium metabolism

P71.0 Cow's milk hypocalcemia in newborn

P71.1 Other neonatal hypocalcemia
EXCLUDES 1 *neonatal hypoparathyroidism (P71.4)*

P71.2 Neonatal hypomagnesemia

P71.3 Neonatal tetany without calcium or magnesium deficiency
Neonatal tetany NOS

P71.4 Transitory neonatal hypoparathyroidism

P71.8 Other transitory neonatal disorders of calcium and magnesium metabolism

P71.9 Transitory neonatal disorder of calcium and magnesium metabolism, unspecified

P72 Other transitory neonatal endocrine disorders
EXCLUDES 1 *congenital hypothyroidism with or without goiter (E03.0-E03.1)*
dyshormogenetic goiter (E07.1)
Pendred's syndrome (E07.1)

P72.0 Neonatal goiter, not elsewhere classified
Transitory congenital goiter with normal functioning

P72.1 Transitory neonatal hyperthyroidism
Neonatal thyrotoxicosis

P72.2 Other transitory neonatal disorders of thyroid function, not elsewhere classified
Transitory neonatal hypothyroidism

P72.8 Other specified transitory neonatal endocrine disorders

P72.9 Transitory neonatal endocrine disorder, unspecified

P74 Other transitory neonatal electrolyte and metabolic disturbances

P74.0 Late metabolic acidosis of newborn
EXCLUDES 1 *(fetal) metabolic acidosis of newborn (P19)*

P74.1 Dehydration of newborn

P74.2 Disturbances of sodium balance of newborn

P74.3 Disturbances of potassium balance of newborn

P74.4 Other transitory electrolyte disturbances of newborn

P74.5 Transitory tyrosinemia of newborn

P74.6 Transitory hyperammonemia of newborn

P74.8 Other transitory metabolic disturbances of newborn
Amino-acid metabolic disorders described as transitory

P74.9 Transitory metabolic disturbance of newborn, unspecified

Digestive system disorders of newborn (P76-P78)

P76 Other intestinal obstruction of newborn

P76.0 Meconium plug syndrome
Meconium ileus NOS
EXCLUDES 1 *meconium ileus in cystic fibrosis (E84.11)*

P76.1 Transitory ileus of newborn
EXCLUDES 1 *Hirschsprung's disease (Q43.1)*

P76.2 Intestinal obstruction due to inspissated milk

P76.8 Other specified intestinal obstruction of newborn
EXCLUDES 1 *intestinal obstruction classifiable to K56-*

P76.9 Intestinal obstruction of newborn, unspecified

P77 Necrotizing enterocolitis of newborn

P77.1 Stage 1 necrotizing enterocolitis in newborn
Necrotizing enterocolitis without pneumatosis, without perforation

P77.2 Stage 2 necrotizing enterocolitis in newborn
Necrotizing enterocolitis with pneumatosis, without perforation

P77.3 Stage 3 necrotizing enterocolitis in newborn
Necrotizing enterocolitis with perforation
Necrotizing enterocolitis with pneumatosis and perforation

P77.9 Necrotizing enterocolitis in newborn, unspecified
Necrotizing enterocolitis in newborn, NOS

P78 Other perinatal digestive system disorders
EXCLUDES 1 *cystic fibrosis (E84.0-E84.9)*
neonatal gastrointestinal hemorrhages (P54.0-P54.3)

P78.0 Perinatal intestinal perforation
Meconium peritonitis

P78.1 Other neonatal peritonitis
Neonatal peritonitis NOS

P78.2 Neonatal hematemesis and melena due to swallowed maternal blood

P78.3 Noninfective neonatal diarrhea
Neonatal diarrhea NOS

P78.8 Other specified perinatal digestive system disorders

P78.81 Congenital cirrhosis (of liver)

P78.82 Peptic ulcer of newborn

P78.83 Newborn esophageal reflux
Neonatal esophageal reflux

P78.89 Other specified perinatal digestive system disorders

P78.9 Perinatal digestive system disorder, unspecified

Conditions involving the integument and temperature regulation of newborn (P80-P83)

P80 Hypothermia of newborn

P80.0 Cold injury syndrome
Severe and usually chronic hypothermia associated with a pink flushed appearance, edema and neurological and biochemical abnormalities.
EXCLUDES 1 *mild hypothermia of newborn (P80.8)*

P80.8 Other hypothermia of newborn
Mild hypothermia of newborn

P80.9 Hypothermia of newborn, unspecified

P81 Other disturbances of temperature regulation of newborn

P81.0 Environmental hyperthermia of newborn

P81.8 Other specified disturbances of temperature regulation of newborn

P81.9 Disturbance of temperature regulation of newborn, unspecified
Fever of newborn NOS

P83 Other conditions of integument specific to newborn
EXCLUDES 1 *congenital malformations of skin and integument (Q80-Q84)*
hydrops fetalis due to hemolytic disease (P56.-)
neonatal skin infection (P39.4)
staphylococcal scalded skin syndrome (L00)
EXCLUDES 2 *cradle cap (L21.0)*
diaper [napkin] dermatitis (L22)

P83.0 Sclerema neonatorum

P83.1 Neonatal erythema toxicum

P83.2 Hydrops fetalis not due to hemolytic disease
Hydrops fetalis NOS

P83.3 Other and unspecified edema specific to newborn

P83.30 Unspecified edema specific to newborn

P83.39 Other edema specific to newborn

P83.4 Breast engorgement of newborn
Noninfective mastitis of newborn

P83.5 Congenital hydrocele

P83.6 Umbilical polyp of newborn

P83.8 Other specified conditions of integument specific to newborn
Bronze baby syndrome
Neonatal scleroderma
Urticaria neonatorum

P83.9 Condition of the integument specific to newborn, unspecified

Other problems with newborn (P84)

P84 Other problems with newborn
Acidemia of newborn
Acidosis of newborn
Anoxia of newborn NOS
Asphyxia of newborn NOS
Hypercapnia of newborn
Hypoxemia of newborn
Hypoxia of newborn NOS
Mixed metabolic and respiratory acidosis of newborn
EXCLUDES 1 *intracranial hemorrhage due to anoxia or hypoxia (P52.-)*
hypoxic ischemic encephalopathy [HIE] (P91.6-)
late metabolic acidosis of newborn (P74.0)

Other disorders originating in the perinatal period (P90-P96)

P90 Convulsions of newborn
EXCLUDES 1 *benign myoclonic epilepsy in infancy (G40.3-)*
benign neonatal convulsions (familial) (G40.3-)

✓4th **P91 Other disturbances of cerebral status of newborn**

P91.0 Neonatal cerebral ischemia

P91.1 Acquired periventricular cysts of newborn

P91.2 Neonatal cerebral leukomalacia
Periventricular leukomalacia

P91.3 Neonatal cerebral irritability

P91.4 Neonatal cerebral depression

P91.5 Neonatal coma

✓5th **P91.6 Hypoxic ischemic encephalopathy [HIE]**

P91.60 Hypoxic ischemic encephalopathy [HIE], unspecified

P91.61 Mild hypoxic ischemic encephalopathy [HIE]

P91.62 Moderate hypoxic ischemic encephalopathy [HIE]

P91.63 Severe hypoxic ischemic encephalopathy [HIE]

P91.8 Other specified disturbances of cerebral status of newborn

P91.9 Disturbance of cerebral status of newborn, unspecified

✓4th **P92 Feeding problems of newborn**
EXCLUDES 1 *feeding problems in child over 28 days old (R63.3)*

✓5th **P92.0 Vomiting of newborn**
EXCLUDES 1 *vomiting of child over 28 days old (R11.-)*

P92.01 Bilious vomiting of newborn
EXCLUDES 1 *bilious vomiting in child over 28 days old (R11.4)*

P92.09 Other vomiting of newborn
EXCLUDES 1 *regurgitation of food in newborn (P92.1)*

P92.1 Regurgitation and rumination of newborn

P92.2 Slow feeding of newborn

P92.3 Underfeeding of newborn

P92.4 Overfeeding of newborn

P92.5 Neonatal difficulty in feeding at breast

P92.6 Failure to thrive in newborn
EXCLUDES 1 *failure to thrive in child over 28 days old (R62.51)*

P92.8 Other feeding problems of newborn

P92.9 Feeding problem of newborn, unspecified

✓4th **P93 Reactions and intoxications due to drugs administered to newborn**
INCLUDES reactions and intoxications due to drugs administered to fetus affecting newborn
EXCLUDES 1 *jaundice due to drugs or toxins transmitted from mother or given to newborn (P58.4-)*
reactions and intoxications from maternal opiates, tranquilizers and other medication (P04.0-P04.1, P04.4)
withdrawal symptoms from maternal use of drugs of addiction (P96.1)
withdrawal symptoms from therapeutic use of drugs in newborn (P96.2)

P93.0 Grey baby syndrome
Grey syndrome from chloramphenicol administration in newborn

P93.8 Other reactions and intoxications due to drugs administered to newborn
Use additional code for adverse effect, if applicable, to identify drug (T36-T50 with fifth or sixth character 5)

✓4th **P94 Disorders of muscle tone of newborn**

P94.0 Transient neonatal myasthenia gravis
EXCLUDES 1 *myasthenia gravis (G70.0)*

P94.1 Congenital hypertonia

P94.2 Congenital hypotonia
Floppy baby syndrome, unspecified

P94.8 Other disorders of muscle tone of newborn

P94.9 Disorder of muscle tone of newborn, unspecified

P95 Stillbirth
Deadborn fetus NOS
Fetal death of unspecified cause
Stillbirth NOS
EXCLUDES 1 *maternal care for intrauterine death (O36.4)*
missed abortion (O02.1)
outcome of delivery, stillbirth (Z37.1, Z37.3, Z37.4, Z37.7)

✓4th **P96 Other conditions originating in the perinatal period**

P96.0 Congenital renal failure
Uremia of newborn

P96.1 Neonatal withdrawal symptoms from maternal use of drugs of addiction
Drug withdrawal syndrome in infant of dependent mother
Neonatal abstinence syndrome
EXCLUDES 1 *reactions and intoxications from maternal opiates and tranquilizers administered during labor and delivery (P04.0)*

P96.2 Withdrawal symptoms from therapeutic use of drugs in newborn

P96.3 Wide cranial sutures of newborn
Neonatal craniotabes

P96.5 Complication to newborn due to (fetal) intrauterine procedure
EXCLUDES 2 *newborn (suspected to be) affected by amniocentesis (P00.6)*

✓5th **P96.8 Other specified conditions originating in the perinatal period**

P96.81 Exposure to (parental) (environmental) tobacco smoke in the perinatal period
EXCLUDES 2 *newborn affected by in utero exposure to tobacco (P04.2)*
exposure to environmental tobacco smoke after the perinatal period (Z77.22)

P96.82 Delayed separation of umbilical cord

P96.83 Meconium staining
EXCLUDES 1 *meconium aspiration (P24.00, P24.01)*
meconium passage during delivery (P03.82)

P96.89 Other specified conditions originating in the perinatal period
Use additional code to specify condition

P96.9 Condition originating in the perinatal period, unspecified
Congenital debility NOS

Chapter 17. Congenital Malformations, Deformations and Chromosomal Abnormalities (Q00-Q99)

NOTE Codes from this chapter are not for use on maternal or fetal records

EXCLUDES 1 *inborn errors of metabolism (E70-E88)*

This chapter contains the following blocks:

- Q00-Q07 Congenital malformations of the nervous system
- Q10-Q18 Congenital malformations of eye, ear, face and neck
- Q20-Q28 Congenital malformations of the circulatory system
- Q30-Q34 Congenital malformations of the respiratory system
- Q35-Q37 Cleft lip and cleft palate
- Q38-Q45 Other congenital malformations of the digestive system
- Q50-Q56 Congenital malformations of genital organs
- Q60-Q64 Congenital malformations of the urinary system
- Q65-Q79 Congenital malformations and deformations of the musculoskeletal system
- Q80-Q89 Other congenital malformations
- Q90-Q99 Chromosomal abnormalities, not elsewhere classified

Congenital malformations of the nervous system (Q00-Q07)

✓4th Q00 Anencephaly and similar malformations

Q00.0 Anencephaly
Acephaly
Acrania
Amyelencephaly
Hemianencephaly
Hemicephaly

Q00.1 Craniorachischisis

Q00.2 Iniencephaly

✓4th Q01 Encephalocele

INCLUDES Arnold-Chiari syndrome, type III
encephalocystocele
encephalomyelocele
hydroencephalocele
hydromeningocele, cranial
meningocele, cerebral
meningoencephalocele

EXCLUDES 1 *Meckel-Gruber syndrome (Q61.9)*

Q01.0 Frontal encephalocele

Q01.1 Nasofrontal encephalocele

Q01.2 Occipital encephalocele

Q01.8 Encephalocele of other sites

Q01.9 Encephalocele, unspecified

Q02 Microcephaly

INCLUDES hydromicrocephaly
micrencephalon

EXCLUDES 1 *Meckel-Gruber syndrome (Q61.9)*

✓4th Q03 Congenital hydrocephalus

INCLUDES hydrocephalus in newborn

EXCLUDES 1 *Arnold-Chiari syndrome, type II (Q07.0-)*
acquired hydrocephalus (G91.-)
hydrocephalus due to congenital toxoplasmosis (P37.1)
hydrocephalus with spina bifida (Q05.0-Q05.4)

Q03.0 Malformations of aqueduct of Sylvius
Anomaly of aqueduct of Sylvius
Obstruction of aqueduct of Sylvius, congenital
Stenosis of aqueduct of Sylvius

Q03.1 Atresia of foramina of Magendie and Luschka
Dandy-Walker syndrome

Q03.8 Other congenital hydrocephalus

Q03.9 Congenital hydrocephalus, unspecified

✓4th Q04 Other congenital malformations of brain

EXCLUDES 1 *cyclopia (Q87.0)*
macrocephaly (Q75.3)

Q04.0 Congenital malformations of corpus callosum
Agenesis of corpus callosum

Q04.1 Arhinencephaly

Q04.2 Holoprosencephaly

Q04.3 Other reduction deformities of brain
Absence of part of brain
Agenesis of part of brain
Agyria
Aplasia of part of brain
Hydranencephaly
Hypoplasia of part of brain
Lissencephaly
Microgyria
Pachygyria

EXCLUDES 1 *congenital malformations of corpus callosum (Q04.0)*

Q04.4 Septo-optic dysplasia of brain

Q04.5 Megalencephaly

Q04.6 Congenital cerebral cysts
Porencephaly
Schizencephaly

EXCLUDES 1 *acquired porencephalic cyst (G93.0)*

Q04.8 Other specified congenital malformations of brain
Arnold-Chiari syndrome, type IV
Macrogyria

Q04.9 Congenital malformation of brain, unspecified
Congenital anomaly NOS of brain
Congenital deformity NOS of brain
Congenital disease or lesion NOS of brain
Multiple anomalies NOS of brain, congenital

✓4th Q05 Spina bifida
Hydromeningocele (spinal)
Meningocele (spinal)
Meningomyelocele
Myelocele
Myelomeningocele
Rachischisis
Spina bifida (aperta)(cystica)
Syringomyelocele

Use additional code for any associated paraplegia (paraparesis) (G82.2-)

EXCLUDES 1 *Arnold-Chiari syndrome, type II (Q07.0-)*
spina bifida occulta (Q76.0)

Q05.0 Cervical spina bifida with hydrocephalus

Q05.1 Thoracic spina bifida with hydrocephalus
Dorsal spina bifida with hydrocephalus
Thoracolumbar spina bifida with hydrocephalus

Q05.2 Lumbar spina bifida with hydrocephalus
Lumbosacral spina bifida with hydrocephalus

Q05.3 Sacral spina bifida with hydrocephalus

Q05.4 Unspecified spina bifida with hydrocephalus

Q05.5 Cervical spina bifida without hydrocephalus

Q05.6 Thoracic spina bifida without hydrocephalus
Dorsal spina bifida NOS
Thoracolumbar spina bifida NOS

Q05.7 Lumbar spina bifida without hydrocephalus
Lumbosacral spina bifida NOS

Q05.8 Sacral spina bifida without hydrocephalus

Q05.9 Spina bifida, unspecified

✓4th Q06 Other congenital malformations of spinal cord

Q06.0 Amyelia

Q06.1 Hypoplasia and dysplasia of spinal cord
Atelomyelia
Myelatelia
Myelodysplasia of spinal cord

Q06.2 Diastematomyelia

Q06.3 Other congenital cauda equina malformations

Q06.4 Hydromyelia
Hydrorachis

Q06.8 Other specified congenital malformations of spinal cord

Q06.9 Congenital malformation of spinal cord, unspecified
Congenital anomaly NOS of spinal cord
Congenital deformity NOS of spinal cord
Congenital disease or lesion NOS of spinal cord

✓4th Q07 Other congenital malformations of nervous system
EXCLUDES 2 *congenital central alveolar hypoventilation syndrome (G47.35)*
familial dysautonomia [Riley-Day] (G90.1)
neurofibromatosis (nonmalignant) (Q85.0-)

✓5th Q07.0 Arnold-Chiari syndrome
Arnold-Chiari syndrome, type II
EXCLUDES 1 *Arnold-Chiari syndrome, type III (Q01.-)*
Arnold-Chiari syndrome, type IV (Q04.8)

Q07.00 Arnold-Chiari syndrome without spina bifida or hydrocephalus
Q07.01 Arnold-Chiari syndrome with spina bifida
Q07.02 Arnold-Chiari syndrome with hydrocephalus
Q07.03 Arnold-Chiari syndrome with spina bifida and hydrocephalus

Q07.8 Other specified congenital malformations of nervous system
Agenesis of nerve
Displacement of brachial plexus
Jaw-winking syndrome
Marcus Gunn's syndrome

Q07.9 Congenital malformation of nervous system, unspecified
Congenital anomaly NOS of nervous system
Congenital deformity NOS of nervous system
Congenital disease or lesion NOS of nervous system

Congenital malformations of eye, ear, face and neck (Q10-Q18)

EXCLUDES 2 *cleft lip and cleft palate (Q35-Q37)*
congenital malformation of:
cervical spine (Q05.0, Q05.5, Q67.5, Q76.0-Q76.4)
larynx (Q31.-)
lip NEC (Q38.0)
nose (Q30.-)
parathyroid gland (Q89.2)
thyroid gland (Q89.2)

✓4th Q10 Congenital malformations of eyelid, lacrimal apparatus and orbit
EXCLUDES 1 *cryptophthalmos NOS (Q11.2)*
cryptophthalmos syndrome (Q87.0)

Q10.0 Congenital ptosis
Q10.1 Congenital ectropion
Q10.2 Congenital entropion
Q10.3 Other congenital malformations of eyelid
Ablepharon
Blepharophimosis, congenital
Coloboma of eyelid
Congenital absence or agenesis of cilia
Congenital absence or agenesis of eyelid
Congenital accessory eyelid
Congenital accessory eye muscle
Congenital malformation of eyelid NOS

Q10.4 Absence and agenesis of lacrimal apparatus
Congenital absence of punctum lacrimale

Q10.5 Congenital stenosis and stricture of lacrimal duct
Q10.6 Other congenital malformations of lacrimal apparatus
Congenital malformation of lacrimal apparatus NOS

Q10.7 Congenital malformation of orbit

✓4th Q11 Anophthalmos, microphthalmos and macrophthalmos
Q11.0 Cystic eyeball
Q11.1 Other anophthalmos
Anophthalmos NOS
Agenesis of eye
Aplasia of eye

Q11.2 Microphthalmos
Cryptophthalmos NOS
Dysplasia of eye
Hypoplasia of eye
Rudimentary eye
EXCLUDES 1 *cryptophthalmos syndrome (Q87.0)*

Q11.3 Macrophthalmos
EXCLUDES 1 *macrophthalmos in congenital glaucoma (Q15.0)*

✓4th Q12 Congenital lens malformations
Q12.0 Congenital cataract
Q12.1 Congenital displaced lens
Q12.2 Coloboma of lens
Q12.3 Congenital aphakia
Q12.4 Spherophakia
Q12.8 Other congenital lens malformations
Microphakia

Q12.9 Congenital lens malformation, unspecified

✓4th Q13 Congenital malformations of anterior segment of eye
Q13.0 Coloboma of iris
Coloboma NOS

Q13.1 Absence of iris
Aniridia
Use additional code for associated glaucoma (H42)

Q13.2 Other congenital malformations of iris
Anisocoria, congenital
Atresia of pupil
Congenital malformation of iris NOS
Corectopia

Q13.3 Congenital corneal opacity
Q13.4 Other congenital corneal malformations
Congenital malformation of cornea NOS
Microcornea
Peter's anomaly

Q13.5 Blue sclera
✓5th Q13.8 Other congenital malformations of anterior segment of eye
Q13.81 Rieger's anomaly
Use additional code for associated glaucoma (H42)

Q13.89 Other congenital malformations of anterior segment of eye

Q13.9 Congenital malformation of anterior segment of eye, unspecified

✓4th Q14 Congenital malformations of posterior segment of eye
EXCLUDES 2 *optic nerve hypoplasia (H47.03-)*

Q14.0 Congenital malformation of vitreous humor
Congenital vitreous opacity

Q14.1 Congenital malformation of retina
Congenital retinal aneurysm

Q14.2 Congenital malformation of optic disc
Coloboma of optic disc

Q14.3 Congenital malformation of choroid
Q14.8 Other congenital malformations of posterior segment of eye
Coloboma of the fundus

Q14.9 Congenital malformation of posterior segment of eye, unspecified

✓4th Q15 Other congenital malformations of eye
EXCLUDES 1 *congenital nystagmus (H55.01)*
ocular albinism (E70.31-)
optic nerve hypoplasia (H47.03-)
retinitis pigmentosa (H35.52)

Q15.0 Congenital glaucoma
Axenfeld's anomaly
Buphthalmos
Glaucoma of childhood
Glaucoma of newborn
Hydrophthalmos
Keratoglobus, congenital, with glaucoma
Macrocornea with glaucoma
Macrophthalmos in congenital glaucoma
Megalocornea with glaucoma

Q15.8 Other specified congenital malformations of eye
Q15.9 Congenital malformation of eye, unspecified
Congenital anomaly of eye
Congenital deformity of eye

✓4th Q16 Congenital malformations of ear causing impairment of hearing
EXCLUDES 1 *congenital deafness (H90.-)*

Q16.0 Congenital absence of (ear) auricle
Q16.1 Congenital absence, atresia and stricture of auditory canal (external)
Congenital atresia or stricture of osseous meatus

Q16.2 Absence of eustachian tube
Q16.3 Congenital malformation of ear ossicles
Congenital fusion of ear ossicles

Q16.4 Other congenital malformations of middle ear
Congenital malformation of middle ear NOS

Q16.5 Congenital malformation of inner ear
Congenital anomaly of membranous labyrinth
Congenital anomaly of organ of Corti

Q16.9 Congenital malformation of ear causing impairment of hearing, unspecified
Congenital absence of ear NOS

✓4th Q17 Other congenital malformations of ear
EXCLUDES 1 *congenital malformations of ear with impairment of hearing (Q16.0-Q16.9)*
preauricular sinus (Q18.1)

Q17.0 Accessory auricle
Accessory tragus
Polyotia
Preauricular appendage or tag
Supernumerary ear
Supernumerary lobule

Q17.1 Macrotia

Q17.2 Microtia

Q17.3 Other misshapen ear
Pointed ear

Q17.4 Misplaced ear
Low-set ears
EXCLUDES 1 *cervical auricle (Q18.2)*

Q17.5 Prominent ear
Bat ear

Q17.8 Other specified congenital malformations of ear
Congenital absence of lobe of ear

Q17.9 Congenital malformation of ear, unspecified
Congenital anomaly of ear NOS

✓4th Q18 Other congenital malformations of face and neck
EXCLUDES 1 *cleft lip and cleft palate (Q35-Q37)*
conditions classified to Q67.0-Q67.4
congenital malformations of skull and face bones (Q75.-)
cyclopia (Q87.0)
dentofacial anomalies [including malocclusion] (M26.-)
malformation syndromes affecting facial appearance (Q87.0)
persistent thyroglossal duct (Q89.2)

Q18.0 Sinus, fistula and cyst of branchial cleft
Branchial vestige

Q18.1 Preauricular sinus and cyst
Fistula of auricle, congenital
Cervicoaural fistula

Q18.2 Other branchial cleft malformations
Branchial cleft malformation NOS
Cervical auricle
Otocephaly

Q18.3 Webbing of neck
Pterygium colli

Q18.4 Macrostomia

Q18.5 Microstomia

Q18.6 Macrocheilia
Hypertrophy of lip, congenital

Q18.7 Microcheilia

Q18.8 Other specified congenital malformations of face and neck
Medial cyst of face and neck
Medial fistula of face and neck
Medial sinus of face and neck

Q18.9 Congenital malformation of face and neck, unspecified
Congenital anomaly NOS of face and neck

Congenital malformations of the circulatory system (Q20-Q28)

✓4th Q20 Congenital malformations of cardiac chambers and connections
EXCLUDES 1 *dextrocardia with situs inversus (Q89.3)*
mirror-image atrial arrangement with situs inversus (Q89.3)

Q20.0 Common arterial trunk
Persistent truncus arteriosus
EXCLUDES 1 *aortic septal defect (Q21.4)*

Q20.1 Double outlet right ventricle
Taussig-Bing syndrome

Q20.2 Double outlet left ventricle

Q20.3 Discordant ventriculoarterial connection
Dextrotransposition of aorta
Transposition of great vessels (complete)

Q20.4 Double inlet ventricle
Common ventricle
Cor triloculare biatriatum
Single ventricle

Q20.5 Discordant atrioventricular connection
Corrected transposition
Levotransposition
Ventricular inversion

Q20.6 Isomerism of atrial appendages
Isomerism of atrial appendages with asplenia or polysplenia

Q20.8 Other congenital malformations of cardiac chambers and connections
Cor binoculare

Q20.9 Congenital malformation of cardiac chambers and connections, unspecified

✓4th Q21 Congenital malformations of cardiac septa
EXCLUDES 1 *acquired cardiac septal defect (I51.0)*

Q21.0 Ventricular septal defect
Roger's disease

Q21.1 Atrial septal defect
Coronary sinus defect
Patent or persistent foramen ovale
Patent or persistent ostium secundum defect (type II)
Patent or persistent sinus venosus defect

Q21.2 Atrioventricular septal defect
Common atrioventricular canal
Endocardial cushion defect
Ostium primum atrial septal defect (type I)

Q21.3 Tetralogy of Fallot
Ventricular septal defect with pulmonary stenosis or atresia, dextroposition of aorta and hypertrophy of right ventricle.

Q21.4 Aortopulmonary septal defect
Aortic septal defect
Aortopulmonary window

Q21.8 Other congenital malformations of cardiac septa
Eisenmenger's defect
Pentalogy of Fallot
EXCLUDES 1 *Eisenmenger's complex (I27.8)*
Eisenmenger's syndrome (I27.8)

Q21.9 Congenital malformation of cardiac septum, unspecified
Septal (heart) defect NOS

✓4th Q22 Congenital malformations of pulmonary and tricuspid valves

Q22.0 Pulmonary valve atresia

Q22.1 Congenital pulmonary valve stenosis

Q22.2 Congenital pulmonary valve insufficiency
Congenital pulmonary valve regurgitation

Q22.3 Other congenital malformations of pulmonary valve
Congenital malformation of pulmonary valve NOS
Supernumerary cusps of pulmonary valve

Q22.4 Congenital tricuspid stenosis
Congenital tricuspid atresia

Q22.5 Ebstein's anomaly

Q22.6 Hypoplastic right heart syndrome

Q22.8 Other congenital malformations of tricuspid valve

Q22.9 Congenital malformation of tricuspid valve, unspecified

✓4th Q23 Congenital malformations of aortic and mitral valves

Q23.0 Congenital stenosis of aortic valve
Congenital aortic atresia
Congenital aortic stenosis NOS
EXCLUDES 1 *congenital stenosis of aortic valve in hypoplastic left heart syndrome (Q23.4)*
congenital subaortic stenosis (Q24.4)
supravalvular aortic stenosis (congenital) (Q25.3)

Q23.1 Congenital insufficiency of aortic valve
Bicuspid aortic valve
Congenital aortic insufficiency

Q23.2 Congenital mitral stenosis
Congenital mitral atresia

Q23.3 Congenital mitral insufficiency

Q23.4 Hypoplastic left heart syndrome

Q23.8 Other congenital malformations of aortic and mitral valves

Q23.9 Congenital malformation of aortic and mitral valves, unspecified

Q24 Other congenital malformations of heart
EXCLUDES 1 *endocardial fibroelastosis (I42.4)*

Q24.0 Dextrocardia
EXCLUDES 1 *dextrocardia with situs inversus (Q89.3)*
isomerism of atrial appendages (with asplenia or polysplenia) (Q20.6)
mirror-image atrial arrangement with situs inversus (Q89.3)

Q24.1 Levocardia

Q24.2 Cor triatriatum

Q24.3 Pulmonary infundibular stenosis
Subvalvular pulmonic stenosis

Q24.4 Congenital subaortic stenosis

Q24.5 Malformation of coronary vessels
Congenital coronary (artery) aneurysm

Q24.6 Congenital heart block

Q24.8 Other specified congenital malformations of heart
Congenital diverticulum of left ventricle
Congenital malformation of myocardium
Congenital malformation of pericardium
Malposition of heart
Uhl's disease

Q24.9 Congenital malformation of heart, unspecified
Congenital anomaly of heart
Congenital disease of heart

Q25 Congenital malformations of great arteries

Q25.0 Patent ductus arteriosus
Patent ductus Botallo
Persistent ductus arteriosus

Q25.1 Coarctation of aorta
Coarctation of aorta (preductal) (postductal)

Q25.2 Atresia of aorta

Q25.3 Supravalvular aortic stenosis
EXCLUDES 1 *congenital aortic stenosis NOS (Q23.0)*
congenital stenosis of aortic valve (Q23.0)

Q25.4 Other congenital malformations of aorta
Absence of aorta
Aneurysm of sinus of Valsalva (ruptured)
Aplasia of aorta
Congenital aneurysm of aorta
Congenital malformations of aorta
Congenital dilatation of aorta
Double aortic arch [vascular ring of aorta]
Hypoplasia of aorta
Persistent convolutions of aortic arch
Persistent right aortic arch
EXCLUDES 1 *hypoplasia of aorta in hypoplastic left heart syndrome (Q23.4)*

Q25.5 Atresia of pulmonary artery

Q25.6 Stenosis of pulmonary artery
Supravalvular pulmonary stenosis

Q25.7 Other congenital malformations of pulmonary artery

Q25.71 Coarctation of pulmonary artery

Q25.72 Congenital pulmonary arteriovenous malformation
Congenital pulmonary arteriovenous aneurysm

Q25.79 Other congenital malformations of pulmonary artery
Aberrant pulmonary artery
Agenesis of pulmonary artery
Congenital aneurysm of pulmonary artery
Congenital anomaly of pulmonary artery
Hypoplasia of pulmonary artery

Q25.8 Other congenital malformations of other great arteries

Q25.9 Congenital malformation of great arteries, unspecified

Q26 Congenital malformations of great veins

Q26.0 Congenital stenosis of vena cava
Congenital stenosis of vena cava (inferior)(superior)

Q26.1 Persistent left superior vena cava

Q26.2 Total anomalous pulmonary venous connection
Total anomalous pulmonary venous return [TAPVR], subdiaphragmatic
Total anomalous pulmonary venous return [TAPVR], supradiaphragmatic

Q26.3 Partial anomalous pulmonary venous connection
Partial anomalous pulmonary venous return

Q26.4 Anomalous pulmonary venous connection, unspecified

Q26.5 Anomalous portal venous connection

Q26.6 Portal vein-hepatic artery fistula

Q26.8 Other congenital malformations of great veins
Absence of vena cava (inferior) (superior)
Azygos continuation of inferior vena cava
Persistent left posterior cardinal vein
Scimitar syndrome

Q26.9 Congenital malformation of great vein, unspecified
Congenital anomaly of vena cava (inferior) (superior) NOS

Q27 Other congenital malformations of peripheral vascular system
EXCLUDES 2 *anomalies of cerebral and precerebral vessels (Q28.0-Q28.3)*
anomalies of coronary vessels (Q24.5)
anomalies of pulmonary artery (Q25.5-Q25.7)
congenital retinal aneurysm (Q14.1)
hemangioma and lymphangioma (D18.-)

Q27.0 Congenital absence and hypoplasia of umbilical artery
Single umbilical artery

Q27.1 Congenital renal artery stenosis

Q27.2 Other congenital malformations of renal artery
Congenital malformation of renal artery NOS
Multiple renal arteries

Q27.3 Arteriovenous malformation (peripheral)
Arteriovenous aneurysm
EXCLUDES 1 *acquired arteriovenous aneurysm (I77.0)*
EXCLUDES 2 *arteriovenous malformation of cerebral vessels (Q28.2)*
arteriovenous malformation of precerebral vessels (Q28.0)

Q27.30 Arteriovenous malformation, site unspecified

Q27.31 Arteriovenous malformation of vessel of upper limb

Q27.32 Arteriovenous malformation of vessel of lower limb

Q27.33 Arteriovenous malformation of digestive system vessel

Q27.34 Arteriovenous malformation of renal vessel

Q27.39 Arteriovenous malformation, other site

Q27.4 Congenital phlebectasia

Q27.8 Other specified congenital malformations of peripheral vascular system
Absence of peripheral vascular system
Atresia of peripheral vascular system
Congenital aneurysm (peripheral)
Congenital stricture, artery
Congenital varix
EXCLUDES 1 *arteriovenous malformation (Q27.3-)*

Q27.9 Congenital malformation of peripheral vascular system, unspecified
Anomaly of artery or vein NOS

Q28 Other congenital malformations of circulatory system
EXCLUDES 1 *congenital aneurysm NOS (Q27.8)*
congenital coronary aneurysm (Q24.5)
ruptured cerebral arteriovenous malformation (I60.8)
ruptured malformation of precerebral vessels (I72.0)
EXCLUDES 2 *congenital peripheral aneurysm (Q27.8)*
congenital pulmonary aneurysm (Q25.79)
congenital retinal aneurysm (Q14.1)

Q28.0 Arteriovenous malformation of precerebral vessels
Congenital arteriovenous precerebral aneurysm (nonruptured)

Q28.1 Other malformations of precerebral vessels
Congenital malformation of precerebral vessels NOS
Congenital precerebral aneurysm (nonruptured)

Q28.2 Arteriovenous malformation of cerebral vessels
Arteriovenous malformation of brain NOS
Congenital arteriovenous cerebral aneurysm (nonruptured)

Q28.3 Other malformations of cerebral vessels
Congenital cerebral aneurysm (nonruptured)
Congenital malformation of cerebral vessels NOS
Developmental venous anomaly

Q28.8 Other specified congenital malformations of circulatory system
Congenital aneurysm, specified site NEC
Spinal vessel anomaly

Q28.9 Congenital malformation of circulatory system, unspecified

Congenital malformations of the respiratory system (Q30-Q34)

Q30 Congenital malformations of nose
EXCLUDES 1 *congenital deviation of nasal septum (Q67.4)*

Q30.0 Choanal atresia
Atresia of nares (anterior) (posterior)
Congenital stenosis of nares (anterior) (posterior)

Q30.1 Agenesis and underdevelopment of nose
Congenital absent of nose

Q30.2 Fissured, notched and cleft nose

Q30.3 Congenital perforated nasal septum

Q30.8 Other congenital malformations of nose
Accessory nose
Congenital anomaly of nasal sinus wall

Q30.9 Congenital malformation of nose, unspecified

Q31 Congenital malformations of larynx
EXCLUDES 1 *congenital laryngeal stridor NOS (P28.89)*

Q31.0 Web of larynx
Glottic web of larynx
Subglottic web of larynx
Web of larynx NOS

Q31.1 Congenital subglottic stenosis

Q31.2 Laryngeal hypoplasia

Q31.3 Laryngocele

Q31.5 Congenital laryngomalacia

Q31.8 Other congenital malformations of larynx
Absence of larynx
Agenesis of larynx
Atresia of larynx
Congenital cleft thyroid cartilage
Congenital fissure of epiglottis
Congenital stenosis of larynx NEC
Posterior cleft of cricoid cartilage

Q31.9 Congenital malformation of larynx, unspecified

Q32 Congenital malformations of trachea and bronchus
EXCLUDES 1 *congenital bronchiectasis (Q33.4)*

Q32.0 Congenital tracheomalacia

Q32.1 Other congenital malformations of trachea
Atresia of trachea
Congenital anomaly of tracheal cartilage
Congenital dilatation of trachea
Congenital malformation of trachea
Congenital stenosis of trachea
Congenital tracheocele

Q32.2 Congenital bronchomalacia

Q32.3 Congenital stenosis of bronchus

Q32.4 Other congenital malformations of bronchus
Absence of bronchus
Agenesis of bronchus
Atresia of bronchus
Congenital diverticulum of bronchus
Congenital malformation of bronchus NOS

Q33 Congenital malformations of lung

Q33.0 Congenital cystic lung
Congenital cystic lung disease
Congenital honeycomb lung
Congenital polycystic lung disease
EXCLUDES 1 *cystic fibrosis (E84.0)*
cystic lung disease, acquired or unspecified (J98.4)

Q33.1 Accessory lobe of lung
Azygos lobe (fissured), lung

Q33.2 Sequestration of lung

Q33.3 Agenesis of lung
Congenital absence of lung (lobe)

Q33.4 Congenital bronchiectasis

Q33.5 Ectopic tissue in lung

Q33.6 Congenital hypoplasia and dysplasia of lung
EXCLUDES 1 *pulmonary hypoplasia associated with short gestation (P28.0)*

Q33.8 Other congenital malformations of lung

Q33.9 Congenital malformation of lung, unspecified

Q34 Other congenital malformations of respiratory system
EXCLUDES 2 *congenital central alveolar hypoventilation syndrome (G47.35)*

Q34.0 Anomaly of pleura

Q34.1 Congenital cyst of mediastinum

Q34.8 Other specified congenital malformations of respiratory system
Atresia of nasopharynx

Q34.9 Congenital malformation of respiratory system, unspecified
Congenital absence of respiratory system
Congenital anomaly of respiratory system NOS

Cleft lip and cleft palate (Q35-Q37)

Use additional code to identify associated malformation of the nose (Q30.2)
EXCLUDES 1 *Robin syndrome (Q87.0)*

Q35 Cleft palate
INCLUDES fissure of palate
palatoschisis
EXCLUDES 1 *cleft palate with cleft lip (Q37.-)*

Q35.1 Cleft hard palate

Q35.3 Cleft soft palate

Q35.5 Cleft hard palate with cleft soft palate

Q35.7 Cleft uvula

Q35.9 Cleft palate, unspecified
Cleft palate NOS

Q36 Cleft lip
Cheiloschisis
Congenital fissure of lip
Harelip
Labium leporinum
EXCLUDES 1 *cleft lip with cleft palate (Q37.-)*

Q36.0 Cleft lip, bilateral

Q36.1 Cleft lip, median

Q36.9 Cleft lip, unilateral
Cleft lip NOS

Q37 Cleft palate with cleft lip
Cheilopalatoschisis

Q37.0 Cleft hard palate with bilateral cleft lip

Q37.1 Cleft hard palate with unilateral cleft lip
Cleft hard palate with cleft lip NOS

Q37.2 Cleft soft palate with bilateral cleft lip

Q37.3 Cleft soft palate with unilateral cleft lip
Cleft soft palate with cleft lip NOS

Q37.4 Cleft hard and soft palate with bilateral cleft lip

Q37.5 Cleft hard and soft palate with unilateral cleft lip
Cleft hard and soft palate with cleft lip NOS

Q37.8 Unspecified cleft palate with bilateral cleft lip

Q37.9 Unspecified cleft palate with unilateral cleft lip
Cleft palate with cleft lip NOS

Other congenital malformations of the digestive system (Q38-Q45)

Q38 Other congenital malformations of tongue, mouth and pharynx
EXCLUDES 1 *dentofacial anomalies (M26.-)*
macrostomia (Q18.4)
microstomia (Q18.5)

Q38.0 Congenital malformations of lips, not elsewhere classified
Congenital fistula of lip
Congenital malformation of lip NOS
Van der Woude's syndrome
EXCLUDES 1 *cleft lip (Q36.-)*
cleft lip with cleft palate (Q37.-)
macrocheilia (Q18.6)
microcheilia (Q18.7)

Q38.1 Ankyloglossia
Tongue tie

Q38.2 Macroglossia
Congenital hypertrophy of tongue

Q38.3 Other congenital malformations of tongue
Aglossia
Bifid tongue
Congenital adhesion of tongue
Congenital fissure of tongue
Congenital malformation of tongue NOS
Double tongue
Hypoglossia
Hypoplasia of tongue
Microglossia

Q38.4 Congenital malformations of salivary glands and ducts
Atresia of salivary glands and ducts
Congenital absence of salivary glands and ducts
Congenital accessory salivary glands and ducts
Congenital fistula of salivary gland

Q38.5 Congenital malformations of palate, not elsewhere classified
Congenital absence of uvula
Congenital malformation of palate NOS
Congenital high arched palate
EXCLUDES 1 *cleft palate (Q35.-)*
cleft palate with cleft lip (Q37.-)

Q38.6 Other congenital malformations of mouth
Congenital malformation of mouth NOS

Q38.7 Congenital pharyngeal pouch
Congenital diverticulum of pharynx
EXCLUDES 1 *pharyngeal pouch syndrome (D82.1)*

Q38.8 Other congenital malformations of pharynx
Congenital malformation of pharynx NOS
Imperforate pharynx

4th Q39 Congenital malformations of esophagus

Q39.0 Atresia of esophagus without fistula
Atresia of esophagus NOS

Q39.1 Atresia of esophagus with tracheo-esophageal fistula
Atresia of esophagus with broncho-esophageal fistula

Q39.2 Congenital tracheo-esophageal fistula without atresia
Congenital tracheo-esophageal fistula NOS

Q39.3 Congenital stenosis and stricture of esophagus

Q39.4 Esophageal web

Q39.5 Congenital dilatation of esophagus
Congenital cardiospasm

Q39.6 Congenital diverticulum of esophagus
Congenital esophageal pouch

Q39.8 Other congenital malformations of esophagus
Congenital absence of esophagus
Congenital displacement of esophagus
Congenital duplication of esophagus

Q39.9 Congenital malformation of esophagus, unspecified

4th Q40 Other congenital malformations of upper alimentary tract

Q40.0 Congenital hypertrophic pyloric stenosis
Congenital or infantile constriction
Congenital or infantile hypertrophy
Congenital or infantile spasm
Congenital or infantile stenosis
Congenital or infantile stricture

Q40.1 Congenital hiatus hernia
Congenital displacement of cardia through esophageal hiatus
EXCLUDES 1 *congenital diaphragmatic hernia (Q79.0)*

Q40.2 Other specified congenital malformations of stomach
Congenital displacement of stomach
Congenital diverticulum of stomach
Congenital hourglass stomach
Congenital duplication of stomach
Megalogastria
Microgastria

Q40.3 Congenital malformation of stomach, unspecified

Q40.8 Other specified congenital malformations of upper alimentary tract

Q40.9 Congenital malformation of upper alimentary tract, unspecified
Congenital anomaly of upper alimentary tract
Congenital deformity of upper alimentary tract

4th Q41 Congenital absence, atresia and stenosis of small intestine
Congenital obstruction, occlusion or stricture of small intestine or intestine NOS
EXCLUDES 1 *cystic fibrosis with intestinal manifestation (E84.11)*
meconium ileus NOS (without cystic fibrosis) (P76.0)

Q41.0 Congenital absence, atresia and stenosis of duodenum

Q41.1 Congenital absence, atresia and stenosis of jejunum
Apple peel syndrome
Imperforate jejunum

Q41.2 Congenital absence, atresia and stenosis of ileum

Q41.8 Congenital absence, atresia and stenosis of other specified parts of small intestine

Q41.9 Congenital absence, atresia and stenosis of small intestine, part unspecified
Congenital absence, atresia and stenosis of intestine NOS

4th Q42 Congenital absence, atresia and stenosis of large intestine
Congenital obstruction, occlusion and stricture of large intestine

Q42.0 Congenital absence, atresia and stenosis of rectum with fistula

Q42.1 Congenital absence, atresia and stenosis of rectum without fistula
Imperforate rectum

Q42.2 Congenital absence, atresia and stenosis of anus with fistula

Q42.3 Congenital absence, atresia and stenosis of anus without fistula
Imperforate anus

Q42.8 Congenital absence, atresia and stenosis of other parts of large intestine

Q42.9 Congenital absence, atresia and stenosis of large intestine, part unspecified

4th Q43 Other congenital malformations of intestine

Q43.0 Meckel's diverticulum (displaced) (hypertrophic)
Persistent omphalomesenteric duct
Persistent vitelline duct

Q43.1 Hirschsprung's disease
Aganglionosis
Congenital (aganglionic) megacolon

Q43.2 Other congenital functional disorders of colon
Congenital dilatation of colon

Q43.3 Congenital malformations of intestinal fixation
Congenital omental, anomalous adhesions [bands]
Congenital peritoneal adhesions [bands]
Incomplete rotation of cecum and colon
Insufficient rotation of cecum and colon
Jackson's membrane
Malrotation of colon
Rotation failure of cecum and colon
Universal mesentery

Q43.4 Duplication of intestine

Q43.5 Ectopic anus

Q43.6 Congenital fistula of rectum and anus
EXCLUDES 1 *congenital fistula of anus with absence, atresia and stenosis (Q42.2)*
congenital fistula of rectum with absence, atresia and stenosis (Q42.0)
congenital rectovaginal fistula (Q52.2)
congenital urethrorectal fistula (Q64.7)
pilonidal fistula or sinus (L05.-)

Q43.7 Persistent cloaca
Cloaca NOS

Q43.8 Other specified congenital malformations of intestine
Congenital blind loop syndrome
Congenital diverticulitis, colon
Congenital diverticulum, intestine
Dolichocolon
Megaloappendix
Megaloduodenum
Microcolon
Transposition of appendix
Transposition of colon
Transposition of intestine

Q43.9 Congenital malformation of intestine, unspecified

4th Q44 Congenital malformations of gallbladder, bile ducts and liver

Q44.0 Agenesis, aplasia and hypoplasia of gallbladder
Congenital absence of gallbladder

Q44.1 Other congenital malformations of gallbladder
Congenital malformation of gallbladder NOS
Intrahepatic gallbladder

Q44.2 Atresia of bile ducts

Q44.3 Congenital stenosis and stricture of bile ducts

Q44.4 Choledochal cyst

Q44.5 Other congenital malformations of bile ducts
Accessory hepatic duct
Biliary duct duplication
Congenital malformation of bile duct NOS
Cystic duct duplication

Q44.6 Cystic disease of liver
Fibrocystic disease of liver

DRAFT

Q44.7 Other congenital malformations of liver
Accessory liver
Alagille's syndrome
Congenital absence of liver
Congenital hepatomegaly
Congenital malformation of liver NOS

✓4th **Q45 Other congenital malformations of digestive system**
EXCLUDES 2 *congenital diaphragmatic hernia (Q79.0)*
congenital hiatus hernia (Q40.1)

Q45.0 Agenesis, aplasia and hypoplasia of pancreas
Congenital absence of pancreas

Q45.1 Annular pancreas

Q45.2 Congenital pancreatic cyst

Q45.3 Other congenital malformations of pancreas and pancreatic duct
Accessory pancreas
Congenital malformation of pancreas or pancreatic duct NOS
EXCLUDES 1 *congenital diabetes mellitus (E10.-)*
cystic fibrosis (E84.0-E84.9)
fibrocystic disease of pancreas (E84.-)
neonatal diabetes mellitus (P70.2)

Q45.8 Other specified congenital malformations of digestive system
Absence (complete) (partial) of alimentary tract NOS
Duplication of digestive system
Malposition, congenital of digestive system

Q45.9 Congenital malformation of digestive system, unspecified
Congenital anomaly of digestive system
Congenital deformity of digestive system

Congenital malformations of genital organs (Q50-Q56)

EXCLUDES 1 *androgen insensitivity syndrome (E34.5-)*
syndromes associated with anomalies in the number and form of chromosomes (Q90-Q99)

✓4th **Q50 Congenital malformations of ovaries, fallopian tubes and broad ligaments**

✓5th **Q50.0 Congenital absence of ovary**
EXCLUDES 1 *Turner's syndrome (Q96.-)*

Q50.01 Congenital absence of ovary, unilateral

Q50.02 Congenital absence of ovary, bilateral

Q50.1 Developmental ovarian cyst

Q50.2 Congenital torsion of ovary

✓5th **Q50.3 Other congenital malformations of ovary**

Q50.31 Accessory ovary

Q50.32 Ovarian streak
46, XX with streak gonads

Q50.39 Other congenital malformation of ovary
Congenital malformation of ovary NOS

Q50.4 Embryonic cyst of fallopian tube
Fimbrial cyst

Q50.5 Embryonic cyst of broad ligament
Epoophoron cyst
Parovarian cyst

Q50.6 Other congenital malformations of fallopian tube and broad ligament
Absence of fallopian tube and broad ligament
Accessory fallopian tube and broad ligament
Atresia of fallopian tube and broad ligament
Congenital malformation of fallopian tube or broad ligament NOS

✓4th **Q51 Congenital malformations of uterus and cervix**

Q51.0 Agenesis and aplasia of uterus
Congenital absence of uterus

✓5th **Q51.1 Doubling of uterus with doubling of cervix and vagina**

Q51.10 Doubling of uterus with doubling of cervix and vagina without obstruction
Doubling of uterus with doubling of cervix and vagina NOS

Q51.11 Doubling of uterus with doubling of cervix and vagina with obstruction

Q51.2 Other doubling of uterus
Doubling of uterus NOS
Septate uterus, complete or partial

Q51.3 Bicornate uterus
Bicornate uterus, complete or partial

Q51.4 Unicornate uterus
Unicornate uterus with or without a separate uterine horn
Uterus with only one functioning horn

Q51.5 Agenesis and aplasia of cervix
Congenital absence of cervix

Q51.6 Embryonic cyst of cervix

Q51.7 Congenital fistulae between uterus and digestive and urinary tracts

✓5th **Q51.8 Other congenital malformations of uterus and cervix**

✓6th **Q51.81 Other congenital malformations of uterus**

Q51.810 Arcuate uterus
Arcuatus uterus

Q51.811 Hypoplasia of uterus

Q51.818 Other congenital malformations of uterus
Müllerian anomaly of uterus NEC

✓6th **Q51.82 Other congenital malformations of cervix**

Q51.820 Cervical duplication

Q51.821 Hypoplasia of cervix

Q51.828 Other congenital malformations of cervix

Q51.9 Congenital malformation of uterus and cervix, unspecified

✓4th **Q52 Other congenital malformations of female genitalia**

Q52.0 Congenital absence of vagina
Vaginal agenesis, total or partial

✓5th **Q52.1 Doubling of vagina**
EXCLUDES 1 *doubling of vagina with doubling of uterus and cervix (Q51.1-)*

Q52.10 Doubling of vagina, unspecified
Septate vagina NOS

Q52.11 Transverse vaginal septum

Q52.12 Longitudinal vaginal septum
Longitudinal vaginal septum with or without obstruction

Q52.2 Congenital rectovaginal fistula
EXCLUDES 1 *cloaca (Q43.7)*

Q52.3 Imperforate hymen

Q52.4 Other congenital malformations of vagina
Canal of Nuck cyst, congenital
Congenital malformation of vagina NOS
Embryonic vaginal cyst
Gartner's duct cyst

Q52.5 Fusion of labia

Q52.6 Congenital malformation of clitoris

✓5th **Q52.7 Other and unspecified congenital malformations of vulva**

Q52.70 Unspecified congenital malformations of vulva
Congenital malformation of vulva NOS

Q52.71 Congenital absence of vulva

Q52.79 Other congenital malformations of vulva
Congenital cyst of vulva

Q52.8 Other specified congenital malformations of female genitalia

Q52.9 Congenital malformation of female genitalia, unspecified

✓4th **Q53 Undescended and ectopic testicle**

✓5th **Q53.0 Ectopic testis**

Q53.00 Ectopic testis, unspecified

Q53.01 Ectopic testis, unilateral

Q53.02 Ectopic testes, bilateral

✓5th **Q53.1 Undescended testicle, unilateral**

Q53.10 Unspecified undescended testicle, unilateral

Q53.11 Abdominal testis, unilateral

Q53.12 Ectopic perineal testis, unilateral

✓5th **Q53.2 Undescended testicle, bilateral**

Q53.20 Undescended testicle, unspecified, bilateral

Q53.21 Abdominal testis, bilateral

Q53.22 Ectopic perineal testis, bilateral

Q53.9 Undescended testicle, unspecified
Cryptorchism NOS

✓4th **Q54 Hypospadias**
EXCLUDES 1 *epispadias (Q64.0)*

Q54.0 Hypospadias, balanic
Hypospadias, coronal
Hypospadias, glandular

Q54.1 Hypospadias, penile

Q54.2 Hypospadias, penoscrotal

Q54.3 Hypospadias, perineal

Q54.4 **Congenital chordee**
Chordee without hypospadias
Q54.8 **Other hypospadias**
Hypospadias with intersex state
Q54.9 **Hypospadias, unspecified**

✓4th **Q55 Other congenital malformations of male genital organs**
EXCLUDES 1 *congenital hydrocele (P83.5)*
hypospadias (Q54.-)
Q55.0 **Absence and aplasia of testis**
Monorchism
Q55.1 **Hypoplasia of testis and scrotum**
Fusion of testes
✓5th Q55.2 **Other and unspecified congenital malformations of testis and scrotum**
Q55.20 **Unspecified congenital malformations of testis and scrotum**
Congenital malformation of testis or scrotum NOS
Q55.21 **Polyorchism**
Q55.22 **Retractile testis**
Q55.23 **Scrotal transposition**
Q55.29 **Other congenital malformations of testis and scrotum**
Q55.3 **Atresia of vas deferens**
Code first any associated cystic fibrosis (E84.-)
Q55.4 **Other congenital malformations of vas deferens, epididymis, seminal vesicles and prostate**
Absence or aplasia of prostate
Absence or aplasia of spermatic cord
Congenital malformation of vas deferens, epididymis, seminal vesicles or prostate NOS
Q55.5 **Congenital absence and aplasia of penis**
✓5th Q55.6 **Other congenital malformations of penis**
Q55.61 **Curvature of penis (lateral)**
Q55.62 **Hypoplasia of penis**
Micropenis
Q55.63 **Congenital torsion of penis**
EXCLUDES 1 *acquired torsion of penis (N48.82)*
Q55.64 **Hidden penis**
Buried penis
Concealed penis
EXCLUDES 1 *acquired buried penis (N48.83)*
Q55.69 **Other congenital malformation of penis**
Congenital malformation of penis NOS
Q55.7 **Congenital vasocutaneous fistula**
Q55.8 **Other specified congenital malformations of male genital organs**
Q55.9 **Congenital malformation of male genital organ, unspecified**
Congenital anomaly of male genital organ
Congenital deformity of male genital organ

✓4th **Q56 Indeterminate sex and pseudohermaphroditism**
EXCLUDES 1 *46, XX true hermaphrodite (Q99.1)*
androgen insensitivity syndrome (E34.5-)
chimera 46, XX/46, XY true hermaphrodite (Q99.0)
female pseudohermaphroditism with adrenocortical disorder (E25.-)
pseudohermaphroditism with specified chromosomal anomaly (Q96-Q99)
pure gonadal dysgenesis (Q99.1)
Q56.0 **Hermaphroditism, not elsewhere classified**
Ovotestis
Q56.1 **Male pseudohermaphroditism, not elsewhere classified**
46, XY with streak gonads
Male pseudohermaphroditism NOS
Q56.2 **Female pseudohermaphroditism, not elsewhere classified**
Female pseudohermaphroditism NOS
Q56.3 **Pseudohermaphroditism, unspecified**
Q56.4 **Indeterminate sex, unspecified**
Ambiguous genitalia

Congenital malformations of the urinary system (Q60-Q64)

✓4th **Q60 Renal agenesis and other reduction defects of kidney**
Congenital absence of kidney
Congenital atrophy of kidney
Infantile atrophy of kidney
Q60.0 **Renal agenesis, unilateral**
Q60.1 **Renal agenesis, bilateral**
Q60.2 **Renal agenesis, unspecified**
Q60.3 **Renal hypoplasia, unilateral**
Q60.4 **Renal hypoplasia, bilateral**
Q60.5 **Renal hypoplasia, unspecified**
Q60.6 **Potter's syndrome**

✓4th **Q61 Cystic kidney disease**
EXCLUDES 1 *acquired cyst of kidney (N28.1)*
Potter's syndrome (Q60.6)
✓5th Q61.0 **Congenital renal cyst**
Q61.00 **Congenital renal cyst, unspecified**
Cyst of kidney NOS (congenital)
Q61.01 **Congenital single renal cyst**
Q61.02 **Congenital multiple renal cysts**
✓5th Q61.1 **Polycystic kidney, infantile type**
Polycystic kidney, autosomal recessive
Q61.11 **Cystic dilatation of collecting ducts**
Q61.19 **Other polycystic kidney, infantile type**
Q61.2 **Polycystic kidney, adult type**
Polycystic kidney, autosomal dominant
Q61.3 **Polycystic kidney, unspecified**
Q61.4 **Renal dysplasia**
Multicystic dysplastic kidney
Multicystic kidney (development)
Multicystic kidney disease
Multicystic renal dysplasia
EXCLUDES 1 *polycystic kidney disease (Q61.11-Q61.3)*
Q61.5 **Medullary cystic kidney**
Nephronopthisis
Sponge kidney NOS
Q61.8 **Other cystic kidney diseases**
Fibrocystic kidney
Fibrocystic renal degeneration or disease
Q61.9 **Cystic kidney disease, unspecified**
Meckel-Gruber syndrome

✓4th **Q62 Congenital obstructive defects of renal pelvis and congenital malformations of ureter**
Q62.0 **Congenital hydronephrosis**
✓5th Q62.1 **Congenital occlusion of ureter**
Atresia and stenosis of ureter
Q62.10 **Congenital occlusion of ureter, unspecified**
Q62.11 **Congenital occlusion of ureteropelvic junction**
Q62.12 **Congenital occlusion of ureterovesical orifice**
Q62.2 **Congenital megaureter**
Congenital dilatation of ureter
✓5th Q62.3 **Other obstructive defects of renal pelvis and ureter**
Q62.31 **Congenital ureterocele, orthotopic**
Q62.32 **Cecoureterocele**
Ectopic ureterocele
Q62.39 **Other obstructive defects of renal pelvis and ureter**
Ureteropelvic junction obstruction NOS
Q62.4 **Agenesis of ureter**
Congenital absence ureter
Q62.5 **Duplication of ureter**
Accessory ureter
Double ureter
✓5th Q62.6 **Malposition of ureter**
Q62.60 **Malposition of ureter, unspecified**
Q62.61 **Deviation of ureter**
Q62.62 **Displacement of ureter**
Q62.63 **Anomalous implantation of ureter**
Ectopia of ureter
Ectopic ureter
Q62.69 **Other malposition of ureter**
Q62.7 **Congenital vesico-uretero-renal reflux**
Q62.8 **Other congenital malformations of ureter**
Anomaly of ureter NOS

✓4th **Q63 Other congenital malformations of kidney**
EXCLUDES 1 *congenital nephrotic syndrome (N04.-)*
Q63.0 **Accessory kidney**
Q63.1 **Lobulated, fused and horseshoe kidney**
Q63.2 **Ectopic kidney**
Congenital displaced kidney
Malrotation of kidney
Q63.3 **Hyperplastic and giant kidney**
Compensatory hypertrophy of kidney

Q63.8 Other specified congenital malformations of kidney
Congenital renal calculi
Q63.9 Congenital malformation of kidney, unspecified

4th **Q64 Other congenital malformations of urinary system**
Q64.0 Epispadias
EXCLUDES 1 *hypospadias (Q54.-)*
5th **Q64.1 Exstrophy of urinary bladder**
Q64.10 Exstrophy of urinary bladder, unspecified
Ectopia vesicae
Q64.11 Supravesical fissure of urinary bladder
Q64.12 Cloacal extrophy of urinary bladder
Q64.19 Other exstrophy of urinary bladder
Extroversion of bladder
Q64.2 Congenital posterior urethral valves
5th **Q64.3 Other atresia and stenosis of urethra and bladder neck**
Q64.31 Congenital bladder neck obstruction
Congenital obstruction of vesicourethral orifice
Q64.32 Congenital stricture of urethra
Q64.33 Congenital stricture of urinary meatus
Q64.39 Other atresia and stenosis of urethra and bladder neck
Atresia and stenosis of urethra and bladder neck NOS
Q64.4 Malformation of urachus
Cyst of urachus
Patent urachus
Prolapse of urachus
Q64.5 Congenital absence of bladder and urethra
Q64.6 Congenital diverticulum of bladder
5th **Q64.7 Other and unspecified congenital malformations of bladder and urethra**
EXCLUDES 1 *congenital prolapse of bladder (mucosa) (Q79.4)*
Q64.70 Unspecified congenital malformation of bladder and urethra
Malformation of bladder or urethra NOS
Q64.71 Congenital prolapse of urethra
Q64.72 Congenital prolapse of urinary meatus
Q64.73 Congenital urethrorectal fistula
Q64.74 Double urethra
Q64.75 Double urinary meatus
Q64.79 Other congenital malformations of bladder and urethra
Q64.8 Other specified congenital malformations of urinary system
Q64.9 Congenital malformation of urinary system, unspecified
Congenital anomaly NOS of urinary system
Congenital deformity NOS of urinary system

Congenital malformations and deformations of the musculoskeletal system (Q65-Q79)

4th **Q65 Congenital deformities of hip**
EXCLUDES 1 *clicking hip (R29.4)*
5th **Q65.0 Congenital dislocation of hip, unilateral**
Q65.00 Congenital dislocation of unspecified hip, unilateral
Q65.01 Congenital dislocation of right hip, unilateral
Q65.02 Congenital dislocation of left hip, unilateral
Q65.1 Congenital dislocation of hip, bilateral
Q65.2 Congenital dislocation of hip, unspecified
5th **Q65.3 Congenital partial dislocation of hip, unilateral**
Q65.30 Congenital partial dislocation of unspecified hip, unilateral
Q65.31 Congenital partial dislocation of right hip, unilateral
Q65.32 Congenital partial dislocation of left hip, unilateral
Q65.4 Congenital partial dislocation of hip, bilateral
Q65.5 Congenital partial dislocation of hip, unspecified
Q65.6 Congenital unstable hip
Congenital dislocatable hip
5th **Q65.8 Other congenital deformities of hip**
Q65.81 Congenital coxa valga
Q65.82 Congenital coxa vara
Q65.89 Other specified congenital deformities of hip
Anteversion of femoral neck
Congenital acetabular dysplasia
Q65.9 Congenital deformity of hip, unspecified

4th **Q66 Congenital deformities of feet**
EXCLUDES 1 *reduction defects of feet (Q72.-)*
valgus deformities (acquired) (M21.0-)
varus deformities (acquired) (M21.1-)
Q66.0 Congenital talipes equinovarus
Q66.1 Congenital talipes calcaneovarus
Q66.2 Congenital metatarsus (primus) varus
Q66.3 Other congenital varus deformities of feet
Hallux varus, congenital
Q66.4 Congenital talipes calcaneovalgus
5th **Q66.5 Congenital pes planus**
Congenital flat foot
Congenital rigid flat foot
Congenital spastic (everted) flat foot
EXCLUDES 1 *pes planus, acquired (M21.4)*
Q66.50 Congenital pes planus, unspecified foot
Q66.51 Congenital pes planus, right foot
Q66.52 Congenital pes planus, left foot
Q66.6 Other congenital valgus deformities of feet
Congenital metatarsus valgus
Q66.7 Congenital pes cavus
5th **Q66.8 Other congenital deformities of feet**
Q66.80 Congenital vertical talus deformity, unspecified foot
Q66.81 Congenital vertical talus deformity, right foot
Q66.82 Congenital vertical talus deformity, left foot
Q66.89 Other specified congenital deformities of feet
Congenital asymmetric talipes
Congenital clubfoot NOS
Congenital talipes NOS
Congenital tarsal coalition
Hammer toe, congenital
Q66.9 Congenital deformity of feet, unspecified

4th **Q67 Congenital musculoskeletal deformities of head, face, spine and chest**
EXCLUDES 1 *congenital malformation syndromes classified to Q87-*
Potter's syndrome (Q60.6)
Q67.0 Congenital facial asymmetry
Q67.1 Congenital compression facies
Q67.2 Dolichocephaly
Q67.3 Plagiocephaly
Q67.4 Other congenital deformities of skull, face and jaw
Congenital depressions in skull
Congenital hemifacial atrophy or hypertrophy
Deviation of nasal septum, congenital
Squashed or bent nose, congenital
EXCLUDES 1 *dentofacial anomalies [including malocclusion] (M26.-)*
syphilitic saddle nose (A50.5)
Q67.5 Congenital deformity of spine
Congenital postural scoliosis
Congenital scoliosis NOS
EXCLUDES 1 *infantile idiopathic scoliosis (M41.0)*
scoliosis due to congenital bony malformation (Q76.3)
Q67.6 Pectus excavatum
Congenital funnel chest
Q67.7 Pectus carinatum
Congenital pigeon chest
Q67.8 Other congenital deformities of chest
Congenital deformity of chest wall NOS

4th **Q68 Other congenital musculoskeletal deformities**
EXCLUDES 1 *reduction defects of limb(s) (Q71-Q73)*
EXCLUDES 2 *congenital myotonic chondrodystrophy (G71.13)*
Q68.0 Congenital deformity of sternocleidomastoid muscle
Congenital contracture of sternocleidomastoid (muscle)
Congenital (sternomastoid) torticollis
Sternomastoid tumor (congenital)
Q68.1 Congenital deformity of finger(s) and hand
Congenital clubfinger
Spade-like hand (congenital)
Q68.2 Congenital deformity of knee
Congenital dislocation of knee
Congenital genu recurvatum
Q68.3 Congenital bowing of femur
EXCLUDES 1 *anteversion of femur (neck) (Q65.89)*
Q68.4 Congenital bowing of tibia and fibula

EXCLUDES 1 Not coded here EXCLUDES 2 Not included here ***Manifestation Code***

Q68.5 Congenital bowing of long bones of leg, unspecified
Q68.6 Discoid meniscus
Q68.8 Other specified congenital musculoskeletal deformities
Congenital deformity of clavicle
Congenital deformity of elbow
Congenital deformity of forearm
Congenital deformity of scapula
Congenital deformity of wrist
Congenital dislocation of elbow
Congenital dislocation of shoulder
Congenital dislocation of wrist

✓4th **Q69 Polydactyly**
Q69.0 Accessory finger(s)
Q69.1 Accessory thumb(s)
Q69.2 Accessory toe(s)
Accessory hallux
Q69.9 Polydactyly, unspecified
Supernumerary digit(s) NOS

✓4th **Q70 Syndactyly**
✓5th **Q70.0 Fused fingers**
Complex syndactyly of fingers with synostosis
Q70.00 Fused fingers, unspecified hand
Q70.01 Fused fingers, right hand
Q70.02 Fused fingers, left hand
Q70.03 Fused fingers, bilateral
✓5th **Q70.1 Webbed fingers**
Simple syndactyly of fingers without synostosis
Q70.10 Webbed fingers, unspecified hand
Q70.11 Webbed fingers, right hand
Q70.12 Webbed fingers, left hand
Q70.13 Webbed fingers, bilateral
✓5th **Q70.2 Fused toes**
Complex syndactyly of toes with synostosis
Q70.20 Fused toes, unspecified foot
Q70.21 Fused toes, right foot
Q70.22 Fused toes, left foot
Q70.23 Fused toes, bilateral
✓5th **Q70.3 Webbed toes**
Simple syndactyly of toes without synostosis
Q70.30 Webbed toes, unspecified foot
Q70.31 Webbed toes, right foot
Q70.32 Webbed toes, left foot
Q70.33 Webbed toes, bilateral
Q70.4 Polysyndactyly, unspecified
EXCLUDES1 *specified syndactyly of hand and feet - code to specified conditions (Q70.0- - Q70.3-)*
Q70.9 Syndactyly, unspecified
Symphalangy NOS

✓4th **Q71 Reduction defects of upper limb**
✓5th **Q71.0 Congenital complete absence of upper limb**
Q71.00 Congenital complete absence of unspecified upper limb
Q71.01 Congenital complete absence of right upper limb
Q71.02 Congenital complete absence of left upper limb
Q71.03 Congenital complete absence of upper limb, bilateral
✓5th **Q71.1 Congenital absence of upper arm and forearm with hand present**
Q71.10 Congenital absence of unspecified upper arm and forearm with hand present
Q71.11 Congenital absence of right upper arm and forearm with hand present
Q71.12 Congenital absence of left upper arm and forearm with hand present
Q71.13 Congenital absence of upper arm and forearm with hand present, bilateral
✓5th **Q71.2 Congenital absence of both forearm and hand**
Q71.20 Congenital absence of both forearm and hand, unspecified upper limb
Q71.21 Congenital absence of both forearm and hand, right upper limb
Q71.22 Congenital absence of both forearm and hand, left upper limb
Q71.23 Congenital absence of both forearm and hand, bilateral
✓5th **Q71.3 Congenital absence of hand and finger**
Q71.30 Congenital absence of unspecified hand and finger
Q71.31 Congenital absence of right hand and finger
Q71.32 Congenital absence of left hand and finger
Q71.33 Congenital absence of hand and finger, bilateral
✓5th **Q71.4 Longitudinal reduction defect of radius**
Clubhand (congenital)
Radial clubhand
Q71.40 Longitudinal reduction defect of unspecified radius
Q71.41 Longitudinal reduction defect of right radius
Q71.42 Longitudinal reduction defect of left radius
Q71.43 Longitudinal reduction defect of radius, bilateral
✓5th **Q71.5 Longitudinal reduction defect of ulna**
Q71.50 Longitudinal reduction defect of unspecified ulna
Q71.51 Longitudinal reduction defect of right ulna
Q71.52 Longitudinal reduction defect of left ulna
Q71.53 Longitudinal reduction defect of ulna, bilateral
✓5th **Q71.6 Lobster-claw hand**
Q71.60 Lobster-claw hand, unspecified hand
Q71.61 Lobster-claw right hand
Q71.62 Lobster-claw left hand
Q71.63 Lobster-claw hand, bilateral
✓5th **Q71.8 Other reduction defects of upper limb**
✓6th **Q71.81 Congenital shortening of upper limb**
Q71.811 Congenital shortening of right upper limb
Q71.812 Congenital shortening of left upper limb
Q71.813 Congenital shortening of upper limb, bilateral
Q71.819 Congenital shortening of unspecified upper limb
✓6th **Q71.89 Other reduction defects of upper limb**
Q71.891 Other reduction defects of right upper limb
Q71.892 Other reduction defects of left upper limb
Q71.893 Other reduction defects of upper limb, bilateral
Q71.899 Other reduction defects of unspecified upper limb
✓5th **Q71.9 Unspecified reduction defect of upper limb**
Q71.90 Unspecified reduction defect of upper limb
Q71.91 Unspecified reduction defect of right upper limb
Q71.92 Unspecified reduction defect of left upper limb
Q71.93 Unspecified reduction defect of upper limb, bilateral

✓4th **Q72 Reduction defects of lower limb**
✓5th **Q72.0 Congenital complete absence of lower limb**
Q72.00 Congenital complete absence of unspecified lower limb
Q72.01 Congenital complete absence of right lower limb
Q72.02 Congenital complete absence of left lower limb
Q72.03 Congenital complete absence of lower limb, bilateral
✓5th **Q72.1 Congenital absence of thigh and lower leg with foot present**
Q72.10 Congenital absence of unspecified thigh and lower leg with foot present
Q72.11 Congenital absence of right thigh and lower leg with foot present
Q72.12 Congenital absence of left thigh and lower leg with foot present
Q72.13 Congenital absence of thigh and lower leg with foot present, bilateral
✓5th **Q72.2 Congenital absence of both lower leg and foot**
Q72.20 Congenital absence of both lower leg and foot, unspecified lower limb
Q72.21 Congenital absence of both lower leg and foot, right lower limb
Q72.22 Congenital absence of both lower leg and foot, left lower limb
Q72.23 Congenital absence of both lower leg and foot, bilateral
✓5th **Q72.3 Congenital absence of foot and toe(s)**
Q72.30 Congenital absence of unspecified foot and toe(s)
Q72.31 Congenital absence of right foot and toe(s)

Q72.32 Congenital absence of left foot and toe(s)
Q72.33 Congenital absence of foot and toe(s), bilateral
Q72.4 Longitudinal reduction defect of femur
Proximal femoral focal deficiency
Q72.40 Longitudinal reduction defect of unspecified femur
Q72.41 Longitudinal reduction defect of right femur
Q72.42 Longitudinal reduction defect of left femur
Q72.43 Longitudinal reduction defect of femur, bilateral
Q72.5 Longitudinal reduction defect of tibia
Q72.50 Longitudinal reduction defect of unspecified tibia
Q72.51 Longitudinal reduction defect of right tibia
Q72.52 Longitudinal reduction defect of left tibia
Q72.53 Longitudinal reduction defect of tibia, bilateral
Q72.6 Longitudinal reduction defect of fibula
Q72.60 Longitudinal reduction defect of unspecified fibula
Q72.61 Longitudinal reduction defect of right fibula
Q72.62 Longitudinal reduction defect of left fibula
Q72.63 Longitudinal reduction defect of fibula, bilateral
Q72.7 Split foot
Q72.70 Split foot, unspecified lower limb
Q72.71 Split foot, right lower limb
Q72.72 Split foot, left lower limb
Q72.73 Split foot, bilateral
Q72.8 Other reduction defects of lower limb
Q72.81 Congenital shortening of lower limb
Q72.811 Congenital shortening of right lower limb
Q72.812 Congenital shortening of left lower limb
Q72.813 Congenital shortening of lower limb, bilateral
Q72.819 Congenital shortening of unspecified lower limb
Q72.89 Other reduction defects of lower limb
Q72.891 Other reduction defects of right lower limb
Q72.892 Other reduction defects of left lower limb
Q72.893 Other reduction defects of lower limb, bilateral
Q72.899 Other reduction defects of unspecified lower limb
Q72.9 Unspecified reduction defect of lower limb
Q72.90 Unspecified reduction defect of unspecified lower limb
Q72.91 Unspecified reduction defect of right lower limb
Q72.92 Unspecified reduction defect of left lower limb
Q72.93 Unspecified reduction defect of lower limb, bilateral

Q73 Reduction defects of unspecified limb

Q73.0 Congenital absence of unspecified limb(s)
Amelia NOS
Q73.1 Phocomelia, unspecified limb(s)
Phocomelia NOS
Q73.8 Other reduction defects of unspecified limb(s)
Longitudinal reduction deformity of unspecified limb(s)
Ectromelia of limb NOS
Hemimelia of limb NOS
Reduction defect of limb NOS

Q74 Other congenital malformations of limb(s)

EXCLUDES 1 *polydactyly (Q69.-)*
reduction defect of limb (Q71-Q73)
syndactyly (Q70.-)

Q74.0 Other congenital malformations of upper limb(s), including shoulder girdle
Accessory carpal bones
Cleidocranial dysostosis
Congenital pseudarthrosis of clavicle
Macrodactylia (fingers)
Madelung's deformity
Radioulnar synostosis
Sprengel's deformity
Triphalangeal thumb
Q74.1 Congenital malformation of knee
Congenital absence of patella
Congenital dislocation of patella
Congenital genu valgum
Congenital genu varum
Rudimentary patella
EXCLUDES 1 *congenital dislocation of knee (Q68.2)*
congenital genu recurvatum (Q68.2)
nail patella syndrome (Q87.2)
Q74.2 Other congenital malformations of lower limb(s), including pelvic girdle
Congenital fusion of sacroiliac joint
Congenital malformation of ankle joint
Congenital malformation of sacroiliac joint
EXCLUDES 1 *anteversion of femur (neck) (Q65.89)*
Q74.3 Arthrogryposis multiplex congenita
Q74.8 Other specified congenital malformations of limb(s)
Q74.9 Unspecified congenital malformation of limb(s)
Congenital anomaly of limb(s) NOS

Q75 Other congenital malformations of skull and face bones

EXCLUDES 1 *congenital malformation of face NOS (Q18.-)*
congenital malformation syndromes classified to Q87.-
dentofacial anomalies [including malocclusion] (M26.-)
musculoskeletal deformities of head and face (Q67.0-Q67.4)
skull defects associated with congenital anomalies of brain such as:
anencephaly (Q00.0)
encephalocele (Q01.-)
hydrocephalus (Q03.-)
microcephaly (Q02)

Q75.0 Craniosynostosis
Acrocephaly
Imperfect fusion of skull
Oxycephaly
Trigonocephaly
Q75.1 Craniofacial dysostosis
Crouzon's disease
Q75.2 Hypertelorism
Q75.3 Macrocephaly
Q75.4 Mandibulofacial dysostosis
Franceschetti syndrome
Treacher Collins syndrome
Q75.5 Oculomandibular dysostosis
Q75.8 Other specified congenital malformations of skull and face bones
Absence of skull bone, congenital
Congenital deformity of forehead
Platybasia
Q75.9 Congenital malformation of skull and face bones, unspecified
Congenital anomaly of face bones NOS
Congenital anomaly of skull NOS

Q76 Congenital malformations of spine and bony thorax

EXCLUDES 1 *congenital musculoskeletal deformities of spine and chest (Q67.5-Q67.8)*

Q76.0 Spina bifida occulta
EXCLUDES 1 *meningocele (spinal) (Q05.-)*
spina bifida (aperta) (cystica) (Q05.-)
Q76.1 Klippel-Feil syndrome
Cervical fusion syndrome
Q76.2 Congenital spondylolisthesis
Congenital spondylolysis
EXCLUDES 1 *spondylolisthesis (acquired) (M43.1-)*
spondylolysis (acquired) (M43.0-)
Q76.3 Congenital scoliosis due to congenital bony malformation
Hemivertebra fusion or failure of segmentation with scoliosis
Q76.4 Other congenital malformations of spine, not associated with scoliosis
Q76.41 Congenital kyphosis
Q76.411 Congenital kyphosis, occipito-atlanto-axial region
Q76.412 Congenital kyphosis, cervical region
Q76.413 Congenital kyphosis, cervicothoracic region
Q76.414 Congenital kyphosis, thoracic region
Q76.415 Congenital kyphosis, thoracolumbar region
Q76.419 Congenital kyphosis, unspecified region

√6th **Q76.42 Congenital lordosis**
Q76.425 Congenital lordosis, thoracolumbar region
Q76.426 Congenital lordosis, lumbar region
Q76.427 Congenital lordosis, lumbosacral region
Q76.428 Congenital lordosis, sacral and sacrococcygeal region
Q76.429 Congenital lordosis, unspecified region
Q76.49 Other congenital malformations of spine, not associated with scoliosis
Congenital absence of vertebra NOS
Congenital fusion of spine NOS
Congenital malformation of lumbosacral (joint) (region) NOS
Congenital malformation of spine NOS
Hemivertebra NOS
Malformation of spine NOS
Platyspondylisis NOS
Supernumerary vertebra NOS
Q76.5 Cervical rib
Supernumerary rib in cervical region
Q76.6 Other congenital malformations of ribs
Accessory rib
Congenital absence of rib
Congenital fusion of ribs
Congenital malformation of ribs NOS
EXCLUDES 1 *short rib syndrome (Q77.2)*
Q76.7 Congenital malformation of sternum
Congenital absence of sternum
Sternum bifidum
Q76.8 Other congenital malformations of bony thorax
Q76.9 Congenital malformation of bony thorax, unspecified

√4th **Q77 Osteochondrodysplasia with defects of growth of tubular bones and spine**
EXCLUDES 1 *mucopolysaccharidosis (E76.0-E76.3)*
EXCLUDES 2 *congenital myotonic chondrodystrophy (G71.13)*
Q77.0 Achondrogenesis
Hypochondrogenesis
Q77.1 Thanatophoric short stature
Q77.2 Short rib syndrome
Asphyxiating thoracic dysplasia [Jeune]
Q77.3 Chondrodysplasia punctata
EXCLUDES 1 *Rhizomelic chondrodysplasia punctata (E71.43)*
Q77.4 Achondroplasia
Hypochondroplasia
Osteosclerosis congenita
Q77.5 Diastrophic dysplasia
Q77.6 Chondroectodermal dysplasia
Ellis-van Creveld syndrome
Q77.7 Spondyloepiphyseal dysplasia
Q77.8 Other osteochondrodysplasia with defects of growth of tubular bones and spine
Q77.9 Osteochondrodysplasia with defects of growth of tubular bones and spine, unspecified

√4th **Q78 Other osteochondrodysplasias**
EXCLUDES 2 *congenital myotonic chondrodystrophy (G71.13)*
Q78.0 Osteogenesis imperfecta
Fragilitas ossium
Osteopsathyrosis
Q78.1 Polyostotic fibrous dysplasia
Albright(-McCune)(-Sternberg) syndrome
Q78.2 Osteopetrosis
Albers-Schönberg syndrome
Osteosclerosis NOS
Q78.3 Progressive diaphyseal dysplasia
Camurati-Engelmann syndrome
Q78.4 Enchondromatosis
Maffucci's syndrome
Ollier's disease
Q78.5 Metaphyseal dysplasia
Pyle's syndrome
Q78.6 Multiple congenital exostoses
Diaphyseal aclasis
Q78.8 Other specified osteochondrodysplasias
Osteopoikilosis
Q78.9 Osteochondrodysplasia, unspecified
Chondrodystrophy NOS
Osteodystrophy NOS

√4th **Q79 Congenital malformations of musculoskeletal system, not elsewhere classified**
EXCLUDES 2 *congenital (sternomastoid) torticollis (Q68.0)*
Q79.0 Congenital diaphragmatic hernia
EXCLUDES 1 *congenital hiatus hernia (Q40.1)*
Q79.1 Other congenital malformations of diaphragm
Absence of diaphragm
Congenital malformation of diaphragm NOS
Eventration of diaphragm
Q79.2 Exomphalos
Omphalocele
EXCLUDES 1 *umbilical hernia (K42.-)*
Q79.3 Gastroschisis
Q79.4 Prune belly syndrome
Congenital prolapse of bladder mucosa
Eagle-Barrett syndrome
√5th **Q79.5 Other congenital malformations of abdominal wall**
EXCLUDES 1 *umbilical hernia (K42.-)*
Q79.51 Congenital hernia of bladder
Q79.59 Other congenital malformations of abdominal wall
Q79.6 Ehlers-Danlos syndrome
Q79.8 Other congenital malformations of musculoskeletal system
Absence of muscle
Absence of tendon
Accessory muscle
Amyotrophia congenita
Congenital constricting bands
Congenital shortening of tendon
Poland syndrome
Q79.9 Congenital malformation of musculoskeletal system, unspecified
Congenital anomaly of musculoskeletal system NOS
Congenital deformity of musculoskeletal system NOS

Other congenital malformations (Q80-Q89)

√4th **Q80 Congenital ichthyosis**
EXCLUDES 1 *Refsum's disease (G60.1)*
Q80.0 Ichthyosis vulgaris
Q80.1 X-linked ichthyosis
Q80.2 Lamellar ichthyosis
Collodion baby
Q80.3 Congenital bullous ichthyosiform erythroderma
Q80.4 Harlequin fetus
Q80.8 Other congenital ichthyosis
Q80.9 Congenital ichthyosis, unspecified

√4th **Q81 Epidermolysis bullosa**
Q81.0 Epidermolysis bullosa simplex
EXCLUDES 1 *Cockayne's syndrome (Q87.1)*
Q81.1 Epidermolysis bullosa letalis
Herlitz' syndrome
Q81.2 Epidermolysis bullosa dystrophica
Q81.8 Other epidermolysis bullosa
Q81.9 Epidermolysis bullosa, unspecified

√4th **Q82 Other congenital malformations of skin**
EXCLUDES 1 *acrodermatitis enteropathica (E83.2)*
congenital erythropoietic porphyria (E80.0)
pilonidal cyst or sinus (L05.-)
Sturge-Weber (-Dimitri) syndrome (Q85.8)
Q82.0 Hereditary lymphedema
Q82.1 Xeroderma pigmentosum
Q82.2 Mastocytosis
Urticaria pigmentosa
EXCLUDES 1 *malignant mastocytosis (C96.2)*
Q82.3 Incontinentia pigmenti
Q82.4 Ectodermal dysplasia (anhidrotic)
EXCLUDES 1 *Ellis-van Creveld syndrome (Q77.6)*

Q82.5 Congenital non-neoplastic nevus
Birthmark NOS
Flammeus Nevus
Portwine Nevus
Sanguineous Nevus
Strawberry Nevus
Vascular Nevus NOS
Verrucous Nevus
EXCLUDES 2 *araneus nevus (I78.1)*
café au lait spots (L81.3)
lentigo (L81.4)
melanocytic nevus (D22.-)
nevus NOS (D22.-)
pigmented nevus (D22.-)
spider nevus (I78.1)
stellar nevus (I78.1)

Q82.8 Other specified congenital malformations of skin
Abnormal palmar creases
Accessory skin tags
Benign familial pemphigus [Hailey-Hailey]
Congenital poikiloderma
Cutis laxa (hyperelastica)
Dermatoglyphic anomalies
Inherited keratosis palmaris et plantaris
Keratosis follicularis [Darier-White]
EXCLUDES 1 *Ehlers-Danlos syndrome (Q79.6)*

Q82.9 Congenital malformation of skin, unspecified

✓4th **Q83 Congenital malformations of breast**
EXCLUDES 2 *absence of pectoral muscle (Q79.8)*
hypoplasia of breast (N64.82)
micromastia (N64.82)

Q83.0 Congenital absence of breast with absent nipple
Q83.1 Accessory breast
Supernumerary breast
Q83.2 Absent nipple
Q83.3 Accessory nipple
Supernumerary nipple
Q83.8 Other congenital malformations of breast
Q83.9 Congenital malformation of breast, unspecified

✓4th **Q84 Other congenital malformations of integument**
Q84.0 Congenital alopecia
Congenital atrichosis
Q84.1 Congenital morphological disturbances of hair, not elsewhere classified
Beaded hair
Monilethrix
Pili annulati
EXCLUDES 1 *Menkes' kinky hair syndrome (E83.0)*
Q84.2 Other congenital malformations of hair
Congenital hypertrichosis
Congenital malformation of hair NOS
Persistent lanugo
Q84.3 Anonychia
EXCLUDES 1 *nail patella syndrome (Q87.2)*
Q84.4 Congenital leukonychia
Q84.5 Enlarged and hypertrophic nails
Congenital onychauxis
Pachyonychia
Q84.6 Other congenital malformations of nails
Congenital clubnail
Congenital koilonychia
Congenital malformation of nail NOS
Q84.8 Other specified congenital malformations of integument
Aplasia cutis congenita
Q84.9 Congenital malformation of integument, unspecified
Congenital anomaly of integument NOS
Congenital deformity of integument NOS

✓4th **Q85 Phakomatoses, not elsewhere classified**
EXCLUDES 1 *ataxia telangiectasia [Louis-Bar] (G11.3)*
familial dysautonomia [Riley-Day] (G90.1)

✓5th **Q85.0 Neurofibromatosis (nonmalignant)**
Q85.00 Neurofibromatosis, unspecified
Q85.01 Neurofibromatosis, type 1
Von Recklinghausen disease
Q85.02 Neurofibromatosis, type 2
Acoustic neurofibromatosis
Q85.03 Schwannomatosis
Q85.09 Other neurofibromatosis

Q85.1 Tuberous sclerosis
Bourneville's disease
Epiloia
Q85.8 Other phakomatoses, not elsewhere classified
Peutz-Jeghers Syndrome
Sturge-Weber(-Dimitri) syndrome
von Hippel-Lindau syndrome
EXCLUDES 1 *Meckel-Gruber syndrome (Q61.9)*
Q85.9 Phakomatosis, unspecified
Hamartosis NOS

✓4th **Q86 Congenital malformation syndromes due to known exogenous causes, not elsewhere classified**
EXCLUDES 2 *iodine-deficiency-related hypothyroidism (E00-E02)*
nonteratogenic effects of substances transmitted via placenta or breast milk (P04.-)

Q86.0 Fetal alcohol syndrome (dysmorphic)
Q86.1 Fetal hydantoin syndrome
Meadow's syndrome
Q86.2 Dysmorphism due to warfarin
Q86.8 Other congenital malformation syndromes due to known exogenous causes

✓4th **Q87 Other specified congenital malformation syndromes affecting multiple systems**
Use additional code(s) to identify all associated manifestations

Q87.0 Congenital malformation syndromes predominantly affecting facial appearance
Acrocephalopolysyndactyly
Acrocephalosyndactyly [Apert]
Cryptophthalmos syndrome
Cyclopia
Goldenhar syndrome
Moebius syndrome
Oro-facial-digital syndrome
Robin syndrome
Whistling face
Q87.1 Congenital malformation syndromes predominantly associated with short stature
Aarskog syndrome
Cockayne syndrome
De Lange syndrome
Dubowitz syndrome
Noonan syndrome
Prader-Willi syndrome
Robinow-Silverman-Smith syndrome
Russell-Silver syndrome
Seckel syndrome
EXCLUDES 1 *Ellis-van Creveld syndrome (Q77.6)*
Smith-Lemli-Opitz syndrome (E78.72)
Q87.2 Congenital malformation syndromes predominantly involving limbs
Holt-Oram syndrome
Klippel-Trenaunay-Weber syndrome
Nail patella syndrome
Rubinstein-Taybi syndrome
Sirenomelia syndrome
Thrombocytopenia with absent radius [TAR] syndrome
VATER syndrome
Q87.3 Congenital malformation syndromes involving early overgrowth
Beckwith-Wiedemann syndrome
Sotos syndrome
Weaver syndrome

✓5th **Q87.4 Marfan's syndrome**
Q87.40 Marfan's syndrome, unspecified
✓6th **Q87.41 Marfan's syndrome with cardiovascular manifestations**
Q87.410 Marfan's syndrome with aortic dilation
Q87.418 Marfan's syndrome with other cardiovascular manifestations
Q87.42 Marfan's syndrome with ocular manifestations
Q87.43 Marfan's syndrome with skeletal manifestation

Q87.5 Other congenital malformation syndromes with other skeletal changes

✓5th **Q87.8 Other specified congenital malformation syndromes, not elsewhere classified**
EXCLUDES 1 *Zellweger syndrome (E71.510)*
Q87.81 Alport syndrome
Use additional code to identify stage of chronic kidney disease (N18.1-N18.6)

Q87.89 Other specified congenital malformation syndromes, not elsewhere classified
Laurence-Moon (-Bardet)-Biedl syndrome

Q89 Other congenital malformations, not elsewhere classified

Q89.0 Congenital absence and malformations of spleen
EXCLUDES 1 *isomerism of atrial appendages (with asplenia or polysplenia) (Q20.6)*

Q89.01 Asplenia (congenital)

Q89.09 Congenital malformations of spleen
Congenital splenomegaly

Q89.1 Congenital malformations of adrenal gland
EXCLUDES 1 *adrenogenital disorders (E25.-)*
congenital adrenal hyperplasia (E25.0)

Q89.2 Congenital malformations of other endocrine glands
Congenital malformation of parathyroid or thyroid gland
Persistent thyroglossal duct
Thyroglossal cyst
EXCLUDES 1 *congenital goiter (E03.0)*
congenital hypothyroidism (E03.1)

Q89.3 Situs inversus
Dextrocardia with situs inversus
Mirror-image atrial arrangement with situs inversus
Situs inversus or transversus abdominalis
Situs inversus or transversus thoracis
Transposition of abdominal viscera
Transposition of thoracic viscera
EXCLUDES 1 *dextrocardia NOS (Q24.0)*

Q89.4 Conjoined twins
Craniopagus
Dicephaly
Pygopagus
Thoracopagus

Q89.7 Multiple congenital malformations, not elsewhere classified
Multiple congenital anomalies NOS
Multiple congenital deformities NOS
EXCLUDES 1 *congenital malformation syndromes affecting multiple systems (Q87.-)*

Q89.8 Other specified congenital malformations
Use additional code(s) to identify all associated manifestations

Q89.9 Congenital malformation, unspecified
Congenital anomaly NOS
Congenital deformity NOS

Chromosomal abnormalities, not elsewhere classified (Q90-Q99)

EXCLUDES 2 *mitochondrial metabolic disorders (E88.4-)*

Q90 Down syndrome
Use additional code(s) to identify any associated physical conditions and degree of intellectual disabilities (F70-F79)

Q90.0 Trisomy 21, nonmosaicism (meiotic nondisjunction)
Q90.1 Trisomy 21, mosaicism (mitotic nondisjunction)
Q90.2 Trisomy 21, translocation
Q90.9 Down syndrome, unspecified
Trisomy 21 NOS

Q91 Trisomy 18 and Trisomy 13

Q91.0 Trisomy 18, nonmosaicism (meiotic nondisjunction)
Q91.1 Trisomy 18, mosaicism (mitotic nondisjunction)
Q91.2 Trisomy 18, translocation
Q91.3 Trisomy 18, unspecified
Q91.4 Trisomy 13, nonmosaicism (meiotic nondisjunction)
Q91.5 Trisomy 13, mosaicism (mitotic nondisjunction)
Q91.6 Trisomy 13, translocation
Q91.7 Trisomy 13, unspecified

Q92 Other trisomies and partial trisomies of the autosomes, not elsewhere classified
INCLUDES unbalanced translocations and insertions
EXCLUDES 1 *trisomies of chromosomes 13, 18, 21 (Q90-Q91)*

Q92.0 Whole chromosome trisomy, nonmosaicism (meiotic nondisjunction)
Q92.1 Whole chromosome trisomy, mosaicism (mitotic nondisjunction)
Q92.2 Partial trisomy
Less than whole arm duplicated
Whole arm or more duplicated
EXCLUDES 1 *partial trisomy due to unbalanced translocation (Q92.5)*

Q92.5 Duplications with other complex rearrangements
Partial trisomy due to unbalanced translocations
Code also any associated deletions due to unbalanced translocations, inversions and insertions (Q93.7)

Q92.6 Marker chromosomes
Trisomies due to dicentrics
Trisomies due to extra rings
Trisomies due to isochromosomes
Individual with marker heterochromatin

Q92.61 Marker chromosomes in normal individual
Q92.62 Marker chromosomes in abnormal individual

Q92.7 Triploidy and polyploidy
Q92.8 Other specified trisomies and partial trisomies of autosomes
Duplications identified by fluorescence in situ hybridization (FISH)
Duplications identified by in situ hybridization (ISH)
Duplications seen only at prometaphase
Q92.9 Trisomy and partial trisomy of autosomes, unspecified

Q93 Monosomies and deletions from the autosomes, not elsewhere classified

Q93.0 Whole chromosome monosomy, nonmosaicism (meiotic nondisjunction)
Q93.1 Whole chromosome monosomy, mosaicism (mitotic nondisjunction)
Q93.2 Chromosome replaced with ring, dicentric or isochromosome
Q93.3 Deletion of short arm of chromosome 4
Wolff-Hirschorn syndrome
Q93.4 Deletion of short arm of chromosome 5
Cri-du-chat syndrome
Q93.5 Other deletions of part of a chromosome
Angelman syndrome
Q93.7 Deletions with other complex rearrangements
Deletions due to unbalanced translocations, inversions and insertions
Code also any associated duplications due to unbalanced translocations, inversions and insertions (Q92.5)
Q93.8 Other deletions from the autosomes

Q93.81 Velo-cardio-facial syndrome
Deletion 22q11.2
Q93.88 Other microdeletions
Miller-Dieker syndrome
Smith-Magenis syndrome
Q93.89 Other deletions from the autosomes
Deletions identified by fluorescence in situ hybridization (FISH)
Deletions identified by in situ hybridization (ISH)
Deletions seen only at prometaphase

Q93.9 Deletion from autosomes, unspecified

Q95 Balanced rearrangements and structural markers, not elsewhere classified
INCLUDES Robertsonian and balanced reciprocal translocations and insertions

Q95.0 Balanced translocation and insertion in normal individual
Q95.1 Chromosome inversion in normal individual
Q95.2 Balanced autosomal rearrangement in abnormal individual
Q95.3 Balanced sex/autosomal rearrangement in abnormal individual
Q95.5 Individual with autosomal fragile site
Q95.8 Other balanced rearrangements and structural markers
Q95.9 Balanced rearrangement and structural marker, unspecified

Q96 Turner's syndrome
EXCLUDES 1 *Noonan syndrome (Q87.1)*

Q96.0 Karyotype 45, X
Q96.1 Karyotype 46, X iso (Xq)
Karyotype 46, isochromosome Xq
Q96.2 Karyotype 46, X with abnormal sex chromosome, except iso (Xq)
Karyotype 46, X with abnormal sex chromosome, except isochromosome Xq
Q96.3 Mosaicism, 45, X/46, XX or XY
Q96.4 Mosaicism, 45, X/other cell line(s) with abnormal sex chromosome
Q96.8 Other variants of Turner's syndrome
Q96.9 Turner's syndrome, unspecified

4th Q97 Other sex chromosome abnormalities, female phenotype, not elsewhere classified

EXCLUDES 1 *Turner's syndrome (Q96.-)*

Q97.0 Karyotype 47, XXX

Q97.1 Female with more than three X chromosomes

Q97.2 Mosaicism, lines with various numbers of X chromosomes

Q97.3 Female with 46, XY karyotype

Q97.8 Other specified sex chromosome abnormalities, female phenotype

Q97.9 Sex chromosome abnormality, female phenotype, unspecified

4th Q98 Other sex chromosome abnormalities, male phenotype, not elsewhere classified

Q98.0 Klinefelter syndrome karyotype 47, XXY

Q98.1 Klinefelter syndrome, male with more than two X chromosomes

Q98.3 Other male with 46, XX karyotype

Q98.4 Klinefelter syndrome, unspecified

Q98.5 Karyotype 47, XYY

Q98.6 Male with structurally abnormal sex chromosome

Q98.7 Male with sex chromosome mosaicism

Q98.8 Other specified sex chromosome abnormalities, male phenotype

Q98.9 Sex chromosome abnormality, male phenotype, unspecified

4th Q99 Other chromosome abnormalities, not elsewhere classified

Q99.0 Chimera 46, XX/46, XY

Chimera 46, XX/46, XY true hermaphrodite

Q99.1 46, XX true hermaphrodite

46, XX with streak gonads

46, XY with streak gonads

Pure gonadal dysgenesis

Q99.2 Fragile X chromosome

Fragile X syndrome

Q99.8 Other specified chromosome abnormalities

Q99.9 Chromosomal abnormality, unspecified

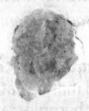

Chapter 18. Symptoms, Signs and Abnormal Clinical and Laboratory Findings, Not Elsewhere Classified (RØØ-R99)

This chapter includes symptoms, signs, abnormal results of clinical or other investigative procedures, and ill-defined conditions regarding which no diagnosis classifiable elsewhere is recorded.

Signs and symptoms that point rather definitely to a given diagnosis have been assigned to a category in other chapters of the classification. In general, categories in this chapter include the less well-defined conditions and symptoms that, without the necessary study of the case to establish a final diagnosis, point perhaps equally to two or more diseases or to two or more systems of the body. Practically all categories in the chapter could be designated "not otherwise specified", "unknown etiology" or "transient". The Alphabetical Index should be consulted to determine which symptoms and signs are to be allocated here and which to other chapters. The residual subcategories, numbered .8, are generally provided for other relevant symptoms that cannot be allocated elsewhere in the classification.

The conditions and signs or symptoms included in categories RØØ-R94 consist of:

(a) cases for which no more specific diagnosis can be made even after all the facts bearing on the case have been investigated:
(b) signs or symptoms existing at the time of initial encounter that proved to be transient and whose causes could not be determined;
(c) provisional diagnosis in a patient who failed to return for further investigation or care;
(d) cases referred elsewhere for investigation or treatment before the diagnosis was made;
(e) cases in which a more precise diagnosis was not available for any other reason;
(f) certain symptoms, for which supplementary information is provided, that represent important problems in medical care in their own right.

EXCLUDES 2 *abnormal findings on antenatal screening of mother (O28.-)*
certain conditions originating in the perinatal period (PØ4-P96)
signs and symptoms classified in the body system chapters
signs and symptoms of breast (N63, N64.5)

This chapter contains the following blocks:

RØØ-RØ9	Symptoms and signs involving the circulatory and respiratory systems
R1Ø-R19	Symptoms and signs involving the digestive system and abdomen
R2Ø-R23	Symptoms and signs involving the skin and subcutaneous tissue
R25-R29	Symptoms and signs involving the nervous and musculoskeletal systems
R3Ø-R39	Symptoms and signs involving the genitourinary system
R4Ø-R46	Symptoms and signs involving cognition, perception, emotional state and behavior
R47-R49	Symptoms and signs involving speech and voice
R5Ø-R69	General symptoms and signs
R7Ø-R79	Abnormal findings on examination of blood, without diagnosis
R8Ø-R82	Abnormal findings on examination of urine, without diagnosis
R83-R89	Abnormal findings on examination of other body fluids, substances and tissues, without diagnosis
R9Ø-R94	Abnormal findings on diagnostic imaging and in function studies, without diagnosis
R97	Abnormal tumor markers
R99	Ill-defined and unknown cause of mortality

Symptoms and signs involving the circulatory and respiratory systems (RØØ-RØ9)

✓4th **RØØ Abnormalities of heart beat**
EXCLUDES 1 *abnormalities originating in the perinatal period (P29.1-)*
specified arrhythmias (I47-I49)

RØØ.Ø Tachycardia, unspecified
Rapid heart beat
Sinoauricular tachycardia NOS
Sinus [sinusal] tachycardia NOS
EXCLUDES 1 *neonatal tachycardia (P29.11)*
paroxysmal tachycardia (I47.-)

RØØ.1 Bradycardia, unspecified
Sinoatrial bradycardia
Sinus bradycardia
Slow heart beat
Vagal bradycardia
Use additional code for adverse effect, if applicable, to identify drug (T36-T5Ø with fifth or sixth character 5)
EXCLUDES 1 *neonatal bradycardia (P29.12)*

RØØ.2 Palpitations
Awareness of heart beat

RØØ.8 Other abnormalities of heart beat

RØØ.9 Unspecified abnormalities of heart beat

✓4th **RØ1 Cardiac murmurs and other cardiac sounds**
EXCLUDES 1 *cardiac murmurs and sounds originating in the perinatal period (P29.8)*

RØ1.Ø Benign and innocent cardiac murmurs
Functional cardiac murmur

RØ1.1 Cardiac murmur, unspecified
Cardiac bruit NOS
Heart murmur NOS

RØ1.2 Other cardiac sounds
Cardiac dullness, increased or decreased
Precordial friction

✓4th **RØ3 Abnormal blood-pressure reading, without diagnosis**

RØ3.Ø Elevated blood-pressure reading, without diagnosis of hypertension
NOTE This category is to be used to record an episode of elevated blood pressure in a patient in whom no formal diagnosis of hypertension has been made, or as an isolated incidental finding.

RØ3.1 Nonspecific low blood-pressure reading
EXCLUDES 1 *hypotension (I95.-)*
maternal hypotension syndrome (O26.5-)
neurogenic orthostatic hypotension (G9Ø.3)

✓4th **RØ4 Hemorrhage from respiratory passages**

RØ4.Ø Epistaxis
Hemorrhage from nose
Nosebleed

RØ4.1 Hemorrhage from throat
EXCLUDES 2 *hemoptysis (RØ4.2)*

RØ4.2 Hemoptysis
Blood-stained sputum
Cough with hemorrhage

✓5th **RØ4.8 Hemorrhage from other sites in respiratory passages**

RØ4.81 Acute idiopathic pulmonary hemorrhage in infants
AIPHI
Acute idiopathic hemorrhage in infants over 28 days old
EXCLUDES 1 *perinatal pulmonary hemorrhage (P26.-)*
von Willebrand's disease (D68.Ø)

RØ4.89 Hemorrhage from other sites in respiratory passages
Pulmonary hemorrhage NOS

RØ4.9 Hemorrhage from respiratory passages, unspecified

RØ5 Cough
EXCLUDES 1 *cough with hemorrhage (RØ4.2)*
smoker's cough (J41.Ø)

✓4th **RØ6 Abnormalities of breathing**
EXCLUDES 1 *acute respiratory distress syndrome (J8Ø)*
respiratory arrest (RØ9.2)
respiratory arrest of newborn (P28.81)
respiratory distress syndrome of newborn (P22.-)
respiratory failure (J96.-)
respiratory failure of newborn (P28.5)

✓5th **RØ6.Ø Dyspnea**
EXCLUDES 1 *tachypnea NOS (RØ6.82)*
transient tachypnea of newborn (P22.1)

RØ6.ØØ Dyspnea, unspecified

RØ6.Ø1 Orthopnea

RØ6.Ø2 Shortness of breath

RØ6.Ø9 Other forms of dyspnea

RØ6.1 Stridor
EXCLUDES 1 *congenital laryngeal stridor (P28.89)*
laryngismus (stridulus) (J38.5)

RØ6.2 Wheezing
EXCLUDES 1 *asthma (J45.-)*

RØ6.3 Periodic breathing
Cheyne-Stokes breathing

RØ6.4 Hyperventilation
EXCLUDES 1 *psychogenic hyperventilation (F45.8)*

RØ6.5 Mouth breathing
EXCLUDES 2 *dry mouth NOS (R68.2)*

RØ6.6 Hiccough
EXCLUDES 1 *psychogenic hiccough (F45.8)*

RØ6.7 Sneezing

✓5th **RØ6.8 Other abnormalities of breathing**

RØ6.81 Apnea, not elsewhere classified
Apnea NOS
EXCLUDES 1 *apnea (of) newborn (P28.4)*
sleep apnea (G47.3-)
sleep apnea of newborn (primary) (P28.3)

RØ6.82 Tachypnea, not elsewhere classified
Tachypnea NOS
EXCLUDES 1 *transitory tachypnea of newborn (P22.1)*

RØ6.83 Snoring

RØ6.89 Other abnormalities of breathing
Breath-holding (spells)
Sighing

RØ6.9 Unspecified abnormalities of breathing

✓4th **RØ7 Pain in throat and chest**
EXCLUDES 1 *epidemic myalgia (B33.Ø)*
EXCLUDES 2 *jaw pain (R68.84)*
pain in breast (N64.4)

RØ7.Ø Pain in throat
EXCLUDES 1 *chronic sore throat (J31.2)*
sore throat (acute) NOS (JØ2.9)
EXCLUDES 2 *dysphagia (R13.1-)*
pain in neck (M54.2)

RØ7.1 Chest pain on breathing
Painful respiration

RØ7.2 Precordial pain

✓5th **RØ7.8 Other chest pain**

RØ7.81 Pleurodynia
Pleurodynia NOS
EXCLUDES 1 *epidemic pleurodynia (B33.Ø)*

RØ7.82 Intercostal pain

RØ7.89 Other chest pain
Anterior chest-wall pain NOS

RØ7.9 Chest pain, unspecified

✓4th **RØ9 Other symptoms and signs involving the circulatory and respiratory system**
EXCLUDES 1 *acute respiratory distress syndrome (J8Ø)*
respiratory arrest of newborn (P28.81)
respiratory distress syndrome of newborn (P22.Ø)
respiratory failure (J96.-)
respiratory failure of newborn (P28.5)

✓5th **RØ9.Ø Asphyxia and hypoxemia**
EXCLUDES 1 *asphyxia due to carbon monoxide (T58.-)*
asphyxia due to foreign body in respiratory tract (T17.-)
birth (intrauterine) asphyxia (P84)
hypercapnia (RØ6.4)
hyperventilation (RØ6.4)
traumatic asphyxia (T71.-)

RØ9.Ø1 Asphyxia

RØ9.Ø2 Hypoxemia

RØ9.1 Pleurisy
EXCLUDES 1 *pleurisy with effusion (J9Ø)*

RØ9.2 Respiratory arrest
Cardiorespiratory failure
EXCLUDES 1 *cardiac arrest (I46.-)*
respiratory arrest of newborn (P28.81)
respiratory distress of newborn (P22.Ø)
respiratory failure (J96.-)
respiratory failure of newborn (P28.5)
respiratory insufficiency (RØ6.89)
respiratory insufficiency of newborn (P28.5)

RØ9.3 Abnormal sputum
Abnormal amount of sputum
Abnormal color of sputum
Abnormal odor of sputum
Excessive sputum
EXCLUDES 1 *blood-stained sputum (RØ4.2)*

✓5th **RØ9.8 Other specified symptoms and signs involving the circulatory and respiratory systems**

RØ9.81 Nasal congestion

RØ9.82 Postnasal drip

RØ9.89 Other specified symptoms and signs involving the circulatory and respiratory systems
Abnormal chest percussion
Bruit (arterial)
Chest tympany
Choking sensation
Feeling of foreign body in throat
Friction sounds in chest
Rales
Weak pulse
EXCLUDES 2 *foreign body in throat (T17.2-)*
wheezing (RØ6.2)

Symptoms and signs involving the digestive system and abdomen (R1Ø-R19)

EXCLUDES 1 *congenital or infantile pylorospasm (Q4Ø.Ø)*
gastrointestinal hemorrhage (K92.Ø-K92.2)
intestinal obstruction (K56.-)
newborn gastrointestinal hemorrhage (P54.Ø-P54.3)
newborn intestinal obstruction (P76.-)
pylorospasm (K31.3)
signs and symptoms involving the urinary system (R3Ø-R39)
symptoms referable to female genital organs (N94.-)
symptoms referable to male genital organs male (N48-N5Ø)

✓4th **R1Ø Abdominal and pelvic pain**
EXCLUDES 1 *renal colic (N23)*
EXCLUDES 2 *dorsalgia (M54.-)*
flatulence and related conditions (R14.-)

R1Ø.Ø Acute abdomen
Severe abdominal pain (generalized) (with abdominal rigidity)
EXCLUDES 1 *abdominal rigidity NOS (R19.3)*
generalized abdominal pain NOS (R1Ø.84)
localized abdominal pain (R1Ø.1-R1Ø.3-)

✓5th **R1Ø.1 Pain localized to upper abdomen**

R1Ø.1Ø Upper abdominal pain, unspecified

R1Ø.11 Right upper quadrant pain

R1Ø.12 Left upper quadrant pain

R1Ø.13 Epigastric pain
Dyspepsia
EXCLUDES 1 *functional dyspepsia (K3Ø)*

R1Ø.2 Pelvic and perineal pain
EXCLUDES 1 *vulvodynia (N94.81)*

✓5th **R1Ø.3 Pain localized to other parts of lower abdomen**

R1Ø.3Ø Lower abdominal pain, unspecified

R1Ø.31 Right lower quadrant pain

R1Ø.32 Left lower quadrant pain

R1Ø.33 Periumbilical pain

✓5th **R1Ø.8 Other abdominal pain**

✓6th **R1Ø.81 Abdominal tenderness**
Abdominal tenderness NOS

R1Ø.811 Right upper quadrant abdominal tenderness

R1Ø.812 Left upper quadrant abdominal tenderness

R1Ø.813 Right lower quadrant abdominal tenderness

R1Ø.814 Left lower quadrant abdominal tenderness

R1Ø.815 Periumbilic abdominal tenderness

R1Ø.816 Epigastric abdominal tenderness

R1Ø.817 Generalized abdominal tenderness

R1Ø.819 Abdominal tenderness, unspecified site

✓6th **R1Ø.82 Rebound abdominal tenderness**

R1Ø.821 Right upper quadrant rebound abdominal tenderness

R1Ø.822 Left upper quadrant rebound abdominal tenderness

R1Ø.823 Right lower quadrant rebound abdominal tenderness

R1Ø.824 Left lower quadrant rebound abdominal tenderness

R1Ø.825 Periumbilic rebound abdominal tenderness

R1Ø.826 Epigastric rebound abdominal tenderness

R1Ø.827 Generalized rebound abdominal tenderness

R10.829 Rebound abdominal tenderness, unspecified site

R10.83 Colic
Colic NOS
Infantile colic
EXCLUDES 1 *colic in adult and child over 12 months old (R10.84)*

R10.84 Generalized abdominal pain
EXCLUDES 1 *generalized abdominal pain associated with acute abdomen (R10.0)*

R10.9 Unspecified abdominal pain

✓4th **R11 Nausea and vomiting**
EXCLUDES 1 *cyclical vomiting associated with migraine (G43.A-)*
excessive vomiting in pregnancy (O21.-)
hematemesis (K92.0)
neonatal hematemesis (P54.0)
newborn vomiting (P92.0-)
psychogenic vomiting (F50.8)
vomiting associated with bulimia nervosa (F50.2)
vomiting following gastrointestinal surgery (K91.0)

R11.0 Nausea
Nausea NOS
Nausea without vomiting

✓5th **R11.1 Vomiting**

R11.10 Vomiting, unspecified
Vomiting NOS

R11.11 Vomiting without nausea

R11.12 Projectile vomiting

R11.13 Vomiting of fecal matter

R11.14 Bilious vomiting
Bilious emesis

R11.2 Nausea with vomiting, unspecified
Persistent nausea with vomiting NOS

R12 Heartburn
EXCLUDES 1 *dyspepsia NOS (R10.13)*
functional dyspepsia (K30)

✓4th **R13 Aphagia and dysphagia**

R13.0 Aphagia
Inability to swallow
EXCLUDES 1 *psychogenic aphagia (F50.9)*

✓5th **R13.1 Dysphagia**
Code first, if applicable, dysphagia following cerebrovascular disease (I69. with final characters -91)
EXCLUDES 1 *psychogenic dysphagia (F45.8)*

R13.10 Dysphagia, unspecified
Difficulty in swallowing NOS

R13.11 Dysphagia, oral phase

R13.12 Dysphagia, oropharyngeal phase

R13.13 Dysphagia, pharyngeal phase

R13.14 Dysphagia, pharyngoesophageal phase

R13.19 Other dysphagia
Cervical dysphagia
Neurogenic dysphagia

✓4th **R14 Flatulence and related conditions**
EXCLUDES 1 *psychogenic aerophagy (F45.8)*

R14.0 Abdominal distension (gaseous)
Bloating
Tympanites (abdominal) (intestinal)

R14.1 Gas pain

R14.2 Eructation

R14.3 Flatulence

✓4th **R15 Fecal incontinence**
Encopresis NOS
EXCLUDES 1 *fecal incontinence of nonorganic origin (F98.1)*

R15.0 Incomplete defecation
EXCLUDES 1 *constipation (K59.0-)*
fecal impaction (K56.41)

R15.1 Fecal smearing
Fecal soiling

R15.2 Fecal urgency

R15.9 Full incontinence of feces
Fecal incontinence NOS

✓4th **R16 Hepatomegaly and splenomegaly, not elsewhere classified**

R16.0 Hepatomegaly, not elsewhere classified
Hepatomegaly NOS

R16.1 Splenomegaly, not elsewhere classified
Splenomegaly NOS

R16.2 Hepatomegaly with splenomegaly, not elsewhere classified
Hepatosplenomegaly NOS

R17 Unspecified jaundice
EXCLUDES 1 *neonatal jaundice (P55, P57-P59)*

✓4th **R18 Ascites**
INCLUDES fluid in peritoneal cavity
EXCLUDES 1 *ascites in alcoholic cirrhosis (K70.31)*
ascites in alcoholic hepatitis (K70.11)
ascites in toxic liver disease with chronic active hepatitis (K71.51)

R18.0 Malignant ascites
Code first malignancy, such as:
malignant neoplasm of ovary (C56.-)
secondary malignant neoplasm of retroperitoneum and peritoneum (C78.6)

R18.8 Other ascites
Ascites NOS
Peritoneal effusion (chronic)

✓4th **R19 Other symptoms and signs involving the digestive system and abdomen**
EXCLUDES 1 *acute abdomen (R10.0)*

✓5th **R19.0 Intra-abdominal and pelvic swelling, mass and lump**
EXCLUDES 1 *abdominal distension (gaseous) (R14.-)*
ascites (R18.-)

R19.00 Intra-abdominal and pelvic swelling, mass and lump, unspecified site

R19.01 Right upper quadrant abdominal swelling, mass and lump

R19.02 Left upper quadrant abdominal swelling, mass and lump

R19.03 Right lower quadrant abdominal swelling, mass and lump

R19.04 Left lower quadrant abdominal swelling, mass and lump

R19.05 Periumbilic swelling, mass or lump
Diffuse or generalized umbilical swelling or mass

R19.06 Epigastric swelling, mass or lump

R19.07 Generalized intra-abdominal and pelvic swelling, mass and lump
Diffuse or generalized intra-abdominal swelling or mass NOS
Diffuse or generalized pelvic swelling or mass NOS

R19.09 Other intra-abdominal and pelvic swelling, mass and lump

✓5th **R19.1 Abnormal bowel sounds**

R19.11 Absent bowel sounds

R19.12 Hyperactive bowel sounds

R19.15 Other abnormal bowel sounds
Abnormal bowel sounds NOS

R19.2 Visible peristalsis
Hyperperistalsis

✓5th **R19.3 Abdominal rigidity**
EXCLUDES 1 *abdominal rigidity with severe abdominal pain (R10.0)*

R19.30 Abdominal rigidity, unspecified site

R19.31 Right upper quadrant abdominal rigidity

R19.32 Left upper quadrant abdominal rigidity

R19.33 Right lower quadrant abdominal rigidity

R19.34 Left lower quadrant abdominal rigidity

R19.35 Periumbilic abdominal rigidity

R19.36 Epigastric abdominal rigidity

R19.37 Generalized abdominal rigidity

R19.4 Change in bowel habit
EXCLUDES 1 *constipation (K59.0-)*
functional diarrhea (K59.1)

R19.5 Other fecal abnormalities
Abnormal stool color
Bulky stools
Mucus in stools
Occult blood in feces
Occult blood in stools
EXCLUDES 1 *melena (K92.1)*
neonatal melena (P54.1)

R19.6 Halitosis

R19.7 Diarrhea, unspecified
Diarrhea NOS
EXCLUDES 1 *functional diarrhea (K59.1)*
neonatal diarrhea (P78.3)
psychogenic diarrhea (F45.8)

R19.8 Other specified symptoms and signs involving the digestive system and abdomen

Symptoms and signs involving the skin and subcutaneous tissue (R20-R23)

EXCLUDES 2 *symptoms relating to breast (N64.4-N64.5)*

✓4th R20 Disturbances of skin sensation
EXCLUDES 1 *dissociative anesthesia and sensory loss (F44.6)*
psychogenic disturbances (F45.8)

R20.0 Anesthesia of skin
R20.1 Hypoesthesia of skin
R20.2 Paresthesia of skin
Formication
Pins and needles
Tingling skin
EXCLUDES 1 *acroparesthesia (I73.8)*

R20.3 Hyperesthesia
R20.8 Other disturbances of skin sensation
R20.9 Unspecified disturbances of skin sensation

R21 Rash and other nonspecific skin eruption
Rash NOS
EXCLUDES 1 *specified type of rash—code to condition*
vesicular eruption (R23.8)

✓4th R22 Localized swelling, mass and lump of skin and subcutaneous tissue
Subcutaneous nodules (localized)(superficial)
EXCLUDES 1 *abnormal findings on diagnostic imaging (R90-R93)*
edema (R60.-)
enlarged lymph nodes (R59.-)
localized adiposity (E65)
swelling of joint (M25.4-)

R22.0 Localized swelling, mass and lump, head
R22.1 Localized swelling, mass and lump, neck
R22.2 Localized swelling, mass and lump, trunk
EXCLUDES 1 *intra-abdominal or pelvic mass and lump (R19.0-)*
intra-abdominal or pelvic swelling (R19.0-)
EXCLUDES 2 *breast mass and lump (N63)*

✓5th R22.3 Localized swelling, mass and lump, upper limb
R22.30 Localized swelling, mass and lump, unspecified upper limb
R22.31 Localized swelling, mass and lump, right upper limb
R22.32 Localized swelling, mass and lump, left upper limb
R22.33 Localized swelling, mass and lump, upper limb, bilateral

✓5th R22.4 Localized swelling, mass and lump, lower limb
R22.40 Localized swelling, mass and lump, unspecified lower limb
R22.41 Localized swelling, mass and lump, right lower limb
R22.42 Localized swelling, mass and lump, left lower limb
R22.43 Localized swelling, mass and lump, lower limb, bilateral

R22.9 Localized swelling, mass and lump, unspecified

✓4th R23 Other skin changes
R23.0 Cyanosis
EXCLUDES 1 *acrocyanosis (I73.8)*
cyanotic attacks of newborn (P28.2)

R23.1 Pallor
Clammy skin

R23.2 Flushing
Excessive blushing
Code first, if applicable, menopausal and female climacteric states (N95.1)

R23.3 Spontaneous ecchymoses
Petechiae
EXCLUDES 1 *ecchymoses of newborn (P54.5)*
purpura (D69.-)

R23.4 Changes in skin texture
Desquamation of skin
Induration of skin
Scaling of skin
EXCLUDES 1 *epidermal thickening NOS (L85.9)*

R23.8 Other skin changes
R23.9 Unspecified skin changes

Symptoms and signs involving the nervous and musculoskeletal systems (R25-R29)

✓4th R25 Abnormal involuntary movements
EXCLUDES 1 *specific movement disorders (G20-G26)*
stereotyped movement disorders (F98.4)
tic disorders (F95.-)

R25.0 Abnormal head movements
R25.1 Tremor, unspecified
EXCLUDES 1 *chorea NOS (G25.5)*
essential tremor (G25.0)
hysterical tremor (F44.4)
intention tremor (G25.2)

R25.2 Cramp and spasm
EXCLUDES 2 *carpopedal spasm (R29.0)*
charley-horse (M62.831)
infantile spasms (G40.4-)
muscle spasm of back (M62.830)
muscle spasm of calf (M62.831)

R25.3 Fasciculation
Twitching NOS

R25.8 Other abnormal involuntary movements
R25.9 Unspecified abnormal involuntary movements

✓4th R26 Abnormalities of gait and mobility
EXCLUDES 1 *ataxia NOS (R27.0)*
hereditary ataxia (G11.-)
locomotor (syphilitic) ataxia (A52.11)
immobility syndrome (paraplegic) (M62.3)

R26.0 Ataxic gait
Staggering gait

R26.1 Paralytic gait
Spastic gait

R26.2 Difficulty in walking, not elsewhere classified
EXCLUDES 1 *falling (R29.6)*
unsteadiness on feet (R26.81)

✓5th R26.8 Other abnormalities of gait and mobility
R26.81 Unsteadiness on feet
R26.89 Other abnormalities of gait and mobility

R26.9 Unspecified abnormalities of gait and mobility

✓4th R27 Other lack of coordination
EXCLUDES 1 *ataxic gait (R26.0)*
hereditary ataxia (G11.-)
vertigo NOS (R42)

R27.0 Ataxia, unspecified
EXCLUDES 1 *ataxia following cerebrovascular disease (I69. with final characters -93)*

R27.8 Other lack of coordination
R27.9 Unspecified lack of coordination

✓4th R29 Other symptoms and signs involving the nervous and musculoskeletal systems
R29.0 Tetany
Carpopedal spasm
EXCLUDES 1 *hysterical tetany (F44.5)*
neonatal tetany (P71.3)
parathyroid tetany (E20.9)
post-thyroidectomy tetany (E89.2)

R29.1 Meningismus
R29.2 Abnormal reflex
EXCLUDES 2 *abnormal pupillary reflex (H57.0)*
hyperactive gag reflex (J39.2)
vasovagal reaction or syncope (R55)

R29.3 Abnormal posture
R29.4 Clicking hip
EXCLUDES 1 *congenital deformities of hip (Q65.-)*

R29.5 Transient paralysis
Code first any associated spinal cord injury (S14.0, S14.1-, S24.0, S24.1-, S34.0-, S34.1-)
EXCLUDES 1 *transient ischemic attack (G45.9)*

R29.6 Repeated falls
Falling
Tendency to fall
EXCLUDES 2 *at risk for falling (Z91.81)*
history of falling (Z91.81)

✓5th **R29.8 Other symptoms and signs involving the nervous and musculoskeletal systems**

✓6th **R29.81 Other symptoms and signs involving the nervous system**

R29.810 Facial weakness
Facial droop
EXCLUDES 1 *Bell's palsy (G51.0)*
facial weakness following cerebrovascular disease (I69. with final characters -92)

R29.818 Other symptoms and signs involving the nervous system

✓6th **R29.89 Other symptoms and signs involving the musculoskeletal system**
EXCLUDES 2 *pain in limb (M79.6-)*

R29.890 Loss of height
EXCLUDES 1 *osteoporosis (M80-M81)*

R29.891 Ocular torticollis
EXCLUDES 1 *congenital (sternomastoid) torticollis Q68.0*
psychogenic torticollis (F45.8)
spasmodic torticollis (G24.3)
torticollis due to birth injury (P15.8)
torticollis NOS M43.6

R29.898 Other symptoms and signs involving the musculoskeletal system

✓5th **R29.9 Unspecified symptoms and signs involving the nervous and musculoskeletal systems**

R29.90 Unspecified symptoms and signs involving the nervous system

R29.91 Unspecified symptoms and signs involving the musculoskeletal system

Symptoms and signs involving the genitourinary system (R30-R39)

✓4th **R30 Pain associated with micturition**
EXCLUDES 1 *psychogenic pain associated with micturition (F45.8)*

R30.0 Dysuria
Strangury

R30.1 Vesical tenesmus

R30.9 Painful micturition, unspecified
Painful urination NOS

✓4th **R31 Hematuria**
EXCLUDES 1 *hematuria included with underlying conditions, such as:*
acute cystitis with hematuria (N30.01)
acute prostatitis with hematuria (N41.01)
recurrent and persistent hematuria in glomerular diseases (N02.-)

R31.0 Gross hematuria

R31.1 Benign essential microscopic hematuria

R31.2 Other microscopic hematuria

R31.9 Hematuria, unspecified

R32 Unspecified urinary incontinence
Enuresis NOS
EXCLUDES 1 *functional urinary incontinence (R39.81)*
nonorganic enuresis (F98.0)
stress incontinence and other specified urinary incontinence (N39.3-N39.4-)
urinary incontinence associated with cognitive impairment (R39.81)

✓4th **R33 Retention of urine**
EXCLUDES 1 *psychogenic retention of urine (F45.8)*

R33.0 Drug induced retention of urine
Use additional code for adverse effect, if applicable, to identify drug (T36-T50 with fifth or sixth character 5)

R33.8 Other retention of urine
Code first, if applicable, any causal condition, such as:
enlarged prostate (N40.1)

R33.9 Retention of urine, unspecified

R34 Anuria and oliguria
EXCLUDES 1 *anuria and oliguria complicating abortion or ectopic or molar pregnancy (O00-O07, O08.4)*
anuria and oliguria complicating pregnancy (O26.83-)
anuria and oliguria complicating the puerperium (O90.4)

✓4th **R35 Polyuria**
Code first, if applicable, any causal condition, such as:
enlarged prostate (N40.1)
EXCLUDES 1 *psychogenic polyuria (F45.8)*

R35.0 Frequency of micturition

R35.1 Nocturia

R35.8 Other polyuria
Polyuria NOS

✓4th **R36 Urethral discharge**

R36.0 Urethral discharge without blood

R36.1 Hematospermia

R36.9 Urethral discharge, unspecified
Penile discharge NOS
Urethrorrhea

R37 Sexual dysfunction, unspecified

✓4th **R39 Other and unspecified symptoms and signs involving the genitourinary system**

R39.0 Extravasation of urine

✓5th **R39.1 Other difficulties with micturition**
Code first, if applicable, any causal condition, such as:
enlarged prostate (N40.1)

R39.11 Hesitancy of micturition

R39.12 Poor urinary stream
Weak urinary steam

R39.13 Splitting of urinary stream

R39.14 Feeling of incomplete bladder emptying

R39.15 Urgency of urination
EXCLUDES 1 *urge incontinence (N39.41, N39.46)*

R39.16 Straining to void

R39.19 Other difficulties with micturition

R39.2 Extrarenal uremia
Prerenal uremia
EXCLUDES 1 *uremia NOS (N19)*

✓5th **R39.8 Other symptoms and signs involving the genitourinary system**

R39.81 Functional urinary incontinence
Urinary incontinence due to cognitive impairment, or severe physical disability or immobility
EXCLUDES 1 *stress incontinence and other specified urinary incontinence (N39.3-N39.4-)*
urinary incontinence NOS (R32)

R39.89 Other symptoms and signs involving the genitourinary system

R39.9 Unspecified symptoms and signs involving the genitourinary system

Symptoms and signs involving cognition, perception, emotional state and behavior (R40-R46)

EXCLUDES 1 *symptoms and signs constituting part of a pattern of mental disorder (F01-F99)*

✓4th **R40 Somnolence, stupor and coma**
EXCLUDES 1 *neonatal coma (P91.5)*
somnolence, stupor and coma in diabetes (E08-E13)
somnolence, stupor and coma in hepatic failure (K72.-)
somnolence, stupor and coma in hypoglycemia (nondiabetic) (E15)

R40.0 Somnolence
Drowsiness
EXCLUDES 1 *coma (R40.2-)*

R40.1 Stupor
Catatonic stupor
Semicoma
EXCLUDES 1 *catatonic schizophrenia (F20.2)*
coma (R40.2-)
depressive stupor (F31-F33)
dissociative stupor (F44.2)
manic stupor (F30.2)

5th **R40.2 Coma**

Codes first any associated:
coma in fracture of skull (S02.-)
coma in intracranial injury (S06.-)

The appropriate 7th character is to be added to each code from subcategory R40.21-, R40.22-, R40.23-.
0 unspecified time
1 in the field [EMT or ambulance]
2 at arrival to emergency department
3 at hospital admission
4 24 hours or more after hospital admission

NOTE A code from each subcategory is required to complete the coma scale

R40.20 Unspecified coma
Coma NOS
Unconsciousness NOS

6th **R40.21 Coma scale, eyes open**
7th **R40.211 Coma scale, eyes open, never**
7th **R40.212 Coma scale, eyes open, to pain**
7th **R40.213 Coma scale, eyes open, to sound**
7th **R40.214 Coma scale, eyes open, spontaneous**

6th **R40.22 Coma scale, best verbal response**
7th **R40.221 Coma scale, best verbal response, none**
7th **R40.222 Coma scale, best verbal response, incomprehensible words**
7th **R40.223 Coma scale, best verbal response, inappropriate words**
7th **R40.224 Coma scale, best verbal response, confused conversation**
7th **R40.225 Coma scale, best verbal response, oriented**

6th **R40.23 Coma scale, best motor response**
7th **R40.231 Coma scale, best motor response, none**
7th **R40.232 Coma scale, best motor response, extension**
7th **R40.233 Coma scale, best motor response, abnormal**
7th **R40.234 Coma scale, best motor response, flexion withdrawal**
7th **R40.235 Coma scale, best motor response, localizes pain**
7th **R40.236 Coma scale, best motor response, obeys commands**

6th **R40.24 Glasgow coma scale, total score**
Use codes R40.21- through R40.23- only when the individual score(s) are documented
R40.241 Glasgow coma scale score 13-15
R40.242 Glasgow coma scale score 9-12
R40.243 Glasgow coma scale score 3-8
R40.244 Other coma, without documented Glasgow coma scale score, or with partial score reported

R40.3 Persistent vegetative state

R40.4 Transient alteration of awareness

4th **R41 Other symptoms and signs involving cognitive functions and awareness**

EXCLUDES 1 *dissociative [conversion] disorders (F44.-)*
mild cognitive impairment, so stated (G31.84)

R41.0 Disorientation, unspecified
Confusion NOS
Delirium NOS

R41.1 Anterograde amnesia

R41.2 Retrograde amnesia

R41.3 Other amnesia
Amnesia NOS
Memory loss NOS
EXCLUDES 1 *amnestic disorder due to known physiologic condition (F04)*
amnestic syndrome due to psychoactive substance use (F10-F19 with 5th character .6)
mild memory disturbance due to known physiological condition (F06.8)
transient global amnesia (G45.4)

R41.4 Neurologic neglect syndrome
Asomatognosia
Hemi-akinesia
Hemi-inattention
Hemispatial neglect
Left-sided neglect
Sensory neglect
Visuospatial neglect
EXCLUDES 1 *visuospatial deficit (R41.842)*

5th **R41.8 Other symptoms and signs involving cognitive functions and awareness**

R41.81 Age-related cognitive decline
Senility NOS

R41.82 Altered mental status, unspecified
Change in mental status NOS
EXCLUDES 1 *altered level of consciousness (R40.-)*
altered mental status due to known condition—code to condition
delirium NOS (R41.0)

R41.83 Borderline intellectual functioning
IQ level 71 to 84
EXCLUDES 1 *intellectual disabilities (F70-F79)*

6th **R41.84 Other specified cognitive deficit**
R41.840 Attention and concentration deficit
EXCLUDES 1 *attention-deficit hyperactivity disorders (F90.-)*
R41.841 Cognitive communication deficit
R41.842 Visuospatial deficit
R41.843 Psychomotor deficit
R41.844 Frontal lobe and executive function deficit

R41.89 Other symptoms and signs involving cognitive functions and awareness
Anosognosia

R41.9 Unspecified symptoms and signs involving cognitive functions and awareness

R42 Dizziness and giddiness
Light-headedness
Vertigo NOS
EXCLUDES 1 *vertiginous syndromes (H81.-)*
vertigo from infrasound (T75.23)

4th **R43 Disturbances of smell and taste**

R43.0 Anosmia

R43.1 Parosmia

R43.2 Parageusia

R43.8 Other disturbances of smell and taste
Mixed disturbance of smell and taste

R43.9 Unspecified disturbances of smell and taste

4th **R44 Other symptoms and signs involving general sensations and perceptions**

EXCLUDES 1 *alcoholic hallucinations (F1.5)*
hallucinations in drug psychosis (F11-F19 with .5)
hallucinations in mood disorders with psychotic symptoms (F30.2, F31.5, F32.3, F33.3)
hallucinations in schizophrenia, schizotypal and delusional disorders (F20-F29)
EXCLUDES 2 *disturbances of skin sensation (R20.-)*

R44.0 Auditory hallucinations

R44.1 Visual hallucinations

R44.2 Other hallucinations

R44.3 Hallucinations, unspecified

R44.8 Other symptoms and signs involving general sensations and perceptions

R44.9 Unspecified symptoms and signs involving general sensations and perceptions

4th **R45 Symptoms and signs involving emotional state**

R45.0 Nervousness
Nervous tension

R45.1 Restlessness and agitation

R45.2 Unhappiness

R45.3 Demoralization and apathy
EXCLUDES 1 *anhedonia (R45.84)*

R45.4 Irritability and anger

R45.5 Hostility

R45.6 Violent behavior

R45.7 State of emotional shock and stress, unspecified

√5th **R45.8 Other symptoms and signs involving emotional state**
R45.81 Low self-esteem
R45.82 Worries
R45.83 Excessive crying of child, adolescent or adult
EXCLUDES 1 *excessive crying of infant (baby) R68.11*
R45.84 Anhedonia
√6th **R45.85 Homicidal and suicidal ideations**
EXCLUDES 1 *suicide attempt (T14.91)*
R45.850 Homicidal ideations
R45.851 Suicidal ideations
R45.86 Emotional lability
R45.87 Impulsiveness
R45.89 Other symptoms and signs involving emotional state

√4th **R46 Symptoms and signs involving appearance and behavior**
EXCLUDES 1 *appearance and behavior in schizophrenia, schizotypal and delusional disorders (F20-F29)*
mental and behavioral disorders (F01-F99)
R46.0 Very low level of personal hygiene
R46.1 Bizarre personal appearance
R46.2 Strange and inexplicable behavior
R46.3 Overactivity
R46.4 Slowness and poor responsiveness
EXCLUDES 1 *stupor (R40.1)*
R46.5 Suspiciousness and marked evasiveness
R46.6 Undue concern and preoccupation with stressful events
R46.7 Verbosity and circumstantial detail obscuring reason for contact
√5th **R46.8 Other symptoms and signs involving appearance and behavior**
R46.81 Obsessive-compulsive behavior
EXCLUDES 1 *obsessive-compulsive disorder (F42)*
R46.89 Other symptoms and signs involving appearance and behavior

Symptoms and signs involving speech and voice (R47-R49)

√4th **R47 Speech disturbances, not elsewhere classified**
EXCLUDES 1 *autism (F84.0)*
cluttering (F80.81)
specific developmental disorders of speech and language (F80.-)
stuttering (F80.81)
√5th **R47.0 Dysphasia and aphasia**
R47.01 Aphasia
EXCLUDES 1 *aphasia following cerebrovascular disease (I69. with final characters -20)*
progressive isolated aphasia (G31.01)
R47.02 Dysphasia
EXCLUDES 1 *dysphasia following cerebrovascular disease (I69. with final characters -21)*
R47.1 Dysarthria and anarthria
EXCLUDES 1 *dysarthria following cerebrovascular disease (I69. with final characters -22)*
√5th **R47.8 Other speech disturbances**
EXCLUDES 1 *dysarthria following cerebrovascular disease (I69. with final characters -28)*
R47.81 Slurred speech
R47.82 Fluency disorder in conditions classified elsewhere
Stuttering in conditions classified elsewhere
Code first underlying disease or condition, such as:
Parkinson's disease (G20)
EXCLUDES 1 *adult onset fluency disorder (F98.5)*
childhood onset fluency disorder (F80.81)
fluency disorder (stuttering) following cerebrovascular disease (I69. with final characters-23)
R47.89 Other speech disturbances
R47.9 Unspecified speech disturbances

√4th **R48 Dyslexia and other symbolic dysfunctions, not elsewhere classified**
EXCLUDES 1 *specific developmental disorders of scholastic skills (F81.-)*
R48.0 Dyslexia and alexia
R48.1 Agnosia
Astereognosia (astereognosis)
Autotopagnosia
EXCLUDES 1 *visual object agnosia (R48.3)*
R48.2 Apraxia
EXCLUDES 1 *apraxia following cerebrovascular disease (I69. with final characters -90)*
R48.3 Visual agnosia
Prosopagnosia
Simultanagnosia (asimultagnosia)
R48.8 Other symbolic dysfunctions
Acalculia
Agraphia
R48.9 Unspecified symbolic dysfunctions

√4th **R49 Voice and resonance disorders**
EXCLUDES 1 *psychogenic voice and resonance disorders (F44.4)*
R49.0 Dysphonia
Hoarseness
R49.1 Aphonia
Loss of voice
√5th **R49.2 Hypernasality and hyponasality**
R49.21 Hypernasality
R49.22 Hyponasality
R49.8 Other voice and resonance disorders
R49.9 Unspecified voice and resonance disorder
Change in voice NOS
Resonance disorder NOS

General symptoms and signs (R50-R69)

√4th **R50 Fever of other and unknown origin**
EXCLUDES 1 *chills without fever (R68.83)*
febrile convulsions (R56.0-)
fever of unknown origin during labor (O75.2)
fever of unknown origin in newborn (P81.9)
hypothermia due to illness (R68.0)
malignant hyperthermia due to anesthesia (T88.3)
puerperal pyrexia NOS (O86.4)
R50.2 Drug induced fever
Use additional code for adverse effect, if applicable, to identify drug (T36-T50 with fifth or sixth character 5)
EXCLUDES 1 *postvaccination (postimmunization) fever (R50.83)*
√5th **R50.8 Other specified fever**
R50.81 Fever presenting with conditions classified elsewhere
Code first underlying condition when associated fever is present, such as with:
leukemia (C91-C95)
neutropenia (D70.-)
sickle-cell disease (D57.-)
R50.82 Postprocedural fever
EXCLUDES 1 *postprocedural infection (T81.4)*
posttransfusion fever (R50.84)
postvaccination (postimmunization) fever (R50.83)
R50.83 Postvaccination fever
Postimmunization fever
R50.84 Febrile nonhemolytic transfusion reaction
FNHTR
Posttransfusion fever
R50.9 Fever, unspecified
Fever NOS
Fever of unknown origin [FUO]
Fever with chills
Fever with rigors
Hyperpyrexia NOS
Persistent fever
Pyrexia NOS

R51 Headache
Facial pain NOS
EXCLUDES 1 *atypical face pain (G50.1)*
migraine and other headache syndromes (G43-G44)
trigeminal neuralgia (G50.0)

R52 Pain, unspecified
Acute pain NOS
Generalized pain NOS
Pain NOS
EXCLUDES 1 *acute and chronic pain, not elsewhere classified (G89.-)*
localized pain, unspecified type—code to pain by site, such as:
abdomen pain (R10.-)
back pain (M54.9)
breast pain (N64.4)
chest pain (R07.1-R07.9)
ear pain (H92.0-)
eye pain (H57.1)
headache (R51)
joint pain (M25.5-)
limb pain (M79.6-)
lumbar region pain (M54.5)
pelvic and perineal pain (R10.2)
shoulder pain (M25.51-)
spine pain (M54.-)
throat pain (R07.0)
tongue pain (K14.6)
tooth pain (K08.8)
renal colic (N23)
pain disorders exclusively related to psychological factors (F45.41)

✓4th **R53 Malaise and fatigue**

R53.0 Neoplastic (malignant) related fatigue
Code first associated neoplasm

R53.1 Weakness
Asthenia NOS
EXCLUDES 1 *age-related weakness (R54)*
muscle weakness (M62.8-)
senile asthenia (R54)

R53.2 Functional quadriplegia
Complete immobility due to severe physical disability or frailty
EXCLUDES 1 *frailty NOS (R54)*
hysterical paralysis (F44.4)
immobility syndrome (M62.3)
neurologic quadriplegia (G82.5-)
quadriplegia (G82.50)

✓5th **R53.8 Other malaise and fatigue**
EXCLUDES 1 *combat exhaustion and fatigue (F43.0)*
congenital debility (P96.9)
exhaustion and fatigue due to:
depressive episode (F32.-)
excessive exertion (T73.3)
exposure (T73.2)
heat (T67.-)
pregnancy (O26.8-)
recurrent depressive episode (F33)
senile debility (R54)

R53.81 Other malaise
Chronic debility
Debility NOS
General physical deterioration
Malaise NOS
Nervous debility
EXCLUDES 1 *age-related physical debility (R54)*

R53.82 Chronic fatigue, unspecified
Chronic fatigue syndrome NOS
EXCLUDES 1 *postviral fatigue syndrome (G93.3)*

R53.83 Other fatigue
Fatigue NOS
Lack of energy
Lethargy
Tiredness

R54 Age-related physical debility
Frailty
Old age
Senescence
Senile asthenia
Senile debility
EXCLUDES 1 *age-related cognitive decline (R41.81)*
senile psychosis (F03)
senility NOS (R41.81)

R55 Syncope and collapse
Blackout
Fainting
Vasovagal attack
EXCLUDES 1 *cardiogenic shock (R57.0)*
carotid sinus syncope (G90.01)
heat syncope (T67.1)
neurocirculatory asthenia (F45.8)
neurogenic orthostatic hypotension (G90.3)
orthostatic hypotension (I95.1)
postprocedural shock (T81.1-)
psychogenic syncope (F48.8)
shock NOS (R57.9)
shock complicating or following abortion or ectopic or molar pregnancy (O00-O07, O08.3)
shock complicating or following labor and delivery (O75.1)
Stokes-Adams attack (I45.9)
unconsciousness NOS (R40.2-)

✓4th **R56 Convulsions, not elsewhere classified**
EXCLUDES 1 *dissociative convulsions and seizures (F44.5)*
epileptic convulsions and seizures (G40.-)
newborn convulsions and seizures (P90)

✓5th **R56.0 Febrile convulsions**

R56.00 Simple febrile convulsions
Febrile convulsion NOS
Febrile seizure NOS

R56.01 Complex febrile convulsions
Atypical febrile seizure
Complex febrile seizure
Complicated febrile seizure
EXCLUDES 1 *status epilepticus (G40.901)*

R56.1 Post traumatic seizures
EXCLUDES 1 *post traumatic epilepsy (G40.-)*

R56.9 Unspecified convulsions
Convulsion disorder
Fit NOS
Recurrent convulsions
Seizure(s) (convulsive) NOS

✓4th **R57 Shock, not elsewhere classified**
EXCLUDES 1 *anaphylactic shock NOS (T78.2)*
anaphylactic reaction or shock due to adverse food reaction (T78.0-)
anaphylactic shock due to adverse effect of correct drug or medicament properly administered (T88.6)
anaphylactic shock due to serum (T80.5-)
anesthetic shock (T88.3)
electric shock (T75.4)
obstetric shock (O75.1)
postprocedural shock (T81.1-)
psychic shock (F43.0)
septic shock (R65.21)
shock complicating or following ectopic or molar pregnancy (O00-O07, O08.3)
shock due to lightning (T75.01)
traumatic shock (T79.4)
toxic shock syndrome (A48.3)

R57.0 Cardiogenic shock
R57.1 Hypovolemic shock
R57.8 Other shock
R57.9 Shock, unspecified
Failure of peripheral circulation NOS

R58 Hemorrhage, not elsewhere classified
Hemorrhage NOS
EXCLUDES 1 *hemorrhage included with underlying conditions, such as:*
acute duodenal ulcer with hemorrhage (K26.0)
acute gastritis with bleeding (K29.01)
ulcerative enterocolitis with rectal bleeding (K51.01)

✓4th **R59 Enlarged lymph nodes**
INCLUDES swollen glands
EXCLUDES 1 *acute lymphadenitis (L04.-)*
chronic lymphadenitis (I88.1)
lymphadenitis NOS (I88.9)
mesenteric (acute) (chronic) lymphadenitis (I88.0)

R59.0 Localized enlarged lymph nodes
R59.1 Generalized enlarged lymph nodes
Lymphadenopathy NOS
R59.9 Enlarged lymph nodes, unspecified

R60 Edema, not elsewhere classified
EXCLUDES 1 *angioneurotic edema (T78.3)*
ascites (R18.-)
cerebral edema (G93.6)
cerebral edema due to birth injury (P11.0)
edema of larynx (J38.4)
edema of nasopharynx (J39.2)
edema of pharynx (J39.2)
gestational edema (O12.0-)
hereditary edema (Q82.0)
hydrops fetalis NOS (P83.2)
hydrothorax (J94.8)
nutritional edema (E40-E46)
hydrops fetalis NOS (P83.2)
newborn edema (P83.3)
pulmonary edema (J81.-)

R60.0 Localized edema
R60.1 Generalized edema
R60.9 Edema, unspecified
Fluid retention NOS

R61 Generalized hyperhidrosis
Excessive sweating
Night sweats
Secondary hyperhidrosis
Code first, if applicable, menopausal and female climacteric states (N95.1)
EXCLUDES 1 *focal (primary) (secondary) hyperhidrosis (L74.5-)*
Frey's syndrome (L74.52)
localized (primary) (secondary) hyperhidrosis (L74.5-)

R62 Lack of expected normal physiological development in childhood and adults
EXCLUDES 1 *delayed puberty (E30.0)*
gonadal dysgenesis (Q99.1)
hypopituitarism (E23.0)

R62.0 Delayed milestone in childhood
Delayed attainment of expected physiological developmental stage
Late talker
Late walker

R62.5 Other and unspecified lack of expected normal physiological development in childhood
EXCLUDES 1 *HIV disease resulting in failure to thrive (B20)*
physical retardation due to malnutrition (E45)

R62.50 Unspecified lack of expected normal physiological development in childhood
Infantilism NOS

R62.51 Failure to thrive (child)
Failure to gain weight
EXCLUDES 1 *failure to thrive in child under 28 days old (P92.6)*

R62.52 Short stature (child)
Lack of growth
Physical retardation
Short stature NOS
EXCLUDES 1 *short stature due to endocrine disorder (E34.3)*

R62.59 Other lack of expected normal physiological development in childhood

R62.7 Adult failure to thrive

R63 Symptoms and signs concerning food and fluid intake
EXCLUDES 1 *bulimia NOS (F50.2)*
eating disorders of nonorganic origin (F50.-)
malnutrition (E40-E46)

R63.0 Anorexia
Loss of appetite
EXCLUDES 1 *anorexia nervosa (F50.0-)*
loss of appetite of nonorganic origin (F50.8)

R63.1 Polydipsia
Excessive thirst

R63.2 Polyphagia
Excessive eating
Hyperalimentation NOS

R63.3 Feeding difficulties
Feeding problem (elderly) (infant) NOS
EXCLUDES 1 *feeding problems of newborn (P92.-)*
infant feeding disorder of nonorganic origin (F98.2-)

R63.4 Abnormal weight loss

R63.5 Abnormal weight gain
EXCLUDES 1 *excessive weight gain in pregnancy (O26.0-)*
obesity (E66.-)

R63.6 Underweight
Use additional code to identify body mass index (BMI), if known (Z68.-)
EXCLUDES 1 *abnormal weight loss (R63.4)*
anorexia nervosa (F50.0-)
malnutrition (E40-E46)

R63.8 Other symptoms and signs concerning food and fluid intake

R64 Cachexia
Wasting syndrome
Code first underlying condition, if known
EXCLUDES 1 *abnormal weight loss (R63.4)*
nutritional marasmus (E41)

R65 Symptoms and signs specifically associated with systemic inflammation and infection

R65.1 Systemic inflammatory response syndrome [SIRS] of non-infectious origin
Code first underlying condition, such as:
heatstroke (T67.0)
injury and trauma (S00-T88)
EXCLUDES 1 *sepsis—code to infection*
severe sepsis (R65.2)

R65.10 Systemic inflammatory response syndrome [SIRS] of non-infectious origin without acute organ dysfunction
Systemic inflammatory response syndrome (SIRS) NOS

R65.11 Systemic inflammatory response syndrome [SIRS] of non-infectious origin with acute organ dysfunction
Use additional code to identify specific acute organ dysfunction, such as:
acute kidney failure (N17.-)
acute respiratory failure (J96.0-)
critical illness myopathy (G72.81)
critical illness polyneuropathy (G62.81)
disseminated intravascular coagulopathy [DIC] (D65)
encephalopathy (metabolic) (septic) (G93.41)
hepatic failure (K72.0-)

R65.2 Severe sepsis
Infection with associated acute organ dysfunction
Sepsis with acute organ dysfunction
Sepsis with multiple organ dysfunction
Systemic inflammatory response syndrome due to infectious process with acute organ dysfunction
Code first underlying infection, such as:
infection following a procedure (T81.4)
infections following infusion, transfusion and therapeutic injection (T80.2-)
puerperal sepsis (O85)
sepsis following complete or unspecified spontaneous abortion (O03.87)
sepsis following ectopic and molar pregnancy (O08.82)
sepsis following incomplete spontaneous abortion (O03.37)
sepsis following (induced) termination of pregnancy (O04.87)
sepsis NOS A41.9
Use additional code to identify specific acute organ dysfunction, such as:
acute kidney failure (N17.-)
acute respiratory failure (J96.0-)
critical illness myopathy (G72.81)
critical illness polyneuropathy (G62.81)
disseminated intravascular coagulopathy [DIC] (D65)
encephalopathy (metabolic) (septic) (G93.41)
hepatic failure (K72.0-)

R65.20 Severe sepsis without septic shock
Severe sepsis NOS

R65.21 Severe sepsis with septic shock

R68 Other general symptoms and signs

R68.0 Hypothermia, not associated with low environmental temperature

EXCLUDES 1 *hypothermia NOS (accidental) (T68)*
hypothermia due to anesthesia (T88.51)
hypothermia due to low environmental temperature (T68)
newborn hypothermia (P80.-)

R68.1 Nonspecific symptoms peculiar to infancy

EXCLUDES 1 *colic, infantile (R10.83)*
neonatal cerebral irritability (P91.3)
teething syndrome (K00.7)

R68.11 Excessive crying of infant (baby)

EXCLUDES 1 *excessive crying of child, adolescent, or adult (R45.83)*

R68.12 Fussy infant (baby)

Irritable infant

R68.13 Apparent life threatening event in infant [ALTE]

Apparent life threatening event in newborn
Code first confirmed diagnosis, if known
Use additional code(s) for associated signs and symptoms if no confirmed diagnosis established, or if signs and symptoms are not associated routinely with confirmed diagnosis, or provide additional information for cause of ALTE

R68.19 Other nonspecific symptoms peculiar to infancy

R68.2 Dry mouth, unspecified

EXCLUDES 1 *dry mouth due to dehydration (E86.0)*
dry mouth due to sicca syndrome [Sjögren] (M35.0-)
salivary gland hyposecretion (K11.7)

R68.3 Clubbing of fingers

Clubbing of nails

EXCLUDES 1 *congenital clubfinger (Q68.1)*

R68.8 Other general symptoms and signs

R68.81 Early satiety

R68.82 Decreased libido

Decreased sexual desire

R68.83 Chills (without fever)

Chills NOS

EXCLUDES 1 *chills with fever (R50.9)*

R68.84 Jaw pain

Mandibular pain
Maxilla pain

EXCLUDES 1 *temporomandibular joint arthralgia (M26.62)*

R68.89 Other general symptoms and signs

R69 Illness, unspecified

Unknown and unspecified cases of morbidity

Abnormal findings on examination of blood, without diagnosis (R70-R79)

EXCLUDES 1 *abnormalities (of)(on):*
abnormal findings on antenatal screening of mother (O28.-)
coagulation hemorrhagic disorders (D65-D68)
lipids (E78.-)
platelets and thrombocytes (D69.-)
white blood cells classified elsewhere (D70-D72)
diagnostic abnormal findings classified elsewhere—see Alphabetical Index
hemorrhagic and hematological disorders of newborn (P50-P61)

R70 Elevated erythrocyte sedimentation rate and abnormality of plasma viscosity

R70.0 Elevated erythrocyte sedimentation rate

R70.1 Abnormal plasma viscosity

R71 Abnormality of red blood cells

EXCLUDES 1 *anemias (D50-D64)*
anemia of premature infant (P61.2)
benign (familial) polycythemia (D75.0)
congenital anemias (P61.2-P61.4)
newborn anemia due to isoimmunization (P55.-)
polycythemia neonatorum (P61.1)
polycythemia NOS (D75.1)
polycythemia vera (D45)
secondary polycythemia (D75.1)

R71.0 Precipitous drop in hematocrit

Drop (precipitous) in hemoglobin
Drop in hematocrit

R71.8 Other abnormality of red blood cells

Abnormal red-cell morphology NOS
Abnormal red-cell volume NOS
Anisocytosis
Poikilocytosis

R73 Elevated blood glucose level

EXCLUDES 1 *diabetes mellitus (E08-E13)*
diabetes mellitus in pregnancy, childbirth and the puerperium (O24.-)
neonatal disorders (P70.0-P70.2)
postsurgical hypoinsulinemia (E89.1)

R73.0 Abnormal glucose

EXCLUDES 1 *abnormal glucose in pregnancy (O99.81-)*
diabetes mellitus (E08-E13)
dysmetabolic syndrome X (E88.81)
gestational diabetes (O24.4-)
glycosuria (R81)
hypoglycemia (E16.2)

R73.01 Impaired fasting glucose

Elevated fasting glucose

R73.02 Impaired glucose tolerance (oral)

Elevated glucose tolerance

R73.09 Other abnormal glucose

Abnormal glucose NOS
Abnormal non-fasting glucose tolerance
Latent diabetes
Prediabetes

R73.9 Hyperglycemia, unspecified

R74 Abnormal serum enzyme levels

R74.0 Nonspecific elevation of levels of transaminase and lactic acid dehydrogenase [LDH]

R74.8 Abnormal levels of other serum enzymes

Abnormal level of acid phosphatase
Abnormal level of alkaline phosphatase
Abnormal level of amylase
Abnormal level of lipase [triacylglycerol lipase]

R74.9 Abnormal serum enzyme level, unspecified

R75 Inconclusive laboratory evidence of human immunodeficiency virus [HIV]

Nonconclusive HIV-test finding in infants

EXCLUDES 1 *asymptomatic human immunodeficiency virus [HIV] infection status (Z21)*
human immunodeficiency virus [HIV] disease (B20)

R76 Other abnormal immunological findings in serum

R76.0 Raised antibody titer

EXCLUDES 1 *isoimmunization in pregnancy (O36.0-O36.1)*
isoimmunization affecting newborn (P55.-)

R76.1 Nonspecific reaction to test for tuberculosis

R76.11 Nonspecific reaction to tuberculin skin test without active tuberculosis

Abnormal result of Mantoux test
PPD positive
Tuberculin (skin test) positive
Tuberculin (skin test) reactor

EXCLUDES 1 *nonspecific reaction to cell mediated immunity measurement of gamma interferon antigen response without active tuberculosis (R76.12)*

R76.12 Nonspecific reaction to cell mediated immunity measurement of gamma interferon antigen response without active tuberculosis

Nonspecific reaction to QuantiFERON-TB test (QFT) without active tuberculosis

EXCLUDES 1 *nonspecific reaction to tuberculin skin test without active tuberculosis (R76.11)*
positive tuberculin skin test (R76.11)

R76.8 Other specified abnormal immunological findings in serum
Raised level of immunoglobulins NOS

R76.9 Abnormal immunological finding in serum, unspecified

✓4th **R77 Other abnormalities of plasma proteins**
EXCLUDES 1 *disorders of plasma-protein metabolism (E88.0)*

R77.0 Abnormality of albumin

R77.1 Abnormality of globulin
Hyperglobulinemia NOS

R77.2 Abnormality of alphafetoprotein

R77.8 Other specified abnormalities of plasma proteins

R77.9 Abnormality of plasma protein, unspecified

✓4th **R78 Findings of drugs and other substances, not normally found in blood**
Use additional code to identify any retained foreign body, if applicable (Z18.-)
EXCLUDES 1 *mental or behavioral disorders due to psychoactive substance use (F10-F19)*

R78.0 Finding of alcohol in blood
Use additional external cause code (Y90.-), for detail regarding alcohol level

R78.1 Finding of opiate drug in blood

R78.2 Finding of cocaine in blood

R78.3 Finding of hallucinogen in blood

R78.4 Finding of other drugs of addictive potential in blood

R78.5 Finding of other psychotropic drug in blood

R78.6 Finding of steroid agent in blood

✓5th **R78.7 Finding of abnormal level of heavy metals in blood**

R78.71 Abnormal lead level in blood
EXCLUDES 1 *lead poisoning (T56.0-)*

R78.79 Finding of abnormal level of heavy metals in blood

✓5th **R78.8 Finding of other specified substances, not normally found in blood**

R78.81 Bacteremia
EXCLUDES 1 *sepsis—code to specified infection (A00-B99)*

R78.89 Finding of other specified substances, not normally found in blood
Finding of abnormal level of lithium in blood

R78.9 Finding of unspecified substance, not normally found in blood

✓4th **R79 Other abnormal findings of blood chemistry**
Use additional code to identify any retained foreign body, if applicable (Z18.-)
EXCLUDES 1 *abnormality of fluid, electrolyte or acid-base balance (E86-E87)*
asymptomatic hyperuricemia (E79.0)
hyperglycemia NOS (R73.9)
hypoglycemia NOS (E16.2)
neonatal hypoglycemia (P70.3-P70.4)
specific findings indicating disorder of:
amino-acid metabolism (E70-E72)
carbohydrate metabolism (E73-E74)
lipid metabolism (E75.-)

R79.0 Abnormal level of blood mineral
Abnormal blood level of cobalt
Abnormal blood level of copper
Abnormal blood level of iron
Abnormal blood level of magnesium
Abnormal blood level of mineral NEC
Abnormal blood level of zinc
EXCLUDES 1 *abnormal level of lithium (R78.89)*
disorders of mineral metabolism (E83.-)
neonatal hypomagnesemia (P71.2)
nutritional mineral deficiency (E58-E61)

R79.1 Abnormal coagulation profile
Abnormal or prolonged bleeding time
Abnormal or prolonged coagulation time
Abnormal or prolonged partial thromboplastin time [PTT]
Abnormal or prolonged prothrombin time [PT]
EXCLUDES 1 *coagulation defects (D68.-)*

✓5th **R79.8 Other specified abnormal findings of blood chemistry**

R79.81 Abnormal blood-gas level

R79.82 Elevated C-reactive protein [CRP]

R79.89 Other specified abnormal findings of blood chemistry

R79.9 Abnormal finding of blood chemistry, unspecified

Abnormal findings on examination of urine, without diagnosis (R80-R82)

EXCLUDES 1 *abnormal findings on antenatal screening of mother (O28.-)*
diagnostic abnormal findings classified elsewhere—see Alphabetical Index
specific findings indicating disorder of:
amino-acid metabolism (E70-E72)
carbohydrate metabolism (E73-E74)

✓4th **R80 Proteinuria**
EXCLUDES 1 *gestational proteinuria (O12.1-)*

R80.0 Isolated proteinuria
Idiopathic proteinuria
EXCLUDES 1 *isolated proteinuria with specific morphological lesion (N06.-)*

R80.1 Persistent proteinuria, unspecified

R80.2 Orthostatic proteinuria, unspecified
Postural proteinuria

R80.3 Bence Jones proteinuria

R80.8 Other proteinuria

R80.9 Proteinuria, unspecified
Albuminuria NOS

R81 Glycosuria
EXCLUDES 1 *renal glycosuria (E74.8)*

✓4th **R82 Other and unspecified abnormal findings in urine**
Chromoabnormalities in urine
Use additional code to identify any retained foreign body, if applicable (Z18.-)
EXCLUDES 2 *hematuria (R31.-)*

R82.0 Chyluria
EXCLUDES 1 *filarial chyluria (B74.-)*

R82.1 Myoglobinuria

R82.2 Biliuria

R82.3 Hemoglobinuria
EXCLUDES 1 *hemoglobinuria due to hemolysis from external causes NEC (D59.6)*
hemoglobinuria due to paroxysmal nocturnal [Marchiafava-Micheli] (D59.5)

R82.4 Acetonuria
Ketonuria

R82.5 Elevated urine levels of drugs, medicaments and biological substances
Elevated urine levels of catecholamines
Elevated urine levels of indoleacetic acid
Elevated urine levels of 17-ketosteroids
Elevated urine levels of steroids

R82.6 Abnormal urine levels of substances chiefly nonmedicinal as to source
Abnormal urine level of heavy metals

R82.7 Abnormal findings on microbiological examination of urine
Positive culture findings of urine
EXCLUDES 1 *colonization status (Z22.-)*

R82.8 Abnormal findings on cytological and histological examination of urine

✓5th **R82.9 Other and unspecified abnormal findings in urine**

R82.90 Unspecified abnormal findings in urine

R82.91 Other chromoabnormalities of urine
Chromoconversion (dipstick)
Idiopathic dipstick converts positive for blood with no cellular forms in sediment
EXCLUDES 1 *hemoglobinuria (R82.3)*
myoglobinuria (R82.1)

R82.99 Other abnormal findings in urine
Cells and casts in urine
Crystalluria
Melanuria

DRAFT

Abnormal findings on examination of other body fluids, substances and tissues, without diagnosis (R83-R89)

EXCLUDES 1 *abnormal findings on antenatal screening of mother (O28.-)*
diagnostic abnormal findings classified elsewhere—see Alphabetical Index

EXCLUDES 2 *abnormal findings on examination of blood, without diagnosis (R70-R79)*
abnormal findings on examination of urine, without diagnosis (R80-R82)
abnormal tumor markers (R97.-)

✓4th **R83 Abnormal findings in cerebrospinal fluid**

R83.0 Abnormal level of enzymes in cerebrospinal fluid

R83.1 Abnormal level of hormones in cerebrospinal fluid

R83.2 Abnormal level of other drugs, medicaments and biological substances in cerebrospinal fluid

R83.3 Abnormal level of substances chiefly nonmedicinal as to source in cerebrospinal fluid

R83.4 Abnormal immunological findings in cerebrospinal fluid

R83.5 Abnormal microbiological findings in cerebrospinal fluid
Positive culture findings in cerebrospinal fluid
EXCLUDES 1 *colonization status (Z22.-)*

R83.6 Abnormal cytological findings in cerebrospinal fluid

R83.8 Other abnormal findings in cerebrospinal fluid
Abnormal chromosomal findings in cerebrospinal fluid

R83.9 Unspecified abnormal finding in cerebrospinal fluid

✓4th **R84 Abnormal findings in specimens from respiratory organs and thorax**
Abnormal findings in bronchial washings
Abnormal findings in nasal secretions
Abnormal findings in pleural fluid
Abnormal findings in sputum
Abnormal findings in throat scrapings
EXCLUDES 1 *blood-stained sputum (R04.2)*

R84.0 Abnormal level of enzymes in specimens from respiratory organs and thorax

R84.1 Abnormal level of hormones in specimens from respiratory organs and thorax

R84.2 Abnormal level of other drugs, medicaments and biological substances in specimens from respiratory organs and thorax

R84.3 Abnormal level of substances chiefly nonmedicinal as to source in specimens from respiratory organs and thorax

R84.4 Abnormal immunological findings in specimens from respiratory organs and thorax

R84.5 Abnormal microbiological findings in specimens from respiratory organs and thorax
Positive culture findings in specimens from respiratory organs and thorax
EXCLUDES 1 *colonization status (Z22.-)*

R84.6 Abnormal cytological findings in specimens from respiratory organs and thorax

R84.7 Abnormal histological findings in specimens from respiratory organs and thorax

R84.8 Other abnormal findings in specimens from respiratory organs and thorax
Abnormal chromosomal findings in specimens from respiratory organs and thorax

R84.9 Unspecified abnormal finding in specimens from respiratory organs and thorax

✓4th **R85 Abnormal findings in specimens from digestive organs and abdominal cavity**
INCLUDES abnormal findings in peritoneal fluid
abnormal findings in saliva
EXCLUDES 1 *cloudy peritoneal dialysis effluent (R88.0)*
fecal abnormalities (R19.5)

R85.0 Abnormal level of enzymes in specimens from digestive organs and abdominal cavity

R85.1 Abnormal level of hormones in specimens from digestive organs and abdominal cavity

R85.2 Abnormal level of other drugs, medicaments and biological substances in specimens from digestive organs and abdominal cavity

R85.3 Abnormal level of substances chiefly nonmedicinal as to source in specimens from digestive organs and abdominal cavity

R85.4 Abnormal immunological findings in specimens from digestive organs and abdominal cavity

R85.5 Abnormal microbiological findings in specimens from digestive organs and abdominal cavity
Positive culture findings in specimens from digestive organs and abdominal cavity
EXCLUDES 1 *colonization status (Z22.-)*

✓5th **R85.6 Abnormal cytological findings in specimens from digestive organs and abdominal cavity**

✓6th **R85.61 Abnormal cytologic smear of anus**
EXCLUDES 1 *abnormal cytological findings in specimens from other digestive organs and abdominal cavity (R85.69)*
carcinoma in situ of anus (histologically confirmed) (D01.3)
anal intraepithelial neoplasia I [AIN I] (K62.82)
anal intraepithelial neoplasia II [AIN II] (K62.82)
anal intraepithelial neoplasia III [AIN III] (D01.3)
dysplasia (mild) (moderate) of anus (histologically confirmed) (K62.82)
severe dysplasia of anus (histologically confirmed) (D01.3)
EXCLUDES 2 *anal high risk human papillomavirus (HPV) DNA test positive (R85.81)*
anal low risk human papillomavirus (HPV) DNA test positive (R85.82)

R85.610 Atypical squamous cells of undetermined significance on cytologic smear of anus [ASC-US]

R85.611 Atypical squamous cells cannot exclude high grade squamous intraepithelial lesion on cytologic smear of anus [ASC-H]

R85.612 Low grade squamous intraepithelial lesion on cytologic smear of anus [LGSIL]

R85.613 High grade squamous intraepithelial lesion on cytologic smear of anus [HGSIL]

R85.614 Cytologic evidence of malignancy on smear of anus

R85.615 Unsatisfactory cytologic smear of anus
Inadequate sample of cytologic smear of anus

R85.616 Satisfactory anal smear but lacking transformation zone

R85.618 Other abnormal cytological findings on specimens from anus

R85.619 Unspecified abnormal cytological findings in specimens from anus
Abnormal anal cytology NOS
Atypical glandular cells of anus NOS

R85.69 Abnormal cytological findings in specimens from other digestive organs and abdominal cavity

R85.7 Abnormal histological findings in specimens from digestive organs and abdominal cavity

✓5th **R85.8 Other abnormal findings in specimens from digestive organs and abdominal cavity**

R85.81 Anal high risk human papillomavirus [HPV] DNA test positive
EXCLUDES 1 *anogenital warts due to human papillomavirus (HPV) (A63.0)*
condyloma acuminatum (A63.0)

R85.82 Anal low risk human papillomavirus [HPV] DNA test positive
Use additional code for associated human papillomavirus (B97.7)

R85.89 Other abnormal findings in specimens from digestive organs and abdominal cavity
Abnormal chromosomal findings in specimens from digestive organs and abdominal cavity

R85.9 Unspecified abnormal finding in specimens from digestive organs and abdominal cavity

R86 Abnormal findings in specimens from male genital organs

INCLUDES abnormal findings in prostatic secretions
abnormal findings in semen, seminal fluid
abnormal spermatozoa

EXCLUDES 1 *azoospermia (N46.0-)*
oligospermia (N46.1-)

R86.0 Abnormal level of enzymes in specimens from male genital organs

R86.1 Abnormal level of hormones in specimens from male genital organs

R86.2 Abnormal level of other drugs, medicaments and biological substances in specimens from male genital organs

R86.3 Abnormal level of substances chiefly nonmedicinal as to source in specimens from male genital organs

R86.4 Abnormal immunological findings in specimens from male genital organs

R86.5 Abnormal microbiological findings in specimens from male genital organs

Positive culture findings in specimens from male genital organs

EXCLUDES 1 *colonization status (Z22.-)*

R86.6 Abnormal cytological findings in specimens from male genital organs

R86.7 Abnormal histological findings in specimens from male genital organs

R86.8 Other abnormal findings in specimens from male genital organs

Abnormal chromosomal findings in specimens from male genital organs

R86.9 Unspecified abnormal finding in specimens from male genital organs

R87 Abnormal findings in specimens from female genital organs

Abnormal findings in secretion and smears from cervix uteri
Abnormal findings in secretion and smears from vagina
Abnormal findings in secretion and smears from vulva

R87.0 Abnormal level of enzymes in specimens from female genital organs

R87.1 Abnormal level of hormones in specimens from female genital organs

R87.2 Abnormal level of other drugs, medicaments and biological substances in specimens from female genital organs

R87.3 Abnormal level of substances chiefly nonmedicinal as to source in specimens from female genital organs

R87.4 Abnormal immunological findings in specimens from female genital organs

R87.5 Abnormal microbiological findings in specimens from female genital organs

Positive culture findings in specimens from female genital organs

EXCLUDES 1 *colonization status (Z22.-)*

R87.6 Abnormal cytological findings in specimens from female genital organs

R87.61 Abnormal cytological findings in specimens from cervix uteri

EXCLUDES 1 *abnormal cytological findings in specimens from other female genital organs (R87.69)*
abnormal cytological findings in specimens from vagina (R87.62-)
carcinoma in situ of cervix uteri (histologically confirmed) (D06.-)
cervical intraepithelial neoplasia I [CIN I] (N87.0)
cervical intraepithelial neoplasia II [CIN II] (N87.1)
cervical intraepithelial neoplasia III [CIN III] (D06.-)
dysplasia (mild) (moderate) of cervix uteri (histologically confirmed) (N87.-)
severe dysplasia of cervix uteri (histologically confirmed) (D06.-)

EXCLUDES 2 *cervical high risk human papillomavirus (HPV) DNA test positive (R87.810)*
cervical low risk human papillomavirus (HPV) DNA test positive (R87.820)

R87.610 Atypical squamous cells of undetermined significance on cytologic smear of cervix [ASC-US]

R87.611 Atypical squamous cells cannot exclude high grade squamous intraepithelial lesion on cytologic smear of cervix [ASC-H]

R87.612 Low grade squamous intraepithelial lesion on cytologic smear of cervix [LGSIL]

R87.613 High grade squamous intraepithelial lesion on cytologic smear of cervix [HGSIL]

R87.614 Cytologic evidence of malignancy on smear of cervix

R87.615 Unsatisfactory cytologic smear of cervix

Inadequate sample of cytologic smear of cervix

R87.616 Satisfactory cervical smear but lacking transformation zone

R87.618 Other abnormal cytological findings on specimens from cervix uteri

R87.619 Unspecified abnormal cytological findings in specimens from cervix uteri

Abnormal cervical cytology NOS
Abnormal Papanicolaou smear of cervix NOS
Abnormal thin preparation smear of cervix NOS
Atypical endocervial cells of cervix NOS
Atypical endometrial cells of cervix NOS
Atypical glandular cells of cervix NOS

R87.62 Abnormal cytological findings in specimens from vagina

Use additional code to identify acquired absence of uterus and cervix, if applicable (Z90.71-)

EXCLUDES 1 *abnormal cytological findings in specimens from cervix uteri (R87.61-)*
abnormal cytological findings in specimens from other female genital organs (R87.69)
carcinoma in situ of vagina (histologically confirmed) (D07.2)
dysplasia (mild) (moderate) of vagina (histologically confirmed) (N89.-)
severe dysplasia of vagina (histologically confirmed) (D07.2)
vaginal intraepithelial neoplasia I [VAIN I] (N89.0)
vaginal intraepithelial neoplasia II [VAIN II] (N89.1)
vaginal intraepithelial neoplasia III [VAIN III] (D07.2)

EXCLUDES 2 *vaginal high risk human papillomavirus (HPV) DNA test positive (R87.811)*
vaginal low risk human papillomavirus (HPV) DNA test positive (R87.821)

R87.620 Atypical squamous cells of undetermined significance on cytologic smear of vagina [ASC-US]

R87.621 Atypical squamous cells cannot exclude high grade squamous intraepithelial lesion on cytologic smear of vagina [ASC-H]

R87.622 Low grade squamous intraepithelial lesion on cytologic smear of vagina [LGSIL]

R87.623 High grade squamous intraepithelial lesion on cytologic smear of vagina [HGSIL]

R87.624 Cytologic evidence of malignancy on smear of vagina

R87.625 Unsatisfactory cytologic smear of vagina

Inadequate sample of cytologic smear of vagina

R87.628 Other abnormal cytological findings on specimens from vagina

R87.629 Unspecified abnormal cytological findings in specimens from vagina
Abnormal Papanicolaou smear of vagina NOS
Abnormal thin preparation smear of vagina NOS
Abnormal vaginal cytology NOS
Atypical endocervical cells of vagina NOS
Atypical endometrial cells of vagina NOS
Atypical glandular cells of vagina NOS

R87.69 Abnormal cytological findings in specimens from other female genital organs
Abnormal cytological findings in specimens from female genital organs NOS
EXCLUDES 1 *dysplasia of vulva (histologically confirmed) (N9Ø.Ø-N9Ø.3)*

R87.7 Abnormal histological findings in specimens from female genital organs
EXCLUDES 1 *carcinoma in situ (histologically confirmed) of female genital organs (DØ6-DØ7.3)*
cervical intraepithelial neoplasia I [CIN I] (N87.Ø)
cervical intraepithelial neoplasia II [CIN II] (N87.1)
cervical intraepithelial neoplasia III [CIN III] (DØ6.-)
dysplasia (mild) (moderate) of cervix uteri (histologically confirmed) (N87.-)
dysplasia (mild) (moderate) of vagina (histologically confirmed) (N89.-)
severe dysplasia of cervix uteri (histologically confirmed) (DØ6.-)
severe dysplasia of vagina (histologically confirmed) (DØ7.2)
vaginal intraepithelial neoplasia I [VAIN I] (N89.Ø)
vaginal intraepithelial neoplasia II [VAIN II] (N89.1)
vaginal intraepithelial neoplasia III [VAIN III] (DØ7.2)

✓5th **R87.8 Other abnormal findings in specimens from female genital organs**

✓6th **R87.81 High risk human papillomavirus [HPV] DNA test positive from female genital organs**
EXCLUDES 1 *anogenital warts due to human papillomavirus (HPV) (A63.Ø)*
condyloma acuminatum (A63.Ø)

R87.81Ø Cervical high risk human papillomavirus [HPV] DNA test positive

R87.811 Vaginal high risk human papillomavirus [HPV] DNA test positive

✓6th **R87.82 Low risk human papillomavirus [HPV] DNA test positive from female genital organs**
Use additional code for associated human papillomavirus (B97.7)

R87.82Ø Cervical low risk human papillomavirus [HPV] DNA test positive

R87.821 Vaginal low risk human papillomavirus [HPV] DNA test positive

R87.89 Other abnormal findings in specimens from female genital organs
Abnormal chromosomal findings in specimens from female genital organs

R87.9 Unspecified abnormal finding in specimens from female genital organs

✓4th **R88 Abnormal findings in other body fluids and substances**

R88.Ø Cloudy (hemodialysis) (peritoneal) dialysis effluent

R88.8 Abnormal findings in other body fluids and substances

✓4th **R89 Abnormal findings in specimens from other organs, systems and tissues**
INCLUDES abnormal findings in nipple discharge
abnormal findings in synovial fluid
abnormal findings in wound secretions

R89.Ø Abnormal level of enzymes in specimens from other organs, systems and tissues

R89.1 Abnormal level of hormones in specimens from other organs, systems and tissues

R89.2 Abnormal level of other drugs, medicaments and biological substances in specimens from other organs, systems and tissues

R89.3 Abnormal level of substances chiefly nonmedicinal as to source in specimens from other organs, systems and tissues

R89.4 Abnormal immunological findings in specimens from other organs, systems and tissues

R89.5 Abnormal microbiological findings in specimens from other organs, systems and tissues
Positive culture findings in specimens from other organs, systems and tissues
EXCLUDES 1 *colonization status (Z22.-)*

R89.6 Abnormal cytological findings in specimens from other organs, systems and tissues

R89.7 Abnormal histological findings in specimens from other organs, systems and tissues

R89.8 Other abnormal findings in specimens from other organs, systems and tissues
Abnormal chromosomal findings in specimens from other organs, systems and tissues

R89.9 Unspecified abnormal finding in specimens from other organs, systems and tissues

Abnormal findings on diagnostic imaging and in function studies, without diagnosis (R9Ø-R94)

INCLUDES nonspecific abnormal findings on diagnostic imaging by computerized axial tomography [CAT scan]
nonspecific abnormal findings on diagnostic imaging by magnetic resonance imaging [MRI][NMR]
nonspecific abnormal findings on diagnostic imaging by positron emission tomography [PET scan]
nonspecific abnormal findings on diagnostic imaging by thermography
nonspecific abnormal findings on diagnostic imaging by ultrasound [echogram]
nonspecific abnormal findings on diagnostic imaging by X-ray examination
EXCLUDES 1 *abnormal findings on antenatal screening of mother (O28.-)*
diagnostic abnormal findings classified elsewhere—see Alphabetical Index

✓4th **R9Ø Abnormal findings on diagnostic imaging of central nervous system**

R9Ø.Ø Intracranial space-occupying lesion found on diagnostic imaging of central nervous system

✓5th **R9Ø.8 Other abnormal findings on diagnostic imaging of central nervous system**

R9Ø.81 Abnormal echoencephalogram

R9Ø.82 White matter disease, unspecified

R9Ø.89 Other abnormal findings on diagnostic imaging of central nervous system
Other cerebrovascular abnormality found on diagnostic imaging of central nervous system

✓4th **R91 Abnormal findings on diagnostic imaging of lung**

R91.1 Solitary pulmonary nodule
Coin lesion lung
Solitary pulmonary nodule, subsegmental branch of the bronchial tree

R91.8 Other nonspecific abnormal finding of lung field
Lung mass NOS found on diagnostic imaging of lung
Pulmonary infiltrate NOS
Shadow, lung

✓4th **R92 Abnormal and inconclusive findings on diagnostic imaging of breast**

R92.Ø Mammographic microcalcification found on diagnostic imaging of breast
EXCLUDES 2 *mammographic calcification (calculus) found on diagnostic imaging of breast (R92.1)*

R92.1 Mammographic calcification found on diagnostic imaging of breast
Mammographic calculus found on diagnostic imaging of breast

R92.2 Inconclusive mammogram
Dense breasts NOS
Inconclusive mammogram NEC
Inconclusive mammography due to dense breasts
Inconclusive mammography NEC

R92.8 Other abnormal and inconclusive findings on diagnostic imaging of breast

✓4th **R93 Abnormal findings on diagnostic imaging of other body structures**

R93.Ø Abnormal findings on diagnostic imaging of skull and head, not elsewhere classified
EXCLUDES 1 *intracranial space-occupying lesion found on diagnostic imaging (R9Ø.Ø)*

R93.1 Abnormal findings on diagnostic imaging of heart and coronary circulation
Abnormal echocardiogram NOS
Abnormal heart shadow

R93.2 Abnormal findings on diagnostic imaging of liver and biliary tract
Nonvisualization of gallbladder

R93.3 Abnormal findings on diagnostic imaging of other parts of digestive tract

R93.4 Abnormal findings on diagnostic imaging of urinary organs
Filling defect of bladder found on diagnostic imaging
Filling defect of kidney found on diagnostic imaging
Filling defect of ureter found on diagnostic imaging
EXCLUDES 1 *hypertrophy of kidney (N28.81)*

R93.5 Abnormal findings on diagnostic imaging of other abdominal regions, including retroperitoneum

R93.6 Abnormal findings on diagnostic imaging of limbs
EXCLUDES 2 *abnormal finding in skin and subcutaneous tissue (R93.8)*

R93.7 Abnormal findings on diagnostic imaging of other parts of musculoskeletal system
EXCLUDES 2 *abnormal findings on diagnostic imaging of skull (R93.0)*

R93.8 Abnormal findings on diagnostic imaging of other specified body structures
Abnormal finding by radioisotope localization of placenta
Abnormal radiological finding in skin and subcutaneous tissue
Mediastinal shift

R93.9 Diagnostic imaging inconclusive due to excess body fat of patient

✓4th **R94 Abnormal results of function studies**
INCLUDES abnormal results of radionuclide [radioisotope] uptake studies
abnormal results of scintigraphy

✓5th **R94.0 Abnormal results of function studies of central nervous system**
R94.01 Abnormal electroencephalogram [EEG]
R94.02 Abnormal brain scan
R94.09 Abnormal results of other function studies of central nervous system

✓5th **R94.1 Abnormal results of function studies of peripheral nervous system and special senses**
✓6th **R94.11 Abnormal results of function studies of eye**
R94.110 Abnormal electro-oculogram [EOG]
R94.111 Abnormal electroretinogram [ERG]
Abnormal retinal function study
R94.112 Abnormal visually evoked potential [VEP]
R94.113 Abnormal oculomotor study
R94.118 Abnormal results of other function studies of eye
✓6th **R94.12 Abnormal results of function studies of ear and other special senses**
R94.120 Abnormal auditory function study
R94.121 Abnormal vestibular function study
R94.128 Abnormal results of other function studies of ear and other special senses
✓6th **R94.13 Abnormal results of function studies of peripheral nervous system**
R94.130 Abnormal response to nerve stimulation, unspecified
R94.131 Abnormal electromyogram [EMG]
EXCLUDES 1 *electromyogram of eye (R94.113)*
R94.138 Abnormal results of other function studies of peripheral nervous system

R94.2 Abnormal results of pulmonary function studies
Reduced ventilatory capacity
Reduced vital capacity

✓5th **R94.3 Abnormal results of cardiovascular function studies**
R94.30 Abnormal result of cardiovascular function study, unspecified
R94.31 Abnormal electrocardiogram [ECG] [EKG]
EXCLUDES 1 *long QT syndrome (I45.81)*
R94.39 Abnormal result of other cardiovascular function study
Abnormal electrophysiological intracardiac studies
Abnormal phonocardiogram
Abnormal vectorcardiogram

R94.4 Abnormal results of kidney function studies
Abnormal renal function test

R94.5 Abnormal results of liver function studies

R94.6 Abnormal results of thyroid function studies

R94.7 Abnormal results of other endocrine function studies
EXCLUDES 2 *abnormal glucose (R73.0-)*

R94.8 Abnormal results of function studies of other organs and systems
Abnormal basal metabolic rate [BMR]
Abnormal bladder function test
Abnormal splenic function test

Abnormal tumor markers (R97)

✓4th **R97 Abnormal tumor markers**
Elevated tumor associated antigens [TAA]
Elevated tumor specific antigens [TSA]
R97.0 Elevated carcinoembryonic antigen [CEA]
R97.1 Elevated cancer antigen 125 [CA 125]
R97.2 Elevated prostate specific antigen [PSA]
R97.8 Other abnormal tumor markers

Ill-defined and unknown cause of mortality (R99)

R99 Ill-defined and unknown cause of mortality
Death (unexplained) NOS
Unspecified cause of mortality

Chapter 19. Injury, Poisoning and Certain Other Consequences of External Causes (S00-T88)

NOTE Use secondary code(s) from Chapter 20, External causes of morbidity, to indicate cause of injury. Codes within the T section that include the external cause do not require an additional external cause code

Use additional code to identify any retained foreign body, if applicable (Z18.-)

EXCLUDES 1 *birth trauma (P10-P15)*
obstetric trauma (O70-O71)

This chapter contains the following blocks:

S00-S09	Injuries to the head
S10-S19	Injuries to the neck
S20-S29	Injuries to the thorax
S30-S39	Injuries to the abdomen, lower back, lumbar spine, pelvis and external genitals
S40-S49	Injuries to the shoulder and upper arm
S50-S59	Injuries to the elbow and forearm
S60-S69	Injuries to the wrist, hand and fingers
S70-S79	Injuries to the hip and thigh
S80-S89	Injuries to the knee and lower leg
S90-S99	Injuries to the ankle and foot
T07	Injuries involving multiple body regions
T14	Injury of unspecified body region
T15-T19	Effects of foreign body entering through natural orifice
T20-T25	Burns and corrosions of external body surface, specified by site
T26-T28	Burns and corrosions confined to eye and internal organs
T30-T32	Burns and corrosions of multiple and unspecified body regions
T33-T34	Frostbite
T36-T50	Poisoning by, adverse effect of and underdosing of drugs, medicaments and biological substances
T51-T65	Toxic effects of substances chiefly nonmedicinal as to source
T66-T78	Other and unspecified effects of external causes
T79	Certain early complications of trauma
T80-T88	Complications of surgical and medical care, not elsewhere classified

The chapter uses the S-section for coding different types of injuries related to single body regions and the T-section to cover injuries to unspecified body regions as well as poisoning and certain other consequences of external causes.

Injuries to the head (S00-S09)

INCLUDES injuries of ear
injuries of eye
injuries of face [any part]
injuries of gum
injuries of jaw
injuries of oral cavity
injuries of palate
injuries of periocular area
injuries of scalp
injuries of temporomandibular joint area
injuries of tongue
injuries of tooth

Code also for any associated infection

EXCLUDES 2 *burns and corrosions (T20-T32)*
effects of foreign body in ear (T16)
effects of foreign body in larynx (T17.3)
effects of foreign body in mouth NOS (T18.0)
effects of foreign body in nose (T17.0-T17.1)
effects of foreign body in pharynx (T17.2)
effects of foreign body on external eye (T15.-)
frostbite (T33-T34)
insect bite or sting, venomous (T63.4)

√4th **S00 Superficial injury of head**
EXCLUDES 1 *diffuse cerebral contusion (S06.2-)*
focal cerebral contusion (S06.3-)
injury of eye and orbit (S05.-)
open wound of head (S01.-)

The appropriate 7th character is to be added to each code from category S00.
A initial encounter
D subsequent encounter
S sequela

√5th **S00.0 Superficial injury of scalp**
√x7th **S00.00 Unspecified superficial injury of scalp**
√x7th **S00.01 Abrasion of scalp**
√x7th **S00.02 Blister (nonthermal) of scalp**
√x7th **S00.03 Contusion of scalp**
Bruise of scalp
Hematoma of scalp
√x7th **S00.04 External constriction of part of scalp**
√x7th **S00.05 Superficial foreign body of scalp**
Splinter in the scalp
√x7th **S00.06 Insect bite (nonvenomous) of scalp**
√x7th **S00.07 Other superficial bite of scalp**
EXCLUDES 1 *open bite of scalp (S01.05)*

√5th **S00.1 Contusion of eyelid and periocular area**
Black eye
EXCLUDES 2 *contusion of eyeball and orbital tissues (S05.1)*
√x7th **S00.10 Contusion of unspecified eyelid and periocular area**
√x7th **S00.11 Contusion of right eyelid and periocular area**
√x7th **S00.12 Contusion of left eyelid and periocular area**

√5th **S00.2 Other and unspecified superficial injuries of eyelid and periocular area**
EXCLUDES 2 *superficial injury of conjunctiva and cornea (S05.0-)*
√6th **S00.20 Unspecified superficial injury of eyelid and periocular area**
√7th **S00.201 Unspecified superficial injury of right eyelid and periocular area**
√7th **S00.202 Unspecified superficial injury of left eyelid and periocular area**
√7th **S00.209 Unspecified superficial injury of unspecified eyelid and periocular area**
√6th **S00.21 Abrasion of eyelid and periocular area**
√7th **S00.211 Abrasion of right eyelid and periocular area**
√7th **S00.212 Abrasion of left eyelid and periocular area**
√7th **S00.219 Abrasion of unspecified eyelid and periocular area**
√6th **S00.22 Blister (nonthermal) of eyelid and periocular area**
√7th **S00.221 Blister (nonthermal) of right eyelid and periocular area**
√7th **S00.222 Blister (nonthermal) of left eyelid and periocular area**
√7th **S00.229 Blister (nonthermal) of unspecified eyelid and periocular area**
√6th **S00.24 External constriction of eyelid and periocular area**
√7th **S00.241 External constriction of right eyelid and periocular area**
√7th **S00.242 External constriction of left eyelid and periocular area**
√7th **S00.249 External constriction of unspecified eyelid and periocular area**
√6th **S00.25 Superficial foreign body of eyelid and periocular area**
Splinter of eyelid and periocular area
EXCLUDES 2 *retained foreign body in eyelid (H02.81-)*
√7th **S00.251 Superficial foreign body of right eyelid and periocular area**
√7th **S00.252 Superficial foreign body of left eyelid and periocular area**
√7th **S00.259 Superficial foreign body of unspecified eyelid and periocular area**
√6th **S00.26 Insect bite (nonvenomous) of eyelid and periocular area**
√7th **S00.261 Insect bite (nonvenomous) of right eyelid and periocular area**
√7th **S00.262 Insect bite (nonvenomous) of left eyelid and periocular area**
√7th **S00.269 Insect bite (nonvenomous) of unspecified eyelid and periocular area**
√6th **S00.27 Other superficial bite of eyelid and periocular area**
EXCLUDES 1 *open bite of eyelid and periocular area (S01.15)*
√7th **S00.271 Other superficial bite of right eyelid and periocular area**
√7th **S00.272 Other superficial bite of left eyelid and periocular area**

✓7th S00.279 **Other superficial bite of unspecified eyelid and periocular area**

✓5th **S00.3 Superficial injury of nose**

✓x7th **S00.30 Unspecified superficial injury of nose**

✓x7th **S00.31 Abrasion of nose**

✓x7th **S00.32 Blister (nonthermal) of nose**

✓x7th **S00.33 Contusion of nose**

Bruise of nose
Hematoma of nose

✓x7th **S00.34 External constriction of nose**

✓x7th **S00.35 Superficial foreign body of nose**

Splinter in the nose

✓x7th **S00.36 Insect bite (nonvenomous) of nose**

✓x7th **S00.37 Other superficial bite of nose**

EXCLUDES 1 *open bite of nose (S01.25)*

✓5th **S00.4 Superficial injury of ear**

✓6th **S00.40 Unspecified superficial injury of ear**

✓7th **S00.401 Unspecified superficial injury of right ear**

✓7th **S00.402 Unspecified superficial injury of left ear**

✓7th **S00.409 Unspecified superficial injury of unspecified ear**

✓6th **S00.41 Abrasion of ear**

✓7th **S00.411 Abrasion of right ear**

✓7th **S00.412 Abrasion of left ear**

✓7th **S00.419 Abrasion of unspecified ear**

✓6th **S00.42 Blister (nonthermal) of ear**

✓7th **S00.421 Blister (nonthermal) of right ear**

✓7th **S00.422 Blister (nonthermal) of left ear**

✓7th **S00.429 Blister (nonthermal) of unspecified ear**

✓6th **S00.43 Contusion of ear**

Bruise of ear
Hematoma of ear

✓7th **S00.431 Contusion of right ear**

✓7th **S00.432 Contusion of left ear**

✓7th **S00.439 Contusion of unspecified ear**

✓6th **S00.44 External constriction of ear**

✓7th **S00.441 External constriction of right ear**

✓7th **S00.442 External constriction of left ear**

✓7th **S00.449 External constriction of unspecified ear**

✓6th **S00.45 Superficial foreign body of ear**

Splinter in the ear

✓7th **S00.451 Superficial foreign body of right ear**

✓7th **S00.452 Superficial foreign body of left ear**

✓7th **S00.459 Superficial foreign body of unspecified ear**

✓6th **S00.46 Insect bite (nonvenomous) of ear**

✓7th **S00.461 Insect bite (nonvenomous) of right ear**

✓7th **S00.462 Insect bite (nonvenomous) of left ear**

✓7th **S00.469 Insect bite (nonvenomous) of unspecified ear**

✓6th **S00.47 Other superficial bite of ear**

EXCLUDES 1 *open bite of ear (S01.35)*

✓7th **S00.471 Other superficial bite of right ear**

✓7th **S00.472 Other superficial bite of left ear**

✓7th **S00.479 Other superficial bite of unspecified ear**

✓5th **S00.5 Superficial injury of lip and oral cavity**

✓6th **S00.50 Unspecified superficial injury of lip and oral cavity**

✓7th **S00.501 Unspecified superficial injury of lip**

✓7th **S00.502 Unspecified superficial injury of oral cavity**

✓6th **S00.51 Abrasion of lip and oral cavity**

✓7th **S00.511 Abrasion of lip**

✓7th **S00.512 Abrasion of oral cavity**

✓6th **S00.52 Blister (nonthermal) of lip and oral cavity**

✓7th **S00.521 Blister (nonthermal) of lip**

✓7th **S00.522 Blister (nonthermal) of oral cavity**

✓6th **S00.53 Contusion of lip and oral cavity**

✓7th **S00.531 Contusion of lip**

Bruise of lip
Hematoma of oral cavity

✓7th **S00.532 Contusion of oral cavity**

Bruise of lip
Hematoma of oral cavity

✓6th **S00.54 External constriction of lip and oral cavity**

✓7th **S00.541 External constriction of lip**

✓7th **S00.542 External constriction of oral cavity**

✓6th **S00.55 Superficial foreign body of lip and oral cavity**

✓7th **S00.551 Superficial foreign body of lip**

Splinter of lip and oral cavity

✓7th **S00.552 Superficial foreign body of oral cavity**

Splinter of lip and oral cavity

✓6th **S00.56 Insect bite (nonvenomous) of lip and oral cavity**

✓7th **S00.561 Insect bite (nonvenomous) of lip**

✓7th **S00.562 Insect bite (nonvenomous) of oral cavity**

✓6th **S00.57 Other superficial bite of lip and oral cavity**

✓7th **S00.571 Other superficial bite of lip**

EXCLUDES 1 *open bite of lip (S01.551)*

✓7th **S00.572 Other superficial bite of oral cavity**

EXCLUDES 1 *open bite of oral cavity (S01.552)*

✓5th **S00.8 Superficial injury of other parts of head**

✓x7th **S00.80 Unspecified superficial injury of other part of head**

✓x7th **S00.81 Abrasion of other part of head**

✓x7th **S00.82 Blister (nonthermal) of other part of head**

✓x7th **S00.83 Contusion of other part of head**

Bruise of other part of head
Hematoma of other part of head

✓x7th **S00.84 External constriction of other part of head**

✓x7th **S00.85 Superficial foreign body of other part of head**

Splinter in other part of head

✓x7th **S00.86 Insect bite (nonvenomous) of other part of head**

✓x7th **S00.87 Other superficial bite of other part of head**

EXCLUDES 1 *open bite of other part of head (S01.85)*

✓5th **S00.9 Superficial injury of unspecified part of head**

✓x7th **S00.90 Unspecified superficial injury of unspecified part of head**

✓x7th **S00.91 Abrasion of unspecified part of head**

✓x7th **S00.92 Blister (nonthermal) of unspecified part of head**

✓x7th **S00.93 Contusion of unspecified part of head**

Bruise of head
Hematoma of head

✓x7th **S00.94 External constriction of unspecified part of head**

✓x7th **S00.95 Superficial foreign body of unspecified part of head**

Splinter of head

✓x7th **S00.96 Insect bite (nonvenomous) of unspecified part of head**

✓x7th **S00.97 Other superficial bite of unspecified part of head**

EXCLUDES 1 *open bite of head (S01.95)*

✓4th **S01 Open wound of head**

Code also any associated:
- injury of cranial nerve (S04.-)
- injury of muscle and tendon of head (S09.1-)
- intracranial injury (S06.-)
- wound infection

EXCLUDES 1 *open skull fracture (S02- with 7th character B)*

EXCLUDES 2 *injury of eye and orbit (S05.-)*
traumatic amputation of part of head (S08.-)

The appropriate 7th character is to be added to each code from category S01.
A initial encounter
D subsequent encounter
S sequela

✓5th **S01.0 Open wound of scalp**

EXCLUDES 1 *avulsion of scalp (S08.0)*

✓x7th **S01.00 Unspecified open wound of scalp**

✓x7th **S01.01 Laceration without foreign body of scalp**

✓x7th **S01.02 Laceration with foreign body of scalp**

✓x7th **S01.03 Puncture wound without foreign body of scalp**

✓x7th **S01.04 Puncture wound with foreign body of scalp**

✓x7th **S01.05 Open bite of scalp**

Bite of scalp NOS

EXCLUDES 1 *superficial bite of scalp (S00.06, S00.07-)*

✓5th **SØ1.1 Open wound of eyelid and periocular area**
Open wound of eyelid and periocular area with or without involvement of lacrimal passages

✓6th **SØ1.1Ø Unspecified open wound of eyelid and periocular area**
✓7th **SØ1.1Ø1 Unspecified open wound of right eyelid and periocular area**
✓7th **SØ1.1Ø2 Unspecified open wound of left eyelid and periocular area**
✓7th **SØ1.1Ø9 Unspecified open wound of unspecified eyelid and periocular area**

✓6th **SØ1.11 Laceration without foreign body of eyelid and periocular area**
✓7th **SØ1.111 Laceration without foreign body of right eyelid and periocular area**
✓7th **SØ1.112 Laceration without foreign body of left eyelid and periocular area**
✓7th **SØ1.119 Laceration without foreign body of unspecified eyelid and periocular area**

✓6th **SØ1.12 Laceration with foreign body of eyelid and periocular area**
✓7th **SØ1.121 Laceration with foreign body of right eyelid and periocular area**
✓7th **SØ1.122 Laceration with foreign body of left eyelid and periocular area**
✓7th **SØ1.129 Laceration with foreign body of unspecified eyelid and periocular area**

✓6th **SØ1.13 Puncture wound without foreign body of eyelid and periocular area**
✓7th **SØ1.131 Puncture wound without foreign body of right eyelid and periocular area**
✓7th **SØ1.132 Puncture wound without foreign body of left eyelid and periocular area**
✓7th **SØ1.139 Puncture wound without foreign body of unspecified eyelid and periocular area**

✓6th **SØ1.14 Puncture wound with foreign body of eyelid and periocular area**
✓7th **SØ1.141 Puncture wound with foreign body of right eyelid and periocular area**
✓7th **SØ1.142 Puncture wound with foreign body of left eyelid and periocular area**
✓7th **SØ1.149 Puncture wound with foreign body of unspecified eyelid and periocular area**

✓6th **SØ1.15 Open bite of eyelid and periocular area**
Bite of eyelid and periocular area NOS
EXCLUDES 1 *superficial bite of eyelid and periocular area (SØØ.26, SØØ.27)*
✓7th **SØ1.151 Open bite of right eyelid and periocular area**
✓7th **SØ1.152 Open bite of left eyelid and periocular area**
✓7th **SØ1.159 Open bite of unspecified eyelid and periocular area**

✓5th **SØ1.2 Open wound of nose**
✓x7th **SØ1.2Ø Unspecified open wound of nose**
✓x7th **SØ1.21 Laceration without foreign body of nose**
✓x7th **SØ1.22 Laceration with foreign body of nose**
✓x7th **SØ1.23 Puncture wound without foreign body of nose**
✓x7th **SØ1.24 Puncture wound with foreign body of nose**
✓x7th **SØ1.25 Open bite of nose**
Bite of nose NOS
EXCLUDES 1 *superficial bite of nose (SØØ.36, SØØ.37)*

✓5th **SØ1.3 Open wound of ear**
✓6th **SØ1.3Ø Unspecified open wound of ear**
✓7th **SØ1.3Ø1 Unspecified open wound of right ear**
✓7th **SØ1.3Ø2 Unspecified open wound of left ear**
✓7th **SØ1.3Ø9 Unspecified open wound of unspecified ear**

✓6th **SØ1.31 Laceration without foreign body of ear**
✓7th **SØ1.311 Laceration without foreign body of right ear**
✓7th **SØ1.312 Laceration without foreign body of left ear**
✓7th **SØ1.319 Laceration without foreign body of unspecified ear**

✓6th **SØ1.32 Laceration with foreign body of ear**
✓7th **SØ1.321 Laceration with foreign body of right ear**
✓7th **SØ1.322 Laceration with foreign body of left ear**
✓7th **SØ1.329 Laceration with foreign body of unspecified ear**

✓6th **SØ1.33 Puncture wound without foreign body of ear**
✓7th **SØ1.331 Puncture wound without foreign body of right ear**
✓7th **SØ1.332 Puncture wound without foreign body of left ear**
✓7th **SØ1.339 Puncture wound without foreign body of unspecified ear**

✓6th **SØ1.34 Puncture wound with foreign body of ear**
✓7th **SØ1.341 Puncture wound with foreign body of right ear**
✓7th **SØ1.342 Puncture wound with foreign body of left ear**
✓7th **SØ1.349 Puncture wound with foreign body of unspecified ear**

✓6th **SØ1.35 Open bite of ear**
Bite of ear NOS
EXCLUDES 1 *superficial bite of ear (SØØ.46, SØØ.47)*
✓7th **SØ1.351 Open bite of right ear**
✓7th **SØ1.352 Open bite of left ear**
✓7th **SØ1.359 Open bite of unspecified ear**

✓5th **SØ1.4 Open wound of cheek and temporomandibular area**
✓6th **SØ1.4Ø Unspecified open wound of cheek and temporomandibular area**
✓7th **SØ1.4Ø1 Unspecified open wound of right cheek and temporomandibular area**
✓7th **SØ1.4Ø2 Unspecified open wound of left cheek and temporomandibular area**
✓7th **SØ1.4Ø9 Unspecified open wound of unspecified cheek and temporomandibular area**

✓6th **SØ1.41 Laceration without foreign body of cheek and temporomandibular area**
✓7th **SØ1.411 Laceration without foreign body of right cheek and temporomandibular area**
✓7th **SØ1.412 Laceration without foreign body of left cheek and temporomandibular area**
✓7th **SØ1.419 Laceration without foreign body of unspecified cheek and temporomandibular area**

✓6th **SØ1.42 Laceration with foreign body of cheek and temporomandibular area**
✓7th **SØ1.421 Laceration with foreign body of right cheek and temporomandibular area**
✓7th **SØ1.422 Laceration with foreign body of left cheek and temporomandibular area**
✓7th **SØ1.429 Laceration with foreign body of unspecified cheek and temporomandibular area**

✓6th **SØ1.43 Puncture wound without foreign body of cheek and temporomandibular area**
✓7th **SØ1.431 Puncture wound without foreign body of right cheek and temporomandibular area**
✓7th **SØ1.432 Puncture wound without foreign body of left cheek and temporomandibular area**
✓7th **SØ1.439 Puncture wound without foreign body of unspecified cheek and temporomandibular area**

✓6th **SØ1.44 Puncture wound with foreign body of cheek and temporomandibular area**
✓7th **SØ1.441 Puncture wound with foreign body of right cheek and temporomandibular area**
✓7th **SØ1.442 Puncture wound with foreign body of left cheek and temporomandibular area**
✓7th **SØ1.449 Puncture wound with foreign body of unspecified cheek and temporomandibular area**

√6th **S01.45 Open bite of cheek and temporomandibular area**
Bite of cheek and temporomandibular area NOS
EXCLUDES 2 *superficial bite of cheek and temporomandibular area (S00.86, S00.87)*
√7th **S01.451 Open bite of right cheek and temporomandibular area**
√7th **S01.452 Open bite of left cheek and temporomandibular area**
√7th **S01.459 Open bite of unspecified cheek and temporomandibular area**

√5th **S01.5 Open wound of lip and oral cavity**
EXCLUDES 2 *tooth dislocation (S03.2)*
tooth fracture (S02.5)
√6th **S01.50 Unspecified open wound of lip and oral cavity**
√7th **S01.501 Unspecified open wound of lip**
√7th **S01.502 Unspecified open wound of oral cavity**
√6th **S01.51 Laceration of lip and oral cavity without foreign body**
√7th **S01.511 Laceration without foreign body of lip**
√7th **S01.512 Laceration without foreign body of oral cavity**
√6th **S01.52 Laceration of lip and oral cavity with foreign body**
√7th **S01.521 Laceration with foreign body of lip**
√7th **S01.522 Laceration with foreign body of oral cavity**
√6th **S01.53 Puncture wound of lip and oral cavity without foreign body**
√7th **S01.531 Puncture wound without foreign body of lip**
√7th **S01.532 Puncture wound without foreign body of oral cavity**
√6th **S01.54 Puncture wound of lip and oral cavity with foreign body**
√7th **S01.541 Puncture wound with foreign body of lip**
√7th **S01.542 Puncture wound with foreign body of oral cavity**
√6th **S01.55 Open bite of lip and oral cavity**
√7th **S01.551 Open bite of lip**
Bite of lip NOS
EXCLUDES 1 *superficial bite of lip (S00.571)*
√7th **S01.552 Open bite of oral cavity**
Bite of oral cavity NOS
EXCLUDES 1 *superficial bite of oral cavity (S00.572)*

√5th **S01.8 Open wound of other parts of head**
√x7th **S01.80 Unspecified open wound of other part of head**
√x7th **S01.81 Laceration without foreign body of other part of head**
√x7th **S01.82 Laceration with foreign body of other part of head**
√x7th **S01.83 Puncture wound without foreign body of other part of head**
√x7th **S01.84 Puncture wound with foreign body of other part of head**
√x7th **S01.85 Open bite of other part of head**
Bite of other part of head NOS
EXCLUDES 1 *superficial bite of other part of head (S00.85)*

√5th **S01.9 Open wound of unspecified part of head**
√x7th **S01.90 Unspecified open wound of unspecified part of head**
√x7th **S01.91 Laceration without foreign body of unspecified part of head**
√x7th **S01.92 Laceration with foreign body of unspecified part of head**
√x7th **S01.93 Puncture wound without foreign body of unspecified part of head**
√x7th **S01.94 Puncture wound with foreign body of unspecified part of head**
√x7th **S01.95 Open bite of unspecified part of head**
Bite of head NOS
EXCLUDES 1 *superficial bite of head NOS (S00.97)*

√4th **S02 Fracture of skull and facial bones**
NOTE A fracture not indicated as open or closed should be coded to closed
Code also any associated intracranial injury (S06.-).

The appropriate 7th character is to be added to each code from category S02.
A initial encounter for closed fracture
B initial encounter for open fracture
D subsequent encounter for fracture with routine healing
G subsequent encounter for fracture with delayed healing
K subsequent encounter for fracture with nonunion
S sequela

√x7th **S02.0 Fracture of vault of skull**
Fracture of frontal bone
Fracture of parietal bone
√5th **S02.1 Fracture of base of skull**
EXCLUDES 1 *orbit NOS (S02.8)*
EXCLUDES 2 *orbital floor (S02.3-)*
√x7th **S02.10 Unspecified fracture of base of skull**
√6th **S02.11 Fracture of occiput**
√7th **S02.110 Type I occipital condyle fracture**
√7th **S02.111 Type II occipital condyle fracture**
√7th **S02.112 Type III occipital condyle fracture**
√7th **S02.113 Unspecified occipital condyle fracture**
√7th **S02.118 Other fracture of occiput**
√7th **S02.119 Unspecified fracture of occiput**
√x7th **S02.19 Other fracture of base of skull**
Fracture of anterior fossa of base of skull
Fracture of ethmoid sinus
Fracture of frontal sinus
Fracture of middle fossa of base of skull
Fracture of orbital roof
Fracture of posterior fossa of base of skull
Fracture of sphenoid
Fracture of temporal bone
√x7th **S02.2 Fracture of nasal bones**
√x7th **S02.3 Fracture of orbital floor**
EXCLUDES 1 *orbit NOS (S02.8)*
EXCLUDES 2 *orbital roof (S02.1-)*
√5th **S02.4 Fracture of malar, maxillary and zygoma bones**
Fracture of superior maxilla
Fracture of upper jaw (bone)
Fracture of zygomatic process of temporal bone
√6th **S02.40 Fracture of malar, maxillary and zygoma bones, unspecified**
√7th **S02.400 Malar fracture unspecified**
√7th **S02.401 Maxillary fracture, unspecified**
√7th **S02.402 Zygomatic fracture, unspecified**
√6th **S02.41 LeFort fracture**
√7th **S02.411 LeFort I fracture**
√7th **S02.412 LeFort II fracture**
√7th **S02.413 LeFort III fracture**
√x7th **S02.42 Fracture of alveolus of maxilla**
√x7th **S02.5 Fracture of tooth (traumatic)**
Broken tooth
EXCLUDES 1 *cracked tooth (nontraumatic) (K03.81)*
√5th **S02.6 Fracture of mandible**
Fracture of lower jaw (bone)
√6th **S02.60 Fracture of mandible, unspecified**
√7th **S02.600 Fracture of unspecified part of body of mandible**
√7th **S02.609 Fracture of mandible, unspecified**
√x7th **S02.61 Fracture of condylar process of mandible**
√x7th **S02.62 Fracture of subcondylar process of mandible**
√x7th **S02.63 Fracture of coronoid process of mandible**
√x7th **S02.64 Fracture of ramus of mandible**
√x7th **S02.65 Fracture of angle of mandible**
√x7th **S02.66 Fracture of symphysis of mandible**
√x7th **S02.67 Fracture of alveolus of mandible**
√x7th **S02.69 Fracture of mandible of other specified site**
√x7th **S02.8 Fractures of other specified skull and facial bones**
Fracture of orbit NOS
Fracture of palate
EXCLUDES 1 *fracture of orbital floor (S02.3-)*
fracture of orbital roof (S02.1-)

5th **SØ2.9 Fracture of unspecified skull and facial bones**
x7th **SØ2.91 Unspecified fracture of skull**
x7th **SØ2.92 Unspecified fracture of facial bones**

4th **SØ3 Dislocation and sprain of joints and ligaments of head**
INCLUDES avulsion of joint (capsule) or ligament of head
laceration of cartilage, joint (capsule) or ligament of head
sprain of cartilage, joint (capsule) or ligament of head
traumatic hemarthrosis of joint or ligament of head
traumatic rupture of joint or ligament of head
traumatic subluxation of joint or ligament of head
traumatic tear of joint or ligament of head
Code also any associated open wound
EXCLUDES 2 *strain of muscle or tendon of head (SØ9.1)*

The appropriate 7th character is to be added to each code from category SØ3.
A initial encounter
D subsequent encounter
S sequela

x7th **SØ3.Ø Dislocation of jaw**
Dislocation of jaw (cartilage) (meniscus)
Dislocation of mandible
Dislocation of temporomandibular (joint)
x7th **SØ3.1 Dislocation of septal cartilage of nose**
x7th **SØ3.2 Dislocation of tooth**
x7th **SØ3.4 Sprain of jaw**
Sprain of temporomandibular (joint) (ligament)
x7th **SØ3.8 Sprain of joints and ligaments of other parts of head**
x7th **SØ3.9 Sprain of joints and ligaments of unspecified parts of head**

4th **SØ4 Injury of cranial nerve**
The selection of side should be based on the side of the body being affected
Codes first any associated intracranial injury (SØ6.-)
Code also any associated:
open wound of head (SØ1.-)
skull fracture (SØ2.-)

The appropriate 7th character is to be added to each code from category SØ4.
A initial encounter
D subsequent encounter
S sequela

5th **SØ4.Ø Injury of optic nerve and pathways**
Use additional code to identify any visual field defect or blindness (H53.4-, H54)
6th **SØ4.Ø1 Injury of optic nerve**
Injury of 2nd cranial nerve
7th **SØ4.Ø11 Injury of optic nerve, right eye**
7th **SØ4.Ø12 Injury of optic nerve, left eye**
7th **SØ4.Ø19 Injury of optic nerve, unspecified eye**
Injury of optic nerve NOS
x7th **SØ4.Ø2 Injury of optic chiasm**
6th **SØ4.Ø3 Injury of optic tract and pathways**
Injury of optic radiation
7th **SØ4.Ø31 Injury of optic tract and pathways, right eye**
7th **SØ4.Ø32 Injury of optic tract and pathways, left eye**
7th **SØ4.Ø39 Injury of optic tract and pathways, unspecified eye**
Injury of optic tract and pathways NOS
6th **SØ4.Ø4 Injury of visual cortex**
7th **SØ4.Ø41 Injury of visual cortex, right eye**
7th **SØ4.Ø42 Injury of visual cortex, left eye**
7th **SØ4.Ø49 Injury of visual cortex, unspecified eye**
Injury of visual cortex NOS
5th **SØ4.1 Injury of oculomotor nerve**
Injury of 3rd cranial nerve
x7th **SØ4.1Ø Injury of oculomotor nerve, unspecified side**
x7th **SØ4.11 Injury of oculomotor nerve, right side**
x7th **SØ4.12 Injury of oculomotor nerve, left side**
5th **SØ4.2 Injury of trochlear nerve**
Injury of 4th cranial nerve
x7th **SØ4.2Ø Injury of trochlear nerve, unspecified side**
x7th **SØ4.21 Injury of trochlear nerve, right side**
x7th **SØ4.22 Injury of trochlear nerve, left side**
5th **SØ4.3 Injury of trigeminal nerve**
Injury of 5th cranial nerve
x7th **SØ4.3Ø Injury of trigeminal nerve, unspecified side**
x7th **SØ4.31 Injury of trigeminal nerve, right side**
x7th **SØ4.32 Injury of trigeminal nerve, left side**
5th **SØ4.4 Injury of abducent nerve**
Injury of 6th cranial nerve
x7th **SØ4.4Ø Injury of abducent nerve, unspecified side**
x7th **SØ4.41 Injury of abducent nerve, right side**
x7th **SØ4.42 Injury of abducent nerve, left side**
5th **SØ4.5 Injury of facial nerve**
Injury of 7th cranial nerve
x7th **SØ4.5Ø Injury of facial nerve, unspecified side**
x7th **SØ4.51 Injury of facial nerve, right side**
x7th **SØ4.52 Injury of facial nerve, left side**
5th **SØ4.6 Injury of acoustic nerve**
Injury of auditory nerve
Injury of 8th cranial nerve
x7th **SØ4.6Ø Injury of acoustic nerve, unspecified side**
x7th **SØ4.61 Injury of acoustic nerve, right side**
x7th **SØ4.62 Injury of acoustic nerve, left side**
5th **SØ4.7 Injury of accessory nerve**
Injury of 11th cranial nerve
x7th **SØ4.7Ø Injury of accessory nerve, unspecified side**
x7th **SØ4.71 Injury of accessory nerve, right side**
x7th **SØ4.72 Injury of accessory nerve, left side**
5th **SØ4.8 Injury of other cranial nerves**
6th **SØ4.81 Injury of olfactory [1st] nerve**
7th **SØ4.811 Injury of olfactory [1st] nerve, right side**
7th **SØ4.812 Injury of olfactory [1st] nerve, left side**
7th **SØ4.819 Injury of olfactory [1st] nerve, unspecified side**
6th **SØ4.89 Injury of other cranial nerves**
Injury of vagus [1Øth] nerve
7th **SØ4.891 Injury of other cranial nerves, right side**
7th **SØ4.892 Injury of other cranial nerves, left side**
7th **SØ4.899 Injury of other cranial nerves, unspecified side**
SØ4.9 Injury of unspecified cranial nerve

4th **SØ5 Injury of eye and orbit**
Open wound of eye and orbit
EXCLUDES 2 *2nd cranial [optic] nerve injury (SØ4.Ø-)*
3rd cranial [oculomotor] nerve injury (SØ4.1-)
open wound of eyelid and periocular area (SØ1.1-)
orbital bone fracture (SØ2.1-, SØ2.3-, SØ2.8-)
superficial injury of eyelid (SØØ.1-SØØ.2)

The appropriate 7th character is to be added to each code from category SØ5.
A initial encounter
D subsequent encounter
S sequela

5th **SØ5.Ø Injury of conjunctiva and corneal abrasion without foreign body**
EXCLUDES 1 *foreign body in conjunctival sac (T15.1)*
foreign body in cornea (T15.Ø)
x7th **SØ5.ØØ Injury of conjunctiva and corneal abrasion without foreign body, unspecified eye**
x7th **SØ5.Ø1 Injury of conjunctiva and corneal abrasion without foreign body, right eye**
x7th **SØ5.Ø2 Injury of conjunctiva and corneal abrasion without foreign body, left eye**
5th **SØ5.1 Contusion of eyeball and orbital tissues**
Traumatic hyphema
EXCLUDES 2 *black eye NOS (SØØ.1)*
contusion of eyelid and periocular area (SØØ.1)
x7th **SØ5.1Ø Contusion of eyeball and orbital tissues, unspecified eye**
x7th **SØ5.11 Contusion of eyeball and orbital tissues, right eye**
x7th **SØ5.12 Contusion of eyeball and orbital tissues, left eye**
5th **SØ5.2 Ocular laceration and rupture with prolapse or loss of intraocular tissue**
x7th **SØ5.2Ø Ocular laceration and rupture with prolapse or loss of intraocular tissue, unspecified eye**
x7th **SØ5.21 Ocular laceration and rupture with prolapse or loss of intraocular tissue, right eye**

√x7th **S05.22 Ocular laceration and rupture with prolapse or loss of intraocular tissue, left eye**

√5th **S05.3 Ocular laceration without prolapse or loss of intraocular tissue**
Laceration of eye NOS

√x7th **S05.30 Ocular laceration without prolapse or loss of intraocular tissue, unspecified eye**

√x7th **S05.31 Ocular laceration without prolapse or loss of intraocular tissue, right eye**

√x7th **S05.32 Ocular laceration without prolapse or loss of intraocular tissue, left eye**

√5th **S05.4 Penetrating wound of orbit with or without foreign body**
EXCLUDES 2 *retained (old) foreign body following penetrating wound in orbit (H05.5-)*

√x7th **S05.40 Penetrating wound of orbit with or without foreign body, unspecified eye**

√x7th **S05.41 Penetrating wound of orbit with or without foreign body, right eye**

√x7th **S05.42 Penetrating wound of orbit with or without foreign body, left eye**

√5th **S05.5 Penetrating wound with foreign body of eyeball**
EXCLUDES 2 *retained (old) intraocular foreign body (H44.6-, H44.7)*

√x7th **S05.50 Penetrating wound with foreign body of unspecified eyeball**

√x7th **S05.51 Penetrating wound with foreign body of right eyeball**

√x7th **S05.52 Penetrating wound with foreign body of left eyeball**

√5th **S05.6 Penetrating wound without foreign body of eyeball**
Ocular penetration NOS

√x7th **S05.60 Penetrating wound without foreign body of unspecified eyeball**

√x7th **S05.61 Penetrating wound without foreign body of right eyeball**

√x7th **S05.62 Penetrating wound without foreign body of left eyeball**

√5th **S05.7 Avulsion of eye**
Traumatic enucleation

√x7th **S05.70 Avulsion of unspecified eye**

√x7th **S05.71 Avulsion of right eye**

√x7th **S05.72 Avulsion of left eye**

√5th **S05.8 Other injuries of eye and orbit**
Lacrimal duct injury

√6th **S05.8X Other injuries of eye and orbit**

√7th **S05.8X1 Other injuries of right eye and orbit**

√7th **S05.8X2 Other injuries of left eye and orbit**

√7th **S05.8X9 Other injuries of unspecified eye and orbit**

√5th **S05.9 Unspecified injury of eye and orbit**
Injury of eye NOS

√x7th **S05.90 Unspecified injury of unspecified eye and orbit**

√x7th **S05.91 Unspecified injury of right eye and orbit**

√x7th **S05.92 Unspecified injury of left eye and orbit**

√4th **S06 Intracranial injury**
Traumatic brain injury
Code also any associated:
open wound of head (S01.-)
skull fracture (S02.-)
EXCLUDES 1 *head injury NOS (S09.90)*

The appropriate 7th character is to be added to each code from category S06.
A initial encounter
D subsequent encounter
S sequela

√5th **S06.0 Concussion**
Commotio cerebri
EXCLUDES 1 *concussion with other intracranial injuries classified in category S06—code to specified intracranial injury*

√6th **S06.0X Concussion**

√7th **S06.0X0 Concussion without loss of consciousness**

√7th **S06.0X1 Concussion with loss of consciousness of 30 minutes or less**

√7th **S06.0X2 Concussion with loss of consciousness of 31 minutes to 59 minutes**

√7th **S06.0X3 Concussion with loss of consciousness of 1 hour to 5 hours 59 minutes**

√7th **S06.0X4 Concussion with loss of consciousness of 6 hours to 24 hours**

√7th **S06.0X5 Concussion with loss of consciousness greater than 24 hours with return to pre-existing conscious level**

√7th **S06.0X6 Concussion with loss of consciousness greater than 24 hours without return to pre-existing conscious level with patient surviving**

√7th **S06.0X7 Concussion with loss of consciousness of any duration with death due to brain injury prior to regaining consciousness**

√7th **S06.0X8 Concussion with loss of consciousness of any duration with death due to other cause prior to regaining consciousness**

√7th **S06.0X9 Concussion with loss of consciousness of unspecified duration**
Concussion NOS

√5th **S06.1 Traumatic cerebral edema**
Diffuse traumatic cerebral edema
Focal traumatic cerebral edema

√6th **S06.1X Traumatic cerebral edema**

√7th **S06.1X0 Traumatic cerebral edema without loss of consciousness**

√7th **S06.1X1 Traumatic cerebral edema with loss of consciousness of 30 minutes or less**

√7th **S06.1X2 Traumatic cerebral edema with loss of consciousness of 31 minutes to 59 minutes**

√7th **S06.1X3 Traumatic cerebral edema with loss of consciousness of 1 hour to 5 hours 59 minutes**

√7th **S06.1X4 Traumatic cerebral edema with loss of consciousness of 6 hours to 24 hours**

√7th **S06.1X5 Traumatic cerebral edema with loss of consciousness greater than 24 hours with return to pre-existing conscious level**

√7th **S06.1X6 Traumatic cerebral edema with loss of consciousness greater than 24 hours without return to pre-existing conscious level with patient surviving**

√7th **S06.1X7 Traumatic cerebral edema with loss of consciousness of any duration with death due to brain injury prior to regaining consciousness**

√7th **S06.1X8 Traumatic cerebral edema with loss of consciousness of any duration with death due to other cause prior to regaining consciousness**

√7th **S06.1X9 Traumatic cerebral edema with loss of consciousness of unspecified duration**
Traumatic cerebral edema NOS

√5th **S06.2 Diffuse traumatic brain injury**
Diffuse axonal brain injury
EXCLUDES 1 *traumatic diffuse cerebral edema (S06.1X)*

√6th **S06.2X Diffuse traumatic brain injury**

√7th **S06.2X0 Diffuse traumatic brain injury without loss of consciousness**

√7th **S06.2X1 Diffuse traumatic brain injury with loss of consciousness of 30 minutes or less**

√7th **S06.2X2 Diffuse traumatic brain injury with loss of consciousness of 31 minutes to 59 minutes**

√7th **S06.2X3 Diffuse traumatic brain injury with loss of consciousness of 1 hour to 5 hours 59 minutes**

√7th **S06.2X4 Diffuse traumatic brain injury with loss of consciousness of 6 hours to 24 hours**

7th **S06.2X5 Diffuse traumatic brain injury with loss of consciousness greater than 24 hours with return to pre-existing conscious levels**

7th **S06.2X6 Diffuse traumatic brain injury with loss of consciousness greater than 24 hours without return to pre-existing conscious level with patient surviving**

7th **S06.2X7 Diffuse traumatic brain injury with loss of consciousness of any duration with death due to brain injury prior to regaining consciousness**

7th **S06.2X8 Diffuse traumatic brain injury with loss of consciousness of any duration with death due to other cause prior to regaining consciousness**

7th **S06.2X9 Diffuse traumatic brain injury with loss of consciousness of unspecified duration**
Diffuse traumatic brain injury NOS

5th **S06.3 Focal traumatic brain injury**
EXCLUDES 1 *any condition classifiable to S06.4-S06.6*
focal cerebral edema (S06.1)

6th **S06.30 Unspecified focal traumatic brain injury**

7th **S06.300 Unspecified focal traumatic brain injury without loss of consciousness**

7th **S06.301 Unspecified focal traumatic brain injury with loss of consciousness of 30 minutes or less**

7th **S06.302 Unspecified focal traumatic brain injury with loss of consciousness of 31 minutes to 59 minutes**

7th **S06.303 Unspecified focal traumatic brain injury with loss of consciousness of 1 hour to 5 hours 59 minutes**

7th **S06.304 Unspecified focal traumatic brain injury with loss of consciousness of 6 hours to 24 hours**

7th **S06.305 Unspecified focal traumatic brain injury with loss of consciousness greater than 24 hours with return to pre-existing conscious level**

7th **S06.306 Unspecified focal traumatic brain injury with loss of consciousness greater than 24 hours without return to pre-existing conscious level with patient surviving**

7th **S06.307 Unspecified focal traumatic brain injury with loss of consciousness of any duration with death due to brain injury prior to regaining consciousness**

7th **S06.308 Unspecified focal traumatic brain injury with loss of consciousness of any duration with death due to other cause prior to regaining consciousness**

7th **S06.309 Unspecified focal traumatic brain injury with loss of consciousness of unspecified duration**
Unspecified focal traumatic brain injury NOS

6th **S06.31 Contusion and laceration of right cerebrum**

7th **S06.310 Contusion and laceration of right cerebrum without loss of consciousness**

7th **S06.311 Contusion and laceration of right cerebrum with loss of consciousness of 30 minutes or less**

7th **S06.312 Contusion and laceration of right cerebrum with loss of consciousness of 31 minutes to 59 minutes**

7th **S06.313 Contusion and laceration of right cerebrum with loss of consciousness of 1 hour to 5 hours 59 minutes**

7th **S06.314 Contusion and laceration of right cerebrum with loss of consciousness of 6 hours to 24 hours**

7th **S06.315 Contusion and laceration of right cerebrum with loss of consciousness greater than 24 hours with return to pre-existing conscious level**

7th **S06.316 Contusion and laceration of right cerebrum with loss of consciousness greater than 24 hours without return to pre-existing conscious level with patient surviving**

7th **S06.317 Contusion and laceration of right cerebrum with loss of consciousness of any duration with death due to brain injury prior to regaining consciousness**

7th **S06.318 Contusion and laceration of right cerebrum with loss of consciousness of any duration with death due to other cause prior to regaining consciousness**

7th **S06.319 Contusion and laceration of right cerebrum with loss of consciousness of unspecified duration**
Contusion and laceration of right cerebrum NOS

6th **S06.32 Contusion and laceration of left cerebrum**

7th **S06.320 Contusion and laceration of left cerebrum without loss of consciousness**

7th **S06.321 Contusion and laceration of left cerebrum with loss of consciousness of 30 minutes or less**

7th **S06.322 Contusion and laceration of left cerebrum with loss of consciousness of 31 minutes to 59 minutes**

7th **S06.323 Contusion and laceration of left cerebrum with loss of consciousness of 1 hour to 5 hours 59 minutes**

7th **S06.324 Contusion and laceration of left cerebrum with loss of consciousness of 6 hours to 24 hours**

7th **S06.325 Contusion and laceration of left cerebrum with loss of consciousness greater than 24 hours with return to pre-existing conscious level**

7th **S06.326 Contusion and laceration of left cerebrum with loss of consciousness greater than 24 hours without return to pre-existing conscious level with patient surviving**

7th **S06.327 Contusion and laceration of left cerebrum with loss of consciousness of any duration with death due to brain injury prior to regaining consciousness**

7th **S06.328 Contusion and laceration of left cerebrum with loss of consciousness of any duration with death due to other cause prior to regaining consciousness**

7th **S06.329 Contusion and laceration of left cerebrum with loss of consciousness of unspecified duration**
Contusion and laceration of left cerebrum NOS

6th **S06.33 Contusion and laceration of cerebrum, unspecified**

7th **S06.330 Contusion and laceration of cerebrum, unspecified, without loss of consciousness**

7th **S06.331 Contusion and laceration of cerebrum, unspecified, with loss of consciousness of 30 minutes or less**

7th **S06.332 Contusion and laceration of cerebrum, unspecified, with loss of consciousness of 31 minutes to 59 minutes**

7th **S06.333 Contusion and laceration of cerebrum, unspecified, with loss of consciousness of 1 hour to 5 hours 59 minutes**

7th **S06.334 Contusion and laceration of cerebrum, unspecified, with loss of consciousness of 6 hours to 24 hours**

7th **S06.335 Contusion and laceration of cerebrum, unspecified, with loss of consciousness greater than 24 hours with return to pre-existing conscious level**

S06.336 Contusion and laceration of cerebrum, unspecified, with loss of consciousness greater than 24 hours without return to pre-existing conscious level with patient surviving

S06.337 Contusion and laceration of cerebrum, unspecified, with loss of consciousness of any duration with death due to brain injury prior to regaining consciousness

S06.338 Contusion and laceration of cerebrum, unspecified, with loss of consciousness of any duration with death due to other cause prior to regaining consciousness

S06.339 Contusion and laceration of cerebrum, unspecified, with loss of consciousness of unspecified duration
Contusion and laceration of cerebrum NOS

S06.34 Traumatic hemorrhage of right cerebrum
Traumatic intracerebral hemorrhage and hematoma of right cerebrum

S06.340 Traumatic hemorrhage of right cerebrum without loss of consciousness

S06.341 Traumatic hemorrhage of right cerebrum with loss of consciousness of 30 minutes or less

S06.342 Traumatic hemorrhage of right cerebrum with loss of consciousness of 31 minutes to 59 minutes

S06.343 Traumatic hemorrhage of right cerebrum with loss of consciousness of 1 hours to 5 hours 59 minutes

S06.344 Traumatic hemorrhage of right cerebrum with loss of consciousness of 6 hours to 24 hours

S06.345 Traumatic hemorrhage of right cerebrum with loss of consciousness greater than 24 hours with return to pre-existing conscious level

S06.346 Traumatic hemorrhage of right cerebrum with loss of consciousness greater than 24 hours without return to pre-existing conscious level with patient surviving

S06.347 Traumatic hemorrhage of right cerebrum with loss of consciousness of any duration with death due to brain injury prior to regaining consciousness

S06.348 Traumatic hemorrhage of right cerebrum with loss of consciousness of any duration with death due to other cause prior to regaining consciousness

S06.349 Traumatic hemorrhage of right cerebrum with loss of consciousness of unspecified duration
Traumatic hemorrhage of right cerebrum NOS

S06.35 Traumatic hemorrhage of left cerebrum
Traumatic intracerebral hemorrhage and hematoma of left cerebrum

S06.350 Traumatic hemorrhage of left cerebrum without loss of consciousness

S06.351 Traumatic hemorrhage of left cerebrum with loss of consciousness of 30 minutes or less

S06.352 Traumatic hemorrhage of left cerebrum with loss of consciousness of 31 minutes to 59 minutes

S06.353 Traumatic hemorrhage of left cerebrum with loss of consciousness of 1 hours to 5 hours 59 minutes

S06.354 Traumatic hemorrhage of left cerebrum with loss of consciousness of 6 hours to 24 hours

S06.355 Traumatic hemorrhage of left cerebrum with loss of consciousness greater than 24 hours with return to pre-existing conscious level

S06.356 Traumatic hemorrhage of left cerebrum with loss of consciousness greater than 24 hours without return to pre-existing conscious level with patient surviving

S06.357 Traumatic hemorrhage of left cerebrum with loss of consciousness of any duration with death due to brain injury prior to regaining consciousness

S06.358 Traumatic hemorrhage of left cerebrum with loss of consciousness of any duration with death due to other cause prior to regaining consciousness

S06.359 Traumatic hemorrhage of left cerebrum with loss of consciousness of unspecified duration
Traumatic hemorrhage of left cerebrum NOS

S06.36 Traumatic hemorrhage of cerebrum, unspecified
Traumatic intracerebral hemorrhage and hematoma, unspecified

S06.360 Traumatic hemorrhage of cerebrum, unspecified, without loss of consciousness

S06.361 Traumatic hemorrhage of cerebrum, unspecified, with loss of consciousness of 30 minutes or less

S06.362 Traumatic hemorrhage of cerebrum, unspecified, with loss of consciousness of 31 minutes to 59 minutes

S06.363 Traumatic hemorrhage of cerebrum, unspecified, with loss of consciousness of 1 hours to 5 hours 59 minutes

S06.364 Traumatic hemorrhage of cerebrum, unspecified, with loss of consciousness of 6 hours to 24 hours

S06.365 Traumatic hemorrhage of cerebrum, unspecified, with loss of consciousness greater than 24 hours with return to pre-existing conscious level

S06.366 Traumatic hemorrhage of cerebrum, unspecified, with loss of consciousness greater than 24 hours without return to pre-existing conscious level with patient surviving

S06.367 Traumatic hemorrhage of cerebrum, unspecified, with loss of consciousness of any duration with death due to brain injury prior to regaining consciousness

S06.368 Traumatic hemorrhage of cerebrum, unspecified, with loss of consciousness of any duration with death due to other cause prior to regaining consciousness

S06.369 Traumatic hemorrhage of cerebrum, unspecified, with loss of consciousness of unspecified duration
Traumatic hemorrhage of cerebrum NOS

S06.37 Contusion, laceration, and hemorrhage of cerebellum

S06.370 Contusion, laceration, and hemorrhage of cerebellum without loss of consciousness

S06.371 Contusion, laceration, and hemorrhage of cerebellum with loss of consciousness of 30 minutes or less

S06.372 Contusion, laceration, and hemorrhage of cerebellum with loss of consciousness of 31 minutes to 59 minutes

S06.373 Contusion, laceration, and hemorrhage of cerebellum with loss of consciousness of 1 hour to 5 hours 59 minutes

S06.374 Contusion, laceration, and hemorrhage of cerebellum with loss of consciousness of 6 hours to 24 hours

S06.375 Contusion, laceration, and hemorrhage of cerebellum with loss of consciousness greater than 24 hours with return to pre-existing conscious level

7th **SØ6.376 Contusion, laceration, and hemorrhage of cerebellum with loss of consciousness greater than 24 hours without return to pre-existing conscious level with patient surviving**

7th **SØ6.377 Contusion, laceration, and hemorrhage of cerebellum with loss of consciousness of any duration with death due to brain injury prior to regaining consciousness**

7th **SØ6.378 Contusion, laceration, and hemorrhage of cerebellum with loss of consciousness of any duration with death due to other cause prior to regaining consciousness**

7th **SØ6.379 Contusion, laceration, and hemorrhage of cerebellum with loss of consciousness of unspecified duration**
Contusion, laceration, and hemorrhage of cerebellum NOS

6th **SØ6.38 Contusion, laceration, and hemorrhage of brainstem**

7th **SØ6.380 Contusion, laceration, and hemorrhage of brainstem without loss of consciousness**

7th **SØ6.381 Contusion, laceration, and hemorrhage of brainstem with loss of consciousness of 3Ø minutes or less**

7th **SØ6.382 Contusion, laceration, and hemorrhage of brainstem with loss of consciousness of 31 minutes to 59 minutes**

7th **SØ6.383 Contusion, laceration, and hemorrhage of brainstem with loss of consciousness of 1 hour to 5 hours 59 minutes**

7th **SØ6.384 Contusion, laceration, and hemorrhage of brainstem with loss of consciousness of 6 hours to 24 hours**

7th **SØ6.385 Contusion, laceration, and hemorrhage of brainstem with loss of consciousness greater than 24 hours with return to pre-existing conscious level**

7th **SØ6.386 Contusion, laceration, and hemorrhage of brainstem with loss of consciousness greater than 24 hours without return to pre-existing conscious level with patient surviving**

7th **SØ6.387 Contusion, laceration, and hemorrhage of brainstem with loss of consciousness of any duration with death due to brain injury prior to regaining consciousness**

7th **SØ6.388 Contusion, laceration, and hemorrhage of brainstem with loss of consciousness of any duration with death due to other cause prior to regaining consciousness**

7th **SØ6.389 Contusion, laceration, and hemorrhage of brainstem with loss of consciousness of unspecified duration**
Contusion, laceration, and hemorrhage of brainstem NOS

5th **SØ6.4 Epidural hemorrhage**
Extradural hemorrhage NOS
Extradural hemorrhage (traumatic)

6th **SØ6.4X Epidural hemorrhage**

7th **SØ6.4XØ Epidural hemorrhage without loss of consciousness**

7th **SØ6.4X1 Epidural hemorrhage with loss of consciousness of 3Ø minutes or less**

7th **SØ6.4X2 Epidural hemorrhage with loss of consciousness of 31 minutes to 59 minutes**

7th **SØ6.4X3 Epidural hemorrhage with loss of consciousness of 1 hour to 5 hours 59 minutes**

7th **SØ6.4X4 Epidural hemorrhage with loss of consciousness of 6 hours to 24 hours**

7th **SØ6.4X5 Epidural hemorrhage with loss of consciousness greater than 24 hours with return to pre-existing conscious level**

7th **SØ6.4X6 Epidural hemorrhage with loss of consciousness greater than 24 hours without return to pre-existing conscious level with patient surviving**

7th **SØ6.4X7 Epidural hemorrhage with loss of consciousness of any duration with death due to brain injury prior to regaining consciousness**

7th **SØ6.4X8 Epidural hemorrhage with loss of consciousness of any duration with death due to other causes prior to regaining consciousness**

7th **SØ6.4X9 Epidural hemorrhage with loss of consciousness of unspecified duration**
Epidural hemorrhage NOS

5th **SØ6.5 Traumatic subdural hemorrhage**

6th **SØ6.5X Traumatic subdural hemorrhage**

7th **SØ6.5XØ Traumatic subdural hemorrhage without loss of consciousness**

7th **SØ6.5X1 Traumatic subdural hemorrhage with loss of consciousness of 3Ø minutes or less**

7th **SØ6.5X2 Traumatic subdural hemorrhage with loss of consciousness of 31 minutes to 59 minutes**

7th **SØ6.5X3 Traumatic subdural hemorrhage with loss of consciousness of 1 hour to 5 hours 59 minutes**

7th **SØ6.5X4 Traumatic subdural hemorrhage with loss of consciousness of 6 hours to 24 hours**

7th **SØ6.5X5 Traumatic subdural hemorrhage with loss of consciousness greater than 24 hours with return to pre-existing conscious level**

7th **SØ6.5X6 Traumatic subdural hemorrhage with loss of consciousness greater than 24 hours without return to pre-existing conscious level with patient surviving**

7th **SØ6.5X7 Traumatic subdural hemorrhage with loss of consciousness of any duration with death due to brain injury before regaining consciousness**

7th **SØ6.5X8 Traumatic subdural hemorrhage with loss of consciousness of any duration with death due to other cause before regaining consciousness**

7th **SØ6.5X9 Traumatic subdural hemorrhage with loss of consciousness of unspecified duration**
Traumatic subdural hemorrhage NOS

5th **SØ6.6 Traumatic subarachnoid hemorrhage**

6th **SØ6.6X Traumatic subarachnoid hemorrhage**

7th **SØ6.6XØ Traumatic subarachnoid hemorrhage without loss of consciousness**

7th **SØ6.6X1 Traumatic subarachnoid hemorrhage with loss of consciousness of 3Ø minutes or less**

7th **SØ6.6X2 Traumatic subarachnoid hemorrhage with loss of consciousness of 31 minutes to 59 minutes**

7th **SØ6.6X3 Traumatic subarachnoid hemorrhage with loss of consciousness of 1 hour to 5 hours 59 minutes**

7th **SØ6.6X4 Traumatic subarachnoid hemorrhage with loss of consciousness of 6 hours to 24 hours**

7th **SØ6.6X5 Traumatic subarachnoid hemorrhage with loss of consciousness greater than 24 hours with return to pre-existing conscious level**

7th **SØ6.6X6 Traumatic subarachnoid hemorrhage with loss of consciousness greater than 24 hours without return to pre-existing conscious level with patient surviving**

7th **SØ6.6X7 Traumatic subarachnoid hemorrhage with loss of consciousness of any duration with death due to brain injury prior to regaining consciousness**

√7th **S06.6X8 Traumatic subarachnoid hemorrhage with loss of consciousness of any duration with death due to other cause prior to regaining consciousness**

√7th **S06.6X9 Traumatic subarachnoid hemorrhage with loss of consciousness of unspecified duration**
Traumatic subarachnoid hemorrhage NOS

√5th **S06.8 Other specified intracranial injuries**

√6th **S06.81 Injury of right internal carotid artery, intracranial portion, not elsewhere classified**

√7th **S06.810 Injury of right internal carotid artery, intracranial portion, not elsewhere classified without loss of consciousness**

√7th **S06.811 Injury of right internal carotid artery, intracranial portion, not elsewhere classified with loss of consciousness of 30 minutes or less**

√7th **S06.812 Injury of right internal carotid artery, intracranial portion, not elsewhere classified with loss of consciousness of 31 minutes to 59 minutes**

√7th **S06.813 Injury of right internal carotid artery, intracranial portion, not elsewhere classified with loss of consciousness of 1 hour to 5 hours 59 minutes**

√7th **S06.814 Injury of right internal carotid artery, intracranial portion, not elsewhere classified with loss of consciousness of 6 hours to 24 hours**

√7th **S06.815 Injury of right internal carotid artery, intracranial portion, not elsewhere classified with loss of consciousness greater than 24 hours with return to pre-existing conscious level**

√7th **S06.816 Injury of right internal carotid artery, intracranial portion, not elsewhere classified with loss of consciousness greater than 24 hours without return to pre-existing conscious level with patient surviving**

√7th **S06.817 Injury of right internal carotid artery, intracranial portion, not elsewhere classified with loss of consciousness of any duration with death due to brain injury prior to regaining consciousness**

√7th **S06.818 Injury of right internal carotid artery, intracranial portion, not elsewhere classified with loss of consciousness of any duration with death due to other cause prior to regaining consciousness**

√7th **S06.819 Injury of right internal carotid artery, intracranial portion, not elsewhere classified with loss of consciousness of unspecified duration**
Injury of right internal carotid artery, intracranial portion, not elsewhere classified NOS

√6th **S06.82 Injury of left internal carotid artery, intracranial portion, not elsewhere classified**

√7th **S06.820 Injury of left internal carotid artery, intracranial portion, not elsewhere classified without loss of consciousness**

√7th **S06.821 Injury of left internal carotid artery, intracranial portion, not elsewhere classified with loss of consciousness of 30 minutes or less**

√7th **S06.822 Injury of left internal carotid artery, intracranial portion, not elsewhere classified with loss of consciousness of 31 minutes to 59 minutes**

√7th **S06.823 Injury of left internal carotid artery, intracranial portion, not elsewhere classified with loss of consciousness of 1 hour to 5 hours 59 minutes**

√7th **S06.824 Injury of left internal carotid artery, intracranial portion, not elsewhere classified with loss of consciousness of 6 hours to 24 hours**

√7th **S06.825 Injury of left internal carotid artery, intracranial portion, not elsewhere classified with loss of consciousness greater than 24 hours with return to pre-existing conscious level**

√7th **S06.826 Injury of left internal carotid artery, intracranial portion, not elsewhere classified with loss of consciousness greater than 24 hours without return to pre-existing conscious level with patient surviving**

√7th **S06.827 Injury of left internal carotid artery, intracranial portion, not elsewhere classified with loss of consciousness of any duration with death due to brain injury prior to regaining consciousness**

√7th **S06.828 Injury of left internal carotid artery, intracranial portion, not elsewhere classified with loss of consciousness of any duration with death due to other cause prior to regaining consciousness**

√7th **S06.829 Injury of left internal carotid artery, intracranial portion, not elsewhere classified with loss of consciousness of unspecified duration**
Injury of left internal carotid artery, intracranial portion, not elsewhere classified NOS

√6th **S06.89 Other specified intracranial injury**

√7th **S06.890 Other specified intracranial injury without loss of consciousness**

√7th **S06.891 Other specified intracranial injury with loss of consciousness of 30 minutes or less**

√7th **S06.892 Other specified intracranial injury with loss of consciousness of 31 minutes to 59 minutes**

√7th **S06.893 Other specified intracranial injury with loss of consciousness of 1 hour to 5 hours 59 minutes**

√7th **S06.894 Other specified intracranial injury with loss of consciousness of 6 hours to 24 hours**

√7th **S06.895 Other specified intracranial injury with loss of consciousness greater than 24 hours with return to pre-existing conscious level**

√7th **S06.896 Other specified intracranial injury with loss of consciousness greater than 24 hours without return to pre-existing conscious level with patient surviving**

√7th **S06.897 Other specified intracranial injury with loss of consciousness of any duration with death due to brain injury prior to regaining consciousness**

√7th **S06.898 Other specified intracranial injury with loss of consciousness of any duration with death due to other cause prior to regaining consciousness**

√7th **S06.899 Other specified intracranial injury with loss of consciousness of unspecified duration**

√5th **S06.9 Unspecified intracranial injury**
Brain injury NOS
Head injury NOS with loss of consciousness
EXCLUDES 1 *head injury NOS (S09.90)*

√6th **S06.9X Unspecified intracranial injury**

√7th **S06.9X0 Unspecified intracranial injury without loss of consciousness**

√7th **S06.9X1 Unspecified intracranial injury with loss of consciousness of 30 minutes or less**

√7th **S06.9X2 Unspecified intracranial injury with loss of consciousness of 31 minutes to 59 minutes**

SØ6.9X3 Unspecified intracranial injury with loss of consciousness of 1 hour to 5 hours 59 minutes

SØ6.9X4 Unspecified intracranial injury with loss of consciousness of 6 hours to 24 hours

SØ6.9X5 Unspecified intracranial injury with loss of consciousness greater than 24 hours with return to pre-existing conscious level

SØ6.9X6 Unspecified intracranial injury with loss of consciousness greater than 24 hours without return to pre-existing conscious level with patient surviving

SØ6.9X7 Unspecified intracranial injury with loss of consciousness of any duration with death due to brain injury prior to regaining consciousness

SØ6.9X8 Unspecified intracranial injury with loss of consciousness of any duration with death due to other cause prior to regaining consciousness

SØ6.9X9 Unspecified intracranial injury with loss of consciousness of unspecified duration

SØ7 Crushing injury of head

Use additional code for all associated injuries, such as:
intracranial injuries (SØ6.-)
skull fractures (SØ2.-)

The appropriate 7th character is to be added to each code from category SØ7.
A initial encounter
D subsequent encounter
S sequela

SØ7.Ø Crushing injury of face

SØ7.1 Crushing injury of skull

SØ7.8 Crushing injury of other parts of head

SØ7.9 Crushing injury of head, part unspecified

SØ8 Avulsion and traumatic amputation of part of head

NOTE An amputation not identified as partial or complete should be coded to complete

The appropriate 7th character is to be added to each code from category SØ8.
A initial encounter
D subsequent encounter
S sequela

SØ8.Ø Avulsion of scalp

SØ8.1 Traumatic amputation of ear

SØ8.11 Complete traumatic amputation of ear

SØ8.111 Complete traumatic amputation of right ear

SØ8.112 Complete traumatic amputation of left ear

SØ8.119 Complete traumatic amputation of unspecified ear

SØ8.12 Partial traumatic amputation of ear

SØ8.121 Partial traumatic amputation of right ear

SØ8.122 Partial traumatic amputation of left ear

SØ8.129 Partial traumatic amputation of unspecified ear

SØ8.8 Traumatic amputation of other parts of head

SØ8.81 Traumatic amputation of nose

SØ8.811 Complete traumatic amputation of nose

SØ8.812 Partial traumatic amputation of nose

SØ8.89 Traumatic amputation of other parts of head

SØ9 Other and unspecified injuries of head

The appropriate 7th character is to be added to each code from category SØ9.
A initial encounter
D subsequent encounter
S sequela

SØ9.Ø Injury of blood vessels of head, not elsewhere classified

EXCLUDES 1 *injury of cerebral blood vessels (SØ6.-)*
injury of precerebral blood vessels (S15.-)

SØ9.1 Injury of muscle and tendon of head

Code also any associated open wound (SØ1.-)

EXCLUDES 2 *sprain to joints and ligament of head (SØ3.9)*

SØ9.1Ø Unspecified injury of muscle and tendon of head

Injury of muscle and tendon of head NOS

SØ9.11 Strain of muscle and tendon of head

SØ9.12 Laceration of muscle and tendon of head

SØ9.19 Other specified injury of muscle and tendon of head

SØ9.2 Traumatic rupture of ear drum

EXCLUDES 1 *traumatic rupture of ear drum due to blast injury (SØ9.31-)*

SØ9.2Ø Traumatic rupture of unspecified ear drum

SØ9.21 Traumatic rupture of right ear drum

SØ9.22 Traumatic rupture of left ear drum

SØ9.3 Other specified and unspecified injury of middle and inner ear

EXCLUDES 1 *injury to ear NOS (SØ9.91-)*

EXCLUDES 2 *injury to external ear (SØØ.4-, SØ1.3-, SØ8.1-)*

SØ9.3Ø Unspecified injury of middle and inner ear

SØ9.3Ø1 Unspecified injury of right middle and inner ear

SØ9.3Ø2 Unspecified injury of left middle and inner ear

SØ9.3Ø9 Unspecified injury of unspecified middle and inner ear

SØ9.31 Primary blast injury of ear

Blast injury of ear NOS

SØ9.311 Primary blast injury of right ear

SØ9.312 Primary blast injury of left ear

SØ9.313 Primary blast injury of ear, bilateral

SØ9.319 Primary blast injury of unspecified ear

SØ9.39 Other specified injury of middle and inner ear

Secondary blast injury to ear

SØ9.391 Other specified injury of right middle and inner ear

SØ9.392 Other specified injury of left middle and inner ear

SØ9.399 Other specified injury of unspecified middle and inner ear

SØ9.8 Other specified injuries of head

SØ9.9 Unspecified injury of face and head

SØ9.9Ø Unspecified injury of head

Head injury NOS

EXCLUDES 1 *brain injury NOS (SØ6.9-)*
head injury NOS with loss of consciousness (SØ6.9-)
intracranial injury NOS (SØ6.9-)

SØ9.91 Unspecified injury of ear

Injury of ear NOS

SØ9.92 Unspecified injury of nose

Injury of nose NOS

SØ9.93 Unspecified injury of face

Injury of face NOS

Injuries to the neck (S10-S19)

INCLUDES injuries of nape
injuries of supraclavicular region
injuries of throat

EXCLUDES 2 *burns and corrosions (T20-T32)*
effects of foreign body in esophagus (T18.1)
effects of foreign body in larynx (T17.3)
effects of foreign body in pharynx (T17.2)
effects of foreign body in trachea (T17.4)
frostbite (T33-T34)
insect bite or sting, venomous (T63.4)

✓4th **S10 Superficial injury of neck**

The appropriate 7th character is to be added to each code from category S10.
A initial encounter
D subsequent encounter
S sequela

✓x7th **S10.0 Contusion of throat**
Contusion of cervical esophagus
Contusion of larynx
Contusion of pharynx
Contusion of trachea

✓5th **S10.1 Other and unspecified superficial injuries of throat**
✓x7th **S10.10 Unspecified superficial injuries of throat**
✓x7th **S10.11 Abrasion of throat**
✓x7th **S10.12 Blister (nonthermal) of throat**
✓x7th **S10.14 External constriction of part of throat**
✓x7th **S10.15 Superficial foreign body of throat**
Splinter in the throat
✓x7th **S10.16 Insect bite (nonvenomous) of throat**
✓x7th **S10.17 Other superficial bite of throat**
EXCLUDES 1 *open bite of throat (S11.85)*

✓5th **S10.8 Superficial injury of other specified parts of neck**
✓x7th **S10.80 Unspecified superficial injury of other specified part of neck**
✓x7th **S10.81 Abrasion of other specified part of neck**
✓x7th **S10.82 Blister (nonthermal) of other specified part of neck**
✓x7th **S10.83 Contusion of other specified part of neck**
✓x7th **S10.84 External constriction of other specified part of neck**
✓x7th **S10.85 Superficial foreign body of other specified part of neck**
Splinter in other specified part of neck
✓x7th **S10.86 Insect bite of other specified part of neck**
✓x7th **S10.87 Other superficial bite of other specified part of neck**
EXCLUDES 1 *open bite of other specified parts of neck (S11.85)*

✓5th **S10.9 Superficial injury of unspecified part of neck**
✓x7th **S10.90 Unspecified superficial injury of unspecified part of neck**
✓x7th **S10.91 Abrasion of unspecified part of neck**
✓x7th **S10.92 Blister (nonthermal) of unspecified part of neck**
✓x7th **S10.93 Contusion of unspecified part of neck**
✓x7th **S10.94 External constriction of unspecified part of neck**
✓x7th **S10.95 Superficial foreign body of unspecified part of neck**
✓x7th **S10.96 Insect bite of unspecified part of neck**
✓x7th **S10.97 Other superficial bite of unspecified part of neck**

✓4th **S11 Open wound of neck**
Code also any associated:
spinal cord injury (S14.0, S14.1-)
wound infection
EXCLUDES 2 *open fracture of vertebra (S12- with 7th character B)*

The appropriate 7th character is to be added to each code from category S11.
A initial encounter
D subsequent encounter
S sequela

✓5th **S11.0 Open wound of larynx and trachea**
✓6th **S11.01 Open wound of larynx**
EXCLUDES 2 *open wound of vocal cord (S11.03)*
✓7th **S11.011 Laceration without foreign body of larynx**
✓7th **S11.012 Laceration with foreign body of larynx**
✓7th **S11.013 Puncture wound without foreign body of larynx**
✓7th **S11.014 Puncture wound with foreign body of larynx**
✓7th **S11.015 Open bite of larynx**
Bite of larynx NOS
✓7th **S11.019 Unspecified open wound of larynx**
✓6th **S11.02 Open wound of trachea**
Open wound of cervical trachea
Open wound of trachea NOS
EXCLUDES 2 *open wound of thoracic trachea (S27.5-)*
✓7th **S11.021 Laceration without foreign body of trachea**
✓7th **S11.022 Laceration with foreign body of trachea**
✓7th **S11.023 Puncture wound without foreign body of trachea**
✓7th **S11.024 Puncture wound with foreign body of trachea**
✓7th **S11.025 Open bite of trachea**
Bite of trachea NOS
✓7th **S11.029 Unspecified open wound of trachea**
✓6th **S11.03 Open wound of vocal cord**
✓7th **S11.031 Laceration without foreign body of vocal cord**
✓7th **S11.032 Laceration with foreign body of vocal cord**
✓7th **S11.033 Puncture wound without foreign body of vocal cord**
✓7th **S11.034 Puncture wound with foreign body of vocal cord**
✓7th **S11.035 Open bite of vocal cord**
Bite of vocal cord NOS
✓7th **S11.039 Unspecified open wound of vocal cord**

✓5th **S11.1 Open wound of thyroid gland**
✓x7th **S11.10 Unspecified open wound of thyroid gland**
✓x7th **S11.11 Laceration without foreign body of thyroid gland**
✓x7th **S11.12 Laceration with foreign body of thyroid gland**
✓x7th **S11.13 Puncture wound without foreign body of thyroid gland**
✓x7th **S11.14 Puncture wound with foreign body of thyroid gland**
✓x7th **S11.15 Open bite of thyroid gland**
Bite of thyroid gland NOS

✓5th **S11.2 Open wound of pharynx and cervical esophagus**
EXCLUDES 1 *open wound of esophagus NOS (S27.8-)*
✓x7th **S11.20 Unspecified open wound of pharynx and cervical esophagus**
✓x7th **S11.21 Laceration without foreign body of pharynx and cervical esophagus**
✓x7th **S11.22 Laceration with foreign body of pharynx and cervical esophagus**
✓x7th **S11.23 Puncture wound without foreign body of pharynx and cervical esophagus**
✓x7th **S11.24 Puncture wound with foreign body of pharynx and cervical esophagus**
✓x7th **S11.25 Open bite of pharynx and cervical esophagus**
Bite of pharynx and cervical esophagus NOS

✓5th **S11.8 Open wound of other specified parts of neck**
✓x7th **S11.80 Unspecified open wound of other specified part of neck**
✓x7th **S11.81 Laceration without foreign body of other specified part of neck**
✓x7th **S11.82 Laceration with foreign body of other specified part of neck**
✓x7th **S11.83 Puncture wound without foreign body of other specified part of neck**
✓x7th **S11.84 Puncture wound with foreign body of other specified part of neck**
✓x7th **S11.85 Open bite of other specified part of neck**
Bite of other specified part of neck NOS
EXCLUDES 1 *superficial bite of other specified part of neck (S10.87)*
✓x7th **S11.89 Other open wound of other specified part of neck**

S11.9 Open wound of unspecified part of neck
S11.9Ø Unspecified open wound of unspecified part of neck
S11.91 Laceration without foreign body of unspecified part of neck
S11.92 Laceration with foreign body of unspecified part of neck
S11.93 Puncture wound without foreign body of unspecified part of neck
S11.94 Puncture wound with foreign body of unspecified part of neck
S11.95 Open bite of unspecified part of neck
Bite of neck NOS
EXCLUDES 1 *superficial bite of neck (S1Ø.97)*

S12 Fracture of cervical vertebra and other parts of neck
NOTE A fracture not indicated as nondisplaced or displaced should be classified to displaced
A fracture not indicated as open or closed should be coded to closed.
INCLUDES fracture of cervical neural arch
fracture of cervical spine
fracture of cervical spinous process
fracture of cervical transverse process
fracture of cervical vertebral arch
fracture of neck
Code also any associated cervical spinal cord injury (S14.Ø, S14.1-)

The appropriate 7th character is to be added to all codes from subcategories S12.Ø-S12.6.
A initial encounter for closed fracture
B initial encounter for open fracture
D subsequent encounter for fracture with routine healing
G subsequent encounter for fracture with delayed healing
K subsequent encounter for fracture with nonunion
S sequela

S12.Ø Fracture of first cervical vertebra
Atlas
S12.ØØ Unspecified fracture of first cervical vertebra
S12.ØØØ Unspecified displaced fracture of first cervical vertebra
S12.ØØ1 Unspecified nondisplaced fracture of first cervical vertebra
S12.Ø1 Stable burst fracture of first cervical vertebra
S12.Ø2 Unstable burst fracture of first cervical vertebra
S12.Ø3 Posterior arch fracture of first cervical vertebra
S12.Ø3Ø Displaced posterior arch fracture of first cervical vertebra
S12.Ø31 Nondisplaced posterior arch fracture of first cervical vertebra
S12.Ø4 Lateral mass fracture of first cervical vertebra
S12.Ø4Ø Displaced lateral mass fracture of first cervical vertebra
S12.Ø41 Nondisplaced lateral mass fracture of first cervical vertebra
S12.Ø9 Other fracture of first cervical vertebra
S12.Ø9Ø Other displaced fracture of first cervical vertebra
S12.Ø91 Other nondisplaced fracture of first cervical vertebra
S12.1 Fracture of second cervical vertebra
Axis
S12.1Ø Unspecified fracture of second cervical vertebra
S12.1ØØ Unspecified displaced fracture of second cervical vertebra
S12.1Ø1 Unspecified nondisplaced fracture of second cervical vertebra
S12.11 Type II dens fracture
S12.11Ø Anterior displaced Type II dens fracture
S12.111 Posterior displaced Type II dens fracture
S12.112 Nondisplaced Type II dens fracture
S12.12 Other dens fracture
S12.12Ø Other displaced dens fracture
S12.121 Other nondisplaced dens fracture
S12.13 Unspecified traumatic spondylolisthesis of second cervical vertebra
S12.13Ø Unspecified traumatic displaced spondylolisthesis of second cervical vertebra
S12.131 Unspecified traumatic nondisplaced spondylolisthesis of second cervical vertebra
S12.14 Type III traumatic spondylolisthesis of second cervical vertebra
S12.15 Other traumatic spondylolisthesis of second cervical vertebra
S12.15Ø Other traumatic displaced spondylolisthesis of second cervical vertebra
S12.151 Other traumatic nondisplaced spondylolisthesis of second cervical vertebra
S12.19 Other fracture of second cervical vertebra
S12.19Ø Other displaced fracture of second cervical vertebra
S12.191 Other nondisplaced fracture of second cervical vertebra
S12.2 Fracture of third cervical vertebra
S12.2Ø Unspecified fracture of third cervical vertebra
S12.2ØØ Unspecified displaced fracture of third cervical vertebra
S12.2Ø1 Unspecified nondisplaced fracture of third cervical vertebra
S12.23 Unspecified traumatic spondylolisthesis of third cervical vertebra
S12.23Ø Unspecified traumatic displaced spondylolisthesis of third cervical vertebra
S12.231 Unspecified traumatic nondisplaced spondylolisthesis of third cervical vertebra
S12.24 Type III traumatic spondylolisthesis of third cervical vertebra
S12.25 Other traumatic spondylolisthesis of third cervical vertebra
S12.25Ø Other traumatic displaced spondylolisthesis of third cervical vertebra
S12.251 Other traumatic nondisplaced spondylolisthesis of third cervical vertebra
S12.29 Other fracture of third cervical vertebra
S12.29Ø Other displaced fracture of third cervical vertebra
S12.291 Other nondisplaced fracture of third cervical vertebra
S12.3 Fracture of fourth cervical vertebra
S12.3Ø Unspecified fracture of fourth cervical vertebra
S12.3ØØ Unspecified displaced fracture of fourth cervical vertebra
S12.3Ø1 Unspecified nondisplaced fracture of fourth cervical vertebra
S12.33 Unspecified traumatic spondylolisthesis of fourth cervical vertebra
S12.33Ø Unspecified traumatic displaced spondylolisthesis of fourth cervical vertebra
S12.331 Unspecified traumatic nondisplaced spondylolisthesis of fourth cervical vertebra
S12.34 Type III traumatic spondylolisthesis of fourth cervical vertebra
S12.35 Other traumatic spondylolisthesis of fourth cervical vertebra
S12.35Ø Other traumatic displaced spondylolisthesis of fourth cervical vertebra
S12.351 Other traumatic nondisplaced spondylolisthesis of fourth cervical vertebra
S12.39 Other fracture of fourth cervical vertebra
S12.39Ø Other displaced fracture of fourth cervical vertebra

S12.391 Other nondisplaced fracture of fourth cervical vertebra

S12.4 Fracture of fifth cervical vertebra

S12.40 Unspecified fracture of fifth cervical vertebra

S12.400 Unspecified displaced fracture of fifth cervical vertebra

S12.401 Unspecified nondisplaced fracture of fifth cervical vertebra

S12.43 Unspecified traumatic spondylolisthesis of fifth cervical vertebra

S12.430 Unspecified traumatic displaced spondylolisthesis of fifth cervical vertebra

S12.431 Unspecified traumatic nondisplaced spondylolisthesis of fifth cervical vertebra

S12.44 Type III traumatic spondylolisthesis of fifth cervical vertebra

S12.45 Other traumatic spondylolisthesis of fifth cervical vertebra

S12.450 Other traumatic displaced spondylolisthesis of fifth cervical vertebra

S12.451 Other traumatic nondisplaced spondylolisthesis of fifth cervical vertebra

S12.49 Other fracture of fifth cervical vertebra

S12.490 Other displaced fracture of fifth cervical vertebra

S12.491 Other nondisplaced fracture of fifth cervical vertebra

S12.5 Fracture of sixth cervical vertebra

S12.50 Unspecified fracture of sixth cervical vertebra

S12.500 Unspecified displaced fracture of sixth cervical vertebra

S12.501 Unspecified nondisplaced fracture of sixth cervical vertebra

S12.53 Unspecified traumatic spondylolisthesis of sixth cervical vertebra

S12.530 Unspecified traumatic displaced spondylolisthesis of sixth cervical vertebra

S12.531 Unspecified traumatic nondisplaced spondylolisthesis of sixth cervical vertebra

S12.54 Type III traumatic spondylolisthesis of sixth cervical vertebra

S12.55 Other traumatic spondylolisthesis of sixth cervical vertebra

S12.550 Other traumatic displaced spondylolisthesis of sixth cervical vertebra

S12.551 Other traumatic nondisplaced spondylolisthesis of sixth cervical vertebra

S12.59 Other fracture of sixth cervical vertebra

S12.590 Other displaced fracture of sixth cervical vertebra

S12.591 Other nondisplaced fracture of sixth cervical vertebra

S12.6 Fracture of seventh cervical vertebra

S12.60 Unspecified fracture of seventh cervical vertebra

S12.600 Unspecified displaced fracture of seventh cervical vertebra

S12.601 Unspecified nondisplaced fracture of seventh cervical vertebra

S12.63 Unspecified traumatic spondylolisthesis of seventh cervical vertebra

S12.630 Unspecified traumatic displaced spondylolisthesis of seventh cervical vertebra

S12.631 Unspecified traumatic nondisplaced spondylolisthesis of seventh cervical vertebra

S12.64 Type III traumatic spondylolisthesis of seventh cervical vertebra

S12.65 Other traumatic spondylolisthesis of seventh cervical vertebra

S12.650 Other traumatic displaced spondylolisthesis of seventh cervical vertebra

S12.651 Other traumatic nondisplaced spondylolisthesis of seventh cervical vertebra

S12.69 Other fracture of seventh cervical vertebra

S12.690 Other displaced fracture of seventh cervical vertebra

S12.691 Other nondisplaced fracture of seventh cervical vertebra

S12.8 Fracture of other parts of neck

The appropriate 7th character is to be added to code S12.8.
A initial encounter
D subsequent encounter
S sequela

Hyoid bone
Larynx
Thyroid cartilage
Trachea

S12.9 Fracture of neck, unspecified

The appropriate 7th character is to be added to code S12.9.
A initial encounter
D subsequent encounter
S sequela

Fracture of neck NOS
Fracture of cervical spine NOS
Fracture of cervical vertebra NOS

S13 Dislocation and sprain of joints and ligaments at neck level

INCLUDES avulsion of joint or ligament at neck level
laceration of cartilage, joint or ligament at neck level
sprain of cartilage, joint or ligament at neck level
traumatic hemarthrosis of joint or ligament at neck level
traumatic rupture of joint or ligament at neck level
traumatic subluxation of joint or ligament at neck level
traumatic tear of joint or ligament at neck level

Code also: any associated open wound

EXCLUDES 2 *strain of muscle or tendon at neck level (S16.1)*

The appropriate 7th character is to be added to each code from category S13.
A initial encounter
D subsequent encounter
S sequela

S13.0 Traumatic rupture of cervical intervertebral disc

EXCLUDES 1 *rupture or displacement (nontraumatic) of cervical intervertebral disc NOS (M50.-)*

S13.1 Subluxation and dislocation of cervical vertebrae

Code also any associated:
open wound of neck (S11.-)
spinal cord injury (S14.1-)

EXCLUDES 2 *fracture of cervical vertebrae (S12.0--S12.3-)*

S13.10 Subluxation and dislocation of unspecified cervical vertebrae

S13.100 Subluxation of unspecified cervical vertebrae

S13.101 Dislocation of unspecified cervical vertebrae

S13.11 Subluxation and dislocation of C0/C1 cervical vertebrae

Subluxation and dislocation of atlantooccipital joint
Subluxation and dislocation of atloidooccipital joint
Subluxation and dislocation of occipitoatloid joint

S13.110 Subluxation of C0/C1 cervical vertebrae

S13.111 Dislocation of C0/C1 cervical vertebrae

S13.12 Subluxation and dislocation of C1/C2 cervical vertebrae

Subluxation and dislocation of atlantoaxial joint

S13.120 Subluxation of C1/C2 cervical vertebrae

S13.121 Dislocation of C1/C2 cervical vertebrae

S13.13 Subluxation and dislocation of C2/C3 cervical vertebrae

S13.130 Subluxation of C2/C3 cervical vertebrae

√7th S13.131 **Dislocation of C2/C3 cervical vertebrae**

√6th S13.14 **Subluxation and dislocation of C3/C4 cervical vertebrae**

√7th S13.140 **Subluxation of C3/C4 cervical vertebrae**

√7th S13.141 **Dislocation of C3/C4 cervical vertebrae**

√6th S13.15 **Subluxation and dislocation of C4/C5 cervical vertebrae**

√7th S13.150 **Subluxation of C4/C5 cervical vertebrae**

√7th S13.151 **Dislocation of C4/C5 cervical vertebrae**

√6th S13.16 **Subluxation and dislocation of C5/C6 cervical vertebrae**

√7th S13.160 **Subluxation of C5/C6 cervical vertebrae**

√7th S13.161 **Dislocation of C5/C6 cervical vertebrae**

√6th S13.17 **Subluxation and dislocation of C6/C7 cervical vertebrae**

√7th S13.170 **Subluxation of C6/C7 cervical vertebrae**

√7th S13.171 **Dislocation of C6/C7 cervical vertebrae**

√6th S13.18 **Subluxation and dislocation of C7/T1 cervical vertebrae**

√7th S13.180 **Subluxation of C7/T1 cervical vertebrae**

√7th S13.181 **Dislocation of C7/T1 cervical vertebrae**

√5th S13.2 **Dislocation of other and unspecified parts of neck**

S13.20 **Dislocation of unspecified parts of neck**

S13.29 **Dislocation of other parts of neck**

√x7th S13.4 **Sprain of ligaments of cervical spine**

Sprain of anterior longitudinal (ligament), cervical
Sprain of atlanto-axial (joints)
Sprain of atlanto-occipital (joints)
Whiplash injury of cervical spine

√x7th S13.5 **Sprain of thyroid region**

Sprain of cricoarytenoid (joint) (ligament)
Sprain of cricothyroid (joint) (ligament)
Sprain of thyroid cartilage

√x7th S13.8 **Sprain of joints and ligaments of other parts of neck**

√x7th S13.9 **Sprain of joints and ligaments of unspecified parts of neck**

√4th **S14 Injury of nerves and spinal cord at neck level**

NOTE Code to highest level of cervical cord injury

Code also any associated:
fracture of cervical vertebra (S12.0--S12.6-)
open wound of neck (S11.-)
transient paralysis (R29.5)

The appropriate 7th character is to be added to each code from category S14.
A initial encounter
D subsequent encounter
S sequela

√x7th S14.0 **Concussion and edema of cervical spinal cord**

√5th S14.1 **Other and unspecified injuries of cervical spinal cord**

√6th S14.10 **Unspecified injury of cervical spinal cord**

√7th S14.101 **Unspecified injury at C1 level of cervical spinal cord**

√7th S14.102 **Unspecified injury at C2 level of cervical spinal cord**

√7th S14.103 **Unspecified injury at C3 level of cervical spinal cord**

√7th S14.104 **Unspecified injury at C4 level of cervical spinal cord**

√7th S14.105 **Unspecified injury at C5 level of cervical spinal cord**

√7th S14.106 **Unspecified injury at C6 level of cervical spinal cord**

√7th S14.107 **Unspecified injury at C7 level of cervical spinal cord**

√7th S14.108 **Unspecified injury at C8 level of cervical spinal cord**

√7th S14.109 **Unspecified injury at unspecified level of cervical spinal cord**

Injury of cervical spinal cord NOS

√6th S14.11 **Complete lesion of cervical spinal cord**

√7th S14.111 **Complete lesion at C1 level of cervical spinal cord**

√7th S14.112 **Complete lesion at C2 level of cervical spinal cord**

√7th S14.113 **Complete lesion at C3 level of cervical spinal cord**

√7th S14.114 **Complete lesion at C4 level of cervical spinal cord**

√7th S14.115 **Complete lesion at C5 level of cervical spinal cord**

√7th S14.116 **Complete lesion at C6 level of cervical spinal cord**

√7th S14.117 **Complete lesion at C7 level of cervical spinal cord**

√7th S14.118 **Complete lesion at C8 level of cervical spinal cord**

√7th S14.119 **Complete lesion at unspecified level of cervical spinal cord**

√6th S14.12 **Central cord syndrome of cervical spinal cord**

√7th S14.121 **Central cord syndrome at C1 level of cervical spinal cord**

√7th S14.122 **Central cord syndrome at C2 level of cervical spinal cord**

√7th S14.123 **Central cord syndrome at C3 level of cervical spinal cord**

√7th S14.124 **Central cord syndrome at C4 level of cervical spinal cord**

√7th S14.125 **Central cord syndrome at C5 level of cervical spinal cord**

√7th S14.126 **Central cord syndrome at C6 level of cervical spinal cord**

√7th S14.127 **Central cord syndrome at C7 level of cervical spinal cord**

√7th S14.128 **Central cord syndrome at C8 level of cervical spinal cord**

√7th S14.129 **Central cord syndrome at unspecified level of cervical spinal cord**

√6th S14.13 **Anterior cord syndrome of cervical spinal cord**

√7th S14.131 **Anterior cord syndrome at C1 level of cervical spinal cord**

√7th S14.132 **Anterior cord syndrome at C2 level of cervical spinal cord**

√7th S14.133 **Anterior cord syndrome at C3 level of cervical spinal cord**

√7th S14.134 **Anterior cord syndrome at C4 level of cervical spinal cord**

√7th S14.135 **Anterior cord syndrome at C5 level of cervical spinal cord**

√7th S14.136 **Anterior cord syndrome at C6 level of cervical spinal cord**

√7th S14.137 **Anterior cord syndrome at C7 level of cervical spinal cord**

√7th S14.138 **Anterior cord syndrome at C8 level of cervical spinal cord**

√7th S14.139 **Anterior cord syndrome at unspecified level of cervical spinal cord**

√6th S14.14 **Brown-Séquard syndrome of cervical spinal cord**

√7th S14.141 **Brown-Séquard syndrome at C1 level of cervical spinal cord**

√7th S14.142 **Brown-Séquard syndrome at C2 level of cervical spinal cord**

√7th S14.143 **Brown-Séquard syndrome at C3 level of cervical spinal cord**

√7th S14.144 **Brown-Séquard syndrome at C4 level of cervical spinal cord**

√7th S14.145 **Brown-Séquard syndrome at C5 level of cervical spinal cord**

√7th S14.146 **Brown-Séquard syndrome at C6 level of cervical spinal cord**

√7th S14.147 **Brown-Séquard syndrome at C7 level of cervical spinal cord**

√7th S14.148 **Brown-Séquard syndrome at C8 level of cervical spinal cord**

√7th S14.149 **Brown-Séquard syndrome at unspecified level of cervical spinal cord**

√6th S14.15 **Other incomplete lesions of cervical spinal cord**

Incomplete lesion of cervical spinal cord NOS
Posterior cord syndrome of cervical spinal cord

√7th S14.151 **Other incomplete lesion at C1 level of cervical spinal cord**

√7th **S14.152 Other incomplete lesion at C2 level of cervical spinal cord**
√7th **S14.153 Other incomplete lesion at C3 level of cervical spinal cord**
√7th **S14.154 Other incomplete lesion at C4 level of cervical spinal cord**
√7th **S14.155 Other incomplete lesion at C5 level of cervical spinal cord**
√7th **S14.156 Other incomplete lesion at C6 level of cervical spinal cord**
√7th **S14.157 Other incomplete lesion at C7 level of cervical spinal cord**
√7th **S14.158 Other incomplete lesion at C8 level of cervical spinal cord**
√7th **S14.159 Other incomplete lesion at unspecified level of cervical spinal cord**

√x7th **S14.2 Injury of nerve root of cervical spine**
√x7th **S14.3 Injury of brachial plexus**
√x7th **S14.4 Injury of peripheral nerves of neck**
√x7th **S14.5 Injury of cervical sympathetic nerves**
√x7th **S14.8 Injury of other specified nerves of neck**
√x7th **S14.9 Injury of unspecified nerves of neck**

√4th **S15 Injury of blood vessels at neck level**
Code also any associated open wound (S11.-)

The appropriate 7th character is to be added to each code from category S15.
A initial encounter
D subsequent encounter
S sequela

√5th **S15.0 Injury of carotid artery of neck**
Injury of carotid artery (common) (external) (internal, extracranial portion)
Injury of carotid artery NOS
EXCLUDES 1 *injury of internal carotid artery, intracranial portion (S06.8)*

√6th **S15.00 Unspecified injury of carotid artery**
√7th **S15.001 Unspecified injury of right carotid artery**
√7th **S15.002 Unspecified injury of left carotid artery**
√7th **S15.009 Unspecified injury of unspecified carotid artery**

√6th **S15.01 Minor laceration of carotid artery**
Incomplete transection of carotid artery
Laceration of carotid artery NOS
Superficial laceration of carotid artery
√7th **S15.011 Minor laceration of right carotid artery**
√7th **S15.012 Minor laceration of left carotid artery**
√7th **S15.019 Minor laceration of unspecified carotid artery**

√6th **S15.02 Major laceration of carotid artery**
Complete transection of carotid artery
Traumatic rupture of carotid artery
√7th **S15.021 Major laceration of right carotid artery**
√7th **S15.022 Major laceration of left carotid artery**
√7th **S15.029 Major laceration of unspecified carotid artery**

√6th **S15.09 Other specified injury of carotid artery**
√7th **S15.091 Other specified injury of right carotid artery**
√7th **S15.092 Other specified injury of left carotid artery**
√7th **S15.099 Other specified injury of unspecified carotid artery**

√5th **S15.1 Injury of vertebral artery**
√6th **S15.10 Unspecified injury of vertebral artery**
√7th **S15.101 Unspecified injury of right vertebral artery**
√7th **S15.102 Unspecified injury of left vertebral artery**
√7th **S15.109 Unspecified injury of unspecified vertebral artery**

√6th **S15.11 Minor laceration of vertebral artery**
Incomplete transection of vertebral artery
Laceration of vertebral artery NOS
Superficial laceration of vertebral artery
√7th **S15.111 Minor laceration of right vertebral artery**
√7th **S15.112 Minor laceration of left vertebral artery**
√7th **S15.119 Minor laceration of unspecified vertebral artery**

√6th **S15.12 Major laceration of vertebral artery**
Complete transection of vertebral artery
Traumatic rupture of vertebral artery
√7th **S15.121 Major laceration of right vertebral artery**
√7th **S15.122 Major laceration of left vertebral artery**
√7th **S15.129 Major laceration of unspecified vertebral artery**

√6th **S15.19 Other specified injury of vertebral artery**
√7th **S15.191 Other specified injury of right vertebral artery**
√7th **S15.192 Other specified injury of left vertebral artery**
√7th **S15.199 Other specified injury of unspecified vertebral artery**

√5th **S15.2 Injury of external jugular vein**
√6th **S15.20 Unspecified injury of external jugular vein**
√7th **S15.201 Unspecified injury of right external jugular vein**
√7th **S15.202 Unspecified injury of left external jugular vein**
√7th **S15.209 Unspecified injury of unspecified external jugular vein**

√6th **S15.21 Minor laceration of external jugular vein**
Incomplete transection of external jugular vein
Laceration of external jugular vein NOS
Superficial laceration of external jugular vein
√7th **S15.211 Minor laceration of right external jugular vein**
√7th **S15.212 Minor laceration of left external jugular vein**
√7th **S15.219 Minor laceration of unspecified external jugular vein**

√6th **S15.22 Major laceration of external jugular vein**
Complete transection of external jugular vein
Traumatic rupture of external jugular vein
√7th **S15.221 Major laceration of right external jugular vein**
√7th **S15.222 Major laceration of left external jugular vein**
√7th **S15.229 Major laceration of unspecified external jugular vein**

√6th **S15.29 Other specified injury of external jugular vein**
√7th **S15.291 Other specified injury of right external jugular vein**
√7th **S15.292 Other specified injury of left external jugular vein**
√7th **S15.299 Other specified injury of unspecified external jugular vein**

√5th **S15.3 Injury of internal jugular vein**
√6th **S15.30 Unspecified injury of internal jugular vein**
√7th **S15.301 Unspecified injury of right internal jugular vein**
√7th **S15.302 Unspecified injury of left internal jugular vein**
√7th **S15.309 Unspecified injury of unspecified internal jugular vein**

√6th **S15.31 Minor laceration of internal jugular vein**
Incomplete transection of internal jugular vein
Laceration of internal jugular vein NOS
Superficial laceration of internal jugular vein
√7th **S15.311 Minor laceration of right internal jugular vein**
√7th **S15.312 Minor laceration of left internal jugular vein**
√7th **S15.319 Minor laceration of unspecified internal jugular vein**

√6th **S15.32 Major laceration of internal jugular vein**
Complete transection of internal jugular vein
Traumatic rupture of internal jugular vein
√7th **S15.321 Major laceration of right internal jugular vein**

DRAFT

√ Appropriate additional character required
√x7th Requires 7th character, placeholder x must fill empty characters

7th **S15.322 Major laceration of left internal jugular vein**

7th **S15.329 Major laceration of unspecified internal jugular vein**

6th **S15.39 Other specified injury of internal jugular vein**

7th **S15.391 Other specified injury of right internal jugular vein**

7th **S15.392 Other specified injury of left internal jugular vein**

7th **S15.399 Other specified injury of unspecified internal jugular vein**

x7th **S15.8 Injury of other specified blood vessels at neck level**

x7th **S15.9 Injury of unspecified blood vessel at neck level**

4th **S16 Injury of muscle, fascia and tendon at neck level**

Code also any associated open wound (S11.-)

EXCLUDES 2 *sprain of joint or ligament at neck level (S13.9)*

The appropriate 7th character is to be added to each code from category S16.
A initial encounter
D subsequent encounter
S sequela

x7th **S16.1 Strain of muscle, fascia and tendon at neck level**

x7th **S16.2 Laceration of muscle, fascia and tendon at neck level**

x7th **S16.8 Other specified injury of muscle, fascia and tendon at neck level**

x7th **S16.9 Unspecified injury of muscle, fascia and tendon at neck level**

4th **S17 Crushing injury of neck**

Use additional code for all associated injuries, such as:
injury of blood vessels (S15.-)
open wound of neck (S11.-)
spinal cord injury (S14.0, S14.1-)
vertebral fracture (S12.0--S12.3-)

The appropriate 7th character is to be added to each code from category S17.
A initial encounter
D subsequent encounter
S sequela

x7th **S17.0 Crushing injury of larynx and trachea**

x7th **S17.8 Crushing injury of other specified parts of neck**

x7th **S17.9 Crushing injury of neck, part unspecified**

4th **S19 Other specified and unspecified injuries of neck**

The appropriate 7th character is to be added to each code from category S19.
A initial encounter
D subsequent encounter
S sequela

5th **S19.8 Other specified injuries of neck**

x7th **S19.80 Other specified injuries of unspecified part of neck**

x7th **S19.81 Other specified injuries of larynx**

x7th **S19.82 Other specified injuries of cervical trachea**

EXCLUDES 2 *other specified injury of thoracic trachea (S27.5-)*

x7th **S19.83 Other specified injuries of vocal cord**

x7th **S19.84 Other specified injuries of thyroid gland**

x7th **S19.85 Other specified injuries of pharynx and cervical esophagus**

x7th **S19.89 Other specified injuries of other specified part of neck**

x7th **S19.9 Unspecified injury of neck**

Injuries to the thorax (S20-S29)

INCLUDES injuries of breast
injuries of chest (wall)
injuries of interscapular area

EXCLUDES 2 *burns and corrosions (T20-T32)*
effects of foreign body in bronchus (T17.5)
effects of foreign body in esophagus (T18.1)
effects of foreign body in lung (T17.8)
effects of foreign body in trachea (T17.4)
frostbite (T33-T34)
injuries of axilla
injuries of clavicle
injuries of scapular region
injuries of shoulder
insect bite or sting, venomous (T63.4)

4th **S20 Superficial injury of thorax**

The appropriate 7th character is to be added to each code from category S20.
A initial encounter
D subsequent encounter
S sequela

5th **S20.0 Contusion of breast**

x7th **S20.00 Contusion of breast, unspecified breast**

x7th **S20.01 Contusion of right breast**

x7th **S20.02 Contusion of left breast**

5th **S20.1 Other and unspecified superficial injuries of breast**

6th **S20.10 Unspecified superficial injuries of breast**

7th **S20.101 Unspecified superficial injuries of breast, right breast**

7th **S20.102 Unspecified superficial injuries of breast, left breast**

7th **S20.109 Unspecified superficial injuries of breast, unspecified breast**

6th **S20.11 Abrasion of breast**

7th **S20.111 Abrasion of breast, right breast**

7th **S20.112 Abrasion of breast, left breast**

7th **S20.119 Abrasion of breast, unspecified breast**

6th **S20.12 Blister (nonthermal) of breast**

7th **S20.121 Blister (nonthermal) of breast, right breast**

7th **S20.122 Blister (nonthermal) of breast, left breast**

7th **S20.129 Blister (nonthermal) of breast, unspecified breast**

6th **S20.14 External constriction of part of breast**

7th **S20.141 External constriction of part of breast, right breast**

7th **S20.142 External constriction of part of breast, left breast**

7th **S20.149 External constriction of part of breast, unspecified breast**

6th **S20.15 Superficial foreign body of breast**

Splinter in the breast

7th **S20.151 Superficial foreign body of breast, right breast**

7th **S20.152 Superficial foreign body of breast, left breast**

7th **S20.159 Superficial foreign body of breast, unspecified breast**

6th **S20.16 Insect bite (nonvenomous) of breast**

7th **S20.161 Insect bite (nonvenomous) of breast, right breast**

7th **S20.162 Insect bite (nonvenomous) of breast, left breast**

7th **S20.169 Insect bite (nonvenomous) of breast, unspecified breast**

6th **S20.17 Other superficial bite of breast**

EXCLUDES 1 *open bite of breast (S21.05-)*

7th **S20.171 Other superficial bite of breast, right breast**

7th **S20.172 Other superficial bite of breast, left breast**

7th **S20.179 Other superficial bite of breast, unspecified breast**

5th **S20.2 Contusion of thorax**

x7th **S20.20 Contusion of thorax, unspecified**

✓6th **S2Ø.21 Contusion of front wall of thorax**
✓7th **S2Ø.211 Contusion of right front wall of thorax**
✓7th **S2Ø.212 Contusion of left front wall of thorax**
✓7th **S2Ø.219 Contusion of unspecified front wall of thorax**
✓6th **S2Ø.22 Contusion of back wall of thorax**
✓7th **S2Ø.221 Contusion of right back wall of thorax**
✓7th **S2Ø.222 Contusion of left back wall of thorax**
✓7th **S2Ø.229 Contusion of unspecified back wall of thorax**
✓5th **S2Ø.3 Other and unspecified superficial injuries of front wall of thorax**
✓6th **S2Ø.3Ø Unspecified superficial injuries of front wall of thorax**
✓7th **S2Ø.3Ø1 Unspecified superficial injuries of right front wall of thorax**
✓7th **S2Ø.3Ø2 Unspecified superficial injuries of left front wall of thorax**
✓7th **S2Ø.3Ø9 Unspecified superficial injuries of unspecified front wall of thorax**
✓6th **S2Ø.31 Abrasion of front wall of thorax**
✓7th **S2Ø.311 Abrasion of right front wall of thorax**
✓7th **S2Ø.312 Abrasion of left front wall of thorax**
✓7th **S2Ø.319 Abrasion of unspecified front wall of thorax**
✓6th **S2Ø.32 Blister (nonthermal) of front wall of thorax**
✓7th **S2Ø.321 Blister (nonthermal) of right front wall of thorax**
✓7th **S2Ø.322 Blister (nonthermal) of left front wall of thorax**
✓7th **S2Ø.329 Blister (nonthermal) of unspecified front wall of thorax**
✓6th **S2Ø.34 External constriction of front wall of thorax**
✓7th **S2Ø.341 External constriction of right front wall of thorax**
✓7th **S2Ø.342 External constriction of left front wall of thorax**
✓7th **S2Ø.349 External constriction of unspecified front wall of thorax**
✓6th **S2Ø.35 Superficial foreign body of front wall of thorax**
Splinter in front wall of thorax
✓7th **S2Ø.351 Superficial foreign body of right front wall of thorax**
✓7th **S2Ø.352 Superficial foreign body of left front wall of thorax**
✓7th **S2Ø.359 Superficial foreign body of unspecified front wall of thorax**
✓6th **S2Ø.36 Insect bite (nonvenomous) of front wall of thorax**
✓7th **S2Ø.361 Insect bite (nonvenomous) of right front wall of thorax**
✓7th **S2Ø.362 Insect bite (nonvenomous) of left front wall of thorax**
✓7th **S2Ø.369 Insect bite (nonvenomous) of unspecified front wall of thorax**
✓6th **S2Ø.37 Other superficial bite of front wall of thorax**
EXCLUDES 1 *open bite of front wall of thorax (S21.15)*
✓7th **S2Ø.371 Other superficial bite of right front wall of thorax**
✓7th **S2Ø.372 Other superficial bite of left front wall of thorax**
✓7th **S2Ø.379 Other superficial bite of unspecified front wall of thorax**
✓5th **S2Ø.4 Other and unspecified superficial injuries of back wall of thorax**
✓6th **S2Ø.4Ø Unspecified superficial injuries of back wall of thorax**
✓7th **S2Ø.4Ø1 Unspecified superficial injuries of right back wall of thorax**
✓7th **S2Ø.4Ø2 Unspecified superficial injuries of left back wall of thorax**
✓7th **S2Ø.4Ø9 Unspecified superficial injuries of unspecified back wall of thorax**
✓6th **S2Ø.41 Abrasion of back wall of thorax**
✓7th **S2Ø.411 Abrasion of right back wall of thorax**
✓7th **S2Ø.412 Abrasion of left back wall of thorax**
✓7th **S2Ø.419 Abrasion of unspecified back wall of thorax**
✓6th **S2Ø.42 Blister (nonthermal) of back wall of thorax**
✓7th **S2Ø.421 Blister (nonthermal) of right back wall of thorax**
✓7th **S2Ø.422 Blister (nonthermal) of left back wall of thorax**
✓7th **S2Ø.429 Blister (nonthermal) of unspecified back wall of thorax**
✓6th **S2Ø.44 External constriction of back wall of thorax**
✓7th **SS2Ø.441 External constriction of right back wall of thorax**
✓7th **S2Ø.442 External constriction of left back wall of thorax**
✓7th **S2Ø.449 External constriction of unspecified back wall of thorax**
✓6th **S2Ø.45 Superficial foreign body of back wall of thorax**
Splinter of back wall of thorax
✓7th **S2Ø.451 Superficial foreign body of right back wall of thorax**
✓7th **S2Ø.452 Superficial foreign body of left back wall of thorax**
✓7th **S2Ø.459 Superficial foreign body of unspecified back wall of thorax**
✓6th **S2Ø.46 Insect bite (nonvenomous) of back wall of thorax**
✓7th **S2Ø.461 Insect bite (nonvenomous) of right back wall of thorax**
✓7th **S2Ø.462 Insect bite (nonvenomous) of left back wall of thorax**
✓7th **S2Ø.469 Insect bite (nonvenomous) of unspecified back wall of thorax**
✓6th **S2Ø.47 Other superficial bite of back wall of thorax**
EXCLUDES 1 *open bite of back wall of thorax (S21.25)*
✓7th **S2Ø.471 Other superficial bite of right back wall of thorax**
✓7th **S2Ø.472 Other superficial bite of left back wall of thorax**
✓7th **S2Ø.479 Other superficial bite of unspecified back wall of thorax**
✓5th **S2Ø.9 Superficial injury of unspecified parts of thorax**
EXCLUDES 1 *contusion of thorax NOS (S2Ø.2Ø)*
✓x7th **S2Ø.9Ø Unspecified superficial injury of unspecified parts of thorax**
Superficial injury of thoracic wall NOS
✓x7th **S2Ø.91 Abrasion of unspecified parts of thorax**
✓x7th **S2Ø.92 Blister (nonthermal) of unspecified parts of thorax**
✓x7th **S2Ø.94 External constriction of unspecified parts of thorax**
✓x7th **S2Ø.95 Superficial foreign body of unspecified parts of thorax**
Splinter in thorax NOS
✓x7th **S2Ø.96 Insect bite (nonvenomous) of unspecified parts of thorax**
✓x7th **S2Ø.97 Other superficial bite of unspecified parts of thorax**
EXCLUDES 1 *open bite of thorax NOS (S21.95)*

✓4th **S21 Open wound of thorax**
Code also any associated injury (to) (such as) :
heart (S26.-)
intrathoracic organs (S27.-)
rib fracture (S22.3-, S22.4-)
spinal cord injury (S24.Ø-, S24.1-)
traumatic hemothorax (S27.1)
traumatic hemopneumothorax (S27.3)
traumatic pneumothorax (S27.Ø)
wound infection
EXCLUDES 1 *traumatic amputation (partial) of thorax (S28.1)*

The appropriate 7th character is to be added to each code from category S21.
A initial encounter
D subsequent encounter
S sequela

✓5th **S21.Ø Open wound of breast**
✓6th **S21.ØØ Unspecified open wound of breast**
✓7th **S21.ØØ1 Unspecified open wound of right breast**
✓7th **S21.ØØ2 Unspecified open wound of left breast**

✓7th S21.009 Unspecified open wound of unspecified breast

✓6th S21.01 Laceration without foreign body of breast

✓7th S21.011 Laceration without foreign body of right breast

✓7th S21.012 Laceration without foreign body of left breast

✓7th S21.019 Laceration without foreign body of unspecified breast

✓6th S21.02 Laceration with foreign body of breast

✓7th S21.021 Laceration with foreign body of right breast

✓7th S21.022 Laceration with foreign body of left breast

✓7th S21.029 Laceration with foreign body of unspecified breast

✓6th S21.03 Puncture wound without foreign body of breast

✓7th S21.031 Puncture wound without foreign body of right breast

✓7th S21.032 Puncture wound without foreign body of left breast

✓7th S21.039 Puncture wound without foreign body of unspecified breast

✓6th S21.04 Puncture wound with foreign body of breast

✓7th S21.041 Puncture wound with foreign body of right breast

✓7th S21.042 Puncture wound with foreign body of left breast

✓7th S21.049 Puncture wound with foreign body of unspecified breast

✓6th S21.05 Open bite of breast

Bite of breast NOS

EXCLUDES 1 *superficial bite of breast (S20.17)*

✓7th S21.051 Open bite of right breast

✓7th S21.052 Open bite of left breast

✓7th S21.059 Open bite of unspecified breast

✓5th S21.1 Open wound of front wall of thorax without penetration into thoracic cavity

Open wound of chest without penetration into thoracic cavity

✓6th S21.10 Unspecified open wound of front wall of thorax without penetration into thoracic cavity

✓7th S21.101 Unspecified open wound of right front wall of thorax without penetration into thoracic cavity

✓7th S21.102 Unspecified open wound of left front wall of thorax without penetration into thoracic cavity

✓7th S21.109 Unspecified open wound of unspecified front wall of thorax without penetration into thoracic cavity

✓6th S21.11 Laceration without foreign body of front wall of thorax without penetration into thoracic cavity

✓7th S21.111 Laceration without foreign body of right front wall of thorax without penetration into thoracic cavity

✓7th S21.112 Laceration without foreign body of left front wall of thorax without penetration into thoracic cavity

✓7th S21.119 Laceration without foreign body of unspecified front wall of thorax without penetration into thoracic cavity

✓6th S21.12 Laceration with foreign body of front wall of thorax without penetration into thoracic cavity

✓7th S21.121 Laceration with foreign body of right front wall of thorax without penetration into thoracic cavity

✓7th S21.122 Laceration with foreign body of left front wall of thorax without penetration into thoracic cavity

✓7th S21.129 Laceration with foreign body of unspecified front wall of thorax without penetration into thoracic cavity

✓6th S21.13 Puncture wound without foreign body of front wall of thorax without penetration into thoracic cavity

✓7th S21.131 Puncture wound without foreign body of right front wall of thorax without penetration into thoracic cavity

✓7th S21.132 Puncture wound without foreign body of left front wall of thorax without penetration into thoracic cavity

✓7th S21.139 Puncture wound without foreign body of unspecified front wall of thorax without penetration into thoracic cavity

✓6th S21.14 Puncture wound with foreign body of front wall of thorax without penetration into thoracic cavity

✓7th S21.141 Puncture wound with foreign body of right front wall of thorax without penetration into thoracic cavity

✓7th S21.142 Puncture wound with foreign body of left front wall of thorax without penetration into thoracic cavity

✓7th S21.149 Puncture wound with foreign body of unspecified front wall of thorax without penetration into thoracic cavity

✓6th S21.15 Open bite of front wall of thorax without penetration into thoracic cavity

Bite of front wall of thorax NOS

EXCLUDES 1 *superficial bite of front wall of thorax (S20.37)*

✓7th S21.151 Open bite of right front wall of thorax without penetration into thoracic cavity

✓7th S21.152 Open bite of left front wall of thorax without penetration into thoracic cavity

✓7th S21.159 Open bite of unspecified front wall of thorax without penetration into thoracic cavity

✓5th S21.2 Open wound of back wall of thorax without penetration into thoracic cavity

✓6th S21.20 Unspecified open wound of back wall of thorax without penetration into thoracic cavity

✓7th S21.201 Unspecified open wound of right back wall of thorax without penetration into thoracic cavity

✓7th S21.202 Unspecified open wound of left back wall of thorax without penetration into thoracic cavity

✓7th S21.209 Unspecified open wound of unspecified back wall of thorax without penetration into thoracic cavity

✓6th S21.21 Laceration without foreign body of back wall of thorax without penetration into thoracic cavity

✓7th S21.211 Laceration without foreign body of right back wall of thorax without penetration into thoracic cavity

✓7th S21.212 Laceration without foreign body of left back wall of thorax without penetration into thoracic cavity

✓7th S21.219 Laceration without foreign body of unspecified back wall of thorax without penetration into thoracic cavity

✓6th S21.22 Laceration with foreign body of back wall of thorax without penetration into thoracic cavity

✓7th S21.221 Laceration with foreign body of right back wall of thorax without penetration into thoracic cavity

✓7th S21.222 Laceration with foreign body of left back wall of thorax without penetration into thoracic cavity

✓7th S21.229 Laceration with foreign body of unspecified back wall of thorax without penetration into thoracic cavity

✓6th S21.23 Puncture wound without foreign body of back wall of thorax without penetration into thoracic cavity

✓7th S21.231 Puncture wound without foreign body of right back wall of thorax without penetration into thoracic cavity

✓7th S21.232 Puncture wound without foreign body of left back wall of thorax without penetration into thoracic cavity

✓7th S21.239 **Puncture wound without foreign body of unspecified back wall of thorax without penetration into thoracic cavity**

✓6th S21.24 **Puncture wound with foreign body of back wall of thorax without penetration into thoracic cavity**

✓7th S21.241 **Puncture wound with foreign body of right back wall of thorax without penetration into thoracic cavity**

✓7th S21.242 **Puncture wound with foreign body of left back wall of thorax without penetration into thoracic cavity**

✓7th S21.249 **Puncture wound with foreign body of unspecified back wall of thorax without penetration into thoracic cavity**

✓6th S21.25 **Open bite of back wall of thorax without penetration into thoracic cavity**

Bite of back wall of thorax NOS

EXCLUDES 1 *superficial bite of back wall of thorax (S20.47)*

✓7th S21.251 **Open bite of right back wall of thorax without penetration into thoracic cavity**

✓7th S21.252 **Open bite of left back wall of thorax without penetration into thoracic cavity**

✓7th S21.259 **Open bite of unspecified back wall of thorax without penetration into thoracic cavity**

✓5th S21.3 **Open wound of front wall of thorax with penetration into thoracic cavity**

Open wound of chest with penetration into thoracic cavity

✓6th S21.30 **Unspecified open wound of front wall of thorax with penetration into thoracic cavity**

✓7th S21.301 **Unspecified open wound of right front wall of thorax with penetration into thoracic cavity**

✓7th S21.302 **Unspecified open wound of left front wall of thorax with penetration into thoracic cavity**

✓7th S21.309 **Unspecified open wound of unspecified front wall of thorax with penetration into thoracic cavity**

✓6th S21.31 **Laceration without foreign body of front wall of thorax with penetration into thoracic cavity**

✓7th S21.311 **Laceration without foreign body of right front wall of thorax with penetration into thoracic cavity**

✓7th S21.312 **Laceration without foreign body of left front wall of thorax with penetration into thoracic cavity**

✓7th S21.319 **Laceration without foreign body of unspecified front wall of thorax with penetration into thoracic cavity**

✓6th S21.32 **Laceration with foreign body of front wall of thorax with penetration into thoracic cavity**

✓7th S21.321 **Laceration with foreign body of right front wall of thorax with penetration into thoracic cavity**

✓7th S21.322 **Laceration with foreign body of left front wall of thorax with penetration into thoracic cavity**

✓7th S21.329 **Laceration with foreign body of unspecified front wall of thorax with penetration into thoracic cavity**

✓6th S21.33 **Puncture wound without foreign body of front wall of thorax with penetration into thoracic cavity**

✓7th S21.331 **Puncture wound without foreign body of right front wall of thorax with penetration into thoracic cavity**

✓7th S21.332 **Puncture wound without foreign body of left front wall of thorax with penetration into thoracic cavity**

✓7th S21.339 **Puncture wound without foreign body of unspecified front wall of thorax with penetration into thoracic cavity**

✓6th S21.34 **Puncture wound with foreign body of front wall of thorax with penetration into thoracic cavity**

✓7th S21.341 **Puncture wound with foreign body of right front wall of thorax with penetration into thoracic cavity**

✓7th S21.342 **Puncture wound with foreign body of left front wall of thorax with penetration into thoracic cavity**

✓7th S21.349 **Puncture wound with foreign body of unspecified front wall of thorax with penetration into thoracic cavity**

✓6th S21.35 **Open bite of front wall of thorax with penetration into thoracic cavity**

EXCLUDES 1 *superficial bite of front wall of thorax (S20.37)*

✓7th S21.351 **Open bite of right front wall of thorax with penetration into thoracic cavity**

✓7th S21.352 **Open bite of left front wall of thorax with penetration into thoracic cavity**

✓7th S21.359 **Open bite of unspecified front wall of thorax with penetration into thoracic cavity**

✓5th S21.4 **Open wound of back wall of thorax with penetration into thoracic cavity**

✓6th S21.40 **Unspecified open wound of back wall of thorax with penetration into thoracic cavity**

✓7th S21.401 **Unspecified open wound of right back wall of thorax with penetration into thoracic cavity**

✓7th S21.402 **Unspecified open wound of left back wall of thorax with penetration into thoracic cavity**

✓7th S21.409 **Unspecified open wound of unspecified back wall of thorax with penetration into thoracic cavity**

✓6th S21.41 **Laceration without foreign body of back wall of thorax with penetration into thoracic cavity**

✓7th S21.411 **Laceration without foreign body of right back wall of thorax with penetration into thoracic cavity**

✓7th S21.412 **Laceration without foreign body of left back wall of thorax with penetration into thoracic cavity**

✓7th S21.419 **Laceration without foreign body of unspecified back wall of thorax with penetration into thoracic cavity**

✓6th S21.42 **Laceration with foreign body of back wall of thorax with penetration into thoracic cavity**

✓7th S21.421 **Laceration with foreign body of right back wall of thorax with penetration into thoracic cavity**

✓7th S21.422 **Laceration with foreign body of left back wall of thorax with penetration into thoracic cavity**

✓7th S21.429 **Laceration with foreign body of unspecified back wall of thorax with penetration into thoracic cavity**

✓6th S21.43 **Puncture wound without foreign body of back wall of thorax with penetration into thoracic cavity**

✓7th S21.431 **Puncture wound without foreign body of right back wall of thorax with penetration into thoracic cavity**

✓7th S21.432 **Puncture wound without foreign body of left back wall of thorax with penetration into thoracic cavity**

✓7th S21.439 **Puncture wound without foreign body of unspecified back wall of thorax with penetration into thoracic cavity**

✓6th S21.44 **Puncture wound with foreign body of back wall of thorax with penetration into thoracic cavity**

✓7th S21.441 **Puncture wound with foreign body of right back wall of thorax with penetration into thoracic cavity**

✓7th S21.442 **Puncture wound with foreign body of left back wall of thorax with penetration into thoracic cavity**

✓7th S21.449 **Puncture wound with foreign body of unspecified back wall of thorax with penetration into thoracic cavity**

✓6th **S21.45 Open bite of back wall of thorax with penetration into thoracic cavity**
Bite of back wall of thorax NOS
EXCLUDES 1 *superficial bite of back wall of thorax (S20.47)*
✓7th **S21.451 Open bite of right back wall of thorax with penetration into thoracic cavity**
✓7th **S21.452 Open bite of left back wall of thorax with penetration into thoracic cavity**
✓7th **S21.459 Open bite of unspecified back wall of thorax with penetration into thoracic cavity**

✓5th **S21.9 Open wound of unspecified part of thorax**
Open wound of thoracic wall NOS
✓x7th **S21.90 Unspecified open wound of unspecified part of thorax**
✓x7th **S21.91 Laceration without foreign body of unspecified part of thorax**
✓x7th **S21.92 Laceration with foreign body of unspecified part of thorax**
✓x7th **S21.93 Puncture wound without foreign body of unspecified part of thorax**
✓x7th **S21.94 Puncture wound with foreign body of unspecified part of thorax**
✓x7th **S21.95 Open bite of unspecified part of thorax**
EXCLUDES 1 *superficial bite of thorax (S20.97)*

✓4th **S22 Fracture of rib(s), sternum and thoracic spine**
NOTE A fracture not indicated as nondisplaced or displaced should be classified to displaced
A fracture not indicated as open or closed should be coded to closed
Fracture of thoracic neural arch
Fracture of thoracic spinous process
Fracture of thoracic transverse process
Fracture of thoracic vertebra
Fracture of thoracic vertebral arch
Codes first any associated:
injury of intrathoracic organ (S27.-)
spinal cord injury (S24.0-, S24.1-)
EXCLUDES 1 *transection of thorax (S28.1)*
EXCLUDES 2 *fracture of clavicle (S42.0-)*
fracture of scapula (S42.1-)

The appropriate 7th character is to be added to each code from category S22.
A initial encounter for closed fracture
B initial encounter for open fracture
D subsequent encounter for fracture with routine healing
G subsequent encounter for fracture with delayed healing
K subsequent encounter for fracture with nonunion
S sequela

✓5th **S22.0 Fracture of thoracic vertebra**
✓6th **S22.00 Fracture of unspecified thoracic vertebra**
✓7th **S22.000 Wedge compression fracture of unspecified thoracic vertebra**
✓7th **S22.001 Stable burst fracture of unspecified thoracic vertebra**
✓7th **S22.002 Unstable burst fracture of unspecified thoracic vertebra**
✓7th **S22.008 Other fracture of unspecified thoracic vertebra**
✓7th **S22.009 Unspecified fracture of unspecified thoracic vertebra**
✓6th **S22.01 Fracture of first thoracic vertebra**
✓7th **S22.010 Wedge compression fracture of first thoracic vertebra**
✓7th **S22.011 Stable burst fracture of first thoracic vertebra**
✓7th **S22.012 Unstable burst fracture of first thoracic vertebra**
✓7th **S22.018 Other fracture of first thoracic vertebra**
✓7th **S22.019 Unspecified fracture of first thoracic vertebra**
✓6th **S22.02 Fracture of second thoracic vertebra**
✓7th **S22.020 Wedge compression fracture of second thoracic vertebra**
✓7th **S22.021 Stable burst fracture of second thoracic vertebra**
✓7th **S22.022 Unstable burst fracture of second thoracic vertebra**
✓7th **S22.028 Other fracture of second thoracic vertebra**
✓7th **S22.029 Unspecified fracture of second thoracic vertebra**
✓6th **S22.03 Fracture of third thoracic vertebra**
✓7th **S22.030 Wedge compression fracture of third thoracic vertebra**
✓7th **S22.031 Stable burst fracture of third thoracic vertebra**
✓7th **S22.032 Unstable burst fracture of third thoracic vertebra**
✓7th **S22.038 Other fracture of third thoracic vertebra**
✓7th **S22.039 Unspecified fracture of third thoracic vertebra**
✓6th **S22.04 Fracture of fourth thoracic vertebra**
✓7th **S22.040 Wedge compression fracture of fourth thoracic vertebra**
✓7th **S22.041 Stable burst fracture of fourth thoracic vertebra**
✓7th **S22.042 Unstable burst fracture of fourth thoracic vertebra**
✓7th **S22.048 Other fracture of fourth thoracic vertebra**
✓7th **S22.049 Unspecified fracture of fourth thoracic vertebra**
✓6th **S22.05 Fracture of T5-T6 vertebra**
✓7th **S22.050 Wedge compression fracture of T5-T6 vertebra**
✓7th **S22.051 Stable burst fracture of T5-T6 vertebra**
✓7th **S22.052 Unstable burst fracture of T5-T6 vertebra**
✓7th **S22.058 Other fracture of T5-T6 vertebra**
✓7th **S22.059 Unspecified fracture of T5-T6 vertebra**
✓6th **S22.06 Fracture of T7-T8 vertebra**
✓7th **S22.060 Wedge compression fracture of T7-T8 vertebra**
✓7th **S22.061 Stable burst fracture of T7-T8 vertebra**
✓7th **S22.062 Unstable burst fracture of T7-T8 vertebra**
✓7th **S22.068 Other fracture of T7-T8 thoracic vertebra**
✓7th **S22.069 Unspecified fracture of T7-T8 vertebra**
✓6th **S22.07 Fracture of T9-T10 vertebra**
✓7th **S22.070 Wedge compression fracture of T9-T10 vertebra**
✓7th **S22.071 Stable burst fracture of T9-T10 vertebra**
✓7th **S22.072 Unstable burst fracture of T9-T10 vertebra**
✓7th **S22.078 Other fracture of T9-T10 vertebra**
✓7th **S22.079 Unspecified fracture of T9-T10 vertebra**
✓6th **S22.08 Fracture of T11-T12 vertebra**
✓7th **S22.080 Wedge compression fracture of T11-T12 vertebra**
✓7th **S22.081 Stable burst fracture of T11-T12 vertebra**
✓7th **S22.082 Unstable burst fracture of T11-T12 vertebra**
✓7th **S22.088 Other fracture of T11-T12 vertebra**
✓7th **S22.089 Unspecified fracture of T11-T12 vertebra**
✓5th **S22.2 Fracture of sternum**
✓x7th **S22.20 Unspecified fracture of sternum**
✓x7th **S22.21 Fracture of manubrium**
✓x7th **S22.22 Fracture of body of sternum**
✓x7th **S22.23 Sternal manubrial dissociation**
✓x7th **S22.24 Fracture of xiphoid process**
✓5th **S22.3 Fracture of one rib**
✓x7th **S22.31 Fracture of one rib, right side**
✓x7th **S22.32 Fracture of one rib, left side**
✓x7th **S22.39 Fracture of one rib, unspecified side**
✓5th **S22.4 Multiple fractures of ribs**
Fractures of two or more ribs
EXCLUDES 1 *flail chest (S22.5-)*
✓x7th **S22.41 Multiple fractures of ribs, right side**
✓x7th **S22.42 Multiple fractures of ribs, left side**

S22.43 Multiple fractures of ribs, bilateral
S22.49 Multiple fractures of ribs, unspecified side
S22.5 Flail chest
S22.9 Fracture of bony thorax, part unspecified

S23 Dislocation and sprain of joints and ligaments of thorax

INCLUDES avulsion of joint or ligament of thorax
laceration of cartilage, joint or ligament of thorax
sprain of cartilage, joint or ligament of thorax
traumatic hemarthrosis of joint or ligament of thorax
traumatic rupture of joint or ligament of thorax
traumatic subluxation of joint or ligament of thorax
traumatic tear of joint or ligament of thorax

Code also any associated open wound

EXCLUDES 2 *dislocation, sprain of sternoclavicular joint (S43.2, S43.6)*
strain of muscle or tendon of thorax (S29.01-)

The appropriate 7th character is to be added to each code from category S23.
A initial encounter
D subsequent encounter
S sequela

S23.0 Traumatic rupture of thoracic intervertebral disc
EXCLUDES 1 *rupture or displacement (nontraumatic) of thoracic intervertebral disc NOS (M51- with fifth character 4)*

S23.1 Subluxation and dislocation of thoracic vertebra
Code also any associated
open wound of thorax (S21.-)
spinal cord injury (S24.0-, S24.1-)
EXCLUDES 2 *fracture of thoracic vertebrae (S22.0-)*

S23.10 Subluxation and dislocation of unspecified thoracic vertebra
S23.100 Subluxation of unspecified thoracic vertebra
S23.101 Dislocation of unspecified thoracic vertebra

S23.11 Subluxation and dislocation of T1/T2 thoracic vertebra
S23.110 Subluxation of T1/T2 thoracic vertebra
S23.111 Dislocation of T1/T2 thoracic vertebra

S23.12 Subluxation and dislocation of T2/T3-T3/T4 thoracic vertebra
S23.120 Subluxation of T2/T3 thoracic vertebra
S23.121 Dislocation of T2/T3 thoracic vertebra
S23.122 Subluxation of T3/T4 thoracic vertebra
S23.123 Dislocation of T3/T4 thoracic vertebra

S23.13 Subluxation and dislocation of T4/T5-T5/T6 thoracic vertebra
S23.130 Subluxation of T4/T5 thoracic vertebra
S23.131 Dislocation of T4/T5 thoracic vertebra
S23.132 Subluxation of T5/T6 thoracic vertebra
S23.133 Dislocation of T5/T6 thoracic vertebra

S23.14 Subluxation and dislocation of T6/T7-T7/T8 thoracic vertebra
S23.140 Subluxation of T6/T7 thoracic vertebra
S23.141 Dislocation of T6/T7 thoracic vertebra
S23.142 Subluxation of T7/T8 thoracic vertebra
S23.143 Dislocation of T7/T8 thoracic vertebra

S23.15 Subluxation and dislocation of T8/T9-T9/T10 thoracic vertebra
S23.150 Subluxation of T8/T9 thoracic vertebra
S23.151 Dislocation of T8/T9 thoracic vertebra
S23.152 Subluxation of T9/T10 thoracic vertebra
S23.153 Dislocation of T9/T10 thoracic vertebra

S23.16 Subluxation and dislocation of T10/T11-T11/T12 thoracic vertebra
S23.160 Subluxation of T10/T11 thoracic vertebra
S23.161 Dislocation of T10/T11 thoracic vertebra
S23.162 Subluxation of T11/T12 thoracic vertebra
S23.163 Dislocation of T11/T12 thoracic vertebra

S23.17 Subluxation and dislocation of T12/L1 thoracic vertebra
S23.170 Subluxation of T12/L1 thoracic vertebra
S23.171 Dislocation of T12/L1 thoracic vertebra

S23.2 Dislocation of other and unspecified parts of thorax
S23.20 Dislocation of unspecified part of thorax
S23.29 Dislocation of other parts of thorax

S23.3 Sprain of ligaments of thoracic spine

S23.4 Sprain of ribs and sternum
S23.41 Sprain of ribs
S23.42 Sprain of sternum
S23.420 Sprain of sternoclavicular (joint) (ligament)
S23.421 Sprain of chondrosternal joint
S23.428 Other sprain of sternum
S23.429 Unspecified sprain of sternum

S23.8 Sprain of other specified parts of thorax
S23.9 Sprain of unspecified parts of thorax

S24 Injury of nerves and spinal cord at thorax level

NOTE Code to highest level of thoracic spinal cord injury

Code also any associated:
fracture of thoracic vertebra (S22.0-)
open wound of thorax (S21.-)
transient paralysis (R29.5)

EXCLUDES 2 *injury of brachial plexus (S14.3)*

The appropriate 7th character is to be added to each code from category S24.
A initial encounter
D subsequent encounter
S sequela

S24.0 Concussion and edema of thoracic spinal cord

S24.1 Other and unspecified injuries of thoracic spinal cord
S24.10 Unspecified injury of thoracic spinal cord
S24.101 Unspecified injury at T1 level of thoracic spinal cord
S24.102 Unspecified injury at T2-T6 level of thoracic spinal cord
S24.103 Unspecified injury at T7-T10 level of thoracic spinal cord
S24.104 Unspecified injury at T11-T12 level of thoracic spinal cord
S24.109 Unspecified injury at unspecified level of thoracic spinal cord
Injury of thoracic spinal cord NOS

S24.11 Complete lesion of thoracic spinal cord
S24.111 Complete lesion at T1 level of thoracic spinal cord
S24.112 Complete lesion at T2-T6 level of thoracic spinal cord
S24.113 Complete lesion at T7-T10 level of thoracic spinal cord
S24.114 Complete lesion at T11-T12 level of thoracic spinal cord
S24.119 Complete lesion at unspecified level of thoracic spinal cord

S24.13 Anterior cord syndrome of thoracic spinal cord
S24.131 Anterior cord syndrome at T1 level of thoracic spinal cord
S24.132 Anterior cord syndrome at T2-T6 level of thoracic spinal cord
S24.133 Anterior cord syndrome at T7-T10 level of thoracic spinal cord
S24.134 Anterior cord syndrome at T11-T12 level of thoracic spinal cord
S24.139 Anterior cord syndrome at unspecified level of thoracic spinal cord

S24.14 Brown-Séquard syndrome of thoracic spinal cord
S24.141 Brown-Séquard syndrome at T1 level of thoracic spinal cord
S24.142 Brown-Séquard syndrome at T2-T6 level of thoracic spinal cord
S24.143 Brown-Séquard syndrome at T7-T10 level of thoracic spinal cord
S24.144 Brown-Séquard syndrome at T11-T12 level of thoracic spinal cord
S24.149 Brown-Séquard syndrome at unspecified level of thoracic spinal cord

✓6th **S24.15 Other incomplete lesions of thoracic spinal cord**
Incomplete lesion of thoracic spinal cord NOS
Posterior cord syndrome of thoracic spinal cord

✓7th **S24.151 Other incomplete lesion at T1 level of thoracic spinal cord**

✓7th **S24.152 Other incomplete lesion at T2-T6 level of thoracic spinal cord**

✓7th **S24.153 Other incomplete lesion at T7-T10 level of thoracic spinal cord**

✓7th **S24.154 Other incomplete lesion at T11-T12 level of thoracic spinal cord**

✓7th **S24.159 Other incomplete lesion at unspecified level of thoracic spinal cord**

✓x7th **S24.2 Injury of nerve root of thoracic spine**

✓x7th **S24.3 Injury of peripheral nerves of thorax**

✓x7th **S24.4 Injury of thoracic sympathetic nervous system**
Injury of cardiac plexus
Injury of esophageal plexus
Injury of pulmonary plexus
Injury of stellate ganglion
Injury of thoracic sympathetic ganglion

✓x7th **S24.8 Injury of other specified nerves of thorax**

✓x7th **S24.9 Injury of unspecified nerve of thorax**

✓4th **S25 Injury of blood vessels of thorax**
Code also any associated open wound (S21.-)

The appropriate 7th character is to be added to each code from category S25.
A initial encounter
D subsequent encounter
S sequela

✓5th **S25.0 Injury of thoracic aorta**
Injury of aorta NOS

✓x7th **S25.00 Unspecified injury of thoracic aorta**

✓x7th **S25.01 Minor laceration of thoracic aorta**
Incomplete transection of thoracic aorta
Laceration of thoracic aorta NOS
Superficial laceration of thoracic aorta

✓x7th **S25.02 Major laceration of thoracic aorta**
Complete transection of thoracic aorta
Traumatic rupture of thoracic aorta

✓x7th **S25.09 Other specified injury of thoracic aorta**

✓5th **S25.1 Injury of innominate or subclavian artery**

✓6th **S25.10 Unspecified injury of innominate or subclavian artery**

✓7th **S25.101 Unspecified injury of right innominate or subclavian artery**

✓7th **S25.102 Unspecified injury of left innominate or subclavian artery**

✓7th **S25.109 Unspecified injury of unspecified innominate or subclavian artery**

✓6th **S25.11 Minor laceration of innominate or subclavian artery**
Incomplete transection of innominate or subclavian artery
Laceration of innominate or subclavian artery NOS
Superficial laceration of innominate or subclavian artery

✓7th **S25.111 Minor laceration of right innominate or subclavian artery**

✓7th **S25.112 Minor laceration of left innominate or subclavian artery**

✓7th **S25.119 Minor laceration of unspecified innominate or subclavian artery**

✓6th **S25.12 Major laceration of innominate or subclavian artery**
Complete transection of innominate or subclavian artery
Traumatic rupture of innominate or subclavian artery

✓7th **S25.121 Major laceration of right innominate or subclavian artery**

✓7th **S25.122 Major laceration of left innominate or subclavian artery**

✓7th **S25.129 Major laceration of unspecified innominate or subclavian artery**

✓6th **S25.19 Other specified injury of innominate or subclavian artery**

✓7th **S25.191 Other specified injury of right innominate or subclavian artery**

✓7th **S25.192 Other specified injury of left innominate or subclavian artery**

✓7th **S25.199 Other specified injury of unspecified innominate or subclavian artery**

✓5th **S25.2 Injury of superior vena cava**
Injury of vena cava NOS

✓x7th **S25.20 Unspecified injury of superior vena cava**

✓x7th **S25.21 Minor laceration of superior vena cava**
Incomplete transection of superior vena cava
Laceration of superior vena cava NOS
Superficial laceration of superior vena cava

✓x7th **S25.22 Major laceration of superior vena cava**
Complete transection of superior vena cava
Traumatic rupture of superior vena cava

✓x7th **S25.29 Other specified injury of superior vena cava**

✓5th **S25.3 Injury of innominate or subclavian vein**

✓6th **S25.30 Unspecified injury of innominate or subclavian vein**

✓7th **S25.301 Unspecified injury of right innominate or subclavian vein**

✓7th **S25.302 Unspecified injury of left innominate or subclavian vein**

✓7th **S25.309 Unspecified injury of unspecified innominate or subclavian vein**

✓6th **S25.31 Minor laceration of innominate or subclavian vein**
Incomplete transection of innominate or subclavian vein
Laceration of innominate or subclavian vein NOS
Superficial laceration of innominate or subclavian vein

✓7th **S25.311 Minor laceration of right innominate or subclavian vein**

✓7th **S25.312 Minor laceration of left innominate or subclavian vein**

✓7th **S25.319 Minor laceration of unspecified innominate or subclavian vein**

✓6th **S25.32 Major laceration of innominate or subclavian vein**
Complete transection of innominate or subclavian vein
Traumatic rupture of innominate or subclavian vein

✓7th **S25.321 Major laceration of right innominate or subclavian vein**

✓7th **S25.322 Major laceration of left innominate or subclavian vein**

✓7th **S25.329 Major laceration of unspecified innominate or subclavian vein**

✓6th **S25.39 Other specified injury of innominate or subclavian vein**

✓7th **S25.391 Other specified injury of right innominate or subclavian vein**

✓7th **S25.392 Other specified injury of left innominate or subclavian vein**

✓7th **S25.399 Other specified injury of unspecified innominate or subclavian vein**

✓5th **S25.4 Injury of pulmonary blood vessels**

✓6th **S25.40 Unspecified injury of pulmonary blood vessels**

✓7th **S25.401 Unspecified injury of right pulmonary blood vessels**

✓7th **S25.402 Unspecified injury of left pulmonary blood vessels**

✓7th **S25.409 Unspecified injury of unspecified pulmonary blood vessels**

✓6th **S25.41 Minor laceration of pulmonary blood vessels**
Incomplete transection of pulmonary blood vessels
Laceration of pulmonary blood vessels NOS
Superficial laceration of pulmonary blood vessels

✓7th **S25.411 Minor laceration of right pulmonary blood vessels**

✓7th **S25.412 Minor laceration of left pulmonary blood vessels**

✓7th **S25.419 Minor laceration of unspecified pulmonary blood vessels**

S25.42 Major laceration of pulmonary blood vessels
Complete transection of pulmonary blood vessels
Traumatic rupture of pulmonary blood vessels
S25.421 Major laceration of right pulmonary blood vessels
S25.422 Major laceration of left pulmonary blood vessels
S25.429 Major laceration of unspecified pulmonary blood vessels
S25.49 Other specified injury of pulmonary blood vessels
S25.491 Other specified injury of right pulmonary blood vessels
S25.492 Other specified injury of left pulmonary blood vessels
S25.499 Other specified injury of unspecified pulmonary blood vessels
S25.5 Injury of intercostal blood vessels
S25.50 Unspecified injury of intercostal blood vessels
S25.501 Unspecified injury of intercostal blood vessels, right side
S25.502 Unspecified injury of intercostal blood vessels, left side
S25.509 Unspecified injury of intercostal blood vessels, unspecified side
S25.51 Laceration of intercostal blood vessels
S25.511 Laceration of intercostal blood vessels, right side
S25.512 Laceration of intercostal blood vessels, left side
S25.519 Laceration of intercostal blood vessels, unspecified side
S25.59 Other specified injury of intercostal blood vessels
S25.591 Other specified injury of intercostal blood vessels, right side
S25.592 Other specified injury of intercostal blood vessels, left side
S25.599 Other specified injury of intercostal blood vessels, unspecified side
S25.8 Injury of other blood vessels of thorax
Injury of azygos vein
Injury of mammary artery or vein
S25.80 Unspecified injury of other blood vessels of thorax
S25.801 Unspecified injury of other blood vessels of thorax, right side
S25.802 Unspecified injury of other blood vessels of thorax, left side
S25.809 Unspecified injury of other blood vessels of thorax, unspecified side
S25.81 Laceration of other blood vessels of thorax
S25.811 Laceration of other blood vessels of thorax, right side
S25.812 Laceration of other blood vessels of thorax, left side
S25.819 Laceration of other blood vessels of thorax, unspecified side
S25.89 Other specified injury of other blood vessels of thorax
S25.891 Other specified injury of other blood vessels of thorax, right side
S25.892 Other specified injury of other blood vessels of thorax, left side
S25.899 Other specified injury of other blood vessels of thorax, unspecified side
S25.9 Injury of unspecified blood vessel of thorax
S25.90 Unspecified injury of unspecified blood vessel of thorax
S25.91 Laceration of unspecified blood vessel of thorax
S25.99 Other specified injury of unspecified blood vessel of thorax

S26 Injury of heart
Code also any associated:
open wound of thorax (S21.-)
traumatic hemopneumothorax (S27.2)
traumatic hemothorax (S27.1)
traumatic pneumothorax (S27.0)

The appropriate 7th character is to be added to each code from category S26.
A initial encounter
D subsequent encounter
S sequela

S26.0 Injury of heart with hemopericardium
S26.00 Unspecified injury of heart with hemopericardium
S26.01 Contusion of heart with hemopericardium
S26.02 Laceration of heart with hemopericardium
S26.020 Mild laceration of heart with hemopericardium
Laceration of heart without penetration of heart chamber
S26.021 Moderate laceration of heart with hemopericardium
Laceration of heart with penetration of heart chamber
S26.022 Major laceration of heart with hemopericardium
Laceration of heart with penetration of multiple heart chambers
S26.09 Other injury of heart with hemopericardium
S26.1 Injury of heart without hemopericardium
S26.10 Unspecified injury of heart without hemopericardium
S26.11 Contusion of heart without hemopericardium
S26.12 Laceration of heart without hemopericardium
S26.19 Other injury of heart without hemopericardium
S26.9 Injury of heart, unspecified with or without hemopericardium
S26.90 Unspecified injury of heart, unspecified with or without hemopericardium
S26.91 Contusion of heart, unspecified with or without hemopericardium
S26.92 Laceration of heart, unspecified with or without hemopericardium
Laceration of heart NOS
S26.99 Other injury of heart, unspecified with or without hemopericardium

S27 Injury of other and unspecified intrathoracic organs
Code also any associated open wound of thorax (S21.-)
EXCLUDES 2 *injury of cervical esophagus (S10-S19)*
injury of trachea (cervical) (S10-S19)

The appropriate 7th character is to be added to each code from category S27.
A initial encounter
D subsequent encounter
S sequela

S27.0 Traumatic pneumothorax
EXCLUDES 1 *spontaneous pneumothorax (J93.-)*
S27.1 Traumatic hemothorax
S27.2 Traumatic hemopneumothorax
S27.3 Other and unspecified injuries of lung
S27.30 Unspecified injury of lung
S27.301 Unspecified injury of lung, unilateral
S27.302 Unspecified injury of lung, bilateral
S27.309 Unspecified injury of lung, unspecified
S27.31 Primary blast injury of lung
Blast injury of lung NOS
S27.311 Primary blast injury of lung, unilateral
S27.312 Primary blast injury of lung, bilateral
S27.319 Primary blast injury of lung, unspecified
S27.32 Contusion of lung
S27.321 Contusion of lung, unilateral
S27.322 Contusion of lung, bilateral
S27.329 Contusion of lung, unspecified

Appropriate additional character required — x7th Requires 7th character, placeholder x must fill empty characters

S27.33 Laceration of lung
S27.331 Laceration of lung, unilateral
S27.332 Laceration of lung, bilateral
S27.339 Laceration of lung, unspecified
S27.39 Other injuries of lung
Secondary blast injury of lung
S27.391 Other injuries of lung, unilateral
S27.392 Other injuries of lung, bilateral
S27.399 Other injuries of lung, unspecified
S27.4 Injury of bronchus
S27.40 Unspecified injury of bronchus
S27.401 Unspecified injury of bronchus, unilateral
S27.402 Unspecified injury of bronchus, bilateral
S27.409 Unspecified injury of bronchus, unspecified
S27.41 Primary blast injury of bronchus
Blast injury of bronchus NOS
S27.411 Primary blast injury of bronchus, unilateral
S27.412 Primary blast injury of bronchus, bilateral
S27.419 Primary blast injury of bronchus, unspecified
S27.42 Contusion of bronchus
S27.421 Contusion of bronchus, unilateral
S27.422 Contusion of bronchus, bilateral
S27.429 Contusion of bronchus, unspecified
S27.43 Laceration of bronchus
S27.431 Laceration of bronchus, unilateral
S27.432 Laceration of bronchus, bilateral
S27.439 Laceration of bronchus, unspecified
S27.49 Other injury of bronchus
Secondary blast injury of bronchus
S27.491 Other injury of bronchus, unilateral
S27.492 Other injury of bronchus, bilateral
S27.499 Other injury of bronchus, unspecified
S27.5 Injury of thoracic trachea
S27.50 Unspecified injury of thoracic trachea
S27.51 Primary blast injury of thoracic trachea
Blast injury of thoracic trachea NOS
S27.52 Contusion of thoracic trachea
S27.53 Laceration of thoracic trachea
S27.59 Other injury of thoracic trachea
Secondary blast injury of thoracic trachea
S27.6 Injury of pleura
S27.60 Unspecified injury of pleura
S27.63 Laceration of pleura
S27.69 Other injury of pleura
S27.8 Injury of other specified intrathoracic organs
S27.80 Injury of diaphragm
S27.802 Contusion of diaphragm
S27.803 Laceration of diaphragm
S27.808 Other injury of diaphragm
S27.809 Unspecified injury of diaphragm
S27.81 Injury of esophagus (thoracic part)
S27.812 Contusion of esophagus (thoracic part)
S27.813 Laceration of esophagus (thoracic part)
S27.818 Other injury of esophagus (thoracic part)
S27.819 Unspecified injury of esophagus (thoracic part)
S27.89 Injury of other specified intrathoracic organs
Injury of lymphatic thoracic duct
Injury of thymus gland
S27.892 Contusion of other specified intrathoracic organs
S27.893 Laceration of other specified intrathoracic organs
S27.898 Other injury of other specified intrathoracic organs
S27.899 Unspecified injury of other specified intrathoracic organs
S27.9 Injury of unspecified intrathoracic organ

S28 Crushing injury of thorax, and traumatic amputation of part of thorax

The appropriate 7th character is to be added to each code from category S28.
A initial encounter
D subsequent encounter
S sequela

S28.0 Crushed chest
Use additional code for all associated injuries
EXCLUDES1 *flail chest (S22.5)*
S28.1 Traumatic amputation (partial) of part of thorax, except breast
S28.2 Traumatic amputation of breast
S28.21 Complete traumatic amputation of breast
Traumatic amputation of breast NOS
S28.211 Complete traumatic amputation of right breast
S28.212 Complete traumatic amputation of left breast
S28.219 Complete traumatic amputation of unspecified breast
S28.22 Partial traumatic amputation of breast
S28.221 Partial traumatic amputation of right breast
S28.222 Partial traumatic amputation of left breast
S28.229 Partial traumatic amputation of unspecified breast

S29 Other and unspecified injuries of thorax
Code also any associated open wound (S21.-)

The appropriate 7th character is to be added to each code from category S29.
A initial encounter
D subsequent encounter
S sequela

S29.0 Injury of muscle and tendon at thorax level
S29.00 Unspecified injury of muscle and tendon of thorax
S29.001 Unspecified injury of muscle and tendon of front wall of thorax
S29.002 Unspecified injury of muscle and tendon of back wall of thorax
S29.009 Unspecified injury of muscle and tendon of unspecified wall of thorax
S29.01 Strain of muscle and tendon of thorax
S29.011 Strain of muscle and tendon of front wall of thorax
S29.012 Strain of muscle and tendon of back wall of thorax
S29.019 Strain of muscle and tendon of unspecified wall of thorax
S29.02 Laceration of muscle and tendon of thorax
S29.021 Laceration of muscle and tendon of front wall of thorax
S29.022 Laceration of muscle and tendon of back wall of thorax
S29.029 Laceration of muscle and tendon of unspecified wall of thorax
S29.09 Other injury of muscle and tendon of thorax
S29.091 Other injury of muscle and tendon of front wall of thorax
S29.092 Other injury of muscle and tendon of back wall of thorax
S29.099 Other injury of muscle and tendon of unspecified wall of thorax
S29.8 Other specified injuries of thorax
S29.9 Unspecified injury of thorax

Injuries to the abdomen, lower back, lumbar spine, pelvis and external genitals (S30-S39)

INCLUDES injuries to the abdominal wall
injuries to the anus
injuries to the buttock
injuries to the external genitalia
injuries to the flank
injuries to the groin

EXCLUDES 2 *burns and corrosions (T20-T32)*
effects of foreign body in anus and rectum (T18.5)
effects of foreign body in genitourinary tract (T19.-)
effects of foreign body in stomach, small intestine and colon (T18.2-T18.4)
frostbite (T33-T34)
insect bite or sting, venomous (T63.4)

S30 Superficial injury of abdomen, lower back, pelvis and external genitals

EXCLUDES 2 *superficial injury of hip (S70.-)*

The appropriate 7th character is to be added to each code from category S30.
A initial encounter
D subsequent encounter
S sequela

S30.0 Contusion of lower back and pelvis
Contusion of buttock

S30.1 Contusion of abdominal wall
Contusion of flank
Contusion of groin

S30.2 Contusion of external genital organs

S30.20 Contusion of unspecified external genital organ

S30.201 Contusion of unspecified external genital organ, male

S30.202 Contusion of unspecified external genital organ, female

S30.21 Contusion of penis

S30.22 Contusion of scrotum and testes

S30.23 Contusion of vagina and vulva

S30.3 Contusion of anus

S30.8 Other superficial injuries of abdomen, lower back, pelvis and external genitals

S30.81 Abrasion of abdomen, lower back, pelvis and external genitals

S30.810 Abrasion of lower back and pelvis

S30.811 Abrasion of abdominal wall

S30.812 Abrasion of penis

S30.813 Abrasion of scrotum and testes

S30.814 Abrasion of vagina and vulva

S30.815 Abrasion of unspecified external genital organs, male

S30.816 Abrasion of unspecified external genital organs, female

S30.817 Abrasion of anus

S30.82 Blister (nonthermal) of abdomen, lower back, pelvis and external genitals

S30.820 Blister (nonthermal) of lower back and pelvis

S30.821 Blister (nonthermal) of abdominal wall

S30.822 Blister (nonthermal) of penis

S30.823 Blister (nonthermal) of scrotum and testes

S30.824 Blister (nonthermal) of vagina and vulva

S30.825 Blister (nonthermal) of unspecified external genital organs, male

S30.826 Blister (nonthermal) of unspecified external genital organs, female

S30.827 Blister (nonthermal) of anus

S30.84 External constriction of abdomen, lower back, pelvis and external genitals

S30.840 External constriction of lower back and pelvis

S30.841 External constriction of abdominal wall

S30.842 External constriction of penis
Hair tourniquet syndrome of penis
Use additional cause code to identify the constricting item (W49.0-)

S30.843 External constriction of scrotum and testes

S30.844 External constriction of vagina and vulva

S30.845 External constriction of unspecified external genital organs, male

S30.846 External constriction of unspecified external genital organs, female

S30.85 Superficial foreign body of abdomen, lower back, pelvis and external genitals
Splinter in the abdomen, lower back, pelvis and external genitals

S30.850 Superficial foreign body of lower back and pelvis

S30.851 Superficial foreign body of abdominal wall

S30.852 Superficial foreign body of penis

S30.853 Superficial foreign body of scrotum and testes

S30.854 Superficial foreign body of vagina and vulva

S30.855 Superficial foreign body of unspecified external genital organs, male

S30.856 Superficial foreign body of unspecified external genital organs, female

S30.857 Superficial foreign body of anus

S30.86 Insect bite (nonvenomous) of abdomen, lower back, pelvis and external genitals

S30.860 Insect bite (nonvenomous) of lower back and pelvis

S30.861 Insect bite (nonvenomous) of abdominal wall

S30.862 Insect bite (nonvenomous) of penis

S30.863 Insect bite (nonvenomous) of scrotum and testes

S30.864 Insect bite (nonvenomous) of vagina and vulva

S30.865 Insect bite (nonvenomous) of unspecified external genital organs, male

S30.866 Insect bite (nonvenomous) of unspecified external genital organs, female

S30.867 Insect bite (nonvenomous) of anus

S30.87 Other superficial bite of abdomen, lower back, pelvis and external genitals

EXCLUDES 1 *open bite of abdomen, lower back, pelvis and external genitals (S31.05, S31.15, S31.25, S31.35, S31.45, S31.55)*

S30.870 Other superficial bite of lower back and pelvis

S30.871 Other superficial bite of abdominal wall

S30.872 Other superficial bite of penis

S30.873 Other superficial bite of scrotum and testes

S30.874 Other superficial bite of vagina and vulva

S30.875 Other superficial bite of unspecified external genital organs, male

S30.876 Other superficial bite of unspecified external genital organs, female

S30.877 Other superficial bite of anus

S30.9 Unspecified superficial injury of abdomen, lower back, pelvis and external genitals

S30.91 Unspecified superficial injury of lower back and pelvis

S30.92 Unspecified superficial injury of abdominal wall

S30.93 Unspecified superficial injury of penis

S30.94 Unspecified superficial injury of scrotum and testes

S30.95 Unspecified superficial injury of vagina and vulva

S30.96 Unspecified superficial injury of unspecified external genital organs, male

S30.97 Unspecified superficial injury of unspecified external genital organs, female

S30.98 Unspecified superficial injury of anus

4th S31 Open wound of abdomen, lower back, pelvis and external genitals

Code also any associated:
spinal cord injury (S24.0, S24.1-, S34.0-, S34.1-)
wound infection

EXCLUDES 1 *traumatic amputation of part of abdomen, lower back and pelvis (S38.2-, S38.3)*

EXCLUDES 2 *open wound of hip (S71.00-S71.02)*
open fracture of pelvis (S32.1--S32.9 with 7th character B)

The appropriate 7th character is to be added to each code from category S31.
A initial encounter
D subsequent encounter
S sequela

5th S31.0 Open wound of lower back and pelvis

6th S31.00 Unspecified open wound of lower back and pelvis

7th S31.000 Unspecified open wound of lower back and pelvis without penetration into retroperitoneum
Unspecified open wound of lower back and pelvis NOS

7th S31.001 Unspecified open wound of lower back and pelvis with penetration into retroperitoneum

6th S31.01 Laceration without foreign body of lower back and pelvis

7th S31.010 Laceration without foreign body of lower back and pelvis without penetration into retroperitoneum
Laceration without foreign body of lower back and pelvis NOS

7th S31.011 Laceration without foreign body of lower back and pelvis with penetration into retroperitoneum

6th S31.02 Laceration with foreign body of lower back and pelvis

7th S31.020 Laceration with foreign body of lower back and pelvis without penetration into retroperitoneum
Laceration with foreign body of lower back and pelvis NOS

7th S31.021 Laceration with foreign body of lower back and pelvis with penetration into retroperitoneum

6th S31.03 Puncture wound without foreign body of lower back and pelvis

7th S31.030 Puncture wound without foreign body of lower back and pelvis without penetration into retroperitoneum
Puncture wound without foreign body of lower back and pelvis NOS

7th S31.031 Puncture wound without foreign body of lower back and pelvis with penetration into retroperitoneum

6th S31.04 Puncture wound with foreign body of lower back and pelvis

7th S31.040 Puncture wound with foreign body of lower back and pelvis without penetration into retroperitoneum
Puncture wound with foreign body of lower back and pelvis NOS

7th S31.041 Puncture wound with foreign body of lower back and pelvis with penetration into retroperitoneum

6th S31.05 Open bite of lower back and pelvis
Bite of lower back and pelvis NOS

EXCLUDES 1 *superficial bite of lower back and pelvis (S30.860, S30.870)*

7th S31.050 Open bite of lower back and pelvis without penetration into retroperitoneum
Open bite of lower back and pelvis NOS

7th S31.051 Open bite of lower back and pelvis with penetration into retroperitoneum

5th S31.1 Open wound of abdominal wall without penetration into peritoneal cavity
Open wound of abdominal wall NOS

EXCLUDES 2 *open wound of abdominal wall with penetration into peritoneal cavity (S31.6-)*

6th S31.10 Unspecified open wound of abdominal wall without penetration into peritoneal cavity

7th S31.100 Unspecified open wound of abdominal wall, right upper quadrant without penetration into peritoneal cavity

7th S31.101 Unspecified open wound of abdominal wall, left upper quadrant without penetration into peritoneal cavity

7th S31.102 Unspecified open wound of abdominal wall, epigastric region without penetration into peritoneal cavity

7th S31.103 Unspecified open wound of abdominal wall, right lower quadrant without penetration into peritoneal cavity

7th S31.104 Unspecified open wound of abdominal wall, left lower quadrant without penetration into peritoneal cavity

7th S31.105 Unspecified open wound of abdominal wall, periumbilic region without penetration into peritoneal cavity

7th S31.109 Unspecified open wound of abdominal wall, unspecified quadrant without penetration into peritoneal cavity
Unspecified open wound of abdominal wall NOS

6th S31.11 Laceration without foreign body of abdominal wall without penetration into peritoneal cavity

7th S31.110 Laceration without foreign body of abdominal wall, right upper quadrant without penetration into peritoneal cavity

7th S31.111 Laceration without foreign body of abdominal wall, left upper quadrant without penetration into peritoneal cavity

7th S31.112 Laceration without foreign body of abdominal wall, epigastric region without penetration into peritoneal cavity

7th S31.113 Laceration without foreign body of abdominal wall, right lower quadrant without penetration into peritoneal cavity

7th S31.114 Laceration without foreign body of abdominal wall, left lower quadrant without penetration into peritoneal cavity

7th S31.115 Laceration without foreign body of abdominal wall, periumbilic region without penetration into peritoneal cavity

7th S31.119 Laceration without foreign body of abdominal wall, unspecified quadrant without penetration into peritoneal cavity

6th S31.12 Laceration with foreign body of abdominal wall without penetration into peritoneal cavity

7th S31.120 Laceration of abdominal wall with foreign body, right upper quadrant without penetration into peritoneal cavity

7th S31.121 Laceration of abdominal wall with foreign body, left upper quadrant without penetration into peritoneal cavity

7th S31.122 Laceration of abdominal wall with foreign body, epigastric region without penetration into peritoneal cavity

7th S31.123 Laceration of abdominal wall with foreign body, right lower quadrant without penetration into peritoneal cavity

✓7th **S31.124 Laceration of abdominal wall with foreign body, left lower quadrant without penetration into peritoneal cavity**

✓7th **S31.125 Laceration of abdominal wall with foreign body, periumbilic region without penetration into peritoneal cavity**

✓7th **S31.129 Laceration of abdominal wall with foreign body, unspecified quadrant without penetration into peritoneal cavity**

✓6th **S31.13 Puncture wound of abdominal wall without foreign body without penetration into peritoneal cavity**

✓7th **S31.130 Puncture wound of abdominal wall without foreign body, right upper quadrant without penetration into peritoneal cavity**

✓7th **S31.131 Puncture wound of abdominal wall without foreign body, left upper quadrant without penetration into peritoneal cavity**

✓7th **S31.132 Puncture wound of abdominal wall without foreign body, epigastric region without penetration into peritoneal cavity**

✓7th **S31.133 Puncture wound of abdominal wall without foreign body, right lower quadrant without penetration into peritoneal cavity**

✓7th **S31.134 Puncture wound of abdominal wall without foreign body, left lower quadrant without penetration into peritoneal cavity**

✓7th **S31.135 Puncture wound of abdominal wall without foreign body, periumbilic region without penetration into peritoneal cavity**

✓7th **S31.139 Puncture wound of abdominal wall without foreign body, unspecified quadrant without penetration into peritoneal cavity**

✓6th **S31.14 Puncture wound of abdominal wall with foreign body without penetration into peritoneal cavity**

✓7th **S31.140 Puncture wound of abdominal wall with foreign body, right upper quadrant without penetration into peritoneal cavity**

✓7th **S31.141 Puncture wound of abdominal wall with foreign body, left upper quadrant without penetration into peritoneal cavity**

✓7th **S31.142 Puncture wound of abdominal wall with foreign body, epigastric region without penetration into peritoneal cavity**

✓7th **S31.143 Puncture wound of abdominal wall with foreign body, right lower quadrant without penetration into peritoneal cavity**

✓7th **S31.144 Puncture wound of abdominal wall with foreign body, left lower quadrant without penetration into peritoneal cavity**

✓7th **S31.145 Puncture wound of abdominal wall with foreign body, periumbilic region without penetration into peritoneal cavity**

✓7th **S31.149 Puncture wound of abdominal wall with foreign body, unspecified quadrant without penetration into peritoneal cavity**

✓6th **S31.15 Open bite of abdominal wall without penetration into peritoneal cavity**

Bite of abdominal wall NOS

EXCLUDES 1 *superficial bite of abdominal wall (S30.871)*

✓7th **S31.150 Open bite of abdominal wall, right upper quadrant without penetration into peritoneal cavity**

✓7th **S31.151 Open bite of abdominal wall, left upper quadrant without penetration into peritoneal cavity**

✓7th **S31.152 Open bite of abdominal wall, epigastric region without penetration into peritoneal cavity**

✓7th **S31.153 Open bite of abdominal wall, right lower quadrant without penetration into peritoneal cavity**

✓7th **S31.154 Open bite of abdominal wall, left lower quadrant without penetration into peritoneal cavity**

✓7th **S31.155 Open bite of abdominal wall, periumbilic region without penetration into peritoneal cavity**

✓7th **S31.159 Open bite of abdominal wall, unspecified quadrant without penetration into peritoneal cavity**

✓5th **S31.2 Open wound of penis**

✓x7th **S31.20 Unspecified open wound of penis**

✓x7th **S31.21 Laceration without foreign body of penis**

✓x7th **S31.22 Laceration with foreign body of penis**

✓x7th **S31.23 Puncture wound without foreign body of penis**

✓x7th **S31.24 Puncture wound with foreign body of penis**

✓x7th **S31.25 Open bite of penis**

Bite of penis NOS

EXCLUDES 1 *superficial bite of penis (S30.862, S30.872)*

✓5th **S31.3 Open wound of scrotum and testes**

✓x7th **S31.30 Unspecified open wound of scrotum and testes**

✓x7th **S31.31 Laceration without foreign body of scrotum and testes**

✓x7th **S31.32 Laceration with foreign body of scrotum and testes**

✓x7th **S31.33 Puncture wound without foreign body of scrotum and testes**

✓x7th **S31.34 Puncture wound with foreign body of scrotum and testes**

✓x7th **S31.35 Open bite of scrotum and testes**

Bite of scrotum and testes NOS

EXCLUDES 1 *superficial bite of scrotum and testes (S30.863, S30.873)*

✓5th **S31.4 Open wound of vagina and vulva**

EXCLUDES 1 *injury to vagina and vulva during delivery (O70-, O71.4)*

✓x7th **S31.40 Unspecified open wound of vagina and vulva**

✓x7th **S31.41 Laceration without foreign body of vagina and vulva**

✓x7th **S31.42 Laceration with foreign body of vagina and vulva**

✓x7th **S31.43 Puncture wound without foreign body of vagina and vulva**

✓x7th **S31.44 Puncture wound with foreign body of vagina and vulva**

✓x7th **S31.45 Open bite of vagina and vulva**

Bite of vagina and vulva NOS

EXCLUDES 1 *superficial bite of vagina and vulva (S30.864, S30.874)*

✓5th **S31.5 Open wound of unspecified external genital organs**

EXCLUDES 1 *traumatic amputation of external genital organs (S38.21, S38.22)*

✓6th **S31.50 Unspecified open wound of unspecified external genital organs**

✓7th **S31.501 Unspecified open wound of unspecified external genital organs, male**

✓7th **S31.502 Unspecified open wound of unspecified external genital organs, female**

✓6th **S31.51 Laceration without foreign body of unspecified external genital organs**

✓7th **S31.511 Laceration without foreign body of unspecified external genital organs, male**

✓7th **S31.512 Laceration without foreign body of unspecified external genital organs, female**

✓6th **S31.52 Laceration with foreign body of unspecified external genital organs**

✓7th **S31.521 Laceration with foreign body of unspecified external genital organs, male**

✓7th **S31.522 Laceration with foreign body of unspecified external genital organs, female**

✓6th **S31.53 Puncture wound without foreign body of unspecified external genital organs**

✓7th **S31.531 Puncture wound without foreign body of unspecified external genital organs, male**

✓7th **S31.532 Puncture wound without foreign body of unspecified external genital organs, female**

✓6th **S31.54 Puncture wound with foreign body of unspecified external genital organs**

✓7th **S31.541 Puncture wound with foreign body of unspecified external genital organs, male**

✓7th **S31.542 Puncture wound with foreign body of unspecified external genital organs, female**

✓6th **S31.55 Open bite of unspecified external genital organs**

Bite of unspecified external genital organs NOS

EXCLUDES 1 *superficial bite of unspecified external genital organs (S30.865, S30.866, S30.875, S30.876)*

✓7th **S31.551 Open bite of unspecified external genital organs, male**

✓7th **S31.552 Open bite of unspecified external genital organs, female**

✓5th **S31.6 Open wound of abdominal wall with penetration into peritoneal cavity**

✓6th **S31.60 Unspecified open wound of abdominal wall with penetration into peritoneal cavity**

✓7th **S31.600 Unspecified open wound of abdominal wall, right upper quadrant with penetration into peritoneal cavity**

✓7th **S31.601 Unspecified open wound of abdominal wall, left upper quadrant with penetration into peritoneal cavity**

✓7th **S31.602 Unspecified open wound of abdominal wall, epigastric region with penetration into peritoneal cavity**

✓7th **S31.603 Unspecified open wound of abdominal wall, right lower quadrant with penetration into peritoneal cavity**

✓7th **S31.604 Unspecified open wound of abdominal wall, left lower quadrant with penetration into peritoneal cavity**

✓7th **S31.605 Unspecified open wound of abdominal wall, periumbilic region with penetration into peritoneal cavity**

✓7th **S31.609 Unspecified open wound of abdominal wall, unspecified quadrant with penetration into peritoneal cavity**

✓6th **S31.61 Laceration without foreign body of abdominal wall with penetration into peritoneal cavity**

✓7th **S31.610 Laceration without foreign body of abdominal wall, right upper quadrant with penetration into peritoneal cavity**

✓7th **S31.611 Laceration without foreign body of abdominal wall, left upper quadrant with penetration into peritoneal cavity**

✓7th **S31.612 Laceration without foreign body of abdominal wall, epigastric region with penetration into peritoneal cavity**

✓7th **S31.613 Laceration without foreign body of abdominal wall, right lower quadrant with penetration into peritoneal cavity**

✓7th **S31.614 Laceration without foreign body of abdominal wall, left lower quadrant with penetration into peritoneal cavity**

✓7th **S31.615 Laceration without foreign body of abdominal wall, periumbilic region with penetration into peritoneal cavity**

✓7th **S31.619 Laceration without foreign body of abdominal wall, unspecified quadrant with penetration into peritoneal cavity**

✓6th **S31.62 Laceration with foreign body of abdominal wall with penetration into peritoneal cavity**

✓7th **S31.620 Laceration with foreign body of abdominal wall, right upper quadrant with penetration into peritoneal cavity**

✓7th **S31.621 Laceration with foreign body of abdominal wall, left upper quadrant with penetration into peritoneal cavity**

✓7th **S31.622 Laceration with foreign body of abdominal wall, epigastric region with penetration into peritoneal cavity**

✓7th **S31.623 Laceration with foreign body of abdominal wall, right lower quadrant with penetration into peritoneal cavity**

✓7th **S31.624 Laceration with foreign body of abdominal wall, left lower quadrant with penetration into peritoneal cavity**

✓7th **S31.625 Laceration with foreign body of abdominal wall, periumbilic region with penetration into peritoneal cavity**

✓7th **S31.629 Laceration with foreign body of abdominal wall, unspecified quadrant with penetration into peritoneal cavity**

✓6th **S31.63 Puncture wound without foreign body of abdominal wall with penetration into peritoneal cavity**

✓7th **S31.630 Puncture wound without foreign body of abdominal wall, right upper quadrant with penetration into peritoneal cavity**

✓7th **S31.631 Puncture wound without foreign body of abdominal wall, left upper quadrant with penetration into peritoneal cavity**

✓7th **S31.632 Puncture wound without foreign body of abdominal wall, epigastric region with penetration into peritoneal cavity**

✓7th **S31.633 Puncture wound without foreign body of abdominal wall, right lower quadrant with penetration into peritoneal cavity**

✓7th **S31.634 Puncture wound without foreign body of abdominal wall, left lower quadrant with penetration into peritoneal cavity**

✓7th **S31.635 Puncture wound without foreign body of abdominal wall, periumbilic region with penetration into peritoneal cavity**

✓7th **S31.639 Puncture wound without foreign body of abdominal wall, unspecified quadrant with penetration into peritoneal cavity**

✓6th **S31.64 Puncture wound with foreign body of abdominal wall with penetration into peritoneal cavity**

✓7th **S31.640 Puncture wound with foreign body of abdominal wall, right upper quadrant with penetration into peritoneal cavity**

✓7th **S31.641 Puncture wound with foreign body of abdominal wall, left upper quadrant with penetration into peritoneal cavity**

✓7th **S31.642 Puncture wound with foreign body of abdominal wall, epigastric region with penetration into peritoneal cavity**

✓7th **S31.643 Puncture wound with foreign body of abdominal wall, right lower quadrant with penetration into peritoneal cavity**

✓7th **S31.644 Puncture wound with foreign body of abdominal wall, left lower quadrant with penetration into peritoneal cavity**

✓7th **S31.645 Puncture wound with foreign body of abdominal wall, periumbilic region with penetration into peritoneal cavity**

✓7th **S31.649 Puncture wound with foreign body of abdominal wall, unspecified quadrant with penetration into peritoneal cavity**

S31.65 Open bite of abdominal wall with penetration into peritoneal cavity
EXCLUDES 1 *superficial bite of abdominal wall (S30.861, S30.871)*
S31.650 Open bite of abdominal wall, right upper quadrant with penetration into peritoneal cavity
S31.651 Open bite of abdominal wall, left upper quadrant with penetration into peritoneal cavity
S31.652 Open bite of abdominal wall, epigastric region with penetration into peritoneal cavity
S31.653 Open bite of abdominal wall, right lower quadrant with penetration into peritoneal cavity
S31.654 Open bite of abdominal wall, left lower quadrant with penetration into peritoneal cavity
S31.655 Open bite of abdominal wall, periumbilic region with penetration into peritoneal cavity
S31.659 Open bite of abdominal wall, unspecified quadrant with penetration into peritoneal cavity

S31.8 Open wound of other parts of abdomen, lower back and pelvis
S31.80 Open wound of unspecified buttock
S31.801 Laceration without foreign body of unspecified buttock
S31.802 Laceration with foreign body of unspecified buttock
S31.803 Puncture wound without foreign body of unspecified buttock
S31.804 Puncture wound with foreign body of unspecified buttock
S31.805 Open bite of unspecified buttock
Bite of buttock NOS
EXCLUDES 1 *superficial bite of buttock (S30.870)*
S31.809 Unspecified open wound of unspecified buttock
S31.81 Open wound of right buttock
S31.811 Laceration without foreign body of right buttock
S31.812 Laceration with foreign body of right buttock
S31.813 Puncture wound without foreign body of right buttock
S31.814 Puncture wound with foreign body of right buttock
S31.815 Open bite of right buttock
Bite of right buttock NOS
EXCLUDES 1 *superficial bite of buttock (S30.870)*
S31.819 Unspecified open wound of right buttock
S31.82 Open wound of left buttock
S31.821 Laceration without foreign body of left buttock
S31.822 Laceration with foreign body of left buttock
S31.823 Puncture wound without foreign body of left buttock
S31.824 Puncture wound with foreign body of left buttock
S31.825 Open bite of left buttock
Bite of left buttock NOS
EXCLUDES 1 *superficial bite of buttock (S30.870)*
S31.829 Unspecified open wound of left buttock
S31.83 Open wound of anus
S31.831 Laceration without foreign body of anus
S31.832 Laceration with foreign body of anus
S31.833 Puncture wound without foreign body of anus
S31.834 Puncture wound with foreign body of anus
S31.835 Open bite of anus
Bite of anus NOS
EXCLUDES 1 *superficial bite of anus (S30.877)*
S31.839 Unspecified open wound of anus

S32 Fracture of lumbar spine and pelvis

NOTE A fracture not indicated as displaced or nondisplaced should be coded to displaced
A fracture not indicated as opened or closed should be coded to closed

INCLUDES fracture of lumbosacral neural arch
fracture of lumbosacral spinous process
fracture of lumbosacral transverse process
fracture of lumbosacral vertebra
fracture of lumbosacral vertebral arch

Codes first any associated spinal cord and spinal nerve injury (S34.-)
EXCLUDES 1 *transection of abdomen (S38.3)*
EXCLUDES 2 *fracture of hip NOS (S72.0-)*

The appropriate 7th character is to be added to each code from category S32.
A initial encounter for closed fracture
B initial encounter for open fracture
D subsequent encounter for fracture with routine healing
G subsequent encounter for fracture with delayed healing
K subsequent encounter for fracture with nonunion
S sequela

S32.0 Fracture of lumbar vertebra
Fracture of lumbar spine NOS
S32.00 Fracture of unspecified lumbar vertebra
S32.000 Wedge compression fracture of unspecified lumbar vertebra
S32.001 Stable burst fracture of unspecified lumbar vertebra
S32.002 Unstable burst fracture of unspecified lumbar vertebra
S32.008 Other fracture of unspecified lumbar vertebra
S32.009 Unspecified fracture of unspecified lumbar vertebra
S32.01 Fracture of first lumbar vertebra
S32.010 Wedge compression fracture of first lumbar vertebra
S32.011 Stable burst fracture of first lumbar vertebra
S32.012 Unstable burst fracture of first lumbar vertebra
S32.018 Other fracture of first lumbar vertebra
S32.019 Unspecified fracture of first lumbar vertebra
S32.02 Fracture of second lumbar vertebra
S32.020 Wedge compression fracture of second lumbar vertebra
S32.021 Stable burst fracture of second lumbar vertebra
S32.022 Unstable burst fracture of second lumbar vertebra
S32.028 Other fracture of second lumbar vertebra
S32.029 Unspecified fracture of second lumbar vertebra
S32.03 Fracture of third lumbar vertebra
S32.030 Wedge compression fracture of third lumbar vertebra
S32.031 Stable burst fracture of third lumbar vertebra
S32.032 Unstable burst fracture of third lumbar vertebra
S32.038 Other fracture of third lumbar vertebra
S32.039 Unspecified fracture of third lumbar vertebra

√6th S32.04 **Fracture of fourth lumbar vertebra**
- √7th S32.040 **Wedge compression fracture of fourth lumbar vertebra**
- √7th S32.041 **Stable burst fracture of fourth lumbar vertebra**
- √7th S32.042 **Unstable burst fracture of fourth lumbar vertebra**
- √7th S32.048 **Other fracture of fourth lumbar vertebra**
- √7th S32.049 **Unspecified fracture of fourth lumbar vertebra**

√6th S32.05 **Fracture of fifth lumbar vertebra**
- √7th S32.050 **Wedge compression fracture of fifth lumbar vertebra**
- √7th S32.051 **Stable burst fracture of fifth lumbar vertebra**
- √7th S32.052 **Unstable burst fracture of fifth lumbar vertebra**
- √7th S32.058 **Other fracture of fifth lumbar vertebra**
- √7th S32.059 **Unspecified fracture of fifth lumbar vertebra**

√5th S32.1 **Fracture of sacrum**

NOTE For vertical fractures, code to most medial fracture extension
Use two codes if both a vertical and transverse fracture are present

Code also any associated fracture of pelvic ring (S32.8-)

√x7th S32.10 **Unspecified fracture of sacrum**

√6th S32.11 **Zone I fracture of sacrum**
Vertical sacral ala fracture of sacrum
- √7th S32.110 **Nondisplaced Zone I fracture of sacrum**
- √7th S32.111 **Minimally displaced Zone I fracture of sacrum**
- √7th S32.112 **Severely displaced Zone I fracture of sacrum**
- √7th S32.119 **Unspecified Zone I fracture of sacrum**

√6th S32.12 **Zone II fracture of sacrum**
Vertical foraminal region fracture of sacrum
- √7th S32.120 **Nondisplaced Zone II fracture of sacrum**
- √7th S32.121 **Minimally displaced Zone II fracture of sacrum**
- √7th S32.122 **Severely displaced Zone II fracture of sacrum**
- √7th S32.129 **Unspecified Zone II fracture of sacrum**

√6th S32.13 **Zone III fracture of sacrum**
Vertical fracture into spinal canal region of sacrum
- √7th S32.130 **Nondisplaced Zone III fracture of sacrum**
- √7th S32.131 **Minimally displaced Zone III fracture of sacrum**
- √7th S32.132 **Severely displaced Zone III fracture of sacrum**
- √7th S32.139 **Unspecified Zone III fracture of sacrum**

√x7th S32.14 **Type 1 fracture of sacrum**
Transverse flexion fracture of sacrum without displacement

√x7th S32.15 **Type 2 fracture of sacrum**
Transverse flexion fracture of sacrum with posterior displacement

√x7th S32.16 **Type 3 fracture of sacrum**
Transverse extension fracture of sacrum with anterior displacement

√x7th S32.17 **Type 4 fracture of sacrum**
Transverse segmental comminution of upper sacrum

√x7th S32.19 **Other fracture of sacrum**

√x7th S32.2 **Fracture of coccyx**

√5th S32.3 **Fracture of ilium**

EXCLUDES1 *fracture of ilium with associated disruption of pelvic ring (S32.8-)*

√6th S32.30 **Unspecified fracture of ilium**
- √7th S32.301 **Unspecified fracture of right ilium**
- √7th S32.302 **Unspecified fracture of left ilium**
- √7th S32.309 **Unspecified fracture of unspecified ilium**

√6th S32.31 **Avulsion fracture of ilium**
- √7th S32.311 **Displaced avulsion fracture of right ilium**
- √7th S32.312 **Displaced avulsion fracture of left ilium**
- √7th S32.313 **Displaced avulsion fracture of unspecified ilium**
- √7th S32.314 **Nondisplaced avulsion fracture of right ilium**
- √7th S32.315 **Nondisplaced avulsion fracture of left ilium**
- √7th S32.316 **Nondisplaced avulsion fracture of unspecified ilium**

√6th S32.39 **Other fracture of ilium**
- √7th S32.391 **Other fracture of right ilium**
- √7th S32.392 **Other fracture of left ilium**
- √7th S32.399 **Other fracture of unspecified ilium**

√5th S32.4 **Fracture of acetabulum**

Code also any associated fracture of pelvic ring (S32.8-)

√6th S32.40 **Unspecified fracture of acetabulum**
- √7th S32.401 **Unspecified fracture of right acetabulum**
- √7th S32.402 **Unspecified fracture of left acetabulum**
- √7th S32.409 **Unspecified fracture of unspecified acetabulum**

√6th S32.41 **Fracture of anterior wall of acetabulum**
- √7th S32.411 **Displaced fracture of anterior wall of right acetabulum**
- √7th S32.412 **Displaced fracture of anterior wall of left acetabulum**
- √7th S32.413 **Displaced fracture of anterior wall of unspecified acetabulum**
- √7th S32.414 **Nondisplaced fracture of anterior wall of right acetabulum**
- √7th S32.415 **Nondisplaced fracture of anterior wall of left acetabulum**
- √7th S32.416 **Nondisplaced fracture of anterior wall of unspecified acetabulum**

√6th S32.42 **Fracture of posterior wall of acetabulum**
- √7th S32.421 **Displaced fracture of posterior wall of right acetabulum**
- √7th S32.422 **Displaced fracture of posterior wall of left acetabulum**
- √7th S32.423 **Displaced fracture of posterior wall of unspecified acetabulum**
- √7th S32.424 **Nondisplaced fracture of posterior wall of right acetabulum**
- √7th S32.425 **Nondisplaced fracture of posterior wall of left acetabulum**
- √7th S32.426 **Nondisplaced fracture of posterior wall of unspecified acetabulum**

√6th S32.43 **Fracture of anterior column [iliopubic] of acetabulum**
- √7th S32.431 **Displaced fracture of anterior column [iliopubic] of right acetabulum**
- √7th S32.432 **Displaced fracture of anterior column [iliopubic] of left acetabulum**
- √7th S32.433 **Displaced fracture of anterior column [iliopubic] of unspecified acetabulum**
- √7th S32.434 **Nondisplaced fracture of anterior column [iliopubic] of right acetabulum**
- √7th S32.435 **Nondisplaced fracture of anterior column [iliopubic] of left acetabulum**
- √7th S32.436 **Nondisplaced fracture of anterior column [iliopubic] of unspecified acetabulum**

√6th S32.44 **Fracture of posterior column [ilioischial] of acetabulum**
- √7th S32.441 **Displaced fracture of posterior column [ilioischial] of right acetabulum**
- √7th S32.442 **Displaced fracture of posterior column [ilioischial] of left acetabulum**
- √7th S32.443 **Displaced fracture of posterior column [ilioischial] of unspecified acetabulum**
- √7th S32.444 **Nondisplaced fracture of posterior column [ilioischial] of right acetabulum**
- √7th S32.445 **Nondisplaced fracture of posterior column [ilioischial] of left acetabulum**

√7th **S32.446 Nondisplaced fracture of posterior column [ilioischial] of unspecified acetabulum**

√6th **S32.45 Transverse fracture of acetabulum**

√7th **S32.451 Displaced transverse fracture of right acetabulum**

√7th **S32.452 Displaced transverse fracture of left acetabulum**

√7th **S32.453 Displaced transverse fracture of unspecified acetabulum**

√7th **S32.454 Nondisplaced transverse fracture of right acetabulum**

√7th **S32.455 Nondisplaced transverse fracture of left acetabulum**

√7th **S32.456 Nondisplaced transverse fracture of unspecified acetabulum**

√6th **S32.46 Associated transverse-posterior fracture of acetabulum**

√7th **S32.461 Displaced associated transverse-posterior fracture of right acetabulum**

√7th **S32.462 Displaced associated transverse-posterior fracture of left acetabulum**

√7th **S32.463 Displaced associated transverse-posterior fracture of unspecified acetabulum**

√7th **S32.464 Nondisplaced associated transverse-posterior fracture of right acetabulum**

√7th **S32.465 Nondisplaced associated transverse-posterior fracture of left acetabulum**

√7th **S32.466 Nondisplaced associated transverse-posterior fracture of unspecified acetabulum**

√6th **S32.47 Fracture of medial wall of acetabulum**

√7th **S32.471 Displaced fracture of medial wall of right acetabulum**

√7th **S32.472 Displaced fracture of medial wall of left acetabulum**

√7th **S32.473 Displaced fracture of medial wall of unspecified acetabulum**

√7th **S32.474 Nondisplaced fracture of medial wall of right acetabulum**

√7th **S32.475 Nondisplaced fracture of medial wall of left acetabulum**

√7th **S32.476 Nondisplaced fracture of medial wall of unspecified acetabulum**

√6th **S32.48 Dome fracture of acetabulum**

√7th **S32.481 Displaced dome fracture of right acetabulum**

√7th **S32.482 Displaced dome fracture of left acetabulum**

√7th **S32.483 Displaced dome fracture of unspecified acetabulum**

√7th **S32.484 Nondisplaced dome fracture of right acetabulum**

√7th **S32.485 Nondisplaced dome fracture of left acetabulum**

√7th **S32.486 Nondisplaced dome fracture of unspecified acetabulum**

√6th **S32.49 Other specified fracture of acetabulum**

√7th **S32.491 Other specified fracture of right acetabulum**

√7th **S32.492 Other specified fracture of left acetabulum**

√7th **S32.499 Other specified fracture of unspecified acetabulum**

√5th **S32.5 Fracture of pubis**

EXCLUDES 1 *fracture of pubis with associated disruption of pelvic ring (S32.8-)*

√6th **S32.50 Unspecified fracture of pubis**

√7th **S32.501 Unspecified fracture of right pubis**

√7th **S32.502 Unspecified fracture of left pubis**

√7th **S32.509 Unspecified fracture of unspecified pubis**

√6th **S32.51 Fracture of superior rim of pubis**

√7th **S32.511 Fracture of superior rim of right pubis**

√7th **S32.512 Fracture of superior rim of left pubis**

√7th **S32.519 Fracture of superior rim of unspecified pubis**

√6th **S32.59 Other specified fracture of pubis**

√7th **S32.591 Other specified fracture of right pubis**

√7th **S32.592 Other specified fracture of left pubis**

√7th **S32.599 Other specified fracture of unspecified pubis**

√5th **S32.6 Fracture of ischium**

EXCLUDES 1 *fracture of ischium with associated disruption of pelvic ring (S32.8-)*

√6th **S32.60 Unspecified fracture of ischium**

√7th **S32.601 Unspecified fracture of right ischium**

√7th **S32.602 Unspecified fracture of left ischium**

√7th **S32.609 Unspecified fracture of unspecified ischium**

√6th **S32.61 Avulsion fracture of ischium**

√7th **S32.611 Displaced avulsion fracture of right ischium**

√7th **S32.612 Displaced avulsion fracture of left ischium**

√7th **S32.613 Displaced avulsion fracture of unspecified ischium**

√7th **S32.614 Nondisplaced avulsion fracture of right ischium**

√7th **S32.615 Nondisplaced avulsion fracture of left ischium**

√7th **S32.616 Nondisplaced avulsion fracture of unspecified ischium**

√6th **S32.69 Other specified fracture of ischium**

√7th **S32.691 Other specified fracture of right ischium**

√7th **S32.692 Other specified fracture of left ischium**

√7th **S32.699 Other specified fracture of unspecified ischium**

√5th **S32.8 Fracture of other parts of pelvis**

Code also any associated:
fracture of acetabulum (S32.4-)
sacral fracture (S32.1-)

√6th **S32.81 Multiple fractures of pelvis with disruption of pelvic ring**

Multiple pelvic fractures with disruption of pelvic circle

√7th **S32.810 Multiple fractures of pelvis with stable disruption of pelvic ring**

√7th **S32.811 Multiple fractures of pelvis with unstable disruption of pelvic ring**

√x7th **S32.82 Multiple fractures of pelvis without disruption of pelvic ring**

Multiple pelvic fractures without disruption of pelvic circle

√x7th **S32.89 Fracture of other parts of pelvis**

√x7th **S32.9 Fracture of unspecified parts of lumbosacral spine and pelvis**

Fracture of lumbosacral spine NOS
Fracture of pelvis NOS

√4th **S33 Dislocation and sprain of joints and ligaments of lumbar spine and pelvis**

INCLUDES avulsion of joint or ligament of lumbar spine and pelvis
laceration of cartilage, joint or ligament of lumbar spine and pelvis
sprain of cartilage, joint or ligament of lumbar spine and pelvis
traumatic hemarthrosis of joint or ligament of lumbar spine and pelvis
traumatic rupture of joint or ligament of lumbar spine and pelvis
traumatic subluxation of joint or ligament of lumbar spine and pelvis
traumatic tear of joint or ligament of lumbar spine and pelvis

Code also any associated open wound

EXCLUDES 1 *nontraumatic rupture or displacement of lumbar intervertebral disc NOS (M51.-)*
obstetric damage to pelvic joints and ligaments (O71.6)

EXCLUDES 2 *dislocation and sprain of joints and ligaments of hip (S73.-)*
strain of muscle of lower back and pelvis (S39.01-)

The appropriate 7th character is to be added to each code from category S33.
A initial encounter
D subsequent encounter
S sequela

√x7th **S33.0 Traumatic rupture of lumbar intervertebral disc**
EXCLUDES 1 *rupture or displacement (nontraumatic) of lumbar intervertebral disc NOS (M51- with fifth character 6)*

√5th **S33.1 Subluxation and dislocation of lumbar vertebra**
Code also any associated:
open wound of abdomen, lower back and pelvis (S31)
spinal cord injury (S24.0, S24.1-, S34.0-, S34.1-)
EXCLUDES 2 *fracture of lumbar vertebrae (S32.0-)*

√6th **S33.10 Subluxation and dislocation of unspecified lumbar vertebra**
√7th **S33.100 Subluxation of unspecified lumbar vertebra**
√7th **S33.101 Dislocation of unspecified lumbar vertebra**

√6th **S33.11 Subluxation and dislocation of L1/L2 lumbar vertebra**
√7th **S33.110 Subluxation of L1/L2 lumbar vertebra**
√7th **S33.111 Dislocation of L1/L2 lumbar vertebra**

√6th **S33.12 Subluxation and dislocation of L2/L3 lumbar vertebra**
√7th **S33.120 Subluxation of L2/L3 lumbar vertebra**
√7th **S33.121 Dislocation of L2/L3 lumbar vertebra**

√6th **S33.13 Subluxation and dislocation of L3/L4 lumbar vertebra**
√7th **S33.130 Subluxation of L3/L4 lumbar vertebra**
√7th **S33.131 Dislocation of L3/L4 lumbar vertebra**

√6th **S33.14 Subluxation and dislocation of L4/L5 lumbar vertebra**
√7th **S33.140 Subluxation of L4/L5 lumbar vertebra**
√7th **S33.141 Dislocation of L4/L5 lumbar vertebra**

√x7th **S33.2 Dislocation of sacroiliac and sacrococcygeal joint**

√5th **S33.3 Dislocation of other and unspecified parts of lumbar spine and pelvis**
√x7th **S33.30 Dislocation of unspecified parts of lumbar spine and pelvis**
√x7th **S33.39 Dislocation of other parts of lumbar spine and pelvis**

√x7th **S33.4 Traumatic rupture of symphysis pubis**
√x7th **S33.5 Sprain of ligaments of lumbar spine**
√x7th **S33.6 Sprain of sacroiliac joint**
√x7th **S33.8 Sprain of other parts of lumbar spine and pelvis**
√x7th **S33.9 Sprain of unspecified parts of lumbar spine and pelvis**

√4th **S34 Injury of lumbar and sacral spinal cord and nerves at abdomen, lower back and pelvis level**

NOTE Code to highest level of lumbar cord injury

Code also any associated:
fracture of vertebra (S22.0-, S32.0-)
open wound of abdomen, lower back and pelvis (S31.-)
transient paralysis (R29.5)

The appropriate 7th character is to be added to each code from category S34.
A initial encounter
D subsequent encounter
S sequela

√5th **S34.0 Concussion and edema of lumbar and sacral spinal cord**
√x7th **S34.01 Concussion and edema of lumbar spinal cord**
√x7th **S34.02 Concussion and edema of sacral spinal cord**
Concussion and edema of conus medullaris

√5th **S34.1 Other and unspecified injury of lumbar and sacral spinal cord**

√6th **S34.10 Unspecified injury to lumbar spinal cord**
√7th **S34.101 Unspecified injury to L1 level of lumbar spinal cord**
√7th **S34.102 Unspecified injury to L2 level of lumbar spinal cord**
√7th **S34.103 Unspecified injury to L3 level of lumbar spinal cord**
√7th **S34.104 Unspecified injury to L4 level of lumbar spinal cord**
√7th **S34.105 Unspecified injury to L5 level of lumbar spinal cord**
√7th **S34.109 Unspecified injury to unspecified level of lumbar spinal cord**

√6th **S34.11 Complete lesion of lumbar spinal cord**
√7th **S34.111 Complete lesion of L1 level of lumbar spinal cord**
√7th **S34.112 Complete lesion of L2 level of lumbar spinal cord**
√7th **S34.113 Complete lesion of L3 level of lumbar spinal cord**
√7th **S34.114 Complete lesion of L4 level of lumbar spinal cord**
√7th **S34.115 Complete lesion of L5 level of lumbar spinal cord**
√7th **S34.119 Complete lesion of unspecified level of lumbar spinal cord**

√6th **S34.12 Incomplete lesion of lumbar spinal cord**
√7th **S34.121 Incomplete lesion of L1 level of lumbar spinal cord**
√7th **S34.122 Incomplete lesion of L2 level of lumbar spinal cord**
√7th **S34.123 Incomplete lesion of L3 level of lumbar spinal cord**
√7th **S34.124 Incomplete lesion of L4 level of lumbar spinal cord**
√7th **S34.125 Incomplete lesion of L5 level of lumbar spinal cord**
√7th **S34.129 Incomplete lesion of unspecified level of lumbar spinal cord**

√6th **S34.13 Other and unspecified injury to sacral spinal cord**
Other injury to conus medullaris
√7th **S34.131 Complete lesion of sacral spinal cord**
Complete lesion of conus medullaris
√7th **S34.132 Incomplete lesion of sacral spinal cord**
Incomplete lesion of conus medullaris
√7th **S34.139 Unspecified injury to sacral spinal cord**
Unspecified injury of conus medullaris

√5th **S34.2 Injury of nerve root of lumbar and sacral spine**
√x7th **S34.21 Injury of nerve root of lumbar spine**
√x7th **S34.22 Injury of nerve root of sacral spine**

√x7th **S34.3 Injury of cauda equina**
√x7th **S34.4 Injury of lumbosacral plexus**
√x7th **S34.5 Injury of lumbar, sacral and pelvic sympathetic nerves**
Injury of celiac ganglion or plexus
Injury of hypogastric plexus
Injury of mesenteric plexus (inferior) (superior)
Injury of splanchnic nerve

√x7th **S34.6 Injury of peripheral nerve(s) at abdomen, lower back and pelvis level**

√x7th **S34.8 Injury of other nerves at abdomen, lower back and pelvis level**

√x7th **S34.9 Injury of unspecified nerves at abdomen, lower back and pelvis level**

√4th **S35 Injury of blood vessels at abdomen, lower back and pelvis level**

Code also any associated open wound (S31.-)

> The appropriate 7th character is to be added to each code from category S35.
> A initial encounter
> D subsequent encounter
> S sequela

√5th **S35.0 Injury of abdominal aorta**

EXCLUDES 1 *injury of aorta NOS (S25.0)*

√x7th **S35.00 Unspecified injury of abdominal aorta**

√x7th **S35.01 Minor laceration of abdominal aorta**
Incomplete transection of abdominal aorta
Laceration of abdominal aorta NOS
Superficial laceration of abdominal aorta

√x7th **S35.02 Major laceration of abdominal aorta**
Complete transection of abdominal aorta
Traumatic rupture of abdominal aorta

√x7th **S35.09 Other injury of abdominal aorta**

√5th **S35.1 Injury of inferior vena cava**
Injury of hepatic vein

EXCLUDES 1 *injury of vena cava NOS (S25.2)*

√x7th **S35.10 Unspecified injury of inferior vena cava**

√x7th **S35.11 Minor laceration of inferior vena cava**
Incomplete transection of inferior vena cava
Laceration of inferior vena cava NOS
Superficial laceration of inferior vena cava

√x7th **S35.12 Major laceration of inferior vena cava**
Complete transection of inferior vena cava
Traumatic rupture of inferior vena cava

√x7th **S35.19 Other injury of inferior vena cava**

√5th **S35.2 Injury of celiac or mesenteric artery and branches**

√6th **S35.21 Injury of celiac artery**

√7th **S35.211 Minor laceration of celiac artery**
Incomplete transection of celiac artery
Laceration of celiac artery NOS
Superficial laceration of celiac artery

√7th **S35.212 Major laceration of celiac artery**
Complete transection of celiac artery
Traumatic rupture of celiac artery

√7th **S35.218 Other injury of celiac artery**

√7th **S35.219 Unspecified injury of celiac artery**

√6th **S35.22 Injury of superior mesenteric artery**

√7th **S35.221 Minor laceration of superior mesenteric artery**
Incomplete transection of superior mesenteric artery
Laceration of superior mesenteric artery NOS
Superficial laceration of superior mesenteric artery

√7th **S35.222 Major laceration of superior mesenteric artery**
Complete transection of superior mesenteric artery
Traumatic rupture of superior mesenteric artery

√7th **S35.228 Other injury of superior mesenteric artery**

√7th **S35.229 Unspecified injury of superior mesenteric artery**

√6th **S35.23 Injury of inferior mesenteric artery**

√7th **S35.231 Minor laceration of inferior mesenteric artery**
Incomplete transection of inferior mesenteric artery
Laceration of inferior mesenteric artery NOS
Superficial laceration of inferior mesenteric artery

√7th **S35.232 Major laceration of inferior mesenteric artery**
Complete transection of inferior mesenteric artery
Traumatic rupture of inferior mesenteric artery

√7th **S35.238 Other injury of inferior mesenteric artery**

√7th **S35.239 Unspecified injury of inferior mesenteric artery**

√6th **S35.29 Injury of branches of celiac and mesenteric artery**
Injury of gastric artery
Injury of gastroduodenal artery
Injury of hepatic artery
Injury of splenic artery

√7th **S35.291 Minor laceration of branches of celiac and mesenteric artery**
Incomplete transection of branches of celiac and mesenteric artery
Laceration of branches of celiac and mesenteric artery NOS
Superficial laceration of branches of celiac and mesenteric artery

√7th **S35.292 Major laceration of branches of celiac and mesenteric artery**
Complete transection of branches of celiac and mesenteric artery
Traumatic rupture of branches of celiac and mesenteric artery

√7th **S35.298 Other injury of branches of celiac and mesenteric artery**

√7th **S35.299 Unspecified injury of branches of celiac and mesenteric artery**

√5th **S35.3 Injury of portal or splenic vein and branches**

√6th **S35.31 Injury of portal vein**

√7th **S35.311 Laceration of portal vein**

√7th **S35.318 Other specified injury of portal vein**

√7th **S35.319 Unspecified injury of portal vein**

√6th **S35.32 Injury of splenic vein**

√7th **S35.321 Laceration of splenic vein**

√7th **S35.328 Other specified injury of splenic vein**

√7th **S35.329 Unspecified injury of splenic vein**

√6th **S35.33 Injury of superior mesenteric vein**

√7th **S35.331 Laceration of superior mesenteric vein**

√7th **S35.338 Other specified injury of superior mesenteric vein**

√7th **S35.339 Unspecified injury of superior mesenteric vein**

√6th **S35.34 Injury of inferior mesenteric vein**

√7th **S35.341 Laceration of inferior mesenteric vein**

√7th **S35.348 Other specified injury of inferior mesenteric vein**

√7th **S35.349 Unspecified injury of inferior mesenteric vein**

√5th **S35.4 Injury of renal blood vessels**

√6th **S35.40 Unspecified injury of renal blood vessel**

√7th **S35.401 Unspecified injury of right renal artery**

√7th **S35.402 Unspecified injury of left renal artery**

√7th **S35.403 Unspecified injury of unspecified renal artery**

√7th **S35.404 Unspecified injury of right renal vein**

√7th **S35.405 Unspecified injury of left renal vein**

√7th **S35.406 Unspecified injury of unspecified renal vein**

√6th **S35.41 Laceration of renal blood vessel**

√7th **S35.411 Laceration of right renal artery**

√7th **S35.412 Laceration of left renal artery**

√7th **S35.413 Laceration of unspecified renal artery**

√7th **S35.414 Laceration of right renal vein**

√7th **S35.415 Laceration of left renal vein**

√7th **S35.416 Laceration of unspecified renal vein**

√6th **S35.49 Other specified injury of renal blood vessel**

√7th **S35.491 Other specified injury of right renal artery**

√7th **S35.492 Other specified injury of left renal artery**

S35.493 Other specified injury of unspecified renal artery
S35.494 Other specified injury of right renal vein
S35.495 Other specified injury of left renal vein
S35.496 Other specified injury of unspecified renal vein

S35.5 Injury of iliac blood vessels
S35.50 Injury of unspecified iliac blood vessel(s)
S35.51 Injury of iliac artery or vein
Injury of hypogastric artery or vein
S35.511 Injury of right iliac artery
S35.512 Injury of left iliac artery
S35.513 Injury of unspecified iliac artery
S35.514 Injury of right iliac vein
S35.515 Injury of left iliac vein
S35.516 Injury of unspecified iliac vein
S35.53 Injury of uterine artery or vein
S35.531 Injury of right uterine artery
S35.532 Injury of left uterine artery
S35.533 Injury of unspecified uterine artery
S35.534 Injury of right uterine vein
S35.535 Injury of left uterine vein
S35.536 Injury of unspecified uterine vein
S35.59 Injury of other iliac blood vessels

S35.8 Injury of other blood vessels at abdomen, lower back and pelvis level
Injury of ovarian artery or vein
S35.8X Injury of other blood vessels at abdomen, lower back and pelvis level
S35.8X1 Laceration of other blood vessels at abdomen, lower back and pelvis level
S35.8X8 Other specified injury of other blood vessels at abdomen, lower back and pelvis level
S35.8X9 Unspecified injury of other blood vessels at abdomen, lower back and pelvis level

S35.9 Injury of unspecified blood vessel at abdomen, lower back and pelvis level
S35.90 Unspecified injury of unspecified blood vessel at abdomen, lower back and pelvis level
S35.91 Laceration of unspecified blood vessel at abdomen, lower back and pelvis level
S35.99 Other specified injury of unspecified blood vessel at abdomen, lower back and pelvis level

S36 Injury of intra-abdominal organs
Code also any associated open wound (S31.-)

The appropriate 7th character is to be added to each code from category S36.
A initial encounter
D subsequent encounter
S sequela

S36.0 Injury of spleen
S36.00 Unspecified injury of spleen
S36.02 Contusion of spleen
S36.020 Minor contusion of spleen
Contusion of spleen less than 2 cm
S36.021 Major contusion of spleen
Contusion of spleen greater than 2 cm
S36.029 Unspecified contusion of spleen
S36.03 Laceration of spleen
S36.030 Superficial (capsular) laceration of spleen
Laceration of spleen less than 1 cm
Minor laceration of spleen
S36.031 Moderate laceration of spleen
Laceration of spleen 1 to 3 cm
S36.032 Major laceration of spleen
Avulsion of spleen
Laceration of spleen greater than 3 cm
Massive laceration of spleen
Multiple moderate lacerations of spleen
Stellate laceration of spleen
S36.039 Unspecified laceration of spleen
S36.09 Other injury of spleen

S36.1 Injury of liver and gallbladder and bile duct
S36.11 Injury of liver
S36.112 Contusion of liver
S36.113 Laceration of liver, unspecified degree
S36.114 Minor laceration of liver
Laceration involving capsule only, or, without significant involvement of hepatic parenchyma [i.e., less than 1 cm deep]
S36.115 Moderate laceration of liver
Laceration involving parenchyma but without major disruption of parenchyma [i.e., less than 10 cm long and less than 3 cm deep]
S36.116 Major laceration of liver
Laceration with significant disruption of hepatic parenchyma [i.e., greater than 10 cm long and 3 cm deep]
Multiple moderate lacerations, with or without hematoma
Stellate laceration of liver
S36.118 Other injury of liver
S36.119 Unspecified injury of liver
S36.12 Injury of gallbladder
S36.122 Contusion of gallbladder
S36.123 Laceration of gallbladder
S36.128 Other injury of gallbladder
S36.129 Unspecified injury of gallbladder
S36.13 Injury of bile duct

S36.2 Injury of pancreas
S36.20 Unspecified injury of pancreas
S36.200 Unspecified injury of head of pancreas
S36.201 Unspecified injury of body of pancreas
S36.202 Unspecified injury of tail of pancreas
S36.209 Unspecified injury of unspecified part of pancreas
S36.22 Contusion of pancreas
S36.220 Contusion of head of pancreas
S36.221 Contusion of body of pancreas
S36.222 Contusion of tail of pancreas
S36.229 Contusion of unspecified part of pancreas
S36.23 Laceration of pancreas, unspecified degree
S36.230 Laceration of head of pancreas, unspecified degree
S36.231 Laceration of body of pancreas, unspecified degree
S36.232 Laceration of tail of pancreas, unspecified degree
S36.239 Laceration of unspecified part of pancreas, unspecified degree
S36.24 Minor laceration of pancreas
S36.240 Minor laceration of head of pancreas
S36.241 Minor laceration of body of pancreas
S36.242 Minor laceration of tail of pancreas
S36.249 Minor laceration of unspecified part of pancreas
S36.25 Moderate laceration of pancreas
S36.250 Moderate laceration of head of pancreas
S36.251 Moderate laceration of body of pancreas
S36.252 Moderate laceration of tail of pancreas
S36.259 Moderate laceration of unspecified part of pancreas
S36.26 Major laceration of pancreas
S36.260 Major laceration of head of pancreas
S36.261 Major laceration of body of pancreas
S36.262 Major laceration of tail of pancreas
S36.269 Major laceration of unspecified part of pancreas
S36.29 Other injury of pancreas
S36.290 Other injury of head of pancreas
S36.291 Other injury of body of pancreas
S36.292 Other injury of tail of pancreas
S36.299 Other injury of unspecified part of pancreas

S36.3 Injury of stomach
- S36.30 Unspecified injury of stomach
- S36.32 Contusion of stomach
- S36.33 Laceration of stomach
- S36.39 Other injury of stomach

S36.4 Injury of small intestine
- S36.40 Unspecified injury of small intestine
  - S36.400 Unspecified injury of duodenum
  - S36.408 Unspecified injury of other part of small intestine
  - S36.409 Unspecified injury of unspecified part of small intestine
- S36.41 Primary blast injury of small intestine
  Blast injury of small intestine NOS
  - S36.410 Primary blast injury of duodenum
  - S36.418 Primary blast injury of other part of small intestine
  - S36.419 Primary blast injury of unspecified part of small intestine
- S36.42 Contusion of small intestine
  - S36.420 Contusion of duodenum
  - S36.428 Contusion of other part of small intestine
  - S36.429 Contusion of unspecified part of small intestine
- S36.43 Laceration of small intestine
  - S36.430 Laceration of duodenum
  - S36.438 Laceration of other part of small intestine
  - S36.439 Laceration of unspecified part of small intestine
- S36.49 Other injury of small intestine
  - S36.490 Other injury of duodenum
  - S36.498 Other injury of other part of small intestine
  - S36.499 Other injury of unspecified part of small intestine

S36.5 Injury of colon
EXCLUDES 2 *injury of rectum (S36.6-)*
- S36.50 Unspecified injury of colon
  - S36.500 Unspecified injury of ascending [right] colon
  - S36.501 Unspecified injury of transverse colon
  - S36.502 Unspecified injury of descending [left] colon
  - S36.503 Unspecified injury of sigmoid colon
  - S36.508 Unspecified injury of other part of colon
  - S36.509 Unspecified injury of unspecified part of colon
- S36.51 Primary blast injury of colon
  Blast injury of colon NOS
  - S36.510 Primary blast injury of ascending [right] colon
  - S36.511 Primary blast injury of transverse colon
  - S36.512 Primary blast injury of descending [left] colon
  - S36.513 Primary blast injury of sigmoid colon
  - S36.518 Primary blast injury of other part of colon
  - S36.519 Primary blast injury of unspecified part of colon
- S36.52 Contusion of colon
  - S36.520 Contusion of ascending [right] colon
  - S36.521 Contusion of transverse colon
  - S36.522 Contusion of descending [left] colon
  - S36.523 Contusion of sigmoid colon
  - S36.528 Contusion of other part of colon
  - S36.529 Contusion of unspecified part of colon
- S36.53 Laceration of colon
  - S36.530 Laceration of ascending [right] colon
  - S36.531 Laceration of transverse colon
  - S36.532 Laceration of descending [left] colon
  - S36.533 Laceration of sigmoid colon
  - S36.538 Laceration of other part of colon
  - S36.539 Laceration of unspecified part of colon
- S36.59 Other injury of colon
  Secondary blast injury of colon
  - S36.590 Other injury of ascending [right] colon
  - S36.591 Other injury of transverse colon
  - S36.592 Other injury of descending [left] colon
  - S36.593 Other injury of sigmoid colon
  - S36.598 Other injury of other part of colon
  - S36.599 Other injury of unspecified part of colon

S36.6 Injury of rectum
- S36.60 Unspecified injury of rectum
- S36.61 Primary blast injury of rectum
  Blast injury of rectum NOS
- S36.62 Contusion of rectum
- S36.63 Laceration of rectum
- S36.69 Other injury of rectum
  Secondary blast injury of rectum

S36.8 Injury of other intra-abdominal organs
- S36.81 Injury of peritoneum
- S36.89 Injury of other intra-abdominal organs
  Injury of retroperitoneum
  - S36.892 Contusion of other intra-abdominal organs
  - S36.893 Laceration of other intra-abdominal organs
  - S36.898 Other injury of other intra-abdominal organs
  - S36.899 Unspecified injury of other intra-abdominal organs

S36.9 Injury of unspecified intra-abdominal organ
- S36.90 Unspecified injury of unspecified intra-abdominal organ
- S36.92 Contusion of unspecified intra-abdominal organ
- S36.93 Laceration of unspecified intra-abdominal organ
- S36.99 Other injury of unspecified intra-abdominal organ

S37 Injury of urinary and pelvic organs

Code also any associated open wound (S31.-)

EXCLUDES 1 *obstetric trauma to pelvic organs (O71.-)*

EXCLUDES 2 *injury of peritoneum (S36.81)*
injury of retroperitoneum (S36.89-)

The appropriate 7th character is to be added to each code from category S37.
- A initial encounter
- D subsequent encounter
- S sequela

S37.0 Injury of kidney
EXCLUDES 2 *acute kidney injury (nontraumatic) (N17.9)*
- S37.00 Unspecified injury of kidney
  - S37.001 Unspecified injury of right kidney
  - S37.002 Unspecified injury of left kidney
  - S37.009 Unspecified injury of unspecified kidney
- S37.01 Minor contusion of kidney
  Contusion of kidney less than 2 cm
  Contusion of kidney NOS
  - S37.011 Minor contusion of right kidney
  - S37.012 Minor contusion of left kidney
  - S37.019 Minor contusion of unspecified kidney
- S37.02 Major contusion of kidney
  Contusion of kidney greater than 2 cm
  - S37.021 Major contusion of right kidney
  - S37.022 Major contusion of left kidney
  - S37.029 Major contusion of unspecified kidney
- S37.03 Laceration of kidney, unspecified degree
  - S37.031 Laceration of right kidney, unspecified degree
  - S37.032 Laceration of left kidney, unspecified degree
  - S37.039 Laceration of unspecified kidney, unspecified degree
- S37.04 Minor laceration of kidney
  Laceration of kidney less than 1 cm
  - S37.041 Minor laceration of right kidney
  - S37.042 Minor laceration of left kidney
  - S37.049 Minor laceration of unspecified kidney

✓ Appropriate additional character required   ✓x7th Requires 7th character, placeholder x must fill empty characters

6th **S37.05 Moderate laceration of kidney**
Laceration of kidney 1 to 3 cm
7th **S37.051 Moderate laceration of right kidney**
7th **S37.052 Moderate laceration of left kidney**
7th **S37.059 Moderate laceration of unspecified kidney**
6th **S37.06 Major laceration of kidney**
Avulsion of kidney
Laceration of kidney greater than 3 cm
Massive laceration of kidney
Multiple moderate lacerations of kidney
Stellate laceration of kidney
7th **S37.061 Major laceration of right kidney**
7th **S37.062 Major laceration of left kidney**
7th **S37.069 Major laceration of unspecified kidney**
6th **S37.09 Other injury of kidney**
7th **S37.091 Other injury of right kidney**
7th **S37.092 Other injury of left kidney**
7th **S37.099 Other injury of unspecified kidney**
5th **S37.1 Injury of ureter**
x7th **S37.10 Unspecified injury of ureter**
x7th **S37.12 Contusion of ureter**
x7th **S37.13 Laceration of ureter**
x7th **S37.19 Other injury of ureter**
5th **S37.2 Injury of bladder**
x7th **S37.20 Unspecified injury of bladder**
x7th **S37.22 Contusion of bladder**
x7th **S37.23 Laceration of bladder**
x7th **S37.29 Other injury of bladder**
5th **S37.3 Injury of urethra**
x7th **S37.30 Unspecified injury of urethra**
x7th **S37.32 Contusion of urethra**
x7th **S37.33 Laceration of urethra**
x7th **S37.39 Other injury of urethra**
5th **S37.4 Injury of ovary**
6th **S37.40 Unspecified injury of ovary**
7th **S37.401 Unspecified injury of ovary, unilateral**
7th **S37.402 Unspecified injury of ovary, bilateral**
7th **S37.409 Unspecified injury of ovary, unspecified**
6th **S37.42 Contusion of ovary**
7th **S37.421 Contusion of ovary, unilateral**
7th **S37.422 Contusion of ovary, bilateral**
7th **S37.429 Contusion of ovary, unspecified**
6th **S37.43 Laceration of ovary**
7th **S37.431 Laceration of ovary, unilateral**
7th **S37.432 Laceration of ovary, bilateral**
7th **S37.439 Laceration of ovary, unspecified**
6th **S37.49 Other injury of ovary**
7th **S37.491 Other injury of ovary, unilateral**
7th **S37.492 Other injury of ovary, bilateral**
7th **S37.499 Other injury of ovary, unspecified**
5th **S37.5 Injury of fallopian tube**
6th **S37.50 Unspecified injury of fallopian tube**
7th **S37.501 Unspecified injury of fallopian tube, unilateral**
7th **S37.502 Unspecified injury of fallopian tube, bilateral**
7th **S37.509 Unspecified injury of fallopian tube, unspecified**
6th **S37.51 Primary blast injury of fallopian tube**
Blast injury of fallopian tube NOS
7th **S37.511 Primary blast injury of fallopian tube, unilateral**
7th **S37.512 Primary blast injury of fallopian tube, bilateral**
7th **S37.519 Primary blast injury of fallopian tube, unspecified**
6th **S37.52 Contusion of fallopian tube**
7th **S37.521 Contusion of fallopian tube, unilateral**
7th **S37.522 Contusion of fallopian tube, bilateral**
7th **S37.529 Contusion of fallopian tube, unspecified**
6th **S37.53 Laceration of fallopian tube**
7th **S37.531 Laceration of fallopian tube, unilateral**
7th **S37.532 Laceration of fallopian tube, bilateral**
7th **S37.539 Laceration of fallopian tube, unspecified**
6th **S37.59 Other injury of fallopian tube**
Secondary blast injury of fallopian tube
7th **S37.591 Other injury of fallopian tube, unilateral**
7th **S37.592 Other injury of fallopian tube, bilateral**
7th **S37.599 Other injury of fallopian tube, unspecified**
5th **S37.6 Injury of uterus**
EXCLUDES 1 *injury to gravid uterus (O9A.2-)*
injury to uterus during delivery (O71.-)
x7th **S37.60 Unspecified injury of uterus**
x7th **S37.62 Contusion of uterus**
x7th **S37.63 Laceration of uterus**
x7th **S37.69 Other injury of uterus**
5th **S37.8 Injury of other urinary and pelvic organs**
6th **S37.81 Injury of adrenal gland**
7th **S37.812 Contusion of adrenal gland**
7th **S37.813 Laceration of adrenal gland**
7th **S37.818 Other injury of adrenal gland**
7th **S37.819 Unspecified injury of adrenal gland**
6th **S37.82 Injury of prostate**
7th **S37.822 Contusion of prostate**
7th **S37.823 Laceration of prostate**
7th **S37.828 Other injury of prostate**
7th **S37.829 Unspecified injury of prostate**
6th **S37.89 Injury of other urinary and pelvic organ**
7th **S37.892 Contusion of other urinary and pelvic organ**
7th **S37.893 Laceration of other urinary and pelvic organ**
7th **S37.898 Other injury of other urinary and pelvic organ**
7th **S37.899 Unspecified injury of other urinary and pelvic organ**
5th **S37.9 Injury of unspecified urinary and pelvic organ**
x7th **S37.90 Unspecified injury of unspecified urinary and pelvic organ**
x7th **S37.92 Contusion of unspecified urinary and pelvic organ**
x7th **S37.93 Laceration of unspecified urinary and pelvic organ**
x7th **S37.99 Other injury of unspecified urinary and pelvic organ**

4th **S38 Crushing injury and traumatic amputation of abdomen, lower back, pelvis and external genitals**
NOTE An amputation not identified as partial or complete should be coded to complete

The appropriate 7th character is to be added to each code from category S38.
A initial encounter
D subsequent encounter
S sequela

5th **S38.0 Crushing injury of external genital organs**
Use additional code for any associated injuries
6th **S38.00 Crushing injury of unspecified external genital organs**
7th **S38.001 Crushing injury of unspecified external genital organs, male**
7th **S38.002 Crushing injury of unspecified external genital organs, female**
x7th **S38.01 Crushing injury of penis**
x7th **S38.02 Crushing injury of scrotum and testis**
x7th **S38.03 Crushing injury of vulva**
x7th **S38.1 Crushing injury of abdomen, lower back, and pelvis**
Use additional code for all associated injuries, such as:
fracture of thoracic or lumbar spine and pelvis (S22.0-, S32-)
injury to intra-abdominal organs (S36.-)
injury to urinary and pelvic organs (S37.-)
open wound of abdominal wall (S31.-)
spinal cord injury (S34.0, S34.1-)
EXCLUDES 2 *crushing injury of external genital organs (S38.2-)*

✓5th **S38.2 Traumatic amputation of external genital organs**
✓6th **S38.21 Traumatic amputation of female external genital organs**
Traumatic amputation of clitoris
Traumatic amputation of labium (majus) (minus)
Traumatic amputation of vulva
✓7th **S38.211 Complete traumatic amputation of female external genital organs**
✓7th **S38.212 Partial traumatic amputation of female external genital organs**
✓6th **S38.22 Traumatic amputation of penis**
✓7th **S38.221 Complete traumatic amputation of penis**
✓7th **S38.222 Partial traumatic amputation of penis**
✓6th **S38.23 Traumatic amputation of scrotum and testis**
✓7th **S38.231 Complete traumatic amputation of scrotum and testis**
✓7th **S38.232 Partial traumatic amputation of scrotum and testis**
✓x7th **S38.3 Transection (partial) of abdomen**

✓4th **S39 Other and unspecified injuries of abdomen, lower back, pelvis and external genitals**
Code also any associated open wound (S31.-)
EXCLUDES 2 *sprain of joints and ligaments of lumbar spine and pelvis (S33.-)*

The appropriate 7th character is to be added to each code from category S39.
A initial encounter
D subsequent encounter
S sequela

✓5th **S39.0 Injury of muscle, fascia and tendon of abdomen, lower back and pelvis**
✓6th **S39.00 Unspecified injury of muscle, fascia and tendon of abdomen, lower back and pelvis**
✓7th **S39.001 Unspecified injury of muscle, fascia and tendon of abdomen**
✓7th **S39.002 Unspecified injury of muscle, fascia and tendon of lower back**
✓7th **S39.003 Unspecified injury of muscle, fascia and tendon of pelvis**
✓6th **S39.01 Strain of muscle, fascia and tendon of abdomen, lower back and pelvis**
✓7th **S39.011 Strain of muscle, fascia and tendon of abdomen**
✓7th **S39.012 Strain of muscle, fascia and tendon of lower back**
✓7th **S39.013 Strain of muscle, fascia and tendon of pelvis**
✓6th **S39.02 Laceration of muscle, fascia and tendon of abdomen, lower back and pelvis**
✓7th **S39.021 Laceration of muscle, fascia and tendon of abdomen**
✓7th **S39.022 Laceration of muscle, fascia and tendon of lower back**
✓7th **S39.023 Laceration of muscle, fascia and tendon of pelvis**
✓6th **S39.09 Other injury of muscle, fascia and tendon of abdomen, lower back and pelvis**
✓7th **S39.091 Other injury of muscle, fascia and tendon of abdomen**
✓7th **S39.092 Other injury of muscle, fascia and tendon of lower back**
✓7th **S39.093 Other injury of muscle, fascia and tendon of pelvis**
✓5th **S39.8 Other specified injuries of abdomen, lower back, pelvis and external genitals**
✓x7th **S39.81 Other specified injuries of abdomen**
✓x7th **S39.82 Other specified injuries of lower back**
✓x7th **S39.83 Other specified injuries of pelvis**
✓6th **S39.84 Other specified injuries of external genitals**
✓7th **S39.840 Fracture of corpus cavernosum penis**
✓7th **S39.848 Other specified injuries of external genitals**
✓5th **S39.9 Unspecified injury of abdomen, lower back, pelvis and external genitals**
✓x7th **S39.91 Unspecified injury of abdomen**
✓x7th **S39.92 Unspecified injury of lower back**
✓x7th **S39.93 Unspecified injury of pelvis**
✓x7th **S39.94 Unspecified injury of external genitals**

Injuries to the shoulder and upper arm (S40-S49)

INCLUDES injuries of axilla
injuries of scapular region
EXCLUDES 2 *burns and corrosions (T20-T32)*
frostbite (T33-T34)
injuries of elbow (S50-S59)
insect bite or sting, venomous (T63.4)

✓4th **S40 Superficial injury of shoulder and upper arm**

The appropriate 7th character is to be added to each code from category S40.
A initial encounter
D subsequent encounter
S sequela

✓5th **S40.0 Contusion of shoulder and upper arm**
✓6th **S40.01 Contusion of shoulder**
✓7th **S40.011 Contusion of right shoulder**
✓7th **S40.012 Contusion of left shoulder**
✓7th **S40.019 Contusion of unspecified shoulder**
✓6th **S40.02 Contusion of upper arm**
✓7th **S40.021 Contusion of right upper arm**
✓7th **S40.022 Contusion of left upper arm**
✓7th **S40.029 Contusion of unspecified upper arm**
✓5th **S40.2 Other superficial injuries of shoulder**
✓6th **S40.21 Abrasion of shoulder**
✓7th **S40.211 Abrasion of right shoulder**
✓7th **S40.212 Abrasion of left shoulder**
✓7th **S40.219 Abrasion of unspecified shoulder**
✓6th **S40.22 Blister (nonthermal) of shoulder**
✓7th **S40.221 Blister (nonthermal) of right shoulder**
✓7th **S40.222 Blister (nonthermal) of left shoulder**
✓7th **S40.229 Blister (nonthermal) of unspecified shoulder**
✓6th **S40.24 External constriction of shoulder**
✓7th **S40.241 External constriction of right shoulder**
✓7th **S40.242 External constriction of left shoulder**
✓7th **S40.249 External constriction of unspecified shoulder**
✓6th **S40.25 Superficial foreign body of shoulder**
Splinter in the shoulder
✓7th **S40.251 Superficial foreign body of right shoulder**
✓7th **S40.252 Superficial foreign body of left shoulder**
✓7th **S40.259 Superficial foreign body of unspecified shoulder**
✓6th **S40.26 Insect bite (nonvenomous) of shoulder**
✓7th **S40.261 Insect bite (nonvenomous) of right shoulder**
✓7th **S40.262 Insect bite (nonvenomous) of left shoulder**
✓7th **S40.269 Insect bite (nonvenomous) of unspecified shoulder**
✓6th **S40.27 Other superficial bite of shoulder**
EXCLUDES 1 *open bite of shoulder (S41.05)*
✓7th **S40.271 Other superficial bite of right shoulder**
✓7th **S40.272 Other superficial bite of left shoulder**
✓7th **S40.279 Other superficial bite of unspecified shoulder**
✓5th **S40.8 Other superficial injuries of upper arm**
✓6th **S40.81 Abrasion of upper arm**
✓7th **S40.811 Abrasion of right upper arm**
✓7th **S40.812 Abrasion of left upper arm**
✓7th **S40.819 Abrasion of unspecified upper arm**
✓6th **S40.82 Blister (nonthermal) of upper arm**
✓7th **S40.821 Blister (nonthermal) of right upper arm**
✓7th **S40.822 Blister (nonthermal) of left upper arm**

- 7th **S4Ø.829 Blister (nonthermal) of unspecified upper arm**
- 6th **S4Ø.84 External constriction of upper arm**
  - 7th **S4Ø.841 External constriction of right upper arm**
  - 7th **S4Ø.842 External constriction of left upper arm**
  - 7th **S4Ø.849 External constriction of unspecified upper arm**
- 6th **S4Ø.85 Superficial foreign body of upper arm**
  Splinter in the upper arm
  - 7th **S4Ø.851 Superficial foreign body of right upper arm**
  - 7th **S4Ø.852 Superficial foreign body of left upper arm**
  - 7th **S4Ø.859 Superficial foreign body of unspecified upper arm**
- 6th **S4Ø.86 Insect bite (nonvenomous) of upper arm**
  - 7th **S4Ø.861 Insect bite (nonvenomous) of right upper arm**
  - 7th **S4Ø.862 Insect bite (nonvenomous) of left upper arm**
  - 7th **S4Ø.869 Insect bite (nonvenomous) of unspecified upper arm**
- 6th **S4Ø.87 Other superficial bite of upper arm**
  EXCLUDES 1 *open bite of upper arm (S41.14)*
  EXCLUDES 2 *other superficial bite of shoulder (S4Ø.27-)*
  - 7th **S4Ø.871 Other superficial bite of right upper arm**
  - 7th **S4Ø.872 Other superficial bite of left upper arm**
  - 7th **S4Ø.879 Other superficial bite of unspecified upper arm**

5th **S4Ø.9 Unspecified superficial injury of shoulder and upper arm**
- 6th **S4Ø.91 Unspecified superficial injury of shoulder**
  - 7th **S4Ø.911 Unspecified superficial injury of right shoulder**
  - 7th **S4Ø.912 Unspecified superficial injury of left shoulder**
  - 7th **S4Ø.919 Unspecified superficial injury of unspecified shoulder**
- 6th **S4Ø.92 Unspecified superficial injury of upper arm**
  - 7th **S4Ø.921 Unspecified superficial injury of right upper arm**
  - 7th **S4Ø.922 Unspecified superficial injury of left upper arm**
  - 7th **S4Ø.929 Unspecified superficial injury of unspecified upper arm**

4th S41 Open wound of shoulder and upper arm

Code also any associated wound infection

EXCLUDES 1 *traumatic amputation of shoulder and upper arm (S48.-)*
EXCLUDES 2 *open fracture of shoulder and upper arm (S42.- with 7th character B)*

The appropriate 7th character is to be added to each code from category S41.
A initial encounter
D subsequent encounter
S sequela

5th **S41.Ø Open wound of shoulder**
- 6th **S41.ØØ Unspecified open wound of shoulder**
  - 7th **S41.ØØ1 Unspecified open wound of right shoulder**
  - 7th **S41.ØØ2 Unspecified open wound of left shoulder**
  - 7th **S41.ØØ9 Unspecified open wound of unspecified shoulder**
- 6th **S41.Ø1 Laceration without foreign body of shoulder**
  - 7th **S41.Ø11 Laceration without foreign body of right shoulder**
  - 7th **S41.Ø12 Laceration without foreign body of left shoulder**
  - 7th **S41.Ø19 Laceration without foreign body of unspecified shoulder**
- 6th **S41.Ø2 Laceration with foreign body of shoulder**
  - 7th **S41.Ø21 Laceration with foreign body of right shoulder**
  - 7th **S41.Ø22 Laceration with foreign body of left shoulder**
  - 7th **S41.Ø29 Laceration with foreign body of unspecified shoulder**
- 6th **S41.Ø3 Puncture wound without foreign body of shoulder**
  - 7th **S41.Ø31 Puncture wound without foreign body of right shoulder**
  - 7th **S41.Ø32 Puncture wound without foreign body of left shoulder**
  - 7th **S41.Ø39 Puncture wound without foreign body of unspecified shoulder**
- 6th **S41.Ø4 Puncture wound with foreign body of shoulder**
  - 7th **S41.Ø41 Puncture wound with foreign body of right shoulder**
  - 7th **S41.Ø42 Puncture wound with foreign body of left shoulder**
  - 7th **S41.Ø49 Puncture wound with foreign body of unspecified shoulder**
- 6th **S41.Ø5 Open bite of shoulder**
  Bite of shoulder NOS
  EXCLUDES 1 *superficial bite of shoulder (S4Ø.27)*
  - 7th **S41.Ø51 Open bite of right shoulder**
  - 7th **S41.Ø52 Open bite of left shoulder**
  - 7th **S41.Ø59 Open bite of unspecified shoulder**

5th **S41.1 Open wound of upper arm**
- 6th **S41.1Ø Unspecified open wound of upper arm**
  - 7th **S41.1Ø1 Unspecified open wound of right upper arm**
  - 7th **S41.1Ø2 Unspecified open wound of left upper arm**
  - 7th **S41.1Ø9 Unspecified open wound of unspecified upper arm**
- 6th **S41.11 Laceration without foreign body of upper arm**
  - 7th **S41.111 Laceration without foreign body of right upper arm**
  - 7th **S41.112 Laceration without foreign body of left upper arm**
  - 7th **S41.119 Laceration without foreign body of unspecified upper arm**
- 6th **S41.12 Laceration with foreign body of upper arm**
  - 7th **S41.121 Laceration with foreign body of right upper arm**
  - 7th **S41.122 Laceration with foreign body of left upper arm**
  - 7th **S41.129 Laceration with foreign body of unspecified upper arm**
- 6th **S41.13 Puncture wound without foreign body of upper arm**
  - 7th **S41.131 Puncture wound without foreign body of right upper arm**
  - 7th **S41.132 Puncture wound without foreign body of left upper arm**
  - 7th **S41.139 Puncture wound without foreign body of unspecified upper arm**
- 6th **S41.14 Puncture wound with foreign body of upper arm**
  - 7th **S41.141 Puncture wound with foreign body of right upper arm**
  - 7th **S41.142 Puncture wound with foreign body of left upper arm**
  - 7th **S41.149 Puncture wound with foreign body of unspecified upper arm**
- 6th **S41.15 Open bite of upper arm**
  Bite of upper arm NOS
  EXCLUDES 1 *superficial bite of upper arm (S4Ø.87)*
  - 7th **S41.151 Open bite of right upper arm**
  - 7th **S41.152 Open bite of left upper arm**
  - 7th **S41.159 Open bite of unspecified upper arm**

√4th S42 Fracture of shoulder and upper arm

NOTE A fracture not indicated as displaced or nondisplaced should be coded to displaced

A fracture not indicated as open or closed should be coded to closed

EXCLUDES 1 *traumatic amputation of shoulder and upper arm (S48.-)*

The appropriate 7th character is to be added to all codes from category S42 [unless otherwise indicated].
- A initial encounter for closed fracture
- B initial encounter for open fracture
- D subsequent encounter for fracture with routine healing
- G subsequent encounter for fracture with delayed healing
- K subsequent encounter for fracture with nonunion
- P subsequent encounter for fracture with malunion
- S sequela

√5th S42.0 Fracture of clavicle
√6th S42.00 Fracture of unspecified part of clavicle
√7th S42.001 Fracture of unspecified part of right clavicle
√7th S42.002 Fracture of unspecified part of left clavicle
√7th S42.009 Fracture of unspecified part of unspecified clavicle
√6th S42.01 Fracture of sternal end of clavicle
√7th S42.011 Anterior displaced fracture of sternal end of right clavicle
√7th S42.012 Anterior displaced fracture of sternal end of left clavicle
√7th S42.013 Anterior displaced fracture of sternal end of unspecified clavicle
Displaced fracture of sternal end of clavicle NOS
√7th S42.014 Posterior displaced fracture of sternal end of right clavicle
√7th S42.015 Posterior displaced fracture of sternal end of left clavicle
√7th S42.016 Posterior displaced fracture of sternal end of unspecified clavicle
√7th S42.017 Nondisplaced fracture of sternal end of right clavicle
√7th S42.018 Nondisplaced fracture of sternal end of left clavicle
√7th S42.019 Nondisplaced fracture of sternal end of unspecified clavicle
√6th S42.02 Fracture of shaft of clavicle
√7th S42.021 Displaced fracture of shaft of right clavicle
√7th S42.022 Displaced fracture of shaft of left clavicle
√7th S42.023 Displaced fracture of shaft of unspecified clavicle
√7th S42.024 Nondisplaced fracture of shaft of right clavicle
√7th S42.025 Nondisplaced fracture of shaft of left clavicle
√7th S42.026 Nondisplaced fracture of shaft of unspecified clavicle
√6th S42.03 Fracture of lateral end of clavicle
Fracture of acromial end of clavicle
√7th S42.031 Displaced fracture of lateral end of right clavicle
√7th S42.032 Displaced fracture of lateral end of left clavicle
√7th S42.033 Displaced fracture of lateral end of unspecified clavicle
√7th S42.034 Nondisplaced fracture of lateral end of right clavicle
√7th S42.035 Nondisplaced fracture of lateral end of left clavicle
√7th S42.036 Nondisplaced fracture of lateral end of unspecified clavicle
√5th S42.1 Fracture of scapula
√6th S42.10 Fracture of unspecified part of scapula
√7th S42.101 Fracture of unspecified part of scapula, right shoulder
√7th S42.102 Fracture of unspecified part of scapula, left shoulder
√7th S42.109 Fracture of unspecified part of scapula, unspecified shoulder
√6th S42.11 Fracture of body of scapula
√7th S42.111 Displaced fracture of body of scapula, right shoulder
√7th S42.112 Displaced fracture of body of scapula, left shoulder
√7th S42.113 Displaced fracture of body of scapula, unspecified shoulder
√7th S42.114 Nondisplaced fracture of body of scapula, right shoulder
√7th S42.115 Nondisplaced fracture of body of scapula, left shoulder
√7th S42.116 Nondisplaced fracture of body of scapula, unspecified shoulder
√6th S42.12 Fracture of acromial process
√7th S42.121 Displaced fracture of acromial process, right shoulder
√7th S42.122 Displaced fracture of acromial process, left shoulder
√7th S42.123 Displaced fracture of acromial process, unspecified shoulder
√7th S42.124 Nondisplaced fracture of acromial process, right shoulder
√7th S42.125 Nondisplaced fracture of acromial process, left shoulder
√7th S42.126 Nondisplaced fracture of acromial process, unspecified shoulder
√6th S42.13 Fracture of coracoid process
√7th S42.131 Displaced fracture of coracoid process, right shoulder
√7th S42.132 Displaced fracture of coracoid process, left shoulder
√7th S42.133 Displaced fracture of coracoid process, unspecified shoulder
√7th S42.134 Nondisplaced fracture of coracoid process, right shoulder
√7th S42.135 Nondisplaced fracture of coracoid process, left shoulder
√7th S42.136 Nondisplaced fracture of coracoid process, unspecified shoulder
√6th S42.14 Fracture of glenoid cavity of scapula
√7th S42.141 Displaced fracture of glenoid cavity of scapula, right shoulder
√7th S42.142 Displaced fracture of glenoid cavity of scapula, left shoulder
√7th S42.143 Displaced fracture of glenoid cavity of scapula, unspecified shoulder
√7th S42.144 Nondisplaced fracture of glenoid cavity of scapula, right shoulder
√7th S42.145 Nondisplaced fracture of glenoid cavity of scapula, left shoulder
√7th S42.146 Nondisplaced fracture of glenoid cavity of scapula, unspecified shoulder
√6th S42.15 Fracture of neck of scapula
√7th S42.151 Displaced fracture of neck of scapula, right shoulder
√7th S42.152 Displaced fracture of neck of scapula, left shoulder
√7th S42.153 Displaced fracture of neck of scapula, unspecified shoulder
√7th S42.154 Nondisplaced fracture of neck of scapula, right shoulder
√7th S42.155 Nondisplaced fracture of neck of scapula, left shoulder
√7th S42.156 Nondisplaced fracture of neck of scapula, unspecified shoulder
√6th S42.19 Fracture of other part of scapula
√7th S42.191 Fracture of other part of scapula, right shoulder
√7th S42.192 Fracture of other part of scapula, left shoulder
√7th S42.199 Fracture of other part of scapula, unspecified shoulder

5th S42.2 Fracture of upper end of humerus
Fracture of proximal end of humerus
EXCLUDES 2 *fracture of shaft of humerus (S42.3-)*
physeal fracture of upper end of humerus (S49.0-)

6th S42.20 Unspecified fracture of upper end of humerus
7th S42.201 Unspecified fracture of upper end of right humerus
7th S42.202 Unspecified fracture of upper end of left humerus
7th S42.209 Unspecified fracture of upper end of unspecified humerus

6th S42.21 Unspecified fracture of surgical neck of humerus
Fracture of neck of humerus NOS
7th S42.211 Unspecified displaced fracture of surgical neck of right humerus
7th S42.212 Unspecified displaced fracture of surgical neck of left humerus
7th S42.213 Unspecified displaced fracture of surgical neck of unspecified humerus
7th S42.214 Unspecified nondisplaced fracture of surgical neck of right humerus
7th S42.215 Unspecified nondisplaced fracture of surgical neck of left humerus
7th S42.216 Unspecified nondisplaced fracture of surgical neck of unspecified humerus

6th S42.22 2-part fracture of surgical neck of humerus
7th S42.221 2-part displaced fracture of surgical neck of right humerus
7th S42.222 2-part displaced fracture of surgical neck of left humerus
7th S42.223 2-part displaced fracture of surgical neck of unspecified humerus
7th S42.224 2-part nondisplaced fracture of surgical neck of right humerus
7th S42.225 2-part nondisplaced fracture of surgical neck of left humerus
7th S42.226 2-part nondisplaced fracture of surgical neck of unspecified humerus

6th S42.23 3-part fracture of surgical neck of humerus
7th S42.231 3-part fracture of surgical neck of right humerus
7th S42.232 3-part fracture of surgical neck of left humerus
7th S42.239 3-part fracture of surgical neck of unspecified humerus

6th S42.24 4-part fracture of surgical neck of humerus
7th S42.241 4-part fracture of surgical neck of right humerus
7th S42.242 4-part fracture of surgical neck of left humerus
7th S42.249 4-part fracture of surgical neck of unspecified humerus

6th S42.25 Fracture of greater tuberosity of humerus
7th S42.251 Displaced fracture of greater tuberosity of right humerus
7th S42.252 Displaced fracture of greater tuberosity of left humerus
7th S42.253 Displaced fracture of greater tuberosity of unspecified humerus
7th S42.254 Nondisplaced fracture of greater tuberosity of right humerus
7th S42.255 Nondisplaced fracture of greater tuberosity of left humerus
7th S42.256 Nondisplaced fracture of greater tuberosity of unspecified humerus

6th S42.26 Fracture of lesser tuberosity of humerus
7th S42.261 Displaced fracture of lesser tuberosity of right humerus
7th S42.262 Displaced fracture of lesser tuberosity of left humerus
7th S42.263 Displaced fracture of lesser tuberosity of unspecified humerus
7th S42.264 Nondisplaced fracture of lesser tuberosity of right humerus
7th S42.265 Nondisplaced fracture of lesser tuberosity of left humerus
7th S42.266 Nondisplaced fracture of lesser tuberosity of unspecified humerus

6th S42.27 Torus fracture of upper end of humerus

The appropriate 7th character is to be added to all codes in subcategory S42.27.
A initial encounter for closed fracture
D subsequent encounter for fracture with routine healing
G subsequent encounter for fracture with delayed healing
K subsequent encounter for fracture with nonunion
P subsequent encounter for fracture with malunion
S sequela

7th S42.271 Torus fracture of upper end of right humerus
7th S42.272 Torus fracture of upper end of left humerus
7th S42.279 Torus fracture of upper end of unspecified humerus

6th S42.29 Other fracture of upper end of humerus
Fracture of anatomical neck of humerus
Fracture of articular head of humerus
7th S42.291 Other displaced fracture of upper end of right humerus
7th S42.292 Other displaced fracture of upper end of left humerus
7th S42.293 Other displaced fracture of upper end of unspecified humerus
7th S42.294 Other nondisplaced fracture of upper end of right humerus
7th S42.295 Other nondisplaced fracture of upper end of left humerus
7th S42.296 Other nondisplaced fracture of upper end of unspecified humerus

5th S42.3 Fracture of shaft of humerus
Fracture of humerus NOS
Fracture of upper arm NOS
EXCLUDES 2 *physeal fractures of upper end of humerus (S49.0-)*
physeal fractures of lower end of humerus (S49.1-)

6th S42.30 Unspecified fracture of shaft of humerus
7th S42.301 Unspecified fracture of shaft of humerus, right arm
7th S42.302 Unspecified fracture of shaft of humerus, left arm
7th S42.309 Unspecified fracture of shaft of humerus, unspecified arm

6th S42.31 Greenstick fracture of shaft of humerus

The appropriate 7th character is to be added to all codes in subcategory S42.31.
A initial encounter for closed fracture
D subsequent encounter for fracture with routine healing
G subsequent encounter for fracture with delayed healing
K subsequent encounter for fracture with nonunion
P subsequent encounter for fracture with malunion
S sequela

7th S42.311 Greenstick fracture of shaft of humerus, right arm
7th S42.312 Greenstick fracture of shaft of humerus, left arm
7th S42.319 Greenstick fracture of shaft of humerus, unspecified arm

6th S42.32 Transverse fracture of shaft of humerus
7th S42.321 Displaced transverse fracture of shaft of humerus, right arm
7th S42.322 Displaced transverse fracture of shaft of humerus, left arm
7th S42.323 Displaced transverse fracture of shaft of humerus, unspecified arm
7th S42.324 Nondisplaced transverse fracture of shaft of humerus, right arm

✓7th **S42.325 Nondisplaced transverse fracture of shaft of humerus, left arm**
✓7th **S42.326 Nondisplaced transverse fracture of shaft of humerus, unspecified arm**
✓6th **S42.33 Oblique fracture of shaft of humerus**
✓7th **S42.331 Displaced oblique fracture of shaft of humerus, right arm**
✓7th **S42.332 Displaced oblique fracture of shaft of humerus, left arm**
✓7th **S42.333 Displaced oblique fracture of shaft of humerus, unspecified arm**
✓7th **S42.334 Nondisplaced oblique fracture of shaft of humerus, right arm**
✓7th **S42.335 Nondisplaced oblique fracture of shaft of humerus, left arm**
✓7th **S42.336 Nondisplaced oblique fracture of shaft of humerus, unspecified arm**
✓6th **S42.34 Spiral fracture of shaft of humerus**
✓7th **S42.341 Displaced spiral fracture of shaft of humerus, right arm**
✓7th **S42.342 Displaced spiral fracture of shaft of humerus, left arm**
✓7th **S42.343 Displaced spiral fracture of shaft of humerus, unspecified arm**
✓7th **S42.344 Nondisplaced spiral fracture of shaft of humerus, right arm**
✓7th **S42.345 Nondisplaced spiral fracture of shaft of humerus, left arm**
✓7th **S42.346 Nondisplaced spiral fracture of shaft of humerus, unspecified arm**
✓6th **S42.35 Comminuted fracture of shaft of humerus**
✓7th **S42.351 Displaced comminuted fracture of shaft of humerus, right arm**
✓7th **S42.352 Displaced comminuted fracture of shaft of humerus, left arm**
✓7th **S42.353 Displaced comminuted fracture of shaft of humerus, unspecified arm**
✓7th **S42.354 Nondisplaced comminuted fracture of shaft of humerus, right arm**
✓7th **S42.355 Nondisplaced comminuted fracture of shaft of humerus, left arm**
✓7th **S42.356 Nondisplaced comminuted fracture of shaft of humerus, unspecified arm**
✓6th **S42.36 Segmental fracture of shaft of humerus**
✓7th **S42.361 Displaced segmental fracture of shaft of humerus, right arm**
✓7th **S42.362 Displaced segmental fracture of shaft of humerus, left arm**
✓7th **S42.363 Displaced segmental fracture of shaft of humerus, unspecified arm**
✓7th **S42.364 Nondisplaced segmental fracture of shaft of humerus, right arm**
✓7th **S42.365 Nondisplaced segmental fracture of shaft of humerus, left arm**
✓7th **S42.366 Nondisplaced segmental fracture of shaft of humerus, unspecified arm**
✓6th **S42.39 Other fracture of shaft of humerus**
✓7th **S42.391 Other fracture of shaft of right humerus**
✓7th **S42.392 Other fracture of shaft of left humerus**
✓7th **S42.399 Other fracture of shaft of unspecified humerus**
✓5th **S42.4 Fracture of lower end of humerus**
Fracture of distal end of humerus
EXCLUDES 2 *fracture of shaft of humerus (S42.3-)*
physeal fracture of lower end of humerus (S49.1-)
✓6th **S42.40 Unspecified fracture of lower end of humerus**
Fracture of elbow NOS
✓7th **S42.401 Unspecified fracture of lower end of right humerus**
✓7th **S42.402 Unspecified fracture of lower end of left humerus**
✓7th **S42.409 Unspecified fracture of lower end of unspecified humerus**
✓6th **S42.41 Simple supracondylar fracture without intercondylar fracture of humerus**
✓7th **S42.411 Displaced simple supracondylar fracture without intercondylar fracture of right humerus**
✓7th **S42.412 Displaced simple supracondylar fracture without intercondylar fracture of left humerus**
✓7th **S42.413 Displaced simple supracondylar fracture without intercondylar fracture of unspecified humerus**
✓7th **S42.414 Nondisplaced simple supracondylar fracture without intercondylar fracture of right humerus**
✓7th **S42.415 Nondisplaced simple supracondylar fracture without intercondylar fracture of left humerus**
✓7th **S42.416 Nondisplaced simple supracondylar fracture without intercondylar fracture of unspecified humerus**
✓6th **S42.42 Comminuted supracondylar fracture without intercondylar fracture of humerus**
✓7th **S42.421 Displaced comminuted supracondylar fracture without intercondylar fracture of right humerus**
✓7th **S42.422 Displaced comminuted supracondylar fracture without intercondylar fracture of left humerus**
✓7th **S42.423 Displaced comminuted supracondylar fracture without intercondylar fracture of unspecified humerus**
✓7th **S42.424 Nondisplaced comminuted supracondylar fracture without intercondylar fracture of right humerus**
✓7th **S42.425 Nondisplaced comminuted supracondylar fracture without intercondylar fracture of left humerus**
✓7th **S42.426 Nondisplaced comminuted supracondylar fracture without intercondylar fracture of unspecified humerus**
✓6th **S42.43 Fracture (avulsion) of lateral epicondyle of humerus**
✓7th **S42.431 Displaced fracture (avulsion) of lateral epicondyle of right humerus**
✓7th **S42.432 Displaced fracture (avulsion) of lateral epicondyle of left humerus**
✓7th **S42.433 Displaced fracture (avulsion) of lateral epicondyle of unspecified humerus**
✓7th **S42.434 Nondisplaced fracture (avulsion) of lateral epicondyle of right humerus**
✓7th **S42.435 Nondisplaced fracture (avulsion) of lateral epicondyle of left humerus**
✓7th **S42.436 Nondisplaced fracture (avulsion) of lateral epicondyle of unspecified humerus**
✓6th **S42.44 Fracture (avulsion) of medial epicondyle of humerus**
✓7th **S42.441 Displaced fracture (avulsion) of medial epicondyle of right humerus**
✓7th **S42.442 Displaced fracture (avulsion) of medial epicondyle of left humerus**
✓7th **S42.443 Displaced fracture (avulsion) of medial epicondyle of unspecified humerus**
✓7th **S42.444 Nondisplaced fracture (avulsion) of medial epicondyle of right humerus**
✓7th **S42.445 Nondisplaced fracture (avulsion) of medial epicondyle of left humerus**
✓7th **S42.446 Nondisplaced fracture (avulsion) of medial epicondyle of unspecified humerus**
✓7th **S42.447 Incarcerated fracture (avulsion) of medial epicondyle of right humerus**
✓7th **S42.448 Incarcerated fracture (avulsion) of medial epicondyle of left humerus**
✓7th **S42.449 Incarcerated fracture (avulsion) of medial epicondyle of unspecified humerus**

✓6th **S42.45 Fracture of lateral condyle of humerus**
Fracture of capitellum of humerus
- ✓7th **S42.451 Displaced fracture of lateral condyle of right humerus**
- ✓7th **S42.452 Displaced fracture of lateral condyle of left humerus**
- ✓7th **S42.453 Displaced fracture of lateral condyle of unspecified humerus**
- ✓7th **S42.454 Nondisplaced fracture of lateral condyle of right humerus**
- ✓7th **S42.455 Nondisplaced fracture of lateral condyle of left humerus**
- ✓7th **S42.456 Nondisplaced fracture of lateral condyle of unspecified humerus**

✓6th **S42.46 Fracture of medial condyle of humerus**
Trochlea fracture of humerus
- ✓7th **S42.461 Displaced fracture of medial condyle of right humerus**
- ✓7th **S42.462 Displaced fracture of medial condyle of left humerus**
- ✓7th **S42.463 Displaced fracture of medial condyle of unspecified humerus**
- ✓7th **S42.464 Nondisplaced fracture of medial condyle of right humerus**
- ✓7th **S42.465 Nondisplaced fracture of medial condyle of left humerus**
- ✓7th **S42.466 Nondisplaced fracture of medial condyle of unspecified humerus**

✓6th **S42.47 Transcondylar fracture of humerus**
- ✓7th **S42.471 Displaced transcondylar fracture of right humerus**
- ✓7th **S42.472 Displaced transcondylar fracture of left humerus**
- ✓7th **S42.473 Displaced transcondylar fracture of unspecified humerus**
- ✓7th **S42.474 Nondisplaced transcondylar fracture of right humerus**
- ✓7th **S42.475 Nondisplaced transcondylar fracture of left humerus**
- ✓7th **S42.476 Nondisplaced transcondylar fracture of unspecified humerus**

✓6th **S42.48 Torus fracture of lower end of humerus**

The appropriate 7th character is to be added to all codes in subcategory S42.48.
- A initial encounter for closed fracture
- D subsequent encounter for fracture with routine healing
- G subsequent encounter for fracture with delayed healing
- K subsequent encounter for fracture with nonunion
- P subsequent encounter for fracture with malunion
- S sequela

- ✓7th **S42.481 Torus fracture of lower end of right humerus**
- ✓7th **S42.482 Torus fracture of lower end of left humerus**
- ✓7th **S42.489 Torus fracture of lower end of unspecified humerus**

✓6th **S42.49 Other fracture of lower end of humerus**
- ✓7th **S42.491 Other displaced fracture of lower end of right humerus**
- ✓7th **S42.492 Other displaced fracture of lower end of left humerus**
- ✓7th **S42.493 Other displaced fracture of lower end of unspecified humerus**
- ✓7th **S42.494 Other nondisplaced fracture of lower end of right humerus**
- ✓7th **S42.495 Other nondisplaced fracture of lower end of left humerus**
- ✓7th **S42.496 Other nondisplaced fracture of lower end of unspecified humerus**

✓5th **S42.9 Fracture of shoulder girdle, part unspecified**
Fracture of shoulder NOS
- ✓x7th **S42.9Ø Fracture of unspecified shoulder girdle, part unspecified**
- ✓x7th **S42.91 Fracture of right shoulder girdle, part unspecified**
- ✓x7th **S42.92 Fracture of left shoulder girdle, part unspecified**

✓4th **S43 Dislocation and sprain of joints and ligaments of shoulder girdle**

INCLUDES avulsion of joint or ligament of shoulder girdle
laceration of cartilage, joint or ligament of shoulder girdle
sprain of cartilage, joint or ligament of shoulder girdle
traumatic hemarthrosis of joint or ligament of shoulder girdle
traumatic rupture of joint or ligament of shoulder girdle
traumatic subluxation of joint or ligament of shoulder girdle
traumatic tear of joint or ligament of shoulder girdle

Code also any associated open wound

EXCLUDES 2 *strain of muscle, fascia and tendon of shoulder and upper arm (S46.-)*

The appropriate 7th character is to be added to each code from category S43.
- A initial encounter
- D subsequent encounter
- S sequela

✓5th **S43.Ø Subluxation and dislocation of shoulder joint**
Dislocation of glenohumeral joint
Subluxation of glenohumeral joint

✓6th **S43.ØØ Unspecified subluxation and dislocation of shoulder joint**
Dislocation of humerus NOS
Subluxation of humerus NOS
- ✓7th **S43.ØØ1 Unspecified subluxation of right shoulder joint**
- ✓7th **S43.ØØ2 Unspecified subluxation of left shoulder joint**
- ✓7th **S43.ØØ3 Unspecified subluxation of unspecified shoulder joint**
- ✓7th **S43.ØØ4 Unspecified dislocation of right shoulder joint**
- ✓7th **S43.ØØ5 Unspecified dislocation of left shoulder joint**
- ✓7th **S43.ØØ6 Unspecified dislocation of unspecified shoulder joint**

✓6th **S43.Ø1 Anterior subluxation and dislocation of humerus**
- ✓7th **S43.Ø11 Anterior subluxation of right humerus**
- ✓7th **S43.Ø12 Anterior subluxation of left humerus**
- ✓7th **S43.Ø13 Anterior subluxation of unspecified humerus**
- ✓7th **S43.Ø14 Anterior dislocation of right humerus**
- ✓7th **S43.Ø15 Anterior dislocation of left humerus**
- ✓7th **S43.Ø16 Anterior dislocation of unspecified humerus**

✓6th **S43.Ø2 Posterior subluxation and dislocation of humerus**
- ✓7th **S43.Ø21 Posterior subluxation of right humerus**
- ✓7th **S43.Ø22 Posterior subluxation of left humerus**
- ✓7th **S43.Ø23 Posterior subluxation of unspecified humerus**
- ✓7th **S43.Ø24 Posterior dislocation of right humerus**
- ✓7th **S43.Ø25 Posterior dislocation of left humerus**
- ✓7th **S43.Ø26 Posterior dislocation of unspecified humerus**

✓6th **S43.Ø3 Inferior subluxation and dislocation of humerus**
- ✓7th **S43.Ø31 Inferior subluxation of right humerus**
- ✓7th **S43.Ø32 Inferior subluxation of left humerus**
- ✓7th **S43.Ø33 Inferior subluxation of unspecified humerus**
- ✓7th **S43.Ø34 Inferior dislocation of right humerus**
- ✓7th **S43.Ø35 Inferior dislocation of left humerus**
- ✓7th **S43.Ø36 Inferior dislocation of unspecified humerus**

✓6th **S43.Ø8 Other subluxation and dislocation of shoulder joint**
- ✓7th **S43.Ø81 Other subluxation of right shoulder joint**

S43.082 Other subluxation of left shoulder joint
S43.083 Other subluxation of unspecified shoulder joint
S43.084 Other dislocation of right shoulder joint
S43.085 Other dislocation of left shoulder joint
S43.086 Other dislocation of unspecified shoulder joint
S43.1 Subluxation and dislocation of acromioclavicular joint
S43.10 Unspecified dislocation of acromioclavicular joint
S43.101 Unspecified dislocation of right acromioclavicular joint
S43.102 Unspecified dislocation of left acromioclavicular joint
S43.109 Unspecified dislocation of unspecified acromioclavicular joint
S43.11 Subluxation of acromioclavicular joint
S43.111 Subluxation of right acromioclavicular joint
S43.112 Subluxation of left acromioclavicular joint
S43.119 Subluxation of unspecified acromioclavicular joint
S43.12 Dislocation of acromioclavicular joint, 100%-200% displacement
S43.121 Dislocation of right acromioclavicular joint, 100%-200% displacement
S43.122 Dislocation of left acromioclavicular joint, 100%-200% displacement
S43.129 Dislocation of unspecified acromioclavicular joint, 100%-200% displacement
S43.13 Dislocation of acromioclavicular joint, greater than 200% displacement
S43.131 Dislocation of right acromioclavicular joint, greater than 200% displacement
S43.132 Dislocation of left acromioclavicular joint, greater than 200% displacement
S43.139 Dislocation of unspecified acromioclavicular joint, greater than 200% displacement
S43.14 Inferior dislocation of acromioclavicular joint
S43.141 Inferior dislocation of right acromioclavicular joint
S43.142 Inferior dislocation of left acromioclavicular joint
S43.149 Inferior dislocation of unspecified acromioclavicular joint
S43.15 Posterior dislocation of acromioclavicular joint
S43.151 Posterior dislocation of right acromioclavicular joint
S43.152 Posterior dislocation of left acromioclavicular joint
S43.159 Posterior dislocation of unspecified acromioclavicular joint
S43.2 Subluxation and dislocation of sternoclavicular joint
S43.20 Unspecified subluxation and dislocation of sternoclavicular joint
S43.201 Unspecified subluxation of right sternoclavicular joint
S43.202 Unspecified subluxation of left sternoclavicular joint
S43.203 Unspecified subluxation of unspecified sternoclavicular joint
S43.204 Unspecified dislocation of right sternoclavicular joint
S43.205 Unspecified dislocation of left sternoclavicular joint
S43.206 Unspecified dislocation of unspecified sternoclavicular joint
S43.21 Anterior subluxation and dislocation of sternoclavicular joint
S43.211 Anterior subluxation of right sternoclavicular joint
S43.212 Anterior subluxation of left sternoclavicular joint
S43.213 Anterior subluxation of unspecified sternoclavicular joint
S43.214 Anterior dislocation of right sternoclavicular joint
S43.215 Anterior dislocation of left sternoclavicular joint
S43.216 Anterior dislocation of unspecified sternoclavicular joint
S43.22 Posterior subluxation and dislocation of sternoclavicular joint
S43.221 Posterior subluxation of right sternoclavicular joint
S43.222 Posterior subluxation of left sternoclavicular joint
S43.223 Posterior subluxation of unspecified sternoclavicular joint
S43.224 Posterior dislocation of right sternoclavicular joint
S43.225 Posterior dislocation of left sternoclavicular joint
S43.226 Posterior dislocation of unspecified sternoclavicular joint
S43.3 Subluxation and dislocation of other and unspecified parts of shoulder girdle
S43.30 Subluxation and dislocation of unspecified parts of shoulder girdle
Dislocation of shoulder girdle NOS
Subluxation of shoulder girdle NOS
S43.301 Subluxation of unspecified parts of right shoulder girdle
S43.302 Subluxation of unspecified parts of left shoulder girdle
S43.303 Subluxation of unspecified parts of unspecified shoulder girdle
S43.304 Dislocation of unspecified parts of right shoulder girdle
S43.305 Dislocation of unspecified parts of left shoulder girdle
S43.306 Dislocation of unspecified parts of unspecified shoulder girdle
S43.31 Subluxation and dislocation of scapula
S43.311 Subluxation of right scapula
S43.312 Subluxation of left scapula
S43.313 Subluxation of unspecified scapula
S43.314 Dislocation of right scapula
S43.315 Dislocation of left scapula
S43.316 Dislocation of unspecified scapula
S43.39 Subluxation and dislocation of other parts of shoulder girdle
S43.391 Subluxation of other parts of right shoulder girdle
S43.392 Subluxation of other parts of left shoulder girdle
S43.393 Subluxation of other parts of unspecified shoulder girdle
S43.394 Dislocation of other parts of right shoulder girdle
S43.395 Dislocation of other parts of left shoulder girdle
S43.396 Dislocation of other parts of unspecified shoulder girdle
S43.4 Sprain of shoulder joint
S43.40 Unspecified sprain of shoulder joint
S43.401 Unspecified sprain of right shoulder joint
S43.402 Unspecified sprain of left shoulder joint
S43.409 Unspecified sprain of unspecified shoulder joint
S43.41 Sprain of coracohumeral (ligament)
S43.411 Sprain of right coracohumeral (ligament)
S43.412 Sprain of left coracohumeral (ligament)
S43.419 Sprain of unspecified coracohumeral (ligament)

Appropriate additional character required
Requires 7th character, placeholder x must fill empty characters

✓6th **S43.42 Sprain of rotator cuff capsule**
EXCLUDES 1 *rotator cuff syndrome (complete) (incomplete), not specified as traumatic (M75.1-)*
EXCLUDES 2 *injury of tendon of rotator cuff (S46.Ø-)*
✓7th **S43.421 Sprain of right rotator cuff capsule**
✓7th **S43.422 Sprain of left rotator cuff capsule**
✓7th **S43.429 Sprain of unspecified rotator cuff capsule**

✓6th **S43.43 Superior glenoid labrum lesion**
SLAP lesion
✓7th **S43.431 Superior glenoid labrum lesion of right shoulder**
✓7th **S43.432 Superior glenoid labrum lesion of left shoulder**
✓7th **S43.439 Superior glenoid labrum lesion of unspecified shoulder**

✓6th **S43.49 Other sprain of shoulder joint**
✓7th **S43.491 Other sprain of right shoulder joint**
✓7th **S43.492 Other sprain of left shoulder joint**
✓7th **S43.499 Other sprain of unspecified shoulder joint**

✓5th **S43.5 Sprain of acromioclavicular joint**
Sprain of acromioclavicular ligament
✓x7th **S43.5Ø Sprain of unspecified acromioclavicular joint**
✓x7th **S43.51 Sprain of right acromioclavicular joint**
✓x7th **S43.52 Sprain of left acromioclavicular joint**

✓5th **S43.6 Sprain of sternoclavicular joint**
✓x7th **S43.6Ø Sprain of unspecified sternoclavicular joint**
✓x7th **S43.61 Sprain of right sternoclavicular joint**
✓x7th **S43.62 Sprain of left sternoclavicular joint**

✓5th **S43.8 Sprain of other specified parts of shoulder girdle**
✓x7th **S43.8Ø Sprain of other specified parts of unspecified shoulder girdle**
✓x7th **S43.81 Sprain of other specified parts of right shoulder girdle**
✓x7th **S43.82 Sprain of other specified parts of left shoulder girdle**

✓5th **S43.9 Sprain of unspecified parts of shoulder girdle**
✓x7th **S43.9Ø Sprain of unspecified parts of unspecified shoulder girdle**
Sprain of shoulder girdle NOS
✓x7th **S43.91 Sprain of unspecified parts of right shoulder girdle**
✓x7th **S43.92 Sprain of unspecified parts of left shoulder girdle**

✓4th S44 Injury of nerves at shoulder and upper arm level

Code also any associated open wound (S41.-)
EXCLUDES 2 *injury of brachial plexus (S14.3-)*

The appropriate 7th character is to be added to each code from category S44.
A initial encounter
D subsequent encounter
S sequela

✓5th **S44.Ø Injury of ulnar nerve at upper arm level**
EXCLUDES 1 *ulnar nerve NOS (S54.Ø)*
✓x7th **S44.ØØ Injury of ulnar nerve at upper arm level, unspecified arm**
✓x7th **S44.Ø1 Injury of ulnar nerve at upper arm level, right arm**
✓x7th **S44.Ø2 Injury of ulnar nerve at upper arm level, left arm**

✓5th **S44.1 Injury of median nerve at upper arm level**
EXCLUDES 1 *median nerve NOS (S54.1)*
✓x7th **S44.1Ø Injury of median nerve at upper arm level, unspecified arm**
✓x7th **S44.11 Injury of median nerve at upper arm level, right arm**
✓x7th **S44.12 Injury of median nerve at upper arm level, left arm**

✓5th **S44.2 Injury of radial nerve at upper arm level**
EXCLUDES 1 *radial nerve NOS (S54.2)*
✓x7th **S44.2Ø Injury of radial nerve at upper arm level, unspecified arm**
✓x7th **S44.21 Injury of radial nerve at upper arm level, right arm**
✓x7th **S44.22 Injury of radial nerve at upper arm level, left arm**

✓5th **S44.3 Injury of axillary nerve**
✓x7th **S44.3Ø Injury of axillary nerve, unspecified arm**
✓x7th **S44.31 Injury of axillary nerve, right arm**
✓x7th **S44.32 Injury of axillary nerve, left arm**

✓5th **S44.4 Injury of musculocutaneous nerve**
✓x7th **S44.4Ø Injury of musculocutaneous nerve, unspecified arm**
✓x7th **S44.41 Injury of musculocutaneous nerve, right arm**
✓x7th **S44.42 Injury of musculocutaneous nerve, left arm**

✓5th **S44.5 Injury of cutaneous sensory nerve at shoulder and upper arm level**
✓x7th **S44.5Ø Injury of cutaneous sensory nerve at shoulder and upper arm level, unspecified arm**
✓x7th **S44.51 Injury of cutaneous sensory nerve at shoulder and upper arm level, right arm**
✓x7th **S44.52 Injury of cutaneous sensory nerve at shoulder and upper arm level, left arm**

✓5th **S44.8 Injury of other nerves at shoulder and upper arm level**
✓6th **S44.8X Injury of other nerves at shoulder and upper arm level**
✓7th **S44.8X1 Injury of other nerves at shoulder and upper arm level, right arm**
✓7th **S44.8X2 Injury of other nerves at shoulder and upper arm level, left arm**
✓7th **S44.8X9 Injury of other nerves at shoulder and upper arm level, unspecified arm**

✓5th **S44.9 Injury of unspecified nerve at shoulder and upper arm level**
✓x7th **S44.9Ø Injury of unspecified nerve at shoulder and upper arm level, unspecified arm**
✓x7th **S44.91 Injury of unspecified nerve at shoulder and upper arm level, right arm**
✓x7th **S44.92 Injury of unspecified nerve at shoulder and upper arm level, left arm**

✓4th S45 Injury of blood vessels at shoulder and upper arm level

Code also any associated open wound (S41.-)
EXCLUDES 2 *injury of subclavian artery (S25.1)*
injury of subclavian vein (S25.3)

The appropriate 7th character is to be added to each code from category S45.
A initial encounter
D subsequent encounter
S sequela

✓5th **S45.Ø Injury of axillary artery**
✓6th **S45.ØØ Unspecified injury of axillary artery**
✓7th **S45.ØØ1 Unspecified injury of axillary artery, right side**
✓7th **S45.ØØ2 Unspecified injury of axillary artery, left side**
✓7th **S45.ØØ9 Unspecified injury of axillary artery, unspecified side**
✓6th **S45.Ø1 Laceration of axillary artery**
✓7th **S45.Ø11 Laceration of axillary artery, right side**
✓7th **S45.Ø12 Laceration of axillary artery, left side**
✓7th **S45.Ø19 Laceration of axillary artery, unspecified side**
✓6th **S45.Ø9 Other specified injury of axillary artery**
✓7th **S45.Ø91 Other specified injury of axillary artery, right side**
✓7th **S45.Ø92 Other specified injury of axillary artery, left side**
✓7th **S45.Ø99 Other specified injury of axillary artery, unspecified side**

✓5th **S45.1 Injury of brachial artery**
✓6th **S45.1Ø Unspecified injury of brachial artery**
✓7th **S45.1Ø1 Unspecified injury of brachial artery, right side**
✓7th **S45.1Ø2 Unspecified injury of brachial artery, left side**
✓7th **S45.1Ø9 Unspecified injury of brachial artery, unspecified side**
✓6th **S45.11 Laceration of brachial artery**
✓7th **S45.111 Laceration of brachial artery, right side**
✓7th **S45.112 Laceration of brachial artery, left side**
✓7th **S45.119 Laceration of brachial artery, unspecified side**
✓6th **S45.19 Other specified injury of brachial artery**
✓7th **S45.191 Other specified injury of brachial artery, right side**

√7th S45.192 Other specified injury of brachial artery, left side
√7th S45.199 Other specified injury of brachial artery, unspecified side

√5th S45.2 Injury of axillary or brachial vein
√6th S45.20 Unspecified injury of axillary or brachial vein
√7th S45.201 Unspecified injury of axillary or brachial vein, right side
√7th S45.202 Unspecified injury of axillary or brachial vein, left side
√7th S45.209 Unspecified injury of axillary or brachial vein, unspecified side
√6th S45.21 Laceration of axillary or brachial vein
√7th S45.211 Laceration of axillary or brachial vein, right side
√7th S45.212 Laceration of axillary or brachial vein, left side
√7th S45.219 Laceration of axillary or brachial vein, unspecified side
√6th S45.29 Other specified injury of axillary or brachial vein
√7th S45.291 Other specified injury of axillary or brachial vein, right side
√7th S45.292 Other specified injury of axillary or brachial vein, left side
√7th S45.299 Other specified injury of axillary or brachial vein, unspecified side

√5th S45.3 Injury of superficial vein at shoulder and upper arm level
√6th S45.30 Unspecified injury of superficial vein at shoulder and upper arm level
√7th S45.301 Unspecified injury of superficial vein at shoulder and upper arm level, right arm
√7th S45.302 Unspecified injury of superficial vein at shoulder and upper arm level, left arm
√7th S45.309 Unspecified injury of superficial vein at shoulder and upper arm level, unspecified arm
√6th S45.31 Laceration of superficial vein at shoulder and upper arm level
√7th S45.311 Laceration of superficial vein at shoulder and upper arm level, right arm
√7th S45.312 Laceration of superficial vein at shoulder and upper arm level, left arm
√7th S45.319 Laceration of superficial vein at shoulder and upper arm level, unspecified arm
√6th S45.39 Other specified injury of superficial vein at shoulder and upper arm level
√7th S45.391 Other specified injury of superficial vein at shoulder and upper arm level, right arm
√7th S45.392 Other specified injury of superficial vein at shoulder and upper arm level, left arm
√7th S45.399 Other specified injury of superficial vein at shoulder and upper arm level, unspecified arm

√5th S45.8 Injury of other specified blood vessels at shoulder and upper arm level
√6th S45.80 Unspecified injury of other specified blood vessels at shoulder and upper arm level
√7th S45.801 Unspecified injury of other specified blood vessels at shoulder and upper arm level, right arm
√7th S45.802 Unspecified injury of other specified blood vessels at shoulder and upper arm level, left arm
√7th S45.809 Unspecified injury of other specified blood vessels at shoulder and upper arm level, unspecified arm
√6th S45.81 Laceration of other specified blood vessels at shoulder and upper arm level
√7th S45.811 Laceration of other specified blood vessels at shoulder and upper arm level, right arm
√7th S45.812 Laceration of other specified blood vessels at shoulder and upper arm level, left arm
√7th S45.819 Laceration of other specified blood vessels at shoulder and upper arm level, unspecified arm
√6th S45.89 Other specified injury of other specified blood vessels at shoulder and upper arm level
√7th S45.891 Other specified injury of other specified blood vessels at shoulder and upper arm level, right arm
√7th S45.892 Other specified injury of other specified blood vessels at shoulder and upper arm level, left arm
√7th S45.899 Other specified injury of other specified blood vessels at shoulder and upper arm level, unspecified arm

√5th S45.9 Injury of unspecified blood vessel at shoulder and upper arm level
√6th S45.90 Unspecified injury of unspecified blood vessel at shoulder and upper arm level
√7th S45.901 Unspecified injury of unspecified blood vessel at shoulder and upper arm level, right arm
√7th S45.902 Unspecified injury of unspecified blood vessel at shoulder and upper arm level, left arm
√7th S45.909 Unspecified injury of unspecified blood vessel at shoulder and upper arm level, unspecified arm
√6th S45.91 Laceration of unspecified blood vessel at shoulder and upper arm level
√7th S45.911 Laceration of unspecified blood vessel at shoulder and upper arm level, right arm
√7th S45.912 Laceration of unspecified blood vessel at shoulder and upper arm level, left arm
√7th S45.919 Laceration of unspecified blood vessel at shoulder and upper arm level, unspecified arm
√6th S45.99 Other specified injury of unspecified blood vessel at shoulder and upper arm level
√7th S45.991 Other specified injury of unspecified blood vessel at shoulder and upper arm level, right arm
√7th S45.992 Other specified injury of unspecified blood vessel at shoulder and upper arm level, left arm
√7th S45.999 Other specified injury of unspecified blood vessel at shoulder and upper arm level, unspecified arm

√4th S46 Injury of muscle, fascia and tendon at shoulder and upper arm level

Code also any associated open wound (S41.-)

EXCLUDES 2 *injury of muscle, fascia and tendon at elbow (S56.-)*
sprain of joints and ligaments of shoulder girdle (S43.9)

The appropriate 7th character is to be added to each code from category S46.
A initial encounter
D subsequent encounter
S sequela

√5th S46.0 Injury of muscle(s) and tendon(s) of the rotator cuff of shoulder
√6th S46.00 Unspecified injury of muscle(s) and tendon(s) of the rotator cuff of shoulder
√7th S46.001 Unspecified injury of muscle(s) and tendon(s) of the rotator cuff of right shoulder
√7th S46.002 Unspecified injury of muscle(s) and tendon(s) of the rotator cuff of left shoulder
√7th S46.009 Unspecified injury of muscle(s) and tendon(s) of the rotator cuff of unspecified shoulder
√6th S46.01 Strain of muscle(s) and tendon(s) of the rotator cuff of shoulder
√7th S46.011 Strain of muscle(s) and tendon(s) of the rotator cuff of right shoulder

✓7th S46.012 Strain of muscle(s) and tendon(s) of the rotator cuff of left shoulder

✓7th S46.019 Strain of muscle(s) and tendon(s) of the rotator cuff of unspecified shoulder

✓6th S46.02 Laceration of muscle(s) and tendon(s) of the rotator cuff of shoulder

✓7th S46.021 Laceration of muscle(s) and tendon(s) of the rotator cuff of right shoulder

✓7th S46.022 Laceration of muscle(s) and tendon(s) of the rotator cuff of left shoulder

✓7th S46.029 Laceration of muscle(s) and tendon(s) of the rotator cuff of unspecified shoulder

✓6th S46.09 Other injury of muscle(s) and tendon(s) of the rotator cuff of shoulder

✓7th S46.091 Other injury of muscle(s) and tendon(s) of the rotator cuff of right shoulder

✓7th S46.092 Other injury of muscle(s) and tendon(s) of the rotator cuff of left shoulder

✓7th S46.099 Other injury of muscle(s) and tendon(s) of the rotator cuff of unspecified shoulder

✓5th S46.1 Injury of muscle, fascia and tendon of long head of biceps

✓6th S46.10 Unspecified injury of muscle, fascia and tendon of long head of biceps

✓7th S46.101 Unspecified injury of muscle, fascia and tendon of long head of biceps, right arm

✓7th S46.102 Unspecified injury of muscle, fascia and tendon of long head of biceps, left arm

✓7th S46.109 Unspecified injury of muscle, fascia and tendon of long head of biceps, unspecified arm

✓6th S46.11 Strain of muscle, fascia and tendon of long head of biceps

✓7th S46.111 Strain of muscle, fascia and tendon of long head of biceps, right arm

✓7th S46.112 Strain of muscle, fascia and tendon of long head of biceps, left arm

✓7th S46.119 Strain of muscle, fascia and tendon of long head of biceps, unspecified arm

✓6th S46.12 Laceration of muscle, fascia and tendon of long head of biceps

✓7th S46.121 Laceration of muscle, fascia and tendon of long head of biceps, right arm

✓7th S46.122 Laceration of muscle, fascia and tendon of long head of biceps, left arm

✓7th S46.129 Laceration of muscle, fascia and tendon of long head of biceps, unspecified arm

✓6th S46.19 Other injury of muscle, fascia and tendon of long head of biceps

✓7th S46.191 Other injury of muscle, fascia and tendon of long head of biceps, right arm

✓7th S46.192 Other injury of muscle, fascia and tendon of long head of biceps, left arm

✓7th S46.199 Other injury of muscle, fascia and tendon of long head of biceps, unspecified arm

✓5th S46.2 Injury of muscle, fascia and tendon of other parts of biceps

✓6th S46.20 Unspecified injury of muscle, fascia and tendon of other parts of biceps

✓7th S46.201 Unspecified injury of muscle, fascia and tendon of other parts of biceps, right arm

✓7th S46.202 Unspecified injury of muscle, fascia and tendon of other parts of biceps, left arm

✓7th S46.209 Unspecified injury of muscle, fascia and tendon of other parts of biceps, unspecified arm

✓6th S46.21 Strain of muscle, fascia and tendon of other parts of biceps

✓7th S46.211 Strain of muscle, fascia and tendon of other parts of biceps, right arm

✓7th S46.212 Strain of muscle, fascia and tendon of other parts of biceps, left arm

✓7th S46.219 Strain of muscle, fascia and tendon of other parts of biceps, unspecified arm

✓6th S46.22 Laceration of muscle, fascia and tendon of other parts of biceps

✓7th S46.221 Laceration of muscle, fascia and tendon of other parts of biceps, right arm

✓7th S46.222 Laceration of muscle, fascia and tendon of other parts of biceps, left arm

✓7th S46.229 Laceration of muscle, fascia and tendon of other parts of biceps, unspecified arm

✓6th S46.29 Other injury of muscle, fascia and tendon of other parts of biceps

✓7th S46.291 Other injury of muscle, fascia and tendon of other parts of biceps, right arm

✓7th S46.292 Other injury of muscle, fascia and tendon of other parts of biceps, left arm

✓7th S46.299 Other injury of muscle, fascia and tendon of other parts of biceps, unspecified arm

✓5th S46.3 Injury of muscle, fascia and tendon of triceps

✓6th S46.30 Unspecified injury of muscle, fascia and tendon of triceps

✓7th S46.301 Unspecified injury of muscle, fascia and tendon of triceps, right arm

✓7th S46.302 Unspecified injury of muscle, fascia and tendon of triceps, left arm

✓7th S46.309 Unspecified injury of muscle, fascia and tendon of triceps, unspecified arm

✓6th S46.31 Strain of muscle, fascia and tendon of triceps

✓7th S46.311 Strain of muscle, fascia and tendon of triceps, right arm

✓7th S46.312 Strain of muscle, fascia and tendon of triceps, left arm

✓7th S46.319 Strain of muscle, fascia and tendon of triceps, unspecified arm

✓6th S46.32 Laceration of muscle, fascia and tendon of triceps

✓7th S46.321 Laceration of muscle, fascia and tendon of triceps, right arm

✓7th S46.322 Laceration of muscle, fascia and tendon of triceps, left arm

✓7th S46.329 Laceration of muscle, fascia and tendon of triceps, unspecified arm

✓6th S46.39 Other injury of muscle, fascia and tendon of triceps

✓7th S46.391 Other injury of muscle, fascia and tendon of triceps, right arm

✓7th S46.392 Other injury of muscle, fascia and tendon of triceps, left arm

✓7th S46.399 Other injury of muscle, fascia and tendon of triceps, unspecified arm

✓5th S46.8 Injury of other muscles, fascia and tendons at shoulder and upper arm level

✓6th S46.80 Unspecified injury of other muscles, fascia and tendons at shoulder and upper arm level

✓7th S46.801 Unspecified injury of other muscles, fascia and tendons at shoulder and upper arm level, right arm

✓7th S46.802 Unspecified injury of other muscles, fascia and tendons at shoulder and upper arm level, left arm

✓7th S46.809 Unspecified injury of other muscles, fascia and tendons at shoulder and upper arm level, unspecified arm

✓6th S46.81 Strain of other muscles, fascia and tendons at shoulder and upper arm level

✓7th S46.811 Strain of other muscles, fascia and tendons at shoulder and upper arm level, right arm

✓7th S46.812 Strain of other muscles, fascia and tendons at shoulder and upper arm level, left arm

✓7th S46.819 Strain of other muscles, fascia and tendons at shoulder and upper arm level, unspecified arm

✓6th S46.82 Laceration of other muscles, fascia and tendons at shoulder and upper arm level

✓7th S46.821 Laceration of other muscles, fascia and tendons at shoulder and upper arm level, right arm

7th S46.822 **Laceration of other muscles, fascia and tendons at shoulder and upper arm level, left arm**
7th S46.829 **Laceration of other muscles, fascia and tendons at shoulder and upper arm level, unspecified arm**
6th S46.89 **Other injury of other muscles, fascia and tendons at shoulder and upper arm level**
7th S46.891 **Other injury of other muscles, fascia and tendons at shoulder and upper arm level, right arm**
7th S46.892 **Other injury of other muscles, fascia and tendons at shoulder and upper arm level, left arm**
7th S46.899 **Other injury of other muscles, fascia and tendons at shoulder and upper arm level, unspecified arm**
5th S46.9 **Injury of unspecified muscle, fascia and tendon at shoulder and upper arm level**
6th S46.90 **Unspecified injury of unspecified muscle, fascia and tendon at shoulder and upper arm level**
7th S46.901 **Unspecified injury of unspecified muscle, fascia and tendon at shoulder and upper arm level, right arm**
7th S46.902 **Unspecified injury of unspecified muscle, fascia and tendon at shoulder and upper arm level, left arm**
7th S46.909 **Unspecified injury of unspecified muscle, fascia and tendon at shoulder and upper arm level, unspecified arm**
6th S46.91 **Strain of unspecified muscle, fascia and tendon at shoulder and upper arm level**
7th S46.911 **Strain of unspecified muscle, fascia and tendon at shoulder and upper arm level, right arm**
7th S46.912 **Strain of unspecified muscle, fascia and tendon at shoulder and upper arm level, left arm**
7th S46.919 **Strain of unspecified muscle, fascia and tendon at shoulder and upper arm level, unspecified arm**
6th S46.92 **Laceration of unspecified muscle, fascia and tendon at shoulder and upper arm level**
7th S46.921 **Laceration of unspecified muscle, fascia and tendon at shoulder and upper arm level, right arm**
7th S46.922 **Laceration of unspecified muscle, fascia and tendon at shoulder and upper arm level, left arm**
7th S46.929 **Laceration of unspecified muscle, fascia and tendon at shoulder and upper arm level, unspecified arm**
6th S46.99 **Other injury of unspecified muscle, fascia and tendon at shoulder and upper arm level**
7th S46.991 **Other injury of unspecified muscle, fascia and tendon at shoulder and upper arm level, right arm**
7th S46.992 **Other injury of unspecified muscle, fascia and tendon at shoulder and upper arm level, left arm**
7th S46.999 **Other injury of unspecified muscle, fascia and tendon at shoulder and upper arm level, unspecified arm**

4th **S47 Crushing injury of shoulder and upper arm**

Use additional code for all associated injuries

EXCLUDES 2 *crushing injury of elbow (S57.0-)*

The appropriate 7th character is to be added to each code from category S47.
A initial encounter
D subsequent encounter
S sequela

x7th S47.1 **Crushing injury of right shoulder and upper arm**
x7th S47.2 **Crushing injury of left shoulder and upper arm**
x7th S47.9 **Crushing injury of shoulder and upper arm, unspecified arm**

4th **S48 Traumatic amputation of shoulder and upper arm**

NOTE An amputation not identified as partial or complete should be coded to complete

EXCLUDES 1 *traumatic amputation at elbow level (S58.0)*

The appropriate 7th character is to be added to each code from category S48.
A initial encounter
D subsequent encounter
S sequela

5th S48.0 **Traumatic amputation at shoulder joint**
6th S48.01 **Complete traumatic amputation at shoulder joint**
7th S48.011 **Complete traumatic amputation at right shoulder joint**
7th S48.012 **Complete traumatic amputation at left shoulder joint**
7th S48.019 **Complete traumatic amputation at unspecified shoulder joint**
6th S48.02 **Partial traumatic amputation at shoulder joint**
7th S48.021 **Partial traumatic amputation at right shoulder joint**
7th S48.022 **Partial traumatic amputation at left shoulder joint**
7th S48.029 **Partial traumatic amputation at unspecified shoulder joint**
5th S48.1 **Traumatic amputation at level between shoulder and elbow**
6th S48.11 **Complete traumatic amputation at level between shoulder and elbow**
7th S48.111 **Complete traumatic amputation at level between right shoulder and elbow**
7th S48.112 **Complete traumatic amputation at level between left shoulder and elbow**
7th S48.119 **Complete traumatic amputation at level between unspecified shoulder and elbow**
6th S48.12 **Partial traumatic amputation at level between shoulder and elbow**
7th S48.121 **Partial traumatic amputation at level between right shoulder and elbow**
7th S48.122 **Partial traumatic amputation at level between left shoulder and elbow**
7th S48.129 **Partial traumatic amputation at level between unspecified shoulder and elbow**
5th S48.9 **Traumatic amputation of shoulder and upper arm, level unspecified**
6th S48.91 **Complete traumatic amputation of shoulder and upper arm, level unspecified**
7th S48.911 **Complete traumatic amputation of right shoulder and upper arm, level unspecified**
7th S48.912 **Complete traumatic amputation of left shoulder and upper arm, level unspecified**
7th S48.919 **Complete traumatic amputation of unspecified shoulder and upper arm, level unspecified**
6th S48.92 **Partial traumatic amputation of shoulder and upper arm, level unspecified**
7th S48.921 **Partial traumatic amputation of right shoulder and upper arm, level unspecified**
7th S48.922 **Partial traumatic amputation of left shoulder and upper arm, level unspecified**
7th S48.929 **Partial traumatic amputation of unspecified shoulder and upper arm, level unspecified**

S49 Other and unspecified injuries of shoulder and upper arm

The appropriate 7th character is to be added to each code from subcategories S49.Ø and S49.1.
A initial encounter for closed fracture
D subsequent encounter for fracture with routine healing
G subsequent encounter for fracture with delayed healing
K subsequent encounter for fracture with nonunion
P subsequent encounter for fracture with malunion
S sequela

S49.Ø Physeal fracture of upper end of humerus
S49.ØØ Unspecified physeal fracture of upper end of humerus
S49.ØØ1 Unspecified physeal fracture of upper end of humerus, right arm
S49.ØØ2 Unspecified physeal fracture of upper end of humerus, left arm
S49.ØØ9 Unspecified physeal fracture of upper end of humerus, unspecified arm
S49.Ø1 Salter-Harris Type I physeal fracture of upper end of humerus
S49.Ø11 Salter-Harris Type I physeal fracture of upper end of humerus, right arm
S49.Ø12 Salter-Harris Type I physeal fracture of upper end of humerus, left arm
S49.Ø19 Salter-Harris Type I physeal fracture of upper end of humerus, unspecified arm
S49.Ø2 Salter-Harris Type II physeal fracture of upper end of humerus
S49.Ø21 Salter-Harris Type II physeal fracture of upper end of humerus, right arm
S49.Ø22 Salter-Harris Type II physeal fracture of upper end of humerus, left arm
S49.Ø29 Salter-Harris Type II physeal fracture of upper end of humerus, unspecified arm
S49.Ø3 Salter-Harris Type III physeal fracture of upper end of humerus
S49.Ø31 Salter Harris Type III physeal fracture of upper end of humerus, right arm
S49.Ø32 Salter Harris Type III physeal fracture of upper end of humerus, left arm
S49.Ø39 Salter Harris Type III physeal fracture of upper end of humerus, unspecified arm
S49.Ø4 Salter-Harris Type IV physeal fracture of upper end of humerus
S49.Ø41 Salter-Harris Type IV physeal fracture of upper end of humerus, right arm
S49.Ø42 Salter-Harris Type IV physeal fracture of upper end of humerus, left arm
S49.Ø49 Salter-Harris Type IV physeal fracture of upper end of humerus, unspecified arm
S49.Ø9 Other physeal fracture of upper end of humerus
S49.Ø91 Other physeal fracture of upper end of humerus, right arm
S49.Ø92 Other physeal fracture of upper end of humerus, left arm
S49.Ø99 Other physeal fracture of upper end of humerus, unspecified arm
S49.1 Physeal fracture of lower end of humerus
S49.1Ø Unspecified physeal fracture of lower end of humerus
S49.1Ø1 Unspecified physeal fracture of lower end of humerus, right arm
S49.1Ø2 Unspecified physeal fracture of lower end of humerus, left arm
S49.1Ø9 Unspecified physeal fracture of lower end of humerus, unspecified arm
S49.11 Salter-Harris Type I physeal fracture of lower end of humerus
S49.111 Salter-Harris Type I physeal fracture of lower end of humerus, right arm
S49.112 Salter-Harris Type I physeal fracture of lower end of humerus, left arm
S49.119 Salter-Harris Type I physeal fracture of lower end of humerus, unspecified arm
S49.12 Salter-Harris Type II physeal fracture of lower end of humerus
S49.121 Salter-Harris Type II physeal fracture of lower end of humerus, right arm
S49.122 Salter-Harris Type II physeal fracture of lower end of humerus, left arm
S49.129 Salter-Harris Type II physeal fracture of lower end of humerus, unspecified arm
S49.13 Salter Harris Type III physeal fracture of lower end of humerus
S49.131 Salter Harris Type III physeal fracture of lower end of humerus, right arm
S49.132 Salter Harris Type III physeal fracture of lower end of humerus, left arm
S49.139 Salter Harris Type III physeal fracture of lower end of humerus, unspecified arm
S49.14 Salter-Harris Type IV physeal fracture of lower end of humerus
S49.141 Salter-Harris Type IV physeal fracture of lower end of humerus, right arm
S49.142 Salter-Harris Type IV physeal fracture of lower end of humerus, left arm
S49.149 Salter-Harris Type IV physeal fracture of lower end of humerus, unspecified arm
S49.19 Other physeal fracture of lower end of humerus
S49.191 Other physeal fracture of lower end of humerus, right arm
S49.192 Other physeal fracture of lower end of humerus, left arm
S49.199 Other physeal fracture of lower end of humerus, unspecified arm
S49.8 Other specified injuries of shoulder and upper arm

The appropriate 7th character is to be added to each code in subcategory S49.8.
A initial encounter
D subsequent encounter
S sequela

S49.8Ø Other specified injuries of shoulder and upper arm, unspecified arm
S49.81 Other specified injuries of right shoulder and upper arm
S49.82 Other specified injuries of left shoulder and upper arm
S49.9 Unspecified injury of shoulder and upper arm

The appropriate 7th character is to be added to each code in subcategory S49.9.
A initial encounter
D subsequent encounter
S sequela

S49.9Ø Unspecified injury of shoulder and upper arm, unspecified arm
S49.91 Unspecified injury of right shoulder and upper arm
S49.92 Unspecified injury of left shoulder and upper arm

Injuries to the elbow and forearm (S5Ø-S59)

EXCLUDES 2 *burns and corrosions (T2Ø-T32)*
frostbite (T33-T34)
injuries of wrist and hand (S6Ø-S69)
insect bite or sting, venomous (T63.4)

S5Ø Superficial injury of elbow and forearm

EXCLUDES 2 *superficial injury of wrist and hand (S6Ø.-)*

The appropriate 7th character is to be added to each code from category S5Ø.
A initial encounter
D subsequent encounter
S sequela

S5Ø.Ø Contusion of elbow
S5Ø.ØØ Contusion of unspecified elbow
S5Ø.Ø1 Contusion of right elbow
S5Ø.Ø2 Contusion of left elbow
S5Ø.1 Contusion of forearm
S5Ø.1Ø Contusion of unspecified forearm
S5Ø.11 Contusion of right forearm

✓x7th S50.12 Contusion of left forearm

✓5th S50.3 Other superficial injuries of elbow

✓6th S50.31 Abrasion of elbow

✓7th S50.311 Abrasion of right elbow

✓7th S50.312 Abrasion of left elbow

✓7th S50.319 Abrasion of unspecified elbow

✓6th S50.32 Blister (nonthermal) of elbow

✓7th S50.321 Blister (nonthermal) of right elbow

✓7th S50.322 Blister (nonthermal) of left elbow

✓7th S50.329 Blister (nonthermal) of unspecified elbow

✓6th S50.34 External constriction of elbow

✓7th S50.341 External constriction of right elbow

✓7th S50.342 External constriction of left elbow

✓7th S50.349 External constriction of unspecified elbow

✓6th S50.35 Superficial foreign body of elbow

Splinter in the elbow

✓7th S50.351 Superficial foreign body of right elbow

✓7th S50.352 Superficial foreign body of left elbow

✓7th S50.359 Superficial foreign body of unspecified elbow

✓6th S50.36 Insect bite (nonvenomous) of elbow

✓7th S50.361 Insect bite (nonvenomous) of right elbow

✓7th S50.362 Insect bite (nonvenomous) of left elbow

✓7th S50.369 Insect bite (nonvenomous) of unspecified elbow

✓6th S50.37 Other superficial bite of elbow

EXCLUDES 1 *open bite of elbow (S51.05)*

✓7th S50.371 Other superficial bite of right elbow

✓7th S50.372 Other superficial bite of left elbow

✓7th S50.379 Other superficial bite of unspecified elbow

✓5th S50.8 Other superficial injuries of forearm

✓6th S50.81 Abrasion of forearm

✓7th S50.811 Abrasion of right forearm

✓7th S50.812 Abrasion of left forearm

✓7th S50.819 Abrasion of unspecified forearm

✓6th S50.82 Blister (nonthermal) of forearm

✓7th S50.821 Blister (nonthermal) of right forearm

✓7th S50.822 Blister (nonthermal) of left forearm

✓7th S50.829 Blister (nonthermal) of unspecified forearm

✓6th S50.84 External constriction of forearm

✓7th S50.841 External constriction of right forearm

✓7th S50.842 External constriction of left forearm

✓7th S50.849 External constriction of unspecified forearm

✓6th S50.85 Superficial foreign body of forearm

Splinter in the forearm

✓7th S50.851 Superficial foreign body of right forearm

✓7th S50.852 Superficial foreign body of left forearm

✓7th S50.859 Superficial foreign body of unspecified forearm

✓6th S50.86 Insect bite (nonvenomous) of forearm

✓7th S50.861 Insect bite (nonvenomous) of right forearm

✓7th S50.862 Insect bite (nonvenomous) of left forearm

✓7th S50.869 Insect bite (nonvenomous) of unspecified forearm

✓6th S50.87 Other superficial bite of forearm

EXCLUDES 1 *open bite of forearm (S51.85)*

✓7th S50.871 Other superficial bite of right forearm

✓7th S50.872 Other superficial bite of left forearm

✓7th S50.879 Other superficial bite of unspecified forearm

✓5th S50.9 Unspecified superficial injury of elbow and forearm

✓6th S50.90 Unspecified superficial injury of elbow

✓7th S50.901 Unspecified superficial injury of right elbow

✓7th S50.902 Unspecified superficial injury of left elbow

✓7th S50.909 Unspecified superficial injury of unspecified elbow

✓6th S50.91 Unspecified superficial injury of forearm

✓7th S50.911 Unspecified superficial injury of right forearm

✓7th S50.912 Unspecified superficial injury of left forearm

✓7th S50.919 Unspecified superficial injury of unspecified forearm

✓4th **S51 Open wound of elbow and forearm**

Code also any associated wound infection

EXCLUDES 1 *open fracture of elbow and forearm (S52- with open fracture 7th character)*

traumatic amputation of elbow and forearm (S58.-)

EXCLUDES 2 *open wound of wrist and hand (S61.-)*

The appropriate 7th character is to be added to each code from category S51.

A initial encounter

D subsequent encounter

S sequela

✓5th S51.0 Open wound of elbow

✓6th S51.00 Unspecified open wound of elbow

✓7th S51.001 Unspecified open wound of right elbow

✓7th S51.002 Unspecified open wound of left elbow

✓7th S51.009 Unspecified open wound of unspecified elbow

Open wound of elbow NOS

✓6th S51.01 Laceration without foreign body of elbow

✓7th S51.011 Laceration without foreign body of right elbow

✓7th S51.012 Laceration without foreign body of left elbow

✓7th S51.019 Laceration without foreign body of unspecified elbow

✓6th S51.02 Laceration with foreign body of elbow

✓7th S51.021 Laceration with foreign body of right elbow

✓7th S51.022 Laceration with foreign body of left elbow

✓7th S51.029 Laceration with foreign body of unspecified elbow

✓6th S51.03 Puncture wound without foreign body of elbow

✓7th S51.031 Puncture wound without foreign body of right elbow

✓7th S51.032 Puncture wound without foreign body of left elbow

✓7th S51.039 Puncture wound without foreign body of unspecified elbow

✓6th S51.04 Puncture wound with foreign body of elbow

✓7th S51.041 Puncture wound with foreign body of right elbow

✓7th S51.042 Puncture wound with foreign body of left elbow

✓7th S51.049 Puncture wound with foreign body of unspecified elbow

✓6th S51.05 Open bite of elbow

Bite of elbow NOS

EXCLUDES 1 *superficial bite of elbow (S50.36, S50.37)*

✓7th S51.051 Open bite, right elbow

✓7th S51.052 Open bite, left elbow

✓7th S51.059 Open bite, unspecified elbow

✓5th S51.8 Open wound of forearm

EXCLUDES 2 *open wound of elbow (S51.0-)*

✓6th S51.80 Unspecified open wound of forearm

✓7th S51.801 Unspecified open wound of right forearm

✓7th S51.802 Unspecified open wound of left forearm

✓7th S51.809 Unspecified open wound of unspecified forearm

Open wound of forearm NOS

✓6th S51.81 Laceration without foreign body of forearm

✓7th S51.811 Laceration without foreign body of right forearm

✓7th S51.812 Laceration without foreign body of left forearm

✓ Appropriate additional character required ✓x7th Requires 7th character, placeholder x must fill empty characters

√7th **S51.819 Laceration without foreign body of unspecified forearm**

√6th **S51.82 Laceration with foreign body of forearm**

√7th **S51.821 Laceration with foreign body of right forearm**

√7th **S51.822 Laceration with foreign body of left forearm**

√7th **S51.829 Laceration with foreign body of unspecified forearm**

√6th **S51.83 Puncture wound without foreign body of forearm**

√7th **S51.831 Puncture wound without foreign body of right forearm**

√7th **S51.832 Puncture wound without foreign body of left forearm**

√7th **S51.839 Puncture wound without foreign body of unspecified forearm**

√6th **S51.84 Puncture wound with foreign body of forearm**

√7th **S51.841 Puncture wound with foreign body of right forearm**

√7th **S51.842 Puncture wound with foreign body of left forearm**

√7th **S51.849 Puncture wound with foreign body of unspecified forearm**

√6th **S51.85 Open bite of forearm**

Bite of forearm NOS

EXCLUDES 1 *superficial bite of forearm (S5Ø.86, S5Ø.87)*

√7th **S51.851 Open bite of right forearm**

√7th **S51.852 Open bite of left forearm**

√7th **S51.859 Open bite of unspecified forearm**

√4th **S52 Fracture of forearm**

NOTE A fracture not indicated as displaced or nondisplaced should be coded to displaced

A fracture not indicated as open or closed should be coded to closed.

The open fracture designations are based on the Gustilo open fracture classification.

EXCLUDES 1 *traumatic amputation of forearm (S58.-)*

EXCLUDES 2 *fracture at wrist and hand level (S62.-)*

The appropriate 7th character is to be added to all codes from category S52 [unless otherwise indicated].

- A initial encounter for closed fracture
- B initial encounter for open fracture type I or II
  initial encounter for open fracture NOS
- C initial encounter for open fracture type IIIA, IIIB, or IIIC
- D subsequent encounter for closed fracture with routine healing
- E subsequent encounter for open fracture type I or II with routine healing
- F subsequent encounter for open fracture type IIIA, IIIB, or IIIC with routine healing
- G subsequent encounter for closed fracture with delayed healing
- H subsequent encounter for open fracture type I or II with delayed healing
- J subsequent encounter for open fracture type IIIA, IIIB, or IIIC with delayed healing
- K subsequent encounter for closed fracture with nonunion
- M subsequent encounter for open fracture type I or II with nonunion
- N subsequent encounter for open fracture type IIIA, IIIB, or IIIC with nonunion
- P subsequent encounter for closed fracture with malunion
- Q subsequent encounter for open fracture type I or II with malunion
- R subsequent encounter for open fracture type IIIA, IIIB, or IIIC with malunion
- S sequela

√5th **S52.Ø Fracture of upper end of ulna**

Fracture of proximal end of ulna

EXCLUDES 2 *fracture of elbow NOS (S42.4Ø-)*
fractures of shaft of ulna (S52.2-)

√6th **S52.ØØ Unspecified fracture of upper end of ulna**

√7th **S52.ØØ1 Unspecified fracture of upper end of right ulna**

√7th **S52.ØØ2 Unspecified fracture of upper end of left ulna**

√7th **S52.ØØ9 Unspecified fracture of upper end of unspecified ulna**

√6th **S52.Ø1 Torus fracture of upper end of ulna**

The appropriate 7th character is to be added to all codes in subcategory S52.Ø1.

- A initial encounter for closed fracture
- D subsequent encounter for fracture with routine healing
- G subsequent encounter for fracture with delayed healing
- K subsequent encounter for fracture with nonunion
- P subsequent encounter for fracture with malunion
- S sequela

√7th **S52.Ø11 Torus fracture of upper end of right ulna**

√7th **S52.Ø12 Torus fracture of upper end of left ulna**

√7th **S52.Ø19 Torus fracture of upper end of unspecified ulna**

√6th **S52.Ø2 Fracture of olecranon process without intraarticular extension of ulna**

√7th **S52.Ø21 Displaced fracture of olecranon process without intraarticular extension of right ulna**

√7th **S52.Ø22 Displaced fracture of olecranon process without intraarticular extension of left ulna**

√7th **S52.Ø23 Displaced fracture of olecranon process without intraarticular extension of unspecified ulna**

√7th **S52.Ø24 Nondisplaced fracture of olecranon process without intraarticular extension of right ulna**

√7th **S52.Ø25 Nondisplaced fracture of olecranon process without intraarticular extension of left ulna**

√7th **S52.Ø26 Nondisplaced fracture of olecranon process without intraarticular extension of unspecified ulna**

√6th **S52.Ø3 Fracture of olecranon process with intraarticular extension of ulna**

√7th **S52.Ø31 Displaced fracture of olecranon process with intraarticular extension of right ulna**

√7th **S52.Ø32 Displaced fracture of olecranon process with intraarticular extension of left ulna**

√7th **S52.Ø33 Displaced fracture of olecranon process with intraarticular extension of unspecified ulna**

√7th **S52.Ø34 Nondisplaced fracture of olecranon process with intraarticular extension of right ulna**

√7th **S52.Ø35 Nondisplaced fracture of olecranon process with intraarticular extension of left ulna**

√7th **S52.Ø36 Nondisplaced fracture of olecranon process with intraarticular extension of unspecified ulna**

√6th **S52.Ø4 Fracture of coronoid process of ulna**

√7th **S52.Ø41 Displaced fracture of coronoid process of right ulna**

√7th **S52.Ø42 Displaced fracture of coronoid process of left ulna**

√7th **S52.Ø43 Displaced fracture of coronoid process of unspecified ulna**

√7th **S52.Ø44 Nondisplaced fracture of coronoid process of right ulna**

√7th **S52.Ø45 Nondisplaced fracture of coronoid process of left ulna**

√7th **S52.Ø46 Nondisplaced fracture of coronoid process of unspecified ulna**

√6th **S52.Ø9 Other fracture of upper end of ulna**

√7th **S52.Ø91 Other fracture of upper end of right ulna**

√7th **S52.Ø92 Other fracture of upper end of left ulna**

√7th **S52.Ø99 Other fracture of upper end of unspecified ulna**

✓5th **S52.1 Fracture of upper end of radius**
Fracture of proximal end of radius
EXCLUDES 2 *physeal fractures of upper end of radius (S59.2-)*
fracture of shaft of radius (S52.3-)

✓6th **S52.10 Unspecified fracture of upper end of radius**
✓7th **S52.101 Unspecified fracture of upper end of right radius**
✓7th **S52.102 Unspecified fracture of upper end of left radius**
✓7th **S52.109 Unspecified fracture of upper end of unspecified radius**

✓6th **S52.11 Torus fracture of upper end of radius**

The appropriate 7th character is to be added to all codes in subcategory S52.11.
A initial encounter for closed fracture
D subsequent encounter for fracture with routine healing
G subsequent encounter for fracture with delayed healing
K subsequent encounter for fracture with nonunion
P subsequent encounter for fracture with malunion
S sequela

✓7th **S52.111 Torus fracture of upper end of right radius**
✓7th **S52.112 Torus fracture of upper end of left radius**
✓7th **S52.119 Torus fracture of upper end of unspecified radius**

✓6th **S52.12 Fracture of head of radius**
✓7th **S52.121 Displaced fracture of head of right radius**
✓7th **S52.122 Displaced fracture of head of left radius**
✓7th **S52.123 Displaced fracture of head of unspecified radius**
✓7th **S52.124 Nondisplaced fracture of head of right radius**
✓7th **S52.125 Nondisplaced fracture of head of left radius**
✓7th **S52.126 Nondisplaced fracture of head of unspecified radius**

✓6th **S52.13 Fracture of neck of radius**
✓7th **S52.131 Displaced fracture of neck of right radius**
✓7th **S52.132 Displaced fracture of neck of left radius**
✓7th **S52.133 Displaced fracture of neck of unspecified radius**
✓7th **S52.134 Nondisplaced fracture of neck of right radius**
✓7th **S52.135 Nondisplaced fracture of neck of left radius**
✓7th **S52.136 Nondisplaced fracture of neck of unspecified radius**

✓6th **S52.18 Other fracture of upper end of radius**
✓7th **S52.181 Other fracture of upper end of right radius**
✓7th **S52.182 Other fracture of upper end of left radius**
✓7th **S52.189 Other fracture of upper end of unspecified radius**

✓5th **S52.2 Fracture of shaft of ulna**

✓6th **S52.20 Unspecified fracture of shaft of ulna**
Fracture of ulna NOS
✓7th **S52.201 Unspecified fracture of shaft of right ulna**
✓7th **S52.202 Unspecified fracture of shaft of left ulna**
✓7th **S52.209 Unspecified fracture of shaft of unspecified ulna**

✓6th **S52.21 Greenstick fracture of shaft of ulna**

The appropriate 7th character is to be added to all codes in subcategory S52.21.
A initial encounter for closed fracture
D subsequent encounter for fracture with routine healing
G subsequent encounter for fracture with delayed healing
K subsequent encounter for fracture with nonunion
P subsequent encounter for fracture with malunion
S sequela

✓7th **S52.211 Greenstick fracture of shaft of right ulna**
✓7th **S52.212 Greenstick fracture of shaft of left ulna**
✓7th **S52.219 Greenstick fracture of shaft of unspecified ulna**

✓6th **S52.22 Transverse fracture of shaft of ulna**
✓7th **S52.221 Displaced transverse fracture of shaft of right ulna**
✓7th **S52.222 Displaced transverse fracture of shaft of left ulna**
✓7th **S52.223 Displaced transverse fracture of shaft of unspecified ulna**
✓7th **S52.224 Nondisplaced transverse fracture of shaft of right ulna**
✓7th **S52.225 Nondisplaced transverse fracture of shaft of left ulna**
✓7th **S52.226 Nondisplaced transverse fracture of shaft of unspecified ulna**

✓6th **S52.23 Oblique fracture of shaft of ulna**
✓7th **S52.231 Displaced oblique fracture of shaft of right ulna**
✓7th **S52.232 Displaced oblique fracture of shaft of left ulna**
✓7th **S52.233 Displaced oblique fracture of shaft of unspecified ulna**
✓7th **S52.234 Nondisplaced oblique fracture of shaft of right ulna**
✓7th **S52.235 Nondisplaced oblique fracture of shaft of left ulna**
✓7th **S52.236 Nondisplaced oblique fracture of shaft of unspecified ulna**

✓6th **S52.24 Spiral fracture of shaft of ulna**
✓7th **S52.241 Displaced spiral fracture of shaft of ulna, right arm**
✓7th **S52.242 Displaced spiral fracture of shaft of ulna, left arm**
✓7th **S52.243 Displaced spiral fracture of shaft of ulna, unspecified arm**
✓7th **S52.244 Nondisplaced spiral fracture of shaft of ulna, right arm**
✓7th **S52.245 Nondisplaced spiral fracture of shaft of ulna, left arm**
✓7th **S52.246 Nondisplaced spiral fracture of shaft of ulna, unspecified arm**

✓6th **S52.25 Comminuted fracture of shaft of ulna**
✓7th **S52.251 Displaced comminuted fracture of shaft of ulna, right arm**
✓7th **S52.252 Displaced comminuted fracture of shaft of ulna, left arm**
✓7th **S52.253 Displaced comminuted fracture of shaft of ulna, unspecified arm**
✓7th **S52.254 Nondisplaced comminuted fracture of shaft of ulna, right arm**
✓7th **S52.255 Nondisplaced comminuted fracture of shaft of ulna, left arm**
✓7th **S52.256 Nondisplaced comminuted fracture of shaft of ulna, unspecified arm**

✓6th **S52.26 Segmental fracture of shaft of ulna**
✓7th **S52.261 Displaced segmental fracture of shaft of ulna, right arm**
✓7th **S52.262 Displaced segmental fracture of shaft of ulna, left arm**
✓7th **S52.263 Displaced segmental fracture of shaft of ulna, unspecified arm**

✓7th **S52.264 Nondisplaced segmental fracture of shaft of ulna, right arm**
✓7th **S52.265 Nondisplaced segmental fracture of shaft of ulna, left arm**
✓7th **S52.266 Nondisplaced segmental fracture of shaft of ulna, unspecified arm**

✓6th **S52.27 Monteggia's fracture of ulna**
Fracture of upper shaft of ulna with dislocation of radial head
✓7th **S52.271 Monteggia's fracture of right ulna**
✓7th **S52.272 Monteggia's fracture of left ulna**
✓7th **S52.279 Monteggia's fracture of unspecified ulna**

✓6th **S52.28 Bent bone of ulna**
✓7th **S52.281 Bent bone of right ulna**
✓7th **S52.282 Bent bone of left ulna**
✓7th **S52.283 Bent bone of unspecified ulna**

✓6th **S52.29 Other fracture of shaft of ulna**
✓7th **S52.291 Other fracture of shaft of right ulna**
✓7th **S52.292 Other fracture of shaft of left ulna**
✓7th **S52.299 Other fracture of shaft of unspecified ulna**

✓5th **S52.3 Fracture of shaft of radius**

✓6th **S52.30 Unspecified fracture of shaft of radius**
✓7th **S52.301 Unspecified fracture of shaft of right radius**
✓7th **S52.302 Unspecified fracture of shaft of left radius**
✓7th **S52.309 Unspecified fracture of shaft of unspecified radius**

✓6th **S52.31 Greenstick fracture of shaft of radius**

The appropriate 7th character is to be added to all codes in subcategory S52.31.
A initial encounter for closed fracture
D subsequent encounter for fracture with routine healing
G subsequent encounter for fracture with delayed healing
K subsequent encounter for fracture with nonunion
P subsequent encounter for fracture with malunion
S sequela

✓7th **S52.311 Greenstick fracture of shaft of radius, right arm**
✓7th **S52.312 Greenstick fracture of shaft of radius, left arm**
✓7th **S52.319 Greenstick fracture of shaft of radius, unspecified arm**

✓6th **S52.32 Transverse fracture of shaft of radius**
✓7th **S52.321 Displaced transverse fracture of shaft of right radius**
✓7th **S52.322 Displaced transverse fracture of shaft of left radius**
✓7th **S52.323 Displaced transverse fracture of shaft of unspecified radius**
✓7th **S52.324 Nondisplaced transverse fracture of shaft of right radius**
✓7th **S52.325 Nondisplaced transverse fracture of shaft of left radius**
✓7th **S52.326 Nondisplaced transverse fracture of shaft of unspecified radius**

✓6th **S52.33 Oblique fracture of shaft of radius**
✓7th **S52.331 Displaced oblique fracture of shaft of right radius**
✓7th **S52.332 Displaced oblique fracture of shaft of left radius**
✓7th **S52.333 Displaced oblique fracture of shaft of unspecified radius**
✓7th **S52.334 Nondisplaced oblique fracture of shaft of right radius**
✓7th **S52.335 Nondisplaced oblique fracture of shaft of left radius**
✓7th **S52.336 Nondisplaced oblique fracture of shaft of unspecified radius**

✓6th **S52.34 Spiral fracture of shaft of radius**
✓7th **S52.341 Displaced spiral fracture of shaft of radius, right arm**
✓7th **S52.342 Displaced spiral fracture of shaft of radius, left arm**
✓7th **S52.343 Displaced spiral fracture of shaft of radius, unspecified arm**
✓7th **S52.344 Nondisplaced spiral fracture of shaft of radius, right arm**
✓7th **S52.345 Nondisplaced spiral fracture of shaft of radius, left arm**
✓7th **S52.346 Nondisplaced spiral fracture of shaft of radius, unspecified arm**

✓6th **S52.35 Comminuted fracture of shaft of radius**
✓7th **S52.351 Displaced comminuted fracture of shaft of radius, right arm**
✓7th **S52.352 Displaced comminuted fracture of shaft of radius, left arm**
✓7th **S52.353 Displaced comminuted fracture of shaft of radius, unspecified arm**
✓7th **S52.354 Nondisplaced comminuted fracture of shaft of radius, right arm**
✓7th **S52.355 Nondisplaced comminuted fracture of shaft of radius, left arm**
✓7th **S52.356 Nondisplaced comminuted fracture of shaft of radius, unspecified arm**

✓6th **S52.36 Segmental fracture of shaft of radius**
✓7th **S52.361 Displaced segmental fracture of shaft of radius, right arm**
✓7th **S52.362 Displaced segmental fracture of shaft of radius, left arm**
✓7th **S52.363 Displaced segmental fracture of shaft of radius, unspecified arm**
✓7th **S52.364 Nondisplaced segmental fracture of shaft of radius, right arm**
✓7th **S52.365 Nondisplaced segmental fracture of shaft of radius, left arm**
✓7th **S52.366 Nondisplaced segmental fracture of shaft of radius, unspecified arm**

✓6th **S52.37 Galeazzi's fracture**
Fracture of lower shaft of radius with radioulnar joint dislocation
✓7th **S52.371 Galeazzi's fracture of right radius**
✓7th **S52.372 Galeazzi's fracture of left radius**
✓7th **S52.379 Galeazzi's fracture of unspecified radius**

✓6th **S52.38 Bent bone of radius**
✓7th **S52.381 Bent bone of right radius**
✓7th **S52.382 Bent bone of left radius**
✓7th **S52.389 Bent bone of unspecified radius**

✓6th **S52.39 Other fracture of shaft of radius**
✓7th **S52.391 Other fracture of shaft of radius, right arm**
✓7th **S52.392 Other fracture of shaft of radius, left arm**
✓7th **S52.399 Other fracture of shaft of radius, unspecified arm**

✓5th **S52.5 Fracture of lower end of radius**
Fracture of distal end of radius
EXCLUDES 2 *physeal fractures of lower end of radius (S59.2-)*

✓6th **S52.50 Unspecified fracture of the lower end of radius**
✓7th **S52.501 Unspecified fracture of the lower end of right radius**
✓7th **S52.502 Unspecified fracture of the lower end of left radius**
✓7th **S52.509 Unspecified fracture of the lower end of unspecified radius**

✓6th **S52.51 Fracture of radial styloid process**
✓7th **S52.511 Displaced fracture of right radial styloid process**
✓7th **S52.512 Displaced fracture of left radial styloid process**
✓7th **S52.513 Displaced fracture of unspecified radial styloid process**
✓7th **S52.514 Nondisplaced fracture of right radial styloid process**
✓7th **S52.515 Nondisplaced fracture of left radial styloid process**

✓7th **S52.516 Nondisplaced fracture of unspecified radial styloid process**

✓6th **S52.52 Torus fracture of lower end of radius**

The appropriate 7th character is to be added to all codes in subcategory S52.52.
A initial encounter for closed fracture
D subsequent encounter for fracture with routine healing
G subsequent encounter for fracture with delayed healing
K subsequent encounter for fracture with nonunion
P subsequent encounter for fracture with malunion
S sequela

✓7th **S52.521 Torus fracture of lower end of right radius**
✓7th **S52.522 Torus fracture of lower end of left radius**
✓7th **S52.529 Torus fracture of lower end of unspecified radius**

✓6th **S52.53 Colles' fracture**
✓7th **S52.531 Colles' fracture of right radius**
✓7th **S52.532 Colles' fracture of left radius**
✓7th **S52.539 Colles' fracture of unspecified radius**

✓6th **S52.54 Smith's fracture**
✓7th **S52.541 Smith's fracture of right radius**
✓7th **S52.542 Smith's fracture of left radius**
✓7th **S52.549 Smith's fracture of unspecified radius**

✓6th **S52.55 Other extraarticular fracture of lower end of radius**
✓7th **S52.551 Other extraarticular fracture of lower end of right radius**
✓7th **S52.552 Other extraarticular fracture of lower end of left radius**
✓7th **S52.559 Other extraarticular fracture of lower end of unspecified radius**

✓6th **S52.56 Barton's fracture**
✓7th **S52.561 Barton's fracture of right radius**
✓7th **S52.562 Barton's fracture of left radius**
✓7th **S52.569 Barton's fracture of unspecified radius**

✓6th **S52.57 Other intraarticular fracture of lower end of radius**
✓7th **S52.571 Other intraarticular fracture of lower end of right radius**
✓7th **S52.572 Other intraarticular fracture of lower end of left radius**
✓7th **S52.579 Other intraarticular fracture of lower end of unspecified radius**

✓6th **S52.59 Other fractures of lower end of radius**
✓7th **S52.591 Other fractures of lower end of right radius**
✓7th **S52.592 Other fractures of lower end of left radius**
✓7th **S52.599 Other fractures of lower end of unspecified radius**

✓5th **S52.6 Fracture of lower end of ulna**

✓6th **S52.60 Unspecified fracture of lower end of ulna**
✓7th **S52.601 Unspecified fracture of lower end of right ulna**
✓7th **S52.602 Unspecified fracture of lower end of left ulna**
✓7th **S52.609 Unspecified fracture of lower end of unspecified ulna**

✓6th **S52.61 Fracture of ulna styloid process**
✓7th **S52.611 Displaced fracture of right ulna styloid process**
✓7th **S52.612 Displaced fracture of left ulna styloid process**
✓7th **S52.613 Displaced fracture of unspecified ulna styloid process**
✓7th **S52.614 Nondisplaced fracture of right ulna styloid process**
✓7th **S52.615 Nondisplaced fracture of left ulna styloid process**
✓7th **S52.616 Nondisplaced fracture of unspecified ulna styloid process**

✓6th **S52.62 Torus fracture of lower end of ulna**

The appropriate 7th character is to be added to all codes in subcategory S52.62.
A initial encounter for closed fracture
D subsequent encounter for fracture with routine healing
G subsequent encounter for fracture with delayed healing
K subsequent encounter for fracture with nonunion
P subsequent encounter for fracture with malunion
S sequela

✓7th **S52.621 Torus fracture of lower end of right ulna**
✓7th **S52.622 Torus fracture of lower end of left ulna**
✓7th **S52.629 Torus fracture of lower end of unspecified ulna**

✓6th **S52.69 Other fracture of lower end of ulna**
✓7th **S52.691 Other fracture of lower end of right ulna**
✓7th **S52.692 Other fracture of lower end of left ulna**
✓7th **S52.699 Other fracture of lower end of unspecified ulna**

✓5th **S52.9 Unspecified fracture of forearm**
✓x7th **S52.90 Unspecified fracture of unspecified forearm**
✓x7th **S52.91 Unspecified fracture of right forearm**
✓x7th **S52.92 Unspecified fracture of left forearm**

✓4th **S53 Dislocation and sprain of joints and ligaments of elbow**

INCLUDES avulsion of joint or ligament of elbow
laceration of cartilage, joint or ligament of elbow
sprain of cartilage, joint or ligament of elbow
traumatic hemarthrosis of joint or ligament of elbow
traumatic rupture of joint or ligament of elbow
traumatic subluxation of joint or ligament of elbow
traumatic tear of joint or ligament of elbow

Code also any associated open wound

EXCLUDES 2 *strain of muscle, fascia and tendon at forearm level (S56.-)*

The appropriate 7th character is to be added to each code from category S53.
A initial encounter
D subsequent encounter
S sequela

✓5th **S53.0 Subluxation and dislocation of radial head**
Dislocation of radiohumeral joint
Subluxation of radiohumeral joint

EXCLUDES 1 *Monteggia's fracture-dislocation (S52.27-)*

✓6th **S53.00 Unspecified subluxation and dislocation of radial head**
✓7th **S53.001 Unspecified subluxation of right radial head**
✓7th **S53.002 Unspecified subluxation of left radial head**
✓7th **S53.003 Unspecified subluxation of unspecified radial head**
✓7th **S53.004 Unspecified dislocation of right radial head**
✓7th **S53.005 Unspecified dislocation of left radial head**
✓7th **S53.006 Unspecified dislocation of unspecified radial head**

✓6th **S53.01 Anterior subluxation and dislocation of radial head**
Anteriomedial subluxation and dislocation of radial head
✓7th **S53.011 Anterior subluxation of right radial head**
✓7th **S53.012 Anterior subluxation of left radial head**
✓7th **S53.013 Anterior subluxation of unspecified radial head**
✓7th **S53.014 Anterior dislocation of right radial head**
✓7th **S53.015 Anterior dislocation of left radial head**
✓7th **S53.016 Anterior dislocation of unspecified radial head**

√6th **S53.02 Posterior subluxation and dislocation of radial head**
Posteriolateral subluxation and dislocation of radial head
√7th **S53.021 Posterior subluxation of right radial head**
√7th **S53.022 Posterior subluxation of left radial head**
√7th **S53.023 Posterior subluxation of unspecified radial head**
√7th **S53.024 Posterior dislocation of right radial head**
√7th **S53.025 Posterior dislocation of left radial head**
√7th **S53.026 Posterior dislocation of unspecified radial head**
√6th **S53.03 Nursemaid's elbow**
√7th **S53.031 Nursemaid's elbow, right elbow**
√7th **S53.032 Nursemaid's elbow, left elbow**
√7th **S53.033 Nursemaid's elbow, unspecified elbow**
√6th **S53.09 Other subluxation and dislocation of radial head**
√7th **S53.091 Other subluxation of right radial head**
√7th **S53.092 Other subluxation of left radial head**
√7th **S53.093 Other subluxation of unspecified radial head**
√7th **S53.094 Other dislocation of right radial head**
√7th **S53.095 Other dislocation of left radial head**
√7th **S53.096 Other dislocation of unspecified radial head**
√5th **S53.1 Subluxation and dislocation of ulnohumeral joint**
Subluxation and dislocation of elbow NOS
EXCLUDES 1 *dislocation of radial head alone (S53.0-)*
√6th **S53.10 Unspecified subluxation and dislocation of ulnohumeral joint**
√7th **S53.101 Unspecified subluxation of right ulnohumeral joint**
√7th **S53.102 Unspecified subluxation of left ulnohumeral joint**
√7th **S53.103 Unspecified subluxation of unspecified ulnohumeral joint**
√7th **S53.104 Unspecified dislocation of right ulnohumeral joint**
√7th **S53.105 Unspecified dislocation of left ulnohumeral joint**
√7th **S53.106 Unspecified dislocation of unspecified ulnohumeral joint**
√6th **S53.11 Anterior subluxation and dislocation of ulnohumeral joint**
√7th **S53.111 Anterior subluxation of right ulnohumeral joint**
√7th **S53.112 Anterior subluxation of left ulnohumeral joint**
√7th **S53.113 Anterior subluxation of unspecified ulnohumeral joint**
√7th **S53.114 Anterior dislocation of right ulnohumeral joint**
√7th **S53.115 Anterior dislocation of left ulnohumeral joint**
√7th **S53.116 Anterior dislocation of unspecified ulnohumeral joint**
√6th **S53.12 Posterior subluxation and dislocation of ulnohumeral joint**
√7th **S53.121 Posterior subluxation of right ulnohumeral joint**
√7th **S53.122 Posterior subluxation of left ulnohumeral joint**
√7th **S53.123 Posterior subluxation of unspecified ulnohumeral joint**
√7th **S53.124 Posterior dislocation of right ulnohumeral joint**
√7th **S53.125 Posterior dislocation of left ulnohumeral joint**
√7th **S53.126 Posterior dislocation of unspecified ulnohumeral joint**
√6th **S53.13 Medial subluxation and dislocation of ulnohumeral joint**
√7th **S53.131 Medial subluxation of right ulnohumeral joint**
√7th **S53.132 Medial subluxation of left ulnohumeral joint**
√7th **S53.133 Medial subluxation of unspecified ulnohumeral joint**
√7th **S53.134 Medial dislocation of right ulnohumeral joint**
√7th **S53.135 Medial dislocation of left ulnohumeral joint**
√7th **S53.136 Medial dislocation of unspecified ulnohumeral joint**
√6th **S53.14 Lateral subluxation and dislocation of ulnohumeral joint**
√7th **S53.141 Lateral subluxation of right ulnohumeral joint**
√7th **S53.142 Lateral subluxation of left ulnohumeral joint**
√7th **S53.143 Lateral subluxation of unspecified ulnohumeral joint**
√7th **S53.144 Lateral dislocation of right ulnohumeral joint**
√7th **S53.145 Lateral dislocation of left ulnohumeral joint**
√7th **S53.146 Lateral dislocation of unspecified ulnohumeral joint**
√6th **S53.19 Other subluxation and dislocation of ulnohumeral joint**
√7th **S53.191 Other subluxation of right ulnohumeral joint**
√7th **S53.192 Other subluxation of left ulnohumeral joint**
√7th **S53.193 Other subluxation of unspecified ulnohumeral joint**
√7th **S53.194 Other dislocation of right ulnohumeral joint**
√7th **S53.195 Other dislocation of left ulnohumeral joint**
√7th **S53.196 Other dislocation of unspecified ulnohumeral joint**
√5th **S53.2 Traumatic rupture of radial collateral ligament**
EXCLUDES 1 *sprain of radial collateral ligament NOS (S53.43-)*
√x7th **S53.20 Traumatic rupture of unspecified radial collateral ligament**
√x7th **S53.21 Traumatic rupture of right radial collateral ligament**
√x7th **S53.22 Traumatic rupture of left radial collateral ligament**
√5th **S53.3 Traumatic rupture of ulnar collateral ligament**
EXCLUDES 1 *sprain of ulnar collateral ligament (S53.44-)*
√x7th **S53.30 Traumatic rupture of unspecified ulnar collateral ligament**
√x7th **S53.31 Traumatic rupture of right ulnar collateral ligament**
√x7th **S53.32 Traumatic rupture of left ulnar collateral ligament**
√5th **S53.4 Sprain of elbow**
EXCLUDES 2 *traumatic rupture of radial collateral ligament (S53.2-)*
traumatic rupture of ulnar collateral ligament (S53.3-)
√6th **S53.40 Unspecified sprain of elbow**
√7th **S53.401 Unspecified sprain of right elbow**
√7th **S53.402 Unspecified sprain of left elbow**
√7th **S53.409 Unspecified sprain of unspecified elbow**
Sprain of elbow NOS
√6th **S53.41 Radiohumeral (joint) sprain**
√7th **S53.411 Radiohumeral (joint) sprain of right elbow**
√7th **S53.412 Radiohumeral (joint) sprain of left elbow**
√7th **S53.419 Radiohumeral (joint) sprain of unspecified elbow**
√6th **S53.42 Ulnohumeral (joint) sprain**
√7th **S53.421 Ulnohumeral (joint) sprain of right elbow**
√7th **S53.422 Ulnohumeral (joint) sprain of left elbow**
√7th **S53.429 Ulnohumeral (joint) sprain of unspecified elbow**

S53.43 Radial collateral ligament sprain
S53.431 Radial collateral ligament sprain of right elbow
S53.432 Radial collateral ligament sprain of left elbow
S53.439 Radial collateral ligament sprain of unspecified elbow
S53.44 Ulnar collateral ligament sprain
S53.441 Ulnar collateral ligament sprain of right elbow
S53.442 Ulnar collateral ligament sprain of left elbow
S53.449 Ulnar collateral ligament sprain of unspecified elbow
S53.49 Other sprain of elbow
S53.491 Other sprain of right elbow
S53.492 Other sprain of left elbow
S53.499 Other sprain of unspecified elbow

S54 Injury of nerves at forearm level

Code also any associated open wound (S51.-)

EXCLUDES 2 *injury of nerves at wrist and hand level (S64.-)*

The appropriate 7th character is to be added to each code from category S54.
A initial encounter
D subsequent encounter
S sequela

S54.0 Injury of ulnar nerve at forearm level
Injury of ulnar nerve NOS
S54.00 Injury of ulnar nerve at forearm level, unspecified arm
S54.01 Injury of ulnar nerve at forearm level, right arm
S54.02 Injury of ulnar nerve at forearm level, left arm
S54.1 Injury of median nerve at forearm level
Injury of median nerve NOS
S54.10 Injury of median nerve at forearm level, unspecified arm
S54.11 Injury of median nerve at forearm level, right arm
S54.12 Injury of median nerve at forearm level, left arm
S54.2 Injury of radial nerve at forearm level
Injury of radial nerve NOS
S54.20 Injury of radial nerve at forearm level, unspecified arm
S54.21 Injury of radial nerve at forearm level, right arm
S54.22 Injury of radial nerve at forearm level, left arm
S54.3 Injury of cutaneous sensory nerve at forearm level
S54.30 Injury of cutaneous sensory nerve at forearm level, unspecified arm
S54.31 Injury of cutaneous sensory nerve at forearm level, right arm
S54.32 Injury of cutaneous sensory nerve at forearm level, left arm
S54.8 Injury of other nerves at forearm level
S54.8X Injury of other nerves at forearm level
S54.8X1 Unspecified injury of other nerves at forearm level, right ar
S54.8X2 Unspecified injury of other nerves at forearm level, left arm
S54.8X9 Unspecified injury of other nerves at forearm level, unspecified arm
S54.9 Injury of unspecified nerve at forearm level
S54.90 Injury of unspecified nerve at forearm level, unspecified arm
S54.91 Injury of unspecified nerve at forearm level, right arm
S54.92 Injury of unspecified nerve at forearm level, left arm

S55 Injury of blood vessels at forearm level

Code also any associated open wound (S51.-)

EXCLUDES 2 *injury of blood vessels at wrist and hand level (S65.-)*
injury of brachial vessels (S45.1-S45.2)

The appropriate 7th character is to be added to each code from category S55.
A initial encounter
D subsequent encounter
S sequela

S55.0 Injury of ulnar artery at forearm level
S55.00 Unspecified injury of ulnar artery at forearm level
S55.001 Unspecified injury of ulnar artery at forearm level, right arm
S55.002 Unspecified injury of ulnar artery at forearm level, left arm
S55.009 Unspecified injury of ulnar artery at forearm level, unspecified arm
S55.01 Laceration of ulnar artery at forearm level
S55.011 Laceration of ulnar artery at forearm level, right arm
S55.012 Laceration of ulnar artery at forearm level, left arm
S55.019 Laceration of ulnar artery at forearm level, unspecified arm
S55.09 Other specified injury of ulnar artery at forearm level
S55.091 Other specified injury of ulnar artery at forearm level, right arm
S55.092 Other specified injury of ulnar artery at forearm level, left arm
S55.099 Other specified injury of ulnar artery at forearm level, unspecified arm
S55.1 Injury of radial artery at forearm level
S55.10 Unspecified injury of radial artery at forearm level
S55.101 Unspecified injury of radial artery at forearm level, right arm
S55.102 Unspecified injury of radial artery at forearm level, left arm
S55.109 Unspecified injury of radial artery at forearm level, unspecified arm
S55.11 Laceration of radial artery at forearm level
S55.111 Laceration of radial artery at forearm level, right arm
S55.112 Laceration of radial artery at forearm level, left arm
S55.119 Laceration of radial artery at forearm level, unspecified arm
S55.19 Other specified injury of radial artery at forearm level
S55.191 Other specified injury of radial artery at forearm level, right arm
S55.192 Other specified injury of radial artery at forearm level, left arm
S55.199 Other specified injury of radial artery at forearm level, unspecified arm
S55.2 Injury of vein at forearm level
S55.20 Unspecified injury of vein at forearm level
S55.201 Unspecified injury of vein at forearm level, right arm
S55.202 Unspecified injury of vein at forearm level, left arm
S55.209 Unspecified injury of vein at forearm level, unspecified arm
S55.21 Laceration of vein at forearm level
S55.211 Laceration of vein at forearm level, right arm
S55.212 Laceration of vein at forearm level, left arm
S55.219 Laceration of vein at forearm level, unspecified arm
S55.29 Other specified injury of vein at forearm level
S55.291 Other specified injury of vein at forearm level, right arm
S55.292 Other specified injury of vein at forearm level, left arm

7th **S55.299 Other specified injury of vein at forearm level, unspecified arm**

5th **S55.8 Injury of other blood vessels at forearm level**

6th **S55.80 Unspecified injury of other blood vessels at forearm level**

7th **S55.801 Unspecified injury of other blood vessels at forearm level, right arm**

7th **S55.802 Unspecified injury of other blood vessels at forearm level, left arm**

7th **S55.809 Unspecified injury of other blood vessels at forearm level, unspecified arm**

6th **S55.81 Laceration of other blood vessels at forearm level**

7th **S55.811 Laceration of other blood vessels at forearm level, right arm**

7th **S55.812 Laceration of other blood vessels at forearm level, left arm**

7th **S55.819 Laceration of other blood vessels at forearm level, unspecified arm**

6th **S55.89 Other specified injury of other blood vessels at forearm level**

7th **S55.891 Other specified injury of other blood vessels at forearm level, right arm**

7th **S55.892 Other specified injury of other blood vessels at forearm level, left arm**

7th **S55.899 Other specified injury of other blood vessels at forearm level, unspecified arm**

5th **S55.9 Injury of unspecified blood vessel at forearm level**

6th **S55.90 Unspecified injury of unspecified blood vessel at forearm level**

7th **S55.901 Unspecified injury of unspecified blood vessel at forearm level, right arm**

7th **S55.902 Unspecified injury of unspecified blood vessel at forearm level, left arm**

7th **S55.909 Unspecified injury of unspecified blood vessel at forearm level, unspecified arm**

6th **S55.91 Laceration of unspecified blood vessel at forearm level**

7th **S55.911 Laceration of unspecified blood vessel at forearm level, right arm**

7th **S55.912 Laceration of unspecified blood vessel at forearm level, left arm**

7th **S55.919 Laceration of unspecified blood vessel at forearm level, unspecified arm**

6th **S55.99 Other specified injury of unspecified blood vessel at forearm level**

7th **S55.991 Other specified injury of unspecified blood vessel at forearm level, right arm**

7th **S55.992 Other specified injury of unspecified blood vessel at forearm level, left arm**

7th **S55.999 Other specified injury of unspecified blood vessel at forearm level, unspecified arm**

4th **S56 Injury of muscle, fascia and tendon at forearm level**

Code also any associated open wound (S51.-)

EXCLUDES 2 *injury of muscle, fascia and tendon at or below wrist (S66.-)*
sprain of joints and ligaments of elbow (S53.4-)

The appropriate 7th character is to be added to each code from category S56.
A initial encounter
D subsequent encounter
S sequela

5th **S56.0 Injury of flexor muscle, fascia and tendon of thumb at forearm level**

6th **S56.00 Unspecified injury of flexor muscle, fascia and tendon of thumb at forearm level**

7th **S56.001 Unspecified injury of flexor muscle, fascia and tendon of right thumb at forearm level**

7th **S56.002 Unspecified injury of flexor muscle, fascia and tendon of left thumb at forearm level**

7th **S56.009 Unspecified injury of flexor muscle, fascia and tendon of unspecified thumb at forearm level**

6th **S56.01 Strain of flexor muscle, fascia and tendon of thumb at forearm level**

7th **S56.011 Strain of flexor muscle, fascia and tendon of right thumb at forearm level**

7th **S56.012 Strain of flexor muscle, fascia and tendon of left thumb at forearm level**

7th **S56.019 Strain of flexor muscle, fascia and tendon of unspecified thumb at forearm level**

6th **S56.02 Laceration of flexor muscle, fascia and tendon of thumb at forearm level**

7th **S56.021 Laceration of flexor muscle, fascia and tendon of right thumb at forearm level**

7th **S56.022 Laceration of flexor muscle, fascia and tendon of left thumb at forearm level**

7th **S56.029 Laceration of flexor muscle, fascia and tendon of unspecified thumb at forearm level**

6th **S56.09 Other injury of flexor muscle, fascia and tendon of thumb at forearm level**

7th **S56.091 Other injury of flexor muscle, fascia and tendon of right thumb at forearm level**

7th **S56.092 Other injury of flexor muscle, fascia and tendon of left thumb at forearm level**

7th **S56.099 Other injury of flexor muscle, fascia and tendon of unspecified thumb at forearm level**

5th **S56.1 Injury of flexor muscle, fascia and tendon of other and unspecified finger at forearm level**

6th **S56.10 Unspecified injury of flexor muscle, fascia and tendon of other and unspecified finger at forearm level**

7th **S56.101 Unspecified injury of flexor muscle, fascia and tendon of right index finger at forearm level**

7th **S56.102 Unspecified injury of flexor muscle, fascia and tendon of left index finger at forearm level**

7th **S56.103 Unspecified injury of flexor muscle, fascia and tendon of right middle finger at forearm level**

7th **S56.104 Unspecified injury of flexor muscle, fascia and tendon of left middle finger at forearm level**

7th **S56.105 Unspecified injury of flexor muscle, fascia and tendon of right ring finger at forearm level**

7th **S56.106 Unspecified injury of flexor muscle, fascia and tendon of left ring finger at forearm level**

7th **S56.107 Unspecified injury of flexor muscle, fascia and tendon of right little finger at forearm level**

7th **S56.108 Unspecified injury of flexor muscle, fascia and tendon of left little finger at forearm level**

7th **S56.109 Unspecified injury of flexor muscle, fascia and tendon of unspecified finger at forearm level**

6th **S56.11 Strain of flexor muscle, fascia and tendon of other and unspecified finger at forearm level**

7th **S56.111 Strain of flexor muscle, fascia and tendon of right index finger at forearm level**

7th **S56.112 Strain of flexor muscle, fascia and tendon of left index finger at forearm level**

7th **S56.113 Strain of flexor muscle, fascia and tendon of right middle finger at forearm level**

7th **S56.114 Strain of flexor muscle, fascia and tendon of left middle finger at forearm level**

7th **S56.115 Strain of flexor muscle, fascia and tendon of right ring finger at forearm level**

- ✓7th **S56.116 Strain of flexor muscle, fascia and tendon of left ring finger at forearm level**
- ✓7th **S56.117 Strain of flexor muscle, fascia and tendon of right little finger at forearm level**
- ✓7th **S56.118 Strain of flexor muscle, fascia and tendon of left little finger at forearm level**
- ✓7th **S56.119 Strain of flexor muscle, fascia and tendon of finger of unspecified finger at forearm level**

✓6th **S56.12 Laceration of flexor muscle, fascia and tendon of other and unspecified finger at forearm level**

- ✓7th **S56.121 Laceration of flexor muscle, fascia and tendon of right index finger at forearm level**
- ✓7th **S56.122 Laceration of flexor muscle, fascia and tendon of left index finger at forearm level**
- ✓7th **S56.123 Laceration of flexor muscle, fascia and tendon of right middle finger at forearm level**
- ✓7th **S56.124 Laceration of flexor muscle, fascia and tendon of left middle finger at forearm level**
- ✓7th **S56.125 Laceration of flexor muscle, fascia and tendon of right ring finger at forearm level**
- ✓7th **S56.126 Laceration of flexor muscle, fascia and tendon of left ring finger at forearm level**
- ✓7th **S56.127 Laceration of flexor muscle, fascia and tendon of right little finger at forearm level**
- ✓7th **S56.128 Laceration of flexor muscle, fascia and tendon of left little finger at forearm level**
- ✓7th **S56.129 Laceration of flexor muscle, fascia and tendon of unspecified finger at forearm level**

✓6th **S56.19 Other injury of flexor muscle, fascia and tendon of other and unspecified finger at forearm level**

- ✓7th **S56.191 Other injury of flexor muscle, fascia and tendon of right index finger at forearm level**
- ✓7th **S56.192 Other injury of flexor muscle, fascia and tendon of left index finger at forearm level**
- ✓7th **S56.193 Other injury of flexor muscle, fascia and tendon of right middle finger at forearm level**
- ✓7th **S56.194 Other injury of flexor muscle, fascia and tendon of left middle finger at forearm level**
- ✓7th **S56.195 Other injury of flexor muscle, fascia and tendon of right ring finger at forearm level**
- ✓7th **S56.196 Other injury of flexor muscle, fascia and tendon of left ring finger at forearm level**
- ✓7th **S56.197 Other injury of flexor muscle, fascia and tendon of right little finger at forearm level**
- ✓7th **S56.198 Other injury of flexor muscle, fascia and tendon of left little finger at forearm level**
- ✓7th **S56.199 Other injury of flexor muscle, fascia and tendon of unspecified finger at forearm level**

✓5th **S56.2 Injury of other flexor muscle, fascia and tendon at forearm level**

✓6th **S56.20 Unspecified injury of other flexor muscle, fascia and tendon at forearm level**

- ✓7th **S56.201 Unspecified injury of other flexor muscle, fascia and tendon at forearm level, right arm**
- ✓7th **S56.202 Unspecified injury of other flexor muscle, fascia and tendon at forearm level, left arm**
- ✓7th **S56.209 Unspecified injury of other flexor muscle, fascia and tendon at forearm level, unspecified arm**

✓6th **S56.21 Strain of other flexor muscle, fascia and tendon at forearm level**

- ✓7th **S56.211 Strain of other flexor muscle, fascia and tendon at forearm level, right arm**
- ✓7th **S56.212 Strain of other flexor muscle, fascia and tendon at forearm level, left arm**
- ✓7th **S56.219 Strain of other flexor muscle, fascia and tendon at forearm level, unspecified arm**

✓6th **S56.22 Laceration of other flexor muscle, fascia and tendon at forearm level**

- ✓7th **S56.221 Laceration of other flexor muscle, fascia and tendon at forearm level, right arm**
- ✓7th **S56.222 Laceration of other flexor muscle, fascia and tendon at forearm level, left arm**
- ✓7th **S56.229 Laceration of other flexor muscle, fascia and tendon at forearm level, unspecified arm**

✓6th **S56.29 Other injury of other flexor muscle, fascia and tendon at forearm level**

- ✓7th **S56.291 Other injury of other flexor muscle, fascia and tendon at forearm level, right arm**
- ✓7th **S56.292 Other injury of other flexor muscle, fascia and tendon at forearm level, left arm**
- ✓7th **S56.299 Other injury of other flexor muscle, fascia and tendon at forearm level, unspecified arm**

✓5th **S56.3 Injury of extensor or abductor muscles, fascia and tendons of thumb at forearm level**

✓6th **S56.30 Unspecified injury of extensor or abductor muscles, fascia and tendons of thumb at forearm level**

- ✓7th **S56.301 Unspecified injury of extensor or abductor muscles, fascia and tendons of right thumb at forearm level**
- ✓7th **S56.302 Unspecified injury of extensor or abductor muscles, fascia and tendons of left thumb at forearm level**
- ✓7th **S56.309 Unspecified injury of extensor or abductor muscles, fascia and tendons of unspecified thumb at forearm level**

✓6th **S56.31 Strain of extensor or abductor muscles, fascia and tendons of thumb at forearm level**

- ✓7th **S56.311 Strain of extensor or abductor muscles, fascia and tendons of right thumb at forearm level**
- ✓7th **S56.312 Strain of extensor or abductor muscles, fascia and tendons of left thumb at forearm level**
- ✓7th **S56.319 Strain of extensor or abductor muscles, fascia and tendons of unspecified thumb at forearm level**

✓6th **S56.32 Laceration of extensor or abductor muscles, fascia and tendons of thumb at forearm level**

- ✓7th **S56.321 Laceration of extensor or abductor muscles, fascia and tendons of right thumb at forearm level**
- ✓7th **S56.322 Laceration of extensor or abductor muscles, fascia and tendons of left thumb at forearm level**
- ✓7th **S56.329 Laceration of extensor or abductor muscles, fascia and tendons of unspecified thumb at forearm level**

✓6th **S56.39 Other injury of extensor or abductor muscles, fascia and tendons of thumb at forearm level**

- ✓7th **S56.391 Other injury of extensor or abductor muscles, fascia and tendons of right thumb at forearm level**

S56.392 Other injury of extensor or abductor muscles, fascia and tendons of left thumb at forearm level

S56.399 Other injury of extensor or abductor muscles, fascia and tendons of unspecified thumb at forearm level

S56.4 Injury of extensor muscle, fascia and tendon of other and unspecified finger at forearm level

S56.40 Unspecified injury of extensor muscle, fascia and tendon of other and unspecified finger at forearm level

S56.401 Unspecified injury of extensor muscle, fascia and tendon of right index finger at forearm level

S56.402 Unspecified injury of extensor muscle, fascia and tendon of left index finger at forearm level

S56.403 Unspecified injury of extensor muscle, fascia and tendon of right middle finger at forearm level

S56.404 Unspecified injury of extensor muscle, fascia and tendon of left middle finger at forearm level

S56.405 Unspecified injury of extensor muscle, fascia and tendon of right ring finger at forearm level

S56.406 Unspecified injury of extensor muscle, fascia and tendon of left ring finger at forearm level

S56.407 Unspecified injury of extensor muscle, fascia and tendon of right little finger at forearm level

S56.408 Unspecified injury of extensor muscle, fascia and tendon of left little finger at forearm level

S56.409 Unspecified injury of extensor muscle, fascia and tendon of unspecified finger at forearm level

S56.41 Strain of extensor muscle, fascia and tendon of other and unspecified finger at forearm level

S56.411 Strain of extensor muscle, fascia and tendon of right index finger at forearm level

S56.412 Strain of extensor muscle, fascia and tendon of left index finger at forearm level

S56.413 Strain of extensor muscle, fascia and tendon of right middle finger at forearm level

S56.414 Strain of extensor muscle, fascia and tendon of left middle finger at forearm level

S56.415 Strain of extensor muscle, fascia and tendon of right ring finger at forearm level

S56.416 Strain of extensor muscle, fascia and tendon of left ring finger at forearm level

S56.417 Strain of extensor muscle, fascia and tendon of right little finger at forearm level

S56.418 Strain of extensor muscle, fascia and tendon of left little finger at forearm level

S56.419 Strain of extensor muscle, fascia and tendon of finger, unspecified finger at forearm level

S56.42 Laceration of extensor muscle, fascia and tendon of other and unspecified finger at forearm level

S56.421 Laceration of extensor muscle, fascia and tendon of right index finger at forearm level

S56.422 Laceration of extensor muscle, fascia and tendon of left index finger at forearm level

S56.423 Laceration of extensor muscle, fascia and tendon of right middle finger at forearm level

S56.424 Laceration of extensor muscle, fascia and tendon of left middle finger at forearm level

S56.425 Laceration of extensor muscle, fascia and tendon of right ring finger at forearm level

S56.426 Laceration of extensor muscle, fascia and tendon of left ring finger at forearm level

S56.427 Laceration of extensor muscle, fascia and tendon of right little finger at forearm level

S56.428 Laceration of extensor muscle, fascia and tendon of left little finger at forearm level

S56.429 Laceration of extensor muscle, fascia and tendon of unspecified finger at forearm level

S56.49 Other injury of extensor muscle, fascia and tendon of other and unspecified finger at forearm level

S56.491 Other injury of extensor muscle, fascia and tendon of right index finger at forearm level

S56.492 Other injury of extensor muscle, fascia and tendon of left index finger at forearm level

S56.493 Other injury of extensor muscle, fascia and tendon of right middle finger at forearm level

S56.494 Other injury of extensor muscle, fascia and tendon of left middle finger at forearm level

S56.495 Other injury of extensor muscle, fascia and tendon of right ring finger at forearm level

S56.496 Other injury of extensor muscle, fascia and tendon of left ring finger at forearm level

S56.497 Other injury of extensor muscle, fascia and tendon of right little finger at forearm level

S56.498 Other injury of extensor muscle, fascia and tendon of left little finger at forearm level

S56.499 Other injury of extensor muscle, fascia and tendon of unspecified finger at forearm level

S56.5 Injury of other extensor muscle, fascia and tendon at forearm level

S56.50 Unspecified injury of other extensor muscle, fascia and tendon at forearm level

S56.501 Unspecified injury of other extensor muscle, fascia and tendon at forearm level, right arm

S56.502 Unspecified injury of other extensor muscle, fascia and tendon at forearm level, left arm

S56.509 Unspecified injury of other extensor muscle, fascia and tendon at forearm level, unspecified arm

S56.51 Strain of other extensor muscle, fascia and tendon at forearm level

S56.511 Strain of other extensor muscle, fascia and tendon at forearm level, right arm

S56.512 Strain of other extensor muscle, fascia and tendon at forearm level, left arm

S56.519 Strain of other extensor muscle, fascia and tendon at forearm level, unspecified arm

S56.52 Laceration of other extensor muscle, fascia and tendon at forearm level

S56.521 Laceration of other extensor muscle, fascia and tendon at forearm level, right arm

S56.522 Laceration of other extensor muscle, fascia and tendon at forearm level, left arm

7th S56.529 Laceration of other extensor muscle, fascia and tendon at forearm level, unspecified arm
6th S56.59 Other injury of other extensor muscle, fascia and tendon at forearm level
7th S56.591 Other injury of other extensor muscle, fascia and tendon at forearm level, right arm
7th S56.592 Other injury of other extensor muscle, fascia and tendon at forearm level, left arm
7th S56.599 Other injury of other extensor muscle, fascia and tendon at forearm level, unspecified arm
5th S56.8 Injury of other muscles, fascia and tendons at forearm level
6th S56.80 Unspecified injury of other muscles, fascia and tendons at forearm level
7th S56.801 Unspecified injury of other muscles, fascia and tendons at forearm level, right arm
7th S56.802 Unspecified injury of other muscles, fascia and tendons at forearm level, left arm
7th S56.809 Unspecified injury of other muscles, fascia and tendons at forearm level, unspecified arm
6th S56.81 Strain of other muscles, fascia and tendons at forearm level
7th S56.811 Strain of other muscles, fascia and tendons at forearm level, right arm
7th S56.812 Strain of other muscles, fascia and tendons at forearm level, left arm
7th S56.819 Strain of other muscles, fascia and tendons at forearm level, unspecified arm
6th S56.82 Laceration of other muscles, fascia and tendons at forearm level
7th S56.821 Laceration of other muscles, fascia and tendons at forearm level, right arm
7th S56.822 Laceration of other muscles, fascia and tendons at forearm level, left arm
7th S56.829 Laceration of other muscles, fascia and tendons at forearm level, unspecified arm
6th S56.89 Other injury of other muscles, fascia and tendons at forearm level
7th S56.891 Other injury of other muscles, fascia and tendons at forearm level, right arm
7th S56.892 Other injury of other muscles, fascia and tendons at forearm level, left arm
7th S56.899 Other injury of other muscles, fascia and tendons at forearm level, unspecified arm
5th S56.9 Injury of unspecified muscles, fascia and tendons at forearm level
6th S56.90 Unspecified injury of unspecified muscles, fascia and tendons at forearm level
7th S56.901 Unspecified injury of unspecified muscles, fascia and tendons at forearm level, right arm
7th S56.902 Unspecified injury of unspecified muscles, fascia and tendons at forearm level, left arm
7th S56.909 Unspecified injury of unspecified muscles, fascia and tendons at forearm level, unspecified arm
6th S56.91 Strain of unspecified muscles, fascia and tendons at forearm level
7th S56.911 Strain of unspecified muscles, fascia and tendons at forearm level, right arm
7th S56.912 Strain of unspecified muscles, fascia and tendons at forearm level, left arm
7th S56.919 Strain of unspecified muscles, fascia and tendons at forearm level, unspecified arm
6th S56.92 Laceration of unspecified muscles, fascia and tendons at forearm level
7th S56.921 Laceration of unspecified muscles, fascia and tendons at forearm level, right arm
7th S56.922 Laceration of unspecified muscles, fascia and tendons at forearm level, left arm
7th S56.929 Laceration of unspecified muscles, fascia and tendons at forearm level, unspecified arm
6th S56.99 Other injury of unspecified muscles, fascia and tendons at forearm level
7th S56.991 Other injury of unspecified muscles, fascia and tendons at forearm level, right arm
7th S56.992 Other injury of unspecified muscles, fascia and tendons at forearm level, left arm
7th S56.999 Other injury of unspecified muscles, fascia and tendons at forearm level, unspecified arm

4th **S57 Crushing injury of elbow and forearm**

Use additional code(s) for all associated injuries

EXCLUDES 2 *crushing injury of wrist and hand (S67.-)*

The appropriate 7th character is to be added to each code from category S57.
A initial encounter
D subsequent encounter
S sequela

5th S57.0 Crushing injury of elbow
x7th S57.00 Crushing injury of unspecified elbow
x7th S57.01 Crushing injury of right elbow
x7th S57.02 Crushing injury of left elbow
5th S57.8 Crushing injury of forearm
x7th S57.80 Crushing injury of unspecified forearm
x7th S57.81 Crushing injury of right forearm
x7th S57.82 Crushing injury of left forearm

4th **S58 Traumatic amputation of elbow and forearm**

NOTE An amputation not identified as partial or complete should be coded to complete

EXCLUDES 1 *traumatic amputation of wrist and hand (S68.-)*

The appropriate 7th character is to be added to each code from category S58.
A initial encounter
D subsequent encounter
S sequela

5th S58.0 Traumatic amputation at elbow level
6th S58.01 Complete traumatic amputation at elbow level
7th S58.011 Complete traumatic amputation at elbow level, right arm
7th S58.012 Complete traumatic amputation at elbow level, left arm
7th S58.019 Complete traumatic amputation at elbow level, unspecified arm
6th S58.02 Partial traumatic amputation at elbow level
7th S58.021 Partial traumatic amputation at elbow level, right arm
7th S58.022 Partial traumatic amputation at elbow level, left arm
7th S58.029 Partial traumatic amputation at elbow level, unspecified arm
5th S58.1 Traumatic amputation at level between elbow and wrist
6th S58.11 Complete traumatic amputation at level between elbow and wrist
7th S58.111 Complete traumatic amputation at level between elbow and wrist, right arm
7th S58.112 Complete traumatic amputation at level between elbow and wrist, left arm
7th S58.119 Complete traumatic amputation at level between elbow and wrist, unspecified arm
6th S58.12 Partial traumatic amputation at level between elbow and wrist
7th S58.121 Partial traumatic amputation at level between elbow and wrist, right arm

7th S58.122 **Partial traumatic amputation at level between elbow and wrist, left arm**

7th S58.129 **Partial traumatic amputation at level between elbow and wrist, unspecified arm**

5th S58.9 **Traumatic amputation of forearm, level unspecified**

EXCLUDES 1 *traumatic amputation of wrist (S68.-)*

6th S58.91 **Complete traumatic amputation of forearm, level unspecified**

7th S58.911 **Complete traumatic amputation of right forearm, level unspecified**

7th S58.912 **Complete traumatic amputation of left forearm, level unspecified**

7th S58.919 **Complete traumatic amputation of unspecified forearm, level unspecified**

6th S58.92 **Partial traumatic amputation of forearm, level unspecified**

7th S58.921 **Partial traumatic amputation of right forearm, level unspecified**

7th S58.922 **Partial traumatic amputation of left forearm, level unspecified**

7th S58.929 **Partial traumatic amputation of unspecified forearm, level unspecified**

4th **S59 Other and unspecified injuries of elbow and forearm**

EXCLUDES 2 *other and unspecified injuries of wrist and hand (S69.-)*

The appropriate 7th character is to be added to each code from subcategories S59.0, S59.1, and S59.2.

A	initial encounter for closed fracture
D	subsequent encounter for fracture with routine healing
G	subsequent encounter for fracture with delayed healing
K	subsequent encounter for fracture with nonunion
P	subsequent encounter for fracture with malunion
S	sequela

5th S59.0 **Physeal fracture of lower end of ulna**

6th S59.00 **Unspecified physeal fracture of lower end of ulna**

7th S59.001 **Unspecified physeal fracture of lower end of ulna, right arm**

7th S59.002 **Unspecified physeal fracture of lower end of ulna, left arm**

7th S59.009 **Unspecified physeal fracture of lower end of ulna, unspecified arm**

6th S59.01 **Salter-Harris Type I physeal fracture of lower end of ulna**

7th S59.011 **Salter-Harris Type I physeal fracture of lower end of ulna, right arm**

7th S59.012 **Salter-Harris Type I physeal fracture of lower end of ulna, left arm**

7th S59.019 **Salter-Harris Type I physeal fracture of lower end of ulna, unspecified arm**

6th S59.02 **Salter-Harris Type II physeal fracture of lower end of ulna**

7th S59.021 **Salter-Harris Type II physeal fracture of lower end of ulna, right arm**

7th S59.022 **Salter-Harris Type II physeal fracture of lower end of ulna, left arm**

7th S59.029 **Salter-Harris Type II physeal fracture of lower end of ulna, unspecified arm**

6th S59.03 **Salter-Harris Type III physeal fracture of lower end of ulna**

7th S59.031 **Salter-Harris Type III physeal fracture of lower end of ulna, right arm**

7th S59.032 **Salter-Harris Type III physeal fracture of lower end of ulna, left arm**

7th S59.039 **Salter-Harris Type III physeal fracture of lower end of ulna, unspecified arm**

6th S59.04 **Salter-Harris Type IV physeal fracture of lower end of ulna**

7th S59.041 **Salter-Harris Type IV physeal fracture of lower end of ulna, right arm**

7th S59.042 **Salter-Harris Type IV physeal fracture of lower end of ulna, left arm**

7th S59.049 **Salter-Harris Type IV physeal fracture of lower end of ulna, unspecified arm**

6th S59.09 **Other physeal fracture of lower end of ulna**

7th S59.091 **Other physeal fracture of lower end of ulna, right arm**

7th S59.092 **Other physeal fracture of lower end of ulna, left arm**

7th S59.099 **Other physeal fracture of lower end of ulna, unspecified arm**

5th S59.1 **Physeal fracture of upper end of radius**

6th S59.10 **Unspecified physeal fracture of upper end of radius**

7th S59.101 **Unspecified physeal fracture of upper end of radius, right arm**

7th S59.102 **Unspecified physeal fracture of upper end of radius, left arm**

7th S59.109 **Unspecified physeal fracture of upper end of radius, unspecified arm**

6th S59.11 **Salter-Harris Type I physeal fracture of upper end of radius**

7th S59.111 **Salter-Harris Type I physeal fracture of upper end of radius, right arm**

7th S59.112 **Salter-Harris Type I physeal fracture of upper end of radius, left arm**

7th S59.119 **Salter-Harris Type I physeal fracture of upper end of radius, unspecified arm**

6th S59.12 **Salter-Harris Type II physeal fracture of upper end of radius**

7th S59.121 **Salter-Harris Type II physeal fracture of upper end of radius, right arm**

7th S59.122 **Salter-Harris Type II physeal fracture of upper end of radius, left arm**

7th S59.129 **Salter-Harris Type II physeal fracture of upper end of radius, unspecified arm**

6th S59.13 **Salter-Harris Type III physeal fracture of upper end of radius**

7th S59.131 **Salter-Harris Type III physeal fracture of upper end of radius, right arm**

7th S59.132 **Salter-Harris Type III physeal fracture of upper end of radius, left arm**

7th S59.139 **Salter-Harris Type III physeal fracture of upper end of radius, unspecified arm**

6th S59.14 **Salter-Harris Type IV physeal fracture of upper end of radius**

7th S59.141 **Salter-Harris Type IV physeal fracture of upper end of radius, right arm**

7th S59.142 **Salter-Harris Type IV physeal fracture of upper end of radius, left arm**

7th S59.149 **Salter-Harris Type IV physeal fracture of upper end of radius, unspecified arm**

6th S59.19 **Other physeal fracture of upper end of radius**

7th S59.191 **Other physeal fracture of upper end of radius, right arm**

7th S59.192 **Other physeal fracture of upper end of radius, left arm**

7th S59.199 **Other physeal fracture of upper end of radius, unspecified arm**

5th S59.2 **Physeal fracture of lower end of radius**

6th S59.20 **Unspecified physeal fracture of lower end of radius**

7th S59.201 **Unspecified physeal fracture of lower end of radius, right arm**

7th S59.202 **Unspecified physeal fracture of lower end of radius, left arm**

7th S59.209 **Unspecified physeal fracture of lower end of radius, unspecified arm**

6th S59.21 **Salter-Harris Type I physeal fracture of lower end of radius**

7th S59.211 **Salter-Harris Type I physeal fracture of lower end of radius, right arm**

7th S59.212 **Salter-Harris Type I physeal fracture of lower end of radius, left arm**

7th S59.219 **Salter-Harris Type I physeal fracture of lower end of radius, unspecified arm**

6th S59.22 **Salter-Harris Type II physeal fracture of lower end of radius**

7th S59.221 **Salter-Harris Type II physeal fracture of lower end of radius, right arm**

7th S59.222 **Salter-Harris Type II physeal fracture of lower end of radius, left arm**

7th S59.229 **Salter-Harris Type II physeal fracture of lower end of radius, unspecified arm**

✓6th **S59.23 Salter-Harris Type III physeal fracture of lower end of radius**

✓7th **S59.231 Salter-Harris Type III physeal fracture of lower end of radius, right arm**

✓7th **S59.232 Salter-Harris Type III physeal fracture of lower end of radius, left arm**

✓7th **S59.239 Salter-Harris Type III physeal fracture of lower end of radius, unspecified arm**

✓6th **S59.24 Salter-Harris Type IV physeal fracture of lower end of radius**

✓7th **S59.241 Salter-Harris Type IV physeal fracture of lower end of radius, right arm**

✓7th **S59.242 Salter-Harris Type IV physeal fracture of lower end of radius, left arm**

✓7th **S59.249 Salter-Harris Type IV physeal fracture of lower end of radius, unspecified arm**

✓6th **S59.29 Other physeal fracture of lower end of radius**

✓7th **S59.291 Other physeal fracture of lower end of radius, right arm**

✓7th **S59.292 Other physeal fracture of lower end of radius, left arm**

✓7th **S59.299 Other physeal fracture of lower end of radius, unspecified arm**

✓5th **S59.8 Other specified injuries of elbow and forearm**

The appropriate 7th character is to be added to each code in subcategory S59.8.
A initial encounter
D subsequent encounter
S sequela

✓6th **S59.80 Other specified injuries of elbow**

✓7th **S59.801 Other specified injuries of right elbow**

✓7th **S59.802 Other specified injuries of left elbow**

✓7th **S59.809 Other specified injuries of unspecified elbow**

✓6th **S59.81 Other specified injuries of forearm**

✓7th **S59.811 Other specified injuries right forearm**

✓7th **S59.812 Other specified injuries left forearm**

✓7th **S59.819 Other specified injuries unspecified forearm**

✓5th **S59.9 Unspecified injury of elbow and forearm**

The appropriate 7th character is to be added to each code in subcategory S59.9.
A initial encounter
D subsequent encounter
S sequela

✓6th **S59.90 Unspecified injury of elbow**

✓7th **S59.901 Unspecified injury of right elbow**

✓7th **S59.902 Unspecified injury of left elbow**

✓7th **S59.909 Unspecified injury of unspecified elbow**

✓6th **S59.91 Unspecified injury of forearm**

✓7th **S59.911 Unspecified injury of right forearm**

✓7th **S59.912 Unspecified injury of left forearm**

✓7th **S59.919 Unspecified injury of unspecified forearm**

Injuries to the wrist, hand and fingers (S60-S69)

EXCLUDES 2 *burns and corrosions (T20-T32)*
frostbite (T33-T34)
insect bite or sting, venomous (T63.4)

✓4th **S60 Superficial injury of wrist, hand and fingers**

The appropriate 7th character is to be added to each code from category S60.
A initial encounter
D subsequent encounter
S sequela

✓5th **S60.0 Contusion of finger without damage to nail**

EXCLUDES 1 *contusion involving nail (matrix) (S60.1)*

✓x7th **S60.00 Contusion of unspecified finger without damage to nail**

Contusion of finger(s) NOS

✓6th **S60.01 Contusion of thumb without damage to nail**

✓7th **S60.011 Contusion of right thumb without damage to nail**

✓7th **S60.012 Contusion of left thumb without damage to nail**

✓7th **S60.019 Contusion of unspecified thumb without damage to nail**

✓6th **S60.02 Contusion of index finger without damage to nail**

✓7th **S60.021 Contusion of right index finger without damage to nail**

✓7th **S60.022 Contusion of left index finger without damage to nail**

✓7th **S60.029 Contusion of unspecified index finger without damage to nail**

✓6th **S60.03 Contusion of middle finger without damage to nail**

✓7th **S60.031 Contusion of right middle finger without damage to nail**

✓7th **S60.032 Contusion of left middle finger without damage to nail**

✓7th **S60.039 Contusion of unspecified middle finger without damage to nail**

✓6th **S60.04 Contusion of ring finger without damage to nail**

✓7th **S60.041 Contusion of right ring finger without damage to nail**

✓7th **S60.042 Contusion of left ring finger without damage to nail**

✓7th **S60.049 Contusion of unspecified ring finger without damage to nail**

✓6th **S60.05 Contusion of little finger without damage to nail**

✓7th **S60.051 Contusion of right little finger without damage to nail**

✓7th **S60.052 Contusion of left little finger without damage to nail**

✓7th **S60.059 Contusion of unspecified little finger without damage to nail**

✓5th **S60.1 Contusion of finger with damage to nail**

✓x7th **S60.10 Contusion of unspecified finger with damage to nail**

✓6th **S60.11 Contusion of thumb with damage to nail**

✓7th **S60.111 Contusion of right thumb with damage to nail**

✓7th **S60.112 Contusion of left thumb with damage to nail**

✓7th **S60.119 Contusion of unspecified thumb with damage to nail**

✓6th **S60.12 Contusion of index finger with damage to nail**

✓7th **S60.121 Contusion of right index finger with damage to nail**

✓7th **S60.122 Contusion of left index finger with damage to nail**

✓7th **S60.129 Contusion of unspecified index finger with damage to nail**

✓6th **S60.13 Contusion of middle finger with damage to nail**

✓7th **S60.131 Contusion of right middle finger with damage to nail**

✓7th **S60.132 Contusion of left middle finger with damage to nail**

✓7th **S60.139 Contusion of unspecified middle finger with damage to nail**

✓6th **S60.14 Contusion of ring finger with damage to nail**

✓7th **S60.141 Contusion of right ring finger with damage to nail**

✓7th **S60.142 Contusion of left ring finger with damage to nail**

✓7th **S60.149 Contusion of unspecified ring finger with damage to nail**

✓6th **S60.15 Contusion of little finger with damage to nail**

✓7th **S60.151 Contusion of right little finger with damage to nail**

✓7th **S60.152 Contusion of left little finger with damage to nail**

✓7th **S60.159 Contusion of unspecified little finger with damage to nail**

✓5th **S60.2 Contusion of wrist and hand**

EXCLUDES 2 *contusion of fingers (S60.0-, S60.1-)*

✓6th **S60.21 Contusion of wrist**

✓7th **S60.211 Contusion of right wrist**

- ✓7th **S6Ø.212 Contusion of left wrist**
- ✓7th **S6Ø.219 Contusion of unspecified wrist**
- ✓6th **S6Ø.22 Contusion of hand**
  - ✓7th **S6Ø.221 Contusion of right hand**
  - ✓7th **S6Ø.222 Contusion of left hand**
  - ✓7th **S6Ø.229 Contusion of unspecified hand**

✓5th **S6Ø.3 Other superficial injuries of thumb**

- ✓6th **S6Ø.31 Abrasion of thumb**
  - ✓7th **S6Ø.311 Abrasion of right thumb**
  - ✓7th **S6Ø.312 Abrasion of left thumb**
  - ✓7th **S6Ø.319 Abrasion of unspecified thumb**
- ✓6th **S6Ø.32 Blister (nonthermal) of thumb**
  - ✓7th **S6Ø.321 Blister (nonthermal) of right thumb**
  - ✓7th **S6Ø.322 Blister (nonthermal) of left thumb**
  - ✓7th **S6Ø.329 Blister (nonthermal) of unspecified thumb**
- ✓6th **S6Ø.34 External constriction of thumb**
  Hair tourniquet syndrome of thumb
  Use additional cause code to identify the constricting item (W49.Ø-)
  - ✓7th **S6Ø.341 External constriction of right thumb**
  - ✓7th **S6Ø.342 External constriction of left thumb**
  - ✓7th **S6Ø.349 External constriction of unspecified thumb**
- ✓6th **S6Ø.35 Superficial foreign body of thumb**
  Splinter in the thumb
  - ✓7th **S6Ø.351 Superficial foreign body of right thumb**
  - ✓7th **S6Ø.352 Superficial foreign body of left thumb**
  - ✓7th **S6Ø.359 Superficial foreign body of unspecified thumb**
- ✓6th **S6Ø.36 Insect bite (nonvenomous) of thumb**
  - ✓7th **S6Ø.361 Insect bite (nonvenomous) of right thumb**
  - ✓7th **S6Ø.362 Insect bite (nonvenomous) of left thumb**
  - ✓7th **S6Ø.369 Insect bite (nonvenomous) of unspecified thumb**
- ✓6th **S6Ø.37 Other superficial bite of thumb**
  EXCLUDES 1 *open bite of thumb (S61.Ø5-, S61.15-)*
  - ✓7th **S6Ø.371 Other superficial bite of right thumb**
  - ✓7th **S6Ø.372 Other superficial bite of left thumb**
  - ✓7th **S6Ø.379 Other superficial bite of unspecified thumb**
- ✓6th **S6Ø.39 Other superficial injuries of thumb**
  - ✓7th **S6Ø.391 Other superficial injuries of right thumb**
  - ✓7th **S6Ø.392 Other superficial injuries of left thumb**
  - ✓7th **S6Ø.399 Other superficial injuries of unspecified thumb**

✓5th **S6Ø.4 Other superficial injuries of other fingers**

- ✓6th **S6Ø.41 Abrasion of fingers**
  - ✓7th **S6Ø.41Ø Abrasion of right index finger**
  - ✓7th **S6Ø.411 Abrasion of left index finger**
  - ✓7th **S6Ø.412 Abrasion of right middle finger**
  - ✓7th **S6Ø.413 Abrasion of left middle finger**
  - ✓7th **S6Ø.414 Abrasion of right ring finger**
  - ✓7th **S6Ø.415 Abrasion of left ring finger**
  - ✓7th **S6Ø.416 Abrasion of right little finger**
  - ✓7th **S6Ø.417 Abrasion of left little finger**
  - ✓7th **S6Ø.418 Abrasion of other finger**
    Abrasion of specified finger with unspecified laterality
  - ✓7th **S6Ø.419 Abrasion of unspecified finger**
- ✓6th **S6Ø.42 Blister (nonthermal) of fingers**
  - ✓7th **S6Ø.42Ø Blister (nonthermal) of right index finger**
  - ✓7th **S6Ø.421 Blister (nonthermal) of left index finger**
  - ✓7th **S6Ø.422 Blister (nonthermal) of right middle finger**
  - ✓7th **S6Ø.423 Blister (nonthermal) of left middle finger**
  - ✓7th **S6Ø.424 Blister (nonthermal) of right ring finger**
  - ✓7th **S6Ø.425 Blister (nonthermal) of left ring finger**
  - ✓7th **S6Ø.426 Blister (nonthermal) of right little finger**
  - ✓7th **S6Ø.427 Blister (nonthermal) of left little finger**
  - ✓7th **S6Ø.428 Blister (nonthermal) of other finger**
    Blister (nonthermal) of specified finger with unspecified laterality
  - ✓7th **S6Ø.429 Blister (nonthermal) of unspecified finger**
- ✓6th **S6Ø.44 External constriction of fingers**
  Hair tourniquet syndrome of finger
  Use additional cause code to identify the constricting item (W49.Ø-)
  - ✓7th **S6Ø.44Ø External constriction of right index finger**
  - ✓7th **S6Ø.441 External constriction of left index finger**
  - ✓7th **S6Ø.442 External constriction of right middle finger**
  - ✓7th **S6Ø.443 External constriction of left middle finger**
  - ✓7th **S6Ø.444 External constriction of right ring finger**
  - ✓7th **S6Ø.445 External constriction of left ring finger**
  - ✓7th **S6Ø.446 External constriction of right little finger**
  - ✓7th **S6Ø.447 External constriction of left little finger**
  - ✓7th **S6Ø.448 External constriction of other finger**
    External constriction of specified finger with unspecified laterality
  - ✓7th **S6Ø.449 External constriction of unspecified finger**
- ✓6th **S6Ø.45 Superficial foreign body of fingers**
  Splinter in the finger(s)
  - ✓7th **S6Ø.45Ø Superficial foreign body of right index finger**
  - ✓7th **S6Ø.451 Superficial foreign body of left index finger**
  - ✓7th **S6Ø.452 Superficial foreign body of right middle finger**
  - ✓7th **S6Ø.453 Superficial foreign body of left middle finger**
  - ✓7th **S6Ø.454 Superficial foreign body of right ring finger**
  - ✓7th **S6Ø.455 Superficial foreign body of left ring finger**
  - ✓7th **S6Ø.456 Superficial foreign body of right little finger**
  - ✓7th **S6Ø.457 Superficial foreign body of left little finger**
  - ✓7th **S6Ø.458 Superficial foreign body of other finger**
    Superficial foreign body of specified finger with unspecified laterality
  - ✓7th **S6Ø.459 Superficial foreign body of unspecified finger**
- ✓6th **S6Ø.46 Insect bite (nonvenomous) of fingers**
  - ✓7th **S6Ø.46Ø Insect bite (nonvenomous) of right index finger**
  - ✓7th **S6Ø.461 Insect bite (nonvenomous) of left index finger**
  - ✓7th **S6Ø.462 Insect bite (nonvenomous) of right middle finger**
  - ✓7th **S6Ø.463 Insect bite (nonvenomous) of left middle finger**
  - ✓7th **S6Ø.464 Insect bite (nonvenomous) of right ring finger**
  - ✓7th **S6Ø.465 Insect bite (nonvenomous) of left ring finger**
  - ✓7th **S6Ø.466 Insect bite (nonvenomous) of right little finger**
  - ✓7th **S6Ø.467 Insect bite (nonvenomous) of left little finger**
  - ✓7th **S6Ø.468 Insect bite (nonvenomous) of other finger**
    Insect bite (nonvenomous) of specified finger with unspecified laterality
  - ✓7th **S6Ø.469 Insect bite (nonvenomous) of unspecified finger**
- ✓6th **S6Ø.47 Other superficial bite of fingers**
  EXCLUDES 1 *open bite of fingers (S61.25-, S61.35-)*
  - ✓7th **S6Ø.47Ø Other superficial bite of right index finger**
  - ✓7th **S6Ø.471 Other superficial bite of left index finger**

✓7th S60.472 Other superficial bite of right middle finger
✓7th S60.473 Other superficial bite of left middle finger
✓7th S60.474 Other superficial bite of right ring finger
✓7th S60.475 Other superficial bite of left ring finger
✓7th S60.476 Other superficial bite of right little finger
✓7th S60.477 Other superficial bite of left little finger
✓7th S60.478 Other superficial bite of other finger
Other superficial bite of specified finger with unspecified laterality
✓7th S60.479 Other superficial bite of unspecified finger

✓5th **S60.5 Other superficial injuries of hand**
EXCLUDES 2 *superficial injuries of fingers (S60.3-, S60.4-)*

✓6th **S60.51 Abrasion of hand**
✓7th S60.511 Abrasion of right hand
✓7th S60.512 Abrasion of left hand
✓7th S60.519 Abrasion of unspecified hand

✓6th **S60.52 Blister (nonthermal) of hand**
✓7th S60.521 Blister (nonthermal) of right hand
✓7th S60.522 Blister (nonthermal) of left hand
✓7th S60.529 Blister (nonthermal) of unspecified hand

✓6th **S60.54 External constriction of hand**
✓7th S60.541 External constriction of right hand
✓7th S60.542 External constriction of left hand
✓7th S60.549 External constriction of unspecified hand

✓6th **S60.55 Superficial foreign body of hand**
Splinter in the hand
✓7th S60.551 Superficial foreign body of right hand
✓7th S60.552 Superficial foreign body of left hand
✓7th S60.559 Superficial foreign body of unspecified hand

✓6th **S60.56 Insect bite (nonvenomous) of hand**
✓7th S60.561 Insect bite (nonvenomous) of right hand
✓7th S60.562 Insect bite (nonvenomous) of left hand
✓7th S60.569 Insect bite (nonvenomous) of unspecified hand

✓6th **S60.57 Other superficial bite of hand**
EXCLUDES 1 *open bite of hand (S61.45-)*
✓7th S60.571 Other superficial bite of hand of right hand
✓7th S60.572 Other superficial bite of hand of left hand
✓7th S60.579 Other superficial bite of hand of unspecified hand

✓5th **S60.8 Other superficial injuries of wrist**

✓6th **S60.81 Abrasion of wrist**
✓7th S60.811 Abrasion of right wrist
✓7th S60.812 Abrasion of left wrist
✓7th S60.819 Abrasion of unspecified wrist

✓6th **S60.82 Blister (nonthermal) of wrist**
✓7th S60.821 Blister (nonthermal) of right wrist
✓7th S60.822 Blister (nonthermal) of left wrist
✓7th S60.829 Blister (nonthermal) of unspecified wrist

✓6th **S60.84 External constriction of wrist**
✓7th S60.841 External constriction of right wrist
✓7th S60.842 External constriction of left wrist
✓7th S60.849 External constriction of unspecified wrist

✓6th **S60.85 Superficial foreign body of wrist**
Splinter in the wrist
✓7th S60.851 Superficial foreign body of right wrist
✓7th S60.852 Superficial foreign body of left wrist
✓7th S60.859 Superficial foreign body of unspecified wrist

✓6th **S60.86 Insect bite (nonvenomous) of wrist**
✓7th S60.861 Insect bite (nonvenomous) of right wrist
✓7th S60.862 Insect bite (nonvenomous) of left wrist
✓7th S60.869 Insect bite (nonvenomous) of unspecified wrist

✓6th **S60.87 Other superficial bite of wrist**
EXCLUDES 1 *open bite of wrist (S61.55)*
✓7th S60.871 Other superficial bite of right wrist
✓7th S60.872 Other superficial bite of left wrist
✓7th S60.879 Other superficial bite of unspecified wrist

✓5th **S60.9 Unspecified superficial injury of wrist, hand and fingers**

✓6th **S60.91 Unspecified superficial injury of wrist**
✓7th S60.911 Unspecified superficial injury of right wrist
✓7th S60.912 Unspecified superficial injury of left wrist
✓7th S60.919 Unspecified superficial injury of unspecified wrist

✓6th **S60.92 Unspecified superficial injury of hand**
✓7th S60.921 Unspecified superficial injury of right hand
✓7th S60.922 Unspecified superficial injury of left hand
✓7th S60.929 Unspecified superficial injury of unspecified hand

✓6th **S60.93 Unspecified superficial injury of thumb**
✓7th S60.931 Unspecified superficial injury of right thumb
✓7th S60.932 Unspecified superficial injury of left thumb
✓7th S60.939 Unspecified superficial injury of unspecified thumb

✓6th **S60.94 Unspecified superficial injury of other fingers**
✓7th S60.940 Unspecified superficial injury of right index finger
✓7th S60.941 Unspecified superficial injury of left index finger
✓7th S60.942 Unspecified superficial injury of right middle finger
✓7th S60.943 Unspecified superficial injury of left middle finger
✓7th S60.944 Unspecified superficial injury of right ring finger
✓7th S60.945 Unspecified superficial injury of left ring finger
✓7th S60.946 Unspecified superficial injury of right little finger
✓7th S60.947 Unspecified superficial injury of left little finger
✓7th S60.948 Unspecified superficial injury of other finger
Unspecified superficial injury of specified finger with unspecified laterality
✓7th S60.949 Unspecified superficial injury of unspecified finger

✓4th S61 Open wound of wrist, hand and fingers

Code also any associated wound infection
EXCLUDES 1 *open fracture of wrist, hand and finger (S62- with 7th character B)*
traumatic amputation of wrist and hand (S68.-)

The appropriate 7th character is to be added to each code from category S61.
A initial encounter
D subsequent encounter
S sequela

✓5th **S61.0 Open wound of thumb without damage to nail**
EXCLUDES 1 *open wound of thumb with damage to nail (S61.1-)*

✓6th **S61.00 Unspecified open wound of thumb without damage to nail**
✓7th S61.001 Unspecified open wound of right thumb without damage to nail
✓7th S61.002 Unspecified open wound of left thumb without damage to nail
✓7th S61.009 Unspecified open wound of unspecified thumb without damage to nail

✓6th **S61.01 Laceration without foreign body of thumb without damage to nail**
✓7th S61.011 Laceration without foreign body of right thumb without damage to nail

√7th **S61.Ø12 Laceration without foreign body of left thumb without damage to nail**
√7th **S61.Ø19 Laceration without foreign body of unspecified thumb without damage to nail**
√6th **S61.Ø2 Laceration with foreign body of thumb without damage to nail**
√7th **S61.Ø21 Laceration with foreign body of right thumb without damage to nail**
√7th **S61.Ø22 Laceration with foreign body of left thumb without damage to nail**
√7th **S61.Ø29 Laceration with foreign body of unspecified thumb without damage to nail**
√6th **S61.Ø3 Puncture wound without foreign body of thumb without damage to nail**
√7th **S61.Ø31 Puncture wound without foreign body of right thumb without damage to nail**
√7th **S61.Ø32 Puncture wound without foreign body of left thumb without damage to nail**
√7th **S61.Ø39 Puncture wound without foreign body of unspecified thumb without damage to nail**
√6th **S61.Ø4 Puncture wound with foreign body of thumb without damage to nail**
√7th **S61.Ø41 Puncture wound with foreign body of right thumb without damage to nail**
√7th **S61.Ø42 Puncture wound with foreign body of left thumb without damage to nail**
√7th **S61.Ø49 Puncture wound with foreign body of unspecified thumb without damage to nail**
√6th **S61.Ø5 Open bite of thumb without damage to nail**
Bite of thumb NOS
EXCLUDES 1 *superficial bite of thumb (S6Ø.36-, S6Ø.37-)*
√7th **S61.Ø51 Open bite of right thumb without damage to nail**
√7th **S61.Ø52 Open bite of left thumb without damage to nail**
√7th **S61.Ø59 Open bite of unspecified thumb without damage to nail**
√5th **S61.1 Open wound of thumb with damage to nail**
√6th **S61.1Ø Unspecified open wound of thumb with damage to nail**
√7th **S61.1Ø1 Unspecified open wound of right thumb with damage to nail**
√7th **S61.1Ø2 Unspecified open wound of left thumb with damage to nail**
√7th **S61.1Ø9 Unspecified open wound of unspecified thumb with damage to nail**
√6th **S61.11 Laceration without foreign body of thumb with damage to nail**
√7th **S61.111 Laceration without foreign body of right thumb with damage to nail**
√7th **S61.112 Laceration without foreign body of left thumb with damage to nail**
√7th **S61.119 Laceration without foreign body of unspecified thumb with damage to nail**
√6th **S61.12 Laceration with foreign body of thumb with damage to nail**
√7th **S61.121 Laceration with foreign body of right thumb with damage to nail**
√7th **S61.122 Laceration with foreign body of left thumb with damage to nail**
√7th **S61.129 Laceration with foreign body of unspecified thumb with damage to nail**
√6th **S61.13 Puncture wound without foreign body of thumb with damage to nail**
√7th **S61.131 Puncture wound without foreign body of right thumb with damage to nail**
√7th **S61.132 Puncture wound without foreign body of left thumb with damage to nail**
√7th **S61.139 Puncture wound without foreign body of unspecified thumb with damage to nail**
√6th **S61.14 Puncture wound with foreign body of thumb with damage to nail**
√7th **S61.141 Puncture wound with foreign body of right thumb with damage to nail**
√7th **S61.142 Puncture wound with foreign body of left thumb with damage to nail**
√7th **S61.149 Puncture wound with foreign body of unspecified thumb with damage to nail**
√6th **S61.15 Open bite of thumb with damage to nail**
Bite of thumb with damage to nail NOS
EXCLUDES 1 *superficial bite of thumb (S6Ø.36-, S6Ø.37-)*
√7th **S61.151 Open bite of right thumb with damage to nail**
√7th **S61.152 Open bite of left thumb with damage to nail**
√7th **S61.159 Open bite of unspecified thumb with damage to nail**
√5th **S61.2 Open wound of other finger without damage to nail**
EXCLUDES 1 *open wound of finger involving nail (matrix) (S61.3-)*
EXCLUDES 2 *open wound of thumb without damage to nail (S61.Ø-)*
√6th **S61.2Ø Unspecified open wound of other finger without damage to nail**
√7th **S61.2ØØ Unspecified open wound of right index finger without damage to nail**
√7th **S61.2Ø1 Unspecified open wound of left index finger without damage to nail**
√7th **S61.2Ø2 Unspecified open wound of right middle finger without damage to nail**
√7th **S61.2Ø3 Unspecified open wound of left middle finger without damage to nail**
√7th **S61.2Ø4 Unspecified open wound of right ring finger without damage to nail**
√7th **S61.2Ø5 Unspecified open wound of left ring finger without damage to nail**
√7th **S61.2Ø6 Unspecified open wound of right little finger without damage to nail**
√7th **S61.2Ø7 Unspecified open wound of left little finger without damage to nail**
√7th **S61.2Ø8 Unspecified open wound of other finger without damage to nail**
Unspecified open wound of specified finger with unspecified laterality without damage to nail
√7th **S61.2Ø9 Unspecified open wound of unspecified finger without damage to nail**
√6th **S61.21 Laceration without foreign body of finger without damage to nail**
√7th **S61.21Ø Laceration without foreign body of right index finger without damage to nail**
√7th **S61.211 Laceration without foreign body of left index finger without damage to nail**
√7th **S61.212 Laceration without foreign body of right middle finger without damage to nail**
√7th **S61.213 Laceration without foreign body of left middle finger without damage to nail**
√7th **S61.214 Laceration without foreign body of right ring finger without damage to nail**
√7th **S61.215 Laceration without foreign body of left ring finger without damage to nail**
√7th **S61.216 Laceration without foreign body of right little finger without damage to nail**
√7th **S61.217 Laceration without foreign body of left little finger without damage to nail**
√7th **S61.218 Laceration without foreign body of other finger without damage to nail**
Laceration without foreign body of specified finger with unspecified laterality without damage to nail
√7th **S61.219 Laceration without foreign body of unspecified finger without damage to nail**
√6th **S61.22 Laceration with foreign body of finger without damage to nail**
√7th **S61.22Ø Laceration with foreign body of right index finger without damage to nail**

S61.221 Laceration with foreign body of left index finger without damage to nail

S61.222 Laceration with foreign body of right middle finger without damage to nail

S61.223 Laceration with foreign body of left middle finger without damage to nail

S61.224 Laceration with foreign body of right ring finger without damage to nail

S61.225 Laceration with foreign body of left ring finger without damage to nail

S61.226 Laceration with foreign body of right little finger without damage to nail

S61.227 Laceration with foreign body of left little finger without damage to nail

S61.228 Laceration with foreign body of other finger without damage to nail
Laceration with foreign body of specified finger with unspecified laterality without damage to nail

S61.229 Laceration with foreign body of unspecified finger without damage to nail

S61.23 Puncture wound without foreign body of finger without damage to nail

S61.230 Puncture wound without foreign body of right index finger without damage to nail

S61.231 Puncture wound without foreign body of left index finger without damage to nail

S61.232 Puncture wound without foreign body of right middle finger without damage to nail

S61.233 Puncture wound without foreign body of left middle finger without damage to nail

S61.234 Puncture wound without foreign body of right ring finger without damage to nail

S61.235 Puncture wound without foreign body of left ring finger without damage to nail

S61.236 Puncture wound without foreign body of right little finger without damage to nail

S61.237 Puncture wound without foreign body of left little finger without damage to nail

S61.238 Puncture wound without foreign body of other finger without damage to nail
Puncture wound without foreign body of specified finger with unspecified laterality without damage to nail

S61.239 Puncture wound without foreign body of unspecified finger without damage to nail

S61.24 Puncture wound with foreign body of finger without damage to nail

S61.240 Puncture wound with foreign body of right index finger without damage to nail

S61.241 Puncture wound with foreign body of left index finger without damage to nail

S61.242 Puncture wound with foreign body of right middle finger without damage to nail

S61.243 Puncture wound with foreign body of left middle finger without damage to nail

S61.244 Puncture wound with foreign body of right ring finger without damage to nail

S61.245 Puncture wound with foreign body of left ring finger without damage to nail

S61.246 Puncture wound with foreign body of right little finger without damage to nail

S61.247 Puncture wound with foreign body of left little finger without damage to nail

S61.248 Puncture wound with foreign body of other finger without damage to nail
Puncture wound with foreign body of specified finger with unspecified laterality without damage to nail

S61.249 Puncture wound with foreign body of unspecified finger without damage to nail

S61.25 Open bite of finger without damage to nail
Bite of finger without damage to nail NOS
EXCLUDES 1 *superficial bite of finger (S60.46-, S60.47-)*

S61.250 Open bite of right index finger without damage to nail

S61.251 Open bite of left index finger without damage to nail

S61.252 Open bite of right middle finger without damage to nail

S61.253 Open bite of left middle finger without damage to nail

S61.254 Open bite of right ring finger without damage to nail

S61.255 Open bite of left ring finger without damage to nail

S61.256 Open bite of right little finger without damage to nail

S61.257 Open bite of left little finger without damage to nail

S61.258 Open bite of other finger without damage to nail
Open bite of specified finger with unspecified laterality without damage to nail

S61.259 Open bite of unspecified finger without damage to nail

S61.3 Open wound of other finger with damage to nail

S61.30 Unspecified open wound of finger with damage to nail

S61.300 Unspecified open wound of right index finger with damage to nail

S61.301 Unspecified open wound of left index finger with damage to nail

S61.302 Unspecified open wound of right middle finger with damage to nail

S61.303 Unspecified open wound of left middle finger with damage to nail

S61.304 Unspecified open wound of right ring finger with damage to nail

S61.305 Unspecified open wound of left ring finger with damage to nail

S61.306 Unspecified open wound of right little finger with damage to nail

S61.307 Unspecified open wound of left little finger with damage to nail

S61.308 Unspecified open wound of other finger with damage to nail
Unspecified open wound of specified finger with unspecified laterality with damage to nail

S61.309 Unspecified open wound of unspecified finger with damage to nail

S61.31 Laceration without foreign body of finger with damage to nail

S61.310 Laceration without foreign body of right index finger with damage to nail

S61.311 Laceration without foreign body of left index finger with damage to nail

S61.312 Laceration without foreign body of right middle finger with damage to nail

S61.313 Laceration without foreign body of left middle finger with damage to nail

S61.314 Laceration without foreign body of right ring finger with damage to nail

S61.315 Laceration without foreign body of left ring finger with damage to nail

S61.316 Laceration without foreign body of right little finger with damage to nail

Appropriate additional character required   Requires 7th character, placeholder x must fill empty characters

S61.317 Laceration without foreign body of left little finger with damage to nail
S61.318 Laceration without foreign body of other finger with damage to nail
Laceration without foreign body of specified finger with unspecified laterality with damage to nail
S61.319 Laceration without foreign body of unspecified finger with damage to nail
S61.32 Laceration with foreign body of finger with damage to nail
S61.320 Laceration with foreign body of right index finger with damage to nail
S61.321 Laceration with foreign body of left index finger with damage to nail
S61.322 Laceration with foreign body of right middle finger with damage to nail
S61.323 Laceration with foreign body of left middle finger with damage to nail
S61.324 Laceration with foreign body of right ring finger with damage to nail
S61.325 Laceration with foreign body of left ring finger with damage to nail
S61.326 Laceration with foreign body of right little finger with damage to nail
S61.327 Laceration with foreign body of left little finger with damage to nail
S61.328 Laceration with foreign body of other finger with damage to nail
Laceration with foreign body of specified finger with unspecified laterality with damage to nail
S61.329 Laceration with foreign body of unspecified finger with damage to nail
S61.33 Puncture wound without foreign body of finger with damage to nail
S61.330 Puncture wound without foreign body of right index finger with damage to nail
S61.331 Puncture wound without foreign body of left index finger with damage to nail
S61.332 Puncture wound without foreign body of right middle finger with damage to nail
S61.333 Puncture wound without foreign body of left middle finger with damage to nail
S61.334 Puncture wound without foreign body of right ring finger with damage to nail
S61.335 Puncture wound without foreign body of left ring finger with damage to nail
S61.336 Puncture wound without foreign body of right little finger with damage to nail
S61.337 Puncture wound without foreign body of left little finger with damage to nail
S61.338 Puncture wound without foreign body of other finger with damage to nail
Puncture wound without foreign body of specified finger with unspecified laterality with damage to nail
S61.339 Puncture wound without foreign body of unspecified finger with damage to nail
S61.34 Puncture wound with foreign body of finger with damage to nail
S61.340 Puncture wound with foreign body of right index finger with damage to nail
S61.341 Puncture wound with foreign body of left index finger with damage to nail
S61.342 Puncture wound with foreign body of right middle finger with damage to nail
S61.343 Puncture wound with foreign body of left middle finger with damage to nail
S61.344 Puncture wound with foreign body of right ring finger with damage to nail
S61.345 Puncture wound with foreign body of left ring finger with damage to nail
S61.346 Puncture wound with foreign body of right little finger with damage to nail
S61.347 Puncture wound with foreign body of left little finger with damage to nail
S61.348 Puncture wound with foreign body of other finger with damage to nail
Puncture wound with foreign body of specified finger with unspecified laterality with damage to nail
S61.349 Puncture wound with foreign body of unspecified finger with damage to nail
S61.35 Open bite of finger with damage to nail
Bite of finger with damage to nail NOS
EXCLUDES 1 *superficial bite of finger (S60.46-, S60.47-)*
S61.350 Open bite of right index finger with damage to nail
S61.351 Open bite of left index finger with damage to nail
S61.352 Open bite of right middle finger with damage to nail
S61.353 Open bite of left middle finger with damage to nail
S61.354 Open bite of right ring finger with damage to nail
S61.355 Open bite of left ring finger with damage to nail
S61.356 Open bite of right little finger with damage to nail
S61.357 Open bite of left little finger with damage to nail
S61.358 Open bite of other finger with damage to nail
Open bite of specified finger with unspecified laterality with damage to nail
S61.359 Open bite of unspecified finger with damage to nail
S61.4 Open wound of hand
S61.40 Unspecified open wound of hand
S61.401 Unspecified open wound of right hand
S61.402 Unspecified open wound of left hand
S61.409 Unspecified open wound of unspecified hand
S61.41 Laceration without foreign body of hand
S61.411 Laceration without foreign body of right hand
S61.412 Laceration without foreign body of left hand
S61.419 Laceration without foreign body of unspecified hand
S61.42 Laceration with foreign body of hand
S61.421 Laceration with foreign body of right hand
S61.422 Laceration with foreign body of left hand
S61.429 Laceration with foreign body of unspecified hand
S61.43 Puncture wound without foreign body of hand
S61.431 Puncture wound without foreign body of right hand
S61.432 Puncture wound without foreign body of left hand
S61.439 Puncture wound without foreign body of unspecified hand
S61.44 Puncture wound with foreign body of hand
S61.441 Puncture wound with foreign body of right hand
S61.442 Puncture wound with foreign body of left hand
S61.449 Puncture wound with foreign body of unspecified hand
S61.45 Open bite of hand
Bite of hand NOS
EXCLUDES 1 *superficial bite of hand (S60.56-, S60.57-)*
S61.451 Open bite of right hand
S61.452 Open bite of left hand
S61.459 Open bite of unspecified hand

S61.5 Open wound of wrist
S61.50 Unspecified open wound of wrist
S61.501 Unspecified open wound of right wrist
S61.502 Unspecified open wound of left wrist
S61.509 Unspecified open wound of unspecified wrist
S61.51 Laceration without foreign body of wrist
S61.511 Laceration without foreign body of right wrist
S61.512 Laceration without foreign body of left wrist
S61.519 Laceration without foreign body of unspecified wrist
S61.52 Laceration with foreign body of wrist
S61.521 Laceration with foreign body of right wrist
S61.522 Laceration with foreign body of left wrist
S61.529 Laceration with foreign body of unspecified wrist
S61.53 Puncture wound without foreign body of wrist
S61.531 Puncture wound without foreign body of right wrist
S61.532 Puncture wound without foreign body of left wrist
S61.539 Puncture wound without foreign body of unspecified wrist
S61.54 Puncture wound with foreign body of wrist
S61.541 Puncture wound with foreign body of right wrist
S61.542 Puncture wound with foreign body of left wrist
S61.549 Puncture wound with foreign body of unspecified wrist
S61.55 Open bite of wrist
Bite of wrist NOS
EXCLUDES 1 *superficial bite of wrist (S60.86-, S60.87-)*
S61.551 Open bite of right wrist
S61.552 Open bite of left wrist
S61.559 Open bite of unspecified wrist

S62 Fracture at wrist and hand level
NOTE A fracture not indicated as displaced or nondisplaced should be coded to displaced
A fracture not indicated as open or closed should be coded to closed.
EXCLUDES 1 *traumatic amputation of wrist and hand (S68.-)*
EXCLUDES 2 *fracture of distal parts of ulna and radius (S52.-)*

The appropriate 7th character is to be added to each code from category S62.
A initial encounter for closed fracture
B initial encounter for open fracture
D subsequent encounter for fracture with routine healing
G subsequent encounter for fracture with delayed healing
K subsequent encounter for fracture with nonunion
P subsequent encounter for fracture with malunion
S sequela

S62.0 Fracture of navicular [scaphoid] bone of wrist
S62.00 Unspecified fracture of navicular [scaphoid] bone of wrist
S62.001 Unspecified fracture of navicular [scaphoid] bone of right wrist
S62.002 Unspecified fracture of navicular [scaphoid] bone of left wrist
S62.009 Unspecified fracture of navicular [scaphoid] bone of unspecified wrist
S62.01 Fracture of distal pole of navicular [scaphoid] bone of wrist
Fracture of volar tuberosity of navicular [scaphoid] bone of wrist
S62.011 Displaced fracture of distal pole of navicular [scaphoid] bone of right wrist
S62.012 Displaced fracture of distal pole of navicular [scaphoid] bone of left wrist
S62.013 Displaced fracture of distal pole of navicular [scaphoid] bone of unspecified wrist
S62.014 Nondisplaced fracture of distal pole of navicular [scaphoid] bone of right wrist
S62.015 Nondisplaced fracture of distal pole of navicular [scaphoid] bone of left wrist
S62.016 Nondisplaced fracture of distal pole of navicular [scaphoid] bone of unspecified wrist
S62.02 Fracture of middle third of navicular [scaphoid] bone of wrist
S62.021 Displaced fracture of middle third of navicular [scaphoid] bone of right wrist
S62.022 Displaced fracture of middle third of navicular [scaphoid] bone of left wrist
S62.023 Displaced fracture of middle third of navicular [scaphoid] bone of unspecified wrist
S62.024 Nondisplaced fracture of middle third of navicular [scaphoid] bone of right wrist
S62.025 Nondisplaced fracture of middle third of navicular [scaphoid] bone of left wrist
S62.026 Nondisplaced fracture of middle third of navicular [scaphoid] bone of unspecified wrist
S62.03 Fracture of proximal third of navicular [scaphoid] bone of wrist
S62.031 Displaced fracture of proximal third of navicular [scaphoid] bone of right wrist
S62.032 Displaced fracture of proximal third of navicular [scaphoid] bone of left wrist
S62.033 Displaced fracture of proximal third of navicular [scaphoid] bone of unspecified wrist
S62.034 Nondisplaced fracture of proximal third of navicular [scaphoid] bone of right wrist
S62.035 Nondisplaced fracture of proximal third of navicular [scaphoid] bone of left wrist
S62.036 Nondisplaced fracture of proximal third of navicular [scaphoid] bone of unspecified wrist
S62.1 Fracture of other and unspecified carpal bone(s)
EXCLUDES 2 *fracture of scaphoid of wrist (S62.0-)*
S62.10 Fracture of unspecified carpal bone
Fracture of wrist NOS
S62.101 Fracture of unspecified carpal bone, right wrist
S62.102 Fracture of unspecified carpal bone, left wrist
S62.109 Fracture of unspecified carpal bone, unspecified wrist
S62.11 Fracture of triquetrum [cuneiform] bone of wrist
S62.111 Displaced fracture of triquetrum [cuneiform] bone, right wrist
S62.112 Displaced fracture of triquetrum [cuneiform] bone, left wrist
S62.113 Displaced fracture of triquetrum [cuneiform] bone, unspecified wrist
S62.114 Nondisplaced fracture of triquetrum [cuneiform] bone, right wrist
S62.115 Nondisplaced fracture of triquetrum [cuneiform] bone, left wrist
S62.116 Nondisplaced fracture of triquetrum [cuneiform] bone, unspecified wrist
S62.12 Fracture of lunate [semilunar]
S62.121 Displaced fracture of lunate [semilunar], right wrist
S62.122 Displaced fracture of lunate [semilunar], left wrist
S62.123 Displaced fracture of lunate [semilunar], unspecified wrist
S62.124 Nondisplaced fracture of lunate [semilunar], right wrist
S62.125 Nondisplaced fracture of lunate [semilunar], left wrist
S62.126 Nondisplaced fracture of lunate [semilunar], unspecified wrist

- 6th **S62.13 Fracture of capitate [os magnum] bone**
  - 7th **S62.131 Displaced fracture of capitate [os magnum] bone, right wrist**
  - 7th **S62.132 Displaced fracture of capitate [os magnum] bone, left wrist**
  - 7th **S62.133 Displaced fracture of capitate [os magnum] bone, unspecified wrist**
  - 7th **S62.134 Nondisplaced fracture of capitate [os magnum] bone, right wrist**
  - 7th **S62.135 Nondisplaced fracture of capitate [os magnum] bone, left wrist**
  - 7th **S62.136 Nondisplaced fracture of capitate [os magnum] bone, unspecified wrist**
- 6th **S62.14 Fracture of body of hamate [unciform] bone**
  Fracture of hamate [unciform] bone NOS
  - 7th **S62.141 Displaced fracture of body of hamate [unciform] bone, right wrist**
  - 7th **S62.142 Displaced fracture of body of hamate [unciform] bone, left wrist**
  - 7th **S62.143 Displaced fracture of body of hamate [unciform] bone, unspecified wrist**
  - 7th **S62.144 Nondisplaced fracture of body of hamate [unciform] bone, right wrist**
  - 7th **S62.145 Nondisplaced fracture of body of hamate [unciform] bone, left wrist**
  - 7th **S62.146 Nondisplaced fracture of body of hamate [unciform] bone, unspecified wrist**
- 6th **S62.15 Fracture of hook process of hamate [unciform] bone**
  Fracture of unciform process of hamate [unciform] bone
  - 7th **S62.151 Displaced fracture of hook process of hamate [unciform] bone, right wrist**
  - 7th **S62.152 Displaced fracture of hook process of hamate [unciform] bone, left wrist**
  - 7th **S62.153 Displaced fracture of hook process of hamate [unciform] bone, unspecified wrist**
  - 7th **S62.154 Nondisplaced fracture of hook process of hamate [unciform] bone, right wrist**
  - 7th **S62.155 Nondisplaced fracture of hook process of hamate [unciform] bone, left wrist**
  - 7th **S62.156 Nondisplaced fracture of hook process of hamate [unciform] bone, unspecified wrist**
- 6th **S62.16 Fracture of pisiform**
  - 7th **S62.161 Displaced fracture of pisiform, right wrist**
  - 7th **S62.162 Displaced fracture of pisiform, left wrist**
  - 7th **S62.163 Displaced fracture of pisiform, unspecified wrist**
  - 7th **S62.164 Nondisplaced fracture of pisiform, right wrist**
  - 7th **S62.165 Nondisplaced fracture of pisiform, left wrist**
  - 7th **S62.166 Nondisplaced fracture of pisiform, unspecified wrist**
- 6th **S62.17 Fracture of trapezium [larger multangular]**
  - 7th **S62.171 Displaced fracture of trapezium [larger multangular], right wrist**
  - 7th **S62.172 Displaced fracture of trapezium [larger multangular], left wrist**
  - 7th **S62.173 Displaced fracture of trapezium [larger multangular], unspecified wrist**
  - 7th **S62.174 Nondisplaced fracture of trapezium [larger multangular], right wrist**
  - 7th **S62.175 Nondisplaced fracture of trapezium [larger multangular], left wrist**
  - 7th **S62.176 Nondisplaced fracture of trapezium [larger multangular], unspecified wrist**
- 6th **S62.18 Fracture of trapezoid [smaller multangular]**
  - 7th **S62.181 Displaced fracture of trapezoid [smaller multangular], right wrist**
  - 7th **S62.182 Displaced fracture of trapezoid [smaller multangular], left wrist**
  - 7th **S62.183 Displaced fracture of trapezoid [smaller multangular], unspecified wrist**
  - 7th **S62.184 Nondisplaced fracture of trapezoid [smaller multangular], right wrist**
  - 7th **S62.185 Nondisplaced fracture of trapezoid [smaller multangular], left wrist**
  - 7th **S62.186 Nondisplaced fracture of trapezoid [smaller multangular], unspecified wrist**

5th **S62.2 Fracture of first metacarpal bone**

- 6th **S62.20 Unspecified fracture of first metacarpal bone**
  - 7th **S62.201 Unspecified fracture of first metacarpal bone, right hand**
  - 7th **S62.202 Unspecified fracture of first metacarpal bone, left hand**
  - 7th **S62.209 Unspecified fracture of first metacarpal bone, unspecified hand**
- 6th **S62.21 Bennett's fracture**
  - 7th **S62.211 Bennett's fracture, right hand**
  - 7th **S62.212 Bennett's fracture, left hand**
  - 7th **S62.213 Bennett's fracture, unspecified hand**
- 6th **S62.22 Rolando's fracture**
  - 7th **S62.221 Displaced Rolando's fracture, right hand**
  - 7th **S62.222 Displaced Rolando's fracture, left hand**
  - 7th **S62.223 Displaced Rolando's fracture, unspecified hand**
  - 7th **S62.224 Nondisplaced Rolando's fracture, right hand**
  - 7th **S62.225 Nondisplaced Rolando's fracture, left hand**
  - 7th **S62.226 Nondisplaced Rolando's fracture, unspecified hand**
- 6th **S62.23 Other fracture of base of first metacarpal bone**
  - 7th **S62.231 Other displaced fracture of base of first metacarpal bone, right hand**
  - 7th **S62.232 Other displaced fracture of base of first metacarpal bone, left hand**
  - 7th **S62.233 Other displaced fracture of base of first metacarpal bone, unspecified hand**
  - 7th **S62.234 Other nondisplaced fracture of base of first metacarpal bone, right hand**
  - 7th **S62.235 Other nondisplaced fracture of base of first metacarpal bone, left hand**
  - 7th **S62.236 Other nondisplaced fracture of base of first metacarpal bone, unspecified hand**
- 6th **S62.24 Fracture of shaft of first metacarpal bone**
  - 7th **S62.241 Displaced fracture of shaft of first metacarpal bone, right hand**
  - 7th **S62.242 Displaced fracture of shaft of first metacarpal bone, left hand**
  - 7th **S62.243 Displaced fracture of shaft of first metacarpal bone, unspecified hand**
  - 7th **S62.244 Nondisplaced fracture of shaft of first metacarpal bone, right hand**
  - 7th **S62.245 Nondisplaced fracture of shaft of first metacarpal bone, left hand**
  - 7th **S62.246 Nondisplaced fracture of shaft of first metacarpal bone, unspecified hand**
- 6th **S62.25 Fracture of neck of first metacarpal bone**
  - 7th **S62.251 Displaced fracture of neck of first metacarpal bone, right hand**
  - 7th **S62.252 Displaced fracture of neck of first metacarpal bone, left hand**
  - 7th **S62.253 Displaced fracture of neck of first metacarpal bone, unspecified hand**
  - 7th **S62.254 Nondisplaced fracture of neck of first metacarpal bone, right hand**
  - 7th **S62.255 Nondisplaced fracture of neck of first metacarpal bone, left hand**
  - 7th **S62.256 Nondisplaced fracture of neck of first metacarpal bone, unspecified hand**
- 6th **S62.29 Other fracture of first metacarpal bone**
  - 7th **S62.291 Other fracture of first metacarpal bone, right hand**
  - 7th **S62.292 Other fracture of first metacarpal bone, left hand**

S62.299 Other fracture of first metacarpal bone, unspecified hand

S62.3 Fracture of other and unspecified metacarpal bone
EXCLUDES 2 *fracture of first metacarpal bone (S62.2-)*

S62.30 Unspecified fracture of other metacarpal bone
S62.300 Unspecified fracture of second metacarpal bone, right hand
S62.301 Unspecified fracture of second metacarpal bone, left hand
S62.302 Unspecified fracture of third metacarpal bone, right hand
S62.303 Unspecified fracture of third metacarpal bone, left hand
S62.304 Unspecified fracture of fourth metacarpal bone, right hand
S62.305 Unspecified fracture of fourth metacarpal bone, left hand
S62.306 Unspecified fracture of fifth metacarpal bone, right hand
S62.307 Unspecified fracture of fifth metacarpal bone, left hand
S62.308 Unspecified fracture of other metacarpal bone
Unspecified fracture of specified metacarpal bone with unspecified laterality
S62.309 Unspecified fracture of unspecified metacarpal bone

S62.31 Displaced fracture of base of other metacarpal bone
S62.310 Displaced fracture of base of second metacarpal bone, right hand
S62.311 Displaced fracture of base of second metacarpal bone. left hand
S62.312 Displaced fracture of base of third metacarpal bone, right hand
S62.313 Displaced fracture of base of third metacarpal bone, left hand
S62.314 Displaced fracture of base of fourth metacarpal bone, right hand
S62.315 Displaced fracture of base of fourth metacarpal bone, left hand
S62.316 Displaced fracture of base of fifth metacarpal bone, right hand
S62.317 Displaced fracture of base of fifth metacarpal bone. left hand
S62.318 Displaced fracture of base of other metacarpal bone
Displaced fracture of base of specified metacarpal bone with unspecified laterality
S62.319 Displaced fracture of base of unspecified metacarpal bone

S62.32 Displaced fracture of shaft of other metacarpal bone
S62.320 Displaced fracture of shaft of second metacarpal bone, right hand
S62.321 Displaced fracture of shaft of second metacarpal bone, left hand
S62.322 Displaced fracture of shaft of third metacarpal bone, right hand
S62.323 Displaced fracture of shaft of third metacarpal bone, left hand
S62.324 Displaced fracture of shaft of fourth metacarpal bone, right hand
S62.325 Displaced fracture of shaft of fourth metacarpal bone, left hand
S62.326 Displaced fracture of shaft of fifth metacarpal bone, right hand
S62.327 Displaced fracture of shaft of fifth metacarpal bone, left hand
S62.328 Displaced fracture of shaft of other metacarpal bone
Displaced fracture of shaft of specified metacarpal bone with unspecified laterality
S62.329 Displaced fracture of shaft of unspecified metacarpal bone

S62.33 Displaced fracture of neck of other metacarpal bone
S62.330 Displaced fracture of neck of second metacarpal bone, right hand
S62.331 Displaced fracture of neck of second metacarpal bone, left hand
S62.332 Displaced fracture of neck of third metacarpal bone, right hand
S62.333 Displaced fracture of neck of third metacarpal bone, left hand
S62.334 Displaced fracture of neck of fourth metacarpal bone, right hand
S62.335 Displaced fracture of neck of fourth metacarpal bone, left hand
S62.336 Displaced fracture of neck of fifth metacarpal bone, right hand
S62.337 Displaced fracture of neck of fifth metacarpal bone, left hand
S62.338 Displaced fracture of neck of other metacarpal bone
Displaced fracture of neck of specified metacarpal bone with unspecified laterality
S62.339 Displaced fracture of neck of unspecified metacarpal bone

S62.34 Nondisplaced fracture of base of other metacarpal bone
S62.340 Nondisplaced fracture of base of second metacarpal bone, right hand
S62.341 Nondisplaced fracture of base of second metacarpal bone. left hand
S62.342 Nondisplaced fracture of base of third metacarpal bone, right hand
S62.343 Nondisplaced fracture of base of third metacarpal bone, left hand
S62.344 Nondisplaced fracture of base of fourth metacarpal bone, right hand
S62.345 Nondisplaced fracture of base of fourth metacarpal bone, left hand
S62.346 Nondisplaced fracture of base of fifth metacarpal bone, right hand
S62.347 Nondisplaced fracture of base of fifth metacarpal bone. left hand
S62.348 Nondisplaced fracture of base of other metacarpal bone
Nondisplaced fracture of base of specified metacarpal bone with unspecified laterality
S62.349 Nondisplaced fracture of base of unspecified metacarpal bone

S62.35 Nondisplaced fracture of shaft of other metacarpal bone
S62.350 Nondisplaced fracture of shaft of second metacarpal bone, right hand
S62.351 Nondisplaced fracture of shaft of second metacarpal bone, left hand
S62.352 Nondisplaced fracture of shaft of third metacarpal bone, right hand
S62.353 Nondisplaced fracture of shaft of third metacarpal bone, left hand
S62.354 Nondisplaced fracture of shaft of fourth metacarpal bone, right hand
S62.355 Nondisplaced fracture of shaft of fourth metacarpal bone, left hand
S62.356 Nondisplaced fracture of shaft of fifth metacarpal bone, right hand
S62.357 Nondisplaced fracture of shaft of fifth metacarpal bone, left hand
S62.358 Nondisplaced fracture of shaft of other metacarpal bone
Nondisplaced fracture of shaft of specified metacarpal bone with unspecified laterality
S62.359 Nondisplaced fracture of shaft of unspecified metacarpal bone

6th S62.36 Nondisplaced fracture of neck of other metacarpal bone

7th S62.360 Nondisplaced fracture of neck of second metacarpal bone, right hand

7th S62.361 Nondisplaced fracture of neck of second metacarpal bone, left hand

7th S62.362 Nondisplaced fracture of neck of third metacarpal bone, right hand

7th S62.363 Nondisplaced fracture of neck of third metacarpal bone, left hand

7th S62.364 Nondisplaced fracture of neck of fourth metacarpal bone, right hand

7th S62.365 Nondisplaced fracture of neck of fourth metacarpal bone, left hand

7th S62.366 Nondisplaced fracture of neck of fifth metacarpal bone, right hand

7th S62.367 Nondisplaced fracture of neck of fifth metacarpal bone, left hand

7th S62.368 Nondisplaced fracture of neck of other metacarpal bone

Nondisplaced fracture of neck of specified metacarpal bone with unspecified laterality

7th S62.369 Nondisplaced fracture of neck of unspecified metacarpal bone

6th S62.39 Other fracture of other metacarpal bone

7th S62.390 Other fracture of second metacarpal bone, right hand

7th S62.391 Other fracture of second metacarpal bone, left hand

7th S62.392 Other fracture of third metacarpal bone, right hand

7th S62.393 Other fracture of third metacarpal bone, left hand

7th S62.394 Other fracture of fourth metacarpal bone, right hand

7th S62.395 Other fracture of fourth metacarpal bone, left hand

7th S62.396 Other fracture of fifth metacarpal bone, right hand

7th S62.397 Other fracture of fifth metacarpal bone, left hand

7th S62.398 Other fracture of other metacarpal bone

Other fracture of specified metacarpal bone with unspecified laterality

7th S62.399 Other fracture of unspecified metacarpal bone

5th S62.5 Fracture of thumb

6th S62.50 Fracture of unspecified phalanx of thumb

7th S62.501 Fracture of unspecified phalanx of right thumb

7th S62.502 Fracture of unspecified phalanx of left thumb

7th S62.509 Fracture of unspecified phalanx of unspecified thumb

6th S62.51 Fracture of proximal phalanx of thumb

7th S62.511 Displaced fracture of proximal phalanx of right thumb

7th S62.512 Displaced fracture of proximal phalanx of left thumb

7th S62.513 Displaced fracture of proximal phalanx of unspecified thumb

7th S62.514 Nondisplaced fracture of proximal phalanx of right thumb

7th S62.515 Nondisplaced fracture of proximal phalanx of left thumb

7th S62.516 Nondisplaced fracture of proximal phalanx of unspecified thumb

6th S62.52 Fracture of distal phalanx of thumb

7th S62.521 Displaced fracture of distal phalanx of right thumb

7th S62.522 Displaced fracture of distal phalanx of left thumb

7th S62.523 Displaced fracture of distal phalanx of unspecified thumb

7th S62.524 Nondisplaced fracture of distal phalanx of right thumb

7th S62.525 Nondisplaced fracture of distal phalanx of left thumb

7th S62.526 Nondisplaced fracture of distal phalanx of unspecified thumb

5th S62.6 Fracture of other and unspecified finger(s)

EXCLUDES 2 *fracture of thumb (S62.5-)*

6th S62.60 Fracture of unspecified phalanx of finger

7th S62.600 Fracture of unspecified phalanx of right index finger

7th S62.601 Fracture of unspecified phalanx of left index finger

7th S62.602 Fracture of unspecified phalanx of right middle finger

7th S62.603 Fracture of unspecified phalanx of left middle finger

7th S62.604 Fracture of unspecified phalanx of right ring finger

7th S62.605 Fracture of unspecified phalanx of left ring finger

7th S62.606 Fracture of unspecified phalanx of right little finger

7th S62.607 Fracture of unspecified phalanx of left little finger

7th S62.608 Fracture of unspecified phalanx of other finger

Fracture of unspecified phalanx of specified finger with unspecified laterality

7th S62.609 Fracture of unspecified phalanx of unspecified finger

6th S62.61 Displaced fracture of proximal phalanx of finger

7th S62.610 Displaced fracture of proximal phalanx of right index finger

7th S62.611 Displaced fracture of proximal phalanx of left index finger

7th S62.612 Displaced fracture of proximal phalanx of right middle finger

7th S62.613 Displaced fracture of proximal phalanx of left middle finger

7th S62.614 Displaced fracture of proximal phalanx of right ring finger

7th S62.615 Displaced fracture of proximal phalanx of left ring finger

7th S62.616 Displaced fracture of proximal phalanx of right little finger

7th S62.617 Displaced fracture of proximal phalanx of left little finger

7th S62.618 Displaced fracture of proximal phalanx of other finger

Displaced fracture of proximal phalanx of specified finger with unspecified laterality

7th S62.619 Displaced fracture of proximal phalanx of unspecified finger

6th S62.62 Displaced fracture of medial phalanx of finger

7th S62.620 Displaced fracture of medial phalanx of right index finger

7th S62.621 Displaced fracture of medial phalanx of left index finger

7th S62.622 Displaced fracture of medial phalanx of right middle finger

7th S62.623 Displaced fracture of medial phalanx of left middle finger

7th S62.624 Displaced fracture of medial phalanx of right ring finger

7th S62.625 Displaced fracture of medial phalanx of left ring finger

7th S62.626 Displaced fracture of medial phalanx of right little finger

7th S62.627 Displaced fracture of medial phalanx of left little finger

7th S62.628 Displaced fracture of medial phalanx of other finger

Displaced fracture of medial phalanx of specified finger with unspecified laterality

S62.629 Displaced fracture of medial phalanx of unspecified finger

S62.63 Displaced fracture of distal phalanx of finger

S62.630 Displaced fracture of distal phalanx of right index finger

S62.631 Displaced fracture of distal phalanx of left index finger

S62.632 Displaced fracture of distal phalanx of right middle finger

S62.633 Displaced fracture of distal phalanx of left middle finger

S62.634 Displaced fracture of distal phalanx of right ring finger

S62.635 Displaced fracture of distal phalanx of left ring finger

S62.636 Displaced fracture of distal phalanx of right little finger

S62.637 Displaced fracture of distal phalanx of left little finger

S62.638 Displaced fracture of distal phalanx of other finger
Displaced fracture of distal phalanx of specified finger with unspecified laterality

S62.639 Displaced fracture of distal phalanx of unspecified finger

S62.64 Nondisplaced fracture of proximal phalanx of finger

S62.640 Nondisplaced fracture of proximal phalanx of right index finger

S62.641 Nondisplaced fracture of proximal phalanx of left index finger

S62.642 Nondisplaced fracture of proximal phalanx of right middle finger

S62.643 Nondisplaced fracture of proximal phalanx of left middle finger

S62.644 Nondisplaced fracture of proximal phalanx of right ring finger

S62.645 Nondisplaced fracture of proximal phalanx of left ring finger

S62.646 Nondisplaced fracture of proximal phalanx of right little finger

S62.647 Nondisplaced fracture of proximal phalanx of left little finger

S62.648 Nondisplaced fracture of proximal phalanx of other finger
Nondisplaced fracture of proximal phalanx of specified finger with unspecified laterality

S62.649 Nondisplaced fracture of proximal phalanx of unspecified finger

S62.65 Nondisplaced fracture of medial phalanx of finger

S62.650 Nondisplaced fracture of medial phalanx of right index finger

S62.651 Nondisplaced fracture of medial phalanx of left index finger

S62.652 Nondisplaced fracture of medial phalanx of right middle finger

S62.653 Nondisplaced fracture of medial phalanx of left middle finger

S62.654 Nondisplaced fracture of medial phalanx of right ring finger

S62.655 Nondisplaced fracture of medial phalanx of left ring finger

S62.656 Nondisplaced fracture of medial phalanx of right little finger

S62.657 Nondisplaced fracture of medial phalanx of left little finger

S62.658 Nondisplaced fracture of medial phalanx of other finger
Nondisplaced fracture of medial phalanx of specified finger with unspecified laterality

S62.659 Nondisplaced fracture of medial phalanx of unspecified finger

S62.66 Nondisplaced fracture of distal phalanx of finger

S62.660 Nondisplaced fracture of distal phalanx of right index finger

S62.661 Nondisplaced fracture of distal phalanx of left index finger

S62.662 Nondisplaced fracture of distal phalanx of right middle finger

S62.663 Nondisplaced fracture of distal phalanx of left middle finger

S62.664 Nondisplaced fracture of distal phalanx of right ring finger

S62.665 Nondisplaced fracture of distal phalanx of left ring finger

S62.666 Nondisplaced fracture of distal phalanx of right little finger

S62.667 Nondisplaced fracture of distal phalanx of left little finger

S62.668 Nondisplaced fracture of distal phalanx of other finger
Nondisplaced fracture of distal phalanx of specified finger with unspecified laterality

S62.669 Nondisplaced fracture of distal phalanx of unspecified finger

S62.9 Unspecified fracture of wrist and hand

S62.90 Unspecified fracture of unspecified wrist and hand

S62.91 Unspecified fracture of right wrist and hand

S62.92 Unspecified fracture of left wrist and hand

S63 Dislocation and sprain of joints and ligaments at wrist and hand level

INCLUDES avulsion of joint or ligament at wrist and hand level
laceration of cartilage, joint or ligament at wrist and hand level
sprain of cartilage, joint or ligament at wrist and hand level
traumatic hemarthrosis of joint or ligament at wrist and hand level
traumatic rupture of joint or ligament at wrist and hand level
traumatic subluxation of joint or ligament at wrist and hand level
traumatic tear of joint or ligament at wrist and hand level

Code also any associated open wound

EXCLUDES 2 *strain of muscle, fascia and tendon of wrist and hand (S66.-)*

The appropriate 7th character is to be added to each code from category S63.
A initial encounter
D subsequent encounter
S sequela

S63.0 Subluxation and dislocation of wrist and hand joints

S63.00 Unspecified subluxation and dislocation of wrist and hand
Dislocation of carpal bone NOS
Dislocation of distal end of radius NOS
Subluxation of carpal bone NOS
Subluxation of distal end of radius NOS

S63.001 Unspecified subluxation of right wrist and hand

S63.002 Unspecified subluxation of left wrist and hand

S63.003 Unspecified subluxation of unspecified wrist and hand

S63.004 Unspecified dislocation of right wrist and hand

S63.005 Unspecified dislocation of left wrist and hand

S63.006 Unspecified dislocation of unspecified wrist and hand

S63.01 Subluxation and dislocation of distal radioulnar joint

S63.011 Subluxation of distal radioulnar joint of right wrist

S63.012 Subluxation of distal radioulnar joint of left wrist

S63.013 Subluxation of distal radioulnar joint of unspecified wrist

✓7th S63.014 Dislocation of distal radioulnar joint of right wrist
✓7th S63.015 Dislocation of distal radioulnar joint of left wrist
✓7th S63.016 Dislocation of distal radioulnar joint of unspecified wrist
✓6th S63.02 Subluxation and dislocation of radiocarpal joint
✓7th S63.021 Subluxation of radiocarpal joint of right wrist
✓7th S63.022 Subluxation of radiocarpal joint of left wrist
✓7th S63.023 Subluxation of radiocarpal joint of unspecified wrist
✓7th S63.024 Dislocation of radiocarpal joint of right wrist
✓7th S63.025 Dislocation of radiocarpal joint of left wrist
✓7th S63.026 Dislocation of radiocarpal joint of unspecified wrist
✓6th S63.03 Subluxation and dislocation of midcarpal joint
✓7th S63.031 Subluxation of midcarpal joint of right wrist
✓7th S63.032 Subluxation of midcarpal joint of left wrist
✓7th S63.033 Subluxation of midcarpal joint of unspecified wrist
✓7th S63.034 Dislocation of midcarpal joint of right wrist
✓7th S63.035 Dislocation of midcarpal joint of left wrist
✓7th S63.036 Dislocation of midcarpal joint of unspecified wrist
✓6th S63.04 Subluxation and dislocation of carpometacarpal joint of thumb
EXCLUDES 2 *interphalangeal subluxation and dislocation of thumb (S63.1-)*
✓7th S63.041 Subluxation of carpometacarpal joint of right thumb
✓7th S63.042 Subluxation of carpometacarpal joint of left thumb
✓7th S63.043 Subluxation of carpometacarpal joint of unspecified thumb
✓7th S63.044 Dislocation of carpometacarpal joint of right thumb
✓7th S63.045 Dislocation of carpometacarpal joint of left thumb
✓7th S63.046 Dislocation of carpometacarpal joint of unspecified thumb
✓6th S63.05 Subluxation and dislocation of other carpometacarpal joint
EXCLUDES 2 *subluxation and dislocation of carpometacarpal joint of thumb (S63.04-)*
✓7th S63.051 Subluxation of other carpometacarpal joint of right hand
✓7th S63.052 Subluxation of other carpometacarpal joint of left hand
✓7th S63.053 Subluxation of other carpometacarpal joint of unspecified hand
✓7th S63.054 Dislocation of other carpometacarpal joint of right hand
✓7th S63.055 Dislocation of other carpometacarpal joint of left hand
✓7th S63.056 Dislocation of other carpometacarpal joint of unspecified hand
✓6th S63.06 Subluxation and dislocation of metacarpal (bone), proximal end
✓7th S63.061 Subluxation of metacarpal (bone), proximal end of right hand
✓7th S63.062 Subluxation of metacarpal (bone), proximal end of left hand
✓7th S63.063 Subluxation of metacarpal (bone), proximal end of unspecified hand
✓7th S63.064 Dislocation of metacarpal (bone), proximal end of right hand
✓7th S63.065 Dislocation of metacarpal (bone), proximal end of left hand
✓7th S63.066 Dislocation of metacarpal (bone), proximal end of unspecified hand
✓6th S63.07 Subluxation and dislocation of distal end of ulna
✓7th S63.071 Subluxation of distal end of right ulna
✓7th S63.072 Subluxation of distal end of left ulna
✓7th S63.073 Subluxation of distal end of unspecified ulna
✓7th S63.074 Dislocation of distal end of right ulna
✓7th S63.075 Dislocation of distal end of left ulna
✓7th S63.076 Dislocation of distal end of unspecified ulna
✓6th S63.09 Other subluxation and dislocation of wrist and hand
✓7th S63.091 Other subluxation of right wrist and hand
✓7th S63.092 Other subluxation of left wrist and hand
✓7th S63.093 Other subluxation of unspecified wrist and hand
✓7th S63.094 Other dislocation of right wrist and hand
✓7th S63.095 Other dislocation of left wrist and hand
✓7th S63.096 Other dislocation of unspecified wrist and hand
✓5th S63.1 Subluxation and dislocation of thumb
✓6th S63.10 Unspecified subluxation and dislocation of thumb
✓7th S63.101 Unspecified subluxation of right thumb
✓7th S63.102 Unspecified subluxation of left thumb
✓7th S63.103 Unspecified subluxation of unspecified thumb
✓7th S63.104 Unspecified dislocation of right thumb
✓7th S63.105 Unspecified dislocation of left thumb
✓7th S63.106 Unspecified dislocation of unspecified thumb
✓6th S63.11 Subluxation and dislocation of metacarpophalangeal joint of thumb
✓7th S63.111 Subluxation of metacarpophalangeal joint of right thumb
✓7th S63.112 Subluxation of metacarpophalangeal joint of left thumb
✓7th S63.113 Subluxation of metacarpophalangeal joint of unspecified thumb
✓7th S63.114 Dislocation of metacarpophalangeal joint of right thumb
✓7th S63.115 Dislocation of metacarpophalangeal joint of left thumb
✓7th S63.116 Dislocation of metacarpophalangeal joint of unspecified thumb
✓6th S63.12 Subluxation and dislocation of unspecified interphalangeal joint of thumb
✓7th S63.121 Subluxation of unspecified interphalangeal joint of right thumb
✓7th S63.122 Subluxation of unspecified interphalangeal joint of left thumb
✓7th S63.123 Subluxation of unspecified interphalangeal joint of unspecified thumb
✓7th S63.124 Dislocation of unspecified interphalangeal joint of right thumb
✓7th S63.125 Dislocation of unspecified interphalangeal joint of left thumb
✓7th S63.126 Dislocation of unspecified interphalangeal joint of unspecified thumb
✓6th S63.13 Subluxation and dislocation of proximal interphalangeal joint of thumb
✓7th S63.131 Subluxation of proximal interphalangeal joint of right thumb
✓7th S63.132 Subluxation of proximal interphalangeal joint of left thumb
✓7th S63.133 Subluxation of proximal interphalangeal joint of unspecified thumb
✓7th S63.134 Dislocation of proximal interphalangeal joint of right thumb
✓7th S63.135 Dislocation of proximal interphalangeal joint of left thumb

7th S63.136 **Dislocation of proximal interphalangeal joint of unspecified thumb**

6th S63.14 **Subluxation and dislocation of distal interphalangeal joint of thumb**

7th S63.141 **Subluxation of distal interphalangeal joint of right thumb**

7th S63.142 **Subluxation of distal interphalangeal joint of left thumb**

7th S63.143 **Subluxation of distal interphalangeal joint of unspecified thumb**

7th S63.144 **Dislocation of distal interphalangeal joint of right thumb**

7th S63.145 **Dislocation of distal interphalangeal joint of left thumb**

7th S63.146 **Dislocation of distal interphalangeal joint of unspecified thumb**

5th S63.2 **Subluxation and dislocation of other finger(s)**

EXCLUDES 2 *subluxation and dislocation of thumb (S63.1-)*

6th S63.20 **Unspecified subluxation of other finger**

7th S63.200 **Unspecified subluxation of right index finger**

7th S63.201 **Unspecified subluxation of left index finger**

7th S63.202 **Unspecified subluxation of right middle finger**

7th S63.203 **Unspecified subluxation of left middle finger**

7th S63.204 **Unspecified subluxation of right ring finger**

7th S63.205 **Unspecified subluxation of left ring finger**

7th S63.206 **Unspecified subluxation of right little finger**

7th S63.207 **Unspecified subluxation of left little finger**

7th S63.208 **Unspecified subluxation of other finger**

Unspecified subluxation of specified finger with unspecified laterality

7th S63.209 **Unspecified subluxation of unspecified finger**

6th S63.21 **Subluxation of metacarpophalangeal joint of finger**

7th S63.210 **Subluxation of metacarpophalangeal joint of right index finger**

7th S63.211 **Subluxation of metacarpophalangeal joint of left index finger**

7th S63.212 **Subluxation of metacarpophalangeal joint of right middle finger**

7th S63.213 **Subluxation of metacarpophalangeal joint of left middle finger**

7th S63.214 **Subluxation of metacarpophalangeal joint of right ring finger**

7th S63.215 **Subluxation of metacarpophalangeal joint of left ring finger**

7th S63.216 **Subluxation of metacarpophalangeal joint of right little finger**

7th S63.217 **Subluxation of metacarpophalangeal joint of left little finger**

7th S63.218 **Subluxation of metacarpophalangeal joint of other finger**

Subluxation of metacarpophalangeal joint of specified finger with unspecified laterality

7th S63.219 **Subluxation of metacarpophalangeal joint of unspecified finger**

6th S63.22 **Subluxation of unspecified interphalangeal joint of finger**

7th S63.220 **Subluxation of unspecified interphalangeal joint of right index finger**

7th S63.221 **Subluxation of unspecified interphalangeal joint of left index finger**

7th S63.222 **Subluxation of unspecified interphalangeal joint of right middle finger**

7th S63.223 **Subluxation of unspecified interphalangeal joint of left middle finger**

7th S63.224 **Subluxation of unspecified interphalangeal joint of right ring finger**

7th S63.225 **Subluxation of unspecified interphalangeal joint of left ring finger**

7th S63.226 **Subluxation of unspecified interphalangeal joint of right little finger**

7th S63.227 **Subluxation of unspecified interphalangeal joint of left little finger**

7th S63.228 **Subluxation of unspecified interphalangeal joint of other finger**

Subluxation of unspecified interphalangeal joint of specified finger with unspecified laterality

7th S63.229 **Subluxation of unspecified interphalangeal joint of unspecified finger**

6th S63.23 **Subluxation of proximal interphalangeal joint of finger**

7th S63.230 **Subluxation of proximal interphalangeal joint of right index finger**

7th S63.231 **Subluxation of proximal interphalangeal joint of left index finger**

7th S63.232 **Subluxation of proximal interphalangeal joint of right middle finger**

7th S63.233 **Subluxation of proximal interphalangeal joint of left middle finger**

7th S63.234 **Subluxation of proximal interphalangeal joint of right ring finger**

7th S63.235 **Subluxation of proximal interphalangeal joint of left ring finger**

7th S63.236 **Subluxation of proximal interphalangeal joint of right little finger**

7th S63.237 **Subluxation of proximal interphalangeal joint of left little finger**

7th S63.238 **Subluxation of proximal interphalangeal joint of other finger**

Subluxation of proximal interphalangeal joint of specified finger with unspecified laterality

7th S63.239 **Subluxation of proximal interphalangeal joint of unspecified finger**

6th S63.24 **Subluxation of distal interphalangeal joint of finger**

7th S63.240 **Subluxation of distal interphalangeal joint of right index finger**

7th S63.241 **Subluxation of distal interphalangeal joint of left index finger**

7th S63.242 **Subluxation of distal interphalangeal joint of right middle finger**

7th S63.243 **Subluxation of distal interphalangeal joint of left middle finger**

7th S63.244 **Subluxation of distal interphalangeal joint of right ring finger**

7th S63.245 **Subluxation of distal interphalangeal joint of left ring finger**

7th S63.246 **Subluxation of distal interphalangeal joint of right little finger**

7th S63.247 **Subluxation of distal interphalangeal joint of left little finger**

7th S63.248 **Subluxation of distal interphalangeal joint of other finger**

Subluxation of distal interphalangeal joint of specified finger with unspecified laterality

7th S63.249 **Subluxation of distal interphalangeal joint of unspecified finger**

✓6th **S63.25 Unspecified dislocation of other finger**

✓7th **S63.250 Unspecified dislocation of right index finger**

✓7th **S63.251 Unspecified dislocation of left index finger**

✓7th **S63.252 Unspecified dislocation of right middle finger**

✓7th **S63.253 Unspecified dislocation of left middle finger**

✓7th **S63.254 Unspecified dislocation of right ring finger**

✓7th **S63.255 Unspecified dislocation of left ring finger**

✓7th **S63.256 Unspecified dislocation of right little finger**

✓7th **S63.257 Unspecified dislocation of left little finger**

✓7th **S63.258 Unspecified dislocation of other finger**
Unspecified dislocation of specified finger with unspecified laterality

✓7th **S63.259 Unspecified dislocation of unspecified finger**
Unspecified dislocation of specified finger with unspecified laterality

✓6th **S63.26 Dislocation of metacarpophalangeal joint of finger**

✓7th **S63.260 Dislocation of metacarpophalangeal joint of right index finger**

✓7th **S63.261 Dislocation of metacarpophalangeal joint of left index finger**

✓7th **S63.262 Dislocation of metacarpophalangeal joint of right middle finger**

✓7th **S63.263 Dislocation of metacarpophalangeal joint of left middle finger**

✓7th **S63.264 Dislocation of metacarpophalangeal joint of right ring finger**

✓7th **S63.265 Dislocation of metacarpophalangeal joint of left ring finger**

✓7th **S63.266 Dislocation of metacarpophalangeal joint of right little finger**

✓7th **S63.267 Dislocation of metacarpophalangeal joint of left little finger**

✓7th **S63.268 Dislocation of metacarpophalangeal joint of other finger**
Dislocation of metacarpophalangeal joint of specified finger with unspecified laterality

✓7th **S63.269 Dislocation of metacarpophalangeal joint of unspecified finger**

✓6th **S63.27 Dislocation of unspecified interphalangeal joint of finger**

✓7th **S63.270 Dislocation of unspecified interphalangeal joint of right index finger**

✓7th **S63.271 Dislocation of unspecified interphalangeal joint of left index finger**

✓7th **S63.272 Dislocation of unspecified interphalangeal joint of right middle finger**

✓7th **S63.273 Dislocation of unspecified interphalangeal joint of left middle finger**

✓7th **S63.274 Dislocation of unspecified interphalangeal joint of right ring finger**

✓7th **S63.275 Dislocation of unspecified interphalangeal joint of left ring finger**

✓7th **S63.276 Dislocation of unspecified interphalangeal joint of right little finger**

✓7th **S63.277 Dislocation of unspecified interphalangeal joint of left little finger**

✓7th **S63.278 Dislocation of unspecified interphalangeal joint of other finger**
Dislocation of unspecified interphalangeal joint of specified finger with unspecified laterality

✓7th **S63.279 Dislocation of unspecified interphalangeal joint of unspecified finger**
Dislocation of unspecified interphalangeal joint of specified finger without specified laterality

✓6th **S63.28 Dislocation of proximal interphalangeal joint of finger**

✓7th **S63.280 Dislocation of proximal interphalangeal joint of right index finger**

✓7th **S63.281 Dislocation of proximal interphalangeal joint of left index finger**

✓7th **S63.282 Dislocation of proximal interphalangeal joint of right middle finger**

✓7th **S63.283 Dislocation of proximal interphalangeal joint of left middle finger**

✓7th **S63.284 Dislocation of proximal interphalangeal joint of right ring finger**

✓7th **S63.285 Dislocation of proximal interphalangeal joint of left ring finger**

✓7th **S63.286 Dislocation of proximal interphalangeal joint of right little finger**

✓7th **S63.287 Dislocation of proximal interphalangeal joint of left little finger**

✓7th **S63.288 Dislocation of proximal interphalangeal joint of other finger**
Dislocation of proximal interphalangeal joint of specified finger with unspecified laterality

✓7th **S63.289 Dislocation of proximal interphalangeal joint of unspecified finger**

✓6th **S63.29 Dislocation of distal interphalangeal joint of finger**

✓7th **S63.290 Dislocation of distal interphalangeal joint of right index finger**

✓7th **S63.291 Dislocation of distal interphalangeal joint of left index finger**

✓7th **S63.292 Dislocation of distal interphalangeal joint of right middle finger**

✓7th **S63.293 Dislocation of distal interphalangeal joint of left middle finger**

✓7th **S63.294 Dislocation of distal interphalangeal joint of right ring finger**

✓7th **S63.295 Dislocation of distal interphalangeal joint of left ring finger**

✓7th **S63.296 Dislocation of distal interphalangeal joint of right little finger**

✓7th **S63.297 Dislocation of distal interphalangeal joint of left little finger**

✓7th **S63.298 Dislocation of distal interphalangeal joint of other finger**
Dislocation of distal interphalangeal joint of specified finger with unspecified laterality

✓7th **S63.299 Dislocation of distal interphalangeal joint of unspecified finger**

✓5th **S63.3 Traumatic rupture of ligament of wrist**

✓6th **S63.30 Traumatic rupture of unspecified ligament of wrist**

✓7th **S63.301 Traumatic rupture of unspecified ligament of right wrist**

✓7th **S63.302 Traumatic rupture of unspecified ligament of left wrist**

✓7th **S63.309 Traumatic rupture of unspecified ligament of unspecified wrist**

✓6th **S63.31 Traumatic rupture of collateral ligament of wrist**

✓7th **S63.311 Traumatic rupture of collateral ligament of right wrist**

✓7th **S63.312 Traumatic rupture of collateral ligament of left wrist**

✓7th **S63.319 Traumatic rupture of collateral ligament of unspecified wrist**

✓6th **S63.32 Traumatic rupture of radiocarpal ligament**

✓7th **S63.321 Traumatic rupture of right radiocarpal ligament**

✓7th **S63.322 Traumatic rupture of left radiocarpal ligament**

✓7th **S63.329 Traumatic rupture of unspecified radiocarpal ligament**

✓6th **S63.33 Traumatic rupture of ulnocarpal (palmar) ligament**
✓7th **S63.331 Traumatic rupture of right ulnocarpal (palmar) ligament**
✓7th **S63.332 Traumatic rupture of left ulnocarpal (palmar) ligament**
✓7th **S63.339 Traumatic rupture of unspecified ulnocarpal (palmar) ligament**

✓6th **S63.39 Traumatic rupture of other ligament of wrist**
✓7th **S63.391 Traumatic rupture of other ligament of right wrist**
✓7th **S63.392 Traumatic rupture of other ligament of left wrist**
✓7th **S63.399 Traumatic rupture of other ligament of unspecified wrist**

✓5th **S63.4 Traumatic rupture of ligament of finger at metacarpophalangeal and interphalangeal joint(s)**

✓6th **S63.40 Traumatic rupture of unspecified ligament of finger at metacarpophalangeal and interphalangeal joint**
✓7th **S63.400 Traumatic rupture of unspecified ligament of right index finger at metacarpophalangeal and interphalangeal joint**
✓7th **S63.401 Traumatic rupture of unspecified ligament of left index finger at metacarpophalangeal and interphalangeal joint**
✓7th **S63.402 Traumatic rupture of unspecified ligament of right middle finger at metacarpophalangeal and interphalangeal joint**
✓7th **S63.403 Traumatic rupture of unspecified ligament of left middle finger at metacarpophalangeal and interphalangeal joint**
✓7th **S63.404 Traumatic rupture of unspecified ligament of right ring finger at metacarpophalangeal and interphalangeal joint**
✓7th **S63.405 Traumatic rupture of unspecified ligament of left ring finger at metacarpophalangeal and interphalangeal joint**
✓7th **S63.406 Traumatic rupture of unspecified ligament of right little finger at metacarpophalangeal and interphalangeal joint**
✓7th **S63.407 Traumatic rupture of unspecified ligament of left little finger at metacarpophalangeal and interphalangeal joint**
✓7th **S63.408 Traumatic rupture of unspecified ligament of other finger at metacarpophalangeal and interphalangeal joint**
Traumatic rupture of unspecified ligament of specified finger with unspecified laterality at metacarpophalangeal and interphalangeal joint
✓7th **S63.409 Traumatic rupture of unspecified ligament of unspecified finger at metacarpophalangeal and interphalangeal joint**

✓6th **S63.41 Traumatic rupture of collateral ligament of finger at metacarpophalangeal and interphalangeal joint**
✓7th **S63.410 Traumatic rupture of collateral ligament of right index finger at metacarpophalangeal and interphalangeal joint**
✓7th **S63.411 Traumatic rupture of collateral ligament of left index finger at metacarpophalangeal and interphalangeal joint**
✓7th **S63.412 Traumatic rupture of collateral ligament of right middle finger at metacarpophalangeal and interphalangeal joint**
✓7th **S63.413 Traumatic rupture of collateral ligament of left middle finger at metacarpophalangeal and interphalangeal joint**
✓7th **S63.414 Traumatic rupture of collateral ligament of right ring finger at metacarpophalangeal and interphalangeal joint**
✓7th **S63.415 Traumatic rupture of collateral ligament of left ring finger at metacarpophalangeal and interphalangeal joint**
✓7th **S63.416 Traumatic rupture of collateral ligament of right little finger at metacarpophalangeal and interphalangeal joint**
✓7th **S63.417 Traumatic rupture of collateral ligament of left little finger at metacarpophalangeal and interphalangeal joint**
✓7th **S63.418 Traumatic rupture of collateral ligament of other finger at metacarpophalangeal and interphalangeal joint**
Traumatic rupture of collateral ligament of specified finger with unspecified laterality at metacarpophalangeal and interphalangeal joint
✓7th **S63.419 Traumatic rupture of collateral ligament of unspecified finger at metacarpophalangeal and interphalangeal joint**

✓6th **S63.42 Traumatic rupture of palmar ligament of finger at metacarpophalangeal and interphalangeal joint**
✓7th **S63.420 Traumatic rupture of palmar ligament of right index finger at metacarpophalangeal and interphalangeal joint**
✓7th **S63.421 Traumatic rupture of palmar ligament of left index finger at metacarpophalangeal and interphalangeal joint**
✓7th **S63.422 Traumatic rupture of palmar ligament of right middle finger at metacarpophalangeal and interphalangeal joint**
✓7th **S63.423 Traumatic rupture of palmar ligament of left middle finger at metacarpophalangeal and interphalangeal joint**
✓7th **S63.424 Traumatic rupture of palmar ligament of right ring finger at metacarpophalangeal and interphalangeal joint**
✓7th **S63.425 Traumatic rupture of palmar ligament of left ring finger at metacarpophalangeal and interphalangeal joint**
✓7th **S63.426 Traumatic rupture of palmar ligament of right little finger at metacarpophalangeal and interphalangeal joint**
✓7th **S63.427 Traumatic rupture of palmar ligament of left little finger at metacarpophalangeal and interphalangeal joint**
✓7th **S63.428 Traumatic rupture of palmar ligament of other finger at metacarpophalangeal and interphalangeal joint**
Traumatic rupture of palmar ligament of specified finger with unspecified laterality at metacarpophalangeal and interphalangeal joint
✓7th **S63.429 Traumatic rupture of palmar ligament of unspecified finger at metacarpophalangeal and interphalangeal joint**

✓6th **S63.43 Traumatic rupture of volar plate of finger at metacarpophalangeal and interphalangeal joint**
✓7th **S63.430 Traumatic rupture of volar plate of right index finger at metacarpophalangeal and interphalangeal joint**

- ✓7th **S63.431 Traumatic rupture of volar plate of left index finger at metacarpophalangeal and interphalangeal joint**
- ✓7th **S63.432 Traumatic rupture of volar plate of right middle finger at metacarpophalangeal and interphalangeal joint**
- ✓7th **S63.433 Traumatic rupture of volar plate of left middle finger at metacarpophalangeal and interphalangeal joint**
- ✓7th **S63.434 Traumatic rupture of volar plate of right ring finger at metacarpophalangeal and interphalangeal joint**
- ✓7th **S63.435 Traumatic rupture of volar plate of left ring finger at metacarpophalangeal and interphalangeal joint**
- ✓7th **S63.436 Traumatic rupture of volar plate of right little finger at metacarpophalangeal and interphalangeal joint**
- ✓7th **S63.437 Traumatic rupture of volar plate of left little finger at metacarpophalangeal and interphalangeal joint**
- ✓7th **S63.438 Traumatic rupture of volar plate of other finger at metacarpophalangeal and interphalangeal joint**
  Traumatic rupture of volar plate of specified finger with unspecified laterality at metacarpophalangeal and interphalangeal joint
- ✓7th **S63.439 Traumatic rupture of volar plate of unspecified finger at metacarpophalangeal and interphalangeal joint**

✓6th **S63.49 Traumatic rupture of other ligament of finger at metacarpophalangeal and interphalangeal joint**

- ✓7th **S63.490 Traumatic rupture of other ligament of right index finger at metacarpophalangeal and interphalangeal joint**
- ✓7th **S63.491 Traumatic rupture of other ligament of left index finger at metacarpophalangeal and interphalangeal joint**
- ✓7th **S63.492 Traumatic rupture of other ligament of right middle finger at metacarpophalangeal and interphalangeal joint**
- ✓7th **S63.493 Traumatic rupture of other ligament of left middle finger at metacarpophalangeal and interphalangeal joint**
- ✓7th **S63.494 Traumatic rupture of other ligament of right ring finger at metacarpophalangeal and interphalangeal joint**
- ✓7th **S63.495 Traumatic rupture of other ligament of left ring finger at metacarpophalangeal and interphalangeal joint**
- ✓7th **S63.496 Traumatic rupture of other ligament of right little finger at metacarpophalangeal and interphalangeal joint**
- ✓7th **S63.497 Traumatic rupture of other ligament of left little finger at metacarpophalangeal and interphalangeal joint**
- ✓7th **S63.498 Traumatic rupture of other ligament of other finger at metacarpophalangeal and interphalangeal joint**
  Traumatic rupture of ligament of specified finger with unspecified laterality at metacarpophalangeal and interphalangeal joint
- ✓7th **S63.499 Traumatic rupture of other ligament of unspecified finger at metacarpophalangeal and interphalangeal joint**

✓5th **S63.5 Other and unspecified sprain of wrist**

✓6th **S63.50 Unspecified sprain of wrist**

- ✓7th **S63.501 Unspecified sprain of right wrist**
- ✓7th **S63.502 Unspecified sprain of left wrist**
- ✓7th **S63.509 Unspecified sprain of unspecified wrist**

✓6th **S63.51 Sprain of carpal (joint)**

- ✓7th **S63.511 Sprain of carpal joint of right wrist**
- ✓7th **S63.512 Sprain of carpal joint of left wrist**
- ✓7th **S63.519 Sprain of carpal joint of unspecified wrist**

✓6th **S63.52 Sprain of radiocarpal joint**

EXCLUDES 1 *traumatic rupture of radiocarpal ligament (S63.32-)*

- ✓7th **S63.521 Sprain of radiocarpal joint of right wrist**
- ✓7th **S63.522 Sprain of radiocarpal joint of left wrist**
- ✓7th **S63.529 Sprain of radiocarpal joint of unspecified wrist**

✓6th **S63.59 Other specified sprain of wrist**

- ✓7th **S63.591 Other specified sprain of right wrist**
- ✓7th **S63.592 Other specified sprain of left wrist**
- ✓7th **S63.599 Other specified sprain of unspecified wrist**

✓5th **S63.6 Other and unspecified sprain of finger(s)**

EXCLUDES 1 *traumatic rupture of ligament of finger at metacarpophalangeal and interphalangeal joint(s) (S63.4-)*

✓6th **S63.60 Unspecified sprain of thumb**

- ✓7th **S63.601 Unspecified sprain of right thumb**
- ✓7th **S63.602 Unspecified sprain of left thumb**
- ✓7th **S63.609 Unspecified sprain of unspecified thumb**

✓6th **S63.61 Unspecified sprain of other and unspecified finger(s)**

- ✓7th **S63.610 Unspecified sprain of right index finger**
- ✓7th **S63.611 Unspecified sprain of left index finger**
- ✓7th **S63.612 Unspecified sprain of right middle finger**
- ✓7th **S63.613 Unspecified sprain of left middle finger**
- ✓7th **S63.614 Unspecified sprain of right ring finger**
- ✓7th **S63.615 Unspecified sprain of left ring finger**
- ✓7th **S63.616 Unspecified sprain of right little finger**
- ✓7th **S63.617 Unspecified sprain of left little finger**
- ✓7th **S63.618 Unspecified sprain of other finger**
  Unspecified sprain of specified finger with unspecified laterality
- ✓7th **S63.619 Unspecified sprain of unspecified finger**

✓6th **S63.62 Sprain of interphalangeal joint of thumb**

- ✓7th **S63.621 Sprain of interphalangeal joint of right thumb**
- ✓7th **S63.622 Sprain of interphalangeal joint of left thumb**
- ✓7th **S63.629 Sprain of interphalangeal joint of unspecified thumb**

✓6th **S63.63 Sprain of interphalangeal joint of other and unspecified finger(s)**

- ✓7th **S63.630 Sprain of interphalangeal joint of right index finger**
- ✓7th **S63.631 Sprain of interphalangeal joint of left index finger**
- ✓7th **S63.632 Sprain of interphalangeal joint of right middle finger**
- ✓7th **S63.633 Sprain of interphalangeal joint of left middle finger**
- ✓7th **S63.634 Sprain of interphalangeal joint of right ring finger**
- ✓7th **S63.635 Sprain of interphalangeal joint of left ring finger**
- ✓7th **S63.636 Sprain of interphalangeal joint of right little finger**
- ✓7th **S63.637 Sprain of interphalangeal joint of left little finger**
- ✓7th **S63.638 Sprain of interphalangeal joint of other finger**
- ✓7th **S63.639 Sprain of interphalangeal joint of unspecified finger**

✓6th **S63.64 Sprain of metacarpophalangeal joint of thumb**

- ✓7th **S63.641 Sprain of metacarpophalangeal joint of right thumb**
- ✓7th **S63.642 Sprain of metacarpophalangeal joint of left thumb**

✓7th S63.649 **Sprain of metacarpophalangeal joint of unspecified thumb**

✓6th S63.65 **Sprain of metacarpophalangeal joint of other and unspecified finger(s)**

✓7th S63.65Ø **Sprain of metacarpophalangeal joint of right index finger**

✓7th S63.651 **Sprain of metacarpophalangeal joint of left index finger**

✓7th S63.652 **Sprain of metacarpophalangeal joint of right middle finger**

✓7th S63.653 **Sprain of metacarpophalangeal joint of left middle finger**

✓7th S63.654 **Sprain of metacarpophalangeal joint of right ring finger**

✓7th S63.655 **Sprain of metacarpophalangeal joint of left ring finger**

✓7th S63.656 **Sprain of metacarpophalangeal joint of right little finger**

✓7th S63.657 **Sprain of metacarpophalangeal joint of left little finger**

✓7th S63.658 **Sprain of metacarpophalangeal joint of other finger**
Sprain of metacarpophalangeal joint of specified finger with unspecified laterality

✓7th S63.659 **Sprain of metacarpophalangeal joint of unspecified finger**

✓6th S63.68 **Other sprain of thumb**

✓7th S63.681 **Other sprain of right thumb**

✓7th S63.682 **Other sprain of left thumb**

✓7th S63.689 **Other sprain of unspecified thumb**

✓6th S63.69 **Other sprain of other and unspecified finger(s)**

✓7th S63.69Ø **Other sprain of right index finger**

✓7th S63.691 **Other sprain of left index finger**

✓7th S63.692 **Other sprain of right middle finger**

✓7th S63.693 **Other sprain of left middle finger**

✓7th S63.694 **Other sprain of right ring finger**

✓7th S63.695 **Other sprain of left ring finger**

✓7th S63.696 **Other sprain of right little finger**

✓7th S63.697 **Other sprain of left little finger**

✓7th S63.698 **Other sprain of other finger**
Other sprain of specified finger with unspecified laterality

✓7th S63.699 **Other sprain of unspecified finger**

✓5th S63.8 **Sprain of other part of wrist and hand**

✓6th S63.8X **Sprain of other part of wrist and hand**

✓7th S63.8X1 **Sprain of other part of right wrist and hand**

✓7th S63.8X2 **Sprain of other part of left wrist and hand**

✓7th S63.8X9 **Sprain of other part of unspecified wrist and hand**

✓5th S63.9 **Sprain of unspecified part of wrist and hand**

✓x7th S63.9Ø **Sprain of unspecified part of unspecified wrist and hand**

✓x7th S63.91 **Sprain of unspecified part of right wrist and hand**

✓x7th S63.92 **Sprain of unspecified part of left wrist and hand**

✓4th **S64 Injury of nerves at wrist and hand level**
Code also any associated open wound (S61.-)

> The appropriate 7th character is to be added to each code from category S64.
> A initial encounter
> D subsequent encounter
> S sequela

✓5th S64.Ø **Injury of ulnar nerve at wrist and hand level**

✓x7th S64.ØØ **Injury of ulnar nerve at wrist and hand level of unspecified arm**

✓x7th S64.Ø1 **Injury of ulnar nerve at wrist and hand level of right arm**

✓x7th S64.Ø2 **Injury of ulnar nerve at wrist and hand level of left arm**

✓5th S64.1 **Injury of median nerve at wrist and hand level**

✓x7th S64.1Ø **Injury of median nerve at wrist and hand level of unspecified arm**

✓x7th S64.11 **Injury of median nerve at wrist and hand level of right arm**

✓x7th S64.12 **Injury of median nerve at wrist and hand level of left arm**

✓5th S64.2 **Injury of radial nerve at wrist and hand level**

✓x7th S64.2Ø **Injury of radial nerve at wrist and hand level of unspecified arm**

✓x7th S64.21 **Injury of radial nerve at wrist and hand level of right arm**

✓x7th S64.22 **Injury of radial nerve at wrist and hand level of left arm**

✓5th S64.3 **Injury of digital nerve of thumb**

✓x7th S64.3Ø **Injury of digital nerve of unspecified thumb**

✓x7th S64.31 **Injury of digital nerve of right thumb**

✓x7th S64.32 **Injury of digital nerve of left thumb**

✓5th S64.4 **Injury of digital nerve of other and unspecified finger**

✓x7th S64.4Ø **Injury of digital nerve of unspecified finger**

✓6th S64.49 **Injury of digital nerve of other finger**

✓7th S64.49Ø **Injury of digital nerve of right index finger**

✓7th S64.491 **Injury of digital nerve of left index finger**

✓7th S64.492 **Injury of digital nerve of right middle finger**

✓7th S64.493 **Injury of digital nerve of left middle finger**

✓7th S64.494 **Injury of digital nerve of right ring finger**

✓7th S64.495 **Injury of digital nerve of left ring finger**

✓7th S64.496 **Injury of digital nerve of right little finger**

✓7th S64.497 **Injury of digital nerve of left little finger**

✓7th S64.498 **Injury of digital nerve of other finger**
Injury of digital nerve of specified finger with unspecified laterality

✓5th S64.8 **Injury of other nerves at wrist and hand level**

✓6th S64.8X **Injury of other nerves at wrist and hand level**

✓7th S64.8X1 **Injury of other nerves at wrist and hand level of right arm**

✓7th S64.8X2 **Injury of other nerves at wrist and hand level of left arm**

✓7th S64.8X9 **Injury of other nerves at wrist and hand level of unspecified arm**

✓5th S64.9 **Injury of unspecified nerve at wrist and hand level**

✓x7th S64.9Ø **Injury of unspecified nerve at wrist and hand level of unspecified arm**

✓x7th S64.91 **Injury of unspecified nerve at wrist and hand level of right arm**

✓x7th S64.92 **Injury of unspecified nerve at wrist and hand level of left arm**

✓4th **S65 Injury of blood vessels at wrist and hand level**
Code also any associated open wound (S61.-)

> The appropriate 7th character is to be added to each code from category S65.
> A initial encounter
> D subsequent encounter
> S sequela

✓5th S65.Ø **Injury of ulnar artery at wrist and hand level**

✓6th S65.ØØ **Unspecified injury of ulnar artery at wrist and hand level**

✓7th S65.ØØ1 **Unspecified injury of ulnar artery at wrist and hand level of right arm**

✓7th S65.ØØ2 **Unspecified injury of ulnar artery at wrist and hand level of left arm**

✓7th S65.ØØ9 **Unspecified injury of ulnar artery at wrist and hand level of unspecified arm**

✓6th S65.Ø1 **Laceration of ulnar artery at wrist and hand level**

✓7th S65.Ø11 **Laceration of ulnar artery at wrist and hand level of right arm**

✓7th S65.Ø12 **Laceration of ulnar artery at wrist and hand level of left arm**

✓7th S65.Ø19 **Laceration of ulnar artery at wrist and hand level of unspecified arm**

✓6th **S65.09 Other specified injury of ulnar artery at wrist and hand level**
✓7th **S65.091 Other specified injury of ulnar artery at wrist and hand level of right arm**
✓7th **S65.092 Other specified injury of ulnar artery at wrist and hand level of left arm**
✓7th **S65.099 Other specified injury of ulnar artery at wrist and hand level of unspecified arm**

✓5th **S65.1 Injury of radial artery at wrist and hand level**
✓6th **S65.10 Unspecified injury of radial artery at wrist and hand level**
✓7th **S65.101 Unspecified injury of radial artery at wrist and hand level of right arm**
✓7th **S65.102 Unspecified injury of radial artery at wrist and hand level of left arm**
✓7th **S65.109 Unspecified injury of radial artery at wrist and hand level of unspecified arm**
✓6th **S65.11 Laceration of radial artery at wrist and hand level**
✓7th **S65.111 Laceration of radial artery at wrist and hand level of right arm**
✓7th **S65.112 Laceration of radial artery at wrist and hand level of left arm**
✓7th **S65.119 Laceration of radial artery at wrist and hand level of unspecified arm**
✓6th **S65.19 Other specified injury of radial artery at wrist and hand level**
✓7th **S65.191 Other specified injury of radial artery at wrist and hand level of right arm**
✓7th **S65.192 Other specified injury of radial artery at wrist and hand level of left arm**
✓7th **S65.199 Other specified injury of radial artery at wrist and hand level of unspecified arm**

✓5th **S65.2 Injury of superficial palmar arch**
✓6th **S65.20 Unspecified injury of superficial palmar arch**
✓7th **S65.201 Unspecified injury of superficial palmar arch of right hand**
✓7th **S65.202 Unspecified injury of superficial palmar arch of left hand**
✓7th **S65.209 Unspecified injury of superficial palmar arch of unspecified hand**
✓6th **S65.21 Laceration of superficial palmar arch**
✓7th **S65.211 Laceration of superficial palmar arch of right hand**
✓7th **S65.212 Laceration of superficial palmar arch of left hand**
✓7th **S65.219 Laceration of superficial palmar arch of unspecified hand**
✓6th **S65.29 Other specified injury of superficial palmar arch**
✓7th **S65.291 Other specified injury of superficial palmar arch of right hand**
✓7th **S65.292 Other specified injury of superficial palmar arch of left hand**
✓7th **S65.299 Other specified injury of superficial palmar arch of unspecified hand**

✓5th **S65.3 Injury of deep palmar arch**
✓6th **S65.30 Unspecified injury of deep palmar arch**
✓7th **S65.301 Unspecified injury of deep palmar arch of right hand**
✓7th **S65.302 Unspecified injury of deep palmar arch of left hand**
✓7th **S65.309 Unspecified injury of deep palmar arch of unspecified hand**
✓6th **S65.31 Laceration of deep palmar arch**
✓7th **S65.311 Laceration of deep palmar arch of right hand**
✓7th **S65.312 Laceration of deep palmar arch of left hand**
✓7th **S65.319 Laceration of deep palmar arch of unspecified hand**
✓6th **S65.39 Other specified injury of deep palmar arch**
✓7th **S65.391 Other specified injury of deep palmar arch of right hand**
✓7th **S65.392 Other specified injury of deep palmar arch of left hand**
✓7th **S65.399 Other specified injury of deep palmar arch of unspecified hand**

✓5th **S65.4 Injury of blood vessel of thumb**
✓6th **S65.40 Unspecified injury of blood vessel of thumb**
✓7th **S65.401 Unspecified injury of blood vessel of right thumb**
✓7th **S65.402 Unspecified injury of blood vessel of left thumb**
✓7th **S65.409 Unspecified injury of blood vessel of unspecified thumb**
✓6th **S65.41 Laceration of blood vessel of thumb**
✓7th **S65.411 Laceration of blood vessel of right thumb**
✓7th **S65.412 Laceration of blood vessel of left thumb**
✓7th **S65.419 Laceration of blood vessel of unspecified thumb**
✓6th **S65.49 Other specified injury of blood vessel of thumb**
✓7th **S65.491 Other specified injury of blood vessel of right thumb**
✓7th **S65.492 Other specified injury of blood vessel of left thumb**
✓7th **S65.499 Other specified injury of blood vessel of unspecified thumb**

✓5th **S65.5 Injury of blood vessel of other and unspecified finger**
✓6th **S65.50 Unspecified injury of blood vessel of other and unspecified finger**
✓7th **S65.500 Unspecified injury of blood vessel of right index finger**
✓7th **S65.501 Unspecified injury of blood vessel of left index finger**
✓7th **S65.502 Unspecified injury of blood vessel of right middle finger**
✓7th **S65.503 Unspecified injury of blood vessel of left middle finger**
✓7th **S65.504 Unspecified injury of blood vessel of right ring finger**
✓7th **S65.505 Unspecified injury of blood vessel of left ring finger**
✓7th **S65.506 Unspecified injury of blood vessel of right little finger**
✓7th **S65.507 Unspecified injury of blood vessel of left little finger**
✓7th **S65.508 Unspecified injury of blood vessel of other finger**
Unspecified injury of blood vessel of specified finger with unspecified laterality
✓7th **S65.509 Unspecified injury of blood vessel of unspecified finger**
✓6th **S65.51 Laceration of blood vessel of other and unspecified finger**
✓7th **S65.510 Laceration of blood vessel of right index finger**
✓7th **S65.511 Laceration of blood vessel of left index finger**
✓7th **S65.512 Laceration of blood vessel of right middle finger**
✓7th **S65.513 Laceration of blood vessel of left middle finger**
✓7th **S65.514 Laceration of blood vessel of right ring finger**
✓7th **S65.515 Laceration of blood vessel of left ring finger**
✓7th **S65.516 Laceration of blood vessel of right little finger**
✓7th **S65.517 Laceration of blood vessel of left little finger**
✓7th **S65.518 Laceration of blood vessel of other finger**
Laceration of blood vessel of specified finger with unspecified laterality
✓7th **S65.519 Laceration of blood vessel of unspecified finger**
✓6th **S65.59 Other specified injury of blood vessel of other and unspecified finger**
✓7th **S65.590 Other specified injury of blood vessel of right index finger**
✓7th **S65.591 Other specified injury of blood vessel of left index finger**

S65.592 Other specified injury of blood vessel of right middle finger
S65.593 Other specified injury of blood vessel of left middle finger
S65.594 Other specified injury of blood vessel of right ring finger
S65.595 Other specified injury of blood vessel of left ring finger
S65.596 Other specified injury of blood vessel of right little finger
S65.597 Other specified injury of blood vessel of left little finger
S65.598 Other specified injury of blood vessel of other finger
Other specified injury of blood vessel of specified finger with unspecified laterality
S65.599 Other specified injury of blood vessel of unspecified finger
S65.8 Injury of other blood vessels at wrist and hand level
S65.80 Unspecified injury of other blood vessels at wrist and hand level
S65.801 Unspecified injury of other blood vessels at wrist and hand level of right arm
S65.802 Unspecified injury of other blood vessels at wrist and hand level of left arm
S65.809 Unspecified injury of other blood vessels at wrist and hand level of unspecified arm
S65.81 Laceration of other blood vessels at wrist and hand level
S65.811 Laceration of other blood vessels at wrist and hand level of right arm
S65.812 Laceration of other blood vessels at wrist and hand level of left arm
S65.819 Laceration of other blood vessels at wrist and hand level of unspecified arm
S65.89 Other specified injury of other blood vessels at wrist and hand level
S65.891 Other specified injury of other blood vessels at wrist and hand level of right arm
S65.892 Other specified injury of other blood vessels at wrist and hand level of left arm
S65.899 Other specified injury of other blood vessels at wrist and hand level of unspecified arm
S65.9 Injury of unspecified blood vessel at wrist and hand level
S65.90 Unspecified injury of unspecified blood vessel at wrist and hand level
S65.901 Unspecified injury of unspecified blood vessel at wrist and hand level of right arm
S65.902 Unspecified injury of unspecified blood vessel at wrist and hand level of left arm
S65.909 Unspecified injury of unspecified blood vessel at wrist and hand level of unspecified arm
S65.91 Laceration of unspecified blood vessel at wrist and hand level
S65.911 Laceration of unspecified blood vessel at wrist and hand level of right arm
S65.912 Laceration of unspecified blood vessel at wrist and hand level of left arm
S65.919 Laceration of unspecified blood vessel at wrist and hand level of unspecified arm
S65.99 Other specified injury of unspecified blood vessel at wrist and hand level
S65.991 Other specified injury of unspecified blood vessel at wrist and hand of right arm
S65.992 Other specified injury of unspecified blood vessel at wrist and hand of left arm
S65.999 Other specified injury of unspecified blood vessel at wrist and hand of unspecified arm

S66 Injury of muscle, fascia and tendon at wrist and hand level
Code also any associated open wound (S61.-)
EXCLUDES 2 *sprain of joints and ligaments of wrist and hand (S63.-)*

The appropriate 7th character is to be added to each code from category S66.
A initial encounter
D subsequent encounter
S sequela

S66.0 Injury of long flexor muscle, fascia and tendon of thumb at wrist and hand level
S66.00 Unspecified injury of long flexor muscle, fascia and tendon of thumb at wrist and hand level
S66.001 Unspecified injury of long flexor muscle, fascia and tendon of right thumb at wrist and hand level
S66.002 Unspecified injury of long flexor muscle, fascia and tendon of left thumb at wrist and hand level
S66.009 Unspecified injury of long flexor muscle, fascia and tendon of unspecified thumb at wrist and hand level
S66.01 Strain of long flexor muscle, fascia and tendon of thumb at wrist and hand level
S66.011 Strain of long flexor muscle, fascia and tendon of right thumb at wrist and hand level
S66.012 Strain of long flexor muscle, fascia and tendon of left thumb at wrist and hand level
S66.019 Strain of long flexor muscle, fascia and tendon of unspecified thumb at wrist and hand level
S66.02 Laceration of long flexor muscle, fascia and tendon of thumb at wrist and hand level
S66.021 Laceration of long flexor muscle, fascia and tendon of right thumb at wrist and hand level
S66.022 Laceration of long flexor muscle, fascia and tendon of left thumb at wrist and hand level
S66.029 Laceration of long flexor muscle, fascia and tendon of unspecified thumb at wrist and hand level
S66.09 Other specified injury of long flexor muscle, fascia and tendon of thumb at wrist and hand level
S66.091 Other specified injury of long flexor muscle, fascia and tendon of right thumb at wrist and hand level
S66.092 Other specified injury of long flexor muscle, fascia and tendon of left thumb at wrist and hand level
S66.099 Other specified injury of long flexor muscle, fascia and tendon of unspecified thumb at wrist and hand level
S66.1 Injury of flexor muscle, fascia and tendon of other and unspecified finger at wrist and hand level
EXCLUDES 2 *Injury of long flexor muscle, fascia and tendon of thumb at wrist and hand level (S66.0-)*
S66.10 Unspecified injury of flexor muscle, fascia and tendon of other and unspecified finger at wrist and hand level
S66.100 Unspecified injury of flexor muscle, fascia and tendon of right index finger at wrist and hand level
S66.101 Unspecified injury of flexor muscle, fascia and tendon of left index finger at wrist and hand level
S66.102 Unspecified injury of flexor muscle, fascia and tendon of right middle finger at wrist and hand level
S66.103 Unspecified injury of flexor muscle, fascia and tendon of left middle finger at wrist and hand level

7th **S66.104 Unspecified injury of flexor muscle, fascia and tendon of right ring finger at wrist and hand level**

7th **S66.105 Unspecified injury of flexor muscle, fascia and tendon of left ring finger at wrist and hand level**

7th **S66.106 Unspecified injury of flexor muscle, fascia and tendon of right little finger at wrist and hand level**

7th **S66.107 Unspecified injury of flexor muscle, fascia and tendon of left little finger at wrist and hand level**

7th **S66.108 Unspecified injury of flexor muscle, fascia and tendon of other finger at wrist and hand level**

Unspecified injury of flexor muscle, fascia and tendon of specified finger with unspecified laterality at wrist and hand level

7th **S66.109 Unspecified injury of flexor muscle, fascia and tendon of unspecified finger at wrist and hand level**

6th **S66.11 Strain of flexor muscle, fascia and tendon of other and unspecified finger at wrist and hand level**

7th **S66.110 Strain of flexor muscle, fascia and tendon of right index finger at wrist and hand level**

7th **S66.111 Strain of flexor muscle, fascia and tendon of left index finger at wrist and hand level**

7th **S66.112 Strain of flexor muscle, fascia and tendon of right middle finger at wrist and hand level**

7th **S66.113 Strain of flexor muscle, fascia and tendon of left middle finger at wrist and hand level**

7th **S66.114 Strain of flexor muscle, fascia and tendon of right ring finger at wrist and hand level**

7th **S66.115 Strain of flexor muscle, fascia and tendon of left ring finger at wrist and hand level**

7th **S66.116 Strain of flexor muscle, fascia and tendon of right little finger at wrist and hand level**

7th **S66.117 Strain of flexor muscle, fascia and tendon of left little finger at wrist and hand level**

7th **S66.118 Strain of flexor muscle, fascia and tendon of other finger at wrist and hand level**

Strain of flexor muscle, fascia and tendon of specified finger with unspecified laterality at wrist and hand level

7th **S66.119 Strain of flexor muscle, fascia and tendon of unspecified finger at wrist and hand level**

6th **S66.12 Laceration of flexor muscle, fascia and tendon of other and unspecified finger at wrist and hand level**

7th **S66.120 Laceration of flexor muscle, fascia and tendon of right index finger at wrist and hand level**

7th **S66.121 Laceration of flexor muscle, fascia and tendon of left index finger at wrist and hand level**

7th **S66.122 Laceration of flexor muscle, fascia and tendon of right middle finger at wrist and hand level**

7th **S66.123 Laceration of flexor muscle, fascia and tendon of left middle finger at wrist and hand level**

7th **S66.124 Laceration of flexor muscle, fascia and tendon of right ring finger at wrist and hand level**

7th **S66.125 Laceration of flexor muscle, fascia and tendon of left ring finger at wrist and hand level**

7th **S66.126 Laceration of flexor muscle, fascia and tendon of right little finger at wrist and hand level**

7th **S66.127 Laceration of flexor muscle, fascia and tendon of left little finger at wrist and hand level**

7th **S66.128 Laceration of flexor muscle, fascia and tendon of other finger at wrist and hand level**

Laceration of flexor muscle, fascia and tendon of specified finger with unspecified laterality at wrist and hand level

7th **S66.129 Laceration of flexor muscle, fascia and tendon of unspecified finger at wrist and hand level**

6th **S66.19 Other injury of flexor muscle, fascia and tendon of other and unspecified finger at wrist and hand level**

7th **S66.190 Other injury of flexor muscle, fascia and tendon of right index finger at wrist and hand level**

7th **S66.191 Other injury of flexor muscle, fascia and tendon of left index finger at wrist and hand level**

7th **S66.192 Other injury of flexor muscle, fascia and tendon of right middle finger at wrist and hand level**

7th **S66.193 Other injury of flexor muscle, fascia and tendon of left middle finger at wrist and hand level**

7th **S66.194 Other injury of flexor muscle, fascia and tendon of right ring finger at wrist and hand level**

7th **S66.195 Other injury of flexor muscle, fascia and tendon of left ring finger at wrist and hand level**

7th **S66.196 Other injury of flexor muscle, fascia and tendon of right little finger at wrist and hand level**

7th **S66.197 Other injury of flexor muscle, fascia and tendon of left little finger at wrist and hand level**

7th **S66.198 Other injury of flexor muscle, fascia and tendon of other finger at wrist and hand level**

Other injury of flexor muscle, fascia and tendon of specified finger with unspecified laterality at wrist and hand level

7th **S66.199 Other injury of flexor muscle, fascia and tendon of unspecified finger at wrist and hand level**

5th **S66.2 Injury of extensor muscle, fascia and tendon of thumb at wrist and hand level**

6th **S66.20 Unspecified injury of extensor muscle, fascia and tendon of thumb at wrist and hand level**

7th **S66.201 Unspecified injury of extensor muscle, fascia and tendon of right thumb at wrist and hand level**

7th **S66.202 Unspecified injury of extensor muscle, fascia and tendon of left thumb at wrist and hand level**

7th **S66.209 Unspecified injury of extensor muscle, fascia and tendon of unspecified thumb at wrist and hand level**

6th **S66.21 Strain of extensor muscle, fascia and tendon of thumb at wrist and hand level**

7th **S66.211 Strain of extensor muscle, fascia and tendon of right thumb at wrist and hand level**

7th **S66.212 Strain of extensor muscle, fascia and tendon of left thumb at wrist and hand level**

7th **S66.219 Strain of extensor muscle, fascia and tendon of unspecified thumb at wrist and hand level**

6th **S66.22 Laceration of extensor muscle, fascia and tendon of thumb at wrist and hand level**

✓7th **S66.221 Laceration of extensor muscle, fascia and tendon of right thumb at wrist and hand level**

✓7th **S66.222 Laceration of extensor muscle, fascia and tendon of left thumb at wrist and hand level**

✓7th **S66.229 Laceration of extensor muscle, fascia and tendon of unspecified thumb at wrist and hand level**

✓6th **S66.29 Other specified injury of extensor muscle, fascia and tendon of thumb at wrist and hand level**

✓7th **S66.291 Other specified injury of extensor muscle, fascia and tendon of right thumb at wrist and hand level**

✓7th **S66.292 Other specified injury of extensor muscle, fascia and tendon of left thumb at wrist and hand level**

✓7th **S66.299 Other specified injury of extensor muscle, fascia and tendon of unspecified thumb at wrist and hand level**

✓5th **S66.3 Injury of extensor muscle, fascia and tendon of other and unspecified finger at wrist and hand level**

EXCLUDES 2 *Injury of extensor muscle, fascia and tendon of thumb at wrist and hand level (S66.2-)*

✓6th **S66.30 Unspecified injury of extensor muscle, fascia and tendon of other and unspecified finger at wrist and hand level**

✓7th **S66.300 Unspecified injury of extensor muscle, fascia and tendon of right index finger at wrist and hand level**

✓7th **S66.301 Unspecified injury of extensor muscle, fascia and tendon of left index finger at wrist and hand level**

✓7th **S66.302 Unspecified injury of extensor muscle, fascia and tendon of right middle finger at wrist and hand level**

✓7th **S66.303 Unspecified injury of extensor muscle, fascia and tendon of left middle finger at wrist and hand level**

✓7th **S66.304 Unspecified injury of extensor muscle, fascia and tendon of right ring finger at wrist and hand level**

✓7th **S66.305 Unspecified injury of extensor muscle, fascia and tendon of left ring finger at wrist and hand level**

✓7th **S66.306 Unspecified injury of extensor muscle, fascia and tendon of right little finger at wrist and hand level**

✓7th **S66.307 Unspecified injury of extensor muscle, fascia and tendon of left little finger at wrist and hand level**

✓7th **S66.308 Unspecified injury of extensor muscle, fascia and tendon of other finger at wrist and hand level**

Unspecified injury of extensor muscle, fascia and tendon of specified finger with unspecified laterality at wrist and hand level

✓7th **S66.309 Unspecified injury of extensor muscle, fascia and tendon of unspecified finger at wrist and hand level**

✓6th **S66.31 Strain of extensor muscle, fascia and tendon of other and unspecified finger at wrist and hand level**

✓7th **S66.310 Strain of extensor muscle, fascia and tendon of right index finger at wrist and hand level**

✓7th **S66.311 Strain of extensor muscle, fascia and tendon of left index finger at wrist and hand level**

✓7th **S66.312 Strain of extensor muscle, fascia and tendon of right middle finger at wrist and hand level**

✓7th **S66.313 Strain of extensor muscle, fascia and tendon of left middle finger at wrist and hand level**

✓7th **S66.314 Strain of extensor muscle, fascia and tendon of right ring finger at wrist and hand level**

✓7th **S66.315 Strain of extensor muscle, fascia and tendon of left ring finger at wrist and hand level**

✓7th **S66.316 Strain of extensor muscle, fascia and tendon of right little finger at wrist and hand level**

✓7th **S66.317 Strain of extensor muscle, fascia and tendon of left little finger at wrist and hand level**

✓7th **S66.318 Strain of extensor muscle, fascia and tendon of other finger at wrist and hand level**

Strain of extensor muscle, fascia and tendon of specified finger with unspecified laterality at wrist and hand level

✓7th **S66.319 Strain of extensor muscle, fascia and tendon of unspecified finger at wrist and hand level**

✓6th **S66.32 Laceration of extensor muscle, fascia and tendon of other and unspecified finger at wrist and hand level**

✓7th **S66.320 Laceration of extensor muscle, fascia and tendon of right index finger at wrist and hand level**

✓7th **S66.321 Laceration of extensor muscle, fascia and tendon of left index finger at wrist and hand level**

✓7th **S66.322 Laceration of extensor muscle, fascia and tendon of right middle finger at wrist and hand level**

✓7th **S66.323 Laceration of extensor muscle, fascia and tendon of left middle finger at wrist and hand level**

✓7th **S66.324 Laceration of extensor muscle, fascia and tendon of right ring finger at wrist and hand level**

✓7th **S66.325 Laceration of extensor muscle, fascia and tendon of left ring finger at wrist and hand level**

✓7th **S66.326 Laceration of extensor muscle, fascia and tendon of right little finger at wrist and hand level**

✓7th **S66.327 Laceration of extensor muscle, fascia and tendon of left little finger at wrist and hand level**

✓7th **S66.328 Laceration of extensor muscle, fascia and tendon of other finger at wrist and hand level**

Laceration of extensor muscle, fascia and tendon of specified finger with unspecified laterality at wrist and hand level

✓7th **S66.329 Laceration of extensor muscle, fascia and tendon of unspecified finger at wrist and hand level**

✓6th **S66.39 Other injury of extensor muscle, fascia and tendon of other and unspecified finger at wrist and hand level**

✓7th **S66.390 Other injury of extensor muscle, fascia and tendon of right index finger at wrist and hand level**

✓7th **S66.391 Other injury of extensor muscle, fascia and tendon of left index finger at wrist and hand level**

✓7th **S66.392 Other injury of extensor muscle, fascia and tendon of right middle finger at wrist and hand level**

✓7th **S66.393 Other injury of extensor muscle, fascia and tendon of left middle finger at wrist and hand level**

✓7th **S66.394 Other injury of extensor muscle, fascia and tendon of right ring finger at wrist and hand level**

✓7th **S66.395 Other injury of extensor muscle, fascia and tendon of left ring finger at wrist and hand level**

√7th **S66.396 Other injury of extensor muscle, fascia and tendon of right little finger at wrist and hand level**

√7th **S66.397 Other injury of extensor muscle, fascia and tendon of left little finger at wrist and hand level**

√7th **S66.398 Other injury of extensor muscle, fascia and tendon of other finger at wrist and hand level**

Other injury of extensor muscle, fascia and tendon of specified finger with unspecified laterality at wrist and hand level

√7th **S66.399 Other injury of extensor muscle, fascia and tendon of unspecified finger at wrist and hand level**

√5th **S66.4 Injury of intrinsic muscle, fascia and tendon of thumb at wrist and hand level**

√6th **S66.40 Unspecified injury of intrinsic muscle, fascia and tendon of thumb at wrist and hand level**

√7th **S66.401 Unspecified injury of intrinsic muscle, fascia and tendon of right thumb at wrist and hand level**

√7th **S66.402 Unspecified injury of intrinsic muscle, fascia and tendon of left thumb at wrist and hand level**

√7th **S66.409 Unspecified injury of intrinsic muscle, fascia and tendon of unspecified thumb at wrist and hand level**

√6th **S66.41 Strain of intrinsic muscle, fascia and tendon of thumb at wrist and hand level**

√7th **S66.411 Strain of intrinsic muscle, fascia and tendon of right thumb at wrist and hand level**

√7th **S66.412 Strain of intrinsic muscle, fascia and tendon of left thumb at wrist and hand level**

√7th **S66.419 Strain of intrinsic muscle, fascia and tendon of unspecified thumb at wrist and hand level**

√6th **S66.42 Laceration of intrinsic muscle, fascia and tendon of thumb at wrist and hand level**

√7th **S66.421 Laceration of intrinsic muscle, fascia and tendon of right thumb at wrist and hand level**

√7th **S66.422 Laceration of intrinsic muscle, fascia and tendon of left thumb at wrist and hand**

√7th **S66.429 Laceration of intrinsic muscle, fascia and tendon of unspecified thumb at wrist and hand level of side**

√6th **S66.49 Other specified injury of intrinsic muscle, fascia and tendon of thumb at wrist and hand level**

√7th **S66.491 Other specified injury of intrinsic muscle, fascia and tendon of right thumb at wrist and hand level**

√7th **S66.492 Other specified injury of intrinsic muscle, fascia and tendon of left thumb at wrist and hand level**

√7th **S66.499 Other specified injury of intrinsic muscle, fascia and tendon of unspecified thumb at wrist and hand level**

√5th **S66.5 Injury of intrinsic muscle, fascia and tendon of other and unspecified finger at wrist and hand level**

EXCLUDES 2 *injury of intrinsic muscle, fascia and tendon of thumb at wrist and hand level (S66.4-)*

√6th **S66.50 Unspecified injury of intrinsic muscle, fascia and tendon of other and unspecified finger at wrist and hand level**

√7th **S66.500 Unspecified injury of intrinsic muscle, fascia and tendon of right index finger at wrist and hand level**

√7th **S66.501 Unspecified injury of intrinsic muscle, fascia and tendon of left index finger at wrist and hand level**

√7th **S66.502 Unspecified injury of intrinsic muscle, fascia and tendon of right middle finger at wrist and hand level**

√7th **S66.503 Unspecified injury of intrinsic muscle, fascia and tendon of left middle finger at wrist and hand level**

√7th **S66.504 Unspecified injury of intrinsic muscle, fascia and tendon of right ring finger at wrist and hand level**

√7th **S66.505 Unspecified injury of intrinsic muscle, fascia and tendon of left ring finger at wrist and hand level**

√7th **S66.506 Unspecified injury of intrinsic muscle, fascia and tendon of right little finger at wrist and hand level**

√7th **S66.507 Unspecified injury of intrinsic muscle, fascia and tendon of left little finger at wrist and hand level**

√7th **S66.508 Unspecified injury of intrinsic muscle, fascia and tendon of other finger at wrist and hand level**

Unspecified injury of intrinsic muscle, fascia and tendon of specified finger with unspecified laterality at wrist and hand level

√7th **S66.509 Unspecified injury of intrinsic muscle, fascia and tendon of unspecified finger at wrist and hand level**

√6th **S66.51 Strain of intrinsic muscle, fascia and tendon of other and unspecified finger at wrist and hand level**

√7th **S66.510 Strain of intrinsic muscle, fascia and tendon of right index finger at wrist and hand level**

√7th **S66.511 Strain of intrinsic muscle, fascia and tendon of left index finger at wrist and hand level**

√7th **S66.512 Strain of intrinsic muscle, fascia and tendon of right middle finger at wrist and hand level**

√7th **S66.513 Strain of intrinsic muscle, fascia and tendon of left middle finger at wrist and hand level**

√7th **S66.514 Strain of intrinsic muscle, fascia and tendon of right ring finger at wrist and hand level**

√7th **S66.515 Strain of intrinsic muscle, fascia and tendon of left ring finger at wrist and hand level**

√7th **S66.516 Strain of intrinsic muscle, fascia and tendon of right little finger at wrist and hand level**

√7th **S66.517 Strain of intrinsic muscle, fascia and tendon of left little finger at wrist and hand level**

√7th **S66.518 Strain of intrinsic muscle, fascia and tendon of other finger at wrist and hand level**

Strain of intrinsic muscle, fascia and tendon of specified finger with unspecified laterality at wrist and hand level

√7th **S66.519 Strain of intrinsic muscle, fascia and tendon of unspecified finger at wrist and hand level**

√6th **S66.52 Laceration of intrinsic muscle, fascia and tendon of other and unspecified finger at wrist and hand level**

√7th **S66.520 Laceration of intrinsic muscle, fascia and tendon of right index finger at wrist and hand level**

√7th **S66.521 Laceration of intrinsic muscle, fascia and tendon of left index finger at wrist and hand level**

√7th **S66.522 Laceration of intrinsic muscle, fascia and tendon of right middle finger at wrist and hand level**

√7th **S66.523 Laceration of intrinsic muscle, fascia and tendon of left middle finger at wrist and hand level**

S66.524 Laceration of intrinsic muscle, fascia and tendon of right ring finger at wrist and hand level

S66.525 Laceration of intrinsic muscle, fascia and tendon of left ring finger at wrist and hand level

S66.526 Laceration of intrinsic muscle, fascia and tendon of right little finger at wrist and hand level

S66.527 Laceration of intrinsic muscle, fascia and tendon of left little finger at wrist and hand level

S66.528 Laceration of intrinsic muscle, fascia and tendon of other finger at wrist and hand level

Laceration of intrinsic muscle, fascia and tendon of specified finger with unspecified laterality at wrist and hand level

S66.529 Laceration of intrinsic muscle, fascia and tendon of unspecified finger at wrist and hand level

S66.59 Other injury of intrinsic muscle, fascia and tendon of other and unspecified finger at wrist and hand level

S66.590 Other injury of intrinsic muscle, fascia and tendon of right index finger at wrist and hand level

S66.591 Other injury of intrinsic muscle, fascia and tendon of left index finger at wrist and hand level

S66.592 Other injury of intrinsic muscle, fascia and tendon of right middle finger at wrist and hand level

S66.593 Other injury of intrinsic muscle, fascia and tendon of left middle finger at wrist and hand level

S66.594 Other injury of intrinsic muscle, fascia and tendon of right ring finger at wrist and hand level

S66.595 Other injury of intrinsic muscle, fascia and tendon of left ring finger at wrist and hand level

S66.596 Other injury of intrinsic muscle, fascia and tendon of right little finger at wrist and hand level

S66.597 Other injury of intrinsic muscle, fascia and tendon of left little finger at wrist and hand level

S66.598 Other injury of intrinsic muscle, fascia and tendon of other finger at wrist and hand level

Other injury of intrinsic muscle, fascia and tendon of specified finger with unspecified laterality at wrist and hand level

S66.599 Other injury of intrinsic muscle, fascia and tendon of unspecified finger at wrist and hand level

S66.8 Injury of other specified muscles, fascia and tendons at wrist and hand level

S66.80 Unspecified injury of other specified muscles, fascia and tendons at wrist and hand level

S66.801 Unspecified injury of other specified muscles, fascia and tendons at wrist and hand level, right hand

S66.802 Unspecified injury of other specified muscles, fascia and tendons at wrist and hand level, left hand

S66.809 Unspecified injury of other specified muscles, fascia and tendons at wrist and hand level, unspecified hand

S66.81 Strain of other specified muscles, fascia and tendons at wrist and hand level

S66.811 Strain of other specified muscles, fascia and tendons at wrist and hand level, right hand

S66.812 Strain of other specified muscles, fascia and tendons at wrist and hand level, left hand

S66.819 Strain of other specified muscles, fascia and tendons at wrist and hand level, unspecified hand

S66.82 Laceration of other specified muscles, fascia and tendons at wrist and hand level

S66.821 Laceration of other specifed muscles, fascia and tendons at wrist and hand level, right hand

S66.822 Laceration of other specified muscles, fascia and tendons at wrist and hand level, left hand

S66.829 Laceration of other specified muscles, fascia and tendons at wrist and hand level, unspecified hand

S66.89 Other injury of other specified muscles, fascia and tendons at wrist and hand level

S66.891 Other injury of other specified muscles, fascia and tendons at wrist and hand level, right hand

S66.892 Other injury of other specified muscles, fascia and tendons at wrist and hand level, left hand

S66.899 Other injury of other specified muscles, fascia and tendons at wrist and hand level, unspecified hand

S66.9 Injury of unspecified muscle, fascia and tendon at wrist and hand level

S66.90 Unspecified injury of unspecified muscle, fascia and tendon at wrist and hand level

S66.901 Unspecified injury of unspecified muscle, fascia and tendon at wrist and hand level, right hand

S66.902 Unspecified injury of unspecified muscle, fascia and tendon at wrist and hand level, left hand

S66.909 Unspecified injury of unspecified muscle, fascia and tendon at wrist and hand level, unspecified hand

S66.91 Strain of unspecified muscle, fascia and tendon at wrist and hand level

S66.911 Strain of unspecified muscle, fascia and tendon at wrist and hand level, right hand

S66.912 Strain of unspecified muscle, fascia and tendon at wrist and hand level, left hand

S66.919 Strain of unspecified muscle, fascia and tendon at wrist and hand level, unspecified hand

S66.92 Laceration of unspecified muscle, fascia and tendon at wrist and hand level

S66.921 Laceration of unspecified muscle, fascia and tendon at wrist and hand level, right hand

S66.922 Laceration of unspecified muscle, fascia and tendon at wrist and hand level, left hand

S66.929 Laceration of unspecified muscle, fascia and tendon at wrist and hand level, unspecified hand

S66.99 Other injury of unspecified muscle, fascia and tendon at wrist and hand level

S66.991 Other injury of unspecified muscle, fascia and tendon at wrist and hand level, right hand

S66.992 Other injury of unspecified muscle, fascia and tendon at wrist and hand level, left hand

S66.999 Other injury of unspecified muscle, fascia and tendon at wrist and hand level, unspecified hand

S67 Crushing injury of wrist, hand and fingers
Use additional code for all associated injuries, such as:
fracture of wrist and hand (S62.-)
open wound of wrist and hand (S61.-)

The appropriate 7th character is to be added to each code from category S67.
A initial encounter
D subsequent encounter
S sequela

S67.0 Crushing injury of thumb
S67.00 Crushing injury of unspecified thumb
S67.01 Crushing injury of right thumb
S67.02 Crushing injury of left thumb
S67.1 Crushing injury of other and unspecified finger(s)
EXCLUDES 2 *crushing injury of thumb (S67.0-)*
S67.10 Crushing injury of unspecified finger(s)
S67.19 Crushing injury of other finger(s)
S67.190 Crushing injury of right index finger
S67.191 Crushing injury of left index finger
S67.192 Crushing injury of right middle finger
S67.193 Crushing injury of left middle finger
S67.194 Crushing injury of right ring finger
S67.195 Crushing injury of left ring finger
S67.196 Crushing injury of right little finger
S67.197 Crushing injury of left little finger
S67.198 Crushing injury of other finger
Crushing injury of specified finger with unspecified laterality
S67.2 Crushing injury of hand
EXCLUDES 2 *crushing injury of fingers (S67.1-)*
crushing injury of thumb (S67.0-)
S67.20 Crushing injury of unspecified hand
S67.21 Crushing injury of right hand
S67.22 Crushing injury of left hand
S67.3 Crushing injury of wrist
S67.30 Crushing injury of unspecified wrist
S67.31 Crushing injury of right wrist
S67.32 Crushing injury of left wrist
S67.4 Crushing injury of wrist and hand
EXCLUDES 1 *crushing injury of hand alone (S67.2-)*
crushing injury of wrist alone (S67.3-)
EXCLUDES 2 *crushing injury of fingers (S67.1-)*
crushing injury of thumb (S67.0-)
S67.40 Crushing injury of unspecified wrist and hand
S67.41 Crushing injury of right wrist and hand
S67.42 Crushing injury of left wrist and hand
S67.9 Crushing injury of unspecified part(s) of wrist, hand and fingers
S67.90 Crushing injury of unspecified part(s) of unspecified wrist, hand and fingers
S67.91 Crushing injury of unspecified part(s) of right wrist, hand and fingers
S67.92 Crushing injury of unspecified part(s) of left wrist, hand and fingers

S68 Traumatic amputation of wrist, hand and fingers
NOTE An amputation not identified as partial or complete should be coded to complete

The appropriate 7th character is to be added to each code from category S68.
A initial encounter
D subsequent encounter
S sequela

S68.0 Traumatic metacarpophalangeal amputation of thumb
Traumatic amputation of thumb NOS
S68.01 Complete traumatic metacarpophalangeal amputation of thumb
S68.011 Complete traumatic metacarpophalangeal amputation of right thumb
S68.012 Complete traumatic metacarpophalangeal amputation of left thumb
S68.019 Complete traumatic metacarpophalangeal amputation of unspecified thumb
S68.02 Partial traumatic metacarpophalangeal amputation of thumb
S68.021 Partial traumatic metacarpophalangeal amputation of right thumb
S68.022 Partial traumatic metacarpophalangeal amputation of left thumb
S68.029 Partial traumatic metacarpophalangeal amputation of unspecified thumb
S68.1 Traumatic metacarpophalangeal amputation of other and unspecified finger
Traumatic amputation of finger NOS
EXCLUDES 2 *traumatic metacarpophalangeal amputation of thumb (S68.0-)*
S68.11 Complete traumatic metacarpophalangeal amputation of other and unspecified finger
S68.110 Complete traumatic metacarpophalangeal amputation of right index finger
S68.111 Complete traumatic metacarpophalangeal amputation of left index finger
S68.112 Complete traumatic metacarpophalangeal amputation of right middle finger
S68.113 Complete traumatic metacarpophalangeal amputation of left middle finger
S68.114 Complete traumatic metacarpophalangeal amputation of right ring finger
S68.115 Complete traumatic metacarpophalangeal amputation of left ring finger
S68.116 Complete traumatic metacarpophalangeal amputation of right little finger
S68.117 Complete traumatic metacarpophalangeal amputation of left little finger
S68.118 Complete traumatic metacarpophalangeal amputation of other finger
Complete traumatic metacarpophalangeal amputation of specified finger with unspecified laterality
S68.119 Complete traumatic metacarpophalangeal amputation of unspecified finger
S68.12 Partial traumatic metacarpophalangeal amputation of other and unspecified finger
S68.120 Partial traumatic metacarpophalangeal amputation of right index finger
S68.121 Partial traumatic metacarpophalangeal amputation of left index finger
S68.122 Partial traumatic metacarpophalangeal amputation of right middle finger
S68.123 Partial traumatic metacarpophalangeal amputation of left middle finger
S68.124 Partial traumatic metacarpophalangeal amputation of right ring finger
S68.125 Partial traumatic metacarpophalangeal amputation of left ring finger
S68.126 Partial traumatic metacarpophalangeal amputation of right little finger
S68.127 Partial traumatic metacarpophalangeal amputation of left little finger
S68.128 Partial traumatic metacarpophalangeal amputation of other finger
Partial traumatic metacarpophalangeal amputation of specified finger with unspecified laterality
S68.129 Partial traumatic metacarpophalangeal amputation of unspecified finger

✓5th **S68.4 Traumatic amputation of hand at wrist level**
Traumatic amputation of hand NOS
Traumatic amputation of wrist
✓6th **S68.41 Complete traumatic amputation of hand at wrist level**
✓7th **S68.411 Complete traumatic amputation of right hand at wrist level**
✓7th **S68.412 Complete traumatic amputation of left hand at wrist level**
✓7th **S68.419 Complete traumatic amputation of unspecified hand at wrist level**
✓6th **S68.42 Partial traumatic amputation of hand at wrist level**
✓7th **S68.421 Partial traumatic amputation of right hand at wrist level**
✓7th **S68.422 Partial traumatic amputation of left hand at wrist level**
✓7th **S68.429 Partial traumatic amputation of unspecified hand at wrist level**
S68.5 Traumatic transphalangeal amputation of thumb
Traumatic interphalangeal joint amputation of thumb
✓6th **S68.51 Complete traumatic transphalangeal amputation of thumb**
✓7th **S68.511 Complete traumatic transphalangeal amputation of right thumb**
✓7th **S68.512 Complete traumatic transphalangeal amputation of left thumb**
✓7th **S68.519 Complete traumatic transphalangeal amputation of unspecified thumb**
✓6th **S68.52 Partial traumatic transphalangeal amputation of thumb**
✓7th **S68.521 Partial traumatic transphalangeal amputation of right thumb**
✓7th **S68.522 Partial traumatic transphalangeal amputation of left thumb**
✓7th **S68.529 Partial traumatic transphalangeal amputation of unspecified thumb**
✓5th **S68.6 Traumatic transphalangeal amputation of other and unspecified finger**
✓6th **S68.61 Complete traumatic transphalangeal amputation of other and unspecified finger(s)**
✓7th **S68.610 Complete traumatic transphalangeal amputation of right index finger**
✓7th **S68.611 Complete traumatic transphalangeal amputation of left index finger**
✓7th **S68.612 Complete traumatic transphalangeal amputation of right middle finger**
✓7th **S68.613 Complete traumatic transphalangeal amputation of left middle finger**
✓7th **S68.614 Complete traumatic transphalangeal amputation of right ring finger**
✓7th **S68.615 Complete traumatic transphalangeal amputation of left ring finger**
✓7th **S68.616 Complete traumatic transphalangeal amputation of right little finger**
✓7th **S68.617 Complete traumatic transphalangeal amputation of left little finger**
✓7th **S68.618 Complete traumatic transphalangeal amputation of other finger**
Complete traumatic transphalangeal amputation of specified finger with unspecified laterality
✓7th **S68.619 Complete traumatic transphalangeal amputation of unspecified finger**
✓6th **S68.62 Partial traumatic transphalangeal amputation of other and unspecified finger**
✓7th **S68.620 Partial traumatic transphalangeal amputation of right index finger**
✓7th **S68.621 Partial traumatic transphalangeal amputation of left index finger**
✓7th **S68.622 Partial traumatic transphalangeal amputation of right middle finger**
✓7th **S68.623 Partial traumatic transphalangeal amputation of left middle finger**
✓7th **S68.624 Partial traumatic transphalangeal amputation of right ring finger**
✓7th **S68.625 Partial traumatic transphalangeal amputation of left ring finger**
✓7th **S68.626 Partial traumatic transphalangeal amputation of right little finger**
✓7th **S68.627 Partial traumatic transphalangeal amputation of left little finger**
✓7th **S68.628 Partial traumatic transphalangeal amputation of other finger**
Partial traumatic transphalangeal amputation of specified finger with unspecified laterality
✓7th **S68.629 Partial traumatic transphalangeal amputation of unspecified finger**
✓5th **S68.7 Traumatic transmetacarpal amputation of hand**
✓6th **S68.71 Complete traumatic transmetacarpal amputation of hand**
✓7th **S68.711 Complete traumatic transmetacarpal amputation of right hand**
✓7th **S68.712 Complete traumatic transmetacarpal amputation of left hand**
✓7th **S68.719 Complete traumatic transmetacarpal amputation of unspecified hand**
✓6th **S68.72 Partial traumatic transmetacarpal amputation of hand**
✓7th **S68.721 Partial traumatic transmetacarpal amputation of right hand**
✓7th **S68.722 Partial traumatic transmetacarpal amputation of left hand**
✓7th **S68.729 Partial traumatic transmetacarpal amputation of unspecified hand**

✓4th **S69 Other and unspecified injuries of wrist, hand and finger(s)**

The appropriate 7th character is to be added to each code from category S69.
A initial encounter
D subsequent encounter
S sequela

✓5th **S69.8 Other specified injuries of wrist, hand and finger(s)**
✓x7th **S69.80 Other specified injuries of unspecified wrist, hand and finger(s)**
✓x7th **S69.81 Other specified injuries of right wrist, hand and finger(s)**
✓x7th **S69.82 Other specified injuries of left wrist, hand and finger(s)**
✓5th **S69.9 Unspecified injury of wrist, hand and finger(s)**
✓x7th **S69.90 Unspecified injury of unspecified wrist, hand and finger(s)**
✓x7th **S69.91 Unspecified injury of right wrist, hand and finger(s)**
✓x7th **S69.92 Unspecified injury of left wrist, hand and finger(s)**

Injuries to the hip and thigh (S70-S79)

EXCLUDES 2 *burns and corrosions (T20-T32)*
frostbite (T33-T34)
snake bite (T63.0-)
venomous insect bite or sting (T63.4-)

✓4th **S70 Superficial injury of hip and thigh**

The appropriate 7th character is to be added to each code from category S70.
A initial encounter
D subsequent encounter
S sequela

✓5th **S70.0 Contusion of hip**
✓x7th **S70.00 Contusion of unspecified hip**
✓x7th **S70.01 Contusion of right hip**
✓x7th **S70.02 Contusion of left hip**
✓5th **S70.1 Contusion of thigh**
✓x7th **S70.10 Contusion of unspecified thigh**
✓x7th **S70.11 Contusion of right thigh**
✓x7th **S70.12 Contusion of left thigh**
✓5th **S70.2 Other superficial injuries of hip**
✓6th **S70.21 Abrasion of hip**
✓7th **S70.211 Abrasion, right hip**
✓7th **S70.212 Abrasion, left hip**
✓7th **S70.219 Abrasion, unspecified hip**
✓6th **S70.22 Blister (nonthermal) of hip**
✓7th **S70.221 Blister (nonthermal), right hip**

✓ Appropriate additional character required ✓x7th Requires 7th character, placeholder x must fill empty characters

√7th **S70.222 Blister (nonthermal), left hip**
√7th **S70.229 Blister (nonthermal), unspecified hip**
√6th **S70.24 External constriction of hip**
√7th **S70.241 External constriction, right hip**
√7th **S70.242 External constriction, left hip**
√7th **S70.249 External constriction, unspecified hip**
√6th **S70.25 Superficial foreign body of hip**
Splinter in the hip
√7th **S70.251 Superficial foreign body, right hip**
√7th **S70.252 Superficial foreign body, left hip**
√7th **S70.259 Superficial foreign body, unspecified hip**
√6th **S70.26 Insect bite (nonvenomous) of hip**
√7th **S70.261 Insect bite (nonvenomous), right hip**
√7th **S70.262 Insect bite (nonvenomous), left hip**
√7th **S70.269 Insect bite (nonvenomous), unspecified hip**
√6th **S70.27 Other superficial bite of hip**
EXCLUDES 1 *open bite of hip (S71.05-)*
√7th **S70.271 Other superficial bite of hip, right hip**
√7th **S70.272 Other superficial bite of hip, left hip**
√7th **S70.279 Other superficial bite of hip, unspecified hip**
√5th **S70.3 Other superficial injuries of thigh**
√6th **S70.31 Abrasion of thigh**
√7th **S70.311 Abrasion, right thigh**
√7th **S70.312 Abrasion, left thigh**
√7th **S70.319 Abrasion, unspecified thigh**
√6th **S70.32 Blister (nonthermal) of thigh**
√7th **S70.321 Blister (nonthermal), right thigh**
√7th **S70.322 Blister (nonthermal), left thigh**
√7th **S70.329 Blister (nonthermal), unspecified thigh**
√6th **S70.34 External constriction of thigh**
√7th **S70.341 External constriction, right thigh**
√7th **S70.342 External constriction, left thigh**
√7th **S70.349 External constriction, unspecified thigh**
√6th **S70.35 Superficial foreign body of thigh**
Splinter in the thigh
√7th **S70.351 Superficial foreign body, right thigh**
√7th **S70.352 Superficial foreign body, left thigh**
√7th **S70.359 Superficial foreign body, unspecified thigh**
√6th **S70.36 Insect bite (nonvenomous) of thigh**
√7th **S70.361 Insect bite (nonvenomous), right thigh**
√7th **S70.362 Insect bite (nonvenomous), left thigh**
√7th **S70.369 Insect bite (nonvenomous), unspecified thigh**
√6th **S70.37 Other superficial bite of thigh**
EXCLUDES 1 *open bite of thigh (S71.15)*
√7th **S70.371 Other superficial bite of right thigh**
√7th **S70.372 Other superficial bite of left thigh**
√7th **S70.379 Other superficial bite of unspecified thigh**
√5th **S70.9 Unspecified superficial injury of hip and thigh**
√6th **S70.91 Unspecified superficial injury of hip**
√7th **S70.911 Unspecified superficial injury of right hip**
√7th **S70.912 Unspecified superficial injury of left hip**
√7th **S70.919 Unspecified superficial injury of unspecified hip**
√6th **S70.92 Unspecified superficial injury of thigh**
√7th **S70.921 Unspecified superficial injury of right thigh**
√7th **S70.922 Unspecified superficial injury of left thigh**
√7th **S70.929 Unspecified superficial injury of unspecified thigh**

√4th **S71 Open wound of hip and thigh**
Code also any associated wound infection
EXCLUDES 1 *open fracture of hip and thigh (S72.-)*
traumatic amputation of hip and thigh (S78.-)
EXCLUDES 2 *bite of venomous animal (T63.-)*
open wound of ankle, foot and toes (S91.-)
open wound of knee and lower leg (S81.-)

The appropriate 7th character is to be added to each code from category S71.
A initial encounter
D subsequent encounter
S sequela

√5th **S71.0 Open wound of hip**
√6th **S71.00 Unspecified open wound of hip**
√7th **S71.001 Unspecified open wound, right hip**
√7th **S71.002 Unspecified open wound, left hip**
√7th **S71.009 Unspecified open wound, unspecified hip**
√6th **S71.01 Laceration without foreign body of hip**
√7th **S71.011 Laceration without foreign body, right hip**
√7th **S71.012 Laceration without foreign body, left hip**
√7th **S71.019 Laceration without foreign body, unspecified hip**
√6th **S71.02 Laceration with foreign body of hip**
√7th **S71.021 Laceration with foreign body, right hip**
√7th **S71.022 Laceration with foreign body, left hip**
√7th **S71.029 Laceration with foreign body, unspecified hip**
√6th **S71.03 Puncture wound without foreign body of hip**
√7th **S71.031 Puncture wound without foreign body, right hip**
√7th **S71.032 Puncture wound without foreign body, left hip**
√7th **S71.039 Puncture wound without foreign body, unspecified hip**
√6th **S71.04 Puncture wound with foreign body of hip**
√7th **S71.041 Puncture wound with foreign body, right hip**
√7th **S71.042 Puncture wound with foreign body, left hip**
√7th **S71.049 Puncture wound with foreign body, unspecified hip**
√6th **S71.05 Open bite of hip**
Bite of hip NOS
EXCLUDES 1 *superficial bite of hip (S70.26, S70.27)*
√7th **S71.051 Open bite, right hip**
√7th **S71.052 Open bite, left hip**
√7th **S71.059 Open bite, unspecified hip**
√5th **S71.1 Open wound of thigh**
√6th **S71.10 Unspecified open wound of thigh**
√7th **S71.101 Unspecified open wound, right thigh**
√7th **S71.102 Unspecified open wound, left thigh**
√7th **S71.109 Unspecified open wound, unspecified thigh**
√6th **S71.11 Laceration without foreign body of thigh**
√7th **S71.111 Laceration without foreign body, right thigh**
√7th **S71.112 Laceration without foreign body, left thigh**
√7th **S71.119 Laceration without foreign body, unspecified thigh**
√6th **S71.12 Laceration with foreign body of thigh**
√7th **S71.121 Laceration with foreign body, right thigh**
√7th **S71.122 Laceration with foreign body, left thigh**
√7th **S71.129 Laceration with foreign body, unspecified thigh**
√6th **S71.13 Puncture wound without foreign body of thigh**
√7th **S71.131 Puncture wound without foreign body, right thigh**
√7th **S71.132 Puncture wound without foreign body, left thigh**

S71.139 Puncture wound without foreign body, unspecified thigh

S71.14 Puncture wound with foreign body of thigh

S71.141 Puncture wound with foreign body, right thigh

S71.142 Puncture wound with foreign body, left thigh

S71.149 Puncture wound with foreign body, unspecified thigh

S71.15 Open bite of thigh

Bite of thigh NOS

EXCLUDES 1 *superficial bite of thigh (S70.37-)*

S71.151 Open bite, right thigh

S71.152 Open bite, left thigh

S71.159 Open bite, unspecified thigh

S72 Fracture of femur

NOTE A fracture not indicated as displaced or nondisplaced should be coded to displaced

The open fracture designations are based on the Gustilo open fracture classification A fracture not indicated as open or closed should be coded to closed

EXCLUDES 1 *traumatic amputation of hip and thigh (S78.-)*

EXCLUDES 2 *fracture of lower leg and ankle (S82.-)*

fracture of foot (S92.-)

periprosthetic fracture of prosthetic implant of hip (T84.040, T84.041)

The appropriate 7th character is to be added to all codes from category S72 [unless otherwise indicated].

- A initial encounter for closed fracture
- B initial encounter for open fracture type I or II
  initial encounter for open fracture NOS
- C initial encounter for open fracture type IIIA, IIIB, or IIIC
- D subsequent encounter for closed fracture with routine healing
- E subsequent encounter for open fracture type I or II with routine healing
- F subsequent encounter for open fracture type IIIA, IIIB, or IIIC with routine healing
- G subsequent encounter for closed fracture with delayed healing
- H subsequent encounter for open fracture type I or II with delayed healing
- J subsequent encounter for open fracture type IIIA, IIIB, or IIIC with delayed healing
- K subsequent encounter for closed fracture with nonunion
- M subsequent encounter for open fracture type I or I with nonunion
- N subsequent encounter for open fracture type IIIA, IIIB, or IIIC with nonunion
- P subsequent encounter for closed fracture with malunion
- Q subsequent encounter for open fracture type I or II with malunion
- R subsequent encounter for open fracture type IIIA, IIIB, or IIIC with malunion
- S sequela

S72.0 Fracture of head and neck of femur

EXCLUDES 2 *physeal fracture of upper end of femur (S79.0-)*

S72.00 Fracture of unspecified part of neck of femur

Fracture of hip NOS

Fracture of neck of femur NOS

S72.001 Fracture of unspecified part of neck of right femur

S72.002 Fracture of unspecified part of neck of left femur

S72.009 Fracture of unspecified part of neck of unspecified femur

S72.01 Unspecified intracapsular fracture of femur

Subcapital fracture of femur

S72.011 Unspecified intracapsular fracture of right femur

S72.012 Unspecified intracapsular fracture of left femur

S72.019 Unspecified intracapsular fracture of unspecified femur

S72.02 Fracture of epiphysis (separation) (upper) of femur

Transepiphyseal fracture of femur

EXCLUDES 1 *capital femoral epiphyseal fracture (pediatric) of femur (S79.01-)*

Salter-Harris Type I physeal fracture of upper end of femur (S79.01-)

S72.021 Displaced fracture of epiphysis (separation) (upper) of right femur

S72.022 Displaced fracture of epiphysis (separation) (upper) of left femur

S72.023 Displaced fracture of epiphysis (separation) (upper) of unspecified femur

S72.024 Nondisplaced fracture of epiphysis (separation) (upper) of right femur

S72.025 Nondisplaced fracture of epiphysis (separation) (upper) of left femur

S72.026 Nondisplaced fracture of epiphysis (separation) (upper) of unspecified femur

S72.03 Midcervical fracture of femur

Transcervical fracture of femur NOS

S72.031 Displaced midcervical fracture of right femur

S72.032 Displaced midcervical fracture of left femur

S72.033 Displaced midcervical fracture of unspecified femur

S72.034 Nondisplaced midcervical fracture of right femur

S72.035 Nondisplaced midcervical fracture of left femur

S72.036 Nondisplaced midcervical fracture of unspecified femur

S72.04 Fracture of base of neck of femur

Cervicotrochanteric fracture of femur

S72.041 Displaced fracture of base of neck of right femur

S72.042 Displaced fracture of base of neck of left femur

S72.043 Displaced fracture of base of neck of unspecified femur

S72.044 Nondisplaced fracture of base of neck of right femur

S72.045 Nondisplaced fracture of base of neck of left femur

S72.046 Nondisplaced fracture of base of neck of unspecified femur

S72.05 Unspecified fracture of head of femur

Fracture of head of femur NOS

S72.051 Unspecified fracture of head of right femur

S72.052 Unspecified fracture of head of left femur

S72.059 Unspecified fracture of head of unspecified femur

S72.06 Articular fracture of head of femur

S72.061 Displaced articular fracture of head of right femur

S72.062 Displaced articular fracture of head of left femur

S72.063 Displaced articular fracture of head of unspecified femur

S72.064 Nondisplaced articular fracture of head of right femur

S72.065 Nondisplaced articular fracture of head of left femur

S72.066 Nondisplaced articular fracture of head of unspecified femur

S72.09 Other fracture of head and neck of femur

S72.091 Other fracture of head and neck of right femur

S72.092 Other fracture of head and neck of left femur

S72.099 Other fracture of head and neck of unspecified femur

S72.1 Pertrochanteric fracture

S72.10 Unspecified trochanteric fracture of femur

Fracture of trochanter NOS

S72.101 Unspecified trochanteric fracture of right femur

S72.102 Unspecified trochanteric fracture of left femur

S72.109 Unspecified trochanteric fracture of unspecified femur

S72.11 Fracture of greater trochanter of femur

S72.111 Displaced fracture of greater trochanter of right femur

S72.112 Displaced fracture of greater trochanter of left femur

S72.113 Displaced fracture of greater trochanter of unspecified femur

S72.114 Nondisplaced fracture of greater trochanter of right femur

S72.115 Nondisplaced fracture of greater trochanter of left femur

S72.116 Nondisplaced fracture of greater trochanter of unspecified femur

S72.12 Fracture of lesser trochanter of femur

S72.121 Displaced fracture of lesser trochanter of right femur

S72.122 Displaced fracture of lesser trochanter of left femur

S72.123 Displaced fracture of lesser trochanter of unspecified femur

S72.124 Nondisplaced fracture of lesser trochanter of right femur

S72.125 Nondisplaced fracture of lesser trochanter of left femur

S72.126 Nondisplaced fracture of lesser trochanter of unspecified femur

S72.13 Apophyseal fracture of femur

EXCLUDES 1 *chronic (nontraumatic) slipped upper femoral epiphysis (M93.0-)*

S72.131 Displaced apophyseal fracture of right femur

S72.132 Displaced apophyseal fracture of left femur

S72.133 Displaced apophyseal fracture of unspecified femur

S72.134 Nondisplaced apophyseal fracture of right femur

S72.135 Nondisplaced apophyseal fracture of left femur

S72.136 Nondisplaced apophyseal fracture of unspecified femur

S72.14 Intertrochanteric fracture of femur

S72.141 Displaced intertrochanteric fracture of right femur

S72.142 Displaced intertrochanteric fracture of left femur

S72.143 Displaced intertrochanteric fracture of unspecified femur

S72.144 Nondisplaced intertrochanteric fracture of right femur

S72.145 Nondisplaced intertrochanteric fracture of left femur

S72.146 Nondisplaced intertrochanteric fracture of unspecified femur

S72.2 Subtrochanteric fracture of femur

S72.21 Displaced subtrochanteric fracture of right femur

S72.22 Displaced subtrochanteric fracture of left femur

S72.23 Displaced subtrochanteric fracture of unspecified femur

S72.24 Nondisplaced subtrochanteric fracture of right femur

S72.25 Nondisplaced subtrochanteric fracture of left femur

S72.26 Nondisplaced subtrochanteric fracture of unspecified femur

S72.3 Fracture of shaft of femur

S72.30 Unspecified fracture of shaft of femur

S72.301 Unspecified fracture of shaft of right femur

S72.302 Unspecified fracture of shaft of left femur

S72.309 Unspecified fracture of shaft of unspecified femur

S72.32 Transverse fracture of shaft of femur

S72.321 Displaced transverse fracture of shaft of right femur

S72.322 Displaced transverse fracture of shaft of left femur

S72.323 Displaced transverse fracture of shaft of unspecified femur

S72.324 Nondisplaced transverse fracture of shaft of right femur

S72.325 Nondisplaced transverse fracture of shaft of left femur

S72.326 Nondisplaced transverse fracture of shaft of unspecified femur

S72.33 Oblique fracture of shaft of femur

S72.331 Displaced oblique fracture of shaft of right femur

S72.332 Displaced oblique fracture of shaft of left femur

S72.333 Displaced oblique fracture of shaft of unspecified femur

S72.334 Nondisplaced oblique fracture of shaft of right femur

S72.335 Nondisplaced oblique fracture of shaft of left femur

S72.336 Nondisplaced oblique fracture of shaft of unspecified femur

S72.34 Spiral fracture of shaft of femur

S72.341 Displaced spiral fracture of shaft of right femur

S72.342 Displaced spiral fracture of shaft of left femur

S72.343 Displaced spiral fracture of shaft of unspecified femur

S72.344 Nondisplaced spiral fracture of shaft of right femur

S72.345 Nondisplaced spiral fracture of shaft of left femur

S72.346 Nondisplaced spiral fracture of shaft of unspecified femur

S72.35 Comminuted fracture of shaft of femur

S72.351 Displaced comminuted fracture of shaft of right femur

S72.352 Displaced comminuted fracture of shaft of left femur

S72.353 Displaced comminuted fracture of shaft of unspecified femur

S72.354 Nondisplaced comminuted fracture of shaft of right femur

S72.355 Nondisplaced comminuted fracture of shaft of left femur

S72.356 Nondisplaced comminuted fracture of shaft of unspecified femur

S72.36 Segmental fracture of shaft of femur

S72.361 Displaced segmental fracture of shaft of right femur

S72.362 Displaced segmental fracture of shaft of left femur

S72.363 Displaced segmental fracture of shaft of unspecified femur

S72.364 Nondisplaced segmental fracture of shaft of right femur

S72.365 Nondisplaced segmental fracture of shaft of left femur

S72.366 Nondisplaced segmental fracture of shaft of unspecified femur

S72.39 Other fracture of shaft of femur

S72.391 Other fracture of shaft of right femur

S72.392 Other fracture of shaft of left femur

S72.399 Other fracture of shaft of unspecified femur

S72.4 Fracture of lower end of femur
Fracture of distal end of femur
EXCLUDES 2 *fracture of shaft of femur (S72.3-)*
physeal fracture of lower end of femur (S79.1-)

S72.40 Unspecified fracture of lower end of femur
S72.401 Unspecified fracture of lower end of right femur
S72.402 Unspecified fracture of lower end of left femur
S72.409 Unspecified fracture of lower end of unspecified femur

S72.41 Unspecified condyle fracture of lower end of femur
Condyle fracture of femur NOS
S72.411 Displaced unspecified condyle fracture of lower end of right femur
S72.412 Displaced unspecified condyle fracture of lower end of left femur
S72.413 Displaced unspecified condyle fracture of lower end of unspecified femur
S72.414 Nondisplaced unspecified condyle fracture of lower end of right femur
S72.415 Nondisplaced unspecified condyle fracture of lower end of left femur
S72.416 Nondisplaced unspecified condyle fracture of lower end of unspecified femur

S72.42 Fracture of lateral condyle of femur
S72.421 Displaced fracture of lateral condyle of right femur
S72.422 Displaced fracture of lateral condyle of left femur
S72.423 Displaced fracture of lateral condyle of unspecified femur
S72.424 Nondisplaced fracture of lateral condyle of right femur
S72.425 Nondisplaced fracture of lateral condyle of left femur
S72.426 Nondisplaced fracture of lateral condyle of unspecified femur

S72.43 Fracture of medial condyle of femur
S72.431 Displaced fracture of medial condyle of right femur
S72.432 Displaced fracture of medial condyle of left femur
S72.433 Displaced fracture of medial condyle of unspecified femur
S72.434 Nondisplaced fracture of medial condyle of right femur
S72.435 Nondisplaced fracture of medial condyle of left femur
S72.436 Nondisplaced fracture of medial condyle of unspecified femur

S72.44 Fracture of lower epiphysis (separation) of femur
EXCLUDES 1 *Salter-Harris Type I physeal fracture of lower end of femur (S79.11-)*
S72.441 Displaced fracture of lower epiphysis (separation) of right femur
S72.442 Displaced fracture of lower epiphysis (separation) of left femur
S72.443 Displaced fracture of lower epiphysis (separation) of unspecified femur
S72.444 Nondisplaced fracture of lower epiphysis (separation) of right femur
S72.445 Nondisplaced fracture of lower epiphysis (separation) of left femur
S72.446 Nondisplaced fracture of lower epiphysis (separation) of unspecified femur

S72.45 Supracondylar fracture without intracondylar extension of lower end of femur
Supracondylar fracture of lower end of femur NOS
EXCLUDES 1 *supracondylar fracture with intracondylar extension of lower end of femur (S72.46-)*
S72.451 Displaced supracondylar fracture without intracondylar extension of lower end of right femur
S72.452 Displaced supracondylar fracture without intracondylar extension of lower end of left femur
S72.453 Displaced supracondylar fracture without intracondylar extension of lower end of unspecified femur
S72.454 Nondisplaced supracondylar fracture without intracondylar extension of lower end of right femur
S72.455 Nondisplaced supracondylar fracture without intracondylar extension of lower end of left femur
S72.456 Nondisplaced supracondylar fracture without intracondylar extension of lower end of unspecified femur

S72.46 Supracondylar fracture with intracondylar extension of lower end of femur
EXCLUDES 1 *supracondylar fracture without intracondylar extension of lower end of femur (S72.45-)*
S72.461 Displaced supracondylar fracture with intracondylar extension of lower end of right femur
S72.462 Displaced supracondylar fracture with intracondylar extension of lower end of left femur
S72.463 Displaced supracondylar fracture with intracondylar extension of lower end of unspecified femur
S72.464 Nondisplaced supracondylar fracture with intracondylar extension of lower end of right femur
S72.465 Nondisplaced supracondylar fracture with intracondylar extension of lower end of left femur
S72.466 Nondisplaced supracondylar fracture with intracondylar extension of lower end of unspecified femur

S72.47 Torus fracture of lower end of femur

The appropriate 7th character is to be added to all codes in subcategory S72.47.
- A initial encounter for closed fracture
- D subsequent encounter for fracture with routine healing
- G subsequent encounter for fracture with delayed healing
- K subsequent encounter for fracture with nonunion
- P subsequent encounter for fracture with malunion
- S sequela

S72.471 Torus fracture of lower end of right femur
S72.472 Torus fracture of lower end of left femur
S72.479 Torus fracture of lower end of unspecified femur

S72.49 Other fracture of lower end of femur
S72.491 Other fracture of lower end of right femur
S72.492 Other fracture of lower end of left femur
S72.499 Other fracture of lower end of unspecified femur

S72.8 Other fracture of femur
S72.8X Other fracture of femur
S72.8X1 Other fracture of right femur
S72.8X2 Other fracture of left femur
S72.8X9 Other fracture of unspecified femur

Appropriate additional character required   x7th Requires 7th character, placeholder x must fill empty characters

S72.9 Unspecified fracture of femur
Fracture of thigh NOS
Fracture of upper leg NOS
EXCLUDES 1 *fracture of hip NOS (S72.00-, S72.01-)*
S72.90 Unspecified fracture of unspecified femur
S72.91 Unspecified fracture of right femur
S72.92 Unspecified fracture of left femur

S73 Dislocation and sprain of joint and ligaments of hip
INCLUDES avulsion of joint or ligament of hip
laceration of cartilage, joint or ligament of hip
sprain of cartilage, joint or ligament of hip
traumatic hemarthrosis of joint or ligament of hip
traumatic rupture of joint or ligament of hip
traumatic subluxation of joint or ligament of hip
traumatic tear of joint or ligament of hip
Code also any associated open wound
EXCLUDES 2 *strain of muscle, fascia and tendon of hip and thigh (S76.-)*

The appropriate 7th character is to be added to each code from category S73.
A initial encounter
D subsequent encounter
S sequela

S73.0 Subluxation and dislocation of hip
EXCLUDES 2 *dislocation and subluxation of hip prosthesis (T84.020, T84.021)*
S73.00 Unspecified subluxation and dislocation of hip
Dislocation of hip NOS
Subluxation of hip NOS
S73.001 Unspecified subluxation of right hip
S73.002 Unspecified subluxation of left hip
S73.003 Unspecified subluxation of unspecified hip
S73.004 Unspecified dislocation of right hip
S73.005 Unspecified dislocation of left hip
S73.006 Unspecified dislocation of unspecified hip
S73.01 Posterior subluxation and dislocation of hip
S73.011 Posterior subluxation of right hip
S73.012 Posterior subluxation of left hip
S73.013 Posterior subluxation of unspecified hip
S73.014 Posterior dislocation of right hip
S73.015 Posterior dislocation of left hip
S73.016 Posterior dislocation of unspecified hip
S73.02 Obturator subluxation and dislocation of hip
S73.021 Obturator subluxation of right hip
S73.022 Obturator subluxation of left hip
S73.023 Obturator subluxation of unspecified hip
S73.024 Obturator dislocation of right hip
S73.025 Obturator dislocation of left hip
S73.026 Obturator dislocation of unspecified hip
S73.03 Other anterior dislocation of hip
S73.031 Other anterior subluxation of right hip
S73.032 Other anterior subluxation of left hip
S73.033 Other anterior subluxation of unspecified hip
S73.034 Other anterior dislocation of right hip
S73.035 Other anterior dislocation of left hip
S73.036 Other anterior dislocation of unspecified hip
S73.04 Central dislocation of hip
S73.041 Central subluxation of right hip
S73.042 Central subluxation of left hip
S73.043 Central subluxation of unspecified hip
S73.044 Central dislocation of right hip
S73.045 Central dislocation of left hip
S73.046 Central dislocation of unspecified hip
S73.1 Sprain of hip
S73.10 Unspecified sprain of hip
S73.101 Unspecified sprain of right hip
S73.102 Unspecified sprain of left hip
S73.109 Unspecified sprain of unspecified hip
S73.11 Iliofemoral ligament sprain of hip
S73.111 Iliofemoral ligament sprain of right hip
S73.112 Iliofemoral ligament sprain of left hip
S73.119 Iliofemoral ligament sprain of unspecified hip
S73.12 Ischiocapsular (ligament) sprain of hip
S73.121 Ischiocapsular ligament sprain of right hip
S73.122 Ischiocapsular ligament sprain of left hip
S73.129 Ischiocapsular ligament sprain of unspecified hip
S73.19 Other sprain of hip
S73.191 Other sprain of right hip
S73.192 Other sprain of left hip
S73.199 Other sprain of unspecified hip

S74 Injury of nerves at hip and thigh level
Code also any associated open wound (S71.-)
EXCLUDES 2 *injury of nerves at ankle and foot level (S94.-)*
injury of nerves at lower leg level (S84.-)

The appropriate 7th character is to be added to each code from category S74.
A initial encounter
D subsequent encounter
S sequela

S74.0 Injury of sciatic nerve at hip and thigh level
S74.00 Injury of sciatic nerve at hip and thigh level, unspecified leg
S74.01 Injury of sciatic nerve at hip and thigh level, right leg
S74.02 Injury of sciatic nerve at hip and thigh level, left leg
S74.1 Injury of femoral nerve at hip and thigh level
S74.10 Injury of femoral nerve at hip and thigh level, unspecified leg
S74.11 Injury of femoral nerve at hip and thigh level, right leg
S74.12 Injury of femoral nerve at hip and thigh level, left leg
S74.2 Injury of cutaneous sensory nerve at hip and thigh level
S74.20 Injury of cutaneous sensory nerve at hip and thigh level, unspecified leg
S74.21 Injury of cutaneous sensory nerve at hip and high level, right leg
S74.22 Injury of cutaneous sensory nerve at hip and thigh level, left leg
S74.8 Injury of other nerves at hip and thigh level
S74.8X Injury of other nerves at hip and thigh level
S74.8X1 Injury of other nerves at hip and thigh level, right leg
S74.8X2 Injury of other nerves at hip and thigh level, left leg
S74.8X9 Injury of other nerves at hip and thigh level, unspecified leg
S74.9 Injury of unspecified nerve at hip and thigh level
S74.90 Injury of unspecified nerve at hip and thigh level, unspecified leg
S74.91 Injury of unspecified nerve at hip and thigh level, right leg
S74.92 Injury of unspecified nerve at hip and thigh level, left leg

S75 Injury of blood vessels at hip and thigh level
Code also any associated open wound (S71.-)
EXCLUDES 2 *injury of blood vessels at lower leg level (S85.-)*
injury of popliteal artery (S85.0)

The appropriate 7th character is to be added to each code from category S75.
A initial encounter
D subsequent encounter
S sequela

S75.0 Injury of femoral artery
S75.00 Unspecified injury of femoral artery
S75.001 Unspecified injury of femoral artery, right leg
S75.002 Unspecified injury of femoral artery, left leg

7th S75.009 **Unspecified injury of femoral artery, unspecified leg**

6th S75.01 **Minor laceration of femoral artery**
Incomplete transection of femoral artery
Laceration of femoral artery NOS
Superficial laceration of femoral artery

7th S75.011 **Minor laceration of femoral artery, right leg**

7th S75.012 **Minor laceration of femoral artery, left leg**

7th S75.019 **Minor laceration of femoral artery, unspecified leg**

6th S75.02 **Major laceration of femoral artery**
Complete transection of femoral artery
Traumatic rupture of femoral artery

7th S75.021 **Major laceration of femoral artery, right leg**

7th S75.022 **Major laceration of femoral artery, left leg**

7th S75.029 **Major laceration of femoral artery, unspecified leg**

6th S75.09 **Other specified injury of femoral artery**

7th S75.091 **Other specified injury of femoral artery, right leg**

7th S75.092 **Other specified injury of femoral artery, left leg**

7th S75.099 **Other specified injury of femoral artery, unspecified leg**

5th S75.1 **Injury of femoral vein at hip and thigh level**

6th S75.10 **Unspecified injury of femoral vein at hip and thigh level**

7th S75.101 **Unspecified injury of femoral vein at hip and thigh level, right leg**

7th S75.102 **Unspecified injury of femoral vein at hip and thigh level, left leg**

7th S75.109 **Unspecified injury of femoral vein at hip and thigh level, unspecified leg**

6th S75.11 **Minor laceration of femoral vein at hip and thigh level**
Incomplete transection of femoral vein at hip and thigh level
Laceration of femoral vein at hip and thigh level NOS
Superficial laceration of femoral vein at hip and thigh level

7th S75.111 **Minor laceration of femoral vein at hip and thigh level, right leg**

7th S75.112 **Minor laceration of femoral vein at hip and thigh level, left leg**

7th S75.119 **Minor laceration of femoral vein at hip and thigh level, unspecified leg**

6th S75.12 **Major laceration of femoral vein at hip and thigh level**
Complete transection of femoral vein at hip and thigh level
Traumatic rupture of femoral vein at hip and thigh level

7th S75.121 **Major laceration of femoral vein at hip and thigh level, right leg**

7th S75.122 **Major laceration of femoral vein at hip and thigh level, left leg**

7th S75.129 **Major laceration of femoral vein at hip and thigh level, unspecified leg**

6th S75.19 **Other specified injury of femoral vein at hip and thigh level**

7th S75.191 **Other specified injury of femoral vein at hip and thigh level, right leg**

7th S75.192 **Other specified injury of femoral vein at hip and thigh level, left leg**

7th S75.199 **Other specified injury of femoral vein at hip and thigh level, unspecified leg**

5th S75.2 **Injury of greater saphenous vein at hip and thigh level**
EXCLUDES1 *greater saphenous vein NOS (S85.3)*

6th S75.20 **Unspecified injury of greater saphenous vein at hip and thigh level**

7th S75.201 **Unspecified injury of greater saphenous vein at hip and thigh level, right leg**

7th S75.202 **Unspecified injury of greater saphenous vein at hip and thigh level, left leg**

7th S75.209 **Unspecified injury of greater saphenous vein at hip and thigh level, unspecified leg**

6th S75.21 **Minor laceration of greater saphenous vein at hip and thigh level**
Incomplete transection of greater saphenous vein at hip and thigh level
Laceration of greater saphenous vein at hip and thigh level NOS
Superficial laceration of greater saphenous vein at hip and thigh level

7th S75.211 **Minor laceration of greater saphenous vein at hip and thigh level, right leg**

7th S75.212 **Minor laceration of greater saphenous vein at hip and thigh level, left leg**

7th S75.219 **Minor laceration of greater saphenous vein at hip and thigh level, unspecified leg**

6th S75.22 **Major laceration of greater saphenous vein at hip and thigh level**
Complete transection of greater saphenous vein at hip and thigh level
Traumatic rupture of greater saphenous vein at hip and thigh level

7th S75.221 **Major laceration of greater saphenous vein at hip and thigh level, right leg**

7th S75.222 **Major laceration of greater saphenous vein at hip and thigh level, left leg**

7th S75.229 **Major laceration of greater saphenous vein at hip and thigh level, unspecified leg**

6th S75.29 **Other specified injury of greater saphenous vein at hip and thigh level**

7th S75.291 **Other specified injury of greater saphenous vein at hip and thigh level, right leg**

7th S75.292 **Other specified injury of greater saphenous vein at hip and thigh level, left leg**

7th S75.299 **Other specified injury of greater saphenous vein at hip and thigh level, unspecified leg**

5th S75.8 **Injury of other blood vessels at hip and thigh level**

6th S75.80 **Unspecified injury of other blood vessels at hip and thigh level**

7th S75.801 **Unspecified injury of other blood vessels at hip and thigh level, right leg**

7th S75.802 **Unspecified injury of other blood vessels at hip and thigh level, left leg**

7th S75.809 **Unspecified injury of other blood vessels at hip and thigh level, unspecified leg**

6th S75.81 **Laceration of other blood vessels at hip and thigh level**

7th S75.811 **Laceration of other blood vessels at hip and thigh level, right leg**

7th S75.812 **Laceration of other blood vessels at hip and thigh level, left leg**

7th S75.819 **Laceration of other blood vessels at hip and thigh level, unspecified leg**

6th S75.89 **Other specified injury of other blood vessels at hip and thigh level**

7th S75.891 **Other specified injury of other blood vessels at hip and thigh level, right leg**

7th S75.892 **Other specified injury of other blood vessels at hip and thigh level, left leg**

7th S75.899 **Other specified injury of other blood vessels at hip and thigh level, unspecified leg**

5th S75.9 **Injury of unspecified blood vessel at hip and thigh level**

6th S75.90 **Unspecified injury of unspecified blood vessel at hip and thigh level**

7th S75.901 **Unspecified injury of unspecified blood vessel at hip and thigh level, right leg**

7th S75.902 **Unspecified injury of unspecified blood vessel at hip and thigh level, left leg**

7th S75.909 **Unspecified injury of unspecified blood vessel at hip and thigh level, unspecified leg**

✓ Appropriate additional character required   x7th Requires 7th character, placeholder x must fill empty characters

√6th **S75.91 Laceration of unspecified blood vessel at hip and thigh level**
- √7th **S75.911 Laceration of unspecified blood vessel at hip and thigh level, right leg**
- √7th **S75.912 Laceration of unspecified blood vessel at hip and thigh level, left leg**
- √7th **S75.919 Laceration of unspecified blood vessel at hip and thigh level, unspecified leg**

√6th **S75.99 Other specified injury of unspecified blood vessel at hip and thigh level**
- √7th **S75.991 Other specified injury of unspecified blood vessel at hip and thigh level, right leg**
- √7th **S75.992 Other specified injury of unspecified blood vessel at hip and thigh level, left leg**
- √7th **S75.999 Other specified injury of unspecified blood vessel at hip and thigh level, unspecified leg**

√4th **S76 Injury of muscle, fascia and tendon at hip and thigh level**

Code also any associated open wound (S71.-)

EXCLUDES 2 *injury of muscle, fascia and tendon at lower leg level (S86)*
sprain of joint and ligament of hip (S73.1)

The appropriate 7th character is to be added to each code from category S76.
- A initial encounter
- D subsequent encounter
- S sequela

√5th **S76.0 Injury of muscle, fascia and tendon of hip**

√6th **S76.00 Unspecified injury of muscle, fascia and tendon of hip**
- √7th **S76.001 Unspecified injury of muscle, fascia and tendon of right hip**
- √7th **S76.002 Unspecified injury of muscle, fascia and tendon of left hip**
- √7th **S76.009 Unspecified injury of muscle, fascia and tendon of unspecified hip**

√6th **S76.01 Strain of muscle, fascia and tendon of hip**
- √7th **S76.011 Strain of muscle, fascia and tendon of right hip**
- √7th **S76.012 Strain of muscle, fascia and tendon of left hip**
- √7th **S76.019 Strain of muscle, fascia and tendon of unspecified hip**

√6th **S76.02 Laceration of muscle, fascia and tendon of hip**
- √7th **S76.021 Laceration of muscle, fascia and tendon of right hip**
- √7th **S76.022 Laceration of muscle, fascia and tendon of left hip**
- √7th **S76.029 Laceration of muscle, fascia and tendon of unspecified hip**

√6th **S76.09 Other specified injury of muscle, fascia and tendon of hip**
- √7th **S76.091 Other specified injury of muscle, fascia and tendon of right hip**
- √7th **S76.092 Other specified injury of muscle, fascia and tendon of left hip**
- √7th **S76.099 Other specified injury of muscle, fascia and tendon of unspecified hip**

√5th **S76.1 Injury of quadriceps muscle, fascia and tendon**

Injury of patellar ligament (tendon)

√6th **S76.10 Unspecified injury of quadriceps muscle, fascia and tendon**
- √7th **S76.101 Unspecified injury of right quadriceps muscle, fascia and tendon**
- √7th **S76.102 Unspecified injury of left quadriceps muscle, fascia and tendon**
- √7th **S76.109 Unspecified injury of unspecified quadriceps muscle, fascia and tendon**

√6th **S76.11 Strain of quadriceps muscle, fascia and tendon**
- √7th **S76.111 Strain of right quadriceps muscle, fascia and tendon**
- √7th **S76.112 Strain of left quadriceps muscle, fascia and tendon**
- √7th **S76.119 Strain of unspecified quadriceps muscle, fascia and tendon**

√6th **S76.12 Laceration of quadriceps muscle, fascia and tendon**
- √7th **S76.121 Laceration of right quadriceps muscle, fascia and tendon**
- √7th **S76.122 Laceration of left quadriceps muscle, fascia and tendon**
- √7th **S76.129 Laceration of unspecified quadriceps muscle, fascia and tendon**

√6th **S76.19 Other specified injury of quadriceps muscle, fascia and tendon**
- √7th **S76.191 Other specified injury of right quadriceps muscle, fascia and tendon**
- √7th **S76.192 Other specified injury of left quadriceps muscle, fascia and tendon**
- √7th **S76.199 Other specified injury of unspecified quadriceps muscle, fascia and tendon**

√5th **S76.2 Injury of adductor muscle, fascia and tendon of thigh**

√6th **S76.20 Unspecified injury of adductor muscle, fascia and tendon of thigh**
- √7th **S76.201 Unspecified injury of adductor muscle, fascia and tendon of right thigh**
- √7th **S76.202 Unspecified injury of adductor muscle, fascia and tendon of left thigh**
- √7th **S76.209 Unspecified injury of adductor muscle, fascia and tendon of unspecified thigh**

√6th **S76.21 Strain of adductor muscle, fascia and tendon of thigh**
- √7th **S76.211 Strain of adductor muscle, fascia and tendon of right thigh**
- √7th **S76.212 Strain of adductor muscle, fascia and tendon of left thigh**
- √7th **S76.219 Strain of adductor muscle, fascia and tendon of unspecified thigh**

√6th **S76.22 Laceration of adductor muscle, fascia and tendon of thigh**
- √7th **S76.221 Laceration of adductor muscle, fascia and tendon of right thigh**
- √7th **S76.222 Laceration of adductor muscle, fascia and tendon of left thigh**
- √7th **S76.229 Laceration of adductor muscle, fascia and tendon of unspecified thigh**

√6th **S76.29 Other injury of adductor muscle, fascia and tendon of thigh**
- √7th **S76.291 Other injury of adductor muscle, fascia and tendon of right thigh**
- √7th **S76.292 Other injury of adductor muscle, fascia and tendon of left thigh**
- √7th **S76.299 Other injury of adductor muscle, fascia and tendon of unspecified thigh**

√5th **S76.3 Injury of muscle, fascia and tendon of the posterior muscle group at thigh level**

√6th **S76.30 Unspecified injury of muscle, fascia and tendon of the posterior muscle group at thigh level**
- √7th **S76.301 Unspecified injury of muscle, fascia and tendon of the posterior muscle group at thigh level, right thigh**
- √7th **S76.302 Unspecified injury of muscle, fascia and tendon of the posterior muscle group at thigh level, left thigh**
- √7th **S76.309 Unspecified injury of muscle, fascia and tendon of the posterior muscle group at thigh level, unspecified thigh**

√6th **S76.31 Strain of muscle, fascia and tendon of the posterior muscle group at thigh level**
- √7th **S76.311 Strain of muscle, fascia and tendon of the posterior muscle group at thigh level, right thigh**
- √7th **S76.312 Strain of muscle, fascia and tendon of the posterior muscle group at thigh level, left thigh**
- √7th **S76.319 Strain of muscle, fascia and tendon of the posterior muscle group at thigh level, unspecified thigh**

√6th **S76.32 Laceration of muscle, fascia and tendon of the posterior muscle group at thigh level**
- √7th **S76.321 Laceration of muscle, fascia and tendon of the posterior muscle group at thigh level, right thigh**

S76.322 Laceration of muscle, fascia and tendon of the posterior muscle group at thigh level, left thigh
S76.329 Laceration of muscle, fascia and tendon of the posterior muscle group at thigh level, unspecified thigh
S76.39 Other specified injury of muscle, fascia and tendon of the posterior muscle group at thigh level
S76.391 Other specified injury of muscle, fascia and tendon of the posterior muscle group at thigh level, right thigh
S76.392 Other secified injury of muscle, fascia and tendon of the posterior muscle group at thigh level, left thigh
S76.399 Other specified injury of muscle, fascia and tendon of the posterior muscle group at thigh level, unspecified thigh
S76.8 Injury of other specified muscles, fascia and tendons at thigh level
S76.80 Unspecified injury of other specified muscles, fascia and tendons at thigh level
S76.801 Unspecified injury of other specified muscles, fascia and tendons at thigh level, right thigh
S76.802 Unspecified injury of other specified muscles, fascia and tendons at thigh level, left thigh
S76.809 Unspecified injury of other specified muscles, fascia and tendons at thigh level, unspecified thigh
S76.81 Strain of other specified muscles, fascia and tendons at thigh level
S76.811 Strain of other specified muscles, fascia and tendons at thigh level, right thigh
S76.812 Strain of other specified muscles, fascia and tendons at thigh level, left thigh
S76.819 Strain of other specified muscles, fascia and tendons at thigh level, unspecified thigh
S76.82 Laceration of other specified muscles, fascia and tendons at thigh level
S76.821 Laceration of other specified muscles, fascia and tendons at thigh level, right thigh
S76.822 Laceration of other specified muscles, fascia and tendons at thigh level, left thigh
S76.829 Laceration of other specified muscles, fascia and tendons at thigh level, unspecified thigh
S76.89 Other injury of other specified muscles, fascia and tendons at thigh level
S76.891 Other injury of other specified muscles, fascia and tendons at thigh level, right thigh
S76.892 Other injury of other specified muscles, fascia and tendons at thigh level, left thigh
S76.899 Other injury of other specified muscles, fascia and tendons at thigh level, unspecified thigh
S76.9 Injury of unspecified muscles, fascia and tendons at thigh level
S76.90 Unspecified injury of unspecified muscles, fascia and tendons at thigh level
S76.901 Unspecified injury of unspecified muscles, fascia and tendons at thigh level, right thigh
S76.902 Unspecified injury of unspecified muscles, fascia and tendons at thigh level, left thigh
S76.909 Unspecified injury of unspecified muscles, fascia and tendons at thigh level, unspecified thigh
S76.91 Strain of unspecified muscles, fascia and tendons at thigh level
S76.911 Strain of unspecified muscles, fascia and tendons at thigh level, right thigh
S76.912 Strain of unspecified muscles, fascia and tendons at thigh level, left thigh
S76.919 Strain of unspecified muscles, fascia and tendons at thigh level, unspecified thigh
S76.92 Laceration of unspecified muscles, fascia and tendons at thigh level
S76.921 Laceration of unspecified muscles, fascia and tendons at thigh level, right thigh
S76.922 Laceration of unspecified muscles, fascia and tendons at thigh level, left thigh
S76.929 Laceration of unspecified muscles, fascia and tendons at thigh level, unspecified thigh
S76.99 Other specified injury of unspecified muscles, fascia and tendons at thigh level
S76.991 Other specified injury of unspecified muscles, fascia and tendons at thigh level, right thigh
S76.992 Other specified injury of unspecified muscles, fascia and tendons at thigh level, left thigh
S76.999 Other specified injury of unspecified muscles, fascia and tendons at thigh level, unspecified thigh

S77 Crushing injury of hip and thigh

Use additional code(s) for all associated injuries

EXCLUDES 2 *crushing injury of ankle and foot (S97.-)*
crushing injury of lower leg (S87.-)

The appropriate 7th character is to be added to each code from category S77.
A initial encounter
D subsequent encounter
S sequela

S77.0 Crushing injury of hip
S77.00 Crushing injury of unspecified hip
S77.01 Crushing injury of right hip
S77.02 Crushing injury of left hip
S77.1 Crushing injury of thigh
S77.10 Crushing injury of unspecified thigh
S77.11 Crushing injury of right thigh
S77.12 Crushing injury of left thigh
S77.2 Crushing injury of hip with thigh
S77.20 Crushing injury of unspecified hip with thigh
S77.21 Crushing injury of right hip with thigh
S77.22 Crushing injury of left hip with thigh

S78 Traumatic amputation of hip and thigh

NOTE An amputation not identified as partial or complete should be coded to complete.

EXCLUDES 1 *traumatic amputation of knee (S88.0-)*

The appropriate 7th character is to be added to each code from category S78.
A initial encounter
D subsequent encounter
S sequela

S78.0 Traumatic amputation at hip joint
S78.01 Complete traumatic amputation at hip joint
S78.011 Complete traumatic amputation at right hip joint
S78.012 Complete traumatic amputation at left hip joint
S78.019 Complete traumatic amputation at unspecified hip joint
S78.02 Partial traumatic amputation at hip joint
S78.021 Partial traumatic amputation at right hip joint
S78.022 Partial traumatic amputation at left hip joint
S78.029 Partial traumatic amputation at unspecified hip joint

√5th **S78.1 Traumatic amputation at level between hip and knee**
EXCLUDES 1 *traumatic amputation of knee (S88.0-)*
√6th **S78.11 Complete traumatic amputation at level between hip and knee**
√7th **S78.111 Complete traumatic amputation at level between right hip and knee**
√7th **S78.112 Complete traumatic amputation at level between left hip and knee**
√7th **S78.119 Complete traumatic amputation at level between unspecified hip and knee**
√6th **S78.12 Partial traumatic amputation at level between hip and knee**
√7th **S78.121 Partial traumatic amputation at level between right hip and knee**
√7th **S78.122 Partial traumatic amputation at level between left hip and knee**
√7th **S78.129 Partial traumatic amputation at level between unspecified hip and knee**
√5th **S78.9 Traumatic amputation of hip and thigh, level unspecified**
√6th **S78.91 Complete traumatic amputation of hip and thigh, level unspecified**
√7th **S78.911 Complete traumatic amputation of right hip and thigh, level unspecified**
√7th **S78.912 Complete traumatic amputation of left hip and thigh, level unspecified**
√7th **S78.919 Complete traumatic amputation of unspecified hip and thigh, level unspecified**
√6th **S78.92 Partial traumatic amputation of hip and thigh, level unspecified**
√7th **S78.921 Partial traumatic amputation of right hip and thigh, level unspecified**
√7th **S78.922 Partial traumatic amputation of left hip and thigh, level unspecified**
√7th **S78.929 Partial traumatic amputation of unspecified hip and thigh, level unspecified**

√4th **S79 Other and unspecified injuries of hip and thigh**
√5th **S79.0 Physeal fracture of upper end of femur**
NOTE A fracture not indicated as open or closed should be coded to closed.
EXCLUDES 1 *apophyseal fracture of upper end of femur (S72.13-)*
nontraumatic slipped upper femoral epiphysis (M93.0-)

The appropriate 7th character is to be added to each code from subcategory S79.0.
A initial encounter for closed fracture
D subsequent encounter for fracture with routine healing
G subsequent encounter for fracture with delayed healing
K subsequent encounter for fracture with nonunion
P subsequent encounter for fracture with malunion
S sequela

√6th **S79.00 Unspecified physeal fracture of upper end of femur**
√7th **S79.001 Unspecified physeal fracture of upper end of right femur**
√7th **S79.002 Unspecified physeal fracture of upper end of left femur**
√7th **S79.009 Unspecified physeal fracture of upper end of unspecified femur**
√6th **S79.01 Salter-Harris Type I physeal fracture of upper end of femur**
Acute on chronic slipped capital femoral epiphysis (traumatic)
Acute slipped capital femoral epiphysis (traumatic)
Capital femoral epiphyseal fracture
EXCLUDES 1 *chronic slipped upper femoral epiphysis (nontraumatic) (M93.02-)*
√7th **S79.011 Salter-Harris Type I physeal fracture of upper end of right femur**
√7th **S79.012 Salter-Harris Type I physeal fracture of upper end of left femur**
√7th **S79.019 Salter-Harris Type I physeal fracture of upper end of unspecified femur**
√6th **S79.09 Other physeal fracture of upper end of femur**
√7th **S79.091 Other physeal fracture of upper end of right femur**
√7th **S79.092 Other physeal fracture of upper end of left femur**
√7th **S79.099 Other physeal fracture of upper end of unspecified femur**
√5th **S79.1 Physeal fracture of lower end of femur**
NOTE A fracture not indicated as open or closed should be coded to closed.

The appropriate 7th character is to be added to each code from subcategory S79.1.
A initial encounter for closed fracture
D subsequent encounter for fracture with routine healing
G subsequent encounter for fracture with delayed healing
K subsequent encounter for fracture with nonunion
P subsequent encounter for fracture with malunion
S sequela

√6th **S79.10 Unspecified physeal fracture of lower end of femur**
√7th **S79.101 Unspecified physeal fracture of lower end of right femur**
√7th **S79.102 Unspecified physeal fracture of lower end of left femur**
√7th **S79.109 Unspecified physeal fracture of lower end of unspecified femur**
√6th **S79.11 Salter-Harris Type I physeal fracture of lower end of femur**
√7th **S79.111 Salter-Harris Type I physeal fracture of lower end of right femur**
√7th **S79.112 Salter-Harris Type I physeal fracture of lower end of left femur**
√7th **S79.119 Salter-Harris Type I physeal fracture of lower end of unspecified femur**
√6th **S79.12 Salter-Harris Type II physeal fracture of lower end of femur**
√7th **S79.121 Salter-Harris Type II physeal fracture of lower end of right femur**
√7th **S79.122 Salter-Harris Type II physeal fracture of lower end of left femur**
√7th **S79.129 Salter-Harris Type II physeal fracture of lower end of unspecified femur**
√6th **S79.13 Salter-Harris Type III physeal fracture of lower end of femur**
√7th **S79.131 Salter-Harris Type III physeal fracture of lower end of right femur**
√7th **S79.132 Salter-Harris Type III physeal fracture of lower end of left femur**
√7th **S79.139 Salter-Harris Type III physeal fracture of lower end of unspecified femur**
√6th **S79.14 Salter-Harris Type IV physeal fracture of lower end of femur**
√7th **S79.141 Salter-Harris Type IV physeal fracture of lower end of right femur**
√7th **S79.142 Salter-Harris Type IV physeal fracture of lower end of left femur**
√7th **S79.149 Salter-Harris Type IV physeal fracture of lower end of unspecified femur**
√6th **S79.19 Other physeal fracture of lower end of femur**
√7th **S79.191 Other physeal fracture of lower end of right femur**
√7th **S79.192 Other physeal fracture of lower end of left femur**
√7th **S79.199 Other physeal fracture of lower end of unspecified femur**
√5th **S79.8 Other specified injuries of hip and thigh**

The appropriate 7th character is to be added to each code in subcategory S79.8.
A initial encounter
D subsequent encounter
S sequela

√6th **S79.81 Other specified injuries of hip**
√7th **S79.811 Other specified injuries of right hip**
√7th **S79.812 Other specified injuries of left hip**

S79.819 Other specified injuries of unspecified hip
S79.82 Other specified injuries of thigh
S79.821 Other specified injuries of right thigh
S79.822 Other specified injuries of left thigh
S79.829 Other specified injuries of unspecified thigh
S79.9 Unspecified injury of hip and thigh

The appropriate 7th character is to be added to each code in subcategory S79.9.
A initial encounter
D subsequent encounter
S sequela

S79.91 Unspecified injury of hip
S79.911 Unspecified injury of right hip
S79.912 Unspecified injury of left hip
S79.919 Unspecified injury of unspecified hip
S79.92 Unspecified injury of thigh
S79.921 Unspecified injury of right thigh
S79.922 Unspecified injury of left thigh
S79.929 Unspecified injury of unspecified thigh

Injuries to the knee and lower leg (S80-S89)

EXCLUDES 2 *burns and corrosions (T20-T32)*
frostbite (T33-T34)
injuries of ankle and foot, except fracture of ankle and malleolus (S90-S99)
insect bite or sting, venomous (T63.4)

S80 Superficial injury of knee and lower leg

EXCLUDES 2 *superficial injury of ankle and foot (S90.-)*

The appropriate 7th character is to be added to each code from category S80.
A initial encounter
D subsequent encounter
S sequela

S80.0 Contusion of knee
S80.00 Contusion of unspecified knee
S80.01 Contusion of right knee
S80.02 Contusion of left knee
S80.1 Contusion of lower leg
S80.10 Contusion of unspecified lower leg
S80.11 Contusion of right lower leg
S80.12 Contusion of left lower leg
S80.2 Other superficial injuries of knee
S80.21 Abrasion of knee
S80.211 Abrasion, right knee
S80.212 Abrasion, left knee
S80.219 Abrasion, unspecified knee
S80.22 Blister (nonthermal) of knee
S80.221 Blister (nonthermal), right knee
S80.222 Blister (nonthermal), left knee
S80.229 Blister (nonthermal), unspecified knee
S80.24 External constriction of knee
S80.241 External constriction, right knee
S80.242 External constriction, left knee
S80.249 External constriction, unspecified knee
S80.25 Superficial foreign body of knee
Splinter in the knee
S80.251 Superficial foreign body, right knee
S80.252 Superficial foreign body, left knee
S80.259 Superficial foreign body, unspecified knee
S80.26 Insect bite (nonvenomous) of knee
S80.261 Insect bite (nonvenomous), right knee
S80.262 Insect bite (nonvenomous), left knee
S80.269 Insect bite (nonvenomous), unspecified knee
S80.27 Other superficial bite of knee
EXCLUDES 1 *open bite of knee (S81.05-)*
S80.271 Other superficial bite of right knee
S80.272 Other superficial bite of left knee
S80.279 Other superficial bite of unspecified knee
S80.8 Other superficial injuries of lower leg
S80.81 Abrasion of lower leg
S80.811 Abrasion, right lower leg
S80.812 Abrasion, left lower leg
S80.819 Abrasion, unspecified lower leg
S80.82 Blister (nonthermal) of lower leg
S80.821 Blister (nonthermal), right lower leg
S80.822 Blister (nonthermal), left lower leg
S80.829 Blister (nonthermal), unspecified lower leg
S80.84 External constriction of lower leg
S80.841 External constriction, right lower leg
S80.842 External constriction, left lower leg
S80.849 External constriction, unspecified lower leg
S80.85 Superficial foreign body of lower leg
Splinter in the lower leg
S80.851 Superficial foreign body, right lower leg
S80.852 Superficial foreign body, left lower leg
S80.859 Superficial foreign body, unspecified lower leg
S80.86 Insect bite (nonvenomous) of lower leg
S80.861 Insect bite (nonvenomous), right lower leg
S80.862 Insect bite (nonvenomous), left lower leg
S80.869 Insect bite (nonvenomous), unspecified lower leg
S80.87 Other superficial bite of lower leg
EXCLUDES 1 *open bite of lower leg (S81.85-)*
S80.871 Other superficial bite, right lower leg
S80.872 Other superficial bite, left lower leg
S80.879 Other superficial bite, unspecified lower leg
S80.9 Unspecified superficial injury of knee and lower leg
S80.91 Unspecified superficial injury of knee
S80.911 Unspecified superficial injury of right knee
S80.912 Unspecified superficial injury of left knee
S80.919 Unspecified superficial injury of unspecified knee
S80.92 Unspecified superficial injury of lower leg
S80.921 Unspecified superficial injury of right lower leg
S80.922 Unspecified superficial injury of left lower leg
S80.929 Unspecified superficial injury of unspecified lower leg

S81 Open wound of knee and lower leg

Code also any associated wound infection
EXCLUDES 1 *open fracture of knee and lower leg (S82.-)*
traumatic amputation of lower leg (S88.-)
EXCLUDES 2 *open wound of ankle and foot (S91.-)*

The appropriate 7th character is to be added to each code from category S81.
A initial encounter
D subsequent encounter
S sequela

S81.0 Open wound of knee
S81.00 Unspecified open wound of knee
S81.001 Unspecified open wound, right knee
S81.002 Unspecified open wound, left knee
S81.009 Unspecified open wound, unspecified knee
S81.01 Laceration without foreign body of knee
S81.011 Laceration without foreign body, right knee
S81.012 Laceration without foreign body, left knee
S81.019 Laceration without foreign body, unspecified knee

6th **S81.02 Laceration with foreign body of knee**
- 7th **S81.021 Laceration with foreign body, right knee**
- 7th **S81.022 Laceration with foreign body, left knee**
- 7th **S81.029 Laceration with foreign body, unspecified knee**

6th **S81.03 Puncture wound without foreign body of knee**
- 7th **S81.031 Puncture wound without foreign body, right knee**
- 7th **S81.032 Puncture wound without foreign body, left knee**
- 7th **S81.039 Puncture wound without foreign body, unspecified knee**

6th **S81.04 Puncture wound with foreign body of knee**
- 7th **S81.041 Puncture wound with foreign body, right knee**
- 7th **S81.042 Puncture wound with foreign body, left knee**
- 7th **S81.049 Puncture wound with foreign body, unspecified knee**

6th **S81.05 Open bite of knee**
Bite of knee NOS
EXCLUDES 1 *superficial bite of knee (S80.27-)*
- 7th **S81.051 Open bite, right knee**
- 7th **S81.052 Open bite, left knee**
- 7th **S81.059 Open bite, unspecified knee**

5th **S81.8 Open wound of lower leg**

6th **S81.80 Unspecified open wound of lower leg**
- 7th **S81.801 Unspecified open wound, right lower leg**
- 7th **S81.802 Unspecified open wound, left lower leg**
- 7th **S81.809 Unspecified open wound, unspecified lower leg**

6th **S81.81 Laceration without foreign body of lower leg**
- 7th **S81.811 Laceration without foreign body, right lower leg**
- 7th **S81.812 Laceration without foreign body, left lower leg**
- 7th **S81.819 Laceration without foreign body, unspecified lower leg**

6th **S81.82 Laceration with foreign body of lower leg**
- 7th **S81.821 Laceration with foreign body, right lower leg**
- 7th **S81.822 Laceration with foreign body, left lower leg**
- 7th **S81.829 Laceration with foreign body, unspecified lower leg**

6th **S81.83 Puncture wound without foreign body of lower leg**
- 7th **S81.831 Puncture wound without foreign body, right lower leg**
- 7th **S81.832 Puncture wound without foreign body, left lower leg**
- 7th **S81.839 Puncture wound without foreign body, unspecified lower leg**

6th **S81.84 Puncture wound with foreign body of lower leg**
- 7th **S81.841 Puncture wound with foreign body, right lower leg**
- 7th **S81.842 Puncture wound with foreign body, left lower leg**
- 7th **S81.849 Puncture wound with foreign body, unspecified lower leg**

6th **S81.85 Open bite of lower leg**
Bite of lower leg NOS
EXCLUDES 1 *superficial bite of lower leg (S80.86-, S80.87-)*
- 7th **S81.851 Open bite, right lower leg**
- 7th **S81.852 Open bite, left lower leg**
- 7th **S81.859 Open bite, unspecified lower leg**

4th **S82 Fracture of lower leg, including ankle**

NOTE A fracture not indicated as displaced or nondisplaced should be coded to displaced.
A fracture not designated as open or closed should be coded to closed.
The open fracture designations are based on the Gustilo open fracture classification.

INCLUDES fracture of malleolus

EXCLUDES 1 *traumatic amputation of lower leg (S88.-)*

EXCLUDES 2 *fracture of foot, except ankle (S92.-)*
periprosthetic fracture of prosthetic implant of knee (T84.042, T84.043)

The appropriate 7th character is to be added to all codes from category S82 [unless otherwise indicated].
- A initial encounter for closed fracture
- B initial encounter for open fracture type I or II
  initial encounter for open fracture NOS
- C initial encounter for open fracture type IIIA, IIIB, or IIIC
- D subsequent encounter for closed fracture with routine healing
- E subsequent encounter for open fracture type I or II with routine healing
- F subsequent encounter for open fracture type IIIA, IIIB, or IIIC with routine healing
- G subsequent encounter for closed fracture with delayed healing
- H subsequent encounter for open fracture type I or II with delayed healing
- J subsequent encounter for open fracture type IIIA, IIIB or IIIC with delayed healing
- K subsequent encounter for closed fracture with nonunion
- M subsequent encounter for open fracture type I or II with nonunion
- N subsequent encounter for open fracture type IIIA, IIIB or IIIC with nonunion
- P subsequent encounter for closed fracture with malunion
- Q subsequent encounter for open fracture type I or II with malunion
- R subsequent encounter for open fracture type IIIA, IIIB or IIIC with malunion
- S sequela

5th **S82.0 Fracture of patella**
Knee cap

6th **S82.00 Unspecified fracture of patella**
- 7th **S82.001 Unspecified fracture of right patella**
- 7th **S82.002 Unspecified fracture of left patella**
- 7th **S82.009 Unspecified fracture of unspecified patella**

6th **S82.01 Osteochondral fracture of patella**
- 7th **S82.011 Displaced osteochondral fracture of right patella**
- 7th **S82.012 Displaced osteochondral fracture of left patella**
- 7th **S82.013 Displaced osteochondral fracture of unspecified patella**
- 7th **S82.014 Nondisplaced osteochondral fracture of right patella**
- 7th **S82.015 Nondisplaced osteochondral fracture of left patella**
- 7th **S82.016 Nondisplaced osteochondral fracture of unspecified patella**

6th **S82.02 Longitudinal fracture of patella**
- 7th **S82.021 Displaced longitudinal fracture of right patella**
- 7th **S82.022 Displaced longitudinal fracture of left patella**
- 7th **S82.023 Displaced longitudinal fracture of unspecified patella**
- 7th **S82.024 Nondisplaced longitudinal fracture of right patella**
- 7th **S82.025 Nondisplaced longitudinal fracture of left patella**
- 7th **S82.026 Nondisplaced longitudinal fracture of unspecified patella**

6th **S82.03 Transverse fracture of patella**
- 7th **S82.031 Displaced transverse fracture of right patella**

7th S82.032 **Displaced transverse fracture of left patella**
7th S82.033 **Displaced transverse fracture of unspecified patella**
7th S82.034 **Nondisplaced transverse fracture of right patella**
7th S82.035 **Nondisplaced transverse fracture of left patella**
7th S82.036 **Nondisplaced transverse fracture of unspecified patella**
6th S82.04 **Comminuted fracture of patella**
7th S82.041 **Displaced comminuted fracture of right patella**
7th S82.042 **Displaced comminuted fracture of left patella**
7th S82.043 **Displaced comminuted fracture of unspecified patella**
7th S82.044 **Nondisplaced comminuted fracture of right patella**
7th S82.045 **Nondisplaced comminuted fracture of left patella**
7th S82.046 **Nondisplaced comminuted fracture of unspecified patella**
6th S82.09 **Other fracture of patella**
7th S82.091 **Other fracture of right patella**
7th S82.092 **Other fracture of left patella**
7th S82.099 **Other fracture of unspecified patella**
5th S82.1 **Fracture of upper end of tibia**
Fracture of proximal end of tibia
EXCLUDES 2 *fracture of shaft of tibia (S82.2-)*
physeal fracture of upper end of tibia (S89.0-)
6th S82.10 **Unspecified fracture of upper end of tibia**
7th S82.101 **Unspecified fracture of upper end of right tibia**
7th S82.102 **Unspecified fracture of upper end of left tibia**
7th S82.109 **Unspecified fracture of upper end of unspecified tibia**
6th S82.11 **Fracture of tibial spine**
7th S82.111 **Displaced fracture of right tibial spine**
7th S82.112 **Displaced fracture of left tibial spine**
7th S82.113 **Displaced fracture of unspecified tibial spine**
7th S82.114 **Nondisplaced fracture of right tibial spine**
7th S82.115 **Nondisplaced fracture of left tibial spine**
7th S82.116 **Nondisplaced fracture of unspecified tibial spine**
6th S82.12 **Fracture of lateral condyle of tibia**
7th S82.121 **Displaced fracture of lateral condyle of right tibia**
7th S82.122 **Displaced fracture of lateral condyle of left tibia**
7th S82.123 **Displaced fracture of lateral condyle of unspecified tibia**
7th S82.124 **Nondisplaced fracture of lateral condyle of right tibia**
7th S82.125 **Nondisplaced fracture of lateral condyle of left tibia**
7th S82.126 **Nondisplaced fracture of lateral condyle of unspecified tibia**
6th S82.13 **Fracture of medial condyle of tibia**
7th S82.131 **Displaced fracture of medial condyle of right tibia**
7th S82.132 **Displaced fracture of medial condyle of left tibia**
7th S82.133 **Displaced fracture of medial condyle of unspecified tibia**
7th S82.134 **Nondisplaced fracture of medial condyle of right tibia**
7th S82.135 **Nondisplaced fracture of medial condyle of left tibia**
7th S82.136 **Nondisplaced fracture of medial condyle of unspecified tibia**
6th S82.14 **Bicondylar fracture of tibia**
Fracture of tibial plateau NOS
7th S82.141 **Displaced bicondylar fracture of right tibia**
7th S82.142 **Displaced bicondylar fracture of left tibia**
7th S82.143 **Displaced bicondylar fracture of unspecified tibia**
7th S82.144 **Nondisplaced bicondylar fracture of right tibia**
7th S82.145 **Nondisplaced bicondylar fracture of left tibia**
7th S82.146 **Nondisplaced bicondylar fracture of unspecified tibia**
6th S82.15 **Fracture of tibial tuberosity**
7th S82.151 **Displaced fracture of right tibial tuberosity**
7th S82.152 **Displaced fracture of left tibial tuberosity**
7th S82.153 **Displaced fracture of unspecified tibial tuberosity**
7th S82.154 **Nondisplaced fracture of right tibial tuberosity**
7th S82.155 **Nondisplaced fracture of left tibial tuberosity**
7th S82.156 **Nondisplaced fracture of unspecified tibial tuberosity**
6th S82.16 **Torus fracture of upper end of tibia)**

The appropriate 7th character is to be added to all codes in subcategory S82.16.
A initial encounter for closed fracture
D subsequent encounter for fracture with routine healing
G subsequent encounter for fracture with delayed healing
K subsequent encounter for fracture with nonunion
P subsequent encounter for fracture with malunion
S sequela

7th S82.161 **Torus fracture of upper end of right tibia**
7th S82.162 **Torus fracture of upper end of left tibia**
7th S82.169 **Torus fracture of upper end of unspecified tibia**
6th S82.19 **Other fracture of upper end of tibia**
7th S82.191 **Other fracture of upper end of right tibia**
7th S82.192 **Other fracture of upper end of left tibia**
7th S82.199 **Other fracture of upper end of unspecified tibia**
5th S82.2 **Fracture of shaft of tibia**
6th S82.20 **Unspecified fracture of shaft of tibia**
Fracture of tibia NOS
7th S82.201 **Unspecified fracture of shaft of right tibia**
7th S82.202 **Unspecified fracture of shaft of left tibia**
7th S82.209 **Unspecified fracture of shaft of unspecified tibia**
6th S82.22 **Transverse fracture of shaft of tibia**
7th S82.221 **Displaced transverse fracture of shaft of right tibia**
7th S82.222 **Displaced transverse fracture of shaft of left tibia**
7th S82.223 **Displaced transverse fracture of shaft of unspecified tibia**
7th S82.224 **Nondisplaced transverse fracture of shaft of right tibia**
7th S82.225 **Nondisplaced transverse fracture of shaft of left tibia**
7th S82.226 **Nondisplaced transverse fracture of shaft of unspecified tibia**
6th S82.23 **Oblique fracture of shaft of tibia**
7th S82.231 **Displaced oblique fracture of shaft of right tibia**
7th S82.232 **Displaced oblique fracture of shaft of left tibia**

√7th S82.233 **Displaced oblique fracture of shaft of unspecified tibia**
√7th S82.234 **Nondisplaced oblique fracture of shaft of right tibia**
√7th S82.235 **Nondisplaced oblique fracture of shaft of left tibia**
√7th S82.236 **Nondisplaced oblique fracture of shaft of unspecified tibia**

√6th S82.24 **Spiral fracture of shaft of tibia**
Toddler fracture
√7th S82.241 **Displaced spiral fracture of shaft of right tibia**
√7th S82.242 **Displaced spiral fracture of shaft of left tibia**
√7th S82.243 **Displaced spiral fracture of shaft of unspecified tibia**
√7th S82.244 **Nondisplaced spiral fracture of shaft of right tibia**
√7th S82.245 **Nondisplaced spiral fracture of shaft of left tibia**
√7th S82.246 **Nondisplaced spiral fracture of shaft of unspecified tibia**

√6th S82.25 **Comminuted fracture of shaft of tibia**
√7th S82.251 **Displaced comminuted fracture of shaft of right tibia**
√7th S82.252 **Displaced comminuted fracture of shaft of left tibia**
√7th S82.253 **Displaced comminuted fracture of shaft of unspecified tibia**
√7th S82.254 **Nondisplaced comminuted fracture of shaft of right tibia**
√7th S82.255 **Nondisplaced comminuted fracture of shaft of left tibia**
√7th S82.256 **Nondisplaced comminuted fracture of shaft of unspecified tibia**

√6th S82.26 **Segmental fracture of shaft of tibia**
√7th S82.261 **Displaced segmental fracture of shaft of right tibia**
√7th S82.262 **Displaced segmental fracture of shaft of left tibia**
√7th S82.263 **Displaced segmental fracture of shaft of unspecified tibia**
√7th S82.264 **Nondisplaced segmental fracture of shaft of right tibia**
√7th S82.265 **Nondisplaced segmental fracture of shaft of left tibia**
√7th S82.266 **Nondisplaced segmental fracture of shaft of unspecified tibia**

√6th S82.29 **Other fracture of shaft of tibia**
√7th S82.291 **Other fracture of shaft of right tibia**
√7th S82.292 **Other fracture of shaft of left tibia**
√7th S82.299 **Other fracture of shaft of unspecified tibia**

√5th S82.3 **Fracture of lower end of tibia**
EXCLUDES 1 *bimalleolar fracture of lower leg (S82.84-)*
fracture of medial malleolus alone (S82.5-)
Maisonneuve's fracture (S82.86-)
pilon fracture of distal tibia (S82.87-)
trimalleolar fractures of lower leg (S82.85-)

√6th S82.30 **Unspecified fracture of lower end of tibia**
√7th S82.301 **Unspecified fracture of lower end of right tibia**
√7th S82.302 **Unspecified fracture of lower end of left tibia**
√7th S82.309 **Unspecified fracture of lower end of unspecified tibia**

√6th S82.31 **Torus fracture of lower end of tibia)**

The appropriate 7th character is to be added to all codes in subcategory S82.31.
A initial encounter for closed fracture
D subsequent encounter for fracture with routine healing
G subsequent encounter for fracture with delayed healing
K subsequent encounter for fracture with nonunion
P subsequent encounter for fracture with malunion
S sequela

√7th S82.311 **Torus fracture of lower end of right tibia**
√7th S82.312 **Torus fracture of lower end of left tibia**
√7th S82.319 **Torus fracture of lower end of unspecified tibia**

√6th S82.39 **Other fracture of lower end of tibia**
√7th S82.391 **Other fracture of lower end of right tibia**
√7th S82.392 **Other fracture of lower end of left tibia**
√7th S82.399 **Other fracture of lower end of unspecified tibia**

√5th S82.4 **Fracture of shaft of fibula**
EXCLUDES 2 *fracture of lateral malleolus alone (S82.6-)*

√6th S82.40 **Unspecified fracture of shaft of fibula**
√7th S82.401 **Unspecified fracture of shaft of right fibula**
√7th S82.402 **Unspecified fracture of shaft of left fibula**
√7th S82.409 **Unspecified fracture of shaft of unspecified fibula**

√6th S82.42 **Transverse fracture of shaft of fibula**
√7th S82.421 **Displaced transverse fracture of shaft of right fibula**
√7th S82.422 **Displaced transverse fracture of shaft of left fibula**
√7th S82.423 **Displaced transverse fracture of shaft of unspecified fibula**
√7th S82.424 **Nondisplaced transverse fracture of shaft of right fibula**
√7th S82.425 **Nondisplaced transverse fracture of shaft of left fibula**
√7th S82.426 **Nondisplaced transverse fracture of shaft of unspecified fibula**

√6th S82.43 **Oblique fracture of shaft of fibula**
√7th S82.431 **Displaced oblique fracture of shaft of right fibula**
√7th S82.432 **Displaced oblique fracture of shaft of left fibula**
√7th S82.433 **Displaced oblique fracture of shaft of unspecified fibula**
√7th S82.434 **Nondisplaced oblique fracture of shaft of right fibula**
√7th S82.435 **Nondisplaced oblique fracture of shaft of left fibula**
√7th S82.436 **Nondisplaced oblique fracture of shaft of unspecified fibula**

√6th S82.44 **Spiral fracture of shaft of fibula**
√7th S82.441 **Displaced spiral fracture of shaft of right fibula**
√7th S82.442 **Displaced spiral fracture of shaft of left fibula**
√7th S82.443 **Displaced spiral fracture of shaft of unspecified fibula**
√7th S82.444 **Nondisplaced spiral fracture of shaft of right fibula**
√7th S82.445 **Nondisplaced spiral fracture of shaft of left fibula**
√7th S82.446 **Nondisplaced spiral fracture of shaft of unspecified fibula**

√6th S82.45 **Comminuted fracture of shaft of fibula**
√7th S82.451 **Displaced comminuted fracture of shaft of right fibula**
√7th S82.452 **Displaced comminuted fracture of shaft of left fibula**

S82.453 Displaced comminuted fracture of shaft of unspecified fibula
S82.454 Nondisplaced comminuted fracture of shaft of right fibula
S82.455 Nondisplaced comminuted fracture of shaft of left fibula
S82.456 Nondisplaced comminuted fracture of shaft of unspecified fibula
S82.46 Segmental fracture of shaft of fibula
S82.461 Displaced segmental fracture of shaft of right fibula
S82.462 Displaced segmental fracture of shaft of left fibula
S82.463 Displaced segmental fracture of shaft of unspecified fibula
S82.464 Nondisplaced segmental fracture of shaft of right fibula
S82.465 Nondisplaced segmental fracture of shaft of left fibula
S82.466 Nondisplaced segmental fracture of shaft of unspecified fibula
S82.49 Other fracture of shaft of fibula
S82.491 Other fracture of shaft of right fibula
S82.492 Other fracture of shaft of left fibula
S82.499 Other fracture of shaft of unspecified fibula
S82.5 Fracture of medial malleolus
EXCLUDES 1 *pilon fracture of distal tibia (S82.87-)*
Salter-Harris type III of lower end of tibia (S89.13-)
Salter-Harris type IV of lower end of tibia (S89.14-)
S82.51 Displaced fracture of medial malleolus of right tibia
S82.52 Displaced fracture of medial malleolus of left tibia
S82.53 Displaced fracture of medial malleolus of unspecified tibia
S82.54 Nondisplaced fracture of medial malleolus of right tibia
S82.55 Nondisplaced fracture of medial malleolus of left tibia
S82.56 Nondisplaced fracture of medial malleolus of unspecified tibia
S82.6 Fracture of lateral malleolus
EXCLUDES 1 *pilon fracture of distal tibia (S82.87-)*
S82.61 Displaced fracture of lateral malleolus of right fibula
S82.62 Displaced fracture of lateral malleolus of left fibula
S82.63 Displaced fracture of lateral malleolus of unspecified fibula
S82.64 Nondisplaced fracture of lateral malleolus of right fibula
S82.65 Nondisplaced fracture of lateral malleolus of left fibula
S82.66 Nondisplaced fracture of lateral malleolus of unspecified fibula
S82.8 Other fractures of lower leg
S82.81 Torus fracture of upper end of fibula

The appropriate 7th character is to be added to all codes in subcategory S82.81.
A initial encounter for closed fracture
D subsequent encounter for fracture with routine healing
G subsequent encounter for fracture with delayed healing
K subsequent encounter for fracture wit nonunion
P subsequent encounter for fracture with malunion
S sequela

S82.811 Torus fracture of upper end of right fibula
S82.812 Torus fracture of upper end of left fibula
S82.819 Torus fracture of upper end of unspecified fibula
S82.82 Torus fracture of lower end of fibula

The appropriate 7th character is to be added to all codes in subcategory S82.82.
A initial encounter for closed fracture
D subsequent encounter for fracture with routine healing
G subsequent encounter for fracture with delayed healing
K subsequent encounter for fracture with nonunion
P subsequent encounter for fracture with malunion
S sequela

S82.821 Torus fracture of lower end of right fibula
S82.822 Torus fracture of lower end of left fibula
S82.829 Torus fracture of lower end of unspecified fibula
S82.83 Other fracture of upper and lower end of fibula
S82.831 Other fracture of upper and lower end of right fibula
S82.832 Other fracture of upper and lower end of left fibula
S82.839 Other fracture of upper and lower end of unspecified fibula
S82.84 Bimalleolar fracture of lower leg
S82.841 Displaced bimalleolar fracture of right lower leg
S82.842 Displaced bimalleolar fracture of left lower leg
S82.843 Displaced bimalleolar fracture of unspecified lower leg
S82.844 Nondisplaced bimalleolar fracture of right lower leg
S82.845 Nondisplaced bimalleolar fracture of left lower leg
S82.846 Nondisplaced bimalleolar fracture of unspecified lower leg
S82.85 Trimalleolar fracture of lower leg
S82.851 Displaced trimalleolar fracture of right lower leg
S82.852 Displaced trimalleolar fracture of left lower leg
S82.853 Displaced trimalleolar fracture of unspecified lower leg
S82.854 Nondisplaced trimalleolar fracture of right lower leg
S82.855 Nondisplaced trimalleolar fracture of left lower leg
S82.856 Nondisplaced trimalleolar fracture of unspecified lower leg
S82.86 Maisonneuve's fracture
S82.861 Displaced Maisonneuve's fracture of right leg
S82.862 Displaced Maisonneuve's fracture of left leg
S82.863 Displaced Maisonneuve's fracture of unspecified leg
S82.864 Nondisplaced Maisonneuve's fracture of right leg
S82.865 Nondisplaced Maisonneuve's fracture of left leg
S82.866 Nondisplaced Maisonneuve's fracture of unspecified leg
S82.87 Pilon fracture of tibia
S82.871 Displaced pilon fracture of right tibia
S82.872 Displaced pilon fracture of left tibia
S82.873 Displaced pilon fracture of unspecified tibia
S82.874 Nondisplaced pilon fracture of right tibia
S82.875 Nondisplaced pilon fracture of left tibia
S82.876 Nondisplaced pilon fracture of unspecified tibia

6th **S82.89 Other fractures of lower leg**
Fracture of ankle NOS
7th **S82.891 Other fracture of right lower leg**
7th **S82.892 Other fracture of left lower leg**
7th **S82.899 Other fracture of unspecified lower leg**
5th **S82.9 Unspecified fracture of lower leg**
x7th **S82.90 Unspecified fracture of unspecified lower leg**
x7th **S82.91 Unspecified fracture of right lower leg**
x7th **S82.92 Unspecified fracture of left lower leg**

4th **S83 Dislocation and sprain of joints and ligaments of knee**
INCLUDES avulsion of joint or ligament of knee
laceration of cartilage, joint or ligament of knee
sprain of cartilage, joint or ligament of knee
traumatic hemarthrosis of joint or ligament of knee
traumatic rupture of joint or ligament of knee
traumatic subluxation of joint or ligament of knee
traumatic tear of joint or ligament of knee
Code also any associated open wound
EXCLUDES 1 *derangement of patella (M22.0-M22.3)*
injury of patellar ligament (tendon) (S76.1-)
internal derangement of knee (M23.-)
old dislocation of knee (M23.8X-)
pathological dislocation of knee (M24.36)
recurrent dislocation of knee (M22.0)
EXCLUDES 2 *strain of muscle, fascia and tendon of lower leg (S86.-)*

The appropriate 7th character is to be added to each code from category S83.
A initial encounter
D subsequent encounter
S sequela

5th **S83.0 Subluxation and dislocation of patella**
6th **S83.00 Unspecified subluxation and dislocation of patella**
7th **S83.001 Unspecified subluxation of right patella**
7th **S83.002 Unspecified subluxation of left patella**
7th **S83.003 Unspecified subluxation of unspecified patella**
7th **S83.004 Unspecified dislocation of right patella**
7th **S83.005 Unspecified dislocation of left patella**
7th **S83.006 Unspecified dislocation of unspecified patella**
6th **S83.01 Lateral subluxation and dislocation of patella**
7th **S83.011 Lateral subluxation of right patella**
7th **S83.012 Lateral subluxation of left patella**
7th **S83.013 Lateral subluxation of unspecified patella**
7th **S83.014 Lateral dislocation of right patella**
7th **S83.015 Lateral dislocation of left patella**
7th **S83.016 Lateral dislocation of unspecified patella**
6th **S83.09 Other subluxation and dislocation of patella**
7th **S83.091 Other subluxation of right patella**
7th **S83.092 Other subluxation of left patella**
7th **S83.093 Other subluxation of unspecified patella**
7th **S83.094 Other dislocation of right patella**
7th **S83.095 Other dislocation of left patella**
7th **S83.096 Other dislocation of unspecified patella**
5th **S83.1 Subluxation and dislocation of knee**
EXCLUDES 2 *instability of knee prosthesis (T84.022, T84.023)*
6th **S83.10 Unspecified subluxation and dislocation of knee**
7th **S83.101 Unspecified subluxation of right knee**
7th **S83.102 Unspecified subluxation of left knee**
7th **S83.103 Unspecified subluxation of unspecified knee**
7th **S83.104 Unspecified dislocation of right knee**
7th **S83.105 Unspecified dislocation of left knee**
7th **S83.106 Unspecified dislocation of unspecified knee**
6th **S83.11 Anterior subluxation and dislocation of proximal end of tibia**
Posterior subluxation and dislocation of distal end of femur
7th **S83.111 Anterior subluxation of proximal end of tibia, right knee**
7th **S83.112 Anterior subluxation of proximal end of tibia, left knee**
7th **S83.113 Anterior subluxation of proximal end of tibia, unspecified knee**
7th **S83.114 Anterior dislocation of proximal end of tibia, right knee**
7th **S83.115 Anterior dislocation of proximal end of tibia, left knee**
7th **S83.116 Anterior dislocation of proximal end of tibia, unspecified knee**
6th **S83.12 Posterior subluxation and dislocation of proximal end of tibia**
Anterior dislocation of distal end of femur
7th **S83.121 Posterior subluxation of proximal end of tibia, right knee**
7th **S83.122 Posterior subluxation of proximal end of tibia, left knee**
7th **S83.123 Posterior subluxation of proximal end of tibia, unspecified knee**
7th **S83.124 Posterior dislocation of proximal end of tibia, right knee**
7th **S83.125 Posterior dislocation of proximal end of tibia, left knee**
7th **S83.126 Posterior dislocation of proximal end of tibia, unspecified knee**
6th **S83.13 Medial subluxation and dislocation of proximal end of tibia**
7th **S83.131 Medial subluxation of proximal end of tibia, right knee**
7th **S83.132 Medial subluxation of proximal end of tibia, left knee**
7th **S83.133 Medial subluxation of proximal end of tibia, unspecified knee**
7th **S83.134 Medial dislocation of proximal end of tibia, right knee**
7th **S83.135 Medial dislocation of proximal end of tibia, left knee**
7th **S83.136 Medial dislocation of proximal end of tibia, unspecified knee**
6th **S83.14 Lateral subluxation and dislocation of proximal end of tibia**
7th **S83.141 Lateral subluxation of proximal end of tibia, right knee**
7th **S83.142 Lateral subluxation of proximal end of tibia, left knee**
7th **S83.143 Lateral subluxation of proximal end of tibia, unspecified knee**
7th **S83.144 Lateral dislocation of proximal end of tibia, right knee**
7th **S83.145 Lateral dislocation of proximal end of tibia, left knee**
7th **S83.146 Lateral dislocation of proximal end of tibia, unspecified knee**
6th **S83.19 Other subluxation and dislocation of knee**
7th **S83.191 Other subluxation of right knee**
7th **S83.192 Other subluxation of left knee**
7th **S83.193 Other subluxation of unspecified knee**
7th **S83.194 Other dislocation of right knee**
7th **S83.195 Other dislocation of left knee**
7th **S83.196 Other dislocation of unspecified knee**
5th **S83.2 Tear of meniscus, current injury**
EXCLUDES 1 *old bucket-handle tear (M23.2)*
6th **S83.20 Tear of unspecified meniscus, current injury**
Tear of meniscus of knee NOS
7th **S83.200 Bucket-handle tear of unspecified meniscus, current injury, right knee**
7th **S83.201 Bucket-handle tear of unspecified meniscus, current injury, left knee**
7th **S83.202 Bucket-handle tear of unspecified meniscus, current injury, unspecified knee**
7th **S83.203 Other tear of unspecified meniscus, current injury, right knee**
7th **S83.204 Other tear of unspecified meniscus, current injury, left knee**

✓7th **S83.2Ø5 Other tear of unspecified meniscus, current injury, unspecified knee**
✓7th **S83.2Ø6 Unspecified tear of unspecified meniscus, current injury, right knee**
✓7th **S83.2Ø7 Unspecified tear of unspecified meniscus, current injury, left knee**
✓7th **S83.2Ø9 Unspecified tear of unspecified meniscus, current injury, unspecified knee**
✓6th **S83.21 Bucket-handle tear of medial meniscus, current injury**
✓7th **S83.211 Bucket-handle tear of medial meniscus, current injury, right knee**
✓7th **S83.212 Bucket-handle tear of medial meniscus, current injury, left knee**
✓7th **S83.219 Bucket-handle tear of medial meniscus, current injury, unspecified knee**
✓6th **S83.22 Peripheral tear of medial meniscus, current injury**
✓7th **S83.221 Peripheral tear of medial meniscus, current injury, right knee**
✓7th **S83.222 Peripheral tear of medial meniscus, current injury, left knee**
✓7th **S83.229 Peripheral tear of medial meniscus, current injury, unspecified knee**
✓6th **S83.23 Complex tear of medial meniscus, current injury**
✓7th **S83.231 Complex tear of medial meniscus, current injury, right knee**
✓7th **S83.232 Complex tear of medial meniscus, current injury, left knee**
✓7th **S83.239 Complex tear of medial meniscus, current injury, unspecified knee**
✓6th **S83.24 Other tear of medial meniscus, current injury**
✓7th **S83.241 Other tear of medial meniscus, current injury, right knee**
✓7th **S83.242 Other tear of medial meniscus, current injury, left knee**
✓7th **S83.249 Other tear of medial meniscus, current injury, unspecified knee**
✓6th **S83.25 Bucket-handle tear of lateral meniscus, current injury**
✓7th **S83.251 Bucket-handle tear of lateral meniscus, current injury, right knee**
✓7th **S83.252 Bucket-handle tear of lateral meniscus, current injury, left knee**
✓7th **S83.259 Bucket-handle tear of lateral meniscus, current injury, unspecified knee**
✓6th **S83.26 Peripheral tear of lateral meniscus, current injury**
✓7th **S83.261 Peripheral tear of lateral meniscus, current injury, right knee**
✓7th **S83.262 Peripheral tear of lateral meniscus, current injury, left knee**
✓7th **S83.269 Peripheral tear of lateral meniscus, current injury, unspecified knee**
✓6th **S83.27 Complex tear of lateral meniscus, current injury**
✓7th **S83.271 Complex tear of lateral meniscus, current injury, right knee**
✓7th **S83.272 Complex tear of lateral meniscus, current injury, left knee**
✓7th **S83.279 Complex tear of lateral meniscus, current injury, unspecified knee**
✓6th **S83.28 Other tear of lateral meniscus, current injury**
✓7th **S83.281 Other tear of lateral meniscus, current injury, right knee**
✓7th **S83.282 Other tear of lateral meniscus, current injury, left knee**
✓7th **S83.289 Other tear of lateral meniscus, current injury, unspecified knee**
✓5th **S83.3 Tear of articular cartilage of knee, current**
✓x7th **S83.3Ø Tear of articular cartilage of unspecified knee, current**
✓x7th **S83.31 Tear of articular cartilage of right knee, current**
✓x7th **S83.32 Tear of articular cartilage of left knee, current**
✓5th **S83.4 Sprain of collateral ligament of knee**
✓6th **S83.4Ø Sprain of unspecified collateral ligament of knee**
✓7th **S83.4Ø1 Sprain of unspecified collateral ligament of right knee**
✓7th **S83.4Ø2 Sprain of unspecified collateral ligament of left knee**
✓7th **S83.4Ø9 Sprain of unspecified collateral ligament of unspecified knee**
✓6th **S83.41 Sprain of medial collateral ligament of knee**
Sprain of tibial collateral ligament
✓7th **S83.411 Sprain of medial collateral ligament of right knee**
✓7th **S83.412 Sprain of medial collateral ligament of left knee**
✓7th **S83.419 Sprain of medial collateral ligament of unspecified knee**
✓6th **S83.42 Sprain of lateral collateral ligament of knee**
Sprain of fibular collateral ligament
✓7th **S83.421 Sprain of lateral collateral ligament of right knee**
✓7th **S83.422 Sprain of lateral collateral ligament of left knee**
✓7th **S83.429 Sprain of lateral collateral ligament of unspecified knee**
✓5th **S83.5 Sprain of cruciate ligament of knee**
✓6th **S83.5Ø Sprain of unspecified cruciate ligament of knee**
✓7th **S83.5Ø1 Sprain of unspecified cruciate ligament of right knee**
✓7th **S83.5Ø2 Sprain of unspecified cruciate ligament of left knee**
✓7th **S83.5Ø9 Sprain of unspecified cruciate ligament of unspecified knee**
✓6th **S83.51 Sprain of anterior cruciate ligament of knee**
✓7th **S83.511 Sprain of anterior cruciate ligament of right knee**
✓7th **S83.512 Sprain of anterior cruciate ligament of left knee**
✓7th **S83.519 Sprain of anterior cruciate ligament of unspecified knee**
✓6th **S83.52 Sprain of posterior cruciate ligament of knee**
✓7th **S83.521 Sprain of posterior cruciate ligament of right knee**
✓7th **S83.522 Sprain of posterior cruciate ligament of left knee**
✓7th **S83.529 Sprain of posterior cruciate ligament of unspecified knee**
✓5th **S83.6 Sprain of the superior tibiofibular joint and ligament**
✓x7th **S83.6Ø Sprain of the superior tibiofibular joint and ligament, unspecified knee**
✓x7th **S83.61 Sprain of the superior tibiofibular joint and ligament, right knee**
✓x7th **S83.62 Sprain of the superior tibiofibular joint and ligament, left knee**
✓5th **S83.8 Sprain of other specified parts of knee**
✓6th **S83.8X Sprain of other specified parts of knee**
✓7th **S83.8X1 Sprain of other specified parts of right knee**
✓7th **S83.8X2 Sprain of other specified parts of left knee**
✓7th **S83.8X9 Sprain of other specified parts of unspecified knee**
✓5th **S83.9 Sprain of unspecified site of knee**
✓x7th **S83.9Ø Sprain of unspecified site of unspecified knee**
✓x7th **S83.91 Sprain of unspecified site of right knee**
✓x7th **S83.92 Sprain of unspecified site of left knee**

✓4th **S84 Injury of nerves at lower leg level**
Code also any associated open wound (S81.-)
EXCLUDES 2 *injury of nerves at ankle and foot level (S94.-)*

The appropriate 7th character is to be added to each code from category S84.
A initial encounter
D subsequent encounter
S sequela

✓5th **S84.Ø Injury of tibial nerve at lower leg level**
✓x7th **S84.ØØ Injury of tibial nerve at lower leg level, unspecified leg**
✓x7th **S84.Ø1 Injury of tibial nerve at lower leg level, right leg**
✓x7th **S84.Ø2 Injury of tibial nerve at lower leg level, left leg**

✓5th **S84.1 Injury of peroneal nerve at lower leg level**
- ✓x7th **S84.1Ø Injury of peroneal nerve at lower leg level, unspecified leg**
- ✓x7th **S84.11 Injury of peroneal nerve at lower leg level, right leg**
- ✓x7th **S84.12 Injury of peroneal nerve at lower leg level, left leg**

✓5th **S84.2 Injury of cutaneous sensory nerve at lower leg level**
- ✓x7th **S84.2Ø Injury of cutaneous sensory nerve at lower leg level, unspecified leg**
- ✓x7th **S84.21 Injury of cutaneous sensory nerve at lower leg level, right leg**
- ✓x7th **S84.22 Injury of cutaneous sensory nerve at lower leg level, left leg**

✓5th **S84.8 Injury of other nerves at lower leg level**
- ✓6th **S84.8Ø Injury of other nerves at lower leg level**
  - ✓7th **S84.8Ø1 Injury of other nerves at lower leg level, right leg**
  - ✓7th **S84.8Ø2 Injury of other nerves at lower leg level, left leg**
  - ✓7th **S84.8Ø9 Injury of other nerves at lower leg level, unspecified leg**

✓5th **S84.9 Injury of unspecified nerve at lower leg level**
- ✓x7th **S84.9Ø Injury of unspecified nerve at lower leg level, unspecified leg**
- ✓x7th **S84.91 Injury of unspecified nerve at lower leg level, right leg**
- ✓x7th **S84.92 Injury of unspecified nerve at lower leg level, left leg**

✓4th S85 Injury of blood vessels at lower leg level

Code also any associated open wound (S81.-)

EXCLUDES 2 *injury of blood vessels at ankle and foot level (S95.-)*

The appropriate 7th character is to be added to each code from category S85.
A initial encounter
D subsequent encounter
S sequela

✓5th **S85.Ø Injury of popliteal artery**
- ✓6th **S85.ØØ Unspecified injury of popliteal artery**
  - ✓7th **S85.ØØ1 Unspecified injury of popliteal artery, right leg**
  - ✓7th **S85.ØØ2 Unspecified injury of popliteal artery, left leg**
  - ✓7th **S85.ØØ9 Unspecified injury of popliteal artery, unspecified leg**
- ✓6th **S85.Ø1 Laceration of popliteal artery**
  - ✓7th **S85.Ø11 Laceration of popliteal artery, right leg**
  - ✓7th **S85.Ø12 Laceration of popliteal artery, left leg**
  - ✓7th **S85.Ø19 Laceration of popliteal artery, unspecified leg**
- ✓6th **S85.Ø9 Other specified injury of popliteal artery**
  - ✓7th **S85.Ø91 Other specified injury of popliteal artery, right leg**
  - ✓7th **S85.Ø92 Other specified injury of popliteal artery, left leg**
  - ✓7th **S85.Ø99 Other specified injury of popliteal artery, unspecified leg**

✓5th **S85.1 Injury of tibial artery**
- ✓6th **S85.1Ø Unspecified injury of unspecified tibial artery**
  Injury of tibial artery NOS
  - ✓7th **S85.1Ø1 Unspecified injury of unspecified tibial artery, right leg**
  - ✓7th **S85.1Ø2 Unspecified injury of unspecified tibial artery, left leg**
  - ✓7th **S85.1Ø9 Unspecified injury of unspecified tibial artery, unspecified leg**
- ✓6th **S85.11 Laceration of unspecified tibial artery**
  - ✓7th **S85.111 Laceration of unspecified tibial artery, right leg**
  - ✓7th **S85.112 Laceration of unspecified tibial artery, left leg**
  - ✓7th **S85.119 Laceration of unspecified tibial artery, unspecified leg**
- ✓6th **S85.12 Other specified injury of unspecified tibial artery**
  - ✓7th **S85.121 Other specified injury of unspecified tibial artery, right leg**
  - ✓7th **S85.122 Other specified injury of unspecified tibial artery, left leg**
  - ✓7th **S85.129 Other specified injury of unspecified tibial artery, unspecified leg**
- ✓6th **S85.13 Unspecified injury of anterior tibial artery**
  - ✓7th **S85.131 Unspecified injury of anterior tibial artery, right leg**
  - ✓7th **S85.132 Unspecified injury of anterior tibial artery, left leg**
  - ✓7th **S85.139 Unspecified injury of anterior tibial artery, unspecified leg**
- ✓6th **S85.14 Laceration of anterior tibial artery**
  - ✓7th **S85.141 Laceration of anterior tibial artery, right leg**
  - ✓7th **S85.142 Laceration of anterior tibial artery, left leg**
  - ✓7th **S85.149 Laceration of anterior tibial artery, unspecified leg**
- ✓6th **S85.15 Other specified injury of anterior tibial artery**
  - ✓7th **S85.151 Other specified injury of anterior tibial artery, right leg**
  - ✓7th **S85.152 Other specified injury of anterior tibial artery, left leg**
  - ✓7th **S85.159 Other specified injury of anterior tibial artery, unspecified leg**
- ✓6th **S85.16 Unspecified injury of posterior tibial artery**
  - ✓7th **S85.161 Unspecified injury of posterior tibial artery, right leg**
  - ✓7th **S85.162 Unspecified injury of posterior tibial artery, left leg**
  - ✓7th **S85.169 Unspecified injury of posterior tibial artery, unspecified leg**
- ✓6th **S85.17 Laceration of posterior tibial artery**
  - ✓7th **S85.171 Laceration of posterior tibial artery, right leg**
  - ✓7th **S85.172 Laceration of posterior tibial artery, left leg**
  - ✓7th **S85.179 Laceration of posterior tibial artery, unspecified leg**
- ✓6th **S85.18 Other specified injury of posterior tibial artery**
  - ✓7th **S85.181 Other specified injury of posterior tibial artery, right leg**
  - ✓7th **S85.182 Other specified injury of posterior tibial artery, left leg**
  - ✓7th **S85.189 Other specified injury of posterior tibial artery, unspecified leg**

✓5th **S85.2 Injury of peroneal artery**
- ✓6th **S85.2Ø Unspecified injury of peroneal artery**
  - ✓7th **S85.2Ø1 Unspecified injury of peroneal artery, right leg**
  - ✓7th **S85.2Ø2 Unspecified injury of peroneal artery, left leg**
  - ✓7th **S85.2Ø9 Unspecified injury of peroneal artery, unspecified leg**
- ✓6th **S85.21 Laceration of peroneal artery**
  - ✓7th **S85.211 Laceration of peroneal artery, right leg**
  - ✓7th **S85.212 Laceration of peroneal artery, left leg**
  - ✓7th **S85.219 Laceration of peroneal artery, unspecified leg**
- ✓6th **S85.29 Other specified injury of peroneal artery**
  - ✓7th **S85.291 Other specified injury of peroneal artery, right leg**
  - ✓7th **S85.292 Other specified injury of peroneal artery, left leg**
  - ✓7th **S85.299 Other specified injury of peroneal artery, unspecified leg**

✓5th **S85.3 Injury of greater saphenous vein at lower leg level**
Injury of greater saphenous vein NOS
Injury of saphenous vein NOS
- ✓6th **S85.3Ø Unspecified injury of greater saphenous vein at lower leg level**
  - ✓7th **S85.3Ø1 Unspecified injury of greater saphenous vein at lower leg level, right leg**
  - ✓7th **S85.3Ø2 Unspecified injury of greater saphenous vein at lower leg level, left leg**

S85.309 Unspecified injury of greater saphenous vein at lower leg level, unspecified leg
S85.31 Laceration of greater saphenous vein at lower leg level
S85.311 Laceration of greater saphenous vein at lower leg level, right leg
S85.312 Laceration of greater saphenous vein at lower leg level, left leg
S85.319 Laceration of greater saphenous vein at lower leg level, unspecified leg
S85.39 Other specified injury of greater saphenous vein at lower leg level
S85.391 Other specified injury of greater saphenous vein at lower leg level, right leg
S85.392 Other specified injury of greater saphenous vein at lower leg level, left leg
S85.399 Other specified injury of greater saphenous vein at lower leg level, unspecified leg
S85.4 Injury of lesser saphenous vein at lower leg level
S85.40 Unspecified injury of lesser saphenous vein at lower leg level
S85.401 Unspecified injury of lesser saphenous vein at lower leg level, right leg
S85.402 Unspecified injury of lesser saphenous vein at lower leg level, left leg
S85.409 Unspecified injury of lesser saphenous vein at lower leg level, unspecified leg
S85.41 Laceration of lesser saphenous vein at lower leg level
S85.411 Laceration of lesser saphenous vein at lower leg level, right leg
S85.412 Laceration of lesser saphenous vein at lower leg level, left leg
S85.419 Laceration of lesser saphenous vein at lower leg level, unspecified leg
S85.49 Other specified injury of lesser saphenous vein at lower leg level
S85.491 Other specified injury of lesser saphenous vein at lower leg level, right leg
S85.492 Other specified injury of lesser saphenous vein at lower leg level, left leg
S85.499 Other specified injury of lesser saphenous vein at lower leg level, unspecified leg
S85.5 Injury of popliteal vein
S85.50 Unspecified injury of popliteal vein
S85.501 Unspecified injury of popliteal vein, right leg
S85.502 Unspecified injury of popliteal vein, left leg
S85.509 Unspecified injury of popliteal vein, unspecified leg
S85.51 Laceration of popliteal vein
S85.511 Laceration of popliteal vein, right leg
S85.512 Laceration of popliteal vein, left leg
S85.519 Laceration of popliteal vein, unspecified leg
S85.59 Other specified injury of popliteal vein
S85.591 Other specified injury of popliteal vein, right leg
S85.592 Other specified injury of popliteal vein, left leg
S85.599 Other specified injury of popliteal vein, unspecified leg
S85.8 Injury of other blood vessels at lower leg level
S85.80 Unspecified injury of other blood vessels at lower leg level
S85.801 Unspecified injury of other blood vessels at lower leg level, right leg
S85.802 Unspecified injury of other blood vessels at lower leg level, left leg
S85.809 Unspecified injury of other blood vessels at lower leg level, unspecified leg
S85.81 Laceration of other blood vessels at lower leg level
S85.811 Laceration of other blood vessels at lower leg level, right leg
S85.812 Laceration of other blood vessels at lower leg level, left leg
S85.819 Laceration of other blood vessels at lower leg level, unspecified leg
S85.89 Other specified injury of other blood vessels at lower leg level
S85.891 Other specified injury of other blood vessels at lower leg level, right leg
S85.892 Other specified injury of other blood vessels at lower leg level, left leg
S85.899 Other specified injury of other blood vessels at lower leg level, unspecified leg
S85.9 Injury of unspecified blood vessel at lower leg level
S85.90 Unspecified injury of unspecified blood vessel at lower leg level
S85.901 Unspecified injury of unspecified blood vessel at lower leg level, right leg
S85.902 Unspecified injury of unspecified blood vessel at lower leg level, left leg
S85.909 Unspecified injury of unspecified blood vessel at lower leg level, unspecified leg
S85.91 Laceration of unspecified blood vessel at lower leg level
S85.911 Laceration of unspecified blood vessel at lower leg level, right leg
S85.912 Laceration of unspecified blood vessel at lower leg level, left leg
S85.919 Laceration of unspecified blood vessel at lower leg level, unspecified leg
S85.99 Other specified injury of unspecified blood vessel at lower leg level
S85.991 Other specified injury of unspecified blood vessel at lower leg level, right leg
S85.992 Other specified injury of unspecified blood vessel at lower leg level, left leg
S85.999 Other specified injury of unspecified blood vessel at lower leg level, unspecified leg

S86 Injury of muscle, fascia and tendon at lower leg level

Code also any associated open wound (S81.-)

EXCLUDES 2 *injury of muscle, fascia and tendon at ankle (S96.-)*
injury of patellar ligament (tendon) (S76.1-)
sprain of joints and ligaments of knee (S83.-)

The appropriate 7th character is to be added to each code from category S86.
A initial encounter
D subsequent encounter
S sequela

S86.0 Injury of Achilles tendon
S86.00 Unspecified injury of Achilles tendon
S86.001 Unspecified injury of right Achilles tendon
S86.002 Unspecified injury of left Achilles tendon
S86.009 Unspecified injury of unspecified Achilles tendon
S86.01 Strain of Achilles tendon
S86.011 Strain of right Achilles tendon
S86.012 Strain of left Achilles tendon
S86.019 Strain of unspecified Achilles tendon
S86.02 Laceration of Achilles tendon
S86.021 Laceration of right Achilles tendon
S86.022 Laceration of left Achilles tendon
S86.029 Laceration of unspecified Achilles tendon
S86.09 Other specified injury of Achilles tendon
S86.091 Other specified injury of right Achilles tendon

7th S86.092 Other specified injury of left Achilles tendon
7th S86.099 Other specified injury of unspecified Achilles tendon
5th S86.1 Injury of other muscle(s) and tendon(s) of posterior muscle group at lower leg level
6th S86.10 Unspecified injury of other muscle(s) and tendon(s) of posterior muscle group at lower leg level
7th S86.101 Unspecified injury of other muscle(s) and tendon(s) of posterior muscle group at lower leg level, right leg
7th S86.102 Unspecified injury of other muscle(s) and tendon(s) of posterior muscle group at lower leg level, left leg
7th S86.109 Unspecified injury of other muscle(s) and tendon(s) of posterior muscle group at lower leg level, unspecified leg
6th S86.11 Strain of other muscle(s) and tendon(s) of posterior muscle group at lower leg level
7th S86.111 Strain of other muscle(s) and tendon(s) of posterior muscle group at lower leg level, right leg
7th S86.112 Strain of other muscle(s) and tendon(s) of posterior muscle group at lower leg level, left leg
7th S86.119 Strain of other muscle(s) and tendon(s) of posterior muscle group at lower leg level, unspecified leg
6th S86.12 Laceration of other muscle(s) and tendon(s) of posterior muscle group at lower leg level
7th S86.121 Laceration of other muscle(s) and tendon(s) of posterior muscle group at lower leg level, right leg
7th S86.122 Laceration of other muscle(s) and tendon(s) of posterior muscle group at lower leg level, left leg
7th S86.129 Laceration of other muscle(s) and tendon(s) of posterior muscle group at lower leg level, unspecified leg
6th S86.19 Other injury of other muscle(s) and tendon(s) of posterior muscle group at lower leg level
7th S86.191 Other injury of other muscle(s) and tendon(s) of posterior muscle group at lower leg level, right leg
7th S86.192 Other injury of other muscle(s) and tendon(s) of posterior muscle group at lower leg level, left leg
7th S86.199 Other injury of other muscle(s) and tendon(s) of posterior muscle group at lower leg level, unspecified leg
5th S86.2 Injury of muscle(s) and tendon(s) of anterior muscle group at lower leg level
6th S86.20 Unspecified injury of muscle(s) and tendon(s) of anterior muscle group at lower leg level
7th S86.201 Unspecified injury of muscle(s) and tendon(s) of anterior muscle group at lower leg level, right leg
7th S86.202 Unspecified injury of muscle(s) and tendon(s) of anterior muscle group at lower leg level, left leg
7th S86.209 Unspecified injury of muscle(s) and tendon(s) of anterior muscle group at lower leg level, unspecified leg
6th S86.21 Strain of muscle(s) and tendon(s) of anterior muscle group at lower leg level
7th S86.211 Strain of muscle(s) and tendon(s) of anterior muscle group at lower leg level, right leg
7th S86.212 Strain of muscle(s) and tendon(s) of anterior muscle group at lower leg level, left leg
7th S86.219 Strain of muscle(s) and tendon(s) of anterior muscle group at lower leg level, unspecified leg
6th S86.22 Laceration of muscle(s) and tendon(s) of anterior muscle group at lower leg level
7th S86.221 Laceration of muscle(s) and tendon(s) of anterior muscle group at lower leg level, right leg
7th S86.222 Laceration of muscle(s) and tendon(s) of anterior muscle group at lower leg level, left leg
7th S86.229 Laceration of muscle(s) and tendon(s) of anterior muscle group at lower leg level, unspecified leg
6th S86.29 Other injury of muscle(s) and tendon(s) of anterior muscle group at lower leg level
7th S86.291 Other injury of muscle(s) and tendon(s) of anterior muscle group at lower leg level, right leg
7th S86.292 Other injury of muscle(s) and tendon(s) of anterior muscle group at lower leg level, left leg
7th S86.299 Other injury of muscle(s) and tendon(s) of anterior muscle group at lower leg level, unspecified leg
5th S86.3 Injury of muscle(s) and tendon(s) of peroneal muscle group at lower leg level
6th S86.30 Unspecified injury of muscle(s) and tendon(s) of peroneal muscle group at lower leg level
7th S86.301 Unspecified injury of muscle(s) and tendon(s) of peroneal muscle group at lower leg level, right leg
7th S86.302 Unspecified injury of muscle(s) and tendon(s) of peroneal muscle group at lower leg level, left leg
7th S86.309 Unspecified injury of muscle(s) and tendon(s) of peroneal muscle group at lower leg level, unspecified leg
6th S86.31 Strain of muscle(s) and tendon(s) of peroneal muscle group at lower leg level
7th S86.311 Strain of muscle(s) and tendon(s) of peroneal muscle group at lower leg level, right leg
7th S86.312 Strain of muscle(s) and tendon(s) of peroneal muscle group at lower leg level, left leg
7th S86.319 Strain of muscle(s) and tendon(s) of peroneal muscle group at lower leg level, unspecified leg
6th S86.32 Laceration of muscle(s) and tendon(s) of peroneal muscle group at lower leg level
7th S86.321 Laceration of muscle(s) and tendon(s) of peroneal muscle group at lower leg level, right leg
7th S86.322 Laceration of muscle(s) and tendon(s) of peroneal muscle group at lower leg level, left leg
7th S86.329 Laceration of muscle(s) and tendon(s) of peroneal muscle group at lower leg level, unspecified leg
6th S86.39 Other injury of muscle(s) and tendon(s) of peroneal muscle group at lower leg level
7th S86.391 Other injury of muscle(s) and tendon(s) of peroneal muscle group at lower leg level, right leg
7th S86.392 Other injury of muscle(s) and tendon(s) of peroneal muscle group at lower leg level, left leg
7th S86.399 Other injury of muscle(s) and tendon(s) of peroneal muscle group at lower leg level, unspecified leg
5th S86.8 Injury of other muscles and tendons at lower leg level
6th S86.80 Unspecified injury of other muscles and tendons at lower leg level
7th S86.801 Unspecified injury of other muscle(s) and tendon(s) at lower leg level, right leg
7th S86.802 Unspecified injury of other muscle(s) and tendon(s) at lower leg level, left leg

✓7th S86.809 **Unspecified injury of other muscle(s) and tendon(s) at lower leg level, unspecified leg**

✓6th S86.81 **Strain of other muscles and tendons at lower leg level**

✓7th S86.811 **Strain of other muscle(s) and tendon(s) at lower leg level, right leg**

✓7th S86.812 **Strain of other muscle(s) and tendon(s) at lower leg level, left leg**

✓7th S86.819 **Strain of other muscle(s) and tendon(s) at lower leg level, unspecified leg**

✓6th S86.82 **Laceration of other muscles and tendons at lower leg level**

✓7th S86.821 **Laceration of other muscle(s) and tendon(s) at lower leg level, right leg**

✓7th S86.822 **Laceration of other muscle(s) and tendon(s) at lower leg level, left leg**

✓7th S86.829 **Laceration of other muscle(s) and tendon(s) at lower leg level, unspecified leg**

✓6th S86.89 **Other injury of other muscles and tendons at lower leg level**

✓7th S86.891 **Other injury of other muscle(s) and tendon(s) at lower leg level, right leg**

✓7th S86.892 **Other injury of other muscle(s) and tendon(s) at lower leg level, left leg**

✓7th S86.899 **Other injury of other muscle(s) and tendon(s) at lower leg level, unspecified leg**

✓5th S86.9 **Injury of unspecified muscle and tendon at lower leg level**

✓6th S86.90 **Unspecified injury of unspecified muscle and tendon at lower leg level**

✓7th S86.901 **Unspecified injury of unspecified muscle(s) and tendon(s) at lower leg level, right leg**

✓7th S86.902 **Unspecified injury of unspecified muscle(s) and tendon(s) at lower leg level, left leg**

✓7th S86.909 **Unspecified injury of unspecified muscle(s) and tendon(s) at lower leg level, unspecified leg**

✓6th S86.91 **Strain of unspecified muscle and tendon at lower leg level**

✓7th S86.911 **Strain of unspecified muscle(s) and tendon(s) at lower leg level, right leg**

✓7th S86.912 **Strain of unspecified muscle(s) and tendon(s) at lower leg level, left leg**

✓7th S86.919 **Strain of unspecified muscle(s) and tendon(s) at lower leg level, unspecified leg**

✓6th S86.92 **Laceration of unspecified muscle and tendon at lower leg level**

✓7th S86.921 **Laceration of unspecified muscle(s) and tendon(s) at lower leg level, right leg**

✓7th S86.922 **Laceration of unspecified muscle(s) and tendon(s) at lower leg level, left leg**

✓7th S86.929 **Laceration of unspecified muscle(s) and tendon(s) at lower leg level, unspecified leg**

✓6th S86.99 **Other injury of unspecified muscle and tendon at lower leg level**

✓7th S86.991 **Other injury of unspecified muscle(s) and tendon(s) at lower leg level, right leg**

✓7th S86.992 **Other injury of unspecified muscle(s) and tendon(s) at lower leg level, left leg**

✓7th S86.999 **Other injury of unspecified muscle(s) and tendon(s) at lower leg level, unspecified leg**

✓4th **S87 Crushing injury of lower leg**

Use additional code(s) for all associated injuries

EXCLUDES 2 *crushing injury of ankle and foot (S97.-)*

> The appropriate 7th character is to be added to each code from category S87.
> A initial encounter
> D subsequent encounter
> S sequela

✓5th S87.0 **Crushing injury of knee**

✓x7th S87.00 **Crushing injury of unspecified knee**

✓x7th S87.01 **Crushing injury of right knee**

✓x7th S87.02 **Crushing injury of left knee**

✓5th S87.8 **Crushing injury of lower leg**

✓x7th S87.80 **Crushing injury of unspecified lower leg**

✓x7th S87.81 **Crushing injury of right lower leg**

✓x7th S87.82 **Crushing injury of left lower leg**

✓4th **S88 Traumatic amputation of lower leg**

NOTE An amputation not identified as partial or complete should be coded to complete

EXCLUDES 1 *traumatic amputation of ankle and foot (S98.-)*

> The appropriate 7th character is to be added to each code from category S88.
> A initial encounter
> D subsequent encounter
> S sequela

✓5th S88.0 **Traumatic amputation at knee level**

✓6th S88.01 **Complete traumatic amputation at knee level**

✓7th S88.011 **Complete traumatic amputation at knee level, right lower leg**

✓7th S88.012 **Complete traumatic amputation at knee level, left lower leg**

✓7th S88.019 **Complete traumatic amputation at knee level, unspecified lower leg**

✓6th S88.02 **Partial traumatic amputation at knee level**

✓7th S88.021 **Partial traumatic amputation at knee level, right lower leg**

✓7th S88.022 **Partial traumatic amputation at knee level, left lower leg**

✓7th S88.029 **Partial traumatic amputation at knee level, unspecified lower leg**

✓5th S88.1 **Traumatic amputation at level between knee and ankle**

✓6th S88.11 **Complete traumatic amputation at level between knee and ankle**

✓7th S88.111 **Complete traumatic amputation at level between knee and ankle, right lower leg**

✓7th S88.112 **Complete traumatic amputation at level between knee and ankle, left lower leg**

✓7th S88.119 **Complete traumatic amputation at level between knee and ankle, unspecified lower leg**

✓6th S88.12 **Partial traumatic amputation at level between knee and ankle**

✓7th S88.121 **Partial traumatic amputation at level between knee and ankle, right lower leg**

✓7th S88.122 **Partial traumatic amputation at level between knee and ankle, left lower leg**

✓7th S88.129 **Partial traumatic amputation at level between knee and ankle, unspecified lower leg**

✓5th S88.9 **Traumatic amputation of lower leg, level unspecified**

✓6th S88.91 **Complete traumatic amputation of lower leg, level unspecified**

✓7th S88.911 **Complete traumatic amputation of right lower leg, level unspecified**

✓7th S88.912 **Complete traumatic amputation of left lower leg, level unspecified**

✓7th S88.919 **Complete traumatic amputation of unspecified lower leg, level unspecified**

✓6th S88.92 **Partial traumatic amputation of lower leg, level unspecified**

✓7th S88.921 **Partial traumatic amputation of right lower leg, level unspecified**

✓7th S88.922 **Partial traumatic amputation of left lower leg, level unspecified**

7th **S88.929 Partial traumatic amputation of unspecified lower leg, level unspecified**

4th **S89 Other and unspecified injuries of lower leg**

NOTE A fracture not indicated as open or closed should be coded to closed.

EXCLUDES 2 *other and unspecified injuries of ankle and foot (S99.-)*

The appropriate 7th character is to be added to each code from subcategories S89.0, S89.1, S89.2, and S89.3.
A initial encounter for closed fracture
D subsequent encounter for fracture with routine healing
G subsequent encounter for fracture with delayed healing
K subsequent encounter for fracture with nonunion
P subsequent encounter for fracture with malunion
S sequela

5th **S89.0 Physeal fracture of upper end of tibia**
6th **S89.00 Unspecified physeal fracture of upper end of tibia**
7th **S89.001 Unspecified physeal fracture of upper end of right tibia**
7th **S89.002 Unspecified physeal fracture of upper end of left tibia**
7th **S89.009 Unspecified physeal fracture of upper end of unspecified tibia**
6th **S89.01 Salter-Harris Type I physeal fracture of upper end of tibia**
7th **S89.011 Salter-Harris Type I physeal fracture of upper end of right tibia**
7th **S89.012 Salter-Harris Type I physeal fracture of upper end of left tibia**
7th **S89.019 Salter-Harris Type I physeal fracture of upper end of unspecified tibia**
6th **S89.02 Salter-Harris Type II physeal fracture of upper end of tibia**
7th **S89.021 Salter-Harris Type II physeal fracture of upper end of right tibia**
7th **S89.022 Salter-Harris Type II physeal fracture of upper end of left tibia**
7th **S89.029 Salter-Harris Type II physeal fracture of upper end of unspecified tibia**
6th **S89.03 Salter-Harris Type III physeal fracture of upper end of tibia**
7th **S89.031 Salter-Harris Type III physeal fracture of upper end of right tibia**
7th **S89.032 Salter-Harris Type III physeal fracture of upper end of left tibia**
7th **S89.039 Salter-Harris Type III physeal fracture of upper end of unspecified tibia**
6th **S89.04 Salter-Harris Type IV physeal fracture of upper end of tibia**
7th **S89.041 Salter-Harris Type IV physeal fracture of upper end of right tibia**
7th **S89.042 Salter-Harris Type IV physeal fracture of upper end of left tibia**
7th **S89.049 Salter-Harris Type IV physeal fracture of upper end of unspecified tibia**
6th **S89.09 Other physeal fracture of upper end of tibia**
7th **S89.091 Other physeal fracture of upper end of right tibia**
7th **S89.092 Other physeal fracture of upper end of left tibia**
7th **S89.099 Other physeal fracture of upper end of unspecified tibia**

5th **S89.1 Physeal fracture of lower end of tibia**
6th **S89.10 Unspecified physeal fracture of lower end of tibia**
7th **S89.101 Unspecified physeal fracture of lower end of right tibia**
7th **S89.102 Unspecified physeal fracture of lower end of left tibia**
7th **S89.109 Unspecified physeal fracture of lower end of unspecified tibia**
6th **S89.11 Salter-Harris Type I lphyseal fracture of ower end of tibia**
7th **S89.111 Salter-Harris Type I physeal fracture of lower end of right tibia**
7th **S89.112 Salter-Harris Type I physeal fracture of lower end of left tibia**
7th **S89.119 Salter-Harris Type I physeal fracture of lower end of unspecified tibia**
6th **S89.12 Salter-Harris Type II physeal fracture of lower end of tibia**
7th **S89.121 Salter-Harris Type II physeal fracture of lower end of right tibia**
7th **S89.122 Salter-Harris Type II physeal fracture of lower end of left tibia**
7th **S89.129 Salter-Harris Type II physeal fracture of lower end of unspecified tibia**
6th **S89.13 Salter-Harris Type III physeal fracture of lower end of tibia**

EXCLUDES 1 *fracture of medial malleolus (adult) (S82.5-)*

7th **S89.131 Salter-Harris Type III physeal fracture of lower end of right tibia**
7th **S89.132 Salter-Harris Type III physeal fracture of lower end of left tibia**
7th **S89.139 Salter-Harris Type III physeal fracture of lower end of unspecified tibia**
6th **S89.14 Salter-Harris Type IV physeal fracture of lower end of tibia**

EXCLUDES 1 *fracture of medial malleolus (adult) (S82.5-)*

7th **S89.141 Salter-Harris Type IV physeal fracture of lower end of right tibia**
7th **S89.142 Salter-Harris Type IV physeal fracture of lower end of left tibia**
7th **S89.149 Salter-Harris Type IV physeal fracture of lower end of unspecified tibia**
6th **S89.19 Other physeal fracture of lower end of tibia**
7th **S89.191 Other physeal fracture of lower end of right tibia**
7th **S89.192 Other physeal fracture of lower end of left tibia**
7th **S89.199 Other physeal fracture of lower end of unspecified tibia**

5th **S89.2 Physeal fracture of upper end of fibula**
6th **S89.20 Unspecified physeal fracture of upper end of fibula**
7th **S89.201 Unspecified physeal fracture of upper end of right fibula**
7th **S89.202 Unspecified physeal fracture of upper end of left fibula**
7th **S89.209 Unspecified physeal fracture of upper end of unspecified fibula**
6th **S89.21 Salter-Harris Type I physeal fracture of upper end of fibula**
7th **S89.211 Salter-Harris Type I physeal fracture of upper end of right fibula**
7th **S89.212 Salter-Harris Type I physeal fracture of upper end of left fibula**
7th **S89.219 Salter-Harris Type I physeal fracture of upper end of unspecified fibula**
6th **S89.22 Salter-Harris Type II physeal fracture of upper end of fibula**
7th **S89.221 Salter-Harris Type II physeal fracture of upper end of right fibula**
7th **S89.222 Salter-Harris Type II physeal fracture of upper end of left fibula**
7th **S89.229 Salter-Harris Type II physeal fracture of upper end of unspecified fibula**
6th **S89.29 Other physeal fracture of upper end of fibula**
7th **S89.291 Other physeal fracture of upper end of right fibula**
7th **S89.292 Other physeal fracture of upper end of left fibula**
7th **S89.299 Other physeal fracture of upper end of unspecified fibula**

5th **S89.3 Physeal fracture of lower end of fibula**
6th **S89.30 Unspecified physeal fracture of lower end of fibula**
7th **S89.301 Unspecified physeal fracture of lower end of right fibula**
7th **S89.302 Unspecified physeal fracture of lower end of left fibula**
7th **S89.309 Unspecified physeal fracture of lower end of unspecified fibula**

√6th S89.31 Salter-Harris Type I physeal fracture of lower end of fibula
√7th S89.311 Salter-Harris Type I physeal fracture of lower end of right fibula
√7th S89.312 Salter-Harris Type I physeal fracture of lower end of left fibula
√7th S89.319 Salter-Harris Type I physeal fracture of lower end of unspecified fibula
√6th S89.32 Salter-Harris Type II physeal fracture of lower end of fibula
√7th S89.321 Salter-Harris Type II physeal fracture of lower end of right fibula
√7th S89.322 Salter-Harris Type II physeal fracture of lower end of left fibula
√7th S89.329 Salter-Harris Type II physeal fracture of lower end of unspecified fibula
√6th S89.39 Other physeal fracture of lower end of fibula
√7th S89.391 Other physeal fracture of lower end of right fibula
√7th S89.392 Other physeal fracture of lower end of left fibula
√7th S89.399 Other physeal fracture of lower end of unspecified fibula
√5th S89.8 Other specified injuries of lower leg

The appropriate 7th character is to be added to each code in subcategory S89.8.
A initial encounter
D subsequent encounter
S sequela

√x7th S89.80 Other specified injuries of unspecified lower leg
√x7th S89.81 Other specified injuries of right lower leg
√x7th S89.82 Other specified injuries of left lower leg
√5th S89.9 Unspecified injury of lower leg

The appropriate 7th character is to be added to each code in subcategory S89.9.
A initial encounter
D subsequent encounter
S sequela

√x7th S89.90 Unspecified injury of unspecified lower leg
√x7th S89.91 Unspecified injury of right lower leg
√x7th S89.92 Unspecified injury of left lower leg

Injuries to the ankle and foot (S90-S99)

EXCLUDES 2 *burns and corrosions (T20-T32)*
fracture of ankle and malleolus (S82.-)
frostbite (T33-T34)
insect bite or sting, venomous (T63.4)

√4th **S90 Superficial injury of ankle, foot and toes**

The appropriate 7th character is to be added to each code from category S90.
A initial encounter
D subsequent encounter
S sequela

√5th S90.0 Contusion of ankle
√x7th S90.00 Contusion of unspecified ankle
√x7th S90.01 Contusion of right ankle
√x7th S90.02 Contusion of left ankle
√5th S90.1 Contusion of toe without damage to nail
√6th S90.11 Contusion of great toe without damage to nail
√7th S90.111 Contusion of right great toe without damage to nail
√7th S90.112 Contusion of left great toe without damage to nail
√7th S90.119 Contusion of unspecified great toe without damage to nail
√6th S90.12 Contusion of lesser toe without damage to nail
√7th S90.121 Contusion of right lesser toe(s) without damage to nail
√7th S90.122 Contusion of left lesser toe(s) without damage to nail
√7th S90.129 Contusion of unspecified lesser toe(s) without damage to nail
Contusion of toe NOS
√5th S90.2 Contusion of toe with damage to nail
√6th S90.21 Contusion of great toe with damage to nail
√7th S90.211 Contusion of right great toe with damage to nail
√7th S90.212 Contusion of left great toe with damage to nail
√7th S90.219 Contusion of unspecified great toe with damage to nail
√6th S90.22 Contusion of lesser toe with damage to nail
√7th S90.221 Contusion of right lesser toe(s) with damage to nail
√7th S90.222 Contusion of left lesser toe(s) with damage to nail
√7th S90.229 Contusion of unspecified lesser toe(s) with damage to nail
√5th S90.3 Contusion of foot
EXCLUDES 2 *contusion of toes (S90.1-, S90.2-)*
√x7th S90.30 Contusion of unspecified foot
Contusion of foot NOS
√x7th S90.31 Contusion of right foot
√x7th S90.32 Contusion of left foot
√5th S90.4 Other superficial injuries of toe
√6th S90.41 Abrasion of toe
√7th S90.411 Abrasion, right great toe
√7th S90.412 Abrasion, left great toe
√7th S90.413 Abrasion, unspecified great toe
√7th S90.414 Abrasion, right lesser toe(s)
√7th S90.415 Abrasion, left lesser toe(s)
√7th S90.416 Abrasion, unspecified lesser toe(s)
√6th S90.42 Blister (nonthermal) of toe
√7th S90.421 Blister (nonthermal), right great toe
√7th S90.422 Blister (nonthermal), left great toe
√7th S90.423 Blister (nonthermal), unspecified great toe
√7th S90.424 Blister (nonthermal), right lesser toe(s)
√7th S90.425 Blister (nonthermal), left lesser toe(s)
√7th S90.426 Blister (nonthermal), unspecified lesser toe(s)
√6th S90.44 External constriction of toe
Hair tourniquet syndrome of toe
√7th S90.441 External constriction, right great toe
√7th S90.442 External constriction, left great toe
√7th S90.443 External constriction, unspecified great toe
√7th S90.444 External constriction, right lesser toe(s)
√7th S90.445 External constriction, left lesser toe(s)
√7th S90.446 External constriction, unspecified lesser toe(s)
√6th S90.45 Superficial foreign body of toe
Splinter in the toe
√7th S90.451 Superficial foreign body, right great toe
√7th S90.452 Superficial foreign body, left great toe
√7th S90.453 Superficial foreign body, unspecified great toe
√7th S90.454 Superficial foreign body, right lesser toe(s)
√7th S90.455 Superficial foreign body, left lesser toe(s)
√7th S90.456 Superficial foreign body, unspecified lesser toe(s)
√6th S90.46 Insect bite (nonvenomous) of toe
√7th S90.461 Insect bite (nonvenomous), right great toe
√7th S90.462 Insect bite (nonvenomous), left great toe
√7th S90.463 Insect bite (nonvenomous), unspecified great toe
√7th S90.464 Insect bite (nonvenomous), right lesser toe(s)
√7th S90.465 Insect bite (nonvenomous), left lesser toe(s)
√7th S90.466 Insect bite (nonvenomous), unspecified lesser toe(s)

√ Appropriate additional character required
√x7th Requires 7th character, placeholder x must fill empty characters

√6th **S90.47 Other superficial bite of toe**
EXCLUDES 1 *open bite of toe (S91.15-, S91.25-)*
√7th **S90.471 Other superficial bite of right great toe**
√7th **S90.472 Other superficial bite of left great toe**
√7th **S90.473 Other superficial bite of unspecified great toe**
√7th **S90.474 Other superficial bite of right lesser toe(s)**
√7th **S90.475 Other superficial bite of left lesser toe(s)**
√7th **S90.476 Other superficial bite of unspecified lesser toe(s)**
√5th **S90.5 Other superficial injuries of ankle**
√6th **S90.51 Abrasion of ankle**
√7th **S90.511 Abrasion, right ankle**
√7th **S90.512 Abrasion, left ankle**
√7th **S90.519 Abrasion, unspecified ankle**
√6th **S90.52 Blister (nonthermal) of ankle**
√7th **S90.521 Blister (nonthermal), right ankle**
√7th **S90.522 Blister (nonthermal), left ankle**
√7th **S90.529 Blister (nonthermal), unspecified ankle**
√6th **S90.54 External constriction of ankle**
√7th **S90.541 External constriction, right ankle**
√7th **S90.542 External constriction, left ankle**
√7th **S90.549 External constriction, unspecified ankle**
√6th **S90.55 Superficial foreign body of ankle**
Splinter in the ankle
√7th **S90.551 Superficial foreign body, right ankle**
√7th **S90.552 Superficial foreign body, left ankle**
√7th **S90.559 Superficial foreign body, unspecified ankle**
√6th **S90.56 Insect bite (nonvenomous) of ankle**
√7th **S90.561 Insect bite (nonvenomous), right ankle**
√7th **S90.562 Insect bite (nonvenomous), left ankle**
√7th **S90.569 Insect bite (nonvenomous), unspecified ankle**
√6th **S90.57 Other superficial bite of ankle**
EXCLUDES 1 *open bite of ankle (S91.05-)*
√7th **S90.571 Other superficial bite of ankle, right ankle**
√7th **S90.572 Other superficial bite of ankle, left ankle**
√7th **S90.579 Other superficial bite of ankle, unspecified ankle**
√5th **S90.8 Other superficial injuries of foot**
√6th **S90.81 Abrasion of foot**
√7th **S90.811 Abrasion, right foot**
√7th **S90.812 Abrasion, left foot**
√7th **S90.819 Abrasion, unspecified foot**
√6th **S90.82 Blister (nonthermal) of foot**
√7th **S90.821 Blister (nonthermal), right foot**
√7th **S90.822 Blister (nonthermal), left foot**
√7th **S90.829 Blister (nonthermal), unspecified foot**
√6th **S90.84 External constriction of foot**
√7th **S90.841 External constriction, right foot**
√7th **S90.842 External constriction, left foot**
√7th **S90.849 External constriction, unspecified foot**
√6th **S90.85 Superficial foreign body of foot**
Splinter in the foot
√7th **S90.851 Superficial foreign body, right foot**
√7th **S90.852 Superficial foreign body, left foot**
√7th **S90.859 Superficial foreign body, unspecified foot**
√6th **S90.86 Insect bite (nonvenomous) of foot**
√7th **S90.861 Insect bite (nonvenomous), right foot**
√7th **S90.862 Insect bite (nonvenomous), left foot**
√7th **S90.869 Insect bite (nonvenomous), unspecified foot**
√6th **S90.87 Other superficial bite of foot**
EXCLUDES 1 *open bite of foot (S91.35-)*
√7th **S90.871 Other superficial bite of right foot**
√7th **S90.872 Other superficial bite of left foot**
√7th **S90.879 Other superficial bite of unspecified foot**

√5th **S90.9 Unspecified superficial injury of ankle, foot and toe**
√6th **S90.91 Unspecified superficial injury of ankle**
√7th **S90.911 Unspecified superficial injury of right ankle**
√7th **S90.912 Unspecified superficial injury of left ankle**
√7th **S90.919 Unspecified superficial injury of unspecified ankle**
√6th **S90.92 Unspecified superficial injury of foot**
√7th **S90.921 Unspecified superficial injury of right foot**
√7th **S90.922 Unspecified superficial injury of left foot**
√7th **S90.929 Unspecified superficial injury of unspecified foot**
√6th **S90.93 Unspecified superficial injury of toes**
√7th **S90.931 Unspecified superficial injury of right great toe**
√7th **S90.932 Unspecified superficial injury of left great toe**
√7th **S90.933 Unspecified superficial injury of unspecified great toe**
√7th **S90.934 Unspecified superficial injury of right lesser toe(s)**
√7th **S90.935 Unspecified superficial injury of left lesser toe(s)**
√7th **S90.936 Unspecified superficial injury of unspecified lesser toe(s)**

√4th **S91 Open wound of ankle, foot and toes**
Code also any associated wound infection
EXCLUDES 1 *open fracture of ankle, foot and toes (S92-with 7th character B)*
traumatic amputation of ankle and foot (S98.-)

The appropriate 7th character is to be added to each code from category S91.
A initial encounter
D subsequent encounter
S sequela

√5th **S91.0 Open wound of ankle**
√6th **S91.00 Unspecified open wound of ankle**
√7th **S91.001 Unspecified open wound, right ankle**
√7th **S91.002 Unspecified open wound, left ankle**
√7th **S91.009 Unspecified open wound, unspecified ankle**
√6th **S91.01 Laceration without foreign body of ankle**
√7th **S91.011 Laceration without foreign body, right ankle**
√7th **S91.012 Laceration without foreign body, left ankle**
√7th **S91.019 Laceration without foreign body, unspecified ankle**
√6th **S91.02 Laceration with foreign body of ankle**
√7th **S91.021 Laceration with foreign body, right ankle**
√7th **S91.022 Laceration with foreign body, left ankle**
√7th **S91.029 Laceration with foreign body, unspecified ankle**
√6th **S91.03 Puncture wound without foreign body of ankle**
√7th **S91.031 Puncture wound without foreign body, right ankle**
√7th **S91.032 Puncture wound without foreign body, left ankle**
√7th **S91.039 Puncture wound without foreign body, unspecified ankle**
√6th **S91.04 Puncture wound with foreign body of ankle**
√7th **S91.041 Puncture wound with foreign body, right ankle**
√7th **S91.042 Puncture wound with foreign body, left ankle**
√7th **S91.049 Puncture wound with foreign body, unspecified ankle**
√6th **S91.05 Open bite of ankle**
EXCLUDES 1 *superficial bite of ankle (S90.56-, S90.57-)*
√7th **S91.051 Open bite, right ankle**
√7th **S91.052 Open bite, left ankle**

✓7th S91.059 Open bite, unspecified ankle

✓5th **S91.1 Open wound of toe without damage to nail**

✓6th **S91.10 Unspecified open wound of toe without damage to nail**

✓7th S91.101 Unspecified open wound of right great toe without damage to nail

✓7th S91.102 Unspecified open wound of left great toe without damage to nail

✓7th S91.103 Unspecified open wound of unspecified great toe without damage to nail

✓7th S91.104 Unspecified open wound of right lesser toe(s) without damage to nail

✓7th S91.105 Unspecified open wound of left lesser toe(s) without damage to nail

✓7th S91.106 Unspecified open wound of unspecified lesser toe(s) without damage to nail

✓7th S91.109 Unspecified open wound of unspecified toe(s) without damage to nail

✓6th **S91.11 Laceration without foreign body of toe without damage to nail**

✓7th S91.111 Laceration without foreign body of right great toe without damage to nail

✓7th S91.112 Laceration without foreign body of left great toe without damage to nail

✓7th S91.113 Laceration without foreign body of unspecified great toe without damage to nail

✓7th S91.114 Laceration without foreign body of right lesser toe(s) without damage to nail

✓7th S91.115 Laceration without foreign body of left lesser toe(s) without damage to nail

✓7th S91.116 Laceration without foreign body of unspecified lesser toe(s) without damage to nail

✓7th S91.119 Laceration without foreign body of unspecified toe without damage to nail

✓6th **S91.12 Laceration with foreign body of toe without damage to nail**

✓7th S91.121 Laceration with foreign body of right great toe without damage to nail

✓7th S91.122 Laceration with foreign body of left great toe without damage to nail

✓7th S91.123 Laceration with foreign body of unspecified great toe without damage to nail

✓7th S91.124 Laceration with foreign body of right lesser toe(s) without damage to nail

✓7th S91.125 Laceration with foreign body of left lesser toe(s) without damage to nail

✓7th S91.126 Laceration with foreign body of unspecified lesser toe(s) without damage to nail

✓7th S91.129 Laceration with foreign body of unspecified toe(s) without damage to nail

✓6th **S91.13 Puncture wound without foreign body of toe without damage to nail**

✓7th S91.131 Puncture wound without foreign body of right great toe without damage to nail

✓7th S91.132 Puncture wound without foreign body of left great toe without damage to nail

✓7th S91.133 Puncture wound without foreign body of unspecified great toe without damage to nail

✓7th S91.134 Puncture wound without foreign body of right lesser toe(s) without damage to nail

✓7th S91.135 Puncture wound without foreign body of left lesser toe(s) without damage to nail

✓7th S91.136 Puncture wound without foreign body of unspecified lesser toe(s) without damage to nail

✓7th S91.139 Puncture wound without foreign body of unspecified toe(s) without damage to nail

✓6th **S91.14 Puncture wound with foreign body of toe without damage to nail**

✓7th S91.141 Puncture wound with foreign body of right great toe without damage to nail

✓7th S91.142 Puncture wound with foreign body of left great toe without damage to nail

✓7th S91.143 Puncture wound with foreign body of unspecified great toe without damage to nail

✓7th S91.144 Puncture wound with foreign body of right lesser toe(s) without damage to nail

✓7th S91.145 Puncture wound with foreign body of left lesser toe(s) without damage to nail

✓7th S91.146 Puncture wound with foreign body of unspecified lesser toe(s) without damage to nail

✓7th S91.149 Puncture wound with foreign body of unspecified toe(s) without damage to nail

✓6th **S91.15 Open bite of toe without damage to nail**

Bite of toe NOS

EXCLUDES1 *superficial bite of toe (S90.46-, S90.47-)*

✓7th S91.151 Open bite of right great toe without damage to nail

✓7th S91.152 Open bite of left great toe without damage to nail

✓7th S91.153 Open bite of unspecified great toe without damage to nail

✓7th S91.154 Open bite of right lesser toe(s) without damage to nail

✓7th S91.155 Open bite of left lesser toe(s) without damage to nail

✓7th S91.156 Open bite of unspecified lesser toe(s) without damage to nail

✓7th S91.159 Open bite of unspecified toe(s) without damage to nail

✓5th **S91.2 Open wound of toe with damage to nail**

✓6th **S91.20 Unspecified open wound of toe with damage to nail**

✓7th S91.201 Unspecified open wound of right great toe with damage to nail

✓7th S91.202 Unspecified open wound of left great toe with damage to nail

✓7th S91.203 Unspecified open wound of unspecified great toe with damage to nail

✓7th S91.204 Unspecified open wound of right lesser toe(s) with damage to nail

✓7th S91.205 Unspecified open wound of left lesser toe(s) with damage to nail

✓7th S91.206 Unspecified open wound of unspecified lesser toe(s) with damage to nail

✓7th S91.209 Unspecified open wound of unspecified toe(s) with damage to nail

✓6th **S91.21 Laceration without foreign body of toe with damage to nail**

✓7th S91.211 Laceration without foreign body of right great toe with damage to nail

✓7th S91.212 Laceration without foreign body of left great toe with damage to nail

✓7th S91.213 Laceration without foreign body of unspecified great toe with damage to nail

✓7th S91.214 Laceration without foreign body of right lesser toe(s) with damage to nail

✓7th S91.215 Laceration without foreign body of left lesser toe(s) with damage to nail

✓7th S91.216 Laceration without foreign body of unspecified lesser toe(s) with damage to nail

✓7th S91.219 Laceration without foreign body of unspecified toe(s) with damage to nail

✓6th **S91.22 Laceration with foreign body of toe with damage to nail**

✓7th S91.221 Laceration with foreign body of right great toe with damage to nail

✓7th **S91.222 Laceration with foreign body of left great toe with damage to nail**

✓7th **S91.223 Laceration with foreign body of unspecified great toe with damage to nail**

✓7th **S91.224 Laceration with foreign body of right lesser toe(s) with damage to nail**

✓7th **S91.225 Laceration with foreign body of left lesser toe(s) with damage to nail**

✓7th **S91.226 Laceration with foreign body of unspecified lesser toe(s) with damage to nail**

✓7th **S91.229 Laceration with foreign body of unspecified toe(s) with damage to nail**

✓6th **S91.23 Puncture wound without foreign body of toe with damage to nail**

✓7th **S91.231 Puncture wound without foreign body of right great toe with damage to nail**

✓7th **S91.232 Puncture wound without foreign body of left great toe with damage to nail**

✓7th **S91.233 Puncture wound without foreign body of unspecified great toe with damage to nail**

✓7th **S91.234 Puncture wound without foreign body of right lesser toe(s) with damage to nail**

✓7th **S91.235 Puncture wound without foreign body of left lesser toe(s) with damage to nail**

✓7th **S91.236 Puncture wound without foreign body of unspecified lesser toe(s) with damage to nail**

✓7th **S91.239 Puncture wound without foreign body of unspecified toe(s) with damage to nail**

✓6th **S91.24 Puncture wound with foreign body of toe with damage to nail**

✓7th **S91.241 Puncture wound with foreign body of right great toe with damage to nail**

✓7th **S91.242 Puncture wound with foreign body of left great toe with damage to nail**

✓7th **S91.243 Puncture wound with foreign body of unspecified great toe with damage to nail**

✓7th **S91.244 Puncture wound with foreign body of right lesser toe(s) with damage to nail**

✓7th **S91.245 Puncture wound with foreign body of left lesser toe(s) with damage to nail**

✓7th **S91.246 Puncture wound with foreign body of unspecified lesser toe(s) with damage to nail**

✓7th **S91.249 Puncture wound with foreign body of unspecified toe(s) with damage to nail**

✓6th **S91.25 Open bite of toe with damage to nail**

Bite of toe with damage to nail NOS

EXCLUDES 1 *superficial bite of toe (S90.46-, S90.47-)*

✓7th **S91.251 Open bite of right great toe with damage to nail**

✓7th **S91.252 Open bite of left great toe with damage to nail**

✓7th **S91.253 Open bite of unspecified great toe with damage to nail**

✓7th **S91.254 Open bite of right lesser toe(s) with damage to nail**

✓7th **S91.255 Open bite of left lesser toe(s) with damage to nail**

✓7th **S91.256 Open bite of unspecified lesser toe(s) with damage to nail**

✓7th **S91.259 Open bite of unspecified toe(s) with damage to nail**

✓5th **S91.3 Open wound of foot**

✓6th **S91.30 Unspecified open wound of foot**

✓7th **S91.301 Unspecified open wound, right foot**

✓7th **S91.302 Unspecified open wound, left foot**

✓7th **S91.309 Unspecified open wound, unspecified foot**

✓6th **S91.31 Laceration without foreign body of foot**

✓7th **S91.311 Laceration without foreign body, right foot**

✓7th **S91.312 Laceration without foreign body, left foot**

✓7th **S91.319 Laceration without foreign body, unspecified foot**

✓6th **S91.32 Laceration with foreign body of foot**

✓7th **S91.321 Laceration with foreign body, right foot**

✓7th **S91.322 Laceration with foreign body, left foot**

✓7th **S91.329 Laceration with foreign body, unspecified foot**

✓6th **S91.33 Puncture wound without foreign body of foot**

✓7th **S91.331 Puncture wound without foreign body, right foot**

✓7th **S91.332 Puncture wound without foreign body, left foot**

✓7th **S91.339 Puncture wound without foreign body, unspecified foot**

✓6th **S91.34 Puncture wound with foreign body of foot**

✓7th **S91.341 Puncture wound with foreign body, right foot**

✓7th **S91.342 Puncture wound with foreign body, left foot**

✓7th **S91.349 Puncture wound with foreign body, unspecified foot**

✓6th **S91.35 Open bite of foot**

EXCLUDES 1 *superficial bite of foot (S90.86-, S90.87-)*

✓7th **S91.351 Open bite, right foot**

✓7th **S91.352 Open bite, left foot**

✓7th **S91.359 Open bite, unspecified foot**

✓4th **S92 Fracture of foot and toe, except ankle**

NOTE A fracture not indicated as displaced or nondisplaced should be coded to displaced

A fracture not indicated as open or closed should be coded to closed.

EXCLUDES 1 *traumatic amputation of ankle and foot (S98.-)*

EXCLUDES 2 *fracture of ankle (S82.-)*
fracture of malleolus (S82.-)

The appropriate 7th character is to be added to each code from category S92.

A initial encounter for closed fracture
B initial encounter for open fracture
D subsequent encounter for fracture with routine healing
G subsequent encounter for fracture with delayed healing
K subsequent encounter for fracture with nonunion
P subsequent encounter for fracture with malunion
S sequela

✓5th **S92.0 Fracture of calcaneus**

Heel bone
Os calcis

✓6th **S92.00 Unspecified fracture of calcaneus**

✓7th **S92.001 Unspecified fracture of right calcaneus**

✓7th **S92.002 Unspecified fracture of left calcaneus**

✓7th **S92.009 Unspecified fracture of unspecified calcaneus**

✓6th **S92.01 Fracture of body of calcaneus**

✓7th **S92.011 Displaced fracture of body of right calcaneus**

✓7th **S92.012 Displaced fracture of body of left calcaneus**

✓7th **S92.013 Displaced fracture of body of unspecified calcaneus**

✓7th **S92.014 Nondisplaced fracture of body of right calcaneus**

✓7th **S92.015 Nondisplaced fracture of body of left calcaneus**

✓7th **S92.016 Nondisplaced fracture of body of unspecified calcaneus**

✓6th **S92.02 Fracture of anterior process of calcaneus**

✓7th **S92.021 Displaced fracture of anterior process of right calcaneus**

✓7th **S92.022 Displaced fracture of anterior process of left calcaneus**

✓7th **S92.023 Displaced fracture of anterior process of unspecified calcaneus**

✓7th **S92.024 Nondisplaced fracture of anterior process of right calcaneus**

✓7th S92.025 **Nondisplaced fracture of anterior process of left calcaneus**
✓7th S92.026 **Nondisplaced fracture of anterior process of unspecified calcaneus**
✓6th S92.03 **Avulsion fracture of tuberosity of calcaneus**
✓7th S92.031 **Displaced avulsion fracture of tuberosity of right calcaneus**
✓7th S92.032 **Displaced avulsion fracture of tuberosity of left calcaneus**
✓7th S92.033 **Displaced avulsion fracture of tuberosity of unspecified calcaneus**
✓7th S92.034 **Nondisplaced avulsion fracture of tuberosity of right calcaneus**
✓7th S92.035 **Nondisplaced avulsion fracture of tuberosity of left calcaneus**
✓7th S92.036 **Nondisplaced avulsion fracture of tuberosity of unspecified calcaneus**
✓6th S92.04 **Other fracture of tuberosity of calcaneus**
✓7th S92.041 **Displaced other fracture of tuberosity of right calcaneus**
✓7th S92.042 **Displaced other fracture of tuberosity of left calcaneus**
✓7th S92.043 **Displaced other fracture of tuberosity of unspecified calcaneus**
✓7th S92.044 **Nondisplaced other fracture of tuberosity of right calcaneus**
✓7th S92.045 **Nondisplaced other fracture of tuberosity of left calcaneus**
✓7th S92.046 **Nondisplaced other fracture of tuberosity of unspecified calcaneus**
✓6th S92.05 **Other extraarticular fracture of calcaneus**
✓7th S92.051 **Displaced other extraarticular fracture of right calcaneus**
✓7th S92.052 **Displaced other extraarticular fracture of left calcaneus**
✓7th S92.053 **Displaced other extraarticular fracture of unspecified calcaneus**
✓7th S92.054 **Nondisplaced other extraarticular fracture of right calcaneus**
✓7th S92.055 **Nondisplaced other extraarticular fracture of left calcaneus**
✓7th S92.056 **Nondisplaced other extraarticular fracture of unspecified calcaneus**
✓6th S92.06 **Intraarticular fracture of calcaneus**
✓7th S92.061 **Displaced intraarticular fracture of right calcaneus**
✓7th S92.062 **Displaced intraarticular fracture of left calcaneus**
✓7th S92.063 **Displaced intraarticular fracture of unspecified calcaneus**
✓7th S92.064 **Nondisplaced intraarticular fracture of right calcaneus**
✓7th S92.065 **Nondisplaced intraarticular fracture of left calcaneus**
✓7th S92.066 **Nondisplaced intraarticular fracture of unspecified calcaneus**
✓5th S92.1 **Fracture of talus**
Astragalus
✓6th S92.10 **Unspecified fracture of talus**
✓7th S92.101 **Unspecified fracture of right talus**
✓7th S92.102 **Unspecified fracture of left talus**
✓7th S92.109 **Unspecified fracture of unspecified talus**
✓6th S92.11 **Fracture of neck of talus**
✓7th S92.111 **Displaced fracture of neck of right talus**
✓7th S92.112 **Displaced fracture of neck of left talus**
✓7th S92.113 **Displaced fracture of neck of unspecified talus**
✓7th S92.114 **Nondisplaced fracture of neck of right talus**
✓7th S92.115 **Nondisplaced fracture of neck of left talus**
✓7th S92.116 **Nondisplaced fracture of neck of unspecified talus**
✓6th S92.12 **Fracture of body of talus**
✓7th S92.121 **Displaced fracture of body of right talus**
✓7th S92.122 **Displaced fracture of body of left talus**
✓7th S92.123 **Displaced fracture of body of unspecified talus**
✓7th S92.124 **Nondisplaced fracture of body of right talus**
✓7th S92.125 **Nondisplaced fracture of body of left talus**
✓7th S92.126 **Nondisplaced fracture of body of unspecified talus**
✓6th S92.13 **Fracture of posterior process of talus**
✓7th S92.131 **Displaced fracture of posterior process of right talus**
✓7th S92.132 **Displaced fracture of posterior process of left talus**
✓7th S92.133 **Displaced fracture of posterior process of unspecified talus**
✓7th S92.134 **Nondisplaced fracture of posterior process of right talus**
✓7th S92.135 **Nondisplaced fracture of posterior process of left talus**
✓7th S92.136 **Nondisplaced fracture of posterior process of unspecified talus**
✓6th S92.14 **Dome fracture of talus**
EXCLUDES1 *osteochondritis dissecans (M93.2)*
✓7th S92.141 **Displaced dome fracture of right talus**
✓7th S92.142 **Displaced dome fracture of left talus**
✓7th S92.143 **Displaced dome fracture of unspecified talus**
✓7th S92.144 **Nondisplaced dome fracture of right talus**
✓7th S92.145 **Nondisplaced dome fracture of left talus**
✓7th S92.146 **Nondisplaced dome fracture of unspecified talus**
✓6th S92.15 **Avulsion fracture (chip fracture) of talus**
✓7th S92.151 **Displaced avulsion fracture (chip fracture) of right talus**
✓7th S92.152 **Displaced avulsion fracture (chip fracture) of left talus**
✓7th S92.153 **Displaced avulsion fracture (chip fracture) of unspecified talus**
✓7th S92.154 **Nondisplaced avulsion fracture (chip fracture) of right talus**
✓7th S92.155 **Nondisplaced avulsion fracture (chip fracture) of left talus**
✓7th S92.156 **Nondisplaced avulsion fracture (chip fracture) of unspecified talus**
✓6th S92.19 **Other fracture of talus**
✓7th S92.191 **Other fracture of right talus**
✓7th S92.192 **Other fracture of left talus**
✓7th S92.199 **Other fracture of unspecified talus**
✓5th S92.2 **Fracture of other and unspecified tarsal bone(s)**
✓6th S92.20 **Fracture of unspecified tarsal bone(s)**
✓7th S92.201 **Fracture of unspecified tarsal bone(s) of right foot**
✓7th S92.202 **Fracture of unspecified tarsal bone(s) of left foot**
✓7th S92.209 **Fracture of unspecified tarsal bone(s) of unspecified foot**
✓6th S92.21 **Fracture of cuboid bone**
✓7th S92.211 **Displaced fracture of cuboid bone of right foot**
✓7th S92.212 **Displaced fracture of cuboid bone of left foot**
✓7th S92.213 **Displaced fracture of cuboid bone of unspecified foot**
✓7th S92.214 **Nondisplaced fracture of cuboid bone of right foot**
✓7th S92.215 **Nondisplaced fracture of cuboid bone of left foot**
✓7th S92.216 **Nondisplaced fracture of cuboid bone of unspecified foot**
✓6th S92.22 **Fracture of lateral cuneiform**
✓7th S92.221 **Displaced fracture of lateral cuneiform of right foot**
✓7th S92.222 **Displaced fracture of lateral cuneiform of left foot**

✓7th **S92.223 Displaced fracture of lateral cuneiform of unspecified foot**
✓7th **S92.224 Nondisplaced fracture of lateral cuneiform of right foot**
✓7th **S92.225 Nondisplaced fracture of lateral cuneiform of left foot**
✓7th **S92.226 Nondisplaced fracture of lateral cuneiform of unspecified foot**
✓6th **S92.23 Fracture of intermediate cuneiform**
✓7th **S92.231 Displaced fracture of intermediate cuneiform of right foot**
✓7th **S92.232 Displaced fracture of intermediate cuneiform of left foot**
✓7th **S92.233 Displaced fracture of intermediate cuneiform of unspecified foot**
✓7th **S92.234 Nondisplaced fracture of intermediate cuneiform of right foot**
✓7th **S92.235 Nondisplaced fracture of intermediate cuneiform of left foot**
✓7th **S92.236 Nondisplaced fracture of intermediate cuneiform of unspecified foot**
✓6th **S92.24 Fracture of medial cuneiform**
✓7th **S92.241 Displaced fracture of medial cuneiform of right foot**
✓7th **S92.242 Displaced fracture of medial cuneiform of left foot**
✓7th **S92.243 Displaced fracture of medial cuneiform of unspecified foot**
✓7th **S92.244 Nondisplaced fracture of medial cuneiform of right foot**
✓7th **S92.245 Nondisplaced fracture of medial cuneiform of left foot**
✓7th **S92.246 Nondisplaced fracture of medial cuneiform of unspecified foot**
✓6th **S92.25 Fracture of navicular [scaphoid] of foot**
✓7th **S92.251 Displaced fracture of navicular [scaphoid] of right foot**
✓7th **S92.252 Displaced fracture of navicular [scaphoid] of left foot**
✓7th **S92.253 Displaced fracture of navicular [scaphoid] of unspecified foot**
✓7th **S92.254 Nondisplaced fracture of navicular [scaphoid] of right foot**
✓7th **S92.255 Nondisplaced fracture of navicular [scaphoid] of left foot**
✓7th **S92.256 Nondisplaced fracture of navicular [scaphoid] of unspecified foot**
✓5th **S92.3 Fracture of metatarsal bone(s)**
✓6th **S92.3Ø Fracture of unspecified metatarsal bone(s)**
✓7th **S92.3Ø1 Fracture of unspecified metatarsal bone(s), right foot**
✓7th **S92.3Ø2 Fracture of unspecified metatarsal bone(s), left foot**
✓7th **S92.3Ø9 Fracture of unspecified metatarsal bone(s), unspecified foot**
✓6th **S92.31 Fracture of first metatarsal bone**
✓7th **S92.311 Displaced fracture of first metatarsal bone, right foot**
✓7th **S92.312 Displaced fracture of first metatarsal bone, left foot**
✓7th **S92.313 Displaced fracture of first metatarsal bone, unspecified foot**
✓7th **S92.314 Nondisplaced fracture of first metatarsal bone, right foot**
✓7th **S92.315 Nondisplaced fracture of first metatarsal bone, left foot**
✓7th **S92.316 Nondisplaced fracture of first metatarsal bone, unspecified foot**
✓6th **S92.32 Fracture of second metatarsal bone**
✓7th **S92.321 Displaced fracture of second metatarsal bone, right foot**
✓7th **S92.322 Displaced fracture of second metatarsal bone, left foot**
✓7th **S92.323 Displaced fracture of second metatarsal bone, unspecified foot**
✓7th **S92.324 Nondisplaced fracture of second metatarsal bone, right foot**
✓7th **S92.325 Nondisplaced fracture of second metatarsal bone, left foot**
✓7th **S92.326 Nondisplaced fracture of second metatarsal bone, unspecified foot**
✓6th **S92.33 Fracture of third metatarsal bone**
✓7th **S92.331 Displaced fracture of third metatarsal bone, right foot**
✓7th **S92.332 Displaced fracture of third metatarsal bone, left foot**
✓7th **S92.333 Displaced fracture of third metatarsal bone, unspecified foot**
✓7th **S92.334 Nondisplaced fracture of third metatarsal bone, right foot**
✓7th **S92.335 Nondisplaced fracture of third metatarsal bone, left foot**
✓7th **S92.336 Nondisplaced fracture of third metatarsal bone, unspecified foot**
✓6th **S92.34 Fracture of fourth metatarsal bone**
✓7th **S92.341 Displaced fracture of fourth metatarsal bone, right foot**
✓7th **S92.342 Displaced fracture of fourth metatarsal bone, left foot**
✓7th **S92.343 Displaced fracture of fourth metatarsal bone, unspecified foot**
✓7th **S92.344 Nondisplaced fracture of fourth metatarsal bone, right foot**
✓7th **S92.345 Nondisplaced fracture of fourth metatarsal bone, left foot**
✓7th **S92.346 Nondisplaced fracture of fourth metatarsal bone, unspecified foot**
✓6th **S92.35 Fracture of fifth metatarsal bone**
✓7th **S92.351 Displaced fracture of fifth metatarsal bone, right foot**
✓7th **S92.352 Displaced fracture of fifth metatarsal bone, left foot**
✓7th **S92.353 Displaced fracture of fifth metatarsal bone, unspecified foot**
✓7th **S92.354 Nondisplaced fracture of fifth metatarsal bone, right foot**
✓7th **S92.355 Nondisplaced fracture of fifth metatarsal bone, left foot**
✓7th **S92.356 Nondisplaced fracture of fifth metatarsal bone, unspecified foot**
✓5th **S92.4 Fracture of great toe**
✓6th **S92.4Ø Unspecified fracture of great toe**
✓7th **S92.4Ø1 Displaced unspecified fracture of right great toe**
✓7th **S92.4Ø2 Displaced unspecified fracture of left great toe**
✓7th **S92.4Ø3 Displaced unspecified fracture of unspecified great toe**
✓7th **S92.4Ø4 Nondisplaced unspecified fracture of right great toe**
✓7th **S92.4Ø5 Nondisplaced unspecified fracture of left great toe**
✓7th **S92.4Ø6 Nondisplaced unspecified fracture of unspecified great toe**
✓6th **S92.41 Fracture of proximal phalanx of great toe**
✓7th **S92.411 Displaced fracture of proximal phalanx of right great toe**
✓7th **S92.412 Displaced fracture of proximal phalanx of left great toe**
✓7th **S92.413 Displaced fracture of proximal phalanx of unspecified great toe**
✓7th **S92.414 Nondisplaced fracture of proximal phalanx of right great toe**
✓7th **S92.415 Nondisplaced fracture of proximal phalanx of left great toe**
✓7th **S92.416 Nondisplaced fracture of proximal phalanx of unspecified great toe**
✓6th **S92.42 Fracture of distal phalanx of great toe**
✓7th **S92.421 Displaced fracture of distal phalanx of right great toe**

✓7th **S92.422 Displaced fracture of distal phalanx of left great toe**
✓7th **S92.423 Displaced fracture of distal phalanx of unspecified great toe**
✓7th **S92.424 Nondisplaced fracture of distal phalanx of right great toe**
✓7th **S92.425 Nondisplaced fracture of distal phalanx of left great toe**
✓7th **S92.426 Nondisplaced fracture of distal phalanx of unspecified great toe**
✓6th **S92.49 Other fracture of great toe**
✓7th **S92.491 Other fracture of right great toe**
✓7th **S92.492 Other fracture of left great toe**
✓7th **S92.499 Other fracture of unspecified great toe**
✓5th **S92.5 Fracture of lesser toe(s)**
✓6th **S92.50 Unspecified fracture of lesser toe(s)**
✓7th **S92.501 Displaced unspecified fracture of right lesser toe(s)**
✓7th **S92.502 Displaced unspecified fracture of left lesser toe(s)**
✓7th **S92.503 Displaced unspecified fracture of unspecified lesser toe(s)**
✓7th **S92.504 Nondisplaced unspecified fracture of right lesser toe(s)**
✓7th **S92.505 Nondisplaced unspecified fracture of left lesser toe(s)**
✓7th **S92.506 Nondisplaced unspecified fracture of unspecified lesser toe(s)**
✓6th **S92.51 Fracture of proximal phalanx of lesser toe(s)**
✓7th **S92.511 Displaced fracture of proximal phalanx of right lesser toe(s)**
✓7th **S92.512 Displaced fracture of proximal phalanx of left lesser toe(s)**
✓7th **S92.513 Displaced fracture of proximal phalanx of unspecified lesser toe(s)**
✓7th **S92.514 Nondisplaced fracture of proximal phalanx of right lesser toe(s)**
✓7th **S92.515 Nondisplaced fracture of proximal phalanx of left lesser toe(s)**
✓7th **S92.516 Nondisplaced fracture of proximal phalanx of unspecified lesser toe(s)**
✓6th **S92.52 Fracture of medial phalanx of lesser toe(s)**
✓7th **S92.521 Displaced fracture of medial phalanx of right lesser toe(s)**
✓7th **S92.522 Displaced fracture of medial phalanx of left lesser toe(s)**
✓7th **S92.523 Displaced fracture of medial phalanx of unspecified lesser toe(s)**
✓7th **S92.524 Nondisplaced fracture of medial phalanx of right lesser toe(s)**
✓7th **S92.525 Nondisplaced fracture of medial phalanx of left lesser toe(s)**
✓7th **S92.526 Nondisplaced fracture of medial phalanx of unspecified lesser toe(s)**
✓6th **S92.53 Fracture of distal phalanx of lesser toe(s)**
✓7th **S92.531 Displaced fracture of distal phalanx of right lesser toe(s)**
✓7th **S92.532 Displaced fracture of distal phalanx of left lesser toe(s)**
✓7th **S92.533 Displaced fracture of distal phalanx of unspecified lesser toe(s)**
✓7th **S92.534 Nondisplaced fracture of distal phalanx of right lesser toe(s)**
✓7th **S92.535 Nondisplaced fracture of distal phalanx of left lesser toe(s)**
✓7th **S92.536 Nondisplaced fracture of distal phalanx of unspecified lesser toe(s)**
✓6th **S92.59 Other fracture of lesser toe(s)**
✓7th **S92.591 Other fracture of right lesser toe(s)**
✓7th **S92.592 Other fracture of left lesser toe(s)**
✓7th **S92.599 Other fracture of unspecified lesser toe(s)**
✓5th **S92.9 Unspecified fracture of foot and toe**
✓6th **S92.90 Unspecified fracture of foot**
✓7th **S92.901 Unspecified fracture of right foot**
✓7th **S92.902 Unspecified fracture of left foot**
✓7th **S92.909 Unspecified fracture of unspecified foot**
✓6th **S92.91 Unspecified fracture of toe**
✓7th **S92.911 Unspecified fracture of right toe(s)**
✓7th **S92.912 Unspecified fracture of left toe(s)**
✓7th **S92.919 Unspecified fracture of unspecified toe(s)**

✓4th **S93 Dislocation and sprain of joints and ligaments at ankle, foot and toe level**

INCLUDES avulsion of joint or ligament of ankle, foot and toe
laceration of cartilage, joint or ligament of ankle, foot and toe
sprain of cartilage, joint or ligament of ankle, foot and toe
traumatic hemarthrosis of joint or ligament of ankle, foot and toe
traumatic rupture of joint or ligament of ankle, foot and toe
traumatic subluxation of joint or ligament of ankle, foot and toe
traumatic tear of joint or ligament of ankle, foot and toe

Code also any associated open wound

EXCLUDES 2 *strain of muscle and tendon of ankle and foot (S96.-)*

The appropriate 7th character is to be added to each code from category S93.
A initial encounter
D subsequent encounter
S sequela

✓5th **S93.0 Subluxation and dislocation of ankle joint**
Subluxation and dislocation of astragalus
Subluxation and dislocation of fibula, lower end
Subluxation and dislocation of talus
Subluxation and dislocation of tibia, lower end
✓x7th **S93.01 Subluxation of right ankle joint**
✓x7th **S93.02 Subluxation of left ankle joint**
✓x7th **S93.03 Subluxation of unspecified ankle joint**
✓x7th **S93.04 Dislocation of right ankle joint**
✓x7th **S93.05 Dislocation of left ankle joint**
✓x7th **S93.06 Dislocation of unspecified ankle joint**
✓5th **S93.1 Subluxation and dislocation of toe**
✓6th **S93.10 Unspecified subluxation and dislocation of toe**
Dislocation of toe NOS
Subluxation of toe NOS
✓7th **S93.101 Unspecified subluxation of right toe(s)**
✓7th **S93.102 Unspecified subluxation of left toe(s)**
✓7th **S93.103 Unspecified subluxation of unspecified toe(s)**
✓7th **S93.104 Unspecified dislocation of right toe(s)**
✓7th **S93.105 Unspecified dislocation of left toe(s)**
✓7th **S93.106 Unspecified dislocation of unspecified toe(s)**
✓6th **S93.11 Dislocation of interphalangeal joint**
✓7th **S93.111 Dislocation of interphalangeal joint of right great toe**
✓7th **S93.112 Dislocation of interphalangeal joint of left great toe**
✓7th **S93.113 Dislocation of interphalangeal joint of unspecified great toe**
✓7th **S93.114 Dislocation of interphalangeal joint of right lesser toe(s)**
✓7th **S93.115 Dislocation of interphalangeal joint of left lesser toe(s)**
✓7th **S93.116 Dislocation of interphalangeal joint of unspecified lesser toe(s)**
✓7th **S93.119 Dislocation of interphalangeal joint of unspecified toe(s)**
✓6th **S93.12 Dislocation of metatarsophalangeal joint**
✓7th **S93.121 Dislocation of metatarsophalangeal joint of right great toe**
✓7th **S93.122 Dislocation of metatarsophalangeal joint of left great toe**
✓7th **S93.123 Dislocation of metatarsophalangeal joint of unspecified great toe**
✓7th **S93.124 Dislocation of metatarsophalangeal joint of right lesser toe(s)**
✓7th **S93.125 Dislocation of metatarsophalangeal joint of left lesser toe(s)**
✓7th **S93.126 Dislocation of metatarsophalangeal joint of unspecified lesser toe(s)**

√7th **S93.129 Dislocation of metatarsophalangeal joint of unspecified toe(s)**

√6th **S93.13 Subluxation of interphalangeal joint**

√7th **S93.131 Subluxation of interphalangeal joint of right great toe**

√7th **S93.132 Subluxation of interphalangeal joint of left great toe**

√7th **S93.133 Subluxation of interphalangeal joint of unspecified great toe**

√7th **S93.134 Subluxation of interphalangeal joint of right lesser toe(s)**

√7th **S93.135 Subluxation of interphalangeal joint of left lesser toe(s)**

√7th **S93.136 Subluxation of interphalangeal joint of unspecified lesser toe(s)**

√7th **S93.139 Subluxation of interphalangeal joint of unspecified toe(s)**

√6th **S93.14 Subluxation of metatarsophalangeal joint**

√7th **S93.141 Subluxation of metatarsophalangeal joint of right great toe**

√7th **S93.142 Subluxation of metatarsophalangeal joint of left great toe**

√7th **S93.143 Subluxation of metatarsophalangeal joint of unspecified great toe**

√7th **S93.144 Subluxation of metatarsophalangeal joint of right lesser toe(s)**

√7th **S93.145 Subluxation of metatarsophalangeal joint of left lesser toe(s)**

√7th **S93.146 Subluxation of metatarsophalangeal joint of unspecified lesser toe(s)**

√7th **S93.149 Subluxation of metatarsophalangeal joint of unspecified toe(s)**

√5th **S93.3 Subluxation and dislocation of foot**

EXCLUDES 2 *dislocation of toe (S93.1-)*

√6th **S93.30 Unspecified subluxation and dislocation of foot**

Dislocation of foot NOS

Subluxation of foot NOS

√7th **S93.301 Unspecified subluxation of right foot**

√7th **S93.302 Unspecified subluxation of left foot**

√7th **S93.303 Unspecified subluxation of unspecified foot**

√7th **S93.304 Unspecified dislocation of right foot**

√7th **S93.305 Unspecified dislocation of left foot**

√7th **S93.306 Unspecified dislocation of unspecified foot**

√6th **S93.31 Subluxation and dislocation of tarsal joint**

√7th **S93.311 Subluxation of tarsal joint of right foot**

√7th **S93.312 Subluxation of tarsal joint of left foot**

√7th **S93.313 Subluxation of tarsal joint of unspecified foot**

√7th **S93.314 Dislocation of tarsal joint of right foot**

√7th **S93.315 Dislocation of tarsal joint of left foot**

√7th **S93.316 Dislocation of tarsal joint of unspecified foot**

√6th **S93.32 Subluxation and dislocation of tarsometatarsal joint**

√7th **S93.321 Subluxation of tarsometatarsal joint of right foot**

√7th **S93.322 Subluxation of tarsometatarsal joint of left foot**

√7th **S93.323 Subluxation of tarsometatarsal joint of unspecified foot**

√7th **S93.324 Dislocation of tarsometatarsal joint of right foot**

√7th **S93.325 Dislocation of tarsometatarsal joint of left foot**

√7th **S93.326 Dislocation of tarsometatarsal joint of unspecified foot**

√6th **S93.33 Other subluxation and dislocation of foot**

√7th **S93.331 Other subluxation of right foot**

√7th **S93.332 Other subluxation of left foot**

√7th **S93.333 Other subluxation of unspecified foot**

√7th **S93.334 Other dislocation of right foot**

√7th **S93.335 Other dislocation of left foot**

√7th **S93.336 Other dislocation of unspecified foot**

√5th **S93.4 Sprain of ankle**

EXCLUDES 2 *injury of Achilles tendon (S86.0-)*

√6th **S93.40 Sprain of unspecified ligament of ankle**

Sprain of ankle NOS

Sprained ankle NOS

√7th **S93.401 Sprain of unspecified ligament of right ankle**

√7th **S93.402 Sprain of unspecified ligament of left ankle**

√7th **S93.409 Sprain of unspecified ligament of unspecified ankle**

√6th **S93.41 Sprain of calcaneofibular ligament**

√7th **S93.411 Sprain of calcaneofibular ligament of right ankle**

√7th **S93.412 Sprain of calcaneofibular ligament of left ankle**

√7th **S93.419 Sprain of calcaneofibular ligament of unspecified ankle**

√6th **S93.42 Sprain of deltoid ligament**

√7th **S93.421 Sprain of deltoid ligament of right ankle**

√7th **S93.422 Sprain of deltoid ligament of left ankle**

√7th **S93.429 Sprain of deltoid ligament of unspecified ankle**

√6th **S93.43 Sprain of tibiofibular ligament**

√7th **S93.431 Sprain of tibiofibular ligament of right ankle**

√7th **S93.432 Sprain of tibiofibular ligament of left ankle**

√7th **S93.439 Sprain of tibiofibular ligament of unspecified ankle**

√6th **S93.49 Sprain of other ligament of ankle**

Sprain of internal collateral ligament

Sprain of talofibular ligament

√7th **S93.491 Sprain of other ligament of right ankle**

√7th **S93.492 Sprain of other ligament of left ankle**

√7th **S93.499 Sprain of other ligament of unspecified ankle**

√5th **S93.5 Sprain of toe**

√6th **S93.50 Unspecified sprain of toe**

√7th **S93.501 Unspecified sprain of right great toe**

√7th **S93.502 Unspecified sprain of left great toe**

√7th **S93.503 Unspecified sprain of unspecified great toe**

√7th **S93.504 Unspecified sprain of right lesser toe(s)**

√7th **S93.505 Unspecified sprain of left lesser toe(s)**

√7th **S93.506 Unspecified sprain of unspecified lesser toe(s)**

√7th **S93.509 Unspecified sprain of unspecified toe(s)**

√6th **S93.51 Sprain of interphalangeal joint of toe**

√7th **S93.511 Sprain of interphalangeal joint of right great toe**

√7th **S93.512 Sprain of interphalangeal joint of left great toe**

√7th **S93.513 Sprain of interphalangeal joint of unspecified great toe**

√7th **S93.514 Sprain of interphalangeal joint of right lesser toe(s)**

√7th **S93.515 Sprain of interphalangeal joint of left lesser toe(s)**

√7th **S93.516 Sprain of interphalangeal joint of unspecified lesser toe(s)**

√7th **S93.519 Sprain of interphalangeal joint of unspecified toe(s)**

√6th **S93.52 Sprain of metatarsophalangeal joint of toe**

√7th **S93.521 Sprain of metatarsophalangeal joint of right great toe**

√7th **S93.522 Sprain of metatarsophalangeal joint of left great toe**

√7th **S93.523 Sprain of metatarsophalangeal joint of unspecified great toe**

√7th **S93.524 Sprain of metatarsophalangeal joint of right lesser toe(s)**

√7th **S93.525 Sprain of metatarsophalangeal joint of left lesser toe(s)**

√7th **S93.526 Sprain of metatarsophalangeal joint of unspecified lesser toe(s)**

S93.529 Sprain of metatarsophalangeal joint of unspecified toe(s)

S93.6 Sprain of foot
EXCLUDES 2 *sprain of metatarsophalangeal joint of toe (S93.52-)*
sprain of toe (S93.5-)

S93.60 Unspecified sprain of foot
S93.601 Unspecified sprain of right foot
S93.602 Unspecified sprain of left foot
S93.609 Unspecified sprain of unspecified foot

S93.61 Sprain of tarsal ligament of foot
S93.611 Sprain of tarsal ligament of right foot
S93.612 Sprain of tarsal ligament of left foot
S93.619 Sprain of tarsal ligament of unspecified foot

S93.62 Sprain of tarsometatarsal ligament of foot
S93.621 Sprain of tarsometatarsal ligament of right foot
S93.622 Sprain of tarsometatarsal ligament of left foot
S93.629 Sprain of tarsometatarsal ligament of unspecified foot

S93.69 Other sprain of foot
S93.691 Other sprain of right foot
S93.692 Other sprain of left foot
S93.699 Other sprain of unspecified foot

S94 Injury of nerves at ankle and foot level

Code also any associated open wound (S91.-)

The appropriate 7th character is to be added to each code from category S94.
A initial encounter
D subsequent encounter
S sequela

S94.0 Injury of lateral plantar nerve
S94.00 Injury of lateral plantar nerve, unspecified leg
S94.01 Injury of lateral plantar nerve, right leg
S94.02 Injury of lateral plantar nerve, left leg

S94.1 Injury of medial plantar nerve
S94.10 Injury of medial plantar nerve, unspecified leg
S94.11 Injury of medial plantar nerve, right leg
S94.12 Injury of medial plantar nerve, left leg

S94.2 Injury of deep peroneal nerve at ankle and foot level
Injury of terminal, lateral branch of deep peroneal nerve
S94.20 Injury of deep peroneal nerve at ankle and foot level, unspecified leg
S94.21 Injury of deep peroneal nerve at ankle and foot level, right leg
S94.22 Injury of deep peroneal nerve at ankle and foot level, left leg

S94.3 Injury of cutaneous sensory nerve at ankle and foot level
S94.30 Injury of cutaneous sensory nerve at ankle and foot level, unspecified leg
S94.31 Injury of cutaneous sensory nerve at ankle and foot level, right leg
S94.32 Injury of cutaneous sensory nerve at ankle and foot level, left leg

S94.8 Injury of other nerves at ankle and foot level
S94.8X Injury of other nerves at ankle and foot level
S94.8X1 Injury of other nerves at ankle and foot level, right leg
S94.8X2 Injury of other nerves at ankle and foot level, left leg
S94.8X9 Injury of other nerves at ankle and foot level, unspecified leg

S94.9 Injury of unspecified nerve at ankle and foot level
S94.90 Injury of unspecified nerve at ankle and foot level, unspecified leg
S94.91 Injury of unspecified nerve at ankle and foot level, right leg
S94.92 Injury of unspecified nerve at ankle and foot level, left leg

S95 Injury of blood vessels at ankle and foot level

Code also any associated open wound (S91.-)
EXCLUDES 2 *injury of posterior tibial artery and vein (S85.1-, S85.8-)*

The appropriate 7th character is to be added to each code from category S95.
A initial encounter
D subsequent encounter
S sequela

S95.0 Injury of dorsal artery of foot
S95.00 Unspecified injury of dorsal artery of foot
S95.001 Unspecified injury of dorsal artery of right foot
S95.002 Unspecified injury of dorsal artery of left foot
S95.009 Unspecified injury of dorsal artery of unspecified foot

S95.01 Laceration of dorsal artery of foot
S95.011 Laceration of dorsal artery of right foot
S95.012 Laceration of dorsal artery of left foot
S95.019 Laceration of dorsal artery of unspecified foot

S95.09 Other specified injury of dorsal artery of foot
S95.091 Other specified injury of dorsal artery of right foot
S95.092 Other specified injury of dorsal artery of left foot
S95.099 Other specified injury of dorsal artery of unspecified foot

S95.1 Injury of plantar artery of foot
S95.10 Unspecified injury of plantar artery of foot
S95.101 Unspecified injury of plantar artery of right foot
S95.102 Unspecified injury of plantar artery of left foot
S95.109 Unspecified injury of plantar artery of unspecified foot

S95.11 Laceration of plantar artery of foot
S95.111 Laceration of plantar artery of right foot
S95.112 Laceration of plantar artery of left foot
S95.119 Laceration of plantar artery of unspecified foot

S95.19 Other specified injury of plantar artery of foot
S95.191 Other specified injury of plantar artery of right foot
S95.192 Other specified injury of plantar artery of left foot
S95.199 Other specified injury of plantar artery of unspecified foot

S95.2 Injury of dorsal vein of foot
S95.20 Unspecified injury of dorsal vein of foot
S95.201 Unspecified injury of dorsal vein of right foot
S95.202 Unspecified injury of dorsal vein of left foot
S95.209 Unspecified injury of dorsal vein of unspecified foot

S95.21 Laceration of dorsal vein of foot
S95.211 Laceration of dorsal vein of right foot
S95.212 Laceration of dorsal vein of left foot
S95.219 Laceration of dorsal vein of unspecified foot

S95.29 Other specified injury of dorsal vein of foot
S95.291 Other specified injury of dorsal vein of right foot
S95.292 Other specified injury of dorsal vein of left foot
S95.299 Other specified injury of dorsal vein of unspecified foot

S95.8 Injury of other blood vessels at ankle and foot level
S95.80 Unspecified injury of other blood vessels at ankle and foot level
S95.801 Unspecified injury of other blood vessels at ankle and foot level, right leg
S95.802 Unspecified injury of other blood vessels at ankle and foot level, left leg

- 7th **S95.809 Unspecified injury of other blood vessels at ankle and foot level, unspecified leg**
- 6th **S95.81 Laceration of other blood vessels at ankle and foot level**
  - 7th **S95.811 Laceration of other blood vessels at ankle and foot level, right leg**
  - 7th **S95.812 Laceration of other blood vessels at ankle and foot level, left leg**
  - 7th **S95.819 Laceration of other blood vessels at ankle and foot level, unspecified leg**
- 6th **S95.89 Other specified injury of other blood vessels at ankle and foot level**
  - 7th **S95.891 Other specified injury of other blood vessels at ankle and foot level, right leg**
  - 7th **S95.892 Other specified injury of other blood vessels at ankle and foot level, left leg**
  - 7th **S95.899 Other specified injury of other blood vessels at ankle and foot level, unspecified leg**

5th **S95.9 Injury of unspecified blood vessel at ankle and foot level**

- 6th **S95.90 Unspecified injury of unspecified blood vessel at ankle and foot level**
  - 7th **S95.901 Unspecified injury of unspecified blood vessel at ankle and foot level, right leg**
  - 7th **S95.902 Unspecified injury of unspecified blood vessel at ankle and foot level, left leg**
  - 7th **S95.909 Unspecified injury of unspecified blood vessel at ankle and foot level, unspecified leg**
- 6th **S95.91 Laceration of unspecified blood vessel at ankle and foot level**
  - 7th **S95.911 Laceration of unspecified blood vessel at ankle and foot level, right leg**
  - 7th **S95.912 Laceration of unspecified blood vessel at ankle and foot level, left leg**
  - 7th **S95.919 Laceration of unspecified blood vessel at ankle and foot level, unspecified leg**
- 6th **S95.99 Other specified injury of unspecified blood vessel at ankle and foot level**
  - 7th **S95.991 Other specified injury of unspecified blood vessel at ankle and foot level, right leg**
  - 7th **S95.992 Other specified injury of unspecified blood vessel at ankle and foot level, left leg**
  - 7th **S95.999 Other specified injury of unspecified blood vessel at ankle and foot level, unspecified leg**

4th **S96 Injury of muscle and tendon at ankle and foot level**

Code also any associated open wound (S91.-)

EXCLUDES 2 *injury of Achilles tendon (S86.0-)*
sprain of joints and ligaments of ankle and foot (S93.-)

The appropriate 7th character is to be added to each code from category S96.
A initial encounter
D subsequent encounter
S sequela

5th **S96.0 Injury of muscle and tendon of long flexor muscle of toe at ankle and foot level**

- 6th **S96.00 Unspecified injury of muscle and tendon of long flexor muscle of toe at ankle and foot level**
  - 7th **S96.001 Unspecified injury of muscle and tendon of long flexor muscle of toe at ankle and foot level, right foot**
  - 7th **S96.002 Unspecified injury of muscle and tendon of long flexor muscle of toe at ankle and foot level, left foot**
  - 7th **S96.009 Unspecified injury of muscle and tendon of long flexor muscle of toe at ankle and foot level, unspecified foot**
- 6th **S96.01 Strain of muscle and tendon of long flexor muscle of toe at ankle and foot level**
  - 7th **S96.011 Strain of muscle and tendon of long flexor muscle of toe at ankle and foot level, right foot**
  - 7th **S96.012 Strain of muscle and tendon of long flexor muscle of toe at ankle and foot level, left foot**
  - 7th **S96.019 Strain of muscle and tendon of long flexor muscle of toe at ankle and foot level, unspecified foot**
- 6th **S96.02 Laceration of muscle and tendon of long flexor muscle of toe at ankle and foot level**
  - 7th **S96.021 Laceration of muscle and tendon of long flexor muscle of toe at ankle and foot level, right foot**
  - 7th **S96.022 Laceration of muscle and tendon of long flexor muscle of toe at ankle and foot level, left foot**
  - 7th **S96.029 Laceration of muscle and tendon of long flexor muscle of toe at ankle and foot level, unspecified foot**
- 6th **S96.09 Other injury of muscle and tendon of long flexor muscle of toe at ankle and foot level**
  - 7th **S96.091 Other injury of muscle and tendon of long flexor muscle of toe at ankle and foot level, right foot**
  - 7th **S96.092 Other injury of muscle and tendon of long flexor muscle of toe at ankle and foot level, left foot**
  - 7th **S96.099 Other injury of muscle and tendon of long flexor muscle of toe at ankle and foot level, unspecified foot**

5th **S96.1 Injury of muscle and tendon of long extensor muscle of toe at ankle and foot level**

- 6th **S96.10 Unspecified injury of muscle and tendon of long extensor muscle of toe at ankle and foot level**
  - 7th **S96.101 Unspecified injury of muscle and tendon of long extensor muscle of toe at ankle and foot level, right foot**
  - 7th **S96.102 Unspecified injury of muscle and tendon of long extensor muscle of toe at ankle and foot level, left foot**
  - 7th **S96.109 Unspecified injury of muscle and tendon of long extensor muscle of toe at ankle and foot level, unspecified foot**
- 6th **S96.11 Strain of muscle and tendon of long extensor muscle of toe at ankle and foot level**
  - 7th **S96.111 Strain of muscle and tendon of long extensor muscle of toe at ankle and foot level, right foot**
  - 7th **S96.112 Strain of muscle and tendon of long extensor muscle of toe at ankle and foot level, left foot**
  - 7th **S96.119 Strain of muscle and tendon of long extensor muscle of toe at ankle and foot level, unspecified foot**
- 6th **S96.12 Laceration of muscle and tendon of long extensor muscle of toe at ankle and foot level**
  - 7th **S96.121 Laceration of muscle and tendon of long extensor muscle of toe at ankle and foot level, right foot**
  - 7th **S96.122 Laceration of muscle and tendon of long extensor muscle of toe at ankle and foot level, left foot**
  - 7th **S96.129 Laceration of muscle and tendon of long extensor muscle of toe at ankle and foot level, unspecified foot**
- 6th **S96.19 Other specified injury of muscle and tendon of long extensor muscle of toe at ankle and foot level**
  - 7th **S96.191 Other specified injury of muscle and tendon of long extensor muscle of toe at ankle and foot level, right foot**
  - 7th **S96.192 Other specified injury of muscle and tendon of long extensor muscle of toe at ankle and foot level, left foot**
  - 7th **S96.199 Other specified injury of muscle and tendon of long extensor muscle of toe at ankle and foot level, unspecified foot**

✓5th **S96.2 Injury of intrinsic muscle and tendon at ankle and foot level**
✓6th **S96.20 Unspecified injury of intrinsic muscle and tendon at ankle and foot level**
✓7th **S96.201 Unspecified injury of intrinsic muscle and tendon at ankle and foot level, right foot**
✓7th **S96.202 Unspecified injury of intrinsic muscle and tendon at ankle and foot level, left foot**
✓7th **S96.209 Unspecified injury of intrinsic muscle and tendon at ankle and foot level, unspecified foot**
✓6th **S96.21 Strain of intrinsic muscle and tendon at ankle and foot level**
✓7th **S96.211 Strain of intrinsic muscle and tendon at ankle and foot level, right foot**
✓7th **S96.212 Strain of intrinsic muscle and tendon at ankle and foot level, left foot**
✓7th **S96.219 Strain of intrinsic muscle and tendon at ankle and foot level, unspecified foot**
✓6th **S96.22 Laceration of intrinsic muscle and tendon at ankle and foot level**
✓7th **S96.221 Laceration of intrinsic muscle and tendon at ankle and foot level, right foot**
✓7th **S96.222 Laceration of intrinsic muscle and tendon at ankle and foot level, left foot**
✓7th **S96.229 Laceration of intrinsic muscle and tendon at ankle and foot level, unspecified foot**
✓6th **S96.29 Other specified injury of intrinsic muscle and tendon at ankle and foot level**
✓7th **S96.291 Other specified injury of intrinsic muscle and tendon at ankle and foot level, right foot**
✓7th **S96.292 Other specified injury of intrinsic muscle and tendon at ankle and foot level, left foot**
✓7th **S96.299 Other specified injury of intrinsic muscle and tendon at ankle and foot level, unspecified foot**

✓5th **S96.8 Injury of other specified muscles and tendons at ankle and foot level**
✓6th **S96.80 Unspecified injury of other specified muscles and tendons at ankle and foot level**
✓7th **S96.801 Unspecified injury of other specified muscles and tendons at ankle and foot level, right foot**
✓7th **S96.802 Unspecified injury of other specified muscles and tendons at ankle and foot level, left foot**
✓7th **S96.809 Unspecified injury of other specified muscles and tendons at ankle and foot level, unspecified foot**
✓6th **S96.81 Strain of other specified muscles and tendons at ankle and foot level**
✓7th **S96.811 Strain of other specified muscles and tendons at ankle and foot level, right foot**
✓7th **S96.812 Strain of other specified muscles and tendons at ankle and foot level, left foot**
✓7th **S96.819 Strain of other specified muscles and tendons at ankle and foot level, unspecified foot**
✓6th **S96.82 Laceration of other specified muscles and tendons at ankle and foot level**
✓7th **S96.821 Laceration of other specified muscles and tendons at ankle and foot level, right foot**
✓7th **S96.822 Laceration of other specified muscles and tendons at ankle and foot level, left foot**
✓7th **S96.829 Laceration of other specified muscles and tendons at ankle and foot level, unspecified foot**
✓6th **S96.89 Other specified injury of other specified muscles and tendons at ankle and foot level**
✓7th **S96.891 Other specified injury of other specified muscles and tendons at ankle and foot level, right foot**
✓7th **S96.892 Other specified injury of other specified muscles and tendons at ankle and foot level, left foot**
✓7th **S96.899 Other specified injury of other specified muscles and tendons at ankle and foot level, unspecified foot**

✓5th **S96.9 Injury of unspecified muscle and tendon at ankle and foot level**
✓6th **S96.90 Unspecified injury of unspecified muscle and tendon at ankle and foot level**
✓7th **S96.901 Unspecified injury of unspecified muscle and tendon at ankle and foot level, right foot**
✓7th **S96.902 Unspecified injury of unspecified muscle and tendon at ankle and foot level, left foot**
✓7th **S96.909 Unspecified injury of unspecified muscle and tendon at ankle and foot level, unspecified foot**
✓6th **S96.91 Strain of unspecified muscle and tendon at ankle and foot level**
✓7th **S96.911 Strain of unspecified muscle and tendon at ankle and foot level, right foot**
✓7th **S96.912 Strain of unspecified muscle and tendon at ankle and foot level, left foot**
✓7th **S96.919 Strain of unspecified muscle and tendon at ankle and foot level, unspecified foot**
✓6th **S96.92 Laceration of unspecified muscle and tendon at ankle and foot level**
✓7th **S96.921 Laceration of unspecified muscle and tendon at ankle and foot level, right foot**
✓7th **S96.922 Laceration of unspecified muscle and tendon at ankle and foot level, left foot**
✓7th **S96.929 Laceration of unspecified muscle and tendon at ankle and foot level, unspecified foot**
✓6th **S96.99 Other specified injury of unspecified muscle and tendon at ankle and foot level**
✓7th **S96.991 Other specified injury of unspecified muscle and tendon at ankle and foot level, right foot**
✓7th **S96.992 Other specified injury of unspecified muscle and tendon at ankle and foot level, left foot**
✓7th **S96.999 Other specified injury of unspecified muscle and tendon at ankle and foot level, unspecified foot**

✓4th **S97 Crushing injury of ankle and foot**
Use additional code(s) for all associated injuries

The appropriate 7th character is to be added to each code from category S97.
A initial encounter
D subsequent encounter
S sequela

✓5th **S97.0 Crushing injury of ankle**
✓x7th **S97.00 Crushing injury of unspecified ankle**
✓x7th **S97.01 Crushing injury of right ankle**
✓x7th **S97.02 Crushing injury of left ankle**
✓5th **S97.1 Crushing injury of toe**
✓6th **S97.10 Crushing injury of unspecified toe(s)**
✓7th **S97.101 Crushing injury of unspecified right toe(s)**
✓7th **S97.102 Crushing injury of unspecified left toe(s)**
✓7th **S97.109 Crushing injury of unspecified toe(s)**
Crushing injury of toe NOS
✓6th **S97.11 Crushing injury of great toe**
✓7th **S97.111 Crushing injury of right great toe**
✓7th **S97.112 Crushing injury of left great toe**
✓7th **S97.119 Crushing injury of unspecified great toe**
✓6th **S97.12 Crushing injury of lesser toe(s)**
✓7th **S97.121 Crushing injury of right lesser toe(s)**

S97.122 Crushing injury of left lesser toe(s)
S97.129 Crushing injury of unspecified lesser toe(s)
S97.8 Crushing injury of foot
S97.80 Crushing injury of unspecified foot
Crushing injury of foot NOS
S97.81 Crushing injury of right foot
S97.82 Crushing injury of left foot

S98 Traumatic amputation of ankle and foot
An amputation not identified as partial or complete should be coded to complete

The appropriate 7th character is to be added to each code from category S98.
A initial encounter
D subsequent encounter
S sequela

S98.0 Traumatic amputation of foot at ankle level
S98.01 Complete traumatic amputation of foot at ankle level
S98.011 Complete traumatic amputation of right foot at ankle level
S98.012 Complete traumatic amputation of left foot at ankle level
S98.019 Complete traumatic amputation of unspecified foot at ankle level
S98.02 Partial traumatic amputation of foot at ankle level
S98.021 Partial traumatic amputation of right foot at ankle level
S98.022 Partial traumatic amputation of left foot at ankle level
S98.029 Partial traumatic amputation of unspecified foot at ankle level
S98.1 Traumatic amputation of one toe
S98.11 Complete traumatic amputation of great toe
S98.111 Complete traumatic amputation of right great toe
S98.112 Complete traumatic amputation of left great toe
S98.119 Complete traumatic amputation of unspecified great toe
S98.12 Partial traumatic amputation of great toe
S98.121 Partial traumatic amputation of right great toe
S98.122 Partial traumatic amputation of left great toe
S98.129 Partial traumatic amputation of unspecified great toe
S98.13 Complete traumatic amputation of one lesser toe
Traumatic amputation of toe NOS
S98.131 Complete traumatic amputation of one right lesser toe
S98.132 Complete traumatic amputation of one left lesser toe
S98.139 Complete traumatic amputation of one unspecified lesser toe
S98.14 Partial traumatic amputation of one lesser toe
S98.141 Partial traumatic amputation of one right lesser toe
S98.142 Partial traumatic amputation of one left lesser toe
S98.149 Partial traumatic amputation of one unspecified lesser toe
S98.2 Traumatic amputation of two or more lesser toes
S98.21 Complete traumatic amputation of two or more lesser toes
S98.211 Complete traumatic amputation of two or more right lesser toes
S98.212 Complete traumatic amputation of two or more left lesser toes
S98.219 Complete traumatic amputation of two or more unspecified lesser toes
S98.22 Partial traumatic amputation of two or more lesser toes
S98.221 Partial traumatic amputation of two or more right lesser toes
S98.222 Partial traumatic amputation of two or more left lesser toes
S98.229 Partial traumatic amputation of two or more unspecified lesser toes
S98.3 Traumatic amputation of midfoot
S98.31 Complete traumatic amputation of midfoot
S98.311 Complete traumatic amputation of right midfoot
S98.312 Complete traumatic amputation of left midfoot
S98.319 Complete traumatic amputation of unspecified midfoot
S98.32 Partial traumatic amputation of midfoot
S98.321 Partial traumatic amputation of right midfoot
S98.322 Partial traumatic amputation of left midfoot
S98.329 Partial traumatic amputation of unspecified midfoot
S98.9 Traumatic amputation of foot, level unspecified
S98.91 Complete traumatic amputation of foot, level unspecified
S98.911 Complete traumatic amputation of right foot, level unspecified
S98.912 Complete traumatic amputation of left foot, level unspecified
S98.919 Complete traumatic amputation of unspecified foot, level unspecified
S98.92 Partial traumatic amputation of foot, level unspecified
S98.921 Partial traumatic amputation of right foot, level unspecified
S98.922 Partial traumatic amputation of left foot, level unspecified
S98.929 Partial traumatic amputation of unspecified foot, level unspecified

S99 Other and unspecified injuries of ankle and foot

The appropriate 7th character is to be added to each code from category S99.
A initial encounter
D subsequent encounter
S sequela

S99.8 Other specified injuries of ankle and foot
S99.81 Other specified injuries of ankle
S99.811 Other specified injuries of right ankle
S99.812 Other specified injuries of left ankle
S99.819 Other specified injuries of unspecified ankle
S99.82 Other specified injuries of foot
S99.821 Other specified injuries of right foot
S99.822 Other specified injuries of left foot
S99.829 Other specified injuries of unspecified foot
S99.9 Unspecified injury of ankle and foot
S99.91 Unspecified injury of ankle
S99.911 Unspecified injury of right ankle
S99.912 Unspecified injury of left ankle
S99.919 Unspecified injury of unspecified ankle
S99.92 Unspecified injury of foot
S99.921 Unspecified injury of right foot
S99.922 Unspecified injury of left foot
S99.929 Unspecified injury of unspecified foot

Injury, Poisoning And Certain Other Consequences Of External Causes (T07-T88)

Injuries involving multiple body regions (T07)

EXCLUDES 1 *burns and corrosions (T20-T32)*
frostbite (T33-T34)
insect bite or sting, venomous (T63.4)
sunburn (L55.-)

T07 Unspecified multiple injuries
EXCLUDES 1 *injury NOS (T14)*

Injury of unspecified body region (T14)

✓4th **T14 Injury of unspecified body region**
EXCLUDES 1 *multiple unspecified injuries (T07)*

T14.8 Other injury of unspecified body region
Abrasion NOS
Contusion NOS
Crush injury NOS
Fracture NOS
Skin injury NOS
Vascular injury NOS

✓5th **T14.9 Unspecified injury**
T14.90 Injury, unspecified
Injury NOS
T14.91 Suicide attempt
Attempted suicide NOS

Effects of foreign body entering through natural orifice (T15-T19)

EXCLUDES 2 *foreign body accidentally left in operation wound (T81.5-)*
foreign body in penetrating wound—See open wound by body region
residual foreign body in soft tissue (M79.5)
splinter, without open wound—See superficial injury by body region

✓4th **T15 Foreign body on external eye**
EXCLUDES 2 *foreign body in penetrating wound of orbit and eye ball (S05.4-, S05.5-)*
open wound of eyelid and periocular area (S01.1-)
retained foreign body in eyelid (H02.8-)
retained (old) foreign body in penetrating wound of orbit and eye ball (H05.5-, H44.6-, H44.7-)
superficial foreign body of eyelid and periocular area (S00.25-)

The appropriate 7th character is to be added to each code from category T15.
A initial encounter
D subsequent encounter
S sequela

✓5th **T15.0 Foreign body in cornea**
✓x7th **T15.00 Foreign body in cornea, unspecified eye**
✓x7th **T15.01 Foreign body in cornea, right eye**
✓x7th **T15.02 Foreign body in cornea, left eye**

✓5th **T15.1 Foreign body in conjunctival sac**
✓x7th **T15.10 Foreign body in conjunctival sac, unspecified eye**
✓x7th **T15.11 Foreign body in conjunctival sac, right eye**
✓x7th **T15.12 Foreign body in conjunctival sac, left eye**

✓5th **T15.8 Foreign body in other and multiple parts of external eye**
Foreign body in lacrimal punctum
✓x7th **T15.80 Foreign body in other and multiple parts of external eye, unspecified eye**
✓x7th **T15.81 Foreign body in other and multiple parts of external eye, right eye**
✓x7th **T15.82 Foreign body in other and multiple parts of external eye, left eye**

✓5th **T15.9 Foreign body on external eye, part unspecified**
✓x7th **T15.90 Foreign body on external eye, part unspecified, unspecified eye**
✓x7th **T15.91 Foreign body on external eye, part unspecified, right eye**
✓x7th **T15.92 Foreign body on external eye, part unspecified, left eye**

✓4th **T16 Foreign body in ear**
Foreign body in auditory canal

The appropriate 7th character is to be added to each code from category T16.
A initial encounter
D subsequent encounter
S sequela

✓x7th **T16.1 Foreign body in right ear**
✓x7th **T16.2 Foreign body in left ear**
✓x7th **T16.9 Foreign body in ear, unspecified ear**

✓4th **T17 Foreign body in respiratory tract**

The appropriate 7th character is to be added to each code from category T17.
A initial encounter
D subsequent encounter
S sequela

✓x7th **T17.0 Foreign body in nasal sinus**
✓x7th **T17.1 Foreign body in nostril**
Foreign body in nose NOS

✓5th **T17.2 Foreign body in pharynx**
Foreign body in nasopharynx
Foreign body in throat NOS
✓6th **T17.20 Unspecified foreign body in pharynx**
✓7th **T17.200 Unspecified foreign body in pharynx causing asphyxiation**
✓7th **T17.208 Unspecified foreign body in pharynx causing other injury**
✓6th **T17.21 Gastric contents in pharynx**
Aspiration of gastric contents into pharynx
Vomitus in pharynx
✓7th **T17.210 Gastric contents in pharynx causing asphyxiation**
✓7th **T17.218 Gastric contents in pharynx causing other injury**
✓6th **T17.22 Food in pharynx**
Bones in pharynx
Seeds in pharynx
✓7th **T17.220 Food in pharynx causing asphyxiation**
✓7th **T17.228 Food in pharynx causing other injury**
✓6th **T17.29 Other foreign object in pharynx**
✓7th **T17.290 Other foreign object in pharynx causing asphyxiation**
✓7th **T17.298 Other foreign object in pharynx causing other injury**

✓5th **T17.3 Foreign body in larynx**
✓6th **T17.30 Unspecified foreign body in larynx**
✓7th **T17.300 Unspecified foreign body in larynx causing asphyxiation**
✓7th **T17.308 Unspecified foreign body in larynx causing other injury**
✓6th **T17.31 Gastric contents in larynx**
Aspiration of gastric contents into larynx
Vomitus in larynx
✓7th **T17.310 Gastric contents in larynx causing asphyxiation**
✓7th **T17.318 Gastric contents in larynx causing other injury**
✓6th **T17.32 Food in larynx**
Bones in larynx
Seeds in larynx
✓7th **T17.320 Food in larynx causing asphyxiation**
✓7th **T17.328 Food in larynx causing other injury**
✓6th **T17.39 Other foreign object in larynx**
✓7th **T17.390 Other foreign object in larynx causing asphyxiation**
✓7th **T17.398 Other foreign object in larynx causing other injury**

✓5th **T17.4 Foreign body in trachea**
✓6th **T17.40 Unspecified foreign body in trachea**
✓7th **T17.400 Unspecified foreign body in trachea causing asphyxiation**
✓7th **T17.408 Unspecified foreign body in trachea causing other injury**

6th **T17.41 Gastric contents in trachea**
Aspiration of gastric contents into trachea
Vomitus in trachea
7th **T17.410 Gastric contents in trachea causing asphyxiation**
7th **T17.418 Gastric contents in trachea causing other injury**
6th **T17.42 Food in trachea**
Bones in trachea
Seeds in trachea
7th **T17.420 Food in trachea causing asphyxiation**
7th **T17.428 Food in trachea causing other injury**
6th **T17.49 Other foreign object in trachea**
7th **T17.490 Other foreign object in trachea causing asphyxiation**
7th **T17.498 Other foreign object in trachea causing other injury**
5th **T17.5 Foreign body in bronchus**
6th **T17.50 Unspecified foreign body in bronchus**
7th **T17.500 Unspecified foreign body in bronchus causing asphyxiation**
7th **T17.508 Unspecified foreign body in bronchus causing other injury**
6th **T17.51 Gastric contents in bronchus**
Aspiration of gastric contents into bronchus
Vomitus in bronchus
7th **T17.510 Gastric contents in bronchus causing asphyxiation**
7th **T17.518 Gastric contents in bronchus causing other injury**
6th **T17.52 Food in bronchus**
Bones in bronchus
Seeds in bronchus
7th **T17.520 Food in bronchus causing asphyxiation**
7th **T17.528 Food in bronchus causing other injury**
6th **T17.59 Other foreign object in bronchus**
7th **T17.590 Other foreign object in bronchus causing asphyxiation**
7th **T17.598 Other foreign object in bronchus causing other injury**
5th **T17.8 Foreign body in other parts of respiratory tract**
Foreign body in bronchioles
Foreign body in lung
6th **T17.80 Unspecified foreign body in other parts of respiratory tract**
7th **T17.800 Unspecified foreign body in other parts of respiratory tract causing asphyxiation**
7th **T17.808 Unspecified foreign body in other parts of respiratory tract causing other injury**
6th **T17.81 Gastric contents in other parts of respiratory tract**
Aspiration of gastric contents into other parts of respiratory tract
Vomitus in other parts of respiratory tract
7th **T17.810 Gastric contents in other parts of respiratory tract causing asphyxiation**
7th **T17.818 Gastric contents in other parts of respiratory tract causing other injury**
6th **T17.82 Food in other parts of respiratory tract**
Bones in other parts of respiratory tract
Seeds in other parts of respiratory tract
7th **T17.820 Food in other parts of respiratory tract causing asphyxiation**
7th **T17.828 Food in other parts of respiratory tract causing other injury**
6th **T17.89 Other foreign object in other parts of respiratory tract**
7th **T17.890 Other foreign object in other parts of respiratory tract causing asphyxiation**
7th **T17.898 Other foreign object in other parts of respiratory tract causing other injury**
5th **T17.9 Foreign body in respiratory tract, part unspecified**
6th **T17.90 Unspecified foreign body in respiratory tract, part unspecified**
7th **T17.900 Unspecified foreign body in respiratory tract, part unspecified causing asphyxiation**
7th **T17.908 Unspecified foreign body in respiratory tract, part unspecified causing other injury**
6th **T17.91 Gastric contents in respiratory tract, part unspecified**
Aspiration of gastric contents into respiratory tract, part unspecified
Vomitus in trachea respiratory tract, part unspecified
7th **T17.910 Gastric contents in respiratory tract, part unspecified causing asphyxiation**
7th **T17.918 Gastric contents in respiratory tract, part unspecified causing other injury**
6th **T17.92 Food in respiratory tract, part unspecified**
Bones in respiratory tract, part unspecified
Seeds in respiratory tract, part unspecified
7th **T17.920 Food in respiratory tract, part unspecified causing asphyxiation**
7th **T17.928 Food in respiratory tract, part unspecified causing other injury**
6th **T17.99 Other foreign object in respiratory tract, part unspecified**
7th **T17.990 Other foreign object in respiratory tract, part unspecified in causing asphyxiation**
7th **T17.998 Other foreign object in respiratory tract, part unspecified causing other injury**

4th **T18 Foreign body in alimentary tract**
EXCLUDES 2 *foreign body in pharynx (T17.2-)*

The appropriate 7th character is to be added to each code from category T18.
A initial encounter
D subsequent encounter
S sequela

x7th **T18.0 Foreign body in mouth**
5th **T18.1 Foreign body in esophagus**
EXCLUDES 2 *foreign body in respiratory tract (T17.-)*
6th **T18.10 Unspecified foreign body in esophagus**
7th **T18.100 Unspecified foreign body in esophagus causing compression of trachea**
Unspecified foreign body in esophagus causing obstruction of respiration
7th **T18.108 Unspecified foreign body in esophagus causing other injury**
6th **T18.11 Gastric contents in esophagus**
Vomitus in esophagus
7th **T18.110 Gastric contents in esophagus causing compression of trachea**
Gastric contents in esophagus causing obstruction of respiration
7th **T18.118 Gastric contents in esophagus causing other injury**
6th **T18.12 Food in esophagus**
Bones in esophagus
Seeds in esophagus
7th **T18.120 Food in esophagus causing compression of trachea**
Food in esophagus causing obstruction of respiration
7th **T18.128 Food in esophagus causing other injury**
6th **T18.19 Other foreign object in esophagus**
7th **T18.190 Other foreign object in esophagus causing compression of trachea**
Other foreign body in esophagus causing obstruction of respiration
7th **T18.198 Other foreign object in esophagus causing other injury**
x7th **T18.2 Foreign body in stomach**
x7th **T18.3 Foreign body in small intestine**
x7th **T18.4 Foreign body in colon**
x7th **T18.5 Foreign body in anus and rectum**
Foreign body in rectosigmoid (junction)
x7th **T18.8 Foreign body in other parts of alimentary tract**
x7th **T18.9 Foreign body of alimentary tract, part unspecified**
Foreign body in digestive system NOS
Swallowed foreign body NOS

DRAFT

T19 Foreign body in genitourinary tract

EXCLUDES 2 *complications due to implanted mesh (T83.7-)*
mechanical complications of contraceptive device (intrauterine) (vaginal) (T83.3-)
presence of contraceptive device (intrauterine) (vaginal) (Z97.5)

The appropriate 7th character is to be added to each code from category T19.
A initial encounter
D subsequent encounter
S sequela

T19.0 Foreign body in urethra
T19.1 Foreign body in bladder
T19.2 Foreign body in vulva and vagina
T19.3 Foreign body in uterus
T19.4 Foreign body in penis
T19.8 Foreign body in other parts of genitourinary tract
T19.9 Foreign body in genitourinary tract, part unspecified

Burns and corrosions (T20-T32)

INCLUDES burns (thermal) from electrical heating appliances
burns (thermal) from electricity
burns (thermal) from flame
burns (thermal) from friction
burns (thermal) from hot air and hot gases
burns (thermal) from hot objects
burns (thermal) from lightning
burns (thermal) from radiation
chemical burn [corrosion] (external) (internal)
scalds

EXCLUDES 2 *erythema [dermatitis] ab igne (L59.0)*
radiation-related disorders of the skin and subcutaneous tissue (L55-L59)
sunburn (L55.-)

Burns and corrosions of external body surface, specified by site (T20-T25)

INCLUDES burns and corrosions of first degree [erythema]
burns and corrosions of second degree [blisters][epidermal loss]
burns and corrosions of third degree [deep necrosis of underlying tissue] [full-thickness skin loss]

Use additional code from category T31 or T32 to identify extent of body surface involved

T20 Burn and corrosion of head, face, and neck

EXCLUDES 2 *burn and corrosion of ear drum (T28.41, T28.91)*
burn and corrosion of eye and adnexa (T26.-)
burn and corrosion of mouth and pharynx (T28.0)

The appropriate 7th character is to be added to each code from category T20.
A initial encounter
D subsequent encounter
S sequela

T20.0 Burn of unspecified degree of head, face, and neck
Use additional external cause code to identify the source, place and intent of the burn (X00-X19, X75-X77, X96-X98, Y92)

T20.00 Burn of unspecified degree of head, face, and neck, unspecified site
T20.01 Burn of unspecified degree of ear [any part, except ear drum]
EXCLUDES 2 *burn of ear drum (T28.41-)*
T20.011 Burn of unspecified degree of right ear [any part, except ear drum]
T20.012 Burn of unspecified degree of left ear [any part, except ear drum]
T20.019 Burn of unspecified degree of unspecified ear [any part, except ear drum]
T20.02 Burn of unspecified degree of lip(s)
T20.03 Burn of unspecified degree of chin
T20.04 Burn of unspecified degree of nose (septum)
T20.05 Burn of unspecified degree of scalp [any part]
T20.06 Burn of unspecified degree of forehead and cheek
T20.07 Burn of unspecified degree of neck
T20.09 Burn of unspecified degree of multiple sites of head, face, and neck

T20.1 Burn of first degree of head, face, and neck
Use additional external cause code to identify the source, place and intent of the burn (X00-X19, X75-X77, X96-X98, Y92)

T20.10 Burn of first degree of head, face, and neck, unspecified site
T20.11 Burn of first degree of ear [any part, except ear drum]
EXCLUDES 2 *burn of ear drum (T28.41-)*
T20.111 Burn of first degree of right ear [any part, except ear drum]
T20.112 Burn of first degree of left ear [any part, except ear drum]
T20.119 Burn of first degree of unspecified ear [any part, except ear drum]
T20.12 Burn of first degree of lip(s)
T20.13 Burn of first degree of chin
T20.14 Burn of first degree of nose (septum)
T20.15 Burn of first degree of scalp [any part]
T20.16 Burn of first degree of forehead and cheek
T20.17 Burn of first degree of neck
T20.19 Burn of first degree of multiple sites of head, face, and neck

T20.2 Burn of second degree of head, face, and neck
Use additional external cause code to identify the source, place and intent of the burn (X00-X19, X75-X77, X96-X98, Y92)

T20.20 Burn of second degree of head, face, and neck, unspecified site
T20.21 Burn of second degree of ear [any part, except ear drum]
EXCLUDES 2 *burn of ear drum (T28.41-)*
T20.211 Burn of second degree of right ear [any part, except ear drum]
T20.212 Burn of second degree of left ear [any part, except ear drum]
T20.219 Burn of second degree of unspecified ear [any part, except ear drum]
T20.22 Burn of second degree of lip(s)
T20.23 Burn of second degree of chin
T20.24 Burn of second degree of nose (septum)
T20.25 Burn of second degree of scalp [any part]
T20.26 Burn of second degree of forehead and cheek
T20.27 Burn of second degree of neck
T20.29 Burn of second degree of multiple sites of head, face, and neck

T20.3 Burn of third degree of head, face, and neck
Use additional external cause code to identify the source, place and intent of the burn (X00-X19, X75-X77, X96-X98, Y92)

T20.30 Burn of third degree of head, face, and neck, unspecified site
T20.31 Burn of third degree of ear [any part, except ear drum]
EXCLUDES 2 *burn of ear drum (T28.41-)*
T20.311 Burn of third degree of right ear [any part, except ear drum]
T20.312 Burn of third degree of left ear [any part, except ear drum]
T20.319 Burn of third degree of unspecified ear [any part, except ear drum]
T20.32 Burn of third degree of lip(s)
T20.33 Burn of third degree of chin
T20.34 Burn of third degree of nose (septum)
T20.35 Burn of third degree of scalp [any part]
T20.36 Burn of third degree of forehead and cheek
T20.37 Burn of third degree of neck
T20.39 Burn of third degree of multiple sites of head, face, and neck

T20.4 Corrosion of unspecified degree of head, face, and neck
Code first (T51-T65) to identify chemical and intent
Use additional external cause code to identify place (Y92)

T20.40 Corrosion of unspecified degree of head, face, and neck, unspecified site

T20.41 Corrosion of unspecified degree of ear [any part, except ear drum]
EXCLUDES2 *corrosion of ear drum (T28.91-)*

T20.411 Corrosion of unspecified degree of right ear [any part, except ear drum]

T20.412 Corrosion of unspecified degree of left ear [any part, except ear drum]

T20.419 Corrosion of unspecified degree of unspecified ear [any part, except ear drum]

T20.42 Corrosion of unspecified degree of lip(s)

T20.43 Corrosion of unspecified degree of chin

T20.44 Corrosion of unspecified degree of nose (septum)

T20.45 Corrosion of unspecified degree of scalp [any part]

T20.46 Corrosion of unspecified degree of forehead and cheek

T20.47 Corrosion of unspecified degree of neck

T20.49 Corrosion of unspecified degree of multiple sites of head, face, and neck

T20.5 Corrosion of first degree of head, face, and neck
Code first (T51-T65) to identify chemical and intent
Use additional external cause code to identify place (Y92)

T20.50 Corrosion of first degree of head, face, and neck, unspecified site

T20.51 Corrosion of first degree of ear [any part, except ear drum]
EXCLUDES2 *corrosion of ear drum (T28.91-)*

T20.511 Corrosion of first degree of right ear [any part, except ear drum]

T20.512 Corrosion of first degree of left ear [any part, except ear drum]

T20.519 Corrosion of first degree of unspecified ear [any part, except ear drum]

T20.52 Corrosion of first degree of lip(s)

T20.53 Corrosion of first degree of chin

T20.54 Corrosion of first degree of nose (septum)

T20.55 Corrosion of first degree of scalp [any part]

T20.56 Corrosion of first degree of cheek

T20.57 Corrosion of first degree of neck

T20.59 Corrosion of first degree of multiple sites of head, face, and neck

T20.6 Corrosion of second degree of head, face, and neck
Code first (T51-T65) to identify chemical and intent
Use additional external cause code to identify place (Y92)

T20.60 Corrosion of second degree of head, face, and neck, unspecified site

T20.61 Corrosion of second degree of ear [any part, except ear drum]
EXCLUDES2 *corrosion of ear drum (T28.91-)*

T20.611 Corrosion of second degree of right ear [any part, except ear drum]

T20.612 Corrosion of second degree of left ear [any part, except ear drum]

T20.619 Corrosion of second degree of unspecified ear [any part, except ear drum]

T20.62 Corrosion of second degree of lip(s)

T20.63 Corrosion of second degree of chin

T20.64 Corrosion of second degree of nose (septum)

T20.65 Corrosion of second degree of scalp [any part]

T20.66 Corrosion of second degree of forehead and cheek

T20.67 Corrosion of second degree of neck

T20.69 Corrosion of second degree of multiple sites of head, face, and neck

T20.7 Corrosion of third degree of head, face, and neck
Code first (T51-T65) to identify chemical and intent
Use additional external cause code to identify place (Y92)

T20.70 Corrosion of third degree of head, face, and neck, unspecified site

T20.71 Corrosion of third degree of ear [any part, except ear drum]
EXCLUDES2 *corrosion of ear drum (T28.91-)*

T20.711 Corrosion of third degree of right ear [any part, except ear drum]

T20.712 Corrosion of third degree of left ear [any part, except ear drum]

T20.719 Corrosion of third degree of unspecified ear [any part, except ear drum]

T20.72 Corrosion of third degree of lip(s)

T20.73 Corrosion of third degree of chin

T20.74 Corrosion of third degree of nose (septum)

T20.75 Corrosion of third degree of scalp [any part]

T20.76 Corrosion of third degree of forehead and cheek

T20.77 Corrosion of third degree of neck

T20.79 Corrosion of third degree of multiple sites of head, face, and neck

T21 Burn and corrosion of trunk
Burns and corrosion of hip region
EXCLUDES2 *burns and corrosion of:*
axilla (T22- with fifth character 4)
scapular region (T22- with fifth character 6)
shoulder (T22. with fifth character 5)

The appropriate 7th character is to be added to each code from category T21.
A initial encounter
D subsequent encounter
S sequela

T21.0 Burn of unspecified degree of trunk
Use additional external cause code to identify the source, place and intent of the burn (X00-X19, X75-X77, X96-X98, Y92)

T21.00 Burn of unspecified degree of trunk, unspecified site

T21.01 Burn of unspecified degree of chest wall
Burn of of unspecified degree of breast

T21.02 Burn of unspecified degree of abdominal wall
Burn of unspecified degree of flank
Burn of unspecified degree of groin

T21.03 Burn of unspecified degree of upper back
Burn of unspecified degree of interscapular region

T21.04 Burn of unspecified degree of lower back

T21.05 Burn of unspecified degree of buttock
Burn of unspecified degree of anus

T21.06 Burn of unspecified degree of male genital region
Burn of unspecified degree of penis
Burn of unspecified degree of scrotum
Burn of unspecified degree of testis

T21.07 Burn of unspecified degree of female genital region
Burn of unspecified degree of labium (majus) (minus)
Burn of unspecified degree of perineum
Burn of unspecified degree of vulva
EXCLUDES2 *burn of vagina (T28.3)*

T21.09 Burn of unspecified degree of other site of trunk

T21.1 Burn of first degree of trunk
Use additional external cause code to identify the source, place and intent of the burn (X00-X19, X75-X77, X96-X98, Y92)

T21.10 Burn of first degree of trunk, unspecified site

T21.11 Burn of first degree of chest wall
Burn of first degree of breast

T21.12 Burn of first degree of abdominal wall
Burn of first degree of flank
Burn of first degree of groin

T21.13 Burn of first degree of upper back
Burn of first degree of interscapular region

T21.14 Burn of first degree of lower back

T21.15 Burn of first degree of buttock
Burn of first degree of anus

T21.16 Burn of first degree of male genital region
Burn of first degree of penis
Burn of first degree of scrotum
Burn of first degree of testis

T21.17 Burn of first degree of female genital region
Burn of first degree of labium (majus) (minus)
Burn of first degree of perineum
Burn of first degree of vulva
EXCLUDES2 *burn of vagina (T28.3)*

T21.19 Burn of first degree of other site of trunk

√5th **T21.2 Burn of second degree of trunk**
Use additional external cause code to identify the source, place and intent of the burn (X00-X19, X75-X77, X96-X98, Y92)
√x7th **T21.20 Burn of second degree of trunk, unspecified site**
√x7th **T21.21 Burn of second degree of chest wall**
Burn of second degree of breast
√x7th **T21.22 Burn of second degree of abdominal wall**
Burn of second degree of flank
Burn of second degree of groin
√x7th **T21.23 Burn of second degree of upper back**
Burn of second degree of interscapular region
√x7th **T21.24 Burn of second degree of lower back**
√x7th **T21.25 Burn of second degree of buttock**
Burn of second degree of anus
√x7th **T21.26 Burn of second degree of male genital region**
Burn of second degree of penis
Burn of second degree of scrotum
Burn of second degree of testis
√x7th **T21.27 Burn of second degree of female genital region**
Burn of second degree of labium (majus) (minus)
Burn of second degree of perineum
Burn of second degree of vulva
EXCLUDES 2 *burn of vagina (T28.3)*
√x7th **T21.29 Burn of second degree of other site of trunk**
√5th **T21.3 Burn of third degree of trunk**
Use additional external cause code to identify the source, place and intent of the burn (X00-X19, X75-X77, X96-X98, Y92)
√x7th **T21.30 Burn of third degree of trunk, unspecified site**
√x7th **T21.31 Burn of third degree of chest wall**
Burn of third degree of breast
√x7th **T21.32 Burn of third degree of abdominal wall**
Burn of third degree of flank
Burn of third degree of groin
√x7th **T21.33 Burn of third degree of upper back**
Burn of third degree of interscapular region
√x7th **T21.34 Burn of third degree of lower back**
√x7th **T21.35 Burn of third degree of buttock**
Burn of third degree of anus
√x7th **T21.36 Burn of third degree of male genital region**
Burn of third degree of penis
Burn of third degree of scrotum
Burn of third degree of testis
√x7th **T21.37 Burn of third degree of female genital region**
Burn of third degree of labium (majus) (minus)
Burn of third degree of perineum
Burn of third degree of vulva
EXCLUDES 2 *burn of vagina (T28.3)*
√x7th **T21.39 Burn of third degree of other site of trunk**
√5th **T21.4 Corrosion of unspecified degree of trunk**
Code first (T51-T65) to identify chemical and intent
Use additional external cause code to identify place (Y92)
√x7th **T21.40 Corrosion of unspecified degree of trunk, unspecified site**
√x7th **T21.41 Corrosion of unspecified degree of chest wall**
Corrosion of unspecified degree of breast
√x7th **T21.42 Corrosion of unspecified degree of abdominal wall**
Corrosion of unspecified degree of flank
Corrosion of unspecified degree of groin
√x7th **T21.43 Corrosion of unspecified degree of upper back**
Corrosion of unspecified degree of interscapular region
√x7th **T21.44 Corrosion of unspecified degree of lower back**
√x7th **T21.45 Corrosion of unspecified degree of buttock**
Corrosion of unspecified degree of anus
√x7th **T21.46 Corrosion of unspecified degree of male genital region**
Corrosion of unspecified degree of penis
Corrosion of unspecified degree of scrotum
Corrosion of unspecified degree of testis
√x7th **T21.47 Corrosion of unspecified degree of female genital region**
Corrosion of unspecified degree of labium (majus) (minus)
Corrosion of unspecified degree of perineum
Corrosion of unspecified degree of vulva
EXCLUDES 2 *corrosion of vagina (T28.8)*
√x7th **T21.49 Corrosion of unspecified degree of other site of trunk**
√5th **T21.5 Corrosion of first degree of trunk**
Code first (T51-T65) to identify chemical and intent
Use additional external cause code to identify place (Y92)
√x7th **T21.50 Corrosion of first degree of trunk, unspecified site**
√x7th **T21.51 Corrosion of first degree of chest wall**
Corrosion of first degree of breast
√x7th **T21.52 Corrosion of first degree of abdominal wall**
Corrosion of first degree of flank
Corrosion of first degree of groin
√x7th **T21.53 Corrosion of first degree of upper back**
Corrosion of first degree of interscapular region
√x7th **T21.54 Corrosion of first degree of lower back**
√x7th **T21.55 Corrosion of first degree of buttock**
Corrosion of first degree of anus
√x7th **T21.56 Corrosion of first degree of male genital region**
Corrosion of first degree of penis
Corrosion of first degree of scrotum
Corrosion of first degree of testis
√x7th **T21.57 Corrosion of first degree of female genital region**
Corrosion of first degree of labium (majus) (minus)
Corrosion of first degree of perineum
Corrosion of first degree of vulva
EXCLUDES 2 *corrosion of vagina (T28.8)*
√x7th **T21.59 Corrosion of first degree of other site of trunk**
√5th **T21.6 Corrosion of second degree of trunk**
Code first (T51-T65) to identify chemical and intent
Use additional external cause code to identify place (Y92)
√x7th **T21.60 Corrosion of second degree of trunk, unspecified site**
√x7th **T21.61 Corrosion of second degree of chest wall**
Corrosion of second degree of breast
√x7th **T21.62 Corrosion of second degree of abdominal wall**
Corrosion of second degree of flank
Corrosion of second degree of groin
√x7th **T21.63 Corrosion of second degree of upper back**
Corrosion of second degree of interscapular region
√x7th **T21.64 Corrosion of second degree of lower back**
√x7th **T21.65 Corrosion of second degree of buttock**
Corrosion of second degree of anus
√x7th **T21.66 Corrosion of second degree of male genital region**
Corrosion of second degree of penis
Corrosion of second degree of scrotum
Corrosion of second degree of testis
√x7th **T21.67 Corrosion of second degree of female genital region**
Corrosion of second degree of labium (majus) (minus)
Corrosion of second degree of perineum
Corrosion of second degree of vulva
EXCLUDES 2 *corrosion of vagina (T28.8)*
√x7th **T21.69 Corrosion of second degree of other site of trunk**
√5th **T21.7 Corrosion of third degree of trunk**
Code first (T51-T65) to identify chemical and intent
Use additional external cause code to identify place (Y92)
√x7th **T21.70 Corrosion of third degree of trunk, unspecified site**
√x7th **T21.71 Corrosion of third degree of chest wall**
Corrosion of third degree of breast
√x7th **T21.72 Corrosion of third degree of abdominal wall**
Corrosion of third degree of flank
Corrosion of third degree of groin
√x7th **T21.73 Corrosion of third degree of upper back**
Corrosion of third degree of interscapular region
√x7th **T21.74 Corrosion of third degree of lower back**
√x7th **T21.75 Corrosion of third degree of buttock**
Corrosion of third degree of anus
√x7th **T21.76 Corrosion of third degree of male genital region**
Corrosion of third degree of penis
Corrosion of third degree of scrotum
Corrosion of third degree of testis
√x7th **T21.77 Corrosion of third degree of female genital region**
Corrosion of third degree of labium (majus) (minus)
Corrosion of third degree of perineum
Corrosion of third degree of vulva
EXCLUDES 2 *corrosion of vagina (T28.8)*
√x7th **T21.79 Corrosion of third degree of other site of trunk**

T22 Burn and corrosion of shoulder and upper limb, except wrist and hand

EXCLUDES 2 *burn and corrosion of interscapular region (T21.-)*
burn and corrosion of wrist and hand (T23.-)

The appropriate 7th character is to be added to each code from category T22.
- A initial encounter
- D subsequent encounter
- S sequela

T22.0 Burn of unspecified degree of shoulder and upper limb, except wrist and hand
Use additional external cause code to identify the source, place and intent of the burn (X00-X19, X75-X77, X96-X98, Y92)
- **T22.00 Burn of unspecified degree of shoulder and upper limb, except wrist and hand, unspecified site**
- **T22.01 Burn of unspecified degree of forearm**
  - **T22.011 Burn of unspecified degree of right forearm**
  - **T22.012 Burn of unspecified degree of left forearm**
  - **T22.019 Burn of unspecified degree of unspecified forearm**
- **T22.02 Burn of unspecified degree of elbow**
  - **T22.021 Burn of unspecified degree of right elbow**
  - **T22.022 Burn of unspecified degree of left elbow**
  - **T22.029 Burn of unspecified degree of unspecified elbow**
- **T22.03 Burn of unspecified degree of upper arm**
  - **T22.031 Burn of unspecified degree of right upper arm**
  - **T22.032 Burn of unspecified degree of left upper arm**
  - **T22.039 Burn of unspecified degree of unspecified upper arm**
- **T22.04 Burn of unspecified degree of axilla**
  - **T22.041 Burn of unspecified degree of right axilla**
  - **T22.042 Burn of unspecified degree of left axilla**
  - **T22.049 Burn of unspecified degree of unspecified axilla**
- **T22.05 Burn of unspecified degree of shoulder**
  - **T22.051 Burn of unspecified degree of right shoulder**
  - **T22.052 Burn of unspecified degree of left shoulder**
  - **T22.059 Burn of unspecified degree of unspecified shoulder**
- **T22.06 Burn of unspecified degree of scapular region**
  - **T22.061 Burn of unspecified degree of right scapular region**
  - **T22.062 Burn of unspecified degree of left scapular region**
  - **T22.069 Burn of unspecified degree of unspecified scapular region**
- **T22.09 Burn of unspecified degree of multiple sites of shoulder and upper limb, except wrist and hand**
  - **T22.091 Burn of unspecified degree of multiple sites of right shoulder and upper limb, except wrist and hand**
  - **T22.092 Burn of unspecified degree of multiple sites of left shoulder and upper limb, except wrist and hand**
  - **T22.099 Burn of unspecified degree of multiple sites of unspecified shoulder and upper limb, except wrist and hand**

T22.1 Burn of first degree of shoulder and upper limb, except wrist and hand
Use additional external cause code to identify the source, place and intent of the burn (X00-X19, X75-X77, X96-X98, Y92)
- **T22.10 Burn of first degree of shoulder and upper limb, except wrist and hand, unspecified site**
- **T22.11 Burn of first degree of forearm**
  - **T22.111 Burn of first degree of right forearm**
  - **T22.112 Burn of first degree of left forearm**
  - **T22.119 Burn of first degree of unspecified forearm**
- **T22.12 Burn of first degree of elbow**
  - **T22.121 Burn of first degree of right elbow**
  - **T22.122 Burn of first degree of left elbow**
  - **T22.129 Burn of first degree of unspecified elbow**
- **T22.13 Burn of first degree of upper arm**
  - **T22.131 Burn of first degree of right upper arm**
  - **T22.132 Burn of first degree of left upper arm**
  - **T22.139 Burn of first degree of unspecified upper arm**
- **T22.14 Burn of first degree of axilla**
  - **T22.141 Burn of first degree of right axilla**
  - **T22.142 Burn of first degree of left axilla**
  - **T22.149 Burn of first degree of unspecified axilla**
- **T22.15 Burn of first degree of shoulder**
  - **T22.151 Burn of first degree of right shoulder**
  - **T22.152 Burn of first degree of left shoulder**
  - **T22.159 Burn of first degree of unspecified shoulder**
- **T22.16 Burn of first degree of scapular region**
  - **T22.161 Burn of first degree of right scapular region**
  - **T22.162 Burn of first degree of left scapular region**
  - **T22.169 Burn of first degree of unspecified scapular region**
- **T22.19 Burn of first degree of multiple sites of shoulder and upper limb, except wrist and hand**
  - **T22.191 Burn of first degree of multiple sites of right shoulder and upper limb, except wrist and hand**
  - **T22.192 Burn of first degree of multiple sites of left shoulder and upper limb, except wrist and hand**
  - **T22.199 Burn of first degree of multiple sites of unspecified shoulder and upper limb, except wrist and hand**

T22.2 Burn of second degree of shoulder and upper limb, except wrist and hand
Use additional external cause code to identify the source, place and intent of the burn (X00-X19, X75-X77, X96-X98, Y92)
- **T22.20 Burn of second degree of shoulder and upper limb, except wrist and hand, unspecified site**
- **T22.21 Burn of second degree of forearm**
  - **T22.211 Burn of second degree of right forearm**
  - **T22.212 Burn of second degree of left forearm**
  - **T22.219 Burn of second degree of unspecified forearm**
- **T22.22 Burn of second degree of elbow**
  - **T22.221 Burn of second degree of right elbow**
  - **T22.222 Burn of second degree of left elbow**
  - **T22.229 Burn of second degree of unspecified elbow**
- **T22.23 Burn of second degree of upper arm**
  - **T22.231 Burn of second degree of right upper arm**
  - **T22.232 Burn of second degree of left upper arm**
  - **T22.239 Burn of second degree of unspecified upper arm**
- **T22.24 Burn of second degree of axilla**
  - **T22.241 Burn of second degree of right axilla**
  - **T22.242 Burn of second degree of left axilla**
  - **T22.249 Burn of second degree of unspecified axilla**
- **T22.25 Burn of second degree of shoulder**
  - **T22.251 Burn of second degree of right shoulder**
  - **T22.252 Burn of second degree of left shoulder**
  - **T22.259 Burn of second degree of unspecified shoulder**

6th T22.26 **Burn of second degree of scapular region**
7th T22.261 **Burn of second degree of right scapular region**
7th T22.262 **Burn of second degree of left scapular region**
7th T22.269 **Burn of second degree of unspecified scapular region**
6th T22.29 **Burn of second degree of multiple sites of shoulder and upper limb, except wrist and hand**
7th T22.291 **Burn of second degree of multiple sites of right shoulder and upper limb, except wrist and hand**
7th T22.292 **Burn of second degree of multiple sites of left shoulder and upper limb, except wrist and hand**
7th T22.299 **Burn of second degree of multiple sites of unspecified shoulder and upper limb, except wrist and hand**
5th T22.3 **Burn of third degree of shoulder and upper limb, except wrist and hand**
Use additional external cause code to identify the source, place and intent of the burn (X00-X19, X75-X77, X96-X98, Y92)
x7th T22.30 **Burn of third degree of shoulder and upper limb, except wrist and hand, unspecified site**
6th T22.31 **Burn of third degree of forearm**
7th T22.311 **Burn of third degree of right forearm**
7th T22.312 **Burn of third degree of left forearm**
7th T22.319 **Burn of third degree of unspecified forearm**
6th T22.32 **Burn of third degree of elbow**
7th T22.321 **Burn of third degree of right elbow**
7th T22.322 **Burn of third degree of left elbow**
7th T22.329 **Burn of third degree of unspecified elbow**
6th T22.33 **Burn of third degree of upper arm**
7th T22.331 **Burn of third degree of right upper arm**
7th T22.332 **Burn of third degree of left upper arm**
7th T22.339 **Burn of third degree of unspecified upper arm**
6th T22.34 **Burn of third degree of axilla**
7th T22.341 **Burn of third degree of right axilla**
7th T22.342 **Burn of third degree of left axilla**
7th T22.349 **Burn of third degree of unspecified axilla**
6th T22.35 **Burn of third degree of shoulder**
7th T22.351 **Burn of third degree of right shoulder**
7th T22.352 **Burn of third degree of left shoulder**
7th T22.359 **Burn of third degree of unspecified shoulder**
6th T22.36 **Burn of third degree of scapular region**
7th T22.361 **Burn of third degree of right scapular region**
7th T22.362 **Burn of third degree of left scapular region**
7th T22.369 **Burn of third degree of unspecified scapular region**
6th T22.39 **Burn of third degree of multiple sites of shoulder and upper limb, except wrist and hand**
7th T22.391 **Burn of third degree of multiple sites of right shoulder and upper limb, except wrist and hand**
7th T22.392 **Burn of third degree of multiple sites of left shoulder and upper limb, except wrist and hand**
7th T22.399 **Burn of third degree of multiple sites of unspecified shoulder and upper limb, except wrist and hand**
5th T22.4 **Corrosion of unspecified degree of shoulder and upper limb, except wrist and hand**
Code first (T51-T65) to identify chemical and intent
Use additional external cause code to identify place (Y92)
x7th T22.40 **Corrosion of unspecified degree of shoulder and upper limb, except wrist and hand, unspecified site**
6th T22.41 **Corrosion of unspecified degree of forearm**
7th T22.411 **Corrosion of unspecified degree of right forearm**
7th T22.412 **Corrosion of unspecified degree of left forearm**
7th T22.419 **Corrosion of unspecified degree of unspecified forearm**
6th T22.42 **Corrosion of unspecified degree of elbow**
7th T22.421 **Corrosion of unspecified degree of right elbow**
7th T22.422 **Corrosion of unspecified degree of left elbow**
7th T22.429 **Corrosion of unspecified degree of unspecified elbow**
6th T22.43 **Corrosion of unspecified degree of upper arm**
7th T22.431 **Corrosion of unspecified degree of right upper arm**
7th T22.432 **Corrosion of unspecified degree of left upper arm**
7th T22.439 **Corrosion of unspecified degree of unspecified upper arm**
6th T22.44 **Corrosion of unspecified degree of axilla**
7th T22.441 **Corrosion of unspecified degree of right axilla**
7th T22.442 **Corrosion of unspecified degree of left axilla**
7th T22.449 **Corrosion of unspecified degree of unspecified axilla**
6th T22.45 **Corrosion of unspecified degree of shoulder**
7th T22.451 **Corrosion of unspecified degree of right shoulder**
7th T22.452 **Corrosion of unspecified degree of left shoulder**
7th T22.459 **Corrosion of unspecified degree of unspecified shoulder**
6th T22.46 **Corrosion of unspecified degree of scapular region**
7th T22.461 **Corrosion of unspecified degree of right scapular region**
7th T22.462 **Corrosion of unspecified degree of left scapular region**
7th T22.469 **Corrosion of unspecified degree of unspecified scapular region**
6th T22.49 **Corrosion of unspecified degree of multiple sites of shoulder and upper limb, except wrist and hand**
7th T22.491 **Corrosion of unspecified degree of multiple sites of right shoulder and upper limb, except wrist and hand**
7th T22.492 **Corrosion of unspecified degree of multiple sites of left shoulder and upper limb, except wrist and hand**
7th T22.499 **Corrosion of unspecified degree of multiple sites of unspecified shoulder and upper limb, except wrist and hand**
5th T22.5 **Corrosion of first degree of shoulder and upper limb, except wrist and hand**
Code first (T51-T65) to identify chemical and intent
Use additional external cause code to identify place (Y92)
x7th T22.50 **Corrosion of first degree of shoulder and upper limb, except wrist and hand unspecified site**
6th T22.51 **Corrosion of first degree of forearm**
7th T22.511 **Corrosion of first degree of right forearm**
7th T22.512 **Corrosion of first degree of left forearm**
7th T22.519 **Corrosion of first degree of unspecified forearm**
6th T22.52 **Corrosion of first degree of elbow**
7th T22.521 **Corrosion of first degree of right elbow**
7th T22.522 **Corrosion of first degree of left elbow**
7th T22.529 **Corrosion of first degree of unspecified elbow**
6th T22.53 **Corrosion of first degree of upper arm**
7th T22.531 **Corrosion of first degree of right upper arm**
7th T22.532 **Corrosion of first degree of left upper arm**

- ✓7th T22.539 Corrosion of first degree of unspecified upper arm
- ✓6th T22.54 Corrosion of first degree of axilla
  - ✓7th T22.541 Corrosion of first degree of right axilla
  - ✓7th T22.542 Corrosion of first degree of left axilla
  - ✓7th T22.549 Corrosion of first degree of unspecified axilla
- ✓6th T22.55 Corrosion of first degree of shoulder
  - ✓7th T22.551 Corrosion of first degree of right shoulder
  - ✓7th T22.552 Corrosion of first degree of left shoulder
  - ✓7th T22.559 Corrosion of first degree of unspecified shoulder
- ✓6th T22.56 Corrosion of first degree of scapular region
  - ✓7th T22.561 Corrosion of first degree of right scapular region
  - ✓7th T22.562 Corrosion of first degree of left scapular region
  - ✓7th T22.569 Corrosion of first degree of unspecified scapular region
- ✓6th T22.59 Corrosion of first degree of multiple sites of shoulder and upper limb, except wrist and hand
  - ✓7th T22.591 Corrosion of first degree of multiple sites of right shoulder and upper limb, except wrist and hand
  - ✓7th T22.592 Corrosion of first degree of multiple sites of left shoulder and upper limb, except wrist and hand
  - ✓7th T22.599 Corrosion of first degree of multiple sites of unspecified shoulder and upper limb, except wrist and hand

✓5th **T22.6 Corrosion of second degree of shoulder and upper limb, except wrist and hand**

Code first (T51-T65) to identify chemical and intent

Use additional external cause code to identify place (Y92)

- ✓x7th T22.60 Corrosion of second degree of shoulder and upper limb, except wrist and hand, unspecified site
- ✓6th T22.61 Corrosion of second degree of forearm
  - ✓7th T22.611 Corrosion of second degree of right forearm
  - ✓7th T22.612 Corrosion of second degree of left forearm
  - ✓7th T22.619 Corrosion of second degree of unspecified forearm
- ✓6th T22.62 Corrosion of second degree of elbow
  - ✓7th T22.621 Corrosion of second degree of right elbow
  - ✓7th T22.622 Corrosion of second degree of left elbow
  - ✓7th T22.629 Corrosion of second degree of unspecified elbow
- ✓6th T22.63 Corrosion of second degree of upper arm
  - ✓7th T22.631 Corrosion of second degree of right upper arm
  - ✓7th T22.632 Corrosion of second degree of left upper arm
  - ✓7th T22.639 Corrosion of second degree of unspecified upper arm
- ✓6th T22.64 Corrosion of second degree of axilla
  - ✓7th T22.641 Corrosion of second degree of right axilla
  - ✓7th T22.642 Corrosion of second degree of left axilla
  - ✓7th T22.649 Corrosion of second degree of unspecified axilla
- ✓6th T22.65 Corrosion of second degree of shoulder
  - ✓7th T22.651 Corrosion of second degree of right shoulder
  - ✓7th T22.652 Corrosion of second degree of left shoulder
  - ✓7th T22.659 Corrosion of second degree of unspecified shoulder
- ✓6th T22.66 Corrosion of second degree of scapular region
  - ✓7th T22.661 Corrosion of second degree of right scapular region
  - ✓7th T22.662 Corrosion of second degree of left scapular region
  - ✓7th T22.669 Corrosion of second degree of unspecified scapular region
- ✓6th T22.69 Corrosion of second degree of multiple sites of shoulder and upper limb, except wrist and hand
  - ✓7th T22.691 Corrosion of second degree of multiple sites of right shoulder and upper limb, except wrist and hand
  - ✓7th T22.692 Corrosion of second degree of multiple sites of left shoulder and upper limb, except wrist and hand
  - ✓7th T22.699 Corrosion of second degree of multiple sites of unspecified shoulder and upper limb, except wrist and hand

✓5th **T22.7 Corrosion of third degree of shoulder and upper limb, except wrist and hand**

Code first (T51-T65) to identify chemical and intent

Use additional external cause code to identify place (Y92)

- ✓x7th T22.70 Corrosion of third degree of shoulder and upper limb, except wrist and hand, unspecified site
- ✓6th T22.71 Corrosion of third degree of forearm
  - ✓7th T22.711 Corrosion of third degree of right forearm
  - ✓7th T22.712 Corrosion of third degree of left forearm
  - ✓7th T22.719 Corrosion of third degree of unspecified forearm
- ✓6th T22.72 Corrosion of third degree of elbow
  - ✓7th T22.721 Corrosion of third degree of right elbow
  - ✓7th T22.722 Corrosion of third degree of left elbow
  - ✓7th T22.729 Corrosion of third degree of unspecified elbow
- ✓6th T22.73 Corrosion of third degree of upper arm
  - ✓7th T22.731 Corrosion of third degree of right upper arm
  - ✓7th T22.732 Corrosion of third degree of left upper arm
  - ✓7th T22.739 Corrosion of third degree of unspecified upper arm
- ✓6th T22.74 Corrosion of third degree of axilla
  - ✓7th T22.741 Corrosion of third degree of right axilla
  - ✓7th T22.742 Corrosion of third degree of left axilla
  - ✓7th T22.749 Corrosion of third degree of unspecified axilla
- ✓6th T22.75 Corrosion of third degree of shoulder
  - ✓7th T22.751 Corrosion of third degree of right shoulder
  - ✓7th T22.752 Corrosion of third degree of left shoulder
  - ✓7th T22.759 Corrosion of third degree of unspecified shoulder
- ✓6th T22.76 Corrosion of third degree of scapular region
  - ✓7th T22.761 Corrosion of third degree of right scapular region
  - ✓7th T22.762 Corrosion of third degree of left scapular region
  - ✓7th T22.769 Corrosion of third degree of unspecified scapular region
- ✓6th T22.79 Corrosion of third degree of multiple sites of shoulder and upper limb, except wrist and hand
  - ✓7th T22.791 Corrosion of third degree of multiple sites of right shoulder and upper limb, except wrist and hand
  - ✓7th T22.792 Corrosion of third degree of multiple sites of left shoulder and upper limb, except wrist and hand
  - ✓7th T22.799 Corrosion of third degree of multiple sites of unspecified shoulder and upper limb, except wrist and hand

T23 Burn and corrosion of wrist and hand

The appropriate 7th character is to be added to each code from category T23.
A initial encounter
D subsequent encounter
S sequela

T23.0 Burn of unspecified degree of wrist and hand
Use additional external cause code to identify the source, place and intent of the burn (X00-X19, X75-X77, X96-X98, Y92)

T23.00 Burn of unspecified degree of hand, unspecified site
T23.001 Burn of unspecified degree of right hand, unspecified site
T23.002 Burn of unspecified degree of left hand, unspecified site
T23.009 Burn of unspecified degree of unspecified hand, unspecified site
T23.01 Burn of unspecified degree of thumb (nail)
T23.011 Burn of unspecified degree of right thumb (nail)
T23.012 Burn of unspecified degree of left thumb (nail)
T23.019 Burn of unspecified degree of unspecified thumb (nail)
T23.02 Burn of unspecified degree of single finger (nail) except thumb
T23.021 Burn of unspecified degree of single right finger (nail) except thumb
T23.022 Burn of unspecified degree of single left finger (nail) except thumb
T23.029 Burn of unspecified degree of unspecified single finger (nail) except thumb
T23.03 Burn of unspecified degree of multiple fingers (nail), not including thumb
T23.031 Burn of unspecified degree of multiple right fingers (nail), not including thumb
T23.032 Burn of unspecified degree of multiple left fingers (nail), not including thumb
T23.039 Burn of unspecified degree of unspecified multiple fingers (nail), not including thumb
T23.04 Burn of unspecified degree of multiple fingers (nail), including thumb
T23.041 Burn of unspecified degree of multiple right fingers (nail), including thumb
T23.042 Burn of unspecified degree of multiple left fingers (nail), including thumb
T23.049 Burn of unspecified degree of unspecified multiple fingers (nail), including thumb
T23.05 Burn of unspecified degree of palm
T23.051 Burn of unspecified degree of right palm
T23.052 Burn of unspecified degree of left palm
T23.059 Burn of unspecified degree of unspecified palm
T23.06 Burn of unspecified degree of back of hand
T23.061 Burn of unspecified degree of back of right hand
T23.062 Burn of unspecified degree of back of left hand
T23.069 Burn of unspecified degree of back of unspecified hand
T23.07 Burn of unspecified degree of wrist
T23.071 Burn of unspecified degree of right wrist
T23.072 Burn of unspecified degree of left wrist
T23.079 Burn of unspecified degree of unspecified wrist
T23.09 Burn of unspecified degree of multiple sites of wrist and hand
T23.091 Burn of unspecified degree of multiple sites of right wrist and hand
T23.092 Burn of unspecified degree of multiple sites of left wrist and hand
T23.099 Burn of unspecified degree of multiple sites of unspecified wrist and hand

T23.1 Burn of first degree of wrist and hand
Use additional external cause code to identify the source, place and intent of the burn (X00-X19, X75-X77, X96-X98, Y92)

T23.10 Burn of first degree of hand, unspecified site
T23.101 Burn of first degree of right hand, unspecified site
T23.102 Burn of first degree of left hand, unspecified site
T23.109 Burn of first degree of unspecified hand, unspecified site
T23.11 Burn of first degree of thumb (nail)
T23.111 Burn of first degree of right thumb (nail)
T23.112 Burn of first degree of left thumb (nail)
T23.119 Burn of first degree of unspecified thumb (nail)
T23.12 Burn of first degree of single finger (nail) except thumb
T23.121 Burn of first degree of single right finger (nail) except thumb
T23.122 Burn of first degree of single left finger (nail) except thumb
T23.129 Burn of first degree of unspecified single finger (nail) except thumb
T23.13 Burn of first degree of multiple fingers (nail), not including thumb
T23.131 Burn of first degree of multiple right fingers (nail), not including thumb
T23.132 Burn of first degree of multiple left fingers (nail), not including thumb
T23.139 Burn of first degree of unspecified multiple fingers (nail), not including thumb
T23.14 Burn of first degree of multiple fingers (nail), including thumb
T23.141 Burn of first degree of multiple right fingers (nail), including thumb
T23.142 Burn of first degree of multiple left fingers (nail), including thumb
T23.149 Burn of first degree of unspecified multiple fingers (nail), including thumb
T23.15 Burn of first degree of palm
T23.151 Burn of first degree of right palm
T23.152 Burn of first degree of left palm
T23.159 Burn of first degree of unspecified palm
T23.16 Burn of first degree of back of hand
T23.161 Burn of first degree of back of right hand
T23.162 Burn of first degree of back of left hand
T23.169 Burn of first degree of back of unspecified hand
T23.17 Burn of first degree of wrist
T23.171 Burn of first degree of right wrist
T23.172 Burn of first degree of left wrist
T23.179 Burn of first degree of unspecified wrist
T23.19 Burn of first degree of multiple sites of wrist and hand
T23.191 Burn of first degree of multiple sites of right wrist and hand
T23.192 Burn of first degree of multiple sites of left wrist and hand
T23.199 Burn of first degree of multiple sites of unspecified wrist and hand

T23.2 Burn of second degree of wrist and hand
Use additional external cause code to identify the source, place and intent of the burn (X00-X19, X75-X77, X96-X98, Y92)

T23.20 Burn of second degree of hand, unspecified site
T23.201 Burn of second degree of right hand, unspecified site
T23.202 Burn of second degree of left hand, unspecified site
T23.209 Burn of second degree of unspecified hand, unspecified site

✓6th **T23.21 Burn of second degree of thumb (nail)**
✓7th **T23.211 Burn of second degree of right thumb (nail)**
✓7th **T23.212 Burn of second degree of left thumb (nail)**
✓7th **T23.219 Burn of second degree of unspecified thumb (nail)**
✓6th **T23.22 Burn of second degree of single finger (nail) except thumb**
✓7th **T23.221 Burn of second degree of single right finger (nail) except thumb**
✓7th **T23.222 Burn of second degree of single left finger (nail) except thumb**
✓7th **T23.229 Burn of second degree of unspecified single finger (nail) except thumb**
✓6th **T23.23 Burn of second degree of multiple fingers (nail), not including thumb**
✓7th **T23.231 Burn of second degree of multiple right fingers (nail), not including thumb**
✓7th **T23.232 Burn of second degree of multiple left fingers (nail), not including thumb**
✓7th **T23.239 Burn of second degree of unspecified multiple fingers (nail), not including thumb**
✓6th **T23.24 Burn of second degree of multiple fingers (nail), including thumb**
✓7th **T23.241 Burn of second degree of multiple right fingers (nail), including thumb**
✓7th **T23.242 Burn of second degree of multiple left fingers (nail), including thumb**
✓7th **T23.249 Burn of second degree of unspecified multiple fingers (nail), including thumb**
✓6th **T23.25 Burn of second degree of palm**
✓7th **T23.251 Burn of second degree of right palm**
✓7th **T23.252 Burn of second degree of left palm**
✓7th **T23.259 Burn of second degree of unspecified palm**
✓6th **T23.26 Burn of second degree of back of hand**
✓7th **T23.261 Burn of second degree of back of right hand**
✓7th **T23.262 Burn of second degree of back of left hand**
✓7th **T23.269 Burn of second degree of back of unspecified hand**
✓6th **T23.27 Burn of second degree of wrist**
✓7th **T23.271 Burn of second degree of right wrist**
✓7th **T23.272 Burn of second degree of left wrist**
✓7th **T23.279 Burn of second degree of unspecified wrist**
✓6th **T23.29 Burn of second degree of multiple sites of wrist and hand**
✓7th **T23.291 Burn of second degree of multiple sites of right wrist and hand**
✓7th **T23.292 Burn of second degree of multiple sites of left wrist and hand**
✓7th **T23.299 Burn of second degree of multiple sites of unspecified wrist and hand**
✓5th **T23.3 Burn of third degree of wrist and hand**
Use additional external cause code to identify the source, place and intent of the burn (X00-X19, X75-X77, X96-X98, Y92)
✓6th **T23.30 Burn of third degree of hand, unspecified site**
✓7th **T23.301 Burn of third degree of right hand, unspecified site**
✓7th **T23.302 Burn of third degree of left hand, unspecified site**
✓7th **T23.309 Burn of third degree of unspecified hand, unspecified site**
✓6th **T23.31 Burn of third degree of thumb (nail)**
✓7th **T23.311 Burn of third degree of right thumb (nail)**
✓7th **T23.312 Burn of third degree of left thumb (nail)**
✓7th **T23.319 Burn of third degree of unspecified thumb (nail)**
✓6th **T23.32 Burn of third degree of single finger (nail) except thumb**
✓7th **T23.321 Burn of third degree of single right finger (nail) except thumb**
✓7th **T23.322 Burn of third degree of single left finger (nail) except thumb**
✓7th **T23.329 Burn of third degree of unspecified single finger (nail) except thumb**
✓6th **T23.33 Burn of third degree of multiple fingers (nail), not including thumb**
✓7th **T23.331 Burn of third degree of multiple right fingers (nail), not including thumb**
✓7th **T23.332 Burn of third degree of multiple left fingers (nail), not including thumb**
✓7th **T23.339 Burn of third degree of unspecified multiple fingers (nail), not including thumb**
✓6th **T23.34 Burn of third degree of multiple fingers (nail), including thumb**
✓7th **T23.341 Burn of third degree of multiple right fingers (nail), including thumb**
✓7th **T23.342 Burn of third degree of multiple left fingers (nail), including thumb**
✓7th **T23.349 Burn of third degree of unspecified multiple fingers (nail), including thumb**
✓6th **T23.35 Burn of third degree of palm**
✓7th **T23.351 Burn of third degree of right palm**
✓7th **T23.352 Burn of third degree of left palm**
✓7th **T23.359 Burn of third degree of unspecified palm**
✓6th **T23.36 Burn of third degree of back of hand**
✓7th **T23.361 Burn of third degree of back of right hand**
✓7th **T23.362 Burn of third degree of back of left hand**
✓7th **T23.369 Burn of third degree of back of unspecified hand**
✓6th **T23.37 Burn of third degree of wrist**
✓7th **T23.371 Burn of third degree of right wrist**
✓7th **T23.372 Burn of third degree of left wrist**
✓7th **T23.379 Burn of third degree of unspecified wrist**
✓6th **T23.39 Burn of third degree of multiple sites of wrist and hand**
✓7th **T23.391 Burn of third degree of multiple sites of right wrist and hand**
✓7th **T23.392 Burn of third degree of multiple sites of left wrist and hand**
✓7th **T23.399 Burn of third degree of multiple sites of unspecified wrist and hand**
✓5th **T23.4 Corrosion of unspecified degree of wrist and hand**
Code first (T51-T65) to identify chemical and intent
Use additional external cause code to identify place (Y92)
✓6th **T23.40 Corrosion of unspecified degree of hand, unspecified site**
✓7th **T23.401 Corrosion of unspecified degree of right hand, unspecified site**
✓7th **T23.402 Corrosion of unspecified degree of left hand, unspecified site**
✓7th **T23.409 Corrosion of unspecified degree of unspecified hand, unspecified site**
✓6th **T23.41 Corrosion of unspecified degree of thumb (nail)**
✓7th **T23.411 Corrosion of unspecified degree of right thumb (nail)**
✓7th **T23.412 Corrosion of unspecified degree of left thumb (nail)**
✓7th **T23.419 Corrosion of unspecified degree of unspecified thumb (nail)**
✓6th **T23.42 Corrosion of unspecified degree of single finger (nail) except thumb**
✓7th **T23.421 Corrosion of unspecified degree of single right finger (nail) except thumb**
✓7th **T23.422 Corrosion of unspecified degree of single left finger (nail) except thumb**
✓7th **T23.429 Corrosion of unspecified degree of unspecified single finger (nail) except thumb**

6th T23.43 **Corrosion of unspecified degree of multiple fingers (nail), not including thumb**
- 7th T23.431 **Corrosion of unspecified degree of multiple right fingers (nail), not including thumb**
- 7th T23.432 **Corrosion of unspecified degree of multiple left fingers (nail), not including thumb**
- 7th T23.439 **Corrosion of unspecified degree of unspecified multiple fingers (nail), not including thumb**

6th T23.44 **Corrosion of unspecified degree of multiple fingers (nail), including thumb**
- 7th T23.441 **Corrosion of unspecified degree of multiple right fingers (nail), including thumb**
- 7th T23.442 **Corrosion of unspecified degree of multiple left fingers (nail), including thumb**
- 7th T23.449 **Corrosion of unspecified degree of unspecified multiple fingers (nail), including thumb**

6th T23.45 **Corrosion of unspecified degree of palm**
- 7th T23.451 **Corrosion of unspecified degree of right palm**
- 7th T23.452 **Corrosion of unspecified degree of left palm**
- 7th T23.459 **Corrosion of unspecified degree of unspecified palm**

6th T23.46 **Corrosion of unspecified degree of back of hand**
- 7th T23.461 **Corrosion of unspecified degree of back of right hand**
- 7th T23.462 **Corrosion of unspecified degree of back of left hand**
- 7th T23.469 **Corrosion of unspecified degree of back of unspecified hand**

6th T23.47 **Corrosion of unspecified degree of wrist**
- 7th T23.471 **Corrosion of unspecified degree of right wrist**
- 7th T23.472 **Corrosion of unspecified degree of left wrist**
- 7th T23.479 **Corrosion of unspecified degree of unspecified wrist**

6th T23.49 **Corrosion of unspecified degree of multiple sites of wrist and hand**
- 7th T23.491 **Corrosion of unspecified degree of multiple sites of right wrist and hand**
- 7th T23.492 **Corrosion of unspecified degree of multiple sites of left wrist and hand**
- 7th T23.499 **Corrosion of unspecified degree of multiple sites of unspecified wrist and hand**

5th T23.5 **Corrosion of first degree of wrist and hand**

Code first (T51-T65) to identify chemical and intent

Use additional external cause code to identify place (Y92)

6th T23.50 **Corrosion of first degree of hand, unspecified site**
- 7th T23.501 **Corrosion of first degree of right hand, unspecified site**
- 7th T23.502 **Corrosion of first degree of left hand, unspecified site**
- 7th T23.509 **Corrosion of first degree of unspecified hand, unspecified site**

6th T23.51 **Corrosion of first degree of thumb (nail)**
- 7th T23.511 **Corrosion of first degree of right thumb (nail)**
- 7th T23.512 **Corrosion of first degree of left thumb (nail)**
- 7th T23.519 **Corrosion of first degree of unspecified thumb (nail)**

6th T23.52 **Corrosion of first degree of single finger (nail) except thumb**
- 7th T23.521 **Corrosion of first degree of single right finger (nail) except thumb**
- 7th T23.522 **Corrosion of first degree of single left finger (nail) except thumb**
- 7th T23.529 **Corrosion of first degree of unspecified single finger (nail) except thumb**

6th T23.53 **Corrosion of first degree of multiple fingers (nail), not including thumb**
- 7th T23.531 **Corrosion of first degree of multiple right fingers (nail), not including thumb**
- 7th T23.532 **Corrosion of first degree of multiple left fingers (nail), not including thumb**
- 7th T23.539 **Corrosion of first degree of unspecified multiple fingers (nail), not including thumb**

6th T23.54 **Corrosion of first degree of multiple fingers (nail), including thumb**
- 7th T23.541 **Corrosion of first degree of multiple right fingers (nail), including thumb**
- 7th T23.542 **Corrosion of first degree of multiple left fingers (nail), including thumb**
- 7th T23.549 **Corrosion of first degree of unspecified multiple fingers (nail), including thumb**

6th T23.55 **Corrosion of first degree of palm**
- 7th T23.551 **Corrosion of first degree of right palm**
- 7th T23.552 **Corrosion of first degree of left palm**
- 7th T23.559 **Corrosion of first degree of unspecified palm**

6th T23.56 **Corrosion of first degree of back of hand**
- 7th T23.561 **Corrosion of first degree of back of right hand**
- 7th T23.562 **Corrosion of first degree of back of left hand**
- 7th T23.569 **Corrosion of first degree of back of unspecified hand**

6th T23.57 **Corrosion of first degree of wrist**
- 7th T23.571 **Corrosion of first degree of right wrist**
- 7th T23.572 **Corrosion of first degree of left wrist**
- 7th T23.579 **Corrosion of first degree of unspecified wrist**

6th T23.59 **Corrosion of first degree of multiple sites of wrist and hand**
- 7th T23.591 **Corrosion of first degree of multiple sites of right wrist and hand**
- 7th T23.592 **Corrosion of first degree of multiple sites of left wrist and hand**
- 7th T23.599 **Corrosion of first degree of multiple sites of unspecified wrist and hand**

5th T23.6 **Corrosion of second degree of wrist and hand**

Code first (T51-T65) to identify chemical and intent

Use additional external cause code to identify place (Y92)

6th T23.60 **Corrosion of second degree of hand, unspecified site**
- 7th T23.601 **Corrosion of second degree of right hand, unspecified site**
- 7th T23.602 **Corrosion of second degree of left hand, unspecified site**
- 7th T23.609 **Corrosion of second degree of unspecified hand, unspecified site**

6th T23.61 **Corrosion of second degree of thumb (nail)**
- 7th T23.611 **Corrosion of second degree of right thumb (nail)**
- 7th T23.612 **Corrosion of second degree of left thumb (nail)**
- 7th T23.619 **Corrosion of second degree of unspecified thumb (nail)**

6th T23.62 **Corrosion of second degree of single finger (nail) except thumb**
- 7th T23.621 **Corrosion of second degree of single right finger (nail) except thumb**
- 7th T23.622 **Corrosion of second degree of single left finger (nail) except thumb**
- 7th T23.629 **Corrosion of second degree of unspecified single finger (nail) except thumb**

6th T23.63 **Corrosion of second degree of multiple fingers (nail), not including thumb**
- 7th T23.631 **Corrosion of second degree of multiple right fingers (nail), not including thumb**
- 7th T23.632 **Corrosion of second degree of multiple left fingers (nail), not including thumb**

7th T23.639 **Corrosion of second degree of unspecified multiple fingers (nail), not including thumb**

6th T23.64 **Corrosion of second degree of multiple fingers (nail), including thumb**

7th T23.641 **Corrosion of second degree of multiple right fingers (nail), including thumb**

7th T23.642 **Corrosion of second degree of multiple left fingers (nail), including thumb**

7th T23.649 **Corrosion of second degree of unspecified multiple fingers (nail), including thumb**

6th T23.65 **Corrosion of second degree of palm**

7th T23.651 **Corrosion of second degree of right palm**

7th T23.652 **Corrosion of second degree of left palm**

7th T23.659 **Corrosion of second degree of unspecified palm**

6th T23.66 **Corrosion of second degree of back of hand**

7th T23.661 **Corrosion of second degree back of right hand**

7th T23.662 **Corrosion of second degree back of left hand**

7th T23.669 **Corrosion of second degree back of unspecified hand**

6th T23.67 **Corrosion of second degree of wrist**

7th T23.671 **Corrosion of second degree of right wrist**

7th T23.672 **Corrosion of second degree of left wrist**

7th T23.679 **Corrosion of second degree of unspecified wrist**

6th T23.69 **Corrosion of second degree of multiple sites of wrist and hand**

7th T23.691 **Corrosion of second degree of multiple sites of right wrist and hand**

7th T23.692 **Corrosion of second degree of multiple sites of left wrist and hand**

7th T23.699 **Corrosion of second degree of multiple sites of unspecified wrist and hand**

5th T23.7 **Corrosion of third degree of wrist and hand**

Code first (T51-T65) to identify chemical and intent

Use additional external cause code to identify place (Y92)

6th T23.70 **Corrosion of third degree of hand, unspecified site**

7th T23.701 **Corrosion of third degree of right hand, unspecified site**

7th T23.702 **Corrosion of third degree of left hand, unspecified site**

7th T23.709 **Corrosion of third degree of unspecified hand, unspecified site**

6th T23.71 **Corrosion of third degree of thumb (nail)**

7th T23.711 **Corrosion of third degree of right thumb (nail)**

7th T23.712 **Corrosion of third degree of left thumb (nail)**

7th T23.719 **Corrosion of third degree of unspecified thumb (nail)**

6th T23.72 **Corrosion of third degree of single finger (nail) except thumb**

7th T23.721 **Corrosion of third degree of single right finger (nail) except thumb**

7th T23.722 **Corrosion of third degree of single left finger (nail) except thumb**

7th T23.729 **Corrosion of third degree of unspecified single finger (nail) except thumb**

6th T23.73 **Corrosion of third degree of multiple fingers (nail), not including thumb**

7th T23.731 **Corrosion of third degree of multiple right fingers (nail), not including thumb**

7th T23.732 **Corrosion of third degree of multiple left fingers (nail), not including thumb**

7th T23.739 **Corrosion of third degree of unspecified multiple fingers (nail), not including thumb**

6th T23.74 **Corrosion of third degree of multiple fingers (nail), including thumb**

7th T23.741 **Corrosion of third degree of multiple right fingers (nail), including thumb**

7th T23.742 **Corrosion of third degree of multiple left fingers (nail), including thumb**

7th T23.749 **Corrosion of third degree of unspecified multiple fingers (nail), including thumb**

6th T23.75 **Corrosion of third degree of palm**

7th T23.751 **Corrosion of third degree of right palm**

7th T23.752 **Corrosion of third degree of left palm**

7th T23.759 **Corrosion of third degree of unspecified palm**

6th T23.76 **Corrosion of third degree of back of hand**

7th T23.761 **Corrosion of third degree of back of right hand**

7th T23.762 **Corrosion of third degree of back of left hand**

7th T23.769 **Corrosion of third degree back of unspecified hand**

6th T23.77 **Corrosion of third degree of wrist**

7th T23.771 **Corrosion of third degree of right wrist**

7th T23.772 **Corrosion of third degree of left wrist**

7th T23.779 **Corrosion of third degree of unspecified wrist**

6th T23.79 **Corrosion of third degree of multiple sites of wrist and hand**

7th T23.791 **Corrosion of third degree of multiple sites of right wrist and hand**

7th T23.792 **Corrosion of third degree of multiple sites of left wrist and hand**

7th T23.799 **Corrosion of third degree of multiple sites of unspecified wrist and hand**

4th **T24 Burn and corrosion of lower limb, except ankle and foot**

EXCLUDES 2 *burn and corrosion of ankle and foot (T25.-)*
burn and corrosion of hip region (T21.-)

The appropriate 7th character is to be added to each code from category T24.
A initial encounter
D subsequent encounter
S sequela

5th T24.0 **Burn of unspecified degree of lower limb, except ankle and foot**

Use additional external cause code to identify the source, place and intent of the burn (X00-X19, X75-X77, X96-X98, Y92)

6th T24.00 **Burn of unspecified degree of unspecified site of lower limb, except ankle and foot**

7th T24.001 **Burn of unspecified degree of unspecified site of right lower limb, except ankle and foot**

7th T24.002 **Burn of unspecified degree of unspecified site of left lower limb, except ankle and foot**

7th T24.009 **Burn of unspecified degree of unspecified site of unspecified lower limb, except ankle and foot**

6th T24.01 **Burn of unspecified degree of thigh**

7th T24.011 **Burn of unspecified degree of right thigh**

7th T24.012 **Burn of unspecified degree of left thigh**

7th T24.019 **Burn of unspecified degree of unspecified thigh**

6th T24.02 **Burn of unspecified degree of knee**

7th T24.021 **Burn of unspecified degree of right knee**

7th T24.022 **Burn of unspecified degree of left knee**

7th T24.029 **Burn of unspecified degree of unspecified knee**

6th T24.03 **Burn of unspecified degree of lower leg**

7th T24.031 **Burn of unspecified degree of right lower leg**

7th T24.032 **Burn of unspecified degree of left lower leg**

7th T24.039 **Burn of unspecified degree of unspecified lower leg**

6th **T24.09 Burn of unspecified degree of multiple sites of lower limb, except ankle and foot**
7th **T24.091 Burn of unspecified degree of multiple sites of right lower limb, except ankle and foot**
7th **T24.092 Burn of unspecified degree of multiple sites of left lower limb, except ankle and foot**
7th **T24.099 Burn of unspecified degree of multiple sites of unspecified lower limb, except ankle and foot**

5th **T24.1 Burn of first degree of lower limb, except ankle and foot**
Use additional external cause code to identify the source, place and intent of the burn (X00-X19, X75-X77, X96-X98, Y92)

6th **T24.10 Burn of first degree of unspecified site of lower limb, except ankle and foot**
7th **T24.101 Burn of first degree of unspecified site of right lower limb, except ankle and foot**
7th **T24.102 Burn of first degree of unspecified site of left lower limb, except ankle and foot**
7th **T24.109 Burn of first degree of unspecified site of unspecified lower limb, except ankle and foot**

6th **T24.11 Burn of first degree of thigh**
7th **T24.111 Burn of first degree of right thigh**
7th **T24.112 Burn of first degree of left thigh**
7th **T24.119 Burn of first degree of unspecified thigh**

6th **T24.12 Burn of first degree of knee**
7th **T24.121 Burn of first degree of right knee**
7th **T24.122 Burn of first degree of left knee**
7th **T24.129 Burn of first degree of unspecified knee**

6th **T24.13 Burn of first degree of lower leg**
7th **T24.131 Burn of first degree of right lower leg**
7th **T24.132 Burn of first degree of left lower leg**
7th **T24.139 Burn of first degree of unspecified lower leg**

6th **T24.19 Burn of first degree of multiple sites of lower limb, except ankle and foot**
7th **T24.191 Burn of first degree of multiple sites of right lower limb, except ankle and foot**
7th **T24.192 Burn of first degree of multiple sites of left lower limb, except ankle and foot**
7th **T24.199 Burn of first degree of multiple sites of unspecified lower limb, except ankle and foot**

5th **T24.2 Burn of second degree of lower limb, except ankle and foot**
Use additional external cause code to identify the source, place and intent of the burn (X00-X19, X75-X77, X96-X98, Y92)

6th **T24.20 Burn of second degree of unspecified site of lower limb, except ankle and foot**
7th **T24.201 Burn of second degree of unspecified site of right lower limb, except ankle and foot**
7th **T24.202 Burn of second degree of unspecified site of left lower limb, except ankle and foot**
7th **T24.209 Burn of second degree of unspecified site of unspecified lower limb, except ankle and foot**

6th **T24.21 Burn of second degree of thigh**
7th **T24.211 Burn of second degree of right thigh**
7th **T24.212 Burn of second degree of left thigh**
7th **T24.219 Burn of second degree of unspecified thigh**

6th **T24.22 Burn of second degree of knee**
7th **T24.221 Burn of second degree of right knee**
7th **T24.222 Burn of second degree of left knee**
7th **T24.229 Burn of second degree of unspecified knee**

6th **T24.23 Burn of second degree of lower leg**
7th **T24.231 Burn of second degree of right lower leg**
7th **T24.232 Burn of second degree of left lower leg**
7th **T24.239 Burn of second degree of unspecified lower leg**

6th **T24.29 Burn of second degree of multiple sites of lower limb, except ankle and foot**
7th **T24.291 Burn of second degree of multiple sites of right lower limb, except ankle and foot**
7th **T24.292 Burn of second degree of multiple sites of left lower limb, except ankle and foot**
7th **T24.299 Burn of second degree of multiple sites of unspecified lower limb, except ankle and foot**

5th **T24.3 Burn of third degree of lower limb, except ankle and foot**
Use additional external cause code to identify the source, place and intent of the burn (X00-X19, X75-X77, X96-X98, Y92)

6th **T24.30 Burn of third degree of unspecified site of lower limb, except ankle and foot**
7th **T24.301 Burn of third degree of unspecified site of right lower limb, except ankle and foot**
7th **T24.302 Burn of third degree of unspecified site of left lower limb, except ankle and foot**
7th **T24.309 Burn of third degree of unspecified site of unspecified lower limb, except ankle and foot**

6th **T24.31 Burn of third degree of thigh**
7th **T24.311 Burn of third degree of right thigh**
7th **T24.312 Burn of third degree of left thigh**
7th **T24.319 Burn of third degree of unspecified thigh**

6th **T24.32 Burn of third degree of knee**
7th **T24.321 Burn of third degree of right knee**
7th **T24.322 Burn of third degree of left knee**
7th **T24.329 Burn of third degree of unspecified knee**

6th **T24.33 Burn of third degree of lower leg**
7th **T24.331 Burn of third degree of right lower leg**
7th **T24.332 Burn of third degree of left lower leg**
7th **T24.339 Burn of third degree of unspecified lower leg**

6th **T24.39 Burn of third degree of multiple sites of lower limb, except ankle and foot**
7th **T24.391 Burn of third degree of multiple sites of right lower limb, except ankle and foot**
7th **T24.392 Burn of third degree of multiple sites of left lower limb, except ankle and foot**
7th **T24.399 Burn of third degree of multiple sites of unspecified lower limb, except ankle and foot**

5th **T24.4 Corrosion of unspecified degree of lower limb, except ankle and foot**
Code first (T51-T65) to identify chemical and intent
Use additional external cause code to identify place (Y92)

6th **T24.40 Corrosion of unspecified degree of unspecified site of lower limb, except ankle and foot**
7th **T24.401 Corrosion of unspecified degree of unspecified site of right lower limb, except ankle and foot**
7th **T24.402 Corrosion of unspecified degree of unspecified site of left lower limb, except ankle and foot**
7th **T24.409 Corrosion of unspecified degree of unspecified site of unspecified lower limb, except ankle and foot**

6th **T24.41 Corrosion of unspecified degree of thigh**
7th **T24.411 Corrosion of unspecified degree of right thigh**
7th **T24.412 Corrosion of unspecified degree of left thigh**
7th **T24.419 Corrosion of unspecified degree of unspecified thigh**

6th **T24.42 Corrosion of unspecified degree of knee**
7th **T24.421 Corrosion of unspecified degree of right knee**
7th **T24.422 Corrosion of unspecified degree of left knee**
7th **T24.429 Corrosion of unspecified degree of unspecified knee**

Appropriate additional character required
x7th Requires 7th character, placeholder x must fill empty characters

✓6th **T24.43 Corrosion of unspecified degree of lower leg**
- ✓7th **T24.431 Corrosion of unspecified degree of right lower leg**
- ✓7th **T24.432 Corrosion of unspecified degree of left lower leg**
- ✓7th **T24.439 Corrosion of unspecified degree of unspecified lower leg**

✓6th **T24.49 Corrosion of unspecified degree of multiple sites of lower limb, except ankle and foot**
- ✓7th **T24.491 Corrosion of unspecified degree of multiple sites of right lower limb, except ankle and foot**
- ✓7th **T24.492 Corrosion of unspecified degree of multiple sites of left lower limb, except ankle and foot**
- ✓7th **T24.499 Corrosion of unspecified degree of multiple sites of unspecified lower limb, except ankle and foot**

✓5th **T24.5 Corrosion of first degree of lower limb, except ankle and foot**

Code first (T51-T65) to identify chemical and intent

Use additional external cause code to identify place (Y92)

✓6th **T24.50 Corrosion of first degree of unspecified site of lower limb, except ankle and foot**
- ✓7th **T24.501 Corrosion of first degree of unspecified site of right lower limb, except ankle and foot**
- ✓7th **T24.502 Corrosion of first degree of unspecified site of left lower limb, except ankle and foot**
- ✓7th **T24.509 Corrosion of first degree of unspecified site of unspecified lower limb, except ankle and foot**

✓6th **T24.51 Corrosion of first degree of thigh**
- ✓7th **T24.511 Corrosion of first degree of right thigh**
- ✓7th **T24.512 Corrosion of first degree of left thigh**
- ✓7th **T24.519 Corrosion of first degree of unspecified thigh**

✓6th **T24.52 Corrosion of first degree of knee**
- ✓7th **T24.521 Corrosion of first degree of right knee**
- ✓7th **T24.522 Corrosion of first degree of left knee**
- ✓7th **T24.529 Corrosion of first degree of unspecified knee**

✓6th **T24.53 Corrosion of first degree of lower leg**
- ✓7th **T24.531 Corrosion of first degree of right lower leg**
- ✓7th **T24.532 Corrosion of first degree of left lower leg**
- ✓7th **T24.539 Corrosion of first degree of unspecified lower leg**

✓6th **T24.59 Corrosion of first degree of multiple sites of lower limb, except ankle and foot**
- ✓7th **T24.591 Corrosion of first degree of multiple sites of right lower limb, except ankle and foot**
- ✓7th **T24.592 Corrosion of first degree of multiple sites of left lower limb, except ankle and foot**
- ✓7th **T24.599 Corrosion of first degree of multiple sites of unspecified lower limb, except ankle and foot**

✓5th **T24.6 Corrosion of second degree of lower limb, except ankle and foot**

Code first (T51-T65) to identify chemical and intent

Use additional external cause code to identify place (Y92)

✓6th **T24.60 Corrosion of second degree of unspecified site of lower limb, except ankle and foot**
- ✓7th **T24.601 Corrosion of second degree of unspecified site of right lower limb, except ankle and foot**
- ✓7th **T24.602 Corrosion of second degree of unspecified site of left lower limb, except ankle and foot**
- ✓7th **T24.609 Corrosion of second degree of unspecified site of unspecified lower limb, except ankle and foot**

✓6th **T24.61 Corrosion of second degree of thigh**
- ✓7th **T24.611 Corrosion of second degree of right thigh**
- ✓7th **T24.612 Corrosion of second degree of left thigh**
- ✓7th **T24.619 Corrosion of second degree of unspecified thigh**

✓6th **T24.62 Corrosion of second degree of knee**
- ✓7th **T24.621 Corrosion of second degree of right knee**
- ✓7th **T24.622 Corrosion of second degree of left knee**
- ✓7th **T24.629 Corrosion of second degree of unspecified knee**

✓6th **T24.63 Corrosion of second degree of lower leg**
- ✓7th **T24.631 Corrosion of second degree of right lower leg**
- ✓7th **T24.632 Corrosion of second degree of left lower leg**
- ✓7th **T24.639 Corrosion of second degree of unspecified lower leg**

✓6th **T24.69 Corrosion of second degree of multiple sites of lower limb, except ankle and foot**
- ✓7th **T24.691 Corrosion of second degree of multiple sites of right lower limb, except ankle and foot**
- ✓7th **T24.692 Corrosion of second degree of multiple sites of left lower limb, except ankle and foot**
- ✓7th **T24.699 Corrosion of second degree of multiple sites of unspecified lower limb, except ankle and foot**

✓5th **T24.7 Corrosion of third degree of lower limb, except ankle and foot**

Code first (T51-T65) to identify chemical and intent

Use additional external cause code to identify place (Y92)

✓6th **T24.70 Corrosion of third degree of unspecified site of lower limb, except ankle and foot**
- ✓7th **T24.701 Corrosion of third degree of unspecified site of right lower limb, except ankle and foot**
- ✓7th **T24.702 Corrosion of third degree of unspecified site of left lower limb, except ankle and foot**
- ✓7th **T24.709 Corrosion of third degree of unspecified site of unspecified lower limb, except ankle and foot**

✓6th **T24.71 Corrosion of third degree of thigh**
- ✓7th **T24.711 Corrosion of third degree of right thigh**
- ✓7th **T24.712 Corrosion of third degree of left thigh**
- ✓7th **T24.719 Corrosion of third degree of unspecified thigh**

✓6th **T24.72 Corrosion of third degree of knee**
- ✓7th **T24.721 Corrosion of third degree of right knee**
- ✓7th **T24.722 Corrosion of third degree of left knee**
- ✓7th **T24.729 Corrosion of third degree of unspecified knee**

✓6th **T24.73 Corrosion of third degree of lower leg**
- ✓7th **T24.731 Corrosion of third degree of right lower leg**
- ✓7th **T24.732 Corrosion of third degree of left lower leg**
- ✓7th **T24.739 Corrosion of third degree of unspecified lower leg**

✓6th **T24.79 Corrosion of third degree of multiple sites of lower limb, except ankle and foot**
- ✓7th **T24.791 Corrosion of third degree of multiple sites of right lower limb, except ankle and foot**
- ✓7th **T24.792 Corrosion of third degree of multiple sites of left lower limb, except ankle and foot**
- ✓7th **T24.799 Corrosion of third degree of multiple sites of unspecified lower limb, except ankle and foot**

4th T25 Burn and corrosion of ankle and foot

The appropriate 7th character is to be added to each code from category T25.
A initial encounter
D subsequent encounter
S sequela

5th T25.0 Burn of unspecified degree of ankle and foot
Use additional external cause code to identify the source, place and intent of the burn (X00-X19, X75-X77, X96-X98, Y92)
6th T25.01 Burn of unspecified degree of ankle
7th T25.011 Burn of unspecified degree of right ankle
7th T25.012 Burn of unspecified degree of left ankle
7th T25.019 Burn of unspecified degree of unspecified ankle
6th T25.02 Burn of unspecified degree of foot
EXCLUDES 2 *burn of unspecified degree of toe(s) (nail) (T25.03-)*
7th T25.021 Burn of unspecified degree of right foot
7th T25.022 Burn of unspecified degree of left foot
7th T25.029 Burn of unspecified degree of unspecified foot
6th T25.03 Burn of unspecified degree of toe(s) (nail)
7th T25.031 Burn of unspecified degree of right toe(s) (nail)
7th T25.032 Burn of unspecified degree of left toe(s) (nail)
7th T25.039 Burn of unspecified degree of unspecified toe(s) (nail)
6th T25.09 Burn of unspecified degree of multiple sites of ankle and foot
7th T25.091 Burn of unspecified degree of multiple sites of right ankle and foot
7th T25.092 Burn of unspecified degree of multiple sites of left ankle and foot
7th T25.099 Burn of unspecified degree of multiple sites of unspecified ankle and foot

5th T25.1 Burn of first degree of ankle and foot
Use additional external cause code to identify the source, place and intent of the burn (X00-X19, X75-X77, X96-X98, Y92)
6th T25.11 Burn of first degree of ankle
7th T25.111 Burn of first degree of right ankle
7th T25.112 Burn of first degree of left ankle
7th T25.119 Burn of first degree of unspecified ankle
6th T25.12 Burn of first degree of foot
EXCLUDES 2 *burn of first degree of toe(s) (nail) (T25.13-)*
7th T25.121 Burn of first degree of right foot
7th T25.122 Burn of first degree of left foot
7th T25.129 Burn of first degree of unspecified foot
6th T25.13 Burn of first degree of toe(s) (nail)
7th T25.131 Burn of first degree of right toe(s) (nail)
7th T25.132 Burn of first degree of left toe(s) (nail)
7th T25.139 Burn of first degree of unspecified toe(s) (nail)
6th T25.19 Burn of first degree of multiple sites of ankle and foot
7th T25.191 Burn of first degree of multiple sites of right ankle and foot
7th T25.192 Burn of first degree of multiple sites of left ankle and foot
7th T25.199 Burn of first degree of multiple sites of unspecified ankle and foot

5th T25.2 Burn of second degree of ankle and foot
Use additional external cause code to identify the source, place and intent of the burn (X00-X19, X75-X77, X96-X98, Y92)
6th T25.21 Burn of second degree of ankle
7th T25.211 Burn of second degree of right ankle
7th T25.212 Burn of second degree of left ankle
7th T25.219 Burn of second degree of unspecified ankle
6th T25.22 Burn of second degree of foot
EXCLUDES 2 *burn of second degree of toe(s) (nail) (T25.23-)*
7th T25.221 Burn of second degree of right foot
7th T25.222 Burn of second degree of left foot
7th T25.229 Burn of second degree of unspecified foot
6th T25.23 Burn of second degree of toe(s) (nail)
7th T25.231 Burn of second degree of right toe(s) (nail)
7th T25.232 Burn of second degree of left toe(s) (nail)
7th T25.239 Burn of second degree of unspecified toe(s) (nail)
6th T25.29 Burn of second degree of multiple sites of ankle and foot
7th T25.291 Burn of second degree of multiple sites of right ankle and foot
7th T25.292 Burn of second degree of multiple sites of left ankle and foot
7th T25.299 Burn of second degree of multiple sites of unspecified ankle and foot

5th T25.3 Burn of third degree of ankle and foot
Use additional external cause code to identify the source, place and intent of the burn (X00-X19, X75-X77, X96-X98, Y92)
6th T25.31 Burn of third degree of ankle
7th T25.311 Burn of third degree of right ankle
7th T25.312 Burn of third degree of left ankle
7th T25.319 Burn of third degree of unspecified ankle
6th T25.32 Burn of third degree of foot
EXCLUDES 2 *burn of third degree of toe(s) (nail) (T25.33-)*
7th T25.321 Burn of third degree of right foot
7th T25.322 Burn of third degree of left foot
7th T25.329 Burn of third degree of unspecified foot
6th T25.33 Burn of third degree of toe(s) (nail)
7th T25.331 Burn of third degree of right toe(s) (nail)
7th T25.332 Burn of third degree of left toe(s) (nail)
7th T25.339 Burn of third degree of unspecified toe(s) (nail)
6th T25.39 Burn of third degree of multiple sites of ankle and foot
7th T25.391 Burn of third degree of multiple sites of right ankle and foot
7th T25.392 Burn of third degree of multiple sites of left ankle and foot
7th T25.399 Burn of third degree of multiple sites of unspecified ankle and foot

5th T25.4 Corrosion of unspecified degree of ankle and foot
Code first (T51-T65) to identify chemical and intent
Use additional external cause code to identify place (Y92)
6th T25.41 Corrosion of unspecified degree of ankle
7th T25.411 Corrosion of unspecified degree of right ankle
7th T25.412 Corrosion of unspecified degree of left ankle
7th T25.419 Corrosion of unspecified degree of unspecified ankle
6th T25.42 Corrosion of unspecified degree of foot
EXCLUDES 2 *corrosion of unspecified degree of toe(s) (nail) (T25.43-)*
7th T25.421 Corrosion of unspecified degree of right foot
7th T25.422 Corrosion of unspecified degree of left foot
7th T25.429 Corrosion of unspecified degree of unspecified foot
6th T25.43 Corrosion of unspecified degree of toe(s) (nail)
7th T25.431 Corrosion of unspecified degree of right toe(s) (nail)
7th T25.432 Corrosion of unspecified degree of left toe(s) (nail)
7th T25.439 Corrosion of unspecified degree of unspecified toe(s) (nail)

✓6th **T25.49 Corrosion of unspecified degree of multiple sites of ankle and foot**

✓7th **T25.491 Corrosion of unspecified degree of multiple sites of right ankle and foot**

✓7th **T25.492 Corrosion of unspecified degree of multiple sites of left ankle and foot**

✓7th **T25.499 Corrosion of unspecified degree of multiple sites of unspecified ankle and foot**

✓5th **T25.5 Corrosion of first degree of ankle and foot**

Code first (T51-T65) to identify chemical and intent

Use additional external cause code to identify place (Y92)

✓6th **T25.51 Corrosion of first degree of ankle**

✓7th **T25.511 Corrosion of first degree of right ankle**

✓7th **T25.512 Corrosion of first degree of left ankle**

✓7th **T25.519 Corrosion of first degree of unspecified ankle**

✓6th **T25.52 Corrosion of first degree of foot**

EXCLUDES 2 *corrosion of first degree of toe(s) (nail) (T25.53-)*

✓7th **T25.521 Corrosion of first degree of right foot**

✓7th **T25.522 Corrosion of first degree of left foot**

✓7th **T25.529 Corrosion of first degree of unspecified foot**

✓6th **T25.53 Corrosion of first degree of toe(s) (nail)**

✓7th **T25.531 Corrosion of first degree of right toe(s) (nail)**

✓7th **T25.532 Corrosion of first degree of left toe(s) (nail)**

✓7th **T25.539 Corrosion of first degree of unspecified toe(s) (nail)**

✓6th **T25.59 Corrosion of first degree of multiple sites of ankle and foot**

✓7th **T25.591 Corrosion of first degree of multiple sites of right ankle and foot**

✓7th **T25.592 Corrosion of first degree of multiple sites of left ankle and foot**

✓7th **T25.599 Corrosion of first degree of multiple sites of unspecified ankle and foot**

✓5th **T25.6 Corrosion of second degree of ankle and foot**

Code first (T51-T65) to identify chemical and intent

Use additional external cause code to identify place (Y92)

✓6th **T25.61 Corrosion of second degree of ankle**

✓7th **T25.611 Corrosion of second degree of right ankle**

✓7th **T25.612 Corrosion of second degree of left ankle**

✓7th **T25.619 Corrosion of second degree of unspecified ankle**

✓6th **T25.62 Corrosion of second degree of foot**

EXCLUDES 2 *corrosion of second degree of toe(s) (nail) (T25.63-)*

✓7th **T25.621 Corrosion of second degree of right foot**

✓7th **T25.622 Corrosion of second degree of left foot**

✓7th **T25.629 Corrosion of second degree of unspecified foot**

✓6th **T25.63 Corrosion of second degree of toe(s) (nail)**

✓7th **T25.631 Corrosion of second degree of right toe(s) (nail)**

✓7th **T25.632 Corrosion of second degree of left toe(s) (nail)**

✓7th **T25.639 Corrosion of second degree of unspecified toe(s) (nail)**

✓6th **T25.69 Corrosion of second degree of multiple sites of ankle and foot**

✓7th **T25.691 Corrosion of second degree of right ankle and foot**

✓7th **T25.692 Corrosion of second degree of left ankle and foot**

✓7th **T25.699 Corrosion of second degree of unspecified ankle and foot**

✓5th **T25.7 Corrosion of third degree of ankle and foot**

Code first (T51-T65) to identify chemical and intent

Use additional external cause code to identify place (Y92)

✓6th **T25.71 Corrosion of third degree of ankle**

✓7th **T25.711 Corrosion of third degree of right ankle**

✓7th **T25.712 Corrosion of third degree of left ankle**

✓7th **T25.719 Corrosion of third degree of unspecified ankle**

✓6th **T25.72 Corrosion of third degree of foot**

EXCLUDES 2 *corrosion of third degree of toe(s) (nail) (T25.73-)*

✓7th **T25.721 Corrosion of third degree of right foot**

✓7th **T25.722 Corrosion of third degree of left foot**

✓7th **T25.729 Corrosion of third degree of unspecified foot**

✓6th **T25.73 Corrosion of third degree of toe(s) (nail)**

✓7th **T25.731 Corrosion of third degree of right toe(s) (nail)**

✓7th **T25.732 Corrosion of third degree of left toe(s) (nail)**

✓7th **T25.739 Corrosion of third degree of unspecified toe(s) (nail)**

✓6th **T25.79 Corrosion of third degree of multiple sites of ankle and foot**

✓7th **T25.791 Corrosion of third degree of multiple sites of right ankle and foot**

✓7th **T25.792 Corrosion of third degree of multiple sites of left ankle and foot**

✓7th **T25.799 Corrosion of third degree of multiple sites of unspecified ankle and foot**

Burns and corrosions confined to eye and internal organs (T26-T28)

✓4th **T26 Burn and corrosion confined to eye and adnexa**

The appropriate 7th character is to be added to each code from category T26.
A initial encounter
D subsequent encounter
S sequela

✓5th **T26.0 Burn of eyelid and periocular area**

Use additional external cause code to identify the source, place and intent of the burn (X00-X19, X75-X77, X96-X98, Y92)

✓x7th **T26.00 Burn of unspecified eyelid and periocular area**

✓x7th **T26.01 Burn of right eyelid and periocular area**

✓x7th **T26.02 Burn of left eyelid and periocular area**

✓5th **T26.1 Burn of cornea and conjunctival sac**

Use additional external cause code to identify the source, place and intent of the burn (X00-X19, X75-X77, X96-X98, Y92)

✓x7th **T26.10 Burn of cornea and conjunctival sac, unspecified eye**

✓x7th **T26.11 Burn of cornea and conjunctival sac, right eye**

✓x7th **T26.12 Burn of cornea and conjunctival sac, left eye**

✓5th **T26.2 Burn with resulting rupture and destruction of eyeball**

Use additional external cause code to identify the source, place and intent of the burn (X00-X19, X75-X77, X96-X98, Y92)

✓x7th **T26.20 Burn with resulting rupture and destruction of unspecified eyeball**

✓x7th **T26.21 Burn with resulting rupture and destruction of right eyeball**

✓x7th **T26.22 Burn with resulting rupture and destruction of left eyeball**

✓5th **T26.3 Burns of other specified parts of eye and adnexa**

Use additional external cause code to identify the source, place and intent of the burn (X00-X19, X75-X77, X96-X98, Y92)

✓x7th **T26.30 Burns of other specified parts of unspecified eye and adnexa**

✓x7th **T26.31 Burns of other specified parts of right eye and adnexa**

✓x7th **T26.32 Burns of other specified parts of left eye and adnexa**

✓5th **T26.4 Burn of eye and adnexa, part unspecified**

Use additional external cause code to identify the source, place and intent of the burn (X00-X19, X75-X77, X96-X98, Y92)

✓x7th **T26.40 Burn of unspecified eye and adnexa, part unspecified**

✓x7th **T26.41 Burn of right eye and adnexa, part unspecified**

T26.42 Burn of left eye and adnexa, part unspecified

T26.5 Corrosion of eyelid and periocular area
Code first (T51-T65) to identify chemical and intent
Use additional external cause code to identify place (Y92)

T26.50 Corrosion of unspecified eyelid and periocular area

T26.51 Corrosion of right eyelid and periocular area

T26.52 Corrosion of left eyelid and periocular area

T26.6 Corrosion of cornea and conjunctival sac
Code first (T51-T65) to identify chemical and intent
Use additional external cause code to identify place (Y92)

T26.60 Corrosion of cornea and conjunctival sac, unspecified eye

T26.61 Corrosion of cornea and conjunctival sac, right eye

T26.62 Corrosion of cornea and conjunctival sac, left eye

T26.7 Corrosion with resulting rupture and destruction of eyeball
Code first (T51-T65) to identify chemical and intent
Use additional external cause code to identify place (Y92)

T26.70 Corrosion with resulting rupture and destruction of unspecified eyeball

T26.71 Corrosion with resulting rupture and destruction of right eyeball

T26.72 Corrosion with resulting rupture and destruction of left eyeball

T26.8 Corrosions of other specified parts of eye and adnexa
Code first (T51-T65) to identify chemical and intent
Use additional external cause code to identify place (Y92)

T26.80 Corrosions of other specified parts of unspecified eye and adnexa

T26.81 Corrosions of other specified parts of right eye and adnexa

T26.82 Corrosions of other specified parts of left eye and adnexa

T26.9 Corrosion of eye and adnexa, part unspecified
Code first (T51-T65) to identify chemical and intent
Use additional external cause code to identify place (Y92)

T26.90 Corrosion of unspecified eye and adnexa, part unspecified

T26.91 Corrosion of right eye and adnexa, part unspecified

T26.92 Corrosion of left eye and adnexa, part unspecified

T27 Burn and corrosion of respiratory tract
Use additional external cause code to identify the source and intent of the burn (X00- X19, X75-X77, X96-X98)
Use additional external cause code to identify place (Y92)

The appropriate 7th character is to be added to each code from category T27.
A initial encounter
D subsequent encounter
S sequela

T27.0 Burn of larynx and trachea

T27.1 Burn involving larynx and trachea with lung

T27.2 Burn of other parts of respiratory tract
Burn of thoracic cavity

T27.3 Burn of respiratory tract, part unspecified
Code first (T51-T65) to identify chemical and intent for codes T27.4-T27.7

T27.4 Corrosion of larynx and trachea

T27.5 Corrosion involving larynx and trachea with lung

T27.6 Corrosion of other parts of respiratory tract

T27.7 Corrosion of respiratory tract, part unspecified

T28 Burn and corrosion of other internal organs
Use additional external cause code to identify the source and intent of the burn (X00- X19, X75-X77, X96-X98)
Use additional external cause code to identify place (Y92)

The appropriate 7th character is to be added to each code from category T28.
A initial encounter
D subsequent encounter
S sequela

T28.0 Burn of mouth and pharynx

T28.1 Burn of esophagus

T28.2 Burn of other parts of alimentary tract

T28.3 Burn of internal genitourinary organs

T28.4 Burns of other and unspecified internal organs

T28.40 Burn of unspecified internal organ

T28.41 Burn of ear drum

T28.411 Burn of right ear drum

T28.412 Burn of left ear drum

T28.419 Burn of unspecified ear drum

T28.49 Burn of other internal organ
Code first (T51-T65) to identify chemical and intent for T28.5-T28.9-

T28.5 Corrosion of mouth and pharynx

T28.6 Corrosion of esophagus

T28.7 Corrosion of other parts of alimentary tract

T28.8 Corrosion of internal genitourinary organs

T28.9 Corrosions of other and unspecified internal organs

T28.90 Corrosions of unspecified internal organs

T28.91 Corrosions of ear drum

T28.911 Corrosions of right ear drum

T28.912 Corrosions of left ear drum

T28.919 Corrosions of unspecified ear drum

T28.99 Corrosions of other internal organs

Burns and corrosions of multiple and unspecified body regions (T30-T32)

T30 Burn and corrosion, body region unspecified

T30.0 Burn of unspecified body region, unspecified degree
NOTE This code is not for inpatient use. Code to specified site and degree of burns
Burn NOS
Multiple burns NOS

T30.4 Corrosion of unspecified body region, unspecified degree
NOTE This code is not for inpatient use. Code to specified site and degree of corrosion
Corrosion NOS
Multiple corrosion NOS

T31 Burns classified according to extent of body surface involved
NOTE This category is to be used as the primary code only when the site of the burn is unspecified. It should be used as a supplementary code with categories T20-T25 when the site is specified.

T31.0 Burns involving less than 10% of body surface

T31.1 Burns involving 10-19% of body surface

T31.10 Burns involving 10-19% of body surface with 0% to 9% third degree burns
Burns involving 10-19% of body surface NOS

T31.11 Burns involving 10-19% of body surface with 10-19% third degree burns

T31.2 Burns involving 20-29% of body surface

T31.20 Burns involving 20-29% of body surface with 0% to 9% third degree burns
Burns involving 20-29% of body surface NOS

T31.21 Burns involving 20-29% of body surface with 10-19% third degree burns

T31.22 Burns involving 20-29% of body surface with 20-29% third degree burns

T31.3 Burns involving 30-39% of body surface

T31.30 Burns involving 30-39% of body surface with 0% to 9% third degree burns
Burns involving 30-39% of body surface NOS

T31.31 Burns involving 30-39% of body surface with 10-19% third degree burns

T31.32 Burns involving 30-39% of body surface with 20-29% third degree burns

T31.33 Burns involving 30-39% of body surface with 30-39% third degree burns

T31.4 Burns involving 40-49% of body surface

T31.40 Burns involving 40-49% of body surface with 0% to 9% third degree burns
Burns involving 40-49% of body surface NOS

T31.41 Burns involving 40-49% of body surface with 10-19% third degree burns

T31.42 Burns involving 40-49% of body surface with 20-29% third degree burns

T31.43 Burns involving 40-49% of body surface with 30-39% third degree burns

T31.44 Burns involving 40-49% of body surface with 40-49% third degree burns

✓5th **T31.5 Burns involving 50-59% of body surface**
- **T31.50 Burns involving 50-59% of body surface with 0% to 9% third degree burns**
  Burns involving 50-59% of body surface NOS
- **T31.51 Burns involving 50-59% of body surface with 10-19% third degree burns**
- **T31.52 Burns involving 50-59% of body surface with 20-29% third degree burns**
- **T31.53 Burns involving 50-59% of body surface with 30-39% third degree burns**
- **T31.54 Burns involving 50-59% of body surface with 40-49% third degree burns**
- **T31.55 Burns involving 50-59% of body surface with 50-59% third degree burns**

✓5th **T31.6 Burns involving 60-69% of body surface**
- **T31.60 Burns involving 60-69% of body surface with 0% to 9% third degree burns**
  Burns involving 60-69% of body surface NOS
- **T31.61 Burns involving 60-69% of body surface with 10-19% third degree burns**
- **T31.62 Burns involving 60-69% of body surface with 20-29% third degree burns**
- **T31.63 Burns involving 60-69% of body surface with 30-39% third degree burns**
- **T31.64 Burns involving 60-69% of body surface with 40-49% third degree burns**
- **T31.65 Burns involving 60-69% of body surface with 50-59% third degree burns**
- **T31.66 Burns involving 60-69% of body surface with 60-69% third degree burns**

✓5th **T31.7 Burns involving 70-79% of body surface**
- **T31.70 Burns involving 70-79% of body surface with 0% to 9% third degree burns**
  Burns involving 70-79% of body surface NOS
- **T31.71 Burns involving 70-79% of body surface with 10-19% third degree burns**
- **T31.72 Burns involving 70-79% of body surface with 20-29% third degree burns**
- **T31.73 Burns involving 70-79% of body surface with 30-39% third degree burns**
- **T31.74 Burns involving 70-79% of body surface with 40-49% third degree burns**
- **T31.75 Burns involving 70-79% of body surface with 50-59% third degree burns**
- **T31.76 Burns involving 70-79% of body surface with 60-69% third degree burns**
- **T31.77 Burns involving 70-79% of body surface with 70-79% third degree burns**

✓5th **T31.8 Burns involving 80-89% of body surface**
- **T31.80 Burns involving 80-89% of body surface with 0% to 9% third degree burns**
  Burns involving 80-89% of body surface NOS
- **T31.81 Burns involving 80-89% of body surface with 10-19% third degree burns**
- **T31.82 Burns involving 80-89% of body surface with 20-29% third degree burns**
- **T31.83 Burns involving 80-89% of body surface with 30-39% third degree burns**
- **T31.84 Burns involving 80-89% of body surface with 40-49% third degree burns**
- **T31.85 Burns involving 80-89% of body surface with 50-59% third degree burns**
- **T31.86 Burns involving 80-89% of body surface with 60-69% third degree burns**
- **T31.87 Burns involving 80-89% of body surface with 70-79% third degree burns**
- **T31.88 Burns involving 80-89% of body surface with 80-89% third degree burns**

✓5th **T31.9 Burns involving 90% or more of body surface**
- **T31.90 Burns involving 90% or more of body surface with 0% to 9% third degree burns**
  Burns involving 90% or more of body surface NOS
- **T31.91 Burns involving 90% or more of body surface with 10-19% third degree burns**
- **T31.92 Burns involving 90% or more of body surface with 20-29% third degree burns**
- **T31.93 Burns involving 90% or more of body surface with 30-39% third degree burns**
- **T31.94 Burns involving 90% or more of body surface with 40-49% third degree burns**
- **T31.95 Burns involving 90% or more of body surface with 50-59% third degree burns**
- **T31.96 Burns involving 90% or more of body surface with 60-69% third degree burns**
- **T31.97 Burns involving 90% or more of body surface with 70-79% third degree burns**
- **T31.98 Burns involving 90% or more of body surface with 80-89% third degree burns**
- **T31.99 Burns involving 90% or more of body surface with 90% or more third degree burns**

✓4th **T32 Corrosions classified according to extent of body surface involved**

NOTE This category is to be used as the primary code only when the site of the corrosion is unspecified. It may be used as a supplementary code with categories T20-T25 when the site is specified.

T32.0 Corrosions involving less than 10% of body surface

✓5th **T32.1 Corrosions involving 10-19% of body surface**
- **T32.10 Corrosions involving 10-19% of body surface with 0% to 9% third degree corrosion**
  Corrosions involving 10-19% of body surface NOS
- **T32.11 Corrosions involving 10-19% of body surface with 10-19% third degree corrosion**

✓5th **T32.2 Corrosions involving 20-29% of body surface**
- **T32.20 Corrosions involving 20-29% of body surface with 0% to 9% third degree corrosion**
- **T32.21 Corrosions involving 20-29% of body surface with 10-19% third degree corrosion**
- **T32.22 Corrosions involving 20-29% of body surface with 20-29% third degree corrosion**

✓5th **T32.3 Corrosions involving 30-39% of body surface**
- **T32.30 Corrosions involving 30-39% of body surface with 0% to 9% third degree corrosion**
- **T32.31 Corrosions involving 30-39% of body surface with 10-19% third degree corrosion**
- **T32.32 Corrosions involving 30-39% of body surface with 20-29% third degree corrosion**
- **T32.33 Corrosions involving 30-39% of body surface with 30-39% third degree corrosion**

✓5th **T32.4 Corrosions involving 40-49% of body surface**
- **T32.40 Corrosions involving 40-49% of body surface with 0% to 9% third degree corrosion**
- **T32.41 Corrosions involving 40-49% of body surface with 10-19% third degree corrosion**
- **T32.42 Corrosions involving 40-49% of body surface with 20-29% third degree corrosion**
- **T32.43 Corrosions involving 40-49% of body surface with 30-39% third degree corrosion**
- **T32.44 Corrosions involving 40-49% of body surface with 40-49% third degree corrosion**

✓5th **T32.5 Corrosions involving 50-59% of body surface**
- **T32.50 Corrosions involving 50-59% of body surface with 0% to 9% third degree corrosion**
- **T32.51 Corrosions involving 50-59% of body surface with 10-19% third degree corrosion**
- **T32.52 Corrosions involving 50-59% of body surface with 20-29% third degree corrosion**
- **T32.53 Corrosions involving 50-59% of body surface with 30-39% third degree corrosion**
- **T32.54 Corrosions involving 50-59% of body surface with 40-49% third degree corrosion**
- **T32.55 Corrosions involving 50-59% of body surface with 50-59% third degree corrosion**

✓5th **T32.6 Corrosions involving 60-69% of body surface**
- **T32.60 Corrosions involving 60-69% of body surface with 0% to 9% third degree corrosion**
- **T32.61 Corrosions involving 60-69% of body surface with 10-19% third degree corrosion**
- **T32.62 Corrosions involving 60-69% of body surface with 20-29% third degree corrosion**
- **T32.63 Corrosions involving 60-69% of body surface with 30-39% third degree corrosion**
- **T32.64 Corrosions involving 60-69% of body surface with 40-49% third degree corrosion**
- **T32.65 Corrosions involving 60-69% of body surface with 50-59% third degree corrosion**

T32.66 Corrosions involving 60-69% of body surface with 60-69% third degree corrosion

✓5th T32.7 Corrosions involving 70-79% of body surface

T32.70 Corrosions involving 70-79% of body surface with 0% to 9% third degree corrosion

T32.71 Corrosions involving 70-79% of body surface with 10-19% third degree corrosion

T32.72 Corrosions involving 70-79% of body surface with 20-29% third degree corrosion

T32.73 Corrosions involving 70-79% of body surface with 30-39% third degree corrosion

T32.74 Corrosions involving 70-79% of body surface with 40-49% third degree corrosion

T32.75 Corrosions involving 70-79% of body surface with 50-59% third degree corrosion

T32.76 Corrosions involving 70-79% of body surface with 60-69% third degree corrosion

T32.77 Corrosions involving 70-79% of body surface with 70-79% third degree corrosion

✓5th T32.8 Corrosions involving 80-89% of body surface

T32.80 Corrosions involving 80-89% of body surface with 0% to 9% third degree corrosion

T32.81 Corrosions involving 80-89% of body surface with 10-19% third degree corrosion

T32.82 Corrosions involving 80-89% of body surface with 20-29% third degree corrosion

T32.83 Corrosions involving 80-89% of body surface with 30-39% third degree corrosion

T32.84 Corrosions involving 80-89% of body surface with 40-49% third degree corrosion

T32.85 Corrosions involving 80-89% of body surface with 50-59% third degree corrosion

T32.86 Corrosions involving 80-89% of body surface with 60-69% third degree corrosion

T32.87 Corrosions involving 80-89% of body surface with 70-79% third degree corrosion

T32.88 Corrosions involving 80-89% of body surface with 80-89% third degree corrosion

✓5th T32.9 Corrosions involving 90% or more of body surface

T32.90 Corrosions involving 90% or more of body surface with 0% to 9% third degree corrosion

T32.91 Corrosions involving 90% or more of body surface with 10-19% third degree corrosion

T32.92 Corrosions involving 90% or more of body surface with 20-29% third degree corrosion

T32.93 Corrosions involving 90% or more of body surface with 30-39% third degree corrosion

T32.94 Corrosions involving 90% or more of body surface with 40-49% third degree corrosion

T32.95 Corrosions involving 90% or more of body surface with 50-59% third degree corrosion

T32.96 Corrosions involving 90% or more of body surface with 60-69% third degree corrosion

T32.97 Corrosions involving 90% or more of body surface with 70-79% third degree corrosion

T32.98 Corrosions involving 90% or more of body surface with 80-89% third degree corrosion

T32.99 Corrosions involving 90% or more of body surface with 90% or more third degree corrosion

Frostbite (T33-T34)

EXCLUDES 2 *hypothermia and other effects of reduced temperature (T68, T69-)*

✓4th **T33 Superficial frostbite**

INCLUDES frostbite with partial thickness skin loss

The appropriate 7th character is to be added to each code from category T33.
A initial encounter
D subsequent encounter
S sequela

✓5th T33.0 Superficial frostbite of head

✓6th T33.01 Superficial frostbite of ear

✓7th T33.011 Superficial frostbite of right ear

✓7th T33.012 Superficial frostbite of left ear

✓7th T33.019 Superficial frostbite of unspecified ear

✓x7th T33.02 Superficial frostbite of nose

✓x7th T33.09 Superficial frostbite of other part of head

✓x7th T33.1 Superficial frostbite of neck

✓x7th T33.2 Superficial frostbite of thorax

✓x7th T33.3 Superficial frostbite of abdominal wall, lower back and pelvis

✓5th T33.4 Superficial frostbite of arm

EXCLUDES 2 *superficial frostbite of wrist and hand (T33.5-)*

✓x7th T33.40 Superficial frostbite of unspecified arm

✓x7th T33.41 Superficial frostbite of right arm

✓x7th T33.42 Superficial frostbite of left arm

✓5th T33.5 Superficial frostbite of wrist, hand, and fingers

✓6th T33.51 Superficial frostbite of wrist

✓7th T33.511 Superficial frostbite of right wrist

✓7th T33.512 Superficial frostbite of left wrist

✓7th T33.519 Superficial frostbite of unspecified wrist

✓6th T33.52 Superficial frostbite of hand

EXCLUDES 2 *superficial frostbite of fingers (T33.53-)*

✓7th T33.521 Superficial frostbite of right hand

✓7th T33.522 Superficial frostbite of left hand

✓7th T33.529 Superficial frostbite of unspecified hand

✓6th T33.53 Superficial frostbite of finger(s)

✓7th T33.531 Superficial frostbite of right finger(s)

✓7th T33.532 Superficial frostbite of left finger(s)

✓7th T33.539 Superficial frostbite of unspecified finger(s)

✓5th T33.6 Superficial frostbite of hip and thigh

✓x7th T33.60 Superficial frostbite of unspecified hip and thigh

✓x7th T33.61 Superficial frostbite of right hip and thigh

✓x7th T33.62 Superficial frostbite of left hip and thigh

✓5th T33.7 Superficial frostbite of knee and lower leg

EXCLUDES 2 *superficial frostbite of ankle and foot (T33.8-)*

✓x7th T33.70 Superficial frostbite of unspecified knee and lower leg

✓x7th T33.71 Superficial frostbite of right knee and lower leg

✓x7th T33.72 Superficial frostbite of left knee and lower leg

✓5th T33.8 Superficial frostbite of ankle, foot, and toe(s)

✓6th T33.81 Superficial frostbite of ankle

✓7th T33.811 Superficial frostbite of right ankle

✓7th T33.812 Superficial frostbite of left ankle

✓7th T33.819 Superficial frostbite of unspecified ankle

✓6th T33.82 Superficial frostbite of foot

✓7th T33.821 Superficial frostbite of right foot

✓7th T33.822 Superficial frostbite of left foot

✓7th T33.829 Superficial frostbite of unspecified foot

✓6th T33.83 Superficial frostbite of toe(s)

✓7th T33.831 Superficial frostbite of right toe(s)

✓7th T33.832 Superficial frostbite of left toe(s)

✓7th T33.839 Superficial frostbite of unspecified toe(s)

✓5th T33.9 Superficial frostbite of other and unspecified sites

✓x7th T33.90 Superficial frostbite of unspecified sites
Superficial frostbite NOS

✓x7th T33.99 Superficial frostbite of other sites
Superficial frostbite of leg NOS
Superficial frostbite of trunk NOS

✓4th **T34 Frostbite with tissue necrosis**

The appropriate 7th character is to be added to each code from category T34.
A initial encounter
D subsequent encounter
S sequela

✓5th T34.0 Frostbite with tissue necrosis of head

✓6th T34.01 Frostbite with tissue necrosis of ear

✓7th T34.011 Frostbite with tissue necrosis of right ear

✓7th T34.012 Frostbite with tissue necrosis of left ear

✓7th T34.019 Frostbite with tissue necrosis of unspecified ear

✓x7th T34.02 Frostbite with tissue necrosis of nose

✓x7th T34.09 Frostbite with tissue necrosis of other part of head

✓x7th T34.1 Frostbite with tissue necrosis of neck

✓x7th T34.2 Frostbite with tissue necrosis of thorax

✓x7th T34.3 Frostbite with tissue necrosis of abdominal wall, lower back and pelvis

✓5th **T34.4 Frostbite with tissue necrosis of arm**
EXCLUDES 2 *frostbite with tissue necrosis of wrist and hand (T34.5-)*
✓x7th **T34.40 Frostbite with tissue necrosis of unspecified arm**
✓x7th **T34.41 Frostbite with tissue necrosis of right arm**
✓x7th **T34.42 Frostbite with tissue necrosis of left arm**

✓5th **T34.5 Frostbite with tissue necrosis of wrist, hand, and finger(s)**
✓6th **T34.51 Frostbite with tissue necrosis of wrist**
✓7th **T34.511 Frostbite with tissue necrosis of right wrist**
✓7th **T34.512 Frostbite with tissue necrosis of left wrist**
✓7th **T34.519 Frostbite with tissue necrosis of unspecified wrist**
✓6th **T34.52 Frostbite with tissue necrosis of hand**
EXCLUDES 2 *frostbite with tissue necrosis of finger(s) (T34.53-)*
✓7th **T34.521 Frostbite with tissue necrosis of right hand**
✓7th **T34.522 Frostbite with tissue necrosis of left hand**
✓7th **T34.529 Frostbite with tissue necrosis of unspecified hand**
✓6th **T34.53 Frostbite with tissue necrosis of finger(s)**
✓7th **T34.531 Frostbite with tissue necrosis of right finger(s)**
✓7th **T34.532 Frostbite with tissue necrosis of left finger(s)**
✓7th **T34.539 Frostbite with tissue necrosis of unspecified finger(s)**

✓5th **T34.6 Frostbite with tissue necrosis of hip and thigh**
✓x7th **T34.60 Frostbite with tissue necrosis of unspecified hip and thigh**
✓x7th **T34.61 Frostbite with tissue necrosis of right hip and thigh**
✓x7th **T34.62 Frostbite with tissue necrosis of left hip and thigh**

✓5th **T34.7 Frostbite with tissue necrosis of knee and lower leg**
EXCLUDES 2 *frostbite with tissue necrosis of ankle and foot (T34.8-)*
✓x7th **T34.70 Frostbite with tissue necrosis of unspecified knee and lower leg**
✓x7th **T34.71 Frostbite with tissue necrosis of right knee and lower leg**
✓x7th **T34.72 Frostbite with tissue necrosis of left knee and lower leg**

✓5th **T34.8 Frostbite with tissue necrosis of ankle, foot, and toe(s)**
✓6th **T34.81 Frostbite with tissue necrosis of ankle**
✓7th **T34.811 Frostbite with tissue necrosis of right ankle**
✓7th **T34.812 Frostbite with tissue necrosis of left ankle**
✓7th **T34.819 Frostbite with tissue necrosis of unspecified ankle**
✓6th **T34.82 Frostbite with tissue necrosis of foot**
✓7th **T34.821 Frostbite with tissue necrosis of right foot**
✓7th **T34.822 Frostbite with tissue necrosis of left foot**
✓7th **T34.829 Frostbite with tissue necrosis of unspecified foot**
✓6th **T34.83 Frostbite with tissue necrosis of toe(s)**
✓7th **T34.831 Frostbite with tissue necrosis of right toe(s)**
✓7th **T34.832 Frostbite with tissue necrosis of left toe(s)**
✓7th **T34.839 Frostbite with tissue necrosis of unspecified toe(s)**

✓5th **T34.9 Frostbite with tissue necrosis of other and unspecified sites**
✓x7th **T34.90 Frostbite with tissue necrosis of unspecified sites**
Frostbite with tissue necrosis NOS
✓x7th **T34.99 Frostbite with tissue necrosis of other sites**
Frostbite with tissue necrosis of leg NOS
Frostbite with tissue necrosis of trunk NOS

Poisoning by, adverse effects of and underdosing of drugs, medicaments and biological substances (T36-T50)

INCLUDES adverse effect of correct substance properly administered
poisoning by overdose of substance
poisoning by wrong substance given or taken in error
underdosing by (inadvertently) (deliberately) taking less substance than prescribed or instructed

Code first, for adverse effects, the nature of the adverse effect, such as:
adverse effect NOS (T88.7)
aspirin gastritis (K29.-)
blood disorders (D56-D76)
contact dermatitis (L23-L25)
dermatitis due to substances taken internally (L27.-)
nephropathy (N14.0-N14.2)

NOTE The drug giving rise to the adverse effect should be identified by use of codes from categories T36-T50 with fifth or sixth character 5.

Use additional code(s) to specify:
manifestations of poisoning
underdosing or failure in dosage during medical and surgical care (Y63.6, Y63.8-Y63.9)
underdosing of medication regimen (Z91.12-, Z91.13-)

EXCLUDES 1 *toxic reaction to local anesthesia in pregnancy (O29.3-)*
EXCLUDES 2 *abuse and dependence of psychoactive substances (F10-F19)*
abuse of non-dependence-producing substances (F55.-)
drug reaction and poisoning affecting newborn (P00-P96)
pathological drug intoxication (inebriation) (F10-F19)

✓4th **T36 Poisoning by, adverse effect of and underdosing of systemic antibiotics**
EXCLUDES 1 *antineoplastic antibiotics (T45.1-)*
locally applied antibiotic NEC (T49.0)
topically used antibiotic for ear, nose and throat (T49.6)
topically used antibiotic for eye (T49.5)

The appropriate 7th character is to be added to each code from category T36.
A initial encounter
D subsequent encounter
S sequela

✓5th **T36.0 Poisoning by, adverse effect of and underdosing of penicillins**
✓6th **T36.0X Poisoning by, adverse effect of and underdosing of penicillins**
✓7th **T36.0X1 Poisoning by penicillins, accidental (utentional)**
Poisoning by penicillins NOS
✓7th **T36.0X2 Poisoning by penicillins, intentional self-harm**
✓7th **T36.0X3 Poisoning by penicillins, assault**
✓7th **T36.0X4 Poisoning by penicillins, undetermined**
✓7th **T36.0X5 Adverse effect of penicillins**
✓7th **T36.0X6 Underdosing of penicillins**

✓5th **T36.1 Poisoning by, adverse effect of and underdosing of cephalosporins and other beta-lactam antibiotics**
✓6th **T36.1X Poisoning by, adverse effect of and underdosing of cephalosporins and other beta-lactam antibiotics**
✓7th **T36.1X1 Poisoning by cephalosporins and other beta-lactam antibiotics, accidental (unintentional)**
Poisoning by cephalosporins and other beta-lactam antibiotics NOS
✓7th **T36.1X2 Poisoning by cephalosporins and other beta-lactam antibiotics, intentional self-harm**
✓7th **T36.1X3 Poisoning by cephalosporins and other beta-lactam antibiotics, assault**
✓7th **T36.1X4 Poisoning by cephalosporins and other beta-lactam antibiotics, undetermined**
✓7th **T36.1X5 Adverse effect of cephalosporins and other beta-lactam antibiotics**
✓7th **T36.1X6 Underdosing of cephalosporins and other beta-lactam antibiotics**

✓5th **T36.2 Poisoning by, adverse effect of and underdosing of chloramphenicol group**

✓6th **T36.2X Poisoning by, adverse effect of and underdosing of chloramphenicol group**

✓7th **T36.2X1 Poisoning by chloramphenicol group, accidental (unintentional)**
Poisoning by chloramphenicol group NOS

✓7th **T36.2X2 Poisoning by chloramphenicol group, intentional self-harm**

✓7th **T36.2X3 Poisoning by chloramphenicol group, assault**

✓7th **T36.2X4 Poisoning by chloramphenicol group, undetermined**

✓7th **T36.2X5 Adverse effect of chloramphenicol group**

✓7th **T36.2X6 Underdosing of chloramphenicol group**

✓5th **T36.3 Poisoning by, adverse effect of and underdosing of macrolides**

✓6th **T36.3X Poisoning by, adverse effect of and underdosing of macrolides**

✓7th **T36.3X1 Poisoning by macrolides, accidental (unintentional)**
Poisoning by macrolides NOS

✓7th **T36.3X2 Poisoning by macrolides, intentional self-harm**

✓7th **T36.3X3 Poisoning by macrolides, assault**

✓7th **T36.3X4 Poisoning by macrolides, undetermined**

✓7th **T36.3X5 Adverse effect of macrolides**

✓7th **T36.3X6 Underdosing of macrolides**

✓5th **T36.4 Poisoning by, adverse effect of and underdosing of tetracyclines**

✓6th **T36.4X Poisoning by, adverse effect of and underdosing of tetracyclines**

✓7th **T36.4X1 Poisoning by tetracyclines, accidental (unintentional)**
Poisoning by tetracyclines NOS

✓7th **T36.4X2 Poisoning by tetracyclines, intentional self-harm**

✓7th **T36.4X3 Poisoning by tetracyclines, assault**

✓7th **T36.4X4 Poisoning by tetracyclines, undetermined**

✓7th **T36.4X5 Adverse effect of tetracyclines**

✓7th **T36.4X6 Underdosing of tetracyclines**

✓5th **T36.5 Poisoning by, adverse effect of and underdosing of aminoglycosides**
Poisoning by, adverse effect of and underdosing of streptomycin

✓6th **T36.5X Poisoning by, adverse effect of and underdosing of aminoglycosides**

✓7th **T36.5X1 Poisoning by aminoglycosides, accidental (unintentional)**
Poisoning by aminoglycosides NOS

✓7th **T36.5X2 Poisoning by aminoglycosides, intentional self-harm**

✓7th **T36.5X3 Poisoning by aminoglycosides, assault**

✓7th **T36.5X4 Poisoning by aminoglycosides, undetermined**

✓7th **T36.5X5 Adverse effect of aminoglycosides**

✓7th **T36.5X6 Underdosing of aminoglycosides**

✓5th **T36.6 Poisoning by, adverse effect of and underdosing of rifampicins**

✓6th **T36.6X Poisoning by, adverse effect of and underdosing of rifampicins**

✓7th **T36.6X1 Poisoning by rifampicins, accidental (unintentional)**
Poisoning by rifampicins NOS

✓7th **T36.6X2 Poisoning by rifampicins, intentional self-harm**

✓7th **T36.6X3 Poisoning by rifampicins, assault**

✓7th **T36.6X4 Poisoning by rifampicins, undetermined**

✓7th **T36.6X5 Adverse effect of rifampicins**

✓7th **T36.6X6 Underdosing of rifampicins**

✓5th **T36.7 Poisoning by, adverse effect of and underdosing of antifungal antibiotics, systemically used**

✓6th **T36.7X Poisoning by, adverse effect of and underdosing of antifungal antibiotics, systemically used**

✓7th **T36.7X1 Poisoning by antifungal antibiotics, systemically used, accidental (unintentional)**
Poisoning by antifungal antibiotics, systemically used NOS

✓7th **T36.7X2 Poisoning by antifungal antibiotics, systemically used, intentional self-harm**

✓7th **T36.7X3 Poisoning by antifungal antibiotics, systemically used, assault**

✓7th **T36.7X4 Poisoning by antifungal antibiotics, systemically used, undetermined**

✓7th **T36.7X5 Adverse effect of antifungal antibiotics, systemically used**

✓7th **T36.7X6 Underdosing of antifungal antibiotics, systemically used**

✓5th **T36.8 Poisoning by, adverse effect of and underdosing of other systemic antibiotics**

✓6th **T36.8X Poisoning by, adverse effect of and underdosing of other systemic antibiotics**

✓7th **T36.8X1 Poisoning by other systemic antibiotics, accidental (unintentional)**
Poisoning by other systemic antibiotics NOS

✓7th **T36.8X2 Poisoning by other systemic antibiotics, intentional self-harm**

✓7th **T36.8X3 Poisoning by other systemic antibiotics, assault**

✓7th **T36.8X4 Poisoning by other systemic antibiotics, undetermined**

✓7th **T36.8X5 Adverse effect of other systemic antibiotics**

✓7th **T36.8X6 Underdosing of other systemic antibiotics**

✓5th **T36.9 Poisoning by, adverse effect of and underdosing of unspecified systemic antibiotic**

✓x7th **T36.91 Poisoning by unspecified systemic antibiotic, accidental (unintentional)**
Poisoning by systemic antibiotic NOS

✓x7th **T36.92 Poisoning by unspecified systemic antibiotic, intentional self-harm**

✓x7th **T36.93 Poisoning by unspecified systemic antibiotic, assault**

✓x7th **T36.94 Poisoning by unspecified systemic antibiotic, undetermined**

✓x7th **T36.95 Adverse effect of unspecified systemic antibiotic**

✓x7th **T36.96 Underdosing of unspecified systemic antibiotic**

✓4th **T37 Poisoning by, adverse effect of and underdosing of other systemic anti- infectives and antiparasitics**

EXCLUDES 1 *anti-infectives topically used for ear, nose and throat (T49.6-)*
anti-infectives topically used for eye (T49.5-)
locally applied anti-infectives NEC (T49.0-)

The appropriate 7th character is to be added to each code from category T37.
A initial encounter
D subsequent encounter
S sequela

✓5th **T37.0 Poisoning by, adverse effect of and underdosing of sulfonamides**

✓6th **T37.0X Poisoning by, adverse effect of and underdosing of sulfonamides**

✓7th **T37.0X1 Poisoning by sulfonamides, accidental (unintentional)**
Poisoning by sulfonamides NOS

✓7th **T37.0X2 Poisoning by sulfonamides, intentional self-harm**

✓7th **T37.0X3 Poisoning by sulfonamides, assault**

✓7th **T37.0X4 Poisoning by sulfonamides, undetermined**

✓7th **T37.0X5 Adverse effect of sulfonamides**

✓7th **T37.0X6 Underdosing of sulfonamides**

✓5th **T37.1 Poisoning by, adverse effect of and underdosing of antimycobacterial drugs**

EXCLUDES 1 *rifampicins (T36.6-)*
streptomycin (T36.5-)

✓6th **T37.1X Poisoning by, adverse effect of and underdosing of antimycobacterial drugs**

√7th **T37.1X1 Poisoning by antimycobacterial drugs, accidental (unintentional)**
Poisoning by antimycobacterial drugs NOS

√7th **T37.1X2 Poisoning by antimycobacterial drugs, intentional self-harm**

√7th **T37.1X3 Poisoning by antimycobacterial drugs, assault**

√7th **T37.1X4 Poisoning by antimycobacterial drugs, undetermined**

√7th **T37.1X5 Adverse effect of antimycobacterial drugs**

√7th **T37.1X6 Underdosing of antimycobacterial drugs**

√5th **T37.2 Poisoning by, adverse effect of and underdosing of antimalarials and drugs acting on other blood protozoa**
EXCLUDES 1 *hydroxyquinoline derivatives (T37.8-)*

√6th **T37.2X Poisoning by, adverse effect of and underdosing of antimalarials and drugs acting on other blood protozoa**

√7th **T37.2X1 Poisoning by antimalarials and drugs acting on other blood protozoa, accidental (unintentional)**
Poisoning by antimalarials and drugs acting on other blood protozoa NOS

√7th **T37.2X2 Poisoning by antimalarials and drugs acting on other blood protozoa, intentional self-harm**

√7th **T37.2X3 Poisoning by antimalarials and drugs acting on other blood protozoa, assault**

√7th **T37.2X4 Poisoning by antimalarials and drugs acting on other blood protozoa, undetermined**

√7th **T37.2X5 Adverse effect of antimalarials and drugs acting on other blood protozoa**

√7th **T37.2X6 Underdosing of antimalarials and drugs acting on other blood protozoa**

√5th **T37.3 Poisoning by, adverse effect of and underdosing of other antiprotozoal drugs**

√6th **T37.3X Poisoning by, adverse effect of and underdosing of other antiprotozoal drugs**

√7th **T37.3X1 Poisoning by other antiprotozoal drugs, accidental (unintentional)**
Poisoning by other antiprotozoal drugs NOS

√7th **T37.3X2 Poisoning by other antiprotozoal drugs, intentional self-harm**

√7th **T37.3X3 Poisoning by other antiprotozoal drugs, assault**

√7th **T37.3X4 Poisoning by other antiprotozoal drugs, undetermined**

√7th **T37.3X5 Adverse effect of other antiprotozoal drugs**

√7th **T37.3X6 Underdosing of other antiprotozoal drugs**

√5th **T37.4 Poisoning by, adverse effect of and underdosing of anthelminthics**

√6th **T37.4X Poisoning by, adverse effect of and underdosing of anthelminthics**

√7th **T37.4X1 Poisoning by anthelminthics, accidental (unintentional)**
Poisoning by anthelminthics NOS

√7th **T37.4X2 Poisoning by anthelminthics, intentional self-harm**

√7th **T37.4X3 Poisoning by anthelminthics, assault**

√7th **T37.4X4 Poisoning by anthelminthics, undetermined**

√7th **T37.4X5 Adverse effect of anthelminthics**

√7th **T37.4X6 Underdosing of anthelminthics**

√5th **T37.5 Poisoning by, adverse effect of and underdosing of antiviral drugs**
EXCLUDES 1 *amantadine (T42.8-)*
cytarabine (T45.1-)

√6th **T37.5X Poisoning by, adverse effect of and underdosing of antiviral drugs**

√7th **T37.5X1 Poisoning by antiviral drugs, accidental (unintentional)**
Poisoning by antiviral drugs NOS

√7th **T37.5X2 Poisoning by antiviral drugs, intentional self-harm**

√7th **T37.5X3 Poisoning by antiviral drugs, assault**

√7th **T37.5X4 Poisoning by antiviral drugs, undetermined**

√7th **T37.5X5 Adverse effect of antiviral drugs**

√7th **T37.5X6 Underdosing of antiviral drugs**

√5th **T37.8 Poisoning by, adverse effect of and underdosing of other specified systemic anti-infectives and antiparasitics**
Poisoning by, adverse effect of and underdosing of hydroxyquinoline derivatives
EXCLUDES 1 *antimalarial drugs (T37.2-)*

√6th **T37.8X Poisoning by, adverse effect of and underdosing of other specified systemic anti-infectives and antiparasitics**

√7th **T37.8X1 Poisoning by other specified systemic anti-infectives and antiparasitics, accidental (unintentional)**
Poisoning by other specified systemic anti-infectives and antiparasitics NOS

√7th **T37.8X2 Poisoning by other specified systemic anti-infectives and antiparasitics, intentional self-harm**

√7th **T37.8X3 Poisoning by other specified systemic anti-infectives and antiparasitics, assault**

√7th **T37.8X4 Poisoning by other specified systemic anti-infectives and antiparasitics, undetermined**

√7th **T37.8X5 Adverse effect of other specified systemic anti-infectives and antiparasitics**

√7th **T37.8X6 Underdosing of other specified systemic anti-infectives and antiparasitics**

√5th **T37.9 Poisoning by, adverse effect of and underdosing of unspecified systemic anti-infective and antiparasitics**

√x7th **T37.91 Poisoning by unspecified systemic anti-infective and antiparasitics, accidental (unintentional)**
Poisoning by, adverse effect of and underdosing of systemic anti-infective and antiparasitics NOS

√x7th **T37.92 Poisoning by unspecified systemic anti-infective and antiparasitics, intentional self-harm**

√x7th **T37.93 Poisoning by unspecified systemic anti-infective and antiparasitics, assault**

√x7th **T37.94 Poisoning by unspecified systemic anti-infective and antiparasitics, undetermined**

√x7th **T37.95 Adverse effect of unspecified systemic anti-infective and antiparasitic**

√x7th **T37.96 Underdosing of unspecified systemic anti-infectives and antiparasitics**

√4th **T38 Poisoning by, adverse effect of and underdosing of hormones and their synthetic substitutes and antagonists, not elsewhere classified**
EXCLUDES 1 *mineralocorticoids and their antagonists (T5Ø.Ø-)*
oxytocic hormones (T48.Ø-)
parathyroid hormones and derivatives (T5Ø.9-)

The appropriate 7th character is to be added to each code from category T38.
A initial encounter
D subsequent encounter
S sequela

√5th **T38.Ø Poisoning by, adverse effect of and underdosing of glucocorticoids and synthetic analogues**
EXCLUDES 1 *glucocorticoids, topically used (T49.-)*

√6th **T38.ØX Poisoning by, adverse effect of and underdosing of glucocorticoids and synthetic analogues**

√7th **T38.ØX1 Poisoning by glucocorticoids and synthetic analogues, accidental (unintentional)**
Poisoning by glucocorticoids and synthetic analogues NOS

√7th **T38.ØX2 Poisoning by glucocorticoids and synthetic analogues, intentional self-harm**

√7th **T38.ØX3 Poisoning by glucocorticoids and synthetic analogues, assault**

T38.0X4 Poisoning by glucocorticoids and synthetic analogues, undetermined

T38.0X5 Adverse effect of glucocorticoids and synthetic analogues

T38.0X6 Underdosing of glucocorticoids and synthetic analogues

T38.1 Poisoning by, adverse effect of and underdosing of thyroid hormones and substitutes

T38.1X Poisoning by, adverse effect of and underdosing of thyroid hormones and substitutes

T38.1X1 Poisoning by thyroid hormones and substitutes, accidental (unintentional)
Poisoning by thyroid hormones and substitutes NOS

T38.1X2 Poisoning by thyroid hormones and substitutes, intentional self-harm

T38.1X3 Poisoning by thyroid hormones and substitutes, assault

T38.1X4 Poisoning by thyroid hormones and substitutes, undetermined

T38.1X5 Adverse effect of thyroid hormones and substitutes

T38.1X6 Underdosing of thyroid hormones and substitutes

T38.2 Poisoning by, adverse effect of and underdosing of antithyroid drugs

T38.2X Poisoning by, adverse effect of and underdosing of antithyroid drugs

T38.2X1 Poisoning by antithyroid drugs, accidental (unintentional)
Poisoning by antithyroid drugs NOS

T38.2X2 Poisoning by antithyroid drugs, intentional self-harm

T38.2X3 Poisoning by antithyroid drugs, assault

T38.2X4 Poisoning by antithyroid drugs, undetermined

T38.2X5 Adverse effect of antithyroid drugs

T38.2X6 Underdosing of antithyroid drugs

T38.3 Poisoning by, adverse effect of and underdosing of insulin and oral hypoglycemic [antidiabetic] drugs

T38.3X Poisoning by, adverse effect of and underdosing of insulin and oral hypoglycemic [antidiabetic] drugs

T38.3X1 Poisoning by insulin and oral hypoglycemic [antidiabetic] drugs, accidental (unintentional)
Poisoning by insulin and oral hypoglycemic [antidiabetic] drugs NOS

T38.3X2 Poisoning by insulin and oral hypoglycemic [antidiabetic] drugs, intentional self-harm

T38.3X3 Poisoning by insulin and oral hypoglycemic [antidiabetic] drugs, assault

T38.3X4 Poisoning by insulin and oral hypoglycemic [antidiabetic] drugs, undetermined

T38.3X5 Adverse effect of insulin and oral hypoglycemic [antidiabetic] drugs

T38.3X6 Underdosing of insulin and oral hypoglycemic [antidiabetic] drugs

T38.4 Poisoning by, adverse effect of and underdosing of oral contraceptives
Poisoning by, adverse effect of and underdosing of multiple- and single-ingredient oral contraceptive preparations

T38.4X Poisoning by, adverse effect of and underdosing of oral contraceptives

T38.4X1 Poisoning by oral contraceptives, accidental (unintentional)
Poisoning by oral contraceptives NOS

T38.4X2 Poisoning by oral contraceptives, intentional self-harm

T38.4X3 Poisoning by oral contraceptives, assault

T38.4X4 Poisoning by oral contraceptives, undetermined

T38.4X5 Adverse effect of oral contraceptives

T38.4X6 Underdosing of oral contraceptives

T38.5 Poisoning by, adverse effect of and underdosing of other estrogens and progestogens
Poisoning by, adverse effect of and underdosing of estrogens and progestogens mixtures and substitutes

T38.5X Poisoning by, adverse effect of and underdosing of other estrogens and progestogens

T38.5X1 Poisoning by other estrogens and progestogens, accidental (unintentional)
Poisoning by other estrogens and progestogens NOS

T38.5X2 Poisoning by other estrogens and progestogens, intentional self-harm

T38.5X3 Poisoning by other estrogens and progestogens, assault

T38.5X4 Poisoning by other estrogens and progestogens, undetermined

T38.5X5 Adverse effect of other estrogens and progestogens

T38.5X6 Underdosing of other estrogens and progestogens

T38.6 Poisoning by, adverse effect of and underdosing of antigonadotrophins, antiestrogens, antiandrogens, not elsewhere classified
Poisoning by, adverse effect of and underdosing of tamoxifen

T38.6X Poisoning by, adverse effect of and underdosing of antigonadotrophins, antiestrogens, antiandrogens, not elsewhere classified

T38.6X1 Poisoning by antigonadotrophins, antiestrogens, antiandrogens, not elsewhere classified, accidental (unintentional)
Poisoning by antigonadotrophins, antiestrogens, antiandrogens, not elsewhere classified NOS

T38.6X2 Poisoning by antigonadotrophins, antiestrogens, antiandrogens, not elsewhere classified, intentional self-harm

T38.6X3 Poisoning by antigonadotrophins, antiestrogens, antiandrogens, not elsewhere classified, assault

T38.6X4 Poisoning by antigonadotrophins, antiestrogens, antiandrogens, not elsewhere classified, undetermined

T38.6X5 Adverse effect of antigonadotrophins, antiestrogens, antiandrogens, not elsewhere classified

T38.6X6 Underdosing of antigonadotrophins, antiestrogens, antiandrogens, not elsewhere classified

T38.7 Poisoning by, adverse effect of and underdosing of androgens and anabolic congeners

T38.7X Poisoning by, adverse effect of and underdosing of androgens and anabolic congeners

T38.7X1 Poisoning by androgens and anabolic congeners, accidental (unintentional)
Poisoning by androgens and anabolic congeners NOS

T38.7X2 Poisoning by androgens and anabolic congeners, intentional self-harm

T38.7X3 Poisoning by androgens and anabolic congeners, assault

T38.7X4 Poisoning by androgens and anabolic congeners, undetermined

T38.7X5 Adverse effect of androgens and anabolic congeners

T38.7X6 Underdosing of androgens and anabolic congeners

T38.8 Poisoning by, adverse effect of and underdosing of other and unspecified hormones and synthetic substitutes

T38.80 Poisoning by, adverse effect of and underdosing of unspecified hormones and synthetic substitutes

T38.801 Poisoning by unspecified hormones and synthetic substitutes, accidental (unintentional)
Poisoning by unspecified hormones and synthetic substitutes NOS

✓7th T38.802 **Poisoning by unspecified hormones and synthetic substitutes, intentional self-harm**

✓7th T38.803 **Poisoning by unspecified hormones and synthetic substitutes, assault**

✓7th T38.804 **Poisoning by unspecified hormones and synthetic substitutes, undetermined**

✓7th T38.805 **Adverse effect of unspecified hormones and synthetic substitutes**

✓7th T38.806 **Underdosing of unspecified hormones and synthetic substitutes**

✓6th T38.81 **Poisoning by, adverse effect of and underdosing of anterior pituitary [adenohypophyseal] hormones**

✓7th T38.811 **Poisoning by anterior pituitary [adenohypophyseal] hormones, accidental (unintentional)**

Poisoning by anterior pituitary [adenohypophyseal] hormones NOS

✓7th T38.812 **Poisoning by anterior pituitary [adenohypophyseal] hormones, intentional self-harm**

✓7th T38.813 **Poisoning by anterior pituitary [adenohypophyseal] hormones, assault**

✓7th T38.814 **Poisoning by anterior pituitary [adenohypophyseal] hormones, undetermined**

✓7th T38.815 **Adverse effect of anterior pituitary [adenohypophyseal] hormones**

✓7th T38.816 **Underdosing of anterior pituitary [adenohypophyseal] hormones**

✓6th T38.89 **Poisoning by, adverse effect of and underdosing of other hormones and synthetic substitutes**

✓7th T38.891 **Poisoning by other hormones and synthetic substitutes, accidental (unintentional)**

Poisoning by other hormones and synthetic substitutes NOS

✓7th T38.892 **Poisoning by other hormones and synthetic substitutes, intentional self-harm**

✓7th T38.893 **Poisoning by other hormones and synthetic substitutes, assault**

✓7th T38.894 **Poisoning by other hormones and synthetic substitutes, undetermined**

✓7th T38.895 **Adverse effect of other hormones and synthetic substitutes**

✓7th T38.896 **Underdosing of other hormones and synthetic substitutes**

✓5th T38.9 **Poisoning by, adverse effect of and underdosing of other and unspecified hormone antagonists**

✓6th T38.90 **Poisoning by, adverse effect of and underdosing of unspecified hormone antagonists**

✓7th T38.901 **Poisoning by unspecified hormone antagonists, accidental (unintentional)**

Poisoning by unspecified hormone antagonists NOS

✓7th T38.902 **Poisoning by unspecified hormone antagonists, intentional self-harm**

✓7th T38.903 **Poisoning by unspecified hormone antagonists, assault**

✓7th T38.904 **Poisoning by unspecified hormone antagonists, undetermined**

✓7th T38.905 **Adverse effect of unspecified hormone antagonists**

✓7th T38.906 **Underdosing of unspecified hormone antagonists**

✓6th T38.99 **Poisoning by, adverse effect of and underdosing of other hormone antagonists**

✓7th T38.991 **Poisoning by other hormone antagonists, accidental (unintentional)**

Poisoning by other hormone antagonists NOS

✓7th T38.992 **Poisoning by other hormone antagonists, intentional self-harm**

✓7th T38.993 **Poisoning by other hormone antagonists, assault**

✓7th T38.994 **Poisoning by other hormone antagonists, undetermined**

✓7th T38.995 **Adverse effect of other hormone antagonists**

✓7th T38.996 **Underdosing of other hormone antagonists**

✓4th **T39 Poisoning by, adverse effect of and underdosing of nonopioid analgesics, antipyretics and antirheumatics**

The appropriate 7th character is to be added to each code from category T39.
A initial encounter
D subsequent encounter
S sequela

✓5th T39.0 **Poisoning by, adverse effect of and underdosing of salicylates**

✓6th T39.01 **Poisoning by, adverse effect of and underdosing of aspirin**

Poisoning by, adverse effect of and underdosing of acetylsalicylic acid

✓7th T39.011 **Poisoning by aspirin, accidental (unintentional)**

✓7th T39.012 **Poisoning by aspirin, intentional self-harm**

✓7th T39.013 **Poisoning by aspirin, assault**

✓7th T39.014 **Poisoning by aspirin, undetermined**

✓7th T39.015 **Adverse effect of aspirin**

✓7th T39.016 **Underdosing of aspirin**

✓6th T39.09 **Poisoning by, adverse effect of and underdosing of other salicylates**

✓7th T39.091 **Poisoning by salicylates, accidental (unintentional)**

Poisoning by salicylates NOS

✓7th T39.092 **Poisoning by salicylates, intentional self-harm**

✓7th T39.093 **Poisoning by salicylates, assault**

✓7th T39.094 **Poisoning by salicylates, undetermined**

✓7th T39.095 **Adverse effect of salicylates**

✓7th T39.096 **Underdosing of salicylates**

✓5th T39.1 **Poisoning by, adverse effect of and underdosing of 4-Aminophenol derivatives**

✓6th T39.1X **Poisoning by, adverse effect of and underdosing of 4-Aminophenol derivatives**

✓7th T39.1X1 **Poisoning by 4-Aminophenol derivatives, accidental (unintentional)**

Poisoning by 4-Aminophenol derivatives NOS

✓7th T39.1X2 **Poisoning by 4-Aminophenol derivatives, intentional self-harm**

✓7th T39.1X3 **Poisoning by 4-Aminophenol derivatives, assault**

✓7th T39.1X4 **Poisoning by 4-Aminophenol derivatives, undetermined**

✓7th T39.1X5 **Adverse effect of 4-Aminophenol derivatives**

✓7th T39.1X6 **Underdosing of 4-Aminophenol derivatives**

✓5th T39.2 **Poisoning by, adverse effect of and underdosing of pyrazolone derivatives**

✓6th T39.2X **Poisoning by, adverse effect of and underdosing of pyrazolone derivatives**

✓7th T39.2X1 **Poisoning by pyrazolone derivatives, accidental (unintentional)**

Poisoning by pyrazolone derivatives NOS

✓7th T39.2X2 **Poisoning by pyrazolone derivatives, intentional self-harm**

✓7th T39.2X3 **Poisoning by pyrazolone derivatives, assault**

✓7th T39.2X4 **Poisoning by pyrazolone derivatives, undetermined**

✓7th T39.2X5 **Adverse effect of pyrazolone derivatives**

✓7th T39.2X6 **Underdosing of pyrazolone derivatives**

√5th **T39.3 Poisoning by, adverse effect of and underdosing of other nonsteroidal anti-inflammatory drugs [NSAID]**

√6th **T39.31 Poisoning by, adverse effect of and underdosing of propionic acid derivatives**

Poisoning by, adverse effect of and underdosing of fenoprofen

Poisoning by, adverse effect of and underdosing of flurbiprofen

Poisoning by, adverse effect of and underdosing of ibuprofen

Poisoning by, adverse effect of and underdosing of ketoprofen

Poisoning by, adverse effect of and underdosing of naproxen

Poisoning by, adverse effect of and underdosing of oxaprozin

√7th **T39.311 Poisoning by propionic acid derivatives, accidental (unintentional)**

√7th **T39.312 Poisoning by propionic acid derivatives, intentional self-harm**

√7th **T39.313 Poisoning by propionic acid derivatives, assault**

√7th **T39.314 Poisoning by propionic acid derivatives, undetermined**

√7th **T39.315 Adverse effect of propionic acid derivatives**

√7th **T39.316 Underdosing of propionic acid derivatives**

√6th **T39.39 Poisoning by, adverse effect of and underdosing of other nonsteroidal anti-inflammatory drugs [NSAID]**

√7th **T39.391 Poisoning by other nonsteroidal anti-inflammatory drugs [NSAID], accidental (unintentional)**

Poisoning by other nonsteroidal anti-inflammatory drugs NOS

√7th **T39.392 Poisoning by other nonsteroidal anti-inflammatory drugs [NSAID], intentional self-harm**

√7th **T39.393 Poisoning by other nonsteroidal anti-inflammatory drugs [NSAID], assault**

√7th **T39.394 Poisoning by other nonsteroidal anti-inflammatory drugs [NSAID], undetermined**

√7th **T39.395 Adverse effect of other nonsteroidal anti-inflammatory drugs [NSAID]**

√7th **T39.396 Underdosing of other nonsteroidal anti-inflammatory drugs [NSAID]**

√5th **T39.4 Poisoning by, adverse effect of and underdosing of antirheumatics, not elsewhere classified**

EXCLUDES 1 *poisoning by, adverse effect of and underdosing of glucocorticoids (T38.0-)*

poisoning by, adverse effect of and underdosing of salicylates (T39.0-)

√6th **T39.4X Poisoning by, adverse effect of and underdosing of antirheumatics, not elsewhere classified**

√7th **T39.4X1 Poisoning by antirheumatics, not elsewhere classified, accidental (unintentional)**

Poisoning by antirheumatics, not elsewhere classified NOS

√7th **T39.4X2 Poisoning by antirheumatics, not elsewhere classified, intentional self-harm**

√7th **T39.4X3 Poisoning by antirheumatics, not elsewhere classified, assault**

√7th **T39.4X4 Poisoning by antirheumatics, not elsewhere classified, undetermined**

√7th **T39.4X5 Adverse effect of antirheumatics, not elsewhere classified**

√7th **T39.4X6 Underdosing of antirheumatics, not elsewhere classified**

√5th **T39.8 Poisoning by, adverse effect of and underdosing of other nonopioid analgesics and antipyretics, not elsewhere classified**

√6th **T39.8X Poisoning by, adverse effect of and underdosing of other nonopioid analgesics and antipyretics, not elsewhere classified**

√7th **T39.8X1 Poisoning by other nonopioid analgesics and antipyretics, not elsewhere classified, accidental (unintentional)**

Poisoning by other nonopioid analgesics and antipyretics, not elsewhere classified NOS

√7th **T39.8X2 Poisoning by other nonopioid analgesics and antipyretics, not elsewhere classified, intentional self-harm**

√7th **T39.8X3 Poisoning by other nonopioid analgesics and antipyretics, not elsewhere classified, assault**

√7th **T39.8X4 Poisoning by other nonopioid analgesics and antipyretics, not elsewhere classified, undetermined**

√7th **T39.8X5 Adverse effect of other nonopioid analgesics and antipyretics, not elsewhere classified**

√7th **T39.8X6 Underdosing of other nonopioid analgesics and antipyretics, not elsewhere classified**

√5th **T39.9 Poisoning by, adverse effect of and underdosing of unspecified nonopioid analgesic, antipyretic and antirheumatic**

√x7th **T39.91 Poisoning by unspecified nonopioid analgesic, antipyretic and antirheumatic, accidental (unintentional)**

Poisoning by nonopioid analgesic, antipyretic and antirheumatic NOS

√x7th **T39.92 Poisoning by unspecified nonopioid analgesic, antipyretic and antirheumatic, intentional self-harm**

√x7th **T39.93 Poisoning by unspecified nonopioid analgesic, antipyretic and antirheumatic, assault**

√x7th **T39.94 Poisoning by unspecified nonopioid analgesic, antipyretic and antirheumatic, undetermined**

√x7th **T39.95 Adverse effect of unspecified nonopioid analgesic, antipyretic and antirheumatic**

√x7th **T39.96 Underdosing of unspecified nonopioid analgesic, antipyretic and antirheumatic**

√4th **T40 Poisoning by, adverse effect of and underdosing of narcotics and psychodysleptics [hallucinogens]**

EXCLUDES 2 *drug dependence and related mental and behavioral disorders due to psychoactive substance use (F10-F19-)*

The appropriate 7th character is to be added to each code from category T40.
A initial encounter
D subsequent encounter
S sequela

√5th **T40.0 Poisoning by, adverse effect of and underdosing of opium**

√6th **T40.0X Poisoning by, adverse effect of and underdosing of opium**

√7th **T40.0X1 Poisoning by opium, accidental (unintentional)**

Poisoning by opium NOS

√7th **T40.0X2 Poisoning by opium, intentional self-harm**

√7th **T40.0X3 Poisoning by opium, assault**

√7th **T40.0X4 Poisoning by opium, undetermined**

√7th **T40.0X5 Adverse effect of opium**

√7th **T40.0X6 Underdosing of opium**

√5th **T40.1 Poisoning by and adverse effect of heroin**

√6th **T40.1X Poisoning by and adverse effect of heroin**

√7th **T40.1X1 Poisoning by heroin, accidental (unintentional)**

Poisoning by heroin NOS

√7th **T40.1X2 Poisoning by heroin, intentional self-harm**

√7th **T40.1X3 Poisoning by heroin, assault**

7th **T40.1X4 Poisoning by heroin, undetermined**
7th **T40.1X5 Adverse effect of heroin**

5th **T40.2 Poisoning by, adverse effect of and underdosing of other opioids**
6th **T40.2X Poisoning by, adverse effect of and underdosing of other opioids**
7th **T40.2X1 Poisoning by other opioids, accidental (unintentional)**
Poisoning by other opioids NOS
7th **T40.2X2 Poisoning by other opioids, intentional self-harm**
7th **T40.2X3 Poisoning by other opioids, assault**
7th **T40.2X4 Poisoning by other opioids, undetermined**
7th **T40.2X5 Adverse effect of other opioids**
7th **T40.2X6 Underdosing of other opioids**

5th **T40.3 Poisoning by, adverse effect of and underdosing of methadone**
6th **T40.3X Poisoning by, adverse effect of and underdosing of methadone**
7th **T40.3X1 Poisoning by methadone, accidental (unintentional)**
Poisoning by methadone NOS
7th **T40.3X2 Poisoning by methadone, intentional self-harm**
7th **T40.3X3 Poisoning by methadone, assault**
7th **T40.3X4 Poisoning by methadone, undetermined**
7th **T40.3X5 Adverse effect of methadone**
7th **T40.3X6 Underdosing of methadone**

5th **T40.4 Poisoning by, adverse effect of and underdosing of other synthetic narcotics**
6th **T40.4X Poisoning by, adverse effect of and underdosing of other synthetic narcotics**
7th **T40.4X1 Poisoning by other synthetic narcotics, accidental (unintentional)**
Poisoning by other synthetic narcotics NOS
7th **T40.4X2 Poisoning by other synthetic narcotics, intentional self-harm**
7th **T40.4X3 Poisoning by other synthetic narcotics, assault**
7th **T40.4X4 Poisoning by other synthetic narcotics, undetermined**
7th **T40.4X5 Adverse effect of other synthetic narcotics**
7th **T40.4X6 Underdosing of other synthetic narcotics**

5th **T40.5 Poisoning by, adverse effect of and underdosing of cocaine**
6th **T40.5X Poisoning by, adverse effect of and underdosing of cocaine**
7th **T40.5X1 Poisoning by cocaine, accidental (unintentional)**
Poisoning by cocaine NOS
7th **T40.5X2 Poisoning by cocaine, intentional self-harm**
7th **T40.5X3 Poisoning by cocaine, assault**
7th **T40.5X4 Poisoning by cocaine, undetermined**
7th **T40.5X5 Adverse effect of cocaine**
7th **T40.5X6 Underdosing of cocaine**

5th **T40.6 Poisoning by, adverse effect of and underdosing of other and unspecified narcotics**
6th **T40.60 Poisoning by, adverse effect of and underdosing of unspecified narcotics**
7th **T40.601 Poisoning by unspecified narcotics, accidental (unintentional)**
Poisoning by narcotics NOS
7th **T40.602 Poisoning by unspecified narcotics, intentional self-harm**
7th **T40.603 Poisoning by unspecified narcotics, assault**
7th **T40.604 Poisoning by unspecified narcotics, undetermined**
7th **T40.605 Adverse effect of unspecified narcotics**
7th **T40.606 Underdosing of unspecified narcotics**
6th **T40.69 Poisoning by, adverse effect of and underdosing of other narcotics**
7th **T40.691 Poisoning by other narcotics, accidental (unintentional)**
Poisoning by other narcotics NOS
7th **T40.692 Poisoning by other narcotics, intentional self-harm**
7th **T40.693 Poisoning by other narcotics, assault**
7th **T40.694 Poisoning by other narcotics, undetermined**
7th **T40.695 Adverse effect of other narcotics**
7th **T40.696 Underdosing of other narcotics**

5th **T40.7 Poisoning by, adverse effect of and underdosing of cannabis (derivatives)**
6th **T40.7X Poisoning by, adverse effect of and underdosing of cannabis (derivatives)**
7th **T40.7X1 Poisoning by cannabis (derivatives), accidental (unintentional)**
Poisoning by cannabis NOS
7th **T40.7X2 Poisoning by cannabis (derivatives), intentional self-harm**
7th **T40.7X3 Poisoning by cannabis (derivatives), assault**
7th **T40.7X4 Poisoning by cannabis (derivatives), undetermined**
7th **T40.7X5 Adverse effect of cannabis (derivatives)**
7th **T40.7X6 Underdosing of cannabis (derivatives)**

5th **T40.8 Poisoning by and adverse effect of lysergide [LSD]**
6th **T40.8X Poisoning by and adverse effect of lysergide [LSD]**
7th **T40.8X1 Poisoning by lysergide [LSD], accidental (unintentional)**
Poisoning by lysergide [LSD]NOS
7th **T40.8X2 Poisoning by lysergide [LSD], intentional self-harm**
7th **T40.8X3 Poisoning by lysergide [LSD], assault**
7th **T40.8X4 Poisoning by lysergide [LSD], undetermined**
7th **T40.8X5 Adverse effect of lysergide [LSD]**

5th **T40.9 Poisoning by, adverse effect of and underdosing of other and unspecified psychodysleptics [hallucinogens]**
6th **T40.90 Poisoning by, adverse effect of and underdosing of unspecified psychodysleptics [hallucinogens]**
7th **T40.901 Poisoning by unspecified psychodysleptics [hallucinogens], accidental (unintentional)**
7th **T40.902 Poisoning by unspecified psychodysleptics [hallucinogens], intentional self-harm**
7th **T40.903 Poisoning by unspecified psychodysleptics [hallucinogens], assault**
7th **T40.904 Poisoning by unspecified psychodysleptics [hallucinogens], undetermined**
7th **T40.905 Adverse effect of unspecified psychodysleptics [hallucinogens]**
7th **T40.906 Underdosing of unspecified psychodysleptics**
6th **T40.99 Poisoning by, adverse effect of and underdosing of other psychodysleptics [hallucinogens]**
7th **T40.991 Poisoning by other psychodysleptics [hallucinogens], accidental (unintentional)**
Poisoning by other psychodysleptics [hallucinogens] NOS
7th **T40.992 Poisoning by other psychodysleptics [hallucinogens], intentional self-harm**
7th **T40.993 Poisoning by other psychodysleptics [hallucinogens], assault**
7th **T40.994 Poisoning by other psychodysleptics [hallucinogens], undetermined**
7th **T40.995 Adverse effect of other psychodysleptics [hallucinogens]**
7th **T40.996 Underdosing of other psychodysleptics**

T41 Poisoning by, adverse effect of and underdosing of anesthetics and therapeutic gases

EXCLUDES 1 *benzodiazepines (T42.4-)*
cocaine (T40.5-)
complications of anesthesia during pregnancy (O29.-)
complications of anesthesia during labor and delivery (O74.-)
complications of anesthesia during the puerperium (O89.-)
opioids (T40.0-T40.2-)

The appropriate 7th character is to be added to each code from category T41.
A initial encounter
D subsequent encounter
S sequela

T41.0 Poisoning by, adverse effect of and underdosing of inhaled anesthetics
EXCLUDES 1 *oxygen (T41.5-)*
T41.0X Poisoning by, adverse effect of and underdosing of inhaled anesthetics
T41.0X1 Poisoning by inhaled anesthetics, accidental (unintentional)
Poisoning by inhaled anesthetics NOS
T41.0X2 Poisoning by inhaled anesthetics, intentional self-harm
T41.0X3 Poisoning by inhaled anesthetics, assault
T41.0X4 Poisoning by inhaled anesthetics, undetermined
T41.0X5 Adverse effect of inhaled anesthetics
T41.0X6 Underdosing of inhaled anesthetics

T41.1 Poisoning by, adverse effect of and underdosing of intravenous anesthetics
Poisoning by, adverse effect of and underdosing of thiobarbiturates
T41.1X Poisoning by, adverse effect of and underdosing of intravenous anesthetics
T41.1X1 Poisoning by intravenous anesthetics, accidental (unintentional)
Poisoning by intravenous anesthetics NOS
T41.1X2 Poisoning by intravenous anesthetics, intentional self-harm
T41.1X3 Poisoning by intravenous anesthetics, assault
T41.1X4 Poisoning by intravenous anesthetics, undetermined
T41.1X5 Adverse effect of intravenous anesthetics
T41.1X6 Underdosing of intravenous anesthetics

T41.2 Poisoning by, adverse effect of and underdosing of other and unspecified general anesthetics
T41.20 Poisoning by, adverse effect of and underdosing of unspecified general anesthetics
T41.201 Poisoning by unspecified general anesthetics, accidental (unintentional)
Poisoning by general anesthetics NOS
T41.202 Poisoning by unspecified general anesthetics, intentional self-harm
T41.203 Poisoning by unspecified general anesthetics, assault
T41.204 Poisoning by unspecified general anesthetics, undetermined
T41.205 Adverse effect of unspecified general anesthetics
T41.206 Underdosing of unspecified general anesthetics
T41.29 Poisoning by, adverse effect of and underdosing of other general anesthetics
T41.291 Poisoning by other general anesthetics, accidental (unintentional)
Poisoning by other general anesthetics NOS
T41.292 Poisoning by other general anesthetics, intentional self-harm
T41.293 Poisoning by other general anesthetics, assault
T41.294 Poisoning by other general anesthetics, undetermined
T41.295 Adverse effect of other general anesthetics
T41.296 Underdosing of other general anesthetics

T41.3 Poisoning by, adverse effect of and underdosing of local anesthetics
Cocaine (topical)
EXCLUDES 2 *poisoning by cocaine used as a central nervous system stimulant (T40.5X1-T40.5X4)*
T41.3X Poisoning by, adverse effect of and underdosing of local anesthetics
T41.3X1 Poisoning by local anesthetics, accidental (unintentional)
Poisoning by local anesthetics NOS
T41.3X2 Poisoning by local anesthetics, intentional self-harm
T41.3X3 Poisoning by local anesthetics, assault
T41.3X4 Poisoning by local anesthetics, undetermined
T41.3X5 Adverse effect of local anesthetics
T41.3X6 Underdosing of local anesthetics

T41.4 Poisoning by, adverse effect of and underdosing of unspecified anesthetic
T41.41 Poisoning by unspecified anesthetic, accidental (unintentional)
Poisoning by anesthetic NOS
T41.42 Poisoning by unspecified anesthetic, intentional self-harm
T41.43 Poisoning by unspecified anesthetic, assault
T41.44 Poisoning by unspecified anesthetic, undetermined
T41.45 Adverse effect of unspecified anesthetic
T41.46 Underdosing of unspecified anesthetics

T41.5 Poisoning by, adverse effect of and underdosing of therapeutic gases
T41.5X Poisoning by, adverse effect of and underdosing of therapeutic gases
T41.5X1 Poisoning by therapeutic gases, accidental (unintentional)
Poisoning by therapeutic gases NOS
T41.5X2 Poisoning by therapeutic gases, intentional self-harm
T41.5X3 Poisoning by therapeutic gases, assault
T41.5X4 Poisoning by therapeutic gases, undetermined
T41.5X5 Adverse effect of therapeutic gases
T41.5X6 Underdosing of therapeutic gases

T42 Poisoning by, adverse effect of and underdosing of antiepileptic, sedative- hypnotic and antiparkinsonism drugs
EXCLUDES 2 *drug dependence and related mental and behavioral disorders due to psychoactive substance use (F10--F19-)*

The appropriate 7th character is to be added to each code from category T42.
A initial encounter
D subsequent encounter
S sequela

T42.0 Poisoning by, adverse effect of and underdosing of hydantoin derivatives
T42.0X Poisoning by, adverse effect of and underdosing of hydantoin derivatives
T42.0X1 Poisoning by hydantoin derivatives, accidental (unintentional)
Poisoning by hydantoin derivatives NOS
T42.0X2 Poisoning by hydantoin derivatives, intentional self-harm
T42.0X3 Poisoning by hydantoin derivatives, assault
T42.0X4 Poisoning by hydantoin derivatives, undetermined
T42.0X5 Adverse effect of hydantoin derivatives
T42.0X6 Underdosing of hydantoin derivatives

T42.1 Poisoning by, adverse effect of and underdosing of iminostilbenes
Poisoning by, adverse effect of and underdosing of carbamazepine

T42.1X Poisoning by, adverse effect of and underdosing of iminostilbenes

T42.1X1 Poisoning by iminostilbenes, accidental (unintentional)
Poisoning by iminostilbenes NOS

T42.1X2 Poisoning by iminostilbenes, intentional self-harm

T42.1X3 Poisoning by iminostilbenes, assault

T42.1X4 Poisoning by iminostilbenes, undetermined

T42.1X5 Adverse effect of iminostilbenes

T42.1X6 Underdosing of iminostilbenes

T42.2 Poisoning by, adverse effect of and underdosing of succinimides and oxazolidinediones

T42.2X Poisoning by, adverse effect of and underdosing of succinimides and oxazolidinediones

T42.2X1 Poisoning by succinimides and oxazolidinediones, accidental (unintentional)
Poisoning by succinimides and oxazolidinediones NOS

T42.2X2 Poisoning by succinimides and oxazolidinediones, intentional self-harm

T42.2X3 Poisoning by succinimides and oxazolidinediones, assault

T42.2X4 Poisoning by succinimides and oxazolidinediones, undetermined

T42.2X5 Adverse effect of succinimides and oxazolidinediones

T42.2X6 Underdosing of succinimides and oxazolidinediones

T42.3 Poisoning by, adverse effect of and underdosing of barbiturates
EXCLUDES 1 *poisoning by, adverse effect of and underdosing of thiobarbiturates (T41.1-)*

T42.3X Poisoning by, adverse effect of and underdosing of barbiturates

T42.3X1 Poisoning by barbiturates, accidental (unintentional)
Poisoning by barbiturates NOS

T42.3X2 Poisoning by barbiturates, intentional self-harm

T42.3X3 Poisoning by barbiturates, assault

T42.3X4 Poisoning by barbiturates, undetermined

T42.3X5 Adverse effect of barbiturates

T42.3X6 Underdosing of barbiturates

T42.4 Poisoning by, adverse effect of and underdosing of benzodiazepines

T42.4X Poisoning by, adverse effect of and underdosing of benzodiazepines

T42.4X1 Poisoning by benzodiazepines, accidental (unintentional)
Poisoning by benzodiazepines NOS

T42.4X2 Poisoning by benzodiazepines, intentional self-harm

T42.4X3 Poisoning by benzodiazepines, assault

T42.4X4 Poisoning by benzodiazepines, undetermined

T42.4X5 Adverse effect of benzodiazepines

T42.4X6 Underdosing of benzodiazepines

T42.5 Poisoning by, adverse effect of and underdosing of mixed antiepileptics

T42.5X Poisoning by, adverse effect of and underdosing of antiepileptics

T42.5X1 Poisoning by mixed antiepileptics, accidental (unintentional)
Poisoning by mixed antiepileptics NOS

T42.5X2 Poisoning by mixed antiepileptics, intentional self-harm

T42.5X3 Poisoning by mixed antiepileptics, assault

T42.5X4 Poisoning by mixed antiepileptics, undetermined

T42.5X5 Adverse effect of mixed antiepileptics

T42.5X6 Underdosing of mixed antiepileptics

T42.6 Poisoning by, adverse effect of and underdosing of other antiepileptic and sedative-hypnotic drugs
Poisoning by, adverse effect of and underdosing of methaqualone
Poisoning by, adverse effect of and underdosing of valproic acid
EXCLUDES 1 *poisoning by, adverse effect of and underdosing of carbamazepine (T42.1-)*

T42.6X Poisoning by, adverse effect of and underdosing of other antiepileptic and sedative-hypnotic drugs

T42.6X1 Poisoning by other antiepileptic and sedative-hypnotic drugs, accidental (unintentional)
Poisoning by other antiepileptic and sedative-hypnotic drugs NOS

T42.6X2 Poisoning by other antiepileptic and sedative-hypnotic drugs, intentional self-harm

T42.6X3 Poisoning by other antiepileptic and sedative-hypnotic drugs, assault

T42.6X4 Poisoning by other antiepileptic and sedative-hypnotic drugs, undetermined

T42.6X5 Adverse effect of other antiepileptic and sedative-hypnotic drugs

T42.6X6 Underdosing of other antiepileptic and sedative-hypnotic drugs

T42.7 Poisoning by, adverse effect of and underdosing of unspecified antiepileptic and sedative-hypnotic drugs

T42.71 Poisoning by unspecified antiepileptic and sedative-hypnotic drugs, accidental (unintentional)
Poisoning by antiepileptic and sedative-hypnotic drugs NOS

T42.72 Poisoning by unspecified antiepileptic and sedative-hypnotic drugs, intentional self-harm

T42.73 Poisoning by unspecified antiepileptic and sedative-hypnotic drugs, assault

T42.74 Poisoning by unspecified antiepileptic and sedative-hypnotic drugs, undetermined

T42.75 Adverse effect of unspecified antiepileptic and sedative-hypnotic drugs

T42.76 Underdosing of unspecified antiepileptic and sedative-hypnotic drugs

T42.8 Poisoning by, adverse effect of and underdosing of antiparkinsonism drugs and other central muscle-tone depressants
Poisoning by, adverse effect of and underdosing of amantadine

T42.8X Poisoning by, adverse effect of and underdosing of antiparkinsonism drugs and other central muscle-tone depressants

T42.8X1 Poisoning by antiparkinsonism drugs and other central muscle-tone depressants, accidental (unintentional)
Poisoning by antiparkinsonism drugs and other central muscle-tone depressants NOS

T42.8X2 Poisoning by antiparkinsonism drugs and other central muscle-tone depressants, intentional self-harm

T42.8X3 Poisoning by antiparkinsonism drugs and other central muscle-tone depressants, assault

T42.8X4 Poisoning by antiparkinsonism drugs and other central muscle-tone depressants, undetermined

T42.8X5 Adverse effect of antiparkinsonism drugs and other central muscle-tone depressants

T42.8X6 Underdosing of antiparkinsonism drugs and other central muscle-tone depressants

✓4th **T43 Poisoning by, adverse effect of and underdosing of psychotropic drugs, not elsewhere classified**

EXCLUDES 1 *appetite depressants (T50.5-)*
barbiturates (T42.3-)
benzodiazepines (T42.4-)
methaqualone (T42.6-)
psychodysleptics [hallucinogens] (T40.7-T40.9-)

EXCLUDES 2 *drug dependence and related mental and behavioral disorders due to psychoactive substance use (F10--F19-)*

The appropriate 7th character is to be added to each code from category T43.
A initial encounter
D subsequent encounter
S sequela

✓5th **T43.0 Poisoning by, adverse effect of and underdosing of tricyclic and tetracyclic antidepressants**

✓6th **T43.01 Poisoning by, adverse effect of and underdosing of tricyclic antidepressants**

✓7th **T43.011 Poisoning by tricyclic antidepressants, accidental (unintentional)**
Poisoning by tricyclic antidepressants NOS

✓7th **T43.012 Poisoning by tricyclic antidepressants, intentional self-harm**

✓7th **T43.013 Poisoning by tricyclic antidepressants, assault**

✓7th **T43.014 Poisoning by tricyclic antidepressants, undetermined**

✓7th **T43.015 Adverse effect of tricyclic antidepressants**

✓7th **T43.016 Underdosing of tricyclic antidepressants**

✓6th **T43.02 Poisoning by, adverse effect of and underdosing of tetracyclic antidepressants**

✓7th **T43.021 Poisoning by tetracyclic antidepressants, accidental (unintentional)**
Poisoning by tetracyclic antidepressants NOS

✓7th **T43.022 Poisoning by tetracyclic antidepressants, intentional self-harm**

✓7th **T43.023 Poisoning by tetracyclic antidepressants, assault**

✓7th **T43.024 Poisoning by tetracyclic antidepressants, undetermined**

✓7th **T43.025 Adverse effect of tetracyclic antidepressants**

✓7th **T43.026 Underdosing of tetracyclic antidepressants**

✓5th **T43.1 Poisoning by, adverse effect of and underdosing of monoamine-oxidase-inhibitor antidepressants**

✓6th **T43.1X Poisoning by, adverse effect of and underdosing of monoamine-oxidase-inhibitor antidepressants**

✓7th **T43.1X1 Poisoning by monoamine-oxidase-inhibitor antidepressants, accidental (unintentional)**
Poisoning by monoamine-oxidase-inhibitor antidepressants NOS

✓7th **T43.1X2 Poisoning by monoamine-oxidase-inhibitor antidepressants, intentional self-harm**

✓7th **T43.1X3 Poisoning by monoamine-oxidase-inhibitor antidepressants, assault**

✓7th **T43.1X4 Poisoning by monoamine-oxidase-inhibitor antidepressants, undetermined**

✓7th **T43.1X5 Adverse effect of monoamine-oxidase-inhibitor antidepressants**

✓7th **T43.1X6 Underdosing of monoamine-oxidase-inhibitor antidepressants**

✓5th **T43.2 Poisoning by, adverse effect of and underdosing of other and unspecified antidepressants**

✓6th **T43.20 Poisoning by, adverse effect of and underdosing of unspecified antidepressants**

✓7th **T43.201 Poisoning by unspecified antidepressants, accidental (unintentional)**
Poisoning by antidepressants NOS

✓7th **T43.202 Poisoning by unspecified antidepressants, intentional self-harm**

✓7th **T43.203 Poisoning by unspecified antidepressants, assault**

✓7th **T43.204 Poisoning by unspecified antidepressants, undetermined**

✓7th **T43.205 Adverse effect of unspecified antidepressants**

✓7th **T43.206 Underdosing of unspecified antidepressants**

✓6th **T43.21 Poisoning by, adverse effect of and underdosing of selective serotonin and norepinephrine reuptake inhibitors**
Poisoning by, adverse effect of and underdosing of SSNRI antidepressants

✓7th **T43.211 Poisoning by selective serotonin and norepinephrine reuptake inhibitors, accidental (unintentional)**

✓7th **T43.212 Poisoning by selective serotonin and norepinephrine reuptake inhibitors, intentional self-harm**

✓7th **T43.213 Poisoning by selective serotonin and norepinephrine reuptake inhibitors, assault**

✓7th **T43.214 Poisoning by selective serotonin and norepinephrine reuptake inhibitors, undetermined**

✓7th **T43.215 Adverse effect of selective serotonin and norepinephrine reuptake inhibitors**

✓7th **T43.216 Underdosing of selective serotonin and norepinephrine reuptake inhibitors**

✓6th **T43.22 Poisoning by, adverse effect of and underdosing of selective serotonin reuptake inhibitors**
Poisoning by, adverse effect of and underdosing of SSRI antidepressants

✓7th **T43.221 Poisoning by selective serotonin reuptake inhibitors, accidental (unintentional)**

✓7th **T43.222 Poisoning by selective serotonin reuptake inhibitors, intentional self-harm**

✓7th **T43.223 Poisoning by selective serotonin reuptake inhibitors, assault**

✓7th **T43.224 Poisoning by selective serotonin reuptake inhibitors, undetermined**

✓7th **T43.225 Adverse effect of selective serotonin reuptake inhibitors**

✓7th **T43.226 Underdosing of selective serotonin reuptake inhibitors**

✓6th **T43.29 Poisoning by, adverse effect of and underdosing of other antidepressants**

✓7th **T43.291 Poisoning by other antidepressants, accidental (unintentional)**
Poisoning by other antidepressants NOS

✓7th **T43.292 Poisoning by other antidepressants, intentional self-harm**

✓7th **T43.293 Poisoning by other antidepressants, assault**

✓7th **T43.294 Poisoning by other antidepressants, undetermined**

✓7th **T43.295 Adverse effect of other antidepressants**

✓7th **T43.296 Underdosing of other antidepressants**

✓5th **T43.3 Poisoning by, adverse effect of and underdosing of phenothiazine antipsychotics and neuroleptics**

✓6th **T43.3X Poisoning by, adverse effect of and underdosing of phenothiazine antipsychotics and neuroleptics**

✓7th **T43.3X1 Poisoning by phenothiazine antipsychotics and neuroleptics, accidental (unintentional)**
Poisoning by phenothiazine antipsychotics and neuroleptics NOS

✓7th **T43.3X2 Poisoning by phenothiazine antipsychotics and neuroleptics, intentional self-harm**

✓7th **T43.3X3 Poisoning by phenothiazine antipsychotics and neuroleptics, assault**

✓7th **T43.3X4 Poisoning by phenothiazine antipsychotics and neuroleptics, undetermined**

✓7th **T43.3X5 Adverse effect of phenothiazine antipsychotics and neuroleptics**

✓7th **T43.3X6 Underdosing of phenothiazine antipsychotics and neuroleptics**

✓5th **T43.4 Poisoning by, adverse effect of and underdosing of butyrophenone and thiothixene neuroleptics**

✓6th **T43.4X Poisoning by, adverse effect of and underdosing of butyrophenone and thiothixene neuroleptics**

✓7th **T43.4X1 Poisoning by butyrophenone and thiothixene neuroleptics, accidental (unintentional)**
Poisoning by butyrophenone and thiothixene neuroleptics NOS

✓7th **T43.4X2 Poisoning by butyrophenone and thiothixene neuroleptics, intentional self-harm**

✓7th **T43.4X3 Poisoning by butyrophenone and thiothixene neuroleptics, assault**

✓7th **T43.4X4 Poisoning by butyrophenone and thiothixene neuroleptics, undetermined**

✓7th **T43.4X5 Adverse effect of butyrophenone and thiothixene neuroleptics**

✓7th **T43.4X6 Underdosing of butyrophenone and thiothixene neuroleptics**

✓5th **T43.5 Poisoning by, adverse effect of and underdosing of other and unspecified antipsychotics and neuroleptics**
EXCLUDES 1 *poisoning by, adverse effect of and underdosing of rauwolfia (T46.5-)*

✓6th **T43.50 Poisoning by, adverse effect of and underdosing of unspecified antipsychotics and neuroleptics**

✓7th **T43.501 Poisoning by unspecified antipsychotics and neuroleptics, accidental (unintentional)**
Poisoning by antipsychotics and neuroleptics NOS

✓7th **T43.502 Poisoning by unspecified antipsychotics and neuroleptics, intentional self-harm**

✓7th **T43.503 Poisoning by unspecified antipsychotics and neuroleptics, assault**

✓7th **T43.504 Poisoning by unspecified antipsychotics and neuroleptics, undetermined**

✓7th **T43.505 Adverse effect of unspecified antipsychotics and neuroleptics**

✓7th **T43.506 Underdosing of unspecified antipsychotics and neuroleptics**

✓6th **T43.59 Poisoning by, adverse effect of and underdosing of other antipsychotics and neuroleptics**

✓7th **T43.591 Poisoning by other antipsychotics and neuroleptics, accidental (unintentional)**
Poisoning by other antipsychotics and neuroleptics NOS

✓7th **T43.592 Poisoning by other antipsychotics and neuroleptics, intentional self-harm**

✓7th **T43.593 Poisoning by other antipsychotics and neuroleptics, assault**

✓7th **T43.594 Poisoning by other antipsychotics and neuroleptics, undetermined**

✓7th **T43.595 Adverse effect of other antipsychotics and neuroleptics**

✓7th **T43.596 Underdosing of other antipsychotics and neuroleptics**

✓5th **T43.6 Poisoning by, adverse effect of and underdosing of psychostimulants**
EXCLUDES 1 *poisoning by, adverse effect of and underdosing of cocaine (T40.5-)*

✓6th **T43.60 Poisoning by, adverse effect of and underdosing of unspecified psychostimulant**

✓7th **T43.601 Poisoning by unspecified psychostimulants, accidental (unintentional)**
Poisoning by psychostimulants NOS

✓7th **T43.602 Poisoning by unspecified psychostimulants, intentional self-harm**

✓7th **T43.603 Poisoning by unspecified psychostimulants, assault**

✓7th **T43.604 Poisoning by unspecified psychostimulants, undetermined**

✓7th **T43.605 Adverse effect of unspecified psychostimulants**

✓7th **T43.606 Underdosing of unspecified psychostimulants**

✓6th **T43.61 Poisoning by, adverse effect of and underdosing of caffeine**

✓7th **T43.611 Poisoning by caffeine, accidental (unintentional)**
Poisoning by caffeine NOS

✓7th **T43.612 Poisoning by caffeine, intentional self-harm**

✓7th **T43.613 Poisoning by caffeine, assault**

✓7th **T43.614 Poisoning by caffeine, undetermined**

✓7th **T43.615 Adverse effect of caffeine**

✓7th **T43.616 Underdosing of caffeine**

✓6th **T43.62 Poisoning by, adverse effect of and underdosing of amphetamines**
Poisoning by, adverse effect of and underdosing of methamphetamines

✓7th **T43.621 Poisoning by amphetamines, accidental (unintentional)**
Poisoning by amphetamines NOS

✓7th **T43.622 Poisoning by amphetamines, intentional self-harm**

✓7th **T43.623 Poisoning by amphetamines, assault**

✓7th **T43.624 Poisoning by amphetamines, undetermined**

✓7th **T43.625 Adverse effect of amphetamines**

✓7th **T43.626 Underdosing of amphetamines**

✓6th **T43.63 Poisoning by, adverse effect of and underdosing of methylphenidate**

✓7th **T43.631 Poisoning by methylphenidate, accidental (unintentional)**
Poisoning by methylphenidate NOS

✓7th **T43.632 Poisoning by methylphenidate, intentional self-harm**

✓7th **T43.633 Poisoning by methylphenidate, assault**

✓7th **T43.634 Poisoning by methylphenidate, undetermined**

✓7th **T43.635 Adverse effect of methylphenidate**

✓7th **T43.636 Underdosing of methylphenidate**

✓6th **T43.69 Poisoning by, adverse effect of and underdosing of other psychostimulants**

✓7th **T43.691 Poisoning by other psychostimulants, accidental (unintentional)**
Poisoning by other psychostimulants NOS

✓7th **T43.692 Poisoning by other psychostimulants, intentional self-harm**

✓7th **T43.693 Poisoning by other psychostimulants, assault**

✓7th **T43.694 Poisoning by other psychostimulants, undetermined**

✓7th **T43.695 Adverse effect of other psychostimulants**

✓7th **T43.696 Underdosing of other psychostimulants**

✓5th **T43.8 Poisoning by, adverse effect of and underdosing of other psychotropic drugs**

✓6th **T43.8X Poisoning by, adverse effect of and underdosing of other psychotropic drugs**

✓7th **T43.8X1 Poisoning by other psychotropic drugs, accidental (unintentional)**
Poisoning by other psychotropic drugs NOS

✓7th **T43.8X2 Poisoning by other psychotropic drugs, intentional self-harm**

✓7th **T43.8X3 Poisoning by other psychotropic drugs, assault**

✓7th **T43.8X4 Poisoning by other psychotropic drugs, undetermined**

✓7th **T43.8X5 Adverse effect of other psychotropic drugs**

✓7th **T43.8X6 Underdosing of other psychotropic drugs**

T43.9 Poisoning by, adverse effect of and underdosing of unspecified psychotropic drug

T43.91 Poisoning by unspecified psychotropic drug, accidental (unintentional)
Poisoning by psychotropic drug NOS

T43.92 Poisoning by unspecified psychotropic drug, intentional self-harm

T43.93 Poisoning by unspecified psychotropic drug, assault

T43.94 Poisoning by unspecified psychotropic drug, undetermined

T43.95 Adverse effect of unspecified psychotropic drug

T43.96 Underdosing of unspecified psychotropic drug

T44 Poisoning by, adverse effect of and underdosing of drugs primarily affecting the autonomic nervous system

The appropriate 7th character is to be added to each code from category T44.
A initial encounter
D subsequent encounter
S sequela

T44.0 Poisoning by, adverse effect of and underdosing of anticholinesterase agents

T44.0X Poisoning by, adverse effect of and underdosing of anticholinesterase agents

T44.0X1 Poisoning by anticholinesterase agents, accidental (unintentional)
Poisoning by anticholinesterase agents NOS

T44.0X2 Poisoning by anticholinesterase agents, intentional self-harm

T44.0X3 Poisoning by anticholinesterase agents, assault

T44.0X4 Poisoning by anticholinesterase agents, undetermined

T44.0X5 Adverse effect of anticholinesterase agents

T44.0X6 Underdosing of anticholinesterase agents

T44.1 Poisoning by, adverse effect of and underdosing of other parasympathomimetics [cholinergics]

T44.1X Poisoning by, adverse effect of and underdosing of other parasympathomimetics [cholinergics]

T44.1X1 Poisoning by other parasympathomimetics [cholinergics], accidental (unintentional)
Poisoning by other parasympathomimetics [cholinergics] NOS

T44.1X2 Poisoning by other parasympathomimetics [cholinergics], intentional self-harm

T44.1X3 Poisoning by other parasympathomimetics [cholinergics], assault

T44.1X4 Poisoning by other parasympathomimetics [cholinergics], undetermined

T44.1X5 Adverse effect of other parasympathomimetics [cholinergics]

T44.1X6 Underdosing of other parasympathomimetics

T44.2 Poisoning by, adverse effect of and underdosing of ganglionic blocking drugs

T44.2X Poisoning by, adverse effect of and underdosing of ganglionic blocking drugs

T44.2X1 Poisoning by ganglionic blocking drugs, accidental (unintentional)
Poisoning by ganglionic blocking drugs NOS

T44.2X2 Poisoning by ganglionic blocking drugs, intentional self-harm

T44.2X3 Poisoning by ganglionic blocking drugs, assault

T44.2X4 Poisoning by ganglionic blocking drugs, undetermined

T44.2X5 Adverse effect of ganglionic blocking drugs

T44.2X6 Underdosing of ganglionic blocking drugs

T44.3 Poisoning by, adverse effect of and underdosing of other parasympatholytics [anticholinergics and antimuscarinics] and spasmolytics
Poisoning by, adverse effect of and underdosing of papaverine

T44.3X Poisoning by, adverse effect of and underdosing of other parasympatholytics [anticholinergics and antimuscarinics] and spasmolytics

T44.3X1 Poisoning by other parasympatholytics [anticholinergics and antimuscarinics] and spasmolytics, accidental (unintentional)
Poisoning by other parasympatholytics [anticholinergics and antimuscarinics] and spasmolytics NOS

T44.3X2 Poisoning by other parasympatholytics [anticholinergics and antimuscarinics] and spasmolytics, intentional self-harm

T44.3X3 Poisoning by other parasympatholytics [anticholinergics and antimuscarinics] and spasmolytics, assault

T44.3X4 Poisoning by other parasympatholytics [anticholinergics and antimuscarinics] and spasmolytics, undetermined

T44.3X5 Adverse effect of other parasympatholytics [anticholinergics and antimuscarinics] and spasmolytics

T44.3X6 Underdosing of other parasympatholytics [anticholinergics and antimuscarinics] and spasmolytics

T44.4 Poisoning by, adverse effect of and underdosing of predominantly alpha-adrenoreceptor agonists
Poisoning by, adverse effect of and underdosing of metaraminol

T44.4X Poisoning by, adverse effect of and underdosing of predominantly alpha-adrenoreceptor agonists

T44.4X1 Poisoning by predominantly alpha-adrenoreceptor agonists, accidental (unintentional)
Poisoning by predominantly alpha-adrenoreceptor agonists NOS

T44.4X2 Poisoning by predominantly alpha-adrenoreceptor agonists, intentional self-harm

T44.4X3 Poisoning by predominantly alpha-adrenoreceptor agonists, assault

T44.4X4 Poisoning by predominantly alpha-adrenoreceptor agonists, undetermined

T44.4X5 Adverse effect of predominantly alpha-adrenoreceptor agonists

T44.4X6 Underdosing of predominantly alpha-adrenoreceptor agonists

T44.5 Poisoning by, adverse effect of and underdosing of predominantly beta-adrenoreceptor agonists

EXCLUDES1 *poisoning by, adverse effect of and underdosing of beta-adrenoreceptor agonists used in asthma therapy (T48.6-)*

T44.5X Poisoning by, adverse effect of and underdosing of predominantly beta-adrenoreceptor agonists

T44.5X1 Poisoning by predominantly beta-adrenoreceptor agonists, accidental (unintentional)
Poisoning by predominantly beta-adrenoreceptor agonists NOS

T44.5X2 Poisoning by predominantly beta-adrenoreceptor agonists, intentional self-harm

T44.5X3 Poisoning by predominantly beta-adrenoreceptor agonists, assault

T44.5X4 Poisoning by predominantly beta-adrenoreceptor agonists, undetermined

T44.5X5 Adverse effect of predominantly beta-adrenoreceptor agonists

7th T44.5X6 **Underdosing of predominantly beta-adrenoreceptor agonists**

5th T44.6 **Poisoning by, adverse effect of and underdosing of alpha-adrenoreceptor antagonists**

EXCLUDES 1 *poisoning by, adverse effect of and underdosing of ergot alkaloids (T48.Ø)*

6th T44.6X **Poisoning by, adverse effect of and underdosing of alpha-adrenoreceptor antagonists**

7th T44.6X1 **Poisoning by alpha-adrenoreceptor antagonists, accidental (unintentional)**
Poisoning by alpha-adrenoreceptor antagonists NOS

7th T44.6X2 **Poisoning by alpha-adrenoreceptor antagonists, intentional self-harm**

7th T44.6X3 **Poisoning by alpha-adrenoreceptor antagonists, assault**

7th T44.6X4 **Poisoning by alpha-adrenoreceptor antagonists, undetermined**

7th T44.6X5 **Adverse effect of alpha-adrenoreceptor antagonists**

7th T44.6X6 **Underdosing of alpha-adrenoreceptor antagonists**

5th T44.7 **Poisoning by, adverse effect of and underdosing of beta-adrenoreceptor antagonists**

6th T44.7X **Poisoning by, adverse effect of and underdosing of beta-adrenoreceptor antagonists**

7th T44.7X1 **Poisoning by beta-adrenoreceptor antagonists, accidental (unintentional)**
Poisoning by beta-adrenoreceptor antagonists NOS

7th T44.7X2 **Poisoning by beta-adrenoreceptor antagonists, intentional self-harm**

7th T44.7X3 **Poisoning by beta-adrenoreceptor antagonists, assault**

7th T44.7X4 **Poisoning by beta-adrenoreceptor antagonists, undetermined**

7th T44.7X5 **Adverse effect of beta-adrenoreceptor antagonists**

7th T44.7X6 **Underdosing of beta-adrenoreceptor antagonists**

5th T44.8 **Poisoning by, adverse effect of and underdosing of centrally-acting and adrenergic-neuron- blocking agents**

EXCLUDES 1 *poisoning by, adverse effect of and underdosing of clonidine (T46.5)*
poisoning by, adverse effect of and underdosing of guanethidine (T46.5)

6th T44.8X **Poisoning by, adverse effect of and underdosing of centrally-acting and adrenergic-neuron-blocking agents**

7th T44.8X1 **Poisoning by centrally-acting and adrenergic-neuron-blocking agents, accidental (unintentional)**
Poisoning by centrally-acting and adrenergic-neuron-blocking agents NOS

7th T44.8X2 **Poisoning by centrally-acting and adrenergic-neuron-blocking agents, intentional self-harm**

7th T44.8X3 **Poisoning by centrally-acting and adrenergic-neuron-blocking agents, assault**

7th T44.8X4 **Poisoning by centrally-acting and adrenergic-neuron-blocking agents, undetermined**

7th T44.8X5 **Adverse effect of centrally-acting and adrenergic-neuron-blocking agents**

7th T44.8X6 **Underdosing of centrally-acting and adrenergic-neuron-blocking agents**

5th T44.9 **Poisoning by, adverse effect of and underdosing of other and unspecified drugs primarily affecting the autonomic nervous system**
Poisoning by, adverse effect of and underdosing of drug stimulating both alpha and beta-adrenoreceptors

6th T44.90 **Poisoning by, adverse effect of and underdosing of unspecified drugs primarily affecting the autonomic nervous system**

7th T44.901 **Poisoning by unspecified drugs primarily affecting the autonomic nervous system, accidental (unintentional)**
Poisoning by unspecified drugs primarily affecting the autonomic nervous system NOS

7th T44.902 **Poisoning by unspecified drugs primarily affecting the autonomic nervous system, intentional self-harm**

7th T44.903 **Poisoning by unspecified drugs primarily affecting the autonomic nervous system, assault**

7th T44.904 **Poisoning by unspecified drugs primarily affecting the autonomic nervous system, undetermined**

7th T44.905 **Adverse effect of unspecified drugs primarily affecting the autonomic nervous system**

7th T44.906 **Underdosing of unspecified drugs primarily affecting the autonomic nervous system**

6th T44.99 **Poisoning by, adverse effect of and underdosing of other drugs primarily affecting the autonomic nervous system**

7th T44.991 **Poisoning by other drug primarily affecting the autonomic nervous system, accidental (unintentional)**
Poisoning by other drugs primarily affecting the autonomic nervous system NOS

7th T44.992 **Poisoning by other drug primarily affecting the autonomic nervous system, intentional self-harm**

7th T44.993 **Poisoning by other drug primarily affecting the autonomic nervous system, assault**

7th T44.994 **Poisoning by other drug primarily affecting the autonomic nervous system, undetermined**

7th T44.995 **Adverse effect of other drug primarily affecting the autonomic nervous system**

7th T44.996 **Underdosing of other drug primarily affecting the autonomic nervous system**

4th **T45 Poisoning by, adverse effect of and underdosing of primarily systemic and hematological agents, not elsewhere classified**

The appropriate 7th character is to be added to each code from category T45.
A initial encounter
D subsequent encounter
S sequela

5th T45.Ø **Poisoning by, adverse effect of and underdosing of antiallergic and antiemetic drugs**

EXCLUDES 1 *poisoning by, adverse effect of and underdosing of phenothiazine-based neuroleptics (T43.3)*

6th T45.ØX **Poisoning by, adverse effect of and underdosing of antiallergic and antiemetic drugs**

7th T45.ØX1 **Poisoning by antiallergic and antiemetic drugs, accidental (unintentional)**
Poisoning by antiallergic and antiemetic drugs NOS

7th T45.ØX2 **Poisoning by antiallergic and antiemetic drugs, intentional self-harm**

7th T45.ØX3 **Poisoning by antiallergic and antiemetic drugs, assault**

7th T45.ØX4 **Poisoning by antiallergic and antiemetic drugs, undetermined**

7th T45.ØX5 **Adverse effect of antiallergic and antiemetic drugs**

T45.0X6 Underdosing of antiallergic and antiemetic drugs

T45.1 Poisoning by, adverse effect of and underdosing of antineoplastic and immunosuppressive drugs
EXCLUDES 1 *poisoning by, adverse effect of and underdosing of tamoxifen (T38.6)*

T45.1X Poisoning by, adverse effect of and underdosing of antineoplastic and immunosuppressive drugs

T45.1X1 Poisoning by antineoplastic and immunosuppressive drugs, accidental (unintentional)
Poisoning by antineoplastic and immunosuppressive drugs NOS

T45.1X2 Poisoning by antineoplastic and immunosuppressive drugs, intentional self-harm

T45.1X3 Poisoning by antineoplastic and immunosuppressive drugs, assault

T45.1X4 Poisoning by antineoplastic and immunosuppressive drugs, undetermined

T45.1X5 Adverse effect of antineoplastic and immunosuppressive drugs

T45.1X6 Underdosing of antineoplastic and immunosuppressive drugs

T45.2 Poisoning by, adverse effect of and underdosing of vitamins
EXCLUDES 2 *poisoning by, adverse effect of and underdosing of nicotinic acid (derivatives) (T46.7)*
poisoning by, adverse effect of and underdosing of iron (T45.4)
poisoning by, adverse effect of and underdosing of vitamin K (T45.7)

T45.2X Poisoning by, adverse effect of and underdosing of vitamins

T45.2X1 Poisoning by vitamins, accidental (unintentional)
Poisoning by vitamins NOS

T45.2X2 Poisoning by vitamins, intentional self-harm

T45.2X3 Poisoning by vitamins, assault

T45.2X4 Poisoning by vitamins, undetermined

T45.2X5 Adverse effect of vitamins

T45.2X6 Underdosing of vitamins
EXCLUDES 1 *vitamin deficiencies (E50-E56)*

T45.3 Poisoning by, adverse effect of and underdosing of enzymes

T45.3X Poisoning by, adverse effect of and underdosing of enzymes

T45.3X1 Poisoning by enzymes, accidental (unintentional)
Poisoning by enzymes NOS

T45.3X2 Poisoning by enzymes, intentional self-harm

T45.3X3 Poisoning by enzymes, assault

T45.3X4 Poisoning by enzymes, undetermined

T45.3X5 Adverse effect of enzymes

T45.3X6 Underdosing of enzymes

T45.4 Poisoning by, adverse effect of and underdosing of iron and its compounds

T45.4X Poisoning by, adverse effect of and underdosing of iron and its compounds

T45.4X1 Poisoning by iron and its compounds, accidental (unintentional)
Poisoning by iron and its compounds NOS

T45.4X2 Poisoning by iron and its compounds, intentional self-harm

T45.4X3 Poisoning by iron and its compounds, assault

T45.4X4 Poisoning by iron and its compounds, undetermined

T45.4X5 Adverse effect of iron and its compounds

T45.4X6 Underdosing of iron and its compounds
EXCLUDES 1 *iron deficiency (E61.1)*

T45.5 Poisoning by, adverse effect of and underdosing of anticoagulants and antithrombotic drugs

T45.51 Poisoning by, adverse effect of and underdosing of anticoagulants

T45.511 Poisoning by anticoagulants, accidental (unintentional)
Poisoning by anticoagulants NOS

T45.512 Poisoning by anticoagulants, intentional self-harm

T45.513 Poisoning by anticoagulants, assault

T45.514 Poisoning by anticoagulants, undetermined

T45.515 Adverse effect of anticoagulants

T45.516 Underdosing of anticoagulants

T45.52 Poisoning by, adverse effect of and underdosing of antithrombotic drugs
Poisoning by, adverse effect of and underdosing of antiplatelet drugs
EXCLUDES 2 *poisoning by, adverse effect of and underdosing of aspirin (T39.01-)*
poisoning by, adverse effect of and underdosing of acetylsalicylic acid (T39.01-)

T45.521 Poisoning by antithrombotic drugs, accidental (unintentional)
Poisoning by antithrombotic drug NOS

T45.522 Poisoning by antithrombotic drugs, intentional self-harm

T45.523 Poisoning by antithrombotic drugs, assault

T45.524 Poisoning by antithrombotic drugs, undetermined

T45.525 Adverse effect of antithrombotic drugs

T45.526 Underdosing of antithrombotic drugs

T45.6 Poisoning by, adverse effect of and underdosing of fibrinolysis-affecting drugs

T45.60 Poisoning by, adverse effect of and underdosing of unspecified fibrinolysis-affecting drugs

T45.601 Poisoning by unspecified fibrinolysis-affecting drugs, accidental (unintentional)
Poisoning by fibrinolysis-affecting drug NOS

T45.602 Poisoning by unspecified fibrinolysis-affecting drugs, intentional self-harm

T45.603 Poisoning by unspecified fibrinolysis-affecting drugs, assault

T45.604 Poisoning by unspecified fibrinolysis-affecting drugs, undetermined

T45.605 Adverse effect of unspecified fibrinolysis-affecting drugs

T45.606 Underdosing of unspecified fibrinolysis-affecting drugs

T45.61 Poisoning by, adverse effect of and underdosing of thrombolytic drugs

T45.611 Poisoning by thrombolytic drug, accidental (unintentional)
Poisoning by thrombolytic drug NOS

T45.612 Poisoning by thrombolytic drug, intentional self-harm

T45.613 Poisoning by thrombolytic drug, assault

T45.614 Poisoning by thrombolytic drug, undetermined

T45.615 Adverse effect of thrombolytic drugs

T45.616 Underdosing of thrombolytic drugs

T45.62 Poisoning by, adverse effect of and underdosing of hemostatic drugs

T45.621 Poisoning by hemostatic drug, accidental (unintentional)
Poisoning by hemostatic drug NOS

T45.622 Poisoning by hemostatic drug, intentional self-harm

T45.623 Poisoning by hemostatic drug, assault

T45.624 Poisoning by hemostatic drug, undetermined

✓7th **T45.625 Adverse effect of hemostatic drug**

✓7th **T45.626 Underdosing of hemostatic drugs**

✓6th **T45.69 Poisoning by, adverse effect of and underdosing of other fibrinolysis-affecting drugs**

✓7th **T45.691 Poisoning by other fibrinolysis-affecting drugs, accidental (unintentional)**
Poisoning by other fibrinolysis-affecting drug NOS

✓7th **T45.692 Poisoning by other fibrinolysis-affecting drugs, intentional self-harm**

✓7th **T45.693 Poisoning by other fibrinolysis-affecting drugs, assault**

✓7th **T45.694 Poisoning by other fibrinolysis-affecting drugs, undetermined**

✓7th **T45.695 Adverse effect of other fibrinolysis-affecting drugs**

✓7th **T45.696 Underdosing of other fibrinolysis-affecting drugs**

✓5th **T45.7 Poisoning by, adverse effect of and underdosing of anticoagulant antagonists, vitamin K and other coagulants**

✓6th **T45.7X Poisoning by, adverse effect of and underdosing of anticoagulant antagonists, vitamin K and other coagulants**

✓7th **T45.7X1 Poisoning by anticoagulant antagonists, vitamin K and other coagulants, accidental (unintentional)**
Poisoning by anticoagulant antagonists, vitamin K and other coagulants NOS

✓7th **T45.7X2 Poisoning by anticoagulant antagonists, vitamin K and other coagulants, intentional self-harm**

✓7th **T45.7X3 Poisoning by anticoagulant antagonists, vitamin K and other coagulants, assault**

✓7th **T45.7X4 Poisoning by anticoagulant antagonists, vitamin K and other coagulants, undetermined**

✓7th **T45.7X5 Adverse effect of anticoagulant antagonists, vitamin K and other coagulants**

✓7th **T45.7X6 Underdosing of anticoagulant antagonist, vitamin K and other coagulants**
EXCLUDES1 *vitamin K deficiency (E56.1)*

✓5th **T45.8 Poisoning by, adverse effect of and underdosing of other primarily systemic and hematological agents**
Poisoning by, adverse effect of and underdosing of liver preparations and other antianemic agents
Poisoning by, adverse effect of and underdosing of natural blood and blood products
Poisoning by, adverse effect of and underdosing of plasma substitute
EXCLUDES2 *poisoning by, adverse effect of and underdosing of immunoglobulin (T5Ø.Z1)*
poisoning by, adverse effect of and underdosing of iron (T45.4)
transfusion reactions (T8Ø.-)

✓6th **T45.8X Poisoning by, adverse effect of and underdosing of other primarily systemic and hematological agents**

✓7th **T45.8X1 Poisoning by other primarily systemic and hematological agents, accidental (unintentional)**
Poisoning by other primarily systemic and hematological agents NOS

✓7th **T45.8X2 Poisoning by other primarily systemic and hematological agents, intentional self-harm**

✓7th **T45.8X3 Poisoning by other primarily systemic and hematological agents, assault**

✓7th **T45.8X4 Poisoning by other primarily systemic and hematological agents, undetermined**

✓7th **T45.8X5 Adverse effect of other primarily systemic and hematological agents**

✓7th **T45.8X6 Underdosing of other primarily systemic and hematological agents**

✓5th **T45.9 Poisoning by, adverse effect of and underdosing of unspecified primarily systemic and hematological agent**

✓x7th **T45.91 Poisoning by unspecified primarily systemic and hematological agent, accidental (unintentional)**
Poisoning by primarily systemic and hematological agent NOS

✓x7th **T45.92 Poisoning by unspecified primarily systemic and hematological agent, intentional self-harm**

✓x7th **T45.93 Poisoning by unspecified primarily systemic and hematological agent, assault**

✓x7th **T45.94 Poisoning by unspecified primarily systemic and hematological agent, undetermined**

✓x7th **T45.95 Adverse effect of unspecified primarily systemic and hematological agent**

✓x7th **T45.96 Underdosing of unspecified primarily systemic and hematological agent**

✓4th **T46 Poisoning by, adverse effect of and underdosing of agents primarily affecting the cardiovascular system**
EXCLUDES1 *poisoning by, adverse effect of and underdosing of metaraminol (T44.4)*

The appropriate 7th character is to be added to each code from category T46.
A initial encounter
D subsequent encounter
S sequela

✓5th **T46.Ø Poisoning by, adverse effect of and underdosing of cardiac-stimulant glycosides and drugs of similar action**

✓6th **T46.ØX Poisoning by, adverse effect of and underdosing of cardiac-stimulant glycosides and drugs of similar action**

✓7th **T46.ØX1 Poisoning by cardiac-stimulant glycosides and drugs of similar action, accidental (unintentional)**
Poisoning by cardiac-stimulant glycosides and drugs of similar action NOS

✓7th **T46.ØX2 Poisoning by cardiac-stimulant glycosides and drugs of similar action, intentional self-harm**

✓7th **T46.ØX3 Poisoning by cardiac-stimulant glycosides and drugs of similar action, assault**

✓7th **T46.ØX4 Poisoning by cardiac-stimulant glycosides and drugs of similar action, undetermined**

✓7th **T46.ØX5 Adverse effect of cardiac-stimulant glycosides and drugs of similar action**

✓7th **T46.ØX6 Underdosing of cardiac-stimulant glycosides and drugs of similar action**

T46.1 Poisoning by, adverse effect of and underdosing of calcium-channel blockers

✓6th **T46.1X Poisoning by, adverse effect of and underdosing of calcium-channel blockers**

✓7th **T46.1X1 Poisoning by calcium-channel blockers, accidental (unintentional)**
Poisoning by calcium-channel blockers NOS

✓7th **T46.1X2 Poisoning by calcium-channel blockers, intentional self-harm**

✓7th **T46.1X3 Poisoning by calcium-channel blockers, assault**

✓7th **T46.1X4 Poisoning by calcium-channel blockers, undetermined**

✓7th **T46.1X5 Adverse effect of calcium-channel blockers**

✓7th **T46.1X6 Underdosing of calcium-channel blockers**

✓5th **T46.2 Poisoning by, adverse effect of and underdosing of other antidysrhythmic drugs, not elsewhere classified**
EXCLUDES1 *poisoning by, adverse effect of and underdosing of beta-adrenoreceptor antagonists (T44.7-)*

✓6th **T46.2X Poisoning by, adverse effect of and underdosing of other antidysrhythmic drugs**

✓7th **T46.2X1 Poisoning by other antidysrhythmic drugs, accidental (unintentional)**
Poisoning by other antidysrhythmic drugs NOS

√7th T46.2X2 **Poisoning by other antidysrhythmic drugs, intentional self-harm**

√7th T46.2X3 **Poisoning by other antidysrhythmic drugs, assault**

√7th T46.2X4 **Poisoning by other antidysrhythmic drugs, undetermined**

√7th T46.2X5 **Adverse effect of other antidysrhythmic drugs**

√7th T46.2X6 **Underdosing of other antidysrhythmic drugs**

√5th **T46.3 Poisoning by, adverse effect of and underdosing of coronary vasodilators**

Poisoning by, adverse effect of and underdosing of dipyridamole

EXCLUDES 1 *poisoning by, adverse effect of and underdosing of calcium-channel blockers (T46.1)*

√6th **T46.3X Poisoning by, adverse effect of and underdosing of coronary vasodilators**

√7th T46.3X1 **Poisoning by coronary vasodilators, accidental (unintentional)**

Poisoning by coronary vasodilators NOS

√7th T46.3X2 **Poisoning by coronary vasodilators, intentional self-harm**

√7th T46.3X3 **Poisoning by coronary vasodilators, assault**

√7th T46.3X4 **Poisoning by coronary vasodilators, undetermined**

√7th T46.3X5 **Adverse effect of coronary vasodilators**

√7th T46.3X6 **Underdosing of coronary vasodilators**

√5th **T46.4 Poisoning by, adverse effect of and underdosing of angiotensin-converting-enzyme inhibitors**

√6th **T46.4X Poisoning by, adverse effect of and underdosing of angiotensin-converting-enzyme inhibitors**

√7th T46.4X1 **Poisoning by angiotensin-converting-enzyme inhibitors, accidental (unintentional)**

Poisoning by angiotensin-converting-enzyme inhibitors NOS

√7th T46.4X2 **Poisoning by angiotensin-converting-enzyme inhibitors, intentional self-harm**

√7th T46.4X3 **Poisoning by angiotensin-converting-enzyme inhibitors, assault**

√7th T46.4X4 **Poisoning by angiotensin-converting-enzyme inhibitors, undetermined**

√7th T46.4X5 **Adverse effect of angiotensin-converting- enzyme inhibitors**

√7th T46.4X6 **Underdosing of angiotensin-converting-enzyme inhibitors**

√5th **T46.5 Poisoning by, adverse effect of and underdosing of other antihypertensive drugs**

EXCLUDES 2 *poisoning by, adverse effect of and underdosing of beta-adrenoreceptor antagonists (T44.7)*
poisoning by, adverse effect of and underdosing of calcium-channel blockers (T46.1)
poisoning by, adverse effect of and underdosing of diuretics (T50.0-T50.2)

√6th **T46.5X Poisoning by, adverse effect of and underdosing of other antihypertensive drugs**

√7th T46.5X1 **Poisoning by other antihypertensive drugs, accidental (unintentional)**

Poisoning by other antihypertensive drugs NOS

√7th T46.5X2 **Poisoning by other antihypertensive drugs, intentional self-harm**

√7th T46.5X3 **Poisoning by other antihypertensive drugs, assault**

√7th T46.5X4 **Poisoning by other antihypertensive drugs, undetermined**

√7th T46.5X5 **Adverse effect of other antihypertensive drugs**

√7th T46.5X6 **Underdosing of other antihypertensive drugs**

√5th **T46.6 Poisoning by, adverse effect of and underdosing of antihyperlipidemic and antiarteriosclerotic drugs**

√6th **T46.6X Poisoning by, adverse effect of and underdosing of antihyperlipidemic and antiarteriosclerotic drugs**

√7th T46.6X1 **Poisoning by antihyperlipidemic and antiarteriosclerotic drugs, accidental (unintentional)**

Poisoning by antihyperlipidemic and antiarteriosclerotic drugs NOS

√7th T46.6X2 **Poisoning by antihyperlipidemic and antiarteriosclerotic drugs, intentional self-harm**

√7th T46.6X3 **Poisoning by antihyperlipidemic and antiarteriosclerotic drugs, assault**

√7th T46.6X4 **Poisoning by antihyperlipidemic and antiarteriosclerotic drugs, undetermined**

√7th T46.6X5 **Adverse effect of antihyperlipidemic and antiarteriosclerotic drugs**

√7th T46.6X6 **Underdosing of antihyperlipidemic and antiarteriosclerotic drugs**

√5th **T46.7 Poisoning by, adverse effect of and underdosing of peripheral vasodilators**

Poisoning by, adverse effect of and underdosing of nicotinic acid (derivatives)

EXCLUDES 1 *poisoning by, adverse effect of and underdosing of papaverine (T44.3)*

√6th **T46.7X Poisoning by, adverse effect of and underdosing of peripheral vasodilators**

√7th T46.7X1 **Poisoning by peripheral vasodilators, accidental (unintentional)**

Poisoning by peripheral vasodilators NOS

√7th T46.7X2 **Poisoning by peripheral vasodilators, intentional self-harm**

√7th T46.7X3 **Poisoning by peripheral vasodilators, assault**

√7th T46.7X4 **Poisoning by peripheral vasodilators, undetermined**

√7th T46.7X5 **Adverse effect of peripheral vasodilators**

√7th T46.7X6 **Underdosing of peripheral vasodilators**

√5th **T46.8 Poisoning by, adverse effect of and underdosing of antivaricose drugs, including sclerosing agents**

√6th **T46.8X Poisoning by, adverse effect of and underdosing of antivaricose drugs, including sclerosing agents**

√7th T46.8X1 **Poisoning by antivaricose drugs, including sclerosing agents, accidental (unintentional)**

Poisoning by antivaricose drugs, including sclerosing agents NOS

√7th T46.8X2 **Poisoning by antivaricose drugs, including sclerosing agents, intentional self-harm**

√7th T46.8X3 **Poisoning by antivaricose drugs, including sclerosing agents, assault**

√7th T46.8X4 **Poisoning by antivaricose drugs, including sclerosing agents, undetermined**

√7th T46.8X5 **Adverse effect of antivaricose drugs, including sclerosing agents**

√7th T46.8X6 **Underdosing of antivaricose drugs, including sclerosing agents**

√5th **T46.9 Poisoning by, adverse effect of and underdosing of other and unspecified agents primarily affecting the cardiovascular system**

√6th **T46.90 Poisoning by, adverse effect of and underdosing of unspecified agents primarily affecting the cardiovascular system**

√7th T46.901 **Poisoning by unspecified agents primarily affecting the cardiovascular system, accidental (unintentional)**

√7th T46.902 **Poisoning by unspecified agents primarily affecting the cardiovascular system, intentional self-harm**

√7th T46.903 **Poisoning by unspecified agents primarily affecting the cardiovascular system, assault**

✓7th **T46.9Ø4 Poisoning by unspecified agents primarily affecting the cardiovascular system, undetermined**

✓7th **T46.9Ø5 Adverse effect of unspecified agents primarily affecting the cardiovascular system**

✓7th **T46.9Ø6 Underdosing of unspecified agents primarily affecting the cardiovascular system**

✓6th **T46.99 Poisoning by, adverse effect of and underdosing of other agents primarily affecting the cardiovascular system**

✓7th **T46.991 Poisoning by other agents primarily affecting the cardiovascular system, accidental (unintentional)**

✓7th **T46.992 Poisoning by other agents primarily affecting the cardiovascular system, intentional self-harm**

✓7th **T46.993 Poisoning by other agents primarily affecting the cardiovascular system, assault**

✓7th **T46.994 Poisoning by other agents primarily affecting the cardiovascular system, undetermined**

✓7th **T46.995 Adverse effect of other agents primarily affecting the cardiovascular system**

✓7th **T46.996 Underdosing of other agents primarily affecting the cardiovascular system**

✓4th **T47 Poisoning by, adverse effect of and underdosing of agents primarily affecting the gastrointestinal system**

The appropriate 7th character is to be added to each code from category T47.
A initial encounter
D subsequent encounter
S sequela

✓5th **T47.Ø Poisoning by, adverse effect of and underdosing of histamine H2-receptor blockers**

✓6th **T47.ØX Poisoning by, adverse effect of and underdosing of histamine H2-receptor blockers**

✓7th **T47.ØX1 Poisoning by histamine H2-receptor blockers, accidental (unintentional)**
Poisoning by histamine H2-receptor blockers NOS

✓7th **T47.ØX2 Poisoning by histamine H2-receptor blockers, intentional self-harm**

✓7th **T47.ØX3 Poisoning by histamine H2-receptor blockers, assault**

✓7th **T47.ØX4 Poisoning by histamine H2-receptor blockers, undetermined**

✓7th **T47.ØX5 Adverse effect of histamine H2-receptor blockers**

✓7th **T47.ØX6 Underdosing of histamine H2-receptor blockers**

✓5th **T47.1 Poisoning by, adverse effect of and underdosing of other antacids and anti-gastric-secretion drugs**

✓6th **T47.1X Poisoning by, adverse effect of and underdosing of other antacids and anti-gastric-secretion drugs**

✓7th **T47.1X1 Poisoning by other antacids and anti-gastric-secretion drugs, accidental (unintentional)**
Poisoning by other antacids and anti-gastric-secretion drugs NOS

✓7th **T47.1X2 Poisoning by other antacids and anti-gastric-secretion drugs, intentional self-harm**

✓7th **T47.1X3 Poisoning by other antacids and anti-gastric-secretion drugs, assault**

✓7th **T47.1X4 Poisoning by other antacids and anti-gastric-secretion drugs, undetermined**

✓7th **T47.1X5 Adverse effect of other antacids and anti-gastric-secretion drugs**

✓7th **T47.1X6 Underdosing of other antacids and anti-gastric-secretion drugs**

✓5th **T47.2 Poisoning by, adverse effect of and underdosing of stimulant laxatives**

✓6th **T47.2X Poisoning by, adverse effect of and underdosing of stimulant laxatives**

✓7th **T47.2X1 Poisoning by stimulant laxatives, accidental (unintentional)**
Poisoning by stimulant laxatives NOS

✓7th **T47.2X2 Poisoning by stimulant laxatives, intentional self-harm**

✓7th **T47.2X3 Poisoning by stimulant laxatives, assault**

✓7th **T47.2X4 Poisoning by stimulant laxatives, undetermined**

✓7th **T47.2X5 Adverse effect of stimulant laxatives**

✓7th **T47.2X6 Underdosing of stimulant laxatives**

✓5th **T47.3 Poisoning by, adverse effect of and underdosing of saline and osmotic laxatives**

✓6th **T47.3X Poisoning by and adverse effect of saline and osmotic laxatives**

✓7th **T47.3X1 Poisoning by saline and osmotic laxatives, accidental (unintentional)**
Poisoning by saline and osmotic laxatives NOS

✓7th **T47.3X2 Poisoning by saline and osmotic laxatives, intentional self-harm**

✓7th **T47.3X3 Poisoning by saline and osmotic laxatives, assault**

✓7th **T47.3X4 Poisoning by saline and osmotic laxatives, undetermined**

✓7th **T47.3X5 Adverse effect of saline and osmotic laxatives**

✓7th **T47.3X6 Underdosing of saline and osmotic laxatives**

✓5th **T47.4 Poisoning by, adverse effect of and underdosing of other laxatives**

✓6th **T47.4X Poisoning by, adverse effect of and underdosing of other laxatives**

✓7th **T47.4X1 Poisoning by other laxatives, accidental (unintentional)**
Poisoning by other laxatives NOS

✓7th **T47.4X2 Poisoning by other laxatives, intentional self-harm**

✓7th **T47.4X3 Poisoning by other laxatives, assault**

✓7th **T47.4X4 Poisoning by other laxatives, undetermined**

✓7th **T47.4X5 Adverse effect of other laxatives**

✓7th **T47.4X6 Underdosing of other laxatives**

✓5th **T47.5 Poisoning by, adverse effect of and underdosing of digestants**

✓6th **T47.5X Poisoning by, adverse effect of and underdosing of digestants**

✓7th **T47.5X1 Poisoning by digestants, accidental (unintentional)**
Poisoning by digestants NOS

✓7th **T47.5X2 Poisoning by digestants, intentional self-harm**

✓7th **T47.5X3 Poisoning by digestants, assault**

✓7th **T47.5X4 Poisoning by digestants, undetermined**

✓7th **T47.5X5 Adverse effect of digestants**

✓7th **T47.5X6 Underdosing of digestants**

✓5th **T47.6 Poisoning by, adverse effect of and underdosing of antidiarrheal drugs**

EXCLUDES 2 *poisoning by, adverse effect of and underdosing of systemic antibiotics and other anti-infectives (T36-T37)*

✓6th **T47.6X Poisoning by, adverse effect of and underdosing of antidiarrheal drugs**

✓7th **T47.6X1 Poisoning by antidiarrheal drugs, accidental (unintentional)**
Poisoning by antidiarrheal drugs NOS

✓7th **T47.6X2 Poisoning by antidiarrheal drugs, intentional self-harm**

✓7th **T47.6X3 Poisoning by antidiarrheal drugs, assault**

✓7th **T47.6X4 Poisoning by antidiarrheal drugs, undetermined**

✓7th **T47.6X5 Adverse effect of antidiarrheal drugs**

√7th **T47.6X6 Underdosing of antidiarrheal drugs**

√5th **T47.7 Poisoning by, adverse effect of and underdosing of emetics**

√6th **T47.7X Poisoning by, adverse effect of and underdosing of emetics**

√7th **T47.7X1 Poisoning by emetics, accidental (unintentional)**
Poisoning by emetics NOS

√7th **T47.7X2 Poisoning by emetics, intentional self-harm**

√7th **T47.7X3 Poisoning by emetics, assault**

√7th **T47.7X4 Poisoning by emetics, undetermined**

√7th **T47.7X5 Adverse effect of emetics**

√7th **T47.7X6 Underdosing of emetics**

√5th **T47.8 Poisoning by, adverse effect of and underdosing of other agents primarily affecting gastrointestinal system**

√6th **T47.8X Poisoning by, adverse effect of and underdosing of other agents primarily affecting gastrointestinal system**

√7th **T47.8X1 Poisoning by other agents primarily affecting gastrointestinal system, accidental (unintentional)**
Poisoning by other agents primarily affecting gastrointestinal system NOS

√7th **T47.8X2 Poisoning by other agents primarily affecting gastrointestinal system, intentional self-harm**

√7th **T47.8X3 Poisoning by other agents primarily affecting gastrointestinal system, assault**

√7th **T47.8X4 Poisoning by other agents primarily affecting gastrointestinal system, undetermined**

√7th **T47.8X5 Adverse effect of other agents primarily affecting gastrointestinal system**

√7th **T47.8X6 Underdosing of other agents primarily affecting gastrointestinal system**

√5th **T47.9 Poisoning by, adverse effect of and underdosing of unspecified agents primarily affecting the gastrointestinal system**

√x7th **T47.91 Poisoning by unspecified agents primarily affecting the gastrointestinal system, accidental (unintentional)**
Poisoning by agents primarily affecting the gastrointestinal system NOS

√x7th **T47.92 Poisoning by unspecified agents primarily affecting the gastrointestinal system, intentional self-harm**

√x7th **T47.93 Poisoning by unspecified agents primarily affecting the gastrointestinal system, assault**

√x7th **T47.94 Poisoning by unspecified agents primarily affecting the gastrointestinal system, undetermined**

√x7th **T47.95 Adverse effect of unspecified agents primarily affecting the gastrointestinal system**

√x7th **T47.96 Underdosing of unspecified agents primarily affecting the gastrointestinal system**

√4th **T48 Poisoning by, adverse effect of and underdosing of agents primarily acting on smooth and skeletal muscles and the respiratory system**

The appropriate 7th character is to be added to each code from category T48.
A initial encounter
D subsequent encounter
S sequela

√5th **T48.0 Poisoning by, adverse effect of and underdosing of oxytocic drugs**

EXCLUDES 1 *poisoning by, adverse effect of and underdosing of estrogens, progestogens and antagonists (T38.4-T38.6)*

√6th **T48.0X Poisoning by, adverse effect of and underdosing of oxytocic drugs**

√7th **T48.0X1 Poisoning by oxytocic drugs, accidental (unintentional)**
Poisoning by oxytocic drugs NOS

√7th **T48.0X2 Poisoning by oxytocic drugs, intentional self-harm**

√7th **T48.0X3 Poisoning by oxytocic drugs, assault**

√7th **T48.0X4 Poisoning by oxytocic drugs, undetermined**

√7th **T48.0X5 Adverse effect of oxytocic drugs**

√7th **T48.0X6 Underdosing of oxytocic drugs**

√5th **T48.1 Poisoning by, adverse effect of and underdosing of skeletal muscle relaxants [neuromuscular blocking agents]**

√6th **T48.1X Poisoning by, adverse effect of and underdosing of skeletal muscle relaxants [neuromuscular blocking agents]**

√7th **T48.1X1 Poisoning by skeletal muscle relaxants [neuromuscular blocking agents], accidental (unintentional)**
Poisoning by skeletal muscle relaxants [neuromuscular blocking agents] NOS

√7th **T48.1X2 Poisoning by skeletal muscle relaxants [neuromuscular blocking agents], intentional self-harm**

√7th **T48.1X3 Poisoning by skeletal muscle relaxants [neuromuscular blocking agents], assault**

√7th **T48.1X4 Poisoning by skeletal muscle relaxants [neuromuscular blocking agents], undetermined**

√7th **T48.1X5 Adverse effect of skeletal muscle relaxants [neuromuscular blocking agents]**

√7th **T48.1X6 Underdosing of skeletal muscle relaxants [neuromuscular blocking agents]**

√5th **T48.2 Poisoning by, adverse effect of and underdosing of other and unspecified drugs acting on muscles**

√6th **T48.20 Poisoning by, adverse effect of and underdosing of unspecified drugs acting on muscles**

√7th **T48.201 Poisoning by unspecified drugs acting on muscles, accidental (unintentional)**
Poisoning by unspecified drugs acting on muscles NOS

√7th **T48.202 Poisoning by unspecified drugs acting on muscles, intentional self-harm**

√7th **T48.203 Poisoning by unspecified drugs acting on muscles, assault**

√7th **T48.204 Poisoning by unspecified drugs acting on muscles, undetermined**

√7th **T48.205 Adverse effect of unspecified drugs acting on muscles**

√7th **T48.206 Underdosing of unspecified drugs acting on muscles**

√6th **T48.29 Poisoning by, adverse effect of and underdosing of other drugs acting on muscles**

√7th **T48.291 Poisoning by other drugs acting on muscles, accidental (unintentional)**
Poisoning by other drugs acting on muscles NOS

√7th **T48.292 Poisoning by other drugs acting on muscles, intentional self-harm**

√7th **T48.293 Poisoning by other drugs acting on muscles, assault**

√7th **T48.294 Poisoning by other drugs acting on muscles, undetermined**

√7th **T48.295 Adverse effect of other drugs acting on muscles**

√7th **T48.296 Underdosing of other drugs acting on muscles**

√5th **T48.3 Poisoning by, adverse effect of and underdosing of antitussives**

√6th **T48.3X Poisoning by, adverse effect of and underdosing of antitussives**

√7th **T48.3X1 Poisoning by antitussives, accidental (unintentional)**
Poisoning by antitussives NOS

√7th **T48.3X2 Poisoning by antitussives, intentional self-harm**

√7th **T48.3X3 Poisoning by antitussives, assault**

√7th **T48.3X4 Poisoning by antitussives, undetermined**

√7th **T48.3X5 Adverse effect of antitussives**

√ Appropriate additional character required √x7th Requires 7th character, placeholder x must fill empty characters

7th T48.3X6 **Underdosing of antitussives**

5th T48.4 **Poisoning by, adverse effect of and underdosing of expectorants**

6th T48.4X **Poisoning by, adverse effect of and underdosing of expectorants**

7th T48.4X1 **Poisoning by expectorants, accidental (unintentional)**
Poisoning by expectorants NOS

7th T48.4X2 **Poisoning by expectorants, intentional self-harm**

7th T48.4X3 **Poisoning by expectorants, assault**

7th T48.4X4 **Poisoning by expectorants, undetermined**

7th T48.4X5 **Adverse effect of expectorants**

7th T48.4X6 **Underdosing of expectorants**

5th T48.5 **Poisoning by, adverse effect of and underdosing of other anti-common-cold drugs**
Poisoning by, adverse effect of and underdosing of decongestants

EXCLUDES 2 *poisoning by, adverse effect of and underdosing of antipyretics, NEC (T39.9-)*
poisoning by, adverse effect of and underdosing of non-steroidal antiinflammatory drugs (T39.3-)
poisoning by, adverse effect of and underdosing of salicylates (T39.0-)

6th T48.5X **Poisoning by, adverse effect of and underdosing of other anti-common-cold drugs**

7th T48.5X1 **Poisoning by other anti-common-cold drugs, accidental (unintentional)**
Poisoning by other anti-common-cold drugs NOS

7th T48.5X2 **Poisoning by other anti-common-cold drugs, intentional self-harm**

7th T48.5X3 **Poisoning by other anti-common-cold drugs, assault**

7th T48.5X4 **Poisoning by other anti-common-cold drugs, undetermined**

7th T48.5X5 **Adverse effect of other anti-common-cold drugs**

7th T48.5X6 **Underdosing of other anti-common-cold drugs**

5th T48.6 **Poisoning by, adverse effect of and underdosing of antiasthmatics, not elsewhere classified**
Poisoning by, adverse effect of and underdosing of beta-adrenoreceptor agonists used in asthma therapy

EXCLUDES 1 *poisoning by, adverse effect of and underdosing of beta-adrenoreceptor agonists not used in asthma therapy (T44.5)*
poisoning by, adverse effect of and underdosing of anterior pituitary [adenohypophyseal] hormones (T38.8)

6th T48.6X **Poisoning by, adverse effect of and underdosing of antiasthmatics**

7th T48.6X1 **Poisoning by antiasthmatics, accidental (unintentional)**
Poisoning by antiasthmatics NOS

7th T48.6X2 **Poisoning by antiasthmatics, intentional self-harm**

7th T48.6X3 **Poisoning by antiasthmatics, assault**

7th T48.6X4 **Poisoning by antiasthmatics, undetermined**

7th T48.6X5 **Adverse effect of antiasthmatics**

7th T48.6X6 **Underdosing of antiasthmatics**

5th T48.9 **Poisoning by, adverse effect of and underdosing of other and unspecified agents primarily acting on the respiratory system**

6th T48.90 **Poisoning by, adverse effect of and underdosing of unspecified agents primarily acting on the respiratory system**

7th T48.901 **Poisoning by unspecified agents primarily acting on the respiratory system, accidental (unintentional)**

7th T48.902 **Poisoning by unspecified agents primarily acting on the respiratory system, intentional self-harm**

7th T48.903 **Poisoning by unspecified agents primarily acting on the respiratory system, assault**

7th T48.904 **Poisoning by unspecified agents primarily acting on the respiratory system, undetermined**

7th T48.905 **Adverse effect of unspecified agents primarily acting on the respiratory system**

7th T48.906 **Underdosing of unspecified agents primarily acting on the respiratory system**

6th T48.99 **Poisoning by, adverse effect of and underdosing of other agents primarily acting on the respiratory system**

7th T48.991 **Poisoning by other agents primarily acting on the respiratory system, accidental (unintentional)**

7th T48.992 **Poisoning by other agents primarily acting on the respiratory system, intentional self-harm**

7th T48.993 **Poisoning by other agents primarily acting on the respiratory system, assault**

7th T48.994 **Poisoning by other agents primarily acting on the respiratory system, undetermined**

7th T48.995 **Adverse effect of other agents primarily acting on the respiratory system**

7th T48.996 **Underdosing of other agents primarily acting on the respiratory system**

4th **T49 Poisoning by, adverse effect of and underdosing of topical agents primarily affecting skin and mucous membrane and by ophthalmological, otorhinolaryngological and dental drugs**
Poisoning by, adverse effect of and underdosing of glucocorticoids, topically used

The appropriate 7th character is to be added to each code from category T49.
A initial encounter
D subsequent encounter
S sequela

5th T49.0 **Poisoning by, adverse effect of and underdosing of local antifungal, anti-infective and anti-inflammatory drugs**

6th T49.0X **Poisoning by, adverse effect of and underdosing of local antifungal, anti-infective and anti-inflammatory drugs**

7th T49.0X1 **Poisoning by local antifungal, anti-infective and anti-inflammatory drugs, accidental (unintentional)**
Poisoning by local antifungal, anti-infective and anti-inflammatory drugs NOS

7th T49.0X2 **Poisoning by local antifungal, anti-infective and anti-inflammatory drugs, intentional self-harm**

7th T49.0X3 **Poisoning by local antifungal, anti-infective and anti-inflammatory drugs, assault**

7th T49.0X4 **Poisoning by local antifungal, anti-infective and anti-inflammatory drugs, undetermined**

7th T49.0X5 **Adverse effect of local antifungal, anti-infective and anti-inflammatory drugs**

7th T49.0X6 **Underdosing of local antifungal, anti-infective and anti-inflammatory drugs**

5th T49.1 **Poisoning by, adverse effect of and underdosing of antipruritics**

6th T49.1X **Poisoning by, adverse effect of and underdosing of antipruritics**

7th T49.1X1 **Poisoning by antipruritics, accidental (unintentional)**
Poisoning by antipruritics NOS

7th T49.1X2 **Poisoning by antipruritics, intentional self-harm**

7th T49.1X3 **Poisoning by antipruritics, assault**

7th T49.1X4 **Poisoning by antipruritics, undetermined**

7th T49.1X5 **Adverse effect of antipruritics**

7th T49.1X6 **Underdosing of antipruritics**

✓5th **T49.2 Poisoning by, adverse effect of and underdosing of local astringents and local detergents**

✓6th **T49.2X Poisoning by, adverse effect of and underdosing of local astringents and local detergents**

✓7th **T49.2X1 Poisoning by local astringents and local detergents, accidental (unintentional)**
Poisoning by local astringents and local detergents NOS

✓7th **T49.2X2 Poisoning by local astringents and local detergents, intentional self-harm**

✓7th **T49.2X3 Poisoning by local astringents and local detergents, assault**

✓7th **T49.2X4 Poisoning by local astringents and local detergents, undetermined**

✓7th **T49.2X5 Adverse effect of local astringents and local detergents**

✓7th **T49.2X6 Underdosing of local astringents and local detergents**

✓5th **T49.3 Poisoning by, adverse effect of and underdosing of emollients, demulcents and protectants**

✓6th **T49.3X Poisoning by, adverse effect of and underdosing of emollients, demulcents and protectants**

✓7th **T49.3X1 Poisoning by emollients, demulcents and protectants, accidental (unintentional)**
Poisoning by emollients, demulcents and protectants NOS

✓7th **T49.3X2 Poisoning by emollients, demulcents and protectants, intentional self-harm**

✓7th **T49.3X3 Poisoning by emollients, demulcents and protectants, assault**

✓7th **T49.3X4 Poisoning by emollients, demulcents and protectants, undetermined**

✓7th **T49.3X5 Adverse effect of emollients, demulcents and protectants**

✓7th **T49.3X6 Underdosing of emollients, demulcents and protectants**

✓5th **T49.4 Poisoning by, adverse effect of and underdosing of keratolytics, keratoplastics, and other hair treatment drugs and preparations**

✓6th **T49.4X Poisoning by, adverse effect of and underdosing of keratolytics, keratoplastics, and other hair treatment drugs and preparations**

✓7th **T49.4X1 Poisoning by keratolytics, keratoplastics, and other hair treatment drugs and preparations, accidental (unintentional)**
Poisoning by keratolytics, keratoplastics, and other hair treatment drugs and preparations NOS

✓7th **T49.4X2 Poisoning by keratolytics, keratoplastics, and other hair treatment drugs and preparations, intentional self-harm**

✓7th **T49.4X3 Poisoning by keratolytics, keratoplastics, and other hair treatment drugs and preparations, assault**

✓7th **T49.4X4 Poisoning by keratolytics, keratoplastics, and other hair treatment drugs and preparations, undetermined**

✓7th **T49.4X5 Adverse effect of keratolytics, keratoplastics, and other hair treatment drugs and preparations**

✓7th **T49.4X6 Underdosing of keratolytics, keratoplastics, and other hair treatment drugs and preparations**

✓5th **T49.5 Poisoning by, adverse effect of and underdosing of ophthalmological drugs and preparations**

✓6th **T49.5X Poisoning by, adverse effect of and underdosing of ophthalmological drugs and preparations**

✓7th **T49.5X1 Poisoning by ophthalmological drugs and preparations, accidental (unintentional)**
Poisoning by ophthalmological drugs and preparations NOS

✓7th **T49.5X2 Poisoning by ophthalmological drugs and preparations, intentional self-harm**

✓7th **T49.5X3 Poisoning by ophthalmological drugs and preparations, assault**

✓7th **T49.5X4 Poisoning by ophthalmological drugs and preparations, undetermined**

✓7th **T49.5X5 Adverse effect of ophthalmological drugs and preparations**

✓7th **T49.5X6 Underdosing of ophthalmological drugs and preparations**

✓5th **T49.6 Poisoning by, adverse effect of and underdosing of otorhinolaryngological drugs and preparations**

✓6th **T49.6X Poisoning by, adverse effect of and underdosing of otorhinolaryngological drugs and preparations**

✓7th **T49.6X1 Poisoning by otorhinolaryngological drugs and preparations, accidental (unintentional)**
Poisoning by otorhinolaryngological drugs and preparations NOS

✓7th **T49.6X2 Poisoning by otorhinolaryngological drugs and preparations, intentional self-harm**

✓7th **T49.6X3 Poisoning by otorhinolaryngological drugs and preparations, assault**

✓7th **T49.6X4 Poisoning by otorhinolaryngological drugs and preparations, undetermined**

✓7th **T49.6X5 Adverse effect of otorhinolaryngological drugs and preparations**

✓7th **T49.6X6 Underdosing of otorhinolaryngological drugs and preparations**

✓5th **T49.7 Poisoning by, adverse effect of and underdosing of dental drugs, topically applied**

✓6th **T49.7X Poisoning by, adverse effect of and underdosing of dental drugs, topically applied**

✓7th **T49.7X1 Poisoning by dental drugs, topically applied, accidental (unintentional)**
Poisoning by dental drugs, topically applied NOS

✓7th **T49.7X2 Poisoning by dental drugs, topically applied, intentional self-harm**

✓7th **T49.7X3 Poisoning by dental drugs, topically applied, assault**

✓7th **T49.7X4 Poisoning by dental drugs, topically applied, undetermined**

✓7th **T49.7X5 Adverse effect of dental drugs, topically applied**

✓7th **T49.7X6 Underdosing of dental drugs, topically applied**

✓5th **T49.8 Poisoning by, adverse effect of and underdosing of other topical agents**
Poisoning by, adverse effect of and underdosing of spermicides

✓6th **T49.8X Poisoning by, adverse effect of and underdosing of other topical agents**

✓7th **T49.8X1 Poisoning by other topical agents, accidental (unintentional)**
Poisoning by other topical agents NOS

✓7th **T49.8X2 Poisoning by other topical agents, intentional self-harm**

✓7th **T49.8X3 Poisoning by other topical agents, assault**

✓7th **T49.8X4 Poisoning by other topical agents, undetermined**

✓7th **T49.8X5 Adverse effect of other topical agents**

✓7th **T49.8X6 Underdosing of other topical agents**

✓5th **T49.9 Poisoning by, adverse effect of and underdosing of unspecified topical agent**

✓x7th **T49.91 Poisoning by unspecified topical agent, accidental (unintentional)**

✓x7th **T49.92 Poisoning by unspecified topical agent, intentional self-harm**

✓x7th **T49.93 Poisoning by unspecified topical agent, assault**

✓x7th **T49.94 Poisoning by unspecified topical agent, undetermined**

✓x7th **T49.95 Adverse effect of unspecified topical agent**

✓x7th **T49.96 Underdosing of unspecified topical agent**

✓ Appropriate additional character required
✓x7th Requires 7th character, placeholder x must fill empty characters

4th T50 Poisoning by, adverse effect of and underdosing of diuretics and other and unspecified drugs, medicaments and biological substances

The appropriate 7th character is to be added to each code from category T50.
A initial encounter
D subsequent encounter
S sequela

5th T50.0 Poisoning by, adverse effect of and underdosing of mineralocorticoids and their antagonists

6th T50.0X Poisoning by, adverse effect of and underdosing of mineralocorticoids and their antagonists

7th T50.0X1 Poisoning by mineralocorticoids and their antagonists, accidental (unintentional)
Poisoning by mineralocorticoids and their antagonists NOS

7th T50.0X2 Poisoning by mineralocorticoids and their antagonists, intentional self-harm

7th T50.0X3 Poisoning by mineralocorticoids and their antagonists, assault

7th T50.0X4 Poisoning by mineralocorticoids and their antagonists, undetermined

7th T50.0X5 Adverse effect of mineralocorticoids and their antagonists

7th T50.0X6 Underdosing of mineralocorticoids and their antagonists

5th T50.1 Poisoning by, adverse effect of and underdosing of loop [high-ceiling] diuretics

6th T50.1X Poisoning by, adverse effect of and underdosing of loop [high-ceiling] diuretics

7th T50.1X1 Poisoning by loop [high-ceiling] diuretics, accidental (unintentional)
Poisoning by loop [high-ceiling] diuretics NOS

7th T50.1X2 Poisoning by loop [high-ceiling] diuretics, intentional self-harm

7th T50.1X3 Poisoning by loop [high-ceiling] diuretics, assault

7th T50.1X4 Poisoning by loop [high-ceiling] diuretics, undetermined

7th T50.1X5 Adverse effect of loop [high-ceiling] diuretics

7th T50.1X6 Underdosing of loop [high-ceiling] diuretics

5th T50.2 Poisoning by, adverse effect of and underdosing of carbonic-anhydrase inhibitors, benzothiadiazides and other diuretics
Poisoning by, adverse effect of and underdosing of acetazolamide

6th T50.2X Poisoning by, adverse effect of and underdosing of carbonic-anhydrase inhibitors, benzothiadiazides and other diuretics

7th T50.2X1 Poisoning by carbonic-anhydrase inhibitors, benzothiadiazides and other diuretics, accidental (unintentional)
Poisoning by carbonic-anhydrase inhibitors, benzothiadiazides and other diuretics NOS

7th T50.2X2 Poisoning by carbonic-anhydrase inhibitors, benzothiadiazides and other diuretics, intentional self-harm

7th T50.2X3 Poisoning by carbonic-anhydrase inhibitors, benzothiadiazides and other diuretics, assault

7th T50.2X4 Poisoning by carbonic-anhydrase inhibitors, benzothiadiazides and other diuretics, undetermined

7th T50.2X5 Adverse effect of carbonic-anhydrase inhibitors, benzothiadiazides and other diuretics

7th T50.2X6 Underdosing of carbonic-anhydrase inhibitors, benzothiadiazides and other diuretics

5th T50.3 Poisoning by, adverse effect of and underdosing of electrolytic, caloric and water-balance agents
Poisoning by, adverse effect of and underdosing of oral rehydration salts

6th T50.3X Poisoning by, adverse effect of and underdosing of electrolytic, caloric and water-balance agents

7th T50.3X1 Poisoning by electrolytic, caloric and water-balance agents, accidental (unintentional)
Poisoning by electrolytic, caloric and water-balance agents NOS

7th T50.3X2 Poisoning by electrolytic, caloric and water-balance agents, intentional self-harm

7th T50.3X3 Poisoning by electrolytic, caloric and water-balance agents, assault

7th T50.3X4 Poisoning by electrolytic, caloric and water-balance agents, undetermined

7th T50.3X5 Adverse effect of electrolytic, caloric and water-balance agents

7th T50.3X6 Underdosing of electrolytic, caloric and water-balance agents

5th T50.4 Poisoning by, adverse effect of and underdosing of drugs affecting uric acid metabolism

6th T50.4X Poisoning by, adverse effect of and underdosing of drugs affecting uric acid metabolism

7th T50.4X1 Poisoning by drugs affecting uric acid metabolism, accidental (unintentional)
Poisoning by drugs affecting uric acid metabolism NOS

7th T50.4X2 Poisoning by drugs affecting uric acid metabolism, intentional self-harm

7th T50.4X3 Poisoning by drugs affecting uric acid metabolism, assault

7th T50.4X4 Poisoning by drugs affecting uric acid metabolism, undetermined

7th T50.4X5 Adverse effect of drugs affecting uric acid metabolism

7th T50.4X6 Underdosing of drugs affecting uric acid metabolism

5th T50.5 Poisoning by, adverse effect of and underdosing of appetite depressants

6th T50.5X Poisoning by, adverse effect of and underdosing of appetite depressants

7th T50.5X1 Poisoning by appetite depressants, accidental (unintentional)
Poisoning by appetite depressants NOS

7th T50.5X2 Poisoning by appetite depressants, intentional self-harm

7th T50.5X3 Poisoning by appetite depressants, assault

7th T50.5X4 Poisoning by appetite depressants, undetermined

7th T50.5X5 Adverse effect of appetite depressants

7th T50.5X6 Underdosing of appetite depressants

5th T50.6 Poisoning by, adverse effect of and underdosing of antidotes and chelating agents
Poisoning by, adverse effect of and underdosing of alcohol deterrents

6th T50.6X Poisoning by, adverse effect of and underdosing of antidotes and chelating agents

7th T50.6X1 Poisoning by antidotes and chelating agents, accidental (unintentional)
Poisoning by antidotes and chelating agents NOS

7th T50.6X2 Poisoning by antidotes and chelating agents, intentional self-harm

7th T50.6X3 Poisoning by antidotes and chelating agents, assault

7th T50.6X4 Poisoning by antidotes and chelating agents, undetermined

7th T50.6X5 Adverse effect of antidotes and chelating agents

7th T50.6X6 Underdosing of antidotes and chelating agents

✓5th **T5Ø.7 Poisoning by, adverse effect of and underdosing of analeptics and opioid receptor antagonists**

✓6th **T5Ø.7X Poisoning by, adverse effect of and underdosing of analeptics and opioid receptor antagonists**

✓7th **T5Ø.7X1 Poisoning by analeptics and opioid receptor antagonists, accidental (unintentional)**
Poisoning by analeptics and opioid receptor antagonists NOS

✓7th **T5Ø.7X2 Poisoning by analeptics and opioid receptor antagonists, intentional self-harm**

✓7th **T5Ø.7X3 Poisoning by analeptics and opioid receptor antagonists, assault**

✓7th **T5Ø.7X4 Poisoning by analeptics and opioid receptor antagonists, undetermined**

✓7th **T5Ø.7X5 Adverse effect of analeptics and opioid receptor antagonists**

✓7th **T5Ø.7X6 Underdosing of analeptics and opioid receptor antagonists**

✓5th **T5Ø.8 Poisoning by, adverse effect of and underdosing of diagnostic agents**

✓6th **T5Ø.8X Poisoning by, adverse effect of and underdosing of diagnostic agents**

✓7th **T5Ø.8X1 Poisoning by diagnostic agents, accidental (unintentional)**
Poisoning by diagnostic agents NOS

✓7th **T5Ø.8X2 Poisoning by diagnostic agents, intentional self-harm**

✓7th **T5Ø.8X3 Poisoning by diagnostic agents, assault**

✓7th **T5Ø.8X4 Poisoning by diagnostic agents, undetermined**

✓7th **T5Ø.8X5 Adverse effect of diagnostic agents**

✓7th **T5Ø.8X6 Underdosing of diagnostic agents**

✓5th **T5Ø.A Poisoning by, adverse effect of and underdosing of bacterial vaccines**

✓6th **T5Ø.A1 Poisoning by, adverse effect of and underdosing of pertussis vaccine, including combinations with a pertussis component**

✓7th **T5Ø.A11 Poisoning by pertussis vaccine, including combinations with a pertussis component, accidental (unintentional)**

✓7th **T5Ø.A12 Poisoning by pertussis vaccine, including combinations with a pertussis component, intentional self-harm**

✓7th **T5Ø.A13 Poisoning by pertussis vaccine, including combinations with a pertussis component, assault**

✓7th **T5Ø.A14 Poisoning by pertussis vaccine, including combinations with a pertussis component, undetermined**

✓7th **T5Ø.A15 Adverse effect of pertussis vaccine, including combinations with a pertussis component**

✓7th **T5Ø.A16 Underdosing of pertussis vaccine, including combinations with a pertussis component**

✓6th **T5Ø.A2 Poisoning by, adverse effect of and underdosing of mixed bacterial vaccines without a pertussis component**

✓7th **T5Ø.A21 Poisoning by mixed bacterial vaccines without a pertussis component, accidental (unintentional)**

✓7th **T5Ø.A22 Poisoning by mixed bacterial vaccines without a pertussis component, intentional self-harm**

✓7th **T5Ø.A23 Poisoning by mixed bacterial vaccines without a pertussis component, assault**

✓7th **T5Ø.A24 Poisoning by mixed bacterial vaccines without a pertussis component, undetermined**

✓7th **T5Ø.A25 Adverse effect of mixed bacterial vaccines without a pertussis component**

✓7th **T5Ø.A26 Underdosing of mixed bacterial vaccines without a pertussis component**

✓6th **T5Ø.A9 Poisoning by, adverse effect of and underdosing of other bacterial vaccines**

✓7th **T5Ø.A91 Poisoning by other bacterial vaccines, accidental (unintentional)**

✓7th **T5Ø.A92 Poisoning by other bacterial vaccines, intentional self-harm**

✓7th **T5Ø.A93 Poisoning by other bacterial vaccines, assault**

✓7th **T5Ø.A94 Poisoning by other bacterial vaccines, undetermined**

✓7th **T5Ø.A95 Adverse effect of other bacterial vaccines**

✓7th **T5Ø.A96 Underdosing of other bacterial vaccines**

✓5th **T5Ø.B Poisoning by, adverse effect of and underdosing of viral vaccines**

✓6th **T5Ø.B1 Poisoning by, adverse effect of and underdosing of smallpox vaccines**

✓7th **T5Ø.B11 Poisoning by smallpox vaccines, accidental (unintentional)**

✓7th **T5Ø.B12 Poisoning by smallpox vaccines, intentional self-harm**

✓7th **T5Ø.B13 Poisoning by smallpox vaccines, assault**

✓7th **T5Ø.B14 Poisoning by smallpox vaccines, undetermined**

✓7th **T5Ø.B15 Adverse effect of smallpox vaccines**

✓7th **T5Ø.B16 Underdosing of smallpox vaccines**

✓6th **T5Ø.B9 Poisoning by, adverse effect of and underdosing of other viral vaccines**

✓7th **T5Ø.B91 Poisoning by other viral vaccines, accidental (unintentional)**

✓7th **T5Ø.B92 Poisoning by other viral vaccines, intentional self-harm**

✓7th **T5Ø.B93 Poisoning by other viral vaccines, assault**

✓7th **T5Ø.B94 Poisoning by other viral vaccines, undetermined**

✓7th **T5Ø.B95 Adverse effect of other viral vaccines**

✓7th **T5Ø.B96 Underdosing of other viral vaccines**

✓5th **T5Ø.Z Poisoning by, adverse effect of and underdosing of other vaccines and biological substances**

✓6th **T5Ø.Z1 Poisoning by, adverse effect of and underdosing of immunoglobulin**

✓7th **T5Ø.Z11 Poisoning by immunoglobulin, accidental (unintentional)**

✓7th **T5Ø.Z12 Poisoning by immunoglobulin, intentional self-harm**

✓7th **T5Ø.Z13 Poisoning by immunoglobulin, assault**

✓7th **T5Ø.Z14 Poisoning by immunoglobulin, undetermined**

✓7th **T5Ø.Z15 Adverse effect of immunoglobulin**

✓7th **T5Ø.Z16 Underdosing of immunoglobulin**

✓6th **T5Ø.Z9 Poisoning by, adverse effect of and underdosing of other vaccines and biological substances**

✓7th **T5Ø.Z91 Poisoning by other vaccines and biological substances, accidental (unintentional)**

✓7th **T5Ø.Z92 Poisoning by other vaccines and biological substances, intentional self-harm**

✓7th **T5Ø.Z93 Poisoning by other vaccines and biological substances, assault**

✓7th **T5Ø.Z94 Poisoning by other vaccines and biological substances, undetermined**

✓7th **T5Ø.Z95 Adverse effect of other vaccines and biological substances**

✓7th **T5Ø.Z96 Underdosing of other vaccines and biological substances**

✓5th **T5Ø.9 Poisoning by, adverse effect of and underdosing of other and unspecified drugs, medicaments and biological substances**

✓6th **T5Ø.9Ø Poisoning by, adverse effect of and underdosing of unspecified drugs, medicaments and biological substances**

✓7th **T5Ø.9Ø1 Poisoning by unspecified drugs, medicaments and biological substances, accidental (unintentional)**

7th **T50.902 Poisoning by unspecified drugs, medicaments and biological substances, intentional self-harm**

7th **T50.903 Poisoning by unspecified drugs, medicaments and biological substances, assault**

7th **T50.904 Poisoning by unspecified drugs, medicaments and biological substances, undetermined**

7th **T50.905 Adverse effect of unspecified drugs, medicaments and biological substances**

7th **T50.906 Underdosing of unspecified drugs, medicaments and biological substances**

6th **T50.99 Poisoning by, adverse effect of and underdosing of other drugs, medicaments and biological substances**

7th **T50.991 Poisoning by other drugs, medicaments and biological substances, accidental (unintentional)**

7th **T50.992 Poisoning by other drugs, medicaments and biological substances, intentional self-harm**

7th **T50.993 Poisoning by other drugs, medicaments and biological substances, assault**

7th **T50.994 Poisoning by other drugs, medicaments and biological substances, undetermined**

7th **T50.995 Adverse effect of other drugs, medicaments and biological substances**

7th **T50.996 Underdosing of other drugs, medicaments and biological substances**

Toxic effects of substances chiefly nonmedicinal as to source (T51-T65)

Use additional code(s) for all associated manifestations of toxic effect, such as:
personal history of foreign body fully removed (Z87.821)
respiratory conditions due to external agents (J60-J70)
to identify any retained foreign body, if applicable (Z18.-)

NOTE When no intent is indicated code to accidental. Undetermined intent is only for use when there is specific documentation in the record that the intent of the toxic effect cannot be determined

EXCLUDES 1 *contact with and (suspected) exposure to toxic substances (Z77.-)*

4th **T51 Toxic effect of alcohol**

The appropriate 7th character is to be added to each code from category T51.
A initial encounter
D subsequent encounter
S sequela

5th **T51.0 Toxic effect of ethanol**
Toxic effect of ethyl alcohol
EXCLUDES 2 *acute alcohol intoxication or 'hangover' effects (F10.129, F10.229, F10.929)*
drunkenness (F10.129, F10.229, F10.929)
pathological alcohol intoxication (F10.129, F10.229, F10.929)

6th **T51.0X Toxic effect of ethanol**

7th **T51.0X1 Toxic effect of ethanol, accidental (unintentional)**
Toxic effect of ethanol NOS

7th **T51.0X2 Toxic effect of ethanol, intentional self-harm**

7th **T51.0X3 Toxic effect of ethanol, assault**

7th **T51.0X4 Toxic effect of ethanol, undetermined**

5th **T51.1 Toxic effect of methanol**
Toxic effect of methyl alcohol

6th **T51.1X Toxic effect of methanol**

7th **T51.1X1 Toxic effect of methanol, accidental (unintentional)**
Toxic effect of methanol NOS

7th **T51.1X2 Toxic effect of methanol, intentional self-harm**

7th **T51.1X3 Toxic effect of methanol, assault**

7th **T51.1X4 Toxic effect of methanol, undetermined**

5th **T51.2 Toxic effect of 2-Propanol**
Toxic effect of isopropyl alcohol

6th **T51.2X Toxic effect of 2-Propanol**

7th **T51.2X1 Toxic effect of 2-Propanol, accidental (unintentional)**
Toxic effect of 2-Propanol NOS

7th **T51.2X2 Toxic effect of 2-Propanol, intentional self-harm**

7th **T51.2X3 Toxic effect of 2-Propanol, assault**

7th **T51.2X4 Toxic effect of 2-Propanol, undetermined**

5th **T51.3 Toxic effect of fusel oil**
Toxic effect of amyl alcohol
Toxic effect of butyl [1-butanol] alcohol
Toxic effect of propyl [1-propanol] alcohol

6th **T51.3X Toxic effect of fusel oil**

7th **T51.3X1 Toxic effect of fusel oil, accidental (unintentional)**
Toxic effect of fusel oil NOS

7th **T51.3X2 Toxic effect of fusel oil, intentional self-harm**

7th **T51.3X3 Toxic effect of fusel oil, assault**

7th **T51.3X4 Toxic effect of fusel oil, undetermined**

5th **T51.8 Toxic effect of other alcohols**

6th **T51.8X Toxic effect of other alcohols**

7th **T51.8X1 Toxic effect of other alcohols, accidental (unintentional)**
Toxic effect of other alcohols NOS

7th **T51.8X2 Toxic effect of other alcohols, intentional self-harm**

7th **T51.8X3 Toxic effect of other alcohols, assault**

7th **T51.8X4 Toxic effect of other alcohols, undetermined**

5th **T51.9 Toxic effect of unspecified alcohol**

x7th **T51.91 Toxic effect of unspecified alcohol, accidental (unintentional)**

x7th **T51.92 Toxic effect of unspecified alcohol, intentional self-harm**

x7th **T51.93 Toxic effect of unspecified alcohol, assault**

x7th **T51.94 Toxic effect of unspecified alcohol, undetermined**

4th **T52 Toxic effect of organic solvents**
EXCLUDES 1 *halogen derivatives of aliphatic and aromatic hydrocarbons (T53.-)*

The appropriate 7th character is to be added to each code from category T52.
A initial encounter
D subsequent encounter
S sequela

5th **T52.0 Toxic effects of petroleum products**
Toxic effects of gasoline [petrol]
Toxic effects of kerosene [paraffin oil]
Toxic effects of paraffin wax
Toxic effects of ether petroleum
Toxic effects of naphtha petroleum
Toxic effects of spirit petroleum

6th **T52.0X Toxic effects of petroleum products**

7th **T52.0X1 Toxic effect of petroleum products, accidental (unintentional)**
Toxic effects of petroleum products NOS

7th **T52.0X2 Toxic effect of petroleum products, intentional self-harm**

7th **T52.0X3 Toxic effect of petroleum products, assault**

7th **T52.0X4 Toxic effect of petroleum products, undetermined**

5th **T52.1 Toxic effects of benzene**
EXCLUDES 1 *homologues of benzene (T52.2)*
nitroderivatives and aminoderivatives of benzene and its homologues (T65.3)

6th **T52.1X Toxic effects of benzene**

7th **T52.1X1 Toxic effect of benzene, accidental (unintentional)**
Toxic effects of benzene NOS

7th **T52.1X2 Toxic effect of benzene, intentional self-harm**

7th **T52.1X3 Toxic effect of benzene, assault**

T52.1X4 Toxic effect of benzene, undetermined

T52.2 Toxic effects of homologues of benzene
Toxic effects of toluene [methylbenzene]
Toxic effects of xylene [dimethylbenzene]

T52.2X Toxic effects of homologues of benzene
- T52.2X1 Toxic effect of homologues of benzene, accidental (unintentional)
  Toxic effects of homologues of benzene NOS
- T52.2X2 Toxic effect of homologues of benzene, intentional self-harm
- T52.2X3 Toxic effect of homologues of benzene, assault
- T52.2X4 Toxic effect of homologues of benzene, undetermined

T52.3 Toxic effects of glycols

T52.3X Toxic effects of glycols
- T52.3X1 Toxic effect of glycols, accidental (unintentional)
  Toxic effects of glycols NOS
- T52.3X2 Toxic effect of glycols, intentional self-harm
- T52.3X3 Toxic effect of glycols, assault
- T52.3X4 Toxic effect of glycols, undetermined

T52.4 Toxic effects of ketones

T52.4X Toxic effects of ketones
- T52.4X1 Toxic effect of ketones, accidental (unintentional)
  Toxic effects of ketones NOS
- T52.4X2 Toxic effect of ketones, intentional self-harm
- T52.4X3 Toxic effect of ketones, assault
- T52.4X4 Toxic effect of ketones, undetermined

T52.8 Toxic effects of other organic solvents

T52.8X Toxic effects of other organic solvents
- T52.8X1 Toxic effect of other organic solvents, accidental (unintentional)
  Toxic effects of other organic solvents NOS
- T52.8X2 Toxic effect of other organic solvents, intentional self-harm
- T52.8X3 Toxic effect of other organic solvents, assault
- T52.8X4 Toxic effect of other organic solvents, undetermined

T52.9 Toxic effects of unspecified organic solvent
- T52.91 Toxic effect of unspecified organic solvent, accidental (unintentional)
- T52.92 Toxic effect of unspecified organic solvent, intentional self-harm
- T52.93 Toxic effect of unspecified organic solvent, assault
- T52.94 Toxic effect of unspecified organic solvent, undetermined

T53 Toxic effect of halogen derivatives of aliphatic and aromatic hydrocarbons

The appropriate 7th character is to be added to each code from category T53.
A initial encounter
D subsequent encounter
S sequela

T53.0 Toxic effects of carbon tetrachloride
Toxic effects of tetrachloromethane

T53.0X Toxic effects of carbon tetrachloride
- T53.0X1 Toxic effect of carbon tetrachloride, accidental (unintentional)
  Toxic effects of carbon tetrachloride NOS
- T53.0X2 Toxic effect of carbon tetrachloride, intentional self-harm
- T53.0X3 Toxic effect of carbon tetrachloride, assault
- T53.0X4 Toxic effect of carbon tetrachloride, undetermined

T53.1 Toxic effects of chloroform
Toxic effects of trichloromethane

T53.1X Toxic effects of chloroform
- T53.1X1 Toxic effect of chloroform, accidental (unintentional)
  Toxic effects of chloroform NOS
- T53.1X2 Toxic effect of chloroform, intentional self-harm
- T53.1X3 Toxic effect of chloroform, assault
- T53.1X4 Toxic effect of chloroform, undetermined

T53.2 Toxic effects of trichloroethylene
Toxic effects of trichloroethene

T53.2X Toxic effects of trichloroethylene
- T53.2X1 Toxic effect of trichloroethylene, accidental (unintentional)
  Toxic effects of trichloroethylene NOS
- T53.2X2 Toxic effect of trichloroethylene, intentional self-harm
- T53.2X3 Toxic effect of trichloroethylene, assault
- T53.2X4 Toxic effect of trichloroethylene, undetermined

T53.3 Toxic effects of tetrachloroethylene
Toxic effects of perchloroethylene
Toxic effect of tetrachloroethene

T53.3X Toxic effects of tetrachloroethylene
- T53.3X1 Toxic effect of tetrachloroethylene, accidental (unintentional)
  Toxic effects of tetrachloroethylene NOS
- T53.3X2 Toxic effect of tetrachloroethylene, intentional self-harm
- T53.3X3 Toxic effect of tetrachloroethylene, assault
- T53.3X4 Toxic effect of tetrachloroethylene, undetermined

T53.4 Toxic effects of dichloromethane
Toxic effects of methylene chloride

T53.4X Toxic effects of dichloromethane
- T53.4X1 Toxic effect of dichloromethane, accidental (unintentional)
  Toxic effects of dichloromethane NOS
- T53.4X2 Toxic effect of dichloromethane, intentional self-harm
- T53.4X3 Toxic effect of dichloromethane, assault
- T53.4X4 Toxic effect of dichloromethane, undetermined

T53.5 Toxic effects of chlorofluorocarbons

T53.5X Toxic effects of chlorofluorocarbons
- T53.5X1 Toxic effect of chlorofluorocarbons, accidental (unintentional)
  Toxic effects of chlorofluorocarbons NOS
- T53.5X2 Toxic effect of chlorofluorocarbons, intentional self-harm
- T53.5X3 Toxic effect of chlorofluorocarbons, assault
- T53.5X4 Toxic effect of chlorofluorocarbons, undetermined

T53.6 Toxic effects of other halogen derivatives of aliphatic hydrocarbons

T53.6X Toxic effects of other halogen derivatives of aliphatic hydrocarbons
- T53.6X1 Toxic effect of other halogen derivatives of aliphatic hydrocarbons, accidental (unintentional)
  Toxic effects of other halogen derivatives of aliphatic hydrocarbons NOS
- T53.6X2 Toxic effect of other halogen derivatives of aliphatic hydrocarbons, intentional self-harm
- T53.6X3 Toxic effect of other halogen derivatives of aliphatic hydrocarbons, assault
- T53.6X4 Toxic effect of other halogen derivatives of aliphatic hydrocarbons, undetermined

√5th **T53.7 Toxic effects of other halogen derivatives of aromatic hydrocarbons**

√6th **T53.7X Toxic effects of other halogen derivatives of aromatic hydrocarbons**

√7th **T53.7X1 Toxic effect of other halogen derivatives of aromatic hydrocarbons, accidental (unintentional)**
Toxic effects of other halogen derivatives of aromatic hydrocarbons NOS

√7th **T53.7X2 Toxic effect of other halogen derivatives of aromatic hydrocarbons, intentional self-harm**

√7th **T53.7X3 Toxic effect of other halogen derivatives of aromatic hydrocarbons, assault**

√7th **T53.7X4 Toxic effect of other halogen derivatives of aromatic hydrocarbons, undetermined**

√5th **T53.9 Toxic effects of unspecified halogen derivatives of aliphatic and aromatic hydrocarbons**

√x7th **T53.91 Toxic effect of unspecified halogen derivatives of aliphatic and aromatic hydrocarbons, accidental (unintentional)**

√x7th **T53.92 Toxic effect of unspecified halogen derivatives of aliphatic and aromatic hydrocarbons, intentional self-harm**

√x7th **T53.93 Toxic effect of unspecified halogen derivatives of aliphatic and aromatic hydrocarbons, assault**

√x7th **T53.94 Toxic effect of unspecified halogen derivatives of aliphatic and aromatic hydrocarbons, undetermined**

√4th **T54 Toxic effect of corrosive substances**

The appropriate 7th character is to be added to each code from category T54.
A initial encounter
D subsequent encounter
S sequela

√5th **T54.Ø Toxic effects of phenol and phenol homologues**

√6th **T54.ØX Toxic effects of phenol and phenol homologues**

√7th **T54.ØX1 Toxic effect of phenol and phenol homologues, accidental (unintentional)**
Toxic effects of phenol and phenol homologues NOS

√7th **T54.ØX2 Toxic effect of phenol and phenol homologues, intentional self-harm**

√7th **T54.ØX3 Toxic effect of phenol and phenol homologues, assault**

√7th **T54.ØX4 Toxic effect of phenol and phenol homologues, undetermined**

√5th **T54.1 Toxic effects of other corrosive organic compounds**

√6th **T54.1X Toxic effects of other corrosive organic compounds**

√7th **T54.1X1 Toxic effect of other corrosive organic compounds, accidental (unintentional)**
Toxic effects of other corrosive organic compounds NOS

√7th **T54.1X2 Toxic effect of other corrosive organic compounds, intentional self-harm**

√7th **T54.1X3 Toxic effect of other corrosive organic compounds, assault**

√7th **T54.1X4 Toxic effect of other corrosive organic compounds, undetermined**

√5th **T54.2 Toxic effects of corrosive acids and acid-like substances**
Toxic effects of hydrochloric acid
Toxic effects of sulfuric acid

√6th **T54.2X Toxic effects of corrosive acids and acid-like substances**

√7th **T54.2X1 Toxic effect of corrosive acids and acid-like substances, accidental (unintentional)**
Toxic effects of corrosive acids and acid-like substances NOS

√7th **T54.2X2 Toxic effect of corrosive acids and acid-like substances, intentional self-harm**

√7th **T54.2X3 Toxic effect of corrosive acids and acid-like substances, assault**

√7th **T54.2X4 Toxic effect of corrosive acids and acid-like substances, undetermined**

√5th **T54.3 Toxic effects of corrosive alkalis and alkali-like substances**
Toxic effects of potassium hydroxide
Toxic effects of sodium hydroxide

√6th **T54.3X Toxic effects of corrosive alkalis and alkali-like substances**

√7th **T54.3X1 Toxic effect of corrosive alkalis and alkali-like substances, accidental (unintentional)**
Toxic effects of corrosive alkalis and alkali-like substances NOS

√7th **T54.3X2 Toxic effect of corrosive alkalis and alkali-like substances, intentional self-harm**

√7th **T54.3X3 Toxic effect of corrosive alkalis and alkali-like substances, assault**

√7th **T54.3X4 Toxic effect of corrosive alkalis and alkali-like substances, undetermined**

√5th **T54.9 Toxic effects of unspecified corrosive substance**

√x7th **T54.91 Toxic effect of unspecified corrosive substance, accidental (unintentional)**

√x7th **T54.92 Toxic effect of unspecified corrosive substance, intentional self-harm**

√x7th **T54.93 Toxic effect of unspecified corrosive substance, assault**

√x7th **T54.94 Toxic effect of unspecified corrosive substance, undetermined**

√4th **T55 Toxic effect of soaps and detergents**

The appropriate 7th character is to be added to each code from category T55.
A initial encounter
D subsequent encounter
S sequela

√5th **T55.Ø Toxic effect of soaps**

√6th **T55.ØX Toxic effect of soaps**

√7th **T55.ØX1 Toxic effect of soaps, accidental (unintentional)**
Toxic effect of soaps NOS

√7th **T55.ØX2 Toxic effect of soaps, intentional self-harm**

√7th **T55.ØX3 Toxic effect of soaps, assault**

√7th **T55.ØX4 Toxic effect of soaps, undetermined**

√5th **T55.1 Toxic effect of detergents**

√6th **T55.1X Toxic effect of detergents**

√7th **T55.1X1 Toxic effect of detergents, accidental (unintentional)**
Toxic effect of detergents NOS

√7th **T55.1X2 Toxic effect of detergents, intentional self-harm**

√7th **T55.1X3 Toxic effect of detergents, assault**

√7th **T55.1X4 Toxic effect of detergents, undetermined**

√4th **T56 Toxic effect of metals**

INCLUDES toxic effects of fumes and vapors of metals
toxic effects of metals from all sources, except medicinal substances

Use additional code to identify any retained metal foreign body, if applicable (Z18.Ø-, T18.1-)

EXCLUDES 1 *arsenic and its compounds (T57.Ø)*
manganese and its compounds (T57.2)

The appropriate 7th character is to be added to each code from category T56.
A initial encounter
D subsequent encounter
S sequela

√5th **T56.Ø Toxic effects of lead and its compounds**

√6th **T56.ØX Toxic effects of lead and its compounds**

√7th **T56.ØX1 Toxic effect of lead and its compounds, accidental (unintentional)**
Toxic effects of lead and its compounds NOS

√7th **T56.ØX2 Toxic effect of lead and its compounds, intentional self-harm**

- T56.0X3 **Toxic effect of lead and its compounds, assault**
- T56.0X4 **Toxic effect of lead and its compounds, undetermined**

T56.1 Toxic effects of mercury and its compounds

T56.1X Toxic effects of mercury and its compounds

- T56.1X1 **Toxic effect of mercury and its compounds, accidental (unintentional)**
  Toxic effects of mercury and its compounds NOS
- T56.1X2 **Toxic effect of mercury and its compounds, intentional self-harm**
- T56.1X3 **Toxic effect of mercury and its compounds, assault**
- T56.1X4 **Toxic effect of mercury and its compounds, undetermined**

T56.2 Toxic effects of chromium and its compounds

T56.2X Toxic effects of chromium and its compounds

- T56.2X1 **Toxic effect of chromium and its compounds, accidental (unintentional)**
  Toxic effects of chromium and its compounds NOS
- T56.2X2 **Toxic effect of chromium and its compounds, intentional self-harm**
- T56.2X3 **Toxic effect of chromium and its compounds, assault**
- T56.2X4 **Toxic effect of chromium and its compounds, undetermined**

T56.3 Toxic effects of cadmium and its compounds

T56.3X Toxic effects of cadmium and its compounds

- T56.3X1 **Toxic effect of cadmium and its compounds, accidental (unintentional)**
  Toxic effects of cadmium and its compounds NOS
- T56.3X2 **Toxic effect of cadmium and its compounds, intentional self-harm**
- T56.3X3 **Toxic effect of cadmium and its compounds, assault**
- T56.3X4 **Toxic effect of cadmium and its compounds, undetermined**

T56.4 Toxic effects of copper and its compounds

T56.4X Toxic effects of copper and its compounds

- T56.4X1 **Toxic effect of copper and its compounds, accidental (unintentional)**
  Toxic effects of copper and its compounds NOS
- T56.4X2 **Toxic effect of copper and its compounds, intentional self-harm**
- T56.4X3 **Toxic effect of copper and its compounds, assault**
- T56.4X4 **Toxic effect of copper and its compounds, undetermined**

T56.5 Toxic effects of zinc and its compounds

T56.5X Toxic effects of zinc and its compounds

- T56.5X1 **Toxic effect of zinc and its compounds, accidental (unintentional)**
  Toxic effects of zinc and its compounds NOS
- T56.5X2 **Toxic effect of zinc and its compounds, intentional self-harm**
- T56.5X3 **Toxic effect of zinc and its compounds, assault**
- T56.5X4 **Toxic effect of zinc and its compounds, undetermined**

T56.6 Toxic effects of tin and its compounds

T56.6X Toxic effects of tin and its compounds

- T56.6X1 **Toxic effect of tin and its compounds, accidental (unintentional)**
  Toxic effects of tin and its compounds NOS
- T56.6X2 **Toxic effect of tin and its compounds, intentional self-harm**
- T56.6X3 **Toxic effect of tin and its compounds, assault**
- T56.6X4 **Toxic effect of tin and its compounds, undetermined**

T56.7 Toxic effects of beryllium and its compounds

T56.7X Toxic effects of beryllium and its compounds

- T56.7X1 **Toxic effect of beryllium and its compounds, accidental (unintentional)**
  Toxic effects of beryllium and its compounds NOS
- T56.7X2 **Toxic effect of beryllium and its compounds, intentional self-harm**
- T56.7X3 **Toxic effect of beryllium and its compounds, assault**
- T56.7X4 **Toxic effect of beryllium and its compounds, undetermined**

T56.8 Toxic effects of other metals

T56.81 Toxic effect of thallium

- T56.811 **Toxic effect of thallium, accidental (unintentional)**
  Toxic effect of thallium NOS
- T56.812 **Toxic effect of thallium, intentional self-harm**
- T56.813 **Toxic effect of thallium, assault**
- T56.814 **Toxic effect of thallium, undetermined**

T56.89 Toxic effects of other metals

- T56.891 **Toxic effect of other metals, accidental (unintentional)**
  Toxic effects of other metals NOS
- T56.892 **Toxic effect of other metals, intentional self-harm**
- T56.893 **Toxic effect of other metals, assault**
- T56.894 **Toxic effect of other metals, undetermined**

T56.9 Toxic effects of unspecified metal

- T56.91 **Toxic effect of unspecified metal, accidental (unintentional)**
- T56.92 **Toxic effect of unspecified metal, intentional self-harm**
- T56.93 **Toxic effect of unspecified metal, assault**
- T56.94 **Toxic effect of unspecified metal, undetermined**

T57 Toxic effect of other inorganic substances

The appropriate 7th character is to be added to each code from category T57.
A initial encounter
D subsequent encounter
S sequela

T57.0 Toxic effect of arsenic and its compounds

T57.0X Toxic effect of arsenic and its compounds

- T57.0X1 **Toxic effect of arsenic and its compounds, accidental (unintentional)**
  Toxic effect of arsenic and its compounds NOS
- T57.0X2 **Toxic effect of arsenic and its compounds, intentional self-harm**
- T57.0X3 **Toxic effect of arsenic and its compounds, assault**
- T57.0X4 **Toxic effect of arsenic and its compounds, undetermined**

T57.1 Toxic effect of phosphorus and its compounds

EXCLUDES 1 *organophosphate insecticides (T60.0)*

T57.1X Toxic effect of phosphorus and its compounds

- T57.1X1 **Toxic effect of phosphorus and its compounds, accidental (unintentional)**
  Toxic effect of phosphorus and its compounds NOS
- T57.1X2 **Toxic effect of phosphorus and its compounds, intentional self-harm**
- T57.1X3 **Toxic effect of phosphorus and its compounds, assault**
- T57.1X4 **Toxic effect of phosphorus and its compounds, undetermined**

T57.2 Toxic effect of manganese and its compounds

T57.2X Toxic effect of manganese and its compounds

- T57.2X1 **Toxic effect of manganese and its compounds, accidental (unintentional)**
  Toxic effect of manganese and its compounds NOS

T57.2X2 Toxic effect of manganese and its compounds, intentional self-harm

T57.2X3 Toxic effect of manganese and its compounds, assault

T57.2X4 Toxic effect of manganese and its compounds, undetermined

T57.3 Toxic effect of hydrogen cyanide

T57.3X Toxic effect of hydrogen cyanide

T57.3X1 Toxic effect of hydrogen cyanide, accidental (unintentional)

Toxic effect of hydrogen cyanide NOS

T57.3X2 Toxic effect of hydrogen cyanide, intentional self-harm

T57.3X3 Toxic effect of hydrogen cyanide, assault

T57.3X4 Toxic effect of hydrogen cyanide, undetermined

T57.8 Toxic effect of other specified inorganic substances

T57.8X Toxic effect of other specified inorganic substances

T57.8X1 Toxic effect of other specified inorganic substances, accidental (unintentional)

Toxic effect of other specified inorganic substances NOS

T57.8X2 Toxic effect of other specified inorganic substances, intentional self-harm

T57.8X3 Toxic effect of other specified inorganic substances, assault

T57.8X4 Toxic effect of other specified inorganic substances, undetermined

T57.9 Toxic effect of unspecified inorganic substance

T57.91 Toxic effect of unspecified inorganic substance, accidental (unintentional)

T57.92 Toxic effect of unspecified inorganic substance, intentional self-harm

T57.93 Toxic effect of unspecified inorganic substance, assault

T57.94 Toxic effect of unspecified inorganic substance, undetermined

T58 Toxic effect of carbon monoxide

INCLUDES asphyxiation from carbon monoxide
toxic effect of carbon monoxide from all sources

The appropriate 7th character is to be added to each code from category T58.
A initial encounter
D subsequent encounter
S sequela

T58.0 Toxic effect of carbon monoxide from motor vehicle exhaust

Toxic effect of exhaust gas from gas engine
Toxic effect of exhaust gas from motor pump

T58.01 Toxic effect of carbon monoxide from motor vehicle exhaust, accidental (unintentional)

T58.02 Toxic effect of carbon monoxide from motor vehicle exhaust, intentional self-harm

T58.03 Toxic effect of carbon monoxide from motor vehicle exhaust, assault

T58.04 Toxic effect of carbon monoxide from motor vehicle exhaust, undetermined

T58.1 Toxic effect of carbon monoxide from utility gas

Toxic effect of acetylene
Toxic effect of gas NOS used for lighting, heating, cooking
Toxic effect of water gas

T58.11 Toxic effect of carbon monoxide from utility gas, accidental (unintentional)

T58.12 Toxic effect of carbon monoxide from utility gas, intentional self-harm

T58.13 Toxic effect of carbon monoxide from utility gas, assault

T58.14 Toxic effect of carbon monoxide from utility gas, undetermined

T58.2 Toxic effect of carbon monoxide from incomplete combustion of other domestic fuels

Toxic effect of carbon monoxide from incomplete combustion of coal, coke, kerosene, wood

T58.2X Toxic effect of carbon monoxide from incomplete combustion of other domestic fuels

T58.2X1 Toxic effect of carbon monoxide from incomplete combustion of other domestic fuels, accidental (unintentional)

T58.2X2 Toxic effect of carbon monoxide from incomplete combustion of other domestic fuels, intentional self-harm

T58.2X3 Toxic effect of carbon monoxide from incomplete combustion of other domestic fuels, assault

T58.2X4 Toxic effect of carbon monoxide from incomplete combustion of other domestic fuels, undetermined

T58.8 Toxic effect of carbon monoxide from other source

Toxic effect of carbon monoxide from blast furnace gas
Toxic effect of carbon monoxide from fuels in industrial use
Toxic effect of carbon monoxide from kiln vapor

T58.8X Toxic effect of carbon monoxide from other source

T58.8X1 Toxic effect of carbon monoxide from other source, accidental (unintentional)

T58.8X2 Toxic effect of carbon monoxide from other source, intentional self-harm

T58.8X3 Toxic effect of carbon monoxide from other source, assault

T58.8X4 Toxic effect of carbon monoxide from other source, undetermined

T58.9 Toxic effect of carbon monoxide from unspecified source

T58.91 Toxic effect of carbon monoxide from unspecified source, accidental (unintentional)

T58.92 Toxic effect of carbon monoxide from unspecified source, intentional self-harm

T58.93 Toxic effect of carbon monoxide from unspecified source, assault

T58.94 Toxic effect of carbon monoxide from unspecified source, undetermined

T59 Toxic effect of other gases, fumes and vapors

INCLUDES aerosol propellants
EXCLUDES 1 *chlorofluorocarbons (T53.5)*

The appropriate 7th character is to be added to each code from category T59.
A initial encounter
D subsequent encounter
S sequela

T59.0 Toxic effect of nitrogen oxides

T59.0X Toxic effect of nitrogen oxides

T59.0X1 Toxic effect of nitrogen oxides, accidental (unintentional)

Toxic effect of nitrogen oxides NOS

T59.0X2 Toxic effect of nitrogen oxides, intentional self-harm

T59.0X3 Toxic effect of nitrogen oxides, assault

T59.0X4 Toxic effect of nitrogen oxides, undetermined

T59.1 Toxic effect of sulfur dioxide

T59.1X Toxic effect of sulfur dioxide

T59.1X1 Toxic effect of sulfur dioxide, accidental (unintentional)

Toxic effect of sulfur dioxide NOS

T59.1X2 Toxic effect of sulfur dioxide, intentional self-harm

T59.1X3 Toxic effect of sulfur dioxide, assault

T59.1X4 Toxic effect of sulfur dioxide, undetermined

T59.2 Toxic effect of formaldehyde

T59.2X Toxic effect of formaldehyde

T59.2X1 Toxic effect of formaldehyde, accidental (unintentional)

Toxic effect of formaldehyde NOS

T59.2X2 Toxic effect of formaldehyde, intentional self-harm

T59.2X3 Toxic effect of formaldehyde, assault
T59.2X4 Toxic effect of formaldehyde, undetermined
T59.3 Toxic effect of lacrimogenic gas
Toxic effect of tear gas
T59.3X Toxic effect of lacrimogenic gas
T59.3X1 Toxic effect of lacrimogenic gas, accidental (unintentional)
Toxic effect of lacrimogenic gas NOS
T59.3X2 Toxic effect of lacrimogenic gas, intentional self-harm
T59.3X3 Toxic effect of lacrimogenic gas, assault
T59.3X4 Toxic effect of lacrimogenic gas, undetermined
T59.4 Toxic effect of chlorine gas
T59.4X Toxic effect of chlorine gas
T59.4X1 Toxic effect of chlorine gas, accidental (unintentional)
Toxic effect of chlorine gas NOS
T59.4X2 Toxic effect of chlorine gas, intentional self-harm
T59.4X3 Toxic effect of chlorine gas, assault
T59.4X4 Toxic effect of chlorine gas, undetermined
T59.5 Toxic effect of fluorine gas and hydrogen fluoride
T59.5X Toxic effect of fluorine gas and hydrogen fluoride
T59.5X1 Toxic effect of fluorine gas and hydrogen fluoride, accidental (unintentional)
Toxic effect of fluorine gas and hydrogen fluoride NOS
T59.5X2 Toxic effect of fluorine gas and hydrogen fluoride, intentional self-harm
T59.5X3 Toxic effect of fluorine gas and hydrogen fluoride, assault
T59.5X4 Toxic effect of fluorine gas and hydrogen fluoride, undetermined
T59.6 Toxic effect of hydrogen sulfide
T59.6X Toxic effect of hydrogen sulfide
T59.6X1 Toxic effect of hydrogen sulfide, accidental (unintentional)
Toxic effect of hydrogen sulfide NOS
T59.6X2 Toxic effect of hydrogen sulfide, intentional self-harm
T59.6X3 Toxic effect of hydrogen sulfide, assault
T59.6X4 Toxic effect of hydrogen sulfide, undetermined
T59.7 Toxic effect of carbon dioxide
T59.7X Toxic effect of carbon dioxide
T59.7X1 Toxic effect of carbon dioxide, accidental (unintentional)
Toxic effect of carbon dioxide NOS
T59.7X2 Toxic effect of carbon dioxide, intentional self-harm
T59.7X3 Toxic effect of carbon dioxide, assault
T59.7X4 Toxic effect of carbon dioxide, undetermined
T59.8 Toxic effect of other specified gases, fumes and vapors
T59.81 Toxic effect of smoke
Smoke inhalation
EXCLUDES 2 *toxic effect of cigarette (tobacco) smoke (T65.22-)*
T59.811 Toxic effect of smoke, accidental (unintentional)
Toxic effect of smoke NOS
T59.812 Toxic effect of smoke, intentional self-harm
T59.813 Toxic effect of smoke, assault
T59.814 Toxic effect of smoke, undetermined
T59.89 Toxic effect of other specified gases, fumes and vapors
T59.891 Toxic effect of other specified gases, fumes and vapors, accidental (unintentional)
T59.892 Toxic effect of other specified gases, fumes and vapors, intentional self-harm
T59.893 Toxic effect of other specified gases, fumes and vapors, assault
T59.894 Toxic effect of other specified gases, fumes and vapors, undetermined
T59.9 Toxic effect of unspecified gases, fumes and vapors
T59.91 Toxic effect of unspecified gases, fumes and vapors, accidental (unintentional)
T59.92 Toxic effect of unspecified gases, fumes and vapors, intentional self-harm
T59.93 Toxic effect of unspecified gases, fumes and vapors, assault
T59.94 Toxic effect of unspecified gases, fumes and vapors, undetermined

T60 Toxic effect of pesticides
INCLUDES toxic effect of wood preservatives

The appropriate 7th character is to be added to each code from category T60.
A initial encounter
D subsequent encounter
S sequela

T60.0 Toxic effect of organophosphate and carbamate insecticides
T60.0X Toxic effect of organophosphate and carbamate insecticides
T60.0X1 Toxic effect of organophosphate and carbamate insecticides, accidental (unintentional)
Toxic effect of organophosphate and carbamate insecticides NOS
T60.0X2 Toxic effect of organophosphate and carbamate insecticides, intentional self-harm
T60.0X3 Toxic effect of organophosphate and carbamate insecticides, assault
T60.0X4 Toxic effect of organophosphate and carbamate insecticides, undetermined
T60.1 Toxic effect of halogenated insecticides
EXCLUDES 1 *chlorinated hydrocarbon (T53.-)*
T60.1X Toxic effect of halogenated insecticides
T60.1X1 Toxic effect of halogenated insecticides, accidental (unintentional)
Toxic effect of halogenated insecticides NOS
T60.1X2 Toxic effect of halogenated insecticides, intentional self-harm
T60.1X3 Toxic effect of halogenated insecticides, assault
T60.1X4 Toxic effect of halogenated insecticides, undetermined
T60.2 Toxic effect of other insecticides
T60.2X Toxic effect of other insecticides
T60.2X1 Toxic effect of other insecticides, accidental (unintentional)
Toxic effect of other insecticides NOS
T60.2X2 Toxic effect of other insecticides, intentional self-harm
T60.2X3 Toxic effect of other insecticides, assault
T60.2X4 Toxic effect of other insecticides, undetermined
T60.3 Toxic effect of herbicides and fungicides
T60.3X Toxic effect of herbicides and fungicides
T60.3X1 Toxic effect of herbicides and fungicides, accidental (unintentional)
Toxic effect of herbicides and fungicides NOS
T60.3X2 Toxic effect of herbicides and fungicides, intentional self-harm
T60.3X3 Toxic effect of herbicides and fungicides, assault
T60.3X4 Toxic effect of herbicides and fungicides, undetermined

T60.4 Toxic effect of rodenticides
EXCLUDES 1 *strychnine and its salts (T65.1)*
thallium (T56.81-)
T60.4X Toxic effect of rodenticides
T60.4X1 Toxic effect of rodenticides, accidental (unintentional)
Toxic effect of rodenticides NOS
T60.4X2 Toxic effect of rodenticides, intentional self-harm
T60.4X3 Toxic effect of rodenticides, assault
T60.4X4 Toxic effect of rodenticides, undetermined
T60.8 Toxic effect of other pesticides
T60.8X Toxic effect of other pesticides
T60.8X1 Toxic effect of other pesticides, accidental (unintentional)
Toxic effect of other pesticides NOS
T60.8X2 Toxic effect of other pesticides, intentional self-harm
T60.8X3 Toxic effect of other pesticides, assault
T60.8X4 Toxic effect of other pesticides, undetermined
T60.9 Toxic effect of unspecified pesticide
T60.91 Toxic effect of unspecified pesticide, accidental (unintentional)
T60.92 Toxic effect of unspecified pesticide, intentional self-harm
T60.93 Toxic effect of unspecified pesticide, assault
T60.94 Toxic effect of unspecified pesticide, undetermined

T61 Toxic effect of noxious substances eaten as seafood
EXCLUDES 1 *allergic reaction to food, such as:*
anaphylactic reaction or shock due to adverse food reaction (T78.0-)
dermatitis (L23.6, L25.4, L27.2)
gastroenteritis (noninfective) (K52.2)
anaphylactic shock (T78.02, T78.05)
bacterial foodborne intoxications (A05.-)
toxic effect of food contaminants, such as:
aflatoxin and other mycotoxins (T64)
cyanides (T65.0-)
harmful algae bloom (T65.82-)
hydrogen cyanide (T57.3-)
mercury (T56.1-)
red tide (T65.82-)

The appropriate 7th character is to be added to each code from category T61.
A initial encounter
D subsequent encounter
S sequela

T61.0 Ciguatera fish poisoning
T61.01 Ciguatera fish poisoning, accidental (unintentional)
T61.02 Ciguatera fish poisoning, intentional self-harm
T61.03 Ciguatera fish poisoning, assault
T61.04 Ciguatera fish poisoning, undetermined
T61.1 Scombroid fish poisoning
Histamine-like syndrome
T61.11 Scombroid fish poisoning, accidental (unintentional)
T61.12 Scombroid fish poisoning, intentional self-harm
T61.13 Scombroid fish poisoning, assault
T61.14 Scombroid fish poisoning, undetermined
T61.7 Other fish and shellfish poisoning
T61.77 Other fish poisoning
T61.771 Other fish poisoning, accidental (unintentional)
T61.772 Other fish poisoning, intentional self-harm
T61.773 Other fish poisoning, assault
T61.774 Other fish poisoning, undetermined
T61.78 Other shellfish poisoning
T61.781 Other shellfish poisoning, accidental (unintentional)
T61.782 Other shellfish poisoning, intentional self-harm
T61.783 Other shellfish poisoning, assault
T61.784 Other shellfish poisoning, undetermined
T61.8 Toxic effect of other seafood
T61.8X Toxic effect of other seafood
T61.8X1 Toxic effect of other seafood, accidental (unintentional)
T61.8X2 Toxic effect of other seafood, intentional self-harm
T61.8X3 Toxic effect of other seafood, assault
T61.8X4 Toxic effect of other seafood, undetermined
T61.9 Toxic effect of unspecified seafood
T61.91 Toxic effect of unspecified seafood, accidental (unintentional)
T61.92 Toxic effect of unspecified seafood, intentional self-harm
T61.93 Toxic effect of unspecified seafood, assault
T61.94 Toxic effect of unspecified seafood, undetermined

T62 Toxic effect of other noxious substances eaten as food
EXCLUDES 1 *allergic reaction to food, such as:*
anaphylactic shock (reaction) due to adverse food reaction (T78.0-)
dermatitis (L23.6, L25.4, L27.2)
gastroenteritis (noninfective) (K52.2)
bacterial food borne intoxications (A05.-)
toxic effect of food contaminants, such as:
aflatoxin and other mycotoxins (T64)
cyanides (T65.0-)
hydrogen cyanide (T57.3-)
mercury (T56.1-)

The appropriate 7th character is to be added to each code from category T62.
A initial encounter
D subsequent encounter
S sequela

T62.0 Toxic effect of ingested mushrooms
T62.0X Toxic effect of ingested mushrooms
T62.0X1 Toxic effect of ingested mushrooms, accidental (unintentional)
Toxic effect of ingested mushrooms NOS
T62.0X2 Toxic effect of ingested mushrooms, intentional self-harm
T62.0X3 Toxic effect of ingested mushrooms, assault
T62.0X4 Toxic effect of ingested mushrooms, undetermined
T62.1 Toxic effect of ingested berries
T62.1X Toxic effect of ingested berries
T62.1X1 Toxic effect of ingested berries, accidental (unintentional)
Toxic effect of ingested berries NOS
T62.1X2 Toxic effect of ingested berries, intentional self-harm
T62.1X3 Toxic effect of ingested berries, assault
T62.1X4 Toxic effect of ingested berries, undetermined
T62.2 Toxic effect of other ingested (parts of) plant(s)
T62.2X Toxic effect of other ingested (parts of) plant(s)
T62.2X1 Toxic effect of other ingested (parts of) plant(s), accidental (unintentional)
Toxic effect of other ingested (parts of) plant(s) NOS
T62.2X2 Toxic effect of other ingested (parts of) plant(s), intentional self-harm
T62.2X3 Toxic effect of other ingested (parts of) plant(s), assault
T62.2X4 Toxic effect of other ingested (parts of) plant(s), undetermined

✓5th **T62.8 Toxic effect of other specified noxious substances eaten as food**

✓6th **T62.8X Toxic effect of other specified noxious substances eaten as food**

✓7th **T62.8X1 Toxic effect of other specified noxious substances eaten as food, accidental (unintentional)**
Toxic effect of other specified noxious substances eaten as food NOS

✓7th **T62.8X2 Toxic effect of other specified noxious substances eaten as food, intentional self-harm**

✓7th **T62.8X3 Toxic effect of other specified noxious substances eaten as food, assault**

✓7th **T62.8X4 Toxic effect of other specified noxious substances eaten as food, undetermined**

✓5th **T62.9 Toxic effect of unspecified noxious substance eaten as food**

✓x7th **T62.91 Toxic effect of unspecified noxious substance eaten as food, accidental (unintentional)**
Toxic effect of unspecified noxious substance eaten as food NOS

✓x7th **T62.92 Toxic effect of unspecified noxious substance eaten as food, intentional self-harm**

✓x7th **T62.93 Toxic effect of unspecified noxious substance eaten as food, assault**

✓x7th **T62.94 Toxic effect of unspecified noxious substance eaten as food, undetermined**

✓4th **T63 Toxic effect of contact with venomous animals and plants**

INCLUDES bite or touch of venomous animal
pricked or stuck by thorn or leaf

EXCLUDES 2 *ingestion of toxic animal or plant (T61-, T62-)*

The appropriate 7th character is to be added to each code from category T63.
A initial encounter
D subsequent encounter
S sequela

✓5th **T63.0 Toxic effect of snake venom**

✓6th **T63.00 Toxic effect of unspecified snake venom**

✓7th **T63.001 Toxic effect of unspecified snake venom, accidental (unintentional)**
Toxic effect of unspecified snake venom NOS

✓7th **T63.002 Toxic effect of unspecified snake venom, intentional self-harm**

✓7th **T63.003 Toxic effect of unspecified snake venom, assault**

✓7th **T63.004 Toxic effect of unspecified snake venom, undetermined**

✓6th **T63.01 Toxic effect of rattlesnake venom**

✓7th **T63.011 Toxic effect of rattlesnake venom, accidental (unintentional)**
Toxic effect of rattlesnake venom NOS

✓7th **T63.012 Toxic effect of rattlesnake venom, intentional self-harm**

✓7th **T63.013 Toxic effect of rattlesnake venom, assault**

✓7th **T63.014 Toxic effect of rattlesnake venom, undetermined**

✓6th **T63.02 Toxic effect of coral snake venom**

✓7th **T63.021 Toxic effect of coral snake venom, accidental (unintentional)**
Toxic effect of coral snake venom NOS

✓7th **T63.022 Toxic effect of coral snake venom, intentional self-harm**

✓7th **T63.023 Toxic effect of coral snake venom, assault**

✓7th **T63.024 Toxic effect of coral snake venom, undetermined**

✓6th **T63.03 Toxic effect of taipan venom**

✓7th **T63.031 Toxic effect of taipan venom, accidental (unintentional)**
Toxic effect of taipan venom NOS

✓7th **T63.032 Toxic effect of taipan venom, intentional self-harm**

✓7th **T63.033 Toxic effect of taipan venom, assault**

✓7th **T63.034 Toxic effect of taipan venom, undetermined**

✓6th **T63.04 Toxic effect of cobra venom**

✓7th **T63.041 Toxic effect of cobra venom, accidental (unintentional)**
Toxic effect of cobra venom NOS

✓7th **T63.042 Toxic effect of cobra venom, intentional self-harm**

✓7th **T63.043 Toxic effect of cobra venom, assault**

✓7th **T63.044 Toxic effect of cobra venom, undetermined**

✓6th **T63.06 Toxic effect of venom of other North and South American snake**

✓7th **T63.061 Toxic effect of venom of other North and South American snake, accidental (unintentional)**
Toxic effect of venom of other North and South American snake NOS

✓7th **T63.062 Toxic effect of venom of other North and South American snake, intentional self-harm**

✓7th **T63.063 Toxic effect of venom of other North and South American snake, assault**

✓7th **T63.064 Toxic effect of venom of other North and South American snake, undetermined**

✓6th **T63.07 Toxic effect of venom of other Australian snake**

✓7th **T63.071 Toxic effect of venom of other Australian snake, accidental (unintentional)**
Toxic effect of venom of other Australian snake NOS

✓7th **T63.072 Toxic effect of venom of other Australian snake, intentional self-harm**

✓7th **T63.073 Toxic effect of venom of other Australian snake, assault**

✓7th **T63.074 Toxic effect of venom of other Australian snake, undetermined**

✓6th **T63.08 Toxic effect of venom of other African and Asian snake**

✓7th **T63.081 Toxic effect of venom of other African and Asian snake, accidental (unintentional)**
Toxic effect of venom of other African and Asian snake NOS

✓7th **T63.082 Toxic effect of venom of other African and Asian snake, intentional self-harm**

✓7th **T63.083 Toxic effect of venom of other African and Asian snake, assault**

✓7th **T63.084 Toxic effect of venom of other African and Asian snake, undetermined**

✓6th **T63.09 Toxic effect of venom of other snake**

✓7th **T63.091 Toxic effect of venom of other snake, accidental (unintentional)**
Toxic effect of venom of other snake NOS

✓7th **T63.092 Toxic effect of venom of other snake, intentional self-harm**

✓7th **T63.093 Toxic effect of venom of other snake, assault**

✓7th **T63.094 Toxic effect of venom of other snake, undetermined**

✓5th **T63.1 Toxic effect of venom of other reptiles**

✓6th **T63.11 Toxic effect of venom of gila monster**

✓7th **T63.111 Toxic effect of venom of gila monster, accidental (unintentional)**
Toxic effect of venom of gila monster NOS

✓7th **T63.112 Toxic effect of venom of gila monster, intentional self-harm**

✓7th **T63.113 Toxic effect of venom of gila monster, assault**

✓7th **T63.114 Toxic effect of venom of gila monster, undetermined**

✓6th **T63.12 Toxic effect of venom of other venomous lizard**

✓7th **T63.121 Toxic effect of venom of other venomous lizard, accidental (unintentional)**
Toxic effect of venom of other venomous lizard NOS

√7th **T63.122 Toxic effect of venom of other venomous lizard, intentional self-harm**

√7th **T63.123 Toxic effect of venom of other venomous lizard, assault**

√7th **T63.124 Toxic effect of venom of other venomous lizard, undetermined**

√6th **T63.19 Toxic effect of venom of other reptiles**

√7th **T63.191 Toxic effect of venom of other reptiles, accidental (unintentional)**
Toxic effect of venom of other reptiles NOS

√7th **T63.192 Toxic effect of venom of other reptiles, intentional self-harm**

√7th **T63.193 Toxic effect of venom of other reptiles, assault**

√7th **T63.194 Toxic effect of venom of other reptiles, undetermined**

√5th **T63.2 Toxic effect of venom of scorpion**

√6th **T63.2X Toxic effect of venom of scorpion**

√7th **T63.2X1 Toxic effect of venom of scorpion, accidental (unintentional)**
Toxic effect of venom of scorpion NOS

√7th **T63.2X2 Toxic effect of venom of scorpion, intentional self-harm**

√7th **T63.2X3 Toxic effect of venom of scorpion, assault**

√7th **T63.2X4 Toxic effect of venom of scorpion, undetermined**

√5th **T63.3 Toxic effect of venom of spider**

√6th **T63.30 Toxic effect of unspecified spider venom**

√7th **T63.301 Toxic effect of unspecified spider venom, accidental (unintentional)**

√7th **T63.302 Toxic effect of unspecified spider venom, intentional self-harm**

√7th **T63.303 Toxic effect of unspecified spider venom, assault**

√7th **T63.304 Toxic effect of unspecified spider venom, undetermined**

√6th **T63.31 Toxic effect of venom of black widow spider**

√7th **T63.311 Toxic effect of venom of black widow spider, accidental (unintentional)**

√7th **T63.312 Toxic effect of venom of black widow spider, intentional self-harm**

√7th **T63.313 Toxic effect of venom of black widow spider, assault**

√7th **T63.314 Toxic effect of venom of black widow spider, undetermined**

√6th **T63.32 Toxic effect of venom of tarantula**

√7th **T63.321 Toxic effect of venom of tarantula, accidental (unintentional)**

√7th **T63.322 Toxic effect of venom of tarantula, intentional self-harm**

√7th **T63.323 Toxic effect of venom of tarantula, assault**

√7th **T63.324 Toxic effect of venom of tarantula, undetermined**

√6th **T63.33 Toxic effect of venom of brown recluse spider**

√7th **T63.331 Toxic effect of venom of brown recluse spider, accidental (unintentional)**

√7th **T63.332 Toxic effect of venom of brown recluse spider, intentional self-harm**

√7th **T63.333 Toxic effect of venom of brown recluse spider, assault**

√7th **T63.334 Toxic effect of venom of brown recluse spider, undetermined**

√6th **T63.39 Toxic effect of venom of other spider**

√7th **T63.391 Toxic effect of venom of other spider, accidental (unintentional)**

√7th **T63.392 Toxic effect of venom of other spider, intentional self-harm**

√7th **T63.393 Toxic effect of venom of other spider, assault**

√7th **T63.394 Toxic effect of venom of other spider, undetermined**

√5th **T63.4 Toxic effect of venom of other arthropods**

√6th **T63.41 Toxic effect of venom of centipedes and venomous millipedes**

√7th **T63.411 Toxic effect of venom of centipedes and venomous millipedes, accidental (unintentional)**

√7th **T63.412 Toxic effect of venom of centipedes and venomous millipedes, intentional self-harm**

√7th **T63.413 Toxic effect of venom of centipedes and venomous millipedes, assault**

√7th **T63.414 Toxic effect of venom of centipedes and venomous millipedes, undetermined**

√6th **T63.42 Toxic effect of venom of ants**

√7th **T63.421 Toxic effect of venom of ants, accidental (unintentional)**

√7th **T63.422 Toxic effect of venom of ants, intentional self-harm**

√7th **T63.423 Toxic effect of venom of ants, assault**

√7th **T63.424 Toxic effect of venom of ants, undetermined**

√6th **T63.43 Toxic effect of venom of caterpillars**

√7th **T63.431 Toxic effect of venom of caterpillars, accidental (unintentional)**

√7th **T63.432 Toxic effect of venom of caterpillars, intentional self-harm**

√7th **T63.433 Toxic effect of venom of caterpillars, assault**

√7th **T63.434 Toxic effect of venom of caterpillars, undetermined**

√6th **T63.44 Toxic effect of venom of bees**

√7th **T63.441 Toxic effect of venom of bees, accidental (unintentional)**

√7th **T63.442 Toxic effect of venom of bees, intentional self-harm**

√7th **T63.443 Toxic effect of venom of bees, assault**

√7th **T63.444 Toxic effect of venom of bees, undetermined**

√6th **T63.45 Toxic effect of venom of hornets**

√7th **T63.451 Toxic effect of venom of hornets, accidental (unintentional)**

√7th **T63.452 Toxic effect of venom of hornets, intentional self-harm**

√7th **T63.453 Toxic effect of venom of hornets, assault**

√7th **T63.454 Toxic effect of venom of hornets, undetermined**

√6th **T63.46 Toxic effect of venom of wasps**
Toxic effect of yellow jacket

√7th **T63.461 Toxic effect of venom of wasps, accidental (unintentional)**

√7th **T63.462 Toxic effect of venom of wasps, intentional self-harm**

√7th **T63.463 Toxic effect of venom of wasps, assault**

√7th **T63.464 Toxic effect of venom of wasps, undetermined**

√6th **T63.48 Toxic effect of venom of other arthropod**

√7th **T63.481 Toxic effect of venom of other arthropod, accidental (unintentional)**

√7th **T63.482 Toxic effect of venom of other arthropod, intentional self-harm**

√7th **T63.483 Toxic effect of venom of other arthropod, assault**

√7th **T63.484 Toxic effect of venom of other arthropod, undetermined**

√5th **T63.5 Toxic effect of contact with venomous fish**
EXCLUDES 2 *poisoning by ingestion of fish (T61.-)*

√6th **T63.51 Toxic effect of contact with stingray**

√7th **T63.511 Toxic effect of contact with stingray, accidental (unintentional)**

√7th **T63.512 Toxic effect of contact with stingray, intentional self-harm**

√7th **T63.513 Toxic effect of contact with stingray, assault**

√7th **T63.514 Toxic effect of contact with stingray, undetermined**

√6th T63.59 Toxic effect of contact with other venomous fish
√7th T63.591 Toxic effect of contact with other venomous fish, accidental (unintentional)
√7th T63.592 Toxic effect of contact with other venomous fish, intentional self-harm
√7th T63.593 Toxic effect of contact with other venomous fish, assault
√7th T63.594 Toxic effect of contact with other venomous fish, undetermined

√5th T63.6 Toxic effect of contact with other venomous marine animals
EXCLUDES 1 *sea-snake venom (T63.09)*
EXCLUDES 2 *poisoning by ingestion of shellfish (T61.78-)*

√6th T63.61 Toxic effect of contact with Portugese Man-o-war
Toxic effect of contact with bluebottle
√7th T63.611 Toxic effect of contact with Portugese Man-o-war, accidental (unintentional)
√7th T63.612 Toxic effect of contact with Portugese Man-o-war, intentional self-harm
√7th T63.613 Toxic effect of contact with Portugese Man-o-war, assault
√7th T63.614 Toxic effect of contact with Portugese Man-o-war, undetermined

√6th T63.62 Toxic effect of contact with other jellyfish
√7th T63.621 Toxic effect of contact with other jellyfish, accidental (unintentional)
√7th T63.622 Toxic effect of contact with other jellyfish, intentional self-harm
√7th T63.623 Toxic effect of contact with other jellyfish, assault
√7th T63.624 Toxic effect of contact with other jellyfish, undetermined

√6th T63.63 Toxic effect of contact with sea anemone
√7th T63.631 Toxic effect of contact with sea anemone, accidental (unintentional)
√7th T63.632 Toxic effect of contact with sea anemone, intentional self-harm
√7th T63.633 Toxic effect of contact with sea anemone, assault
√7th T63.634 Toxic effect of contact with sea anemone, undetermined

√6th T63.69 Toxic effect of contact with other venomous marine animals
√7th T63.691 Toxic effect of contact with other venomous marine animals, accidental (unintentional)
√7th T63.692 Toxic effect of contact with other venomous marine animals, intentional self-harm
√7th T63.693 Toxic effect of contact with other venomous marine animals, assault
√7th T63.694 Toxic effect of contact with other venomous marine animals, undetermined

√5th T63.7 Toxic effect of contact with venomous plant
√6th T63.71 Toxic effect of contact with venomous marine plant
√7th T63.711 Toxic effect of contact with venomous marine plant, accidental (unintentional)
√7th T63.712 Toxic effect of contact with venomous marine plant, intentional self-harm
√7th T63.713 Toxic effect of contact with venomous marine plant, assault
√7th T63.714 Toxic effect of contact with venomous marine plant, undetermined

√6th T63.79 Toxic effect of contact with other venomous plant
√7th T63.791 Toxic effect of contact with other venomous plant, accidental (unintentional)
√7th T63.792 Toxic effect of contact with other venomous plant, intentional self-harm
√7th T63.793 Toxic effect of contact with other venomous plant, assault
√7th T63.794 Toxic effect of contact with other venomous plant, undetermined

√5th T63.8 Toxic effect of contact with other venomous animals
√6th T63.81 Toxic effect of contact with venomous frog
EXCLUDES 1 *contact with nonvenomous frog (W62.0)*
√7th T63.811 Toxic effect of contact with venomous frog, accidental (unintentional)
√7th T63.812 Toxic effect of contact with venomous frog, intentional self-harm
√7th T63.813 Toxic effect of contact with venomous frog, assault
√7th T63.814 Toxic effect of contact with venomous frog, undetermined

√6th T63.82 Toxic effect of contact with venomous toad
EXCLUDES 1 *contact with nonvenomous toad (W62.1)*
√7th T63.821 Toxic effect of contact with venomous toad, accidental (unintentional)
√7th T63.822 Toxic effect of contact with venomous toad, intentional self-harm
√7th T63.823 Toxic effect of contact with venomous toad, assault
√7th T63.824 Toxic effect of contact with venomous toad, undetermined

√6th T63.83 Toxic effect of contact with other venomous amphibian
EXCLUDES 1 *contact with nonvenomous amphibian (W62.9)*
√7th T63.831 Toxic effect of contact with other venomous amphibian, accidental (unintentional)
√7th T63.832 Toxic effect of contact with other venomous amphibian, intentional self-harm
√7th T63.833 Toxic effect of contact with other venomous amphibian, assault
√7th T63.834 Toxic effect of contact with other venomous amphibian, undetermined

√6th T63.89 Toxic effect of contact with other venomous animals
√7th T63.891 Toxic effect of contact with other venomous animals, accidental (unintentional)
√7th T63.892 Toxic effect of contact with other venomous animals, intentional self-harm
√7th T63.893 Toxic effect of contact with other venomous animals, assault
√7th T63.894 Toxic effect of contact with other venomous animals, undetermined

√5th T63.9 Toxic effect of contact with unspecified venomous animal
√x7th T63.91 Toxic effect of contact with unspecified venomous animal, accidental (unintentional)
√x7th T63.92 Toxic effect of contact with unspecified venomous animal, intentional self-harm
√x7th T63.93 Toxic effect of contact with unspecified venomous animal, assault
√x7th T63.94 Toxic effect of contact with unspecified venomous animal, undetermined

√4th **T64 Toxic effect of aflatoxin and other mycotoxin food contaminants**

The appropriate 7th character is to be added to each code from category T64.
A initial encounter
D subsequent encounter
S sequela

√5th T64.0 Toxic effect of aflatoxin
√x7th T64.01 Toxic effect of aflatoxin, accidental (unintentional)
√x7th T64.02 Toxic effect of aflatoxin, intentional self-harm
√x7th T64.03 Toxic effect of aflatoxin, assault
√x7th T64.04 Toxic effect of aflatoxin, undetermined

√5th T64.8 Toxic effect of other mycotoxin food contaminants
√x7th T64.81 Toxic effect of other mycotoxin food contaminants, accidental (unintentional)
√x7th T64.82 Toxic effect of other mycotoxin food contaminants, intentional self-harm
√x7th T64.83 Toxic effect of other mycotoxin food contaminants, assault

✓x7th **T64.84 Toxic effect of other mycotoxin food contaminants, undetermined**

✓4th **T65 Toxic effect of other and unspecified substances**

The appropriate 7th character is to be added to each code from category T65.
A initial encounter
D subsequent encounter
S sequela

✓5th **T65.0 Toxic effect of cyanides**
EXCLUDES1 *hydrogen cyanide (T57.3-)*

✓6th **T65.0X Toxic effect of cyanides**

✓7th **T65.0X1 Toxic effect of cyanides, accidental (unintentional)**
Toxic effect of cyanides NOS

✓7th **T65.0X2 Toxic effect of cyanides, intentional self-harm**

✓7th **T65.0X3 Toxic effect of cyanides, assault**

✓7th **T65.0X4 Toxic effect of cyanides, undetermined**

✓5th **T65.1 Toxic effect of strychnine and its salts**

✓6th **T65.1X Toxic effect of strychnine and its salts**

✓7th **T65.1X1 Toxic effect of strychnine and its salts, accidental (unintentional)**
Toxic effect of strychnine and its salts NOS

✓7th **T65.1X2 Toxic effect of strychnine and its salts, intentional self-harm**

✓7th **T65.1X3 Toxic effect of strychnine and its salts, assault**

✓7th **T65.1X4 Toxic effect of strychnine and its salts, undetermined**

✓5th **T65.2 Toxic effect of tobacco and nicotine**
EXCLUDES2 *nicotine dependence (F17.-)*

✓6th **T65.21 Toxic effect of chewing tobacco**

✓7th **T65.211 Toxic effect of chewing tobacco, accidental (unintentional)**
Toxic effect of chewing tobacco NOS

✓7th **T65.212 Toxic effect of chewing tobacco, intentional self-harm**

✓7th **T65.213 Toxic effect of chewing tobacco, assault**

✓7th **T65.214 Toxic effect of chewing tobacco, undetermined**

✓6th **T65.22 Toxic effect of tobacco cigarettes**
Toxic effect of tobacco smoke
Use additional code for exposure to second hand tobacco smoke (Z57.31, Z77.22)

✓7th **T65.221 Toxic effect of tobacco cigarettes, accidental (unintentional)**
Toxic effect of tobacco cigarettes NOS

✓7th **T65.222 Toxic effect of tobacco cigarettes, intentional self-harm**

✓7th **T65.223 Toxic effect of tobacco cigarettes, assault**

✓7th **T65.224 Toxic effect of tobacco cigarettes, undetermined**

✓6th **T65.29 Toxic effect of other tobacco and nicotine**

✓7th **T65.291 Toxic effect of other tobacco and nicotine, accidental (unintentional)**
Toxic effect of other tobacco and nicotine NOS

✓7th **T65.292 Toxic effect of other tobacco and nicotine, intentional self-harm**

✓7th **T65.293 Toxic effect of other tobacco and nicotine, assault**

✓7th **T65.294 Toxic effect of other tobacco and nicotine, undetermined**

✓5th **T65.3 Toxic effect of nitroderivatives and aminoderivatives of benzene and its homologues**
Toxic effect of anilin [benzenamine]
Toxic effect of nitrobenzene
Toxic effect of trinitrotoluene

✓6th **T65.3X Toxic effect of nitroderivatives and aminoderivatives of benzene and its homologues**

✓7th **T65.3X1 Toxic effect of nitroderivatives and aminoderivatives of benzene and its homologues, accidental (unintentional)**
Toxic effect of nitroderivatives and aminoderivatives of benzene and its homologues NOS

✓7th **T65.3X2 Toxic effect of nitroderivatives and aminoderivatives of benzene and its homologues, intentional self-harm**

✓7th **T65.3X3 Toxic effect of nitroderivatives and aminoderivatives of benzene and its homologues, assault**

✓7th **T65.3X4 Toxic effect of nitroderivatives and aminoderivatives of benzene and its homologues, undetermined**

✓5th **T65.4 Toxic effect of carbon disulfide**

✓6th **T65.4X Toxic effect of carbon disulfide**

✓7th **T65.4X1 Toxic effect of carbon disulfide, accidental (unintentional)**
Toxic effect of carbon disulfide NOS

✓7th **T65.4X2 Toxic effect of carbon disulfide, intentional self-harm**

✓7th **T65.4X3 Toxic effect of carbon disulfide, assault**

✓7th **T65.4X4 Toxic effect of carbon disulfide, undetermined**

✓5th **T65.5 Toxic effect of nitroglycerin and other nitric acids and esters**
Toxic effect of 1,2,3-Propanetriol trinitrate

✓6th **T65.5X Toxic effect of nitroglycerin and other nitric acids and esters**

✓7th **T65.5X1 Toxic effect of nitroglycerin and other nitric acids and esters, accidental (unintentional)**
Toxic effect of nitroglycerin and other nitric acids and esters NOS

✓7th **T65.5X2 Toxic effect of nitroglycerin and other nitric acids and esters, intentional self-harm**

✓7th **T65.5X3 Toxic effect of nitroglycerin and other nitric acids and esters, assault**

✓7th **T65.5X4 Toxic effect of nitroglycerin and other nitric acids and esters, undetermined**

✓5th **T65.6 Toxic effect of paints and dyes, not elsewhere classified**

✓6th **T65.6X Toxic effect of paints and dyes, not elsewhere classified**

✓7th **T65.6X1 Toxic effect of paints and dyes, not elsewhere classified, accidental (unintentional)**
Toxic effect of paints and dyes NOS

✓7th **T65.6X2 Toxic effect of paints and dyes, not elsewhere classified, intentional self-harm**

✓7th **T65.6X3 Toxic effect of paints and dyes, not elsewhere classified, assault**

✓7th **T65.6X4 Toxic effect of paints and dyes, not elsewhere classified, undetermined**

✓5th **T65.8 Toxic effect of other specified substances**

✓6th **T65.81 Toxic effect of latex**

✓7th **T65.811 Toxic effect of latex, accidental (unintentional)**
Toxic effect of latex NOS

✓7th **T65.812 Toxic effect of latex, intentional self-harm**

✓7th **T65.813 Toxic effect of latex, assault**

✓7th **T65.814 Toxic effect of latex, undetermined**

T65.82 Toxic effect of harmful algae and algae toxins
Toxic effect of (harmful) algae bloom NOS
Toxic effect of blue-green algae bloom
Toxic effect of brown tide
Toxic effect of cyanobacteria bloom
Toxic effect of Florida red tide
Toxic effect of pfiesteria piscicida
Toxic effect of red tide

T65.821 Toxic effect of harmful algae and algae toxins, accidental (unintentional)
Toxic effect of harmful algae and algae toxins NOS

T65.822 Toxic effect of harmful algae and algae toxins, intentional self-harm

T65.823 Toxic effect of harmful algae and algae toxins, assault

T65.824 Toxic effect of harmful algae and algae toxins, undetermined

T65.83 Toxic effect of fiberglass

T65.831 Toxic effect of fiberglass, accidental (unintentional)
Toxic effect of fiberglass NOS

T65.832 Toxic effect of fiberglass, intentional self-harm

T65.833 Toxic effect of fiberglass, assault

T65.834 Toxic effect of fiberglass, undetermined

T65.89 Toxic effect of other specified substances

T65.891 Toxic effect of other specified substances, accidental (unintentional)
Toxic effect of other specified substances NOS

T65.892 Toxic effect of other specified substances, intentional self-harm

T65.893 Toxic effect of other specified substances, assault

T65.894 Toxic effect of other specified substances, undetermined

T65.9 Toxic effect of unspecified substance

T65.91 Toxic effect of unspecified substance, accidental (unintentional)
Poisoning NOS

T65.92 Toxic effect of unspecified substance, intentional self-harm

T65.93 Toxic effect of unspecified substance, assault

T65.94 Toxic effect of unspecified substance, undetermined

Other and unspecified effects of external causes (T66-T78)

T66 Radiation sickness, unspecified
EXCLUDES 1 *specified adverse effects of radiation, such as:*
burns (T20-T31)
leukemia (C91-C95)
radiation gastroenteritis and colitis (K52.0)
radiation pneumonitis (J70.0)
radiation related disorders of the skin and subcutaneous tissue (L55-L59)
radiation sunburn (L55.-)

The appropriate 7th character is to be added to code T66.
A initial encounter
D subsequent encounter
S sequela

T67 Effects of heat and light
EXCLUDES 1 *erythema [dermatitis] ab igne (L59.0)*
malignant hyperpyrexia due to anesthesia (T88.3)
radiation-related disorders of the skin and subcutaneous tissue (L55-L59)
EXCLUDES 2 *burns (T20-T31)*
sunburn (L55.-)
sweat disorder due to heat (L74-L75))

The appropriate 7th character is to be added to each code from category T67.
A initial encounter
D subsequent encounter
S sequela

T67.0 Heatstroke and sunstroke
Heat apoplexy
Heat pyrexia
Siriasis
Thermoplegia
Use additional code(s) to identify any associated complications of heatstroke, such as:
coma and stupor (R40.-)
systemic inflammatory response syndrome (R65.1-)

T67.1 Heat syncope
Heat collapse

T67.2 Heat cramp

T67.3 Heat exhaustion, anhydrotic
Heat prostration due to water depletion
EXCLUDES 1 *heat exhaustion due to salt depletion (T67.4)*

T67.4 Heat exhaustion due to salt depletion
Heat prostration due to salt (and water) depletion

T67.5 Heat exhaustion, unspecified
Heat prostration NOS

T67.6 Heat fatigue, transient

T67.7 Heat edema

T67.8 Other effects of heat and light

T67.9 Effect of heat and light, unspecified

T68 Hypothermia
Accidental hypothermia
Hypothermia NOS
EXCLUDES 1 *hypothermia following anesthesia (T88.51)*
hypothermia not associated with low environmental temperature (R68.0)
hypothermia of newborn (P80.-)
EXCLUDES 2 *frostbite (T33-T34)*
Use additional code to identify source of exposure:
exposure to excessive cold of man-made origin (W93)
exposure to excessive cold of natural origin (X31)

The appropriate 7th character is to be added to code T68.
A initial encounter
D subsequent encounter
S sequela

T69 Other effects of reduced temperature
EXCLUDES 2 *frostbite (T33-T34)*
Use additional code to identify source of exposure:
exposure to excessive cold of man-made origin (W93)
exposure to excessive cold of natural origin (X31)

The appropriate 7th character is to be added to each code from category T69.
A initial encounter
D subsequent encounter
S sequela

T69.0 Immersion hand and foot

T69.01 Immersion hand

T69.011 Immersion hand, right hand

T69.012 Immersion hand, left hand

T69.019 Immersion hand, unspecified hand

T69.02 Immersion foot
Trench foot

T69.021 Immersion foot, right foot

T69.022 Immersion foot, left foot

T69.029 Immersion foot, unspecified foot

T69.1 Chilblains

T69.8 Other specified effects of reduced temperature

T69.9 Effect of reduced temperature, unspecified

T70 Effects of air pressure and water pressure

The appropriate 7th character is to be added to each code from category T70.
A initial encounter
D subsequent encounter
S sequela

T70.0 Otitic barotrauma
Aero-otitis media
Effects of change in ambient atmospheric pressure or water pressure on ears

T70.1 Sinus barotrauma
Aerosinusitis
Effects of change in ambient atmospheric pressure on sinuses

T70.2 Other and unspecified effects of high altitude
EXCLUDES 2 *polycythemia due to high altitude (D75.1)*
T70.20 Unspecified effects of high altitude
T70.29 Other effects of high altitude
Alpine sickness
Anoxia due to high altitude
Barotrauma NOS
Hypobaropathy
Mountain sickness
T70.3 Caisson disease [decompression sickness]
Compressed-air disease
Diver's palsy or paralysis
T70.4 Effects of high-pressure fluids
Hydraulic jet injection (industrial)
Pneumatic jet injection (industrial)
Traumatic jet injection (industrial)
T70.8 Other effects of air pressure and water pressure
T70.9 Effect of air pressure and water pressure, unspecified

T71 Asphyxiation
Mechanical suffocation
Traumatic suffocation
EXCLUDES 1 *acute respiratory distress (syndrome) (J80)*
anoxia due to high altitude (T70.2)
asphyxia NOS (R09.01)
asphyxia from carbon monoxide (T58.-)
asphyxia from inhalation of food or foreign body (T17.-)
asphyxia from other gases, fumes and vapors (T59.-)
respiratory distress (syndrome) in newborn (P22.-)

The appropriate 7th character is to be added to each code from category T71.
A initial encounter
D subsequent encounter
S sequela

T71.1 Asphyxiation due to mechanical threat to breathing
Suffocation due to mechanical threat to breathing
T71.11 Asphyxiation due to smothering under pillow
T71.111 Asphyxiation due to smothering under pillow, accidental
Asphyxiation due to smothering under pillow NOS
T71.112 Asphyxiation due to smothering under pillow, intentional self-harm
T71.113 Asphyxiation due to smothering under pillow, assault
T71.114 Asphyxiation due to smothering under pillow, undetermined
T71.12 Asphyxiation due to plastic bag
T71.121 Asphyxiation due to plastic bag, accidental
Asphyxiation due to plastic bag NOS
T71.122 Asphyxiation due to plastic bag, intentional self-harm
T71.123 Asphyxiation due to plastic bag, assault
T71.124 Asphyxiation due to plastic bag, undetermined
T71.13 Asphyxiation due to being trapped in bed linens
T71.131 Asphyxiation due to being trapped in bed linens, accidental
Asphyxiation due to being trapped in bed linens NOS
T71.132 Asphyxiation due to being trapped in bed linens, intentional self-harm
T71.133 Asphyxiation due to being trapped in bed linens, assault
T71.134 Asphyxiation due to being trapped in bed linens, undetermined
T71.14 Asphyxiation due to smothering under another person's body (in bed)
T71.141 Asphyxiation due to smothering under another person's body (in bed), accidental
Asphyxiation due to smothering under another person's body (in bed) NOS
T71.143 Asphyxiation due to smothering under another person's body (in bed), assault
T71.144 Asphyxiation due to smothering under another person's body (in bed), undetermined
T71.15 Asphyxiation due to smothering in furniture
T71.151 Asphyxiation due to smothering in furniture, accidental
Asphyxiation due to smothering in furniture NOS
T71.152 Asphyxiation due to smothering in furniture, intentional self-harm
T71.153 Asphyxiation due to smothering in furniture, assault
T71.154 Asphyxiation due to smothering in furniture, undetermined
T71.16 Asphyxiation due to hanging
Hanging by window shade cord
Use additional code for any associated injuries, such as:
crushing injury of neck (S17.-)
fracture of cervical vertebrae (S12.0-S12.2-)
open wound of neck (S11.-)
T71.161 Asphyxiation due to hanging, accidental
Asphyxiation due to hanging NOS
Hanging NOS
T71.162 Asphyxiation due to hanging, intentional self-harm
T71.163 Asphyxiation due to hanging, assault
T71.164 Asphyxiation due to hanging, undetermined
T71.19 Asphyxiation due to mechanical threat to breathing due to other causes
T71.191 Asphyxiation due to mechanical threat to breathing due to other causes, accidental
Asphyxiation due to other causes NOS
T71.192 Asphyxiation due to mechanical threat to breathing due to other causes, intentional self-harm
T71.193 Asphyxiation due to mechanical threat to breathing due to other causes, assault
T71.194 Asphyxiation due to mechanical threat to breathing due to other causes, undetermined
T71.2 Asphyxiation due to systemic oxygen deficiency due to low oxygen content in ambient air
Suffocation due to systemic oxygen deficiency due to low oxygen content in ambient air
T71.20 Asphyxiation due to systemic oxygen deficiency due to low oxygen content in ambient air due to unspecified cause
T71.21 Asphyxiation due to cave-in or falling earth
Use additional code for any associated cataclysm (X34-X38)
T71.22 Asphyxiation due to being trapped in a car trunk
T71.221 Asphyxiation due to being trapped in a car trunk, accidental
T71.222 Asphyxiation due to being trapped in a car trunk, intentional self-harm
T71.223 Asphyxiation due to being trapped in a car trunk, assault
T71.224 Asphyxiation due to being trapped in a car trunk, undetermined
T71.23 Asphyxiation due to being trapped in a (discarded) refrigerator
T71.231 Asphyxiation due to being trapped in a (discarded) refrigerator, accidental
T71.232 Asphyxiation due to being trapped in a (discarded) refrigerator, intentional self-harm
T71.233 Asphyxiation due to being trapped in a (discarded) refrigerator, assault
T71.234 Asphyxiation due to being trapped in a (discarded) refrigerator, undetermined
T71.29 Asphyxiation due to being trapped in other low oxygen environment

T71.9 Asphyxiation due to unspecified cause
Suffocation (by strangulation) due to unspecified cause
Suffocation NOS
Systemic oxygen deficiency due to low oxygen content in ambient air due to unspecified cause
Systemic oxygen deficiency due to mechanical threat to breathing due to unspecified cause
Traumatic asphyxia NOS

T73 Effects of other deprivation

The appropriate 7th character is to be added to each code from category T73.
A initial encounter
D subsequent encounter
S sequela

T73.0 Starvation
Deprivation of food
T73.1 Deprivation of water
T73.2 Exhaustion due to exposure
T73.3 Exhaustion due to excessive exertion
Exhaustion due to overexertion
T73.8 Other effects of deprivation
T73.9 Effect of deprivation, unspecified

T74 Adult and child abuse, neglect and other maltreatment, confirmed
EXCLUDES 1 *abuse and maltreatment in pregnancy (O9A.3-, O9A.4-, O9A.5-)*
adult and child maltreatment, suspected (T76.-)
Use additional code, if applicable, to identify any associated current injury
Use additional external cause code to identify perpetrator, if known (Y07.-)

The appropriate 7th character is to be added to each code from category T74.
A initial encounter
D subsequent encounter
S sequela

T74.0 Neglect or abandonment, confirmed
T74.01 Adult neglect or abandonment, confirmed
T74.02 Child neglect or abandonment, confirmed
T74.1 Physical abuse, confirmed
EXCLUDES 2 *sexual abuse (T74.2-)*
T74.11 Adult physical abuse, confirmed
T74.12 Child physical abuse, confirmed
EXCLUDES 2 *shaken infant syndrome (T74.4)*
T74.2 Sexual abuse, confirmed
Rape, confirmed
Sexual assault, confirmed
T74.21 Adult sexual abuse, confirmed
T74.22 Child sexual abuse, confirmed
T74.3 Psychological abuse, confirmed
T74.31 Adult psychological abuse, confirmed
T74.32 Child psychological abuse, confirmed
T74.4 Shaken infant syndrome
T74.9 Unspecified maltreatment, confirmed
T74.91 Unspecified adult maltreatment, confirmed
T74.92 Unspecified child maltreatment, confirmed

T75 Other and unspecified effects of other external causes
EXCLUDES 1 *adverse effects NEC (T78.-)*
EXCLUDES 2 *burns (electric) (T20-T31)*

The appropriate 7th character is to be added to each code from category T75.
A initial encounter
D subsequent encounter
S sequela

T75.0 Effects of lightning
Struck by lightning
T75.00 Unspecified effects of lightning
Struck by lightning NOS
T75.01 Shock due to being struck by lightning
T75.09 Other effects of lightning
Use additional code for other effects of lightning
T75.1 Unspecified effects of drowning and nonfatal submersion
Immersion
EXCLUDES 1 *specified effects of drowning—code to effects*
T75.2 Effects of vibration
T75.20 Unspecified effects of vibration
T75.21 Pneumatic hammer syndrome
T75.22 Traumatic vasospastic syndrome
T75.23 Vertigo from infrasound
EXCLUDES 1 *vertigo NOS (R42)*
T75.29 Other effects of vibration
T75.3 Motion sickness
Airsickness
Seasickness
Travel sickness
Use additional external cause code to identify vehicle or type of motion (Y92.81-, Y93.5-)
T75.4 Electrocution
Shock from electric current
Shock from electroshock gun (taser)
T75.8 Other specified effects of external causes
T75.81 Effects of abnormal gravitation [G] forces
T75.82 Effects of weightlessness
T75.89 Other specified effects of external causes

T76 Adult and child abuse, neglect and other maltreatment, suspected
EXCLUDES 1 *adult and child maltreatment, confirmed (T74.-)*
suspected abuse and maltreatment in pregnancy (O9A.3-, O9A.4-, O9A.5-)
suspected adult physical and sexual abuse, ruled out (Z04.71)
suspected child physical and sexual abuse, ruled out (Z04.72)
Use additional code, if applicable, to identify any associated current injury

The appropriate 7th character is to be added to each code from category T76.
A initial encounter
D subsequent encounter
S sequela

T76.0 Neglect or abandonment, suspected
T76.01 Adult neglect or abandonment, suspected
T76.02 Child neglect or abandonment, suspected
T76.1 Physical abuse, suspected
T76.11 Adult physical abuse, suspected
T76.12 Child physical abuse, suspected
T76.2 Sexual abuse, suspected
Rape, suspected
Sexual abuse, suspected
EXCLUDES 1 *alleged abuse, ruled out (Z04.7)*
T76.21 Adult sexual abuse, suspected
T76.22 Child sexual abuse, suspected
T76.3 Psychological abuse, suspected
T76.31 Adult psychological abuse, suspected
T76.32 Child psychological abuse, suspected
T76.9 Unspecified maltreatment, suspected
T76.91 Unspecified adult maltreatment, suspected
T76.92 Unspecified child maltreatment, suspected

T78 Adverse effects, not elsewhere classified
EXCLUDES 2 *complications of surgical and medical care NEC (T80-T88)*

The appropriate 7th character is to be added to each code from category T78.
A initial encounter
D subsequent encounter
S sequela

T78.0 Anaphylactic reaction due to food
Anaphylactic reaction due to adverse food reaction
Anaphylactic shock or reaction due to nonpoisonous foods
Anaphylactoid reaction due to food
T78.00 Anaphylactic reaction due to unspecified food
T78.01 Anaphylactic reaction due to peanuts
T78.02 Anaphylactic reaction due to shellfish (crustaceans)
T78.03 Anaphylactic reaction due to other fish
T78.04 Anaphylactic reaction due to fruits and vegetables

Appropriate additional character required
Requires 7th character, placeholder x must fill empty characters

√x7th **T78.05 Anaphylactic reaction due to tree nuts and seeds**
EXCLUDES 1 *anaphylactic reaction due to peanuts (T78.01)*

√x7th **T78.06 Anaphylactic reaction due to food additives**

√x7th **T78.07 Anaphylactic reaction due to milk and dairy products**

√x7th **T78.08 Anaphylactic reaction due to eggs**

√x7th **T78.09 Anaphylactic reaction due to other food products**

√x7th **T78.1 Other adverse food reactions, not elsewhere classified**
Use additional code to identify the type of reaction
EXCLUDES 1 *anaphylactic reaction or shock due to adverse food reaction (T78.0-)*
anaphylactic reaction due to food (T78.0-)
bacterial food borne intoxications (A05.-)
EXCLUDES 2 *allergic and dietetic gastroenteritis and colitis (K52.2)*
allergic rhinitis due to food (J30.5)
dermatitis due to food in contact with skin (L23.6, L24.6, L25.4)
dermatitis due to ingested food (L27.2)

√x7th **T78.2 Anaphylactic shock, unspecified**
Allergic shock
Anaphylactic reaction
Anaphylaxis
EXCLUDES 1 *anaphylactic reaction or shock due to adverse effect of correct medicinal substance properly administered (T88.6)*
anaphylactic reaction or shock due to adverse food reaction (T78.0-)
anaphylactic reaction or shock due to serum (T80.5-)

√x7th **T78.3 Angioneurotic edema**
Allergic angioedema
Giant urticaria
Quincke's edema
EXCLUDES 1 *serum urticaria (T80.6-)*
urticaria (L50.-)

√5th **T78.4 Other and unspecified allergy**
EXCLUDES 1 *specified types of allergic reaction such as:*
allergic diarrhea (K52.2)
allergic gastroenteritis and colitis (K52.2)
dermatitis (L23-L25, L27-)
hay fever (J30.1)

√x7th **T78.40 Allergy, unspecified**
Allergic reaction NOS
Hypersensitivity NOS

√x7th **T78.41 Arthus phenomenon**
Arthus reaction

√x7th **T78.49 Other allergy**

√x7th **T78.8 Other adverse effects, not elsewhere classified**

Certain early complications of trauma (T79)

√4th **T79 Certain early complications of trauma, not elsewhere classified**
EXCLUDES 2 *acute respiratory distress syndrome (J80)*
complications occurring during or following medical procedures (T80-T88)
complications of surgical and medical care NEC (T80-T88)
newborn respiratory distress syndrome (P22.0)

The appropriate 7th character is to be added to each code from category T79.
A initial encounter
D subsequent encounter
S sequela

√x7th **T79.0 Air embolism (traumatic)**
EXCLUDES 1 *air embolism complicating:*
abortion or ectopic or molar pregnancy (O00-O07, O08.2)
pregnancy, childbirth and the puerperium (O88.0)
air embolism following:
infusion, transfusion, and therapeutic injection (T80.0)
procedure NEC (T81.7-)

√x7th **T79.1 Fat embolism (traumatic)**
EXCLUDES 1 *fat embolism complicating:*
abortion or ectopic or molar pregnancy (O00-O07, O08.2)
pregnancy, childbirth and the puerperium (O88.8)

√x7th **T79.2 Traumatic secondary and recurrent hemorrhage and seroma**

√x7th **T79.4 Traumatic shock**
Shock (immediate) (delayed) following injury
EXCLUDES 1 *anaphylactic shock due to adverse food reaction (T78.0-)*
anaphylactic shock due to correct medicinal substance properly administered (T88.6)
anaphylactic shock due to serum (T80.5-)
anaphylactic shock NOS (T78.2)
anesthetic shock (T88.2)
electric shock (T75.4)
nontraumatic shock NEC (R57.-)
obstetric shock (O75.1)
postprocedural shock (T81.1-)
septic shock (R65.21)
shock complicating abortion or ectopic or molar pregnancy (O00-O07, O08.3)
shock due to lightning (T75.01)
shock NOS (R57.9)

√x7th **T79.5 Traumatic anuria**
Crush syndrome
Renal failure following crushing

√x7th **T79.6 Traumatic ischemia of muscle**
Traumatic rhabdomyolysis
Volkmann's ischemic contracture
EXCLUDES 2 *anterior tibial syndrome (M76.8)*
compartment syndrome (traumatic) (T79.A-)
nontraumatic ischemia of muscle (M62.2-)

√x7th **T79.7 Traumatic subcutaneous emphysema**
EXCLUDES 1 *emphysema NOS (J43)*
emphysema (subcutaneous) resulting from a procedure (T81.82)

√5th **T79.A Traumatic compartment syndrome**
EXCLUDES 1 *fibromyalgia (M79.7)*
nontraumatic compartment syndrome (M79.A-)
traumatic ischemic infarction of muscle (T79.6)

√x7th **T79.A0 Compartment syndrome, unspecified**
Compartment syndrome NOS

√6th **T79.A1 Traumatic compartment syndrome of upper extremity**
Traumatic compartment syndrome of shoulder, arm, forearm, wrist, hand, and fingers

√7th **T79.A11 Traumatic compartment syndrome of right upper extremity**

√7th **T79.A12 Traumatic compartment syndrome of left upper extremity**

√7th **T79.A19 Traumatic compartment syndrome of unspecified upper extremity**

√6th **T79.A2 Traumatic compartment syndrome of lower extremity**
Traumatic compartment syndrome of hip, buttock, thigh, leg, foot, and toes

√7th **T79.A21 Traumatic compartment syndrome of right lower extremity**

√7th **T79.A22 Traumatic compartment syndrome of left lower extremity**

√7th **T79.A29 Traumatic compartment syndrome of unspecified lower extremity**

√x7th **T79.A3 Traumatic compartment syndrome of abdomen**

√x7th **T79.A9 Traumatic compartment syndrome of other sites**

√x7th **T79.8 Other early complications of trauma**

√x7th **T79.9 Unspecified early complication of trauma**

Complications of surgical and medical care, not elsewhere classified (T80-T88)

Use additional code for adverse effect, if applicable, to identify drug (T36-T50 with fifth or sixth character 5)

Use additional code(s) to identify the specified condition resulting from the complication

Use additional code to identify devices involved and details of circumstances (Y62-Y82)

EXCLUDES 2 *any encounters with medical care for postprocedural conditions in which no complications are present, such as:*
artificial opening status (Z93.-)
closure of external stoma (Z43.-)
fitting and adjustment of external prosthetic device (Z44.-)
burns and corrosions from local applications and irradiation (T20-T32)
complications of surgical procedures during pregnancy, childbirth and the puerperium (O00-O9A)
mechanical complication of respirator [ventilator] (J95.850)
poisoning and toxic effects of drugs and chemicals (T36-T65 with fifth or sixth character 1-4 or 6)
postprocedural fever (R50.82)
specified complications classified elsewhere, such as:
cerebrospinal fluid leak from spinal puncture (G97.0)
colostomy malfunction (K94.0-)
disorders of fluid and electrolyte imbalance (E86- E87)
functional disturbances following cardiac surgery (I97.0-I97.1)
intraoperative and postprocedural complications of specified body systems (D78-, E36-, E89-, G97.3-, G97.4, H59.3-, H59-, H95.2-, H95.3, I97.4-, I97.5, J95.6-, J95.7, K91.6-, L76-, M96-, N99-)
ostomy complications (J95.0-, K94-, N99.5-)
postgastric surgery syndromes (K91.1)
postlaminectomy syndrome NEC (M96.1)
postmastectomy lymphedema syndrome (I97.2)
postsurgical blind-loop syndrome (K91.2)
ventilator associated pneumonia (J95.851)

✓4th **T80 Complications following infusion, transfusion and therapeutic injection**

INCLUDES complications following perfusion

EXCLUDES 2 *bone marrow transplant rejection (T86.01)*
febrile nonhemolytic transfusion reaction (R50.84)
fluid overload due to transfusion (E87.71)
posttransfusion purpura (D69.51)
transfusion associated circulatory overload (TACO) (E87.71)
transfusion (red blood cell) associated hemochromatosis (E83.111)
transfusion related acute lung injury (TRALI) (J95.84)

The appropriate 7th character is to be added to each code from category T80.
A initial encounter
D subsequent encounter
S sequela

✓x7th **T80.0 Air embolism following infusion, transfusion and therapeutic injection**

✓x7th **T80.1 Vascular complications following infusion, transfusion and therapeutic injection**

Use additional code to identify the vascular complication

EXCLUDES 2 *extravasation of vesicant agent (T80.81-)*
infiltration of vesicant agent (T80.81-)
vascular complications specified as due to prosthetic devices, implants and grafts (T82.8-, T83.8, T84.8-, T85.8)
postprocedural vascular complications (T81.7-)

✓5th **T80.2 Infections following infusion, transfusion and therapeutic injection**

Use additional code to identify the specific infection, such as: sepsis (A41.9)

Use additional code (R65.2-) to identify severe sepsis, if applicable

EXCLUDES 2 *infections specified as due to prosthetic devices, implants and grafts (T82.6-T82.7, T83.5-T83.6, T84.5-T84.7, T85.7)*
postprocedural infections (T81.4)

✓6th **T80.21 Infection due to central venous catheter**

✓7th **T80.211 Bloodstream infection due to central venous catheter**
Catheter-related bloodstream infection (CRBSI) NOS
Central line-associated bloodstream infection (CLABSI)
Bloodstream infection due to Hickman catheter
Bloodstream infection due to peripherally inserted central catheter (PICC)
Bloodstream infection due to portacath (port-a-cath)
Bloodstream infection due to triple lumen catheter
Bloodstream infection due to umbilical venous catheter

✓7th **T80.212 Local infection due to central venous catheter**
Exit or insertion site infection
Local infection due to Hickman catheter
Local infection due to peripherally inserted central catheter (PICC)
Local infection due to portacath (port-a-cath)
Local infection due to triple lumen catheter
Local infection due to umbilical venous catheter
Port or reservoir infection
Tunnel infection

✓7th **T80.218 Other infection due to central venous catheter**
Other central line-associated infection
Other infection due to Hickman catheter
Other infection due to peripherally inserted central catheter (PICC)
Other infection due to portacath (port-a-cath)
Other infection due to triple lumen catheter
Other infection due to umbilical venous catheter

✓7th **T80.219 Unspecified infection due to central venous catheter**
Central line-associated infection NOS
Unspecified infection due to Hickman catheter
Unspecified infection due to peripherally inserted central catheter (PICC)
Unspecified infection due to portacath (port-a-cath)
Unspecified infection due to triple lumen catheter
Unspecified infection due to umbilical venous catheter

✓x7th **T80.22 Acute infection following transfusion, infusion, or injection of blood and blood products**

✓x7th **T80.29 Infection following other infusion, transfusion and therapeutic injection**

✓5th **T80.3 ABO incompatibility reaction due to transfusion of blood or blood products**

EXCLUDES 1 *minor blood group antigens reactions (Duffy) (E) (K(ell)) (Kidd) (Lewis) (M) (N) (P) (S) (T80.A)*

✓x7th **T80.30 ABO incompatibility reaction due to transfusion of blood or blood products, unspecified**
ABO incompatibility blood transfusion NOS
Reaction to ABO incompatibility from transfusion NOS

√6th **T80.31 ABO incompatibility with hemolytic transfusion reaction**

√7th **T80.310 ABO incompatibility with acute hemolytic transfusion reaction**
ABO incompatibility with hemolytic transfusion reaction less than 24 hours after transfusion
Acute hemolytic transfusion reaction (AHTR) due to ABO incompatibility

√7th **T80.311 ABO incompatibility with delayed hemolytic transfusion reaction**
ABO incompatibility with hemolytic transfusion reaction 24 hours or more after transfusion
Delayed hemolytic transfusion reaction (DHTR) due to ABO incompatibility

√7th **T80.319 ABO incompatibility with hemolytic transfusion reaction, unspecified**
ABO incompatibility with hemolytic transfusion reaction at unspecified time after transfusion
Hemolytic transfusion reaction (HTR) due to ABO incompatibility NOS

√x7th **T80.39 Other ABO incompatibility reaction due to transfusion of blood or blood products**
Delayed serologic transfusion reaction (DSTR) from ABO incompatibility
Other ABO incompatible blood transfusion
Other reaction to ABO incompatible blood transfusion

√x7th **T80.4 Rh incompatibility reaction due to transfusion of blood or blood products**
Reaction due to incompatibility of Rh antigens (C) (c) (D) (E) (e)

√x7th **T80.40 Rh incompatibility reaction due to transfusion of blood or blood products, unspecified**
Reaction due to Rh factor in transfusion NOS
Rh incompatible blood transfusion NOS

√6th **T80.41 Rh incompatibility with hemolytic transfusion reaction**

√7th **T80.410 Rh incompatibility with acute hemolytic transfusion reaction**
Acute hemolytic transfusion reaction (AHTR) due to Rh incompatibility
Rh incompatibility with hemolytic transfusion reaction less than 24 hours after transfusion

√7th **T80.411 Rh incompatibility with delayed hemolytic transfusion reaction**
Delayed hemolytic transfusion reaction (DHTR) due to Rh incompatibility
Rh incompatibility with hemolytic transfusion reaction 24 hours or more after transfusion

√7th **T80.419 Rh incompatibility with hemolytic transfusion reaction, unspecified**
Hemolytic transfusion reaction (HTR) due to Rh incompatibility NOS
Rh incompatibility with hemolytic transfusion reaction at unspecified time after transfusion

√x7th **T80.49 Other Rh incompatibility reaction due to transfusion of blood or blood products**
Delayed serologic transfusion reaction (DSTR) from Rh incompatibility
Other reaction to Rh incompatible blood transfusion

√5th **T80.A Non-ABO incompatibility reaction due to transfusion of blood or blood products**
Reaction due to incompatibility of minor antigens (Duffy) (Kell) (Kidd) (Lewis) (M) (N) (P) (S)

√x7th **T80.A0 Non-ABO incompatibility reaction due to transfusion of blood or blood products, unspecified**
Non-ABO antigen incompatibility reaction from transfusion NOS

√6th **T80.A1 Non-ABO incompatibility with hemolytic transfusion reaction**

√7th **T80.A10 Non-ABO incompatibility with acute hemolytic transfusion reaction**
Acute hemolytic transfusion reaction (AHTR) due to non-ABO incompatibility
Non-ABO incompatibility with hemolytic transfusion reaction less than 24 hours after transfusion

√7th **T80.A11 Non-ABO incompatibility with delayed hemolytic transfusion reaction**
Delayed hemolytic transfusion reaction (DHTR) due to non-ABO incompatibility
Non-ABO incompatibility with hemolytic transfusion reaction 24 or more hours after transfusion

√7th **T80.A19 Non-ABO incompatibility with hemolytic transfusion reaction, unspecified**
Hemolytic transfusion reaction (HTR) due to non-ABO incompatibility NOS
Non-ABO incompatibility with hemolytic transfusion reaction at unspecified time after transfusion

√x7th **T80.A9 Other non-ABO incompatibility reaction due to transfusion of blood or blood products**
Delayed serologic transfusion reaction (DSTR) from non-ABO incompatibility
Other reaction to non-ABO incompatible blood transfusion

√5th **T80.5 Anaphylactic reaction due to serum**
Allergic shock due to serum
Anaphylactic shock due to serum
Anaphylactoid reaction due to serum
Anaphylaxis due to serum

EXCLUDES 1 *ABO incompatibility reaction due to transfusion of blood or blood products (T80.3-)*
allergic reaction or shock NOS (T78.2)
anaphylactic reaction or shock NOS (T78.2)
anaphylactic reaction or shock due to adverse effect of correct medicinal substance properly administered (T88.6)
other serum reaction (T80.6-)

√x7th **T80.51 Anaphylactic reaction due to administration of blood and blood products**

√x7th **T80.52 Anaphylactic reaction due to vaccination**

√x7th **T80.59 Anaphylactic reaction due to other serum**

√5th **T80.6 Other serum reactions**
Intoxication by serum
Protein sickness
Serum rash
Serum sickness
Serum urticaria

EXCLUDES 2 *serum hepatitis (B16.-)*

√x7th **T80.61 Other serum reaction due to administration of blood and blood products**

√x7th **T80.62 Other serum reaction due to vaccination**

√x7th **T80.69 Other serum reaction due to other serum**

√5th **T80.8 Other complications following infusion, transfusion and therapeutic injection**

√6th **T80.81 Extravasation of vesicant agent**
Infiltration of vesicant agent

√7th **T80.810 Extravasation of vesicant antineoplastic chemotherapy**
Infiltration of vesicant antineoplastic chemotherapy

√7th **T80.818 Extravasation of other vesicant agent**
Infiltration of other vesicant agent

√x7th **T80.89 Other complications following infusion, transfusion and therapeutic injection**
Delayed serologic transfusion reaction (DSTR), unspecified incompatibility
Use additional code to identify graft-versus-host reaction, if applicable, (D89.81-)

√5th **T80.9 Unspecified complication following infusion, transfusion and therapeutic injection**

√x7th **T80.90 Unspecified complication following infusion and therapeutic injection**

✓6th **T80.91 Hemolytic transfusion reaction, unspecified incompatibility**
EXCLUDES 1 *ABO incompatibility with hemolytic transfusion reaction (T80.31-)*
Non-ABO incompatibility with hemolytic transfusion reaction (T80.A1-)
Rh incompatibility with hemolytic transfusion reaction (T80.41-)
✓7th **T80.910 Acute hemolytic transfusion reaction, unspecified incompatibility**
✓7th **T80.911 Delayed hemolytic transfusion reaction, unspecified incompatibility**
✓7th **T80.919 Hemolytic transfusion reaction, unspecified incompatibility, unspecified as acute or delayed**
Hemolytic transfusion reaction NOS
✓x7th **T80.92 Unspecified transfusion reaction**
Transfusion reaction NOS

✓4th **T81 Complications of procedures, not elsewhere classified**
Use additional code for adverse effect, if applicable, to identify drug (T36-T50 with fifth or sixth character 5)
EXCLUDES 2 *complications following immunization (T88.0-T88.1)*
complications following infusion, transfusion and therapeutic injection (T80.-)
complications of transplanted organs and tissue (T86.-)
specified complications classified elsewhere, such as:
complication of prosthetic devices, implants and grafts (T82-T85)
dermatitis due to drugs and medicaments (L23.3, L24.4, L25.1, L27.0-L27.1)
endosseous dental implant failure (M27.6-)
floppy iris syndrome (IFIS) (intraoperative) H21.81
intraoperative and postprocedural complications of specific body system (D78-, E36-, E89-, G97.3-, G97.4, H59.3-, H59-, H95.2-, H95.3, I97.4-, I97.5, J95, K91-, L76-, M96-, N99-)
ostomy complications (J95.0-, K94-, N99.5-)
plateau iris syndrome (post-iridectomy) (postprocedural) H21.82
poisoning and toxic effects of drugs and chemicals (T36-T65 with fifth or sixth character 1-4 or 6)

The appropriate 7th character is to be added to each code from category T81.
A initial encounter
D subsequent encounter
S sequela

✓5th **T81.1 Postprocedural shock**
Shock during or resulting from a procedure, not elsewhere classified
EXCLUDES 1 *anaphylactic shock NOS (T78.2)*
anaphylactic shock due to correct substance properly administered (T88.6)
anaphylactic shock due to serum (T80.5-)
anesthetic shock (T88.2)
electric shock (T75.4)
obstetric shock (O75.1)
septic shock (R65.21)
shock following abortion or ectopic or molar pregnancy (O00-O07, O08.3)
traumatic shock (T79.4)
✓x7th **T81.10 Postprocedural shock unspecified**
Collapse NOS during or resulting from a procedure, not elsewhere classified
Postprocedural failure of peripheral circulation
Postprocedural shock NOS
✓x7th **T81.11 Postprocedural cardiogenic shock**
✓x7th **T81.12 Postprocedural septic shock**
Postprocedural endotoxic shock during or resulting from a procedure, not elsewhere classified
Postprocedural gram-negative shock during or resulting from a procedure, not elsewhere classified
Code first underlying infection
Use additional code, to identify any associated acute organ dysfunction, if applicable
✓x7th **T81.19 Other postprocedural shock**
Postprocedural hypovolemic shock

✓5th **T81.3 Disruption of wound, not elsewhere classified**
Disruption of any suture materials or other closure methods
EXCLUDES 1 *breakdown (mechanical) of permanent sutures (T85.612)*
displacement of permanent sutures (T85.622)
disruption of cesarean delivery wound (O90.0)
disruption of perineal obstetric wound (O90.1)
mechanical complication of permanent sutures NEC (T85.692)
✓x7th **T81.30 Disruption of wound, unspecified**
Disruption of wound NOS
✓x7th **T81.31 Disruption of external operation (surgical) wound, not elsewhere classified**
Dehiscence of operation wound NOS
Disruption of operation wound NOS
Disruption or dehiscence of closure of cornea
Disruption or dehiscence of closure of mucosa
Disruption or dehiscence of closure of skin and subcutaneous tissue
Full-thickness skin disruption or dehiscence
Superficial disruption or dehiscence of operation wound
EXCLUDES 1 *dehiscence of amputation stump (T87.81)*
✓x7th **T81.32 Disruption of internal operation (surgical) wound, not elsewhere classified**
Deep disruption or dehiscence of operation wound NOS
Disruption or dehiscence of closure of internal organ or other internal tissue
Disruption or dehiscence of closure of muscle or muscle flap
Disruption or dehiscence of closure of ribs or rib cage
Disruption or dehiscence of closure of skull or craniotomy
Disruption or dehiscence of closure of sternum or sternotomy
Disruption or dehiscence of closure of tendon or ligament
Disruption or dehiscence of closure of superficial or muscular fascia
✓x7th **T81.33 Disruption of traumatic injury wound repair**
Disruption or dehiscence of closure of traumatic laceration (external) (internal)
✓x7th **T81.4 Infection following a procedure**
Intra-abdominal abscess following a procedure
Postprocedural infection, not elsewhere classified
Sepsis following a procedure
Stitch abscess following a procedure
Subphrenic abscess following a procedure
Wound abscess following a procedure
Use additional code to identify infection
Use additional code (R65.2-) to identify severe sepsis, if applicable
EXCLUDES 1 *obstetric surgical wound infection (O86.0)*
postprocedural fever NOS (R50.82)
postprocedural retroperitoneal abscess (K68.11)
EXCLUDES 2 *bleb associated endophthalmitis (H59.4-)*
infection due to infusion, transfusion and therapeutic injection (T80.2-)
infection due to prosthetic devices, implants and grafts (T82.6-T82.7, T83.5-T83.6, T84.5-T84.7, T85.7)
✓5th **T81.5 Complications of foreign body accidentally left in body following procedure**
✓6th **T81.50 Unspecified complication of foreign body accidentally left in body following procedure**
✓7th **T81.500 Unspecified complication of foreign body accidentally left in body following surgical operation**
✓7th **T81.501 Unspecified complication of foreign body accidentally left in body following infusion or transfusion**
✓7th **T81.502 Unspecified complication of foreign body accidentally left in body following kidney dialysis**
✓7th **T81.503 Unspecified complication of foreign body accidentally left in body following injection or immunization**

DRAFT

✓ Appropriate additional character required
✓x7th Requires 7th character, placeholder x must fill empty characters

✓7th T81.504 Unspecified complication of foreign body accidentally left in body following endoscopic examination

✓7th T81.505 Unspecified complication of foreign body accidentally left in body following heart catheterization

✓7th T81.506 Unspecified complication of foreign body accidentally left in body following aspiration, puncture or other catheterization

✓7th T81.507 Unspecified complication of foreign body accidentally left in body following removal of catheter or packing

✓7th T81.508 Unspecified complication of foreign body accidentally left in body following other procedure

✓7th T81.509 Unspecified complication of foreign body accidentally left in body following unspecified procedure

✓6th T81.51 Adhesions due to foreign body accidentally left in body following procedure

✓7th T81.510 Adhesions due to foreign body accidentally left in body following surgical operation

✓7th T81.511 Adhesions due to foreign body accidentally left in body following infusion or transfusion

✓7th T81.512 Adhesions due to foreign body accidentally left in body following kidney dialysis

✓7th T81.513 Adhesions due to foreign body accidentally left in body following injection or immunization

✓7th T81.514 Adhesions due to foreign body accidentally left in body following endoscopic examination

✓7th T81.515 Adhesions due to foreign body accidentally left in body following heart catheterization

✓7th T81.516 Adhesions due to foreign body accidentally left in body following aspiration, puncture or other catheterization

✓7th T81.517 Adhesions due to foreign body accidentally left in body following removal of catheter or packing

✓7th T81.518 Adhesions due to foreign body accidentally left in body following other procedure

✓7th T81.519 Adhesions due to foreign body accidentally left in body following unspecified procedure

✓6th T81.52 Obstruction due to foreign body accidentally left in body following procedure

✓7th T81.520 Obstruction due to foreign body accidentally left in body following surgical operation

✓7th T81.521 Obstruction due to foreign body accidentally left in body following infusion or transfusion

✓7th T81.522 Obstruction due to foreign body accidentally left in body following kidney dialysis

✓7th T81.523 Obstruction due to foreign body accidentally left in body following injection or immunization

✓7th T81.524 Obstruction due to foreign body accidentally left in body following endoscopic examination

✓7th T81.525 Obstruction due to foreign body accidentally left in body following heart catheterization

✓7th T81.526 Obstruction due to foreign body accidentally left in body following aspiration, puncture or other catheterization

✓7th T81.527 Obstruction due to foreign body accidentally left in body following removal of catheter or packing

✓7th T81.528 Obstruction due to foreign body accidentally left in body following other procedure

✓7th T81.529 Obstruction due to foreign body accidentally left in body following unspecified procedure

✓6th T81.53 Perforation due to foreign body accidentally left in body following procedure

✓7th T81.530 Perforation due to foreign body accidentally left in body following surgical operation

✓7th T81.531 Perforation due to foreign body accidentally left in body following infusion or transfusion

✓7th T81.532 Perforation due to foreign body accidentally left in body following kidney dialysis

✓7th T81.533 Perforation due to foreign body accidentally left in body following injection or immunization

✓7th T81.534 Perforation due to foreign body accidentally left in body following endoscopic examination

✓7th T81.535 Perforation due to foreign body accidentally left in body following heart catheterization

✓7th T81.536 Perforation due to foreign body accidentally left in body following aspiration, puncture or other catheterization

✓7th T81.537 Perforation due to foreign body accidentally left in body following removal of catheter or packing

✓7th T81.538 Perforation due to foreign body accidentally left in body following other procedure

✓7th T81.539 Perforation due to foreign body accidentally left in body following unspecified procedure

✓6th T81.59 Other complications of foreign body accidentally left in body following procedure

EXCLUDES 2 *obstruction or perforation due to prosthetic devices and implants intentionally left in body (T82.0-T82.5, T83.0-T83.4, T83.7, T84.0-T84.4, T85.0-T85.6)*

✓7th T81.590 Other complications of foreign body accidentally left in body following surgical operation

✓7th T81.591 Other complications of foreign body accidentally left in body following infusion or transfusion

✓7th T81.592 Other complications of foreign body accidentally left in body following kidney dialysis

✓7th T81.593 Other complications of foreign body accidentally left in body following injection or immunization

✓7th T81.594 Other complications of foreign body accidentally left in body following endoscopic examination

✓7th T81.595 Other complications of foreign body accidentally left in body following heart catheterization

✓7th T81.596 Other complications of foreign body accidentally left in body following aspiration, puncture or other catheterization

✓7th T81.597 Other complications of foreign body accidentally left in body following removal of catheter or packing

✓7th T81.598 Other complications of foreign body accidentally left in body following other procedure

✓7th T81.599 Other complications of foreign body accidentally left in body following unspecified procedure

5th **T81.6 Acute reaction to foreign substance accidentally left during a procedure**
EXCLUDES 2 *complications of foreign body accidentally left in body cavity or operation wound following procedure (T81.5-)*
x7th **T81.60 Unspecified acute reaction to foreign substance accidentally left during a procedure**
x7th **T81.61 Aseptic peritonitis due to foreign substance accidentally left during a procedure**
Chemical peritonitis
x7th **T81.69 Other acute reaction to foreign substance accidentally left during a procedure**
5th **T81.7 Vascular complications following a procedure, not elsewhere classified**
Air embolism following procedure NEC
Phlebitis or thrombophlebitis resulting from a procedure
EXCLUDES 1 *embolism complicating abortion or ectopic or molar pregnancy (O00-O07, O08.2)*
embolism complicating pregnancy, childbirth and the puerperium (O88.-)
traumatic embolism (T79.0)
EXCLUDES 2 *embolism due to prosthetic devices, implants and grafts (T82.8-, T83.8, T84.8-, T85.8)*
embolism following infusion, transfusion and therapeutic injection (T80.0)
6th **T81.71 Complication of artery following a procedure, not elsewhere classified**
7th **T81.710 Complication of mesenteric artery following a procedure, not elsewhere classified**
7th **T81.711 Complication of renal artery following a procedure, not elsewhere classified**
7th **T81.718 Complication of other artery following a procedure, not elsewhere classified**
7th **T81.719 Complication of unspecified artery following a procedure, not elsewhere classified**
x7th **T81.72 Complication of vein following a procedure, not elsewhere classified**
5th **T81.8 Other complications of procedures, not elsewhere classified**
EXCLUDES 2 *hypothermia following anesthesia (T88.51)*
malignant hyperpyrexia due to anesthesia (T88.3)
x7th **T81.81 Complication of inhalation therapy**
x7th **T81.82 Emphysema (subcutaneous) resulting from a procedure**
x7th **T81.83 Persistent postprocedural fistula**
x7th **T81.89 Other complications of procedures, not elsewhere classified**
Use additional code to specify complication, such as: postprocedural delirium (F05)
x7th **T81.9 Unspecified complication of procedure**

4th **T82 Complications of cardiac and vascular prosthetic devices, implants and grafts**
EXCLUDES 2 *failure and rejection of transplanted organs and tissue (T86.-)*

The appropriate 7th character is to be added to each code from category T82.
A initial encounter
D subsequent encounter
S sequela

5th **T82.0 Mechanical complication of heart valve prosthesis**
Mechanical complication of artificial heart valve
EXCLUDES 1 *mechanical complication of biological heart valve graft (T82.22-)*
x7th **T82.01 Breakdown (mechanical) of heart valve prosthesis**
x7th **T82.02 Displacement of heart valve prosthesis**
Malposition of heart valve prosthesis
x7th **T82.03 Leakage of heart valve prosthesis**
x7th **T82.09 Other mechanical complication of heart valve prosthesis**
Obstruction (mechanical) of heart valve prosthesis
Perforation of heart valve prosthesis
Protrusion of heart valve prosthesis
5th **T82.1 Mechanical complication of cardiac electronic device**
6th **T82.11 Breakdown (mechanical) of cardiac electronic device**
7th **T82.110 Breakdown (mechanical) of cardiac electrode**
7th **T82.111 Breakdown (mechanical) of cardiac pulse generator (battery)**
7th **T82.118 Breakdown (mechanical) of other cardiac electronic device**
7th **T82.119 Breakdown (mechanical) of unspecified cardiac electronic device**
6th **T82.12 Displacement of cardiac electronic device**
Malposition of cardiac electronic device
7th **T82.120 Displacement of cardiac electrode**
7th **T82.121 Displacement of cardiac pulse generator (battery)**
7th **T82.128 Displacement of other cardiac electronic device**
7th **T82.129 Displacement of unspecified cardiac electronic device**
6th **T82.19 Other mechanical complication of cardiac electronic device**
Leakage of cardiac electronic device
Obstruction of cardiac electronic device
Perforation of cardiac electronic device
Protrusion of cardiac electronic device
7th **T82.190 Other mechanical complication of cardiac electrode**
7th **T82.191 Other mechanical complication of cardiac pulse generator (battery)**
7th **T82.198 Other mechanical complication of other cardiac electronic device**
7th **T82.199 Other mechanical complication of unspecified cardiac device**
5th **T82.2 Mechanical complication of coronary artery bypass graft and biological heart valve graft**
EXCLUDES 1 *mechanical complication of artificial heart valve prosthesis (T82.0-)*
6th **T82.21 Mechanical complication of coronary artery bypass graft**
7th **T82.211 Breakdown (mechanical) of coronary artery bypass graft**
7th **T82.212 Displacement of coronary artery bypass graft**
Malposition of coronary artery bypass graft
7th **T82.213 Leakage of coronary artery bypass graft**
7th **T82.218 Other mechanical complication of coronary artery bypass graft**
Obstruction, mechanical of coronary artery bypass graft
Perforation of coronary artery bypass graft
Protrusion of coronary artery bypass graft
6th **T82.22 Mechanical complication of biological heart valve graft**
7th **T82.221 Breakdown (mechanical) of biological heart valve graft**
7th **T82.222 Displacement of biological heart valve graft**
Malposition of biological heart valve graft
7th **T82.223 Leakage of biological heart valve graft**
7th **T82.228 Other mechanical complication of biological heart valve graft**
Obstruction of biological heart valve graft
Perforation of biological heart valve graft
Protrusion of biological heart valve graft
5th **T82.3 Mechanical complication of other vascular grafts**
6th **T82.31 Breakdown (mechanical) of other vascular grafts**
7th **T82.310 Breakdown (mechanical) of aortic (bifurcation) graft (replacement)**
7th **T82.311 Breakdown (mechanical) of carotid arterial graft (bypass)**
7th **T82.312 Breakdown (mechanical) of femoral arterial graft (bypass)**
7th **T82.318 Breakdown (mechanical) of other vascular grafts**
7th **T82.319 Breakdown (mechanical) of unspecified vascular grafts**

✓6th **T82.32 Displacement of other vascular grafts**
Malposition of other vascular grafts
✓7th **T82.320 Displacement of aortic (bifurcation) graft (replacement)**
✓7th **T82.321 Displacement of carotid arterial graft (bypass)**
✓7th **T82.322 Displacement of femoral arterial graft (bypass)**
✓7th **T82.328 Displacement of other vascular grafts**
✓7th **T82.329 Displacement of unspecified vascular grafts**

✓6th **T82.33 Leakage of other vascular grafts**
✓7th **T82.330 Leakage of aortic (bifurcation) graft (replacement)**
✓7th **T82.331 Leakage of carotid arterial graft (bypass)**
✓7th **T82.332 Leakage of femoral arterial graft (bypass)**
✓7th **T82.338 Leakage of other vascular grafts**
✓7th **T82.339 Leakage of unspecified vascular graft**

✓6th **T82.39 Other mechanical complication of other vascular grafts**
Obstruction (mechanical) of other vascular grafts
Perforation of other vascular grafts
Protrusion of other vascular grafts
✓7th **T82.390 Other mechanical complication of aortic (bifurcation) graft (replacement)**
✓7th **T82.391 Other mechanical complication of carotid arterial graft (bypass)**
✓7th **T82.392 Other mechanical complication of femoral arterial graft (bypass)**
✓7th **T82.398 Other mechanical complication of other vascular grafts**
✓7th **T82.399 Other mechanical complication of unspecified vascular grafts**

✓5th **T82.4 Mechanical complication of vascular dialysis catheter**
Mechanical complication of hemodialysis catheter
EXCLUDES 1 *mechanical complication of intraperitoneal dialysis catheter (T85.62)*

✓x7th **T82.41 Breakdown (mechanical) of vascular dialysis catheter**
✓x7th **T82.42 Displacement of vascular dialysis catheter**
Malposition of vascular dialysis catheter
✓x7th **T82.43 Leakage of vascular dialysis catheter**
✓x7th **T82.49 Other complication of vascular dialysis catheter**
Obstruction (mechanical) of vascular dialysis catheter
Perforation of vascular dialysis catheter
Protrusion of vascular dialysis catheter

✓5th **T82.5 Mechanical complication of other cardiac and vascular devices and implants**
EXCLUDES 2 *mechanical complication of epidural and subdural infusion catheter (T85.61)*

✓6th **T82.51 Breakdown (mechanical) of other cardiac and vascular devices and implants**
✓7th **T82.510 Breakdown (mechanical) of surgically created arteriovenous fistula**
✓7th **T82.511 Breakdown (mechanical) of surgically created arteriovenous shunt**
✓7th **T82.512 Breakdown (mechanical) of artificial heart**
✓7th **T82.513 Breakdown (mechanical) of balloon (counterpulsation) device**
✓7th **T82.514 Breakdown (mechanical) of infusion catheter**
✓7th **T82.515 Breakdown (mechanical) of umbrella device**
✓7th **T82.518 Breakdown (mechanical) of other cardiac and vascular devices and implants**
✓7th **T82.519 Breakdown (mechanical) of unspecified cardiac and vascular devices and implants**

✓6th **T82.52 Displacement of other cardiac and vascular devices and implants**
Malposition of other cardiac and vascular devices and implants
✓7th **T82.520 Displacement of surgically created arteriovenous fistula**
✓7th **T82.521 Displacement of surgically created arteriovenous shunt**
✓7th **T82.522 Displacement of artificial heart**
✓7th **T82.523 Displacement of balloon (counterpulsation) device**
✓7th **T82.524 Displacement of infusion catheter**
✓7th **T82.525 Displacement of umbrella device**
✓7th **T82.528 Displacement of other cardiac and vascular devices and implants**
✓7th **T82.529 Displacement of unspecified cardiac and vascular devices and implants**

✓6th **T82.53 Leakage of other cardiac and vascular devices and implants**
✓7th **T82.530 Leakage of surgically created arteriovenous fistula**
✓7th **T82.531 Leakage of surgically created arteriovenous shunt**
✓7th **T82.532 Leakage of artificial heart**
✓7th **T82.533 Leakage of balloon (counterpulsation) device**
✓7th **T82.534 Leakage of infusion catheter**
✓7th **T82.535 Leakage of umbrella device**
✓7th **T82.538 Leakage of other cardiac and vascular devices and implants**
✓7th **T82.539 Leakage of unspecified cardiac and vascular devices and implants**

✓6th **T82.59 Other mechanical complication of other cardiac and vascular devices and implants**
Obstruction (mechanical) of other cardiac and vascular devices and implants
Perforation of other cardiac and vascular devices and implants
Protrusion of other cardiac and vascular devices and implants
✓7th **T82.590 Other mechanical complication of surgically created arteriovenous fistula**
✓7th **T82.591 Other mechanical complication of surgically created arteriovenous shunt**
✓7th **T82.592 Other mechanical complication of artificial heart**
✓7th **T82.593 Other mechanical complication of balloon (counterpulsation) device**
✓7th **T82.594 Other mechanical complication of infusion catheter**
✓7th **T82.595 Other mechanical complication of umbrella device**
✓7th **T82.598 Other mechanical complication of other cardiac and vascular devices and implants**
✓7th **T82.599 Other mechanical complication of unspecified cardiac and vascular devices and implants**

✓x7th **T82.6 Infection and inflammatory reaction due to cardiac valve prosthesis**
Use additional code to identify infection

✓x7th **T82.7 Infection and inflammatory reaction due to other cardiac and vascular devices, implants and grafts**
Use additional code to identify infection

✓5th **T82.8 Other specified complications of cardiac and vascular prosthetic devices, implants and grafts**

✓6th **T82.81 Embolism of cardiac and vascular prosthetic devices, implants and grafts**
✓7th **T82.817 Embolism of cardiac prosthetic devices, implants and grafts**
✓7th **T82.818 Embolism of vascular prosthetic devices, implants and grafts**

✓6th **T82.82 Fibrosis of cardiac and vascular prosthetic devices, implants and grafts**
✓7th **T82.827 Fibrosis of cardiac prosthetic devices, implants and grafts**

T82.828 Fibrosis of vascular prosthetic devices, implants and grafts

T82.83 Hemorrhage of cardiac and vascular prosthetic devices, implants and grafts

T82.837 Hemorrhage of cardiac prosthetic devices, implants and grafts

T82.838 Hemorrhage of vascular prosthetic devices, implants and grafts

T82.84 Pain from cardiac and vascular prosthetic devices, implants and grafts

T82.847 Pain from cardiac prosthetic devices, implants and grafts

T82.848 Pain from vascular prosthetic devices, implants and grafts

T82.85 Stenosis of cardiac and vascular prosthetic devices, implants and grafts

T82.857 Stenosis of cardiac prosthetic devices, implants and grafts

T82.858 Stenosis of vascular prosthetic devices, implants and grafts

T82.86 Thrombosis of cardiac and vascular prosthetic devices, implants and grafts

T82.867 Thrombosis of cardiac prosthetic devices, implants and grafts

T82.868 Thrombosis of vascular prosthetic devices, implants and grafts

T82.89 Other specified complication of cardiac and vascular prosthetic devices, implants and grafts

T82.897 Other specified complication of cardiac prosthetic devices, implants and grafts

T82.898 Other specified complication of vascular prosthetic devices, implants and grafts

T82.9 Unspecified complication of cardiac and vascular prosthetic device, implant and graft

T83 Complications of genitourinary prosthetic devices, implants and grafts

EXCLUDES 2 *failure and rejection of transplanted organs and tissue (T86.-)*

The appropriate 7th character is to be added to each code from category T83.
A initial encounter
D subsequent encounter
S sequela

T83.0 Mechanical complication of urinary (indwelling) catheter

EXCLUDES 2 *complications of stoma of urinary tract (N99.5-)*

T83.01 Breakdown (mechanical) of urinary (indwelling) catheter

T83.010 Breakdown (mechanical) of cystostomy catheter

T83.018 Breakdown (mechanical) of other indwelling urethral catheter

T83.02 Displacement of urinary (indwelling) catheter

Malposition of urinary (indwelling) catheter

T83.020 Displacement of cystostomy catheter

T83.028 Displacement of other indwelling urethral catheter

T83.03 Leakage of urinary (indwelling) catheter

T83.030 Leakage of cystostomy catheter

T83.038 Leakage of other indwelling urethral catheter

T83.09 Other mechanical complication of urinary (indwelling) catheter

Obstruction (mechanical) of urinary (indwelling) catheter
Perforation of urinary (indwelling) catheter
Protrusion of urinary (indwelling) catheter

T83.090 Other mechanical complication of cystostomy catheter

T83.098 Other mechanical complication of other indwelling urethral catheter

T83.1 Mechanical complication of other urinary devices and implants

T83.11 Breakdown (mechanical) of other urinary devices and implants

T83.110 Breakdown (mechanical) of urinary electronic stimulator device

T83.111 Breakdown (mechanical) of urinary sphincter implant

T83.112 Breakdown (mechanical) of urinary stent

T83.118 Breakdown (mechanical) of other urinary devices and implants

T83.12 Displacement of other urinary devices and implants

Malposition of other urinary devices and implants

T83.120 Displacement of urinary electronic stimulator device

T83.121 Displacement of urinary sphincter implant

T83.122 Displacement of urinary stent

T83.128 Displacement of other urinary devices and implants

T83.19 Other mechanical complication of other urinary devices and implants

Leakage of other urinary devices and implants
Obstruction (mechanical) of other urinary devices and implants
Perforation of other urinary devices and implants
Protrusion of other urinary devices and implants

T83.190 Other mechanical complication of urinary electronic stimulator device

T83.191 Other mechanical complication of urinary sphincter implant

T83.192 Other mechanical complication of urinary stent

T83.198 Other mechanical complication of other urinary devices and implants

T83.2 Mechanical complication of graft of urinary organ

T83.21 Breakdown (mechanical) of graft of urinary organ

T83.22 Displacement of graft of urinary organ

Malposition of graft of urinary organ

T83.23 Leakage of graft of urinary organ

T83.29 Other mechanical complication of graft of urinary organ

Obstruction (mechanical) of graft of urinary organ
Perforation of graft of urinary organ
Protrusion of graft of urinary organ

T83.3 Mechanical complication of intrauterine contraceptive device

T83.31 Breakdown (mechanical) of intrauterine contraceptive device

T83.32 Displacement of intrauterine contraceptive device

Malposition of intrauterine contraceptive device

T83.39 Other mechanical complication of intrauterine contraceptive device

Leakage of intrauterine contraceptive device
Obstruction (mechanical) of intrauterine contraceptive device
Perforation of intrauterine contraceptive device
Protrusion of intrauterine contraceptive device

T83.4 Mechanical complication of other prosthetic devices, implants and grafts of genital tract

T83.41 Breakdown (mechanical) of other prosthetic devices, implants and grafts of genital tract

T83.410 Breakdown (mechanical) of penile (implanted) prosthesis

T83.418 Breakdown (mechanical) of other prosthetic devices, implants and grafts of genital tract

T83.42 Displacement of other prosthetic devices, implants and grafts of genital tract

Malposition of other prosthetic devices, implants and grafts of genital tract

T83.420 Displacement of penile (implanted) prosthesis

T83.428 Displacement of other prosthetic devices, implants and grafts of genital tract

√6th **T83.49 Other mechanical complication of other prosthetic devices, implants and grafts of genital tract**
Leakage of other prosthetic devices, implants and grafts of genital tract
Obstruction, mechanical of other prosthetic devices, implants and grafts of genital tract
Perforation of other prosthetic devices, implants and grafts of genital tract
Protrusion of other prosthetic devices, implants and grafts of genital tract

√7th **T83.490 Other mechanical complication of penile (implanted) prosthesis**

√7th **T83.498 Other mechanical complication of other prosthetic devices, implants and grafts of genital tract**

√5th **T83.5 Infection and inflammatory reaction due to prosthetic device, implant and graft in urinary system**
Use additional code to identify infection

√x7th **T83.51 Infection and inflammatory reaction due to indwelling urinary catheter**
EXCLUDES 2 *complications of stoma of urinary tract (N99.5-)*

√x7th **T83.59 Infection and inflammatory reaction due to prosthetic device, implant and graft in urinary system**

√x7th **T83.6 Infection and inflammatory reaction due to prosthetic device, implant and graft in genital tract**
Use additional code to identify infection

√5th **T83.7 Complications due to implanted mesh and other prosthetic materials**

√6th **T83.71 Erosion of implanted mesh and other prosthetic materials to surrounding organ or tissue**

√7th **T83.711 Erosion of implanted vaginal mesh and other prosthetic materials to surrounding organ or tissue**
Erosion of implanted vaginal mesh and other prosthetic materials into pelvic floor muscles

√7th **T83.718 Erosion of other implanted mesh and other prosthetic materials to surrounding organ or tissue**

√6th **T83.72 Exposure of implanted mesh and other prosthetic materials into surrounding organ or tissue**

√7th **T83.721 Exposure of implanted vaginal mesh and other prosthetic materials into vagina**
Exposure of implanted vaginal mesh and other prosthetic materials through vaginal wall

√7th **T83.728 Exposure of other implanted mesh and other prosthetic materials to surrounding organ or tissue**

√5th **T83.8 Other specified complications of genitourinary prosthetic devices, implants and grafts**

√x7th **T83.81 Embolism of genitourinary prosthetic devices, implants and grafts**

√x7th **T83.82 Fibrosis of genitourinary prosthetic devices, implants and grafts**

√x7th **T83.83 Hemorrhage of genitourinary prosthetic devices, implants and grafts**

√x7th **T83.84 Pain from genitourinary prosthetic devices, implants and grafts**

√x7th **T83.85 Stenosis of genitourinary prosthetic devices, implants and grafts**

√x7th **T83.86 Thrombosis of genitourinary prosthetic devices, implants and grafts**

√x7th **T83.89 Other specified complication of genitourinary prosthetic devices, implants and grafts**

√x7th **T83.9 Unspecified complication of genitourinary prosthetic device, implant and graft**

√4th **T84 Complications of internal orthopedic prosthetic devices, implants and grafts**
EXCLUDES 2 *failure and rejection of transplanted organs and tissues (T86.-)*
fracture of bone following insertion of orthopedic implant, joint prosthesis or bone plate (M96.6)

The appropriate 7th character is to be added to each code from category T84.
A initial encounter
D subsequent encounter
S sequela

√5th **T84.0 Mechanical complication of internal joint prosthesis**

√6th **T84.01 Broken internal joint prosthesis**
Breakage (fracture) of prosthetic joint
Broken prosthetic joint implant
EXCLUDES 1 *periprosthetic joint implant fracture (T84.04)*

√7th **T84.010 Broken internal right hip prosthesis**

√7th **T84.011 Broken internal left hip prosthesis**

√7th **T84.012 Broken internal right knee prosthesis**

√7th **T84.013 Broken internal left knee prosthesis**

√7th **T84.018 Broken internal joint prosthesis, other site**
Use additional code to identify the joint (Z96.6-)

√7th **T84.019 Broken internal joint prosthesis, unspecified site**

√6th **T84.02 Dislocation of internal joint prosthesis**
Instability of internal joint prosthesis
Subluxation of internal joint prosthesis

√7th **T84.020 Dislocation of internal right hip prosthesis**

√7th **T84.021 Dislocation of internal left hip prosthesis**

√7th **T84.022 Instability of internal right knee prosthesis**

√7th **T84.023 Instability of internal left knee prosthesis**

√7th **T84.028 Dislocation of other internal joint prosthesis**
Use additional code to identify the joint (Z96.6-)

√7th **T84.029 Dislocation of unspecified internal joint prosthesis**

√6th **T84.03 Mechanical loosening of internal prosthetic joint**
Aseptic loosening of prosthetic joint

√7th **T84.030 Mechanical loosening of internal right hip prosthetic joint**

√7th **T84.031 Mechanical loosening of internal left hip prosthetic joint**

√7th **T84.032 Mechanical loosening of internal right knee prosthetic joint**

√7th **T84.033 Mechanical loosening of internal left knee prosthetic joint**

√7th **T84.038 Mechanical loosening of other internal prosthetic joint**
Use additional code to identify the joint (Z96.6-)

√7th **T84.039 Mechanical loosening of unspecified internal prosthetic joint**

√6th **T84.04 Periprosthetic fracture around internal prosthetic joint**
EXCLUDES 2 *breakage (fracture) of prosthetic joint (T84.01)*

√7th **T84.040 Periprosthetic fracture around internal prosthetic right hip joint**

√7th **T84.041 Periprosthetic fracture around internal prosthetic left hip joint**

√7th **T84.042 Periprosthetic fracture around internal prosthetic right knee joint**

√7th **T84.043 Periprosthetic fracture around internal prosthetic left knee joint**

√7th **T84.048 Periprosthetic fracture around other internal prosthetic joint**
Use additional code to identify the joint (Z96.6-)

√7th **T84.049 Periprosthetic fracture around unspecified internal prosthetic joint**

✓6th T84.05 **Periprosthetic osteolysis of internal prosthetic joint**
Use additional code to identify major osseous defect, if applicable (M89.7-)
✓7th T84.050 **Periprosthetic osteolysis of internal prosthetic right hip joint**
✓7th T84.051 **Periprosthetic osteolysis of internal prosthetic left hip joint**
✓7th T84.052 **Periprosthetic osteolysis of internal prosthetic right knee joint**
✓7th T84.053 **Periprosthetic osteolysis of internal prosthetic left knee joint**
✓7th T84.058 **Periprosthetic osteolysis of other internal prosthetic joint**
Use additional code to identify the joint (Z96.6-)
✓7th T84.059 **Periprosthetic osteolysis of unspecified internal prosthetic joint**
✓6th T84.06 **Wear of articular bearing surface of internal prosthetic joint**
✓7th T84.060 **Wear of articular bearing surface of internal prosthetic right hip joint**
✓7th T84.061 **Wear of articular bearing surface of internal prosthetic left hip joint**
✓7th T84.062 **Wear of articular bearing surface of internal prosthetic right knee joint**
✓7th T84.063 **Wear of articular bearing surface of internal prosthetic left knee joint**
✓7th T84.068 **Wear of articular bearing surface of other internal prosthetic joint**
Use additional code to identify the joint (Z96.6-)
✓7th T84.069 **Wear of articular bearing surface of unspecified internal prosthetic joint**
✓6th T84.09 **Other mechanical complication of internal joint prosthesis**
Prosthetic joint implant failure NOS
✓7th T84.090 **Other mechanical complication of internal right hip prosthesis**
✓7th T84.091 **Other mechanical complication of internal left hip prosthesis**
✓7th T84.092 **Other mechanical complication of internal right knee prosthesis**
✓7th T84.093 **Other mechanical complication of internal left knee prosthesis**
✓7th T84.098 **Other mechanical complication of other internal joint prosthesis**
Use additional code to identify the joint (Z96.6-)
✓7th T84.099 **Other mechanical complication of unspecified internal joint prosthesis**
✓5th T84.1 **Mechanical complication of internal fixation device of bones of limb**
EXCLUDES 2 *mechanical complication of internal fixation device of bones of feet (T84.2-)*
mechanical complication of internal fixation device of bones of fingers (T84.2-)
mechanical complication of internal fixation device of bones of hands (T84.2-)
mechanical complication of internal fixation device of bones of toes (T84.2-)
✓6th T84.11 **Breakdown (mechanical) of internal fixation device of bones of limb**
✓7th T84.110 **Breakdown (mechanical) of internal fixation device of right humerus**
✓7th T84.111 **Breakdown (mechanical) of internal fixation device of left humerus**
✓7th T84.112 **Breakdown (mechanical) of internal fixation device of bone of right forearm**
✓7th T84.113 **Breakdown (mechanical) of internal fixation device of bone of left forearm**
✓7th T84.114 **Breakdown (mechanical) of internal fixation device of right femur**
✓7th T84.115 **Breakdown (mechanical) of internal fixation device of left femur**
✓7th T84.116 **Breakdown (mechanical) of internal fixation device of bone of right lower leg**
✓7th T84.117 **Breakdown (mechanical) of internal fixation device of bone of left lower leg**
✓7th T84.119 **Breakdown (mechanical) of internal fixation device of unspecified bone of limb**
✓6th T84.12 **Displacement of internal fixation device of bones of limb**
Malposition of internal fixation device of bones of limb
✓7th T84.120 **Displacement of internal fixation device of right humerus**
✓7th T84.121 **Displacement of internal fixation device of left humerus**
✓7th T84.122 **Displacement of internal fixation device of bone of right forearm**
✓7th T84.123 **Displacement of internal fixation device of bone of left forearm**
✓7th T84.124 **Displacement of internal fixation device of right femur**
✓7th T84.125 **Displacement of internal fixation device of left femur**
✓7th T84.126 **Displacement of internal fixation device of bone of right lower leg**
✓7th T84.127 **Displacement of internal fixation device of bone of left lower leg**
✓7th T84.129 **Displacement of internal fixation device of unspecified bone of limb**
✓6th T84.19 **Other mechanical complication of internal fixation device of bones of limb**
Obstruction (mechanical) of internal fixation device of bones of limb
Perforation of internal fixation device of bones of limb
Protrusion of internal fixation device of bones of limb
✓7th T84.190 **Other mechanical complication of internal fixation device of right humerus**
✓7th T84.191 **Other mechanical complication of internal fixation device of left humerus**
✓7th T84.192 **Other mechanical complication of internal fixation device of bone of right forearm**
✓7th T84.193 **Other mechanical complication of internal fixation device of bone of left forearm**
✓7th T84.194 **Other mechanical complication of internal fixation device of right femur**
✓7th T84.195 **Other mechanical complication of internal fixation device of left femur**
✓7th T84.196 **Other mechanical complication of internal fixation device of bone of right lower leg**
✓7th T84.197 **Other mechanical complication of internal fixation device of bone of left lower leg**
✓7th T84.199 **Other mechanical complication of internal fixation device of unspecified bone of limb**
✓5th T84.2 **Mechanical complication of internal fixation device of other bones**
✓6th T84.21 **Breakdown (mechanical) of internal fixation device of other bones**
✓7th T84.210 **Breakdown (mechanical) of internal fixation device of bones of hand and fingers**
✓7th T84.213 **Breakdown (mechanical) of internal fixation device of bones of foot and toes**
✓7th T84.216 **Breakdown (mechanical) of internal fixation device of vertebrae**
✓7th T84.218 **Breakdown (mechanical) of internal fixation device of other bones**
✓6th T84.22 **Displacement of internal fixation device of other bones**
Malposition of internal fixation device of other bones
✓7th T84.220 **Displacement of internal fixation device of bones of hand and fingers**

✓7th **T84.223 Displacement of internal fixation device of bones of foot and toes**

✓7th **T84.226 Displacement of internal fixation device of vertebrae**

✓7th **T84.228 Displacement of internal fixation device of other bones**

✓6th **T84.29 Other mechanical complication of internal fixation device of other bones**

Obstruction (mechanical) of internal fixation device of other bones

Perforation of internal fixation device of other bones

Protrusion of internal fixation device of other bones

✓7th **T84.290 Other mechanical complication of internal fixation device of bones of hand and fingers**

✓7th **T84.293 Other mechanical complication of internal fixation device of bones of foot and toes**

✓7th **T84.296 Other mechanical complication of internal fixation device of vertebrae**

✓7th **T84.298 Other mechanical complication of internal fixation device of other bones**

✓5th **T84.3 Mechanical complication of other bone devices, implants and grafts**

EXCLUDES 2 *other complications of bone graft (T86.83-)*

✓6th **T84.31 Breakdown (mechanical) of other bone devices, implants and grafts**

✓7th **T84.310 Breakdown (mechanical) of electronic bone stimulator**

✓7th **T84.318 Breakdown (mechanical) of other bone devices, implants and grafts**

✓6th **T84.32 Displacement of other bone devices, implants and grafts**

Malposition of other bone devices, implants and grafts

✓7th **T84.320 Displacement of electronic bone stimulator**

✓7th **T84.328 Displacement of other bone devices, implants and grafts**

✓6th **T84.39 Other mechanical complication of other bone devices, implants and grafts**

Obstruction (mechanical) of other bone devices, implants and grafts

Perforation of other bone devices, implants and grafts

Protrusion of other bone devices, implants and grafts

✓7th **T84.390 Other mechanical complication of electronic bone stimulator**

✓7th **T84.398 Other mechanical complication of other bone devices, implants and grafts**

✓5th **T84.4 Mechanical complication of other internal orthopedic devices, implants and grafts**

✓6th **T84.41 Breakdown (mechanical) of other internal orthopedic devices, implants and grafts**

✓7th **T84.410 Breakdown (mechanical) of muscle and tendon graft**

✓7th **T84.418 Breakdown (mechanical) of other internal orthopedic devices, implants and grafts**

✓6th **T84.42 Displacement of other internal orthopedic devices, implants and grafts**

Malposition of other internal orthopedic devices, implants and grafts

✓7th **T84.420 Displacement of muscle and tendon graft**

✓7th **T84.428 Displacement of other internal orthopedic devices, implants and grafts**

✓6th **T84.49 Other mechanical complication of other internal orthopedic devices, implants and grafts**

Mechanical complication of other internal orthopedic devices, implants and grafts NOS

Obstruction (mechanical) of other internal orthopedic devices, implants and grafts

Perforation of other internal orthopedic devices, implants and grafts

Protrusion of other internal orthopedic devices, implants and grafts

✓7th **T84.490 Other mechanical complication of muscle and tendon graft**

✓7th **T84.498 Other mechanical complication of other internal orthopedic devices, implants and grafts**

✓5th **T84.5 Infection and inflammatory reaction due to internal joint prosthesis**

Use additional code to identify infection

✓x7th **T84.50 Infection and inflammatory reaction due to unspecified internal joint prosthesis**

✓x7th **T84.51 Infection and inflammatory reaction due to internal right hip prosthesis**

✓x7th **T84.52 Infection and inflammatory reaction due to internal left hip prosthesis**

✓x7th **T84.53 Infection and inflammatory reaction due to internal right knee prosthesis**

✓x7th **T84.54 Infection and inflammatory reaction due to internal left knee prosthesis**

✓x7th **T84.59 Infection and inflammatory reaction due to other internal joint prosthesis**

✓5th **T84.6 Infection and inflammatory reaction due to internal fixation device**

Use additional code to identify infection

✓x7th **T84.60 Infection and inflammatory reaction due to internal fixation device of unspecified site**

✓6th **T84.61 Infection and inflammatory reaction due to internal fixation device of arm**

✓7th **T84.610 Infection and inflammatory reaction due to internal fixation device of right humerus**

✓7th **T84.611 Infection and inflammatory reaction due to internal fixation device of left humerus**

✓7th **T84.612 Infection and inflammatory reaction due to internal fixation device of right radius**

✓7th **T84.613 Infection and inflammatory reaction due to internal fixation device of left radius**

✓7th **T84.614 Infection and inflammatory reaction due to internal fixation device of right ulna**

✓7th **T84.615 Infection and inflammatory reaction due to internal fixation device of left ulna**

✓7th **T84.619 Infection and inflammatory reaction due to internal fixation device of unspecified bone of arm**

✓6th **T84.62 Infection and inflammatory reaction due to internal fixation device of leg**

✓7th **T84.620 Infection and inflammatory reaction due to internal fixation device of right femur**

✓7th **T84.621 Infection and inflammatory reaction due to internal fixation device of left femur**

✓7th **T84.622 Infection and inflammatory reaction due to internal fixation device of right tibia**

✓7th **T84.623 Infection and inflammatory reaction due to internal fixation device of left tibia**

✓7th **T84.624 Infection and inflammatory reaction due to internal fixation device of right fibula**

✓7th **T84.625 Infection and inflammatory reaction due to internal fixation device of left fibula**

✓7th **T84.629 Infection and inflammatory reaction due to internal fixation device of unspecified bone of leg**

✓x7th **T84.63 Infection and inflammatory reaction due to internal fixation device of spine**

✓x7th **T84.69 Infection and inflammatory reaction due to internal fixation device of other site**

✓x7th **T84.7 Infection and inflammatory reaction due to other internal orthopedic prosthetic devices, implants and grafts**

Use additional code to identify infection

√5th **T84.8 Other specified complications of internal orthopedic prosthetic devices, implants and grafts**

√x7th **T84.81 Embolism due to internal orthopedic prosthetic devices, implants and grafts**

√x7th **T84.82 Fibrosis due to internal orthopedic prosthetic devices, implants and grafts**

√x7th **T84.83 Hemorrhage due to internal orthopedic prosthetic devices, implants and grafts**

√x7th **T84.84 Pain due to internal orthopedic prosthetic devices, implants and grafts**

√x7th **T84.85 Stenosis due to internal orthopedic prosthetic devices, implants and grafts**

√x7th **T84.86 Thrombosis due to internal orthopedic prosthetic devices, implants and grafts**

√x7th **T84.89 Other specified complication of internal orthopedic prosthetic devices, implants and grafts**

√x7th **T84.9 Unspecified complication of internal orthopedic prosthetic device, implant and graft**

√4th **T85 Complications of other internal prosthetic devices, implants and grafts**

EXCLUDES 2 *failure and rejection of transplanted organs and tissue (T86.-)*

The appropriate 7th character is to be added to each code from category T85.
A initial encounter
D subsequent encounter
S sequela

√5th **T85.0 Mechanical complication of ventricular intracranial (communicating) shunt**

√x7th **T85.01 Breakdown (mechanical) of ventricular intracranial (communicating) shunt**

√x7th **T85.02 Displacement of ventricular intracranial (communicating) shunt**
Malposition of ventricular intracranial (communicating) shunt

√x7th **T85.03 Leakage of ventricular intracranial (communicating) shunt**

√x7th **T85.09 Other mechanical complication of ventricular intracranial (communicating) shunt**
Obstruction (mechanical) of ventricular intracranial (communicating) shunt
Perforation of ventricular intracranial (communicating) shunt
Protrusion of ventricular intracranial (communicating) shunt

√5th **T85.1 Mechanical complication of implanted electronic stimulator of nervous system**

√6th **T85.11 Breakdown (mechanical) of implanted electronic stimulator of nervous system**

√7th **T85.110 Breakdown (mechanical) of implanted electronic neurostimulator (electrode) of brain**

√7th **T85.111 Breakdown (mechanical) of implanted electronic neurostimulator (electrode) of peripheral nerve**

√7th **T85.112 Breakdown (mechanical) of implanted electronic neurostimulator (electrode) of spinal cord**

√7th **T85.118 Breakdown (mechanical) of other implanted electronic stimulator of nervous system**

√6th **T85.12 Displacement of implanted electronic stimulator of nervous system**
Malposition of implanted electronic stimulator of nervous system

√7th **T85.120 Displacement of implanted electronic neurostimulator (electrode) of brain**

√7th **T85.121 Displacement of implanted electronic neurostimulator (electrode) of peripheral nerve**

√7th **T85.122 Displacement of implanted electronic neurostimulator (electrode) of spinal cord**

√7th **T85.128 Displacement of other implanted electronic stimulator of nervous system**

√6th **T85.19 Other mechanical complication of implanted electronic stimulator of nervous system**
Leakage of implanted electronic stimulator of nervous system
Obstruction (mechanical) of implanted electronic stimulator of nervous system
Perforation of implanted electronic stimulator of nervous system
Protrusion of implanted electronic stimulator of nervous system

√7th **T85.190 Other mechanical complication of implanted electronic neurostimulator (electrode) of brain**

√7th **T85.191 Other mechanical complication of implanted electronic neurostimulator (electrode) of peripheral nerve**

√7th **T85.192 Other mechanical complication of implanted electronic neurostimulator (electrode) of spinal cord**

√7th **T85.199 Other mechanical complication of other implanted electronic stimulator of nervous system**

√5th **T85.2 Mechanical complication of intraocular lens**

√x7th **T85.21 Breakdown (mechanical) of intraocular lens**

√x7th **T85.22 Displacement of intraocular lens**
Malposition of intraocular lens

√x7th **T85.29 Other mechanical complication of intraocular lens**
Obstruction (mechanical) of intraocular lens
Perforation of intraocular lens
Protrusion of intraocular lens

√5th **T85.3 Mechanical complication of other ocular prosthetic devices, implants and grafts**

EXCLUDES 2 *other complications of corneal graft (T86.84-)*

√6th **T85.31 Breakdown (mechanical) of other ocular prosthetic devices, implants and grafts**

√7th **T85.310 Breakdown (mechanical) of prosthetic orbit of right eye**

√7th **T85.311 Breakdown (mechanical) of prosthetic orbit of left eye**

√7th **T85.318 Breakdown (mechanical) of other ocular prosthetic devices, implants and grafts**

√6th **T85.32 Displacement of other ocular prosthetic devices, implants and grafts**
Malposition of other ocular prosthetic devices, implants and grafts

√7th **T85.320 Displacement of prosthetic orbit of right eye**

√7th **T85.321 Displacement of prosthetic orbit of left eye**

√7th **T85.328 Displacement of other ocular prosthetic devices, implants and grafts**

√6th **T85.39 Other mechanical complication of other ocular prosthetic devices, implants and grafts**
Obstruction (mechanical) of other ocular prosthetic devices, implants and grafts
Perforation of other ocular prosthetic devices, implants and grafts
Protrusion of other ocular prosthetic devices, implants and grafts

√7th **T85.390 Other mechanical complication of prosthetic orbit of right eye**

√7th **T85.391 Other mechanical complication of prosthetic orbit of left eye**

√7th **T85.398 Other mechanical complication of other ocular prosthetic devices, implants and grafts**

√5th **T85.4 Mechanical complication of breast prosthesis and implant**

√x7th **T85.41 Breakdown (mechanical) of breast prosthesis and implant**

√x7th **T85.42 Displacement of breast prosthesis and implant**
Malposition of breast prosthesis and implant

√x7th **T85.43 Leakage of breast prosthesis and implant**

√x7th **T85.44 Capsular contracture of breast implant**

√x7th **T85.49 Other mechanical complication of breast prosthesis and implant**
Obstruction (mechanical) of breast prosthesis and implant
Perforation of breast prosthesis and implant
Protrusion of breast prosthesis and implant

✓5th **T85.5 Mechanical complication of gastrointestinal prosthetic devices, implants and grafts**

✓6th **T85.51 Breakdown (mechanical) of gastrointestinal prosthetic devices, implants and grafts**

✓7th **T85.510 Breakdown (mechanical) of bile duct prosthesis**

✓7th **T85.511 Breakdown (mechanical) of esophageal anti-reflux device**

✓7th **T85.518 Breakdown (mechanical) of other gastrointestinal prosthetic devices, implants and grafts**

✓6th **T85.52 Displacement of gastrointestinal prosthetic devices, implants and grafts**
Malposition of gastrointestinal prosthetic devices, implants and grafts

✓7th **T85.520 Displacement of bile duct prosthesis**

✓7th **T85.521 Displacement of esophageal anti-reflux device**

✓7th **T85.528 Displacement of other gastrointestinal prosthetic devices, implants and grafts**

✓6th **T85.59 Other mechanical complication of gastrointestinal prosthetic devices, implants and**
Obstruction, mechanical of gastrointestinal prosthetic devices, implants and grafts
Perforation of gastrointestinal prosthetic devices, implants and grafts
Protrusion of gastrointestinal prosthetic devices, implants and grafts

✓7th **T85.590 Other mechanical complication of bile duct prosthesis**

✓7th **T85.591 Other mechanical complication of esophageal anti-reflux device**

✓7th **T85.598 Other mechanical complication of other gastrointestinal prosthetic devices, implants and grafts**

✓5th **T85.6 Mechanical complication of other specified internal and external prosthetic devices, implants and grafts**

✓6th **T85.61 Breakdown (mechanical) of other specified internal prosthetic devices, implants and grafts**

✓7th **T85.610 Breakdown (mechanical) of epidural and subdural infusion catheter**

✓7th **T85.611 Breakdown (mechanical) of intraperitoneal dialysis catheter**
EXCLUDES1 *mechanical complication of vascular dialysis catheter (T82.4-)*

✓7th **T85.612 Breakdown (mechanical) of permanent sutures**
EXCLUDES1 *mechanical complication of permanent (wire) suture used in bone repair (T84.1-T84.2)*

✓7th **T85.613 Breakdown (mechanical) of artificial skin graft and decellularized allodermis**
Failure of artificial skin graft and decellularized allodermis
Non-adherence of artificial skin graft and decellularized allodermis
Poor incorporation of artificial skin graft and decellularized allodermis
Shearing of artificial skin graft and decellularized allodermis

✓7th **T85.614 Breakdown (mechanical) of insulin pump**

✓7th **T85.618 Breakdown (mechanical) of other specified internal prosthetic devices, implants and grafts**

✓6th **T85.62 Displacement of other specified internal prosthetic devices, implants and grafts**
Malposition of other specified internal prosthetic devices, implants and grafts

✓7th **T85.620 Displacement of epidural and subdural infusion catheter**

✓7th **T85.621 Displacement of intraperitoneal dialysis catheter**
EXCLUDES1 *mechanical complication of vascular dialysis catheter (T82.4-)*

✓7th **T85.622 Displacement of permanent sutures**
EXCLUDES1 *mechanical complication of permanent (wire) suture used in bone repair (T84.1-T84.2)*

✓7th **T85.623 Displacement of artificial skin graft and decellularized allodermis**
Dislodgement of artificial skin graft and decellularized allodermis
Displacement of artificial skin graft and decellularized allodermis

✓7th **T85.624 Displacement of insulin pump**

✓7th **T85.628 Displacement of other specified internal prosthetic devices, implants and grafts**

✓6th **T85.63 Leakage of other specified internal prosthetic devices, implants and grafts**

✓7th **T85.630 Leakage of epidural and subdural infusion catheter**

✓7th **T85.631 Leakage of intraperitoneal dialysis catheter**
EXCLUDES1 *mechanical complication of vascular dialysis catheter (T82.4)*

✓7th **T85.633 Leakage of insulin pump**

✓7th **T85.638 Leakage of other specified internal prosthetic devices, implants and grafts**

✓6th **T85.69 Other mechanical complication of other specified internal prosthetic devices, implants and grafts**
Obstruction, mechanical of other specified internal prosthetic devices, implants and grafts
Perforation of other specified internal prosthetic devices, implants and grafts
Protrusion of other specified internal prosthetic devices, implants and grafts

✓7th **T85.690 Other mechanical complication of epidural and subdural infusion catheter**

✓7th **T85.691 Other mechanical complication of intraperitoneal dialysis catheter**
EXCLUDES1 *mechanical complication of vascular dialysis catheter (T82.4)*

✓7th **T85.692 Other mechanical complication of permanent sutures**
EXCLUDES1 *mechanical complication of permanent (wire) suture used in bone repair (T84.1-T84.2)*

✓7th **T85.693 Other mechanical complication of artificial skin graft and decellularized allodermis**

✓7th **T85.694 Other mechanical complication of insulin pump**

✓7th **T85.698 Other mechanical complication of other specified internal prosthetic devices, implants and grafts**
Mechanical complication of nonabsorbable surgical material NOS

✓5th **T85.7 Infection and inflammatory reaction due to other internal prosthetic devices, implants and grafts**
Use additional code to identify infection

✓x7th **T85.71 Infection and inflammatory reaction due to peritoneal dialysis catheter**

✓x7th **T85.72 Infection and inflammatory reaction due to insulin pump**

✓x7th **T85.79 Infection and inflammatory reaction due to other internal prosthetic devices, implants and grafts**

✓5th **T85.8 Other specified complications of internal prosthetic devices, implants and grafts, not elsewhere classified**

✓x7th **T85.81 Embolism due to internal prosthetic devices, implants and grafts, not elsewhere classified**

✓x7th **T85.82 Fibrosis due to internal prosthetic devices, implants and grafts, not elsewhere classified**

✓x7th **T85.83 Hemorrhage due to internal prosthetic devices, implants and grafts, not elsewhere classified**

✓x7th **T85.84 Pain due to internal prosthetic devices, implants and grafts, not elsewhere classified**

✓x7th **T85.85 Stenosis due to internal prosthetic devices, implants and grafts, not elsewhere classified**

√x7th **T85.86 Thrombosis due to internal prosthetic devices, implants and grafts, not elsewhere classified**

√x7th **T85.89 Other specified complication of internal prosthetic devices, implants and grafts, not elsewhere classified**

√x7th **T85.9 Unspecified complication of internal prosthetic device, implant and graft**
Complication of internal prosthetic device, implant and graft NOS

√4th **T86 Complications of transplanted organs and tissue**
Use additional code to identify other transplant complications, such as:
graft-versus-host disease (D89.81-)
malignancy associated with organ transplant (C80.2)
post-transplant lymphoproliferative disorders (PTLD) (D47.Z1)

√5th **T86.0 Complications of bone marrow transplant**
T86.00 Unspecified complication of bone marrow transplant
T86.01 Bone marrow transplant rejection
T86.02 Bone marrow transplant failure
T86.03 Bone marrow transplant infection
T86.09 Other complications of bone marrow transplant

√5th **T86.1 Complications of kidney transplant**
T86.10 Unspecified complication of kidney transplant
T86.11 Kidney transplant rejection
T86.12 Kidney transplant failure
T86.13 Kidney transplant infection
Use additional code to specify infection
T86.19 Other complication of kidney transplant

√5th **T86.2 Complications of heart transplant**
EXCLUDES 1 *complication of:*
artificial heart device (T82.5)
heart-lung transplant (T86.3)
T86.20 Unspecified complication of heart transplant
T86.21 Heart transplant rejection
T86.22 Heart transplant failure
T86.23 Heart transplant infection
Use additional code to specify infection
√6th **T86.29 Other complications of heart transplant**
T86.290 Cardiac allograft vasculopathy
EXCLUDES 1 *atherosclerosis of coronary arteries (I25.75-, I25.76-, I25.81-)*
T86.298 Other complications of heart transplant

√5th **T86.3 Complications of heart-lung transplant**
T86.30 Unspecified complication of heart-lung transplant
T86.31 Heart-lung transplant rejection
T86.32 Heart-lung transplant failure
T86.33 Heart-lung transplant infection
Use additional code to specify infection
T86.39 Other complications of heart-lung transplant

√5th **T86.4 Complications of liver transplant**
T86.40 Unspecified complication of liver transplant
T86.41 Liver transplant rejection
T86.42 Liver transplant failure
T86.43 Liver transplant infection
Use additional code to identify infection, such as:
cytomegalovirus (CMV) infection (B25.-)
T86.49 Other complications of liver transplant

T86.5 Complications of stem cell transplant
Complications from stem cells from peripheral blood
Complications from stem cells from umbilical cord

√5th **T86.8 Complications of other transplanted organs and tissues**
√6th **T86.81 Complications of lung transplant**
EXCLUDES 1 *complication of heart-lung transplant (T86.3-)*
T86.810 Lung transplant rejection
T86.811 Lung transplant failure
T86.812 Lung transplant infection
Use additional code to specify infection
T86.818 Other complications of lung transplant
T86.819 Unspecified complication of lung transplant
√6th **T86.82 Complications of skin graft (allograft) (autograft)**
EXCLUDES 2 *complication of artificial skin graft (T85.64)*
T86.820 Skin graft (allograft) rejection
T86.821 Skin graft (allograft) (autograft) failure
T86.822 Skin graft (allograft) (autograft) infection
Use additional code to specify infection
T86.828 Other complications of skin graft (allograft) (autograft)
T86.829 Unspecified complication of skin graft (allograft) (autograft)
√6th **T86.83 Complications of bone graft**
EXCLUDES 2 *mechanical complications of bone graft (T84.3-)*
T86.830 Bone graft rejection
T86.831 Bone graft failure
T86.832 Bone graft infection
Use additional code to specify infection
T86.838 Other complications of bone graft
T86.839 Unspecified complication of bone graft
√6th **T86.84 Complications of corneal transplant**
EXCLUDES 2 *mechanical complications of corneal graft (T85.3-)*
T86.840 Corneal transplant rejection
T86.841 Corneal transplant failure
T86.842 Corneal transplant infection
Use additional code to specify infection
T86.848 Other complications of corneal transplant
T86.849 Unspecified complication of corneal transplant
√6th **T86.85 Complication of intestine transplant**
T86.850 Intestine transplant rejection
T86.851 Intestine transplant failure
T86.852 Intestine transplant infection
Use additional code to specify infection
T86.858 Other complications of intestine transplant
T86.859 Unspecified complication of intestine transplant
√6th **T86.89 Complications of other transplanted tissue**
Transplant failure or rejection of pancreas
T86.890 Other transplanted tissue rejection
T86.891 Other transplanted tissue failure
T86.892 Other transplanted tissue infection
Use additional code to specify infection
T86.898 Other complications of other transplanted tissue
T86.899 Unspecified complication of other transplanted tissue

√5th **T86.9 Complication of unspecified transplanted organ and tissue**
T86.90 Unspecified complication of unspecified transplanted organ and tissue
T86.91 Unspecified transplanted organ and tissue rejection
T86.92 Unspecified transplanted organ and tissue failure
T86.93 Unspecified transplanted organ and tissue infection
Use additional code to specify infection
T86.99 Other complications of unspecified transplanted organ and tissue

√4th **T87 Complications peculiar to reattachment and amputation**

√5th **T87.0 Complications of reattached (part of) upper extremity**
√6th **T87.0X Complications of reattached (part of) upper extremity**
T87.0X1 Complications of reattached (part of) right upper extremity
T87.0X2 Complications of reattached (part of) left upper extremity
T87.0X9 Complications of reattached (part of) unspecified upper extremity

√5th **T87.1 Complications of reattached (part of) lower extremity**
√6th **T87.1X Complications of reattached (part of) lower extremity**
T87.1X1 Complications of reattached (part of) right lower extremity
T87.1X2 Complications of reattached (part of) left lower extremity
T87.1X9 Complications of reattached (part of) unspecified lower extremity

T87.2 Complications of other reattached body part

√5th **T87.3 Neuroma of amputation stump**

T87.3Ø Neuroma of amputation stump, unspecified extremity

T87.31 Neuroma of amputation stump, right upper extremity

T87.32 Neuroma of amputation stump, left upper extremity

T87.33 Neuroma of amputation stump, right lower extremity

T87.34 Neuroma of amputation stump, left lower extremity

√5th **T87.4 Infection of amputation stump**

T87.4Ø Infection of amputation stump, unspecified extremity

T87.41 Infection of amputation stump, right upper extremity

T87.42 Infection of amputation stump, left upper extremity

T87.43 Infection of amputation stump, right lower extremity

T87.44 Infection of amputation stump, left lower extremity

√5th **T87.5 Necrosis of amputation stump**

T87.5Ø Necrosis of amputation stump, unspecified extremity

T87.51 Necrosis of amputation stump, right upper extremity

T87.52 Necrosis of amputation stump, left upper extremity

T87.53 Necrosis of amputation stump, right lower extremity

T87.54 Necrosis of amputation stump, left lower extremity

√5th **T87.8 Other complications of amputation stump**

T87.81 Dehiscence of amputation stump

T87.89 Other complications of amputation stump

Amputation stump contracture

Amputation stump contracture of next proximal joint

Amputation stump flexion

Amputation stump edema

Amputation stump hematoma

EXCLUDES 2 *phantom limb syndrome (G54.6-G54.7)*

T87.9 Unspecified complications of amputation stump

√4th **T88 Other complications of surgical and medical care, not elsewhere classified**

EXCLUDES 2 *complication following infusion, transfusion and therapeutic injection (T8Ø.-)*
complication following procedure NEC (T81.-)
complications of anesthesia in labor and delivery (O74.-)
complications of anesthesia in pregnancy (O29.-)
complications of anesthesia in puerperium (O89.-)
complications of devices, implants and grafts (T82-T85)
complications of obstetric surgery and procedure (O75.4)
dermatitis due to drugs and medicaments (L23.3, L24.4, L25.1, L27.Ø-L27.1)
poisoning and toxic effects of drugs and chemicals (T36-T65 with fifth or sixth character 1-4 or 6)
specified complications classified elsewhere

The appropriate 7th character is to be added to each code from category T88.
A initial encounter
D subsequent encounter
S sequela

√x7th **T88.Ø Infection following immunization**

Sepsis following immunization

√x7th **T88.1 Other complications following immunization, not elsewhere classified**

Generalized vaccinia

Rash following immunization

EXCLUDES 1 *vaccinia not from vaccine (BØ8.Ø11)*

EXCLUDES 2 *anaphylactic shock due to serum (T8Ø.5-)*
other serum reactions (T8Ø.6-)
postimmunization arthropathy (MØ2.2)
postimmunization encephalitis (GØ4.Ø2)
postimmunization fever (R5Ø.83)

√x7th **T88.2 Shock due to anesthesia**

Use additional code for adverse effect, if applicable, to identify drug (T41.- with fifth or sixth character 5)

EXCLUDES 1 *complications of anesthesia (in):*
labor and delivery (O74.-)
pregnancy (O29.-)
puerperium (O89.-)
postprocedural shock NOS (T81.1-)

√x7th **T88.3 Malignant hyperthermia due to anesthesia**

Use additional code for adverse effect, if applicable, to identify drug (T41.- with fifth or sixth character 5)

√x7th **T88.4 Failed or difficult intubation**

√5th **T88.5 Other complications of anesthesia**

Use additional code for adverse effect, if applicable, to identify drug (T41.- with fifth or sixth character 5)

√x7th **T88.51 Hypothermia following anesthesia**

√x7th **T88.52 Failed moderate sedation during procedure**

Failed conscious sedation during procedure

EXCLUDES 2 *personal history of failed moderate sedation (Z92.83)*

√x7th **T88.59 Other complications of anesthesia**

√x7th **T88.6 Anaphylactic reaction due to adverse effect of correct drug or medicament properly administered**

Anaphylactic shock due to adverse effect of correct drug or medicament properly administered

Anaphylactoid reaction NOS

Use additional code for adverse effect, if applicable, to identify drug (T41.- with fifth or sixth character 5)

EXCLUDES 1 *anaphylactic reaction due to serum (T8Ø.5-)*
anaphylactic shock or reaction due to adverse food reaction (T78.Ø-)

√x7th **T88.7 Unspecified adverse effect of drug or medicament**

Use additional code for adverse effect, if applicable, to identify drug (T41.- with fifth or sixth character 5)

Drug hypersensitivity NOS

Drug reaction NOS

EXCLUDES 1 *specified adverse effects of drugs and medicaments (AØØ-R94 and T8Ø-T88.6, T88.8)*

√x7th **T88.8 Other specified complications of surgical and medical care, not elsewhere classified**

Use additional code to identify the complication

√x7th **T88.9 Complication of surgical and medical care, unspecified**

Chapter 20. External Causes of Morbidity (V00-Y99)

NOTE This chapter permits the classification of environmental events and circumstances as the cause of injury, and other adverse effects. Where a code from this section is applicable, it is intended that it shall be used secondary to a code from another chapter of the Classification indicating the nature of the condition. Most often, the condition will be classifiable to Chapter 19, Injury, poisoning and certain other consequences of external causes (S00-T88). Other conditions that may be stated to be due to external causes are classified in Chapters I to XVIII. For these conditions, codes from Chapter 20 should be used to provide additional information as to the cause of the condition.

This chapter contains the following blocks:

V00-V09 Pedestrian injured in transport accident
V10-V19 Pedal cycle rider injured in transport accident
V20-V29 Motorcycle rider injured in transport accident
V30-V39 Occupant of three-wheeled motor vehicle injured in transport accident
V40-V49 Car occupant injured in transport accident
V50-V59 Occupant of pick-up truck or van injured in transport accident
V60-V69 Occupant of heavy transport vehicle injured in transport accident
V70-V79 Bus occupant injured in transport accident
V80-V89 Other land transport accidents
V90-V94 Water transport accidents
V95-V97 Air and space transport accidents
V98-V99 Other and unspecified transport accidents
W00-X58 Other external causes of accidental injury
W00-W19 Slipping, tripping, stumbling and falls
W20-W49 Exposure to inanimate mechanical forces
W50-W64 Exposure to animate mechanical forces
W65-W74 Accidental non-transport drowning and submersion
W85-W99 Exposure to electric current, radiation and extreme ambient air temperature and pressure
X00-X08 Exposure to smoke, fire and flames
X10-X19 Contact with heat and hot substances
X30-X39 Exposure to forces of nature
X52, X58 Accidental exposure to other specified factors
X71-X83 Intentional self-harm
X92-Y08 Assault
Y21-Y33 Event of undetermined intent
Y35-Y38 Legal intervention, operations of war, military operations, and terrorism
Y62-Y84 Complications of medical and surgical care
Y62-Y69 Misadventures to patients during surgical and medical care
Y70-Y82 Medical devices associated with adverse incidents in diagnostic and therapeutic use
Y83-Y84 Surgical and other medical procedures as the cause of abnormal reaction of the patient, or of later complication, without mention of misadventure at the time of the procedure
Y90-Y99 Supplementary factors related to causes of morbidity classified elsewhere

Transport accidents (V00-V99)

Use additional code to identify:
airbag injury (W22.1)
type of street or road (Y92.4-)
use of cellular telephone and other electronic equipment at the time of the transport accident (Y93.C-)

EXCLUDES 1 *agricultural vehicles in stationary use or maintenance (W31.-)*
assault by crashing of motor vehicle (Y03.-)
automobile or motor cycle in stationary use or maintenance—code to type of accident
crashing of motor vehicle, undetermined intent (Y32)
intentional self-harm by crashing of motor vehicle (X82)

EXCLUDES 2 *transport accidents due to cataclysm (X34-X38)*

Definitions of transport vehicles:

(a) A transport accident is any accident involving a device designed primarily for, or used at the time primarily for, conveying persons or good from one place to another.

(b) A public highway [trafficway] or street is the entire width between property lines (or other boundary lines) ofland open to the public as a matter of right or custom for purposes of moving persons or property from one place toanother. A roadway is that part of the public highway designed, improved and customarily used for vehicular traffic.

(c) A traffic accident is any vehicle accident occurring on the public highway [i.e. originating on, terminating on, orinvolving a vehicle partially on the highway]. A vehicle accident is assumed to have occurred on the public highway unless another place is specified, except in the case of accidents involving only off-road motor vehicles, which are classified as nontraffic accidents unless the contrary is stated.

(d) A nontraffic accident is any vehicle accident that occurs entirely in any place other than a public highway.

(e) A pedestrian is any person involved in an accident who was not at the time of the accident riding in or on a motor vehicle, railway train, streetcar or animal-drawn or other vehicle, or on a pedal cycle or animal. This includes, a person changing a tire or working on a parked car. It also includes the use of a pedestrian conveyance such as a baby carriage, ice-skates, roller skates, a skateboard, nonmotorized or motorized wheelchair, motorized mobility scooter, or nonmotorized scooter.

(f) A driver is an occupant of a transport vehicle who is operating or intending to operate it.

(g) A passenger is any occupant of a transport vehicle other than the driver, except a person traveling on the outsideof the vehicle.

(h) A person on the outside of a vehicle is any person being transported by a vehicle but not occupying the space normally reserved for the driver or passengers, or the space intended for the transport of property. This includes the body, bumper, fender, roof, running board or step of a vehicle.

(i) A pedal cycle is any land transport vehicle operated solely by nonmotorized pedals including a bicycle or tricycle.

(j) A pedal cyclist is any person riding a pedal cycle or in a sidecar or trailer attached to a pedal cycle.

(k) A motorcycle is a two-wheeled motor vehicle with one or two riding saddles and sometimes with a third wheel for the support of a sidecar. The sidecar is considered part of the motorcycle.

(l) A motorcycle rider is any person riding a motorcycle or in a sidecar or trailer attached to the motorcycle.

(m) A three-wheeled motor vehicle is a motorized tricycle designed primarily for on-road use. This includes a motor-driven tricycle, a motorized rickshaw, or a three-wheeled motor car.

(n) A car [automobile] is a four-wheeled motor vehicle designed primarily for carrying up to 7 persons. A trailer being towed by the car is considered part of the car.

(o) A pick-up truck or van is a four or six-wheeled motor vehicle designed for carrying passengers as well as property or cargo weighing less than the local limit for classification as a heavy goods vehicle, and not requiring a special driver's license. This includes a minivan and a sport-utility vehicle (SUV).

(p) A heavy transport vehicle is a motor vehicle designed primarily for carrying property, meeting local criteria for classification as a heavy goods vehicle in terms of weight and requiring a special driver's license.

(q) A bus (coach) is a motor vehicle designed or adapted primarily for carrying more than 10 passengers, and requiring a special driver's license.

(r) A railway train or railway vehicle is any device, with or without freight or passenger cars couple to it, designed for traffic on a railway track. This includes subterranean (subways) or elevated trains.

(s) A streetcar, is a device designed and used primarily for transporting passengers within a municipality, running on rails, usually subject to normal traffic control signals, and operated principally on a right-of-way that forms part of the roadway. This includes a tram or trolley that runs on rails. A trailer being towed by a streetcar is considered part of the streetcar.

(t) A special vehicle mainly used on industrial premises is a motor vehicle designed primarily for use within the buildings and premises of industrial or commercial establishments. This includes battery-powered trucks, forklifts, coal-cars in a coal mine, logging cars and trucks used in mines or quarries.

(u) A special vehicle mainly used in agriculture is a motor vehicle designed specifically for use in farming and agriculture (horticulture), to work the land, tend and harvest crops and transport materials on the farm. This includes harvesters, farm machinery and tractor and trailers.

(v) A special construction vehicle is a motor vehicle designed specifically for use on construction and demolition sites. This includes bulldozers, diggers, earth levelers, dump trucks. backhoes, front-end loaders, pavers, and mechanical shovels.

(w) A special all-terrain vehicle is a motor vehicle of special design to enable it to negotiate over rough or soft terrain , snow or sand. This includes snow mobiles, All-terrain vehicles (ATV), and dune buggies. It does not include passenger vehicle designated as Sport Utility Vehicles (SUV).

(x) A watercraft is any device designed for transporting passengers or goods on water. This includes motor or sailboats, ships, and hovercraft.

(y) An aircraft is any device for transporting passengers or goods in the air. This includes hot-air balloons, gliders, helicopters and airplanes.

(z) A military vehicle is any motorized vehicle operating on a public roadway owned by the military and being operated by a member of the military.

Pedestrian injured in transport accident (V00-V09)

INCLUDES person changing tire on transport vehicle
person examining engine of vehicle broken down in (on side of) road

EXCLUDES 1 *fall due to non-transport collision with other person (W03)*
pedestrian on foot falling (slipping) on ice and snow (W00.-)
struck or bumped by another person (W51)

✓4th V00 Pedestrian conveyance accident

Use additional place of occurrence and activity external cause codes, if known (Y92-, Y93-)

EXCLUDES 1 *collision with another person without fall (W51)*
fall due to person on foot colliding with another person on foot (W03)
fall from non-moving wheelchair, nonmotorized scooter and motorized mobility scooter without collision (W05.-)
pedestrian (conveyance) collision with other land transport vehicle (V01-V09)
pedestrian on foot falling (slipping) on ice and snow (W00.-)

The appropriate 7th character is to be added to each code from category V00.
A initial encounter
D subsequent encounter
S sequela

✓5th V00.0 Pedestrian on foot injured in collision with pedestrian conveyance

✓x7th V00.01 Pedestrian on foot injured in collision with roller-skater

✓x7th V00.02 Pedestrian on foot injured in collision with skateboarder

✓x7th V00.09 Pedestrian on foot injured in collision with other pedestrian conveyance

✓5th V00.1 Rolling-type pedestrian conveyance accident

EXCLUDES 1 *accident with babystroller (V00.82-)*
accident with motorized mobility scooter (V00.83-)
accident with wheelchair (powered) (V00.81-)

✓6th V00.11 In-line roller-skate accident

✓7th V00.111 Fall from in-line roller-skates

✓7th V00.112 In-line roller-skater colliding with stationary object

✓7th V00.118 Other in-line roller-skate accident

EXCLUDES 1 *roller-skater collision with other land transport vehicle (V01-V09 with 5th character 1)*

✓6th V00.12 Non-in- line roller-skate accident

✓7th V00.121 Fall from non-in-line roller-skates

✓7th V00.122 Non-in-line roller-skater colliding with stationary object

✓7th V00.128 Other non-in-line roller-skating accident

EXCLUDES 1 *roller-skater collision with other land transport vehicle (V01-V09 with 5th character 1)*

✓6th V00.13 Skateboard accident

✓7th V00.131 Fall from skateboard

✓7th V00.132 Skateboarder colliding with stationary object

✓7th V00.138 Other skateboard accident

EXCLUDES 1 *skateboarder collision with other land transport vehicle (V01-V09 with 5th character 2)*

✓6th V00.14 Scooter (nonmotorized) accident

EXCLUDES 1 *motorscooter accident (V20-V29)*

✓7th V00.141 Fall from scooter (nonmotorized)

✓7th V00.142 Scooter (nonmotorized) colliding with stationary object

✓7th V00.148 Other scooter (nonmotorized) accident

EXCLUDES 1 *scooter (nonmotorized) collision with other land transport vehicle (V01-V09 with fifth character 9)*

✓6th V00.15 Heelies accident

Rolling shoe
Wheeled shoe
Wheelies accident

✓7th V00.151 Fall from heelies

✓7th V00.152 Heelies colliding with stationary object

✓7th V00.158 Other heelies accident

✓6th V00.18 Accident on other rolling-type pedestrian conveyance

✓7th V00.181 Fall from other rolling-type pedestrian conveyance

✓7th V00.182 Pedestrian on other rolling-type pedestrian conveyance colliding with stationary object

✓7th V00.188 Other accident on other rolling-type pedestrian conveyance

✓5th V00.2 Gliding-type pedestrian conveyance accident

✓6th V00.21 Ice-skates accident

✓7th V00.211 Fall from ice-skates

✓7th V00.212 Ice-skater colliding with stationary object

✓7th V00.218 Other ice-skates accident

EXCLUDES 1 *ice-skater collision with other land transport vehicle (V01-V09 with 5th digit 9)*

✓6th V00.22 Sled accident

✓7th V00.221 Fall from sled

✓7th V00.222 Sledder colliding with stationary object

✓7th V00.228 Other sled accident

EXCLUDES 1 *sled collision with other land transport vehicle (V01-V09 with 5th digit 9)*

✓6th V00.28 Other gliding-type pedestrian conveyance accident

✓7th V00.281 Fall from other gliding-type pedestrian conveyance

✓7th V00.282 Pedestrian on other gliding-type pedestrian conveyance colliding with stationary object

✓7th V00.288 Other accident on other gliding-type pedestrian conveyance

EXCLUDES 1 *gliding-type pedestrian conveyance collision with other land transport vehicle (V01-V09 with 5th digit 9)*

✓5th V00.3 Flat-bottomed pedestrian conveyance accident

✓6th V00.31 Snowboard accident

✓7th V00.311 Fall from snowboard

✓7th V00.312 Snowboarder colliding with stationary object

✓7th V00.318 Other snowboard accident

EXCLUDES 1 *snowboarder collision with other land transport vehicle (V01-V09 with 5th digit 9)*

✓6th V00.32 Snow-ski accident

✓7th V00.321 Fall from snow-skis

✓7th V00.322 Snow-skier colliding with stationary object

✓7th V00.328 Other snow-ski accident

EXCLUDES 1 *snow-skier collision with other land transport vehicle (V01-V09 with 5th digit 9)*

✓6th V00.38 Other flat-bottomed pedestrian conveyance accident

✓7th V00.381 Fall from other flat-bottomed pedestrian conveyance

✓7th V00.382 Pedestrian on other flat-bottomed pedestrian conveyance colliding with stationary object

✓7th V00.388 Other accident on other flat-bottomed pedestrian conveyance

✓5th V00.8 Accident on other pedestrian conveyance

✓6th V00.81 Accident with wheelchair (powered)

✓7th V00.811 Fall from moving wheelchair (powered)

EXCLUDES 1 *fall from non-moving wheelchair (W05.0)*

✓7th **VØØ.812 Wheelchair (powered) colliding with stationary object**

✓7th **VØØ.818 Other accident with wheelchair (powered)**

✓6th **VØØ.82 Accident with babystroller**

✓7th **VØØ.821 Fall from babystroller**

✓7th **VØØ.822 Babystroller colliding with stationary object**

✓7th **VØØ.828 Other accident with babystroller**

✓6th **VØØ.83 Accident with motorized mobility scooter**

VØØ.831 Fall from motorized mobility scooter

EXCLUDES 1 *fall from non-moving motorized mobility scooter (WØ5.2)*

VØØ.832 Motorized mobility scooter colliding with stationary object

VØØ.838 Other accident with motorized mobility scooter

✓6th **VØØ.89 Accident on other pedestrian conveyance**

✓7th **VØØ.891 Fall from other pedestrian conveyance**

✓7th **VØØ.892 Pedestrian on other pedestrian conveyance colliding with stationary object**

✓7th **VØØ.898 Other accident on other pedestrian conveyance**

EXCLUDES 1 *other pedestrian (conveyance) collision with other land transport vehicle (VØ1-VØ9 with 5th digit 9)*

✓4th **VØ1 Pedestrian injured in collision with pedal cycle**

The appropriate 7th character is to be added to each code from category VØ1.

A initial encounter
D subsequent encounter
S sequela

✓5th **VØ1.Ø Pedestrian injured in collision with pedal cycle in nontraffic accident**

✓x7th **VØ1.ØØ Pedestrian on foot injured in collision with pedal cycle in nontraffic accident**

Pedestrian NOS injured in collision with pedal cycle in nontraffic accident

✓x7th **VØ1.Ø1 Pedestrian on roller-skates injured in collision with pedal cycle in nontraffic accident**

✓x7th **VØ1.Ø2 Pedestrian on skateboard injured in collision with pedal cycle in nontraffic accident**

✓x7th **VØ1.Ø9 Pedestrian with other conveyance injured in collision with pedal cycle in nontraffic accident**

Pedestrian with babystroller injured in collision with pedal cycle in nontraffic accident
Pedestrian on ice-skates injured in collision with pedal cycle in nontraffic accident
Pedestrian on nonmotorized scooter injured in collision with pedal cycle in nontraffic accident
Pedestrian on sled injured in collision with pedal cycle in nontraffic accident
Pedestrian on snowboard injured in collision with pedal cycle in nontraffic accident
Pedestrian on snow-skis injured in collision with pedal cycle in nontraffic accident
Pedestrian in wheelchair (powered) injured in collision with pedal cycle in nontraffic accident
Pedestrian in motorized mobility scooter injured in collision with pedal cycle in nontraffic accident

✓5th **VØ1.1 Pedestrian injured in collision with pedal cycle in traffic accident**

✓x7th **VØ1.1Ø Pedestrian on foot injured in collision with pedal cycle in traffic accident**

Pedestrian NOS injured in collision with pedal cycle in traffic accident

✓x7th **VØ1.11 Pedestrian on roller-skates injured in collision with pedal cycle in traffic accident**

✓x7th **VØ1.12 Pedestrian on skateboard injured in collision with pedal cycle in traffic accident**

✓x7th **VØ1.19 Pedestrian with other conveyance injured in collision with pedal cycle in traffic accident**

Pedestrian with babystroller injured in collision with pedal cycle in traffic accident
Pedestrian on ice-skates injured in collision with pedal cycle in traffic accident
Pedestrian on nonmotorized scooter injured in collision with pedal cycle in traffic accident
Pedestrian on sled injured in collision with pedal cycle in traffic accident
Pedestrian on snowboard injured in collision with pedal cycle in traffic accident
Pedestrian on snow-skis injured in collision with pedal cycle in traffic accident
Pedestrian in wheelchair (powered) injured in collision with pedal cycle in traffic accident
Pedestrian in motorized mobility scooter injured in collision with pedal cycle in traffic accident

✓5th **VØ1.9 Pedestrian injured in collision with pedal cycle, unspecified whether traffic or nontraffic accident**

✓x7th **VØ1.9Ø Pedestrian on foot injured in collision with pedal cycle, unspecified whether traffic or nontraffic accident**

Pedestrian NOS injured in collision with pedal cycle, unspecified whether traffic or nontraffic accident

✓x7th **VØ1.91 Pedestrian on roller-skates injured in collision with pedal cycle, unspecified whether traffic or nontraffic accident**

✓x7th **VØ1.92 Pedestrian on skateboard injured in collision with pedal cycle, unspecified whether traffic or nontraffic accident**

✓x7th **VØ1.99 Pedestrian with other conveyance injured in collision with pedal cycle, unspecified whether traffic or nontraffic accident**

Pedestrian with babystroller injured in collision with pedal cycle, unspecified whether traffic or nontraffic accident
Pedestrian on ice-skates injured in collision with pedal cycle unspecified, whether traffic or nontraffic accident
Pedestrian on nonmotorized scooter injured in collision with pedal cycle, unspecified whether traffic or nontraffic accident
Pedestrian on sled injured in collision with pedal cycle unspecified, whether traffic or nontraffic accident
Pedestrian on snowboard injured in collision with pedal cycle, unspecified whether traffic or nontraffic accident
Pedestrian on snow-skis injured in collision with pedal cycle, unspecified whether traffic or nontraffic accident
Pedestrian in wheelchair (powered) injured in collision with pedal cycle, unspecified whether traffic or nontraffic accident
Pedestrian in motorized mobility scooter injured in collision with pedal cycle, unspecified whether traffic or nontraffic accident

✓4th **VØ2 Pedestrian injured in collision with two- or three-wheeled motor vehicle**

The appropriate 7th character is to be added to each code from category VØ2.

A initial encounter
D subsequent encounter
S sequela

✓5th **VØ2.Ø Pedestrian injured in collision with two- or three-wheeled motor vehicle in nontraffic accident**

✓x7th **VØ2.ØØ Pedestrian on foot injured in collision with two- or three-wheeled motor vehicle in nontraffic accident**

Pedestrian NOS injured in collision with two- or three-wheeled motor vehicle in nontraffic accident

✓x7th **VØ2.Ø1 Pedestrian on roller-skates injured in collision with two- or three-wheeled motor vehicle in nontraffic accident**

✓x7th **VØ2.Ø2 Pedestrian on skateboard injured in collision with two- or three-wheeled motor vehicle in nontraffic accident**

√x7th **V02.09 Pedestrian with other conveyance injured in collision with two- or three-wheeled motor vehicle in nontraffic accident**
Pedestrian with babystroller injured in collision with two- or three-wheeled motor vehicle in nontraffic accident
Pedestrian on ice-skates injured in collision with two- or three-wheeled motor vehicle in nontraffic accident
Pedestrian on nonmotorized scooter injured in collision with two- or three-wheeled motor vehicle in nontraffic accident
Pedestrian on sled injured in collision with two- or three-wheeled motor vehicle in nontraffic accident
Pedestrian on snowboard injured in collision with two- or three-wheeled motor vehicle in nontraffic accident
Pedestrian on snow-skis injured in collision with two- or three-wheeled motor vehicle in nontraffic accident
Pedestrian in wheelchair (powered) injured in collision with two- or three-wheeled motor vehicle in nontraffic accident
Pedestrian in motorized mobility scooter injured in collision with two- or three-wheeled motor vehicle in nontraffic accident

√5th **V02.1 Pedestrian injured in collision with two- or three-wheeled motor vehicle in traffic accident**

√x7th **V02.10 Pedestrian on foot injured in collision with two- or three-wheeled motor vehicle in traffic accident**
Pedestrian NOS injured in collision with two- or three-wheeled motor vehicle in traffic accident

√x7th **V02.11 Pedestrian on roller-skates injured in collision with two- or three-wheeled motor vehicle in traffic accident**

√x7th **V02.12 Pedestrian on skateboard injured in collision with two- or three-wheeled motor vehicle in traffic accident**

√x7th **V02.19 Pedestrian with other conveyance injured in collision with two- or three-wheeled motor vehicle in traffic accident**
Pedestrian with babystroller injured in collision with two- or three-wheeled motor vehicle in traffic accident
Pedestrian on ice-skates injured in collision with two- or three-wheeled motor vehicle in traffic accident
Pedestrian on nonmotorized scooter injured in collision with two- or three-wheeled motor vehicle in traffic accident
Pedestrian on sled injured in collision with two- or three-wheeled motor vehicle in traffic accident
Pedestrian on snowboard injured in collision with two- or three-wheeled motor vehicle in traffic accident
Pedestrian on snow-skis injured in collision with two- or three-wheeled motor vehicle in traffic accident
Pedestrian in wheelchair (powered) injured in collision with two- or three-wheeled motor vehicle in traffic accident
Pedestrian in motorized mobility scooter injured in collision with two- or three-wheeled motor vehicle in traffic accident

√5th **V02.9 Pedestrian injured in collision with two- or three-wheeled motor vehicle, unspecified whether traffic or nontraffic accident**

√x7th **V02.90 Pedestrian on foot injured in collision with two- or three-wheeled motor vehicle, unspecified whether traffic or nontraffic accident**
Pedestrian NOS injured in collision with two- or three-wheeled motor vehicle, unspecified whether traffic or nontraffic accident

√x7th **V02.91 Pedestrian on roller-skates injured in collision with two- or three-wheeled motor vehicle, unspecified whether traffic or nontraffic accident**

√x7th **V02.92 Pedestrian on skateboard injured in collision with two- or three-wheeled motor vehicle, unspecified whether traffic or nontraffic accident**

√x7th **V02.99 Pedestrian with other conveyance injured in collision with two- or three-wheeled motor vehicle, unspecified whether traffic or nontraffic accident**
Pedestrian with babystroller injured in collision with two- or three-wheeled motor vehicle, unspecified whether traffic or nontraffic accident
Pedestrian on ice-skates injured in collision with two- or three-wheeled motor vehicle, unspecified whether traffic or nontraffic accident
Pedestrian on nonmotorized scooter injured in collision with two- or three-wheeled motor vehicle, unspecified whether traffic or nontraffic accident
Pedestrian on sled injured in collision with two- or three-wheeled motor vehicle, unspecified whether traffic or nontraffic accident
Pedestrian on snowboard injured in collision with two- or three-wheeled motor vehicle, unspecified whether traffic or nontraffic accident
Pedestrian on snow-skis injured in collision with two- or three-wheeled motor vehicle, unspecified whether traffic or nontraffic accident
Pedestrian in wheelchair (powered) injured in collision with two- or three-wheeled motor vehicle, unspecified whether traffic or nontraffic accident
Pedestrian in motorized mobility scooter injured in collision with two- or three-wheeled motor vehicle, unspecified whether traffic or nontraffic accident

√4th **V03 Pedestrian injured in collision with car, pick-up truck or van**

The appropriate 7th character is to be added to each code from category V03.
A initial encounter
D subsequent encounter
S sequela

√5th **V03.0 Pedestrian injured in collision with car, pick-up truck or van in nontraffic accident**

√x7th **V03.00 Pedestrian on foot injured in collision with car, pick-up truck or van in nontraffic accident**
Pedestrian NOS injured in collision with car, pick-up truck or van in nontraffic accident

√x7th **V03.01 Pedestrian on roller-skates injured in collision with car, pick-up truck or van in nontraffic accident**

√x7th **V03.02 Pedestrian on skateboard injured in collision with car, pick-up truck or van in nontraffic accident**

√x7th **V03.09 Pedestrian with other conveyance injured in collision with car, pick-up truck or van in nontraffic accident**
Pedestrian with babystroller injured in collision with car, pick-up truck or van in nontraffic accident
Pedestrian on ice-skates injured in collision with car, pick-up truck or van in nontraffic accident
Pedestrian on nonmotorized scooter injured in collision with car, pick-up truck or van in nontraffic accident
Pedestrian on sled injured in collision with car, pick-up truck or van in nontraffic accident
Pedestrian on snowboard injured in collision with car, pick-up truck or van in nontraffic accident
Pedestrian on snow-skis injured in collision with car, pick-up truck or van in nontraffic accident
Pedestrian in wheelchair (powered) injured in collision with car, pick-up truck or van in nontraffic accident
Pedestrian in motorized mobility scooter injured in collision with car, pick-up truck or van in nontraffic accident

√5th **V03.1 Pedestrian injured in collision with car, pick-up truck or van in traffic accident**

√x7th **V03.10 Pedestrian on foot injured in collision with car, pick-up truck or van in traffic accident**
Pedestrian NOS injured in collision with car, pick-up truck or van in traffic accident

√x7th **V03.11 Pedestrian on roller-skates injured in collision with car, pick-up truck or van in traffic accident**

√x7th **V03.12 Pedestrian on skateboard injured in collision with car, pick-up truck or van in traffic accident**

√x7th **V03.19 Pedestrian with other conveyance injured in collision with car, pick-up truck or van in traffic accident**
Pedestrian with babystroller injured in collision with car, pick-up truck or van in traffic accident
Pedestrian on ice-skates injured in collision with car, pick-up truck or van in traffic accident
Pedestrian on nonmotorized scooter injured in collision with car, pick-up truck or van in traffic accident
Pedestrian on sled injured in collision with car, pick-up truck or van in traffic accident
Pedestrian on snowboard injured in collision with car, pick-up truck or van in traffic accident
Pedestrian on snow-skis injured in collision with car, pick-up truck or van in traffic accident
Pedestrian in wheelchair (powered) injured in collision with car, pick-up truck or van in traffic accident
Pedestrian in motorized mobility scooter injured in collision with car, pick-up truck or van in traffic accident

√5th **V03.9 Pedestrian injured in collision with car, pick-up truck or van, unspecified whether traffic or nontraffic accident**

√x7th **V03.90 Pedestrian on foot injured in collision with car, pick-up truck or van, unspecified whether traffic or nontraffic accident**
Pedestrian NOS injured in collision with car, pick-up truck or van, unspecified whether traffic or nontraffic accident

√x7th **V03.91 Pedestrian on roller-skates injured in collision with car, pick-up truck or van, unspecified whether traffic or nontraffic accident**

√x7th **V03.92 Pedestrian on skateboard injured in collision with car, pick-up truck or van, unspecified whether traffic or nontraffic accident**

√x7th **V03.99 Pedestrian with other conveyance injured in collision with car, pick-up truck or van, unspecified whether traffic or nontraffic accident**
Pedestrian with babystroller injured in collision with car, pick-up truck or van, unspecified whether traffic or nontraffic accident
Pedestrian on ice-skates injured in collision with car, pick-up truck or van, unspecified whether traffic or nontraffic accident
Pedestrian on nonmotorized scooter injured in collision with car, pick-up truck or van, unspecified whether traffic or nontraffic accident
Pedestrian on sled injured in collision with car, pick-up truck or van in nontraffic accident
Pedestrian on snowboard injured in collision with car, pick-up truck or van, unspecified whether traffic or nontraffic accident
Pedestrian on snow-skis injured in collision with car, pick-up truck or van, unspecified whether traffic or nontraffic accident
Pedestrian in wheelchair (powered) injured in collision with car, pick-up truck or van, unspecified whether traffic or nontraffic accident
Pedestrian in motorized mobility scooter injured in collision with car, pick-up truck or van, unspecified whether traffic or nontraffic accident

√4th **V04 Pedestrian injured in collision with heavy transport vehicle or bus**

EXCLUDES 1 *pedestrian injured in collision with military vehicle (V09.01, V09.21)*

The appropriate 7th character is to be added to each code from category V04.
A initial encounter
D subsequent encounter
S sequela

√5th **V04.0 Pedestrian injured in collision with heavy transport vehicle or bus in nontraffic accident**

√x7th **V04.00 Pedestrian on foot injured in collision with heavy transport vehicle or bus in nontraffic accident**
Pedestrian NOS injured in collision with heavy transport vehicle or bus in nontraffic accident

√x7th **V04.01 Pedestrian on roller-skates injured in collision with heavy transport vehicle or bus in nontraffic accident**

√x7th **V04.02 Pedestrian on skateboard injured in collision with heavy transport vehicle or bus in nontraffic accident**

√x7th **V04.09 Pedestrian with other conveyance injured in collision with heavy transport vehicle or bus in nontraffic accident**
Pedestrian with babystroller injured in collision with heavy transport vehicle or bus in nontraffic accident
Pedestrian on ice-skates injured in collision with heavy transport vehicle or bus in nontraffic accident
Pedestrian on nonmotorized scooter injured in collision with heavy transport vehicle or bus in nontraffic accident
Pedestrian on sled injured in collision with heavy transport vehicle or bus in nontraffic accident
Pedestrian on snowboard injured in collision with heavy transport vehicle or bus in nontraffic accident
Pedestrian on snow-skis injured in collision with heavy transport vehicle or bus in nontraffic accident
Pedestrian in wheelchair (powered) injured in collision with heavy transport vehicle or bus in nontraffic accident
Pedestrian in motorized mobility scooter injured in collision with heavy transport vehicle or bus in nontraffic accident

√5th **V04.1 Pedestrian injured in collision with heavy transport vehicle or bus in traffic accident**

√x7th **V04.10 Pedestrian on foot injured in collision with heavy transport vehicle or bus in traffic accident**
Pedestrian NOS injured in collision with heavy transport vehicle or bus in traffic accident

√x7th **V04.11 Pedestrian on roller-skates injured in collision with heavy transport vehicle or bus in traffic accident**

√x7th **V04.12 Pedestrian on skateboard injured in collision with heavy transport vehicle or bus in traffic accident**

√x7th **V04.19 Pedestrian with other conveyance injured in collision with heavy transport vehicle or bus in traffic accident**
Pedestrian with babystroller injured in collision with heavy transport vehicle or bus in traffic accident
Pedestrian on ice-skates injured in collision with heavy transport vehicle or bus in traffic accident
Pedestrian on nonmotorized scooter injured in collision with heavy transport vehicle or bus in traffic accident
Pedestrian on sled injured in collision with heavy transport vehicle or bus in traffic accident
Pedestrian on snowboard injured in collision with heavy transport vehicle or bus in traffic accident
Pedestrian on snow-skis injured in collision with heavy transport vehicle or bus in traffic accident
Pedestrian in wheelchair (powered) injured in collision with heavy transport vehicle or bus in traffic accident
Pedestrian in motorized mobility scooter injured in collision with heavy transport vehicle or bus in traffic accident

√5th **V04.9 Pedestrian injured in collision with heavy transport vehicle or bus, unspecified whether traffic or nontraffic accident**

√x7th **V04.90 Pedestrian on foot injured in collision with heavy transport vehicle or bus, unspecified whether traffic or nontraffic accident**

Pedestrian NOS injured in collision with heavy transport vehicle or bus, unspecified whether traffic or nontraffic accident

√x7th **V04.91 Pedestrian on roller-skates injured in collision with heavy transport vehicle or bus, unspecified whether traffic or nontraffic accident**

√x7th **V04.92 Pedestrian on skateboard injured in collision with heavy transport vehicle or bus, unspecified whether traffic or nontraffic accident**

√x7th **V04.99 Pedestrian with other conveyance injured in collision with heavy transport vehicle or bus, unspecified whether traffic or nontraffic accident**

Pedestrian with babystroller injured in collision with heavy transport vehicle or bus, unspecified whether traffic or nontraffic accident

Pedestrian on ice-skates injured in collision with heavy transport vehicle or bus, unspecified whether traffic or nontraffic accident

Pedestrian on nonmotorized scooter injured in collision with heavy transport vehicle or bus, unspecified whether traffic or nontraffic accident

Pedestrian on sled injured in collision with heavy transport vehicle or bus, unspecified whether traffic or nontraffic accident

Pedestrian on snowboard injured in collision with heavy transport vehicle or bus, unspecified whether traffic or nontraffic accident

Pedestrian on snow-skis injured in collision with heavy transport vehicle or bus, unspecified whether traffic or nontraffic accident

Pedestrian in wheelchair (powered) injured in collision with heavy transport vehicle or bus, unspecified whether traffic or nontraffic accident

Pedestrian in motorized mobility scooter injured in collision with heavy transport vehicle or bus, unspecified whether traffic or nontraffic accident

√4th **V05 Pedestrian injured in collision with railway train or railway vehicle**

The appropriate 7th character is to be added to each code from category V05.

A initial encounter
D subsequent encounter
S sequela

√5th **V05.0 Pedestrian injured in collision with railway train or railway vehicle in nontraffic accident**

√x7th **V05.00 Pedestrian on foot injured in collision with railway train or railway vehicle in nontraffic accident**

Pedestrian NOS injured in collision with railway train or railway vehicle in nontraffic accident

√x7th **V05.01 Pedestrian on roller-skates injured in collision with railway train or railway vehicle in nontraffic accident**

√x7th **V05.02 Pedestrian on skateboard injured in collision with railway train or railway vehicle in nontraffic accident**

√x7th **V05.09 Pedestrian with other conveyance injured in collision with railway train or railway vehicle in nontraffic accident**

Pedestrian with babystroller injured in collision with railway train or railway vehicle in nontraffic accident

Pedestrian on ice-skates injured in collision with railway train or railway vehicle in nontraffic accident

Pedestrian on nonmotorized scooter injured in collision with railway train or railway vehicle in nontraffic accident

Pedestrian on sled injured in collision with railway train or railway vehicle in nontraffic accident

Pedestrian on snowboard injured in collision with railway train or railway vehicle in nontraffic accident

Pedestrian on snow-skis injured in collision with railway train or railway vehicle in nontraffic accident

Pedestrian in wheelchair (powered) injured in collision with railway train or railway vehicle in nontraffic accident

Pedestrian in motorized mobility scooter injured in collision with railway train or railway vehicle in nontraffic accident

√5th **V05.1 Pedestrian injured in collision with railway train or railway vehicle in traffic accident**

√x7th **V05.10 Pedestrian on foot injured in collision with railway train or railway vehicle in traffic accident**

Pedestrian NOS injured in collision with railway train or railway vehicle in traffic accident

√x7th **V05.11 Pedestrian on roller-skates injured in collision with railway train or railway vehicle in traffic accident**

√x7th **V05.12 Pedestrian on skateboard injured in collision with railway train or railway vehicle in traffic accident**

√x7th **V05.19 Pedestrian with other conveyance injured in collision with railway train or railway vehicle in traffic accident**

Pedestrian with babystroller injured in collision with railway train or railway vehicle in traffic accident

Pedestrian on ice-skates injured in collision with railway train or railway vehicle in traffic accident

Pedestrian on nonmotorized scooter injured in collision with railway train or railway vehicle in traffic accident

Pedestrian on sled injured in collision with railway train or railway vehicle in traffic accident

Pedestrian on snowboard injured in collision with railway train or railway vehicle in traffic accident

Pedestrian on snow-skis injured in collision with railway train or railway vehicle in traffic accident

Pedestrian in wheelchair (powered) injured in collision with railway train or railway vehicle in traffic accident

Pedestrian in motorized mobility scooter injured in collision with railway train or railway vehicle in traffic accident

√5th **V05.9 Pedestrian injured in collision with railway train or railway vehicle, unspecified whether traffic or nontraffic accident**

√x7th **V05.90 Pedestrian on foot injured in collision with railway train or railway vehicle, unspecified whether traffic or nontraffic accident**

Pedestrian NOS injured in collision with railway train or railway vehicle, unspecified whether traffic or nontraffic accident

√x7th **V05.91 Pedestrian on roller-skates injured in collision with railway train or railway vehicle, unspecified whether traffic or nontraffic accident**

√x7th **V05.92 Pedestrian on skateboard injured in collision with railway train or railway vehicle, unspecified whether traffic or nontraffic accident**

√x7th **V05.99 Pedestrian with other conveyance injured in collision with railway train or railway vehicle, unspecified whether traffic or nontraffic accident**
Pedestrian with babystroller injured in collision with railway train or railway vehicle, unspecified whether traffic or nontraffic
Pedestrian on ice-skates injured in collision with railway train or railway vehicle, unspecified whether traffic or nontraffic
Pedestrian on nonmotorized scooter injured in collision with railway train or railway vehicle, unspecified whether traffic or nontraffic
Pedestrian on sled injured in collision with railway train or railway vehicle, unspecified whether traffic or nontraffic
Pedestrian on snowboard injured in collision with railway train or railway vehicle, unspecified whether traffic or nontraffic
Pedestrian on snow-skis injured in collision with railway train or railway vehicle, unspecified whether traffic or nontraffic
Pedestrian in wheelchair (powered) injured in collision with railway train or railway vehicle, unspecified whether traffic or nontraffic
Pedestrian in motorized mobility scooter injured in collision with railway train or railway vehicle, unspecified whether traffic or nontraffic

√4th **V06 Pedestrian injured in collision with other nonmotor vehicle**
INCLUDES collision with animal-drawn vehicle, animal being ridden, nonpowered streetcar
EXCLUDES 1 *pedestrian injured in collision with pedestrian conveyance (V00.0-)*

The appropriate 7th character is to be added to each code from category V06.
A initial encounter
D subsequent encounter
S sequela

√5th **V06.0 Pedestrian injured in collision with other nonmotor vehicle in nontraffic accident**
√x7th **V06.00 Pedestrian on foot injured in collision with other nonmotor vehicle in nontraffic accident**
Pedestrian NOS injured in collision with other nonmotor vehicle in nontraffic accident
√x7th **V06.01 Pedestrian on roller-skates injured in collision with other nonmotor vehicle in nontraffic accident**
√x7th **V06.02 Pedestrian on skateboard injured in collision with other nonmotor vehicle in nontraffic accident**
√x7th **V06.09 Pedestrian with other conveyance injured in collision with other nonmotor vehicle in nontraffic accident**
Pedestrian with babystroller injured in collision with other nonmotor vehicle in nontraffic accident
Pedestrian on ice-skates injured in collision with other nonmotor vehicle in nontraffic accident
Pedestrian on nonmotorized scooter injured in collision with other nonmotor vehicle in nontraffic accident
Pedestrian on sled injured in collision with other nonmotor vehicle in nontraffic accident
Pedestrian on snowboard injured in collision with other nonmotor vehicle in nontraffic accident
Pedestrian on snow-skis injured in collision with other nonmotor vehicle in nontraffic accident
Pedestrian in wheelchair (powered) injured in collision with other nonmotor vehicle in nontraffic accident
Pedestrian in motorized mobility scooter injured in collision with other nonmotor vehicle in nontraffic accident

√5th **V06.1 Pedestrian injured in collision with other nonmotor vehicle in traffic accident**
√x7th **V06.10 Pedestrian on foot injured in collision with other nonmotor vehicle in traffic accident**
Pedestrian NOS injured in collision with other nonmotor vehicle in traffic accident
√x7th **V06.11 Pedestrian on roller-skates injured in collision with other nonmotor vehicle in traffic accident**
√x7th **V06.12 Pedestrian on skateboard injured in collision with other nonmotor vehicle in traffic accident**
√x7th **V06.19 Pedestrian with other conveyance injured in collision with other nonmotor vehicle in traffic accident**
Pedestrian with babystroller injured in collision with other nonmotor vehicle in nontraffic accident
Pedestrian on ice-skates injured in collision with other nonmotor vehicle in traffic accident
Pedestrian on nonmotorized scooter injured in collision with other nonmotor vehicle in traffic accident
Pedestrian on sled injured in collision with other nonmotor vehicle in traffic accident
Pedestrian on snowboard injured in collision with other nonmotor vehicle in traffic accident
Pedestrian on snow-skis injured in collision with other nonmotor vehicle in traffic accident
Pedestrian in wheelchair (powered) injured in collision with other nonmotor vehicle in traffic accident
Pedestrian in motorized mobility scooter injured in collision with other nonmotor vehicle in traffic accident

√5th **V06.9 Pedestrian injured in collision with other nonmotor vehicle, unspecified whether traffic or nontraffic accident**
√x7th **V06.90 Pedestrian on foot injured in collision with other nonmotor vehicle, unspecified whether traffic or nontraffic accident**
Pedestrian NOS injured in collision with other nonmotor vehicle, unspecified whether traffic or nontraffic accident
√x7th **V06.91 Pedestrian on roller-skates injured in collision with other nonmotor vehicle, unspecified whether traffic or nontraffic accident**
√x7th **V06.92 Pedestrian on skateboard injured in collision with other nonmotor vehicle, unspecified whether traffic or nontraffic accident**
√x7th **V06.99 Pedestrian with other conveyance injured in collision with other nonmotor vehicle, unspecified whether traffic or nontraffic accident**
Pedestrian with babystroller injured in collision with other nonmotor vehicle, unspecified whether traffic or nontraffic accident
Pedestrian on ice-skates injured in collision with other nonmotor vehicle, unspecified whether traffic or nontraffic accident
Pedestrian on nonmotorized scooter injured in collision with other nonmotor vehicle, unspecified whether traffic or nontraffic accident
Pedestrian on sled injured in collision with other nonmotor vehicle, unspecified whether traffic or nontraffic accident
Pedestrian on snowboard injured in collision with other nonmotor vehicle, unspecified whether traffic or nontraffic accident
Pedestrian on snow-skis injured in collision with other nonmotor vehicle, unspecified whether traffic or nontraffic accident
Pedestrian in wheelchair (powered) injured in collision with other nonmotor vehicle, unspecified whether traffic or nontraffic accident
Pedestrian in motorized mobility scooter injured in collision with other nonmotor vehicle, unspecified whether traffic or nontraffic accident

√4th **V09 Pedestrian injured in other and unspecified transport accidents**

The appropriate 7th character is to be added to each code from category V09.
A initial encounter
D subsequent encounter
S sequela

√5th **V09.0 Pedestrian injured in nontraffic accident involving other and unspecified motor vehicles**
√x7th **V09.00 Pedestrian injured in nontraffic accident involving unspecified motor vehicles**
√x7th **V09.01 Pedestrian injured in nontraffic accident involving military vehicle**

√x7th **V09.09 Pedestrian injured in nontraffic accident involving other motor vehicles**
Pedestrian injured in nontraffic accident by special vehicle

√x7th **V09.1 Pedestrian injured in unspecified nontraffic accident**

√5th **V09.2 Pedestrian injured in traffic accident involving other and unspecified motor vehicles**

√x7th **V09.20 Pedestrian injured in traffic accident involving unspecified motor vehicles**

√x7th **V09.21 Pedestrian injured in traffic accident involving military vehicle**

√x7th **V09.29 Pedestrian injured in traffic accident involving other motor vehicles**

√x7th **V09.3 Pedestrian injured in unspecified traffic accident**

√x7th **V09.9 Pedestrian injured in unspecified transport accident**

Pedal cycle rider injured in transport accident (V10-V19)

INCLUDES any non-motorized vehicle, excluding an animal-drawn vehicle, or a sidecar or trailer attached to the pedal cycle

EXCLUDES 2 *rupture of pedal cycle tire (W37.0)*

√4th **V10 Pedal cycle rider injured in collision with pedestrian or animal**

EXCLUDES 1 *pedal cycle rider collision with animal-drawn vehicle or animal being ridden (V16.-)*

The appropriate 7th character is to be added to each code from category V10.
A initial encounter
D subsequent encounter
S sequela

√x7th **V10.0 Pedal cycle driver injured in collision with pedestrian or animal in nontraffic accident**

√x7th **V10.1 Pedal cycle passenger injured in collision with pedestrian or animal in nontraffic accident**

√x7th **V10.2 Unspecified pedal cyclist injured in collision with pedestrian or animal in nontraffic accident**

√x7th **V10.3 Person boarding or alighting a pedal cycle injured in collision with pedestrian or animal**

√x7th **V10.4 Pedal cycle driver injured in collision with pedestrian or animal in traffic accident**

√x7th **V10.5 Pedal cycle passenger injured in collision with pedestrian or animal in traffic accident**

√x7th **V10.9 Unspecified pedal cyclist injured in collision with pedestrian or animal in traffic accident**

√4th **V11 Pedal cycle rider injured in collision with other pedal cycle**

The appropriate 7th character is to be added to each code from category V11.
A initial encounter
D subsequent encounter
S sequela

√x7th **V11.0 Pedal cycle driver injured in collision with other pedal cycle in nontraffic accident**

√x7th **V11.1 Pedal cycle passenger injured in collision with other pedal cycle in nontraffic accident**

√x7th **V11.2 Unspecified pedal cyclist injured in collision with other pedal cycle in nontraffic accident**

√x7th **V11.3 Person boarding or alighting a pedal cycle injured in collision with other pedal cycle**

√x7th **V11.4 Pedal cycle driver injured in collision with other pedal cycle in traffic accident**

√x7th **V11.5 Pedal cycle passenger injured in collision with other pedal cycle in traffic accident**

√x7th **V11.9 Unspecified pedal cyclist injured in collision with other pedal cycle in traffic accident**

√4th **V12 Pedal cycle rider injured in collision with two- or three-wheeled motor vehicle**

The appropriate 7th character is to be added to each code from category V12.
A initial encounter
D subsequent encounter
S sequela

√x7th **V12.0 Pedal cycle driver injured in collision with two- or three-wheeled motor vehicle in nontraffic accident**

√x7th **V12.1 Pedal cycle passenger injured in collision with two- or three-wheeled motor vehicle in nontraffic accident**

√x7th **V12.2 Unspecified pedal cyclist injured in collision with two- or three-wheeled motor vehicle in nontraffic accident**

√x7th **V12.3 Person boarding or alighting a pedal cycle injured in collision with two- or three-wheeled motor vehicle**

√x7th **V12.4 Pedal cycle driver injured in collision with two- or three-wheeled motor vehicle in traffic accident**

√x7th **V12.5 Pedal cycle passenger injured in collision with two- or three-wheeled motor vehicle in traffic accident**

√x7th **V12.9 Unspecified pedal cyclist injured in collision with two- or three-wheeled motor vehicle in traffic accident**

√4th **V13 Pedal cycle rider injured in collision with car, pick-up truck or van**

The appropriate 7th character is to be added to each code from category V13.
A initial encounter
D subsequent encounter
S sequela

√x7th **V13.0 Pedal cycle driver injured in collision with car, pick-up truck or van in nontraffic accident**

√x7th **V13.1 Pedal cycle passenger injured in collision with car, pick-up truck or van in nontraffic accident**

√x7th **V13.2 Unspecified pedal cyclist injured in collision with car, pick-up truck or van in nontraffic accident**

√x7th **V13.3 Person boarding or alighting a pedal cycle injured in collision with car, pick-up truck or van**

√x7th **V13.4 Pedal cycle driver injured in collision with car, pick-up truck or van in traffic accident**

√x7th **V13.5 Pedal cycle passenger injured in collision with car, pick-up truck or van in traffic accident**

√x7th **V13.9 Unspecified pedal cyclist injured in collision with car, pick-up truck or van in traffic accident**

√4th **V14 Pedal cycle rider injured in collision with heavy transport vehicle or bus**

EXCLUDES 1 *pedal cycle rider injured in collision with military vehicle (V19.81)*

The appropriate 7th character is to be added to each code from category V14.
A initial encounter
D subsequent encounter
S sequela

√x7th **V14.0 Pedal cycle driver injured in collision with heavy transport vehicle or bus in nontraffic accident**

√x7th **V14.1 Pedal cycle passenger injured in collision with heavy transport vehicle or bus in nontraffic accident**

√x7th **V14.2 Unspecified pedal cyclist injured in collision with heavy transport vehicle or bus in nontraffic accident**

√x7th **V14.3 Person boarding or alighting a pedal cycle injured in collision with heavy transport vehicle or bus**

√x7th **V14.4 Pedal cycle driver injured in collision with heavy transport vehicle or bus in traffic accident**

√x7th **V14.5 Pedal cycle passenger injured in collision with heavy transport vehicle or bus in traffic accident**

√x7th **V14.9 Unspecified pedal cyclist injured in collision with heavy transport vehicle or bus in traffic accident**

√4th **V15 Pedal cycle rider injured in collision with railway train or railway vehicle**

The appropriate 7th character is to be added to each code from category V15.
A initial encounter
D subsequent encounter
S sequela

√x7th **V15.0 Pedal cycle driver injured in collision with railway train or railway vehicle in nontraffic accident**

√x7th **V15.1 Pedal cycle passenger injured in collision with railway train or railway vehicle in nontraffic accident**

√x7th **V15.2 Unspecified pedal cyclist injured in collision with railway train or railway vehicle in nontraffic accident**

√x7th **V15.3 Person boarding or alighting a pedal cycle injured in collision with railway train or railway vehicle**

√x7th **V15.4 Pedal cycle driver injured in collision with railway train or railway vehicle in traffic accident**

√x7th **V15.5 Pedal cycle passenger injured in collision with railway train or railway vehicle in traffic accident**

√x7th **V15.9 Unspecified pedal cyclist injured in collision with railway train or railway vehicle in traffic accident**

√4th **V16 Pedal cycle rider injured in collision with other nonmotor vehicle**

INCLUDES collision with animal-drawn vehicle, animal being ridden, streetcar

The appropriate 7th character is to be added to each code from category V16.
A initial encounter
D subsequent encounter
S sequela

√x7th **V16.0 Pedal cycle driver injured in collision with other nonmotor vehicle in nontraffic accident**

√x7th **V16.1 Pedal cycle passenger injured in collision with other nonmotor vehicle in nontraffic accident**

√x7th **V16.2 Unspecified pedal cyclist injured in collision with other nonmotor vehicle in nontraffic accident**

√x7th **V16.3 Person boarding or alighting a pedal cycle injured in collision with other nonmotor vehicle in nontraffic accident**

√x7th **V16.4 Pedal cycle driver injured in collision with other nonmotor vehicle in traffic accident**

√x7th **V16.5 Pedal cycle passenger injured in collision with other nonmotor vehicle in traffic accident**

√x7th **V16.9 Unspecified pedal cyclist injured in collision with other nonmotor vehicle in traffic accident**

√4th **V17 Pedal cycle rider injured in collision with fixed or stationary object**

The appropriate 7th character is to be added to each code from category V17.
A initial encounter
D subsequent encounter
S sequela

√x7th **V17.0 Pedal cycle driver injured in collision with fixed or stationary object in nontraffic accident**

√x7th **V17.1 Pedal cycle passenger injured in collision with fixed or stationary object in nontraffic accident**

√x7th **V17.2 Unspecified pedal cyclist injured in collision with fixed or stationary object in nontraffic accident**

√x7th **V17.3 Person boarding or alighting a pedal cycle injured in collision with fixed or stationary object**

√x7th **V17.4 Pedal cycle driver injured in collision with fixed or stationary object in traffic accident**

√x7th **V17.5 Pedal cycle passenger injured in collision with fixed or stationary object in traffic accident**

√x7th **V17.9 Unspecified pedal cyclist injured in collision with fixed or stationary object in traffic accident**

√4th **V18 Pedal cycle rider injured in noncollision transport accident**

INCLUDES fall or thrown from pedal cycle (without antecedent collision)
overturning pedal cycle NOS
overturning pedal cycle without collision

The appropriate 7th character is to be added to each code from category V18.
A initial encounter
D subsequent encounter
S sequela

√x7th **V18.0 Pedal cycle driver injured in noncollision transport accident in nontraffic accident**

√x7th **V18.1 Pedal cycle passenger injured in noncollision transport accident in nontraffic accident**

√x7th **V18.2 Unspecified pedal cyclist injured in noncollision transport accident in nontraffic accident**

√x7th **V18.3 Person boarding or alighting a pedal cycle injured in noncollision transport accident**

√x7th **V18.4 Pedal cycle driver injured in noncollision transport accident in traffic accident**

√x7th **V18.5 Pedal cycle passenger injured in noncollision transport accident in traffic accident**

√x7th **V18.9 Unspecified pedal cyclist injured in noncollision transport accident in traffic accident**

√4th **V19 Pedal cycle rider injured in other and unspecified transport accidents**

The appropriate 7th character is to be added to each code from category V19.
A initial encounter
D subsequent encounter
S sequela

√5th **V19.0 Pedal cycle driver injured in collision with other and unspecified motor vehicles in nontraffic accident**

√x7th **V19.00 Pedal cycle driver injured in collision with unspecified motor vehicles in nontraffic accident**

√x7th **V19.09 Pedal cycle driver injured in collision with other motor vehicles in nontraffic accident**

√5th **V19.1 Pedal cycle passenger injured in collision with other and unspecified motor vehicles in nontraffic accident**

√x7th **V19.10 Pedal cycle passenger injured in collision with unspecified motor vehicles in nontraffic accident**

√x7th **V19.19 Pedal cycle passenger injured in collision with other motor vehicles in nontraffic accident**

√5th **V19.2 Unspecified pedal cyclist injured in collision with other and unspecified motor vehicles in nontraffic accident**

√x7th **V19.20 Unspecified pedal cyclist injured in collision with unspecified motor vehicles in nontraffic accident**
Pedal cycle collision NOS, nontraffic

√x7th **V19.29 Unspecified pedal cyclist injured in collision with other motor vehicles in nontraffic accident**

√x7th **V19.3 Pedal cyclist (driver) (passenger) injured in unspecified nontraffic accident**
Pedal cycle accident NOS, nontraffic
Pedal cyclist injured in nontraffic accident NOS

√5th **V19.4 Pedal cycle driver injured in collision with other and unspecified motor vehicles in traffic accident**

√x7th **V19.40 Pedal cycle driver injured in collision with unspecified motor vehicles in traffic accident**

√x7th **V19.49 Pedal cycle driver injured in collision with other motor vehicles in traffic accident**

√5th **V19.5 Pedal cycle passenger injured in collision with other and unspecified motor vehicles in traffic accident**

√x7th **V19.50 Pedal cycle passenger injured in collision with unspecified motor vehicles in traffic accident**

√x7th **V19.59 Pedal cycle passenger injured in collision with other motor vehicles in traffic accident**

√5th **V19.6 Unspecified pedal cyclist injured in collision with other and unspecified motor vehicles in traffic accident**

√x7th **V19.60 Unspecified pedal cyclist injured in collision with unspecified motor vehicles in traffic accident**
Pedal cycle collision NOS (traffic)

√x7th **V19.69 Unspecified pedal cyclist injured in collision with other motor vehicles in traffic accident**

√5th **V19.8 Pedal cyclist (driver) (passenger) injured in other specified transport accidents**

√x7th **V19.81 Pedal cyclist (driver) (passenger) injured in transport accident with military vehicle**

√x7th **V19.88 Pedal cyclist (driver) (passenger) injured in other specified transport accidents**

√x7th **V19.9 Pedal cyclist (driver) (passenger) injured in unspecified traffic accident**
Pedal cycle accident NOS

Motorcycle rider injured in transport accident (V20-V29)

INCLUDES moped
motorcycle with sidecar
motorized bicycle
motor scooter

EXCLUDES1 *three-wheeled motor vehicle (V30-V39)*

√4th **V20 Motorcycle rider injured in collision with pedestrian or animal**

EXCLUDES1 *motorcycle rider collision with animal-drawn vehicle or animal being ridden (V26.-)*

The appropriate 7th character is to be added to each code from category V20.
A initial encounter
D subsequent encounter
S sequela

√x7th **V20.0 Motorcycle driver injured in collision with pedestrian or animal in nontraffic accident**

√x7th **V20.1 Motorcycle passenger injured in collision with pedestrian or animal in nontraffic accident**

√x7th **V20.2 Unspecified motorcycle rider injured in collision with pedestrian or animal in nontraffic accident**

√x7th **V20.3 Person boarding or alighting a motorcycle injured in collision with pedestrian or animal**

√x7th **V20.4 Motorcycle driver injured in collision with pedestrian or animal in traffic accident**

√x7th **V20.5 Motorcycle passenger injured in collision with pedestrian or animal in traffic accident**

√x7th **V20.9 Unspecified motorcycle rider injured in collision with pedestrian or animal in traffic accident**

√4th **V21 Motorcycle rider injured in collision with pedal cycle**

The appropriate 7th character is to be added to each code from category V21.
A initial encounter
D subsequent encounter
S sequela

√x7th **V21.0 Motorcycle driver injured in collision with pedal cycle in nontraffic accident**

√x7th **V21.1 Motorcycle passenger injured in collision with pedal cycle in nontraffic accident**

√x7th **V21.2 Unspecified motorcycle rider injured in collision with pedal cycle in nontraffic accident**

√x7th **V21.3 Person boarding or alighting a motorcycle injured in collision with pedal cycle**

√x7th **V21.4 Motorcycle driver injured in collision with pedal cycle in traffic accident**

√x7th **V21.5 Motorcycle passenger injured in collision with pedal cycle in traffic accident**

√x7th **V21.9 Unspecified motorcycle rider injured in collision with pedal cycle in traffic accident**

√4th **V22 Motorcycle rider injured in collision with two- or three-wheeled motor vehicle**

The appropriate 7th character is to be added to each code from category V22.
A initial encounter
D subsequent encounter
S sequela

√x7th **V22.0 Motorcycle driver injured in collision with two- or three-wheeled motor vehicle in nontraffic accident**

√x7th **V22.1 Motorcycle passenger injured in collision with two- or three-wheeled motor vehicle in nontraffic accident**

√x7th **V22.2 Unspecified motorcycle rider injured in collision with two- or three-wheeled motor vehicle in nontraffic accident**

√x7th **V22.3 Person boarding or alighting a motorcycle injured in collision with two- or three-wheeled motor vehicle**

√x7th **V22.4 Motorcycle driver injured in collision with two- or three-wheeled motor vehicle in traffic accident**

√x7th **V22.5 Motorcycle passenger injured in collision with two- or three-wheeled motor vehicle in traffic accident**

√x7th **V22.9 Unspecified motorcycle rider injured in collision with two- or three-wheeled motor vehicle in traffic accident**

√4th **V23 Motorcycle rider injured in collision with car, pick-up truck or van**

The appropriate 7th character is to be added to each code from category V23.
A initial encounter
D subsequent encounter
S sequela

√x7th **V23.0 Motorcycle driver injured in collision with car, pick-up truck or van in nontraffic accident**

√x7th **V23.1 Motorcycle passenger injured in collision with car, pick-up truck or van in nontraffic accident**

√x7th **V23.2 Unspecified motorcycle rider injured in collision with car, pick-up truck or van in nontraffic accident**

√x7th **V23.3 Person boarding or alighting a motorcycle injured in collision with car, pick-up truck or van**

√x7th **V23.4 Motorcycle driver injured in collision with car, pick-up truck or van in traffic accident**

√x7th **V23.5 Motorcycle passenger injured in collision with car, pick-up truck or van in traffic accident**

√x7th **V23.9 Unspecified motorcycle rider injured in collision with car, pick-up truck or van in traffic accident**

√4th **V24 Motorcycle rider injured in collision with heavy transport vehicle or bus**

EXCLUDES 1 *motorcycle rider injured in collision with military vehicle (V29.81)*

The appropriate 7th character is to be added to each code from category V24.
A initial encounter
D subsequent encounter
S sequela

√x7th **V24.0 Motorcycle driver injured in collision with heavy transport vehicle or bus in nontraffic accident**

√x7th **V24.1 Motorcycle passenger injured in collision with heavy transport vehicle or bus in nontraffic accident**

√x7th **V24.2 Unspecified motorcycle rider injured in collision with heavy transport vehicle or bus in nontraffic accident**

√x7th **V24.3 Person boarding or alighting a motorcycle injured in collision with heavy transport vehicle or bus**

√x7th **V24.4 Motorcycle driver injured in collision with heavy transport vehicle or bus in traffic accident**

√x7th **V24.5 Motorcycle passenger injured in collision with heavy transport vehicle or bus in traffic accident**

√x7th **V24.9 Unspecified motorcycle rider injured in collision with heavy transport vehicle or bus in traffic accident**

√4th **V25 Motorcycle rider injured in collision with railway train or railway vehicle**

The appropriate 7th character is to be added to each code from category V25.
A initial encounter
D subsequent encounter
S sequela

√x7th **V25.0 Motorcycle driver injured in collision with railway train or railway vehicle in nontraffic accident**

√x7th **V25.1 Motorcycle passenger injured in collision with railway train or railway vehicle in nontraffic accident**

√x7th **V25.2 Unspecified motorcycle rider injured in collision with railway train or railway vehicle in nontraffic accident**

√x7th **V25.3 Person boarding or alighting a motorcycle injured in collision with railway train or railway vehicle**

√x7th **V25.4 Motorcycle driver injured in collision with railway train or railway vehicle in traffic accident**

√x7th **V25.5 Motorcycle passenger injured in collision with railway train or railway vehicle in traffic accident**

√x7th **V25.9 Unspecified motorcycle rider injured in collision with railway train or railway vehicle in traffic accident**

√4th **V26 Motorcycle rider injured in collision with other nonmotor vehicle**

INCLUDES collision with animal-drawn vehicle, animal being ridden, streetcar

The appropriate 7th character is to be added to each code from category V26.
A initial encounter
D subsequent encounter
S sequela

√x7th **V26.0 Motorcycle driver injured in collision with other nonmotor vehicle in nontraffic accident**

√x7th **V26.1 Motorcycle passenger injured in collision with other nonmotor vehicle in nontraffic accident**

√x7th **V26.2 Unspecified motorcycle rider injured in collision with other nonmotor vehicle in nontraffic accident**

√x7th **V26.3 Person boarding or alighting a motorcycle injured in collision with other nonmotor vehicle**

√x7th **V26.4 Motorcycle driver injured in collision with other nonmotor vehicle in traffic accident**

√x7th **V26.5 Motorcycle passenger injured in collision with other nonmotor vehicle in traffic accident**

√x7th **V26.9 Unspecified motorcycle rider injured in collision with other nonmotor vehicle in traffic accident**

V27 Motorcycle rider injured in collision with fixed or stationary object

The appropriate 7th character is to be added to each code from category V27.
A initial encounter
D subsequent encounter
S sequela

V27.0 Motorcycle driver injured in collision with fixed or stationary object in nontraffic accident
V27.1 Motorcycle passenger injured in collision with fixed or stationary object in nontraffic accident
V27.2 Unspecified motorcycle rider injured in collision with fixed or stationary object in nontraffic accident
V27.3 Person boarding or alighting a motorcycle injured in collision with fixed or stationary object
V27.4 Motorcycle driver injured in collision with fixed or stationary object in traffic accident
V27.5 Motorcycle passenger injured in collision with fixed or stationary object in traffic accident
V27.9 Unspecified motorcycle rider injured in collision with fixed or stationary object in traffic accident

V28 Motorcycle rider injured in noncollision transport accident

INCLUDES fall or thrown from motorcycle (without antecedent collision)
overturning motorcycle NOS
overturning motorcycle without collision

The appropriate 7th character is to be added to each code from category V28.
A initial encounter
D subsequent encounter
S sequela

V28.0 Motorcycle driver injured in noncollision transport accident in nontraffic accident
V28.1 Motorcycle passenger injured in noncollision transport accident in nontraffic accident
V28.2 Unspecified motorcycle rider injured in noncollision transport accident in nontraffic accident
V28.3 Person boarding or alighting a motorcycle injured in noncollision transport accident
V28.4 Motorcycle driver injured in noncollision transport accident in traffic accident
V28.5 Motorcycle passenger injured in noncollision transport accident in traffic accident
V28.9 Unspecified motorcycle rider injured in noncollision transport accident in traffic accident

V29 Motorcycle rider injured in other and unspecified transport accidents

The appropriate 7th character is to be added to each code from category V29.
A initial encounter
D subsequent encounter
S sequela

V29.0 Motorcycle driver injured in collision with other and unspecified motor vehicles in nontraffic accident
V29.00 Motorcycle driver injured in collision with unspecified motor vehicles in nontraffic accident
V29.09 Motorcycle driver injured in collision with other motor vehicles in nontraffic accident
V29.1 Motorcycle passenger injured in collision with other and unspecified motor vehicles in nontraffic accident
V29.10 Motorcycle passenger injured in collision with unspecified motor vehicles in nontraffic accident
V29.19 Motorcycle passenger injured in collision with other motor vehicles in nontraffic accident
V29.2 Unspecified motorcycle rider injured in collision with other and unspecified motor vehicles in nontraffic accident
V29.20 Unspecified motorcycle rider injured in collision with unspecified motor vehicles in nontraffic accident
Motorcycle collision NOS, nontraffic
V29.29 Unspecified motorcycle rider injured in collision with other motor vehicles in nontraffic accident
V29.3 Motorcycle rider (driver) (passenger) injured in unspecified nontraffic accident
Motorcycle accident NOS, nontraffic
Motorcycle rider injured in nontraffic accident NOS
V29.4 Motorcycle driver injured in collision with other and unspecified motor vehicles in traffic accident
V29.40 Motorcycle driver injured in collision with unspecified motor vehicles in traffic accident
V29.49 Motorcycle driver injured in collision with other motor vehicles in traffic accident
V29.5 Motorcycle passenger injured in collision with other and unspecified motor vehicles in traffic accident
V29.50 Motorcycle passenger injured in collision with unspecified motor vehicles in traffic accident
V29.59 Motorcycle passenger injured in collision with other motor vehicles in traffic accident
V29.6 Unspecified motorcycle rider injured in collision with other and unspecified motor vehicles in traffic accident
V29.60 Unspecified motorcycle rider injured in collision with unspecified motor vehicles in traffic accident
Motorcycle collision NOS (traffic)
V29.69 Unspecified motorcycle rider injured in collision with other motor vehicles in traffic accident
V29.8 Motorcycle rider (driver) (passenger) injured in other specified transport accidents
V29.81 Motorcycle rider (driver) (passenger) injured in transport accident with military vehicle
V29.88 Motorcycle rider (driver) (passenger) injured in other specified transport accidents
V29.9 Motorcycle rider (driver) (passenger) injured in unspecified traffic accident
Motorcycle accident NOS

Occupant of three-wheeled motor vehicle injured in transport accident (V30-V39)

INCLUDES motorized tricycle
motorized rickshaw
three-wheeled motor car
EXCLUDES 1 *all-terrain vehicles (V86.-)*
motorcycle with sidecar (V20-V29)
vehicle designed primarily for off-road use (V86.-)

V30 Occupant of three-wheeled motor vehicle injured in collision with pedestrian or animal

EXCLUDES 1 *three-wheeled motor vehicle collision with animal-drawn vehicle or animal being ridden (V36.-)*

The appropriate 7th character is to be added to each code from category V30.
A initial encounter
D subsequent encounter
S sequela

V30.0 Driver of three-wheeled motor vehicle injured in collision with pedestrian or animal in nontraffic accident
V30.1 Passenger in three-wheeled motor vehicle injured in collision with pedestrian or animal in nontraffic accident
V30.2 Person on outside of three-wheeled motor vehicle injured in collision with pedestrian or animal in nontraffic accident
V30.3 Unspecified occupant of three-wheeled motor vehicle injured in collision with pedestrian or animal in nontraffic accident
V30.4 Person boarding or alighting a three-wheeled motor vehicle injured in collision with pedestrian or animal
V30.5 Driver of three-wheeled motor vehicle injured in collision with pedestrian or animal in traffic accident
V30.6 Passenger in three-wheeled motor vehicle injured in collision with pedestrian or animal in traffic accident
V30.7 Person on outside of three-wheeled motor vehicle injured in collision with pedestrian or animal in traffic accident
V30.9 Unspecified occupant of three-wheeled motor vehicle injured in collision with pedestrian or animal in traffic accident

√4th V31 Occupant of three-wheeled motor vehicle injured in collision with pedal cycle

The appropriate 7th character is to be added to each code from category V31.
A initial encounter
D subsequent encounter
S sequela

√x7th V31.0 Driver of three-wheeled motor vehicle injured in collision with pedal cycle in nontraffic accident

√x7th V31.1 Passenger in three-wheeled motor vehicle injured in collision with pedal cycle in nontraffic accident

√x7th V31.2 Person on outside of three-wheeled motor vehicle injured in collision with pedal cycle in nontraffic accident

√x7th V31.3 Unspecified occupant of three-wheeled motor vehicle injured in collision with pedal cycle in nontraffic accident

√x7th V31.4 Person boarding or alighting a three-wheeled motor vehicle injured in collision with pedal cycle

√x7th V31.5 Driver of three-wheeled motor vehicle injured in collision with pedal cycle in traffic accident

√x7th V31.6 Passenger in three-wheeled motor vehicle injured in collision with pedal cycle in traffic accident

√x7th V31.7 Person on outside of three-wheeled motor vehicle injured in collision with pedal cycle in traffic accident

√x7th V31.9 Unspecified occupant of three-wheeled motor vehicle injured in collision with pedal cycle in traffic accident

√4th V32 Occupant of three-wheeled motor vehicle injured in collision with two- or three-wheeled motor vehicle

The appropriate 7th character is to be added to each code from category V32.
A initial encounter
D subsequent encounter
S sequela

√x7th V32.0 Driver of three-wheeled motor vehicle injured in collision with two- or three-wheeled motor vehicle in nontraffic accident

√x7th V32.1 Passenger in three-wheeled motor vehicle injured in collision with two- or three-wheeled motor vehicle in nontraffic accident

√x7th V32.2 Person on outside of three-wheeled motor vehicle injured in collision with two- or three-wheeled motor vehicle in nontraffic accident

√x7th V32.3 Unspecified occupant of three-wheeled motor vehicle injured in collision with two- or three-wheeled motor vehicle in nontraffic accident

√x7th V32.4 Person boarding or alighting a three-wheeled motor vehicle injured in collision with two- or three-wheeled motor vehicle

√x7th V32.5 Driver of three-wheeled motor vehicle injured in collision with two- or three-wheeled motor vehicle in traffic accident

√x7th V32.6 Passenger in three-wheeled motor vehicle injured in collision with two- or three-wheeled motor vehicle in traffic accident

√x7th V32.7 Person on outside of three-wheeled motor vehicle injured in collision with two- or three-wheeled motor vehicle in traffic accident

√x7th V32.9 Unspecified occupant of three-wheeled motor vehicle injured in collision with two- or three-wheeled motor vehicle in traffic accident

√4th V33 Occupant of three-wheeled motor vehicle injured in collision with car, pick-up truck or van

The appropriate 7th character is to be added to each code from category V33.
A initial encounter
D subsequent encounter
S sequela

√x7th V33.0 Driver of three-wheeled motor vehicle injured in collision with car, pick-up truck or van in nontraffic accident

√x7th V33.1 Passenger in three-wheeled motor vehicle injured in collision with car, pick-up truck or van in nontraffic accident

√x7th V33.2 Person on outside of three-wheeled motor vehicle injured in collision with car, pick-up truck or van in nontraffic accident

√x7th V33.3 Unspecified occupant of three-wheeled motor vehicle injured in collision with car, pick-up truck or van in nontraffic accident

√x7th V33.4 Person boarding or alighting a three-wheeled motor vehicle injured in collision with car, pick-up truck or van

√x7th V33.5 Driver of three-wheeled motor vehicle injured in collision with car, pick-up truck or van in traffic accident

√x7th V33.6 Passenger in three-wheeled motor vehicle injured in collision with car, pick-up truck or van in traffic accident

√x7th V33.7 Person on outside of three-wheeled motor vehicle injured in collision with car, pick-up truck or van in traffic accident

√x7th V33.9 Unspecified occupant of three-wheeled motor vehicle injured in collision with car, pick-up truck or van in traffic accident

√4th V34 Occupant of three-wheeled motor vehicle injured in collision with heavy transport vehicle or bus

EXCLUDES1 *occupant of three-wheeled motor vehicle injured in collision with military vehicle (V39.81)*

The appropriate 7th character is to be added to each code from category V34.
A initial encounter
D subsequent encounter
S sequela

√x7th V34.0 Driver of three-wheeled motor vehicle injured in collision with heavy transport vehicle or bus in nontraffic accident

√x7th V34.1 Passenger in three-wheeled motor vehicle injured in collision with heavy transport vehicle or bus in nontraffic accident

√x7th V34.2 Person on outside of three-wheeled motor vehicle injured in collision with heavy transport vehicle or bus in nontraffic accident

√x7th V34.3 Unspecified occupant of three-wheeled motor vehicle injured in collision with heavy transport vehicle or bus in nontraffic accident

√x7th V34.4 Person boarding or alighting a three-wheeled motor vehicle injured in collision with heavy transport vehicle or bus

√x7th V34.5 Driver of three-wheeled motor vehicle injured in collision with heavy transport vehicle or bus in traffic accident

√x7th V34.6 Passenger in three-wheeled motor vehicle injured in collision with heavy transport vehicle or bus in traffic accident

√x7th V34.7 Person on outside of three-wheeled motor vehicle injured in collision with heavy transport vehicle or bus in traffic accident

√x7th V34.9 Unspecified occupant of three-wheeled motor vehicle injured in collision with heavy transport vehicle or bus in traffic accident

√4th V35 Occupant of three-wheeled motor vehicle injured in collision with railway train or railway vehicle

The appropriate 7th character is to be added to each code from category V35.
A initial encounter
D subsequent encounter
S sequela

√x7th V35.0 Driver of three-wheeled motor vehicle injured in collision with railway train or railway vehicle in nontraffic accident

√x7th V35.1 Passenger in three-wheeled motor vehicle injured in collision with railway train or railway vehicle in nontraffic accident

√x7th V35.2 Person on outside of three-wheeled motor vehicle injured in collision with railway train or railway vehicle in nontraffic accident

√x7th V35.3 Unspecified occupant of three-wheeled motor vehicle injured in collision with railway train or railway vehicle in nontraffic accident

√x7th V35.4 Person boarding or alighting a three-wheeled motor vehicle injured in collision with railway train or railway vehicle

√x7th V35.5 Driver of three-wheeled motor vehicle injured in collision with railway train or railway vehicle in traffic accident

√x7th V35.6 Passenger in three-wheeled motor vehicle injured in collision with railway train or railway vehicle in traffic accident

√x7th V35.7 Person on outside of three-wheeled motor vehicle injured in collision with railway train or railway vehicle in traffic accident

√x7th **V35.9 Unspecified occupant of three-wheeled motor vehicle injured in collision with railway train or railway vehicle in traffic accident**

√4th **V36 Occupant of three-wheeled motor vehicle injured in collision with other nonmotor vehicle**

INCLUDES collision with animal-drawn vehicle, animal being ridden, streetcar

The appropriate 7th character is to be added to each code from category V36.
A initial encounter
D subsequent encounter
S sequela

√x7th **V36.0 Driver of three-wheeled motor vehicle injured in collision with other nonmotor vehicle in nontraffic accident**

√x7th **V36.1 Passenger in three-wheeled motor vehicle injured in collision with other nonmotor vehicle in nontraffic accident**

√x7th **V36.2 Person on outside of three-wheeled motor vehicle injured in collision with other nonmotor vehicle in nontraffic accident**

√x7th **V36.3 Unspecified occupant of three-wheeled motor vehicle injured in collision with other nonmotor vehicle in nontraffic accident**

√x7th **V36.4 Person boarding or alighting a three-wheeled motor vehicle injured in collision with other nonmotor vehicle**

√x7th **V36.5 Driver of three-wheeled motor vehicle injured in collision with other nonmotor vehicle in traffic accident**

√x7th **V36.6 Passenger in three-wheeled motor vehicle injured in collision with other nonmotor vehicle in traffic accident**

√x7th **V36.7 Person on outside of three-wheeled motor vehicle injured in collision with other nonmotor vehicle in traffic accident**

√x7th **V36.9 Unspecified occupant of three-wheeled motor vehicle injured in collision with other nonmotor vehicle in traffic accident**

√4th **V37 Occupant of three-wheeled motor vehicle injured in collision with fixed or stationary object**

The appropriate 7th character is to be added to each code from category V37.
A initial encounter
D subsequent encounter
S sequela

√x7th **V37.0 Driver of three-wheeled motor vehicle injured in collision with fixed or stationary object in nontraffic accident**

√x7th **V37.1 Passenger in three-wheeled motor vehicle injured in collision with fixed or stationary object in nontraffic accident**

√x7th **V37.2 Person on outside of three-wheeled motor vehicle injured in collision with fixed or stationary object in nontraffic accident**

√x7th **V37.3 Unspecified occupant of three-wheeled motor vehicle injured in collision with fixed or stationary object in nontraffic accident**

√x7th **V37.4 Person boarding or alighting a three-wheeled motor vehicle injured in collision with fixed or stationary object**

√x7th **V37.5 Driver of three-wheeled motor vehicle injured in collision with fixed or stationary object in traffic accident**

√x7th **V37.6 Passenger in three-wheeled motor vehicle injured in collision with fixed or stationary object in traffic accident**

√x7th **V37.7 Person on outside of three-wheeled motor vehicle injured in collision with fixed or stationary object in traffic accident**

√x7th **V37.9 Unspecified occupant of three-wheeled motor vehicle injured in collision with fixed or stationary object in traffic accident**

V38 Occupant of three-wheeled motor vehicle injured in noncollision transport accident

INCLUDES fall or thrown from three-wheeled motor vehicle
overturning of three-wheeled motor vehicle NOS
overturning of three-wheeled motor vehicle without collision

The appropriate 7th character is to be added to each code from category V38.
A initial encounter
D subsequent encounter
S sequela

√x7th **V38.0 Driver of three-wheeled motor vehicle injured in noncollision transport accident in nontraffic accident**

√x7th **V38.1 Passenger in three-wheeled motor vehicle injured in noncollision transport accident in nontraffic accident**

√x7th **V38.2 Person on outside of three-wheeled motor vehicle injured in noncollision transport accident in nontraffic accident**

√x7th **V38.3 Unspecified occupant of three-wheeled motor vehicle injured in noncollision transport accident in nontraffic accident**

√x7th **V38.4 Person boarding or alighting a three-wheeled motor vehicle injured in noncollision transport accident**

√x7th **V38.5 Driver of three-wheeled motor vehicle injured in noncollision transport accident in traffic accident**

√x7th **V38.6 Passenger in three-wheeled motor vehicle injured in noncollision transport accident in traffic accident**

√x7th **V38.7 Person on outside of three-wheeled motor vehicle injured in noncollision transport accident in traffic accident**

√x7th **V38.9 Unspecified occupant of three-wheeled motor vehicle injured in noncollision transport accident in traffic accident**

√4th **V39 Occupant of three-wheeled motor vehicle injured in other and unspecified transport accidents**

The appropriate 7th character is to be added to each code from category V39.
A initial encounter
D subsequent encounter
S sequela

√5th **V39.0 Driver of three-wheeled motor vehicle injured in collision with other and unspecified motor vehicles in nontraffic accident**

√x7th **V39.00 Driver of three-wheeled motor vehicle injured in collision with unspecified motor vehicles in nontraffic accident**

√x7th **V39.09 Driver of three-wheeled motor vehicle injured in collision with other motor vehicles in nontraffic accident**

√5th **V39.1 Passenger in three-wheeled motor vehicle injured in collision with other and unspecified motor vehicles in nontraffic accident**

√x7th **V39.10 Passenger in three-wheeled motor vehicle injured in collision with unspecified motor vehicles in nontraffic accident**

√x7th **V39.19 Passenger in three-wheeled motor vehicle injured in collision with other motor vehicles in nontraffic accident**

√5th **V39.2 Unspecified occupant of three-wheeled motor vehicle injured in collision with other and unspecified motor vehicles in nontraffic accident**

√x7th **V39.20 Unspecified occupant of three-wheeled motor vehicle injured in collision with unspecified motor vehicles in nontraffic accident**
Collision NOS involving three-wheeled motor vehicle, nontraffic

√x7th **V39.29 Unspecified occupant of three-wheeled motor vehicle injured in collision with other motor vehicles in nontraffic accident**

√x7th **V39.3 Occupant (driver) (passenger) of three-wheeled motor vehicle injured in unspecified nontraffic accident**
Accident NOS involving three-wheeled motor vehicle, nontraffic
Occupant of three-wheeled motor vehicle injured in nontraffic accident NOS

√5th **V39.4 Driver of three-wheeled motor vehicle injured in collision with other and unspecified motor vehicles in traffic accident**

√x7th **V39.40 Driver of three-wheeled motor vehicle injured in collision with unspecified motor vehicles in traffic accident**

√x7th **V39.49 Driver of three-wheeled motor vehicle injured in collision with other motor vehicles in traffic accident**

√5th **V39.5 Passenger in three-wheeled motor vehicle injured in collision with other and unspecified motor vehicles in traffic accident**

√x7th **V39.50 Passenger in three-wheeled motor vehicle injured in collision with unspecified motor vehicles in traffic accident**

√x7th **V39.59 Passenger in three-wheeled motor vehicle injured in collision with other motor vehicles in traffic accident**

✓5th **V39.6 Unspecified occupant of three-wheeled motor vehicle injured in collision with other and unspecified motor vehicles in traffic accident**

✓x7th **V39.60 Unspecified occupant of three-wheeled motor vehicle injured in collision with unspecified motor vehicles in traffic accident**

Collision NOS involving three-wheeled motor vehicle (traffic)

✓x7th **V39.69 Unspecified occupant of three-wheeled motor vehicle injured in collision with other motor vehicles in traffic accident**

✓5th **V39.8 Occupant (driver) (passenger) of three-wheeled motor vehicle injured in other specified transport accidents**

✓x7th **V39.81 Occupant (driver) (passenger) of three-wheeled motor vehicle injured in transport accident with military vehicle**

✓x7th **V39.89 Occupant (driver) (passenger) of three-wheeled motor vehicle injured in other specified transport accidents**

✓x7th **V39.9 Occupant (driver) (passenger) of three-wheeled motor vehicle injured in unspecified traffic accident**

Accident NOS involving three-wheeled motor vehicle

Car occupant injured in transport accident (V40-V49)

INCLUDES a four-wheeled motor vehicle designed primarily for carrying passengers

automobile (pulling a trailer or camper)

EXCLUDES 1 *bus (V50-V59)*

minibus (V50-V59)

minivan (V50-V59)

motorcoach (V70-V79)

pick-up truck (V50-V59)

sport utility vehicle (SUV) (V50-V59)

✓4th **V40 Car occupant injured in collision with pedestrian or animal**

EXCLUDES 1 *car collision with animal-drawn vehicle or animal being ridden (V46.-)*

The appropriate 7th character is to be added to each code from category V40.
A initial encounter
D subsequent encounter
S sequela

✓x7th **V40.0 Car driver injured in collision with pedestrian or animal in nontraffic accident**

✓x7th **V40.1 Car passenger injured in collision with pedestrian or animal in nontraffic accident**

✓x7th **V40.2 Person on outside of car injured in collision with pedestrian or animal in nontraffic accident**

✓x7th **V40.3 Unspecified car occupant injured in collision with pedestrian or animal in nontraffic accident**

✓x7th **V40.4 Person boarding or alighting a car injured in collision with pedestrian or animal**

✓x7th **V40.5 Car driver injured in collision with pedestrian or animal in traffic accident**

✓x7th **V40.6 Car passenger injured in collision with pedestrian or animal in traffic accident**

✓x7th **V40.7 Person on outside of car injured in collision with pedestrian or animal in traffic accident**

✓x7th **V40.9 Unspecified car occupant injured in collision with pedestrian or animal in traffic accident**

✓4th **V41 Car occupant injured in collision with pedal cycle**

The appropriate 7th character is to be added to each code from category V41.
A initial encounter
D subsequent encounter
S sequela

✓x7th **V41.0 Car driver injured in collision with pedal cycle in nontraffic accident**

✓x7th **V41.1 Car passenger injured in collision with pedal cycle in nontraffic accident**

✓x7th **V41.2 Person on outside of car injured in collision with pedal cycle in nontraffic accident**

✓x7th **V41.3 Unspecified car occupant injured in collision with pedal cycle in nontraffic accident**

✓x7th **V41.4 Person boarding or alighting a car injured in collision with pedal cycle**

✓x7th **V41.5 Car driver injured in collision with pedal cycle in traffic accident**

✓x7th **V41.6 Car passenger injured in collision with pedal cycle in traffic accident**

✓x7th **V41.7 Person on outside of car injured in collision with pedal cycle in traffic accident**

✓x7th **V41.9 Unspecified car occupant injured in collision with pedal cycle in traffic accident**

✓4th **V42 Car occupant injured in collision with two- or three-wheeled motor vehicle**

The appropriate 7th character is to be added to each code from category V42.
A initial encounter
D subsequent encounter
S sequela

✓x7th **V42.0 Car driver injured in collision with two- or three-wheeled motor vehicle in nontraffic accident**

✓x7th **V42.1 Car passenger injured in collision with two- or three-wheeled motor vehicle in nontraffic accident**

✓x7th **V42.2 Person on outside of car injured in collision with two- or three-wheeled motor vehicle in nontraffic accident**

✓x7th **V42.3 Unspecified car occupant injured in collision with two- or three-wheeled motor vehicle in nontraffic accident**

✓x7th **V42.4 Person boarding or alighting a car injured in collision with two- or three-wheeled motor vehicle**

✓x7th **V42.5 Car driver injured in collision with two- or three-wheeled motor vehicle in traffic accident**

✓x7th **V42.6 Car passenger injured in collision with two- or three-wheeled motor vehicle in traffic accident**

✓x7th **V42.7 Person on outside of car injured in collision with two- or three-wheeled motor vehicle in traffic accident**

✓x7th **V42.9 Unspecified car occupant injured in collision with two- or three-wheeled motor vehicle in traffic accident**

✓4th **V43 Car occupant injured in collision with car, pick-up truck or van**

The appropriate 7th character is to be added to each code from category V43.
A initial encounter
D subsequent encounter
S sequela

✓5th **V43.0 Car driver injured in collision with car, pick-up truck or van in nontraffic accident**

✓x7th **V43.01 Car driver injured in collision with sport utility vehicle in nontraffic accident**

✓x7th **V43.02 Car driver injured in collision with other type car in nontraffic accident**

✓x7th **V43.03 Car driver injured in collision with pick-up truck in nontraffic accident**

✓x7th **V43.04 Car driver injured in collision with van in nontraffic accident**

✓5th **V43.1 Car passenger injured in collision with car, pick-up truck or van in nontraffic accident**

✓x7th **V43.11 Car passenger injured in collision with sport utility vehicle in nontraffic accident**

✓x7th **V43.12 Car passenger injured in collision with other type car in nontraffic accident**

✓x7th **V43.13 Car passenger injured in collision with pick-up in nontraffic accident**

✓x7th **V43.14 Car passenger injured in collision with van in nontraffic accident**

✓5th **V43.2 Person on outside of car injured in collision with car, pick-up truck or van in nontraffic accident**

✓x7th **V43.21 Person on outside of car injured in collision with sport utility vehicle in nontraffic accident**

✓x7th **V43.22 Person on outside of car injured in collision with other type car in nontraffic accident**

✓x7th **V43.23 Person on outside of car injured in collision with pick-up truck in nontraffic accident**

✓x7th **V43.24 Person on outside of car injured in collision with van in nontraffic accident**

✓5th **V43.3 Unspecified car occupant injured in collision with car, pick-up truck or van in nontraffic accident**

✓x7th **V43.31 Unspecified car occupant injured in collision with sport utility vehicle in nontraffic accident**

✓x7th **V43.32 Unspecified car occupant injured in collision with other type car in nontraffic accident**

√x7th V43.33 **Unspecified car occupant injured in collision with pick-up truck in nontraffic accident**
√x7th V43.34 **Unspecified car occupant injured in collision with van in nontraffic accident**

√5th V43.4 **Person boarding or alighting a car injured in collision with car, pick-up truck or van**
√x7th V43.41 **Person boarding or alighting a car injured in collision with sport utility vehicle**
√x7th V43.42 **Person boarding or alighting a car injured in collision with other type car**
√x7th V43.43 **Person boarding or alighting a car injured in collision with pick-up truck**
√x7th V43.44 **Person boarding or alighting a car injured in collision with van**

√5th V43.5 **Car driver injured in collision with car, pick-up truck or van in traffic accident**
√x7th V43.51 **Car driver injured in collision with sport utility vehicle in traffic accident**
√x7th V43.52 **Car driver injured in collision with other type car in traffic accident**
√x7th V43.53 **Car driver injured in collision with pick-up truck in traffic accident**
√x7th V43.54 **Car driver injured in collision with van in traffic accident**

√5th V43.6 **Car passenger injured in collision with car, pick-up truck or van in traffic accident**
√x7th V43.61 **Car passenger injured in collision with sport utility vehicle in traffic accident**
√x7th V43.62 **Car passenger injured in collision with other type car in traffic accident**
√x7th V43.63 **Car passenger injured in collision with pick-up truck in traffic accident**
√x7th V43.64 **Car passenger injured in collision with van in traffic accident**

√5th V43.7 **Person on outside of car injured in collision with car, pick-up truck or van in traffic accident**
√x7th V43.71 **Person on outside of car injured in collision with sport utility vehicle in traffic accident**
√x7th V43.72 **Person on outside of car injured in collision with other type car in traffic accident**
√x7th V43.73 **Person on outside of car injured in collision with pick-up truck in traffic accident**
√x7th V43.74 **Person on outside of car injured in collision with van in traffic accident**

√5th V43.9 **Unspecified car occupant injured in collision with car, pick-up truck or van in traffic accident**
√x7th V43.91 **Unspecified car occupant injured in collision with sport utility vehicle in traffic accident**
√x7th V43.92 **Unspecified car occupant injured in collision with other type car in traffic accident**
√x7th V43.93 **Unspecified car occupant injured in collision with pick-up truck in traffic accident**
√x7th V43.94 **Unspecified car occupant injured in collision with van in traffic accident**

√4th V44 Car occupant injured in collision with heavy transport vehicle or bus

EXCLUDES 1 *car occupant injured in collision with military vehicle (V49.81)*

The appropriate 7th character is to be added to each code from category V44.
A initial encounter
D subsequent encounter
S sequela

√x7th V44.0 **Car driver injured in collision with heavy transport vehicle or bus in nontraffic accident**
√x7th V44.1 **Car passenger injured in collision with heavy transport vehicle or bus in nontraffic accident**
√x7th V44.2 **Person on outside of car injured in collision with heavy transport vehicle or bus in nontraffic accident**
√x7th V44.3 **Unspecified car occupant injured in collision with heavy transport vehicle or bus in nontraffic accident**
√x7th V44.4 **Person boarding or alighting a car injured in collision with heavy transport vehicle or bus**
√x7th V44.5 **Car driver injured in collision with heavy transport vehicle or bus in traffic accident**
√x7th V44.6 **Car passenger injured in collision with heavy transport vehicle or bus in traffic accident**
√x7th V44.7 **Person on outside of car injured in collision with heavy transport vehicle or bus in traffic accident**
√x7th V44.9 **Unspecified car occupant injured in collision with heavy transport vehicle or bus in traffic accident**

√4th V45 Car occupant injured in collision with railway train or railway vehicle

The appropriate 7th character is to be added to each code from category V45.
A initial encounter
D subsequent encounter
S sequela

√x7th V45.0 **Car driver injured in collision with railway train or railway vehicle in nontraffic accident**
√x7th V45.1 **Car passenger injured in collision with railway train or railway vehicle in nontraffic accident**
√x7th V45.2 **Person on outside of car injured in collision with railway train or railway vehicle in nontraffic accident**
√x7th V45.3 **Unspecified car occupant injured in collision with railway train or railway vehicle in nontraffic accident**
√x7th V45.4 **Person boarding or alighting a car injured in collision with railway train or railway vehicle**
√x7th V45.5 **Car driver injured in collision with railway train or railway vehicle in traffic accident**
√x7th V45.6 **Car passenger injured in collision with railway train or railway vehicle in traffic accident**
√x7th V45.7 **Person on outside of car injured in collision with railway train or railway vehicle in traffic accident**
√x7th V45.9 **Unspecified car occupant injured in collision with railway train or railway vehicle in traffic accident**

√4th V46 Car occupant injured in collision with other nonmotor vehicle

INCLUDES collision with animal-drawn vehicle, animal being ridden, streetcar

The appropriate 7th character is to be added to each code from category V46.
A initial encounter
D subsequent encounter
S sequela

√x7th V46.0 **Car driver injured in collision with other nonmotor vehicle in nontraffic accident**
√x7th V46.1 **Car passenger injured in collision with other nonmotor vehicle in nontraffic accident**
√x7th V46.2 **Person on outside of car injured in collision with other nonmotor vehicle in nontraffic accident**
√x7th V46.3 **Unspecified car occupant injured in collision with other nonmotor vehicle in nontraffic accident**
√x7th V46.4 **Person boarding or alighting a car injured in collision with other nonmotor vehicle**
√x7th V46.5 **Car driver injured in collision with other nonmotor vehicle in traffic accident**
√x7th V46.6 **Car passenger injured in collision with other nonmotor vehicle in traffic accident**
√x7th V46.7 **Person on outside of car injured in collision with other nonmotor vehicle in traffic accident**
√x7th V46.9 **Unspecified car occupant injured in collision with other nonmotor vehicle in traffic accident**

√4th V47 Car occupant injured in collision with fixed or stationary object

The appropriate 7th character is to be added to each code from category V47.
A initial encounter
D subsequent encounter
S sequela

√5th V47.0 **Car driver injured in collision with fixed or stationary object in nontraffic accident**
√x7th V47.01 **Driver of sport utility vehicle injured in collision with fixed or stationary object in nontraffic accident**
√x7th V47.02 **Driver of other type car injured in collision with fixed or stationary object in nontraffic accident**

√5th V47.1 **Car passenger injured in collision with fixed or stationary object in nontraffic accident**
√x7th V47.11 **Passenger of sport utility vehicle injured in collision with fixed or stationary object in nontraffic accident**

√ Appropriate additional character required
√x7th Requires 7th character, placeholder x must fill empty characters

✓x7th V47.12 Passenger of other type car injured in collision with fixed or stationary object in nontraffic accident

✓x7th V47.2 Person on outside of car injured in collision with fixed or stationary object in nontraffic accident

✓5th V47.3 Unspecified car occupant injured in collision with fixed or stationary object in nontraffic accident

✓x7th V47.31 Unspecified occupant of sport utility vehicle injured in collision with fixed or stationary object in nontraffic accident

✓x7th V47.32 Unspecified occupant of other type car injured in collision with fixed or stationary object in nontraffic accident

✓x7th V47.4 Person boarding or alighting a car injured in collision with fixed or stationary object

✓5th V47.5 Car driver injured in collision with fixed or stationary object in traffic accident

✓x7th V47.51 Driver of sport utility vehicle injured in collision with fixed or stationary object in traffic accident

✓x7th V47.52 Driver of other type car injured in collision with fixed or stationary object in traffic accident

✓5th V47.6 Car passenger injured in collision with fixed or stationary object in traffic accident

✓x7th V47.61 Passenger of sport utility vehicle injured in collision with fixed or stationary object in traffic accident

✓x7th V47.62 Passenger of other type car injured in collision with fixed or stationary object in traffic accident

✓x7th V47.7 Person on outside of car injured in collision with fixed or stationary object in traffic accident

✓5th V47.9 Unspecified car occupant injured in collision with fixed or stationary object in traffic accident

✓x7th V47.91 Unspecified occupant of sport utility vehicle injured in collision with fixed or stationary object in traffic accident

✓x7th V47.92 Unspecified occupant of other type car injured in collision with fixed or stationary object in traffic accident

✓4th V48 Car occupant injured in noncollision transport accident

INCLUDES overturning car NOS
overturning car without collision

The appropriate 7th character is to be added to each code from category V48.
A initial encounter
D subsequent encounter
S sequela

✓x7th V48.Ø Car driver injured in noncollision transport accident in nontraffic accident

✓x7th V48.1 Car passenger injured in noncollision transport accident in nontraffic accident

✓x7th V48.2 Person on outside of car injured in noncollision transport accident in nontraffic accident

✓x7th V48.3 Unspecified car occupant injured in noncollision transport accident in nontraffic accident

✓x7th V48.4 Person boarding or alighting a car injured in noncollision transport accident

✓x7th V48.5 Car driver injured in noncollision transport accident in traffic accident

✓x7th V48.6 Car passenger injured in noncollision transport accident in traffic accident

✓x7th V48.7 Person on outside of car injured in noncollision transport accident in traffic accident

✓x7th V48.9 Unspecified car occupant injured in noncollision transport accident in traffic accident

✓4th V49 Car occupant injured in other and unspecified transport accidents

The appropriate 7th character is to be added to each code from category V49.
A initial encounter
D subsequent encounter
S sequela

✓5th V49.Ø Driver injured in collision with other and unspecified motor vehicles in nontraffic accident

✓x7th V49.ØØ Driver injured in collision with unspecified motor vehicles in nontraffic accident

✓x7th V49.Ø9 Driver injured in collision with other motor vehicles in nontraffic accident

✓5th V49.1 Passenger injured in collision with other and unspecified motor vehicles in nontraffic accident

✓x7th V49.1Ø Passenger injured in collision with unspecified motor vehicles in nontraffic accident

✓x7th V49.19 Passenger injured in collision with other motor vehicles in nontraffic accident

✓5th V49.2 Unspecified car occupant injured in collision with other and unspecified motor vehicles in nontraffic accident

✓x7th V49.2Ø Unspecified car occupant injured in collision with unspecified motor vehicles in nontraffic accident
Car collision NOS, nontraffic

✓x7th V49.29 Unspecified car occupant injured in collision with other motor vehicles in nontraffic accident

✓x7th V49.3 Car occupant (driver) (passenger) injured in unspecified nontraffic accident
Car accident NOS, nontraffic
Car occupant injured in nontraffic accident NOS

✓5th V49.4 Driver injured in collision with other and unspecified motor vehicles in traffic accident

✓x7th V49.4Ø Driver injured in collision with unspecified motor vehicles in traffic accident

✓x7th V49.49 Driver injured in collision with other motor vehicles in traffic accident

✓5th V49.5 Passenger injured in collision with other and unspecified motor vehicles in traffic accident

✓x7th V49.5Ø Passenger injured in collision with unspecified motor vehicles in traffic accident

✓x7th V49.59 Passenger injured in collision with other motor vehicles in traffic accident

✓5th V49.6 Unspecified car occupant injured in collision with other and unspecified motor vehicles in traffic accident

✓x7th V49.6Ø Unspecified car occupant injured in collision with unspecified motor vehicles in traffic accident
Car collision NOS (traffic)

✓x7th V49.69 Unspecified car occupant injured in collision with other motor vehicles in traffic accident

✓5th V49.8 Car occupant (driver) (passenger) injured in other specified transport accidents

✓x7th V49.81 Car occupant (driver) (passenger) injured in transport accident with military vehicle

✓x7th V49.88 Car occupant (driver) (passenger) injured in other specified transport accidents

✓x7th V49.9 Car occupant (driver) (passenger) injured in unspecified traffic accident
Car accident NOS

Occupant of pick-up truck or van injured in transport accident (V5Ø-V59)

INCLUDES a four or six wheel motor vehicle designed primarily for carrying passengers and property but weighing less than the local limit for classification as a heavy goods vehicle
minibus
minivan
sport utility vehicle (SUV)
truck
van

EXCLUDES 1 *heavy transport vehicle (V6Ø-V69)*

✓4th V5Ø Occupant of pick-up truck or van injured in collision with pedestrian or animal

EXCLUDES 1 *pick-up truck or van collision with animal-drawn vehicle or animal being ridden (V56.-)*

The appropriate 7th character is to be added to each code from category V5Ø.
A initial encounter
D subsequent encounter
S sequela

✓x7th V5Ø.Ø Driver of pick-up truck or van injured in collision with pedestrian or animal in nontraffic accident

✓x7th V5Ø.1 Passenger in pick-up truck or van injured in collision with pedestrian or animal in nontraffic accident

✓x7th V5Ø.2 Person on outside of pick-up truck or van injured in collision with pedestrian or animal in nontraffic accident

✓x7th V5Ø.3 Unspecified occupant of pick-up truck or van injured in collision with pedestrian or animal in nontraffic accident

✓x7th V50.4 **Person boarding or alighting a pick-up truck or van injured in collision with pedestrian or animal**
✓x7th V50.5 **Driver of pick-up truck or van injured in collision with pedestrian or animal in traffic accident**
✓x7th V50.6 **Passenger in pick-up truck or van injured in collision with pedestrian or animal in traffic accident**
✓x7th V50.7 **Person on outside of pick-up truck or van injured in collision with pedestrian or animal in traffic accident**
✓x7th V50.9 **Unspecified occupant of pick-up truck or van injured in collision with pedestrian or animal in traffic accident**

✓4th **V51 Occupant of pick-up truck or van injured in collision with pedal cycle**

The appropriate 7th character is to be added to each code from category V51.
A initial encounter
D subsequent encounter
S sequela

✓x7th V51.0 **Driver of pick-up truck or van injured in collision with pedal cycle in nontraffic accident**
✓x7th V51.1 **Passenger in pick-up truck or van injured in collision with pedal cycle in nontraffic accident**
✓x7th V51.2 **Person on outside of pick-up truck or van injured in collision with pedal cycle in nontraffic accident**
✓x7th V51.3 **Unspecified occupant of pick-up truck or van injured in collision with pedal cycle in nontraffic accident**
✓x7th V51.4 **Person boarding or alighting a pick-up truck or van injured in collision with pedal cycle**
✓x7th V51.5 **Driver of pick-up truck or van injured in collision with pedal cycle in traffic accident**
✓x7th V51.6 **Passenger in pick-up truck or van injured in collision with pedal cycle in traffic accident**
✓x7th V51.7 **Person on outside of pick-up truck or van injured in collision with pedal cycle in traffic accident**
✓x7th V51.9 **Unspecified occupant of pick-up truck or van injured in collision with pedal cycle in traffic accident**

✓4th **V52 Occupant of pick-up truck or van injured in collision with two- or three-wheeled motor vehicle**

The appropriate 7th character is to be added to each code from category V52.
A initial encounter
D subsequent encounter
S sequela

✓x7th V52.0 **Driver of pick-up truck or van injured in collision with two- or three-wheeled motor vehicle in nontraffic accident**
✓x7th V52.1 **Passenger in pick-up truck or van injured in collision with two- or three-wheeled motor vehicle in nontraffic accident**
✓x7th V52.2 **Person on outside of pick-up truck or van injured in collision with two- or three-wheeled motor vehicle in nontraffic accident**
✓x7th V52.3 **Unspecified occupant of pick-up truck or van injured in collision with two- or three-wheeled motor vehicle in nontraffic accident**
✓x7th V52.4 **Person boarding or alighting a pick-up truck or van injured in collision with two- or three-wheeled motor vehicle**
✓x7th V52.5 **Driver of pick-up truck or van injured in collision with two- or three-wheeled motor vehicle in traffic accident**
✓x7th V52.6 **Passenger in pick-up truck or van injured in collision with two- or three-wheeled motor vehicle in traffic accident**
✓x7th V52.7 **Person on outside of pick-up truck or van injured in collision with two- or three-wheeled motor vehicle in traffic accident**
✓x7th V52.9 **Unspecified occupant of pick-up truck or van injured in collision with two- or three-wheeled motor vehicle in traffic accident**

✓4th **V53 Occupant of pick-up truck or van injured in collision with car, pick-up truck or van**

The appropriate 7th character is to be added to each code from category V53.
A initial encounter
D subsequent encounter
S sequela

✓x7th V53.0 **Driver of pick-up truck or van injured in collision with car, pick-up truck or van in nontraffic accident**
✓x7th V53.1 **Passenger in pick-up truck or van injured in collision with car, pick-up truck or van in nontraffic accident**
✓x7th V53.2 **Person on outside of pick-up truck or van injured in collision with car, pick-up truck or van in nontraffic accident**
✓x7th V53.3 **Unspecified occupant of pick-up truck or van injured in collision with car, pick-up truck or van in nontraffic accident**
✓x7th V53.4 **Person boarding or alighting a pick-up truck or van injured in collision with car, pick-up truck or van**
✓x7th V53.5 **Driver of pick-up truck or van injured in collision with car, pick-up truck or van in traffic accident**
✓x7th V53.6 **Passenger in pick-up truck or van injured in collision with car, pick-up truck or van in traffic accident**
✓x7th V53.7 **Person on outside of pick-up truck or van injured in collision with car, pick-up truck or van in traffic accident**
✓x7th V53.9 **Unspecified occupant of pick-up truck or van injured in collision with car, pick-up truck or van in traffic accident**

✓4th **V54 Occupant of pick-up truck or van injured in collision with heavy transport vehicle or bus**

EXCLUDES 1 *occupant of pick-up truck or van injured in collision with military vehicle (V59.81)*

The appropriate 7th character is to be added to each code from category V54.
A initial encounter
D subsequent encounter
S sequela

✓x7th V54.0 **Driver of pick-up truck or van injured in collision with heavy transport vehicle or bus in nontraffic accident**
✓x7th V54.1 **Passenger in pick-up truck or van injured in collision with heavy transport vehicle or bus in nontraffic accident**
✓x7th V54.2 **Person on outside of pick-up truck or van injured in collision with heavy transport vehicle or bus in nontraffic accident**
✓x7th V54.3 **Unspecified occupant of pick-up truck or van injured in collision with heavy transport vehicle or bus in nontraffic accident**
✓x7th V54.4 **Person boarding or alighting a pick-up truck or van injured in collision with heavy transport vehicle or bus**
✓x7th V54.5 **Driver of pick-up truck or van injured in collision with heavy transport vehicle or bus in traffic accident**
✓x7th V54.6 **Passenger in pick-up truck or van injured in collision with heavy transport vehicle or bus in traffic accident**
✓x7th V54.7 **Person on outside of pick-up truck or van injured in collision with heavy transport vehicle or bus in traffic accident**
✓x7th V54.9 **Unspecified occupant of pick-up truck or van injured in collision with heavy transport vehicle or bus in traffic accident**

✓4th **V55 Occupant of pick-up truck or van injured in collision with railway train or railway vehicle**

The appropriate 7th character is to be added to each code from category V55.
A initial encounter
D subsequent encounter
S sequela

✓x7th V55.0 **Driver of pick-up truck or van injured in collision with railway train or railway vehicle in nontraffic accident**
✓x7th V55.1 **Passenger in pick-up truck or van injured in collision with railway train or railway vehicle in nontraffic accident**
✓x7th V55.2 **Person on outside of pick-up truck or van injured in collision with railway train or railway vehicle in nontraffic accident**
✓x7th V55.3 **Unspecified occupant of pick-up truck or van injured in collision with railway train or railway vehicle in nontraffic accident**
✓x7th V55.4 **Person boarding or alighting a pick-up truck or van injured in collision with railway train or railway vehicle**
✓x7th V55.5 **Driver of pick-up truck or van injured in collision with railway train or railway vehicle in traffic accident**
✓x7th V55.6 **Passenger in pick-up truck or van injured in collision with railway train or railway vehicle in traffic accident**
✓x7th V55.7 **Person on outside of pick-up truck or van injured in collision with railway train or railway vehicle in traffic accident**
✓x7th V55.9 **Unspecified occupant of pick-up truck or van injured in collision with railway train or railway vehicle in traffic accident**

✓4th V56 Occupant of pick-up truck or van injured in collision with other nonmotor vehicle

INCLUDES collision with animal-drawn vehicle, animal being ridden, streetcar

The appropriate 7th character is to be added to each code from category V56.
A initial encounter
D subsequent encounter
S sequela

✓x7th V56.Ø Driver of pick-up truck or van injured in collision with other nonmotor vehicle in nontraffic accident

✓x7th V56.1 Passenger in pick-up truck or van injured in collision with other nonmotor vehicle in nontraffic accident

✓x7th V56.2 Person on outside of pick-up truck or van injured in collision with other nonmotor vehicle in nontraffic accident

✓x7th V56.3 Unspecified occupant of pick-up truck or van injured in collision with other nonmotor vehicle in nontraffic accident

✓x7th V56.4 Person boarding or alighting a pick-up truck or van injured in collision with other nonmotor vehicle

✓x7th V56.5 Driver of pick-up truck or van injured in collision with other nonmotor vehicle in traffic accident

✓x7th V56.6 Passenger in pick-up truck or van injured in collision with other nonmotor vehicle in traffic accident

✓x7th V56.7 Person on outside of pick-up truck or van injured in collision with other nonmotor vehicle in traffic accident

✓x7th V56.9 Unspecified occupant of pick-up truck or van injured in collision with other nonmotor vehicle in traffic accident

✓4th V57 Occupant of pick-up truck or van injured in collision with fixed or stationary object

The appropriate 7th character is to be added to each code from category V57.
A initial encounter
D subsequent encounter
S sequela

✓x7th V57.Ø Driver of pick-up truck or van injured in collision with fixed or stationary object in nontraffic accident

✓x7th V57.1 Passenger in pick-up truck or van injured in collision with fixed or stationary object in nontraffic accident

✓x7th V57.2 Person on outside of pick-up truck or van injured in collision with fixed or stationary object in nontraffic accident

✓x7th V57.3 Unspecified occupant of pick-up truck or van injured in collision with fixed or stationary object in nontraffic accident

✓x7th V57.4 Person boarding or alighting a pick-up truck or van injured in collision with fixed or stationary object

✓x7th V57.5 Driver of pick-up truck or van injured in collision with fixed or stationary object in traffic accident

✓x7th V57.6 Passenger in pick-up truck or van injured in collision with fixed or stationary object in traffic accident

✓x7th V57.7 Person on outside of pick-up truck or van injured in collision with fixed or stationary object in traffic accident

✓x7th V57.9 Unspecified occupant of pick-up truck or van injured in collision with fixed or stationary object in traffic accident

✓4th V58 Occupant of pick-up truck or van injured in noncollision transport accident

INCLUDES overturning pick-up truck or van NOS
overturning pick-up truck or van without collision

The appropriate 7th character is to be added to each code from category V58.
A initial encounter
D subsequent encounter
S sequela

✓x7th V58.Ø Driver of pick-up truck or van injured in noncollision transport accident in nontraffic accident

✓x7th V58.1 Passenger in pick-up truck or van injured in noncollision transport accident in nontraffic accident

✓x7th V58.2 Person on outside of pick-up truck or van injured in noncollision transport accident in nontraffic accident

✓x7th V58.3 Unspecified occupant of pick-up truck or van injured in noncollision transport accident in nontraffic accident

✓x7th V58.4 Person boarding or alighting a pick-up truck or van injured in noncollision transport accident

✓x7th V58.5 Driver of pick-up truck or van injured in noncollision transport accident in traffic accident

✓x7th V58.6 Passenger in pick-up truck or van injured in noncollision transport accident in traffic accident

✓x7th V58.7 Person on outside of pick-up truck or van injured in noncollision transport accident in traffic accident

✓x7th V58.9 Unspecified occupant of pick-up truck or van injured in noncollision transport accident in traffic accident

✓4th V59 Occupant of pick-up truck or van injured in other and unspecified transport accidents

The appropriate 7th character is to be added to each code from category V59.
A initial encounter
D subsequent encounter
S sequela

✓5th V59.Ø Driver of pick-up truck or van injured in collision with other and unspecified motor vehicles in nontraffic accident

✓7th V59.ØØ Driver of pick-up truck or van injured in collision with unspecified motor vehicles in nontraffic accident

✓7th V59.Ø9 Driver of pick-up truck or van injured in collision with other motor vehicles in nontraffic accident

✓5th V59.1 Passenger in pick-up truck or van injured in collision with other and unspecified motor vehicles in nontraffic accident

✓7th V59.1Ø Passenger in pick-up truck or van injured in collision with unspecified motor vehicles in nontraffic accident

✓7th V59.19 Passenger in pick-up truck or van injured in collision with other motor vehicles in nontraffic accident

✓5th V59.2 Unspecified occupant of pick-up truck or van injured in collision with other and unspecified motor vehicles in nontraffic accident

✓7th V59.2Ø Unspecified occupant of pick-up truck or van injured in collision with unspecified motor vehicles in nontraffic accident

Collision NOS involving pick-up truck or van, nontraffic

✓7th V59.29 Unspecified occupant of pick-up truck or van injured in collision with other motor vehicles in nontraffic accident

✓x7th V59.3 Occupant (driver) (passenger) of pick-up truck or van injured in unspecified nontraffic accident

Accident NOS involving pick-up truck or van, nontraffic
Occupant of pick-up truck or van injured in nontraffic accident NOS

✓5th V59.4 Driver of pick-up truck or van injured in collision with other and unspecified motor vehicles in traffic accident

✓7th V59.4Ø Driver of pick-up truck or van injured in collision with unspecified motor vehicles in traffic accident

✓7th V59.49 Driver of pick-up truck or van injured in collision with other motor vehicles in traffic accident

✓5th V59.5 Passenger in pick-up truck or van injured in collision with other and unspecified motor vehicles in traffic accident

✓7th V59.5Ø Passenger in pick-up truck or van injured in collision with unspecified motor vehicles in traffic accident

✓7th V59.59 Passenger in pick-up truck or van injured in collision with other motor vehicles in traffic accident

✓5th V59.6 Unspecified occupant of pick-up truck or van injured in collision with other and unspecified motor vehicles in traffic accident

✓7th V59.6Ø Unspecified occupant of pick-up truck or van injured in collision with unspecified motor vehicles in traffic accident

Collision NOS involving pick-up truck or van (traffic)

✓7th V59.69 Unspecified occupant of pick-up truck or van injured in collision with other motor vehicles in traffic accident

✓5th V59.8 Occupant (driver) (passenger) of pick-up truck or van injured in other specified transport accidents

✓7th V59.81 Occupant (driver) (passenger) of pick-up truck or van injured in transport accident with military vehicle

✓7th V59.88 Occupant (driver) (passenger) of pick-up truck or van injured in other specified transport accidents

✓x7th V59.9 Occupant (driver) (passenger) of pick-up truck or van injured in unspecified traffic accident

Accident NOS involving pick-up truck or van

Occupant of heavy transport vehicle injured in transport accident (V60-V69)

INCLUDES 18 wheeler
armored car
panel truck

EXCLUDES 1 *bus*
motorcoach

V60 Occupant of heavy transport vehicle injured in collision with pedestrian or animal

EXCLUDES 1 *heavy transport vehicle collision with animal-drawn vehicle or animal being ridden (V66.-)*

The appropriate 7th character is to be added to each code from category V60.
A initial encounter
D subsequent encounter
S sequela

V60.0 Driver of heavy transport vehicle injured in collision with pedestrian or animal in nontraffic accident
V60.1 Passenger in heavy transport vehicle injured in collision with pedestrian or animal in nontraffic accident
V60.2 Person on outside of heavy transport vehicle injured in collision with pedestrian or animal in nontraffic accident
V60.3 Unspecified occupant of heavy transport vehicle injured in collision with pedestrian or animal in nontraffic accident
V60.4 Person boarding or alighting a heavy transport vehicle injured in collision with pedestrian or animal
V60.5 Driver of heavy transport vehicle injured in collision with pedestrian or animal in traffic accident
V60.6 Passenger in heavy transport vehicle injured in collision with pedestrian or animal in traffic accident
V60.7 Person on outside of heavy transport vehicle injured in collision with pedestrian or animal in traffic accident
V60.9 Unspecified occupant of heavy transport vehicle injured in collision with pedestrian or animal in traffic accident

V61 Occupant of heavy transport vehicle injured in collision with pedal cycle

The appropriate 7th character is to be added to each code from category V61.
A initial encounter
D subsequent encounter
S sequela

V61.0 Driver of heavy transport vehicle injured in collision with pedal cycle in nontraffic accident
V61.1 Passenger in heavy transport vehicle injured in collision with pedal cycle in nontraffic accident
V61.2 Person on outside of heavy transport vehicle injured in collision with pedal cycle in nontraffic accident
V61.3 Unspecified occupant of heavy transport vehicle injured in collision with pedal cycle in nontraffic accident
V61.4 Person boarding or alighting a heavy transport vehicle injured in collision with pedal cycle while boarding or alighting
V61.5 Driver of heavy transport vehicle injured in collision with pedal cycle in traffic accident
V61.6 Passenger in heavy transport vehicle injured in collision with pedal cycle in traffic accident
V61.7 Person on outside of heavy transport vehicle injured in collision with pedal cycle in traffic accident
V61.9 Unspecified occupant of heavy transport vehicle injured in collision with pedal cycle in traffic accident

V62 Occupant of heavy transport vehicle injured in collision with two- or three-wheeled motor vehicle

The appropriate 7th character is to be added to each code from category V62.
A initial encounter
D subsequent encounter
S sequela

V62.0 Driver of heavy transport vehicle injured in collision with two- or three-wheeled motor vehicle in nontraffic accident
V62.1 Passenger in heavy transport vehicle injured in collision with two- or three-wheeled motor vehicle in nontraffic accident
V62.2 Person on outside of heavy transport vehicle injured in collision with two- or three-wheeled motor vehicle in nontraffic accident
V62.3 Unspecified occupant of heavy transport vehicle injured in collision with two- or three-wheeled motor vehicle in nontraffic accident
V62.4 Person boarding or alighting a heavy transport vehicle injured in collision with two- or three-wheeled motor vehicle
V62.5 Driver of heavy transport vehicle injured in collision with two- or three-wheeled motor vehicle in traffic accident
V62.6 Passenger in heavy transport vehicle injured in collision with two- or three-wheeled motor vehicle in traffic accident
V62.7 Person on outside of heavy transport vehicle injured in collision with two- or three-wheeled motor vehicle in traffic accident
V62.9 Unspecified occupant of heavy transport vehicle injured in collision with two- or three-wheeled motor vehicle in traffic accident

V63 Occupant of heavy transport vehicle injured in collision with car, pick-up truck or van

The appropriate 7th character is to be added to each code from category V63.
A initial encounter
D subsequent encounter
S sequela

V63.0 Driver of heavy transport vehicle injured in collision with car, pick-up truck or van in nontraffic accident
V63.1 Passenger in heavy transport vehicle injured in collision with car, pick-up truck or van in nontraffic accident
V63.2 Person on outside of heavy transport vehicle injured in collision with car, pick-up truck or van in nontraffic accident
V63.3 Unspecified occupant of heavy transport vehicle injured in collision with car, pick-up truck or van in nontraffic accident
V63.4 Person boarding or alighting a heavy transport vehicle injured in collision with car, pick-up truck or van
V63.5 Driver of heavy transport vehicle injured in collision with car, pick-up truck or van in traffic accident
V63.6 Passenger in heavy transport vehicle injured in collision with car, pick-up truck or van in traffic accident
V63.7 Person on outside of heavy transport vehicle injured in collision with car, pick-up truck or van in traffic accident
V63.9 Unspecified occupant of heavy transport vehicle injured in collision with car, pick-up truck or van in traffic accident

V64 Occupant of heavy transport vehicle injured in collision with heavy transport vehicle or bus

EXCLUDES 1 *occupant of heavy transport vehicle injured in collision with military vehicle (V69.81)*

The appropriate 7th character is to be added to each code from category V64.
A initial encounter
D subsequent encounter
S sequela

V64.0 Driver of heavy transport vehicle injured in collision with heavy transport vehicle or bus in nontraffic accident
V64.1 Passenger in heavy transport vehicle injured in collision with heavy transport vehicle or bus in nontraffic accident
V64.2 Person on outside of heavy transport vehicle injured in collision with heavy transport vehicle or bus in nontraffic accident
V64.3 Unspecified occupant of heavy transport vehicle injured in collision with heavy transport vehicle or bus in nontraffic accident
V64.4 Person boarding or alighting a heavy transport vehicle injured in collision with heavy transport vehicle or bus while boarding or alighting
V64.5 Driver of heavy transport vehicle injured in collision with heavy transport vehicle or bus in traffic accident
V64.6 Passenger in heavy transport vehicle injured in collision with heavy transport vehicle or bus in traffic accident
V64.7 Person on outside of heavy transport vehicle injured in collision with heavy transport vehicle or bus in traffic accident
V64.9 Unspecified occupant of heavy transport vehicle injured in collision with heavy transport vehicle or bus in traffic accident

√4th V65 Occupant of heavy transport vehicle injured in collision with railway train or railway vehicle

The appropriate 7th character is to be added to each code from category V65.
A initial encounter
D subsequent encounter
S sequela

√x7th V65.0 Driver of heavy transport vehicle injured in collision with railway train or railway vehicle in nontraffic accident
√x7th V65.1 Passenger in heavy transport vehicle injured in collision with railway train or railway vehicle in nontraffic accident
√x7th V65.2 Person on outside of heavy transport vehicle injured in collision with railway train or railway vehicle in nontraffic accident
√x7th V65.3 Unspecified occupant of heavy transport vehicle injured in collision with railway train or railway vehicle in nontraffic accident
√x7th V65.4 Person boarding or alighting a heavy transport vehicle injured in collision with railway train or railway vehicle
√x7th V65.5 Driver of heavy transport vehicle injured in collision with railway train or railway vehicle in traffic accident
√x7th V65.6 Passenger in heavy transport vehicle injured in collision with railway train or railway vehicle in traffic accident
√x7th V65.7 Person on outside of heavy transport vehicle injured in collision with railway train or railway vehicle in traffic accident
√x7th V65.9 Unspecified occupant of heavy transport vehicle injured in collision with railway train or railway vehicle in traffic accident

√4th V66 Occupant of heavy transport vehicle injured in collision with other nonmotor vehicle

INCLUDES collision with animal-drawn vehicle, animal being ridden, streetcar

The appropriate 7th character is to be added to each code from category V66.
A initial encounter
D subsequent encounter
S sequela

√x7th V66.0 Driver of heavy transport vehicle injured in collision with other nonmotor vehicle in nontraffic accident
√x7th V66.1 Passenger in heavy transport vehicle injured in collision with other nonmotor vehicle in nontraffic accident
√x7th V66.2 Person on outside of heavy transport vehicle injured in collision with other nonmotor vehicle in nontraffic accident
√x7th V66.3 Unspecified occupant of heavy transport vehicle injured in collision with other nonmotor vehicle in nontraffic accident
√x7th V66.4 Person boarding or alighting a heavy transport vehicle injured in collision with other nonmotor vehicle
√x7th V66.5 Driver of heavy transport vehicle injured in collision with other nonmotor vehicle in traffic accident
√x7th V66.6 Passenger in heavy transport vehicle injured in collision with other nonmotor vehicle in traffic accident
√x7th V66.7 Person on outside of heavy transport vehicle injured in collision with other nonmotor vehicle in traffic accident
√x7th V66.9 Unspecified occupant of heavy transport vehicle injured in collision with other nonmotor vehicle in traffic accident

√4th V67 Occupant of heavy transport vehicle injured in collision with fixed or stationary object

The appropriate 7th character is to be added to each code from category V67.
A initial encounter
D subsequent encounter
S sequela

√x7th V67.0 Driver of heavy transport vehicle injured in collision with fixed or stationary object in nontraffic accident
√x7th V67.1 Passenger in heavy transport vehicle injured in collision with fixed or stationary object in nontraffic accident
√x7th V67.2 Person on outside of heavy transport vehicle injured in collision with fixed or stationary object in nontraffic accident
√x7th V67.3 Unspecified occupant of heavy transport vehicle injured in collision with fixed or stationary object in nontraffic accident
√x7th V67.4 Person boarding or alighting a heavy transport vehicle injured in collision with fixed or stationary object
√x7th V67.5 Driver of heavy transport vehicle injured in collision with fixed or stationary object in traffic accident
√x7th V67.6 Passenger in heavy transport vehicle injured in collision with fixed or stationary object in traffic accident
√x7th V67.7 Person on outside of heavy transport vehicle injured in collision with fixed or stationary object in traffic accident
√x7th V67.9 Unspecified occupant of heavy transport vehicle injured in collision with fixed or stationary object in traffic accident

√4th V68 Occupant of heavy transport vehicle injured in noncollision transport accident

INCLUDES overturning heavy transport vehicle NOS
overturning heavy transport vehicle without collision

The appropriate 7th character is to be added to each code from category V68.
A initial encounter
D subsequent encounter
S sequela

√x7th V68.0 Driver of heavy transport vehicle injured in noncollision transport accident in nontraffic accident
√x7th V68.1 Passenger in heavy transport vehicle injured in noncollision transport accident in nontraffic accident
√x7th V68.2 Person on outside of heavy transport vehicle injured in noncollision transport accident in nontraffic accident
√x7th V68.3 Unspecified occupant of heavy transport vehicle injured in noncollision transport accident in nontraffic accident
√x7th V68.4 Person boarding or alighting a heavy transport vehicle injured in noncollision transport accident
√x7th V68.5 Driver of heavy transport vehicle injured in noncollision transport accident in traffic accident
√x7th V68.6 Passenger in heavy transport vehicle injured in noncollision transport accident in traffic accident
√x7th V68.7 Person on outside of heavy transport vehicle injured in noncollision transport accident in traffic accident
√x7th V68.9 Unspecified occupant of heavy transport vehicle injured in noncollision transport accident in traffic accident

√4th V69 Occupant of heavy transport vehicle injured in other and unspecified transport accidents

The appropriate 7th character is to be added to each code from category V69.
A initial encounter
D subsequent encounter
S sequela

√5th V69.0 Driver of heavy transport vehicle injured in collision with other and unspecified motor vehicles in nontraffic accident
√x7th V69.00 Driver of heavy transport vehicle injured in collision with unspecified motor vehicles in nontraffic accident
√x7th V69.09 Driver of heavy transport vehicle injured in collision with other motor vehicles in nontraffic accident
√5th V69.1 Passenger in heavy transport vehicle injured in collision with other and unspecified motor vehicles in nontraffic accident
√x7th V69.10 Passenger in heavy transport vehicle injured in collision with unspecified motor vehicles in nontraffic accident
√x7th V69.19 Passenger in heavy transport vehicle injured in collision with other motor vehicles in nontraffic accident
√5th V69.2 Unspecified occupant of heavy transport vehicle injured in collision with other and unspecified motor vehicles in nontraffic accident
√x7th V69.20 Unspecified occupant of heavy transport vehicle injured in collision with unspecified motor vehicles in nontraffic accident
Collision NOS involving heavy transport vehicle, nontraffic
√x7th V69.29 Unspecified occupant of heavy transport vehicle injured in collision with other motor vehicles in nontraffic accident
√x7th V69.3 Occupant (driver) (passenger) of heavy transport vehicle injured in unspecified nontraffic accident
Accident NOS involving heavy transport vehicle, nontraffic
Occupant of heavy transport vehicle injured in nontraffic accident NOS

√5th **V69.4 Driver of heavy transport vehicle injured in collision with other and unspecified motor vehicles in traffic accident**

√x7th **V69.40 Driver of heavy transport vehicle injured in collision with unspecified motor vehicles in traffic accident**

√x7th **V69.49 Driver of heavy transport vehicle injured in collision with other motor vehicles in traffic accident**

√5th **V69.5 Passenger in heavy transport vehicle injured in collision with other and unspecified motor vehicles in traffic accident**

√x7th **V69.50 Passenger in heavy transport vehicle injured in collision with unspecified motor vehicles in traffic accident**

√x7th **V69.59 Passenger in heavy transport vehicle injured in collision with other motor vehicles in traffic accident**

√5th **V69.6 Unspecified occupant of heavy transport vehicle injured in collision with other and unspecified motor vehicles in traffic accident**

√x7th **V69.60 Unspecified occupant of heavy transport vehicle injured in collision with unspecified motor vehicles in traffic accident**

Collision NOS involving heavy transport vehicle (traffic)

√x7th **V69.69 Unspecified occupant of heavy transport vehicle injured in collision with other motor vehicles in traffic accident**

√5th **V69.8 Occupant (driver) (passenger) of heavy transport vehicle injured in other specified transport accidents**

√x7th **V69.81 Occupant (driver) (passenger) of heavy transport vehicle injured in transport accidents with military vehicle**

√x7th **V69.88 Occupant (driver) (passenger) of heavy transport vehicle injured in other specified transport accidents**

√x7th **V69.9 Occupant (driver) (passenger) of heavy transport vehicle injured in unspecified traffic accident**

Accident NOS involving heavy transport vehicle

Bus occupant injured in transport accident (V70-V79)

INCLUDES motorcoach

EXCLUDES 1 *minibus (V50-V59)*

√4th **V70 Bus occupant injured in collision with pedestrian or animal**

The appropriate 7th character is to be added to each code from category V70.
A initial encounter
D subsequent encounter
S sequela

EXCLUDES 1 *bus collision with animal-drawn vehicle or animal being ridden (V76.-)*

√x7th **V70.0 Driver of bus injured in collision with pedestrian or animal in nontraffic accident**

√x7th **V70.1 Passenger on bus injured in collision with pedestrian or animal in nontraffic accident**

√x7th **V70.2 Person on outside of bus injured in collision with pedestrian or animal in nontraffic accident**

√x7th **V70.3 Unspecified occupant of bus injured in collision with pedestrian or animal in nontraffic accident**

√x7th **V70.4 Person boarding or alighting from bus injured in collision with pedestrian or animal**

√x7th **V70.5 Driver of bus injured in collision with pedestrian or animal in traffic accident**

√x7th **V70.6 Passenger on bus injured in collision with pedestrian or animal in traffic accident**

√x7th **V70.7 Person on outside of bus injured in collision with pedestrian or animal in traffic accident**

√x7th **V70.9 Unspecified occupant of bus injured in collision with pedestrian or animal in traffic accident**

√4th **V71 Bus occupant injured in collision with pedal cycle**

The appropriate 7th character is to be added to each code from category V71.
A initial encounter
D subsequent encounter
S sequela

√x7th **V71.0 Driver of bus injured in collision with pedal cycle in nontraffic accident**

√x7th **V71.1 Passenger on bus injured in collision with pedal cycle in nontraffic accident**

√x7th **V71.2 Person on outside of bus injured in collision with pedal cycle in nontraffic accident**

√x7th **V71.3 Unspecified occupant of bus injured in collision with pedal cycle in nontraffic accident**

√x7th **V71.4 Person boarding or alighting from bus injured in collision with pedal cycle**

√x7th **V71.5 Driver of bus injured in collision with pedal cycle in traffic accident**

√x7th **V71.6 Passenger on bus injured in collision with pedal cycle in traffic accident**

√x7th **V71.7 Person on outside of bus injured in collision with pedal cycle in traffic accident**

√x7th **V71.9 Unspecified occupant of bus injured in collision with pedal cycle in traffic accident**

√4th **V72 Bus occupant injured in collision with two- or three-wheeled motor vehicle**

The appropriate 7th character is to be added to each code from category V72.
A initial encounter
D subsequent encounter
S sequela

√x7th **V72.0 Driver of bus injured in collision with two- or three-wheeled motor vehicle in nontraffic accident**

√x7th **V72.1 Passenger on bus injured in collision with two- or three-wheeled motor vehicle in nontraffic accident**

√x7th **V72.2 Person on outside of bus injured in collision with two- or three-wheeled motor vehicle in nontraffic accident**

√x7th **V72.3 Unspecified occupant of bus injured in collision with two- or three-wheeled motor vehicle in nontraffic accident**

√x7th **V72.4 Person boarding or alighting from bus injured in collision with two- or three-wheeled motor vehicle**

√x7th **V72.5 Driver of bus injured in collision with two- or three-wheeled motor vehicle in traffic accident**

√x7th **V72.6 Passenger on bus injured in collision with two- or three-wheeled motor vehicle in traffic accident**

√x7th **V72.7 Person on outside of bus injured in collision with two- or three-wheeled motor vehicle in traffic accident**

√x7th **V72.9 Unspecified occupant of bus injured in collision with two- or three-wheeled motor vehicle in traffic accident**

√4th **V73 Bus occupant injured in collision with car, pick-up truck or van**

The appropriate 7th character is to be added to each code from category V73.
A initial encounter
D subsequent encounter
S sequela

√x7th **V73.0 Driver of bus injured in collision with car, pick-up truck or van in nontraffic accident**

√x7th **V73.1 Passenger on bus injured in collision with car, pick-up truck or van in nontraffic accident**

√x7th **V73.2 Person on outside of bus injured in collision with car, pick-up truck or van in nontraffic accident**

√x7th **V73.3 Unspecified occupant of bus injured in collision with car, pick-up truck or van in nontraffic accident**

√x7th **V73.4 Person boarding or alighting from bus injured in collision with car, pick-up truck or van**

√x7th **V73.5 Driver of bus injured in collision with car, pick-up truck or van in traffic accident**

√x7th **V73.6 Passenger on bus injured in collision with car, pick-up truck or van in traffic accident**

√x7th **V73.7 Person on outside of bus injured in collision with car, pick-up truck or van in traffic accident**

√x7th **V73.9 Unspecified occupant of bus injured in collision with car, pick-up truck or van in traffic accident**

V74 Bus occupant injured in collision with heavy transport vehicle or bus

EXCLUDES1 bus occupant injured in collision with military vehicle (V79.81)

The appropriate 7th character is to be added to each code from category V74.
A initial encounter
D subsequent encounter
S sequela

V74.0 Driver of bus injured in collision with heavy transport vehicle or bus in nontraffic accident

V74.1 Passenger on bus injured in collision with heavy transport vehicle or bus in nontraffic accident

V74.2 Person on outside of bus injured in collision with heavy transport vehicle or bus in nontraffic accident

V74.3 Unspecified occupant of bus injured in collision with heavy transport vehicle or bus in nontraffic accident

V74.4 Person boarding or alighting from bus injured in collision with heavy transport vehicle or bus

V74.5 Driver of bus injured in collision with heavy transport vehicle or bus in traffic accident

V74.6 Passenger on bus injured in collision with heavy transport vehicle or bus in traffic accident

V74.7 Person on outside of bus injured in collision with heavy transport vehicle or bus in traffic accident

V74.9 Unspecified occupant of bus injured in collision with heavy transport vehicle or bus in traffic accident

V75 Bus occupant injured in collision with railway train or railway vehicle

The appropriate 7th character is to be added to each code from category V75.
A initial encounter
D subsequent encounter
S sequela

V75.0 Driver of bus injured in collision with railway train or railway vehicle in nontraffic accident

V75.1 Passenger on bus injured in collision with railway train or railway vehicle in nontraffic accident

V75.2 Person on outside of bus injured in collision with railway train or railway vehicle in nontraffic accident

V75.3 Unspecified occupant of bus injured in collision with railway train or railway vehicle in nontraffic accident

V75.4 Person boarding or alighting from bus injured in collision with railway train or railway vehicle

V75.5 Driver of bus injured in collision with railway train or railway vehicle in traffic accident

V75.6 Passenger on bus injured in collision with railway train or railway vehicle in traffic accident

V75.7 Person on outside of bus injured in collision with railway train or railway vehicle in traffic accident

V75.9 Unspecified occupant of bus injured in collision with railway train or railway vehicle in traffic accident

V76 Bus occupant injured in collision with other nonmotor vehicle

INCLUDES collision with animal-drawn vehicle, animal being ridden, streetcar

The appropriate 7th character is to be added to each code from category V76.
A initial encounter
D subsequent encounter
S sequela

V76.0 Driver of bus injured in collision with other nonmotor vehicle in nontraffic accident

V76.1 Passenger on bus injured in collision with other nonmotor vehicle in nontraffic accident

V76.2 Person on outside of bus injured in collision with other nonmotor vehicle in nontraffic accident

V76.3 Unspecified occupant of bus injured in collision with other nonmotor vehicle in nontraffic accident

V76.4 Person boarding or alighting from bus injured in collision with other nonmotor vehicle

V76.5 Driver of bus injured in collision with other nonmotor vehicle in traffic accident

V76.6 Passenger on bus injured in collision with other nonmotor vehicle in traffic accident

V76.7 Person on outside of bus injured in collision with other nonmotor vehicle in traffic accident

V76.9 Unspecified occupant of bus injured in collision with other nonmotor vehicle in traffic accident

V77 Bus occupant injured in collision with fixed or stationary object

The appropriate 7th character is to be added to each code from category V77.
A initial encounter
D subsequent encounter
S sequela

V77.0 Driver of bus injured in collision with fixed or stationary object in nontraffic accident

V77.1 Passenger on bus injured in collision with fixed or stationary object in nontraffic accident

V77.2 Person on outside of bus injured in collision with fixed or stationary object in nontraffic accident

V77.3 Unspecified occupant of bus injured in collision with fixed or stationary object in nontraffic accident

V77.4 Person boarding or alighting from bus injured in collision with fixed or stationary object

V77.5 Driver of bus injured in collision with fixed or stationary object in traffic accident

V77.6 Passenger on bus injured in collision with fixed or stationary object in traffic accident

V77.7 Person on outside of bus injured in collision with fixed or stationary object in traffic accident

V77.9 Unspecified occupant of bus injured in collision with fixed or stationary object in traffic accident

V78 Bus occupant injured in noncollision transport accident

INCLUDES overturning bus NOS
overturning bus without collision

The appropriate 7th character is to be added to each code from category V78.
A initial encounter
D subsequent encounter
S sequela

V78.0 Driver of bus injured in noncollision transport accident in nontraffic accident

V78.1 Passenger on bus injured in noncollision transport accident in nontraffic accident

V78.2 Person on outside of bus injured in noncollision transport accident in nontraffic accident

V78.3 Unspecified occupant of bus injured in noncollision transport accident in nontraffic accident

V78.4 Person boarding or alighting from bus injured in noncollision transport accident

V78.5 Driver of bus injured in noncollision transport accident in traffic accident

V78.6 Passenger on bus injured in noncollision transport accident in traffic accident

V78.7 Person on outside of bus injured in noncollision transport accident in traffic accident

V78.9 Unspecified occupant of bus injured in noncollision transport accident in traffic accident

V79 Bus occupant injured in other and unspecified transport accidents

The appropriate 7th character is to be added to each code from category V79.
A initial encounter
D subsequent encounter
S sequela

V79.0 Driver of bus injured in collision with other and unspecified motor vehicles in nontraffic accident

V79.00 Driver of bus injured in collision with unspecified motor vehicles in nontraffic accident

V79.09 Driver of bus injured in collision with other motor vehicles in nontraffic accident

V79.1 Passenger on bus injured in collision with other and unspecified motor vehicles in nontraffic accident

V79.10 Passenger on bus injured in collision with unspecified motor vehicles in nontraffic accident

V79.19 Passenger on bus injured in collision with other motor vehicles in nontraffic accident

V79.2 Unspecified bus occupant injured in collision with other and unspecified motor vehicles in nontraffic accident

V79.20 Unspecified bus occupant injured in collision with unspecified motor vehicles in nontraffic accident
Bus collision NOS, nontraffic

V79.29 Unspecified bus occupant injured in collision with other motor vehicles in nontraffic accident

V79.3 Bus occupant (driver) (passenger) injured in unspecified nontraffic accident
Bus accident NOS, nontraffic
Bus occupant injured in nontraffic accident NOS

V79.4 Driver of bus injured in collision with other and unspecified motor vehicles in traffic accident

V79.40 Driver of bus injured in collision with unspecified motor vehicles in traffic accident

V79.49 Driver of bus injured in collision with other motor vehicles in traffic accident

V79.5 Passenger on bus injured in collision with other and unspecified motor vehicles in traffic accident

V79.50 Passenger on bus injured in collision with unspecified motor vehicles in traffic accident

V79.59 Passenger on bus injured in collision with other motor vehicles in traffic accident

V79.6 Unspecified bus occupant injured in collision with other and unspecified motor vehicles in traffic accident

V79.60 Unspecified bus occupant injured in collision with unspecified motor vehicles in traffic accident
Bus collision NOS (traffic)

V79.69 Unspecified bus occupant injured in collision with other motor vehicles in traffic accident

V79.8 Bus occupant (driver) (passenger) injured in other specified transport accidents

V79.81 Bus occupant (driver) (passenger) injured in transport accidents with military vehicle

V79.88 Bus occupant (driver) (passenger) injured in other specified transport accidents

V79.9 Bus occupant (driver) (passenger) injured in unspecified traffic accident
Bus accident NOS

Other land transport accidents (V80-V89)

V80 Animal-rider or occupant of animal-drawn vehicle injured in transport accident

The appropriate 7th character is to be added to each code from category V80.
A initial encounter
D subsequent encounter
S sequela

V80.0 Animal-rider or occupant of animal drawn vehicle injured by fall from or being thrown from animal or animal-drawn vehicle in noncollision accident

V80.01 Animal-rider injured by fall from or being thrown from animal in noncollision accident

V80.010 Animal-rider injured by fall from or being thrown from horse in noncollision accident

V80.018 Animal-rider injured by fall from or being thrown from other animal in noncollision accident

V80.02 Occupant of animal-drawn vehicle injured by fall from or being thrown from animal-drawn vehicle in noncollision accident
Overturning animal-drawn vehicle NOS
Overturning animal-drawn vehicle without collision

V80.1 Animal-rider or occupant of animal-drawn vehicle injured in collision with pedestrian or animal
EXCLUDES 1 *animal-rider or animal-drawn vehicle collision with animal-drawn vehicle or animal being ridden (V80.7)*

V80.11 Animal-rider injured in collision with pedestrian or animal

V80.12 Occupant of animal-drawn vehicle injured in collision with pedestrian or animal

V80.2 Animal-rider or occupant of animal-drawn vehicle injured in collision with pedal cycle

V80.21 Animal-rider injured in collision with pedal cycle

V80.22 Occupant of animal-drawn vehicle injured in collision with pedal cycle

V80.3 Animal-rider or occupant of animal-drawn vehicle injured in collision with two- or three-wheeled motor vehicle

V80.31 Animal-rider injured in collision with two- or three-wheeled motor vehicle

V80.32 Occupant of animal-drawn vehicle injured in collision with two- or three-wheeled motor vehicle

V80.4 Animal-rider or occupant of animal-drawn vehicle injured in collision with car, pick-up truck, van, heavy transport vehicle or bus
EXCLUDES 1 *animal-rider injured in collision with military vehicle (V80.910)*
occupant of animal-drawn vehicle injured in collision with military vehicle (V80.920)

V80.41 Animal-rider injured in collision with car, pick-up truck, van, heavy transport vehicle or bus

V80.42 Occupant of animal-drawn vehicle injured in collision with car, pick-up truck, van, heavy transport vehicle or bus

V80.5 Animal-rider or occupant of animal-drawn vehicle injured in collision with other specified motor vehicle

V80.51 Animal-rider injured in collision with other specified motor vehicle

V80.52 Occupant of animal-drawn vehicle injured in collision with other specified motor vehicle

V80.6 Animal-rider or occupant of animal-drawn vehicle injured in collision with railway train or railway vehicle

V80.61 Animal-rider injured in collision with railway train or railway vehicle

V80.62 Occupant of animal-drawn vehicle injured in collision with railway train or railway vehicle

V80.7 Animal-rider or occupant of animal-drawn vehicle injured in collision with other nonmotor vehicles

V80.71 Animal-rider or occupant of animal-drawn vehicle injured in collision with animal being ridden

V80.710 Animal-rider injured in collision with other animal being ridden

V80.711 Occupant of animal-drawn vehicle injured in collision with animal being ridden

V80.72 Animal-rider or occupant of animal-drawn vehicle injured in collision with other animal-drawn vehicle

V80.720 Animal-rider injured in collision with animal-drawn vehicle

V80.721 Occupant of animal-drawn vehicle injured in collision with other animal-drawn vehicle

V80.73 Animal-rider or occupant of animal-drawn vehicle injured in collision with streetcar

V80.730 Animal-rider injured in collision with streetcar

V80.731 Occupant of animal-drawn vehicle injured in collision with streetcar

V80.79 Animal-rider or occupant of animal-drawn vehicle injured in collision with other nonmotor vehicles

V80.790 Animal-rider injured in collision with other nonmotor vehicles

V80.791 Occupant of animal-drawn vehicle injured in collision with other nonmotor vehicles

V80.8 Animal-rider or occupant of animal-drawn vehicle injured in collision with fixed or stationary object

V80.81 Animal-rider injured in collision with fixed or stationary object

V80.82 Occupant of animal-drawn vehicle injured in collision with fixed or stationary object

V80.9 Animal-rider or occupant of animal-drawn vehicle injured in other and unspecified transport accidents

V80.91 Animal-rider injured in other and unspecified transport accidents

V80.910 Animal-rider injured in transport accident with military vehicle

V80.918 Animal-rider injured in other transport accident

✓7th **V80.919 Animal-rider injured in unspecified transport accident**
Animal rider accident NOS

✓6th **V80.92 Occupant of animal-drawn vehicle injured in other and unspecified transport accidents**

✓7th **V80.920 Occupant of animal-drawn vehicle injured in transport accident with military vehicle**

✓7th **V80.928 Occupant of animal-drawn vehicle injured in other transport accident**

✓7th **V80.929 Occupant of animal-drawn vehicle injured in unspecified transport accident**
Animal-drawn vehicle accident NOS

✓4th **V81 Occupant of railway train or railway vehicle injured in transport accident**

INCLUDES derailment of railway train or railway vehicle
person on outside of train

EXCLUDES1 *streetcar (V82.-)*

The appropriate 7th character is to be added to each code from category V81.
A initial encounter
D subsequent encounter
S sequela

✓x7th **V81.0 Occupant of railway train or railway vehicle injured in collision with motor vehicle in nontraffic accident**
EXCLUDES1 *occupant of railway train or railway vehicle injured due to collision with military vehicle (V81.83)*

✓x7th **V81.1 Occupant of railway train or railway vehicle injured in collision with motor vehicle in traffic accident**
EXCLUDES1 *occupant of railway train or railway vehicle injured due to collision with military vehicle (V81.83)*

✓x7th **V81.2 Occupant of railway train or railway vehicle injured in collision with or hit by rolling stock**

✓x7th **V81.3 Occupant of railway train or railway vehicle injured in collision with other object**
Railway collision NOS

✓x7th **V81.4 Person injured while boarding or alighting from railway train or railway vehicle**

✓x7th **V81.5 Occupant of railway train or railway vehicle injured by fall in railway train or railway vehicle**

✓x7th **V81.6 Occupant of railway train or railway vehicle injured by fall from railway train or railway vehicle**

✓x7th **V81.7 Occupant of railway train or railway vehicle injured in derailment without antecedent collision**

✓5th **V81.8 Occupant of railway train or railway vehicle injured in other specified railway accidents**

✓x7th **V81.81 Occupant of railway train or railway vehicle injured due to explosion or fire on train**

✓x7th **V81.82 Occupant of railway train or railway vehicle injured due to object falling onto train**
Occupant of railway train or railway vehicle injured due to falling earth onto train
Occupant of railway train or railway vehicle injured due to falling rocks onto train
Occupant of railway train or railway vehicle injured due to falling snow onto train
Occupant of railway train or railway vehicle injured due to falling trees onto train

✓x7th **V81.83 Occupant of railway train or railway vehicle injured due to collision with military vehicle**

✓x7th **V81.89 Occupant of railway train or railway vehicle injured due to other specified railway accident**

✓x7th **V81.9 Occupant of railway train or railway vehicle injured in unspecified railway accident**
Railway accident NOS

✓4th **V82 Occupant of powered streetcar injured in transport accident**

INCLUDES interurban electric car
person on outside of streetcar
tram (car)
trolley (car)

EXCLUDES1 *bus (V70-V79)*
motorcoach (V70-V79)
nonpowered streetcar (V76.-)
train (V81.-)

The appropriate 7th character is to be added to each code from category V82.
A initial encounter
D subsequent encounter
S sequela

✓x7th **V82.0 Occupant of streetcar injured in collision with motor vehicle in nontraffic accident**

✓x7th **V82.1 Occupant of streetcar injured in collision with motor vehicle in traffic accident**

✓x7th **V82.2 Occupant of streetcar injured in collision with or hit by rolling stock**

✓x7th **V82.3 Occupant of streetcar injured in collision with other object**
EXCLUDES1 *collision with animal-drawn vehicle or animal being ridden (V82.8)*

✓x7th **V82.4 Person injured while boarding or alighting from streetcar**

✓x7th **V82.5 Occupant of streetcar injured by fall in streetcar**
EXCLUDES1 *fall in streetcar:*
while boarding or alighting (V82.4)
with antecedent collision (V82.0-V82.3)

✓x7th **V82.6 Occupant of streetcar injured by fall from streetcar**
EXCLUDES1 *fall from streetcar:*
while boarding or alighting (V82.4)
with antecedent collision (V82.0-V82.3)

✓x7th **V82.7 Occupant of streetcar injured in derailment without antecedent collision**
EXCLUDES1 *occupant of streetcar injured in derailment with antecedent collision (V82.0-V82.3)*

✓x7th **V82.8 Occupant of streetcar injured in other specified transport accidents**
Streetcar collision with military vehicle
Streetcar collision with train or nonmotor vehicles

✓x7th **V82.9 Occupant of streetcar injured in unspecified traffic accident**
Streetcar accident NOS

✓4th **V83 Occupant of special vehicle mainly used on industrial premises injured in transport accident**

INCLUDES battery-powered airport passenger vehicle
battery-powered truck (baggage) (mail)
coal-car in mine
forklift (truck)
logging car
self-propelled industrial truck
station baggage truck (powered)
tram, truck, or tub (powered) in mine or quarry

EXCLUDES1 *special construction vehicles (V85.-)*
special industrial vehicle in stationary use or maintenance (W31.-)

The appropriate 7th character is to be added to each code from category V83.
A initial encounter
D subsequent encounter
S sequela

✓x7th **V83.0 Driver of special industrial vehicle injured in traffic accident**

✓x7th **V83.1 Passenger of special industrial vehicle injured in traffic accident**

✓x7th **V83.2 Person on outside of special industrial vehicle injured in traffic accident**

✓x7th **V83.3 Unspecified occupant of special industrial vehicle injured in traffic accident**

✓x7th **V83.4 Person injured while boarding or alighting from special industrial vehicle**

✓x7th **V83.5 Driver of special industrial vehicle injured in nontraffic accident**

✓x7th **V83.6 Passenger of special industrial vehicle injured in nontraffic accident**

✓x7th **V83.7 Person on outside of special industrial vehicle injured in nontraffic accident**

V83.9 Unspecified occupant of special industrial vehicle injured in nontraffic accident
Special-industrial-vehicle accident NOS

V84 Occupant of special vehicle mainly used in agriculture injured in transport accident
INCLUDES self-propelled farm machinery
tractor (and trailer)
EXCLUDES 1 *animal-powered farm machinery accident (W30.8-)*
contact with combine harvester (W30.0)
special agricultural vehicle in stationary use or maintenance (W30.-)

The appropriate 7th character is to be added to each code from category V84.
A initial encounter
D subsequent encounter
S sequela

V84.0 Driver of special agricultural vehicle injured in traffic accident
V84.1 Passenger of special agricultural vehicle injured in traffic accident
V84.2 Person on outside of special agricultural vehicle injured in traffic accident
V84.3 Unspecified occupant of special agricultural vehicle injured in traffic accident
V84.4 Person injured while boarding or alighting from special agricultural vehicle
V84.5 Driver of special agricultural vehicle injured in nontraffic accident
V84.6 Passenger of special agricultural vehicle injured in nontraffic accident
V84.7 Person on outside of special agricultural vehicle injured in nontraffic accident
V84.9 Unspecified occupant of special agricultural vehicle injured in nontraffic accident
Special-agricultural vehicle accident NOS

V85 Occupant of special construction vehicle injured in transport accident
INCLUDES bulldozer
digger
dump truck
earth-leveller
mechanical shovel
road-roller
EXCLUDES 1 *special industrial vehicle (V83.-)*
special construction vehicle in stationary use or maintenance (W31.-)

The appropriate 7th character is to be added to each code from category V85.
A initial encounter
D subsequent encounter
S sequela

V85.0 Driver of special construction vehicle injured in traffic accident
V85.1 Passenger of special construction vehicle injured in traffic accident
V85.2 Person on outside of special construction vehicle injured in traffic accident
V85.3 Unspecified occupant of special construction vehicle injured in traffic accident
V85.4 Person injured while boarding or alighting from special construction vehicle
V85.5 Driver of special construction vehicle injured in nontraffic accident
V85.6 Passenger of special construction vehicle injured in nontraffic accident
V85.7 Person on outside of special construction vehicle injured in nontraffic accident
V85.9 Unspecified occupant of special construction vehicle injured in nontraffic accident
Special-construction-vehicle accident NOS

V86 Occupant of special all-terrain or other off-road motor vehicle, injured in transport accident
EXCLUDES 1 *special all-terrain vehicle in stationary use or maintenance (W31.-)*
sport-utility vehicle (V50-V59)
three-wheeled motor vehicle designed for on-road use (V30-V39)

The appropriate 7th character is to be added to each code from category V86.
A initial encounter
D subsequent encounter
S sequela

V86.0 Driver of special all-terrain or other off-road motor vehicle injured in traffic accident
V86.01 Driver of ambulance or fire engine injured in traffic accident
V86.02 Driver of snowmobile injured in traffic accident
V86.03 Driver of dune buggy injured in traffic accident
V86.04 Driver of military vehicle injured in traffic accident
V86.09 Driver of other special all-terrain or other off-road motor vehicle injured in traffic accident
Driver of dirt bike injured in traffic accident
Driver of go cart injured in traffic accident
Driver of golf cart injured in traffic accident

V86.1 Passenger of special all-terrain or other off-road motor vehicle injured in traffic accident
V86.11 Passenger of ambulance or fire engine injured in traffic accident
V86.12 Passenger of snowmobile injured in traffic accident
V86.13 Passenger of dune buggy injured in traffic accident
V86.14 Passenger of military vehicle injured in traffic accident
V86.19 Passenger of other special all-terrain or other off-road motor vehicle injured in traffic accident
Passenger of dirt bike injured in traffic accident
Passenger of go cart injured in traffic accident
Passenger of golf cart injured in traffic accident

V86.2 Person on outside of special all-terrain or other off-road motor vehicle injured in traffic accident
V86.21 Person on outside of ambulance or fire engine injured in traffic accident
V86.22 Person on outside of snowmobile injured in traffic accident
V86.23 Person on outside of dune buggy injured in traffic accident
V86.24 Person on outside of military vehicle injured in traffic accident
V86.29 Person on outside of other special all-terrain or other off-road motor vehicle injured in traffic accident
Person on outside of dirt bike injured in traffic accident
Person on outside of go cart in traffic accident
Person on outside of golf cart injured in traffic accident

V86.3 Unspecified occupant of special all-terrain or other off-road motor vehicle injured in traffic accident
V86.31 Unspecified occupant of ambulance or fire engine injured in traffic accident
V86.32 Unspecified occupant of snowmobile injured in traffic accident
V86.33 Unspecified occupant of dune buggy injured in traffic accident
V86.34 Unspecified occupant of military vehicle injured in traffic accident
V86.39 Unspecified occupant of other special all-terrain or other off-road motor vehicle injured in traffic accident
Unspecified occupant of dirt bike injured in traffic accident
Unspecified occupant of go cart injured in traffic accident
Unspecified occupant of golf cart injured in traffic accident

✓5th **V86.4 Person injured while boarding or alighting from special all-terrain or other off-road motor vehicle**

✓x7th **V86.41 Person injured while boarding or alighting from ambulance or fire engine**

✓x7th **V86.42 Person injured while boarding or alighting from snowmobile**

✓x7th **V86.43 Person injured while boarding or alighting from dune buggy**

✓x7th **V86.44 Person injured while boarding or alighting from military vehicle**

✓x7th **V86.49 Person injured while boarding or alighting from other special all-terrain or other off-road motor vehicle**

Person injured while boarding or alighting from dirt bike
Person injured while boarding or alighting from go cart
Person injured while boarding or alighting from golf cart

✓5th **V86.5 Driver of special all-terrain or other off-road motor vehicle injured in nontraffic accident**

✓x7th **V86.51 Driver of ambulance or fire engine injured in nontraffic accident**

✓x7th **V86.52 Driver of snowmobile injured in nontraffic accident**

✓x7th **V86.53 Driver of dune buggy injured in nontraffic accident**

✓x7th **V86.54 Driver of military vehicle injured in nontraffic accident**

✓x7th **V86.59 Driver of other special all-terrain or other off-road motor vehicle injured in nontraffic accident**

Driver of dirt bike injured in nontraffic accident
Driver of go cart injured in nontraffic accident
Driver of golf cart injured in nontraffic accident

✓5th **V86.6 Passenger of special all-terrain or other off-road motor vehicle injured in nontraffic accident**

✓x7th **V86.61 Passenger of ambulance or fire engine injured in nontraffic accident**

✓x7th **V86.62 Passenger of snowmobile injured in nontraffic accident**

✓x7th **V86.63 Passenger of dune buggy injured in nontraffic accident**

✓x7th **V86.64 Passenger of military vehicle injured in nontraffic accident**

✓x7th **V86.69 Passenger of other special all-terrain or other off-road motor vehicle injured in nontraffic accident**

Passenger of dirt bike injured in nontraffic accident
Passenger of go cart injured in nontraffic accident
Passenger of golf cart injured in nontraffic accident

✓5th **V86.7 Person on outside of special all-terrain or other off-road motor vehicle injured in nontraffic accident**

✓x7th **V86.71 Person on outside of ambulance or fire engine injured in nontraffic accident**

✓x7th **V86.72 Person on outside of snowmobile injured in nontraffic accident**

✓x7th **V86.73 Person on outside of dune buggy injured in nontraffic accident**

✓x7th **V86.74 Person on outside of military vehicle injured in nontraffic accident**

✓x7th **V86.79 Person on outside of other special all-terrain or other off-road motor vehicles injured in nontraffic accident**

Person on outside of dirt bike injured in nontraffic accident
Person on outside of go cart injured in nontraffic accident
Person on outside of golf cart injured in nontraffic accident

✓5th **V86.9 Unspecified occupant of special all-terrain or other off-road motor vehicle injured in nontraffic accident**

✓x7th **V86.91 Unspecified occupant of ambulance or fire engine injured in nontraffic accident**

✓x7th **V86.92 Unspecified occupant of snowmobile injured in nontraffic accident**

✓x7th **V86.93 Unspecified occupant of dune buggy injured in nontraffic accident**

✓x7th **V86.94 Unspecified occupant of military vehicle injured in nontraffic accident**

✓x7th **V86.99 Unspecified occupant of other special all-terrain or other off-road motor vehicle injured in nontraffic accident**

All-terrain motor-vehicle accident NOS
Off-road motor-vehicle accident NOS
Other motor-vehicle accident NOS
Unspecified occupant of dirt bike injured in nontraffic accident
Unspecified occupant of go cart injured in nontraffic accident
Unspecified occupant of golf cart injured in nontraffic accident

✓4th **V87 Traffic accident of specified type but victim's mode of transport unknown**

EXCLUDES1 *collision involving:*
pedal cycle (V10-V19)
pedestrian (V01-V09)

The appropriate 7th character is to be added to each code from category V87.
A initial encounter
D subsequent encounter
S sequela

✓x7th **V87.0 Person injured in collision between car and two- or three-wheeled powered vehicle (traffic)**

✓x7th **V87.1 Person injured in collision between other motor vehicle and two- or three-wheeled motor vehicle (traffic)**

✓x7th **V87.2 Person injured in collision between car and pick-up truck or van (traffic)**

✓x7th **V87.3 Person injured in collision between car and bus (traffic)**

✓x7th **V87.4 Person injured in collision between car and heavy transport vehicle (traffic)**

✓x7th **V87.5 Person injured in collision between heavy transport vehicle and bus (traffic)**

✓x7th **V87.6 Person injured in collision between railway train or railway vehicle and car (traffic)**

✓x7th **V87.7 Person injured in collision between other specified motor vehicles (traffic)**

✓x7th **V87.8 Person injured in other specified noncollision transport accidents involving motor vehicle (traffic)**

✓x7th **V87.9 Person injured in other specified (collision)(noncollision) transport accidents involving nonmotor vehicle (traffic)**

✓4th **V88 Nontraffic accident of specified type but victim's mode of transport unknown**

EXCLUDES1 *collision involving:*
pedal cycle (V10-V19)
pedestrian (V01-V09)

The appropriate 7th character is to be added to each code from category V88.
A initial encounter
D subsequent encounter
S sequela

✓x7th **V88.0 Person injured in collision between car and two- or three-wheeled motor vehicle, nontraffic**

✓x7th **V88.1 Person injured in collision between other motor vehicle and two- or three-wheeled motor vehicle, nontraffic**

✓x7th **V88.2 Person injured in collision between car and pick-up truck or van, nontraffic**

✓x7th **V88.3 Person injured in collision between car and bus, nontraffic**

✓x7th **V88.4 Person injured in collision between car and heavy transport vehicle, nontraffic**

✓x7th **V88.5 Person injured in collision between heavy transport vehicle and bus, nontraffic**

✓x7th **V88.6 Person injured in collision between railway train or railway vehicle and car, nontraffic**

✓x7th **V88.7 Person injured in collision between other specified motor vehicle, nontraffic**

✓x7th **V88.8 Person injured in other specified noncollision transport accidents involving motor vehicle, nontraffic**

✓x7th **V88.9 Person injured in other specified (collision)(noncollision) transport accidents involving nonmotor vehicle, nontraffic**

V89 Motor- or nonmotor-vehicle accident, type of vehicle unspecified

The appropriate 7th character is to be added to each code from category V89.
A initial encounter
D subsequent encounter
S sequela

V89.0 Person injured in unspecified motor-vehicle accident, nontraffic
Motor-vehicle accident NOS, nontraffic

V89.1 Person injured in unspecified nonmotor-vehicle accident, nontraffic
Nonmotor-vehicle accident NOS (nontraffic)

V89.2 Person injured in unspecified motor-vehicle accident, traffic
Motor-vehicle accident [MVA] NOS
Road (traffic) accident [RTA] NOS

V89.3 Person injured in unspecified nonmotor-vehicle accident, traffic
Nonmotor-vehicle traffic accident NOS

V89.9 Person injured in unspecified vehicle accident
Collision NOS

Water transport accidents (V90-V94)

V90 Drowning and submersion due to accident to watercraft

EXCLUDES 1 *civilian water transport accident involving military watercraft (V94.81-)*
fall into water not from watercraft (W16.-)
military watercraft accident in military or war operations (Y36.0-, Y37.0-)
water-transport-related drowning or submersion without accident to watercraft (V92.-)

The appropriate 7th character is to be added to each code from category V90.
A initial encounter
D subsequent encounter
S sequela

V90.0 Drowning and submersion due to watercraft overturning

V90.00 Drowning and submersion due to merchant ship overturning

V90.01 Drowning and submersion due to passenger ship overturning
Drowning and submersion due to Ferry-boat overturning
Drowning and submersion due to Liner overturning

V90.02 Drowning and submersion due to fishing boat overturning

V90.03 Drowning and submersion due to other powered watercraft overturning
Drowning and submersion due to Hovercraft (on open water) overturning
Drowning and submersion due to Jet ski overturning

V90.04 Drowning and submersion due to sailboat overturning

V90.05 Drowning and submersion due to canoe or kayak overturning

V90.06 Drowning and submersion due to (nonpowered) inflatable craft overturning

V90.08 Drowning and submersion due to other unpowered watercraft overturning
Drowning and submersion due to windsurfer overturning

V90.09 Drowning and submersion due to unspecified watercraft overturning
Drowning and submersion due to boat NOS overturning
Drowning and submersion due to ship NOS overturning
Drowning and submersion due to watercraft NOS overturning

V90.1 Drowning and submersion due to watercraft sinking

V90.10 Drowning and submersion due to merchant ship sinking

V90.11 Drowning and submersion due to passenger ship sinking
Drowning and submersion due to Ferry-boat sinking
Drowning and submersion due to Liner sinking

V90.12 Drowning and submersion due to fishing boat sinking

V90.13 Drowning and submersion due to other powered watercraft sinking
Drowning and submersion due to Hovercraft (on open water) sinking
Drowning and submersion due to Jet ski sinking

V90.14 Drowning and submersion due to sailboat sinking

V90.15 Drowning and submersion due to canoe or kayak sinking

V90.16 Drowning and submersion due to (nonpowered) inflatable craft sinking

V90.18 Drowning and submersion due to other unpowered watercraft sinking

V90.19 Drowning and submersion due to unspecified watercraft sinking
Drowning and submersion due to boat NOS sinking
Drowning and submersion due to ship NOS sinking
Drowning and submersion due to watercraft NOS sinking

V90.2 Drowning and submersion due to falling or jumping from burning watercraft

V90.20 Drowning and submersion due to falling or jumping from burning merchant ship

V90.21 Drowning and submersion due to falling or jumping from burning passenger ship
Drowning and submersion due to falling or jumping from burning Ferry-boat
Drowning and submersion due to falling or jumping from burning Liner

V90.22 Drowning and submersion due to falling or jumping from burning fishing boat

V90.23 Drowning and submersion due to falling or jumping from other burning powered watercraft
Drowning and submersion due to falling and jumping from burning Hovercraft (on open water)
Drowning and submersion due to falling and jumping from burning Jet ski

V90.24 Drowning and submersion due to falling or jumping from burning sailboat

V90.25 Drowning and submersion due to falling or jumping from burning canoe or kayak

V90.26 Drowning and submersion due to falling or jumping from burning (nonpowered) inflatable craft

V90.27 Drowning and submersion due to falling or jumping from burning water-skis

V90.28 Drowning and submersion due to falling or jumping from other burning unpowered watercraft
Drowning and submersion due to falling and jumping from burning surf-board
Drowning and submersion due to falling and jumping from burning windsurfer

V90.29 Drowning and submersion due to falling or jumping from unspecified burning watercraft
Drowning and submersion due to falling or jumping from burning boat NOS
Drowning and submersion due to falling or jumping from burning ship NOS
Drowning and submersion due to falling or jumping from burning watercraft NOS

V90.3 Drowning and submersion due to falling or jumping from crushed watercraft

V90.30 Drowning and submersion due to falling or jumping from crushed merchant ship

V90.31 Drowning and submersion due to falling or jumping from crushed passenger ship
Drowning and submersion due to falling and jumping from crushed Ferry boat
Drowning and submersion due to falling and jumping from crushed Liner

V90.32 Drowning and submersion due to falling or jumping from crushed fishing boat

V90.33 Drowning and submersion due to falling or jumping from other crushed powered watercraft
Drowning and submersion due to falling and jumping from crushed Hovercraft
Drowning and submersion due to falling and jumping from crushed Jet ski

V90.34 Drowning and submersion due to falling or jumping from crushed sailboat

V90.35 Drowning and submersion due to falling or jumping from crushed canoe or kayak

V90.36 Drowning and submersion due to falling or jumping from crushed (nonpowered) inflatable craft

V90.37 Drowning and submersion due to falling or jumping from crushed water-skis

V90.38 Drowning and submersion due to falling or jumping from other crushed unpowered watercraft
Drowning and submersion due to falling and jumping from crushed surf-board
Drowning and submersion due to falling and jumping from crushed windsurfer

V90.39 Drowning and submersion due to falling or jumping from crushed unspecified watercraft
Drowning and submersion due to falling and jumping from crushed boat NOS
Drowning and submersion due to falling and jumping from crushed ship NOS
Drowning and submersion due to falling and jumping from crushed watercraft NOS

V90.8 Drowning and submersion due to other accident to watercraft

V90.80 Drowning and submersion due to other accident to merchant ship

V90.81 Drowning and submersion due to other accident to passenger ship
Drowning and submersion due to other accident to Ferry-boat
Drowning and submersion due to other accident to Liner

V90.82 Drowning and submersion due to other accident to fishing boat

V90.83 Drowning and submersion due to other accident to other powered watercraft
Drowning and submersion due to other accident to Hovercraft (on open water)
Drowning and submersion due to other accident to Jet ski

V90.84 Drowning and submersion due to other accident to sailboat

V90.85 Drowning and submersion due to other accident to canoe or kayak

V90.86 Drowning and submersion due to other accident to (nonpowered) inflatable craft

V90.87 Drowning and submersion due to other accident to water-skis

V90.88 Drowning and submersion due to other accident to other unpowered watercraft
Drowning and submersion due to other accident to surf-board
Drowning and submersion due to other accident to windsurfer

V90.89 Drowning and submersion due to other accident to unspecified watercraft
Drowning and submersion due to other accident to boat NOS
Drowning and submersion due to other accident to ship NOS
Drowning and submersion due to other accident to watercraft NOS

V91 Other injury due to accident to watercraft
INCLUDES any injury except drowning and submersion as a result of an accident to watercraft
EXCLUDES 1 *civilian water transport accident involving military watercraft (V94.81-)*
military watercraft accident in military or war operations (Y36, Y37-)
EXCLUDES 2 *drowning and submersion due to accident to watercraft (V90.-)*

The appropriate 7th character is to be added to each code from category V91.
A initial encounter
D subsequent encounter
S sequela

V91.0 Burn due to watercraft on fire
EXCLUDES 1 *burn from localized fire or explosion on board ship without accident to watercraft (V93.-)*

V91.00 Burn due to merchant ship on fire

V91.01 Burn due to passenger ship on fire
Burn due to Ferry-boat on fire
Burn due to Liner on fire

V91.02 Burn due to fishing boat on fire

V91.03 Burn due to other powered watercraft on fire
Burn due to Hovercraft (on open water) on fire
Burn due to Jet ski on fire

V91.04 Burn due to sailboat on fire

V91.05 Burn due to canoe or kayak on fire

V91.06 Burn due to (nonpowered) inflatable craft on fire

V91.07 Burn due to water-skis on fire

V91.08 Burn due to other unpowered watercraft on fire

V91.09 Burn due to unspecified watercraft on fire
Burn due to boat NOS on fire
Burn due to ship NOS on fire
Burn due to watercraft NOS on fire

V91.1 Crushed between watercraft and other watercraft or other object due to collision
Crushed by lifeboat after abandoning ship in a collision
NOTE select the specified type of watercraft that the victim was on at the time of the collision

V91.10 Crushed between merchant ship and other watercraft or other object due to collision

V91.11 Crushed between passenger ship and other watercraft or other object due to collision
Crushed between Ferry-boat and other watercraft or other object due to collision
Crushed between Liner and other watercraft or other object due to collision

V91.12 Crushed between fishing boat and other watercraft or other object due to collision

V91.13 Crushed between other powered watercraft and other watercraft or other object due to collision
Crushed between Hovercraft (on open water) and other watercraft or other object due to collision
Crushed between Jet ski and other watercraft or other object due to collision

V91.14 Crushed between sailboat and other watercraft or other object due to collision

V91.15 Crushed between canoe or kayak and other watercraft or other object due to collision

V91.16 Crushed between (nonpowered) inflatable craft and other watercraft or other object due to collision

V91.18 Crushed between other unpowered watercraft and other watercraft or other object due to collision
Crushed between surfboard and other watercraft or other object due to collision
Crushed between windsurfer and other watercraft or other object due to collision

V91.19 Crushed between unspecified watercraft and other watercraft or other object due to collision
Crushed between boat NOS and other watercraft or other object due to collision
Crushed between ship NOS and other watercraft or other object due to collision
Crushed between watercraft NOS and other watercraft or other object due to collision

V91.2 Fall due to collision between watercraft and other watercraft or other object
Fall while remaining on watercraft after collision
NOTE Select the specified type of watercraft that the victim was on at the time of the collision
EXCLUDES1 *crushed between watercraft and other watercraft and other object due to collision (V91.1-)*
drowning and submersion due to falling from crushed watercraft (V90.3-)

V91.20 Fall due to collision between merchant ship and other watercraft or other object

V91.21 Fall due to collision between passenger ship and other watercraft or other object
Fall due to collision between Ferry-boat and other watercraft or other object
Fall due to collision between Liner and other watercraft or other object

V91.22 Fall due to collision between fishing boat and other watercraft or other object

V91.23 Fall due to collision between other powered watercraft and other watercraft or other object
Fall due to collision between Hovercraft (on open water) and other watercraft or other object
Fall due to collision between Jet ski and other watercraft or other object

V91.24 Fall due to collision between sailboat and other watercraft or other object

V91.25 Fall due to collision between canoe or kayak and other watercraft or other object

V91.26 Fall due to collision between (nonpowered) inflatable craft and other watercraft or other object

V91.29 Fall due to collision between unspecified watercraft and other watercraft or other object
Fall due to collision between boat NOS and other watercraft or other object
Fall due to collision between ship NOS and other watercraft or other object
Fall due to collision between watercraft NOS and other watercraft or other object

V91.3 Hit or struck by falling object due to accident to watercraft
Hit or struck by falling object (part of damaged watercraft or other object) after falling or jumping from damaged watercraft
EXCLUDES2 *drowning or submersion due to fall or jumping from damaged watercraft (V90.2-, V90.3-)*

V91.30 Hit or struck by falling object due to accident to merchant ship

V91.31 Hit or struck by falling object due to accident to passenger ship
Hit or struck by falling object due to accident to Ferry-boat
Hit or struck by falling object due to accident to Liner

V91.32 Hit or struck by falling object due to accident to fishing boat

V91.33 Hit or struck by falling object due to accident to other powered watercraft
Hit or struck by falling object due to accident to Hovercraft (on open water)
Hit or struck by falling object due to accident to Jet ski

V91.34 Hit or struck by falling object due to accident to sailboat

V91.35 Hit or struck by falling object due to accident to canoe or kayak

V91.36 Hit or struck by falling object due to accident to (nonpowered) inflatable craft

V91.37 Hit or struck by falling object due to accident to water-skis
Hit by water-skis after jumping off of waterskis

V91.38 Hit or struck by falling object due to accident to other unpowered watercraft
Hit or struck by surf-board after falling off damaged surf-board
Hit or struck by object after falling off damaged windsurfer

V91.39 Hit or struck by falling object due to accident to unspecified watercraft
Hit or struck by falling object due to accident to boat NOS
Hit or struck by falling object due to accident to ship NOS
Hit or struck by falling object due to accident to watercraft NOS

V91.8 Other injury due to other accident to watercraft

V91.80 Other injury due to other accident to merchant ship

V91.81 Other injury due to other accident to passenger ship
Other injury due to other accident to Ferry-boat
Other injury due to other accident to Liner

V91.82 Other injury due to other accident to fishing boat

V91.83 Other injury due to other accident to other powered watercraft
Other injury due to other accident to Hovercraft (on open water)
Other injury due to other accident to Jet ski

V91.84 Other injury due to other accident to sailboat

V91.85 Other injury due to other accident to canoe or kayak

V91.86 Other injury due to other accident to (nonpowered) inflatable craft

V91.87 Other injury due to other accident to water-skis

V91.88 Other injury due to other accident to other unpowered watercraft
Other injury due to other accident to surf-board
Other injury due to other accident to windsurfer

V91.89 Other injury due to other accident to unspecified watercraft
Other injury due to other accident to boat NOS
Other injury due to other accident to ship NOS
Other injury due to other accident to watercraft NOS

V92 Drowning and submersion due to accident on board watercraft, without accident to watercraft
EXCLUDES1 *civilian water transport accident involving military watercraft (V94.81-)*
drowning or submersion due to accident to watercraft (V90-V91)
drowning or submersion of diver who voluntarily jumps from boat not involved in an accident (W16.711, W16.721)
fall into water without watercraft (W16.-)
military watercraft accident in military or war operations (Y36, Y37)

The appropriate 7th character is to be added to each code from category V92.
A initial encounter
D subsequent encounter
S sequela

V92.0 Drowning and submersion due to fall off watercraft
Drowning and submersion due to fall from gangplank of watercraft
Drowning and submersion due to fall overboard watercraft
EXCLUDES2 *hitting head on object or bottom of body of water due to fall from watercraft (V94.0-)*

V92.00 Drowning and submersion due to fall off merchant ship

V92.01 Drowning and submersion due to fall off passenger ship
Drowning and submersion due to fall off Ferry-boat
Drowning and submersion due to fall off Liner

V92.02 Drowning and submersion due to fall off fishing boat

V92.03 Drowning and submersion due to fall off other powered watercraft
Drowning and submersion due to fall off Hovercraft (on open water)
Drowning and submersion due to fall off Jet ski

V92.04 Drowning and submersion due to fall off sailboat

V92.05 Drowning and submersion due to fall off canoe or kayak

V92.06 Drowning and submersion due to fall off (nonpowered) inflatable craft

√x7th **V92.07 Drowning and submersion due to fall off water-skis**
EXCLUDES 1 *drowning and submersion due to falling off burning water-skis (V90.27)*
drowning and submersion due to falling off crushed water-skis (V90.37)
hit by boat while water-skiing NOS (V94.X)

√x7th **V92.08 Drowning and submersion due to fall off other unpowered watercraft**
Drowning and submersion due to fall off surf-board
Drowning and submersion due to fall off windsurfer
EXCLUDES 1 *drowning and submersion due to fall off burning unpowered watercraft (V90.28)*
drowning and submersion due to fall off crushed unpowered watercraft (V90.38)
drowning and submersion due to fall off damaged unpowered watercraft (V90.88)
drowning and submersion due to rider of nonpowered watercraft being hit by other watercraft (V94.21)
other injury due to rider of nonpowered watercraft being hit by other watercraft (V94.22)

√x7th **V92.09 Drowning and submersion due to fall off unspecified watercraft**
Drowning and submersion due to fall off boat NOS
Drowning and submersion due to fall off ship
Drowning and submersion due to fall off watercraft NOS

√5th **V92.1 Drowning and submersion due to being thrown overboard by motion of watercraft**
EXCLUDES 1 *drowning and submersion due to fall off surf-board (V92.08)*
drowning and submersion due to fall off water-skis (V92.07)
drowning and submersion due to fall off windsurfer (V92.08)

√x7th **V92.10 Drowning and submersion due to being thrown overboard by motion of merchant ship**

√x7th **V92.11 Drowning and submersion due to being thrown overboard by motion of passenger ship**
Drowning and submersion due to being thrown overboard by motion of Ferry-boat
Drowning and submersion due to being thrown overboard by motion of Liner

√x7th **V92.12 Drowning and submersion due to being thrown overboard by motion of fishing boat**

√x7th **V92.13 Drowning and submersion due to being thrown overboard by motion of other powered watercraft**
Drowning and submersion due to being thrown overboard by motion of Hovercraft

√x7th **V92.14 Drowning and submersion due to being thrown overboard by motion of sailboat**

√x7th **V92.15 Drowning and submersion due to being thrown overboard by motion of canoe or kayak**

√x7th **V92.16 Drowning and submersion due to being thrown overboard by motion of (nonpowered) inflatable craft**

√x7th **V92.19 Drowning and submersion due to being thrown overboard by motion of unspecified watercraft**
Drowning and submersion due to being thrown overboard by motion of boat NOS
Drowning and submersion due to being thrown overboard by motion of ship NOS
Drowning and submersion due to being thrown overboard by motion of watercraft NOS

√5th **V92.2 Drowning and submersion due to being washed overboard from watercraft**
Code first any associated cataclysm (X37.0-)

√x7th **V92.20 Drowning and submersion due to being washed overboard from merchant ship**

√x7th **V92.21 Drowning and submersion due to being washed overboard from passenger ship**
Drowning and submersion due to being washed overboard from Ferry-boat
Drowning and submersion due to being washed overboard from Liner

√x7th **V92.22 Drowning and submersion due to being washed overboard from fishing boat**

√x7th **V92.23 Drowning and submersion due to being washed overboard from other powered watercraft**
Drowning and submersion due to being washed overboard from Hovercraft (on open water)
Drowning and submersion due to being washed overboard from Jet ski

√x7th **V92.24 Drowning and submersion due to being washed overboard from sailboat**

√x7th **V92.25 Drowning and submersion due to being washed overboard from canoe or kayak**

√x7th **V92.26 Drowning and submersion due to being washed overboard from (nonpowered) inflatable craft**

√x7th **V92.27 Drowning and submersion due to being washed overboard from water-skis**
EXCLUDES 1 *drowning and submersion due to fall off water-skis (V92.07)*

√x7th **V92.28 Drowning and submersion due to being washed overboard from other unpowered watercraft**
Drowning and submersion due to being washed overboard from surf-board
Drowning and submersion due to being washed overboard from windsurfer

√x7th **V92.29 Drowning and submersion due to being washed overboard from unspecified watercraft**
Drowning and submersion due to being washed overboard from boat NOS
Drowning and submersion due to being washed overboard from ship NOS
Drowning and submersion due to being washed overboard from watercraft NOS

√4th **V93 Other injury due to accident on board watercraft, without accident to watercraft**
EXCLUDES 1 *civilian water transport accident involving military watercraft (V94.81-)*
other injury due to accident to watercraft (V91.-)
military watercraft accident in military or war operations (Y36, Y37-)
EXCLUDES 2 *drowning and submersion due to accident on board watercraft, without accident to watercraft (V92.-)*

The appropriate 7th character is to be added to each code from category V93.
A initial encounter
D subsequent encounter
S sequela

√5th **V93.0 Burn due to localized fire on board watercraft**
EXCLUDES 1 *burn due to watercraft on fire (V91.0-)*

√x7th **V93.00 Burn due to localized fire on board merchant vessel**

√x7th **V93.01 Burn due to localized fire on board passenger vessel**
Burn due to localized fire on board Ferry-boat
Burn due to localized fire on board Liner

√x7th **V93.02 Burn due to localized fire on board fishing boat**

√x7th **V93.03 Burn due to localized fire on board other powered watercraft**
Burn due to localized fire on board Hovercraft
Burn due to localized fire on board Jet ski

√x7th **V93.04 Burn due to localized fire on board sailboat**

√x7th **V93.09 Burn due to localized fire on board unspecified watercraft**
Burn due to localized fire on board boat NOS
Burn due to localized fire on board ship NOS
Burn due to localized fire on board watercraft NOS

√5th **V93.1 Other burn on board watercraft**
Burn due to source other than fire on board watercraft
EXCLUDES 1 *burn due to watercraft on fire (V91.0-)*

√x7th **V93.10 Other burn on board merchant vessel**

√x7th **V93.11 Other burn on board passenger vessel**
Other burn on board Ferry-boat
Other burn on board Liner

√x7th **V93.12 Other burn on board fishing boat**

√x7th **V93.13 Other burn on board other powered watercraft**
Other burn on board Hovercraft
Other burn on board Jet ski

√x7th **V93.14 Other burn on board sailboat**

√x7th **V93.19 Other burn on board unspecified watercraft**
Other burn on board boat NOS
Other burn on board ship NOS
Other burn on board watercraft NOS

√5th **V93.2 Heat exposure on board watercraft**
EXCLUDES 1 *exposure to man-made heat not aboard watercraft (W92)*
exposure to natural heat while on board watercraft (X30)
exposure to sunlight while on board watercraft (X32)
EXCLUDES 2 *burn due to fire on board watercraft (V93.0-)*

√x7th **V93.20 Heat exposure on board merchant ship**
√x7th **V93.21 Heat exposure on board passenger ship**
Heat exposure on board Ferry-boat
Heat exposure on board Liner
√x7th **V93.22 Heat exposure on board fishing boat**
√x7th **V93.23 Heat exposure on board other powered watercraft**
Heat exposure on board hovercraft
√x7th **V93.24 Heat exposure on board sailboat**
√x7th **V93.29 Heat exposure on board unspecified watercraft**
Heat exposure on board boat NOS
Heat exposure on board ship NOS
Heat exposure on board watercraft NOS

√5th **V93.3 Fall on board watercraft**
EXCLUDES 1 *fall due to collision of watercraft (V91.2-)*

√x7th **V93.30 Fall on board merchant ship**
√x7th **V93.31 Fall on board passenger ship**
Fall on board Ferry-boat
Fall on board Liner
√x7th **V93.32 Fall on board fishing boat**
√x7th **V93.33 Fall on board other powered watercraft**
Fall on board Hovercraft (on open water)
Fall on board Jet ski
√x7th **V93.34 Fall on board sailboat**
√x7th **V93.35 Fall on board canoe or kayak**
√x7th **V93.36 Fall on board (nonpowered) inflatable craft**
√x7th **V93.38 Fall on board other unpowered watercraft**
√x7th **V93.39 Fall on board unspecified watercraft**
Fall on board boat NOS
Fall on board ship NOS
Fall on board watercraft NOS

√5th **V93.4 Struck by falling object on board watercraft**
Hit by falling object on board watercraft
EXCLUDES 1 *struck by falling object due to accident to watercraft (V91.3)*

√x7th **V93.40 Struck by falling object on merchant ship**
√x7th **V93.41 Struck by falling object on passenger ship**
Struck by falling object on Ferry-boat
Struck by falling object on Liner
√x7th **V93.42 Struck by falling object on fishing boat**
√x7th **V93.43 Struck by falling object on other powered watercraft**
Struck by falling object on Hovercraft
√x7th **V93.44 Struck by falling object on sailboat**
√x7th **V93.48 Struck by falling object on other unpowered watercraft**
√x7th **V93.49 Struck by falling object on unspecified watercraft**

√5th **V93.5 Explosion on board watercraft**
Boiler explosion on steamship
EXCLUDES 2 *fire on board watercraft (V93.0-)*

√x7th **V93.50 Explosion on board merchant ship**
√x7th **V93.51 Explosion on board passenger ship**
Explosion on board Ferry-boat
Explosion on board Liner
√x7th **V93.52 Explosion on board fishing boat**
√x7th **V93.53 Explosion on board other powered watercraft**
Explosion on board Hovercraft
Explosion on board Jet ski
√x7th **V93.54 Explosion on board sailboat**
√x7th **V93.59 Explosion on board unspecified watercraft**
Explosion on board boat NOS
Explosion on board ship NOS
Explosion on board watercraft NOS

√5th **V93.6 Machinery accident on board watercraft**
EXCLUDES 1 *machinery explosion on board watercraft (V93.4-)*
machinery fire on board watercraft (V93.0-)

√x7th **V93.60 Machinery accident on board merchant ship**
√x7th **V93.61 Machinery accident on board passenger ship**
Machinery accident on board Ferry-boat
Machinery accident on board Liner
√x7th **V93.62 Machinery accident on board fishing boat**
√x7th **V93.63 Machinery accident on board other powered watercraft**
Machinery accident on board Hovercraft
√x7th **V93.64 Machinery accident on board sailboat**
√x7th **V93.69 Machinery accident on board unspecified watercraft**
Machinery accident on board boat NOS
Machinery accident on board ship NOS
Machinery accident on board watercraft NOS

√5th **V93.8 Other injury due to other accident on board watercraft**
Accidental poisoning by gases or fumes on watercraft

√x7th **V93.80 Other injury due to other accident on board merchant ship**
√x7th **V93.81 Other injury due to other accident on board passenger ship**
Other injury due to other accident on board Ferry-boat
Other injury due to other accident on board Liner
√x7th **V93.82 Other injury due to other accident on board fishing boat**
√x7th **V93.83 Other injury due to other accident on board other powered watercraft**
Other injury due to other accident on board Hovercraft
Other injury due to other accident on board Jet ski
√x7th **V93.84 Other injury due to other accident on board sailboat**
√x7th **V93.85 Other injury due to other accident on board canoe or kayak**
√x7th **V93.86 Other injury due to other accident on board (nonpowered) inflatable craft**
√x7th **V93.87 Other injury due to other accident on board water-skis**
Hit or struck by object while waterskiing
√x7th **V93.88 Other injury due to other accident on board other unpowered watercraft**
Hit or struck by object while surfing
Hit or struck by object while on board windsurfer
√x7th **V93.89 Other injury due to other accident on board unspecified watercraft**
Other injury due to other accident on board boat NOS
Other injury due to other accident on board ship NOS
Other injury due to other accident on board watercraft NOS

√4th **V94 Other and unspecified water transport accidents**
EXCLUDES 1 *military watercraft accidents in military or war operations (Y36, Y37)*

The appropriate 7th character is to be added to each code from category V94.
A initial encounter
D subsequent encounter
S sequela

√x7th **V94.0 Hitting object or bottom of body of water due to fall from watercraft**
EXCLUDES 2 *drowning and submersion due to fall from watercraft (V92.0-)*

√5th **V94.1 Bather struck by watercraft**
Swimmer hit by watercraft
√x7th **V94.11 Bather struck by powered watercraft**
√x7th **V94.12 Bather struck by nonpowered watercraft**

√5th **V94.2 Rider of nonpowered watercraft struck by other watercraft**
√x7th **V94.21 Rider of nonpowered watercraft struck by other nonpowered watercraft**
Canoer hit by other nonpowered watercraft
Surfer hit by other nonpowered watercraft
Windsurfer hit by other nonpowered watercraft
√x7th **V94.22 Rider of nonpowered watercraft struck by powered watercraft**
Canoer hit by motorboat
Surfer hit by motorboat
Windsurfer hit by motorboat

√5th **V94.3 Injury to rider of (inflatable) watercraft being pulled behind other watercraft**
√x7th **V94.31 Injury to rider of (inflatable) recreational watercraft being pulled behind other watercraft**
Injury to rider of inner-tube pulled behind motor boat
√x7th **V94.32 Injury to rider of non-recreational watercraft being pulled behind other watercraft**
Injury to occupant of dingy being pulled behind boat or ship
Injury to occupant of life-raft being pulled behind boat or ship
√x7th **V94.4 Injury to barefoot water-skier**
Injury to person being pulled behind boat or ship
√5th **V94.8 Other water transport accident**
√6th **V94.81 Water transport accident involving military watercraft**
√7th **V94.810 Civilian watercraft involved in water transport accident with military watercraft**
Passenger on civilian watercraft injured due to accident with military watercraft
√7th **V94.811 Civilian in water injured by military watercraft**
√7th **V94.818 Other water transport accident involving military watercraft**
√x7th **V94.89 Other water transport accident**
√x7th **V94.9 Unspecified water transport accident**
Water transport accident NOS

Air and space transport accidents (V95-V97)

EXCLUDES 1 *military aircraft accidents in military or war operations (Y36, Y37)*

√4th **V95 Accident to powered aircraft causing injury to occupant**

The appropriate 7th character is to be added to each code from category V95.
A initial encounter
D subsequent encounter
S sequela

√5th **V95.0 Helicopter accident injuring occupant**
√x7th **V95.00 Unspecified helicopter accident injuring occupant**
√x7th **V95.01 Helicopter crash injuring occupant**
√x7th **V95.02 Forced landing of helicopter injuring occupant**
√x7th **V95.03 Helicopter collision injuring occupant**
Helicopter collision with any object, fixed, movable or moving
√x7th **V95.04 Helicopter fire injuring occupant**
√x7th **V95.05 Helicopter explosion injuring occupant**
√x7th **V95.09 Other helicopter accident injuring occupant**
√5th **V95.1 Ultralight, microlight or powered-glider accident injuring occupant**
√x7th **V95.10 Unspecified ultralight, microlight or powered-glider accident injuring occupant**
√x7th **V95.11 Ultralight, microlight or powered-glider crash injuring occupant**
√x7th **V95.12 Forced landing of ultralight, microlight or powered-glider injuring occupant**
√x7th **V95.13 Ultralight, microlight or powered-glider collision injuring occupant**
Ultralight, microlight or powered-glider collision with any object, fixed, movable or moving
√x7th **V95.14 Ultralight, microlight or powered-glider fire injuring occupant**
√x7th **V95.15 Ultralight, microlight or powered-glider explosion injuring occupant**
√x7th **V95.19 Other ultralight, microlight or powered-glider accident injuring occupant**
√5th **V95.2 Other private fixed-wing aircraft accident injuring occupant**
√x7th **V95.20 Unspecified accident to other private fixed-wing aircraft, injuring occupant**
√x7th **V95.21 Other private fixed-wing aircraft crash injuring occupant**
√x7th **V95.22 Forced landing of other private fixed-wing aircraft injuring occupant**
√x7th **V95.23 Other private fixed-wing aircraft collision injuring occupant**
Other private fixed-wing aircraft collision with any object, fixed, movable or moving
√x7th **V95.24 Other private fixed-wing aircraft fire injuring occupant**
√x7th **V95.25 Other private fixed-wing aircraft explosion injuring occupant**
√x7th **V95.29 Other accident to other private fixed-wing aircraft injuring occupant**
√5th **V95.3 Commercial fixed-wing aircraft accident injuring occupant**
√x7th **V95.30 Unspecified accident to commercial fixed-wing aircraft injuring occupant**
√x7th **V95.31 Commercial fixed-wing aircraft crash injuring occupant**
√x7th **V95.32 Forced landing of commercial fixed-wing aircraft injuring occupant**
√x7th **V95.33 Commercial fixed-wing aircraft collision injuring occupant**
Commercial fixed-wing aircraft collision with any object, fixed, movable or moving
√x7th **V95.34 Commercial fixed-wing aircraft fire injuring occupant**
√x7th **V95.35 Commercial fixed-wing aircraft explosion injuring occupant**
√x7th **V95.39 Other accident to commercial fixed-wing aircraft injuring occupant**
√5th **V95.4 Spacecraft accident injuring occupant**
√x7th **V95.40 Unspecified spacecraft accident injuring occupant**
√x7th **V95.41 Spacecraft crash injuring occupant**
√x7th **V95.42 Forced landing of spacecraft injuring occupant**
√x7th **V95.43 Spacecraft collision injuring occupant**
Spacecraft collision with any object, fixed, moveable or moving
√x7th **V95.44 Spacecraft fire injuring occupant**
√x7th **V95.45 Spacecraft explosion injuring occupant**
√x7th **V95.49 Other spacecraft accident injuring occupant**
√x7th **V95.8 Other powered aircraft accidents injuring occupant**
√x7th **V95.9 Unspecified aircraft accident injuring occupant**
Aircraft accident NOS
Air transport accident NOS

√4th **V96 Accident to nonpowered aircraft causing injury to occupant**

The appropriate 7th character is to be added to each code from category V96.
A initial encounter
D subsequent encounter
S sequela

√5th **V96.0 Balloon accident injuring occupant**
√x7th **V96.00 Unspecified balloon accident injuring occupant**
√x7th **V96.01 Balloon crash injuring occupant**
√x7th **V96.02 Forced landing of balloon injuring occupant**
√x7th **V96.03 Balloon collision injuring occupant**
Balloon collision with any object, fixed, moveable or moving
√x7th **V96.04 Balloon fire injuring occupant**
√x7th **V96.05 Balloon explosion injuring occupant**
√x7th **V96.09 Other balloon accident injuring occupant**
√5th **V96.1 Hang-glider accident injuring occupant**
√x7th **V96.10 Unspecified hang-glider accident injuring occupant**
√x7th **V96.11 Hang-glider crash injuring occupant**
√x7th **V96.12 Forced landing of hang-glider injuring occupant**
√x7th **V96.13 Hang-glider collision injuring occupant**
Hang-glider collision with any object, fixed, moveable or moving
√x7th **V96.14 Hang-glider fire injuring occupant**
√x7th **V96.15 Hang-glider explosion injuring occupant**
√x7th **V96.19 Other hang-glider accident injuring occupant**
√5th **V96.2 Glider (nonpowered) accident injuring occupant**
√x7th **V96.20 Unspecified glider (nonpowered) accident injuring occupant**
√x7th **V96.21 Glider (nonpowered) crash injuring occupant**
√x7th **V96.22 Forced landing of glider (nonpowered) injuring occupant**

√x7th **V96.23 Glider (nonpowered) collision injuring occupant**
Glider (nonpowered) collision with any object, fixed, moveable or moving
√x7th **V96.24 Glider (nonpowered) fire injuring occupant**
√x7th **V96.25 Glider (nonpowered) explosion injuring occupant**
√x7th **V96.29 Other glider (nonpowered) accident injuring occupant**
√x7th **V96.8 Other nonpowered-aircraft accidents injuring occupant**
Kite carrying a person accident injuring occupant
√x7th **V96.9 Unspecified nonpowered-aircraft accident injuring occupant**
Nonpowered-aircraft accident NOS

√4th **V97 Other specified air transport accidents**

The appropriate 7th character is to be added to each code from category V97.
A initial encounter
D subsequent encounter
S sequela

√x7th **V97.0 Occupant of aircraft injured in other specified air transport accidents**
Fall in, on or from aircraft in air transport accident
EXCLUDES 1 *accident while boarding or alighting aircraft (V97.1)*
√x7th **V97.1 Person injured while boarding or alighting from aircraft**
√5th **V97.2 Parachutist accident**
√x7th **V97.21 Parachutist entangled in object**
Parachutist landing in tree
√x7th **V97.22 Parachutist injured on landing**
√x7th **V97.29 Other parachutist accident**
√5th **V97.3 Person on ground injured in air transport accident**
√x7th **V97.31 Hit by object falling from aircraft**
Hit by crashing aircraft
Injured by aircraft hitting house
Injured by aircraft hitting car
√x7th **V97.32 Injured by rotating propeller**
√x7th **V97.33 Sucked into jet engine**
√x7th **V97.39 Other injury to person on ground due to air transport accident**
√5th **V97.8 Other air transport accidents, not elsewhere classified**
EXCLUDES 1 *aircraft accident NOS (V95.9)*
exposure to changes in air pressure during ascent or descent (W94.-)
√6th **V97.81 Air transport accident involving military aircraft**
√7th **V97.810 Civilian aircraft involved in air transport accident with military aircraft**
Passenger in civilian aircraft injured due to accident with military aircraft
√7th **V97.811 Civilian injured by military aircraft**
√7th **V97.818 Other air transport accident involving military aircraft**
√x7th **V97.89 Other air transport accidents, not elsewhere classified**
Injury from machinery on aircraft

Other and unspecified transport accidents (V98-V99)

EXCLUDES 1 *vehicle accident, type of vehicle unspecified (V89.-)*

√4th **V98 Other specified transport accidents**

The appropriate 7th character is to be added to each code from category V98.
A initial encounter
D subsequent encounter
S sequela

√x7th **V98.0 Accident to, on or involving cable-car, not on rails**
Caught or dragged by cable-car, not on rails
Fall or jump from cable-car, not on rails
Object thrown from or in cable-car, not on rails
√x7th **V98.1 Accident to, on or involving land-yacht**
√x7th **V98.2 Accident to, on or involving ice yacht**
√x7th **V98.3 Accident to, on or involving ski lift**
Accident to, on or involving ski chair-lift
Accident to, on or involving ski-lift with gondola
√x7th **V98.8 Other specified transport accidents**

√x7th **V99 Unspecified transport accident**

The appropriate 7th character is to be added to code V99.
A initial encounter
D subsequent encounter
S sequela

OTHER EXTERNAL CAUSES OF ACCIDENTAL INJURY (W00-X58)

Slipping, tripping, stumbling and falls (W00-W19)

EXCLUDES 1 *assault involving a fall (Y01-Y02)*
fall (in) (from):
animal (V80.-)
machinery (in operation) (W28-W31)
transport vehicle (V01-V99)
intentional self-harm involving a fall (X80-X81)
EXCLUDES 2 *at risk for fall (history of fall) Z91.81*
fall (in) (from):
burning building (X00-.)
into fire (X00-X04, X08-X09)

√4th **W00 Fall due to ice and snow**
INCLUDES pedestrian on foot falling (slipping) on ice and snow
EXCLUDES 1 *fall on (from) ice and snow involving pedestrian conveyance (V00.-)*
fall from stairs and steps not due to ice and snow (W10.-)

The appropriate 7th character is to be added to each code from category W00.
A initial encounter
D subsequent encounter
S sequela

√x7th **W00.0 Fall on same level due to ice and snow**
√x7th **W00.1 Fall from stairs and steps due to ice and snow**
√x7th **W00.2 Other fall from one level to another due to ice and snow**
√x7th **W00.9 Unspecified fall due to ice and snow**

√4th **W01 Fall on same level from slipping, tripping and stumbling**
INCLUDES fall on moving sidewalk
EXCLUDES 1 *fall due to bumping (striking) against object (W18.0-)*
fall in shower or bathtub (W18.2-)
fall on same level NOS (W18.30)
fall on same level from slipping, tripping and stumbling due to ice or snow (W00.0)
fall off or from toilet (W18.1-)
slipping, tripping and stumbling NOS (W18.40)
slipping, tripping and stumbling without falling (W18.4-)

The appropriate 7th character is to be added to each code from category W01.
A initial encounter
D subsequent encounter
S sequela

√x7th **W01.0 Fall on same level from slipping, tripping and stumbling without subsequent striking against object**
Falling over animal
√5th **W01.1 Fall on same level from slipping, tripping and stumbling with subsequent striking against object**
√x7th **W01.10 Fall on same level from slipping, tripping and stumbling with subsequent striking against unspecified object**
√6th **W01.11 Fall on same level from slipping, tripping and stumbling with subsequent striking against sharp object**
√7th **W01.110 Fall on same level from slipping, tripping and stumbling with subsequent striking against sharp glass**
√7th **W01.111 Fall on same level from slipping, tripping and stumbling with subsequent striking against power tool or machine**
√7th **W01.118 Fall on same level from slipping, tripping and stumbling with subsequent striking against other sharp object**
√7th **W01.119 Fall on same level from slipping, tripping and stumbling with subsequent striking against unspecified sharp object**

W01.19 Fall on same level from slipping, tripping and stumbling with subsequent striking against other object

W01.190 Fall on same level from slipping, tripping and stumbling with subsequent striking against furniture

W01.198 Fall on same level from slipping, tripping and stumbling with subsequent striking against other object

W03 Other fall on same level due to collision with another person

Fall due to non-transport collision with other person

EXCLUDES 1 *collision with another person without fall (W51)*
crushed or pushed by a crowd or human stampede (W52)
fall involving pedestrian conveyance (V00-V09)
fall due to ice or snow (W00)
fall on same level NOS (W18.30)

The appropriate 7th character is to be added to code W03.
A initial encounter
D subsequent encounter
S sequela

W04 Fall while being carried or supported by other persons

Accidentally dropped while being carried

The appropriate 7th character is to be added to code W04.
A initial encounter
D subsequent encounter
S sequela

W05 Fall from non-moving wheelchair, nonmotorized scooter and motorized mobility scooter

EXCLUDES 1 *fall from moving wheelchair (powered) (V00.811)*
fall from moving motorized mobility scooter (V00.831)
fall from nonmotorized scooter (V00.141)

The appropriate 7th character is to be added to each code from category W05.
A initial encounter
D subsequent encounter
S sequela

W05.0 Fall from non-moving wheelchair

W05.1 Fall from non-moving nonmotorized scooter

W05.2 Fall from non-moving motorized mobility scooter

W06 Fall from bed

The appropriate 7th character is to be added to code W06.
A initial encounter
D subsequent encounter
S sequela

W07 Fall from chair

The appropriate 7th character is to be added to code W07.
A initial encounter
D subsequent encounter
S sequela

W08 Fall from other furniture

The appropriate 7th character is to be added to code W08.
A initial encounter
D subsequent encounter
S sequela

W09 Fall on and from playground equipment

EXCLUDES 1 *fall involving recreational machinery (W31)*

The appropriate 7th character is to be added to each code from category W09.
A initial encounter
D subsequent encounter
S sequela

W09.0 Fall on or from playground slide

W09.1 Fall from playground swing

W09.2 Fall on or from jungle gym

W09.8 Fall on or from other playground equipment

W10 Fall on and from stairs and steps

EXCLUDES 1 *Fall from stairs and steps due to ice and snow (W00.1)*

The appropriate 7th character is to be added to each code from category W10.
A initial encounter
D subsequent encounter
S sequela

W10.0 Fall (on)(from) escalator

W10.1 Fall (on)(from) sidewalk curb

W10.2 Fall (on)(from) incline

Fall (on) (from) ramp

W10.8 Fall (on) (from) other stairs and steps

W10.9 Fall (on) (from) unspecified stairs and steps

W11 Fall on and from ladder

The appropriate 7th character is to be added code W11.
A initial encounter
D subsequent encounter
S sequela

W12 Fall on and from scaffolding

The appropriate 7th character is to be added code W12.
A initial encounter
D subsequent encounter
S sequela

W13 Fall from, out of or through building or structure

The appropriate 7th character is to be added to each code from category W13.
A initial encounter
D subsequent encounter
S sequela

W13.0 Fall from, out of or through balcony

Fall from, out of or through railing

W13.1 Fall from, out of or through bridge

W13.2 Fall from, out of or through roof

W13.3 Fall through floor

W13.4 Fall from, out of or through window

EXCLUDES 2 *fall with subsequent striking against sharp glass (W01.110)*

W13.8 Fall from, out of or through other building or structure

Fall from, out of or through viaduct
Fall from, out of or through wall
Fall from, out of or through flag-pole

W13.9 Fall from, out of or through building, not otherwise specified

EXCLUDES 1 *collapse of a building or structure (W20.-)*
fall or jump from burning building or structure (X00.-)

W14 Fall from tree

The appropriate 7th character is to be added to code W14.
A initial encounter
D subsequent encounter
S sequela

W15 Fall from cliff

The appropriate 7th character is to be added to code W15.
A initial encounter
D subsequent encounter
S sequela

W16 Fall, jump or diving into water
EXCLUDES 1 *accidental non-watercraft drowning and submersion not involving fall (W65-W74)*
effects of air pressure from diving (W94.-)
fall into water from watercraft (V90-V94)
hitting an object or against bottom when falling from watercraft (V94.0)
EXCLUDES 2 *striking or hitting diving board (W21.3)*

The appropriate 7th character is to be added to each code from category W16.
A initial encounter
D subsequent encounter
S sequela

W16.0 Fall into swimming pool
Fall into swimming pool NOS
EXCLUDES 1 *fall into empty swimming pool (W17.3)*
W16.01 Fall into swimming pool striking water surface
W16.011 Fall into swimming pool striking water surface causing drowning and submersion
EXCLUDES 1 *drowning and submersion while in swimming pool without fall (W67)*
W16.012 Fall into swimming pool striking water surface causing other injury
W16.02 Fall into swimming pool striking bottom
W16.021 Fall into swimming pool striking bottom causing drowning and submersion
EXCLUDES 1 *drowning and submersion while in swimming pool without fall (W67)*
W16.022 Fall into swimming pool striking bottom causing other injury
W16.03 Fall into swimming pool striking wall
W16.031 Fall into swimming pool striking wall causing drowning and submersion
EXCLUDES 1 *drowning and submersion while in swimming pool without fall (W67)*
W16.032 Fall into swimming pool striking wall causing other injury
W16.1 Fall into natural body of water
Fall into lake
Fall into open sea
Fall into river
Fall into stream
W16.11 Fall into natural body of water striking water surface
W16.111 Fall into natural body of water striking water surface causing drowning and submersion
EXCLUDES 1 *drowning and submersion while in natural body of water without fall (W69)*
W16.112 Fall into natural body of water striking water surface causing other injury
W16.12 Fall into natural body of water striking bottom
W16.121 Fall into natural body of water striking bottom causing drowning and submersion
EXCLUDES 1 *drowning and submersion while in natural body of water without fall (W69)*
W16.122 Fall into natural body of water striking bottom causing other injury
W16.13 Fall into natural body of water striking side
W16.131 Fall into natural body of water striking side causing drowning and submersion
EXCLUDES 1 *drowning and submersion while in natural body of water without fall (W69)*
W16.132 Fall into natural body of water striking side causing other injury
W16.2 Fall in (into) filled bathtub or bucket of water
W16.21 Fall in (into) filled bathtub
EXCLUDES 1 *fall into empty bathtub (W18.2)*
W16.211 Fall in (into) filled bathtub causing drowning and submersion
EXCLUDES 1 *drowning and submersion while in filled bathtub without fall (W65)*
W16.212 Fall in (into) filled bathtub causing other injury
W16.22 Fall in (into) bucket of water
W16.221 Fall in (into) bucket of water causing drowning and submersion
W16.222 Fall in (into) bucket of water causing other injury
W16.3 Fall into other water
Fall into fountain
Fall into reservoir
W16.31 Fall into other water striking water surface
W16.311 Fall into other water striking water surface causing drowning and submersion
EXCLUDES 1 *drowning and submersion while in other water without fall (W73)*
W16.312 Fall into other water striking water surface causing other injury
W16.32 Fall into other water striking bottom
W16.321 Fall into other water striking bottom causing drowning and submersion
EXCLUDES 1 *drowning and submersion while in other water without fall (W73)*
W16.322 Fall into other water striking bottom causing other injury
W16.33 Fall into other water striking wall
W16.331 Fall into other water striking wall causing drowning and submersion
EXCLUDES 1 *drowning and submersion while in other water without fall (W73)*
W16.332 Fall into other water striking wall causing other injury
W16.4 Fall into unspecified water
W16.41 Fall into unspecified water causing drowning and submersion
W16.42 Fall into unspecified water causing other injury
W16.5 Jumping or diving into swimming pool
W16.51 Jumping or diving into swimming pool striking water surface
W16.511 Jumping or diving into swimming pool striking water surface causing drowning and submersion
EXCLUDES 1 *drowning and submersion while in swimming pool without jumping or diving (W67)*
W16.512 Jumping or diving into swimming pool striking water surface causing other injury
W16.52 Jumping or diving into swimming pool striking bottom
W16.521 Jumping or diving into swimming pool striking bottom causing drowning and submersion
EXCLUDES 1 *drowning and submersion while in swimming pool without jumping or diving (W67)*
W16.522 Jumping or diving into swimming pool striking bottom causing other injury
W16.53 Jumping or diving into swimming pool striking wall
W16.531 Jumping or diving into swimming pool striking wall causing drowning and submersion
EXCLUDES 1 *drowning and submersion while in swimming pool without jumping or diving (W67)*
W16.532 Jumping or diving into swimming pool striking wall causing other injury

✓5th **W16.6 Jumping or diving into natural body of water**
Jumping or diving into lake
Jumping or diving into open sea
Jumping or diving into river
Jumping or diving into stream

✓6th **W16.61 Jumping or diving into natural body of water striking water surface**

✓7th **W16.611 Jumping or diving into natural body of water striking water surface causing drowning and submersion**
EXCLUDES 1 *drowning and submersion while in natural body of water without jumping or diving (W69)*

✓7th **W16.612 Jumping or diving into natural body of water striking water surface causing other injury**

✓6th **W16.62 Jumping or diving into natural body of water striking bottom**

✓7th **W16.621 Jumping or diving into natural body of water striking bottom causing drowning and submersion**
EXCLUDES 1 *drowning and submersion while in natural body of water without jumping or diving (W69)*

✓7th **W16.622 Jumping or diving into natural body of water striking bottom causing other injury**

✓5th **W16.7 Jumping or diving from boat**
EXCLUDES 1 *Fall from boat into water—see watercraft accident (V90-V94)*

✓6th **W16.71 Jumping or diving from boat striking water surface**

✓7th **W16.711 Jumping or diving from boat striking water surface causing drowning and submersion**

✓7th **W16.712 Jumping or diving from boat striking water surface causing other injury**

✓6th **W16.72 Jumping or diving from boat striking bottom**

✓7th **W16.721 Jumping or diving from boat striking bottom causing drowning and submersion**

✓7th **W16.722 Jumping or diving from boat striking bottom causing other injury**

✓5th **W16.8 Jumping or diving into other water**
Jumping or diving into fountain
Jumping or diving into reservoir

✓6th **W16.81 Jumping or diving into other water striking water surface**

✓7th **W16.811 Jumping or diving into other water striking water surface causing drowning and submersion**
EXCLUDES 1 *drowning and submersion while in other water without jumping or diving (W73)*

✓7th **W16.812 Jumping or diving into other water striking water surface causing other injury**

✓6th **W16.82 Jumping or diving into other water striking bottom**

✓7th **W16.821 Jumping or diving into other water striking bottom causing drowning and submersion**
EXCLUDES 1 *drowning and submersion while in other water without jumping or diving (W73)*

✓7th **W16.822 Jumping or diving into other water striking bottom causing other injury**

✓6th **W16.83 Jumping or diving into other water striking wall**

✓7th **W16.831 Jumping or diving into other water striking wall causing drowning and submersion**
EXCLUDES 1 *drowning and submersion while in other water without jumping or diving (W73)*

✓7th **W16.832 Jumping or diving into other water striking wall causing other injury**

✓5th **W16.9 Jumping or diving into unspecified water**

✓x7th **W16.91 Jumping or diving into unspecified water causing drowning and submersion**

✓x7th **W16.92 Jumping or diving into unspecified water causing other injury**

✓4th **W17 Other fall from one level to another**

The appropriate 7th character is to be added to each code from category W17.
A initial encounter
D subsequent encounter
S sequela

✓x7th **W17.0 Fall into well**

✓x7th **W17.1 Fall into storm drain or manhole**

✓x7th **W17.2 Fall into hole**
Fall into pit

✓x7th **W17.3 Fall into empty swimming pool**
EXCLUDES 1 *fall into filled swimming pool (W16.0-)*

✓x7th **W17.4 Fall from dock**

✓5th **W17.8 Other fall from one level to another**

✓x7th **W17.81 Fall down embankment (hill)**

✓x7th **W17.82 Fall from (out of) grocery cart**
Fall due to grocery cart tipping over

✓x7th **W17.89 Other fall from one level to another**
Fall from cherry picker
Fall from lifting device
Fall from mobile elevated work platform [MEWP]
Fall from sky lift

✓4th **W18 Other slipping, tripping and stumbling and falls**

The appropriate 7th character is to be added to each code from category W18.
A initial encounter
D subsequent encounter
S sequela

✓5th **W18.0 Fall due to bumping against object**
Striking against object with subsequent fall
EXCLUDES 1 *fall on same level due to slipping, tripping, or stumbling with subsequent striking against object (W01.1-)*

✓x7th **W18.00 Striking against unspecified object with subsequent fall**

✓x7th **W18.01 Striking against sports equipment with subsequent fall**

✓x7th **W18.02 Striking against glass with subsequent fall**

✓x7th **W18.09 Striking against other object with subsequent fall**

✓5th **W18.1 Fall from or off toilet**

✓x7th **W18.11 Fall from or off toilet without subsequent striking against object**
Fall from (off) toilet NOS

✓x7th **W18.12 Fall from or off toilet with subsequent striking against object**

✓x7th **W18.2 Fall in (into) shower or empty bathtub**
EXCLUDES 1 *fall in full bathtub causing drowning or submersion (W16.21-)*

✓5th **W18.3 Other and unspecified fall on same level**

✓x7th **W18.30 Fall on same level, unspecified**

✓x7th **W18.31 Fall on same level due to stepping on an object**
Fall on same level due to stepping on an animal
EXCLUDES 1 *slipping, tripping and stumbling without fall due to stepping on animal (W18.41)*

✓x7th **W18.39 Other fall on same level**

✓5th **W18.4 Slipping, tripping and stumbling without falling**
EXCLUDES 1 *collision with another person without fall (W51)*

✓x7th **W18.40 Slipping, tripping and stumbling without falling, unspecified**

✓x7th **W18.41 Slipping, tripping and stumbling without falling due to stepping on object**
Slipping, tripping and stumbling without falling due to stepping on animal
EXCLUDES 1 *slipping, tripping and stumbling with fall due to stepping on animal (W18.31)*

✓x7th **W18.42 Slipping, tripping and stumbling without falling due to stepping into hole or opening**

W18.43 Slipping, tripping and stumbling without falling due to stepping from one level to another

W18.49 Other slipping, tripping and stumbling without falling

W19 Unspecified fall
Accidental fall NOS

The appropriate 7th character is to be added to code W19.
A initial encounter
D subsequent encounter
S sequela

Exposure to inanimate mechanical forces (W20-W49)

EXCLUDES 1 *assault (X91-Y08)*
contact or collision with animals or persons (W50-W64)
exposure to inanimate mechanical forces involving military or war operations (Y36-, Y37-)
intentional self-harm (X70-X83)

W20 Struck by thrown, projected or falling object
Code first any associated:
cataclysm (X34-X39)
lightning strike (T75.00)
EXCLUDES 1 *falling object in:*
machinery accident (W24, W28-W31)
transport accident (V01-V99)
object set in motion by:
explosion (W35-W40)
firearm (W32-W34)
struck by thrown sports equipment (W21.-)

The appropriate 7th character is to be added to each code from category W20.
A initial encounter
D subsequent encounter
S sequela

W20.0 Struck by falling object in cave-in
EXCLUDES 2 *asphyxiation due to cave-in (T71.21)*

W20.1 Struck by object due to collapse of building
EXCLUDES 1 *struck by object due to collapse of burning building (X00.2, X02.2)*

W20.8 Other cause of strike by thrown, projected or falling object
EXCLUDES 1 *struck by thrown sports equipment (W21.-)*

W21 Striking against or struck by sports equipment
EXCLUDES 1 *assault with sports equipment (Y08.0-)*
striking against or struck by sports equipment with subsequent fall (W18.01)

The appropriate 7th character is to be added to each code from category W21.
A initial encounter
D subsequent encounter
S sequela

W21.0 Struck by hit or thrown ball
W21.00 Struck by hit or thrown ball, unspecified type
W21.01 Struck by football
W21.02 Struck by soccer ball
W21.03 Struck by baseball
W21.04 Struck by golf ball
W21.05 Struck by basketball
W21.06 Struck by volleyball
W21.07 Struck by softball
W21.09 Struck by other hit or thrown ball

W21.1 Struck by bat, racquet or club
W21.11 Struck by baseball bat
W21.12 Struck by tennis racquet
W21.13 Struck by golf club
W21.19 Struck by other bat, racquet or club

W21.2 Struck by hockey stick or puck
W21.21 Struck by hockey stick
W21.210 Struck by ice hockey stick
W21.211 Struck by field hockey stick
W21.22 Struck by hockey puck
W21.220 Struck by ice hockey puck
W21.221 Struck by field hockey puck

W21.3 Struck by sports foot wear
W21.31 Struck by shoe cleats
Stepped on by shoe cleats
W21.32 Struck by skate blades
Skated over by skate blades
W21.39 Struck by other sports foot wear

W21.4 Striking against diving board
Use additional code for subsequent falling into water, if applicable (W16.-)

W21.8 Striking against or struck by other sports equipment
W21.81 Striking against or struck by football helmet
W21.89 Striking against or struck by other sports equipment

W21.9 Striking against or struck by unspecified sports equipment

W22 Striking against or struck by other objects
EXCLUDES 1 *striking against or struck by object with subsequent fall (W18.09)*

The appropriate 7th character is to be added to each code from category W22.
A initial encounter
D subsequent encounter
S sequela

W22.0 Striking against stationary object
EXCLUDES 1 *striking against stationary sports equipment (W21.8)*
W22.01 Walked into wall
W22.02 Walked into lamppost
W22.03 Walked into furniture
W22.04 Striking against wall of swimming pool
W22.041 Striking against wall of swimming pool causing drowning and submersion
EXCLUDES 1 *drowning and submersion while swimming without striking against wall (W67)*
W22.042 Striking against wall of swimming pool causing other injury
W22.09 Striking against other stationary object

W22.1 Striking against or struck by automobile airbag
W22.10 Striking against or struck by unspecified automobile airbag
W22.11 Striking against or struck by driver side automobile airbag
W22.12 Striking against or struck by front passenger side automobile airbag
W22.19 Striking against or struck by other automobile airbag

W22.8 Striking against or struck by other objects
Striking against or struck by object NOS
EXCLUDES 1 *struck by thrown, projected or falling object (W20.-)*

W23 Caught, crushed, jammed or pinched in or between objects
EXCLUDES 1 *injury caused by cutting or piercing instruments (W25-W27)*
injury caused by firearms malfunction (W32.1, W33.1-, W34.1-)
injury caused by lifting and transmission devices (W24.-)
injury caused by machinery (W28-W31)
injury caused by nonpowered hand tools (W27.-)
injury caused by transport vehicle being used as a means of transportation (V01-V99)
injury caused by struck by thrown, projected or falling object (W20.-)

The appropriate 7th character is to be added to each code from category W23.
A initial encounter
D subsequent encounter
S sequela

W23.0 Caught, crushed, jammed, or pinched between moving objects

W23.1 Caught, crushed, jammed, or pinched between stationary objects

Appropriate additional character required
Requires 7th character, placeholder x must fill empty characters

✓4th **W24 Contact with lifting and transmission devices, not elsewhere classified**

EXCLUDES 1 *transport accidents (V01-V99)*

The appropriate 7th character is to be added to each code from category W24.
A initial encounter
D subsequent encounter
S sequela

✓x7th **W24.0 Contact with lifting devices, not elsewhere classified**
Contact with chain hoist
Contact with drive belt
Contact with pulley (block)

✓x7th **W24.1 Contact with transmission devices, not elsewhere classified**
Contact with transmission belt or cable

✓x7th **W25 Contact with sharp glass**
Code first any associated:
injury due to flying glass from explosion or firearm discharge (W32-W40)
transport accident (V00-V99)

EXCLUDES 1 *fall on same level due to slipping, tripping and stumbling with subsequent striking against sharp glass (W01.10)*
striking against sharp glass with subsequent fall (W18.02)

The appropriate 7th character is to be added to code W25.
A initial encounter
D subsequent encounter
S sequela

✓4th **W26 Contact with knife, sword or dagger**

The appropriate 7th character is to be added to each code from category W26.
A initial encounter
D subsequent encounter
S sequela

✓x7th **W26.0 Contact with knife**
EXCLUDES 1 *contact with electric knife (W29.1)*

✓x7th **W26.1 Contact with sword or dagger**

✓4th **W27 Contact with nonpowered hand tool**

The appropriate 7th character is to be added to each code from category W27.
A initial encounter
D subsequent encounter
S sequela

✓x7th **W27.0 Contact with workbench tool**
Contact with auger
Contact with axe
Contact with chisel
Contact with handsaw
Contact with screwdriver

✓x7th **W27.1 Contact with garden tool**
Contact with hoe
Contact with nonpowered lawn mower
Contact with pitchfork
Contact with rake

✓x7th **W27.2 Contact with scissors**

✓x7th **W27.3 Contact with needle (sewing)**
EXCLUDES 1 *contact with hypodermic needle (W46.-)*

✓x7th **W27.4 Contact with kitchen utensil**
Contact with fork
Contact with ice-pick
Contact with can-opener NOS

✓x7th **W27.5 Contact with paper-cutter**

✓x7th **W27.8 Contact with other nonpowered hand tool**
Contact with nonpowered sewing machine
Contact with shovel

✓x7th **W28 Contact with powered lawn mower**
Powered lawn mower (commercial) (residential)

EXCLUDES 1 *contact with nonpowered lawn mower (W27.1)*
EXCLUDES 2 *exposure to electric current (W86.-)*

The appropriate 7th character is to be added to code W28.
A initial encounter
D subsequent encounter
S sequela

✓4th **W29 Contact with other powered hand tools and household machinery**

EXCLUDES 1 *contact with commercial machinery (W31.82)*
contact with hot household appliance (X15)
contact with nonpowered hand tool (W27.-)
exposure to electric current (W86)

The appropriate 7th character is to be added to each code from category W29.
A initial encounter
D subsequent encounter
S sequela

✓x7th **W29.0 Contact with powered kitchen appliance**
Contact with blender
Contact with can-opener
Contact with garbage disposal
Contact with mixer

✓x7th **W29.1 Contact with electric knife**

✓x7th **W29.2 Contact with other powered household machinery**
Contact with electric fan
Contact with powered dryer (clothes) (powered) (spin)
Contact with washing-machine
Contact with sewing machine

✓x7th **W29.3 Contact with powered garden and outdoor hand tools and machinery**
Contact with chainsaw
Contact with edger
Contact with garden cultivator (tiller)
Contact with hedge trimmer
Contact with other powered garden tool
EXCLUDES 1 *contact with powered lawn mower (W28)*

✓x7th **W29.4 Contact with nail gun**

✓x7th **W29.8 Contact with other powered powered hand tools and household machinery**
Contact with do-it-yourself tool NOS

✓4th **W30 Contact with agricultural machinery**

INCLUDES animal-powered farm machine
EXCLUDES 1 *agricultural transport vehicle accident (V01-V99)*
explosion of grain store (W40.8)
exposure to electric current (W86.-)

The appropriate 7th character is to be added to each code from category W30.
A initial encounter
D subsequent encounter
S sequela

✓x7th **W30.0 Contact with combine harvester**
Contact with reaper
Contact with thresher

✓x7th **W30.1 Contact with power take-off devices (PTO)**

✓x7th **W30.2 Contact with hay derrick**

✓x7th **W30.3 Contact with grain storage elevator**
EXCLUDES 1 *explosion of grain store (W40.8)*

✓5th **W30.8 Contact with other specified agricultural machinery**

✓x7th **W30.81 Contact with agricultural transport vehicle in stationary use**
Contact with agricultural transport vehicle under repair, not on public roadway
EXCLUDES 1 *agricultural transport vehicle accident (V01-V99)*

✓x7th **W30.89 Contact with other specified agricultural machinery**

✓x7th **W30.9 Contact with unspecified agricultural machinery**
Contact with farm machinery NOS

✓4th **W31 Contact with other and unspecified machinery**

EXCLUDES 1 *contact with agricultural machinery (W30.-)*
contact with machinery in transport under own power or being towed by a vehicle (V01-V99)
exposure to electric current (W86)

The appropriate 7th character is to be added to each code from category W31.
A initial encounter
D subsequent encounter
S sequela

W31.0 Contact with mining and earth-drilling machinery
Contact with bore or drill (land) (seabed)
Contact with shaft hoist
Contact with shaft lift
Contact with undercutter

W31.1 Contact with metalworking machines
Contact with abrasive wheel
Contact with forging machine
Contact with lathe
Contact with mechanical shears
Contact with metal drilling machine
Contact with milling machine
Contact with power press
Contact with rolling-mill
Contact with metal sawing machine

W31.2 Contact with powered woodworking and forming machines
Contact with band saw
Contact with bench saw
Contact with circular saw
Contact with molding machine
Contact with overhead plane
Contact with powered saw
Contact with radial saw
Contact with sander
EXCLUDES 1 *nonpowered woodworking tools (W27.0)*

W31.3 Contact with prime movers
Contact with gas turbine
Contact with internal combustion engine
Contact with steam engine
Contact with water driven turbine

W31.8 Contact with other specified machinery

W31.81 Contact with recreational machinery
Contact with roller coaster

W31.82 Contact with other commercial machinery
Contact with commercial electric fan
Contact with commercial kitchen appliances
Contact with commercial powered dryer (clothes) (powered) (spin)
Contact with commercial washing-machine
Contact with commercial sewing machine
EXCLUDES 1 *contact with household machinery (W29.-)*
contact with powered lawn mower (W28)

W31.83 Contact with special construction vehicle in stationary use
Contact with special construction vehicle under repair, not on public roadway
EXCLUDES 1 *special construction vehicle accident (V01-V99)*

W31.89 Contact with other specified machinery

W31.9 Contact with unspecified machinery
Contact with machinery NOS

W32 Accidental handgun discharge and malfunction
INCLUDES Accidental discharge and malfunction of gun for single hand use
Accidental discharge and malfunction of pistol
Accidental discharge and malfunction of revolver
Handgun discharge and malfunction NOS
EXCLUDES 1 *accidental airgun discharge and malfunction (W34.010, W34.110)*
accidental BB gun discharge and malfunction (W34.010, W34.110)
accidental pellet gun discharge and malfunction (W34.010, W34.110)
accidental shotgun discharge and malfunction (W33.01, W33.11)
assault by handgun discharge (X93)
handgun discharge involving legal intervention (Y35.0-)
handgun discharge involving military or war operations (Y36.4-)
intentional self-harm by handgun discharge (X72)
Very pistol discharge and malfunction (W34.09, W34.19)

The appropriate 7th character is to be added to each code from category W32.
A initial encounter
D subsequent encounter
S sequela

W32.0 Accidental handgun discharge

W32.1 Accidental handgun malfunction
Injury due to explosion of handgun (parts)
Injury due to malfunction of mechanism or component of handgun
Injury due to recoil of handgun
Powder burn from handgun

W33 Accidental rifle, shotgun and larger firearm discharge and malfunction
INCLUDES rifle, shotgun and larger firearm discharge and malfunction NOS
EXCLUDES 1 *accidental airgun discharge and malfunction (W34.010, W34.110)*
accidental BB gun discharge and malfunction (W34.010, W34.110)
accidental handgun discharge and malfunction (W32.-)
accidental pellet gun discharge and malfunction (W34.010, W34.110)
assault by rifle, shotgun and larger firearm discharge (X94)
firearm discharge involving legal intervention (Y35.0-)
firearm discharge involving military or war operations (Y36.4-)
intentional self-harm by rifle, shotgun and larger firearm discharge (X73)

The appropriate 7th character is to be added to each code from category W33.
A initial encounter
D subsequent encounter
S sequela

W33.0 Accidental rifle, shotgun and larger firearm discharge

W33.00 Accidental discharge of unspecified larger firearm
Discharge of unspecified larger firearm NOS

W33.01 Accidental discharge of shotgun
Discharge of shotgun NOS

W33.02 Accidental discharge of hunting rifle
Discharge of hunting rifle NOS

W33.03 Accidental discharge of machine gun
Discharge of machine gun NOS

W33.09 Accidental discharge of other larger firearm
Discharge of other larger firearm NOS

W33.1 Accidental rifle, shotgun and larger firearm malfunction
Injury due to explosion of rifle, shotgun and larger firearm (parts)
Injury due to malfunction of mechanism or component of rifle, shotgun and larger firearm
Injury due to piercing, cutting, crushing or pinching due to (by) slide trigger mechanism, scope or other gun part
Injury due to recoil of rifle, shotgun and larger firearm
Powder burn from rifle, shotgun and larger firearm

W33.10 Accidental malfunction of unspecified larger firearm
Malfunction of unspecified larger firearm NOS

W33.11 Accidental malfunction of shotgun
Malfunction of shotgun NOS

W33.12 Accidental malfunction of hunting rifle
Malfunction of hunting rifle NOS

W33.13 Accidental malfunction of machine gun
Malfunction of machine gun NOS

W33.19 Accidental malfunction of other larger firearm
Malfunction of other larger firearm NOS

W34 Accidental discharge and malfunction from other and unspecified firearms and guns

The appropriate 7th character is to be added to each code from category W34.
A initial encounter
D subsequent encounter
S sequela

W34.0 Accidental discharge from other and unspecified firearms and guns

W34.00 Accidental discharge from unspecified firearms or gun
Discharge from firearm NOS
Gunshot wound NOS
Shot NOS

W34.01 Accidental discharge of gas, air or spring-operated guns

W34.010 Accidental discharge of airgun
Accidental discharge of BB gun
Accidental discharge of pellet gun

Appropriate additional character required — Requires 7th character, placeholder x must fill empty characters

√7th **W34.011 Accidental discharge of paintball gun**
Accidental injury due to paintball discharge

√7th **W34.018 Accidental discharge of other gas, air or spring-operated gun**

√x7th **W34.09 Accidental discharge from other specified firearms**
Accidental discharge from Very pistol [flare]

√5th **W34.1 Accidental malfunction from other and unspecified firearms and guns**

√x7th **W34.10 Accidental malfunction from unspecified firearms or gun**
Firearm malfunction NOS

√6th **W34.11 Accidental malfunction of gas, air or spring-operated guns**

√7th **W34.110 Accidental malfunction of airgun**
Accidental malfunction of BB gun
Accidental malfunction of pellet gun

√7th **W34.111 Accidental malfunction of paintball gun**
Accidental injury due to paintball gun malfunction

√7th **W34.118 Accidental malfunction of other gas, air or spring-operated gun**

√x7th **W34.19 Accidental malfunction from other specified firearms**
Accidental malfunction from Very pistol [flare]

√x7th **W35 Explosion and rupture of boiler**
EXCLUDES 1 *explosion and rupture of boiler on watercraft (V93.4)*

The appropriate 7th character is to be added to code W35.
A initial encounter
D subsequent encounter
S sequela

√4th **W36 Explosion and rupture of gas cylinder**

The appropriate 7th character is to be added to each code from category W36.
A initial encounter
D subsequent encounter
S sequela

√x7th **W36.1 Explosion and rupture of aerosol can**
√x7th **W36.2 Explosion and rupture of air tank**
√x7th **W36.3 Explosion and rupture of pressurized-gas tank**
√x7th **W36.8 Explosion and rupture of other gas cylinder**
√x7th **W36.9 Explosion and rupture of unspecified gas cylinder**

√4th **W37 Explosion and rupture of pressurized tire, pipe or hose**

The appropriate 7th character is to be added to each code from category W37.
A initial encounter
D subsequent encounter
S sequela

√x7th **W37.0 Explosion of bicycle tire**
√x7th **W37.8 Explosion and rupture of other pressurized tire, pipe or hose**

√x7th **W38 Explosion and rupture of other specified pressurized devices**

The appropriate 7th character is to be added to code W38.
A initial encounter
D subsequent encounter
S sequela

√x7th **W39 Discharge of firework**

The appropriate 7th character is to be added to code W39.
A initial encounter
D subsequent encounter
S sequela

√4th **W40 Explosion of other materials**
EXCLUDES 1 *assault by explosive material (X96)*
explosion involving legal intervention (Y35.1-)
explosion involving military or war operations (Y36.0-, Y36.2-)
intentional self-harm by explosive material (X75)

The appropriate 7th character is to be added to each code from category W40.
A initial encounter
D subsequent encounter
S sequela

√x7th **W40.0 Explosion of blasting material**
Explosion of blasting cap
Explosion of detonator
Explosion of dynamite
Explosion of explosive (any) used in blasting operations

√x7th **W40.1 Explosion of explosive gases**
Explosion of acetylene
Explosion of butane
Explosion of coal gas
Explosion in mine NOS
Explosion of explosive gas
Explosion of fire damp
Explosion of gasoline fumes
Explosion of methane
Explosion of propane

√x7th **W40.8 Explosion of other specified explosive materials**
Explosion in dump NOS
Explosion in factory NOS
Explosion in grain store
Explosion in munitions
EXCLUDES 1 *explosion involving legal intervention (Y35.1-)*
explosion involving military or war operations (Y36.0-, Y36.2-)

√x7th **W40.9 Explosion of unspecified explosive materials**
Explosion NOS

√4th **W42 Exposure to noise**

The appropriate 7th character is to be added to each code from category W42.
A initial encounter
D subsequent encounter
S sequela

√x7th **W42.0 Exposure to supersonic waves**
√x7th **W42.9 Exposure to other noise**
Exposure to sound waves NOS

√4th **W45 Foreign body or object entering through skin**
EXCLUDES 2 *contact with hand tools (nonpowered) (powered) (W27-W29)*
contact with knife, sword or dagger (W26.-)
contact with sharp glass (W25.-)
struck by objects (W20-W22)

The appropriate 7th character is to be added to each code from category W45.
A initial encounter
D subsequent encounter
S sequela

√x7th **W45.0 Nail entering through skin**
√x7th **W45.1 Paper entering through skin**
Paper cut
√x7th **W45.2 Lid of can entering through skin**
√x7th **W45.8 Other foreign body or object entering through skin**
Splinter in skin NOS

√4th **W46 Contact with hypodermic needle**

The appropriate 7th character is to be added to each code from category W46.
A initial encounter
D subsequent encounter
S sequela

√x7th **W46.0 Contact with hypodermic needle**
Hypodermic needle stick NOS
√x7th **W46.1 Contact with contaminated hypodermic needle**

√4th **W49 Exposure to other inanimate mechanical forces**
INCLUDES exposure to abnormal gravitational [G] forces
exposure to inanimate mechanical forces NEC
EXCLUDES 1 *exposure to inanimate mechanical forces involving military or war operations (Y36-, Y37-)*

The appropriate 7th character is to be added to each code from category W49.
A initial encounter
D subsequent encounter
S sequela

√5th **W49.0 Item causing external constriction**
√x7th **W49.01 Hair causing external constriction**
√x7th **W49.02 String or thread causing external constriction**
√x7th **W49.03 Rubber band causing external constriction**

W49.04 Ring or other jewelry causing external constriction
W49.09 Other specified item causing external constriction
W49.9 Exposure to other inanimate mechanical forces

Exposure to animate mechanical forces (W50-W64)

EXCLUDES 1 *Toxic effect of contact with venomous animals and plants (T63.-)*

W50 Accidental hit, strike, kick, twist, bite or scratch by another person
Hit, strike, kick, twist, bite, or scratch by another person NOS
EXCLUDES 1 *assault by bodily force (Y04)*
struck by objects (W20-W22)

The appropriate 7th character is to be added to each code from category W50.
A initial encounter
D subsequent encounter
S sequela

W50.0 Accidental hit or strike by another person
Hit or strike by another person NOS
W50.1 Accidental kick by another person
Kick by another person NOS
W50.2 Accidental twist by another person
Twist by another person NOS
W50.3 Accidental bite by another person
Human bite
Bite by another person NOS
W50.4 Accidental scratch by another person
Scratch by another person NOS

W51 Accidental striking against or bumped into by another person
EXCLUDES 1 *assault by striking against or bumping into by another person (Y04.2)*
fall due to collision with another person (W03)

The appropriate 7th character is to be added to code W51.
A initial encounter
D subsequent encounter
S sequela

W52 Crushed, pushed or stepped on by crowd or human stampede
Crushed, pushed or stepped on by crowd or human stampede with or without fall

The appropriate 7th character is to be added to code W52.
A initial encounter
D subsequent encounter
S sequela

W53 Contact with rodent
Contact with saliva, feces or urine of rodent

The appropriate 7th character is to be added to each code from category W53.
A initial encounter
D subsequent encounter
S sequela

W53.0 Contact with mouse
W53.01 Bitten by mouse
W53.09 Other contact with mouse
W53.1 Contact with rat
W53.11 Bitten by rat
W53.19 Other contact with rat
W53.2 Contact with squirrel
W53.21 Bitten by squirrel
W53.29 Other contact with squirrel
W53.8 Contact with other rodent
W53.81 Bitten by other rodent
W53.89 Other contact with other rodent

W54 Contact with dog
Contact with saliva, feces or urine of dog

The appropriate 7th character is to be added to each code from category W54.
A initial encounter
D subsequent encounter
S sequela

W54.0 Bitten by dog
W54.1 Struck by dog
Knocked over by dog
W54.8 Other contact with dog

W55 Contact with other mammals
Contact with saliva, feces or urine of mammal
EXCLUDES 1 *animal being ridden—see transport accidents*
bitten or struck by dog (W54)
bitten or struck by rodent (W53.-)
contact with marine mammals (W56.X-)

The appropriate 7th character is to be added to each code from category W55.
A initial encounter
D subsequent encounter
S sequela

W55.0 Contact with cat
W55.01 Bitten by cat
W55.03 Scratched by cat
W55.09 Other contact with cat
W55.1 Contact with horse
W55.11 Bitten by horse
W55.12 Struck by horse
W55.19 Other contact with horse
W55.2 Contact with cow
Contact with bull
W55.21 Bitten by cow
W55.22 Struck by cow
Gored by bull
W55.29 Other contact with cow
W55.3 Contact with other hoof stock
Contact with goats
Contact with sheep
W55.31 Bitten by other hoof stock
W55.32 Struck by other hoof stock
Gored by goat
Gored by ram
W55.39 Other contact with other hoof stock
W55.4 Contact with pig
W55.41 Bitten by pig
W55.42 Struck by pig
W55.49 Other contact with pig
W55.5 Contact with raccoon
W55.51 Bitten by raccoon
W55.52 Struck by raccoon
W55.59 Other contact with raccoon
W55.8 Contact with other mammals
W55.81 Bitten by other mammals
W55.82 Struck by other mammals
W55.89 Other contact with other mammals

W56 Contact with nonvenomous marine animal
EXCLUDES 1 *contact with venomous marine animal (T63.-)*

The appropriate 7th character is to be added to each code from category W56.
A initial encounter
D subsequent encounter
S sequela

W56.0 Contact with dolphin
W56.01 Bitten by dolphin
W56.02 Struck by dolphin
W56.09 Other contact with dolphin
W56.1 Contact with sea lion
W56.11 Bitten by sea lion
W56.12 Struck by sea lion
W56.19 Other contact with sea lion
W56.2 Contact with orca
Contact with killer whale
W56.21 Bitten by orca
W56.22 Struck by orca
W56.29 Other contact with orca
W56.3 Contact with other marine mammals
W56.31 Bitten by other marine mammals
W56.32 Struck by other marine mammals
W56.39 Other contact with other marine mammals
W56.4 Contact with shark
W56.41 Bitten by shark
W56.42 Struck by shark

√x7th **W56.49 Other contact with shark**

√5th **W56.5 Contact with other fish**

√x7th **W56.51 Bitten by other fish**

√x7th **W56.52 Struck by other fish**

√x7th **W56.59 Other contact with other fish**

√5th **W56.8 Contact with other nonvenomous marine animals**

√x7th **W56.81 Bitten by other nonvenomous marine animals**

√x7th **W56.82 Struck by other nonvenomous marine animals**

√x7th **W56.89 Other contact with other nonvenomous marine animals**

√x7th **W57 Bitten or stung by nonvenomous insect and other nonvenomous arthropods**

EXCLUDES 1 *contact with venomous insects and arthropods (T63.2-, T63.3-, T63.4-)*

The appropriate 7th character is to be added to code W57.
A initial encounter
D subsequent encounter
S sequela

√4th **W58 Contact with crocodile or alligator**

The appropriate 7th character is to be added to each code from category W58.
A initial encounter
D subsequent encounter
S sequela

√5th **W58.0 Contact with alligator**

√x7th **W58.01 Bitten by alligator**

√x7th **W58.02 Struck by alligator**

√x7th **W58.03 Crushed by alligator**

√x7th **W58.09 Other contact with alligator**

√5th **W58.1 Contact with crocodile**

√x7th **W58.11 Bitten by crocodile**

√x7th **W58.12 Struck by crocodile**

√x7th **W58.13 Crushed by crocodile**

√x7th **W58.19 Other contact with crocodile**

√4th **W59 Contact with other nonvenomous reptiles**

EXCLUDES 1 *contact with venomous reptile (T63.0-, T63.1-)*

The appropriate 7th character is to be added to each code from category W59.
A initial encounter
D subsequent encounter
S sequela

√5th **W59.0 Contact with nonvenomous lizards**

√x7th **W59.01 Bitten by nonvenomous lizards**

√x7th **W59.02 Struck by nonvenomous lizards**

√x7th **W59.09 Other contact with nonvenomous lizards**
Exposure to nonvenomous lizards

√5th **W59.1 Contact with nonvenomous snakes**

√x7th **W59.11 Bitten by nonvenomous snake**

√x7th **W59.12 Struck by nonvenomous snake**

√x7th **W59.13 Crushed by nonvenomous snake**

√x7th **W59.19 Other contact with nonvenomous snake**

√5th **W59.2 Contact with turtles**

EXCLUDES 1 *contact with tortoises (W59.8-)*

√x7th **W59.21 Bitten by turtle**

√x7th **W59.22 Struck by turtle**

√x7th **W59.29 Other contact with turtle**
Exposure to turtles

√5th **W59.8 Contact with other nonvenomous reptiles**

√x7th **W59.81 Bitten by other nonvenomous reptiles**

√x7th **W59.82 Struck by other nonvenomous reptiles**

√x7th **W59.83 Crushed by other nonvenomous reptiles**

√x7th **W59.89 Other contact with other nonvenomous reptiles**

√x7th **W60 Contact with nonvenomous plant thorns and spines and sharp leaves**

EXCLUDES 1 *contact with venomous plants (T63.X-)*

The appropriate 7th character is to be added to code W60.
A initial encounter
D subsequent encounter
S sequela

√4th **W61 Contact with birds (domestic) (wild)**
Contact with excreta of birds

The appropriate 7th character is to be added to each code from category W61.
A initial encounter
D subsequent encounter
S sequela

√5th **W61.0 Contact with parrot**

√x7th **W61.01 Bitten by parrot**

√x7th **W61.02 Struck by parrot**

√x7th **W61.09 Other contact with parrot**
Exposure to parrots

√5th **W61.1 Contact with macaw**

√x7th **W61.11 Bitten by macaw**

√x7th **W61.12 Struck by macaw**

√x7th **W61.19 Other contact with macaw**
Exposure to macaws

√5th **W61.2 Contact with other psittacines**

√x7th **W61.21 Bitten by other psittacines**

√x7th **W61.22 Struck by other psittacines**

√x7th **W61.29 Other contact with other psittacines**
Exposure to other psittacines

√5th **W61.3 Contact with chicken**

√x7th **W61.32 Struck by chicken**

√x7th **W61.33 Pecked by chicken**

√x7th **W61.39 Other contact with chicken**
Exposure to chickens

√5th **W61.4 Contact with turkey**

√x7th **W61.42 Struck by turkey**

√x7th **W61.43 Pecked by turkey**

√x7th **W61.49 Other contact with turkey**

√5th **W61.5 Contact with goose**

√x7th **W61.51 Bitten by goose**

√x7th **W61.52 Struck by goose**

√x7th **W61.59 Other contact with goose**

√5th **W61.6 Contact with duck**

√x7th **W61.61 Bitten by duck**

√x7th **W61.62 Struck by duck**

√x7th **W61.69 Other contact with duck**

√5th **W61.9 Contact with other birds**

√x7th **W61.91 Bitten by other birds**

√x7th **W61.92 Struck by other birds**

√x7th **W61.99 Other contact with other birds**
Contact with bird NOS

√4th **W62 Contact with nonvenomous amphibians**

EXCLUDES 1 *contact with venomous amphibians (T63.81-R63.83)*

The appropriate 7th character is to be added to each code from category W62.
A initial encounter
D subsequent encounter
S sequela

√x7th **W62.0 Contact with nonvenomous frogs**

√x7th **W62.1 Contact with nonvenomous toads**

√x7th **W62.9 Contact with other nonvenomous amphibians**

√x7th **W64 Exposure to other animate mechanical forces**
Exposure to nonvenomous animal NOS

EXCLUDES 1 *contact with venomous animal (T63.-)*

The appropriate 7th character is to be added to code W64.
A initial encounter
D subsequent encounter
S sequela

Accidental non-transport drowning and submersion (W65-W74)

EXCLUDES 1 *accidental drowning and submersion due to fall into water (W16.-)*
accidental drowning and submersion due to water transport accident (V90-, V92-)
EXCLUDES 2 *accidental drowning and submersion due to cataclysm (X34-X39)*

W65 Accidental drowning and submersion while in bath-tub
EXCLUDES 1 *accidental drowning and submersion due to fall in (into) bathtub (W16.211)*

The appropriate 7th character is to be added to code W65.
A initial encounter
D subsequent encounter
S sequela

W67 Accidental drowning and submersion while in swimming-pool
EXCLUDES 1 *accidental drowning and submersion due to fall into swimming pool (W16.011, W16.021, W16.031)*
accidental drowning and submersion due to striking into wall of swimming pool (W22.041)

The appropriate 7th character is to be added to code W67.
A initial encounter
D subsequent encounter
S sequela

W69 Accidental drowning and submersion while in natural water
Accidental drowning and submersion while in lake
Accidental drowning and submersion while in open sea
Accidental drowning and submersion while in river
Accidental drowning and submersion while in stream
EXCLUDES 1 *accidental drowning and submersion due to fall into natural body of water (W16.111, W16.121, W16.131)*

The appropriate 7th character is to be added to code W69.
A initial encounter
D subsequent encounter
S sequela

W73 Other specified cause of accidental non-transport drowning and submersion
Accidental drowning and submersion while in quenching tank
Accidental drowning and submersion while in reservoir
EXCLUDES 1 *accidental drowning and submersion due to fall into other water (W16.311, W16.321, W16.331)*

The appropriate 7th character is to be added to code W73.
A initial encounter
D subsequent encounter
S sequela

W74 Unspecified cause of accidental drowning and submersion
Drowning NOS

The appropriate 7th character is to be added to code W74.
A initial encounter
D subsequent encounter
S sequela

Exposure to electric current, radiation and extreme ambient air temperature and pressure (W85-W99)

EXCLUDES 1 *exposure to:*
failure in dosage of radiation or temperature during surgical and medical care (Y63.2-Y63.5)
lightning (T75.0-)
natural cold (X31)
natural heat (X30)
natural radiation NOS (X39)
radiological procedure and radiotherapy (Y84.2)
sunlight (X32)

W85 Exposure to electric transmission lines
Broken power line

The appropriate 7th character is to be added to code W85.
A initial encounter
D subsequent encounter
S sequela

W86 Exposure to other specified electric current

The appropriate 7th character is to be added to each code from category W86.
A initial encounter
D subsequent encounter
S sequela

W86.0 Exposure to domestic wiring and appliances
W86.1 Exposure to industrial wiring, appliances and electrical machinery
Exposure to conductors
Exposure to control apparatus
Exposure to electrical equipment and machinery
Exposure to transformers
W86.8 Exposure to other electric current
Exposure to wiring and appliances in or on farm (not farmhouse)
Exposure to wiring and appliances outdoors
Exposure to wiring and appliances in or on public building
Exposure to wiring and appliances in or on residential institutions
Exposure to wiring and appliances in or on schools

W88 Exposure to ionizing radiation
EXCLUDES 1 *exposure to sunlight (X32)*

The appropriate 7th character is to be added to each code from category W88.
A initial encounter
D subsequent encounter
S sequela

W88.0 Exposure to X-rays
W88.1 Exposure to radioactive isotopes
W88.8 Exposure to other ionizing radiation

W89 Exposure to man-made visible and ultraviolet light
Exposure to welding light (arc)
EXCLUDES 2 *exposure to sunlight (X32)*

The appropriate 7th character is to be added to each code from category W89.
A initial encounter
D subsequent encounter
S sequela

W89.0 Exposure to welding light (arc)
W89.1 Exposure to tanning bed
W89.8 Exposure to other man-made visible and ultraviolet light
W89.9 Exposure to unspecified man-made visible and ultraviolet light

W90 Exposure to other nonionizing radiation
EXCLUDES 1 *exposure to sunlight (X32)*

The appropriate 7th character is to be added to each code from category W90.
A initial encounter
D subsequent encounter
S sequela

W90.0 Exposure to radiofrequency
W90.1 Exposure to infrared radiation
W90.2 Exposure to laser radiation
W90.8 Exposure to other nonionizing radiation

W92 Exposure to excessive heat of man-made origin

The appropriate 7th character is to be added to code W92.
A initial encounter
D subsequent encounter
S sequela

W93 Exposure to excessive cold of man-made origin

The appropriate 7th character is to be added to each code from category W93.
A initial encounter
D subsequent encounter
S sequela

W93.0 Contact with or inhalation of dry ice
W93.01 Contact with dry ice
W93.02 Inhalation of dry ice

√5th **W93.1 Contact with or inhalation of liquid air**

√x7th **W93.11 Contact with liquid air**
Contact with liquid hydrogen
Contact with liquid nitrogen

√x7th **W93.12 Inhalation of liquid air**
Inhalation of liquid hydrogen
Inhalation of liquid nitrogen

√x7th **W93.2 Prolonged exposure in deep freeze unit or refrigerator**

√x7th **W93.8 Exposure to other excessive cold of man-made origin**

√4th **W94 Exposure to high and low air pressure and changes in air pressure**

The appropriate 7th character is to be added to each code from category W94.
A initial encounter
D subsequent encounter
S sequela

√x7th **W94.Ø Exposure to prolonged high air pressure**

√5th **W94.1 Exposure to prolonged low air pressure**

√x7th **W94.11 Exposure to residence or prolonged visit at high altitude**

√x7th **W94.12 Exposure to other prolonged low air pressure**

√5th **W94.2 Exposure to rapid changes in air pressure during ascent**

√x7th **W94.21 Exposure to reduction in atmospheric pressure while surfacing from deep-water diving**

√x7th **W94.22 Exposure to reduction in atmospheric pressure while surfacing from underground**

√x7th **W94.23 Exposure to sudden change in air pressure in aircraft during ascent**

√x7th **W94.29 Exposure to other rapid changes in air pressure during ascent**

√5th **W94.3 Exposure to rapid changes in air pressure during descent**

√x7th **W94.31 Exposure to sudden change in air pressure in aircraft during ascent or descent**

√x7th **W94.32 Exposure to high air pressure from rapid descent in water**

√x7th **W94.39 Exposure to other rapid changes in air pressure during descent**

√x7th **W99 Exposure to other man-made environmental factors**

The appropriate 7th character is to be added to code W99.
A initial encounter
D subsequent encounter
S sequela

Exposure to smoke, fire and flames (XØØ-XØ8)

EXCLUDES 1 *arson (X97)*

EXCLUDES 2 *explosions (W35-W4Ø)*
lightning (T75.Ø-)
transport accident (VØ1-V99)

√4th **XØØ Exposure to uncontrolled fire in building or structure**
Conflagration in building or structure
Code first any associated cataclysm

EXCLUDES 2 *exposure to ignition or melting of nightwear (XØ5)*
exposure to ignition or melting of other clothing and apparel (XØ6.-)
exposure to other specified smoke, fire and flames (XØ8.-)

The appropriate 7th character is to be added to each code from category XØØ.
A initial encounter
D subsequent encounter
S sequela

√x7th **XØØ.Ø Exposure to flames in uncontrolled fire in building or structure**

√x7th **XØØ.1 Exposure to smoke in uncontrolled fire in building or structure**

√x7th **XØØ.2 Injury due to collapse of burning building or structure in uncontrolled fire**
EXCLUDES 1 *injury due to collapse of building not on fire (W2Ø.1)*

√x7th **XØØ.3 Fall from burning building or structure in uncontrolled fire**

√x7th **XØØ.4 Hit by object from burning building or structure in uncontrolled fire**

√x7th **XØØ.5 Jump from burning building or structure in uncontrolled fire**

√x7th **XØØ.8 Other exposure to uncontrolled fire in building or structure**

√4th **XØ1 Exposure to uncontrolled fire, not in building or structure**
Exposure to forest fire

The appropriate 7th character is to be added to each code from category XØ1.
A initial encounter
D subsequent encounter
S sequela

√x7th **XØ1.Ø Exposure to flames in uncontrolled fire, not in building or structure**

√x7th **XØ1.1 Exposure to smoke in uncontrolled fire, not in building or structure**

√x7th **XØ1.3 Fall due to uncontrolled fire, not in building or structure**

√x7th **XØ1.4 Hit by object due to uncontrolled fire, not in building or structure**

√x7th **XØ1.8 Other exposure to uncontrolled fire, not in building or structure**

√4th **XØ2 Exposure to controlled fire in building or structure**
Exposure to fire in fireplace
Exposure to fire in stove

The appropriate 7th character is to be added to each code from category XØ2.
A initial encounter
D subsequent encounter
S sequela

√x7th **XØ2.Ø Exposure to flames in controlled fire in building or structure**

√x7th **XØ2.1 Exposure to smoke in controlled fire in building or structure**

√x7th **XØ2.2 Injury due to collapse of burning building or structure in controlled fire**
EXCLUDES 1 *injury due to collapse of building not on fire (W2Ø.1)*

√x7th **XØ2.3 Fall from burning building or structure in controlled fire**

√x7th **XØ2.4 Hit by object from burning building or structure in controlled fire**

√x7th **XØ2.5 Jump from burning building or structure in controlled fire**

√x7th **XØ2.8 Other exposure to controlled fire in building or structure**

√4th **XØ3 Exposure to controlled fire, not in building or structure**
Exposure to bon fire
Exposure to camp-fire
Exposure to trash fire

The appropriate 7th character is to be added to each code from category XØ3.
A initial encounter
D subsequent encounter
S sequela

√x7th **XØ3.Ø Exposure to flames in controlled fire, not in building or structure**

√x7th **XØ3.1 Exposure to smoke in controlled fire, not in building or structure**

√x7th **XØ3.3 Fall due to controlled fire, not in building or structure**

√x7th **XØ3.4 Hit by object due to controlled fire, not in building or structure**

√x7th **XØ3.8 Other exposure to controlled fire, not in building or structure**

√x7th **XØ4 Exposure to ignition of highly flammable material**
Exposure to ignition of gasoline
Exposure to ignition of kerosene
Exposure to ignition of petrol

EXCLUDES 2 *exposure to ignition or melting of nightwear (XØ5)*
exposure to ignition or melting of other clothing and apparel (XØ6)

The appropriate 7th character is to be added to code XØ4.
A initial encounter
D subsequent encounter
S sequela

X05 Exposure to ignition or melting of nightwear
EXCLUDES 2 *exposure to uncontrolled fire in building or structure (X00.-)*
exposure to uncontrolled fire, not in building or structure (X01.-)
exposure to controlled fire in building or structure (X02.-)
exposure to controlled fire, not in building or structure (X03.-)
exposure to ignition of highly flammable materials (X04.-)

The appropriate 7th character is to be added to code X05.
A initial encounter
D subsequent encounter
S sequela

X06 Exposure to ignition or melting of other clothing and apparel
EXCLUDES 2 *exposure to uncontrolled fire in building or structure (X00.-)*
exposure to uncontrolled fire, not in building or structure (X01.-)
exposure to controlled fire in building or structure (X02.-)
exposure to controlled fire, not in building or structure (X03.-)
exposure to ignition of highly flammable materials (X04.-)

The appropriate 7th character is to be added to each code from category X06.
A initial encounter
D subsequent encounter
S sequela

X06.0 Exposure to ignition of plastic jewelry
X06.1 Exposure to melting of plastic jewelry
X06.2 Exposure to ignition of other clothing and apparel
X06.3 Exposure to melting of other clothing and apparel

X08 Exposure to other specified smoke, fire and flames

The appropriate 7th character is to be added to each code from category X08.
A initial encounter
D subsequent encounter
S sequela

X08.0 Exposure to bed fire
Exposure to mattress fire
X08.00 Exposure to bed fire due to unspecified burning material
X08.01 Exposure to bed fire due to burning cigarette
X08.09 Exposure to bed fire due to other burning material
X08.1 Exposure to sofa fire
X08.10 Exposure to sofa fire due to unspecified burning material
X08.11 Exposure to sofa fire due to burning cigarette
X08.19 Exposure to sofa fire due to other burning material
X08.2 Exposure to other furniture fire
X08.20 Exposure to other furniture fire due to unspecified burning material
X08.21 Exposure to other furniture fire due to burning cigarette
X08.29 Exposure to other furniture fire due to other burning material
X08.8 Exposure to other specified smoke, fire and flames

Contact with heat and hot substances (X10-X19)

EXCLUDES 1 *exposure to excessive natural heat (X30)*
exposure to fire and flames (X00-X09)

X10 Contact with hot drinks, food, fats and cooking oils

The appropriate 7th character is to be added to each code from category X10.
A initial encounter
D subsequent encounter
S sequela

X10.0 Contact with hot drinks
X10.1 Contact with hot food
X10.2 Contact with fats and cooking oils

X11 Contact with hot tap-water
Contact with boiling tap-water
Contact with boiling water NOS
EXCLUDES 1 *contact with water heated on stove (X12)*

The appropriate 7th character is to be added to each code from category X11.
A initial encounter
D subsequent encounter
S sequela

X11.0 Contact with hot water in bath or tub
EXCLUDES 1 *contact with running hot water in bath or tub (X11.1)*
X11.1 Contact with running hot water
Contact with hot water running out of hose
Contact with hot water running out of tap
X11.8 Contact with other hot tap-water
Contact with hot water in bucket
Contact with hot tap-water NOS

X12 Contact with other hot fluids
Contact with water heated on stove
EXCLUDES 1 *hot (liquid) metals (X18)*

The appropriate 7th character is to be added to code X12.
A initial encounter
D subsequent encounter
S sequela

X13 Contact with steam and other hot vapors

The appropriate 7th character is to be added to each code from category X13.
A initial encounter
D subsequent encounter
S sequela

X13.0 Inhalation of steam and other hot vapors
X13.1 Other contact with steam and other hot vapors

X14 Contact with hot air and other hot gases

The appropriate 7th character is to be added to each code from category X14.
A initial encounter
D subsequent encounter
S sequela

X14.0 Inhalation of hot air and gases
X14.1 Other contact with hot air and other hot gases

X15 Contact with hot household appliances
EXCLUDES 1 *contact with heating appliances (X16)*
contact with powered household appliances (W29.-)
exposure to controlled fire in building or structure due to household appliance (X02.8)
exposure to household appliances electrical current (W86.0)

The appropriate 7th character is to be added to each code from category X15.
A initial encounter
D subsequent encounter
S sequela

X15.0 Contact with hot stove (kitchen)
X15.1 Contact with hot toaster
X15.2 Contact with hotplate
X15.3 Contact with hot saucepan or skillet
X15.8 Contact with other hot household appliances
Contact with cooker
Contact with kettle
Contact with light bulbs

X16 Contact with hot heating appliances, radiators and pipes
EXCLUDES 1 *contact with powered appliances (W29.-)*
exposure to controlled fire in building or structure due to appliance (X02.8)
exposure to industrial appliances electrical current (W86.1)

The appropriate 7th character is to be added to code X16.
A initial encounter
D subsequent encounter
S sequela

✓x7th X17 Contact with hot engines, machinery and tools

EXCLUDES 1 *contact with hot heating appliances, radiators and pipes (X16)*
contact with hot household appliances (X15)

The appropriate 7th character is to be added to code X17.
A initial encounter
D subsequent encounter
S sequela

✓x7th X18 Contact with other hot metals

Contact with liquid metal

The appropriate 7th character is to be added to code X18.
A initial encounter
D subsequent encounter
S sequela

✓x7th X19 Contact with other heat and hot substances

EXCLUDES 1 *objects that are not normally hot, e.g., an object made hot by a house fire (X00-X09)*

The appropriate 7th character is to be added to code X19.
A initial encounter
D subsequent encounter
S sequela

Exposure to forces of nature (X30-X39)

✓x7th X30 Exposure to excessive natural heat

Exposure to excessive heat as the cause of sunstroke
Exposure to heat NOS

EXCLUDES 1 *excessive heat of man-made origin (W92)*
exposure to man-made radiation (W89)
exposure to sunlight (X32)
exposure to tanning bed (W89)

The appropriate 7th character is to be added to code X30.
A initial encounter
D subsequent encounter
S sequela

✓x7th X31 Exposure to excessive natural cold

Excessive cold as the cause of chilblains NOS
Excessive cold as the cause of immersion foot or hand
Exposure to cold NOS
Exposure to weather conditions

EXCLUDES 1 *cold of man-made origin (W93.-)*
contact with or inhalation of:
dry ice (W93.-)
liquefied gas (W93.-)

The appropriate 7th character is to be added to code X31.
A initial encounter
D subsequent encounter
S sequela

✓x7th X32 Exposure to sunlight

EXCLUDES 1 *radiation-related disorders of the skin and subcutaneous tissue (L55-L59)*
man-made radiation (tanning bed) (W89)

The appropriate 7th character is to be added to code X32.
A initial encounter
D subsequent encounter
S sequela

✓x7th X34 Earthquake

EXCLUDES 2 *tidal wave (tsunami) due to earthquake (X37.41)*

The appropriate 7th character is to be added to code X34.
A initial encounter
D subsequent encounter
S sequela

✓x7th X35 Volcanic eruption

EXCLUDES 2 *tidal wave (tsunami) due to volcanic eruption (X37.41)*

The appropriate 7th character is to be added to code X35.
A initial encounter
D subsequent encounter
S sequela

✓4th X36 Avalanche, landslide and other earth movements

INCLUDES victim of mudslide of cataclysmic nature

EXCLUDES 1 *earthquake (X34)*

EXCLUDES 2 *transport accident involving collision with avalanche or landslide not in motion (V01-V99)*

The appropriate 7th character is to be added to each code from category X36.
A initial encounter
D subsequent encounter
S sequela

✓x7th **X36.0 Collapse of dam or man-made structure causing earth movement**

✓x7th **X36.1 Avalanche, landslide, or mudslide**

✓4th X37 Cataclysmic storm

The appropriate 7th character is to be added to each code from category X37.
A initial encounter
D subsequent encounter
S sequela

✓x7th **X37.0 Hurricane**
Storm surge
Typhoon

✓x7th **X37.1 Tornado**
Cyclone
Twister

✓x7th **X37.2 Blizzard (snow)(ice)**

✓x7th **X37.3 Dust storm**

✓5th **X37.4 Tidalwave**

✓x7th **X37.41 Tidal wave due to earthquake or volcanic eruption**
Tidal wave NOS
Tsunami

✓x7th **X37.42 Tidal wave due to storm**

✓x7th **X37.43 Tidal wave due to landslide**

✓x7th **X37.8 Other cataclysmic storms**
Cloudburst
Torrential rain
EXCLUDES 2 *flood (X38)*

✓x7th **X37.9 Unspecified cataclysmic storm**
Storm NOS
EXCLUDES 1 *collapse of dam or man-made structure causing earth movement (X36.0)*

✓x7th X38 Flood

Flood arising from remote storm
Flood of cataclysmic nature arising from melting snow
Flood resulting directly from storm

EXCLUDES 1 *collapse of dam or man-made structure causing earth movement (X36.0)*
tidal wave NOS (X37.41)
tidal wave caused by storm (X37.42)

The appropriate 7th character is to be added to code X38.
A initial encounter
D subsequent encounter
S sequela

✓4th X39 Exposure to other forces of nature

The appropriate 7th character is to be added to each code from category X39.
A initial encounter
D subsequent encounter
S sequela

✓5th **X39.0 Exposure to natural radiation**
EXCLUDES 1 *contact with and (suspected) exposure to radon and other naturally occuring radiation (Z77.123)*
exposure to man-made radiation (W88-W90)
exposure to sunlight (X32)

✓x7th **X39.01 Exposure to radon**

✓x7th **X39.08 Exposure to other natural radiation**

✓x7th **X39.8 Other exposure to forces of nature**

Accidental exposure to other specified factors (X52, X58)

√x7th **X52 Prolonged stay in weightless environment**
Weightlessness in spacecraft (simulator)

> The appropriate 7th character is to be added to code X52.
> A initial encounter
> D subsequent encounter
> S sequela

√x7th **X58 Exposure to other specified factors**
Accident NOS
Exposure NOS

> The appropriate 7th character is to be added to code X58.
> A initial encounter
> D subsequent encounter
> S sequela

Intentional self-harm (X71-X83)

Purposely self-inflicted injury
Suicide (attempted)

√4th **X71 Intentional self-harm by drowning and submersion**

> The appropriate 7th character is to be added to each code from category X71.
> A initial encounter
> D subsequent encounter
> S sequela

√x7th **X71.0 Intentional self-harm by drowning and submersion while in bathtub**
√x7th **X71.1 Intentional self-harm by drowning and submersion while in swimming pool**
√x7th **X71.2 Intentional self-harm by drowning and submersion after jump into swimming pool**
√x7th **X71.3 Intentional self-harm by drowning and submersion in natural water**
√x7th **X71.8 Other intentional self-harm by drowning and submersion**
√x7th **X71.9 Intentional self-harm by drowning and submersion, unspecified**

√x7th **X72 Intentional self-harm by handgun discharge**
Intentional self-harm by gun for single hand use
Intentional self-harm by pistol
Intentional self-harm by revolver
EXCLUDES 1 *Very pistol (X74.8)*

> The appropriate 7th character is to be added to code X72.
> A initial encounter
> D subsequent encounter
> S sequela

√4th **X73 Intentional self-harm by rifle, shotgun and larger firearm discharge**
EXCLUDES 1 *airgun (X74.01)*

> The appropriate 7th character is to be added to each code from category X73.
> A initial encounter
> D subsequent encounter
> S sequela

√x7th **X73.0 Intentional self-harm by shotgun discharge**
√x7th **X73.1 Intentional self-harm by hunting rifle discharge**
√x7th **X73.2 Intentional self-harm by machine gun discharge**
√x7th **X73.8 Intentional self-harm by other larger firearm discharge**
√x7th **X73.9 Intentional self-harm by unspecified larger firearm discharge**

√4th **X74 Intentional self-harm by other and unspecified firearm and gun discharge**

> The appropriate 7th character is to be added to each code from category X74.
> A initial encounter
> D subsequent encounter
> S sequela

√5th **X74.0 Intentional self-harm by gas, air or spring-operated guns**
√x7th **X74.01 Intentional self-harm by airgun**
Intentional self-harm by BB gun discharge
Intentional self-harm by pellet gun discharge
√x7th **X74.02 Intentional self-harm by paintball gun**
√x7th **X74.09 Intentional self-harm by other gas, air or spring-operated gun**
√x7th **X74.8 Intentional self-harm by other firearm discharge**
Intentional self-harm by Very pistol [flare] discharge
√x7th **X74.9 Intentional self-harm by unspecified firearm discharge**

√x7th **X75 Intentional self-harm by explosive material**

> The appropriate 7th character is to be added to code X75.
> A initial encounter
> D subsequent encounter
> S sequela

√x7th **X76 Intentional self-harm by smoke, fire and flames**

> The appropriate 7th character is to be added to code X76.
> A initial encounter
> D subsequent encounter
> S sequela

√4th **X77 Intentional self-harm by steam, hot vapors and hot objects**

> The appropriate 7th character is to be added to each code from category X77.
> A initial encounter
> D subsequent encounter
> S sequela

√x7th **X77.0 Intentional self-harm by steam or hot vapors**
√x7th **X77.1 Intentional self-harm by hot tap water**
√x7th **X77.2 Intentional self-harm by other hot fluids**
√x7th **X77.3 Intentional self-harm by hot household appliances**
√x7th **X77.8 Intentional self-harm by other hot objects**
√x7th **X77.9 Intentional self-harm by unspecified hot objects**

√4th **X78 Intentional self-harm by sharp object**

> The appropriate 7th character is to be added to each code from category X78.
> A initial encounter
> D subsequent encounter
> S sequela

√x7th **X78.0 Intentional self-harm by sharp glass**
√x7th **X78.1 Intentional self-harm by knife**
√x7th **X78.2 Intentional self-harm by sword or dagger**
√x7th **X78.8 Intentional self-harm by other sharp object**
√x7th **X78.9 Intentional self-harm by unspecified sharp object**

√x7th **X79 Intentional self-harm by blunt object**

> The appropriate 7th character is to be added to code X79.
> A initial encounter
> D subsequent encounter
> S sequela

√x7th **X80 Intentional self-harm by jumping from a high place**
Intentional fall from one level to another

> The appropriate 7th character is to be added to code X80.
> A initial encounter
> D subsequent encounter
> S sequela

√4th **X81 Intentional self-harm by jumping or lying in front of moving object**

> The appropriate 7th character is to be added to each code from category X81.
> A initial encounter
> D subsequent encounter
> S sequela

√x7th **X81.0 Intentional self-harm by jumping or lying in front of motor vehicle**
√x7th **X81.1 Intentional self-harm by jumping or lying in front of (subway) train**
√x7th **X81.8 Intentional self-harm by jumping or lying in front of other moving object**

√4th X82 Intentional self-harm by crashing of motor vehicle

The appropriate 7th character is to be added to each code from category X82.
A initial encounter
D subsequent encounter
S sequela

√x7th X82.Ø Intentional collision of motor vehicle with other motor vehicle
√x7th X82.1 Intentional collision of motor vehicle with train
√x7th X82.2 Intentional collision of motor vehicle with tree
√x7th X82.8 Other intentional self-harm by crashing of motor vehicle

√4th X83 Intentional self-harm by other specified means
EXCLUDES1 *intentional self-harm by poisoning or contact with toxic substance—see Table of Drugs and Chemicals*

The appropriate 7th character is to be added to each code from category X83.
A initial encounter
D subsequent encounter
S sequela

√x7th X83.Ø Intentional self-harm by crashing of aircraft
√x7th X83.1 Intentional self-harm by electrocution
√x7th X83.2 Intentional self-harm by exposure to extremes of cold
√x7th X83.8 Intentional self-harm by other specified means

Assault (X92-YØ8)

INCLUDES homicide
injuries inflicted by another person with intent to injure or kill, by any means
EXCLUDES1 *injuries due to legal intervention (Y35.-)*
injuries due to operations of war (Y36.-)
injuries due to terrorism (Y38.-)

√4th X92 Assault by drowning and submersion

The appropriate 7th character is to be added to each code from category X92.
A initial encounter
D subsequent encounter
S sequela

√x7th X92.Ø Assault by drowning and submersion while in bathtub
√x7th X92.1 Assault by drowning and submersion while in swimming pool
√x7th X92.2 Assault by drowning and submersion after push into swimming pool
√x7th X92.3 Assault by drowning and submersion in natural water
√x7th X92.8 Other assault by drowning and submersion
√x7th X92.9 Assault by drowning and submersion, unspecified

√x7th X93 Assault by handgun discharge
Assault by discharge of gun for single hand use
Assault by discharge of pistol
Assault by discharge of revolver
EXCLUDES1 *Very pistol (X95.8)*

The appropriate 7th character is to be added to code X93.
A initial encounter
D subsequent encounter
S sequela

√4th X94 Assault by rifle, shotgun and larger firearm discharge
EXCLUDES1 *airgun (X95.Ø1)*

The appropriate 7th character is to be added to each code from category X94.
A initial encounter
D subsequent encounter
S sequela

√x7th X94.Ø Assault by shotgun
√x7th X94.1 Assault by hunting rifle
√x7th X94.2 Assault by machine gun
√x7th X94.8 Assault by other larger firearm discharge
√x7th X94.9 Assault by unspecified larger firearm discharge

√4th X95 Assault by other and unspecified firearm and gun discharge

The appropriate 7th character is to be added to each code from category X95.
A initial encounter
D subsequent encounter
S sequela

√5th X95.Ø Assault by gas, air or spring-operated guns
√x7th X95.Ø1 Assault by airgun discharge
Assault by BB gun discharge
Assault by pellet gun discharge
√x7th X95.Ø2 Assault by paintball gun discharge
√x7th X95.Ø9 Assault by other gas, air or spring-operated gun
√x7th X95.8 Assault by other firearm discharge
Assault by Very pistol [flare] discharge
√x7th X95.9 Assault by unspecified firearm discharge

√4th X96 Assault by explosive material
EXCLUDES1 *incendiary device (X97)*
terrorism involving explosive material (Y38.2-)

The appropriate 7th character is to be added to each code from category X96.
A initial encounter
D subsequent encounter
S sequela

√x7th X96.Ø Assault by antipersonnel bomb
EXCLUDES1 *antipersonnel bomb use in military or war (Y36.2-)*
√x7th X96.1 Assault by gasoline bomb
√x7th X96.2 Assault by letter bomb
√x7th X96.3 Assault by fertilizer bomb
√x7th X96.4 Assault by pipe bomb
√x7th X96.8 Assault by other specified explosive
√x7th X96.9 Assault by unspecified explosive

√x7th X97 Assault by smoke, fire and flames
Assault by arson
Assault by cigarettes
Assault by incendiary device

The appropriate 7th character is to be added to code X97.
A initial encounter
D subsequent encounter
S sequela

√4th X98 Assault by steam, hot vapors and hot objects

The appropriate 7th character is to be added to each code from category X98.
A initial encounter
D subsequent encounter
S sequela

√x7th X98.Ø Assault by steam or hot vapors
√x7th X98.1 Assault by hot tap water
√x7th X98.2 Assault by hot fluids
√x7th X98.3 Assault by hot household appliances
√x7th X98.8 Assault by other hot objects
√x7th X98.9 Assault by unspecified hot objects

√4th X99 Assault by sharp object
EXCLUDES1 *assault by strike by sports equipment (YØ8.Ø-)*

The appropriate 7th character is to be added to each code from category X99.
A initial encounter
D subsequent encounter
S sequela

√x7th X99.Ø Assault by sharp glass
√x7th X99.1 Assault by knife
√x7th X99.2 Assault by sword or dagger
√x7th X99.8 Assault by other sharp object
√x7th X99.9 Assault by unspecified sharp object
Assault by stabbing NOS

√x7th YØØ Assault by blunt object
EXCLUDES1 *assault by strike by sports equipment (YØ8.Ø-)*

The appropriate 7th character is to be added to code YØØ.
A initial encounter
D subsequent encounter
S sequela

Y01 Assault by pushing from high place

The appropriate 7th character is to be added to code Y01.
A initial encounter
D subsequent encounter
S sequela

Y02 Assault by pushing or placing victim in front of moving object

The appropriate 7th character is to be added to each code from category Y02.
A initial encounter
D subsequent encounter
S sequela

Y02.0 Assault by pushing or placing victim in front of motor vehicle
Y02.1 Assault by pushing or placing victim in front of (subway) train
Y02.8 Assault by pushing or placing victim in front of other moving object

Y03 Assault by crashing of motor vehicle

The appropriate 7th character is to be added to each code from category Y03.
A initial encounter
D subsequent encounter
S sequela

Y03.0 Assault by being hit or run over by motor vehicle
Y03.8 Other assault by crashing of motor vehicle

Y04 Assault by bodily force
EXCLUDES 1 *assault by:*
submersion (X92.-)
use of weapon (X93-X95, X99, Y00)

The appropriate 7th character is to be added to each code from category Y04.
A initial encounter
D subsequent encounter
S sequela

Y04.0 Assault by unarmed brawl or fight
Y04.1 Assault by human bite
Y04.2 Assault by strike against or bumped into by another person
Y04.8 Assault by other bodily force
Assault by bodily force NOS

Y07 Perpetrator of assault, maltreatment and neglect
NOTE Codes from this category are for use only in cases of confirmed abuse (T74.-)
Selection of the correct perpetrator code is based on the relationship between the perpetrator and the victim
INCLUDES perpetrator of abandonment
perpetrator of emotional neglect
perpetrator of mental cruelty
perpetrator of physical abuse
perpetrator of physical neglect
perpetrator of sexual abuse
perpetrator of torture

Y07.0 Spouse or partner, perpetrator of maltreatment and neglect
NOTE Spouse or partner, perpetrator of maltreatment and neglect against spouse or partner
Y07.01 Husband, perpetrator of maltreatment and neglect
Y07.02 Wife, perpetrator of maltreatment and neglect
Y07.03 Male partner, perpetrator of maltreatment and neglect
Y07.04 Female partner, perpetrator of maltreatment and neglect

Y07.1 Parent (adoptive) (biological), perpetrator of maltreatment and neglect
Y07.11 Biological father, perpetrator of maltreatment and neglect
Y07.12 Biological mother, perpetrator of maltreatment and neglect
Y07.13 Adoptive father, perpetrator of maltreatment and neglect
Y07.14 Adoptive mother, perpetrator of maltreatment and neglect

Y07.4 Other family member, perpetrator of maltreatment and neglect
Y07.41 Sibling, perpetrator of maltreatment and neglect
EXCLUDES 1 *stepsibling, perpetrator of maltreatment and neglect (Y07.435, Y07.436)*
Y07.410 Brother, perpetrator of maltreatment and neglect
Y07.411 Sister, perpetrator of maltreatment and neglect
Y07.42 Foster parent, perpetrator of maltreatment and neglect
Y07.420 Foster father, perpetrator of maltreatment and neglect
Y07.421 Foster mother, perpetrator of maltreatment and neglect
Y07.43 Stepparent or stepsibling, perpetrator of maltreatment and neglect
Y07.430 Stepfather, perpetrator of maltreatment and neglect
Y07.432 Male friend of parent (co-residing in household), perpetrator of maltreatment and neglect
Y07.433 Stepmother, perpetrator of maltreatment and neglect
Y07.434 Female friend of parent (co-residing in household), perpetrator of maltreatment and neglect
Y07.435 Stepbrother, perpetrator or maltreatment and neglect
Y07.436 Stepsister, perpetrator of maltreatment and neglect
Y07.49 Other family member, perpetrator of maltreatment and neglect
Y07.490 Male cousin, perpetrator of maltreatment and neglect
Y07.491 Female cousin, perpetrator of maltreatment and neglect
Y07.499 Other family member, perpetrator of maltreatment and neglect

Y07.5 Non-family member, perpetrator of maltreatment and neglect
Y07.50 Unspecified non-family member, perpetrator of maltreatment and neglect
Y07.51 Daycare provider, perpetrator of maltreatment and neglect
Y07.510 At-home childcare provider, perpetrator of maltreatment and neglect
Y07.511 Daycare center childcare provider, perpetrator of maltreatment and neglect
Y07.512 At-home adultcare provider, perpetrator of maltreatment and neglect
Y07.513 Adultcare center provider, perpetrator of maltreatment and neglect
Y07.519 Unspecified daycare provider, perpetrator of maltreatment and neglect
Y07.52 Healthcare provider, perpetrator of maltreatment and neglect
Y07.521 Mental health provider, perpetrator of maltreatment and neglect
Y07.528 Other therapist or healthcare provider, perpetrator of maltreatment and neglect
Nurse, perpetrator of maltreatment and neglect
Occupational therapist, perpetrator of maltreatment and neglect
Physical therapist, perpetrator of maltreatment and neglect
Speech therapist, perpetrator of maltreatment and neglect
Y07.529 Unspecified healthcare provider, perpetrator of maltreatment and neglect
Y07.53 Teacher or instructor, perpetrator of maltreatment and neglect
Coach, perpetrator of maltreatment and neglect

Y07.59 Other non-family member, perpetrator of maltreatment and neglect

Y07.9 Unspecified perpetrator of maltreatment and neglect

✓4th **Y08 Assault by other specified means**

The appropriate 7th character is to be added to each code from category Y08.
A initial encounter
D subsequent encounter
S sequela

✓5th **Y08.0 Assault by strike by sport equipment**

✓x7th **Y08.01 Assault by strike by hockey stick**

✓x7th **Y08.02 Assault by strike by baseball bat**

✓x7th **Y08.09 Assault by strike by other specified type of sport equipment**

✓5th **Y08.8 Assault by other specified means**

✓x7th **Y08.81 Assault by crashing of aircraft**

✓x7th **Y08.89 Assault by other specified means**

Y09 Assault by unspecified means
Assassination (attempted) NOS
Homicide (attempted) NOS
Manslaughter (attempted) NOS
Murder (attempted) NOS

Event of undetermined intent (Y21-Y33)

Undetermined intent is only for use when there is specific documentation in the record that the intent of the injury cannot be determined. If no such documentation is present, code to accidental (unintentional)

✓4th **Y21 Drowning and submersion, undetermined intent**

The appropriate 7th character is to be added to each code from category Y21.
A initial encounter
D subsequent encounter
S sequela

✓x7th **Y21.0 Drowning and submersion while in bathtub, undetermined intent**

✓x7th **Y21.1 Drowning and submersion after fall into bathtub, undetermined intent**

✓x7th **Y21.2 Drowning and submersion while in swimming pool, undetermined intent**

✓x7th **Y21.3 Drowning and submersion after fall into swimming pool, undetermined intent**

✓x7th **Y21.4 Drowning and submersion in natural water, undetermined intent**

✓x7th **Y21.8 Other drowning and submersion, undetermined intent**

✓x7th **Y21.9 Unspecified drowning and submersion, undetermined intent**

✓x7th **Y22 Handgun discharge, undetermined intent**
Discharge of gun for single hand use, undetermined intent
Discharge of pistol, undetermined intent
Discharge of revolver, undetermined intent
EXCLUDES 2 *Very pistol (Y24.8)*

The appropriate 7th character is to be added to code Y22.
A initial encounter
D subsequent encounter
S sequela

✓4th **Y23 Rifle, shotgun and larger firearm discharge, undetermined intent**
EXCLUDES 2 *airgun (Y24.0)*

The appropriate 7th character is to be added to each code from category Y23.
A initial encounter
D subsequent encounter
S sequela

✓x7th **Y23.0 Shotgun discharge, undetermined intent**

✓x7th **Y23.1 Hunting rifle discharge, undetermined intent**

✓x7th **Y23.2 Military firearm discharge, undetermined intent**

✓x7th **Y23.3 Machine gun discharge, undetermined intent**

✓x7th **Y23.8 Other larger firearm discharge, undetermined intent**

✓x7th **Y23.9 Unspecified larger firearm discharge, undetermined intent**

✓4th **Y24 Other and unspecified firearm discharge, undetermined intent**

The appropriate 7th character is to be added to each code from category Y24.
A initial encounter
D subsequent encounter
S sequela

✓x7th **Y24.0 Airgun discharge, undetermined intent**
BB gun discharge, undetermined intent
Pellet gun discharge, undetermined intent

✓x7th **Y24.8 Other firearm discharge, undetermined intent**
Paintball gun discharge, undetermined intent
Very pistol [flare] discharge, undetermined intent

✓x7th **Y24.9 Unspecified firearm discharge, undetermined intent**

✓x7th **Y25 Contact with explosive material, undetermined intent**

The appropriate 7th character is to be added to code Y25.
A initial encounter
D subsequent encounter
S sequela

✓x7th **Y26 Exposure to smoke, fire and flames, undetermined intent**

The appropriate 7th character is to be added to code Y26.
A initial encounter
D subsequent encounter
S sequela

✓4th **Y27 Contact with steam, hot vapors and hot objects, undetermined intent**

The appropriate 7th character is to be added to each code from category Y27.
A initial encounter
D subsequent encounter
S sequela

✓x7th **Y27.0 Contact with steam and hot vapors, undetermined intent**

✓x7th **Y27.1 Contact with hot tap water, undetermined intent**

✓x7th **Y27.2 Contact with hot fluids, undetermined intent**

✓x7th **Y27.3 Contact with hot household appliance, undetermined intent**

✓x7th **Y27.8 Contact with other hot objects, undetermined intent**

✓x7th **Y27.9 Contact with unspecified hot objects, undetermined intent**

✓4th **Y28 Contact with sharp object, undetermined intent**

The appropriate 7th character is to be added to each code from category Y28.
A initial encounter
D subsequent encounter
S sequela

✓x7th **Y28.0 Contact with sharp glass, undetermined intent**

✓x7th **Y28.1 Contact with knife, undetermined intent**

✓x7th **Y28.2 Contact with sword or dagger, undetermined intent**

✓x7th **Y28.8 Contact with other sharp object, undetermined intent**

✓x7th **Y28.9 Contact with unspecified sharp object, undetermined intent**

✓x7th **Y29 Contact with blunt object, undetermined intent**

The appropriate 7th character is to be added to code Y29.
A initial encounter
D subsequent encounter
S sequela

✓x7th **Y30 Falling, jumping or pushed from a high place, undetermined intent**
Victim falling from one level to another, undetermined intent

The appropriate 7th character is to be added to code Y30.
A initial encounter
D subsequent encounter
S sequela

✓x7th Y31 Falling, lying or running before or into moving object, undetermined intent

The appropriate 7th character is to be added to code Y31.
A initial encounter
D subsequent encounter
S sequela

✓x7th Y32 Crashing of motor vehicle, undetermined intent

The appropriate 7th character is to be added to code Y32.
A initial encounter
D subsequent encounter
S sequela

✓x7th Y33 Other specified events, undetermined intent

The appropriate 7th character is to be added to code Y33.
A initial encounter
D subsequent encounter
S sequela

Legal intervention, operations of war, military operations, and terrorism (Y35-Y38)

✓4th Y35 Legal intervention

INCLUDES any injury sustained as a result of an encounter with any law enforcement official, serving in any capacity at the time of the encounter, whether on-duty or off-duty. Includes injury to law enforcement official, suspect and bystander

The appropriate 7th character is to be added to each code from category Y35.
A initial encounter
D subsequent encounter
S sequela

✓5th Y35.0 Legal intervention involving firearm discharge

✓6th Y35.00 Legal intervention involving unspecified firearm discharge
Legal intervention involving gunshot wound
Legal intervention involving shot NOS

✓7th Y35.001 Legal intervention involving unspecified firearm discharge, law enforcement official injured

✓7th Y35.002 Legal intervention involving unspecified firearm discharge, bystander injured

✓7th Y35.003 Legal intervention involving unspecified firearm discharge, suspect injured

✓6th Y35.01 Legal intervention involving injury by machine gun

✓7th Y35.011 Legal intervention involving injury by machine gun, law enforcement official injured

✓7th Y35.012 Legal intervention involving injury by machine gun, bystander injured

✓7th Y35.013 Legal intervention involving injury by machine gun, suspect injured

✓6th Y35.02 Legal intervention involving injury by handgun

✓7th Y35.021 Legal intervention involving injury by handgun, law enforcement official injured

✓7th Y35.022 Legal intervention involving injury by handgun, bystander injured

✓7th Y35.023 Legal intervention involving injury by handgun, suspect injured

✓6th Y35.03 Legal intervention involving injury by rifle pellet

✓7th Y35.031 Legal intervention involving injury by rifle pellet, law enforcement official injured

✓7th Y35.032 Legal intervention involving injury by rifle pellet, bystander injured

✓7th Y35.033 Legal intervention involving injury by rifle pellet, suspect injured

✓6th Y35.04 Legal intervention involving injury by rubber bullet

✓7th Y35.041 Legal intervention involving injury by rubber bullet, law enforcement official injured

✓7th Y35.042 Legal intervention involving injury by rubber bullet, bystander injured

✓7th Y35.043 Legal intervention involving injury by rubber bullet, suspect injured

✓6th Y35.09 Legal intervention involving other firearm discharge

✓7th Y35.091 Legal intervention involving other firearm discharge, law enforcement official injured

✓7th Y35.092 Legal intervention involving other firearm discharge, bystander injured

✓7th Y35.093 Legal intervention involving other firearm discharge, suspect injured

✓5th Y35.1 Legal intervention involving explosives

✓6th Y35.10 Legal intervention involving unspecified explosives

✓7th Y35.101 Legal intervention involving unspecified explosives, law enforcement official injured

✓7th Y35.102 Legal intervention involving unspecified explosives, bystander injured

✓7th Y35.103 Legal intervention involving unspecified explosives, suspect injured

✓6th Y35.11 Legal intervention involving injury by dynamite

✓7th Y35.111 Legal intervention involving injury by dynamite, law enforcement official injured

✓7th Y35.112 Legal intervention involving injury by dynamite, bystander injured

✓7th Y35.113 Legal intervention involving injury by dynamite, suspect injured

✓6th Y35.12 Legal intervention involving injury by explosive shell

✓7th Y35.121 Legal intervention involving injury by explosive shell, law enforcement official injured

✓7th Y35.122 Legal intervention involving injury by explosive shell, bystander injured

✓7th Y35.123 Legal intervention involving injury by explosive shell, suspect injured

✓6th Y35.19 Legal intervention involving other explosives
Legal intervention involving injury by grenade
Legal intervention involving injury by mortar bomb

✓7th Y35.191 Legal intervention involving other explosives, law enforcement official injured

✓7th Y35.192 Legal intervention involving other explosives, bystander injured

✓7th Y35.193 Legal intervention involving other explosives, suspect injured

✓5th Y35.2 Legal intervention involving gas
Legal intervention involving asphyxiation by gas
Legal intervention involving poisoning by gas

✓6th Y35.20 Legal intervention involving unspecified gas

✓7th Y35.201 Legal intervention involving unspecified gas, law enforcement official injured

✓7th Y35.202 Legal intervention involving unspecified gas, bystander injured

✓7th Y35.203 Legal intervention involving unspecified gas, suspect injured

✓6th Y35.21 Legal intervention involving injury by tear gas

✓7th Y35.211 Legal intervention involving injury by tear gas, law enforcement official injured

✓7th Y35.212 Legal intervention involving injury by tear gas, bystander injured

✓7th Y35.213 Legal intervention involving injury by tear gas, suspect injured

✓ Appropriate additional character required
✓x7th Requires 7th character, placeholder x must fill empty characters

√6th Y35.29 **Legal intervention involving other gas**
- √7th Y35.291 **Legal intervention involving other gas, law enforcement official injured**
- √7th Y35.292 **Legal intervention involving other gas, bystander injured**
- √7th Y35.293 **Legal intervention involving other gas, suspect injured**

√5th Y35.3 **Legal intervention involving blunt objects**
Legal intervention involving being hit or struck by blunt object

√6th Y35.30 **Legal intervention involving unspecified blunt objects**
- √7th Y35.301 **Legal intervention involving unspecified blunt objects, law enforcement official injured**
- √7th Y35.302 **Legal intervention involving unspecified blunt objects, bystander injured**
- √7th Y35.303 **Legal intervention involving unspecified blunt objects, suspect injured**

√6th Y35.31 **Legal intervention involving baton**
- √7th Y35.311 **Legal intervention involving baton, law enforcement official injured**
- √7th Y35.312 **Legal intervention involving baton, bystander injured**
- √7th Y35.313 **Legal intervention involving baton, suspect injured**

√6th Y35.39 **Legal intervention involving other blunt objects**
- √7th Y35.391 **Legal intervention involving other blunt objects, law enforcement official injured**
- √7th Y35.392 **Legal intervention involving other blunt objects, bystander injured**
- √7th Y35.393 **Legal intervention involving other blunt objects, suspect injured**

√5th Y35.4 **Legal intervention involving sharp objects**
Legal intervention involving being cut by sharp objects
Legal intervention involving being stabbed by sharp objects

√6th Y35.40 **Legal intervention involving unspecified sharp objects**
- √7th Y35.401 **Legal intervention involving unspecified sharp objects, law enforcement official injured**
- √7th Y35.402 **Legal intervention involving unspecified sharp objects, bystander injured**
- √7th Y35.403 **Legal intervention involving unspecified sharp objects, suspect injured**

√6th Y35.41 **Legal intervention involving bayonet**
- √7th Y35.411 **Legal intervention involving bayonet, law enforcement official injured**
- √7th Y35.412 **Legal intervention involving bayonet, bystander injured**
- √7th Y35.413 **Legal intervention involving bayonet, suspect injured**

√6th Y35.49 **Legal intervention involving other sharp objects**
- √7th Y35.491 **Legal intervention involving other sharp objects, law enforcement official injured**
- √7th Y35.492 **Legal intervention involving other sharp objects, bystander injured**
- √7th Y35.493 **Legal intervention involving other sharp objects, suspect injured**

√5th Y35.8 **Legal intervention involving other specified means**

√6th Y35.81 **Legal intervention involving manhandling**
- √7th Y35.811 **Legal intervention involving manhandling, law enforcement official injured**
- √7th Y35.812 **Legal intervention involving manhandling, bystander injured**
- √7th Y35.813 **Legal intervention involving manhandling, suspect injured**

√6th Y35.89 **Legal intervention involving other specified means**
- √7th Y35.891 **Legal intervention involving other specified means, law enforcement official injured**
- √7th Y35.892 **Legal intervention involving other specified means, bystander injured**
- √7th Y35.893 **Legal intervention involving other specified means, suspect injured**

√5th Y35.9 **Legal intervention, means unspecified**
- √x7th Y35.91 **Legal intervention, means unspecified, law enforcement official injured**
- √x7th Y35.92 **Legal intervention, means unspecified, bystander injured**
- √x7th Y35.93 **Legal intervention, means unspecified, suspect injured**

√4th Y36 Operations of war

INCLUDES injuries to military personnel and civilians caused by war, civil insurrection, and peacekeeping missions

EXCLUDES 1 *injury to military personnel occurring during peacetime military operations (Y37.-)*
military vehicles involved in transport accidents with non-military vehicle during peacetime (V09.01, V09.21, V19.81, V29.81, V39.81, V49.81, V59.81, V69.81, V79.81)

The appropriate 7th character is to be added to each code from category Y36.
- A initial encounter
- D subsequent encounter
- S sequela

√5th Y36.0 **War operations involving explosion of marine weapons**

√6th Y36.00 **War operations involving explosion of unspecified marine weapon**
War operations involving underwater blast NOS
- √7th Y36.000 **War operations involving explosion of unspecified marine weapon, military personnel**
- √7th Y36.001 **War operations involving explosion of unspecified marine weapon, civilian**

√6th Y36.01 **War operations involving explosion of depth-charge**
- √7th Y36.010 **War operations involving explosion of depth-charge, military personnel**
- √7th Y36.011 **War operations involving explosion of depth-charge, civilian**

√6th Y36.02 **War operations involving explosion of marine mine**
War operations involving explosion of marine mine, at sea or in harbor
- √7th Y36.020 **War operations involving explosion of marine mine, military personnel**
- √7th Y36.021 **War operations involving explosion of marine mine, civilian**

√6th Y36.03 **War operations involving explosion of sea-based artillery shell**
- √7th Y36.030 **War operations involving explosion of sea-based artillery shell, military personnel**
- √7th Y36.031 **War operations involving explosion of sea-based artillery shell, civilian**

√6th Y36.04 **War operations involving explosion of torpedo**
- √7th Y36.040 **War operations involving explosion of torpedo, military personnel**
- √7th Y36.041 **War operations involving explosion of torpedo, civilian**

√6th Y36.05 **War operations involving accidental detonation of onboard marine weapons**
- √7th Y36.050 **War operations involving accidental detonation of onboard marine weapons, military personnel**
- √7th Y36.051 **War operations involving accidental detonation of onboard marine weapons, civilian**

√6th Y36.09 **War operations involving explosion of other marine weapons**
- √7th Y36.090 **War operations involving explosion of other marine weapons, military personnel**
- √7th Y36.091 **War operations involving explosion of other marine weapons, civilian**

5th Y36.1 War operations involving destruction of aircraft

6th Y36.10 War operations involving unspecified destruction of aircraft

7th Y36.100 War operations involving unspecified destruction of aircraft, military personnel

7th Y36.101 War operations involving unspecified destruction of aircraft, civilian

6th Y36.11 War operations involving destruction of aircraft due to enemy fire or explosives

War operations involving destruction of aircraft due to air to air missile

War operations involving destruction of aircraft due to explosive placed on aircraft

War operations involving destruction of aircraft due to rocket propelled grenade [RPG]

War operations involving destruction of aircraft due to small arms fire

War operations involving destruction of aircraft due to surface to air missile

7th Y36.110 War operations involving destruction of aircraft due to enemy fire or explosives, military personnel

7th Y36.111 War operations involving destruction of aircraft due to enemy fire or explosives, civilian

6th Y36.12 War operations involving destruction of aircraft due to collision with other aircraft

7th Y36.120 War operations involving destruction of aircraft due to collision with other aircraft, military personnel

7th Y36.121 War operations involving destruction of aircraft due to collision with other aircraft, civilian

6th Y36.13 War operations involving destruction of aircraft due to onboard fire

7th Y36.130 War operations involving destruction of aircraft due to onboard fire, military personnel

7th Y36.131 War operations involving destruction of aircraft due to onboard fire, civilian

6th Y36.14 War operations involving destruction of aircraft due to accidental detonation of onboard munitions and explosives

7th Y36.140 War operations involving destruction of aircraft due to accidental detonation of onboard munitions and explosives, military personnel

7th Y36.141 War operations involving destruction of aircraft due to accidental detonation of onboard munitions and explosives, civilian

6th Y36.19 War operations involving other destruction of aircraft

7th Y36.190 War operations involving other destruction of aircraft, military personnel

7th Y36.191 War operations involving other destruction of aircraft, civilian

5th Y36.2 War operations involving other explosions and fragments

EXCLUDES 1 *war operations involving explosion of aircraft (Y36.1-)*

war operations involving explosion of marine weapons (Y36.0-)

war operations involving explosion of nuclear weapons (Y36.5-)

war operations involving explosion occurring after cessation of hostilities (Y36.8-)

6th Y36.20 War operations involving unspecified explosion and fragments

War operations involving air blast NOS

War operations involving blast NOS

War operations involving blast fragments NOS

War operations involving blast wave NOS

War operations involving blast wind NOS

War operations involving explosion NOS

War operations involving explosion of bomb NOS

7th Y36.200 War operations involving unspecified explosion and fragments, military personnel

7th Y36.201 War operations involving unspecified explosion and fragments, civilian

6th Y36.21 War operations involving explosion of aerial bomb

7th Y36.210 War operations involving explosion of aerial bomb, military personnel

7th Y36.211 War operations involving explosion of aerial bomb, civilian

6th Y36.22 War operations involving explosion of guided missile

7th Y36.220 War operations involving explosion of guided missile, military personnel

7th Y36.221 War operations involving explosion of guided missile, civilian

6th Y36.23 War operations involving explosion of improvised explosive device [IED]

War operations involving explosion of person-borne improvised explosive device [IED]

War operations involving explosion of vehicle-borne improvised explosive device [IED]

War operations involving explosion of roadside improvised explosive device [IED]

7th Y36.230 War operations involving explosion of improvised explosive device [IED], military personnel

7th Y36.231 War operations involving explosion of improvised explosive device [IED], civilian

6th Y36.24 War operations involving explosion due to accidental detonation and discharge of own munitions or munitions launch device

7th Y36.240 War operations involving explosion due to accidental detonation and discharge of own munitions or munitions launch device, military personnel

7th Y36.241 War operations involving explosion due to accidental detonation and discharge of own munitions or munitions launch device, civilian

6th Y36.25 War operations involving fragments from munitions

7th Y36.250 War operations involving fragments from munitions, military personnel

7th Y36.251 War operations involving fragments from munitions, civilian

6th Y36.26 War operations involving fragments of improvised explosive device [IED]

War operations involving fragments of person-borne improvised explosive device [IED]

War operations involving fragments of vehicle-borne improvised explosive device [IED]

War operations involving fragments of roadside improvised explosive device [IED]

7th Y36.260 War operations involving fragments of improvised explosive device [IED], military personnel

7th Y36.261 War operations involving fragments of improvised explosive device [IED], civilian

6th Y36.27 War operations involving fragments from weapons

7th Y36.270 War operations involving fragments from weapons, military personnel

7th Y36.271 War operations involving fragments from weapons, civilian

6th Y36.29 War operations involving other explosions and fragments

War operations involving explosion of grenade

War operations involving explosions of land mine

War operations involving shrapnel NOS

7th Y36.290 War operations involving other explosions and fragments, military personnel

7th Y36.291 War operations involving other explosions and fragments, civilian

5th Y36.3 War operations involving fires, conflagrations and hot substances
War operations involving smoke, fumes, and heat from fires, conflagrations and hot substances
EXCLUDES1 *war operations involving fires and conflagrations aboard military aircraft (Y36.1-)*
war operations involving fires and conflagrations aboard military watercraft (Y36.0-)
war operations involving fires and conflagrations caused indirectly by conventional weapons (Y36.2-)
war operations involving fires and thermal effects of nuclear weapons (Y36.53-)

6th Y36.30 War operations involving unspecified fire, conflagration and hot substance
7th Y36.300 War operations involving unspecified fire, conflagration and hot substance, military personnel
7th Y36.301 War operations involving unspecified fire, conflagration and hot substance, civilian

6th Y36.31 War operations involving gasoline bomb
War operations involving incendiary bomb
War operations involving petrol bomb
7th Y36.310 War operations involving gasoline bomb, military personnel
7th Y36.311 War operations involving gasoline bomb, civilian

6th Y36.32 War operations involving incendiary bullet
7th Y36.320 War operations involving incendiary bullet, military personnel
7th Y36.321 War operations involving incendiary bullet, civilian

6th Y36.33 War operations involving flamethrower
7th Y36.330 War operations involving flamethrower, military personnel
7th Y36.331 War operations involving flamethrower, civilian

6th Y36.39 War operations involving other fires, conflagrations and hot substances
7th Y36.390 War operations involving other fires, conflagrations and hot substances, military personnel
7th Y36.391 War operations involving other fires, conflagrations and hot substances, civilian

5th Y36.4 War operations involving firearm discharge and other forms of conventional warfare

6th Y36.41 War operations involving rubber bullets
7th Y36.410 War operations involving rubber bullets, military personnel
7th Y36.411 War operations involving rubber bullets, civilian

6th Y36.42 War operations involving firearms pellets
7th Y36.420 War operations involving firearms pellets, military personnel
7th Y36.421 War operations involving firearms pellets, civilian

6th Y36.43 War operations involving other firearms discharge
War operations involving bullets NOS
EXCLUDES1 *war operations involving munitions fragments (Y36.25-)*
war operations involving incendiary bullets (Y36.32-)
7th Y36.430 War operations involving other firearms discharge, military personnel
7th Y36.431 War operations involving other firearms discharge, civilian

6th Y36.44 War operations involving unarmed hand to hand combat
EXCLUDES1 *war operations involving combat using blunt or piercing object (Y36.45-)*
war operations involving intentional restriction of air and airway (Y36.46-)
war operations involving unintentional restriction of air and airway (Y36.47-)
7th Y36.440 War operations involving unarmed hand to hand combat, military personnel
7th Y36.441 War operations involving unarmed hand to hand combat, civilian

6th Y36.45 War operations involving combat using blunt or piercing object
7th Y36.450 War operations involving combat using blunt or piercing object, military personnel
7th Y36.451 War operations involving combat using blunt or piercing object, civilian

6th Y36.46 War operations involving intentional restriction of air and airway
7th Y36.460 War operations involving intentional restriction of air and airway, military personnel
7th Y36.461 War operations involving intentional restriction of air and airway, civilian

6th Y36.47 War operations involving unintentional restriction of air and airway
7th Y36.470 War operations involving unintentional restriction of air and airway, military personnel
7th Y36.471 War operations involving unintentional restriction of air and airway, civilian

6th Y36.49 War operations involving other forms of conventional warfare
7th Y36.490 War operations involving other forms of conventional warfare, military personnel
7th Y36.491 War operations involving other forms of conventional warfare, civilian

5th Y36.5 War operations involving nuclear weapons
War operations involving dirty bomb NOS

6th Y36.50 War operations involving unspecified effect of nuclear weapon
7th Y36.500 War operations involving unspecified effect of nuclear weapon, military personnel
7th Y36.501 War operations involving unspecified effect of nuclear weapon, civilian

6th Y36.51 War operations involving direct blast effect of nuclear weapon
War operations involving blast pressure of nuclear weapon
7th Y36.510 War operations involving direct blast effect of nuclear weapon, military personnel
7th Y36.511 War operations involving direct blast effect of nuclear weapon, civilian

6th Y36.52 War operations involving indirect blast effect of nuclear weapon
War operations involving being thrown by blast of nuclear weapon
War operations involving being struck or crushed by blast debris of nuclear weapon
7th Y36.520 War operations involving indirect blast effect of nuclear weapon, military personnel
7th Y36.521 War operations involving indirect blast effect of nuclear weapon, civilian

6th Y36.53 War operations involving thermal radiation effect of nuclear weapon
War operations involving direct heat from nuclear weapon
War operation involving fireball effects from nuclear weapon
7th Y36.530 War operations involving thermal radiation effect of nuclear weapon, military personnel
7th Y36.531 War operations involving thermal radiation effect of nuclear weapon, civilian

Y36.54 War operation involving nuclear radiation effects of nuclear weapon
War operation involving acute radiation exposure from nuclear weapon
War operation involving exposure to immediate ionizing radiation from nuclear weapon
War operation involving fallout exposure from nuclear weapon
War operation involving secondary effects of nuclear weapons

Y36.540 War operation involving nuclear radiation effects of nuclear weapon, military personnel

Y36.541 War operation involving nuclear radiation effects of nuclear weapon, civilian

Y36.59 War operation involving other effects of nuclear weapons

Y36.590 War operation involving other effects of nuclear weapons, military personnel

Y36.591 War operation involving other effects of nuclear weapons, civilian

Y36.6 War operations involving biological weapons

Y36.6X War operations involving biological weapons

Y36.6X0 War operations involving biological weapons, military personnel

Y36.6X1 War operations involving biological weapons, civilian

Y36.7 War operations involving chemical weapons and other forms of unconventional warfare
EXCLUDES 1 *war operations involving incendiary devices (Y36.3-, Y36.5-)*

Y36.7X War operations involving chemical weapons and other forms of unconventional warfare

Y36.7X0 War operations involving chemical weapons and other forms of unconventional warfare, military personnel

Y36.7X1 War operations involving chemical weapons and other forms of unconventional warfare, civilian

Y36.8 War operations occurring after cessation of hostilities
War operations classifiable to categories Y36.0-Y36.8 but occurring after cessation of hostilities

Y36.81 Explosion of mine placed during war operations but exploding after cessation of hostilities

Y36.810 Explosion of mine placed during war operations but exploding after cessation of hostilities, military personnel

Y36.811 Explosion of mine placed during war operations but exploding after cessation of hostilities, civilian

Y36.82 Explosion of bomb placed during war operations but exploding after cessation of hostilities

Y36.820 Explosion of bomb placed during war operations but exploding after cessation of hostilities, military personnel

Y36.821 Explosion of bomb placed during war operations but exploding after cessation of hostilities, civilian

Y36.88 Other war operations occurring after cessation of hostilities

Y36.880 Other war operations occurring after cessation of hostilities, military personnel

Y36.881 Other war operations occurring after cessation of hostilities, civilian

Y36.89 Unspecified war operations occurring after cessation of hostilities

Y36.890 Unspecified war operations occurring after cessation of hostilities, military personnel

Y36.891 Unspecified war operations occurring after cessation of hostilities, civilian

Y36.9 Other and unspecified war operations

Y36.90 War operations, unspecified

Y36.91 War operations involving unspecified weapon of mass destruction [WMD]

Y36.92 War operations involving friendly fire

Y37 Military operations
INCLUDES injuries to military personnel and civilians occurring during peacetime on military property and during routine military exercises and operations
EXCLUDES 1 *military aircraft involved in aircraft accident with civilian aircraft (V97.81-)*
military vehicles involved in transport accident with civilian vehicle (V09.01, V09.21, V19.81, V29.81, V39.81, V49.81, V59.81, V69.81, V79.81)
military watercraft involved in water transport accident with civilian watercraft (V94.81-)
war operations (Y36.-)

The appropriate 7th character is to be added to each code from category Y37.
A initial encounter
D subsequent encounter
S sequela

Y37.0 Military operations involving explosion of marine weapons

Y37.00 Military operations involving explosion of unspecified marine weapon
Military operations involving underwater blast NOS

Y37.000 Military operations involving explosion of unspecified marine weapon, military personnel

Y37.001 Military operations involving explosion of unspecified marine weapon, civilian

Y37.01 Military operations involving explosion of depth-charge

Y37.010 Military operations involving explosion of depth-charge, military personnel

Y37.011 Military operations involving explosion of depth-charge, civilian

Y37.02 Military operations involving explosion of marine mine
Military operations involving explosion of marine mine, at sea or in harbor

Y37.020 Military operations involving explosion of marine mine, military personnel

Y37.021 Military operations involving explosion of marine mine, civilian

Y37.03 Military operations involving explosion of sea-based artillery shell

Y37.030 Military operations involving explosion of sea-based artillery shell, military personnel

Y37.031 Military operations involving explosion of sea-based artillery shell, civilian

Y37.04 Military operations involving explosion of torpedo

Y37.040 Military operations involving explosion of torpedo, military personnel

Y37.041 Military operations involving explosion of torpedo, civilian

Y37.05 Military operations involving accidental detonation of onboard marine weapons

Y37.050 Military operations involving accidental detonation of onboard marine weapons, military personnel

Y37.051 Military operations involving accidental detonation of onboard marine weapons, civilian

Y37.09 Military operations involving explosion of other marine weapons

Y37.090 Military operations involving explosion of other marine weapons, military personnel

Y37.091 Military operations involving explosion of other marine weapons, civilian

Y37.1 Military operations involving destruction of aircraft

Y37.10 Military operations involving unspecified destruction of aircraft

7th **Y37.100 Military operations involving unspecified destruction of aircraft, military personnel**

7th **Y37.101 Military operations involving unspecified destruction of aircraft, civilian**

6th **Y37.11 Military operations involving destruction of aircraft due to enemy fire or explosives**

Military operations involving destruction of aircraft due to air to air missile
Military operations involving destruction of aircraft due to explosive placed on aircraft
Military operations involving destruction of aircraft due to rocket propelled grenade [RPG]
Military operations involving destruction of aircraft due to small arms fire
Military operations involving destruction of aircraft due to surface to air missile

7th **Y37.110 Military operations involving destruction of aircraft due to enemy fire or explosives, military personnel**

7th **Y37.111 Military operations involving destruction of aircraft due to enemy fire or explosives, civilian**

6th **Y37.12 Military operations involving destruction of aircraft due to collision with other aircraft**

7th **Y37.120 Military operations involving destruction of aircraft due to collision with other aircraft, military personnel**

7th **Y37.121 Military operations involving destruction of aircraft due to collision with other aircraft, civilian**

6th **Y37.13 Military operations involving destruction of aircraft due to onboard fire**

7th **Y37.130 Military operations involving destruction of aircraft due to onboard fire, military personnel**

7th **Y37.131 Military operations involving destruction of aircraft due to onboard fire, civilian**

6th **Y37.14 Military operations involving destruction of aircraft due to accidental detonation of onboard munitions and explosives**

7th **Y37.140 Military operations involving destruction of aircraft due to accidental detonation of onboard munitions and explosives, military personnel**

7th **Y37.141 Military operations involving destruction of aircraft due to accidental detonation of onboard munitions and explosives, civilian**

6th **Y37.19 Military operations involving other destruction of aircraft**

7th **Y37.190 Military operations involving other destruction of aircraft, military personnel**

7th **Y37.191 Military operations involving other destruction of aircraft, civilian**

5th **Y37.2 Military operations involving other explosions and fragments**

EXCLUDES1 *military operations involving explosion of aircraft (Y37.1-)*
military operations involving explosion of marine weapons (Y37.0-)
military operations involving explosion of nuclear weapons (Y37.5-)

6th **Y37.20 Military operations involving unspecified explosion and fragments**

Military operations involving air blast NOS
Military operations involving blast NOS
Military operations involving blast fragments NOS
Military operations involving blast wave NOS
Military operations involving blast wind NOS
Military operations involving explosion NOS
Military operations involving explosion of bomb NOS

7th **Y37.200 Military operations involving unspecified explosion and fragments, military personnel**

7th **Y37.201 Military operations involving unspecified explosion and fragments, civilian**

6th **Y37.21 Military operations involving explosion of aerial bomb**

7th **Y37.210 Military operations involving explosion of aerial bomb, military personnel**

7th **Y37.211 Military operations involving explosion of aerial bomb, civilian**

6th **Y37.22 Military operations involving explosion of guided missile**

7th **Y37.220 Military operations involving explosion of guided missile, military personnel**

7th **Y37.221 Military operations involving explosion of guided missile, civilian**

6th **Y37.23 Military operations involving explosion of improvised explosive device [IED]**

Military operations involving explosion of person-borne improvised explosive device [IED]
Military operations involving explosion of vehicle-borne improvised explosive device [IED]
Military operations involving explosion of roadside improvised explosive device [IED]

7th **Y37.230 Military operations involving explosion of improvised explosive device [IED], military personnel**

7th **Y37.231 Military operations involving explosion of improvised explosive device [IED], civilian**

6th **Y37.24 Military operations involving explosion due to accidental detonation and discharge of own munitions or munitions launch device**

7th **Y37.240 Military operations involving explosion due to accidental detonation and discharge of own munitions or munitions launch device, military personnel**

7th **Y37.241 Military operations involving explosion due to accidental detonation and discharge of own munitions or munitions launch device, civilian**

6th **Y37.25 Military operations involving fragments from munitions**

7th **Y37.250 Military operations involving fragments from munitions, military personnel**

7th **Y37.251 Military operations involving fragments from munitions, civilian**

6th **Y37.26 Military operations involving fragments of improvised explosive device [IED]**

Military operations involving fragments of person-borne improvised explosive device [IED]
Military operations involving fragments of vehicle-borne improvised explosive device [IED]
Military operations involving fragments of roadside improvised explosive device [IED]

7th **Y37.260 Military operations involving fragments of improvised explosive device [IED], military personnel**

7th **Y37.261 Military operations involving fragments of improvised explosive device [IED], civilian**

6th **Y37.27 Military operations involving fragments from weapons**

7th **Y37.270 Military operations involving fragments from weapons, military personnel**

7th **Y37.271 Military operations involving fragments from weapons, civilian**

6th **Y37.29 Military operations involving other explosions and fragments**

Military operations involving explosion of grenade
Military operations involving explosions of land mine
Military operations involving shrapnel NOS

✓7th **Y37.290 Military operations involving other explosions and fragments, military personnel**

✓7th **Y37.291 Military operations involving other explosions and fragments, civilian**

✓5th **Y37.3 Military operations involving fires, conflagrations and hot substances**

Military operations involving smoke, fumes, and heat from fires, conflagrations and hot substances

EXCLUDES 1 *military operations involving fires and conflagrations aboard military aircraft (Y37.1-)*

military operations involving fires and conflagrations aboard military watercraft (Y37.0-)

military operations involving fires and conflagrations caused indirectly by conventional weapons (Y37.2-)

military operations involving fires and thermal effects of nuclear weapons (Y36.53-)

✓6th **Y37.30 Military operations involving unspecified fire, conflagration and hot substance**

✓7th **Y37.300 Military operations involving unspecified fire, conflagration and hot substance, military personnel**

✓7th **Y37.301 Military operations involving unspecified fire, conflagration and hot substance, civilian**

✓6th **Y37.31 Military operations involving gasoline bomb**

Military operations involving incendiary bomb

Military operations involving petrol bomb

✓7th **Y37.310 Military operations involving gasoline bomb, military personnel**

✓7th **Y37.311 Military operations involving gasoline bomb, civilian**

✓6th **Y37.32 Military operations involving incendiary bullet**

✓7th **Y37.320 Military operations involving incendiary bullet, military personnel**

✓7th **Y37.321 Military operations involving incendiary bullet, civilian**

✓6th **Y37.33 Military operations involving flamethrower**

✓7th **Y37.330 Military operations involving flamethrower, military personnel**

✓7th **Y37.331 Military operations involving flamethrower, civilian**

✓6th **Y37.39 Military operations involving other fires, conflagrations and hot substances**

✓7th **Y37.390 Military operations involving other fires, conflagrations and hot substances, military personnel**

✓7th **Y37.391 Military operations involving other fires, conflagrations and hot substances, civilian**

✓5th **Y37.4 Military operations involving firearm discharge and other forms of conventional warfare**

✓6th **Y37.41 Military operations involving rubber bullets**

✓7th **Y37.410 Military operations involving rubber bullets, military personnel**

✓7th **Y37.411 Military operations involving rubber bullets, civilian**

✓6th **Y37.42 Military operations involving firearms pellets**

✓7th **Y37.420 Military operations involving firearms pellets, military personnel**

✓7th **Y37.421 Military operations involving firearms pellets, civilian**

✓6th **Y37.43 Military operations involving other firearms discharge**

Military operations involving bullets NOS

EXCLUDES 1 *military operations involving munitions fragments (Y37.25-)*

military operations involving incendiary bullets (Y37.32-)

✓7th **Y37.430 Military operations involving other firearms discharge, military personnel**

✓7th **Y37.431 Military operations involving other firearms discharge, civilian**

✓6th **Y37.44 Military operations involving unarmed hand to hand combat**

EXCLUDES 1 *military operations involving combat using blunt or piercing object (Y37.45-)*

military operations involving intentional restriction of air and airway (Y37.46-)

military operations involving unintentional restriction of air and airway (Y37.47-)

✓7th **Y37.440 Military operations involving unarmed hand to hand combat, military personnel**

✓7th **Y37.441 Military operations involving unarmed hand to hand combat, civilian**

✓6th **Y37.45 Military operations involving combat using blunt or piercing object**

✓7th **Y37.450 Military operations involving combat using blunt or piercing object, military personnel**

✓7th **Y37.451 Military operations involving combat using blunt or piercing object, civilian**

✓6th **Y37.46 Military operations involving intentional restriction of air and airway**

✓7th **Y37.460 Military operations involving intentional restriction of air and airway, military personnel**

✓7th **Y37.461 Military operations involving intentional restriction of air and airway, civilian**

✓6th **Y37.47 Military operations involving unintentional restriction of air and airway**

✓7th **Y37.470 Military operations involving unintentional restriction of air and airway, military personnel**

✓7th **Y37.471 Military operations involving unintentional restriction of air and airway, civilian**

✓6th **Y37.49 Military operations involving other forms of conventional warfare**

✓7th **Y37.490 Military operations involving other forms of conventional warfare, military personnel**

✓7th **Y37.491 Military operations involving other forms of conventional warfare, civilian**

✓5th **Y37.5 Military operations involving nuclear weapons**

Military operation involving dirty bomb NOS

✓6th **Y37.50 Military operations involving unspecified effect of nuclear weapon**

✓7th **Y37.500 Military operations involving unspecified effect of nuclear weapon, military personnel**

✓7th **Y37.501 Military operations involving unspecified effect of nuclear weapon, civilian**

✓6th **Y37.51 Military operations involving direct blast effect of nuclear weapon**

Military operations involving blast pressure of nuclear weapon

✓7th **Y37.510 Military operations involving direct blast effect of nuclear weapon, military personnel**

✓7th **Y37.511 Military operations involving direct blast effect of nuclear weapon, civilian**

✓6th **Y37.52 Military operations involving indirect blast effect of nuclear weapon**

Military operations involving being thrown by blast of nuclear weapon

Military operations involving being struck or crushed by blast debris of nuclear weapon

✓7th **Y37.520 Military operations involving indirect blast effect of nuclear weapon, military personnel**

✓7th **Y37.521 Military operations involving indirect blast effect of nuclear weapon, civilian**

✓6th **Y37.53 Military operations involving thermal radiation effect of nuclear weapon**

Military operations involving direct heat from nuclear weapon

Military operation involving fireball effects from nuclear weapon

Y37.530 Military operations involving thermal radiation effect of nuclear weapon, military personnel

Y37.531 Military operations involving thermal radiation effect of nuclear weapon, civilian

Y37.54 Military operation involving nuclear radiation effects of nuclear weapon
Military operation involving acute radiation exposure from nuclear weapon
Military operation involving exposure to immediate ionizing radiation from nuclear weapon
Military operation involving fallout exposure from nuclear weapon
Military operation involving secondary effects of nuclear weapons

Y37.540 Military operation involving nuclear radiation effects of nuclear weapon, military personnel

Y37.541 Military operation involving nuclear radiation effects of nuclear weapon, civilian

Y37.59 Military operation involving other effects of nuclear weapons

Y37.590 Military operation involving other effects of nuclear weapons, military personnel

Y37.591 Military operation involving other effects of nuclear weapons, civilian

Y37.6 Military operations involving biological weapons

Y37.6X Military operations involving biological weapons

Y37.6X0 Military operations involving biological weapons, military personnel

Y37.6X1 Military operations involving biological weapons, civilian

Y37.7 Military operations involving chemical weapons and other forms of unconventional warfare
EXCLUDES 1 *military operations involving incendiary devices (Y36.3-, Y36.5-)*

Y37.7X Military operations involving chemical weapons and other forms of unconventional warfare

Y37.7X0 Military operations involving chemical weapons and other forms of unconventional warfare, military personnel

Y37.7X1 Military operations involving chemical weapons and other forms of unconventional warfare, civilian

Y37.9 Other and unspecified military operations

Y37.90 Military operations, unspecified

Y37.91 Military operations involving unspecified weapon of mass destruction [WMD]

Y37.92 Military operations involving friendly fire

Y38 Terrorism

NOTE These codes are for use to identify injuries resulting from the unlawful use of force or violence against persons or property to intimidate or coerce a Government, the civilian population, or any segment thereof, in furtherance of political or social objective

Use additional code for place of occurrence (Y92.-)

The appropriate 7th character is to be added to each code from category Y38.
A initial encounter
D subsequent encounter
S sequela

Y38.0 Terrorism involving explosion of marine weapons
Terrorism involving depth-charge
Terrorism involving marine mine
Terrorism involving mine NOS, at sea or in harbor
Terrorism involving sea-based artillery shell
Terrorism involving torpedo
Terrorism involving underwater blast

Y38.0X Terrorism involving explosion of marine weapons

Y38.0X1 Terrorism involving explosion of marine weapons, public safety official injured

Y38.0X2 Terrorism involving explosion of marine weapons, civilian injured

Y38.0X3 Terrorism involving explosion of marine weapons, terrorist injured

Y38.1 Terrorism involving destruction of aircraft
Terrorism involving aircraft burned
Terrorism involving aircraft exploded
Terrorism involving aircraft being shot down
Terrorism involving aircraft used as a weapon

Y38.1X Terrorism involving destruction of aircraft

Y38.1X1 Terrorism involving destruction of aircraft, public safety official injured

Y38.1X2 Terrorism involving destruction of aircraft, civilian injured

Y38.1X3 Terrorism involving destruction of aircraft, terrorist injured

Y38.2 Terrorism involving other explosions and fragments
Terrorism involving antipersonnel (fragments) bomb
Terrorism involving blast NOS
Terrorism involving explosion NOS
Terrorism involving explosion of breech block
Terrorism involving explosion of cannon block
Terrorism involving explosion (fragments) of artillery shell
Terrorism involving explosion (fragments) of bomb
Terrorism involving explosion (fragments) of grenade
Terrorism involving explosion (fragments) of guided missile
Terrorism involving explosion (fragments) of land mine
Terrorism involving explosion of mortar bomb
Terrorism involving explosion of munitions
Terrorism involving explosion (fragments) of rocket
Terrorism involving explosion (fragments) of shell
Terrorism involving shrapnel
Terrorism involving mine NOS, on land
EXCLUDES 1 *terrorism involving explosion of nuclear weapon (Y38.5)*
terrorism involving suicide bomber (Y38.81)

Y38.2X Terrorism involving other explosions and fragments

Y38.2X1 Terrorism involving other explosions and fragments, public safety official injured

Y38.2X2 Terrorism involving other explosions and fragments, civilian injured

Y38.2X3 Terrorism involving other explosions and fragments, terrorist injured

Y38.3 Terrorism involving fires, conflagration and hot substances
Terrorism involving conflagration NOS
Terrorism involving fire NOS
Terrorism involving petrol bomb
EXCLUDES 1 *terrorism involving fire or heat of nuclear weapon (Y38.5)*

Y38.3X Terrorism involving fires, conflagration and hot substances

Y38.3X1 Terrorism involving fires, conflagration and hot substances, public safety official injured

Y38.3X2 Terrorism involving fires, conflagration and hot substances, civilian injured

Y38.3X3 Terrorism involving fires, conflagration and hot substances, terrorist injured

Y38.4 Terrorism involving firearms
Terrorism involving carbine bullet
Terrorism involving machine gun bullet
Terrorism involving pellets (shotgun)
Terrorism involving pistol bullet
Terrorism involving rifle bullet
Terrorism involving rubber (rifle) bullet

Y38.4X Terrorism involving firearms

Y38.4X1 Terrorism involving firearms, public safety official injured

Y38.4X2 Terrorism involving firearms, civilian injured

Y38.4X3 Terrorism involving firearms, terrorist injured

Y38.5 Terrorism involving nuclear weapons
Terrorism involving blast effects of nuclear weapon
Terrorism involving exposure to ionizing radiation from nuclear weapon
Terrorism involving fireball effect of nuclear weapon
Terrorism involving heat from nuclear weapon

Y38.5X Terrorism involving nuclear weapons

Y38.5X1 **Terrorism involving nuclear weapons, public safety official injured**
Y38.5X2 **Terrorism involving nuclear weapons, civilian injured**
Y38.5X3 **Terrorism involving nuclear weapons, terrorist injured**

Y38.6 Terrorism involving biological weapons
Terrorism involving anthrax
Terrorism involving cholera
Terrorism involving smallpox

Y38.6X Terrorism involving biological weapons
Y38.6X1 **Terrorism involving biological weapons, public safety official injured**
Y38.6X2 **Terrorism involving biological weapons, civilian injured**
Y38.6X3 **Terrorism involving biological weapons, terrorist injured**

Y38.7 Terrorism involving chemical weapons
Terrorism involving gases, fumes, chemicals
Terrorism involving hydrogen cyanide
Terrorism involving phosgene
Terrorism involving sarin

Y38.7X Terrorism involving chemical weapons
Y38.7X1 **Terrorism involving chemical weapons, public safety official injured**
Y38.7X2 **Terrorism involving chemical weapons, civilian injured**
Y38.7X3 **Terrorism involving chemical weapons, terrorist injured**

Y38.8 Terrorism involving other and unspecified means
Y38.80 Terrorism involving unspecified means
Terrorism NOS
Y38.81 Terrorism involving suicide bomber
Y38.811 **Terrorism involving suicide bomber, public safety official injured**
Y38.812 **Terrorism involving suicide bomber, civilian injured**
Y38.89 Terrorism involving other means
Terrorism involving drowning and submersion
Terrorism involving lasers
Terrorism involving piercing or stabbing instruments
Y38.891 **Terrorism involving other means, public safety official injured**
Y38.892 **Terrorism involving other means, civilian injured**
Y38.893 **Terrorism involving other means, terrorist injured**

Y38.9 Terrorism, secondary effects
NOTE This code is for use to identify injuries occurring subsequent to a terrorist attack, not those that are due to the initial terrorist attack.
Y38.9X Terrorism, secondary effects
Y38.9X1 **Terrorism, secondary effects, public safety official injured**
Y38.9X2 **Terrorism, secondary effects, civilian injured**

Complications of medical and surgical care (Y62-Y84)

INCLUDES complications of medical devices
surgical and medical procedures as the cause of abnormal reaction of the patient, or of later complication, without mention of misadventure at the time of the procedure

Misadventures to patients during surgical and medical care (Y62-Y69)

EXCLUDES 2 *breakdown or malfunctioning of medical device (during procedure) (after implantation) (ongoing use) (Y70-Y82)*
surgical and medical procedures as the cause of abnormal reaction of the patient, without mention of misadventure at the time of the procedure (Y83-Y84)

Y62 Failure of sterile precautions during surgical and medical care
Y62.0 Failure of sterile precautions during surgical operation
Y62.1 Failure of sterile precautions during infusion or transfusion
Y62.2 Failure of sterile precautions during kidney dialysis and other perfusion
Y62.3 Failure of sterile precautions during injection or immunization
Y62.4 Failure of sterile precautions during endoscopic examination
Y62.5 Failure of sterile precautions during heart catheterization
Y62.6 Failure of sterile precautions during aspiration, puncture and other catheterization
Y62.8 Failure of sterile precautions during other surgical and medical care
Y62.9 Failure of sterile precautions during unspecified surgical and medical care

Y63 Failure in dosage during surgical and medical care
EXCLUDES 2 *accidental overdose of drug or wrong drug given in error (T36-T50)*
Y63.0 Excessive amount of blood or other fluid given during transfusion or infusion
Y63.1 Incorrect dilution of fluid used during infusion
Y63.2 Overdose of radiation given during therapy
Y63.3 Inadvertent exposure of patient to radiation during medical care
Y63.4 Failure in dosage in electroshock or insulin-shock therapy
Y63.5 Inappropriate temperature in local application and packing
Y63.6 Underdosing and nonadministration of necessary drug, medicament or biological substance
Y63.8 Failure in dosage during other surgical and medical care
Y63.9 Failure in dosage during unspecified surgical and medical care

Y64 Contaminated medical or biological substances
Y64.0 Contaminated medical or biological substance, transfused or infused
Y64.1 Contaminated medical or biological substance, injected or used for immunization
Y64.8 Contaminated medical or biological substance administered by other means
Y64.9 Contaminated medical or biological substance administered by unspecified means
Administered contaminated medical or biological substance NOS

Y65 Other misadventures during surgical and medical care
Y65.0 Mismatched blood in transfusion
Y65.1 Wrong fluid used in infusion
Y65.2 Failure in suture or ligature during surgical operation
Y65.3 Endotracheal tube wrongly placed during anesthetic procedure
Y65.4 Failure to introduce or to remove other tube or instrument
Y65.5 Performance of wrong procedure (operation)
Y65.51 Performance of wrong procedure (operation) on correct patient
Wrong device implanted into correct surgical site
EXCLUDES 1 *performance of correct procedure (operation) on wrong side or body part (Y65.53)*
Y65.52 Performance of procedure (operation) on patient not scheduled for surgery
Performance of procedure (operation) intended for another patient
Performance of procedure (operation) on wrong patient
Y65.53 Performance of correct procedure (operation) on wrong side or body part
Performance of correct procedure (operation) on wrong side
Performance of correct procedure (operation) on wrong site
Y65.8 Other specified misadventures during surgical and medical care

Y66 Nonadministration of surgical and medical care
Premature cessation of surgical and medical care
EXCLUDES 1 *DNR status (Z66)*
palliative care (Z51.5)

Y69 Unspecified misadventure during surgical and medical care

Medical devices associated with adverse incidents in diagnostic and therapeutic use (Y70-Y82)

INCLUDES breakdown or malfunction of medical devices (during use) (after implantation) (ongoing use)

EXCLUDES 1 *misadventure to patients during surgical and medical care, classifiable to (Y62-Y69)*

later complications following use of medical devices without breakdown or malfunctioning of device (Y83-Y84)

4th Y70 Anesthesiology devices associated with adverse incidents

Y70.0 Diagnostic and monitoring anesthesiology devices associated with adverse incidents

Y70.1 Therapeutic (nonsurgical) and rehabilitative anesthesiology devices associated with adverse incidents

Y70.2 Prosthetic and other implants, materials and accessory anesthesiology devices associated with adverse incidents

Y70.3 Surgical instruments, materials and anesthesiology devices (including sutures) associated with adverse incidents

Y70.8 Miscellaneous anesthesiology devices associated with adverse incidents, not elsewhere classified

4th Y71 Cardiovascular devices associated with adverse incidents

Y71.0 Diagnostic and monitoring cardiovascular devices associated with adverse incidents

Y71.1 Therapeutic (nonsurgical) and rehabilitative cardiovascular devices associated with adverse incidents

Y71.2 Prosthetic and other implants, materials and accessory cardiovascular devices associated with adverse incidents

Y71.3 Surgical instruments, materials and cardiovascular devices (including sutures) associated with adverse incidents

Y71.8 Miscellaneous cardiovascular devices associated with adverse incidents, not elsewhere classified

4th Y72 Otorhinolaryngological devices associated with adverse incidents

Y72.0 Diagnostic and monitoring otorhinolaryngological devices associated with adverse incidents

Y72.1 Therapeutic (nonsurgical) and rehabilitative otorhinolaryngological devices associated with adverse incidents

Y72.2 Prosthetic and other implants, materials and accessory otorhinolaryngological devices associated with adverse incidents

Y72.3 Surgical instruments, materials and otorhinolaryngological devices (including sutures) associated with adverse incidents

Y72.8 Miscellaneous otorhinolaryngological devices associated with adverse incidents, not elsewhere classified

4th Y73 Gastroenterology and urology devices associated with adverse incidents

Y73.0 Diagnostic and monitoring gastroenterology and urology devices associated with adverse incidents

Y73.1 Therapeutic (nonsurgical) and rehabilitative gastroenterology and urology devices associated with adverse incidents

Y73.2 Prosthetic and other implants, materials and accessory gastroenterology and urology devices associated with adverse incidents

Y73.3 Surgical instruments, materials and gastroenterology and urology devices (including sutures) associated with adverse incidents

Y73.8 Miscellaneous gastroenterology and urology devices associated with adverse incidents, not elsewhere classified

4th Y74 General hospital and personal-use devices associated with adverse incidents

Y74.0 Diagnostic and monitoring general hospital and personal-use devices associated with adverse incidents

Y74.1 Therapeutic (nonsurgical) and rehabilitative general hospital and personal-use devices associated with adverse incidents

Y74.2 Prosthetic and other implants, materials and accessory general hospital and personal-use devices associated with adverse incidents

Y74.3 Surgical instruments, materials and general hospital and personal-use devices (including sutures) associated with adverse incidents

Y74.8 Miscellaneous general hospital and personal-use devices associated with adverse incidents, not elsewhere classified

4th Y75 Neurological devices associated with adverse incidents

Y75.0 Diagnostic and monitoring neurological devices associated with adverse incidents

Y75.1 Therapeutic (nonsurgical) and rehabilitative neurological devices associated with adverse incidents

Y75.2 Prosthetic and other implants, materials and neurological devices associated with adverse incidents

Y75.3 Surgical instruments, materials and neurological devices (including sutures) associated with adverse incidents

Y75.8 Miscellaneous neurological devices associated with adverse incidents, not elsewhere classified

4th Y76 Obstetric and gynecological devices associated with adverse incidents

Y76.0 Diagnostic and monitoring obstetric and gynecological devices associated with adverse incidents

Y76.1 Therapeutic (nonsurgical) and rehabilitative obstetric and gynecological devices associated with adverse incidents

Y76.2 Prosthetic and other implants, materials and accessory obstetric and gynecological devices associated with adverse incidents

Y76.3 Surgical instruments, materials and obstetric and gynecological devices (including sutures) associated with adverse incidents

Y76.8 Miscellaneous obstetric and gynecological devices associated with adverse incidents, not elsewhere classified

4th Y77 Ophthalmic devices associated with adverse incidents

Y77.0 Diagnostic and monitoring ophthalmic devices associated with adverse incidents

Y77.1 Therapeutic (nonsurgical) and rehabilitative ophthalmic devices associated with adverse incidents

Y77.2 Prosthetic and other implants, materials and accessory ophthalmic devices associated with adverse incidents

Y77.3 Surgical instruments, materials and ophthalmic devices (including sutures) associated with adverse incidents

Y77.8 Miscellaneous ophthalmic devices associated with adverse incidents, not elsewhere classified

4th Y78 Radiological devices associated with adverse incidents

Y78.0 Diagnostic and monitoring radiological devices associated with adverse incidents

Y78.1 Therapeutic (nonsurgical) and rehabilitative radiological devices associated with adverse incidents

Y78.2 Prosthetic and other implants, materials and accessory radiological devices associated with adverse incidents

Y78.3 Surgical instruments, materials and radiological devices (including sutures) associated with adverse incidents

Y78.8 Miscellaneous radiological devices associated with adverse incidents, not elsewhere classified

4th Y79 Orthopedic devices associated with adverse incidents

Y79.0 Diagnostic and monitoring orthopedic devices associated with adverse incidents

Y79.1 Therapeutic (nonsurgical) and rehabilitative orthopedic devices associated with adverse incidents

Y79.2 Prosthetic and other implants, materials and accessory orthopedic devices associated with adverse incidents

Y79.3 Surgical instruments, materials and orthopedic devices (including sutures) associated with adverse incidents

Y79.8 Miscellaneous orthopedic devices associated with adverse incidents, not elsewhere classified

4th Y80 Physical medicine devices associated with adverse incidents

Y80.0 Diagnostic and monitoring physical medicine devices associated with adverse incidents

Y80.1 Therapeutic (nonsurgical) and rehabilitative physical medicine devices associated with adverse incidents

Y80.2 Prosthetic and other implants, materials and accessory physical medicine devices associated with adverse incidents

Y80.3 Surgical instruments, materials and physical medicine devices (including sutures) associated with adverse incidents

Y80.8 Miscellaneous physical medicine devices associated with adverse incidents, not elsewhere classified

Y81 General- and plastic-surgery devices associated with adverse incidents

Y81.Ø Diagnostic and monitoring general- and plastic-surgery devices associated with adverse incidents

Y81.1 Therapeutic (nonsurgical) and rehabilitative general- and plastic-surgery devices associated with adverse incidents

Y81.2 Prosthetic and other implants, materials and accessory general- and plastic-surgery devices associated with adverse incidents

Y81.3 Surgical instruments, materials and general- and plastic-surgery devices (including sutures) associated with adverse incidents

Y81.8 Miscellaneous general- and plastic-surgery devices associated with adverse incidents, not elsewhere classified

Y82 Other and unspecified medical devices associated with adverse incidents

Y82.8 Other medical devices associated with adverse incidents

Y82.9 Unspecified medical devices associated with adverse incidents

Surgical and other medical procedures as the cause of abnormal reaction of the patient, or of later complication, without mention of misadventure at the time of the procedure (Y83-Y84)

EXCLUDES 1 *misadventures to patients during surgical and medical care, classifiable to (Y62-Y69)*

Y83 Surgical operation and other surgical procedures as the cause of abnormal reaction of the patient, or of later complication, without mention of misadventure at the time of the procedure

Y83.Ø Surgical operation with transplant of whole organ as the cause of abnormal reaction of the patient, or of later complication, without mention of misadventure at the time of the procedure

Y83.1 Surgical operation with implant of artificial internal device as the cause of abnormal reaction of the patient, or of later complication, without mention of misadventure at the time of the procedure

Y83.2 Surgical operation with anastomosis, bypass or graft as the cause of abnormal reaction of the patient, or of later complication, without mention of misadventure at the time of the procedure

Y83.3 Surgical operation with formation of external stoma as the cause of abnormal reaction of the patient, or of later complication, without mention of misadventure at the time of the procedure

Y83.4 Other reconstructive surgery as the cause of abnormal reaction of the patient, or of later complication, without mention of misadventure at the time of the procedure

Y83.5 Amputation of limb(s) as the cause of abnormal reaction of the patient, or of later complication, without mention of misadventure at the time of the procedure

Y83.6 Removal of other organ (partial) (total) as the cause of abnormal reaction of the patient, or of later complication, without mention of misadventure at the time of the procedure

Y83.8 Other surgical procedures as the cause of abnormal reaction of the patient, or of later complication, without mention of misadventure at the time of the procedure

Y83.9 Surgical procedure, unspecified as the cause of abnormal reaction of the patient, or of later complication, without mention of misadventure at the time of the procedure

Y84 Other medical procedures as the cause of abnormal reaction of the patient, or of later complication, without mention of misadventure at the time of the procedure

Y84.Ø Cardiac catheterization as the cause of abnormal reaction of the patient, or of later complication, without mention of misadventure at the time of the procedure

Y84.1 Kidney dialysis as the cause of abnormal reaction of the patient, or of later complication, without mention of misadventure at the time of the procedure

Y84.2 Radiological procedure and radiotherapy as the cause of abnormal reaction of the patient, or of later complication, without mention of misadventure at the time of the procedure

Y84.3 Shock therapy as the cause of abnormal reaction of the patient, or of later complication, without mention of misadventure at the time of the procedure

Y84.4 Aspiration of fluid as the cause of abnormal reaction of the patient, or of later complication, without mention of misadventure at the time of the procedure

Y84.5 Insertion of gastric or duodenal sound as the cause of abnormal reaction of the patient, or of later complication, without mention of misadventure at the time of the procedure

Y84.6 Urinary catheterization as the cause of abnormal reaction of the patient, or of later complication, without mention of misadventure at the time of the procedure

Y84.7 Blood-sampling as the cause of abnormal reaction of the patient, or of later complication, without mention of misadventure at the time of the procedure

Y84.8 Other medical procedures as the cause of abnormal reaction of the patient, or of later complication, without mention of misadventure at the time of the procedure

Y84.9 Medical procedure, unspecified as the cause of abnormal reaction of the patient, or of later complication, without mention of misadventure at the time of the procedure

Supplementary factors related to causes of morbidity classified elsewhere (Y9Ø-Y99)

NOTE These categories may be used to provide supplementary information concerning causes of morbidity. They are not to be used for single-condition coding.

Y9Ø Evidence of alcohol involvement determined by blood alcohol level

Code first any associated alcohol related disorders (F1Ø)

Y9Ø.Ø Blood alcohol level of less than 2Ø mg/1ØØ ml

Y9Ø.1 Blood alcohol level of 2Ø-39 mg/1ØØ ml

Y9Ø.2 Blood alcohol level of 4Ø-59 mg/1ØØ ml

Y9Ø.3 Blood alcohol level of 6Ø-79 mg/1ØØ ml

Y9Ø.4 Blood alcohol level of 8Ø-99 mg/1ØØ ml

Y9Ø.5 Blood alcohol level of 1ØØ-119 mg/1ØØ ml

Y9Ø.6 Blood alcohol level of 12Ø-199 mg/1ØØ ml

Y9Ø.7 Blood alcohol level of 2ØØ-239 mg/1ØØ ml

Y9Ø.8 Blood alcohol level of 24Ø mg/1ØØ ml or more

Y9Ø.9 Presence of alcohol in blood, level not specified

Y92 Place of occurrence of the external cause

The following category is for use, when relevant, to identify the place of occurrence of the external cause. Use in conjunction with an activity code.

Place of occurrence should be recorded only at the initial encounter for treatment

Y92.Ø Non-institutional (private) residence as the place of occurrence of the external cause

EXCLUDES 1 *abandoned or derelict house (Y92.89)*
home under construction but not yet occupied (Y92.6-)
institutional place of residence (Y92.1-)

Y92.ØØ Unspecified non-institutional (private) residence as the place of occurrence of the external cause

Y92.ØØØ Kitchen of unspecified non-institutional (private) residence as the place of occurrence of the external cause

Y92.ØØ1 Dining room of unspecified non-institutional (private) residence as the place of occurrence of the external cause

Y92.ØØ2 Bathroom of unspecified non-institutional (private) residence single-family (private) house as the place of occurrence of the external cause

Y92.ØØ3 Bedroom of unspecified non-institutional (private) residence as the place of occurrence of the external cause

Y92.ØØ7 Garden or yard of unspecified non-institutional (private) residence as the place of occurrence of the external cause

Y92.ØØ8 Other place in unspecified non-institutional (private) residence as the place of occurrence of the external cause

Y92.009 Unspecified place in unspecified non-institutional (private) residence as the place of occurrence of the external cause
Home (NOS) as the place of occurrence of the external cause

✓6th **Y92.01 Single-family non-institutional (private) house as the place of occurrence of the external cause**
Farmhouse as the place of occurrence of the external cause
EXCLUDES 1 *barn (Y92.71)*
chicken coop or hen house (Y92.72)
farm field (Y92.73)
orchard (Y92.74)
single family mobile home or trailer (Y92.02-)
slaughter house (Y92.86)

Y92.010 Kitchen of single-family (private) house as the place of occurrence of the external cause
Y92.011 Dining room of single-family (private) house as the place of occurrence of the external cause
Y92.012 Bathroom of single-family (private) house as the place of occurrence of the external cause
Y92.013 Bedroom of single-family (private) house as the place of occurrence of the external cause
Y92.014 Private driveway to single-family (private) house as the place of occurrence of the external cause
Y92.015 Private garage of single-family (private) house as the place of occurrence of the external cause
Y92.016 Swimming-pool in single-family (private) house or garden as the place of occurrence of the external cause
Y92.017 Garden or yard in single-family (private) house as the place of occurrence of the external cause
Y92.018 Other place in single-family (private) house as the place of occurrence of the external cause
Y92.019 Unspecified place in single-family (private) house as the place of occurrence of the external cause

✓6th **Y92.02 Mobile home as the place of occurrence of the external cause**
Y92.020 Kitchen in mobile home as the place of occurrence of the external cause
Y92.021 Dining room in mobile home as the place of occurrence of the external cause
Y92.022 Bathroom in mobile home as the place of occurrence of the external cause
Y92.023 Bedroom in mobile home as the place of occurrence of the external cause
Y92.024 Driveway of mobile home as the place of occurrence of the external cause
Y92.025 Garage of mobile home as the place of occurrence of the external cause
Y92.026 Swimming-pool of mobile home as the place of occurrence of the external cause
Y92.027 Garden or yard of mobile home as the place of occurrence of the external cause
Y92.028 Other place in mobile home as the place of occurrence of the external cause
Y92.029 Unspecified place in mobile home as the place of occurrence of the external cause

✓6th **Y92.03 Apartment as the place of occurrence of the external cause**
Condominium as the place of occurrence of the external cause
Co-op apartment as the place of occurrence of the external cause
Y92.030 Kitchen in apartment as the place of occurrence of the external cause
Y92.031 Bathroom in apartment as the place of occurrence of the external cause
Y92.032 Bedroom in apartment as the place of occurrence of the external cause
Y92.038 Other place in apartment as the place of occurrence of the external cause
Y92.039 Unspecified place in apartment as the place of occurrence of the external cause

✓6th **Y92.04 Boarding-house as the place of occurrence of the external cause**
Y92.040 Kitchen in boarding-house as the place of occurrence of the external cause
Y92.041 Bathroom in boarding-house as the place of occurrence of the external cause
Y92.042 Bedroom in boarding-house as the place of occurrence of the external cause
Y92.043 Driveway of boarding-house as the place of occurrence of the external cause
Y92.044 Garage of boarding-house as the place of occurrence of the external cause
Y92.045 Swimming-pool of boarding-house as the place of occurrence of the external cause
Y92.046 Garden or yard of boarding-house as the place of occurrence of the external cause
Y92.048 Other place in boarding-house as the place of occurrence of the external cause
Y92.049 Unspecified place in boarding-house as the place of occurrence of the external cause

✓6th **Y92.09 Other non-institutional residence as the place of occurrence of the external cause**
Y92.090 Kitchen in other non-institutional residence as the place of occurrence of the external cause
Y92.091 Bathroom in other non-institutional residence as the place of occurrence of the external cause
Y92.092 Bedroom in other non-institutional residence as the place of occurrence of the external cause
Y92.093 Driveway of other non-institutional residence as the place of occurrence of the external cause
Y92.094 Garage of other non-institutional residence as the place of occurrence of the external cause
Y92.095 Swimming-pool of other non-institutional residence as the place of occurrence of the external cause
Y92.096 Garden or yard of other non-institutional residence as the place of occurrence of the external cause
Y92.098 Other place in other non-institutional residence as the place of occurrence of the external cause
Y92.099 Unspecified place in other non-institutional residence as the place of occurrence of the external cause

✓5th **Y92.1 Institutional (nonprivate) residence as the place of occurrence of the external cause**
Y92.10 Unspecified residential institution as the place of occurrence of the external cause

✓6th **Y92.11 Children's home and orphanage as the place of occurrence of the external cause**
Y92.110 Kitchen in children's home and orphanage as the place of occurrence of the external cause
Y92.111 Bathroom in children's home and orphanage as the place of occurrence of the external cause
Y92.112 Bedroom in children's home and orphanage as the place of occurrence of the external cause
Y92.113 Driveway of children's home and orphanage as the place of occurrence of the external cause

Y92.114 Garage of children's home and orphanage as the place of occurrence of the external cause

Y92.115 Swimming-pool of children's home and orphanage as the place of occurrence of the external cause

Y92.116 Garden or yard of children's home and orphanage as the place of occurrence of the external cause

Y92.118 Other place in children's home and orphanage as the place of occurrence of the external cause

Y92.119 Unspecified place in children's home and orphanage as the place of occurrence of the external cause

✓6th **Y92.12 Nursing home as the place of occurrence of the external cause**

Home for the sick as the place of occurrence of the external cause

Hospice as the place of occurrence of the external cause

Y92.120 Kitchen in nursing home as the place of occurrence of the external cause

Y92.121 Bathroom in nursing home as the place of occurrence of the external cause

Y92.122 Bedroom in nursing home as the place of occurrence of the external cause

Y92.123 Driveway of nursing home as the place of occurrence of the external cause

Y92.124 Garage of nursing home as the place of occurrence of the external cause

Y92.125 Swimming-pool of nursing home as the place of occurrence of the external cause

Y92.126 Garden or yard of nursing home as the place of occurrence of the external cause

Y92.128 Other place in nursing home as the place of occurrence of the external cause

Y92.129 Unspecified place in nursing home as the place of occurrence of the external cause

✓6th **Y92.13 Military base as the place of occurrence of the external cause**

EXCLUDES1 *military training grounds (Y92.84)*

Y92.130 Kitchen on military base as the place of occurrence of the external cause

Y92.131 Mess hall on military base as the place of occurrence of the external cause

Y92.133 Barracks on military base as the place of occurrence of the external cause

Y92.135 Garage on military base as the place of occurrence of the external cause

Y92.136 Swimming-pool on military base as the place of occurrence of the external cause

Y92.137 Garden or yard on military base as the place of occurrence of the external cause

Y92.138 Other place on military base as the place of occurrence of the external cause

Y92.139 Unspecified place military base as the place of occurrence of the external cause

✓6th **Y92.14 Prison as the place of occurrence of the external cause**

Y92.140 Kitchen in prison as the place of occurrence of the external cause

Y92.141 Dining room in prison as the place of occurrence of the external cause

Y92.142 Bathroom in prison as the place of occurrence of the external cause

Y92.143 Cell of prison as the place of occurrence of the external cause

Y92.146 Swimming-pool of prison as the place of occurrence of the external cause

Y92.147 Courtyard of prison as the place of occurrence of the external cause

Y92.148 Other place in prison as the place of occurrence of the external cause

Y92.149 Unspecified place in prison as the place of occurrence of the external cause

✓6th **Y92.15 Reform school as the place of occurrence of the external cause**

Y92.150 Kitchen in reform school as the place of occurrence of the external cause

Y92.151 Dining room in reform school as the place of occurrence of the external cause

Y92.152 Bathroom in reform school as the place of occurrence of the external cause

Y92.153 Bedroom in reform school as the place of occurrence of the external cause

Y92.154 Driveway of reform school as the place of occurrence of the external cause

Y92.155 Garage of reform school as the place of occurrence of the external cause

Y92.156 Swimming-pool of reform school as the place of occurrence of the external cause

Y92.157 Garden or yard of reform school as the place of occurrence of the external cause

Y92.158 Other place in reform school as the place of occurrence of the external cause

Y92.159 Unspecified place in reform school as the place of occurrence of the external cause

✓6th **Y92.16 School dormitory as the place of occurrence of the external cause**

EXCLUDES1 *reform school as the place of occurrence of the external cause (Y92.15-)*

school buildings and grounds as the place of occurrence of the external cause (Y92.2-)

school sports and athletic areas as the place of occurrence of the external cause (Y92.3-)

Y92.160 Kitchen in school dormitory as the place of occurrence of the external cause

Y92.161 Dining room in school dormitory as the place of occurrence of the external cause

Y92.162 Bathroom in school dormitory as the place of occurrence of the external cause

Y92.163 Bedroom in school dormitory as the place of occurrence of the external cause

Y92.168 Other place in school dormitory as the place of occurrence of the external cause

Y92.169 Unspecified place in school dormitory as the place of occurrence of the external cause

✓6th **Y92.19 Other specified residential institution as the place of occurrence of the external cause**

Y92.190 Kitchen in other specified residential institution as the place of occurrence of the external cause

Y92.191 Dining room in other specified residential institution as the place of occurrence of the external cause

Y92.192 Bathroom in other specified residential institution as the place of occurrence of the external cause

Y92.193 Bedroom in other specified residential institution as the place of occurrence of the external cause

Y92.194 Driveway of other specified residential institution as the place of occurrence of the external cause

Y92.195 Garage of other specified residential institution as the place of occurrence of the external cause

Y92.196 Pool of other specified residential institution as the place of occurrence of the external cause

Y92.197 Garden or yard of other specified residential institution as the place of occurrence of the external cause

Y92.198 Other place in other specified residential institution as the place of occurrence of the external cause

Y92.199 Unspecified place in other specified residential institution as the place of occurrence of the external cause

✓5th **Y92.2 School, other institution and public administrative area as the place of occurrence of the external cause**
Building and adjacent grounds used by the general public or by a particular group of the public
EXCLUDES 1 *building under construction as the place of occurrence of the external cause (Y92.6)*
residential institution as the place of occurrence of the external cause (Y92.1)
school dormitory as the place of occurrence of the external cause (Y92.16-)
sports and athletics area of schools as the place of occurrence of the external cause (Y92.3-)

✓6th **Y92.21 School (private) (public) (state) as the place of occurrence of the external cause**
Y92.210 Daycare center as the place of occurrence of the external cause
Y92.211 Elementary school as the place of occurrence of the external cause
Kindergarten as the place of occurrence of the external cause
Y92.212 Middle school as the place of occurrence of the external cause
Y92.213 High school as the place of occurrence of the external cause
Y92.214 College as the place of occurrence of the external cause
University as the place of occurrence of the external cause
Y92.215 Trade school as the place of occurrence of the external cause
Y92.218 Other school as the place of occurrence of the external cause
Y92.219 Unspecified school as the place of occurrence of the external cause

Y92.22 Religious institution as the place of occurrence of the external cause
Church as the place of occurrence of the external cause
Mosque as the place of occurrence of the external cause
Synagogue as the place of occurrence of the external cause

✓6th **Y92.23 Hospital as the place of occurrence of the external cause**
EXCLUDES 1 *ambulatory (outpatient) health services establishments (Y92.53-)*
home for the sick as the place of occurrence of the external cause (Y92.12-)
hospice as the place of occurrence of the external cause (Y92.12-)
nursing home as the place of occurrence of the external cause (Y92.12-)
Y92.230 Patient room in hospital as the place of occurrence of the external cause
Y92.231 Patient bathroom in hospital as the place of occurrence of the external cause
Y92.232 Corridor of hospital as the place of occurrence of the external cause
Y92.233 Cafeteria of hospital as the place of occurrence of the external cause
Y92.234 Operating room of hospital as the place of occurrence of the external cause
Y92.238 Other place in hospital as the place of occurrence of the external cause
Y92.239 Unspecified place in hospital as the place of occurrence of the external cause

✓6th **Y92.24 Public administrative building as the place of occurrence of the external cause**
Y92.240 Courthouse as the place of occurrence of the external cause
Y92.241 Library as the place of occurrence of the external cause
Y92.242 Post office as the place of occurrence of the external cause
Y92.243 City hall as the place of occurrence of the external cause
Y92.248 Other public administrative building as the place of occurrence of the external cause

✓6th **Y92.25 Cultural building as the place of occurrence of the external cause**
Y92.250 Art Gallery as the place of occurrence of the external cause
Y92.251 Museum as the place of occurrence of the external cause
Y92.252 Music hall as the place of occurrence of the external cause
Y92.253 Opera house as the place of occurrence of the external cause
Y92.254 Theater (live) as the place of occurrence of the external cause
Y92.258 Other cultural public building as the place of occurrence of the external cause

Y92.26 Movie house or cinema as the place of occurrence of the external cause

Y92.29 Other specified public building as the place of occurrence of the external cause
Assembly hall as the place of occurrence of the external cause
Clubhouse as the place of occurrence of the external cause

✓5th **Y92.3 Sports and athletics area as the place of occurrence of the external cause**

✓6th **Y92.31 Athletic court as the place of occurrence of the external cause**
EXCLUDES 1 *tennis court in private home or garden (Y92.09)*
Y92.310 Basketball court as the place of occurrence of the external cause
Y92.311 Squash court as the place of occurrence of the external cause
Y92.312 Tennis court as the place of occurrence of the external cause
Y92.318 Other athletic court as the place of occurrence of the external cause

✓6th **Y92.32 Athletic field as the place of occurrence of the external cause**
Y92.320 Baseball field as the place of occurrence of the external cause
Y92.321 Football field as the place of occurrence of the external cause
Y92.322 Soccer field as the place of occurrence of the external cause
Y92.328 Other athletic field as the place of occurrence of the external cause
Cricket field as the place of occurrence of the external cause
Hockey field as the place of occurrence of the external cause

✓6th **Y92.33 Skating rink as the place of occurrence of the external cause**
Y92.330 Ice skating rink (indoor) (outdoor) as the place of occurrence of the external cause
Y92.331 Roller skating rink as the place of occurrence of the external cause

Y92.34 Swimming pool (public) as the place of occurrence of the external cause
EXCLUDES 1 *swimming pool in private home or garden (Y92.016)*

Y92.39 Other specified sports and athletic area as the place of occurrence of the external cause
Golf-course as the place of occurrence of the external cause
Gymnasium as the place of occurrence of the external cause
Riding-school as the place of occurrence of the external cause
Stadium as the place of occurrence of the external cause

Y92.4 Street, highway and other paved roadways as the place of occurrence of the external cause [5th]

EXCLUDES 1 *private driveway of residence (Y92.014, Y92.024, Y92.043)*

Y92.41 Street and highway as the place of occurrence of the external cause [6th]

Y92.410 Unspecified street and highway as the place of occurrence of the external cause

Road NOS as the place of occurrence of the external cause

Y92.411 Interstate highway as the place of occurrence of the external cause

Freeway as the place of occurrence of the external cause

Motorway as the place of occurrence of the external cause

Y92.412 Parkway as the place of occurrence of the external cause

Y92.413 State road as the place of occurrence of the external cause

Y92.414 Local residential or business street as the place of occurrence of the external cause

Y92.415 Exit ramp or entrance ramp of street or highway as the place of occurrence of the external cause

Y92.48 Other paved roadways as the place of occurrence of the external cause [6th]

Y92.480 Sidewalk as the place of occurrence of the external cause

Y92.481 Parking lot as the place of occurrence of the external cause

Y92.482 Bike path as the place of occurrence of the external cause

Y92.488 Other paved roadways as the place of occurrence of the external cause

Y92.5 Trade and service area as the place of occurrence of the external cause [5th]

EXCLUDES 1 *garage in private home (Y92.015)*

schools and other public administration buildings (Y92.2-)

Y92.51 Private commercial establishments as the place of occurrence of the external cause [6th]

Y92.510 Bank as the place of occurrence of the external cause

Y92.511 Restaurant or café as the place of occurrence of the external cause

Y92.512 Supermarket, store or market as the place of occurrence of the external cause

Y92.513 Shop (commercial) as the place of occurrence of the external cause

Y92.52 Service areas as the place of occurrence of the external cause [6th]

Y92.520 Airport as the place of occurrence of the external cause

Y92.521 Bus station as the place of occurrence of the external cause

Y92.522 Railway station as the place of occurrence of the external cause

Y92.523 Highway rest stop as the place of occurrence of the external cause

Y92.524 Gas station as the place of occurrence of the external cause

Petroleum station as the place of occurrence of the external cause

Service station as the place of occurrence of the external cause

Y92.53 Ambulatory health services establishments as the place of occurrence of the external cause [6th]

Y92.530 Ambulatory surgery center as the place of occurrence of the external cause

Outpatient surgery center, including that connected with a hospital as the place of occurrence of the external cause

Same day surgery center, including that connected with a hospital as the place of occurrence of the external cause

Y92.531 Health care provider office as the place of occurrence of the external cause

Physician office as the place of occurrence of the external cause

Y92.532 Urgent care center as the place of occurrence of the external cause

Y92.538 Other ambulatory health services establishments as the place of occurrence of the external cause

Y92.59 Other trade areas as the place of occurrence of the external cause

Office building as the place of occurrence of the external cause

Casino as the place of occurrence of the external cause

Garage (commercial) as the place of occurrence of the external cause

Hotel as the place of occurrence of the external cause

Radio or television station as the place of occurrence of the external cause

Shopping mall as the place of occurrence of the external cause

Warehouse as the place of occurrence of the external cause

Y92.6 Industrial and construction area as the place of occurrence of the external cause [5th]

Y92.61 Building [any] under construction as the place of occurrence of the external cause

Y92.62 Dock or shipyard as the place of occurrence of the external cause

Dockyard as the place of occurrence of the external cause

Dry dock as the place of occurrence of the external cause

Shipyard as the place of occurrence of the external cause

Y92.63 Factory as the place of occurrence of the external cause

Factory building as the place of occurrence of the external cause

Factory premises as the place of occurrence of the external cause

Industrial yard as the place of occurrence of the external cause

Y92.64 Mine or pit as the place of occurrence of the external cause

Mine as the place of occurrence of the external cause

Y92.65 Oil rig as the place of occurrence of the external cause

Pit (coal) (gravel) (sand) as the place of occurrence of the external cause

Y92.69 Other specified industrial and construction area as the place of occurrence of the external cause

Gasworks as the place of occurrence of the external cause

Power-station (coal) (nuclear) (oil) as the place of occurrence of the external cause

Tunnel under construction as the place of occurrence of the external cause

Workshop as the place of occurrence of the external cause

Y92.7 Farm as the place of occurrence of the external cause [5th]

Ranch as the place of occurrence of the external cause

EXCLUDES 1 *farmhouse and home premises of farm (Y92.01-)*

Y92.71 Barn as the place of occurrence of the external cause

Y92.72 Chicken coop as the place of occurrence of the external cause

Hen house as the place of occurrence of the external cause

Y92.73 Farm field as the place of occurrence of the external cause

Y92.74 Orchard as the place of occurrence of the external cause

Y92.79 Other farm location as the place of occurrence of the external cause

Y92.8 Other places as the place of occurrence of the external cause

Y92.81 Transport vehicle as the place of occurrence of the external cause

EXCLUDES 1 *transport accidents (V00-V99)*

Y92.810 Car as the place of occurrence of the external cause

Y92.811 Bus as the place of occurrence of the external cause

Y92.812 Truck as the place of occurrence of the external cause

Y92.813 Airplane as the place of occurrence of the external cause

Y92.814 Boat as the place of occurrence of the external cause

Y92.815 Train as the place of occurrence of the external cause

Y92.816 Subway car as the place of occurrence of the external cause

Y92.818 Other transport vehicle as the place of occurrence of the external cause

Y92.82 Wilderness area

Y92.820 Desert as the place of occurrence of the external cause

Y92.821 Forest as the place of occurrence of the external cause

Y92.828 Other wilderness area as the place of occurrence of the external cause

Swamp as the place of occurrence of the external cause

Mountain as the place of occurrence of the external cause

Marsh as the place of occurrence of the external cause

Prairie as the place of occurrence of the external cause

Y92.83 Recreation area as the place of occurrence of the external cause

Y92.830 Public park as the place of occurrence of the external cause

Y92.831 Amusement park as the place of occurrence of the external cause

Y92.832 Beach as the place of occurrence of the external cause

Seashore as the place of occurrence of the external cause

Y92.833 Campsite as the place of occurrence of the external cause

Y92.834 Zoological garden (Zoo) as the place of occurrence of the external cause

Y92.838 Other recreation area as the place of occurrence of the external cause

Y92.84 Military training ground as the place of occurrence of the external cause

Y92.85 Railroad track as the place of occurrence of the external cause

Y92.86 Slaughter house as the place of occurrence of the external cause

Y92.89 Other specified places as the place of occurrence of the external cause

Derelict house as the place of occurrence of the external cause

Y92.9 Unspecified place or not applicable

Y93 Activity codes

NOTE Category Y93 is provided for use to indicate the activity of the person seeking healthcare for an injury or health condition, such as a heart attack while shoveling snow, which resulted from, or was contributed to, by the activity. These codes are appropriate for use for both acute injuries, such as those from chapter 19, and conditions that are due to the long-term, cumulative effects of an activity, such as those from chapter 13. They are also appropriate for use with external cause codes for cause and intent if identifying the activity provides additional information on the event. These codes should be used in conjunction with codes for external cause status (Y99) and place of occurrence (Y92). This section contains the following broad activity categories:

Y93.0 Activities involving walking and running
Y93.1 Activities involving water and water craft
Y93.2 Activities involving ice and snow
Y93.3 Activities involving climbing, rappelling, and jumping off
Y93.4 Activities involving dancing and other rhythmic movement
Y93.5 Activities involving other sports and athletics played individually
Y93.6 Activities involving other sports and athletics played as a team or group
Y93.7 Activities involving other specified sports and athletics
Y93.A Activities involving other cardiorespiratory exercise
Y93.B Activities involving other muscle strengthening exercises
Y93.C Activities involving computer technology and electronic devices
Y93.D Activities involving arts and handcrafts
Y93.E Activities involving personal hygiene and interior property and clothing maintenance
Y93.F Activities involving caregiving
Y93.G Activities involving food preparation, cooking and grilling
Y93.H Activities involving exterior property and land maintenance, building and construction
Y93.I Activities involving roller coasters and other types of external motion
Y93.J Activities involving playing musical instrument
Y93.K Activities involving animal care
Y93.8 Activities, other specified
Y93.9 Activity, unspecified

Y93.0 Activities involving walking and running

EXCLUDES 1 *activity, walking an animal (Y93.K1)*
activity, walking or running on a treadmill (Y93.A1)

Y93.01 Activity, walking, marching and hiking

Activity, walking, marching and hiking on level or elevated terrain

EXCLUDES 1 *activity, mountain climbing (Y93.31)*

Y93.02 Activity, running

Y93.1 Activities involving water and water craft

EXCLUDES 1 *activities involving ice (Y93.2-)*

Y93.11 Activity, swimming

Y93.12 Activity, springboard and platform diving

Y93.13 Activity, water polo

Y93.14 Activity, water aerobics and water exercise

Y93.15 Activity, underwater diving and snorkeling

Activity, SCUBA diving

Y93.16 Activity, rowing, canoeing, kayaking, rafting and tubing

Activity, canoeing, kayaking, rafting and tubing in calm and turbulent water

Y93.17 Activity, water skiing and wake boarding

Y93.18 Activity, surfing, windsurfing and boogie boarding

Activity, water sliding

Y93.19 Activity, other activity involving water and watercraft

Activity involving water NOS
Activity, parasailing
Activity, water survival training and testing

Y93.2 Activities involving ice and snow [5th]
EXCLUDES 1 *activity, shoveling ice and snow (Y93.H1)*

Y93.21 Activity, ice skating
Activity, figure skating (singles) (pairs)
Activity, ice dancing
EXCLUDES 1 *activity, ice hockey (Y93.22)*

Y93.22 Activity, ice hockey

Y93.23 Activity, snow (alpine) (downhill) skiing, snow boarding, sledding, tobogganing and snow tubing
EXCLUDES 1 *activity, cross country skiing (Y93.24)*

Y93.24 Activity, cross country skiing
Activity, nordic skiing

Y93.29 Activity, other involving ice and snow
Activity involving ice and snow NOS

Y93.3 Activities involving climbing, rappelling and jumping off [5th]
EXCLUDES 1 *activity, hiking on level or elevated terrain (Y93.01)*
activity, jumping rope (Y93.56)
activity, trampoline jumping (Y93.44)

Y93.31 Activity, mountain climbing, rock climbing and wall climbing

Y93.32 Activity, rappelling

Y93.33 Activity, BASE jumping
Activity, Building, Antenna, Span, Earth jumping

Y93.34 Activity, bungee jumping

Y93.35 Activity, hang gliding

Y93.39 Activity, other involving climbing, rappelling and jumping off

Y93.4 Activities involving dancing and other rhythmic movement [5th]
EXCLUDES 1 *activity, martial arts (Y93.75)*

Y93.41 Activity, dancing

Y93.42 Activity, yoga

Y93.43 Activity, gymnastics
Activity, rhythmic gymnastics
EXCLUDES 1 *activity, trampolining (Y93.44)*

Y93.44 Activity, trampolining

Y93.45 Activity, cheerleading

Y93.49 Activity, other involving dancing and other rhythmic movements

Y93.5 Activities involving other sports and athletics played individually [5th]
EXCLUDES 1 *activity, dancing (Y93.41)*
activity, gymnastic (Y93.43)
activity, trampolining (Y93.44)
activity, yoga (Y93.42)

Y93.51 Activity, roller skating (inline) and skateboarding

Y93.52 Activity, horseback riding

Y93.53 Activity, golf

Y93.54 Activity, bowling

Y93.55 Activity, bike riding

Y93.56 Activity, jumping rope

Y93.57 Activity, non-running track and field events
EXCLUDES 1 *activity, running (any form) (Y93.02)*

Y93.59 Activity, other involving other sports and athletics played individually
EXCLUDES 1 *activities involving climbing, rappelling, and jumping (Y93.3-)*
activities involving ice and snow (Y93.2-)
activities involving walking and running (Y93.0-)
activities involving water and watercraft (Y93.1-)

Y93.6 Activities involving other sports and athletics played as a team or group [5th]
EXCLUDES 1 *activity, ice hockey (Y93.22)*
activity, water polo (Y93.13)

Y93.61 Activity, American tackle football
Activity, football NOS

Y93.62 Activity, American flag or touch football

Y93.63 Activity, rugby

Y93.64 Activity, baseball
Activity, softball

Y93.65 Activity, lacrosse and field hockey

Y93.66 Activity, soccer

Y93.67 Activity, basketball

Y93.68 Activity, volleyball (beach) (court)

Y93.6A Activity, physical games generally associated with school recess, summer camp and children
Activity, capture the flag
Activity, dodge ball
Activity, four square
Activity, kickball

Y93.69 Activity, other involving other sports and athletics played as a team or group
Activity, cricket

Y93.7 Activities involving other specified sports and athletics [5th]

Y93.71 Activity, boxing

Y93.72 Activity, wrestling

Y93.73 Activity, racquet and hand sports
Activity, handball
Activity, racquetball
Activity, squash
Activity, tennis

Y93.74 Activity, frisbee
Activity, ultimate frisbee

Y93.75 Activity, martial arts
Activity, combatives

Y93.79 Activity, other specified sports and athletics
EXCLUDES 1 *sports and athletics activities specified in categories Y93.0-Y93.6*

Y93.A Activities involving other cardiorespiratory exercise [5th]
Activities involving physical training

Y93.A1 Activity, exercise machines primarily for cardiorespiratory conditioning
Activity, elliptical and stepper machines
Activity, stationary bike
Activity, treadmill

Y93.A2 Activity, calisthenics
Activity, jumping jacks
Activity, warm up and cool down

Y93.A3 Activity, aerobic and step exercise

Y93.A4 Activity, circuit training

Y93.A5 Activity, obstacle course
Activity, challenge course
Activity, confidence course

Y93.A6 Activity, grass drills
Activity, guerilla drills

Y93.A9 Activity, other involving other cardiorespiratory exercise
EXCLUDES 1 *activities involving cardiorespiratory exercise specified in categories Y93.0-Y93.7*

Y93.B Activities involving other muscle strengthening exercises [5th]

Y93.B1 Activity, exercise machines primarily for muscle strengthening

Y93.B2 Activity, push-ups, pull-ups, sit-ups

Y93.B3 Activity, free weights
Activity, barbells
Activity, dumbbells

Y93.B4 Activity, pilates

Y93.B9 Activity, other involving other muscle strengthening exercises
EXCLUDES 1 *activities involving muscle strengthening specified in categories Y93.0-Y93.A*

Y93.C Activities involving computer technology and electronic devices [5th]
EXCLUDES 1 *activity, electronic musical keyboard or instruments (Y93.J-)*

Y93.C1 Activity, computer keyboarding
Activity, electronic game playing using keyboard or other stationary device

Y93.C2 Activity, hand held interactive electronic device
Activity, cellular telephone and communication device
Activity, electronic game playing using interactive device
EXCLUDES 1 *activity, electronic game playing using keyboard or other stationary device (Y93.C1)*

Y93.C9 Activity, other involving computer technology and electronic devices

Y93.D Activities involving arts and handcrafts [5th]
EXCLUDES 1 *activities involving playing musical instrument (Y93.J-)*

Y93.D1 Activity, knitting and crocheting

DRAFT

Appropriate additional character required
[x7th] Requires 7th character, placeholder x must fill empty characters

Y93.D2 Activity, sewing

Y93.D3 Activity, furniture building and finishing
Activity, furniture repair

Y93.D9 Activity, involving other arts and handcrafts

✓5th **Y93.E Activities involving personal hygiene and interior property and clothing maintenance**
EXCLUDES 1 *activities involving cooking and grilling (Y93.G-)*
activities involving exterior property and land maintenance, building and construction (Y93.H-)
activities involving caregiving (Y93.F-)
activity, dishwashing (Y93.G1)
activity, food preparation (Y93.G1)
activity, gardening (Y93.H2)

Y93.E1 Activity, personal bathing and showering

Y93.E2 Activity, laundry

Y93.E3 Activity, vacuuming

Y93.E4 Activity, ironing

Y93.E5 Activity, floor mopping and cleaning

Y93.E6 Activity, residential relocation
Activity, packing up and unpacking involved in moving to a new residence

Y93.E8 Activity, other personal hygiene

Y93.E9 Activity, other interior property and clothing maintenance

✓5th **Y93.F Activities involving caregiving**
Activity involving the provider of caregiving

Y93.F1 Activity, caregiving, bathing

Y93.F2 Activity, caregiving, lifting

Y93.F9 Activity, other caregiving

✓5th **Y93.G Activities involving food preparation, cooking and grilling**

Y93.G1 Activity, food preparation and clean up
Activity, dishwashing

Y93.G2 Activity, grilling and smoking food

Y93.G3 Activity, cooking and baking
Activity, use of stove, oven and microwave oven

Y93.G9 Activity, other involving cooking and grilling

✓5th **Y93.H Activities involving exterior property and land maintenance, building and construction**

Y93.H1 Activity, digging, shoveling and raking
Activity, dirt digging
Activity, raking leaves
Activity, snow shoveling

Y93.H2 Activity, gardening and landscaping
Activity, pruning, trimming shrubs, weeding

Y93.H3 Activity, building and construction

Y93.H9 Activity, other involving exterior property and land maintenance, building and construction

✓5th **Y93.I Activities involving roller coasters and other types of external motion**

Y93.I1 Activity, rollercoaster riding

Y93.I9 Activity, other involving external motion

✓5th **Y93.J Activities involving playing musical instrument**
Activity involving playing electric musical instrument

Y93.J1 Activity, piano playing
Activity, musical keyboard (electronic) playing

Y93.J2 Activity, drum and other percussion instrument playing

Y93.J3 Activity, string instrument playing

Y93.J4 Activity, winds and brass instrument playing

✓5th **Y93.K Activities involving animal care**
EXCLUDES 1 *activity, horseback riding (Y93.52)*

Y93.K1 Activity, walking an animal

Y93.K2 Activity, milking an animal

Y93.K3 Activity, grooming and shearing an animal

Y93.K9 Activity, other involving animal care

✓5th **Y93.8 Activities, other specified**

Y93.81 Activity, refereeing a sports activity

Y93.82 Activity, spectator at an event

Y93.83 Activity, rough housing and horseplay

Y93.84 Activity, sleeping

Y93.89 Activity, other specified

Y93.9 Activity, unspecified

Y95 Nosocomial condition

✓4th **Y99 External cause status**
NOTE A single code from category Y99 should be used in conjunction with the external cause code(s) assigned to a record to indicate the status of the person at the time the event occurred.

Y99.0 Civilian activity done for income or pay
Civilian activity done for financial or other compensation
EXCLUDES 1 *military activity (Y99.1)*
volunteer activity (Y99.2)

Y99.1 Military activity
EXCLUDES 2 *activity of off duty military personnel (Y99.8)*

Y99.2 Volunteer activity
EXCLUDES 1 *activity of child or other family member assisting in compensated work of other family member (Y99.8)*

Y99.8 Other external cause status
Activity NEC
Activity of child or other family member assisting in compensated work of other family member
Hobby not done for income
Leisure activity
Off-duty activity of military personnel
Recreation or sport not for income or while a student
Student activity
EXCLUDES 1 *civilian activity done for income or compensation (Y99.0)*
military activity (Y99.1)

Y99.9 Unspecified external cause status

Chapter 21. Factors Influencing Health Status and Contact With Health Services (Z00-Z99)

NOTE Z codes represent reasons for encounters. A corresponding procedure code must accompany a Z code if a procedure is performed. Categories Z00-Z99 are provided for occasions when circumstances other than a disease, injury or external cause classifiable to categories A00-Y89 are recorded as "diagnoses" or "problems". This can arise in two main ways:

(a) When a person who may or may not be sick encounters the health services for some specific purpose, such as to receive limited care or service for a current condition, to donate an organ or tissue, to receive prophylactic vaccination (immunization), or to discuss a problem which is in itself not a disease or injury.

(b) When some circumstance or problem is present which influences the person's health status but is not in itself a current illness or injury.

This chapter contains the following blocks:

Z00-Z13	Persons encountering health services for examinations
Z14-Z15	Genetic carrier and genetic susceptibility to disease
Z16	Resistance to antimicrobial drugs
Z17	Estrogen receptor status
Z18	Retained foreign body fragments
Z20-Z28	Persons with potential health hazards related to communicable diseases
Z30-Z39	Persons encountering health services in circumstances related to reproduction
Z40-Z53	Encounters for other specific health care
Z55-Z65	Persons with potential health hazards related to socioeconomic and psychosocial circumstances
Z66	Do not resuscitate status
Z67	Blood type
Z68	Body mass index (BMI)
Z69-Z76	Persons encountering health services in other circumstances
Z77-Z99	Persons with potential health hazards related to family and personal history and certain conditions influencing health status

Persons encountering health services for examinations (Z00-Z13)

NOTE Nonspecific abnormal findings disclosed at the time of these examinations are classified to categories R70-R94.

EXCLUDES 1 *examinations related to pregnancy and reproduction (Z30-Z36, Z39-)*

✓4th **Z00 Encounter for general examination without complaint, suspected or reported diagnosis**

EXCLUDES 1 *encounter for examination for administrative purposes (Z02.-)*

EXCLUDES 2 *encounter for pre-procedural examinations (Z01.81-)*
special screening examinations (Z11-Z13)

✓5th **Z00.0 Encounter for general adult medical examination**

Encounter for adult periodic examination (annual) (physical) and any associated laboratory and radiologic examinations

EXCLUDES 1 *encounter for examination of sign or symptom—code to sign or symptom*
general health check-up of infant or child (Z00.12-)

Z00.00 Encounter for general adult medical examination without abnormal findings

Encounter for adult health check-up NOS

Z00.01 Encounter for general adult medical examination with abnormal findings

Use additional code to identify abnormal findings

✓5th **Z00.1 Encounter for newborn, infant and child health examinations**

✓6th **Z00.11 Newborn health examination**

Health check for child under 29 days old

Use additional code to identify any abnormal findings

EXCLUDES 1 *health check for child over 28 days old (Z00.12-)*

Z00.110 Health examination for newborn under 8 days old

Health check for newborn under 8 days old

Z00.111 Health examination for newborn 8 to 28 days old

Health check for newborn 8 to 28 days old

Newborn weight check

✓6th **Z00.12 Encounter for routine child health examination**

Encounter for development testing of infant or child

Health check (routine) for child over 28 days old

EXCLUDES 1 *health check for child under 29 days old (Z00.11-)*
health supervision of foundling or other healthy infant or child (Z76.1-Z76.2)
newborn health examination (Z00.11-)

Z00.121 Encounter for routine child health examination with abnormal findings

Use additional code to identify abnormal findings

Z00.129 Encounter for routine child health examination without abnormal findings

Encounter for routine child health examination NOS

Z00.2 Encounter for examination for period of rapid growth in childhood

Z00.3 Encounter for examination for adolescent development state

Encounter for puberty development state

Z00.5 Encounter for examination of potential donor of organ and tissue

Z00.6 Encounter for examination for normal comparison and control in clinical research program

Examination of participant or control in clinical research program

✓5th **Z00.7 Encounter for examination for period of delayed growth in childhood**

Z00.70 Encounter for examination for period of delayed growth in childhood without abnormal findings

Z00.71 Encounter for examination for period of delayed growth in childhood with abnormal findings

Use additional code to identify abnormal findings

Z00.8 Encounter for other general examination

Encounter for health examination in population surveys

✓4th **Z01 Encounter for other special examination without complaint, suspected or reported diagnosis**

INCLUDES routine examination of specific system

NOTE Codes from category Z01 represent the reason for the encounter. A separate procedure code is required to identify any examinations or procedures performed

EXCLUDES 1 *encounter for examination for administrative purposes (Z02.-)*
encounter for examination for suspected conditions, proven not to exist (Z03.-)
encounter for laboratory and radiologic examinations as a component of general medical examinations (Z00.0-)
encounter for laboratory, radiologic and imaging examinations for sign(s) and symptom(s)—code to the sign(s) or symptom(s)

EXCLUDES 2 *screening examinations (Z11-Z13)*

✓5th **Z01.0 Encounter for examination of eyes and vision**

EXCLUDES 1 *examination for driving license (Z02.4)*

Z01.00 Encounter for examination of eyes and vision without abnormal findings

Encounter for examination of eyes and vision NOS

Z01.01 Encounter for examination of eyes and vision with abnormal findings

Use additional code to identify abnormal findings

✓5th **Z01.1 Encounter for examination of ears and hearing**

Z01.10 Encounter for examination of ears and hearing without abnormal findings

Encounter for examination of ears and hearing NOS

✓6th **Z01.11 Encounter for examination of ears and hearing with abnormal findings**

Z01.110 Encounter for hearing examination following failed hearing screening

Z01.118 Encounter for examination of ears and hearing with other abnormal findings

Use additional code to identify abnormal findings

Z01.12 Encounter for hearing conservation and treatment

Factors Influencing Health Status and Contact With Health Services Z00–Z01.12

✓5th **Z01.2 Encounter for dental examination and cleaning**

Z01.20 Encounter for dental examination and cleaning without abnormal findings
Encounter for dental examination and cleaning NOS

Z01.21 Encounter for dental examination and cleaning with abnormal findings
Use additional code to identify abnormal findings

✓5th **Z01.3 Encounter for examination of blood pressure**

Z01.30 Encounter for examination of blood pressure without abnormal findings
Encounter for examination of blood pressure NOS

Z01.31 Encounter for examination of blood pressure with abnormal findings
Use additional code to identify abnormal findings

✓5th **Z01.4 Encounter for gynecological examination**
EXCLUDES 2 *pregnancy examination or test (Z32.0-)*
routine examination for contraceptive maintenance (Z30.4-)

✓6th **Z01.41 Encounter for routine gynecological examination**
Encounter for general gynecological examination with or without cervical smear
Encounter for gynecological examination (general) (routine) NOS
Encounter for pelvic examination (annual) (periodic)
Use additional code:
for screening for human papillomavirus, if applicable, (Z11.51)
for screening vaginal pap smear, if applicable (Z12.72)
to identify acquired absence of uterus, if applicable (Z90.71-)
EXCLUDES 1 *gynecologic examination status-post hysterectomy for malignant condition (Z08)*
screening cervical pap smear not a part of a routine gynecological examination (Z12.4)

Z01.411 Encounter for gynecological examination (general) (routine) with abnormal findings
Use additional code to identify abnormal findings

Z01.419 Encounter for gynecological examination (general) (routine) without abnormal findings

Z01.42 Encounter for cervical smear to confirm findings of recent normal smear following initial abnormal smear

✓5th **Z01.8 Encounter for other specified special examinations**

✓6th **Z01.81 Encounter for preprocedural examinations**
Encounter for preoperative examinations
Encounter for radiological and imaging examinations as part of preprocedural examination

Z01.810 Encounter for preprocedural cardiovascular examination

Z01.811 Encounter for preprocedural respiratory examination

Z01.812 Encounter for preprocedural laboratory examination
Blood and urine tests prior to treatment or procedure

Z01.818 Encounter for other preprocedural examination
Encounter for preprocedural examination NOS
Encounter for examinations prior to antineoplastic chemotherapy

Z01.82 Encounter for allergy testing
EXCLUDES 1 *encounter for antibody response examination (Z01.84)*

Z01.83 Encounter for blood typing
Encounter for Rh typing

Z01.84 Encounter for antibody response examination
Encounter for immunity status testing
EXCLUDES 1 *encounter for allergy testing (Z01.82)*

Z01.89 Encounter for other specified special examinations

✓4th **Z02 Encounter for administrative examination**

Z02.0 Encounter for examination for admission to educational institution
Encounter for examination for admission to preschool (education)
Encounter for examination for re-admission to school following illness or medical treatment

Z02.1 Encounter for pre-employment examination

Z02.2 Encounter for examination for admission to residential institution
EXCLUDES 1 *examination for admission to prison (Z02.89)*

Z02.3 Encounter for examination for recruitment to armed forces

Z02.4 Encounter for examination for driving license

Z02.5 Encounter for examination for participation in sport
EXCLUDES 1 *blood-alcohol and blood-drug test (Z02.83)*

Z02.6 Encounter for examination for insurance purposes

✓5th **Z02.7 Encounter for issue of medical certificate**
EXCLUDES 1 *encounter for general medical examination (Z00-Z01, Z02.0-Z02.6, Z02.8-Z02.9,)*

Z02.71 Encounter for disability determination
Encounter for issue of medical certificate of incapacity
Encounter for issue of medical certificate of invalidity

Z02.79 Encounter for issue of other medical certificate

✓5th **Z02.8 Encounter for other administrative examinations**

Z02.81 Encounter for paternity testing

Z02.82 Encounter for adoption services

Z02.83 Encounter for blood-alcohol and blood-drug test
Use additional code for findings of alcohol or drugs in blood (R78.-)

Z02.89 Encounter for other administrative examinations
Encounter for examination for admission to prison
Encounter for examination for admission to summer camp
Encounter for immigration examination
Encounter for naturalization examination
Encounter for premarital examination
EXCLUDES 1 *health supervision of foundling or other healthy infant or child (Z76.1-Z76.2)*

Z02.9 Encounter for administrative examinations, unspecified

✓4th **Z03 Encounter for medical observation for suspected diseases and conditions ruled out**
NOTE This category is to be used when a person without a diagnosis is suspected of having an abnormal condition, without signs or symptoms, which requires study, but after examination and observation, is ruled out. This category is also for use for administrative and legal observation status.
EXCLUDES 1 *contact with and (suspected) exposures hazardous to health (Z77.-)*
newborn observation for suspected condition, ruled out (P00-P04)
person with feared complaint in whom no diagnosis is made (Z71.1)
signs or symptoms under study—code to signs or symptoms

Z03.6 Encounter for observation for suspected toxic effect from ingested substance ruled out
Encounter for observation for suspected adverse effect from drug
Encounter for observation for suspected poisoning

✓5th **Z03.7 Encounter for suspected maternal and fetal conditions ruled out**
Encounter for suspected maternal and fetal conditions not found
EXCLUDES 1 *known or suspected fetal anomalies affecting management of mother, not ruled out (O26-, O35-, O36-, O40-, O41-)*

Z03.71 Encounter for suspected problem with amniotic cavity and membrane ruled out
Encounter for suspected oligohydramnios ruled out
Encounter for suspected polyhydramnios ruled out

Z03.72 Encounter for suspected placental problem ruled out

Z03.73 Encounter for suspected fetal anomaly ruled out

Z03.74 Encounter for suspected problem with fetal growth ruled out

Z03.75 Encounter for suspected cervical shortening ruled out

Z03.79 Encounter for other suspected maternal and fetal conditions ruled out

5th Z03.8 Encounter for observation for other suspected diseases and conditions ruled out

6th Z03.81 Encounter for observation for suspected exposure to biological agents ruled out

Z03.810 Encounter for observation for suspected exposure to anthrax ruled out

Z03.818 Encounter for observation for suspected exposure to other biological agents ruled out

Z03.89 Encounter for observation for other suspected diseases and conditions ruled out

4th Z04 Encounter for examination and observation for other reasons

INCLUDES encounter for examination for medicolegal reasons

NOTE This category is to be used when a person without a diagnosis is suspected of having an abnormal condition, without signs or symptoms, which requires study, but after examination and observation, is ruled-out. This category is also for use for administrative and legal observation status.

Z04.1 Encounter for examination and observation following transport accident

EXCLUDES 1 *encounter for examination and observation following work accident (Z04.2)*

Z04.2 Encounter for examination and observation following work accident

Z04.3 Encounter for examination and observation following other accident

5th Z04.4 Encounter for examination and observation following alleged rape

Encounter for examination and observation of victim following alleged rape

Encounter for examination and observation of victim following alleged sexual abuse

Z04.41 Encounter for examination and observation following alleged adult rape

Suspected adult rape, ruled out

Suspected adult sexual abuse, ruled out

Z04.42 Encounter for examination and observation following alleged child rape

Suspected child rape, ruled out

Suspected child sexual abuse, ruled out

Z04.6 Encounter for general psychiatric examination, requested by authority

5th Z04.7 Encounter for examination and observation following alleged physical abuse

Z04.71 Encounter for examination and observation following alleged adult physical abuse

Suspected adult physical abuse, ruled out

EXCLUDES 1 *confirmed case of adult physical abuse (T74.-)*

encounter for examination and observation following alleged adult sexual abuse (Z04.41)

suspected case of adult physical abuse, not ruled out (T76.-)

Z04.72 Encounter for examination and observation following alleged child physical abuse

Suspected child physical abuse, ruled out

EXCLUDES 1 *confirmed case of child physical abuse (T74.-)*

encounter for examination and observation following alleged child sexual abuse (Z04.42)

suspected case of child physical abuse, not ruled out (T76.-)

Z04.8 Encounter for examination and observation for other specified reasons

Encounter for examination and observation for request for expert evidence

Z04.9 Encounter for examination and observation for unspecified reason

Encounter for observation NOS

Z08 Encounter for follow-up examination after completed treatment for malignant neoplasm

Medical surveillance following completed treatment

Use additional code to identify any acquired absence of organs (Z90.-)

Use additional code to identify the personal history of malignant neoplasm (Z85.-)

EXCLUDES 1 *aftercare following medical care (Z43-Z49, Z51)*

Z09 Encounter for follow-up examination after completed treatment for conditions other than malignant neoplasm

Medical surveillance following completed treatment

Use additional code to identify any applicable history of disease code (Z86-, Z87-)

EXCLUDES 1 *aftercare following medical care (Z43-Z49, Z51)*

surveillance of contraception (Z30.4-)

surveillance of prosthetic and other medical devices (Z44-Z46)

4th Z11 Encounter for screening for infectious and parasitic diseases

NOTE Screening is the testing for disease or disease precursors in asymptomatic individuals so that early detection and treatment can be provided for those who test positive for the disease.

EXCLUDES 1 *encounter for diagnostic examination—code to sign or symptom*

Z11.0 Encounter for screening for intestinal infectious diseases

Z11.1 Encounter for screening for respiratory tuberculosis

Z11.2 Encounter for screening for other bacterial diseases

Z11.3 Encounter for screening for infections with a predominantly sexual mode of transmission

EXCLUDES 2 *encounter for screening for human immunodeficiency virus [HIV] (Z11.4)*

encounter for screening for human papillomavirus (Z11.51)

Z11.4 Encounter for screening for human immunodeficiency virus [HIV]

5th Z11.5 Encounter for screening for other viral diseases

EXCLUDES 2 *encounter for screening for viral intestinal disease (Z11.0)*

Z11.51 Encounter for screening for human papillomavirus (HPV)

Z11.59 Encounter for screening for other viral diseases

Z11.6 Encounter for screening for other protozoal diseases and helminthiases

EXCLUDES 2 *encounter for screening for protozoal intestinal disease (Z11.0)*

Z11.8 Encounter for screening for other infectious and parasitic diseases

Encounter for screening for chlamydia

Encounter for screening for rickettsial

Encounter for screening for spirochetal

Encounter for screening for mycoses

Z11.9 Encounter for screening for infectious and parasitic diseases, unspecified

4th Z12 Encounter for screening for malignant neoplasms

NOTE Screening is the testing for disease or disease precursors in asymptomatic individuals so that early detection and treatment can be provided for those who test positive for the disease.

Use additional code to identify any family history of malignant neoplasm (Z80.-)

EXCLUDES 1 *encounter for diagnostic examination—code to sign or symptom*

Z12.0 Encounter for screening for malignant neoplasm of stomach

5th Z12.1 Encounter for screening for malignant neoplasm of intestinal tract

Z12.10 Encounter for screening for malignant neoplasm of intestinal tract, unspecified

Z12.11 Encounter for screening for malignant neoplasm of colon

Encounter for screening colonoscopy NOS

Z12.12 Encounter for screening for malignant neoplasm of rectum

Z12.13 Encounter for screening for malignant neoplasm of small intestine

Z12.2 Encounter for screening for malignant neoplasm of respiratory organs

√5th **Z12.3 Encounter for screening for malignant neoplasm of breast**
- **Z12.31 Encounter for screening mammogram for malignant neoplasm of breast**
  - EXCLUDES 1 *inconclusive mammogram (R92.2)*
- **Z12.39 Encounter for other screening for malignant neoplasm of breast**

Z12.4 Encounter for screening for malignant neoplasm of cervix
Encounter for screening pap smear for malignant neoplasm of cervix
EXCLUDES 1 *encounter for screening for human papillomavirus (Z11.51)*
when screening is part of general gynecological examination (Z01.4-)

Z12.5 Encounter for screening for malignant neoplasm of prostate

Z12.6 Encounter for screening for malignant neoplasm of bladder

√5th **Z12.7 Encounter for screening for malignant neoplasm of other genitourinary organs**
- **Z12.71 Encounter for screening for malignant neoplasm of testis**
- **Z12.72 Encounter for screening for malignant neoplasm of vagina**
  - Vaginal pap smear status-post hysterectomy for non-malignant condition
  - Use additional code to identify acquired absence of uterus (Z90.71-)
  - EXCLUDES 1 *vaginal pap smear status-post hysterectomy for malignant conditions (Z08)*
- **Z12.73 Encounter for screening for malignant neoplasm of ovary**
- **Z12.79 Encounter for screening for malignant neoplasm of other genitourinary organs**

√5th **Z12.8 Encounter for screening for malignant neoplasm of other sites**
- **Z12.81 Encounter for screening for malignant neoplasm of oral cavity**
- **Z12.82 Encounter for screening for malignant neoplasm of nervous system**
- **Z12.83 Encounter for screening for malignant neoplasm of skin**
- **Z12.89 Encounter for screening for malignant neoplasm of other sites**

Z12.9 Encounter for screening for malignant neoplasm, site unspecified

√4th **Z13 Encounter for screening for other diseases and disorders**
NOTE Screening is the testing for disease or disease precursors in asymptomatic individuals so that early detection and treatment can be provided for those who test positive for the disease.
EXCLUDES 1 *encounter for diagnostic examination—code to sign or symptom*

Z13.0 Encounter for screening for diseases of the blood and blood-forming organs and certain disorders involving the immune mechanism

Z13.1 Encounter for screening for diabetes mellitus

√5th **Z13.2 Encounter for screening for nutritional, metabolic and other endocrine disorders**
- **Z13.21 Encounter for screening for nutritional disorder**
- √6th **Z13.22 Encounter for screening for metabolic disorder**
  - **Z13.220 Encounter for screening for lipoid disorders**
    - Encounter for screening for cholesterol level
    - Encounter for screening for hypercholesterolemia
    - Encounter for screening for hyperlipidemia
  - **Z13.228 Encounter for screening for other metabolic disorders**
- **Z13.29 Encounter for screening for other suspected endocrine disorder**
  - EXCLUDES 1 *encounter for screening for diabetes mellitus (Z13.1)*

Z13.4 Encounter for screening for certain developmental disorders in childhood
Encounter for screening for developmental handicaps in early childhood
EXCLUDES 1 *routine development testing of infant or child (Z00.1-)*

Z13.5 Encounter for screening for eye and ear disorders
EXCLUDES 2 *encounter for general hearing examination (Z01.1-)*
encounter for general vision examination (Z01.0-)

Z13.6 Encounter for screening for cardiovascular disorders

√5th **Z13.7 Encounter for screening for genetic and chromosomal anomalies**
EXCLUDES 1 *genetic testing for procreative management (Z31.4-)*
- **Z13.71 Encounter for nonprocreative screening for genetic disease carrier status**
- **Z13.79 Encounter for other screening for genetic and chromosomal anomalies**

√5th **Z13.8 Encounter for screening for other specified diseases and disorders**
EXCLUDES 2 *screening for malignant neoplasms (Z12.-)*
- √6th **Z13.81 Encounter for screening for digestive system disorders**
  - **Z13.810 Encounter for screening for upper gastrointestinal disorder**
  - **Z13.811 Encounter for screening for lower gastrointestinal disorder**
    - EXCLUDES 1 *encounter for screening for intestinal infectious disease (Z11.0)*
  - **Z13.818 Encounter for screening for other digestive system disorders**
- √6th **Z13.82 Encounter for screening for musculoskeletal disorder**
  - **Z13.820 Encounter for screening for osteoporosis**
  - **Z13.828 Encounter for screening for other musculoskeletal disorder**
- **Z13.83 Encounter for screening for respiratory disorder NEC**
  - EXCLUDES 1 *encounter for screening for respiratory tuberculosis (Z11.1)*
- **Z13.84 Encounter for screening for dental disorders**
- √6th **Z13.85 Encounter for screening for nervous system disorders**
  - **Z13.850 Encounter for screening for traumatic brain injury**
  - **Z13.858 Encounter for screening for other nervous system disorders**
- **Z13.88 Encounter for screening for disorder due to exposure to contaminants**
  - EXCLUDES 1 *those exposed to contaminants without suspected disorders (Z57-Z77-)*
- **Z13.89 Encounter for screening for other disorder**
  - Encounter for screening for genitourinary disorders

Z13.9 Encounter for screening, unspecified

Genetic carrier and genetic susceptibility to disease (Z14-Z15)

√4th **Z14 Genetic carrier**

√5th **Z14.0 Hemophilia A carrier**
- **Z14.01 Asymptomatic hemophilia A carrier**
- **Z14.02 Symptomatic hemophilia A carrier**

Z14.1 Cystic fibrosis carrier

Z14.8 Genetic carrier of other disease

√4th **Z15 Genetic susceptibility to disease**
Confirmed abnormal gene
Use additional code, if applicable, for any associated family history of the disease (Z80-Z84)
EXCLUDES 1 *chromosomal anomalies (Q90-Q99)*

√5th **Z15.0 Genetic susceptibility to malignant neoplasm**
Code first, if applicable, any current malignant neoplasm (C00-C75, C81-C96)
Use additional code, if applicable, for any personal history of malignant neoplasm (Z85.-)
- **Z15.01 Genetic susceptibility to malignant neoplasm of breast**
- **Z15.02 Genetic susceptibility to malignant neoplasm of ovary**

Z15.03 Genetic susceptibility to malignant neoplasm of prostate
Z15.04 Genetic susceptibility to malignant neoplasm of endometrium
Z15.09 Genetic susceptibility to other malignant neoplasm
✓5th **Z15.8 Genetic susceptibility to other disease**
Z15.81 Genetic susceptibility to multiple endocrine neoplasia [MEN]
EXCLUDES 1 *multiple endocrine neoplasia [MEN] syndromes (E31.2-)*
Z15.89 Genetic susceptibility to other disease

Resistance to antimicrobial drugs (Z16)

✓4th **Z16 Resistance to antimicrobial drugs**
NOTE The codes in this category are provided for use as additional codes to identify the resistance and non-responsiveness of a condition to antimicrobial drugs.
Code first the infection
EXCLUDES 1 *Methicillin resistant Staphylococcus aureus infection (A49.02)*
Methicillin resistant Staphylococcus aureus infection in diseases classified elsewhere (B95.62)
Methicillin resistant Staphylococcus aureus pneumonia (J15.212)
Sepsis due to Methicillin resistant Staphylococcus aureus (A41.02)
✓5th **Z16.1 Resistance to beta lactam antibiotics**
Z16.10 Resistance to unspecified beta lactam antibiotics
Z16.11 Resistance to penicillins
Resistance to amoxicillin
Resistance to ampicillin
Z16.12 Extended spectrum beta lactamase (ESBL) resistance
Z16.19 Resistance to other specified beta lactam antibiotics
Resistance to cephalosporins
✓5th **Z16.2 Resistance to other antibiotics**
Z16.20 Resistance to unspecified antibiotic
Resistance to antibiotics NOS
Z16.21 Resistance to vancomycin
Z16.22 Resistance to vancomycin related antibiotics
Z16.23 Resistance to quinolones and fluoroquinolones
Z16.24 Resistance to multiple antibiotics
Z16.29 Resistance to other single specified antibiotic
Resistance to aminoglycosides
Resistance to macrolides
Resistance to sulfonamides
Resistance to tetracyclines
✓5th **Z16.3 Resistance to other antimicrobial drugs**
EXCLUDES 1 *resistance to antibiotics (Z16.1-, Z16.2-)*
Z16.30 Resistance to unspecified antimicrobial drugs
Drug resistance NOS
Z16.31 Resistance to antiparasitic drug(s)
Resistance to quinine and related compounds
Z16.32 Resistance to antifungal drug(s)
Z16.33 Resistance to antiviral drug(s)
✓6th **Z16.34 Resistance to antimycobacterial drug(s)**
Resistance to tuberculostatics
Z16.341 Resistance to single antimycobacterial drug
Resistance to antimycobacterial drug NOS
Z16.342 Resistance to multiple antimycobacterial drugs
Z16.35 Resistance to multiple antimicrobial drugs
EXCLUDES 1 *Resistance to multiple antibiotics only (Z16.24)*
Z16.39 Resistance to other specified antimicrobial drug

Estrogen receptor status (Z17)

✓4th **Z17 Estrogen receptor status**
Code first malignant neoplasm of breast (C50.-)
Z17.0 Estrogen receptor positive status [ER+]
Z17.1 Estrogen receptor negative status [ER-]

Retained foreign body fragment (Z18)

✓4th **Z18 Retained foreign body fragments**
Embedded fragment (status)
Embedded splinter (status)
Retained foreign body status
EXCLUDES 1 *artificial joint prosthesis status (Z96.6-)*
foreign body accidentally left during a procedure (T81.5-)
foreign body entering through orifice (T15-T19)
in situ cardiac device (Z95.-)
organ or tissue replaced by means other than transplant (Z96.-, Z97.-)
organ or tissue replaced by transplant (Z94.-)
personal history of retained foreign body fully removed (Z87.821)
superficial foreign body (non-embedded splinter)—code to superficial foreign body, by site
✓5th **Z18.0 Retained radioactive fragments**
Z18.01 Retained depleted uranium fragments
Z18.09 Other retained radioactive fragments
Other retained depleted isotope fragments
Retained nontherapeutic radioactive fragments
✓5th **Z18.1 Retained metal fragments**
EXCLUDES 1 *retained radioactive metal fragments (Z18.01-Z18.09)*
Z18.10 Retained metal fragments, unspecified
Retained metal fragment NOS
Z18.11 Retained magnetic metal fragments
Z18.12 Retained nonmagnetic metal fragments
Z18.2 Retained plastic fragments
Acrylics fragments
Diethylhexylphthalates fragments
Isocyanate fragments
✓5th **Z18.3 Retained organic fragments**
Z18.31 Retained animal quills or spines
Z18.32 Retained tooth
Z18.33 Retained wood fragments
Z18.39 Other retained organic fragments
✓5th **Z18.8 Other specified retained foreign body**
Z18.81 Retained glass fragments
Z18.83 Retained stone or crystalline fragments
Retained concrete or cement fragments
Z18.89 Other specified retained foreign body fragments
Z18.9 Retained foreign body fragments, unspecified material

Persons with potential health hazards related to communicable diseases (Z20-Z28)

✓4th **Z20 Contact with and (suspected) exposure to communicable diseases**
EXCLUDES 1 *carrier of infectious disease (Z22.-)*
diagnosed current infectious or parasitic disease—see Alphabetic Index
EXCLUDES 2 *personal history of infectious and parasitic diseases (Z86.1-)*
✓5th **Z20.0 Contact with and (suspected) exposure to intestinal infectious diseases**
Z20.01 Contact with and (suspected) exposure to intestinal infectious diseases due to Escherichia coli (E. coli)
Z20.09 Contact with and (suspected) exposure to other intestinal infectious diseases
Z20.1 Contact with and (suspected) exposure to tuberculosis
Z20.2 Contact with and (suspected) exposure to infections with a predominantly sexual mode of transmission
Z20.3 Contact with and (suspected) exposure to rabies
Z20.4 Contact with and (suspected) exposure to rubella
Z20.5 Contact with and (suspected) exposure to viral hepatitis
Z20.6 Contact with and (suspected) exposure to human immunodeficiency virus [HIV]
EXCLUDES 1 *asymptomatic human immunodeficiency virus [HIV] HIV infection status (Z21)*
Z20.7 Contact with and (suspected) exposure to pediculosis, acariasis and other infestations

√5th **Z20.8 Contact with and (suspected) exposure to other communicable diseases**

√6th **Z20.81 Contact with and (suspected) exposure to other bacterial communicable diseases**

Z20.810 Contact with and (suspected) exposure to anthrax

Z20.811 Contact with and (suspected) exposure to meningococcus

Z20.818 Contact with and (suspected) exposure to other bacterial communicable diseases

√6th **Z20.82 Contact with and (suspected) exposure to other viral communicable diseases**

Z20.820 Contact with and (suspected) exposure to varicella

Z20.828 Contact with and (suspected) exposure to other viral communicable diseases

Z20.89 Contact with and (suspected) exposure to other communicable diseases

Z20.9 Contact with and (suspected) exposure to unspecified communicable disease

Z21 Asymptomatic human immunodeficiency virus [HIV] infection status

HIV positive NOS

Code first human immunodeficiency virus [HIV] disease complicating pregnancy, childbirth and the puerperium, if applicable (O98.7-)

EXCLUDES 1 *acquired immunodeficiency syndrome (B20)*
contact with human immunodeficiency virus [HIV] (Z20.6)
exposure to human immunodeficiency virus [HIV] (Z20.6)
human immunodeficiency virus [HIV] disease (B20)
inconclusive laboratory evidence of human immunodeficiency virus [HIV] (R75)

√4th **Z22 Carrier of infectious disease**

Colonization status
Suspected carrier

Z22.0 Carrier of typhoid

Z22.1 Carrier of other intestinal infectious diseases

Z22.2 Carrier of diphtheria

√5th **Z22.3 Carrier of other specified bacterial diseases**

Z22.31 Carrier of bacterial disease due to meningococci

√6th **Z22.32 Carrier of bacterial disease due to staphylococci**

Z22.321 Carrier or suspected carrier of Methicillin susceptible Staphylococcus aureus

MSSA colonization

Z22.322 Carrier or suspected carrier of Methicillin resistant Staphylococcus aureus

MRSA colonization

√6th **Z22.33 Carrier of bacterial disease due to streptococci**

Z22.330 Carrier of Group B streptococcus

Z22.338 Carrier of other streptococcus

Z22.39 Carrier of other specified bacterial diseases

Z22.4 Carrier of infections with a predominantly sexual mode of transmission

√5th **Z22.5 Carrier of viral hepatitis**

Z22.50 Carrier of unspecified viral hepatitis

Z22.51 Carrier of viral hepatitis B

Hepatitis B surface antigen [HBsAg] carrier

Z22.52 Carrier of viral hepatitis C

Z22.59 Carrier of other viral hepatitis

Z22.6 Carrier of human T-lymphotropic virus type-1 [HTLV-1] infection

Z22.8 Carrier of other infectious diseases

Z22.9 Carrier of infectious disease, unspecified

Z23 Encounter for immunization

Code first any routine childhood examination

NOTE Procedure codes are required to identify the types of immunizations given

√4th **Z28 Immunization not carried out and underimmunization status**

Vaccination not carried out

√5th **Z28.0 Immunization not carried out because of contraindication**

Z28.01 Immunization not carried out because of acute illness of patient

Z28.02 Immunization not carried out because of chronic illness or condition of patient

Z28.03 Immunization not carried out because of immune compromised state of patient

Z28.04 Immunization not carried out because of patient allergy to vaccine or component

Z28.09 Immunization not carried out because of other contraindication

Z28.1 Immunization not carried out because of patient decision for reasons of belief or group pressure

Immunization not carried out because of religious belief

√5th **Z28.2 Immunization not carried out because of patient decision for other and unspecified reason**

Z28.20 Immunization not carried out because of patient decision for unspecified reason

Z28.21 Immunization not carried out because of patient refusal

Z28.29 Immunization not carried out because of patient decision for other reason

Z28.3 Underimmunization status

Delinquent immunization status
Lapsed immunization schedule status

√5th **Z28.8 Immunization not carried out for other reason**

Z28.81 Immunization not carried out due to patient having had the disease

Z28.82 Immunization not carried out because of caregiver refusal

Immunization not carried out because of guardian refusal
Immunization not carried out because of parent refusal

EXCLUDES 1 *immunization not carried out because of caregiver refusal because of religious belief (Z28.1)*

Z28.89 Immunization not carried out for other reason

Z28.9 Immunization not carried out for unspecified reason

Persons encountering health services in circumstances related to reproduction (Z30-Z39)

√4th **Z30 Encounter for contraceptive management**

√5th **Z30.0 Encounter for general counseling and advice on contraception**

√6th **Z30.01 Encounter for initial prescription of contraceptives**

EXCLUDES 1 *encounter for surveillance of contraceptives (Z30.4-)*

Z30.011 Encounter for initial prescription of contraceptive pills

Z30.012 Encounter for prescription of emergency contraception

Encounter for postcoital contraception

Z30.013 Encounter for initial prescription of injectable contraceptive

Z30.014 Encounter for initial prescription of intrauterine contraceptive device

EXCLUDES 1 *encounter for insertion of intrauterine contraceptive device (Z30.430, Z30.432)*

Z30.018 Encounter for initial prescription of other contraceptives

Z30.019 Encounter for initial prescription of contraceptives, unspecified

Z30.02 Counseling and instruction in natural family planning to avoid pregnancy

Z30.09 Encounter for other general counseling and advice on contraception

Encounter for family planning advice NOS

Z30.2 Encounter for sterilization

√5th **Z30.4 Encounter for surveillance of contraceptives**

Z30.40 Encounter for surveillance of contraceptives, unspecified

Z30.41 Encounter for surveillance of contraceptive pills

Encounter for repeat prescription for contraceptive pill

Z30.42 Encounter for surveillance of injectable contraceptive

√6th **Z30.43 Encounter for surveillance of intrauterine contraceptive device**

Z30.430 Encounter for insertion of intrauterine contraceptive device

Z30.431 Encounter for routine checking of intrauterine contraceptive device

Z30.432 Encounter for removal of intrauterine contraceptive device

Z30.433 Encounter for removal and reinsertion of intrauterine contraceptive device
Encounter for replacement of intrauterine contraceptive device

Z30.49 Encounter for surveillance of other contraceptives

Z30.8 Encounter for other contraceptive management
Encounter for postvasectomy sperm count
Encounter for routine examination for contraceptive maintenance
EXCLUDES 1 *sperm count following sterilization reversal (Z31.42)*
sperm count for fertility testing (Z31.41)

Z30.9 Encounter for contraceptive management, unspecified

✓4th **Z31 Encounter for procreative management**
EXCLUDES 1 *complications associated with artificial fertilization (N98.-)*
female infertility (N97.-)
male infertility (N46.-)

Z31.0 Encounter for reversal of previous sterilization

✓5th **Z31.4 Encounter for procreative investigation and testing**
EXCLUDES 1 *postvasectomy sperm count (Z30.8)*

Z31.41 Encounter for fertility testing
Encounter for fallopian tube patency testing
Encounter for sperm count for fertility testing

Z31.42 Aftercare following sterilization reversal
Sperm count following sterilization reversal

✓6th **Z31.43 Encounter for genetic testing of female for procreative management**
Use additional code for recurrent pregnancy loss, if applicable (N96, O26.2-)
EXCLUDES 1 *nonprocreative genetic testing (Z13.7-)*

Z31.430 Encounter of female for testing for genetic disease carrier status for procreative management

Z31.438 Encounter for other genetic testing of female for procreative management

✓6th **Z31.44 Encounter for genetic testing of male for procreative management**
EXCLUDES 1 *nonprocreative genetic testing (Z13.7-)*

Z31.440 Encounter of male for testing for genetic disease carrier status for procreative management

Z31.441 Encounter for testing of male partner of patient with recurrent pregnancy loss

Z31.448 Encounter for other genetic testing of male for procreative management

Z31.49 Encounter for other procreative investigation and testing

Z31.5 Encounter for genetic counseling

✓5th **Z31.6 Encounter for general counseling and advice on procreation**

Z31.61 Procreative counseling and advice using natural family planning

Z31.62 Encounter for fertility preservation counseling
Encounter for fertility preservation counseling prior to cancer therapy
Encounter for fertility preservation counseling prior to surgical removal of gonads

Z31.69 Encounter for other general counseling and advice on procreation

✓5th **Z31.8 Encounter for other procreative management**

Z31.81 Encounter for male factor infertility in female patient

Z31.82 Encounter for Rh incompatibility status

Z31.83 Encounter for assisted reproductive fertility procedure cycle
Patient undergoing in vitro fertilization cycle
Use additional code to identify the type of infertility
EXCLUDES 1 *pre-cycle diagnosis and testing—code to reason for encounter*

Z31.84 Encounter for fertility preservation procedure
Encounter for fertility preservation procedure prior to cancer therapy
Encounter for fertility preservation procedure prior to surgical removal of gonads

Z31.89 Encounter for other procreative management

Z31.9 Encounter for procreative management, unspecified

✓4th **Z32 Encounter for pregnancy test and childbirth and childcare instruction**

✓5th **Z32.0 Encounter for pregnancy test**

Z32.00 Encounter for pregnancy test, result unknown
Encounter for pregnancy test NOS

Z32.01 Encounter for pregnancy test, result positive

Z32.02 Encounter for pregnancy test, result negative

Z32.2 Encounter for childbirth instruction

Z32.3 Encounter for childcare instruction
Encounter for prenatal or postpartum childcare instruction

✓4th **Z33 Pregnant state**

Z33.1 Pregnant state, incidental
Pregnant state NOS
EXCLUDES 1 *complications of pregnancy (O00-O9A)*

Z33.2 Encounter for elective termination of pregnancy
EXCLUDES 1 *early fetal death with retention of dead fetus (O02.1)*
late fetal death (O36.4)
spontaneous abortion (O03)

✓4th **Z34 Encounter for supervision of normal pregnancy**
EXCLUDES 1 *any complication of pregnancy (O00-O9A)*
encounter for pregnancy test (Z32.0-)
encounter for supervision of high risk pregnancy (O09.-)

✓5th **Z34.0 Encounter for supervision of normal first pregnancy**

Z34.00 Encounter for supervision of normal first pregnancy, unspecified trimester

Z34.01 Encounter for supervision of normal first pregnancy, first trimester

Z34.02 Encounter for supervision of normal first pregnancy, second trimester

Z34.03 Encounter for supervision of normal first pregnancy, third trimester

✓5th **Z34.8 Encounter for supervision of other normal pregnancy**

Z34.80 Encounter for supervision of other normal pregnancy, unspecified trimester

Z34.81 Encounter for supervision of other normal pregnancy, first trimester

Z34.82 Encounter for supervision of other normal pregnancy, second trimester

Z34.83 Encounter for supervision of other normal pregnancy, third trimester

✓5th **Z34.9 Encounter for supervision of normal pregnancy, unspecified**

Z34.90 Encounter for supervision of normal pregnancy, unspecified, unspecified trimester

Z34.91 Encounter for supervision of normal pregnancy, unspecified, first trimester

Z34.92 Encounter for supervision of normal pregnancy, unspecified, second trimester

Z34.93 Encounter for supervision of normal pregnancy, unspecified, third trimester

Z36 Encounter for antenatal screening of mother
EXCLUDES 1 *abnormal findings on antenatal screening of mother (O28.-)*
diagnostic examination—code to sign or symptom
encounter for suspected maternal and fetal conditions ruled out (Z03.7-)
suspected fetal condition affecting management of pregnancy—code to condition in Chapter 15
EXCLUDES 2 *genetic counseling and testing (Z31.43-, Z31.5)*
routine prenatal care (Z34)

✓4th **Z3A Weeks of gestation**
NOTE Codes from category Z3A are for use, only on the maternal record, to indicate the weeks of gestation of the pregnancy.
Code first complications of pregnancy, childbirth and the puerperium (O00-O9A)

✓5th **Z3A.0 Weeks of gestation of pregnancy, unspecified or less than 10 weeks**

Z3A.00 Weeks of gestation of pregnancy not specified

Z3A.01 Less than 8 weeks gestation of pregnancy

Z3A.08 8 weeks gestation of pregnancy

Z3A.09 9 weeks gestation of pregnancy

✓5th **Z3A.1 Weeks of gestation of pregnancy, weeks 10-19**

Z3A.10 10 weeks gestation of pregnancy

Z3A.11 11 weeks gestation of pregnancy

Z3A.12 12 weeks gestation of pregnancy

Z3A.13 13 weeks gestation of pregnancy

Z3A.14 14 weeks gestation of pregnancy
Z3A.15 15 weeks gestation of pregnancy
Z3A.16 16 weeks gestation of pregnancy
Z3A.17 17 weeks gestation of pregnancy
Z3A.18 18 weeks gestation of pregnancy
Z3A.19 19 weeks gestation of pregnancy

✓5th **Z3A.2 Weeks of gestation of pregnancy, weeks 20-29**
Z3A.20 20 weeks gestation of pregnancy
Z3A.21 21 weeks gestation of pregnancy
Z3A.22 22 weeks gestation of pregnancy
Z3A.23 23 weeks gestation of pregnancy
Z3A.24 24 weeks gestation of pregnancy
Z3A.25 25 weeks gestation of pregnancy
Z3A.26 26 weeks gestation of pregnancy
Z3A.27 27 weeks gestation of pregnancy
Z3A.28 28 weeks gestation of pregnancy
Z3A.29 29 weeks gestation of pregnancy

✓5th **Z3A.3 Weeks of gestation of pregnancy, weeks 30-39**
Z3A.30 30 weeks gestation of pregnancy
Z3A.31 31 weeks gestation of pregnancy
Z3A.32 32 weeks gestation of pregnancy
Z3A.33 33 weeks gestation of pregnancy
Z3A.34 34 weeks gestation of pregnancy
Z3A.35 35 weeks gestation of pregnancy
Z3A.36 36 weeks gestation of pregnancy
Z3A.37 37 weeks gestation of pregnancy
Z3A.38 38 weeks gestation of pregnancy
Z3A.39 39 weeks gestation of pregnancy

✓5th **Z3A.4 Weeks of gestation of pregnancy, weeks 40 or greater**
Z3A.40 40 weeks gestation of pregnancy
Z3A.41 41 weeks gestation of pregnancy
Z3A.42 42 weeks gestation of pregnancy
Z3A.49 Greater than 42 weeks gestation of pregnancy

✓4th **Z37 Outcome of delivery**

NOTE This category is intended for use as an additional code to identify the outcome of delivery on the mother's record. It is not for use on the newborn record.

EXCLUDES1 *stillbirth (P95)*

Z37.0 Single live birth
Z37.1 Single stillbirth
Z37.2 Twins, both liveborn
Z37.3 Twins, one liveborn and one stillborn
Z37.4 Twins, both stillborn

✓5th **Z37.5 Other multiple births, all liveborn**
Z37.50 Multiple births, unspecified, all liveborn
Z37.51 Triplets, all liveborn
Z37.52 Quadruplets, all liveborn
Z37.53 Quintuplets, all liveborn
Z37.54 Sextuplets, all liveborn
Z37.59 Other multiple births, all liveborn

✓5th **Z37.6 Other multiple births, some liveborn**
Z37.60 Multiple births, unspecified, some liveborn
Z37.61 Triplets, some liveborn
Z37.62 Quadruplets, some liveborn
Z37.63 Quintuplets, some liveborn
Z37.64 Sextuplets, some liveborn
Z37.69 Other multiple births, some liveborn

Z37.7 Other multiple births, all stillborn
Z37.9 Outcome of delivery, unspecified
Multiple birth NOS
Single birth NOS

✓4th **Z38 Liveborn infants according to place of birth and type of delivery**

NOTE This category is for use as the principal code on the initial record of a newborn baby. It is to be used for the initial birth record only. It is not to be used on the mother's record.

✓5th **Z38.0 Single liveborn infant, born in hospital**
Single liveborn infant, born in birthing center or other health care facility
Z38.00 Single liveborn infant, delivered vaginally
Z38.01 Single liveborn infant, delivered by cesarean

Z38.1 Single liveborn infant, born outside hospital
Z38.2 Single liveborn infant, unspecified as to place of birth
Single liveborn infant NOS

✓5th **Z38.3 Twin liveborn infant, born in hospital**
Z38.30 Twin liveborn infant, delivered vaginally
Z38.31 Twin liveborn infant, delivered by cesarean

Z38.4 Twin liveborn infant, born outside hospital
Z38.5 Twin liveborn infant, unspecified as to place of birth

✓5th **Z38.6 Other multiple liveborn infant, born in hospital**
Z38.61 Triplet liveborn infant, delivered vaginally
Z38.62 Triplet liveborn infant, delivered by cesarean
Z38.63 Quadruplet liveborn infant, delivered vaginally
Z38.64 Quadruplet liveborn infant, delivered by cesarean
Z38.65 Quintuplet liveborn infant, delivered vaginally
Z38.66 Quintuplet liveborn infant, delivered by cesarean
Z38.68 Other multiple liveborn infant, delivered vaginally
Z38.69 Other multiple liveborn infant, delivered by cesarean

Z38.7 Other multiple liveborn infant, born outside hospital
Z38.8 Other multiple liveborn infant, unspecified as to place of birth

✓4th **Z39 Encounter for maternal postpartum care and examination**

Z39.0 Encounter for care and examination of mother immediately after delivery
Care and observation in uncomplicated cases when the delivery occurs outside a healthcare facility
EXCLUDES1 *care for postpartum complication—see Alphabetic index*

Z39.1 Encounter for care and examination of lactating mother
Encounter for supervision of lactation
EXCLUDES1 *disorders of lactation (O92.-)*

Z39.2 Encounter for routine postpartum follow-up

Encounters for other specific health care (Z40-Z53)

NOTE Categories Z40-Z53 are intended for use to indicate a reason for care. They may be used for patients who have already been treated for a disease or injury, but who are receiving aftercare or prophylactic care, or care to consolidate the treatment, or to deal with a residual state

EXCLUDES2 *follow-up examination for medical surveillance after treatment (Z08-Z09)*

✓4th **Z40 Encounter for prophylactic surgery**
EXCLUDES1 *organ donations (Z52.-)*
therapeutic organ removal—code to condition

✓5th **Z40.0 Encounter for prophylactic surgery for risk factors related to malignant neoplasms**
Admission for prophylactic organ removal
Use additional code to identify risk factor
Z40.00 Encounter for prophylactic removal of unspecified organ
Z40.01 Encounter for prophylactic removal of breast
Z40.02 Encounter for prophylactic removal of ovary
Z40.09 Encounter for prophylactic removal of other organ

Z40.8 Encounter for other prophylactic surgery
Z40.9 Encounter for prophylactic surgery, unspecified

✓4th **Z41 Encounter for procedures for purposes other than remedying health state**

Z41.1 Encounter for cosmetic surgery
Encounter for cosmetic breast implant
Encounter for cosmetic procedure
EXCLUDES1 *encounter for plastic and reconstructive surgery following medical procedure or healed injury (Z42.-)*
encounter for post-mastectomy breast implantation (Z42.1)

Z41.2 Encounter for routine and ritual male circumcision
Z41.3 Encounter for ear piercing
Z41.8 Encounter for other procedures for purposes other than remedying health state
Z41.9 Encounter for procedure for purposes other than remedying health state, unspecified

Z42 Encounter for plastic and reconstructive surgery following medical procedure or healed injury
EXCLUDES 1 *encounter for cosmetic plastic surgery (Z41.1)*
encounter for plastic surgery for treatment of current injury—code to relevent injury

Z42.1 Encounter for breast reconstruction following mastectomy
EXCLUDES 1 *deformity and disproportion of reconstructed breast (N65.1-)*

Z42.8 Encounter for other plastic and reconstructive surgery following medical procedure or healed injury

Z43 Encounter for attention to artificial openings
INCLUDES closure of artificial openings
passage of sounds or bougies through artificial openings
reforming artificial openings
removal of catheter from artificial openings
toilet or cleansing of artificial openings
EXCLUDES 1 *artificial opening status only, without need for care (Z93.-)*
complications of external stoma (J95.0-, K94.-, N99.5-)
EXCLUDES 2 *fitting and adjustment of prosthetic and other devices (Z44-Z46)*

Z43.0 Encounter for attention to tracheostomy
Z43.1 Encounter for attention to gastrostomy
Z43.2 Encounter for attention to ileostomy
Z43.3 Encounter for attention to colostomy
Z43.4 Encounter for attention to other artificial openings of digestive tract
Z43.5 Encounter for attention to cystostomy
Z43.6 Encounter for attention to other artificial openings of urinary tract
Encounter for attention to nephrostomy
Encounter for attention to ureterostomy
Encounter for attention to urethrostomy
Z43.7 Encounter for attention to artificial vagina
Z43.8 Encounter for attention to other artificial openings
Z43.9 Encounter for attention to unspecified artificial opening

Z44 Encounter for fitting and adjustment of external prosthetic device
INCLUDES removal or replacement of external prosthetic device
EXCLUDES 1 *malfunction or other complications of device—see Alphabetical Index*
presence of prosthetic device (Z97.-)

Z44.0 Encounter for fitting and adjustment of artificial arm
Z44.00 Encounter for fitting and adjustment of unspecified artificial arm
Z44.001 Encounter for fitting and adjustment of unspecified right artificial arm
Z44.002 Encounter for fitting and adjustment of unspecified left artificial arm
Z44.009 Encounter for fitting and adjustment of unspecified artificial arm, unspecified arm
Z44.01 Encounter for fitting and adjustment of complete artificial arm
Z44.011 Encounter for fitting and adjustment of complete right artificial arm
Z44.012 Encounter for fitting and adjustment of complete left artificial arm
Z44.019 Encounter for fitting and adjustment of complete artificial arm, unspecified arm
Z44.02 Encounter for fitting and adjustment of partial artificial arm
Z44.021 Encounter for fitting and adjustment of partial artificial right arm
Z44.022 Encounter for fitting and adjustment of partial artificial left arm
Z44.029 Encounter for fitting and adjustment of partial artificial arm, unspecified arm
Z44.1 Encounter for fitting and adjustment of artificial leg
Z44.10 Encounter for fitting and adjustment of unspecified artificial leg
Z44.101 Encounter for fitting and adjustment of unspecified right artificial leg
Z44.102 Encounter for fitting and adjustment of unspecified left artificial leg
Z44.109 Encounter for fitting and adjustment of unspecified artificial leg, unspecified leg
Z44.11 Encounter for fitting and adjustment of complete artificial leg
Z44.111 Encounter for fitting and adjustment of complete right artificial leg
Z44.112 Encounter for fitting and adjustment of complete left artificial leg
Z44.119 Encounter for fitting and adjustment of complete artificial leg, unspecified leg
Z44.12 Encounter for fitting and adjustment of partial artificial leg
Z44.121 Encounter for fitting and adjustment of partial artificial right leg
Z44.122 Encounter for fitting and adjustment of partial artificial left leg
Z44.129 Encounter for fitting and adjustment of partial artificial leg, unspecified leg
Z44.2 Encounter for fitting and adjustment of artificial eye
EXCLUDES 1 *mechanical complication of ocular prosthesis (T85.3)*
Z44.20 Encounter for fitting and adjustment of artificial eye, unspecified
Z44.21 Encounter for fitting and adjustment of artificial right eye
Z44.22 Encounter for fitting and adjustment of artificial left eye
Z44.3 Encounter for fitting and adjustment of external breast prosthesis
EXCLUDES 1 *complications of breast implant (T85.4-)*
encounter for adjustment or removal of breast implant (Z45.81-)
encounter for initial breast implant insertion for cosmetic breast augmentation (Z41.1)
encounter for breast reconstruction following mastectomy (Z42.1)
Z44.30 Encounter for fitting and adjustment of external breast prosthesis, unspecified breast
Z44.31 Encounter for fitting and adjustment of external right breast prosthesis
Z44.32 Encounter for fitting and adjustment of external left breast prosthesis
Z44.8 Encounter for fitting and adjustment of other external prosthetic devices
Z44.9 Encounter for fitting and adjustment of unspecified external prosthetic device

Z45 Encounter for adjustment and management of implanted device
INCLUDES removal or replacement of implanted device
EXCLUDES 1 *malfunction or other complications of device—see Alphabetical Index*
presence of prosthetic and other devices (Z95-Z97)
EXCLUDES 2 *encounter for fitting and adjustment of non-implanted device (Z46.-)*

Z45.0 Encounter for adjustment and management of cardiac device
Z45.01 Encounter for adjustment and management of cardiac pacemaker
EXCLUDES 1 *encounter for adjustment and management of automatic implantable cardiac defibrillator with synchronous cardiac pacemaker (Z45.02)*
Z45.010 Encounter for checking and testing of cardiac pacemaker pulse generator [battery]
Encounter for replacing cardiac pacemaker pulse generator [battery]
Z45.018 Encounter for adjustment and management of other part of cardiac pacemaker
Z45.02 Encounter for adjustment and management of automatic implantable cardiac defibrillator
Encounter for adjustment and management of automatic implantable cardiac defibrillator with synchronous cardiac pacemaker
Z45.09 Encounter for adjustment and management of other cardiac device
Z45.1 Encounter for adjustment and management of infusion pump

Z45.2 Encounter for adjustment and management of vascular access device
Encounter for adjustment and management of vascular catheters
EXCLUDES 1 *encounter for adjustment and management of renal dialysis catheter (Z49.01)*

✓5th **Z45.3 Encounter for adjustment and management of implanted devices of the special senses**

Z45.31 Encounter for adjustment and management of implanted visual substitution device

✓6th **Z45.32 Encounter for adjustment and management of implanted hearing device**
EXCLUDES 1 *Encounter for fitting and adjustment of hearing aide (Z46.1)*

Z45.320 Encounter for adjustment and management of bone conduction device

Z45.321 Encounter for adjustment and management of cochlear device

Z45.328 Encounter for adjustment and management of other implanted hearing device

✓5th **Z45.4 Encounter for adjustment and management of implanted nervous system device**

Z45.41 Encounter for adjustment and management of cerebrospinal fluid drainage device
Encounter for adjustment and management of cerebral ventricular (communicating) shunt

Z45.42 Encounter for adjustment and management of neuropacemaker (brain) (peripheral nerve) (spinal cord)

Z45.49 Encounter for adjustment and management of other implanted nervous system device

✓5th **Z45.8 Encounter for adjustment and management of other implanted devices**

✓6th **Z45.81 Encounter for adjustment or removal of breast implant**
Encounter for elective implant exchange (different material) (different size)
Encounter removal of tissue expander without synchronous insertion of permanent implant
EXCLUDES 1 *complications of breast implant (T85.4-)*
encounter for initial breast implant insertion for cosmetic breast augmentation (Z41.1)
encounter for breast reconstruction following mastectomy (Z42.1)

Z45.811 Encounter for adjustment or removal of right breast implant

Z45.812 Encounter for adjustment or removal of left breast implant

Z45.819 Encounter for adjustment or removal of unspecified breast implant

Z45.82 Encounter for adjustment or removal of myringotomy device (stent) (tube)

Z45.89 Encounter for adjustment and management of other implanted devices

Z45.9 Encounter for adjustment and management of unspecified implanted device

✓4th **Z46 Encounter for fitting and adjustment of other devices**
INCLUDES removal or replacement of other device
EXCLUDES 1 *malfunction or other complications of device—see Alphabetical Index*
EXCLUDES 2 *encounter for fitting and management of implanted devices (Z45.-)*
issue of repeat prescription only (Z76.0)
presence of prosthetic and other devices (Z95-Z97)

Z46.0 Encounter for fitting and adjustment of spectacles and contact lenses

Z46.1 Encounter for fitting and adjustment of hearing aid
EXCLUDES 1 *encounter for adjustment and management of implanted hearing device (Z45.32-)*

Z46.2 Encounter for fitting and adjustment of other devices related to nervous system and special senses
EXCLUDES 2 *encounter for adjustment and management of implanted nervous system device (Z45.4-)*
encounter for adjustment and management of implanted visual substitution device (Z45.31)

Z46.3 Encounter for fitting and adjustment of dental prosthetic device
Encounter for fitting and adjustment of dentures

Z46.4 Encounter for fitting and adjustment of orthodontic device

✓5th **Z46.5 Encounter for fitting and adjustment of other gastrointestinal appliance and device**
EXCLUDES 1 *encounter for attention to artificial openings of digestive tract (Z43.1-Z43.4)*

Z46.51 Encounter for fitting and adjustment of gastric lap band

Z46.59 Encounter for fitting and adjustment of other gastrointestinal appliance and device

Z46.6 Encounter for fitting and adjustment of urinary device
EXCLUDES 2 *attention to artificial openings of urinary tract (Z43.5, Z43.6)*

✓5th **Z46.8 Encounter for fitting and adjustment of other specified devices**

Z46.81 Encounter for fitting and adjustment of insulin pump
Encounter for insulin pump titration
Encounter for insulin pump instruction and training

Z46.82 Encounter for fitting and adjustment of non-vascular catheter

Z46.89 Encounter for fitting and adjustment of other specified devices
Encounter for fitting and adjustment of wheelchair

Z46.9 Encounter for fitting and adjustment of unspecified device

✓4th **Z47 Orthopedic aftercare**
EXCLUDES 1 *aftercare for healing fracture—code to fracture with 7th character D*

Z47.1 Aftercare following joint replacement surgery
Use additional code to identify the joint (Z96.6-)

Z47.2 Encounter for removal of internal fixation device
EXCLUDES 1 *encounter for adjustment of internal fixation device for fracture treatment—code to fracture with appropriate 7th character*
encounter for removal of external fixation device—code to fracture with 7th character D
infection or inflammatory reaction to internal fixation device (T84.6-)
mechanical complication of internal fixation device (T84.1-)

✓5th **Z47.3 Aftercare following explantation of joint prosthesis**
Aftercare following explantation of joint prosthesis, staged procedure
Encounter for joint prosthesis insertion following prior explantation of joint prosthesis

Z47.31 Aftercare following explantation of shoulder joint prosthesis
EXCLUDES 1 *acquired absence of shoulder joint following prior explantation of shoulder joint prosthesis (Z89.23-)*
shoulder joint prosthesis explantation status (Z89.23-)

Z47.32 Aftercare following explantation of hip joint prosthesis
EXCLUDES 1 *acquired absence of hip joint following prior explantation of hip joint prosthesis (Z89.62-)*
hip joint prosthesis explantation status (Z89.62-)

Z47.33 Aftercare following explantation of knee joint prosthesis
EXCLUDES 1 *acquired absence of knee joint following prior explantation of knee prosthesis (Z89.52-)*
knee joint prosthesis explantation status (Z89.52-)

✓5th **Z47.8 Encounter for other orthopedic aftercare**

Z47.81 Encounter for orthopedic aftercare following surgical amputation
Use additional code to identify the limb amputated (Z89.-)

Z47.82 Encounter for orthopedic aftercare following scoliosis surgery

Z47.89 Encounter for other orthopedic aftercare

Z48 Encounter for other postprocedural aftercare
EXCLUDES 1 *encounter for follow-up examination after completed treatment (Z08-Z09)*
EXCLUDES 2 *encounter for attention to artificial openings (Z43.-)*
encounter for fitting and adjustment of prosthetic and other devices (Z44-Z46)

Z48.0 Encounter for attention to dressings, sutures and drains
EXCLUDES 1 *encounter for planned postprocedural wound closure (Z48.1)*
Z48.00 Encounter for change or removal of nonsurgical wound dressing
Encounter for change or removal of wound dressing NOS
Z48.01 Encounter for change or removal of surgical wound dressing
Z48.02 Encounter for removal of sutures
Encounter for removal of staples
Z48.03 Encounter for change or removal of drains

Z48.1 Encounter for planned postprocedural wound closure
EXCLUDES 1 *encounter for attention to dressings and sutures (Z48.0-)*

Z48.2 Encounter for aftercare following organ transplant
Z48.21 Encounter for aftercare following heart transplant
Z48.22 Encounter for aftercare following kidney transplant
Z48.23 Encounter for aftercare following liver transplant
Z48.24 Encounter for aftercare following lung transplant
Z48.28 Encounter for aftercare following multiple organ transplant
Z48.280 Encounter for aftercare following heart-lung transplant
Z48.288 Encounter for aftercare following multiple organ transplant
Z48.29 Encounter for aftercare following other organ transplant
Z48.290 Encounter for aftercare following bone marrow transplant
Z48.298 Encounter for aftercare following other organ transplant

Z48.3 Aftercare following surgery for neoplasm
Use additional code to identify the neoplasm

Z48.8 Encounter for other specified postprocedural aftercare
Z48.81 Encounter for surgical aftercare following surgery on specified body systems
NOTE These codes identify the body system requiring aftercare. They are for use in conjunction with other aftercare codes to fully explain the aftercare encounter. The condition treated should also be coded if still present.
EXCLUDES 1 *aftercare for injury—code the injury with 7th character D*
aftercare following surgery for neoplasm (Z48.3)
EXCLUDES 2 *aftercare following organ transplant (Z48.2-)*
orthopedic aftercare (Z47.-)
Z48.810 Encounter for surgical aftercare following surgery on the sense organs
Z48.811 Encounter for surgical aftercare following surgery on the nervous system
EXCLUDES 2 *encounter for surgical aftercare following surgery on the sense organs (Z48.810)*
Z48.812 Encounter for surgical aftercare following surgery on the circulatory system
Z48.813 Encounter for surgical aftercare following surgery on the respiratory system
Z48.814 Encounter for surgical aftercare following surgery on the teeth or oral cavity
Z48.815 Encounter for surgical aftercare following surgery on the digestive system
Z48.816 Encounter for surgical aftercare following surgery on the genitourinary system
EXCLUDES 1 *encounter for aftercare following sterilization reversal (Z31.42)*
Z48.817 Encounter for surgical aftercare following surgery on the skin and subcutaneous tissue
Z48.89 Encounter for other specified surgical aftercare

Z49 Encounter for care involving renal dialysis
Code also associated end stage renal disease (N18.6)

Z49.0 Preparatory care for renal dialysis
Encounter for dialysis instruction and training
Z49.01 Encounter for fitting and adjustment of extracorporeal dialysis catheter
Removal or replacement of renal dialysis catheter
Toilet or cleansing of renal dialysis catheter
Z49.02 Encounter for fitting and adjustment of peritoneal dialysis catheter

Z49.3 Encounter for adequacy testing for dialysis
Z49.31 Encounter for adequacy testing for hemodialysis
Z49.32 Encounter for adequacy testing for peritoneal dialysis
Encounter for peritoneal equilibration test

Z51 Encounter for other aftercare
Code also condition requiring care
EXCLUDES 1 *follow-up examination after treatment (Z08-Z09)*

Z51.0 Encounter for antineoplastic radiation therapy

Z51.1 Encounter for antineoplastic chemotherapy and immunotherapy
EXCLUDES 2 *encounter for chemotherapy and immunotherapy for nonneoplastic condition—code to condition*
Z51.11 Encounter for antineoplastic chemotherapy
Z51.12 Encounter for antineoplastic immunotherapy

Z51.5 Encounter for palliative care

Z51.8 Encounter for other specified aftercare
EXCLUDES 1 *holiday relief care (Z75.5)*
Z51.81 Encounter for therapeutic drug level monitoring
Code also any long-term (current) drug therapy (Z79.-)
EXCLUDES 1 *encounter for blood-drug test for administrative or medicolegal reasons (Z02.83)*
Z51.89 Encounter for other specified aftercare

Z52 Donors of organs and tissues
INCLUDES autologous and other living donors
EXCLUDES 1 *cadaveric donor—omit code*
examination of potential donor (Z00.5)

Z52.0 Blood donor
Z52.00 Unspecified blood donor
Z52.000 Unspecified donor, whole blood
Z52.001 Unspecified donor, stem cells
Z52.008 Unspecified donor, other blood
Z52.01 Autologous blood donor
Z52.010 Autologous donor, whole blood
Z52.011 Autologous donor, stem cells
Z52.018 Autologous donor, other blood
Z52.09 Other blood donor
Volunteer donor
Z52.090 Other blood donor, whole blood
Z52.091 Other blood donor, stem cells
Z52.098 Other blood donor, other blood

Z52.1 Skin donor
Z52.10 Skin donor, unspecified
Z52.11 Skin donor, autologous
Z52.19 Skin donor, other

Z52.2 Bone donor
Z52.20 Bone donor, unspecified
Z52.21 Bone donor, autologous
Z52.29 Bone donor, other

Z52.3 Bone marrow donor
Z52.4 Kidney donor
Z52.5 Cornea donor
Z52.6 Liver donor

Z52.8 Donor of other specified organs or tissues
Z52.81 Egg (Oocyte) donor
Z52.810 Egg (Oocyte) donor under age 35, anonymous recipient
Egg donor under age 35 NOS
Z52.811 Egg (Oocyte) donor under age 35, designated recipient
Z52.812 Egg (Oocyte) donor age 35 and over, anonymous recipient
Egg donor age 35 and over NOS
Z52.813 Egg (Oocyte) donor age 35 and over, designated recipient
Z52.819 Egg (Oocyte) donor, unspecified
Z52.89 Donor of other specified organs or tissues
Z52.9 Donor of unspecified organ or tissue
Donor NOS

Z53 Persons encountering health services for specific procedures and treatment, not carried out
Z53.0 Procedure and treatment not carried out because of contraindication
Z53.01 Procedure and treatment not carried out due to patient smoking
Z53.09 Procedure and treatment not carried out because of other contraindication
Z53.1 Procedure and treatment not carried out because of patient's decision for reasons of belief and group pressure
Z53.2 Procedure and treatment not carried out because of patient's decision for other and unspecified reasons
Z53.20 Procedure and treatment not carried out because of patient's decision for unspecified reasons
Z53.21 Procedure and treatment not carried out due to patient leaving prior to being seen by health care provider
Z53.29 Procedure and treatment not carried out because of patient's decision for other reasons
Z53.8 Procedure and treatment not carried out for other reasons
Z53.9 Procedure and treatment not carried out, unspecified reason

Persons with potential health hazards related to socioeconomic and psychosocial circumstances (Z55-Z65)

Z55 Problems related to education and literacy
EXCLUDES 1 *disorders of psychological development (F80-F89)*
Z55.0 Illiteracy and low-level literacy
Z55.1 Schooling unavailable and unattainable
Z55.2 Failed school examinations
Z55.3 Underachievement in school
Z55.4 Educational maladjustment and discord with teachers and classmates
Z55.8 Other problems related to education and literacy
Problems related to inadequate teaching
Z55.9 Problems related to education and literacy, unspecified
Academic problems NOS

Z56 Problems related to employment and unemployment
EXCLUDES 2 *occupational exposure to risk factors (Z57.-)*
problems related to housing and economic circumstances (Z59.-)
Z56.0 Unemployment, unspecified
Z56.1 Change of job
Z56.2 Threat of job loss
Z56.3 Stressful work schedule
Z56.4 Discord with boss and workmates
Z56.5 Uncongenial work environment
Difficult conditions at work
Z56.6 Other physical and mental strain related to work
Z56.8 Other problems related to employment
Z56.81 Sexual harassment on the job
Z56.82 Military deployment status
Individual (civilian or military) currently deployed in theater or in support of military war, peacekeeping and humanitarian operations
Z56.89 Other problems related to employment
Z56.9 Unspecified problems related to employment
Occupational problems NOS

Z57 Occupational exposure to risk factors
Z57.0 Occupational exposure to noise
Z57.1 Occupational exposure to radiation
Z57.2 Occupational exposure to dust
Z57.3 Occupational exposure to other air contaminants
Z57.31 Occupational exposure to environmental tobacco smoke
EXCLUDES 2 *exposure to environmental tobacco smoke (Z77.22)*
Z57.39 Occupational exposure to other air contaminants
Z57.4 Occupational exposure to toxic agents in agriculture
Occupational exposure to solids, liquids, gases or vapors in agriculture
Z57.5 Occupational exposure to toxic agents in other industries
Occupational exposure to solids, liquids, gases or vapors in other industries
Z57.6 Occupational exposure to extreme temperature
Z57.7 Occupational exposure to vibration
Z57.8 Occupational exposure to other risk factors
Z57.9 Occupational exposure to unspecified risk factor

Z59 Problems related to housing and economic circumstances
EXCLUDES 2 *problems related to upbringing (Z62.-)*
Z59.0 Homelessness
Z59.1 Inadequate housing
Lack of heating
Restriction of space
Technical defects in home preventing adequate care
Unsatisfactory surroundings
EXCLUDES 1 *problems related to the natural and physical environment (Z77.1-)*
Z59.2 Discord with neighbors, lodgers and landlord
Z59.3 Problems related to living in residential institution
Boarding-school resident
EXCLUDES 1 *institutional upbringing (Z62.2)*
Z59.4 Lack of adequate food and safe drinking water
Inadequate drinking water supply
EXCLUDES 1 *effects of hunger (T73.0)*
inappropriate diet or eating habits (Z72.4)
malnutrition (E40-E46)
Z59.5 Extreme poverty
Z59.6 Low income
Z59.7 Insufficient social insurance and welfare support
Z59.8 Other problems related to housing and economic circumstances
Foreclosure on loan
Isolated dwelling
Problems with creditors
Z59.9 Problem related to housing and economic circumstances, unspecified

Z60 Problems related to social environment
Z60.0 Problems of adjustment to life-cycle transitions
Empty nest syndrome
Phase of life problem
Problem with adjustment to retirement [pension]
Z60.2 Problems related to living alone
Z60.3 Acculturation difficulty
Problem with migration
Problem with social transplantation
Z60.4 Social exclusion and rejection
Exclusion and rejection on the basis of personal characteristics, such as unusual physical appearance, illness or behavior.
EXCLUDES 1 *target of adverse discrimination such as for racial or religious reasons (Z60.5)*
Z60.5 Target of (perceived) adverse discrimination and persecution
EXCLUDES 1 *social exclusion and rejection (Z60.4)*
Z60.8 Other problems related to social environment
Z60.9 Problem related to social environment, unspecified

Z62 Problems related to upbringing
Current and past negative life events in childhood
Current and past problems of a child related to upbringing
EXCLUDES 2 *maltreatment syndrome (T74.-)*
problems related to housing and economic circumstances (Z59.-)
Z62.0 Inadequate parental supervision and control
Z62.1 Parental overprotection

✓5th **Z62.2 Upbringing away from parents**
EXCLUDES 1 *problems with boarding school (Z59.3)*
Z62.21 Child in welfare custody
Child in care of non-parental family member
Child in foster care
EXCLUDES 2 *problem for parent due to child in welfare custody (Z63.5)*
Z62.22 Institutional upbringing
Child living in orphanage or group home
Z62.29 Other upbringing away from parents
Z62.3 Hostility towards and scapegoating of child
Z62.6 Inappropriate (excessive) parental pressure
✓5th **Z62.8 Other specified problems related to upbringing**
✓6th **Z62.81 Personal history of abuse in childhood**
Z62.810 Personal history of physical and sexual abuse in childhood
EXCLUDES 1 *current child physical abuse (T74.12, T76.12)*
current child sexual abuse (T74.22, T76.22)
Z62.811 Personal history of psychological abuse in childhood
EXCLUDES 1 *current child psychological abuse (T74.32, T76.32)*
Z62.812 Personal history of neglect in childhood
EXCLUDES 1 *current child neglect (T74.02, T76.02)*
Z62.819 Personal history of unspecified abuse in childhood
EXCLUDES 1 *current child abuse NOS (T74.92, T76.92)*
✓6th **Z62.82 Parent-child conflict**
Z62.820 Parent-biological child conflict
Parent-child problem NOS
Z62.821 Parent-adopted child conflict
Z62.822 Parent-foster child conflict
✓6th **Z62.89 Other specified problems related to upbringing**
Z62.890 Parent-child estrangement NEC
Z62.891 Sibling rivalry
Z62.898 Other specified problems related to upbringing
Z62.9 Problem related to upbringing, unspecified

✓4th **Z63 Other problems related to primary support group, including family circumstances**
EXCLUDES 2 *maltreatment syndrome (T74-, T76)*
parent-child problems (Z62.-)
problems related to negative life events in childhood (Z62.-)
problems related to upbringing (Z62.-)
Z63.0 Problems in relationship with spouse or partner
EXCLUDES 1 *counseling for spousal or partner abuse problems (Z69.1)*
counseling related to sexual attitude, behavior, and orientation (Z70.-)
Z63.1 Problems in relationship with in-laws
✓5th **Z63.3 Absence of family member**
EXCLUDES 1 *absence of family member due to disappearance and death (Z63.4)*
absence of family member due to separation and divorce (Z63.5)
Z63.31 Absence of family member due to military deployment
Individual or family affected by other family member being on military deployment
EXCLUDES 1 *family disruption due to return of family member from military deployment (Z63.71)*
Z63.32 Other absence of family member
Z63.4 Disappearance and death of family member
Assumed death of family member
Bereavement
Z63.5 Disruption of family by separation and divorce
Marital estrangement
Z63.6 Dependent relative needing care at home
✓5th **Z63.7 Other stressful life events affecting family and household**
Z63.71 Stress on family due to return of family member from military deployment
Individual or family affected by family member having returned from military deployment (current or past conflict)
Z63.72 Alcoholism and drug addiction in family
Z63.79 Other stressful life events affecting family and household
Anxiety (normal) about sick person in family
Health problems within family
Ill or disturbed family member
Isolated family
Z63.8 Other specified problems related to primary support group
Family discord NOS
Family estrangement NOS
High expressed emotional level within family
Inadequate family support NOS
Inadequate or distorted communication within family
Z63.9 Problem related to primary support group, unspecified
Relationship disorder NOS

✓4th **Z64 Problems related to certain psychosocial circumstances**
Z64.0 Problems related to unwanted pregnancy
Z64.1 Problems related to multiparity
Z64.4 Discord with counselors
Discord with probation officer
Discord with social worker

✓4th **Z65 Problems related to other psychosocial circumstances**
Z65.0 Conviction in civil and criminal proceedings without imprisonment
Z65.1 Imprisonment and other incarceration
Z65.2 Problems related to release from prison
Z65.3 Problems related to other legal circumstances
Arrest
Child custody or support proceedings
Litigation
Prosecution
Z65.4 Victim of crime and terrorism
Victim of torture
Z65.5 Exposure to disaster, war and other hostilities
EXCLUDES 1 *target of perceived discrimination or persecution (Z60.5)*
Z65.8 Other specified problems related to psychosocial circumstances
Z65.9 Problem related to unspecified psychosocial circumstances

Do not resuscitate status (Z66)

Z66 Do not resuscitate
DNR status

Blood type (Z67)

✓4th **Z67 Blood type**
✓5th **Z67.1 Type A blood**
Z67.10 Type A blood, Rh positive
Z67.11 Type A blood, Rh negative
✓5th **Z67.2 Type B blood**
Z67.20 Type B blood, Rh positive
Z67.21 Type B blood, Rh negative
✓5th **Z67.3 Type AB blood**
Z67.30 Type AB blood, Rh positive
Z67.31 Type AB blood, Rh negative
✓5th **Z67.4 Type O blood**
Z67.40 Type O blood, Rh positive
Z67.41 Type O blood, Rh negative
✓5th **Z67.9 Unspecified blood type**
Z67.90 Unspecified blood type, Rh positive
Z67.91 Unspecified blood type, Rh negative

Body mass index [BMI] (Z68)

Z68 Body mass index [BMI]
Kilograms per meters squared
NOTE BMI adult codes are for use for persons 21 years of age or older
BMI pediatric codes are for use for persons 2-20 years of age. These percentiles are based on the growth charts published by the Centers for Disease Control and Prevention (CDC)

Z68.1 Body mass index [BMI] 19 or less, adult
Z68.2 Body mass index [BMI] 20-29, adult
Z68.20 Body mass index [BMI] 20.0-20.9, adult
Z68.21 Body mass index [BMI] 21.0-21.9, adult
Z68.22 Body mass index [BMI] 22.0-22.9, adult
Z68.23 Body mass index [BMI] 23.0-23.9, adult
Z68.24 Body mass index [BMI] 24.0-24.9, adult
Z68.25 Body mass index [BMI] 25.0-25.9, adult
Z68.26 Body mass index [BMI] 26.0-26.9, adult
Z68.27 Body mass index [BMI] 27.0-27.9, adult
Z68.28 Body mass index [BMI] 28.0-28.9, adult
Z68.29 Body mass index [BMI] 29.0-29.9, adult
Z68.3 Body mass index [BMI] 30-39, adult
Z68.30 Body mass index [BMI] 30.0-30.9, adult
Z68.31 Body mass index [BMI] 31.0-31.9, adult
Z68.32 Body mass index [BMI] 32.0-32.9, adult
Z68.33 Body mass index [BMI] 33.0-33.9, adult
Z68.34 Body mass index [BMI] 34.0-34.9, adult
Z68.35 Body mass index [BMI] 35.0-35.9, adult
Z68.36 Body mass index [BMI] 36.0-36.9, adult
Z68.37 Body mass index [BMI] 37.0-37.9, adult
Z68.38 Body mass index [BMI] 38.0-38.9, adult
Z68.39 Body mass index [BMI] 39.0-39.9, adult
Z68.4 Body mass index [BMI] 40 or greater, adult
Z68.41 Body mass index [BMI] 40.0-44.9, adult
Z68.42 Body mass index [BMI] 45.0-49.9, adult
Z68.43 Body mass index [BMI] 50-59.9 , adult
Z68.44 Body mass index [BMI] 60.0-69.9, adult
Z68.45 Body mass index [BMI] 70 or greater, adult
Z68.5 Body mass index [BMI] pediatric
Z68.51 Body mass index [BMI] pediatric, less than 5th percentile for age
Z68.52 Body mass index [BMI] pediatric, 5th percentile to less than 85th percentile for age
Z68.53 Body mass index [BMI] pediatric, 85th percentile to less than 95th percentile for age
Z68.54 Body mass index [BMI] pediatric, greater than or equal to 95th percentile for age

Persons encountering health services in other circumstances (Z69-Z76)

Z69 Encounter for mental health services for victim and perpetrator of abuse
Counseling for victims and perpetrators of abuse
Z69.0 Encounter for mental health services for child abuse problems
Z69.01 Encounter for mental health services for parental child abuse
Z69.010 Encounter for mental health services for victim of parental child abuse
Z69.011 Encounter for mental health services for perpetrator of parental child abuse
EXCLUDES 1 *encounter for mental health services for non-parental child abuse (Z69.02-)*
Z69.02 Encounter for mental health services for non-parental child abuse
Z69.020 Encounter for mental health services for victim of non-parental child abuse
Z69.021 Encounter for mental health services for perpetrator of non-parental child abuse
Z69.1 Encounter for mental health services for spousal or partner abuse problems
Z69.11 Encounter for mental health services for victim of spousal or partner abuse
Z69.12 Encounter for mental health services for perpetrator of spousal or partner abuse
Z69.8 Encounter for mental health services for victim or perpetrator of other abuse
Z69.81 Encounter for mental health services for victim of other abuse
Encounter for rape victim counseling
Z69.82 Encounter for mental health services for perpetrator of other abuse

Z70 Counseling related to sexual attitude, behavior and orientation
Encounter for mental health services for sexual attitude, behavior and orientation
EXCLUDES 2 *contraceptive or procreative counseling (Z30-Z31)*
Z70.0 Counseling related to sexual attitude
Z70.1 Counseling related to patient's sexual behavior and orientation
Patient concerned regarding impotence
Patient concerned regarding non-responsiveness
Patient concerned regarding promiscuity
Patient concerned regarding sexual orientation
Z70.2 Counseling related to sexual behavior and orientation of third party
Advice sought regarding sexual behavior and orientation of child
Advice sought regarding sexual behavior and orientation of partner
Advice sought regarding sexual behavior and orientation of spouse
Z70.3 Counseling related to combined concerns regarding sexual attitude, behavior and orientation
Z70.8 Other sex counseling
Encounter for sex education
Z70.9 Sex counseling, unspecified

Z71 Persons encountering health services for other counseling and medical advice, not elsewhere classified
EXCLUDES 2 *contraceptive or procreation counseling (Z30-Z31)*
sex counseling (Z70.-)
Z71.0 Person encountering health services to consult on behalf of another person
Person encountering health services to seek advice or treatment for non-attending third party
EXCLUDES 2 *anxiety (normal) about sick person in family (Z63.7)*
expectant (adoptive) parent(s) pre-birth pediatrician visit (Z76.81)
Z71.1 Person with feared health complaint in whom no diagnosis is made
Person encountering health services with feared condition which was not demonstrated
Person encountering health services in which problem was normal state
"Worried well"
EXCLUDES 1 *medical observation for suspected diseases and conditions proven not to exist (Z03.-)*
Z71.2 Person consulting for explanation of examination or test findings
Z71.3 Dietary counseling and surveillance
Use additional code for any associated underlying medical condition
Use additional code to identify body mass index (BMI), if known (Z68.-)
Z71.4 Alcohol abuse counseling and surveillance
Use additional code for alcohol abuse or dependence (F10.-)
Z71.41 Alcohol abuse counseling and surveillance of alcoholic
Z71.42 Counseling for family member of alcoholic
Counseling for significant other, partner, or friend of alcoholic
Z71.5 Drug abuse counseling and surveillance
Use additional code for drug abuse or dependence (F11-F16, F18-F19)
Z71.51 Drug abuse counseling and surveillance of drug abuser
Z71.52 Counseling for family member of drug abuser
Counseling for significant other, partner, or friend of drug abuser
Z71.6 Tobacco abuse counseling
Use additional code for nicotine dependence (F17.-)

Z71.7 Human immunodeficiency virus [HIV] counseling

5th Z71.8 Other specified counseling

EXCLUDES 2 *counseling for contraception (Z30.0-)*
counseling for genetics (Z31.5)
counseling for procreative management (Z31.6-)

Z71.81 Spiritual or religious counseling

Z71.89 Other specified counseling

Z71.9 Counseling, unspecified

Encounter for medical advice NOS

4th Z72 Problems related to lifestyle

EXCLUDES 2 *problems related to life-management difficulty (Z73.-)*
problems related to socioeconomic and psychosocial circumstances (Z55-Z65)

Z72.0 Tobacco use

Tobacco use NOS

EXCLUDES 1 *history of tobacco dependence (Z87.891)*
nicotine dependence (F17.2-)
tobacco dependence (F17.2-)
tobacco use during pregnancy (O99.33-)

Z72.3 Lack of physical exercise

Z72.4 Inappropriate diet and eating habits

EXCLUDES 1 *behavioral eating disorders of infancy or childhood (F98.2- F98.3)*
eating disorders (F50.-)
lack of adequate food (Z59.4)
malnutrition and other nutritional deficiencies (E40-E64)

5th Z72.5 High risk sexual behavior

Promiscuity

EXCLUDES 1 *paraphilias (F65)*

Z72.51 High risk heterosexual behavior

Z72.52 High risk homosexual behavior

Z72.53 High risk bisexual behavior

Z72.6 Gambling and betting

EXCLUDES 1 *compulsive or pathological gambling (F63.0)*

Z72.8 Other problems related to lifestyle

6th Z72.81 Antisocial behavior

EXCLUDES 1 *conduct disorders (F91.-)*

Z72.810 Child and adolescent antisocial behavior

Antisocial behavior (child) (adolescent) without manifest psychiatric disorder
Delinquency NOS
Group delinquency
Offenses in the context of gang membership
Stealing in company with others
Truancy from school

Z72.811 Adult antisocial behavior

Adult antisocial behavior without manifest psychiatric disorder

6th Z72.82 Problems related to sleep

Z72.820 Sleep deprivation

Lack of adequate sleep

EXCLUDES 1 *insomnia (G47.0-)*

Z72.821 Inadequate sleep hygiene

Bad sleep habits
Irregular sleep habits
Unhealthy sleep wake schedule

EXCLUDES 1 *insomnia (F51.0-, G47.0-)*

Z72.89 Other problems related to lifestyle

Self-damaging behavior

Z72.9 Problem related to lifestyle, unspecified

4th Z73 Problems related to life management difficulty

EXCLUDES 2 *problems related to socioeconomic and psychosocial circumstances (Z55-Z65)*

Z73.0 Burn-out

Z73.1 Type A behavior pattern

Z73.2 Lack of relaxation and leisure

Z73.3 Stress, not elsewhere classified

Physical and mental strain NOS

EXCLUDES 1 *stress related to employment or unemployment (Z56.-)*

Z73.4 Inadequate social skills, not elsewhere classified

Z73.5 Social role conflict, not elsewhere classified

Z73.6 Limitation of activities due to disability

EXCLUDES 1 *care-provider dependency (Z74.-)*

5th Z73.8 Other problems related to life management difficulty

6th Z73.81 Behavioral insomnia of childhood

Z73.810 Behavioral insomnia of childhood, sleep-onset association type

Z73.811 Behavioral insomnia of childhood, limit setting type

Z73.812 Behavioral insomnia of childhood, combined type

Z73.819 Behavioral insomnia of childhood, unspecified type

Z73.82 Dual sensory impairment

Z73.89 Other problems related to life management difficulty

Z73.9 Problem related to life management difficulty, unspecified

4th Z74 Problems related to care provider dependency

EXCLUDES 2 *dependence on enabling machines or devices NEC (Z99.-)*

5th Z74.0 Reduced mobility

Z74.01 Bed confinement status

Bedridden

Z74.09 Other reduced mobility

Chair ridden
Reduced mobility NOS

EXCLUDES 2 *wheelchair dependence (Z99.3)*

Z74.1 Need for assistance with personal care

Z74.2 Need for assistance at home and no other household member able to render care

Z74.3 Need for continuous supervision

Z74.8 Other problems related to care provider dependency

Z74.9 Problem related to care provider dependency, unspecified

4th Z75 Problems related to medical facilities and other health care

Z75.0 Medical services not available in home

EXCLUDES 1 *no other household member able to render care (Z74.2)*

Z75.1 Person awaiting admission to adequate facility elsewhere

Z75.2 Other waiting period for investigation and treatment

Z75.3 Unavailability and inaccessibility of health-care facilities

EXCLUDES 1 *bed unavailable (Z75.1)*

Z75.4 Unavailability and inaccessibility of other helping agencies

Z75.5 Holiday relief care

Z75.8 Other problems related to medical facilities and other health care

Z75.9 Unspecified problem related to medical facilities and other health care

4th Z76 Persons encountering health services in other circumstances

Z76.0 Encounter for issue of repeat prescription

Encounter for issue of repeat prescription for appliance
Encounter for issue of repeat prescription for medicaments
Encounter for issue of repeat prescription for spectacles

EXCLUDES 2 *issue of medical certificate (Z02.7)*
repeat prescription for contraceptive (Z30.4-)

Z76.1 Encounter for health supervision and care of foundling

Z76.2 Encounter for health supervision and care of other healthy infant and child

Encounter for medical or nursing care or supervision of healthy infant under circumstances such as adverse socioeconomic conditions at home
Encounter for medical or nursing care or supervision of healthy infant under circumstances such as awaiting foster or adoptive placement
Encounter for medical or nursing care or supervision of healthy infant under circumstances such as maternal illness
Encounter for medical or nursing care or supervision of healthy infant under circumstances such as number of children at home preventing or interfering with normal care

Z76.3 Healthy person accompanying sick person

Z76.4 Other boarder to healthcare facility

EXCLUDES 1 *homelessness (Z59.0)*

Z76.5 Malingerer [conscious simulation]

Person feigning illness (with obvious motivation)

EXCLUDES 1 *factitious disorder (F68.1-)*
peregrinating patient (F68.1-)

5th Z76.8 Persons encountering health services in other specified circumstances

Z76.81 Expectant parent(s) prebirth pediatrician visit

Pre-adoption pediatrician visit for adoptive parent(s)

☑ Appropriate additional character required   x7th Requires 7th character, placeholder x must fill empty characters

Z76.82 Awaiting organ transplant status
Patient waiting for organ availability

Z76.89 Persons encountering health services in other specified circumstances
Persons encountering health services NOS

Persons with potential health hazards related to family and personal history and certain conditions influencing health status (Z77-Z99)

Code also any follow-up examination (Z08-Z09)

✓4th **Z77 Other contact with and (suspected) exposures hazardous to health**
INCLUDES contact with and (suspected) exposures to potential hazards to health
EXCLUDES 2 *contact with and (suspected) exposure to communicable diseases (Z20.-)*
exposure to (parental) (environmental) tobacco smoke in the perinatal period (P96.81)
newborn (suspected to be) affected by noxious substances transmitted via placenta or breast milk (P04.-)
occupational exposure to risk factors (Z57.-)
retained foreign body (Z18.-)
retained foreign body fully removed (Z87.821)
toxic effects of substances chiefly nonmedicinal as to source (T51-T65)

✓5th **Z77.0 Contact with and (suspected) exposure to hazardous, chiefly nonmedicinal, chemicals**

✓6th **Z77.01 Contact with and (suspected) exposure to hazardous metals**

Z77.010 Contact with and (suspected) exposure to arsenic

Z77.011 Contact with and (suspected) exposure to lead

Z77.012 Contact with and (suspected) exposure to uranium
EXCLUDES 1 *retained depleted uranium fragments (Z18.01)*

Z77.018 Contact with and (suspected) exposure to other hazardous metals
Contact with and (suspected) exposure to chromium compounds
Contact with and (suspected) exposure to nickel dust

✓6th **Z77.02 Contact with and (suspected) exposure to hazardous aromatic compounds**

Z77.020 Contact with and (suspected) exposure to aromatic amines

Z77.021 Contact with and (suspected) exposure to benzene

Z77.028 Contact with and (suspected) exposure to other hazardous aromatic compounds
Aromatic dyes NOS
Polycyclic aromatic hydrocarbons

✓6th **Z77.09 Contact with and (suspected) exposure to other hazardous, chiefly nonmedicinal, chemicals**

Z77.090 Contact with and (suspected) exposure to asbestos

Z77.098 Contact with and (suspected) exposure to other hazardous, chiefly nonmedicinal, chemicals
Dyes NOS

✓5th **Z77.1 Contact with and (suspected) exposure to environmental pollution and hazards in the physical environment**

✓6th **Z77.11 Contact with and (suspected) exposure to environmental pollution**

Z77.110 Contact with and (suspected) exposure to air pollution

Z77.111 Contact with and (suspected) exposure to water pollution

Z77.112 Contact with and (suspected) exposure to soil pollution

Z77.118 Contact with and (suspected) exposure to other environmental pollution

✓6th **Z77.12 Contact with and (suspected) exposure to hazards in the physical environment**

Z77.120 Contact with and (suspected) exposure to mold (toxic)

Z77.121 Contact with and (suspected) exposure to harmful algae and algae toxins
Contact with and (suspected) exposure to (harmful) algae bloom NOS
Contact with and (suspected) exposure to blue-green algae bloom
Contact with and (suspected) exposure to brown tide
Contact with and (suspected) exposure to cyanobacteria bloom
Contact with and (suspected) exposure to Florida red tide
Contact with and (suspected) exposure to pfiesteria piscicida
Contact with and (suspected) exposure to red tide

Z77.122 Contact with and (suspected) exposure to noise

Z77.123 Contact with and (suspected) exposure to radon and other naturally occuring radiation
EXCLUDES 2 *radiation exposure as the cause of a confirmed condition (W88-W90, X39.0-)*
radiation sickness NOS (T66)

Z77.128 Contact with and (suspected) exposure to other hazards in the physical environment

✓5th **Z77.2 Contact with and (suspected) exposure to other hazardous substances**

Z77.21 Contact with and (suspected) exposure to potentially hazardous body fluids

Z77.22 Contact with and (suspected) exposure to environmental tobacco smoke (acute) (chronic)
Exposure to second hand tobacco smoke (acute) (chronic)
Passive smoking (acute) (chronic)
EXCLUDES 1 *nicotine dependence (F17.-)*
tobacco use (Z72.0)
EXCLUDES 2 *occupational exposure to environmental tobacco smoke (Z57.31)*

Z77.29 Contact with and (suspected) exposure to other hazardous substances

Z77.9 Other contact with and (suspected) exposures hazardous to health

✓4th **Z78 Other specified health status**
EXCLUDES 2 *asymptomatic human immunodeficiency virus [HIV] infection status (Z21)*
postprocedural status (Z93- Z99)
sex reassignment status (Z87.890)

Z78.0 Asymptomatic menopausal state
Menopausal state NOS
Postmenopausal status NOS
EXCLUDES 2 *symptomatic menopausal state (N95.1)*

Z78.1 Physical restraint status
EXCLUDES 1 *physical restraint due to a procedure - omit code*

Z78.9 Other specified health status

✓4th **Z79 Long term (current) drug therapy**
INCLUDES long term (current) drug use for prophylactic purposes
Code also any therapeutic drug level monitoring (Z51.81)
EXCLUDES 2 *drug abuse and dependence (F11-F19)*
drug use complicating pregnancy, childbirth, and the puerperium (O99.32-)

✓5th **Z79.0 Long term (current) use of anticoagulants and antithrombotics/antiplatelets**
EXCLUDES 2 *long term (current) use of aspirin (Z79.82)*

Z79.01 Long term (current) use of anticoagulants

Z79.02 Long term (current) use of antithrombotics/antiplatelets

Z79.1 Long term (current) use of non-steroidal anti-inflammatories (NSAID)
EXCLUDES 2 *long term (current) use of aspirin (Z79.82)*

Z79.2 Long term (current) use of antibiotics

Z79.3 Long term (current) use of hormonal contraceptives
Long term (current) use of birth control pill or patch

Z79.4 Long term (current) use of insulin

√5th **Z79.5 Long term (current) use of steroids**
Z79.51 Long term (current) use of inhaled steroids
Z79.52 Long term (current) use of systemic steroids

√5th **Z79.8 Other long term (current) drug therapy**

√6th **Z79.81 Long term (current) use of agents affecting estrogen receptors and estrogen levels**
Code first, if applicable:
malignant neoplasm of breast (C50.-)
malignant neoplasm of prostate (C61)
Use additional code, if applicable, to identify:
estrogen receptor positive status (Z17.0)
family history of breast cancer (Z80.3)
genetic susceptibility to malignant neoplasm (cancer) (Z15.0-)
personal history of breast cancer (Z85.3)
personal history of prostate cancer (Z85.46)
postmenopausal status (Z78.0)
EXCLUDES 1 *hormone replacement therapy (postmenopausal) (Z79.890)*

Z79.810 Long term (current) use of selective estrogen receptor modulators (SERMs)
Long term (current) use of raloxifene (Evista)
Long term (current) use of tamoxifen (Nolvadex)
Long term (current) use of toremifene (Fareston)

Z79.811 Long term (current) use of aromatase inhibitors
Long term (current) use of anastrozole (Arimidex)
Long term (current) use of exemestane (Aromasin)
Long term (current) use of letrozole (Femara)

Z79.818 Long term (current) use of other agents affecting estrogen receptors and estrogen levels
Long term (current) use of estrogen receptor downregulators
Long term (current) use of fulvestrant (Faslodex)
Long term (current) use of gonadotropin-releasing hormone (GnRH) agonist
Long term (current) use of goserelin acetate (Zoladex)
Long term (current) use of leuprolide acetate (leuprorelin) (Lupron)
Long term (current) use of megestrol acetate (Megace)

Z79.82 Long term (current) use of aspirin
Z79.83 Long term (current) use of bisphosphonates

√6th **Z79.89 Other long term (current) drug therapy**
Z79.890 Hormone replacement therapy (postmenopausal)
Z79.891 Long term (current) use of opiate analgesic
Long term (current) use of methadone for pain management
EXCLUDES 1 *methodone use NOS (F11.2-)*
use of methodone for treatment of heroin addiction (F11.2-)
Z79.899 Other long term (current) drug therapy

√4th **Z80 Family history of primary malignant neoplasm**

Z80.0 Family history of malignant neoplasm of digestive organs
Conditions classifiable to C15-C26

Z80.1 Family history of malignant neoplasm of trachea, bronchus and lung
Conditions classifiable to C33-C34

Z80.2 Family history of malignant neoplasm of other respiratory and intrathoracic organs
Conditions classifiable to C30-C32, C37-C39

Z80.3 Family history of malignant neoplasm of breast
Conditions classifiable to C50-

√5th **Z80.4 Family history of malignant neoplasm of genital organs**
Conditions classifiable to C51-C63
Z80.41 Family history of malignant neoplasm of ovary
Z80.42 Family history of malignant neoplasm of prostate
Z80.43 Family history of malignant neoplasm of testis
Z80.49 Family history of malignant neoplasm of other genital organs

√5th **Z80.5 Family history of malignant neoplasm of urinary tract**
Conditions classifiable to C64-C68
Z80.51 Family history of malignant neoplasm of kidney
Z80.52 Family history of malignant neoplasm of bladder
Z80.59 Family history of malignant neoplasm of other urinary tract organ

Z80.6 Family history of leukemia
Conditions classifiable to C91-C95

Z80.7 Family history of other malignant neoplasms of lymphoid, hematopoietic and related tissues
Conditions classifiable to C81-C90, C96-

Z80.8 Family history of malignant neoplasm of other organs or systems
Conditions classifiable to C00-C14, C40-C49, C69-C79

Z80.9 Family history of malignant neoplasm, unspecified
Conditions classifiable to C80.1

√4th **Z81 Family history of mental and behavioral disorders**

Z81.0 Family history of intellectual disabilities
Conditions classifiable to F70-F79

Z81.1 Family history of alcohol abuse and dependence
Conditions classifiable to F10-

Z81.2 Family history of tobacco abuse and dependence
Conditions classifiable to F17-

Z81.3 Family history of other psychoactive substance abuse and dependence
Conditions classifiable to F11-F16, F18-F19

Z81.4 Family history of other substance abuse and dependence
Conditions classifiable to F55

Z81.8 Family history of other mental and behavioral disorders
Conditions classifiable elsewhere in F01-F99

√4th **Z82 Family history of certain disabilities and chronic diseases (leading to disablement)**

Z82.0 Family history of epilepsy and other diseases of the nervous system
Conditions classifiable to G00-G99

Z82.1 Family history of blindness and visual loss
Conditions classifiable to H54-

Z82.2 Family history of deafness and hearing loss
Conditions classifiable to H90-H91

Z82.3 Family history of stroke
Conditions classifiable to I60-I64

√5th **Z82.4 Family history of ischemic heart disease and other diseases of the circulatory system**
Conditions classifiable to I00-I52, I65-I99
Z82.41 Family history of sudden cardiac death
Z82.49 Family history of ischemic heart disease and other diseases of the circulatory system

Z82.5 Family history of asthma and other chronic lower respiratory diseases
Conditions classifiable to J40-J47
EXCLUDES 2 *family history of other diseases of the respiratory system (Z83.6)*

√5th **Z82.6 Family history of arthritis and other diseases of the musculoskeletal system and connective tissue**
Conditions classifiable to M00-M99
Z82.61 Family history of arthritis
Z82.62 Family history of osteoporosis
Z82.69 Family history of other diseases of the musculoskeletal system and connective tissue

√5th **Z82.7 Family history of congenital malformations, deformations and chromosomal abnormalities**
Conditions classifiable to Q00-Q99
Z82.71 Family history of polycystic kidney
Z82.79 Family history of other congenital malformations, deformations and chromosomal abnormalities

Z82.8 Family history of other disabilities and chronic diseases leading to disablement, not elsewhere classified

√4th **Z83 Family history of other specific disorders**
EXCLUDES 2 *contact with and (suspected) exposure to communicable disease in the family (Z20.-)*

Z83.0 Family history of human immunodeficiency virus [HIV] disease
Conditions classifiable to B20

DRAFT

Z83.1 Family history of other infectious and parasitic diseases
Conditions classifiable to A00-B19, B25-B94, B99

Z83.2 Family history of diseases of the blood and blood-forming organs and certain disorders involving the immune mechanism
Conditions classifiable to D50-D89

Z83.3 Family history of diabetes mellitus
Conditions classifiable to E08-E13

✓5th **Z83.4 Family history of other endocrine, nutritional and metabolic diseases**
Conditions classifiable to E00-E07, E15-E88

Z83.41 Family history of multiple endocrine neoplasia [MEN] syndrome

Z83.49 Family history of other endocrine, nutritional and metabolic diseases

✓5th **Z83.5 Family history of eye and ear disorders**

✓6th **Z83.51 Family history of eye disorders**
Conditions classifiable to H00-H53, H55-H59
EXCLUDES 2 *family history of blindness and visual loss (Z82.1)*

Z83.511 Family history of glaucoma

Z83.518 Family history of other specified eye disorder

Z83.52 Family history of ear disorders
Conditions classifiable to H60-H83, H92-H95
EXCLUDES 2 *family history of deafness and hearing loss (Z82.2)*

Z83.6 Family history of other diseases of the respiratory system
Conditions classifiable to J00-J39, J60-J99
EXCLUDES 2 *family history of asthma and other chronic lower respiratory diseases (Z82.5)*

✓5th **Z83.7 Family history of diseases of the digestive system**
Conditions classifiable to K00-K93

Z83.71 Family history of colonic polyps
EXCLUDES 1 *family history of malignant neoplasm of digestive organs (Z80.0)*

Z83.79 Family history of other diseases of the digestive system

✓4th **Z84 Family history of other conditions**

Z84.0 Family history of diseases of the skin and subcutaneous tissue
Conditions classifiable to L00-L99

Z84.1 Family history of disorders of kidney and ureter
Conditions classifiable to N00-N29

Z84.2 Family history of other diseases of the genitourinary system
Conditions classifiable to N30-N99

Z84.3 Family history of consanguinity

✓5th **Z84.8 Family history of other specified conditions**

Z84.81 Family history of carrier of genetic disease

Z84.89 Family history of other specified conditions

✓4th **Z85 Personal history of malignant neoplasm**

Code first any follow-up examination after treatment of malignant neoplasm (Z08)

Use additional code to identify:
- alcohol use and dependence (F10.-)
- exposure to environmental tobacco smoke (Z77.22)
- history of tobacco use (Z87.891)
- occupational exposure to environmental tobacco smoke (Z57.31)
- tobacco dependence (F17.-)
- tobacco use (Z72.0)

EXCLUDES 2 *personal history of benign neoplasm (Z86.01-)*
personal history of carcinoma-in-situ (Z86.00-)

✓5th **Z85.0 Personal history of malignant neoplasm of digestive organs**

Z85.00 Personal history of malignant neoplasm of unspecified digestive organ

Z85.01 Personal history of malignant neoplasm of esophagus
Conditions classifiable to C15

✓6th **Z85.02 Personal history of malignant neoplasm of stomach**

Z85.020 Personal history of malignant carcinoid tumor of stomach
Conditions classifiable to C7A.092

Z85.028 Personal history of other malignant neoplasm of stomach
Conditions classifiable to C16

✓6th **Z85.03 Personal history of malignant neoplasm of large intestine**

Z85.030 Personal history of malignant carcinoid tumor of large intestine
Conditions classifiable to C7A.022-C7A.025, C7A.029

Z85.038 Personal history of other malignant neoplasm of large intestine
Conditions classifiable to C18

✓6th **Z85.04 Personal history of malignant neoplasm of rectum, rectosigmoid junction, and anus**

Z85.040 Personal history of malignant carcinoid tumor of rectum
Conditions classifiable to C7A.026

Z85.048 Personal history of other malignant neoplasm of rectum, rectosigmoid junction, and anus
Conditions classifiable to C19-C21

Z85.05 Personal history of malignant neoplasm of liver
Conditions classifiable to C22

✓6th **Z85.06 Personal history of malignant neoplasm of small intestine**

Z85.060 Personal history of malignant carcinoid tumor of small intestine
Conditions classifiable to C7A.01-

Z85.068 Personal history of other malignant neoplasm of small intestine
Conditions classifiable to C17

Z85.07 Personal history of malignant neoplasm of pancreas
Conditions classifiable to C25

Z85.09 Personal history of malignant neoplasm of other digestive organs

✓5th **Z85.1 Personal history of malignant neoplasm of trachea, bronchus and lung**

✓6th **Z85.11 Personal history of malignant neoplasm of bronchus and lung**

Z85.110 Personal history of malignant carcinoid tumor of bronchus and lung
Conditions classifiable to C7A.090

Z85.118 Personal history of other malignant neoplasm of bronchus and lung
Conditions classifiable to C34

Z85.12 Personal history of malignant neoplasm of trachea
Conditions classifiable to C33

✓5th **Z85.2 Personal history of malignant neoplasm of other respiratory and intrathoracic organs**

Z85.20 Personal history of malignant neoplasm of unspecified respiratory organ

Z85.21 Personal history of malignant neoplasm of larynx
Conditions classifiable to C32

Z85.22 Personal history of malignant neoplasm of nasal cavities, middle ear, and accessory sinuses
Conditions classifiable to C30-C31

✓6th **Z85.23 Personal history of malignant neoplasm of thymus**

Z85.230 Personal history of malignant carcinoid tumor of thymus
Conditions classifiable to C7A.091

Z85.238 Personal history of other malignant neoplasm of thymus
Conditions classifiable to C37

Z85.29 Personal history of malignant neoplasm of other respiratory and intrathoracic organs

Z85.3 Personal history of malignant neoplasm of breast
Conditions classifiable to C50-

✓5th **Z85.4 Personal history of malignant neoplasm of genital organs**
Conditions classifiable to C51-C63

Z85.40 Personal history of malignant neoplasm of unspecified female genital organ

Z85.41 Personal history of malignant neoplasm of cervix uteri

Z85.42 Personal history of malignant neoplasm of other parts of uterus

Z85.43 Personal history of malignant neoplasm of ovary

Z85.44 Personal history of malignant neoplasm of other female genital organs

Z85.45 Personal history of malignant neoplasm of unspecified male genital organ

Z85.46 Personal history of malignant neoplasm of prostate
Z85.47 Personal history of malignant neoplasm of testis
Z85.48 Personal history of malignant neoplasm of epididymis
Z85.49 Personal history of malignant neoplasm of other male genital organs

✓5th **Z85.5 Personal history of malignant neoplasm of urinary tract**
Conditions classifiable to C64-C68
Z85.50 Personal history of malignant neoplasm of unspecified urinary tract organ
Z85.51 Personal history of malignant neoplasm of bladder
✓6th **Z85.52 Personal history of malignant neoplasm of kidney**
EXCLUDES 1 *personal history of malignant neoplasm of renal pelvis (Z85.53)*
Z85.520 Personal history of malignant carcinoid tumor of kidney
Conditions classifiable to C7A.093
Z85.528 Personal history of other malignant neoplasm of kidney
Conditions classifiable to C64
Z85.53 Personal history of malignant neoplasm of renal pelvis
Z85.54 Personal history of malignant neoplasm of ureter
Z85.59 Personal history of malignant neoplasm of other urinary tract organ

Z85.6 Personal history of leukemia
Conditions classifiable to C91-C95
EXCLUDES 1 *leukemia in remission C91.0-C95.9 with 5th character 1*

✓5th **Z85.7 Personal history of other malignant neoplasms of lymphoid, hematopoietic and related tissues**
Z85.71 Personal history of Hodgkin lymphoma
Conditions classifiable to C81
Z85.72 Personal history of non-Hodgkin lymphomas
Conditions classifiable to C82-C85
Z85.79 Personal history of other malignant neoplasms of lymphoid, hematopoietic and related tissues
Conditions classifiable to C88-C90, C96
EXCLUDES 1 *multiple myeloma in remission (C90.01)*
plasma cell leukemia in remission (C90.11)
plasmacytoma in remission (C90.21)

✓5th **Z85.8 Personal history of malignant neoplasms of other organs and systems**
Conditions classifiable to C00-C14, C40-C49, C69-C79, C7A.098
✓6th **Z85.81 Personal history of malignant neoplasm of lip, oral cavity, and pharynx**
Z85.810 Personal history of malignant neoplasm of tongue
Z85.818 Personal history of malignant neoplasm of other sites of lip, oral cavity, and pharynx
Z85.819 Personal history of malignant neoplasm of unspecified site of lip, oral cavity, and pharynx
✓6th **Z85.82 Personal history of malignant neoplasm of skin**
Z85.820 Personal history of malignant melanoma of skin
Conditions classifiable to C43
Z85.821 Personal history of Merkel cell carcinoma
Conditions classifiable to C4A
Z85.828 Personal history of other malignant neoplasm of skin
Conditions classifiable to C44
✓6th **Z85.83 Personal history of malignant neoplasm of bone and soft tissue**
Z85.830 Personal history of malignant neoplasm of bone
Z85.831 Personal history of malignant neoplasm of soft tissue
EXCLUDES 2 *personal history of malignant neoplasm of skin (Z85.82-)*
✓6th **Z85.84 Personal history of malignant neoplasm of eye and nervous tissue**
Z85.840 Personal history of malignant neoplasm of eye
Z85.841 Personal history of malignant neoplasm of brain
Z85.848 Personal history of malignant neoplasm of other parts of nervous tissue
✓6th **Z85.85 Personal history of malignant neoplasm of endocrine glands**
Z85.850 Personal history of malignant neoplasm of thyroid
Z85.858 Personal history of malignant neoplasm of other endocrine glands
Z85.89 Personal history of malignant neoplasm of other organs and systems

Z85.9 Personal history of malignant neoplasm, unspecified
Conditions classifiable to C7A.00, C80.1

✓4th **Z86 Personal history of certain other diseases**
Code first any follow-up examination after treatment (Z09)

✓5th **Z86.0 Personal history of in-situ and benign neoplasms and neoplasms of uncertain behavior**
EXCLUDES 2 *personal history of malignant neoplasms (Z85.-)*
✓6th **Z86.00 Personal history of in-situ neoplasm**
Z86.000 Personal history of in-situ neoplasm of breast
Z86.001 Personal history of in-situ neoplasm of cervix uteri
Z86.008 Personal history of in-situ neoplasm of other site
✓6th **Z86.01 Personal history of benign neoplasm**
Z86.010 Personal history of colonic polyps
Z86.011 Personal history of benign neoplasm of the brain
Z86.012 Personal history of benign carcinoid tumor
Z86.018 Personal history of other benign neoplasm
Z86.03 Personal history of neoplasm of uncertain behavior

✓5th **Z86.1 Personal history of infectious and parasitic diseases**
Conditions classifiable to A00-B89, B99
EXCLUDES 1 *personal history of infectious diseases specific to a body system*
sequelae of infectious and parasitic diseases (B90-B94)
Z86.11 Personal history of tuberculosis
Z86.12 Personal history of poliomyelitis
Z86.13 Personal history of malaria
Z86.14 Personal history of Methicillin resistant Staphylococcus aureus infection
Personal history of MRSA infection
Z86.19 Personal history of other infectious and parasitic diseases

Z86.2 Personal history of diseases of the blood and blood-forming organs and certain disorders involving the immune mechanism
Conditions classifiable to D50-D89

✓5th **Z86.3 Personal history of endocrine, nutritional and metabolic diseases**
Conditions classifiable to E00-E88
Z86.31 Personal history of diabetic foot ulcer
EXCLUDES 2 *current diabetic foot ulcer (E08.621, E09.621, E10.621, E11.621, E13.621)*
Z86.32 Personal history of gestational diabetes
Personal history of conditions classifiable to O24.4-
EXCLUDES 1 *gestational diabetes mellitus in current pregnancy (O24.4-)*
Z86.39 Personal history of other endocrine, nutritional and metabolic disease

✓5th **Z86.5 Personal history of mental and behavioral disorders**
Conditions classifiable to F40-F59
Z86.51 Personal history of combat and operational stress reaction
Z86.59 Personal history of other mental and behavioral disorders

5th **Z86.6 Personal history of diseases of the nervous system and sense organs**
Conditions classifiable to G00-G99, H00-H95
EXCLUDES 2 *personal history of anaphylactic shock (Z87.892)*

Z86.61 Personal history of infections of the central nervous system
Personal history of encephalitis
Personal history of meningitis

Z86.69 Personal history of other diseases of the nervous system and sense organs

5th **Z86.7 Personal history of diseases of the circulatory system**
Conditions classifiable to I00-I99
EXCLUDES 2 *old myocardial infarction (I25.2)*
personal history of anaphylactic shock (Z87.892)
postmyocardial infarction syndrome (I24.1)

6th **Z86.71 Personal history of venous thrombosis and embolism**

Z86.711 Personal history of pulmonary embolism

Z86.718 Personal history of other venous thrombosis and embolism

Z86.72 Personal history of thrombophlebitis

Z86.73 Personal history of transient ischemic attack (TIA), and cerebral infarction without residual deficits
Personal history of prolonged reversible ischemic neurological deficit (PRIND)
Personal history of stroke NOS without residual deficits
EXCLUDES 1 *personal history of traumatic brain injury (Z87.820)*
sequelae of cerebrovascular disease (I69.-)

Z86.74 Personal history of sudden cardiac arrest
Personal history of sudden cardiac death successfully resuscitated

Z86.79 Personal history of other diseases of the circulatory system

4th **Z87 Personal history of other diseases and conditions**
Code first any follow-up examination after treatment (Z09)

5th **Z87.0 Personal history of diseases of the respiratory system**
Conditions classifiable to J00-J99

Z87.01 Personal history of pneumonia (recurrent)

Z87.09 Personal history of other diseases of the respiratory system

5th **Z87.1 Personal history of diseases of the digestive system**
Conditions classifiable to K00-K93

Z87.11 Personal history of peptic ulcer disease

Z87.19 Personal history of other diseases of the digestive system

Z87.2 Personal history of diseases of the skin and subcutaneous tissue
Conditions classifiable to L00-L99
EXCLUDES 2 *personal history of diabetic foot ulcer (Z86.31)*

5th **Z87.3 Personal history of diseases of the musculoskeletal system and connective tissue**
Conditions classifiable to M00-M99
EXCLUDES 2 *personal history of (healed) traumatic fracture (Z87.81)*

6th **Z87.31 Personal history of (healed) nontraumatic fracture**

Z87.310 Personal history of (healed) osteoporosis fracture
Personal history of (healed) fragility fracture
Personal history of (healed) collapsed vertebra due to osteoporosis

Z87.311 Personal history of (healed) other pathological fracture
Personal history of (healed) collapsed vertebra NOS
EXCLUDES 2 *personal history of osteoporosis fracture (Z87.310)*

Z87.312 Personal history of (healed) stress fracture
Personal history of (healed) fatigue fracture

Z87.39 Personal history of other diseases of the musculoskeletal system and connective tissue

5th **Z87.4 Personal history of diseases of the genitourinary system**
Conditions classifiable to N00-N99

6th **Z87.41 Personal history of dysplasia of the female genital tract**
EXCLUDES 1 *personal history of malignant neoplasm of female genital tract (Z85.40-Z85.44)*

Z87.410 Personal history of cervical dysplasia

Z87.411 Personal history of vaginal dysplasia

Z87.412 Personal history of vulvar dysplasia

Z87.42 Personal history of other diseases of the female genital tract

6th **Z87.43 Personal history of diseases of the male genital organs**

Z87.430 Personal history of prostatic dysplasia
EXCLUDES 1 *personal history of malignant neoplasm of prostate (Z85.46)*

Z87.438 Personal history of other diseases of male genital organs

6th **Z87.44 Personal history of diseases of the urinary system**
EXCLUDES 1 *personal history of malignant neoplasm of cervix uteri (Z85.41)*

Z87.440 Personal history of urinary (tract) infections

Z87.441 Personal history of nephrotic syndrome

Z87.442 Personal history of urinary calculi
Personal history of kidney stones

Z87.448 Personal history of other diseases of urinary system

5th **Z87.5 Personal history of complications of pregnancy, childbirth and the puerperium**
Conditions classifiable to O00-O9A
EXCLUDES 2 *recurrent pregnancy loss (N96)*

Z87.51 Personal history of pre-term labor
EXCLUDES 1 *current pregnancy with history of pre-term labor (O09.21-)*

Z87.59 Personal history of other complications of pregnancy, childbirth and the puerperium
Personal history of trophoblastic disease

5th **Z87.7 Personal history of (corrected) congenital malformations**
Conditions classifiable to Q00-Q89 that have been repaired or corrected
EXCLUDES 1 *congenital malformations that have been partially corrected or repaired but which still require medical treatment—code to condition*
EXCLUDES 2 *other postprocedural states (Z98.-)*
personal history of medical treatment (Z92.-)
presence of cardiac and vascular implants and grafts (Z95.-)
presence of other devices (Z97.-)
presence of other functional implants (Z96.-)
transplanted organ and tissue status (Z94.-)

6th **Z87.71 Personal history of (corrected) congenital malformations of genitourinary system**

Z87.710 Personal history of (corrected) hypospadias

Z87.718 Personal history of other specified (corrected) congenital malformations of genitourinary system

6th **Z87.72 Personal history of (corrected) congenital malformations of nervous system and sense organs**

Z87.720 Personal history of (corrected) congenital malformations of eye

Z87.721 Personal history of (corrected) congenital malformations of ear

Z87.728 Personal history of other specified (corrected) congenital malformations of nervous system and sense organs

6th **Z87.73 Personal history of (corrected) congenital malformations of digestive system**

Z87.730 Personal history of (corrected) cleft lip and palate

Z87.738 Personal history of other specified (corrected) congenital malformations of digestive system

Z87.74 Personal history of (corrected) congenital malformations of heart and circulatory system

Z87.75 Personal history of (corrected) congenital malformations of respiratory system
Z87.76 Personal history of (corrected) congenital malformations of integument, limbs and musculoskeletal system
✓6th Z87.79 Personal history of other (corrected) congenital malformations
Z87.790 Personal history of (corrected) congenital malformations of face and neck
Z87.798 Personal history of other (corrected) congenital malformations
✓5th Z87.8 Personal history of other specified conditions
EXCLUDES 2 *personal history of self harm (Z91.5)*
Z87.81 Personal history of (healed) traumatic fracture
EXCLUDES 2 *personal history of (healed) nontraumatic fracture (Z87.31-)*
✓6th Z87.82 Personal history of other (healed) physical injury and trauma
Conditions classifiable to S00-T88, except traumatic fractures
Z87.820 Personal history of traumatic brain injury
EXCLUDES 1 *personal history of transient ischemic attack (TIA), and cerebral infarction without residual deficits (Z86.73)*
Z87.821 Personal history of retained foreign body fully removed
Z87.828 Personal history of other (healed) physical injury and trauma
✓6th Z87.89 Personal history of other specified conditions
Z87.890 Personal history of sex reassignment
Z87.891 Personal history of nicotine dependence
EXCLUDES 1 *current nicotine dependence (F17.2-)*
Z87.892 Personal history of anaphylaxis
Code also allergy status such as:
allergy status to drugs, medicaments and biological substances (Z88.-)
allergy status, other than to drugs and biological substances (Z91.0-)
Z87.898 Personal history of other specified conditions

✓4th **Z88 Allergy status to drugs, medicaments and biological substances**
EXCLUDES 2 *allergy status, other than to drugs and biological substances (Z91.0-)*
Z88.0 Allergy status to penicillin
Z88.1 Allergy status to other antibiotic agents status
Z88.2 Allergy status to sulfonamides status
Z88.3 Allergy status to other anti-infective agents status
Z88.4 Allergy status to anesthetic agent status
Z88.5 Allergy status to narcotic agent status
Z88.6 Allergy status to analgesic agent status
Z88.7 Allergy status to serum and vaccine status
Z88.8 Allergy status to other drugs, medicaments and biological substances status
Z88.9 Allergy status to unspecified drugs, medicaments and biological substances status

✓4th **Z89 Acquired absence of limb**
INCLUDES amputation status
postprocedural loss of limb
post-traumatic loss of limb
EXCLUDES 1 *acquired deformities of limbs (M20-M21)*
congenital absence of limbs (Q71-Q73)
✓5th Z89.0 Acquired absence of thumb and other finger(s)
✓6th Z89.01 Acquired absence of thumb
Z89.011 Acquired absence of right thumb
Z89.012 Acquired absence of left thumb
Z89.019 Acquired absence of unspecified thumb
✓6th Z89.02 Acquired absence of other finger(s)
EXCLUDES 2 *acquired absence of thumb (Z89.01-)*
Z89.021 Acquired absence of right finger(s)
Z89.022 Acquired absence of left finger(s)
Z89.029 Acquired absence of unspecified finger(s)
✓5th Z89.1 Acquired absence of hand and wrist
✓6th Z89.11 Acquired absence of hand
Z89.111 Acquired absence of right hand
Z89.112 Acquired absence of left hand
Z89.119 Acquired absence of unspecified hand
✓6th Z89.12 Acquired absence of wrist
Disarticulation at wrist
Z89.121 Acquired absence of right wrist
Z89.122 Acquired absence of left wrist
Z89.129 Acquired absence of unspecified wrist
✓5th Z89.2 Acquired absence of upper limb above wrist
✓6th Z89.20 Acquired absence of upper limb, unspecified level
Z89.201 Acquired absence of right upper limb, unspecified level
Z89.202 Acquired absence of left upper limb, unspecified level
Z89.209 Acquired absence of unspecified upper limb, unspecified level
Acquired absence of arm NOS
✓6th Z89.21 Acquired absence of upper limb below elbow
Z89.211 Acquired absence of right upper limb below elbow
Z89.212 Acquired absence of left upper limb below elbow
Z89.219 Acquired absence of unspecified upper limb below elbow
✓6th Z89.22 Acquired absence of upper limb above elbow
Disarticulation at elbow
Z89.221 Acquired absence of right upper limb above elbow
Z89.222 Acquired absence of left upper limb above elbow
Z89.229 Acquired absence of unspecified upper limb above elbow
✓6th Z89.23 Acquired absence of shoulder
Acquired absence of shoulder joint following explantation of shoulder joint prosthesis, with or without presence of antibiotic-impregnated cement spacer
Z89.231 Acquired absence of right shoulder
Z89.232 Acquired absence of left shoulder
Z89.239 Acquired absence of unspecified shoulder
✓5th Z89.4 Acquired absence of toe(s), foot, and ankle
✓6th Z89.41 Acquired absence of great toe
Z89.411 Acquired absence of right great toe
Z89.412 Acquired absence of left great toe
Z89.419 Acquired absence of unspecified great toe
✓6th Z89.42 Acquired absence of other toe(s)
EXCLUDES 2 *acquired absence of great toe (Z89.41-)*
Z89.421 Acquired absence of other right toe(s)
Z89.422 Acquired absence of other left toe(s)
Z89.429 Acquired absence of other toe(s), unspecified side
✓6th Z89.43 Acquired absence of foot
Z89.431 Acquired absence of right foot
Z89.432 Acquired absence of left foot
Z89.439 Acquired absence of unspecified foot
✓6th Z89.44 Acquired absence of ankle
Disarticulation of ankle
Z89.441 Acquired absence of right ankle
Z89.442 Acquired absence of left ankle
Z89.449 Acquired absence of unspecified ankle
✓5th Z89.5 Acquired absence of leg below knee
✓6th Z89.51 Acquired absence of leg below knee
Z89.511 Acquired absence of right leg below knee
Z89.512 Acquired absence of left leg below knee
Z89.519 Acquired absence of unspecified leg below knee

✓6th **Z89.52 Acquired absence of knee**
Acquired absence of knee joint following explantation of knee joint prosthesis, with or without presence of antibiotic-impregnated cement spacer
Z89.521 Acquired absence of right knee
Z89.522 Acquired absence of left knee
Z89.529 Acquired absence of unspecified knee

✓5th **Z89.6 Acquired absence of leg above knee**
✓6th **Z89.61 Acquired absence of leg above knee**
Acquired absence of leg NOS
Disarticulation at knee
Z89.611 Acquired absence of right leg above knee
Z89.612 Acquired absence of left leg above knee
Z89.619 Acquired absence of unspecified leg above knee
✓6th **Z89.62 Acquired absence of hip**
Acquired absence of hip joint following explantation of hip joint prosthesis, with or without presence of antibiotic-impregnated cement spacer
Disarticulation at hip
Z89.621 Acquired absence of right hip joint
Z89.622 Acquired absence of left hip joint
Z89.629 Acquired absence of unspecified hip joint
Z89.9 Acquired absence of limb, unspecified

✓4th **Z90 Acquired absence of organs, not elsewhere classified**
INCLUDES postprocedural or post-traumatic loss of body part NEC
EXCLUDES 1 *congenital absence—see Alphabetical Index*
EXCLUDES 2 *postprocedural absence of endocrine glands (E89.-)*

✓5th **Z90.0 Acquired absence of part of head and neck**
Z90.01 Acquired absence of eye
Z90.02 Acquired absence of larynx
Z90.09 Acquired absence of other part of head and neck
Acquired absence of nose
EXCLUDES 2 *teeth (K08.1)*

✓5th **Z90.1 Acquired absence of breast and nipple**
Z90.10 Acquired absence of unspecified breast and nipple
Z90.11 Acquired absence of right breast and nipple
Z90.12 Acquired absence of left breast and nipple
Z90.13 Acquired absence of bilateral breasts and nipples
Z90.2 Acquired absence of lung [part of]
Z90.3 Acquired absence of stomach [part of]

✓5th **Z90.4 Acquired absence of other specified parts of digestive tract**
✓6th **Z90.41 Acquired absence of pancreas**
Use additional code to identify any associated:
insulin use (Z79.4)
diabetes mellitus, postpancreatectomy (E13.-)
Z90.410 Acquired total absence of pancreas
Acquired absence of pancreas NOS
Z90.411 Acquired partial absence of pancreas
Z90.49 Acquired absence of other specified parts of digestive tract
Z90.5 Acquired absence of kidney
Z90.6 Acquired absence of other parts of urinary tract
Acquired absence of bladder

✓5th **Z90.7 Acquired absence of genital organ(s)**
EXCLUDES 1 *personal history of sex reassignment (Z87.890)*
EXCLUDES 2 *female genital mutilation status (N90.81-)*
✓6th **Z90.71 Acquired absence of cervix and uterus**
Z90.710 Acquired absence of both cervix and uterus
Acquired absence of uterus NOS
Status post total hysterectomy
Z90.711 Acquired absence of uterus with remaining cervical stump
Status post partial hysterectomy with remaining cervical stump
Z90.712 Acquired absence of cervix with remaining uterus
✓6th **Z90.72 Acquired absence of ovaries**
Z90.721 Acquired absence of ovaries, unilateral
Z90.722 Acquired absence of ovaries, bilateral
Z90.79 Acquired absence of other genital organ(s)

✓5th **Z90.8 Acquired absence of other organs**
Z90.81 Acquired absence of spleen
Z90.89 Acquired absence of other organs

✓4th **Z91 Personal risk factors, not elsewhere classified**
EXCLUDES 2 *contact with and (suspected) exposures hazardous to health (Z77.-)*
exposure to pollution and other problems related to physical environment (Z77.1-)
personal history of physical injury and trauma (Z87.81, Z87.82-)
occupational exposure to risk factors (Z57.-)

✓5th **Z91.0 Allergy status, other than to drugs and biological substances**
EXCLUDES 2 *allergy status to drugs, medicaments, and biological substances (Z88.-)*
✓6th **Z91.01 Food allergy status**
EXCLUDES 2 *food additives allergy status (Z91.02)*
Z91.010 Allergy to peanuts
Z91.011 Allergy to milk products
EXCLUDES 1 *lactose intolerance (E73.-)*
Z91.012 Allergy to eggs
Z91.013 Allergy to seafood
Allergy to shellfish
Allergy to octopus or squid ink
Z91.018 Allergy to other foods
Allergy to nuts other than peanuts
Z91.02 Food additives allergy status
✓6th **Z91.03 Insect allergy status**
Z91.030 Bee allergy status
Z91.038 Other insect allergy status
✓6th **Z91.04 Nonmedicinal substance allergy status**
Z91.040 Latex allergy status
Latex sensitivity status
Z91.041 Radiographic dye allergy status
Allergy status to contrast media used for diagnostic X-ray procedure
Z91.048 Other nonmedicinal substance allergy status
Z91.09 Other allergy status, other than to drugs and biological substances

✓5th **Z91.1 Patient's noncompliance with medical treatment and regimen**
Z91.11 Patient's noncompliance with dietary regimen
✓6th **Z91.12 Patient's intentional underdosing of medication regimen**
Code first underdosing of medication (T36-T50) with fifth or sixth character 6
EXCLUDES 1 *adverse effect of prescribed drug taken as directed—code to adverse effect*
poisoning (overdose)—code to poisoning
Z91.120 Patient's intentional underdosing of medication regimen due to financial hardship
Z91.128 Patient's intentional underdosing of medication regimen for other reason
✓6th **Z91.13 Patient's unintentional underdosing of medication regimen**
Code first underdosing of medication (T36-T50) with fifth or sixth character 6
EXCLUDES 1 *adverse effect of prescribed drug taken as directed—code to adverse effect*
poisoning (overdose)—code to poisoning
Z91.130 Patient's unintentional underdosing of medication regimen due to age-related debility
Z91.138 Patient's unintentional underdosing of medication regimen for other reason
Z91.14 Patient's other noncompliance with medication regimen
Patient's underdosing of medication NOS
Z91.15 Patient's noncompliance with renal dialysis
Z91.19 Patient's noncompliance with other medical treatment and

√5th **Z91.4 Personal history of psychological trauma, not elsewhere classified**

√6th **Z91.41 Personal history of adult abuse**

EXCLUDES 2 *personal history of abuse in childhood (Z62.81-)*

Z91.410 Personal history of adult physical and sexual abuse

EXCLUDES 1 *current adult physical abuse (T74.11, T76.11)*
current adult sexual abuse (T74. 21, T76.21)

Z91.411 Personal history of adult psychological abuse

Z91.412 Personal history of adult neglect

EXCLUDES 1 *current adult neglect (T74.01, T76.01)*

Z91.419 Personal history of unspecified adult abuse

Z91.49 Other personal history of psychological trauma, not elsewhere classified

Z91.5 Personal history of self-harm

Personal history of parasuicide
Personal history of self-poisoning
Personal history of suicide attempt

√5th **Z91.8 Other specified personal risk factors, not elsewhere classified**

Z91.81 History of falling

At risk for falling

Z91.82 Personal history of military deployment

Individual (civilian or military) with past history of military war, peacekeeping and humanitarian deployment (current or past conflict)
Returned from military deployment

Z91.83 Wandering in diseases classified elsewhere

Code first underlying disorder such as:
Alzheimer's disease (G30-)
autism or pervasive developmental disorder (F84-)
intellectual disabilities (F70-F79)
unspecified dementia with behavioral disturbance (F03.9-)

Z91.89 Other specified personal risk factors, not elsewhere classified

√4th **Z92 Personal history of medical treatment**

EXCLUDES 2 *postprocedural states (Z98.-)*

Z92.0 Personal history of contraception

EXCLUDES 1 *counseling or management of current contraceptive practices (Z30.-)*
long term (current) use of contraception (Z79.3)
presence of (intrauterine) contraceptive device (Z97.5)

√5th **Z92.2 Personal history of drug therapy**

EXCLUDES 2 *long term (current) drug therapy (Z79.-)*

Z92.21 Personal history of antineoplastic chemotherapy

Z92.22 Personal history of monoclonal drug therapy

Z92.23 Personal history of estrogen therapy

√6th **Z92.24 Personal history of steroid therapy**

Z92.240 Personal history of inhaled steroid therapy

Z92.241 Personal history of systemic steroid therapy

Personal history of steroid therapy NOS

Z92.25 Personal history of immunosupression therapy

EXCLUDES 2 *personal history of steroid therapy (Z92.24)*

Z92.29 Personal history of other drug therapy

Z92.3 Personal history of irradiation

Personal history of exposure to therapeutic radiation

EXCLUDES 1 *exposure to radiation in the physical environment (Z77.12)*
occupational exposure to radiation (Z57.1)

√5th **Z92.8 Personal history of other medical treatment**

Z92.81 Personal history of extracorporeal membrane oxygenation (ECMO)

Z92.82 Status post administration of tPA (rtPA) in a different facility within the last 24 hours prior to admission to current facility

Code first condition requiring tPA administration, such as:
acute cerebral infarction (I63.-)
acute myocardial infarction (I21-, I22-)

Z92.83 Personal history of failed moderate sedation

Personal history of failed conscious sedation

EXCLUDES 2 *failed moderate sedation during procedure (T88.52)*

Z92.89 Personal history of other medical treatment

√4th **Z93 Artificial opening status**

EXCLUDES 1 *artificial openings requiring attention or management (Z43.-)*
complications of external stoma (J95.0-, K94.-, N99.5-)

Z93.0 Tracheostomy status

Z93.1 Gastrostomy status

Z93.2 Ileostomy status

Z93.3 Colostomy status

Z93.4 Other artificial openings of gastrointestinal tract status

√5th **Z93.5 Cystostomy status**

Z93.50 Unspecified cystostomy status

Z93.51 Cutaneous-vesicostomy status

Z93.52 Appendico-vesicostomy status

Z93.59 Other cystostomy status

Z93.6 Other artificial openings of urinary tract status

Nephrostomy status
Ureterostomy status
Urethrostomy status

Z93.8 Other artificial opening status

Z93.9 Artificial opening status, unspecified

√4th **Z94 Transplanted organ and tissue status**

INCLUDES organ or tissue replaced by heterogenous or homogenous transplant

EXCLUDES 1 *complications of transplanted organ or tissue—see Alphabetical Index*

EXCLUDES 2 *presence of vascular grafts (Z95.-)*

Z94.0 Kidney transplant status

Z94.1 Heart transplant status

EXCLUDES 1 *artificial heart status (Z95.811)*
heart-valve replacement status (Z95.2-Z95.4)

Z94.2 Lung transplant status

Z94.3 Heart and lungs transplant status

Z94.4 Liver transplant status

Z94.5 Skin transplant status

Autogenous skin transplant status

Z94.6 Bone transplant status

Z94.7 Corneal transplant status

√5th **Z94.8 Other transplanted organ and tissue status**

Z94.81 Bone marrow transplant status

Z94.82 Intestine transplant status

Z94.83 Pancreas transplant status

Z94.84 Stem cells transplant status

Z94.89 Other transplanted organ and tissue status

Z94.9 Transplanted organ and tissue status, unspecified

√4th **Z95 Presence of cardiac and vascular implants and grafts**

EXCLUDES 1 *complications of cardiac and vascular devices, implants and grafts (T82.-)*

Z95.0 Presence of cardiac pacemaker

EXCLUDES 1 *adjustment or management of cardiac pacemaker (Z45.0)*
presence of automatic (implantable) cardiac defibrillator with synchronous cardiac pacemaker (Z95.810)

Z95.1 Presence of aortocoronary bypass graft

Z95.2 Presence of prosthetic heart valve

Presence of heart valve NOS

Z95.3 Presence of xenogenic heart valve

Z95.4 Presence of other heart-valve replacement

Z95.5 Presence of coronary angioplasty implant and graft

EXCLUDES 1 *coronary angioplasty status without implant and graft (Z98.61)*

Z95.8 Presence of other cardiac and vascular implants and grafts

Z95.81 Presence of other cardiac implants and grafts

Z95.810 Presence of automatic (implantable) cardiac defibrillator

Presence of automatic (implantable) cardiac defibrillator with synchronous cardiac pacemaker

Z95.811 Presence of heart assist device

Z95.812 Presence of fully implantable artificial heart

Z95.818 Presence of other cardiac implants and grafts

Z95.82 Presence of other vascular implants and grafts

Z95.820 Peripheral vascular angioplasty status with implants and grafts

EXCLUDES 1 *peripheral vascular angioplasty without implant and graft (Z98.62)*

Z95.828 Presence of other vascular implants and grafts

Presence of intravascular prosthesis NEC

Z95.9 Presence of cardiac and vascular implant and graft, unspecified

Z96 Presence of other functional implants

EXCLUDES 2 *complications of internal prosthetic devices, implants and grafts (T82-T85)*

fitting and adjustment of prosthetic and other devices (Z44-Z46)

Z96.0 Presence of urogenital implants

Z96.1 Presence of intraocular lens

Presence of pseudophakia

Z96.2 Presence of otological and audiological implants

Z96.20 Presence of otological and audiological implant, unspecified

Z96.21 Cochlear implant status

Z96.22 Myringotomy tube(s) status

Z96.29 Presence of other otological and audiological implants

Presence of bone-conduction hearing device

Presence of eustachian tube stent

Stapes replacement

Z96.3 Presence of artificial larynx

Z96.4 Presence of endocrine implants

Z96.41 Presence of insulin pump (external) (internal)

Z96.49 Presence of other endocrine implants

Z96.5 Presence of tooth-root and mandibular implants

Z96.6 Presence of orthopedic joint implants

Z96.60 Presence of unspecified orthopedic joint implant

Z96.61 Presence of artificial shoulder joint

Z96.611 Presence of right artificial shoulder joint

Z96.612 Presence of left artificial shoulder joint

Z96.619 Presence of unspecified artificial shoulder joint

Z96.62 Presence of artificial elbow joint

Z96.621 Presence of right artificial elbow joint

Z96.622 Presence of left artificial elbow joint

Z96.629 Presence of unspecified artificial elbow joint

Z96.63 Presence of artificial wrist joint

Z96.631 Presence of right artificial wrist joint

Z96.632 Presence of left artificial wrist joint

Z96.639 Presence of unspecified artificial wrist joint

Z96.64 Presence of artificial hip joint

Hip-joint replacement (partial) (total)

Z96.641 Presence of right artificial hip joint

Z96.642 Presence of left artificial hip joint

Z96.643 Presence of artificial hip joint, bilateral

Z96.649 Presence of unspecified artificial hip joint

Z96.65 Presence of artificial knee joint

Z96.651 Presence of right artificial knee joint

Z96.652 Presence of left artificial knee joint

Z96.653 Presence of artificial knee joint, bilateral

Z96.659 Presence of unspecified artificial knee joint

Z96.66 Presence of artificial ankle joint

Z96.661 Presence of right artificial ankle joint

Z96.662 Presence of left artificial ankle joint

Z96.669 Presence of unspecified artificial ankle joint

Z96.69 Presence of other orthopedic joint implants

Z96.691 Finger-joint replacement of right hand

Z96.692 Finger-joint replacement of left hand

Z96.693 Finger-joint replacement, bilateral

Z96.698 Presence of other orthopedic joint implants

Z96.7 Presence of other bone and tendon implants

Presence of skull plate

Z96.8 Presence of other specified functional implants

Z96.81 Presence of artificial skin

Z96.89 Presence of other specified functional implants

Z96.9 Presence of functional implant, unspecified

Z97 Presence of other devices

EXCLUDES 1 *complications of internal prosthetic devices, implants and grafts (T82-T85)*

fitting and adjustment of prosthetic and other devices (Z44-Z46)

EXCLUDES 2 *presence of cerebrospinal fluid drainage device (Z98.2)*

Z97.0 Presence of artificial eye

Z97.1 Presence of artificial limb (complete) (partial)

Z97.10 Presence of artificial limb (complete) (partial), unspecified

Z97.11 Presence of artificial right arm (complete) (partial)

Z97.12 Presence of artificial left arm (complete) (partial)

Z97.13 Presence of artificial right leg (complete) (partial)

Z97.14 Presence of artificial left leg (complete) (partial)

Z97.15 Presence of artificial arms, bilateral (complete) (partial)

Z97.16 Presence of artificial legs, bilateral (complete) (partial)

Z97.2 Presence of dental prosthetic device (complete) (partial)

Presence of dentures (complete) (partial)

Z97.3 Presence of spectacles and contact lenses

Z97.4 Presence of external hearing-aid

Z97.5 Presence of (intrauterine) contraceptive device

EXCLUDES 1 *checking, reinsertion or removal of contraceptive device (Z30.43)*

Z97.8 Presence of other specified devices

Z98 Other postprocedural states

EXCLUDES 2 *aftercare (Z43-Z49, Z51)*

follow-up medical care (Z08-Z09)

postprocedural complication—see Alphabetical Index

Z98.0 Intestinal bypass and anastomosis status

EXCLUDES 2 *bariatric surgery status (Z98.84)*

gastric bypass status (Z98.84)

obesity surgery status (Z98.84)

Z98.1 Arthrodesis status

Z98.2 Presence of cerebrospinal fluid drainage device

Presence of CSF shunt

Z98.3 Post therapeutic collapse of lung status

Code first underlying disease

Z98.4 Cataract extraction status

Use additional code to identify intraocular lens implant status (Z96.1)

EXCLUDES 1 *aphakia (H27.0)*

Z98.41 Cataract extraction status, right eye

Z98.42 Cataract extraction status, left eye

Z98.49 Cataract extraction status, unspecified eye

Z98.5 Sterilization status

EXCLUDES 1 *female infertility (N97.-)*

male infertility (N46.-)

Z98.51 Tubal ligation status

Z98.52 Vasectomy status

Z98.6 Angioplasty status

Z98.61 Coronary angioplasty status

EXCLUDES 1 *coronary angioplasty status with implant and graft (Z95.5)*

Z98.62 Peripheral vascular angioplasty status

EXCLUDES 1 *peripheral vascular angioplasty status with implant and graft (Z95.820)*

✓5th **Z98.8 Other specified postprocedural states**

✓6th **Z98.81 Dental procedure status**

Z98.810 Dental sealant status

Z98.811 Dental restoration status
Dental crown status
Dental fillings status

Z98.818 Other dental procedure status

Z98.82 Breast implant status
EXCLUDES 1 *breast implant removal status (Z98.86)*

Z98.83 Filtering (vitreous) bleb after glaucoma surgery status
EXCLUDES 1 *inflammation (infection) of postprocedural bleb (H59.4-)*

Z98.84 Bariatric surgery status
Gastric banding status
Gastric bypass status for obesity
Obesity surgery status
EXCLUDES 1 *bariatric surgery status complicating pregnancy, childbirth, or the puerperium (O99.84)*
EXCLUDES 2 *intestinal bypass and anastomosis status (Z98.0)*

Z98.85 Transplanted organ removal status
Transplanted organ previously removed due to complication, failure, rejection or infection
EXCLUDES 1 *encounter for removal of transplanted organ—code to complication of transplanted organ (T86.-)*

Z98.86 Personal history of breast implant removal

✓6th **Z98.87 Personal history of in utero procedure**

Z98.870 Personal history of in utero procedure during pregnancy
EXCLUDES 2 *complications from in utero procedure for current pregnancy (O35.7)*
supervision of current pregnancy with history of in utero procedure during previous pregnancy (O09.82-)

Z98.871 Personal history of in utero procedure while a fetus

Z98.89 Other specified postprocedural states
Personal history of surgery, not elsewhere classified

✓4th **Z99 Dependence on enabling machines and devices, not elsewhere classified**
EXCLUDES 1 *cardiac pacemaker status (Z95.0)*

Z99.0 Dependence on aspirator

✓5th **Z99.1 Dependence on respirator**
Dependence on ventilator

Z99.11 Dependence on respirator [ventilator] status

Z99.12 Encounter for respirator [ventilator] dependence during power failure
EXCLUDES 1 *mechanical complication of respirator [ventilator] (J95.850)*

Z99.2 Dependence on renal dialysis
Hemodialysis status
Peritoneal dialysis status
Presence of arteriovenous shunt for dialysis
Renal dialysis status NOS
EXCLUDES 1 *encounter for fitting and adjustment of dialysis catheter (Z49.0-)*
noncompliance with renal dialysis (Z91.15)

Z99.3 Dependence on wheelchair
Wheelchair confinement status
Code first cause of dependence, such as:
muscular dystrophy (G71.0)
obesity (E66.-)

✓5th **Z99.8 Dependence on other enabling machines and devices**

Z99.81 Dependence on supplemental oxygen
Dependence on long-term oxygen

Z99.89 Dependence on other enabling machines and devices
Dependence on machine or device NOS